Miller's Anesthesia

Miller's Anesthesia

NINTH EDITION

Editor-in-Chief

Michael A. Gropper, MD, PhD

Professor and Chair
Department of Anesthesia and Perioperative Care
Professor of Physiology
Investigator, Cardiovascular Research Institute
University of California, San Francisco, School of Medicine
San Francisco, California

Honorary Editor

Ronald D. Miller, MD

Professor Emeritus of Anesthesia and Perioperative Care
Department of Anesthesia and Perioperative Care
University of California, San Francisco, School of Medicine
San Francisco, California

Co-Editors

Neal H. Cohen, MD, MPH, MS

Professor of Anesthesia and Perioperative Care
Professor of Medicine
Vice Dean
University of California, San Francisco, School of Medicine
San Francisco, California

Lars I. Eriksson, MD, PhD, FRCA

Professor and Academic Chair
Department of Physiology and Pharmacology
Section for Anaesthesiology and Intensive Care Medicine
Function Preoperative Medicine and Intensive Care
Karolinska Institutet and Karolinska University Hospital
Stockholm, Sweden

Lee A. Fleisher, MD

Robert D. Dripps Professor and Chair
Department of Anesthesiology and Critical Care
Professor of Medicine
Perelman School of Medicine
Senior Fellow, Leonard Davis Institute of Health Economics
University of Pennsylvania
Philadelphia, Pennsylvania

Kate Leslie, MBBS, MD, MEpid, MHlthServMt, Hon DMedSci, FANZCA

Professor and Head of Research
Department of Anaesthesia and Pain Management
Royal Melbourne Hospital
Melbourne, Australia

Jeanine P. Wiener-Kronish, MD

Henry Isaiah Dorr Professor of Research and Teaching in Anaesthetics and Anaesthesia
Department of Anesthesia, Critical Care and Pain Medicine
Harvard Medical School
Anesthetist-in-Chief
Massachusetts General Hospital
Boston, Massachusetts

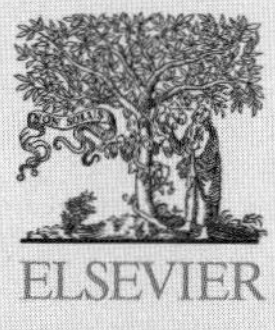

1600 John F. Kennedy Blvd.
Ste 1600
Philadelphia, PA 19103-2899

MILLER'S ANESTHESIA, NINTH EDITION

ISBN: 978-0-323-59604-6
Volume 1 PN: 9996128113
Volume 2 PN: 9996128172

INTERNATIONAL EDITION

ISBN: 978-0-323-61263-0
Volume 1 PN: 9996128415
Volume 2 PN: 9996128474

Copyright © 2020 by Elsevier, Inc. All rights reserved.

Cover image: Opioid analgesics like morphine and fentanyl act by turning on the μ-opioid receptor. Recent advances have enabled visualization of the three-dimensional shape of the μ-opioid receptor *(blue)* and the pocket where endorphins and opioids *(yellow)* bind.
Courtesy Aashish Manglik, MD, PhD, Assistant Professor, Departments of Pharmaceutical Chemistry and Anesthesia and Perioperative Care, University of California, San Francisco.

Chapters 6 and 7: Stephanie M. Oberfrank, Marcus Rall, Peter Dieckmann, Michaela Kolbe, and David M. Gaba retain copyright for their original figures/images.

No part of this publication may be reproduced or transmitted in any form or by any means, electronic or mechanical, including photocopying, recording, or any information storage and retrieval system, without permission in writing from the publisher. Details on how to seek permission, further information about the Publisher's permissions policies and our arrangements with organizations such as the Copyright Clearance Center and the Copyright Licensing Agency, can be found at our website: www.elsevier.com/permissions.

This book and the individual contributions contained in it are protected under copyright by the Publisher (other than as may be noted herein).

Notice

Practitioners and researchers must always rely on their own experience and knowledge in evaluating and using any information, methods, compounds or experiments described herein. Because of rapid advances in the medical sciences, in particular, independent verification of diagnoses and drug dosages should be made. To the fullest extent of the law, no responsibility is assumed by Elsevier, authors, editors or contributors for any injury and/or damage to persons or property as a matter of products liability, negligence or otherwise, or from any use or operation of any methods, products, instructions, or ideas contained in the material herein.

Previous editions copyrighted 2015, 2010, 2005, 2000, 1994, 1990, 1986, 1981

Library of Congress Control Number: 2019948954

Senior Content Strategist: Sarah Barth
Senior Content Development Specialist: Ann Ruzycka Anderson
Publishing Services Manager: Julie Eddy
Senior Project Manager: Cindy Thoms
Senior Book Designer: Amy Buxton

Printed in Canada

Last digit is the print number: 9 8 7 6 5 4 3

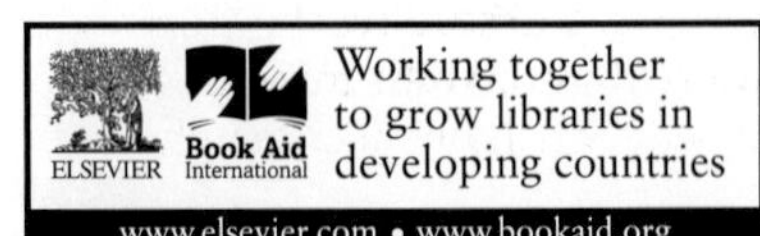

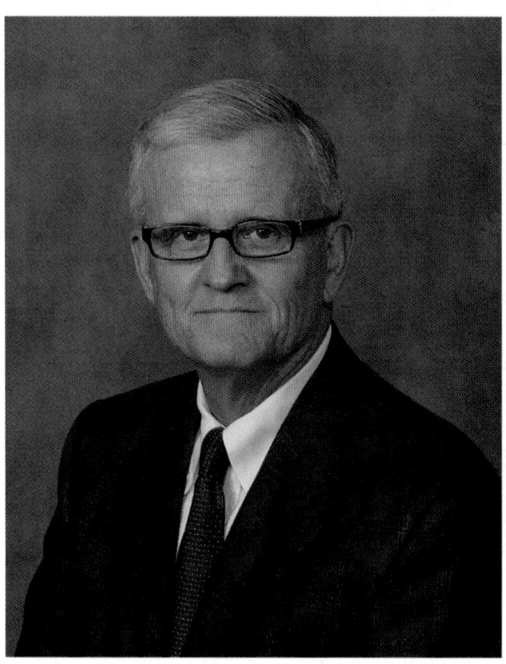

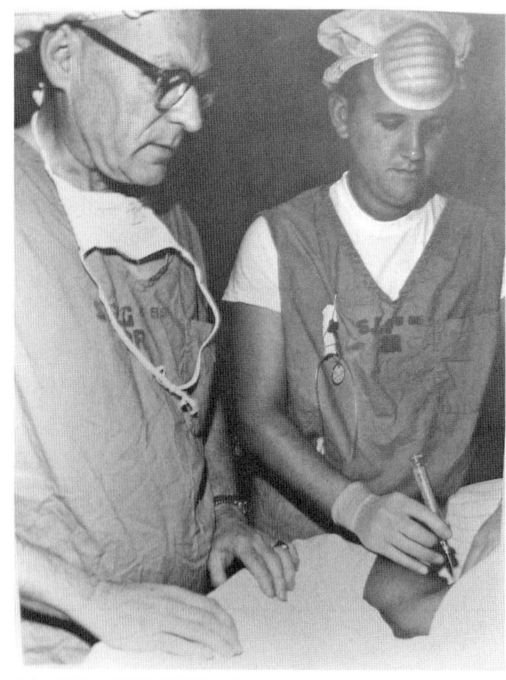

Dr. Stuart Cullen, inaugural chair of the Department of Anesthesia, observes Dr. Ronald Miller performing a regional block.

There are few texts so closely identified with an individual as *Miller's Anesthesia*. Since publication of the first edition in 1981, it is difficult to imagine anyone training in anesthesia, regardless of country of origin or location of training, not having been affected by this book. *Miller's Anesthesia* serves as the definitive source for those practicing or studying anesthesia and its various subspecialties.

Ronald Miller arrived from Indiana and completed his anesthesia training at the University of California, San Francisco (UCSF) in 1968, which included a master's degree in Pharmacology, an experience that would inform his lifelong dedication to academic anesthesia. Soon thereafter, Miller left San Francisco to serve his country in Vietnam, where he cared for wounded soldiers at the Naval Hospital in Da Nang, receiving the Bronze Star for Meritorious Service. He returned with more than a prestigious medal, as it was during this experience that his interest in transfusion medicine began, and while serving, he collected data and pursued both the mechanisms of coagulopathy with massive transfusion. This seminal work led to important practice changes in transfusion medicine. Shortly after returning to UCSF, he began his acclaimed work on neuromuscular blockade, which also led to significant practice change around the world.

As Chair of Anesthesia at UCSF for 25 years, Miller built a legendary department, training hundreds of anesthesiologists and seeding the world with leaders in our specialty. More than 20 alumni of the residency (including two of the co-editors) have become chairs of anesthesia in academic departments. He has had an illustrious career as an academic, publishing nearly 400 papers and accumulating accolades from national and international organizations, including perhaps the highest honor of being inducted into the Institute of Medicine of the National Academy of Sciences (now the National Academy of Medicine). In addition to establishing and leading this text, from 1991-2006, Miller served as Editor-in-Chief of *Anesthesia and Analgesia*, completely re-envisioning the journal and turning it into one of the leading journals in our specialty, drawing from editors and authors from around the world.

While *Miller's Anesthesia* is a team effort, it was the inspired vision of Ron Miller to create this "deep dive" into our specialty. As other texts became smaller and more concise, Miller had the vision to keep his text comprehensive, even spanning three volumes before transitioning to the two volumes in the current form. Each edition over nearly 40 years has defined our specialty. We also celebrate the international flavor of the book, with authors and editors from around the globe giving a diverse perspective on our specialty. As we publish the ninth edition, we are deeply aware of the history of the book, and our obligation to preserve and grow its excellence. We therefore dedicate the ninth edition of the book to a visionary leader of our specialty, Ron Miller.

Associate Editors

Matthew T.V. Chan, MBBS, FANZCA, FHKCA, FHKAM
The Chinese University of Hong Kong

Kristin Engelhard, MD, PhD
University Medical Center, Johannes Gutenberg-University

Malin Jonsson Fagerlund, MD, PhD
Karolinska University Hospital and Karolinska Institutet

Kathryn Hagen
Aukland District Health Board

Meghan Brooks Lane-Fall, MD, MSHP
University of Pennsylvania Perelman School of Medicine

Lisa R. Leffert, MD
Massachusetts General Hospital

Linda L. Liu, MD
University of California, San Francisco

Vivek K. Moitra, MD
Columbia University Medical Center

Ala Nozari, MD, PhD
Harvard Medical School

Andrew Patterson, MD, PhD
Emory University School of Medicine

Marc P. Steurer, MD, MHA, DESA
University of California, San Francisco

Tracey L. Stierer, MD
Johns Hopkins University School of Medicine

Contributors

Anthony Ray Absalom, MBChB, FRCA, MD
Professor, Anesthesiology
University Medical Center Groningen
University of Groningen
Groningen, Netherlands

Leah Acker, MD, PhD
Department of Anesthesiology
Duke University Medical Center
Durham, North Carolina
United States

Oluwaseun Akeju, MD, MMSc
Associate Professor
Harvard Medical School
Department of Anesthesia, Critical Care and Pain Medicine
Massachusetts General Hospital
Boston, Massachusetts
United States

Meredith A. Albrecht, MD, PhD
Chief of Obstetric Anesthesia
Associate Professor
Department of Anesthesiology
Medical College of Wisconsin
Milwaukee, Wisconsin
United States

J. Matthew Aldrich, MD
Medical Director, Critical Care Medicine
Clinical Professor
Anesthesia and Perioperative Care
University of California, San Francisco
San Francisco, California
United States

Paul Denney Allen, MD, PhD
Professor, Anesthesia
University of Leeds
Leeds, United Kingdom
Professor Emeritus
Anesthesia
Harvard Medical School
Boston, Massachusetts
United States

Katherine W. Arendt, MD
Associate Professor of Anesthesiology
Department of Anesthesiology and Perioperative Medicine
Mayo Clinic College of Medicine
Rochester, Minnesota
United States

Carlos A. Artime, MD
Associate Professor and Vice Chair of Finance and Operations
Department of Anesthesiology
McGovern Medical School at University of Texas Health Science Center
Houston, Texas
United States

Atilio Barbeito, MD, MPH
Associate Professor
Department of Anesthesiology
Duke University
Durham, North Carolina
United States

Brian Bateman, MD, MSc
Associate Professor of Anesthesia
Department of Anesthesiology, Perioperative and Pain Medicine
Brigham and Women's Hospital
Harvard Medical School
Boston, Massachusetts
United States

Charles B. Berde, MD, PhD
Sara Page Mayo Chair, Pediatric Pain Medicine
Department of Anesthesiology, Critical Care, and Pain Medicine
Boston Children's Hospital
Professor of Anesthesia and Pediatrics
Harvard Medical School
Boston, Massachusetts
United States

Sheri Berg, MD
Medical Director of the Post-Anesthesia Care Units
Director of Anesthesia, ECT Service
Director of Anesthesia, MGH Ketamine Clinic
Department of Anesthesia, Critical Care and Pain Medicine
Massachusetts General Hospital
Boston, Massachusetts
United States

Miles Berger, MD, PhD
Duke Anesthesiology Department
Neuroanesthesiology Division
Adjunct Faculty
Duke Center for Cognitive Neuroscience Senior Fellow
Duke Center for the Study of Aging and Human Development
Duke University Medical Center
Durham, North Carolina
United States

Edward A. Bittner, MD, PhD, MSEd, FCCM
Associate Professor of Anaesthesia
Harvard Medical School
Program Director, Critical Care-Anesthesiology Fellowship
Associate Director, Surgical Intensive Care Unit
Massachusetts General Hospital
Department of Anesthesia, Critical Care and Pain Medicine
Boston, Massachusetts
United States

James L. Blair, DO
Assistant Professor
Anesthesiology
Vanderbilt University Medical Center
Nashville, Tennessee
United States

Michael P. Bokoch, MD, PhD
Assistant Clinical Professor
Anesthesia and Perioperative Care
University of California, San Francisco
San Francisco, California
United States

Matthias R. Braehler, MD, PhD
Professor, Anesthesia and Perioperative Care
Medical Director, Post Anesthesia Care Unit
University of California, San Francisco, School of Medicine
San Francisco, California
United States

Kristine E.W. Breyer, MD
Associate Professor
Anesthesia
University of California, San Francisco
San Francisco, California
United States

Emery N. Brown, MD, PhD
Warren M. Zapol Professor of Anesthesia
Harvard Medical School
Department of Anesthesia, Critical Care and Pain Medicine
Massachusetts General Hospital
Edward Hood Taplin Professor of Medical Engineering
Professor of Computational Neuroscience
Institute for Medical Engineering and Science
Picower Institute for Learning and Memory
Institute for Data Systems and Society
Department of Brain and Cognitive Sciences
Massachusetts Institute of Technology
Boston, Massachusetts
United States

Richard Brull, MD, FRCPC
Professor
Anesthesia
University of Toronto
Toronto, Ontario
Canada

Sorin J. Brull, MD, FCARCSI (Hon)
Professor
Mayo Clinic College of Medicine and Science
Consultant
Anesthesiology and Perioperative Medicine
Mayo Clinic Florida
Jacksonville, Florida
United States

David Winthrop Buck, MD, MBA
Associate Professor
Anesthesiology
Cincinnati Children's Hospital
Cincinnati, Ohio
United States

Daniel H. Burkhardt III, MD
Associate Professor
Anesthesia and Perioperative Care
University of California, San Francisco
San Francisco, California
United States

Enrico M. Camporesi, MD
Emeritus Professor of Surgery and Molecular Pharmacology/Physiology
University of South Florida
Attending Anesthesiologist and Director of Research
TEAMHealth Anesthesia
Tampa, Florida
United States

Javier H. Campos, MD
Professor
Anesthesia
University of Iowa Health Care
Iowa City, Iowa
United States

Vincent W.S. Chan, MD, FRCPC, FRCA
Professor
Anesthesia
University of Toronto
Toronto, Ontario
Canada

Joyce Chang, MD
Assistant Clinical Professor
Anesthesia and Perioperative Care
University of California, San Francisco
San Francisco, California
United States

Catherine L. Chen, MD, MPH
Assistant Professor
Department of Anesthesia and Perioperative Care
University of California, San Francisco
San Francisco, California
United States

Lucy Lin Chen, MD
Associate Professor
Department of Anesthesia, Critical Care and Pain Medicine
Massachusetts General Hospital
Harvard Medical School
Boston, Massachusetts
United States

Anne D. Cherry, MD
Assistant Professor
Department of Anesthesiology
Duke University Medical Center
Durham, North Carolina
United States

Hovig V. Chitilian, MD
Assistant Professor of Anesthesia
Department of Anesthesia, Critical Care and Pain Medicine
Massachusetts General Hospital
Harvard Medical School
Boston, Massachusetts
United States

Christopher Choukalas, MD, MS
Associate Clinical Professor
Department of Anesthesia and Perioperative Care
University of California, San Francisco
San Francisco, California
United States

Mabel Chung, MD
Instructor in Anesthesia
Department of Anesthesia, Critical Care and Pain Medicine
Massachusetts General Hospital
Boston, Massachusetts
United States

Casper Claudius, MD, PhD
Head of Anesthesia Section
Department of Anesthesia and Intensive Care
Bispebjerg and Frederiksberg Hospital
University of Copenhagen
Copenhagen, Denmark

Neal H. Cohen, MD, MPH, MS
Professor of Anesthesia and Perioperative Care
Professor of Medicine
Vice Dean
University of California, San Francisco, School of Medicine
San Francisco, California
United States

Douglas A. Colquhoun, MB ChB, MSc, MPH
Clinical Lecturer of Anesthesiology
Department of Anesthesiology
University of Michigan Medical School
Ann Arbor, Michigan
United States

Lane C. Crawford, MD
Assistant Professor
Anesthesiology
Vanderbilt University Medical Center
Nashville, Tennessee
United States

Jerome C. Crowley, MD, MPH
Clinical Fellow in Anesthesia
Anesthesia, Critical Care and Pain Medicine
Massachusetts General Hospital
Boston, Massachusetts
United States

Gaston Cudemus, MD
Assistant Professor of Anesthesia
Cardiothoracic Anesthesiology and Critical Care
Harvard Medical School
Heart Center ECMO Director
Massachusetts General Hospital
Boston, Massachusetts
United States

Deborah J. Culley, MD
Assistant Professor
Anesthesia and Pain Management
Harvard Medical School
Department of Anesthesiology
Perioperative and Pain Medicine
Brigham and Women's Hospital
Boston, Massachusetts
United States

Andrew F. Cumpstey, MA(Cantab), BM BCh, DiMM
NIHR BRC Clinical Research Fellow and Specialty Trainee
Anesthesia and Critical Care Research Unit
University Hospital Southampton
Southampton, United Kingdom

Andrew Davidson, MBBS, MD, FANZCA, FAHMS
Staff Anaesthetist
Anaesthesia and Pain Management
Royal Children's Hospital
Medical Director, Melbourne Children's Trials Centre
Murdoch Children's Research Institute
Professor, Department of Paediatrics
University of Melbourne
Melbourne, Victoria
Australia

Nicholas A. Davis, MD
Assistant Professor of Anesthesiology
Department of Anesthesiology
Columbia University Medical Center
New York, New York
United States

Hans D. de Boer, MD PhD
Anesthesiology, Pain Medicine, and Procedural Sedation and Analgesia
Martini General Hospital Groningen
Groningen, Netherlands

Stacie Deiner, MS, MD
Vice Chair for Research
Professor
Departments of Anesthesiology, Geriatrics and Palliative Care, and Neurosurgery
Icahn School of Medicine at Mount Sinai
New York, New York
United States

Peter Dieckmann, PhD, Dipl-Psych
Senior Scientist
Copenhagen Academy for Medical Education and Simulation
Center for Human Resources, Capital Region of Denmark
Herlev Hospital
Herlev, Denmark
Professor for Healthcare Education and Patient Safety
Department of Quality and Health Technology
Faculty of Health Sciences
University of Stavanger
Stavanger, Norway
External Lecturer
Department of Clinical Medicine
Copenhagen University
Copenhagen, Denmark

Anne L. Donovan, MD
Associate Clinical Professor
Anesthesia and Perioperative Care, Division of Critical Care Medicine
University of California, San Francisco
San Francisco, California
United States

John C. Drummond, MD, FRCPC
Emeritus Professor of Anesthesiology
University of California, San Diego
San Diego, California
Staff Anesthesiologist
VA San Diego Healthcare System
La Jolla, California
United States

Matthew Dudley, MD
Assistant Clinical Professor
Anesthesia and Perioperative Care
University of California, San Francisco
San Francisco, California
United States

Roderic G. Eckenhoff, MD
Austin Lamont Professor
Anesthesiology and Critical Care
University of Pennsylvania Perelman School of Medicine
Philadelphia, Pennsylvania
United States

David M. Eckmann, PhD, MD
Horatio C. Wood Professor of Anesthesiology and Critical Care
Professor of Bioengineering
University of Pennsylvania
Philadelphia, Pennsylvania
United States

Mark R. Edwards, BMedSci, BMBS, MRCP, FRCA
Consultant in Anaesthesia and Perioperative Medicine
Department of Anaesthesia
University Hospital Southampton NHS Foundation Trust
Honorary Senior Clinical Lecturer
University of Southampton
Southampton, United Kingdom

Matthias Eikermann, MD, PhD
Professor
Anaesthesia, Critical Care, and Pain Medicine
Beth Israel Deaconess Medical Center
Boston, Massachusetts
United States

Nabil M. Elkassabany, MD, MSCE
Associate Professor
Director; Sections of Orthopedic and Regional Anesthesiology
Department of Anesthesiology and Critical Care
University of Pennsylvania
Philadelphia, Pennsylvania
United States

Dan B. Ellis, MD
Assistant Division Chief, General Surgery Anesthesia
Department of Anesthesia, Critical Care and Pain Medicine
Massachusetts General Hospital
Boston, Massachusetts
United States

Kristin Engelhard, MD, PhD
Professor
Department of Anesthesiology
University Medical Center, Johannes Gutenberg-University
Mainz, Germany

Lars I. Eriksson, MD, PhD, FRCA
Professor and Academic Chair
Department of Physiology and Pharmacology
Section for Anaesthesiology and Intensive Care Medicine
Function Preoperative Medicine and Intensive Care
Karolinska Institutet and Karolinska University Hospital
Stockholm, Sweden

Lisbeth Evered, BSc, MBiostat, PhD
Associate Professor
Anaesthesia and Acute Pain Medicine
St Vincent's Hospital, Melbourne
Associate Professor
Anaesthesia, Perioperative and Pain Medicine Unit
University of Melbourne
Melbourne, Australia

Oleg V. Evgenov, MD, PhD
Clinical Associate Professor
Department of Anesthesiology, Perioperative Care, and Pain Medicine
New York University Langone Medical Center
New York University School of Medicine
New York, New York
United States

Malin Jonsson Fagerlund, MD, PhD
Associate Professor, Senior Consultant
Function Perioperative Medicine and Intensive Care
Karolinska University Hospital and Karolinska Institutet
Stockholm, Sweden

Zhuang T. Fang, MD, MSPH, FASA
Clinical Professor
Department of Anesthesiology and Perioperative Medicine
Associate Director, Jules Stein Operating Room
David Geffen School of Medicine at UCLA
Los Angeles, California

Marla B. Ferschl, MD
Associate Professor of Pediatric Anesthesia
Department of Anesthesia and Perioperative Care
University of California, San Francisco
San Francisco, California
United States

Emily Finlayson, MD, MSc, FACS
Professor of Surgery, Medicine, and Health Policy
University of California, San Francisco
San Francisco, California
United States

Michael Fitzsimons, MD
Director, Division of Cardiac Anesthesia
Department of Anesthesia, Critical Care and Pain Medicine
Massachusetts General Hospital
Associate Professor
Harvard Medical School
Boston, Massachusetts
United States

Lee A. Fleisher, MD
Robert D. Dripps Professor and Chair
Department of Anesthesiology and Critical Care
Professor of Medicine
Perelman School of Medicine
Senior Fellow, Leonard Davis Institute of Health Economics
University of Pennsylvania
Philadelphia, Pennsylvania
United States

Stuart A. Forman, MD, PhD
Professor of Anaesthesia
Anaesthesiology
Harvard Medical School
Anesthetist
Anesthesia Critical Care and Pain Medicine
Massachusetts General Hospital
Boston, Massachusetts
United States

Nicholas P. Franks, BSc, PhD
Professor
Life Sciences
Imperial College London
London, United Kingdom

Thomas Fuchs-Buder, MD, PhD
Professor
Anaesthesia and Critical Care
University Hospital Nancy/University of Lorraine
Head of the Department
OR Department
University Hospital
Nancy, France

Kazuhiko Fukuda, MD, PhD
Kyoto University Hospital
Department of Anesthesia
Kyoto University Hospital
Kyoto, Japan

David M. Gaba, MD
Associate Dean for Immersive and Simulation-based Learning
Professor of Anesthesiology, Perioperative and Pain Medicine
Stanford University School of Medicine
Stanford, California
Founder and Co-Director, Simulation Center
Anesthesia
VA Palo Alto Health Care System
Palo Alto, California
United States

Daniel Gainsburg, MD, MS
Professor
Anesthesiology, Perioperative and Pain Medicine
Professor, Urology
Icahn School of Medicine at Mount Sinai
New York, New York
United States

Samuel Michael Galvagno Jr., DO, PhD, MS
Associate Professor
Anesthesiology
University of Maryland/Shock Trauma Center
Baltimore, Maryland
United States

Sarah Gebauer, BA, MD
Anesthesiologist, Elk River Anesthesia Associates
Chair, Perioperative Service Line
Yampa Valley Medical Center
Steamboat Springs, Colorado
United States

Adrian W. Gelb, MBChB
Professor
Anesthesia and Perioperative Care
University of California, San Francisco
San Francisco, California
United States

Andrew T. Gray, MD, PhD
Professor of Clinical Anesthesia
Anesthesia and Perioperative Care
University of California, San Francisco
San Francisco, California
United States

William J. Greeley, MD, MBA
Professor
Anesthesiology and Critical Care Medicine
The Children's Hospital of Philadelphia
Philadelphia, Pennsylvania
United States

Thomas E. Grissom, MD
Associate Professor
Anesthesiology
University of Maryland School of Medicine
Baltimore, Maryland
United States

Michael P.W. Grocott, BSc, MBBS, MD, FRCA, FRCP, FFICM
Professor of Anaesthesia and Critical Care Medicine
Head, Integrative Physiology and Critical Illness Group
CES Lead, Critical Care Research Area
University of Southampton
Southampton, United Kingdom

Michael A. Gropper, MD, PhD
Professor and Chair
Department of Anesthesia and Perioperative Care
Professor of Physiology
Investigator, Cardiovascular Research Institute
University of California, San Francisco, School of Medicine
San Francisco, California
United States

Rachel A. Hadler, MD
Assistant Professor
Anesthesiology and Critical Care
University of Pennsylvania Perelman School of Medicine
Philadelphia, Pennsylvania
United States

Carin A. Hagberg, MD, FASA
Chief Academic Officer
Division Head, Anesthesiology, Critical Care, and Pain Medicine
Helen Shaffer Fly Distinguished Professor of Anesthesiology
Department of Anesthesiology and Perioperative Medicine
University of Texas MD Anderson Cancer Center
Houston, Texas
United States

Dusan Hanidziar, MD, PhD
Instructor in Anesthesia
Harvard Medical School
Department of Anesthesia, Critical Care and Pain Medicine
Massachusetts General Hospital
Boston, Massachusetts
United States

Göran Hedenstierna, MD, PhD
Senior Professor
Uppsala University, Medical Sciences
Clinical Physiology
Uppsala, Sweden

Eugenie S. Heitmiller, MD, FAAP
Joseph E. Robert, Jr. Professor and Chief
Anesthesiology, Pain and Perioperative Medicine
Children's National Medical Center
Professor of Anesthesiology and Pediatrics
Anesthesiology
George Washington University School of Medicine and Health Sciences
Washington, District of Columbia
United States

Hugh C. Hemmings, MD, PhD
Professor, Anesthesiology and Pharmacology
Weill Cornell Medicine
Attending Anesthesiologist
Anesthesiology
New York Presbyterian Hospital
Senior Associate Dean for Research
Weill Cornell Medicine
New York, New York
United States

Simon Andrew Hendel, MBBS (Hons), FANZCA, GDip Journalism
Specialist Anaesthetist
Anaesthesia and Perioperative Medicine
Trauma Consultant
Trauma Service and National Trauma Research Institute
The Alfred Hospital
Lecturer
Anaesthesia and Perioperative Medicine
Monash University
Retrieval Physician
Adult Retrieval Victoria
Ambulance Victoria
Melbourne, Victoria
Australia

Robert W. Hurley, MD, PhD, FASA
Professor
Department of Anesthesiology and Public Health Sciences
Wake Forest School of Medicine
Executive Director
Pain Shared Service Line
Wake Forest Baptist Health
Winston Salem, North Carolina
United States

Samuel A. Irefin, MD, FCCM
Associate Professor
Anesthesiology and Intensive Care Medicine
Cleveland Clinic
Cleveland, Ohio
United States

Yumiko Ishizawa, MD, MPH, PhD
Assistant Professor of Anaesthesia
Harvard Medical School
Assistant Anesthetist, Critical Care and Pain Medicine
Massachusetts General Hospital
Boston, Massachusetts
United States

Alexander I.R. Jackson, BMedSci (Hons), MBChB
NIHR Academic Clinical Fellow and Specialty Trainee
Anaesthesia and Critical Care Research Unit
University of Southampton
Southampton, United Kingdom

Yandong Jiang, MD, PhD
Professor
Anesthesiology
McGovern Medical School
University of Texas
Houston, Texas
United States

Daniel W. Johnson, MD
Associate Professor
Division Chief, Critical Care
Fellowship Director, Critical Care
Medical Director, Cardiovascular ICU
Department of Anesthesiology
University of Nebraska Medical Center
Omaha, Nebraska
United States

Ken B. Johnson, MD
Professor
Anesthesiology
University of Utah
Salt Lake City, Utah
United States

Rebecca L. Johnson, MD
Associate Professor of Anesthesiology
Department of Anesthesiology and Perioperative Medicine
Mayo Clinic
Rochester, Minnesota
United States

Edmund H. Jooste, MBChB
Associate Professor
Department of Anesthesiology
Duke University School of Medicine
Clinical Director
Pediatric Cardiac Anesthesiology
Duke Children's Hospital and Health Center
Durham, North Carolina
United States

David W. Kaczka, MD, PhD
Associate Professor
Anesthesia, Biomedical Engineering, and Radiology
University of Iowa
Iowa City, Iowa
United States

Cor J. Kalkman, MD, PhD
Professor
Division of Anesthesiology, Intensive Care, and Emergency Medicine
University Medical Center Utrecht
Utrecht, Netherlands

Brian P. Kavanagh, MB FRCPC †
Professor of Anesthesia, Physiology, and Medicine
Departments of Critical Care Medicine and Anesthesia
Hospital for Sick Children
University of Toronto
Toronto, Ontario
Canada

Jens Kessler, MD
Department of Anesthesiology
University Hospital Heidelberg
Heidelberg, Germany

Mary A. Keyes, MD
Clinical Professor
Department of Anesthesiology and Perioperative Medicine
David Geffen School of Medicine at UCLA
Director, Jules Stein Operating Room
University of California, Los Angeles
Los Angeles, California
United States

Sachin K. Kheterpal, MD, MBA
Associate Professor of Anesthesiology
Department of Anesthesiology
University of Michigan Medical School
Ann Arbor, Michigan
United States

Jesse Kiefer, MD
Assistant Professor
Anesthesiology and Critical Care
University of Pennsylvania
Philadelphia, Pennsylvania
United States

Todd J. Kilbaugh, MD
Associate Professor of Anesthesiology, Critical Care, and Pediatrics
Department of Anesthesiology and Critical Care Medicine
Children's Hospital of Philadelphia
University of Pennsylvania School of Medicine
Philadelphia, Pennsylvania
United States

Tae Kyun Kim, MD, PhD
Professor
Anesthesia and Pain Medicine
Pusan National University School of Medicine
Busan, Republic of Korea

Christoph H. Kindler, MD
Professor and Chairman
Department of Anesthesia and Perioperative Medicine
Kantonsspital Aarau
Aarau, Switzerland

---
†Deceased

John R. Klinck, MD
Consultant Anaesthetist
Division of Perioperative Care
Addenbrooke's Hospital
Cambridge, United Kingdom

Nerissa U. Ko, MD, MAS
Professor
Department of Neurology
University of California, San Francisco
San Francisco, California
United States

Michaela Kolbe, PD, Dr rer nat
Psychologist, Director
Simulation Center
University Hospital Zurich
Management, Technology, Economics
Faculty ETH Zurich
Zurich, Switzerland

Andreas Kopf, Dr med
Anesthesiology and Critical Care Medicine
Freie Universität Berlin - Charité Campus Benjamin Franklin
Professor
International Graduate Program Medical Neurosciences
Charité, Berlin
Germany

Sandra L. Kopp, MD
Professor of Anesthesiology
Department of Anesthesiology and Perioperative Medicine
Mayo Clinic
Rochester, Minnesota
United States

Megan L. Krajewski, MD
Instructor in Anaesthesia
Harvard Medical School
Department of Anesthesia, Critical Care and Pain Medicine
Beth Israel Deaconess Medical Center
Boston, Massachusetts
United States

Kate Kronish, MD
Anesthesiology and Perioperative Care
University of California, San Francisco
San Francisco, California
United States

Avinash B. Kumar, MD, FCCM, FCCP
Professor
Anesthesiology and Critical Care
Vanderbilt University Medical Center
Brentwood, Tennessee
United States

Alexander S. Kuo, MS, MD
Assistant Professor
Harvard Medical School
Assistant in Anesthesia
Massachusetts General Hospital
Boston, Massachusetts
United States

Yvonne Y. Lai, MD
Instructor in Anesthesia
Anesthesia, Critical Care and Pain Medicine
Massachusetts General Hospital
Boston, Massachusetts
United States

Arthur Lam, MD
Professor of Anesthesiology
University of California, San Diego
San Diego, California
United States

Benn Morrie Lancman, MBBS, MHumFac, FANZCA
Assistant Professor
Director of Trauma Anesthesia
Department of Anesthesia
University of California, San Francisco
San Francisco, California
United States

Meghan Brooks Lane-Fall, MD, MSHP
Assistant Professor
Anesthesiology and Critical Care
University of Pennsylvania Perelman School of Medicine
Co-Director
Center for Perioperative Outcomes Research and Transformation
University of Pennsylvania Perelman School of Medicine
Senior Fellow
Leonard Davis Institute of Health Economics
University of Pennsylvania
Philadelphia, Pennsylvania
United States

Brian P. Lemkuil, MD
Associate Clinical Professor of Anesthesiology
University of California, San Diego
San Diego, California
United States

Kate Leslie, MBBS, MD, MEpid, MHlthServMt, Hon DMedSci, FANZCA
Professor and Head of Research
Department of Anaesthesia and Pain Management
Royal Melbourne Hospital
Melbourne, Australia

Jason M. Lewis, MD
Assistant Division Chief, Orthopedic Anesthesia Division
Anesthesia, Critical Care, and Pain Medicine
Massachusetts General Hospital
Boston, Massachusetts
United States

Yafen Liang, MD, PhD
Visiting Associate Professor
Cardiovascular Anesthesiology
Director of Advanced Heart Failure Anesthesiology
McGovern Medical School
University of Texas
Houston, Texas
United States

Elaine Chiewlin Liew, MD, FRCA
Assistant Clinical Professor
Department of Anesthesiology and Perioperative Medicine
David Geffen School of Medicine at UCLA
Los Angeles, California
United States

Michael S. Lipnick, MD
Assistant Professor
Anesthesia and Perioperative Care
University of California, San Francisco
San Francisco, California
United States

Philipp Lirk, MD, PhD
Attending Anesthesiologist
Department of Anesthesiology, Perioperative and Pain Medicine
Brigham and Women's Hospital
Associate Professor
Harvard Medical School
Boston, Massachusetts
United States

Steven J. Lisco, MD
Chairman
Newland Professor of Anesthesiology
Department of Anesthesiology
University of Nebraska Medical Center
Omaha, Nebraska
United States

Kathleen D. Liu, MD, PhD, MAS
Professor
Departments of Medicine and Anesthesia
University of California, San Francisco
San Francisco, California
United States

Linda L. Liu, MD
Professor
Department of Anesthesia and Perioperative Care
University of California, San Francisco
San Francisco, California
United States

Per-Anne Lönnqvist, MD, FRCA, DEAA, PhD
Professor
Department of Physiology and Pharmacology
Karolinska Institutet
Senior Consultant
Pediatrics Anesthesia and Intensive Care
Karolinska University Hospital
Stockholm, Sweden

Alan J.R. Macfarlane, BSc (Hons), MBChB, MRCP, FRCA, EDRA
Consultant Anaesthetist
Department of Anaesthesia
Glasgow Royal Infirmary
Honorary Clinical Associate Professor
Anaesthesia, Critical Care and Pain Medicine
University of Glasgow
Glasgow, United Kingdom

Kelly Machovec, MD, MPH
Assistant Professor
Department of Anesthesiology
Duke University Hospital
Durham, North Carolina
United States

Aman Mahajan, MD, PhD
Peter and Eva Safar Professor and Chair
University of Pittsburgh School of Medicine
Pittsburgh, Pennsylvania
United States

Michael Mahla, MD
Professor and Chair
Anesthesiology
Sidney Kimmel Medical College of Thomas Jefferson University
Philadelphia, Pennsylvania
United States

Feroze Mahmood, MD
Professor of Anaesthesia
Harvard Medical School
Department of Anesthesia, Critical Care and Pain Medicine
Beth Israel Deaconess Medical Center
Boston, Massachusetts
United States

Anuj Malhotra, MD
Assistant Professor
Associate Program Director, Pain Medicine
Department of Anesthesiology, Perioperative, and Pain Medicine
Icahn School of Medicine at Mount Sinai
New York, New York
United States

Gaurav Malhotra, MD
Assistant Professor
Anesthesiology and Critical Care
Perelman School of Medicine
Philadelphia, Pennsylvania
United States

Vinod Malhotra, MD
Professor and Vice Chair, Clinical Affairs
Anesthesiology
Professor of Anesthesiology in Clinical Urology
Weill Cornell Medicine
Clinical Director of Operating Rooms
Medical Director
David H. Koch Ambulatory Care Center
Weill Cornell Medicine-New York Presbyterian Hospital
New York, New York
United States

Jianren Mao, MD, PhD
Richard J. Kitz Professor of Anesthesia Research
Anesthesia, Critical Care, and Pain Medicine
Massachusetts General Hospital, Harvard Medical School
Harvard University
Boston, Massachusetts
United States

Jonathan Mark, MD
Professor of Anesthesiology
Assistant Professor in Medicine
Duke University School of Medicine
Durham, North Carolina
United States

Laurie O. Mark, MD
Assistant Professor of Anesthesiology
Department of Anesthesiology
Rush University Medical Center
Chicago, Illinois
United States

J.A. Jeevendra Martyn, MD, FRCA, FCCM
Professor of Anesthesiology
Director, Clinical & Biochemical Pharmacology Laboratory
Department of Anesthesia, Critical Care and Pain Medicine
Massachusetts General Hospital
Anesthetist-in-Chief at the Shriners Hospital for Children
Professor of Anaesthesia
Harvard Medical School
Boston, Massachusetts
United States

George A. Mashour, MD, PhD
Bert N. La Du Professor of Anesthesiology
Director, Center for Consciousness Science
Department of Anesthesiology
University of Michigan
Ann Arbor, Michigan
United States

John J. McAuliffe III, MD, CM, MBA
Professor of Clinical Anesthesiology
Department of Anesthesiology
Cincinnati Children's Hospital Medical Center
University of Cincinnati College of Medicine
Cincinnati, Ohio
United States

Claude Meistelman, MD
Professor and Chair
Anesthesiology and Intensive Care Medicine
CHU de Nancy Brabois
Université de Lorraine
Vandoeuvre, Lorraine
France

Marcos F. Vidal Melo, MD, PhD
Professor of Anaesthesia
Department of Anesthesia, Critical Care and Pain Medicine
Massachusetts General Hospital
Boston, Massachusetts
United States

Marilyn Michelow, MD
Assistant Clinical Professor
Department of Anesthesia and Perioperative Care
University of California, San Francisco
Staff Physician, Anesthesia
San Francisco VA Medical Center
San Francisco, California
United States

Ronald D. Miller, MD
Professor Emeritus of Anesthesia and Perioperative Care
Department of Anesthesia and Perioperative Care
University of California, San Francisco, School of Medicine
San Francisco, California
United States

Richard E. Moon, MD, FACP, FCCP, FRCPC
Professor of Anesthesiology
Professor of Medicine
Medical Director
Center for Hyperbaric Medicine and Environmental Physiology
Duke University Medical Center
Durham, North Carolina
United States

William P. Mulvoy III, MD, MBA
Major, U.S. Army Medical Corps
Assistant Professor
Division of Critical Care and Division of Cardiovascular Anesthesiology
Department of Anesthesiology
University of Nebraska Medical Center
Omaha, Nebraska
United States

Glenn Murphy, MD
Director, Cardiac Anesthesia and Clinical Research
Anesthesiology
NorthShore University Health System
Evanston, Illinois
Clinical Professor
Anesthesiology
University of Chicago Pritzker School of Medicine
Chicago, Illinois
United States

Monty Mythen, MBBS, FRCA, MD, FFICM
Smiths Medical Professor of Anaesthesia and Critical Care
Centre for Anaesthesia
University College London
London, United Kingdom

Jacques Prince Neelankavil, MD
Associate Professor
Department of Anesthesiology
University of California, Los Angeles
Los Angeles, California
United States

Patrick Neligan, MA, MB, FCARCSI
Professor
Department of Anaesthesia and Intensive Care
Galway University Hospitals and National University of Ireland
Galway, Ireland

Mark D. Neuman, MD, MSc
Associate Professor
Anesthesiology and Critical Care
University of Pennsylvania Perelman School of Medicine
Philadelphia, Pennsylvania
United States

Dolores B. Njoku, MD
Associate Professor
Anesthesiology and Critical Care Medicine, Pediatrics and Pathology
Johns Hopkins University
Baltimore, Maryland
United States

Ala Nozari, MD, PhD
Associate Professor of Anaesthesia
Harvard Medical School
Director of Neuroanesthesia and Neurocritical Care
Beth Israel Deaconess Medical Center
Boston, Massachusetts
United States

Shinju Obara, MD
Associate Professor
Surgical Operation Department
Department of Anesthesiology
Fukushima Medical University Hospital
Fukushima, Japan

Stephanie Maria Oberfrank, MD, Dr med, MBA
Marienhospital Stuttgart
Academic Teaching Hospital of the University of Tübingen, Germany
Department of Anesthesia, Intensive Care and Pain Medicine
Stuttgart, Germany
InPASS GmbH
Institute for Patient Safety and Simulation Team Training
Reutlingen, Germany

Anup Pamnani, MD
Assistant Professor of Anesthesiology
Department of Anesthesiology
Weill Cornell Medicine
New York, New York
United States

Anil K. Panigrahi, MD, PhD
Clinical Assistant Professor
Department of Anesthesiology, Perioperative and Pain Medicine
Department of Pathology, Division of Transfusion Medicine
Stanford University School of Medicine
Stanford, California
United States

Anil Patel, MBBS, FRCA
Anaesthesia and Perioperative Medicine
Royal National Throat, Nose and Ear Hospital
University College Hospital
London, United Kingdom

Piyush M. Patel, MD
Professor of Anesthesiology
University of California, San Diego
San Diego, California
Staff Anesthesiologist
VA San Diego Healthcare System
La Jolla, California
United States

Robert A. Pearce, MD, PhD
Professor
Anesthesiology
University of Wisconsin-Madison
Madison, Wisconsin
United States

Rupert M. Pearse, MBBS, BSc, MD(Res), FRCA, FFICM
Professor of Intensive Care Medicine
Queen Mary University
Adult Critical Care Unit
Royal London Hospital
London, United Kingdom

Misha Perouansky, MD
Professor
Anesthesiology and Perioperative Care
University of Wisconsin SMPH
Madison, Wisconsin
United States

Isaac Ness Pessah, MS, PhD
Professor and Chair
Molecular Biosciences
School of Veterinary Medicine
University of California, Davis
Davis, California
United States

Beverly K. Philip, MD
Founding Director, Day Surgery Unit
Department of Anesthesiology, Perioperative and Pain Medicine
Brigham and Women's Hospital
Professor of Anesthesia
Harvard Medical School
President
International Association for Ambulatory Surgery
Boston, Massachusetts
United States

Richard M. Pino, MD, PhD, FCCM
Associate Anesthetist
Department of Anesthesia, Critical Care and Pain Medicine
Massachusetts General Hospital
Associate Professor
Anesthesia
Harvard Medical School
Boston, Massachusetts
United States

Kane O. Pryor, MD
Vice Chair for Academic Affairs
Associate Professor of Clinical Anesthesiology
Associate Professor of Clinical Anesthesiology in Psychiatry
Weill Cornell Medicine
New York, New York
United States

Patrick L. Purdon, PhD
Associate Professor of Anaesthesia
Harvard Medical School
Nathaniel M. Sims Endowed Chair in Anesthesia Innovation and Bioengineering
Department of Anesthesia, Critical Care and Pain Medicine
Massachusetts General Hospital
Boston, Massachusetts
United States

Marcus Rall, MD, Dr med
CEO and Founder, InPASS GmbH
Institute for Patient Safety and Simulation Team Training
Prehospital Emergency Physician
Academic Teach Hospital
Founding President, DGSiM
German Society for Simulation in Healthcare
Reutlingen, Germany

James G. Ramsay, MD
Professor of Anesthesiology
Department of Anesthesia and Perioperative Care
University of California, San Francisco
San Francisco, California
United States

Marije Reekers, MD, PhD, MSc
Associate Professor
Anesthesiology
Leiden University Medical Center
Leiden, Netherlands

Michael F. Roizen, MD
Chair, Wellness Institute
Cleveland Clinic
Professor, Anesthesiology
Cleveland Clinic Learner College of Medicine
Cleveland, Ohio
United States

Mark D. Rollins, MD, PhD
Professor
Anesthesiology
University of Utah
Salt Lake City, Utah
United States

Stanley H. Rosenbaum, MA, MD
Professor of Anesthesiology, Internal Medicine, and Surgery
Department of Anesthesiology
Yale University School of Medicine
New Haven, Connecticut
United States

Patrick Ross, MD
Associate Professor of Anesthesiology and Critical Care Medicine
Children's Hospital of Los Angeles
University of Southern California School of Medicine
Los Angeles, California,
United States

Steven Roth, BA, MD
Michael Reese Endowed Professor of Anesthesiology
Professor, Ophthalmology and Visual Science
Professor Emeritus, Anesthesia and Critical Care
University of Chicago
Vice Head for Research and Faculty Development
Anesthesiology
University of Illinois College of Medicine
Chicago, Illinois
United States

Sten Rubertsson, MD, PhD
Professor
Department of Anesthesiology and Intensive Care Medicine
Uppsala University
Uppsala, Sweden

A. Sassan Sabouri, MD
Assistant Professor of Anesthesiology
Department of Anesthesia, Critical Care and Pain Medicine
Massachusetts General Hospital
Boston, Massachusetts
United States

Muhammad F. Sarwar, MD
Associate Professor of Anesthesiology
Director, Division of Cardiac Anesthesia
Department of Anesthesiology
SUNY Upstate Medical University
Syracuse, New York
United States

Becky Schroeder, MD, MMCi
Associate Professor
Anesthesiology
Duke University
Durham, North Carolina
United States

Mark Schumacher, MD, PhD
Professor and Chief
Division of Pain Medicine
Department of Anesthesia and Perioperative Care
University of California, San Francisco
San Francisco, California
United States

Bruce E. Searles, MS, CCP
Associate Professor and Department Chair
Department of Cardiovascular Perfusion
SUNY Upstate Medical University
Syracuse, New York
United States

Christoph N. Seubert, MD, PhD, DABNM
Professor of Anesthesiology
Anesthesiology
Chief, Division of Neuroanesthesia
Anesthesiology
University of Florida College of Medicine
Gainesville, Florida
United States

Steven L. Shafer, MD
Professor of Anesthesiology
Perioperative and Pain Medicine
Stanford University Medical Center
Stanford, California
United States

Ann Cai Shah, MD
Assistant Clinical Professor
Anesthesia and Perioperative Care
Division of Pain Medicine
University of California, San Francisco
San Francisco, California
United States

Nirav J. Shah, MD
Assistant Professor of Anesthesiology
Department of Anesthesiology
University of Michigan Medical School
Ann Arbor, Michigan
United States

Ahmed Shalabi, MBBCH, MSC
Associate Professor
Anesthesia and Perioperative Care
University of California, San Francisco
San Francisco, California
United States

Emily E. Sharpe, MD
Assistant Professor of Anesthesiology
Department of Anesthesiology and Perioperative Medicine
Mayo Clinic College of Medicine
Rochester, Minnesota
United States

Kenneth Shelton, MD
Assistant Professor of Anesthesiology
Medical Co-Director of the Heart Center ICU
Lead Intensivist of the Heart Center ICU
Director of Perioperative Echocardiography/Ultrasonography
Department of Anesthesia, Critical Care and Pain Medicine
Massachusetts General Hospital
Boston, Massachusetts
United States

Shiqian Shen, MD
Assistant Professor
Department of Anesthesia, Critical Care and Pain Medicine
Massachusetts General Hospital
Boston, Massachusetts
United States

Linda Shore-Lesserson, MD, FAHA, FASE
Professor of Anesthesiology
Zucker School of Medicine at Hofstra Northwell
Vice Chair for Academic Affairs
Director, Cardiovascular Anesthesiology
Northwell Health System, Northshore
Manhasset, New York
United States

Elske Sitsen, MD
Anesthesiology
Leiden University Medical Center
Leiden, Netherlands

Folke Sjöberg, MD, PhD
Professor, Consultant, and Director
The Burn Center
Department of Hand and Plastic Surgery and Intensive Care
Linköping University Hospital
Co-Chair, Division of Research
Department of Clinical and Experimental Medicine
Linköping University
Linköping, Sweden

Mark A. Skues, B Med Sci (Hons), BM, BS, FRCA
Editor-in-Chief
Ambulatory Surgery
Chester, United Kingdom
Chairman
Scientific Subcommittee Ambulatory Anaesthesia
European Society of Anaesthesiology
Belgium

Peter Slinger, MD, FRCPC
Professor
Anesthesia
University of Toronto
Toronto, Ontario
Canada

Ian Smith, FRCA, MD
Retired Senior Lecturer in Anaesthesia
Directorate of Anaesthesia
University Hospital of North Staffordshire
Stoke-on-Trent, United Kingdom

Ken Solt, MD
Associate Professor of Anaesthesia
Harvard Medical School
Department of Anesthesia, Critical Care and Pain Medicine
Massachusetts General Hospital
Boston, Massachusetts
United States

Abraham Sonny, MD
Assistant Anesthetist
Department of Anesthesia, Critical Care and Pain Medicine
Massachusetts General Hospital
Assistant Professor
Anesthesia
Harvard Medical School
Boston, Massachusetts
United States

Randolph H. Steadman, MD, MS
Professor and Vice Chair
Department of Anesthesiology and Perioperative Medicine
David Geffen School of Medicine at UCLA
University of California, Los Angeles
Los Angeles, California
United States

Christoph Stein, Prof, Dr med
Professor and Chair
Anesthesiology and Critical Care Medicine
Freie Universität Berlin - Charité Campus Benjamin Franklin
Professor
International Graduate Program Medical Neurosciences
Charité, Berlin
Germany

Marc P. Steurer, MD, MHA, DESA
Professor of Anesthesia and Perioperative Care
University of California, San Francisco
President, Trauma Anesthesiology Society
Vice-Chair
Committee on Trauma and Emergency Preparedness
American Society of Anesthesiologists
Associate Chair for Finance
UCSF Department of Anesthesia and Perioperative Care
Associate Chief
Department of Anesthesia
Zuckerberg San Francisco General Hospital and Trauma Center
San Francisco, California
United States

Marc E. Stone, MD
Professor of Anesthesiology
Program Director, Fellowship in Cardiothoracic Anesthesiology
Icahn School of Medicine at Mount Sinai
New York, New York
United States

Michel MRF Struys, MD, PhD
Professor and Chair, Department of Anesthesia
University of Groningen and University Medical Center Groningen
Groningen, Netherlands
Professor, Department of Anesthesia
Ghent University
Ghent, Belgium

Lena S. Sun, MD
E.M. Papper Professor of Pediatric Anesthesiology
Anesthesiology and Pediatrics
Columbia University Medical Center
New York, New York
United States

Santhanam Suresh, MD, FAAP
Professor and Chair, Pediatric Anesthesiology
Ann and Robert H Lurie Children's Hospital of Chicago
Arthur C. King Professor in Anesthesiology
Northwestern Feinberg School of Medicine
Chicago, Illinois
United States

John H. Turnbull, MD
Associate Professor
Anesthesia and Perioperative Care
University of California, San Francisco
San Francisco, California
United States

Gail A. Van Norman, MD
Professor
Anesthesiology and Pain Medicine
University of Washington
Adjunct Professor
Bioethics
University of Washington
Seattle, Washington
United States

Anna Mary Varughese, MD, FRCA, MPH
Director, Perioperative Quality and Safety
Associate Chief Quality Officer
Johns Hopkins All Children's Hospital
St. Petersburg, Florida
Associate Professor (PAR)
Anesthesiology
Johns Hopkins University School of Medicine
Baltimore, Maryland
United States

Rafael Vazquez, MD
Assistant Professor of Anesthesia
Harvard Medical School
Director of Anesthesia for Interventional Radiology
Department of Anesthesia, Critical Care and Pain Medicine
Massachusetts General Hospital
Boston, Massachusetts
United States

Laszlo Vutskits, MD, PhD
Head of Pediatric Anesthesia
Department of Anesthesiology
Clinical Pharmacology, Intensive Care, and Emergency Medicine
University Hospitals of Geneva
Geneva, Switzerland

Jaap Vuyk, MD, PhD
Associate Professor in Anesthesia
Vice-Chair, Anesthesiology
Leiden University Medical Center
Leiden, Netherlands

Stephen D. Weston, MD
Assistant Clinical Professor
Anesthesia and Perioperative Care
University of California, San Francisco
San Francisco, California
United States

Elizabeth L. Whitlock, MD, MSc
Assistant Professor
Department of Anesthesia and Perioperative Care
University of California, San Francisco
San Francisco, California
United States

Jeanine P. Wiener-Kronish, MD
Henry Isaiah Dorr Professor of Research and Teaching in Anaesthetics and Anaesthesia
Department of Anesthesia, Critical Care and Pain Medicine
Harvard Medical School
Anesthetist-in-Chief
Massachusetts General Hospital
Boston, Massachusetts
United States

Duminda N. Wijeysundera, MD, PhD, FRCPC
Associate Professor
Department of Anesthesia; and Institute of Health Policy, Management, and Evaluation
University of Toronto
Staff Physician
Department of Anesthesia
St. Michael's Hospital
Scientist
Li Ka Shing Knowledge Institute of St. Michael's Hospital
Toronto, Ontario
Canada

Christopher L. Wray, MD
Associate Professor
Department of Anesthesiology and Perioperative Medicine
University of California Los Angeles
Los Angeles, California
United States

Christopher L. Wu, MD
Clinical Professor of Anesthesiology
Department of Anesthesiology
The Hospital for Special Surgery/Cornell
New York, New York
United States

Victor W. Xia, MD
Clinical Professor
Department of Anesthesiology and Perioperative Medicine
David Geffen School of Medicine at UCLA
University of California, Los Angeles
Los Angeles, California
United States

Sebastian Zaremba, MD
Vice Head of Sleep Disorders Program
Department of Neurology
Rheinische Friedrich-Wilhelms University
Bonn, Germany

Jie Zhou, MD, MS, MBA
Assistant Professor of Anaesthesia
Department of Anesthesiology, Perioperative and Pain Medicine
Brigham and Women's Hospital
Harvard Medical School
Boston, Massachusetts
United States

Maurice S. Zwass, MD
Professor of Anesthesia and Pediatrics
Chief Pediatric Anesthesia
Department of Anesthesia
University of California, San Francisco
San Francisco, California
United States

Preface

There are few textbooks that are so clearly identified as the definitive source for a medical specialty as is *Miller's Anesthesia*. First published in 1981, the book has grown in scope and influence in the specialty and is an international resource for a "deep dive" into anesthesia practice. The 9th edition marks a transition. The book was founded by Ronald Miller, MD, Chair of the Department of Anesthesia at UCSF, and editions 1-8 were all edited by him, along with internationally acclaimed associate editors. For this edition, Dr. Miller began a handoff of the book, recognizing the extraordinary commitment of time necessary to maintain the excellence the book. There is a new editor, Michael A. Gropper, MD, PhD, who serves as Chair of the Department of Anesthesia and Perioperative Care at UCSF, a position held by Ron Miller for more than 25 years. In place of associate editors, there are now co-editors, recognizing their singular contributions to the book. This group of internationally known experts and academic leaders have ensured that the 9th edition will be a worthy successor of its predecessors. William Young, MD, PhD, an outstanding associate editor in past editions passed away prior to publication of the 8th edition, and Kate Leslie, MD, FANZCA, a leading anesthesia clinician scientist from Australia, has joined the team. Our other co-editors include Jeanine P. Wiener-Kronish, MD, Anesthetist in Chief at Massachusetts General Hospital and Professor of Anesthesia at Harvard Medical School; Lars I. Eriksson, MD, PhD, FRCA, Professor and Academic Chair at Karolinska University Hospital in Stockholm; Neal H. Cohen, MD, MPH, MS, Professor of Anesthesia and Vice Dean at UCSF; and Lee A. Fleisher, MD, Professor and Chair of Anesthesiology and Critical Care at the University of Pennsylvania.

While the 9th edition represents the next stage in the evolution of the book, we have made substantial changes in an effort to make the text relevant and representative of textbooks of the time frame. As the content of the text has grown, we made a concerted effort to ensure a coordinated approach and to focus on topics relevant to the current practice of anesthesiology. The reorganization incudes integration of several chapters; the 8th edition had 112 chapters, and the 9th edition has 90. This reduction in the number of chapters does not represent a limitation on topics representing the scope of current anesthesia practice. For example, some chapters were eliminated where content was redundant or could be easily found elsewhere. Other chapters were combined to better focus discussion about specific topics (e.g., Perioperative and Anesthesia Neurotoxicity has been combined with previous chapters on Pediatric Anesthesia and Cognitive. Two new, exciting chapters focusing on improving the ability of clinicians and researchers to interpret medical literature have been added, including a chapter devoted to Clinical Research authored by Kate Leslie, Cor J. Kalkman, and Duminda N. Wijeysundera, and a new chapter on Interpreting the Medical Literature, authored by Elizabeth L. Whitlock and Catherine L. Chen.

Ultimately, the success of the book lies in its breadth and depth of topics of importance to the science and practice of anesthesia globally. We have made a concerted effort to have an international perspective, with some chapters written entirely by international authors, and others in a collaborative manner along with American authors. This perspective is highlighted in Chapter 2, "Anesthesia and Analgesia in the Global Context." This chapter brings together 20 authors from around the world, providing keen insights into the practice of our specialty under a wide array of conditions.

Finally, the editors wish to express our appreciation to all of the authors and associate editors and acknowledge the authors of previous versions of chapters that were updated for the 9th edition. We also want to acknowledge the publisher, Elsevier, and the expert guidance provided by Ann Anderson, Sarah Barth, and Cindy Thoms. We also want to thank Tula Gourdin, who has worked on this and previous editions, providing thoughtful editing and coordinating communication between the editors, authors, and publishers, and Morgen Ahearn, whose editorial and design help has been invaluable. We hope you will find this definitive textbook to be of value to practicing anesthesiologists as well as trainees who are beginning their careers in anesthesiology.

Contents

SECTION III
Anesthesia Management

VOLUME 2
SECTION IV
Adult Subspecialty Management

Video Contents

SECTION I

INTRODUCTION

1 The Scope of Modern Anesthetic Practice

KATE LESLIE, LARS I. ERIKSSON, JEANINE P. WIENER-KRONISH, NEAL H. COHEN, LEE A. FLEISHER, and MICHAEL A. GROPPER

KEY POINTS

- The scope of modern anesthesia practice includes preoperative evaluation and preparation; intraprocedural care; postoperative care including acute pain management; critical care, resuscitation, and retrieval; chronic pain management; and palliative care. Anesthesia plays a key role in health service delivery and has a significant impact on population health and the burden of disease.
- Global and national forces for change include changing patient populations, locations of care, workforce, costs, quality and safety initiatives, research capability, and the availability of data. These forces have major implications for the delivery of care, evaluation and organization of the anesthesia practice, and education and training of physician anesthesiologists.
- The volume of patients presenting for perioperative and obstetric care continues to grow. Increasingly more patients at extremes of age are requiring anesthesia services. Many of the patients are elderly and have significant comorbidities, including obesity and opioid use disorder. This has important implications for delivery of care and health system issues.
- Anesthesia care is shifting from the traditional surgical suite to other procedural areas, ambulatory sites, office-based facilities, and home environments. As anesthesia care expands, anesthesiologists must focus on maintaining the safety and quality of care in these diverse settings.
- Global and regional deficits in the availability of high-quality anesthesia care must be managed by improving the supply of both physician and non-physician anesthesia providers, by better use of technology, and by limiting demand through health promotion and disease prevention strategies.
- Internationally, the costs of health care continue to escalate; unfortunately the increased spending has not consistently translated into improved health outcomes. Health policy initiatives including alternative approaches to healthcare financing and payment systems are increasingly being implemented to encourage efficient and effective team-based anesthesia care.
- Anesthesiology was among the first medical specialties to focus on improving the safety of patient care. As anesthesia has become safer, attention has intensified on quality improvement, a process designed to improve patient experience and outcomes through systematic change and evaluation.
- Basic, translational, clinical, and implementation research is vital to continuous improvement in outcomes. Opportunities to optimize care are supported by the availability of large datasets generated using electronic health records as well as novel analytic techniques. These changes create new opportunities for anesthesiologists to collaborate with basic and translational scientists to better understand current practices and define better ways to deliver care. As always the provision of resources to support these research initiatives is a challenge.
- The scope of modern anesthetic practice is continually expanding and changing. The changes occurring in health care in the 21st century create opportunities for anesthesiologists to assume a broader role in clinical practice and health policy, providing exciting opportunities for the next generation of physicians in our specialty.

Introduction

Anesthesia is fundamental to the overall practice of medicine worldwide. Hundreds of millions of patients receive anesthesia care each year in association with a wide range of medical, surgical, and obstetric procedures. In addition to direct delivery of anesthesia to patients undergoing a surgical procedure, the scope of anesthesia practice extends beyond the traditional surgical suite to include preoperative evaluation and management of underlying clinical conditions (see Chapter 31); postoperative care including acute pain management (see Chapter 81); critical care, resuscitation, and retrieval (see Chapter 67); chronic pain management (see Chapter 51); and palliative care (see Chapter 52). Anesthesia therefore plays an essential role in health service delivery (see Chapter 3) and has a significant impact on global health and the burden of disease (see Chapter 2). The purpose of *Miller's Anesthesia* is to cover the full scope of contemporary anesthesia practice, from fundamental principles to advanced subspecialty procedures.

Every edition of this textbook begins with comments about the novel diagnostic and therapeutic procedures that have been developed since the last edition and the increasing complexity of patients presenting for anesthesia and perioperative care, especially those at the extremes of life. Each edition also provides descriptions about advances in anesthesiology that have facilitated patient care, including improved understanding of the processes that underlie disease and injury, the increasing sophistication of the pharmacologic and technical resources available, and the improvements in systems designed to promote safety and quality in health care. The 9th edition is no exception: in the last decade the advances in anesthesia and surgical care, especially for patients receiving complex clinical care, have been truly remarkable.

None of these advances would have been possible without the commitment of anesthesiologists to leadership, teaching, and research. Evidence of their contributions can be found in every chapter of the book, extending from improved understanding of the mechanisms of anesthesia and the processes that regulate organ function and drive organ failure; through new technologies, drugs, and systems of care and education; to improved understanding and acknowledgement of the critical role patients and their families play in decision making about healthcare and end-of-life issues.

The future of anesthesiology is filled with opportunities and challenges. Global and national forces will drive evidence-based, cost-effective perioperative and obstetric care by multiprofessional and multidisciplinary teams. These changes will be supported by integrated electronic medical records and large databases and registries of healthcare outputs and outcomes. Increasingly, anesthesia care has expanded outside the operating room, into preoperative clinics, intervention suites, extended postanesthesia care units, and even into patients' homes. As is true for other medical specialties, anesthesiologists have adopted telehealth strategies to extend the care provided to patients and colleagues beyond face-to-face encounters. Technological advances have and will continue to facilitate less invasive interventions and improved anesthesia delivery and monitoring systems. As a result, seriously ill and injured patients and those at the extremes of age, often with associated comorbidities now have access to care previously not available to them. Care is also becoming more personalized, in large part because of the availability of genetic testing and an improved understanding of the unique needs of each patient based on disease severity and his or her probability of responding to specific treatment modalities. Partially as a result of these improvements in care, the costs of caring for an aging population with progressively sophisticated therapies challenge all nations. These forces will likely have a major effect on the scope of perioperative care in general and anesthesia services in particular. Therefore, anesthesiologists must be involved in health policy decisions about the distribution of resources and the need for high-quality evidence to guide practice. In the rest of this chapter we will deal with some of these forces in detail.

Forces That Will Change Practice (Fig. 1.1)

CHANGING PATIENT POPULATIONS

The volume of patients having surgical procedures each year is large and growing. In 2012, more than 300 million patients had surgery worldwide.[1] This number probably underestimates the overall volume of patients requiring anesthesia services, in large part because much of anesthesia care is now provided outside of traditional surgical suite environments. Global initiatives aimed at delivering universal health coverage and safe and affordable surgery and anesthesia care will result in further increases in the number of patients requiring anesthesia care in coming decades (see Chapter 2).

Increasingly many of the patients requiring anesthesia services will be older and have multiple health problems, including obesity and chronic pain associated with opioid use.

The World Health Organization has estimated that by the year 2050 nearly one-quarter of the world's population will be over 60 years of age.[2] In the United States the number of people aged 65 years and over, and therefore eligible for treatment under Medicare, is expected to exceed 78 million by 2030. In high income countries the increase in the numbers of older patients will result from improved preventative care and management of chronic disease and injury. In low- and middle-income countries this change will result from improvements in maternal and child health and the eradication or control of infectious diseases. Concurrently, improvements in anesthetic and surgical care in many countries are increasing medical care options for older patients, who are now receiving more surgical services—many complicated procedures—than ever before. However, the accessibility of these additional options is presenting new challenges for both patients and providers. Aging is associated with a decline in physiologic reserve and organ function and an increase in the risk of disease, injury, and disability (both physical and cognitive). The aging process is highly variable, with significant influence from genetic, environmental, and societal factors. Aging is also associated with considerable changes in social and economic circumstances. Overall these factors lead the older adult to greater dependence on health and social care and challenges in the provision of safe surgery and anesthesia (see Chapters 65 and 82).

One significant public health issue that is accelerating internationally is obesity. It has emerged as a global health epidemic. In 2016, 39% of adults and 18% of children and adolescents worldwide were overweight.[3] In the United States the prevalence of overweight populations was 67.9% and 41.8% in adults and children, respectively. Although the rate of increase in the number of overweight and obese populations have slowed in some high-income nations, this is not the case in low- and middle-income countries. Poor access to healthy diets and limited exercise contribute to the problem. Obesity is associated with an increased burden of disease and injury, including diabetes and hypertension that result in the need for more interactions with the health system, high costs, and significant challenges in the provision of safe and high-quality surgical and anesthetic care (see Chapter 58).

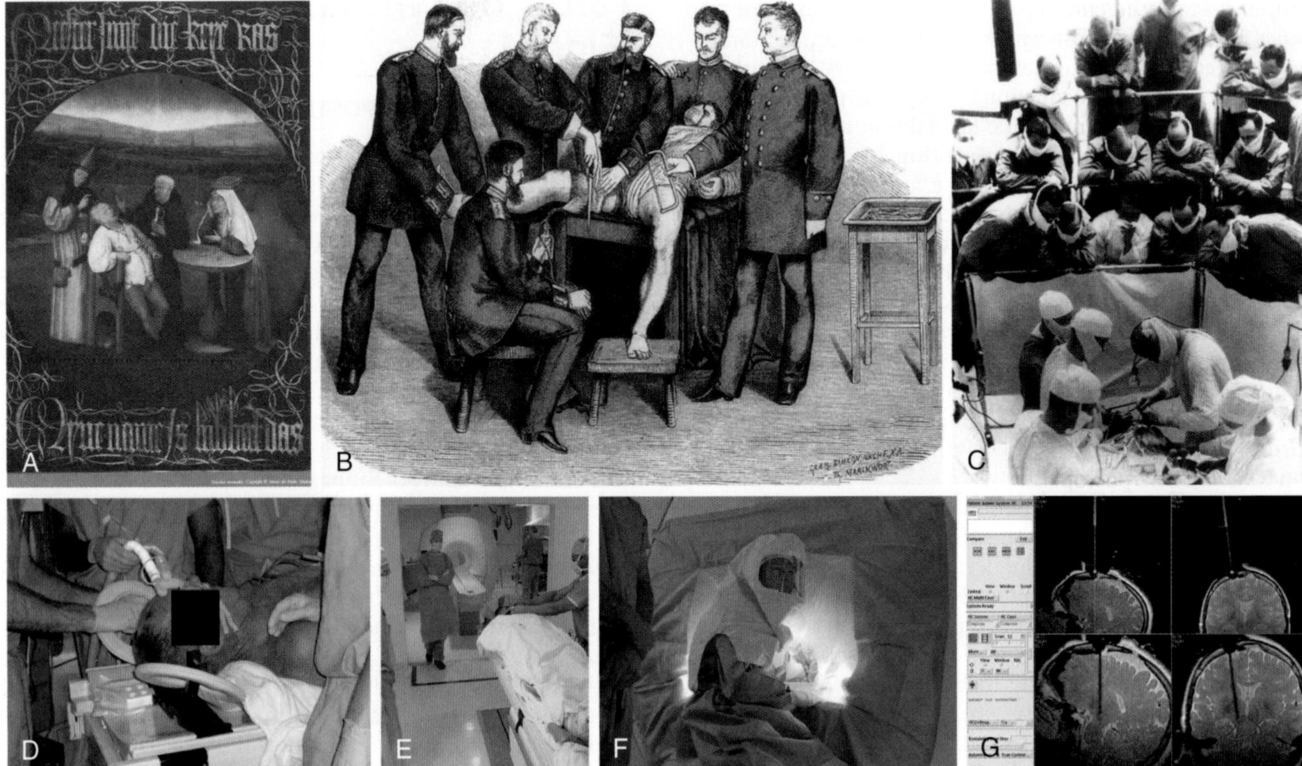

Fig. 1.1 Changing scope and settings of anesthesia and perioperative medicine. (A) *The Cure of Folly,* by Hieronymus Bosch (c.1450–1516), depicting the removal of stones in the head, thought to be a cure for madness. (B) Friedrich Esmarch amputating with the use of anesthesia and antisepsis. (C) Harvey Cushing performing an operation. The Harvey Cushing Society is observing (1932). (D) Placement of a deep brain stimulator for the treatment of Parkinson disease using a real-time magnetic resonance (MR) imaging technology (MR fluoroscopy). The procedure occurs in the MR suite of the radiology department. The patient is anesthetized and (E) moved into the bore of the magnet. (F) A sterile field is created for intracranial instrumentation, and (G) electrodes are placed using real-time guidance. (A, Museo Nacional del Prado, Madrid. B, Woodcut from Esmarch's *Handbuch Der Kriegschirurgischen Technik* [1877]; Jeremy Norman & Co. C, Photograph by Richard Upjohn Light (Boston Medical Library). D to G, Courtesy Paul Larson, University of California–San Francisco, San Francisco Veterans Administration Medical Center.)

Pain management strategies have also had impact on anesthesia practice and perioperative care. The current opioid epidemic arose from increased prescription of opioid drugs to treat all types of acute and chronic pain, including postoperative pain. This crisis has been exacerbated by diversion of prescribed medication (i.e., diverting a medication from its original licit medical purpose) and use of "street" drugs, including opioids. The consequences are significant for individual patients and society as a whole. Opioid use has resulted in addiction, overdoses, homelessness, excessive emergency room visits, increased infections, and neonatal abstinence syndrome. The Centers for Disease Control and Prevention (CDC) estimated that more than 191 million prescriptions (58.7 prescriptions per 100 persons) were filled in the United States in 2017, with marked regional variation characterized with adverse physical, economic, and social circumstances.[4] Opioids were involved in 42,249 overdose deaths in 2016 (66.4% of all drug overdose deaths). The situation is similar in other nations, with the World Health Organization estimating that 27 million people worldwide suffered opioid use disorder in 2015.[5] Recent government action has been substantial, particularly in the United States. The Department of Health and Human Services has implemented a five-point plan to combat the crisis including: (1) improved access to prevention, treatment, and recovery support services; (2) targeted availability and distribution of overdose-reversing (narcotic antagonist) drugs; (3) strengthened public health data reporting and collection; (4) support for cutting-edge research on addiction and pain; and (5) advances in pain management practice.[6] As experts in the pharmacology and clinical use of opioid drugs (see Chapters 24, 51, and 81), anesthesiologists and pain medicine specialists have and must continue their essential role in resolving this crisis.

CHANGING LOCATIONS OF CARE

Anesthesia practice has expanded to a variety of locations. A number of factors account for this shift in anesthesia and perioperative care (see Chapter 73). The costs of traditional operating room care are high and the services available may be unnecessarily comprehensive and complex for the planned episode of care. With advances in clinical care, the need for inpatient perioperative care is reduced for many surgical procedures. As a result more and more procedures are being performed in hospital outpatient settings, ambulatory surgery centers, and office-based practices. The focus of accrediting bodies and anesthesiology societies has been on maintaining the safety and quality of anesthesia care in outpatient settings, including providing for extended admission and escalation of care when clinically necessary to ensure patient safety.[7] At the same time, the payment models have not necessarily kept pace with these advances in clinical care. In the United States, the growth in nonhospital-based care has occurred despite curbs in reimbursement for ambulatory surgery by governmental and private payers.

The clinical practice for surgical patients has also changed because of changes in sites of care and inpatient management. For most patients, many aspects of perioperative care have shifted from the hospital or other healthcare facility to outpatient or home settings. As one example, the elimination of preoperative hospital admission to day-of-surgery admission is virtually complete in high-income nations. Hospital lengths of stay are also much shorter. As a result, postoperative care is increasingly undertaken in the home as well, often as part of enhanced recovery after surgery programs.[8] Advances in monitoring technology and pain management techniques create opportunities for anesthesiologists in which to not only participate, but also manage many aspects of postoperative care in the home. Although these changes have been beneficial to many patients with improved outcomes and reduced costs, for some families the transition to short hospital lengths of stay has created significant clinical and social problems. Anesthesiologists must have an understanding of patients perioperative and postoperative support needs and should be actively engaged in determining the most appropriate setting for a procedure and how to manage the transitions of care.[9]

In addition to the changes taking place for surgical patients, anesthesia care is also shifting outside the operating room as a result of the advances in minimally invasive techniques provided by cardiologists, radiologists, endoscopists, and pain medicine specialists (see Chapters 51, 55, 57, and 73). As the volume of these services increases, anesthesiologists may be asked to provide care in procedural areas that were not designed for delivery of anesthesia services, and often not properly equipped to support patient and provider needs. The locations are frequently remote from the operating suite and may lack the usual support available for the care of patients with complex cases and the management of crises. Anesthesiologists therefore must participate in planning for these services and provide leadership in defining and maintaining the same standards of operating room practice to other areas of the hospital.[10,11]

Another example of the advances in clinical care and implications is the remarkable increase in referrals for colonoscopy for colon cancer screening.[12] Although the sedation provider for colonoscopy widely varies internationally and regionally within the United States, anesthesiologists are now more commonly participating in the care of these patients, in part due to medical needs related to comorbidities, but also because of documented complications associated with the use of sedation that have resulted in airway compromise or respiratory failure. These complications have caused providers and payers to reevaluate patient needs, the appropriate training of practitioners delivering procedural sedation, and when to optimize care by having an anesthesia practitioner monitor the patient and administer sedation. American[11,13] and international[14,15] sedation guidelines recognize that for many patients, nonanesthesiologist physicians and independent or semi-independent nonmedical practitioners can provide deep sedation for endoscopy; however, all guidelines emphasize that anesthesiologists should be involved in the care of high-risk patients or those with significant comorbidities.

CHANGES IN THE ANESTHESIA WORKFORCE

As a result of advances in perioperative care and the many other changes that impact the need for anesthesia practitioners, global and regional workforce shortages have been identified in recent years and are expected to increase (see Chapter 2). There are a number of reasons for these deficits including an insufficient number of medical graduates (in some places exacerbated by outward migration and an aging workforce), duty hour restrictions for practicing physicians (due to regulation of work hours, changing lifestyle preferences, and desire for better work-life balance), and increased demand for medical services (due to population growth and on a per capita basis). In addition to the impact of these societal changes, demand for physician care in the United States has increased in part due to the Patient Protection and Affordable Care Act (Affordable Care Act) with more patients having medical insurance and seeking care. To respond to the shortages, many countries within the Organisation for Economic Co-operation and Development (there are 36 member countries, including the United States) have increased medical school admissions in recent years.[16] Unfortunately, even this increase in number of trainees is insufficient to meet future needs. In 2017, the United States produced 7.55 medical graduates per 100,000 population, well below average (12 per 100,000 inhabitants). The Association of American Medical Colleges (AAMC) projects a shortage of up to 121,000 physicians by 2030.[14] At the same time, despite the increases in medical student enrollment, in the United States, most residency positions are funded by the Medicare program. As the medical school intakes have increased, this federal funding for residency positions (including anesthesiology) has not kept pace resulting in a bottleneck in the training pipeline. Along with reconsidering the cap on federally-funded positions, the AAMC has proposed alternative ways to leverage the skills and experience of physicians to advance care with improved use of technology and more interdisciplinary, team-based care as potential solutions.

Team-based care (anesthesia care team model) is already common in anesthesia practice, particularly in the United States. In the United States, the number of physician and nonphysician anesthesia providers are approaching parity, with the number of nurse anesthetists and anesthesia assistants increasing more rapidly than the number of physician anesthesiologists. In 2017, the American Society of Anesthesiologists (ASA) released a statement on the anesthesia care team that enunciated its vision for physician-led teams where anesthesiologists have a particular role in governance, planning, and oversight of anesthesia care, advanced airway management, and resuscitation.[17] This oversight includes defining and monitoring sedation provided in non-operating room locations and other requirements for the credentialing of providers to optimize care of the patient who requires deep sedation. Similar team-based approaches to care associated with physician supervision are commonplace or emerging in other countries around the world.

The number of women in medical schools has increased to over 50% of the student cohort in many countries. At the same time, until recently, United States anesthesiology training programs have recruited a smaller proportion of women (37%). In academic departments, few women have reached the rank of professor, or become department chairs, or been elected to leadership positions in representative anesthesia organizations.[18] Programs to improve recruitment and advancement of women in academic medicine and anesthesiology have gained traction in the last decade (e.g., Athena Scientific Women's Academic Network[19]). In addition, all academic programs are paying more attention to diversity in the workforce, particularly among women and underrepresented minorities. With the increased understanding of the inequities, programs can be developed to more effectively address the disparities and broaden the diversity of the anesthesia workforce. It is essential that the anesthesia workforce reflect the diversity of the patient population that is served.

INCREASING COSTS OF CARE

The costs of health care continue to grow internationally, with health care consuming 8% of gross domestic product (GDP) on average in most countries, whereas in the United States the costs are as high as 18% of GDP.[20] Unfortunately the increased healthcare expenditures have not translated into improved health outcomes, particularly for Americans. Despite the Affordable Care Act, the United States continues to have a large uninsured or underinsured population, lapses in quality and safety of care inside and outside the hospital, and high rates of drug abuse, violence, and use of firearms.[21] The National Academy of Medicine concluded that healthcare funding in the United States needs to "reorient competition in the healthcare system around the value of services provided rather than the volume of services provided." This transition from volume to value is creating many new challenges and opportunities for anesthesiologists. As the health system adopts practices that provide documented improved outcomes at reduced costs, anesthesiologists must both understand the implications of these changes in clinical practices and also take a leadership role in identifying opportunities to reengineer care if the specialty is to retain its leadership role in quality and safety (see Chapter 3).

Payment for physician services is being modified to better align health systems, providers, and payers with respect to delivery of high-quality, patient-centered care. Compensation for clinical care continues to have a fee-for-service component, particularly in the United States; however, more compensation is becoming incentive-based to encourage changes in practice that improve efficiency and effectiveness. In contrast to fee-for-service models (which reward inputs), pay-for-performance models reward medical care that is consistent with published evidence and that improves the processes of care (e.g., timely administration of perioperative antibiotics), output (e.g., meeting targets for urgent surgery), or outcome (e.g., fewer central-line associated blood stream infections) measures. In the United States, recent pay-for-performance programs have included the Premier Hospital Quality Incentive Demonstration program of the Centers for Medicare and Medicaid Services (2003–2009) and the national Hospital Value-Based Purchasing Program, adopted after the passage of the Affordable Care Act (2011). This initial attempt to modify anesthesia practice has had limited impact on outcomes, possibly because financial incentives are too small, payment is delayed, and/or the costs associated with implementing the programs is greater.[22] Nonetheless, incentive-based pay-for-performance programs (which are widespread in other nations with high-cost healthcare systems) will continue to expand.[23]

In addition to paying for high-quality performance, in the United States and other high-income nations there has been increasing emphasis on not paying for poor outcomes of errors in care. For example, some payers withhold payment for "never" events (e.g., wrong-sided surgery, pressure ulcers, retained foreign objects, mismatched blood transfusion) unless they are present on admission to the hospital. This approach may be expanded to withhold payment associated with treatment of preventable complications. A number of anesthesia-specific activities have been identified that impact outcomes and, if these are not provided, the consequence could be either no payment or penalties. For example, monitoring and maintaining body temperature during surgery as promoted by the Surgical Care Improvement Project is but one example of an anesthesia metric that affects outcomes and costs of care.[24] At the same time, identification of some of the interventions or monitoring techniques that impact outcome is challenging. As a result, it is critically important for anesthesiologists to continue to evaluate practices and do additional research to both optimize care and reduce costs.

Other changes in payment for clinical care have and will continue to have significant impact on compensation for anesthesia services. Some payers are providing "bundled" payments to compensate providers for episodes of care. This approach to payment is an integral part of the reforms introduced under the Affordable Care Act, although some of the incentives may be redefined by subsequent legislation. The Bundled Payments for Care Improvement initiative introduced by the Centers for Medicare and Medicaid Services tested the ability of bundling payments as a method for improving quality and lowering costs. The program has been most successful for selected clinical services such as total joint arthroplasty for which participation by anesthesiologists through the continuum of care can be most significant.[25] The ASA has proposed the Perioperative Surgical Home as an anesthesiologist-managed structure to coordinate perioperative team-based care. This model of coordinated care throughout the perioperative period should be amenable to bundled payments or other new approaches to compensating providers.[26]

INCREASING FOCUS ON SAFETY AND QUALITY

Anesthesiology was among the first medical specialties to focus on improving patient safety.[27] A number of initiatives have had major impact on outcomes of care, including improved monitoring techniques, airway management options, and new improved drugs. Anesthesiologists have been actively assessing clinical care through the use of incident reporting systems, morbidity and mortality conferences, and "near-miss" reports. Incident reporting, which was initiated in the United States more than 50 years ago, has documented a decline in anesthesia-related mortality to less than 1 per 1 million population.[28] In recent years national incident reporting programs have been initiated by the Anesthesia Quality Institute (Anesthesia Incident Reporting System[29]) and the Society of Pediatric Anesthesia (Wake Up Safe[30]). In addition to helping identify areas in which to improve clinical care, these programs provide legal protection to practitioners under the Patient Safety and Quality Improvement Act (2005). A number of programs have developed based on the experiences identified through these reporting mechanisms. Recognition of the human factors associated with adverse events has spawned a national and international movement directed at improving situational awareness and team functioning through simulation training (see Chapter 6). More recently programs to encourage healthcare providers and consumers to speak up about traditional patient safety concerns (e.g., commencing a wrong-side procedure) and unsafe professional behaviors (e.g., bullying and sexual harassment) have been integrated into workplaces nationwide and internationally.[31]

Anesthesiologists also led the way in the development of practice standards and checklists to improve clinical care. In some cases, the implementation of checklists has become a requirement for accreditation. In the last decade anesthesiologists were pivotal in the development, implementation, and evaluation of the World Health Organization's Surgical Safety Checklist.[32] Although the uptake of the Checklist has been patchy and its effect on outcomes has been inconsistent, the Checklist is widely implemented in the United States and other countries (see Chapter 2) in the belief that it will enable effective communication and a culture of safety.[33]

As anesthesia has become more and more safe, our attention has increasingly been focused on quality improvement, a process designed to improve patient experience and outcomes through systematic change and evaluation. In the United States, the Anesthesia Quality Institute established the National Anesthesia Clinical Outcomes Registry to enable systematic collection of quality information for use in quality improvement processes both nationally and locally.[34] Recently greater emphasis has been placed on longer-term and patient-centered or patient-reported outcomes. Many of these outcome measures have been incorporated into quality improvement programs and publicly reported metrics.[35] Anesthesiologists have identified the importance of assessing outcomes beyond the immediate perioperative period. As anesthesiologists assume a greater role in overall periprocedural care and outcomes, they will undoubtedly continue to advance the safety and quality agenda in large part due to their longstanding history in safety and quality as well as their training and pivotal role in perioperative care.

NEW OPPORTUNITIES AND CHALLENGES IN RESEARCH

Academic anesthesia departments are committed to advancing the scientific underpinning of anesthesiology. Basic, translational, clinical, and implementation research is vital to the continuous improvement in patient and health service outcomes (see Chapter 89). Fortunately, overall funding for biomedical and health services research in the United States more than doubled between 1994 and 2012. Although overall research funding has increased, since 2004 the overall growth of NIH funding for medical research has declined by 1.8%.[36] Private sources of funding have been important to supplement government-sponsored research support. Industry support is valuable and has been critical to the research agenda for academic departments. It also creates both real and perceived conflicts of interest that can be difficult to manage. Over the past decade, there has been a decline in early-stage research in favor of device development and clinical trials, poor mapping of research effort to the global burden of disease, and limited funding for critically important health services research.[36]

The implications of these changes in research support on anesthesia are significant. Academic anesthesia departments in the United States, as well as many other countries, continue to compete for government funding. Most benchmarks suggest that the specialty of anesthesiology in the United States fares poorly in National Institutes of Health funding when compared with other disciplines.[37] As a result, anesthesia departments, particularly in the United States have had to identify other funding sources, including foundations, industry, and philanthropy, particularly for early-career investigators.[38] For example the Foundation for Anesthesia Education and Research (FAER) has awarded more than $40 million in grants since 1986 and has demonstrated the leverage that these grants provide in achieving federal funding ($17 in funding for every $1 investment). Similar programs are funded by the International Anesthesia Research Society and by other anesthesiology organizations and foundations worldwide. At the same time, and in many respects related to the funding challenges and competing clinical needs, research support and peer-reviewed publications, which have increased in other countries, have not kept pace in the United States. As a result, an increasing number of publications in peer-reviewed journals are from authors outside the United States.

Other factors have impact on what resources are available for research. The clinical demands put on the faculty in academic departments make it difficult for clinician scientists to pursue research activities. Associated with the increasing clinical volume, supervised residents cannot provide all of the clinical care without compromising their educational experiences and fulfilling duty hour and other requirements. As a result, the faculty members are delivering a larger percentage of care on their own. At the same time, the complexity of some of the basic and translational research requires significant dedicated time and skills that are difficult to maintain when the investigator is also encumbered with a high clinical demand. Historically, clinically generated income was used to support research in general and young investigators in particular. As labor and other costs increase (including those associated with quality of care initiatives, clinical and research compliance, and other activities), fewer funds are available to support research. As a result of the high cost of developing new drugs with insufficient incentives for the pharmaceutical industry to develop new anesthetic agents, there is a reduced pipeline of anesthesia drugs.[39]

Despite these challenges, basic science, as well as clinical and translational research, is being performed by anesthesiologists and advances in the specialty are taking place. New models for research have contributed to advances in our understanding of basic concepts of anesthesia care as well as clinical advances. As is true for clinical care, collaboration has always been vital in biomedical research. In recent years anesthesiology research has increasingly been conducted by multiprofessional, multidisciplinary teams including biostatisticians, health informaticians, and health economists. Translation from discovery to practice has been facilitated by partnerships among basic scientists, clinical scientists, and implementation scientists.[40] In addition to collaborations among colleagues within one institution, increasingly clinical trials are being conducted by large, multicenter networks because of the recognition that single-center studies take too long and cannot recruit enough patients to answer the really important questions in anesthesiology.[41-44] Research based on electronic medical records and databases also requires collaboration between institutions, clinicians, and database experts (see later).

One of the primary motivators to support the research agenda for anesthesiology is the need to define reliable and peer-reviewed data upon which to advance the specialty. Although the volume of anesthesiology information and its ease of access have increased exponentially in the last decade, particularly through social media, anesthesiologists are progressively challenged to find reliable information to guide their practice. In addition to the difficulty of assessing the quality of some of the information posted on various web sites, anesthesiology has also been plagued by high-profile cases of research misconduct, including fabrication, falsification, and misleading reporting of research findings.[45] This has damaged the reputation of anesthesiology research and, as a result of unreliable data upon which to make clinical decisions, put patients at risk. Each anesthesiologist must be diligent in selecting a source of information that takes into consideration the standards of peer review of the material and the financial relationships between the authors and publishers.[46]

INCREASING AVAILABILITY OF DATA

One of the areas of opportunity with respect to better understanding our clinical practices and defining ways to improve care is the increasing amount of data that can inform us. The last decade has seen unprecedented growth in the volume and availability of healthcare data. Electronic health record (EHR) systems (see Chapter 4) facilitate complete data capture and integration from multiple sources, including surgical equipment, anesthesia delivery systems, and physiologic monitors. The EHR has greatly facilitated documentation of individual patient care and provided aggregate data for healthcare services and populations. Other sources of routinely-collected data include health service billing systems, government and insurance databases, disease registries, and public health reporting. In addition, data specifically collected for research and quality improvement is increasingly shared, including research databases and biobanks (including genetic databanks). Meta-data related to the use of electronic resources and social media is also available for interrogation. These data require new management and analysis techniques that are beyond the scope of the practicing anesthesiologist or researcher (see Chapter 4). Truly "big" data includes terabytes of information, is generated and analyzed at high speed, and includes data in a wide variety of formats and from a wide variety of sources.[47]

These large data sets are increasingly being used to answer important research questions, to develop evidence-based clinical guidelines, and to assess the safety and quality of anesthesia and perioperative care, within and across different clinical environments and regions. Although technologic resources are not replacing randomized clinical trials, the information gleaned from large databases can be used to address important questions about how to most effectively deliver cost-effective care. At the same time, it is important to acknowledge the limitations of large databases, which may have missing critical elements of care or outcomes, could misclassify data, or in some cases, lack verification.[48]

Conclusions

The scope of modern anesthetic practice is continually changing and expanding. The forces for change include changes in our patient population, locations of care, workforce, costs, quality and safety initiatives, research, and the availability of data. This chapter emphasizes the implications for these forces on the specialty as well as the influence they have on the delivery of health care in general. The changes occurring in health care in the 21st century obviously have implications for the role of anesthesiology in both the practice and delivery of medicine overall, and provide exciting opportunities for the next generation of practitioners and leaders in our specialty.

Acknowledgment

The editors and publisher recognize the contributions of Ronald D. Miller, who was a contributing author to this topic in previous editions of this work. It has served as the foundation for the current chapter.

 **Complete references available online at expertconsult.com.**

References

1. Weiser TG, et al. *Lancet*. 2015;385(suppl 2):S11.
2. World Health Organisation. World report on ageing and health. Geneva. https://www.who.int/ageing/events/world-report-2015-launch/en/. Accessed October 18 2018.
3. World Health Organisation. Fact sheet on overweight and obesity. http://www.who.int/en/news-room/fact-sheets/detail/obesity-and-overweight. Accessed October 18 2018.
4. Centers for Disease Control and Prevention. U.S. opioid prescribing rate maps. Atlanta. https://www.cdc.gov/drugoverdose/maps/rxrate-maps.html. Accessed October 18 2018.
5. World Health Organisation. Information sheet on opioid overdose. Geneva. http://www.who.int/substance_abuse/information-sheet/en/. Accessed October 18 2018.
6. Department of Health and Human Services. Help, resources and information. National opioid crisis. Washington. https://www.hhs.gov/opioids/. Accessed October 18 2018.
7. American Society of Anesthesiologists. Guidelines for office-based anesthesia. Schaumberg. https://www.asahq.org/quality-and-practice-management/standards-guidelines-and-related-resources-search. Accessed October 18 2018.
8. Kehlet H. *Br J Anaesth*. 1997;78:606.
9. Fleisher LA, et al. *Arch Surg*. 2004;139:67.
10. American Society of Anesthesiologists. Statement on non-operating room anesthetizing locations. Schaumberg. https://www.asahq.org/quality-and-practice-management/standards-guidelines-and-related-resources-search. Accessed.

11. American Society of Anesthesiologists task force on moderate procedural sedation and analgesia. *Anesthesiology*. 2018;128:437.
12. National Cancer Institute. Colorectal cancer screening. Bethesda. https://progressreport.cancer.gov/detection/colorectal_cancer. Accessed October 18 2018.
13. Quality Management and Departmental Administration Committee. Advisory on granting privileges for deep sedation to non-anesthesiologist physicians (amended October 25, 2017). Schaumburg. http://www.asahq.org/quality-and-practice-management/standards-guidelines-and-related-resources. Accessed March 5 2018.
14. The Academy of Medical Royal Colleges. Safe sedation practice for healthcare procedures. London. https://www.rcoa.ac.uk/system/files/PUB-SafeSedPrac2013.pdf. Accessed March 5 2018.
15. Hinkelbein J, et al. *Eur J Anaesthesiol*. 2017;35:6.
16. Organisation for Economic Co-operation and Development. Medical graduates. Paris. https://data.oecd.org/healthres/medical-graduates.htm. Accessed October 18 2018.
17. American Society of Anesthesiologists. Statement on the anesthesia care team. Schaumberg. http://www.asahq.org/quality-and-practice-management/standards-guidelines-and-related-resources/statement-on-anesthesia-care-team. Accessed October 18 2018.
18. Leslie K, et al. *Anesth Analg*. 2017;124:1394.
19. Equality Challenge Unit. Athena SWAN Charter. London. https://www.ecu.ac.uk/equality-charters/athena-swan/. Accessed October 18 2018.
20. Organisation for Economic Co-operation and Development. Health spending. Paris. https://data.oecd.org/healthres/health-spending.htm. Accessed October 18 2018.
21. National Research Council and Institute of Medicine. U.S. *Health in International Perspective: shorter Lives, Poorer Health*. Washington: National Academies Press. 2013.
22. Bonfrer I, et al. *BMJ*. 2018;360:j5622.
23. European Observatory on Health Systems and Policies. Paying for performance in healthcare. Implications for health system performance and accountability. Maidenhead. http://www.euro.who.int/__data/assets/pdf_file/0020/271073/Paying-for-Performance-in-Health-Care.pdf. Accessed October 18 2018.
24. Scott AV, et al. *Anesthesiology*. 2015;123:116.
25. Centers for Medicare & Medicaid Services. Bundled Payments for Care Improvement (BPCI) Initiative: General Information. Washington DC. https://innovation.cms.gov/initiatives/bundled-payments/. Accessed October 18 2018.
26. American Society of Anesthesiologists. Perioperative surgical home. Schaumberg. https://www.asahq.org/psh. Accessed October 18 2018.
27. Kohn L, Corrigan J, Donaldson M. *To Err Is Human: Building a Safer Health System*. Washington DC: National Academy Press; 1999.
28. Li G, et al. *Anesthesiology*. 2009;110:759.
29. Anesthesia Quality Institute. Anesthesia incident reporting system (AIRS). Schaumberg. https://qualityportal.aqihq.org/AIRSMain/AIRSSelectType/0. Accessed October 18 2018.
30. Society for Pediatric Anesthesia. Wake up safe. Richmond. http://www.wakeupsafe.org/. Accessed October 18 2018.
31. Webb LE, et al. *Jt Comm J Qual Patient Saf*. 2016;42:149.
32. Haynes A, et al. *N Engl J Med*. 2009;360:491.
33. de Jager E, et al. *World J Surg*. 2016;40:1842.
34. Liau A, et al. *Anesth Analg*. 2015;121:1604.
35. Peden CJ, et al. *Br J Anaesth*. 2017;119:i5.
36. Moses H 3rd, et al. *JAMA*. 2015;313:174.
37. Reves JG. *Anesthesiology*. 2007;106:826.
38. Speck RM, et al. *Anesth Analg*. 2018;126:2116.
39. Vlassakov KV, Kissin I. *Trends Pharmacol Sci*. 2016;37:344.
40. Kharasch ED. *Anesthesiology*. 2018;128:693.
41. Myles P, et al. *BMJ Open*. 2017;7:e015358.
42. Pearse RM, et al. *JAMA*. 2014;311:2181.
43. Wijeysundera DN, et al. *Lancet*. 2018;391:2631.
44. Devereaux P, et al. *N Engl J Med*. 2014;370:1494.
45. Moylan EC, Kowalczuk MK. *BMJ Open*. 2016;6:e012047.
46. Shen C, Bjork BC. *BMC Med*. 2015;13:230.
47. Levin MA, et al. *Anesth Analg*. 2015;121:1661.
48. Fleischut PM, et al. *Br J Anaesth*. 2013;111:532.

2 *Anesthesia and Analgesia in the Global Context*

MICHAEL S. LIPNICK, RONALD D. MILLER, and ADRIAN W. GELB, EDITORS.
SEE CHAPTER OUTLINE FOR CO-AUTHORS.

CHAPTER OUTLINE

KEY POINTS

- More than 5 of the world's 7 billion people lack access to safe anesthesia and surgical services. Surgical disease accounts for 30% of global disease burden, yet less than 1% of development assistance for health supports delivery of anesthesia and surgical care. Lack of access to safe, timely, and affordable anesthesia and surgery kills more than 4 times as many as acquired immunodeficiency syndrome (AIDS), tuberculosis (TB), and malaria combined.
- Lack of access to safe anesthesia and surgical services are among the most neglected crises in global health. Anesthesia-related mortality in some low-income countries (LICs) is reported in the 1:100s and is mostly avoidable. The burden of surgical disease is growing and disproportionately affects low- and middle-income countries.
- Pain is one of the top causes of morbidity worldwide, and inadequate access to analgesia is among the most inequitable global public health crises the world faces today. Five and a half billion people have limited or no access to narcotic medications for analgesia. Six high-income countries (HICs) account for 80% of the world's opioid consumption. Key drug control policies, organizations, and politics continue to influence issues of access and abuse, with disproportionately negative impacts for underserved populations.
- Critical shortages and the inequitable distribution of anesthesia providers are significant barriers to increasing access to safe anesthesia and surgical care. The density of surgery, anesthesia, and obstetric providers is 0.7 per 100,000 population for LICs as compared with 57 per 100,000 population for HICs.

KEY POINTS—cont'd

- Modern anesthesia workforce training and practice models vary widely from country to country. Innovative workforce solutions are needed to increase provider numbers while simultaneously ensuring quality and promoting access for underserved populations.
- Anesthesia, analgesia, and surgical services are feasible in resource-constrained settings and are as cost-effective as many other public health interventions (e.g., vaccinations).
- Issues of access, safety, and resource utilization are relevant to all anesthesia providers. Equipping anesthesia providers with knowledge and skills needed to address global challenges in anesthesia will become increasingly important in order to expand access to safe and affordable anesthesia care worldwide.
- Health care providers from multiple disciplines (nursing, surgery, obstetrics, anesthesia, and many more) are needed to effectively provide surgical and perioperative care. Anesthesiologists routinely work across the perioperative disciplines and can play a significant role to improve cohesive advocacy efforts and lead progress in global health equity for surgical disease and analgesia.
- The global anesthesia community is lagging behind other health disciplines in addressing global health challenges and must rapidly expand investment in initiatives to help characterize (research), address (implementation and policy), and support (financing) global anesthesia challenges.
- Developing infrastructure, expanding workforce, improving data to drive policy, providing financial risk protection mechanisms for surgical patients, improving referral and prehospital systems, and providing essential medicines are actions the global anesthesia community must prioritize. The need to act promptly is immense and must be balanced but not overshadowed by research agendas.

Introduction

There have been considerable efforts in recent years to define a global "standard" or "optimal" practice of anesthesia.[1-4] These debates, investigations, and innovations have most often been framed in the context of maximizing patient safety. More recently the focus of these efforts has expanded to also incorporate the important goals of maximizing not only safety, but also accessibility and affordability of anesthesia services.[5]

With scientific advancement and economic development, anesthesia—like much of medicine—has changed dramatically since the first public display of ether anesthesia in October of 1846. However, over the past 150-plus years, advances in anesthesia have been neither uniform nor universal, resulting in vastly heterogeneous anesthesia practice models and massive inequities in access to safe anesthesia care worldwide. The majority of the world's population does not have access to safe, affordable surgical, anesthesia, or pain services, and relatively few resources are being invested by governments, donors, or the global anesthesia community to address this crisis.

In this chapter we build off the work of Dr. Miller and colleagues' to explore not only the evolution and diversity of anesthesia practice models from around the world, but also challenges facing the global anesthesia community. A better understanding of the evolution of modern anesthesia care models, as well as the challenges they face and have overcome, is a key step to improving access and patient safety worldwide.

The first section of this chapter describes the scope and magnitude of the ongoing global surgical, anesthesia, and pain crises. This section also explores reasons why these crises have been relatively neglected by the global public health community, and reviews potential areas for intervention, advocacy, and change.

TABLE 2.1 World Bank Income Classifications by Gross National Income per Capita

	GNI per Capita (US $)
Low income	<1,005
Lower-middle income	1,006-3,955
Upper-middle income	3,956-12,235
High income	>12,235

GNI, Gross national income.
Source: https://blogs.worldbank.org/opendata/new-country-classifications-income-level-2017-2018.

The second section of this chapter presents examples of different anesthesia care models from around the world, including select historical milestones and snapshots of current challenges from regional and country-level perspectives.

The final section of this chapter provides a primer on essential clinical and nonclinical knowledge relevant for anesthesia practice in resource-constrained settings. The chapter concludes by discussing the role of anesthesia providers beyond the confines of the operating room or hospital setting, who increasingly will be called upon for solutions that increase access to safe anesthesia, surgery, and analgesia in the global context.

Section 1: Anesthesia and "Global Health"

The terms anesthesia and global health, when used together, often invoke thoughts of providers from high-income countries (HICs) providing clinical care in low- and middle-income countries (LMICs) as part of humanitarian outreach or "mission trips" (Table 2.1). Although such initiatives comprise a substantial proportion of efforts that

TABLE 2.2 Definitions of Global Health and Global Surgery

	Global Health*	Global Surgery†
Approach	Field of study, research, practice and advocacy. Emphasizes global perspective and a scientific approach to health promotion and disease prevention, including broad determinants of health.	Area for study, research, practice, and advocacy that places priority on improving health outcomes and achieving health equity for all people worldwide who are affected by surgical conditions or have a need for surgical care.
Geography	Focuses on issues that directly or indirectly affect health but that can transcend national boundaries.	Global surgery emphasizes supraterritorial and transnational issues, determinants, and solutions.
Level of cooperation	Development and implementation of solutions often require global cooperation.	Recognizes that the determinants of inadequate or inequitable surgical care are often the result of common and interdependent global structures and processes, and require global cooperation for global solutions.
Individuals or populations	Embraces both prevention in populations and clinical care of individuals.	Encompasses surgical care for underserved populations in all countries with special emphasis on those affected by conflict, displacement, and disaster.
Access to health	Health equity among nations and for all people is a major objective.	Equitable access to safe and affordable anesthesia, analgesia, and surgical care is a major objective.
Range of disciplines	Highly interdisciplinary and multidisciplinary within and beyond health sciences.	Incorporates all surgical specialties including obstetric and gynecological surgery, anesthesia, perioperative care, aspects of emergency medicine, rehabilitation, and palliative care, and nursing and the allied health professions involved in the care of the surgical patient. Engages non-clinical stakeholders including health economists, governments, and policymakers.

*Modified from Koplan JP, Bond TC, Merson MH, et al. Towards a common definition of global health. *Lancet*. 2009;(9679);1993–1995; Fried LP, Bentley ME, Buekens P, et al. Global health is public health. *Lancet*. 2010;375(9714):535–537.

†Modified from Dare AJ, Grimes CE, Gillies R, et al. Global surgery: defining an emerging global heath field. *Lancet*. 2014;384(9961):2245–2247.

aim to increase access to surgical and anesthesia services in resource-constrained settings, they represent only a fraction of the ever-expanding role of the anesthesia community in global health.

In this chapter, the term "global health" refers to a multidisciplinary field of study, research, practice, and advocacy that develops and implements solutions to promote health equity. Global health transcends national boundaries, requires global cooperation, and utilizes both population-level (e.g., injury prevention) and individual-level (e.g., clinical care) strategies (Table 2.2). Although some debate exists over the optimal definition of global health and its distinction, or lack thereof, from public health, it is worth highlighting that global health is not synonymous with international aid (i.e., going abroad from one's own country) or the transfer of technologies or interventions from HICs to LMICs.[6,7] Global health encompasses much more, including local providers working in the local environment (whether that is a low-, middle-, or high-income setting), and increasing emphasis on health equity.[8]

Global health has received unprecedented levels of interest in recent decades, expanding from its infectious disease origins to now incorporate a wider range of diseases, including the social and environmental factors affecting health.[9,10] Despite this expanded scope, surgery and anesthesia have remained relatively forgotten by the global health community.

In June of 1980, then Director-General of the World Health Organization (WHO), Dr. Halfdan Mahler, gave a presentation to the International College of Surgeons in Mexico City entitled "Surgery and Health for All." In this speech, Dr. Mahler stated that "*Surgery clearly has an important role to play in primary health care and in the services supporting it. Yet, the vast majority of the world's population has no access whatsoever to skilled surgical care, and little is being done to find a solution. I beg of you to give serious consideration to this most serious manifestation of social inequity in health care.*"[11]

Despite recognition of the global anesthesia and surgical crises several decades ago, it has been only recently that the global health community has begun to take notice and action.[12–17] In 2004, the WHO created the Emergency and Essential Surgical Care Program (EESC) and in 2005, the WHO Global Initiative for Emergency and Essential Surgical Care (GIEESC) was formed to convene multidisciplinary stakeholders interested in surgical disease. In 2007, the Bellagio Essential Surgery Group and Burden of Surgical Disease Working Group (later renamed the Alliance for Surgery and Anesthesia Presence [ASAP]) formed as two of the earliest concerted efforts to raise international awareness for surgical disease by advocating for the integration of surgery into health systems and the promotion of research and collaboration across disciplines.[18] These efforts followed in the wake of a seminal chapter on surgery in the Second Edition of the Disease Control Priorities in Developing Countries (DCP2) book in 2006.[19] In 2008, the WHO launched the Safe Surgery Saves Lives initiative along with the WHO Safe Surgery Checklist.[20,21] Also in 2008 multiple leaders in global health highlighted surgery as the "neglected stepchild" and as the "other neglected disease" in global health, drawing comparison with the then emerging term, "neglected tropical diseases."[22,23]

Despite these pleas and consistent, albeit limited, data demonstrating the massive scale of the surgical disease crisis, it was not until 2014–15 that greater attention began to be realized. In 2014, the Amsterdam Declaration on Essential Surgical Care was created, and in 2015, the 68th World Health Assembly (WHA) unanimously passed resolution 68.15 (WHA68.15) to strengthen emergency and essential

BOX 2.1 Key Messages From the Disease Control Priorities 3rd Edition

- Provision of essential surgical procedures would avert an estimated 1.5 million deaths a year, or 6%-7% of all avertable deaths in low- and middle-income countries (LMICs).
- Essential surgical procedures rank among the most cost-effective of all health interventions. The surgical platform of first-level hospitals delivers 28 of the 44 essential procedures, making investment in this platform also highly cost-effective.
- Measures to expand access to surgery, such as task-sharing, have been shown to be safe and effective while countries make long-term investments in building surgical and anesthesia workforces.
- Because emergency procedures constitute 23 of the 28 procedures provided at first-level hospitals, such facilities must be widely geographically available.
- Substantial disparities remain in the safety of surgical care, driven by high perioperative mortality rates and anesthesia-related deaths in LMICs. Feasible measures, such as the World Health Organization's (WHO's) Surgical Safety Checklist,[27a] have led to improvements in safety and quality.
- The large burden of surgical conditions, the cost-effectiveness of essential surgery, and the strong public demand for surgical services suggest that universal coverage of essential surgery (UCES) should be financed early on the path to universal health coverage.
- We point to estimates that full coverage of the component of UCES applicable to first-level hospitals would require slightly more than $3 billion annually of additional spending and yield a benefit to cost ratio of better than 10:1. It would efficiently and equitably provide health benefits and financial protection, and it would contribute to stronger health systems.

From Jemison DT, Alwan A, Mock CN, et al: Universal health coverage and intersectoral action for health: key messages from Disease Control Priorities, 3rd edition. The Lancet 391, Issue 10125, 2018:1108–1120.

BOX 2.2 Key Messages From The Lancet Commission on Global Surgery

- 5 billion people do not have access to safe, affordable surgical and anesthesia care when needed. Access is worst in low-income and lower-middle-income countries (LMICs), where 9 of 10 people cannot access basic surgical care. 143 Million additional surgical procedures are needed in LMICs each year to save lives and prevent disability. Of the 313 million procedures undertaken worldwide each year, only 6% occur in the poorest countries, where over a third of the world's population lives. Low operative volumes are associated with high case-fatality rates from common, treatable surgical conditions. Unmet need is greatest in eastern, western, and central sub-Saharan Africa, and South Asia.
- 33 Million individuals face catastrophic health expenditure due to payment for surgery and anesthesia care each year. An additional 48 million cases of catastrophic expenditure are attributable to the nonmedical costs of accessing surgical care. A quarter of people who have a surgical procedure will incur financial catastrophe as a result of seeking care. The burden of catastrophic expenditure for surgery is highest in low-income and lower-middle-income countries and, within any country, lands most heavily on poor people.
- Investing in surgical services in LMICs is affordable, saves lives, and promotes economic growth. To meet present and projected population demands, urgent investment in human and physical resources for surgical and anesthesia care is needed. If LMICs were to scale-up surgical services at rates achieved by the present best-performing LMICs, two thirds of countries would be able to reach a minimum operative volume of 5000 surgical procedures per 100,000 population by 2030. Without urgent and accelerated investment in surgical scale-up, LMICs will continue to have losses in economic productivity, estimated cumulatively at US$12.3 trillion (2010 US$, purchasing power parity) between 2015 and 2030.
- Surgery is an "indivisible, indispensable part of health care."[1] Surgical and anesthesia care should be an integral component of a national health system in countries at all levels of development. Surgical services are a prerequisite for the full attainment of local and global health goals in areas as diverse as cancer, injury, cardiovascular disease, infection, and reproductive, maternal, neonatal, and child health. Universal health coverage and the health aspirations set out in the post-2015 Sustainable Development Goals will be impossible to achieve without ensuring that surgical and anesthesia care is available, accessible, safe, timely, and affordable.

Mock CN, Donkor P, Gawande A, et al: Essential surgery: key messages from Disease Control Priorities, 3rd edition. The Lancet 385, Issue 9983, 2015: 2209–2219.

surgical and anesthesia care as a component of universal health coverage.[24,25] Also in 2015, publication of DCP3 and the Lancet Commission on Global Surgery (LCOGS) "Global Surgery 2030" report significantly expanded the body of data characterizing the global surgical and anesthesia crises, and also outlined strategies for addressing some of these challenges (Boxes 2.1and 2.2).[5,26] During the LCOGS development, Jim Kim, President of the World Bank, echoed the words of Dr. Mahler from 35 years earlier by stating, "...surgery is an indivisible, indispensable part of health care and of progress towards universal health coverage."[27]

These events provided a much needed boost to efforts aimed at improving the accessibility, affordability, and safety of surgical, obstetric, and anesthesia care worldwide. They also helped provide a framework for including surgery and anesthesia as global health priorities by linking surgery and anesthesia care to universal health coverage. Surgery and anesthesia were not included in previous priority-setting efforts, in part, because it was not clear how to incorporate them. Limited data about the scale of the crises, as well as misperceptions around complexity and cost-effectiveness (as discussed in the next section) resulted in surgery and anesthesia care being peripheral to global health priority-setting efforts like the Millennium Development Goals (MDGs). Although surgery and anesthesia are not explicitly a focus of more recent global health priority initiatives like the Global Health 2035 report and the United Nations (UN) Sustainable Development Goals (SDGs), these reports emphasize noncommunicable diseases, injuries, healthcare workforce expansion, and universal health coverage, which incontrovertibly depend on surgery and anesthesia.[28,29]

Milestones like LCOGS, the WHA resolution 68.15, and the Lancet Commission on Palliative Care and Pain Relief have helped call attention to the global anesthesia, analgesia, and surgery crises at hand.[30] Entities like the World Federation of Societies of Anaesthesiologists (WFSA), Association of Anesthetists of Great Britain and Ireland (AAGBI), Canadian Anesthesiologists' Society International Education Foundation (CASIEF), and Lifebox are among the increasing number of anesthesia organizations working on system-level changes, research, and large-scale education initiatives in LMICs. Many national anesthesia societies, such as the United Kingdom's Royal College of Anaesthetists (RCoA), the Royal College of Anesthesiologists of Thailand, and the Chilean Society of Anesthesiologists are also actively engaged in such activities. The number of these global anesthesia efforts is unprecedented, but still nascent and evolving.

If surgery is described as the neglected step-child of global health, then anesthesia is the forgotten relative. Despite significant interdependence, surgery, anesthesia, and obstetrics have yet to harmonize global health efforts and maximize impact. Global health efforts involving either surgery or anesthesia have become known collectively as "global surgery" (see Table 2.2). In 2014, "global surgery" was defined "...as an area for study, research, practice, and advocacy that places priority on improving health outcomes and achieving health equity for all people worldwide who are affected by surgical conditions or have a need for surgical care. Global surgery incorporates all surgical specialties, including obstetric and gynecologic surgery; anesthesia; perioperative care; aspects of emergency medicine; rehabilitation; palliative care; and nursing and the allied health professions involved in the care of the surgical patient. It encompasses surgical care for underserved populations in all countries and for populations affected by conflict, displacement, and disaster, and promotes access to safe, quality care. Global surgery emphasizes supraterritorial and transnational issues, determinants, and solutions, recognizing that the determinants of inadequate or inequitable surgical care are often the result of common and interdependent global structures and processes, even though they are predominantly experienced within individual countries and communities.[31]" This definition was abbreviated to state "global surgery is an area of study, research, practice, and advocacy that seeks to improve health outcomes and achieve health equity for all people who require surgical care, with a special emphasis on underserved populations and populations in crisis. It uses collaborative, cross-sectoral, and transnational approaches and is a synthesis of population-based strategies with individual surgical care." Although anesthesia is not directly mentioned in this definition, "global surgery" has become a rallying point for anesthesia global health efforts.

SCOPE AND SCALE OF THE GLOBAL ANESTHESIA, SURGERY, AND PAIN CRISES

Global Burden of Surgical Disease

Nearly 30% of global morbidity and mortality is surgically treatable, with tens of millions of lives lost each year due to surgical conditions.[5] This burden of surgical disease predominantly affects LMICs and kills 4 times more people than human immunodeficiency virus (HIV), TB, and malaria combined (Fig. 2.1).[32] In addition to negative impacts on health and well-being, there is also significant economic burden associated with surgical morbidity and mortality. By 2030, morbidity and mortality from surgical conditions could reduce annual gross domestic product (GDP) growth by an estimated 2% in LMICs. In the past, similar calculations were used to successfully generate global investment in malaria, but had estimated much lower (1.3%) decreases in GDP due to malaria.[33] Without significant and immediate intervention, surgical disease will produce economic productivity losses of more than US$12 trillion for LMICs between 2015 and 2030. While it is generally agreed that surgical conditions account for a large proportion of global morbidity and mortality, precise data to support this have been lacking. This challenge has been attributed in part to a lack of resources being invested in such research and also to several inherent difficulties in quantifying surgical diseases.

The term "global burden of disease" (GBD) uses the disability-adjusted-life-year (DALY) as a unit to quantify premature death (years of life lost) and disability (years of life lived in a state of less than full health) (Fig. 2.2). The DALY was originally developed for the seminal GBD 1990 Study to quantify the burden of different diseases around the world and has since become commonly used in public health and health economics.[34,35] Because the DALY is routinely used to inform resource allocation, it has been utilized to describe surgical and pain disease burdens as well. The global health community has moved away from using terms such as third world, developed, or developing when describing countries' level of economic development. Leading causes of DALYs are often reported geographically by World Bank income level (see Table 2.1) or more recently by socio-demographic index (SDI) (Figs. 2.3 and 2.4). The SDI is a composite average of three indicators predictive of health outcomes: income per capita, average educational attainment (for population >15 years old), and total fertility rate.

The 2006 DCP2 publication was one of the first attempts to quantify surgical disease burden and did so by asking 18 surgeons for an educated guess, using convenience sampling and an online survey. Although the reported number

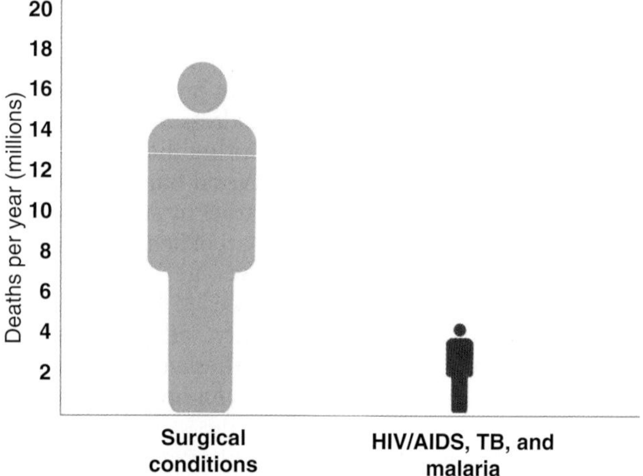

Fig. 2.1 Surgical conditions account for more annual deaths (16.9 million) than HIV/AIDS (1.03 million), TB (1.21 million), and malaria (0.72 million) combined. *AIDS*, Acquired immunodeficiency syndrome; *HIV*, human immune virus, *TB*, tuberculosis. (Data from Shrime MG, Bickler WS, Alkire BC, et al. Global burden of surgical disease: an estimation from the provider perspective. *Lancet Glob Health.* 2015;3:S8–S9; and GBD collaborators 2016. Global, regional, and national age-sex specific mortality for 264 causes of death, 1980–2016: a systematic analysis for the Global Burden of Disease Study 2016. *Lancet.* 2017;390[10100]:1151–1210.)

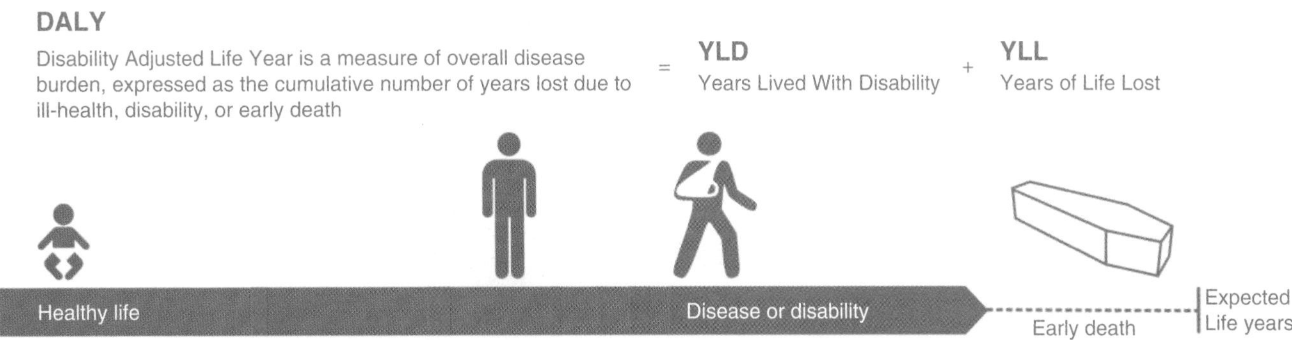

Fig. 2.2 The disability-adjusted life year *(DALY)*. (From Wikipedia. https://en.wikipedia.org/wiki/Disabilityadjusted_life_year#/media/File:DALY_disability_affected_life_year_infographic.svg. Creative commons license: CC BY-SA 3.0.)

(11%) was eye-opening and widely quoted, it was likely a significant underestimation.

In 2015, the DCP3 provided another attempt to assess the public health impact of surgical care by estimating morbidity and mortality averted by scaling up basic surgical and anesthesia services in LMICs (i.e., surgical care for appendicitis, paralytic ileus, intestinal obstruction, hernias, gallbladder and bile duct disease, maternal hemorrhage, obstructed labor, abortion and neonatal encephalopathy, trauma resuscitation, surgical airway, peripheral venous access, suturing, laceration and wound management, chest tube or needle decompression, fracture reduction, escharotomy, fasciotomy, skin grafting, and trauma-related laparotomy and amputation). They concluded that an estimated 1.4 million deaths and 77.2 million DALYs could be prevented each year by scaling up basic surgical and anesthesia services in LMICs.[26]

The LCOGS produced another attempt to estimate global morbidity and mortality from surgical disease by asking 173 surgeons, anesthesiologists, internists, nurses, and public health practitioners from around the world, "What proportion of patients with the following conditions would, in an ideal world, require a surgeon for management?" The result of this survey was 28% to 32% of overall GBD requires a surgeon for management. Based on these results, LCOGS estimated that 30% of GBD is surgically treatable with an estimated 17 million lives lost per year due to surgical conditions.[5]

These reports are consistent with the 1990 GBD Study data, which demonstrate that the morbidity and mortality associated with surgical diseases is significantly larger than that of HIV, TB, and malaria combined.[32] Unintentional injuries are the single largest contributor of DALYs worldwide. The majority of deaths that can be prevented with surgical care are due to injuries (77%), maternal-neonatal

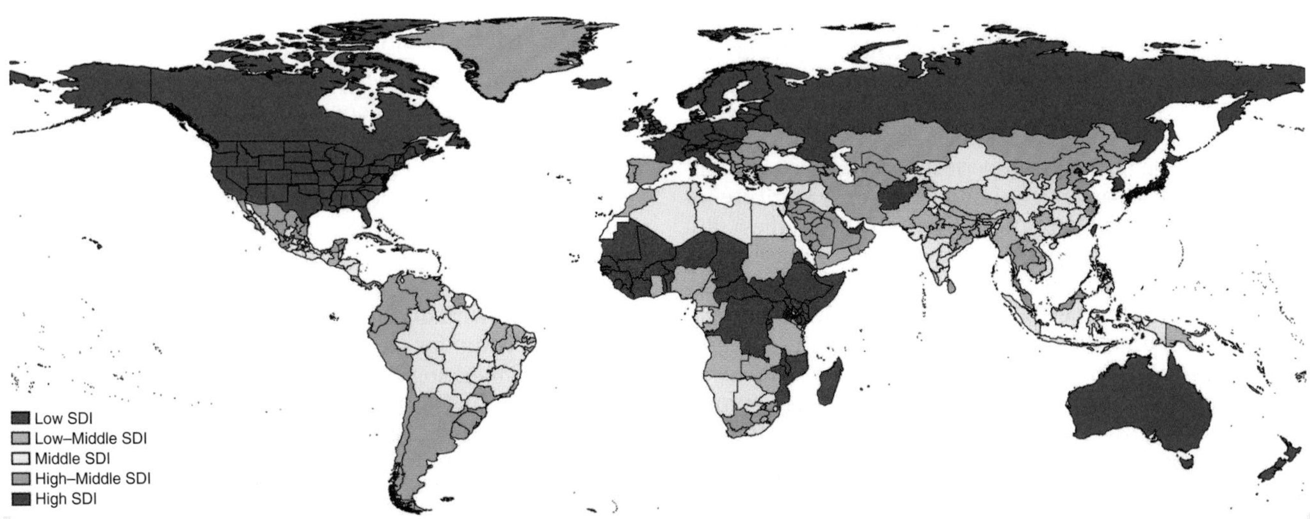

Fig. 2.3 Socio-demographic Index *(SDI)* is calculated for each geography as a function of lag-dependent income per capita, average educational attainment in the population older than age 15 years, and the total fertility rate. SDI units are interpretable; a zero represents the lowest level of income per capita and educational attainment and highest total fertility rate observed during 1980–2015, whereas a one represents the highest income per capita and educational attainment and lowest total fertility rate observed in the same period. Cutoffs on the SDI scale for the quintiles have been selected on the basis of examination of the entire distribution of geographies 1980–2015. ***GBD,*** **Global Burden of Disease.** (From GBD 2015 Mortality and Causes of Death Collaborators. Global, regional, and national life expectancy, all-cause mortality, and cause-specific mortality for 249 causes of death, 1980–2015: a systematic analysis for the Global Burden of Disease Study 2015. *Lancet*. 2016;388[10053]:1459–1544. Copyright © 2017 The Author[s]. Published by Elsevier Ltd. This is an Open Access article under the CC BY 4.0 license.)

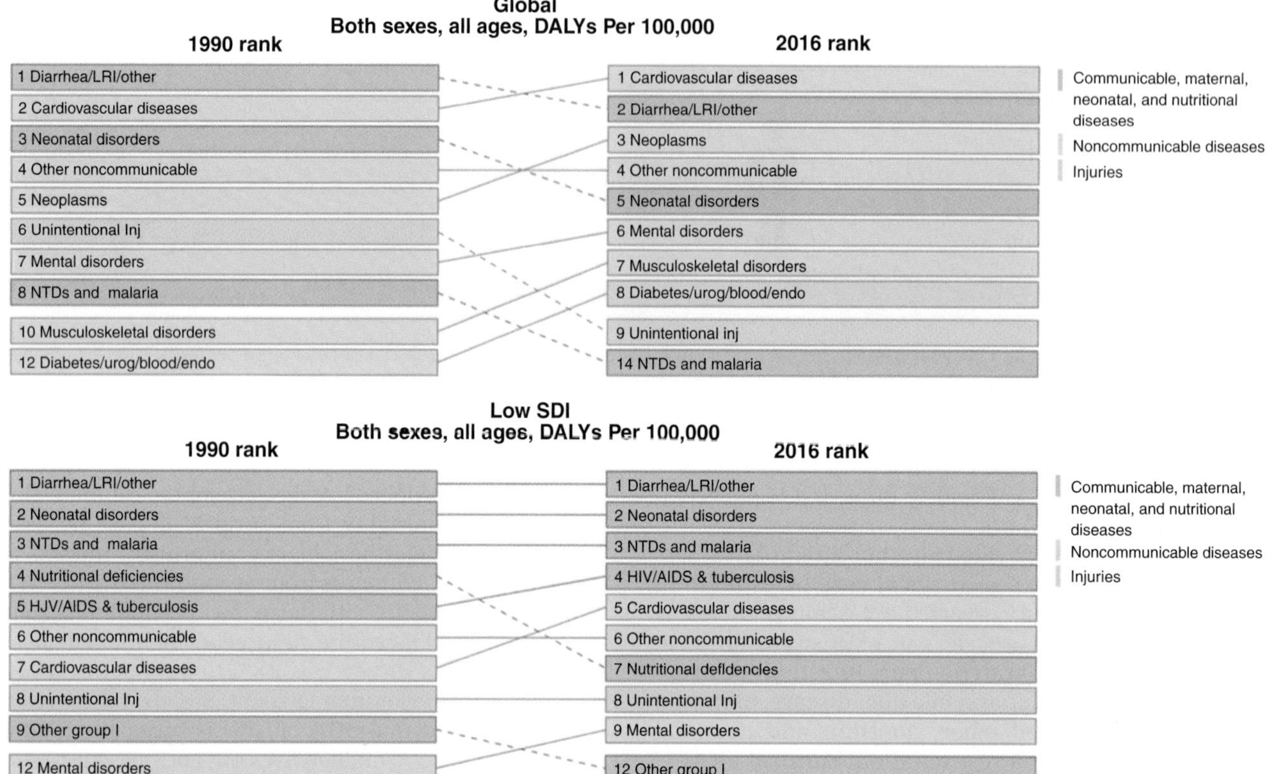

Fig. 2.4 Leading causes of death and disability-adjusted-life-years *(DALYs)*, 1990–2016, global versus low Socio-Demographic Index *(SDI)*. *AIDS*, Acquired immunodeficiency syndrome; *HIV*, human immune virus. (From https://vizhub.healthdata.org/gbd-compare/. Reproduced under Creative Commons Non-Commercial-No Derivatives 4.0 International License.)

conditions (14%), and digestive diseases (9%).[26] Global industrialization and an "epidemiological transition" (i.e., people living longer) in many LMICs have resulted in rising noncommunicable disease and injury burdens (most notably from road traffic crashes) that will likely contribute to increased global surgical disease burden in the coming years.

Each of the methods previously described to estimate surgical disease burden is imperfect. Challenges and limitations include complex methodologies (e.g., Institute for Health Metrics and Evaluation [IHME], GBD Studies), difficulty with measuring and defining surgical diseases (e.g., the same neoplasm in one person may be treated with surgery but in another person may be treated with chemotherapy), and challenges in assigning DALYs to diseases (i.e., disability weighting) and assigning DALYs averted to surgical procedures.[26] To overcome these shortcomings, additional metrics for global surgery and anesthesia have been proposed and include measuring disease prevalence, treatment backlogs for non fatal conditions, morbidity and mortality as a result of delays in care, social benefit, economic benefit, and value of a statistical life (rather than costs per DALY averted).[36]

One significant role for the academic anesthesia community in the global context is working to increase efforts that better quantify the growing surgical disease and pain burdens in order to facilitate appropriate resource allocation and subsequent evaluation of interventions.

Global Burden of Pain

As with surgical disease burden, there is general consensus on the staggering prevalence and incidence of pain worldwide though there are relatively limited data and significant challenges to quantifying pain burden in the global context. Pain is one of the most common reasons for seeking medical attention, is among the top five causes of DALYs worldwide, and directly accounts for four (low back pain, neck pain, musculoskeletal pain, migraine) of the top 10 causes of years lived with disability (YLDs).[32,37] These statistics do not even account for pain secondary to oncology, injury, or postoperative etiologies, which likely increase these numbers substantially. It is estimated that 10% to 25% of the world's population suffer from recurring and chronic pain, with increasing numbers caused by intentional physical harm such as war, violence, and torture.[38] Uncontrolled pain has many potential negative impacts on health, well-being, and economic productivity, including increased risk of myocardial infarction and chronic pain.

The 2017 Lancet Commission on Palliative Care and Pain Relief defined serious health-related suffering (SHS) as suffering associated with illness or injury that compromises physical, social, or emotional functioning, and cannot be relieved without medical intervention.[30] Approximately half of all deaths worldwide involve SHS and more than 80% of people who die with SHS are from LMICs. It is estimated that 2.5 million children die with SHS each year. Ninety-eight percent of these children live in LMICs, and more than 90% of these deaths are avoidable. Among the top 10 conditions associated with SHS are HIV, malignancy, and injury. Though not as obvious as injury or cancer, HIV/AIDS is a major source of pain and analgesia need.[39] Pain related to HIV is not routinely managed by anesthesiologists when compared to other more common pain etiologies, however, the relevance of HIV as a rallying point to advocate for greater access to analgesics in LMICs is discussed further in this chapter. In many countries, conditions such as diabetes, sickle cell, and leprosy are also responsible for significant pain burdens. With increasing longevity and industrialization, the disease burden for malignancy and injury are expected to increase significantly in LMICs. As providers with often the most experience administering analgesics, anesthesia providers play an expanded and critical role in pain management, especially in resource-constrained settings.

Disparities in Access, Affordability, and Safety

The exact level of disease burden attributable to surgical disease or pain is a focus of ongoing debate and research, yet it is generally accepted that the surgical, anesthesia, and pain crises are massive, largely avoidable, and disproportionately affect LMICs. Of the roughly 300,000 maternal deaths worldwide, 99% occur in low-resource settings (66% in sub-Saharan Africa) and the majority are preventable with relatively basic surgical, anesthesia, and perioperative care.[40] Approximately 70% of global cancer deaths occur in LMICs, with the majority requiring surgical, anesthesia, or analgesia services.[41] Scaling access to basic surgical and anesthesia services in LMICs could avert 77 million DALYs and 1.5 million deaths per year.[26] Injury represents the majority (77%) of this avoidable morbidity and mortality, followed by maternal and neonatal conditions (14%). Approximately 90% of deaths and DALYs that are lost due to road traffic accidents occur in LMICs.

Based solely on the inequitable distribution of operating theatres, more than two billion people have no access to surgical services.[42] When also accounting for timeliness, facility capacity, safety, and affordability, nearly 5 billion people—the majority of the world's population—lack access to surgical and anesthesia care. The Global Initiative for Children's Surgery (GICS) estimates that 1.7 billion children lack access to surgical care.[42a] It is estimated that approximately 143 million additional surgeries are required each year.[5] Of the 234 million major surgical procedures performed annually, only 3% to 6% of them are estimated to occur in LIMCs.[5,43] Disparities in access disproportionally affect lower-income areas like sub-Saharan Africa or South Asia, where more than 95% of the population do not have access to surgical and anesthesia care. In some higher-income areas like North America and Europe, access varies considerably, but generally more than 95% of the population has access (Fig. 2.5).[44] Even in HIC like the United States, access to anesthesia, surgical, and analgesia care can be limited for rural and underserved populations.[45,46] It is estimated that universal access to "essential" surgical procedures (which include treatments for injury, obstetric complications, abdominal emergencies, cataracts, and congenital anomalies) would prevent approximately 1.5 million deaths per year or 6% to 7% of all preventable deaths in LMICs.[26]

Inadequate access to analgesia is among the most neglected and inequitable global public health challenges. The global burden of pain disproportionately affects the world's poor due to the high-burden conditions associated with pain (e.g., HIV, malignancy, and injury) in LMICs, and the general lack of access to analgesics. Although pain is the most common reason for seeking medical attention, and analgesia is considered a basic human right, gaps in access to analgesia are significant and among the most striking global health disparities worldwide.[47–49] Injury and malignancy, two conditions with significant analgesia needs, represent a significant proportion of surgical disease burden in LMICs, yet the vast majority of LMIC populations have limited or nonexistent access to opiate analgesia. Six HICs account for 80% of the world's opiate consumption, and countries that contain 17% of the world's population (Canada, United States, Western Europe, Australia, and New Zealand) are responsible for 92% of the world's opiate consumption (Figs. 2.6 and 2.7).[30,50-52] Pain and palliative care remain relatively neglected by the global health community and disproportionately affect vulnerable populations in LMICs.[30,53] In recent decades, access to opiates has improved in some LMICs, but not all (e.g., consumption in Africa and South Asia has declined).[52] Inequitable access to analgesia is not unique to LMICs and has been repeatedly described in many HICs, including the United States.[54-56] Reasons for the inequitable distribution of analgesia are discussed further in the next section of this chapter.

For the proportion of the world's population that has access to surgical and anesthesia care, they must confront significant disparities in safety. In the last half-century perioperative patient safety has improved by more than 10-fold, though the majority of the gains have been seen in HICs.[57] In the United States during the 21st century, anesthesia-related mortality decreased from 1:1560 around 1950 to less than 1:13,000, and is significantly better than this in healthy patients.[58,59] Worldwide, approximately 32 million people per year receive anesthesia without adequate monitoring, and more than 77,000 operating rooms (19%) worldwide lack pulse oximetry. In some regions, more than 70% of operating rooms lack pulse oximetry.[42] Data on surgical outcomes in LMICs remain limited but have expanded significantly in the early part of the 21st century. Reports of perioperative mortality rates (POMRs) from low-income countries (LICs) have varied widely in both methodology and results, ranging from 0.2% to 6% overall, with significantly higher mortality for emergent procedures (10% overall, 20% for typhoid intestinal perforations).[60–64] One international, prospective, observational cohort study of adults undergoing inpatient surgery in 247 hospitals from 25 African countries reported a 30-day in-hospital mortality rate (2.1%) that was twice the reported global average, despite a significantly younger and lower American Society of Anesthesiologists (ASA) physical classification patient population.[65]

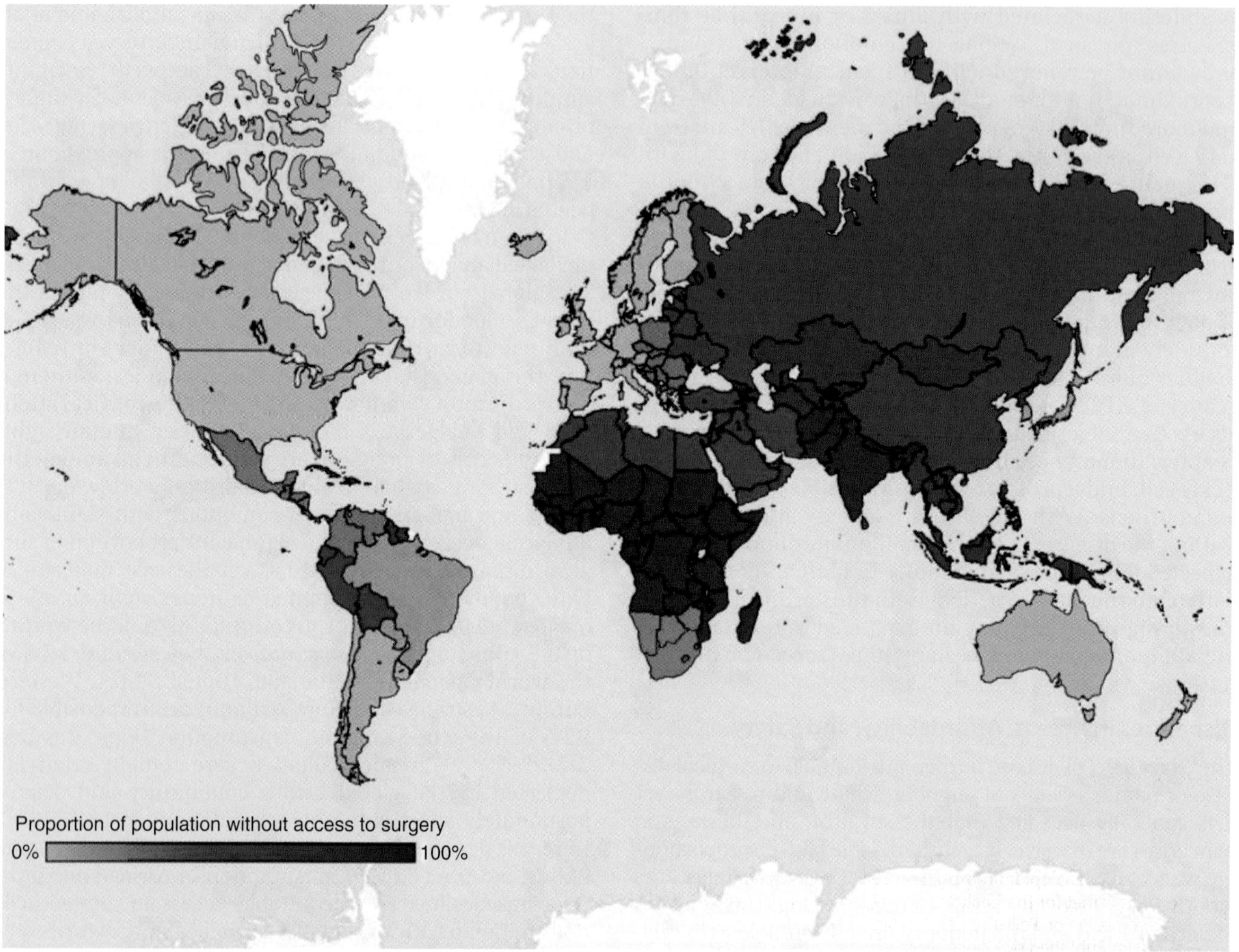

Proportion of population without access to surgery

0% 100%

Fig. 2.5 The proportion of population without access to surgery. (From Alkire BC, Raykar NP, Shrime MG, et al. Global access to surgical care: a modelling study. *Lancet Glob Health.* 2015;3:e316–e323. doi: 10.1016/S2214-109X(15)70115-4. Epub 2015 Apr 27. Copyright © 2015 Alkire et al. Open Access article distributed under the terms of CC.)

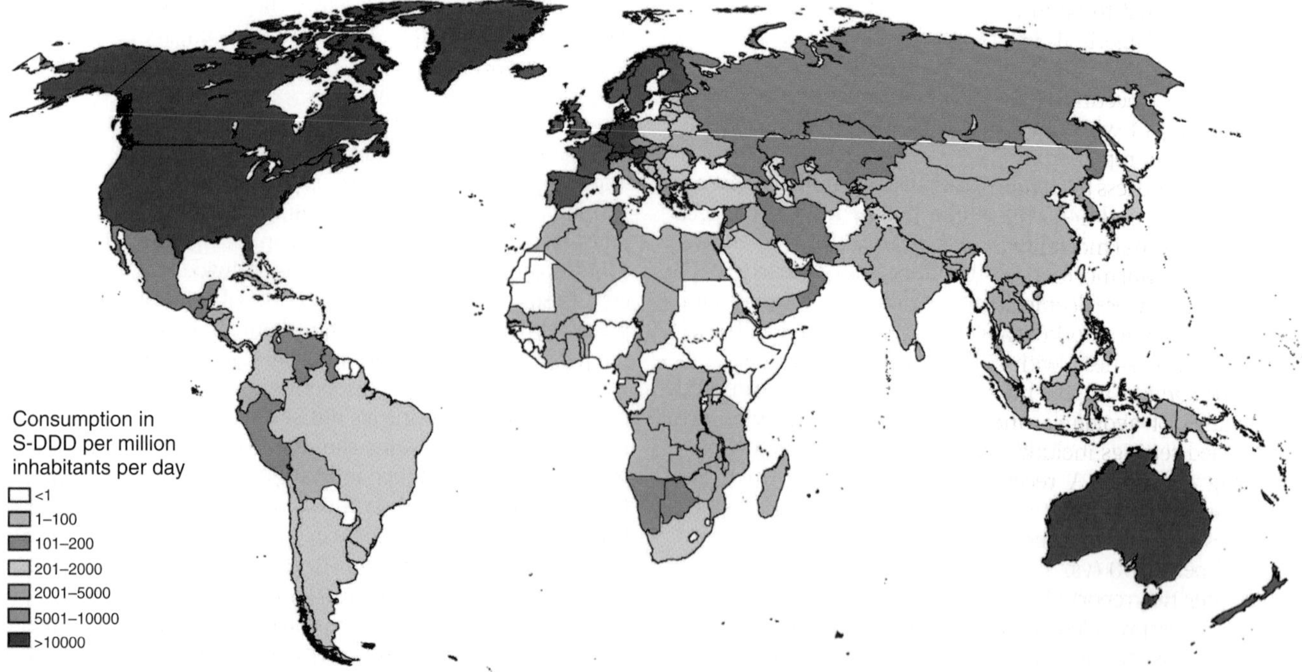

Fig. 2.6 Mean availability of opioids for pain management in 2011–2013. *S-DDD*, Defined daily doses for statistical purposes. (From Berterame S, Erthal J, Thomas J, et al. Use of and barriers to access to opioid analgesics: a worldwide, regional, and national study. *Lancet.* 2016;387:1644–1656. https://doi.org/10.1016/S0140-6736[16]00161-6. Copyright © 2015 Berterame et al. Open Access article distributed under the terms of CC.)

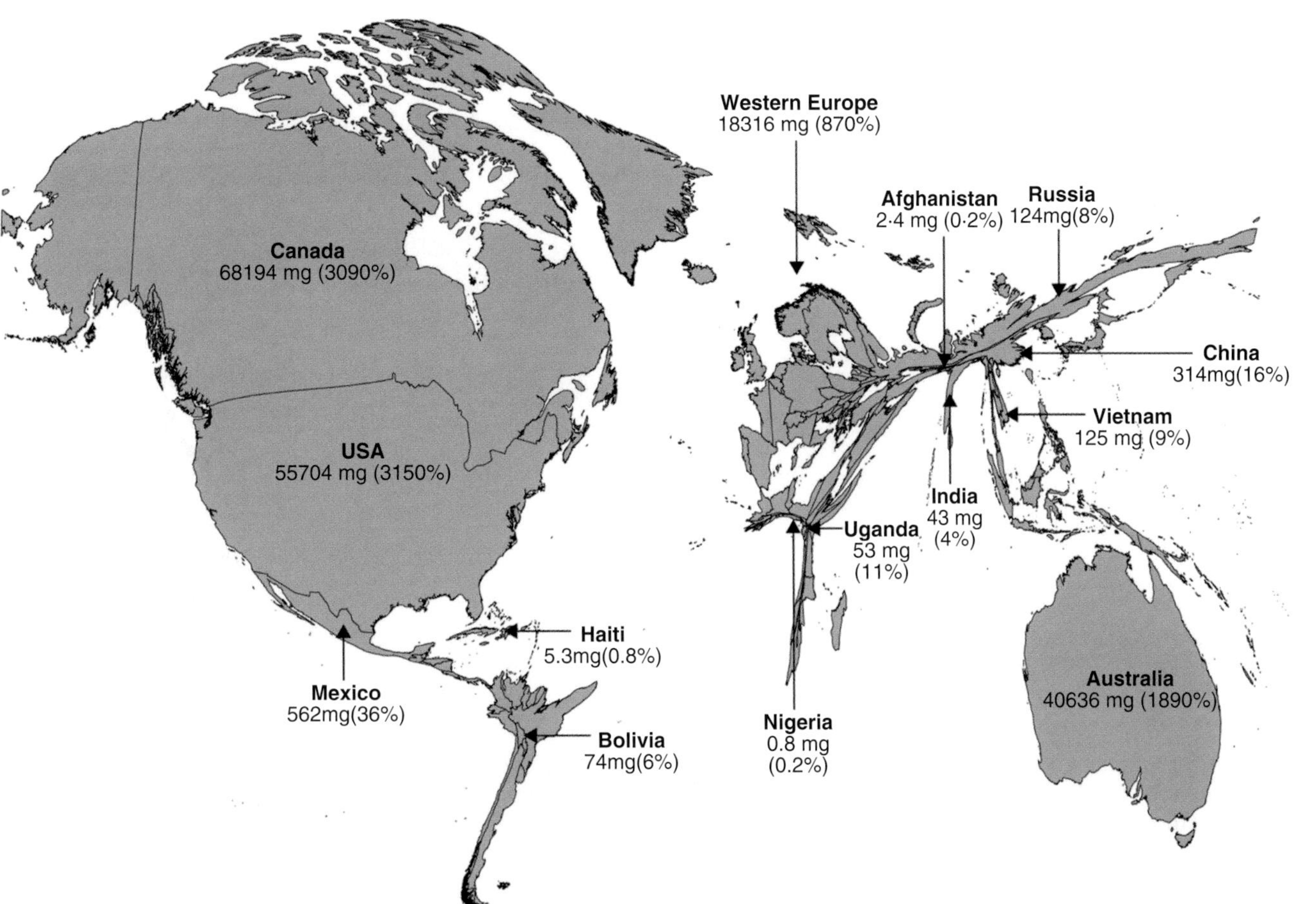

Fig. 2.7 Distributed opioid morphine-equivalent (morphine in mg/patient in need of palliative care, average 2010–2013), and estimated percentage of need that is met for the health conditions most associated with serious health-related suffering. (From Knaul FM, Bhadelia A, Rodriguez NM, et al. The *Lancet* Commission on Palliative Care and Pain Relief—findings, recommendations, and future directions. *Lancet Glob Health*. 2018;6:S5–S6. Copyright © 2018 The Author(s). Published by Elsevier Ltd. This is an open access article under the CC BY 4.0 license.)

In several African countries, anesthesia-related mortality has been reported to be in the 1:100s (Malawi 1:504; Zimbabwe 1:482; Nigeria 1:387 for C-sections; Togo 1:133 to 1:250).[66–69] In one report of 24-hour surgical outcomes in Togo, 30 deaths occurred (total cases 1464), 22 were deemed avoidable, and 11 were due to avoidable anesthesia complications.[15] Another report from Togo reported a mortality rate of 1:250 and found less than half of the 26 facilities surveyed had pulse oximetry, and none had capnography.[70] In a national report on maternal mortality in South Africa, nearly 2.35% of recorded maternal mortalities were anesthesia related, and the majority (93%) were deemed avoidable. One of the most common causes of anesthesia death in this report was the provision of spinal anesthesia without skills necessary to manage an airway or convert to general anesthesia.[71] Other commonly cited causes of avoidable anesthesia mortality in resource-constrained settings include inadequate staffing, monitoring, and drug overdose. A recent meta-analysis of anesthesia-related maternal mortality in LMICs found the risk of death from anesthesia for women undergoing obstetric procedures to be 1.2 per 1000 (vs. 3.8 per million in the United States), with higher risk reported if general anesthesia was used or if anesthesia was provided by a nonphysician[72]. In this analysis, anesthesia was the cause in 2.8% of maternal deaths in LMICs and 13.8% of all deaths during or after C-section in LMICs. To state this differently, anesthesia-related maternal mortality is 300-fold higher for neuraxial and 900-fold higher for general anesthesia than is reported in the United States.

It is important to note that the relationship between hospital-based perioperative morbidity and mortality and surgical disease morbidity and mortality must be interpreted with caution in settings where patients lack access to hospitals. In other words, in an HIC a patient's chances of dying from a ruptured viscous are roughly the same as the chances of dying from surgery for a ruptured viscous because more than 95% of the population has access to care. However, in an LIC, while the perioperative mortality for a ruptured viscous may be 10%, the majority of patients with this condition never make it to surgery and have mortality rates that are dramatically higher.

Affordability is another significant barrier to accessing surgical and anesthesia services. Each year, approximately 33 million people face catastrophic out-of-pocket expenditure due to payment for surgery and anesthesia (Fig. 2.8) with an additional 48 million people facing catastrophic expenditure related to non medical costs of accessing surgical care (e.g., transportation, lodging, and food).[5,73] Nearly half (3.7 billion) of the world's population is at risk of catastrophic expenditure if they were to have surgical and anesthesia care. The majority of those at risk live in

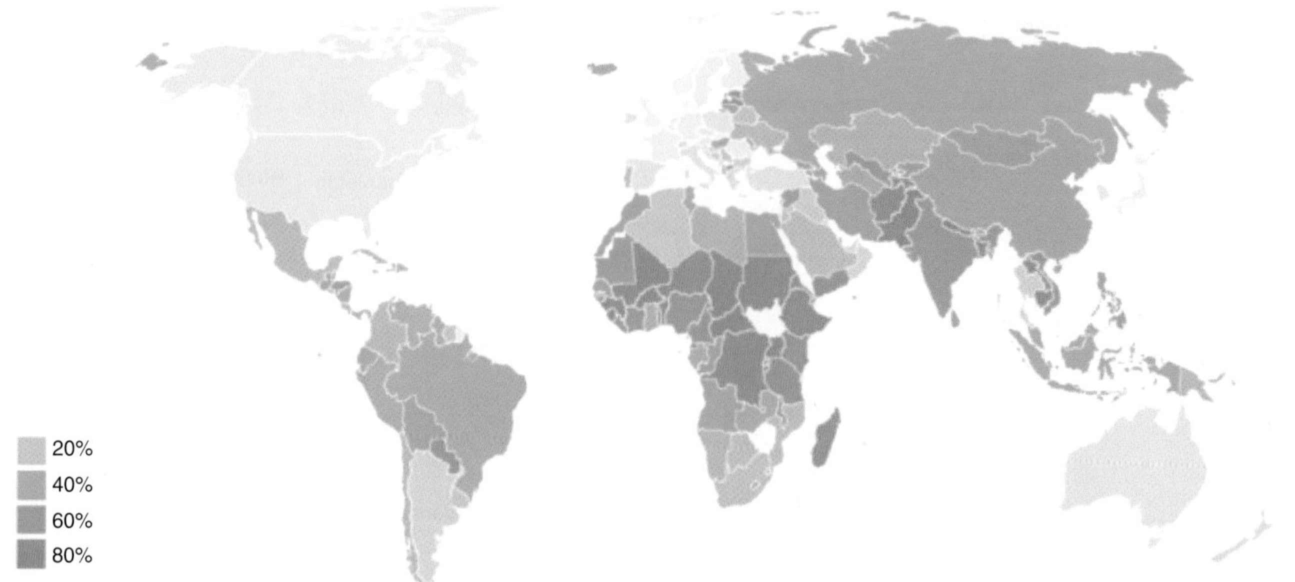

Fig. 2.8 Risk of catastrophic expenditure for surgical care in 2014 (% of people at risk). (Data from http://databank.worldbank.org/data/home.aspx. Originally printed: http://blogs.worldbank.org/opendata/africacan/pt/comment/reply/2341. Copyright © 2018 The World Bank. Reproduced under CC BY 4.0 license.)

sub-Saharan Africa, and South and Southeast Asia. The issue of affordability applies not only to surgery itself but also to components of perioperative care including analgesia and transfusions.[74] For example, in South America, a monthly prescription of opiate for chronic pain may cost 200% of annual income.[57] In India (where nominal gross national income per capita is $1670), a unit of blood often costs up to $247 despite a legal limit of $25.[75,76] Global health and development leaders including the WHO and World Bank prioritize financial risk protection as a key component of achieving universal health coverage goals for all countries. Despite relatively high out-of-pocket costs at the individual level for some procedures, surgery is a highly cost-effective public health intervention as discussed further in the following sections.

GLOBAL ANESTHESIA, SURGERY, AND PAIN CRISES: ORIGINS AND AREAS FOR INTERVENTION

Workforce shortages, inadequate infrastructure, lack of policy and prioritization, and increasing burden of surgical disease are among many factors contributing to current limitations in access, affordability, and safety of anesthesia and surgical services worldwide.[77] As previously discussed, global industrialization and an "epidemiological transition" in many LMICs have resulted in rising noncommunicable disease and injury burdens with lagging investment to address these issues. While these fundamental imbalances between healthcare needs and healthcare resources underlie much of the current global surgery, anesthesia, and pain crises, several additional factors have also contributed.

Misperceptions and Limited Data

Two common misperceptions about surgery and anesthesia have contributed to the delayed recognition of these fields as global public health priorities: (1) the scope and scale of surgical disease and pain burdens were vastly underestimated; and (2) surgical and anesthesia care were erroneously assumed to be too expensive and technology dependent to be done safely or cost-effectively in resource-constrained environments. In this section we discuss reasons why the surgical disease and pain burdens are historically poorly characterized. Misperceptions about cost-effectiveness and feasibility of safe surgery and anesthesia care also have roots in a historical data void, especially from LMICs.

Several innovative service delivery models in the public and private sectors of LMICs (e.g., Indus hospital, Aravind Eye Hospitals, and Narayana Hrudayalaya Heart Hospital) have demonstrated that it is feasible to provide cost-effective, safe, and affordable surgical and anesthesia care in resource-constrained countries.[78–81]

Recent data have consistently demonstrated that surgical services are among the most cost-effective public health interventions (Fig. 2.9). There are several methods to define cost-effectiveness thresholds, each with pros and cons.[82] One of the most commonly cited methods uses GDP-based thresholds. This approach was suggested by the WHO Commission on Macroeconomics and Health and has been defined by authors from the WHO's Choosing Interventions that are Cost–Effective project (WHO-CHOICE) as, "interventions that avert one DALY for less than average per capita income for a given country or region are considered very cost–effective; interventions that cost less than three times average per capita income per DALY averted are still considered cost–effective; and those that exceed this level are considered not cost–effective."[83]

In 2003 in Bangladesh, one of the earliest cost-effectiveness studies on surgical care reported the cost of emergency obstetric care at less than $11 per DALY averted.[16] This was 3 times more cost-effective than the measles vaccine (in 2003 dollars). The DCP2 and DCP3 demonstrated cost-effectiveness of the first-level surgical hospital, with essential surgical services all being highly cost effective and many

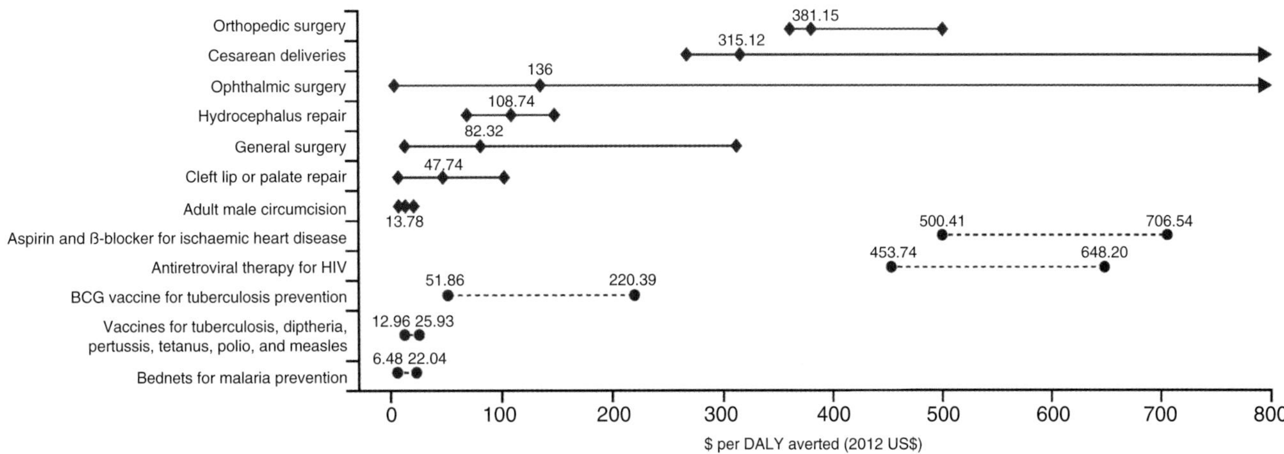

Fig. 2.9 Cost-effectiveness of surgery in low-income and middle-income countries compared with other public health interventions. Data points are medians, error bars show range. Surgical interventions are denoted by the diamonds and solid lines, public health interventions by the circles and dashed lines. *BCG*, Bacillus Calmette–Guérin; *DALY*, disability-adjusted life-year; *HIV*, human immune virus. (Source: Chao TE, Sharma K, Mandigo M, et al. Cost-effectiveness of surgery and its policy implications for global health: a systematic review and analysis. *Lancet Glob Health*. 2014;2:e334–e345. Copyright © 2015 Elsevier Ltd. Creative Commons Attribution License [CC BY].)

costing $10 to $100 per DALY averted. This is comparable to the cost-effectiveness of other public health interventions such as immunizations ($13-$26 per DALY) or bed nets for malaria prevention ($6-$22 per DALY), and much more cost-effective than other high-priority public health interventions such as HIV treatment ($500 per DALY).[84] A recent analysis of the cost-effectiveness of a pediatric operating room in Uganda found a cost of $6.39 per DALY averted and $397.95 per life saved, with a net economic benefit of over US$5 million per year (cost of $41,000 per year).[85]

In a 2012 forum hosted by the Copenhagen Consensus, five leading health economists, including four Nobel laureates, were asked how best to spend US$75 billion over 4 years to "advance global welfare," especially in LMICs. The leading priority identified by the group was the expansion of surgical care capacity (US$3 billion per year).[86]

In the past 5 years the global surgery and anesthesia communities have expanded the volume of data that dispel prior misconceptions and support prioritization of surgical and anesthesia care in the global health agenda. During this timeframe, there has also been an explosion of articles that expand available data on a wide range of global anesthesia and surgical topics. The majority of these articles have been published in the surgical journals though recently anesthesia publications have begun to actively support global anesthesia research. The global anesthesia community must increase research productivity in global health and also invest in advocacy, policy, and implementation sciences in order to ensure impact.

Advocacy and Policy

There are many reasons why surgery, anesthesia, and pain have historically not been prioritized by national health systems, donors, or the broader global health community. Although surgical disease accounts for 30% of global disease burden, less than 1% of development assistance for health supports delivery of anesthesia and surgical care.[87] Imbalance between resource allocation and disease burden is found in many health conditions, though the degree of this disparity for surgical disease and pain is particularly striking.

As discussed previously, lack of disease burden data and misperceptions about safety and cost-effectiveness have significantly hindered advocacy efforts for global anesthesia and surgery. In a qualitative analysis of factors that have hindered political prioritization for global surgery, several additional factors were identified including: fragmentation of the global surgery community, lack of leadership and consensus, and inadequate political strategy (e.g., not capitalizing on opportunities such as the MDGs).[88] In another analysis to determine why certain disease-specific global health networks are relatively more or less effective than others, four common challenges were highlighted, each with relevance to global anesthesia and surgery: (1) defining the problem and how it should be addressed; (2) positioning the issue in a way to inspire action by external audiences; (3) building coalitions that include stakeholders outside the healthcare sector (coalitions are too often dominated by HIC providers); and (4) creating governance institutions that facilitate collective action (Fig. 2.10).[89] Another study that examined factors influencing prioritization of surgery in national health systems concluded that sustained advocacy, effective framing of problems and solutions, robust country-level data, and support from regional and international partners were critical for success but often lacking.[90]

Advocacy efforts for surgery, anesthesia, and pain face a few additional and relatively unique challenges. Unlike infectious diseases such as HIV or Ebola, surgical disease and pain are not pandemic and do not incite similar action by the HIC donor community. Furthermore, most surgical conditions and pain are difficult to advertise and are not disease specific. While select pediatric conditions (e.g., cleft lips) are easily marketable, other conditions like trauma, hernias, and cesarean section are more difficult to compassionately portray in media in attempts to improve public awareness.

The WHA resolution 68.15 emphasized advocacy and resource development in five key focus areas for global surgery (workforce, essential medicines, information management,

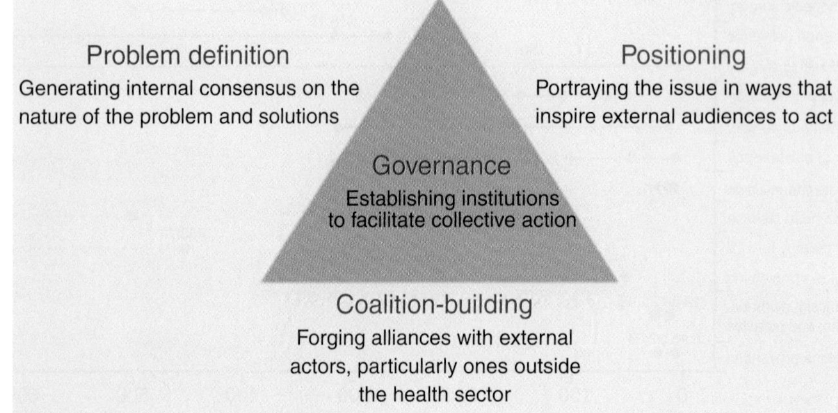

Fig. 2.10 Four challenges that global health networks face. (From Shiffman J. Four challenges that global health networks face. *Int J Health Policy Manag.* 2017;6[4]:183–189. Copyright © 2018 The Author[s]. Published by Kerman University of Medical Sciences. This is an open access article under the CC BY 4.0 license.)

service delivery, and advocacy). The LCOGS provided clear framing of problems (see Box 2.2), outlined priorities for country-level data collection, and helped to provide frameworks for national surgical, obstetric, and anesthesia plans (NSOAPs) in LMICs. As more NSOAPs are produced, they have the potential to serve as key rallying points for national advocacy efforts.

Anesthesia, surgery, and pain need global champions. Only recently has advocacy by leading global organization (e.g., the World Bank, WHO) and select local governments in LMICs focused attention on anesthesia and surgery in the global context. This is in part due to advocacy efforts by several relatively recent initiatives (e.g., LCOGS, The Global Alliance for Surgical, Obstetric, Trauma, and Anaesthesia Care [G4 Alliance], WFSA, GICS, and several more). These multidisciplinary efforts must be expanded and sustained in order to reach the critical mass needed to overcome prior misperceptions and affect change. It is essential that advocacy efforts for surgery, anesthesia, and pain be consistent with the key messages of LCOGS, the Global Health 2035 Report, WHA resolution 68.15, and the SDGs, and emphasize that anesthesia, surgery, and analgesia are indispensable components of "universal health coverage." No longer can surgery be seen as a vertical (i.e., disease-specific) program.

One key objective for advocacy efforts will be to identify new streams of funding from global donors, national budgets, private sectors, and innovative models. Similar to the large-scale funding initiatives to combat HIV/AIDS and other infectious diseases (e.g., the U.S. President's Emergency Plan for AIDS relief, Gavi Vaccine Alliance, The Global Fund), surgery and pain require comparable attention and support. In addition to domestic and international financing mechanisms to support health system scale-up, public-private partnerships and innovative patient-level financial risk protection strategies must be integral components to advocacy efforts.[5]

As leaders in safety, pain, perioperative care, and more, the global anesthesia community must actively engage in policy, research, and innovative global initiatives to expand access to quality care. Academic institutions from all countries can play a significant role in supporting a coordinated research agenda, creating a global voice for advocacy, sharing information, and harmonizing educational standards and opportunities. Anesthesia must follow the lead of other medical disciplines to not only cultivate but also support faculty and trainees with interests in global public health careers. Such advocacy will likely require coordination and partnership with multiple disciplines, including nonphysician provider cadres who perform a significant proportion of anesthesia services, especially in LICs.[91]

Workforce Shortages and Strategies for Expansion

The critical shortage of trained anesthesia providers in resource-constrained settings is one of the most significant barriers to expanding access to safe surgical, anesthesia, and pain services for billions of people worldwide. Although shortages of many key members of the surgical workforce exist (including surgeons, obstetricians, pathologists, radiologists, laboratory technicians, nurses, biomedical engineers, and more), anesthesia provider shortages in LMICs are particularly striking and relatively neglected. Countries like the Central African Republic have no physician anesthesiologists and only 24 nonphysician anesthesia providers (NPAPs) for a population of nearly 5 million. Ethiopia, with a population of over 100 million people, has only 35 physician specialist anesthesiologists. A survey of emergency obstetric care capacity at facilities in Uganda found that lack of staff had the greatest correlation with observed mortality rates.[92] In a survey of 64 public and private hospitals in Uganda, 84% did not have a physician specialist anesthesiologist, and 8% had no trained anesthesia providers at all.[93] In another survey of anesthesia providers from five main referral hospitals in East Africa (Uganda, Kenya, Tanzania, Rwanda, and Burundi), only 7% reported adequate anesthesia staffing.[94] In settings where providers exist but in small numbers, the workforce shortage is compounded by heavy administrative burdens and non-clinical duties.

While the anesthesia workforce shortage is most severe in LICs and particularly pronounced in sub-Saharan Africa, regional workforce shortages also exist in HICs and can significantly limit access to care for rural populations.[95,96] In one survey of rural hospitals in the United States, 36% reported delay or cancellation of surgery due to a lack of anesthesia providers.[97] Data from HICs demonstrate differences in trauma

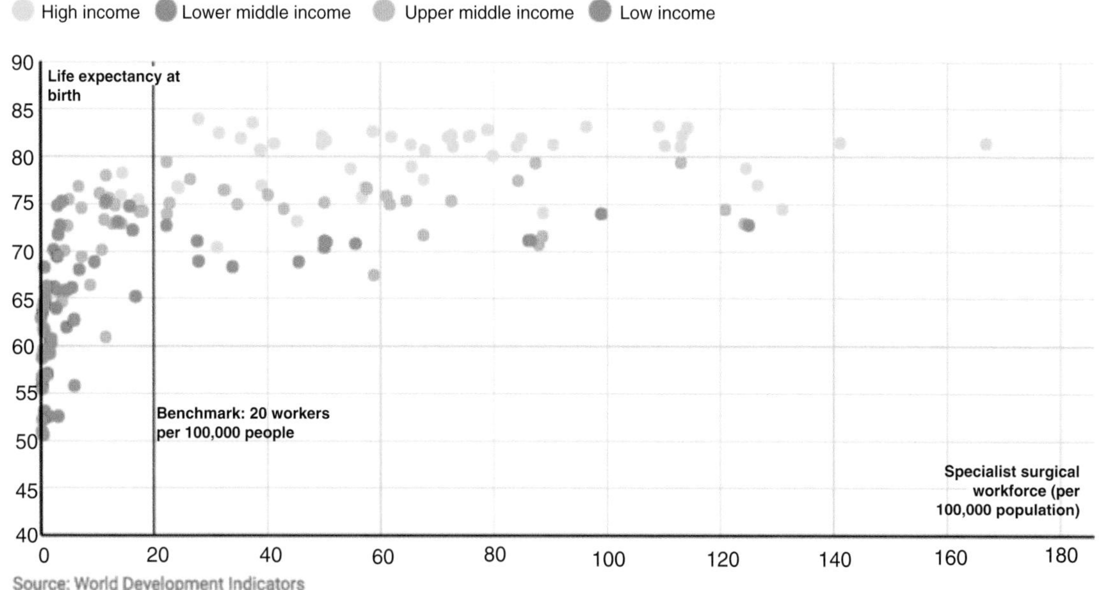

Fig. 2.11 Life expectancy tends to be higher in countries with a surgical workforce larger than 20 workers per 100,000 people. (Data source: http://databank.worldbank.org/data/home.aspx. Originally printed: http://blogs.worldbank.org/opendata/africacan/pt/comment/reply/2341. Copyright © 2018 The World Bank. Reproduced under CC BY 4.0 license.)

mortality are significantly worse starting at five miles from a trauma center in a major urban city.[98] One can only imagine outcome differences in settings where there may be no surgical or anesthesia provider for tens or even hundreds of miles.

The optimal number of specialist surgical, anesthetic, and obstetric workforce (SAO) providers needed to give access to safe surgery is unknown and likely to vary significantly based on local resources and needs. The SAO density correlates with life-expectancy and in one study, as SAO providers increased from 0 to 20 per 100,000 population, maternal mortality decreased by 13.1% for each 10 unit increase in provider density (Fig. 2.11). These benefits were also observed with workforce expansion beyond 20, though with less magnitude beyond 30 and 40 providers per 100,000 (Fig. 2.12).[99] Based on these findings, the LCOGS recommended prioritizing expansion of the SAO workforce to 20 per 100,000 population by 2030, with anesthesia-specific targets of 5 to 10 anesthesia providers per 100,000.[100]

The density of SAO providers has been estimated at 0.7 per 100,000 population for LICs as compared with 56.9 per 100,000 population for HICs.[101] Worldwide, 77 countries report an anesthesia provider density less than 5 per 100,000, with a 90-fold difference between the average physician workforce density in HICs as compared to LICs. The anesthesia workforce crisis is most severe in sub-Saharan Africa, where most countries have approximately 1.0 physician anesthesiologist per 100,000 population as compared to approximately 19 in Europe or 21 per 100,000 in the United States (Fig. 2.13).[100] Twenty-six countries in sub-Saharan Africa reported less than 0.5 physician anesthesia providers (PAPs) per 100,000. In many LICs, NPAPs provide the majority of anesthesia care. When NPAPs are included in calculations of total anesthesia provider density, 16 countries in sub-Saharan Africa still report less than 1 anesthesia provider per 100,000, and worldwide 70 countries still report less than 5 anesthesia providers per 100,000 population. Estimates from the WHO Global Surgical Workforce database demonstrate that 12% of the SAO workforce provides care for approximately a third of the world's population.[101] Worldwide, LICs and LMICs have 48% of the world's population but only 20% of the SAO workforce.

Multiple factors have contributed to the ongoing surgical and anesthesia workforce crises in LMICs, including limited training infrastructure, relatively low professional status, lack of career advancement (especially for NPAPs), perceived limited job opportunities relative to other professions (e.g., infectious disease in LMICs), cost of training, inefficient hiring mechanisms, provider burnout, as well as internal (e.g., private practice in urban settings) and external brain drain (e.g., leaving the country).[102,103] Lack of consensus on anesthesia practice models and polarized views on who should provide anesthesia care (i.e., physician versus nonphysician, supervised versus independent) are additional factors limiting a clear path for rapidly scaling the global anesthesia workforce (Table 2.3).[91] Task-sharing is a prominent and controversial component of many surgical workforce expansion efforts.

Each of the aforementioned challenges must be addressed as part of any national or international effort to expand the anesthesia workforce. The long-term goal of building robust training infrastructures in low-resource settings requires locally led plans for national advocacy, implementation, and evaluation. Such efforts can benefit from international investment and collaboration.[104-108]

Significant heterogeneity in anesthesia care models exists worldwide. Although the varied anesthesia practice and training models have evolved to address different local needs and challenges, excess heterogeneity and lack of consensus on anesthesia workforce strategy may provide an additional challenge to global workforce expansion. For example, within sub-Saharan Africa, formal nonphysician training programs range from 3 to 72 months in duration with widely different entry requirements, no standardized curricula or assessment tools, and different scopes of practice. For countries seeking

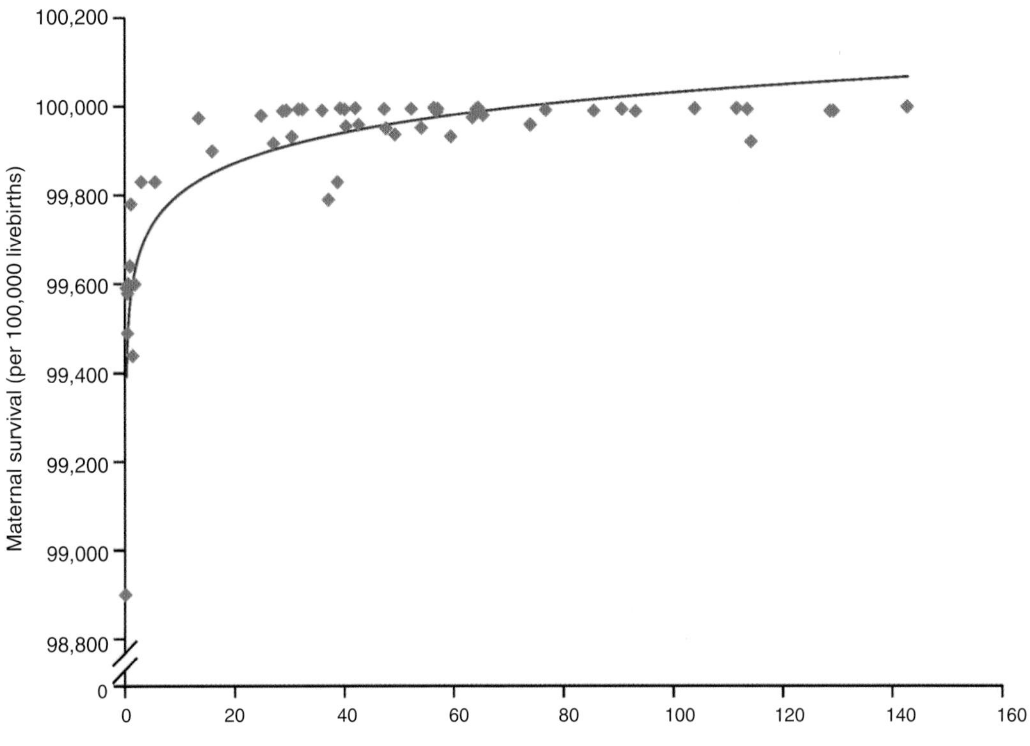

Fig. 2.12 Specialist surgical workforce density and maternal survival. A surgical workforce density of less than 20 per 100,000 specialist surgeons, anesthesiologists, and obstetricians correlates with lower rates of maternal survival. Maternal survival per 100,000 livebirths = 98,292 × ln (workforce density) + 99,579. (From Meara JG, Leather AJ, Hagander L, et al. Global Surgery 2030: evidence and solutions for achieving health, welfare, and economic development. *Lancet.* 2015;386:569–624. Data from Holmer H, Shrime MG, Riesel JN, et al. Towards closing the gap of the global surgeon, anaesthesiologist and obstetrician workforce: thresholds and projections towards 2030. *Lancet.* 2015;385(suppl 2):S40. Copyright © 2018 The Author(s). Published by Elsevier Ltd. This is an open access article under the CC BY 4.0 license.)

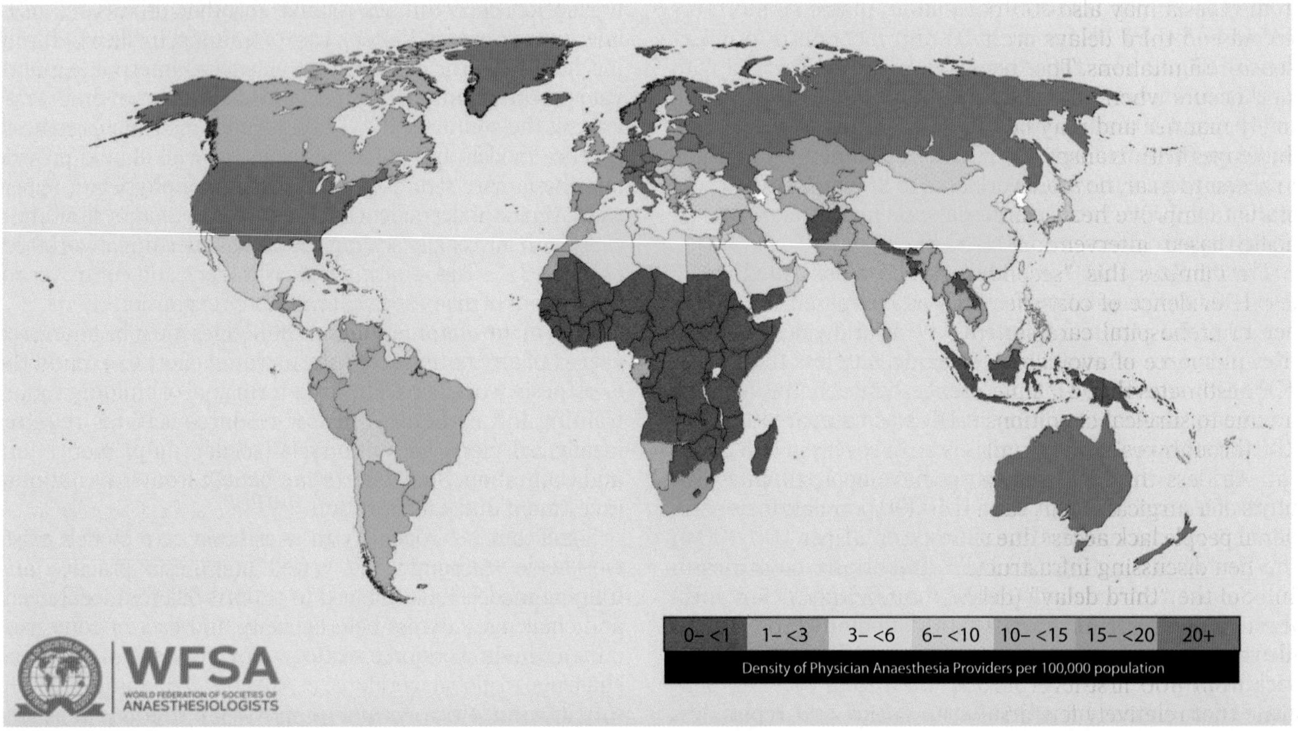

Fig. 2.13 World Federation of Societies of Anaesthesiologists Workforce Map. Image accessed at https://www.wfsahq.org/workforce-map (Data published: Kempthorne P, Morriss WW, Mellin-Olsen J, et al. The WFSA Global Anesthesia Workforce Survey. *Anesth Analg.* 2017;125[3]:981–990. Copyright © 2018 The WFSA. This image is reproduced under the CC BY 4.0 license.)

to increase anesthesia provider numbers, no clear roadmap exists. In most of these countries, task-sharing with NPAPs will likely play a key role in workforce expansion efforts. Collaborative efforts involving stakeholders from different countries and different anesthesia provider cadres can support anesthesia workforce expansion efforts by offering frameworks for anesthesia training, competency assessments, and potential practice models that are feasible with local resources and that meet local needs. Initiatives that ensure quality (e.g., education programs, credentialing bodies, and licensing exams) are as important as those that focus on increasing absolute numbers. The global anesthesia community can play a significant role via advocacy, research, education, and partnership to address many of the challenges that have created the current global anesthesia workforce crisis.

Infrastructure Challenges

The provision of surgical and anesthesia care requires infrastructure that is often lacking in many LMICs. As discussed elsewhere in this chapter, such infrastructure does not necessarily need to be high-cost or based on advanced technologies to provide safe care. In addition to the provider shortages already discussed, additional infrastructure challenges that frequently limit surgical and anesthesia service delivery include: underdeveloped patient referral and prehospital systems, medication and equipment shortages, and inadequate supply chains and facility resources.

In maternal health, and more recently for surgery and anesthesia, a "three delays framework" has been used to describe factors delaying timely access to safe healthcare services.[5] The "first delay" in this model (delay in seeking care) may occur due to financial, cultural, education, or other patient factors. Anecdotally, fear of bad surgical outcomes (whether true or not) and more specifically a fear of anesthesia may also contribute to the "first delay." The second and third delays are more directly linked to infrastructure limitations. The "second delay" (delay in reaching care) occurs when health facilities cannot be reached in a timely manner and may be due to geographic distance or challenges with transportation (e.g., bad road conditions, no access to a car, no money for public transport). Although efforts to improve healthcare infrastructure often focus on facility-based interventions, emphasis on infrastructure that minimizes this "second delay" is underappreciated despite evidence of cost-effectiveness.[109] For example, the lack of prehospital care systems in many LMICs is a significant source of avoidable morbidity and mortality. The DCP3 estimates that 4.7 million deaths in LMICs each year are due to surgical conditions that are potentially addressable through prehospital and emergency care systems. In Uganda, less than 25% of the population lives within 2 hours of a surgical facility, and worldwide approximately 2 billion people lack access due to this second delay.

When discussing infrastructure limitations, most people think of the "third delay" (delay in receiving care), which occurs when patients reach a facility but may not receive adequate care because of limitations in facility resources. Data from 800 first-level health facilities in LICs demonstrate that relatively few first-level hospitals could provide C-sections (64%), laparotomies (58%), or open fracture repairs (40%), and most did not have reliable electricity (31%), running water (22%), oxygen (24%), or Internet access. Without reliable utilities, standard equipment like monitors, ventilators, anesthesia machines, and autoclaves are often not functional, assuming they are even present at all. In recent years, the number of surgical and anesthesia capacity assessment tools increased significantly, although most tools have focused on surgical care with limited ability to assess anesthesia or analgesia capacity.[110–117]

The WHO Surgical Safety Checklist includes requirements for pulse oximetry, anesthesia machine check, and confirmation of instrument sterility, yet these may not currently be feasible in many LMIC health facilities. As the consensus on what constitutes "essential" or "standard" anesthesia and surgical safety equipment is evolving, it is universally agreed that far too many health facilities face routine shortages of even the most basic anesthesia equipment.

Inadequate access to indicator strips, maintenance support, power, and distilled water result in low compliance with the 2016 WHO/Pan American Health Organization (PAHO) standards for cleaning, disinfection, and sterilization in most LMICs.[118,119] In a survey of 28 district hospitals in Zambia, 35% did not have a laryngoscope.[120] A study from Nigeria found that most facilities could not provide general anesthesia (53%); another survey in the Democratic Republic of Congo demonstrated 40% of hospitals lack suction, and in Guatemala only 17% of facilities surveyed had capnography.[121,122] In Uganda, a 2014 survey of health facilities that offer emergency services and surgical care revealed only 22% had pediatric airway equipment, 41% adult airway equipment, and 28% a pulse oximeter.[123] In one survey about obstetric operating room capacity in the five main referral hospitals in East Africa (Uganda, Kenya, Tanzania, Rwanda, and Burundi), only 4% of the providers surveyed reported the presence of electrocardiograph (ECG), pulse oximetry, continuous blood pressure monitoring, capnography, thermometer, stethoscope, difficult airway cart, suction machine, recovery room, and intensive care unit (ICU) facilities.[94] Access to reliable oxygen is a common problem in resource-constrained health systems. In such settings, oxygen is rarely available through central pressurized gas lines and more often provided via tanks or oxygen concentrators, the latter of which has been shown to offer long-term cost savings and increased reliability.[124] (Further discussion of oxygen supply challenges in resource-limited settings is provided in the section, Essentials for Practice in Resource-Constrained Settings of this chapter)

Equipment donations are common in LMICs, however, they often have limited long-term impact and multiple unintended consequences. Donations are frequently made with limited understanding of local needs, lack of communication between donor and recipient, and absence of ongoing technical support or access to consumables. Well-intentioned donors are often unaware of WHO Guidelines for Medical Device Donation, or of the fact that purchase costs account for only 20% of total lifetime costs for a piece of equipment.[125] As a result, up to 30% of donated equipment may only transiently or never become operational, and commonly accumulates in equipment graveyards because of a sense of obligation by recipients to not throw anything away. For example, donations of modern anesthesia machines from HICs is commonly encountered in many LMICs. Without reliable power, pressurized gas supplies, biomedical support, or access to disposables (e.g., carbon

TABLE 2.3 Heterogeneity in Global Anesthesia Workforce

	Australia	Canada	China	Colombia	Fiji	India	Lebanon
Population (millions)	24.1	36.3	1,379	45.5	0.9	1,324	6
GNI per capita (USD)	$54,230	$43,880	$8,250	$6,310	$4,780	$1,670	$7,980
Year formed as a specialty	1952	1910	1989	1963	1970	1964	1954
*Specialist physician anesthesiologists	5,535	3,318	71,698	3,600	18	25,000	500
*Nonphysician anesthetists	0	0	0	0	0	0	70
Anesthesia providers per 100,000 people†	23.0	9.1	5.2	7.9	2.0	1.9	9.5
Years of post-secondary education to qualify as specialist physician anesthesiologist	12	13	11	10	13	8	11
Duration of physician specialist training	5	5	3	3	4	4†	4
Members of anesthesia care team							
Physician specialist	Yes	Yes	Yes	Yes	Yes	Yes	Yes
Physician non-specialist	Yes	Yes	No	No	No	No	No
Nurse anesthetist	No	No	No	No	No	No	Yes
Non-nurse, nonphysician anesthetist	No	No**	No	No	No	No	Yes
Key national challenges	Rural staffing and training, salaries at risk from governmental defunding	Rural staffing, large rural population	Inconsistent medical training, workforce shortage limiting obstetric and NORA coverage	Rural staffing and inequity, low salaries, high workload	Workforce shortage, few specialist job posts, limited postgraduate funding, limited access to resources	Workforce shortage, rural staffing, polarized views on task-sharing, poverty	Regional instability, limited resources and workforce, large refugee population (~1/3 population)
Subspecialty training programs							
Critical care	Yes	Yes	No	Yes	Yes	Yes	No
Cardiac anesthesia	No	Yes	Yes	Yes	No	Yes	Yes
Pediatric anesthesia	No	Yes	Yes	No	No	Yes	No
Regional anesthesia	No	Yes	Yes	No	No	Yes	No
Obstetric anesthesia	No	Yes	Yes	No	No	Yes	No

GNI, Gross national income.

*In many countries (e.g., South Africa) large numbers of physician non-specialists provide anesthesia, but accurate counts of these cadres are unavailable.

†Physician specialist anesthesia training in India includes 3 years anesthesia training after 1 year as a "house surgeon."

**In Canada, Anesthesia Assistants are trained to perform many of the anesthesia tasks including intubation, extubation, maintenance of anesthesia (including administering drugs) as directed by the anesthesiologist, but are not designated as the primary anesthesia provider for a given case.

Mexico	Norway	Pakistan	Paraguay	Romania	South Africa	Uganda	USA	Vietnam
127.5	5.3	193.2	6.7	19.7	55.9	41.5	325.7	92.7
$9,040	$81,980	$1,500	$4,060	$9,480	$5,480	$630	$56,850	$2,060
1934	1949	1960	1973	1957	1935	1985	1940	1960
13,000	1,138	3,000	258	1,400	1,500	72	50,000	1,000
10	2,000	0	497	0	0	430	50,000	2,000
10.2	59.2	1.6	11.3	7.1	2.7	1.2	30.7	3.2
10	11	10	10	11	13	9	12	11
3	5	4	3	5	4	3	4	5
Yes	Yes	Yes	Yes	Yes	Yes	Yes	Yes	Yes
No	Yes	No	No	No	Yes	No	No	No
No	Yes	No	No	No	No	Yes	Yes	Yes
No	No	No	Yes	No	No	Yes	Yes	No
Rural staffing, large rural population, political and civil stability	Inadequate time for non-clinical activities during training	Medication and workforce shortages, geographic distribution and inconsistent quality of care	Inconsistent training standards for non-physicians	Workforce shortages, regional staffing shortages, no standardized nurse curriculum	Workforce shortage, large poor and rural population, inequitable access to care	Workforce shortage, rural staffing, high workload, low remuneration, medication and equipment access, polarized views on task-sharing	Rural access to specialists, high cost of care, polarized views on task-sharing, maternal mortality	Inconsistent medication and equipment access, geographic distribution of workforce
Yes	Yes	Yes	No	Yes	Yes	No	Yes	Yes
Yes	Yes	Yes	No	No	No	No	Yes	No
Yes	Yes	No	No	No	No	No	Yes	Yes
Yes	No	No	No	No	No	No	Yes	Yes
Yes	Yes	No	No	No	No	No	Yes	Yes

BOX 2.3 World Health Organization Essential Medicines List—Anesthesia Medications

General Anesthetics and Oxygen

- Halothane, isoflurane, nitrous oxide
- Oxygen
- Ketamine
- Propofol (or thiopental)
- Bupivacaine
- Lidocaine

Muscle Relaxants

- Atracurium
- Neostigmine
- Suxamethonium
- Vecuronium
- Pyridostigmine*

Preoperative Medication and Sedation for Short-Term Procedures

- Atropine
- Midazolam
- Morphine

Medicines for Pain and Palliative Care

- Acetylsalicylic acid
- Ibuprofen
- Paracetamol
- Codeine
- Fentanyl transdermal (for cancer pain)
- Morphine
- Methadone
- Dexamethasone
- Amitriptyline
- Diazepam
- Haloperidol
- Ondansetron

Additional Medications†

- Epinephrine
- Hydrocortisone
- Naloxone
- Lorazepam
- Enoxaparin
- Heparin
- Tranexamic acid
- Digoxin
- Verapamil
- Amiodarone*
- Hydralazine
- Lasix
- Sodium nitroprusside*
- Dopamine*
- Mannitol
- Insulin
- Glucose
- Ergometrine
- Misoprostol
- Oxytocin
- Misoprostol*

Notable deletions

- Ether (2005)
- Ephedrine (1995)*
- Magnesium sulfate (1988)
- Pethidine (2003)

*Ephedrine is listed in the complementary list of medications in the 2017 20th Edition EML. The complementary list presents essential medicines for priority diseases, for which specialized diagnostic or monitoring facilities, and/or specialist medical care, and/or specialist training are needed.

†Blood products, antiseptics, and antibiotics are included in the EML and not listed here.

Data from http://www.who.int/selection_medicines/committees/DELETIONS.pdf?ua=1.https://www.who.int/medicines/publications/essentialmedicines/20th_EML2017.pdf?ua=1/.

dioxide absorbent, humidity filters, circuit tubing), it is sometimes hard to argue in favor of these machines.

Reliable access to medications and blood are two additional common infrastructure challenges limiting access to safe surgery and anesthesia services worldwide. The WHO Essential Medicines List includes medications to safely perform general anesthesia, monitored anesthesia care (MAC), neuraxial, regional, local anesthesia, as well as acute and chronic pain management (Box 2.3).[126] Despite the existence of the list for more than 40 years, critical shortages of many medications persist. A WHO survey of all health facilities in Uganda examined availability of twelve anesthetic drugs (atracurium, bupivacaine, halothane, isoflurane, desflurane, sevoflurane, ketamine, lidocaine 2%, lidocaine 5% heavy spinal injection, midazolam, nitrous oxide, and suxamethonium) and found that only 2% of the surgical health facilities had all of these medications and only 19% had half.[123] The same WHO survey in the Democratic Republic of Congo found that only 33% of hospitals had bupivacaine, 21% thiopental, and 16% halothane. Factors specifically affecting access to analgesics are discussed further in the next section, though supply chain, cold storage, and cost are common challenges that limit availability for many drugs. Drug quality is also a factor in some LMICs where variable manufacturing quality and fraud (i.e., counterfeiting) are commonly encountered.[127] It is estimated that 1 in 10 medical products (e.g., medications) found in LMICs are substandard or falsified and result in hundreds of thousands of deaths each year.[128,129]

The WHO Essential Medicines List also includes blood products. Despite more than four decades of global advocacy (1975 WHA28.72) for universal access to safe blood, limited transfusion capacity significantly impacts the ability to provide safe surgery and anesthesia care, especially for rural and LMIC populations. Most rural surgical facilities are unable to provide consistent access to safe blood. Patients lack timely access to safe blood as a result of several common challenges including inadequate blood supply, distribution networks, rural blood banking capacity, safety protocols, workforce (e.g., pathologists, laboratory technicians), testing supplies, and policy implementation, as well as high costs of blood and high prevalence of infectious diseases.[75,130,131] The whole blood donation rate is used as an indicator of blood availability. The LCOGS recommends a minimum of 15 blood donations per 1000 people per year, yet this rate is 4.6 per 1000 people per year in LICs (compared with 32.1 per 1000 people per year in HICs).[5,132] Most LMICs cannot maintain adequate supply from voluntary non-remunerated donors (VNRDs) alone (as advocated by WHO), and the use of paid donors or family donors poses numerous logistic and safety concerns.[75] According to WHO data, 71 countries collect the majority of their blood supply from family or paid donors, 50% lack capacity to separate blood components, and 23.5% of countries have less than 100% screening for at least one of these transfusion-transmissible infections: HIV, hepatitis B, hepatitis C , or syphilis.[132] For many LMICs, investment in transfusion infrastructure, expansion of transfusion research, and advocacy (including rethinking of well-intentioned but context-limited policies such as VNRD-only mandates, requirements for onsite pathologists, and mandatory replacement units) are critical areas for engagement by anesthesia providers in the greater global health community.[75,133]

There is an evolving consensus on global standards for anesthesia equipment, medications, and other infrastructure.[3,117] As a result, most assessments of facility or national capacity capture different data that may over- or underestimate current infrastructure limitations. For example, lack of access to rocuronium, sevoflurane, or propofol does not necessarily indicate inability to safely perform anesthesia if suxamethonium, halothane, isoflurane, or thiopental are available. Currently efforts are underway by the WFSA, GICS, and other organizations to develop anesthesia-specific research tools to assist LMICs in monitoring and evaluation of anesthesia capacity.[116,117] The global anesthesia and surgical communities are likely to benefit from continued collaboration and harmonization of efforts that assess global anesthesia infrastructure.

Inequities in Analgesia

Five billion people worldwide have little or no access to analgesia. As with the surgical disease crisis, inequities in analgesia access are in part a result of the limited availability of data that quantify the problem. Unlike most traditional global health metrics that focus on extending healthy life and productivity, alleviating pain may not always target these same goals (e.g., acute surgical pain relief and palliative care), thus adding to the complexity of quantifying pain burden. Massive inequities in access to analgesia are also attributed to several additional factors including advocacy challenges (pain is not disease specific or easy to associate with a "face"), limited training opportunities for healthcare professions, fear of addiction and diversion, financing, supply chain limitations, cultural attitudes, and regulatory and legal barriers (Box 2.4).[52,53] In the ensuing discussion, we consider some of these barriers and potential areas for intervention by the global anesthesia community.

Limited financial resources and infrastructure hinder the ability of healthcare systems to deliver analgesia (i.e., effective supply chains) and limit the ability of patients to afford such care. Countries with a lower GDP or human development index have less access and use of opiates.[53] Opiate prices in LMICs are often significantly higher relative to GDP. In the recent past in Argentina and Mexico, the monthly cost of an opioid prescription for oncologic pain was reported to be more than 200% the average monthly income.[74,134] In Rwanda, the reported price of injectable morphine is 6 times the lowest cost reported in the International Drug Price Indicator Guide.[30,135] Drivers of these inflated prices include import costs, taxes, licensing fees, storage and sales restrictions, and limited public finance programs. International regulations and misconceptions about pain treatment and addiction form the basis for many of these interventions.

BOX 2.4 Factors Affecting Access to and Availability of Analgesia

Knowledge and Attitudes

- Providers—limited training
- Patients—limited health literacy
- Opiophobia—fear of addiction, diversion, or side effects
- Cultural attitudes and beliefs about pain
- Limited data to estimate pain burden or accurate national analgesia needs
- Challenging advocacy (pain is not disease specific or easy to associate with a "face")

Regulations and Policy

- Prohibitionist bias
- Implementation requires significant resources
- Onerous regulations (e.g., limits on who can prescribe, duration, dose and indication)
- Complex regulations create fear of prosecution among providers
- Limited global advocacy efforts to expand analgesia access

Economics and Financing

- Poverty
- Relatively high analgesic costs in LMICs
- Costs of implementing/enforcing international regulations
- Few mechanisms for financial protection from analgesic costs (e.g., subsidies or UHC)

Health Systems

- Supply chains (timely import, procurement, storage, and distribution)
- Limited analgesic options
- Few providers trained/skilled to provide adequate analgesia
- Inadequate number/distribution of facilities providing analgesia care
- Limited national government capacity

LMIC, Low- and middle-income countries; *UHC*, universal health coverage.
Modified from: Berterame S, Erthal J, Thomas J, et al. Use of and barriers to access to opioid analgesics: a worldwide, regional, and national study. *Lancet*. 2016;387(10028):1644–1656.
Goucke CR, Chaudakshetrin P. Pain: a neglected problem in the low-resource setting. *Anesth Analg*. 2018;126(4):1283–1286.
INCB 2017 report https://www.incb.org/documents/Publications/AnnualReports/AR2017/Annual_Report/E_2017_AR_ebook.pdf.

Misinformation about analgesia has biased knowledge and attitudes among providers, patients, and policymakers, and has resulted in significant undertreatment of pain. Several studies have demonstrated that the risk of addiction associated with appropriate analgesic administration is significantly exaggerated and especially low for acute, oncologic, or end-of-life pain.[136] Nonetheless, widespread and excessive fears over diversion and addiction have resulted in unnecessarily onerous regulatory barriers that often confuse tolerance and dependence, users and addicts, and disproportionately affect poor and marginalized populations.[137] In China, for example, a domestic ketamine abuse problem has led to repeat lobbying of the International Narcotics Control Board (INCB) by the Chinese government to reschedule ketamine as a schedule I drug for all countries. Such regulation would effectively remove the nearly ubiquitous access to ketamine in LMICs, and further exacerbate the ongoing global pain crisis.[138] Ketamine is inexpensive, accessible, and safe, and as a result has become a critical resource for the provision of safe and accessible anesthesia and analgesia services worldwide. Fortunately, attempts to restrict ketamine have been promptly recognized as heartless and a violation of international regulatory policies.

Tramadol is another analgesic with frequently misunderstood pharmacology that is commonly found in LMICs. Tramadol is not controlled by international regulations, which has led to its widespread availability for analgesia but also to its abuse.[139] Abuse is widely reported in many HICs (e.g., Canada) and LMICs (e.g., many countries in Africa and the Middle East) and is so severe that in countries like Cameroon, it can literally be found in the groundwater as a result of human excretion.[140] Tramadol is not considered an adequate substitute for opiates and is not included in the WHO Essential Medicines List.

Contemporary legal and regulatory/policy frameworks have significantly exacerbated disparities in access to analgesia care. In the wake of several key events in the 1800s that fueled skyrocketing opioid abuse, including the Opium Wars and invention of the hypodermic syringe, the beginning of the 20th century produced several of the first national and international efforts to restrict and regulate narcotics. This included the first international conference on narcotics in 1909 (International Opium Convention in Shanghai) and the first multilateral drug treaty in 1912 (The Hague Opium Convention). One of the most notable regulations of the 20th century is the 1961 UN Single Convention on Narcotic Drugs. The opening sentence of the "Single Convention" recognizes, "…that the medical use of narcotic drugs continues to be indispensable for the relief of pain and suffering and that adequate provision must be made to ensure the availability of narcotic drugs for such purposes…" The Single Convention set out to control the use and trade of plant-based drugs (opium, cannabis, and cocaine) while also assuring availability for medical purposes.[141] This regulation mandated government participation (reporting national estimates of narcotic needs, meticulous record keeping), regulated drug cultivation, restricted trade to authorized international parties, and created the INCB. The INCB was tasked with monitoring UN drug convention implementation and required each country to designate an enforcement office (e.g., the Drug Enforcement Administration [DEA] in the United States). While most countries adopted this onerous regulation, most poor countries did not have the extensive resources needed to enact all of these changes. The Single Convention's "global estimates" system has been particularly difficult for many countries to implement. This system requires all countries to provide an estimate of opiate need (for medical purposes) in order to inform global production goals and limit excess opiate supplies that are at risk for illicit use. Accurate estimates require significant resources, and for many LMICs, inability to provide accurate estimates translates directly to inadequate supply. For example, 2017 opiate estimates for Chad (population 14.5 million) predicted 341 g fentanyl, 249 g morphine, and 105 g codeine. When compared to estimates from Canada (population 36.3 million: 150,000 g fentanyl, 4,750,000 g morphine, 40,020,000 g codeine, and 70 other controlled substances) the disparity and gross underestimation is apparent.[142] By approving such gross underestimates, the INCB effectively is legally prohibiting patients from having access to opiates. In times of humanitarian crisis, the Single Convention impedes the ability to emergently augment local analgesia capacity as became evident in the wake of the 2010 Haiti earthquake.[143]

Global regulations to curb illicit use have dominated efforts to ensure access to analgesics for medical purposes (or to ensure access to substance abuse treatment). In 1985, the Parliament of India passed the Narcotic Drugs and Psychotropic Substances Act to enforce international drug policy (e.g., the Single Convention). The Act's onerous regulations and extreme penalties (including the death penalty for certain drug-related crimes) resulted in more than a 90% decrease in the medicinal use of morphine.[144,145] This imbalance, referred to by some as "collateral damage from the war on drugs," disproportionately affects LMICs and continues to cripple access to analgesics for the majority of the world's population.[143] Such bias has also impaired scaleup of addiction treatment initiatives. For example, addiction treatment (methadone and buprenorphine) was not added to the WHO Essential Medicines List until 2006, approximately 100 years after the passage of the earliest narcotic regulations and 40 years after the list's creation.

The prohibitory biases of prior international drug policy has resulted in numerous national regulatory barriers that include limitations on who can prescribe, dispense, or administer opiates, as well as limitations on indications (e.g., postoperative but not cancer pain), dosages, or duration of therapy.[137] For example, in Armenia only oncologists with the approval of multiple providers can prescribe outpatient opiates, whereas in the Ukraine, healthcare providers must travel to the patients' homes to administer outpatient opiates. In Jordan, the maximum duration of an opiate prescription for oncologic pain is 10 days, and only three days for all other conditions.[146] These myriad regulations create an additional barrier by inducing fear of prosecution for noncompliance among health professionals, thereby reducing provider willingness to prescribe. Lack of adequate training opportunities for healthcare providers, especially in LMICs, coupled with the rare use of analgesics in clinical practice, create a cycle whereby fewer and fewer providers feel comfortable prescribing opiates.

Several amendments to the Single Convention have been enacted including the 1971 Convention of Psychotropic Substances, the 1988 UN Convention Against Illicit Traffic in Narcotic Drugs and Psychotropic Substances, the inclusion of morphine in the first WHO Essential Medicines List in 1977, and introduction of the WHO Pain Ladder in 1986. Despite these efforts most of the world's population remains without reliable access to analgesia. Nearly 60 years after the Single Convention, the number of drug abusers in many countries is near all-time highs while 150 countries still lack reliable access to analgesia. Even the UN's SDGs, which aim to set development priorities for the world, reflect the prohibitory bias of prior international policies. SDG 3.5 calls for improved prevention and treatment for substance abuse, including narcotics, but fails to mention pain or palliative care anywhere else in the SDGs.[29]

Advocacy and education efforts by the global stakeholders, including the anesthesia community, as well as rethinking of international analgesic policy (including the Single Convention) are essential for progress in addressing the global pain crisis.[125,147] Education for healthcare providers, policymakers, and the public can play a significant role in expanding access to analgesia. Such efforts should focus on pharmacologic treatment strategies, but should also emphasize better understanding and management of causes and contributors to pain, including social and economic determinants. Efforts by numerous Ministry of Health agencies have had small successes. In Vietnam and India, grassroots- and civil-society-led

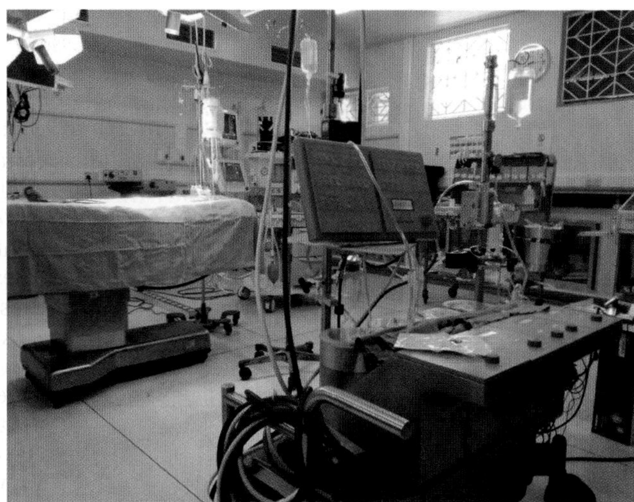
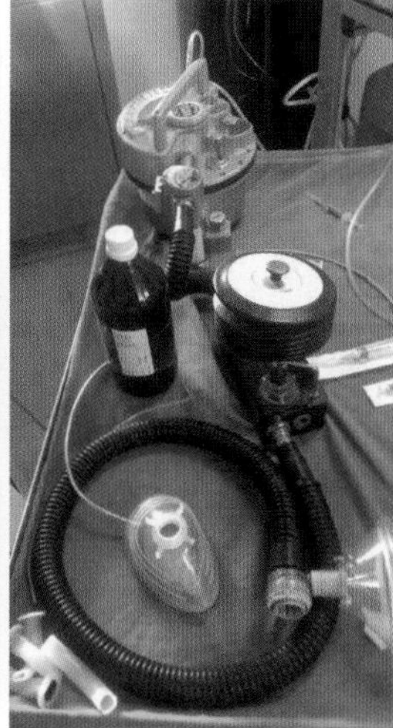

Fig. 2.14 Two operating theatre setups in Uganda, 2018. *Left,* The Ugandan Heart Institute. *Right,* Epstein, Macintosh, Oxford *(EMO)* ether vaporizer at a first-level hospital providing surgical services. (Copyright © 2018 Cornelius Sendagire, reproduced with permission.)

policy initiatives to allay opiophobia and reduce institutional licensing regulations have significantly increased access to analgesia without an increased diversion.[148–151] In Uganda, advocacy efforts by the nongovernmental organization Hospice Africa Uganda helped convince the Uganda Ministry of Health in 1993 to import morphine powder and to provide domestically made morphine liquid free to all cancer or HIV/AIDS patients. In 2004, the Uganda Ministry of Health legalized opioid prescribing by nurses and clinical officers with palliative care training, which significantly expanded access to analgesia especially in rural communities. The import and domestic packaging of oral morphine for palliative care has translated into greater access to oral morphine for the anesthesia and surgical communities. A similar model is currently being adopted in Rwanda, Nigeria, Kenya, Swaziland, and Malawi.[152]

Section 2: Evolution of Anesthesia Care Models and Challenges Around the World

In the mid-19th century the use of inhaled anesthetics (e.g., most notably ether) began in HICs and spread relatively quickly even to many relatively less resourced countries as a consequence of colonial systems. Today, more than 170 years later, ether is still used in some LICs (Fig. 2.14). The practice of anesthesia has changed significantly, though these changes—including large improvements in patient safety—disproportionately occurred in HICs. The practice of anesthesia varies widely between, and even within, countries. Of the numerous challenges and factors that have shaped this heterogeneity, many are shared by multiple countries regardless of income level. These include common challenges such as inadequate workforce (number, composition, or distribution); high cost of care; limited access for rural and poor populations; and lack of standards for practice and training.

This section explores anesthesiology in six geographic regions of the world, providing examples from countries of diverse economic, political, and population backgrounds. Regional variation in anesthesia care models including key milestones in the development of these systems as well as current challenges they face for providing access to safe, affordable anesthesia care are highlighted. This section is not intended to be comprehensive but to provide examples that are representative of the diversity in anesthesiology despite shared common objectives and many similar challenges.

AFRICA

Africa is the second largest continent, with 1.2 billion people, and the youngest population of all the continents (median age ~19 years vs. 38 years in the United States). Africa is also the poorest continent. Recent estimates by the World Bank demonstrate that 11% of the world's population lives on less than US$1.90 per day, and most of the world's extreme poor (over 400 million people) live in Africa (Fig. 2.15).[153]

Economically, Africa is growing fast with an annual change in GDP for most countries of approximately 3% to 6% (Uganda—an LIC 6.3%, South Africa—an upper middle-income country 1.2%).[154] Total health expenditure (THE) has grown more rapidly than GDP with average increases in THE/GDP from 4.8% in 1995 to 5.9% in 2014 for the continent. Out-of-pocket payments as a proportion of THE have also been decreasing (South Africa decreased from around 17% in 1995 to approximately 5% in 2014, and in Uganda from around 45% to around 40%).[155]

African countries have widely disparate health systems. According to a recently published study on outcomes after surgery in Africa, countries participating in the study reported poor outcomes relative to higher-income regions (despite healthier patients) and attributed worse outcomes to limited resources and lack of access to surgical care.[65] The public healthcare sectors of Uganda and South Africa are, in many ways, representative of the current state of anesthesia and surgical care in Africa.

Uganda (Mary T. Nabukenya and Sarah Hodges)

Uganda (population ~40 million) is one the youngest and most rapidly growing nations in the world (fertility rate

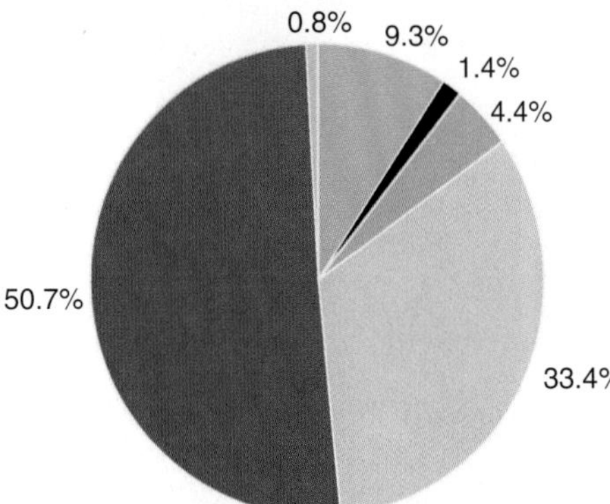

Fig. 2.15 Where are the global poor living? The global poor, by region, 2013. (Source: Most recent estimates, based on 2013 data using PovcalNet [online analysis tool], World Bank, Washington, DC, http://iresearch.worldbank.org/PovcalNet/. [Figure originally appeared in The World Bank Group. Taking on Inequality, Poverty and Shared Prosperity 2016. Copyright © 2016 The World Bank. This image is reproduced under the CC BY 4.0 license.])

~6). Uganda has a gross national income per capita of $630 (see Table 2.1) and despite recent increases in THE/GDP (7.2% vs. 17.10% in the United States), many healthcare challenges exist (life expectancy 56 years), especially with regard to anesthesia and surgery.[76,156]

The first recorded anesthetic in Uganda was a cesarean delivery in 1879 with the use of banana wine as the anesthetic.[157] The first modern anesthetic (chloroform) was given by Sir Albert Cook in 1897.[158]

Anesthesia was initially most commonly given by surgeons. Theater attendants and medical assistants were also trained on the job to administer anesthesia. In the 1970s and early 1980s, a 2-year anesthesia diploma program (anesthetic assistants) was created. In 1985, during a meeting of the Commonwealth Health Ministers of the East, Central, and Southern Africa region, it was established that a medical background was vital for anesthesia provider training. This resulted in abolishment of the "anesthetic assistant" programs and creation of a 2-year diploma (anesthetic officers) in 1986 that required a diploma in clinical medicine, nursing, or midwifery as a prerequisite.

Until the 1980s, training of Ugandan physician anesthesiologists was primarily foreign-based, and due to political turmoil, few returned to Uganda to practice. One anesthesiologist returned in the mid-1970s and started the Department of Anesthesia at Mulago Hospital (Kampala, Uganda). Together, with an Australian anesthesiologist, they established a 1-year Diploma in Anesthesia in 1985, and the following year the Anesthesia Master of Medicine (MMED), a 3-year residency program at the Makerere University Medical School. In 1990, with a total of 4 physician anesthesiologists and roughly 100 nonphysician anesthetists in the country, the Uganda Society of Anesthetists was founded.

Today there are two physician MMED and three nonphysician diploma programs in Uganda. A new nonphysician, 4-year Bachelor's in Anesthesia program was also started in 2017. Each institution awards a qualification to its graduates, as currently there is no accrediting body for anesthesia in Uganda. Regionally, the College of Anesthesiologists for East, Central, and Southern Africa (CANECSA) was founded in 2014 but has not started accreditations.

From 2000–18, the number of physician anesthesiologists in Uganda has increased from less than 10 to over 80, with the majority working near the capital (Kampala). Nonphysician anesthetists outnumber the physician anesthesiologists by almost 6 times and are distributed widely throughout the country where they usually practice without supervision or team support. Despite increasing numbers in recent years, vast shortages in the anesthesia workforce limit access to care throughout the country. Over the past decade, about 10% of physician anesthesiologists have moved to other countries in Africa. This brain drain has been reported in many other countries, including Francophone Africa under the Cotonou program, where brain drain was reported at nearly 18%.[108] In addition to this external brain drain (i.e., emigrating to another country), internal brain drain (e.g., leaving the public sector for private practice, staying in urban centers, or leaving the field of anesthesiology) is also a significant challenge throughout the region. These moves are motivated by economic incentives and political changes.

In 2007, the Ugandan health ministry established health sub-districts in each county (about 150 countrywide), each with an operating theater for provision of emergency obstetric and surgical care. Unfortunately, they were ill-equipped, and many are nonfunctional. None of the 33 district hospitals have a physician anesthesiologist (despite position vacancies), and only 4 of 13 regional referral hospitals have an anesthesiologist on staff. There are currently 25 anesthesiologists in the national referral hospital together with the teaching faculty in the two MMED programs. All other physician anesthesiologists in Uganda are working in private hospitals and universities.

Safety standards in Uganda are based mainly on WFSA guidelines, however, these are not strictly enforced.[3] Compliance rates with the WHO Surgical Safety Checklist are low as is capacity to comply with the checklist requirements. A survey of utilization of the checklist in major East African hospitals showed variable compliance (19% to 65%).[94]

Administration of ether anesthesia with the Epstein, Macintosh, Oxford (EMO) vaporizer is still used in remote locations of Uganda, although its use has declined significantly in recent years. Throughout the country there are a wide range of configurations ranging from EMO drawover setups to modern anesthesia machines for cardiac bypass surgery (see Fig. 2.14). Limitations in reliable power, disposables, and oxygen are among the many infrastructure challenges that affect daily anesthesia care in almost all locations. Even with monitoring, there are significant differences in what is available ranging from a basic stethoscope and blood pressure cuff to monitors allowing for invasive monitoring. In recent years, the scope of practice has expanded as more providers are completing subspecialty training abroad (e.g., pediatrics, cardiac, obstetrics, critical care, and regional) and returning to practice and teach locally.

Besides the nearly universal problem of remuneration, the greatest challenge for anesthesia in Uganda is the massive imbalance between the workforce and the workload. This imbalance coupled with ill-equipped workplaces makes the provision of safe care difficult, and provider burnout is commonplace.

South Africa (Hyla Kluyts)

South Africa is home to approximately 56.5 million people of diverse ethnicity and culture.[159] Since the first democratic election in 1994 and the adoption of the South African Constitution in 1996, the country has been struggling to address its inequalities. In health care, there have been successes such as the decreasing incidence of HIV infections and increasing life expectancy (from 55.2 years in 2002 to 62.4 years in 2016). South Africa has a gross national income per capita of $5,480 (upper middle-income country), yet approximately 19% of the population live below the World Bank poverty line (US$1.90 per day) and only 17% of the population have private medical insurance.[76] The proportion of the population living below the extreme poverty line is much higher than that of many other middle-income countries. A recent collaborative report by the World Bank denotes South Africa as "one of the most unequal countries in the world."[160] The South African Department of Health is working toward universal health coverage and a draft National Health Insurance Bill was published in June 2018.[160a]

Ether was first used for dental extractions in Cape Town in April 1847, and the first major operation under anesthesia was performed in June of the same year. The first specialist anesthetist, British-born and -trained Dr. Bampfylde Daniel, was appointed at Johannesburg Hospital in 1907. The South African Society of Anaesthesiologists (SASA) was founded in 1943 and was a founding member of the WFSA in 1955. SASA published its first Practice Guidelines in 1987, with five subsequent revisions, including 2012 and 2018 revisions that adhere to the WHO-WFSA International Standards on the Practice of Safe Anaesthesia.[161]

Physicians are trained and accredited to provide anesthesia care as general practitioners or specialists. General practitioners are registered as independent practitioners after completing 6 years of undergraduate study and 3 years of supervised training as interns and subsequent community-service medical officers. A general practitioner can obtain a Diploma in Anaesthesia after 6 months of full-time supervised practice in an accredited institution. Specialists can register as such after completing a 4-year postgraduate training period, completing of a research project, and successfully passing the South African College of Anaesthetists' final Fellowship examination.

The Health Professionals Council of South Africa (HPCSA) certifies medical professionals and is the accreditation body for anesthesia training. Eight university departments across the country are responsible for the academic input and implementation of training pathways, whereas the Provincial Departments of Health dictate the number of posts within these training pathways. The curricula are determined by the Colleges of Medicine of South Africa, which also is responsible for assessments and examinations.

Anesthesia providers in South Africa consist of independent practitioners (general practitioners or specialists in both private and public sectors) supplemented by interns, community service medical officers, specialist trainees, and foreign physicians who do not qualify for registration as independent practitioners and must work under supervision in the public sector. Anesthetists in private practice in South Africa are not hospital based and travel between hospitals according to demand from surgical colleagues. The SASA therefore plays a significant role in the private sector as a representative body for clinician interaction with other stakeholders. In contrast, all public sector anesthetists are employed by the provincial Departments of Health at specific hospitals.

The already limited specialist anesthesia workforce is also unequally distributed between the private and the public sector, and between rural and urban areas in South Africa. For example, approximately 1800 specialist anesthesiologists were registered with the HPCSA in 2017, of which around 1100 specialists are SASA members, and of these, 790 work in the private sector. Roughly 9 million patients are insured and cared for in the private sector.[161] Unsatisfactory working conditions and remuneration are the most commonly quoted reasons for anaesthetists leaving the public sector for the private sector after registering as specialists.

There is limited information available regarding the number, distribution and training of non-specialist anesthesia providers in South Africa. The number of non-specialists choosing full-time anesthesia practice as a career is relatively low and likely does not significantly address the lack of anesthesia services available to the population in either sectors of the healthcare system. At best, the estimated total number of anesthesia providers per 100,000 of the population is half of the minimum required for safe care. No non-physicians provide anesthesia in South Africa. Attempts have been made to train more doctors and to recruit doctors to areas of need (e.g., implementation of rural allowance payments). Anesthetists also form part of the District Clinical Specialist Teams alongside the family physicians, primary healthcare nurses, and specialist obstetricians. These teams were created to improve maternal and neonatal mortality and morbidity at a district level, though anesthesia posts within these teams remain largely unfilled and are not considered mandatory for "minimal team" standards.

Access is a major barrier because of the country's geography and distribution of available resources. About one third of the poorest population in South Africa have to travel at least 20 km to the nearest hospital.[160] Often these level 1 facilities provide obstetric surgery services but not surgical services for the bellwether procedures largely because of the failure to recognize basic surgical care as a public health issue.

Information on anesthesia-related outcomes is not available on a national level, but some useful data are obtained through reports from the National Committee for the Confidential Enquiry into Maternal Deaths.[71] Surgical outcomes for South Africa and Africa have been reported following recent multicenter studies.[65] Regulation of healthcare expenditure, improving access to essential surgical care in rural parts of the country, and increasing data perioperative care and on resource distribution will be critical to improving anesthesia and surgical care in South Africa.

NORTH AMERICA

North American countries have widely different economic, political, and healthcare systems. This section describes examples from two HICs (Canada and the United States) and one middle-income country (Mexico). These two HICs have extremely different models of health care as well as anesthesia services. Canada has a predominantly physician-based system and universal health coverage, while the United States is split nearly equally between physician and nonphysician providers. Mexico is physician-based, but with a novel and controversial rural physician anesthesia program. Haiti is the only LIC in North America and suffers from shortages of healthcare providers that are orders of magnitude worse than other countries in the region. There are fewer than 100 anesthesiologists for the country's population of 10.85 million, and most only work in the capital city. In 1998 Médecins Sans Frontières began a nurse anesthetist training program in collaboration with the Ministry of Public Health and Population (independent from The Haitian Medical Association and the Haitian Society of Anesthesiologists), though numbers of nurse anesthetists remain critically low.[100,162]

Canada (Tyler Law)

The first reported anesthetic in Canada was administered in 1847, just after Morton's demonstration in Boston, as a result of the ship carrying the news from Boston to London, via Halifax.[163] The first formal anesthetic training program began in 1910 in Toronto, and anesthesia as a profession became formalized with the creation of the Canadian Anesthesiologists Association in 1943.[164]

PAPs undertake a 5-year specialist anesthesia residency directly from medical school, or through the International Medical Graduate program designed to train practicing physicians from other countries to national standards. This training focuses on the progressive, successful demonstration of task competency (termed entrustable professional activities [EPAs]), rather than time-based rotation training. The EPAs are consistent across residency programs, and residents receive frequent feedback on their performance. Residents must demonstrate competency in EPAs before advancing to the next phase of training.[165,166]

The Royal College of Physicians and Surgeons of Canada sets accreditation standards and required competencies for anesthesiologists in conjunction with the training programs. In conjunction with EPAs, the Royal College certifies a national examination with written and oral components that tests knowledge, application of knowledge, and clinical judgment. Standardized simulation scenarios are being gradually introduced as a component of specialty certification.

The count of physician anesthesiologists in Canada has increased significantly from 2500 in 2005 to 3300 in 2018, resulting in a provider density of 9 anesthesiologists per 100,000 population. In Canada, anesthetics are largely given by specialist physicians, with several additional healthcare provider cadres also administering anesthesia care. Graduates of the two-year Family Medicine residency may opt to take a 1-year "added skill" training program in anesthesia. They practice anesthesia independently for less acute patients and procedures, often in a community or low-volume setting.

A small number of dentists administer both general anesthesia and sedation for dental procedures, typically in ambulatory settings in the clinic or hospital. A 3-year training program undertaken after the completion of dental school enables them to care for ASA physical classification 1, 2, and stable 3 patients.[167] The anesthesia care team also includes anesthesia assistants, who undertake a prescribed educational program (most often 1 year in duration) and provide technical assistance with equipment and perform clinical tasks (such as intubation or intraoperative medical management) under the supervision of an anesthesiologist.

Guidelines for anesthesia practice have been established by the Canadian Anesthesiologists Association and are regularly updated for the core elements of anesthesia practice in Canada, and guidelines from the ASA and other international societies are commonly referenced. Notable elements of recent guidelines include encouraging the use of a structured handover protocol, and requiring capnography monitoring for moderate or deeper sedation.[168]

Most anesthesiologists practice in academic health centers and community hospitals.[169] The costs of most surgical, anesthetic, and postoperative inpatient care services are covered under provincially administered public health insurance schemes. Only 0.7% of private health spending is directed toward physicians, so the market for private anesthetic services is small and usually restricted to services not covered under public plans, such as dental and cosmetic procedures.[170]

Despite universal health coverage and a relatively large number of anesthesia providers, Canada still faces several challenges relevant to anesthesia and surgical care. Canada is the second largest country (by land mass) in the world, and while much of the population is geographically clustered, rural areas suffer from the lack of consistent access to health care, particularly lack of access to specialists including anesthesiologists. Many northern communities have sizable First Nations (indigenous) populations, who are disproportionately underserved. Similar to the United States, tension among anesthesia provider roles is an ongoing issue.

Mexico (Gerardo Prieto)

The Aztec and Maya were among the earliest anesthetists in Mexico and known for using herbal beverages to produce analgesia, with adjuncts such as rattlesnake fangs, leeches, porcupine needles, and the maguey needles to produce local numbness.[171] The Maya witch doctors were divided into specialty groups according to the diseases that they either cured or produced. The first mention is a witch doctor who produced *"sleepiness"* called Ah Pul Uenel, who used plants that produce hallucinations and nervous system stimulants. Also mentioned is Pul-Yahob who treated wounds and pain with different rituals, plants, and animals.

As in many countries, surgeons provided the first contemporary anesthetics in Mexico. The first ether anesthesia in Mexico was performed in 1847 by the military surgeons E. H. Barton and Pedro Vander Linden for a cannon ball wound amputation, during the U.S. Intervention War in Veracruz.[172] In 1852, Dr. Pablo Martinez Del Rio used ether in an obstetric patient during a session of the Medical Society. Dr. Ramos Alfaro is attributed as the founder of Mexican anesthesia with his introduction of chloroform anesthesia in 1852.[173] In 1900, Dr. Juan Ramon Pardo Galindo performed the first spinal anesthetic in Mexico and Latin America. In 1934, the first formal diploma in anesthesiology (DA) was awarded, and The Mexican Society of Anesthesiology (Sociedad Mexicana de Anestesistas) was formed. In 1957 the first contemporary anesthesia residency programs were formed, and in 1973 the Mexican Council of Anesthesia was registered and was active until 2013 when it became the National Council of Certification in Anesthesia (CNCA).

In Mexico, anesthesia training programs are 3 to 4 years in duration after medical school and authorized by a university and a recognized institute of medicine. Once this program is completed, trainees must pass the National Council of Certification in Anesthesia to receive a 5-year license. Mexico has subspecialty training in cardiac, pediatric, neuro, obstetrics and gynecology, and trauma anesthesia.

Mexico City is one of the most populated cities in the world, absorbing an estimated 70% of all Mexican anesthesiologists in a 300-mile radius. Many factors make medical access extremely difficult for large parts of the population, such as the broad geographic distribution of the Mexican population, rural indigenous tribes speaking different dialects, low per-capita income (gross national income per capita US$16,176), and the concentration of healthcare resources in urban areas.

In the wake of Mexico's economic crisis in 1994, the country was forced to evaluate how to improve access for the most impoverished and marginalized parts of the population. The program that emerged was called PROGRESA (Programa de Educación, Salud, y Alimenación) and was designed to alleviate poverty by developing human capital. Part of this program aimed to fill the shortage of specialists working in rural environments. The government and Mexican Social Security Institute established the idea of training "rural specialists" in surgery, obstetrics, pediatrics, and anesthesiology. Medical school graduates who did not pass the national examinations for admission to residency programs were enrolled and trained to work in rural areas for as little as 6 months to 2 years (often with limited educational resources). In many instances these providers migrated to the larger cities or towns. Approximately 500 graduates have been trained by this program, and in 2016 the government ordered the National Council of Certification in Anesthesia to allow rural anesthesia graduates to take the national examination. If these providers pass, they are given a certificate for rural practice only. If they do not pass the written examination in three attempts, they are given the opportunity to complete a practical examination. The efficacy of this training and impact of the program overall remain controversial.

In Mexico there are approximately 13,000 certified anesthesia practitioners for 128 million people (7 per 100,000 population), with 70% located in central Mexico. Approximately 85% of surgical procedures are performed in Government Social Hospitals and 15% in private practice. The Mexican Social Security Institute estimated that 2.5 million procedures were performed in 2015, and when including all the government hospitals and private practices, it is estimated that well over 5 million anesthetic procedures are performed each year.[8]

Mexico faces significant challenges providing access to anesthesia services outside of a few urban settings. In 2012, it was estimated that 21.5% of the population (~25 million people) lacked access to health services. The country has relatively sufficient anesthesia training capacity and increasing numbers of specialist anesthesiologists, yet provider maldistribution is currently the dominant factor limiting access. Additional challenges facing the anesthesia community in Mexico include provider burnout, addiction, and limited data on anesthesia safety.

A number of anesthesia patient safety initiatives are ongoing in Mexico, including legal mandates (the "Norma Oficial Mexicana de Anestesiologia 006") that specify practice requirements for anesthesiologists and hospitals. Success of these efforts will be contingent on addressing each of the challenges discussed previously.

United States (Ronald D. Miller and Adrian W. Gelb)

Anesthesia slowly gained acceptance as a medical specialty in the United States after the initial ether demonstrations by Morton in 1846. It was taught irregularly and informally throughout the early 1900s as a task performed by medical students, interns, or nurses. A large proportion of anesthesia in the United States was provided by nurses, even though the designation of Certified Registered Nurse Anesthetist (CRNA) was not formalized until 1956.

The first anesthesia society in the United States was the Long Island Society of Anesthetists, established in 1905, and the first department of anesthesia and residency program was established by Ralph Waters at the University of Wisconsin in 1927. This program produced several key leaders in anesthesiology directly (e.g., Cullen, Apgar, and Rovenstein) and indirectly (Stoelting, Miller) (Fig. 2.16). The American Board of Anesthesia (ABA) was formed in 1938 to serve as the certification body for anesthesiologists. Anesthesia was recognized as a specialty by the American Medical Association (AMA) in 1940, and the ASA was established in its current form in 1945.[163]

Physician anesthesiologists in the United States must obtain a medical degree (Doctor of Medicine or Doctor of Osteopathic Medicine) followed by specialty (residency) training in anesthesia. An undergraduate bachelor's degree (3-4 years) is required before entering medical school.[174] Residency in anesthesia lasts 4 years: 1 year of general medical internship and 3 years of anesthesia and perioperative medicine training. Residents rotate through the operating room (including subspecialty cases), pain medicine, and at least 4 months of intensive care. Residency training requirements are prescribed by the Accreditation Council for Graduate Medical Education (ACGME). Graduates of an ACGME-approved program are eligible for ABA certification after passing two written examinations (BASIC and ADVANCED), a standardized oral examination, and an objective structured clinical examination. Board

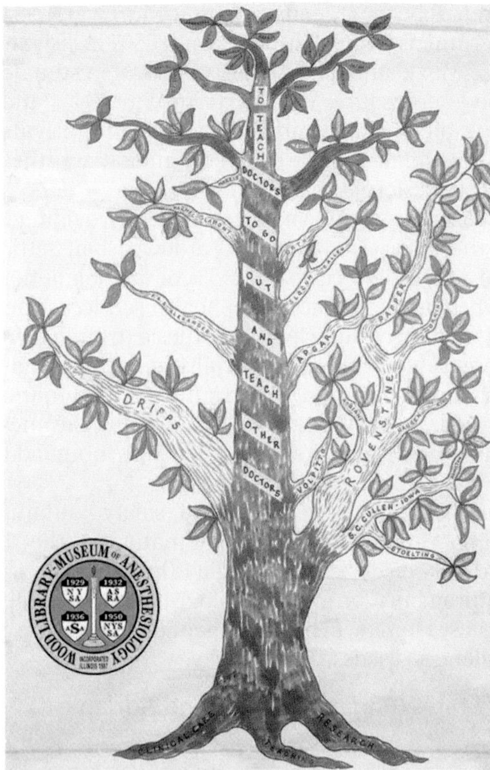

Fig. 2.16 The Aqualumni tree (created by Lucien E. Morris, Ralph M., and Jean P. Morris) depicting names of chairpersons or heads of academic anesthesia centers that came from the lineage of the world's first postgraduate academic residency program in anesthesiology led by Dr. Ralph Waters at the University of Wisconsin. (Copyright © 2018 https://www.woodlibrarymuseum.org. Image reproduced courtesy of the Wood Library-Museum of Anesthesiology, Schaumburg, IL.)

certification is a prerequisite for most hospital-based jobs in anesthesia.

Nurses with at least 1 year of practice in critical care are eligible to train as CRNAs. Training ranges from 24 to 42 months and confers a master's-level degree or higher. Training guidelines are specified by the Council on Accreditation of Nurse Anesthesia Educational Programs and mandate at least 465 hours of classroom education, exposure to a minimum of 600 clinical cases, and 2000 clinical hours.[175] Like physicians, CRNAs who complete an accredited program may take the National Certification Exam administered by the National Board of Certification and Recertification for Nurse Anesthetists.

Certified Anesthesiologist Assistants are a relatively new anesthesia provider group in the United States. Although the first training program opened in 1969 in an attempt to address significant provider shortages that existed in the United States at that time, the cadre has been relatively slow to increase numbers. Certified Anesthesiologist Assistants complete an undergraduate degree with pre-medical studies and then enter a 2.5-year anesthesia training program that is done in collaboration with an anesthesiology department. They conduct anesthesia as directed by a supervising anesthesiologist, and work in close collaboration with the anesthesiologist who leads the care team.

Physician anesthesiologists in the United States are involved in all aspects of perioperative care, including preoperative optimization in outpatient clinics, management of acute postoperative pain, obstetrical anesthesia services, and responding to traumas and inpatient emergencies. They also frequently manage ICUs after completing subspecialty training in critical care.

There are approximately 50,000 physician anesthesiologists, and 50,000 registered CRNAs in the United States, for a combined density of approximately 31 providers per 100,000 people.[176,177] The composition of the anesthesia care team may include from physician anesthesiologists only, to physician anesthesiologists supervising either CRNAs or anesthesia assistants, to CRNA-only models. Federal regulations mandate physician supervision of CRNAs, but 17 states have opted out of this requirement following the introduction of legislation in 2001.[178] Among the 17 states that have opted out, 14 require some degree of physician oversight (not necessarily by an anesthesiologist) and only 3 allow completely independent CRNA practice.

While it is unproven if nonphysician cadres in the United States increase access to anesthesia or provide care with different quality outcomes, data demonstrates that CRNAs are more likely to practice in rural locations and perform more anesthetics under sedation (i.e., MAC) than physician anesthesiologists.[179,180]

Although overall provider density is high in the United States, there is stark geographic maldistribution with providers concentrated in urban areas. Many less populated areas report significant surgical delays due to the lack of anesthesiologists.[95] Access to subspecialists is also limited. For example, nearly one third of the United States pediatric population lives more than 50 miles from the nearest pediatric anesthesiologist.[181]

Maternal mortality has increased in the United States in the last 10 years, though anesthetic-related maternal mortality has declined.[182] The causes are multifactorial, may be attributable to the changing risk profile of obstetric patients, and pose a dynamic challenge to anesthetists.

The high costs of care and incomplete financial coverage (insurance) are two additional, evolving challenges in the United States with significant repercussions and relevance for anesthesia care. Lastly, significant ongoing debate exists over anesthesia provider roles.

EUROPE

Although Europe and the European Union (EU) may appear as one entity, the countries represented are diverse with regard to population, economic situation, culture, and political leadership. Similar diversity is also seen for the training and organization of anesthesiology services in these countries. The official EU title of the specialty is "Anaesthetics," and the only EU training requirement is that its duration should be 3 years.[183] In reality, the duration of training is anything from 3 to 7 years, and the involvement in anesthesia, intensive care, pain, and critical emergency medicine varies to a great extent among countries.[184] The European Section and Board of Anaesthesiology (EBA) of the European Union of Medical Specialists (UEMS) is the political branch of European anesthesiology. The UEMS aims to promote and harmonize the highest level of training of the medical specialists, medical practice, and health care within the EU, and to promote free movement of specialist medical doctors within the EU. The EBA/UEMS has published training guidelines to encourage countries to aim for an agreed standard.[185] In cooperation with the scientific branch of European anesthesiology, the European Society of Anaesthesiology (ESA), the UEMS offers the European Diploma of Anaesthesia and Intensive Care (EDAIC). Another building block for European Anaesthesiology is the Helsinki Declaration on Patient Safety in Anaesthesiology, which was introduced in 2010.[186] In the following paragraphs we describe the situation in two countries—Romania, a middle-income EU member state with a population of 19.7 million and physician-only service, and Norway, a high-income, non-EU member state with a population of 5.2 million and where the team approach is the anesthesia service model.

Norway (Jannicke Mellin-Olsen)

In Norway, the first ether anesthetic was provided at Rikshospitalet (the National Hospital) in Oslo on March 4, 1847.[187] In April, the first ether inhalation for labor followed. At that time, younger surgeons and GPs and later nurses were in charge of anesthesia delivery. In the 1930s two surgeons (Carl Semb and Johan Holst) facilitated anesthesia training opportunities for physicians Otto Mollestad and Ivar Lund in London and Boston (Massachusetts General Hospital), respectively. Dr. Mollestad was hired without salary in 1939, and as the first consultant in anesthesiology in 1947.

The Norwegian Society of Anaesthesiology was founded in January 1949 with only seven members. The founding members faced significant difficulties promoting the specialty, but the anesthesia nurses welcomed physician involvement and leadership.

Physician specialty training is 5 years. There is no final examination, but there are course exams and procedure checklists, in addition to continuous individual assessment. Trainees are encouraged to take exams for the EDAIC. The nurse anesthetist training program is 1.5 years after 3 years of nursing education. Both physician anesthesiologists and nurse anesthetists are accredited by the Directorate of Health.

The first guidelines that described the scope of practice and dynamics of the anesthesia team were authored by both physicians and nurses in 1993.[188,189] It was agreed that anesthesiology is a medical specialty. A physician is responsible for all anesthetic procedures, although nurses are allowed to provide anesthesia for ASA physical classification 1 and 2 adults with indirect supervision. At induction and emergence, there must always be two anesthesia-trained persons immediately available. The "flexible anesthesia team" usually consists of one physician and one nurse.

Anesthesiology is an attractive and prestigious specialty in Norway (second to thoracic and neurosurgery only), and works closely with almost all other hospital specialists, including the surgeons.[190] In contrast to many other countries, anesthesiologists in Norway are highly respected by the general public. This is partly due to increased visibility, as anesthesiologists provide leadership not only in anesthesia, but also perioperative medicine, pain management, intensive care, and critical emergency medicine (including prehospital services). There are currently 1329 physician anesthesia providers (25.5 per 100,000 population) and 2000 nurse anesthesia providers.[100] Anesthesiology is among the medical specialties with the lowest female representation (30%). As Norway has generous paid maternity and paternity leave, the norm is that both sexes stay in the profession and work full-time.

Health care in Norway benefits from the country's economic prosperity, robust public programs, and emphasis on patient safety. The Norwegian Society of Anaesthesiology was among the first signatories of the Helsinki Declaration on Patient Safety in Anaesthesiology, and the WHO Surgical Safety Checklist is distributed and used nationwide. Norwegian health care is funded primarily by the government. Hospital care is free of charge for the patient, as are medication costs once a specified amount is surpassed. Private hospitals exist but provide mostly elective surgery.

Current challenges facing the anesthesia community in Norway include concerns about costs and quality, although in general, hospitals are well equipped. In recent years there has been increasing frequency of medicine shortages, mostly due to the lack of domestic production and export policies of drug companies that can have adverse safety consequences.

Romania (Daniela Filipescu)

The first anesthetic in Romania (ether for a limb amputation) was documented in the journal "TemesvarerWochenblatt" and took place on February 13, 1847.[190a] The world's first-ever use of opioids for intrathecal anesthesia was presented by a Romanian in Paris in 1901.[191] Thoma Ionescu further developed the technique and published the first textbook of intrathecal anesthesia—*La rachianesthésie générale.*[191,192]

The first anesthesia training course in Romania was held in 1951, and a formal 1-year training course began in 1959, after the recognition of Anesthesia and Intensive Care Medicine (AICM) as an independent medical specialty.[190a] The first ICU was instituted in 1958, but it was only in 1972 that AICM departments were formally introduced in the Romanian medical health system.

The first AICM study group was founded by Zorel Filipescu in 1958. The study group was included later as part of the Romanian Society of Surgery and separated as an independent Romanian Society of Anaesthesiology and Intensive Care (RSAIC) in 1972. The RSAIC joined the WFSA the same year.

In Romania, specialist physicians are the only formal anesthesia provider cadre. After graduating from medical school (MD), physicians may enter specialty training after passing a written national examination. The number of places for each specialty is decided by the Ministry of Health, and admission to a specialty depends on candidate preference and performance on the written examination. Usually, AICM is among the top specialties chosen for training due to the wide range of opportunities to work abroad. The Romanian MD and specialist diplomas are automatically recognized in EU countries.

The AICM specialty training is five years and includes two years in intensive care medicine. Romania endorsed the competency-based European Board of Anaesthesiology Curriculum for Anaesthesiology, Intensive Care, and Pain Therapy, but this has been only partially implemented. For obtaining the specialist certification, written and oral examinations must be taken at the end of the training period. Romania adopted the EDAIC Part I examination organized by the ESA as the national written examination since 2010. All physicians practicing in Romania have to be evaluated and re-licensed based on a minimum 200 continuing medical education (CME) credits accumulated every 5 years. There are no specialized anesthesia nursing cadres recognized in Romania, but general nurses may apply for posts in AICM departments where they are trained locally for the job.

An estimated 1400 anesthesiologists are currently practicing in Romania, and approximately 180 trainees are entering the specialty each year. Trainees are distributed to 12 academic centers in the country, although most trainees are taught in the five largest academic centers. The majority of anesthesiologists work in public hospitals though a small number work in private centers and some in both.

Safety in AICM is promoted by the RSAIC, which signed the Helsinki Declaration on Patient Safety in Anaesthesiology, endorsed the WHO checklists, the ESA clinical guidelines, and launched national guidelines. Despite this attention to patient safety, the European Surgical Outcomes Study (EuSOS), which included 17 hospitals and 1298 patients from Romania, demonstrated a higher postoperative mortality (6.8%) after nonemergent general surgery in Romania than the European mean value (4%).[193] Subsequently, a national program for critical care was implemented, and the more recent International Surgical Outcomes Study (ISOS), which included 1875 patients from 26 Romanian hospitals, demonstrated improved outcomes.[194]

The anesthesia community in Romania faces several challenges. A key challenge limiting anesthesia access in Romania is the shortage of providers (anesthesiologists and trained AICM nurses) as well as equipment technicians. Reasons for these shortages include internal and external brain drain (mostly to Western Europe).[195] Workforce shortages particularly affect ICU activities as well as operating theaters where a provider may be assigned multiple rooms simultaneously. Another barrier to scaling the workforce is the lack of a nationally standardized AICM nurse curriculum and training. Additional challenges routinely encountered in Romania include the uneven distribution of specialists and equipment as well as significant infrastructure limitations and drug shortages. For example, ultrasound and certain essential medications (e.g., tranexamic acid, amiodarone) are not universally available. Although the practice of AICM includes perioperative care, there are no formal anesthesia preoperative evaluation or pain therapy centers organized in the public hospitals in Romania. A final and significant challenge facing anesthesia providers is the unavailability of adequate malpractice coverage options which has resulted in defensive medical practices.

Despite the current challenges, the AICM is one of the most dynamic specialties in Romania, with a tremendous development led by dedicated RSAIC leadership.

ASIA AND THE MIDDLE EAST

Asia is the largest continent with a population of 4.43 billion. There is a wide socioeconomic variation among the countries with the GDP PPP (at purchasing power parity) per capita income ranging from 1944 International dollars for Afghanistan to 127,480 for countries like Qatar.[76] Anesthesia services also vary widely. Anesthetic societies are functional in the majority of the countries and a number of societies located in the same geographic regions have voluntarily come together to form regional societies. The officially recognized regional sections of the WFSA in Asia are the Pan Arab Federation of Societies of Anesthesia, Intensive Care and Pain Management (PAFSA) founded in 1884, Confederation of ASEAN Societies of Anaesthesiologists (CASA) as part of the Asian Australasian Regional Section founded in the 1970s, and the South Asian Association of Regional Co-operation—Association of Anaesthesiologists, which came into existence in 1991.

India (Bala Krishnan Kanni)

The first administration of ether anesthesia in India was on March 22, 1847, and the first chloroform anesthesia was administered on January 12, 1848. Chloroform and ether continued to be used until the mid-1950s in many hospitals. Halothane was introduced in 1960 and isoflurane in 1992.[196] Regional anesthesia (with cocaine) was first reported in 1894 and spinal anesthesia with hyperbaric Stovaine (amylocaine) was reported in 1908. In 1935, the first Boyle's apparatus machine arrived in India, and the same year the first oxygen plants were established in Calcutta (Kolkata). The Indian Society of Anesthesia (ISA) was established in 1947. The first official Journal of the ISA was published in July 1953, and in 1956 the ISA joined the WFSA as a founding member.

Formal anesthesia training for undergraduates in India officially started in 1906, followed by diploma (1946) and MD/MS degree programs (1955) in anesthesia. The National Academy of Medical Sciences started Diplomate of National Board of Examinations in 1970 followed by PhD programs in anesthesia. Today, all anesthesiologists in India are required to undergo one of three training pathways prior to independent practice. These pathways take place after completing 4 years of medical school (Bachelor of Medicine, Bachelor of Surgery–MBBS) and 1 year as an intern or "house surgeon." The first training pathway requires physicians to complete 3 years of postgraduate anesthesia training with a dissertation at a university hospital. The second potential pathway is called the Diplomate of the National Board (DNB) and requires 3 years of training as well as a dissertation at a hospital approved by the National Board of Examinations. Physicians can also pursue a 2-year postgraduate diploma program at a university hospital without dissertation. Holders of this latter postgraduate Diploma in Anesthesia often practice with supervision of more senior anesthesiologists. There are no nurse anesthetists in India, and the total number of anesthesiologists in the country (population 1.34 billion) is approximately 25,000 (see Table 2.3).

There have been several attempts to train non-anesthesiologists as stop-gaps for the ongoing workforce crisis. In 2002 the Indian government started a short-term training program for doctors but this could not be sustained due to problems in implementation and lack of support from the government. One ongoing program provides 6 months of training to physicians post-medical school to carry out cesarean sections and lifesaving anesthetic skills for emergency obstetric care in rural facilities where no anesthesiologist exists.[197,198] This program is controversial and not universally supported. India also trains Operation Theatre Technologists (OTT) or Assistants who may undergo a 3-year diploma or 6-month to 1-year training program straight from secondary school. These cadres have limited scopes of practice (e.g., can place IVs or administer medications) and must practice under direct supervision of anesthesiologists. Although the OTTs are not permitted by the ISA to perform tasks such as intubation or neuraxial anesthesia, there are significant concerns that such practice takes place in some centers.

In addition to shortages in number, the anesthesia workforce in India also suffers from inequitable distribution, with a disproportionate number of providers in urban areas. Because anesthesiologists in India are also responsible for many services outside of the operating theaters (e.g., preoperative preparation, postoperative care, and critical care), these services are also frequently unavailable.

The ISA is actively engaged in several activities to promote anesthesia safety throughout India. With initial financial assistance from WFSA, the ISA started a CME program for rural anesthetists to update knowledge and techniques. The ISA endorses the WFSA and WHO guidelines for minimum monitoring standards, the WHO Safe Surgery Checklist, as well as many other anesthesia safety practices (e.g., color coding of drugs, syringe labelling, machine checks, and appropriate records of anesthetic care). Significant efforts have also been made to educate the public about anesthesia and its safety by holding public education programs.[199]

Although safe anesthesia services are available in many institutions both public and private throughout India, access to modern equipment and facilities are not universal. Much like providers, anesthesia infrastructure is also concentrated in urban areas. Anesthesia subspecialties such as neuro, cardiac, pain, pediatrics, and obstetrics are available in most urban hospitals but few rural facilities.[200] As a result, many rural facilities lack capacity for safe anesthesia care. Additional challenges limiting access to safe anesthesia care in India include poverty, distance to care, social and cultural barriers, and comorbidity.

Lebanon and The Middle East (Patricia Yazbeck)

The oldest medical writings in the region were found in cuneiform tablets and Eber's papyrus in Mesopotamia and the Nile valley, describing herbal treatments like Belladonna, Cannabis, and Mandragora. Phoenicians also obtained artificial sleep by using calming herbs, opium poppy, and juniper leaves. In the Middle Ages, prominent Arab scholars (Avicenna, Al Razi, Ibn Al Quff, Al Baghdadi, and others) made important contributions to the field of medicine.

In 1835, the first Arab medical school in the Middle East was established by Dr. Clot in Kasr-Al-Aini Hospital, in Cairo. Graduates practiced in all the large cities of the region. In 1860, American, French, and British powers intervened in the region and with the inflow of missionaries, more medical schools and hospitals were established. In Lebanon, the Syrian Protestant College (American University of Beirut) was founded by American missionaries in 1886 while the French Medical School (St Joseph University) was founded by the French Jesuits in 1883. The first use of inhalational anesthesia occurred in 1865 by Dr. George Post, an American missionary surgeon who administered "kulfera" (chloroform) in the village of Abeih-Lebanon. Dr. Post is considered the pioneer of modern anesthesia in the Middle East (Fig. 2.17).[201]

At the end of WWI, the practice of anesthesia still depended on foreign surgeons, and on local and foreign nurses or technicians, administering ether or chloroform. But the beginning of oil production in the region contributed to economic improvement and led to the foundation of many faculties of medicine in Syria, Sudan, and Iraq. After 1950, Middle Eastern countries established fully independent anesthesia departments with their own structure, staff, residency training, research, and certification by international academic institutions. In addition, in the 1960s and 1970s, many countries founded their own national anesthesia societies and in 1985 a Pan Arab Society of Anesthesia, regional section of the WFSA, was founded.

Anesthesia departments in the Middle Eastern countries are staffed by highly qualified faculty certified either by the Arab Board or by foreign academic bodies, such as the American, French, or European Boards of Anesthesiology or by the RCoA.

A residency program of 4 years in a recognized center may be followed by 1 or 2 years of fellowship in pain management, critical care, obstetric anesthesia, cardiopulmonary anesthesia, or others as recognized by the national anesthesia societies, which also track CME.

Anesthesia is routinely administered by a qualified anesthesiologist. Trainee anesthesiologists or anesthesia nurses can administer anesthesia under the supervision of a qualified anesthesiologist. The density of physician anesthesia providers per 100,000 population is less than three in Morocco, Syria, and Iraq, and less than one in Yemen and Sudan while it ranges from six to more than 10 in countries like Egypt, Oman, Jordan, Lebanon, United Arab Emirates, and Kuwait.

The responsibilities of the anesthesiologist include preoperative assessment and preparation, premedication, as well as staffing PACUs and ICUs. Anesthesia is administered in the operating room, delivery suite, radiology department, and as ambulatory anesthesia. In addition, acute or chronic pain management is becoming routinely practiced. Departments and societies of anesthesiology in the Middle Eastern countries are responsible for setting practice guidelines, matching the standards approved by international societies, such as the American, French, or European Societies of Anesthesiologists. Anesthetic machines, monitoring equipment, and agents adhere to the international standards.

The major key challenges and barriers to safe anesthesia in the region are the consequence of the recent turmoil occurring in many Middle Eastern countries (e.g., Syria, Iraq, Libya, Sudan, and Palestine) resulting in limitations of workforce and anesthesia access and safety in parts of these countries.

Pakistan (Fauzia Khan)

From the time Pakistan gained independence (1947) until the late 1950s, the practice of anesthesia was mostly limited to spinal or open-drop ether after induction with ethyl chloride. The first chair of anesthesia was established at the King Edward Medical College, Lahore, in 1959, and a 2-year diploma course (DA) was introduced at the same institution in 1960. The first ICU in Pakistan was established in 1976 at Mayo Hospital, Lahore, and the Pakistan Society of Anesthesia (PSA) was founded in 1971 in Karachi. A higher

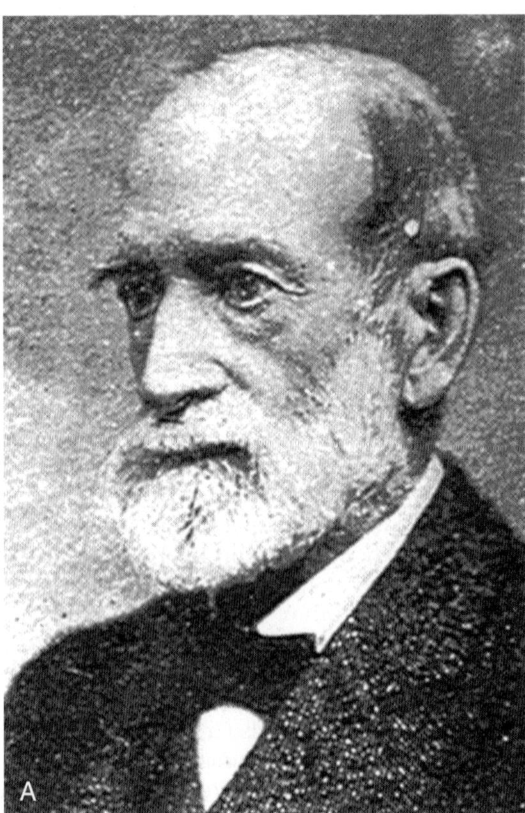

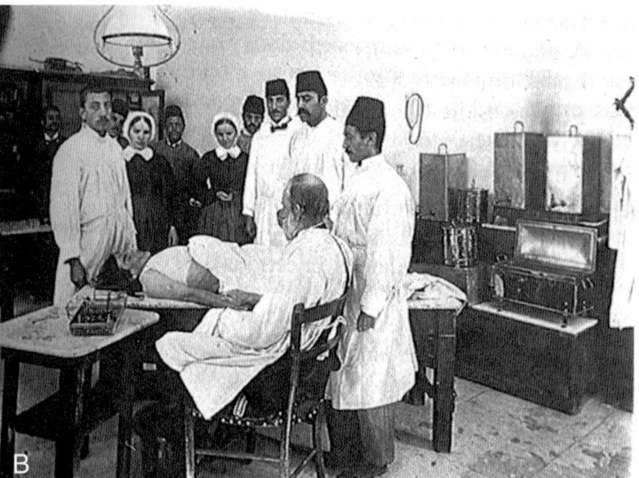

Fig. 2.17 **Dr. George Post (A), in an operating room with a female patient on the table (B).**

diploma, the Fellowship of the College of Physicians and Surgeons of Pakistan (FCPS), was instituted by the College of Physicians and Surgeons of Pakistan (CPSP) in 1972.

The CPSP includes anesthesia faculty and accredits all physician training programs in the country. Two training tracks are offered for anesthesia: (1) a higher professional diploma (FCPS) that requires 4 years of competency-based standardized training; and (2) a Membership of the College (MCPS) that requires 2 years of training after medical school and 1 year of internship. Only FCPS diploma holders can progress in the academic ladder in university anesthesia jobs. Certification in either track requires written, practical, and oral examinations. License to practice is provided by a separate body, the Pakistan Medical and Dental Council.

The anesthetic workforce in Pakistan is comprised of 3100 physician specialists (1.64 physician anesthetists per 100,000 population) (see Table 2.3). Anesthesia almost always is provided by physicians, although in some remote areas surgeons may administer local blocks or even spinal anesthesia. The main clinical responsibility for the majority of anesthesiologists is to provide operating room anesthesia and preoperative assessment, but in several institutions they also lead ICUs and chronic pain management clinics.

Health care in Pakistan is provided mainly by the private sector, with the government contributing only about 20% of services. Government-owned institutions are tiered into teaching, district, and county (taluka) hospitals. A system of basic health units provides primary health care. The majority of anesthesiologists hold two jobs as remuneration from just one is not sufficient. Only a few public institutions allow in-house private work by anesthesiologists. Brain drain is an ongoing issue with a significant proportion of the workforce emigrating to the Middle East or Europe.

There are currently no national guidelines relating to anesthesia and little awareness of international safety standards. There are also limited data on anesthesia outcomes in Pakistan.[202] There is no national body responsible for quality and safety in health care, however, the Punjab Healthcare Commission (PHC) is an autonomous health regulatory body created by the provincial government for the Punjab province (96 million people). The PHC aims to improve quality, safety, and efficiency of healthcare service delivery for the population of Punjab by implementing Minimum Service Delivery Standards (MSDS) in all areas and all disciplines including anesthesia. This model is soon to be replicated in the other provinces.

Anesthesia care varies significantly among health facilities within the country. Larger hospitals in bigger cities have access to modern equipment and monitors comparable to HICs. Many government teaching hospitals and secondary health centers are underfunded and have only basic equipment for monitoring (e.g., ECG and noninvasive blood pressure). Medication shortages are a frequent occurrence as several routine anesthetic medicines like fentanyl, inhalational agents, antiarrhythmics, and vasoactive drugs are imported. Even drugs manufactured within the country like morphine and ephedrine are frequently unavailable. Remifentanil, sufentanil, esmolol, S-ketamine, and clonidine are among many drugs not available at all due to licensing issues.

Additional challenges currently facing the Pakistani anesthesia community include maldistribution of human resources, limited biomedical technician support, and lack of political will. There is great necessity for regional collaboration to collect data on anesthesia and surgical need, resources, and outcomes to help improve safety and better allocate resources.[203]

China (Yugaung Huang)

Modern anesthesia was introduced along with Western medicine into China in the early 20th century. In the 1950s, only simple anesthesia care was available in China, including open-drop ether, tracheal intubation under inhalational anesthesia, and single-shot procaine spinal anesthesia together with peripheral nerve blocks. Because of economic limitations from the 1950s to the 1980s, intravenous procaine combined with opioid anesthesia and even acupuncture anesthesia were common. Anesthesiology in China has evolved in the past 2 decades as a crucial medical specialty that is integral to multidisciplinary surgical care and collaboration. This has resulted in modern anesthesiology shifting from narrowly focused on surgical anesthesia to perioperative medicine.

The training of anesthesia practitioners remains a big challenge. Currently in China, medical school studies range from 5 to 8 years resulting in an inevitable variation in educational quality. The national resident training program was initiated in 2000 and standardized in 2014, which will make the specialty catch up with the international standards of training and help to eliminate disparities due to difference in initial medical education.

To ensure patient safety, it is emphasized that clinical anesthesia is provided by anesthesiologists rather than anesthesia nurses. To meet the rapidly increasing needs outside of the operating room, anesthesiologists are required in nonsurgical diagnostic and therapeutic procedures for endoscopy, painless labor, and delivering optimal care to improve the quality of patient care throughout the hospital. With the economic boom, the majority of Chinese hospitals are equipped with sophisticated anesthetic machines and monitors and have a modern work environment. However, there are obvious variations in the quantity and quality of anesthesia devices and services among the different regions of China. In some small or medium-sized hospitals, there are no anesthetic gas monitors, defibrillators, or target-controlled infusion pumps.[204]

With the support from the National Health Commission (NHC), Chinese anesthesiology has been shifting from only operating room anesthesia to perioperative medicine and moving from a volume-based healthcare system to a value-based healthcare system. Anesthesia safety and quality assurance are of vital significance and great concern. The National Quality Assurance Center for Anesthesia was established with Professor Yuguang Huang as its leader in 2011. Thus far 31 Provincial Quality Assurance Centers have been established throughout mainland China. There have been only sporadic studies so far providing data on anesthesia safety and these have come from several large hospitals, while the current status in resource-limited medical settings remains to be explored.[205,206]

The anesthesia workforce shortage has become one of the greatest challenges in China as the number of surgeries has grown and the anesthesia demand increased without a concomitant increase in the number of anesthesiologists. The density of physician anesthesia providers is only 5.12 per 100,000 population in China, which is approximately 25% of that in the United States. To meet the urgent healthcare needs, Chinese anesthesiologists are struggling with heavy workloads, and thus have high burnout and low job satisfaction.[207] Long working hours, heavy workload, high acuity, and fast work pace are all factors associated with burnout and patient safety. Even with this effort only 10% of pregnant women can receive epidural analgesia during labor, and patients undergoing endoscopy have to be on long waiting lists for analgesia and sedation since anesthesia practitioners are mainly occupied with surgery in the operating rooms. To bridge the workforce gap, the Chinese government has made great efforts to emphasize the importance of anesthesiologists and anesthesiology nationwide with supportive documents focused on improving the perceptions and roles of the anesthesia specialty in medical care not only for patients but also for anesthesia professionals. It is encouraging to see that an increasing number of medical graduates are willing to join the profession of anesthesiology, which prognosticates well for the future.

With great efforts by the Chinese Society of Anesthesiology and Chinese Association of Anesthesiologists, Chinese anesthesiology has developed rapidly to provide patients with safer anesthesia and better quality of life. Challenges include variation in anesthesia safety, shortage of workforce, occupational burnout, and unbalanced working conditions across the country. Further efforts are anticipated to make anesthesia practice even better in China.

Vietnam (Thi Thanh Nguyen and Thang Cong Quyet)

The modern history of anesthesia in Vietnam dates as far back as 1975 only due to the loss of records during the war. During the war, anesthesia was usually administered by surgeons, and only occasionally by an anesthesiologist who had mainly been trained by French or American specialists. During the war, U.S. military anesthesiologists made multiple seminal discoveries that changed modern transfusion practices.[208,209] Following the war, Vietnamese doctors gradually took up anesthesia and in 1979, the Vietnam Society of Anesthesiologists was founded in Hanoi with 100 members and Professor Ton Duc Lang as its first president. The membership continued to expand and currently there are more than 1000 anesthesiologists in Vietnam. In 1980, with the help of Dr. J. Beiboer from The Netherlands, the Vietnam Society of Anesthesiologists joined the WFSA, the CASA, and various other specialist societies throughout the region.

During the past decade, the role of physician anesthesiologists in Southeast Asia has changed remarkably. Physician anesthesiologists have gained recognition by peers and the populace. Training in anesthesia was initially undertaken by surgeons concurrently with surgical training. In 1993 the first department of anesthesia was established at Hanoi Medical University. Other departments were soon established in Ho Chi Minh City, Hue, Can Tho, Thai Nguyen, and Hai Phong. Several different forms of training varying in duration from 1 to 5 years were introduced in order to fulfill different requirements throughout the country, and contemporary anesthesia training is based on both the American and French systems.

Medical school is 6 years in duration, though during times of war a 4-year option has existed for trainees who have already completed a 2-year nursing program. After medical school, graduates can enter a 3-year residency in anesthesia (24 months clinical and 12 months research), for which there are 30 spots per year in the country. Residents do not receive remuneration during training unless they are bonded to a hospital where they worked as a general practitioner between medical school and residency. Upon completing residency, graduates are awarded a Master's degree and can work as a "first specialist" anesthesiologist. Thereafter they can pursue additional training in either an academic pathway (2-year PhD) or a "practical" pathway with "second specialist" training (2 years of apprenticeship and consultant work). The "second specialist" certificate allows these providers to function as a consultant, head of anesthesiology or as a trainer in the practical training system. An additional anesthesia training pathway exists for medical school graduates who are not admitted to residency. These physicians must pass a 1-year anesthesia training program, pursue 2 years of clinical anesthesia practice, and then return to a medical university to complete 2 more years of anesthesia training. At the conclusion of this pathway, these providers receive a "first specialist" anesthesiologist certificate, functionally equivalent to anesthesiologists who have completed the practical pathway previously discussed. There are approximately 100 training spots available per year in the country for this anesthesia training pathway. There are no formal, accredited subspecialty training programs in Vietnam, although several institutions offer 6-month to 1-year certification programs for select subspecialties. Additional training opportunities for Vietnamese anesthesiologists have been introduced in France and Southeast Asia. Numerous Vietnamese anesthesiologists have participated in the Bangkok Anesthesia Regional Training Center (BARTC), a 1-year fellowship supported by the WFSA and the Royal College of Anesthesiologists of Thailand to train anesthesia educators in Asia.[210]

In addition to the courses for physician anesthesiologists, several courses for nurse anesthetists were also introduced, which varied in duration from 1 year for registered nurses to 3 years for new nursing students. Nurse anesthetists are required to always work with a physician anesthesia provider or with permission from the manager of the hospital. Physician and nurse anesthetists are now able to staff over 1000 hospitals and clinics throughout the country where surgery is undertaken. In 2012, the Ministry of Health issued guidelines for anesthesiologists to become involved in pain management and critical care in addition to preoperative, intraoperative, and postoperative care. These specialties require additional training and formal anesthesia subspecialty fellowships do not exist in Vietnam.

Prior to 1990 the major techniques used were inhalational anesthesia, first with ether and subsequently with halothane. Induction was with thiopentone or ketamine and regional anesthesia with spinal or epidural. Since 1990 the responsibilities of anesthetists have expanded to include specialist areas such as extracorporeal circulation for open heart surgery, organ transplantation, ultrasound-guided regional anesthesia, chronic pain management, preoperative assessment clinics, and out of operating room activities such as epidural analgesia for patients in labor, and anesthesia for endoscopic procedures. The WHO Surgical Safety Checklist is commonly applied in every operating room and clinical practice guidelines are selected from ASA or ESA guidelines. There is still a maldistribution of anesthesiologists, a shortage of essential medications, and lack of necessary infrastructure, which can endanger patient safety.

The Vietnam Society of Anesthesiologists is striving to raise standards of education in anesthesia to be at par with international standards in order to enhance the safety of the practice in the country, encourage scientific research among members, establish professional guidelines, and support working with the Ministry of Health to advance the specialty of anesthesia. At present there are no national examinations for certification.

SOUTH AMERICA

South America is a vast continent with a population of 420 million and economies ranging from the eighth largest in the world (Brazil) to some of the poorest in the world (Bolivia).[210a] Some cities or areas of cities have HIC health care including hospitals with top-level research and Joint Commission certification (77 in 6 countries) whereas many others do not even comply with national standards.[211] This is a reflection of the social difficulties of the continent where most countries have poor Gini indexes (measure of distribution of income of a country's residents) ranking among the worst in the world.[212]

Anesthesia workforce density in South America varies by more than 10-fold among countries (Uruguay 13.7 vs. Peru 1.7).[100] Substantial differences exist in practice models, ranging from physician-only anesthesia practice in Colombia to Paraguay where 50% of anesthesia is provided by nonphysicians. This translates into dramatic differences in resources where some hospitals have anesthesia information systems and sophisticated monitoring equipment (e.g., intraoperative transesophageal echocardiography with tissue Doppler, electroencephalograph monitoring), while most still rely on paper records and limited anesthesia machines. Training quality and capacity are also highly variable and few homogenizing mechanisms exist to guarantee a minimal standard of training, as certification mechanisms are virtually absent.

Paraguay (Rodrigo Sosa Argana)

The first reports of anesthesia in Paraguay are of chloroform use during the war Paraguay fought against the Triple Alliance (Brazil, Uruguay, and Argentina) between 1864 and 1870.[213] The country's first recorded physician anesthesia provider was Dr. Roberto Olmedo in 1928, and the first trained anesthesiologist Dr. Luis Ramirez is credited with starting the specialty in Paraguay in 1948. After this time, the number of anesthesiologists who trained abroad began to increase.[214]

The Sociedad Paraguaya de Anestesiología (SPA) was founded in 1973 by the 18 anesthesiologists practicing in the country at the time. The first anesthesia training programs were started in 1982, and the first formal anesthesia residency program (3 years in duration) was created in 1992 by the Hospital de Clinicas of the Universidad Nacional de Asunción.

In addition to physician anesthesiologists, the Ministry of Public Health and Social Welfare also licenses two types of nonphysician providers, technicians and diplomates. Technicians have no formal prerequisites and receive minimal if any formal training (most are taught as apprentices, historically most often by surgeons). Diplomates complete a 3-year anesthesia training program after high school that consists of once-weekly training days. These providers currently administer anesthesia in the most remote areas and public hospitals throughout the country, whereas physician anesthesiologists provide the majority of care in urban settings and the private sector. In the urban and private setting, the nonphysician cadres often work alongside physician anesthesiologists in a supportive role and with close supervision. The Ministry of Public Health has defined a scope of practice for nonphysicians in Paraguay such that they can perform anesthesia independently in remote locations where no anesthesiologists are present. In such circumstances, the nonphysicians are supervised by the surgeon and generally perform cases of lower complexity, most often under spinal anesthesia. There has been significant tension between all anesthesia cadres in the country. The technicians and diplomates consider their training and expertise as equivalent despite significant differences in prerequisites, training, and practice (see Table 2.3). In recent decades the number of physician anesthesiologists has increased relative to the number of nonphysician providers. There are approximately 258 anesthesiologists and 491 nonphysician providers (technicians and diplomates) in Paraguay (10.7 anesthesia providers per 100,000 people).

A major challenge in Paraguay at present is ensuring standards for anesthesia provider training. The SPA has lobbied the government extensively to curb nonphysician training in Paraguay due to ongoing concerns about the quality of training standards. In the last decade the SPA has been successful in enacting high-level education reform to improve anesthesia practice standards and has organized multiple international meetings including a recent large Latin American Anesthesia conference (CLASA 2013).

Colombia (Pedro Ibarra)

The first documented anesthetic in Colombia was provided in 1849 using chloroform.[215] In these early times, underperforming medical students were often relegated to providing anesthesia, and for many years anesthesia services were provided by poorly trained, and often nonmedical, personnel (e.g., technicians, healthcare students, and nurses). Dr. Isaac Rodriguez was the first Colombian physician dedicated to anesthesia, and the first formally trained anesthesiologist was Dr. Juan Jose Salamanca who trained under Dr. Henry Beecher at Massachusetts General Hospital in 1940. The Sociedad Colombiana de Anestesiologia y Reanimacion (SCARE) was founded in 1949 and was one of the founding societies of the WFSA in 1955. The first formal anesthesia training programs in Colombia were established in the 1960s, at Universidad Nacional and Universidad de Antioquia (UdeA). The Universidad Nacional program had input from Dr. Gustavo Delgado, who trained with several pioneers in anesthesia including Dr. Robert Dripps (see Fig. 2.16). The UdeA program was developed by Dr. Nacianceno Valencia, a second-generation "aqualumni" trained by Dr. Perry Volpitto (see Fig. 2.16).[216,217]

The first anesthesia residency programs (2 years in duration) began to increase the number of anesthesiologists in the 1960s, but the large magnitude of the workforce shortage forced several medical schools to introduce strong anesthesia training during medical school. This allowed medical school graduates to provide basic anesthesia care during their mandatory rural service year after graduation. They gradually reduced nonphysician anesthesia care in the 1970s in small towns. Many of these physicians remained in remote towns providing anesthesia care, until 1991 when the first law prohibiting anesthesia practice without a diploma was issued. Since the late 1990s, anesthesia care in Colombia has been exclusively provided by physician anesthesiologists.

Most of the 23 anesthesia residency programs are 3 years in duration (two programs are 4 years in duration) and are overseen by the Ministry of Education, which establishes curricular requirements based on input from the SCARE and the periodic Anesthesia Education Seminars that have been held since 1974. There is no national examination, and license for practice is issued by the Ministry of Health.

Currently there are approximately 3600 anesthesiologists in Colombia for a density of 7.9 anesthesiologists per 100,000 people. Approximately 115 anesthesiology trainees graduate each year, and a nearly matching number of foreigners or foreign-trained Colombians are incorporated into the workforce. In recent years, political and economic uncertainties in Venezuela have increased the influx of foreign-trained anesthesiologists into Colombia. In some cases, this increased supply has driven down remuneration and created tension with locally-trained anesthesiologists.

Rural anesthesia staffing is a significant challenge in Colombia. The needs of remote areas are often met through economic incentives and temporary positions. Rural hospitals pay premium salaries for positions that are difficult to fill and are able to do so because nearly 100% of Colombian citizens have healthcare coverage through the government-funded, multi-institutional insurance scheme. This single-payer approach allows rural hospitals to receive reimbursement comparable to institutions with higher-income, urban patient mixes. Because competition for anesthesia jobs is less in rural than urban settings, some rural hospitals are able to put together competitive compensation packages and recruit more easily than some public institutions in urban settings where reimbursement is lower and competition for jobs is higher.

The first Colombian anesthesia standards were published in 1985, and in 1992 a modern version based on the ASA Standards was published by SCARE and adopted by the Colombian government. The WHO Surgical Safety Checklist was adopted in 2008 and has contributed to the decreasing incidence of malpractice cases involving anesthesiology. Malpractice suits are a significant challenge in Colombia as well as a driver for improved safety. In 1993, SCARE created an anesthesia malpractice defense fund, FEPASDE, which became the major malpractice insurer for the country. To maintain the economic health of the fund, SCARE has adopted national healthcare education strategies for adverse outcome prevention.

Colombia's healthcare system faces several additional challenges. One is economic sustainability, due to healthcare benefits in excess of national resources. A second is regional inequity, where healthcare quality differs dramatically between regions. An additional major challenge is the ongoing workforce shortage. One driver of the health worker shortage is the present training system, which requires residents to pay tuition during specialist training. There is an effort in the Congress of Colombia to eliminate this practice. As with many other LMICs, remuneration is a major challenge for anesthesia providers in Colombia who frequently work more than one full-time position to increase salary. This has expanded anesthesia coverage but also increased the risk of provider burnout.

OCEANIA

There are 16 independent nations in the region of Oceania. This area of the South Western Pacific accounts for approximately 30% of the world's surface area but has less than 40 million people with over 70% of people living in Australia and New Zealand. Of the independent island nations, Papua New Guinea is the most populous with over 8 million people and Tuvalu the least populous with approximately 11,000 people. The region consists of many remote islands and is economically diverse with only Australia and New Zealand being considered as HICs. Australia and New Zealand will be considered together and the independent island nations of Fiji, Solomon Islands, Vanuatu, Tonga, Papua New Guinea, Marshall Islands, Micronesia, Nauru, Samoa, Tuvalu, Palau, and Kiribati will be considered as one group.

Australia and New Zealand (Rob McDougall)

News of the first use of ether for anesthesia reached Australia by sailing ship in May 1847 and soon after, ether was used for a dental procedure in Sydney and general surgery in Launceston.[218] Later that year saw the first use of anesthesia in New Zealand, again following news by ship.[219] In 1888 "chloroformists" were first appointed in Australian hospitals but it was not until 1944 that the first university diploma course in anesthesia was established.[220] The Australian Society of Anaesthetists was established in 1934 and the New Zealand Society of Anaesthetists (NZSA) followed in 1948.

Anesthesia in Australia and New Zealand is provided by physicians. Training, examination, and accreditation of Australian and New Zealand anesthesiologists is the responsibility of the Australian and New Zealand College of Anaesthetists (ANZCA), which was founded in 1992. Prior to this time, specialist training was administered by the Faculty of Anaesthetists of the Royal Australasian College of Surgeons, which was formed in 1952. ANZCA established the Faculty of Pain Medicine in 1998 and pain medicine was recognized as a medical specialty in Australia in 2005. In addition, ANZCA is responsible for the standards of clinical practice of anesthesia and pain medicine in Australia and New Zealand.

Australia and New Zealand have among the highest density of anesthesia providers, in population terms, in the world with 23.09 and 21.79 anesthesia providers per 100,000 population, respectively.[100] A minimum of 7 years of postgraduate training is required to become a specialist anesthesiologist.

Specialist anesthetists account for almost the entire anesthesia workforce in New Zealand, however, Australia has an active body of over 250 GP anesthetists, who predominantly work in regional and remote areas which cannot sustain full-time specialist anesthetists.[221] The training and accreditation of GP anesthetists is overseen by ANZCA and the Royal Australian College of General Practitioners. The provision of high-quality anesthesia in remote areas of Australia continues to be a challenge.

In 2014, the average age of the Australian anesthesiologist workforce was 49 years and 27% of the workforce was female. Australia and New Zealand have publicly funded universal health care but both countries have a private health sector. Just over 50% of work by Australian anesthesiologists was in the public sector.

ANZCA has produced triennial reports on anesthesia-related mortality in Australia and New Zealand since the first comprehensive report for 1985–87. For 2012–14 the anesthesia-related mortality for Australia was 2.96 deaths per million population per annum or 1 death for 57,023 episodes of anesthesia care.[222] In addition, New Zealand is one of the few countries to comprehensively collect and report 30-day POMR. POMR is one of the core indicators recommended by the LCOGS for monitoring safe surgery and anesthesia. Thirty-day POMR in New Zealand for 2010–15 was 0.55% of hospital admissions receiving general anesthesia.[223]

In spite of its huge size, Australia is one of the world's most urbanized countries. This aids centralization of health care but does create equity of access challenges for those living in remote areas. This is a particular problem for indigenous Australians who account for almost half the population of very remote areas.

Australian and New Zealand anesthesiologists are involved in global health activities, particularly in the Asia Pacific region. Both the Australian Society of Anaesthetists and NZSA are active members of the WFSA and also have their own global outreach committees. ANZCA also has a strong Overseas Aid Committee. The Overseas Development and Education Committee of the Australian Society of Anaesthetists has long supported the development of anesthesia in the Pacific, in partnership with the Pacific Society of Anesthetists and the Fiji National University (FNU). ANZCA has similarly supported Papua New Guinea in partnership with the Society of Anesthetists of Papua New Guinea and the University of Papua New Guinea (UPNG). Similar partnerships exist between professional organizations in such countries as Mongolia, Myanmar, Timor-Leste, Micronesia, Solomon Islands, Laos, Cambodia, and other Pacific Island nations. Essential Pain Management, Primary Trauma Care, and Lifebox are examples of programs coordinated by Australian and New Zealand professional bodies in the Asia Pacific region.

Fiji and Pacific Island Nations (Sereima Bale)

The remote geographic locations of the myriad of small and large islands that comprise the Pacific Island nations and their diverse populations make the training and the practice of anesthesia a massive challenge.

In Fiji, Papua New Guinea, and Pacific Island countries, Assistant Medical Practitioners or Anaesthetic Technical Officers were trained as apprentices by expatriate consultant anesthetists during the various colonial eras before each country gained independence. Anesthesia became a recognized specialist discipline in 1970 in Fiji even though doctors (registered as "Native Medical Practitioner") had been practicing as "anesthetists" since the 1920s.

In the early 1970s, many Pacific Island nations (Fiji, Tonga, Kiribati, Niue) sent their doctors for training in the DA program offered by the Anesthesiology Center for the Western Pacific (Manila, Philippines) in collaboration with the WHO Western Pacific Regional Office. Currently the two specialist training institutions in this region are the College of Medicine, Nursing and Health Sciences of the Fiji National University (FNU), which started anesthesia training in 1996, and the University of Papua New Guinea (UPNG), which established anesthesia training in 1989 as the Fiji School of Medicine. These programs offer physicians a 1-year DA, that may be followed by a 3-year anesthesia Master's of Medicine (MMed) as the specialist qualification. Since 1996, FNU has graduated 92 doctors with the DA, and 39 of these have gone on to receive the MMed. There have been 32 anesthesia specialists that have graduated—23 from Fiji and 16 from other Pacific nations.

FNU trains only physicians while UPNG also offers a 1-year diploma course for healthcare workers who train as Anaesthesia Scientific Officers (ASOs). These NPAPs provide 90% of anesthesia services in Papua New Guinea, often in remote provincial and mission hospitals with no physician supervision. Other Pacific Islands that utilize this latter cadre of NPAPs to complement their physician capacity are Vanuatu, Tonga, and Solomon Islands. Other islands in the northern Pacific, including former U.S. territories, employ American-trained nurse anesthetists.[224]

Two issues significantly limit the development of the anesthesia workforce in the Pacific: (1) few students graduate from medical schools in Fiji and Papua New Guinea to supply any specialties and keep pace with growing populations; and (2) few job opportunities are funded by national Ministries of Health. In Fiji for example, there are 23 physician specialist anesthesiologists for a population of 800,000, but only 5 consultant positions supported by the Ministry of Health, which employs all Fijian FNU graduates. Additional challenges routinely faced in the region include limited access to equipment, geographic isolation, and an influx of medical graduates from other regions who may be ill-prepared for postgraduate training or practice in this setting.

In 2018, Fiji (population 800,000) had 18 specialists. Unless there is significant expansion of job opportunities for specialist anesthesiologists, limited access to specialist-level care is likely to continue regardless of numbers of graduates. There is continuing brain drain among graduate specialists in Fiji. Of the 23 MMed graduates, only 17 remain in government employment with minimal opportunities for private practice. Some of these graduates, however, remain in practice in the Pacific, just not in their country of origin.

Other Pacific Islands are continuing to build their capacity and are retaining their graduates: Kiribati (2 MMeds, 1 DA: population 33,000); Solomon Islands (4 MMeds; population 600,000). The volume and range of cases in the smaller island nations pose different challenges. The solo anesthetist who may provide anesthesia for 1 to 2 surgical lists per week may also be required to cover other clinical or administrative services as necessary. In addition, this officer is also expected to cover for emergencies and is permanently on call. Outdated skills and knowledge can develop as can burnout as a result of professional isolation and lack of support.

Papua New Guinea is a LMIC on the eastern half of the island of New Guinea (the second largest island in the world) and has only 19 physician specialist anesthesiologists and 130 ASOs, of which only 50% are currently employed. The challenges of the provision of safe surgery and anesthesia in Papua New Guinea relate to its terrain and poverty. Eighty percent of the population live in remote highland, coastal, and island villages and may be days away from a hospital that can provide the three bellwether procedures. Currently Papua New Guinea has 0.25 PAPs per 100,000 compared with Australia and New Zealand where the anesthesia workforce is 75 times greater.[224]

There are three main anesthesia societies in the western Pacific outside of Australia and New Zealand: The Pacific Society of Anaesthetists (28 members); the Micronesia Society of Anesthetists (7 members); and the Society of Anaesthetists of Papua New Guinea (16 members). All Pacific societies have received varying support from the Australian and New Zealand governments, the ASA, the NZSA, ANZCA, and the WFSA, and hosted joint meetings for the first time in 2014.

Section 3: Essentials for Practice in Resource-Constrained Settings

CLINICAL AND TECHNICAL SKILLS

The practice of anesthesia anywhere in the world is reliant on four principle factors: personnel, equipment, medications, and patients with their comorbidities. Disruption, change, or lack of any of these factors may limit the safe practice of anesthesia. Whether practicing in a rural HIC setting, an LMIC, a military or humanitarian field hospital, or other resource-constrained setting, all of these will be modified. Data guiding practice in these settings are limited and may be interpreted differently. There are numerous instances of well-intentioned, evidence-based practices from HICs producing unintended negative consequences in LMICs.[225]

Clinical practice in resource-constrained settings may be extremely different from what one may be accustomed to, so it is important to understand the local context before attempting to change anything. There is often a logical reason why practice patterns diverge from the "standard," and frequently this has less to do with local providers "not knowing the right way" and more to do with local challenges related to personnel, equipment, medications, or patients. This section will briefly discuss select aspects of anesthesia practice in resource-constrained settings through the lens of these four factors.

Personnel. Limitations in anesthesia workforce are one of the most significant barriers to the safe provision of anesthesia care worldwide. Beyond low absolute numbers of providers, the competencies of existing anesthetic providers may be highly variable. Many practitioners who provide anesthesia in resource-constrained settings may have completed inadequate training and often work in isolation with negligible supervision or colleague support. Many are highly skilled and competent within a narrow spectrum of clinical cases, and often learn to deliver a "recipe" type anesthetic that may not be adaptable or appropriate for more complex cases.

When working in resource-constrained environments, it is important to understand the level of knowledge and experience of the local anesthetic provider. Regardless of training level, there are always opportunities for mutually beneficial bidirectional learning. The role of the anesthetic provider in many resource-constrained settings is often limited to the operating theater, as the concept of perioperative care is underdeveloped and not part of training. Personnel shortages routinely limit capacity for adequate preoperative evaluation (including resuscitation) or routine postoperative monitoring. Staffing (e.g., perioperative nursing) may be entirely lacking, and routine elements of postoperative care such as monitoring or providing regular pain assessments with analgesic administration are rarely available. Thoughtful planning is required especially if higher-level care is needed postoperatively (e.g., ventilation), as this usually will become the responsibility of the anesthesia provider or even family members (who are frequently recruited to help with monitoring or even manual ventilation). The PACU may consist of an unstaffed corridor or a small designated space near the operating room complex exit. In this setting, it is paramount to ensure patients are more fully recovered from their anesthetic when they arrive in the recovery area than may be routine in well-resourced PACUs.

Equipment. Anesthesia Machines: Most modern anesthetic workstations cannot function without pressurized gases and electricity, both of which may be in short supply in many resource-constrained environments. In these settings, familiarity with drawover anesthesia may be essential. In-depth discussion of drawover anesthesia is beyond the scope of this chapter, however, knowledge of drawover anesthesia is highly relevant in many practice settings, and several comprehensive resources for learning drawover are included at the end of this chapter. Here we provide a brief overview of the basics of drawover anesthesia.

An inhalational anesthesia system must be able to deliver accurate concentrations of volatile agent, avoid rebreathing of carbon dioxide, have a provision for intermittent positive-pressure ventilation (IPPV), and provide oxygen-enriched gases. Unlike more complex anesthesia machines, drawover systems do not require compressed gas or power, can function on room air, and cannot deliver hypoxic gas mixtures (which is especially relevant where inspired oxygen monitors may be lacking). A drawover system consists of a temperature-compensated or buffered, low-resistance vaporizer (calibrated to the agent), a self-inflating bag or bellows with a one-way valve upstream to ensure unidirectional gas flow to the patient, and a non-rebreather valve at the patient end to avoid rebreathing of carbon dioxide (Fig. 2.18). Drawover setups that can function with multiple volatile agents are most versatile (i.e., in the event that one volatile agent is unavailable), and providers should be familiar with technical aspects of using the same vaporizer for different volatile agents. The self-inflating bellows (SIB) can be used for IPPV (by hand) and may show movement or a small palpable pressure change with respiration that enables the anesthesia provider to monitor respiratory rate in the spontaneous mode. Air is the "driving" gas (although "sucking" gas might be a more accurate description) in a drawover system, but oxygen supplementation is possible with addition of oxygen at the vaporizer inlet or with the addition of a piece of reservoir tubing or bag. The ability to function on ambient air is a critical safety feature of all drawover setups. Without some form of reservoir, it is impossible to achieve a fraction of inspired oxygen concentration (FiO2) above 0.3 regardless of oxygen flow. With just one meter of standard adult reservoir tubing (22 mm diameter), 4 L per minute can give an FiO_2 of over 0.6 and a flow of 1 L per minute gives an FiO_2 of 0.3. The gas flow, which is dependent on the patient's tidal volume and respiratory rate, is highly variable, but most vaporizers (OMV, DDV, EMO) (see Fig. 2.18) remain extremely accurate as long as the gas flow is intermittent. However, they often lose their accuracy when the system is converted to a continuous flow mode.

Although the drawover system is low resistance, in some situations it may be advisable to convert it to a continuous flow system when anesthetizing babies to overcome the dead space at the level of the non-rebreather valve. This can be done manually by creating a flow using either an Oxford inflating bellows or self-inflating bag. The bellows are jerked up to their full capacity and then released slowly. This is done 6 times per minute to create a continuous flow through the vaporizer. This flow of oxygen-enriched air supplies an Ayre's T-piece attached to the outlet of the bellows. Both valves need to be in use to ensure unidirectional flow as this is still a low-pressure system (Fig. 2.19). If using a self-inflating bag then it must be squeezed and released 12 times per minute. This manual system mimics adult drawover with a more intermittent flow, and the vaporizers tend to still provide an accurate reading as opposed to full continuous flow using either a Farman's entrainer or direct attachment of an oxygen source to the inlet of a vaporizer. Whatever equipment you have at your disposal it is probably simpler to follow these approximate guidelines:

If <5 kg, assisted ventilation for whatever the length of the operation.
If 5-10 kg, spontaneous ventilation for short cases and assisted ventilation for longer procedures.
If >10 kg, spontaneous ventilation for most operations, unless paralysis is required or the procedure is prolonged.

There are a small number of all-in-one drawover anesthetic machines based on the same principles as the portable drawover systems (Fig. 2.20). They are not plenum machines, and supplemental oxygen can be supplied from a cylinder or an integrated oxygen concentrator. These machines are significantly less expensive and relatively easier to maintain than many other anesthesia machines. They can also function without power and without supplemental or pressurized oxygen, making them ideal for some resource-constrained settings. Integrated, uninterruptable power supplies (UPS) provide power for certain functions (e.g., monitors) in the event of power failure, and some versions include integrated ventilators. The companies that manufacture the Universal Anesthesia Machine (Gradian Health) and the Glostavent (Diamedica [UK] Ltd) both invest considerable resources to ensure local expertise for operation, training, and service support. These elements are critical for successful utilization of equipment in resource-constrained settings. Regardless of the anesthesia setup employed, a plan for power or oxygen failure is essential and likely to differ based on the setting.

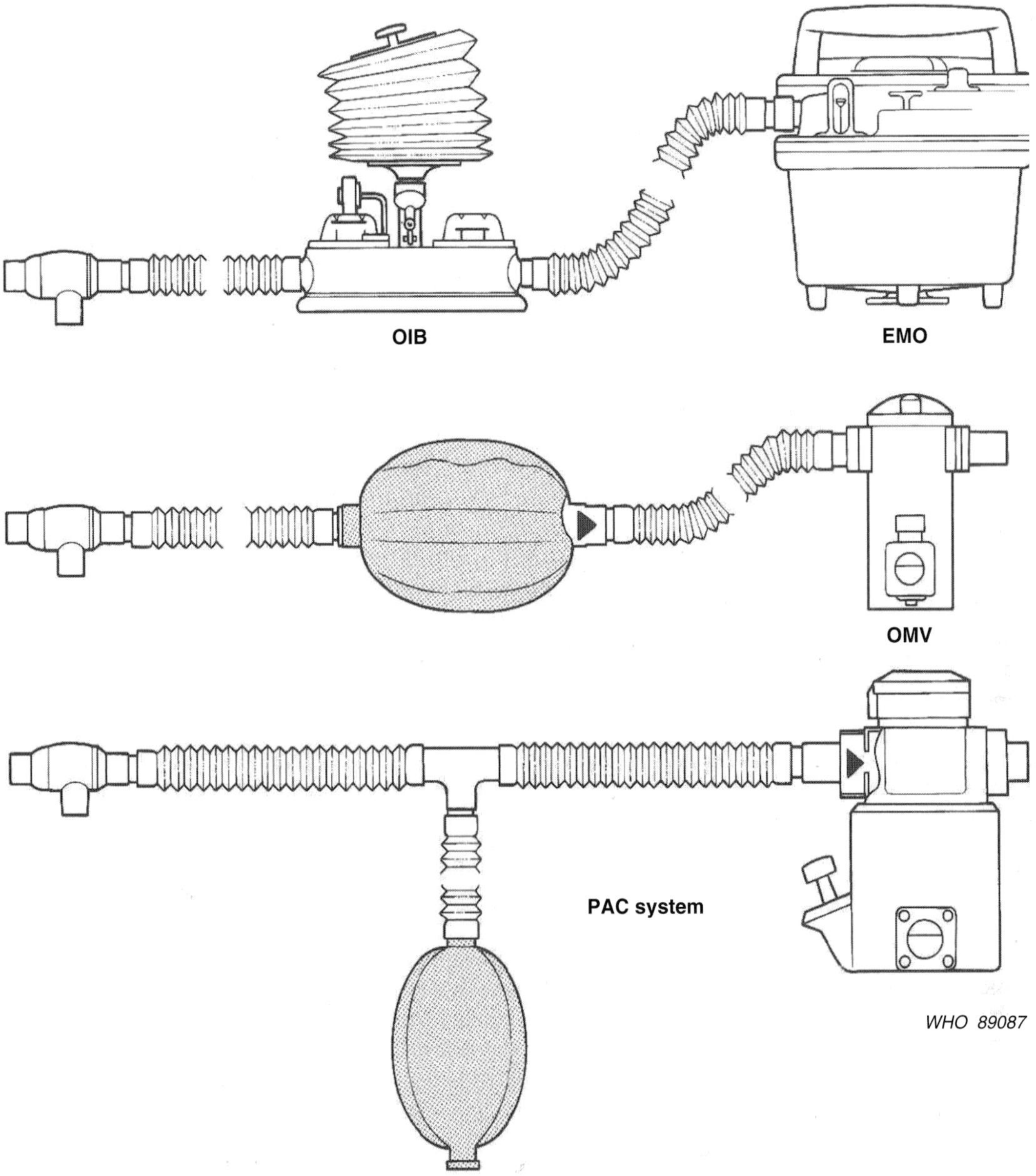

OIB

EMO

OMV

PAC system

WHO 89087

Fig. 2.18 Inhalational drawover anesthesia setups. (Reproduced with permission from the WHO. Dobson MB, World Health Organization. *Anaesthesia at the District Hospital*. 2nd ed. Geneva: World Health Organization. http://www.who.int/iris/handle/10665/42193.)

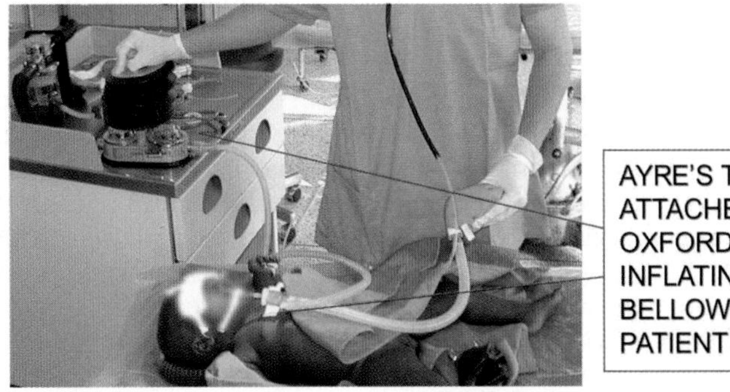

Fig. 2.19 Drawover anesthesia using an Oxford-inflating bellows and Ayre's T-piece with a pediatric patient in Uganda. (Copyright © 2018 Sarah Hodges.)

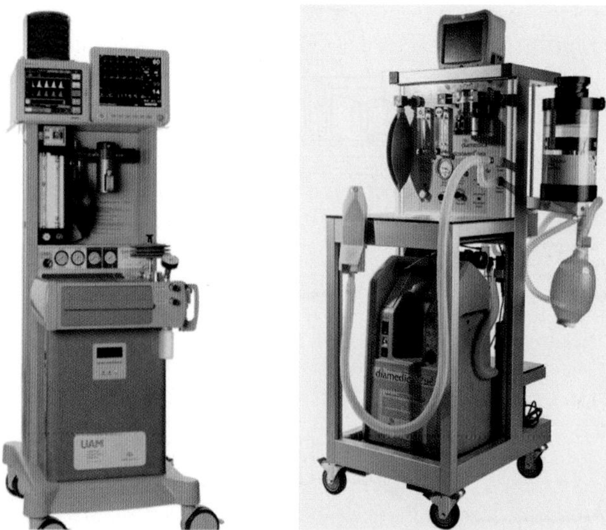

Fig. 2.20 All-in-one drawover anesthesia machines. *Left,* The Universal Anesthesia Machine by Gradian Health (including ventilator module). *Right,* The Glostavent Helix by Diamedica (UK) Ltd. (Copyright © 2018 Gradian Health and Diamedica [UK] Ltd.)

Oxygen Concentrators: In many countries pressurized oxygen is available primarily via cylinders, but the supply may be unreliable or cost prohibitive, and therefore a backup is essential. Providers working in resource-constrained settings should have familiarity with at least the basics of function and maintenance for various oxygen delivery solutions including concentrators. Oxygen concentrators use a technique called pressure swing adsorption and zeolite crystals to extract nitrogen from air to produce oxygen with 90% to 96% purity, although purity drops to around 85% with higher flow rates. In principle, most oxygen concentrators are relatively similar, and non-engineers can often diagnose and fix common problems (e.g., dirty filters, low voltage, compressor or valve system failure, excess flow, or hot ambient temperatures)[226] (see the Appendix 1 for links and useful resources including the WHO guide to oxygen concentrator maintenance). In reality, not all oxygen concentrators are designed to function in all climates, and many do not conform to WHO guidelines.[226,227] In a performance study of eight oxygen concentrators, only two models delivered greater than 82% inspired oxygen concentration at 35°C and 50% relative humidity.[228] Oxygen concentrators can be used to provide supplemental oxygen in the operating theater (via drawover system), the PACU, or the ward. Makeshift splitting of a single oxygen source to supply multiple patients on the ward is a common practice although it can easily result in inadequate inspired oxygen fractions. A small, portable oxygen analyzer can be useful to test the output of concentrators and cylinders as some facilities lack the infrastructure to ensure necessary quality control. Submerging the terminal end of parallel oxygen delivery circuits into cups of water can allow for comparison of gas flow rates.

Monitors: Many operating theaters around the world have minimal monitoring options despite the international standards set out by the WHO and WFSA.[3] In this environment there is increased reliance on clinical skills (e.g., change in palpable pulse volume, degree of chest expansion, pupil size, and change in compliance of bellows, self-inflating bag, or bag on Ayre's T-piece). Because electricity may be unreliable, ideally monitors should have a functional internal battery. Pulse oximetry is invaluable but not universally available. Some inexpensive pulse oximeters meet international quality standards, however, few are designed for harsh environments, and many are extremely inaccurate.[229] The Lifebox initiative is one of the first initiatives to help design and distribute pulse oximeters that meet the demands of LMICs (i.e., affordable, accurate, durable, with audible alarms and specially designed, reusable probes that work with neonates and adults).[230] Precordial stethoscopes are particularly useful and can be made from an ordinary stethoscope with an extension (e.g., suction tube or oxygen tubing). Precordial stethoscopes provide an excellent beat-to-beat heart rate monitor and continuous, audible verification of respiratory rate, airway patency, and endotracheal tube placement. Hypovolemia may be detectable by a decrease in heartbeat tone that is apparent prior to alarms on other monitors.

Airway Equipment: In resource-limited settings it is often absolutely essential to maintain spontaneous respiration and oxygenation with a difficult airway until the airway has been secured. Face mask ventilation with a Guedel or nasopharyngeal airway, regional anesthesia, or ketamine-based anesthetics may be safer than attempting complex airway management. An awake look with direct laryngoscopy can often assist in airway management planning. Safety is key and it may be preferable to opt for a tracheostomy under local anesthesia as the surgical skills may be superior to what is feasible with the limited anesthetic equipment and ability. As advanced airway equipment and experienced assistance is likely to be lacking, excellent technique and positioning for laryngoscopy is crucial for success. Many hospitals providing surgical care will have only a Macintosh size 3 laryngoscope blade, and rarely additional equipment such as a bougie. Retrograde intubation and blind nasal intubation can be useful skills to master. Airway topicalization can be accomplished many ways, including transtracheal lidocaine injection or by gargling or spraying water-based lubricant jelly, lidocaine, and epinephrine. For blind nasal intubation, the tube is pushed forward during inspiration following the base of the nose, listening to the noise of breathing (similar technique to a Patil guide). If the tube enters the esophagus the neck should be extended, and if it impinges on the anterior part of the larynx, the neck should be flexed. Lifting the jaw will stop the endotracheal tube from hitting the epiglottis. Rotating the tube or inflating the cuff slightly may also assist with entering the trachea. If capnography is not available then condensation in the tube, movement of the bag with respiration, auscultation of the chest, and in rare circumstances an esophageal bulb can help verify correct placement. In LMICs, laryngeal mask airways may not be available and face masks, Guedel or nasopharyngeal airways, and endotracheal tubes are often washed and reused. There are a number of products that can be used to easily decontaminate endotracheal tubes, laryngeal mask airways, and other airway equipment, however, access is highly variable. When processing and reusing such equipment, damage to the cuff and increasing stiffness of the plastic are significant challenges.

Endotracheal tube stylets are infrequently available. Improvised endotracheal tube introducers have been crafted by carefully inserting a piece of wire into an appropriately sized suction catheter, taking care that the metal tip is not protruding. Learning safe, sensible techniques that are reproducible without the use of expensive, specialized equipment is fundamental. Where traditional electric suction is unavailable, bulb suction (for neonates) and foot pedal suction devices are invaluable.

Equipment for regional anesthesia: Spinal anesthesia is universally taught and used in many settings though may be used for a wider variety of cases than is commonly done in HICs (e.g., appendectomy). The needles vary in quality and blunt tips can be overcome by using a 21-gauge hypodermic needle as an introducer. The most commonly used local anesthetic is hyperbaric 0.5% bupivacaine. All anesthetic providers are taught to do spinals, but not all are taught how to prevent supine hypotension during spinal anesthesia. Teaching how to fabricate a simple wedge for uterine tilt with pregnant patients, or learning to reposition patients in varying degrees of reverse Trendelendberg position may prevent untoward incidents especially where an adjustable operating table may not exist. Although a spinal might seem like an easier and safer option, appropriate patient selection is critical, especially where preferred vasopressors and fluids may be in short supply. In that situation 0.5 mg epinephrine has been diluted in a 500 mL bottle of 5% dextrose and administered cautiously to treat the hypotension. Epidurals are rarely available in low-resource settings for several reasons: providers may not be proficient with the technique; needles are not commonly found; preservative-free local anesthetic drugs are not readily available for postoperative infusions; and more importantly, the staffing ratio may be inadequate and the knowledge may be insufficient to manage an infusion in the postoperative setting. In some settings where electronic drug infusion pumps are unavailable, low-cost elastomeric bulb pumps can be used to deliver a fixed rate of medication. Caudal blocks using a 22-G cannula are commonly used in children for postoperative pain management although the only safe preparation of local anesthetic may be the spinal bupivacaine.

Ultrasound or nerve stimulators are rarely available but many blocks can be performed using landmark or blind techniques (e.g., ankle, digital, axillary, penile, wrist, fascia iliaca, femoral, and rectus sheath blocks). Local field blocks may be used for a wide variety of procedures, including hernias, which are often done under local anesthesia in the outpatient setting. Where ultrasounds are available, other regional supplies may be lacking such as ultrasound gel, probe covers, echogenic needles, and appropriate local anesthetics. Several workarounds to these common challenges have been well-described. Although many blocks can be done relatively easily and safely without ultrasound or nerve stimulation, serious complications can still occur. Anecdotal reports of local anesthetic toxicity fatalities during penile blocks for circumcision are still encountered in some LICs and attributed to preventable causes (incorrect dosing or technique).[231] In general, distal blocks with lower volume and shorter-acting local anesthetics may be safer options, especially where safety equipment may be limited (e.g., intralipid).

Equipment for venous access: Intravenous cannulas are almost universally obtainable but variable quality may limit use. Needles may be blunt or extend quite a few millimeters beyond the tip of the cannula. Scalp veins are a common site for insertion in critically-ill infants, and with appropriate training, rapid placement of a cannula in the right internal jugular vein or in the peritoneal cavity can be lifesaving in a child dying from hypovolemic shock (e.g., cholera) as you look for a more permanent solution. Intraosseous needles are not easily found, but 18-G or 16-G needles can be used in the tibia of an infant. Butterfly needles, if available, are particularly useful because of the limited length. Twisting is essential to pierce the cortex until a sudden give when entering the medullary cavity. It is feasible to perform anesthesia for an entire operation with such access (Fig. 2.21).

Infusions pumps are often not available in LMICs and when present, are frequently limited by the availability of compatible disposables (i.e., appropriately sized syringes or proprietary tubing). It is important to not only be proficient with calculating infusion rates based on drop factor (drops per mL) but also be aware that infusion sets vary in size and quality, often making accurate calibration challenging.

Drugs. Volatile agents: Ether has now been removed from the WHO Essential Medicines List, and its use has reduced dramatically since 2013. Both isoflurane and halothane are included in the WHO Essential Medicines List, and due to the price differential (e.g., in Uganda 250 mL of halothane ~$21; 250 mL of isoflurane ~$39; 250 mL of sevoflurane ~$250), halothane is the most commonly used agent in many rural or non-teaching hospitals in LICs. Halothane is potent (MAC 0.8%) and sweet smelling, but the blood gas partition coefficient is 2.4 making the onset and offset of anesthesia slower than some agents. This can be useful if managing a difficult airway and intubation under halothane alone. Halothane is a cardio-depressant and arrhythmogenic especially in the presence of an elevated end-tidal carbon dioxide. It is useful for inhalational induction, but it is important to rapidly reduce the inspired concentration once intravenous access is

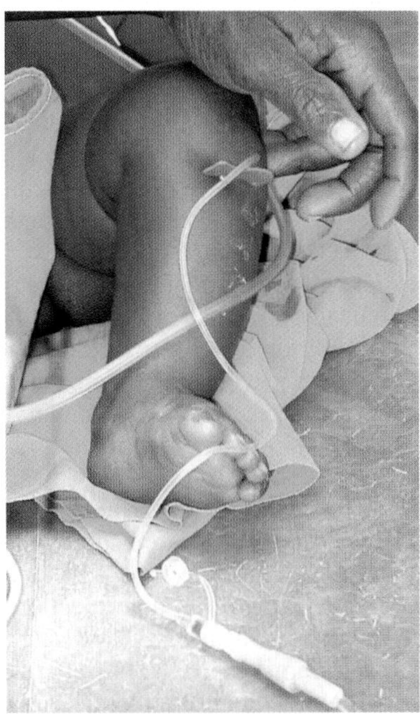

Fig. 2.21 Improvised intraosseous access catheter in a pediatric patient in Uganda. (Copyright © 2018 Sarah Hodges.)

secured. Nitrous oxide may be obtainable in some locations (primarily urban areas) but can be extremely expensive. Because medical-grade air (FiO_2 0.21) is often 4 to 5 times more expensive than oxygen, it is often unavailable and cases may be done on 100% inspired oxygen concentration.

Induction agents: The use of propofol is widespread but ketamine (in addition to volatile agents) remains the most ubiquitous induction agent in many LMICs. Thiopentone (thiopental) is also frequently encountered outside of HICs. Ketamine resembles an intravenous preparation of ether (sympathomimetic, does not depress airway reflexes, causes excessive salivation, and has excellent analgesic properties). S-ketamine is a useful adjunct for regional anesthesia. Ketamine can be used as an infusion (intravenous or subcutaneous injection) postoperatively for the management of pain especially if opioids are in short supply.[232] Ketamine can also be used for total intravenous anesthesia for a variety of procedures (e.g., laparotomies), but the wakeup can be very prolonged, and the patient may experience disturbing hallucinations as benzodiazepines are often not used (provider more likely to encounter diazepam than midazolam in resource-constrained settings). Ketamine is the "go-to" induction agent for any patient in hypovolemic or septic shock, but it can cause cardiac arrest in patients who are maximally sympathetically stimulated. Ketamine may be advised against as the sole anesthetic for pregnant patients undergoing non-obstetric procedures due to its potential oxytocic effects. Ketamine can also cause apnea in neonates, despite the appearance of the neonate moving in response to surgery. Special attention and caution must be emphasized in these patient populations. Because of ketamine's overall safety profile, the drug has been used as the basis for a 5-day course to teach mid-level non-anesthesia providers to administer emergency anesthesia in rural sub-Saharan Africa when no anesthesia provider is available. This program has generated significant controversy and highlights many of the challenges facing the provision of anesthesia in LMICs.[233,234]

Analgesics: Morphine is often the most readily available opioid, although for many LMICs it is frequently challenging to obtain. In some countries where palliative care is more developed (e.g., Uganda), the oral formulation is often available for postoperative analgesia. Pethidine (meperidine) is commonly encountered in LMICs and used routinely for perioperative analgesia. Of note, pethidine is not included in the WHO Essential Medicines List, and it is not recommended for routine acute postoperative pain because of its variable efficacy and side effects. Nonetheless, pethidine may be the only option for analgesia in some LMICs and general familiarity with its pharmacology could be highly useful in select settings (see Chapter 24). As discussed earlier in this chapter, opiophobia and access limitations significantly restrict the use of opiates. As a result, if available, opiates are rarely prescribed beyond 48 hours postoperatively in many resource-constrained settings. Many analgesics (e.g., ketamine, morphine, and pethidine) are frequently given by intramuscular injection, which may have benefits in terms of feasibility and safety, although supporting data are limited.[232] Patient-controlled analgesia is generally unavailable, but in some settings has been substituted by using a small subcutaneous cannula, often placed over the deltoid muscle, used solely for parenteral opiate analgesics. This avoids repeated intramuscular injections especially in children and can remain in place for 48 to 72 hours. Tramadol is pervasive, inexpensive, and often used for perioperative pain management in resource-limited settings. Use of tramadol requires an understanding of its limitations including side effects, abuse potential, and inferiority in many instances to opioid analgesia.

Paracetamol (acetaminophen) is widely available as tablets, suppositories, syrups, and as an intravenous preparation as are nonsteroidal antiinflammatory drugs. Parenteral preparations vary from country to country as does the potency depending on the country of manufacture. Diclofenac is commonly found and intramuscularly injected. One of the major challenges with prescribing analgesics is conveying the concept of multimodal analgesia. Although the full spectrum of analgesic modalities may not be available, multiple analgesic options, including regional anesthesia, are often feasible in low-resource settings.

Muscle relaxants: Suxamethonium (succinylcholine) is a universally available muscle relaxant and may be the safest paralytic to use if there are no means for mechanical ventilation or availability for reversal. It rarely causes malignant hyperpyrexia although it can induce masseter spasm especially in children with neurologic or muscular disorders. Both atracurium and suxamethonium lose potency with exposure to heat and maintaining cold storage is a significant challenge in many settings. For cases where surgeons prefer paralysis for closure (e.g., laparotomy), a small dose of suxamethonium can be administered at the end of the case to facilitate closure of the peritoneum and rectus, while hand ventilating the patient and allowing faster offset of the volatile agent. The availability of nondepolarizing neuromuscular blocking agents is highly variable, and providers should be prepared to use drugs they may not readily use in HICs.

Lack of access to transfusion services (as discussed in the section, Anesthesia and Global Health) is another commonly encountered problem that may require improvisation. Providers in resource-constrained settings may be tasked with ABO typing (e.g., EldonCard) and cross-matching and should be familiar with these techniques. Whole blood transfusion may be more common than component therapy, although there are several notable limitations (including potential loss of platelet and clotting factor activity with refrigeration). Absolute transfusion thresholds are lacking but can create significant dilemmas. For example, is it safe to perform a hernia with a hemoglobin of 9, 8, 7, or lower if no blood products are available? Direct donation from patients or relatives as well as mandatory exchange (i.e., someone must donate in order for units to be released from the blood bank) are variably practiced in LMICs. Other practices such as preoperative normovolemic hemodilution and makeshift intraoperative blood salvaging (e.g., by using a cup, gauze filter, anticoagulant, and a 60 mL syringe) have been reported, but as of yet there is no safe, effective substitute for transfusion services in many settings.[235,236]

Patients. Anesthesia providers in resource-constrained settings must be comfortable with a wide range of potential surgical patients, especially trauma, obstetric (e.g., postpartum hemorrhage), and pediatric patients. In many LMICs, more than 50% of the population is under the age of 18, and most have fewer comorbidities and less polypharmacy than in HICs. On the other hand, patients often present late with advanced pathology. This may be due to a wide range of factors affecting access to care, including physical access to the health unit (unpassable roads in the rainy season, or insecurity on the roads), or they have been consulting the local healer or bone setter and have not seen any improvement, or they are financially destitute and all health care is financially and socially draining.

As relatives often provide most of the in-hospital care (e.g., cook the food, wash the bedding and clothes), an inpatient stay is extremely time consuming and no family will want their patient to be in hospital longer than necessary. Patients will mobilize more rapidly but may also be less compliant with postoperative instructions. Although patients may have lower incidence of chronic cardiac and respiratory comorbidities, many may be anemic, malnourished, or harboring low-grade malaria or helminth infections. If major surgery is being considered, existing maladies may need to be treated first and can prolong the inpatient stay. Multiple preoperative investigations may not be affordable or feasible and many decisions are made solely on clinical judgment.

Anesthesia providers practicing in LMICs must be familiar with perioperative optimization of commonly encountered conditions. Treatment for universally common conditions such as hypertension or diabetes may require context-specific approaches and insights (e.g., where and how to provide temperature-stable, noncounterfeit medications).

The practice of anesthesia in the resource-limited setting is shackled by many issues, and it can be challenging to attempt to administer a high level of care as advocated by many professional entities. Anesthesia safety is an essential component of care. Are there standards of care that are immutable across the globe? If a full term pregnant woman is admitted to hospital with a severe antepartum hemorrhage that requires an emergency cesarean section to save the mother and baby, what is the anesthetic of choice? Is it local anesthetic infiltration alone, intermittent aliquots of intravenous ketamine and oxygen via nasal cannula, rapid sequence induction with ketamine, suxamethonium, and halothane? Then add to that decision the reality that the anesthetic provider may be a nurse with 1 year of training in anesthesia, only 250 mL of compatible blood is available in the hospital, and there is no pediatrician to resuscitate the baby. What is the safest anesthetic technique? It is difficult to answer that question, but for anyone planning to work in an LMIC as an anesthetic provider it is indispensable to learn about the local resources, to listen to the local providers, to have the humility to not have all the answers, but above all to focus on the care and safety of the patient.

GLOBAL HEALTH COMPETENCIES

Although the number of global health opportunities for medical trainees has skyrocketed in recent years, most are short-term, elective-based rotations, and relatively few programs offer structured training in global health competencies.[237]

Although many anesthesia providers may not be directly involved with formal global health initiatives or careers that focus on underserved populations, there are fundamental global health competencies that are relevant to all anesthesia providers (whether in high, middle, or LICs). A broad understanding of key concepts is universally relevant and should be incorporated into anesthesia training for all providers. These include access and affordability, local and global disease burden, structural and social determinants of health, medical ethics, health equity, and social justice. The Consortium of Universities for Global Health (CUGH) has identified 11 competency domains, with four levels of competency per domain (ranging from level I for all providers with any relation to global health, to level IV for providers planning to have significant lifelong engagement in global health) (Box 2.5).[238]

For anesthesia providers who intend to spend a portion of their career focused on global health, additional training should be considered in topics such as: epidemiology, statistics, qualitative research, health policy, health systems, health economics, medical anthropology, demography, ethics, and implementation and management sciences, among others.

Providers from relatively well-resourced settings benefit from preparation before working in resource-constrained settings, even if only for short-term visits.[239] Several nonclinical challenges and pitfalls are routinely encountered in resource-constrained settings, including failure to provide context-appropriate interventions (see discussion on equipment donations in the section on infrastructure challenges), failure to have a follow-up plan, failure to adequately engage local stakeholders, overemphasizing short-term solutions, and draining local resources.[240,241] Certain ethical challenges are also commonly encountered and often relate to the appropriate scope of practice, the equitable distribution of local and external resources, and an inadequate understanding of local social and cultural norms.

In a survey of surgery and anesthesia trainees at a large Ugandan university with numerous visiting international collaborators, most trainees (75%) agreed that visiting groups improve their training. However, 40% of trainees reported that international groups had a neutral or negative impact on patient care. Only 15% felt that research

BOX 2.5 CUGH Global Health Competency Domains

Domain 1—Global Burden of Disease
Domain 2—Globalization of Health and Health Care
Domain 3—Social and Environmental Determinants of Health
Domain 4—Capacity Strengthening
Domain 5—Collaboration, Partnering, and Communication
Domain 6—Ethics
Domain 7—Professional Practice
Domain 8—Health Equity and Social Justice
Domain 9—Program Management
Domain 10—Sociocultural and Political Awareness
Domain 11—Strategic Analysis

CUGH, Consortium of Universities for Global Health.

CUGH Competencies reproduced under Creative Commons 4 Licensing from Jogerst K, Callender B, Adams V, et al. Identifying interprofessional global health competencies for 21st-century health professionals. *Ann Glob Health*. 2015;81:239–247. https://doi.org/10.1016/j.aogh.2015.03.006.

projects conducted by international groups were in local priority areas, and approximately one third of trainees (31%) reported discomfort with the ethics of clinical decisions made by visiting faculty.[242]

It is incumbent upon institutions that offer global health opportunities to provide formal training. Numerous resources exist to help equip trainees, providers, and institutions with the knowledge necessary to manage these challenges and maximize the positive impact of global health efforts (see the Appendix for links and useful resources).[243–246]

In some countries (e.g., the United Kingdom), anesthesia trainees can pursue 6-month to 1-year-long global health experiences, with formal curriculum and relatively long-term clinical, research, and educational components. Trainees are required to complete standardized assessments, including clinical evaluations and case-based discussions as outlined by the RCoA.[247] A relatively small yet increasing number of anesthesia programs in the United States and other countries are providing formal global health tracks for interested residents as well as formal anesthesia global health fellowships.[248] Academic institutions and the global anesthesia community at large must continue to expand training and career development opportunities that increase the number of anesthesiologists interested in and capable of improving equitable access to safe anesthesia worldwide.

Conclusions

Despite dramatic changes in anesthesia around the world over the past century, improvements in safety, access, and affordability have not been universal. At present, the majority of the world does not have access to safe anesthesia, surgical, or analgesia services, and relatively few resources are being devoted to address this growing crisis. The massive and growing surgical and pain crises disproportionately affect LMICs, where severe shortages of workforce and infrastructure, and impractical international regulations limit access to care. Despite many common misperceptions, anesthesia, analgesia, and surgical services are feasible in resource-constrained settings and are as cost-effective as many other public health interventions (e.g., vaccinations).

The neglect of pain and surgical disease by the global health community has resulted in one of the most inequitable global public health crises the world faces today. It has been only in recent years that the surgery, anesthesia, and global health communities have accelerated investment in research, education, and advocacy initiatives that aim to improve access to safe anesthesia and surgical services for the world's poor. These efforts are in their infancy and must be expanded and supported by the global anesthesia community. Factors affecting access to care, safety, and cost are relevant in all countries regardless of income level. All anesthesia providers should maintain awareness of the fundamental challenges facing the global anesthesia community, with the hope that increasing numbers will devote their careers to addressing issues of global health equity. There are many different ways for anesthesia providers to engage in global health at the patient level or system level, including research, advocacy, education, and clinical service.

The role of anesthesia in global health is easy for many to overlook, but the global anesthesia community must quickly increase efforts to actively lead global health initiatives that aim to improve infrastructure, expand workforce, increase translation of data into policy and practice, improve financial risk protection mechanisms for surgical patients, expand referral and prehospital systems, provide essential medicines, and ultimately improve access to safe and affordable anesthesia, surgical, and pain services worldwide.

Acknowledgments

The editors and publisher would like to thank the following collaborators for their contributions to this ever-evolving chapter: Maria Carmona, Deepak Tempe, Naoyuki Hirata, Michiaki Yamakage, Anis Baraka (deceased), Fouad Salim Haddad (deceased), Yury Polushin, Olga Afonin, Guillermo Lema, Florian Nuevo, Lars Eriksson, and D.G. Bogod.
This chapter greatly benefited from the contribution and thoughtful editing of Michael Cooper, Maytinee Lilaonitkul, Fred Bulamba, Cephas Mijumbi, and Doruk Ozgediz.

 **Complete references available online at expertconsult.com.**

References

1. Gelb AW, et al. *World J Surg*. 2015.
2. McQueen K, et al. *World J Surg*. 2015;39(9):2153–2160.
3. Gelb A, et al. *Can J Anaesth*. In Press. 2018.
4. Merry AF, et al. *Can J Anaesth*. 2010;57(11):1027–1034.
5. Meara JG, et al. *Lancet*. 2015.
6. Koplan JP, et al. *Lancet*. 2009;373(9679):1993–1995.
7. Fried LP, et al. *The Lancet*. 2010;375(9714):535–537.
8. Adams LV, et al. *BMC Med Educ*. 2016;16:296.
9. Merson MH. *N Engl J Med*. 2014;370(18):1676–1678.
10. Merson M, Chapman K. *The Dramatic Expansion of University Engagement in Global Health | Center for Strategic and International Studies*. Washington, D.C: Center for Strategic and International Studies; 2009. https://www.csis.org/analysis/dramatic-expansion-university-engagement-global-health. Accessed August 21, 2016.
11. Address by Dr. H. Mahler Director General of the WHO to the World Congress of the International College of Surgeons. 1980. http://www.who.int/surgery/strategies/Mahler1980speech.pdf?ua=1. Accessed March 8, 2018.
12. MacGowan WA. *Bull Am Coll Surg*. 1987;72(6):5–7, 9.
13. Wasunna AE. *Bull Am Coll Surg*. 1987;72(6):18–19.
14. Vaz F, et al. *Bull World Health Organ*. 1999;77(8):688–691.
15. Ouro-Bang'na Maman AF, et al. *Trop Doct*. 2005;35(4):220–222.
16. McCord C, Chowdhury Q. *Int J Gynaecol Obstet Off Organ Int Fed Gynaecol Obstet*. 2003;81(1):83–92.
17. Javitt JC. *Arch Ophthalmol Chic Ill 1960*. 1993;111(12):1615.
18. Luboga S, et al. *PLoS Med*. 2009;6(12):e1000200.
19. Jamison DT, et al., ed. *Disease Control Priorities in Developing Countries*. 2nd ed. Washington (DC): World Bank; 2006. http://www.ncbi.nlm.nih.gov/books/NBK11728/. Accessed January 18, 2016.
20. World Health Organization. *Patient Safety. WHO Guidelines for Safe Surgery 2009: Safe Surgery Saves Lives*; 2009. http://www.ncbi.nlm.nih.gov/books/NBK143243/. Accessed December 14, 2016.
21. Haynes AB, et al. *N Engl J Med*. 2009;360(5):491–499.
22. Farmer PE, Kim JY. *World J Surg*. 2008;32(4):533–536.
23. Ozgediz D, Riviello R. *PLoS Med*. 2008;5(6).
24. 68th World Health Assembly. WHO. http://www.who.int/surgery/wha-eb/en/. Published May 2015. Accessed March 8, 2018.
25. Botman M, et al. *World J Surg*. 2015;39(6):1335–1340.

26. Debas H, et al., ed. *Disease Control Priorities 3. Vol Essential Surgery*. 3rd ed. World Bank Group; 2015. http://dcp-3.org/surgery
27. Jim Yong Kim - Inaugural Lancet Commission on Global Surgery 2014. YouTube; 2014. https://www.youtube.com/watch?v=61iM4Qjk-q4. Accessed March 8, 2018.
28. Jamison DT, et al. *The Lancet*. 2013;382(9908):1898–1955.
29. United Nations Sustainable Development Goals. U N Sustain Dev. http://www.un.org/sustainabledevelopment/health/. Accessed August 25, 2016.
30. Knaul FM, et al. *The Lancet*. 2017;0(0).
31. Dare AJ, et al. *The Lancet*. 2014;384(9961):2245–2247.
32. GBD 2016 DALYs and HALE Collaborators. *Lancet Lond Engl*. 2017;390(10100):1260–1344.
33. Gallup JL, Sachs JD. *The Economic Burden of Malaria*. American Society of Tropical Medicine and Hygiene; 2001. https://www.ncbi.nlm.nih.gov/books/NBK2624/. Accessed April 24, 2018.
34. Murray CJ. *Bull World Health Organ*. 1994;72(3):429–445.
35. Murray CJ, et al. *Bull World Health Organ*. 1994;72(3):495–509.
36. Gosselin R, et al. *World J Surg*. 2013;37(11):2507–2511.
37. Vos T, et al. *The Lancet*. 2017;390(10100):1211–1259.
38. Goldberg DS, McGee SJ. *BMC Public Health*. 2011;11:770.
39. Parker R, et al. *J Int AIDS Soc*. 2014;17(1).
40. Alkema L, et al. *The Lancet*. 2016;387(10017):462–474.
41. WHO cancer fact sheet. World Health Organization. http://www.who.int/news-room/fact-sheets/detail/cancer. Accessed June 24, 2018.
42. Funk LM, et al. *Lancet Lond Engl*. 2010;376(9746):1055–1061.
42a. https://www.who.int/bulletin/online_first/18-216028.pdf. Accessed March 11, 2019.
43. Weiser TG, et al. *The Lancet*. 2008;372(9633):139–144.
44. Alkire BC, et al. *Lancet Glob Health*. 2015;3(6):e316–e323.
45. Khubchandani JA, et al. *Surgery*. 2018;163(2):243–250.
46. Cintron A, Morrison RS. *J Palliat Med*. 2006;9(6):1454–1473.
47. "Please, do not make us suffer any more..." | Access to Pain Treatment as a Human Right. Human Rights Watch. https://www.hrw.org/report/2009/03/03/please-do-not-make-us-suffer-any-more/access-pain-treatment-human-right. Published March 3, 2009. Accessed March 15, 2018.
48. Brennan F, et al. *Anesth Analg*. 2007;105(1):205–221.
49. Lohman D, et al. *BMC Med*. 2010;8:8.
50. Seya M-J, et al. *J Pain Palliat Care Pharmacother*. 2011;25(1):6–18.
51. PPSG Opioid Consumption Map. https://ppsg.medicine.wisc.edu/. Accessed March 5, 2018.
52. International Narcotics Control Board, United Nations. *Availability of Internationally Controlled Drugs: Ensuring Adequate Access for Medical and Scientific Purposes : Indispensable, Adequately Available and Not Unduly Restricted*; 2016.
53. Berterame S, et al. *The Lancet*. 2016;387(10028):1644–1656.
54. Rasu RS, Knell ME. *Pain Med Malden Mass*. 2018;19(3):524–532.
55. Pletcher MJ, et al. *JAMA*. 2008;299(1):70–78.
56. Singhal A, et al. *PloS One*. 2016;11(8):e0159224.
57. Bainbridge D, et al. *Lancet Lond Engl*. 2012;380(9847):1075–1081.
58. Beecher HK, Todd DP. *Ann Surg*. 1954;140(1):2–35.
59. Lagasse RS. *Anesthesiology*. 2002;97(6):1609–1617.
60. Rickard JL, et al. *World J Surg*. 2016;40(4):784–790.
61. Heywood AJ, et al. *Ann R Coll Surg Engl*. 1989;71(6):354–358.
62. Watters DA, et al. *World J Surg*. 2015;39(4):856–864.
63. Ng-Kamstra JS, et al. *The Lancet*. 2015;385:S29.
64. Ng-Kamstra J, et al. *J Am Coll Surg*. 2017;225(4):S107.
65. Biccard BM, et al. *Lancet Lond Engl*. 2018.
66. Walker IA, Wilson IH. *The Lancet*. 2008;371(9617):968–969.
67. Maman AO-B, et al. *Trop Doct*. 2005;35(4):220–222.
68. Hansen D, et al. *Trop Doct*. 2000;30(3):146–149.
69. Glenshaw M, Madzimbamuto FD. *Cent Afr J Med*. 2005;51(3-4):39–44.
70. Sama HD, et al. *Ann Fr Anesth Réanimation*. 2013;32(11):818–819.
71. Saving Mothers 2014-2016: Seventh triennial report on confidential enquiries into maternal deaths in South Africa: short report. 2018. http://www.midwivessociety.co.za/downloads/Short_report_Saving_Mothers_2014-2016_7th_triennial_report.pdf. Accessed May 1, 2018.
72. Sobhy S, et al. *Lancet Glob Health*. 2016;4(5):e320–e327.
73. Shrime MG, et al. *Lancet Glob Health*. 2015;3(suppl 2):S38–44.
74. De Lima L, et al. *J Pain Palliat Care Pharmacother*. 2004;18(1):59–70.
75. Jenny HE, et al. *BMJ Glob Health*. 2017;2(2): bmjgh-2016-000167.
76. Worldbank country data. https://data.worldbank.org/country/india. Published 2018. Accessed April 24, 2018.
77. Albutt K, et al. *PloS One*. 2018;13(4):e0195986.
78. Chu KM, et al. *Arch Surg Chic Ill 1960*. 2010;145(8):721–725.
79. Bhandari A, et al. *Health Aff (Millwood)*. 2008;27(4):964–976.
80. Narayana Hrudayalaya: a model for accessible, affordable health care? knowledge@wharton. http://knowledge.wharton.upenn.edu/article/narayana-hrudayalaya-a-model-for-accessible-affordable-health-care/. Accessed June 22, 2018.
81. Samad L, et al. *World J Surg*. 2015;39(1):21–28.
82. Bertram MY, et al. *Bull World Health Organ*. 2016;94(12):925–930.
83. Hutubessy R, et al. *Cost Eff Resour Alloc CE*. 2003;1:8.
84. Chao TE, et al. *Lancet Glob Health*. 2014;2(6):e334–e345.
85. Yap A, et al. *Surgery*. 2018.
86. Copenhagen Consensus Expert Panel Findings. 2012. http://www.copenhagenconsensus.com/sites/default/files/outcome_document_updated_1105.pdf. Accessed March 6, 2019.
87. Dieleman JL, et al. *Lancet Glob Health*. 2015;3(suppl 2):S2–4.
88. Shawar YR, et al. *Lancet Glob Health*. 2015;3(8):e487–e495.
89. Shiffman J, et al. *Int J Health Policy Manag*. 2017;6(4):183–189.
90. Dare AJ, et al. *PLOS Med*. 2016;13(5):e1002023.
91. Lipnick MS, et al. *Anesth Analg*. 2017;125(3):1049–1052.
92. Mbonye AK, et al. *Int J Gynecol Obstet*. 2007;98(3):285–290.
93. Epiu I, et al. *BMC Pregnancy Childbirth*. 2017;17(1):387.
94. Epiu I, et al. *BMC Anesthesiol*. 2016;16(1):60.
95. Baird M, et al. *The Anesthesiologist Workforce in 2013: A Final Briefing to the American Society of Anesthesiologists*; 2014. https://www.rand.org/content/dam/rand/pubs/research_reports/RR600/RR650/RAND_RR650.pdf. Accessed June 22, 2018.
96. Baird M, et al. *Anesthesiology*. 2015;123(5):997–1012.
97. Abenstein J, et al. *Anesthesiology*. 2002;96(supp 2):A1131.
98. Crandall M, et al. *Am J Public Health*. 2013;103(6):1103–1109.
99. Holmer H, et al. *Lancet Lond Engl*. 2015;385(suppl 2):S40.
100. Kempthorne P, et al. *Anesth Analg*. 2017;125(3):981–990.
101. Holmer H, et al. *Lancet Glob Health*. 2015;3(suppl 2):S9–11.
102. Cherian M, et al. *Bull World Health Organ*. 2010;88(8):637–639.
103. Galukande M, et al. *East Cent Afr J Surg*. 2006;11:11–24.
104. Lipnick M, et al. *World J Surg*. 2012;37(3):488–497.
105. Hewitt-Smith A, et al. *Anaesthesia*. 2018;73(3):284–294.
106. Nurse Anesthetist Training Programs – AIC Kijabe Hospital. http://kijabehospital.org/postgraduate-training/nurse-anesthetist-training-programs. Accessed April 27, 2018.
107. Binagwaho A, et al. *N Engl J Med*. 2013;369(21):2054–2059.
108. Zoumenou E, et al. *Anesth Analg*. 2018;126(4):1321–1328.
109. Thind A, et al. In: Debas HT, Donkor P, Gawande A, Jamison DT, Kruk ME, Mock CN, eds. *Essential Surgery: Disease Control Priorities*. 3rd ed. Vol. 1. Washington (DC): The International Bank for Reconstruction and Development / The World Bank; 2015. http://www.ncbi.nlm.nih.gov/books/NBK333513/. Accessed April 21, 2018.
110. Chao TE, et al. *World J Surg*. 2012;36(11):2545–2553.
111. World Health Organization. Tool for Situational Analysis to Assess Emergency and Essential Surgical Care. http://www.who.int/surgery/publications/QuickSitAnalysisEESCsurvey.pdf. Accessed April 4, 2017.
112. WHO, Harvard PGSSC. WHO-PGSSC surgical assessment tool (SAT) hospital walkthrough tool. http://docs.wixstatic.com/ugd/346076_b9d8e8796eb945fe9bac7e7e35c512b1.pdf. Accessed June 7, 2017.
113. SOS PIPES Surgical Capacity Assessment Tool. Surgeons Overseas. https://www.surgeonsoverseas.org/resources/. Accessed April 4, 2017.
114. Hodges SC, et al. *Anaesthesia*. 2007;62(1):4–11.
115. Evans FM, et al. Availability of essential anesthetic medicines in resource-poor countries in Africa and Central America. Scientific Abstract. American Society of Anesthesiologists.
116. World Federation of Societies of Anaesthesiologists - anesthesia facility assessment tool (AFAT). https://www.wfsahq.org/afat. Published 2018. Accessed June 1, 2018.
117. Global Initiative for Children's Surgery (GICS). *Optimal resources for children's surgical care: guidelines for different levels of care*. Version 2.0. April 2018.
118. Fast O, et al. *BMJ Glob Health*. 2017;2(suppl 4).
119. *Decontamination and Reprocessing of Medical Devices for Health-care Facilities*; 2016. http://apps.who.int/iris/bitstream/handle/10665/250232/9789241549851-eng.pdf;jsessionid=BD6887F06B8291CDBB52A6E5B49357E1?sequence=1. Accessed April 1, 2018.

120. WHO. Zambia - Service Availability and Readiness Assessment 2010, Summary report. http://apps.who.int/healthinfo/systems/datacatalog/index.php/catalog/36/reports. Accessed March 19, 2018.
121. Henry JA, et al. *World J Surg*. 2012;36(12):2811–2818.
122. *Indice de disponibilite et de capacite operationnelle des services (SARA): Republique democratique du Congo*; 2014. http://apps.who.int/healthinfo/systems/datacatalog/index.php/ddibrowser/54/download/165. Accessed April 1, 2018.
123. *Uganda Hospital and Health Centre IV Census Survey*. ; 2014. http://www.who.int/healthinfo/systems/SARA_H_UGA_Results_2014.pdf?ua=1. Accessed April 1, 2018.
124. Bradley BD, et al. *Int J Tuberc Lung Dis Off J Int Union Tuberc Lung Dis*. 2016;20(8):1130–1134.
125. WHO medical device technical series: medical device donations - considerations for solicitation and provision. 2011. http://apps.who.int/iris/bitstream/10665/44568/1/9789241501408_eng.pdf. Accessed March 19, 2018.
126. WHO model list of essential medicines - 20th list. 2017. http://www.who.int/medicines/publications/essentialmedicines/20th_EML2017.pdf?ua=1. Accessed April 1, 2018.
127. Buckley GJ, Gostin LO, eds. Committee on Understanding the Global Public Health Implications of Substandard, Falsified, and Counterfeit Medical Products, Board on Global Health, Institute of Medicine. *Countering the problem of falsified and substandard drugs*. Washington (DC): National Academies Press (US); 2013. http://www.ncbi.nlm.nih.gov/books/NBK202530/. Accessed June 24, 2018.
128. WHO global surveillance and monitoring system for substandard and falsified medical products. 2017. http://www.who.int/medicines/regulation/ssffc/publications/gsms-report-sf/en/. Accessed June 24, 2018.
129. A study on the public health and socioeconomic impact of substandard and falsified medical products. http://www.who.int/medicines/regulation/ssffc/publications/se-study-sf/en/. Accessed June 24, 2018.
130. Roberts DJ, et al. *Hematol Oncol Clin North Am*. 2016;30(2):477–495.
131. Kralievits KE, et al. *The Lancet*. 2015;385:S28.
132. WHO | Blood safety and availability. WHO. http://www.who.int/mediacentre/factsheets/fs279/en/. Accessed April 21, 2018. https://www.who.int/en/news-room/fact-sheets/detail/blood-safety-and-availability. Accessed 3-7-19 TG.
133. Custer B, et al. *Transfusion (Paris)*; 2018.
134. De Lima L. *J Palliat Med*. 2004;7(1):97–103.
135. Frye JE. *International Drug Price Indicator Guide*. 393.
136. Forbes K. *J Pain Palliat Care Pharmacother*. 2006;20(3):33–35.
137. Liliana De Lima MHA, et al. *Health Policy*. 2001;56(2):99–110.
138. Nickerson JW, et al. *Can J Anaesth J Can Anesth*. 2017;64(3):296–307.
139. Scheck J. Tramadol: the opioid crisis for the rest of the world. *Wall Street Journal*. http://www.wsj.com/articles/tramadol-the-opioid-crisis-for-the-rest-of-the-world-1476887401. Published October 20, 2016. Accessed April 24, 2018.
140. Kusari S, et al. *Angew Chem Int Ed*. 55(1):240-243.
141. United Nations. *Single Convention on Narcotics Drugs*; 1961. https://www.unodc.org/pdf/convention_1961_en.pdf.
142. Estimated World Requirements of Narcotic Drugs in Grams for 2017. https://www.incb.org/documents/Narcotic-Drugs/Status-of-Estimates/2017/EstAdv17_Dec._21.pdf. Accessed May 1, 2018. Active 3/7/19.
143. Nickerson JW, Attaran A. *PLoS Med*. 2012;9(1).
144. WHO Regional Office for South-East Asia (SEARO) | Pain & Policy Studies Group. http://www.painpolicy.wisc.edu/who-regional-office-south-east-asia-searo. Accessed May 4, 2018.
145. Shariff U-K. An Epidemic of Pain in India; 2013. *New Yorker* https://www.newyorker.com/tech/elements/an-epidemic-of-pain-in-india. Accessed June 22, 2018.
146. Stjernswärd J, et al. *J Pain Symptom Manage*. 2007;33(5):628–633.
147. Taylor AL. *J Law Med Ethics J Am Soc Law Med Ethics*. 2007;35(4):556–570, 511.
148. Krakauer EL, et al. *J Pain Symptom Manage*. 2015;49(5):916–922.
149. Vallath N, et al. *J Pain Symptom Manage*. 2017;53(3):518–532.
150. Joranson DE, et al. *J Pain Symptom Manage*. 2002;24(2):152–159.
151. Rajagopal M, et al. *The Lancet*. 2001;358(9276):139–143.
152. Jr DGM. 'Opiophobia' Has Left Africa in Agony. *The New York Times*. https://www.nytimes.com/2017/12/04/health/opioids-africa-pain.html. Published December 4, 2017. Accessed April 15, 2018.
153. The World Bank Group. *Taking on Inequality, Poverty and Shared Prosperity 2016*; 2016. https://openknowledge.worldbank.org/bitstream/handle/10986/25078/9781464809583.pdf. Accessed May 1, 2018.
154. The World Monetary Fund. World Economic Outlook (April 2018) - Real GDP growth. http://www.imf.org/external/datamapper/NGDP_RPCH@WEO. Accessed June 24, 2018.
155. *Universal health coverage in Africa: a framework for action*. ; 2016. http://www.who.int/health_financing/documents/uhc-africa-action-framework/en/. Accessed June 24, 2018.
156. The World Factbook — Central Intelligence Agency. https://www.cia.gov/library/publications/the-world-factbook/geos/ug.html. Accessed June 2, 2018.
157. Dunn P. *Arch Dis Child Fetal Neonatal Ed*. 1999;80(3):F250–F251.
158. Billington WR. *Br Med J*. 1970;4(5737):738–740.
159. Statistics South Africa. http://www.statssa.gov.za/. Accessed June 24, 2018.
160. Sulla V, Zikhali P. *Overcoming Poverty and Inequality in South Africa : An Assessment of Drivers, Constraints and Opportunities*. The World Bank; 2018:1–148. http://documents.worldbank.org/curated/en-/530481521735906534/Overcoming-Poverty-and-Inequality-in-South-Africa-An-Assessment-of-Drivers-Constraints-and-Opportunities. Accessed June 24, 2018.
160a. South Africa. Dept of Health. 2018. *National Health Insurance Bill, No. 635:* For broader public comment. Government Gazette No. 41725:636 26 June.
161. SASA - South African Society of Anaesthesiologists Practice Guidelines; 2018. http://sasaweb.com/. Accessed June 24, 2018.
162. Rosseel P, et al. *World J Surg*. 2010;34(3):453–458.
163. Eger II EI, et al., ed. *The Wondrous Story of Anesthesia*. New York: Springer-Verlag; 2014. //www.springer.com/us/book/9781461484400. Accessed June 24, 2018.
164. Chronology of Canadian Anesthesiologists' society events. https://www.cas.ca/English/CAS-Chronology. Accessed June 24, 2018.
165. Fraser AB, et al. *Can J Anaesth J Can Anesth*. 2016;63(12):1364–1373.
166. The Royal College of Physicians and Surgeons of Canada. Specialty education design. http://www.royalcollege.ca/rcsite/cbd/cbd-specialty-education-design-sed-e. Accessed June 24, 2018.
167. *Standard of Practice: Use of Sedation and General Anesthesia in Dental Practice*; 2015. http://www.rcdso.org/Assets/DOCUMENTS/Professional_Practice/Standard_of_Practice/RCDSO_Standard_of_Practice__Use_of_Sedation_and_General_Anesthesia.pdf. Accessed June 1, 2018.
168. Dobson G, et al. *Can J Anaesth J Can Anesth*. 2018;65(1):76–104.
169. CMA Anesthesiology Profile; 2018. https://www.cma.ca/Assets/assets-library/document/en/advocacy/profiles/anesthesiology-e.pdf. Accessed June 1, 2018.
170. *National Health Expenditure Trends, 1975 to 2017*; 2017.
171. Gaspar XC. *Rev Biomed*. 1998;9(1):38–43.
172. Carillo-Esper R, et al. *Rev Mex Anestesiol*. 2017:40:S347–S349.
173. Sanchez-Meneses S. *Gac Med Mex*. 2007;143(6):525–529.
174. *ACGME Program Requirements for Graduate Medical Education in Anesthesiology*; 2017.
175. Accreditation Standards, Policies and Procedures, and Guidelines. Council on Accreditation of Nurse Anesthesia Education Programs. http://home.coa.us.com/accreditation/Pages/Accreditation-Policies-Procedures-and-Standards.aspx. Accessed June 24, 2018.
176. National Board of Certification & Recertification for Nurse Anesthetists. https://www.nbcrna.com/initial-certification. Accessed June 24, 2018.
177. 2016 Anesthesia almanac - analytics and research services - American Society of Anesthesiologists (ASA). https://www.asahq.org/resources/analytics-and-research-services. Accessed June 24, 2018.
178. AANA. Certified Registered Nurse Anesthetists Fact Sheet; 2017. https://www.aana.com/docs/default-source/pr-aana-com-web-documents-(all)/crna-fact-sheet.pdf?sfvrsn=c5f641b1_4.
179. Lewis SR, et al. *Cochrane Database Syst Rev*. 2014;7:CD010357.
180. Daugherty L, et al. An analysis of the labor markets for anesthesiology. https://www.rand.org/pubs/technical_reports/TR688.html. Published 2010. Accessed June 24, 2018.
181. Muffly MK, et al. *Anesth Analg*. 2016;123(1):179–185.
182. Creanga AA, et al. *Obstet Gynecol*. 2017;130(2):366–373.

183. Recognition of professional qualifications in practice - growth - European commission. /growth/single-market/services/free-movement-professionals/qualifications-recognition_en. Accessed June 24, 2018.
184. Egger Halbeis CB, et al. *Eur J Anaesthesiol*. 2007;24(12):991–1007.
185. Van Gessel E, et al. *Eur J Anaesthesiol*. 2012;29(4):165–168.
186. Mellin-Olsen J, et al. *Eur J Anaesthesiol*. 2010;27(7):592–597.
187. Strømskag KE. *Tidsskr Den Nor Laegeforening Tidsskr Prakt Med Ny Raekke*. 2002;122(8):804–805.
188. Gisvold SE, et al. *Acta Anaesthesiol Scand*. 2002;46(8):942–946.
189. Ringvold E-M, et al. *Acta Anaesthesiol Scand*. 2018;62(3):411–417.
190. Aasland OG, et al. *Tidsskr Den Nor Laegeforening Tidsskr Prakt Med Ny Raekke*. 2008;128(16):1833–1837.
190a. Litarczek G, Tecău M. Tabelcronologic cu date din istoriaanesteziei. In: *Bazeleteoretice Ale Anesteziologiei. Bucureşti: Editura Academiei de Ştiinţe Medicale;* 201:15–22.
191. Brill S, et al. *Eur J Anaesthesiol*. 2003;20(9):682–689.
192. Jonnesco T. *Br Med J*. 1909;2(2550):1396–1401.
193. Pearse RM, et al. *Lancet Lond Engl*. 2012;380(9847):1059–1065.
194. International Surgical Outcomes Study Group. *Br J Anaesth*. 2016;117(5):601–609.
195. Mitre C, et al. *Eur J Anaesthesiol*. 2016;33(3):157–159.
196. Divekar VM, Naik LD. *J Postgrad Med*. 2001;47(2):149–152.
197. Mavalankar D, et al. *Int J Gynaecol Obstet Off Organ Int Fed Gynaecol Obstet*. 2009;107(3):283–288.
198. Ashtekar SV, et al. *Indian J Community Med Off Publ Indian Assoc Prev Soc Med*. 2012;37(3):180–184.
199. Ray M. *Indian J Anaesth*. 2010;54(1):6–7.
200. Agarwal A. *Indian J Anaesth*. 2012;56(6):524.
201. Haddad FS. *Middle East J Anaesthesiol*. 1982;6(5):241–280.
202. Khan M, Khan FA. *Middle East J Anaesthesiol*. 2007;19(1):159–172.
203. Abayadeera A. *Anaesth Pain Intensive Care*. 2017;21:125–127.
204. Juan X, et al. *Anesth Analg*. 2012;114(6):1249–1253.
205. Yu X, et al. *BMJ Open*. 2017;7(6):e015147.
206. Zhu B, et al. *Am J Med Qual Off J Am Coll Med Qual*. 2018;33(1):93–99.
207. Li H, et al. *Anesth Analg*. 2018;126(3):1004–1012.
208. Miller RD, et al. *Ann Surg*. 1971;174(5):794–801.
209. Miller RD, et al. *JAMA*. 1971;216(11):1762–1765.
210. Bangkok Anesthesia Regional Training Center | BARTC. http://www.wfsa-bartc.org/. Accessed June 25, 2018.
210a. World Bank. GDP ranking. 2019. https://datacatalog.worldbank.org/dataset/gdp-ranking. Accessed June 10, 2019.
211. JCI-Accredited Organizations. Joint Commission International. https://www.jointcommissioninternational.org/about-jci/jci-accredited-organizations/. Accessed June 25, 2018.
212. The world factbook — Central Intelligence Agency - Gini coefficient. https://www.cia.gov/library/publications/the-world-factbook/rankorder/2172rank.html. Accessed June 25, 2018.
213. Venturini A. *Historia de la anestesia en sudamerica*; 2010. http://files.sld.cu/anestesiologia/files/2012/03/anestesia-sudamerica.pdf. Accessed June 1, 2018.
214. Historia de la Anestesia en Paraguay. http://www.clasa-anestesia.org/search/apendice/comision_historia/paraguay.htm. Accessed June 25, 2018.
215. Ponton JH. *Sociedad Colombiana de Anestesiologia y Reanimacion*. 1999.
216. Ocampo B, Peña JE. *Br J Anaesth*. 2014;112(3):406–409.
217. Bacon DR, Ament R. *J Clin Anesth*. 1995;7(6):534–543.
218. Cooper M. *Anaesth Intensive Care J*. 1997;25(3):221.
219. Newson AJ. *Anaesth Intensive Care*. 2006;34(suppl 1):39–45.
220. Wilson G. *Anaesth Intensive Care*. 1988;16(4):448–456.
221. Department of Health. *Australia's Future Health Workforce - Anaesthesia*; 2016. http://www.health.gov.au/internet/main/publishing.nsf/Content/australias-future-health-workforce-anaesthesia-report. Accessed June 1, 2018.
222. McNicol L. *A review of anaesthesia-related mortality reporting in Australia and New Zealand*; 2017:2012–2014. http://www.anzca.edu.au/documents/soa-mortality-report_p4.pdf. Accessed June 1, 2018.
223. Perioperative Mortality Review Committee. *Perioperative Mortality in New Zealand: Sixth report of the Perioperative Mortality Review Committee*; 2017. https://www.hqsc.govt.nz/assets/POMRC/Publications/POMRC_6th_Report_2017.pdf. Accessed June 1, 2018.
224. Cooper MG, et al. *Anaesth Intensive Care*. 2016;44(3):420–424.
225. Maitland K, et al. *N Engl J Med*. 2011;364(26):2483–2495.
226. Duke T, et al. *Ann Trop Paediatr*. 2010;30(2):87–101.
227. Technical Specifications for Oxygen Concentrators. (WHO medical device technical series). http://apps.who.int/medicinedocs/en/d/Js22194en/. Accessed April 26, 2018.
228. Peel D, et al. *Anaesthesia*. 2013;68(7):706–712.
229. Lipnick, et al. *Anesth Analg*. 2016.
230. Dubowitz G, et al. *Anaesthesia*. 2013;68(12):1220–1223.
231. Gray A. *Atlas of Ultrasound-Guided Regional Anesthesia*. 3rd ed. 2018. https://www.elsevier.com/books/atlas-of-ultrasound-guided-regional-anesthesia/gray/978-1-4557-2819-0. Accessed May 4, 2018.
232. Sacevich C, et al. *Can J Anaesth J Can Anesth*. 2018;65(2):170–177.
233. Burke TF, et al. *World J Surg*. 2017;41(12):2990–2997.
234. Cheng D, et al. *World J Surg. February*. 2018.
235. Shukla P, et al. *J Obstet Gynaecol India*. 2014;64(5):358–361.
236. Nkwabong E, et al. *Med Sante Trop*. 2016;26(1):75–77.
237. Kerry VB, et al. *J Glob Health*. 2013;3(2):020406.
238. Jogerst K, et al. *Ann Glob Health*. 2015;81(2):239–247.
239. Butler M, et al. *J Pediatr Surg*. 2018;53(4):828–836.
240. Welling DR, et al. *World J Surg*. 2010;34(3):466–470.
241. Holm JD, Malete L. Nine problems that hinder partnerships in Africa. *The Chronicle of Higher Education*. http://chronicle.com/article/Nine-Problems-That-Hinder/65892/. Published June 13, 2010. Accessed February 17, 2011.
242. Elobu AE, et al. *Surgery*. 2014;155(4):585–592.
243. DeCamp M, et al. *Ann Intern Med. March*. 2018.
244. Crump JA, Sugarman J. *JAMA*. 2008;300(12):1456–1458.
245. Crump JA, Sugarman J. *Am J Trop Med Hyg*. 2010;83(6):1178–1182.
246. Le Phuoc. Teaching global health ethics using simulation. Poster Presentation. Presented at the: https://interprofessional.ucsf.edu/sites/interprofessional.ucsf.edu/files/wysiwyg/GH_ethics_poster_1-23-14_final_draft.pdf.
247. The Royal College of Anaesthetists. Unit of training for working in a developing country. http://www.rcoa.ac.uk/careers-training/oope-and-oopt/working-training-developing-countries/unit-of-training-working-developing-country. Accessed August 23, 2016.
248. Tabaie S, et al. *Curr Anesthesiol Rep*. 2017;7(1):30–36.

Appendix 1 Links and Useful Resources

- WHO Essential Surgery: http://www.who.int/surgery/en/
- Surgical Care at the District Hospital: http://www.who.int/surgery/en/
- World Federation of Societies of Anaesthesiologists (WFSA): www.wfsahq.org
- WFSA Workforce Map: www.wfsahq.org/workforce-map
- WFSA Anesthesia Facility Assessment Tool: www.wfsahq.org/afat
- Open Anesthesia Global Health: http://www.openanesthesia.org/subspecialty/global-health/
- American Society of Anesthesiologists Global Humanitarian Outreach: https://www.asahq.org/gho
- Consortium of Universities for Global Health: www.cugh.org

- Royal College of Anesthetists e-Learning Anaesthesia: www.rcoa.ac.uk/e-la
- Royal College of Anesthetists Anaesthesia for Austere Environments modules: https://www.rcoa.ac.uk/e-la/anaesthesia-humanitarian-austere-environments
- Institute for Health Metrics and Evaluation: http://ghdx.healthdata.org/
- Global Health Ethics Course (Johns Hopkins): http://ethicsandglobalhealth.org/
- Essential Pain Management Course: www.essentialpainmanagement.org/
- "Anaesthesia at the district hospital" by Mike Dobson: http://apps.who.int/iris/handle/10665/42193
- Developing Anaesthesia Handbook: http://www.developinganaesthesia.org/
- *Primary Anesthesia*, Book by Maurice King
- International Association for the Study of Pain (IASP) Guide to pain management in low-resource settings: http://ebooks.iasp-pain.org/guide_to_pain_management_in_low_resource_settings
- *Developing Global Health Programming: A Guidebook for Medical and Professional Schools.* By Jessica Evert et al: www.cfhi.org/sites/files/files/pages/developingglobalhealthprogramming_0.pdf
- *The Right Stuff*, Michael Dobson, MD Publications, 2017

3 Perioperative Medicine

NEAL H. COHEN, MICHAEL A. GROPPER, and AMAN MAHAJAN

KEY POINTS

- The practice of anesthesiology continues to evolve with health care for patients undergoing new and, in many cases, more complicated procedures in the operating room as well as minimally invasive or interventional procedures performed in other nonoperating room settings. With the rapid growth of nonoperating room anesthesia, traditional operating room anesthesia care no longer dominates most anesthesia practices.
- The number of anesthesia subspecialties has also increased to include pediatric, cardiothoracic, obstetric, neuroanesthesia, critical care medicine, acute and chronic pain management, palliative care, and sleep medicine. Anesthesiologists' skills and expertise in subspecialties have grown paralleling the respective surgical specialties.
- The diversity of anesthesiology skills and clinical capabilities has created opportunities for anesthesiologists to take advantage of the changing healthcare environment and assume a more expansive role in perioperative care in both hospital and nonhospital settings, providing management of patients through the continuum of the perioperative or periprocedural period, and extending to home care and other settings.
- With changes in healthcare delivery, anesthesiologists will have to not only reassess current practices, but also define ways to adapt to new models of care. New approaches to care, while exciting for the specialty will be challenging to implement. While expanding the scope of practice, anesthesiologists must also continue to fulfill the traditional operating room roles and maintain the commitment to safe and high-quality intraoperative anesthesia care.
- To successfully transition to these new models of practice, anesthesiologists must acquire a more comprehensive understanding of the economics of health care and the role their perioperative care has in determining costs of care, outcomes, quality, and safety.
- The electronic health record and access to big data can serve as valuable resources in identifying opportunities to advance care and improve quality. To use the electronic record effectively will require that anesthesiologists acquire skills in biomedical informatics and data sciences to advance perioperative care.
- Public and private insurers are implementing new payment models to replace traditional fee-for-service payment for clinical care. They are transitioning from fee-for-service to "value-based" payment methodologies that better align quality, costs, and goals of care. At the same time, both government (e.g., Medicare) and private payors (e.g., insurance companies) are implementing new alternative payment models including bundled (fixed) payment methodologies designed to transfer the financial risk from patients and payors to providers, both physicians and health systems. Anesthesiologists must understand these new payment models and how they will impact clinical management and compensation for anesthesia services, particularly as anesthesia services and perioperative medicine evolve.
- Providing optimal perioperative care in the current healthcare environment requires implementation of new and creative models of value-based care that encompass the patient's entire clinical course as well as development of new partnerships and collaborations with other providers across the healthcare system. Anesthesiologists are well positioned to take a more prominent role in perioperative management, integrating their understanding of the surgical and medical needs of patients during and after surgical procedures. Concurrently, other physicians, including hospitalists, are partnering with surgeons to optimize perioperative inpatient care. Collaboration with hospitalists, medical specialists, and others is critical to improving perioperative care and in clarifying the roles anesthesiologists can play in providing value-based perioperative care. For some patient populations, co-management agreements can be executed to coordinate perioperative care and optimize transitions through the continuum of care.
- A variety of models for perioperative medicine are being successfully adopted in the United States and other countries. The perioperative surgical home (PSH) and Enhanced Recovery After Surgery (ERAS) protocols are examples of new approaches to collaborative multidisciplinary care that have demonstrated significant benefit for a number of patient populations—aligning goals for patients, providers, hospitals, and payors.

Introduction

The primary focus of anesthesia practice has traditionally been on the intraoperative management of patients undergoing surgical procedures in hospitals or ambulatory settings. Over the past few decades, anesthesiologists have been acknowledged for the significant improvement in perioperative safety and quality.[1] As a result of advances in anesthesia care as well as surgical and diagnostic capabilities, anesthesia services have expanded to include a wide variety of hospital-based and ambulatory settings outside of the operating room. While the diversity of anesthesia services has expanded, the basic elements of anesthesia care remained relatively consistent—preoperative assessment, intraoperative management, and postoperative care provided to ensure safe transition through the perioperative period. With increasing subspecialty training opportunities and changes in healthcare delivery and payment, new opportunities have developed for anesthesiologists to assume a broader role in both perioperative care and management of patients in the operating room and beyond. At the same time, the increasing capabilities and high costs of health care, particularly in the United States, is undergoing significant pressure to improve quality and safety while delivering value-based care consistent with patient wishes.[2,3] The changes create opportunities for anesthesia practices to evolve and for the role of anesthesiologists to extend beyond current clinical practices.

This chapter reviews the changes taking place in healthcare delivery and financing that create challenges and opportunities for anesthesiologists to expand their practices to incorporate concepts of perioperative medicine.

THE ANESTHESIOLOGIST AND PERIOPERATIVE MEDICINE

Perioperative medicine is an evolving field that focuses on optimizing the health and healthcare delivery of patients who will be undergoing surgery, and providing medical care for those patients following surgery. Anesthesiologists are well suited to advance their role as specialists in perioperative medicine and provide better care for surgical patients. New anesthetic techniques, monitoring capabilities, and evidence-based approaches to perioperative management have made anesthesia safer and improved the quality and safety of perioperative care.[1] Advances in surgery and development of minimally invasive techniques have had major impact on how anesthesia care is provided and expanded the locations in which anesthesia services are needed. At the same time, in part as a result of these changes, the patient population presenting for anesthesia has changed. Patients with significant underlying medical conditions who in the past were not considered candidates for surgery are now able to undergo complex surgical procedures successfully. These changes have had major impact on health systems, significantly increasing complexity and costs of care, while also putting pressure on healthcare resources including hospital bed capacity.[4,5]

For anesthesiologists, the advances in care, diversity of patients requiring anesthesia services, and the high costs of care create both new opportunities and challenges. Most significant to the practice of anesthesia has been the expansion in scope of clinical responsibilities in perioperative care of patients beyond the traditional operating room roles, and the need to improve operational efficiency in perioperative/periprocedural care and reduce costs. The challenges also provide the opportunity for anesthesiologists knowledgeable about operating room management to assume health system leadership roles and improve healthcare delivery for the surgical patients.

The change in scope of anesthesia practice is related to a number of different factors. The extension of anesthesia care to other inpatient and outpatient settings is based on management strategies and lessons learned in optimizing care in the operating room. The expansion of anesthesia services to interventional radiology, endoscopy, and cardiology suites has resulted in improved clinical management and, in some cases, better throughput.

Anesthesiologists have also modified clinical practices to optimize clinical care and improve efficiency. For example, preoperative assessment has been refined to improve clinical outcomes, but also reduce costs associated with laboratory testing and other preoperative testing that add no value.[6,7] At the same time, anesthesiologists have had a greater role in optimizing patients prior to surgery. Preoperative *management* of patients with underlying medical conditions, including diabetes, cardiopulmonary disease, and renal insufficiency, has improved the perioperative course and minimized the likelihood of postoperative complications. In some cases consultation with other medical specialists is required, but for most patients, the anesthesiologist's role is critical to optimizing the patient's conditions preoperatively as they best understand the interplay of the various perioperative variables including patient factors, anesthesia, and surgical techniques. As a key aspect of optimal perioperative medicine, anesthesiologists are able to provide postoperative management, including critical care and pain management for many of these patients based on their individual preoperative risk assessment and intraoperative course. In many respects, these changes have redefined anesthesia to encompass perioperative medicine.[8]

The expansion of anesthesia training in multiple subspecialties, as well as critical care medicine and acute and chronic pain management, also provides advanced and diverse skills that allow anesthesiologists, in collaboration with the surgical specialists, to ensure a coordinated approach to perioperative management. As a result, many anesthesia subspecialists have successfully expanded their roles in perioperative care. As one example, transplant anesthesiologists (also see Chapter 60) are often involved in discussions about patient selection, preoperative optimization, and transitions of care from the operating room to the postoperative period. Based on the collaboration of anesthesiologists, transplant surgeons, and medical specialists, anesthesiologists participate in selection discussions to provide their perspective on the perioperative implications of transplantation. For many transplant services, collaboration with the anesthesiologists has resulted in reengineering of care. Many patients who previously required postoperative care in the intensive care unit (ICU) can now bypass the ICU and have reduced hospital lengths of stay.[9] Similar outcomes have been documented for patients who have anesthesiologists participate in their perioperative management for cardiac surgery (also see Chapter 54), pediatric surgery (also see Chapters 77-79), neurosurgery (also see Chapter 57), or other subspecialties. In each of these examples, collaboration among the surgeons, anesthesiologists, and the overall team of providers both within and beyond the operating room environment is critical to realizing improved outcomes and reduced costs of care.

Anesthesiologists with advanced training in pain medicine and critical care are able to facilitate and optimize perioperative management. Pain management strategies have significant positive impact on the care of patients with both acute and chronic pain (also see Chapters 51, 80, and 82). Employing multimodal approaches to perioperative pain management, particularly for patients with longstanding chronic pain, perioperative pain medicine teams have had positive impact on perioperative outcomes, including reduced need for opioid analgesics and in some cases shortened the length of stay in hospital and improved patient satisfaction.[10-12] Similarly, critical care anesthesiologists play a large role in improving perioperative management of patients requiring ICU care. The value of the critical care physician on ICU utilization in reducing complications of mechanical ventilation, providing early diagnosis and treatment of sepsis, and improved management strategies for patients with renal dysfunction are well documented (see Chapters in 80, 84, and 85).[13-15]

An equally important factor contributing to anesthesiologists assuming greater responsibility in perioperative management is related to their knowledge of the overall perioperative environment, its complexities, and associated high costs. Advances in anesthetic management have facilitated implementation of new surgical techniques and allowed patients previously considered poor risks to undergo complex surgical procedures with good outcomes. These advances in care have contributed to the escalating cost of health care, particularly in the United States.[2] Not only are the high costs specifically related to the procedure, there are often substantial additional costs associated with complications of care, postdischarge care, and readmissions.[16,17] Anesthetic management has impact on costs of perioperative care, hospital length of stay, need for prolonged postoperative ICU stay, and other clinical outcomes. For example, intraoperative management can contribute to postoperative complications, such as pressure ulcers, central line infections, renal failure, aspiration and ventilator-associated pneumonia, cognitive dysfunction, and other complications. When these complications occur, hospitalizations are lengthy and rehabilitation (skilled nursing, physical, and rehabilitation services) needs are significant.

The need to address costs associated with managing complications of care is taking on greater importance. Over the past few years in the United States, government and private payors have raised concerns about the costs associated with managing complications of care, some of which are relevant to anesthetic management. These payors are reducing payment for costs associated with complications and denying payment for costs associated with readmissions.[18,19] As part of perioperative medicine, anesthesiologists have to identify these perioperative risks and, when clinically appropriate, identify ways to modify management to improve outcomes and reduce costs.

Another factor that has precipitated a need to address perioperative care in a more coordinated manner is the impact of changes in payment methods being implemented by both government and private payors as a way to control costs of care. In the United States, the primary method of payment to physicians remains fee based. While the implications of fee-for-service (FFS) payment methodology on quality of care and resource utilization are widely debated, FFS payment models are associated with overuse of some services, higher costs, and poor coordination of care.[20] In response to these issues, a number of alternative payment models (APMs) have been implemented including bundled payment methods and incentive-based payments associated with reduced costs of care and penalties when costs remain high. Under the Medicare Access and CHIP Reauthorization Act of 2015, Medicare has implemented a number of APMs and a Quality Payment Program that includes a Merit-Based Incentive Payment System (MIPS), each designed to compensate physicians for improving patient outcomes at reduced cost.[21] Medicare is also encouraging development of accountable care organizations (ACOs) in which health systems assume clinical and financial responsibility for managing a population of patients, improving quality, and reducing overall costs.

These changes in care management and payment methodologies have significant impact on all physicians and health systems. They shift responsibility and risk to the providers and are forcing physicians and health systems to implement value-based care. Anesthesiologists are knowledgeable about the complexities associated with perioperative care and have the ability to manage many aspects of the care and systems needed to optimize it. Consequently, they can help define new models of care and extend their role and assume greater responsibility for managing the perioperative course of some patient populations. For example, if anesthesiologists can help reduce costs during the course of care for a surgical patient, they can benefit financially under bundled payment methodologies, shared savings plans, and when participating in ACOs. Although issues related to payment methodologies are very different from one country to another and are beyond the scope of this chapter, the goals and implications of these newer payment methodologies should be understood by all anesthesiologists, since they have significant implications on the practice of anesthesia and the role for the anesthesiologist in perioperative medicine broadly.

While anesthesiologists are well suited to positively impact perioperative care, anesthesiology departments will need to adjust their focus and priorities to be better engaged in perioperative medicine. When provided in a coordinated way, perioperative care is cost effective and improves outcomes.[22] At the same time, the expansion of anesthesia practices, diversity of roles and responsibilities, and the subspecialization of anesthesia care have in some ways compromised the ability of anesthesiologists to fulfill their potential as perioperative providers. Compartmentalization of perioperative care and subspecialization have the risk of fragmenting care and undermining the development of a coordinated approach to perioperative management. At many hospitals, preoperative care is now provided in a dedicated preoperative evaluation clinic, physically separate from the operating room or other clinical sites. The evaluation is performed at some time prior to the surgical procedure; communication about the patient's status and clinical plans is most often done electronically with no face-to-face dialog or communication with the anesthesiologist who will deliver care during the procedure. Operating room care is provided by an anesthesiologist either personally or as part of the anesthesia care team model. Postoperative management—including care in the postanesthesia care unit, pain management, and ICU care—is often provided by another set of care providers. Perioperative medicine requires collaboration among all anesthesia providers, incorporating the knowledge and skills of each of the participants, including those providing preoperative management, intraoperative care, critical care, pain management, and so on. As much as each of the providers is critical to the care of the patient, the coordination of care among the anesthesiologists as a group is also a critical element in optimizing care, understanding and fulfilling the patient's goals for care, and improving efficiencies.

Perioperative Management

Throughout this text, the role of the anesthesiologist in various aspects of perioperative management is discussed. Each component is critically important to the quality, safety, and costs of care. The overall approach to care from the time a case is scheduled until the patient has recovered from anesthesia and surgery and resumed normal activities should be of concern to the anesthesiologist. Just as anesthesia as a specialty is acknowledged for advances in safety and quality in the intraoperative case, it should extend its focus and responsibility to the entire perioperative period—coordinating assessment, management, and responsibilities with the surgeons, hospitalists, other physicians, and nurses. By optimizing each of them independently and then coordinating the care across the continuum, the benefits of providing perioperative medicine will be achieved—with improved clinical outcomes, safer care, and reduced costs.

PREOPERATIVE ASSESSMENT AND MANAGEMENT

Chapter 31 emphasizes the changing patient needs and role of the anesthesiologist with respect to preoperative assessment and management. The chapter provides a more comprehensive discussion. To summarize current practices, for most healthy patients, a formal preoperative assessment is usually not required.[6,7] In fact, anesthesia providers have been able to reduce preoperative testing and other costs through the implementation of evidence-based protocols to standardize preoperative management for many patients.[7] Rather than requiring a preoperative visit, laboratory testing, and radiologic studies, most patients now have a phone consultation, often performed by a nurse practitioner to assess preoperative status and perioperative needs, and to address a patient's questions or concerns. For other patients, particularly those with underlying medical conditions or complex comorbidities, a more comprehensive evaluation and preoperative management and optimization of underlying conditions may be required.[23] For this subset of complex patients, preoperative assessment and management are an integral part of the continuum of perioperative care for which the anesthesiologist has a significant role. In some cases, additional diagnostic studies, such as an echocardiogram or focused pulmonary function studies, may be helpful in determining how best to manage a patient during the perioperative period. In this situation, interpretation of the studies may be done in coordination with a consultant or physician who has provided care to the patient preoperatively and who will resume care after the procedure is beneficial. The preoperative anesthesiologist may require a formal consultation with another specialist, such as a cardiologist, nephrologist, or pulmonary medicine physician, although these are needed for only a select few patients. For those patients with significant underlying conditions that will influence the perioperative course, particularly the postoperative recovery, referral for additional preoperative management (prehabilitation) can be helpful in optimizing their clinical status prior to proceeding with a major surgical procedure.[24-26] For most patients, the specific management strategies required to optimize the patient for anesthesia and surgery are often best defined when input is provided by the anesthesiologist who is most knowledgeable about the impact of chronic conditions on perioperative care needs as well as the implications of anesthesia on underlying physiology.

INTRAOPERATIVE (INTRAPROCEDURAL) MANAGEMENT

A number of initiatives have been implemented in hospitals throughout the world to improve intraoperative management, minimize complications, and reduce costs. The implementation of checklists has been demonstrated to improve patient safety in the operating room (also see Chapter 5).[27-29] Similarly, the routine briefing (i.e., time out) before beginning a surgical procedure reduces the incidence of wrong-site surgery, facilitates communication among providers, and ensures optimal patient care.[30] Some hospitals and surgical services also conduct debriefings at the end of each surgical procedure to define what procedure has been completed, clarify the postoperative expectations for the patient, and ensure that all supplies and materials have been appropriately retrieved from the surgical field.[31] These initiatives have reduced complications during surgery and, in some cases reduced costs of care. For example, the British National Health Service instituted "The Productive Operating Theatre" to improve productivity and patient outcomes during surgical procedures.[32,33] The program includes both briefings and debriefings to identify critical issues during and after a surgical procedure. This process has reduced errors and facilitated the transition from the operating room after a surgical procedure. Operating room utilization has increased, turnaround times shortened, and waste reduced. Significant financial savings have also resulted from this effort. The National Health Service is implementing similar initiatives in other hospital settings, such as "The Productive Ward" to build on the success achieved in the operating room environment.[34] Anesthesiologists need to be part of such initiatives that ensure there is an integrated approach to management during the intraoperative periods in order to demonstrate a significant and sustained impact on outcomes.

POSTOPERATIVE MANAGEMENT

The transition out of the operating room represents another important opportunity for anesthesiologists to enhance the quality and safety advances achieved in the operating room and improve perioperative patient outcomes. Advances in anesthesia safety have been acknowledged by the Academy of Medicine (formerly the Institute of Medicine) of the National Academy of Sciences[1] and other groups as a result of better anesthetic drugs, new anesthetic techniques, and improved monitoring. Although the incidence of intraoperative complications has been dramatically reduced, complication rates in the postoperative period remain high. The impact of variability in anesthetic practices on postoperative outcomes—beyond the immediate postoperative period—has received increasing attention for both patients who remain hospitalized and those who experience unintended and often unrecognized sequelae of anesthesia and surgery after discharge. For example, after a surgical procedure requiring tracheal intubation, a significant number of patients experience postextubation stridor or dysphagia that may last for days. These findings compromise the ability to protect the airway, particularly during sleep.[35] Does the dysphagia contribute to postoperative pneumonia that may not become clinically apparent until after discharge? Similarly, the most common healthcare–associated infections are pneumonia and surgical site infection, supporting the concept that intraoperative management is an important determinant of postoperative outcome.[36] Many other intraoperative strategies also impact long-term outcomes beyond the immediate postoperative period. Three examples support this conclusion. First is the influence of intraoperative fluid and vasopressor management on postoperative metabolic status and renal function.[37,38] Second, intraoperative glucose control can have a major impact on wound healing.[39] Finally, and more recently, anesthetic management can influence postoperative cognitive dysfunction for both adults and children.[40,41] As a result of these findings, anesthesiologists have a responsibility and an opportunity to understand the causes for these and other complications. We need to understand how anesthetic management contributes to adverse outcomes and how we can modify both intraoperative and postoperative care to reduce them.

COORDINATED PERIOPERATIVE MANAGEMENT STRATEGIES

While each of the components of perioperative care have specific requirements and approaches to optimize management, improve outcome, and potentially to reduce cost, perioperative management strategies must be assessed collectively, often using evidence-based clinical pathways to ensure that the goals of perioperative medicine are met.[42,43] Anesthesiologists have the opportunity to address these needs. To achieve these goals, however, anesthesiologists must reassess current models of care and modify some practices. One critical challenge to effectively coordinate care is the complexity of the perioperative course and management. In most clinical situations, it is no longer possible, nor appropriate, for a single anesthesia provider to participate in all aspects of the perioperative course. Perioperative, intraoperative, and postoperative care are often provided by different anesthesiologists, including pain medicine and critical care anesthesiologists in selected cases. To optimize perioperative management under this model requires improved communication and collaboration *among the anesthesia providers* as well as with others who participate in a patient's care. For some patient populations, such as geriatric patients or those with complex comorbidities, co-management agreements with other specialists can be executed to optimize care across the perioperative continuum, while clarifying roles and responsibilities.[44] The electronic health record is a valuable source of clinical information, but cannot substitute for more direct communication among providers, particularly in the management of complex clinical problems (also see Chapter 6).

The collaborative approach to care may not seem essential for healthy patients undergoing straightforward procedures. However, the value and opportunities for anesthesiologists to take a larger role in perioperative care is clearly evident for almost all patients—and the coordinated approach is appreciated by patients who are often confused about who is managing their care.[45] For example, patients undergoing "simple" procedures often have postoperative clinical issues that are underrecognized and require assessment and management. Anesthesiologists, surgeons, and nurses provide patients with instructions and information to help them manage their postoperative course, often at a time when they are not able to understand or process the information. As a result, even in these cases, the anesthesiologist can be instrumental in addressing postoperative anesthesia-related problems and coordinating the transition of the patient's care back to the primary care provider. The surgeon can provide information about the surgical procedure by forwarding the operative note to the primary care provider, but it rarely addresses any issues related to anesthetic management, concerns about the airway or potential for airway obstruction, or sequelae related to anesthetic agents, narcotics, muscle relaxants, or regional anesthetic blocks. In many cases, a phone consultation or teleconference is sufficient to address clinical needs. In other cases, a formal postoperative office visit may be required, as some anesthesia practices offer. Expansion of the postoperative assessment and management can be very helpful to patients, the surgeons, and other providers at the facilities to purvey a level of support to the patients that is often unavailable. The adoption of information technology resources and continued evolution of medical informatics (see Chapter 4) can enhance communication between patients and physicians during the entire perioperative period.

Besides the desire for a more coordinated approach to the entire perioperative course for every patient, a more formal and robust perioperative management strategy must be available for those patients with underlying medical conditions, those undergoing complex surgical procedures, and those needing prolonged hospitalization. In addition, for patients who require skilled nursing or rehabilitation services after discharge and for those needing home health services, the transitions of care create challenges for ensuring that postoperative management strategies are maintained, responses are assessed, and therapy is modified as needed. By its very nature, perioperative care for these patients is collaborative, requiring input and expertise from a number of different disciplines, including, but not limited to, anesthesia subspecialty expertise, surgeons, and medical subspecialists. Diverse perspectives and clinical expertise are essential, particularly for the more complex procedures in patients with multiple comorbidities. At the same time, the coordination of care must be assumed by a provider who is able to integrate the diverse perspectives into a comprehensive plan of care consistent with each patient's needs and goals. In the distant past, this coordination was provided by the patient's primary care provider, who maintained a role throughout the perioperative period. With the increasing complexity of perioperative care, changing demographics, and need to provide more efficient and coordinated care to reduce overall costs, the anesthesiologist has the opportunity to assume a more involved role in the management of some of these patients. To do so will require the commitment of the anesthesia practice to this new model of care and, in many cases, the acquisition of new clinical and management skills to deliver optimized care that is efficient and consistent with patient expectations.

One of the most prominent barriers for an anesthesia department to assume a greater role in perioperative management is its own members. It is imperative that there be consensus from all members of the department that a coordinated strategy is important and consistent with their expectations. To achieve department support, it is vital to clarify that perioperative management is a comprehensive approach to care that involves a diverse group of providers. Every member of the group must participate in the overall commitment to perioperative care. The care will be provided by a number of different anesthesiologists, each with different clinical expertise. One example of this coordinated approach to perioperative care is the management of a patient with a history of chronic severe pain who undergoes a complex surgical procedure. The patient will undergo extensive evaluation and optimization of care in the preoperative evaluation programs. Intraoperative care will be provided by another anesthesiologist, one who has communicated with the patient and understands all of the clinical issues identified and addressed preoperatively. When the patient is transferred to the ICU for postoperative care, which includes ventilator support, intensive respiratory care, hemodynamic monitoring, and fluid management, the transition from the anesthesiologist who provided intraoperative care to the critical care anesthesiologist is seamless. Pain management is provided by the pain service in collaboration with the critical care anesthesiologist (also see Chapters 51 and 82). The remainder of the patient's course of care will be managed by a member of the anesthesia department to facilitate transition to another care facility or home, and to ensure effective communication with the primary care provider or other caregivers. Although this model is foreign to many practices, it represents one of many approaches to optimizing perioperative management and takes advantage of the expertise of anesthesiologists in the overall care of the patients they anesthetize.

Finally, new approaches to perioperative management also require that each practice acquire the necessary operational, clinical, and financial data, as well as the analytical capability to interpret it. Larger regional and national organizations have the broad expertise available to analyze the practice and determine where improvements in processes can benefit patients and enhance the efficiency of the practice. For smaller practices, it can be challenging to have this broad level of expertise and access to information, although some have very successfully incorporated these strategies. As a consequence, in the United States there has been considerable consolidation of anesthesia practices by large regional and national organizations.[46] This consolidation has enabled the larger, often multi-institutional group to provide the resources needed to help anesthesia practices optimize perioperative management and document the value of the anesthesia services from both a clinical and financial perspective. Some groups have transitioned to multispecialty groups or recruited hospitalists or other providers to the anesthesia practice to supplement the clinical skills of the anesthesiologists so that the department has the diverse clinical and management expertise needed to optimize perioperative care. This multidisciplinary approach to perioperative care enables the group to expand its scope of practice and to develop clinical and administrative databases that allow them to document the value of their services to both patients and the institution. From an administrative perspective, this strategy better positions the practice to negotiate with representatives from the hospital or health system, particularly when advocating for the share of bundled payments. Because the administrative and analytical capabilities are essential to optimize delivery of perioperative care, each practice of whatever size will need to identify the most effective ways to develop this expertise and acquire the data needed to successfully address the many challenges facing anesthesia practices.

Models of Perioperative Care

Most health systems and providers are challenged to identify ways to become more efficient and reduce costs while maintaining or improving the quality of care, particularly perioperative care. Accomplishing these diverse goals is difficult and no single model of care works for every patient population or healthcare setting. As a result, many approaches to delivery of perioperative care have been implemented, some of these successful and some for which the outcome remains unknown. Although models of perioperative management include the anesthesiologist, other providers have participated in the preoperative and postoperative management of complex patient populations, each with variable success. Based on these experiences, the key aspects for any model for perioperative management include: (1) an understanding of the specific patient population included in the model (e.g., specific surgical procedure), (2) sufficient clinical and financial information to allow evaluation of the management strategies and their implications, and (3) coordination and collaboration among all providers participating in the model.[47] As models for perioperative management have evolved, they have taken advantage of the experiences from the hospitalist model for inpatient care and the medical home model for chronic disease management.

PATIENT-CENTERED MEDICAL HOME

The medical home model, also referred to as the "patient-centered medical home" (PCMH) refers to the model of care in which a primary care physician provides comprehensive care to improve health outcomes for a population of patients.[48] The critical element of the PCMH is the coordination of care to reduce emergency room visits and hospitalizations. In managing the patient population, a number of strategies are implemented to reduce costs and improve outcomes. These models often utilize additional providers, including advance practice nurses, respiratory therapists, physical therapists, and patient advocates to manage chronic diseases such as asthma, chronic obstructive pulmonary disease, heart failure, and diabetes mellitus. Payment for the PCMH includes FFS payments for episodes of care as well as payment to coordinate care. This model has been successful in improving care, particularly for patients with selected chronic diseases, although the financial success has not been consistently achieved.[49-51] In some cases, the PCMH actually resulted in increased hospital admissions.[52] Despite the variable success of the PCMH, there are some lessons that can be applied to perioperative care. First, preoperative assessment must be comprehensive enough to identify underlying clinical problems and effectively manage them, both preoperatively and postoperatively (also see Chapter 31). For the anesthesiologist managing the perioperative period, chronic conditions must be addressed; the management of these cannot be deferred to other providers. The implications of the perioperative needs must be taken into account when managing chronic diseases during the course of surgical care. Second, the underlying medical conditions must be considered as part of the proposed procedure and its implications for postoperative management. This broader perspective requires coordination with the surgeon and for some patients, the hospitalist, other specialists, and the primary care provider. For example, a patient with peripheral neuropathy associated with diabetes mellitus may be unable to participate in traditional approaches to rehabilitation; care must be tailored to the specific needs of each patient in consultation with others who can modify care as needed to optimize likelihood of achieving the desired outcome. Third, while participation by anesthesiologists is essential, many aspects of perioperative care can be managed by other providers, including other physicians and advance practice nurses. The keys to successful perioperative management, however, require that there be a single physician responsible for coordinating care among the team of providers, ensuring consistent and ongoing communication about patient care needs, and the availability of data that can be used to analyze clinical and business practices, costs of care, and outcome measures. The responsible provider during the perioperative period may be the anesthesiologist, surgeon, or hospitalist. As the patient recovers, the responsible provider may transition to the primary care provider, as long as there is good communication and appropriate "hand-off."

SURGICAL HOSPITALIST

Another model that has been implemented in many hospitals in the United States and other parts of the world is the surgical hospitalist model, which builds on the hospitalist model of care for inpatient medical patients. Many studies have documented the clinical values and other advantages associated with implementation of a robust hospitalist program.[53,54] Most of the programs have been focused on the care of patients with acute (and perhaps underlying chronic) medical problems rather than patients undergoing surgical procedures. For the surgical patient, the role of the surgeon is evolving for a number of reasons: the percentage of surgical inpatients is increasing, and inpatient clinical needs are becoming more complex and difficult for the surgeon to manage without additional support. As a result, many hospitals are recruiting hospitalists to provide perioperative care for surgical patients.[53,54] In some cases hospitalists work with specific surgical services (or an individual surgeon) to manage overall care and transitions of care into and out of the hospital environment. The models for surgical hospitalist programs vary, in some cases incorporating hospitalists with primary training in internal medicine or pediatrics, and in some cases, having a surgeon with interest in perioperative care take on the hospitalist role. In each model, the clinical management issues are similar, though the knowledge and skill to manage patients with complex comorbidities may differ considerably.

Many of these surgical hospitalist models have been successful in optimizing care of both underlying medical conditions and perioperative needs related to the surgical procedure. Although there is limited experience to document the effect on hospital lengths of stay and readmission rates, the models have been effective at improving timeliness of interventions, and patient and staff satisfaction.[54] For this model to be most effective requires that the surgical hospitalist be knowledgeable about the idiosyncrasies of perioperative management related to the specific surgical procedures. Their effectiveness is most evident when the care of underlying medical conditions is carefully coordinated with the other perioperative needs of the patient. For example, the neurosurgical hospitalist must understand concepts such as cerebral autoregulation and the impact of clinical interventions on cerebral hemodynamics for the patient who has undergone a neurovascular procedure. Similar considerations must be addressed for hospitalists working collaboratively with other surgical services.

The surgical hospitalist model has been very effective in allowing surgeons to concentrate their efforts in the operating room. However, the optimal relationship between the surgical hospitalist (whether a surgeon who has assumed this nonoperative responsibility or a medical hospitalist) and anesthesiologist during the immediate perioperative period has not been standardized. In some cases perioperative care is transferred from the anesthesiologist to the hospitalist in the immediate postoperative period; in other cases, care may be transferred from the anesthesiologist to an intensivist (either a critical care anesthesiologist or another intensive care physician) while the hospitalist maintains responsibility for managing some of the underlying clinical conditions. In the latter case, the roles and responsibilities of the anesthesiologist, critical care provider, and hospitalist need to be clearly defined to ensure appropriate coordination and transitions. Either model can be effective when coordination of responsibilities is clearly delineated. Another important component in the perioperative care of the patient is the transition from the inpatient to outpatient setting. When possible, there should be good communication and coordination of the transfer of care to the outpatient physician who is provided sufficient information about the intraoperative course and its implications, including any issues that arise as part of the anesthetic management that might impact postoperative management.

ENHANCED RECOVERY AFTER SURGERY

Enhanced recovery after surgery (ERAS) is another example of a creative approach to the perioperative management of patients who undergo major surgical procedures.[55,56] ERAS protocols are evidence-based pathways designed to improve care and outcomes as well as efficiency in the perioperative period. ERAS protocols require a multidisciplinary approach to perioperative care with particular emphasis on the entire perioperative course. The most successful ERAS programs are the ones that include participation by all of the healthcare and service providers who have a role in the perioperative course for the patient population.[57,58] Most ERAS protocols include preoperative education, perioperative antimicrobial management, pain management strategies, and early rehabilitation. In some cases, separate protocols have been initiated to address each period in the perioperative course, one to address the immediate perioperative management strategies and another to concentrate on the patient-care needs outside of the immediate postoperative period.[59] Many successful ERAS protocols have been implemented to optimize care of patients undergoing a variety of surgical procedures, including laparoscopic and other colorectal procedures, breast surgery, and urologic surgery.[60,61] Recently an ERAS protocol was implemented to optimize perioperative management of living liver donors[62] and another designed to improve perioperative management of patients undergoing elective craniotomy.[63] Each of these protocols has resulted in improved patient outcomes. For some patients, hospital lengths of stay and postoperative complications were reduced by as much as 30% and 50%, respectively[64,65]; for others postoperative pain management was improved despite administration of less opioids.[60-62,66]

As noted earlier, one of the most important features of the ERAS program, as with other pathways designed to improve perioperative care, is that the protocols are developed by a multidisciplinary group of providers that includes physicians, nurses, respiratory therapists, and others to ensure seamless coordination across the continuum from preoperative, intraoperative, and postoperative (postdischarge) periods.[67] The anesthesiologists offer essential information about key components of anesthetic management that can be modified to improve outcomes.

The outcomes associated with implementation of ERAS protocols have generally been positive for patients, providers, and health systems. In addition, the implementation of the protocols with participation of all providers involved in patient care enables a comprehensive review of the clinical course and outcomes, costs, and resource needs. The participants should be encouraged to review the clinical, financial, and other data regularly and, if appropriate, to modify the protocol to optimize care. One protocol recently implemented to improve care in colorectal surgery identified an increased incidence of acute renal injury.[68] The patients at risk for acute renal injury were those who had longer operative times and an associated diagnosis of diverticulitis. The findings emphasized a need to reassess the management strategies and to implement a goal-directed approach to fluid management intraoperatively and postoperatively. Follow-up will be required to determine if these changes in the protocol will be successful. These findings, however, emphasize the need to not only work collaboratively during the development of the protocol, but also review the experiences after implementation and modify the protocol when adverse outcomes occur.

Based on experiences with many of the ERAS protocols initiated to date, this approach to refining and improving care has been successful in improving outcomes and lowering costs. From a healthcare economic perspective, the ERAS protocols represent a value-based approach to optimizing care.[55] The development of the protocols give anesthesiologists an opportunity to engage in discussions with surgeons and other providers involved in the patients' care about how to optimize perioperative care and how to modify anesthesia practice and pain management strategies to facilitate recovery and potentially reduce complications. At the same time, while the reported improvements in outcome are impressive, anesthesiologists and other providers should ensure that outcome measures of most importance to patients are incorporated into future ERAS protocols in order to enhance their value.[58,69]

PERIOPERATIVE SURGICAL HOME

The expanding roles identified for anesthesiologists provide the foundation and framework upon which they can take on even broader roles as perioperative physicians.[70-72] The American Society of Anesthesiologists (ASA) in collaboration with other medical specialties has developed the perioperative surgical home (PSH) as a model for coordinating care throughout the entire perioperative period.[73-75] Many of the concepts incorporated into the PSH are built on the same foundation as those incorporated into the PCMH model. The PCMH is designed to better manage patients with complex medical problems and comorbidities in the outpatient setting,[49-51] whereas the PSH emphasizes clinical management of the patient from the time of scheduling of a surgical procedure through the entire perioperative period. The PSH is designed to specifically optimize outcomes during and after surgery, and to facilitate the transition of the patient back to the primary care provider. As with PCMH, the concept of the PSH model is to provide patient-focused care, consistent with patient goals and expectations. The goal for the PSH is to develop evidence-based clinical pathways designed to improve outcomes, and reduce overall costs-of-care across the continuum, including costs associated with home care and skilled nursing facilities.[76] Although the goals for implementation of the perioperative surgical home are clear, there is no single model nor list of specific guidelines one can follow when implementing a PSH. For some PSH models, the anesthesiologist assumes primary responsibility, whereas in other cases the surgeon is the lead provider. For some PSH models, co-management agreements with other providers has facilitated coordination of care and resulted in fewer surgical cancellations, less complications, lower lengths of stay, and fewer readmissions. For many PSH experiences, even when the anesthesiologist assumes a major role in the overall care of planning and execution, input from other providers (including hospitalist or medical subspecialist) is obtained based on the clinical needs of the patient. The collaborative relationships that are developed under the PSH extend to the care of other patients and provide the opportunity for other providers to better understand the skills, roles, and responsibilities of the anesthesiologists. These relationships are also critically important in representing the value anesthesiologists have under bundled payment models.

Although the goals for the PSH and ERAS protocols have some similarities, the components and overall goals for the PSH are somewhat broader than the expected outcomes for ERAS protocols. As proposed by the ASA, the PSH has the following major goals:

- identify the patient and proposed plans;
- facilitate communication among the surgeons, anesthesiologists, and others as needed to coordinate care;
- provide thorough preoperative assessment and develop a care plan, including management strategies for associated diseases;
- develop and implement evidence-based protocols for clinical care throughout the perioperative period;
- manage clinical care across the continuum; and
- measure and publicly report outcomes and performance.

The fundamental components of the PSH are clearly desirable goals and build on many of the basic concepts of perioperative medicine. The PSH is generally more comprehensive, requires thoughtful leadership and institutional commitment beyond what is often required for an ERAS protocol designed to reengineer care for a focused surgical procedure.[76,77]

A number of examples of the PSH model have been successfully implemented for selected patient populations with impressive results.[78,79] Some are relatively straightforward evidence-based strategies to optimize perioperative care, whereas others are more comprehensive. The process for developing a PSH can be cumbersome and requires a great deal of coordination across both inpatient and outpatient settings and, in some cases, participation of different healthcare systems. The model requires a designated physician leader who has responsibility for overseeing the continuum of perioperative care. To implement a successful PSH requires that the physician champion have some training and experience in process improvement strategies.[80] The model also requires support from other providers, particularly surgeons and hospital administrators.[81] Although the PSHs have been implemented in a variety of healthcare settings, the most comprehensive models can be successfully implemented in "closed" healthcare systems, such as the Veterans Administration, Kaiser, and other fully integrated delivery models.[79,82-84] The implementation is more challenging when the PSH requires participation of providers and facilities from multiple different environments, as may be required for patients needing rehabilitation, skilled nursing, or home care.

Despite these constraints, the implementation of the PSH has been successful with improved clinical care, reduced costs, shorter lengths of stay, fewer hospital readmissions, and both provider and patient satisfaction. The fundamental components of the PSH are clearly desirable goals and build on many of the basic concepts described for perioperative medicine. The model has promise in addressing the challenges associated with care to patients with complicated medical problems who are scheduled to undergo a complex surgical procedure. How effectively this model can be expanded to address this broader patient population and engage more providers and health systems is still to be determined.[77,85]

Conclusion

Perioperative care continues to evolve, in large part because of the advances made in surgical and anesthesia management of patients undergoing complex procedures in the operating room and nonoperating room settings. Surgical procedures are now commonly performed on patients with underlying medical conditions that impact anesthetic and surgical management. At the same time, and, in part as a result of the changing patient population, the cost of care continues to escalate. Payors are concerned about the increasing costs of care and, in some cases, point to the lack of evidence to support some costly clinical practices. Medicare and some private payors are transitioning to MIPS with associated incentives for providing value-based care and penalties for poor performance.[86] At the same time, providers are being asked to assume greater risk by providing bundled payment for selected diagnoses. To address these dramatic shifts in payment and concerns about the overall costs of surgical care, new models of perioperative care and implementation of clinical pathways based on evidence have evolved. These new models of care require better cooperation and coordination among all providers. The concepts behind perioperative medicine provide the framework upon which to reengineer care to address these challenges. Although no single strategy is appropriate for all clinical settings and patient needs, the one critical component of perioperative medicine is the need to implement a model of care that ensures coordination, collaboration, and improved transitions across the continuum from preoperative assessment and management to postoperative rehabilitation. These elements provide the opportunity for anesthesiologists and anesthesia departments to expand their scope of practice, building on the successes in improving intraoperative quality and safety. A number of alternative approaches to optimizing perioperative care may be appropriate and in all likelihood, multiple strategies will be required to address the idiosyncrasies of each patient population, surgical procedure, and institutional capabilities. The PSH is an example of a new creative model that might have significant benefit for selected patient populations; aligning patient's, provider's, hospital's, and payor's goals; and significantly improving perioperative care by building on the experience and successes of other approaches including ERAS, the surgical hospitalist model, and the PSH. To successfully assume an expanded role, anesthesiologists will have to build on their clinical expertise, and will have to acquire and analyze data on outcomes and costs to document that the new models of perioperative care are fulfilling the needs of all providers, health systems, payors, and, most importantly, patients.

Complete references available online at expertconsult.com.

References

1. Committee on Quality of Care in America. *Institute of Medicine: To Err is Human: Building a Safer Health System*. Washington: National Academy Press; 2000.
2. Papanicolas I, et al. *JAMA*. 2018;319(10):1024–1039.
3. Patel AS, et al. *Appl Health Econ Health Policy*. 2013;11:577.
4. McCrum ML, et al. *Med Care*. 2014;52(3):235–242.
5. Song PH, et al. *J Healthc Manag*. 2017;62(3):186–194.
6. Bader AM, et al. *Cleve Clin J Med*. 2009;76(suppl 4):S104.
7. Correll DJ, et al. *Anesthesiology*. 2006;105:1254.
8. Rock P. *Anesthesiology Clin NA*. 2000;18:495–513.
9. Taner CB, et al. *Liver Transpl*. 2012;18:361–369.
10. Garimella V, Cellini C. *Clin Colon Rectal Surg*. 2013;26:191–196.
11. Ilfeld BM, et al. *Pain*. 2010;150:477–485.
12. Rivard C, et al. *Gynecol Oncol*. 2014.
13. Hashemian SM, et al. *N Engl J Med*. 2014;370:979–980.
14. Shiramizo SC, et al. *PLoS One*. 2011;6:e26790.
15. Ferrer R, Artigas A. *Minerva Anestesiol*. 2011;77:360–365.
16. Deepa C, Muralidhar K. *J Anaesthesiol Clin Pharmacol*. 2012;28:386–396.
17. Bozic KJ. *Clin Orthop Relat Res*. 2014;472:188–193.
18. Mattie AS, Webster BL. *Health Care Manag*. 2008;27:338–349.
19. Teufack SG, et al. *J Neurosurg*. 2010;112:249–256.
20. Vats S, et al. *Med Care*. 2013;51:964–969.
21. Medicare QPP Resource Library. https://qpp.cms.gov/about/resource-library. Accessed December 31, 2018
22. Vetter TR, et al. *Anesth Analg*. 2017;124:1450–1458.
23. Ferschl MB, et al. *Anesthesiology*. 2005;103:855.
24. Carli F, Scheede-Bergdahl C. *Anesthesiol Clin*. 2015;33(1):17–33.
25. Vlisides PE, et al. *J Neurosurg Anesthesiol*. 2018.
26. West MA, et al. *Curr Anesthesiol Rep*. 2017;7(4):340–349.
27. Cullati S, et al. *BMJ Qual Saf*. 2013;22:639–646.
28. Millat B. *J Visc Surg*. 2012;149:369.
29. Rateau F, et al. *Ann Fr Anesth Reanim*. 2011;30:479.
30. Khoshbin A, et al. *Can J Surg*. 2009;52:309.
31. Ahmed M, et al. *Ann Surg*. 2013;258:958.
32. Ahmed K, et al. *Urol Int*. 2013;90:417.
33. Gilmour D. *J Perioper Pract*. 2009;19:196.
34. Bloodworth K. *J Perioper Pract*. 2011;21:97.
35. Skoretz SA, et al. *Chest*. 2010;137:665.
36. Magill SS, et al. *N Engl J Med*. 2014;370:1196.
37. Adanir T, et al. *Int J Surg*. 2010;8:221–224.
38. Canet E, Bellomo R. *Curr Opin Crit Care*. 2018;24(6):568–574.
39. Endara ML, et al. *Plast Reconstr Surg*. 2013;132:996.
40. Monk TG, Price CC. *Curr Opin Crit Care*. 2011;17:376.
41. Millar K, et al. *Paediatr Anaesth*. 2014;24:201.
42. Rieth EF, et al. *Curr Anesthesiol Rep*. 2018;8(4):368–374.
43. Soffin EM, et al. *Anesth Analg*. 2018.
44. Adogwa O, et al. *J Neurosurg Spine*. 2017;27(6):670–675.
45. Wang MC, et al. *J Ambul Care Manage*. 2015;38(1):69–76.
46. https://www.abeo.com/anesthesia-mergers-understand-and-thrive/. Accessed December 31, 2018
47. Martin J, Cheng D. *Can J Anaesth*. 2013;60:918.
48. Robeznieks A. *Mod Healthc*. 2013;43(6):18–19.
49. Graham J, et al. *Patient Saf Surg*. 2014;8(7).
50. Schwenk TL. *JAMA*. 2014;311:802.
51. Kociol RD, et al. *JACC Heart Fail*. 2013;1:445.
52. Kuo YFL, Goodwin JS. *J Am Geriatr Soc*. 2010;58:1649.
53. Auerbach AD, et al. *Arch Intern Med*. 2004;170:2010.
54. Rohatgi N, et al. *Ann Surg*. 2016;264(2):275–282.
55. Ljungqvist O. *JPEN J Parenter Enteral Nutr*. 2014.
56. Oda Y, Kakinohana M. *J Anesth*. 2014;28:141.
57. Ljungqvist O, et al. *JAMA Surg*. 2017;152:292–298.
58. Abola RE, et al. *Anesth Analg*. 2018;126(6):1874–1882.
59. Merchea A, Larson DW. *Surg Clin North Am*. 2018;98(6):1287–1292.
60. Lemini R, et al. *Int J Colorectal Dis*. 2018;33(11):1543–1550.
61. Rojas KE, et al. *Breast Cancer Res Treat*. 2018;171(3):621–626.
62. Khalil A, et al. *Clin Transplant*. 2018;32(8):e13342.
63. Wang Y, et al. *J Neurosurg*. 2018:1–12.
64. Fierens J, et al. *Acta Chir Belg*. 2012;112:355.
65. Lee L, et al. *Ann Surg*. 2014;259:670.
66. Brandal D, et al. *Anesth Analg*. 2017;125(5):1784–1792.
67. Persice M, et al. *J Perianesthe Nurs*. 2018.
68. Marcotte JH, et al. *Int J Colorectal Dis*. 2018;33(9):1259–1267.
69. Fleisher LA, Ko CY. *Anesth Analg*. 2018;126(6):1801–1802.
70. Longnecker DE. *Anesthesiology*. 1997;86:736.
71. Miller RD. *Anesthesiology*. 2009;110:714.
72. Kain ZN, et al. *Anesth Analg*. 2015;120(5):1155–1157.
73. Perioperative surgical home. http://www.periopsurghome.info/index.php. Accessed March 28, 2014.
74. Paloski D: Forum Focus—Perioperative Surgical Home Model AHA Physician Forum 7/3/13. http://www.ahaphysicianforum.org/news/enews/2013/070313.html. Retrieved March 30, 2014.
75. Vetter TR. *Anesthesiol Clin*. 2018;36(4):677–687.
76. Vetter TR, et al. *Anesth Analg*. 2014;118(5):1131–1136.
77. Vetter TR, et al. *Anesth Analg*. 2015;120(5):968–973.
78. Qiu C, et al. *Anesth Analg*. 2016;123:597–606.
79. Walters TL, et al. *Semin Cardiothorac Vasc Anesth*. 2016;20:133–140.
80. Mariano ER, et al. *Anesth Analg*. 2017;125(5):1443–1445.
81. Butterworth JF, Green JA. *Anesth Analg*. 2014;118:896–897.
82. Alvis BD, et al. *Anesth Analg*. 2017;125(5):1526–1531.
83. Mariano ER, et al. *Anesth Analg*. 2015;120:1163–1166.
84. Mahajan A, et al. *Anesth Analg*. 2017;125(1):333–341.
85. Vetter TR, et al. *BMC Anesthesiol*. 2013;13:6.
86. Centers for Medicare & Medicaid Services (CMS). HHS. Medicare Program; Merit-Based Incentive Payment System (MIPS) and Alternative Payment Model (APM) incentive under the physician fee schedule, and criteria for physician-focused payment models. Final rule with comment period. *Fed Regist*. 2016;81(214):77008–77831.

4 Informatics in Perioperative Medicine

DOUGLAS A. COLQUHOUN, NIRAV J. SHAH, and
SACHIN K. KHETERPAL

KEY POINTS

- Individual computers are connected via networks to share information across many users.
- Information security is about ensuring that the correct information is available only to the correct users at the correct time.
- Healthcare information storage and exchange is regulated to protect patient privacy.
- Information regarding the provision of anesthesia care is highly structured and organized compared to most healthcare specialties.
- Anesthesia care documentation systems have evolved in complexity and are now widely adopted in the perioperative care of patients in the United States.
- Benefits of electronic documentation of anesthesia care typically emerge from integration with monitoring, scheduling, billing, and enterprise electronic health record (EHR) systems.
- Active and passive decision-support tools may suggest typical courses of action or call to attention patterns that are not apparent to the clinician.
- Secondary use of EHR data is valuable in understanding the impact of clinical decisions on patient outcomes and the measurement of quality of care.
- Electronic devices may act as distractions within the operating room (OR) care environment.

Introduction

Computers have become ubiquitous in modern life. Their use has penetrated every medical field and the practice of perioperative care is no different. Computers have given rise to the academic discipline of informatics, the study of information creation, storage, handling, manipulation, and presentation. Within health care this is referred to as medical, biomedical, or clinical informatics.

Computer Systems

At their most basic, computer systems are complex electronic circuits that perform mathematical operations (add, subtract, multiply, divide, and compare) on information available to them. Even the most complicated computer systems consist of these operations repeated millions of times per second, which collectively generate the activity specified by the user. Every operation performed within the computer begins with the retrieval of information in the memory, a mathematical operation within the processor, and the storage of the output of that operation back to the memory. This cycle of retrieval, processing, and storage repeats millions of times per second.

Software applications execute the instructions that a computer uses to process information. The operating system is the fundamental software that controls the communication among the components of the computer. The operating system controls the order in which a processor completes tasks, allocates memory among different applications, provides a structure for organizing files in the long-term storage, controls access to files, determines which applications may run, and manages the interaction between the user and the computer. Modern operating systems provide graphic interfaces that act as paradigms to describe the organization of information and methods of user-specified computer action.

A software application is a set of instructions for a computer designed to perform a specific set of tasks. Electronic health record (EHR) software is an example of a software application. Software may (via the operating system) interact with external hardware devices, data held in long-term storage, and the user by way of input devices and display devices.

Because of the proliferation of mobile devices, traditional laptop or desktop computer systems have been supplanted in many environments by tablets or smartphone computers. These devices are structurally similar to traditional computing devices; however, the operating systems and software applications feature user interfaces that have been re-engineered to support use by touch screen or voice control operation. These devices trade off computational power, portability (size- and weight-related), and duration of operation (battery power).

Computer Networks

Networks are the means for the exchange of information among computers, enabling the sharing of resources. These networks may be established using wireless (e.g., microwave radio spectrum) or wired connections (Fig. 4.1). Dedicated hardware (equipment) controls the sending and receiving of information across these links, with specialized devices required to ensure that information is sent correctly

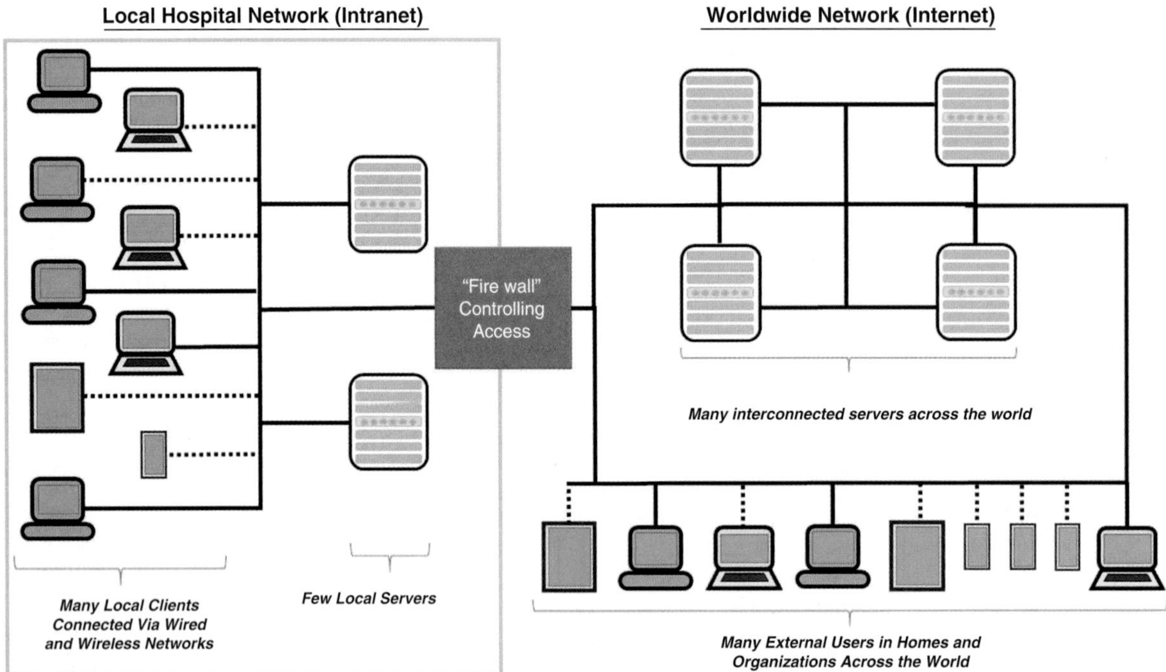

Fig. 4.1 Relationship between a local intranet (within an institution) and the wider Internet. Institutions may choose to use an external vendor to provide certain services hosted on external servers, this is referred to as "cloud" computing or services. Prevention of unauthorized access to the intranet from external parties while allowing users to access the Internet and other remote resources is of paramount concern. "Firewall" devices aid in the separation of the institutional network from the wider Internet and control access.

to the intended computers on the network. Software is used to ensure communication is performed according to predefined standards. In order for a computer to be accessible in the network, each computer must be given a unique address on the network so that information can be identified as destined for that computer. The process of obtaining and maintaining network addresses is performed within the local operating system and network hardware. This allows software applications to specify the information to be sent and the operating system and network hardware to manage how it is exchanged between computers.

Wired networks require the computer system and the receiving hardware to be physically connected by electrical or optical cable. This limits the flexibility in the connection points, which must be placed in preplanned areas, with any subsequent adjustments requiring re-routing of cables. However, information travelling on the network cannot be intercepted or accessed without physical access to the network cables or connection points.

Wireless network systems offer advantages of convenience and the ability to move around a work environment without maintaining a physical connection among the computer systems. However, this usually occurs at the expense of speed of information exchange. Information exchange via wireless links is an order of magnitude slower than the fastest wired connections. Because wireless systems require the availability of strong radio links between the computer and the network equipment, they are subject to issues of poor reception (possibly because of physical barriers) and interference, which manifest as inaccessible or degraded network performance. It is difficult to control the precise limits of where a wireless network is available (i.e., only within a building and not immediately outside of it), therefore processes to limit wireless network access to authorized users and to encrypt data transmitted across wireless links are required.

In practice, healthcare facilities use a blend of both wired and wireless networks to ensure that the advantages of each system are available to support the users.

In most settings, the network is organized as a "client-server" model. The computer that hosts the shared resources is referred to as the "server" and the computer accessing the resources is the "client." The server is responsible for ensuring the client is an authorized user of the shared resource (access control) and ensuring the resource remains available to multiple users, potentially by preventing one client from monopolizing the use of the resource.

The client-server concept stands in contrast to peer-to-peer architecture, whereby resources are distributed across systems, with each computer on the network contributing its resources (e.g., files or specialized hardware). All computers are both clients and servers in this arrangement. There is limited ability to control access in a planned and coordinated manner.

Use of a client-server infrastructure may allow for a significant amount of the computational tasks to be outsourced to the central server. When the client has very limited computational resources this is referred to as a "thin client." Computationally intensive tasks can be performed by the server and the client receives the results of the computation. Fundamentally, the thin client is viewing and interacting with a software application that is running on the server. The client is little more than a means of sending user input to the server and a dynamic display of application results. In order for this arrangement to work, there must be a limited, predictable set of software applications that the client accesses on the server, with a reliable network connection. Without the network connection, the thin client has no functionality. This model may be easier to maintain because any changes are done centrally and need to be made once and then become available to every client connecting in.

An alternative model is the "thick client," where the client is capable of significant computational activities, retains a fully functional state when not connected to the network, accesses only the information required across the network, and processes it independently. However, these clients require individual maintenance.

A hybrid solution is the concept of "application virtualization," whereby a single software application is hosted and uses the computational resources centrally and the client systems access this application regardless of their configurations. This blends the advantages of a thin client—control of the application's availability, ease of maintenance, and ensuring compatibility (by not requiring any level of computational resources aside from running the connection to the server)—with users having a fully functional computer or device to use for the remainder of their tasks. Additionally, this hybrid enforces a separation between the information stored on the server and any applications running on the client and thus information can be secured within the server that is housed within the institutional network.

The Internet

The Internet is a global network of networks. Best known by two of the ways in which it can be used—websites and email—the Internet is at its simplest a method for transferring electronic information across the world. Internet service providers (ISPs) provide access to optical and electrical cables, which transfer information across the world. As these cables are all interconnected, multiple paths are available to transfer data at any one time. Routers control the flow of Internet traffic and ensure that it takes the most direct and fastest routes across the multiple paths available to it. Although the delay that a user may experience in accessing information varies widely and is dependent on many factors, the flow of information around the world can be measured in the order of hundreds of milliseconds or less.

Use of the Internet has led to the development of a series of technologies where computing resources are offered to multiple clients using an Internet connection as a means of distribution and interaction with the clients (see Fig. 4.1). These "cloud" platforms allow on-demand and scalable use of computing resources. Computing resources can be bought and sold based on the variable amount of time they are used or the amount of information stored; additional capacity can be flexibly added. These resources are accessible from anywhere with an Internet connection. Furthermore, cloud platforms give organizations the ability to transfer the management of the specialized computer hardware needed to provide these services to another party.

The integration of mobile phone data networks and the proliferation of increasingly powerful handheld devices (such as smartphones or tablets) has increased further the number of potential clients. For healthcare organizations, there is significant user pressure to be able to access healthcare information systems remotely or from these mobile devices.

The most ubiquitous usage of the Internet is in the delivery of "web pages." Information is stored on a "web server" and upon request from an application being run on a remote client computer (web browser), the information and display formatting instructions (i.e., size, shape, position of text, or graphics) are sent to the client. The web browser then interprets these instructions and displays the information according to the specified instructions. This process is highly dependent on well-defined and accepted standards of information exchange between client and server and rendering by the client.

These web pages have become increasingly sophisticated incorporating text, video, audio, complex animations, stylesheets, and hypertext links. Technologies have evolved into an interactive process that can dispense information specific to only one user (e.g., a record of the user's bank transactions) and that can be supplied in a manner that is generalizable to many different users (so all customers can access their bank transactions this way). When these instructions are assembled to generate specific business processes, they function as software applications that are web based and are referred to as "web applications" or "web apps." Interaction with web pages may lead to complex business processes being undertaken in the physical world. For example, the ability to buy a book over the Internet starts with a web page displaying the information and ends in someone delivering it to the door, with many physical steps in between. Healthcare organizations have embraced these technologies to support their delivery and administration of patient care, including scheduling systems, laboratory result reporting, patient communications, and equipment management systems, all of which are delivered in this manner.

Of note, information which is travelling across the Internet, without additional measures, is not necessarily private. A salient metaphor would be to consider the difference between information being conveyed in an envelope (where the contents are not visible) and information being conveyed on a postcard (where the message is clear to anyone who holds it).

Information Security

Although computing technology has significantly influenced the delivery of medical care, it has also brought a series of challenges that must be addressed. A major consideration is information security. Core to these considerations is ensuring that the correct information is available to the correct users at the correct time.

These threats to information security may come from within or outside an organization. Within organizations, an employee may access information that they are not authorized to so do or by transferring and storing it in an insecure manner. They may introduce security threats by using applications that may transfer information outside of the organization or by modifying an existing network by using a personal device. External threats may seek to improperly access information ("hacking") by obtaining passwords or identities from legitimate users (via "phishing" attacks) or by introducing applications that degrade computer function to extort payment ("ransomware" attacks).

The paradigm used for controlling access to computing resources is users and accounts. Each person who uses the computer is considered to be a user. Users can be identified and mapped to real-world persons. Users may belong to groups that share common attributes. It should be known in advance which resources should be available to which users or groups of users. A group of users (i.e., anesthesia providers) may have access to particular resources (e.g., a document of anesthesia policies) but each user may also have access based on their individual parameters (e.g., an individual anesthesiologist may have sole access to his or her own private files). A group of users with similar functional roles who have a defined set of resource privileges is known as "role-based security." Changes in privileges affect all users in that functional group.

Users should be able to positively identify themselves; commonly this involves the combination of a username and password with the password being known only to the user and the computer system. However, other methods of authentication, such as biometric information (fingerprint, iris scan, or face scan) or physical access tokens (e.g., identification badges) are now commonplace. Password policies that enforce a mandatory level of complexity (minimum length, mixing letters and numbers, or special characters), specific expiry dates, and prevent password reuse are designed to make it harder for passwords to be guessed by an unknown party or to mitigate or minimize the risk of passwords being accessed or used externally. However, requirements for increasing complexity or frequency of changes may pose additional burdens on users that they consider unacceptable and may not decrease risk.

Organizations may also choose to adopt "two-factor authentication" methods, which can be summarized as requiring "something you know and something you have" to gain access to the computer system. The password fulfills the first part of this concept as it is meant to be known only to the user. Devices such as physical token code generators (which provide a predictable response to be entered alongside the password) or an interactive system (authentication via a smartphone application or phone call) may satisfy the second concept. Thus, in order for someone to impersonate the user they must have both the password (that may have been taken without the user's knowledge) and a physical device (that the user is more likely to detect the absence of). This makes remote access less likely because an external user on the other side of the world may be able to obtain or guess a password but is very unlikely to also be able to obtain the token or smartphone required for access.

Physical security is an integral part of information security. Ensuring that an unauthorized person does not have physical access to computer hardware or access to the means of connecting to that computer hardware are important considerations. This can be accomplished by physical measures (such as locked rooms, doors, and devices that prevent movement of computer hardware) and considerations of where computers containing controlled information are placed (to prevent an unauthorized person from having access to a computer that is available in a public area).

However, as alluded to before, these restrictions are balanced against desires for increased usability and portability of computing devices from computer users and the need to make information available to the provider at the point of clinical interaction.

Therefore, it is necessary to ensure secure access to information across wireless links and across the Internet. One method for doing this is to ensure that the information transferred is not readily visible along its means of transmission. This is performed by a group of processes known as encryption. Encryption is the process of transforming a piece of information from its original and accessible state to one that is not accessible and lacks meaning without an additional piece of information (an encryption key).

The transformation to and from encrypted text takes place in a manner that is relatively easy to perform with the known encryption key but is infeasible to do so without knowing this key. Encryption processes are based on mathematics involving multiplication of very large numbers, which creates many possible combinations of different factors that could have led to the same outcome. Therefore, it would be computationally infeasible, with current technology, to attempt to try all possible solutions.

External threats to an organization involve outside entities attempting to access services or applications that are meant for internal use only. Because healthcare organizations must be connected to the Internet to enable many information exchange functions, their data may potentially be available to every Internet-connected device in the world. "Firewalls" are used to ensure that only legitimate transactions and interactions with the external world are exposed to the internal hospital network. These hardware or software tools, collectively known as a firewall, prevent the creation of unauthorized connections from outside the organization to the internal computing systems. Firewalls can also limit the types of network traffic that are allowed to exit from the internal networked system. For example, it may restrict network traffic typically used for the sharing of files.

In order to allow legitimate external access, organizations may allow the creation of virtual private networks (VPNs). After appropriate authentication and verification, VPNs set up an encrypted path for information from an external Internet-connected computer to the organization's internal network. This allows the external computer to act as if it was physically connected to the organization's internal network and to access resources such as specialized software or shared files. This adds an additional layer of access security to the connection and ensures the communication is secure. A healthcare organization may require use of a VPN to access an EHR from outside the organization's network.

Standards for Healthcare Data Exchange

Although not always obvious, the EHR is typically an amalgamation of multiple computer systems and devices of various complexity. These systems exchange data according to common standards, languages, and processes.

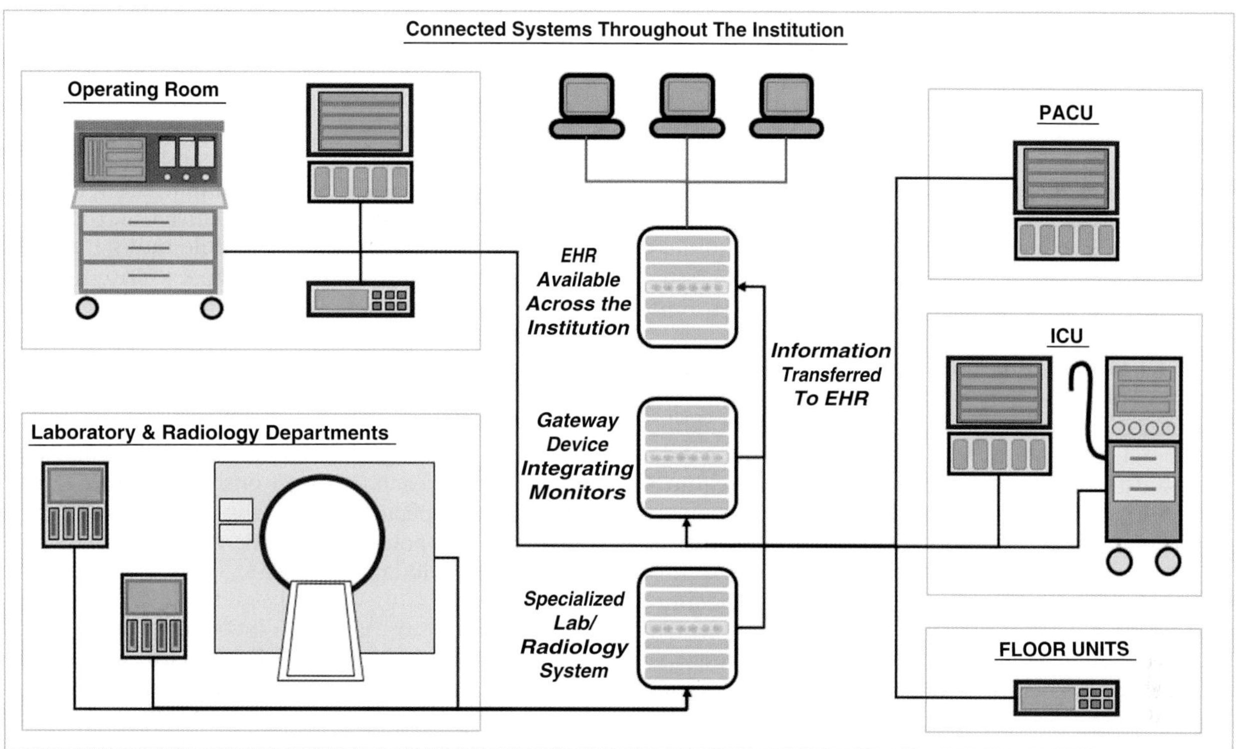

Fig. 4.2 Information flows from connected devices across the institution into the electronic health record (*EHR*). Some departments maintain specialized software to manage the needs specific to their workflow—for example Radiology departments using Picture Archiving and Communication Systems—that are interfaced into the EHR (i.e., to allow a report to be connected to the original CT scan). Similarly networked monitor data is made available by the use of a gateway interface device. *PACU*, Postanesthesia care unit

Common connections include monitoring devices that allow automatic transfer for measured parameters into the electronic chart, infusion pumps (recording programmed settings), laboratory instruments (blood gas machines, cell counters, biochemistry analyzers, point-of-care testing devices), or systems that manage patient admission, identification, and bed occupancy (admission, discharge, and transfer [ADT] system). All of these devices and systems need methods of communicating with the EHR (Fig. 4.2). Although in some situations it may be possible to use a proprietary standard for communication between systems, it can quickly become difficult to manage across an entire institution. As a consequence, a series of commonly used standards have been established that allow the communication of healthcare information.

The Health Level-7 (HL7) standard, originally developed in the late 1980s, is still used widely in the exchange of health information. HL7 allows the transmission of data in a standardized manner among devices and clinical systems. The information can be identified to a specific patient and organized into different data types, indicating laboratory results, monitor data, and billing information. It can also cause the receiving system to perform an action, such as update previously obtained data. The HL7 standard and subsequent derivatives that address the exchange of clinical documents in a structured and identified manner support communication among different clinical systems. However, this standard was based on data exchange within different software application systems within an institution and did not envisage the proliferation of Internet-connected devices remotely accessing shared resources across many healthcare organizations.

This new paradigm led to the development of Fast Health Interoperability Resources (FHIR). This communication standard is analogous to how modern Internet applications exchange data via simple standardized requests to a central resource. FHIR enables easier integration across different types of software and integrates security features necessary due to the proliferation of mobile devices. This standard is designed to facilitate the exchange of data regardless whether it is a single vital sign or a scanned document from a physical chart.

Regulation of Electronic Data Exchange

In the United States, the 1996 passage of the Health Insurance Portability and Accountability Act (HIPAA) established a common regulatory framework that defined health information and the processes by which it should be stored and transferred, and established powers to investigate concerns regarding noncompliance with these rules.

There are four major regulatory rules: the HIPAA Privacy Rule, Security Rule, Enforcement Rule, and the Breach Notification Rule. Each update is a complex regulatory document and professional advice should be sought on the applicability and relevance of each of these to a particular situation.

The HIPAA Privacy Rule details the allowable uses and disclosures of individually identifiable health information, which is referred to as "protected health information" (PHI). Identifiers that are considered PHI are listed in Table 4.1. The privacy rule additionally defines the healthcare agencies covered by the rule. It defines processes that must be taken when working with business partners outside the healthcare agency through the creation of business associate agreements. Further, it establishes the concept of a limited data set, which is a set of identifiable healthcare information that is devoid of direct identifiers and can be shared with certain entities for research purposes, healthcare operations, and public health reasons; use of these is governed by "data use agreements."

The HIPAA Security Rule applies specifically to electronic PHI (e-PHI). The rule requires that e-PHI created, received, maintained, or transmitted by an organization should be done so confidentially and in a manner that ensures data integrity and availability. Additionally, the rule requires that threats to information security be monitored and measures be taken to mitigate these threats; this includes audits of computer systems to ensure unauthorized access has not occurred. The specification includes physical, technical, procedural, and administrative measures, all of which need to be undertaken for compliance. In general, the rule does not specify a particular set of computing resources that should be used, but instead specifies the standards to which they should be verified.

The HIPAA Enforcement Rule established the processes whereby a breach of the privacy rule could be investigated, and sanctions enforced. The Office of Civil Rights (OCR) within the Department of Health and Human Services (HHS) is responsible for receiving and investigating these complaints. Complaints may also be referred to the Department of Justice if it is believed that a criminal breach has occurred. Penalties for noncompliance can involve significant monetary fines or imprisonment in the context of criminal acts.

Finally, the HIPAA Breach Notification Rule defines what a breach of PHI data security is and obligates covered organizations to report to the OCR breaches of PHI that are discovered. Differing timelines for reporting apply, depending on if the breach involved greater or fewer than 500 individuals. Notification must also be provided to affected individuals and potentially to the media, depending on the number of individuals involved.

TABLE 4.1 Data Elements that Allow Patients to Be Identified

HIPAA IDENTIFIERS
Names
All geographic subdivisions smaller than a state, including street address, city, county, precinct, ZIP code
All elements of dates (except year) for dates that are directly related to an individual. Ages over 89 and all elements of dates (including year) indicative of such age
Telephone numbers
Vehicle identifiers and serial numbers, including license plate numbers
Fax numbers
Device identifiers and serial numbers
Email addresses
Web Universal Resource Locators (URLs)
Social security numbers
Internet Protocol (IP) addresses
Medical record numbers
Biometric identifiers, including finger and voice prints
Health plan beneficiary numbers
Full-face photographs and any comparable images
Account numbers
Any other unique identifying number, characteristic, or code
Certificate/license numbers

HIPAA, Health Insurance Portability and Accountability Act.
Adapted from https://www.hhs.gov/hipaa/for-professionals/privacy/special-topics/de-identification/index.html. Accessed March 3, 2019.

The Nature of Healthcare Information in the Anesthesia Encounter

In the conduct of anesthesia care, much of the information gathered could be considered as frequently-occurring structured data. That is, much of the information contained within the encounter can be categorized into one of a relatively small number of groups. This information is present commonly across anesthesia encounters. And the information itself can often be restricted to a small number of possible options—consider the example of an airway assessment.

This applies to information gathered in the preoperative phase of care (i.e., Mallampati classification from an airway examination) and the intraoperative phase of care (i.e., heart rate or systolic blood pressure). Furthermore, the intraoperative phase of care is marked by repetition of information at predefined intervals with measurements that may be taken in an automated manner (e.g., noninvasive blood pressure recordings every 3 minutes).

A majority of data gathered during an anesthesia case is structured, limited, and predictably repeated. However, the data are also voluminous with data generated and captured continuously on monitors, anesthesia machines, and medication pumps. More than 50 different parameters may describe a single minute of anesthesia care.

This is in contrast with the nature of the information captured in many medical specialties that are not easily constrained by content or structure. The documentation of a primary care visit may follow a standard format, however the number of variables captured may not be easily defined in advance or constrained to a standard structure; the range of possible issues to be documented may be too broad.

Anesthesia-derived data is well suited for capture into electronic charting systems. A number of mature commercially available systems are available for undertaking this task. These systems are often not standalone, and we will discuss how they are integrated in the next section.

Development and Deployment of Anesthesia Information Management Systems

Given the suitability for automated capture of recurring high-volume data, the concept of using computerized capture and storage for parts of the anesthesia record is not new. McKesson in 1934 described an early form of monitor that integrated with a vital signs data recorder (Fig. 4.3).[1] Early pioneering systems included the Duke Automatic Monitoring Equipment (DAME) System and its more compact successor, microDAME, which combined an internal monitoring platform with an integrated network architecture for central data recording.[2] Anesthesia Record Keeper Integrating Voice Recognition (ARKIVE) developed commercially in 1982 by Diatek included both a voice and touch screen interface.[3,4] Over time, other systems became available and these progressively morphed from being described as "anesthesia record keeping" (ARK) systems to "anesthesia information management systems" (AIMS) as the range of features and integration with other systems progressed.

Despite extensive development of a number of commercial systems, the use of AIMS was relatively limited in the early 2000s. Survey estimates suggest that by 2007 market penetration in academic medical centers increased from approximately 10% to approximately 75% by the end of 2014. By 2020, it is estimated that market penetration will reach 84% of all medical centers.[5-7] In the United States, the implementation of EHRs has been encouraged by federal government financial incentives including the American Reinvestment and Recovery Act of 2009, which authorized up to $11 million dollars per hospital to finance the adoption of health information technology.[8]

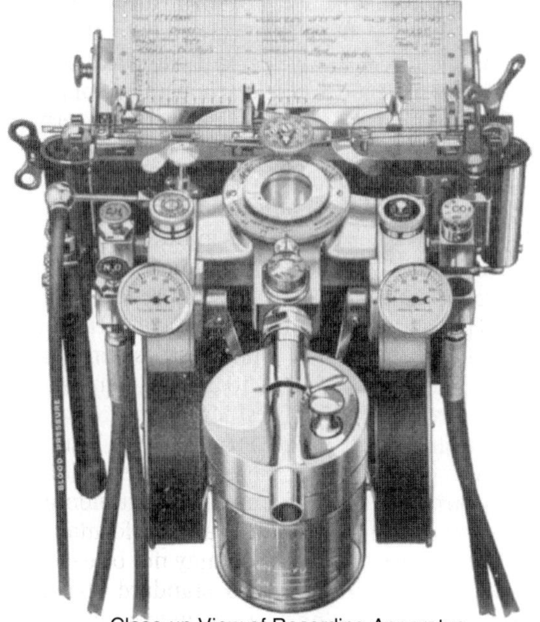

Fig. 4.3 McKesson's apparatus for the automated recording of physiologic recordings and gas mixtures. From 1934. (From McKesson EI. The technique of recording the effects of gas-oxygen mixtures, pressures, rebreathing and carbon-dioxide, with a summary of the effects. *Anesth-Analg.* 1934;13[1]:1–7 ["Apparatus" Page 2])

The adoption of health information technology has resulted in the increasing integration of the anesthesia record with other clinical systems. The American Society of Anesthesiologists (ASA) has produced a statement on the documentation of anesthesia care.[9] Such systems can be used to fulfill clinical documentation needs; however, much of the promise of these systems is in the potential for integration with the broader hospital environment and secondary uses of the data that they potentially facilitate.

ANATOMY OF AN ANESTHESIA INFORMATION MANAGEMENT SYSTEM

A mature AIMS must be capable of (1) recording all aspects of the anesthesia encounter (preoperative, intraoperative, and postanesthesia care unit [PACU]); (2) must automatically gather the high-fidelity physiologic data generated by monitoring platforms and anesthesia machines; and (3) must allow the anesthesia provider to record observations regarding the conduct of the anesthetic. These three simple requirements allow us to closely specify the anatomy of an AIMS.

The first requirement for access of the same patient record during multiple phases of a case suggests the use of a system organized on a computer network, where the computer record is maintained on a central server and accessed by multiple clients. This capability requires accessibility of computer workstations at each patient-care location to facilitate documentation. The computer must be accessible during the clinical interaction but in a way that does not interfere with this interaction, which is both an issue of ergonomics and of provider behavior. In the operating room (OR), the system should be directly accessible at the time of clinical care to allow contemporaneous documentation without the anesthesia provider physically moving away from the patient or care area. In many deployments, this is achieved with a computer mounted to the anesthesia workstation alongside the monitoring equipment. Because the computer hardware is located in clinical environments, these may become contaminated with pathogens and it is important that the hardware can be cleaned in a manner that is compatible with infection control policies.[10,11]

The second requirement for automated capture of data from OR monitors and anesthesia machines is some form of interface device between the computer hardware and the hemodynamic monitors, anesthesia machines, and other patient-connected equipment (infusion pumps or ventilators)—Table 4.2. In most AIMS implementations, this interface occurs at a central level, where a network of the physiologic monitors and the central server hosting the AIMS communicate via a gateway device. Typically, interfaces use standardized data formats, such as those described earlier that transmit communication among devices and software solutions from different manufacturers and developers. Interfacing these devices with a computer network may require specialized hardware and additional cost. However, the interface enables the automated capture of

TABLE 4.2 Examples of Parameters Commonly Included in the Anesthesia Record Gathered Automatically from Different Sources

FROM CORE PHYSIOLOGIC MONITOR
Arterial blood pressure (systolic, diastolic, mean)
Cardiac index
Cardiac output
Central venous pressure
End tidal CO_2
Heart rate (ECG monitoring and SpO_2)
Intracranial pressure (ICP)
Noninvasive blood pressure (systolic, diastolic, mean)
Pulmonary artery pressure (systolic, diastolic, mean)
Pulse pressure variation (PPV) and systolic pressure variation (SPV)
Saturation of peripheral oxygen (SpO_2)
ST segment analysis
Systemic vascular resistance
Temperature (all sources)
FROM STAND-ALONE DEVICES (MAY BE AVAILABLE WITHIN SOME CORE PHYSIOLOGIC MONITORS)
Acceleromyography value
Cerebral oximeter (NIRS)
Continuous cardiac output measurement devices
Level of consciousness monitors
Mixed venous oxygen saturation (SvO_2)
FROM ANESTHESIA WORKSTATION
Fraction of inspired oxygen (FiO_2)
Fresh gas flows: oxygen, air, nitrous oxide
Volatile anesthetic agents (inspired and expired concentrations)
Minute volume
Nitrous oxide (inspired and expired concentrations)
Oxygen (inspired and expired concentrations)
Peak inspiratory pressure (PIP)
Positive end-expiratory pressure (PEEP)
Respiratory rate (ventilator and $ETCO_2$)
Tidal volume
Ventilator mode

monitor and anesthesia machine data, freeing up clinical providers from the recording of these data elements. In light of the cost and practical challenges, some AIMS situated in low-resource settings (e.g., an office-based anesthesia location) may choose to eliminate the data interface feature.

Theoretically all electronically generated data can be recorded in the AIMS. As a consequence, the anesthesia provider must determine how much data should be incorporated into the system. Although some monitoring data is obtained with a defined frequency, such as a noninvasive blood pressure measurement taken every 3 minutes, most

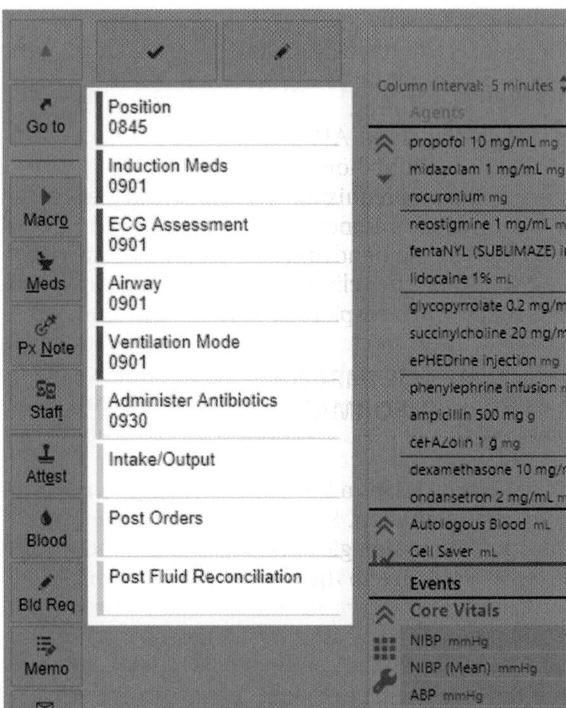

Fig. 4.4 A pre-defined set of charting elements for a given case. These may function as an example of passive decision support built into the EPIC Electronic Health Record Anesthesia Documentation (EPIC Systems, Verona, WI). The macro *(highlighted)* prompts the user to complete next documentation element. The "Administer Antibiotics" acts as an *aide-mémoire* reminding anesthesia providers that this is likely the next step in the process of care. (Image: © 2018 Epic System Corporation. Used with Permission.)

parameters are sampled from continuous data sources. In the OR, a pulse oximeter is not a single parameter checked at a discrete interval, but a continuous source of data. Continuous data sources (e.g., electrocardiogram [ECG], pulse oximeter, invasive blood pressure, or end-tidal carbon dioxide [$EtCO_2$] tracings) are transformed into measures that can be recorded with lower data intensity requirement, a process known as sampling. An ECG tracing may be sampled and interpreted to report heart rate and ST segment analysis results. Although it is technically possible to record continuous sources of data electronically for future review, this usually does not occur because the resulting data stream is difficult to present, archive, and review. Therefore, continuous data sources are usually reported as sampled values at a prespecified frequency.

The third requirement of an AIMS is to allow the user to annotate information (e.g., medications administered, descriptions of procedures performed, annotations to describe significant clinical events, or attestations for regulatory compliance) to the automatically collected data. Because of the similarity of one anesthesia encounter to another, some charting elements may be predefined to facilitate these documentation tasks and minimize the use of nonstructured or "free text" entries. Because of the possibility of similarity among cases, many systems use organized templates (sometimes referred to as "scripts," "templates," or "macros") that give the anesthesia provider easier access to charting elements required for a specific case type (Fig 4.4). For example, a cardiac anesthesia template may make charting elements regarding cardiopulmonary bypass prominent and easily selectable. These charting elements and templates are typically customizable at each installed site, thus providing flexibility in documenting site-specific practices or procedures.

Although the three AIMS requirements described give some specifics about how a system may be constructed, they are minimum requisites. The AIMS that only provides these requirements is not one that would be considered high value. The major advantages of AIMS come from their integration into other clinical systems and healthcare processes, which will be explored in the coming sections.

ADVANTAGES OF IMPLEMENTATION OF AN ANESTHESIA INFORMATION MANAGEMENT SYSTEM

The shift to an AIMS is a key improvement in the quality of clinical documentation. Removing the task of manual documentation of physiologic parameters has not been shown to decrease vigilance to the clinical situation and may free up anesthesia providers to perform other tasks.[12-15] An AIMS also establishes an independent, unbiased record of monitoring and machine data. Finally, legibility issues noted in handwritten charting are resolved by the use of an electronically assembled record.

Early studies compared blood pressure values recorded in handwritten charts and those recorded by automated collection. The blood pressure recordings on handwritten charts had lower maximum systolic pressures and higher minimum diastolic pressures when compared with automated collected values in OR studies.[16-18] This variation has been termed the "smoothing effect" of handwritten charting and may result in loss of clinically meaningful data.[16,19] A subsequent study demonstrated that errors in handwritten charting were clustered during high-intensity periods; that is, induction, emergence, and significant clinical events.[20,21]

Although documentation of physiologic parameters may be more complete in AIMS-charted records compared with handwritten charts other data elements may remain incomplete.[22,23] As AIMS deployments have matured, it has become apparent that documentation quality varies among providers and important clinical fields can often be left incomplete, particularly when completion requires the entry of free text.[24] Medication administration has also been incompletely documented or omitted in the AIMS compared with observed practice with a similar effect of inaccuracies occurring during high intensity periods of care.[25] AIMS support degrees of customization, including designating certain data elements as mandatory prior to completion of the case, but the decision to add more mandatory elements must be traded off against risks of arbitrary data entry ("clicking through") or provider frustration, both of which detract from the aim of improved data quality.[26] It is clear that the system design and decisions made for default values or required data elements have significant influence on the quality of record created.

One solution to the challenge of excessively burdensome documentation requirements is to use an adaptive method that changes the required elements for documentation based on the clinical context—for example, requiring documentation of bilateral breath sounds in cases involving an endotracheal tube, but not with an laryngeal mask airway.[26]

In addition, to improve compliance with the capture of individual, high-priority data elements alternative strategies may be employed. Real-time provider notification by text page for allergy or procedural notes has demonstrated increases in completeness of this documentation.[27,28] Non-real-time feedback, via dashboards, email feedback, or informational campaigns may leverage AIMS data to improve data element completion.[29] These effects may be sustained past the interventional period.[27,29]

Integration with billing processes allows the automated capture of case elements necessary to facilitate anesthesia billing, such as care start and stop times, details of the surgical procedure for which anesthesia care is being provided, the nature of anesthesia care, any separately billable procedures, and the involved providers. This information can be extracted by reporting functions and integrated with the patient identifiers. Compared to solutions that require the manual review of copies of paper records, AIMS-based workflows offer significant overall process efficiency gains; although some designs unfortunately redistribute administrative tasks to point-of-care clinicians. The potential impact of AIMS use on anesthesia procedure includes improving capture of data elements needed for billing, improved documentation to support billing of anesthesia procedures, and billing capture at time of clinical care leading to more rapid processing.[27,28,30,31]

An advantage of an AIMS system is the ability to check concurrency of anesthesia providers across one entire organization in real time. In the United States, an "in-room" anesthesia provider must be physically present when anesthesia care is provided at all times. This is typically documented by "sign in" and "sign out" documentation times. An in-room provider may be supervised by a supervising provider who may supervise a number of ORs up to maximum specified by institutional or payer policy. The AIMS system can, at time of sign-in, check that no in-room provider is documented in more than one OR simultaneously and no supervising provider exceeds the prespecified supervision ratios. Checking at time of sign-in assures that these standards are not violated by documentation errors and prevents delays in the billing process. In certain billing environments, violation of the concurrency rules may cause rejection of claims at the time of billing.

Providing an anesthesia record that can be accessed concurrently by multiple users may facilitate remote monitoring of care being provided by the in-room anesthesia provider by a supervising anesthesia provider. This increased visibility of patient care being provided at each care location allows the supervising provider to maintain a better level of awareness on the course of the case and gives the supervising provider additional guidance on management decisions. OR managers benefit from similar insight and may be able to make decisions about resource utilization based on the documented care.

Integration of Anesthesia Care Information with Operating Room Information Systems

Given the necessity of maintaining information regarding locations of care, case, patient, staffing, and case progress, it is natural to integrate anesthesia information systems with OR management systems. These systems are used in the scheduling of OR cases and assignment of staffing and supplies.

ORs are finite resources. There are a set number of available rooms, set number of available staff for these rooms, set times of availability of these staff, defined experience and specialization of these staff, and finite amount of specialist equipment for use in the rooms. As a result of these factors, ORs create enormous costs prior to any procedure being performed; efficient allocation and utilization of these resources are tied to financial outcomes of a hospital.

Each procedure performed requires allocation of procedural space, staff, and equipment that may be specific to the particular case. Therefore, it makes sense for this to be coordinated in a centralized manner. OR management systems are designed to accomplish this task controlling the allocation of these resources. These systems allow these resources to be allocated both generally (e.g., on Mondays OR 12 is dedicated for thoracic surgery cases [block scheduling]) and also specifically (e.g., John Smith is undergoing a right upper lobectomy by Dr. Jones from 11 AM to 1 PM on August 20), and further allocate staff and equipment to this procedure (case scheduling). Case scheduling may be enhanced by using historical procedural lengths to estimate future time needs stratified by proceduralist and specific procedure to be performed.

Scheduling of a case by a specific proceduralist allows the generation of a specific list of required equipment/instruments to be recalled based on anticipated requirements and proceduralist preferences. These "case pick lists" of "surgeons preference cards" can be used by supply teams to ensure that necessary equipment is available and predict future utilization.

The integration of OR management systems with AIMS provides the cases and procedures against which charting functions can be performed. Furthermore, communication between these systems can create common charting, such as phase of procedure (induction, procedure begun, procedure complete, etc.) which can be useful in understanding utilization of the OR environment for daily management and ascertaining longer-term trends. Given the enormous fixed expense incurred in the OR suite, an extensive literature has developed from the analysis of information derived from these systems regarding variability in procedure time, "turnover time" between sequentially scheduled procedures, and effect of variability of anesthesia-related case timings.[32-37]

A more recent trend is the integration of the AIMS and Operating Room Management Systems with the wider hospital-wide or "enterprise" EHR. This occurs via the development of specialized modules which account for the differences in workflow between the OR environment and the inpatient floor/ward units. These systems leverage common patient information—such as patient identification, demographics, registration, and location—then add specialization discussed above. Furthermore, this allows medical documentation, and laboratory and other diagnostic results to be made available to the perioperative providers on a single computer system.

One of the larger contrasts emerging from the OR workflow versus the rest of the inpatient environment is the process of medication documentation. When using an inpatient EHR, a provider enters a computer-based order for the routine administration of a medication. After pharmacy verification of the order, the medication is delivered to the appropriate unit for administration to the patient by a bedside nurse. In the OR environment, the medication administration decision making, selection of the medication from a pre-stocked cart, and administration is handled by an individual providing anesthesia care. This shortens the time from provider intent to patient administration. Therefore, the documentation needs to reflect the concept of care provided rather than care to be provided in the future (i.e., scheduling a medication to be administered). Given the high intensity of medication administrations, short time interval between administrations and supply from the bedside cart of the medications to be administered, the ideal documentation system should not be burdensome and allow rapid entry.

A number of features of the inpatient EHR are unavailable due to this mode of medication administration and documentation: positive identification of the patient and medication with a specified order—typically performed by "barcode" scanning of medications and patients at time of administration—is not performed as medications are typically documented retrospectively, although patients are positively identified at the beginning of each anesthesia care encounter. Additionally, automated medication interaction, dose, and allergy checking may not function in the context of perioperative administration due the practice of retrospective documentation. As the documentation of anesthesia care is quite different from that of most medical interactions. The differences in workflows must be accounted for in the development of modes of interaction and creation of documentation.

While most medications administered in the OR have a relatively short duration of action, there are important cases where medications which are administered in the OR have important consequences beyond the OR. Examples such as neuromuscular blockade, long-acting opioids, long-acting local anesthetic agents, and antibiotic administrations all may lead to important medication interactions well beyond the OR or need for modifications of postoperative care. Therefore, information regarding these administrations must be available to care providers working in the postoperative period. The use of "standalone" AIMS may contribute to a failure of communication of the use of these important medications. Interfaces between the stand-alone systems and enterprise EHRs allow this information to be communicated, however this poses additional development, maintenance, and deployment burden. Similarly, documentation of difficult airway management in the OR has impact beyond the OR as the patient may require emergent airway management in the intensive care unit or during future visits; information gleaned during the perioperative encounter may have enduring value to many other providers.

Development of Decision Support Tools

One of the most exciting promises of AIMS and enterprise EHRs is their ability to improve patient care by improving the decisions made by providers.[38] While medical decision making must be provided by responsible care providers, it is possible to aid decision making by providing default choices that support particular practice patterns, suggesting options which may be appropriate based on the type of care (see Fig 4.4), providing additional notification of important updated trends or results, and providing alerts based on the integration of multiple pieces of information. The former

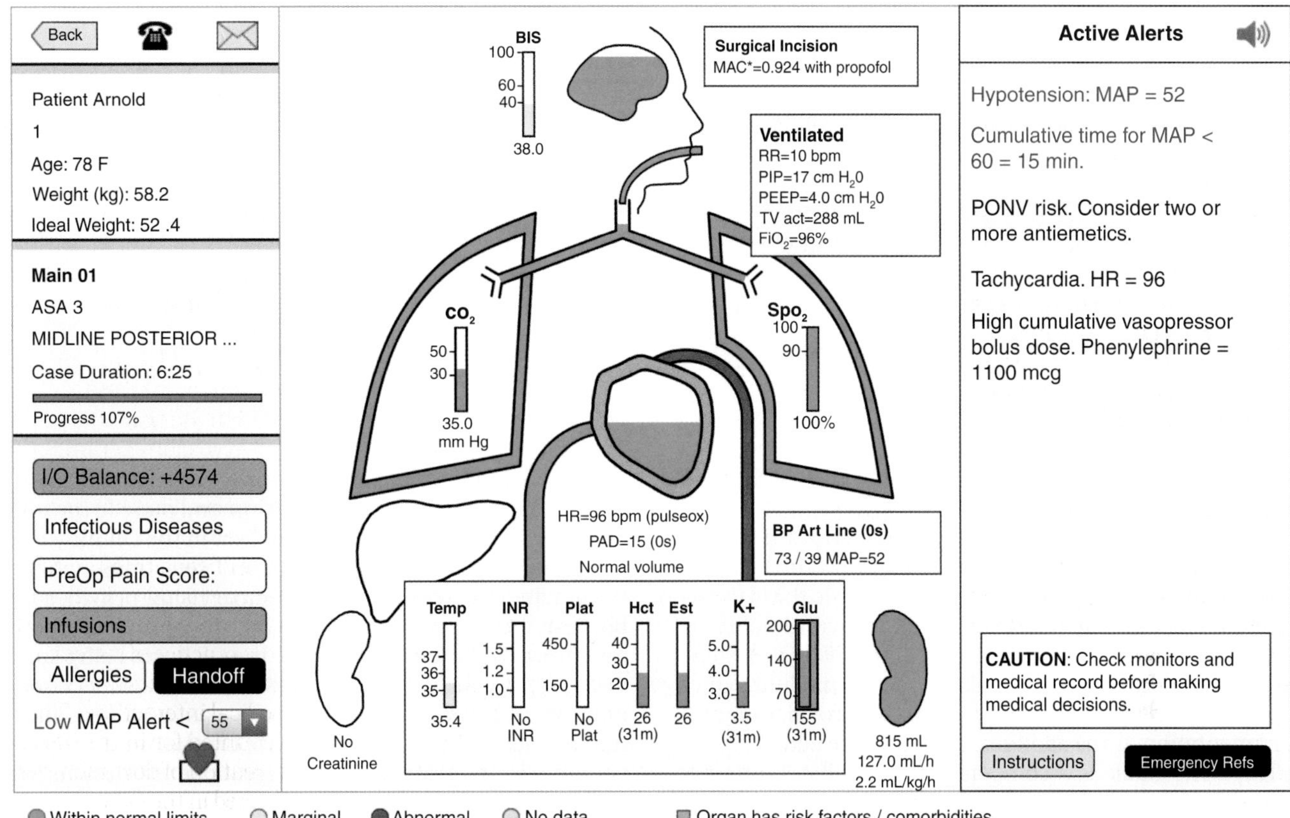

Fig. 4.5 The Alertwatch OR (Alertwatch, Ann Arbor, MI) multiparameter decision support system, illustrating the physiologic status of a patient under anesthetic care. This integrates data from physiologic monitors and electronic health record elements. Based on pre-specified rules it prompts providers to consider a specific course of action or indicates additional markers of patient state. * Indicates a calculated additive MAC value of inhaled agents and propofol and dexmedetomidine infusions.

two are examples of passive decision support, the latter two are examples of active decision support. Collectively these tools are referred to as decision support and are an integral part of the perioperative information system.[39]

PASSIVE DECISION SUPPORT SYSTEMS

In considering these tools it is helpful to move from the simplest to the most complex. At the simplest level in the configuration of the perioperative information system, decisions regarding the choices presented to users (default doses, units, and range checks) may act as prompts for users in their selections—the so-called anchoring effect. This is an example of passive decision support. Over time it is important to continue to assess how usage aligns with users' practice to ensure that the default options presented do indeed capture the typical usage at a particular institution.[40]

Systems for the documentation of anesthetic care typically feature methods for documentation of aspects of clinical care which cluster together based on aspects of the procedure, anesthetic technique employed, or location of service. For example, a template for cases performed via a spinal anesthetic would not be configured to require documentation of the endotracheal intubation technique as these do not frequently overlap. These can form the basis of decision prompts for providers; for example, in a cardiac case, the charting element available immediately after documentation of full cardiopulmonary bypass may be regarding discontinuation of mechanical ventilation. This may act as a reminder to the provider to perform this task. The level of sophistication of these prompts depends on the time devoted to their construction at the time of system installation and configuration.

One feature to improve documentation is the utilization of mandatory documentation elements that are required prior to the completion of case documentation. Extreme care needs should dictate what elements of documentation should be made mandatory. There are likely exceptions to even the most universal documentation element and forcing completion or entry of such items may undermine trust in the entirety of the clinical documentation.

ACTIVE DECISION SUPPORT SYSTEMS

In the intraoperative space, a number of more sophisticated approaches to decision support have been developed (Fig 4.5). These decision support tools continuously evaluate the medical record for incoming information and provide feedback to the user. These tools may be separate from the EHR but access the information being recorded by that software. These tools apply rules to alert providers to aspects of care which may have been overlooked or need to be addressed. This may guide users to re-evaluate patient status (if a blood pressure monitoring gap is detected), or consider additional interventions (prompts to treat extremely elevated blood glucose) or alternative management strategies (e.g., if large tidal volumes are being used).[41-46]

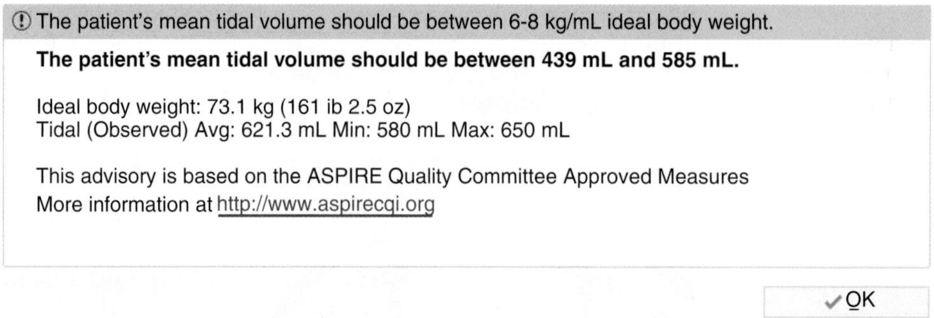

ⓘ The patient's mean tidal volume should be between 6-8 kg/mL ideal body weight.

The patient's mean tidal volume should be between 439 mL and 585 mL.

Ideal body weight: 73.1 kg (161 ib 2.5 oz)
Tidal (Observed) Avg: 621.3 mL Min: 580 mL Max: 650 mL

This advisory is based on the ASPIRE Quality Committee Approved Measures
More information at http://www.aspirecqi.org

✓OK

Fig. 4.6 An example of active decision support. Providers prompted to consider the tidal volume, with information which may allow them to consider change in clinical practice. This alert is triggered in the context of an averaged measured value which is above a predefined threshold. Image: © 2018 Epic System Corporation. Used with Permission.

In order to function, these more sophisticated forms of decision support are designed around a common architecture. They run in parallel with the clinical documentation functions of the EHR. They may be built into the EHR (Fig 4.6) or may run as separate software alongside the EHR (see Fig 4.5). Regardless of the specifics of the software implementation, it is best to consider the construction of these systems as being in components.[39] In addition to the modules which capture incoming device data and enable provider manual documentation, three additional modules are added.

The first module is a component which allows a user to define a series of rules against which the incoming information will be assessed. These rules should define the population to which the rule applies (i.e., patients aged over 18 undergoing surgeries in the main hospital operating rooms), the details of the rule (i.e., determine if blood glucose value is >300 mg/dL), and then the proposed action (i.e., notify provider of this finding by text page or display a pop-up window in the EHR software). The second component is the surveillance process which repeatedly assesses the patient status against the rules using newly updated laboratory results, charting elements, monitor or device data; the process determines when a rule has been triggered. The final component is the notification module; this is the method of interacting with the user. This may be within the EHR (as a pop-up message at the front of the patient's attention), separate to the EHR (in dedicated software running on the anesthesia workstation to display notifications regarding patient status), or alternatively may use a completely separate means of communication such as text paging, text messaging, or even phone calls.

Calibrating the alert to the clinical scenario is important and should take into account the lead time involved in data acquisition and notification. If an EHR obtains updated monitor information every minute, the rules require repeated values (to ensure non-artifact) and the output system has a 1-minute lag time, then this restricts the kinds of clinical events which are best addressed via this system. Second-to-second changes (such as in oxygen saturations) translate poorly through systems which have delays in the order minutes.[47] Therefore it is important in the design of decision support systems to target the correct events and recognize that extreme or rapidly occurring events may best be addressed via alternative notification systems or embedded into clinical monitors at the point of care.

The other key consideration is who is the intended recipient of the clinical decision support alert. In the US practice setting, there may be providers responsible for anesthesia care who are both within and outside the anesthetizing location. Alerts for providers in the OR may focus on supporting clinical decisions and selections, whereas those which are targeted at the supervising provider may be best focused on ensuring that the provider retains awareness of the current state of the OR cases being supervised. A provider in the role of OR anesthesia supervisor or manager may have additional concerns regarding allocation of anesthesia resources to support the anesthesia care being provided; notifications of significant deviations from schedules or occurrence of emergency events may be relevant to this group.

Various tools are available which incorporate these features. As discussed earlier, many passive decision support features are built into the EHR software natively. While more active decision support systems may be integrated into the EHR software it is also possible that this may come as part of stand-alone software which provides a mechanism for delivering these alerts to providers. More sophisticated implementations may additionally attempt to provide information about overall patient state drawing widely from EHR-derived data elements. This may be of use to providers in supervisory or OR manager roles seeking snapshots of the course of care.

IMPACT OF DECISION SUPPORT IN ANESTHESIA CARE

Evaluation of implementation of clinical decision support in anesthesia care has typically been focused around specific aspects of care, usually process measures. Examples include changes in ventilation parameters, perioperative β blockade, antibiotic administration, blood pressure management, administration of postoperative nausea and vomiting (PONV) prophylaxis and decreases in anesthesia agent usage (by reductions in fresh gas flow).[44,48-58] What is less well established is the relationship between clinical decision support and relevant patient outcomes. Perioperative decision support tools in the domain of perioperative glucose management in diabetic patients has been able to demonstrate differences in surgical site infection alongside improvements in perioperative glucose control in a single-center study.[59] It is likely that measurable changes in patient outcome do not come from use of a single decision rule in most circumstances. Therefore, patient outcome impact is more likely in systems which include multiple elements in their decision support; this type of implementation is not widely implemented or studied. This is supported by a single-institution study which has demonstrated that deployment of a multiparameter perioperative decision support system may reduce hospital charges and therefore resources.[45]

Integration with the Enterprise Electronic Health Record

Given the substantial shared pool of information from which the AIMS and the enterprise EHR may draw on and contribute to, it is not surprising that these systems have become integrated at many institutions into a single system. It is important to note that this increases the complexity of the EHR. For organizations where the IT support for an OR or anesthesia information system was supported and maintained through an anesthesia or surgery department relationship, the migration to an enterprise EHR will result in these duties being transferred to the hospital or enterprise-wide support group. This may reduce the customizability of these systems as changes and alterations now become handled by groups with broader responsibilities and competing priorities.

An emerging feature of EHRs, which fulfills an early promise of their utility, is meaningful transmission of data from different EHR platforms across institutions. Typically, each institution maintains an EHR that is unique to that institution. As smaller medical practices have aggregated into larger health systems, providers come under the same umbrella EHR system. This has allowed records from more health interactions to be available in a single location; a satellite clinic in a physically separate location may use a health–systemwide common EHR for documentation, making it available to the anesthesiologist who sees the patient presenting for surgery at main campus. However, when a patient presents to a nonaffiliated practice or hospital, documentation from the other institutions are unavailable and have to be obtained as printed paper, or communicated by the patient manually.

To address this issue, healthcare information exchanges (HIE) have been developed. These exchanges facilitate the transfer of health information between multiple distinct healthcare system's EHRs. This can occur in a directed way: a user at one facility chooses to send imaging data to another and uses the EHR's HIE user interface to discover records available via the HIE. These come in multiple forms but are typically based on a geographic (i.e., at the state or regional level) or a shared EHR platform (i.e., EPIC Systems Care Everywhere functionality).

In order to function, HIEs must be able to correctly match the same patient across different hospitals or clinics. Failures of this process (both incorrectly matching two patients across institutions or failing to match the correct patient across institutions) could have potential for catastrophic consequences in clinical care. Matching must consider different identifiers used at each hospital; a medical record or registration number is usually unique to the institution so is not suitable for this task. Additionally, unique identification assigned for other reasons—such as social security numbers—may not be suitable for this task as their use may shift over time and the accuracy may not match the level of confidence required for medical care. Furthermore, social security numbers may pose risk to patient privacy as they are connected to multiple other datasets including financial records.

Typically, combinations of identifiers are used to uniquely identify patients. This is joined with logic that balances a degree of uncertainty to account for the challenges previously noted with the risks of failure to match and false matches. However, this may still lead to the exchange of patient identifiers. Cryptographic solutions may be employed to prevent the need to exchange patient identifiers.

In some situations, even acknowledging the existence of a record may be revealing and pose risk to patient privacy—for example a record existing in a clinic specializing in the treatment of a particular illness may cause an inference to be drawn about a particular diagnosis. One way to minimize this issue is to limit the links to another health system's records to patients in common at the source health system. Rather than allowing a user at one institution to search freely for patients at another institution, such an approach would allow users to access the "matched" patient records at another institution only. Access to remote systems could further be controlled to limit it to the context of an active patient-provider encounter. Each of these options contains trade-offs with maximizing information availability with patient privacy.

Billing System Interactions

Billing for hospital services involves capturing accurately the resources used in the delivery of care; for example, in the perioperative setting, OR and PACU times, or specific surgical supplies and equipment used. This is recorded via the OR management system and may be linked to a broader process which manages surgical supplies, resource utilization, and scheduling. In this manner, information captured as part of OR clinical care documentation may be reused for billing, supply, and utilization management. The management of information in a centralized EHR accessible by multiple users enables simultaneous use for clinical, operational, and administrative reasons. Automated export of documented parameters may form the basis of these other uses.

In the United States, professional charges for anesthesia care are based on the duration of the care provided and the procedure for which the care is provided. Additional charges may be possible for specialized monitoring, specialized vascular access, or pain management procedures provided for postoperative analgesia. Data necessary to aid the billing process can be extracted from the EHR: for example, basic case information such as duration of anesthesia care, ASA physical status classification, staff providing for anesthesia care, and procedure performed. Reports can be run at or near to the conclusion of the anesthesia care and allow a case to be rapidly turned over to the billing staff for further processing. This may speed up the billing process and make it less dependent on paper billing sheets or other means. The implementation of automated billing alerts via text paging and email have been shown to increase prevention of documentation practices that may have been erroneous and alter reimbursement, reduce time to documentation being complete and ready to be billed, reduce time to correct errors, and increase capture of arterial line placement leading to increased reimbursement.[28,30,60]

Challenges in Anesthesia Information Management System Implementation

Just as the OR must be available for emergencies at all times, the underlying perioperative information systems which capture this activity must also be highly reliable. Despite architecting extensive EHR redundancy, backup processes must be available in cases where the system is unavailable due to hardware and software failures, or in times of planned maintenance. Typically, these result in reverting to a paper-based system for the limited periods of planned or unplanned downtime. Processes must be in place to determine how documentation captured during these downtimes is subsequently handled.

Due to the complexity of these systems it is possible that certain elements fail without the entire system becoming unavailable. For example, if the link between the monitoring platform and the AIMS system becomes unavailable, anesthesia providers may have to respond by manually entering monitoring data. Importantly, this data link failure has to be recognized. Unfortunately, it is unlikely that manual data entry will replicate the degree of completeness of the automatically gathered information. Concerns have been raised of the possibility of legal liability arising from such scenarios.[61]

In all situations where electronic records are created, a plan needs to be created to ensure that access in the future is preserved. Medical records retention requirements vary significantly by state. These typically extend for a period of time past the last contact with the health service, even up to 10 years beyond that period for adult patients. For minor patients, this period typically extends beyond the time in which the patient reaches the age of majority, even up until the patient turns 30 years old. These time periods may extend past the life expectancy of the software which created the records. Operators of EHRs, including those in the perioperative period, need to have a plan in place to ensure that data can be archived, retained, and remain accessible in line with these legal requirements.

Even with the most comprehensive of EHRs there may be a need for a physical medical record to be created as part of care—consent forms may be provided on paper, patients may write letters to their providers, and outside hospitals may send printed or paper records with a transferring patient. Decisions need to be made as to how these physical documents are retained and archived. This may involve making electronic copies which become available within the electronic record.

In situations in which separate systems are used in the perioperative process from the rest of the institution there may be situations where a paper record is printed and placed inside a patient's physical chart. When a paper record and an electronic record exist simultaneously at a given institution, then a decision needs to be made as to which has primacy. If a provider creates a paper record at the end of anesthesia care and then subsequently updates a documentation element at a later time, a process needs to be in place to ensure that this can be transferred to the patient's physical record for the paper record to maintain primacy.

Additionally, if differing systems are used in the perioperative period there may be failure of communication of important information to the entire healthcare team. While specific examples regarding medications with prolonged duration of action and challenges in airway management have been discussed above, the siloing of information in a separate system (potentially with different access requirements) contributes to the appearance of the perioperative period as being one which is completely distinct from the rest of the clinical encounter. This can contribute to failures of communication of events which occur during this important phase of care and thus potentially patient harm.

Ensuring coverage of all locations where an anesthetic may be performed can be challenging. There may be many sites where anesthesia care is provided infrequently. These are likely "non-operating room sites." In such cases the economic justification for the capital investment required to allow these sites to participate in electronic charting may not be justified. In such situations, cases performed in non-connected locations may require traditional paper charting. This creates a significant overhead as business processes need to be maintained to support the documentation of activity in these locations and ensure that the paper documentation is archived as the record of care, available for billing processes and quality assurance review.

Additional Uses for Collected Data

Secondary use of EHR data has become commonplace and is part of the value proposition of the transition to these systems. In addition to the primary purposes of clinical documentation, operational and support tasks, information contained within the EHR may find secondary uses including in the ascertainment of practice quality measures and research endeavors.

USE FOR MEDICAL RESEARCH

The rapid emergence of AIMS led to a proliferation of research into anesthesia care practices and outcomes. This proliferation has occurred because of the improved ease with which study data may be acquired. Queries of the underlying EHR databases are far quicker to perform and may be more extensive in scope than review of paper documentation in the same population. Collectively, this has led to a rapid development of retrospective database research within anesthesiology. This work has allowed quantification and identification of risk factors for both rare events, such as difficult mask ventilation combined with difficult intubation or epidural hematoma after neuraxial anesthesia, and more common perioperative events, such as acute kidney injury.[62-67]

The use of an EHR as a data source for research initiatives has offered advantages of scale in study size but also allows a wide range of risk factors to be considered. It is now routine for observational research studies using EHR data to include thousands of patient records. Given the relatively infrequent occurrence of catastrophic complications or major adverse outcomes in modern anesthetic practice, extremely large sample sizes are necessary for quantification of risk factors and rates of occurrence of significant patient outcomes.

Despite the rarity of intraoperative complications, long-term complications of the surgical procedure remain common. The ability to utilize information drawn from the entire hospital record to characterize patient outcome is extremely important to the perioperative outcome researcher, as postoperative complications may have substantial impact on patient outcome.

It has become apparent that even the largest of single center studies may not be able to generalize well across sites. Substantial heterogeneity in clinical practice exists between institutions and across geographical regions. This has driven the development of multicenter studies, facilitated by the interchange of electronic data. The Multicenter Perioperative Outcomes Group (MPOG)* is one example of such an undertaking, bringing together investigators from over 50 institutions across the United States and Europe who have assembled, standardized, and identified over 10 million perioperative records for research and quality improvement.† By including data from many sites and seeking to include diverse practice locations, such efforts aim to develop generalizable knowledge.

One of the challenges in performing this work is the level of abstraction required to summarize the patient's clinical encounter into a small number of variables for inclusion in any analysis. For example, studies on the relationship of intraoperative hypotension and postoperative outcome need to consider how to develop a measure of hypotension which summarizes multiple hours of highly granular blood pressure information into a small number of variables for inclusion in the research study. A single 3-hour case may have 60 or more non-invasive blood pressure values recorded. To include in any analysis, these need to be summarized in a manner which remains biologically plausible. Many options are available, such as averages of all collected blood pressures or time or fraction of the case above (or below) absolute (i.e., mean arterial pressure [MAP] <65 mm Hg) or relative (<20% drop from baseline MAP) thresholds. Each approach would have very different output values and may alter the results and interpretation of a research finding. With any automatically collected information, methods for handling artifacts should be considered as artifactual values may have been propagated from the monitoring platform to the automated record without clinician intervention. Given the abundance of possible data to be included in any study, it is key that a clear hypothesis and approach be developed a-priori rather than post-hoc decisions that may evaluate particular statistically or clinically significant outcomes.

While most of the research thus far has been in the context of retrospective observational studies, an emerging theme in EHR-derived research is the use of this data in near real time (within days) for prospective interventional trials. These studies attempt to gather much of the information required for the trial as a byproduct of the clinical documentation created in the EHR. Additional information regarding patient progress in the study can be appended via traditional study management software. More novel methodologies such as embedded pragmatic clinical trials where hospitals or clinics choose to standardize their management in a coordinated manner for all patients (i.e., one class of antihypertensive or another as the usual first agent for adult patients without chronic kidney disease) are dependent on EHR data collection for patient follow up and perhaps even delivering the "usual choice" via decision support tools (see Chapter 89).[68]

MEASUREMENT OF QUALITY OF CARE

Information regarding the quality of care delivered and patient outcomes may be obtained from review of the EHR. Traditional models of quality management frequently depended on the use of trained abstractors reviewing medical records and applying standardized definitions. While these systems work well, they do not scale well into high volume clinical settings due to the time-consuming nature of detailed review and the resultant staffing costs. Interest has developed in the use of EHR data for the automated derivation of quality of care information. With careful design, both process of care (i.e., appropriate antibiotic prophylaxis administration) and outcome measures (i.e., surgical site infection) may be tracked using data derived from the EHR. Decision support tools may be used to aid in the alignment of the quality measures and the clinical practice which they seek to measure. Care needs to be taken to ensure the pattern of care which may be promoted is consistent with good clinical practice.

Using automatically derived measures, it is possible to provide feedback to medical providers near the time of clinical care. Automated data extraction and processing is well developed, with feedback being described across provider groups using email, provider and institutional specific "dashboard' reporting tools, and real-time paging alerts (Fig. 4.7).[38,49,51] Various groups have worked to make available tools to enable the widespread deployment of quality measures via submission of data from individual sites to a centralized database.[69] This approach is designed to limit the need for each site to develop the required technical architecture to build and deploy such tools—a significant hurdle for many organizations. However, this likely comes at the expense of flexibility of measurement offered at each site and some degree of delay in processing.

*Multicenter Perioperative Outcomes Group: http://www.mpog.org
†Personal communication, October 2018.

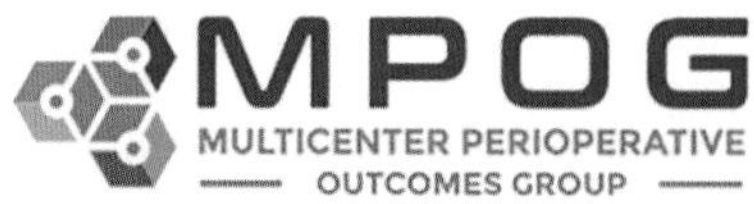

Claim MOCA® Credit

Hello

Below is your new MPOG Quality performance report. For a case-by-case breakdown of each measure's result, click on the graph's label and you will be taken to our reporting website (login required).

If you have any questions, please read our FAQ or send them to anes-aspire@med.umich.edu. Thank you for your participation in MPOG Quality.

Sincerely,
The MPOG Team

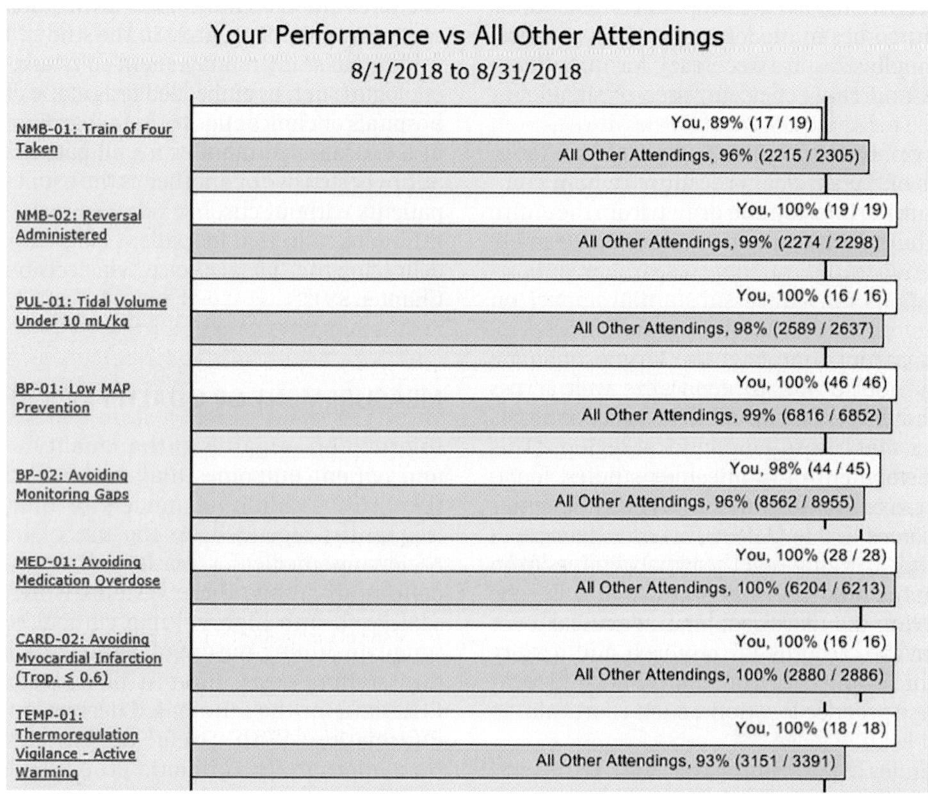

Fig. 4.7 Example of feedback email summarizing performance based on an automated assessment of compliance against predefined measurement instruments using data derived from the electronic health record. This figure has been lightly edited to remove identifying information of the recipient.

Interactions of Electronic Devices with the Delivery of Anesthesia Care

Safe anesthesia care requires the maintenance of a high degree of vigilance to multiple sources of information concurrently. When combined with required clinical tasks, estimates suggest that anesthesia care has high workload requirements.[70] Workload includes the factors related to the nature of the task, the situation in which it is performed, and the operator performing it.[71] In relation to phases of OR care, workload is clearly not uniformly distributed, clustering particularly in the induction and emergence phases of care.[70] The ability of providers to engage in tasks additional to patient care is debated.

Distractions from current patient care may include communication with other team members in the OR unrelated to patient care, preparation for subsequent patients, clinical reference lookup, pursuit of educational activities, and attention to personal issues. Attempts to quantify providers' attentiveness to the clinical situation or impact of a distracting event have been performed and note that distractions are a common feature of anesthesia care.[70,72-75] Given the common occurrence and diverse sources of possible distracting events during anesthesia care, mitigating the effects of distraction to maintain focus on patient care may be a required skill of an anesthesia provider.[74]

In particular, the proliferation of electronic devices in the OR including personally owned devices by providers (such as smartphone and tablet devices) and those that are part of the anesthesia workstation (frequently Internet-connected computers for accessing EHR and documentation purposes) has raised concern for the new sources of distraction in the OR.[76] A study from eight anesthesia workstations in one institution found that the computer attached to the anesthesia workstation was used for non-anesthesia documentation purposes for 16% of the procedure time. Importantly, this study did not differentiate between time spent in this category that was related to patient care (i.e., accessing a separate lab or EHR system) or not.[77] Additional research has observed self-initiated distractions occurred in 54% of anesthesia cases.[78] Distractions related to personal matters were found in 49% of cases and related to educational activities in 24% of cases.[78]

Professional societies have issued guidelines on the role of distractions, including electronic devices, in the OR, some of which recommend the development of local policies to cover usage of electronic devices.[79-81] These policies may differentiate between clinical, educational, and personal usage of electronic devices and resources, and the appropriateness of each during patient care. It should be noted that many aspects of use of perioperative information technology, including use of personal devices, are subject to logging or recording. This may allow medicolegal review of activity performed on electronic devices contemporaneous to anesthesia care being provided in the future.

Conclusion

Information technology is very much part of the perioperative care process. It has significantly impacted clinical care, organizational performance, provider satisfaction, research, and assessment of quality of care. It is important that anesthesiologists understand the principles behind its use and be keenly aware of the benefits and potential shortcomings that applications of these tools may have. It seems likely that the future will hold a more connected perioperative environment with even more information available. The challenge, and the promise, of perioperative informatics still lies in ensuring the right people have access to the right information at the right time to enable them to make the right decision for the patient care they are providing.

Acknowledgment

The editors and publisher would like to thank Dr. C. William Hanson for contributing a chapter on this topic in the prior edition of this work.

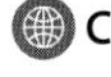 **Complete references available online at expertconsult.com.**

References

1. McKesson EI. *Curr Res Anesth Analg*. 1934;13:1.
2. Block Jr FE, et al. *J Clin Monit*. 1985;1:30.
3. Block Jr FE. *Baillière's Clinical Anaesthesiology*. 1990;4:159.
4. Stonemetz J. *Anesthesiol Clin*. 2011;29:367.
5. Egger Halbeis CB. *Anesth Analg*. 2008;107:1323.
6. Trentman TL, et al. *J Clin Monit Comput*. 2011;25:129.
7. Stol IS. *Anesth Analg*. 2014;118:644.
8. Steinbrook R. *N Engl J Med*. 2009;360:1057.
9. Committee on Quality Management and Departmental Administration. *Statement on Documentation of Anesthesia Care*. Schaumburg, IL: American Society of Anesthesiologists; 2018.
10. Rutala WA, et al. *Infect Control Hosp Epidemiol*. 2006;27:372.
11. Bures S, et al. *Am J Infect Control*. 2000;28:465.
12. Loeb RG. *J Clin Monit*. 1995;11:9.
13. Allard J, et al. *Br J Anaesth*. 1995;74:619.
14. Weinger MB, et al. *Anesthesiology*. 1997;87:144; discussion 29A.
15. Davis TC, et al. *J Clin Monit Comput*. 2012;26:163.
16. Reich DL, et al. *Anesth Analg*. 2000;91:612.
17. Thrush DN. *J Clin Anesth*. 1992;4:386.
18. Cook RI, et al. *Anesthesiology*. 1989;71:385.
19. van Schalkwyk JM, et al. *Br J Anaesth*. 2011;107:546.
20. Lerou JG, et al. *J Clin Monit*. 1988;4:37.
21. Devitt JH, et al. *Can J Anaesth*. 1999;46:122.
22. Edwards KE, et al. *Can J Anaesth*. 2013;60:990.
23. Jang J, et al. *Int J Med Inform*. 2013;82:702.
24. Driscoll WD, et al. *Anesth Analg*. 2007;104:1454; table of contents.
25. Avidan A, et al. *Can J Anaesth*. 2014;61:979.
26. Avidan A, Weissman C. *Int J Med Inform*. 2012;81:173.
27. Sandberg WS, et al. *Anesth Analg*. 2008;106:192; table of contents.
28. Kheterpal S, et al. *Anesth Analg*. 2007;104:592.
29. McCarty LK, et al. *Anesthesiology*. 2014;121:1166.
30. Spring SF, et al. *Anesthesiology*. 2007;106:157.
31. Reich DL, et al. *Anesthesiology*. 2006;105:179; quiz 231.
32. Luedi MM, et al. *Anesth Analg*. 2016;122:1169.
33. Wang J, et al. *Anesth Analg*. 2013;116:1333.
34. Dexter F, et al. *Anesth Analg*. 2009;108:929.
35. Dexter F, et al. *Anesth Analg*. 2003;97:1119; table of contents.
36. Dexter F, et al. *Anesth Analg*. 2013;116:1103.
37. Deal LG, et al. *J Clin Anesth*. 2014;26:264.
38. Epstein RH, et al. *Anesth Analg*. 2015;121:678.
39. Nair BG, et al. *Anesth Analg*. 2017;124:603.
40. Rodriquez LI, et al. *Anesth Analg*. 2017;125:255.
41. Ehrenfeld JM, et al. *Anesth Analg*. 2011;113:356.
42. Nair BG, et al. *J Clin Monit Comput*. 2013;27:265.
43. Sathishkumar S, et al. *Anesthesiology*. 2015;123:29.
44. Blum JM, et al. *Anesthesiology*. 2013;119:295.
45. Kheterpal S, et al. *Anesthesiology*. 2018;128:272.
46. Simpao AF, et al. *J Clin Monit Comput*. 2017;31:885.
47. Epstein RH, Dexter F. *Anesth Analg*. 2012;115:929.
48. Nair BG, et al. *Jt Comm J Qual Patient Saf*. 2012;38:283.
49. O'Reilly M, et al. *Anesth Analg*. 2006;103:908.
50. Nair BG, et al. *Surg Infect (Larchmt)*. 2011;12:57.
51. Nair BG, et al. *Anesth Analg*. 2010;111:1293.
52. St Jacques P, et al. *Surg Infect (Larchmt)*. 2005;6:215.
53. Wax DB, et al. *Anesth Analg*. 2007;104:1462; table of contents.
54. Nair BG, et al. *Anesth Analg*. 2014;118:206.
55. Kooij FO, et al. *Anesth Analg*. 2008;106:893; table of contents.
56. Kooij FO, et al. *Br J Anaesth*. 2012;108:961.
57. Kooij FO, et al. *Appl Clin Inform*. 2017;8:313.
58. Nair BG, et al. *Anesthesiology*. 2013;118:874.
59. Ehrenfeld JM, et al. *Anesthesiology*. 2017;126:431.
60. Freundlich RE, et al. *J Clin Anesth*. 2013;25:110.
61. Vigoda MM, Lubarsky DA. *Anesth Analg*. 2006;102:1798.
62. Kheterpal S, et al. *Anesthesiology*. 2006;105:885.
63. Kheterpal S, et al. *Anesthesiology*. 2013;119:1360.
64. Lee LO, et al. *Anesthesiology*. 2017;126:1053.
65. Ehrenfeld JM, et al. *Reg Anesth Pain Med*. 2013;38:409.
66. Kheterpal S, et al. *Anesthesiology*. 2007;107:892.
67. Sun LY, et al. *Anesthesiology*. 2015;123:515.
68. Weinfurt KP, et al. *BMC Med Res Methodol*. 2017;17:144.
69. Valentine EA, Falk SA. *Anesthesiol Clin*. 2018;36:31.
70. Weinger MB, et al. *Anesth Analg*. 2004;98:1419; table of contents.
71. Leedal JM, Smith AF. *Br J Anaesth*. 2005;94:702.
72. Slagle JM, Weinger MB. *Anesthesiology*. 2009;110:275.
73. Jothiraj H, et al. *Br J Anaesth*. 2013;111:477.
74. Campbell G, et al. *Br J Anaesth*. 2012;109:707.
75. Savoldelli GL, et al. *Eur J Anaesthesiol*. 2010;27:683.
76. Jorm CM, O'Sullivan G, et al. *Anaesth Intensive Care*. 2012;40:71.
77. Wax DB, et al. *Anesthesiology*. 2012;117:1184.
78. Slagle JM, et al. *Anesthesiology*. 2018;128:44.
79. Committee on Quality Management and Departmental Administration. *Statement on Distractions*. Schaumburg, IL: American Society of Anesthesiologists; 2015.
80. Committee on Perioperative Care. *Statement on Distractions in the Operating Room*. Chicago, IL: American College of Surgeons (ACS); 2016.
81. Position Statement. *Mobile Information Technology*. Park Ridge, IL: American Association of Nurse Anesthetists; 2015.

5 Quality Improvement in Anesthesia Practice and Patient Safety

ANNA MARY VARUGHESE, DAVID WINTHROP BUCK, MEGHAN BROOKS LANE-FALL, and EUGENIE S. HEITMILLER

KEY POINTS

- Quality needs to be an integral characteristic of the system in which care is delivered. Improving the quality of care often requires reorganization of the way we work. A challenge to the anesthesia team is to combine efficiency in perioperative care (especially the operating room) with safety and the best quality possible.
- The growing demand from patients, clinicians, insurers, regulators, accreditors, and purchasers for improved quality and safety in health care requires that anesthesiologists and members of the anesthesia team persistently evaluate the quality of care they provide.
- Improving quality of care requires measuring performance. Clinicians have an enhanced ability to obtain feedback regarding performance in their daily work, in part because of the increasing use of information systems. Unfortunately, consensus has not been reached on how to measure quality of care.
- The goal of measurement is to learn and improve. The measurement system must fit into an improvement system; clinicians must have the will to work cooperatively to improve, and they must have ideas or hypotheses about changes to the current system of care. Also, the clinical team must have a model for testing changes and implementing those that result in improvements.
- Outcome measures, including in-hospital mortality rates, have been the basis for evaluating performance and quality. However, hospital mortality alone provides an incomplete picture of quality, does not include all domains of quality, and does not measure the overall success of the full cycle of care for a specific medical condition. A balanced set of structures (how care is organized), processes (what we do), and outcome measures (results of care in terms of patient's health over time) is needed to evaluate the quality of care overall.
- Efforts to improve quality of care require development of valid, reliable, and practical measures of quality. Identification of clinical care that truly achieves excellence would be helpful not only to the administration of anesthesia, but also to health care overall.
- Developing a quality measure requires several steps: prioritizing the clinical area to evaluate; selecting the type of measure; writing definitions and designing specifications; developing data collection tools; pilot-testing data collection tools and evaluating the validity, reliability, and feasibility of measures; developing scoring and analytic specifications; and collecting baseline data.
- The best opportunities to improve quality of care and patient outcomes will most likely come not only from discovering new therapies, but also from discovering how to better deliver therapies that are already known to be effective.
- Safety is an integral part of quality that is focused on the prevention of error and patient harm. The airline industry is often lauded as an exemplar of safety because it has embraced important safety principles, including the standardization of routine tasks, the reduction of unnecessary complexity, and the creation of redundancies. Anesthesia care teams have also adopted these principles, although many opportunities remain to further bolster patient safety.
- Healthcare providers can organize their quality improvement and patient safety efforts around three key areas: (1) translating evidence into practice, (2) identifying and mitigating hazards, and (3) improving culture and communication. Although each of these areas requires different tools, they all help health care organizations evaluate progress in patient safety and quality.

The need for improving quality and reducing the cost of health care has been highlighted repeatedly in the scientific literature and lay press. Improving care, minimizing variation, and reducing costs have increasingly become national priorities in many countries. Quality improvement (QI) programs that address these issues not only improve delivery of care but also have a positive effect on practitioner job satisfaction and organizational commitment.[1]

The goal of this chapter is to present a practical framework for developing and implementing QI programs in anesthesiology and critical care medicine that are both scientifically sound and feasible. To accomplish this goal, we review the science and approaches to QI, present measures that help evaluate whether QI programs have resulted in improvements, and describe examples of successful QI efforts.

What Is Quality?

DEFINITION OF QUALITY

W. Edwards Deming, scholar, professor, author, lecturer, and consultant to business leaders, corporations, and governments defined quality as "a predictable degree of uniformity and dependability with a quality standard suited to the customer."[1] This early definition of quality, in the context of QI, stems from its application to industrial production. However, when the term *quality* is applied to health care, the subtleties and implications of treating a human being are of prime importance, as opposed to the concerns involved in producing consumer goods. Use of the term *quality* in the context of health care can sometimes lead to defensive attitudes, economic concerns, and even ethical debates.

In the healthcare sector, quality can have various meanings to different people. For example, a daughter may evaluate quality by the level of dignity and respect with which her elderly mother is treated by a nurse. A cardiac surgeon may see quality as a percentage of improvement in the function of a heart on which he or she has just operated. A business may judge quality by the timeliness and cost effectiveness of the care delivered to its employees and its effect on the bottom line. Finally, society may evaluate quality by the ability to deliver care to those who need it, regardless of their cultural or socioeconomic backgrounds.

Despite the numerous definitions of quality in both business and medicine, a unified definition of quality in the context of QI should exist in health care. This definition of quality may have implications for both its measurement and its improvement. In order to help standardize the definition of quality in health care, the Institute of Medicine (IOM) published its own definition in a 1990 report titled *Medicare: A Strategy for Quality Assurance.* The IOM, which has since been renamed the National Academy of Medicine (NAM), defined *quality* as "the degree to which health services for individuals and populations increase the likelihood of desired health outcomes and are consistent with current professional knowledge."[2] Inherent in this definition are the elements of measurement, goal orientation, process and outcomes, individual and society preferences, and a dynamic state of professional knowledge. This definition of quality in health care has gained widespread acceptance. A similar definition is offered by the U.S. Government Department of Health and Human Services, which defines quality in public health as "the degree to which policies, programs, services, and research for the population increase desired health outcomes and conditions in which the population can be healthy."

AIMS OF QUALITY IN HEALTH CARE

In the 2001 report, *Crossing the Quality Chasm,* six aims for quality in health care were outlined.[3] These aims of safety, effectiveness, patient-centeredness, timeliness, efficiency, and equity included and extended the issues of patient safety described in their earlier report *To Err Is Human.*[4] The aims have been adopted by many organizations, including the Institute for Healthcare Improvement (IHI), a United States nongovernmental agency devoted to advancing QI and patient safety in health care. These aims serve as a basis on which quality is evaluated and improved and are described as follows.

1. Safety. No patient or healthcare worker should be harmed by the healthcare system at any time, including during transitions of care and "off hours," such as nights or weekends. Errors may be categorized as either failure of an action to occur as planned, such as the administration of a wrong medication to a patient, or having the wrong plan altogether, such as misdiagnosing and subsequently mistreating a patient.[4] As much as possible, patients should be informed about the risks and benefits of medical care in advance. If a complication does occur, medical staff should make full disclosure, provide assistance to the patient and family, and exercise due diligence in preventing any recurrences of the error.
2. Effectiveness. Effective medicine requires evidence-based decisions about treatment for individual patients, when such evidence exists. The best available evidence should be combined with clinical expertise and patient values in forming a treatment plan. With effective care, medical practitioners avoid underuse by providing a treatment to all who will benefit and avoid overuse by refraining from giving treatment to those unlikely to benefit.
3. Patient-centeredness. Patient-centered care is respectful of individual patient preferences, needs, and values and uses these factors to guide clinical decisions.[4] More specifically, according to Gerteis and colleagues,[6] patient-centered care encompasses respect for patients' values; coordination and integration of care; information, communication, and education; physical comfort; emotional support that relieves fear and anxiety; and involvement of family and friends. The dramatic increase in access to health information on the Internet has resulted in more patients who are well informed and proactive in their care. Patient-centered care embraces this trend and shifts more of the power and control to patients and their families. Examples of patient-centered care include shared decision making, patient and family participation in rounds, patient ownership of medical records, schedules that minimize patient inconvenience, and unrestricted visitation hours.[7]
4. Timeliness. Reduced wait time is important to both patients and healthcare practitioners. Long waits signal a lack of respect for a patient's time. Furthermore, delays may not only affect patient satisfaction, but may impair timely diagnosis and treatment. For healthcare workers, delays in availability of equipment or information may decrease job satisfaction and the ability to perform their jobs adequately.
5. Efficiency. Rising costs have increased scrutiny of waste in health care; this includes waste in labor, capital, equipment, supplies, ideas, and energy.[8] Improved efficiency reduces waste and results in an increased output for a given cost. Examples of efficiency measures include mean length of hospital stay, readmission rate, and mean cost of treatment for a diagnosis. The elimination of waste can result in better quality of care for patients at the same or lower cost.
6. Equity. Equitable care does not vary in quality based on personnel. The NAM defines equitable care at two levels. At the population level, equitable care means

reducing or eliminating disparities between subgroups. At the individual level, it means absence of discrimination based on factors such as age, gender, race, ethnicity, nationality, religion, educational attainment, sexual orientation, disability, or geographic location.[3]

Another framing of quality is the "quadruple aim" proposed by Bodenheimer and Sinsky[5] and adopted by the IHI. These four aims include better care, better outcomes, lower cost, and better work life for the healthcare workforce. This last aim was added to the IHI's previous "Triple Aim" in recognition that increasing clinician burnout represents a threat to high-quality care.[5]

DEMING'S SYSTEM OF PROFOUND KNOWLEDGE

Before learning about frameworks and tools for improvement, it helps to have an understanding of the theory behind improvement work. W. Edwards Deming wrote about two different types of knowledge: subject matter knowledge and profound knowledge. Subject matter knowledge is professional expertise, such as expertise in anesthesiology. Profound knowledge is the knowledge of improvement. The most significant improvement occurs where these two types of knowledge overlap. Deming divides profound knowledge into four different categories: appreciation of a system, the theory of knowledge, understanding variation, and psychology.

The first area of profound knowledge is appreciation of a system. A system is a network of interdependent components working together for a common aim.[6] It is often said that "Every system is perfectly designed to get the results it gets." If a system is underperforming, it is because it has unintentionally been designed to underperform. If this is the case, it is our responsibility to manage the system to get the results we want.

The second part of Deming's profound knowledge is the idea that knowledge requires a theory. Information by itself is not knowledge. For example, a dictionary contains information, but it is not knowledge. We must have a theory behind our improvement work, not just data, if we are going to learn.[6]

In order to learn, we must additionally understand variation and how to react to it. Deming says that "life is variation."[6] Common cause variation is variation that is inherent to the process. Special cause variation is variation from causes that are not inherent to the process but arise from specific circumstances. A process which only has common cause variation is in statistical "control." On the other hand, a process that has both common cause and special cause variation is an unstable process.[7] Two common errors in improvement work are acting upon common cause variation as if it were special cause, and acting upon special cause variation as if it were common cause.

The last area of profound knowledge is psychology. This is often the most challenging part of improvement work. Deming believed in intrinsic motivation, and the need to nurture people's joy in work and intrinsic motivation to learn.[6] More recently John P. Kotter describes eight steps to change in his book *The Heart of Change*. These are increase urgency, build the guiding team, get the vision right, communicate for buy-in, empower action, create short-term wins, don't let up, and make change stick.[8]

Approaches to Quality Assessment

QUALITY ASSURANCE VERSUS CONTINUOUS QUALITY IMPROVEMENT

Although the terms *continuous quality improvement (CQI)* and *quality assurance (QA)* were used interchangeably in the past, substantial differences existed between the two. Most medical CQI systems were built on the foundation of a traditional QA system that used *standards* to define quality.[9] Standards can be defined as an "acceptable" level of performance. For example, a standard for overall mortality after cardiac surgery is less than 3%; however, is 3% (vs. 4% or 2%) mortality after cardiac surgery acceptable? Similarly, a standard for head injury evaluation is a computerized tomography (CT) brain scan within 4 hours of admission, but in certain circumstances, patients with head injury may warrant a CT scan sooner than that.

Most standards are inherently arbitrary and often lack consensus among medical professionals.[9] Additionally, QA systems typically react only when a standard is not met. Examples of traditional standard-based QA systems were peer review systems and morbidity and mortality reviews. These systems often exist to flag certain cases or practitioners for intense review. Practitioners may regard this intense review as a punishment because only "failures" or "bad apples" are identified, and process failures are not connected with the outcome on every case. Thus, QA systems are inherently judgmental and, if not carefully administered, can hold practitioners responsible for random causes over which they have no control. CQI systems, on the other hand, recognize that errors occur and require different responses. Often excellence in health care is not identified by analysis of QA systems. Excellence is sometimes defined by the lack of failure. Is there a difference between good (acceptable) and excellent health care?

Systems within health care are a series of interlinked processes, each of which results in one or more outputs. CQI systems, as opposed to QA systems, include an explicit approach to process and the use of specifications to improve a process or outcome. A specification is an explicit, measurable statement regarding an important attribute of a process or the outcome it produces.[9] Specifications identify variables that need to be measured, but typically do not set acceptable limits or standards. Once specifications have been defined in a CQI system, all outputs or cases, not just failures, are evaluated against these specifications. The system then attempts to correct errors by fixing the process rather than the people. Thus, CQI aims to change the process and prevent quality failures before they happen by building improvements into the process. To quote Philip Crosby, "The system for causing quality is prevention, not appraisal."[10]

FRAMEWORKS FOR IMPROVEMENT

Model for Improvement

The journey toward improvement can be made more efficient and more effective with a systematic approach. The Model for Improvement, developed by the training and management consulting company Associates in Process Improvement (http://www.apiweb.org), is one such

TABLE 5.1 Steps of a Plan, Do, Study, Act (PDSA) Cycle

Step	Description
Plan	Make a plan for the test of change. Include predictions of results and how data will be collected.
Do	Test change on a small scale. Document data, observations, and problems that occur.
Study	Use data gathered from previous stages to build new knowledge and make predictions. Knowledge is gained from both successful and unsuccessful changes.
Act	Adopt the change, or use knowledge gained to plan or modify the next test of action.

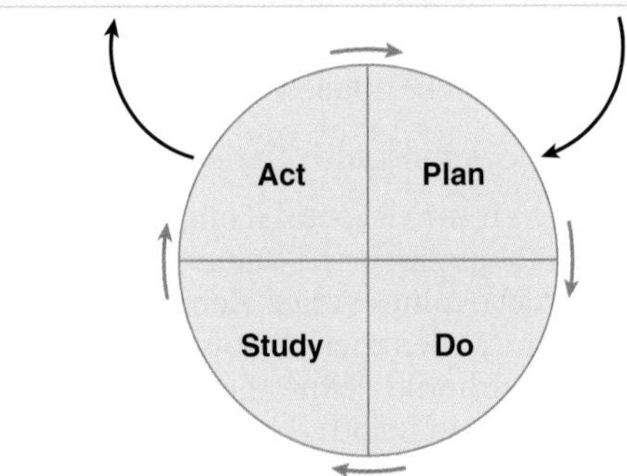

Fig. 5.1 Diagram of model for improvement. (From Langley GJ, Moen RD, Nolan KM, et al. *The Improvement Guide: A Practical Approach to Enhancing Organizational Performance.* San Francisco: Jossey-Bass; 2009. With permission from John Wiley & Sons.)

approach adopted by organizations across varied disciplines and is currently the approach used by IHI. It is a structured, dynamic model that applies the scientific method to testing and implementing a change.[7] In 1939, Walter A. Shewhart, a physicist, engineer, and statistician, introduced the science of modern QI.[11] He introduced a three-step scientific process of specification, production, and inspection, stating that "these three steps must go in a circle instead of in a straight line."[12] In the 1940s, his protégé, W. Edwards Deming, applied these concepts to government and industry and developed the Plan, Do, Study, Act (PDSA) cycle (Table 5.1).[13] A modification of the PDSA by the addition of three fundamental questions (as explained in the next paragraph) resulted in the Model for Improvement (Fig. 5.1).[12]

Beginning an improvement project with the three fundamental questions for improvement helps set a clear direction for the project, define what success will look like, and hypothesize successful interventions. The three fundamental questions for improvement are:

1. Aim: "What are we trying to accomplish?" The aim (or objective) for improvement should be specific, measurable, actionable, relevant, and time-specific (also referred to as a SMART aim). Ideas for improvements may come from interviewing those involved or affected by the process, such as staff or patients. Ideas may also come from examining previous data on operational, clinical, or financial processes.
2. Measure: "How will we know if change is an improvement?" Ideally, measures should be linked directly to the aim or goal of the project and should ensure that the interests of the stakeholders of the process are represented.[7] Quantitative measures should be used when possible to measure change over time. These measures provide the feedback that enables one to know whether or not the change is an improvement. However, not all projects have an easily quantifiable outcome and the outcome may be more qualitative. It is worth the time and effort to identify opportunities to translate goals into quantifiable outcomes if possible. These can be easier to use to communicate success.
3. Changes: "What changes can we make that will result in improvement?" Ideas for changes that result in improvement often start with observations, modeling the success of others, and brainstorming. The more intimate the understanding of a process and its key drivers, the higher the likelihood of generating successful changes.

The three fundamental questions are followed by a PDSA cycle, which is the framework for testing and implementing previously generated ideas for change. Improvement may require multiple cycles of preferably small tests of change over time. By testing changes on a small scale before implementation, risk is mitigated. Small tests of change may also help overcome individuals' resistance to change. Through repeated cycles, increased knowledge is acquired, and actions are continuously modified or changed. Measures defined in the first part of the model help determine whether or not a change is a success. These measures are often plotted over time on run charts or control charts (Figs. 5.2 and 5.3). Knowledge can be gained from both successful and unsuccessful tests! Finally, PDSA cycles both test a change and implement a successful change on a larger scale or in diverse clinical areas.

Lean Methodology and Six Sigma

In addition to the Model for Improvement, CQI initiatives have many other frameworks. Two of these frameworks, Lean Production and Six Sigma, are briefly discussed here. These frameworks are sometimes combined, as in "Lean Six Sigma." Regardless of which framework is employed, benefits are gained by retaining a structured and consistent approach to CQI.

Lean methodology has its roots in Japanese manufacturing, particularly in the Toyota Production System.[14] More recently, Lean has found success in the healthcare industry. Two notable examples of its use are Virginia Mason Medical Center and ThedaCare, Inc., both of which have transformed their organizations through the application of Lean principles. In fact, ThedaCare reported $3.3 million in savings in 2004 with reduced accounts receivable, redeployed staff, reduced phone triage times, reduced time spent on paperwork, and decreased medication distribution time.[14]

Lean methodology is focused on creating more value for the customer (i.e., the patient) with fewer resources. Every step in a process is evaluated to differentiate those steps that add value from those that do not. The ultimate goal is to eliminate all waste so that every step adds value

TABLE 5.2 Steps in the Lean or Six Sigma Process

Step	Description
Define	Define the goals of the improvement project. Obtain necessary support and resources and put together a project team.
Measure	Establish appropriate metrics. Measure baseline performance of the current system.
Analyze	Examine the system for possible areas of improvement.
Improve	Improve the system through implementation of ideas. Statistically validate improvements.
Control	Institutionalize the new system and monitor its stability over time.

to a process. Other key components of Lean include reducing unevenness of workflow—for instance, what we might find in intensive care unit (ICU) admissions or emergency cases—and eliminating the overburdening of people and equipment. Five principles govern Lean improvement:[7]

1. *Define the value* that the customer is seeking. Virginia Mason Medical Center has a "patient-first" focus for all its processes.[14]
2. *Identify and map* the value stream. If evaluating preoperative assessment, map the physical flow of a patient from the scheduling of a procedure through the day of surgery (history and physical, preoperative counseling, laboratory tests, imaging, consultations). In this process, all of the steps are accounted for, including the back-and-forth flow of the patient to the front desk, to the laboratory, and so on. Time spent during each step of the process should be documented.
3. *Smooth the flow* between value-added steps. Eliminate steps that do not add value to the overall process and are likely a poor use of time or effort on the part of the caregivers or the patient. An example of this process might be eliminating unnecessary tests or consultations in a patient's preoperative evaluation and reducing excess wait times that are the result of correctable inefficiencies.
4. *Create pull* between steps. Customer demand should trigger the start of a downstream process. Examples include opening operating rooms (ORs) or increasing staffing based on surgical demand, as opposed to having a fixed amount of time for each surgeon or surgical division.
5. *Pursue perfection* by continuing the process until you have achieved ultimate value with no waste.

The transformation of Motorola in the 1980s from a struggling company to a high-quality, high-profit organization helped give rise to the Six Sigma methodology. Two key fundamental objectives of Six Sigma are a virtually error-free process and a large focus on reducing variation.[15] In fact, a Six Sigma process, or a process whose frequency falls six deviations from the mean, corresponds to just 3.4 errors per million.

Health care often falls far short of this standard. In a 1998 report, Chassin[16] reported that hospitalized patients harmed by negligence were at a four sigma level (10,000/million), patients inadequately treated for depression were at a two sigma level (580,000/million), and eligible heart attack survivors who failed to receive β-adrenergic blockers were at a one sigma level (790,000/million). In contrast, Chassin found that anesthesiology was the one healthcare specialty that approached the six sigma level, with deaths caused by anesthesia as low as 5.4/million.[16] In comparison with health care, airline fatalities were a two sigma process (230/million) and a traditional company operated around four sigma, the equivalent of 6200 errors/million.[16] Considering that errors are often tied directly to cost, this error rate has significant financial implications.

Six Sigma is similar to the Model for Improvement in that it makes use of a simple framework to guide improvement, in this case using Define, Measure, Analyze, Improve, Control (DMAIC).[15] The DMAIC steps are described in Table 5.2. As mentioned earlier, many organizations have found the greatest benefit by combining elements of different methodologies in their CQI work. One popular example of this is Lean Six Sigma, which combines improvements in flow and value with reduction in error and variation. Furthermore, individual tools from these strategies, such as PDSA cycles or DMAIC processes, can be applied where appropriate.

The Value Framework in Health Care

Since quality in health care is focused on patient outcomes, another approach to quality is the value framework. Quality relative to cost determines value. Hence, in health care, value is defined as the patient health outcomes achieved per dollar spent.[17] Value should define the framework for performance improvement in health care. Value includes goals already embraced by health care such as quality, safety, patient centeredness, and cost containment; the value framework allows for a way to integrate these goals.

Because value is always defined around the customer, in the healthcare industry it is what matters most to patients, and unites the interests of all the stakeholders in the healthcare system. Thus, when value improves, not only do patients, payers, providers, and suppliers all benefit, but the economic sustainability of the healthcare system also improves. As such, value should be the overarching goal of healthcare delivery. According to Porter, the failure to adopt value as the central goal in health care and the failure to measure it, are the most serious failures of the medical community.[18]

Value measurement today is limited and highly imperfect. Value should be measured by outputs not inputs. Thus, value is dependent on patient health outcomes and not the volume of services delivered. The only way to accurately measure value is to track individual patient outcomes and costs longitudinally over the full cycle of care, which can vary from 30 to 90 days for hospital care and 1 year for chronic care.

Value is not measured by processes of care utilized by a patient. While process measurement is an important component of improvement, it should not be substituted for measurement of patient outcomes. Outcomes and cost should be measured separately. Outcomes, the numerator of the value equation, refer to the actual results of care in terms of patient health and should consist of a set of multidimensional outcomes that, when considered together, constitute patient benefit. Cost, the denominator of the value equation, should include total costs involved in the full cycle of care for the patient's medical condition. Most physicians do not know the full costs of caring for a patient, thus they lack the information to make real efficiency improvements.

Outcomes measurement is critical to driving rapid improvements in health care. Without a feedback loop that includes the outcomes achieved, providers lack the information they require to learn and improve. Effective outcome measurement is hampered by several problems. First, there is a lack of consensus as to what constitutes an outcome. Second, electronic medical record (EMR) systems often do not facilitate the capture of longitudinal outcomes measures with appropriate scope; these systems may focus too narrowly or too broadly, giving only a partial view of patient outcomes. Third, outcomes such as infection rates may vary substantially by medical condition. Finally, true outcome measurement has been limited because the cost of gathering longitudinal patient results is high, due in part to fragmented organizational structures and poor EMR interoperability.

Cost is the most pressing issue in health care. Current cost measurement approaches have not only hampered our understanding of costs but also contributed to approaches involving cost-containment. A focus on cost-containment rather than value improvement can be dangerous and is often self-defeating. Two major problems associated with cost measurement include: (a) cost aggregation, wherein we often measure and accumulate costs based on how care is organized and billed for, that is, costs for departments, discrete service areas, and line items such as supplies or drugs and (b) cost allocation where the costs of healthcare delivery are shared costs, involving shared resources and as such are normally calculated as the average cost over all patients for a department. A good example of this is the hourly charge for the OR. However, to truly understand costs, they must be aggregated around the patient, rather than discrete services, and shared costs must be allocated to individual patients on the basis of each patient's actual use of the resources involved. Finally, the perspective used to calculate costs matters and patient costs including lost work may not be included in the analysis.

Proper measurement of outcomes and costs is the single most powerful lever for improving healthcare delivery and although current measurements are highly imperfect, the process of measurement has begun. As Michael Porter outlines in the framework papers underpinning his value commentary in the *New England Journal of Medicine*,[18] if all the stakeholders in health care were to embrace value as the central goal and measure it, the resulting improvements would be enormous.

Quality Improvement Measures and Tools

The concept of using measurement to drive improvement has its origins in both medicine and industry. The use of data to improve patient health originated in the mid-1800s with two pioneers, Florence Nightingale and John Snow. Nightingale used data on mortality among British soldiers to drive improvements in sanitation in field hospitals. Similarly, Snow used data on the incidence and geographic location of cholera to make the connection between the incidence of the disease and water obtained from the Broad Street water pump. In the early 20th century, Ernest Codman, a surgeon at Massachusetts General Hospital, was the first to advocate tracking of patient outcomes so that adverse events could be identified and improvements in care made for future patients.[19] In the 1960s, Avedis Donabedian emphasized the importance of measurement and described a model for evaluating quality of health care based on structure, process, and outcomes—*structure* being the environment in which health care is provided, *process* being the method by which it is provided, and *outcomes* being the result of the care provided.[20] More recently, in 1991, Paul Baltaden and Don Berwick developed the IHI, which has become one of the leading organizations in the application of improvement science to health care.[21]

In QI, measurement can serve many purposes. It can be used to identify problems and establish baseline performance, inform and guide QI projects, select and test changes for improvement, and assess and align progress with organizational goals. Selecting and developing measures that are useful can be challenging. Optimal measures must be comprehensive, carefully defined, tailored to the target audience, and involve minimal measurement burden. Target audiences usually include clinical staff, so measures should address and align with clinical targets for specific patient populations with whom the staff work. Measures should pass the face validity test with clinical practitioners delivering care. National or organizational measures, if applicable, can also be used, but they may not always be relevant or credible to the local target audience. Within an organization, target audiences should include system leaders, so measures should also align with organizational priorities and strategic goals.

PROCESS AND OUTCOME MEASURES

Measures should include the following:

1. Process measures that address the processes of healthcare delivery (e.g., perioperative β-adrenergic blocker administration for patients, antibiotic administration for prevention of surgical site infection)
2. Outcome measures that address patient outcomes from delivery of these services, such as clinical and functional outcomes or satisfaction with health (e.g., morbidity, mortality, length of stay, quality of life)
3. Balancing measures that address the possible consequences of changes in the process (e.g., when process improvements are made to improve efficiency, other outcomes, such as patient satisfaction, should not be adversely affected)

Each of these measures has advantages and limitations.[22] A comprehensive set of measures should include at least one process, outcome, and balancing measure. In addition, structural measures, such as ICU nurse-to-physician staffing ratios, can be important to include when appropriate.[23,24]

Healthcare providers readily accept process measures because they demonstrate the degree to which caregivers can influence a process with the intention to improve patient outcomes. Practitioners generally feel more accountable for the process of care than its outcomes, because outcomes may be affected by many other variables.[22] An obstacle to using process as a measure of quality is sustainability; frequent updating is required as the science of medicine advances.

Process measures, which evaluate how care is delivered, may be easier to measure and implement than outcome measures and can provide important insight into care.[25] Process measures can provide immediate feedback regarding performance, allowing for rapid improvements in care. If an outcome occurs infrequently, providers will be unable to obtain meaningful feedback on outcomes on a timely basis. For example, evidence of improved rates of catheter-related bloodstream infections (CRBSI; an outcome measure) may require 12 to 24 months of data (because few patients develop infections), whereas improved adherence to evidence-based practices to reduce infections (process measures) may be observed within a week (because all patients can be evaluated to determine whether they received the intervention).

Process measures have two other important advantages. First, they generally have face validity for providers, meaning that providers believe they can use the data to improve care; and second, because risk adjustment is less important, broad implementation is feasible. Moreover, joint efforts among providers, professional societies, and external government or payer agencies have made process measures more feasible.[25]

To be valid, process measures should have causal links to important outcomes; a change in the process should produce a desired change in outcome. One of the best opportunities to improve patient outcomes may well come from discovering how to deliver therapies (processes) that are known to be effective in producing a desired outcome.[26] For example, hand hygiene and application of chlorhexidine to sterilize the skin site before insertion of a central venous catheter (CVC) are two of five processes known to reduce CRBSI.[27] Process measures such as these are indicators of whether patients reliably receive evidence-based interventions known to prevent complications.

Although process measurement is useful and should continue, there is no substitute for measuring outcomes, whose principal purpose is not comparing providers but enabling innovations in care. Process measurement should largely be an internal effort, but should not be the means of external measurement and reporting of quality and value. As mentioned above, measuring value requires measuring actual outcomes over time.

Outcome measurement refers to the actual results of care in terms of patient health over time; for each medical condition there is a set of multidimensional outcomes that together constitute patient benefit. These include survival, functional status, and sustainability of recovery. Outcome measures relate directly to the health status of the patient. Patient satisfaction with care is a process measure, not an outcome. Patient satisfaction with health is an outcome measure. However, current measures for outcome often focus on the immediate results of particular procedures or interventions rather than on the overall success of the full cycle of care of a medical condition.

The relative focus on outcome and process measures will depend on balancing the collection of data between that which is scientifically sound and that which is feasible. In general, a balanced set of process and outcome measures helps inform improvement efforts and provides evidence that efforts have made a difference in the lives of patients.

For measurement to be effective, the following principles are important. First, measures should focus on something that the improvement team has the power to change and should initially be simple, small-scale measures that focus on the process itself and not on people. Second, measures should be practical, seek usefulness—not perfection—and fit the work environment and cost constraints. Third, data for measurement should be easy to obtain; finding ways to capture data while the work is getting done allows measures to be built into daily work. Fourth, qualitative data (e.g., reasons for patient dissatisfaction in the patients' own words, observations to contextualize quantitative data) are highly informative and should complement quantitative data (e.g., percentage of patients satisfied with care). Finally, when using measures, balance is key; a balanced set of measures can help answer the question, "Are we improving parts of our system at the expense of others?"

Measurement should not overwhelm the change process. Improvement teams should minimize the burden of measurement whenever possible. Measurement can have both direct and indirect consequences on resource use, provider behaviors, and patients.[28] Measurement of performance and outcomes of care can be costly, especially if the data collection process is manual and involves chart reviews. The burden of measurement is reduced with an EMR system and computerized order entry, although these information technology systems are costly to implement and maintain. Additionally, these resources may not be equally available throughout a system or organization, leading to disparities in the care provided.

Measurement fixation is an unintended consequence on healthcare staff behavior that may occur with the use of process measures. For example, when a process measure such as "the percentage of diabetic patients who received an action plan" is used rather than an outcome measure such as "improved patient understanding about diabetic management," the measure is perceived by the clinician as defining what is important. Thus, measurement of the process becomes the priority, rather than the intended outcome.[28] Alternatively, the clinician may become so focused on what is being measured that different aspects of care are not equally prioritized. In addition, a predominance of process rather than outcome measures can stifle innovation by scripting a process, thus inhibiting process-level innovation. Practice variation does have some utility because medical practice is dynamic, and it is through the trial of new methods of care that innovation occurs. Finally, QI performance measures may not match patient preferences for clinical care. Performance measures that do not take patient preference into account can lead to decreased patient satisfaction, trust, and confidence in their healthcare practitioners and system.[28] Thus, selection of a set of appropriate measures with the attributes described previously can be a balancing act that includes weighing the tradeoffs involved.

Consumers, payers, and employers are increasingly requesting outcome measures to both improve care and decrease cost. Even national governmental bodies are influencing the measurement and reporting of quality in health care. In the United States, the Centers for Medicare and Medicaid Services (CMS), the single largest healthcare purchaser, requires hospitals and physicians to participate in the Quality Payment Program (QPP). This program requires providers to demonstrate quality by either participating in an Advanced Alternative Payment Model (akin to a quality collaborative or participants in a bundled payment model) or by accumulating points through the Merit-based Incentive Payment System.[29] The United Kingdom Quality and Outcomes framework[30] is an analogous system. These quality mandates have fundamentally changed the ways that clinicians, hospitals, and health systems engage in and report QI activities.

ANALYSIS AND DISPLAY OF QUALITY IMPROVEMENT DATA

Interpretation of data and understanding of process variation are fundamental to QI work. Data elements central to improvement are first and foremost—those data are collected as a basis for action. Second, interpretation of data is made within the context of the process. Last, the analysis technique should filter out noise in the process. Aggregate data or summary statistics typically do not filter out noise in the system and do not present a broad enough context to point practitioners in the direction of proper action or process improvement.

Shewhart postulated that data contain both signal and noise; to be able to learn, one must separate the signal from the noise.[31] CQI science defines two types of variation within a process: random variation and specific variation. Random variation, also known as common-cause variation, results from differences in the inputs that a process receives or inherent factors in the process itself. Random variation is the random background noise within a system and occurs in the process all the time. Specific variation, also known as special-cause or attributable variation, is not present all of the time as background noise, but rather arises from one or more specific causes that are not part of the system. A process is considered to be unstable when specific variation exists, and efforts should be made to learn about the special causes for this variation. A stable process exists when specific variation no longer occurs, leaving only random or common variation.[9] CQI aims to eliminate specific variation for every process so that only random variation remains. A standards-based QA system fails to distinguish random cause from special cause and attempts to correct all variation. Attempts to correct random variation will necessarily fail—a process CQI defines as "tampering." When a process exhibits only random variation, the process should be evaluated to determine whether it is functioning at an acceptable level. If it is not, the process will need to be changed so that the average is moving in the desired direction. Standardization of a process is often the key to reducing random variation and improving a process.

Run Charts and Control Charts

Run charts and control charts are graphic displays of data that enable observation of trends and patterns over time. They are the best tools for determining whether improvement strategies have had an effect. A run chart (see Fig. 5.2), also called a time series chart, plots the variable or measure being studied on the vertical axis and plots the time on the horizontal axis. The average, or centerline, is the median. At least 12 data points are required to establish a baseline, and at least 20 to 25 data points are required to detect trends and patterns. Run charts should be annotated with tests of change to provide the context within which data can be interpreted. Four rules can be used with run charts to determine whether nonrandom patterns exist or to detect whether the change has led to an improvement:

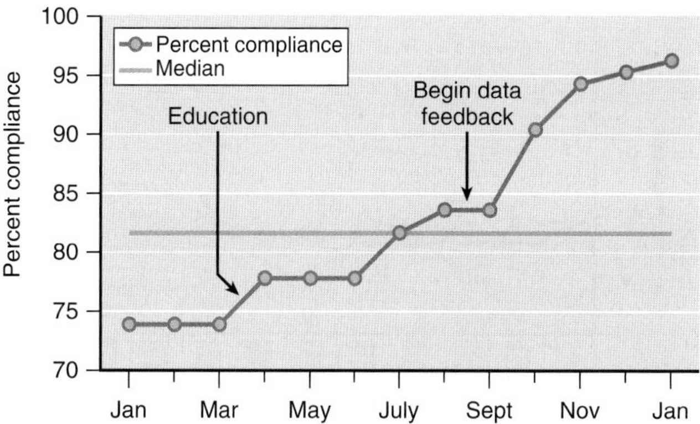

Fig. 5.2 Example of a run chart. This chart shows the plot of a performance measure over time. The horizontal (*x*) axis represents time in months, and the vertical (*y*) axis represents the performance measure—the percentage of compliance with the timing of preoperative antibiotics.

1. A shift is indicated by six or more consecutive points above or below the median.
2. A trend is indicated by five or more points all increasing or all decreasing.
3. A run is defined as a series of consecutive points on the same side of the median line.
4. An astronomical data point is an unusual point that is obviously different in value (an outlier).[7]

Because change is by nature temporal, run charts in which data are presented over time are powerful tools for interpreting data within the context of the process.

A control chart (see Fig. 5.3),[32] also known as a Shewhart chart,[7,11] is an extension of a run chart and is used to distinguish between specific and random variation. As on a run chart, the variable is plotted on the vertical axis and time on the horizontal axis. However, with a control chart the centerline or average is the mean, rather than the median, and the upper control limit (UCL) and lower control limit (LCL) are calculated. The UCL and LCL correspond to ±3 sigma from the mean. A process is considered to be "in control," or stable, when data points are within these control limits.[11] Random variation, or variation that is the result of the regular rhythm of the process, produces a stable process. However, in an unstable process that contains variation from special causes, data points exceed the UCL or LCL.[33]

Failure Modes and Effects Analysis

A failure modes and effects analysis (FMEA) is a tool to help identify problems in a process before they occur and cause harm.[7] An FMEA can help you decide where to target your improvement efforts. In addition, the proactive approach makes it especially useful before implementing a new process.

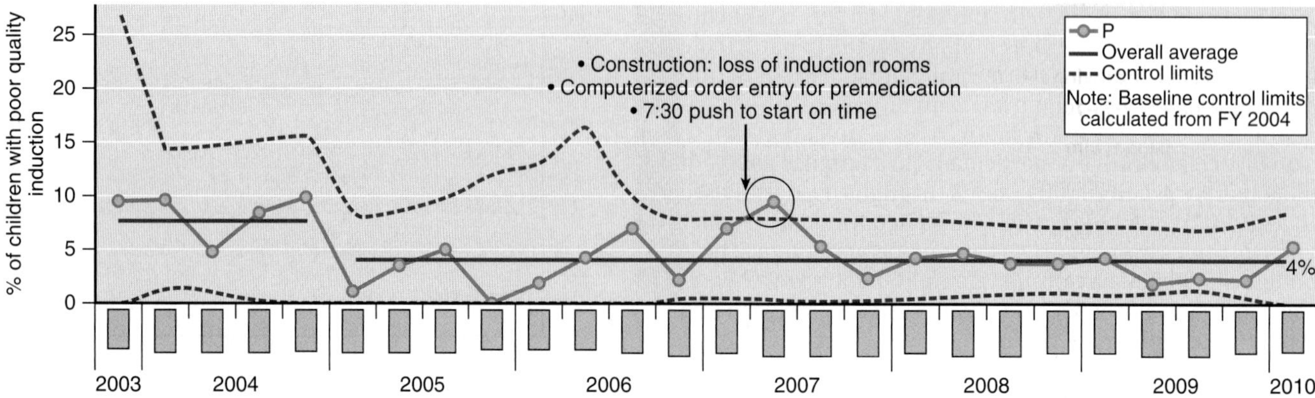

Fig. 5.3 Example of a control chart that monitors the quality of the anesthesia induction process, as measured by an induction compliance checklist. The solid red line marks the mean, and the dashed lines indicate the upper control limit and lower control limit, which are ±3 standard deviations from the mean. The circled point represents a single special cause variation in quality of induction. (From Varughese AM. Quality in pediatric anesthesia. *Paediatr Anaesth.* 2010;20:684–696.)

An FMEA reviews the steps in a process, the potential failure modes (what could go wrong), failure causes (why would the failure happen?), and failure effects (what would be the consequences?). (IHI, QI Essentials Toolkit) After listing the steps in a process, a risk profile number is calculated based on the likelihood of occurrence, likelihood of detection, and severity. Improvement efforts are then targeted at the steps with the highest risk profile number.

A simplified FMEA is a quicker version of the FMEA that can help guide improvement work. A simplified FMEA consists of listing the steps in a process, listing potential failures that could go wrong for each step, and brainstorming interventions for each of those possible failures. Below is an example simplified FMEA for programming infusion pumps that was used in an improvement project to reduce medication errors.

Putting It All Together: An Example Quality Improvement Project

The following is an example of how the QI methodology previously discussed could be used to address a practical problem. A hypothetical example of reducing medication errors in an anesthesiology department is described.

An anesthesia group was concerned over the large number of medication errors that were occurring in their department. They formed a multidisciplinary group including an anesthesiologist, nurse anesthetist, anesthesia resident, and pharmacist. They addressed the first question in the Model for Improvement—"What are we trying to achieve?"—by writing a SMART aim. Their SMART aim was to reduce medication errors in the Department of Anesthesiology from three errors per month to one error per month within 12 months.

The next question in the Model for Improvement is "How will we know that a change will result in an improvement?" In order to monitor their progress, they constructed a run chart of medication errors per month in their department. They captured data through a previously existing self-reporting system.

The last question of the Model for Improvement is "What changes can we make that will result in an improvement?" To better understand the errors that were occurring, the group categorized the medication errors into categories and constructed a Pareto Chart. A Pareto Chart is a bar chart in which categories are listed in descending order. The group learned that three categories of errors accounted for about 80% of the total number of errors. These categories were infusion pump errors, acetaminophen errors, and antibiotic errors. They decided to focus their initial efforts on these three categories. They created process maps for these three categories to better understand the current process and develop possible interventions. Finally, to help organize their theory of improvement, they created a key driver diagram listing the drivers they thought would affect their aim, as well as possible interventions targeting the drivers.

Now that they had a theory of improvement, they started testing their interventions. They tested their ideas using PDSA cycles. They adopted the successful tests, adapted tests with mixed results, and abandoned the failed tests. Some of their tests included requiring a sticker from pharmacy and requiring a two-person double check of infusion pumps. As their testing and implementation continued, they saw the centerline, or median, of the run chart decrease from three to two. The run chart rules indicated this was a significant change. The group was excited that they had decreased the number of medication errors in their department, but they had not yet reached their aim of no more than one medication error per month. They decided to continue testing new ideas until the median decreased to less than one error per month.

Dashboards and Scorecards

A dashboard of measures functions like an instrument panel for an aircraft or automobile and provides real-time feedback on what is happening. Balanced *scorecards*, or "whole system measures," are similar to dashboards and are used to provide a complete picture of quality. Developed by Kaplan and Norton, the balanced scorecard is defined as a "multidimensional framework for describing, implementing, and managing strategy at all levels of an enterprise by linking objectives, initiatives, and measures to an organization's strategy."[34] A set of measures should reflect the culture and mission of an organization. Viewed collectively, this set of measures provides a gauge of current performance and can also guide the direction for future organizational improvement efforts. A balanced set of measures is critical to ensure

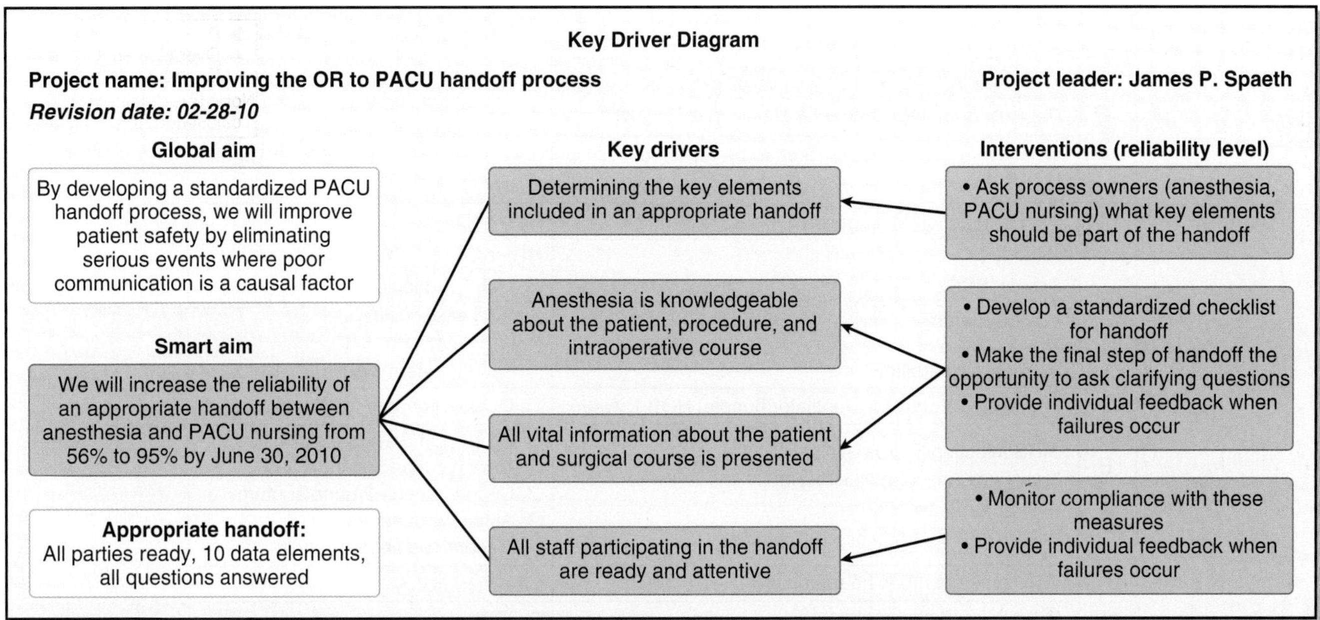

Fig. 5.4 **Example of a key driver diagram developed to improve the operating room *(OR)* to postanesthesia care unit (*PACU*) handoff process. This diagram incorporates the global and smart aim of the project, the key drivers inherent to the process, and specific interventions targeting each of the key drivers.** (From Boat AC, Spaeth JP. Handoff checklists improve the reliability of patient handoffs in the operating room and postanesthesia care unit. *Paediatr Anaesth.* 2013;23(7):647-654.)[93]

that improvement efforts in one area do not adversely affect outcomes in other areas.

Additional Quality Improvement Evaluation and Communication Tools

In most situations, QI frameworks such as the Model for Improvement or Lean Sigma are sufficient to help guide the development, testing, implementation, and spread of improvement. However, to better understand problems within a system or process, QI professionals have developed or adapted a number of methods and tools. Some of these methods and tools help with viewing systems and processes and organizing and communicating information. These are described in the following section.

Understanding how a process or system works is fundamental to improving it. Process mapping is a method to gain this understanding. A flow diagram, or flow chart, is an improvement tool used during process mapping; it provides a visual picture of the process being studied, wherein the series of activities that define a process is graphically represented. Flow charts identify and clarify all steps in the process. They also help the team understand the complexity of the process and identify opportunities for improvement.

Failure mode and effects analysis is a systematic, proactive method of identifying and addressing problems associated with a process. It uses a standardized approach to analysis that includes identifying the various steps in a process and addressing their failure modes, effects, and possible interventions.

A key driver diagram (KDD) (Fig. 5.4)[35] is another approach to organizing the theories and ideas for improvement that a team has developed. The KDD presents the aim or outcome of the project with both the theories (key drivers) behind the improvement and ideas for test of change.[7] Initially, the driver diagram helps lay out the descriptive theory behind the improved outcomes. As these theories are tested, the driver diagram is updated and enhanced to develop a predictive theory. KDDs are extremely useful because they provide a shared mental model for the team during its improvement efforts.

IMPROVEMENT INTERVENTION TOOLS

Efforts in QI and patient safety have produced tools with which to reorganize the way care is delivered. QI intervention tools are used to improve communication and teamwork. Examples of these tools include daily goals sheets, briefings/debriefings, and checklists.

Daily Goals Sheet

For nearly 20 years, documentation of daily goals as either a hand-written sheet or a whiteboard have been used to improve communication during multidisciplinary rounds in adult and pediatric ICUs.[36,37] As a one-page paper checklist, this tool would be completed every morning to establish the care plan, set goals, and review potential safety risks for each patient (Fig. 5.5).

Before implementation of the daily goals sheet in an adult ICU, an initial survey showed that ICU team members were unable to answer two simple questions after rounding at each patient's bedside: "Do you understand the patient's goals for the day?" and "Do you understand what work needs to be accomplished on this patient today?" Fewer than 10% of the residents and nurses knew the care plan for the day—a finding that was not surprising because traditional bedside rounds tended to focus on teaching the staff about disease processes rather than focusing on the work that was necessary to treat the patient. Approximately 4 weeks after the daily goals sheet was implemented, 95% of residents and nurses understood the goals for each patient. Moreover, after the daily goals sheet was implemented, length of stay in the

	Room Number ____________	Shift: ❒ AM / ❒ PM
Safety	What needs to be done to d/c patient from the ICU?	
	Patient's greatest safety risk? How can we ↓ risk?	
	What events or deviations need to be reported? ICUSRS issues?	
Patient Care	Pain & Sedation Management	Pain goal ____ /10
	Cardiac Review ECGs	HR goal ____ ❒ at goal ❒ ↑ ❒ ↓ β-blockade
	Volume status Net goal for midnight	Even ❒ Pos ❒ Neg ___ Net ___ (cc) ❒ Patient determined
	Pulmonary: Ventilator, ventilator bundle, HOB ↑, wean	❒ OOB/pulmonary toilet/ambulation
	SIRS/Infection/Sepsis evaluation Temp >38°C or <36°C; HR >90 RR >20 or $Paco_2$ <32 WBC >12000 < 4000 or >10% bands	❒ No current SIRS/sepsis issues ❒ Known/suspected infection ❒ Culture blood ×2/urine/sputum ❒ Antibiotic changes ❒ Discontinue sepsis bundle
	Can catheters/tubes be removed?	Y/N
	GI/Nutrition/Bowel regimen: TPN catheter, ND tube PEG needed?	❒ TPN ❒ NPO/Advance diet
	Is patient receiving DVT/PUD prophylaxis?	Y/N
	Can meds be discontinued, changed to PO, adjusted?	
To Do	Tests/Procedures today	
	Scheduled labs	
	AM labs needed/CXR?	
	Consultations	
Description	Has primary service been updated?	
	Has family been updated? Social issues addressed? Long-term/Palliative care	

Fig. 5.5 Example of an intensive care unit *(ICU)* daily goals sheet. *CXR*, Chest radiograph; *d/c*, discharge; *DVT*, deep vein thrombosis; *ECG*, electrocardiogram; *GI*, gastrointestinal; *HOB*, head of bed; *HR*, heart rate; *ICUSRS*, ICU self-reporting system; *ND*, naso-duodenal; *NPO*, nothing by mouth; *OOB*, out of bed; *PEG*, percutaneous endoscopic gastrostomy; *PUD*, peptic ulcer disease; *RR*, respiratory rate; *SIRS*, severe infectious respiratory syndrome; *temp*, temperature; *TPN*, total parenteral nutrition; *vent*, ventilator; *WBC*, white blood cell count.

surgical ICU decreased from a mean of 2.2 days to only 1.1 days.[38] These results have been reproduced in ICUs with nurses, physicians, and pharmacists. Interviews supported that communication, patient care, and education were enhanced by providing a structured, thorough, and individualized approach to the patient's care. The daily goals checklist helped to identify new patient care issues and sparked management discussions, especially for sedation, weaning, and medications.[36] Additionally, a QI intervention using daily goals checklists in 118 ICUs in Brazil improved the use of low tidal volumes, avoidance of heavy sedation, use of CVCs, use of urinary catheters, perception of teamwork, and perception of patient safety climate, but did not reduce in-hospital mortality.[37]

A further improvement was implemented in a pediatric cardiac ICU using a whiteboard for visual display of the daily goals.[39] Use of the whiteboard increased the percent agreement among the patient care team for patient goals from 62% to over 87%.[37] The goals were updated as needed and used as an information source for all staff involved in the patient's care as well as for the patient's family. A daily goals display such as this can be modified for use on other nursing units or during OR sign-out or emergency department rounds.

Checklists

Checklists have been used in health care and other industries to ensure that important steps in a process are not forgotten. The Food and Drug Administration recommends that a checklist be used when checking out and inspecting an anesthesia machine before use to ensure that the equipment and monitors are functioning properly.[40,41] Checklists have been shown to be effective in reducing central line associated blood stream infections (CLABSI) by standardizing practice, reducing complexity, and providing a redundant safety check. The idea behind having a person, such as a nurse or another physician, be responsible for actually reading the checklist also empowers that person or anyone involved to stop the procedure if the checklist is not followed or if sterile technique is compromised. An early study showed that use of a central line insertion checklist and bundle resulted in a 66% reduction in the overall CLABSI rate; the median rate was reduced from 2.7 per 1000

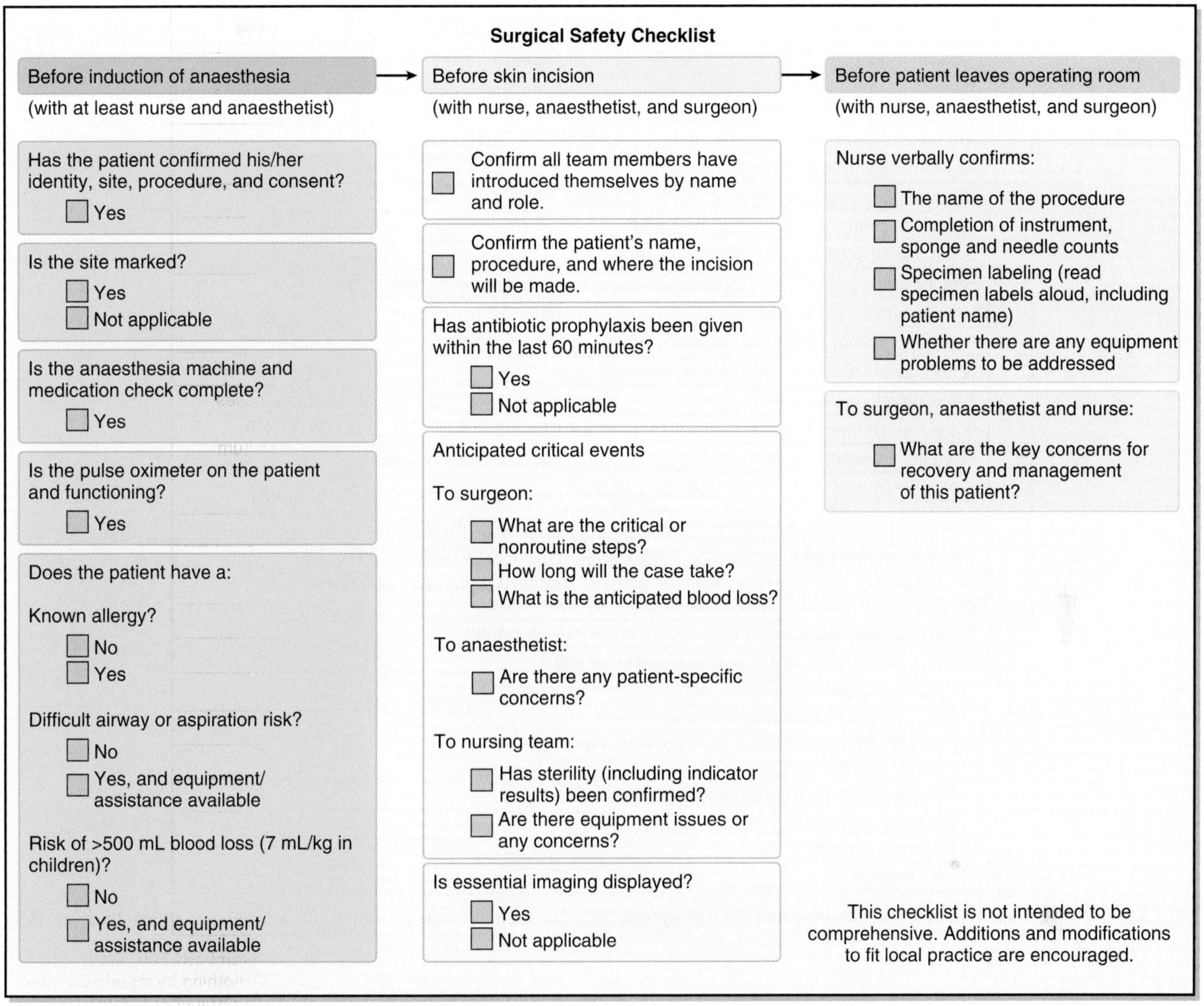

Surgical Safety Checklist

Before induction of anaesthesia (with at least nurse and anaesthetist)

Has the patient confirmed his/her identity, site, procedure, and consent?
- ☐ Yes

Is the site marked?
- ☐ Yes
- ☐ Not applicable

Is the anaesthesia machine and medication check complete?
- ☐ Yes

Is the pulse oximeter on the patient and functioning?
- ☐ Yes

Does the patient have a:

Known allergy?
- ☐ No
- ☐ Yes

Difficult airway or aspiration risk?
- ☐ No
- ☐ Yes, and equipment/assistance available

Risk of >500 mL blood loss (7 mL/kg in children)?
- ☐ No
- ☐ Yes, and equipment/assistance available

→ **Before skin incision** (with nurse, anaesthetist, and surgeon)

- ☐ Confirm all team members have introduced themselves by name and role.
- ☐ Confirm the patient's name, procedure, and where the incision will be made.

Has antibiotic prophylaxis been given within the last 60 minutes?
- ☐ Yes
- ☐ Not applicable

Anticipated critical events

To surgeon:
- ☐ What are the critical or nonroutine steps?
- ☐ How long will the case take?
- ☐ What is the anticipated blood loss?

To anaesthetist:
- ☐ Are there any patient-specific concerns?

To nursing team:
- ☐ Has sterility (including indicator results) been confirmed?
- ☐ Are there equipment issues or any concerns?

Is essential imaging displayed?
- ☐ Yes
- ☐ Not applicable

→ **Before patient leaves operating room** (with nurse, anaesthetist, and surgeon)

Nurse verbally confirms:
- ☐ The name of the procedure
- ☐ Completion of instrument, sponge and needle counts
- ☐ Specimen labeling (read specimen labels aloud, including patient name)
- ☐ Whether there are any equipment problems to be addressed

To surgeon, anaesthetist and nurse:
- ☐ What are the key concerns for recovery and management of this patient?

This checklist is not intended to be comprehensive. Additions and modifications to fit local practice are encouraged.

Fig. 5.6 World Health Organization Safe Surgery Checklist. (Reproduced with permission from World Health Organization. WHO Surgical Safety Checklist.)

catheter days before the intervention to 0 by month 3 and through month 18 of the postintervention.[42] A central line insertion checklist has since been adopted by institutions, safety groups, and regulatory agencies as a tool to ensure compliance with the best practices for CVC placement and prevent CLABSI. Checklists and central line insertion bundles are widely available online; one such resource is the IHI (http://www.ihi.org).

In addition to standardizing technical tasks, checklists are also used to standardize communication. Haynes and colleagues[43] described the use of a checklist to guide the perioperative time-out, briefing, and debriefing process. They showed that implementing the World Health Organization Surgical Safety Checklist (Fig. 5.6) reduced mortality and inpatient complications.[43] The use of surgical checklists is now widespread and is standard of care in most OR settings around the world. Numerous studies related to surgical checklists either as a tool or a process have shown their effectiveness, while some studies have reported limited impact. A review of 25 highly cited research papers on surgical safety checklists from 2009 to 2016 showed the complexity of standardizing, implementing, and sustaining the use of surgical safety checklists.[44] Complexities include variations in the environment, distribution of staff, timing of when the checklist is actually used, relationship between those using the checklist, and the culture of the institution.[44] These complexities may undermine the effectiveness of checklists and should be considered prior to checklist implementation.

Briefings and Debriefings

The surgical checklist is part of the Universal Protocol, which was created to prevent wrong person, wrong procedure, and wrong site surgery. In order to address many of the other important safety issues, such as antibiotic needs, deep vein thrombosis prevention, fire prevention, special equipment needs, and blood product availability, many institutions have implemented OR briefings or huddles, as well as debriefings at the end of surgery. Preoperative briefings have been shown to improve team communication, improve compliance with best practices, and enhance the overall perception of the safety climate in the OR.[45]

Briefing and debriefing tools are designed to promote effective interdisciplinary communication and teamwork.

	Briefing: Before Every Procedure
	Team introductions: First and last names, including roles; write names on board
	Verify: Patient ID band, informed consent (read out loud), site marking, OR posting, patient's verbalization of procedure (if patient awake), H&P or clinic note
	Are there any safety, equipment, instrument, implant, or other concerns?
	Have antibiotics been given, if indicated?
	What are the anticipated times of antibiotic redosing?
	Is glucose control or β-blockade indicated?
	Is the patient positioned to minimize injury?
	Has the prep solution been applied properly, without pooling, and allowed to dry?
	Have the goals and critical steps of the procedure been discussed?
	Is the appropriate amount of blood available?
	Is DVT prophylaxis indicated? If yes, describe.
	Are warmers on the patient?
	Is the time allotted for this procedure an accurate estimate?
	Have the attendings reviewed the latest laboratory and radiology results?
	Debriefing: After Every Procedure
	Could anything have been done to make this case safer or more efficient?
	Has the Surgical Site Infection data collection form been completed?
	Are the patient's name, history number, surgical specimen name, and laterality on the paper work? (must be independently verified by the surgeon)
	Did we have problems with instruments? Were they reported?
	Plan for transition of care to postop unit discussed? ❐ Fluid management? ❐ Blood transfusion paperwork in chart? ❐ Antibiotic dose and interval to be continued postop? ❐ Pain management/PCA plan? ❐ New medications needed immediately postop? ❐ β-blockers needed? ❐ Glucose control? ❐ DVT prophylaxis?

Fig. 5.7 Example of an operating room briefing and debriefing tool. *DVT,* Deep vein thrombosis; *H&P,* history and physical; *ID,* identification; *OR,* operating rooms.

Both have been used in the OR, during sign-out from the ICU nursing staff to the intensivist, and between OR nursing and anesthesia coordinators.[40,46,47] A briefing is a structured review of the case at hand that takes place among all team members before the start of an operative procedure. A debriefing occurs after the procedure; the team reviews what worked well, what failed, and what could be accomplished better in the future (Fig. 5.7).

An example of an OR briefing includes introduction by name (first and last) and role of each team member, confirmation of the correct patient, confirmation of the site/side and procedure (time-out), and a verbal assurance that all team members agree that they understand the procedure and what is required to ensure its success. A check of all necessary equipment, medications (e.g., appropriate antibiotic), and blood availability is performed. The question, "If something were to go wrong, what would it be?" is asked, and plans to mitigate or respond to the potential hazard are discussed.

A collaborative effort by the Agency for Healthcare Research and Quality (AHRQ) and the Department of Defense adopted crew resource management strategies for OR briefings and produced an evidence-based resource called Team Strategies and Tools to Enhance Performance and Patient Safety (TeamSTEPPS) www.ahrq.gov. This team approach in the OR encourages situational awareness and communication among all members of the healthcare team.[48-51]

Sources of Quality Improvement Information

Development of a QI project first requires that an issue be identified. Baseline data are then collected and an improvement intervention instituted, often using one of the approaches described earlier. Data are re-collected after the intervention. If the intervention is found to be effective, ongoing monitoring or audits are instituted to ensure that the change is sustained. As part of the audits, feedback must be given to the providers. Healthcare providers traditionally have had limited ability to obtain feedback regarding performance in their daily work, in part because of a lack of information systems and a lack of agreement on how to measure quality of care.[52]

Ideas for QI projects can be identified from a multitude of sources, but they typically start with surveys and input from local medical staff and reviews of reported incidents. Additional information is gathered from the literature, review of national guidelines and quality metrics, and information obtained from external or internal reviews.

Sources of QI data that span both the clinical and administrative arenas include evidence-based medicine and evidence-based clinical practice guidelines, alerts from accrediting agencies and nonprofit safety organizations, standards and guidelines put forth by medical specialty associations, closed claims databases, and government agency administrative databases. United States governmental agencies, including the AHRQ, CMS, and the National Quality Forum (NQF), promote the development and reporting of healthcare quality measures.[53]

INCIDENT REPORTING

Voluntary incident reporting capturing hazardous conditions has been successfully used to improve patient care and foster QI programs.[54] As the potential of voluntary incident reporting is being realized in health care, this reporting has become less punitive and more focused on systems rather than on individuals. Voluntary incident reporting, when appropriately applied, helps identify hazards to patients that can then become the focus of QI efforts that seek to mitigate those hazards.[55] Unlike other methods that evaluate harmed patients, voluntary incident reporting provides the potential to also learn from near misses—incidents that did not lead to harm but were potentially hazardous. These near misses and potential hazards are a rich source for QI projects highlighting the importance of preventing harm.

All anesthesiology departments should have a process in place for capturing adverse events and near misses. Although most departments have a process for reporting, many incidents go unreported for a variety of reasons. Departments should encourage voluntary reporting without threat of punishment. Electronic capture of adverse events, near misses, and complaints can provide data that can subsequently be analyzed to identify trends and assess the degree of harm that a hazard poses to patients.

Events that occur frequently with low harm can be just as important as an event that occurs rarely with high harm. At the local level, it is more effective to focus on a more frequently occurring adverse event (e.g., perioperative skin abrasions, mislabeling of laboratory specimens) or on a process that can be measured with high frequency (e.g., hand hygiene, administration of antibiotic prophylaxis). For rarely occurring harmful events, a QI initiative may encompass a more expansive analysis of a national adverse-event database with multicenter participation.

With multiinstitutional event reporting systems, events that would rarely be seen in a single institution can be collected in larger numbers. Such systems allow analysis for common causes that increase our knowledge base for prevention initiatives. Larger multiinstitutional data gathering systems include the Vizient collaborative (the former University HealthSystem Consortium), which supports event reporting and databases that can be used to develop QI programs, benchmarking, and evidence-based practice.[56] Reporting systems that have been developed specifically to investigate rarely occurring anesthesia-related events include the Anesthesia Incident Reporting System (AIRS) created by the Anesthesia Quality Institute (AQI)[57] and Wake Up Safe, a QI initiative of the Society for Pediatric Anesthesia.[58] The AIRS program publishes a learning case each month in the *ASA Newsletter*, including a summary of a reported case with learning points.

More expansive international incident-reporting systems that are anonymous and voluntary have also been analyzed in the literature and have provided important information. Examples are the United Kingdom's Serious Incident Reporting and Learning Framework[59] and the Australian Incident Monitoring Study.[60] These incident registries do not require that the events be considered human error or preventable to merit reporting and are a source of ideas for QI projects.

Although voluntary systems often prove fruitful, many events and near misses still frequently go unreported. One way to capture these incidents is to survey local medical staff members to obtain their thoughts on how the last patient was harmed or how the next patient might be harmed. This process of performing a staff safety assessment survey is described in two later sections of this chapter (see "Collaborative Programs" and "Comprehensive Unit-Based Safety Program"). Staff safety assessment surveys can be particularly helpful for identifying issues for QI projects. Additionally, if staff members identify the issue, the likelihood is greater that they will have a vested interest in participating in the QI efforts.

PUBLISHED LITERATURE

Literature reviews offer ideas for QI topics in specific areas and information to guide interventions. For example, if the QI project plan is to reduce hazards in cardiac anesthesia, a literature review will provide reports of various cardiac anesthesia risks. Once a topic within a clinical area is selected, a literature search should be performed again to determine whether similar QI projects have been performed and whether they were successful. Such information will help with the design of a future initiative. The literature also provides published reports that identify guidelines and/or evidence-based practices that can be the basis for future programs.[61,62]

NATIONAL INITIATIVES AND QUALITY METRICS

The AHRQ is the source for both the U.S. National Quality Measures Clearinghouse and the National Guideline Clearinghouse. Professional organizations, such as the American Society of Anesthesiologists (ASA) and the World Federation of Societies of Anesthesiologists, offer field-specific guidelines. The ASA has supported the review and development of many important guidelines that can serve as a rich source of QI initiatives. These guidelines cover a range of practices and include guidelines for the placement of central venous access,[63] management of patients with obstructive sleep apnea,[64] and management of preoperative fasting.[65] For those who are also involved in critical care medicine, guidelines and protocols do improve performance with specific care processes such as sedation and ventilator weaning protocols in ICUs. Such protocols decrease the duration of mechanical ventilation and ICU length of stay.[66,67]

Review of national quality metrics is another source of ideas for QI topics. National initiatives from CMS, such as the QPP (described earlier in "Quality Improvement Measures and Tools") and Surgical Care Improvement Project (SCIP), provide quality metrics and are associated with pay for performance. Most of the SCIP measures, which predominantly

TABLE 5.3 Nonprofit and Governmental Quality Improvement Organizations Pertinent to Anesthesia

Quality Improvement Organization	Website	Description
Agency for Healthcare Research and Quality (AHRQ)	www.ahrq.gov	Lead federal agency charged with improving the quality, safety, efficiency, and effectiveness of health care
American Health Quality Association (AHQA)	www.ahqa.org	Represents quality improvement organizations and professionals working to improve the quality of health care
Anesthesia Patient Safety Foundation (APSF)	www.apsf.org	Promotes investigations and programs that will provide a better understanding of anesthetic injuries
Centers for Disease Control (CDC)	www.cdc.gov	One of the major operating components of the U.S. Department of Health and Human Services
Emergency Care Research Institute (ECRI)	www.ecri.org	Uses applied scientific research to discover which medical procedures, devices, drugs, and processes are best
Institute for Healthcare Improvement (IHI)	www.ihi.org	Health care improvement organization based in Cambridge, Massachusetts
Institute for Safe Medication Practices (ISMP)	www.ismp.org	The nation's only 501(c)(3) organization devoted entirely to medication error prevention and safe medication use
Medicare Quality Improvement Community (MedQIC)	www.medquic.org	A national knowledge forum for health care and quality improvement professionals
National Quality Forum	www.qualityforum.org	Created to develop and implement a national strategy for health care quality and reporting
National Patient Safety Foundation (NPSF)	www.npsf.org	An independent 501(c)(3) organization with a mission to improve the safety of patients

measure processes of care, are topped out (nearly 100% in all hospitals) and have therefore been retired from active surveillance. The Joint Commission (TJC) website (www.jointcommission.org) lists United States National Patient Safety Goals and national quality core measures that are surveyed during site visits for accreditation. In 2004, TJC partnered with CMS to align measures common to both organizations in an initiative called Hospital Quality Measures. These measures are also endorsed by the NQF, a private, nonprofit membership organization created to develop and implement a national strategy for healthcare quality measurement and reporting (www.qualityforum.org). One of NQF's functions is to endorse quality and safety measures (consensus standards), which are then incorporated into other national quality initiatives. The goal for NQF-endorsed standards is that they become the primary standards used to measure the quality of health care in the United States. Increasingly, anesthesia programs are focusing on the standards that are relevant to the specialty because facilities are being evaluated on compliance with regulations and are required to report their performance regarding these standards to the governing bodies.

An increasing number of regional and national organizations are developing initiatives that are stimulating the reporting of specific evidence-based practices and outcomes. These initiatives are also determining the local selection of areas for QI (Table 5.3). As described earlier, reporting of these measures to CMS is being incentivized by performance-based payment. National professional organizations such as the ASA are developing metrics specific to the field.

OUTCOMES RESEARCH

The comparison of outcomes associated with different process decisions, or variations in care delivery, is the basis for outcomes research. Outcomes research offers a potential to identify these variations in care and to determine whether they improve outcomes for patients undergoing anesthesia. One of the key issues in outcomes research is risk adjustment, a challenging goal that requires a robust dataset. Using administrative data to identify patient risk factors has many limitations.[68] Registries designed specifically for research, benchmarking, and QI are good sources for this purpose.

The Society of Thoracic Surgeons (STS) and the National Surgical Quality Improvement Programs (NSQIP) are examples of outcomes research registries. Established in the early 1990s, the STS database now includes participation by nearly all U.S. cardiac surgery centers and has developed robust risk-stratification models. Findings from this database have led to initiatives associated with significant reductions in mortality; examples include the use of β-adrenergic blockers and aspirin perioperatively and the use of internal mammary arteries for coronary artery bypass grafting. NSQIP is a newer registry that was developed by the U.S. Department of Veterans Affairs (VA). Findings from this risk-adjusted outcomes database were used to identify variations in care. The changes that were instituted based on these findings resulted in improved surgical outcomes throughout the VA network. NSQIP has been adopted by the American College of Surgeons to provide comparisons among hospitals. Currently, more than 350 general surgery centers participate.[69] Hospitals that participate submit detailed data on a sample of general surgical patients for a number of common surgical procedures. They then receive a graphic display that compares their outcomes with those of the entire cohort. Surgery centers then use these data to identify areas in which they might be able to make improvements and initiate QI projects with that focus. As an example, the Kaiser Permanente group used this information to develop a QI program focused on reducing the percentage of patients with prolonged perioperative intubation.[69]

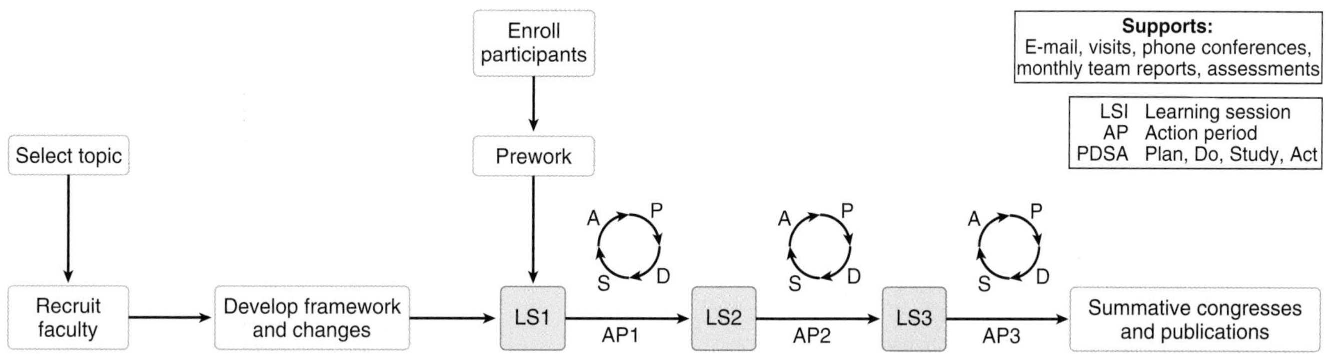

Fig. 5.8 Breakthrough series collaborative model. (Reproduced with permission from Institute for Healthcare Improvement: The Breakthrough Series: IHI's Collaborative Model for Achieving Breakthrough Improvement. IHI Innovation Series white paper, Boston, 2003. *PDSA*, Plan, Do, Study, Act. http://www.ihi.org/knowledge/Pages/IHIWhitePapers/TheBreakthroughSeriesIHIsCollaborativeModelforAchievingBreakthroughImprovement.aspx.)

The ASA created the AQI and the National Anesthesia Clinical Outcomes Registry with the goal of improving anesthesia outcomes through capture of case-specific data directly from electronic anesthesia data systems.[70,71] These resources are still evolving and moving forward to improve outcomes in anesthesia. Another important effort in anesthesia is the Multicenter Perioperative Outcomes Group (MPOG), which is led by researchers at the University of Michigan.[72] MPOG has established a national network of anesthesia practice groups that contribute data to a unified database. The goals of MPOG are to develop a structure for multiinstitutional collaboration and data sharing, to develop the information technology infrastructure to pool a wide variety of perioperative data for patient-centered research, to develop the statistical infrastructure to analyze the data, and to provide an academic venue in which faculty from multiple institutions will be able to collaborate in outcomes research (http://mpog.med.umich.edu).[72]

INTERNAL OR EXTERNAL INSTITUTIONAL REVIEWS

Internal or external institutional reviews of healthcare processes can provide important insights and ideas for QI initiatives. In addition to the external regulatory reviews, institutions are expected to perform internal reviews of quality and identify areas for improvement. These reviews are often used for QI projects at the institutional level.

Examples of Quality Improvement Programs

Examples of QI frameworks and tools have been discussed. This section addresses broad initiatives for quality and safety improvement that have used some of the methodologies and tools detailed earlier in this chapter.

COLLABORATIVE PROGRAMS

Use of a collaborative is one approach to improving broad areas of care. A QI collaborative involves the participation of two or more healthcare teams working toward a shared goal. In healthcare, a set of multidisciplinary representatives (from all of the clinical and administrative areas that are linked to the area of focus) should participate in the collaborative. A collaborative can be developed within a single organization and/or across multiple healthcare organizations. Collaborative programs are typically led by a team that is responsible for the following:

1. Determining the evidence-based interventions to be used and presenting these to the participants (if evidence-based interventions are not available, the team will generate interventions based on local and broad expert consensus)
2. Establishing the data collection approach (defining measures, collection methods, and feedback mechanism)

A key element to the success of collaboratives is an established process for educating members and for sharing interventions and obstacles. Through group discussions (meetings and/or conference calls), teams can learn about best practices and innovative methods used by other teams to approach a problem. In addition, collaboratives bring a shared momentum and enthusiasm that can increase sustainability.[24,73,74]

INSTITUTE FOR HEALTHCARE IMPROVEMENT BREAKTHROUGH SERIES COLLABORATIVES

QI collaboratives provide an opportunity to learn from other teams, work collaboratively, and spread change on a larger scale. The IHI has used a collaborative model for improvement, called the Breakthrough Series Model, for more than a decade. Collaboratives run from 12 to 160 teams across multiple organizations. Successful IHI collaboratives have included reducing waiting times by 50%, reducing ICU costs by 25%, and reducing hospitalizations of heart failure patients by 50%.[75]

In the Breakthrough Series Model, a topic is selected and participating teams are enrolled (Fig. 5.8). Expert faculty from across the country, or even internationally, are recruited for an expert meeting to develop a framework for change called a "change package." The change package describes interventions for improvement based on available evidence. Next, team members from all groups attend collaborative learning sessions where they learn the model for improvement and share their progress implementing the change package. At the end of the collaborative, a summative meeting and publications are used to share the findings with others.

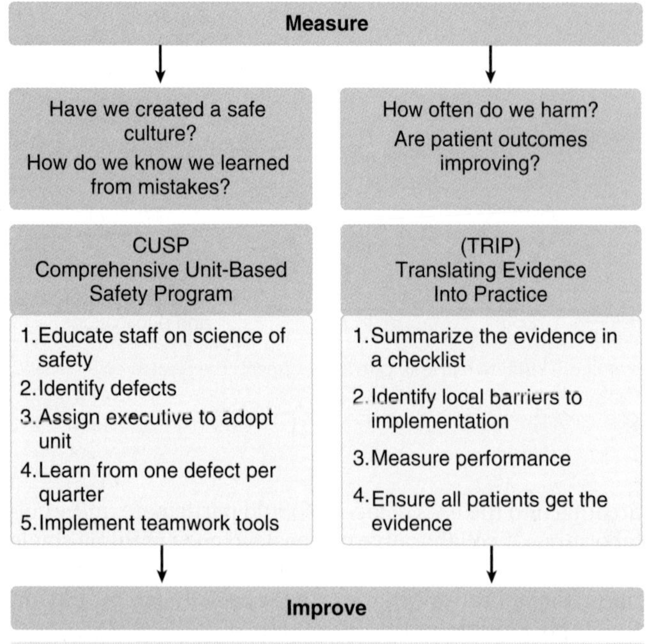

Fig. 5.9 Comprehensive unit-based safety program *(CUSP)* and translating evidence into practice *(TRIP)*: basic steps to ensure patients receive evidence-based care. (Reproduced with permission from Sawyer M. Using evidence, rigorous measurement, and collaboration to eliminate central catheter-associated bloodstream infections. *Crit Care Med.* 2010;38:S292–S298.)

TABLE 5.4 Four Steps That Ensure Patients Receive Evidence-Based Interventions Through a Collaborative Using the Example of Catheter-Related Bloodstream Infections

Step	Action	Example
Engage	Make the problem real	Share information of local CRBSI rate vs. national rate
Educate	Develop an educational plan to reach ALL members of the caregiver team	Present evidence-based practices at grand rounds and multidisciplinary team meetings Present plans to improve care and measure outcome
Execute	Develop a safety culture Reduce complexity of the processes Introduce redundancy in processes Hold regular team meetings	Develop a culture of intolerance for CRBSI Ensure that all equipment and supplies for sterile CVC insertion are in one place and easily available Use checklists that identify key steps to reduce CRBSI Focus on one to two tasks per week and identify team member responsible for task
Evaluate	Measure and provide feedback	Develop data collection plan and database to track progress Give staff real-time feedback; post progress in highly visible location Identify causes of defects

CRBSI, Catheter-related bloodstream infections; *CVC*, central venous catheter.

COMPREHENSIVE UNIT-BASED PROGRAM

Sawyer and associates reported the success of a collaborative that incorporates a "mechanism to move evidence to the bedside and foster a culture where the focus is the patient."[76] The collaborative includes an emphasis on translating evidence into practice (TRIP) and the Comprehensive Unit-Based Safety Program (CUSP). This methodology has been reproduced and validated in several large collaborative efforts (Fig. 5.9).[76-78]

The TRIP model incorporates the following key steps and emphasizes the importance of measurement and feedback of data to teams.

1. Identify evidence-based interventions associated with an improved outcome through review of peer-reviewed publications.
2. Select goal-oriented interventions that have the most impact on outcomes and transform them into behaviors. In selecting behaviors, focus on interventions with the strongest treatment effect (smallest number needed to treat) and the lowest barrier to use.
3. Develop and implement measures that evaluate either the interventions (processes) or the outcomes.
4. Measure baseline performance and establish databases to facilitate accurate data management and timely feedback to teams.
5. Ensure that patients receive evidence-based interventions through four basic steps: engagement, education, execution, and evaluation (Table 5.4).

The format for the collaborative also includes annual face-to-face meetings with the participating teams and periodic conference calls, which focus on education about the actual processes being implemented, the evidence base to support these processes, and the sharing of experiences. First, weekly immersion calls provide an initial overview of the program, describe the roles and responsibilities of each of the individuals, and introduce the tools that are to be used. Once the collaborative is introduced, monthly content calls are held throughout the program and are typified by a slide presentation of the evidence base for the intervention or of other components of the program to be implemented. The monthly coaching calls offer an opportunity for teams to share how well or how poorly they are implementing the interventions and share ideas for overcoming barriers.

Inclusion of the CUSP program in the collaborative provides a structured approach to improve safety culture and identify and mitigate hazards (i.e., learn from mistakes).[38,47] CUSP is a five-step program that has been tested and used successfully to improve quality and safety in ICUs (Table 5.5).[79,80] CUSP programs have been used in many different environments including inpatient units, primary care practices,[81] and in the perioperative period[82] to enhance the safety culture and improve the patient experience.[83]

Safety culture is assessed before the implementation of CUSP and reassessed after 1 year to evaluate the impact of the program. Multiple culture assessment tools are available.[64,65] The AHRQ offers a free survey online (www.ahrq.gov). The initial measure provides a baseline assessment of staff perceptions of safety culture in their clinical areas and their perceptions of the organization's commitment to patient safety.

Education is a crucial aspect of CUSP; it provides staff with a new set of lenses through which to identify hazards and

TABLE 5.5 Five-Step Comprehensive Unit-Based Safety Program

	Step	Description
1	Present educational material	Educate staff on science of safety though lectures and other educational materials
2	Complete forms that identify patient safety issues	Ask the following questions: ▪ How will the next patient be harmed? ▪ How can this harm be prevented? ▪ Establish voluntary incident reporting
3	Assign senior executive responsible for specific area	Senior executive meets with all staff of the clinical area to: ▪ Help prioritize safety efforts ▪ Remove barriers for system changes ▪ Provide resources ▪ Demonstrate hospital commitment to patient safety ▪ Foster relationship between senior leadership and staff
4	Learn from defects	Implement projects focused on two to three safety issues Keep goals simple: ▪ Reduce complexity in the process ▪ Create independent redundancies to ensure critical steps are accomplished
5	Implement teamwork tools	Implement programs such as checklists, training, and daily goals targeted at improving teamwork and communication

recommend system changes to improve care. The objectives of these educational efforts are to ensure that staff: (1) understand that safety is a system property, (2) learn concepts for reliable healthcare design, and (3) understand the basics of change management. After an educational lecture on the science of safety, staff members are requested to identify patient safety hazards in their clinical areas and suggest improvement interventions. For this process, staff members review incident reports, liability claims, and sentinel events from their unit. In addition, two questions are asked: "How do you think the next patient will be harmed?" and "How can we prevent it from happening?"

After the completion of the survey and educational component, a senior leader of the institution (e.g., hospital president, vice president, director) is partnered with a unit or clinical area. This leader attends rounds on the unit monthly to help staff members prioritize safety efforts, to ensure that they have the resources to implement improvements, and to hold them accountable for evaluating whether safety has improved. Staff members are asked to learn from one defect per month and to implement one tool per quarter designed to improve care delivery.[38,47]

CUSP was pilot-tested in ICUs and subsequently implemented throughout Johns Hopkins Hospital and in the Michigan Keystone project.[77] In the pilot, a patient-safety team that consisted of staff from the clinical area was responsible for oversight of the program. To be most effective, this team included the ICU director as the ICU physician safety champion, the nurse manager, another ICU physician and nurse, a risk manager or patient-safety officer, and a senior executive from the institution. The program worked best if the physician and nurse who led the program dedicated at least 20% of their time to improving quality and patient safety. The first unit was the beta site; subsequent teams from other clinical areas would learn from its successes and failures. The ultimate goal was to have every area in the hospital organizing and managing safety through CUSP.

CUSP has been associated with significant improvements in safety culture. The percentage of staff reporting a positive safety climate increased from 35% before CUSP to 60% after CUSP.[80,84] In addition, teams identified and mitigated several specific hazards through CUSP. As a result of asking staff members to speculate on how the next patient might be harmed, the ICU created a dedicated ICU transport team, implemented point-of-care pharmacists, implemented the daily goals sheet, clearly labeled epidural catheters to prevent inadvertent intravenous connection, and standardized the equipment in transvenous pacing kits.[85] Moreover, the use of CUSP decreased the length of stay and nurse turnover.

In summary, CUSP provides several benefits for improving safety culture and is a primer for staff compliance in implementing any safety or QI intervention or project. It provides enough structure to convert the often-vague goals of improving safety into a focused strategy; yet it is flexible enough to allow units to work on issues most important to them. CUSP provides a venue to introduce rigorous research methods, acts as a learning laboratory to identify and mitigate hazards, and has the potential to improve patient outcomes.

CHALLENGES AND BARRIERS TO QUALITY IMPROVEMENT PROJECTS

Multicentered and/or single-hospital projects can fail because of inadequate resources, lack of leadership support, vague expectations and objectives for team members, poor communication, complex study plans, inadequate management of data collection, and wasted efforts to "reinvent the wheel" rather than adopting practices proven to be effective. Successful collaboratives require a local culture (the set of values, attitudes, and beliefs of the group) that is ready for change and participants who have a shared view of safety and who understand the science of patient quality and safety (i.e., the technical components of how care is organized and delivered).

RELATED CONCEPTS: IMPROVEMENT SCIENCE AND IMPLEMENTATION SCIENCE

The focus of this chapter has been QI operations, or the efforts concerned with the measurement and timely improvement of quality in a given setting. QI operations is related to improvement science and implementation science, both of which aim to create generalizable knowledge that has the potential to improve care quality and patient outcomes across settings. These three fields are often confused because they share tools and are all interested in improving patient outcomes, but may use different terms to refer to similar concepts. To provide clarity about the similarities and differences between these fields, Koczwara and colleagues conceptualized a spectrum with QI operations at one end, implementation science at the other, and improvement science in the middle.[86] Understanding the roles for these fields may prove useful to those interested in anesthesia QI.

QI operations. As described at length in this chapter, QI is the systematic approach to improving problems in healthcare delivery that compromise care quality and outcomes. It is a timely, context-dependent team endeavor that has the potential to improve local care in the short, medium, and long term.

Improvement science. A common criticism of QI is that it is "unscientific" and more concerned with action than with understanding the mechanisms through which improvement occurs (or the reasons underlying the failure of improvement efforts). Improvement science draws from QI principles, aiming to "create practical learning that can make a timely difference to patient care."[87] But improvement science is also concerned with the creation of generalizable knowledge. Hence, close attention is paid to both internal and external validity in the design of improvement studies. Rigorously designed improvement science projects may sacrifice some of the timeliness of QI projects, but balance this downside with greater potential utility of the findings outside of a local setting.

Implementation science. Implementation science (known as knowledge translation in Canada) aims to narrow the evidence-to-practice gap evident when proven-effective interventions do not translate into improved care and outcomes.[88] Although the field is characterized as a new one, it draws from psychology, education, management, and related sciences. Two features clearly distinguish implementation science from QI and improvement science: the reliance on evidence-based practices and the use of explicit frameworks, theories, and models. Implementation science is a major focus for research funding agencies in the United States and Canada, as it is seen as one approach to maximize the return on grant dollars allocated to scientific discovery in health care. As with QI and improvement science, the adequate characterization of "real world" contexts is paramount. In contrast, there tends to be greater emphasis on generalizability in implementation science as compared to improvement science.

A key distinction between these three fields is their relationship to evidence. Implementation science relies on evidence-based interventions. However, there is not always evidence to guide our practice in situations with clearly suboptimal quality. In these situations, QI approaches can be useful, as rapid-cycle small-scale tests of change can minimize harm and mitigate risk at the same time as quality is addressed.

The Future: Research, Education, and Ethics

Much remains to be accomplished in QI. The opportunity to improve patient care is substantial, and the pressure to improve the quality of perioperative care continues to increase. Improving quality of care requires the ability to measure and improve performance. Research is needed to develop measures of quality that clinicians believe are valid and to learn how to ensure that all patients reliably receive recommended interventions. Innovation is needed to develop information systems that can be used by multiple disciplines. Anesthesiologists and professional societies may need to partner with experts in quality measurement to develop and implement quality measures. Future efforts should balance the feasibility and validity of quality

TABLE 5.6 Accreditation Council of Graduate Medical Education (ACGME) Six Core Competencies and Institute of Medicine (IOM) Six Aims for Improvement

	ACGME Core Competencies	IOM Aims for Improvement
1	Patient care	Safe
2	Medical knowledge	Timely
3	Interpersonal and communication skills	Effective
4	Professionalism	Efficient
5	System-based practice	Equitable
6	Practice-based learning and improvement	Patient-centered

measures and develop integrated approaches to improving quality, including strategies to develop care bundles, decrease complexity, and create independent redundancies.

Clinicians now need the skills necessary to improve quality. Health care will cross the quality chasm only when all view quality and safety as their primary job, rather than as an added activity, and healthcare organizations provide the infrastructure to monitor and improve performance. Frontline healthcare providers must understand the science of quality and safety and evaluate safety risks as hazardous systems, not incompetent people. Integral to this is the education of our trainees. CQI in anesthesia residency training programs has been touted for more than 25 years.[89] In the United States, residents in training are expected to master six core competencies, as mandated by the Accreditation Council of Graduate Medical Education,[90] competencies that are linked to the NAM's six Aims for Improvement (Table 5.6).[3] In an effort to link these two sets of goals and apply them to the clinical setting for training purposes, Bingham and colleagues[91] developed a framework called the Healthcare Matrix that can be used as both an educational tool and a research tool for improvement.

With the increasing amount of intellectual focus and healthcare resources being directed toward QI programs, the ethics of QI have come to light. QI projects have generally been exempt from the rigorous review of human-subjects research. However, a Hastings Center Report on the ethics of using QI methods to improve health quality and safety suggests that some QI projects may involve risk to patients and should undergo a formal review.[92] This report lists QI initiatives that may trigger the need for a review as those that have a randomized design, use novel treatments, involve researchers, have delayed feedback of monitoring, or are funded by external sources. The reporting of QI activities should be encouraged, as should requiring approval by an internal review board and following a standardized format for reporting the results. All of these practices support the premise that delivery of quality care is a science as well as an art.

Summary

Healthcare organizations need a systematic approach to three areas of patient safety: (1) TRIP, (2) identifying and mitigating hazards, and (3) improving culture and communication. The underlying principle for all of the approaches discussed in this chapter is that improvement of the quality of care dictates that practitioners must be able to measure their performance. Healthcare practitioners traditionally have had limited ability to obtain feedback regarding performance in their daily work, in part because of the absence of information systems and a lack of agreement on how to measure quality of care.[44] As a result, many in health care do not have access to performance data and consequently do not know what results they achieve (or fail to achieve). As consumers, payors, regulators, and accreditors increasingly require evidence regarding quality of care, the demand for quality measures will grow. To meet these demands, anesthesiologists must be prepared to use valid measures to evaluate the quality of care that they provide and to implement evidence-based best practices in the perioperative care of patients.

Acknowledgments

The editors and the publisher would like to acknowledge Dr. Elizabeth Martinez (b. 1966–d. 2013) for her contributions to previous editions of this chapter. Her work served as the foundation for the current chapter.

This chapter greatly benefited from the thoughtful editing of Claire Levine.

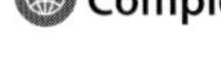 **Complete references available online at expertconsult.com.**

References

1. Chandrupatla TR. *Quality and Reliability in Engineering: Excerpt*. New York: Cambridge University Press; 2009.
2. Lohr KN, Schroeder SA. *N Engl J Med.* 1990;322(10):707.
3. Institute of Medicine. *Crossing the Quality Chasm: A New Health System for the 21st Century*. Washington, DC: The National Academies Press; 2001.
4. Institute of Medicine. *To Err Is Human: Building a Safer Health System*. Washington, DC: The National Academies Press; 2000.
5. Bodenheimer T, Sinsky C. *Ann Fam Med.* 2014;12(6):573.
5a. Kohn L, et al. *To err is Human: Building a Safer Health System*. Washington, DC: The National Academies Press; 2000.
6. Gerteis M. *Picker/Commonwealth Program for Patient-Centered Care: Through the Patient's Eyes: Understanding and Promoting Patient-Centered Care*. 4th ed. San Francisco: Jossey-Bass; 1993.
7. Langley GJ, et al. *The Improvement Guide: A Practical Approach to Enhancing Organizational Performance*. Wiley; 2009.
8. Kotter JP, Cohen DS. *The Heart of Change: Real-life Stories of how People Change Their Organizations*. Harvard Business School Press; 2002.
9. James B. *Quality Management for Health Care Delivery*. Chicago: The Health Research and Educational Trust of the American Hospital Association; 1989.
10. Crosby PB. *Quality is Free: The Art of Making Quality Certain*. McGraw-Hill; 1979.
11. Shewhart WA, Deming WE. *Statistical Method from the Viewpoint of Quality Control*. New York: Dover; 1986.
12. Moen R, Clifford C. *Circling back: Clearing up Myths About the Deming Cycle and Seeing how it Keeps Evolving*. Quality Progress; 2010.
13. Deming WE. *Out of the Crisis*. 1st MIT Press ed. Cambridge, Mass: MIT Press; 2000.
14. Institute for Healthcare Improvement. *Going Lean in Health care*. Boston: IHI Innovation Series white paper; 2005. www.IHI.org
15. Pyzdek T, Keller PA. *The six Sigma Handbook : A Complete Guide for Green Belts, Black Belts, and Managers at all Levels*. 3rd ed. New York: McGraw-Hill; 2010.
16. Chassin MR. *Milbank Q.* 1998;76:565.
17. Porter ME, Teisberg EO. *Redefining Health Care: Creating Value-Based Competition on Results*. Boston, MA: Harvard Business School Press; 2006.
18. Porter ME. *N Engl J Med.* 2010;363(26):2477.
19. Howell J, Ayanian J. *J Health Serv Res Policy*. 2016;21(4):279.
20. Donabedian A. *The Milbank Memorial Fund quarterly*. 1966;44(3): suppl:166.
21. Randolph G, et al. *Pediatr Clin North Am.* 2009;56:779.
22. Rubin HR, et al. *Int J Qual Health Care.* 2001;13:469.
23. Nelson EC, et al. *Jt Comm J Qual Saf.* 2003;29:5.
24. Nelson EC, et al. *Front Health Serv Manage.* 1998;15:3.
25. Pronovost PJ, et al. *Curr Opin Crit Care.* 2001;7:297.
26. Lenfant C. *N Engl J Med.* 2003;349:868.
27. Mermel LA, et al. *Clin Inf Dis.* 2009;49(1):1.
28. Bardach NS, Cabana MD. *Curr Opin Pediatr.* 2009;21:777.
29. Centers for Medicare & Medicaid Services. *Fed Regist.* 2016;81(214): 77008.
30. Roland M, Guthrie B. *BMJ.* 2016;354.
31. Shewhart WA. *Economic Control of Quality of Manufactured Product*. American Society for Quality Control; 1931.
32. Varughese AM, et al. *Paediatr Anaesth.* 2010;20:684.
33. Carey RG, Lloyd RC. *Measuring Quality Improvement in Healthcare: a Guide to Statistical Process Control Applications*. New York: Quality Resources; 1995.
34. Kaplan RS, Norton DP. *The Balanced Scorecard: Translating Strategy into Action*. Boston, Mass: Harvard Business School Press; 1996.
35. Christie CA, Inkelas M, Lemire S. *Improvement Science in Evaluation: Methods and Uses: New Directions for Evaluation*. Wiley; 2017. Number 153.
36. Centofanti JE, et al. *Crit Care Med.* 2014;42(8):1797.
37. Cavalcanti AB, et al. *JAMA.* 2016;315(14):1480.
38. Pronovost P, et al. *J Crit Care.* 2003;18:71.
39. Justice LB, et al. *Pediatr Crit Care Med.* 2016;17(7):677.
40. Makary MA, et al. *Jt Comm J Qual Patient Saf.* 2006;32:357.
41. March MG, Crowley JJ. *Anesthesiology.* 1991;75:724.
42. Berenholtz SM, et al. *Crit Care Med.* 2004;32:2014.
43. Haynes AB, et al. *N Engl J Med.* 2009;360:491.
44. Mitchell B, et al. *BMJ Qual Saf.* 2017;26(10):837.
45. Hicks CW, et al. *JAMA Surg.* 2014;149(8):863.
46. Makary MA, et al. *Jt Comm J Qual Patient Saf.* 2006;32(7):407.
47. Thompson D, et al. *Jt Comm J Qual Patient Saf.* 2005;31(8):476.
48. Baker DP, et al. *Medical Teamwork and Patient Safety: The Evidence-Based Relation*. Rockville, MD 2003.
49. Alonso A, et al. *Hum Res Manage Rev.* 2006;16(3):396.
50. Clancy CM. *Aorn J.* 2007;86(1):18.
51. Weld LR, et al. *Am J Med Qual.* 2016;31(5):408.
52. McGlynn EA, Asch SM. *Am J Prev Med.* 1998;14:14.
53. Miller T, Leatherman S. *Health Affairs (Project Hope)*. 1999;18:233.
54. Leape LL. *N Engl J Med.* 2002;347:1633.
55. Vincent C. *N Engl J Med.* 2003;348:1051.
56. White C. *Am J Med Qual.* 2017;32(1_suppl):3S.
57. Dutton RP. *ASA Monitor.* 2011;75(10). 30.
58. Tjia I, et al. *Anesth Analg.* 2014;119(1):122.
59. Cassidy CJ, et al. *Anaesthesia.* 2011;66:879.
60. Webb RK, et al. *Anaesth Intensive Care.* 1993;21:520.
61. Sackett DL, et al. *BMJ.* 1996;312:71.
62. Shojania KG, et al. *Evid Rep Technol Assess (Summ) i.* 2001;1.
63. Rupp SM, et al. *Anesthesiology.* 2012;116:539.
64. Gross JB, et al. *Anesthesiology.* 2006;104:1081; quiz, p 117.
65. Apfelbaum JL, et al. *Anesthesiology.* 2011;114(3):495.
66. Brook AD, et al. *Crit Care Med.* 1999;27:2609.
67. Marelich GP, et al. *Chest.* 2000;118:459.
68. Freundlich RE, Kheterpal S. *Best Pract Res Clin Anaesthesiol.* 2011; 25:489.
69. Fuchshuber PR, et al. *Perm J.* 2012;16:39.
70. Dutton RP. *Anesth Analg.* 2015;120(3):507.
71. Dutton RP, Dukatz A. *Anesthesiol Clin.* 2011;29(3):439.
72. Kheterpal S. *Anesthesiol Clin.* 2011;29(3):377.
73. Ovretveit J, et al. *Qual Saf Health Care.* 2002;11:345.
74. Mittman BS. *Ann Intern Med.* 2004;140:897.
75. Institute for Healthcare Improvement. Boston: IHI Innovation Series white paper; 2003.
76. Sawyer M, et al. *Crit Care Med.* 2010;38:S292.
77. Pronovost P, et al. *N Engl J Med.* 2006;355:2725.
78. Pronovost PJ, et al. *Health Serv Res.* 2006;41:1599.
79. Pronovost P, Goeschel C. *Healthc Exec.* 2005;20:14.
80. Pronovost PJ, et al. *Jt Comm J Qual Patient Saf.* 2006;32:119.
81. Pitts SI, et al. *Jt Comm J Qual Patient Saf.* 2017;43(11):591.

82. Moloo H, et al. *Can J Surg*. 2016;59(6):422.
83. Pottenger BC, et al. *Qual Manag Health Care*. 2016;25(4):197.
84. Pronovost P, et al. *J Pat Safety*. 2005;1:33.
85. Pronovost PJ, et al. *Jt Comm J Qual Patient Saf*. 2006;32:102.
86. Koczwara B, et al. *J Oncol Pract*. 2018;14(6):335.
87. Marshall M, et al. *Lancet*. 2013;381(9864):419.
88. Lane-Fall MB, et al. *Anesthesiol Clin*. 2018;36(1):1.
89. Dubin SA, et al. *Int Anesthesiol Clin*. 1992;30:29.
90. Accreditation Council for Graduate Medical Education. ACGME Common Program Requirements. 7/29/2013 2016.
91. Bingham JW, et al. *Jt Comm J Qual Patient Saf*. 2005;31:98.
92. Baily MA, et al. *Hastings Cent Rep*. 2006;36:S1.
93. Boat AC, Spaeth JP. *Paediatr Anaesth*. 2013;23(7):647.

6 Avoiding Patient Harm in Anesthesia: Human Performance and Patient Safety

STEPHANIE MARIA OBERFRANK, MARCUS RALL, PETER DIECKMANN, MICHAELA KOLBE, and DAVID M. GABA

KEY POINTS

- Excellent clinical performance is not achieved by the use of sound medical knowledge alone, as clinicians have to face multifaceted challenges not just medical issues. There is an increased awareness that human factors—both on the individual and the team level—as well as organizational factors in the health care system play major roles in providing excellent medical care. Therefore, for anesthesia professionals (1) the study of human performance is fundamental, (2) the knowledge and successful application of efficient safety strategies are highly relevant, and (3) understanding of the pertinent organizational matters is very important.
- The health care system in general, individual clinical institutions, and work units in particular must provide the appropriate organizational characteristics to facilitate safe patient care including: promoting a culture of safety, effective incident reporting and analysis systems, continuous training for professionals, and optimized structures and processes.
- Organizations that provide such characteristics are referred to as high-reliability organizations (HRO). HRO theory describes the key features of systems that conduct complex and hazardous work, but do so with extremely low failure rates and complications. The credo of HROs is not to erase all errors but rather to identify human error mechanisms and make systems more impervious to errors and their sequelae (resilience).
- Several mechanisms of optimal versus poor performance have been demonstrated through human performance research. A particular technique of human performance research called task analysis has been useful in understanding the work of anesthesia professionals. Observing them during routine operations or in the handling of (simulated) adverse events has improved our knowledge on human performance. The findings include the impact of critical and continuous situation awareness and decision making (i.e., core cognitive process model), effective teamwork, leadership, and communication, as well as task management and the use of cognitive aids (e.g., checklists or emergency manuals).
- Organizations and individuals need to fully recognize that the performance of individual anesthesia professionals can—as for all human beings—be adversely influenced by performance-shaping factors, including noise, illness, aging, boredom, distraction, sleep deprivation, and fatigue, as well as by social dynamics within and between crews and teams.
- It is necessary to have a clear understanding of known human performance pitfalls such as fixation errors, ineffective team communication, misunderstandings, medication errors, unclear task management, and erroneous assumptions. While anesthesia professionals' knowledge and skill are key strengths needed for safe patient care, addressing the limitations will help them to actively avoid or mitigate the risk of adverse events.
- One approach to understanding and intervening in human performance issues for anesthesia care, especially focused on challenging situations, is that of crisis resource management (CRM). CRM (as in "cockpit [then crew] resource management") was developed in aviation first but then adapted to health care, initially for anesthesia care, in the early 1990s. There are many formulations of CRM but they typically highlight situation awareness, dynamic decision making, task management, communication, and teamwork. The introduction of CRM in anesthesiology and its spread into many other health care disciplines and domains have typically been associated with the use of realistic simulation-based training of anesthesia professionals in single-discipline or combined team training. It also has helped focus attention on systems' issues that relate to key aspects of human performance highlighted in CRM-oriented training.

- "First do no harm": Every avoidable harm or death to a patient is one tragic event too many. Anesthesia professionals must strive to avoid all harm that they may potentially impose, knowingly or not, on patients. Future progress on patient safety and human performance in anesthesia will require interdisciplinary research and training, improvements in systems thinking and systems safety, organizational learning, and the involvement of all levels of the health care industry.

What this Chapter is About: An Overview

This chapter provides the reader with an overview of key human performance and safety issues concerning anesthesiology and demonstrates the relevance of those topics to the clinical performance of anesthesia professionals. Applying the knowledge of this chapter to patient care can help to avoid unnecessary harm to patients and also prevent psychological harm to the anesthesia professional (as the "second victim"). Hence, this chapter is not only about patient safety, but also about the anesthesia professional's safety and well-being as care provider. The authors provide a set of practical safety concepts and strategies to guide the reader in improving or refreshing case management-related skills and to sensitize the reader to safety-related core issues and competencies in anesthesia.

Because most of the work on human performance has focused on anesthesiology in the operating room (OR), this chapter deals primarily with aspects of performance and safety in that setting. Nevertheless, most of the same principles and issues are relevant to other perioperative settings, to critical care, and to a lesser degree, in pain medicine. They will also largely apply to emergency medicine and other health care domains sharing similar cognitive profiles. For readers with a special interest in intensive care, a selection of references is given as a starting point.[1-8]

The chapter contains references ranging from several decades old to quite recent. The authors have tried to balance retention of classic references, where the intellectual content has only changed slightly over the years, with the introduction of current literature that reflects changes in thinking or evidence, or newer syntheses of knowledge and experience.

In this chapter, the authors use "anesthesia professional" to refer to any anesthesia clinician taking care of a patient, whether a physician, certified registered nurse anesthetist (CRNA), or anesthesia assistant (or to similar positions in other countries).

READERS WILL LEARN

- ... safety relevant aspects of a dynamic and complex work environment and the resulting consequences for clinicians. Several sections highlight the nature of anesthesia as a highly complex and dynamic working environment and the difficulties that arise for human performance and patient safety.
- ... characteristics and risks of different tasks performed by anesthesia professionals and countermeasures to mitigate their potential risks.
- ... the issues of human performance, human limitations, and various relevant safety strategies that address them for both individuals and teams.
- ... aspects of system safety concerning high-reliability organizations (HROs).

WHAT THIS CHAPTER IS NOT ABOUT

The literature related to human performance and patient safety is vast. Standard reference works are available[9-14] as well as several Internet sources (Appendix 6.1). This chapter samples only a portion of this literature as it most closely relates to the work of anesthesia professionals. This chapter does not address in detail human-machine interactions and the physical design of the work environment. These aspects of human factors, or ergonomics, in anesthesiology are important in their own right. The reader is referred to several publications that review these issues in detail.[15-20] Also not part of this chapter are most issues of infection control and medication safety, even as they pertain to the perioperative arena. Here, too, the reader is referred to several publications that review these issues in detail[21-36] and also to other chapters in this book.

Human Performance and Patient Safety in Anesthesia: Why is this Important?

Even though provision of anesthesia has become a "safe" discipline over the last decades through many scientific and technical improvements, anesthesia per se is an intrinsically hazardous undertaking. Many aspects of anesthetic drugs and care can affect vital human functions and are potentially lethal while they are not therapeutic in themselves. Evolution did not intend for human beings to be rendered temporarily insensitive to pain, unconscious, amnestic, and in many cases paralyzed. The surgical procedure itself may cause or trigger a variety of physiologic derangements and some patients needing anesthesia are already severely ill. Thus, in anesthesiology a stable situation can turn into a life-threatening situation in seconds, minutes, or hours, whereas in many arenas of health care changes happen in days, months, or years.

Medical and technical skills alone are not sufficient for excellent medical care. Historically, an adequately trained anesthesia professional was automatically assumed to always perform appropriately. Deviations from optimal outcomes were understood to result from imperfections in the art and science of anesthesiology. This perception led to heavy emphasis on the scientific and technical aspects of anesthesia training and care. Adverse outcomes were mostly ascribed to unavoidable side effects of a medication, underlying patient disease, negligence, or incompetence on the part of the anesthesia professional.

Interestingly, research shows that the etiology of most adverse events is generally not related to intrinsic problems associated with equipment, drugs, or diseases, but rather that 80% of the avoidable events are caused by so-called human factors (HF)—similar to the statistics emanating from the aviation industry. For instance, a review of critical anesthesia incidents by Cooper and associates revealed that human factors were contributory in 82% of the 359 incidents reported.[37] These incidents ranged from simple equipment malfunction in some cases, to death in others, indicating the seriousness and importance of the problems. Data from an earlier evaluation of 2000 incident reports support these findings with 83% of incidents occurring due to human error.[38] The term HF describes the physical and psychological behavior of humans in relation to specific environments, jobs, organizational patterns, machines, products, and individual challenges.

The performance of human beings is incredibly flexible, powerful, and robust in some aspects but limited and vulnerable in others. Today we have a more complete understanding of the human performance of anesthesia professionals than existed decades ago. For example, we know that the successful conduct of an anesthetic depends on having the requisite technical skills and relevant pathophysiologic knowledge. But it has also become clear that the effective real-time implementation of such expertise to a large extent depends on several nonmedical and nontechnical elements of performance. Among HF issues are those that are termed human performance-shaping factors like fatigue, boredom, and distraction.

Human factor-related safety strategies for the individual and the team are indispensable. Lapses, mistakes, and errors have the potential to harm a patient ("first victim"), but can also harm professionals themselves ("second victim"). Professionals suffer as second victims largely from the perceived guilt about an error that led to actual harm.[39] The clinical institution involved may also suffer financially or in reputation from such events, although often the occurrence of these events are not known to the public, and unlike in other industries (e.g., aviation, chemical manufacturing) there is no direct harm to the physical means of production. Nonetheless, the best way to avoid harm to the professional or the organization is to prevent adverse events or mitigate harm to patients.

Organizational safety attitudes are essential to support high individual human performance. More attention should be devoted to training anesthesia professionals in human performance issues so that they can develop and apply core competencies for achieving human performance on a daily basis. Moreover, departmental and organizational leadership must understand the enormous impact their attitudes and behavior have in shaping human performance, safety culture, outcomes, and ultimately (in all likelihood), the level of patient safety.

Even in anesthesiology, still a long way to go. Historically, anesthesiology was the first medical specialty to specifically focus on the promotion of patient safety. As a consequence, anesthesiology is widely recognized as the pioneering leader in patient safety efforts. Compared to other medical disciplines, the track record of anesthesiology is indeed a model of patient safety for the rest of health care.[40] However, safety science teaches us that patient safety and quality improvement are never-ending processes and complacency is dangerous. In addition, the increasing "production pressure" in anesthesia practice from expanding clinical demands in the face of constant or diminishing resources may threaten previously won gains. Any patient harmed by an anesthetic is one patient too many. This approach is aligned with the zero vision statement of the U.S. Anesthesia Patient Safety Foundation (APSF): *"That no one shall be harmed by anesthesia care."* In this regard Cooper and Gaba wrote that anesthesia professionals "... should remain aware of the hazards they still face, take pride in having been the leaders in patient safety efforts, and stay motivated to continue the pursuit of 'no harm from anesthesia' with the passion it still demands" (p. 1336).[40]

Saving hearts, brains, and lives. Several recently published studies demonstrate the benefits of implementing various patient safety strategies.[5,41-44] The authors have experienced the benefit of a more safety- and human performance-focused approach in their own work, as have their colleagues who also work in this field or in other fields that are endeavoring to create a safer health care system. Although it may be challenging to produce undisputable evidence that patient outcomes are improved by addressing the issues and implementing the strategies presented in this chapter, there is strong reason and ongoing research to support the belief that hearts, brains, and lives have indeed been saved by applying them. That belief is reward enough for the efforts of the authors as they share with the reader what is known about human performance and patient safety.

Nature of the Anesthesia Professional's Operational Domain: A Dynamic and Complex Environment

The practice of anesthesiology can be characterized as a dynamic and complex environment that presents the anesthesia professional with challenges that may jeopardize human performance and patient safety.

To better understand these patient safety challenges that are related to human performance, the authors first describe the key characteristics of anesthesia work. In what follows they address (1) critical factors that categorize anesthesiology as a complex and dynamic working environment; (2) the safety challenge of inherent asymmetry between safety and production, and the effects of production pressure; and (3) the safety challenge of complexity and tight coupling in the anesthesia domain.

ANESTHESIOLOGY BY ITS NATURE INVOLVES CRISES

What makes anesthesiology and a few other medical domains (such as intensive care medicine, emergency medicine, obstetrics, neonatology, and surgery, to name a few) different from most other medical fields? The answer is that the clinical environment of anesthesiology is both complex and dynamic which, when combined with the inherent risks of surgery and anesthesia, makes crisis situations frequent and challenging to deal with. These moments of terror necessitate that anesthesia professionals be expert in crisis management.

CRITERIA DEFINING A COMPLEX AND DYNAMIC WORLD

Based on the work of Orasanu and colleagues,[45] the following text describes some of the characteristics of anesthesia that make it a complex and dynamic world.

1. **Ill-structured problems.** In contrast to well-structured problems, the nature and the goal of ill-structured problems are often vague or unclear, and many problem elements remain unknown or ambiguous. In anesthesiology, the patient's physiologic behavior is not an independent random variable but is causally linked to previous decisions and actions. There often is not just a single problem with a single decision to be made, but rather a variety of interrelated problems. Interdependent decisions must be made and actions taken by the anesthesia professional, surgeon, and other perioperative personnel.
2. **Uncertain system.** The patient is the main "system" of immediate interest to the anesthesia professional, just as the aircraft is of immediate interest to the pilot.[46] Patients are intrinsically very complex, and they contain many components with underlying functions that are imperfectly understood. The medical world knows very little about the underlying causes of specific physiologic events, although the general principles involved can be described. Unlike industrial or aviation systems, patients are not designed, built, or tested by humans, nor do they come with an operator's manual. The true state of the patient cannot usually be measured directly. It must be inferred from ambiguous patterns of clinical observations and data from electronic monitors. These data are imperfect because, unlike industrial systems that are designed and built with sensors in key areas to measure the most important variables, patients are typically instrumented to measure the variables that are easiest to monitor, predominantly with the use of noninvasive methods. Most physiologic functions are observed indirectly through weak signals available at the body surface that are prone to various types of electrical and mechanical interference. Invasive measurements are also vulnerable to artifacts and uncertainties of interpretation. Even if the anesthesia professional knew the exact state of the patient, the patient's response to interventions would be unpredictable, as normal patients show genetic or acquired differences in reflex sensitivity, pharmacokinetics, or pharmacodynamics that can yield a wide range of responses to a given dose of a drug or to a routine action (e.g., laryngoscopy). In diseased or traumatized patients, or in the presence of acute abnormalities, these responses may be markedly abnormal, and patients may overreact or underreact to otherwise appropriate actions. Thus, the patient as a system has substantially greater uncertainty than do engineered systems.
3. **Dynamic environment.** Dynamism stems from the frequency of routine and anomalous changes or events, the rapidity with which they evolve, and the unpredictability of the patient's physiology and response to interventions. An anesthetized patient is in a constant state of change during surgery, with many events outside the anesthesia professional's control, such as when the surgeon inadvertently transects a major vessel or when a patient with a previously unknown allergy suffers anaphylaxis. Although preventive measures can reduce the likelihood of some events, other events cannot be totally avoided because they are inevitable side effects of medically necessary procedures (e.g., surgical blood loss). Unpredictable and dynamic occurrences compete with the preplanned aspects of the case and together they drive the anesthesia professional's actions.
4. **Time stress.** Because the OR is a scarce resource, an incessant overall time pressure exists to use the OR efficiently (see section "Production Pressure"). Surgeons or OR managers pressing to start a case may affect the anesthesia professional's decisions and actions that could jeopardize safety standards. Over the long run this can cause a systematic "normalization of deviance" [47-50] (see section "Normalization of Deviance and Flirting with the Margin"), meaning the emergence of new, less stringent standard behaviors that are seen as normal judgments that previously would have been viewed as aberrant. An even more intense time stress occurs within a case when dynamic situations evolve rapidly and become time critical.
5. **Shifting, ill-defined, or competing goals.** Multiple goals of case management may compete with each other. (e.g., hemodynamic stability vs. good operating conditions for the surgeon vs. rapid emergence from anesthesia). The OR manager's administrative goals (high throughput, low cost) may sometimes compete with those of the anesthesia professional. All these goals shift as the patient's situation changes dynamically throughout a procedure and the flow of cases changes throughout the work day. For example, decisions on surgical operation planning are heavily influenced and manipulated by micropolitics and power, as investigated by Engelmann and colleagues.[51] Nurok and colleagues[52] portray this aspect in their survey: *"Are surgeons and anesthesiologists lying to each other or gaming the system?"*
6. **Short action feedback loops.** The time constants of actions and their effects are very short, on the order of seconds to minutes. Complete intermixing of decision making and action occurs; these functions are not performed in separate cycles. Most decisions and actions are implemented incrementally, constantly evaluating the relative success or failure of actions-to-date to determine how best to proceed. Anesthesia professionals often do not jump to conclusions or implement a whole set of actions all at once but try one or two approaches and see how they work, constantly reassessing rather than jumping ahead too far at once.
7. **High stakes.** The decisions and actions taken by anesthesia professionals can determine the outcome for the patient. The stakes are high because even for elective surgery in healthy patients, the risk of catastrophe is ever-present. Death, brain damage, or other permanent injury may be the end result of many pathways that can begin with seemingly innocuous triggering events. Each intervention, even if appropriate, is associated with side effects, some of which are themselves serious. Some risks cannot be anticipated or avoided. Unlike an event such as a commercial flight, which can be delayed or aborted if a problem occurs or if the weather is bad, these options are not always possible in health care. Sometimes immediate surgery (and anesthesia) may be necessary to treat

a medical problem that is itself life threatening. Balancing the risks of anesthesia and surgery against the risk of the patient's underlying diseases can be extremely difficult.

8. **Multiple players.** Perioperative domains involve multiple players from different professional backgrounds. Each profession has its own characteristics. On the one hand, surgeons, anesthesia professionals and OR nurses all want safety and a good outcome for the patient. On the other hand, each discipline and profession has other inherent goals. For example, surgeons may usually seem eager to perform the surgery and may seem to be more willing to take risks and to view the probability of a good outcome with optimism. In contrast, anesthesiologists may tend to be rather risk averse. Also, for a variety of reasons, it seems that surgeons tend to put production pressure on anesthesia professionals and nurses more than the other way around. The idiosyncrasies of interaction among various individual OR team members sometimes dominate the work environment. The OR sometimes offers a unique team structure of action teams, where the members may vary greatly from one day to the next (see later section "Teamwork"). Furthermore, there is a certain individual variation in the performance of each member; on any given day even usually "good" people may not be at their best.
9. **Organizational goals and norms.** The anesthesia professional works within the formal and informal norms of the OR suite, the anesthesia department, the institution, and the professional culture as a whole. Sometimes anesthesia professionals feel pressured to make decisions that they do not believe are best for the patient in order to comply with these norms. Therefore, it is important to face human performance and patient safety pitfalls not only on the individual and team level, but also on a larger departmental and organizational level (see later section "Patient Safety on the Organizational Level: Issues and Strategies").

Although some of these aforementioned characteristics apply to other domains of medicine, anesthesiology is unique in that many of the characteristics are prominent. In particular, what sets anesthesia apart from clinic-based or ward-based medicine is the intensity of the dynamics, time pressure, uncertainty, and extreme variation within the complexity, with danger lurking just below the surface, as well as the unique team constellation of so-called action teams (see section "Human Factors on the Team Level").

Other factors influencing complexity in anesthesia: device variety and tight coupling. The complexity in anesthesia also stems from the variety of devices in use and their interconnections. The challenge is that the equipment often consists of a proliferation of independent devices with multiple, nonstandardized interconnections. Devices seem often to be designed by engineers in isolation. As a consequence, interactions between devices, or among the equipment, the patient, and the human operator, may not be adequately addressed in the design phase.

Furthermore, complexity in anesthesia derives from complex interactions which are highly interdependent (tightly coupled). Coupling describes the notion of relations between parts of a system, which either can be tightly or loosely coupled.[46] Because many body systems affect each other, the patient is a major site of tight coupling. The anesthetic state tends to erode the protective and compensatory physiologic buffers among some of these interconnected systems, thereby forcing the patient's system to become even more connected and strengthening the coupling between them and between the patient and external technologic supports (e.g., ventilator or infusions of hemodynamically active drugs).

PRODUCTION PRESSURE RESULTING IN ASYMMETRY BETWEEN SAFETY AND PRODUCTION

The current trend of increasing production pressure in perioperative care can further strain the working conditions in this demanding work environment.[53] Social and organizational environments may act as a source of production pressure on anesthesia professionals.

Safety attitudes compete against economic thinking. Production pressure encompasses the economic and social pressures placed on workers to consider production, not safety, their primary priority.[54] In anesthesiology, this typically means starting cases early, keeping the OR schedule moving speedily, with few cancellations and minimum time between cases. In principle, safety and efficiency can go hand in hand. Many aspects of high reliability, such as standard operating procedures, preprocedure briefings, and flattening the hierarchy, may smooth operation of the system, as well as make it safer. However, the pressure for throughput as well as the wish to please the surgeon or the OR manager, or the attempt to make up time by skipping essential procedures can erode safety and lead to a normalization of deviance (the new normal, see sections "Normalization of Deviance" and & "Flirting with the Margin").[55] For example, when anesthesia professionals succumb to production pressures, they may skip appropriate preoperative evaluation and planning, or they may not perform adequate pre-use checkout of equipment. Even when preoperative evaluation does take place, overt or covert pressure from surgeons (or others) can cause anesthesia professionals to proceed with elective cases despite the existence of serious or uncontrolled medical problems.

Production pressure as a trigger to depart inappropriately from standard operating procedures and standards. Production pressure can cause anesthesia professionals to choose techniques that they would otherwise believe to be inadvisable. Gaba and associates reported on a survey of a large random sample of California anesthesiologists concerning their experience with production pressure.[56] A nontrivial minority of respondents (20% to 40%) reported meaningful levels of pressure to conform to such pressures, to make decisions against their judgment of optimal safety, and to risk economic consequences if they act as they see appropriate. Generally, the pressures were already internalized after prior unpleasant experiences rather than stemming from blatant external attacks. Although there are anecdotal reports of increasing production pressure, as well as organizational practices that increase it (e.g., scheduling elective cases to start late at night or after midnight without separate shifts of anesthesia professionals), there has been no comparable repeated survey of such pressures in recent years. Fully investigating these aspects of the work environment is difficult because such relationships are driven by economic considerations, as well as by the complex organizational and interpersonal networks linking the different medical cultures. Changing the environment will be equally challenging and calls for organizational action (see section "Patient Safety Strategies on the Individual and Team Level: Crisis Resource Management [CRM] and Other Training Curricula").[57]

The efficiency-thoroughness trade-off (ETTO). Given the limited resources in the health care system, professionals constantly need to prioritize and make trade-offs, the most common being the efficiency-thoroughness trade-off (ETTO) described in detail by Eric Hollnagel in his book *The ETTO Principle: Efficiency-Thoroughness Trade-Off: Why Things that Go Right Sometimes Go Wrong.*[58] One example of a tradeoff is reducing the amount of information sought about individual preoperative patients in order to more efficiently process large numbers of them. Since it rarely is possible to be both effective and thorough at the same time, the balance of the trade-off can get into an unnoticed disequilibrium threatening human performance and patient safety.

Inherent imbalance between signals of safety and signals of production. One of the challenges in achieving optimal safety is the asymmetry of the signals of safety and the signals of production[59]: (1) Investments for production are easy to plan for and measure. Feedback about production is easy to obtain (revenue, earnings, expenses) and to interpret (success, no success). Success is indicated positively (more production, more earnings) and reinforcing. The relationship between the application of resources (money, effort, time) and production goals is relatively certain. (2) On the contrary, investments for safety are more difficult to plan for and the costs and benefits can only be measured indirectly and without continuity, making them difficult to interpret or even deceptive. Feedback about safety is inherently weak and ambiguous. Success is less reinforcing because if indicated negatively (fewer accidents or incidents)—how can one measure the accidents that could have occurred but did not? The relationship between the application of resources (money, effort, time) and safety goals is equally uncertain. There have been many occasions when only after a catastrophe takes place are the signals concerning a safety hazard understood, and often there is evidence that some personnel did recognize the hazards but either did not sufficiently press the issue or else they were systematically ignored or repressed.

Nature of the Anesthesia Professional's Work: Task Variation and Workload Management

As previously described, the operational domain of anesthesia can be considered as a complex and dynamic world, managing different challenges with uncertain systems, competing goals, time pressure, and multiple players with special team constellations. All of these can affect human performance and patient safety. There also exist the challenges of the different specific tasks of conducting an anesthetic, whether manual (i.e., insertion of cannula, intubation), behavioral (i.e., leadership behaviors, communication patterns), or cognitive (i.e., attention, preparedness, dynamic decision making). Safe and efficient performance requires both medical and non-medical skills.[11,60]

Human failure or equipment failure can have disastrous consequences. Errors in cognitive tasks as well as cognitive biases are common in anesthesiology and pose a threat to patient safety.[61,62] In the following section the authors provide insights into the nature of the anesthesiaology professional's many tasks and their various vulnerabilities. This is important not only for individual and team improvements but also for improvements concerning clinical education, training, organizational structures, and equipment design. The focus of the upcoming section is on manual and cognitive tasks. The behavioral non-medical are discussed later (see section "Patient Safety on the Individal and Team Level").

This section briefly highlights the different phases of an anesthetic regimen and summarizes findings of task analysis and task performance studies, provides facts about the anesthesia machine checkout protocol as a safety relevant task, and introduces nonobservable cognitive tasks of administering anesthesia, in particular dynamic decision making. In addition, this section provides an introduction to workload measurement methodologies, gives study results concerning the performance of anesthesia professionals summarizes the benefits and obstacles of human performance measures, and highlights results from task analysis studies.

PROCEDURAL TASKS OF ANESTHESIA PROFESSIONALS AND RELATED VULNERABILITIES

Multiple task analysis studies have investigated what actions and thought processes an anesthesiologist is required to perform to achieve good anesthetic care. Since the 1970s, numerous studies have been done either by direct observation during real cases[63-67] or by indirect observation during cases captured on videotape.[64,68-74] In addition, an increasing number of studies have been performed in realistic simulation environments.[8,64,75-79] Of note, many of the studies cited are pioneering ones that remain valid today.

The early studies of the work of anesthesiologists drew attention to the wide spectrum of tasks in the trajectory of perioperative care. They highlighted that many tasks must be done in close parallel with others (approximating multitasking, see section Task Management), showing not only the different tasks and their substeps that can be prone to error, but also different phases of task intensity during an anesthetic. Subsequent task analysis studies focused on the workload and the performance of the anesthesiologist, at a later time expanding to performance measures based on teamwork,[80-82] communication,[83] and leadership.[82,84,85] More recently, task analysis studies have been performed with respect to ergonomic equipment design questions. Certain very complex issues concerning human-machine interactions and the ways in which technology affects behavior in complex patient-care environments are beyond the scope of this chapter; however a number of publications address these issues.[16,86,87]

The different phases for an anesthetic regimen are commonly classified into (1) preoperative planning, (2) induction, (3) maintenance of, and (4) emergence from anesthesia.[63] Every phase is characterized by manual and cognitive tasks, each of which consists of further subordinated steps and each of which presents with a variable density of tasks and human error pitfalls. For a comprehensive review, the reader is directed to the publication of Phipps and colleagues[63] for detailed information.

Preoperative Planning

The anesthesia professional needs to be prepared for active intervention during the whole anesthetic regimen. Part of this preparedness involves obtaining the necessary equipment and supplies, preparing medications, and conducting pre-use checkouts of life-support equipment and the anesthesia machine before induction (See section "Pre-use Checkout of Equipment/Anesthesia Machine Checkout").

However, with 44 task steps as identified in the task analysis study by Phipps and associates, the equipment check is a lengthy and detailed process, and it is possible that steps may be omitted, either intentionally or unintentionally.

Induction

Task analysis studies demonstrated increased anesthesiologist workload during induction, emergence, and emergency surgery.[63,67,88-94] Phipps and associates identified 73 task steps between the preparation of drugs and transferring the anesthetized patient to the operating room (induction phase), including cognitive and communicative tasks, machine checkouts, as well as a considerable number of manual task steps, such as the insertion of the cannula and airway devices. Pape and Dingman examined the number of unrelated distractions during the induction process (i.e., unrelated questions of other personnel, OR doors opening and closing, noise, answering incoming telephone calls, unrelated communication), discovering an average of 7.5 total interruptions per 9 minutes.[95] They argued that interruptions and distractions can lead to loss of focus and result in errors, and requested further research to determine whether silence during induction is needed as a safety measure. Another study concluded that on average during cases one distractive event occurs every 4 minutes 23 seconds, with approximately 3.4 distractions during induction and 3.0 distractions when moving from the induction room to the OR.[96] In this study while most distracting events had no negative consequences for the patient, 22% had negative consequences (suboptimal management). Interestingly 3% were actually not distractions because they had positive consequences for the patient. In another study, 20% of visual attention during induction was directed to the patient monitor, increasing up to 30% during simulated critical incident induction scenarios.[97] During the observation of real cases, yet another study group found that drug/fluid tasks comprised 20 ± 6% of induction, 15 ± 8% of maintenance, and 12 ± 7% of emergence during routine cases.[91]

Maintenance Phase of Anesthesia

Betza and colleagues found in an observational study that anesthesia providers spent 71% of their time during maintenance doing patient or display monitoring tasks.[98] Transitions between the task categories occurred approximately once every 9 seconds. It appeared that regardless of the task, there was a high frequency of task transitions to look at the visual displays and then from the visual displays toward the patient. Compared with the induction phase, there are fewer (16) task steps during the maintenance phase.[63] However, there is evidence that a relatively high proportion of critical incidents occur during the maintenance phase (59% of incidents during maintenance, 26% during induction).[37] Patients' conditions may vary in an overt or subtle way. Therefore, anesthesia professionals need to continuously monitor several parameters. Their attention may be distracted or misbalanced, as not all parameters need the same level of attention all the time. Sometimes other tasks, such as telephone calls, auscultation, insertion of an arterial cannula, use of transesophageal echocardiography (TEE), and "problem solving," may divert the attention of the anesthesia professional. As attention is a limited resource and susceptible to distractions, it is important to learn how to best allocate one's attention in continuously changing and complex environments like anesthesia (see later section, "Situation Awareness").

Very detailed task analyses took place in a series of studies carried out by the University of California, San Diego (UCSD), Stanford University, the San Diego and Stanford Veterans Administration Medical Centers.[66,67] Generally, studies of workload indicate that induction and, to a lesser degree, emergence are the most intensive. However, it is also argued that many of those tasks performed are part of a routine, which tends to reduce the effort required. Maintenance, in contrast, is typically less physically "action dense" but mental activity continues as a wide range of information is used and processed.[99]

Emergence

With 40 task steps to carry out in a relatively short period of time, the discontinuation of anesthesia and subsequent transfer of the patient to recovery is fairly busy.[63] A study from Broom and associates suggests that emergence is the most distractive period compared with induction and maintenance, finding noise during emergence at 58 decibels (dB) (compared to induction at 46 dB and maintenance at 52 dB), with sudden loud noise (>70 dB) occurring more frequently during emergence than at induction or maintenance.[100] The range of staff entrances and exits were also highest during emergence (10), compared to induction (0) and maintenance (6). Conversations unrelated to the procedure occurred in 93% of emergences. Emergence also was found to be the period of most frequent distractions, occurring on average every 2 minutes.[96] Those findings are acknowledged by the following quotations retrieved from subjective study interviews:

"I don't think people quite appreciate that emergence is as important as induction really and sometimes they're just glad to have finished off their case. They're crashing and banging and moving on and fail to realize." and "(...) [B]asically as far as they're concerned the job's finished. They're there moaning, yelling, or talking about the next case. I do find that distracting because I think: 'we haven't actually finished this case yet'." (p. 711)[96]

PATIENT SAFETY ACTION BOX

The period of the patient's emergence from anesthesia is high risk and a high workload for the anesthesia professional while low stress for other OR personnel. Often they forget and the noise level may rise considerably. If so the anesthesia professional should politely demand thoughtfulness and quiet from the other OR team members. This would also be a possible setting to invoke the auditory "sterile cockpit" protocol (see later section "Distractions and Interruptions in the Operating Room").

PRE-USE CHECKOUT OF EQUIPMENT/ ANESTHESIA MACHINE CHECKOUT

A pre-use check to ensure the correct functioning of anesthetic equipment is essential to patient safety. Failure to check anesthesia equipment prior to use can lead to patient injury or "near misses."[101,102] Based on a retrospective incident analysis of 668 reported incidents, Marcus reported a total of nearly 18% of in-theater incidents in pediatric anesthesia resulted from the failure to check.[102] More recent generations of anesthesia machines have internal computers that can conduct checks of many aspects of machine functioning and alert the anesthesia professional to problems. However, the authors have observed in simulations of embedded machine problems or external equipment faults (e.g., nitrous oxide vs. oxygen swap) that anesthesia professionals may lack a complete understanding of these systems.

In the United States an updated machine checklist was released by the American Society of Anesthesiologists (ASA) in 2008.[103] Because no specific checkout recommendation could be applicable to all modern anesthesia delivery systems and to all anesthetizing locations, the latest recommendation is based on a set of design guidelines for the pre-anesthetic checkout and provides samples of checkout procedures (available at: www.asahq.org/resources/clinical-information/2008-asa-recommendations-for-pre-anesthesia-checkout). The 2008 pre-use anesthesia apparatus checkout recommendation (AACR) contains a list of 15 separate items that should be checked at the beginning of each day (preoperative check) or whenever a machine is moved, serviced, or the vaporizers changed. Eight of these items should be checked prior to each procedure (preinduction check). Some of the steps may be already part of an automated manufacturer's checkout process in the anesthesia machine; others need to be performed individually. Feldman and associates state:

"Following these checklists will typically require <5 minutes at the beginning of the day, and <2 minutes between cases, but will provide you with the confidence that the machine will be able to provide all essential life support functions before you begin a case." (p. 6)[104]

In 2012, the Association of Anaesthetists of Great Britain and Ireland (AAGBI) released a new safety guideline on checking anesthesia equipment that also includes, but is not limited to, the pre-use checkout of the anesthetic machine (available at: https://www.aagbi.org/sites/default/files/checking_anaesthetic_equipment_2012.pdf).[105] Rather recently revised guidelines on pre-use checking of the anesthetic equipment including the anesthesia workstation have been published by the Australian and New Zealand College of Anaesthetists (ANZCA)[106] in 2014 and by the Canadian Anesthesiologists' Society (CAS)[107] in 2016.

PATIENT SAFETY ACTION BOX

There are numerous checkout checklists available. A serious patient safety issue is the non-adherence to standard protocols. The anesthetic checkout of equipment is a method of systematically ensuring the anesthetic professional executes a thorough check of the anesthetic equipment. All professionals should therefore use it as a standard practice for checking the anesthetic machine to provide the best and safest patient care. The implementation of a checklist is an organizational process that needs systematic implementation and, optimally, user training.

COGNITIVE TASKS OF ADMINISTERING ANESTHESIA AND RELATED VULNERABILITIES

The observable tasks do not tell the whole story of what the anesthesia professional is doing. Even when the anesthesia professional appears idle, most of the time mental activity is ongoing. Several investigators have written about the cognitive elements in anesthesiology.[91,108-111] Of those errors made, cognitive errors and cognitive biases in anesthesiology are common and pose a threat to patient safety.[61,62,102] In the following section, (1) the cognitive tasks of dynamic decision making and situation awareness are described and summarized in the anesthesia professional's core cognitive process model; (2) subsequently, the management and coordination of the core cognitive process model are discussed in this section; and (3) several methodologies to measure cognitive workload are touched on.

Introduction of the Anesthesia Professional's Core Cognitive Process Model

Besides the constant check whether anticipated milestones of the anesthetic regimen are achieved and the constant check of incoming data streams, the anesthesia professional must also react to a large number of contingencies, some of which can be predicted in advance based on the patient's history and the type of surgery, whereas others cannot. If so, the existing plan may have to be reactively modified.

Different aspects of decision making and situation awareness are summarized in the anesthesia professional's core cognitive process model. The model was developed by David Gaba and draws heavily on the work of a number of other investigators who studied human performance in a variety of complex, dynamic worlds.[91,112-114] It is described in detail as a framework for understanding the empiric data, and provides a vocabulary for discussing the elements of both successful and unsuccessful performance by anesthesia professionals.

The entire core process model, shown in Fig. 6.1, depicts the anesthesia professional as working at five different interacting cognitive levels (resource management level,

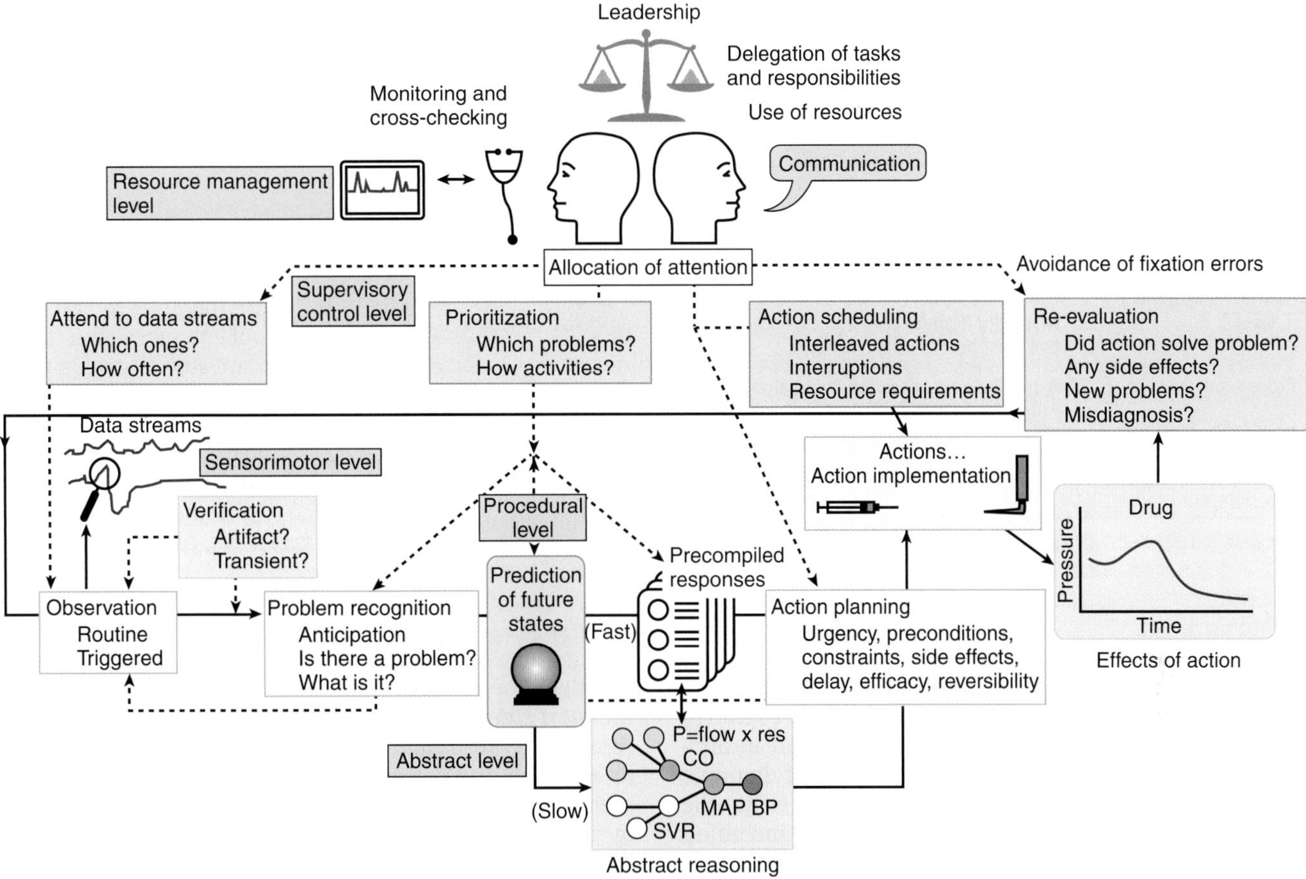

Fig. 6.1 Core cognitive process model of the anesthetist's complex real-time problem-solving behavior (see text for detailed description). Five levels of cognition operate in parallel. The core process involves a main loop (solid arrows) of observation, decision, action, and reevaluation. The core process is managed by two levels of metacognition that involve a second, higher-level loop (both above the core process): supervisor control (allocation of attention) and resource management. Each component of the model requires different cognitive skills. Each component is vulnerable to a different set of performance failures or errors. *BP*, Blood pressure; *CO*, cardiac output; *MAP*, mean arterial pressure; *SVR*, systematic vascular resistance. (From Gaba DM, Fish KJ, Howard SK. *Crisis Management in Anesthesiology*. New York: Churchill Livingstone; 1994.)

BOX 6.1 Elements of the Core Cognitive Process of an Anesthesiologist

1. Observation
2. Verification
3. Problem recognition
4. Prediction of future states
5. Decision making
   a. Application of precompiled responses (recognition-primed decision making)
   b. Decision making using heuristics and probability
   c. Decision making including abstract reasoning
6. Action implementation
7. Reevaluation (avoiding fixation errors)
8. Start again with 1 (loop continues)

procedural level, communication level, abstract reasoning level, supervisory control level) to implement and control a core process of observation, verification, problem recognition, prediction of future states, decision making, action, and reevaluation (Box 6.1). The core process must then be integrated with the behavior of other team members and with the constraints of the work environment. Expert performance in anesthesia involves these features in a repeated loop of the different steps. Errors can occur at each step in this process.

The division of mental activities into levels follows the work of Rasmussen and Reason et al..[113,115] Having multiple levels supports the concepts of parallel processing (performing more than one task at a time but working on different levels of mental activity) and multitasking/multiplexing (performing only one task at a time but switching very rapidly from one task to another), as shown in several task analysis studies.[64,67,89] Table 6.1 gives an overview and a brief explanation of the different mental activity levels.

At the sensorimotor level, activities involving sensory perception or motor actions take place with minimal conscious control; they are smooth, practiced, and highly integrated patterns of behavior. At the procedural level, the anesthesia professional performs regular routines in a familiar work situation. These routines have been derived and internalized from training and from previous work episodes. A level of abstract reasoning is used during preoperative planning, and intraoperatively it is used in unfamiliar situations for which no well-practiced expertise or routine is available from previous encounters. Rasmussen's model[113] was extended by the explicit addition of two additional levels of mental activity—the supervisory and the resource management level—that provide for dynamic adaptation of the anesthesia professional's own thought processes. Supervisory control is concerned with dynamically allocating finite

TABLE 6.1 Levels of Mental Activity

Level of Control	Explanation	Comments
Resource management level	Command and control of all resources, including teamwork and communication	Incident analysis shows a huge contribution of lack of resource management and communication skills to the development of incidents and accidents; the importance of these factors is reflected in the ACRM principles and simulation training courses (see Chapter 7)
Supervisory control level	Metacognition: thinking about thinking	Dynamic adaptation of the thought process, decision making (e.g., avoiding fixation errors), scheduling, and remembering actions (e.g., prospective memory tasks)
Abstract reasoning level	Use of fundamental medical knowledge, search for high-level analogies, deductive reasoning	Often in parallel with other levels; in emergency situations often too slow and too sensitive to distractions in high-workload situations
Procedural level	Precompiled responses, following algorithms, heuristics, "reflexes"	Recognition-primed decision making—experts are more often on this level; special errors may occur as a result of not checking for the appropriateness of the "procedure"; less experienced personnel may misuse this level for ill-considered, unadapted "cookbook medicine"
Sensorimotor level	Use of all senses and manual actions; "feeling, doing, hearing"; sometimes subconscious control of actions	Experts perform smooth action sequences and control their actions by direct feedback from their senses (e.g., action sequences of placing an intravenous line or endotracheal intubation; skill-based errors such as slips and lapses may occur)

ACRM, Anesthesia crisis resource management.

attention between routine and non-routine actions, among multiple problems or themes, and among the five cognitive levels. Attention is such a scarce resource, therefore its allocation is extremely important in every aspect of dynamic decision making. Resource management deals with the command and control of available resources, including teamwork and communication. Expert performance in anesthesia involves these features in a repeated loop. An overview of the core cognitive process and its elements is given in Box 6.1. The elements are explained in detail in the following text sections and include (1) observation; (2) verification; (3) problem recognition; (4) prediction of future states; (5) precompiled responses; (6) action taking/action implementation; and (7) reevaluation.

Observation. Anesthesia professionals use observations to decide whether the patient's course is on track or whether a problem is occurring; this is the first step of the decision making cycle. Data are observed and transformed by interpretation into information, followed by further interpretation into meaning. Data streams typically involve direct visual, auditory, or tactile contact with the patient, the surgical field, routine electronic monitoring, special (sometimes invasive) monitoring systems, contents of suction canisters and sponges, reading of reports of laboratory test results, and communications from other personnel. Loeb showed that anesthesiologists typically observe monitors for approximately 1 to 2 seconds every 10 to 20 seconds and that it usually took several observing cycles before they detected a subtle cue on the monitor.[88] Management of rapidly changing situations requires the anesthesia professional to assess a wide variety of information sources. Because the human mind can attend closely to only one or two items at a time, the anesthesia professional's supervisory control level must decide what information to attend to and how frequently to observe it (as later shown at CRM key point 14 "Allocate attention wisely"). Constant observation and interpretation of the different information systems is executed repeatedly throughout the course of an anesthetic regimen. The plethora of simultaneous data streams in even the most routine cases is a challenge. Vigilance, defined as the capacity to *sustain* attention, plays a crucial role in the observation and detection of problems and is a necessary prerequisite for meaningful care. Vigilance can be degraded by performance-shaping factors (see later section "Performance Shaping Factors") and it can be overwhelmed by the sheer amount of information and the rapidity with which it is changing.

Verification. In the working environment of an anesthesia professional, the available, observed information is not always reliable. Most monitoring is noninvasive and indirect and is susceptible to *artifacts* (false data). Even direct clinical observations such as vision or auscultation can be ambiguous. Brief *transients* (true data of short duration) can occur that quickly correct themselves. To prevent them from skewing the decision making process and triggering precipitous actions that may have significant side effects, critical observations must be verified before the clinician can act on them. This requires the use of all available data and information and cross-checking different related data streams rather than depending solely on any single datum without sensible interpretation (as later shown in CRM key point 8 "Use all available information" and CRM key point 10 "Cross check and double check; never assume anything"). Verification uses a variety of methods, shown in Table 6.2.

PATIENT SAFETY ACTION BOX

Try to be sensitive to changes and do not just explain them away as normal without double-checking or using other information to determine if everything really is okay. Assume there is a big problem unless you can prove otherwise. If in doubt, it should always be assumed that the patient is at risk and that the parameter in question is real (rule out the worst case). The burden of proof is on you. Beware of too easily assuming that it is just a technical artifact.

TABLE 6.2 Methods for Verification of Critical Observations

Method	Explanation and Example
Repeating	The observation or measurement is repeated to rule out a temporary wrong value (e.g., motion artifacts during noninvasive blood pressure measurement)
Checking trend information	The short-term trend is observed for plausibility of the actual value. Trends of physiologic parameters almost always follow curves, not steps
Observing a redundant channel	An existing redundant channel is checked (e.g., invasive arterial pressure and cuff pressure are redundant, or heart rate from an ECG and pulse oximeter)
Correlating	Multiple related (but not redundant) variables are correlated to determine the plausibility of the parameter in question (e.g., if the ECG monitor shows a flat line and "asystole" but the invasive blood pressure curve shows waves)
Activating a new monitoring device	A new monitoring modality is installed (e.g., placing a pulmonary artery catheter). This also adds another parameter for the method of "correlating"
Recalibrating an instrument or testing its function	The quality and reliability of a measurement are checked, and its function is tested (e.g., if the CO_2 detector shows no values, the anesthetist can exhale through it to see whether the device works). Observation of redundant channels can also help verify a value (see above)
Replacing an instrument	If doubt exists about the function of a device, an entirely new instrument or an alternative backup device may be installed
Asking for help	If the decision on the values remains unclear, help should be sought early to obtain a second opinion from other trained personnel

ECG, Electrocardiogram.

Problem Recognition. Having recognized a problem, how does the expert anesthesia professional respond? The classical paradigm of decision making involves a careful comparison of the evidence with various causal hypotheses that could explain the problem. This is followed by a careful analysis of all possible actions and solutions. This approach, although powerful, is relatively slow and does not work well with ambiguous or scanty evidence. Many perioperative problems faced by anesthesia professionals require quick action under uncertainty[116,117] to prevent a rapid cascade to a catastrophic adverse outcome, and solution of these problems through formal deductive reasoning from first principles is just too slow. The process of problem recognition is a central feature of several theories of cognition in complex, dynamic worlds.[110,118,119] Problem recognition involves matching sets of environmental cues to patterns that are known to represent specific types of problems. Given the high uncertainty seen in anesthesia, the available information sources cannot always disclose the existence of a problem, and even if they do, they may not specify its identity or origin. Anesthesia professionals use approximation strategies to handle these ambiguous situations; psychologists term such strategies *heuristics*.[120] Stiegler and Tung give a detailed review of heuristics and other biases that affect problem recognition.[121] One heuristic is to categorize what is happening as one of several generic problems, each of which encompasses many different underlying conditions (similarity/pattern matching). Another is to gamble on a single diagnosis (frequency gambling[115]) by initially choosing the single most frequent candidate event. During preoperative planning, the anesthesia professional may adjust a mental "index of suspicion" for recognizing certain specific problems anticipated for that particular patient or surgical procedure. The anesthesia professional must also decide whether a single underlying diagnosis explains all the data or whether they could come from multiple causes. This decision is important because excessive attempts to refine the diagnosis can be very costly in terms of allocation of attention. By contrast, a premature diagnosis can lead to inadequate or erroneous treatment. The use of heuristics is typical of expert anesthesia professionals and often results in considerable time savings in dealing with problems. However, it is a double-edged sword. Both frequency gambling and inappropriate allocation of attention solely to expected problems can seriously undermine problem solving when these gambles do not pay off or are not corrected in the reevaluation process.

Many of the issues that are related to problem recognition and cognition in general are discussed in more detail in the section on decision making further below, especially when dealing with the models of System I thinking and System II thinking and of recognition-primed decision making.

Prediction of Future States. Problems must be assessed in terms of their significance for the future states of the patient.[110,118] Predicting future states based on the occurrence of seemingly trivial problems is a major part of the anticipatory behaviors that characterize expert crisis managers. Problems that are already critical or that can be predicted to evolve into critical incidents receive the highest priority (as later shown in CRM key point 15 "Set priorities dynamically"). Prediction of future states also influences action planning by defining the timeframe available for required actions. Cook and colleagues described *"going sour"* incidents in which the future state of the patient was not adequately taken into account when early manifestations of problems were apparent.[122] One of the challenges known from research in psychology is that the human mind is not very well suited to predict future states, when things are changing in a nonlinear fashion. Under such circumstances, which are common for natural systems such as the human body, the rate of change is almost invariably underestimated, and people are surprised at the outcome.[123]

PATIENT SAFETY ACTION BOX

Slow but steady and sustained blood loss in a child during surgery might result in few or subtle changes in hemodynamics for some time until rapid decompensation occurs. If the weak signs of the developing problem were not detected or misjudged the ensuing catastrophe may seem to have occurred suddenly. The use of a visible trend monitoring of heart rate or blood pressure over a longer period of time can help the anesthesia professional to be better aware of changes that are not readily apparent if only the last few measurements are compared.

Precompiled Responses. Once a critical event has been observed and verified the anesthesia professional needs to respond. In complex, dynamic domains, the initial responses of experts to the majority of events stem from *precompiled* rules or response plans for dealing with a recognized event.[115] This method is referred to as recognition-primed decision making,[114,124] because once the event is identified, the response is well known (see later section "Decision Making"). In the anesthesia domain, these responses are usually acquired through personal experience alone, although there is a growing realization that critical response protocols must be codified explicitly and taught systematically. Experienced anesthesia professionals have been observed to rearrange, recompile, and rehearse these responses mentally based on the patient's condition, the surgical procedure, and the problems to be expected.[125] Ideally, precompiled responses to common problems are retrieved appropriately and executed rapidly. When the exact nature of the problem is not apparent, a set of *generic* responses appropriate to the overall situation may be invoked. For example, if a problem with ventilation is detected, the anesthesia professional may switch to manual ventilation at a higher fraction of inspired oxygen (FiO_2) while considering further diagnostic actions. However, experiments involving simulation have demonstrated that even experienced anesthesia professionals show great variability in their use of response procedures to critical situations.[75,125-127] This finding led these investigators to target simulator-based training in the systematic training of responses to critical events.[108,128]

Even the ideal use of precompiled responses is destined to fail when the problem does not have the suspected cause or when it does not respond to the usual actions. Anesthesia cannot be administered purely by precompiled "cookbook" procedures. Abstract reasoning about the problem through the use of fundamental medical knowledge still takes place in parallel with precompiled responses, even when quick action must be taken. This seems to involve a search for high-level analogies[115] or true deductive reasoning using deep medical and technical knowledge and a thorough analysis of all possible solutions. Anesthesia professionals managing simulated crises have linked their precompiled actions to abstract medical concepts.[125]

Taking Action/Action Implementation. Anesthesiologists need to share their attention among different cognitive levels, among tasks, and often among problems. The intensive demands on the anesthesia professional's attention could easily swamp the available mental resources. Therefore, the anesthesia professional must strike a balance between acting quickly on every small perturbation (which requires a lot of attention) and adopting a more conservative "wait-and-see" attitude. This balance must be constantly shifted between these extremes as the situation changes. However, during simulated crisis situations, some practitioners showed great reluctance to switch from business as usual to emergency mode even when serious problems were detected.[75] Erring too far in the direction of wait and see is an error that can be particularly catastrophic. Preparedness for active intervention in case of dynamically changing events is a key element of an anesthesiologist's work. But how frequent is this requirement? According to the review of Wacker and Staender, adverse events in the perioperative period continue to be frequent, occur in about 30% of hospital admissions, and may be preventable in more than 50%.[129]

PATIENT SAFETY ACTION BOX

Once you are sure there is a big problem, it is important for the entire team to transition into emergency mode efficiently. One way of doing so is to declare the emergency out loud with appropriate force, such as: *"Ok, everybody, there's a very serious problem with the patient—probably anaphylaxis—this is a major emergency."*

At any time during an anesthetic regimen there may be multiple things to do, each of which is intrinsically appropriate, yet they cannot all be done at once. Simulation experiments have shown that anesthesia professionals sometimes have difficulty selecting, planning, and scheduling actions optimally.[75]

PATIENT SAFETY ACTION BOX

It helps if team members know the actions planned and the schedule of actions preferred (referred to as shared mental models). If the anesthesia professional does not provide the information, team members should check with the anesthesiologist. It also is helpful to distribute actions with clear communicated priorities and/or timeframes (CRM principle 7: "Effective Communication", e.g., *"[Name of receiver of message], prepare xxx first, then I need xxx, and after that bring me xxx,"* or *"After you have done xxx, let's start xxx together"*, or *"In 30 minutes, please check the blood gases/blood sugar level/ etc. again..."*)

A particular hallmark of anesthesiology is that the decision maker does not just decide what action is required but is often involved directly in the implementation of actions. Executing these actions requires substantial attention and may in fact impair the anesthesia professional's mental and physical ability to perform other activities (e.g., when an action requires a sterile procedure). This is particularly an issue when other tasks have been interrupted or temporarily suspended. *Prospective memory,*[130-134] one's ability to remember in the future to perform an action (i.e., to complete a task) can be easily disrupted. In addition, anesthesia professionals engaged in a manual procedure are strongly constrained from performing other manual tasks or from maintaining awareness of incoming information.

Reevaluation. In order to successfully solve dynamic problems and to cope with the rapid changes and profound diagnostic and therapeutic uncertainties seen during anesthesia, the core process must include repetitive reevaluation of the situation. Thus, the reevaluation step, initiated by the supervisory control level, returns the anesthesia professional to the observation phase, but with specific assessments in mind (see also CRM key point 12, "Reevaluate repeatedly"). Only by frequently reassessing the situation can the anesthesia professional adapt to dynamic processes, since the initial diagnosis and situation assessment can be incorrect. Even actions that are appropriate to the problem are not always successful.

BOX 6.2 Reevaluation Questions—Maintaining Situation Awareness

- Did the actions have any effect (e.g., did the drug reach the patient?)?
- Is the problem getting better, or is it getting worse?
- Are there any side effects resulting from previous actions?
- Are there any other problems or new problems that were missed before?
- Was the initial situation assessment/diagnosis correct?
- What further developments can be expected in the (near) future?

The process of continually updating the assessment of the situation and monitoring the efficacy of chosen actions is termed *situation awareness*.[118,119] Situation awareness is a very interesting and important topic in analyzing performance and reasons for errors[110,135,136] and is discussed in detail in a later section. Box 6.2 gives examples of reevaluation questions in order to maintain situation awareness.

Faulty reevaluation, inadequate adaptation of the plan, or loss of situation awareness can result in a type of human error termed *fixation error*.[137,138] Fixation errors have been described in responses of professionals to abnormal situations.[125,126,137-139] Avoiding and recognizing fixation errors in the field of anesthesia is covered more in detail in section "Introduction of the 15 Crisis Resource Management Key Principles."

Management and Coordination of the Core Cognitive Process: Supervisory Control and Resource Management

Anesthesia professionals' abilities to adapt their own thinking (metacognition—thinking about thinking) through supervisory control and resource management are key components of dynamic decision making and therefore of crisis management.

Supervisory Control. The supervisory control allocates the scarce resource of attention during multitasking, and oversees and modulates the core process. For example, determining the frequency of observation of different data streams, prioritizing diagnostic and therapeutic alternatives, actively managing workload, prioritizing and scheduling actions. Supervisory control actively manages the workload by (1) avoiding high-workload situations by anticipation and planning, (2) distributing workload over time or (3) over personnel, (4) changing the nature of the task to reduce work, or (5) minimizing distraction. More details regarding the active management of workload are touched on in the later section on CRM key point 5 "Distribute the Workload."

Resource Management. The highest layer of metacognition and control is known as resource management—the ability to command and control all the resources at hand to care for the patient and to respond to problems. This involves translating the knowledge of what needs to be done into effective team activity by taking into account the limitations of the complex and often ill-structured perioperative domain. Resources include personnel, equipment, and supplies, both in the immediate vicinity and, when necessary, throughout the various levels of the organization. Resource management explicitly demands teamwork and crew coordination. It is not enough for the anesthesia professional to know what to do or even to be able to do each task alone. Only so much can be accomplished in a given time, and some tasks can be performed only by other skilled personnel (e.g., catheterization lab). A key responsibility of the anesthesia professional is to mobilize needed resources and to distribute the relevant goals and tasks among those available. The details of this critical function are described in the section on "Crisis Resource Management."

ANESTHESIA PROFESSIONAL'S WORKLOAD AND METHODOLOGIES TO MEASURE IT

Most anesthesia professionals have significant other responsibilities in addition to the manual, cognitive, and behavioral duties described above, for example in administration, supervision, or teaching. Depending on the task, the task density, the individual's experience and skill, the patient's state, and the given circumstances (production pressure, staff availability, noise, light, space, team, etc.), the workload of the anesthesia professional can change at any time during an anesthetic regimen. Cognitive resources are diminished when the workload is heavy (i.e., during task dense phases like induction, emergence, or during an emergency), leading to lower levels of performance,[76,127] increased response time, [93] decreased vigilance,[90,92] and greater risk of errors.

The concept of workload is tricky to define. Hart and Staveland[140] describe it as follows: "*Workload is not an inherent property, but rather emerges from the interaction between the requirements of a task, the circumstances under which it is performed, and the skills, behaviors, and perceptions of the operator*" (p. 140). Psychology literature suggests that emotions during highly demanding activities impair cognitive processing efficiency.[141] Task analysis studies as described earlier and task (action) density studies (see later) give insights into several aspects of workload, especially facilitating workload measurements by identifying the individual work components or subtasks to be measured. However, those kind of studies do not necessarily give insight into the performance shaping aspects of workload.

Methods to measure workload include task performance via observation, subjective assessments, and physiological measures. They are described below. For a more comprehensive review, see, for example, Leedal and Smith, [142] and Byrne.[143]

Primary Task Performance. The primary task performance measure assesses the subject's performance on standard work tasks (e.g., cases seen, knots tied, etc.) as they are made progressively more difficult by increasing the number of tasks, task density, or task complexity. At first, the subject is able to keep up with the increasing task load, but at some point, the workload exceeds the ability to manage it, and performance on the standard tasks decreases.

Secondary Task Probing. Secondary task probing tests the subject with a minimally intrusive secondary task that is added to the primary work tasks. The secondary task is a simple one for which performance can be objectively measured. Reaction time, finger tapping, mental arithmetic and a vibrotactile device have for example been used for this technique as a secondary task. The anesthesia professional is instructed that the primary tasks of patient care take absolute precedence over the secondary task. Therefore, assuming that the secondary task requires some of the same mental resources as the primary task, the performance of the anesthesiologist on the secondary task is an indirect reflection of the spare capacity available to deal with it: the greater the spare capacity, the lower the primary workload. Depending on the secondary task response channels (manual, voice, gesture, multiple ways) there can exist channel interference. Controversy exists about whether these probes measure "vigilance" or "workload," although the same techniques probably measure both aspects of performance. When probes occur infrequently, are subtle, have multiple response channels, and are performed with a low level of existing workload, they are more likely to measure vigilance; when they are frequent, readily detectable, require a manual response, and are performed during a high-workload period, they probably are more indicative of spare capacity and workload.

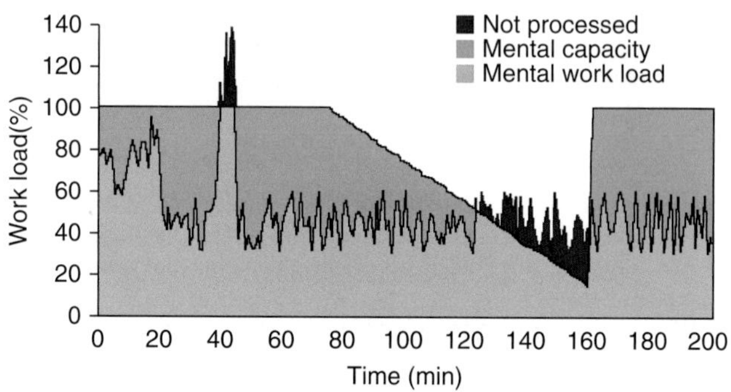

Fig. 6.2 Illustration of how mental workload for the individual and the team may vary during anesthesia. Time is shown on the x-axis. Total workload is shown on the y-axis. During the first 20 minutes of anesthesia induction the workload is high, but does not exceed mental capacity. Then, during the first minutes of maintenance the workload drops. At 35 minutes a crisis leads to a sudden increase in workload, which exceeds mental capacity. As shown, during this time certain information is not processed. Such a sudden overload is a typical feature of critical incidents, known in aviation as "maxing out." Thereafter, the workload of the maintenance phase drops again. But at the same time, after around 80 minutes in the case, the anesthesia professional becomes progressively more tired, resulting in less mental capacity available. So between 120 and 160 minutes workload again exceeds mental capacity and information is not processed. Finally, the anesthesiologist is roused after 160 minutes and workload again lies within capacity until the end of the case. (Figure based on the publication of Byrne A. Measurement of mental workload in clinical medicine: a review study. *Anesth Pain Med.* 2011;1(2):90–94.)

Subjective Measures. In subjective measures, individuals are asked, most commonly in retrospect but sometimes in real time, how much load they were or are under during actual work situations. A common and validated form to assess subjective workload is the NASA TLX form.[140] Subjective measures usually complement objective measurements of external observations, since an anesthesia professional may subjectively underestimate the workload in settings in which objective measurements demonstrate a marked reduction in spare capacity.

Physiologic Measures. The final set of techniques for assessing workload consists of physiologic measures. Visual or auditory evoked potentials have been used successfully to assess mental workload, but this technique can be used only in a static laboratory environment. Heart rate (especially certain aspects of heart rate variability) and blood pressure are other physiologic measures that have been used, but there are challenges in reliable interpretation.

ASSESSING THE PERFORMANCE OF ANESTHESIA PROFESSIONALS

Over the years several study designs investigating manual (i.e., technical aspects of a procedure), cognitive (i.e., dynamic decision making, situation awareness, vigilance) and behavioral/nontechnical (i.e., communication, teamwork, leadership) tasks were used to assess the performance of anesthesiologists. In this section, studies with special focus on anesthesia professional's performance about action density, work experience, teaching/delegation/supervision activity, and critical incidents/emergency treatment are presented. Most of the studies were performed in a simulated medical environment.

Because much of the more recent literature recapitulates findings of the pioneering studies, in this chapter those initial studies are used but the reader also is referred to newer, selected studies, without providing an exhaustive list.[6-8,68,73,74,76,144-149] The latest, large-scale study concerning the performance of anesthesiologists was published by Weinger and co-workers in 2017, examining the performance of board-certified anesthesiologists during four emergency cases.[75] The study is also presented in detail below.

A broader view on general human performance aspects related to anesthesia can be found in the next sections on "human performance, human factors and nontechnical skills" and "system thinking."

Performance as a function of task density

It is generally accepted that there are limits on human ability to process information, and that information overload can lead to poor performance.[150] For example, many people will have experienced the difficulties of simultaneously trying to drive, navigate, read road signs, and listen to passengers. However, the work domain of anesthesia oftentimes seems to require exactly this kind of task density (Fig. 6.2). An interdisciplinary research group performed several task analysis studies, which allowed the analysis of multiple parallel and overlapping actions (action/task density).[89] Figs. 6.3 and 6.4 show examples of observations of 24 real OR studies. The observation data contain many short-term fluctuations *(dots)*; the moving average of action density of the previous 5 minutes was charted as well *(line)*. Fig. 6.3 shows a complete anesthesia procedure with increases in action density during induction and emergence from anesthesia. Fig. 6.4 shows two final phases of cardiac cases

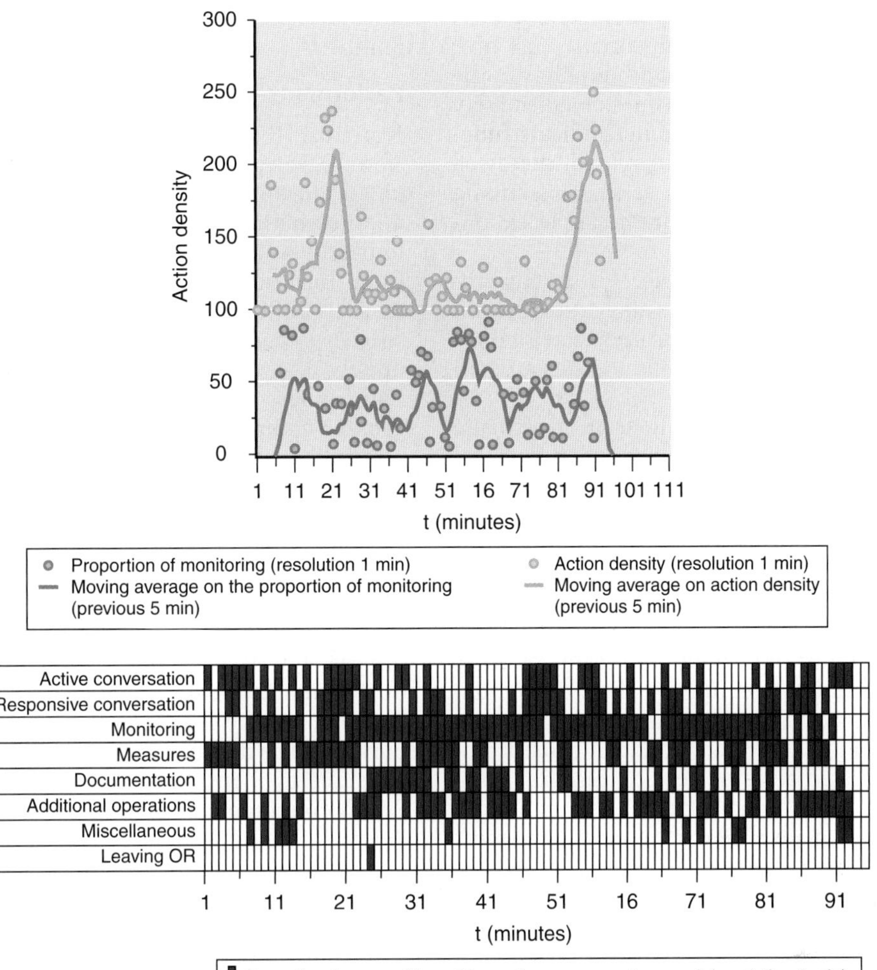

Fig. 6.3 Action density diagram illustrating the derived parameter "action density" from induction of anesthesia to emergence in a real anesthetic case. The *yellow line* in the graph shows the overall action density and the *dots* show the moving average of the density. The *blue line* shows the contribution of one task group, "monitoring," as an example. The table in the lower graph shows the composition of the data for all eight task groups from the same case. *OR,* Operating room.

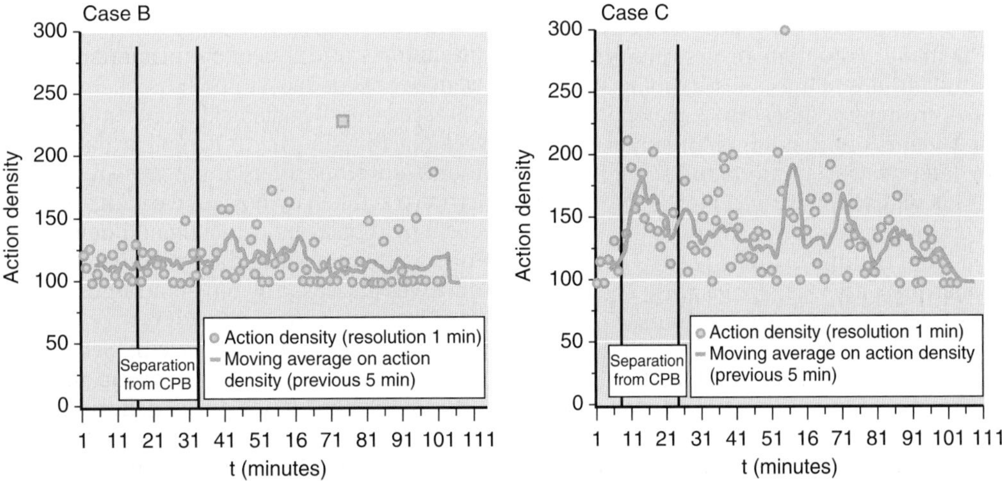

Fig. 6.4 Action density during separation from cardiopulmonary bypass without and with complications. The graph on the *left* is the density diagram of an uncomplicated case (case B) with a "flat" action density diagram during (between the two *vertical lines)* and after separation from cardiopulmonary bypass (CPB). In contrast, case C, shown in the graph on the *right,* had a complicated weaning from CPB; a very high action density is followed by an elevated density with further peaks after separation.

involving cardiopulmonary bypass. The described task analysis technique was also used to study action sequences in simulated cases and compare them with findings in the real OR to demonstrate and evaluate the ecologic validity of simulators (see Chapter 7).[64,89] Findings indicated that as the density of tasks per unit time increased, the dwell time on each task decreased, and vice versa. This finding has important implications for how anesthesia professionals allocate their attention.

Another interesting aspect in this respect is the hypothesis that the mental workload of novices may be lower than that of more experienced staff because they have yet to appreciate the difficulties facing them; this is termed unconscious incompetence.[151]

Xiao and colleagues[70] used simulations to investigate the dimensions of task complexity and their impact on crisis activities and team processes in the trauma room. They identified four components of complexity that affected team coordination in different ways. Multiple concurrent tasks led to goal conflict, task interference, and competition for access to the patient. Uncertainty regarding the case led to differences in opinion when interpreting information and difficulties when trying to anticipate the actions of other team members. The use of contingency plans caused difficulty in knowing when to switch tasks and how then to reallocate activities. Finally, a high workload caused procedures to be compressed and this deviation from normal work further increased the complexity of the situation. They suggested training in explicit communication to meet the challenges of task complexity.

Performance as a Function of Teaching, Delegation, and Supervision

Teaching. Close interaction of experienced anesthesia professionals with inexperienced clinical trainees during actual surgical procedures is a standard approach to training. It can be hypothesized that teaching adds to the workload of the more experienced care provider who is simultaneously responsible for safe and efficient anesthesia care during the procedure. Weinger and co-workers[92] found that teaching teams, involving one-to-one supervision of fourth-year medical students or first-month anesthesia residents by an attending anesthesiologist, had significantly slower response times to a warning light than non-teaching teams of attending(s) of similar experience. Response latency was highest during induction and emergence. This vigilance test was also a procedural (performance) workload assessment measure indicating increased workload and reduced spare capacity. They also found that workload density was significantly increased for teaching as opposed to non-teaching teams. In sum, intraoperative teaching increased workload and decreased vigilance, suggesting the need for caution when educating during patient care.

Delegation and Supervision. Experience suggests that the effect of delegation on workload varies depending on the nature of the task and how confident the delegating anesthesia professional feels about the capability of the person to whom the task is assigned. Delegation must be guided by the supervisor's situation awareness and overall ability to process information on the patients' condition. Several further aspects are presented in the work of Leedal and Smith.[142]

Performance as a Function of Experience

Routine Events. Novice trainee anesthesia professionals were found to perform many of the same tasks as do more experienced personnel at specific phases of an anesthetic regimen, but take longer over tasks, show longer latency of response, and greater task workload than third-year trainees and experienced nurse anesthetists.[90] While task density was generally highest for both subject groups in the period up to, during, and immediately after intubation, the more experienced trainees had higher task densities than the novices, suggesting greater competence among the former in carrying out multiple tasks in a short period of time. Those findings are in line with other studies, including the study of Weinger and associates[67] that evaluated the mean response time of pressing a buzzer at the flashing of a red light (secondary task). The response time was markedly less than 60 seconds for experienced subjects in both the induction and post induction (maintenance) phases, but it was much higher for novice residents during the induction phase. One explanation for those findings may be that the reduction of workload depends partly on the degree to which tasks can become routine, thus freeing mental resources for other tasks. Leedal and Smith conclude concerning this matter in their review: *"Experienced staff appear to show 'spare capacity' in performance during routine cases, which we suggest allows them an attentional 'safety margin' should adverse events occur"* (p. 708) [142]

In contrast, a more recent study presented by Byrne and co-workers found there was limited evidence of a relationship between workload and experience.[152]

Another recent finding indicates that more experienced anesthesia teams may be more likely to attempt to coordinate implicitly, without much overt communication, which makes them more reliant on accurate and shared understandings of the task and their teamwork.[153]

Novice residents also spent more time speaking to their attending staff (11% of preintubation time) than did experienced residents or CRNAs.[90] Experienced personnel observed the surgical field more than did the novices. Novices did take longer to complete patient preparation and induction of anesthesia, but it appeared that some of the extra time taken by novices working under supervision was offset by the efficiency of offloading other concurrent tasks to the attending anesthesiologist such that preintubation time was increased by only 6 minutes for novices.

Critical Events/Emergencies. Schulz and colleagues[97] presented data where more experienced anesthetists (>2 years work experience) increased the amount of time dedicated to manual tasks from 21% to 25% during critical incidents, whereas the less experienced decreased from 20% to 14%. The less experienced anesthesia providers spend more time on monitoring tasks.

A study by Byrne and Jones [76] looked at differences in the performance of experienced and less experienced anesthesia professionals during 180 simulated anesthesia emergency scenarios. The results showed significant differences only between the first and second year. As seen in other studies, significant errors occurred at all levels of experience,[75,76,125,126] and most of the anesthesia professionals deviated from established guidelines.[75,76,154]

A classic simulation study by DeAnda and Gaba investigated the response of anesthesia trainees and experienced anesthesia faculty and private practitioners to six preplanned critical incidents of differing type and severity.[126,155] The incidents included (1) endobronchial intubation (EI) resulting from surgical manipulation of the tube; (2) occlusion of intravenous (IV) tubing; (3) atrial fibrillation (AF) with a rapid ventricular response and hypotension; (4) airway disconnection between the endotracheal tube and the breathing circuit; (5) breathing hoses too short to turn the table 180 degrees, as requested by the surgeon; and (6) ventricular tachycardia or fibrillation. For each incident, considerable interindividual variability was found in detection and correction times, in information sources used, and in actions taken. The average performance of the anesthesia professionals tended to improve with experience, although this varied by incident. The performance of the experienced groups was not better than that of the second-year residents (who were in their final year of training at that time). Many (but not all) novice residents performed indistinguishably from more experienced subjects. Each experience group contained some who required excessive time to solve the problem or who never solved it. In each experience group at least one individual made major errors that could have had a substantial negative impact on a patient's clinical outcome. For example, one faculty member never used electrical countershock to treat ventricular fibrillation. One private practitioner treated the EI as though it were "bronchospasm" and never assessed the symmetry of ventilation. One resident never found the airway disconnection. The elements of suboptimal performance were both technical and cognitive. Technical problems included choosing defibrillation energies appropriate for internal paddles when using external paddles, ampule swap, and failure to inflate the endotracheal tube cuff that resulted in a leak. Cognitive problems included failure to allocate attention to the most critical problems and fixation errors.

Schwid and O'Donnell[125] performed an experiment similar to those of DeAnda and Gaba and received similar results. After working on several practice cases without critical incidents, each subject was asked to manage 3 or 4 cases involving a total of 4 serious critical events (esophageal intubation, myocardial ischemia, anaphylaxis, and cardiac arrest). The anesthesiologists studied had varying experience levels. Significant errors in diagnosis or treatment were made in every experience group. The errors occurred in both diagnosis of problems and in deciding on and implementing appropriate treatment. For example, 60% of subjects did not make the diagnosis of anaphylaxis despite available information on heart rate, blood pressure, wheezing, increased peak inspiratory pressure, and the presence of a rash. In managing myocardial ischemia, multiple failures occurred. 30% of subjects did not compensate for severe abnormalities while considering diagnostic maneuvers. Fixation errors in which initial diagnoses and plans were never revised were frequent, even when they were clearly wrong.

Independent from professionals' experience, Howard and colleagues[127] found a substantial incidence of difficulties during simulated emergencies: managing multiple problems simultaneously, applying attention to the most critical needs, acting as team leader, communicating with personnel, and using all available OR resources to best advantage. Analysis of videotaped trauma and resuscitation cases has revealed inadequacies in the availability and arrangement of monitoring equipment, as well as nonexistent or ambiguous communication.[69] Byrne and Jones [76] evaluated the performance of anesthetists during nine emergency cases, showing that serious errors in both diagnosis and treatment were made and accepted treatment guidelines were not followed. Diagnosis of several common critical incidents, for example, anaphylaxis, was hard to name.[74,125] As described earlier, once diagnosed, no structured plans or algorithms were used.[73,74]

These classic studies date back 25 years or more, yet the most recent studies [75,156] remain completely consistent with older studies. In the 2017 Weinger and colleagues publication, a total of 263 consenting U.S. board-certified anesthesiologists (BCAs—i.e., physicians) participated in two, 20-minute, standardized, high-fidelity simulation scenarios of unanticipated acute events during existing Maintenance of Certification in Anesthesiology simulation courses. The scenarios were from among the following: (1) local anesthetic systemic toxicity with hemodynamic collapse; (2) hemorrhagic shock due to hidden retroperitoneal bleeding during laparoscopy; (3) malignant hyperthermia presenting in the postanesthesia care unit; and (4) acute onset of AF with hemodynamic instability during laparotomy followed by ST elevation myocardial infarction. Performance measurement rubrics were established in advance: a scoresheet of critical clinical performance elements, behavioral anchored ordinal scales of four nontechnical skills, ordinal scales for overall individual and team technical performance and nontechnical performance, and a binary rating as to whether performance met or exceeded that expected of a BCA. The results showed that critical clinical performance elements were commonly omitted, roughly in four broad areas of crisis management, failures to: (1) escalate therapy where first-line options did not work (e.g., using epinephrine or vasopressin when phenylephrine, ephedrine, or fluids did not sufficiently correct hypotension); (2) use available resources (e.g., calling for help when conditions have deteriorated appreciably); (3) speak up and engage other team members, especially when action by them was required (e.g., asking the surgeon to change the surgical approach when it is essential to effective treatment); and (4) follow evidence-based guidelines (e.g., giving dantrolene to a patient with obvious MH). The performance of approximately 25% of subjects was rated in the low portion of the various technical and nontechnical 9-point ordinal scales. In about 30% of encounters, performance was rated as "below the level expected of a BCA."

PATIENT SAFETY ACTION BOX

Experienced anesthetists are not immune to error. Studies show that significant errors can occur at all levels of experience. *Experience is not a substitute for excellence or expertise*, making recurrent training and continuous awareness of possible safety pitfalls important, independent of the experience level.

PATIENT SAFETY ACTION BOX

Do not think this cannot happen to you... In her paper, "Lake Wobegon for anesthesia...where everyone is above average except those who aren't: variability in the management of simulated intraoperative critical incidents," McIntosh[157] discusses the applicability to anesthesiology of the pervasive human tendency to overestimate one's achievements and capabilities in relation to others. Such effects have been documented for drivers, CEOs, stock market analysts, college students, parents, and state education officials, among others.[158] Indeed we may all be living in Lake Wobegon in terms of evaluating our own abilities to manage critical events.

What are the practical implications of performance assessment in Anesthesia?

In summary, simulation studies on performance all showed appreciable performance gaps of anesthesia professionals managing critical incidents and emergencies. The results expand on the few comparable data on real cases.[159-163] Overall, the surprisingly high frequency of mediocre performance represents a patient safety concern for the field of anesthesiology, emphasizing the need for anesthesia professionals and their organizations to:

- be aware of performance shortcomings and pitfalls in everyday work
- regard the knowledge and training of performance-enhancing strategies as one of the core competencies
- focus on the application of and adherence to evidence-based practice guidelines
- focus on the efficient management of the environment (team, resources, equipment, etc.)
- implement case management skills in the education, training, and re-certification, that go beyond only medical/technical knowledge and skill

BENEFITS AND CHALLENGES OF ASSESSING PERFORMANCE

Benefits of the Scientific Study of Tasks and Performance in Anesthesia

The generation of an improved understanding of the human performance of anesthesia professionals can help them to provide patient care more safely, in a wider variety of clinical situations, with greater efficiency, and with increased satisfaction to both patients and practitioners. The possible benefits of studying human performance include, but are not limited to, the following:

1. Improved clinical performance: Behavior observation helps to identify which processes and behaviors are associated with effective and safe performance.[63,83,164] Thus, it provides us with new knowledge on what effective teams do differently compared with ineffective teams and how they do it.[165] Compared with self-reports, behavior observation allows for measuring actual team-level phenomena and dynamics that teams may not even be aware of and that may unfold over time.[166]
2. Improved operational protocols: The way in which individuals conduct anesthesia is based, in part, on knowing the limits of their performance envelope. Anesthetic techniques and OR practices should draw on anesthesia professionals' abilities and should mitigate their weaknesses.
3. Enhanced clinical education and training of anesthesia professionals: Understanding the required performance characteristics and inherent human limitations will lead to improved training, which will most fully develop the strengths and counter the existing vulnerabilities of the anesthesia professional. Identification of performance gaps informs opportunities for improvement. [75] Identification of expert knowledge through elicitation of unaware expertise behavior creates educational gain.[167] Taking this knowledge into action should make patient care safer, less stressful, and more efficient.
4. A more effective work environment: Anesthesia professionals now perform their tasks by using an array of technologies, many of which have not been designed to support the anesthesia professional's work optimally. By understanding the relevant tasks and performance requirements, the workspace and tools could be improved for better support of the most difficult tasks. This, too, can lead to greater safety and to greater efficiency and work satisfaction.
5. A more efficient organizational system: Anesthesiology is embedded within a larger system of organized medical care that involves interactions among numerous people, institutions, organizations, and professional domains. Understanding how the anesthesia professional's work relates to the larger system may enable the development of more rational and efficient flow of information and organizational control.
6. A more rational view of professional work and legal responsibility: Modern health care, especially in the United States, is strongly influenced by medicolegal concerns. The litigation system has a major selection bias in that every case that comes before it involves an adverse outcome for a patient. The duty of the practitioner is to render care as a reasonable and prudent specialist in the area of anesthesia. What is reasonable and prudent? What type of performance is to be expected from appropriately trained human beings in a complex and dynamic environment? By understanding human performance, it may be possible to generate a more rational view of what is and is not within the standard of care.

Challenges of the Scientific Study of Tasks and Performance in Anesthesia

Study of human performance involves research paradigms different from those typically used in the science of anesthesia. Many obstacles exist to obtaining valid data on human performance. There are no animal models for expert human performance and no Sprague-Dawley anesthesia professionals to be studied in detail. Recruiting experienced personnel to be the subjects of study is difficult and raises issues of selection bias concerning those who do volunteer. Especially if conducted during actual patient care, investigations of human performance are strongly influenced by concerns about litigation, credentialing, and confidentiality, thus making it difficult to execute optimal studies. Furthermore, variability among individual anesthesia professionals is quite striking because different anesthesia professionals respond to the same situation in different ways, and each individual may act differently on different days or at different times of the same day. The magnitude of this intraindividual variability is often nearly the same as the interindividual variability. Another challenge is that the performance measures may not be sensitive to an increase or decrease in workload if the subject compensates through increased, or reduced, effort respectively.

Performance itself is an intuitively meaningful concept that is difficult to define precisely. No universal standards are available for the clinical decisions and actions of anesthesia professionals. They depend heavily on the context of specific situations. In addition, determining how anesthesia professionals perform their jobs, whether successfully or unsuccessfully, means delving into their mental processes. This cannot be measured easily. Experimental designs can involve artificial laboratory tasks for which performance can be objectively measured, but these tasks will then be far removed from the real world of administering anesthesia. Conversely, investigating the actual performance of trained practitioners in the real world yields primarily subjective and indirect data. Understanding the anesthesia professional's performance must be seen as analogous to solving a jigsaw puzzle, an analogy introduced by Gaba[128] and extended by McIntosh.[157] Pieces of the puzzle probably come from a variety of sources, none of which by itself captures the entire picture.

Problems faced by all investigators are the lack of an accepted standard for objective or subjective evaluation of anesthesia professional performance and the absence of an agreed-on methodology for analyzing and describing anesthesia professional performance. As one result of the divergent research landscape in human performance, the number, scope, and variety of applied behavior observation taxonomies are growing, making comparison and convergent integration of research findings difficult. Several groups were working on methodologies for evaluating technical and behavioral aspects of performance.[75,89,166,168-170]

Kolbe and colleagues[166] pointed out four methodological challenges when rating behavior. First is identifying the optimal balance between specificity versus generalizability. Researchers must decide whether to investigate processes from a general perspective using methods that capture all teamwork behaviors simultaneously or whether to focus on one single process (e.g., closed-loop communication) to explore it in detail. Second is deciding whether to rate the quality or describe the occurrence of teamwork behavior. Quality of behavior can be measured with an anchored ordinal rating scale (e.g., from excellent to poor). Or alternatively, the occurrences of particular behaviors can be measured such as when?—by whom?—to whom?, etc., delivering different results. Third is linking research findings with team training content, when no common language and no common behavioral codes, respectively, are used in research. Fourth is applying different rating systems (in different studies) without respect to the usability and the different requirements for research, training, and examination purposes.

Patient Safety on the Individual and Team Level

In earlier sections the characteristics of the complex and dynamic working environment in anesthesia were described in detail, as well as the multiple manual, behavioral, and cognitive tasks and related performance assessment studies of the anesthesia professional. Both sections illustrated several human performance and patient safety challenges that personnel face regularly. The knowledge and management of the complex work environment and the various tasks, workload, and performance pitfalls can determine the ultimate success of professionals' intervention. These human factors comprise issues related to perception, memory, problem solving, physiological rhythm, and more. This section focusses on the so-called nontechnical skills and performance-shaping factors [37,38,136,171-174] as they have the most direct practical impact for the work of anesthesia professionals.

The importance of nontechnical skills and performance-shaping factors is also in line with the performance studies of anesthesiologists mentioned earlier in this chapter.[69,70,73-76,125,127] They revealed room for improvement at any level of experience, especially in non-routine and emergency situations. Recent views on nontechnical skills emphasize their relevance also in routine situations to prevent those from becoming critical.[175] Nontechnical skills explain difficulties in applying knowledge and skills that team members possess in stressful moments in a dynamic, complex, and high-workload environment. They are related to challenges in managing and coordinating oneself (e.g., remembering to do tasks, monitoring one's own actions, acting as a team leader), the team (e.g., distributing tasks, managing conflict, sharing mental models), and the equipment (e.g., knowing the application of the equipment, understanding different use modes, troubleshooting).

Therefore, in the upcoming sections the following topics are addressed: (1) General concepts of human factors (HF) and nontechnical skills (NTS) are introduced and discussed in the larger context of human performance. Subsequently, several examples of the impact of HF/NTS are given, indicating that from a safety point of view, HFs and NTS deserve as much attention as medical knowledge [patho-] physiology, diagnosis, treatment) and practical skills, which by tradition have dominated training programs for anesthesia professionals. (2) Two sets of key elements of patient safety: first relating to individual performance (situation awareness and decision making), and second relating to team performance (communication, teamwork, and task management). (3) Additionally, individual performance-shaping factors are discussed, in particular fatigue, interruptions, distractions, and ambient noise.

HUMAN PERFORMANCE, HUMAN FACTORS, AND NONTECHNICAL SKILLS

In the literature, the interrelated terms human performance, human factors, and nontechnical skills are used in a variety of ways and sometimes even synonymously, making it difficult to classify them. They are interconnected and while several models and taxonomies exist there is not always a clear distinction between these terms and concepts. In the upcoming section the authors explain the general underlying principles and give a simplified overview of their interrelationships in order to generate a more systematic understanding of key concepts. The term human error, also used in this context occasionally, is itself a different term, almost the flipside of human factors. One might say that challenges in human factors (and other aspects) can result in human error. For the definition and classification of human error see later section on "System Thinking."

HUMAN PERFORMANCE AND HUMAN FACTORS

What are Human Factors? Human performance is shaped, positively or negatively, by different levels of so-called human factors (HF). Good HF increases and poor HF decreases human performance. The term ergonomics is also used in some contexts. A broad variety of disciplines are involved and many different topics are embraced by both terms; hence, several definitions exist. The Human Factors and Ergonomics Society defines HF as follows: *"Human factors is concerned with the application of what we know about people, their abilities, characteristics, and limitations to the design of equipment they use, environments in which they function, and jobs they perform."*[176] Catchpole and McCulloch define human factors in the medical context as: *"Enhancing clinical performance through an understanding of the effects of teamwork, tasks, equipment, workspace, culture, and organization on human behavior and abilities and application of that knowledge in clinical settings."*[177]

Different Components of Human Factors. Derived from the SEIPS model[178,179] and adapted by the authors, different components of HF are:

- the behavior of individuals and their behavior/knowledge in regard to tasks (individual level)
- the interactions with each other (team level)
- the interactions of professionals with the organizational/sociocultural conditions (organizational level)
- the interactions of professionals with the environment/workspace (environmental level) and
- the interactions of professionals with technology/equipment (technology/engineering/design level)

Those five human factor components are necessary and sufficient to describe and understand the anesthesia professional's entire work system from a HF perspective. The components interact with and influence each other, resulting in a large number of relationships between different levels. At times the components compensate each other (e.g., when professionals work faster to compensate for time pressure or when people collaborate to solve problems that are beyond an individual's abilities). Other times the components resonate with each other and amplify their effects—for the good (e.g., having the right equipment for the task at hand) or the bad (e.g., lacking resources to solve a problem). Given that this chapter cannot deal with human factors in a comprehensive way, many topics can be touched on only briefly. Although the environmental and technology levels can be important—cognition is challenged when there is a power failure or a breakdown of key clinical equipment—in this chapter the focus lies on the most important aspects of human factors directly relevant to anesthesia professionals: the individual level, team level, and organizational level.

HUMAN FACTORS AND NONTECHNICAL SKILLS

What are NonTechnical skills in comparison to Human Factors? When talking specifically about HF that are directly related to actions of a single individual and/or of a team, often this is referred to as the concept of nontechnical skills (NTS). NTS are defined as *"the cognitive, social, and personal resource skills that complement technical skills (which encompass the technical knowledge of health care and its various procedures), and contribute to safe and efficient task performance"*[11] or alternatively as *"attitudes and behaviors not directly related to the use of medical expertise, drugs, or equipment."*[171]

While some authors object to the term nontechnical skills—using a negative to describe something—others have pointed out that not only is this term in wide use already, but that actually a variety of terms involving negation are in common use in science, mathematics, and medicine. One main paper and an editorial discuss this issue.[180,181] For health care, instead of nontechnical skills, the term could also be non-medical skills. However, because of the extensive use of nontechnical skills in the literature of other industries and in health care, this chapter uses that terminology.

Different Ways to Categorize NonTechnical Skills. In general, NTS can be categorized into two broad areas: (1) *cognitive and mental skills* on the individual level, including decision making and situation awareness; and (2) *social and interpersonal skills* on the team level, including teamwork, communication, and leadership. Commercial aviation incorporated such nontechnical skills in the cockpit (later crew) resource management paradigm (CRM, 1980s and continuous later evolution) and the "NOTECHS" paradigm in the late 1990s. In anesthesiology, the anesthesia crisis resource management (ACRM) framework was introduced by Howard and co-workers in 1990[127] as an adaptation of aviation's CRM. The ACRM approach categorizes NTS based on the five key elements of communication, situation awareness, decision making, teamwork (implicitly including leadership), and task management (Fig. 6.5). The anesthesia nontechnical skills (ANTS) framework by Fletcher and colleagues was introduced in 2003; Flin and colleagues give an overview of its history, development, application, use, and emerging is issues.[182, 183] The ANTS approach typically includes the four categories of situation awareness, decision making, teamwork (explicitly including leadership), and task management. Neither of these frameworks, and indeed no usable paradigm, can capture explicitly every important aspect of HF applied to anesthesiology. For example the management of the performance-shaping factors stress and fatigue are also part of the ANTS framework, but are implicit in ACRM. Communication itself is not an explicit skill element of the ANTS framework (which assumes that communication pervades each element), whereas in ACRM it is a specific skill that needs explicit mention and training.[184] Of note, from their start in anesthesiology, nontechnical skills frameworks have been further adapted to several other medical fields, such as for surgeons and intensive care specialists.[8,11,168,169,185-188]

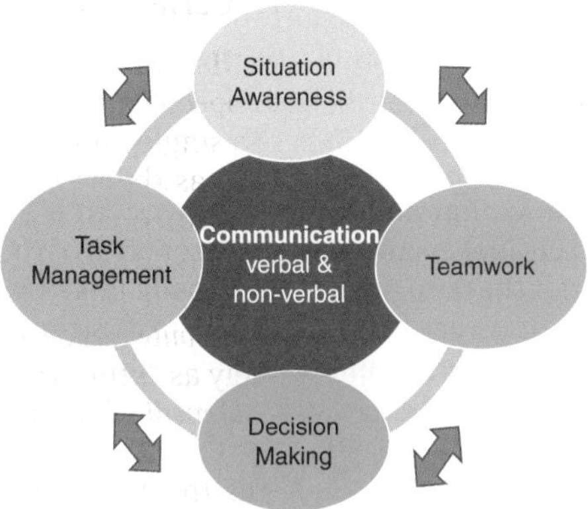

Fig. 6.5 The five main elements of Crisis Resource Management (CRM). The main elements include: Communication, situation awareness, decision making, task management, and teamwork. In this approach, effective communication is like the glue that holds all the other components together. Besides, all the components are intertwined with and related to each other, indicated by the arrows between the elements.

Assessment of NonTechnical Skills. In response to the growing acceptance of human factors and nontechnical skills influencing medical performance, several rubrics to measure NTS have been developed. Gaba and colleagues in 1998 described the direct adaptation for assessment of NTS of a set of CRM-anchored ordinal scale markers from Helmreich et al. concerning aviation.[169,189] In 2004 the ANTS framework was complemented by a behaviorally anchored rating scale in 2004.[182,183] A new set of assessment scales for four markers of NTS was introduced by Weinger and colleagues [75] in 2017 based on the fusion of aspects of a number of prior approaches.

A further, rather new approach for the assessment of nontechnical skills is the Co-ACT framework described by Kolbe and co-workers.[166] The framework serves observing coordination behavior, especially in acute care teams like anesthesia, and consists of four categories, each category obtaining three further subelements that more specifically describe the NTS: (1) *explicit action coordination* with the elements *instruction, speaking up*, and *planning*; (2) *implicit action coordination* with the elements *monitoring, talking to the room* (action-related), and *providing assistance*; (3) *explicit information coordination* with the elements *information request, information evaluation*, and *information upon request*; and (4) *implicit information coordination* with the elements *gathering information, talking to the room (information-related)*, and *information without request*.

Challenges of the Assessment of NonTechnical Skills. The psychometric qualities of measuring NTS have been assessed by the developers of the ANTS system and were considered to be of acceptable level,[182] whereas another study[190] assessed the reliability after a 1-day training for raters and concluded that reliability was poor. A study from Denmark showed good psychometric qualities.[185] Originally developed for educational purposes and used to discuss the NTS of anesthesiologists after training sessions in order to improve in NTS, Zwaan and colleagues assessed the usability and reliability for ANTS in research, finding that the ANTS system was reliable for the total score and usable to measure physicians' NTS in a research setting.[191] However, the investigators found a variation between the reliability of the different elements and recommend excluding elements in advance that are not applicable or observable in the situation of interest. It might not always be easy, however, to identify those elements that should be excluded. On the whole, the ANTS system appears to be a useful tool to enhance assessment of nontechnical skills in anesthesia and other medical fields further, and its careful derivation from an established system of nontechnical assessment in aviation (NOTECHS) may even allow some interdomain comparisons. However, more recently Watkins and colleagues directly compared ANTS with the system used in the Weinger and colleagues 2017 paper [75] and showed that ANTS was more difficult to use but that the two systems otherwise achieved equivalent assessment results.[192]

NonTechnical Skills: The Bad - The Good - The Variable. Good nontechnical skills (i.e., vigilance, efficient communication, team coordination, etc.) reduce the likelihood of active and passive errors and adverse events, and also increase human performance, whereas suboptimal NTS are expected to do the reverse. These effects are variable; for example, a person may communicate very effectively in one instance and fail to do so in the next challenging communication role.

A study from Denmark investigated the relationship between technical and nontechnical skills.[193] Twenty-five video recordings of second-year anesthesiologists managing a simulated difficult airway management scenario were rated with the ANTS instrument[185] and a score for the technical aspect for the procedure. In addition, written descriptions of the NTS performance were collected and content analyzed. The correlation between the two scores was not significant, but the content analysis comparing the NTS description in the best and poorest three scenarios identified what contributed most to good NTS. These were systematically collecting information, thinking ahead, communicating and justifying of decisions, delegating tasks, and vigilantly responding to the evolving situation. Poor NTS were related to: lack of structured approach, lack of articulating plans and decisions, poor resource and task management, lack of considering consequences of treatment, poor response to the evolving situation, and lack of leadership.

What is the Impact of Non-Technical Skills and Human Factors on Poor Performance in Medicine? The impact of poor NTS on poor human performance in the medical field cannot be overestimated. Depending on the literature, it is estimated that up to 80% of all errors in medicine can be attributed to problems with NTS and human factors.[37,38,171-174]

Even though one can argue on the one hand that due to progress in technology the findings and estimates of the pioneer study of Cooper and colleagues[37] performed in 1978 (results relating up to 80% of incidents to human factors) have been outdated for a long time, on the other hand those figures are (1) comparable to findings in other dynamic and complex work environments[171] and (2) newer studies as recent as 2015 still reconfirm those findings (references see below). In the following some illustrative studies are mentioned that link HF and safety challenges.

In 1993 an analysis of 2000 incident reports from the Australian Incident Reporting Study took place, investigating the incidents for relations to human factors and NTS.[38] In 83% of incidents, human factor elements were scored by the reporters. Even though scoring by the incident reporters might not produce results as accurate as those of a systematic scoring by human factor experts and such text descriptions are of limited value for this type of data collection, it still shows the scope of the problem—having also in mind that voluntarily reported incidents only represent the peak of an iceberg, with many incidents not reported at all.

Fletcher and colleagues published a review of studies describing the influence of nontechnical skills in anesthesia in 2002, summarizing that it is clear *"that nontechnical skills play a central role in good anesthesia practice and that a wide range of behaviors are important [...] [including] monitoring, allocation of attention, planning and preparation, situation awareness, prioritization, applying predefined strategies/protocols, flexibility in decision-making, communication, and teamworking"* [p.426].[171]

As increasing evidence suggested that human factors like communication, leadership, and team interaction influence the performance of cardiopulmonary resuscitation (CPR), Hunziker and colleagues[6] presented a study in 2010 reviewing the impact of human factors during simulation-based resuscitation scenarios. Similar to studies in real patients, simulated cardiac arrest scenarios revealed many unnecessary interruptions of CPR as well as significant delays in defibrillation—two outcome-relevant parameters. The studies showed that human factors played a major role in these shortcomings and that medical performance, at least in non-routine situations, depends among others on the quality of leadership and team-structuring.

Jones and co-workers[194] only recently systematically reviewed the literature on the impact of HFs in preventing complications in anesthesia due to poor airway management and highlighted recent national reports and guidelines, including the 4th National Audit Project (NAP4). NAP4 (2011) was the first prospective study of all major airway events occurring throughout the UK, reviewing any complications resulting from airway management that led to either death, brain damage, the need for an emergency surgical airway, unanticipated ICU admission, or prolongation of ICU stay.[173] 184 reports were reviewed. Subsequent in-depth analysis identified HFs as having been a relevant influence in every case, with a median range of 4.5 contributing HFs per case.[195] HFs in the report included for example[173]: casual attitude toward risk/overconfidence, peer tolerance of poor standards, lack of clarity in team structures, poor or dysfunctional communication including incomplete or inadequate handovers, inadequate checking procedures, failure to formulate back-up plans and discuss them with team members, failure to use available equipment, attempts to use unknown equipment in an emergency situation, heavy personal workload, lack of time to undertake thorough assessment, equipment shortage, inexperienced personnel working unsupervised, organizational cultures which induce or tolerate unsafe practices, no formalized requirement to undertake checking procedures, incompatible goals, and reluctance to analyze adverse events and learn from errors.

The Sentinel Event Report of the Joint Commission analyzed the root causes of 764 sentinel events (patient's death, loss in function, unexpected additional care and/or psychological impact) reported voluntarily in 2014.[172] Human-factor-related root causes, including among others communication and leadership, were the leading root causes of sentinel events and made up 65% of root causes. Even though the data are not specifically linked to anesthesia practice, it is very likely that there exist strong parallels.

One of the latest simulation-based studies, performed by Weinger and colleagues [75] in 2017 and explained in detail earlier (section on assessing performance, "Performance as a Function of Experience"), also shows a broad variety of human-factor-related hurdles for anesthesiologists when handling emergencies.

What are the implications of the Impact of Humand Factors and NonTechnical Skills on Human Performance?

- Balancing the importance of technical and non *technical skills during medical education and training.* While technical skills and medical knowledge have always been at the core of medical education and training, the importance of NTS has—despite long growing evidence—only recently been recognized.
- *Acknowledgement of the importance of human factors as individual and team.* One of the first steps for individuals and teams in minimizing and mitigating human frailties and strengthening human strengths—and in consequence reducing medical error and its consequences—is by acknowledging human factors as a part of human performance and thus acknowledging human limitation. The World Health Organization (WHO) states:

"A failure to apply human factors principles is a key aspect of most adverse events in health care. Therefore, all health-care workers need to have a basic understanding of human factors principles. Health-care workers who do not understand the basics of human factors are like infection control professionals not knowing about microbiology." (p. 111)[196]

HUMAN FACTORS ON THE INDIVIDUAL LEVEL

This section will introduce three levels of human factors in more detail: (1) understanding the behavior of individuals (individual level), (2) the interactions between individuals (team level), and (3) their interactions with the organization (organizational level). This first section on the individual level addresses five interrelated elements: (1a) task management, (1b) situation awareness, (1c) decision making, (1d) general individual performance-shaping factors (e.g., fatigue, distractions and noise), and (1e) personal (safety) attitudes.

Task Management

According to the ANTS framework, task management is defined as (p. 8) *"skills for organizing resources and required activities to achieve goals, be they individual case plans or longer-term scheduling issues. It has four skill elements: planning and preparing; prioritizing; providing and maintaining standards; identifying and utilizing resources."*[170]

Anesthesia professionals are often—within the operating room setting—their own phlebotomist, IV inserter, echocardiographer, pharmacist, technician, cleaner, data recorder, patient transporter, as well as performer of activities on behalf of the surgeon (e.g., manipulate the OR table, answer telephone calls, etc.) all while maintaining situation awareness, engaging in decision making, doing administrative tasks, and managing the anesthetic itself. That's a lot of activities! Task management in a team might include the delegation of tasks to appropriate personnel, using effective communication, and closing the loop, both to verify the request was received and understood and then to inform the leader that the task is done, or that there are problems.

Task density can become so high that (1) errors in tasks or their subtasks are more likely; (2) no single person can manage all the tasks alone[89] so that help from team members is needed (teamwork); and (3) tasks may be delayed by interruptions or competing demands, which then require prospective memory[130-134,197] to remember what to do in the future or to correctly resume interrupted actions.

Multitasking and Multiplexing. Sometimes multitasking—doing several things at a time—can be successful, depending on the situation and the tasks at hand. Yet professionals need to be aware that it can be unsuccessful when the situation or the tasks change. When task density becomes high, simple linear performance of tasks becomes impossible; instead more complicated processes of both multitasking and multiplexing are needed. Multitasking—trying to perform two (or more) tasks simultaneously—is frequent in hospital settings,[198] but is virtually impossible to execute if the same cognitive resources are involved. Conducting two or more relatively simple tasks is often possible, such as observing the surgical field while asking the surgeon a straightforward question. Even then there is a risk that one task will be dropped or degraded. However, adjusting an infusion pump while calculating the upcoming dose of antibiotic for an infant would be difficult to do in parallel.

In common use, the term multitasking sometimes refers specifically to media multitasking—everyday attempts to simultaneously work, listen to music, check email and text messages, and search the web. Studies[199,200] have shown that frequent media multitaskers perform worse on psychology laboratory probes of actual multitasking than those who are infrequent media multitaskers. Many suggest that true multitasking is impossible and that almost always there is a decrement of performance on some or all tasks when multitasking is attempted.

The degree to which media multitasking, or laboratory tests, relate to the kinds of multitasking performed by personnel in professional settings of many data streams and many tasks is as yet uncertain; it seems likely that in anesthesia care there are limits to what individuals can safely do on their own.

While simple multitasking in perioperative settings may work, when tasks are complex it may in fact be inefficient. Rather than conducting two (or more) activities in parallel, humans often do things sequentially but shift rapidly between items or back and forth across many simultaneous threads. If the tasks use different cognitive resources, this is referred to as multiplexing.[201] Multiplexing brings the challenges that people (1) have to refocus their concentration each time they switch and (2) are more susceptible to distractions and errors. This is especially true if the tasks at hand involve intensive real-time control as opposed to being cognitively automatic.[201] There is evidence that health care personnel are not aware of the risks of decreased performance when attempting to multitask.[202]

Douglas and co-authors recently reviewed the current literature concerning multitasking in the health care setting.[198] They suggest that multitasking typically results in increased time of task completion, increased stress, risk of memory lapses, and subsequent errors and accidents. Those performance limitations occur more often if one is forced to multitask by the environment and/or if the different tasks compete for the same local cognitive resource. Their review located only two studies on the association between multitasking and errors in the health care setting although nothing definitive was found. Executing two tasks at the same time was found to carry the risk of decreased accuracy and efficiency[203] and to have an increased reaction time to environmental stimuli.[204]

PATIENT SAFETY ACTION BOX

Keep focused. Instead of trying to do several things at once—and maybe none of them well—shift your attention consciously and completely from one task to the next and organize the tasks at hand according to priority. Giving your full attention to what you are doing will help you do it better, with fewer mistakes and less load on your prospective memory. Prevent or modulate avoidable distractions whenever possible.

Multitasking During Handovers?. One study observed different modes of patient handover from the OR to the postanesthesia recovery unit in six hospitals.[205] The researchers compared handovers of (1) *simultaneous* transfer of equipment and information (i.e., a nurse connecting the monitor while at the same time receiving verbal information) to (2) *sequential* transfer (equipment is first connected and lines sorted, then verbal information follows). The findings from 101 observed handovers showed that 65% of them took place simultaneously. Interestingly, simultaneous handovers were not significantly faster than sequential ones (1.8 vs. 2.0 min). In review of postoperative handovers Segall and colleagues[206] recommended: (1) standardize/structure processes (e.g., through the use of checklists and protocols); (2) complete urgent clinical tasks before the information transfer; (3) allow only patient-specific discussions during verbal handovers; (4) require that all relevant team members be present; and (5) provide training in team skills and communication. More information on handoffs is given in the later section on "Communication."

PATIENT SAFETY ACTION BOX

The recommendations given above are helpful for safe postoperative handovers. Another handover type occurs when one anesthesia professional replaces another, temporarily or permanently. And yet another handover is when you have called someone for help or when you are the one coming to help. For this last situation often the person arriving to help concentrates immediately on performing tasks without really listening to the briefing from the original anesthesia professional. Unless the task is critical (e.g., CPR) it is better to wait, assess the situation and the observable information, and then pay full attention to the briefing. For further information on handoffs see section "Effective Communication and Delegation of Tasks."

Situation Awareness

In anesthesia many sources of information need to be scanned in order to get the overview of the situation. These include, but are not limited to: the patient (clinical impression and history), various monitoring equipment, the patient chart, explicit and implicit information by colleagues and OR team members, and workday characteristics (i.e., staff composition, staff shortage, available equipment/time, etc.). Gaba, Howard, and Small introduced the concept of SA in the context of anesthesia in 1995.[110] Schulz and colleagues wrote a review article in 2013 especially on SA in anesthesia. [135]

Situation awareness (SA) describes *"the ability of an individual to maintain an adequate internal representation of the status of the environment in complex and dynamic domains where time constants are short and conditions may change within seconds and minutes"* (p. 729). [135]

SA is a concept drawn from military aviation concerning a variety of aspects of cognition in complex real-time environments. While important itself, situation awareness is influenced by previous decisions, communication patterns, and team dynamics; the level of SA in turn influences team communication and coordination. Situation awareness incorporates the circumstances of the patient at hand (e.g., "Is all required expertise represented?"), the state of the treatment team (e.g., "Is a team member task-overloaded?," "Do team members trust each other?"); and the state of the environment including the rest of the facility (e.g., "Is the problem I'm having also happening elsewhere in my OR suite?").

One of the primary experts on SA, Mica Endsley,[207-209] postulates three different components of individual SA: (1) *Perception* of the elements of a situation/environment within a volume of time and space (= gathering information, detection of cues); (2) *comprehension* of elements and their meaning (= interpretation of information/cues, diagnosis); and (3) *projection* of their status in the near future (= anticipation, prediction). Dekker and Hollnagel challenge this model.[210,211]

Success or failure of SA can occur at each component: gathering, comprehension, and projecting. Some readily available information can be missed, or perceived incorrectly; on the other hand experience makes them sensitive to barely perceptible cues. They also often, but not always, comprehend the meaning of what is perceived by everyone even when others miss its significance.[212] Experts also are usually able to assess the situation not only as it stands but also to project where things are headed, but of course their future projection can be inaccurate or disregarded (including the "everything is OK fixation error").

Schulz and colleagues reviewed 200 incidents in anesthesia and critical care in an in-hospital setting and determined the frequency of situation awareness errors for an individual patient.[136] Admittedly there could be some degree of hindsight bias; nonetheless, situation awareness errors were identified in 81.5% of cases—predominantly in perception (38.0%) and comprehension (31.5%).

Shared Situation Awareness. SA is a concept that can be applied to the individual (personal SA, see above), but also the team (shared SA). Team SA is defined as *"the degree to which every team member possesses the SA required for his or her responsibilities"* (p. 39).[207] Within different professions and different physical positions in the room, the situational awareness and interpretation of the same case can differ substantially within a team, due to variation in experience, involvement, focus point, interest, knowledge, or information. Of course, not every bit of information can be shared with the whole team; doing so would overwhelm everyone. Yet, creating and maintaining an overall shared mental model of the situation across all team members is critical for determining the best plan of action for patient care. Some team communication in the operating room that seemingly does not serve an obvious purpose, might, in fact, be a gauging of shared mental models and therefore shared SA.[213,214] Anesthesia professionals, for example, routinely assess the progress and possible complications of the operation by perceiving nuances in the conversation of the surgeons.[213]

Shared mental models predict good team performance[215] and were, for example, shown to be related to positive performance in trauma teams, with team leaders and followers actively working toward an information exchange.[216] Adapted from psychology and management literature, Schmutz and Eppich[217] introduced the conceptual framework of team reflexivity to health care. They propose that shared SA is fostered by components of team reflexivity, namely (1) pre-action briefing, (2) in-action deliberation, and (3) post-action debriefing. Fioratou and colleagues[218] challenge the common model of individual and team SA and instead introduced the model of distributed situation awareness (DSA) to anesthesia, arguing that cognition actually involves elements of the (physical) environment, for example, the values on a monitor.

A multicenter study from Denmark explored shared mental models of surgical teams during 64 video-assisted thoracoscopic surgery lobectomies to explore familiarity of the people involved in the operation with each other; mutual assessment of technical and nontechnical skills in the other persons present during the operation; assessment of the perceived risk for the patient from the procedure and from the anesthetic; and noting of problems in the present co-works task management. There was poor agreement between team members' risk ratings showing limitations in how much the members of the surgical team share a mental model about the patient and the related risks. A follow-up study demonstrated the connection between relevant clinical markers and shared mental models.

Other aspects of situation awareness have already been introduced within the "core cognitive process model" in an earlier section. Box 6.2 gives examples of reevaluation questions in order to maintain situation awareness.

Decision Making

Decision making is the generic term for the cognitive and emotional processes of determining appropriate information seeking and actions in a changing environment. It involves "*skills for reaching a judgement to select a course of action or make a diagnosis about a situation, in both normal conditions and in time-pressured crisis situations. It … [includes]: identifying options; balancing risks and selecting options [and] re-evaluating"* (p. 13).[170] Many aspects of the anesthesia professional's decision making have already been addressed in the earlier section where the "core cognitive process model" was introduced, so for more information the reader is referred back to that section.

Although decision making in anesthesiology involves many sorts of perioperative decisions, this chapter is particularly interested in the processes used for the non-routine decisions made during the management of problems or crises. This is a very complex process. Although information is sometimes used in what seems to be a purely rational manner,[219,220] decision making is affected strongly by a number of non-rational elements such as group pressure, ingrained habits, cognitive biases, and perceptual illusions. When determining the alternatives and their various pros and cons the set of options available or their perceived value will also vary.

Traditional concepts of decision making in much of medicine (not anesthesiology) have concentrated on relatively static, well-structured decisions. For example, should patient A with an elevated blood pressure be treated for hypertension with drug X, or should no treatment be started? Other studies have looked at diagnosis as an isolated task (specifically, diagnostic explanation) both in internal medicine and in radiology. These approaches to decision making have not captured the unique aspects of dynamism, time pressure, and uncertainty seen in anesthesiology. Since the 1980s, several paradigms have emerged regarding decision making and action in complex real-world situations.

On the one hand there are models that have their basis largely in research done in the psychology laboratory investigating the limits and pitfalls of decision making under controlled conditions, especially delineating cognitive biases. Daniel Kahneman and his colleague Amos Tversky won a Nobel Prize in Economics in 2002 for this kind of research. While Tversky passed away in 1999 Kahneman continued to work on decision making, and he recently synthesized and summarized the topic in the popular book *Thinking Fast and Slow*.[212] Two cognitive systems are described. System I is intuitive (heuristic), very fast, less concerned with the precision of the information processing and decision (as long as it is approximately correct) and more concerned with reducing cognitive load. Research about heuristic decision making shows that reducing the amount of information considered can still lead to equally good or superior decisions.[221] System II is analytical, slow but able to consider in detail the sources of information and the fine points of a decision. Especially in time-critical situations humans tend to run on System I as long as possible, sometimes too long—accepting imprecise results when precision is actually needed. Understanding the pitfalls of System I thinking can help professionals to lower the bar for their activation of System II. Another approach to studying and describing decision making, based on observational research on professionals engaged in doing complex decision-making work in real-world settings (or simulations thereof) is known as naturalistic decision making (NDM), with Gary Klein, Judith Orasanu, and others as the pioneers.[45,114,118] Models in NDM-oriented work also invoke the idea of parallel systems of decision making, one heuristic and fast, the other systematic, precise, and slow, as well as a number of other aspects of iterative consideration of useful actions.

The core cognitive process model including dynamic decision making (see earlier section on "Core Cognitive Process Model of the Anesthesia Professional") is based largely on the NDM model, but is consistent with Kahneman's description of System I and System II. In fact, Klein and Kahnemann have co-written a paper that outlines how their two approaches are in many ways similar, while in a few ways somewhat different. [222] A common (if incomplete) way to describe this is that the work of Kahneman and Tversky emphasizes the pitfalls and errors of decision making, NDM emphasizes how it is often successful despite these risks.

Stiegler and Tung—representing views influenced by the Kahneman-Tversky research—(1) identified current theories of human decision behavior in the context of anesthesia, which are: expected utility, Bayesian probability, formalized pattern matching, heuristics, dual process reasoning, and sensemaking; (2) identified common effects of non-rational cognitive processes on decision making; and (3) suggested strategies to improve anesthesia decision making.[121]

In another publication, Stiegler and co-workers summarized the most common cognitive/non-rational errors detected specific to anesthesiology practice; the leading 10 errors were anchoring, availability bias, premature closure, feedback bias, framing effect, confirmation bias, omission bias, commission bias, overconfidence, and sunk costs.[61] In a simulated emergency setting, the frequency of seven of those errors was over 50%, with premature closure (accepting a diagnosis prematurely, failure to consider reasonable differential of possibilities) and confirmation bias (seeking or acknowledging only information that confirms the desired or suspected diagnosis) being the most common cognitive errors with a frequency of nearly 80% each. In 2016 the Joint Commission also published a paper on the safety issues of cognitive errors and factors that can predispose or increase the likelihood of cognitive biases.[62]

Gigerenzer frames the view on the characteristics of human decision making differently.[223,224] What is called biases in other frameworks is seen as relevant features of human cognition and decision making that allow for functional perception and action in a very complicated world. Perhaps like NDM, this view suggests that theories of decision making do not really describe decision making in the real world. For example, in many situations it will not be possible to collect all relevant decision alternatives, to assess them fully, and to select the best option. There might not be enough data available about the alternatives and/or the evaluation might take too long. The "take-the-best" (also termed "satisficing") heuristic suggests that decision makers consider what they see as a key feature for the decision and only compare any alternatives along this criterion. Further criteria are only considered if the first ones do not identify an acceptable option.

PERFORMANCE-SHAPING FACTORS ON THE INDIVIDUAL LEVEL

The previous discussion about the performance of skilled anesthesia professionals has mostly assumed that they are normally fit, rested, and acting in a standard working environment. However, human performance on the individual level also depends on so-called performance-shaping factors such as interruptions, distractions, fatigue, and stress. Performance-shaping factors can predispose a person to error. Experience in human performance in the laboratory and other domains suggests that internal and external performance-shaping factors exert profound effects on the ability of even highly trained personnel. The degree to which this occurs and to which it affects patient outcome is highly uncertain. In extreme cases, such as profound fatigue, it is obvious these factors result in severe degradation of the anesthesia professional's performance or even complete incapacitation. However, these extreme conditions are quite unusual, and it is still unclear whether the levels of performance decrement most frequently seen in typical work situations have any significant effects.

Several performance-shaping factors are potentially of sufficient magnitude to be of concern. Those include ambient noise, music, distraction by personal electronic devices, distraction by other personnel, fatigue and sleep deprivation, aging, illness, drug use, and relatively fixed hazardous attitudes. These are discussed in the course of this section. A variety of other performance-shaping issues such as the level of illumination and environmental temperature are not dealt with in this chapter.

Currently, the responsibility for ensuring fitness for duty rests solely with the individual clinician. In high-reliability organizations (see later), where the maintenance of organizational safety is one of the key elements, the institution implements measures to mitigate decrements due to performance-shaping factors. As health care systems address issues of human performance and patient safety more seriously, these aspects of work will need to be dealt with.

Distractions and Interruptions in the Operating Room

Several recent publications deal with distractions and interruptions in the OR. For detailed information the reader is referred to further literature,[68,95,96,225-234] as the upcoming section can only give a brief overview on the topic.

Ambient Noise and Music. The workplace of anesthesia professionals—predominantly, but not exclusively, the operating room—is a very complex physical and cognitive setting. Unless there is an unusual effort to reduce sound levels the routine noises of the suction, surgical equipment (electrocautery, pneumatic or electric power tools), and monitoring equipment yield levels considerably higher than in most offices or control rooms. Other sound sources such as conversation and music are controllable. The potential interference of noise with communication and situation awareness[235] among personnel in the OR is particularly worrisome to those concerned with optimizing teamwork in this complex work environment.[68,236]

The use of music in the OR is now widespread. Many health care professionals believe that music enlivens the workday and can build team cohesiveness when all team members enjoy the music. Others note that in some cases the volume level of music makes it harder to hear the rhythm and tone of the pulse oximeter and alarms as well as work-related conversation between team members. A laboratory study by Stevenson and colleagues determined that visual attentional loads and auditory distractions additively reduced anesthesiology residents' ability to detect changes in pulse oximeter tone.[235]

A controversial study by two social psychologists, Allen and Blascovich, suggested that surgeon-selected music improved surgeons' performance on a serial subtraction task and reduced their autonomic reactivity (i.e., "relaxed" them) when compared with control conditions consisting of experimenter-selected music or no music at all.[237] The methodology of this study has been criticized.[238] In response to Allen and Blascovich, several anesthesiologists challenged the notion that the surgeon's preference for the type or volume of music can or should override the needs of other members of the team.[238]

Murthy and colleagues[239] studied the effect of OR noise (80 to 85 dB) and music on knot-tying ability in a laparoscopic skill simulator. They found no difference in time or knot quality in the conditions tested and concluded that surgeons can effectively block out noise and music. The invited commentary that accompanied the article brings up important issues: What impact does noise have on other members of the surgical team? How does noise affect communication between team members? Does noise affect judgment? The question of the proper role of music in the OR has no simple answer. Clearly, optimal patient care is the primary goal. Some surgical or anesthesia personnel explicitly forbid any type of music in the OR. A more common approach of many OR teams is to allow any team member to veto the choice or volume of music if they believe that it interferes with their work.

PATIENT SAFETY ACTION BOX

Distractions include music, social conversation, and jokes. Each of these activities is appropriate under the right circumstances. They can make the work environment more pleasant and promote the development of team spirit, but they can also seriously lessen your ability to detect and correct problems. This issue can be raised during the presurgical time-out to ensure that all personnel agree. During patient care you must take charge of modulating these activities so that they do not become distracting. If the music is too loud, one must insist that the volume be reduced or that it be turned off (a rule of thumb is that the pulse oximeter volume should always be louder than the music or conversation). When a crisis occurs, all distractions should be eliminated or reduced as much as possible.

Reading and Use of Mobile Electronic Devices. The observation that some anesthesia professionals have been seen to read journals or books casually during patient care led to a vigorous debate of the appropriateness of such activity.[240] Although it is indisputable that reading could distract attention from patient care, a study by Slagle and Weinger in 2009 suggested that when the practice of reading is confined to low-workload portions of a case, it has no effect on vigilance.[65] Many comments about the issue were related not to the actual decrement in vigilance induced by reading but rather to the impact of the negative perception of the practice and of those who do it by surgeons and by patients, if they were aware of it.

This issue has been greatly magnified by now-ubiquitous smartphones and social media. Nearly all clinical personnel (other than those scrubbed into surgery) have a smartphone immediately at hand. These provide great temptation for both pull activities—reading email, websites, or social media sites—and push activities, notification of new text messages, mail, or social media posts. The wide variety of channels of information makes it far more likely for people to spend time interacting with their phones than with newspapers, journals, or books. The content available is never ending. In their survey, Soto and colleagues give a current update of the usage patterns, risks, and benefits of personal electronic device use in the operating room.[241]

Distractions Caused by Work Itself. An important source of distraction is actually the work itself. That is, engaging in one task can distract attention from other important tasks. Repositioning the patient on the operating table (or rotating the table itself) can take a surprising amount of time and physical and mental effort. During these tasks it can be difficult, and in some cases impossible, to maintain all usual data streams, or to view, hear, or attend to them. Another highly distracting activity is the use of echocardiography, which requires focused attention on the image and manipulation of the probe and of the device's interface. While it may generate crucial clinical information, it can also distract attention from other important monitors or the surgical field.

Interruptions. Beyond distracting attention from important data streams, various stimuli can also cause "interruptions" in the sequence of conducting a task.[95] Campbell and associates[96] found that slightly more than 20% of distractions—particularly interruptions—were associated with an observable negative impact. Such events are particularly problematic when they disrupt prospective memory which is one's ability to *remember in the future* to perform an action or to resume interrupted tasks in the right spot.[132] It is particularly prone to disruption by concurrent tasks or interruptions. In anesthesia, for example, if the anesthesia professional suspends ventilation temporarily (say to allow a radiograph to be taken), the intention to restart the ventilator depends on prospective memory and can be easily forgotten.

A variety of methods may preserve prospective memory of intentions. Visual or auditory reminders can be used (physiologic monitor alarms often serve this purpose whether intended or not), although the effectiveness of such methods is variable.

PATIENT SAFETY ACTION BOX

Special actions—such as leaving one's finger on the ventilator switch when one has turned off the ventilator for an appropriate reason—can be used to indicate that an important intention is pending. Another strategy is putting a small sign on the ventilator to remind you that it is off. As a last resort in this example, properly set alarms should warn you of apnea should you forget to turn the ventilator back on. Depending on the requested action another strategy can be to accustom oneself to consciously finish tasks entirely before starting the next task (see also section on Task Management). If team members interrupt during a task it can be helpful to let them know that you are busy, something like "One moment please, you'll have my full attention shortly." However, asking others to help you remember ("can you please remind me"), has shown to be a less effective strategy, apparently because it diffuses the responsibility to actually remember.

Resulting Implications. Clearly, for all these distractions and interruptions the pros and cons of policing them need to be balanced. In our opinion—similar to those of Slagle and Weinger[65]—blanket policies against reading nonessential materials or interacting with mobile phones except for patient care needs are both doomed to failure and possibly detrimental. First, because they are hard to enforce and any intensive efforts to eradicate the use of such devices at work is likely to generate a tense work climate despite the best safety intentions of proponents. Second, because reading or phone use might actually counteract boredom in some situations and thus might increase performance. Third, these distractions are not necessarily any different from many other kinds of activities not related to patient care that are routinely accepted, such as social conversation among personnel. Of course, there are reasonable limits for such activities.

The bottom line is, to quote Slagle and Weinger: "*(1) the patient must be the foremost priority and (2) being distracted or performing noncritical tasks during critical or unstable situations is inappropriate and dangerous*" (p. 282).[65] In the end it is important for anesthesia professionals to keep in mind that there are potential pitfalls linked to distractions and that the anesthesia professional is responsible for modulating controllable distractions and for developing work processes that balance the cognitive load of tasks against their personal, clinical, or teambuilding utility. Allowing music during routine work (if all agree) and a modest amount of reading or smartphone use, but emphasizing the need to reduce or eliminate it when it is too distracting, the workload increases, or a situation becomes complex or urgent is one example. The threshold for abandoning any potential distraction to provide maximum attention to patient care should be rather low.

In response to the patient safety concerns related to distractions and interruptions in the OR and other patient care areas from the use of personal electronic devices for non-patient-related purposes, several professional societies and organizations have established position statements and guidelines to define appropriate use of those devices in the OR.[242-245] Some health care settings have implemented a "no interruption zone"[242,246] during critical phases of patient care activities, in the style of a "sterile cockpit" concept,[100] derived from aviation regulations that prohibit crewmembers from engaging in any activity except those duties required for the safe operation of the aircraft during critical phases of flight.

Stress. Stress is a performance-shaping factor that influences human performance. To go into detail about stress is beyond the scope of this chapter. Therefore the reader is referred to other references for more details.[11,247]

Sleep Deprivation and Fatigue

Fatigue is common in the life of anesthesia professionals, whether due to work hours, on-call duties, or the vagaries of life with children and otherwise. Sleep can be thought of as a physiologic drive state similar to hunger or thirst and is necessary for maintenance of alertness, performance, and overall well-being. The amount of sleep required by any individual is genetically determined and is the amount that allows that individual to be awake and alert throughout the day. The average sleep time for young adults is 7 to 8 hours per 24-hour period, with an approximately 15% interindividual variation. These sleep requirements do not change with age, and humans can do little to train their physiology to function optimally on less sleep than required.

The physiology and psychology of sleep and sleep deprivation are well established, and this section can only provide a cursory summary of what is known.

Sleep Debt. Sleep loss is cumulative and results in what is referred to as sleep debt. An individual who has obtained an optimal amount of sleep is better prepared to perform long periods of sustained work than one who is operating from a sleep debt. Because of the additive effects of chronic partial sleep loss, even minor sleep restriction on a nightly basis can insidiously accumulate into a substantial sleep debt. The only way to pay back a sleep debt is with sleep. Sleep debts are commonplace in our culture. The National Sleep Foundation's annual survey continues to reveal that Americans chronically undersleep by 30 to 90 minutes each day.[248] Shift work, long and irregular work hours, and the demands of family and recreation lead to irregular sleep patterns and prevent restful sleep. This is particularly true for health care workers, who often work in shifts, have long duty periods, and must frequently care for patients for long periods. To some degree it seems as if sleep deprivation might have led into a situation that is more dangerous than one thinks.

Circadian Rhythms. Our biological clock, responsible for the human circadian system, is synchronized to the 24-hour day by external stimuli referred to as "zeitgebers," the most influential of which is the light-dark cycle of day and night. The circadian system is biphasic in that it produces a state of increased sleep tendency and decreased performance capacity during two periods throughout the 24-hour day—from 2 a.m. to 6 a.m. and from 2 p.m. to 6 p.m. These are periods when professionals are more vulnerable to incidents and accidents because the body clock is "turned off." The circadian clock is very resistant to alterations, and it does not adjust rapidly to changes such as those produced by jet lag or shift work. Disruption of the normal circadian rhythm or incomplete circadian adaptation leads to acute and chronic sleep deprivation, decreased alertness, increased subjective fatigue, and decreased physical and mental performance.[249]

Sleepiness and Alertness. Sleepiness and alertness are at opposite ends of a continuum. Daytime sleepiness is the most obvious effect of failing to obtain adequate sleep. Data from the U.S. Department of Transportation reveal that the greatest number of single-vehicle accidents takes place during the early morning hours when people are at a circadian lull of alertness. These accidents are thought to result from inadvertent lapses in driver attention brought about by extremes of sleepiness.[250]

Both behavioral and subjective sleepiness can be masked by a stimulating environment. When environmental stimuli wane, physiologic sleepiness manifests itself as an overwhelming propensity to fall asleep. A person who is physiologically alert does not experience sleepiness as environmental stimuli decrease. For example, without physiologic sleepiness, an individual may become bored during a lecture but does not fall asleep.

Microsleep Events. The most extreme cause of impaired vigilance is the occurrence of actual sleep episodes (microsleeps) encroaching into periods of wakefulness. Microsleep events typically last a few seconds to a few minutes. They are intermittent in onset, and their impending occurrence is difficult for the individual to predict. Most individuals underestimate their level of sleepiness when they can be objectively shown to be extremely sleepy, thus making this problem even more insidious. This has significant meaning in the workplace and when driving home after long work periods.

Microsleeps are a sign of extreme sleepiness and are harbingers of the onset of longer sleep periods. Typically, they occur during periods of low workload or stimulation and when an individual is maximally sleepy. In addition, an individual's performance between microsleep episodes is impaired. Frequent and longer microsleeps increase the number of errors of omission.

Evaluation of Physiologic Sleepiness in Anesthesia Residents. Using the Multiple Sleep Latency Test (MSLT), a sleep disorder diagnostic tool, Howard and colleagues evaluated the physiologic (objective) daytime sleepiness of anesthesia residents under three different conditions: (1) baseline (daytime shift, no on-call duty period in the previous 48 hours), (2) post-call (immediately after a 24-hour work and in-house on-call period), and (3) sleep extended.[251,252] In the sleep-extended condition, residents were told to maximize sleep and were allowed to arrive for work at 10 am (3 to 4 hours later than normal) for 4 consecutive days before testing. They were not on call during this time. The sleep-extended condition was included to provide a true control state of maximal rest and optimum alertness. In this study, for anesthesia residents the MSLT scores for baseline as well as for post-call condition revealed the nearly pathologic levels of daytime sleepiness seen in patients with narcolepsy or sleep apnea. The baseline group slept an average of 7.1 ± 1.5 hours per night, whereas the post-call group reported an average of 6.3 ± 1.9 hours of sleep during their night on call. Ironically, although the on-call periods occurred during rotations that often have very busy call nights, only a few subjects were, in fact, awake most of the night. In the sleep-extended condition, the subjects extended their sleep to an average of more than 9 hours per night, and MSLT scores were in the normal range. These results clearly demonstrate that medical personnel who have not been on call cannot be assumed to be rested when compared with fatigued post-call residents. These data also indicate that under normal working conditions, the resident physicians studied were physiologically sleepy to nearly pathologic levels. Notably, these data cast substantial doubt on previous studies of the performance of medical personnel that have relied on the assumption that individuals working under normal conditions are truly rested.

Evaluation of Subjective Sleepiness in Anesthesia Residents. The previously mentioned study also investigated the connection between subjective and physiologic sleepiness. In the previously discussed study, Howard and colleagues also investigated the degree of discrepancy between the residents' subjective sleepiness (how sleepy they felt) and their physiologic sleepiness (how easily they fell asleep). Subjects' self-reported sleepiness immediately before each sleep opportunity did not, in general, correlate with their measured sleepiness. The authors also found that subjects demonstrated little ability to determine whether they had actually fallen asleep. For example, in 51% of trials in which the electroencephalographic and electro-oculographic measurements showed that the subject had fallen asleep, the subjects thought they had remained awake throughout the test. These results support the contention that medical personnel are physiologically vulnerable to degraded alertness yet are unable to perceive this decrement. Thus, an anesthesia professional could, in fact, fall asleep during a case, awaken, and be totally unaware of the lapse in vigilance.

Mood. Long work hours, fatigue, and sleep deprivation have been shown to bring about consistent and dramatic changes in mood and emotions. Depression, anxiety, irritability, anger, and depersonalization have all been shown to increase during testing of chronically fatigued house staff. These emotions are an obvious source of stress between anesthesia professionals and their co-workers, patients, and families. The relationship of mood, performance, and patient safety has yet to be determined.

Sleep Inertia. Sleep inertia corresponds to the period of reduced ability to function optimally immediately on awakening. This phenomenon usually occurs when individuals are awakened out of slow-wave sleep and is manifested as grogginess and impaired performance lasting as long as 15 to 30 minutes after awakening. Sleep inertia can also occur after being awakened from normal sleep and is most common during the early morning circadian trough (2 to 6 am). Depending on the preexisting level of sleepiness, individuals who take naps longer than 40 minutes are at greater risk for sleep inertia on awakening.

PATIENT SAFETY ACTION BOX

Sleep inertia can be important to health care professionals who may be awakened out of deep sleep to provide emergency care to patients (e.g., emergency cesarean section or emergency intubation). If urgent work can be anticipated, the sleeping individual should be awakened with sufficient time (at least 15 minutes) to minimize the fogginess and decrement in performance associated with sleep inertia. Another option is to not sleep longer than short naps in situations where immediate performance is required. If sleep inertia is unavoidable, it would be wise for the affected person to ask for help until the grogginess dissipates.

Effects of Fatigue on Anesthesiologists' Performance and Patient Outcome. It is highly uncertain as to whether, how, or in what circumstances these established psychophysical changes might interact with clinical work processes to affect patient safety in anesthesiology. Various methods are used for assessing an individual's level of sleepiness, including behavioral indicators, subjective measures, and physiologic (objective) measures.

The survey by Gaba and associates revealed that more than 50% of respondents believed that they had made an error in clinical management that they thought was related to fatigue.[56] In another survey of anesthesiologists and CRNAs, 61% of respondents recalled having made an error in the administration of anesthesia that they attributed to fatigue. In a study in 2011, a large, national, random sample of CRNAs in the United States was asked to complete an anonymous survey to quantify sleep activity.[253] Findings of the almost 1300 respondents revealed that nearly 16% have experienced sleep-related behavior during a surgical case, and close to 50% have witnessed a colleague asleep during a case. A similar survey of CRNAs was conducted in 2015, where nearly 30% of the 325 respondents reported they had committed a patient care error because of fatigue.[254]

The challenge of sleep deprivation and fatigue in medical personnel was addressed by the Joint Commission on Accreditation of Healthcare Organizations in 2011 in a Sentinel Event Alert on "Health Care Worker Fatigue and Patient Safety."[255] The Sentinel Event Alert is public and can be retrieved from the homepage of the Joint Commission. Sinha and co-workers ask: *"The fatigued anesthesiologist: A threat to patient safety?"*[256] and Gregory and Edsell picked up the topic in their educational publication in 2014.[257]

Considerable research on fatigue effects has targeted the transportation industries, especially driving which needs both continuous vigilance and psychomotor skill. If a driver has microsleeps lasting many seconds a problem is likely, unless the road is quite straight or there is an autosteering/autospeed autonomy. Even in health care, studies have largely been carried out in hospital ward settings where, during night on-call shifts, they may have responsibility for many patients.[258] The anesthesiology environment is different. Each patient having anesthesia will have at least one anesthesia professional in constant attendance and that individual is not directly responsible for other patients at the same time. Moreover, although vigilance is indeed the slogan of the ASA, there are few situations that require sustained second-by-second attention. The demand for high vigilance and effort does not usually occur at random; such situations are usually present at induction, emergence, and a few key milestones during the surgical procedure. Critical events are uncommon, and even when the chain of accident evolution has begun, the clinical team will likely have multiple opportunities to detect and correct it before any substantive negative impact has occurred. Thus, while anesthesia personnel may be prone to fatigue, and complaints about sleepiness and fatigue are common, the probability of a negative patient outcome during anesthesia directly attributable to sleepiness alone is very small. In health care, there is no formal mechanism for evaluating causation in adverse events, let alone for evaluating sleep-wake issues and fatigue, so one does not know the full contribution of this factor to negative outcomes. As for many aspects of human performance, variables that can be reliably and precisely measured do not capture the complexity or the typical resilience of clinical work. Conversely, measures and techniques that do address such factors are by nature non-quantitative and invasive.

Howard and colleagues conducted a study of rested versus sleep-deprived (awake for 25 hours on a pseudo-on-call period) anesthesiology residents by collecting multiple measures of performance during a 4-hour high-fidelity simulation scenario: Mood questionnaire, PVT psychomotor reaction time, response time to secondary task probes, and response to changing clinical events.[78] Psychomotor tests revealed progressive impairment of alertness, mood, and performance over the course of the pseudo–on-call period, as well as on the experimental day, when compared with the well-rested condition. Secondary task probe response times were slower after sleep deprivation, although this reached statistical significance for just one of three probe types. No statistical difference in case management between conditions was reported—in fact, subjects in both conditions made significant errors. Sleep-deprived subjects cycled (often rapidly) in and out of sleepy behavior, and the most impaired individuals showed such behavior for more than 25% of the experiment (60 minutes).

A key thing learned about fatigue during this study[78] was that highly fatigued anesthesia personnel in simulations are not either awake all the time or asleep all the time. Rather they usually cycled frequently in and out of states of apparent wakefulness, drowsiness, and microsleeps throughout the simulated case. Typically, when awake their performance was at most mildly degraded but when they showed extreme drowsiness or were actually asleep their performance was essentially zero. Participants were observed being totally asleep at one moment but awakening just in time to happen to catch a probe stimulus or clinical event, and respond to it satisfactorily. For most subjects the fraction of time spent in highly impaired states was low as their microsleeps were brief, in part because even a quiet routine clinical setting has a variety of stimuli, including other personnel and their tasks. The intrinsic redundancies in the OR team, the potential benefits of monitor alarms, and the resilience of clinical systems and patients may explain why catastrophes during anesthesia are very rare even though many operations are conducted with personnel suffering from substantial chronic and acute fatigue.

Fatigue Countermeasures. Anesthesia professionals cannot prevent sleepiness by willpower alone because it is a fundamental physiologic drive. Strategies that institutions or practitioners can use to minimize the negative effects of sleepiness and fatigue on performance include: education and promotion of safety culture, improved sleep habits, rest breaks at work, strategic napping, medications and social drugs, and light therapy. Strategies that national bodies and professional societies and organizations can call for are reasonable duty hour requirements.

Duty Hour Requirements. One direct regulatory strategy to minimize sleep deprivation has been to limit the work hours of clinicians. For the most part this has been attempted only for those in training (who traditionally have worked very long hours both during the day and in nighttime on-call). Results of process and outcome studies have varied but there has been no proof that such regulations, by themselves, improve patient safety.[259] Changing work schedules will not eliminate chronic fatigue, and in settings where clinicians at night may cover large numbers of unfamiliar patients the probability of information loss and confusion across the handoffs may outweigh any benefits of greater alertness. Yet, these findings may not apply to the anesthesiologists' operating room environment in the same way. The previous studies provided addressed the effects of sleep deprivation and fatigue on physician performance and well-being.

Back in 2003 the Accreditation Council for Graduate Medical Education (ACGME) instituted the first set of common duty hour requirements for all accredited residency training programs in the United States. Those requirements were revised in 2011[260] in response to the 2009 Institute of Medicine (IOM) report entitled *Resident Duty Hours: Enhancing Sleep, Supervision, and Safety*. A white paper published by Blum and colleagues debates the latest information and innovative practices on the topic and discusses how to best implement the 2009 IOM recommendations.[261] Work hour regulations in the European Union and in Australia or New Zealand are much more stringent than they are for trainees in the United States. For more details on work hour regulations see also further literature.[259,262,263]

Education and Safety Culture. A first and relatively simple and inexpensive step in addressing sleepiness and fatigue of medical personnel is to educate practitioners and the administrators of health care institutions about the impact of sleep issues on work performance, mood, job satisfaction, and health. Educational programs covering sleep deprivation, circadian disruption and fatigue, and countermeasures have been enthusiastically adopted by an increasing fraction of the aviation community. Similar programs should be developed for the health care community. However, it is clear at both the individual and organizational level that education will not be sufficient to address this issue fully. Other competing forces, for example measures of production versus safety, are very powerful and difficult for practitioners to manage.

The organizational framework plays a major role. Only if fatigue is seen as an organizational issue affecting safety negatively and safety is made a high organizational priority with all the resulting consequences, will fatigue-related safety issues be minimized. For an organization that implies, for example, that (a) tired staff are not always implicitly expected to work under all circumstances, (b) opportunities are created for tired staff to rest and to recover (i.e., regular rest breaks, strategic napping, etc.), and (c) an organizational safety culture is fostered that allows anesthesiologists to call for the assistance of a colleague (teamwork, speak up, see next section) when they know that they are impaired (from fatigue or for any other reason), without any negative consequences (cowardice, etc.). For additional countermeasures also see the Sentinel Event Alert of the Joint Commission[255] introduced earlier.

IMPROVED SLEEP HABITS. It is important to obtain adequate sleep. Most adults need at least 8 hours and the amount you need will not change—no matter what you do. Good sleep habits include the following: regularity of bedtime and wake-up time; sufficient time for sustained and individually adequate sleep; restriction of alcohol, caffeine, and nicotine before bedtime; and use of exercise, nutrition, and environmental factors so that they enhance rather than disturb sleep. Also, mobile devices should be put aside about half an hour before sleep—not only because of their (blue) light that signals "wake-up time" to the body, but also because a lot of what you read in them might get your heart-rate up, not down.

A regular sleep schedule is an important part of optimal sleep hygiene, but it is often not possible for medical personnel, given the requirement to cover clinical needs on a 24-hour basis. It helps to maintain as constant a sleep schedule as possible and to maximize sleep opportunities before and after periods of reduced sleep. Social drug use can have profound effects on sleep (see below). Ideally, the sleep setting should be a dark, quiet room devoid of sources of interruption such as pets, telephones, pagers, and children. Psychological stressors increase baseline physiologic arousal and can impair the quality and quantity of sleep. When possible, effort should be made to separate the work of the day with a period of relaxation before attempting to initiate sleep.

Caffeine and other stronger stimulants are known to reduce nocturnal sleep if ingested close to bedtime, hence decreasing sleep quantity and quality. Potent stimulants such as amphetamines do produce increased alertness and performance, but they have significant side effects and are not an option for health care personnel (e.g., the individual must undergo a substantial amount of recovery sleep ["crash"] after their effect is gone).

Rest Breaks, Strategic Napping at Work, and Use of Caffeine

REST BREAKS. Although other industries have openly recognized the reality of decrements in vigilance resulting from fatigue and sleepiness, the health care system has not. Rest breaks and rotation of task duties are mandatory for air traffic controllers and are part of naval ship command procedures in an attempt to prevent potential lapses in vigilance. Short breaks in surgery have been shown to increase productivity and job satisfaction, and they probably also help alleviate boredom.[264] The organizational hurdle in anesthesia: oftentimes an extra anesthesia professional would be necessary to provide these opportunities on a regular basis.

The optimal timing and length of breaks are unknown, but periodic relief from duty should be taken when possible. Cooper and co-workers studied the effects of intraoperative exchange of anesthesia personnel.[265,266] Although in some cases the process of relieving OR personnel caused a problem, it more frequently was associated with the discovery of a preexisting problem. The positive effect of relief of personnel probably depends on the quality of the handover briefing conducted by anesthesia professionals. If anesthesia professionals are unable to obtain a break during long work periods, they can take other measures to remain alert. They can engage other OR personnel in conversation (although this, too, can be distracting), thereby increasing the level of stimulation in the environment. Walking around and standing up are also techniques that decrease subjective (but not physiologic) sleepiness.

STRATEGIC NAPPING AT WORK. If adequate sleep during the night cannot be obtained, naps can be used to decrease sleepiness and improve performance. The optimal nap length for most individuals is about 45 minutes; this duration acutely improves alertness, allows improved performance, and minimizes the possibility of sleep inertia on awakening. Naps as short as 10 minutes have beneficial effects on alertness. A nap of 90 to 120 minutes allows a full sleep cycle and can additionally boost alertness and performance over that of shorter nap periods.

Health care professionals oftentimes have an individual and cultural tendency to ignore or to minimize the effect of fatigue and sleep deprivation and to view work breaks and naps as signs of weakness. The military has addressed similar attitudes with the concept of 10 minute power napping, presenting naps in a positive light as a sign of wisdom and strength rather than one of cowardice and frailty. Again, the predominant organizational safety culture is one of the key elements—how critical safety and quality issues like fatigue are judged and how those obstacles are met (see above and later sections on "Patient Safety at the Organizational Level").

Smith-Coggins and associates studied the effect of naps during the night shift on health care providers working in a busy suburban university emergency department.[267] The investigators found that a nap improved performance on some (but not all) measures. The most important result of this study may be the fact that the subjects were able to (1) use this strategy successfully in the real workplace and (2) improve alertness and performance. At some sites within the Veterans' Affairs system a strategic nap program has been successfully developed and implemented in ICU settings.[268] Components included a formal educational program, guidelines for the individual practitioner and the facility, and other guidance for implementation. No additional staff members were required for the implementation, as the program allows individuals to nap during scheduled break periods. Certain issues complicate the appropriate use of naps by medical professionals. Locating space for the nap has proven to be a major (and continuing) hurdle.

USE OF CAFFEINE. Physicians frequently use caffeine to stay awake and to increase alertness temporarily during on-call periods, but often its use could be more strategic. Strategic use of caffeine includes (1) knowledge of its onset (15 to 30 minutes) and duration of action (3 to 4 hours) and (2) use when alertness is required and the opportunity to sleep is minimal. Besides its alerting effects, caffeine produces an increase in awakenings and decreases the total nocturnal sleep time if ingested close to sleep opportunities. Long-term use of caffeine, common in our culture, produces tolerance to the alerting effect of the drug and hence should be avoided when using caffeine strategically. Nicotine is a stimulant that produces effects similar to those of caffeine.

While anesthesia professionals might get away with working when sleepy without affecting aggregate patient outcome that does not mean that issues of sleep deprivation and fatigue should be ignored. Falling asleep (a long microsleep or full sleep) while taking care of a patient is just not acceptable; it's surely not what any patient or their family has a right to expect. Thus, both the individual anesthesia professional AND the systems and institutions they work within need to address the fatigue issue systematically. It is clear that just placing limits on work hours, either for trainees alone (the current situation in many countries) or for fully certified personnel as well, cannot do so. Only an integrated approach aimed at improving individuals' sleep hygiene along with reorganizing the structure and processes of clinical work will stand any chance of ensuring that anesthesia professionals who are appropriately alert are always there vigilantly protecting their patient.

Aging Anesthesiologists

Human abilities cannot be maintained indefinitely as humans age. On average, performance on laboratory tests of discrete sensory-motor and cognitive skills can be shown to decrease with increasing age.[269] However, large differences are noted among individuals. Again, except at extreme points of performance failure (e.g., severe impairment of vision, hearing, or cognition), the contribution of isolated changes in physiologic or cognitive performance is difficult to relate to real work situations. The work environment is often rich with redundant cues involving multiple sensory modalities, and technologic compensation for physiologic deficits is common (e.g., hearing aids or glasses). Advancing age is associated with worsening performance when tasks involve single-solution or fluency-based definitions of effectiveness.[270] However, along with possible physiologic changes of age typically comes greater experience with a variety of situations. When efficacy is defined in terms of the diversity of strategies used, as well as by the social and emotional impact of solution choice on the individual, performance is remarkably stable and sometimes even improves in the latter half of life.[270]

For many individuals, the lessons learned from experience more than offset the modest degree of physiologic impairment that they face as they grow older. Issues attributed to "age" might instead be related to a longer period away from initial or recurrent systematic training. The originally well-trained practitioner who keeps abreast of the changing standard of care and who exercises emergency skills frequently is less likely to be affected by advancing age than is a marginal practitioner whose knowledge and skills were frozen immediately after completion of initial training. For anesthesia professionals who are enrolled in mandatory maintenance of certification programs this issue might be less serious.

Patient care is a socially-organizationally constructed activity. Aging anesthesiologists may be able to modify their practice type, reducing complexity of cases or eliminating on-call and post-call patient care. Other perioperative team members may also be available to support those who while still competent may be, on any given day, not at their best.

What do other industries do about this issue? In the United States, from 1959 to 2007 there was a limit at 60 years of age for airline pilots; this has since been changed to age 65. Many countries have a higher limit and some have no limit. Moreover, regulations require airline pilots to pass a class I medical examination every 6 to 12 months, aimed at identifying individuals with chronic medical conditions that place them at risk for sudden incapacitation. Simulations show that sudden pilot incapacitation during a high-workload phase of flight (e.g., approach and landing) leads to a significant rate of crashes, even when a second pilot is at the controls. These physical examinations may also weed out pilots with severe cognitive or sensory-motor deficiencies (vision in particular), but they are not designed to assess subtle aspects of changes in performance resulting from age. Airline pilots' flying performance is also formally assessed annually throughout their career both during real flights and in simulation.

For anesthesia professionals, by contrast, there are no statutory requirements for medical examination or formal performance checking, although individual institutions or practice groups may choose to impose testing requirements or to implement age-based reductions in daytime or on-call requirements. No doubt, the issue of age-related effects on anesthesia professional performance is likely to continue to be raised periodically for the foreseeable future.

Illness and Drug Use

Every anesthesia professional is vulnerable to transient illnesses, which in some cases probably reduce performance ability. All personnel are vulnerable to chronic medical conditions that could directly or indirectly affect their fitness and performance capability. The culture of the caring professions often leads individuals to continue to work with illnesses that would cause other professionals to stay at home or to seek medical advice. The performance-shaping effects of the illness can be exacerbated by the use of either over-the-counter or prescribed medications. The degree to which illnesses and medications affect professional performance in anesthesia is unknown.

PATIENT SAFETY ACTION BOX

Pilots use a mnemonic checklist to review the effects of potential performance-shaping factors and are instructed not to fly if they are impaired for any reason. One similar safety strategy in health care is the "I'M SAFE" approach,[271] promoted by the patient safety intervention strategy "TeamSTEPPS," which is explained more in detail later. "I'M SAFE" is a simple personal checklist to determine one's ability to perform safely concerning the factors: **I**llness, **M**edication, **S**tress, **A**lcohol/Drugs, **F**atigue, **E**ating and Elimination. The difficulty in anesthesiology is that the real-world organization and incentives of many practice settings do not provide mechanisms for personnel to excuse themselves if they are temporarily impaired and that there barely exist organizational structures and departmental understanding to promote such approaches (lack of "safety culture").

A more serious problem for anesthesia professionals is that of drug and substance abuse.[272-275] Nearly 15% of all doctors will become substance-dependent over their lifetime, and the incidence in anesthetists is almost 3 times greater than other physician groups. Including alcohol, studies describe up to 3.5% of anesthesiologists being addicted; if alcohol is excluded, drug addiction occurs in about 2.5%.[276,277] The degree to which small doses of alcohol or hangovers affect performance on complex, anesthesia

TABLE 6.3 Examples of Hazardous Attitudes and Antidote Thoughts[279]

Hazardous Attitude	Antidote Thoughts
Antiauthority: *"Don't tell me what to do. The policies are for someone else."*	*"Follow the rules. They are usually right."*
Impulsivity: *"Do something quickly—anything!"*	*"Not so fast. Think first."*
Invulnerability: *"It won't happen to me. It's just a routine case."*	*"It could happen to me. Serious problems can develop even in routine cases."*
Macho: *"I'll show you I can do it. I can intubate the trachea of anyone."*	*"Taking chances is foolish. Plan for failure."*
Resignation: *"What's the use? It's out of my hands. It's up to the surgeon."*	*"I'm not helpless. I can make a difference. There is always something else to try that might help."*

tasks is uncertain. The natural history of serious abuse of alcohol, cocaine, sedatives, or narcotics by anesthesia professionals is such that cognitive performance will at some point be seriously compromised, although addiction specialists frequently report that job performance is one of the last areas of life to become seriously impaired.[273,275,278] The period of time in which an addicted anesthesia professional's performance in the OR is significantly impaired may be a relatively small fraction of the total time during which drugs are abused. Although this in no way excuses the practice of conducting anesthesia while under the influence of drugs, it may account for the fact that reports of addicted anesthesiologists are, unfortunately, common, whereas reports of overt patient risk or harm resulting from an addicted physician's errors are unusual. A host of other threats to patient safety, including production pressure, fatigue, illness, burnout, and distraction will affect far more anesthesia professionals, occur more regularly, and pose greater safety risks to patients, but they do not carry the same level of risk to the professional's own life, nor the same social stigma, as does addiction. On the other hand, diversion of drugs from the patient who needs them to the addicted clinician for use or sale is a growing risk.

Professionals' Attitudes as a Crucial Part of Human Performance and Patient Safety

Attitudes are important components of one's abilities. They can affect performance as strongly as physiologic and cognitive performance-shaping factors. Psychologists studying judgment in aviators have identified five types of attitude as being particularly hazardous, and they have developed specific antidote thoughts for each of these, which are supposed to be verbalized by pilots whenever they find themselves thinking in that way.[279] The authors have adapted these to anesthesiology shown in Table 6.3.

The invulnerable and macho attitudes seem particularly hazardous for anesthesia professionals. They are compounded by production pressures to handle more cases in less time with fewer cancellations and less opportunity for preoperative evaluation. The feeling that a catastrophe "cannot happen to me" and that perfect performance can always be relied on to avert a disaster can lead to cavalier behavior and poor planning. It can alter thresholds for believing that abnormal data represent a problem, thereby leading to the fixation error of "everything's OK."

Expert human performance is the anesthesia professional's most powerful tool to safeguard the patient. However, planning to avoid catastrophe is likely to be more successful than battling to avert it. The economic and social realities of practice can cause these pressures to become internalized by anesthesia professionals, who then develop hazardous attitudes they might otherwise have resisted.

Under these conditions the usual protocols for elective case management must be adapted to seek the best outcome for the patient. In the final analysis, one must ensure that the patient's benefit is the primary criterion in such decisions, and one should establish a bottom line of safe planning, pre-use equipment checks, and patient preparation beyond which one will not be pushed. Even if surgeons, nurses, colleagues, or administrators pressure one to do things that one does not think are safe, no one will thank you if the patient suffers, nor will they come to your defense should litigation arise.

To simplify these decisions, many institutions have developed multidisciplinary written consensus guidelines on the preoperative preparation of patients that address the appropriate workup for patients with various medical conditions in different surgical urgency categories.

PATIENT SAFETY ACTION BOX

Sometimes it might seem appealing for a medical professional to emerge as a hero after a problem is solved or a complication is managed, but the challenge is to realize first that anesthesia professionals cannot rely primarily on heroism to achieve optimal safety, and second that in all likelihood no hero would have been needed at all if proper safety measures had been taken to begin with.

In their review *"Why hospitals don't learn from failures: organizational and psychological dynamics that inhibit system change,"* Tucker and Edmondson[280] describe a further aspect of professionals' attitudes that can have implications on safety: People are creative and they want to make things work for their patient. So, nearly every day they diligently work around problems and obstacles the best they can. However, the very acts of individual resourcefulness by such workarounds may mask the underlying systems issues that expose many patients to risk and thereby delay addressing successfully those very issues.

HUMAN FACTORS AT THE TEAM LEVEL

This section focuses on the human factors at the team level, exploring the key elements (a) effective communication including handoffs and the delegation of tasks; (b) the safety enhancing strategy "speaking up"; (c) aspects of status and hierarchy effects in teams; (d) teamwork including (e) leadership aspects.

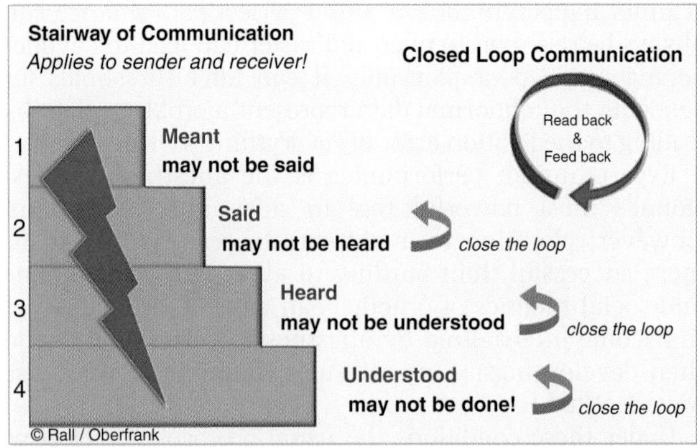

Fig. 6.6 Stairway of Communication and Closed Loop Communication: The importance of proper communication. (1) Especially when dealing with complex situations under time pressure, but also during routine work, people tend to "mean" or "think" a lot, but "say" little. It is important to let other team members know what one thinks in order to create shared mental models of a situation. (2) For several reasons, not everything that is said is necessarily heard by those who should hear it. The sender needs to ensure that the message was heard by the receiver and the receiver needs to confirm the message (= closed loop communication). (3) Acoustic hearing and mental understanding are not the same. "Closely monitor this patient" might be clearly heard, but what is meant is open for interpretation on a large spectrum. Misunderstanding can result, but can be smoothed out. (4) Some tasks may be forgotten, making double checking necessary. Some tasks need time to be completed, some tasks may fail. No matter what, the team needs to know (= closed loop communication).

Effective Communication and Delegation of Tasks

The benefits of effective communication for patient care in anesthesia and the operating room have been repeatedly demonstrated.[281-284] However, the term effective communication is imprecise leaving much room for interpretation. In fact, communication is never a one-way street and effectiveness includes participation of all team members.[285] Based on research showing that teams unfortunately tend to communicate ineffectively, effective communication refers to both content and form.[286] Teams should routinely use and update information from multiple available resources, share key elements between team members, and strive to always communicate as clearly as possible.[286,287]

Closed Loop Communication. For example, addressing team members by name and engaging in closed loop communication (Fig. 6.6) can help avoid misunderstandings.[288-290] Closed loop communication includes (a) when the sender initiates communication, the receiver confirms that the communication has been heard by repeating the content of the communication and (b) when a delegated task is finished, the receiver gets back to the sender and the sender confirms the feedback. For instance, instead of saying *"Can someone call for help, please?"* closed loop communication presents as follows: *"Jeff, can you call for help, please."—"Yes, Megan, I will call for help immediately."—"Megan, I have called for help and they are on their way."—"Ok Jeff, thank you."* El-Shafy and colleagues evaluated the effectiveness of closed loop communication in trauma settings of a level I trauma center in the United States, analyzing all verbal orders issued by the trauma team leader for order audibility, directed responsibility, check-back, and time-to-task-completion.[291] In total, 89 trauma videos were reviewed, with 387 verbal orders identified. Of those, 126 (32.6%) were directed, 372 (96.1%) audible, and 101 (26.1%) closed loop. On average each order required 3.85 minutes to be completed. There was a significant reduction in time-to-task-completion when closed loop communication was utilized. Orders with closed loop communication were completed 3.6 times sooner compared to orders with an open loop. The authors highlighted that closed loop communication not only prevents errors, but has the potential to increase the speed and efficiency with which tasks are completed in the setting of trauma.

ISBAR Tool. Another effective communication tool especially useful for sharing information is the ISBAR concept (Fig. 6.7), often abridged to just SBAR. The acronym stands for **I**ntroduction, **S**ituation, **B**ackground, **A**ssessment, and **R**ecommendation. It originated in U.S. nuclear submarines and has also been used in the airline industry. ISBAR may be used variably by different members of the OR team.[292] Its use is associated with increased accuracy in communication and safety climate[293] and a decrease in communication errors[293] as well as in unexpected death.[294]

In the medical setting, ISBAR is a universally applicable communication tool that is usable in several settings, including for example face-to-face as well as telephone handovers in the OR or in the anesthesia post-anesthesia care unit. It also can be used for the briefing of new team members during emergencies and for briefing senior staff who has been asked for help. In the literature the slogan "Think—Talk—Write—ISBAR" can be found and characterizes the broad field of application of the idea. Shahid and Thomas give an up-to-date narrative review of the current literature on (I)SBAR, the challenges of communication among health care providers, and the proper use of the tool, and compares it to other communication tools that exist in order to assess their strengths and weaknesses.[295] For -detailed information the reader is referred to this review.

Because it assists the transfer of important information in limited time, ISBAR has been adopted by many health care organizations across the world. Medical associations and leading health care organizations, like the German Association of Anesthesiology and Intensive Care Medicine—Deutsche Gesellschaft für Anästhesiologie und Intensivmedizin (DGAI), the Australian Commission for Safety and Quality in Health Care (ACSQHC), the Institute of Healthcare Improvement (IHI), and the WHO have endorsed the (I)SBAR method as a standard communication tool, when appropriate, for health care providers. The experience in the United States is that SBAR has been adopted (in principle if not always in widespread practice) for nurses but is not frequently used by physicians.

PATIENT SAFETY ACTION BOX

Why use ISBAR (or SBAR)? It has the potential to improve patient care by enhancing transfer of information, responsibility, and accountability. It can improve patient safety by encouraging complete communication. ISBAR is an easy-to-remember memory prompt that helps providers (a) to prioritize what needs to be said by preparing consciously for communication, and (b) to set expectations on what will be

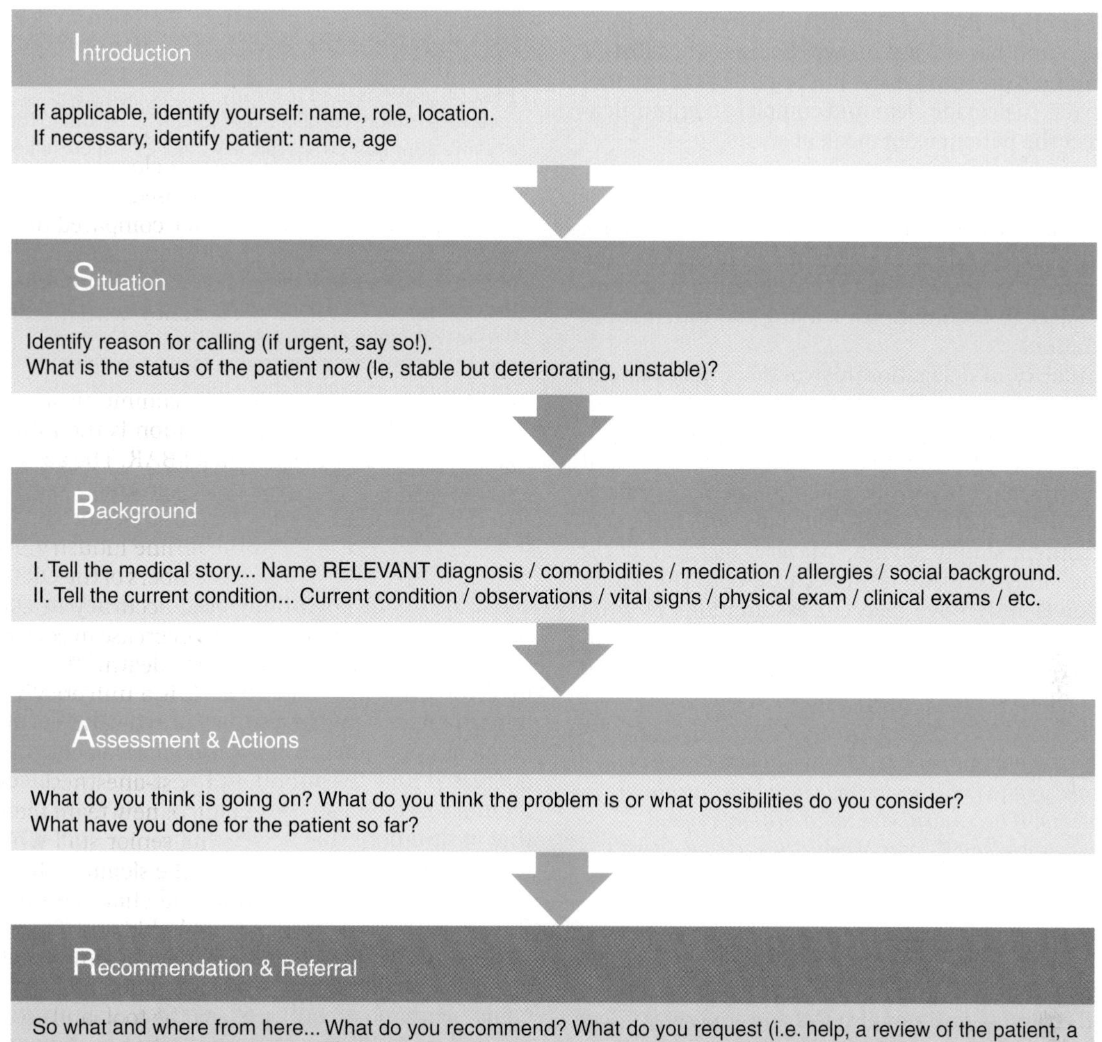

Fig. 6.7 Example of the use of the communication tool ISBAR.

communicated (shared mental models). ISBAR can reduce barriers to effective communication across different levels of staff, professions, and disciplines. Its application should be expected for routine cases, which will then enable its use even during stressful events.

Handoff Protocols[*]. Another aspect of safe and effective communication concerns post-intervention handoffs and intraoperative transitions of care responsibility, which are known settings of risk for critical information to be lost.[296] Intraoperative anesthesia care transitions are known to be associated with adverse postoperative outcomes, with a similar effect size for attendings, residents, and nurse anesthetists.[297] Sometimes though the new person may be able to take a fresh look at the situation, catch errors, or find opportunities to improve care.

Handoff protocols are intended to minimize patient risk by creating a designated time and framework to ensure that crucial information is not missed during care transitions. There is an increased focus on formal protocols because the number of patient care handoffs has markedly increased in some settings due to work hours limits. Protocols can be divided into conceptual models (e.g., IQ—a reminder that the caregiver should inform the receiving provider about the details of the patient and case and then allow them to ask questions before leaving) or scripted models (e.g., I-PASS[298] which stands for **I**llness severity, **P**atient summary, **A**ction list, **S**ituation awareness and contingency plans, and **S**ynthesis by receiver, or I PASS the BATON[271] which stands for Introduction, Patient, Assessment, Situation, Safety Concerns [the] Background, Actions, Timing, Ownership, Next).

Another comparison can be made between verbal and written handoffs and also supplementing a primarily verbal handoff with written information. When a patient's care is being transferred to a different care team, such as when a patient moves between the intensive care unit and the operating room, a team-to-team handoff is beneficial because the report and questions about the patient are consolidated for both teams (e.g., time out for sign out).[299] A good handoff process should be used for every transition, including intraoperative transfers for breaks,[300] dropping

*Acknowledgment: This section on handoffs was contributed by Lisa Sinz, MD (Penn State University School of Medicine).

off the patient in the PACU,[206] or changes from one anesthesiologist to another during a case. Using a checklist or structure can help prevent lapses, but regardless of the tool used, the goal is to provide clear and complete communication to protect the patient from medical errors.

Effective Delegation of Tasks. Delegation of tasks is sometimes ineffective leading to frustration on both sides: the person delegating and the person meant to perform the tasks. A common failing is when the delegation is incomplete and subject to assumptions, leaving too much room for interpretations.

The granularity of delegation instructions may depend on the personnel involved. For peer anesthesia professionals it may work to delegate a whole area of responsibility, such as "Sara, can you handle airway management please?," trusting that person to make the necessary decisions on their own. In other cases, especially with less experienced personnel, simply saying *"Michael, take care of the blood pressure"* may be insufficient because both the leader and the follower may have different assumptions of what that means in practical terms. With such a mismatch both parties may be unhappy. In such settings a more detailed delegation instruction may be needed, such as

"Michael, because our patient has a known hypertension and a risk for stroke, try to keep the diastolic blood pressure at or above 80 mm Hg. If necessary, give up to 500 ml crystalloid and, if necessary, small doses of ephedrine. If that doesn't handle it let me know. Any questions?"

PATIENT SAFETY ACTION BOX

Effective delegation of tasks involves sharing mental models of the situation and oftentimes also sharing concrete orders or suggestions about what one expects the other to do in order to fulfill the task to the other person's satisfaction. One reason why delegators do not use concrete delegation of tasks is because they think that it would take too much time or because they assume that the other person knows or should know what do to. Those few seconds to make it as concrete as the situation requires will probably pay off in the long run.

Asking Open-Ended Questions. A useful and simple means of communication, particularly in interprofessional and interdisciplinary settings, is to ask about other team members' points of view and plans using open-ended questions.[281,301]

Status and Hierarchy: Speaking Up

Speaking up refers to *"discretionary communication of ideas, suggestions, concerns, or opinions about work-related issues with the intent to improve organizational or unit functioning"* (p. 375).[302] Often the notion of speaking up implies doing so from below to above in the authority gradient. Without speaking up, problems cannot be identified, ideas will not be shared, and potential harm will not be prevented. This is particularly important in the multidisciplinary, complex, dynamic, and yet confined environment of operating rooms.[303] Here, a team member's speaking up to raise concerns about potentially risky or inappropriate actions of other team members may often be the final barrier to an emerging adverse event.[10,304-307] Unfortunately, speaking up is rare in teams in general and in operating room crews in particular.[308-310] In a survey of 137 chiefs of medical and surgical departments, 70% said that problems were not addressed and "elephants in the room" were common.[311] Simulation-based studies in anesthesia have demonstrated that in situations that need speaking up, only 40% to 70% of the participants did so.[312,313] For example, one such study showed that faculty anesthesiologists only spoke up: (a) 73% of the time to a surgeon who demonstrated profound sleepiness; (b) 14% of the time to a nurse who put a pathologist on speakerphone while the patient was awake and could hear; and (c) only 24% of the time to an anesthesiologist colleague who ordered the wrong treatment.[303] Creating conditions that encourage speaking up is particularly useful for crews whose composition is constantly changing, so members do not have time to develop as team.[314] This instability impedes the development of both norms to speak up as well as psychological safety, that is, the perception that there is no jeopardy to one's position if they do speak up.[315]

Strong hierarchies, which are prevalent in many hospitals, constitute a barrier to speaking up.[303,316-318] Even formal systems designed to promote it may actually inhibit staff from speaking up.[319] Leadership is a powerful tool in facilitating it: leaders can support speaking up by providing direction and coaching,[320] by using inclusive language,[321] by implementing debriefings to reflect on speaking up, and by establishing and maintaining a norm that considers such actions as socially desirable.[322] New research shows that people who do speak up are seen as more confident, competent, and of higher social status than those who do not speak up.[323]

Two explicit safety strategies that can be used for speaking up are, for example, the CUS tool (Box 6.3) and the two-challenge rule (Box 6.4).[271] But the basic requirement for both tools, for them to work properly and beneficially, like with any tool, is the organizational integration and acceptance of the tools (see section on organizational aspects of patient safety and safety culture).

BOX 6.3 Raising Safety Concerns - the CUS Tool

The CUS tool[271] is used to clearly communicate and escalate a rising level of concern for any issue and to focus a team's attention on specific key phrases that are linked to raising concerns. When a team member uses the phrase *"I am concerned..."* it is to get the team's attention and to ensure that team members are listening. In order to escalate the concern, the team member would use the phrase *"I am uncomfortable because...,"* finally escalating the concern with the phrase *"This is a safety issue...."* Then the current action must be stopped ("Stop the line!") and evaluated before continuing. Having a common framework, consisting of those three escalating key phrases, provides teams with a standardized, easy-to-use, attention-providing communication tool to raise concerns. At the same time, team members have a clear idea of the level of importance associated with the concern, due to the escalating concept.

BOX 6.4 **Raising Safety Concerns - The Two Challenge Rule**

The two-challenge rule[271] is another strategy that also empowers all team members to "Stop the line!" if they sense or discover an essential safety breach.

The two-challenge rule emphasizes the following:

- It is everyone's responsibility to assertively voice concern ***at least 2 times*** to ensure that it has been heard
- The team member being challenged must acknowledge ***with an active verbal response*** that concern has been heard
- If the safety issue still hasn't been addressed: Team members should take a stronger course of action or utilize supervisor or chain of command

PATIENT SAFETY ACTION BOX

Speaking up is never easy. It gets even harder if there is a difference in the hierarchy and experience level or if there is little positive organizational safety culture. Nevertheless, it is important to speak up if patient safety is in danger. The key to speaking up is often how to put things and when to intervene. Speaking up can be misinterpreted as a strategy to always tell colleagues what oneself would do differently. But speaking up should be used only in the case of a patient (or a colleague, or a piece of relevant equipment) at (potential) risk. To initiate speaking up it can help to have (organizationally) standardized phrasing, like for example, *"Excuse me, I see a patient safety issue here…."* Other systematic ways of expressing concern are the use of the CUS tool and the two-challenge rule. It also helps to explain one's thoughts and state a reason for the concern or the objection. For example instead of saying *"Succinylcholine…??? Do you really want to induce with succinylcholine???"* it is more helpful to say: *"Excuse me, in my eyes there is a patient safety issue using succinylcholine for induction. The patient has a potassium of 5.3 mmol/L so I think rocuronium would be better for induction, since the patient could get serious hyperkalemia and suffer cardiac arrest…"*

Teamwork

Teamwork can be defined as "*skills for working in a group context, in any role, to ensure effective joint task completion and team member satisfaction [.... and includes] coordinating activities with team members; exchanging information; using authority and assertiveness; assessing capabilities; supporting others.*"[170]

Unlike teams in aviation, the military, and police and fire services, the OR team is unusual in that the command structure is ambiguous. Physicians (surgeon and anesthesiologist) are nominally superior to nursing and technical staff, but the two sets of physicians are coequally responsible for the patient during the immediate perioperative period.

Although surgeons were historically considered the "captain of the ship," with even a legal doctrine giving them responsibility for the actions of all other OR team members, this has long since formally fallen by the wayside. Nonetheless remnants of this old history remain in aspects of the organizational structure and culture of OR environments. Clearly though when both anesthesiologists and surgeons are jointly caring for a patient, they are both responsible, and this situation can lead to complex issues of command authority, hierarchy, and control. Cooper recently published a paper investigating the critical role of the surgeon-anesthesiologist relationship for patient safety.[324] Even though there is little research about this relationship, Cooper argues that the relationship for each surgeon-anesthesiologist dyad is perhaps the most critical element of overall team performance. His article explores functional and dysfunctional aspects of the relationship, identifies negative stereotypes each profession has of the other, and offers some suggestions on how to improve the working relationship.

Apart from the challenge of the coequal responsibility of the patient, the composition of teams in the OR holds some further challenges. Salas and colleagues defined a team as *"a distinguishable set of two or more people who interact, dynamically, interdependently, and adaptively toward a common and valued goal/ objective/ mission, who have each been assigned specific roles or functions to perform, and who have a limited life-span of membership"* (p. 4).[325] A team is distinct from a group in that a group is an ad hoc collection of individuals without a specific mission and without specific roles. In the OR, all team members have the common goal of a good outcome for the patient. However, considerable disagreement can exist on how to achieve this goal and which elements of patient care have the highest priority. These differences are probably traceable to the fact that the OR team is itself made up of several crews (e.g., surgery, anesthesiology, nursing, as well as sometimes technical personnel from several domains) each of which has its own command hierarchy, its own global properties (professional standing, culture, traditions, and history), and its own set of local goals and objectives for management of the patient. A critical component of the success of this process comprises the establishment and maintenance of a shared mental model of the situation. The greater the overlap in mental models the more likely that team members will predict, coordinate, and adapt.[13] To the degree that these objectives can be accomplished, the different individuals will be able to tailor their efforts toward a common goal.

The quality of teamwork influences clinical performance in anesthesia.[326] Strictly speaking, teams in the operating room and resuscitation teams are not teams in the traditional sense that exist for an extended period of time with a shared goal and fixed team membership. Instead, they are considered action teams: members may be assigned together ad hoc for a rather short tenure, and team membership may change repeatedly.[81]

This has implications for teamwork and training: such teams have limited time to develop and learn as a team.[314] Instead, they must team off the cuff—an ability that has been described as teaming.[285] Teaming includes four pillars: speaking up (see earlier section), collaboration (i.e., adopting a collaborative mindset and collaborative behaviors), experimentation (i.e., working iteratively and considering uncertainty as inherent in interactions), and regular and continuous reflection about teamwork. Briefings and debriefings have been shown to offer an infrastructure for reflection in anesthesia and the OR.[314,327,328] Particularly for action teams such as in the operating room, establishing and updating shared knowledge is challenging. According to Cooke and Salas, team knowledge is more than the sum of individual team members' knowledge.[329] They distinguished between team mental model and team situation model. To judge team knowledge, information is also needed on the broader aspect of team cognition, which involves team knowledge itself, team decision making, team situation awareness, and team perception. Establishing team cognition and adapting to changing requirements requires targeted communication among team members.[215,288,290,330-332] This may be done explicitly to avoid misunderstanding and check mutual assumptions, or implicitly, for example by talking to the room.[153,290,301,333]

Leadership

Whereas in aviation the roles of the captain and the first officer are carefully defined and involve separate but interrelated tasks, in anesthesiology the patient care roles and responsibilities of different members of the crew of anesthesia professionals—whether experienced or in training—are rarely predefined or made explicit. For example, a trainee is often expected to do all tasks with only occasional assistance from the supervisor. Leadership is pivotal in critical, non-routine, and highly complex situations in anesthesiology.[82,334,335] It includes a variety of functions such as composing team, defining mission, establishing expectations and goals, structuring and planning, training and developing, sense making, providing feedback, monitoring the team and managing its boundaries, performing team tasks, challenging the team, solving problems, providing resources, encouraging team self-management, and supporting social climate.[336] Some of these leadership functions may be shared among crew members.[335] A senior leader of a trauma team may dynamically delegate or withdraw certain active leadership roles to junior leaders.[337] While sharing leadership can be effective, it may require the team to know and discuss how to work well in this fashion[338] (see also later section on CRM, section "CRM Key Point 4"). This is important especially in highly dynamic, time-critical situations such as resuscitations in which leadership is critical for performance and has to be adapted to changing task and coordination requirements.[339,340] Behavior observation studies on leadership in acute care have shown that leadership behavior is positively associated with performance during critical and barely standardized situations, but negatively associated with performance during routine and highly standardized situations.[85] In addition, leaders should be role models of civil and respectful interaction as this is important for high and safe performance.[341,342]

PATIENT SAFETY ACTION BOX

There are many kinds of situations where it is not clear who is the team leader in a medical setting. For example, to nurses or even to the physicians involved, it might be unclear who is the team leader when two doctors of the same profession present during an emergency. Leadership may change as personnel of different seniority or expertise enter or exit the scene. It is helpful to clarify roles as necessary. For example: *"Thank you for the handover. Now I will take over" or "Thank you. You stay in charge and I will assist you,"* or if in doubt ask *"Just to double check: Am I still in charge or do you want me to assist you?"* or from the perception of a nurse *"I am sorry, but to better coordinate my work: who is in charge now?"*

A particular issue of hierarchy is known as cue giving and cue taking, in which people give off cues (often without even knowing it) that are taken up by others.[343] People lower in a hierarchy are very sensitive to cues emitted by their superiors, which can inhibit action or even questions from subordinates. Such cues may be read as *"don't bother me," "don't question me," "I know what I'm doing; you don't,"* or *"I just checked on that and it's fine,"* thus inhibiting speaking up. A qualitative, descriptive study on nontechnical skills in Sweden revealed that anesthesia nurses view anesthetists as excellent if they are calm and clear in critical situations, and able to change to a strong leading style.[344] More on leadership in anesthesia can be found later in the associated section of "CRM principle 4."

PATIENT SAFETY STRATEGIES AT THE INDIVIDUAL AND TEAM LEVEL: CRISIS RESOURCE MANAGEMENT AND OTHER TRAINING CURRICULA

This next section is about how to minimize the negative human factors aspects of the anesthesia professional's physical, psychological, and organizational work environments and how to strengthen the positive aspects of individual and team performance. The CRM approach mentioned earlier is a useful organizing principle for tackling these issues. Below the authors (1) give a general explanation of the strategy and its history, (2) introduce the 15 key principles of CRM, (3) discuss the application of CRM in crisis as well as in routine medical situations, (4) cite evidence that CRM is beneficial in health care, and (5) briefly touch on other well-known team training curricula such as TeamSTEPPS and Medical Team Training (MTT).

Crisis/Crew Resource Management

Crisis resource management (CRM) in medicine, sometimes also referred to as crew resource management, is an effective safety strategy concept and tool adapted from the domain of aviation and modified to the needs of health care. Gaba traditionally defines CRM: *"CRM is the ability to translate the knowledge of what needs to be done into effective team activity in the complex and ill-structured real world of medical treatment."*

In overview, CRM means to coordinate, use, and apply all available resources to optimally protect the patient—at an individual as well as at a team level. Resources include all the personnel involved, along with all their skills, abilities, and attitudes—albeit also with their human limitations. Machines, devices, and information sources, including cognitive aids, are also critical resources. In addition, CRM provides effective strategies that cover typical safety pitfalls attributed to the five main elements of human-factor-related behavior as introduced earlier. The underlying scientific basis of CRM is formatted into 15 practical CRM key principles health care professionals can apply during work (Box 6.5).

CRM was introduced in aviation by airlines working with NASA originally as cockpit resource management in the mid-1980s after some sentinel airplane crashes. It later was renamed crew resource management to acknowledge the importance of the crew, not only those in the cockpit. CRM from that time on was and still is considered to be a successful safety strategy in aviation and is also part of safety strategies in other industrial and military settings. Interestingly, even though these industries maintain CRM principles and CRM training as crucial parts of their safety processes, they do so without what evidence-based medicine would call "level 1 evidence"—sound randomized trials—to justify this.[11,345] In fact, such evidence would be impossible to collect.

A similar program for anesthesiology was first developed by Gaba, Howard, and associates at the Veterans Affairs (VA) Palo Alto Health Care System and Stanford School of

BOX 6.5 Crisis Resource Management—Key Points in Health Care

- Know the environment.
- Anticipate and plan.
- Call for help early.
- Establish leadership and followership with appropriate assertiveness.
- Distribute the workload. Use 10 s for 10 min concept.
- Mobilize all available resources.
- Communicate effectively—speak up.
- Use all available information.
- Prevent and manage fixation errors.
- Cross and double check. Never assume anything.
- Use cognitive aids.
- Reevaluate repeatedly. Apply 10 s for 10 min concept.
- Use good teamwork. Coordinate with and support others.
- Allocate attention wisely.
- Set priorities dynamically.

The key points are derived from the publication of Rall and Gaba in the 6th edition of Miller's Anesthesia[559] and presented here in their updated, current version.

Medicine [109,127] originally as anesthesia crisis resource management (ACRM). It was modified from the aviation-based CRM principles to better suit the medical needs. The ACRM-like curricula have since been adopted by training centers worldwide for a variety of health care domains.[346] A detailed description of the ACRM course is provided.[347] More in-depth information on CRM in anesthesiology is provided in related safety literature[11,59,123,127,348] and in both the first (1994) and second edition[14] of the pioneering *Crisis Management in Anesthesiology* textbook by Gaba, Fish, Howard, and now Burden. Note that the term crisis does not mean that these principles only apply in such dire settings; instead, they apply to everything in patient care but are most pronounced in challenging situations. In addition, the pioneers of ACRM wished to retain the CRM acronym without using terms like cockpit or crew that were not familiar in health care.

The 15 Key Principles of Crisis Resource Management

The key points of CRM as they apply to anesthesia care have been steadily updated and expanded over time and are based on the research presented in the earlier sections. The 15 CRM key principles by Rall and Gaba (see Box 6.5) cover the content of the five main elements of human-factor-related behavior as introduced earlier: communication, teamwork, task management, decision making, and situation awareness (see Fig. 6.5). The CRM principles translate the theoretical content of those areas that are known to be important into handy and very applicable action strategies for health care professionals.

Looking closely, one can recognize that the different principles overlap in their content and aim in many cases. This way, different members and professions of a team can apply different CRM principles at different points of time during patient care, minimizing the risk of an error or harm to occur. Clinicians are not expected to memorize these principles; rather, the authors expect that they will be embedded into regular training and practice (see later section "How Can Crisis Resource Management Related Skills be Learned, Trained and Maintained").

Some of the principles may seem obvious or self-evident. However, from our experience in clinical work and simulation team training it is in fact *not* trivial to apply these principles in the real world. In the following sections the 15 CRM key points are introduced in detail.

Know the Environment (CRM Key Point 1). Knowing fully the environment of work is critical. Environment refers to equipment, supplies, processes, and people, as well as how they vary from case to case, or from location to location, time of day or day of the week. This knowledge reduces stress in the case of an emergency and provides more available mental capacity and prudence to deal with the case. It is important to know who can be asked for help, how to mobilize help quickly, and how long it will take help to arrive. Like pilots, anesthesia personnel can be expected to know in detail how to use all equipment and supplies, which in anesthesiology includes anesthesia machine, defibrillator, infusion and blood administration system as well as how to troubleshoot them or switch to backup devices. The experience of the authors as clinicians and teachers in real and simulated anesthetic cases suggests that many anesthesia professionals lack sufficient depth of knowledge or skill in the operation of their equipment. That these systems are not always designed optimally from a human factors standpoint only increases the need for the individual clinician to thoroughly learn about and practice with all their features and pitfalls.

PATIENT SAFETY ACTION BOX

Know Your Environment

- Know how to call for help and how to call a code in the event of a cardiac arrest or other major emergency.
- Know who to call for different kinds of problems or emergencies; learn the emergency numbers (or they may be present on available cognitive aids)—always ask for it if uncertain.
- Use any spare time at work to delve into the details and practice with devices or features that are rarely used. Some equipment (e.g., fiberoptic scopes) can be appropriately used during routine cases to stay in practice with its use.
- Be involved with organizational processes of identifying and implementing needed changes in different aspects of the environment to improve quality and safety.

Anticipate and Plan (CRM Key Point 2). Anticipation is key for goal-oriented behavior and it also helps avoid unpleasant surprises. Anesthesia professionals routinely consider in advance the requirements of a case and plan for its key milestones. In addition, they must imagine what could go wrong and plan ahead for possible difficulties. Savvy anesthesia professionals expect and are prepared for the unexpected. And when it does strike, they then anticipate what could happen next and prepare for the worst. In this context people often talk about "staying ahead of the game" or "not falling behind." Resources can be mobilized and used on the fly, but it is better if their possible need is anticipated and planned for.

For any case, a sound plan matches the anesthetic technique to the patient's disease state, the technical requirements of surgery (e.g., position of the patient), the anesthesia equipment available, and the skills of the anesthesia professional. It also includes specific backup procedures and contingency plans to be used if the original plan fails or needs to be changed. Often, faulty plans can result when underlying disease states are missed or ignored because of inadequate data gathering during preoperative evaluation. Poor planning may also result from the hazardous attitude of invulnerability. Note that a faulty anesthetic plan will expose the patient to risk even if it is carried out perfectly.

For anticipating and planning to be most effective, it should ensure the coordination of all members of the patient care team. One way to do so during routine cases is the use of briefings.[217,328] Over the last 10 years there has been a major movement to formalize such briefings (e.g., mandatory preoperative briefing of the WHO Surgical Safety Checklist, Patient Safety Huddles).

PATIENT SAFETY ACTION BOX

Anticipate and Plan Ahead

- In order to be prepared it is important to know what to potentially expect.
- For proper preparation it helps to imagine possible difficulties or complications before each case and mentally prepare for alternatives or actions. If in doubt it is better to err on the side of extra preparation.
- Perform anticipation and planning with your team: encourage colleagues to speak up; for challenging cases review in depth the primary plan (plan A) as well as the alternate plans B, C, D, etc.

Call for Help Early Early Enough to Make a Difference (CRM Key Point 3). Calling for help is associated with better individual and team performance.[75] Knowing one's own limitations and calling for help early are signs of rationality, strength, and patient-centeredness. Trying to handle everything alone or toughing out a critical situation is dangerous and unfair for everyone. The decision of when to call for help is complicated, but the key point is to do so early enough that the assistance can make a difference. A call so late that the patient is beyond rescue is futile. Knowing in advance who might be available and planning how you would use them will facilitate their utility.

Some typical triggers for calling for help that apply to any anesthesia professional at any level are (1) when there are too many tasks to do, (2) when the situation is already catastrophic (e.g., cardiac arrest, difficulty securing the airway), (3) when serious problems are becoming worse or are not responding to the usual maneuvers (or both), and (4) when you do not know what is going on.

For novice anesthesia professionals, calling for help very early is frequent as they are not expected to handle any critical aspect of a case (e.g., induction of anesthesia) without supervision or assistance. For experienced personnel it will be less frequent, as they are fully able to handle more things alone, but mobilizing help is still critically important. Many situations that would spin out of control can be readily resolved with appropriate and timely assistance.

Whereas prior research on these kinds of backing-up behavior has indicated that it is beneficial to teams, nothing is perfect. Barnes and colleagues published a critique of aspects of backing-up behavior in their article "Harmful help,"[349] citing for example decreased work on subsequent tasks after receiving high amounts of backup. A related concept is that of social shirking in which a task that is typically done separately by two people, to gain redundancy, instead is shirked (dropped) by one or both of them assuming that the other is taking care of it.[350]

PATIENT SAFETY ACTION BOX

Call for Help Early Enough to Make a Difference There are different conceptual categories of help. One can refer to them as hands help (to do things) versus head help (to assist in thinking). Providing bits of key information even during the call for help may assist incoming personnel to be thinking or planning for the possible needs. Calling for help will only succeed in sites with an organizational culture that approves and supports it (see later section on "safety culture"). If someone who calls for help appropriately but early gets criticized or even bullied by colleagues or senior leaders such pro-safety behaviors will likely be extinguished.

Establish Leadership and Followership With Appropriate Assertiveness (CRM Key Point 4). Leadership involves structuring the team, planning, deciding, and distributing tasks. Leadership does not imply knowing more than everyone else, doing everything alone, or putting other people down. Followership is as important as leadership. Team leaders and team followers are jointly responsible for the well-being of the patient (see earlier section on "speaking up"). Since speaking up requires the crossing of many personal and interpersonal hurdles (e.g., fear of repercussions or arising disadvantages),[307] team members may need explicit invitations to contribute and shows of appreciation by the team leader, sometimes referred to as leader inclusiveness.[351,352]

Wacker and Kolbe[82] wrote about leadership, followership, and teamwork in anesthesia:

> *"Intuitively and empirically, leadership and teamwork are essential for team performance, patient safety, and patient outcomes in anesthesia and perioperative care. [...] Current research supports the concept that little explicit leadership is usually required during standardized routine work, but active and even directive leadership is important in unexpected, novel, or stressful situations." (p. 200)*

In their work they give an overview of how leadership practices in anesthesiology optimally change (implicit vs. explicit team coordination) according to clinical work phases and special situations (routine situations with low or high task load; unexpected minor or major events; initiation and maintenance phase). Rosenman and colleagues give a systematic review of leadership and leadership training for health care action teams.[353,354]

PATIENT SAFETY ACTION BOX

Establish Leadership and Followership With Appropriate Assertiveness Whenever people work together, conflict can ensue. Anyone on the team may need to diffuse conflicts to focus the team on care of the patient. One approach is to explicitly ask the team to concentrate on *what* is right (for the patient), not on *who* is right. Conflicts should be settled after the clinical event is resolved. As the leader, strive to have an open ear for the concerns of team members and actively invite them to express their opinion (for example, *"Do you have any other suggestions...?"* or *"The patient is deteriorating—I think we need to intubate him; what do* *you all think?"*). Team members need the confirmation that concerns and encouragement are appreciated. Alternate views may or may not change the leader's approach, but if they are not voiced there is little chance for a modification.

Distribute the Workload. Use the 10-Seconds-for-10-Minutes Principle (CRM Key Point 5). One major aspect of strategic control of attention is the active management of workload. Rather than passively dealing with rising or falling workload, the anesthesia professional actively manages it. Among others, Schneider and Detweiler[240] and Stone et al.[130] described the theoretical basis for a variety of strategies of workload management. These strategies were addressed specifically for anesthesiology by several investigators.[108,111] The anesthesia professional actively manages workload by the following five techniques:

1. *Avoiding excessive workload situations* (i.e., by anticipating and planning, CRM key point 2; calling for help early, CRM key point 3). Experts may choose techniques and plans that reduce the workload (especially when their individual and team resources are limited), even when those plans are otherwise slightly less desirable from a technical standpoint. For example, a single anesthesia professional working alone may opt not to use a high-tech, high-workload monitor (e.g., TEE) for a given case because the effort to use it might outweigh the likely information gained.
2. *Distributing workload over time* (i.e., by setting priorities dynamically, CRM key point 15). The anesthesia professional can prepare for future tasks when the current load is low (preloading) and can delay or shed low-priority tasks when the workload is high (offloading). Resources that require a significant amount of workload to prepare, such as vasopressor infusions, are often made ready before the case starts. Many tasks are made up of several subtasks, each of which has a finite duration. Because close attention may not be required during each of these subtasks, they can sometimes be interleaved with a fixed amount of attention (multitasking/multiplexing, see earlier section).
3. *Distributing workload over personnel* (i.e., by applying the actual CRM key point 5; by coordinating the team, CRM key point 13). When workload cannot be distributed over time and when additional people are available, tasks can be distributed to them with certain considerations: (a) Some resources can be handled by the individual anesthesia professional, whereas others require additional personnel; (b) Some tasks are completely incompatible, for example any activity that requires being gowned and gloved will preclude that individual from performing nearly all other tasks; (c) In very time-sensitive situations distribution over personnel may be needed whereas for more routine situations a single individual may be sufficient for the same set of tasks.
4. *Changing the nature of the task.* The nature of a task is often not fixed. They can be executed to different standards of performance; as standards are loosened, the workload required to perform them is reduced. For example, during periods of massive blood loss, the anesthesia professional focuses primarily on administering blood and fluids and on monitoring blood pressure. The acceptable limits of blood pressure may be widened to reduce the need for more frequent interventions.
5. *Modifying distractions and offloading routine activities.* In addition to the attentional demands of the anesthesia professional's core tasks, any clinical environment may be full of distractions. Expert anesthesia professionals modulate the distractions by eliminating them when the workload is high and allowing them to occur when the workload is low (to improve morale and team building). Similarly certain routine tasks (e.g., entering non-critical information into the anesthesia record) or courtesy activities (e.g., tying the gown of a surgeon or nurse) may be performed by the anesthesia professional only when workload is low, but not when it rises.

PATIENT SAFETY ACTION BOX

Distribute the Workload A team leader should try to stay free of tasks in order to observe, gather information, coordinate, distribute, and delegate tasks. This is because mental capacity of human beings is limited—multitasking leads to often unrecognized errors. Within the operating room this may not be possible until several skilled personnel arrive to help. Even then, there can be some tasks which the leader decides to perform while still being at the center of the team; for example they might choose to be the person administering IV drugs linking decision to action without a communication step. There is no single arrangement of personnel or tasks that is perfect for every situation.

Appropriate assertiveness is important. A frequent observation in simulations and real cases is that anesthesia professionals may be too quiet or too casual, even for situations that demand urgency and assertiveness. But choosing the appropriate level and style of assertiveness is also important because being excessively assertive, especially for non-critical situations, will anger or annoy co-workers and lead to suboptimal results.

Exercising effective followership (see CRM key point 4, exercise leadership and followership with appropriate assertiveness), team members should also look actively for work that needs to be done. The team leader should not have to think of and order every single task or activity. Proper communication will be needed to coordinate the work (see CRM key principle 7, Communicate effectively).

PATIENT SAFETY ACTION BOX

Leaders should try to sensibly prioritize tasks to single individuals or to delegate one task at a time to each person, for example, *"Mary, go and call for help. Peter, go and get the emergency cart. Michael, draw up epinephrine 100 μg per mL."* Team members should speak up if they get too much work allocated at once or when the priorities aren't clear (e.g., *"I can only do one of those things at a time, which should I do first?"*).

We always have 10 seconds! Patient care is very rarely a high-speed discipline where seconds matter—initiating CPR is one example. Usually patients deteriorate in minutes to hours. Despite the stress and intrinsic pressure to perform immediate actions ("do something, do something now!") there is often some time to think of a plan. Trying to be too fast may lead to avoidable errors.

To address this Rall and colleagues developed the 10-seconds-for-10-minutes principle, meaning, metaphorically,

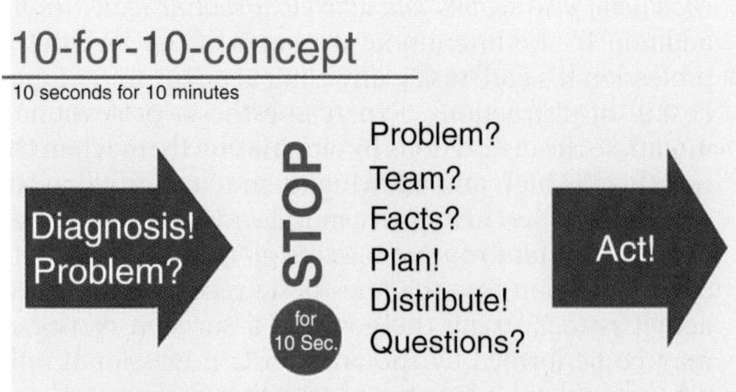

Fig. 6.8 The "10-seconds-for-10-minutes-principle"—"10-for-10."[563] When *making a diagnosis* or *feeling stuck,* perform the 10-seconds-for-10-minutes team timeout and check to see "what the biggest problem is right now" *(Problem)*. Clarify this with all available team members *(Opinions)*. Gather the information available *(Facts)*. Plan the treatment, including the desired sequence of actions. Distribute the workload by assigning tasks and responsibilities. *Check actively* with all team members about any further concerns of suggestions. Then act as an organized team. (Figure provided by M. Rall.)

spending 10 seconds in order to achieve a better coordinated team for the next 10 minutes. Stopping for symbolically 10 seconds in an emergency feels counterintuitive, but once used to it, it is a very effective way to improve performance and patient safety. The 10-for-10 principle has spread to many health care settings (anesthesia, ICU, prehospital, etc.).

The concept can be extended to mean that sometimes an investment of time in an activity—even many minutes—can yield big dividends in various ways (including time saved) in the future. The benefit of strategic investment of time appears to be greatest in key situations, such as (a) the making of a provisional diagnosis and the beginning of treatment, (b) planning for complex interventions, or (c) when the team feels stuck because the initial diagnosis seems incorrect, or when the usual treatment of a known problem is not working (Fig. 6.8).

Research findings show that information sharing (see also CRM key principle 8, Use all available information) can be enhanced by structuring team discussions.[355] The 10-for-10 principle offers one way to encourage and facilitate such deliberations.

PATIENT SAFETY ACTION BOX

When applying the 10-for-10 principle, it helps to use a key word or a key sentence for the team to pause for a moment in order to initiate the 10-for-10 break (e.g., *"Stop, everybody pause for a moment and let's summarize where we stand..."* For the 10-for-10 to work it is important for everyone to stop any non-critical action and for the leader to explicitly invite the whole team to participate (e.g., *"I want you all to stop whatever you are doing and I want to shortly summarize together where we stand. This seems to me like an anaphylactic reaction. What do you all think? Any other diagnoses in the differential?"* The 10-for-10 principle in general can be initiated by any team member, but it remains the decision of the team leader whether or when to execute it.

Mobilize All Available Resources (CRM Key Point 6). In case of an (imminent) emergency, everyone and everything necessary to help the patient should be mobilized, including personnel (CRM key principle 3, Call for help early), equipment, and organizational structures (radiology, other medical specialties, etc.). It is important to know which resources are available and with what delay (CRM key principles 1, Know the environment and 2, Anticipate and plan). On the human side, the anesthesia professional's knowledge and skills, constrained by human factors and one's own human deficiencies, is the most important resource, complemented by the helpers who can be brought to bear.

PATIENT SAFETY ACTION BOX

Mobilize All Available Resources When applicable think of all the team members, not just the anesthesia professionals or technicians. In a tough situation everyone should be willing to help but they do not always know how. The other professionals have many skills, some unique. Even relatively untrained personnel (housekeeping staff or orderlies, for example) may be able to help in some tasks.

Communicate Effectively—Speak Up (CRM Key Point 7). Good teamwork depends on everybody's being on the same page and on coordinating efforts. Communication is a very important vehicle to achieve good teamwork. It is like the glue that holds the disparate members together. Even though anesthesia professionals speak to each other all day long, effective communication is actually challenging, especially in a stressful situation. Based on research showing that teams unfortunately tend to communicate ineffectively,[356-358] effective communication refers to both content and form.[286] Many aspects make communication difficult: for example unspecified assumptions, lack of a shared mental model, hierarchy, acoustics, high mental workload, and time pressure (see earlier sections).

When dealing with complex situations under time pressure, people tend to "mean" a lot, but "say" little. Fig. 6.6 shows the closed loop communication, a systematic model of proper communication, ensuring that other team members know what one means, says, understands, and does in order to create shared mental models.

PATIENT SAFETY ACTION BOX

Communicate Effectively—Speak Up In order to communicate assertively and effectively, these approaches help:

- Do not ordinarily raise your voice, but do so if necessary to get others' attention.
- State your commands or requests as clearly and as precisely as possible. This is very difficult in a crisis, and it takes practice.
- Address people by their names if possible or search for eye contact before speaking. Despite the fact that anesthesia professionals hate to be called "anesthesia" (i.e., address people by function) routinely, there is not much choice but to do likewise to others in a crisis when you do not know their names. Avoid unclear assignments into thin air like *"Can someone monitor the saturation...," "Someone has to call for help...," "I need more propofol...," "We need more fluids..."*
- Use closed loop communication (see also earlier section):
  - Read back —If you received an assignment, repeat what you heard (i.e., Task: "Peter, I need epinephrine 10 μg per mL." Answer: "Ok Mary, I'll draw up epinephrine 10 μg per mL."

- Feedback—Give feedback when you are done with an assignment and also give feedback on what you did, even if it did not work or if it is not satisfying (i.e., "Mary, I got the defibrillator. It's right behind you. Do you want me to set it up?").
- Get back—If someone does not reply or react to you, they might not have heard it or were busy. Ask further questions, wait for acknowledgment, and wait to speak until they are ready to listen.
- Ask back—If you did not hear what the other person was saying or if you did not understand the assigned task, you should clarify matters.

- Accustom yourself to using the correct dosage indication when delegating the drawing up or the administration of medication (i.e., say *"Give 20 mg of propofol"* instead of *"Give 20 of propofol"* or say *"Draw up epinephrine 100 µg per mL"* instead of *"Draw up epinephrine."*
- Ask questions, especially if you do not know how to proceed. *"Ok, team. Right now I don't have any further ideas how to proceed. What should we do next?."*
- If you explain your thoughts or objections, this will help the team to understand better. For example, do not just say *"Get the defibrillator"* (thinking to yourself *"get the defibrillator so that we're prepared if we need it")*. Say instead what you mean: *"Get the defibrillator. We don't need it yet, but I want to be prepared in case we do...."*

Use All Available Information (CRM Key Point 8). Anesthesiology is particularly complex because information must be integrated from many different sources. In emergencies anesthesiologists often have only limited and indirect information on the patient, including those immediately at hand (the patient, non-invasive monitors, the anesthesia record), secondary sources such as the patient's chart, and external sources such as cognitive aids (see CRM key principle 11) or the Internet. Information provided to nurses and physicians who join an ongoing emergency can be unreliable.[355,356] The simulation study of Bogenstätter and co-workers showed that 18% of the information given to newcomers was inaccurate.[356]

Because of the various sources of unreliability of information (artifacts, transients, and miscommunications) various steps of verification and data fusion are needed to provide the best basis for problem recognition, identification, diagnosis, and management (as indicated in the cognitive process model of the anesthesiologist—see earlier section).

PATIENT SAFETY ACTION BOX

Use All Available Information Be aware of the flow of time when considering information streams. Anesthesia can be very dynamic. Vital signs that were satisfactory three minutes ago can change quickly. For periodic noninvasive monitoring—say an automatic blood pressure cuff—we are constantly trading off the rate of recurrence of the measurement against the potential complications of too frequent use. The typical 5-minute interval will leave room for hidden changes should the patient become unstable, a problem exacerbated by the higher likelihood that the next measurement will be more difficult for the device to make adding more time to obtain a reading. This of course is why we sometimes opt to invest time, effort, and a small risk to place an arterial catheter for continuous measurement.

Prevent and Manage Fixation Errors (CRM Key Point 9). Human decisions and actions are based on an instantaneous mental model of the current situation (see earlier section on "core cognitive process model of anesthesia professional"). If the model is erroneous, the decisions and hence the actions will probably be wrong. Faulty reevaluation, inadequate plan adaptation, and loss of situation awareness each can result in the type of human error termed fixation error.[138] A fixation error describes a mental model of a situation that is persistently faulty despite sufficient evidence to correct it. A fixation error therefore leads to a persistent failure to revise a diagnosis or plan, even though readily available evidence suggests that a revision is necessary.

Three main types of fixation errors are recognized[137-139] and described in Box 6.6. Each represents an extreme relative to another; it is usually advantageous to aim for the sweet spot between the extremes. For example, regarding "This and Only This" versus "Everything But This," usually people want to hone in on the one most likely cause of a problem in order to properly address it, while still keeping an open mind for other possibilities. Occasionally the extreme is required—if there is no pulse, initially CPR must happen with no delay (this and only this) regardless of the underlying cause. Conversely, sometimes one must delay treating a possible cause so as to find out what is really going on. And if we never act as if everything is OK every routine case would turn into chaos. One's behavior must be fluid so as to navigate optimally toward or away from the middle ground as needed.

BOX 6.6 Fixation Errors

Three main types of fixation errors[137-139] are recognized and should be understood:

- Fixation Error # 1: *"This and only this" or "cognitive tunnel vision."* In this type of error, attention is focused on only one possibility. Other alternatives (possibly or actually correct) are not taken into account (i.e., There is profound hypotension and tachycardia; the patient must be hypovolemic, there must be bleeding [disregarding anaphylaxis, cardiogenic shock, excessive vasodilator administration, etc.]). The available evidence is interpreted to fit the initial diagnosis or attention is allocated to a minor aspect of a major problem.
- Fixation Error # 2: *"Everything but this."* In this type of error, attention is persistently focused on the search for further (irrelevant) information or diagnosis resulting in the failure to treat a probable cause and commit to the definitive treatment of a major problem. (i.e., Hmm... there is tachycardia, maybe it's light anesthesia, maybe it's hypovolemia, maybe it's... and there's hypercapnia maybe it's the CO_2 absorber, maybe it's... and there's fever, maybe the patient is septic, and... without ever committing to either definitively rule out, or else treat for—"actually all these signs point to malignant hyperthermia so I'm going to treat it as such").
- Fixation Error # 3: *"Everything is OK."* This is the persistent belief that no problem is occurring in spite of plentiful evidence that it is. In this type of error, all abnormalities may be attributed to artifact or transients. Possible (pre-) signs of a catastrophic situation are dismissed. (i.e., "The blood pressure cannot be so low. Probably the blood pressure cuff does not measure right. That is alright."). Another form of this type of fixation error is the failure to actively transition from routine mode into emergency mode when the situation demands it. A failure to declare an emergency or to accept help when facing a major crisis may stem from denial that a serious situation is actually occurring.

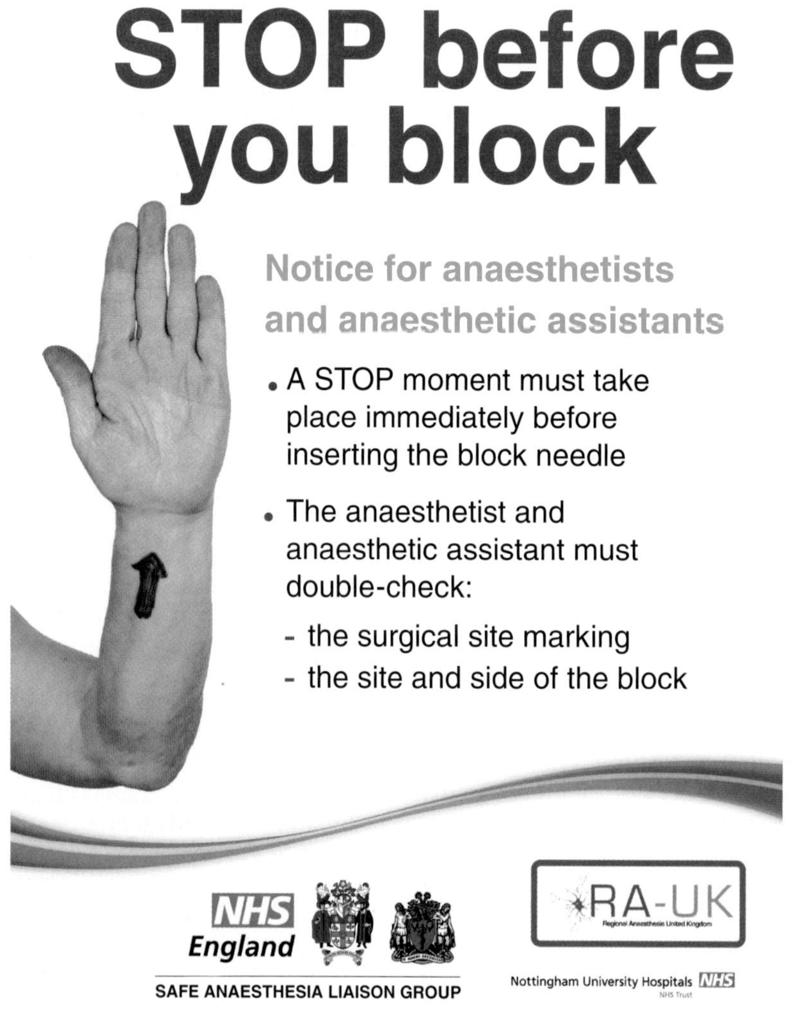

Fig. 6.9 "Stop before you block" to avoid wrong site block. Reproduced here with permission from the Safe Anaesthesia Liaison Group (SALG) and Regional Anaesthesia UK, but SALG has not reviewed this as a whole.

When working alone, an anesthesia professional can deliberately change perspectives (physically or mentally) and look for information not fitting the picture of the situation, as though freshly entering the room. Using the aforementioned 10-for-10 principle (CRM key principle 5) can be helpful by actively involving all team members and facilitating other ideas, diagnoses, and objections. Calling for head help from another anesthesia professional unaware of the previous assumptions can break fixation errors; it is best to try not to excessively bias their view of the situation during their incoming briefing. Remember that the burden of proof is on you. For every abnormality you must assume that the patient is not OK until you satisfy yourself otherwise. Similarly, you must assume that any abnormality represents the worst possible diagnosis until you can determine what is actually going on.

Cross and Double Check—Never Assume Anything (CRM Key Point 10). Cross checking and double checking are error-reduction strategies. Cross checking means correlating information from different sources. For example, there are often three independent sources of information on the patient's heart rate (electrocardiogram [ECG], pulse oximetry, and blood pressure monitor) and two of cardiac rhythm (ECG and pulse oximetry). Cross checking across people can be useful both for information that depends on human perception (e.g., auscultation) and for determining which actions were or were not completed. Human memory of actions delegated and performed is vulnerable, especially when interruptions have occurred.

Double checking means to verify information and/or equipment if it is very critical or if in doubt. In brief: to *never assume anything.* The more important or vital the information, the more certainty is appropriate. When chosen therapies do not seem to be working an important double check is whether the intended processes are really happening. For example to double check the proper performance of a critical infusion pump means to check its settings, operation, source of power, and the lines and stopcocks from it to the patient.

Another safety strategy using double checking in anesthesia is the *"Stop-before-you-block"* (SB4YB) campaign (for more information, free poster, and implementation package see www.rcoa.ac.uk/standards-of-clinical-practice/wrong-site-block). The "block time out" campaign was initiated by the Nottingham University Hospital in the UK in 2010 and by now has been adopted worldwide (poster see Fig. 6.9). Meanwhile, several extensions to this strategy have been published.[359,360]

PATIENT SAFETY ACTION BOX

Cross Check and Double Check—Never Assume Anything A related safety strategy is *"Stop-Inject.—Check!"* (Fig. 6.10). In order to prevent medication errors, this strategy is very applicable. Whenever you intend to give an injection, do not inject ("STOP—INJECT") —and at a crucial point of no return think for a few seconds about the injection ("CHECK")—correct any issues—and only then continue with the injection safely. Because if the drug is in, it's in. This strategy is equally applicable to other interventions which cannot be reversed.

Use Cognitive Aids (CRM Key Point 11). The human factors literature demonstrates conclusively that cognitive functions such as memory and arithmetic calculation are vulnerable to error or even complete failure, especially during periods of stress or time pressure. Cognitive aids—such as posters, algorithms, checklists, handbooks, calculators, personal apps, and advice hotlines—come in different forms but serve similar functions. They offload memory and safeguard the correct recall of critical items. Cognitive aids ensure that critical steps are not missed. And they also help ensure the use of current best practices because during a crisis, people sometimes revert to what they originally learned, not what is the latest recommendation. Cognitive aids make knowledge explicit and applicable in the particular situation rather than only being implicit and in someone's brain.

In anesthesiology and emergency care, emergency manuals/crisis checklists, smartphone apps, electronic health record systems, posters, and algorithms are the most common kinds of cognitive aids used. The Internet has become an increasingly useful cognitive aid and may be available on computer terminals, tablets, and smartphones in hospital settings.

The use of cognitive aids is relatively easy and they help to prevent missing critical steps that can be deadly.

In 2003, the US Department of Veterans Affairs National Center for Patient Safety developed an emergency checklist set of 16 serious perioperative emergencies, in concert with the VA Palo Alto/Stanford group, and placed a set of these checklists on plastic laminated sheets in every OR of 105 hospitals. A study of the use of the VA cognitive aids suggested, that they were beneficial to VA anesthesia professionals.[144] Other research has demonstrated that (1) medical and technical performance is better during simulated crisis when a cognitive aid is used [145,361,362] and (2) it can be very helpful to the anesthesia professional leading the team if a reader is present whose job is to read the relevant aid to the team and keep track of whether the relevant tasks have been performed.[363,364]

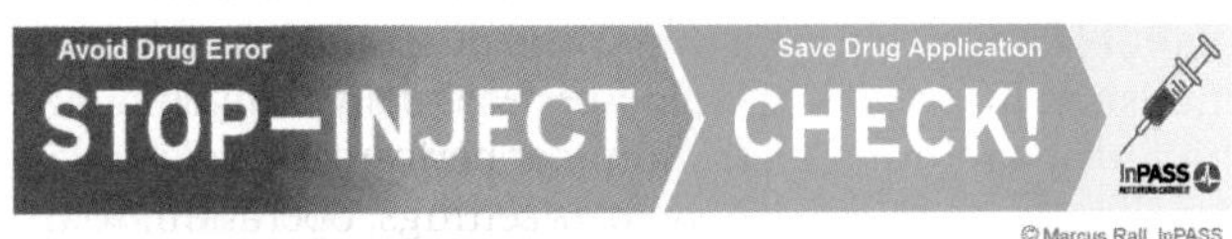
Avoid Drug Error
STOP–INJECT
Save Drug Application
CHECK!
InPASS
©Marcus Rall, InPASS

Fig. 6.10 Using stop moments as a valuable patient safety tool for irreversible, critical points of no return, like for example "Stop-Inject. Check!". To avoid unnecessary drug errors, all who intend to inject drugs should take two seconds before injecting a drug ("Stop-Inject"), then confirm ("Check") that the injection is safe to perform (right patient, right medication, right dose, right route, etc....), and only after this short confirmation inject the drug. The figure shows the slogan printed on a sticker that, for example, can be put on medical equipment carts to serve as a daily patient safety memorizer for medical personnel.

For example, Arriaga and colleagues demonstrated in a high-fidelity simulation study that the use of emergency checklists was associated with significant improvement in the management of operating-room crises, suggesting that checklists for use during operating-room crises have the potential to improve care.[145] In the study, 17 operating-room teams from three institutions (one academic medical center, two community hospitals) participated in 106 simulated surgical-crisis scenarios. Each team was randomly assigned to manage half the scenarios with a set of crisis checklists and the remaining scenarios from memory alone. Every team performed better when the crisis checklists were available than when they were not. Failure to adhere to lifesaving processes was less common when checklists were available (6% of steps missed when checklist available vs. 23% when unavailable). 97% of participants reported that they would want to use a checklist if one of these crises occurred during an operation. Further studies concerning this matter have been undertaken.[300,365-368]

Hepner and colleagues give an up-to-date overview of the history, current role, and future directions of cognitive aids in the operating room.[369] Marshall provides a review of the different cognitive aids existing in anesthesia based on a literature review and summarizes recommendations in cognitive aid design, testing, and implementation for the future.[370]

EXAMPLES OF KNOWN COGNITIVE AIGS. There is a growing movement toward the effective use of cognitive aids like checklists and emergency manuals in the operating room, both for routine and crisis situations. Following those movements there have been some recent large checklist implementation processes in health care:

One movement, for example, is the European "Helsinki Declaration on Patient Safety in Anaesthesiology," a shared European opinion of what currently is both worthy and achievable to improve patient safety in anesthesiology.[371] The declaration demands that *"all institutions providing perioperative anaesthesia care to patients should have protocols [...] for managing [...] difficult/failed intubation, anaphylaxis, local anesthetic toxicity, massive haemorrhage [...]."*

Perhaps the most widely used checklist is the WHO Surgical Safety Checklist that was launched in 2009 by the WHO's World Alliance for Patient Safety accompanying the "Safe Surgery Saves Lives" campaign. A global study[372] showed that the rate of death was 1.5% before the WHO checklist was introduced and declined to 0.8% afterward. Inpatient complications occurred in 11.0% of patients at baseline and in 7.0% after introduction of the WHO checklist. However, there exist several challenges concerning the application of and adherence to the WHO Surgical Safety Checklist, represented by a study that assessed the application attitudes and compliance of the WHO checklist as perceived by anesthesia professionals in Germany.[373] Roughly 60% of participants had knowledge of the theoretical framework. Sign in, patient ID, and surgical site were checked > 95% of the time, allergies addressed in nearly 90%, expected difficult airway in 65%, and availability of blood products by 70%. A total of 85% of participants advocated for the timeout to include all persons present in the operating room, which was the

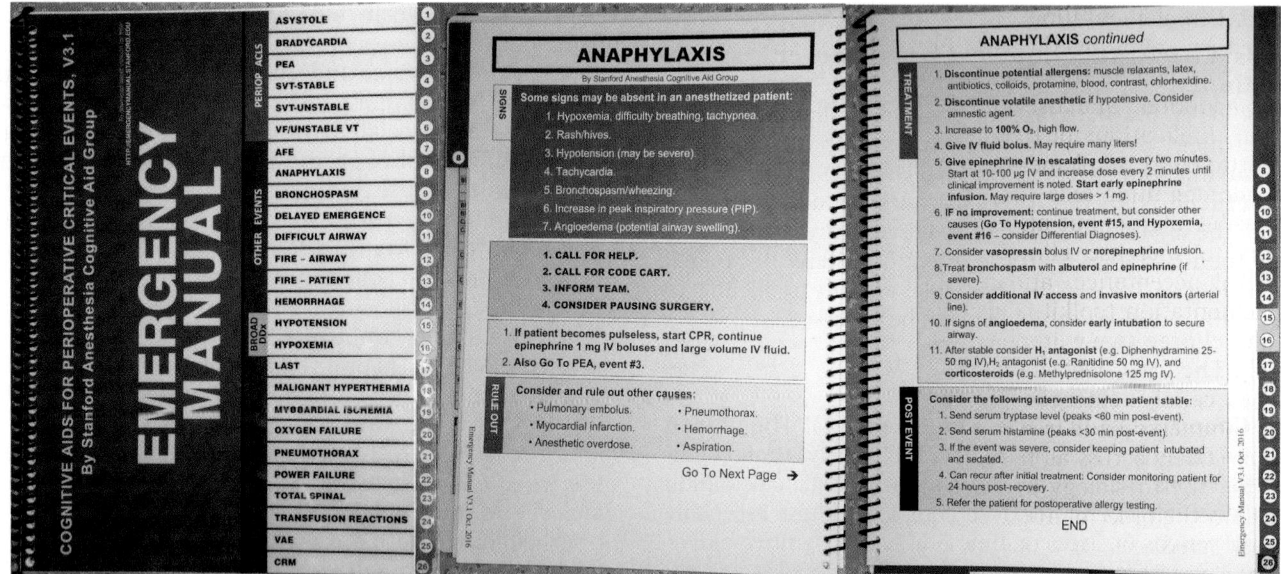

Fig. 6.11 Emergency Manual developed by the Stanford Anesthesia Cognitive Aid Group. (A) Front cover of the emergency manual. On the front page it shows the emergency events, thus making it easy to jump to the right page in the case of an emergency. The manual can be hung by its strong metal grommet. Experience shows that clinicians must be familiarized with the manual in advance for optimal use. (B and C) Two pages of the emergency manual for "Anaphylaxis." The content and the layout have been optimized through graphic layout and careful choice of words for easy and ergonomic use in actual operating room emergencies. (Photographs by David Gaba).

case in 57%. A total of 41% stated that the timeout was only performed between anesthetist and surgeon; in 17% of cases, the patient was simultaneously draped and/or surgically scrubbed.

Furthermore there exists a checklist for the significant reduction of catheter-/central-line-related bloodstream infections (CLABSI) in the ICU from Levy and colleagues.[374] And there exist several checklists for handovers and patient-care transition (see also earlier section "Effective Communication and Delegation of Tasks").[295,298,300] A survey[368] on the perception of anesthesia providers from a large academic U.S. institution revealed that printed or electronic aids for patient care transition and shift handoffs in general were valued (61% and 58%, respectively). To prepare for and perform routine anesthesia care, 40% of providers claimed interest in using checklists, however, the interest differed significantly with clinical experience: while both the least and most experienced providers valued aids for routine anesthesia (54% and 50%), only 29% of providers with 2 to 10 years of anesthesia experience claimed interest in using them. Distraction from patient care and decreased efficiency were concerns expressed for the use of routine checklists (27% and 31%, respectively).

Other checklists used especially in anesthesia are the checklist for the anesthesia machine (see earlier section "Pre-use Checkout of Equipment") and emergency checklists or emergency manuals.

EMERGENCY CHECKLISTS/EMERGENCY MANUALS. One known example of a cognitive aid is the use of emergency checklists or emergency manuals, also known by similar terms including emergency response protocols or critical event algorithms. The Stanford Anesthesia Cognitive Aid Group (SACAG) has conducted many years of simulation testing of cognitive aids meant for real-time intraoperative use,[362,363] with increasing levels of optimization through graphic design. SACAG has produced the *Emergency Manual: Cognitive Aids for Perioperative Critical Events ("Stanford Emergency Manual")* (at the time of this writing in version 3.1, see Fig. 6.11). An earlier version of the emergency manual was published as an appendix in the textbook "Manual of Clinical Anesthesiology."[375] In 2013 these cognitive aids were placed in all anesthetizing locations in the Stanford family of teaching hospitals.

The *Stanford Emergency Manual* is available free electronically throughout the world as a downloadable portable document format (PDF) file under a Creative Commons Attribution; Non-Commercial; No-Derivatives License, allowing free non-commercial use of the document as is, without unauthorized modifications, and with attribution of the author (emergencymanual.stanford.edu). Users are able to choose to print out the *Emergency Manual* locally or using any commercial printer; instructions are given on choices of printing paper (e.g., nonflammable and able to be wiped with disinfectant), binding, and placement in perioperative patient care settings.

An equally well-known emergency checklist was developed by the Ariadne Laboratory affiliated with the Brigham and Women's Hospital; it is also freely available and widely disseminated. The Society for Pediatric Anesthesia has a web-based and iPhone app emergency manual that is widely used in that subspecialty arena. A commercially available anesthesia crisis manual designed as a book was published in 2011 by David Borshoff with support of both the European and Australian Societies of Anesthesiology (for details, see www.theacm.com.au). The textbook *Crisis Management in Anesthesiology* while not optimized for real-time use, can also be used in real-time and contains a rather large number (99) of perioperative events.

A recent study compared the impact of paper versus electronic cognitive aids in a simulation-based study, suggesting that the mode of information does not affect performance.[376] The movement for the dissemination and use of such cognitive aids is growing. An Emergency

Manual Implementation Collaborative (EMIC) has been started, bringing together several leading centers in this arena to facilitate the development, testing, dissemination, adoption, and use of these resources. The most recent publications of the Collaborative emphasize the importance for implementation institutions to not only provide cognitive aids such as emergency manuals in accessible places, but also incorporate training mechanisms to increase clinicians' awareness, familiarity, cultural acceptance, and planned clinical use.[377] An implementation toolkit is provided by the Collaborative free of charge (www.implementingemergencychecklists.org/). The EMIC website provides links to obtain many of the available emergency manuals, most of which are non-commercial and free to download.

Collectively across all the relevant emergency cognitive aids for anesthesiology it is believed [DG] that as of late 2018 on the order of 400,000 have been downloaded or disseminated.

Conflicting data concerning the effectiveness of cognitive aids as described in the literature do not necessarily suggest that there is no benefit but suggest that the success of those tools requires complex cultural and organizational change efforts, not just providing the cognitive aid in perioperative settings. In research where no difference was found, the cognitive aids are almost always found to have been introduced without education (an approach termed "print and plunk" by experts on such aids) or to have flaws in their physical design.[370] In 2013 multiple papers and editorials in a single issue of *Anesthesia and Analgesia* discussed a number of important issues about cognitive aids and their implementation.[370,378-381] In the article "Cognitive aids: Time for a change?," Jenkins [382] among other things, draws attention to the fact that besides having checklists ready to use in OR, using them during OR team training for common emergencies would seem a logical next step.

The key elements of the successful implementation of cognitive aids is (1) a culture that embraces cognitive aids not as a sign of clinical incompetence, but as a tool to improve care (see later section on "Safety Culture"); (2) an organizational implementation process like, for example, suggested emergency checklist implementation toolkit (www.implementingemergencychecklists.org); and (3) a proper checklist development and design. Several publications give an overview of the challenges associated with development and implementation of checklists and cognitive aids in general.[383-390]

Reevaluate Repeatedly—Apply the 10-Seconds-for-10-Minutes Principle (CRM Key Point 12). Anesthesia in critical situations is a very dynamic activity. What is correct now may be wrong in the next minute. Some parameters may change slowly over time, and subtle changes are especially difficult to perceive. Therefore, it is critically important to perform a repeated reevaluation of the patient. Reevaluation describes the continual process of assessing the situation and updating one's individual, and at certain stages also the team's, mental model of the situation.

The process of continually reevaluating in order to update the assessment of the situation and monitoring the efficacy of chosen actions is a major part of situation awareness. No crisis manager can be certain of success at any stage in the event. It is crucial to keep thinking ahead (anticipate and plan, CRM principle 2). Do not assume that anything about the situation is certain—double-check all critical items (CRM principle 10). Trend monitoring can be helpful to detect slow but insidious changes.

Questions that should be raised repeatedly to maintain situation awareness and to check whether one is still treating the most serious problem most effectively include:

- Was the initial assessment of the situation or diagnosis correct?
- Did the actions have any effect?
- Is the problem getting better, or is it getting worse?
- Does the patient have any side effects resulting from previous actions?
- Are there any new problems or other problems that were missed before?
- What further developments can be expected in the (near) future?

One way to reevaluate the situation is the regular application of the 10-seconds-for-10-minutes principle at specific stages during the treatment of a crisis (see Fig. 6.8).

Use Good Teamwork—Coordinate With and Support Others (CRM Key Point 13). Teamwork is a very complex topic. But research demonstrates that quality of teamwork influences clinical performance in anesthesia.[326] Some of the principles of teamwork have already been introduced earlier (see section "Teamwork"). Key principles of teamwork in dynamic situations have been delineated, especially in the work of Eduardo Salas, Nancy Cooke, and colleagues.[391-395] Good teamwork depends on different attitudes and characteristics, some of which were already discussed in CRM principle 4, Exercise Leadership and Followership with Assertiveness, and CRM principle 7, Communicate Effectively—Speak Up.

PATIENT SAFETY ACTION BOX

Implement Principles of Good Teamwork—Coordinate With and Support Others Dream teams are made, not born. Dream teams support each other continuously, with everybody looking after each other in a professional manner, the safety and well-being of the patient being highest priority. In contrast to a widespread opinion, good teamwork does not depend on team members liking each other (although it probably helps). Do all players of champion sports teams like each other, or all the time? Probably not. Nevertheless, they function as a high-performing team because they share the common goal to win. Patients are depending on perioperative personnel to be part of a team with emotionless professionalism, using principles of good teamwork, regardless of their personal affinities.

Coordination within a team ideally begins when it gathers. If all members know about the tasks to be done and their roles during these tasks (briefing, see also CRM principle 7), coordination is easy. Short briefings at the beginning of certain tasks as well as short debriefings afterward are common in other complex and dynamic domains, such as aviation, and they are becoming more common in health care. Research in health care indicates that they seem worth the time spent.[217,328] During the acute phase of a crisis, it is valuable to spend a small amount of time to coordinate the team's activities (see e.g., 10-for-10 principle CRM key point 5). Information sharing in teams is important to team performance, cohesion, decision satisfaction, and knowledge integration.[355]

PATIENT SAFETY ACTION BOX

Surgeons are a key part of the team. Sometimes anesthesia professionals act as though they have only two options in dealing with surgeons when a problem occurs—keep quiet or demand immediate cessation of surgery. Actually there are many options (see also: Communicate Effectively) for coordinating activities and concerns. You should notify the surgeons and nurses of ongoing problems and concisely convey to them the nature of the problem, what you'd like them to do (or not do), and the immediate plan. Conversely, you should be prepared to help the surgeons or nurses in any reasonable way when they encounter problems, as long as you can also maintain safe assessment of the patient and control of the anesthetic course.

Allocate Attention Wisely (CRM Key Point 14). As described earlier, several performance-shaping factors (see section on "performance-shaping factors") and hazardous attitudes (see "Attitudes of Professionals as a Crucial Part of Human Performance and Patient Safety", and Table 6.3) can globally degrade your vigilance. However, there are other factors that can specifically degrade your vigilance whenever they exist in a case: one is distractions and interruptions (see sections on "Interruptions and Distractions"). The other is high task load (see section "Performance as Related to Task Density").

Referring again to the core cognitive process model of the anesthesia professional introduced earlier (see earlier section), empiric studies have clearly demonstrated that attention sharing is needed among cognitive levels, among tasks, and often among problems. The intensive demands on the anesthesia professional's attention could easily swamp the available mental resources. Human attention is very limited, and multitasking as well as multiplexing may become very difficult and unsuccessful in a stressful situation.

Attention must be dynamically allocated where it is needed by a dynamic process of constantly prioritizing the tasks requiring your attention. One should handle critical items quickly and leave the less critical problems for when the patient's status has been stabilized. On the other hand when the task load is low, one should deal even with minor problems because they might otherwise evolve to something more significant. One can also use times when the workload is low to prepare for upcoming high workload periods, such as emergence from anesthesia or termination of cardiopulmonary bypass.

Another way to allocate attention is to develop rhythms and scan patterns. For example, always asking questions during the preoperative evaluation in the same sequence makes it less likely to forget items. The ABC mnemonic that equals airway, breathing, and circulation (now CAB mnemonic per U.S. American Heart Association guidelines) is another example that is based on this principle. Other strategies include alternating between focusing on details and focusing on the big picture, and offloading certain responsibilities, tasks, or information streams to other qualified team members (CRM principle 5), with periodic update to the team leader about the situation (CRM principle 13).

Set Priorities Dynamically (CRM Key Point 15). Dynamic situations demand dynamically changing decisions and actions based on new information and constant reevaluation (CRM principle 12). What was not a right move at one time may become the right move at another. In addition, having one solution to an obvious problem does not guarantee that it is the best solution or that only one problem exists. Some goals are always of the highest priority—ensuring adequate oxygenation and perfusion of critical organs being the most crucial—and can never be neglected. In order for team members to understand changing priorities of the team leader, it is important to communicate dynamic priorities effectively (CRM principle 7) and to support each other the best way possible as a team (CRM principle 4 and 13). Sometimes people stick to their first decisions and actions (CRM principle 9).

Evidence for the Benefit of Crisis Resource Management and Other Human-Factor-Related Team Training Curricula

Improvements Following Implementation of Crisis Resource Management. Recently several studies show evidence that CRM training improves patient safety and patient outcomes. In health care organizations, implementation of programs that deal with the concepts of CRM/NTS have been associated with many improvements following their implementation:

- increased provider satisfaction
- improved safety culture and a heightened culture of teamwork[43]
- increased clinical team performance[396]
- decreased room turnover time[397]
- increased percentage of on-time first case starts[42,397]
- decreased preoperative delays, handoff issues, and equipment issues[42]
- improved patient willingness to recommend[397]
- a decrease in medication and transfusion errors[398]
- increased antibiotic prophylaxis compliance[42]
- an increase of efficiency for clinical processes for multidisciplinary trauma teams[399]
- decreased mortality and morbidity[42,400]

Neily and colleagues[42] investigated in a retrospective study including nearly 182.500 sampled procedures whether there exists an association between a CRM-based team training program and surgical outcomes on a national level. The authors showed an 18% reduction in annual mortality compared with a 7% decrease among non-training facilities.

Haerkens and colleagues[5] introduced CRM successfully in the ICU, with data indicating an association between

CRM implementation and the reduction in serious complications and mortality in critically ill patients. The prospective 3-year cohort study was performed in a 32-bed ICU, admitting 2500 to 3000 patients yearly. At the end of the baseline year, all ICU personnel received a 2-day CRM training in small teams, followed by one year of implementation phase. The third year was defined as the clinical effect year. All 7271 patients admitted to the ICU in the study period were included. The ICU complication rate declined from 67.1/1000 patients to 50.9/1000 patients. The incidence of cardiac arrests decreased from 9.2/1000 patients to 3.5/1000 patients, while CPR success rate increased from 19% to 67%. The standardized mortality ratio decreased from 0.72 to 0.60 in the post-implementation year.

Cost-benefit Analysis of Crisis Resource Management Programs. Moffatt-Bruce and colleagues[41] published an innovative study, not only reporting that the implementation of a CRM program at an academic medical center resulted in a 26% reduction in observed relative to expected events, but also evaluating the program's costs and the return on investment. Costs included training, programmatic fixed costs, time away from work, and leadership time. Cost savings were calculated based on the reduction in avoidable adverse events and cost estimates from the literature. Over a 3-year period, roughly 3000 health system employees across 12 areas were trained, costing $3.6 million. Savings ranged from a conservative estimate of $12.6 million to as much as $28.0 million. Therefore, the study presented an overall return on investment for CRM training in the range of $9.1 to $24.4 million, concluding that CRM presents a financially viable way to systematically organize for quality improvement. This study demonstrates that CRM training not only improves patient outcomes (see above) but is also very cost efficient.

Other Curricula for Team Training: TeamSTEPPS and Clinical Team Training

By now, many different types of training strategies fall under the umbrella of team training in medicine, encompassing a broad range of learning and development strategies, methods, and teamwork competencies. Although each is unique in some aspects many of the principles advocated and behaviors taught are similar, and all draw ultimately from the same pool of underlying literature and experience.[401-408] The adaptation of aviation CRM to health care was first described at length at the beginning in the early 1990s.[348] Another team training curriculum, called TeamSTEPPS, was introduced in 2006 and revised in 2015. TeamSTEPPS originated from work done by the U.S. military and was adapted for health care by the U.S. Agency for Healthcare Research and Quality. The U.S. Department of Veterans Affairs introduced its MTT curriculum (later renamed Clinical Team Training, CTT) in 2007.

In the review of Weaver and colleagues,[409] 9 of the 26 studies reviewed used some form of CRM intervention, 7 reported using components of the TeamSTEPPS curriculum, and 3 studies used VA MTT. Seven studies reported using other team-training curriculums. Another current review is that of Marlow and colleagues.[410]

TeamSTEPPS. The TeamSTEPPS curriculum (Team Strategies and Tools to Enhance Performance and Patient Safety)[411,412] is an evidence-based framework that addresses aspects of the following five key elements: team structure, leadership, situation monitoring/mutual performance monitoring, mutual support/back-up behavior, and communication. For implementation, it involves three continuous organizational phases: (1) assessment; (2) planning, training, implementation; and (3) sustainment. The program consists of multiple, explicit team strategies for each of the above mentioned key elements and it provides a source for ready-to-use materials, monthly webinars, as well as a training curriculum (for details see www.ahrq.gov/teamstepps/index.html). This way the program is intended to be fully or partially implemented in an organizational structure as a holistic organizational safety intervention, composed of several explicit safety strategies. The TeamSTEPPS curriculum is designed for health care professionals in general over a wide set of clinical domains. However, health care professionals working in dynamic arenas of high intrinsic risk, like for example anesthesia, intensive care medicine, emergency medicine, etc., face a cognitive and teamwork environment different from many other medical domains.

Clinical/Medical Team Training. The Clinical Team Training program (CTT - formerly named VA M (medical) TT)[413] of the Veterans Affairs National Center for Patient Safety, originally was a classroom-based CRM training program. However, as the program evolved, simulation-based training came to be a crucial part of the currciulum with multidisciplinary on-site training with integrated simulation conducted by experienced faculty.[414] In the CTT program, principles of aviation's crew resource management (CRM) are introduced in a clinical context to model specific applications in the health care environment. The preparation stage requires two months, top leadership engagement being a crucial part in the concept. For initiation, learning sessions are carried out over two days. The learning session is a one-day session delivered twice to increase attendance from clinical units that cannot be closed for training. Implementation is carried out over six months following the learning sessions, and accompanied by coaching and monitoring of unit-based performance outcomes over 12 months.

In our senior author's [DG] view the key difference between TeamSTEPPS and the (A)CRM approach (see earlier relevant section) is the high focus of TeamSTEPPS on very concrete and relevant behaviors (e.g., SBAR, CUS words, two-challenge rule), whereas (A)CRM addresses a broader set of issues, some of which can encompass the particular TeamSTEPPS behaviors. However, TeamSTEPPS does not address directly the components of dynamic decision making of the individual or of some of the more generic issues of team management and teamwork (e.g., distribution of workload, mobilizing and using resources). Some implementations of TeamSTEPPS may miss the forest for the trees. The focus on concrete behaviors has the benefit of giving a wide variety of personnel specific actions they can practice and then perform in daily work. But the downside is that a variety of complex issues of clinical work and of teamwork may be rarely addressed, if at all.

Actually, it seems evident that all of these curricula, and others, are really complementary approaches to similar issues, drawing from the same underlying principles and practices. No single one of them is demonstrably superior to the other, and hybrids combining two or more of them are possible. TeamSTEPPS is popular in part because it is intended to be neutral as to clinical arena or position in the hierarchy and thus is widely applicable, lending itself to organization-wide implementation as described above. It was formulated and disseminated by the U.S. government's Agency for Healthcare Research and Quality, based on the work of internationally acknowledged experts on teamwork (albeit predominantly from non-medical domains). AHRQ provided a free extensive toolkit for TeamSTEPPS implementation. In contrast (A)CRM does not claim to be widely applicable, neutral as to clinical context, or requiring substantial analysis of or implementation by a clinical organization. It is popular especially in dynamic domains of high intrinsic risk analogous to the original one of anesthesiology. While it is successfully used with interprofessional groups in those domains, it is often aimed at physicians as team leaders. Dissemination of (A)CRM was facilitated by its long-standing existence (begun in 1990 and first described in the literature in 1992), publications on extensions into non-anesthesia domains, and an influential textbook (Crisis Management in Anesthesiology) in print via two editions since 1994.

Further Medical Team Training Programs. Besides these three rather well known team-training programs, there are multiple other team training programs, including Team Performance Plus (TPP), Team Oriented Medical Simulation (TOMS), LifeWings/Dynamic Outcomes Management (DOM), Triad for Optimal Patient Safety (TOPS), MedTeams, and Medical Team Management (MTM). They are mentioned for completeness, but for further details the reader is referred to the summary report of the Canadian Patient Safety Foundation[415] and further literature.

Patient Safety on the Organizational Level

In the following part the authors consider the organizational and systems aspects of human performance in anesthesia care and patient safety. Only the organization can sustain the systematic search for and implementation of cross-cutting and practical solutions for front-line patient care. An extensive overview of organizational aspects of patient safety is given by Charles Vincent in the second edition of his book *Patient Safety*.[9]

Organizations should strive to make it easy for clinicians to follow safety-related processes, essentially turning self-interest to work for patient interest. As pointed out by Reason,[123] as well as by Cook, Woods, and McDonald,[122] what goes on in the operational domain of frontline medicine (the so-called sharp end) is extensively shaped by the organizational and managerial environment in which it is embedded (the so-called blunt end). Of course every level has its own sharp end of deliverables and its blunt end of higher influences. For example, the hospital CEO makes policy and direction and is thus the blunt end for everyone else, but is in turn, shaped by regulators, funders, or patient advocacy groups, etc., constituting the CEO's blunt end.

Ideally, senior management commits not only in spirit but also in deed to patient safety as a primary goal. It encourages individuals and teams to fully engage in system-wide patient safety strategies and to trigger change themselves. Management and managers can do this first by changing their own behavior and that of the team, second by educating and persuading others about key changes, and third by searching for and identifying systems issues and pressing for their resolution.

The upcoming sections address (1) the basic concepts of systematic approaches (system thinking) to patient safety and human performance on the organizational level; (2) four organizational patient safety elements for health care derived from high-reliability organization theory (HROT); and (3) important strategies for organizational implementation of these concepts and principles.

SYSTEMS THINKING

To fully understand many issues in patient safety a broad systems perspective is needed. The actions and failures of individuals and teams usually play a central role, but their thinking and behavior is strongly influenced and constrained by their working environment and by wider organizational processes. The next sections provide systems thinking fundamentals, exploring (1) the definition of human failure and human error; (2) the evolution of accidents and adverse advents in relation to errors; (3) the concepts of hindsight bias and outcome bias as pitfalls in understanding events; (4) three prominent system organizational safety models: normal accident theory (NAT), HROT, and Safety-I/Safety-II; and (5) related concepts of resilience, uncertainty management, and normalization of deviance. More literature for further in-depth engagement with organizational approaches to human performance and patient safety are, for example, the works of René Alamberti, Sidney Dekker, Nancy Leveson, Richard Cook, David D. Woods, Erik Hollnagel, Jens Rasmussen, James Reason, Scott Sagan, Karl Weick, and Kathleen Sutcliffe.

Human Failure: Human Error and Violations

Human error has been conceptualized and investigated for a long time, initially by cataloguing errors and attempting to determine if the myriads of errors could be traced to a small set of causal mechanisms.[132,416] More recently the role of context for understanding error pathways and prevention has become prominent, while research in cognitive neuroscience has contributed to explaining individual vulnerabilities.[417]

Categorization of Human Failure. Different ways to categorize human failure and human error exist. Human failure in general can be categorized into two main types[418]: (1) human error, as an unintentional action

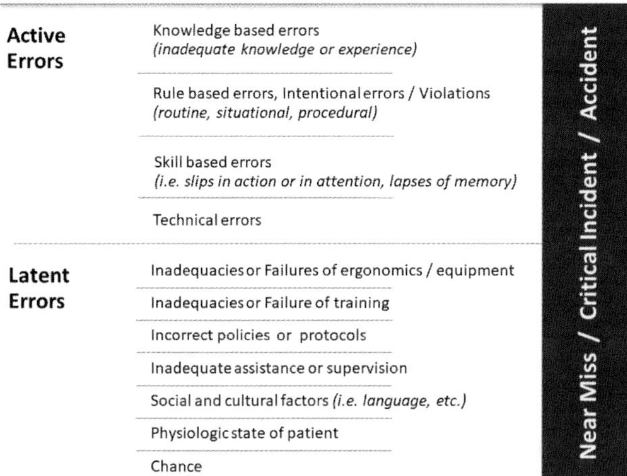

Fig. 6.12 Active and Latent Human Errors. Derived and adapted from the publication *Catalogue of human error* by Arnstein[419] and Rasmussen's performance levels.[420] Skill-based errors, which incorporate slips and lapses, relate to errors in conscious and subconscious (automatic) cognition. They are also summarized under the term "execution errors." Rule- and knowledge-based errors are summarized under the term "planning errors" or "mistakes." For further information see text.

or decision and (2) violations, as an intentional failure, deliberately doing the wrong thing. Derived and adapted from the error models of Arnstein,[419] Norman,[112] and Rasmussen,[420] human failure can be classified as follows (Fig. 6.12): (a) *Active errors*, including knowledge-based errors, skill-based errors, and rule-based errors (violations). (b) *Latent errors*, including, for example, failure of equipment or ergonomics, incorrect policies/protocols, inadequate training/supervision/assistance, social/cultural factors, etc.

Active Errors

SKILL-BASED ERRORS. Those errors incorporate slips (action not as intended) and lapses of memory (forgetting to do something) and relate to errors in conscious and subconscious (automatic) cognition. They are summarized under the term execution errors. Norman has described five types of skill-based errors[112]:

- *capture error*: a common action taking over from the one intended (e.g., force of habit)
- *description error*: performing correct action on wrong target (e.g., flipping wrong switch)
- *memory error*: forgetting an item in a sequence
- *sequence error*: performing an action out of sequence from other actions
- *mode error*: actions appropriate for one mode of operation but incorrect in another mode

Mode errors are possible with simple devices but they are becoming even more frequent with the increased use of computer-based equipment.[86] An example in anesthesiology of a mechanical mode error is the bag/ventilator selector valve in the anesthesia breathing circuit, which selects between two modes of ventilation. Failing to activate the ventilator when in the ventilator mode can be catastrophic. Newer machines may activate the ventilator automatically when ventilator mode is chosen. Mode errors can also occur with monitoring or drug delivery devices if they assign different functions to the same displays or switches depending on the mode of operation selected.

Particularly dangerous slips of execution can be addressed through the use of engineered safety devices that physically prevent incorrect actions.[59] For example, newer anesthesia machines have interlocks that physically prevent the simultaneous administration of more than one volatile anesthetic. Other interlocks physically prevent the selection of a gas mixture containing less than 21% oxygen. However, all this has come at a price, not only in terms of money, but also in terms of complexity and the introduction of new failure mechanisms.

RULE- AND KNOWLEDGE-BASED ERRORS. Those errors (making an intentional decision that is wrong) are summarized by the term planning errors or mistakes. Additionally, three further forms of error are described as fixation errors (see section "Prevent and Manage Fixation Errors [CRM Key Point 9]").[109] These may be seen as cognitive tunnel vision.

Latent Errors. James Reason, who literally wrote the book on human error, introduced the concept of latent errors, for which he also used the metaphor of resident pathogens: "*... whose adverse consequences may lie dormant within the system for a long time, only becoming evident when they combine with other factors to breach the system's defenses. [They are] most likely to be spawned by those whose activities are removed in both time and space from the direct control interface: designers, high-level decision makers, construction workers, managers and maintenance personnel*" (p. 173).[59]

Latent errors evolve from latent threats like organizational culture, professional culture, scheduling, management policies and decisions, organizational processes, etc.

This threat and error model was articulated by the aviation-oriented psychologist Robert Helmreich, distinguishing between (1) latent threats (national and organizational culture, professional culture, scheduling and policies, management decisions, and organizational processes), (2) individual threats (team factors, patient factors, organizational factors, environmental factors, and individual staff factors), and (3) management threats (error management strategies and countermeasures).[421]

A variety of latent failures/threats/errors can exist in the anesthesia environment.[14] They may include such issues as how surgical cases are booked, how cases are assigned to specific anesthesia professionals, what provisions are made for preoperative evaluation of outpatients, and what relative priority is given to rapid turnover between cases or avoiding cancellation of cases as opposed to avoiding risk.[422] Latent errors can also result from the design of anesthesia equipment and its user interfaces, which in some cases lead clinicians to err or are unforgiving of errors. Manufacturing defects and routine maintenance failures are also types of latent failure, as well as training, supervision, etc.

Evolution and Investigation of Accidents: One Error is not the Cause of an Accident

Traditionally, one speaks of errors arising in decisions and actions that lead to a mishap or an accident possibly with patient harm. However, the term error is increasingly considered inappropriate as it typically jumps to

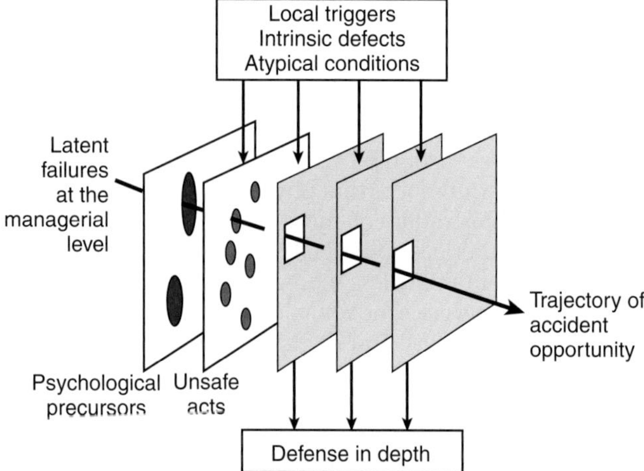

Fig. 6.13 James Reason's model of the causation of accidents. The model shows the different "defense shields" an organization possesses. Those shields prevent accidents at different levels. But each shield has weak spots, envisioned by the holes in the different shields. As work and the work environment in health care are dynamic, the diagram should be envisioned as being three-dimensional and also dynamic—with the shields moving around and holes opening and closing. If now, for example, latent failures at the managerial level combine with psychological precursors and active event triggers at the operational level, an accident sequence can be initiated. As long as there is no direct trajectory through the shields, the accident sequences are trapped at one or more defensive shields of the system. But if there develops a direct trajectory, the unforeseen combination of organizational or performance failures with latent errors and triggers may lead to breach the system's defenses and allow the accident to take place. This model is also known as Reason's "Swiss Cheese Model." Charles Vincent adapted Reason's model and published an extended model named "Organizational Accident Model."[9] (Figure redrawn from Reason JT. *Human Error.* Cambridge: Cambridge University Press; 1990.)

conclusions of attribution and blame. Current organizational accident models indicate that errors are usually the consequence of a combination of several underlying factors and conditions (i.e., root causes and contributing factors) that yield an event (Fig. 6.13).[59] Vincent and colleagues published a framework of contributory factors, called the seven levels of safety.[423] In their work, the error-producing conditions and organizational factors are classified as: patient factors, task factors, staff and team factors, work environment factors, organizational/management factors, and institutional context factors. This classification is used in the London Protocol,[424] an investigation and analysis tool for the processing of incident reports.

Human error—a window to the system. Human error can be seen as a window onto the usually hidden dynamics of the work system.[9,425,426] Sidney Dekker, pilot and human error expert, wrote:

"You can see human error as the cause of a mishap. In this case, 'human error' under whatever label—loss of situation awareness, procedural violation, regulatory shortcomings, managerial deficiencies—is the conclusion of your effort to understand error. [Or] you can see human error as the symptom of deeper trouble. In this case, human error is the starting point for your efforts. Finding 'errors' is only the beginning. You will probe how human error is systematically connected to features of people's tools, tasks, and operational/organizational environment." (p. xi)[427]

Whereas the first statement describes the old view on human error (person approach), the latter describes the new view on human error (system approach), albeit itself being a few decades old.[428] The new view focuses not on finding where people went wrong but rather to understand what triggered their assessment, actions, and decisions at the time, given the circumstances that surrounded them. Errors and violations should be addressed on a systems level as opposed to just with the individual(s) involved.

Investigation. Investigation of untoward events (see later section on "Critical Incident Reporting") should address both latent and active failures, and both the organizational/managerial environment and the operational domain. Focusing primarily on active failures may miss the fact that frontline personnel are often victims of the system in a Catch-22 situation, typically pushed to maximize production while admonished to be safe. Condemning only their actions—and not the latent pressures and conditions under which they work—will make them defensive and uncooperative. Cook and Woods pointed out that if one looks at the chain of events in an accident sequence, one can always find a failure on the part of an operator.[429] If the analysis stops at this point, the operator may be wrongly blamed in part or in whole while the real systemic root causes may not be detected; they will remain to cause other adverse event chains in the future (see later section on "Critical Incident Reporting").

PATIENT SAFETY ACTION BOX

Admonishing personnel to *"Try harder!"/Be more careful!"/" Next time you have to pay more attention!"* is known to be a fruitless way to address safety issues; such situations need explicit practical changes in the way the work is being performed and organized that make it easier to comply.

Evaluation of Errors and Accidents: Hindsight Bias—"I knew it all Along" and Outcome Bias—"No Harm no Foul"

Hindsight Bias. The psychological phenomenon called hindsight bias plays an important role in the attribution of causes to accidents and adverse events. The bias is sometimes called *"Monday morning quarterbacking"* or the *"I knew-it-all-along effect."* After an event, it seems easy to conclude what went wrong, what the people involved did or did not do, what information turned out to be critical, and to recognize exactly the kind of harm that should have been foreseen or prevented: *"There is almost no human action or decision that cannot be made to look flawed and less sensible in the misleading light of hindsight. It is essential that the critic should keep himself constantly aware of that fact"* (p. 147).[430] Similarly Leveson wrote *"Before the event [accident], such insight is difficult and, perhaps, impossible"* (p. 38).[12] Hindsight bias, which typically underestimates complexity and cannot represent a comprehensive analysis of what and how factors interacted to lead to an error or accident, is linked to the old view of human error presented earlier. Hindsight bias still is insidious and very hard to overcome, bearing the danger to impair organizational learning, to contribute to personal overconfidence, and to even to misjudge reasonable actions as medical malpractice.[431,432]

Outcome Bias. A related bias is the outcome bias, sometimes—when the outcome is good—using the sports metaphor of "no harm no foul."[431] It occurs when the judgment of a situation is made dependent on the outcome (known only in hindsight) rather than on the decision-making process itself. Harsher judgments are often made when an outcome is bad, becoming even harsher depending on the severity.[433]

PATIENT SAFETY ACTION BOX

When trying to make sense of events it is important to ask *"Why"* or *"How come?,"* to fully understand the problem and the thought processes in the moment of those involved. Jumping to conclusions prematurely can lead to solutions that are inappropriate or ineffective because they do not address the actual roots of the problem.

System Error Models: Normal Accident Theory and High Reliability Organization Theory

Several schools of thought about organizational safety in highly hazardous activities exist. Two complementary theories, Normal Accident Theory (NAT) and High Reliability Organization Theory (HROT), have dominated the discussion of system safety in many domains and have been applied to health care with increasing frequency since the 1980s.[59,123,434] NAT was originally promulgated by the sociologist Charles Perrow in the wake of the Three Mile Island (Pennsylvania) nuclear accident.[54] It has been applied by him and others to such diverse fields as commercial aviation, maritime transport, and the handling of nuclear weapons. A different theory, HROT, was put forth initially by Todd LaPorte, Gene Rochlin, and Karlene Roberts,[435-437] and later Karl Weick and Kathleen Sutcliffe.[438-441] It has been applied to diverse domains, including aircraft carrier flight decks, offshore oil platforms, air traffic control, nuclear power production, and the financial transaction industry. Both NAT and HROT agree that interactive complexity and tight coupling can lead to a system accident. However, they hold different opinions on whether those system accidents are inevitable or manageable.

In brief, the rather pessimistic view of NAT suggests, that disasters are the unwanted but inevitable (normal) results of complex socio-technical systems one cannot design around; the rather optimistic view of HROT sees disasters as preventable and manageable by certain key design characteristics or response systems of the organization.

A number of comparisons of these theories have been provided, giving an overview of the two theories, their advantages and limitations, and sometimes suggesting approaches that move beyond them.[442-446] Hollnagel and colleagues have promoted another influential error model called resilience engineering,[447-451] which has been compared to HROT by Haavik and colleagues.[452] One can argue that none of the other theories have replaced either NAT or HRO, and nearly all experts now believe that these exist in parallel, each providing a complementary view of the same set of issues.

Normal Accident Theory. NAT focuses primarily on three features of a system: (1) the complexity of interactions in the system, (2) the presence of tight coupling among the system's elements, and (3) the catastrophic potential of the system. Perrow[54] argues that the coexistence of interactive complexity and tight coupling in socio-technological systems leads to unpredictability of interactions and hence system accident is inevitable or normal. NAT suggests that when complexity and tight coupling coexist, abnormal sequences of events can be hidden and have complex or unpredictable consequences. Active errors in the system may not result in an accident only if, they are trapped at some point by the system's multiple layers of checks and defenses (Fig. 6.14; see also Fig. 6.13).

Naive view: error causes accidents

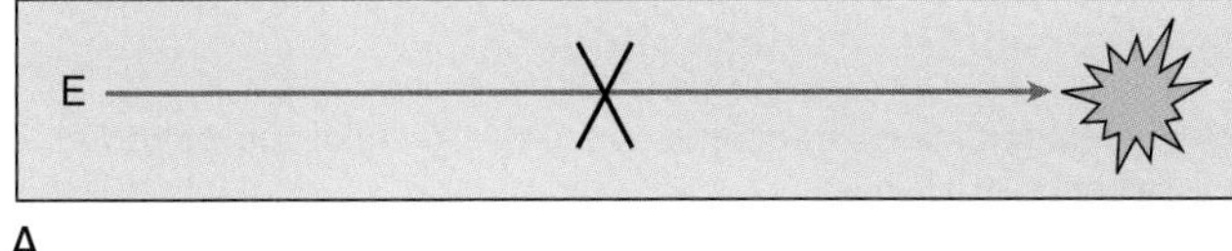

A

Modern view: deeper causes lead to errors that result in accidents

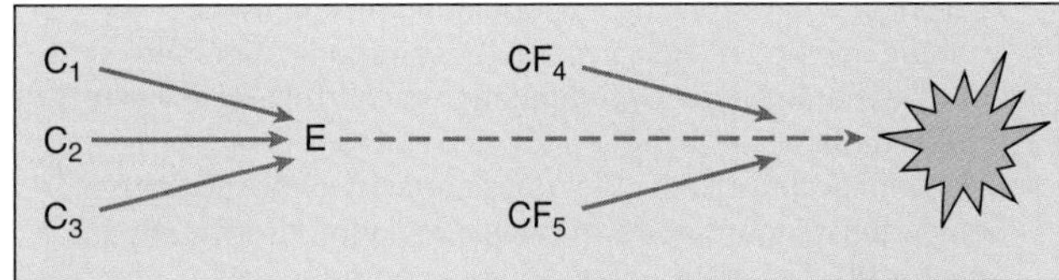

B

Fig. 6.14 Relationship between errors and adverse events. (A) Errors are the cause of accidents. Rather naïve views see the causes of accidents directly and solely linked to errors (*E*), as errors oftentimes lead directly to the accident. But errors are not the cause of accidents alone. (B) Errors are not the cause of accidents. In the more modern view, errors are one part of a multifactorial environment, when accidents occur. Multiple root causes (*C1, C2, C3*) lead to the error (E). For the most part, in an accident sequence additional contributing factors (*CF4, CF5*) are necessary to allow the error to evolve into an accident, explaining why profound analysis of an accident or incident is necessary in order to prevent similar consequences. (Modified from Rall M, Manster T, Guggenberger H, et al. Patient safety and errors in medicine: development, prevention and analyses of incidents [in German]. *Anesthesiol Intensivmed Notfallmed Schmerzther.* 2001;36:321–330 with permission.)

NAT also proposes that professionals delude themselves by believing that they can perfectly control hazardous activities and forestall disaster all the time. In reality, many of the efforts people make at management and design tend only to increase the opacity and complexity of the system (making more holes in the barriers, Fig. 6.13) thereby increasing the likelihood of accidents. The combination of these factors with normal everyday faults, slips, and incidents provides fertile ground for the occurrence of accidents.

NAT considers safety as one of many competing organizational objectives, but often not of sufficiently high priority. For preventing adverse events, Perrow suggested that attention should be directed at strengthening the recovery pathways by which small events can be properly handled before they evolve into a serious accident. In fact, this suggestion by Perrow in the book *Normal Accidents*—plus the apparent success in commercial aviation—were direct inspirations for Gaba and colleagues to develop simulation-based CRM-oriented training, and to create and disseminate emergency manuals (cognitive aids).

BOX 6.7 Characteristics High Reliability Organizations Hold in Common...[454]

- Hypercomplex environment—extreme variety of components, systems, and levels.
- Tight coupling/interdependent teams—reciprocal interdependence across many units and levels.
- Extreme hierarchical differentiation—multiple levels, each with its own elaborate control and regulating mechanisms.
- Multiple decision makers in complex communication networks—characterized by redundancy in control and information systems.
- Degree of accountability that does not exist in most organizations—substandard performance or deviations from standard procedures meet with severe adverse consequences.
- High frequency of immediate feedback about decisions.
- Compressed time constraints—cycles of major activities are measured in seconds.
- More than one critical outcome that must happen simultaneously—simultaneity signifies both the complexity of operations as well as the inability to withdraw or modify operations decisions.

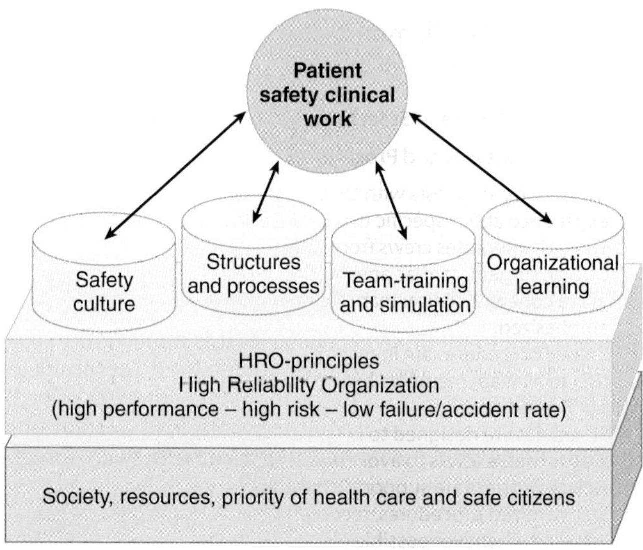

Fig. 6.15 The fundamentals and principles of a high reliability organization.

BOX 6.8 Organizational Strategies[438] that Guide the Thinking of People in High Reliability Organizations:

- Preoccupation with failure
- Reluctance to simplify interpretations
- Sensitivity to (front-line) operations
- Commitment to resilience
- Deference to expertise

BOX 6.9 Elements of a Culture of Safety[437,441,454,560]

Values

- Safety is most important goal, overriding production or efficiency
- Preoccupation is with possible "failures," not past "successes"
- Necessary resources/incentives/rewards are provided for optimal safety, not only for optimal production

Beliefs

- Safety must be actively managed
- Processes and routines of care are as (or more) important to safety as individual dedication, skill, or effort
- Openness about safety and errors is essential; learning from normal and adverse events should be thorough

Norms

- Low-ranking personnel raise safety issues and challenge ambiguity regardless of hierarchy or rank
- Calling for help is encouraged and occurs frequently, even by experienced personnel
- Explicit communication is frequent
- The hierarchy is flat—leaders listen to juniors; juniors speak up; and calling for help is routine regardless of rank
- People are rewarded for rationally erring on the side of safety, even when their credible concerns turn out to be wrong

Modified from Weick KE. Organizational culture as a source of high reliability. *Calif Manage Rev*. 1987;29:112–127.

High-Reliability Organization Theory. In contrast to these rather pessimistic views of NAT concerning the organizational challenges to safety, HROT suggests that proper organization of people, technology, and processes can handle complex and hazardous activities at acceptable levels of performance.[373,453] In fact, consider the many endeavors in which HROs manage to achieve nearly failure-free results despite high intrinsic risk and high throughput.

Box 6.7 shows the common characteristics of HROs.[454] It is important to note that many organizations display some of these characteristics, but true HROs display them all simultaneously. Box 6.8 shows the organizational safety strategies that guide the thinking of people in an HRO. Although these elements point in the right direction, they remain theoretical if not—in our case—translated to health care, and then embedded into the fabric of an organization's operations. An HRO-based safety strategy tool in the form of a reference sheet is available at no cost from the Institute for Healthcare Improvement (IHI).[455] Fig. 6.15 shows four strategic key elements of HROs, which are explained in more detail in Boxes 6.9 and 6.10 and in the following section.

Anesthesiology has traditionally been strong at some elements of HRO, particularly in redundancy and technical safety measures. A movement is growing in anesthesia to implement HRO philosophies and techniques more fully.[456] In fact, anesthesiologists not only have been promoters of the patient safety movement in general but also have been leaders at applying HROT principles to health care. In 2003, the APSF began initiatives in high reliability perioperative health care (see special issue of the *APSF Newsletter*, summer 2003, at www.apsf.org). More recently, HROs have been conceptualized as one of three approaches to safety: ultra-adaptive (which embraces risks, e.g., trauma center), high-reliability (which manages risks, e.g., scheduled surgery), and ultra-safe (which avoids risk, e.g., radiotherapy).[10] Providing anesthesiology to an ASA1 patient is considered between the high-reliability and ultra-safe approach.[10]

BOX 6.10 **Key Elements of a High-Reliability Organization in Medicine**[437,441,454,560]

Established Culture of Safety (see elements Box 6.9)

Optimal Structures and Procedures

- Decision making rests with those with greatest knowledge or experience about specific issues regardless of rank or job type.
- The unit integrates crews from different departments (e.g., cardiac surgery, cardiac anesthesia, OR nursing, perfusion, ICU) into a coherent clinical team. Teamwork and resiliency are emphasized.
- Formal procedures are in place to maximize transfer of information to all team members before a case (e.g., briefings or time-out procedures).
- Schedules are designed to keep work hours and duty periods at reasonable levels to avoid undue fatigue. Personnel under excessive stress are supported or replaced as needed.
- Standardized procedures, techniques, and equipment are adopted whenever possible so that similar tasks or operations are performed similarly regardless of the personnel involved; conversely, when necessary (in an emergency or adverse event), the team is resilient and responds as needed to the situation without slavish dependence on standard routines.
- The use of preplanned algorithms, checklists, and cognitive aids is actively encouraged.
- Easy access to current information systems is available at all times and all locations.

Training and Practice in Routine Procedures and Simulations

- Debriefings are conducted after each case.
- Nonpunitive assessment instruments are used on a regular basis to provide current feedback and identify elements requiring special training.
- Initial and recurrent simulation-based single-discipline and multidisciplinary training in crew resource management occurs (see Chapter 7).
- Actual clinical crews and teams conduct periodic drills or simulations of critical situations in the real OR, PACU, and ICU.
- Resident training uses a guided curriculum; training goals and the level of responsibility assigned to a resident match the current proficiency level of the trainee with the complexity of the procedure.

Organizational Learning

- Robust mechanisms are in regular use for organizational learning, both prospectively (considering in advance how to optimize protocols and procedures, such as failure mode and analysis of effects) and retrospectively (from analyzing reports of adverse events, near misses, or problems such as root cause analysis).
- Problems are analyzed primarily to determine what can be improved, rather than whom to blame. Altered procedures are assessed and adopted as appropriate. Process changes reflect appropriate analysis.

ICU, Intensive care unit; *OR*, operating room; *PACU*, postanesthesia care unit.

Safety I and Safety II: Ensuring that as Few Things as Possible go Wrong or that as Many Things as Possible go Right…?

As indicated above, perspectives on safety are changing. In recent years several scientists questioned the definition of safety as the absence of errors. A new view of safety has evolved, defining it as maximizing the ways that work can evolve in a correct way and focusing primarily on why human performance succeeds most often despite myriad challenges. Erik Hollnagel labelled this new approach Safety-II, as opposed to Safety-I, which denotes the traditional approach investigating errors, incidents, and accidents.[457] *"Safety management should therefore move from ensuring that 'as few things as possible go wrong' [Safety-I] to ensuring that 'as many things as possible go right [Safety-II]'"* (p. 4).[458]

The Safety-II approach aims to understand how good performance is actually produced: how people adapt the workflow, their use of devices, and their organization of tasks to achieve good performance even in challenging circumstances. In this regard it is quite similar to HROT. Safety-II also sees successful performance as a learning space:

> *this "...approach assumes that everyday performance variability provides the adaptations that are needed to respond to varying conditions, and hence is the reason why things go right. Humans are consequently seen as a resource necessary for system flexibility and resilience. In Safety-II the purpose of investigations changes to become an understanding of how things usually go right, since that is the basis for explaining how things occasionally go wrong." (p. 4)*[458]

Perhaps the most important new ideas of Safety-I and -II are the analytical character of the models. The focus on positive performance provides a different lens and rather than emphasizing the individual's success it addresses how and why such success occurs. One specific method that Hollnagel[459] describes is functional resonance analysis, which identifies the different pieces of a system and investigates in detail how they interact with each other dynamically. Many phenomena emerge from the interplay of the system parts, but this emergence might not be easy or possible to explain on a causal basis. A detailed description of the Safety-I and Safety-II approach by Hollnagel, Wears, and Braithwaite is available in PDF format online (*"From Safety-I to Safety-II: A White Paper. The Resilient Health Care Net")*.[458]

Resilience and Uncertainty Management: Safety is a Dynamic State, not all Risks can be Eliminated

System safety is not a static property of hospitals and departments; rather it is dynamic, often on short time scales. Even with the implementation of robust patient safety strategies and regulatory regimes, (1) not all risks can be eliminated in the system and (2) safety, even once established, is not omnipresent or infinitely persistent. Whether risk in any setting can credibly be lowered to zero is widely debated. Admitting that risk cannot be prevented while striving to find more appropriate ways of handling adverse occurrences, for example through improving system resilience [447,448] or the ability to manage uncertainties,[460-465] seems appropriate regardless of the theoretical approach. Whereas some system safety methodologies view even a domain's own professionals as unreliable components, the theories of HRO, Safety-I, and Safety-II view people as core elements in creating reliable systems.

Resilience. The term resilience in respect to patient safety is derived from resilience engineering and is an important characteristic of HROs. The introduction to health care was promoted by Hollnagel and colleagues. Resilience describes the intrinsic ability of individuals, teams, and the system to cope with and adjust to new or changing demands and to respond effectively and safely to unforeseen, unpredicted, and unexpected problems or demands as they occur, even after a major mishap or in the presence of continuous stress. A resilient system owns the ability to produce success despite conditions that could easily lead to failure.

Uncertainty Management. Grote argues that *"in order to improve risk management and safety more generally deliberate increases in uncertainty may be beneficial"* (p. 71).[460] Grote furthermore distinguishes two uncertainty paradigms[461]: (1) Uncertainty may be minimized by high levels of standardization, central planning, automation of work/processes, and high levels of specialization with few degrees of freedom for employees (stability). (2) Newer organization theories in contrast stress the need for flexible adaptation in highly uncertain and networked processes, empowering everyone in the organization to cope with uncertainty by providing them with options for action rather than fixed plans and standards. As a consequence, organizations must find a way to balance stability and flexibility as both can mutually enable each other.[466] It sometimes can be worth tolerating some degree of uncertainty—relying on flexible adaptation of intelligent, well-trained personnel and stability by well-functioning systems—rather than to attempt to eradicate every possible uncertainty by standardization. From an HROT perspective's view one could say to standardize where possible (or sensible) while remaining flexible and resilient. Clearly there is a sweet spot between these extremes, although how to achieve that balance remains under debate.[467]

Normalization of Deviance and Flirting with the Margin

Normalization of Deviance. Normalization of deviance is a term first coined by American sociologist Diane Vaughan who conducted a detailed organizational analysis of the Space Shuttle Challenger disaster.[468] The phenomenon occurs when people within an organization become so insensitive to deviant practices or occurrences that do not cause a problem that the practices themselves no longer seem wrong—essentially creating a *"new normal."* Such normalization of deviance emerges insidiously, sometimes over years. Once this happens on a large scale, no one within an organization is able to see the shortcomings in the behavior. They become resistant to suggestions that they are in fact abnormal and deviant, dismissing allegations that *"the emperor has no clothes."* Because disaster indeed does not happen without a number of critical factors lining up, their resistance is reinforced by the continued good outcomes—until a catastrophe occurs. Many have applied these concepts to health care including anesthesiology.[48-50,445] Banja[47] gives an overview of the topic in health care overall and identifies a number of reasons why normalization of deviance occurs in organizations, including:

- The existing rules are considered stupid and inefficient
- Knowledge is imperfect and uneven
- The work itself, along with new technology, can disrupt work behaviors and rule compliance
- "I'm breaking the rule for the good of my patient!"
- "The rules don't apply to me"/"You can trust me"
- Workers are afraid to speak up
- Leadership is unaware of or downplays reports or findings on system problems

Flirting With the Margin. Cook and Rasmussen published two related models to normalization of deviance that can be understood as flirting with the margin.[469] Their so-called dynamic safety model identifies three different states of a system in which an organization can operate (stable systems, unstable systems, stable but high-risk systems). The model points out that the states can be floating, depending on the set of organizational boundaries (i.e., economic, workload, acceptable performance) and the pressures within the system (i.e., management, safety campaigns/culture, staff). Typically the highest economic yield lies near the margin and the system may be pushed toward or even over the marginal boundary that safeguards systems from errors, accidents, and adverse events. The constitutive flirting with the margin model draws attention to the risk that repeated shifts outside the marginal boundary may lead to the original margin being judged as too conservative, resulting in a shift of the marginal boundary (normalization of deviance). When this happens regular operations in a system take place in an already dangerous marginal zone, implying a false sense of safety and raising the probability of accidents.

ACHIEVING HIGH RELIABILTY AND SYSTEM THINKING: FUNDAMENTAL ELEMENTS FOR A SYSTEMATIC SAFETY APPROACH

How can clinical departments and health care institutions transform into a high-reliability organization? Addressing safety at the individual and team level has yielded some useful improvements in health care. However, more comprehensive improvement will require transforming whole organizations. Altering particular care processes is not enough; the work culture needs to be transformed. The AHRQ published a report in 2008—*"Becoming a High Reliability Organization: Operational advice for Hospital Leaders"*—that summarizes the topic in depth.[470]

As displayed in Fig. 6.15, HROs can be characterized essentially by four key structural pillars: (1) creation and sustainment of a culture of safety; (2) global and profound organizational learning, including incident reporting systems (IRS); (3) continuous training of individuals, teams, and work units including the regular use of simulation; and (4) continuous optimization of safety-relevant structures and processes. The four pillars are intended to provide anchor points for systematic organizational improvement. They are explained in more detail in the subsequent sections.

Culture of Safety

Creating a culture of safety is an important element of enhancing patient safety.[471-473] Safety culture is part of the

BOX 6.11 Key Features of High Reliability Organizations Based on the AHRQ's Definition[561]

- acknowledgment of the high-risk nature of an organization's activities and the determination to achieve consistently safe operations
- a blame-free environment where individuals are able to report errors or near misses without fear of reprimand or punishment
- encouragement of collaboration across ranks and disciplines to seek solutions to patient safety problems
- organizational commitment of resources to address safety concerns

overall culture of an organization. Opposed to the widely spread culture of blame (also called negative safety culture), the culture of safety is also referred to as the culture of no-blame or is reinforced in its meaning by the expression positive safety culture.

One prominent definition of culture is: "*A pattern of shared basic assumptions learned by a group as it solved its problems of external adaptation and internal integration*" (p.12).[474] More simply, culture is "*the way we do things around here,*" or "*what you do when nobody is looking.*" The Joint Commission defines safety culture as follows: "*Safety culture is the sum of what an organization is and does in the pursuit of safety. [...] the product of individual and group beliefs, values, attitudes, perceptions, competencies, and patterns of behavior that determine the organization's commitment to quality and patient safety*" (p. 2).[475]

Edgar Schein described three elements of culture that can be observed: (1) artifacts that are used in the organization (e.g., charts, clothes/uniforms, meetings, rituals), (2) espoused beliefs and values (some measurable in surveys and some by interviews or by watching and listening to everyday work), and (3) underlying assumptions that are so ingrained that they are hardly noticeable any more (e.g., what is meant by a patient vs. a client or partner; by illness vs. health; or by safety vs. quality or outcome). Box 6.9 shows the major elements of a culture of safety based on shared values (what is important), beliefs (how things should work), and norms (the way things work).

The Joint Commission published behaviors that undermine a safety culture and suggests respective counteractions.[476] Two reviews on the current literature of safety culture are available.[477,478]

A health care HRO's commitment to safety needs to start at the top—with full buy-in from chief executives and boards of directors or trustees and palpably extend through all levels of middle managers and fully into frontline personnel (professionals and others). This commitment encompasses the key features (based on AHRQ's formulation) shown in Box 6.11.

When an organization does not promote a culture of safety, staff members often are unwilling to report adverse events and unsafe conditions because they fear reprisal or from prior experience believe reporting rarely results in change (see later sections "Organizational Learning" and "Incident Reporting").[471]

A variety of techniques have been developed to help organizations create and sustain a safety culture. Some of these address getting senior managers and executives more directly in touch with what is happening at the sharp end of work, by activities such as Patient Safety Leadership WalkRounds[479] or Leveraging Frontline Expertise (LFLE).[479,480] Other interventions suggested by the IHI include: designation of a patient safety officer, involvement of patients in safety initiatives, appointment of a safety champion for every unit, safety briefings, and simulation of possible adverse events (see later section on "Periodic Team Training and Simulation Team Training" and Chapter 7).[481] Other widely available guides to address an organization's safety culture come from The American College of Healthcare Executives and IHI/NPSF Lucian Leape Institute[482] and the Joint Commission.[483] It is hard to demonstrate which, if any, of these strategies and techniques are most effective, and it may depend heavily on a variety of local factors in each organization.[484]

It is problematic that, sometimes, safety culture is thought to mean culture of no blame. Safety culture is actually a much broader concept and the notion of no blame or blame-free has widely given way to the concept of a just culture. While no blame is appropriate for many unintended errors, other actions do seem blameworthy and demand individual accountability. A just culture focuses on identifying and addressing systems issues that lead individuals to engage in unsafe behaviors, while maintaining individual accountability by establishing zero tolerance for reckless behavior. It distinguishes between human error (e.g., slips), at-risk behavior (e.g., taking shortcuts), and reckless behavior (e.g., ignoring required safety steps). Gross negligence, behavior violations, and destructive acts are not tolerated.

Nonetheless, unjust cultures of individual blame still appear to be dominant.[476] Khatri and colleagues reported an increased likelihood of a culture of blame in health care organizations that (1) rely predominantly on hierarchical, compliance-based management systems; (2) attach less importance to employee involvement in decision making; and (3) neglect human resource management capabilities to help foster a safety culture.[485]

PATIENT SAFETY ACTION BOX

Mind your language! Ensure that dialogues, interviews, discussions, and reports avoid judgmental or blaming language (e.g., "*You should/could have...,*" "*Why didn't you...?,*" "*Do you think that was a good idea?,*" "*The professional failed to...*"). Instead, use language that encourages systems thinking.[486]

Anesthesiology as a specialty has played a leading role in the attempt to turn the rather predominant culture of blame into a culture of safety—putting safety first and trying to understand how errors, incidents, and adverse events evolve.[11,40,456,487-490]

Measuring Safety Culture. Measuring safety culture is difficult. Strictly speaking, it may only be possible to investigate culture by anthropologic means—embedding ethnographers into the workplace for deep understanding of how work is conducted. This can be supplemented by structured interviews. Such methods are difficult and costly. More frequently safety culture is measured through written surveys of health care personnel. Essentially these measure safety climate—the attitudes of personnel as represented by survey responses. It is difficult to extrapolate from these results to the culture as actually enacted. Nonetheless, surveys are relatively simple and low cost, especially since the advent of online administration of the instruments.

Several validated survey tools are available to measure hospital safety and teamwork safety climates, including, for example, the Patient Safety Culture in Healthcare Organizations (PSCHO),[491-493] the AHRQ Survey on Patient Safety Culture, and the Safety Attitudes Questionnaire (SAQ). Each of the various instruments have a somewhat different focus, and the methods of administration of such surveys can be very important.

Among the issues that influence what can be learned from such surveys are: (a) Who is asked to complete the survey? Is it hospital-wide or just in one or a few work units? Sometimes the work unit is the appropriate unit of analysis but often the target may need to be broader.[494] (b) Are managers and senior leaders sampled in the same fraction as other workers? If so, this will mean that their views will not be well represented because they make up such a small fraction of the overall workforce. Oversampling of important but small populations can compensate for this. (c) Are the surveys truly confidential or anonymous? (d) How are the data interpreted? Looking primarily at the views of the majority of respondents may not be sufficient. If only a modest fraction (the rule of thumb from some experts is about 10% or more) respond in ways antithetical to a culture of safety that may represent a serious lack in its uniformity, and show a problem. For example, elements of the PSCHO survey have been asked also in different surveys of military aviators, acknowledged HRO. The negative safety views almost never were near the 10% level but this was seen substantially more often in the health care population.[495] Teamwork and communication dimensions of safety culture have been significantly related to adverse clinical events.[491,496-498]

Despite the past decade's focus on improving patient safety, most health care organizations are still striving to achieve high-reliability organization status[445,499]—consistently providing high quality care, with substantial load while minimizing adverse events.

In an update of the sentinel event alert from 2009, the Joint Commission 2017 calls again for senior health care leaders to establish a culture of safety within their organizations, use just culture principles to establish transparent and fair policies for addressing errors by clinical personnel in the front lines, and maintain robust structures for analyzing and responding to adverse events. Specific suggested actions include involving hospital boards and patients in safety efforts and making safety performance an explicit part of the evaluation for leaders. Adherence to sentinel event alert recommendations is assessed as part of Joint Commission accreditation surveys.[475]

PATIENT SAFETY ACTION BOX

Mind your attitude! Pursuing a culture of safety oftentimes is about one's attitude and reactions when safety concerns are raised. For example: If a patient's condition is deteriorating and someone else calls the rapid response team (RRT) when you think you might have things under control, don't say *"Why did you call the RRT? It's fine, do you think I'm an idiot?"* Instead it's better to say *"Thanks for calling the RRT—I think I know what's going on and have it under control, but it can't hurt to have them here."* Conversely, when a team arrives, if they find that there is no active crisis, they should not complain (or roll their eyes). Instead they should thank the clinician for calling them and offer to help in any way even though they seem to have things well in hand. In health care, one sometimes rewards people verbally for a good pickup, noticing something that is clearly of importance to the patient's care. Yet one rarely rewards people for raising their credible concerns when they turn out not to be an issue. Providing such rewards regardless of outcome will strengthen the safety culture and foster the desired speaking up.

Organizational Learning

An important strategy for improving patient safety and a core content of HROs is organizational learning. Organizational learning *"is defined as the process of creating and applying valid knowledge to enable an organization to improve."*[500] Such learning should be both prospective (i.e., using Failure Mode and Effect Analysis; FMEA) and retrospective (i.e., using [critical] incident reporting systems; [C]IRS). In analogy to aviation, Donaldson referred to organizational learning in health care as "passing the orange wire test":

> *"Imagine that a Boeing 757 aircraft engine contained an orange-coloured wire essential to its safe functioning. Imagine that an airline engineer doing a preflight inspection spotted that the wire was frayed in a way that suggested a systematic fault rather than routine wear and tear. Imagine what would happen next. It is likely that most 757 engines in the world would be inspected—probably within days—and the orange wire, if faulty, renewed."*[501]

So, what about health care and the orange wire test? Over the last two decades IRS have generated a lot of momentum in enhancing system safety in health care by organizational learning. The next sections focus on: (1) basic information on prospective (FMEA) and retrospective (IRS) organizational learning; (2) more detailed information about the purpose of IRS, their challenges, and their effectiveness; (3) barriers and facilitators for IRS; (4) characteristics of successful IRS; (5) legal issues of IRS; and (6) the linked idea of independent medical accident investigation boards is discussed based on a recent pioneering safety movement in the United Kingdom.

Failure Mode And Effect Analysis. FMEA has been adapted to health care from engineering systems analysis; it is sometimes used as a tool to analyze adverse events in retrospect. The FMEA approach is to lay out comprehensively the possible failure modes and their effects that could have led to the events and the outcome that occurred. This helps define ways in which the chain of accident evolution could have been prevented or thwarted. A prospective approach to safety can use FMEA techniques to identify safety gaps in advance and implement corrective measures. This can be especially useful for assessing proposed changes to the system—such as introducing a new piece of equipment or a new set of surgical procedures (e.g., starting a liver transplant program where none had existed). Contemplating in advance the ways that things might fail will help determine whether the benefits outweigh the risks organizationally, how best to structure the change, as well as how best to prevent or mitigate problems when they inevitably occur.

(Critical) Incident Reporting System†. The retrospective approach to organizational learning means maximizing the learning to be had from understanding incidents or near misses that have already happened. Even though the terms vary in the literature, based on the *WHO Draft Guidelines for Adverse Event Reporting and Learning Systems*[502] an incident is any deviation from usual medical care that causes harm to a patient or presents a risk of harm. It includes (1) adverse events, where harm is caused to a patient, sometimes also referred to as sentinel events (SE) or critical incidents, as well as (2) near misses. A near miss is a situation that potentially could have turned into a critical incident, but was somehow prevented beforehand. Yet another kind of incident is termed a never event, an incident that results in serious patient harm or death, classified as one that is never the natural result of disease or therapeutic side effect.

Apart from certain mandatory legal reporting and disclosure requirements, (critical) IRSs, sometimes also called patient safety reporting systems (PSRS), are usually voluntary. While original IRS were paper-based, technological progress has allowed the development of mostly electronic or web-based systems. Although IRS adopt various formats, most have the same core operating model: frontline staff, usually those directly involved in an event or actions leading to it, anonymously or confidentially provide detailed information about something that has occurred. In the next step, this report is analyzed—usually free of blame to the reporter—by expert analysts to identify contributing system and human factors, and if applicable, develop strategies for preventing such occurrences. A simplified overview of the core processes of IRS is given in Fig. 6.16. IRS aim to provide systematic organizational learning from local to global levels, recognizing that an incident that occurred in one unit might also be a problem in another unit.

Most HROs have made special efforts to create IRS for incidents of various severity and near misses. Despite several limitations, if IRS is used in a successful way, to quote Charles Vincent,[487] it can serve as a powerful *"window on the system,"* enabling understanding of system problems and safety gaps. In order to function well, IRS need to be easy to use, organizationally integrated and coherent, supported by a culture of safety (see earlier correspondent section), free of sanctions, and linked to feedback about what is being done about the issues reported.

Other methods for organizational learning. Neither FMEA nor IRS alone can optimally enhance patient safety. They are just two of many strategies for soliciting input from frontline staff to creating snapshots of safety issues in the patient care arena. Information from many sources needs to be combined through a systematic assessment of error and harm to obtain the full picture. The U.S. Agency for Healthcare Research and Quality provides a detailed discussion of methods of identifying errors and latent safety problems for organizational learning.[503] Walk rounds by senior leaders and executives also offer a way of collecting data from frontline staff about possible safety hazards.[479]

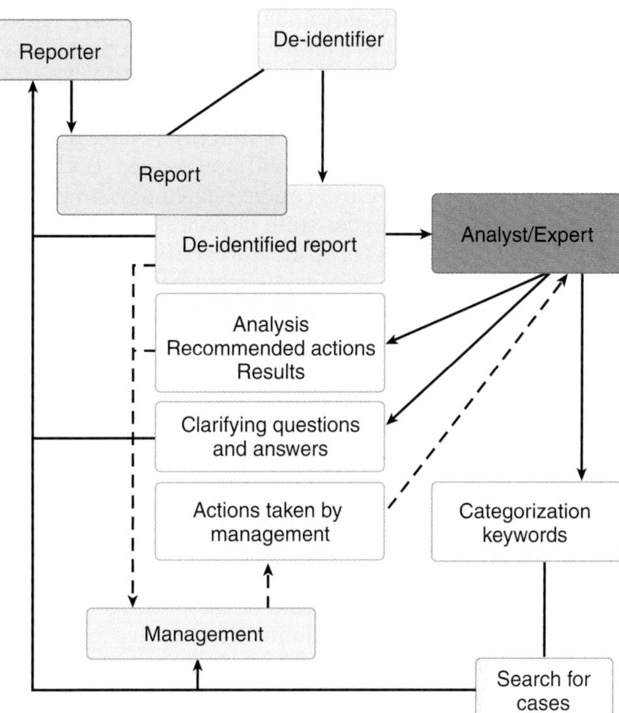

Fig. 6.16 Data handling in a modern incident reporting system with deidentification. The incoming reports are first completely deidentified by a trained deidentifier. Only after this step is the report ready to be analyzed. It is important that the reports are analyzed by a multiprofessional team and that recommendations be fed back to the management of the organization from which the report came. The analysis and feedback should be transparent for all stakeholders.

IRS in health care have drawn their inspiration especially from commercial aviation and the nuclear industry. Unfortunately, the word reporting is a word with a variety of (mostly negative) connotations. In the context of organizational learning it is intended to be regarded as something positive and means communicating safety-relevant information. Anesthesia professionals experience weaknesses and strengths of their work sites during everyday work—valuable information of potential safety gaps that are already out there. By reporting, IRS can help the organization and staff at the rather blunt end of medicine (risk managers, executives, etc.) to extract safety-critical information from frontline staff at first hand, analyze it, and learn from it as an organization. Hence, IRS in a more positive way are often referred to as learning systems, such as the National Reporting and Learning System of the National Patient Safety Agency in the National Health Service (NHS) of the United Kingdom.

Different Operating Modes of Incident Reporting Systems. IRS around the world vary widely in terms of design and operational processes (see Appendix 6.1).[346,502,504-509] IRS can operate at different levels within the health care system: some IRS operate primarily at the local level (i.e., as a

†While reading this section American readers will need to break their ingrained habit of seeing "IRS" as the tax collecting agency of the U.S. federal government (Internal Revenue Service).

tool for local hospital quality and risk management), which may or may not feed into a larger scale; others operate on a larger regional or national scale (i.e., ASA' AIRS). The latter allow (a) a recognition of a pattern of (rare) events that otherwise could not be discerned, and (b) a wider dissemination of lessons learned and solutions created. Both on a local and national level, IRS can be related to a single specialty, or include a broader suite of professional domains. Some IRS accept reports of all kind of events and deviations (i.e., near misses, adverse events, sentinel events, never events, etc.). Others restrict their reports to incidents that match specific narrow criteria.

The Goals of Incident Reporting Systems. The applicable goals of reporting systems are currently under debate with respect to the way in which data can be used, particularly whether for different combinations of the following: (1) help health care organizations learn and improve, (2) benchmark and compare organizations, (3) hold organizations accountable for safety performance, or (4) help regulators and funders make judgments.[502,510-513] Some of these IRS goals, while compatible in theory, may be mutually exclusive in practice. The emphasis applied to each goal influences system design features, such as whether reporting is mandatory or voluntary, whether reports are confidential or made public, and what kind of incidents are allowed to be reported.

Are IRS effective?. In the United States, all hospitals are required to maintain a confidential event reporting system. In Germany, this has been the case since 2013. Almost two decades ago, Lucian Leape wrote: "If reporting is safe and provides useful information from expert analysis, it can measurably improve safety."[504] Despite their current ubiquity, the actual contribution of these systems to any of their stated goals is uncertain and questions about their effectiveness remain.[514,515]

Challenges and Misunderstandings About Incident Reporting Systems. In a recent paper *"The problem with incident reporting,"* Macrae summarizes a variety of issues surrounding IRS.[512] These include, among many others:

1. Underreporting has been recognized as a major limitation of incident reporting. Of the errors and adverse events that occur in hospital settings, reporting systems capture fewer than 10%.[516] A detailed review of causes of underreporting is described in the section on barriers of reporting. While increasing the absolute number of reports can be useful, their quality is of greatest importance. Charles Vincent stresses that analyzing a small number of incidents thoroughly is probably more valuable than a cursory overview of a large number of incidents.[487]
2. Another widespread misunderstanding of IRS is the idea that the goal of reporting is to provide a numerical metric of harm to patients. In contrary, merely counting incidents is largely uninformative and probably a waste of time.[517] It is sometimes described as a box-checking exercise. Many reports can describe similar events and the relative learning per event shrinks markedly after the first few, whereas some kinds of events are not reported and hence the system may be blind to them. All reporting systems, whether voluntary or not, have serious selection-bias issues—many events are never reported both because it takes effort to do so and because doing so seems to expose the individual and the work setting to risk of reputation loss or other negative consequences.
3. Even at best, IRS provide only partial views on the organization. For a variety of reasons 50% to 80% of the reports are filed by nurses. Physicians file only 1% to 3% of incident reports.[518,519] But many issues involve physician care—up to 94% of the events based on a landmark study.[520] It is likely that to fully understand a system it would be necessary for trained observers (ethnographers) to be embedded in it. Moreover, even if all events were known about in detail the tasks of analyzing and understanding them and finding practical but robust solutions to problems uncovered are far more difficult than merely collecting the information.

BOX 6.12 Important Characteristics of Effective Incident Reporting Systems[11,502,523,527]

- Integration of the incident reporting system into the organization and full support by management
- The absence of negative sanctions for reporters and people involved
- Confidential or anonymous reporting option, with active deidentification (domain expertise required)
- Legal protection and state-of-the-art data security
- Independence of the organizational hierarchy: reports are sent to a trusted subunit outside the hierarchy of the organization or outside the organization (external trust center, e.g., NASA for the ASRS)
- Orientation to a system that enables all stakeholders of patient safety, including physicians, nurses, and technicians, to file reports easily
- Easy and fast reporting
- Training of stakeholders to file valuable reports (e.g., focusing on human factor issues, as well as medical-technical aspects)
- Timely feedback about reception of the report, its analysis, and proposed measures to be taken from it
- Analysis of each report by experts (a multiprofessional team that has a background not only in the medical domain but also in issues of human performance and analysis methods)
- Deep analysis of selected cases by using root cause analyses or failure modes and effect analyses with the aim of improving systems safety in the future
- Timely implementation of improvements to confirm the "reactivity" of the system and to *make a difference*
- Evaluation of improvements and special care to avoid "improvements for the worse" (quick fixes without improving the underlying latent dangers)
- Organizational support of reporting and analysis of cases, as well as the implementation of improvements
- Supports continuous improvement of the positive proactive safety culture in the department (systems perspective!)

ASRS, Aviation Safety Reporting System; *NASA,* National Aeronautics and Space Administration.

Characteristics of Successful Incident Reporting Systems

Reporting Environment. The details of successful IRS are covered in a number of publications,[1,502,505-507,521-527], and summarized in Box 6.12. A culture of safety is a prerequisite for an effective IRS.[502,506] If people fear negative consequences from reports or think that nothing will change, they will not file reports.

Additionally, successful IRS need top management to spread the message of a blame-free and non-punitive objective of IRS and to ensure that the actual activities of the organization comply. Furthermore, health care organizations should be accountable for investigating their own reports.[513]

BARRIERS AND FACILITATORS TO REPORTING. IRS live on the willingness of the staff to report. Common barriers reported by health care professionals include[508]: fear of blame; legal penalties; the perception that incident reporting does not improve patient safety; lack of organizational support; inadequate feedback; no incident follow-up; lack of knowledge about IRS; and lack of understanding about what constitutes an error. Additional aspects found by Firth-Cozens and colleagues[528] were a too-narrow definition of reportable errors and the effort of making the report. Lack of feedback appeared also as the most important barrier in another study of doctors and nurses.[529]

Common facilitators included a non-judgmental environment; the perception that incident reporting improves safety; clarifying what to report and how to do it as well as how the system uses reports; role models (such as managers); legislated protection of reporters; ability to report anonymously.[508] Additional aspects found by Firth-Cozens and colleagues were[528]: improved leadership about safety and errors; learning groups and learning timeouts; cultural change to make clear what is acceptable behavior; action by management to bring about change and to support employees; middle-grade staff on policy committees; support for each other and from management.

WHAT SHOULD BE REPORTED IN INCIDENT REPORTING SYSTEMS AND BY WHOM? In aviation, the cradle of IRS, there are separate reporting systems for incidents (deviations without a negative outcome) versus accidents (with negative outcome). Aviation accidents are investigated by an independent national body (see later section on "Accident Investigation Board"). In contrast to aviation, where the occurrence of an accident is usually quite public and events with negative outcomes are never supposed to happen, in the health care setting every human being will become ill and die someday so that most negative outcomes are inherent to the progression of disease. It is often difficult to determine which outcomes are the result of deviations versus those due to disease itself or inherent side effects.

From the authors' point of view, the invitation to staff to report should be very broad with few limitations on reporting criteria. This way, reporting is simpler for clinicians and staff and a wide net can be cast to identify as many safety-relevant occurrences and system gaps as possible. For this reason many experts believe that for health care event reporting systems, all adverse incidents should be reportable to the system regardless of whether there was a negative outcome. Whereas all health care organization staff should be included for reporting,[506] another interesting approach is to also give patients and relatives the opportunity to report.[502]

Recently Macrae[512] and other experts have argued that the "report it all, catch it all" approach misses an important opportunity to use specific reporting criteria to shape attention to certain events and set priorities on key risks. This becomes increasingly important as an IRS becomes established in an organization and receives a higher volume of reports. In their literature review Stavropoulou and colleagues found evidence that IRS seem more effective if there are explicit criteria for what counts as an incident.[515]

A rather new approach to incident reporting is called learning from excellence,[530] an approach that is in line with the idea of Safety-II (see earlier section). Learning from excellence means that analysis of reports of positive events and excellent performance in which the outcome was good despite challenging clinical circumstances may be as useful as analyzing failures.

There is a risk that certain kinds of IRS can end up being dominated by self-interested claims and complaints.[9] This can happen if staff members are not fully introduced to the goals and operating principles of what to report and why. IRS can also be used as a means for one or more individuals to attempt to exert power over other individuals or groups.

WHAT SHOULD REPORT FORMS LOOK LIKE? Typically, incident forms are partly standardized—to collect basic clinical details—while including the possibility to describe the incident in a free-text field. So-called narrative reports provide the opportunity to capture the rich context and storyline that allow the conditions that contributed to the error to be explored and understood. IRS that rely largely on an array of checkboxes for the reporter to choose relevant causes of the incident have not proven to be as useful.[502,506]

While traditional event reporting systems were paper-based, technological enhancements have allowed the development of web-based systems. On the reporting form, staff should be encouraged to also propose solutions for incidents.[513] Ideally, it should not take long for personnel to complete the form.[529] In the future, IRS reporting might use digital resources such as smartphones, enabling staff to report in near real-time using a device that they are accustomed to.[507]

CONFIDENTIALITY AND ANONYMITY. Usually, reports are submitted by staff members who were directly involved in the events; these professionals may have legitimate concerns about potential effects the reporting could have on their reputation or their employment performance record. Some IRS are entirely anonymous—neither the patient nor the reporting professional can be identified. This grants a high level of protection, although unique aspects of clinical events may make them self-identifying. For organizational learning, anonymous reports carry a major disadvantage: analysts cannot go back and ask for further information to clarify the report (which is often incomplete).

Other IRS, in contrast, are confidential but not anonymous, meaning that the identity of the reporter is known to the system but kept as secret as possible. Ideally there will be strong legal protection from disclosing the reporter's identity (sometimes with exclusions about purposeful professional misconduct or criminal acts). In general, confidential reports should be deidentified as fully as possible, once the full story has been elicited by the analyzing team.[9] Experts suggest that confidential systems should also allow for anonymous reports, as obtaining any report is more important than missing it entirely.[502,506]

Deidentifying reports can tricky. It is not always easy during the deidentification process to balance retaining the key information required to understand the situation versus deleting all possibly identifying data. The combination of facts about a case may be unique and may thus be intrinsically identifiable, even when seemingly all objective identifiers are stripped.[531] Those involved in the deidentification process proper need special training and supervision to ensure that the appropriate balance is achieved.

PATIENT SAFETY ACTION BOX

To learn from errors or incidents and to improve system and patient safety systematically, the primary questions of incident reporting should not address *"who was wrong"* but address *"what was wrong and how/why."* In a next step, incident reporting needs to focus on *"who can do what to prevent such things from happening again."*

Another widespread concern in relation to confidentiality and anonymity is fear of repercussions if reported event is disclosed internally to supervisors or managers. This fear likely influences what is reported, generating a counterproductive filter that prevents important information being passed up the hierarchy.[512] A typical model drawn from aviation is that IRS are operated and managed by an independent safety team that has no influence on personnel decisions and performance records.

Incident Categorization. The next step of the IRS is to categorize it to make it easier to find or link to it internally and to compare data across care providers, possibly using a standardized format.[502,506,513] The most commonly used framework for categorization is the WHO Framework of Critical Incidents (www.who.int/patientsafety/implementation/taxonomy/ICPS-report/en/).

Analysis. A structured and defined mechanism should be in place for analyzing reports.[521] A widely used framework for analysis of reported incidents among many others and variants is the London Protocol by Taylor-Adams and Vincent.[424] Reports should be interpreted by someone who knows the work and knows the context.[517] For health care incident reports to be of most value they should be reviewed by clinicians, perhaps working also with people who can identify the human factors and organizational system issues.[532] The value of multidisciplinary and multiprofessional investigating committees for analyzing incidents is stressed by experts.[522,533] Common findings of an analysis should characterize the problem, draw conclusions, and set out an action plan.[506]

Action. One of the major problems with incident reporting in health care as it stands is that *"we collect too much and do too little."*[512] Structured approaches to developing action plans and change may be helpful.[521] Reporting systems, both local and national, are sometimes overwhelmed by the volume of reports filed. As a consequence, they often fall short in defining recommendations for good and sustainable solutions. In the worst case, so-called quick fixes are produced that themselves trigger new risks. Even well-meaning activities of promoting lessons learned as organizational safety alerts, an updated policy, or new clinical recommendations, will not by themselves promote learning.[512] Learning is a complex social and participative process that involves people actively reflecting on and reorganizing shared knowledge, technologies, and practices.

Apart from an optimal organizational embedding, IRS can be particularly effective when they are successfully integrated and intertwined to other safety measures. For example, linking simulation team-training programs with an IRS allows for mutual input. Using reported incidents in anesthesia as a basis for simulation scenarios makes the training experience and message for the anesthesia professional very relevant to everyday clinical work. Conversely simulations can deepen the understanding of how and why things happened the way they did, and the experience of simulations can trigger participating clinicians to be more interested in reporting to the IRS in the future.

Feedback. Timely feedback should be given to the reporter, confirming that the report was received and is being processed so that they do not feel that their report was just tossed aside.[497,504] In the course, the reporter should be individually kept informed of next steps and actions taken. Failure to receive feedback after reporting an event and the perception that incident reporting neither brings change nor improves patient safety frustrates reporters. Summaries of reported events (deidentified) should be disseminated in a timely fashion to staff.[521] A variety of complementary feedback modes have been described.[507,534] Researchers have described a safety action feedback loop. This feedback loop unfortunately receives inadequate attention in many organizations,[512,522] leading to the perception of IRS as black holes (reports go in but nothing useful ever seems to come out). Clinical managers should seek to use action feedback information to motivate their staff.[535]

In the past 15 years, research about IRS have focused primarily on setting the stage for technical infrastructure, report collection forms, and categorization and analysis tools. Although those foundations are important, *"over the next 15 years we must refocus our efforts and develop more sophisticated infrastructures for investigation, learning and sharing, ..."* (p. 74).[512] Leistikow and colleagues controversially argue that "the journey, not the arrival matters," meaning to focus more on how hospitals learn from incidents and less on what hospitals learn.[511]

LEGAL ISSUES OF REPORTING SYSTEMS. Especially in jurisdictions for which medical liability litigation is common, certain legal issues affect reporting systems. For some kinds of events in some settings, legal requirements to report the event to a governmental body may be in place. This is true in the United States for certain kinds of adverse drug events or for certain failures of medical devices. Moreover, some U.S. states have started mandatory reporting programs about certain never events. In general, voluntary IRS operate completely separate from these governmental types of reporting systems.

In the United States there are various aspects of law in individual states and at the federal level that can provide statutory protection (shield) from discovery (in litigation) of certain kinds of reports to certain organizations. The U.S. Congress passed the Patient Safety and Quality Improvement Act of 2005 (Public Law 109-41)—implemented in 2009—providing for the Department of Health and Human Services to certify patient safety organizations (PSOs) to collect confidential reports about events and to analyze the information. The act provides strong legal protection (privilege) from any compelled release of the information, as in the process of discovery in a lawsuit. Separate privilege from discovery may be granted in states that provide it for internal reporting systems within hospitals that are quality improvement activities, but state laws vary widely on this matter. In addition, the quality improvement protections are often challenged during litigation, and whether the privilege will be applied depends on the ruling of a judge in each individual case. Reporting systems in other countries have used different strategies. For example, in Germany, national IRS have constituted themselves as a press office (informing the anesthesia public domain as journalists would); this then brings them under the protection of the free press act and rights, and makes it almost impossible to use its data in litigation.

The Anesthesia Incident Reporting System in the United States. In 2011 the Anesthesia Quality Institute, affiliated with the ASA, initiated the Anesthesia IRS (AIRS) to collect reports of critical events in anesthesia. Incidents can be reported by secure web-based data collection, either confidentially or anonymously. Confidential reporting allows the AIRS analyst to contact the individual for clarification or follow-up. Legal protection is provided by U.S. federal legislation described above. The law also imposes strict guidelines on how confidentiality of the work must be preserved. The AIRS publishes regularly on their Homepage as well a monthly column in the ASA Newsletter, in which it describes—in deidentified form—an interesting case report and its analysis by the AIRS Committee (Lit: https://www.aqihq.org/casereportsandcommittee.aspx). As of October 2018, AIRS has published a case analysis every month since October 2011. AIRS has instituted 4 specialty modules to collect data about events in certain categories of special interest: (1) cases that involved a respiratory depression event; (2) cases that involved a lack of necessary medications (drug shortage); (3) cases that fall under the OB/GYN procedural service type or took place in an institution's OB ward; (4) cases for patients under the age of 18 (pediatrics).

Should Health Care have an Independent Organization for Accident Investigation? As noted, serious incidents and transportation accidents in aviation and other industries are investigated by an entirely independent, interdisciplinary governmental safety investigator. For example the National Transportation Safety Board (NTSB; www.ntsb.gov) in the United States; similar agencies exist in most countries. These generally provide for rapid—usually in well under 24 hours—deployment of expert accident investigators to the scene of accidents with extensive laboratory and analytical facilities and expertise headquarters.

For several decades, suggestions have been made to establish an NTSB-like body to investigate accidents in health care. Especially in the past few years, new calls have been made to establish such an organization.[536] Until 2017, the complexities and pitfalls of such an investigation, including the fact that adverse outcomes are several orders of magnitude more common in health care than in commercial aviation, have obstructed any progress toward creating such a program. In April 2017, the United Kingdom began to operate the first independent investigation body, the Healthcare Safety Investigation Branch (HSIB; www.hsib.org.uk). Even though funded by the Department of Health and hosted by the NHS Improvement, the multidisciplinary team of experienced safety investigators operates independently. Future developments will show what benefit and usage will derive from this activity.

The debate about the feasibility and advisability of such high-level investigating organizations in different jurisdictions will probably continue for a long time. We believe professional investigation of safety critical events and harm, with rapid deployment and expert analysis, will lead to new insights and the implementation of practical, robust, and effective solutions.

Continuous Training including simulation

Small groups of individuals work together throughout perioperative care. Anesthesia professionals, surgeons, nurses, and other health professionals must coordinate their activities in order to make safe and efficient patient care the priority. Whereas teams in the classical sense work together over a longer period of time, the configuration of teams in the dynamic and frequently changing setting of the OR or ICU environment contains particular challenges of so-called action teams (see earlier section on "Teamwork"). Members of action teams are rarely trained together, and to-date, few are trained at all specifically in how to manage challenging situations providing safe care, for example, by applying the CRM concept (see earlier section on "Crisis Resource Management"). Moreover, they come from distinctly different disciplines and diverse educational backgrounds to the extent that they are often described as being in silos or tribes. The varied nature of the work and the necessity for cooperation among those who perform it make team training an ideal tool in the drive to improve patient safety and reduce medical errors.

How the CRM concept can be learned, trained, and implemented best is explained more in detail in the upcoming section. More detailed information on the conduct and modalities of modern simulation team training for health care professionals can be found in Chapter 7.

How Can Crisis Resource Management-related Skills be Learned, Trained, and Sustained? Despite the growing evidence, systematic interventions to improve patient and system safety have only partially penetrated medical thinking and teaching. CRM-oriented training and behavior should be one component of a comprehensive approach to addressing human factors issues in anesthesia safety, but few if any institutions have deployed such integrated approaches. There have been several reviews on the variety of MTTs, the latest published by Weaver and colleagues in 2014.[409] The targeted teamwork competencies of the programs they discuss are similar, but the curricula differ widely: in content, duration, participation frequency of clinicians and staff, delivery strategies (didactic, seminar, simulation/debriefing), maintenance strategies, and evaluation effort. One major question seems to be the degree to which simulation adds to simple classroom activities.

Two Different Approaches of Team Training: Simulation-Based or Classroom-Based? The oldest medical CRM curriculum, namely the ACRM curriculum, relies heavily on high-fidelity simulation-based training, introducing the CRM principles to the participants and then highlighting CRM aspects of medical care in the post-scenario debriefings. A pocket card of the 15 CRM key points is shown in Fig. 6.17.

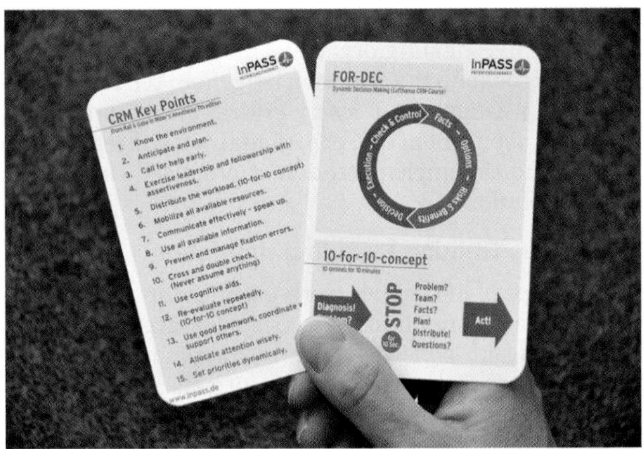

Fig. 6.17 Crisis resource management (CRM) pocket cards. One side of the cards shows the 15 CRM key principles by Rall and Gaba. The other side of the card shows two graphics. One shows a tool for formalizing decision-making and avoiding fixation errors called "FOR-DEC," which is derived from aviation. Another shows the "10-seconds-for-10-minutes" concept, a reminder to take the necessary time to organize into a team, whenever appropriate. The cards are handy and pocket sized, and can be carried around during work as a reminder or can be distributed in the department as reminder, an interest-gaining or a multiplication tool. During the CRM courses or simulation training sessions of the authors, CRM pocket cards are given to each participant. (Photograph by M. Rall.)

Much simpler than simulation-based training is purely seminar-based training about human factors, CRM principles, teamwork, and team communication. Several team training programs, including MedTeams, MTM, and DOM, rely on classroom-based approaches only and use didactic lectures, group exercises and role plays, discussion, and analysis of trigger videos.

The different concepts of these training programs, probably as well as the cost and manpower of high-fidelity simulation and the small number of participants per simulation session, raised the question whether simulation-based CRM training is needed compared to classroom-based training and whether they are equally effective. Only a few studies have investigated the effectiveness of classroom-based team trainings versus simulator-based programs.[537] Weaver's summary of review findings reported similar positive effects on learner reactions, knowledge or skills, and clinical practices, as well as patient outcomes.[409] Riley et al. compared perinatal work areas in three different hospitals; one participated in a didactic team-training program, one participated in an in situ simulation program, and one served as a control.[538] Results indicated that significantly greater reductions in patient harm were achieved by the group that participated in the in situ simulation program compared with both the didactic and control groups (37% reduction vs. 1% reduction vs. 43% increase in harm, respectively). The lessons learned from the implementation of the Veteran Affairs (VA) MTT program introduced earlier also suggest that simulation is a crucial part of CRM-based team training interventions.[414]

Drawing parallels to the translated CRM training curriculum in aviation, the classroom-based approach correlates with what the Federal Aviation Agency (FAA) calls phase I (awareness), whereas the simulation-based approach correlates with phase II (skills practice and feedback), which is followed by phase III for maintenance (recurrence training). This is in accordance with the comprehensive approach to teamwork training of Salas and colleagues.

This didactic approach suggests three elements needed for adult education: (1) convey knowledge about teamwork, (2) develop skills of teamwork, and (3) enhance attitudes concerning teamwork.[539,540] Gaba wrote in a point-counterpoint discussion about the question "What does simulation add to teamwork training"[541] the following, proposing the benefit of simulation-based CRM training:

"Didactic training may address knowledge and can influence attitudes, but to fully develop skills and alter attitudes, experiential training [like simulation-based training] is likely to be the most effective. Thus, given the complexity of the topic, it is likely that multiple approaches will be necessary to maximize learning and transfer to real patient care."

Pratt and Sachs challenge this view, arguing that the rather complex and costly simulation approach is replaceable with classroom-based teaching and intensive coaching of clinicians during and after real patient care activities.[542] A rather new approach is the concept of teaching CRM-related topics with a screen-based interactive virtual simulation featuring typical clinical situations.[543,544] Even though virtual simulations permit flexible, cost-efficient, and asynchronous learning, the role and the effectiveness of such virtual activities away from a physical team intervention have to be further evaluated.

Gaba continued in the aforementioned discussion:

"Moreover, it is also likely that no single course or exercise can change such complex behaviors permanently—only long-term repetitive training and practice, combined with solid reinforcement of the principles and skills in the actual work environment, has any chance of developing new and optimal teamwork patterns that become deeply ingrained in the work culture."[541]

It seems reasonable to combine best practices from classroom-based and simulation-based training for an optimal CRM team-training experience. More and more CRM-related organizational or departmental interventions now do so, following the classical phases I (awareness) and II (practical skills and feedback) of the aviation CRM curriculum: that is, ACRM curriculum, TeamSTEPPS, VA CTT, and several CRM implementation studies. Primarily, staff participates in seminar-based CRM interventions in order to learn about the concepts and to create awareness. Simulation-based training is then used after or during the classroom introduction to apply the theoretical knowledge during practical medical case scenarios and to get feedback or to refresh knowledge in order to reach a sustainable base over time. More details on the simulation-based approach are provided in Chapter 7. More details on different ways of teaching ACRM—both simulation- and classroom-based—can be found in the second edition of the book *Crisis Management in Anesthesiology*.[14]

We believe that practicing the reliable execution of CRM skills in routine and emergency situations requires, among other things, exposure to challenging clinical situations in realistic simulation scenarios, followed by detailed group debriefings led by qualified instructors to analyze what transpired. As discussed in Chapter 7, Such CRM-oriented simulation training may be available in dedicated simulation centers or as in situ simulation training in actual work environments. Many simulation centers offer mobile simulation training whereby a simulation team can bring the simulator and simulation equipment to another facility to train the staff in institutions that do not have a simulator or the relevant instructors. Another way is to prepare a few of a site's own clinicians to conduct CRM-based simulation team trainings by sending them to one of the instructor courses for CRM-based simulation team training. Although there are many such courses, the three best known sites of instructor training in the United States are at the Center for Medical Simulation in Boston, the Center for Immersive and Simulation-based Learning at Stanford School of Medicine, and WISER at University of Pittsburgh. In Europe, among others there is the InPASS InFacT instructor course (by Rall), the instructor courses run by DIMS (by Dieckmann), and the EuSiM instructor course.

When choosing a train-the-trainer course, it is important to understand that simulation is a technique, not a technology. It takes many forms: from nontechnological modalities (e.g. verbal simulation, role-playing) to simple skills training models to computerized full-body mannequins; from training students to training professional teams, from rather simple mega-code training scenarios to complex emergency scenario design. Each training form requires a different amount of manpower, logistics, and costs. But crucial under all circumstances is the special skills of the simulation instructors in course and scenario preparation, scenario execution, and debriefing (see Chapter 7). In order to use simulation successfully, the simulation instructors need to be specially qualified in CRM-based training (see Chapter x), the learning objectives of the simulation training need to be set (see Chapter x), and the needs of learners at each stage of education must be targeted (see Chapter x). Furthermore, for simulation to be effective it needs to be integrated into the strategic concept of an organization in a way that promotes transfer of the ideas and skills learned to clinical practice.

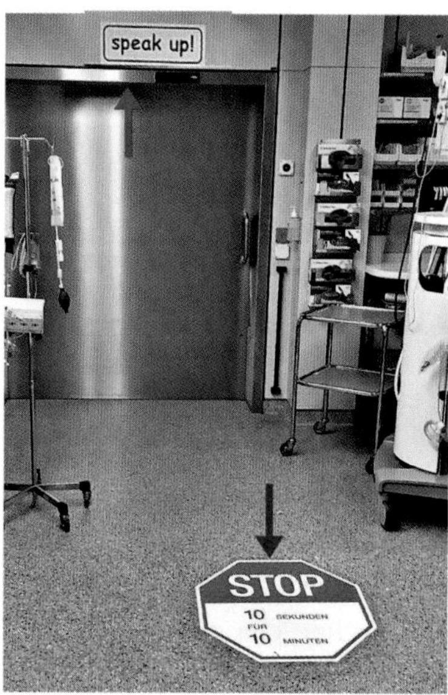

Fig. 6.18 Example of the organizational integration of "Speaking up" and "STOP! 10-seconds-for-10-minutes." The photo shows a laminated sign with the words "Speak up" above the trauma room door (red arrow) and a laminated sign with the words "Stop! 10-seconds-for-10-minutes" on the floor (blue arrow) at the University Hospital of Zurich, Switzerland. The signs are placed as a reminders for safety tools for clinical teams and at the same time show the organizational effort and support for patient safety issues. (Photos published with permission of University Hospital Zurich [USZ], Center for Simulation [Chair: M. Kolbe]).

Reinforcement and Sustainability of Team Training Effects. Sustainability of team training effects over time is a common question among both improvement scientists and practitioners. Many early evaluations of team training limited follow-up evaluations to 6 months post-training or less.[409] Positive responses after a simulation-based CRM intervention have been found to last for up to 6 months after training.[347] Patterson found gains in teamwork knowledge sustained at follow-up conducted 8 to 10 months post-training.[242] In studies examining the implementation of the VA's team training program, results indicated both significant improvements in perceptions of teamwork climate up to 11 months following implementation[545] and statistically significant reductions in surgical mortality 1 year post training.[42] Those numbers mimic the findings of Armour et al. who indicated a decay in gains 1 year post training.[397]

While a great deal of work has been dedicated to examining optimal refresher training intervals for clinical procedural skills (e.g., resuscitation or intubation skills), relatively minimal work has been done to understand optimal refresher intervals for teamwork competencies. Moffatt and colleagues offered a recurrent training two years after the initial training.[41] The VA CTT program conducts mandatory recurrent training one year after the initial training session, viewing this approach *"critical to re-enforcing key CRM concepts in the program."*[546] Nothing is stated in the program about further training frequency after one year. Based on the literature findings and also drawing parallels to the CRM curriculum in aviation (phase III: recurrence training), a refresher interval of one year for CRM team trainings would seem rational, but we do not know of any institutions that do full-day sessions for experienced clinicians this frequently.

It is important not think about simulation as a one-shot thing once or every now and then, but rather about a career-long set of activities. These might sometimes take place in a dedicated simulation center or a hospital simulation area and sometimes in situ, directly where patients are treated and cared for.[547] If simulation activities are combined this way it stands to reason that there will be an accumulation of change in individual and team skills, knowledge, attitudes, and behaviors as well as in systems probing and systems change.

Organizational Aspects of the Implementation and Sustainability of Team Training. As with nearly all patient safety principles, application of CRM key points to patient care must be supported by top leadership and reinforced in the actual work environment (Fig. 6.18). It is of less use to study these principles (or even practice them in simulations) only to find that the pressures and culture of the real OR make them impossible to implement. Fully integrating the concepts underlying the CRM key points into the structures and processes of clinical practice has proven to be a significant challenge. The Joint Commission Journal on Quality and Patient Safety outlined several critical factors for developing successful team training in 2009.[539] In brief, those are:

- Align team training objectives and safety aims with organizational goals.
- Provide organizational support for the team training initiative.
- Get frontline care leaders on board.
- Prepare the environment and trainees for team training.
- Determine required resources and time commitment and ensure their availability.
- Facilitate application of trained teamwork skills on the job.
- Measure the effectiveness of the team training program.

Box 6.13 shows characteristics of the implementation of team training interventions that have proved to be successful characteristics.

Continuous Optimization of Safety-Relevant Structures and Processes

HROs try to continually alter the way that they work to improve safety—the structure of their organization, its work units (sometimes described as microsystems), and teams, as well as the usual processes and protocols of care. Sometimes, but not always, these changes can also improve efficiency as well as safety. Since individual workarounds succeed only one patient at a time, addressing the flow of everyday work, and the preparations for anomalies or crises, will be critical to making lasting improvement.

In order to optimize structures and processes continuously in regard to patient safety, it is important to maintain a culture of safety (see above) so that frontline staff are willing and enabled to contribute actively. Furthermore, when talking about the optimization of structures and processes in regard to safety, it is important to define and generate structured ways to transfer safety-critical information and topics, for example from IRS (see earlier section) and team training events (see earlier section) to those who are in charge of structural changes.

Surely, there are many different ways to optimize structures and processes. Starting points, for example, could be the aforementioned use of walkrounds[479] and closing performance gaps by using debriefing as formative assessment[548] after routine and non-routine events.

In many places, the optimization of structures and processes lies in the hand of quality and risk managers. However, we have observed gaps between what is optimized by those working at the blunt end and what is acknowledged and played out by personnel at the sharp end.[549] In order to master this challenge, from the authors' point of view and based on the view of other experts, it is important to:

- focus on the four main elements of safety culture, organizational learning (i.e., IRS), team training, and optimization of structures and processes in a very balanced manner
- develop and optimize structures and processes together and with close involvement of clinical teams (participatory development and user-centered iterative design)

BOX 6.13 Characteristics of Successful Team Training

Studies[5,41,42,414,546,562] that evaluated the positive impact of the implementation of a CRM team-training program and that were successful, show the following, or part of the following, characteristics for the implementation and training process:

Preparation and Implementation

- Assess measures of collaboration and standardization (i.e., 2 months), followed by planning the implementation (i.e., 1 month) based on individual organizational aspects
- Appointment of a "steering committee" consisting of hospital medical and nursing leadership
- Create leadership support and engage departmental teams for planning and preparation

Initiation

- Administrative Training: Intensive training of the leadership group, for example, chief executive officer, chief financial officer, dean, chief medical officer, chief quality officer, department chairs, division heads (i.e., 2 days)
- Administrative Training: Training of executive and senior leadership, board members, and perioperative departmental leadership attending the same CRM training that all perioperative physicians and staff attend.
- Staff Training: Mandatory CRM training session for all physicians and nurses participating in the intervention. Some programs first started on a voluntary basis ("pilot")
- Interactive training and training in interprofessional teams
- Small groups (i.e., 15 participants/group) and sufficient exposition time for the lectures and interactive training sessions (i.e., 2 day à 9 h[5]; 1 day[42]; 4 h[41])
- Introduction of CRM with en bloc-training (all department staff participates in the training in a short time span, i.e., within 2 or 3 months)
- Team training provided by CRM qualified and experienced instructors; peer-to-peer communication is helpful
- Sufficient Trainer: Participant ratio is 2:15 for moderated interactive group work
- Training is a mixture of lectures and interactive elements (i.e., workshops, discussions, etc.)
- The potential for disturbance is as low as possible (i.e., no duty calls, no pagers, etc.) Eventually ORs must be closed for the training sessions
- Training tailored to organizational/departmental needs

Maintenance

- Creation of a CRM work group consisting of frontline clinicians, giving input to CRM every now and then (posts, bulletin notes, CRM as standard item during morning rounds and staff meetings, etc.), translating CRM into the organizational needs (professional ownership), and organizing several CRM activities (i.e., "week of CRM," refresher lectures, CRM "awards," etc.)
- CRM as part of the yearly individual evaluations
- Nomination of local "champions"
- Coaching and monitoring of unit-based performance outcomes (i.e., over 12 months) or "follow-up support" is provided
- Mandatory team training of all new staff members
- Mandatory "practical training" (i.e., CRM-based simulation team training)
- Mandatory "recurrence training" (after 1 year of initial training, not mandatory after 2 years of initial training)
- Steering committee continues to meet monthly to monitor progress
- Initiation of a "train-the-trainer program" to promote hospital's own CRM facilitators and internalize CRM training and implementation

- introduce and implement new processes and structures systematically, taking whatever time is needed to do this effectively rather than just rolling it out haphazardly. This likely needs change control to determine first how and where the new processes will involve and influence other activities, information that will best come from discussions with clinical personnel and their managers.
- adjust processes and structures in regard to findings from human factors engineering; sometimes it is the work environment or equipment that need to be changed and adapted to the realities of human performance rather than the other way around.

As it is rarely possible to implement or strengthen the four main elements of an HRO all at the same time; it is important to proceed step by step and balance the focus between the elements. Establishing a culture of safety is one of the most important goals as this element is incredibly intertwined with the success of the other elements. Nevertheless, a strong focus on human performance and patient safety within organizations lies in the optimization of structures and processes and IRS. At the same time, organizations should continually train their medical personnel about issues of human performance and patient safety, because there are three related challenges:

- **What do frontline personnel do until all structures and processes are optimized?** The development of strong and safe structures and processes cannot be achieved overnight. Many processes and structures need optimization. While this is going on clinical teams continue to treat patients day after day. They need to hone their skills even while working with outmoded structures and procedures.
- **Even when improved, no system and no process is perfect.** Even optimized processes and structures hold pitfalls; clinical teams will always need to compensate for them and for safety gaps. Only if the individuals and teams have learned and trained together in how to do so can they can operate safely—essentially *"people create safety"* (p. 267).[9]
- **At the very end of any structure or process there always stands a human being.** Regardless of whether the structures and processes are optimized, for the foreseeable future a human professional is at the sharp end of patient care, executing those processes and procedures, and consciously or inadvertently altering or bypassing them. Therefore they need to know and be able to use all relevant safety strategies. These professionals are indeed the last barriers against catastrophe and hence each should individually also exemplify the ideals of HROs, promoting resilience and flexibility at the same time (see earlier sections).

The behavior, commitment, and engagement of frontline staff itself is the crucial key to translate organizational intentions into practice. Our experience is that CRM-based simulation team training (clinical action and clinical relevance) with focus on human performance elements and patient safety can be a good starting point to gain the understanding and buy-in of clinical personnel to organizational changes.

The Bigger Picture: Patient Safety Efforts on the U.S. National and International Level

PATIENT SAFETY MILESTONES AND MOVEMENTS

The field of anesthesiology can rightly be proud of introducing the idea that patient safety is not just a byproduct of clinicians doing a good job, but rather is something to be studied, sought, and fought for as a matter in its own right. This was in large measure achieved by Jeffrey B. Cooper (at Massachusetts General Hospital) and Ellison C. (Jeep) Pierce, Jr., (when president of the ASA), who created a Committee on Patient Safety. Jeff, Jeep, and a few other like-minded innovators created the Anesthesia Patient Safety Foundation. These developments are acknowledged to be the founding milestones of the patient safety endeavor, and the inspiration for further development of similar organizations for all aspects of health care across the world.

In part through the efforts of such PSOs the medical community became more open to taking a harder look at medical human performance, error, and negative outcomes. Since the 1990s, many landmark publications and activities have addressed patient safety and the organizational aspects of reducing errors.[9,11,174,434,550-552]

Although many scholars within and outside of anesthesiology had been addressing these issues for some years, the report of the IOM in 1999, *To Err Is Human*,[174] was a highly publicized awakening in the United States about the problems of patient safety. Summarizing the primary literature, the report stated that *"tens of thousands die each year from errors in their care and hundreds of thousands suffer or barely escape from nonfatal injuries that a truly high-quality care system would largely prevent."* The subsequent report of the IOM Committee on Quality of Health Care in America in 2001, entitled *Crossing the Quality Chasm: A New Health System for the 21st Century*,[434] took a systematic approach to improvement of the entire health care system. It stated that *"between the health care we have and the care we could have, lies not just a gap, but a chasm"* because the health care system today harms too frequently yet routinely fails to deliver its potential benefits. The report concluded: *"The current care system cannot do the job. Trying harder will not work. Changing the systems of care will."*

Various other efforts have taken place, including the *"100,000 Lives Campaign"* (2004) by the IHI; the WHO patient safety program (2004); the patient safety enhancing *TeamSTEPPS* program (2005 and revised 2013); the *Patient Safety and Quality Improvement Act* establishing a voluntary IRS and providing privilege and confidentiality protections for reported patient safety information; the introduction of the *WHO Surgical Safety Checklist* (2008); and the *WHO Patient Safety Curriculum* (2011).

Fifteen years after the IOM report *"To Err is Human,"* the National Patient Safety Foundation (NPSF) convened an expert panel in 2015 to assess the state of the patient safety field and set the stage for the next 15 years of work. Among the recommendations[471] are: establishment of a total systems approach and a culture of safety, and calls for action by government, regulators, health professionals, and others to place higher priority on patient safety science and implementation. The Helsinki Declaration on Patient Safety in Anesthesiology[553] in 2010 from the European Board of Anesthesiology (EBA) and the European Society of Anesthesiology (ESA) emphasized the role of anesthesiology in promoting safe perioperative care in Europe.[371]

Institutions Engaging in Patient Safety

Several governmental and non-governmental patient safety institutions have emerged over the past two decades, including the National Patient Safety Foundation (NPSF), the Agency for Healthcare Research and Quality (AHRQ), and the IHI in the United States; the National Patient Safety Agency (NPSA) in England; the Canadian Patient Safety Institute (CPSI); and many more.

Raising the Awareness for Patient Safety

In 2003 the NPSF initiated a patient safety awareness week that takes place yearly, highlighting different patient safety topics. Two years later, in 2005, the WHO launched a yearly Patient Safety Day for increasing the awareness of patient safety.

Certified Education in Patient Safety for Health Care Professionals

The NPSF created the Certified Professional in Patient Safety (CPPS) credential to establish core standards and benchmarking for the field and set an expected proficiency level for those seeking to become professionally certified in patient safety. By 2018, more than 2000 professionals have achieved the CPPS credential. They represent physicians, nurses, pharmacists, patient safety professionals, quality and risk management professionals, health care executives, nonclinical health care professionals, and others with the requisite background throughout the United States and nine other countries. The content of certification covers knowledge in the following five key elements: safety culture, leadership, patient safety risks and solutions, measuring and improving performance, and systems thinking and design/human factors. The VA National Center for Patient Safety, in cooperation with the VA Office of Academic Affiliations, offers one-year fellowships in patient safety to provide in-depth education in patient safety practice and leadership.

National and International Evaluation of the Benefits of Patient Safety Programs

Over the last years the focus of patient safety initiatives has been put more and more on the question of economy and efficiency. Two major reports demonstrate the cost benefits of patient safety programs: (1) The report provided by the AHRQ in 2016 displays interim data on national efforts from 2010 to 2015 to improve safety in health care.[44,554] The report showed that hospital acquired conditions (HACs) have been declining since 2010 with many fewer deaths and substantial dollar savings. (2) The report launched by the international Organization for Economic Cooperation and Development (OECD) on the economics of patient safety in 2017.[472] The report estimated patient harm being the 14th leading cause of global disease burden and resulting in a considerable cost to patients, health care systems, and societies. Key messages emphasized the important role of leadership and the building of a positive safety culture. Similar economic success, but on the organizational level, was demonstrated in 2017 by Moffatt-Bruce and colleagues at an academic medical center.[41]

Patients for Patient Safety

Furthermore, more and more attention is drawn to the support of patient engagement as a vital contributing component of safe care. The WHO launched the safety program Patients for Patient Safety and provides several toolkits for patients. Several programs in Canada, Australia, and the United States, for example, have been launched, following the idea of patients being the extra sets of eyes and ears that should be integrated into the safety processes.[555-557] Patients are more likely to participate and speak up if they feel authorized and supported to do so by health care workers. As a consequence, the successful setup of patient empowerment strategies requires the understanding of benefit by health care workers to buy in and then requires their full support.

Conclusion and Outlook

Avoiding errors and harm to patients is crucial for every anesthesiologist. For the safety of the patients, but also for the psychological well-being of us as professionals, as professionals commonly suffer from patient harm as a second victim. Clinical knowledge and skills are not sufficient to harm any patient during care. This chapter has summarized, in regard to anesthesiology, how human performance issues matter. As can be gleaned from this chapter, there are many challenges to individual, team, and system performance that can degrade the ability to achieve safe and high-quality care. Knowing and teaching about these is the first of many steps to address them. Recurrent training and practice, with simulation as an important component, organizational learning after both successes and failures, and continuous fostering of a culture of safety and improvement will be needed. As Sir Liam Donaldson stated in 2004 to the Alliance for Patient Safety Conference in Washington: *"To err is human, to cover up is unforgivable, and to fail to learn is inexcusable."*

Anesthesia professionals can and should collaborate with their partners in surgery, nursing, and beyond; however, ultimately anesthesia professionals need to take responsibility for ensuring that we as individuals, the teams we work in, and our workplaces, are ever ready to provide the very best care.

Patient safety has generated a lot of momentum over the last 30 years. Many achievements have been made, although a lot of issues remain to be addressed satisfactorily in part because at their root are fundamental aspects of the way that health care is organized. Even countries that are pioneers in patient safety still struggle. In the developing world and low-resource settings, even basic aspects of patient safety still need to be addressed. Patient safety is a never ending battle, regardless of resources, and as Charles Vincent put it: "Safety in health care is a moving target."[558]

Many patient safety pioneers in medicine, including us (the authors), thought that many of the issues introduced in this chapter would be roughly a decade-long proposition. Now, with many of us being in our fourth decade of the patient safety journey, we know that the road goes ever on...

... and we all just have to keep on trucking.

Acknowledgment

The editors, publisher, and Drs. Marcus Rall, David M. Gaba, and Peter Dieckmann would like to thank Dr. Steven K. Howard for his contribution to this chapter in the prior edition of this work. It has served as the foundation for the current chapter.

Complete references available online at expertconsult.com.

References

1. Valentin A, et al. *BMJ*. 2009;338:b814.
2. Pronovost P, et al. *N Engl J Med*. 2006;355(26):2725–2732.
3. Lipshutz AKM, et al. *BMC Anesthesiology*. 2015;15:93.
4. Steyrer J, et al. *Health Care Manage Rev*. 2013;38(4):306–316.
5. Haerkens MH, et al. *Acta anaesthesiol Scand*. 2015;59(10):1319–1329.
6. Hunziker S, et al. *J Emerg Trauma Shock*. 2010;3(4):389–394.
7. Niles D, et al. *Resuscitation*. 2009;80(8):909–912.
8. Reader TW, et al. *Crit Care Med*. 2009;37(5):1787–1793.
9. Vincent C. *Patient Safety*. 2nd ed. Edinburgh: Wiley-Blackwell & BMJ Books; 2010.
10. Vincent C, Amalberti R. *Safer Healthcare. Strategies for the Real World*. Heidelberg, Germany: Springer; 2016.
11. Flin R, et al. *Safety at the Sharp End: A Guide to Nontechnical Skills*. Farnham, UK: Ashgate; 2008.
12. Leveson NG, et al. *Engineering a Safer World: Systems Thinking Applied to Safety*. Cambridge, Massachusetts & London, England: The MIT Press; 2016 (Reprint).
13. St Pierre M, et al. *Crisis Management in Acute Care Settings: Human Factors and Team Psychology in a High Stakes Environment*. New York: Springer; 2008.
14. Gaba DM, et al. *Crisis Management in Anesthesiology*. 2nd ed. Elsevier; 2014.
15. Carayon P, et al. *BMJ Qual Saf*. 2014;23(3):196–205.
16. Weinger MB, Englund CE. *Anesthesiology*. 1990;73(5):995–1021.
17. Raghavendra Rao RS. *Ind j anaesth*. 2016;60(5):306–311.
18. Decker Bauer. *Min Inv Ther Allied Tech*. 2003;12(6):268–277.
19. Loeb RG, et al. In: Erenwerth J, Eisenkraft JB, Berry J, eds. *Anesthesia Equipment: Principles and Applicaitons*. 2nd ed. Philadelphia, PA: Saunders; 2013:485–509.
20. Davis M, et al. *J Peri Prac*. 2016;26(12):274–280.
21. Cooper L, Nossaman B. *Intl Anesth Clin*. 2013;51(1):1–12.
22. Merry AF, et al. *Best Prac ResClinAnaesth*. 2011;25(2):145–159.
23. Merry AF, Anderson BJ. *Paediatr Anaesth*. 2011;21(7):743–753.
24. Jensen LS, et al. *Anaesthesia*. 2004;59(5):493-504.
25. Orser BA, et al. *Can J Anaesth*. 2013;60(2):127–135.
26. Glavin RJ. *Br J Anaesth*. 2010;105(1):76–82.
27. Prabhakar A, et al. *J Med Prac Mgmt*. 2015;30(6 Spec No):41–43.
28. World Health Organization (WHO). 2007;Volume 1. http://www.-who.int/patientsafety/solutions/patientsafety/PS-Solution1.pdf. Accessed August 13, 2018.
29. World Health Organization (WHO). 2007;Volume 1. http://www.-who.int/patientsafety/solutions/patientsafety/PS-Solution7.pdf. Accessed August 21, 2018.
30. Dolan SA, et al. *Am J Inf Cont*. 2013;41(11):1077–1082.
31. Gariel C, et al. *Br J Anaesth*. 2018;120(3):563–570.
32. Mauger B, et al. *Am J Inf Cont*. 2014;42(suppl 10):S274–283.
33. Nanji KC, et al. *Anesthesiology*. 2016;124(1):25–34.
34. Rothschild JM, et al. *Crit Care Med*. 2005;33(8):1694–1700.
35. Wahr JA, et al. *Br J Anaesth*. 2017;118(1):32–43.
36. Zimlichman E, et al. *JAMAInt Med*. 2013;173(22):2039–2046.
37. Cooper JB, et al. *Qual Saf Hlth Care*. 2002;11(3):277–282.
38. Williamson JA, et al. *Anaesth Intensive Care*. 1993;21(5):678–683.
39. Wu AW. *BMJ*. 2000;320(7237):726–727.
40. Cooper JB, Gaba D. *Anesthesiology*. 2002;97(6):1335–1337.
41. Moffatt-Bruce SD, et al. *Am J Med Qual*. 2017;32(1):5–11.
42. Neily J, et al. *JAMA*. 2010;304(15):1693–1700.
43. Schwartz ME, et al. *J Hlth Risk Mgmt*. 2018;38(1):17–37.
44. *Efforts To Improve Patient Safety Result in 1.3 Million Fewer Patient Harms*. ; 2014. http://www.ahrq.gov/professionals/quality-patient-safety/pfp/interimhacrate2013.html
45. Orasanu J, Connolly T. In: Klein GA, Calderwood R, eds. *Decision Making in Action: Models and Methods*. Norwood, NJ: Ablex Publishing Gorp.; 1993.
46. Gaba DM, et al. *Anesthesiology*. 1987;66(5):670–676.
47. Banja J. *Bus Horiz*. 2010;53(2):139.
48. Odom-Forren J. *J Peri Anesth Nrsg*. 2011;26(3):216–219.
49. Prielipp RC, et al. *Anesth Analg*. 2010;110(5):1499–1502.
50. Price MR, Williams TC. *J Pat Saf*. 2018;14(1):1–2.
51. Engelmann C, et al. *Langenbeck's Arch Surg*. 2017;402(1):187–190.
52. Nurok M, et al. *Pat Saf Surg*. 2015;9(1):34.
53. Eichhorn JH. *Can J Anaesth*. 2013;60(2):111–118.
54. Perrow C. *Normal Accidents: Living with High-Risk Technologies*. New York, US: Princton University Press; 1984.
55. Kirsner K, Biddle C. *Int J Law Hlth Eth*. 2012;8(1).
56. Gaba DM, et al. *Anesthesiology*. 1994;81(2):488–500.
57. *Production Pressures*. Agency for Healthcare Research and Quality (AHRQ); 2007. https://psnet.ahrq.gov/webmm/case/150.
58. Hollnagel E. *The ETTO Principle : Efficiency-Thoroughness Trade-Off. Why Things that go Right Sometimes go Wrong*. Burlington, VT: Ashgate Publishing Company; 2009.
59. Reason JT. *Human Error*. Cambridge: Cambridge University Press; 1990.
60. Riem N, et al. *Br J Anaesth*. 2012;109(5):723–728.
61. Stiegler MP, et al. *Br J Anaesth*. 2012;108(2):229–235.
62. Cognitive biases in health care. *The Joint Commission*. 2016. https://www.jointcommission.org/assets/1/23/Quick_Safety_Issue_28_2016.pdf
63. Phipps D, et al. *Br J Anaesth*. 2008;100(3):333–343.
64. Manser T, et al. *Ergonomics*. 2007;50(2):246–260.
65. Slagle JM, Weinger MB. *Anesthesiology*. 2009;110(2):275–283.
66. Weinger MB, et al. *J Clin Anesth*. 2000;12(4):273–282.
67. Weinger MB, et al. *Anesthesiology*. 1997;87(1):144–155.
68. Slagle JM, et al. *Anesthesiology*. 2018;128(1):44–54.
69. Mackenzie CF, et al. *J Clin Monitor*. 1995;11(5):335–341.
70. Xiao Y, et al. *Hum Factors*. 1996;38(4):636–645.
71. Friedman Z, et al. *Reg Anesth Pain Med*. 2006;31(4):304–310.
72. Weinger MB, et al. *Qual Saf Health Care*. 2004;13(2):136–144.
73. Lindekaer AL, et al. *Acta Anaesth Scan*. 1997;41(10):1280–1284.
74. Jacobsen J, et al. *Acta Anaesth Scan*. 2001;45(3):315–319.
75. Weinger MB, et al. *Anesthesiology*. 2017;127(3):475–489.
76. Byrne AJ, Jones JG. *Br J Anaesth*. 1997;78(5):553–556.
77. Manser T, et al. *Anesth Analg*. 2009;108(5):1606–1615.
78. Howard SK, et al. *Anesthesiology*. 2003;98(6):1345–1355.
79. Marshall SD, et al. *Anaesthesia*. 2016;71(4):389–404.
80. Burtscher MJ, et al. *Hum Factors*. 2010;52(2):282–294.
81. Manser T. *Acta Anaesth Scan*. 2009;53(2):143–151.
82. Wacker J, Kolbe M. *TrendsAnaesth Crit Care*. 2014;4(6):200–205.
83. Lingard L, et al. *Qual Saf Health Care*. 2004;13(5):330–334.
84. Künzle B, et al. *Qual Saf Hlth Care*. 2010;19(6):e46-e46.
85. Künzle B, et al. *Euro J Work Organiz Psych*. 2010;19(5):505–531.
86. Cook RI, Woods DD. *Human Factors*. 1996;38(4):593–613.
87. Cook RI, Woods DD. *J Clin Anaesth*. 1996;8(suppl 3):29s–37s.
88. Loeb RG. *Anesthesiology*. 1994;80(3):527–533.
89. Manser T, Wehner T. *Analysing Action Sequences: Variations in Action Density in the Administration of Anaesthesia*. vol. 4. ; 2002.
90. Weinger MB, et al. *Anesthesiology*. 1994;80(1):77–92.
91. Weinger M, Slagle J. *J Am Med Inform Assoc*. 2002;9(suppl 6):S58–S63.
92. Weinger MB, et al. *Anesth Analg*. 2004;98(5):1419–1425.
93. Byrne AJ, et al. *Br J Anaesth*. 2010;105(6):767–771.
94. Gaba DM, Lee T. *Anesth Analg*. 1990;71(4):354–361.
95. Pape TM, Dingman SK. *Plastic Surg Nrsg*. 2011;31(2):49–56.
96. Campbell G, et al. *Br J Anaesth*. 2012;109(5):707–715.
97. Schulz CM, Schneider E, et al. *Br J Anaesth*. 2011;106(6):807–813.
98. Betza SM, et al. *Proceedings of the Human Factors and Ergonomics Society Annual Meeting*. 2016;60(1):608–612.
99. Smith AF, et al. *Anaesthesia*. 2003;58(11):1070–1078.
100. Broom MA, et al. *Anaesthesia*. 2011;66(3):175–179.
101. Cooper JB, et al. *Anesthesiology*. 1984;60(1):34–42.
102. Marcus R. *Paediatr Anaesth*. 2006;16(3):242–250.
103. American Society of Anesthesiologists. Standards and Guidelines: 2008 ASA Recommendations for Pre Anesthesia Checkout. https://www.asahq.org/resources/clinical-information/2008-asa-recommendations-for-pre-anesthesia-checkout. Accessed November 16, 2018.
104. Feldman JM, et al. *APSF Newsletter*. 2008;23(1):6–7.

105. Association of Anaesthetists of Great Britain and Ireland (AAGBI). *Anaesthesia*. 2012;67(6):660–668.
106. Australian and New Zealand College of Anaesthetists (ANZCA). *Guidelines on Checking Anaesthesia Delivery Systems*; 2014. http://www.anzca.edu.au/documents/ps31-2014-guidelines-on-checking-anaesthesia-deliv.pdf
107. Merchant R, et al. *Can J Anaesth*. 2016;63(1):86–112.
108. Gaba DM. *Dynamic Decision-Making in Anesthesiology: Cognitive Models and Training Approaches*. Berlin, Heidelberg: 1992.
109. Gaba DM. *Intl Anesth Cin*. 1989;27(3):137–147.
110. Gaba DM, et al. *Hum Factors*. 1995;37(1):20–31.
111. Xiao Y, et al. *Incident Evolution And Task Demands: An Analysis And A Field Study Of 'Going Sour' Incidents*. vol. 36.; 1995.
112. Norman DA. *Psychol Rev*. 1981;88(1):1–15.
113. Rasmussen J. *IEEE Trans Syst, Man, and Cybernetics*. 1983;SMC-13(3):257–266.
114. Klein GA. *Adv Man Machine Sys Res*. 1989;5:47–92.
115. Reason J, et al. *Generic Error-Modeling System (GEMS): A Cognitive Framework for Locating Common Human Error Forms*. Chichester, UK: Wiley; 1987.
116. Klemola UM, Norros L. *Med Educ*. 1997;31(6):449–456.
117. Hall KH. *Med Educ*. 2002;36(3):216–224.
118. Sarter NB, Woods DD. *Intl J Aviation Psych*. 1991;1(1):45–57.
119. Hartman BO, Secrist GE. *Aviat Space Environ Med*. 1991;62(11):1084–1089.
120. Tversky A, Kahneman D. *J Science*. 1974;185(4157):1124–1131.
121. Stiegler MP, Tung A. *Anesthesiology*. 2014;120(1):204–217.
122. Cook RI, et al. *Human Performance in Anesthesia: A Corpus of Cases*. Columbus, Ohio: Cognitive Systems Engineering Laboratory Report, prepared for Anesthesia Patient Safety Foundation; 1991.
123. Reason JT, et al. *Qual Health Care*. 2001;10(suppl 2):ii21–25.
124. Klein GA. In: Orasanu J, Calderwood R, Zsambok CE, eds. *Decision Making in Action: Models and Methods*. Norwood: Ablex Publishing Corporation; 1993:138–147.
125. Schwid HA, O'Donnell D. *Anesthesiology*. 1992;76(4):495–501.
126. DeAnda A, Gaba DM. *Anesth Analg*. 1991;72(3):308–315.
127. Howard SK, et al. *Aviat Space Environ Med*. 1992;63(9):763–770.
128. Gaba DM. *Anesthesiology*. 1992;76(4):491–494.
129. Wacker J, Staender S. *Curr Opin Anaesth*. 2014;27(6):649–656.
130. Stone M, et al. *Memory (Hove, England)*. 2001;9(3):165–176.
131. Dodhia RM, Dismukes RK. *Appl Cogn Psych*. 2009;23(1):73–89.
132. Dieckmann P, et al. *Ergonomics*. 2006;49(5-6):526–543.
133. Dismukes RK. *Curr Dir Psych Sci*. 2012;21(4):215–220.
134. Glavin RJ. *Best Prac Res Clin Anaesth*. 2011;25(2):193–206.
135. Schulz CM, et al. *Anesthesiology*. 2013;118(3):729–742.
136. Schulz CM, et al. *BMC Anesthesiology*. 2016;16:4.
137. De Keyser V, et al. *Fixation Errors in Dynamic and Complex Systems: Descriptive Forms, Psychological Mechanisms, Potential Countermeasures*. Brussles: Technical Report for NATO Division of Scientific Affairs. North Atlantic Treaty Organization (NATO); 1988.
138. De Keyser V, Woods DD. In: Colombo AG, Bustamante AS, eds. *Systems Reliability Assessment*. Dordrecht, Germany: Kluwer Academic; 1990:231–251.
139. Xiao Y, et al. *Decision Making in Dynamic Environments: Fixation Errors and Their Causes*. vol. 39.; 1995.
140. Hart SG, Staveland LE. In: Hancock PA, Meshkati N, eds. *Human Mental Workload*. Amsterdam: Elsevier; 1988:139–183.
141. Edwards MS, et al. *Anx Stress Coping*. 2015;28(1):1–16.
142. Leedal JM, Smith AF. *Br J Anaesth*. 2005;94(6):702–709.
143. Byrne A. *Anesth Pain Med*. 2011;1(2):90–94.
144. Neily J, et al. *Jt Comm J Qual Patient Saf*. 2007;33(8):502–511.
145. Arriaga AF, et al. *N Engl J Med*. 2013;368(3):246–253.
146. Yang CW, et al. *Resuscitation*. 2012;83(9):1055–1060.
147. Knudson MM, et al. *J Trauma*. 2008;64(2):255–263. discussion 263-254.
148. Rall M, et al. In: Kyle R, Murra BW, eds. *Clinical Simulation: Operations, Engineering, and Management*. Burlington: Academic Press; 2008:565–581.
149. Kenmoku K. *J Artif Org*. 2009;12(2):67–72.
150. Wickens CD. *Hum Factors*. 2008;50(3):449–455.
151. Regehr G, Mylopoulos M. *J Cont Ed Hlth Prof*. 2008;28(S1):19–23.
152. Byrne AJ, et al. *Anaesthesia*. 2013;68(12):1266–1272.
153. Burtscher MJ, et al. *BMJ Sim Tech Enh Lrng*. 2018;4(4):165–170.
154. Schwid MD, et al. *Anesthesiology*. 2002;97(6):1434–1444.
155. DeAnda A, Gaba DM. *Anesth Analg*. 1990;71(1):77–82.
156. Henrichs B, et al. *Anesth Analg*. 2009;109:255–262.
157. McIntosh CA. *Anesth Analg*. 2009;108(1):6–9.
158. Lake Wobegon. In OxfordReference.com. Retrieved August 21, 2018, from http://www.oxfordreference.com/view/10.1093/oi/authority.20110810105237549.
159. Scherrer V, et al. *A & A Case Reports*. 2013;1(5):75–76.
160. Novick RJ, et al. *J Surg Ed*. 2015;72(2):302–309.
161. Mhyre JM, et al. *Anesthesiology*. 2010;113(4):782–793.
162. Langerman A, et al. *J Am Coll Surg*. 2014;219(6):1181–1186.
163. Dutton RP, et al. *Anesthesiology*. 2014;121(3):450–458.
164. Tschan F, et al. In: Boos M, Kolbe M, Kappeler P, Ellwart T, eds. *Coordination in Human and Primate Groups*. Heidelberg, Germany: Springer; 2011:93–115.
165. Weingart LR. *Res Org Behav*. 1997;19:189–239.
166. Kolbe M,B, et al. *BMJ Qual Saf*. 2013;22(7):596–605.
167. Embrey ED, et al. *Anesthesia eJournal*. 2013;1(2).
168. Lyk-Jensen HT, et al. *AANA J*. 2016;84(2):122–127.
169. Gaba DM, et al. *Anesthesiology*. 1998;89(1):8–18.
170. Fletcher G, et al. *Framework for Observing and Rating Anaesthetists' NonTechnical Skills. Anaesthetists' NonTechnical Skills (ANTS) System Handbook v1.0*. Aberdeen, Scottland: University of Aberdeen; 2012.
171. Fletcher GC, et al. *Br J Anaesth*. 2002;88(3):418–429.
172. The Joint Commission. *Sentinel Event Statistics Released for 2014*; 2015. https://www.jointcommission.org/assets/1/23/jconline_April_29_15.pdf
173. Cook TM, et al. *Br J Anaesth*. 2011;106(5):617–631.
174. Kohn LT, et al. *To Err Is Human: Building a Safer Health System*; 2000.
175. Dieckmann P, et al. *Adv Simul*. 2017;2(1):21.
176. Human Factors and Ergonomics Society (HFES). *Definitions of Human Factors and Ergonomics*; 2016. http://cms.hfes.org/Resources/Educational-and-Professional-Resources/Educational-Resources/Definitions-of-Human-Factors-and-Ergonomics.aspx
177. Catchpole K, McCulloch P. *Curr Opin Crit Care*. 2010;16(6):618–622.
178. Holden RJ, et al. *Ergonomics*. 2013;56(11):1669–1686.
179. Carayon P, et al. *Qual Saf Hlth Care*. 2006;15(suppl 1):i50–i58.
180. Nestel D, et al. *Simul Hlthcare*. 2011;6(1):2–3.
181. Gaba DM. *Simul Hlthcare*. 2011;6(1):8–10.
182. Fletcher G, et al. *Br J Anaesth*. 2003;90(5):580–588.
183. Flin R, et al. *Br J Anaesth*. 2010;105(1):38–44.
184. Salas E, et al. *Human Res Mgmt*. 2014:24. Available at: https://orpca.org/APCM/Salas_et_al-2014-Human_Resource_Management%201%203.pdf.
185. Jepsen RMHG, et al. *Int J Med Ed*. 2015;6:17–25.
186. Spanager L, et al. *Danish Med J*. 2012;59(11):A4526.
187. Shields A, Flin R. *EMJ*. 2013;30(5):350–354.
188. Flin R, et al. *The Surgeon*. 2007;5(2):86–89.
189. Helmreich R, et al. *Vol NASA/UT Technical Manual 90-2, Revision 1*. Austin, TX: NASA/University of Texas Aerospace Crew Performance Project; 1991.
190. Graham J, et al. *Br J Anaesth*. 2010;104(4):440–445.
191. Zwaan L, et al. *Adv Simul*. 2016;1(1):18.
192. Watkins SC, et al. *Simul Hlthcare*. 2017;12(2):69–75.
193. Gjeraa K, et al. *Acta Anaesth Scan*. 2016;60(1):36–47.
194. Jones CPL, et al. *Anaesthesia*. 2018;73(suppl 1):12–24.
195. Flin R, et al. *Anaesthesia*. 2013;68(8):817–825.
196. World Health Organization (WHO). Patient safety curriculum, Topic 2: "Why applying human factors is important for patient safety?". In: *WHO Multi-professional Patient Safety Curriculum Guide*. 2011: 111-107.
197. Brandimonte M, et al. *Prospective Memory: Theory and Applications*. Mahwah, NJ, US: Lawrence Erlbaum Associates Publishers; 1996.
198. Douglas HE, et al. *Appl Ergo*. 2017;59:45–55.
199. Ophir E, et al. *Proc Natl Acad Sci U S A*. 2009;106(37):15583–15587.
200. Uncapher MR, Wagner AD. *Proc Natl Acad Sci U S A*. 2018;115(40):9889–9896.
201. Feng SF, et al. *Cogn Affect Behav Neurosci*. 2014;14(1):129–146.
202. Weigl M, et al. *J Pat Saf*. 2013;9(1):18–23.
203. Rohrer D, Pashler HE. *Psych Bulletin Rev*. 2003;10(1):96–103.
204. Nijboer M, et al. *PLoS ONE*. 2013;8(11).
205. van Rensen ELJ, et al. *Anesth Analg*. 2012;115(5):1183–1187.
206. Segall N, et al. *Anesth Analg*. 2012;115(1):102–115.
207. Endsley MR. *Human Factors*. 1995;37(1):32–64.
208. Endsley MR. *J Cogn Eng Dec Mak*. 2015;9(1):4–32.
209. Endsley MR. *Cogn Tech Work*. 2015;17(2).
210. Dekker S. *Cogn Tech Work*. 2015;17(2):159–161.
211. Dekker S, Hollnagel E. *Cogn Tech Work*. 2003;6:79–86.

212. Kahneman D. *Thinking, Fast and Slow*. New York: Farrar, Straus and Giroux; 2012.
213. Bogdanovic J, et al. *BMC Hlth Serv Resch*. 2015;15:128.
214. Widmer LW, et al. *Wrld J Surg*. 2018;42(7):2011–2017.
215. Burtscher MJ, Manser T. *Safety Sci*. 2012;50:1344–1354.
216. Johnsen BH, et al. *Scand J Trauma Resuc Emg Med*. 2017;25(1):109.
217. Schmutz JB, Eppich WJ. *Acad Med*. 2017;92(11):1555–1563.
218. Fioratou E, et al. *Br J Anaesth*. 2010;105(1):83–90.
219. Gibbs NM. *Anaesth Intev Care*. 2017;45(3):289–290.
220. Fleisher LA. *Euro J Anaesth*. 2012;29(8):357–359.
221. Marewski JN, Gigerenzer G. *Dial Clin Neurosci*. 2012;14(1):77–89.
222. Kahneman D, Klein G. *Am Psychol*. 2009;64:515–526.
223. Gigerenzer G, et al. *Simple Heuristics that Make us Smart*. New York: Oxford University Press; 1999.
224. Gigerenzer G, Gray JA. *Better Doctors, Better Patients, Better Decisions : Envisioning Health Care 2020*. Cambridge, MA: MIT Press; 2011.
225. Schlesinger JJ, et al. *Anesthesiol Clin*. 2018;36(1):99–116.
226. Nurok M, Cohen N. *Intnl Anesth Clin*. 2015;53(3):116–126.
227. Distracted Doctoring. *Returning to Patient-Centered Care in the Digital Age*. Springer; 2017.
228. Jorm CM, O'Sullivan G. *Anaesth Inten Care*. 2012;40(1):71–78.
229. Attri JP, et al. *Saudi J Anaesth*. 2016;10(1):87–94.
230. Ford DA. *AORN journal*. 2018;107(1):P13–P14.
231. Gill PS, et al. *Risk Mgmt Hlthcare Pol*. 2012;5:105–114.
232. van Pelt M, Weinger MB. *Anesth Analg*. 2017;125(1):347–350.
233. Pınar HU, et al. *BMC Anesthesiology*. 2016;16:88.
234. Domino KB, Sessler DI. *Anesthesiology*. 2012;117(6):1156–1158.
235. Stevenson RA, et al. *Anesthesiology*. 2013;118(2):376–381.
236. Weinger MB, van Pelt M. *Anesth Analg*. 2017;125(1):347–350.
237. Allen K, Blascovich J. *JAMA*. 1994;272(11):882–884.
238. Weinger MB. *JAMA*. 1995;273(14):1090–1091.
239. Murthy VS, et al. *Can J Anaesth*. 1995;42(7):608–611.
240. Schneider W, Detweiler M. *Human Factors*. 1988;30(5):539–566.
241. Soto RG, et al. *Euro J Anaesth*. 2017;34(4):246–247.
242. Patterson P. *OR manager*. 2013;29(2):20–22.
243. Statement on use of cell phones in the operating room. *Bulletin of the American College of Surgeons*. 2008;93(9):33–34.
244. (AORN) *Position Statement on Managing Distractions and Noise During Perioperative Patient Care*; 2014. http://www.aorn.org/Clinical_Practice/Position_Statements/Position_Statements.aspx
245. The Joint Commission. Minimizing noise and distractions in the OR and procedural units. *Quick Safety*. 2017;(Issue 35). https://www.jointcommission.org/assets/1/23/Quick_Safety_Issue_35_2017_Noise_in_OR_FINAL.pdf
246. Anthony K, et al. *Crit Care Nurse*. 2010;30(3):21–29.
247. Huber S, et al. 2016.
248. *International Bedroom Poll*. 2013. https://sleepfoundation.org/sleep-polls-data/other-polls/2013-international-bedroom-poll
249. Doran SM, et al. *Arch Italiennes de Biologie*. 2001;139(3):253–267.
250. Akerstedt T, Kecklund G. *J Sleep Research*. 2001;10(2):105–110.
251. Howard SK, et al. *Adad Med*. 2002;77(10):1019–1025.
252. Howard SK, et al. *Anesthesiology*. 2002;97(5):1281–1294.
253. Biddle C, Aker J. *AANA Journal*. 2011;79(4):324–331.
254. Domen R, et al. *AANA Journal*. 2015;83(2):123–131.
255. The Joint Commission. Health care worker fatigue and patient safety. *Sentinel Event Alert*. 2011;48(48):1–4. https://www.jointcommission.org/assets/1/18/SEA_48.pdf
256. Sinha A, et al. *J Anaesth, Clin Pharm*. 2013;29(2):151–159.
257. Gregory P, Edsell M. *Cont Ed Anaesth Crit Care Pain*. 2014;14(1):18–22.
258. Barger LK, et al. *PLoS Med*. 2006;3(12):e487.
259. Fletcher KE, et al. *Ann Intern Med*. 2004;141(11):851–857.
260. Accreditation Council for Graduate Medical Education (ACGME). *The ACGME 2011 Duty Hour Standard: Enhancing Quality of Care*. Supervision and Resident Professional Development; 2011. https://www.acgme.org/Portals/0/PDFs/jgme-monograph[1].pdf
261. Blum AB, et al. *Nat Sci Sleep*. 2011;3:47–85.
262. Philibert I, et al. *Ann Rev Med*. 2013;64:467–483.
263. Landrigan CP, et al. *JAMA*. 2006;296(9):1063–1070.
264. Engelmann C, et al. *Surg Endoscopy*. 2011;25(4):1245–1250.
265. Cooper JB, et al. *Anesthesiology*. 1982;56(6):456–461.
266. Cooper JB. *J Clin Anesth*. 1989;1(3):228–231.
267. Smith-Coggins R, et al. *I Ann Emerg Med*. 2006;48(5):596-604, 604. e591-593.
268. Howard SK. *VA's Strategic Nap Program. TOPICS IN PATIENT SAFETY*. VA Palo Alto Health Care System;MAY/JUNE 2008.
269. Rendell PG, Craik FIM. *Appl Cogn Psych*. 2000;14(7):S43–S62.
270. Mienaltowski A. *Ann New York Acad Sci*. 2011;1235:75–85.
271. Agency for Healthcare Research and Quality (AHRQ). *TeamSTEPPS® 2.0 Pocket Guide*; 2014. 2018 https://www.ahrq.gov/sites/default/files/wysiwyg/professionals/education/curriculum-tools/teamstepps/instructor/essentials/pocketguide.pdf
272. Silverstein JH, et al. *Anesthesiology*. 1993;79(2):354–375.
273. Bryson EO, Silverstein JH. *Anesthesiology*. 2008;109(5):905–917.
274. Jungerman FS, et al. *Braz J Anesth*. 2012;62(3):375–386.
275. Mayall RM. *BJA Educ*. 2016;16(7):236–241.
276. Booth JV, et al. *Anesth Analg*. 2002;95(4):1024–1030.
277. Skipper GE, et al. *Anesth Analg*. 2009;109(3):891–896.
278. Berge KH, et al. *Mayo Clin Proc*. 2009;84(7):625–631.
279. Rossier RN. Hazardous Attitudes. Which one do you have?. https://www.aopa.org/news-and-media/all-news/1999/september/flight-training-magazine/hazardous-attitudes; 1999
280. Tucker AL, Edmondson AC. *Calif Mgmt Rev*. 2003;45(2):55–72.
281. Lingard L, et al. *Acad Med*. 2002;77(3):232–237.
282. Greenberg CC, et al. *J Am Coll Surg*. 2007;204(4):533–540.
283. Kolbe M, et al. *Anesth Analg*. 2012;115:1099–1108.
284. The Joint Commission. Sentinel Event Alert: Inadequate hand-off communication. Issue 58. September 2017; https://www.jointcommission.org/assets/1/18/SEA_58_Hand_off_Comms_9_6_17_FINAL_(1).pdf. Accessed November 16, 2018.
285. Edmondson AC. *Teaming: How Organizations Learn, Innovate, and Compete in the Knowledge Economy*. San Francisco, CA: Jossey-Bass; 2012.
286. Smith-Jentsch KA, et al. *Small Group Research*. 2008;39(3):303–327.
287. Rudolph JW, et al. *Academy Manage J*. 2009;34:733–756.
288. Schmutz J, et al. *Euro J Work Organiz Psych*. 2015;24(5):761–776.
289. Härgestam M, et al. *BMJ Open*. 2013;3(10).
290. Kolbe M. In: Salas E, Tannenbaum S, Cohen D, Latham G, eds. *Developing and Enhancing Teamwork in Organisations: Evidence-Based Best Practices and Guidelines*. San Francisco, CA: Jossey-Bass; 2013: 609–643.
291. El-Shafy IA, et al. *J Surg Educ*. 2018;75(1):58–64.
292. Hunter H, et al. *Periop Care OR Mgmt*. 2017;6:7–10.
293. Randmaa M, et al. *BMJ Open*. 2017;7(8):e015038.
294. De Meester K, et al. *Resuscitation*. 2013;84(9):1192–1196.
295. Shahid S, Thomas S. *Safety in Health*. 2018;4(1):7.
296. Bagian JP, Paull DE. *JAMA*. 2018;319(2):125–127.
297. Saager L, et al. *Anesthesiology*. 2014;121(4):695–706.
298. Starmer AJ, et al. *N Engl J Med*. 2014;371(19):1803–1812.
299. Karamchandani K, et al. *Qual Mgmt Health Care*. 2018;27(4):215–222.
300. Jullia M, et al. *Euro J Anaesth*. 2017;34(7):471–476.
301. Kolbe M, et al. *Anesth Analg*. 2012;115(5):1099–1108.
302. Morrison EW. *Acad Mgmt Ann*. 2011;5(1):373–412.
303. Raemer DB, et al. *Acad Med*. 2016;91(4):530–539.
304. Schwappach DLB, Gehring K. *BMJ Open*. 2014;4(5).
305. Schwappach DL, Gehring K. *PLoS One*. 2014;9(8):e104720.
306. Schwappach DL, Gehring K. *BMC Hlth Serv Res*. 2014;14:303.
307. Okuyama A, et al. *BMC Hlth Serv Res*. 2014;14:61.
308. Detert J, Edmondson A. *Acad Mgmt J*. 2011;54(3):461–488.
309. Morrison EW. *Ann Rev Organiz Psychol*. 2014;1(1):173–197.
310. Kish-Gephart JJ, et al. *Res Organiz Behav*. 2009;29:163–193.
311. Souba W, et al. *Acad Med*. 2011;86(12):1492–1499.
312. St.Pierre M, et al. *Der Anaesthesist*. 2012;61(10):857–866.
313. Weiss M, et al. *Small Group Res*. 2014;45(3):290–313.
314. Vashdi DR, et al. *Acad Mgmt J*. 2013;56(4):945–971.
315. Edmondson AC. *Administrative Science Quarterly*. 1999;44(2):350–383.
316. Bould MD, et al. *Can J Anaesth*. 2015;62(6):576–586.
317. Liu W, et al. *J Appl Psych*. 2013;98(5):841–851.
318. Sydor DT, et al. *Br J Anaesth*. 2013;110(3):463–471.
319. Martin GP, et al. *BMJ Quality Amp; Saf*. 2018.
320. Farh CI, Chen G. *J Appl Psychol*. 2018;103(1):97–110.
321. Weiss M, et al. *We can do It! Inclusive Leader Language Promotes Voice Behavior in Multi-Professional Teams*; 2017.
322. Wei X, et al. *J Appl Psych*. 2015;100(5):1641–1652.
323. Weiss M, Morrison EW. *J Organz Behav*. 2018;0(Special Issue):1–15.
324. Cooper JB. *Anesthesiology*. 2018.
325. Salas E, et al. *Toward an Understanding of Team Performance and Training. Teams: Their Training and Performance*. Westport, CT: Ablex Publishing; 1992:3–29.
326. Schmutz J, Manser T. *Br J Anaesth*. 2013;110(4):529–544.
327. Weiss M, et al. *Euro J Work Organiz Psych*. 2017;26(1):66–80.

328. St Pierre M, et al. *Der Anaesthesist*. 2016;65(9):681–689.
329. Team Cognition. *Understanding the Factors That Drive Process and Performance*. American Psychological Association; 2004.
330. Burtscher MJ, et al. *Br J Anaesth*. 2011;106(6):801–806.
331. Schmutz J, et al. In: Örtenblad A, Abrahamson C, Sheaff R, eds. *Management Innovations for Health Care Organizations. Adopt, Abandon or Adapt?*. New York: Routledge; 2016:359–377.
332. Burtscher MJ, et al. *J Exp Psych: Appl*. 2011;17:257–269.
333. Kolbe M, et al. *J Appl Psych*. 2014;99(6):1254–1267.
334. Künzle B, et al. *Eur J Work Organ Psychol*. 2010;19:505–531.
335. Künzle B, et al. *Safety Science*. 2010;48(1):1–17.
336. Morgeson FP, et al. *J Mgmt*. 2010;36(1):5–39.
337. Klein KJ, et al. *AdminSci Quar*. 2006;51(4):590–621.
338. Seelandt J, et al. *GIO*. 2017;48(1):69–78.
339. Tschan F, et al. *Trends Anaesth Crit Care*. 2014;4:36.
340. Fernandez Castelao E, et al. *J Crit Care*. 2013;28(4):504–521.
341. Foulk T, et al. *J Appl Psych*. 2016;101(1):50–67.
342. Riskin A, et al. *Pediatrics*. 2015;136(3):487–495.
343. Sagan SD. *J Contig Crisis Mgmt*. 1994;2(4):228–240.
344. Larsson J, Holmström IK. *Br J Anaesth*. 2013;110(1):115–121.
345. Helmreich RL, et al. *Intl J Aviat Psych*. 1999;9(1):19–32.
346. Rall M, et al. *AINS*. 2001;36(6):321–330.
347. Gaba D, et al. *Simul Gaming*. 2001;32:175–193.
348. Gaba DM, et al. *Simul Gaming*. 2001;32(2):175–193.
349. Barnes CM, et al. *J Appl Psych*. 2008;93(3):529–539.
350. Sagan SD. *Risk Analysis*. 2004;24(4):935–946.
351. Nembhard IM, Edmondson AC. *J Organiz Behav*. 2006;27(7):941–966.
352. Hirak R, et al. *Leadership Quar*. 2012;23:107–117.
353. Rosenman ED, et al. *J Grad Med Educ*. 2016;8(3):332–340.
354. Rosenman ED, et al. *Acad Med*. 2014;89(9):1295–1306.
355. Mesmer-Magnus JR, Dechurch LA. *J Appl Psych*. 2009;94(2):535–546.
356. Bogenstätter Y, et al. *Human Factors*. 2009;51:115–125.
357. Christensen C, et al. *Med Dec Making*. 2000;20(1):45–50.
358. Larson JRJ, et al. *J Pers Soc Psychol*. 1998;75:93–108.
359. Chikkabbaiah V, et al. *Anaesthesia*. 2015;70(12):1453-1453.
360. Pandit JJ, et al. *Anaesthesia*. 2017;72(2):150–155.
361. Berkenstadt H, et al. *Anesth Analg*. 2006;102(2):530–532.
362. Harrison TK, et al. *Anesth Analg*. 2006;103(3):551–556.
363. Burden AR, et al. *Simul Hlthcare*. 2012;7(1):1–9.
364. Bereknyei Merrell S, et al. *Jt Comm J Qual Patient Saf*. 2018;44(8):477–484.
365. Hilton G, et al. *Intl J Ob Anesth*. 2016;25:9–16.
366. Marshall SD, Mehra R. *Anaesthesia*. 2014;69(7):669–677.
367. Lingard L, et al. *Arch Surg (Chicago, Ill: 1960)*. 2008;143(1):12–17.
368. Krombach JW, et al. *Anesth Pain Med*. 2015;5(4):e26300.
369. Hepner DL, et al. *Anesthesiology*. 2017;127(2):384–392.
370. Marshall S. *Anesth Analg*. 2013;117(5):1162–1171.
371. Mellin-Olsen J, et al. *Euro J Anaesth*. 2010;27(7):592–597.
372. Haynes AB, et al. *New England Journal of Medicine*. 2009;360(5):491–499.
373. Neuhaus C, et al. *J Pat Saf*. 2017.
374. Levy MM, et al. *Crit Care Med*. 2004;32(suppl 11):S595–597.
375. Chu L, Fuller A. *Manual of Clinical Anesthesiology*. Philadelphia: Lippincott Williams & Wilkins; 2011.
376. Watkins SC, et al. *J Clin Monit Comp*. 2016;30(3):275–283.
377. Goldhaber-Fiebert SN, et al. *Jt Comm J Qual Patient Saf*. 2015;41(5):212–220.
378. Gaba DM. *Anesth Analg*. 2013;117(5):1033–1036.
379. Tobin JM, et al. *Anesth Analg*. 2013;117(5):1178–1184.
380. Augoustides JG, et al. *Anesth Analg*. 2013;117(5):1037–1038.
381. Goldhaber-Fiebert SN, Howard SK. *Anesth Analg*. 2013;117(5):1149–1161.
382. Jenkins B. *Anaesthesia*. 2014;69(7):660–664.
383. Walker IA, et al. *Br J Anaesth*. 2012;109(1):47–54.
384. Pugel AE, et al. *J Inf Publ Hlth*. 2015;8(3):219–225.
385. Close KL, et al. *BMJ Global Health*. 2017;2(suppl 4):e000430.
386. Treadwell JR, et al. *BMJ Qual Safety*. 2014;23(4):299–318.
387. Winters BD, et al. *Crit Care*. 2009;13(6):210-210.
388. Gillespie BM, Marshall A. *Implement Sci*. 2015;10:137.
389. Mahajan RP. *Best Prac Res Clin Anaesth*. 2011;25(2):161–168.
390. Clay-Williams R, Colligan L. *BMJ Qual Safety*. 2015;24(7):428–431.
391. Salas E, et al. *Theoret Iss Ergonom*. 2007;8(5):381–394.
392. Cooke NJ, et al. *J Exp Psychol Appl*. 2007;13(3):146–157.
393. Cooke NJ, et al. *Hum Factors*. 2000;42(1):151–173.
394. Cooke NJ. *CurrDir Psycho Sci*. 2015;24(6):415–419.
395. Salas E, et al. *Grp Organ Mgmt*. 2018;43(3):357–381.
396. Gjeraa K, et al. *Acta Anaesth Scand*. 2014;58(7):775–787.
397. Armour Forse R, et al. *Surgery*. 2011;150(4):771–778.
398. Deering S, et al. *Jt Comm J Qual Patient Saf*. 2011;37(8):350–356.
399. Capella J, et al. *J Surg Educ*. 2010;67(6):439–443.
400. Young-Xu Y, et al. *Arch Surg*. 2011;146(12):1368–1373.
401. Risser DT, et al. *Ann Emerg Med*. 1999;34(3):373–383.
402. Morey JC, et al. *Hlth Serv Res*. 2002;37(6):1553–1581.
403. Rosen MA, et al. *Acad Emerg Med*. 2008;15(11):1190–1198.
404. Birnbach DJ, Salas E. *Anesthesiol Clin*. 2008;26(1):159–168. viii.
405. Sundar E, et al. *Anesthesiol Clin*. 2007;25(2):283–300.
406. Nielsen PE, et al. *Ob Gyn*. 2007;109(1):48–55.
407. Marshall DA, Manus DA. *AORN journal*. 2007;86(6):994–1011.
408. Dunn EJ, et al. *Jt Comm J Qual Patient Saf*. 2007;33(6):317–325.
409. Weaver SJ, et al. *BMJ Quality & Safety*. 2014;23(5):359–372.
410. Marlow SL, et al. *Jt Comm J Qual Patient Saf*. 2017;43(4):197–204.
411. Agency for Healthcare Research and Quality. TeamSTEPPS: Curriculum, Toolkit, further information and implementation guidelines, Online Training, Pocket Guide and Pocket Guide App, Webinars, Training Videos, Classroom slides, Measurement Tools. https://www.ahrq.gov/teamstepps/index.html.
412. Agency for Healthcare Research and Quality (AHRQ). *TeamSTEPPS® 2.0*; 2012. https://www.ahrq.gov/teamstepps/index.html
413. Veterans Affairs National Center for Patient Safety. Clinical Team Training (CTT). https://www.patientsafety.va.gov/professionals/training/team.asp. Accessed May, 06 2018.
414. Neily J, et al. *Lessons from the VA's Team Training Program. Perspectives on Safety*; 2011. https://psnet.ahrq.gov/perspectives/perspective/112
415. Canadian Patient Safety Foundation. *Report on Summary of Team Training Programs*; 2010. http://www.patientsafetyinstitute.ca/en/toolsResources/teamworkCommunication/Documents/Teamwork%20and%20Communications%20Final%20Summary%20of%20training%20programs.pdf
416. Moray NP, Senders JW. *Human Error: Cause, Prediction and Reduction*. Lawrence Erlbaum Associates Inc; 2008.
417. Hogan AM, Sanders RD. *Br J Anaesth*. 2014;112(6):960–964.
418. Health and Safety Executive (HSE). Leadership and worker involvement toolkit. http://www.hse.gov.uk/construction/lwit/assets/downloads/human-failure.pdf; 2012
419. Arnstein F. *Br J Anaesth*. 1997;79(5):645–656.
420. Rasmussen J. *Information Processing and Human-Machine Interaction: An Approach to Cognitive Engineering*. New York, USA: Elsevier Science Ltd; 1986.
421. Helmreich RL. *BMJ*. 2000;320(7237):781–785.
422. Engelmann C, et al. *Langenbeck's Arch Surg*. 2017;402(1):187–190.
423. Vincent C, et al. *Br Med J*. 1998;316(7138):1154–1157.
424. Taylor-Adams S, Vincent C. *Clinical Risk*. 2004;10(6):211–220.
425. Nyssen AS, Blavier A. *Ergonomics*. 2006;49(5-6):517–525.
426. Mehl K, Wehner T. In: Bauer J, Harteis C, eds. *Human Fallibility: The Ambiguity of Errors for Work and Learning*. Dordrecht: Springer; 2012:91–106.
427. Dekker S. *The Field Guide to Understanding Human Error*. 2nd New edition. Aldershot (England) & Burlington, VT (USA): Ashgate Publishing Limited; 2006.
428. Reason J. *West J Med*. 2000;172(6):393–396.
429. Cook RI, Woods DD. *Human Error Med*. 1994:255–310.
430. Hidden A. *Clapham Junction Accident Investigation Report*. London: His/Her Majesty's Stationary Office; 1989.
431. Henriksen K, Kaplan H. *Qual Saf Hlth Care*. 2003;12(suppl 2):ii46–ii50.
432. Arkes HR. *Curr Dir Psych Sci*. 2013;22(5):356–360.
433. Hugh TB, Dekker S. Hindsight bias and outcome bias in the social construction of medical negligence. *A Review*. 2009; 16.
434. Institute of Medicine (IOM). *Crossing the Quality Chasm.: A New Health System for the 21st Century*. 2001.
435. Roberts KH. *Ind Crisis Quar*. 1989;3(2):111–125.
436. Laporte T, Consolini P. *Working in Practice But Not in Theory: Theoretical Challenges of "High-Reliability Organizations"*. 1991;1.
437. La Porte TR. *J Cont Crisis Mgmt*. 1996;4(2):60–71.
438. Weick K, Sutcliffe KM. *Managing the Unexpected: Resilient Performance in an Age of Uncertainty*. John Wiley & Sons; 2001.
439. Weick KE. *Calif Mgmt Rev*. 1987;29(2):112–127.
440. Weick KE. In: Staw BM, Cummings LL, eds. *Research in Organizational Behavior*. vol. 21. Greenwich, CT: JAI Press, Inc.; 1999:81–123.
441. Sutcliffe KM. *Best Prac Res Clin Anaesth*. 2011;25(2):133–144.
442. Leveson N, et al. *Organization Studies*. 2009;30(2-3):227–249.
443. Shrivastava S, et al. *Human Relations*. 2009;62(9):1357–1390.

444. Sagan SD. *The Limits of Safety. Organizations, Accidents, and Nuclear Weapons*. Vol 53. Princeton, New Jersey: Princeton University Press; 1993.
445. Gaba DM. Structural and organizational issues in patient safety: a comparison of health care to other high-hazard industries. *California Management Review*. 2000;43(1):83–102.
446. Snook SA. *Friendly Fire: The Accidental Shootdown of U.S. Blackhawks Over Northern Iraq*. Princeton: Princton University Press; 2000.
447. Hollnagel EW, et al. *Resilience Engineering - Concepts and Precepts*. Aldershot: Ashgate; 2006.
448. Fairbanks RJ, et al. *Jt Comm J Qual Patient Safety*. 2014;40(8):376–383.
449. Hollnagel E, et al. *Resilience Engineering in Practice: A Guidebook*. Ashgate: CRC Press; 2010.
450. Hollnagel E. In: Hollnagel E, Braithwaite J, Wears RL, eds. *Resilient Healthcare*. Farnham, UK: Ashgate; 2013:3–17.
451. Hollnagel E, Nemeth CP. In: Nemeth CP, Hollnagel E, Dekker SWA, eds. *Resilience Engineering Perspectives*. vol. 2. Farnham, UK: CRC Press; 2009:310.
452. Haavik TK, et al. *Safety Science*. 2016.
453. Gaba DM. *Anesth Patient Saf Found Newsl (Special Issue)*. 2003;18(13-14).
454. Roberts KH, et al. *J High Tech Mgmt Res*. 1994;5:141–161.
455. Institute for Healthcare Improvement (IHI). High reliability organization (HRO) principles. *Reference Sheet*. 2014. http://app.ihi.org/FacultyDocuments/Events/Event-2491/Presentation-10595/Document-8970/Tools_HRO_Principles.pdf
456. Rall M, Dieckmann P. *Best Pract Res Clin Anaesthesiol*. 2005;19(4):539–557.
457. Hollnagel E. *Safety-I and Safety-II. The Past and Future of Safety Management*. Farnham, UK: Ashgate; 2014.
458. *From Safety-I to Safety-II: A White Paper. The Resilient Health Care Net*. Published simultaneously by the University of Southern Denmark, Australia, University of Florida, USA, and Macquarie University; 2015. https://www.england.nhs.uk/signuptosafety/wp-content/uploads/sites/16/2015/10/safety-1-safety-2-whte-papr.pdf
459. Hollnagel E. *FRAM, The Functional Resonance Analysis Method : Modelling Complex Socio-Technical Systems*. Burlington, VT: Ashgate; 2012.
460. Grote G. *Safety Science*. 2015;71:71–79.
461. Grote G. *Safety Management in Different High-Risk Domains – All the Same?*. 2012;50.
462. Grote G. *Ann Rev Control*. 2004;28:267–274.
463. Gilbert C, et al. *J Risk Research*. 2007;10(7):959–975.
464. Power M. *The Risk Management of Everything: Rethinking the Politics of Uncertainty*. London: Demos; 2004.
465. Grote G. *Management of Uncertainty. Theory and Application in the Design of Systems and Organizations*. London: Springer; 2009.
466. Grote G, et al. *OrganizPsychRev*. 2018;8(2-3):125–148.
467. Pedersen KZ. *Soc Hlth Illness*. 2016;38(7):1180–1193.
468. Vaughan D. *The Challenger Launch Decision: Risky Technology, Culture, and Deviance at NASA*. University of Chicago Press; 1997.
469. Cook R, Rasmussen JJ. *Qual Saf Health Care*. 2005;14:130–134.
470. Hines S, et al. *Becoming a High Reliability Organization: Operational Advice for Hospital Leaders*. Rockville, MD: Agency for Healthcare Research and Quality (AHRQ). AHRQ Publication No. 08-0022; 2008.
471. *Free from Harm: Accelerating Patient Safety Improvement Fifteen Years after To Err Is Human*. National Patient Safety Foundation; 2015. http://www.ihi.org/resources/Pages/Publications/Free-from-Harm-Accelerating-Patient-Safety-Improvement.aspx
472. Slawomirski L, et al. *The Economics of Patient Safety*; 2017.
473. Frankel AS, et al. *Hlth Serv Res*. 2006;41(4 Pt 2):1690–1709.
474. Schein EH. *Organizational Culture and Leadership: A Dynamic View*. San Francisco: Jossey-Bass; 1985:1992.
475. The Joint Commission. *Sentinel Event Alert*. 2017;(57):1–8.
476. Sentinel Event Alert. Behaviors that undermine a culture of safety. *The Joint Commission*. 2008;(Issue 40). https://www.jointcommission.org/assets/1/18/SEA_40.PDF
477. Sammer CE, et al. *J Nrsg Scholar*. 2010;42(2):156–165.
478. Xuanyue M, et al. *J Evidence-Based Med*. 2013;6(1):43–49.
479. Singer SJ, Tucker AL. *BMJ Qual Saf*. 2014;23(10):789–800.
480. Singer SJ, et al. *Jt Comm J Qual Patient Saf*. 2013;39(8):349–360.
481. Institute for Healthcare Improvement (IHI). Develop a Culture of Safety. http://www.ihi.org/resources/Pages/Changes/DevelopaCultureofSafety.aspx. Accessed May 15, 2018.
482. *Leading a Culture of Safety: A Blueprint for Success. Work of an Expert Roundtable Convened by the American College of Healthcare Executives and the IHI/NPSF Lucian Leape Institute. American College of Healthcare Executives, Institute for Healthcare Improvement (IHI), National Patient Safety Foundation (NPSF)*. Lucian Leape Institute; 2017. https://www.npsf.org/page/cultureofsafety.
483. The Joint Commission. *Strategies for Creating, Sustaining, and Improving a Culture of Safety in Health Care. Real-World Solutions to Challenging Safety Culture Implementation Issues*. 2nd ed. ; 2017.
484. Weaver SJ, et al. *Ann Int Med*. 2013;158(5 0 2):369–374.
485. Khatri N, et al. *Health Care Manage Rev*. 2009;34(4):312–322.
486. Shorrock S, et al. *Systems Thinking for Safety: Ten Principles. A White Paper. Moving towards Safety-II*. European Organisation for the Safety of Air Navigation (EUROCONTROL); 2014.
487. Vincent CA. *Qual Saf Health Care*. 2004;13(4):242–243.
488. Pronovost PJ, et al. *J Crit Care*. 2006;21(4):305–315.
489. Vincent C. *N Engl J Med*. 2003;348(11):1051–1056.
490. Pronovost P, et al. *Int Care Med*. 2006;32(10):1467–1469.
491. Singer S, et al. *Health Serv Res*. 2009;44(2 Pt 1):399–421.
492. Singer S, et al. *Hlth Serv Res*. 2007;42(5):1999–2021.
493. Benzer JK, et al. *J Eval Clin Pract*. 2017;23(4):853–859.
494. Gaba DM, et al. *Crit Care Med*. 2007;35(1):314–316.
495. Gaba DM, et al. *Hum Factors*. 2003;45(2):173–185.
496. Flin R. *Safety Sci*. 2007;45:653–667.
497. Mardon RE, et al. *J Patient Saf*. 2010;6(4):226–232.
498. Hogden A, et al. *Safety Culture Assessment in Health Care: A Review of the Literature on Safety Culture Assessment Modes*. Sydney, Australia: Australian Commission on Quality and Safety in Health Care; 2017.
499. Carroll JS, Rudolph JW. *Qual Saf Health Care*. 2006;15(suppl 1):i4–9.
500. Lipshitz R, et al. *J Appl Behav Sci*. 2002;38(1):78–98.
501. Donaldson L. *Lancet*. 2004;364(9445):1567–1568.
502. World Health Organization. *World Alliance for Patient Safety : WHO Draft Guidelines for Adverse Event Reporting and Learning Systems : from Information to Action*. Geneva: World Health Organization; 2005.
503. Patient Safety Primer: Detection of Safety Hazards. Agency for Healthcare Research and Quality (AHRQ); Last updated August 2018. https://psnet.ahrq.gov/primers/primer/24. Accessed October 24, 2018.
504. Leape L. *N Engl J Med*. 2002;347(20):1633–1638.
505. Vincent C. *BMJ*. 2007;334(51).
506. *Key Findings and Recommendations on Reporting and Learning Systems for Patient Safety Incidents Across Europe. Report of the Reporting and Learning Subgroup of the European Commission (PSQCWG)*. European Commission; 2014. https://ec.europa.eu/health/home_en
507. *Patient Safety Reporting Systems: A Literature Review of International Practice*. Health Quality & Safety Commission New Zealand; 2016. https://www.hqsc.govt.nz/assets/Reportable-Events/Publications/Patient-safety-reporting-systems-literature-review-Nov-2016.pdf
508. Health Quality Ontario. *Ontario Health Technology Assessment Series*. 2017;17(3):1–23.
509. Manser T, et al. *Intl J Qual Hlth Care*. 2017;29(3):349–359.
510. Dodds A, Kodate N. *J Pub Policy*. 2012;32(2):117–139.
511. Leistikow I, et al. *BMJ Quality Safety*. 2017;26(3):252–256.
512. Macrae C. *BMJ Qual Saf*. 2016;25(2):71–75.
513. Howell AM, et al. *BMJ Qual Saf*. 2017;26(2):150–163.
514. Mitchell I, et al. *BMJ Qual Saf*. 2016;25(2):92–99.
515. Stavropoulou C, et al. How effective are incident-reporting systems for improving patient safety? *A Systematic Literature Review*. 2015;93.
516. Murff HJ, et al. *J Biomed Inform*. 2003;36(1-2):131–143.
517. Billings C. In: Cook RI, Woods DD, Miller CA, eds. *A Tale of Two Stories: Contrasting Views of Patient Safety*. North Adams, MA: US National Patient Safety Foundation; 1998:52–61.
518. Levtzion-Korach O, et al. *J Pat Safety*. 2009;5(1):9–15.
519. Nuckols TK, et al. *Qual Saf Health Care*. 2007;16(3):164–168.
520. Thomas EJ, et al. *Med Care*. 2000;38(3):261–271.
521. Reporting Patient Safety Events. Agency for Healthcare Research and Quality (AHRQ); Last Updated August 2018. Accessed October 24, 2018.
522. Agency for Healthcare Research and Quality (AHRQ). *Incident Reporting: More Attention to the Safety Action Feedback Loop. Please*; 2011. https://psnet.ahrq.gov/perspectives/perspective/108/Incident-Reporting-More-Attention-to-the-Safety-Action-Feedback-Loop-Please
523. Leape LL. *N Engl J Med*. 2002;347(20):1633–1638.
524. Merry AF. *Anaesthesia*. 2008;63(4):337–339.
525. Mahajan RP. *Br J Anaesth*. 2010;105(1):69–75.

526. Larizgoitia I, et al. *J Pub Hlth Res.* 2013;2(3):e29-e29.
527. Rall M, Dieckmann P. In: Bannister J, ed. *Euroanesthesia 2007.* Munich, Germany: European Society of Anaesthesiology; 2007: 179–186.
528. Firth-Cozens J, et al. *Clinical Risk.* 2004;10(5):184–190.
529. Evans SM, et al. *Qual Saf Health Care.* 2006;15(1):39–43.
530. Kelly N, et al. *Arch Dis Childhood.* 2016;101(9):788–791.
531. Rall M, et al. *[Article in German]*; 2014.
532. Dieckmann P, et al. *Work (Reading, Mass).* 2009;33(2):135–143.
533. Anderson JE, Kodate N. *Safety Sci.* 2015;80.
534. Benn J, et al. *Qual Saf Health Care.* 2009;18(1):11–21.
535. Pham JC, et al. *J Public Health Res.* 2013;2(3):e27.
536. Macrae C, Vincent C. *J Royal Soc Med.* 2014;107(11):439–443.
537. Cook DA, et al. *Simul Hlthcare.* 2012;7(5):308–320.
538. Riley W, et al. *Jt Comm J Qual Patient Saf.* 2011;37(8):357–364.
539. Salas E, et al. *Jt Comm J Qual Patient Saf.* 2009;35(8):398–405.
540. Salas E, et al. In: Kraiger K, ed. *Creating, Implementing, and Managing Effective Training and Development: State-of-the-Art Lessons for Practice.* San Francisco, CA: Jossey-Bass; 2013:234–262.
541. Gaba DM. *Perspectives on Safety.* 2006.
542. Pratt SD, Sachs BP. *Team Training: Classroom Training vs. High-Fidelity Simulation*; 2006. https://psnet.ahrq.gov/perspectives/perspective/21/team-training-classroom-training-vs-high-fidelity-simulation
543. Umoren RA, et al. *Creative Nursing.* 2017;23(3):184–191.
544. Tschannen D. *J Cont Ed Nrsg.* 2017;48(11):525–532.
545. Carney BT, et al. *Am J Med Qual.* 2011;26(6):480–484.
546. VA National Center for Patient Safety. Clinical Team Training. https://www.patientsafety.va.gov/professionals/training/team.asp
547. van de Ven J, et al. *Euro J Ob Gyn Rep Biol.* 2017;216:130–137.
548. Rudolph JW, et al. *Acad Emerg Med.* 2008;15(11):1010–1016.
549. Buist M, Middleton S. *BMJ.* 2013;347:f5800.
550. Landrigan CP, et al. *N Engl J Med.* 2010;363(22):2124–2134.
551. Gaba DM. *BMJ.* 2000;320(7237):785–788.
552. Jha AK, et al. *Qual Saf Health Care.* 2010;19(1):42–47.
553. European Society of Anaesthesiology (ESA). *Helsinki Declaration of Patient Safety*; 2010. https://www.esahq.org/patient-safety/patient-safety/helsinki-declaration/signed-helsinki-declaration/
554. Agency for Healthcare Research and Quality (AHRQ). *National Scorecard on Rates of Hospital-Acquired Conditions 2010 to 2015: Interim Data From National Efforts To Make Health Care Safer.* Rockville, MD; 2016.
555. National Patient Safety Foundation's Lucian Leape Institute. *Safety Is Personal: Partnering with Patients and Families for the Safest Care*; 2014.
556. Canadian Patient Safety Institute (CPSI). Engaging Patients in Patient Safety. A Canadian Guide. http://www.patientsafetyinstitute.ca/en/toolsResources/Patient-Engagement-in-Patient-Safety-Guide/Documents/Engaging%20patients%20as%20partners.pdf
557. Australian Commission on Safety and Quality in Health Care. *National Safety and Quali-ty Health Service Standard 2: Partnering with Consumers. Embedding partnerships in healthcare.* ; 2014. https://www.safetyandquality.gov.au/wp-content/uploads/2014/11/Partnering-with-Consumers-Embedding-partnerships-in-health-care.pdf
558. Vincent C, Amalberti R. *BMJ Quality. Safety.* 2015.
559. Rall M, Gaba DM. In: Miller RD, ed. *Miller's Anesthesia.* 6th ed. Philadelphia, PA: Elsevier Churchill Livingstone; 2005:3021–3072.
560. Roberts KH. *Organization Science.* 1990;1(2):160–176.
561. Agency for Healthcare Research and Quality (AHRQ). Culture of Safety. last updated June 2017 https://psnet.ahrq.gov/primers/primer/5/safety-culture
562. King H, et al. In: Henriksen K, Battles JB, Keyes M, et al., eds. *Advances in Patient Safety: New Directions and Alternative Approaches.* vol. 3. Rockville (MD): Agency for Healthcare Research and Quality (US); 2008. Performance and Tools.
563. Rall M, et al. *Bulletin Royal Coll Anaesth.* 2008;(51):2614–2616.

APPENDIX 6.1 **Online Links and Valuable Public Sources**

- Links to patient safety and crisis resource management resources
  - National Patient Safety Foundation: www.npsf.org/
  - Veterans Affairs National Center for Patient Safety:
    - Patient Safety: www.patientsafety.va.gov
    - VA Clinical Team Training program (CTT): www.patientsafety.va.gov/professionals/training/team.asp
  - The Joint Commission on Accreditation of Healthcare Organizations: www.jointcommission.org/
  - United Kingdom National Health Service National Patient Safety Agency: www.npsa.nhs.uk
  - Stanford School of Medicine, Center for Immersive and Simulation-based Learning https://cisl.stanford.edu/
  - Agency for Healthcare Research and Quality (AHRQ):
    - Patient Safety: www.ahrq.gov/patient-safety/index.html
    - TeamSTEPPS™: www.ahrq.gov/teamstepps/index.html
    - Patient Safety Organization Program: https://pso.ahrq.gov/
  - World Health Organization (WHO)
    - Patient Safety: www.who.int/patientsafety/en/
    - Multiprofessional Patient Safety Curriculum Guide (2011): www.who.int/patientsafety/education/mp_curriculum_guide/en/
    - Patient Safety Curriculum Guide for Medical Schools (2009): www.who.int/patientsafety/education/curriculum_guide_medical_schools/en/
    - The Conceptual Framework for the International Classification for Patient Safety (ICPS): www.who.int/patientsafety/implementation/taxonomy/ICPS-report/en/
    - Surgical Safety Checklist: www.who.int/patientsafety/topics/safe-surgery/checklist/en/
  - Patient Safety Education Program (PSEPTM): www.patientsafetyeducationproject.org/index.php
  - Australian Commission on Safety and Quality in Health Care: www.safetyandquality.gov.au/national-priorities/australian-safety-and-quality-framework-for-health-care/
- Links to different incident reporting systems and related topics
  - The American Society of Anesthesiologists Incident Reporting System (AIRS): www.aqihq.org/airs/airsIntro.aspx
  - United Kingdom National Health Service National Patient Safety Agency reporting system: www.nrls.npsa.nhs.uk/report-a-patient-safety-incident/
  - Pronovost's intensive care unit safety reporting system[85]
  - WHO Draft Guidelines for Adverse Event Reporting and Learning Systems—from Information to Action: www.who.int/iris/handle/10665/69797
  - U.S. Department of Veterans Affairs Patient Safety Reporting System (PSRS): https://psrs.arc.nasa.gov/
- Root Cause Analysis (RCA) Tools
  - United Kingdom National Healthcare Service: www.nrls.npsa.nhs.uk/resources/collections/root-cause-analysis/
  - VA National Center for Patient Safety: www.patientsafety.va.gov/professionals/onthejob/rca.asp
- Failure modes and effects analysis (FMEA) tools https://www.patientsafety.va.gov/professionals/onthejob/HFMEA.asp

7 *Patient Simulation*

STEPHANIE MARIA OBERFRANK, MARCUS RALL, PETER DIECKMANN, MICHAELA KOLBE, and DAVID M. GABA

KEY POINTS

- Led by the discipline of anesthesiology, simulators and the use of simulation have become integral parts of many health care domains for various uses including training of novices, advanced residents, and experienced professionals; research about and with simulation; system probing; and performance assessment. Patient simulation can be part of an organization's patient safety strategy and supports building a culture of safety (see Chapter 6).
- A wide variety of simulators are now available. The pace of technical development and applications is fast. Nevertheless, technology alone does not teach. The use of simulators needs to be consistent with the target population and the learning objectives. Different simulators may be best suited for different purposes; for some scenarios and teaching goals a standardized patient (actor) may be more effective.
- The most widely used simulators in health care are computer screen-based simulators (microsimulators), and part-task trainers mocking parts of a human body or mannequin-based simulators most often used for resuscitation training and complex team training. Complex simulation team training with mannequin-based simulators are often referred to as "high-fidelity" or "full scale" patient simulation training.
- The development of mobile and less expensive simulator models allowed for substantial expansion of simulation training to areas and locales where this training could not previously be afforded or conducted (so-called in situ simulation training).
- When used for education and training, the simulator device alone does not teach. It is merely a tool to accomplish learning objectives that are difficult to achieve during real patient care. The design of programs, curricula, scenarios, and debriefings, as well as the ability of simulation instructors to create appropriate learning opportunities are the crucial factors that determine whether the simulation tool is effective in achieving the relevant goals.
- The greatest obstacles to providing effective and relevant (high-fidelity) patient simulation training are (1) obtaining access to the learner population for the requisite time, and (2) providing appropriately trained and skilled simulation instructors to prepare, conduct, debrief, and evaluate the simulation sessions.
- The most important component of high-fidelity patient simulation training is the self-reflective (often video-assisted) debriefing session after the clinical scenario. The quality of debriefing strongly depends on the training, skills, and experience of the instructors. Thus, special training for developing patient simulation instructors is needed that goes beyond the instructor qualifications for ordinary clinical teaching. Most methods of debriefing emphasize open-ended questions and inquiry to trigger self-reflection and insightful analysis, leading to deep learning by the learner group.
- Simulation scenarios need clear learning objectives for both clinical and nonclinical skills (human factors, see Chapter 6). Scenarios need to take into account the target population, learning goals, relevance, and in-scenario guidance. Maximum realism is not always needed. For high-fidelity patient simulation team training, the *anesthesia crisis resource management* course model (ACRM, often referred to as CRM, developed by one of the authors [David Gaba], see Chapter 6) is a popular approach worldwide for human factor–based simulation training in anesthesiology and health care. The 15 CRM key points help individuals and teams to be aware of human factor–related pitfalls, apply different safety strategies, and enhance human performance and patient safety.
- In terms of research, simulation has proven valuable to study relevant simulation aspects such as debriefing methods, scenario design and conduct, and program development. It also was found to be valuable to study human performance during anesthesia, including human factors and failure modes in care.
- In regard to system probing, simulation can be used successfully for the testing of an organization's structures and processes, such as the early detection of system failure modes and the preparedness for major events, the development of new treatment concepts (e.g., checklist design and use, telemedicine), and the support of bioengineering system development (e.g., device beta-testing, educating the manufacturers' workforce).
- With a view to assessment and evaluation of performance, a variety of assessment tools and behavioral markers have evolved that offer a new window on performance. Nevertheless, when simulation is used to assess and evaluate human performance, the unique constraints of simulation (which is never like the real thing) need to be taken into consideration.

What This Chapter Is About: An Overview

"Simulation training in all its forms will be a vital part of building a safer health care system" [p. 55].[1]

SIR LIAM DONALDSON, CMO ANNUAL REPORT (2008)

In concert with other modalities, simulation can improve patient safety by informing personnel about best practices, guiding established clinical practice, and strengthening human performance. Unfortunately, simulation in health care is still not used as widely and systematically as needed, compared to its use in other high-risk/high-reliability industries. From the authors' point of view, anesthesia professionals, anesthesia departments, and health care organizations need to strive to embrace the use of simulation for the many purposes mentioned in this chapter. Simulation, in combination with human factors training (CRM, see Chapter 6), has the potential to substantially improve the quality and safety of health care.

Anesthesiology has pioneered the field of simulation in health care. The rather new, mannequin-based patient simulators have been in regular use in anesthesiology since the early 1990s. Over the last two decades, there have been many technologic advances in simulation and a wide variety of applications of simulation in anesthesiology have been developed in the domains of education and training, research, system and equipment probing, and assessment. Considerable collective experience has already been achieved with simulation devices, sites, pedagogy, and assessment rubrics. What was once an arcane and small niche activity has expanded enormously. Simulation can be thought of like playing a musical instrument: almost everybody can somehow coax a tone out of it, but to play it well and use it optimally can only come about after considerable practice.

This chapter aims to provide the reader—whether a simulation participant or a novice or experienced instructor—with a solid and nuanced understanding of many aspects of patient simulation in anesthesiology and other parts of health care.

Modern simulation with advanced teaching concepts and the integration of human factors training (CRM) is much more than traditional basic life support and advanced cardiovascular life support ("megacode") training. Modern simulation team training is academically demanding, personally stimulating, and involves many disciplines and lines of thinking. As a simulation instructor, you are operating at the core of our profession!

READERS WILL LEARN

- … about the varying uses of simulation in anesthesiology and health care, mainly focusing on the topics of training and education, research, system equipment probing, and assessment and evaluation.
- … to distinguish and classify different types of patient simulators (e.g., part-task trainers, simulators for low- and high-fidelity simulation, patient actors/standardized patients, hybrid simulation) and to understand their strengths and weaknesses.
- … about the possibilities and limitations of different simulation-based training approaches regarding (1) simulation site (e.g., dedicated simulation center, "in situ" simulation, mobile simulation); (2) simulation time (e.g., scheduled events vs. events on-call); (3) simulation participants (e.g., single discipline, multidiscipline, interprofessional).
- … about educational and psychological factors that enable or inhibit learning in patient simulation, such as scenario design and conduct, the elements or phases of a simulation training, and debriefing techniques.
- … about different multifaceted tasks of a simulation instructor and the need to acquire special skills to teach more complex and nuanced single-discipline or interprofessional activities.
- … about the ecological validity of simulation and what is known about its benefits, costs, and cost-effectiveness.
- … about the use of simulation for assessment of clinician performance and some of the issues and limitations thereof.

To cover those aspects, the authors have tried to balance retaining classic references, where the intellectual content has only changed slightly over the years, with newer ones that reflect either changes in thinking or evidence, or newer reviews and syntheses of knowledge and experience. Since simulation has become a key tool in addressing issues of patient safety and human factors in anesthesiology there is some degree of complementarity between this chapter and Chapter 6.

In this chapter, the authors use "anesthesia professional" to refer to any anesthesia clinician taking care of a patient, whether a physician, certified registered nurse anesthetist (CRNA), or anesthesia assistant (or to similar positions in other countries).

WHAT THIS CHAPTER IS NOT ABOUT

This chapter mainly addresses simulation in anesthesiology and presents the overall picture as seen by anesthesia professionals, intensivists, or others. Simulation devices and activities outside of the scope of perioperative management, that are strictly about psychomotor aspects of invasive procedures or surgery, and part-task screen-based simulators (e.g., Gasman) are at most only touched on briefly.

The chapter describes simulation in anesthesiology generically and does not address separately simulation for specific subspecialties. There is a sizable body of international experience with simulation in pediatric settings now that may be of further interest to some readers.[2-9]

Organizational aspects of simulation training and the topic of organizational implementation and sustainability of simulation programs are covered in Chapter 6, where simulation programs are covered from an organization's view among other organizational improvements to enhance patient and system safety. For more information on this topic, the reader is referred to the back part of Chapter 6 (Box 6.13 in Chapter 6 gives an overview).

Simulation in Anesthesia: Why Is It Important?

See one—do one—teach one? Read one—do one—teach one? Many decades ago anesthesiology trainees might have been "given a long leash" (inadequately supervised) and asked to gain experience by "sink or swim," often with a clinical population of indigent patients. Using actual patients in this way as if they are expendable "simulators" is unethical, and the presumed learning experiences were extremely uneven. In the last few decades unacceptable practices have been eliminated, but it increasingly begs the question of how can clinicians at all levels of experience feel the difficulties of patient care, including managing very difficult situations, without putting patients at undue risk? How does someone go from a total novice to a fully competent independent anesthesia professional? And of increasing importance, how can clinicians—during both initial and recurrent training—learn and hone skills of dynamic decision making, situation awareness, leadership, communication, and teamwork?

Anesthesiology is a "hands-on" discipline. It is not likely for medical students and residents to learn simply by "looking," "time passing," or by "osmosis." The application of (rare) technical skills, the correct use of medical knowledge and algorithms, as well as the reliable utilization of anesthesia nontechnical skills (see Chapter 6)—such as teamwork, communication, and leadership behavior—need to be learned and then trained repeatedly. At the same time, experience is no substitute for excellence (see Chapter 6). This is especially true for nonroutine events, such as emergencies or rare complications. Not only trainees but also experienced clinicians require continuous education and training of their clinical and nontechnical skills in order to stay current and avoid bad habits or the normalization of deviance (see Chapter 6).

Health care, with anesthesiology as the pioneering discipline, borrowed and adapted alternative educational approaches to teach knowledge and gain procedural experience from years of successful service in other industries that faced similar problems. These approaches focused on "simulation." Simulation is a technique well known in the military, aviation, space flight, and nuclear power industries. Simulation refers to the artificial replication of sufficient elements of a real-world domain to achieve a stated goal. The goals include for example education and training of technical and nontechnical skills, system probing, testing of equipment and supplies, and assessment as well as evaluation of students and personnel. These different topics are covered in this chapter, even though there is a focus on simulation as a training and education tool.

In 2000, the National Academy of Medicine (then the Institute of Medicine) released a report, *"To Err Is Human: Building a Safer Health System,"* that suggested the use of simulation training in health care in order to reduce preventable errors.[10] The American College of Critical Care Medicine recommended the use of simulation to improve training in critical care.[11] With anesthesiologists being the pioneers for simulation-based training in health care, simulation in anesthesia already has a long tradition. At the same time, its comprehensive and profound implementation has come a long and rocky way over the last decades and, despite many benefits, still needs further implementation and continuous evaluation. Major recognition of simulation in anesthesia by the clinical world is highlighted by the fact that it is now a highly utilized training course for the practice improvement component of Maintenance of Certification in Anesthesiology (MOCA) in the United States.[12] In Australia and New Zealand, it is an integral part of anesthetic training.[13,14] In their reviews, Lorello and colleagues, [15] LeBlanc and colleagues,[16] and Higham and Baxendale[17] give an overview of simulation-based training in anesthesia. In many parts of the world, including industrial countries, the use of simulation is way behind the United States or Australia.

A fundamental part of the future vision for simulation is that clinical personnel, teams, and systems will undergo periodic and systematic simulation activities across their entire career using various modalities of simulation and for diverse purposes of education, training, performance assessment, refinement in practice, and system probing. This vision is inspired in part by the systems in place in various high-reliability industries, especially commercial aviation and nuclear power (see Chapter 6). Needless to say, using simulation as part of the process of revolutionizing health care is more complex than merely attempting to stick simulation training on top of the current system. Moreover, beyond training, simulation may provide indirect ways to improve safety, including facilitating recruitment and retention of skilled personnel, acting as a lever for culture change, and improving quality and risk management activities.

Application of Simulation in Anesthesia and Health Care

Simulation techniques can be applied across nearly all health care domains.[18] A few books are devoted solely to the topic of simulation and its use in and outside of anesthesiology.[19-24]

In the upcoming section, an overview of the main objectives of simulation in health care and anesthesiology are presented in the following sequence: (1) education and training of technical and nontechnical skills, (2) system probing, (3) testing of equipment and supplies, (4) assessment/evaluation, (5) research, and (6) further purposes.

USE OF PATIENT SIMULATION FOR TRAINING AND EDUCATION

With respect to the first objective—education and training—anesthesiology remains a driving force in the use of simulation in health care,[25] although simulation has spread to nearly every discipline and domain. As used in this chapter, *education* emphasizes conceptual knowledge, basic skills, and an introduction to nontechnical skills and work practices. *Training* emphasizes preparing individuals to perform actual tasks and work of the job.

Disciplines successfully applying simulation for training besides anesthesia[15,26] are, for example, emergency medicine and emergency field responders,[27-29] trauma care,[30,31] neonatology[32-34] and pediatric anaesthesia,[2,3,5,35] labor and delivery,[36-38] surgery,[39,40] radiation oncology,[41] intensive care,[42,43] and infectious disease.[44,45] Simulation serves almost all resuscitation trainings, which have advanced over the years.[46] Fig. 7.1 gives several impressions of simulation training.

Nearly every anesthesia residency program in the United States offers some cogent simulation training experiences,

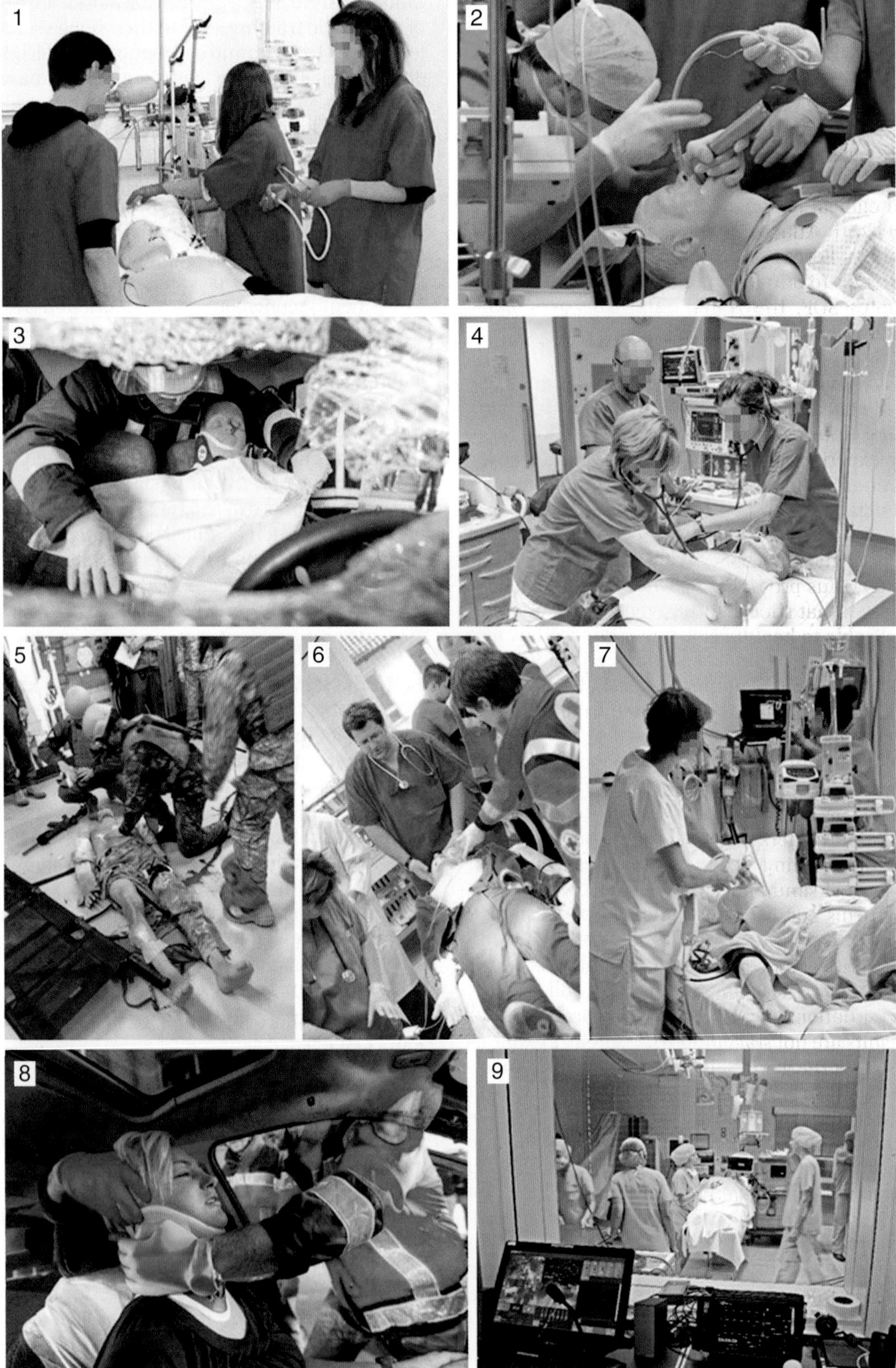

Fig. 7.1 Different impressions of simulation training sessions in different health care environments. Photos from left to right: (1) In situ simulation training on a ward. (2) In situ simulation team training in the anesthesia environment. (3) Simulation exercise during the annual simulation congress INSiM, Frankfurt Main, Germany. The photo shows a simulated patient that is rescued out of a crashed car. (4) Full-scale in situ simulation team training in the emergency department. (5) Military simulation training with Tactical Combat Casualty Training and Care under Fire conditions, *InPASS, Photo with permission by M. Rall.* (6) Simulation Training at the Simulation Center TüPASS in Tübingen, Germany. Shown is a handover moment where a traumatized patient is handed over from the ambulance team to the trauma team. *Photo with permission by director M. Rall 2010.* (7) Simulation training on the intermediate care unit. (8) Simulation exercise with a standardized patient that is rescued out of a crashed car. *Photo provided by M. Rall.* (9) In situ simulation training in an operating room (OR) showing the beginning of a full team obstetric scenario for emergency cesarean. The photo is taken through an OR window from the temporarily established simulation control room outside the OR. (*Photo provided by M. Rall.*)

although the scope, frequency, and target content vary. Other disciplines and other countries may not have adequate simulation training coverage during residency, as evidenced by a study by Hayes and colleagues.[47]

The military and the U.S. Department of Homeland Security also have been heavy users of simulation in health care; simulation has been applied to the initial training of new field medics and to the recurrent training of experienced clinicians and clinical teams.[48] In 2013, a first instructor course for the North Atlantic Treaty Organization (NATO) Special Operations Forces (SOF) was held at NATO headquarters in Brussels to bring together medical experts from the United States SOF, the NATO SOF, and some civilian instructor experts (including authors Rall and later Oberfrank).

Simulation is relevant from the earliest level of vocational or professional education (students) and during apprenticeship training (interns and residents), and it is increasingly used for experienced personnel undergoing periodic refresher training. Simulation can be applied regularly to practicing clinicians (as individuals, teams, or organizations; the latter for example for disaster drills, or for preparing to care for patients with Ebola virus disease[49]) regardless of their seniority, thus providing an integrated accumulation of experiences that should have long-term synergism. Thus, it is applicable to health care providers with a range of experience, including experts,[50] novices, advanced residents,[25] medical, nursing, other health care students,[51-57] and even children.[58-61] Simulation *rehearsals* are now being explored as adjuncts to actual clinical practice; for example, surgeons or an entire operative team can rehearse an unusually complex operation in advance by using a simulation of the specific patient.[62,63]

Many simulation centers offer continuing medical education (CME) and training for experienced practitioners, and many aspects of simulation training for residents can be expanded for this purpose. Several studies have shown that experienced anesthesiologists have deficiencies in the management of critical patient situations and make severe errors comparable to those of anesthesia residents.[64-71] Because crisis situations are rare during routine clinical work, these results are not startling. In addition, experience in terms of years on the job and hierarchy probably do not correspond to expertise and excellence. Crisis management training with patient simulation should be started early in education and training and applied on a recurring basis during practice.

Concerning education of health care professionals about patient safety, patient simulation can be a tool that contributes to changing the culture in an organization bottom-up to create a culture of safety. First, it allows hands-on training of junior and senior clinicians in practices that enact the desired culture of safety based on the principle of high reliability organizations (see Chapter 6).[72] Simulation can be a rallying point about culture change and patient safety that can bring together experienced clinicians from various disciplines and domains (who may be captured because the simulations are clinically challenging and show the need of change in direct relation to patient treatment), along with health care administrators, executives, managers,[73,74] risk managers,[75] and experts on human factors, organizational behavior, or institutional change. For these groups, simulation can convey the complexities of clinical work, and it can be used to exercise and probe the organizational practices of clinical institutions at multiple levels (see section on system probing). Various curricula and recommendations for curricula development for simulation training exist.[76-81]

USE OF PATIENT SIMULATION FOR SYSTEM PROBING AND PROTOCOL TESTING

In regard to the second objective, simulations that are conducted in actual patient treatment locations (referred to as "in situ" simulation, ISS) are powerful tools for testing (system probing) and evaluation of organizational practices (protocol testing).[75]

In a study comparing ISS to center-based simulations, ISS was related to more insights about processes in the organization and challenges with equipment.[82] Another study used simulation as a supplement to a Failure Modes and Effects Analysis (FMEA, see Chapter 6). In order to enhance system safety, FMEA is a risk management tool that proactively tries to enhance organizational learning by experts describing and identifying possible errors and their effects. Whereas adding simulation to that process did not result in more failure modes described, the process resulted in a richer description of how they would actually unfold in practice.[83]

Another way to probe the system is to identify active and latent failures during ISS of the treatment of patients. In Reason's famous error trajectory model to describe incident causation (known as the Swiss cheese model, see Chapter 6), incidents are seen as a combination of active (simplified: human) and latent (simplified: system) failures that interact to cause bad outcomes. Based on this model, a study[84] of 46 sessions of ISS training for handling emergencies was conducted with over 800 participants, with the goal to recognize and remedy active and latent failures in order to suggest where to invest resources. Of the total of 965 breaches, nearly 50% were classified as latent conditions, and the rest was classified as active failures. In another study, simulation was used to discover latent safety threats with the help of unannounced in situ simulation of critical patients in a pediatric emergency department.[85] Similarly, the "hemorrhage project" at Stanford assessed and trained the treatment protocol of life-threatening hemorrhage during several system-probing events using unannounced, simulation-based mock events, and successfully identified areas of improvement after probing.[75]

In 2016 simulation was used to demonstrate gaps in an organization's response system that could expose staff to Ebola once the emergency disaster response had been activated.[86] The simulation center had 12 hours to prepare simulations to evaluate hospital preparedness should a patient screen positive for Ebola exposure. Further simulation cycles were used during the next weeks to identify additional gaps and to evaluate possible solutions.

Furthermore, iterative simulation-based testing and redesign was shown to be of assistance when developing cognitive aids or protocols for all kind of crises, and to eliminate design failure. For instance, McIntosh and colleagues[87] used this approach to develop and test a new cognitive aid for the management of severe local anesthetic toxicity. Utilization of formative usability testing and simulation-based user-centered design resulted in a visually very different cognitive aid, reinforcing the importance of designing aids in the context in which they are to be used.

Simulation has a role in designing new hospitals and departments—whether in terms of the physical layouts or in terms of work processes. Simulation can help in evaluating design ideas. Simulation can be used to facilitate moving into a new location, for example moving with staff and patients into a new intensive care unit (ICU) or a new hospital.[88]

Simulation is increasingly appreciated as a tool for risk management. Driver, Lighthall, and Gaba[75] argue that from a risk management standpoint, simulation has a number of potential ways in which it might prevent claims or mitigate losses. They called simulation *"a data source about clinical performance"* [p. 356]. De Maria[25] and associates demonstrated that a simulation-based approach can identify system-wide practitioner gaps in anesthesiologists and create meaningful improvement plans.

USE OF PATIENT SIMULATION FOR TESTING EQUIPMENT AND SUPPLIES

With respect to the third objective—testing of equipment and supplies—patient simulation is being used in collaboration with biomedical industries. For example, some simulation centers offer training to executives, engineers, and sales representatives of equipment manufacturers. The simulator allows them to gain some understanding of the clinician's task demands during patient care situations (including those of unusual stress) in which their company's devices are useful.

Simulation has been used for research on human factor issues in the development of new monitoring and therapeutic devices. The simulator provides a unique test bed and demonstration modality for pre-procurement evaluation of the usability of medical devices from different manufacturers. In two of our affiliated hospitals (VA Palo Alto [DG] and Tübingen, Germany [MR]), simulation enabled us to conduct evaluations of prototype monitoring systems that were not yet approved for clinical use and could not be evaluated in a pre-procurement clinical trial.

Other industrial uses include training personnel in the use of novel pharmaceuticals. Simulators have been featured in a multifaceted approach to launch the opioid remifentanil in the United States and have been used to teach clinicians in the safe use of drugs, such as for example desflurane. Besides offering important educational benefits, industrial activities are an important source of income for simulation centers to help defray the costs of training students and residents.

USE OF PATIENT SIMULATION FOR PERFORMANCE ASSESSMENT

With respect to the fourth objective, simulations have taken a central role in the evaluation and assessment of the performance and competence of health care students, residents, practicing physicians, and teams—for low-stakes or formative testing (education and training), to a lesser degree to-date for summative testing (certification, recertification, etc.), and for research on clinician decision-making or on care processes. Assessment of performance for both clinical and nonclinical skills can be made in a variety of health care settings.[64,69,89-98]

Anesthesiology has taken a leading role in the development of simulation-based assessment.[99] In a review study in 2012, Boulet and Murray[99] summarized simulation-based assessment for education specifically in anesthesia. In a more recent systematic review in 2016, Ryall and colleagues[100] summarize the use of simulation as an assessment tool of technical skills across health professional education. They concluded that simulation is an effective assessment tool, but pointed out that the effectiveness as a stand-alone assessment tool requires further research.

Assessment with simulation held and still holds several challenges for research and education. Those include: (1) to determine aspects of performance to be measured, (2) to create reliable and valid scores and measurement tools, and (3) to find measures for both clinical and nonclinical performance. Furthermore, simulation itself poses several unique challenges and pitfalls that need to be taken into account, as discussed later in this chapter. Several assessment measures and scoring systems exist.[99-102]

Organizationally, in the United States, the Accreditation Council for Graduate Medical Education made the use of simulation a required component for anesthesiology residency programs. Recognizing its benefits not only for education and teaching of novices and residents, but also for the continuous education of certified practicing anesthesiologists, more recently simulation-based training in managing challenging situations leading to practice improvement was adopted as a favored component of the American Board of Anesthesiology's (ABA's) MOCA program. Whereas simulation as a tool for the formative assessment of performance during training of students and residents is already widely used in anesthesiology, it has still penetrated only modestly for the formative assessment (and less so for summative assessment) of practicing anesthesiologists,[103] raising new questions as described in a study by Weinger and colleagues.[64]

Because performance assessment is closely related to human performance, many results of simulation studies with this focus were already discussed in Chapter 6, and the reader is referred there as well.

USE OF PATIENT SIMULATION FOR RESEARCH

In regard to the fifth objective—research—simulation-based research falls into two categories: (a) research *about* simulation—testing or improving the techniques, technologies, and didactics of simulation; and (b) research *that uses* simulation as a tool to study other things, such as human performance and clinical cognition (see Chapter 6), or clinical care processes.[104] Box 7.1 provides a sampling of these types of questions.

Regarding research about simulation, some examples would include the design of debriefing approaches such as Debriefing with Good Judgement,[105-107] Debriefing-Diamant,[108] PEARLS,[109] TeamGAINS,[110] and others[111-114]; methods for designing simulation scenarios such as PARTS[115]; the efficacy of using videos in debriefings[116-120]; the creation and maintenance of an inviting learning atmosphere[121]; the effective design of specific training interventions such as for resuscitation,[46,122,123] airway

BOX 7.1 Exemplary Research Issues That Can Be Addressed by Using Simulation

Cognitive Science of Dynamic Decision Making (see Chapter 6)

- What is the interaction of precompiled procedural knowledge (Type I thinking) versus deep medical knowledge and abstract reasoning (Type II thinking)?
- How does supervisory control of observation relate to vigilance, data overload, and visual scanning patterns?
- What is the information content and utility of watching the surgical field?
- How are optimal action planning and scheduling implemented?
- How does reevaluation fail and result in fixation errors?

Human-Machine Interactions

- What is the distraction penalty for false alarms?
- Do integrated monitors and displays have an advantage over multiple stand-alone devices and displays?
- How easy to use are the controls and displays of existing anesthesia equipment in standard case situations and in crisis situations?

Teaching Anesthesia in the Operating Room (see Chapter 6)

- How much teaching can be accomplished in the operating room without sacrificing the anesthesia crew's vigilance?
- How well can faculty members detect and categorize the performance of anesthesia trainees?
- What teaching styles are best integrated with case management in the operating room?

Issues of Non-Technical Skills/Teamwork on Anesthesiologist Performance

- How does an anesthesia crew interact during case and crisis management?
- How is workload distributed among individuals?
- How do crew members communicate with each other, and how do they communicate with other members of the operating room team?

Effects of Performance-Shaping Factors on Anesthesiologist Performance

- How do sleep deprivation, fatigue, aging, or the carryover effects of over-the-counter medications, coffee, or alcohol affect the performance of anesthesiologists?
- Can smart alarm systems or artificial intelligence provide correct and clinically meaningful decision support in the operating room or intensive care unit?

Development of New Devices and Applications: Research Regarding Techniques of Simulation

- How well can simulations re-create perioperative clinical settings? Can they provoke the same actions as used in real clinical care (ecologic validity of simulators)?
- How much does debriefing add to learning from simulation? Are specific techniques of debriefing, or combinations thereof, of greater applicability or utility, overall or for particular situations?
- How do various aspects of simulation scenarios influence aspects of perceived reality, and how do they influence transfer of training into the real world?
- Does simulation training lead to better clinical practice and improved clinical outcomes?

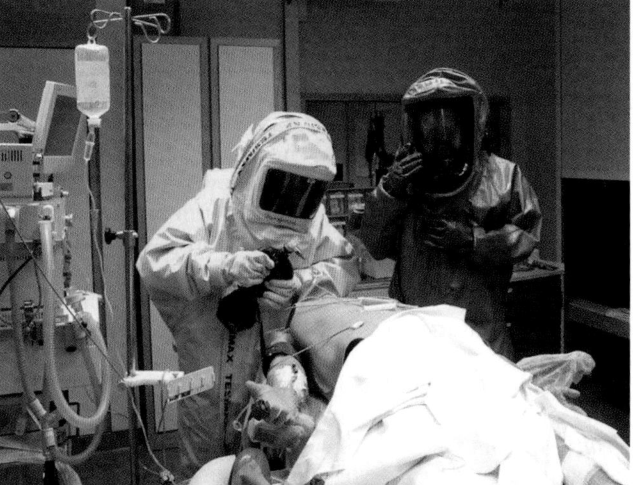

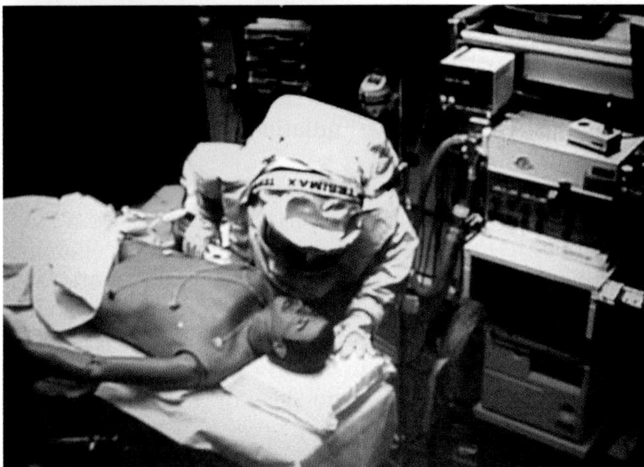

Fig. 7.2 Realistic patient simulation as a test bed for studying the performance of medical rescue teams in full chemical protection gear. Teams wore normal uniforms or full protection suits while performing basic resuscitation actions (e.g., placement of intravenous lines, drawing up drugs, intubation). With full protective gear, communication within the team and with the patient (while still conscious) is difficult. *(Photograph taken by M. Rall at the Center for Patient Safety and Simulation, Tübingen, Germany.)*

management,[124,125] and avoidance of catheter-related infections[126]; and testing of specific training interventions such as for facilitating speaking up,[50,127-129] briefings, [130] and feedback.[131]

Patient simulation is now used sometimes to address the medical management of chemical, biologic, or nuclear threats from accidents, weapons of mass destruction, or terrorism. One group in Germany, used simulation to test the constraints of treating patients in full chemical protection gear to optimize the strategies of the German Ministry of Internal Affairs for dealing with terror attacks or chemical plant disasters (Fig. 7.2). Several investigators have performed multidisciplinary studies with combined simulation modalities (script-based simulators, model-based mannequin simulators, and simulated acted patients) to teach the management of victims of an attack with weapons of mass destruction and terrorism.[132,133] The demand for such training is substantial in nations engaged in active military conflicts or with an ongoing need to prepare for war or terrorist attacks.

Regarding (b) simulation as a research tool, it offers some unique features, and it can be thought of as a complementary window on the clinical world relative to other modalities. It can be applied, for example, when complex phenomena such as medical team processes are studied. Examples are investigations of how teams adapt from routine to non-routine situations and how this adaptation is related to performance,[134-140] communication processes such as information processing,[141] talking to the room[142] and speaking up,[50,129,143-146] problem-solving and decision-making,[142,147-149] and coordination requirements during resuscitation.[139,140,150-154] Important milestones for simulation-based research of both types was the creation by the Society for Simulation in Healthcare (SSH) in 2007 of its flagship peer-reviewed journal, *Simulation in Healthcare* followed in later years by other peer-reviewed journals (e.g., *Advances in Simulation, BMJ Simulation & Technology Enhanced Learning, Clinical Simulation in Nursing*). In addition, for research that is linked tightly to a specific clinical domain, the traditional medical specialty journals have become more welcoming to articles about simulation or that use simulation as an experimental technique.

Cooperation between simulation directors or instructors and psychologists, human factors engineers, or educators has proved useful in research and training. Such collaborations have helped delineate the theoretical foundations of simulation-based experiential learning, improve the understanding of debriefing, and research on work psychology and human performance in health care.[155-161] Many institutions have integrated psychologists or educators, or both, into their simulation center staff.

OTHER USES OF PATIENT SIMULATION

Traditionally, simulation-based training is focused on health care professionals as the recipients. In recent years, simulation was opened up for new types of recipients. These studies are not conducted within anesthesia, but demonstrate innovative ways of thinking about simulation that might be adaptable in some form to anesthesia-oriented simulations. A study showed that the use of "standardized clinicians" to train patients to be more competent in their discharge conversations was feasible.[162] Patients interacted with role players in the role of the discharging clinician, practicing what to say and ask, as well as how to manage the medication they were supposed to take. The group around Kneebone involves patients in the design of simulations, opening simulation activities to them.[163] They use simulation in a demonstration mode that intends, for example, to give citizens an improved insight into what it is like to be in the hospital[164,165] or what care in the clinical context should feel like.[166] The aim is to diversify access to simulation beyond health care professionals.

Other unique applications of simulation have surfaced. Some centers use simulators for conducting outreach programs with high school or college students interested in health care. Patient simulators have been used to help produce educational videos on various patient safety issues. Simulation has sometimes been used to familiarize legislators or regulators with the realities and complexities of dynamic patient care.

Simulation has been used as adjuncts in medicolegal proceedings.[167] While current patient simulators cannot predict the exact physiologic behavior of a specific patient, simulations can be used to illustrate typical perioperative situations and the role of different monitors and therapeutic actions and to provide context for the patient management questions of the litigation.

The use of simulation training for strategic or operational coordination and decision making in health care logistics has been described.[168]

History, Development, and Types of Simulators and Simulation

The following section gives a short, non-exhaustive overview about the history and the development of the main simulators in health care and anesthesia. For a more in-depth examination of the topic, the reader is referred to further literature. Particularly the mannequin-based simulators that are in wide use have been well covered in several review articles[169-171] and a whole book chapter by Rosen written in 2013 is dedicated to the topic in detail.[172] Another comprehensive textbook on the history of simulation in health care tracing it back 1500 years was published by Owen.[173]

Simulation probably is as old as mankind. Simulation has probably been a part of human activity since prehistoric times. Rehearsal for hunting activities and warfare was most likely an occasion for simulating the behavior of prey or enemy warriors. In medieval times soldiers learned the art of swordsmanship on dummy soldiers. Hundreds of years ago, models were used to help teach anatomy and physiology, and simulators were used to train surgical procedures and to help midwives and obstetricians handle complications of childbirth. Italy was the major source of simulators early in the 18th century, but in the 19th century, dominance in clinical simulation moved to France, Britain, and then Germany.[174] In modern times, preparation for warfare has been an equally powerful spur to the development of simulation technologies, especially for aviation, navy and armored vehicles. These technologies have been adopted by their civilian counterparts, but they have attained their most extensive use in commercial aviation. The aircraft simulator achieved its modern form in the late 1960s, but it has been continuously refined.

Mannequin-based simulators (MBSs). In 1969, the first electromechanical mannequin-based simulator in modern health care—Sim One—was produced by an aerospace company working with an educator and an anesthesiologist at the University of Southern California.[175] It consisted of a mannequin comprising an intubatable airway and upper torso and arms, and in many respects was years ahead of its time. It was originally used as an aid for students or residents learning to intubate, as well as to induce anesthesia but the project died out in the early 1970s. In the following years, several other mannequin-based patient simulators were developed and introduced in the middle to late 1980s. Noteworthy among others is Harvey, a cardiology mannequin simulator released in 1976, which is able to simulate the arterial pulse, blood pressure, jugular venous wave, precordial movements, and heart sounds in normal and diseased states.[176] In 1986, a team at Stanford, headed at first by Gaba and DeAnda,[177] developed a full-scale simulator called the Comprehensive Anesthesia Simulation Environment (CASE); they used it initially to study the decision-making processes of anesthesia professionals during critical events,[68,178,179] but they were also interested in its use for training. Over a few years, with their recognition of the parallels with Crew/Crisis/Cockpit Resource Management (CRM) in aviation this team developed their flagship simulation training course Anesthesia Crisis Resource Management (ACRM, see Chapter 6).[180,181] Newer commercially-available mannequin-based patient simulators have been in use in anesthesiology since about 1995, and considerable collective experience with the devices already has been achieved. Currently, full-size mannequin-based simulation devices are used in most simulation centers (available now, for example, from the manufacturers Laerdal, Gaumard, CAE Healthcare, and others). Such devices allow the simulation of rapidly changing physiology and can support a variety of hands-on interventions (e.g., airway management, vascular cannulation, drug administration, electric countershock, or pacing). Some devices allow the system automatically to recognize injection of specific medications or therapeutic maneuvers, such as cardiac massage, and then—with or without instructor input—to respond in an appropriate manner.[182] Even though highly developed, mannequins still miss important features. Box 7.2 shows desirable features of future MBS systems.

BOX 7.2 Desirable Features of Future Mannequin-Based Simulator Systems

- Ability to interface to or to mimic advanced brain monitoring such as: *AEP,* Auditory evoked potential; *BIS,* bispectral index; *EEG,* electroencephalographic; *PSI,* patient state index.
- Advanced skin signs such as: change in skin color to cyanotic or pale, improved diaphoresis, change in skin temperature (e.g., as a result of shock or fever), rash, hives, or generalized edema
- Regurgitation, vomiting, airway bleeding or secretions
- Physical coughing (currently only sounds are simulated)
- Realistic convulsions
- Purposeful movements of extremities
- Improved or possible support for spinal, epidural, or other regional anesthesia procedures
- Improved EEG signals (e.g., for BIS, AEP, PSI)
- Improved intracranial pressure
- Support for physical central venous and arterial cannulation
- Improved fetal and maternal cardiotocogram

Please note: *This list contains features that are not currently incorporated. Some features may be under development and could be available after publication of this book. In addition, some features are currently available as third-party or homemade add-ons.*

PATIENT SIMULATION ACTION BOX

From a patient safety and teaching point of view, it is a mistake to focus too much on complicated and nice-to-have features that the latest device might offer. Those features and add-ons will not necessarily improve simulations or benefit participants. High-fidelity simulation may be useful, but that will not necessarily require a simulation device with complex features. It is critical pedagogically, and economically, to match the simulation device to the target population and objectives of the simulation activity.

(Computer) Screen-based simulators (microsimulators). Beginning in the mid-1980s, several screen-based, also called screen-only simulators (microsimulators), were developed by anesthesiologists. These included (1) screen-based part-task trainers that simulated isolated aspects of anesthesia, such as the uptake and distribution of anesthetic gases in the body given different physiologic and physical chemistry situations (e.g., the well-known Gasman program[183]); and (2) screen-based overall-task trainers that represented nearly all aspects of the patient and clinical environment. Originally, the patient was represented by drawings or animations, but increasingly in these systems the representation of the patient is by photographs or videos. Vital signs appearing on virtual monitors may mimic real clinical devices. Actions are selected typically using a graphic user interface, pointing and clicking on menus and buttons, and using sliders and numeric entry boxes to allow control of most kinds of interventions that clinicians use on a regular basis.

Part-task trainers and virtual procedural simulators. In the 21st century, advancements in engineering and computer science have stimulated a new era of simulator technology, including:

- Part-task trainers in the form of anatomic mock-up devices that are made from synthetic material to represent human body parts, such as models that allow training of central line placement, epidural catheter insertion, cricothyroidotomy, or chest drainage. Over several decades, tissue-based simulation—representing some sort of part-task trainer—has become more common, with trainees no longer learning procedural skills using animal models because of cost and issues of animal rights.
- Virtual simulators for surgical and procedural skills (i.e., hardware and software that provide haptic feedback for performing realistic laparoscopic cholecystectomy, bronchoscopy, colonoscopy, echocardiography, and endovascular procedures).[182] In these systems, the synthetic (virtual) environment exists solely in the computer. The real procedure is performed by using a video display that can be recreated by the simulator. The person simulating the procedure interacts with the video display through the eyes (without or with head-mounted glasses) and the ears, and usually the hands, if the simulator features special instruments, instrumented gloves, or sensors. For anesthesia, for example, there exist VR simulators to train the conduct of fiberoptic intubation[184,185] and regional anesthesia.[186,187] Two systematic reviews are available for more in-depth information on the general use of simulation teaching regional anesthesia.[188,189]

Virtual reality and augmented reality (usually via head-mounted displays). Both immersive *virtual reality* (VR), which fully integrates the human user into the computer's world, and *augmented reality* (AR), which adds computer-generated imagery onto or next to the real-world view, typically use head-mounted displays to either replace ordinary vision or to augment it. Both approaches have been described in the literature, often in prototype or research-only settings. This chapter will discuss only VR and not AR. The authors (DG in particular) have been evaluating commercially available systems for head-mounted display VR. For health care they seem to fall into two categories: (1) *visualization* of objects or spaces—typically for anatomical structures, or for architectural environments, and (2) *physically interactive clinical environments*—meaning the clinicians themselves can move with the space and interact directly with each other and the virtually presented patient, essentially the VR equivalent of physical mannequin-based simulation. Visualization applications are much more common and are direct applications of consumer VR hardware and software (e.g., visualizing the human heart in all its detail inside and out instead of, say, the Taj Mahal). Fully interactive VR makes use of commercial head-mounted displays and other gear but is more complex to create the clinical space, patient, and equipment while providing for multiple physical participants to interact with seamless head and body movements.

Both types of VR are still in quite early stages of practical implementation in health care and how these approaches can best be used in health care remains to be seen, but the tide is now turning away from arcane research or "vaporware" to an era of rapidly improving practical devices and applications. Although Gaba has previously written that VR would soon (by 2020-2025) completely replace all physical simulation, this now seems unlikely in that time frame; in fact, it is likely that VR will join the spectrum of simulation modalities each of which has a set of unique advantages and disadvantages relative to the others.

Virtual Environment/Virtual World. A related type of virtual simulation is the *virtual environment* or *virtual world*. According to Wikipedia, a virtual world is a computer-based simulated environment intended for its users to inhabit and interact through avatars (users' graphic representation of themselves). Such systems typically allow multiple participants to control their own avatars (including speech) simultaneously over a network and to interact verbally and by virtual physical actions within a commonly perceived virtual environment. This technology currently portrays the virtual world as perspective three-dimensional images (or possibly true 3D) on a computer screen with sound. Virtual worlds are most commonly used for computer games. In a medical virtual world, the patient may be an automated avatar controlled by the computer, or the patient may be an avatar inhabited by a human participant. Kleinert and colleagues published a review of such systems in 2015 and concluded that the development and validation of such simulators will need to be the subject of further research.[190]

Standardized patients. Standardized patients (SPs; in some countries referred to as "simulated patients") are actors/role players who are trained to represent a patient's condition (e.g., symptoms or social situation) and may be trained to score a participant's performance and to provide informative feedback. Over the last three decades, students increasingly learn skills in medical history taking and physical examinations using SPs.[170] Overviews of the use and implementation of SPs in anesthesia education are available.[191-193] SP-based simulations are increasingly being used for issues such as disclosure of bad news and other difficult conversation as well as in pain medicine.[194]

Hybrid simulation. Hybrid simulation means combining different types of simulation modalities during a simulation scenario. It can be used in different ways and serves several purposes: (1) *Pairing simulation devices in parallel.* This way, a training atmosphere can be established, in which different professions can have credible clinical work for their role. For example, when training the management of complications in the OR with surgeons and anesthesiologists together, it is helpful if both professions have clear functions during the scenario. For example, Kjellin et al. performed a multidisciplinary OR team training, where training was performed in a mock-up OR equipped with a mannequin-based patient simulator and a laparoscopic simulator.[195] Another option is to integrate manufactured life-like surgical models with the mannequin, as used by Weller et al. for multidisciplinary OR team training.[14] (2) *Pairing simulation devices in sequence.* This way, the best characteristics of each simulation modality can be used in a scenario and create a simulation that is more than the sum of the parts. For example, a scenario can start with a standardized patient/role player presenting in a patient bed or gurney; the simulation can be transferred to a mannequin at a critical point, such as when invasive activities are needed (e.g., intubation or CPR) or when giving birth. Cantrell and Deloney offer suggestions for integrating SPs into high-fidelity simulation scenarios.[192]

Simulation Fidelity and Classification of Simulators

Simulation is becoming more commonly used for education and training purposes as well as for continuing professional development. But people often have very different perceptions of the definition of the term simulation. This highlights the need for definitions of simulation modalities, simulation fidelity, a classification of the relevant technologies and features, and also a brief overview about the methods of teaching.

Simulation fidelity and simulator capability. In the simulation literature the term fidelity—which means how closely something replicates reality—is often used to refer to specific devices or products. In contrast, the authors believe strongly that this is a misnomer and that the concept of fidelity is a property of the simulation *activity* and not primarily of the device(s) or

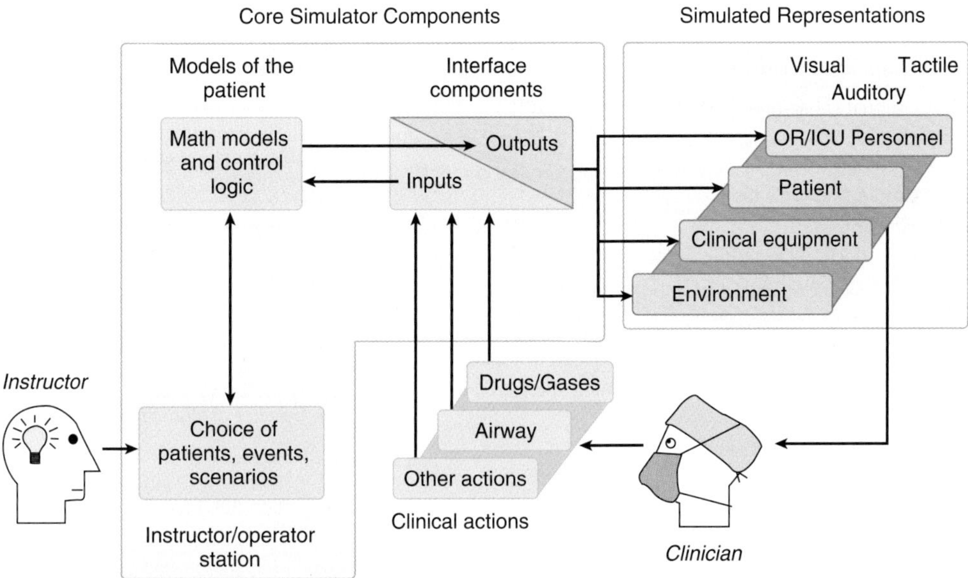

Fig. 7.3 Schematic diagram of the generic architecture of patient simulator systems. The simulator generates a representation of the patient and the work environment with appropriate interface hardware, display technologies, or both. The representation is perceived by the anesthesia professional, whose actions are input to the simulator through physical actions or input devices. The behavior of the simulated scenario is manipulated by the instructor or operator through a workstation that allows selection of different patients, abnormal events, and other features of the simulated patient. The control may be manual, script based, or model based with manual adaptation to reach optimal learning outcomes. *ICU*, Intensive care unit; *OR*, operating room. (*Diagram by D.M. Gaba.*)

products used. That is, fidelity is determined by the number of aspects that are replicated by the simulation (not only physical ones) and the applicable representation of each aspect relative to that of the real world (see subchapter on simulation realism). The fidelity required of a simulation depends on the stated goals and participant population. Some goals can be achieved with minimal and low fidelity, whereas others require very high fidelity.

Classification of simulators. For some purposes it is useful to compare the levels or specifics of the particular technological *capabilities* of simulator devices. There is no universally accepted classification scheme for describing simulators in anesthesia.[169] Any classification involves some overlapping and gray areas.[159] Cumin and Merry describe a classification that is based on the three pillars of (1) user interaction, (2) physiology base, and (3) use.[196] Gaba[171] classifies simulation modalities according to the following scheme: verbal simulation (i.e., "what-if" discussions, storytelling, trigger videos, role playing), SPs, part-task trainers (including realistic mock-up devices and tissue simulation), computer patient (i.e., VR simulation, microsimulators/screen-based simulators), and electronic patient.

In this chapter, a *patient simulator* (as opposed to a part-task trainer) is a system that presents an approximation of a whole patient (not only parts of it) and a clinical work environment of immediate relevance to anesthesiologists (e.g., operating room, postanesthesia care unit, ICU, etc.). A patient simulator system contains several components (Fig. 7.3).[159] Some of the currently available features of typical mannequin-based patient simulators are presented in Table 7.1.

In the following, the major education and teaching purposes of main simulator classifications are presented. The presentation is partly based on the idea of the Miller prism (also pyramid or triangle) of clinical competence. For a more elaborate overview the reader is referred to further literature.[75]

Miller's learning pyramid. For each simulation a variety of different learning objectives exist. Largely they can be aligned to the Miller pyramid[197] shown in Fig. 7.4. On the cognition level, simulations can be used to help learners acquire new knowledge and to better understand conceptual relations and dynamics ("knows," "knows how"). For example, physiologic simulations allow students to watch cardiovascular and respiratory functions unfold over time and how they respond to interventions—in essence, bringing textbooks, diagrams, and graphs to life. The next step on the spectrum is acquisition of isolated skills to accompany knowledge ("knows how," later "shows how"). Some skills follow swiftly from conceptual knowledge (e.g., cardiac auscultation) while others involve intricate and complex psychomotor activities (e.g., catheter placement or intubation). Isolated technical and non-technical skills must then be assembled into care processes and existing workflow concepts, creating a new layer of clinical practices ("shows how," later "does"). Over time those assembled skills get integrated into practice and become part of daily performance ("does"). The expert health care professional performs only in the "does" triangle, except when honing old skills or learning new ones. However, there may be a gap between the level of performance that individuals—or teams or work units—"do" compared to the optimal level. Often, clinicians might be able to demonstrate

TABLE 7.1 Functionality of Typical Current Mannequin-Based Simulator Systems*

Clinical Area	Features and Functions	Remarks
Airway	Appropriate pharyngeal and glottic anatomy Placement of facemask, ETT, supraglottic airway devices, Combitube Laryngospasm, tongue and airway swelling, cervical immobility, jaw closure, breakable teeth Cricothyrotomy Transtracheal jet ventilation Bronchial anatomy (to the lobar bronchus level)	The airway often provides an acceptable seal for ETT; the seal for supraglottic airway devices can be variable, but it generally does allow positive pressure ventilation. The facemask seal is variable (plastic on plastic) Cricothyrotomy of modest anatomic realism; the tissue does not feel like real skin and lacks a subcutaneous fat layer; no bleeding occurs; however, the simulation does allow going through the physical steps of inserting a subglottic surgical airway.
Head	Eyelid movement, pupil dilation, and reaction to light or medications	
	Patient voice and sounds such as coughing and vomiting (through built-in loudspeaker)	A live voice is preferred to the prerecorded audio clips because of higher flexibility in scenarios.
	Palpable carotid pulses	
	Cyanosis represented by blue light at the edge of the mouth	The blue light is a cue that the patient is cyanotic, but it does not physically replicate the appearance of cyanosis.
	Tearing, sweating	
Chest	Physiologic and pathophysiologic heart and breath sounds Spontaneous breathing with chest wall movement	Breath and heart sounds through loudspeakers; sounds contain artifacts and mechanical noise. Often sound level depends on position of stethoscope relative to loudspeaker.
	Bronchospasm	
	Adjustable pulmonary compliance	
	Adjustable airway resistance	
	Pneumothorax	
	Needle thoracotomy and chest tube placement	As for cricothyrotomy the anatomy is not very realistic, but the mannequin may allow performance of these procedures.
	Defibrillation, transthoracic pacing ECG	
	Chest compressions	
Extremities	Palpable pulses (dependent on arterial pressure)	
	Cuff blood pressure by auscultation, palpation, or oscillometry	
	Modules for fractures and wound modules	
	Intravenous line placement	
	Thumb twitch in response to peripheral nerve stimulation	
	Arm movement	Most current simulators do not provide even limited robotic movement of limbs.
	Representations of tonic-clonic seizure activity	These representations are cues that lack anatomic reality.
Monitoring (waveforms or numeric readouts)	ECG (including abnormalities in morphology and rhythm) SpO_2	Most simulators provide a simulated virtual vital signs display; some can interface to actual clinical monitors.
	Invasive blood pressure	
	CVP, PAP, PCWP	
	Cardiac output	
	Temperature	
	CO_2 (may be actual CO_2 exhalation)	
	Anesthetic gases (may have actual uptake and distribution of agents)	
	Cardiopulmonary bypass	Some simulators include(d) a virtual cardiopulmonary bypass machine.
Automation and sensors	Chest compressions Ventilation rate and volume Defibrillation and pacing (including energy measurement) Gas analyzer (inspired O_2, anesthetics) Drug recognition (drug identification and amount)	

CO_2, Carbon monoxide; *CVP*, central venous pressure; *ECG*, electrocardiogram; *ETT*, endotracheal tube; *O_2*, oxygen; *PAP*, positive airway pressure; *PCWP*, pulmonary capillary wedge pressure; *SpO_2*, saturation of peripheral oxygen.

*The features listed are each present in some existing simulators, but not all features are present on any single device. Sets of features depend on the device and model.

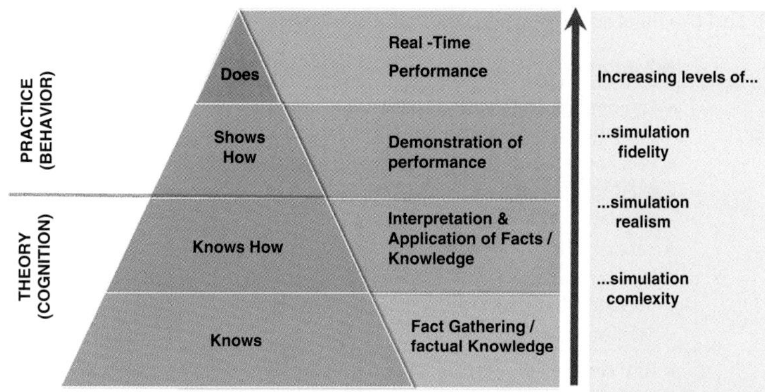

Fig. 7.4 Miller's learning pyramid, also known as Miller's prism of clinical competence.[197] Based on the Miller's learning pyramid, the clinical competence of an anesthesia professional is built on four different competence levels, that can be divided into theory (a person's cognition: "knows"-"knows how") and practice (a person's behavior: "shows how"-"does"). The most relevant clinical competence is the real time performance ("does"). Those four levels need to be considered when addressing learning goals as well as assessment goals of simulation. The figure is modified from a publication of Alinier,[368] indicating that simulation fidelity, simulation realism, and simulation complexity increase with different levels of competency.

"knows how"—"shows how" without necessarily being able to "do" under all relevant circumstances and occasions. Simulation can be a valuable tool to close such gaps.

PATIENT SIMULATION ACTION BOX

In the current health care system, for most invasive procedures, novices' first time performing a task is on a real patient, albeit under supervision, and similarly they will then climb the learning curve by working on real patients. Simulation offers the possibility of having novices practice both before their apprenticeship-like work as well as honing those skills with simulation in parallel with their clinical experiences. This is especially useful because simulation lets them gain experience even with uncommon anatomic or clinical presentations.

Non-technological simulation. Verbal simulations ("what-if" discussions), storytelling, paper and pencil exercises, and experiences with SPs require little or no technology, but can effectively evoke or recreate challenging clinical situations. Similarly, even pieces of fruit or simple dolls can be used for training in some manual tasks. Some education and training on teamwork can be accomplished with role playing or discussion of videos of relevant events.

(Computer) Screen-based simulators (microsimulators) that present the patient on the screen as drawings, photos, or videos, while allowing clinical actions or changes to be chosen can be used to teach basic concepts and technical material, such as the uptake and distribution of inhaled anesthetics or the pharmacokinetics of intravenous drugs. Such programs are inexpensive and easy to use. They allow the presentation of and practice with the concepts and procedures involved in managing normal and abnormal case situations, mostly targeting the parts of the Miller pyramid referred to as "knows" and "knows how," commonly for early learners.

Part-task trainers include artificial (and occasionally animal or human cadaver) models used to teach particular procedural skills, for example intubation, intravenous or intraosseous access, regional anesthesia techniques, thoracic drainage, and use of difficult airway management devices. These target "knows how" and "shows how." Such trainers are most commonly used with novices having little experience with the procedure, or to retrain experienced personnel in the application of the particular tools.

Mannequin-based simulators, representing most or all of a patient, can be used to capture the full complexity of the real task domain, including application of clinical skills and clinical algorithms in combination with human-machine interactions and the complications of working with multiple personnel. They can be used to address "shows how" extending into "does," at least in simulation (see later section on translational research levels). Therefore, MBS are appropriate to teach diagnosis and management of challenging situations as well as non-technical skills and human-factor-based behavior (see Chapter 6). These can be used, with different educational approaches, for all levels of learners. For early learners it is common to use a teacher in the room as an advisor or coach, and to control the simulation by "pause and reflect" allowing the scenario to be stopped and continued or restarted as necessary to maximize their learning.

PATIENT SIMULATION ACTION BOX

Compare to Miller's learning pyramid: If participants are not (yet) familiar with the clinical concepts, procedures, or tasks needed for the mannequin-based training, they should usually be taught those in other ways prior to full-scale simulation.

TABLE 7.2 Site of Simulation and the Related Advantages and Disadvantages

Site of Simulation	Advantages	Disadvantages
Dedicated center *(fixed facility not part of an actual clinical work unit)*	■ Equipment permanently installed, minimized setup time, high level of control and infrastructure ■ Facilitated use of complex audiovisual systems ■ Facilitated conduct of detailed debriefing of simulation involving video review ■ Ease of scheduling ■ No interference with actual clinical work, protects personnel from being pulled into real clinical work ■ Multipurpose use	■ Inability to recreate exact work unit, equipment, supplies of diverse target populations ■ Possible difficulties for clinicians to be off duty to attend training ■ Personnel not readily available for clinical work ■ Eventually remote from site of clinical work ■ Creating and maintaining a dedicated simulation center is expensive ■ Does not probe actual clinical setting
■ Temporary in situ simulation *(Actual work unit; temporary setup and takedown)*	■ Real clinical site ■ Probing/training of personnel in their actual work unit, using real equipment/supplies ■ Ready ability for clinicians to attend in proximity to their work ■ Probes actual clinical site(s) and system(s) ■ Less expensive than operating a dedicated simulation center	■ Vacant clinical space is not always available ■ Difficulties in scheduling—may need site for clinical use ■ Possible interference with actual clinical work; personnel readily drafted to return to clinical work ■ Distractions from onlookers is hard to control ■ Minimal audiovisual system, less audio-video recording capability ■ Great effort of setup and takedown
■ Residential in situ simulation *(Actual work unit; permanent facility)*	■ Same as temporary in situ ■ Minimized setup time ■ Complex audio-video system available ■ Easy scheduling	■ High cost of creating a permanent simulation bed in a clinical work unit ■ Possible interference with actual clinical work; personnel readily drafted to return to clinical work ■ Distractions from onlookers is hard to control
■ Peri-situ/off-site simulation *(simulation in a nonclinical environment such as a conference room, etc.)*	■ Good to schedule ■ Simulation can be used without clinical space or a dedicated simulation center needed ■ Every training is better than no training ■ Many supplies and some equipment can be used as if it was the real thing	■ Lack of ideal realism of bedside or in situ training ■ Minimal audiovisual system, less audio-video recording capability ■ Great effort of setup and takedown ■ No system probing
■ Sequential location simulation/"moving simulation" *(simulated transport of simulator from site to site)*	■ The challenging clinical work of transport itself ■ Replication of natural flow of patients and handoffs between teams	■ Requirement for multiple simulation sites ■ Technologic limitations of portable wireless simulators ■ Great effort of setup and takedown
■ Mobile simulation *(travel of simulation systems and instructor crew to client or neutral sites)*	■ Simulation expertise brought to those who cannot or wish not to invest in it themselves ■ For in situ use, all advantages thereof	■ Possibly high transport costs (driver, fuel, vehicle) ■ For in situ use, all disadvantages thereof plus even greater effort for setup and takedown

PATIENT SIMULATION ACTION BOX

Regardless of the device used, the simulator is only a teaching tool that must be coupled with an effective curriculum for its use.[198] The more complex simulations get (i.e., MBS) and the more a simulator represents a whole patient—to be treated by one or more teams—the more it is important to have qualified instructors with special training.[198]

Sites of Simulation

Some types of simulation such as nontechnological ones and those that use videos or computer programs can be conducted in the privacy of the learners' home or office using their own equipment. Part-task trainers and mannequin-based simulation are often used in a dedicated simulation center, but MBS is increasingly also done "in situ" (in place)—in a real patient room/bed—or "peri-situ" (near the place)—nearby elsewhere in the clinical work unit. For large-scale simulations (e.g., disaster drills[49,86]), the entire organization becomes the site of training, or in the case of a "moving" simulation, different parts of an organization become the site of training. If the simulation training takes place outside the organization, but uses the equipment and personnel of the organization, it is called "mobile" simulation.

Often simulation personnel that work in a dedicated center may either also conduct simulations "in situ," "peri-situ," "mobile," and "moving patients exercises" or may mentor others who do so. The advantages and disadvantages of different simulation sites are discussed in each respective section and summarized in Table 7.2. Sørensen and associates give an overview of the advantages and disadvantages of different simulation sites in a recent publication in 2017.[199]

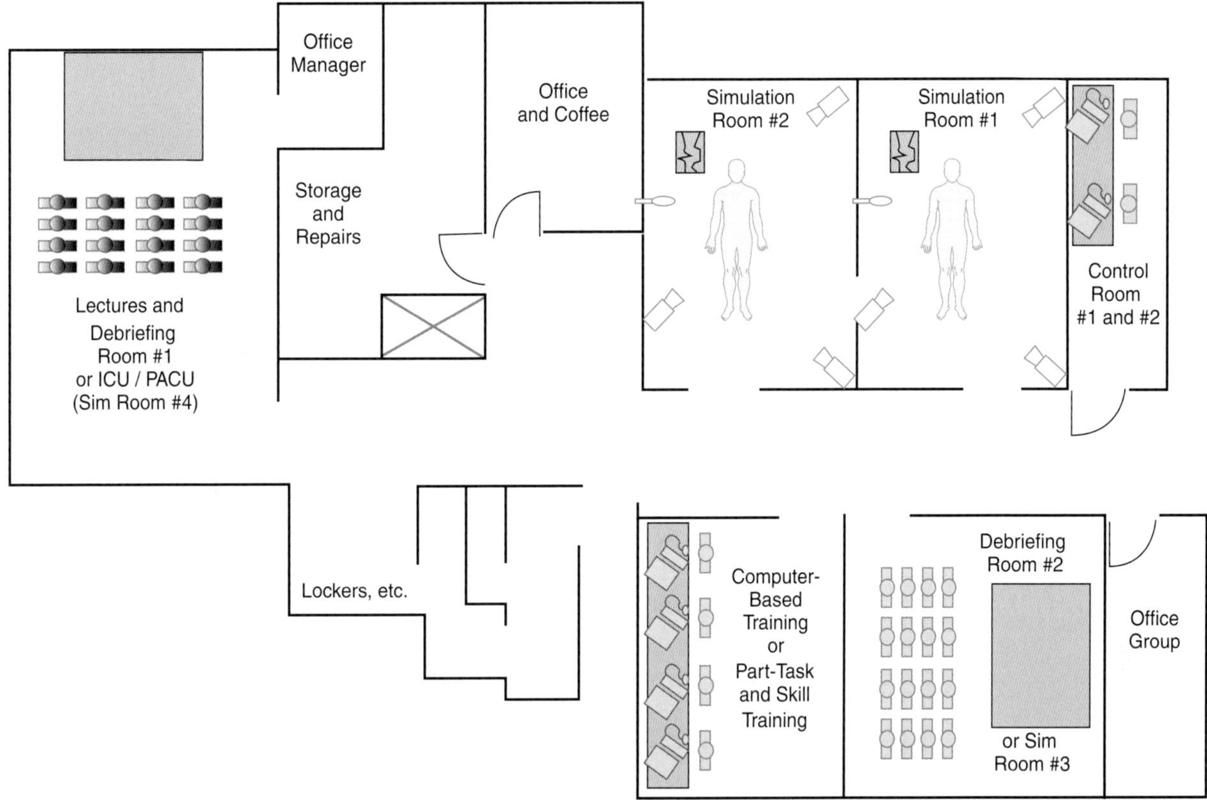

Fig. 7.5 Simulation Center Floor Plan. An intermediate-sized simulation center with four simulation rooms (sim room), a computer-based training room, and several multipurpose rooms, equipped with audio-video patch panels to adjust the room use flexibly to the needs of different training activities (e.g., the large seminar room can be used as a large intensive care unit *[ICU]* or postanesthesia care unit *[PACU]*). *(Figure by M. Rall & E. Stricker, Center for Patient Safety and Simulation [TuPASS], Tübingen, Germany.)*

DEDICATED SIMULATION CENTER

Many institutions have chosen to construct one or more complete simulation centers in which to conduct a variety of education and training sessions. At a few places entire "simulation hospitals" have been created (e.g., Miami, https://simhospital.sonhs.miami.edu/). Some useful websites of simulation centers and other resources are listed at the end of the chapter (Appendix 7.1). The cost structure of a simulation center is a complex issue (see later subchapter). But these programs and their managers in charge have already voted with their feet on the issue of cost versus benefit.

In a dedicated simulation center, one or more simulators may be used, typically in rooms that partially or fully replicate, in a relatively generic fashion, various clinical environments (e.g., operating room, ICU, labor and delivery, emergency department, etc.). Fig. 7.5 and Fig. 7.6 show the floorplan of a medium-sized and a large simulation center. Fig. 7.6 shows the floor plan of the Immersive Learning Center at Stanford University, a pioneering center for health care simulation.

Typically, simulation centers provide a separate control room to allow complex simulations to be presented without an instructor intruding on the simulated case. Fig. 7.7 shows a simulation control room. Many simulation centers have audio-video systems allowing the recording of multiple views during patient simulation. Some centers have computer-based systems to allow annotation of video on the fly and rapid search to the marked portions, but others have found that such mechanisms are not necessary to support debriefing. Dedicated centers typically provide one or more debriefing rooms, often with video replay capability. Ideally a center is located to be easily accessible to a variety of participant populations. Designing, equipping, and overseeing construction of a simulation center may benefit from special knowledge or prior experience.[200,201]

Universities and hospitals or hospital networks are increasingly constructing very large multidisciplinary and multimodal simulation facilities that often still have anesthesiologists in leadership positions. Often, these kind of facilities combine all the types of simulation and immersive learning in one large unit, including actors playing SPs (usually in clinic settings), mannequin-based simulation, part-task and surgical and procedural trainers, wet and dry work (e.g., plaster casting or procedures on food products), and different forms of VR. Sometimes these incorporate facilities for dissection of cadavers or the use of anesthetized animals but often these are in other pre-existing sites. Some institutions have many simulation centers, associated with different learner populations, in different locales, or featuring different kinds of simulation equipment.

Advantages and Disadvantages of Dedicated Simulation Centers. Simulation in a dedicated center facilitates scheduled training and allows the use of complex audiovisual gear and a variety of simulation and clinical equipment, with substantial storage. Devices can be preset, tested, and

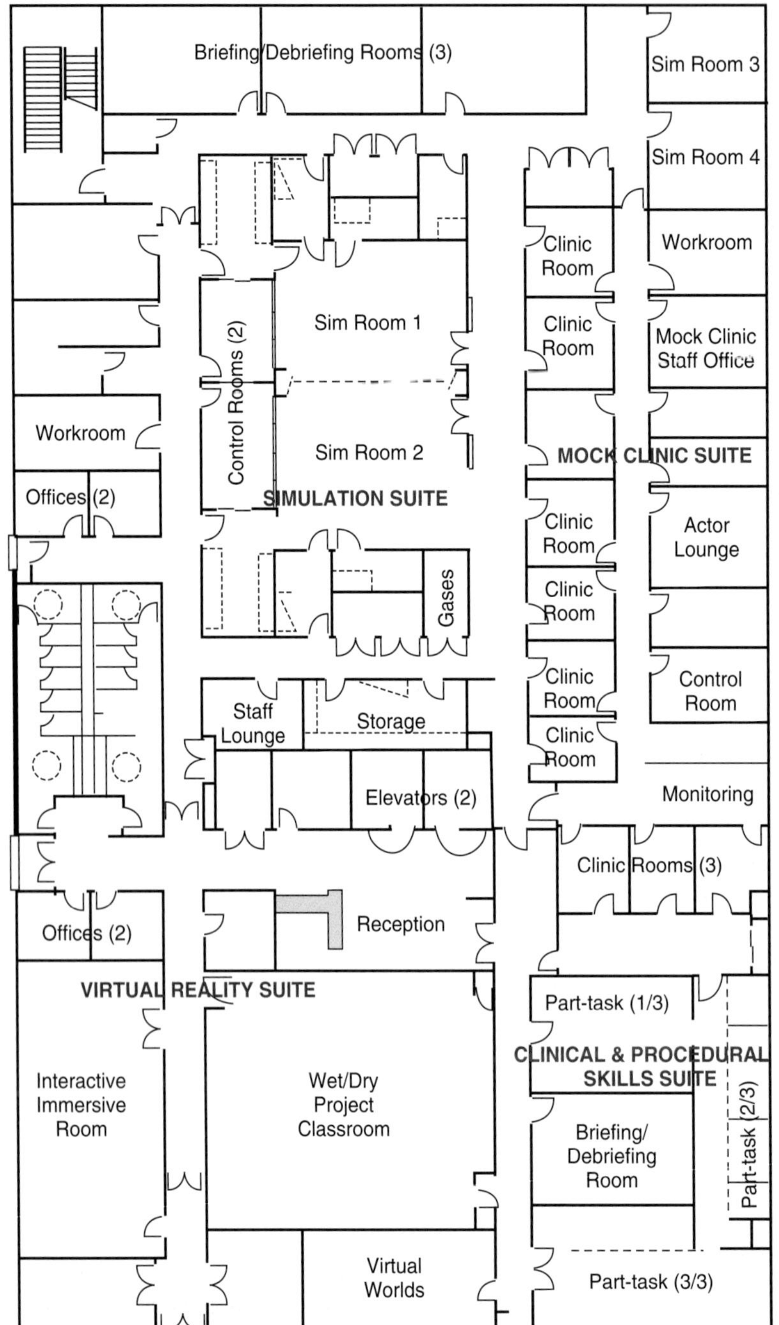

Fig. 7.6 Simulation Center Floor Plan. Floor plan of a large interdisciplinary simulation center for multiple domains (anesthesia, surgery, students) with several multipurpose simulation rooms (sim room) and skills laboratories. (*Figure by D. M. Gaba at the Immersive Learning Center at the Stanford School of Medicine, Stanford, California.*)

ready to go, with briefing and debriefing facilities immediately at hand. In a dedicated center inexpensive discarded, flawed, or outdated clinical equipment and supplies can be safely used. When a center incorporates all modalities of simulation in one place it fosters hybrid techniques, as when an actor playing a standardized patient is combined with a part-task trainer, or when a surgical simulator is combined with a mannequin-based patient simulator.

The main disadvantage of a dedicated center is its cost of construction and outfitting. Moreover, no matter how well equipped it is, it can never replicate the equipment, layout, and clinical processes of any specific clinical workplace. Also, participants know from the very beginning that the activity is a simulation and not the real thing.

TRAINING AND PROBING WHERE CLINICIANS WORK

There are several approaches to conducting simulations in or near actual sites of clinical work. By necessity institutions without a dedicated simulation center must use one of these approaches, but they are useful for many other reasons.

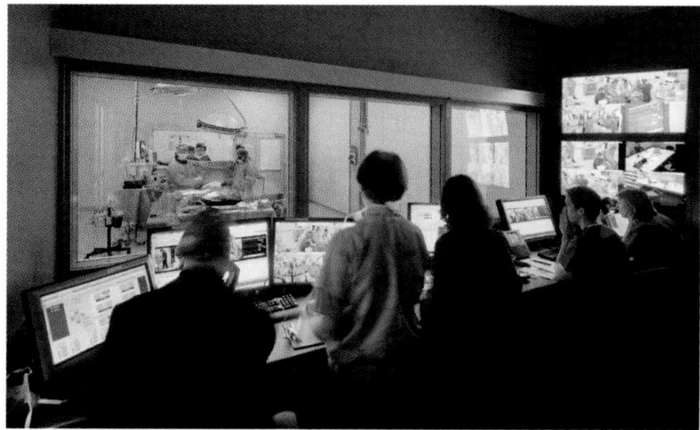

Fig. 7.7 Simulation control room. Through a window wall the simulation control room is separated from the actual simulation room. Several instructors can have a look on the simulation either via the windows, or via one of the several screens that show different views of the simulation room. In front of the instructors the workstation for control of the simulator system itself is placed, including an audio control desk with control of the simulated patient voice, the voice for in-scenario guiding, and several wireless headset channels. (*Photograph provided by D.M. Gab; control room of the Stanford Immersive Learning Center.*)

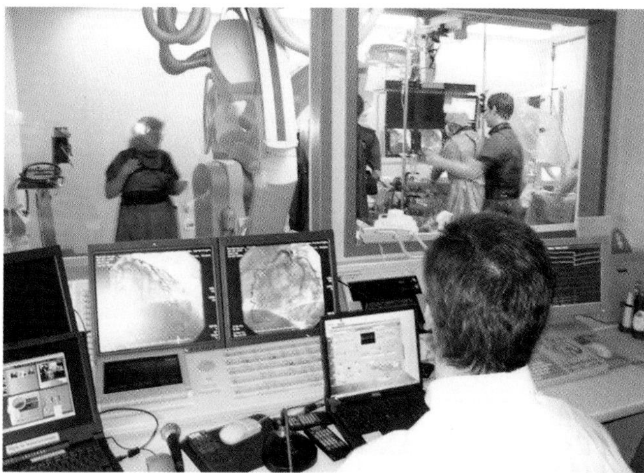

Fig. 7.8 In situ mobile simulation in a catheterization laboratory (cath lab). The simulator is placed on the cath lab table, surrounded by the x-ray equipment, thus complicating treatment of the patient by limiting space. The vital signs monitor provides relevant data to the clinical team. The simulator is controlled from the cath lab control room. Multiple mobile cameras and a scan converter for vital signs provide a live video transmission to a temporary debriefing area for the nonactive part of the training group and allows for crisis resource management–based debriefings. (*Photograph by M. Rall.*)

In Situ Simulation

In situ simulation is conducted in an actual bed/gurney/bay of a real clinical workplace, such as, for example, OR, ICU, trauma room, postanesthesia unit, or ward. ISS training is often used for complex patient simulation scenarios with experienced single-discipline or interprofessional staff. It is typically used for training in order to create high environmental fidelity and/or to probe procedures or the system (see earlier subchapter "Application of Simulation").[4,75,83-87,202] ISS can be a useful training option especially for training in unique workplaces that are difficult to recreate with adequate realism (see later subchapter on simulation realism) in a simulation center or elsewhere, such as a catheterization laboratory, a CT scanner, an ambulance, or an air rescue aircraft (Figs. 7.8 to 7.15).

Rosen and colleagues[203] reviewed the use of in situ simulation in the continuing education for health care professions. They summarized that a positive impact of ISS on learning and organizational performance has been demonstrated in a small number of studies. They also indicated that the evidence surrounding ISS efficacy is still emerging and that existing research is promising.

Most ISS is performed mobile as a temporary setup only for the training sessions. In very few institutions a simulator is permanently installed in a clinical workplace, for example, creating a simulation-specific patient room in the actual ICU.

Advantages and Disadvantages of In Situ Simulation. ISS seems ideal in that it probes and challenges personnel and systems as they actually exist, thus unmasking real issues of patient care. It is available, in principle, to all sites, even those without a dedicated center, and it is conducive to short courses and unannounced mock event drills.

Because it takes place in the actual work unit, it will eliminate travel time to a dedicated center and will put participants at ease. Some substantial disadvantages include potential distractions by ongoing clinical work, lack of privacy, logistics of setup and takedown, reduced availability of AV and simulation equipment, and supply costs (many ISS activities use the unit's real clinical supplies as needed).[204] ISS can be difficult to organize, schedule, and control. The clinical area planned for simulation may not be vacant or may be needed on short notice. Staff members engaged in the simulation are prone to being pulled into clinical duty, and training sessions may be interrupted. Raemer[204] summarized potential risks of ISS and amplified some of the safety hazards of simulation itself including maintaining control of simulated medications and equipment, limiting the use of valuable hospital resources, preventing incorrect learning from simulation shortcuts, and profoundly upsetting patients and their families. In our experience, patients and families are rarely upset and in fact often are pleased to see that such serious training is going on.

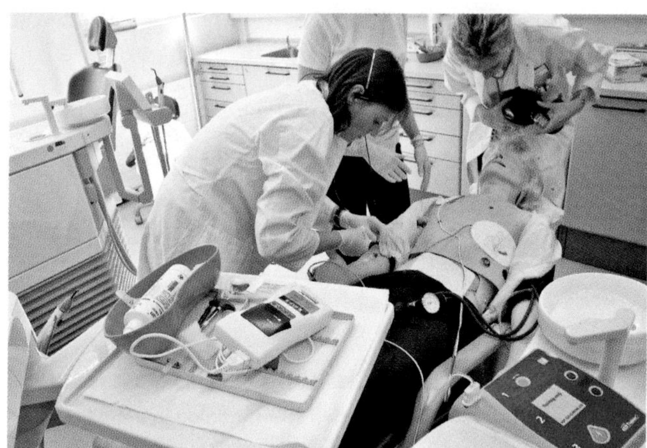

Fig. 7.9 In situ mobile simulation in a dentist chair. The simulator was equipped with artificial teeth gum and a chalk tooth to drill, thereby simulating the dentist's procedures. Then emergencies developed, allowing the team to respond. Training focused on crisis resource management key points and medical aspects including use of an automated external defibrillator. (*Photograph by M. Rall.*)

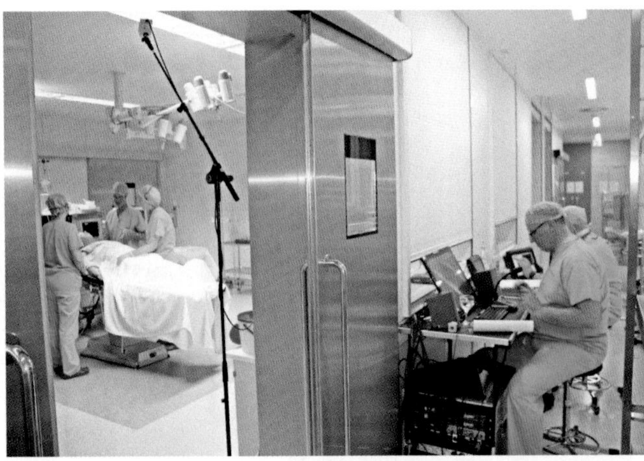

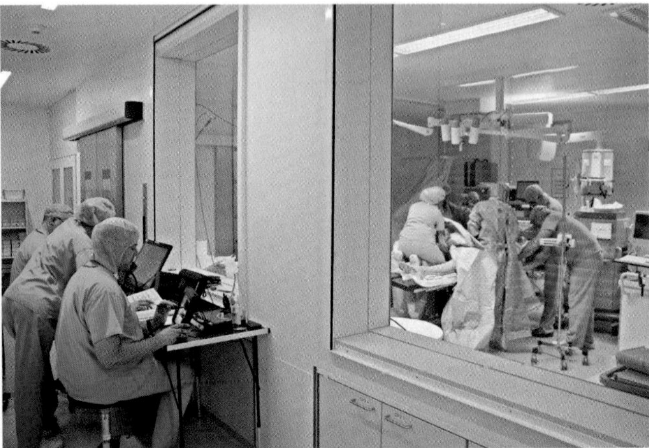

Fig. 7.10 In situ mobile simulation team training in the operating room (OR). The mobile simulation control room is set up outside the OR. The instructors can watch the simulation scenario either indirectly via live video coverage (left photo) or directly via the OR window (right photo). *(Photograph provided by M. Rall, InPASS in situ training in the OR at Scuol Hospital, Switzerland, Chairman: J. Koppenberg.)*

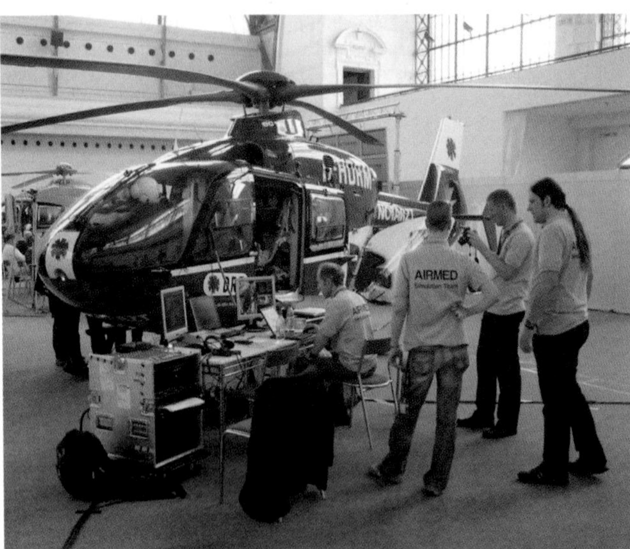

Fig. 7.11 In situ mobile simulation team training in a medical air rescue helicopter. The mobile simulation control room with several cameras and microphones is set up outside the helicopter and provides a multi-perspective view inside to monitor the scenario and react to activities performed. *(Photograph taken by M. Rall at Airmed 2008 with the German Air Rescue (DRF) team.)*

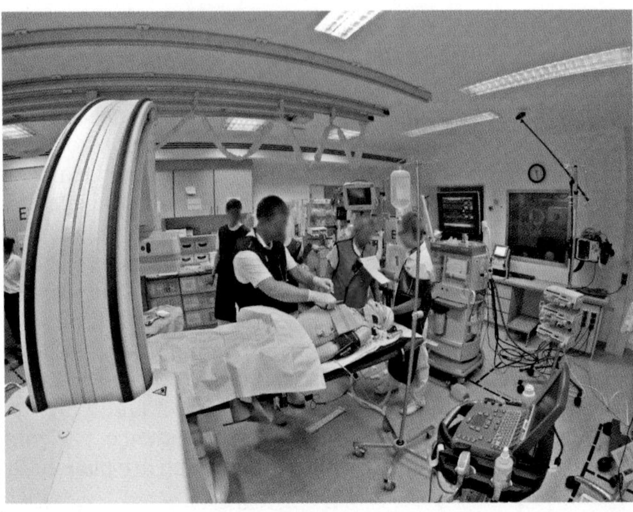

Fig. 7.12 In situ mobile simulation trauma team training at a large trauma center. *(Photo provided by M. Rall.)*

Peri-situ or Off-site Simulation

If simulation is, in principle, worthwhile, then doing simulation anywhere is probably better than not doing it at all. *Peri-situ simulation* (PSS) means simulating in the clinical work unit, but not in an actual patient room/bay/bed—for example in a conference room, or even hallway of the unit. This may be done when an ISS session is planned but there is no actual clinical spot available, or it may be done this way on purpose. PSS has some of the advantages of ISS in terms of locale, systems, and supplies, but it lacks the ideal realism of an actual bedside. When simulation is done outside a clinical unit (say a nonclinical conference room) or in a public area of a hospital it is referred to as *off-site simulation* (OSS).

Sequential Location Simulation

This is sometimes called *moving simulation* and it simulates the patient moving between different sites of care in one scenario, at each stop enacting what might transpire in that location. For example, the patient could be brought to the emergency department by ambulance; assessed and treated; then taken to CT scan, interventional radiology, or OR; and finally transferred to an ICU. Moving simulation may be best accomplished as ISS or PSS, but again, there will be some value to it even if each stop cannot be simulated perfectly. To do it with full veracity requires intensive coordination and complex choreography of simulation equipment and personnel. It is probably only worth it if done occasionally and primarily with a focus on systems probing and improvement. Moving simulations can address different specific issues at each stop, depending on the most important systems probing and learning issues for each.

Advantages and Disadvantages of Moving Simulation. Like all kinds of ISS, moving simulation is a powerful tool to detect latent threats in the system. Apart from a focus on latent threats in certain workspaces, this kind of ISS can detect challenges in the course of transport to those workspaces. As mentioned above, the organizational and technical preparations, the technical challenges, and the movement of the whole simulation gear paired with the clinical staff needed in order to make moving simulations work imply huge effort.

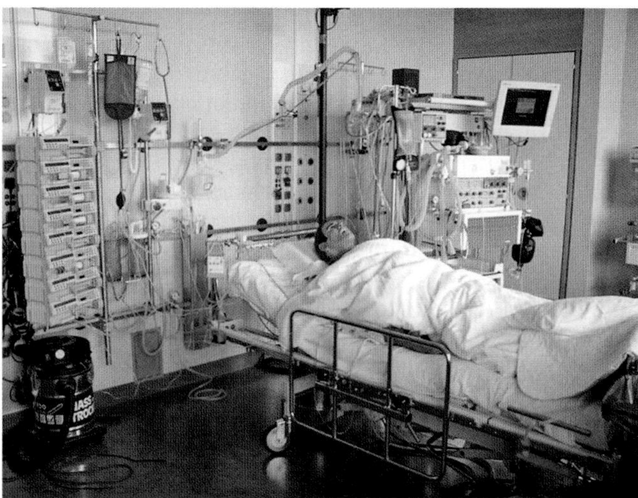

Fig. 7.13 In situ mobile simulation in an intensive care unit (ICU)/intermediate medical care unit location. The training in clinical areas is especially useful for ICU-like surroundings. Crisis resource management–based trainings showcase these highly complex problems and the interactions needed to coordinate high-performing ICU teams. The training allows for checking the local arrangement of equipment and the readiness to react to certain emergencies. There are already a few examples of permanent in situ simulation facilities in ICUs (see text). *(Photograph by M. Rall.)*

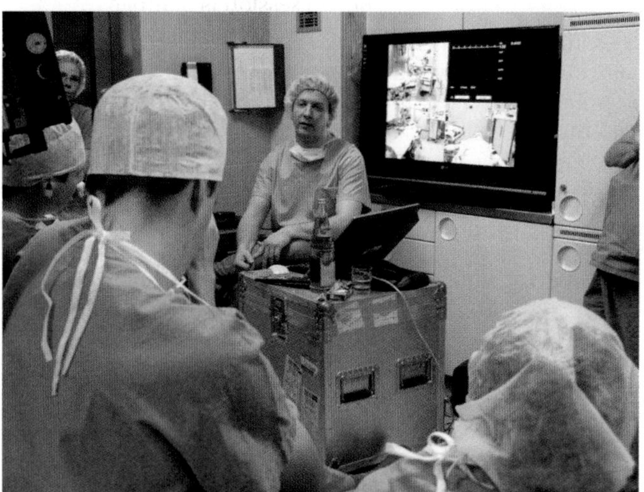

Fig. 7.14 In situ mobile crisis resource management (CRM)–focused simulation team training inside an operating room. This debriefing room is temporarily set up in an induction room. The use of videos for debriefing (here on a 42-inch flat panel placed over the basin) is feasible even in this setting. Training inside a hospital often includes training actual teams with the same setup, if possible conducting training for a large proportion of the relevant personnel. "En-bloc" training sessions may have a greater impact and longer-lasting effects of the lessons learned, including CRM behaviors. *(Photograph by team TuPASS [Center for Patient Safety and Simulation, University Hospital, Tübingen, Germany], who performed a full team training of the anesthesia department at Steinenberg Medical Center, Reutlingen, Germany.)*

MOBILE SIMULATION: "HAVE SIMULATOR, WILL TRAVEL"

Mobile simulation means that the simulator and the audiovisual gear are transported outside the originating institution for purposes of a simulation event. This makes simulation activities an option for clinical sites that lack a dedicated

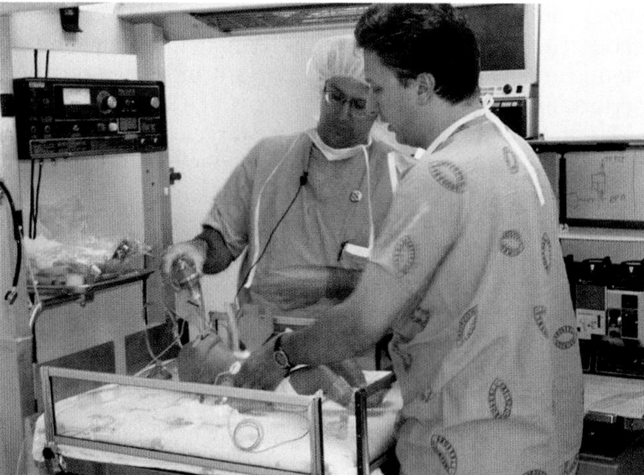

Fig. 7.15 Neonatal crisis resource management and resuscitation training at a neonatal emergency workplace. The experienced instructor (on the right side of the infant) is a confederate acting as part as the team, whereas others in the control room preside over simulation. *(Photograph taken at Stanford Simulation Center, Stanford University, Palo Alto, California; provided by M. Rall.)*

simulation center or the expertise to do ISS/PSS in their own institution.

Mobile simulation can be conducted in clinical settings or in conference rooms, or even hotel meeting rooms. Mobile simulation can be provided by staff from simulation centers that have mobile simulator and audiovisual equipment and are equipped to travel with it. In some places there are small simulation centers built into a truck or bus.

Advantages and Disadvantages of Mobile Simulation. For clients who use mobile simulation, the construct of mobile simulation for sure is a great way to know the promise of simulation training and system probing without extra time and money for staff travelling. At the same time, mobile simulation offers the advantage of external peer feedback. This way normalizations of deviance (see Chapter 6) and pitfalls that are not noticed by internal personnel anymore can be detected by external instructors. Organizations that offer mobile simulation show a greater flexibility for training opportunities. Such organizations can not only offer training at nearly any workspace in their own organization, but also offer simulation to other organizations. This way, the organization's own simulation activities might be funded and vacant equipment and personnel capacities used.

Simulation Team Training Participants: Who Should Be Trained and in What Composition?

Each discipline in health care can be considered a *crew* containing one or more individuals. Several crews may work together closely as a *team*. The operating room team, for example, consists of an anesthesia crew, a surgery crew, and a nursing crew (and crews of technicians and support personnel). The members within a crew are likely to be more familiar with each other than with members of other crews. Such mutual professional (and private) "knowing about each other"—perhaps by enhancing their shared mental model—could be an important influence on their performance.[205]

Many simulation applications are targeted at individuals. These may be especially useful for teaching knowledge and basic skills or for practice on specific psychomotor tasks. As in other high-reliability industries (including anesthesiology, see chapter 6), individual skill is a fundamental building block, but empiric findings show that individual performance is not sufficient to achieve optimal overall performance, and to achieve optimal safety.[206] Performance and safety unfold in the interplay between people and in their interaction with each other, equipment, and organizational structures and processes. That is the reason why in high-reliability organizations a considerable emphasis is applied at higher organizational levels, in various forms of teamwork and communication training, and interpersonal relations. This approach is often summarized under the rubric of *crisis resource management* (see Chapter 6 and later section).[24,207,208] The importance of teamwork and team training is widely accepted in health care and anesthesia,[33,209-216] although team training is still not widely implemented. The prerequisites for effective teamwork (e.g., team leadership, mutual performance monitoring, back-up and speak-up behavior, adaptability and team orientation, the concept of team cognition, etc.) are discussed in Chapter 6. One of the special features of health care teams that poses several challenges is the frequently changing composition of teams with changing crews. Within a discipline, crew membership may fluctuate. For example, in anesthesia or the resuscitation team. Those teams or crews are also referred to as "action teams" (see Chapter 6).

When simulation is intended to go beyond specific medical and technical skills for individuals (as, for example, in CRM-oriented patient simulation) and to involve non-technical skills and teamwork, one can distinguish between single-discipline and multidiscipline approaches. CRM-based "team training" may be addressed first to *crews* (known as *single-discipline teams*), and then to *teams* (known as *multidiscipline teams*).[217] Commonly, in a broader sense and used this way in this chapter, the term "team training" refers to both single-discipline as well as multidiscipline training. For both approaches the best way to train and transfer learning for everyday instances at work is to arrange the training (1) interprofessional (doctors, nurses, allied health personnel, etc.) and (2) in realistic crew/team compositions and roles in regard to the learning objective ("train as you work"—see patient simulation action box below).

PATIENT SIMULATION ACTION BOX

"Train as you work." When conducting patient simulation training with more experienced personnel—beyond "early learners"—those who work together should train together when possible. Although built on a foundation of previous experience and crew-specific training, working together in simulation will hone the skills of coordinating tasks, goals, and strategies in the overall treatment of the patient.

Furthermore, teams exist in actual *work units* in an organization (e.g., a specific ICU), each of which can be its own target for training, and in *organizations* as a whole (e.g., entire hospitals or networks). Each unit can have specific characteristics, culture, etc., that will influence how receptive participants are for training and how easily they can apply in the clinical setting what they learned during simulation. Growing interest and experience have been shown in applying simulation to nonclinical personnel and work units in health care organizations (e.g., to managers, executives, informal leaders).[73,74]

Addressing teamwork in the single-discipline approach in contrast to the multidiscipline approach has advantages and disadvantages.[155] For maximal benefit, these approaches are used in a complementary fashion.

TRAINING INDIVIDUALS

Simulation-based training of individual skills can be used to educate learners (Miller learning pyramid "knows," "knows how," see Fig. 7.4), to promote psychomotor skills ("knows how," "shows how"), and to help integrate different kinds of skills into an effective whole. Usually, early learners need to start somewhere, as do experienced people trying to learn completely new skills or procedures. Whereas screen-based simulators can be used for educational purposes and the acquisition of basic procedural knowledge, part-task trainers promote psychomotor skills, and mannequin-based simulation allows training to bring different concepts together. When mannequin-based simulation is used for the training of individuals (who still perform as a crew!), the focus of patient simulation training lies either (1) on training an individual's clinical skills, for example following a treatment algorithm; or (2) on training non-technical skills such as leadership, communication, task management, etc.; or (3) both.

TRAINING CREWS: INTERPROFESSIONAL SINGLE-DISCIPLINE TEAM TRAINING

Training for crews (e.g., anesthesiologists) involves simulation scenarios, in which all participants are from a single discipline and in which the scenarios are highly relevant to the crew (both in regard to clinical and non-technical skills). The other team members' roles (i.e., surgeons, etc.) are either played by instructor personnel or clinically savvy actors; less critical team roles may be played by participants or, when necessary, not present at all. In this approach the interaction with specific types of behaviors by other crew or team members can be addressed by an instructor or an actor assuming that role as a confederate. These roles can be designed such that participants can be exposed to different kinds of challenges systematically.

This approach allows tailoring simulations to challenge skills, knowledge, and situations specific to the discipline, including material that may be of little relevance to other members of the team and in the context of a wide variety of clinical situations (e.g., cardiac, orthopedic, or general surgery; labor and delivery; intensive care). Single-discipline training can emphasize generic skills of dynamic decision making, resource management, leadership, and teamwork applicable to any challenging clinical situation that is relevant to the particular discipline.

The single-discipline approach may be of particular relevance and value for professionals who work in many different settings and who do not work in permanent crews or teams ("action teams," such as in anesthesia, see Chapter 6), and who therefore must acquire generic teamwork and communication skills that can be used with all co-workers. For dedicated center simulations, single-discipline sessions are simpler logistically because only one discipline needs to be present, rather than scheduling someone from each of the disciplines.

TRAINING TEAMS: INTERPROFESSIONAL MULTIDISCIPLINE TEAM TRAINING

In health care, interdisciplinary teams are becoming ubiquitous. At the same time, experts from each discipline do not necessarily combine to make an expert team.[218] The complementary approach is to conduct *multidiscipline team training* (also called *combined team training* or *interprofessional training [IPE]*). Here, the crews of different disciplines who might work together undergo training together, each acting in their own usual roles, and scenarios designed to challenge all of the disciplines. Multidiscipline team training allows for more natural team interactions and reinforces understanding across the disciplines. Successful examples of such undertakings have been reported in many fields where anesthesia professionals are involved, including the OR,[159,219] obstetrics[220-222] (combining obstetrics, anesthesia, nursing, and neonatology and pediatrics), intensive care (combining physicians from multiple disciplines with nursing, respiratory therapy, and pharmacy),[223] emergency department,[224,225] and trauma management.[30,31,90,226,227]

Depending on the training location (see earlier subchapter), the scheduling of the team training poses several challenges. Multidiscipline training, for example, can be difficult to schedule in a dedicated simulation center. Ideally, the sessions will have instructors from several disciplines especially to handle debriefing. Multidiscipline trainings are typically easier to organize as in situ trainings (see earlier subchapter), or as announced or unannounced "mock events" (see next subchapter) that activate the actual designated team (e.g., ward or unit team, rapid response team, or code team). In the latter situation, the team does not know it is a simulation until they arrive at the scene.

CROSS TRAINING: CHANGING ROLES

The course director of a simulation activity can choose whether to have all participants act in their own regular role, or to assume a different role. Each has its advantages. The philosophy of "train as you work and work as you train" would usually put everyone in their usual role,[82] but cross-training can provide an understanding of and sensitivity to the tasks, decision making, challenges, and responsibilities of another profession or discipline. Study results indicate that cross-training is an important determinant of effective teamwork process, communication, and performance,[228] enhanced shared team-interaction and mental models,[229] and helps to maintain team communication when faced with increased task demands.[230]

PATIENT SIMULATION ACTION BOX

If a cross-training scenario is conducted it is advisable to brief personnel to represent the other professional role in a rational manner without playing out particular personality quirks or go "over the top." The debriefing should emphasize discussion on what individuals can learn from "walking in someone else's shoes." It would be foolish, for example, to debrief anesthesia professionals on their surgical skills or behavior as a surgeon. Acting out may be fun for play but it is disrespectful to others, and wastes valuable simulation time.

EN-BLOC TRAINING: AVOIDING SUB-THRESHOLD TRAINING EFFECTS

If patient simulation is used as an intervention to promote a patient safety initiative, for example the introduction of crisis resource management (see Chapter 6) to crews or teams, or the implementation of a new checklist, algorithm, etc., the organization/curriculum designer may arrange that all crew and team members are trained within a short period of time (i.e. several days or weeks). This would provide a more concentrated and uniform result. On the other hand, this may not be possible logistically or politically within the institution, and may or may not be worth the "political capital" to make it happen. As there are no data to demonstrate the strength of the en-bloc effect, it is necessary to gauge under what circumstances it is worth the effort.

Patient Simulation Timing: Announced in Advance Versus Unannounced in Advance

Regardless of site, simulations can be conducted as prescheduled exercises either for personnel in their regular-duty roles or for personnel on off-duty or education days. Typically, unannounced mock events (announced as if the real thing) would be implemented in a department after making potential participants aware of this possibility on a general level. Again, scheduled and unscheduled ISSs are complementary approaches, each with its own pros and cons. An obvious challenge is that it takes participants away from their actual patient care activities so that ground rules need to be established concerning when and how to abort the exercise when necessary. On the other hand, when done only occasionally and with appropriate safeguards, the clinical system needs to probe its ability to ensure good patient care when an emergency team is called to an event. In summary, the technique has high potential for organizational learning when done carefully.

A number of recent publications discuss the advantages and disadvantages of unannounced mock events as well as issues concerning the implementation of such programs.[199,231-233]

Scopes of Simulation in Health Care: The 12 Dimensions of Simulation

Many different aspects and variations of simulation have been presented so far; they represent examples of combinations of choices from 12 (originally 11[171]) different dimensions of the simulation universe. Each dimension has a variety of choices—a spectrum—to choose from (Fig. 7.16).

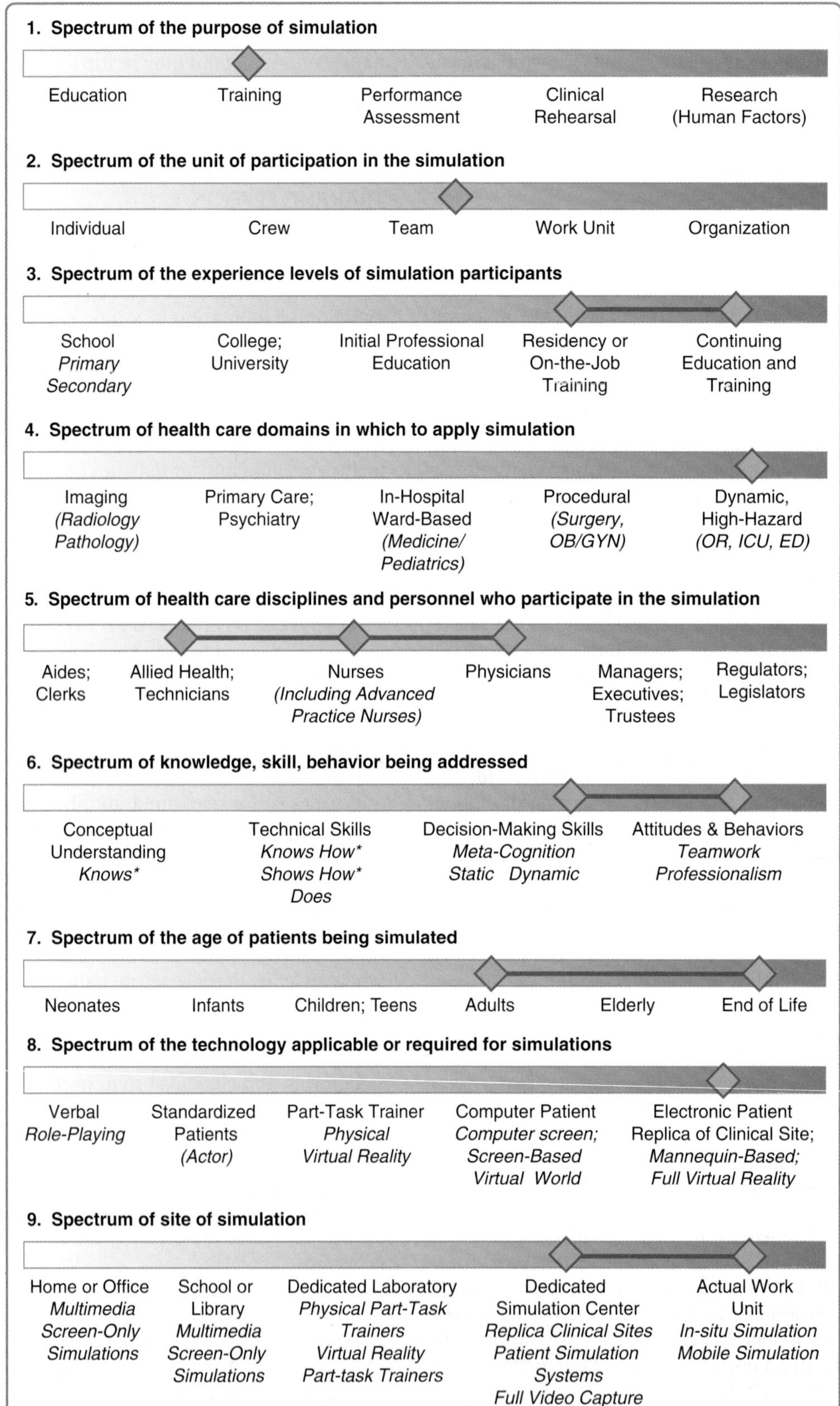

Fig. 7.16 The 12 dimensions of simulation applications. (A) Dimensions 1-9. *These terms are used according to Miller's pyramid of learning.

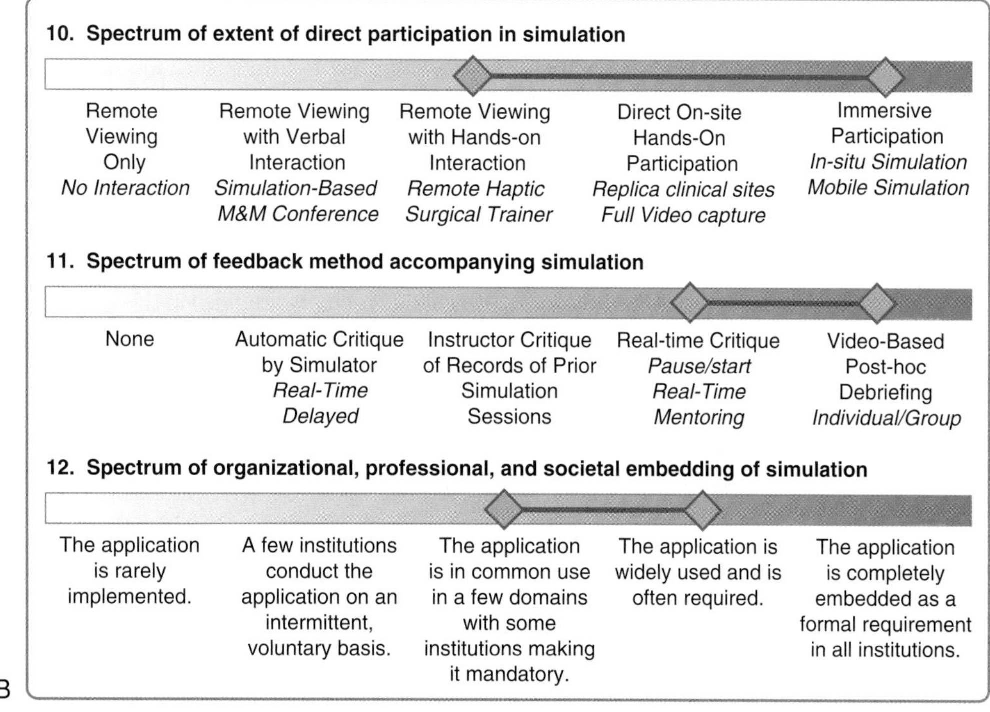

Fig. 7.16, cont'd. (B) Dimensions 10-12. Any particular application can be represented as a point or range on each spectrum (shown by *diamonds*). This figure illustrates a specific application: multidisciplinary crisis resource management (CRM)-oriented decision making and teamwork training for adult intensive care unit *(ICU)* personnel. *ED,* Emergency department; *M&M,* morbidity and mortality; *OB/GYN,* obstetrics and gynecology; *OR,* operating room.

Any particular simulation activity can be classified by delineating one or more characteristics in each of the 12 dimensions. The different attributes can be combined as needed to achieve the pursued objectives. Clearly, some combinations are useless or irrelevant, some are similar to each other, and others are redundant, but the total number of unique combinations across all dimensions is still very large and only some combinations have been implemented. Dimensions of particular relevance are the goals and purposes of the simulation, the target population, the modalities of simulation, and the pedagogical approach that is used.

The content of many dimensions has been addressed in detail in the earlier parts of the chapter. Therefore, for the sake of completeness, only a short description of the dimensions is given here and the reader is referred back to each section for more information. Those who seek a detailed description of the different dimensions are referred to other literature where the model is described as a whole in detail.[75,234]

Dimension 1: Purpose and Aims of the Simulation Activity. The most obvious applications of simulation have been described in the subchapter "Application of Simulators in Anesthesia and Health Care." For more detailed information the reader is referred back to this section. To summarize the main purposes shortly, they are (1) education, (2) training including clinical rehearsal, (3) performance assessment, (4) research about simulation, and (5) research with simulation, including (5a) testing of procedures, (5b) testing of equipment, and (5c) system probing.

Dimension 2: Unit of Participation in the Simulation. The units of participation have been described in the subchapter on the classification of simulation teams. For more detailed information the reader is referred back to this section.

Dimension 3: Experience Level of Simulation Participants. Simulation can be applied along the entire continuum of education of clinical personnel and the public at large. For more information see earlier subchapter on the use of simulation in education and training. As mentioned earlier, simulation training is applicable to health care providers with a range of experience, including experts,[2,50] novices and advanced residents,[2,90,178,235,236] medical/nursing/other healthcare profession students,[51,52,53-57] and even children.[58-61]

Dimension 4: Healthcare Domain in Which Simulation is Applied. Simulation techniques can be applied across nearly all health care domains.[18] A summary of the different domains was given in the earlier subchapter on "Use of simulation."

Dimension 5: Healthcare Disciplines of Personnel Participating in the Simulation. Simulation is applicable to a wide variety of professionals in health care, not only to physicians. In anesthesiology, simulation has been applied to novices and experienced trainees, board certified anesthesiologists, CRNAs, and anesthesia technicians. Simulation is not limited to clinical personnel. It may be directed at managers, executives, hospital trustees, regulators, and legislators.[73,74]

Dimension 6: Type of Knowledge, Skill, Attitudes, or Behavior Addressed in Simulation. Different types of competences can be addressed with simulation: knowledge, skill, attitudes, behavior. Based on the Miller pyramid (see corresponding subchapter), competences can be classified with regard to their level of appearance to "knows," "knows how," "shows how," and "does." Apart from the competences described by Miller,[197] Gaba[234] added cognitive skills such as decision-making processes, attitudes, and behaviors to the competences that can be addressed with the spectrum.

Dimension 7: Age of the Patient Being Simulated. Simulation is applicable to nearly every type and age of patient. Fully interactive neonatal and pediatric patient simulators are available. Simulation can address aspects of end-of-life issues for every age.

Dimension 8: Technology Applicable or Required For Simulations. To accomplish the different simulation goals listed in dimensions 1, 3, 4, 5, 6, and 7 various simulation technologies—including no technology—are relevant for simulation. An overview is given in the earlier subchapters "History and Development of Simulators," "Fidelity and Classification of Simulators," and "So many simulators and simulation options: which one to use…?".

Dimension 9: Site of Simulation Participation. The different sites of simulation have been described in detail in the correspondent subchapter. Video conferencing and advanced networking may allow even advanced types of simulation to be conducted remotely (see dimension 10).

Dimension 10: Extent of Direct Participation in Simulation. Not all learning requires direct participation. Some learning can occur merely by viewing a simulation involving others because the viewer can readily imagine being in the shoes of the participants.[237] A further step is to involve remote viewers with interaction in the simulation itself or verbal interaction in debriefings about what transpired. Several centers have been using videoconferencing to conduct simulation-based exercises, including morbidity and mortality conferences. Because the simulator can be paused, restarted, or otherwise controlled, the remote audience can readily obtain more information from the on-site participants, debate the proper course of action, and discuss with those in the simulator how best to proceed. Further steps of participation are personal involvement ("hands-on") either in a replicated clinical site or immersive personal participation in an in situ simulation.

Dimension 11: Feedback Method Accompanying Simulation. One can learn a great deal just from simulation experiences themselves, without any additional feedback.[238] For many simulations, specific feedback is provided to maximize learning. On-screen-based simulators or VR systems, as well as the simulator (part-task trainer or mannequin) itself, may provide feedback about the participant's actions or decisions, particularly for manual tasks for which clear metrics of performance are readily delineated. More commonly, human instructors provide feedback. This can be as simple as having the instructor review records of previous sessions that the learner has completed alone. For many target populations and applications, an instructor provides real-time guidance and real-time feedback to participants while the simulation is ongoing. The possibility to start, pause, and restart the simulation is valuable in this respect. Alternatively, brief post-hoc feedback is given by the instructor at the end of the simulation. For the most complex uses of simulation, especially when training experienced personnel, the typical form of feedback is provided by an instructor and is included in a detailed post-simulation debriefing session.[105,107,112,113,238] More discussion of debriefing is given later in the subchapter on "Debriefing."

Dimension 12: Embedding of Simulation in Relevant Organizational, Professional, and Societal Contexts. The final important dimension is how the simulation application is embedded into an overall context.[159] Being highly embedded may mean that the simulation is a formal requirement of the institution or is mandated by the governmental regulator. Another aspect of embedding may be that—for early learners—the initial (steep) part of the learning curve is required to occur in a simulation training before the learners are allowed to work on real patients under supervision. In addition, complete embedding of simulation into the workplace means that simulation training is a normal part of the work schedule, rather than being an add-on activity attended in the spare time of clinicians.

Crisis Resource Management (ACRM; CRM): Part of Modern Patient Simulation Team Training

In the last subchapters, the benefits and the effectiveness of simulation-based education were highlighted and its ecologic validity was considered. This subsequent section now explores the idea that simulation-based education for a variety of simulation curricula, especially for team training, needs to take into account not only medical and technical skills, but also what is called anesthesia crisis resource management (ACRM), also referred to as crisis resource management (CRM). For detailed information on CRM see Chapter 6.

THE ROOTS OF ANESTHESIA CRISIS RESOURCE MANAGEMENT TRAINING

In 1989, based on earlier work, Cooper,[239,240] Howard et al.,[181] and Gaba[241,242] of the VA-Stanford and their colleagues identified gaps in the training of anesthesiologists regarding several critical aspects of decision making and crisis management that were not systematically taught during standard residency or postgraduate education. These gaps were inadequate learning and skills of (1) precompiled plans for dealing with perioperative events; (2) metacognition and allocation of attention; and (3) resource management behavior, including leadership, communication, workload management, monitoring, and cross-checking of all available information.

Historically, it had been assumed that anesthesiologists would acquire these plans and non-technical skills (see Chapter 6) by osmosis, solely by experience and by observing role models who had these qualities, rather than specific education and training about them. But similar to aviation, medicine had to learn that those kind of (non-technical) skills were not acquired unless specifically taught. For flight crews, CRM training was originally created to address these issues. Especially for anesthesia, but for other health care domains as well, the VA-Stanford group modeled their training after aviation CRM and named it ACRM.[181] For a broader use in health care, oftentimes ACRM is also referred to solely as CRM. The ACRM approach has been highly influential. ACRM curricula and ACRM-like curricula are taught at simulation centers around the world, not only in anesthesia, but in many other domains of health care, including ICU, emergency medicine, labor and delivery, trauma, and field responders.[3,93,222,243-247]. Fig. 7.17 shows a typical CRM crew training scenario.

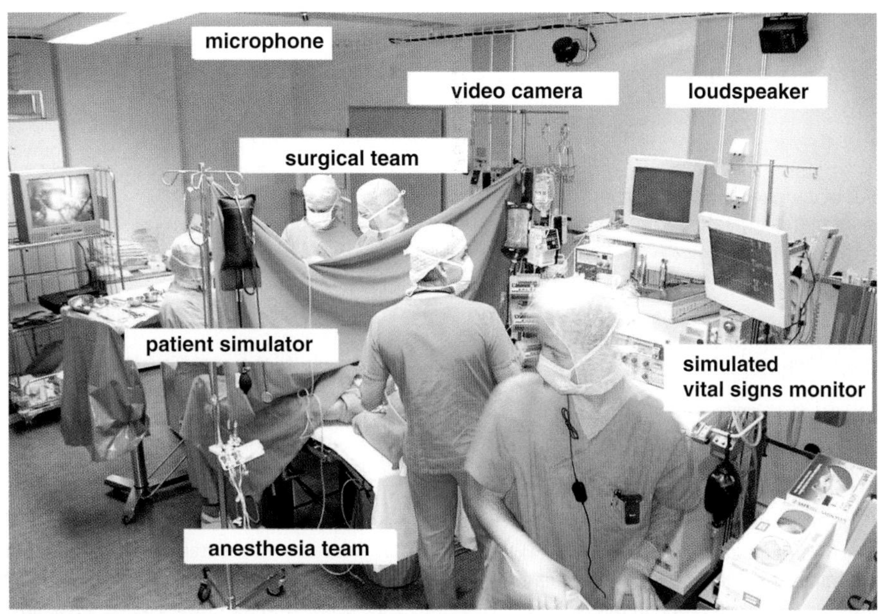

Fig. 7.17 Crisis resource management training scenario during crew training. The surgical team is performing a complicated endoscopic surgical procedure replayed on screen. The anesthesia team must solve a clinical problem and coordinate with the surgical team. Video cameras, microphones, and loudspeakers provide the necessary connectivity and later debriefing tools. *(Photograph taken by M. Rall at the Center for Patient Safety and Simulation, University Hospital, Tübingen, Germany.)*

ANESTHESIA CRISIS RESOURCE MANAGEMENT CURRICULA

A working group of the original ACRM centers (VA-Stanford, Boston CMS, Toronto Sunnybrook) promulgated a set of criteria to be met by a curriculum to be called either ACRM or ACRM-like. Box 7.3 presents an excerpt of the criteria.

Among others, these criteria delineate:

1. To target the above mentioned identified gaps in training, approximately 50% of the emphasis of ACRM is on the medical and technical management of specific high-risk perioperative situations, and about 50% is on generic principles of crisis management that apply to nearly every complex patient care situation. The key teaching points of ACRM are shown in Box 7.4. These points are emphasized during the ACRM simulation course, and their occurrence or omission is highlighted during the debriefing sessions.
2. Special training is needed for instructors in ACRM-like curricula. The authors' experience suggests that the most difficult aspect of ACRM instructing is debriefing, and new instructors require a significant period of experience, preferably under supervision by more senior instructors, before being ready to be fully independent instructors. Several groups working separately or collectively have developed comprehensive training programs on simulation instruction, including substantial modules on debriefing and scenario design (see later subchapter on instructor qualification).
3. ACRM-like curricula employ a variety of teaching modalities to achieve these goals, including the following:
   - Comprehensive textbook on anesthesia crisis management: *Crisis Management in Anesthesiology (now in an expanded second edition)*.[24] This book includes didactic material on ACRM principles and a comprehensive catalog of critical incidents in anesthesia that provides guidelines for preventing, recognizing, and managing 99 perioperative situations in a uniform format. The catalog section of the text is intended to provide study material to increase anesthesiologists' stock of precompiled response plans to common and uncommon situations. This textbook has been translated into Japanese, German (first edition), Spanish, and Portuguese (second edition).
   - Brief presentation and discussion reviewing the principles of CRM and patient safety.
   - Use of trigger videos meant to initiate discussion, sometimes from a non-health care setting (e.g., commercial aviation, British warship during the Napoleonic wars).
   - Group exercises analyzing a patient care event, presented as: (i) an actual patient care event captured on video or a reconstruction thereof; (ii) a video of a presentation as if from a morbidity and mortality conference; or (iii) a written report of the event.
   - The core of simulation activities in ACRM-like curricula will be several hours of different, complex, multifaceted, realistic simulation scenarios in which participants rotate through different roles, including for example primary anesthesiologist, first responder (called cold, with no knowledge of the situation), and scrub tech. Other instructors or actors play the roles of surgeons, nurses, and technicians as in a real perioperative setting. Each situation is followed by a detailed debriefing (see later in discussion on "Debriefing").

Several publications have detailed the response of participants with varying levels of experience to ACRM training or its equivalent.[181,248-250] Participants have

BOX 7.3 Characteristics of Anesthesia Crisis Resource Management-like Simulation Training

Objectives

- Learn generic principles of complex problem solving, decision making, resource management, and teamwork behavior.
- Improve participants' medical and technical, cognitive, and social skills in the recognition and treatment of realistic, complex medical situations.
- Enhance capacity for reflection, self-discovery, and teamwork and for building a personalized tool kit of attitudes, behaviors, and skills.

Aim

- Prevent, ameliorate, and resolve critical incidents.

Course Characteristics

- A realistic simulation environment replicates a relevant work setting (or an actual patient care setting with in situ simulation).
- Personnel will represent those persons found in the typical work environment of the participant, including nurses, surgeons, and technicians.
- The bulk of the training course consists of realistic simulations followed by detailed debriefings.
- Primary participants can request and receive help from other participants.
- Participants may rotate among various roles during different scenarios to gain fresh perspectives.
- Simulation scenarios may be supplemented by additional modalities, including activities such as assigned readings, didactic presentations, analysis of videotapes, role playing, or group discussions.
- Training involves significant time (>4 h, typically ≥8 h) and is conducted with a small group of participants.

Content Characteristics

- Scenarios require participants to engage in appropriate professional interactions.
- At least 50% of the emphasis of the course is on crisis resource management behavior (nontechnical skills) rather than medical or technical issues (non-technical skills are discussed in Chapter 6).
- Observation only is not equivalent to actual participation in one or more scenarios.

Faculty Characteristics

- Training is intense and entails a high level of involvement of faculty with the participants and a low participant-to-faculty ratio.
- Faculty members, especially those leading debriefing, have special training or experience in conducting crisis resource management–oriented training.

Debriefing Characteristics

- Debriefings are performed with the whole group of participants together and use (as appropriate) audio-video recordings of the simulation sessions.
- Debriefings emphasize constructive critique and analysis in which the participants are given the greatest opportunity possible to speak and to critique and to learn from each other.

BOX 7.4 Key Points in Anesthesia Crisis Resource Management

A detailed explanation of the crisis resource management key points is given in *Chapter 6*. The key points are derived from the publication of Rall and Gaba in the sixth edition of Miller's Anesthesia[367] and presented here in their updated, current version.

1. Know the environment.
2. Anticipate and plan.
3. Call for help early.
4. Establish leadership and followership with appropriate assertiveness.
5. Distribute the workload. Use 10 s for 10 min concept.
6. Mobilize all available resources.
7. Communicate effectively—speak up.
8. Use all available information.
9. Prevent and manage fixation errors.
10. Cross and double check. Never assume anything.
11. Use cognitive aids.
12. Reevaluate repeatedly. Apply 10 s for 10 min concept.
13. Use good teamwork. Coordinate with and support others.
14. Allocate attention wisely.
15. Set priorities dynamically.

been extremely positive about their experience in the ACRM course, and most believe that it contributes to their safe practice of anesthesia.[180] In training settings where "practice improvement" is a specific target such courses can trigger credible efforts at personal or system change.[248] At the Stanford residency, ACRM has been extended to a multilevel course conducted over several years (i.e., ACRM 1, 2, 3). As the course levels progress, the scenarios become more complex and involve subspecialties of anesthesia. Besides, additional teaching modules cover other important aspects of organizational safety, such as systems thinking in morbidity and mortality conference settings or peer review settings, follow-up response to severe adverse perioperative events, and disclosure to the patient or family of bad news after an adverse event.

ACRM courses and ACRM-like variants are now offered worldwide and are often mandatory for trainees (and in some cases for experienced personnel). Salas and colleagues published an excellent critical overview about prerequisites for effective CRM training.[251]

BENEFITS OF CRISIS RESOURCE MANAGEMENT-BASED SIMULATION TRAINING

The literature on published benefits of CRM training effects is large; here are a few examples. Knudson and colleagues found a significant improvement in overall and teamwork scores in surgical residents taking care of critically injured simulated trauma patients if the residents had undergone CRM-like simulation training.[90] In a simulation study, no-flow time rates were significantly lower after CRM training paralleled with improved leadership verbalization.[153] A study in a multidisciplinary obstetrical setting involving anesthesia professionals showed a significant improvement in interprofessional teamwork and improved stress recognition after a CRM intervention.[220] In a prospective 3-year cohort study Haerkens and colleagues showed a decline in serious complications and the standardized mortality ratio, decreasing occurrence of cardiac arrests, and improving cardiopulmonary resuscitation success rates

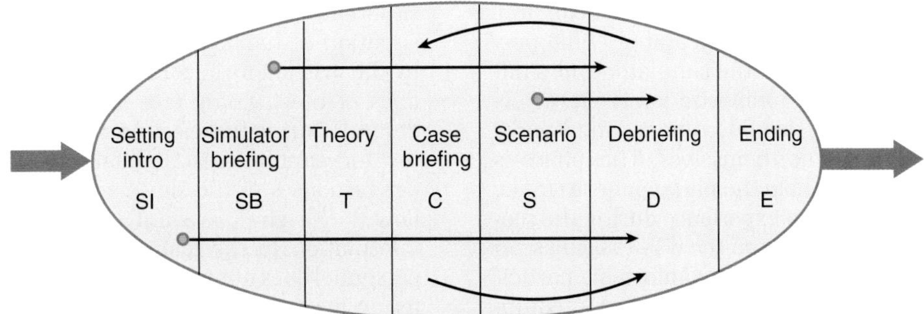

Fig. 7.18 Anatomy of the simulation exercise. A simulation exercise consists of different modules or different phases (e.g., simulation introduction *[SI]*, simulator and clinical environment briefing/"familiarization" *[SB]*, theory input *[T]*, case briefing *[C]*, scenario *[S]*, debriefing *[D]*, ending *[E]*). This figure shows a typical flow for a simulation course. If more than one scenario takes place during the course, the sequence form [C] to [D] is repeated for each scenario. The different modules are interrelated, and problems arising in one module can affect other modules *(thin arrows)*. *(Figure with courtesy of P. Dieckmann.)*

after a CRM-based intervention in a 32-bed ICU.[252] Moffatt-Bruce et al. published a significant reduction rate of adverse events and described return on investment after a system-wide implementation of CRM in 12 different hospital units including perioperative staff.[253]

Anatomy of a Patient Simulation Team Training Exercise

Whenever simulation is used it is important to consider its conceptual basis and the contextual factors that influence its use.[254,255] Therefore, with a focus on (CRM-oriented) mannequin-based patient simulation conducted for health care professionals, the next subchapters (1) give an overview of the training setting and important elements of a simulation exercise; discuss (2) the design of simulation scenarios and their execution; and (3) the modalities of the professionals' debriefing after a simulation scenario. Even though focused on the mannequin-based patient simulation conducted for health care professionals, many of the conceptual approaches presented below are identical or need to be modified only slightly to encompass other choices in the 12 dimensions of simulation.

Simulation activities vary in terms of goals and objectives. Most of the time, simulation scenarios are integrated into a multifaceted curriculum, which itself must be situated relative to the overall educational and training pathway of individuals and groups. Hence, for any given simulation activity both the conceptual and physical setting influence how the exercise is conducted, how it is perceived by participants, what participants learn, and which learned items are applicable in the clinical work domain.[255]

A simulation course/training itself can be divided analytically in different, interconnected phases as shown in Fig. 7.18.[255] Not all phases need to be present at each exercise and conversely some phases—like "scenario" and "debriefing"—may be repeated several times in a longer session.

Optimally the interconnected phases of the simulation exercise should be coordinated. If, for example, the briefing/familiarization is inadequate, participants may not be able to properly immerse themselves in the scenarios and debriefing might be impaired. The role of the simulation instructor changes throughout the different phases of the simulation training—from providing instruction in the beginning of a course to facilitating learning during debriefing. Based to a large extent on the work of Dieckmann,[255] the different phases of a simulation exercise (see Fig. 7.18) are discussed next, using the timeframe and elements of a simulation-based course as an example.

Pre-Briefing (PB). The pre-briefing introduces or reminds participants in advance about the course, its goals, and processes to appropriately situate the activity in their overall training, establish a positive attitude, and review the schedule of activities. An exercise that can be useful (stemming from advice from Ruokamo and Keskitalo from the University of Lapland) is to ask and discuss with participants "what do you want to learn or explore" in today's simulation course?, and similarly to ask the instructors "what are you interested in teaching or exploring?" This conversation engages the participants and demonstrates the instructors' interest in trying to address many of the preferences of the learners.

Simulation introduction (SI). An important aspect at the beginning of a session is to provide an overview about the course and the rules and norms of conduct for the set of exercises.[256] It is also important to provide a shared understanding for the simulation participants of the events that transpire during the course.[111] Besides, it is important to create a positive atmosphere to maximize learning, often referred to as *"psychological safety,"* or as recently published a *"safe container."*[121] Edmondson has defined psychological safety as *"the shared belief that the team is safe for interpersonal risk taking."*[257] Often this has a lot to do with ensuring the confidentiality of the simulation environment (i.e., "what happens here stays here") and that debriefings will "critique the performance, not the performer." Psychological safety *"is not about creating a comfortable space, it is about making it 'ok' to be uncomfortable."*[258]

Simulator and clinical environment briefing (SB) ("familiarization"). Participants need to be familiar with the simulator and the simulated environment in order to perform the closest to reality as possible, and they should not be distracted by technical or procedural uncertainty during the scenario. The participants can best master the scenario and actively engage in it if they know (1) how the simulator works ("normal" breathing sounds, "normal" pulses, intubation, intravenous access, etc.); (2) what it is able to do or not do; (3) how the simulated environment works (how to call for help, how to use the simulated equipment, etc.); and (4) what participants are able to perform on the simulator and what they need to pretend doing. Familiarization is characterized through explanations, demonstrations, and hands-on time for the participants themselves. This phase is very important in order to help the participants to make the best use of the simulation experience during the scenario. The plastic mannequin is on the way to being seen and treated as a patient. The more comfortable participants feel with the simulator and the simulation equipment, the less they will be scared or tense during the scenario. And more reflective learning about medical and non-technical skills can take place during the debriefing because the debriefing will not become about discussing the confusions and challenges regarding the simulation technology or environment. Therefore, it benefits both the instructor and the participants to have enough time for the familiarization process.

Presentation or discussion of theory (T). Theories of human performance or of clinical work processes might or might not be part of the course. Most exercises have didactic or theory components on relevant content information. Those components can either serve for transfer of (new) medical or technical knowledge, or for a refresher lecture on certain algorithms, but also for the introduction of (anesthesia) crisis resource management-related skills (ACRM, CRM) and patient safety issues (Chapter 6). Sometimes educational material is made available in advance through readings or online exercises. Sometimes lectures or group-work modules are put in place at different junctures of the training.

Breaks (B). For complex and long-lasting courses breaks are important for recreation and for socialization among participants and with instructors. Breaks provide a venue for informal sharing and storytelling, one of the many learning opportunities during a simulation training outside of a simulation scenario.

Case briefing (C). Because the simulator is not a real patient itself providing clinical information and because the environment of a simulation imposes several challenges, there are different ways to ensure that participants have certain relevant information concerning the case and the simulation reality before, or at the beginning of, the scenario. Sometimes it is natural for a participant to take over a case from another clinician (in fact in ACRM starting every case from the beginning would waste a lot of time). Such a handoff can be scripted to be complete or cursory as appropriate. In other cases the context information can be presented verbally or in written form by an instructor. Other information that would not be readily available in context might include the look or smell of the patient or the specific location of care (e.g., main OR vs. off-site ambulatory surgery center).

Simulation scenario (S). The scenario and—when possible—the debriefing together form the core of the learning experience during simulation. Simulation scenarios are more than clinical cases. They are the vehicle to reflect on medical knowledge as well as personal and team performance in a safe learning environment that elucidates similar behaviors as during real-world cases. Most simulation exercises involve a scenario that simulates a given clinical situation, challenging the participants to deal with the situation at hand. The scenario is designed in advance by the instructors in accordance with the learning objectives of the training (see later subchapter on scenario design). During the execution of the scenario, the instructor (or simulationist/simulation technician) regulates the responses of the simulator and adapts the scenario flow[259,260]; gives relevant patient, situation, or clinical information to the team that the simulator or clinical personnel does not provide itself[260,261] (see later subchapter on live in-scenario guiding); manages the exercise to enable participants to optimally act as if[259] treating a real patient (see later subchapter on scenario design).

Debriefing (D). Most training scenarios are immediately followed by some form of feedback or debriefing, respectively. Fanning and Gaba give an overview of the origin and background, the role, the models, the structural process, the elements, and several other modalities of debriefing in simulation-based learning in their recommended review.[238] The learning objectives, the target audience, and the simulation modalities drive the decision whether a debriefing is useful and if so how in-depth the debriefing process needs to be. In some courses, feedback is only minimal, whereas other courses have a dedicated debriefing session after each scenario that take as long, or even longer, than the scenario itself (see later subchapter on debriefing techniques). Several different debriefing methods exist.[24,105,109,110,238] Debriefing can be facilitated sometimes by strategically presenting snippets of the recording of the scenario.[117,238]

Ending (E). Especially for multiple-scenario courses, a separate final session may be included to end the course. This phase represents an opportunity to summarize issues that were covered and to reflect on how best to apply these lessons to real patient care.

Scenario Design and Execution: Knowing the Learning Objectives and Making It Real

The design of scenarios for interactive simulation team trainings can be tricky and typically differs from preparing training exercises for traditional curricula.

"The key is the program, not the hardware"[62] was a truth about simulation learned early in aviation simulation and similarly possesses validity for the scenario design and execution with patient simulation. Using simulation in a goal-oriented way is at least as much about the conceptual aspects of the technique as it is about the technology of the simulation devices. An understanding of the conceptual and theoretical aspects of simulation is helpful for determining the right applications of the technique and the important matchups to be made in the design and conduct of simulation exercises to obtain the best results. When used most effectively, simulation can be—to borrow a line from the music band U2—"...even better than the real thing."

In the following sections the design and conduct of scenarios for a patient simulation are touched on more closely, considering (1) establishing learning objectives; (2) applying cognitive load theory to scenario design; (3) pointing out constraints and limitations of the design, discussing

(4) conceptual issues of reality, realism, and relevance; and (5) in-scenario information and guiding.

There is a vast aggregation of literature concerning instructional design for all kinds of simulation applications. For detailed information the reader is referred to further literature.[23,77,115,177,262] The topic is covered extensively in most of the instructor training curricula that are offered at sites around the world. International and regional simulation meetings (e.g., the International Meeting on Simulation in Healthcare [IMSH] of the SSH, or the annual meeting of the Society in Europe for Simulation Applied to Medicine [SESAM]) often provide workshops on scenario design. The user groups of the major simulator manufacturers also have workshops on the topic.

The following sections can only serve as an introduction to the topic and again focus mainly on (CRM) mannequin-based patient simulation conducted for health care professionals.

GOAL ORIENTED: ESTABLISHING LEARNING OBJECTIVES

Learning objectives provide the reason and frame for the simulation scenario. They contain clinical and technical skills, or non-technical skills such as communication, leadership, teamwork, situation awareness, decision making, and task management (see Crisis Resource Management, CRM, Chapter 6). Optimally, scenarios are chosen that stress the individual's diagnostic and problem-solving abilities, the clinical and technical knowledge, and the core aspects of CRM.[75,217]

Learning objectives can be preset by a curriculum, determined via needs analysis, intuitively known by the simulation-savvy clinician educators, or learned about in instructor training or in the literature. Learning objectives operationalize relevant questions by defining who should be able to do what and in what situations.[78]

Simulation scenario design may be thought of in a stepwise, layered fashion. Research in work psychology suggests that, for the purpose of learning, it is helpful to de-construct complex tasks into phases and hierarchical levels. For example, the scenario "resuscitate the patient" includes three main goals: (1) diagnose cardiac arrest (subgoals: check pulse, check breathing, check "brain"), (2) oxygenate brain (subgoals: open airway, cardiac massage, ventilate), and (3) reestablish spontaneous circulation (subgoals: defibrillate, administer epinephrine) which require team members to coordinate (e.g., ensure that all team members know diagnosis, distribute task).[263] This insight into what behaviors are expected of a team during the scenario facilitates not only the design of the scenario as such,[115] but it also helps educators to direct their attention while observing the team's performance and possibly sharing the workload among them by distributing observational tasks in the co-debriefing setting.[264] Furthermore, it helps educators to guide the debriefing.[107] Learning objectives and performance expectations should be considered in advance in order to use the debriefing to close potential gaps and guide teams to maintain good performance.

COGNITIVE LOAD THEORY: NOT TOO MUCH, NOT TOO LITTLE

When designing and conducting simulations the learning opportunity would ideally match the abilities and learning needs of the participants. If the scenario is too difficult, participants' can be overwhelmed and their learning likely compromised. Conversely, if the scenario is too easy, participants will find no challenge, may be bored, and won't learn very much. Cognitive load theory[265] provides a framework to distinguish different aspects in a learning situation that illuminate the "difficulty" of a scenario so as to optimize it for learners. In this theory, three different forms of cognitive load are distinguished. The overall difficulty can be thought of as the sum of the following three parts: (1) Intrinsic cognitive load, which describes the complexity/difficulty of the material to be addressed. This depends somewhat on the learner's prior knowledge but beyond that some issues are just more complex than others for most. (2) Extraneous load, which stems from the presentation of the material to be learned, e.g., a well-structured textbook might make learning easier compared to a chaotic lecture. (3) Germane load, which describes the internal processes and the cognitive energy needed to process information.

Cognitive load theory would suggest, for example, that asking novice anesthesia professionals to manage both a complex clinical situation and a challenging interpersonal one may result in overload. Unfamiliarity with simulation will also raise the extrinsic load—participants have to interpret the pretend situation as if it is the real thing, making it difficult to concentrate on the lessons to be learned. The germane load might be increased when participants are concerned about being observed. They not only need to consider what the best course of action in the scenario might be, but, at the same time, also try to manage the impression that they make on the instructors and observers.

A good simulation scenario will take these different elements into account. Extraneous load can be optimized by carefully designing scenarios and by PB instructions.[255] Germane load might be optimized by helping participants become more familiar and comfortable being in simulations, for example, by well-designed simulation familiarization, or by increasing the complexity of scenarios slowly.

CONSTRAINTS AND LIMITATIONS OF SCENARIO DESIGN IDEAS

It is easy to suggest a scenario on paper but more difficult to translate it into an effective scenario for actual use. Limitations and constraints of the available simulators, personnel resources at hand, the props or external systems that would be needed, and the time needed to set up and run the proposed scenario must be considered. Most scenarios are first generated with a core idea, a "kernel" that is then fleshed out by discussion in an iterative fashion, with creative redesign or minor technical modifications. Ideally the new, redefined scenario is tested out first by instructors and technical staff, or pilot-tested with a volunteer group of participants from the target population. With highly experienced instructors a new scenario may need only a technical walkthrough before it is run for real participants. All scenarios can get better with time as glitches are found and refinements made.

SCENARIO DESIGN TEMPLATES AND SCENARIO TEMPLATES

Many centers have developed design templates for the development of their scenarios. Box 7.5 shows the key questions

BOX 7.5 Key Considerations for Simulation Scenario Scripts

Based on script templates provided by Dieckmann and Rall (https://www.inpass.de/downloadshtml/downloadscenarioscript/), the key information a scenario script should provide includes:

- Scenario name (quick reference)
- Major medical challenge of scenario
- Major cockpit resource management (CRM) challenge of scenario
- Learning goals (medical and [!] CRM)
- Brief narrative description of scenario
- Staffing (instructor/simulation team and participants)
- Case briefing (all participants together or separate briefings for different teams)
- Simulator setup and mannequin preparation
- Props needed
- Scenario "lifesavers"[259] for both excellent and bad performance of participants

Usually, the scenario script contains (1) a summary sheet with brief notes of the above mentioned topics and (2) a more detailed description of the scenario in regard to those questions on several other pages. The proper use of scenario scripts is a regular part of many instructor training courses.

for the design of scenarios. Long scenario templates that are freely available include Dieckmann and Rall's (https://www.inpass.de/downloadshtml/downloadscenarioscript/) and the Duke University template (https://anesthesiology.duke.edu/?page_id=825706). Some journals publish detailed scenario descriptions and some professional societies have created scenario repositories for members; the American Society of Anesthesiologists (ASA) Simulation Committee has a repository for scenarios to be shared among its ASA-endorsed simulation programs. By now, many scenario templates are freely available on the Internet. In general, long and detailed templates are only needed when a scenario is to be shared widely, or when there is a need to formally document it. Simpler templates will likely suffice for in-house use by a single simulation center.

REALITY VERSUS REALISM

Simulation is a complex social undertaking.[155] The concepts discussed in the upcoming section concern the nature and the impact of "fidelity" and "realism" as they apply to simulation and the goals of simulation. Both are terms widely used, and misused, in simulation design. In this chapter the concept of relevance is covered briefly. All three concepts are important components of engaging participants during simulation, an important aspect of conducting meaningful exercises.

A patient simulation exercise is itself a real occurrence that is actually happening. The exercise is a *reality*, but it is intended to represent another reality in the real world of patient care. Hence, it may or may not be perceived that way. *"Realism"* addresses the question of how closely a replication of a situation is needed to meaningfully represent this situation to participants. Aviation simulators, for example, are so realistic now that pilots with experience flying one aircraft are routinely certified to fly a totally new or different aircraft, even though they have never flown the actual aircraft before. Nestel, Krogh, and Kolbe explored realism in health care simulations in detail.[266] In their work, the authors also use the term *"meaningfulness"* in proposing strategies to help simulation educators make sense of decisions about realism.

There is an important distinction between the realism of a *simulator* (a device) and that of a *simulation* (the exercise). For example, a simulator could be indistinguishable from a real human being (e.g., an actor playing a standardized patient) and yet be used in an implausible and useless fashion, so that the simulation itself is not realistic. Conversely, certain kinds of simulation realism can be evoked by exercises that use simple simulators or even no simulator at all (see below).

It is naïve (though frequent) to think that greater realism of a simulation exercise will automatically lead to better achievement of its goals. Maximum "realism" is neither needed nor desired for every type of simulation endeavor. For some applications with some target populations, it can be highly advantageous to reduce the realism to heighten the learning experience.[157] On the other hand, merely creating a realistic simulation does not guarantee meaning or utility (e.g., learning) for the participants.[155,156] The different concepts and explanations with regard to this matter have been discussed repeatedly in the literature.[155-158,260,267-269] However, as "realism" is a complicated set of ideas in simulation, results of studies trying to investigate roots and effects of simulation realism are not conclusive, in part because each study may concentrate on a different aspect of the complex whole. Different fidelities and dimensions are used to describe or achieve the realism of simulation, as described in the following.

Different (practical) fidelities to create simulation realism. Alessi[270] defined fidelity as the "degree to which a simulation replicates reality" (p. 203). Several concepts about simulation fidelity exist.[198,260,271] These include physical fidelity (the device replicates physical aspects of the human body), environmental fidelity (the simulation room looks like the relevant clinical site), equipment fidelity (the clinical equipment works like or is the real thing), and psychological fidelity (the simulation evokes behaviors similar to the real situation). Realism is thought to be achieved by various forms of validity, such as face validity (looks and feels real to participants), content validity (the exercise covers content relevant to the target situation), construct validity (the simulation can replicate performance or behavior according to predefined constructs about work in real situations), and predictive validity (performance during a simulation exercise predicts performance in an analogous real situation.

Different (theoretical) dimensions to create simulation realism. In 2007, Dieckmann, Gaba, and Rall published an article attempting to clarify some issues about realism, reality, relevance, and how they influence the purpose of conducting simulations.[155] In their article, they applied the model of thinking about reality by the German psychologist Laucken to the realism and fidelity of simulation. Laucken described three modes of thinking about reality: physical, semantic, and phenomenal fidelity. Another publication on modes of thinking about reality was published by colleagues from Boston.[158] Apart from those definitions a variety of terms exist to describe conceptual simulation design, in particular with regard to fidelity. To gain a better understanding of the various terms and their meaning, Paige and Morin published a systematic review article on that matter and additionally suggested to divide the concepts of fidelity into physical (including environmental and equipment), conceptual, and psychological.[260] The ideas and concepts presented below are largely contributed by Dieckmann and his adaptation of broader psychological concepts to simulation in medicine:

Physical mode of realism. The physical mode concerns aspects of the simulation that can be measured in fundamental physical and chemical terms and dimensions (e.g., centimeters, grams, and seconds). For example, the weight of the mannequin, the force generated during chest compressions, and the duration of a scenario all are physical aspects of simulation reality. Despite their roughly human shape, existing mannequins have many unrealistic physical elements, for example they are made of plastic, not flesh and bone; they may have unusual mechanical noises detectable during auscultation of the chest; the "skin" does not change color.

The physical mode of simulation also relates to clinical equipment and the clinical environment. (1) Some equipment used in mannequin-based simulation is fully functional and physically identical to the real thing. Labeled syringes may contain only water instead of real medications. (2) An ISS in an actual hospital room and bed has a higher physical realism than does the same equipment in a conference room.

Semantic mode of realism. The semantic mode of realism concerns concepts and their relationships concerning clinical information and its meaning. For example, in a simulation of hemorrhagic shock, how does the participant make sense of what is going on? Within the semantic mode, a simulation of hemorrhage could be described in semantical terms as "bleeding" of flow rate x beginning at time y occurring at site z that is associated with a blood pressure of b that shows a decrease after some time from the prior value of a. It is semantically irrelevant how the information is transmitted or represented. The same pieces of *information* could be represented either using a vital signs monitor, a verbal description, or the tactile perception of decreasingly palpable pulses. The semantic mode allows the simulation exercise to represent a real situation. It allows lifeless, rosy, smiling simulators to be treated as if they were real patients. It allows water-filled syringes to be treated as if they contain effective drugs.

PATIENT SIMULATION ACTION BOX

If the right and sufficient clinical information is given to the participants at the right time, in their minds the inanimate mannequin can become a severely ill patient (see later section on "in-scenario information and guiding"). At the same time it is important for instructors to remember, in particular during the debriefing, that because meaningful simulation depends on interpreting information, it is not always interpreted by participants the way that the instructor imagines it will be.

Phenomenal mode of realism. The *phenomenal mode* deals with the learner's engagement and experience in the simulation including emotions, values, motivation, self-awareness, and beliefs. If participants are fully engaged in the simulation, then they are likely to act as if they are treating a real patient in the real clinical environment. For many purposes, providing high phenomenal realism is the key goal, but sufficient physical and semantic realism are means to this end.

PATIENT SIMULATION ACTION BOX

A good simulation scenario does not necessarily need to be designed as realistic as possible, for example having artificial blood all over the mannequin during a trauma scenario. A good simulation scenario can create the appropriate sense of realism by a combination of the following:

(1) … the simulator and environment used
(2) … the case presented, the team composition, and the professional role of each participant
(3) …clinical equipment used, or sufficient semantic equivalents
(4) … the briefing before the simulation case starts
(5) … instructor feedback when the simulator is examined (see later section, "live in-scenario information and guiding"). The application of those aspects is not trivial; they influence the way the simulation is perceived by clinical professionals.

SIMULATION REALISM AND SIMULATION RELEVANCE

The relevance of a simulation exercise concerns the match between the characteristics of the exercise and the reasons for which the exercise is conducted. Scenarios should be relevant to the trainees, but this depends on many factors, including the trainees' backgrounds and experience, the method of conducting the scenario, and related parts of the simulation course (e.g., familiarization with simulator and simulated environment, case briefing, etc.).

In fact, it is worth utilizing unrealistic elements ("unreality") in order to maximize the learning—a useful slogan is "the point is not to 'fool' them but rather to teach them." So, for example, when training on invasive procedures, it is typical to forego phenomenal realism and emphasize physical and semantic realism so that psychomotor skills can be the focus. Similarly, physical realism may be sacrificed when necessary by time compression or expansion. Boring parts of a case may be skipped for experienced personnel whereas for inexperienced clinicians situations that could become lethal extremely quickly (e.g., swap of N_2O for O_2 in the pipeline) may be slowed down so that inexperienced clinicians can try to think their way out of the problem. If such a situation were allowed to evolve at its normal speed, it would transition to management of cardiac arrest before the participants could deal with the original problem. Other uses of "unreality" include cognitive scaffolding, which provides various forms of assistance—sometimes a teacher or coach in the simulation room—or extra cues to help participants as they struggle with decision making and therapy selection.

IN-SCENARIO INFORMATION AND GUIDING

Although full-scale mannequins mimic a wide range of human features, they differ from the body of an actual patient. This gap implies a need for simulation instructors to provide in-scenario information to help participants understand scenarios. In-scenario information and guiding may also be needed to help (early) learners progress in the scenario if they are stuck or on the wrong path. Different terms such as clues, triggers, prompts, hints, and instructional support have been found in the literature associated with the concept of cueing in a simulation activity.[260] Dieckmann et al. used the unique phrase "scenario life savers."[259] Many cues and "life savers" can be used within the logic of the scenario in ways that do not disrupt the experience.

In general, one good way to feed information to participants in patient simulations about various phenomena that cannot be simulated physically is to announce the missing signs, symptoms, or examination results. Escher and colleagues summarized four methods that instructors used to provide such extra scenario information and how the different methods to convey information affected how scenarios played out.[261] The methods found included cues from (1) confederates, (2) bystanders, (3) loudspeakers from the control room to the scenario room, or via (4) an earpiece. Even though Escher et al. conclude that the mediation of information by a loudspeaker or an earpiece from the adjacent control room could be disturbing for team communication, the authors of this chapter see several advantages in the use of in-scenario audio guidance. In their opinion, audio guidance is especially helpful for feedback in those kind of situations: (a) physical examination results, such as (misleading) auscultation results, or results of abdominal palpation but usually only after the participant has credibly attempted to obtain that result physically; and (b) *immediate* correction of mental models that are not in line with the scenario (i.e., (misleading) auscultation apparently indicates pneumothorax, but there is in fact no pneumothorax).

This kind of in-scenario semantic information is incorporated by participants into their mental model of the situation at hand during the simulation and helps them to "stay in" the simulation despite physically treating a plastic mannequin.

Debriefing: Heart and Soul of Patient Simulation

As introduced in the section on the "anatomy of a simulation course" (see Fig. 7.18), conducting simulation training is not only about running the simulation scenario but equally about how, in debriefing, the participants are facilitated to reflect about what they experienced. The philosophy of teaching and learning in a debriefing of a CRM-based simulation course differs from the traditional clinical teaching style (Table 7.3).[238] For more information on debriefing in health care simulation the reader is referred to further literature.[24,105,109-111,113,238,272-276] This chapter can only serve as an introduction to the topic and focuses mainly on patient simulation with focus on (CRM) team training.

TABLE 7.3 Traditional Teaching Versus Facilitation in Simulation Training Courses

Traditional Teaching: "Teacher"	New way of teaching: "Facilitator"
Focus on theoretical or clinical knowledge only	Focus additionally on human factors/ CRM
Focus on "what" happened/"what" or "who" was *wrong*	Focus on "why" things went wrong (deeper analysis) *and* on "why" things went well
(T) is the (absolute, infallible) expert.	(I) possesses expertise, but moderates different ideas on eye level, uses knowledge and expertise of (P), discusses own views with peers.
(T) tells participants what to do better next time.	(I) helps (P) to find out root causes for their performance, examines possible solutions together.
(T) knows what is right / important for (P).	(I) helps to self-reflect, gain realistic self-awareness / consciousness; (I) guides debriefing toward interesting areas, but is open for topics relevant to (P).
(T) speaks the most during feedback.	(I) stimulates and guides discussion among participants during debriefing, but does not speak the most.
(T) is a domain expert.	(I) additionally is a CRM expert.
(T) has no special training in patient simulation-based learning.	(I) has special training and/or experience in patient simulation-based learning.
(T) makes no video-assisted feedback.	(I) makes strategic use of video when relevant to enhance debriefing.
(T) determines whether (P) has learned the intended lesson.	(I) gauges whether (P) is engaged in discussion and understands relevant issues but (P)'s experience is too complex to assess simply

CRM, Crisis Resource Management; *(I)*, Instructor/Facilitator; *(P)*, Participant; *(T)*, teacher.

SIMULATORS (DEVICES) DON'T TEACH

Most simulation training exercises involve some kind of feedback or debriefing that can be given in many different ways and settings.[111,113,238,272-275] The terms *debriefing* and *feedback* are often used synonymously, but there exists a difference in their meaning. *Feedback* is used with the intention to modify thinking and / or behavior and generally involves comparing the observed performance to a standard (whether formally or informally defined). Usually it is a one-directional flow of information about the performance from the instructor to simulation participants.[111] *Debriefing* refers to a special time and format for discussing an episode of action in the past; it is the counterpoint to a briefing, which occurs before an action or task. In contrast to feedback, debriefing is viewed as a bidirectional, interactive, and reflective discussion or conversation that *"may occur between simulation participants and facilitators [instructors], or among participants themselves, or some combination thereof"* [p. 209].[111]

In medicine, inspired by its use in aviation CRM, the debriefing concept was introduced to simulation training by Gaba and colleagues as part of ACRM simulation training for anesthesia teams.[181,217] Over the years debriefing after simulation training has been refined so that it has become an indispensable component of many simulation curricula.[273]

INSTRUCTION VERSUS FACILITATION—A NEW WAY OF TEACHING

In many learning contexts, the person who is in charge of the training usually is referred to as "instructor." In the debriefing idea described above, the instructor's role changes from an "instructor" to a "facilitator": instead of constantly instructing, the instructor's role is to *facilitate* the learning process. This is accomplished by *directing the participants* to the most interesting and important areas for consideration, *stimulating discussion* among participants to *find underlying issues* for their performance and *seeking individual solutions for future events* of similar type. For most instructors, *facilitation* is a new way of teaching and often must be learned, even if they have many years of traditional instructor teaching experience. In the simulation arena the term instructor refers to an individual who is responsible for overall direction of a simulation scenario; that person is often—but not always—one of the facilitators for the debriefing.

Fruitful discussion and learning can be triggered by reflecting on both aspects of performance that worked well and those that were difficult or problematic (see also "Safety II", chapter 6). In their paper Dieckmann et al.[277] describe the "learning from success" approach to simulation and debriefing drawing on several theoretical frameworks.

PATIENT SIMULATION ACTION BOX

Ideally, the clinical expertise of the simulation participants should be represented in the clinical expertise of the instructors. For an interprofessional trauma team training, for example, it would be best to have instructor(s)/debriefer(s) from each of the relevant professions and disciplines, especially from anesthesiology, nursing, and surgery.

DEBRIEFING TECHNIQUES

Although debriefing styles differ at institutions, sites, and individuals around the world, a common ground is shared by most simulation-based educators: debriefing should *stimulate self-reflection*, and it should unpack *how* and *why* things happened the way they did.

Reviews of debriefing techniques in simulation by Fanning and Gaba,[238] Cheng et al.,[113] and Sawyer et al.[111] indicate the broad range of literature available regarding debriefing, and highlight the many models and approaches that can be used. Debriefing most commonly occurs soon after a scenario run, but the same techniques can be used during pauses in the simulation. Although it is possible for participants to debrief themselves, this would come with limitations due to lack of structure. Usually a post-event debriefing is guided by a facilitator.[111]

A variety of approaches to debriefing exist, each with its own structural phases and several conversational structures.[238] These include Debriefing with Good Judgement,[105-107] The Diamond,[108] SHARP,[278] PEARLS,[109] TeamGAINS,[110] Alternatives and Pros & Cons,[238] and others.[111-114] These conversational structures guide the flow and the context of the debriefing and divide it into various phases, each serving a specific focus and purpose. Whereas the phases differ, Sawyer and colleagues summarize that most frameworks highlight the importance of guiding the conversation from a beginning, through an examination of events, and then relate the aspects most relevant for clinical practice.[111] An example of a debriefing structure is shown in Table 7.4.

Although it is clear that debriefing plays a crucial role in simulation exercises,[119,198,279-281] there is little evidence supporting one format over another. This should not be surprising because the goal is broad, the experience of simulation is intense, and participants' interpretations and discussion are rich.

A qualitative interview study[275] with 24 expert debriefers showed that for experienced debriefers it is not about the specific concept, but about the sets of ideas and beliefs that represent the values and teaching philosophy used: *"the debriefer is a facilitator, who must be dedicated, honest, genuinely curious and possess the abilities to facilitate a reflective debriefing [....] following the learners needs and objectives [...]"* (p. 3).[275]

Apart from applying a similar structure to the debriefing, revealing one's stance and frames, and creating a safe learning environment, most experienced debriefers blend several debriefing models and conversation techniques and adapt them dynamically, depending on personal preferences, the learners' perceived needs, and the scenario as experienced by the debriefer.[275] Asking open-ended questions in order to facilitate the discussion and foster self-reflection and self-assessment on the part of the participants as well as using silence after a question asked by the instructor are other key elements of facilitated debriefing.[111] During this silence, internal thinking processes on the part of the trainees are taking place. Open-ended questions cannot be answered with "yes" or "no" and therefore trigger the participant to explain the situation from his or her point of view. Some facilitators, especially when they are not highly experienced, use a debriefing script or a cognitive aid to help them lead the debriefing conversation effectively. On the other hand, sometimes the debriefer can just sit back and listen; the best debriefings may be when most of the discussion is purely between the participants themselves, addressing issues that are on target for the instructor's purposes, in which case the facilitator will need to use very few specific techniques of debriefing.

For instructors, preparing for a good debriefing starts during the conduct of the scenario. A key skill for the debriefer is to be able to watch and listen carefully to what is happening in the scenario while also attending to the tasks of running it (Fig. 7.19).

For immersive, simulation-based team training, the debriefing sessions usually last approximately as long as the scenarios themselves, although a complex scenario may well generate a nuanced conversation that could go on for much longer. For shorter simulation activities, such as unannounced mock resuscitations, debriefings have to be much shorter. The number of debriefers can vary. Some prefer to have a single debriefer (or there may be only one

TABLE 7.4

Phases of debriefings: Issues relevant to (anesthesia) crisis resource management-based simulation debriefing.

The listed phases do not necessarily all have to be followed in this time sequence and order. Depending on the scenario, the participants' performance, and the debriefing format, several phases have to be repeated within the debriefing, especially during the debriefing center part, as indicated with the circle. Sometimes phases overlap when discussing the scenario.

PHASE OF DEBRIEFING		Explanation
Pre-Debriefing	Ending the scenario	If possible, the (SC) should not be stopped too early. (P) should be allowed to realize the natural end of (SC). Ideally, (SC) should not be terminated when (P) are in the thick of it, e.g., still caring for the patient and applying treatment measures.
	Scenario-to-debriefing transition	Most sites use debriefings immediately following the simulation. This allows the (I) to hear and see (P)s' direct reactions. A variant is to give the (P)s a few minutes to discuss the (SC) itself while the (I) is planning the (D).
Debriefing Start	Emotional venting	All (HS) are given the opportunity to say how they *felt* during the (SC). This vents pent-up feelings and may be a time to deal with anomalies in the (SC) (e.g., simulator malfunction, simulation artifact, etc.). In this phase, (P)s also can critique the (SC)—critique that the (I) should acknowledge and take seriously.
	Descriptive phase	(P)s describe what happened (or portions of the audio-video recordings are replayed) and what the clinical problem in the scenario was. Different points of view are shared (e.g., doctor vs. nurse vs. first responder vs. surgeon, etc.).
	Self-identification of issues	It is sometimes useful to ask (P) to identify issues that did not go well or what they would do differently, in order to give them the opportunity to critique themselves before anyone else does. Nevertheless, the (I) can and should help identify what the underlying causes were and the pros and cons of alternate approaches.
Debriefing Center Part	Discussion of clinical content	Any major issues of clinical treatment and related CRM points should be covered. A (D) should not end without discussing and clarifying any significant clinical errors and ensuring that participants understand the correct clinical management.
	Analysis	(D) should provide considerable analysis of *why* things happened vis-à-vis the intentions of all parties, as well as alternatives and their pros and cons.
	Transfer to the "real world"	Participants can discuss how lessons from the scenario or debriefing can be applied in the real clinical world. They should discuss barriers to improvement and ways to overcome them.
	Opportunities for systems improvement	When applicable, based on the analyses, (P)s can be asked to suggest how the system can be changed to improve handling of similar situations in the future.
Debriefing End	"Take-Home-Message"	A summary of the learned key points of the (D), either by (I) or (P), can be useful.
	Terminating the debriefing	(D) are rich in content and easily can extend beyond the time available. Thus, giving a time frame for the (D) and officially marking its end is a useful transition to preparing for the next (SC) or the end-of-day activities.

"Hot Seats" (HS) = Participants (P) who were actively involved in the scenario (SC); Debriefing Room (DB); Simulation Room (SR); Simulation (S), Instructor (I), Debriefing (D), Crisis Resource Management (CRM).

Provided by M. Rall & P. Dieckmann as used in their own courses, derived from the original ACRM-course structure by D. Gaba and colleagues and used by many others around the world.

instructor) but often there are two or more "co-debriefers." Coordinating multiple facilitators can be tricky (it is sometimes described as being like dancing). Cheng et al.[264] described several effective strategies for co-debriefing.

Generally, faculty members intending to be debriefers in immersive simulation-based education need special training and practice in this teaching method[105,119,238,282,283] and continuous experience and training throughout their career.[275] Several simulation centers conduct instructor training that emphasizes debriefing skills, and debriefing is a frequent topic of workshops at large simulation conferences.

Box 7.6 shows a selection of the learning myths—especially in regard to the debriefing of patient simulation team

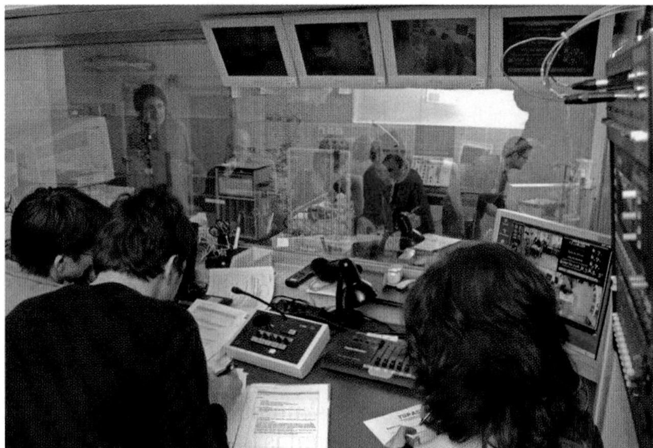

Fig. 7.19 **High workload for instructors during a simulation case.** The photograph shows the instructor team in front of the control panels and monitors in a control room during a simulation scenario. The control room is separated from the simulation room by a one-way mirror. The instructors have to operate the simulator, control the course of the scenario and the vital signs, give live in-scenario guiding, communicate with confederates who support the simulation in the scenario room, and at the same time take notes for the debriefing. These complex tasks need prior training or experience and good organization on the part of the instructor team. *(Photograph by B. Schaedle, Momentum Photo at University Hospital, Tübingen, Germany.)*

training—that seem to spread among medical educators, but are erroneous in the eyes of the authors, especially when training health care professionals.

USE OF RECORDED AUDIO-VIDEO SEQUENCES IN DEBRIEFINGS

In the initial ACRM simulation courses the debriefer and participants viewed the entire recording, pausing at points for discussion. This practice has been abandoned and today most debriefers use the recordings only strategically to trigger discussion of specific points.[111,119,202,283,284] Studies of debriefing provide varying results as to the utility of showing the recordings and there is no definitive proof that this deepens the debriefing experience.[116,118-120,285] Nonetheless, snippets of audio-video recordings are frequently used as a learning and self-awareness experience.[117,119,202,284] Some studies point toward a positive effect, others do not. As the process of debriefing is complex and the effects of simulation and debriefing are expected to be a long-term accumulation of learning, reflection, and change, it is not surprising that teasing out cause and effect is difficult.

One argument for the use of audio-video-triggered reflection is that anesthesia does not support much self-reflection during routine clinical work. Experienced anesthesiologists often work alone, and there is often little feedback from other anesthesia professionals or from other operating room personnel. Most cases are followed as quickly as possible with the next. The lack of peer feedback leaves a large gap between the way individuals think they perform and how they act in reality. Based on the experiential learning cycle of Kolb[286] (Fig. 7.20) the opportunity to witness one's own behavior via a recorded audio-video sequence can be more meaningful to clinicians than described behavior criticized by the instructor. Another argument is that viewing the live transmission of the simulated scenarios is

BOX 7.6 Erroneous Learning Myths in Simulation Training

Learning Myth No. 1: *"Participants always need to figure out themselves what they did wrong."* Although self-reflection can be powerful, instructors can and should be ready to point out examples of problematic decisions or actions that are relevant to the clinical setting and to stimulate discussion of the alternatives and their pros and cons. This may lead to better understanding of possible solutions and how different clinical contexts will affect which are preferred. If participants grasp the situation and possible solutions on their own that is great. But if not, debriefers should not make participants search for the answer they wish to hear (this is called a "guess what I'm thinking" question); rather, they can use their own experience to suggest approaches that have worked for them.

Learning Myth No. 2: *"You always have to say something positive before you criticize."* Educators describe the "sandwich" approach; the full sandwich has a filling of negative comment(s) sandwiched between two positive comments (a simpler "open-face" sandwich is also seen). Since debriefing is not "feedback" this is usually unnecessary. The discussion of what transpired and why should facilitate health care professionals learning from the analysis of all aspects of performance without special cushioning of the blows.

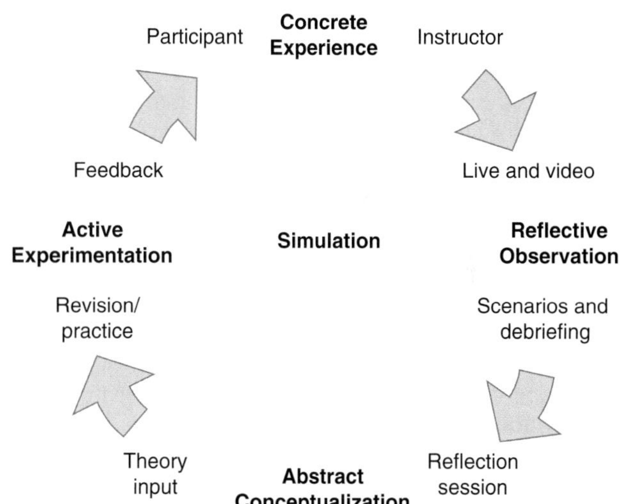

Fig. 7.20 **Kolb's experimental learning cycle.** Simulation team training with live video transmission and a debriefing with audio-video recordings demonstrates an ideal representation of Kolb's learning circle. During the scenario, actively involved trainees have a concrete "hands-on" experience. With the facilitation of the instructor and the own observation of audio-video sequences, the individual behavior can be actively reflected in the debriefing ("reflective observation"). The live video transmission to the non-active group during a scenario allows "reflective observation" during the scenario. During the debriefing, all trainees (active and non-active) have a phase of abstract conceptualization, in which the instructor uses generalizations of factors and root causes to show how behavior developed as it did in the scenario. With the instructor's theory input and the eventually triggered discussions, deep learning can take place and a plan can evolve during the debriefing, for both active and non-active trainees, of how to handle a similar situation next time. Active experimentation with the newly learned input and the drawn conclusions for the active as well as the non-active group can take place either during the next active scenarios or during real patient care. (Modified from Kolb DA. *Experiential learning: experience as the source of learning and development.* Englewood Cliffs, NJ: Prentice-Hall; 1984.)

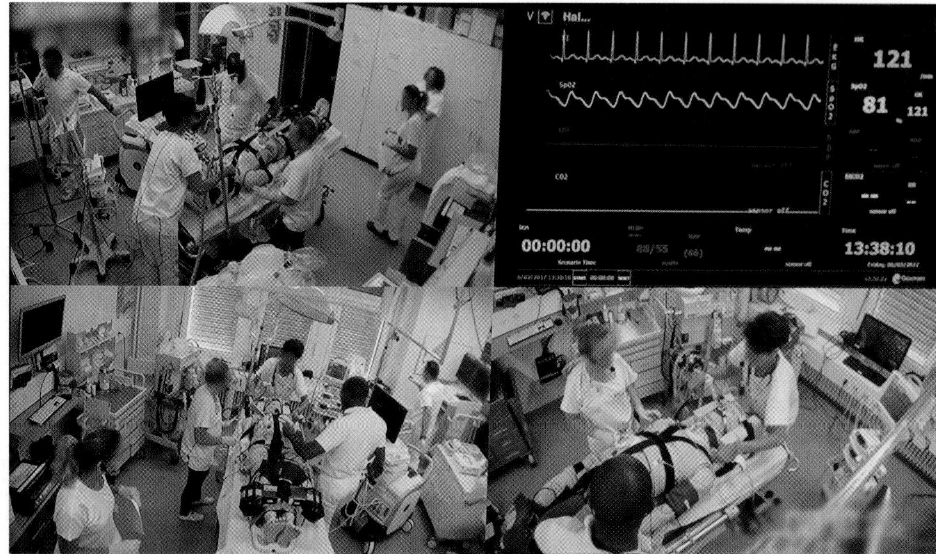

Fig. 7.21 Quad split monitor of a simulation exercise. The quad split of a simulation exercise shows the vital signs during the scenario and usually three different camera perspectives during a simulation scenario. The quad split can be used for the live transmission of the simulation scenario to the participants who are not directly involved in the scenario. And it also serves for the later audio-video-based debriefing to reflect what happened in a certain situation, providing the advantage of different angles of view and an isochronic view of the vital signs. (*Photograph provided by M. Rall, InPASS in-situ-training at Scuol Hospital, Switzerland, Chairman J. Koppenberg.*)

useful for participants who are not actively involved in a given scenario (see Fig. 7.20 and Fig. 7.21). There is evidence that observers of simulations can learn as much as participants.[287]

Advanced simulation course formats generally closely reflect Kolb's circle of adult experiential learning: (1) self-experience (participate in the scenario) or vicarious experience (observe scenario live), (2) reflect on experience (debriefing), (3) abstract conceptualization (debriefing, relate to theoretical material), and (4) active experimentation (future scenarios and use of skills in real cases).

When live transmission is used as an alternative to just watching, the observers can be given special tasks (e.g., look for assigned CRM key points, see Box 7.4) so that they are more engaged in the process. Use of sequences of the scenario recording for debriefing requires additional instructor judgment and high proficiency controlling the replay system.

EXCURSION: DEBRIEFING TECHNIQUES FOR DISCUSSION OF REAL CLINICAL CASES

Techniques of debriefing have also been applied to the analysis of real patient care events. Eppich and colleagues offer a guide to how this can be done in their article *"'Let's talk about it': translating lessons from healthcare simulation to clinical event debriefings and clinical coaching."*[288] Applying the debriefing techniques in short debriefing circles to involved clinical team has also proven quite valuable.[245,276,289-291] Clegg and MacKinnon[292] highlight in their paper *"Strategies for handling the aftermath of intraoperative death"* the need for a debriefing of the OR team after a critical incident in the OR and this concept is in accord with findings of other surveys.[293]

Debriefings after clinical cases can help teams learn.[288,294,295] This is particularly true for crews or action teams with short tenure and changing team membership that have limited time to develop and learn as a team.[296] Here, debriefings offer a useful structure for learning because members may apply the lessons learned from a debriefing of one action team to teamwork of another action team.[296] The advantages of team debriefings include a reduced number of mistakes, higher levels of speaking up and performance, and shorter work duration.[129,296-298]

However, there are barriers to achieving effective debriefings for formative assessment after real cases.[299] For example, teams are typically uncomfortable with explicit communication,[300] they tend to discuss already known instead of new information,[148] and dynamics in organizations foster "undiscussable" topics.[105,301] For example, the various debriefing systems provide useful structures for debriefings after clinical cases, although their particular logistics may have to be adapted to the clinical setting.[302] Unfortunately, most post-clinical event debriefings lack an appropriate setting, a trained debriefing facilitator, and sufficient time. [294] For example, after a cardiac arrest, (1) when resuscitation is successful many of the team members come from the ICU, so they will be busy transporting the patient or otherwise caring for them; or (2) whether or not the event was clinically successful, team members may well have been called away from important activities that need their attention, severely limiting their ability to debrief.

EXCURSION: DEBRIEFING TECHNIQUES FOR MORBIDITY AND MORTALITY CONFERENCES

Much of the philosophy and technique of debriefing applies to discussions of real cases such as morbidity and mortality (M&M) conferences. Both should be about exploring how and why things happened the way they did as opposed to the all-too-common emphasis on who was to blame. Both debriefing and M&M should aim not only to be educational for those participating but also to suggest ways to prevent or mitigate problems in the future, especially by correcting systems issues. Overall, both aim to be constructive, not destructive.

However, both debriefing and M&M conferences face the problem of "hindsight bias" (see also chapter 6). After an event it is often clear what the problem was and how it could have been avoided or best treated, making the original clinicians look foolish. Hindsight bias is very hard to avoid but effort should be made to analyze events from the standpoint of the professionals on the spot in terms of the information they had available at a given moment. Gaba sometimes will explicitly say, *"unfortunately our crystal ball for seeing the future was not operating that day."* Decisions that seem foolish in hindsight will often become totally understandable from this viewpoint.

Another common ground rule is to talk only about observable behaviors—the performance—not about individuals, personality, attitudes, assumptions, or interferences. If someone involved decides to disclose internal thoughts this can then become a topic of discussion. Using such philosophy and technique has a better chance of finding correctable systems issues, fostering a culture of safety, and making personnel comfortable in reporting and discussing problematic cases for the benefit of future patients.

DEBRIEFING IN DIFFERENT CULTURES

While debriefing is widely recognized as an important part of simulation-based training, how it unfolds in practice depends on various contextual considerations. Many of the debriefing models stem from North America and Europe—what might be called the Western cultures. Arguably, the whole idea of debriefing—verbal reflective discussions of actions—might be seen as a Western idea. With simulation spreading more around the world, different national cultures, traditions, habits, and patterns of interpretations become more relevant.[303] The relationship between the learner and the instructor will be influenced by the general customs about how people of different hierarchy levels interact with each other. A recent study, based on interviews with experienced simulation instructors in 28 different countries, showed a strong relation between "power distance" of countries and specific patterns of behavior during the debriefing. The higher the power distance, the more important is the debriefer, the more closed questions are used, and the more difficult it is for participants to discuss issues of non-technical skills and speaking-up.

Qualification and Certification of Simulation Instructors

It has been nearly 30 years since the first major wave of simulation in anesthesiology and other domains began. Over this time a variety of questions have surfaced, in general and at each institution, about how to create and sustain a cadre of simulation instructors. These include: (1) Do simulation instructors need special training? (2) Do they need continuous training after their primary training and if so how much and how often? (3) Do they need to be officially (re-) certified periodically? (4) How can the quality of an instructor be measured or differentiated? This section addresses these questions.

TASKS OF SIMULATION INSTRUCTORS—LEARNING OBJECTIVES FOR SIMULATION INSTRUCTOR COURSES

Sometimes, simulation teaching is completely analogous to bedside teaching, only with a simulated patient, and all the same skills apply. For other uses of simulation new skills may be needed,[112,272,299,304] especially for simulation activity that involves: (1) complex realistic scenarios, (2) with multiple personnel in crews and teams, (3) conducting debriefings in small groups (with or without video), (4) with a focus on human factors and CRM principles and feasible countermeasures. It is widely thought that the quality of the instructors is *the* essential element for any simulation training course, and for complex activities their competence as debriefers is the primary aspect of quality.

Most clinical educators do not necessarily have the skills most needed to be a fully capable simulation instructor. The key tasks include:

- Create relevant, plausible, meaningful clinical scenarios with the necessary realism to reach the intended learning goals (although some instructors who are excellent debriefers leave the design of scenarios to their colleagues).
- Establish an engaging learning context.[121]
- Brief/familiarize simulation participants about the simulator and the unfamiliar simulation environment.[121,299]
- Conduct (complex) clinical scenarios with the need for simultaneous control of (1) the simulator, (2) the simulation environment (i.e., in-scenario information,[261] etc.), (3) the simulation personnel (co-instructors, role-players, simulation technicians, etc.), and (4) the real-time adjustment of scenarios to offer optimal learning for all participants.
- Provide a structured post-scenario debriefing and feedback stimulating self-reflection, facilitating peer-discussion, creating deep and sustainable learning, and promoting transfer lessons to the real world.
- Act on adult learning principles, balancing facilitation and instruction during debriefing (i.e., Kolb's experimental learning cycle, see Fig. 7.20).
- Handle, as necessary, group dynamics as well as individual sensitivities during the training and the debriefing.[272]
- Use recorded audio and video strategically to facilitate debriefing (and/or for feedback especially about technical or procedural skills).
- Teach about crew resource management (CRM) decision making, situation awareness, task and team management, communication, and professionalism in addition to the transfer of medical knowledge.
- Highlight system optimization based on system theory principles of patient safety.

EDUCATION, TRAINING, AND CONTINUOUS DEVELOPMENT OF SIMULATION INSTRUCTORS

Instructor Education and Training

As described by Fanning and Gaba,[238] unlike a traditional teacher, the facilitators can position themselves not as an authority or expert, but rather as a peer and co-learner. Oftentimes, especially for experienced medical teachers,

BOX 7.7 Learning Objectives for Crisis Resource Management–Oriented Simulation Instructor Courses

- Understand how it feels to be a participant in a simulation scenario
- Understand how it feels to be debriefed in a group while others are watching or while seeing oneself on video
- Understand the interdependent influences of the different course phases ("anatomy of a simulation course," see Fig. 7.18) and apply this knowledge to a simulation exercise or course
- Reflect on the changing instructional styles that can be applicable to simulation courses (instruction versus facilitation)
- Understand basic concepts of human factors, crisis resource management (CRM), systems theory, and organizational safety (see Chapter 6)
- Be able to detect, explain, and discuss CRM key points during the debriefing of scenarios
- If using video sequences, use recorded video clips of scenarios well, and select the most relevant portions for replay and discussion
- Be able to conduct a structured debriefing and facilitate a debriefing in a nonjudgmental atmosphere with appropriate boundaries
- Understand how to manage the individual sensitivities and group dynamics of participants during debriefing
- Instead of discussing "who" made "what" "mistake," be able to focus debriefing on the analysis of "what happened," "why did it happen the way it did," "what lessons can be learned," and "how to apply these lessons to real patient care"
- Create a well-designed scenario with learning objectives appropriate for the population

Modified from the learning objectives of instructor courses by Gaba, Rall, and Dieckmann.

the most difficult task in learning this teaching approach is to stop lecturing and start listening and facilitating. At the same time, providing honest critique while holding the learner in high regard—what the authors call "critiquing the *performance* not the *performer*"—seems particularly challenging.[106,304] This is, among other things, why simulation-based educators usually need special education and training. Box 7.7 presents an example of learning objectives for an instructor training course.

Gaba, Howard, and Williams from Veterans Affairs Palo Alto Health Care System /Stanford School of Medicine (VAPAHCS/SU) pioneered CRM-oriented simulation instructor training in 1992, taking their homemade simulation system to Boston for 3 months and teaching approximately a dozen faculty of the Harvard Hospitals anesthesiology programs how to conduct ACRM courses. A few years later a consortium of the Veterans Affairs Palo Alto/Stanford (VAPAHCS/SU), the Boston Anesthesia Simulation Center (the forerunner to the Center for Medical Simulation), and the University of Toronto Sunnybrook Simulation Center created a formal instructor course, spreading the ideas and format of CRM simulation instructor training around the world. Rall has run instructor courses in cooperation with Dieckmann for more than 3000 international participants. Many institutions now offer different instructor courses nationally and internationally (ranging from 2 to 6 days in length, depending on the course and its scope). For further information about such courses the reader is referred to the simulation societies such as SSH or SESAM, or Internet searches targeting well-known simulation centers. In addition, shorter introductory courses on instructor skills are offered every year at the international health care simulation meetings (e.g., SSH's IMSH conference, or the SESAM annual meeting); many workshops at these meetings cover topics such as debriefing, instructor training, and CRM training.

Continuous Faculty Development

Recent research demonstrates the variety of challenges simulation educators perceive when conducting simulation-based training sessions.[272,304] For example, debriefings can include difficult situations such as learners who are unusually quiet, disengaged, or overwhelmed by emotions.[272] Faculty development is important to prepare simulation educators to design and conduct meaningful and respectful training sessions while anticipating potential problems, intervene proactively, and when necessary manage them with good sense and grace.[272,305] Since debriefings are considered particularly challenging, special emphasis is given to continuously improving these skills.[106,306-308]

Reflection can help simulation faculty identify how to improve their debriefing skills.[304] Observation of master debriefers, interactive learning experiences, practice, feedback by peers and experts, and mentoring can foster such improvement.[309-311]

Valid and reliable tools such as the Debriefing Assessment for Simulation in Healthcare (DASH)[307] and Objective Structured Assessment of Debriefing (OSAD)[312] can be used to monitor debriefing quality and provide data for feedback conversations for faculty development. DASH is available in a variety of languages (to date, English, German, French, Japanese, Spanish; https://harvardmedsim.org/debriefing-assessment-for-simulation-in-healthcare-dash/). DASH consists of six rating elements: (1) setting the stage for an engaging learning environment, (2) maintaining an engaging context for learning, (3) structuring the debriefing in an organized way, (4) provoking an in-depth discussion which allows for reflection, (5) identifying performance gaps and their reasons, and (6) helping to see how to improve or sustain good performance. The OSAD consists of eight categories: (1) approach, (2) environment, (3) engagement, (4) reaction, (5) reflection, (6) analysis, (7) diagnosis, and (8) application. Both tools can be applied from various perspectives (i.e., learners, colleagues, educators) which allow for a multifaceted view on debriefing quality.[313]

CERTIFICATION OF SIMULATION INSTRUCTORS

Since being a simulation instructor often requires special skills it is almost universally true that only a small fraction of an institution's faculty or staff are involved in this. For very long-standing simulation groups and centers, informal internal mechanisms have often been used to select and approve instructors. For the bulk of simulation groups and centers there has long been a desire for some formal professional recognition of who is qualified to develop, conduct, and/or debrief health care simulations which has led to different models of certification of qualified individuals. One model is that of the Academy of Medical Educators (AoME),[314] a UK-based organization of educators of medical, dental, or veterinary professionals, for which membership requires satisfying certain levels of achievement in the following five professional standard domains:

- Designing and planning learning
- Teaching and facilitating learning
- Assessment of learning
- Educational research and scholarship
- Educational management and leadership

For each domain, three levels are available that allow assessment and documentation of progress of a person. For more information the reader is referred to the AoME website (https://www.medicaleducators.org/).

The SSH offers a model that addresses more of the simulation-specific aspects of the educator role, and is applicable to all personnel, not just "medical" educators. There is a basic and an advanced level of certification. For more information about the certification for Certified Healthcare Simulation Educator (CHSE) and the Certified Healthcare Simulation Educator—Advanced (CHSE-A) the reader is referred to the society's webpage (https://www.ssih.org/Certification). These programs are rather general and do not fully address the details of qualifications applicable to specific courses. SSH certification has been far more popular for nursing personnel than for physicians; this probably accounts for the fact that few simulation instructors in anesthesiology have obtained formal certification. In another approach, while the U.S. ASA Simulation Education Network (SEN) program endorsement process does not yet certify instructors, when considering a site for endorsement it does examine the simulation background of the site's instructors, as well as the process by which each site trains and approves new instructors for their program.

It is likely that the skills and certification needed (if any) for an instructor will vary greatly with the particular course or curriculum being taught. Competence in conducting a video-based CRM debriefing would not be needed, and would not help, to teach specific manual procedures (e.g., airway management or central venous cannulation) using part-task trainers. Some sites use either a formal or informal system of tiered instructor categorization tied to the specific types of courses and roles each individual is capable of conducting. This also provides a defined process for advancement from novice instructor to grand master as experience and special training are acquired.

Accreditation of Simulation Programs, Sites, and Centers

Besides the qualification of the instructors, the physical and organizational infrastructure is important for the quality of simulation in health care. This aspect is discussed under the label of accreditation. The SESAM wrote: *"By seeking accreditation an institution can demonstrate its quality as having been judged and validated by an independent body who is internationally recognized as an opinion leader in the domain of simulation-based education in healthcare."*[315]

Several systems of program approval have emerged, some of them of particular interest to anesthesia professionals.

SESAM provides a model that has two levels of accreditation (www.sesam-web.org/accreditation/). The basic level is done based on the description of the program's work; the expanded level also includes a site visit.

BOX 7.8 Simulation as Favored Option for Part IV of the U.S. Maintenance of Certification in Anesthesia Program by the American Board of Anesthesiology

The simulation course must be held at a site endorsed by the Simulation Editorial Board of the American Society of Anesthesiologists, with a curriculum meeting minimum standards. Although not specifying anesthesia crisis resource management (ACRM) directly, the standards for the U.S. Maintenance of Certification in Anesthesia (MOCA) simulation are clearly derived from the ACRM simulation courses that have become common around the world:

- A minimum of 6 h of total course instruction
- Active participation in realistic (mannequin-based) simulation scenarios
- Post-scenario instructor-facilitated peer debriefing
- Management of difficult patient-care scenarios, including at least scenarios involving the following: (1) hemodynamic instability and (2) hypoxemia of any cause, including management of the difficult airway
- An emphasis on teamwork and communication
- All participants have at least one opportunity to be the primary anesthesiologist in charge (i.e., the "hot seat")
- The participant-to-instructor ratio must be no greater than 5:1
- At least one instructor must currently be in the MOCA process

The SSH provides an accreditation program, with separate but related accreditations for core standards plus one or more of the following areas of emphasis: teaching/education; assessment; research; systems integration. For more information, the reader is referred to their webpage (https://www.ssih.org/Accreditation/Full-Accreditation).

The U.S. ASA has a process to endorse anesthesia simulation programs (the ASA chose not to use the term accredit) qualifying them to be members of the ASA's SEN. Centers were originally endorsed for their ability to deliver high-quality CME to ASA members. After reaching agreement with the ABA in 2010, this ASA SEN rapidly transformed into a group of programs capable of conducting the semi-standardized Maintenance of Certification in Anesthesia (MOCA) Simulation Course. The course is a component of Part IV (practice improvement) of the ABA MOCA process. Box 7.8 shows the features of the U.S. Maintenance of Certification in Anesthesia (MOCA) simulation program.

As of November 2018, the ASA had endorsed more than 50 programs, each of which was reviewed and approved by the ASA Simulation Education Editorial Board after completion of a detailed application documenting the capability and experience of their simulation instructors, leadership, facilities, and procedures (for ASA members, see http://www.asahq.org/For-Members/Education-and-Events/Simulation-Education.aspx).

The American College of Surgeons (ACS) has a program of Accredited Education Institutes (AEI) that "*...educate and train practicing surgeons, surgical residents, medical students, and members of the surgical team using simulation-based education.*"[316] Many anesthesia simulation programs, especially those endorsed by the ASA-SEB, have a close collaborative relationship with their institution's ACS-AEI.

Benefits, Effectiveness, and Ecological Validity of Simulation Training

In the era of evidence-based medicine everyone wants to know *"does simulation work?"* and *"what is its cost effectiveness?"* This question has now been answered affirmatively, but only for a selected few circumstances. In fact, it seems clear that for many of the common, but most challenging arenas of health care, these questions may not be answerable for all practical purposes.[317] Some argue that the question of whether simulation works needs to be replaced by questions about *"when," "how,"* and *"under what conditions"* simulation "works," and finally *"how 'works' can be defined"* in a given context. In the following, the benefits of simulation are summarized, and some challenges to answer the above raised questions as well as some key findings in settings in which studies were feasible are reviewed.

BENEFITS

Simulation in health care has some fundamental advantages as a training tool. The following were modified and expanded based on the work of Gaba and DeAnda[177]:

- No risk is posed to a patient despite "hands-on" training.
- Routine clinical situations, emergency situations, and those involving uncommon but serious problems can be presented at will.
- Participants can learn to use actual complex devices, often in the relevant clinical context.
- The same situation can be presented independently to multiple subjects for evaluating individual or group performance.
- Errors can be allowed to occur and play out to their likely conclusion, whereas in a clinical setting they would require immediate intervention by a supervisor.
- To a reasonable degree, the training can be standardized and is reproducible.
- Training can be focused and allows for various forms of feedback or discussion that are difficult to embed into real patient care settings.
- "Clinical time" is under the control of the instructor; boring portions can be skipped or sped up while very difficult segments can use time dilation to allow unfamiliar individuals to have a full chance to grasp and handle the situation.
- Simulation can be stopped and restarted for teaching; time of physiological changes can be expanded or compressed, including "death-control."
- Recording, replay, and critique of performance are facilitated because patient safety or confidentiality is not an issue.

Simulation accelerates skill acquisition, improves skill retention, and reduces the extinction of skills.[26] Simulation has been heavily utilized to address non-technical skills (see Chapter 6) such as communication, teamwork, task management, leadership, situation awareness, and decision making. Those non-technical skills and human-factor-based training approaches are vital to conduct safe patient care, taking into account human performance strengths and weaknesses (see Chapter 6). Nevertheless, as mentioned below, such an arena will be the hardest to ever prove that simulation improves patient outcome.

Despite the many advantages of simulation in health care adverse effects of simulation are possible. A stimulating critical overview of medical education in general was written by Hodges and was provocatively titled *"Medical Education and the maintenance of Incompetence."*[318] The article points out that any type of education runs a risk of creating or maintaining incompetence in certain areas, especially areas that are ignored by the actual educational program. The authors recommend that all simulation instructors be especially cognizant of the risks that Hodges articulates.

EFFECTIVENESS

Challenge #1: Comparability of simulation research and evaluation of simulation. For the question of whether simulation works and how effective simulation is in regard to different aspects, evaluation concepts need to be defined and a common ground for the comparison of research in simulation needs to be produced. For the evaluation of learning and later performance outcomes, respectively, oftentimes the four-level model of Kirkpatrick as shown in Fig. 7.22 is cited.[319,320]

Another concept used to evaluate simulation is that of translational science—research designed to accelerate movement of results from the laboratory bench to the patient bedside. The concepts of a continuum of research from fundamental science through clinical trials to widespread use in patient care and of potential translational blocks were articulated originally by Sung and colleagues in 2003.[321] From this publication emerged various nomenclatures for the different levels of the research continuum in terms of increasing level of translation, called T Levels.

For education, translational science addresses how results achieved in the educational laboratory (T1) transfer to improved downstream patient care practices (T2) and improved patient and public health (T3).[322] McGaghie[322-324] first adapted the T levels of translational research to the arenas of medical education and simulation in health care, comprising T1, T2, T3, and T3′ (Table 7.5). The most important T levels for simulation interventions are T1: is performance improved when observed during simulation?; T2: does actual clinical behavior change in the workplace?; T3: is there a change in patient outcome?; and to a lesser extent T3′: is it cost-effective?

Based on those two concepts, for research purposes simple outcomes are Kirkpatrick level 1 (reactions of participants) and Kirkpatrick level 2 (change in self-confidence or of knowledge measurable via multiple choice questions). Both Kirkpatrick levels are represented by level T1. Rall et al.[325] later adapted additional T levels mentioned in other sources,[326,327] adding levels of T0, T4, T5, and T6 (see Table 7.5), and categorizing interventions by their intended outcomes. Researchers in simulation are now starting to use this terminology in describing and comparing their research protocols and results.

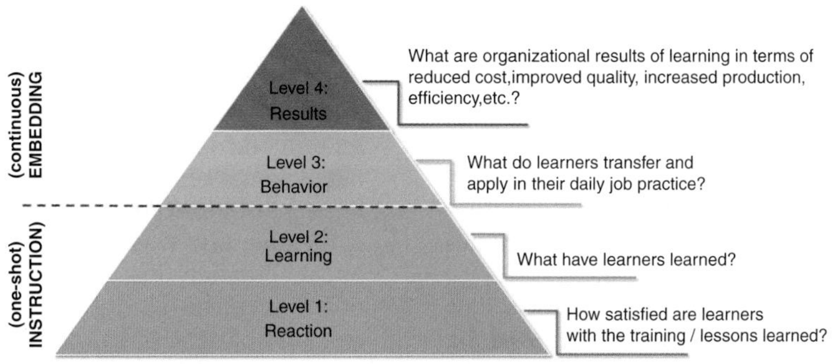

Fig. 7.22 **Kirkpatrick's four-level training evaluation model.** The model is composed of four levels: reaction—learning—behavior—and results.

TABLE 7.5 Translational Research Levels of Simulation-Based Training

Level	Description of Study Methodology	Comments/Examples
0	No measurement of learner performance	Questionnaire or multiple-choice test to assess reaction/change in knowledge
1	Performance measured during simulation only	Do participants do better in a subsequent simulation?
2	Performance measured during actual clinical care	Do participants do better in subsequent clinical practice?
3	Measurement of improvement in patient outcome	Do patients of those who had the training fare better?
3′	Measurement of cost of the intervention, the outcome, and the monetary benefit (= measuring "cost effectiveness")	Does intervention yield a net saving of money (with/without improving outcome)?
4	Measurement of dissemination of the intervention to sites beyond trial sites	Has the intervention spread elsewhere successfully?
5	Measurement of adoption of the intervention in regular practice	Has it been widely adopted?
6	Measurement of population health outcome	Has it made an impact on patient population as a whole?

Challenge #2: To define cost-effectiveness, expenses need to be put in context relative to return on investment. In simulation education the focus of evaluations historically has been mostly on qualitative instead of quantitative measures, and the suite of measurements needed to assess learning outcomes and patient outcomes are still in flux. Bukhari and colleagues published a framework for determining the return on investment of simulation-based education in health care.[328] Unfortunately, so far, evaluations that yield economic information about the return on investment are scarce.[329] And the expenses (see later section) vary (high cost to low cost) depending on many choices regarding the setup of the simulation training (see earlier section on "12 Dimensions of Simulation").

At this point, most studies of simulation-based learning are at level T0 or T1. At lower T levels simulation of various sorts has been shown to have small to medium positive effects.[330] A few studies have been at T2 and only a handful at T3 or T3′ patient outcome. Draycott and colleagues[331] showed positive effects of training that included some simulation components on neonatal outcome. Barsuk and colleagues[126] showed a reduction of central line complications and cost-efficacy after implementing simulation-based training on central venous cannulation. A series of studies from Tanzania shows that positive effects for patients is not necessarily related to the use of high-end simulation equipment.[38,332] Van de Ven and associates[333] concluded in their study that multiprofessional team training for obstetric emergencies in a medical simulation center is cost-effective in a scenario where repetition training sessions are performed on-site. Levels T4 and T5 can be considered implementation science, but few studies of simulation implementation have been performed.

Simulation researchers are encouraged to move toward studies at higher levels of translational research whenever possible. Admittedly, the cost and complexity of studies also rises non-linearly as one climbs the "T ladder." Since many applications of simulation in anesthesiology especially focus on preparing anesthesia professionals to prevent and manage uncommon but serious adverse events more effectively, the rarity of such events and the many confounding variables that affect patient outcome will make intervention studies very difficult to perform.[317]

These studies would per force need to be large, long, and complicated. To date, almost all studies have been too short and too unsystematic, with weak interventions and without adequate control of confounding variables. Unlike many types of clinical trials, which are funded by the pharmaceutical industry—which is willing to invest heavily even in complex trials because of the high direct payoff when a blockbuster drug is found—simulation interventions have no equivalent funding sources. Obtaining level 1A evidence—with multiple randomized controlled trials—of simulation's impact on patient outcome may well take studies of thousands to hundreds of thousands of patients, cared for by hundreds or thousands of clinicians, with simulation interventions that are powerful, comprehensive, sustained, and linked to performance assessment (and remediation) of individual clinicians. As yet, no agency or commercial firm is willing to fund these kinds of large, long, and complex studies.[317] And neither aviation nor nuclear power have assembled "level 1A" evidence that simulation saves airplanes, power plants, or lives. It is unlikely that aviation would ever attempt randomized trials and such studies would be nearly impossible, if not unethical.

Challenge #3: High-fidelity patient simulations can be effective and cost-effective, but work will be educationally effective only, if they meet certain criteria. Flanagan and associates provided a thorough review of the literature on the efficacy of simulation-based training for learning and assessment.[334] They concluded that "simulation makes a valuable contribution to learning for students, trainees, and clinicians. It enables learning of both routine and non-routine procedures and management of patients." In one study the effect between hours of simulation practice and learning outcomes equaled a dose-response relationship.[198]

Similarly to Flanagan, Cook and colleagues[330] concluded in their comparative review that simulation was typically more expensive but also more effective. In their summary, in comparison with other instructional methods, technology-enhanced simulation was associated with small to moderate positive effects. In another comparative review by Cook et al.[335] in which technology-enhanced simulation training in health professions education was compared to "usual practice," simulation was consistently associated with large effects for outcomes of knowledge, skills, and behaviors, and moderate effects for patient-related outcomes. Such findings were confirmed by Lorello et al.[15] in their most recent review; they and other authors[198,334] pointed to the heterogeneity of the studies, the sometimes limited robustness of their methods, and the occasional lack of a suitable control group.

A Best Evidence in Medical Education review by Issenberg and colleagues concluded that high-fidelity medical simulations are educationally effective, but only if the following conditions are met[198]:

- Educational feedback is provided.
- Repetitive practice is used or is allowed.
- Simulation is integrated sensibly into the standard curriculum.
- The range of task difficulty can be adapted to the level of the learner.

Challenge #4: Limitations of research on simulation effectiveness. Even the strongest of results come with caveats. First, it can be difficult to isolate the effects of simulation in the evaluation. In many cases simulation is only a part of a larger bundle of interventions, or concurrent with improvements in the clinical field as a whole ("secular change" as statisticians say). Second, as in the case of central venous cannulation, sometimes the clinical activity is circumscribed, the outcomes are relatively common, there is already ongoing surveillance for them, the relationship of the activity to negative outcomes is well-understood, and the intervention is itself narrow, proving an effect on patient outcome is easy. But for many arenas, especially for the anesthesia professional's management of unexpected adverse situations, the events are relatively rare; there is weak surveillance for negative outcomes, as well as many confounds between anesthesia professionals' actions and the final outcome; and the simulation interventions are complex. Proving an outcome improvement is difficult in such settings and likely would require long, complex trials involving many tens or hundreds of thousands of patients, thousands of clinicians, and a very long time horizon, as mentioned above. Further, it is unrealistic to expect that a single set of training can change complex behaviors and actions or affect patient outcome especially when there is little reinforcement in or linkage to performance assessment in actual clinical practice.

Challenge #5: Assessing the impact of simulation in health care as if it was a pharmaceutical. The assessment of the impact of simulation to date can be seen using the following analogy to drug development and testing that was introduced by Weinger[336] and expanded to address the related policy issues by Gaba.[317] Suppose one wished to test whether a purported antihypertensive drug actually succeeded in reducing blood pressure in patients and, more importantly, whether it reduced the occurrence of adverse cardiovascular events, such as myocardial infarction and stroke. Imagine then that one proceeds as follows: administer a relatively small dose of this drug only a few times per year. Acknowledge variable compliance in taking even these few doses of drug. Immerse all subjects in an environment full of stress and other factors predisposing to cardiovascular events. Use only a few patients, and follow them for a very short time.

Would anyone wonder if no significant effect was found even for a drug otherwise known to be effective? Simulation in health care has so far been tested in this way: very small, short-term studies of infrequent (often short) simulation sessions, whose lessons are not fully reinforced in real clinical environments full of production pressure and stress. In truth, the question is not "*Does one run through a simulation course make a practitioner better?*" To follow the lead of other industries of intrinsic hazard, such as commercial aviation or nuclear power production, the question is "*What is the impact on health care as an industry adopting a comprehensive integrated strategy of intensive simulation-based training and continued performance assessment of clinical personnel, over a long period of time?*" This is the approach in aviation, in which no matter how senior and how experienced pilots are, they still undergo training and assessment in simulation every year, for the entirety of their careers.

It seems unlikely that pilots would forgo simulation training and assessment when their own lives are on the line. For another thing, the public has come to expect a regulatory safety floor imposed by the government to ensure the competence of pilots. The regulator is unlikely to forgo its requirement for mandatory training and testing of pilots. If such requirements continue, there may be only two options: conduct these exercises in real airplanes, with the attendant costs (e.g., fuel) and risks; or conduct them using simulation. With health care heading in that direction,[92,222,226,245,337,338] one may be able to assess the impact of more effective simulation programs, although one may lose a control group that has never experienced simulation.

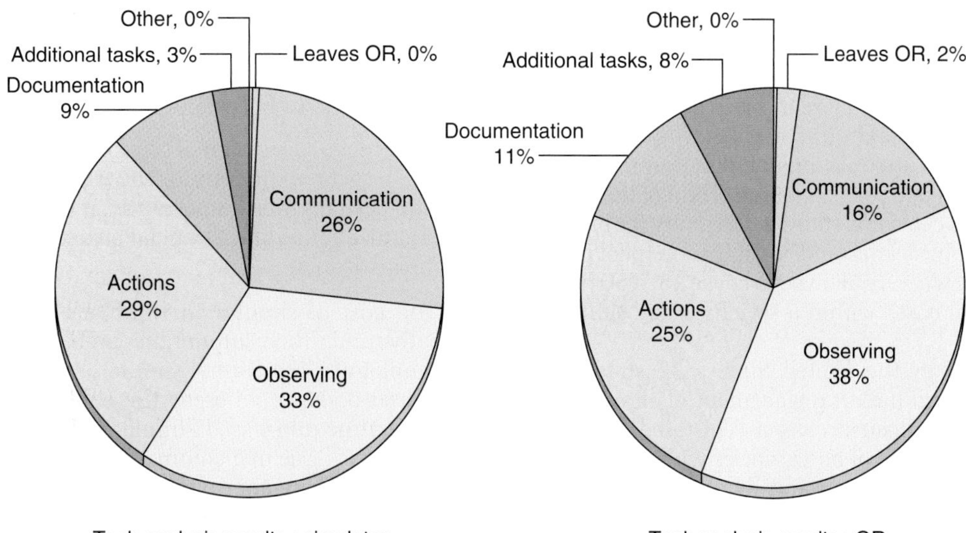

Fig. 7.23 Ecological validity of simulation versus the operating room *(OR)*. For study purposes[160], the same anesthesiologists were observed in the OR and in the simulation environment with full enactment of the OR personnel, surgical team, and anesthesia nurse. Even though the two settings have some interesting differences, the overall ecologic validity of the simulation is good. *(Courtesy of T. Manser, ETH Zurich, and University Hospital, Tübingen, Germany.)*

Other industries have a career-long set of simulation interventions that are considered to have a cumulative effect on ability. Social psychologists Helmreich and Foushee, two of the main architects of CRM training, wrote: "*Data indicate that even intensive initial CRM training constitutes only an awareness phase and introduction to the concepts, and that continuing reinforcement is essential to produce long-term changes in human factors practice.*"[339] Similarly, United Airlines states in its CRM manual: "*Command/Leadership/Resource management [United's terminology for CRM] cannot be a one-shot approach. It has to be a coordinated long range program. It must therefore be an integral part of the entire training effort: new hire training, transition and upgrade programs, and recurrent training.*"[340]

ECOLOGICAL VALIDITY OF PATIENT SIMULATION: IS THERE TRANSFERABILITY TO THE REAL WORLD?

When trying to translate behavior of professionals in the simulation to the behavior professionals might show during real clinical cases, one of the questions raised is the one about whether simulation can engage trainees the same way a real clinical case would. Simplified, in psychological science this is referred to as ecological validity. If actions and behavior in the simulation resemble the actions and behaviors in real-world clinical environments, it is likely that the results of research conducted in a simulation setting or lessons learned in a simulation training will be transferable to the context of actual patient care.

Patient simulation: A valid representation of the clinical reality? The question whether full-scale simulations are a valid representation of the real work environment tasks (e.g., tasks of an anesthetist in the OR, etc.) was investigated by an interdisciplinary research group in Tübingen, Germany and Zurich, Switzerland.[160] Each of the six anesthesiologists participating in the study was observed during two clinical cases and during three comparable simulator cases (one routine and two involving critical incidents). Analysis of the study showed good comparability of the different action categories as shown in Fig. 7.23. The interpretation of the group was that overall comparability between the operating room and the simulator setting is good, thereby indicating high validity for simulators in anesthesia.

Another more recent study by Weller and associates[341] examined the validity of the simulated environment with the question of whether anesthesia professionals show similar verbal communication patterns during a simulated and a real case. Seventeen anesthetists were observed via video-recordings during real cases and two simulated cases. Confirming the findings mentioned by the group in Tübingen and Zurich, the authors of the publication found no significant differences in communication patterns in the OR and the routine simulations. The participants themselves rated communication as realistic and considered their communications occurred with a similar frequency in the simulations as in comparable cases in the OR.

Those findings support the validity of the simulation environment and its value for transferable training and provide further objective confirmation of the favorable subjective impressions of realistic simulation scenarios by anesthesiologists of varying levels of experience.[65,68,69,178,179,181,342] Therefore, the evaluations presented in this chapter suggest that simulator-based training is a powerful technique that novice and experienced anesthesiologists believe to be highly beneficial, and that participants and instructors alike believe may improve clinical performance. As the developers of Sim One[175] pointed out, when simulation provides an opportunity to teach material that cannot be taught in another way, as for the systematic instruction of anesthesiologists in handling severe critical events such as cardiac arrest, anaphylaxis, or malignant hyperthermia, there is nothing with which to compare the simulator.

Simulation replacing clinical hours or case numbers during training? Because simulation offers a valid representation of real health care settings and behaviors, and also offers several advantages, in settings for which a certain number of clinical hours or patient cases are a prerequisite for certification or credentialing, simulations are sometimes allowed to replace some portion of the requirement. This is true in some states in Germany for prehospital emergency physicians (and possibly soon [pilot project] for paramedics) who are allowed to cover 25 of 50 mandatory prehospital cases within a specific 3-day simulation program.

For nursing, in the United States, 22 states allow some degree of simulation replacement of clinical hours required for final licensure as a registered nurse; the number or percentage of hours varies widely as does the specificity of the regulation and whether there are any standards for the intensity or quality of the simulation activities (see https://www.inacsl.org/sim-regulations/). A large and complex study of educational outcome (not patient outcome) provided evidence to support these practices,[343] although from Gaba's view there were some limitations concerning study methodology and the generalizability of the results.

Differences between simulated and real-world cases. Even though the mentioned studies showed high ecological validity of patient simulation, some differences between simulation and real patient care are inherent to simulation and need to be taken into account when debriefing and assessing the performance during a simulated scenario. Based on the findings of Manser and colleagues[160] variations were mostly the result of organizational factors (e.g., fewer additional tasks required in the simulator). At the same time, as described in the literature,[75] subjects (1) eventually become hypervigilant realizing that they are in a simulation, being more attentive or even doing more than they usually do (e.g., participants neglect documentation in the simulation while waiting for a disaster to happen, or scan the patient's documents at length before starting a simulated case so as not to miss an important hidden hint, or jump too quickly on signs of possible trouble); (2) conversely, will not or cannot take the situation serious because it is not a "real patient" and thus do not perform all the actions as they would for a real patient (e.g., acting sloppy, showing cavalier behavior, acting like it is a game).

Careful and creative scenario design and scenario conduct as well as proper introductory briefings may mitigate some of those effects (see earlier sections on those topics).[273]

Cost of Patient Simulation and Simulation Centers

COST OF PATIENT SIMULATION

An important question concerning simulator-based training in anesthesia is its cost effectiveness. This complicated question has two independent components. The first pertains to the impact and benefit of the training on the performance abilities of participants and patient outcome (discussed above), and the second is the cost to achieve that impact.

Although measuring the cost of simulation-based training depends on many factors, the cost may still be more easily estimated than is the impact of the training. Factors affecting the cost include:

- The type (or spectrum of types) of training involved
- The target populations for the training
- And perhaps most importantly, a variety of aspects of the organizational and financial structures and processes of the institution

The cost of simulation hardware and software varies greatly (and much simulation can be done with little to no technology). Screen-only simulators cost very little (a few hundred dollars), whereas the equivalent cost of a complete mannequin-based simulator or VR system is much higher. The price of a commercial mannequin-based simulator ranges from approximately $25,000 for intermediate-capability simulators to more than $150,000, depending on features; only the manufacturers can provide detailed information. This cost does not include any relevant clinical equipment (which, say, for an anesthesia machine is very high) and also of course the building and maintenance of a center's space.[344] Even these large expenditures do not dominate in the operational cost equation, however, because the construction cost is often borne by the institution itself, capital equipment can sometimes be donated or acquired used, and in general is amortized over a relatively long useful life, with appropriate provisions for service and upgrades.

The overall dominant cost for operating a center is likely to be the salary and benefits of its permanent personnel and the effort of expert instructors (which is typically borne directly or indirectly by their clinical department). These costs vary considerably across the spectrum of simulation activities and institutional arrangements. Usually an expert must oversee the curriculum (which may or may not impose direct costs), but the type of training and the target population will determine the amount of expert instruction required. A single faculty member can review the summaries of exercises performed by residents on a screen-based simulator in a few hours per resident per year. Non-physician instructors may be suitable for some task training or for drill and practice sessions. A single instructor can use the simulator to show pulmonary or cardiovascular physiology to a whole class of medical students. For training novice residents in basic anesthesia skills, it may be possible to have senior residents or fellows conduct the sessions at a low marginal cost. For training experienced residents and practitioners in complex material, such as the handling of critical events, it is likely no substitute expert instructors exist. The cost of expert instruction depends on the organizational arrangements of the institution. In a teaching institution where faculty members all have at least some time allocated for teaching or scholarly activities, some faculty may choose to fulfill this requirement by simulation-based teaching or scholarship. When further instructor effort is needed, payment—by the department or the center—for clinical release time may be needed.

Another organizational cost factor relates to providing access to participants for what can be complex, exhausting, and lengthy training sessions. Removing clinical personnel from revenue-producing work for training purposes is expensive. If simulation training could allow them to work more safely and efficiently, the benefit could outweigh the cost. Some research indicates that simulation team training can improve job satisfaction and effectiveness of routine care, as well as contributing to reduced illness leave and job fluctuations.[345] Some residency programs provide protected time for education of residents (e.g., one half day per week). In such cases, residents should already be available for simulation, but it might make faculty time even more scarce. In Australia and Germany, CME requirements are expressed in terms of points to be accrued.

Without question, simulation-based training is more costly than exhorting learners to read or putting them in a room with a lecturer. But when regarding credits for continuous medical education (CME), reading a short article and answering a handful of questions can only generate 1 hour of credit—or as in Australia and Germany only a small amount of CME points, as can sitting through a lecture. Simulation training is generally much more interactive and much more intensive than other activities and therefore professionals earn more credits or points, which may make simulation-based CME financially competitive relative to simpler methods.

Simulation-based training allows a host of issues to be addressed that cannot be easily tackled in other ways. It is the belief of the authors—one that has been borne out by programs "voting with their feet" since the 1990s—that if simulator-based training is deemed to be desirable, innovative changes in the organization will evolve to allow it to occur.

But other emerging aspects also make patient simulation a beneficial tool for addressing future organizations' needs. At the Harvard University hospitals, for example, the captive insurer, Harvard Risk Management Foundation, has taken unprecedented steps to link simulation-based continuous medical education training to discounts for medical malpractice premium rates for experienced clinicians in anesthesia and in obstetrics (J. Cooper, personal communication, 2005). This forward-thinking program is now being adopted by other malpractice carriers. In some jurisdictions, risk managers have chosen to invest directly in simulation activities at their institution, rather than to use the premium discount approach.

COST OF SIMULATION CENTERS

The cost varies greatly depending on the scope of the facility and its programs, the nature of the target populations, and the extent of use by the different possible stakeholder groups. How the costs are allocated to different elements of an institution or consortium is equally complicated and depends highly on local conditions. No one formula for success exists. In some models, the center is wholly responsible for its own costs but is completely free to generate and retain revenue. At the other extreme is a model whereby the host institution bears all costs of operating a central core facility, but it collects any and all revenues and may even tax components of the institution (e.g., departments) to offset the costs. Perhaps most common are mixed models in which the central authority bears the costs of initial construction and outfitting (often funded by philanthropy) and some portion of the ongoing infrastructure (simulation operations personnel, capital refurbishment, utilities), and each user (e.g., department) is responsible for providing instructors and paying for the marginal costs of any specific course or application. To date, few, if any, centers truly generate a profit, but many sites have successfully garnered external funds to offset some of the costs of training their own key target populations.

Using Simulation for Assessment of Clinical Performance

Although the dominant use of simulation is for education and training, the first simulators (both Sim One[175] and CASE[177]) were created to be research tools to assess and understand the performance of clinicians. Such assessment could address routine work in clinical environments[115,134,136,346,347] as well as performance when responding to critical events.[64,68]

Note: the terms "assessment" and "evaluation" are often used interchangeably even though they have slightly different meanings, so the authors chose to do so in this chapter, too.

For further information on the assessment of clinical performance that is related to the topics of human performance and patient safety the reader is referred to Chapter 6, where less simulation-related aspects of this topic are covered in more detail.

Performance can be divided into two components: (a) medical or technical performance, which is the appropriateness and thoroughness of the medical and technical response to the critical event; and (b) behavioral or non-technical[348] performance, which is the appropriate use of sound crisis management behaviors (e.g., leadership, communication, distribution of workload, decision making, etc.)[24,349] (see Chapter 6).

There are a number of potential frameworks that can be referenced when defining clinical and nonclinical competencies for the performance assessment of health care professionals. In different countries, different frameworks are used to describe anesthesiologist's competencies, which provide the ground for assessment measures. Many countries build on the CanMed roles[350] (Canadian Medical Education Directives for Specialists) that describe seven roles for the competent physicians. Those roles are: medical expert, communicator, collaborator, leader/manager, health advocate, scholar, and professional. Other countries build on the six ACGME (Accreditation Council for Graduate Medical Education) core competencies, which include patient care, medical knowledge, practice-based learning and improvement, interpersonal and communication skills, professionalism, and systems-based practice.[102]

Assessment of medical, technical, and non-technical responses in simulation settings has resulted in a variety of tools for assessment and evaluation as suggested by different authors.[64,69,89-93,97,99,101,136,342,349,351-354]

For assessing the non-technical skills of anesthesiologists many investigators use the Anaesthesia Non-Technical Skills (ANTS) system.[91,353] In recent years, the early ANTS evaluation system was adapted to different countries, and modified for different cultures[351] and health care specialties.[355] However, there are other tools for measuring non-technical skills of anesthesia professionals. Of particular note is a rubric developed by Weinger, Gaba, and colleagues[64,356] which is simpler than ANTS but of equivalent capability.

BENEFITS OF SIMULATION-BASED PERFORMANCE ASSESSMENT

Because the nature and cause of a simulated critical incident is known, one can construct in advance a list of appropriate technical activities.[357] Relative weighting of the importance of the different activities can be applied to reflect the fact that different activities, even if appropriate, differ in their importance. This weighting can be done either in advance of data collection, or post hoc (but in an appropriately blinded fashion). For example, when assessing medical or technical performance in managing malignant hyperthermia, termination of the trigger agent and administration of intravenous dantrolene would be highly important, indeed essential, items. Cooling measures, hyperventilation, and bicarbonate therapy would be among many appropriate (but less critical) responses. One can predict in advance specific technical errors to look out for. For example, for malignant hyperthermia management, these could include diluting dantrolene with the wrong diluent or an insufficient quantity of diluent.

Can the clinical outcome of a simulation predict how a real patient would have fared given the same care, and can this outcome be used in assessment? When watching a simulation scenario play out it seems tempting to think that the outcome of the patient—whether calculated by an underlying mathematical model of physiology (for a few simulators) or based on apparent adherence to patient care guidelines—can be the primary determinant of an individual assessment or a definitive prediction of what outcome a real patient would have had. Such a temptation is largely dangerous. Perhaps at the extremes of what transpired the apparent outcome could be reliable. If a patient is portrayed in ventricular fibrillation and nothing is done it is certain that they will die. If a healthy patient with substantial neuromuscular blockade receiving a FiO_2 of 50% oxygen is suddenly not ventilated for 30 seconds it is nearly certain that they will be fine. In between such extremes the exact outcome is very hard to predict. There will be isolated situations in which a mathematical model can predict certain physiologic variables, but the influence of those on other variables may be unknown. Why do some patients suffer an arrhythmia if their blood pressure falls below, say, systolic pressure of 50, 60, or 70 torr for a certain amount of time whereas others tolerate it fine? Why does one patient have return of spontaneous circulation after electric countershock applied at the same interval after dysrhythmia onset and another does not? Perfect decision making in resuscitation of a real patient cannot guarantee that electric countershock would successfully restore a normal cardiac rhythm. For the foreseeable future, any credible performance measurement technique must involve subjective judgments by clinical experts about the care process rather than about the calculated or presumed outcome.

PITFALLS OF SIMULATION-BASED PERFORMANCE ASSESSMENT

Technical versus nontechnical (CRM) skills. As indicated in previous sections, it is feasible (if difficult) to assess a technical response to specific events and generic nontechnical behaviors (CRM). For which kinds of assessments is it appropriate to measure only technical performance, only nontechnical performance, or some combination of the two?

Number of scenarios. How many different scenarios are needed to achieve robust performance assessment of individuals in all relevant aspects (technical and nontechnical) of patient care? The literature suggests that the variability of individual performance across different scenarios is high, in fact greater than the variability across raters. If simulation is to be used to assess an individual a large number of scenarios would need to be conducted for each person. Having a larger number of scenarios is more effective in improving the reliability of ratings than is having a larger number of raters.[64,237,358]

Rating individuals versus rating crews or teams. Anesthesiologists work as individuals and in crews and teams with other anesthesiologists and with surgeons, nurses, technicians, and others. Should the performance of individuals working alone be assessed? Should anesthesiologists be able to call for and use help in solving problems? If so, can one still rate the individual when working with a team?

Performance fluctuation. How can performance that fluctuates substantially over time (i.e., during a simulation scenario) be aggregated into a single rating? This issue was recognized by Gaba and colleagues as a major apparent source of interrater disagreement.[349] It is not addressed by any current rating system.[91,359] One option is to conduct moment-by-moment rating to yield a high-resolution time series of the varying performance. A variety of mathematical techniques could then be applied to the time series to yield appropriate measures of aggregate performance and variation.

Criterion thresholds. What level of performance should be set as criterion thresholds for different purposes? Can benchmarks of performance be established by truly expert clinicians (recognizing that years of experience and hierarchic rank are not surrogates for expertise or skill)? Similarly, how does the rating system deal with single actions or behaviors that were lethal or harmful in the presence of otherwise good performance? If used for formative assessment, a rating system should indicate the successes of the examinee and the failures. If used for summative or high-stakes assessment, however, it may be critical to ensure that the examinee who risks harming a simulated patient cannot outscore another examinee whose overall performance is less strong but who at least did not endanger the patient. Not performing chest compressions in a cardiac arrest situation would be such criterion for exclusion.

Appropriate statistical analysis of validity, interrater reliability, and reproducibility of these assessments. Various statistical tests and approaches have been used to evaluate these characteristics. The data on performance show various levels of interrater variance and high interindividual (and inter-team) variability.[68,69,181,342,349,360] As detailed by Gaba and colleagues,[349] some interrater reliability statistics are more stringent than others, especially in terms of the nature of the "by chance" benchmark. No firm consensus has been reached regarding which tests are most appropriate to answer key questions about simulation-based performance assessment. Some of the rating systems (including ANTS) have used less stringent tests of interrater reliability. Generalizability theory[361] offers a set of statistical techniques to sort out the impact of scenario, subject, rater, number of scenarios, and other facets on such assessments. This technique specifies how comparisons can be made against reference performance levels or as relative comparisons between subjects without a fixed benchmark.

Although simulation should provide a useful window on performance assessment, it remains challenging to develop widely accepted performance measures of anesthesiologists' skills,[362] even if the simulator is used as a tool to present standardized scenarios.[363] Klemola and Norros[364] published a newer way of looking at performance that involves anesthesiologists' habit of actions. These authors distinguished between reactive habits (conservative, self-contained, reluctant to construct subjective evaluations) and interpretative habits (creative, interactive, continuous integrative reasoning). They showed that many issues must be considered when discussing the best method of education and evaluation. Additional issues include defining and assessing professional competence.

USING SIMULATION FOR THE EVALUATION AND TESTING OF ANESTHESIA PROFESSIONALS

The use of simulation as a tool for performance assessment has presumed advantages: scenarios are known, errors can be allowed to occur and play out, and intensive recording and archiving of performance is possible. Simulation provides a unique window on performance that is prospective and about challenging situations, whereas routine observation of real work is prospective but most commonly only sees less challenging situations, and case reports about performance may be of tough cases but are often incomplete and hindsight-based.[365] Scoring or certifying competence by using the simulator is more problematic than using the simulator as a teaching tool, however. Anesthesiologists have long discussed the possibility of using the simulator as a tool for examinations, either for graduation from a residency or for ABA certification. In Israel, a simulation examination has become part of the board certification process.[95]

Despite these difficulties, the use of anesthesia simulation to assist in evaluating performance is likely to increase in the future. Even though simulation is currently used for some high-stakes examinations, the challenges remain the same: (1) It requires independent evaluation of the simulation scenarios and assessment of the predictive power of the subjective judgments made by experts scoring the examinee. (2) There is a lack of any well-accepted standard for performance evaluation.

Another difficulty with using simulation for high-stakes testing at a neutral site is that the operating room equipment would rarely be the same as that used by the candidate, and the operating room staff's operational protocols could differ from the protocols familiar to the candidate. In the training situation, these difficulties can be overlooked as part of the global suspension of disbelief needed to maximize the benefits of simulation training. In the test situation, these differences potentially could skew the results. This issue could be addressed by allowing candidates preparing to take their examination to undergo sufficient practice sessions to familiarize themselves fully with the standard simulation environment used for the test.

Another application of simulation-based performance assessment would be for the evaluation of trainees or experienced clinicians who have been placed on probation or for whom dismissal from their position is already a distinct possibility. For these clinicians, the burden of proof is on them to show their skills. Simulation could offer a more controlled environment for these clinicians to do so. The same could be true for practitioners who wish to return to clinical work after a hiatus.

The existing systems of performance evaluation, which use a haphazard composite of subjective judgment of clinical competency in clinical work along with written and oral examinations, has itself never been validated. Many experts believe that the written examination does not correlate well with clinical ability, and the degree to which the oral examination process tests actual clinical skill is unknown. Simulation could offer candidates the opportunity to show their clinical abilities in a controlled clinical domain; appropriate scenarios can probe language skills and the ability to act as an effective consultant to other clinicians.[226,366]

The ABA transitioned in 2017 to a new format for the Part 2 Examination, named the APPLIED Examination, to include an Objective Standardized Clinical Examination (OSCE) component along with the traditional structured oral examination component. The OSCE stations do not include full-scale mannequin-based simulation but do include performance on task trainers and encounters with actors playing roles as patients or as clinical personnel (e.g., surgeon).

The methods currently used to assess the performance of clinicians in their actual clinical work are weak and inconsistent; systematically incompetent anesthesia professionals are not easily identified or removed from practice. Thus, reasonable arguments can be made that the field of performance assessment has advanced sufficiently to allow consideration of simulation-based examinations, including full mannequin-based simulations, even for high-stakes purposes, especially considering the limitations of the current systems of written and oral examination.[366] Nonetheless, simulation-based performance assessment remains a controversial topic for discussion in the simulation and clinical anesthesiology communities. The anesthesia professions should be careful about how they may introduce simulation-based performance evaluation. The controversy should not divert attention from the most common application of simulation, which is to improve clinical performance through training individuals and teams to prevent and manage adverse clinical events.

Simulation Societies and Simulation Journals

One measure of the evolving maturity of simulation in health care is the formation and growth of professional societies and associated peer-reviewed journals. Organizations such as the Society for Simulation in Health Care (SSH) and the SESAM (www.sesam-web.org) have been constantly striving to promote knowledge and use of simulation in health care. Although anesthesiology was the medical field that initiated work on the fully interactive mannequin-based simulator and that dominated the early developments in the field, simulation is a broad strategy that has now been widely adopted by many different disciplines and domains in health. For the most part, simulation professional societies have sprung up as explicitly multidisciplinary organizations, while clinical societies have also created committees and other bodies to oversee or facilitate the use of simulation in their settings. Major leadership roles in the multidisciplinary societies have been played by anesthesiologists and engineers associated with anesthesiology far more frequently than their prevalence in the clinician population would otherwise predict.

Periodic scientific congresses on simulation such as the Rochester Conferences on Simulation in Anesthesia have been under way since the mid-1990s although attendance was less than 100 people. The largest simulation organization is SSH, which was founded in 2004 as the outgrowth of the group that had operated the International Meeting on Medical Simulation for several years as a satellite to the annual meeting of the Society for Technology in Anesthesia. Under the auspices of SSH, the meeting was transformed into the IMSH, encompassing all health care disciplines and domains, not just medicine. Although starting with far fewer attendees, the annual meeting of SESAM now has around 850 attendees (2018). Similarly, for SSH, whereas the original IMMS had at most 200 attendees, IMSH in 2018 had more than 3000 attendees. For IMSH this number places it in the category of a medium-sized scientific meeting; to put this in the context of anesthesiology, it would rank as the third largest meeting in the United States, falling below only the ASA meeting (about 14,000 attendees) and the New York Postgraduate Assembly in Anesthesiology (PGA) conference (over 4000 attendees), but ranking ahead of the International Anesthesia Research Society (IARS) annual meeting (about 1000 attendees).

Another sign of the growing maturity of simulation in health care is the establishment and growth of peer-reviewed journals for the field. SSH has published *Simulation in Healthcare* in print and online every other month since 2006. This journal was approved for indexing by PubMed in 2008. Many organizations have become affiliates of SSH and most have made *Simulation in Healthcare* their official publication (for example the Australian SSH, and the Association of Standardized Patient Educators). The International Nursing Association for Clinical Simulation and Learning has published (online only) the *Journal of Clinical Simulation in Nursing* since 2006 although it rarely has papers concerning anesthesiology. The BMJ *Simulation and Technology-Enhanced Learning*, the journal of the UK Association for Simulated Practice in Healthcare, has been published (online only) since 2014. *Advances in Simulation*, the official journal of SESAM, has been published (online only) since 2016.

The Future of Patient Simulation in Anesthesia

The future is now—we are it.[234]

More than three decades of consistent development have passed; the field of simulation in health care could be described metaphorically as being in its adolescence or young adulthood. Thousands of simulators are in use around the world in thousands of clinical programs. Anesthesiology and critical care remain important mainstays in simulation, which is now a standard part of the training of anesthesia professionals, although these fields have now become minority users when compared to numerous users across all the rest of health care. Yet even in anesthesiology, with nearly 30 years of simulation under its belt, the fraction of anesthesia professionals who have undergone a serious simulation experience since completing their initial training is relatively small. For example, as of 2018 Gaba estimates that only about 25% of board-certified anesthesiologists in the United States have undergone the MOCA simulation course.

The modalities of simulation have expanded from completely nontechnological to fully virtual. MBS have become more sophisticated, easier to use, and more portable, and available in many different models from multiple manufacturers. On the other hand, considering that it is now nearly 25 years since the first commercial simulators were introduced, the overall improvement in the features, reliability, and clinical or physical realism has not advanced at nearly the rate as for computing equipment over the same period. In part this is due to the fact that improvements in simulators depend heavily on the demand for the devices in general, and for special features in particular. There is a steep tradeoff between features and many otherwise desirable improvements may be too costly for their expected impact or demand. Simulators that use complex mathematical models of physiology and pharmacology have largely retreated from the marketplace since many applications can be managed well with less complicated control systems.

In contrast to aeronautical engineers designing airplanes, anesthesia professionals or biomedical engineers do not design and build human beings. In aviation the fundamental differential equations of fluid mechanics and aerodynamics are firmly established, allowing supercomputers to provide technically meaningful simulations as replacements for many physical tests; furthermore, test flights of prototype aircraft are conducted with sophisticated instrumentation built in to test and carefully capture their behavior. Clinicians will never have this type of knowledge about the human body.

VR and AR are still in an early childhood phase, with rapid development under way but with maturity still far away. Many current (late 2018) VR systems address visualization of anatomy or physical structures. Only a few provide multiparticipant interaction in an immersive virtual environment. As far as the virtual patient is concerned they are only as good as the underlying engines—mathematical or otherwise—that drive their clinical responses. The coming decade(s) will likely see a continued proliferation of VR systems with substantial shakeout of techniques, technologies, and firms. Currently many users of simulation are beginning to try out VR and AR systems but it is still very early in their development and use.

VR proponents imagine a VR so realistic that it rivals, or is indistinguishable from, the real world. This would approach the *Star Trek* holodeck or the "brain in a vat" style of simulation in *The Matrix*. Although we once predicted that interactive VR could take over from physical simulation by 2020 to 2025, and the tide has indeed started to turn, we predict that it will still be a long time—if ever—before this happens. Whether there is indeed something fundamentally different about human professionals working together naturally in a physically realistic clinical environment versus doing the same via some sort of VR remains to be seen.

Patient simulation has now become a regular part of initial and recurrent training of most anesthesia professionals and many other clinicians in many countries in the developed world, and significant penetration into the developing world. Zero to low technology simulations are also being used successfully in low resource areas to address important health issues.

With patient simulation issues of human factors and patient safety, in part via the CRM concept, were introduced to health care as ACRM training and its equivalents in various clinical arenas. This has been an influential complement to traditional methods and content of teaching and learning in a large variety of health care domains, especially those that share the complex and dynamic work profile of anesthesiology—decision making playing out over seconds, minutes, and hours; working with action teams; wielding highly lethal interventions as described in Chapter 6. Since all of the pioneering work on mannequin-based simulation and its key applications was done in anesthesiology, our field can rightly claim to have given one more gift to all of health care, to accompany other gifts such as the Apgar score, modern pulse oximetry and capnography, blood gas analysis, mechanical ventilation, etc. Moreover, despite its wide spread beyond anesthesiology, anesthesia professionals and others working with them continue to play major leadership roles in multidisciplinary and multiprofessional simulation centers and organizations.

Fully integrated simulation team training with a significant focus on human factors and CRM may improve patient safety and quality in acute care settings, and it may increase employee satisfaction and effectiveness of routine work. Simulation team training is becoming more common, but is still not solidly embedded into the fabric of health care as a core part of how we do business as is the case for commercial aviation or nuclear power. While health care has a long way to go to achieve the full impact of simulation on the quality and safety of patient care, the authors no longer fear that the technique of simulation will be rejected in our field, and they believe it is worth it to remain on a path toward the comprehensive industrywide, career-long application of simulation to save as many hearts, brains, and lives as possible.

Appendix 7.1 Online Links and Useful Resources

- American Society of Anesthesiologists (ASA) Simulation Education Network
  - Many resources on simulation and links to ASA-endorsed simulation centers
- Society for Simulation in Healthcare (SSH)
  - Homepage: www.ssih.org
  - Journal *Simulation in Healthcare*, Elsevier:https://journals.lww.com/simulationinhealthcare/pages/default.aspx
  - Website of the Instructor Certification program of SSH: https://www.ssih.org/Certification
  - Criteria for Accreditation of Simulation Centers by SSH: https://www.ssih.org/Accreditation
- Society in Europe for Simulation in Medicine (SESAM): www.sesam-web.org
- Stanford Simulation Site - Center for Immersive and Simulation-based Learning: cisl.stanford.edu
- Center for Advanced Pediatric and Perinatal Education (CAPE): cape.stanford.edu
- Center for Medical Simulation (CMS in Boston): harvardmedsim.org
- WISER Simulation Center—University of Pittsburgh Medical Center: www.wiser.pitt.edu

Acknowledgment

The editors, publisher, and Drs. Marcus Rall, David M. Gaba, and Peter Dieckmann would like to thank Dr. Christoph Bernard Eich for contributing to this chapter on this topic in the prior edition of this work. It has served as the foundation for the current chapter.

 **Complete references available online at expertconsult.com.**

References

1. Donaldson L. London, UK: The Stationary Office. Online available from https://webarchive.nationalarchives.gov.uk/20130105045448/http://www.dh.gov.uk/prod_consum_dh/groups/dh_digitalassets/documents/digitalasset/dh_096231.pdf. Accessed November 28, 2018;2008.
2. Mai CL, et al. In: Coté CJ, Lerman J, Anderson BJ, eds. *A Practice of Anesthesia for Infants and Children*. 6th ed. Philadelphia: Elsevier; 2019:1204–1211.e1202.
3. Eppich WJ, et al. *Curr opinped*. 2006;18(3):266–271.
4. Weinstock PH, et al. *SPediatr Crit Care Med* 2009;10(2):176-181.
5. Everett TC, et al. *Pediatric Anesthesia*. 2017;27(10):984–990.
6. Halamek LP, et al. *Pediatrics*. 2000;106(4):E45.
7. Eich C, et al. *BJA*. 2007;98(4):417–419.
8. Niles D, et al. *Resuscitation*. 2009;80(8):909–912.
9. Sutton RM, et al. *Pediatr Crit Care Med*. 2009;10(3):407–409.
10. Kohn LT, et al. National Academies Press. 2000.
11. Dorman T, et al. *Crit Care Med*. 2004;32(1):263–272.
12. Gallagher CJ, Tan JM. *Int Anesthesiol Clin*. 2010;48(3):83–99.
13. Weller J. In: Riley RH, ed. *Manual of Simulation in Healthcare*. Oxford: Oxford University Press; 2008.
14. Weller J, et al. *N Z Med J*. 2015;128(1418):40–51.
15. Lorello GR, et al. *BJA*. 2014;112(2):231–245.
16. LeBlanc VR, et al. *Simul Healthc*. 2011;6(suppl):S24–S29.
17. Higham H, Baxendale B. *BJA*. 2017;119:i106–i114.
18. Salas E, et al. *BMJ Quality & Safety*. 2013;22(6):449–452.
19. *The Comprehensive Textbook of Healthcare Simulation*. corrected 2nd printing ed. New York, Heidelberg, Dordrecht, London: Springer; 2014.
20. *Defining Excellence in Simulation Programs*. 1st ed. Philadelphia, PA: Society for Simulation in Healthcare; 2014.
21. *Manual of Simulation in Healthcare*. 2nd ed. Oxford University Press; 2015.
22. Gallagher CJ, Issenberg SB. *Simulation in Anesthesia*. Philadelphia: Saunders; 2006.
23. Kyle RR, Murray WB. *Clinical Simulation: Operations, Engineering and Management*. Amsterdam, Sydney, Boston: Academic Press Elsevier; 2008.
24. Gaba DM, et al. *Crisis Management in Anesthesiology*. 2nd ed. Elsevier; 2014.

25. DeMaria S, et al. *BMJ*. 2017.
26. Murray DJ. *Minerva Anestesiol*. 2011;77(5):528–533.
27. Hicks CM, et al. *Acad Emerg Med*. 2008;15(11):1136–1143.
28. Rosen MA, et al. *Acad Emerg Med*. 2008;15(11):1190–1198.
29. Parsons JR, et al. *West J Emerg Med*. 2018;19(1):205–210.
30. Steinemann S, et al. *J Surg Educ*. 2011;68(6):472–477.
31. Härgestam M, et al. *BMJ Open*. 2016;6(1).
32. Rubio-Gurung S, et al. *Pediatrics*. 2014;134(3):e790–e797.
33. Capella J, et al. *J Surg Educ*. 2010;67(6):439–443.
34. Campbell DM, et al. *Paediatr Child Health*. 2009;14(1):19–23.
35. Peacock PJ, et al. *Cureus*. 2016;8(9):e790-e790.
36. Lee MMH, et al. *BMJ*. 2017;3(4):142–148.
37. Gardner R, Raemer DB. *Obstet Gynecol Clin North Am*. 2008;35(1):97–127.
38. Nelissen E, et al. *BMC*. 2017;17(1):301.
39. Fann JI, et al. In: Levine AI, DeMaria Jr S, Schwartz AD, Sim AJ, eds. *The Comprehensive Textbook of Healthcare Simulation*. New York: Springer; 2014:299–313.
40. Maluf MA, et al. *Rev Brasil Cirur Card*. 2015;30(5):562–570.
41. Giuliani M, et al. *Radiation Oncology*. 2014;9:189.
42. Singleton MN, et al. *BMJ*. 2017.
43. Sandahl C, et al. *Int J Health Care Qual Assur*. 2013;26(2):174–188.
44. Phrampus PE, et al. *Simul Healthc*. 2016;11(2):82–88.
45. Walsh K, et al. *BMJ*. 2018;4(1):1–3.
46. Hunt EA, et al. *Resuscitation*. 2014;85:945–951.
47. Hayes CW, et al. *Crit Care Med*. 2007;35(7):1668–1672.
48. Hendrickse AD, et al. *J R Army Med Corps*. 2001;147(2):173–178.
49. Gaba DM. *Simul Healthc*. 2014;9(6):337–338.
50. Raemer DB, et al. *Acad Med*. 2016;91(4):530–539.
51. Szyld D, et al. *Simul Healthc*. 2017;12(6):385–392.
52. Edwards SE, et al. *BMJ*. 2015;1(3):87–93.
53. Jowsey T, et al. *BMJ*. 2018.
54. Beal MD, et al. *Simul Healthc*. 2017;12(2):104–116.
55. Paige JT, et al. *BMJ*. 2017;3(4):127–134.
56. Perdue TO, et al. *Simul Healthc*. 2017;12(5):308–313.
57. Solanki P, et al. *BMJ*. 2017.
58. Stroobants J, et al. *Resuscitation*. 85(12):1769-1774.
59. Wilks J, Pendergast D. *Health Ed J*. 2017;76(8):1009–1023.
60. Böttiger BW, Van Aken H. *The Lancet*. 2015;385(9985):2353.
61. Van de Velde S, et al. *Ann Emerg Med*. 2009;54(3):447–457.e445.
62. Meier AH, et al. *J Am Coll Surg*. 2001;192(3):372–384.
63. Stefanich L, Cruz-Neira C. *BiomedSci Instru*. 1999;35:141–145.
64. Weinger MB, et al. *Anesthesiology*. 2017;127(3):475–489.
65. Schwid HA, O'Donnell D. *Anesthesiology*. 1992;76(4):495–501.
66. Lindekaer AL, et al. *Acta anaesthes Scand*. 1997;41(10):1280–1284.
67. Byrne AJ, Jones JG. *BJA*. 1997;78(5):553–556.
68. DeAnda A, Gaba DM. *Anesth Analg*. 1991;72(3):308–315.
69. Schwid MD, et al. *Anesthesiology*. 2002;97(6):1434–1444.
70. Gardi T, et al. *Acta Anaesth Scand*. 2001;45(8):1032–1035.
71. Jacobsen J, et al. *Acta Anaesth Scand*. 2001;45(3):315–319.
72. Singer SJ, et al. *Qual Saf Health Care*. 2003;12(2):112–118.
73. Cooper JB, et al. *Simul Health*. 2011;6(4):231–238.
74. Singer SJ, et al. *Health Care Manage Rev*. 2011;36(2):188–200.
75. Driver JF, et al. In: Youngberg BJ, ed. *Principles of Risk Management and Patient Safety*. Sudbury, MA: Jones & Bartlett Learning; 2011.
76. Barsuk JH, et al. *Simul Healthc*. 2016;11(1):52–59.
77. Birsner ML, Satin AJ. *Sem Peri*. 2013;37(3):175–178.
78. Thomas PA, eds. *Curriculum Development for Medical Education*. 3rd ed. Baltimore: Johns Hopkins University Press; 2015.
79. Gordon JA, Pawlowski J. *E Acad Med*. 2002;77(7):751–752.
80. Issenberg SB, Scalese RJ. *Perspect Biol Med*. 2008;51(1):31–46.
81. Murray DJ. *Curr Opin Anaesthesiol*. 2014;27(6):610–615.
82. Sørensen JL, et al. *BMJ Open*. 2015;5(10).
83. Nielsen DS, et al. *Simul Healthc*. 2014;9(1):48–55.
84. Riley W, et al. *Qual Safe Health Care*. 2010;19(suppl 3):i53–i56.
85. Patterson MD, et al. *BMJ Qual Saf*. 2013;22(6):468–477.
86. Biddell EA, et al. *Simul Healthc*. 2016;11(2):94–99.
87. McIntosh CA, et al. *BMJ*. 2018;4(1):4–12.
88. Gignon M, et al. *Int J Occup Saf Ergon*. 2017;23(4):589–591.
89. Howard SK, et al. *Anesthesiology*. 2003;98(6):1345–1355.
90. Knudson MM, et al. *J Trauma*. 2008;64(2):255–263.
91. Fletcher G, et al. *Br j Anaesthes*. 2003;90(5):580–588.
92. Barsuk D, et al. *Anesth Analg*. 2005;100(3):803–809. able of contents.
93. Overly FL, et al. *Ped Emerg Care*. 2007;23(1):11–15.
94. Fehr JJ, al dt. *Anesthesiology*. 2011;115(6):1308–1315.
95. Boulet JR, et al. *Anesthesiology*. 2003;99(6):1270–1280.
96. Ottestad E, et al. *Crit Care Med*. 2007;35(3):769–775.
97. Boulet John R, Murray David J. *Anesthesiology*. 2010;112(4):1041–1052.
98. Murray D, Enarson C. *Anesthesiology*. 2007;106(5):895–896.
99. Boulet JR, Murray D. *Can J Anaesthes*. 2012;59(2):182–192.
100. Ryall T, et al. *J Multidisc Healthc*. 2016;9:69–82.
101. Byrne AJ, Greaves JD. *Br J Anaesthes*. 2001;86(3):445–450.
102. Tetzlaff MD, John E. *Anesthesiology*. 2007;106(4):812–825.
103. Lien CA, et al. *Anesthesiology*. 2017;127(3):410–412.
104. Cheng A, et al. *BMJ*. 2016;2(3):51–60.
105. Rudolph JW, et al. *Anesthesiol Clin*. 2007;25:361–376.
106. Rudolph JW, et al. *Simul Healthc*. 2013;8:304–316.
107. Rudolph JW, et al. *Acad Emerg Med*. 2008;15(11):1010–1016.
108. Jaye P, et al. *Clin Teacher*. 2015;12(3):171–175.
109. Eppich W, Cheng A. *Simul Healthc*. 2015;10.
110. Kolbe M, et al. *BMJ Qual Saf*. 2013;22:541–553.
111. Sawyer T, et al. *Simul Healthc*. 2016;11.
112. Eppich WJ, et al. *Acad Med*. 2015;90.
113. Cheng A, et al. *Med Educ*. 2014;48.
114. Kolbe M, et al. *Adv Simul*. 2016;1(1):29.
115. Schick CJ, et al. *Simul in Health*. 2015;10(3):178–187.
116. Farooq O, et al. *BMJ*. 2017;3(2):48–53.
117. Krogh K, et al. *Clin Simul Nursing*. 2015;11(3):180–187.
118. Reed SJ,A, et al. *Clin SimulNursing*. 2013;9:585–591.
119. Savoldelli GL, et al. *Anesthesiology*. 2006;105:279–285.
120. Sawyer T, et al. *Simul Healthc*. 2012;7(4):213–221.
121. Rudolph JW, et al. *Simul Healthc*. 2014;9(6):339–349.
122. Sullivan NJ, et al. *Resuscitation*. 2015;86:6–13.
123. Cheng A, et al. *Resuscitation*. 2015;93:142–149.
124. Grande B, et al. *Curr Opin Anesthes*. 2017;30(6):743–747.
125. Kennedy CC, et al. *Crit Care Med*. 2014;42(1):169–178.
126. Barsuk JH, et al. *BMJ*. 2014;23(9):749–756.
127. Pian-Smith MCM, et al. *Simul Healthc*. 2009;4(2):84–91.
128. O'Connor P, et al. *Jt Comm J Qual Patient Saf*. 2013;39:426–431.
129. Weiss M, et al. *Eur J Work Organ Psychol*. 2017;26(1):66–80.
130. St.Pierre M, et al. *Der Anaesthesist*. 2016;65(9):681–689.
131. Minehart RD, et al. *Anesthesiology*. 2014;120(1):160–171.
132. Kobayashi L, et al. *Simul Healthc*. 2006;1(2):72–78.
133. Kyle RR, et al. *JEPM*. 2004;6(1):E029-E029.
134. Burtscher MJ, et al. *J Exp Psychol Appl*. 2011;17:257–269.
135. Manser T, et al. *Anesth Analg*. 2009;108:1606–1615.
136. Burtscher MJ, et al. *BrJ Anaesth*. 2011;106(6):801–806.
137. Schmutz J, et al. *Eur J Work Organ Psychol*. 2015;24:761–776.
138. Riethmüller M, et al. *Ergonomics*. 2012;55(1):55–68.
139. Künzle B, et al. *Eur J Work Organ Psychol*. 2010;19:505–531.
140. Künzle B, et al. *Qual Saf Health Care*. 2010;19:1–6.
141. Bogenstätter Y, et al. *Hum Factors*. 2009;51:115–125.
142. Tschan F, et al. *Small Group Research*. 2009;40:271–300.
143. Weiss M, et al. *Small Group Research*. 2014;45:290–313.
144. St.Pierre M, et al. *Der Anaesthesist*. 2012;61(10):857–866.
145. Kolbe M, et al. *Anesth Analg*. 2012;115:1099–1108.
146. Minehart RD, et al. *Simul Healthc*. 2012;7:166–170.
147. Rudolph JW, et al. *Acad Manage J*. 2009;34:733–756.
148. Larson JRJ, et al. *J Pers Soc Psychol*. 1998;75:93–108.
149. Christensen C, et al. *Med Dec Making*. 2000;20(1):45–50.
150. Tschan F, et al. *Human Perform*. 2006;19:277–304.
151. Marsch SC, et al. *Eur J Anaesth*. 2005;22.
152. Hunziker S, et al. *BMC Emerg Med*. 2009;9(1):1–10.
153. Fernandez Castelao E, et al. *Resuscitation*. 2011;82:1338–1343.
154. Marsch SCU, et al. *Crit Care Med*. 2005;33:963–967.
155. Dieckmann P. *Simul Healthc*. 2007;2(3):183–193.
156. Dieckmann P, et al. *J Cogn Eng DecMaking*. 2007;1(2):148–168.
157. Scerbo MW, Dawson S. *Simul Healthc*. 2007;2(4):224–230.
158. Rudolph JW, et al. *Simul Healthc*. 2007;2(3):161–163.
159. Dieckmann P, Rall M. In: Cashman JN, Grounds RM, eds. *Recent Advances in Anaesthesia and Intensive Care*. Cambridge, UK: Cambridge University Press; 2007:213–232.
160. Manser T, et al. *Ergonomics*. 2007;50(2):246–260.
161. Dieckmann P, et al. *Ergonomics*. 2006;49(5-6):526–543.
162. Wehbe-Janek H, et al. *Simul Healthc*. 2015;10(1):4–13.
163. Kneebone R, et al. *Adv Simul*. 2016;1(1):19.

164. Huddy JR, et al. *BMJ Open*. 2016;6(9):e011043.
165. Kneebone RL. *Adv Simul*. 2016;1(1):27.
166. Weldon SM, et al. *BMJ*. 2018;4(suppl 2). A21-A21.
167. Kofke WA, et al. *Med Law*. 2001;20(1):79–83.
168. Zhang C, et al. *AdvSimul*. 2018;3:15-15.
169. Cooper JB, Taqueti VR. *Qual SafHealthc*. 2004;13(suppl 1):i11–i18.
170. Rosen KR. *J Crit Care*. 2008;23(2):157–166.
171. Gaba DM. *Simul Healthc*. 2007;2(2):126–135.
172. Rosen K. In: Levine AI, DeMaria Jr S, Schwartz AD, Sim AJ, eds. *The Comprehensive Textbook of Healthcare Simulation*. New York: Springer; 2013:5–49.
173. Owen H. *Simulation in Healthcare Education. An extensive history*. Cham, Heidelberg, New York, Dordrecht, London: Springer International Publishing; 2016.
174. Owen H. *Simul Healthc*. 2012;7(2):102–116.
175. Abrahamson S, et al. *J Med Educ*. 1969;44(6):515–519.
176. Gordon MS, et al. *Am J Cardiol*. 1980;45(4):791–796.
177. Gaba DM, DeAnda A. *Anesthesiology*. 1988;69(3):387–394.
178. DeAnda A, Gaba DM. *Anesth Analg*. 1990;71(1):77–82.
179. Gaba DM, DeAnda A. *Anesth Analg*. 1989;68(4):444–451.
180. Holzman RS, et al. *J Clin Anesthes*. 1995;7(8):675–687.
181. Howard SK, et al. *Aviat Space Environ Med*. 1992;63(9):763–770.
182. Naik VN, Brien SE. *Can J Anaesthes*. 2013;60(2):192–200.
183. Philip JH. *Int J Clin Monit Comp*. 1986;3(3):165–173.
184. De Oliveira Jr GS, et al. *Anaesthesia*. 2013;68(10):1053–1058.
185. Anesthesiology News. *Clinical Anesthesia: Virtual Reality Simulator Improves Intubation Success*; 2017. https://www.anesthesiologynews.com/Clinical-Anesthesiology/Article/12-17/Virtual-Reality-Simulator-Improves-Intubation-Success/45309. Accessed November 11, 2018.
186. Grottke O, et al. *Br J Anaesth*. 2009;103(4):594–600.
187. Ullrich S, et al. *Stud Health Technol Inform*. 2009;142:392–394.
188. Udani AD, et al. *Loc Reg Anesthes*. 2015;8:33–43.
189. Chen XX, et al. *Reg Anesth Pain Med*. 2017;42(6):741–750.
190. Kleinert R, et al. *J Med Internet Res*. 2015;17(4):e91.
191. Levine AI, Swartz MH. *J Crit Care*. 2008;23(2):179–184.
192. Cantrell MJ, Deloney LA. *Anesthes Clin*. 2007;25(2):377–383.
193. Nestel D, Bearman M. *Simulated Patient Methodology. Theory, Evidence and Practice*. Chichester: Wiley; 2015.
194. Hoelzer BC, et al. *Pain Med*. 2015;16(4):680–691.
195. Kjellin A, et al. *Scand J Surg*. 2014;103(4):232–236.
196. Cumin D, Merry AF. *Anaesthesia*. 2007;62(2):151–162.
197. Miller GE. *AcadMed*. 1990;65(suppl 9):S63–67.
198. Issenberg SB, et al. *Med Teach*. 2005;27(1):10–28.
199. Sørensen JL, et al. *BMC Med Ed*. 2017;17(1). 20-20.
200. Eagle A. *Health Facility Management Magazine*. November 1, 2017. https://www.hfmmagazine.com/articles/3184-principles-for-efficient-simulation-center-layouts. Accessed November 12, 2018.
201. Eagle A. *Health Facility Management Magazine*. November 1, 2017. https://www.hfmmagazine.com/articles/3182-the-reality-of-designing-simulation-centers. Accessed November 12, 2018.
202. Rall M, et al. In: Kyle R, Murray BW, eds. *Clinical Simulation: Operations, Engineering, and Management*. Burlington: Academic Press; 2008:565–581.
203. Rosen MA, et al. *J Cont Ed Hlth Prof*. 2012;32(4):243–254.
204. Raemer DB. *Simul Healthc*. 2014;9(3):153–155.
205. Gjeraa K, et al. *Acta Anaesthes Scand*. 2016;60(1):36–47.
206. Billings CE, Reynard WD. *Aviat Space Environ Med*. 1984;55(10):960–965.
207. Helmreich RL, et al. *Int J Aviat Psychol*. 1999;9(1):19–32.
208. Wiener EL, et al., eds. *Cockpit Resource Management*. San Diego: Academic Press; 1993.
209. Manser T. T*Acta Anaesth Scand*. 2009;53(2):143-151.
210. Weaver SJ, et al. *BMJ Qual Saf*. 2014;23(5):359–372.
211. Armour Forse R, et al. *Surgery*. 2011;150(4):771–778.
212. Hughes A, et al. *J Appl Psychol*. 2016;101(9):1266–1304.
213. Baker DP, et al. In: Henriksen K, Battles J, Marks E, et al., eds. *Advances in Patient Safety: From Research to Implementation*. Rockville, MD: Agency for Healthcare Research and Quality (AHRQ); 2005.
214. Salas E, et al. *Human Res Manag*. 2014:24. Available at: https://orpca.org/APCM/Salas_et_al-2014-Human_Resource_Management%201%203.pdf.
215. Weaver SJ, et al. *Jt Comm J Qual Patient Saf*. 2010;36(3):133–142.
216. Salas E, et al. *Acad Emerg Med*. 2008;15(11):1002–1009.
217. Gaba DM, et al. *Simul Gam*. 2001;32(2):175–193.
218. Burke CS, et al. *Qual Saf Health Care*. 2004;13(suppl 1):i96–104.
219. Tan SB, et al. *ANZ J Surg*. 2014;84(7-8):515–522.
220. Haller G, et al. *Int J Qual Health Care*. 2008;20(4):254–263.
221. Hilton G,D, et al. *Int J Ob Anesthes*. 2016;25:9–16.
222. Maslovitz S, et al. *Ob Gyn*. 2007;109(6):1295–1300.
223. Lighthall GK, Barr J. *J Intensiv Care Med*. 2007;22(5):257–269.
224. Shapiro MJ, et al. *Qual Saf Healthc*. 2004;13(6):417–421.
225. Wallin CJ, et al. *Med Educ*. 2007;41(2):173–180.
226. Berkenstadt H, et al. *Anesthesiol Clin*. 2007;25(1):65–74. viii-ix.
227. Murphy M, et al. *Injury*. 2018;49(5):953–958.
228. Volpe CE, et al. *Hum Factors*. 1996;38(1):87–100.
229. Marks MA, et al. *J Appl Psychol*. 2002;87(1):3–13.
230. Strang AJ, et al. *Proc Human Factors Erg Soc Annual Meeting*. 2012;56(1):1581–1585.
231. Walker ST, et al. *BMJ Qual Saf*. 2013;22(6):453–458.
232. Lighthall GK, et al. *Jt Comm J Qual Patient Saf*. 2010;36(5):209–216.
233. Lighthall GK, et al. *Jt Comm J Qual Patient Saf*. 2013;39(4):157–166.
234. Gaba DM. *Qual Saf Health Care*. 2004;13(suppl 1):i2–10.
235. Sidi A, et al. *J Pat Safety*. 2017.
236. Barsuk JH, et al. *Arch Int Med*. 2009;169(15):1420–1423.
237. Murray DJ, et al. *Anesth Analg*. 2005;101(4):1127–1134. table of contents.
238. Fanning RM, Gaba DM. *Simul Healthc*. 2007;2(2):115–125.
239. Cooper JB, et al. *Anesthesiology*. 1984;60(1):34–42.
240. Cooper JB, et al. *Qual Saf Healthc*. 2002;11(3):277–282.
241. Gaba DM. *Int Anesthesiol Clin*. 1989;27(3):137–147.
242. Gaba DM, et al. *Anesthesiology*. 1987;66(5):670–676.
243. Gaba D, et al. *Simul Gaming*. 2001;32:175–193.
244. Dunn EJ, et al. *Jt Comm J Qual Patient Saf*. 2007;33(6):317–325.
245. Weinstock PH, et al. *Ped Crit Care Med*. 2005;6(6):635–641.
246. Cooper JB, et al. *Anesth Analg*. 2008;106(2):574–584.
247. Murphy JG, et al. *J Crit Care*. 2007;22(1):51–55.
248. Steadman RH, et al. *Anesthesiology*. 2015;122(5):1154–1169.
249. Weinger MB, et al. 00.*Anesthesiology*. 2014;121(3):655-659.
250. Kurrek MM, Fish KJ. *An J Anaesthes*. 1996;43(5):430–434.
251. Salas E, et al. *Hum Factors*. 2006;48(2):392–412.
252. Haerkens MH, et al. *Acta Anaesth Scand*. 2015;59(10):1319–1329.
253. Moffatt-Bruce SD, et al. *Am J Med Qual*. 2017;32(1):5–11.
254. Curran I. In: Kyle R, Murray BW, eds. *Clinical Simulation: Operations, Engineering, and Management*. Burlington: Academic Press; 2008:153–161.
255. Dieckmann P. In: Dieckmann P, ed. *Using Simulations for Education, Training and Research*. Lengerich, Germany: Pabst; 2009:40–138.
256. Der Sahakian G, et al. *Simul Gaming*. 2015;46(2):197–208.
257. Edmondson AC. *Admin Sci Qua*. 1999;44(2):350–383.
258. Nickson C. https://litfl.com/the-safe-container-rules-ok/. Accessed November 21, 2018.
259. Dieckmann P, et al. *Simul Healthc*. 2010;5(4):219–225.
260. Paige JB, Morin KH. *Clin Simul Nurs*. 2013;9(11):e481–e489.
261. Escher C, et al. *Adv Simul*. 2017;2:25-25.
262. Choi W, et al. *BMJ*. 2017;3(suppl 1):S23–S32.
263. Tschan F, et al. In: Boos M, Kolbe M, Kappeler P, Ellwart T, eds. *Coordination in Human and Primate Groups*. Heidelberg: Springer; 2011:93–118.
264. Cheng A, et al. *Simul Healthc*. 2015;10(2):69–75.
265. Young JQ, et al. *Med Teach*. 2014;36(5):371–384.
266. Nestel D, et al. In: Nestel D, Kelly M, Jolly B, Watson M, eds. *Healthcare Simulation Education: Evidence, Theory and Practice*. Wiley-Blackwell; 2017.
267. Salas E, et al. *Int J Avia Psychol*. 1998;8(3):197–208.
268. Salas E, Burke CS. *Qual Saf Healthc*. 2002;11(2):119–120.
269. Hays RT, Singer MJ. *Simulation Fidelity in Training System Design: Bridging the Gap Between Reality and Training*. New York: Springer; 1989.
270. Alessi S. In: O'Neil H, Andrews D, eds. *Aircrew Training and Assessment*. Mahwah, NJ: Erlbaum; 2000:197–222.
271. Feinstein AH, Cannon HM. *Simul Gaming*. 2002;33(4):425–440.
272. Grant VJ, et al. *Med Teach*. 2018:1–10.
273. Rall M, et al. *Euro J Anaesthesiol*. 2000;17(8):516–517.
274. Dieckmann P, et al. *MedTeach*. 2009;31(7):e287–e294.
275. Krogh K, et al. *Adv Simul*. 2016;1(1):12.
276. Dismukes RK, et al. *Simul Healthc*. 2006;1(1):23–25.
277. Dieckmann P, et al. *Adv Simul*. 2017;2(1):21.
278. Brindley PG, Reynolds SF. *J Crit Care*. 2011;26(2):155–159.
279. McGaghie WC, et al. *Med Educ*. 2010;44(1):50–63.

280. Cantrell MA. *ClinSimul Nurs*. 2008;4(2):e19–e23.
281. Dreifuerst KT. *Nurs Ed Perspec*. 2009;30(2):109–114.
282. Dieckmann P, Rall M. In: Kyle R, Murray BW, eds. *Clinical Simulation: Operations, Engineering, and Management*. Burlington, MA: Academic Press; 2008:647–652.
283. Dieckmann P, et al. In: Kyle R, Murray BW, eds. *Clinical Simulation: Operations, Engineering, and Management*. Burlington, MA: Academic Press; 2008:667–676.
284. Raemer D, et al. *Simul Healthc*. 2011;6(suppl):S52–57.
285. Ali AA, Miller ET. *J Nurs Ed*. 2018;57(1):14–20.
286. Kolb DA. *Experiential Learning: Experience as the Source of Learning and Development*. Englewood Cliffs, NJ: Prentice-Hall; 1984.
287. Stegmann K, et al. *Med Educ*. 2012;46(10):1001–1008.
288. Eppich W, et al. *Clin Pediatr Emerg Med*. 2016.
289. Marshall DA, Manus DA. *AORN J*. 2007;86(6):994–1011.
290. Makary MA, et al. *Jt Comm J Qual Patient Saf*. 2006;32(7):407–410. 357.
291. Awad SS, et al. *Am J Surg*. 2005;190(5):770–774.
292. Clegg I, MacKinnon R. *Cont Ed Anaesth Crit Care Pain*. 2014;14(4):159–162.
293. Gazoni FM, et al. *Anesth Analg*. 2012;114(3):596–603.
294. Mullan PC, et al. *JAMA*. 2014;312(22):2333–2334.
295. Schmutz JB, Eppich WJ. *Acad Med*. 2017;92(11):1555–1563.
296. Vashdi DR, et al. *Acad Man J*. 2013;56:945–971.
297. Tannenbaum SI, Goldhaber-Fiebert S. In: Salas E, Frush K, eds. *Improving Patient Safety Through Teamwork and Team Training*. New York: Oxford University Press; 2013:249–256.
298. Tannenbaum SI, Cerasoli CP. *Hum Factors*. 2013;55(1):231–245.
299. Kolbe M, et al. *Best Prac Res: Clin Anaesthes*. 2015;29(1):87–96.
300. Hackman JR, Morris CG. In: Berkowitz L, ed. *Adv Exp Soc Psychol*. vol. 8. New York: Academic Press; 1975:45–99.
301. Argyris C. *Pub Admin Rev*. 1980:205–213.
302. Gardner R. *Semin Perinatol*. 2013;37(3):166–174.
303. Chung HS, et al. *Simul Healthc*. 2013;8(3):166–170.
304. Kolbe M, Rudolph JW. *BMJ*. 2018.
305. Palaganas JC, et al., eds. *Defining Excellence in Simulation Programs*. Alphen aan den Rijn, Netherlands: Wolters Kluwer; 2014.
306. Cheng A, et al. *Simul Healthc*. 2015;10(4):217–222.
307. Brett-Fleegler M, et al. *Simul Healthc*. 2012;7:288–294.
308. Loo ME, et al. *Simul Healthc*. 2018;13(1):52–60.
309. Kumar AH, et al. *Simul Healthc*. 2018;13(1):72.
310. Cheng A, et al. *Simul Healthc*. 2017;12(5):319–325.
311. Peterson DT, et al. *Simul Healthc*. 2017;12(4):254–259.
312. Arora S, et al. *Ann Surg*. 2012;256:982–988.
313. Hull L, et al. *BMJ*. 2017;3(1):9–16.
314. *Professional Standards for Medical, Dental and Veterinary Educators*. vol. 21. 3rd ed.. Cardiff, UK: Academy of Medical Educators; 2014.
315. SESAM. Accreditation. https://www.sesam-web.org/accreditation/. Accessed November 27, 2018.
316. American College of Surgeons. Accredited Education Institutes. https://www.facs.org/education/accreditation/aei. Accessed March 26, 2019.
317. Gaba DM. *Simul Healthc*. 2010;5(1):5–7.
318. Hodges B. *Med Teach*. 2006;28(8):690–696.
319. Kirkpatrick DL, Kirkpatrick JD. *Evaluating Training Programs. The Four Levels*. San Francisco, CA: Berrett-Koehler Publishers; 1994.
320. Kirkpatrick DL, Kirkpatrick JD. *Implementing the Four Levels*. San Francisco, CA: Berrett-Koehler Publishers; 2007.
321. Sung NS, et al. *JAMA*. 2003;289(10):1278–1287.
322. McGaghie WC, et al. *Simul Healthc*. 2011;6(suppl):S42–47.
323. McGaghie WC. *Sci Trans Med*. 2010;2(19):19cm8.
324. McGaghie WC, et al. *Chest*. 2012;142(5):1097–1103.
325. Rall M, et al. In: Miller RD, Eriksson L, Fleisher L, Wiener-Kronish J, Neal C, William Y, eds. *Miller's Anesthesia*. 8th ed. Philadelphia, PA: Elsevier Churchill Livingstone; 2014.
326. Translational Research Working Group. *Public Roundtable II - Executive Summary*; 2006. https://www.cancer.gov/images/trwg/trwg-oct06rt-exsum-11-21-06.pdf
327. Khoury MJ, et al. *Gen Med*. 2007;9(10):665–674.
328. Bukhari H, et al. *INQUIRY*. 2017:54.
329. Maloney S, Haines T. *Adv Simul*. 2016;1(1):13.
330. Cook DA, et al. *Simul Healthc*. 2012;7(5):308–320.
331. Draycott T, et al. *BJOG*. 2006;113(2):177–182.
332. Mduma ER, et al. *Int J Qual Healthc*. 2018;30(4):271–275.
333. van de Ven J, et al. *Euro J Ob Gyn Rep Bio*. 2017;216:130–137.
334. Flanagan B, et al. Melbourne, Australia: Department of Health; 2007.
335. Cook DA, et al. *JAMA*. 2011;306(9):978–988.
336. Weinger MB. *Simul Healthc*. 2010;5(1):8–15.
337. Ostergaard HT, et al. *Qual Saf Health Care*. 2004;13(suppl 1):i91–95.
338. Ziv A, Wolpe PR, Small SD, et al. *Acad Med*. 2003;78(8):783–788.
339. Helmreich RL. Paper presented at: Proceeding of the AIAA / NASA / FAA / HFS conference. January 1991; Vienna, VA.
340. Orlady HW. In: Wiener EL, Kanki BG, Helmreich RL, eds. *Cockpit Resource Management*. San Diego, CA: Academic Press; 1993.
341. Weller J, et al. *Anesthesiology*. 2014;120(1):142–148.
342. Forrest FC, et al. *BJA*. 2002;88(3):338–344.
343. Hayden JK, et al. *J Nurs Reg*. 2014;5(2):C1–S64.
344. Kurrek MM, Devitt JH. *Can J Anaesth*. 1997;44(11):1191–1195.
345. Meurling L, et al. *BMJ Qualamp; Safety*. 2013;22(6):485–494.
346. Kolbe M, et al. *J Appl Psychol*. 2014;99(6):1254–1267.
347. Phipps D, et al. *BJA*. 2008;100(3):333–343.
348. Gaba DM. *Simul Healthc*. 2011;6(1):8–10.
349. Gaba DM, et al. *Anesthesiology*. 1998;89(1):8–18.
350. Frank JR, Danoff D. *Med Teach*. 2007;29(7):642–647.
351. Jepsen RM, et al. *Int J Med Ed*. 2015;6:17–25.
352. Lyk-Jensen HT, et al. *AANA journal*. 2016;84(2):122–127.
353. Fletcher G, et al. *Anaesthetists' Non-Technical Skills System Handbook v1.0*. Aberdeen, Scotland: University of Aberdeen; 2012. https://www.rcoa.ac.uk/system/files/AaE-ANTS-HANDBOOK.pdf
354. Scavone BM, et al. *Anesthesiology*. 2006;105(2):260–266.
355. Wisborg T, Manser T. *Acta Anaesth Scan*. 2014;58(7):773–774.
356. Watkins SC, et al. *Simul Healthc*. 2017;12(2):69–75.
357. Schmutz J, et al. *Acad Med*. 2014;89(7):996–1005.
358. Boulet JR, et al. *Simul Healthc*. 2011;6(suppl):S48–51.
359. Yule S, et al. *Med Educ*. 2006;40(11):1098–1104.
360. Weinger MB, et al. *Anesthesiology*. 1994;80(1):77–92.
361. Shavelson R. *Generalizability Theory: A Primer*. Newbury Park, CA: Sage Publications; 1991.
362. Myerson KR. *Anaesthesia*. 1998;53(11):1039–1040.
363. Kapur PA, Steadman RH. *Anesth Analg*. 1998;86(6):1157–1159.
364. Klemola UM, Norros L. *Med Educ*. 2001;35(5):455–464.
365. McIntosh CA. *Anesth Analg*. 2009;108(1):6–9.
366. Holmboe E, et al. *Simul Healthc*. 2011;6(suppl):S58–62.
367. Rall M, Gaba DM. In: Miller RD, ed. *Miller's Anesthesia*. 6th ed. Philadelphia, PA: Elsevier Churchill Livingstone; 2005:3021–3072.
368. Alinier G. *Med Teach*. 2007;29(8):e243–250.

8 Ethical Aspects of Anesthesia Care

GAIL A. VAN NORMAN and STANLEY H. ROSENBAUM

KEY POINTS

- Deontologic ("rules-based") ethical theory and utilitarian (outcome-based) theory clash in clinical scenarios in which the interests of individual patients are pitted against the interests of larger populations.
- In the United States, the predominant medical ethical principle is that of respect for the patient's autonomy, and its expression is in the informed consent of patients for medical therapy.
- Competent and autonomous individuals can make affirmative choices about their medical care and refuse any medical treatments, including lifesaving care. Competence is both functional and relative. Four elements of competent decision making are understanding, appreciation, reasoning, and evidence of a choice.
- Minor patients have varying degrees of decision-making capacity, and they may have legal rights to make certain decisions. Pediatric patients should be involved to the degree that they can be in medical decision making, particularly regarding elective therapy.
- Medical testing should follow the ethical principles of beneficence and nonmaleficence and should be based on clinically validated algorithms whenever possible. Medical tests with special social significance, such as pregnancy and human immunodeficiency virus testing, should be undertaken only with the patient's informed consent and should not be undertaken without sound evidence that they are necessary and beneficial.
- In general, the rights of pregnant women are weighed against the rights of fetuses in a decremental fashion as the fetus approaches and surpasses viable age. Laboring women are able to give informed consent, and the validity of "Ulysses directives" at the time of labor is ethically arguable.
- Use of restraints is antithetical to promotion of autonomy, and anesthesiologists have both ethical and legal obligations to determine whether such extreme intervention is warranted. Coercing or using physical or chemical means to force competent patients to undergo treatment they are refusing is both unethical and illegal.
- Respect for patients' autonomy requires that we disclose mistakes to release patients from misconceptions about their medical past and enhance their ability to share decision making about their medical care.
- An advance directive is a document executed by the patient before incapacity to provide the patient's physicians with guidance in medical decision making when the patient cannot communicate for himself or herself: these directives include, but are not limited to, durable powers of attorney, living wills, transfusion decisions, do-not-attempt-resuscitation (DNAR) directives, and decisions regarding organ donation.
- Surrogate decision makers explicitly act in "substituted judgment" to provide what the patient would have wanted and are not being asked merely for their own preferences. Surrogate decision makers at best only approximate the patient's decisions.
- Patients have moral and legal rights to refuse even life-sustaining therapy, including in the operating room. DNAR orders should not be automatically suspended for anesthesia and/or surgery, but rather require reconsideration of risks and benefits; the goals and decisions of competent patients should generally be honored.
- Terminal care requires special knowledge and experience on the part of the physician. It requires expertise in medically supportive therapy, management of problematic symptoms, knowledge about physiologic changes in the dying patient, support and counseling of patients and families, understanding and respect for the patient's autonomy and religious and cultural practices and beliefs, the ability to work within complex healthcare teams, the ability to communicate well, and empathy.
- Several interventions have special ethical implications—fluid and nutritional management; the administration of sedatives and/or narcotics that have the potential to hasten death; the institution of deep continuous sedation; the administration of neuromuscular blocking agents; and deactivating pacemakers, ventricular assist devices, and implanted cardioverter-defibrillators.

- Physician-assisted suicide (PAS) is the provision of medication and/or prescriptions to patients at their request for the purpose of ending their life. Euthanasia is the administration of medication by someone other than the patient for the express purpose of causing death. PAS and euthanasia are legal only in specific parts of the world, but they are strongly supported by the public.
- Brain death is legally and medically defined as the point at which all cardiorespiratory function irreversibly ceases *or* all function of the whole brain irreversibly stops.
- In donation after cardiac death (DCD), withdrawal of life support occurs with provisions for immediate organ donation after cardiac arrest. Controversies around DCD include concerns about when cardiopulmonary death can be declared and whether medications that preserve organ function but may hasten the donor's death can be administered.
- Research in human subjects must balance many conflicting interests such as the needs and rights of the research subject; the hypothetic interests of future patients; and the physician's financial, professional, and personal goals. The ethical conduct of research in human subjects follows three principles: (1) respect for autonomy, and the obligation to protect subjects with limited autonomy; (2) beneficence, with obligations to minimize risks, maximize benefits, and ensure that the research design is scientifically sound; and (3) justice, the obligation to treat each person with regard to what is morally right and to ensure fair distribution of benefits and burdens.
- Advances in understanding animal cognition have led most biologists to believe that many, if not all, animals are capable of feeling pleasure, pain, anticipation, and fear, and thus they experience both enjoyment and suffering. Allowing animal suffering because of pain, fear, sickness, or poor standards of care is a moral harm that must be avoided, mitigated, and weighed heavily against the benefits it produces.
- U.S. professional organizations for physicians have consistently stated that participation in executions by physicians is unethical, and the American Board of Anesthesiologists states that participation in executions would constitute unprofessional behavior that would result in investigation and possible decertification of anesthesiologists.
- "Conscientious objection" by physician to providing legally allowable medical care that violates their personal moral values is possible, but is limited and counterbalanced by a physician's professional obligations to put the patient's interests first.

Medicine is a respected profession with codes of behavior and definite rules of conduct. Modern medical practitioners have tremendous power, recognized social import, and powerful financial interactions that touch nearly everyone's lives. The American Society of Anesthesiologists (ASA) has established principles for the ethical management of patients.[1] This chapter examines the ethical bases of the practices of medicine and the implications for anesthesiologists.

Ethical Theory

VIRTUE ETHICS, UTILITARIANISM, AND DUTY-DRIVEN ETHICS

The classic "paternalism" of medical practice was derived from *virtue-based ethics*. In this view, the physician is a genuinely virtuous person with inherent qualities of competence, sincerity, confidentiality, and altruism, who naturally knows and does what is correct for the patient. The patient, uneducated about medicine, has to trust the physician to decide what is best. Western society and legal systems have changed substantially since paternalism flourished, giving way to practices based in the four "pillars" of medical ethics: respect for patient autonomy, beneficence, nonmaleficence, and justice. Many different ethical frameworks are applied in modern medicine, but two of the most prominent frameworks relevant to western medicine are utilitarian ethics and deontology.[2]

In *utilitarian ethics*, actions are judged right or wrong on the balance of their good and bad consequences. A "right" action produces the most good, based on a perspective that gives equal weight to the interests of all affected parties. Utilitarian theory is compelling but falls short in defining which benefits are most important. Is it the "good" that all reasonable people want or the "good" defined by the individual patient? What if the only way to maximize good is to commit an entirely immoral act? For example, what if the only way to win a war is to systematically torture children? Outcomes of actions continue to accumulate over time—when on that continuum is it appropriate to determine that an action was right or wrong? The "good" act of saving an individual's life today may be viewed through a completely different lens when, 20 years from now, that same individual is revealed as a mass murderer.

Utilitarian theory may be best when applied to analyzing broad-based policies, in decisions regarding rationing of resources, and when attempting to resolve conflicting ethical obligations between several equally interested parties.

The premise of Kantian-based ethics (also called deontologic—or *duty-based*—theory) is that features of actions other than their consequences make them right or wrong. *Intention* is more important than outcome. Furthermore, no person should use another exclusively as a means to an end, because each person *is* the end for which we should act. No person should be used to further the purposes of another person without that other person's autonomous consent. Kantian philosophy would forbid killing one innocent person to save another innocent person, for example.

Individualism and autonomy are valued highly in Western society, and people tend to turn to Kantian philosophy when ethical questions arise that balance the authority of the physician against the goals and values of individual patients.

Some of the toughest ethical questions in medical practice occur when the rights and desires of individual patients conflict with social policies. Clashes between deontologic and utilitarian principles are common in the intensive care unit (ICU), in managed care settings, in end-of-life care, in transplant medicine, in triage during civilian mass casualty events, and in the care of poor and older patients whose medical management is funded by the government. In each of these settings, the will of the individual patient may conflict with broader principles of minimizing expense, fairly allocating scarce resources, protecting the broader interests of many patients, and determining where and how society's healthcare dollars are best spent.

The political tradition of the United States provides a clear underpinning to individual freedom, and at the beginning of the 20th century, the concept of the autonomy of patients began to emerge.

Clinical Ethics

INFORMED CONSENT AND INFORMED REFUSAL

Legal and moral imperatives for informed consent are based on the ethical principle of respect for patient autonomy. *Autonomy* refers to the ability to choose without controlling interferences by others and without personal limitations that prevent meaningful choices, such as inadequate information or understanding.[2] Individuals have the right to determine what happens to them to the degree to which they are capable. In the United States, this right is rooted in constitutional guarantees of privacy and noninterference.[3] In 1914, the case of *Schloendorff v Society of New York Hospital* established that it was the right of "every human being of adult years and sound mind to determine what shall happen to his own body."[4] In 1957, the term *informed consent* was first used in the case of *Salgo v Trustees of Leland Stanford Hospital*, which established that it is not sufficient for physicians simply to secure consent; physicians have a duty to inform patients about the risks and alternatives to treatment, in addition to the procedures themselves and their consequences.[5]

Respect for the patient's autonomy requires physicians to respect decisions made by competent patients, but also to *promote* autonomy by removing barriers to competent participation in decisions. Such obstacles range from incomplete or inaccurate information to reversible medical conditions that impair a patient's ability to understand the information given to him or her.

Competence and Capacity

Autonomy to make medical decisions cannot exist in the absence of competence. In the United States, *competence* is a legal determination, and *capacity* describes the necessary skills to participate in medical decisions. Most often, the terms are used interchangeably.[3]

Impairments of capacity can be temporary or permanent. Examples include some mental illnesses, dementia, immaturity, anxiety, and pain. Medication effects can variously impede competence, or improve it, depending on their effects and the context in which they are given. Older patients, patients suffering from mental impairment, and children are particularly vulnerable to having their participation in medical decisions inappropriately curtailed or denied because their capacity to participate is frequently underestimated. Hearing loss, expressive aphasia, and other neurologic impairments can create the false impression that capacity is impaired. Many minors have the ability to make medical decisions but may be mistakenly excluded from the decision-making process solely because of their age. Language barriers can present significant challenges to communication.

Capacity is both relative and task specific. Patients may be able to understand and make decisions about medical issues while being unable to manage their financial affairs, for example.

Prejudice and paternalism permeate physician behavior in the informed consent process. Challenges to a patient's competence frequently occur because the patient and the physician have a difference of opinion or values,[3,6,7] and the majority of referred patients are found competent.[3] Unwarranted challenges of a patient's capacity may, intentionally or not, serve to allow the physician to dismiss, rather than solve, a dilemma regarding a difficult patient's wishes, since with a finding of incapacity, the physician's paternalism cannot then be trumped by patient autonomy. In a retrospective study, Katz and associates commented that referrals for urgent or serious treatment put pressure on a consulting psychiatrist to support the medical team's wishes for intervention by simply declaring the patient incompetent.[8] Treatment refusal may simply reflect a patient's prioritization of other things (e.g., dignity, privacy, independence) other than medical outcomes, and not a problem with capacity—or it might reflect manageable emotions and values that disproportionately affect a patient's choices, but do not necessarily rule out capacity.

Doctors are mistaken about patients' preferences regarding life-extending therapies and underestimate older patients' desires for life-extending therapies in 30% to 40% of cases.[9,10] Moreover, surveys indicate that physicians and other healthcare workers are likely to *act* on their personal prejudices regarding handicapped or impaired patients.[11]

Functional capacity for decision making must be judged separately from the perceived quality of the decision itself. Patients have the right to make "bad" decisions (i.e., decisions that *the physician* feels are less than optimal) if they are competent and have appropriate information.[7] Otherwise, the physician would merely prevail whenever a disagreement occurred, and patient autonomy in medical decision making would be nonexistent.

How do we recognize competence? Competence is defined *functionally*, and it *is task specific*.[2] It cannot be defined to be absent by the mere presence of specific diagnoses or medications.[12] Furthermore, evidence of *impairment* is not sufficient to prove *incompetency*. With such high value placed in the United States on autonomy and self-determination, incompetency is, and should be, a difficult bar to leap over, requiring that only persons with impairments "that place them at the very bottom of the performance curve" should be declared incompetent.[12] A "sliding scale" approach to competence determinations, rather than an all-or-none approach, is endorsed by the President's Commission for the Study of Ethical Problems in Medicine and Biomedical and Behavioral Research,[13] and generally reflects how courts deal with competency cases.[12]

Anesthesiologists frequently ask whether valid consent can be obtained after the patient has received premedication. Claims that premedications automatically invalidate consent demonstrate a lack of understanding of the concept of competence. If it were true that benzodiazepines and narcotics, for example, automatically invalidate consent, then we would have to consider the consent of almost all chronic pain patients invalid. In one study, 37.5% of geriatric patients presented for surgery having taken self-prescribed medications and over 25% of these were analgesics and benzodiazepines.[14] If competence were automatically invalidated by the presence of specific medications, then we would be forced to carry out drug testing on all preoperative patients before obtaining consent. While it is true that *sometimes* premedication can interfere with a patient's ability to give consent, in some circumstances, patients cannot give consent *without* premedication. A patient who is in severe pain, for example, is unlikely to be able to focus on detailed risks and alternatives of a proposed procedure without first receiving medication. In that case, treatment of severe pain may actually *improve* competence during the informed consent process.

How does the anesthesiologist determine if they are dealing with a competent patient? Multiple reviews by competency consultants agree that there are several functional elements to competence: (1) *Understanding* - Can the patient receive and understand treatment-related information? (2) *Appreciation* - Does the patient have insight about the disorder and its consequences and potential treatment options? Does the patient understand that treatment could be beneficial in some way? (3) *Reasoning* - Is the patient able to use logic to compare the risks and benefits of treatment alternatives? And, (4) *Evidence of a choice* - Can the patient communicate a choice?[3,12,15]

In respecting and promoting patient autonomy in medical decision making, the anesthesiologist has an ethical duty to treat reversible conditions that interfere with medical decision making when doing so would not delay the medical treatment so much that it becomes irrelevant. Elective surgery may have to be postponed until expert consultation for a determination of mental capacity or treatment of reversible conditions can occur. When surgery in an impaired patient is urgent, the anesthesiologist may have to rely on a surrogate decision maker or proceed with the best determination of the patient's interests in mind. It is important to note that the mere presence of an emergency does not invalidate a *competent* patient's rights to consent to or to refuse treatment. Overriding a competent patient's wishes is unethical, even in emergency situations.[16]

Disclosure

The informed consent process requires honest disclosure of medical information to the patient. U.S. courts generally rely on two standards of disclosure, termed the reasonable person (or objective person) standard and the subjective standard. In the reasonable person standard, the physician must disclose any information that a theoretically reasonable person would want to know, and the risks or cluster of risks to which a reasonable person in the patient's position would attach significance in deciding whether or not to forgo the proposed therapy.[17,18] This standard does not require an exhaustive recitation of facts, and it acknowledges that not all information related to the procedure is integral to making a decision about whether to undergo that procedure. The subjective standard recognizes that some patients may have special needs for specific information, and when that need is obvious or has been brought to the attention of the physician, the information must be disclosed. A concert violinist may have a specific need to know about the potential for nerve damage from an axillary block, while an opera singer may need to know that intubation may adversely affect the voice. In obtaining informed consent, the anesthesiologist should always ask the patient if there are any special concerns regarding the anesthetic, or anything he or she would want the provider to know. In general, legal and ethical standards now require that the physician (1) accurately discuss the therapy and its potential alternative—including no therapy—and (2) disclose the common risks, because they are more likely to happen, and the serious risks, because the consequences are severe.

The doctrine of *therapeutic privilege* is sometimes cited to avoid discussing risks, the reasoning being that discussing risks can psychologically or physically harm the patient by increasing stress. Studies of patients' stress during the informed consent process *do not* support this concept. These studies show that patient stress is generally reduced after risk discussions[19,20] and omission of such conversations is contrary to U.S. law. Although it is ethical to forgo or curtail risk discussions at the patient's request, it is not ethical for the physician to decide to do so unilaterally.

The physician-patient relationship is inherently unequal because of the physician's knowledge and authority and the patient's dependence on the physician for care. Physicians have ethical obligations to avoid exploiting their influence for the purpose of accomplishing their own ends. Although offering a rational basis for a medical choice is acceptable, it is always unethical to coerce or manipulate competent patients into decisions by presenting real or implied threats or by omitting or misrepresenting key information. In fact, such intentional manipulations are morally equivalent to lying to the patient, and thus invalidate the concept of informed consent entirely.[21]

Legal Implications of Informed Consent

The informed consent process does not prevent legal liability when adverse events occur. Flawed informed consent processes have been cited, however, as evidence of a lack of quality of care by the physician, and are associated with poorer litigation outcomes for the physician.[22] The ASA closed-claims database reveals that informed consent is cited in approximately 1% of cases, and cases with inadequate informed consent documentation are associated with larger monetary awards.[23] Studies show that the risk of a malpractice claim is directly related to the patient's perception of his or her relationship with the physician.[24] The informed consent process provides one of the few opportunities anesthesiologists have to establish that relationship, however brief, and the medicolegal importance of that process should not be underestimated.

Informed Refusal

The concept of informed consent is moot if the informed patient cannot refuse medical therapy, because every informed consent process would then have to end with the physician getting his or her way. Examples of informed refusals in anesthesiology include requests to withdraw or withhold life-supporting care in the ICU; do-not-attempt-resuscitation (DNAR) orders in the operating room; refusals of blood transfusions; and cases in which a patient refuses preoperative testing, such as human immunodeficiency virus (HIV) or pregnancy testing.

Informed refusal has concerns and requirements similar to those of informed consent. When patients refuse medical care or insist on what the physician believes to be suboptimal care, disclosure of the risks and benefits becomes even more important because these decisions may veer from options that are already widely accepted and for which the risks are believed to be lowest. It is easier to justify agreeing to the unusual preferences of a well-informed patient than to justify subjecting a poorly informed patient to unorthodox care.

Despite full information, patients may sometimes request or demand care that is unreasonable, either because it will adversely affect the performance of a surgical procedure or because it would be associated with unreasonably high risks. When a patient demands a technique that is inappropriate or outside of the realm of reasonable practice, the anesthesiologist is under no ethical obligation to provide that care. No physician can be compelled by a patient to practice negligently.

Special Issues in Informed Consent and Informed Refusal

THE JEHOVAH'S WITNESS PATIENT

The classic example of a patient who refuses therapy in anesthesia practice is that of Jehovah's Witnesses, many of whom believe that accepting a blood transfusion violates a Biblical injunction. The Jehovah's Witness doctrine has been subject to change over time, with resulting inconsistencies in religious practice regarding which, if any, blood components may be acceptable. Individuals interpret religious doctrines in light of their own spiritual contexts, and not all believers hold to the same tenets with identical fervor. Church doctrines, like medical practices, evolve over time, and practices that are acceptable at one time may not be years later. Anesthesiologists and surgeons have cited individual and doctrinal inconsistencies as justification for ignoring the wishes of Jehovah's Witness patients, but to do so is no more logical than assuming that every hypertensive patient needs or will respond well to identical treatment or that optimal treatments will not evolve over time. Moreover, *any* patient has the right to refuse blood transfusion therapy, regardless of whether this desire is founded in religious preference. Such refusals have become more common in patients who are not Jehovah's Witnesses, as blood transfusion therapy has been connected to infection risk and other complications.

Because of the differing beliefs of Jehovah's Witness patients, the anesthesiologist must have a thorough and detailed preoperative discussion of possible therapies with the patient, and the conclusions should be documented in the patient's chart. A physician who cannot comply with a competent adult patient's desire to forgo transfusion has an ethical obligation to find an alternative caregiver whenever possible.[25,26]

The courts strongly support the rights of most adult patients to refuse blood products for themselves but have been inconsistent and have interfered in cases of some pregnant patients. Transfusion of pediatric Jehovah's Witness patients by court order is common. However, this may become ethically and legally less acceptable as alternative bloodless therapies to maintain oxygen-carrying capacity evolve, as the Jehovah's Witness church further defines its doctrines with regard to children, and as the capacity of children to consent to or refuse therapy is better understood.

THE PEDIATRIC PATIENT AND OTHER PATIENTS WITH IMPAIRED COMPETENCE

The ethical practice of medicine weighs heavily toward adherence to the respect for autonomy of competent patients or advance directives of patients who were previously competent. Medical care of individuals who have never been autonomous relies on principles such as respect for human dignity, beneficence, avoidance of harm, and adherence to the principle of justice.

Children are examples of persons who may or may not yet be autonomous. Laws in each state define the age at which children become legally competent to make medical decisions (usually 18 years), but many younger children have the mental and emotional capacity to make medical decisions. Forcing such individuals to undergo treatments they do not want is unethical and could be illegal as well.

Decision-making capacity in children is variable. Most 2-year-old children are clearly not able to make medical decisions. However, the range of capability in children as young as 7 or 8 years old is wide. In one study, children 6 through 9 years of age who were invited to participate in influenza vaccine research asked pertinent questions about individual risks and benefits and whether their community and other children would benefit.[27] Studies suggest that the average 12-year-old adolescent has capabilities that are required in medical decision-making, but differing influences of the brain's well-developed reward system coupled with underdevelopment of the brain's control systems suggest that decision-making capacity may in fact be diminished in specific contexts in this age group.[28]

Most states recognize "emancipated minor" status, in which a court determines that a minor can legally make medical decisions for himself or herself. Legal exceptions to the age of consent are recognized in most states when treatment is believed to be in the minor's best interest and when a requirement for parental consent would interfere with the child's ability to receive medical help. The law recognizes that, tragically, some conditions for which a minor seeks therapy may even be the result of parental abuse and seeking parental permission for treatment may actually further endanger the minor. One quarter of pregnant teens are at risk for physical or sexual assault, and the most common perpetrator is a member of their family.[29] Thus, minors are allowed in many states to consent for treatment for substance abuse, sexually transmitted disease, mental illness, and medical care affecting pregnancy, including abortion, without seeking parental consent. When a minor has decision-making capacity but is not "emancipated," a judge may declare the child to be a "mature minor" with decision-making rights.

Ideally, individuals of any age should be involved in medical decisions to the degree that their capacity allows. Children ages 7 to 17 have been shown to desire comprehensive perioperative information, including details of the procedure and anesthesia, risks, and complications.[30] A minor with capacity to make decisions should not be coerced or restrained under most circumstances.[31] Determining whether a minor has such capacity may require formal consultation and assessment. The American Academy of Pediatrics has stated that physicians who care for children "should give serious consideration to each patient's developing capacities for participating in decision making, including rationality and autonomy."[32] The term *assent* rather than *consent* is used to refer to agreement to treatment from children who do not fall into legal categories, such as age, that award adult rights. Recently, authors have suggested that informed *consent* rather than *assent* for medical research participation should be applied to children ages 12 and up.[33]

When children dissent from medical care, persistent refusals may be ethically binding, particularly in the case of participation in research. Medical personnel should respect the wishes of a patient who withholds assent and should try to gain a better understanding of the patient's situation or deal with his or her fears. "A patient's reluctance or refusal to assent should also carry considerable weight when the proposed intervention is not essential to his or her welfare and/or can be deferred without substantial risk."[32]

Ethical Challenges of Preoperative Testing

The ethical implications of genetic testing have been widely discussed in the literature, but the ethical implications of routine medical testing have been largely overlooked by professional societies. The performance of diagnostic tests does have ethical dimensions, however. We generally undertake such tests precisely because we intend to help the patient (beneficence) or to use the information to minimize other risks (nonmaleficence). Certain medical tests may also carry implications for the patient's autonomy, privacy, and even social justice.

ROUTINE PREOPERATIVE TESTING PROTOCOLS

Preoperative testing may help identify unrecognized or disguised conditions that could adversely affect anesthetic risk. All medical tests carry risks, however. False-positive and false-negative results may either label patients as having a condition they do not have or inappropriately assure patients that they do not have a condition that they do. Erroneous results may lead either to further testing or to inappropriate and unnecessary therapy associated with further complications. Errors can also cause patients to be deprived of important therapy they would otherwise receive. Tests sometimes have accompanying physical complications, and they are certainly always associated with economic costs. Systematic over-testing increases the costs of health care for entire populations, unnecessarily burdening an already costly system, and diverting badly needed funds to unnecessary enterprise. Medical tests may involve problems of conflicts of interest if the ordering physician has an economic relationship with the entity that carries out the tests. Additionally, not all medical tests are ethically equivalent. Certain tests, such as pregnancy testing and HIV testing, may have complex social consequences and can lead to serious, avoidable harms.

Modern medicine is a science that incorporates theories that are expected to be consistent and generalizable. Although all data are deeply theory laden, the practice of evidence-based medicine (EBM) is founded on the concept that conscientious, judicious, and explicit use of the best available medical evidence should be integrated with clinical experience derived from systematic research in making decisions about the medical care of individual patients. In general, nonsystematic clinical experience, anecdote, and untested theory are not sufficient grounds for clinical decision making.

EBM and medical ethics share common principles and goals: both are aimed at maximizing benefits and minimizing risks, as well as at involving the patient in shared decision making. Using EBM to guide clinical testing and therapy is supported by analysis of traditional therapies that were never subjected to rigorous testing and that, on examination, were shown to be not only unhelpful to patients but possibly harmful. One Cochrane review, for example, found that administration of human albumin, a mainstay of therapy for treatment of shock, may be associated with increased mortality.[34] Another Cochrane review demonstrated that although mammography screening will prolong the life of 1 in 2000 women over a 10-year period, it will lead to the false diagnosis of cancer and the institution of cancer treatment in 10 women during that same period; these findings raise serious questions about the benefits and risks of routine mammography.[35] Using systematic evaluation of medical diagnostic testing to develop principles of preoperative testing not only serves the ethical principles of beneficence and nonmaleficence, but also permits us to provide patients with accurate and up-to-date information on the potential benefits of tests to aid their understanding and input in their medical care—thus honoring the principle of respect for the patient's autonomy.

Conversely, EBM presents potentially significant ethical concerns. In relying on traditional medical experimentation, EBM may not sufficiently account for the role of social and cultural factors (e.g., poverty, ethnicity, spirituality, and gender) in health, and instead may rely too heavily on a narrowly drawn biomedical model of the patient's experience of health and disease. In the words of Rogers, "those with the greatest burden of ill health are disenfranchised, as there is little research that is relevant to them, there is poor access to treatments, and attention is diverted from activities that might have a much greater impact on their health."[36]

Despite its limitations, it nevertheless seems reasonable to believe that in trying to maximize beneficence and minimize nonmaleficence, EBM provides at least an improvement in the search for a rational, cost-effective approach to medical testing over simply adopting "traditional" therapies or protocols without evidence that they will contribute to accomplishing those goals. Applying medical tests inappropriately can cause very real harm to patients. Simply stated, if medical care is not valid, then it is not ethical.

Evidence that routine tests or traditional patterns of preoperative testing enhance perioperative outcomes is scant. Large population studies of many routine preoperative tests, such as coagulation screening,[37] chest radiography,[38] and electrocardiography,[39] have, on the contrary, found that these tests increase costs without necessarily positively affecting outcomes and can even lead to detrimental outcomes. The ASA Task Force for Preanesthesia Evaluation acknowledged that most routine testing is not necessary.[40] When evidence-based algorithms for preoperative testing are available and have been appropriately validated clinically, they should be used to guide clinical decision making.

ROUTINE PREOPERATIVE PREGNANCY AND HUMAN IMMUNODEFICIENCY VIRUS TESTING

Social risks of preoperative testing may not be as obvious to the physician as medical risks, but they can be the source of significant harm. Examples of tests that can produce social harm and are of limited preoperative utility are HIV and pregnancy tests. Both tests have serious ethical consideration; have limited, if any, beneficial impact in the setting of surgery; may have serious social and economic consequences for the patient beyond the operating room; and require the patient's informed consent.

HIV tests are often ordered for the purpose of singling out patients for whom extra universal precautions could be taken to reduce transmission in the operating room. Most surgeons and anesthesiologists believe that compulsory HIV testing would reduce their risk of exposure, and many believe incorrectly that this testing is the physician's prerogative and can be done without the patient's consent.[41]

However, HIV testing does not necessarily yield safer anesthetic management and is more costly than diligent application of universal precautions.[42] In low-prevalence populations, testing is more likely to give false-negative results that wrongly reassure operating room workers that a patient is not infected. This may paradoxically increase the risk of HIV transmission if relaxation in vigilance is the result.

HIV tests can result in loss of employment, insurance coverage, or both. Seropositive women can experience marital breakup, abandonment, verbal abuse, and physical violence if their status is disclosed.[43,44] The threat of compulsory HIV testing almost certainly would prevent some patients from seeking needed surgical care.[41]

Routine preoperative pregnancy testing has ethical ramifications analogous to those of HIV testing. Despite pervasive beliefs to the contrary, studies do not conclusively demonstrate that anesthetic agents lead to early fetal loss, and no anesthetics have been clearly associated with teratogenic effects.[44-47] Studies have also shown that even adolescent girls generally accurately report the possibility of pregnancy when asked privately.[48] Legal ramifications of not routinely testing for pregnancy preoperatively have been virtually nonexistent, and fewer than one third of practices in the United States require such testing.[49] A positive pregnancy test may have extremely negative consequences if a vulnerable patient is in a social situation in which pregnancy is not accepted. Up to two-thirds of sexual assault victims are minors, and some are the result of child rape within the home. Abandonment, negative family interactions, and violence to the patient or her fetus, or both, may all occur, as reactions to revelation of the pregnancy, attempts to hide a sexual domestic crime, or even in some cases as "honor killings."[50] Referral of pregnant adolescents to child protective services should be considered.[49] In many states, it is illegal to disclose or even insinuate a child's pregnancy status to her parents, regardless of her age. Therefore, the anesthesiologist who discovers an adolescent patient's pregnancy has few comfortable or legal options.

Many patients may choose not to undergo an elective surgical procedure if they know they are pregnant. However, *coercing* a female patient to have a test against her wishes and that she may find insulting explicitly violates the principle of the patient's autonomy. The physician's self-interest is not adequate justification for disregarding a patient's autonomy or violating a patient's privacy. The ASA Task Force on Preoperative Testing and the ASA Committee on Ethics jointly recommended that anesthesiologists offer the *choice* of preoperative pregnancy testing to any female patient who may desire it, explain the potential risks and benefits, and obtain informed consent or informed refusal for the test.[40]

Ethics of Anesthesia Involving Pregnant Women

MATERNAL-FETAL CONFLICTS

In general, the rights of pregnant women to refuse therapy, even if it will be detrimental to their fetuses, are protected under right-to-privacy provisions in the U.S. Constitution. Those rights are weighed against potential harms to the fetus in a decremental fashion as the fetus approaches and surpasses viable age. When the fetus is of nonviable age, the mother's rights prevail. Court decisions have consistently upheld the rights of pregnant women to have abortions, to not be subjected to drug testing, and to forgo transfusions early in pregnancy. Attempts to charge women with child abuse, child endangerment, drug trafficking, murder, and attempted murder for activities deemed dangerous to their fetuses have almost uniformly failed.[51] In general, women do not lose their rights to bodily integrity and informed consent when they become pregnant, and neither fetal "rights" nor state interests supersede a pregnant woman's right as medical decision maker.

The American Academy of Pediatrics Committee on Ethics outlined conditions that in their view are necessary to override a mother's refusal of care: (1) the fetus *will* suffer irrevocable harm without the treatment, (2) the treatment is *clearly indicated* and likely to be effective, and (3) the risk to the woman is low.[52] The American College of Obstetricians and Gynecologists condemned the use of coercion in pregnant women and advocated counseling the patient carefully about risks, as well as consultation with an ethics committee.[53]

INFORMED CONSENT IN LABORING WOMEN

The validity of informed consent for epidural anesthesia in laboring women is a topic of concern to anesthesiologists, who periodically raise the question whether laboring women are able to consider and weigh the risks of labor analgesia sufficiently while they are in pain. Although ideal conditions for informed consent are often lacking during labor, it is important to realize that the ideal is seldom achieved even in elective surgical patients; therefore, it is crucial to distinguish between conditions that are not *ideal* from conditions that are not *adequate*.

Despite concerns by anesthesiologists, most studies show that laboring women have the same capacity to give informed consent as the general surgical population,[54,55] are able to recall details of the consent process long after labor is finished, and indicate that labor did not alter their decision making.[56] Furthermore, studies show that the presence or absence of labor pain has minimal effect on a woman's ability to recall analgesia risks and other elements of the informed consent process later.[55,57] Some investigators argue that it is only after the patient enters active labor and she can assess for herself the severity of pain and consequences of proceeding without analgesia that she can be fully informed.[54]

An ethical conflict can arise in the case of so-called Ulysses directives in which, before labor, a woman executes an advance directive that refuses epidural analgesia and instructs doctors to ignore her pleas for epidural anesthesia at the time of labor should she change her mind. Although some experts suggest that ignoring the Ulysses directive disrespects a woman's long-term preferences, others argue that "information and valid experience are critical prerequisites for autonomous decision making" and that only the current wish (to receive an epidural) is ethically relevant.[58] Such cases appear to have no clear and unequivocal ethical ground on which to proceed, and circumstances must guide the physician. However, if an anesthesia practice decides to disregard Ulysses directives routinely, this should obviously be disclosed to patients in advance of labor whenever possible.

The Uncooperative Patient—Coercion and Restraint

The use of physical restraint to control medical research subjects was first directly addressed in the Nuremberg Code following the Doctors' Trial in 1947 to 1949 and is a continuing subject of intense scrutiny.[59] For anesthesiologists, chemical restraints often replace physical ones, but the ethical issues are the same. Anesthesiologists are often asked by medical colleagues to chemically restrain uncooperative patients. Use of restraints is antithetical to promotion of autonomy, and anesthesiologists have both ethical and legal obligations to determine whether such extreme intervention is warranted. Coercing or using physical or chemical means to force a competent patient to undergo treatment that he or she is refusing is both unethical and illegal. Refusal of medical care and angry behavior are not proof of incompetence, intoxication, or inability to make medical decisions.[60]

When faced with the uncooperative adult patient, questions to ask include the following: (1) Is the patient clearly incompetent or merely angry and uncooperative? Does the patient show evidence of neurologic impairment, acute intoxication, or severe mental disability? (2) Is the patient in imminent danger? (3) Does the patient pose a direct threat to staff or other patients? (4) Does a compelling need to treat life-threatening injuries exist? In the absence of any of the foregoing, the use of coercion or physical or chemical restraints is neither ethical nor legal. Physicians may be forced in some situations to act within a time frame that does not permit lengthy evaluation of a patient's competence or a protracted search for a surrogate decision maker. The standard applied in such cases would be to do what a "reasonable" person would wish. Coercion or restraint (or both) in such situations is not ideal, but it may be necessary and ethically permissible.

The uncooperative child presents special ethical concerns. When a patient who does not have the capacity to make healthcare decisions dissents from medical care, the anesthesiologist is ethically required to provide care that is most likely to benefit the patient and prevent harm while preserving the dignity and safety of the patient. Although violation of respect for autonomy is technically not possible in a patient who does not have autonomy, violations of principles of beneficence, nonmaleficence, and respect for dignity certainly are. Indiscriminate use of physical or chemical restraints is not without physical risk, and the fear and anger provoked by such tactics can lead to future aversion of medical care and mistrust of healthcare providers. The American Academy of Pediatrics Committee on Child Abuse and Neglect stated that restraint should not be used in pediatric care "unless it is necessary for proper diagnosis and treatment in a sick child, as in the case of a child with a high fever and potential ear infection, or in emergency situations."[61]

Behavioral control in the uncooperative child or incompetent adult should focus on alternatives to physical restraint, such as offering choices on how to go to sleep and use of fantasy or hypnotic suggestion. Despite many possible social, economic, and scheduling pressures to the contrary, delaying or rescheduling a surgical procedure in a hysterical patient is better than using coercion or force. Delaying elective surgery may reduce stress, allow adequate premedication, and promote safer induction conditions. If medical care is urgent, or if delay is unlikely to result in better conditions for the patient, then the anesthesiologist should proceed in a manner designed to preserve the patient's dignity and safety.

Truth Telling—Disclosure of Errors and Apology

Nonmaleficence has been a foundational principle for the medical profession since the time of Hippocrates, and this principle draws no distinction between deliberate and unintended harms. Medical care is fraught with uncertainty, risk, and error. Harms resulting from unexpected complications, accidents, systems issues, and medical mistakes are to be avoided with equal diligence whenever possible.

Wu and colleagues defined a medical mistake as "a commission or omission with potentially negative consequences for the patient that would have been judged wrong by skilled and knowledgeable peers at the time it occurred, independent of whether there are any negative consequences."[62] Medical errors occur in 3% to 5% of all hospitalizations.[63] More than 40% appear to be preventable, and more than 15% result in patients' deaths.[64] In 1999, the release of the Institute of Medicine's report *To Err Is Human* focused public and political attention on the terrible fallout of medical errors in the United States.[65]

Studies showed that 76% of physicians admitted to a serious medical error that they did not disclose to the patient,[66] and 22% of physicians indicated that they would not disclose an error that caused a patient's death.[67] Reasons cited for a physician's reluctance to disclose errors included personal shame, fear of loss of prestige in the physician's cohort, fear of direct reprisal, lack of experience in disclosing uncomfortable information, fear of causing further harm (emotional or psychological) to the patient and family, and fear of litigation. In many cases, legal advice to physicians has discouraged disclosure and apology in the erroneous belief that these tactics decrease medicolegal liability.

Obfuscating the root cause of a patient's complication when it is caused by a medical error is not difficult in the physician-patient relationship because the physician has unique expertise and is the recipient of unique trust. Furthermore, a minimum standard of disclosure simply does not exist. The Code of Ethics of the American Medical Association (AMA) states that patients have a right to be free of misconceptions about their medical condition and that physicians have ethical obligations to "inform the patient of all the facts necessary to ensure understanding of what has occurred."[68] However, the AMA Code of Ethics addresses only "harms" and not "errors, thus implying no duty to disclose medical errors that do not lead to harm. Although some experts state that physicians may have a lesser obligation to disclose harmless errors and/or "near misses," it is nevertheless arguable that they should consider doing so. The physician has little to lose, and such disclosures may enhance discussion of medical care with the patient and result in a strengthened doctor-patient relationship. Legalistically, some experts consider full disclosure of medical errors to be an extension of the legal principle underlying informed consent: "Clearly, if the patient is entitled to know the risks of a procedure and what could go wrong prior to giving their consent, it follows that they would be entitled to know if something has in fact gone wrong, regardless of whether it was unanticipated."[69]

Respect for patients' autonomy requires that we disclose mistakes that harm patients because in so doing we release patients from misconceptions about their medical past and enhance their ability to share decision making about their medical care. Disclosure prevents mistaken attribution by the patient of adverse consequences to noncontributory causes. Disclosure is usually necessary for informed consent for treatments to address complications of the error. Disclosure may enhance patients' trust in physicians. Moreover, disclosure may facilitate a patient's obtaining just and fair compensation for economic consequences of the injury, such as lost work and pay.

The concern that disclosure of errors to patients will increase litigation or decrease patients' trust, either in the doctor involved or in doctors in general, has not been borne out. Studies have suggested that full disclosure of a medical error reduces the likelihood that patients will change doctors, improves patients' satisfaction, increases trust in the physician, and leads to a more positive emotional response.[70] Studies also have demonstrated that patients take legal action because they want more honesty from their physicians and assurances that the physician has learned from the mistake and that future patients therefore are less likely to suffer.[71]

An often-ignored aspect of medical errors is the effect that errors and disclosures have on physicians and other healthcare workers, who experience anxiety, fear, guilt, shame, self-doubt, anger, and disappointment. Damage to physicians, nurses, and others can be both long-lasting and severe, particularly following serious errors, manifesting as substance abuse and suicide. In a survey of anesthesiologists, 84% had been involved in at least one unanticipated death or serious injury, 88% stated they needed extended time to recover, with 19% stating they never fully recovered after the event. Twelve percent considered a career change. Even though 67% considered their ability to provide care was compromised in the first 4 hours following the event, only 7% were given time off. Five percent admitted to turning to drugs or alcohol as a coping mechanism.[72] Most anesthesiologists report inadequate support from colleagues or their institution in coping with such events.[73]

Physicians benefit from a sense of relief after disclosure and, at least in many cases, the forgiveness of the patient.[74] Disclosure helps physicians learn and improve their practice. Failures to report errors, learn from errors, and communicate errors and their potential solutions within a healthcare system are major causes of medical errors themselves. One could argue that a physician who does not disclose a preventable error, such that it is repeated, bears responsibility for harm not only to his or her own patient, but also to all future patients in whom the error could have been prevented had it been disclosed.

Disclosure can present some harm to the physician: disclosure is stressful, litigation may result, malpractice premiums may increase, and future employment may be adversely affected. However, in the doctor-patient relationship, ethical frameworks hold that benefits and harms to the patient should hold more weight than benefits and harms to the physician.

Do we have an ethical duty to disclose the errors of others? Legally, some North American courts have held that we do not,[69] and social norms about "tattling" on others are powerful deterrents to such disclosures. The reporting physician may hesitate because of a lack of definitive information, potential accusations of interfering in the doctor-patient relationship of another, worry that professional interactions such as patient referrals and performance evaluations may be affected, and fear of libel suits. When a physician observes a medical error committed by another physician, the options include nondisclosure, recommendations to the involved physician to disclose the error, disclosure of the error to a third party such as a risk-management group, or direct disclosure to the patient. Although no strict legal guidelines are in place, ethical principles favor actions that lead the patient to have a full understanding of what has occurred during his or her medical care.

Apology (as opposed to disclosure) remains a controversial aspect of communication following medical errors, largely because of fear that it could be used as an admission of negligence in subsequent litigation. Yet apology appears in many cases to decrease the risk of subsequent litigation, and lack of apology is a commonly cited reason among malpractice plaintiffs for their legal action.[75] Spurred on by a desire to reduce litigation, many states have enacted "apology laws" that prohibit use of various types of apologies in court against physician defendants in malpractice cases. The impact of these laws and the impact of apologies on the incidence and outcomes of malpractice litigation remains unclear, although significant numbers of patients who have sued physicians indicate that an apology would have prevented them from doing so.

ADVANCE DIRECTIVES AND SURROGATE DECISION MAKERS

Critical decisions regarding medical care often arise when patients are too ill to formulate or express decisions regarding medical interventions. *Advance directives* were developed after several legal decisions affirmed that patients can refuse even lifesaving medical care and that clear and convincing evidence of the patient's wishes is needed to allow surrogate decision makers to request withdrawal of life-sustaining therapies.[76] An advance directive is a document executed by the patient before incapacity to provide the patient's physicians with guidance when the patient cannot communicate for himself or herself. Such directives include the following: living wills, which detail the therapies a patient would accept or refuse in the case of terminal incapacity; DNAR orders; and any other preferences regarding medical care decisions.

A surrogate decision maker is someone whom the patient has appointed to make healthcare decisions for him or her (a durable power of attorney [durable POA]) or an individual with other legally recognized authority by virtue of his or her relationship with the patient.

A durable POA for healthcare decisions may be given by the patient to a specific person he or she designates to make healthcare decisions for them if they become incapacitated. The authority vested in a POA supersedes most other decision makers, including family members, except a court-appointed guardian.

When the patient has not designated a durable POA, doctors rely on family members to make decisions for the patient. Many states have a legally defined hierarchy of decision makers. Commonly, the surrogate hierarchy is the spouse or legally recognized domestic partner, followed by the children, if all are in agreement, then parents, if both are in agreement, and then siblings, if all are in agreement. The anesthesiologist should familiarize himself or herself with the specific laws of the state in which they practice.

Surrogate decision makers are explicitly trusted to act in "substituted judgment" to provide what the patient would have wanted and theoretically are not asked merely for their own preferences. However, surrogate decision makers at best only approximate the patient's decisions because their interpretation is subject to their own biases, values, and psychological agendas. Incompetent patients can be emotionally and financially burdensome, and decision makers may have conflicts of interest that distort their beliefs and testimony about what the patient would have wanted.

Studies demonstrate that patients and their proxies only infrequently discuss issues and values involving life-sustaining technologies. Discrepancies between patients and proxies are often significant in the assessment of patients' emotional health and satisfaction. Neither physicians nor proxies can always accurately predict the patient's preferences for life-sustaining therapies.[77,78] Nevertheless, with all the imperfections, proxy decision making may be the only option if a patient has not left specific directives.

Medical Decisions That May Require a Court Order

Some medical treatments have intense cultural connotations, may involve limitation on private freedoms such as reproduction, or may have historically been subject to abuse. Decisions regarding these interventions *cannot* be made by a surrogate decision maker (even if one is available) and require a court review. Examples of such treatments in many states include sterilization and electroshock therapy.

The anesthesiologist should review the patient's record before taking the patient to the operating room and ascertain (1) whether the patient has advance directives, (2) who the patient's surrogate decision makers are, (3) whether the procedure is legally allowed with consent from a surrogate decision maker, and (4) in special cases, whether an appropriate court order has been obtained.

Do-Not-Attempt-Resuscitation Orders in the Operating Room

Up to 60% of anesthesiologists wrongfully believe that DNAR orders are automatically suspended during anesthesia and surgery. The ASA,[25] the American College of Surgeons,[79] the Association of Operating Room Nurses,[80] and The Joint Commission[81] all published practice guidelines requiring reconsideration, not abandonment, of the DNAR orders in the perioperative period.

The causes and outcomes expected with a cardiac arrest in the operating room are different from what may happen outside the operating room, although they are still poor, with a "viable" survival of only about 25%.[82] It is important, therefore, that patients be informed of the risks and benefits of cardiac resuscitation so that they can best determine whether to ask for their DNAR order to be suspended during the perioperative period.

Although the patient's primary care physician may have introduced the idea of DNAR orders to the patient or the surrogate decision maker, it is the anesthesiologist's duty to discuss the risks and benefits of resuscitation in the setting of anesthesia and surgery before undertaking the patient's care. The anesthesiologist should include in this discussion the following steps: (1) determine the patient's goals regarding surgery and resuscitation; (2) establish exactly what is meant by "resuscitation," in contrast to routine anesthetic care; (3) educate the patient about the risks and benefits of resuscitation in the operating room setting; and (4) document the agreements reached with the patient about which interventions commonly associated with resuscitation are acceptable to him or her. Such interventions could include, but are not limited to, intubation, administration of vasoactive drugs, administration of direct current countershock, and institution of chest compressions. Many patients who express reluctance about resuscitation during surgery actually most fear burdensome collateral outcomes, such as permanent neurologic impairment, rather than the process of resuscitation itself. Education and discussion may reassure these patients about the potential outcomes of resuscitation in the operating room and can establish ground rules for discontinuing interventions postoperatively if they do not lead to a chance of meaningful recovery.

Surgery depends on the cooperation of many caregivers with differing expertise, each with independent ethical obligations to the patient. Resuscitation agreements must be discussed with other members of the operating room team. This communication prevents crucial disagreements from occurring during a critical event when treatment decisions must be made quickly. It also allows "conscientious objectors" to withdraw from the healthcare team.

Advance directives are legally and ethically binding. Despite clear, consistent, and forceful legal decisions, physicians have ignored DNAR directives under the false assumption that the legal authority of advance directives and living wills is not binding in the operating room or that the physician has discretion in deciding when to follow or ignore such directives—and families have sued for significant monetary damages for the costs of continued health care and punitive damages for the pain, suffering, and mental anguish of the patients' survivors when DNAR instructions are ignored.[83,84]

In 1990, the U.S. Congress passed the Patient Self-Determination Act that recognizes a competent patient's right to refuse any medical therapy, including life-sustaining therapy, and requires medical institutions and providers to advise patients of these rights and ask about their preferences.[76] Compliance with the act is required in order to participate in Medicare and Medicaid reimbursements. Furthermore, in 2006, the American Civil Liberties Union filed suit against a group of New Mexico orthopedic surgeons who were requiring patients to sign away their rights to DNAR as a requirement of surgery, arguing that this not only violated the 1990 Patient Self-Determination Act, but denied patients their constitutional rights. The surgeons were required to desist in that practice, publicize the change in policy (to respect DNAR), and pay attorneys' fees and various other fines.[85]

Finally, DNAR orders must never be construed as an excuse to not "care" for the patient. A patient's decision to forgo resuscitation does not imply a wish to avoid other beneficial interventions. Placement of a pulmonary artery catheter, for example, may help ensure optimal management of a frail patient who has a DNAR order and enable the anesthesiologist to avoid situations in which the patient's DNAR status becomes pivotal.

END-OF-LIFE DECISION MAKING

A 1996 review by the AMA showed that the following end-of-life issues were of foremost importance to patients: control over the timing and location of death; management of symptoms such as pain, dyspnea, anxiety, and depression; financial management of medical care; and maintenance of therapeutic options, including physician-assisted suicide (PAS).[86]

Withdrawal or Withholding of Medical Therapies

Between 2000 and 2010, about one-third of deaths in the United States occurred in short-stay general hospitals.[87] Patients and doctors alike recognize that aggressive medical therapy may not be desired or even appropriate in the presence of advancing disease, and over time the use of hospice and palliative care facilities has increased.[88] Most deaths in ICUs occur after an explicit decision to withdraw or withhold treatments.[89]

Before the mid-20th century, the concept of beneficence in the eyes of physicians was strongly tied to preventing death. Ethical distinctions between acts of omission ("letting die") and acts of commission ("killing") were and remain confusing at best. Worse, physicians faced threats of criminal punishment if a patient's death resulted from withdrawal of medical treatments.[90] In 1976, the case of Karen Ann Quinlan established that patients have a right to forgo invasive treatments, even if lifesaving, and that surrogate decision makers could ask for withdrawal of lifesaving therapies if the surrogates could show that the patient would not have wanted them.[91] The right to forgo lifesaving treatments was later extended in the cases of Claire Convoy and Nancy Cruzan to include *any* treatment if the patient refused it or if clear and convincing evidence indicated that the patient would have refused therapy if he or she could speak for himself or herself.[76] These decisions were revisited and reconfirmed in the tragic case of Theresa Schiavo in 2005.[92]

Arguments that withdrawing or withholding life-sustaining therapy does not violate rules against killing patients are based on ethical differences between killing and letting die, and between acts of commission (e.g., lethal injection) and acts of omission (e.g., withdrawal or withholding of ventilator therapy).[93] Because such distinctions are confusing to both physicians and patients, a *principle of proportionality* is often applied when withholding or withdrawing treatments.[94] In this principle, treatment is indicated to the extent that it is likely to present more benefits than burdens to the patient based on the patient's perception of such medical, social, and psychological benefits and burdens. Of course, competent patients still always have the right to refuse therapy, even if lifesaving and otherwise indicated.

Two common settings in which anesthesiologists may be involved in withdrawing or withholding life-sustaining interventions are the ICU and the operating room before organ donation after cardiac death (DCD). In both cases, the issues and principles of withdrawing or withholding treatments are the same.

Withdrawal of life-sustaining interventions heralds the final phase of end-of-life care, and it is a socially critical phase in the life of the patient and family. Terminal care requires special knowledge and experience on the part of the physician. It requires expertise in medically supportive therapy, management of problematic symptoms, knowledge about physiologic changes in the dying patient, support and counseling of patients and families, understanding and respect for the patient's autonomy and religious and cultural practices and beliefs, the ability to work within complex healthcare teams, the ability to communicate well, and empathy. Anyone intimately involved in care of the dying patient should also be intimately familiar with ethical and legal standards.

Withdrawal of life-sustaining treatment begins with an assessment of the individual patient's physiology, level of dependence on therapy, degree of consciousness, preferences regarding sedation and analgesia, and preferences regarding privacy and level of involvement of family and other loved ones. All the patient's treatment orders should be reviewed to meet the new treatment goals. Treatments promoting the patient's comfort should generally be continued, whereas those directed only at physiologic maintenance may all be withdrawn. Family members and others attending the patient at the end of life should be educated about physical and mental changes they can expect to see as treatments are scaled back, including the possibility that death will not occur imminently once support is withdrawn.[95]

Several interventions have ethical implications and deserve special consideration—fluid and nutritional management; the administration of sedatives and narcotics that have the potential to hasten death; the administration of neuromuscular blocking drugs; and deactivation of pacemakers, ventricular assist devices, and implantable cardioverter-defibrillators (ICDs).

The issue of fluid and nutritional support is controversial. Burdens associated with continuation of fluid and nutritional support include prolongation of the dying process, and complications and suffering from placement and maintenance of intravenous or enteral access (or both). However, feeding and hydration may have important connotations for family members and members of the healthcare team by allowing a sense of nurturing and mitigating feelings that they are "abandoning" the patient.[95]

Pain, dyspnea, and depression are all common symptoms that cause suffering in the dying patient. Alleviating pain and dyspnea carry the risk of hastening death. Medical, legal, and religious authorities have all clearly accepted the principle of "double effect," in which an action intended to produce a benefit for the patient produces not only the expected benefit but also the potential for significant harm. It is entirely ethical and legal to administer high doses of pain medication and sedatives for the intended effect of relieving suffering, even if the treatment has the side effect of hastening death. However, to administer any medication with the explicit intention of hastening death is euthanasia, and not medical therapy.[95]

TERMINAL SEDATION

"Terminal Sedation," also known as "deep continuous sedation" (DCS), is an ethically controversial end-of-life strategy for patients who are suffering intolerable symptoms in the last stages of dying, and who do not respond well or completely to sedatives or pain medications that are being administered "as needed" in response to symptoms. In DCS, a decision is made with the patient or their appropriate surrogates to forgo reactive treatment of symptoms and to employ intravenous sedative/analgesic infusions with the intention of rendering the patient permanently unconscious until death occurs, but without the intention of causing death. While the goal of DCS—relief of suffering—is a laudable one, ethical questions nevertheless persist: the practice is plagued by vague and nonstandardized terminology and practice, a lack of outcomes research, an uncomfortable confusion with PAS and euthanasia, misunderstanding of the principle of double effect, and culturally diverse philosophies about the role of suffering and transcendence in the meaning of human life.[96] Opponents suggest that DCS is merely euthanasia in disguise, invented to circumvent legal sanctions and moral objections. Some ethicists have argued that DCS permanently deprives the patient of morally relevant aspects of "personhood" and therefore represents a form of killing. Disturbing studies show that many physicians employing DCS actually *do* intend to hasten death.[97,98]

A particularly controversial aspect of DCS is whether it can and should be allowed when the patient is suffering from severe and intractable *existential* suffering: fear, loneliness, anxiety, spiritual crises, and so forth. Professional guidelines regarding DCS and existential suffering at end of life differ greatly in their recommendations: the American Academy of Hospice and Palliative Medicine[99] and the American College of Physicians[100] do not make specific statements about DCS in existential suffering; the AMA Council on Ethical and Judicial Affairs opposes DCS for existential suffering;[101] the Royal Dutch Medical Association[102] and the Harvard University Community Ethics Committee[103] support the use of DCS in cases of existential suffering; and the Veterans Health Administration does not exclude it, but weighed against use of DCS for existential symptoms in their discussions.[104] Even more questions arise when DCS is instituted in pediatric patients.[96]

NEUROMUSCULAR BLOCKING DRUGS

Neuromuscular blocking drugs have no anesthetic, analgesic, or sedative properties. Such drugs should not be initiated if withdrawal of ventilatory support is anticipated. Paralyzing the patient to comfort *the family* so that they see no disturbing movements or respirations as the patient dies is not justifiable. Even worse, it can mask symptoms and signs of distress and can thus prevent relief of suffering during the dying process.[95] When withdrawal of ventilator support is anticipated in a patient already receiving such drugs, they should be withheld in all but extraordinary cases.[105,106]

IMPLANTABLE CARDIAC DEVICES

When a patient who has a cardiac device requests withdrawal of life-sustaining interventions, questions can arise about whether it is ethical to deactivate or even explant such devices at the patient's request. In the case of ICDs, the question might well be whether it is ethical to *continue* such therapy in a patient who has opted for palliative care. Recent studies provide concerning information: in the MADIT II trial, only 15% of patients who died had their ICD deactivated, after receiving "many" shocks at the last days of their lives.[107] A post-mortem device interrogation study indicates that 31% of patients received shocks in the last 24 hours of life.[108] It is likely that patients receiving shocks in the final hours of their lives may be unable to communicate that they are suffering this painful experience and ask to have it stopped. In another study, only 27% of patients had discussed deactivation of the ICD at end-of-life,[109] raising concerns that failure to deactivate the device was due largely to failure of physician-to-patient communication that this was possible and should be considered. In some cases, physicians may lack the expertise or equipment to promptly deactivate such devices when inappropriate shocks are being delivered.[110]

Some experts have said that that these devices must be treated differently from other medical interventions because by virtue of implantation they have become a "biofixture," or literally a part of the patients themselves.[111] Such arguments are difficult to sustain when we consider that many people undergo implantation of medical devices and subsequent explantation of them when the devices are no longer working or do not serve the patient's purpose. Common examples include artificial joints, intraocular lenses, medication delivery devices, and orthopedic hardware. Furthermore, these devices are never uniquely a part of the patient in the same sense as DNA or their native organs. In fact, the ethical distinction between disabling a pacemaker in a pacer-dependent patient and turning off a ventilator for a ventilator-dependent patient is minimal if the request comes from a competent patient or the surrogate decision maker. Both actions involve discontinuance of artificial therapies that the patient no longer desires, and both may be followed by rapid death.

Consensus statements and guidelines by the Resuscitation Council of the UK, British Cardiovascular Society, and National Council for Palliative Care,[112] the European Heart Rhythm Association, and Heart Rhythm Society,[113] and the Canadian Cardiovascular Society[114] all recommend discussion with the patient of deactivation of implantable cardiac devices in end-of-life care.

The presence of a do-not-resuscitate order should not be taken as an automatic request by the patient to discontinue implantable device therapy. As with other end-of-life therapies, discontinuance of such devices should include due consideration of whether the decision is made by a competent patient and with full informed consent. Management of discontinuance of device therapy should always include planning for treatment of distressing symptoms and administration of appropriate comfort measures.

PHYSICIAN-ASSISTED SUICIDE AND EUTHANASIA

PAS is defined as the provision of medication or prescriptions by a physician to a patient at their specific request for the explicit purpose of ending their life. PAS requires a patient who is both competent and capable of communicating the request, as well as capable of self-administration. Euthanasia is defined as the administration of medication by someone other than the patient for the express purpose of causing death in the belief that this would be best for the patient, but not necessarily at the specific request of the patient. Both practices differ ethically from withdrawing or withholding life-supporting medical treatments. In withdrawal or withholding of life-supporting treatment, the primary intention is to discontinue treatments that are causing suffering with an understanding that death may or probably will result. In PAS and euthanasia, the primary intention is to cause death, which secondarily ends suffering.

Currently, euthanasia is legal only in the Netherlands, Belgium, and Luxembourg. Some confusion exists about the status of euthanasia in Colombia, which has been labeled as allowing "euthanasia," but appears in fact to have legalized PAS, reflecting a common misconception in the press about differences between the two practices.[115] In the United States, euthanasia remains illegal regardless of circumstance, but PAS is legal as of 2018 in the states of Oregon, Washington, Montana, Vermont, Colorado, California, and the District of Columbia. It narrowly missed ratification in New Mexico after being passed by both state houses in 2017, and it passed the Hawaii State House of Representatives in March of 2018. It is also under consideration in other states. Thirty-seven states have specific laws that make PAS illegal, and four states have no specific laws regarding PAS.[116] Internationally, PAS is legal only in the Netherlands, Belgium, Luxembourg, Germany, and Switzerland.[117]

Supporters of PAS argue that the right to privacy and respect for autonomy support a patient's right to determine the time, location, and circumstance of his or her own death. Patients consistently rate loss of autonomy and control, inability to pursue previously valued activities, and loss of dignity as the major concerns at the end of life. Adequate control of pain, anxiety, dyspnea, and other symptoms at the end of life remain a challenge to the medical profession, thereby fueling the desire for a means to end life when suffering cannot be controlled. Opponents argue that PAS "medicalizes" death, overly idealizes the physician-patient relationship, ignores possible personal and professional conflicts of interest, and leads to erosion of trust between dying patients and their doctors. Although many ethicists acknowledge that individual circumstances may make assisted suicide an ethically permissible action, most express concerns about potential abuse. Vulnerable members of society, such as the poor, old, and handicapped, could be pressed by financial and social factors into a suicide option in preference to palliative care. An additional argument against PAS or legalized euthanasia is that these approaches could provide solutions to the medical, social, and economic problems common to older and poor patients that are simpler and less expensive than seeking and requiring more difficult but definitive remedies.

Twenty years have passed since Oregon legalized and enacted PAS in 1997 and the Netherlands legalized both PAS and euthanasia, and significant data now provide some insights into whether these concerns about PAS and euthanasia are materializing. In recent polls, more than two thirds of the U.S. population polled favored legalizing PAS, and approximately 70% favored legalization of euthanasia.[118] The percentage of U.S. oncology patients favoring a PAS or euthanasia option in end-of-life care is approximately 65%,[119] whereas physicians frequently involved in end-of-life care, such as intensive care specialists, oncologists, and palliative care specialists, are the most uniformly opposed specialists.[120] This finding represents a significant discordance between physicians and their patients.

In Oregon, where PAS has been legalized for the longest period in the United States, data from 2015 (the most recent year available) remain consistent and show that patients who requested PAS were more likely to be white and had generally higher economic status and education. More than 99.2% were insured, and 92.2% were enrolled in hospice care. Most were more than 65 years old (78%), and 72% were suffering from cancer. As of 2015, 36% of patients receiving prescriptions for PAS (a total of 1545 patients over 20 years) never used them and ultimately died of their underlying disease—with many surviving significantly longer than predicted. More than 92% of patients enrolled in the Oregon program cited loss of autonomy as a primary reason for pursuing the option.[121] Some authors have suggested that the possession of a means to end their lives legally and humanely prevented "preemptive" suicides that could have occurred earlier and thus may have prolonged lives.[122]

Concerns regarding abuses of PAS and euthanasia will undoubtedly continue, but thus far, evidence of systematic abuse is lacking in places where PAS is legalized and regulated. As the population ages and patients desire greater control over end-of-life care and circumstances, debate over PAS and euthanasia in the United States can be expected to continue to grow.

ETHICAL ISSUES IN ORGAN TRANSPLANTATION

Two issues critical to vital organ transplantation that confront anesthesiologists are the concept of brain death and the linkage of withdrawal of life-sustaining therapies with organ retrieval and transplantation after cardiac death (DCD).

Brain Death

Before the 1960s, death was defined as the moment when the heartbeat stopped and respirations ceased. Advances in cardiopulmonary resuscitation and mechanical ventilation then made it possible to postpone death, seemingly indefinitely. In 1968, the Ad Hoc Committee of the Harvard Medical School proposed redefining death as the point at which all cardiorespiratory function had irreversibly ceased, *or* all function of the whole brain had irreversibly stopped (brain death).[123,124] The committee gave two explicit reasons for redefining death. The first was to allow patients to be declared dead and not maintained on machines—thus limiting expense; reallocating medical resources to other, salvageable patients; and allowing the social rituals surrounding death to occur. The second was to allow the donation of vital organs before circulation stopped.

Declaration of death further carries nonmedical consequences, such as the process of mourning, initiation of any criminal prosecutions, inheritance, taxation, and burial concerns. It was thus considered important that determinations of death follow consistent rules across state boundaries, and the National Conference on Uniform State Laws issued the Uniform Definition of Death Act in 1980, which was adopted by the states.[124]

The public has been slow to accept brain death, in part because it requires complete trust in physicians and ignores indicators of death that the public already understands. To nonphysicians, brain-dead donors are superficially indistinguishable in many ways from living persons, and nonphysicians must therefore rely completely on the physician for both accurate and honest information of a loved one's death. Recent court cases challenging declaration of death in patients who clearly did meet standard brain death criteria, such as that of Aden Hailu in Nevada, illustrate continued public uncertainty.[124]

Medical standards in diagnosing brain death are relatively straightforward, although variations in the definition of death itself persist throughout the United States.[124] In the United States, medical standards require demonstration that, in the absence of drugs, paralytic agents, hypothermia, and other reversible conditions that mimic loss of brain function, no cortical or brainstem function is present. The diagnosis is usually made either clinically, by demonstrating that cortical activity and brainstem reflexes are absent, or by radiographic studies demonstrating the complete absence of cerebral blood flow.

Although brain death is a *social* and not a *biologic* definition of death, medical, ethical, theological, and legal experts generally agree that brain death adequately defines a condition in which a person with ethical and legal rights and moral standing ceases to exist and should no longer be treated as though alive. Expensive medical interventions can be discontinued without legal ramifications, and vital organs can be donated for transplantation if the patient or the surrogate decision maker agrees.

Before assuming care of a brain-dead organ donor, the anesthesiologist is obligated to review the chart for documentation of the declaration of brain death and the criteria on which it was based. If any questions exist about the diagnosis, organ donation should be postponed until the anesthesiologist is satisfied that these concerns are addressed.

Donation after Cardiac Death

DCD occurs when a patient wishes to have life-sustaining medical therapies withdrawn and also wishes to proceed with vital organ donation after death. Controlling the time and place of death so that timing of organ donation can be optimized has obvious medical and ethical advantages. The decision to donate organs is made before death, thereby allowing time for discussion and informed consent. Organ ischemia time can be minimized. The dual decision to withdraw life-sustaining interventions and donate vital organs after death can create ethical conflicts, however. When a dying patient becomes an imminent organ donor, the risk is that the patient's interests will be minimized or ignored in favor of the organ recipient.

The National Academy of Medicine reviewed DCD in 1997[125] and 2000[126] and found serious ethical questions, such as determining how quickly after asystole organ donation can begin and whether medications can ethically be administered to the donor before death that are solely for the purpose of organ preservation.

Ethical, theological, and legal principles prohibit us from killing one person to benefit another, but the point at which actual death has occurred in DCD donors is unclear. Although expedient donation is the very purpose of DCD, doctors must never sacrifice any living patient in the process or even take significant risks of doing so; the mistrust this would engender among the public could place the entire concept of DCD at risk by reducing potential donors and ultimately harming future potential organ recipients.[127] Loss of consciousness occurs quickly after asystole, but brain function can continue for some time, and irreversible brain injury may not occur for many minutes. Yet some protocols call for organ retrieval to begin only 2 minutes after circulation has stopped, and in at least one institution, organ harvest is allowed to begin within seconds of cardiac arrest.[128] Scientific and philosophic uncertainty exists about when death is complete—this could even lead to accusations that physicians deliberately kill patients to obtain organs for transplantation. Mistakes have occurred in some cases of brain-dead organ donors for which clear clinical criteria exist; DCD organ donation is potentially even more prone to error because no such clinical guidelines are universally accepted.[129]

Donation of vital organs after brain death and DCD are both ethical and legal, but the interests of the dying patient must be absolutely protected until after death has occurred. Anesthesiologists can play a vital role in the organ donation process by helping hospitals develop reasonable and ethical policies for the management of brain-dead donors and DCD donors. Every anesthesiologist should be thoroughly familiar with brain death criteria and should review the process of brain death determination before accepting care of a brain-dead donor. It is inappropriate for anesthesiologists to be involved in organ DCD unless they have expertise in the relevant ethical, legal, and medical issues and are experienced in end-of-life care.

Research Ethics

HUMAN SUBJECT RESEARCH

The premise that the physician always puts the best interests of the patient first can be jeopardized when research objectives enter the doctor-patient relationship. Human subjects are asked to put aside their own interests to benefit some future, hypothetic group of patients. In extreme cases, the patient becomes a research "object" who will not benefit personally from the experiment at all. Two examples include experiments in healthy subjects and phase I cancer trials in terminally ill patients in which the goal is to determine the toxicity of treatment—not remission, palliation, or cure.

Human subject research must balance many conflicting interests, such as the needs and rights of the research subject, the hypothetic interests of future patients, and the physician's financial, professional, and personal goals. Academic or corporate advancement, personal prestige, and financial incentives may be disincentives to researchers who diligently protect patients' interests or who remain objective in designing protocols and analyzing and reporting their findings. Thus, human subject research is more closely regulated, supervised, and controlled than any other medical endeavor.

Regulation of research began after World War II, with the Nuremburg Code and the Helsinki Declaration outlining the ethical obligations of physicians engaged in human research. The United States was slow to awaken to the parallels between the concentration camp experiments and the sometimes gruesome treatment to which they subjected their own subjects in similar trials.[130] In the years that followed the Doctors' Trial at Nuremburg, Fox[131] and Beecher[132] found that researchers were aware of the standards set at Nuremberg but regularly did not comply with them. In 1974, the National Research Act established the National Commission for the Protection of Human Subjects of Biomedical and Behavioral Research, out of which the modern institutional review board was born.

The ethical conduct of human subject research follows three principles: (1) respect for autonomy and the obligation to protect subjects with limited autonomy; (2) beneficence, with obligations to minimize risks, maximize benefits, and ensure that the research design is scientifically sound; and (3) justice, the obligation to treat each person with regard to what is morally right and to ensure fair distribution of benefits and burdens.

In addition to the comprehensive presentation to research subjects of the risks and benefits of procedures or medications to which they will be subjected, disclosure must include the possibility of commercialization of the results, financial interests of the researchers, and any other actual or perceived conflicts of interest on the part of researchers and their institutions and sponsors. Subjects must be free to refuse or end participation at any time without penalty. *Situational coercion,* in which subjects feel that they are not truly free to refuse, should be avoided or mitigated. Examples of situational coercion include prisoners whose terms and experiences of incarceration may be affected by their decision to participate or refuse, and hospitalized patients who may believe that their care could be compromised if they do not cooperate with researchers.[130]

Monetary or other inducements to participate in research are probably permissible if they do not undermine the freedom of the subject to refuse under reasonable circumstances. Significant monetary awards may have adverse effects on the autonomy of subjects and may negatively affect the scientific quality of the research. If remuneration is high, for example, subjects could conceal factors that would otherwise disqualify them from participating, thus compromising the research results and exposing themselves to greater risks.

Researchers are obligated to maximize benefits and minimize potential harms, including physical, psychological, social, legal, and financial harms. The research must address a question of significant value to justify the level of risk and must follow the approved protocol. Findings must be promptly and accurately reported. The research must be terminated immediately if it is suspected to be harmful to the participants.

Anesthesiology research often involves the treatment or prevention of unpleasant symptoms, such as pain and nausea. When effective treatments are well established, such studies should be restricted to comparison of treatments with known efficacy, not placebo-controlled trials, and "escape" analgesics or antiemetics must be provided on the patient's request.

No population group should be unfairly subjected to research without having equal access to its benefits. Finally, the interests of the individual must always prevail over the interests of society.

Children as Research Subjects

Children are particularly vulnerable as research subjects because they may lack the ability to make mature decisions, are subject to the authority of others, may defer to their parents and others in ways that mask underlying dissent, and may have conditions requiring immediate decisions not consistent with informed consent.[133] Children's rights are frequently undervalued, whereas parental authority may be overvalued. Studies show that even children with decision-making capacity are often excluded from the consent process by both parents and physicians.[134]

If a minor child is "able" to assent, then assent must usually be obtained in addition to the consent of any legal surrogate decision makers. In the United States, federal law requires assent of any minor age 7 years and older to participate in medical research. Particularly for research in which no substantive individual benefit is expected, many ethicists believe that a child's dissent *must always be honored.*[134,135]

ETHICS OF ANIMAL RESEARCH

The animal rights movement in the United States has gained significant momentum since the 1980s, following in the wake of the U.S. civil rights movement and paralleling increasing awareness and concerns about the human impact on the environment and other animal species. In 1959, William Russell and Rex Burch published their sentinel book regarding the ethics of animal research, *The Principles of Humane Experimental Technique*, introducing the concept that humane treatment of animals was not merely an ethical imperative, but absolutely necessary to high-quality research.[136] Federal legislation protecting animal welfare began with the Laboratory Animal Welfare Act of 1966. In 1985, the Health Extension Act and amendments to the Animal Welfare Act required the establishment of Institutional Animal Care and Use Committees, which oversee conditions of laboratory animals; review and approve animal research protocols; educate and train investigators in ethical issues and aspects of animal handling such as anesthesia, analgesia, and euthanasia; and act as community liaisons.

Some researchers deny that animal experimentation could be subject to any moral reservations and assert that medical advances have been and continue to be completely dependent on continued animal research. Many animal welfare activists insist on the moral equivalence of animal experimentation to that of human experimentation and accuse researchers of being blind to or, even worse, actually unmoved by the suffering of animal subjects. The simplicity of these polarized views does not do justice to the complexity of the issues.

Advances in the understanding of animal cognition led most biologists to believe that many, if not all, animals are capable of feeling pleasure, pain, anticipation, and fear, and thus experience both enjoyment and suffering. Many bioethicists state that the higher animals therefore have adequate awareness to possess moral standing, although how much moral standing is intensely debated.[137,138] Allowing animal suffering as a result of pain, fear, sickness, or poor standards of care is a moral harm that must be avoided, mitigated, and weighed heavily against the benefits it produces. Ethicists maintain that cruelty to animals is immoral and that animals should be protected from it, not merely because they have moral standing, but because he who is cruel to animals is more likely to be cruel to humans.[139]

Researchers have obligations to provide clean and humane conditions and appropriate veterinary care for animal subjects. Researchers should mind the "Three Rs"—replacement, reduction, and refinement—that is, use animal subjects only when necessary, minimize any suffering incurred in the study, and seek nonanimate replacements for animal subjects.[99] Mediocre or repetitive research using animal subjects should not be allowed. It is the responsibility of the medical and scientific community to continue aggressively to seek and promote alternatives to the use of animal subjects.[139]

PHYSICIAN PARTICIPATION IN EXECUTIONS

U.S. professional organizations for physicians have consistently stated that physicians' participation in executions is unethical, yet many physicians admit that they would agree to be involved. The role of physicians in euthanasia and executions is of particular concern to anesthesiologists, who have been identified as ideal candidates for duties that involve killing because of their particular professional skills. Arguments in favor of physicians' involvement in executions usually cite the principle of beneficence in allowing a humane death.

Historically, however, beneficence arguments have led to "slippery slope" justifications for physicians to be involved in the killing of persons who have never faced an accuser or had a fair hearing—such killings have included persons with physical or mental handicaps and other "social flaws" for the "benefit" of the individual and of society as a whole. Once physicians accept a beneficence argument for participating in executions, it is difficult ethically to draw the line at participating in other state-sponsored activities, such as torture, coercion, and "medical incarceration," because these activities are also usually defended as being beneficial to society.[140]

When physicians agree to participate in an execution, they act as agents of the state while appearing to act on behalf of the "patient." This situation can lead to eventual erosion of public trust and respect. It also at times undoubtedly leads to physicians' participation in the killing of innocent persons.[141]

To avoid intolerable self-condemnation, virtually all executioners undergo "moral disengagement" in which they dehumanize the convicts and devalue their lives, thereby deflecting moral responsibility for the execution away from themselves by blaming juries, judges, governors, and "the law" rather than accept the responsibility they share in ending the prisoner's life.[142] It is difficult to reconcile the medical profession's overt ethical imperatives of valuing human life, respecting individuals, and accepting personal moral responsibility with participation in a process that requires a rejection of these very values.

In 1980, the AMA issued an opinion that physicians' involvement in capital punishment is unethical and defined "participation" broadly as including not only actions that themselves would lead to the death of the condemned but also any activity that assisted, supervised, or contributed to another's being able to do so.[143] However, no direct sanctions of any participating physician were addressed. In 2010, the American Board of Anesthesiology became the first organization of physicians not only to condemn participation in capital punishment as unethical but also to state that physicians who were certified by their board and who participated in lethal injection would be subject to disciplinary action that could include revocation of their diplomate status.[144]

MORAL INTEGRITY—CAN THE PHYSICIAN BE A CONSCIENTIOUS OBJECTOR IN MEDICINE?

Anesthesia care of patients can involve ethical controversy, legitimate disagreement, and moral ambiguity. How a physician resolves moral conflicts when their personal values run counter to acceptable ethical standards of care is a matter of much concern.[145,146] Medical professional societies recognize the right to conscientious objection in medical practice. The ASA, the British Medical Association, and the bioethics research institute, The Hastings Center, all have issued statements recognizing the physician's right to withdraw from situations in which ethical standards of patient care are in serious conflict with his or her personal values.[147] The ASA specifically recognizes conscientious withdrawal from patient care in the case of patients with DNAR orders or other directives that limit treatment.[25] These rights have limitations, however. Acceptance of moral objections to certain hotly contended issues such as abortion or PAS may be reasonable, but objections to well-established standards, such as informed consent, are not. Moral objections of physicians are also likely to carry more weight if they involve concepts that the physician believes supports him or her as an ethical doctor, and not just as an ethical person, because these concepts are more likely to be founded in professionally established standards than in personal beliefs.[147] When physicians' personal religious and other moral beliefs are allowed to supersede those of patients, the result has almost uniformly been barriers in health care to vulnerable groups, such as women, adolescents, and the elderly.[148,149]

In early 2018, the U.S. Department of Health and Human Services moved under conservative political leadership to strengthen doctors' rights to refuse to refer patients for legal medical treatments that they personally object to, such as abortion, transgender treatments, and birth control, for example. The AMA has raised concerns that the move both combines and illegally broadens laws that have not been subjected to public vote. Dr. Lainie Friedman Ross, physician and ethicist at the University of Chicago, points out that "it is very problematic because it forgets that doctors are powerful individuals and patients are vulnerable. The law is all about protecting doctors, not the individuals who need the protection—those who are sick and frightened."[150] It remains to be seen whether the new rules will withstand inevitable legal challenges. In the meantime, a Canadian court ruled in the opposite direction, that the requirement to refer patients to legal medical treatments in Ontario was "a reasonable limit on the religious freedom of doctors, necessary to prevent harm and inequitable access for patients."[150]

Complete references available online at expertconsult.com.

References

1. Beauchamp TL, et al. The concept of autonomy. In: *Principles of Biomedical Ethics*. Oxford: Oxford University Press; 1994:120.
2. Committee on Ethics. Guidelines for the ethical practice of anesthesiology. American Society of Anesthesiologists. ASA, Schaumburg IL Oct 16, 2013.
3. Leo RJ. *Prim Care Companion J Clin Psychiatry*. 1999;1:131–141.
4. *Schloendorff v Society of New York Hospital*, 311 NY 125, 127, 129; 105 NE 92, 93, 1914.
5. Salgo v Trustees of Leland *Stanford Hospital*, 154 Col App 2d 560, 317 P2d 170 Ct Appl, 1957.
6. Kontos N, et al. *Psychosomatics*. 2013;54:103.
7. Mclivennan CK, Swetz KM. *Amer J Bioeth*. 2016;8:13.
8. Katz M, et al. *Psychosomatics*. 1995;26:33.
9. Hamel M, et al. *Ann Intern Med*. 1999;130:116.
10. DesHarnais S, et al. *J Palliat Med*. 2007;10:728.
11. Madorsky J. *West J Med*. 1997;166(6):410.
12. Appelbaum PS. *N Eng J Med*. 2007;357:1834.
13. President's Commission for the Study of Ethical Problems in Medicine and Biomedical and Behavioral Research. Vol. 1. Washington, DC: Government Printing Office; 1982.
14. Amanor-Boadu D. *Afr Med Med Sci*. 2002;31:49.
15. Grisso T, Appelbaum TS. *Assessing Competence to Treatment: a Guide for Physicians, and Other Health Professionals*. New York: Oxford University Press; 1998.
16. Brach C. *Health Aff (Millwood)*. 2016;35:739.
17. Derse AR. *J Law Med Ethics*. 2017;45:51.
18. Ginsberg MD. *J Law Med Ethics*. 2017;45:106.
19. Kain ZN. *Anesth Analg*. 1999;88(2):237.
20. Bergmann P, et al. *Anesth Analg*. 2001;93:1093.
21. Cox CL, Fritz Z. *J Med Ethics*. 2016;42:632.
22. Vila-Nova de Silva DB, et al. *Aesthet Surg J*. 2015;35:477.
23. Caplan RA, Posner KL. *ASA Newslett*. 1995;59(6):9.
24. Beckman HB, et al. *Arch Intern Med*. 1995;154(12):1365.
25. American Society of Anesthesiologists. *Ethical Guidelines for the Anesthesia Care of Patients with Do-Not-Resuscitate Orders or Other Directives that Limit Treatment. Park Ridge, Ill*: 2013.
26. American Academy of Pediatrics. *Pediatrics*. 2009;124:1689.
27. Lewis CE, et al. *Am J Public Health*. 1978;68(11):1079.
28. Grootens-Wiegers P, et al. *BMC Pediatr*. 2017;17:120.
29. Berenson AB. *J Adolesc Health*. 1992;13:466.
30. Fortier MA, et al. *Anesth Analg*. 2009;109:1085.
31. Mutcherson KM. *Cornell J Law Public Policy*. 2005;14(25):251.
32. American Academy of Pediatrics. *Pediatrics*. 1995;95(2):314.
33. Hein IM, et al. *BMC Med Ethics*. 2015;16:76.
34. Alderson P, et al. *Cochrane Database Syst Rev*. 2002;(1):CD001208.
35. Gotzsche PC, Nielsen M. *Cochrane Database Syst Rev*. 2011;(1):CD001877.
36. Rogers WA. *J Med Ethics*. 2004;30:141.
37. Chee YL, et al. *Br J Haematol*. 2008;140(5):496.
38. Joo HS, et al. *Can J Anaesth*. 2005;52(6):568.
39. Noordzij PG, et al. *Am J Cardiol*. 2006;97(7):1103.
40. American Society of Anesthesiologists Task Force for Preanesthesia Evaluation. *Anesthesiology*. 2012;116(3):1.
41. Chapman K, et al. *AIDS Care*. 1995;7(2):125.
42. Lawrence VA, et al. *J Clin Epidemiol*. 1993;46(11):1219.
43. Lester P, et al. *J Aquir Immune Defic Syndr Hum Retrovirol*. 1995;10(3):341.
44. Gielen AC, et al. *Women Health*. 1997;25(3):19.
45. Canadian Agency for Drugs and Technologies for Health. CADTH; June 8, 2015
46. Mazze RI, Kallen B. *Am J Obstet Gynecol*. 1989;161(5):1178.
47. Reedy MB, et al. *Am J Obstet Gynecol*. 1997;177(3):673.
48. Malviya S, et al. *Anesth Analg*. 1996;83(4):854.
49. Kempen PM. *J Clin Anesth*. 1997;9(7):546.
50. Benagiano G, et al. *Eur J Contracept Reprod Health Care*. 2010;15:220.
51. Harris LH, Paltrow L. *JAMA*. 2003;289:1697.
52. American Academy of Pediatrics. *Committee on Bioethics: Pediatrics*. 1999;103:1061.
53. American College of Obstetricians and Gynecologists. *Obstet Gynecol*. 2005;106:1127.
54. Jackson A, et al. *Can J Anaesth*. 2000;47:1068.
55. Burkle CM, et al. *J Clin Anaesth*. 2017;36:158.
56. Affleck PJ, et al. *J Clin Anesth*. 1998;10:141.
57. Cheng WY, et al. *Anaesth Intensive Care*. 2007;35:68.
58. Davies JM. In: Van Norman G, et al. eds. *Clinical Ethics in Anesthesiology: a Case-Based Textbook*. Cambridge: Cambridge University Press; 2011:44.
59. Shuster E. *N Engl J Med*. 1997;337(20):1436.
60. Clarke JR, et al. *Hastings Cent Rep*. 1980;10(6):20.
61. Krugman RD, et al. *Pediatrics*. 1992;90(4):651.
62. Wu AW, et al. *J Gen Intern Med*. 1997;12(12):770.
63. Brennan TA, et al. *N Engl J Med*. 1991;324(6):370.
64. Baker GR, et al. *CMAJ*. 2004;170(11):1678.
65. Kohn LT, ed. *To err is Human: Building a Safer Health System*. Washington, DC: National Academy Press; 2000.
66. Wu AW, et al. *JAMA*. 1991;265(16):2089.

67. Sweet MP, Bernat JL. *J Clin Ethics*. 1997;8:341.
68. American Medical Association. *Opinion of the Council on Ethical and Judicial Affairs, Ethical Responsibility to Study and Prevent Error and Harm in the Provision of Health care, Opinion 1-I-03*. Chicago: 2003.
69. Waite M. *Health Law J*. 2005;13:1.
70. Mazor KM, et al. *Ann Intern Med*. 2004;140(6):409.
71. Vincent C, et al. *Lancet*. 1994;343(8913):1609.
72. Gazoni F, et al. *Anesth Analg*. 2012;114:596.
73. McLennan SR, et al. *Acta Anaesthesiol Scand*. 2015;59:990.
74. Plews-Ogan M, et al. *Acad Med*. 2016;91:233.
75. McDonnell WM, Guenther E. *Ann Intern Med*. 2008;149(11):811.
76. Jonsen A, et al. *Source Book in Bioethics: a Documentary History*. Washington, DC: Georgetown University Press; 1998.
77. Layde P, et al. *Arch Fam Med*. 1995;4(6):518.
78. Covinsky KE, et al. *J Am Geriatr Soc*. 2000;48(Suppl 5):S187.
79. American College of Surgeons. *ACS Bull*. 1994;79(9):29.
80. AORN Position Statement. *Perioperative Care of Patients with Do-Not-Resuscitate Orders*. Denver: Association of Operating Room Nurses; 1995.
81. Joint Commission on accreditation of healthcare organizations: patient rights. In: *Manual of the Joint Commission on Accreditation of Health Care Organizations*. Chicago: Joint Commission on Accreditation of Healthcare Organizations; 1994.
82. Kalkman S, et al. *Anesthesiology*. 2016;124:723.
83. Lynch AF, Mathes M, Sawicki N. *Compliance with Advance Directives: Wrongful Living and Tort Incentives*. ;17. University of Pennsylvania Law School Legal Scholarship Repository; 2008.
84. Span P. *The New York Times*. 2017.
85. *Following ACLU of New Mexico Lawsuit, Surgical Center Agrees to Honor Patients' end-of-life Wishes*. American Civil Liberties Union; 2006. https://www.aclu.org/news/following-aclu-new-mexico-lawsuit-surgical-center-agrees-honor-patients-end-life-wishes. Accessed 23.03.18.
86. Council on Scientific Affairs: American Medical Association. *JAMA*. 1996;275:474.
87. Hall MJ, et al. NCHS Data Brief No. 118, March 2013.
88. Teno JM, et al. *JAMA*. 2013;309:470.
89. Karlawish J. *Am J Respir Crit Care Med*. 1997;155(1):1.
90. Alpers A. *J Law Med Ethics*. 1998;26:308.
91. *In the matter of Karen Quinlan, an alleged incompetent*, 355 A2d 647 (NJ Super Ct Cir 1976).
92. *Schiavo v Schiavo*, No. 05–11628 (11th Cir, March 25, 2005).
93. Childress J. *Kennedy Inst Ethics J*. 1993;3:203.
94. Jonsen A, et al. *Clinical ethics*. 3rd ed. New York: McGraw-Hill; 1992.
95. Cist A, et al. *Int Anesthesiol Clin*. 2001;39:87.
96. Van Norman G. Ethics and clinical aspects of palliative sedation in the terminally ill child. In: Mason KP, ed. *Pediatric Sedation Outside of the Operating Room*. New York: Springer Science and Business Media; 2014:699–710.
97. Sercu M, et al. *J Pain Symptom Manage*. 2014;47:1054.
98. Anquinet L, et al. *J Am Geriatr Soc*. 2013;61:1768.
99. *American Academy of Hospice and Palliative Medicine Position Statement on Palliative Sedation*; AAHPM Chicago IL; Approved December 2014. http://aahpm.org/positions/palliative-sedation. Accessed 23.03.18.
100. Quill TE, Byock IR. *Ann Intern Med*. 2000;132:408.
101. Sedation to Unconsciousness in End-of-Life Care. Code of Medical Ethics Opinion 5.6. American Medical Association Council on Ethical and Judicial Affairs. 2018. http://aahpm.org/positions/palliative-sedation. Accessed 23.03.18.
102. *Guideline for Palliative Sedation*. The Netherlands: Royal Dutch Medical Association (KNMG). Ultrecht; 2009.
103. Powers CL, McLean PC. *Am J Bioeth*. 2011;11:65.
104. National Ethics Committee Veterans Health Administration. *Am J Hosp Palliat Care*. 2007;23:483.
105. Truog RD, et al. *N Eng J Med*. 2000;342:508.
106. Murray MJ, et al. *Crit Care Med*. 2016;44:2079.
107. Sherazi S, et al. *Pacing Clin Electrophysiol*. 2013:1273.
108. Kinch Westerdahl A, et al. *Circulation*. 2014;129:422.
109. Goldstein NE, et al. *Ann Intern Med*. 2004;141:835.
110. Looi YC. *J Pain Symptom Manage*. 2006;31:1.
111. Morgenweck CJ. Discontinuing pacemakers, ventricular-assist devices, and implanted cardioverter-defibrillators in end-of-life care. In: Van Norman G, Jackson S, Rosenbaum S, Palmer S, eds. *Clinical ethics in Anesthesiology: a Case-Based Textbook*. Cambridge: Cambridge University Press; 2011:103.
112. Pitcher D, et al. *Heart*. 2016;102(suppl 7):A1.
113. Padeletti L, et al. *Europace*. 2010;12:1480.
114. Ezekowitz JA, et al. *Can J Cardiol 2017*. 2017;33:1342.
115. Suarez MP. *Colombian Doctors must now Provide Euthanasia by law Panampost.com*. 2015. https://panampost.com/maria-suarez/2015/06/04/colombian-public-doctors-must-now-provide-euthanasia-by-law/. Accessed 23.03.18.
116. *State-by-State Guide to Physician-Assisted Suicide ProCon.org*; 2017. Available at: https://euthanasia.procon.org/view.resource.php?resourceID=000132. Accessed 23.03.18.
117. *Euthanasia and Physician-Assisted Suicide (PAS) Around the World ProCon.org*; 2017. Available at: https://euthanasia.procon.org/view.resource.php?resourceID=000136. Accessed 28.03.18.
118. McCarthy J. Seven in 10 Americans Back Euthanasia. Gallup News; 2014. Available at: http://news.gallup.com/poll/171704/seven-americans-back-euthanasia.aspx. Accessed 23.03.18.
119. Yun YH, et al. *CMAJ*. 2011;183(10):E673.
120. McCormick R, et al. *Palliat Med*. 2012;26(1):23–33.
121. Oregon death with dignity act: 2015 data summary. Oregon Health Authority. Available at: http://www.oregon.gov/oha/ph/ProviderPartnerResources/EvaluationResearch/DeathwithDignityAct/Documents/year18.pdf. Accessed 23.03.18.
122. Lindsay RA. *Am J Bioeth*. 2009;9(3):19.
123. A definition of irreversible coma: a report of the ad hoc committee of the Harvard School of Medicine to examine the definition of brain death. *JAMA*. 1968;205:337.
124. Lewis A, et al. *J Law Med Ethics*. 2017:45112.
125. Herdman R, Potts J. *Non–Heart Beating Organ Transplantation: Medical and Ethical Issues in Procurement. A report of the Institute of Medicine*. Washington, DC: National Academy Press; 1997.
126. Cassel C, et al. *Non–Heart Beating Organ Transplantation: Practice and Protocols. A Report of the Committee on Non–HEART-Beating Transplantation II. Institute of Medicine*. Washington, DC: 2000. National Academy Press; 2000.
127. Menikoff J. *Issues Law Med*. 2002;18:3.
128. Stein R. *New Trend in Organ Donation Raises Questions*. The Washington Post; 2007.
129. Van Norman G. *Anesthesiology*. 1999;91(1):275.
130. Lerner BH. *N Engl J Med*. 2007;356:1806.
131. *Final report of the Advisory Committee on Human Radiation Experiments*. Washington, DC: U.S. Government Printing Office; 1995.
132. Beecher H. *N Engl J Med*. 1966;74:1354.
133. Brody JL, et al. *Ethics Behav*. 2003;13(1):79.
134. Olechnowicz JQ, et al. *Pediatrics*. 2002;109:806.
135. Wendler DS. *J Med Ethics*. 2006;32(4):229.
136. Russell WMS, et al. *The Principles of Humane Experimental Technique* London: Methuen; 1959.
137. Francione GL. *J Law Med Ethics*. 2007;35(2):241.
138. Pluhar EB. *Theor Med Bioeth*. 2006;27(4):333.
139. Martin J. *J Med Ethics*. 1990;16:160.
140. Krass ME. *Can Med Assoc J*. 1978;119:1340.
141. Harmon TR, Lofquist WS. *Crime Delinquency*. 2005;51(4):498.
142. Osofsky MJ, et al. *Law Hum Behav*. 2005;29:371.
143. American Medical Association Council on Ethical and Judicial Affairs: Code of Medical Ethics opinion 9.7.3. Capital punishment. AMA. Available at: https://www.ama-assn.org/delivering-care/capital-punishment . Accessed 29.03.18.
144. American Board of Anesthesiology. Anesthesiologists and capital punishment. 2010. Available at: http://www.theaba.org/ABOUT/Policies-BOI. Accessed 29.03.18.
145. Hughes JA. *Bioethics*. 2018;32:126.
146. Savulescu J, Schuklenk U. *Bioethics*. 2017;31:162.
147. Wicclair M. *Bioethics*. 2000;14(3):205.
148. Morrel KM, Chaykin W. *Curr Opin Obstet Gynecol*. 2015;27:333.
149. Fiala C, Arthur JH. *Heath Hum Rights*. 2017;19:299.
150. Glauser W. *CMAJ*. 2018;190:E270.

SECTION II

ANESTHETIC PHYSIOLOGY

9 Consciousness, Memory, and Anesthesia

GEORGE A. MASHOUR and KANE O. PRYOR

KEY POINTS

- Mechanisms of consciousness and memory, and their interruption by general anesthetics, are important scientific problems that have clinical relevance for the practice of anesthesiology.
- Consciousness is characterized by both wakefulness (i.e., the brain being aroused) and awareness (i.e., subjective experience).
- Anesthetics act at structures in the brainstem, hypothalamus, and basal forebrain that regulate sleep-wake states, which may account for loss of wakefulness.
- Anesthetics disrupt connectivity and communication across cortical and thalamocortical networks, which may account for loss of awareness.
- Memory can be subdivided into explicit (conscious) and implicit (unconscious) recall; an example of explicit episodic recall is remembering a surgical event.
- Suppression of explicit episodic recall is one of the most potent effects of most general anesthetics.
- Effects on the hippocampus, amygdala, and prefrontal cortex—as well as the connectivity of these structures—may account for anesthetic-induced amnesia, even before loss of consciousness.

Introduction

SCIENTIFIC AND CLINICAL IMPORTANCE

Consciousness and memory are among the most fascinating and complex subjects in all of science. The richness of human consciousness and memory—and the ability to express this richness in language—is a defining characteristic of *homo sapiens*. Consciousness and memory also have clinical relevance for the anesthesiologist; together, the experience and explicit episodic recall of surgical events is known as the problem of "intraoperative awareness." When formally assessed, this complication occurs in approximately 1 to 2 cases per 1000[1-3] and is associated with a high incidence of posttraumatic stress disorder (PTSD).[4,5] The incidence of intraoperative consciousness without recall is substantially higher.[6] To advance the field of perioperative brain monitoring, a detailed understanding of the neurobiology of consciousness, memory, and anesthesia is required.

Consciousness

DEFINITIONS

The field of consciousness studies has been plagued by the indiscriminate use of the term "consciousness." When we refer to consciousness, we mean *subjective experience*. In simple terms, it is what we lose when we have dreamless sleep and what we regain again in the morning upon awakening. There are, however, several important definitions and distinctions that should be considered.

1. **Awareness**: Cognitive neuroscientists and philosophers use the term "awareness" to mean *only* subjective experience. In clinical anesthesiology, we (inaccurately) use the term "awareness" to include *both* consciousness *and* explicit episodic memory[7] (the taxonomy of memory will be discussed in the next major section of the chapter).
2. **Connected versus disconnected consciousness**: Connected consciousness is the experience of environmental stimuli (such as surgery), whereas disconnected consciousness is an endogenous experience (such as a dream state).[8]
3. **Consciousness versus responsiveness**: An individual may fully experience a stimulus (such as the command "Open your eyes!") but not be able to respond (as when a patient is paralyzed but conscious during surgery).[9]

There have been a number of theories proposed to explain the mechanisms of consciousness and general anesthesia. Advances in neuroscience, however, have enabled us to move beyond speculative frameworks and focus on a systems-based approach to both subjects.[10] The remainder of this section on consciousness adopts such an approach by discussing (1) brainstem and hypothalamic nuclei regulating the sleep-wake cycle (and therefore arousal states) (Figs. 9.1 and 9.2); (2) the role of the thalamus in consciousness and anesthesia; (3) cortical-subcortical connectivity, with a focus on the thalamocortical system, which is thought to mediate the experiential component of consciousness; and (4) cortico-cortical communication.

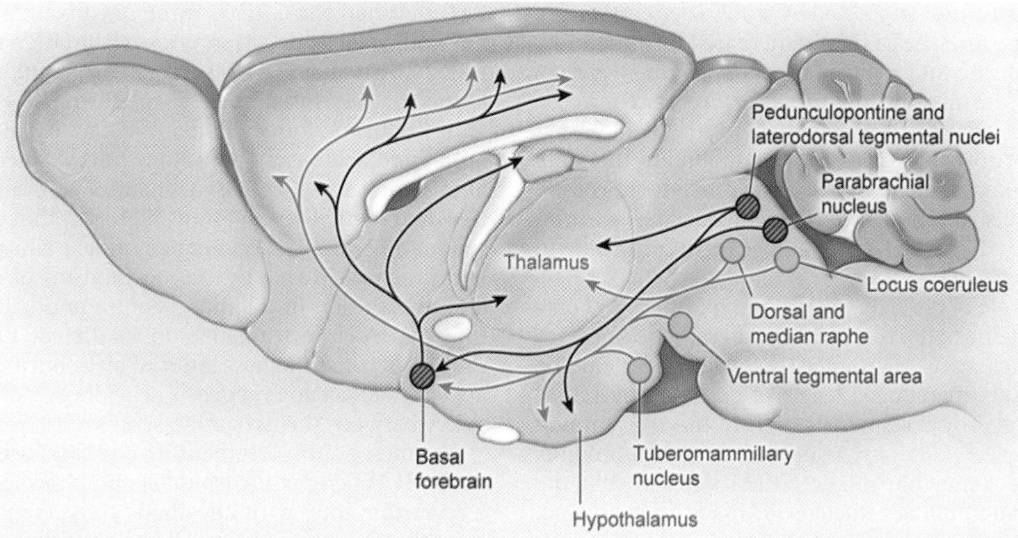

Fig. 9.1 Neurobiology of wakefulness. Multiple neurochemical systems in subcortical regions (shown here in rodent brain) promote arousal and activation of the cortex. Monoaminergic neurons *(light green)* in the rostral brainstem and caudal hypothalamus innervate the cortex as well as many subcortical regions including the hypothalamus and thalamus. These monoaminergic regions include noradrenergic neurons (locus coeruleus), serotonergic neurons (dorsal and median raphe nuclei), dopaminergic neurons (ventral tegmental area), and histaminergic neurons (tuberomammillary nucleus). Wake-promoting signals also arise from cholinergic regions *(dark green with hatching)*, including the pedunculopontine and laterodorsal tegmental nuclei and basal forebrain. General anesthetics have been demonstrated to suppress many of these regions. (Redrawn from Scammell TE, Arrigoni E, Lipton JO. Neural circuitry of wakefulness and sleep. *Neuron.* 2017;93[4]:747–765.)

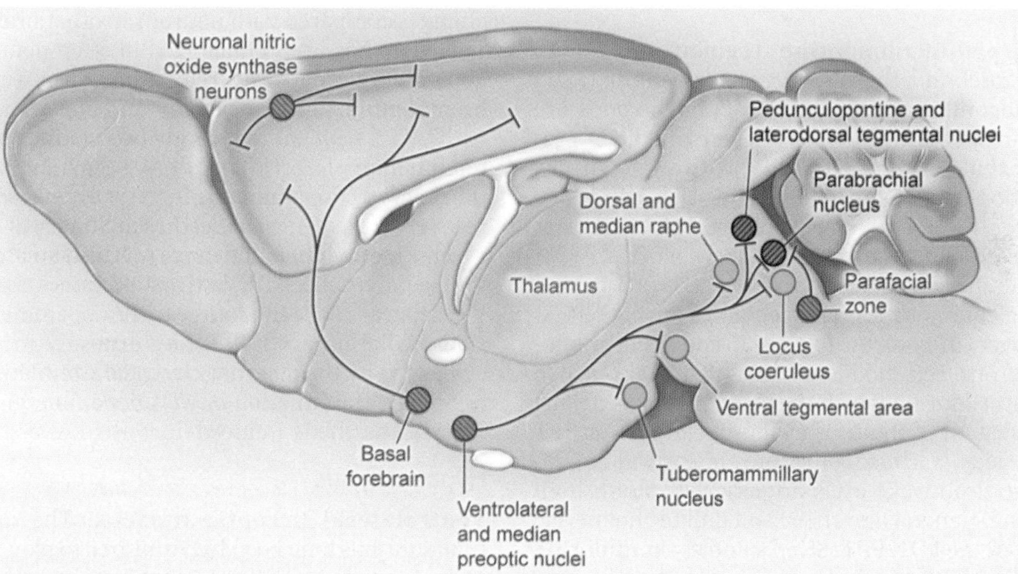

Fig. 9.2 Neurobiology of slow-wave sleep. GABA-ergic neurons in the ventrolateral preoptic area and median preoptic nucleus in the hypothalamus (shown here in rodent brain) promote sleep by inhibiting wake-promoting neurons in the caudal hypothalamus and brainstem. These hypothalamic nuclei are activated by general anesthetics. (Redrawn from Scammell TE, Arrigoni E, Lipton JO. Neural circuitry of wakefulness and sleep. *Neuron.* 2017;93[4]:747–765.)

SUBCORTICAL NUCLEI REGULATING AROUSAL

It was hypothesized in the mid-1990s that anesthetics suppress consciousness by actions at the subcortical nuclei that evolved to control sleep-wake cycles.[11] The past decades have supported the hypothesis that anesthetics interact with a number of these sleep-wake centers,[12,13] although precise interactions and contributions to the state of general anesthesia have yet to be elucidated. The following is a description of select subcortical nuclei in the brainstem and hypothalamus that mediate sleep-wake cycles[14] and, potentially, some traits of anesthesia.

Brainstem

Locus ceruleus. Norepinephrine is synthesized in the locus ceruleus (LC), which is located in the pons and projects widely throughout the cortex.[15] Like other monoaminergic neuronal populations, LC activity is highest during waking consciousness, decreased during nonrapid eye movement (NREM) sleep, and at its nadir during rapid eye movement (REM) sleep.[16,17] Thus LC is associated with cortical arousal only during wakefulness and not with the cortical activation during REM sleep. LC neurons are hyperpolarized by halothane.[18] The role of norepinephrine (generated by LC) in anesthesia is further supported by studies demonstrating that barbiturate anesthesia time is increased by antagonizing norepinephrine and reduced by agonizing it.[19,20] Norepinephrine transmission in the basal forebrain may be of particular relevance to anesthetic depth.[21] It has been found that LC noradrenergic neurons modulate the state of isoflurane anesthesia as well as emergence therefrom.[22] Of note, administration of ketamine is associated with an increase of activity in the LC[23] and appears to contribute to its anesthetic effects.[24]

LC and the role of norepinephrine in hypnosis are of particular interest due to the role of the α-2 agonist dexmedetomidine in clinical care. Microinjection of dexmedetomidine in the LC results in reduced levels of consciousness that can be prevented by coadministration of the α-2 antagonist atipamezole.[25] After exposure to dexmedetomidine, brain changes somewhat mimic NREM sleep in that the LC and tuberomammillary nucleus (TMN) are deactivated, whereas the ventrolateral preoptic nucleus (VLPO) is activated.[26] Data in dopamine-β-hydroxylase knockout mice (which lack the ability to synthesize norepinephrine) demonstrate a *hypersensitivity* to dexmedetomidine, suggesting alternative mechanisms of action.[27] However, selective knockdown of α-2A adrenergic receptors from LC prevent dexmedetomidine-induced loss of righting reflex,[28] a marker of general anesthesia in rodents.

Laterodorsal/pedunculopontine tegmentum. Along with the basal forebrain, the laterodorsal tegmentum (LDT) and pedunculopontine tegmentum (PPT) in the pons are the brain's source of acetylcholine.[29] There are direct projections to the thalamus from LDT/PPT with a known role in the generation of slow oscillations and sleep spindles,[30] which together represent a neurophysiologic sign that information transfer to the cortex is likely blocked.[31] As with the noradrenergic LC, activity of the LDT/PPT is high during waking consciousness and decreases during NREM sleep.[15] However, in contrast to the LC and other monoaminergic neurons, the cholinergic LDT/PPT is also active during REM sleep, during which the cortex is aroused. Furthermore, activation of cholinergic neurons in LDT or PPT induces REM sleep.[32] Thus, both states of cortical activation across the sleep-wake cycle are associated with high cholinergic tone. General anesthetics modulate cholinergic projections from the LDT/PPT. Sleep spindles occur during halothane anesthesia and are associated with decreased cholinergic transmission to the medial pontine reticular formation (PRF).[33,34] There is evidence that synaptic and extrasynaptic γ-aminobutyric acid (GABA) receptors play a role in modulating LDT neurons,[35] which could provide a direct link to molecular mechanisms of numerous general anesthetics. However, there has been relatively little study of the role of LDT/PPT in anesthetic mechanisms, with a greater focus on cholinergic neurons in the basal forebrain.

Pontine reticular formation. The PRF is part of the reticular activating system, which plays an important role in cortical arousal. Although GABA is the primary inhibitory neurotransmitter in the brain, the actions of GABA in the PRF are associated with cortical arousal.[36] For example, there is increased time spent in the waking state when the $GABA_A$ receptor agonist muscimol is microinjected in the PRF.[37] When the $GABA_A$ antagonist bicuculline is microinjected, wakefulness is suppressed, but REM sleep (another state of cortical arousal) is triggered. Vanini and colleagues found that *decreased* levels of GABA in the PRF correlated with isoflurane-induced unconsciousness, muscular hypotonia, and decreased respiratory rate.[38] Since the effects of anesthetics are normally associated with a *potentiation* of GABA activity, these findings highlight that a specific neuroanatomic and neurochemical milieu can play a unique and unexpected role in the mechanisms of consciousness and anesthesia. In addition, Vanini and colleagues found that GABA-ergic transmission in the rat PRF modulates the loss of consciousness induced by isoflurane but does not appear to affect emergence,[39] providing evidence for asymmetry between the two processes.

The mesopontine tegmental anesthesia area is located in the PRF. When pentobarbital is microinjected in this area, a reversible state with anesthetic traits is induced.[40] More recently, this phenomenon has been defined with greater spatial resolution, with the identification of around 1900 neurons in this area that can induce general anesthesia.[41]

Ventral tegmental area. Dopaminergic neurons of the ventral tegmental area (VTA) in the midbrain have not classically been considered key mediators of the sleep-wake cycle because of relatively less evidence of state-dependent changes compared with neurons in other brainstem nuclei. This view has been challenged in sleep neurobiology.[42] A dopaminergic pathway regulating sleep-wake states has been identified in *Drosophila*[43] and dopaminergic neurons of the VTA have more recently been found to play a role in mammalian sleep.[44] There has been renewed interest in the ability of dopaminergic activity to reverse or accelerate recovery from general anesthesia. Studies of the dopamine agonist methylphenidate have revealed an ability to reverse the sedative effects of both isoflurane and propofol.[45,46] VTA appears to be the source of the dopaminergic transmission mediating arousal during exposure to anesthesia, as evidenced by the fact that electrical stimulation of the VTA or selective stimulation of VTA dopaminergic neurons can reverse anesthetic-induced unconsciousness.[47,48]

Hypothalamus

Ventrolateral preoptic nucleus. The anterior hypothalamus has long been hypothesized to play a role in sleep-wake regulation.[49] VLPO is a structure in this region that transmits GABA and galanin.[50] Neurons in VLPO are maximally active during NREM and REM sleep;[51,52] the median preoptic nucleus (MnPO) is also active during sleep. Of note, the activity profile of GABA-ergic neurons in VLPO correlates with sleep amount, whereas the activity of GABA-ergic neurons in MnPO correlates with homeostatic sleep pressure or propensity.[53] Importantly, activity of the VLPO during sleep is correlated with inhibition of other arousal centers in the brainstem and hypothalamus.[51,54] Given its potentially central role as a mediator of sleep, VLPO became an attractive candidate as a mediator of anesthetic-induced unconsciousness. Nelson and colleagues demonstrated activation of VLPO after systemic administration of propofol or pentothal[55]; recent studies have examined the mechanistic significance of these findings. Eikermann and colleagues conducted studies of rats with *chronic* lesions of

VLPO, finding that ablation of VLPO resulted in sleep deprivation (as expected) but conferred *increased sensitivity* to the effects of isoflurane.[56] This finding would argue against a critical role of VLPO in the mechanism of anesthesia. However, Moore and colleagues demonstrated that *acute* lesions of VLPO conferred *resistance* to the effects of isoflurane, an effect that appeared to be mediated specifically through the sleep-active neurons in VLPO.[57] These neurons are actually depolarized (i.e., activated) by isoflurane. Taken together, these data suggest that VLPO plays a role in anesthetic-induced unconsciousness (as evidenced by acute lesion data), but that the effects of sleep deprivation associated with chronic VLPO lesions could overwhelm this role. Curiously, direct administration of dexmedetomidine, an α-2-adrenergic agonist, to the VLPO can destabilize the state of isoflurane anesthesia.[58]

Orexinergic neurons. Orexinergic neurons are found in the lateral hypothalamus and provide an important arousal stimulus for the cortex. There are two types of orexin (A and B), which are also referred to as hypocretins. Orexinergic neurons innervate other arousal centers in the brainstem and basal forebrain, and fire maximally in the waking state, are suppressed during NREM sleep, and show occasional bursts during phasic REM sleep.[59,60] Dysfunction of the orexinergic system is associated with narcolepsy in both human and animal models.[61,62] The often dramatic delay of anesthetic emergence in narcoleptic patients[63] has motivated the study of orexin in anesthetic mechanism. Orexins attenuate the effects of isoflurane,[64] propofol,[65] ketamine,[66] and barbiturates,[67] using various measures. Local infusion of orexin in the basal forebrain is associated with electroencephalographic (EEG) arousal and decreased emergence time in animals anesthetized with sevoflurane[68] and isoflurane.[69] Microinjection of propofol in the perifornical region of the hypothalamus (the locus of orexinergic neurons) is associated with a decrease in cortical acetylcholine, an important mediator of arousal.[70] Importantly, both genetic and pharmacologic studies have demonstrated that orexins play an important role in emergence from sevoflurane and isoflurane anesthesia, but not induction.[71] This seminal study suggested that there is a distinct neurobiology of induction and emergence, and formed the basis for a theory of "neural inertia" across state transitions.[72] Of note, halothane did not show an effect on orexinergic neurons and emergence time was not altered in orexin knockout mice.[73] These findings have been confirmed for propofol anesthesia: propofol reduces activity in orexinergic neurons in rats and infusion of orexin in the basal forebrain affects emergence time, but not induction time.[74] Orexins might facilitate emergence from anesthesia through actions in the basal forebrain.[75]

Tuberomammillary nucleus. The TMN is located in the caudal hypothalamus and is the brain's source of histamine, an arousal-promoting transmitter. TMN activity and histamine levels are highest during wakefulness and lowest during sleep;[76] the TMN is thought to have a relationship of reciprocal inhibition with the sleep-promoting GABAergic neurons of the VLPO.[51,54,77] Histamine release in the anterior hypothalamus is depressed during sleep[78] and halothane anesthesia.[79] Systemic administration of propofol, pentothal, and the GABA agonist muscimol all result in decreased activity in the TMN.[55] Microinjection of histamine in the nucleus basalis magnocellularis of the basal forebrain reverses the depressant effects of isoflurane on the EEG, an effect likely mediated by H1 histamine receptors.[80] A recent study in which $GABA_A$ receptors were genetically removed demonstrated that histaminergic neurons are resistant to the effects of propofol.[81] However, at the behavioral level, there was no effect of propofol on loss-of-righting reflex, a surrogate for anesthetic-induced unconsciousness. Thus the role of TMN and histaminergic transmission in the mechanism of anesthesia is still unclear.

ROLE OF THE THALAMUS

The thalamus is composed of more than 50 nuclei and subnuclei that can be grossly classified as relays for sensory input from the periphery or multimodal, integrative regions that receive input from the cortex. Additionally, the thalamus is critical for transmitting arousal signals from the brainstem and for regulating cortical communication. The involvement of the thalamus in arousal, sensory processing, and cortical computation is likely critical for normal consciousness. As such, the thalamus has been of continued interest to those investigating mechanisms of anesthetic-induced unconsciousness.

The thalamus has been proposed as an ON/OFF switch for anesthetic state transitions.[82] This theory was generated based on the consistent metabolic depression of the thalamus by a number of inhaled and intravenous anesthetics[83-85] (with the exception of ketamine),[86] suggesting that it could serve as an effective OFF switch. The hyperpolarization of the thalamus would shift tonic firing to burst firing that—as with sleep—would prevent afferent sensory stimuli from arousing the cortex. Importantly, however, sensory nuclei in the thalamus (and their connectivity to the cortex) appear to be less involved in anesthetic-induced unconsciousness compared to the higher-order or "nonspecific" nuclei.[87,88]

Evidence for the thalamus as an ON switch has been derived primarily from animal experiments, in which stimulation of the centromedial thalamus by either nicotine or antibodies blocking voltage-gated potassium channels could reverse the effects of inhaled anesthetics.[89,90] Although microinjection of large doses of nicotine into the thalamus could precipitate anesthetic emergence, antagonism of nicotinic acetylcholine receptors in the same location did not appear to contribute to anesthetic-induced unconsciousness. Central thalamic activation results in behavioral improvement in humans with traumatic brain injury.[91] A study in humans demonstrated that (spontaneous) activation of the thalamus along with other subcortical structures is correlated with recovery from anesthesia, suggesting the involvement of the thalamus in the primitive or "core" consciousness observed at emergence.[92]

Nonspecific nuclei of the thalamus have been proposed as a computational blackboard for the cortex.[93] Thus if the mechanism of anesthetic-induced unconsciousness was achieved primarily by a suppression of cortical computation, a depressed thalamus should be the result. To address this question, Velly and colleagues conducted a neurophysiologic study using scalp EEG (reflecting cortical signals) and subthalamic nuclei electrodes (argued to reflect thalamic activity).[94] Induction of anesthesia with either propofol or sevoflurane was associated with cortical rather than subcortical changes, suggesting that the depression of the thalamus identified through neuroimaging studies reflected an effect rather than a cause of anesthetic-induced unconsciousness. Other case studies in humans suggest concurrent suppression of thalamus and cortex during induction of propofol.[95] Furthermore, more precise neurophysiologic recordings of thalamus and cortex in animal models suggest that effects of propofol on central thalamic activity precede effects on the cortex; interestingly this was found during the spontaneous induction of sleep as well.[96] Other animal studies have found that attenuation of high-frequency oscillations by propofol is more pronounced in the thalamus than the cortex.[97]

The prior two possibilities (thalamic switch or computational blackboard for the cortex) treat the thalamus as a passive player in general anesthesia. However, more recent data suggest that it might, instead, play an active role. A computational study using human EEG data and modeling suggested that the action of propofol on GABA receptors in the nucleus reticularis generates a hypersynchronous alpha rhythm (8-13 Hz) with the frontal cortex that blocks sensory input.[98] Hypersynchrony of alpha may block the flexible corticocortical communication required for normal consciousness.[99] A recent animal study identified alpha synchronization between thalamus and medial prefrontal cortex during propofol induction.[100] The potential role of thalamocortical interactions in anesthetic-induced unconsciousness prompts further discussion of the thalamus and its connectivity to the cortex.

CORTICAL-SUBCORTICAL CONNECTIVITY

The closely integrated function of the cortex and thalamus suggests that the two can be treated as a single *thalamocortical system*. The thalamocortical system undergoes state-dependent changes across the sleep-wake cycle, and is thought to play a critical role in consciousness. This role is defined by its ability to integrate the activities of functionally diverse cognitive modules, a property that is critical for subjective experience.[101]

Recent studies using functional magnetic resonance imaging (fMRI) have refined the role of thalamocortical connectivity in anesthesia. One study identified a propofol-induced disruption of connectivity between the thalamus and lateral frontal-parietal networks.[102] Similarly, a study of the specific nuclei (linked to particular sensory modalities) and nonspecific nuclei (linked to integrative functions) found that disrupted connectivity between the nonspecific nuclei and the cortex best accounted for a reduction in the level of consciousness by propofol.[87] Recently, the inhaled anesthetic sevoflurane has been shown to functionally disconnect the thalamus and cortex, especially frontal cortex.[103,104] Notably, a consistent finding of neuroimaging studies is that the thalamocortical connectivity of primary sensory networks is relatively well preserved despite anesthetic-induced unconsciousness.

The finding of impaired thalamocortical connectivity in association with anesthetic-induced unconsciousness has not been universal. An fMRI study of propofol revealed more profound functional disconnections between the cortex and putamen, a subcortical structure in the basal ganglia.[105] In contrast, thalamic connectivity was relatively well preserved. The potential role of the striatum (composed of the putamen and caudate) in anesthetic-induced unconsciousness has been demonstrated in a study of rats undergoing isoflurane anesthesia.[106] This study was conducted with fMRI and found that the functional connection between the frontal cortex and the basal ganglia was disrupted during general anesthesia. A functional disconnection of association cortex and subcortical structures has also been shown by fMRI in a study of propofol-induced unconsciousness in humans.[107] With improved spatial resolution of 7T fMRI machines and templates for brainstem nuclei,[108] future studies can focus on identifying with greater precision the critical subcortical and cortical interactions or functional disconnections that contribute to anesthetic-induced unconsciousness.[109]

CORTICAL CONNECTIVITY AND DYNAMICS

The last three sections were organized according to a bottom-up approach to consciousness and anesthesia, starting with the brainstem, and then moving to the diencephalon and thalamocortical system. Sleep is clearly generated through such bottom-up mechanisms[14]; however, anesthetics may suppress the *level* of consciousness through bottom-up mechanisms and *content* of consciousness through top-down (i.e., cortical) mechanisms.[12]

Early studies using positron emission tomography (PET) demonstrated regional depression in cortical areas, including lateral and medial frontal-parietal networks.[110] Disruption of fMRI-based functional connectivity in frontal-parietal networks has been demonstrated during anesthetic-induced unconsciousness induced by drugs with distinct molecular mechanisms, including propofol,[102,111] sevoflurane,[103] and ketamine.[112] However, the cortex is amenable not only to fMRI but also neurophysiological techniques of assessing connectivity, enabling data on anesthetic-induced unconsciousness with improved temporal resolution. EEG can be used to measure functional connectivity (the statistical covariation of the activities of brain regions), and directional or effective connectivity (the presumed causal influence of one brain region on another).[113] Using such techniques applied to EEG (in some cases with concomitant fMRI), disruption of frontal-parietal connectivity and surrogates of information exchange in humans has been consistently observed after administration of a variety of anesthetics with diverse molecular targets.[104,114-117] It has been suggested that such disruption of frontal-parietal connectivity, with implications for impaired information transfer of relevance to consciousness, might be a common mediator and proximate cause of anesthetic-induced unconsciousness.[118]

The inhibition of frontal-parietal communication is likely representative of a more global disruption of cortical communication. A study using high-density EEG and transcranial magnetic stimulation revealed an inhibition of cortical-effective connectivity after midazolam-induced unconsciousness.[119] After administration of the benzodiazepine, local cortical activation could be observed at the site of magnetic stimulation, but robust evoked potentials

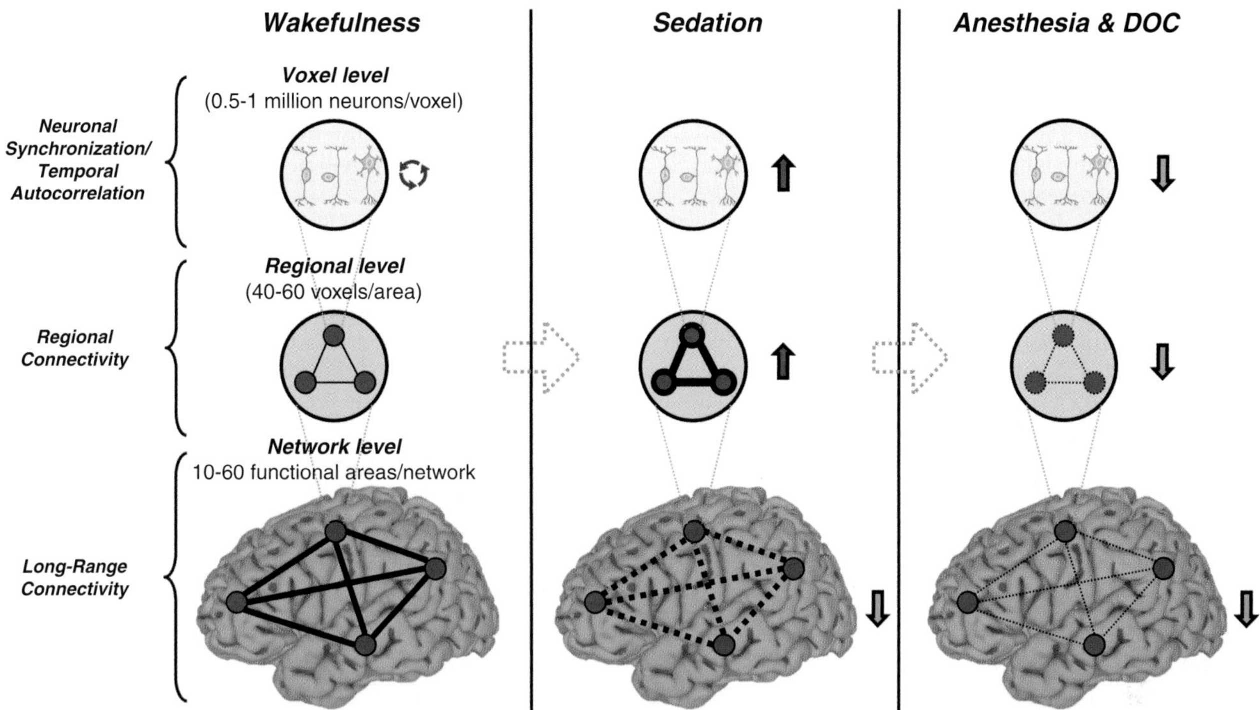

Fig. 9.3 Schematic summary of the consecutive stages of unconsciousness. Relative to the control state of wakefulness *(left column)*, sedation *(middle panel)* is marked by an increase of local/regional signal synchrony and consequent breakdown of global connectivity. Deep surgical anesthesia or disorders of consciousness *(DOC, right column)* is associated with collapse of both local/regional synchrony and global connectivity. (From Huang Z, Liu X, Mashour GA, Hudetz AG. Timescales of intrinsic BOLD signal dynamics and functional connectivity in pharmacologic and neuropathologic states of unconsciousness. *J Neurosci.* 2018;38[9]:2304–2317.)

were terminated at less than 100 milliseconds, and cortical communication was limited. Of note, this finding is consistent with findings in NREM sleep.[120] This perturbational approach determined that the complexity of cortical response to a stimulus decreased during sleep, general anesthesia, and disorders of consciousness.[121] The concordant findings across physiologic (sleep) and pharmacologic (anesthesia) states of unconsciousness may reflect a common neurophysiologic mechanism of disrupted cortical connectivity through slow oscillations, which share a number of characteristics in NREM sleep and general anesthesia.[122] A study of three epilepsy patients with intracranial neurophysiologic monitoring[123] revealed that, within 5 seconds of propofol-induced unconsciousness, there was a dramatic increase in the power of slow oscillations. Although single-unit neuronal activity was initially suppressed, it returned to baseline (or above baseline) but was fragmented into highly active and quiescent periods. Neural firing became coupled with the slow oscillation. However, the slow oscillations themselves demonstrated decay in phase coupling with increased distance across the cortex. Thus neuronal spike activity became fragmented into "on" and "off" periods, which became temporally uncoordinated across the cortex. These neurophysiologic conditions dramatically reduce the probability of meaningful corticocortical communication.

More recent trends of analyzing cortical changes during states of unconsciousness take a dynamic approach that reflects not just connectivity configurations but the repertoire of states that can be accessed during general anesthesia. For example, there is a contraction of dynamic repertoire and neural signal diversity during propofol-induced unconsciousness[124,125] that would preclude the kind of flexibility required for normal conscious experience. Dynamic patterns are impaired during general anesthesia and cortical dynamics are stabilized during general anesthesia.[126] This is likely a discrete, multistage process with distinct dynamic signatures during sedation and general anesthesia (Fig. 9.3).[127,128] Relating dynamics to connectivity, it appears that the repertoire of functional connectivity patterns in the primate brain becomes more tethered to structural/anatomical connectivity patterns during the anesthetized state.[129] Of note, animal studies suggest that the return of consciousness after general anesthesia is defined by discrete neural states that reconfigure during emergence.[130]

In the next section, we discuss memory, the thread that links conscious experiences together to form the narrative of "self."

Memory

HISTORY AND TERMINOLOGY

Modern understanding of the structure, function, and organization of human memory is deeply informed by the study of amnesia. The most renowned demonstration of this principle occurred in 1957, when Brenda Milner reported the remarkable case of Henry Gustav Molaison (1926–2008),[131] an amnesiac who would become known famously as H.M., and who would represent the single most influential case study in the history of neuroscience. In a procedure intended to treat a refractory seizure disorder, significant portions of the medial temporal lobe (MTL) were removed bilaterally—including the hippocampus, amygdala, and adjacent parahippocampal gyrus. H.M. developed profound and enduring anterograde amnesia, and was unable to establish any new conscious memory, irrespective of the sensory modality. He also developed a temporally graded window of retrograde amnesia, with impaired recall of events occurring during the 3 years preceding his surgery. However, most of his associated cognitive functions—perceptual processing, language, attention, access to semantic knowledge, and capacity to retain small packages of information in constant rehearsal—remained largely or entirely intact. Prior to this report, the prevailing theory—articulated by Canadian neuropsychologist Donald Hebb[132]—was that there was no brain region dedicated to memory function. Instead, memory processes were thought to be distributed and integrated into region-specific perceptual and cognitive functions. For example, the visual attribute of a memory would be wholly served within the striate and extrastriate cortical regions responsible for visual perception. The description of H.M. immediately disproved this model. It became clear that the MTL was a specialized and obligatory structure for the establishment and early maintenance of *all* conscious memory, irrespective of the modality. The trajectory of memory research was profoundly transformed. Initially, largely independent branches evolved to focus on the structural-functional organization of the MTL (Fig. 9.4*A*) and the nature of cellular-level neuroplastic processes—the latter notably marked by the description of long-term potentiation (LTP) by Timothy Bliss and Terje Lømo in 1973.[133] Subsequently, emerging technologies enabled the development and investigation of systems-level constructs. Examples include the use of EEG and magnetoencephalography to assess the role of oscillatory phase synchronization in neuronal assemblies,[134] fMRI to identify large-scale networks associated with specific memory functions,[135] and machine learning to classify complex neural network patterns predictive of memory.[136]

Amnesia is the term used to describe one of the cardinal properties of general anesthesia. As understood by most anesthesiologists and laypeople, this description is phenomenological; it states that patients do not recall the events that occur to them while receiving anesthesia. However, this usage confuses a critical mechanistic and semantic distinction. Patients in the deepest states of anesthesia are unable to process and bind perceptual elements into an integrated conscious experience. From the perspective of cognitive neuroscience, the "amnesia" of general anesthesia is not a primary failure of memory, but rather a failure of consciousness. It simply reflects that a conscious experience cannot be reconstructed by memory processes when it does not exist in the first place. Further confusion is added by the frequent use of the term *awareness*—a synonym for conscious perception—to describe the case in which a patient consciously recalls events occurring during the administration of an anesthetic. This ignores the fundamental principle that memory is functionally dissociable from consciousness. Awareness is *necessary* for the establishment of memory under anesthesia, but it is not *sufficient*. Conscious recall can occur only if awareness is accompanied by memory processes in the MTL and elsewhere that establish and preserve a representation that can be reconstructed later.

These important distinctions establish the axiom that patients who form memories while under anesthesia cannot have been truly unconscious; they must have possessed some conscious substrate from which the memory derives. However, the converse inference is not always true: the existence of consciousness will not necessarily lead to the existence of memory if an anesthetic drug is present. Evidence to support this statement is unambiguously encountered in everyday anesthetic practice—patients receiving a small dose of propofol or midazolam who engage in a cogent conversation that they are later unable to recall, or in patients emerging from general anesthesia who follow commands to demonstrate that extubation can proceed safely, yet later cannot recall anything related to this clearly conscious event. Anesthetic drugs must therefore have direct effects on memory processes that are dissociable from those on consciousness—and it is this observation that provides a framework for the systematic study of how anesthetic drugs affect memory.

Organization and Function of Normal Memory

MULTIPLE MEMORY SYSTEMS

When the term *memory* is used in everyday language, it almost always refers to declarative memory. Declarative memory is the representation of prior events and knowledge that is accessible to consciousness and can be manipulated by attention and executive function. It is the form of memory referred to in the context of anesthetic amnesia.

Further important organizational structure exists within declarative memory. The first is the distinction between episodic and semantic memory. *Episodic memory* is the recollection of events with a clear spatiotemporal context (as when recalling autobiographical events with a distinct sense of personal experience, time, and place), whereas *semantic memory* is the capacity to recall and apply meaning, facts, and knowledge without spatiotemporal context (as when recalling that Mount Everest is the tallest mountain in the world without any sense of time and place for the acquisition of that knowledge). The episodic memory system is fast-mapping and highly dependent on the MTL as well as frontal and parietal structures,[137,138] whereas the semantic memory system is slower and involves distributed cortical regions that closely map to the default mode network, a large-scale system that is active during the resting state and flow of spontaneous cognition.[135,139] The second organizational structure within episodic memory is the distinction between recollection and familiarity. *Recollection* involves remembering specific qualitative contextual details about a prior event, whereas in a *familiarity* judgment, there is a sense that an item has been encountered previously, but beyond that there are no added contextual details. The accepted understanding is that recollection and familiarity arise from distinct processes and neural architecture within the MTL. The perirhinal cortex receives input from sensory association areas and supports familiarity judgments through encoding and retrieval of the identifying qualities of an item (the "what" information). The parahippocampal cortex and entorhinal areas receive input from areas

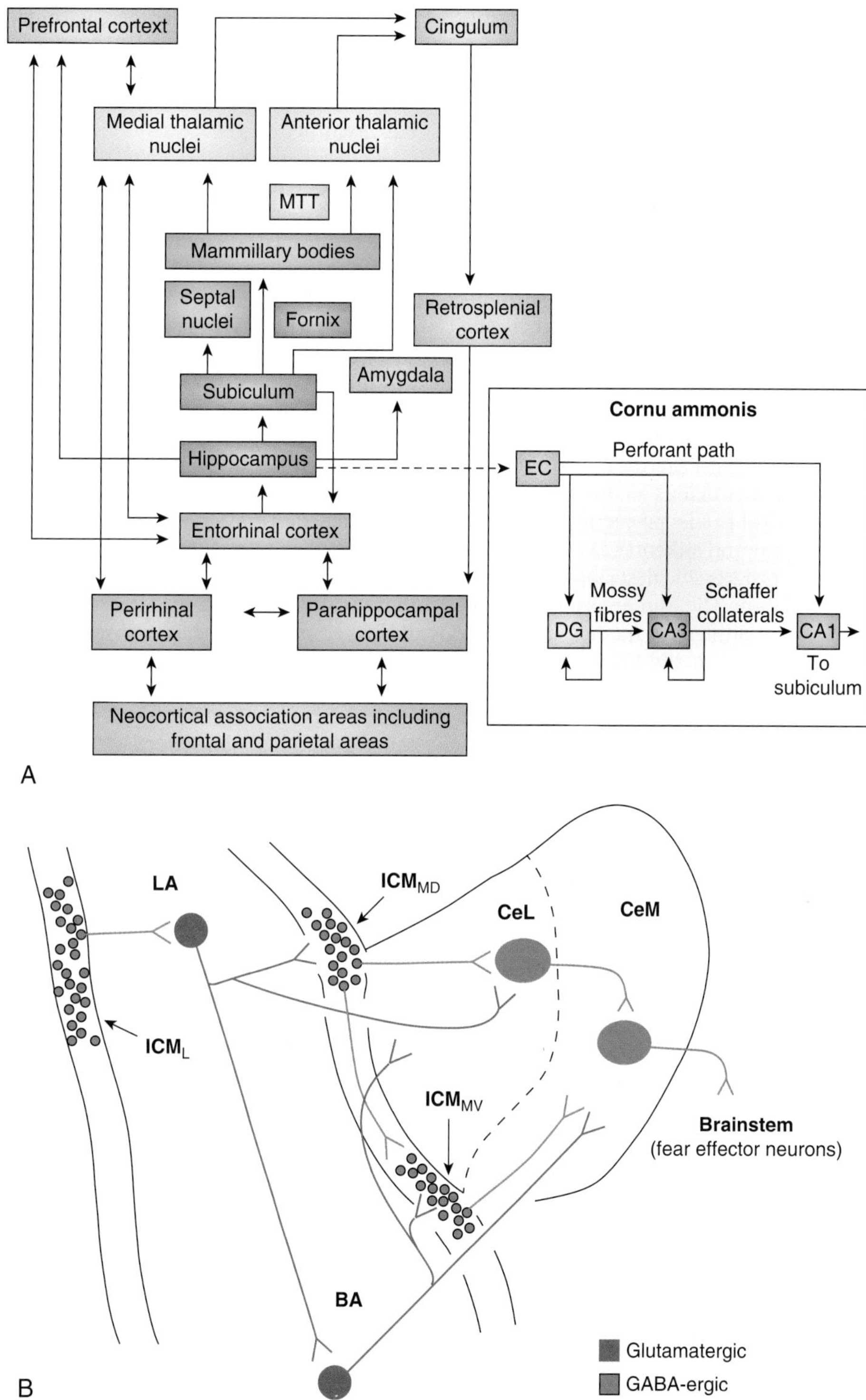

Fig. 9.4 Memory systems in the medial temporal lobe. (A) Representation of unidirectional and bidirectional network connectivity of structures in the medial temporal lobe, diencephalic nuclei, and neocortical association areas. *CA,* Cornu ammonis; *DG,* dentate gyrus; *EC,* entorhinal cortex; *MTT,* mammillothalamic tract. (B) Intrinsic connectivity of the amygdala. *BA,* Basal nucleus; *CeL,* central nucleus lateral segment; *CeM,* central nucleus medial segment; *ICM_L,* lateral intercalated cell mass; *ICM_{MD},* dorsomedial intercalated cell mass; *ICM_{MV},* ventromedial intercalated cell mass; *LA,* lateral nucleus. ([A] Modified from Bartsch T, Butler C. Transient amnesic syndromes. *Nat Rev Neurol.* 2013;9[2]:86–97, Figure 2. [B] Modified from Duvarci S, Pare D. Amygdala microcircuits controlling learned fear. *Neuron.* 2014;82[5]:966–980, Figure 2.)

processing spatial information (the "where" information), and support recollection through encoding and retrieval of context. The hippocampus links these two, binding item and context information, and appears necessary for recollection, but plays little or no role in familiarity.[140,141]

Other forms of memory are dissociable from declarative memory. Findings that amnesiacs could learn a hand-eye coordination skill even while possessing no memory of the task led to the distinction between declarative and *procedural* memory, which is dependent on the caudate nucleus.

Subsequently, memory-impaired patients were also found to have intact *priming*,[142] which is a nonconscious process in which exposure to a stimulus influences the response to a later stimulus—for example, amnesiacs can name pictures 100 milliseconds faster if they have seen them previously, despite having no declarative memory of the exposure.[143] The neural bases for priming effects are thought to arise within regions serving perceptual and contextual processing of the stimulus, and so vary with the nature of the task.[144] Lastly, a large body of work has extensively elucidated the *emotional memory* system. The classic experimental model is Pavlovian fear conditioning and its variants, wherein an emotionally neutral conditioned stimulus is paired with an aversive unconditioned stimulus, leading to an involuntary associative physiologic and/or behavioral response to the conditioned stimulus. The circuitry involves convergence of afferent information from all sensory modalities on the lateral nucleus of the amygdala, and the basolateral and central nuclei projecting widely to modulate processes in cortical and subcortical regions (see Fig. 9. 4*B*).[145,146] With the progressive description of these and other functional distinctions, the framework for understanding memory eventually shifted to models that contained multiple memory systems in the brain, distributed functionally and anatomically.[147]

Working memory refers to the capacity to maintain limited amounts of information in the stream of consciousness, which can be manipulated to perform complex cognitive tasks such as reasoning, comprehension, and learning.[148] The concept evolved from, and has largely replaced, earlier ideas about *short-term memory*, but the terms should not be used interchangeably, as working memory implies both a short-term memory store *and* the capacity for manipulation. The most influential current model, first proposed by Baddeley and Hitch in 1974,[149] divides working memory into capacity-limited component subsystems: a *phonological loop* that maintains information through vocal or subvocal rehearsal, such as when one holds a telephone number in mind; a *visuospatial sketchpad*, which holds and manipulates spatial, visual, and kinesthetic information; and a *central executive*, which is responsible for regulating selective attention and inhibition. A fourth subsystem, the *episodic buffer*, was later added to the model[150] and is responsible for the temporary storage of multidimensional representations and integration with declarative memory.

Working memory has long been understood to not involve the MTL,[151] although the belief that it has no role has recently been questioned in studies of spatial working memory.[152] Notwithstanding, current understanding of working memory suggests that it is served by persistent activity and flexible resource allocation in a distributed cortical network, with a critical hub in the dorsolateral prefrontal cortex (DLPFC) interconnected with parietal cortex, thalamus, caudate, and globus pallidus.[153] The functional and structural distinction between working memory and the MTL does not mean that working memory and declarative memory systems do not interact. Working memory depends on declarative memory representations to provide semantic meaning and context. During working memory tasks, cortical perceptual areas associated with representations of declarative memory become activated and show increased synchrony with prefrontal regions.[154] Reciprocally, encoding of declarative memory is strongly influenced by the nature of processing occurring in working memory, with deeper levels of executive processing resulting in better learning.[155]

The transition of memory from short-term stores through to stable long-term stores is experienced as continuous and was assumed to reflect sequential transfer across systems. However, this model is challenged by rare case examples of patients who have a selective short-term memory deficit but intact declarative memory function, and recent studies have reinforced the view that memories are formed in multiple systems in parallel.[156]

LONG-TERM POTENTIATION, SYNAPTIC TAGGING, AND THE CONSOLIDATION MODEL OF MEMORY

The consolidation hypothesis of memory was first proposed by Müller and Pilzecker in 1900.[157] They noted that memory for new information could be disrupted by learning other information shortly after the initial training. This effect, called *retroactive interference*, is temporally graded such that the susceptibility of the memory is greatest immediately after learning and decreases with time. Müller and Pilzecker proposed that the memory trace must initially exist in a fragile state, but subsequently becomes stable through the process of *consolidation*. The consolidation hypothesis remains the framework for understanding the temporal course of memory processes and behavior.

For a memory trace to be consolidated, it must of course be created. The term used to describe this process is *encoding*. Encoding implies that the networks mediating the neural representation of an event as it is experienced do not immediately return to their previous state and are modified in such a way that potentiates reactivation of that representation. The *synaptic plasticity and memory hypothesis* states that activity-induced synaptic plasticity is both necessary and sufficient for the information storage underlying memory,[158] and within this framework encoding implies that some form of synaptic plasticity has been initiated. However, encoding cannot in itself assure the propagation of a memory trace. Encoding creates the potential for the formation of a long-term memory.

The minimal events that constitute the neural correlates of encoding are incompletely understood. Cellular models demonstrate that functional changes in synaptic strength can occur in the absence of any structural change in dendritic spines.[159] The perpetuation of these initial changes through structural and functional remodeling represents the neural correlate of memory consolidation. The prevailing cellular model for this is LTP,[160] which describes a durable increase in synaptic transmission efficiency following a stimulation protocol. It is now recognized that LTP occurs richly throughout the hippocampus, as well as in other afferent pathways.[161] LTP can be induced by nonphysiologic high-frequency stimulation, but also by stimulation protocols that resemble physiologic activity, the most important being bursts in the theta range (4-8 Hz).[162] This is of notable relevance to memory, as synchronized hippocampal theta oscillations appear critical to successful memory behaviors.[134]

The breadth and depth of literature on the mechanisms of LTP are far too voluminous to summarize here. Nonetheless, certain principles are essential and relevant to anesthesia studies and can be stated succinctly. The induction of most forms of LTP requires activation of postsynaptic *N*-methyl-D-aspartate (NMDA) receptors,[163] followed by influx of Na^+ and Ca^{2+}. This rise in intracellular Ca^{2+} is the critical trigger for LTP. Calcium-calmodulin-dependent kinase II (CaMKII) is then activated and autophosphorylated,[164,165] leading to cytoskeletal reconfiguration.[166] Activation of several other cell-signaling cascades also contribute to LTP. The terminal expression of LTP is protein synthesis, occurring in both the soma and local dendrites, and resulting in enduring structural changes at the synapse.[167] Protein synthesis inhibitors have been demonstrated to consistently prevent sustained LTP in vitro and learning in vivo.[168]

LTP thus proceeds in two phases: early LTP (E-LTP) is independent of protein synthesis and can be sustained across an interval of minutes to a short number of hours, while late LTP (L-LTP) is dependent on intracellular signaling and protein synthesis and can be sustained across many days. The *synaptic tagging and capture hypothesis* provides a mechanistic explanation for the observation that the persistence of synaptic potentiation (and memory) is influenced by events surrounding encoding.[169] In this model, synapses activated during E-LTP become tagged via a protein synthesis-independent mechanism. This tag establishes the potential for sustained L-LTP, but for the cascade to continue the tags must capture plasticity-related proteins (PRPs) synthesized in the soma or dendrites in response to neural activity. The synaptic tagging model explains how the thousands of dendrites of a single neuron can be engaged in memory stabilization processes in various states of evolution, because the tagging and PRP capture need not occur as a singular event.

RECONSOLIDATION

A major shift the in understanding of consolidation occurred in 2000, when Nader et al. reported that an old memory for auditory fear conditioning, which would normally not be sensitive to protein inhibitors, can be made newly sensitive if it is retrieved.[170] The implication is that retrieval of a memory renders it transiently plastic, after which it restabilizes. This process is termed *reconsolidation*, and the period of plasticity is termed the *reconsolidation window*. The mechanism shares many of the LTP processes that are associated with initial consolidation, but also has features that are quite distinct at both the cellular and systems level.[171] Reconsolidation serves as a modulatory process that enables the strengthening of an existing memory, but it is also clear that it provides a window within which an existing memory is malleable and can be updated with the addition of novel information, or diminished through interruption of restabilization processes.[172] These latter properties have generated significant translational interest because of repeated demonstrations of the ability to modify or even eliminate fear memory in animals through pharmacologic and behavioral interventions that interrupt reconsolidation.[173] Indeed, the erasure of fear memory in humans can be demonstrated through performance of a behavioral extinction procedure during the reconsolidation window.[174]

PHASE SYNCHRONIZATION AND COUPLING

The neurons in assemblies and networks undergo oscillatory activation and inhibition. Phase synchronization of these oscillations supports neural communication by creating transient and dynamic associations between different functional brain regions. Phase synchronization appears to be fundamental to neural plasticity and memory,[134] and numerous studies have demonstrated that dynamics of synchrony during memory tasks can be related to both long-term[175] and working memory[176] performance. Gamma-band (30-100 Hz) synchrony is believed to support an important form of Hebbian plasticity, termed spike-timing-dependent plasticity, in the hippocampus. Both computational models and experimental data provide evidence that rapid changes in the frequency and phase of gamma rhythms modulate this form of plasticity through coordination of presynaptic spikes in assemblies of neurons, effectively classifying which assemblies are interpreted as a single event.[177]

Another property of relevance to memory coding is the coupling of gamma oscillations to the phase of slower, synchronized oscillations within the theta-band (4-8 Hz).[178] Theta oscillations, which are prominent in the hippocampus and entorhinal cortex, undergo phase resetting in response to a stimulus. The phase reset involves widely distributed regions, and is thought to serve as an efficient mechanism for the optimization of interregional communication.[179] Theta phase resetting and synchrony in the hippocampal-entorhinal system are implicated in declarative memory,[180] and in the amygdala-hippocampal system in fear-based memory.[181] Coupling between theta phase and gamma amplitude is connected to declarative memory formation,[180,182] and, in an elegant model, is proposed to form a code for representing multiple items and spatial representations in an ordered way.[183] Coupling between theta phase and gamma phase enables a more precise temporal coordination of neuronal spikes, and may code for separated representations of multiple items in working memory.[184]

Effects of Anesthetic Drugs on Declarative Memory Function in Humans

There are multiple potential pathways by which anesthetic drugs could interfere with memory and cause amnesia. Most of these cannot be directly assessed in humans, but the plausibility of candidate mechanisms can be indirectly examined by designing experiments that are informed by the characteristics of known memory processes. Studies of anesthetic effects on memory are most informative when conceptualized and designed with reference to robust methods and findings taken from the larger body of memory research.

BEHAVIORAL STUDIES OF RETROGRADE MEMORY EFFECTS

Notwithstanding some isolated case reports, systematic investigations have found no evidence that anesthetic drugs cause retrograde amnesia in humans. There is no retrograde amnesia associated with induction doses of thiopental,[185] methohexital,[185] or propofol.[186] Adult patients have normal memory for visual stimuli presented 4 minutes before administration of midazolam at doses of 2, 5, and 10 mg.[187] Similarly, memory is normal for word lists learned in the preoperative holding area or operating room immediately before induction.[188] Studies in pediatric patients have shown normal memory for pictures presented immediately before sedation with midazolam,[189] propofol,[190] and dexmedetomidine.[191] In controlled laboratory settings using human volunteers and target-controlled infusions, studies have found no impairment of memory for pictures[192] or words[193,194] presented before sedative infusions of propofol, midazolam, thiopental, or dexmedetomidine.

There is some evidence from controlled studies that anesthetic drugs may instead lead to the opposite effect, in which memory for material presented prior to drug administration is enhanced—a phenomenon termed *retrograde facilitation*. In one study using a mildly sedative dose of propofol,[195] memory for words learned immediately prior to drug administration was enhanced throughout the testing period of 24 hours. Similar effects are described for midazolam and other benzodiazepines in the psychopharmacology literature.[196] The mechanistic explanation for retrograde facilitation can be framed by an understanding of *retrograde interference*—the observation that mental exertion inhibits the consolidation of recently formed memories, with the newest memories being most vulnerable.[197] The induction of new LTP interferes with recently formed LTP and memory performance, even when the tasks are unrelated.[198] However, when the induction of new LTP is blocked by administration of a selective NMDA antagonist after learning, interference with recently formed LTP does not occur, and memory performance improves.[199,200] A parsimonious explanation for the retrograde facilitation seen with propofol and benzodiazepines is that they similarly modulate the induction of new LTP via a GABA-ergic pathway, freeing consolidation resources that enhance survival of recently formed memory.

The findings of retrograde facilitation and absence of retrograde amnesia are suggestive that the key mechanisms of GABA-ergic anesthetic amnesia, at least in humans, involve very early processes in the consolidation cascade. It is more difficult to rationalize that downstream sequences represent principal targets. Were this the case, the expected effect would be interference with ongoing consolidation of memory for events occurring in the past, creating a window of retrograde amnesia. Nonetheless, an alternate model to the induction hypothesis suggests that GABA-ergic anesthetics exert a direct effect on downstream protein transcription processes,[201] based on evidence from rodent studies.[202]

The absence of pharmacologic retrograde amnesia does not dismiss the repeated finding that, in the clinical setting, a percentage of patients will not recall the immediate preanesthetic period—an effect that increases with age.[203] Although not systematically studied, the complex noradrenergic-mediated effects of acute stress and anxiety on memory may be contributory.[204]

MATHEMATICAL MODELING OF ANESTHETIC AMNESIA

Mathematical modeling of memory decay has been used to characterize the amnestic effects of multiple intravenous anesthetic drugs,[193] which are accurately described by a two-parameter power decay function:

$$m_t = \lambda t^{-\Psi}$$

where λ reflects the initial memory strength (an index of encoding), and ψ expresses the rate of decay (an index of consolidation). The drugs are characterized by marked differences in the way they modulate the two coefficients. Propofol is an archetypal amnestic drug—it permits robust encoding of material, but the information undergoes accelerated decay because of a failure of consolidation. In contrast, dexmedetomidine archetypally causes memory impairment because of a failure of information to be strongly encoded but has little or no effect on the subsequent consolidation of memories that are encoded. The benzodiazepine midazolam behaves like propofol at lower doses—selectively causing consolidation failure while leaving encoding intact—but with increasing dose a significant encoding impairment emerges. Thiopental in contrast causes marked encoding failure but demonstrates minimal effect on consolidation. The discrepant patterns observed imply that nonspecific $GABA_A$ agonism is not per se sufficient to explain the ability of a drug to cause consolidation failure.

ANESTHETIC EFFECTS ON ATTENTION AND AROUSAL AS MODULATORS OF ENCODING

The effect of anesthetic drugs on encoding processes is related to the modulation of attention. Selective attention is governed by distinct networks mediating alertness, target orientation, and executive control[205]; involves modulation of neuronal phase synchrony across short- and long-range connections[206]; and is necessary for the successful establishment of declarative memory.[207] The dominant effect of most anesthetic drugs on attention is decreased arousal, with the notable exception being the NMDA antagonist ketamine, which has dominant effects on orienting and selection.[208] Thiopental mimics the effect of an attentional challenge task in decreasing activation in the left inferior prefrontal cortex (LIPFC), an effect that is not seen with propofol.[209] When tested at 225 minutes, arousal is predictive of memory for thiopental and dexmedetomidine, while propofol causes a significantly greater loss of memory than would be predicted by modulation of arousal alone.[194] In mathematical modeling of anesthetic amnesia,[193] arousal predicts the coefficient of encoding strength with precision for a range of sedative concentrations of dexmedetomidine, thiopental, midazolam, and propofol. In sum, arousal is predictive of subsequent memory for drugs that impair memory dominantly through causing encoding failure.

NEUROIMAGING STUDIES OF CORTICAL ENCODING PROCESSES

A limited number of functional neuroimaging studies have evaluated the effect of anesthetics on cortical regional activation during memory encoding. An early PET study investigating sedative doses of propofol using a word memory task[210] identified that activation in LIPFC—a region associated with encoding and subsequent memory for language tasks—was conserved, suggesting that propofol did not block the processes required to support successful encoding. In contrast, activation in DLPFC—a region most associated with executive control functions and cognitive control of motor planning[211]—was decreased. In a subsequent investigation using an auditory depth of processing task, activation of LIPFC was found to be decreased by sedative doses of thiopental, but again was relatively unaffected by propofol.[209] However, other studies have identified decreased activation in encoding areas. An fMRI study of sentence comprehension during light sedation with propofol found that decreased memory for sentences was related to decreased activation in the left inferior frontal gyrus (LIFG, within the LIPFC) and the middle temporal gyrus.[212] Another study using a single-word encoding task showed decreased activation in LIFG at levels of propofol sedation causing memory loss, but also found intact connectivity between LIFG and a number of frontoparietal and temporal regions associated with verbal processing and memory tasks, including the middle temporal gyrus and precuneus.[213]

Some functional neuroimaging studies have used experimental tasks similar to memory encoding tasks while evaluating sedative doses of anesthetic drugs, but have not assessed memory encoding as a primary aim; these are informative, but must be interpreted with caution. An early PET study of sedative doses of midazolam using a tone detection paradigm reported a dose-dependent activation decrease in Brodmann areas 9, 10, and 46, which overlap regions of both DLPFC and LIPFC.[214] An fMRI study of semantic word processing during propofol sedation found a dose-dependent decrease in activation of the LIFG, despite intact behavioral responses.[215] An fMRI study of low-dose dexmedetomidine reported a generalized suppression of bilateral prefrontal activation in Brodmann areas 9 and 10 during an emotional picture memory task, but encoding performance was not specifically analyzed.[216] A recent study using music stimuli found decreased activation in primary and secondary auditory processing areas at sedative doses of dexmedetomidine and midazolam, but not with propofol.[217] Other neuroimaging studies evaluating resting state networks, or passive activation in response to stimuli at nonresponsive levels of sedation, should not be viewed as memory experiments.

Neuroimaging Studies of Medial Temporal Lobe Function

Two methodologically similar studies used event-related fMRI to evaluate MTL activation during low-dose infusions of propofol and dexmedetomidine. The degree of amnesia caused by propofol can be linearly related to decreased activation in the hippocampus bilaterally,[218] an effect that behaviorally corresponded to a failure of consolidation processes. In contrast, dexmedetomidine does not reduce the overall level of hippocampal activity, but the subsequent-memory effect is attenuated, and dynamics of hippocampal activation are less predictive of subsequent memory[216]; one interpretation is that this reflects a downstream effect from weakened cortical encoding processes. An earlier study of the benzodiazepine lorazepam and the cholinergic antagonist scopolamine found decreased memory to be correlated with decreased activation in the anterior hippocampus,[219] accompanied by decreased activation in the encoding-related regions in the fusiform gyrus and inferior frontal cortex. In a largely exploratory investigation, 0.25% sevoflurane was found to reduce hippocampal activation in response to auditory and visual stimuli, but no memory performance was assessed.[220]

A few studies have evaluated anesthetic effects using electrocorticography and depth electrodes implanted in epileptic patients, but none have been dedicated to memory function. One notable study evaluated the effects of mildly sedative concentrations of propofol on hippocampal spectral coherence and power characteristics at rest.[221] The main finding was a significant increase in hippocampal-rhinal spontaneous coherence in the delta-band, but minimal changes in other bands; cortico-hippocampal coherence was not assessed.

STUDIES OF CORTICAL EVENT-RELATED POTENTIALS

A number of memory-dedicated studies have used the event-related potential (ERP)—a small but stereotypic positive and negative signal fluctuation in the EEG time-locked to a stimulus, and which can be isolated through summation over multiple (usually at least 50) identical trials. ERPs are thought to emerge not because new oscillations are induced, but because of a stimulus-induced phase resetting of ongoing oscillations.[222]

An early ERP study[223] of scopolamine, lorazepam, and diphenhydramine suggested that drug-induced effects on arousal and memory may be electrophysiologically dissociable, although memory was not assessed directly. Changes in the P1N1 and N1P2 early complexes, associated with arousal, were seen for all three drugs. However, changes in later complexes associated with memory, notably the P3 and N2P3, were seen only with scopolamine and lorazepam, and not with diphenhydramine, an antihistamine that causes sedation but not amnesia. This work is extended by a series of studies evaluating intravenous anesthetics and using memory-specific experimental paradigms. In a verbal memory task, propofol amnesia was associated with decreased P300 amplitude at the time of the encoding task.[224] In a subsequent study in which multiple drugs were carefully dosed to equivalent levels of sedation,[225] the true amnestic drugs with memory effects independent of sedation—propofol and midazolam—caused decreased amplitude in the P300 and N2P3 components, with the latter being the best predictor of subsequent memory performance. Across all drugs studied, the N2 latency was related to reaction time, a surrogate measure of sedation.

Another study examined early- and mid-latency ERPs originating from the midline parietal precuneal region (Pz), and related them to coefficients describing the extent of encoding and consolidation failure.[226] Across drugs from multiple classes and at multiple doses, consolidation failure was closely correlated with the P2 amplitude and N2 latency observed at the time of encoding. As the visual P2N2 complex is known to originate from synchronous theta oscillations,[227] one possibility is that a common mechanism underlying the effect of anesthetic drugs on consolidation involves changes in theta oscillations across a distributed cortico-hippocampal network occurring at the time of consolidation induction. Further, the P2N2 and memory decay coefficient were also closely correlated with reaction time, which can be related to interregional synchrony.[228] Unfortunately, no direct measures of cortico-hippocampal theta synchrony have yet been performed in studies of pharmacologic amnesia. Another analysis[229] examined the *old-new effect*, a robust phenomenon in the parietal ERP that distinguishes the response to initial item exposure from subsequent exposures as a marker of memory strength. Propofol and midazolam caused a significant decrease in the old-new effect at 27 seconds, even though memory performance was maintained, demonstrating again an early marker of impaired memory processes that precedes behavioral detection.

Studies using very different experimental paradigms have evaluated auditory ERPs at multiple concentrations of propofol.[230,231] Propofol causes a dose-dependent decrease in mismatch negativity and early right anterior negativity, which are elicited in response to specific music signatures and are known to relate to associative memory operations. In contrast, the P1 complex, which derives from primary auditory processing, is not affected even at deep levels of sedation.

Nonhuman Studies of Anesthetic Effects on Memory Processes and Behavior in the Medial Temporal Lobe

ANESTHETIC EFFECTS ON MEDIAL TEMPORAL LOBE PLASTICITY

GABA-ergic interneurons project within and across subregions of the hippocampus,[232] providing an abundant density of possible targets for anesthetic drugs. In an early study using tetanic stimulation of the Schaffer collateral-commissural pathway,[233] isoflurane blocked the induction of LTP, and long-term depression (LTD) by low-frequency stimulation. These effects were reversed by the addition of the $GABA_A$ receptor antagonist picrotoxin, providing strong evidence that the effect of isoflurane on LTP is GABA-ergically mediated. In a similar protocol, amnestic concentrations of sevoflurane caused a failure of LTP which was prevented by the addition of the $GABA_A$ antagonist bicuculline.[234] A recent study of sevoflurane exposure in neonatal rats found reduced spine density of apical dendrites, synaptic ultrastructure damage, elevated expression of synaptic vesicle-associated proteins, and inhibition of LTP but not LTD.[235] One study of isoflurane, in which the hippocampus was studied 24 hours following anesthetic exposure, somewhat unexpectedly found improvement in cognitive performance, accompanied by evidence of upregulation of the 2B subunit of the NMDA receptor and enhanced LTP.[236]

A series of investigations have demonstrated that propofol inhibits the induction, but not the maintenance, of LTP, and has no effect on LTD. The effect is blocked by the addition of picrotoxin, implicating a $GABA_A$ receptor-mediated mechanism.[237,238] Notably, one study found that propofol inhibited LTP only at anesthetic, and not at amnestic concentrations.[238] Propofol has also been demonstrated to inhibit a number of component subprocesses of LTP.[239-241] Propofol reduces expression of activity-related cytoskeleton-associated protein (Arc) in the hippocampus in response to inhibitory avoidance training but does not appear to reduce Arc mRNA,[202] which is notable because it suggests a post-transcriptional mechanism.

The hippocampal $GABA_A$ergic interneuron population is notable for a high density of the α_5-subunit subtype. Of known significance to memory function, the α_5-$GABA_A$ receptor regulates the induction of LTP in response to a narrow range of frequencies in the theta range.[242] These observations have driven a series of anesthesia studies using α_5-$GABA_A$-knockout mice. Etomidate blocks LTP measured in CA1 neurons in wild-type mice, but not in α_5 –/– mutants, and behaviorally the α_5 –/– mutants are resistant to the amnestic effects of etomidate, but not to its general anesthetic effects.[243] Further, the effects of etomidate on LTP and memory behaviors are reversed by the addition of L-655,708, which selectively reduces the activity of α_5-$GABA_A$ receptors.[244] The behavioral findings were later replicated with exposure to 1 MAC of isoflurane, with memory deficits observed in wild-type mice, but not in α_5 –/– mutants or in wild types receiving L-655,708.[245,246] The increase in α_5-$GABA_A$ receptors caused by etomidate and isoflurane does not return to baseline for at least 1 week.[247]

The α_5-subunit subtype is not exclusive in its association with amnesia. α_4-$GABA_A$ receptors are concentrated in the dentate gyrus and dorsal thalamus, and α_4 knockouts are resistant to the amnestic effects of isoflurane but not to its general anesthetic effects.[248] More equivocally, β_3-$GABA_A$ receptor knockout mice have been reported to be resistant to the amnestic effects of isoflurane,[249] while in a study using β_3-$GABA_A$ receptor knock-in mutants, the β_3 subtype was not significantly associated with amnesia.[250] Similar equivocacy has been found in studies of the α_1 subtype.[251,252]

The effects of anesthetics on hippocampal theta oscillations in vivo have been studied. One study used a fear-conditioning paradigm to examine amnestic concentration of isoflurane, nitrous oxide, and halothane, and reported that suppression of hippocampal-dependent contextual conditioning was proportionate to slowing of theta peak frequency.[253] Another study also demonstrated that isoflurane caused slowing of theta oscillations in the CA1 neuronal bundle without changing absolute power,[254] while in contrast the nonimmobilizer F6, which causes amnesia without sedation or a loss of motor activity, caused a loss of theta oscillatory power without slowing. Scopolamine causes amnesia at doses associated with acceleration of theta oscillations, which might otherwise be expected to improve learning.[255] However, a significant loss of absolute power is also observed. Together these findings suggest that individual anesthetics may cause amnesia through distinct forms of hippocampal theta disruption.

Human and Nonhuman Studies of Anesthetic Effects on Fear Memory Systems

THE AMYGDALA-DEPENDENT FEAR SYSTEM

The amygdala is a cluster of interconnected nuclei sitting immediately anterior to the hippocampus, with afferent and efferent projections to a wide distribution of cortical and subcortical structures. It is critical to fear learning and memory, and the systematic study of amygdala-dependent classical (Pavlovian) fear conditioning has produced much information regarding the mechanisms and circuitry.[145,146] The basolateral nucleus of the amygdala (BLA) also modulates the encoding and consolidation of memory in the hippocampus and elsewhere in response to emotion, arousal, and stress.[256] The mechanism is dependent on noradrenergic projections terminating on both α and β receptors within the BLA,[257] and can be triggered by systemic stress mediators—notably glucocorticoids[258] and epinephrine.[259] Amygdalo-hippocampal connectivity occurs via direct and indirect projections, and is dependent on theta oscillatory synchrony.[181,260] The amygdala contains a number of rational targets for GABA-ergic anesthetic drugs.

STUDIES OF ANESTHETIC EFFECTS ON FEAR SYSTEMS IN NONHUMANS

As various forms of fear conditioning represent the dominant experimental method for studying memory in animal models, almost all studies of anesthetic effects on memory offer some insight into their effects on fear systems. Beyond the central conclusion from this sizeable body of literature that GABA-ergic anesthetics in general impair the acquisition of fear memory, a subset of studies are notable for their specific focus on fear circuitry and behavior.

There is substantial evidence that anesthetic effects on fear memory are mediated by GABA-ergic mechanisms in the amygdala. Selective injection of the BLA with midazolam blocks acquisition and stress enhancement of fear memory,[261] while lesions of the BLA block anterograde amnesia for an inhibitory avoidance task in rats receiving diazepam,[262] propofol,[263] and sevoflurane.[264] Further, injection of the BLA with the selective $GABA_A$ antagonist bicuculline blocks the effect of propofol[202] and midazolam.[265]

There are certain conditions under which anesthetic drugs can enhance fear memory. When propofol or ketamine is given immediately following conditioning, retention is enhanced,[266,267] which may represent a form of retrograde facilitation as described earlier, but retention is reduced when dexmedetomidine is similarly administered. In a rat model of PTSD, propofol and ketamine administered immediately after fear learning enhances long-term fear behavior, while dexmedetomidine has a neutral effect.[267] Midazolam given during extinction training, which normally inhibits learned fear expression, blocks the effect of extinction,[261] and also blocks fear-reducing effects when given during preconditioning contextual learning.[268] When sevoflurane is administered at a very low, nonsedating dose (0.11%), fear conditioning is enhanced.[269,270]

STUDIES OF ANESTHETIC EFFECTS ON FEAR SYSTEMS IN HUMANS

Three functional neuroimaging studies have directly addressed anesthetic effects on emotional memory. A study using PET and path analysis (Fig. 9.5 *lower panel*)[271] demonstrated that the superior memorability that negatively arousing emotional items have over neutral items was unaffected by 0.1% and 0.2% sevoflurane, but lost at 0.25%, and was associated with decreased effective connectivity projecting from the right amygdala to hippocampus, and also from the right nucleus basalis to hippocampus. Further, sevoflurane modulated emotional perception such that items were rated more neutrally. An fMRI study demonstrated that sedative doses of propofol do not reduce activation of the amygdala in response to negatively arousing items, but activation of the hippocampus is markedly attenuated (see Fig. 9.5 *upper panel*) and correlates with amnesia and loss of the superior memorability of emotional material.[218] This suggests that cortical and subcortical processes serving emotional interpretative functions and afferent amygdala activation are relatively spared by amnestic levels of propofol, while efferent processes underlying amygdala-dependent modulation of hippocampal plasticity are interrupted. An fMRI study of dexmedetomidine also reported no effect on activation of the amygdala in response to negatively arousing items,[216] but in contrast to propofol, emotional items retained superior memorability, and activation in the left amygdala and hippocampus were correlated with subsequent memory. Taken together, these studies imply that propofol may have a more targeted effect on the amygdalo-hippocampal modulatory axis. One potential explanation is that amygdalo-hippocampal connectivity is markedly interrupted by a loss of theta oscillatory synchrony caused by propofol, whereas α_{2A} antagonism at the LC causes only limited downstream attenuation of noradrenergic signaling in the BLA.

CLINICAL RELEVANCE

Amygdala reactivity is of importance in a number of fear-based psychopathologies, including anxiety, phobia, panic disorder, and PTSD.[272] The neurohumoral stress response to surgery and critical illness can cause complex changes in levels of catecholamines, glucocorticoids, and other potential promoters of plasticity in amygdala-dependent fear processes, occurring within a context that frequently contains emotional stressors. It is unclear under what specific conditions elevated (or depressed) levels of these mediators might contribute to long-term changes in neuropsychological functioning, although multiple studies in the critical care setting relate stress exposure, and exogenous administration of catecholamines, to negative long-term outcomes.[273] In a broad surgical population, the incidence of PTSD-complex symptoms related to surgery was reported to be 16%[5]—similar to that observed in victims of violence. The effect—or lack of effect—of anesthetic drugs on plasticity processes in the perioperative or critical care setting thus has a theoretical potential to impact long-term psychological sequelae, both positively and negatively. However, there is presently insufficient human data to inform specific recommendations.

Anesthetic Effects on Implicit Memory Function

Implicit (nondeclarative) memory processes do not axiomatically require a conscious substrate, and are not dependent on classic hippocampal plasticity. Therefore the effect of anesthetic drugs on implicit memory functions may have important distinction from those on declarative memory, and accordingly a number of investigations have sought evidence for implicit processing in unconscious subjects. Many studies have used auditory adaptations of the *word stem completion task*, or the more rigorous *process dissociation procedure*, in which subjects are asked to exclude items that have been presented; declarative memory will drive avoidance of the target word, while implicit memory will lead to a familiarity response favoring the target word.

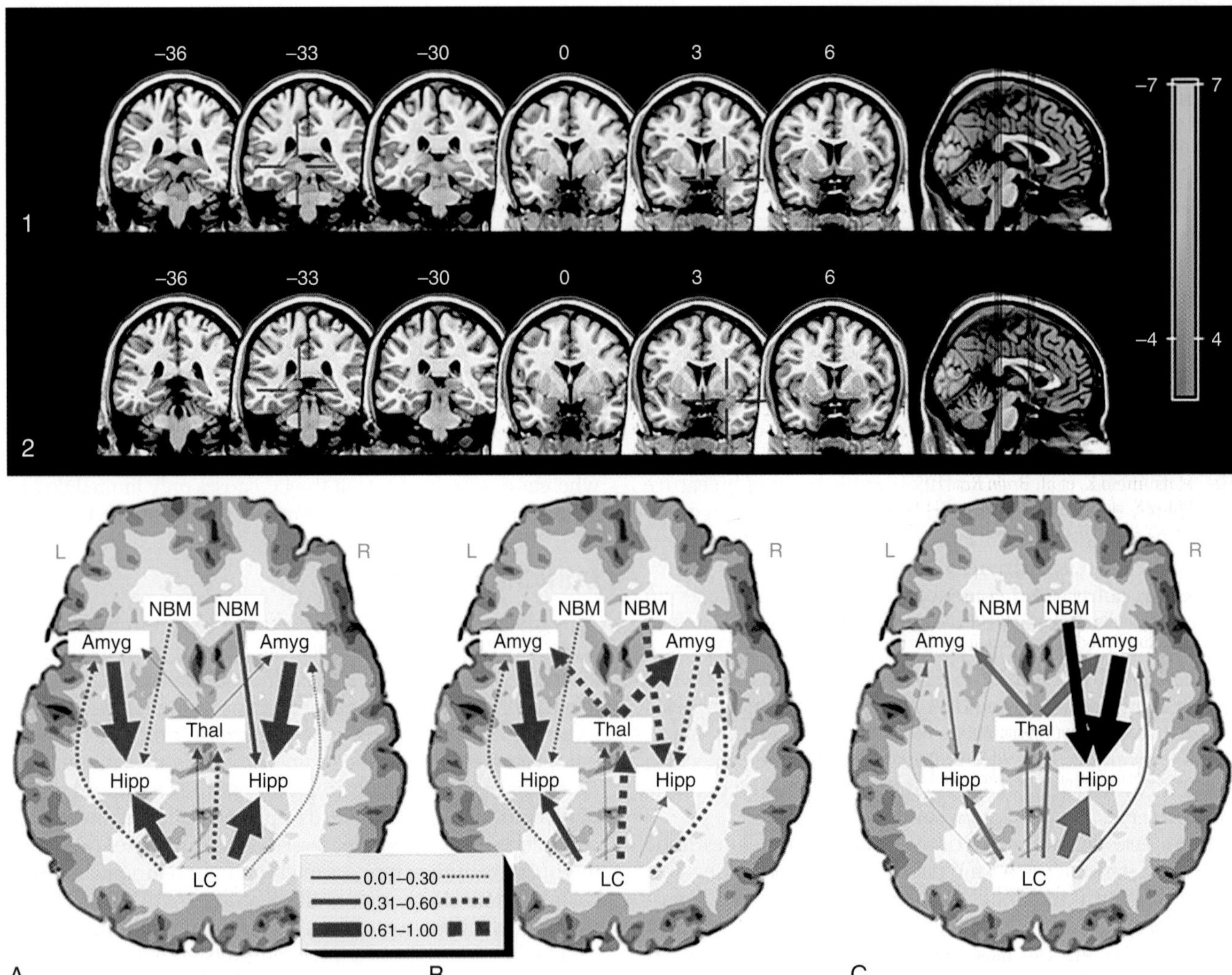

Fig. 9.5 Anesthetic effects on emotional memory systems. (*upper panel*) Functional magnetic resonance imaging scans showing the contrast in response to negatively arousing items relative to neutral items, with coronal slices through the amygdala (0, 3, 6) and hippocampus (−30, −33, −36). The control condition *(top row)* shows enhanced activation of both the amygdala and hippocampus in response to the added emotional information, while in subjects receiving propofol *(bottom row)* there is enhanced activation of the amygdala, but not of the hippocampus. (*lower panel*) Path diagrams of connectivity at rest, with positive influences of one region onto another shown as solid lines, negative influences shown as dotted lines, and width representing magnitude. In the control condition *(A)* there is a significant positive influence of the amygdala onto the hippocampus bilaterally. Administration of sevoflurane 0.25% *(B)* blocks emotional modulation behaviorally, and removes the positive influence of the right amygdala and nucleus basalis of Meynert on the hippocampus. Numerical differences in path weight *(C)* show these two paths to significantly contribute to the network model more in the control than sevoflurane state. *Amyg,* Amygdala; *Hipp,* hippocampus; *LC,* locus ceruleus; *NBM,* nucleus basalis of Meynert; *Thal,* thalamus. ([A] Modified from Pryor KO, Root JC, Mehta M, et al. Effect of propofol on the medial temporal lobe emotional memory system: a functional magnetic resonance imaging study in human subjects. *Br J Anaesth.* 2015;115[suppl 1]:i104–i113, Figure 3; [B] Modified from Alkire MT, Gruver R, Miller J, et al. Neuroimaging analysis of an anesthetic gas that blocks human emotional memory. *Proc Natl Acad Sci U S A.* 2008;105[5]:1722–1727, Figure 5.)

Two early studies in patients undergoing coronary artery[274] and gynecologic[275] procedures showed evidence of implicit learning using word stem completion tasks. Another early study demonstrating implicit recall in cardiac surgery patients correlated performance with preservation of the midlatency auditory evoked potential, and most strongly with the early cortical Pa and Na complexes.[276] Later studies demonstrated implicit memory in both trauma patients[277] and patients undergoing an emergency cesarean section[278] using the process dissociation procedure, and further demonstrated that the degree of processing is related to the bispectral index. However, multiple more recent studies using similar procedures have either failed to show significant implicit priming effects or have been equivocal.[279-281] Synthesis of these disparate results into a cohesive conclusion is difficult. Although differences in patient populations and anesthetic regimens may be of relevance, methodological challenges may have driven both false positive and false negative results. Investigations evaluating implicit memory processes in pediatric patients under anesthesia have also offered conflicting results. One study reported an increased ability to distinguish a primed animal sound from white noise,[282] but other investigations found no evidence of priming.[283–285]

Complete references available online at expertconsult.com.

References

1. Sandin RH, et al. *Lancet*. 2000;355:707.
2. Sebel PS, et al. *Anesth Analg*. 2004;99:833.
3. Mashour GA, et al. *Anesthesiology*. 2012;117:717.
4. Leslie K, et al. *Anesth Analg*. 2010;110:823.
5. Whitlock EL, et al. *Anesth Analg*. 2015;120(1):87.
6. Sanders RD, et al. *Anesthesiology*. 2017;126(2):214.
7. Mashour GA, Avidan MS. *Br J Anaesth*. 2015;115(suppl 1):i20.
8. Sanders RD, et al. *Anesthesiology*. 2012;116:946.
9. Noreika V, et al. *Brain Cogn*. 2011;77:327.
10. Brown EN, et al. *Annu Rev Neurosci*. 2011;34:601.
11. Lydic R, Biebuyck JF. *Br J Anaesth*. 1994;72:506.
12. Mashour GA, Hudetz AG. *Front Neural Circuits*. 2017;11:44.
13. Franks NP. *Nat Rev Neurosci*. 2008;9:370.
14. Scammell TE, et al. *Neuron*. 2017;93(4):747.
15. Jones BE. *Handb Clin Neurol*. 2011;98:131.
16. Aston-Jones G, Bloom FE. *J Neurosci*. 1981;1:876.
17. Takahashi K, et al. *Neurosci*. 2010;169:1115.
18. Sirois JE, et al. *J Neurosci*. 2000;20:6347.
19. Mason ST, Angel A. *Eur J Pharmacol*. 1983;91:29.
20. Matsumoto K, et al. *Brain Res*. 1997;754:325.
21. Pillay S, et al. *Anesthesiology*. 2011;115:733.
22. Vazey EM, Aston-Jones G. *Proc Natl Acad Sci. U S A*. 2014;111(10): 3859.
23. Lu J, et al. *J Comp Neurol*. 2008;508:648.
24. Kushikata T, et al. *Br J Anaesth*. 2011;107(6):924.
25. Correa-Sales C, et al. *Anesthesiology*. 1992;76:948.
26. Nelson LE, et al. *Anesthesiology*. 2003;98:428.
27. Hu FY, et al. *Anesthesiology*. 2012;117:1006.
28. Zhang Z, et al. *Nat Neurosci*. 2015;18(4):553.
29. Woolf NJ, Butcher LL. *Behav Brain Res*. 2011;221:488.
30. Steriade M. *Front Biosci*. 2003;8:d878.
31. Sleigh JW, et al. *Trends in anaesthesia and critical care*. 2011;1:263.
32. Van Dort CJ, et al. *Proc Natl Acad Sci U S A*. 2015;112(2):584.
33. Keifer JC, et al. *Neuroreport*. 1994;5:577.
34. Keifer JC, et al. *Anesthesiology*. 1996;84:945.
35. Kohlmeier KA, et al. *Neurosci*. 2010;171:812.
36. Vanini G, et al. *J Neurosci*. 2011;31:2649.
37. Flint RR, et al. *J Neurosci*. 2010;30:12301.
38. Vanini G, et al. *Anesthesiology*. 2008;109:978.
39. Vanini G, et al. *Eur J Neurosci*. 2014;40(1):2264.
40. Abulafia R, et al. *J Neurosci*. 2009;29:7053.
41. Minert A, et al. *J Neurosci*. 2017;37(38):9320.
42. Dahan L, et al. *Neuropsychopharmacol*. 2007;32:1232.
43. Ueno T, et al. *Nat Neurosci*. 2012;15:1516.
44. Eban-Rothschild A, et al. *Nat Neurosci*. 2016;19(10):1356.
45. Solt K, et al. *Anesthesiology*. 2011;115:791.
46. Chemali JJ, et al. *Anesthesiology*. 2012;116:998.
47. Solt K, et al. *Anesthesiology*. 2014;121(2):311.
48. Taylor NE, et al. *Proc Natl Acad Sci U S A*. 2016.
49. von Economo C. *J Nerv Ment Dis*. 1930;71:248.
50. Gaus SE, et al. *Neurosci*. 2002;115:285.
51. Sherin JE, et al. *Sci*. 1996;271:216.
52. Szymusiak R, et al. *Brain Res*. 1998;803:178.
53. Gong H, et al. *J Physiol*. 2004;556:935.
54. Saper CB, et al. *Nature*. 2005;437:1257.
55. Nelson LE, et al. *Nat Neurosci*. 2002;5:979.
56. Eikermann M, et al. *Brain Res*. 2011;1426:30.
57. Moore JT, et al. *Curr Biol*. 2012;22:2008.
58. McCarren HS, et al. *J Neurosci*. 2014;34(49):16385.
59. Mileykovskiy BY, et al. *Neuron*. 2005;46:787.
60. Lee MG, et al. *J Neurosci*. 2005;25:6716.
61. Nishino S, et al. *Lancet*. 2000;355:39.
62. Lin L, et al. *Cell*. 1999;98:365.
63. Mesa A, et al. *Anesthesiology*. 2000;92:1194.
64. Yasuda Y, et al. *Anesth Analg*. 2003;97:1663.
65. Zecharia AY, et al. *J Neurosci*. 2009;29:2177.
66. Tose R, et al. *Anesth Analg*. 2009;108:491.
67. Kushikata T, et al. *Neurosci*. 2003;121:855.
68. Dong H, et al. *Neuropeptides*. 2009;43:179.
69. Dong HL, et al. *Anesthesiology*. 2006;104:1023.
70. Gamou S, et al. *Anesth Analg*. 2010;111:395.
71. Kelz MB, et al. *Proc Natl Acad Sci U S A*. 2008;105:1309.
72. Friedman EB, et al. *PLoS One*. 2010;5:e11903.
73. Gompf H, et al. *Anesthesiology*. 2009;111:1001.
74. Zhang LN, et al. *Anesth Analg*. 2012;115:789.
75. Zhang LN, et al. *Neuropeptides*. 2016;58:7.
76. Chu M, et al. *Neurosci Res*. 2004;49:417.
77. Liu YW, et al. *J Physiol*. 2010;588:4103.
78. Strecker RE, et al. *Neurosci*. 2002;113:663.
79. Mammoto T, et al. *J Neurochem*. 1997;69:406.
80. Luo T, Leung LS. *Anesthesiology*. 2009;111:725.
81. Zecharia AY, et al. *J Neurosci*. 2012;32:13062.
82. Alkire MT, et al. *Conscious Cogn*. 2000;9(3):370.
83. Alkire MT, et al. *Anesthesiology*. 1997;86:549.
84. Alkire MT, et al. *Anesthesiology*. 1999;90:701.
85. Fiset P, et al. *J Neurosci*. 1999;19:5506.
86. Langsjo JW, et al. *Anesthesiology*. 2005;103:258.
87. Liu X, et al. *Anesthesiology*. 2013;118(1):59.
88. Mashour GA, Alkire MT. *Anesthesiology*. 2013;118(1):13.
89. Alkire MT, et al. *Anesthesiology*. 2007;107:264.
90. Alkire MT, et al. *Anesthesiology*. 2009;110:766.
91. Schiff ND, et al. *Nature*. 2007;448:600.
92. Langsjo JW, et al. *J Neurosci*. 2012;32:4935.
93. Ward LM. *Conscious Cogn*. 2011;20:464.
94. Velly LJ, et al. *Anesthesiology*. 2007;107:202.
95. Verdonck O, et al. *Can J Anaesth*. 2014;61(3):254.
96. Baker R, et al. *J Neurosci*. 2014;34(40):13326.
97. Reed SJ, Plourde G. *PLoS ONE*. 2015;10(4):e0123287.
98. Ching S, et al. *Proc Natl Acad Sci U S A*. 2010;107:22665.
99. Supp GG, et al. *Curr Biol*. 2011;21:1988.
100. Flores FJ, et al. *Proc Natl Acad Sci U S A*. 2017;114(32):E6660.
101. Tononi G. *BMC Neurosci*. 2004;5:42.
102. Boveroux P, et al. *Anesthesiology*. 2010;113:1038.
103. Palanca BJ, et al. *Anesthesiology*. 2015;123(2):346.
104. Ranft A, et al. *Anesthesiology*. 2016;125(5):861.
105. Mhuircheartaigh RN, et al. *J Neurosci*. 2010;30:9095.
106. Liang Z, et al. *J Neurosci*. 2012;32:10183.
107. Schroter MS, et al. *J Neurosci*. 2012;32:12832.
108. Bianciardi M, et al. *Neuroimage*. 2017.
109. Song AH, et al. *J Neurosci*. 2017;37(29):6938.
110. Kaisti KK, et al. *Anesthesiology*. 2002;96:1358.
111. Liu X, et al. *Brain Connect*. 2017;7(6):373.
112. Bonhomme V, et al. *Anesthesiology*. 2016;125(5):873.
113. Friston KJ. *Brain Connect*. 2011;1:13.
114. Lee U, et al. *Anesthesiology*. 2013;118(6):1264.
115. Jordan D, et al. *Anesthesiology*. 2013;119(5):1031.
116. Moon JY, et al. *PLoS Comput Biol*. 2015;11(4):e1004225.
117. Vlisides PE, et al. *Anesthesiology*. 2017;127(1):58.
118. Hudetz AG, Mashour GA. *Anesth Analg*. 2016;123(5):1228.
119. Ferrarelli F, et al. *Proc Natl Acad Sci U S A*. 2010;107:2681.
120. Massimini M, et al. *Sci*. 2005;309:2228.
121. Casali AG, et al. *Sci Transl Med*. 2013;5(198). 198ra105.
122. Murphy M, et al. *Sleep*. 2011;34:283.
123. Lewis LD, et al. *Proc Natl Acad Sci U S A*. 2012;109:E3377.
124. Hudetz AG, et al. *Brain Connect*. 2015;5(1):10.
125. Lee H, et al. *Hum Brain Mapp*. 2017;10.
126. Solovey G, et al. *J Neurosci*. 2015;35(30):10866.
127. Ishizawa Y, et al. *J Neurosci*. 2016;36(29):7718.
128. Huang Z, et al. *J Neurosci*. 2018.
129. Barttfeld P, et al. *Proc Natl Acad Sci U S A*. 2015;112(3):887.
130. Hudson AE, et al. *Proc Natl Acad Sci U S A*. 2014;111(25):9283.
131. Scoville WB, Milner B. *J Neurol Neurosurg Psychiatry*. 1957;20(1):11.
132. Hebb DO. *The Organization of Behavior*. New York: Wiley; 1949.
133. Bliss TV, Lomo T. *J Physiol*. 1973;232(2):331.
134. Fell J, Axmacher N. *Nat Rev Neurosci*. 2011;12(2):105.
135. Binder JR, et al. *Cereb Cortex*. 2009;19(12):2767.
136. Polyn SM, et al. *Science*. 2005;310(5756):1963.
137. Simons JS, Spiers HJ. *Nat Rev Neurosci*. 2003;4:637.
138. Cabeza R, et al. *Nat Rev Neurosci*. 2008;9:613.
139. Raichle ME. *Annu Rev Neurosci*. 2015;38:433.
140. Wixted JT, et al. *Trends Cogn Sci*. 2011;15:210.
141. Eichenbaum H, et al. *Annu Rev Neurosci*. 2007;30:123.
142. Tulving E, Schacter DL. *Sci*. 1990;247:301.
143. Cave CB, Squire LR. *J Exp Psychol Learn Mem Cogn*. 1992;18:509.
144. Henson RN. *Prog Neurobiol*. 2003;70(1):53.
145. Janak PH, Tye KM. *Nature*. 2015;517(7534):284.
146. Duvarci S, Pare D. *Neuron*. 2014;82(5):966.
147. Squire LR, Zola-Morgan S. *Trends Neurosci*. 1988;11:170.
148. Baddeley A. *Annu Rev Psychol*. 2012;63:1.

149. Baddeley A, Hitch GJ. Working memory. In: Bower GA, ed. *Recent advances in learning and motivation*. New York: Academic; 1974.
150. Baddeley A. *Trends Cogn Sci*. 2000;4:417.
151. Shrager Y, et al. *J Neurosci*. 2008;28:4818.
152. Jeneson A, Squire LR. *Learn Mem*. 2012;19(1):15.
153. Ma WJ, et al. *Nat Neurosci*. 2014;17(3):347.
154. Ruchkin DS, et al. *Behav Brain*. 2003;26:709. discussion 28.
155. Craik FIM, et al. *J Verbal Learn Verbal Behav*. 1972;11(671):1972.
156. Kitamura T, et al. *Sci*. 2017;356(6333):73.
157. Dudai Y, et al. *Neuron*. 2015;88(1):20.
158. Neves G, et al. *Nat Rev Neurosci*. 2008;9(1):65.
159. Chater TE, Goda Y. *Front Cell Neurosci*. 2014;8:401.
160. Bliss TV, Collingridge GL. *Nature*. 1993;361(6407):31.
161. Lynch MA. *Physiological reviews*. 2004;84:87.
162. Larson J, et al. *Brain Res*. 1986;368:347.
163. Morris RG, et al. *Nature*. 1986;319:774.
164. Giese KP, et al. *Sci*. 1998;279:870.
165. Malenka RC, et al. *Nature*. 1989;340:554.
166. Cingolani LA, Goda Y. *Nat Rev Neurosci*. 2008;9:344.
167. Costa-Mattioli M, et al. *Neuron*. 2009;61(1):10.
168. Hernandez PJ, Abel T. *Neurobiol Learn Mem*. 2008;89(3):293.
169. Rogerson T, et al. *Nat Rev Neurosci*. 2014;15(3):157.
170. Nader K, et al. *Nature*. 2000;406:722.
171. Tronson NC, Taylor JR. *Nat Rev Neurosci*. 2007;8(4):262.
172. Alberini CM. *Front Behav Neurosci*. 2011;5(12).
173. Monfils MH, et al. *Sci*. 2009;324(5929):951.
174. Agren T, et al. *Sci*. 2012;337(6101):1550.
175. Benchenane K, et al. *Neuron*. 2010;66:921.
176. Spellman T, et al. *Nature*. 2015;522(7556):309.
177. Jutras MJ, et al. *J Neurosci*. 2009;29(40):12521.
178. Canolty RT, et al. *Science*. 2006;313(5793):1626.
179. Mercier MR, et al. *J Neurosci*. 2015;35(22):8546.
180. Burke JF, et al. *J Neurosci*. 2013;33(1):292.
181. Seidenbecher T, et al. *Sci*. 2003;301:846.
182. Igarashi KM, et al. *Nature*. 2014;510(7503):143.
183. Lisman JE, Jensen O. *Neuron*. 2013;77(6):1002.
184. Sauseng P, et al. *Curr Biol*. 2009;19(21):1846.
185. Dundee JW, Pandit SK. *Br J Clin Pract*. 1972;26:164.
186. Hashimoto K, et al. *Masui*. 2007;56:920.
187. Bulach R, et al. *Br J Anaesth*. 2005;94:300.
188. Ghoneim MM, Block RI. *Acta Anaesthesiol Scand*. 2007;51:1054.
189. Twersky RS, et al. *Anesthesiology*. 1993;78:51.
190. Rich JB, et al. *J Clin Exp Neuropsychol*. 1999;21:535.
191. Mason KP, et al. *Br J Anaesth*. 2017;118(2):254.
192. Pryor KO, et al. *Br J Anaesth*. 2004;93:348.
193. Pryor KO, et al. *Anesthesiology*. 2010;113:313.
194. Veselis RA, et al. *Anesthesiology*. 2004;101:831.
195. Pryor KO, et al. *Anesthesiology*. 2012;117:BOC09.
196. Reder LM, et al. *Psychon Bull Rev*. 2007;14:261.
197. Wixted JT. *Annu Rev Psychol*. 2004;55:235.
198. Moser EI, et al. *Sci*. 1998;281:2038.
199. Shinohara K, Hata T. *Neurobiol Learn Mem*. 2018;147:1.
200. Villarreal DM, et al. *Nat Neurosci*. 2002;5:48.
201. Alkire MT, Guzowski JF. *Anesthesiology*. 2008;109:768.
202. Ren Y, et al. *Anesthesiology*. 2008;109(5):775.
203. Chen Y, et al. *Anesth Analg*. 2016;122(4):1158.
204. Hurlemann R, et al. *J Neurosci*. 2005;25(27):6343.
205. Posner MI, Rothbart MK. *Annu Rev Psychol*. 2007;58:1.
206. Womelsdorf T, Fries P. *Curr Opin Neurobiol*. 2007;17(2):154.
207. Muzzio IA, et al. *J Physiol*. 2009;587(12):2837.
208. Musso F, et al. *Neuroimage*. 2011;58(2):508.
209. Veselis RA, et al. *Anesthesiology*. 2008;109:213.
210. Veselis RA, et al. *Anesthesiology*. 2002;97:329.
211. Cieslik EC, et al. *Cereb Cortex*. 2013;23(11):2677.
212. Davis MH, et al. *Proc Natl Acad Sci U S A*. 2007;104(41):16032.
213. Liu X, et al. *Hum Brain Mapp*. 2012;33(10):2487.
214. Reinsel RA, et al. *Int J Neuropsychopharmacol*. 2000;3(2):117.
215. Adapa RM, et al. *Human brain mapping*. 2014;35(7):2935.
216. Hayama HR, et al. *Anesthesiology*. 2012;117(5):981.
217. Frolich MA, et al. *Anesth Analg*. 2017;124(5):1603.
218. Pryor KO, et al. *Br J Anaesth*. 2015;115(suppl 1):i104.
219. Sperling R, et al. *Proc Natl Acad Sci U S A*. 2002;99:455.
220. Ramani R, et al. *Anesth Analg*. 2007;105:648.
221. Fell J, et al. *Biol Cybern*. 2005;92:92.
222. Sauseng P, et al. *Neurosci*. 2007;146:1435.
223. Curran HV, et al. *Psychopharmacol (Berl)*. 1998;135:27.
224. Reinsel RA, et al. *Br J Anaesth*. 1995;74:674.
225. Veselis RA, et al. *Anesthesiology*. 2009;110:295.
226. Pryor KO, et al. *Anesthesiology*. 2010;113(2):313.
227. Freunberger R, et al. *Neurosci Lett*. 2007;426:181.
228. Ghuman AS, et al. *Proc Natl Acad Sci U S A*. 2008;105:8405.
229. Veselis RA, et al. *Anesthesiology*. 2009;110(2):295.
230. Heinke W, et al. *Anesthesiology*. 2004;100(3):617.
231. Simpson TP, et al. *Br J Anaesth*. 2002;89(3):382.
232. Jinno S, et al. *J Neurosci*. 2007;27:8790.
233. Simon W, et al. *Anesthesiology*. 2001;94:1058.
234. Ishizeki J, et al. *Anesthesiology*. 2008;108:447.
235. Xiao H, et al. *Int J Dev Neurosci*. 2016;48:38.
236. Rammes G, et al. *Neuropharmacol*. 2009;56(3):626.
237. Nagashima K, et al. *Anesthesiology*. 2005;103:318.
238. Takamatsu I, et al. *Neurosci Lett*. 2005;389:129.
239. Fibuch EE, Wang JQ. *Neurosci Bull*. 2007;23:119.
240. Kozinn J, et al. *Anesthesiology*. 2006;105(6):1182.
241. Gao J, et al. *Neurosci Lett*. 2014;560:62.
242. Martin LJ, et al. *J Neurosci*. 2010;30(15):5269.
243. Cheng VY, et al. *J Neurosci*. 2006;26(14):3713.
244. Martin LJ, et al. *Anesthesiology*. 2009;111:1025.
245. Saab BJ, et al. *Anesthesiology*. 2010;113:1061.
246. Zurek AA, et al. *Anesth Analg*. 2012;114:845.
247. Zurek AA, et al. *J Clin Invest*. 2014;124(12):5437.
248. Rau V, et al. *Anesth Analg*. 2009;109:1816.
249. Rau V, et al. *Anesth Analg*. 2011;113:500.
250. Liao M, et al. *Anesth Analg*. 2005;101:412. table of contents.
251. Sonner JM, et al. *Anesthesiology*. 2007;106:107.
252. Sonner JM, et al. *Mol Pharmacol*. 2005;68:61.
253. Perouansky M, et al. *Anesthesiology*. 2010;113:1299.
254. Perouansky M, et al. *Anesthesiology*. 2007;106:1168.
255. Markowska AL, et al. *J Neurosci*. 1995;15:2063.
256. Roozendaal B, et al. *Nat Rev Neurosci*. 2009;10:423.
257. Buffalari DM, Grace AA. *J Neurosci*. 2007;27(45):12358.
258. Roozendaal B, et al. *Proc Natl Acad Sci U S A*. 2006;103(17):6741.
259. Chen CC, Williams CL. *Frontiers in behavioral Neurosci*. 2012; 6:35.
260. Tovote P, et al. *Nat Rev Neurosci*. 2015;16(6):317.
261. Hart G, et al. *Learn Mem*. 2010;17(4):210.
262. Tomaz C, et al. *Proc Natl Acad Sci U S A*. 1992;89:3615.
263. Alkire MT, et al. *Anesthesiology*. 2001;95:708.
264. Alkire MT, Nathan SV. *Anesthesiology*. 2005;102:754.
265. Dickinson-Anson H, McGaugh JL. *Brain Res*. 1997;752(1-2):197.
266. Hauer D, et al. *Anesthesiology*. 2011;114(6):1380.
267. Morena M, et al. *Behav Brain Res*. 2017;329:215.
268. Pain L, et al. *Br J Anaesth*. 2002;89(4):614.
269. Zhu QL, et al. *Brain Res*. 2018;1678:174.
270. Alkire MT, et al. *Anesthesiology*. 2005;103(6):1167.
271. Alkire MT, et al. *Proc Natl Acad Sci U S A*. 2008;105:1722.
272. Mahan AL, Ressler KJ. *Trends Neurosci*. 2012;35(1):24.
273. Schelling G, et al. *Crit Care Med*. 2003;31:1971.
274. Bethune DW, et al. *Br J Anaesth*. 1992;69:197.
275. Block RI, et al. *Br J Anaesth*. 1991;66:170.
276. Schwender D, et al. *Anesthesiology*. 1994;80:493.
277. Lubke GH, et al. *Anesthesiology*. 1999;90:670.
278. Lubke GH, et al. *Anesthesiology*. 2000;92:1029.
279. Munte S, et al. *Anesthesiology*. 2002;96:588.
280. Hadzidiakos D, et al. *Anesthesiology*. 2009;111:293.
281. Lequeux PY, et al. *Anesth Analg*. 2014;119(5):1174.
282. Phelan L, et al. *Anaesth Intensive Care*. 2009;37:60.
283. Lopez U, et al. *Br J Anaesth*. 2009;102:379.
284. Pham X, et al. *Anesthesiology*. 2010;112:1097.
285. Bonett E, et al. *Paediatr Anaesth*. 2014;24(3):290.
286. Bartsch T, Butler C. *Nat Rev Neurol*. 2013;9(2):86.

10 Sleep Medicine

MATTHIAS EIKERMANN and SEBASTIAN ZAREMBA

KEY POINTS

- Sleep is a dynamic neuronal and behavioral state that can be characterized using specific electroencephalographic, electrophysiologic, and behavioral findings.
- Characteristics of sleep can be quantified using questionnaires, actigraphy, or respiratory polygraphy. However, polysomnography, including electroencephalogram, electrooculogram, submental electromyogram, and analysis of breathing, is required to describe the cortical characteristics and immediate physiological consequences.
- Activation of hypothalamic sleep-promoting pathways including the ventrolateral preoptic nucleus and the median preoptic nucleus produces the physiological switch from wakefulness to sleep.
- Sleep and anesthesia can look similar. Although small doses of anesthetics can induce sleep by activating sleep-promoting pathways, surgical anesthesia and immobilization cannot be induced by sleep-promoting pathways.
- Control of breathing is altered during sleep and anesthesia, typically leading to a decreased drive to upper airway dilator and respiratory pump muscles.
- Persistent respiratory depressant effects of anesthetics and neuromuscular blocking drugs increase the risk of postoperative respiratory complications, particularly in patients with obstructive sleep apnea.
- Anesthesia and surgery, as well as treatment in the intensive care unit and opioids, affect sleep duration and sleep architecture, which may lead to impaired outcome.

Probably the earliest mention of "overpowering sleep" as a metaphor describing what possibly characterizes anesthesia can be found in Genesis 2:21: "And the Eternal God caused an overpowering sleep to fall upon the man and he slept. He took one of his ribs and shut in flesh instead thereof." Although this "overpowering sleep" allegedly occurred by divine intervention and did not represent the drug-induced unconsciousness and immobility that characterizes anesthesia, the basic narrative is an example of antiquarian history that implicates the concept that deep sleep may be the only viable condition that allows a surgical procedure to be completed successfully.[1]

In the 21st century, an increasing body of knowledge has revealed the common ground between sleep and anesthesia, as well as their fundamental differences in clinical picture and underlying mechanisms.

Sleep is required for survival. Rats deprived of sleep will die within 2 to 3 weeks, a time frame similar to death due to starvation.[2] In humans, sleepiness can be deadly. Approximately 100,000 motor vehicle accidents each year result from drivers who are "asleep at the wheel." In a survey of drivers in New York State, approximately 25% reported they had fallen asleep at the wheel at some time.[3] In addition, sleep deprivation impairs the psychomotor performance of night shift workers, specifically surgeons and residents. In patients, perioperative sleep deprivation occurs frequently, particularly in critically ill patients, and there may be consequences on patients' outcomes. Among sleep disorders, obstructive sleep apnea (OSA) has probably the most meaningful consequences for perioperative treatment.[4]

Therefore, high-quality physiologic sleep is a key domain of public health that needs to be considered in perioperative medicine from both a provider and a patient perspective.

Definition of Sleep

Sleep is the natural periodic suspension of consciousness during which the powers of the body are restored. A behavioral definition of sleep includes a species-specific posture and behavioral quiescence, as well as elevated arousal thresholds. However, sleep is much more than an absence of activity. The brain is highly active during sleep, especially during rapid eye movement (REM) sleep, during which atonia, phasic muscle movements (driven by different activation levels in distinct areas of the brain), and vivid dreaming occur. Sleep is not a simple electrophysiological phenomenon. At different stages of sleep, brain activities can be as distinct from each other as they are from wakefulness.[5] In humans and other vertebrates (see "Evolution"), sleep has two major stages: REM sleep and non-REM (NREM) sleep, with each of these further divided into substates. Most of sleep time is spent in NREM sleep, which is characterized by relatively low electroencephalographic (EEG) frequencies with higher amplitudes compared with awake EEG frequencies (Fig. 10.1). In the transition from wake to NREM sleep, the fast activity of waking disappears (α–θ transition), and then in the deeper stages of NREM large, slow waves (i.e., δ waves) emerge. Thus deep NREM sleep is also referred to as *slow-wave sleep*. NREM sleep is associated with waxing and waning muscle tone, as well as decreased body

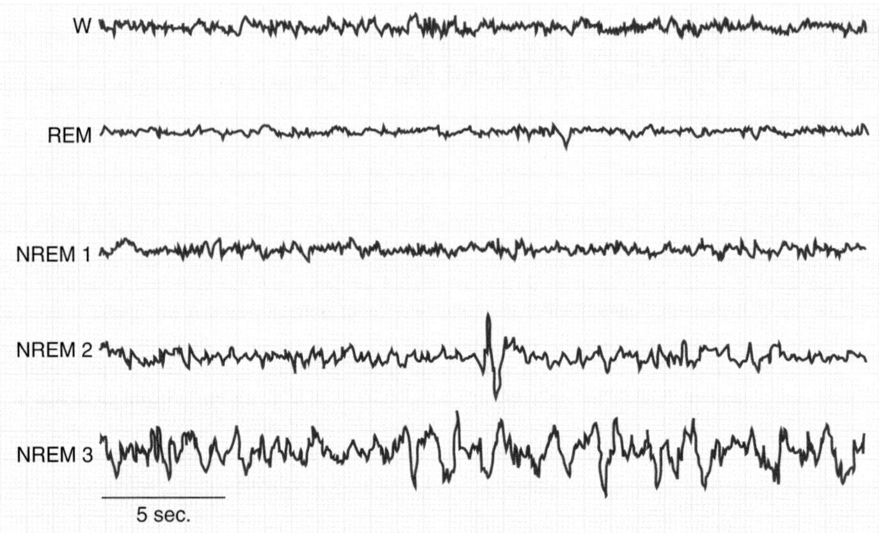

Fig. 10.1 Representative electroencephalogram activity seen during different behavioral states. Electroencephalogram recordings of one patient during wakefulness (eyes closed; *W*), rapid eye movement sleep *(REM)*, and non-REM *(NREM)* sleep stages 1 to 3.

temperature and heart rate. In contrast, REM sleep is characterized by muscle atonia, loss of slow waves in the EEG, and bursts of REMs that give this state its name.[6] Other prominent features of REM include marked irregularities of respiration and heart rate, as well as penile and clitoral erection. REM sleep is associated with the high likelihood of vivid dreaming. A distinct property of REM sleep is the operation of a system that suppresses motor activity, which is responsible for baseline atonia and suppression of motor commands that would otherwise result in acting out of dreams, a phenomenon known as *REM sleep behavior disorder*. This REM atonia system is not constant, as it periodically allows breakthrough muscle activity that comprises REM sleep and twitching of the extremities. REM sleep has therefore been subdivided into *tonic REM sleep* (i.e., a period with muscle atonia and without eye movements) and *phasic REM sleep*, which is interrupted by short phasic events of the eye and other movements.[7] The pattern and amounts of NREM sleep, REM sleep, and wakefulness throughout the night are referred to as *sleep architecture*, and there are many physiologic and pathophysiologic processes that can affect sleep architecture. For example, many antidepressant medications, benzodiazepines, and opioids selectively suppress REM sleep. A disease example is narcolepsy, in which individuals often transition rapidly from wake to REM, whereas normally REM is nearly always entered from a prolonged episode of NREM state.

Physiology

EVOLUTION

It is unknown why we sleep; however, one can imagine that evolutionary pressure would favor systems that are optimized for nature's rhythms.[8,9] In a rhythmic world, organisms must adapt to alternating changes in the environment, such as daily and seasonal rhythms in light intensity, ambient temperature, and humidity.

CIRCADIAN RHYTHMS

Species-dependent temporal behavior can be adapted depending on the environmental conditions: behaviorally, anatomically, and physiologically. Circadian rhythms affect almost every aspect of the body's function, including activity and rest patterns, cognitive function (e.g., learning and memory), cardiovascular and endocrine physiology (e.g., heart rate, metabolism, and hormone secretion), and gene expression (15% of the genes in the human body show daily rhythms).

Virtually all species show circadian rhythms that regulate periodic changes in behavioral and physiologic parameters within a period of approximately 24 hours.[10] These rhythms can be characterized as a synchronization of activity to the external light-dark cycle in the majority of living creatures. Bacteria, plants, animals, and humans exhibit such a behavior that helps them stay in tune with the environmental light-dark cycles.[11] Our sleep timing preference, or chronotype, is a manifestation of our internal biological clock. Variation in chronotype has been linked to sleep disorders, cognitive and physical performance, and chronic disease.[12]

Clock genes generate endogenous clock pulses in most (if not all) cells of the body, synchronized by regulatory pathways across the body to a superior rhythm generator (a so-called master clock). Desynchronization of these rhythms seems to be involved in the pathogenesis of metabolic, psychiatric, and other disorders.[11] The superior rhythm generator in humans is located in the suprachiasmatic nucleus that receives external inputs about light and darkness from the retinal cells and synchronizes inputs of melatonin levels. While this master clock synchronizes the behavioral and biological rhythms of the human body to the changing demands of the environment during the solar day, sleep itself entrains circadian rhythms,[11,13] and the temporal organization of circadian rhythms and nocturnal sleep must be preserved to accomplish a restful and refreshing experience that fulfills the sleep needs produced by the

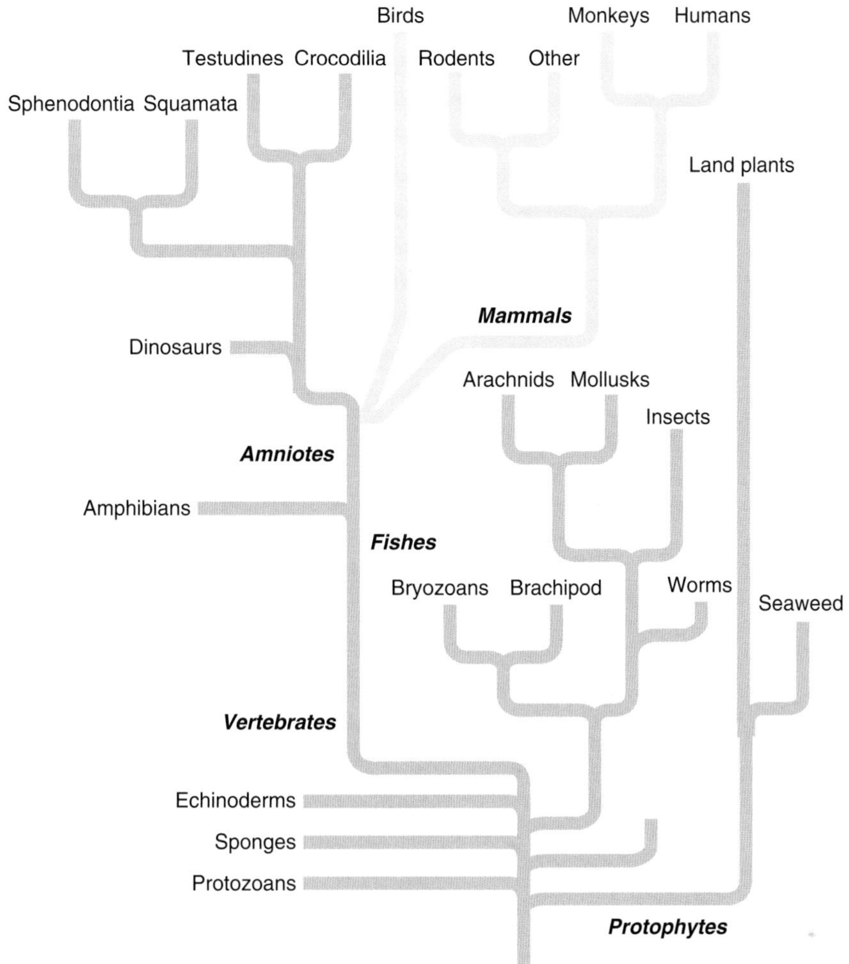

Fig. 10.2 Evolutionary tree. Circadian rhythms are common among all living beings. However, only mammals and birds *(red)* have integrated sleep with different stages. Fish, reptiles, insects, and plants *(blue)* manifest circadian rhythms as periods of activity and rest.

second major regulatory factor, sleep homeostasis. During waking, "sleep pressure" continuously increases, leading to an increased likelihood for the transition from wakefulness to sleep.[14] Increasing homeostatic sleep pressure can be partly offset by a sufficient circadian wakening stimulus during the circadian wake phase, but the circadian wake stimulus disappears in the presence of an overwhelming sleep pressure.[15] In this situation, sleep sufficient in quantity and quality is needed to reestablish proper functioning.

Although circadian and homeostatic regulation of sleep can be observed in almost all living organisms,[16] differentiation of sleep into NREM and REM sleep ("integrated sleep") probably has developed during the last 300 to 350 million years because it appears only in birds and the majority of terrestrial mammals (Fig. 10.2).[17,18]

Sleep Stages and Sleep Cycles

Sleep architecture—a structured temporal order of different sleep stages—is an important determinant of sleep quality. If tired individuals rest in their individual sleeping postures, the increasing level of drowsiness is paralleled by continuous EEG slowing from that seen during attention and cortical activation (16-30 Hz, "β activity") to slower frequencies, predominantly between (7.5 and 11 Hz, "α activity," typically observed in subjects with reduced attention and closed eyes). During this state of vigilance, the individuals do not sleep, and a full level of cognitive function can be established easily even without a strong sensory stimulus. The transition from α state to sleep is paralleled by a further decrease in α and β activity and an increase of EEG activity in the θ band (4.5-7.5 Hz; Fig.10.3).

This transition from α to θ activity is widely accepted as the EEG correlate of sleep onset.[19] At this transition from wakefulness to NREM sleep stage 1, heart rate and heat production decrease, resulting in a slight decrease in body temperature. Furthermore, respiration is regular and deep. As sleep deepens, EEG activity shows low amplitudes and θ activity with intermittent sleep spindles and K-complexes. The latter represents an activation of brainstem and subcortical brain areas during sleep[20,21] for selective processing of unexpected sensory inputs (e.g., sounds) that might require complete arousal and restoration of consciousness to address a potential threat.[22] In accordance with that hypothesis, in comatose patients with brain injury, the presence of K-complexes in response to an acoustic stimulus during coma seems to be a marker of a better outcome compared with comatose patients with no evoked K-complexes.[23] With increasing depth of sleep, during NREM sleep, electrical activity of the cortex measured by EEG is dominated by slower frequencies and high amplitudes, also referred to as *slow-wave sleep*.

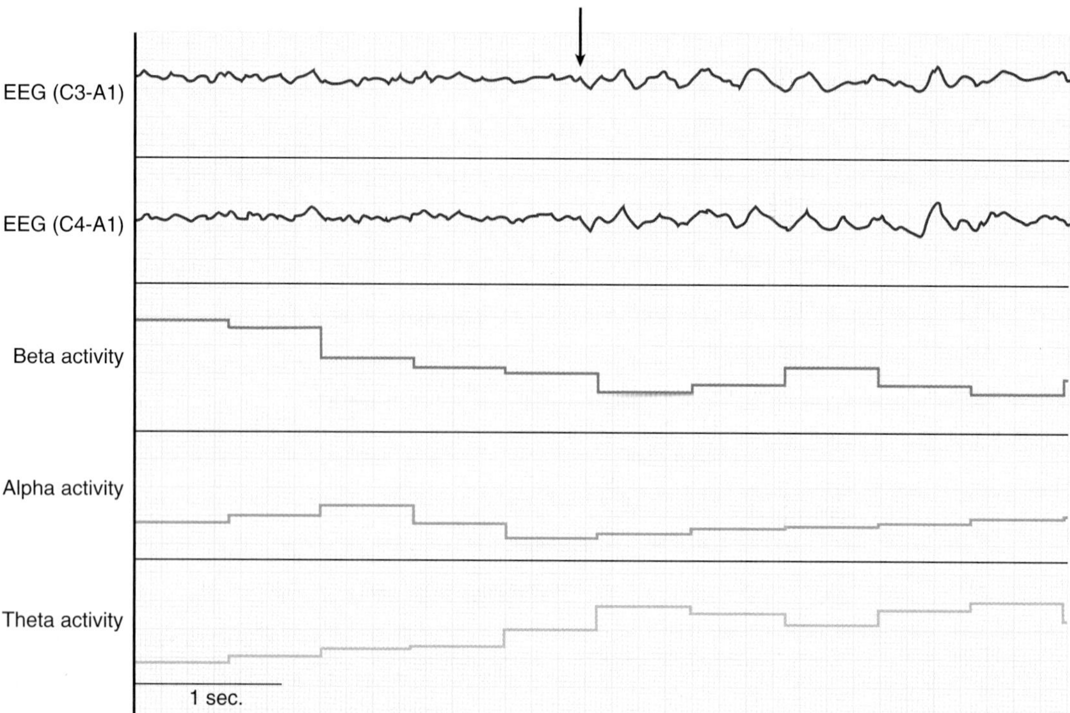

Fig. 10.3 Electroencephalogram recording during sleep onset *(arrow)*. The two top rows show bipolar electroencephalogram *(EEG)* signals from left (C3-A1) and right (C2-A1) frontal leads. Rows 3 to 5 show the relative amount (EEG power) of β, α, and θ activity calculated using fast Fourier transformation.

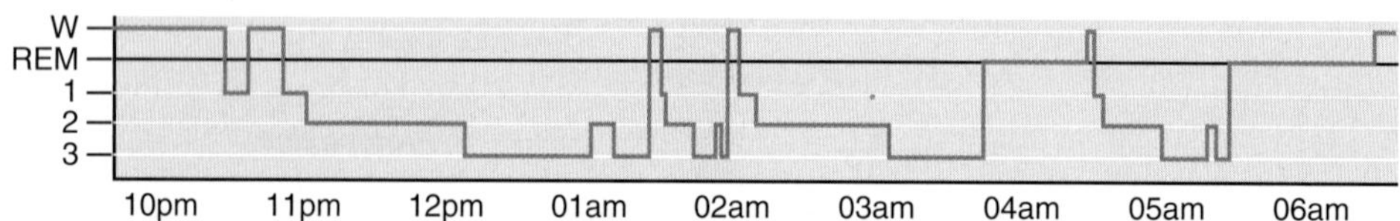

Fig. 10.4 Hypnogram of a night of physiologic sleep. During one night (time on x axis) of sleep, humans transition repetitively from one sleep stage to another with short episodes of occasional wakefulness (indicated on y axis). *REM,* Rapid eye movement sleep; *W,* awake; *1,* non-REM sleep stage 1; *2,* non-REM sleep stage 2; *3,* non-REM sleep stage 3 (slow wave sleep).

REM sleep, or paradoxical sleep, is associated with an alteration of homeostatic regulation, such as increased heart rate variability, irregular respiration, and impaired body temperature control. Brain metabolism increases while EEG recordings show similarities to wakefulness with low-voltage and mixed-frequency power spectra. Prominent θ waves generated by the hippocampus occur. These waves are not apparent in the scalp EEG recording from humans, but in rodents, in which the hippocampus is larger and closer to the brain surface, the EEG is dominated by θ during REM. This sleep state is associated with a decreased tone in skeletal muscles (except for extraocular muscles that control eye movement). Dreaming is a typical experience during REM sleep,[24] but can also happen during NREM sleep.[25] During physiologic sleep, an individual typically switches back and forth across sleep stages, interrupted by occasional arousals from sleep (Fig. 10.4).

NEUROANATOMY OF SLEEP

Sleep-Promoting and Arousal Pathways

Several neuronal pathways have evolved to maintain cortical activation and behavioral arousal during normal waking, and others have evolved to promote and maintain sleep (Fig. 10.5). It is the balance between these two systems that determines whether one is awake or asleep.

Ascending Arousal System. The ascending arousal system (AAS) is the main wakefulness-mediating network in the brain. Main pathways within the network receive cholinergic, monoaminergic, dopaminergic, and glutamatergic inputs. Cholinergic inputs originate from pedunculopontine and laterodorsal tegmental nuclei, innervate the lateral hypothalamus, prefrontal cortex, basal forebrain, and thalamic relay nuclei (i.e., medial and lateral geniculate nuclei; mediodorsal nucleus; pulvinar; anterior, ventral, and lateral thalamic cell groups).[26,27] Glutamatergic neurons that provide inputs to the AAS are mainly located within a small area just ventral of the locus ceruleus (LC), the preceruleus area, as well as in the parabrachial nuclei that mainly project to the basal forebrain and the lateral hypothalamus.[28,29] Monoaminergic inputs mainly come from noradrenergic neurons within the LC, histaminergic neurons of the tuberomammillary nuclei (TMN), serotoninergic neurons of the median and dorsal raphe nuclei,[30,31] as well as dopaminergic neurons adjacent to dorsal raphe nuclei.[24,32] Beside projections to the basal forebrain, multiple inputs are sent to the thalamus, mainly the interlaminar

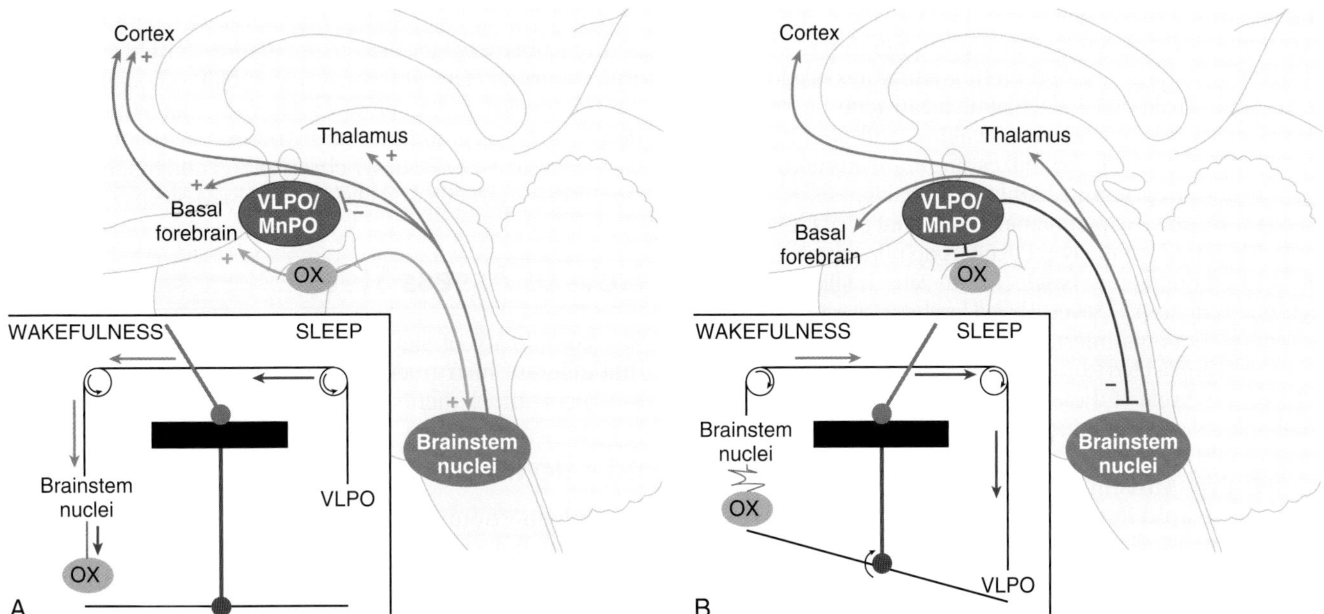

Fig. 10.5 Flip-Flop switch ensuring rapid transitions between wakefulness and sleep. During wakefulness (A), brainstem nuclei of the ascending arousal system (AAS) directly and indirectly provide excitatory input to the thalamus, basal forebrain, and the cerebral cortex, while they inhibit the ventrolateral *(VLPO)* and median *(MnPO)* preoptic nuclei (switch flips to wakefulness). The excitatory, wake-promoting stimulus is enforced by additional excitatory input of orexinergic neurons *(OX)* to the BF and the AAS. During sleep (B), neurons of VLPO and MnPO inhibit the brainstem and orexinergic neurons of the AAS (switch flops to sleep). (Modified from Saper CB, Scammell TE, Lu J. Hypothalamic regulation of sleep and circadian rhythms. *Nature.* 2005;437:1257–1263; and Saper CB, Fuller PM, Pedersen NP, Lu J, Scammell TE. Sleep state switching. *Neuron.* 2010;68:1023–1042.)

and reticular nuclei, as well as the amygdala and cerebral cortex. Furthermore, noradrenergic neurons of the LC project mainly to the posterior part of the lateral hypothalamus. In return, the latter area of the lateral hypothalamus projects to the LC and to the TMN.

Some neurons of the posterior hypothalamus produce orexin A and B, also known as hypocretin (HCRT) 1 and 2. These neurons project to the basal forebrain and the amygdala and cerebral cortex and other important arousal areas, and they are essential for stabilizing the waking state.[32] Orexin deficiency causes narcolepsy (severe daytime sleepiness) with cataplexy (abrupt loss of muscle tone),[33] a disorder showing some characteristics of REM sleep (i.e., REM sleep atonia during wakefulness [discussed later]).

Orexin System. Orexin and its cognate receptors (OX_1R and OX_2R) play a key role in sleep/wake regulation. This neurotransmitter system has a crucial involvement in the pathogenesis of narcolepsy, a disorder associated with chronic excessive daytime sleepiness, sleep attacks, and rapid transitions between vigilance states and sleep in humans.[34] Studies in mice recapitulating the narcolepsy phenotype by targeted mutagenesis of the HCRT gene encoding the prepropeptide precursor of orexin neuropeptides,[35] or the less pervasive phenotype of OX_2R knockout mice,[36] not only demonstrated the role of orexin signaling in sleep/wake regulation but also demonstrated biological proof of concept for the development of orexin receptor antagonists for the treatment of insomnia. In contrast, the activation of orexin pathways, either by exogenous administration of orexin receptor agonists or by optogenetic activation of orexinergic neurons in the lateral hypothalamus, increases arousal.[37,38] Orexinergic neurons are counteracted by inhibitory γ-aminobutyric acid (GABA)-ergic neurons originating from the ventrolateral preoptic nucleus (VLPO). OX_2R is expressed exclusively in the histaminergic TMN, whereas OX_1R is expressed preferentially in the noradrenergic LC, and both receptors are present in cholinergic pedunculopontine and laterodorsal tegmental nuclei.[38,39] Orexinergic tone at these hypothalamic and brainstem nuclei contributes to cortical arousal.[40] TMN, the predominant source of histamine in the brain responsible for cortical arousal, receives a prominent projection from orexinergic neurons[40,41] mediated predominantly by OX_2R. Orexin receptor antagonists promote sleep mainly via inhibition of the OX_2R receptor.[42-45]

Non-Rapid Eye Movement Sleep-Promoting Pathways. About 100 years ago during the epidemic of encephalitis lethargica, it was observed that lesions in the preoptic region around the rostral end of the third ventricle were associated with profound insomnia,[46] which was confirmed in neuroanatomic experiments (lesion studies) in rats and cats.[47,48] Neurons in the preoptic area are active during sleep.[49-51] Two key nuclei within this area are the VLPO as well as the median preoptic nucleus. VLPO neurons fire at a higher frequency during sleep compared with wakefulness.[52] Anatomically, the VLPO consists of a dense core of sleep-active, galanin-positive neurons innervating the TMN (which is part of the AAS) while being surrounded dorsally and medially by a more diffuse population of sleep-active, galanin-positive neurons that project to the dorsal raphe and LC.[53] Physiologically, the VLPO neurons constitute a sleep-promoting pathway that inhibits many components of the arousal system during sleep. Likewise, parts of the arousal system such as the laterodorsal tegmental nucleus and the pedunculopontine tegmental nucleus, as well as the LC, the parabrachial nucleus, the dorsal raphe nucleus, the PC, the ventral periaqueductal gray, and the TMN, are capable of inhibiting the VLPO. The mutually inhibitory relationship of the arousal and sleep-promoting pathways produces the conditions of a flip-flop switch, which can generate rapid and complete transitions between waking and sleeping states (see Fig. 10.5).[53,54] It also makes simultaneous activation of arousal and sleep circuits highly improbable.

Because animal experiments showed that even large lesions of the VLPO substantially reduce but do not completely erase sleep, other brain areas beside this nucleus are likely involved in promoting sleep.[55] Several basal forebrain areas,[49,51] as well as some GABA-ergic interneurons across the cerebral cortex,[56] have been implicated to function as sleep-active neurons. Nevertheless, the role of these brain regions in the promotion or regulation of sleep remains unclear.

Rapid Eye Movement Sleep-Promoting Pathways and Non-Rapid Eye Movement–Rapid Eye Movement Transition. During normal sleep that presents at onset as a sharp α–θ EEG activity transition, a similar sharp transition from NREM to REM sleep can be observed. Two groups of mutually inhibitory neurons located in the pons are involved in mediating the switch between NREM and REM sleep.[28] The first group consists of REM active inhibitory neurons of the sublaterodorsal nucleus and the PC region.[29,54,57] These neurons inhibit but are also inhibited by a second group of neurons that are located in ventrolateral periaqueductal gray and adjacent lateral pontine tegmentum. This mutually inhibitory relationship produces a REM-NREM flip-flop switch, promoting rapid and complete transitions between sleep states.[54]

Within the sublaterodorsal nucleus and PC, glutamatergic neurons are mixed within the population of REM-on GABA-ergic neurons. The glutamatergic sublaterodorsal nucleus neurons project to the spinal cord and are important for REM sleep atonia; the glutamatergic PC neurons activate forebrain pathways driving EEG desynchronization and hippocampal θ rhythms—characteristic EEG signs of REM-sleep.[58]

How to Assess Sleep

The complexity of signs and symptoms of sleep suggests that different instruments need to be applied to capture all the important elements of sleep.

QUESTIONNAIRES

Several questionnaires are used for the assessment of sleep duration, sleep quality, and the related physiologic and pathophysiologic consequences. Quality of sleep is a frequent target of generic health surveys for measuring patient-reported outcomes. Other questionnaires quantify the consequences of sleep deprivation, specific sleep disorders, or both (Table 10.1). The most commonly used instrument in sleep medicine is probably the Epworth Sleepiness Scale, a short questionnaire to assess symptoms of daytime sleepiness, expressed as intolerance to monotony. The questionnaire asks the subject to rate the probability of falling asleep on a scale of increasing probability from 0 to 3 for eight different situations, such as such as watching TV, reading, lying down in the afternoon, and so on.[59] Despite the fact that the Epworth Sleepiness Scale

TABLE 10.1 Sleep Questionnaires: Questionnaires Commonly Used for Clinical and Research Purposes and Their Focus

Questionnaire*	Focus	References
Pittsburgh Sleep Quality Index (PSQI)	Sleep and sleep disorders	60,61
Sleep Quality Scale (SQS)	Sleep quality	66
Functional Outcome of Sleep Questionnaire (FOSQ)	Impact of daytime sleepiness on daily living	12,67
Pediatric Sleep Questionnaire	Sleep and SDB in children	68
Child Sleep Habits Questionnaire (CSHQ)	Sleep	69
Epworth Sleepiness Scale (ESS)	Daytime sleepiness	59,62,63
Sleep Diaries/Sleep Logs	Sleeping times, sleep duration	70,71
Morningness-Eveningness Questionnaire	Sleeping times, sleep duration, circadian rhythm	72
Loughborough Occupational Impact of Sleep Scale (LOISS)	Sleep quality	73
Insomnia Sleep Questionnaire (ISQ)	Insomnia	74
Berlin Questionnaire	SDB in surgical patients	66
STOP/STOP-Bang Questionnaire	Obstructive sleep apnea	75,76
Brief Insomnia Questionnaire (BIQ),	Insomnia	77
International Restless Legs Syndrome Study Group Rating Scale (IRLS)	Restless leg syndrome	78
Clinical Global Impression (CGI) Scale	Restless leg syndrome	67
Richard–Campbell Sleep Questionnaire	Sleep assessment in the ICU	79

*Recommended questionnaires are italicized.

ICU, Intensive care unit; *SDB*, sleep-disordered breathing; *STOP*, snoring, tiredness, observed apneas, and high blood pressure.

is reliable for detection of daytime sleepiness,[60,61] the instrument does not determine the mechanism of daytime sleepiness.[62,63]

Other clinically useful questionnaires that focus on the detection of signs and symptoms of sleep disorders are available,[59-79] which is important because the prevalence of sleep pathologies typically varies in a wide range across populations (see Table 10.1).

An effective process for clinical assessment of sleep-related diseases is a stepwise assessment using a screening tool first (e.g., Epworth Sleepiness Scale), followed by a more specific questionnaire that helps identify individual mechanisms or consequences of sleepiness.

A special form of sleep questionnaires comes in the form of sleep diaries and "morningness-eveningness" questionnaires that evaluate daily sleep habits, including sleep time, sleep duration, number of nocturnal awakenings, and subjective sleep quality.[80]

Although questionnaires allow a quick and easy screening for daytime symptoms of sleep disturbances, they do not quantify sleep architecture. Subjective methods of assessing sleep are influenced by the spectrum of disease within a tested group, actual clinical change over time, the testing conditions, and recall bias.[80] Clearly, a questionnaire cannot replace a medical history or objective assessment for sleep disorders. However, sleep questionnaires are important tools for measuring health improvement or decline, predicting medical expenses, assessing treatment effects, or comparing disease burden across populations.

ACTIGRAPHY

Actigraphy is used to study sleep-wake patterns by detecting motion of the wrist with linear accelerometers in single or multiple axes. Based on movement-derived data, predictions of the time spent during sleep and wakefulness can be made, and even assumptions on sleep staging are made. Actigraphy can be used conveniently in a patient's home for several nights, weeks, or longer,[81] but its validity for detecting transitions from wakefulness to sleep has been debated, especially in patients with high levels of sleep fragmentation.[81,82] In the clinical setting, actigraphy has been used to evaluate sleep patterns in patients with insomnia, for diagnosis of circadian rhythm disorders (including shift work), and in evaluating sleep in individuals who are less likely to tolerate polysomnography (PSG), such as infants and demented elderly. However, its accuracy is limited for patients with reduced mobility, such as nursing home or intensive care unit (ICU) patients. Actigraphy allows for convenient follow-up measurements to evaluate the effects of treatments designed to improve sleep architecture and circadian rhythm disorders.[83] In more recent years, an increasing number of wearable devices for the detection and analysis of activity and rest have been marketed. Although some have claimed to detect sleep accurately, as well as some sleep stages (mainly REM sleep),[84] none of the current models are yet approved or validated for clinical use.

RESPIRATORY POLYGRAPHY

Home respiratory polygraphy (RP) can be a cost-effective alternative to PSG for the diagnosis of sleep apnea-hypopnea syndrome. RP usually calculates airflow through nasal pressure changes taken via nasal cannulae. Thoracic and abdominal movements are measured by piezoelectric bands, which also measure body position and blood oxygen saturation by pulse oximetry. Using these parameters, RP can identify apnea and hypopnea, and categorize the pathophysiology of apnea into obstructive versus central. Furthermore, similar to actigraphy, RP provides some analysis of sleep duration and time spent awake, using its body position and light sensors. However, the quality of the latter can be more precisely evaluated by a combination of sleep diary and actigraphy. Nevertheless, EEG is required to decide whether a subject was awake or sleeping (Table 10.2).

TABLE 10.2 Pros and Cons of Different Methods of Sleep Evaluation

Method	Pros	Cons	Recommendation
Sleep questionnaire	Low cost Good compliance Easy to use	Recall bias Limited reliability in some populations Limited validity	Should be combined with interview
Sleep diary	Less recall bias Easy to administer Low cost Documentation of daily variability	Lower compliance compared with other questionnaires Biased by daily mood and expectations on sleep	Should be combined with other measurement of sleep duration (e.g., actigraphy)
Actigraphy	Provides objective information about daily variability and sleep duration Provides information on sleep habits at home Not influenced by patient expectations, recall bias, or memory impairments Lower cost than laboratory polysomnography	Limited assessment of sleep stages and sleep onset latency Higher cost than questionnaires	Should be combined with other measurement of sleep duration (e.g., sleep diary)

Continued

TABLE 10.2 Pros and Cons of Different Methods of Sleep Evaluation—cont'd

Method	Pros	Cons	Recommendation
Polygraphy	Lower cost than laboratory polysomnography Objective assessment of respiratory events Provide information on sleep habits at home	Limited assessment of sleep Higher cost than questionnaires Limited assessment of sleep disorders other than sleep-disordered breathing	Should be accompanied by questionnaires and clinical interview
Laboratory polysomnography	Objective assessment of sleep, sleep stages, and sleep disorders	High cost First-night effect Limited capacity No information about sleep habits at home	Should be last step in sleep evaluation with previous questionnaires and ambulatory screening (e.g., polygraphy)
Out-of-center polysomnography	Objective assessment of sleep, sleep stages, and sleep disorders Less first-night effect Lower cost than laboratory polysomnography Can provide information about sleep habits at home	Limited observation may lead to decreased recording quality	Good patient education mandatory If possible, surveillance recording preferred

Adapted in part from Martin JL, Hakim AD. Wrist actigraphy. *Chest.* 2011;139(6):1514–1527.

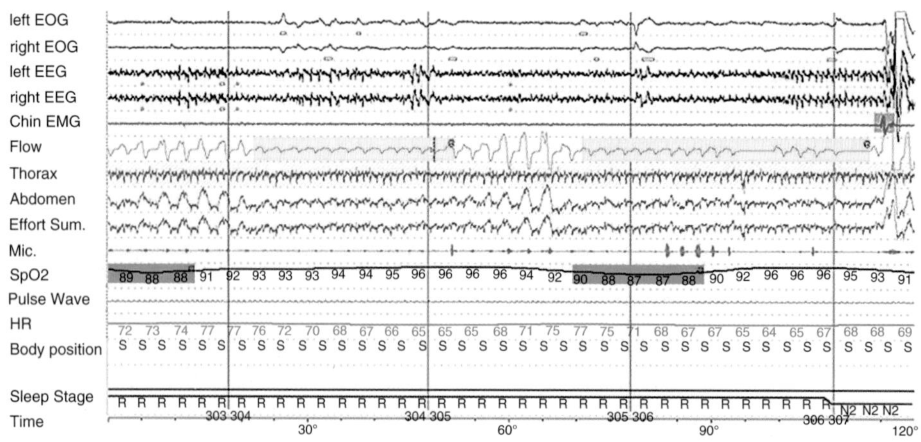

Fig. 10.6 Polysomnographic recording. Left and right electrooculogram *(EOG)*, two electroencephalogram *(EEG)* channels, and mental electromyogram *(Chin EMG)* allow scoring of sleep stage (REM sleep [R] with typical eye movements in the electrooculogram channels). Additional channels (e.g., respiratory flow *[Flow]*, respiratory effort of thorax *[Thorax]* and abdomen *[Abdomen]*, microphone *[Mic.]* oxygen saturation *[SpO$_2$]*) allow diagnosis of sleep disordered breathing. In this patient, apneas *(yellow boxes)* led to oxygen desaturation *(blue boxes)* and finally to arousal *(far right, brown box)*.

POLYSOMNOGRAPHY

PSG is the only method that can precisely determine the actual sleep stage and is a reference diagnostic tool (i.e., gold standard) that is required for the diagnosis of several sleep disorders.[85] PSG measurements include EEG, electrooculography for the measurement of eye movements, and at least electromyographic measurement of muscle activity of the chin.[86] These three measurements are typically supplemented by other channels for the detection of sleep-disordered breathing (SDB), such as a nasal sensor to detect apneas and hypopneas, oximetry, inductance plethysmography for respiratory effort of the chest and abdomen, and a body position sensor and leg electromyogram[87] to identify periodic limb movement syndrome or REM sleep behavior disorder, respectively.[88] A typical PSG recording is shown in Fig. 10.6.

Sleep Laboratory Testing

For several decades, PSG was performed only within a sleep laboratory. Sleep laboratory PSG is attended by a trained technician and is analyzed by a clinician trained in sleep medicine according to the published guidelines.[87,89-91] However, the high cost and requirement of an overnight stay can present socioeconomic challenges that affect the accessibility of this method. In-center PSG provides only a momentary view of the patient's sleep, and the measurements themselves can impair patients' sleep (the so-called first-night effect) and does not provide information about sleep at home. Multiple repeated measurements to tailor treatment over time are challenging or even impossible from a logistic and healthcare economics perspective. Therefore, an increasing number of out-of-center devices

TABLE 10.3 Polysomnographic Characteristic of the Different Behavioral States

	EEG and EOG Characteristics	AASM
Wakefulness	α rhythm (8-13 Hz) present in more than 50% of an epoch	W
Non-REM sleep stage 1	Lower amplitudes and activity in range of 4-7 Hz (vertex sharp waves,* slow eye movements*)	N1
Non-REM sleep stage 2	EEG of sleep stage 1 with additional a sleep spindles and K-complexes; slow waves not fulfilling the criteria for sleep stage 3	N2
Non-REM slow wave sleep	20%-50% of slow wave activity (0.5-2 Hz)	N3
REM sleep	EEG of low amplitude and mixed frequencies, low chin electromyogram activity, rapid eye movements	R

*Not necessary but may be present.
AASM, American Academy of Sleep Medicine criteria (see reference 87); *EEG,* electroencephalography; *EOG,* electrooculogram; *N1,* non-REM sleep stage 1; *N2,* sleep stage 2; *N3,* sleep stage 3; *R,* REM-sleep; *W,* wakefulness.

are now available, offering the possibility of recording PSG in almost every environment, such as at the patient's home, within the hospital or nursing home room, and even within the recovery room or ICU.

Out-of-Center Testing

Portable out-of-center PSG sleep monitors are a reasonable, reliable, and effective method for diagnosing OSA[92] compared with PSG recording performed within a sleep laboratory, when applied in preselected population at risk of moderate-to-severe OSA.[92-94] The Portable Monitoring Task Force of the American Academy of Sleep Medicine (AASM) supports the use of these devices in subjects for clinical and research purposes and indicates a comparable quality of PSG data.[92]

Scoring of Sleep and Sleep Disordered Breathing

More than 40 years ago, Rechtschaffen and Kales[86] standardized the method of scoring PSG recordings—the R&K criteria. Since then, major innovations in technology have transformed the science and clinical practice of sleep medicine. The latest criteria of the AASM[87,95] capture the full potential of innovations resulting from computerization of data, including automation of sleep scoring, recognition of disorders that occur during sleep, and integration with other procedures, such as positive airway pressure titration. Although the R&K criteria are still sufficient for clinical and research purposes, they are less commonly used in sleep centers around the world.

According to these criteria, the arousal states are categorized based on the EEG activity recorded from three different scalp locations and divided into wakefulness (W), REM sleep (R), and three NREM sleep stages (Table 10.3 and see Fig. 10.1).

Respiratory events during sleep are defined as follows:

1. *Apnea* with a decrease in respiratory flow of 90% or more from baseline for at least 10 seconds, whereas a minimum of 90% of the event duration has to meet the criteria of respiratory flow reduction
2. *Hypopneas,* in which the signal of respiratory flow measurement decreases at least 30%, whereas oxygen saturation (SpO_2) decreases by 4% or more compared with pre-event baseline for at least 90% of the duration (minimum of 10 seconds). Hypopneas can also be defined as a decrease in respiratory flow measurement of at least 40% with a decrease in SpO_2 of only 3%.
3. *Respiratory event-related arousal* is defined as a series of breaths not meeting the criteria for apnea or hypopnea lasting at least 10 seconds characterized by increasing respiratory effort or flattening of the nasal pressure waveform leading to an arousal from sleep.
4. *Hypoventilations* are defined as an increase of 10% or more in arterial carbon dioxide tension ($PaCO_2$).

Although the AASM 2007 criteria[87] are commonly used in many sleep centers for clinical and research purposes all over the world, questions about whether the new criteria should be used in children[96] and the scoring of some respiratory events are still unanswered.

Sleep and Breathing

RESPIRATORY REGULATION DURING SLEEP

Sleep puts breathing at risk. The upper airway dilator muscle activity is decreased during sleep compared with wakefulness, particularly at sleep onset and during REM sleep. Furthermore, the ventilatory response to hypoxia can be impaired, such that critical hypoxia levels can occur during sleep that can be offset only by arousal from sleep.

The major determinant of minute ventilation during wakefulness and sleep is $PaCO_2$. In contrast to wakefulness, where $PaCO_2$ is maintained close to 40 mm Hg, the chemo sensitivity to CO_2 decreases during sleep, as does the chemo sensitivity for oxygen. This leads to $PaCO_2$ values of 45 mm Hg commonly occurring during stable sleep, while ventilatory demand is decreased and the arousal threshold varies with sleep stages.

Accordingly, the changes in respiratory muscle activity, ventilatory demand, and arousal threshold observed from wakefulness to sleep and across sleep stages challenge ventilatory control and can lead to instability in breathing. A structured approach to evaluating breathing instabilities is the loop gain. This engineering term is used to describe the stability of a feedback-controlled system (in this case, the chemical feedback loop controlling an individual's ventilation). In the setting of ventilatory control, loop gain reflects the propensity of an individual to develop periodic (unstable) breathing. Patients with a high loop gain caused by a more sensitive respiratory controller (i.e., high controller gain), more effective CO_2 excretion (i.e., high plant gain), or

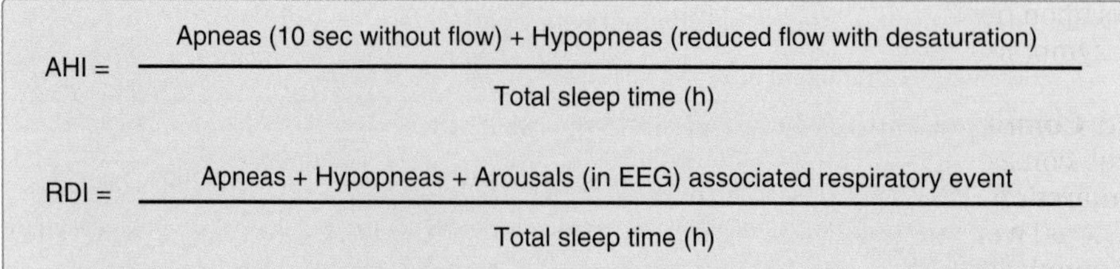

Fig. 10.7 Definition of apnea hypopnea index *(AHI)* and respiratory disturbance index *(RDI)*.

an increased delay because of slowed CO_2 distribution from peripheral tissues to the central chemoreceptors based on, for example, reduced blood circulation (i.e., mixing gain) may be more vulnerable to disturbances of the feedback system, such as slight hypoventilation that occurs as a consequence of decreased upper airway dilator muscle activity during the transition from wakefulness to sleep.

High loop gain may contribute to severity of OSA. Moreover, subjects with a high loop gain have been shown to be more likely to develop breathing instabilities such as Cheyne-Stokes respiration (CSR; see "Central Sleep Apnea").

SLEEP-DISORDERED BREATHING

SDB refers to the respiratory signs and symptoms associated with sleep-associated respiratory dysfunction and is defined by the occurrence of respiratory events, which are cessations in breathing rhythm (apneas) or momentary or sustained reduction in the amplitude of respiratory flow (hypopnea) during the sleeping state, leading to arterial hypoxemia.[97] They are usually caused either by increases in upper-airway resistance due to reduction in intraluminal airway diameter (obstructive event), marked reduction or cessation of brainstem respiratory motor output (central event), or both. A specification of SDB into obstructive or central sleep apneas (CSA) is made based on the predominant type of respiratory events. The severity of SDB is usually quantified by the number of respiratory events per hour of sleep. This is necessary because a low number of short apneas and hypopneas can occur up to about five times per hour in healthy subjects. Two measures can be used for this purpose: the apnea hypopnea index (AHI) and the respiratory disturbance index (RDI). Typically the AHI (number of hypopneas and apneas per hour of sleep; Fig. 10.7, *top*) and RDI (number of hypopneas, apneas, and arousals related to respiratory events per hour of sleep; see Fig. 10.7, *bottom*) are used to quantify the severity of SDB.

Obstructive Sleep Apnea

Definition. OSA is the most common type of SDB and is diagnosed in patients with more than 15 predominantly obstructive events per hour of sleep, or with fewer respiratory events (i.e., 5-15 per hour) if daytime symptoms (i.e., sleepiness) or comorbidities such as hypertension or atrial fibrillation are present. These cutoff values have been used as an indication for treatment by clinicians based on the clinical guidelines and the international classification of sleep disorders.[87,88] The severity of sleep apnea is further characterized as mild in patients with less than 15 events per hour of sleep, as moderate with 15 to 30 or less events per hour of sleep, and as severe sleep apnea with 30 or more events per hour of sleep (Table 10.4).[88,90]

TABLE 10.4 Severity of Sleep Apnea Based on Respiratory Disturbance Index or Apnea Hypopnea Index

	RDI (Events Per Hour)	AHI (Events Per Hour)
No sleep apnea	<5	<5
Mild sleep apnea*	≥5 to <15	≥5 to <15
Moderate sleep apnea	≥15 to <30	≥15 to <30
Severe sleep apnea	≥30	≥30

*Only diagnosed if comorbidities like hypertension, atrial fibrillation of daytime sleepiness are present.

A respiratory disturbance index (RDI) less than 5 per hour is physiologic and found in healthy humans. Sleep apnea is mild with RDI between 5 and 15 per hour, moderate with RDI between 15 and 30 events per hour, and considered severe with an RDI of 30 and greater per hour of sleep. Equal cutoff values are similar for severity based on the apnea hypopnea index (AHI).

Epidemiology. OSA with daytime symptoms affects 0.3% to 5% of the general population.[98,99] As obesity is one of the major risk factors for OSA, the prevalence might continue to increase with higher rates of obesity in the general population.[100-102] The prevalence of SDB without daytime symptoms is even higher, with rates of up to 9% in women and 24% in men between the ages of 30 and 60 years, and is often unrecognized.[103,104]

Furthermore, the prevalence of OSA varies widely between different populations. Individuals with a high susceptibility to OSA include the obese, the elderly, and those with specific comorbidities (e.g., stroke, myocardial infarction). Depending on methodology, the rates of OSA in patients following surgery is between 45%[105] and 75%.[106] A recent study in patients undergoing bariatric surgery revealed an incidence of OSA of as high as 77.5% in this population,[107] while another study showed OSA to be prevalent in 50% of women undergoing gynecologic oncology surgery [108]

Clinical Symptoms. Approximately one-third of patients with OSA complain of typical signs and symptoms occurring during wakefulness. Waking with dry mouth or headache in the morning, daytime sleepiness, falling asleep during monotonous situations (e.g., watching television), as well as subjective impairment of cognitive function are frequently reported. This combination of OSA with daytime symptoms is usually referred to as OSA syndrome.[109,110]

Sleep-associated signs and symptoms of OSA include witnessed pauses in breathing or snoring, and a high number of nocturnal awakenings, mostly reported as pseudo-nocturia. Patients with OSA occasionally complain of tachycardia or respiratory distress upon nocturnal awakening (choking sensation) and other symptoms (Box 10.1).

Consequences and Comorbidities. OSA is associated with serious medical consequences, such as hypertension, myocardial infarction, stroke,[109,111,112] diabetes, diabetic neuropathy, as well as cognitive dysfunction resulting in occupational difficulties and motor vehicle accidents.[113,114] The development of cognitive impairment in patients with OSA[115] is associated with atrophy of brain structures relevant for cognition and memory (hippocampal areas)[116] that can be partially reversed by adequate treatment.[117] Whether the negative effects of OSA are due to impaired sleep architecture or effects of intermittent hypoxia remain unclear,[118] because data investigating the effect of intermittent hypoxia without other symptoms in OSA patients are limited. Nevertheless, recent findings suggest that even asymptomatic OSA might be associated with cardiovascular effects, such as altered daytime autonomic regulation (i.e., heart rate variability).[119]

BOX 10.1 Symptoms of Obstructive Sleep Apnea

Nighttime Symptoms

- Frequent awakening during the night (e.g., pseudo-nocturia)
- Awaking from own snoring with choking sensation
- Tachycardia
- Sleep that is not restorative

Daytime Symptoms

- Awaking with dry mouth
- Dull headache in the morning
- Daytime sleepiness
- Falling asleep during monotonic situations (e.g., watching television)
- Subjective impairment of cognitive function

Symptoms Reported by Bed Partner

- Snoring, especially when loud and arrhythmic
- Observed pauses in breathing during sleep

Given the frequent rate of complications associated with OSA, it is not surprising that OSA leads to increased socioeconomic costs because of significantly more frequent rates of health-related contacts and medication use, and even higher rates of unemployment.[120]

Risk Factors. Predisposing factors for OSA are obesity,[121] age,[121,122] male sex,[121] factors leading to swelling of the superficial tissue of the upper airway (smoking),[123] allergic rhinitis,[124] and decreased muscle tone of upper airway dilator muscles (e.g., central nervous system) caused by respiratory depressants.[125]

Pathophysiology. Respiratory events during OSA are characterized by decreased respiratory flow with persisting respiratory effort due to reduced intraluminal diameter of the upper airway up to complete pharyngeal airway collapse (see Fig. 10.6). The muscles involved in respiration are morphologically and functionally skeletal muscles and can be classified into two groups: upper airway dilator muscles and respiratory pump muscles.

Upper airway dilator muscles counterbalance the negative inspiratory pressure generated by the pump muscle to permit airflow during inspiration. Respiratory pump muscles are the collection of muscles responsible for generating inspiratory and expiratory forces in the thorax across the breathing cycle (Fig. 10.8). The patency of the upper airway is maintained by balancing dilating forces (generated by the upper airway dilator muscles) and collapsing forces (i.e., negative intraluminal pressure generated by the respiratory pump during inspiration and compressive extraluminal forces from the surrounding tissues).[126]

Upper airway dilator muscles. The most extensively studied of the upper airway dilating muscles are the genioglossus and the tensor palatini (Table 10.5). The genioglossus receives a variety of inputs, including phasic (inspiratory) and tonic (noninspiratory) drives, which are distributed differentially across the hypoglossal motoneurons.[127] In response to negative pharyngeal pressure created by the respiratory pump during inspiration, the

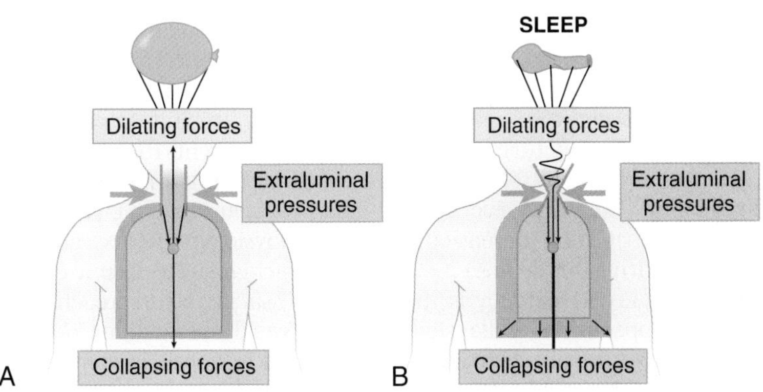

Fig. 10.8 Relationship of upper airway patency and respiratory pump activation. (A) During wakefulness, the force of the upper airway dilator muscles (*green balloon*, dilating forces) counterbalance the collapsing forces imposed on the upper airway by extraluminal pressures and negative inspiratory pressure generated by the respiratory pump muscles (represented by the orange counterweight [collapsing forces]). In obstructive sleep apnea, (B) sleep onset *(blue needle)* leads to decreased upper airway patency by reducing the dilating forces. (Modified from Sasaki N, Meyer MJ, Eikermann M. Postoperative respiratory muscle dysfunction: pathophysiology and preventive strategies. *Anesthesiology*. 2013;118:961–978.)

TABLE 10.5 Some Muscles of the Upper Airway Relevant for Upper Airway Stability

Muscle	Tonic Activity	PHASIC ACTIVITY Insp.	Exp.
Tensor palatini[153]	+	+	–
Levator palatine[153]	+	+	–
Genioglossus[154]	+	+	–
Geniohyoid[155]	+	–	+
Thyrohyoid	X	X	X

+, Present; –, absent; *X*, insufficient data. Major muscles of the upper airway and their activity during breathing. Tonic activity, as well as inspiratory (Insp.) and expiratory (Exp.) muscle activity.

genioglossus reflexively stabilizes the upper airway in animals and humans.[128,129] This reflex is likely a product of signaling from inspiratory modulated motor units. Whereas the genioglossus responds to phasic input on top of its tonic activation, the tensor palatini is considered a tonic muscle with consistent tone throughout the respiratory cycle.[130]

Anatomic vulnerability to collapsing forces. The soft tissues of the pharynx are enclosed and stabilized by bony structures, such as the mandible and the spine, and complete collapse of the pharyngeal airway ordinarily requires extraluminal forces, such as hematoma, edema, peripharyngeal masses, or an airway trauma, for instance, as a consequence of prolonged endotracheal intubation.[131] Pharyngeal manifestation of obesity compresses the airway.[132] Craniofacial abnormalities can further increase the collapsing effects of excessive pharyngeal extraluminal soft tissue in obese patients.[133] The extraluminal soft tissue, as well as size and shape of the bony enclosure, are determinants of the extraluminal pressure that need to be antagonized by the upper airway dilator muscle contraction during inspiration, to avoid an upper airway obstruction–related apnea.[133] In addition, the upper airway is more vulnerable to collapse in the supine position than in the lateral or sitting positions, due to gravitational effects.[134,135]

Excessive intravenous fluid administration can affect upper airway patency. In awake, healthy volunteers, the inflation of antishock trousers displaced fluid from the lower extremities to increase neck circumference,[136] so that the upper airway had a lower threshold to collapse.[137] This concept is reinforced in studies of subjects with lower extremity venous insufficiency[138] and congestive heart failure (CHF).[139] These studies have shown nocturnal redistribution of fluid from the lower extremities into the neck increases upper airway collapsibility[138] and the severity of central apnea and OSA.[139] Similar effects may increase the risk for OSA during pregnancy and early after delivery.[139]

Another important component of airway patency is the interplay between lung volume and upper airway collapsibility. Higher end-expiratory lung volumes are associated with a decrease in upper airway resistance to airflow in awake healthy humans,[140] and an increase in upper airway lumen dimensions in subjects with and without OSA.[141] The mechanism for the interaction between upper airway patency and lung volume is thought to lie in the generation of longitudinal traction forces in the trachea.[142,143] Upon inspiration, the lung inflates and effectively forces the carina into a more caudal position, creating stretching forces on the fixed trachea.[142] These forces are transferred to the side walls of the upper airway.[143] Effectively, tracheal traction allows the respiratory pump muscles to contribute to upper airway opening.

Collapsing intraluminal pressure. The respiratory pump is the motorized action driving inspiration and expiration. It is the force that broadens the thoracic cavity and creates negative intrathoracic pressure to draw a breath in, and when needed, positive intrathoracic pressure to exhale rapidly. Inspiratory pump muscles are an anatomically diverse group, with the most studied being the intercostal muscles and the diaphragm. The diaphragm accounts for 60% to 70% of lung volume change during quiet respiration.[144] During inspiration, the volume of the thoracic cavity increases as a result of contraction of the diaphragm and the external intercostal muscles. The lungs expand secondarily to the increased negative intrathoracic pressure generated by these phasic actions of the inspiratory pump muscles. The negative intrathoracic pressure translates into a negative intraluminal pressure in the upper airway, forcing the airway to collapse as soon as this pressure drops below a critical value.[145]

Although this critical airway pressure (Pcrit) is typically negative (approximately −5 cm H_2O) in healthy controls, the upper airway in patients with OSA during sleep may even collapse at a positive Pcrit. Positive intraluminal pressure is required for reopening the paralyzed airway in patients with OSA.[146] Under normal conditions, the two compressing factors, (1) negative intraluminal pressure and (2) positive extraluminal pressure, need to be actively compensated by muscular activity of the upper airway dilator muscles to maintain airway patency.[97]

Wakefulness stimulus and sleep. Excitatory inputs to the upper airway motoneurons (e.g., hypoglossal motoneurons) include those from serotoninergic and noradrenergic neurons that fire predominantly during wakefulness,[147-150] resulting in a "wakefulness stimulus" that increases the activity of upper airway dilator muscles during this arousal state. With onset of sleep, this arousal-dependent neuronal input (active while awake versus less active, or inactive when asleep) disappears, leading to a decrease in upper airway muscle activity and causing increased upper airway resistance in healthy controls and airway collapse in patients with OSA.[151-153] The resulting retropalatal obstruction of the upper airway is reported to be the most common pathophysiological mechanism in OSA.[146]

One way valves in the upper airway. Observing the respiratory flow tracings in patients with OSA, one can find some respiratory events that do not show the characteristic progressive flow limitation ultimately resulting in complete upper airway occlusion, typically seen as a result of "collapsible tube pathophysiology" with variable compliance. In these cases, the flow tracings show normal expiratory flow and sudden reduction/cessation before reaching maximum inspiratory flow. This "rapid obstruction" only during the inspiratory phase occurred in approximately 20% to 30% of OSA patients.[154] Recent findings suggest that there are two one-way valves in the pharynx. While the epiglottic valve closes during inspiration, the soft palate may function as a second one-way valve limiting flow during expiration.[155]

Similar to the epiglottis, the soft palate hangs from the hard palate like a peninsula in the oropharynx and might

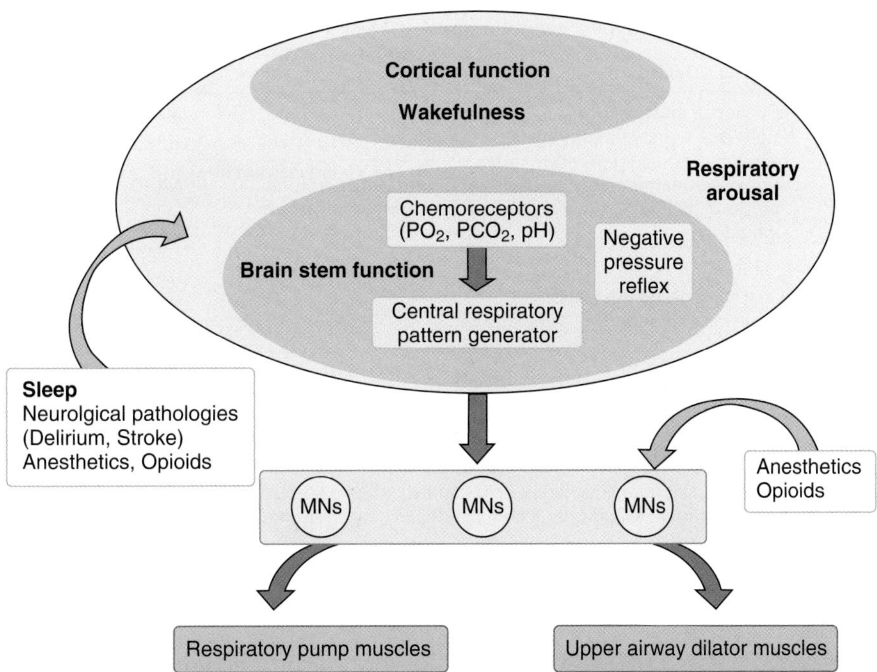

Fig. 10.9 Effects of respiratory arousal on upper airway dilator and respiratory pump muscles. Respiratory arousal is composed of three primary inputs: central respiratory pattern generator processing peripheral and central chemoreceptor afferents, reflex responsiveness to the magnitude of negative pressure in the airway generated by the respiratory pump muscles, and strength of the wakefulness stimulus. Different factors can impair respiratory arousal, such as sleep and neurologic pathologies, anesthetics, and opioids. Blue arrows indicate excitatory effect; yellow arrows indicate inhibitory effect. *MN,* Motor neuron. (Modified from Sasaki N, Meyer MJ, Eikermann M. Postoperative respiratory muscle dysfunction: pathophysiology and preventive strategies. *Anesthesiology*. 2013;118:961–978.)

occlude the upper airway during expiration.[156] A recent study found that sudden reduction of expiratory airflow immediately after peak expiratory flow occurs more often in OSA patients under positive pressure ventilation.[157] Similar expiratory flow limitation pattern was also reported in spontaneously breathing OSA patients, suggesting that this phenomenon is not unique to positive pressure ventilation.[158]

These findings may point to a second, slightly different mechanism underlying OSA than the pure collapsible tube pathophysiology in some OSA patients, which should be particularly important during anesthesia. Correct identification of the closure site in each OSA patient will enable the clinician to provide an individualized OSA treatment.[155]

Respiratory arousal. Respiratory arousal is arousal from sleep owing to cumulative and progressive increases in stimuli related to breathing (hypoxia, hypercapnia, and respiratory effort).[159]

Three primary inputs contribute to arousal-related restoration of breathing following an apnea (Fig. 10.9):

1. Peripheral and central chemoreceptors sensitive to partial pressures of oxygen and carbon dioxide[160]
2. Sensors in the upper airway responsive to negative pressure generated by the respiratory pump[128,129]
3. Cortical inputs directly related to state of consciousness or wakefulness[161]

Any of these inputs can restore respiratory muscle tone if the magnitude of stimulation is sufficient. Cortical awakening from sleep, identified by EEG signs of wakefulness, is an adequate stimulus for ventilation. However, obstructive apneas, such as upper airway collapse in OSA, can be terminated by an increased drive to the respiratory muscles not involving cortical arousal.[162] For example, hypercarbia resulting from sustained hypopnea[160] and elevated upper airway negative pressure[128,129] can independently restore tone to the respiratory muscles. The level of drive provided to the respiratory muscles depends on the summation of stimuli in the central respiratory pattern generator output, including peripheral and central chemo-responsiveness, reflex responsiveness to the negative airway pressure, and strength of the wakefulness drive.

Treatment. Adequate treatment of OSA improves nocturnal oxygen saturation as well as duration and quality of sleep, which translates to reduced daytime sleepiness, improvement of daytime functions, and improved quality of life. Successful treatment of OSA reduces cardiovascular risk, improves insulin sensitivity, and increases neurobehavioral performance.[163-165] Therefore, all patients with a diagnosis of OSA should be offered treatment as soon as the diagnosis of OSA has been established and its severity has been determined by objective testing (i.e., PSG).[88] Although different treatment options for OSA have been developed during the last decades (Table 10.6), continuous positive airway pressure (CPAP) dose dependently increases upper airway diameter and is still the most effective treatment for OSA of all severities.[166-168] However, a recent study has questioned if CPAP treatment is able to prevent the long-term adverse cardiovascular events in OSA.[169]

Positive airway pressure treatment. CPAP as a treatment for SDB is typically applied continuously with a nasal or oronasal mask, and can dose dependently reverse any sleep-associated upper airway obstruction, as outlined in Fig. 10.10. The CPAP level needed for treatment of OSA

TABLE 10.6 Treatment Possibilities for Obstructive Sleep Apnea

Treatment	Procedure/Device	Recommendation	References
Weight reduction	Reduction of body weight Weight-loss surgery (improves success of weight loss)	Medium to high, SU	170,171
Medication	Drug-based treatment (e.g., tricyclic antidepressants, serotonin reuptake inhibitors, cholinergic agonists, carbonic anhydrase inhibitors)	NR, ID	90
Surgical	Nasal surgery Palatal surgery and implants Tongue base surgery	Low, SU Low, MC Low, MC	172,173
Increase of muscle activity	Muscle training Hypoglossal nerve stimulation	ID ID	174
Nonsurgical	Oral appliance Positive airway pressure	High, AT High, GS	175 175

AT, Alternative treatment if positive airway pressure is not tolerated; *GS*, gold standard; *ID*, data not sufficient for recommendation; *MC*, may be concerned in carefully selected patients if conservative treatment fails; *NR*, not recommended; *SU*, supportive treatment.

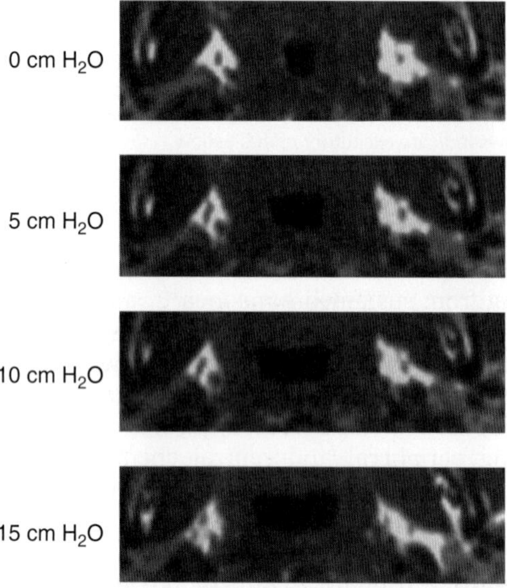

Fig. 10.10 **Magnetic resonance imaging of the human upper airway during different levels of continuous positive airway pressure. Magnetic resonance imaging of the upper airway during continuous positive airway pressure of 0, 5, 10, and 15 cm H_2O shows a dose-dependent increase in upper airway diameter.** (Obtained from Schwab RJ, Pack AI, Gupta KB, et al. Upper airway and soft tissue structural changes induced by CPAP in normal subjects. *Am J Respir Crit Care Med.* 1996;154[4 pt 1]:1106–1116.)

varies mostly between 5 and 20 cm H_2O. However, home RP and titration of CPAP might be similarly effective in some but not all patients with suspected OSA.[176,177] After titration, the prescribed treatment pressure is applied continuously throughout the night. Although this treatment is efficient in reversing the underlying pathology, the impact of CPAP on outcome is limited by patient adherence,[112,178] mostly because of local side-effects at the nose or face, or discomfort caused by the mask.[179] When applied with high pressure, the amount of airflow can prevent the patient from falling asleep while using the treatment device. Some treatment devices offer a ramp or delay function that gradually increases treatment pressure from a low starting pressure to the prescribed pressure over a period of 5 to 45 minutes, allowing the patient to fall asleep more easily. Some patients report difficulties exhaling against high CPAP. To avoid this problem, bilevel treatment with reduced expiratory positive airway pressure and a sufficiently high inspiratory positive airway pressure can be used.

In some cases, one CPAP pressure level is not sufficient to treat sleep apnea. CPAP devices with dynamic pressure levels can improve treatment success, particularly in patients with a variable severity of sleep disordered breathing during different sleep stages. These automatic positive-airway pressure or auto-titrating devices measure different variables associated with hypopnea, such as oropharyngeal wall vibration, snoring, and inspiratory flow limitation, and increase the airway pressure until these signs and symptoms of hypopnea disappear. In addition, it is not entirely clear whether CPAP treatment is able to prevent the increased cardiovascular risk inherited by OSA.

CPAP is sufficient in the treatment of most patients with OSA. However, some patients may need different treatment methods. For example, patients with mixed apneas (obstructive and central) or predominantly central apneas need a more controlled (frequency or time controlled), noninvasive ventilation (NIV) with predefined minimal respiratory frequency or respiratory timing that automatically induces the next inspiration (ventilation) if the patient does not induce the next breath within preset parameters.

Alternative treatment options. Oral appliances (OAs) are possible treatment options in patients with mild to moderate OSA who do not tolerate CPAP therapy. Two major designs are currently used clinically: (1) mandibular repositioning appliance, which holds the mandible in an advanced position (a protrusion of at least 50% of the maximal possible extension is recommended for effective treatment),[179] and (2) tongue-retaining devices, leading to repositioning of the tongue into a forward position without any protrusion of the mandible. A multidisciplinary

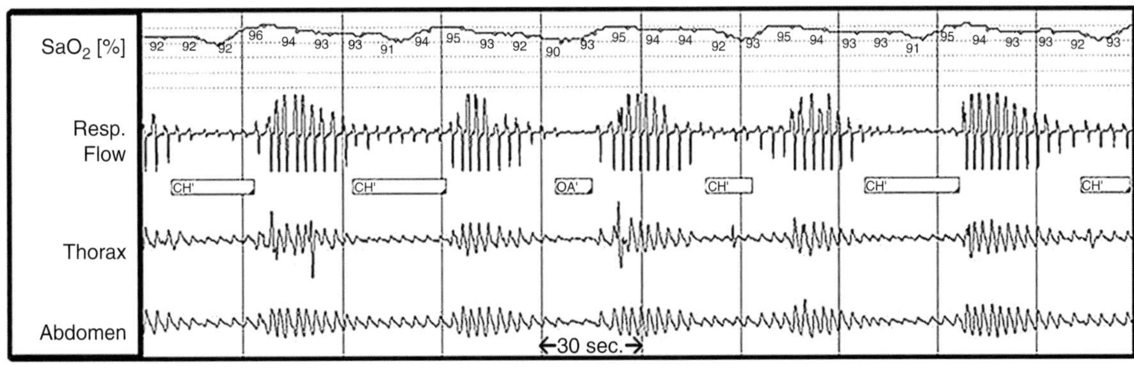

Fig. 10.11 Polysomnographic recording of an episode of Cheyne-Stokes respiration. *CH,* Central hypopnea; *OA,* obstructive apnea.

approach including a sleep physician and a dental technician experienced in OAs has been recommended for this purpose, because both factors are crucial for patient adherence and outcome from OA treatment.[109] OAs are recommended in patients with mild to moderate OSA who do not tolerate,[179] do not respond to, fail, or are not appropriate candidates for CPAP treatment.[88]

Historically, surgical treatment methods were the only approach to treatment of OSA, but the effectiveness of most of the nasopharyngeal surgical approaches for severe OSA remains unclear. However, tonsillectomy is beneficial in adult patients with OSA from tonsillar hypertrophy, and adenotonsillectomy is recommended in children with OSA and adenotonsillar hypertrophy.[180] Repeated sleep testing before and following surgery is recommended to ensure sufficient long-lasting therapeutic effects.[88,179,181]

Electrical stimulation of the upper airway muscles has been explored recently as a new approach to treatment of OSA. Hypoglossal nerve stimulation induces genioglossus muscle contractions, which dose dependently increase inspiratory airflow during OSA,[182] but the invasiveness of the procedure, the cost of the device, and the requirement for preimplantation endoscopy during anesthesia limit its use as a first-line treatment of OSA.[149]

While pharyngeal fat deposits led to a decrease in pharyngeal patency, underlining the risk factor of obesity,[183,184] weight loss leads to a reduction in Pcrit and the severity of OSA[145,171] and is recommended as adjunctive treatment in all overweight patients with OSA.[185] Because long-term weight reduction is more effective when accompanied by weight loss surgery, bariatric surgery may be considered as an adjunctive therapy in very obese patients (body mass index [BMI] ≥ 40 kg/m^2), as well as in those with important comorbidities and BMI of 35 kg/m^2 or greater and in whom dietary attempts at weight control have been ineffective.[88]

Oxygen is currently not recommended as primary treatment of OSA, but may be used as an adjunctive treatment in some patients, particularly in the postoperative period.[88,186]

Although OSA is more common in the older population, it occurs in children with a peak in the incidence between 2 and 5 years of age. Obesity predicts snoring and other signs of obstructive respiratory events in children.[109] Tonsillar and adenoidal hypertrophy is another important cause of OSA in children and can be treated surgically.[187]

Central Sleep Apnea

CSA impairs quality of life[188] and is associated with adverse outcome in heart failure patients.[189,190] CSA is defined as cessation of air flow without respiratory effort,[188] which separates it from OSA, where respiratory effort is maintained or even increased during an apnea. In clinical sleep apnea, considerable overlap between OSA and CSA occur that need to be identified and subsequently treated.[191]

CSA can be found in older patients and in patients with severe comorbidities such as CHF, stroke, or other neurologic disorders (e.g., amyotrophic lateral sclerosis). In a southern Pennsylvania cohort, CSA (AHI ≥ 20/hour) was found in 5% of men aged 65 years and older, but it was not found in younger men or in women of any age. For an AHI of 2.5 per hour and greater, the prevalence estimates in men younger than 45 years remains negligible, while CSA was found in 1.7% of men between 45 and 64 years, and 12% in men older than 65 years,[192] or 9% in individuals between 40 and 97 years, respectively.[193]

CSA mechanisms can be categorized into those with high and low loop gain. The most common subtype of CSA with an increased loop gain is CSR and is commonly seen in patients with CHF and left-ventricular systolic dysfunction. CSR is defined as a crescendo-decrescendo pattern of hyperventilation between 20 and 30 seconds in duration, followed by 10 to 40 seconds of hypopneas or apneas (Fig. 10.11), usually occurring during NREM sleep stage 1 and 2.[194] Nevertheless, CSR can also occur during exercise or wakefulness. Nearly one out of two patients with CHF shows CSR.[195] CSR is more common in men and worse in the supine body position.[161]

Potential respiratory therapies of CSR include oxygen, respiratory stimulants (e.g., CO_2, theophylline, and acetazolamide), and NIV such as bilevel positive airway pressure. The effectiveness of CPAP as therapy is controversial. Optimization of medical therapy is the best treatment, because CSR will often resolve with adequate treatment of CHF (cardiac resynchronization therapy and surgical treatment, such as heart transplant).[194]

Other Forms of Central Breathing Disorders. The term *periodic breathing* refers to altitude-induced breathing instability that occurs in subjects transferred to a high altitude, where ambient hypoxia caused by low barometric pressure leads to an increase in controller gain.[97] Idiopathic CSA, which is a relatively uncommon disorder at sea level, occurs more likely in individuals with an elevated hypercapnic ventilatory response (high controller gain) that leads to hypocapnia and respiratory control instability during sleep. Patients with idiopathic CSA tend to have low $PaCO_2$ levels, even during wakefulness.[196]

Obesity Hypoventilation Syndrome

Alveolar hypoventilation is defined as insufficient ventilation leading to hypercapnia (increased $PaCO_2$). Mechanisms of alveolar hypoventilation include central hypoventilation, chest wall deformities, neuromuscular disorders, chronic obstructive pulmonary disease, as well as severe obesity (obesity hypoventilation syndrome [OHS]). OHS is defined as the combination of nocturnal and daytime hypoventilation, usually leading to hypercapnia in obese subjects (BMI ≥ 30 kg/m^2), in the absence of other causes of hypoventilation.

The prevalence of OHS is estimated to be up to 50% in obese patients with OSA. It can occur in up to 50% of patients with a BMI of 50 kg/m^2 or more,[197] compared with 0.15% to 0.3% in the general adult population. Ninety percent of patients with OHS also suffer from OSA.[198,199] OHS often remains undiagnosed, and the true prevalence remains unclear.

Severe obesity is associated with an increase in respiratory drive that helps maintain eucapnia in the presence of the abnormal chest wall mechanics and high work of breathing.[200,201] In OHS, this compensatory mechanism is abolished,[201,202] which in part might be explained by leptin resistance.[203-205] Typically, OHS manifests as a reduced lung capacity, vital and functional residual capacity, expiratory reserve volume, respiratory system compliance, and inspiratory muscle strength, whereas response to CO_2 might be reduced or normal. In addition, there is an increase in serum bicarbonate and alveolar PCO_2, as well as in the work of breathing and leptin levels.[205,206]

Impairment of the effectiveness of respiratory pump muscle function in patients with OHS can be explained by the effects of low lung volume because of central fat distribution, leading to a cranial displacement of the diaphragm when lying supine.[206,207] In addition, diaphragmatic myopathy might be a contributing factor of OHS.[205] Treatment options include weight loss and NIV.[207,208]

Sleep and Anesthesia: Two Unequal Twins Influencing Perioperative Medicine

CLINICAL PICTURE OF SLEEP AND ANESTHESIA

Although physiologic sleep and anesthesia share some clinical features (loss of consciousness and a modulation of brainstem autonomic function), major differences can be found when closer observations of both behavioral states are undertaken. In contrast to anesthesia, sleep shows spontaneous generation and termination, ready reversibility by noxious stimuli, and homeostatic regulation. Anesthesia does not share the stage-wise structure seen during physiologic sleep. In addition, functional imaging studies underline the fundamental differences during onset of anesthesia and wakefulness-sleep transition.

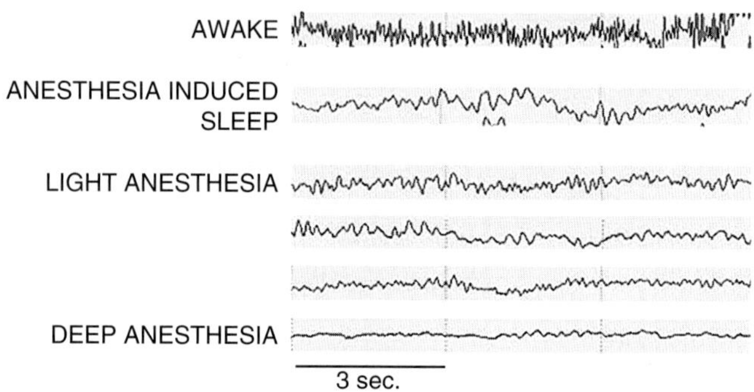

Fig. 10.12 Electroencephalographic recording during sedation and loss of consciousness induced by propofol. Compared with physiologic sleep (see Fig. 10.1), sedation shows electroencephalographic (EEG) traces comparable to slow wave sleep, indicating the sleep-inducing effect of anesthetics. Anesthesia-induced loss of consciousness (lower four traces), shows different EEG activity with reduced amplitudes and burst suppression. (Burst suppression is not shown in these traces.)

Although there are similarities in the EEG patterns between slow-wave sleep and anesthesia-induced unconsciousness, the EEG patterns during sleep and anesthesia are different,[209] with different frequencies and types of activation in EEG recorded during physiologic sleep and the uniform EEG picture observed during anesthesia-induced unconsciousness (Fig. 10.12).[210]

During anesthesia induction, the level of consciousness continuously decreases from fully awake through states of reduced response to external stimuli up to a completely unresponsive state.[211] This is in contrast to the sharp α–θ EEG transitions seen while an individual proceeds from wakefulness to sleep without any transient stages. Individuals in a steady state of physiologic sleep can be aroused with sufficient stimulation, whereas drug-induced unconsciousness needs at least some drug elimination to occur before individuals can be aroused.[212]

ACTIVATION OF SLEEP-PROMOTING PATHWAYS DURING ANESTHESIA

The role of the endogenous sleep-promoting system in the mechanism of action of general anesthetics has recently received much attention. This hypothesis is attractive because of the similarities of sleep and anesthesia and some evidence that anesthetically induced sleep could meet some of the homeostatic need for sleep.[213,214] It is even more attractive because, despite the large database of the molecular effects of anesthetics, how loss of consciousness occurs is still not explained. An important discovery is that some of the neurons that are active during sleep in the VLPO are also activated by certain anesthetics.[213-216] A second key observation is the inhibition of the arousal nuclei, the TMN, contributes to anesthesia.[215] This effect also implicates activation of VLPO because it provides the major source of inhibition of the TMN. The idea has emerged that anesthesia-induced loss of consciousness is mediated by effects of the anesthetics on the flip-flop switch centered in the VLPO that is responsible for the sharp transition from wakefulness to sleep and back (see earlier section).[212,217,218] However, there are a number of problems with this theory, including that rats and mice with complete lesions of the VLPO can still be anesthetized.[216,219] Although lesions of VLPO lead to a transient resistance to volatile anesthetics,[216] if some time elapses following a VLPO lesion, the animals show increased sensitivity to isoflurane anesthesia attributable to increased homeostatic sleep drive.[216,219-221] Another problem with the VLPO-TMN circuit hypothesis of anesthesia is that direct inhibition of the TMN produces sedation but not anesthesia.[215] Animals without VLPO neurons have profound insomnia. Therefore, interaction of anesthetics with these sleep-promoting nuclei alone is not sufficient to produce unconsciousness during anesthesia. During recent years, several studies provided evidence to extend the scientific framework of general anesthetics modulating sleep-promoting regions by the anesthetic depression of arousal-promoting nuclei, including the LC, GABAergic neurons of the pontine reticular formation, the pedunculopontine and laterodorsal tegmentum, the ventral tegmental area, as well as the perifornical area, the tuberomammillary nucleus, and the basal forebrain.[222,223] This "bottom-up" hypothesis of anesthesia-induced unconsciousness may be the result of the simultaneous interaction with the brainstem and diencephalic regions, including the AAS and endogenous sleep circuitry. Although, these mechanisms show similarities with sleep-promoting neuronal interactions, they are unlikely to be the only correlate of anesthesia-induced unconsciousness. Sleep, but not anesthesia, is easily reversed or prevented by real or perceived environmental threats. While interaction with sleep-promoting neurons work by inhibiting these arousal pathways, other neuronal networks crucial for consciousness (e.g., thalamocortical networks) remain active during sleep.[224] However, the finding that many anesthetics engage sleep pathways is still important and meaningful, as this is undoubtedly an important mechanism by which these classes of anesthetics promote sleep. Nevertheless, this effect does not and cannot prevent arousal to sufficient external stimuli. The unique property of anesthesia to do so has to be mediated by an additional mechanism.

PERIOPERATIVE INTERACTIONS BETWEEN ANESTHESIA AND SLEEP

Anesthesia and painful surgical procedures affect sleep and circadian rhythms[225-227] for as long as 6 months, depending on the complexity of the procedure performed.[228] A substantial decrease in REM sleep occurs on the first night after surgery and anesthesia, followed by a profound REM rebound phenomenon on the second to fourth postoperative nights, when REM sleep increases in both intensity and amount.[225,227] Although most anesthetics can lead to an impairment of sleep architecture, such as REM depression and reduced sleep quality during the early postoperative period, the extent of this impairment probably depends on the pharmacokinetics and pharmacodynamics of the anesthetics and opioids used,[229,230] which affect the duration of REM sleep,[231,232] as well as surgery-induced stress.

The effect of propofol on sleep architecture and REM sleep is complex and dose dependent. In long-term ventilated, critically ill patients, propofol sedation abolishes REM sleep and diminishes sleep quality,[233] whereas with low-dose propofol, REM sleep is possible. The effects of ketamine sedation on sleep architecture have not been studied in detail, although it may have rather mild effects on REM duration.[234]

Anesthetics have strong effects on GABA and NMDA receptors, both of which are linked with circadian control. As a result, anesthetics may interfere with entrainment of the circadian rhythm; however, preclinical and human data show inconsistent results. A recent trial in honeybees suggested an anesthetically induced circadian shift. Inside the laboratory with no outdoor cues, daytime anesthesia disturbed the usual activity patterns in the hive for the next several days. In addition, cycles of clock gene activity showed a delay,[235,236] and inhibition of the period circadian protein (per)-2 gene expression (one of the core clock genes) was observed during anesthesia.[237] Of note, psychotropic nonanesthetics, such as opioids, have been shown to affect melatonin secretion indirectly, independent of the behavioral state anesthesia in a pig model.[238] Previous work in humans has shown that 3 hours of anesthetic exposure does not affect the circadian phase of the body temperature rhythm.[239]

In summary, the specific mechanisms of anesthetics effects on circadian rhythm are unclear. The ability to distinguish between effects occurring directly on the circadian pacemaker and those occurring downstream from the pacemaker on other physiologic control systems requires additional research under rigorous experimental conditions.

Surgical treatment itself impairs sleep, expressed as reduced REM sleep duration even in the absence of general anesthesia.[229,230] Pain, inflammation, stress immobility, and anxiety seem to be contributing factors.[240] After surgery, patients show a significant impairment of sleep quality and duration. Eventually, it will be known whether specific anesthetics are preferable to avoid the adverse effects of sleep deprivation.

SLEEP-DISORDERED BREATHING AND AIRWAY PATENCY DURING ANESTHESIA

Perioperative complications occur more often in patients with OSA than in healthy controls,[241,242] but the reasons for this observation are unclear. It is challenging to isolate the effect of OSA from the known adverse effects on perioperative outcome of typical OSA comorbidities, such as hypertension, diabetes, coronary artery disease, neurovascular vulnerability, and obesity. Fortunately, severe postoperative complications are uncommon. As a consequence, large trials are needed to isolate the causal relationship between SDB and perioperative complications, such as severe respiratory failure, thromboembolic complications, increased hospital length of stay, and mortality.

Independent of obesity, OSA is not associated with difficult tracheal intubation or mask ventilation.[243-245] However, recent metaanalyses reported a significantly higher risk of postoperative major cardiac and cerebrovascular events, newly detected postoperative atrial fibrillation and acute postoperative respiratory failure, compared with control subjects.[246-248] These findings need to be confirmed in future prospective studies with a larger sample size and a more homogenous population such that confounding factors can be controlled. OSA is associated with postoperative delirium,[241,249] which is an important perioperative complication associated with increased costs, morbidity, and mortality. However, it is currently unclear if this is due to repetitive hypoxia or sleep fragmentation. In contrast, a

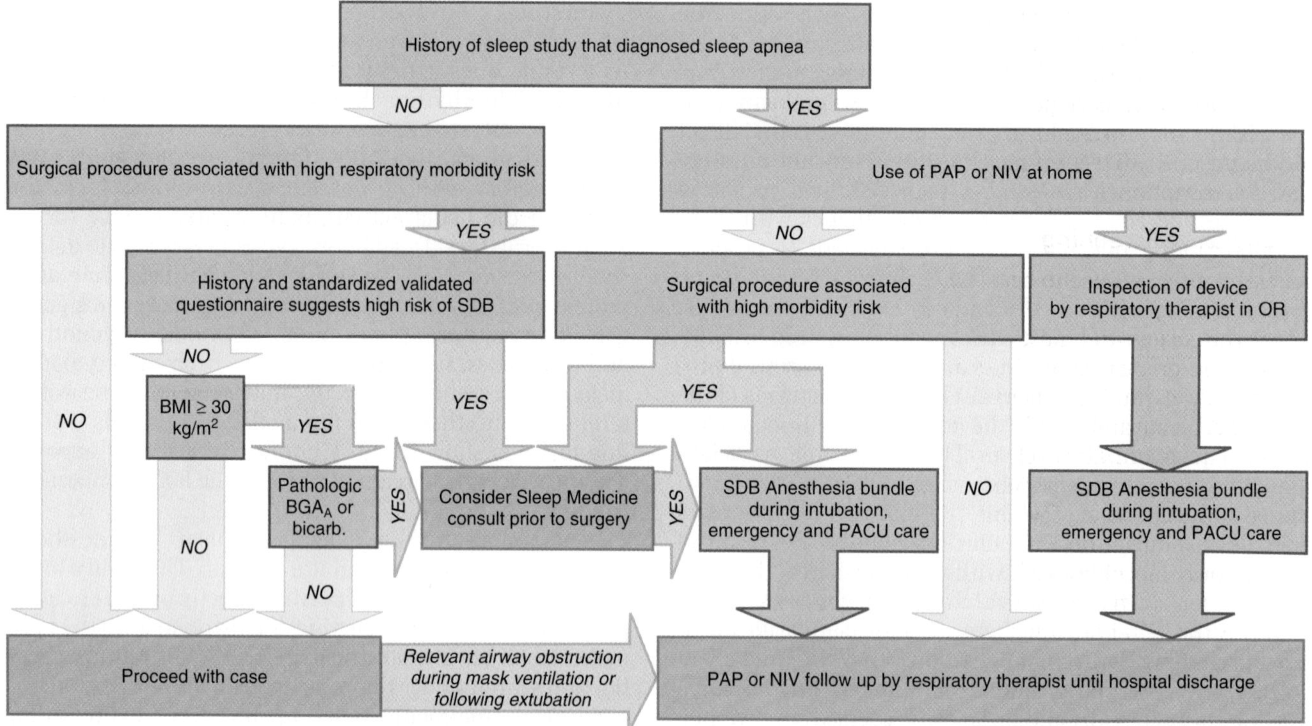

Fig 10.13 Clinical pathway for perioperative management of patients with sleep disordered breathing. *BGA*$_A$, Arterial blood gas analysis; *bicarb*, venous bicarbonate level; *BMI*, body mass index; *NIV*, noninvasive ventilation; *SDB*, sleep-disordered breathing; *PACU*, postanesthesia care unit; *PAP*, positive airway pressure.

recent study using the Nationwide Inpatient Sample database analyzed data from 1,058,710 patients undergoing elective surgery. These authors showed that patients previously diagnosed with SDB had significantly higher rates of emergent mechanical ventilation, use of NIV, and CPAP, as well as increased rates of respiratory failure. Nevertheless, the study also showed that patients with SDB had better outcomes after emergent intubation and had lower care-associated costs compared with their non-SDB counterparts.[250] Similar findings were reported by the same group for data from 91,028 patients undergoing bariatric surgery.[251] In this study, patients with a previous diagnosis of SDB had a shorter hospital length of stay and lower total costs compared with non-SDB patients. The reasons for the differences are unclear. Patients with a known history of sleep apnea may receive more sophisticated perioperative monitoring and more aggressive treatment of their respiratory disease, which might also explain the higher rate of postoperative reintubation in SDB patients reported in the same group.[250] Another possible explanation relates to the consequences of chronic nocturnal desaturation, which can have preventive effects in terms of the consequences of perioperative acute hypoxia. Most importantly, these findings indicate that the association of SDB, and perioperative outcome is likely to be more than a unidirectional relationship. More likely is that SDB could have a dual effect, leading to increased rates of perioperative respiratory complications in patients with SDB, but additionally protecting the same population from the fatal consequences of these complications. The mechanism of the potential link between OSA and postoperative respiratory failure, as well as postoperative delirium, is probably multifactorial. Frequent episodes of airway collapse in OSA lead to hypoxia, disrupted sleep, daytime sleepiness, and increased arousal threshold from sleep, all of which can be considered as potential precipitating or augmenting factors of postoperative complications. It is intriguing to note that patients with OSA appear to be most vulnerable to hypoxia on postoperative night two or three, the time interval during which postoperative delirium most typically manifests.

One population that might deserve additional attention in perioperative care is patients with OHS who, compared with obese patients, are more likely to be admitted to a hospital and require more healthcare resources.[250,252] In addition, higher rates of ICU admission, lengthier long-term care requirements at discharge, and higher mechanical ventilation rates have been reported in patients with OHS compared with severe obese patients without OHS.[251-254]

In summary, patients with SDB are more vulnerable to developing severe perioperative complications. Nevertheless, it is currently unclear whether these complications translate to a poorer overall postoperative outcome for these patients.

PERIOPERATIVE MANAGEMENT IN PATIENTS WITH SLEEP-DISORDERED BREATHING

The standard of care for perioperative management of patients with SDB depends on the severity of the disease, comorbidities, and the threat associated with the planned surgical procedure. It is probably neither feasible nor necessary to conduct a sleep study in all obese patients at risk for sleep apnea who are scheduled for surgery; however, high-risk patients need to be identified and treated perioperatively. Fig. 10.13 shows an algorithm that is being developed by an interdisciplinary international group of clinicians. The algorithm is driven by the idea that patients who have been prescribed CPAP preoperatively should continue to use CPAP perioperatively. Patients who carry several risk factors (procedural and comorbidity-based) may need a preoperative sleep medicine consultation and/or a CPAP prescription.

Preoperative Screening

Several strategies need to be considered to identify patients with SDB adequately.[94,253,254] Although clinical examination is the easiest and most cost-effective method of assessment using predisposing physical characteristics, it has a poor sensitivity and specificity of only 50% to 60% to diagnose OSA accurately.[255,256] However, the clinical value of using questionnaires relates to the fact that they help to identify a high-risk perioperative population, independently of the question of whether an individual patient has OSA. For example, the STOP-Bang questionnaire basically screens for comorbidities of OSA that we know increase the risk of perioperative complications (hypertension, obesity, male sex, older age) rather than direct breathing disorder–associated characteristics. The Score for Prediction of Obstructive Sleep Apnea might also be a helpful tool to predict patients with OSA and its perioperative outcome based on comorbidities and easily available clinical data.[257]

PSG is required to identify SDB specifically, but it cannot be used for preoperative screening of surgical patients. PSG is expensive, may delay surgery, and is inconvenient for the patient. A multistep approach of preoperative screening is required. Preoperative assessment should include a screening for SDB and for the current use of NIV. OSA might not represent real risk in patients scheduled for low-risk procedures from a surgery and anesthesia point of view. The authors believe that patients with no previously diagnosed SDB undergoing a low-risk surgical procedure should receive standard perioperative monitoring and treatment.

Patients undergoing high-risk surgical procedures should receive further workup using a clinical examination combined with standardized and validated questionnaires (e.g., Berlin).[254,258] Although this diagnostic algorithm might be a sufficient screening for OSA, it might be insufficient to detect OHS.[251,253] A blood gas analysis should be considered as a method to detect hypercapnia as a major symptom of OHS (criterion: awake daytime hypercapnia $PaCO_2 \geq 45$ mm Hg). Alternatively, a venous bicarbonate concentration ≥ 27 mmol/L is highly sensitive (92%) for an increased $PaCO_2$, which combined with hypoxemia ($SpO_2 \leq 94\%$) indicates a high risk of OHS in these patients.[251,253,256,259] Of note, OHS is a diagnosis by exclusion. Severe obstructive airway diseases, severe interstitial lung disease, severe chest wall disorders (e.g., kyphoscoliosis), severe hypothyroidism, neuromuscular disease, and congenital central hypoventilation syndrome need to be excluded, and further evaluation of sleep by a sleep medicine specialist before anesthesia should be considered. In these cases, the sleep specialist should determine the optimal diagnostic instruments in cooperation with the perioperative team, prescribe the perioperative auto-titrating CPAP device, and offer in collaboration with respiratory therapy specialists to improve tolerability of perioperative CPAP therapy.

Perioperative Management of Patients with Possible Sleep-Disordered Breathing

Although the data on optimal intraoperative and perioperative management are still limited, and mainly based on studies with low sample size, the techniques and procedures summarized in Box 10.2 might be considered during the perioperative management of patients with SDB.[258] Patients with a history of SDB who are undergoing surgery and anesthesia with high risk of morbidity should receive an "OSA anesthesia bundle" (see Box 10.2) that includes special procedures and preparations during tracheal intubation, extubation, pain therapy, and perioperative CPAP therapy.

Tracheal Intubation. Patients with OSA are frequently obese, and obesity is a risk factor for difficult intubation.[244,259-261] Patients should be preoxygenated efficiently before injection of the anesthetic drug. Sniffing and reverse Trendelenburg position are preferred before intubation, which improves maintenance of the passive (i.e., paralyzed) pharyngeal airway in patients with OSA[260,262] and increases functional residual capacity. To reduce the duration of paralysis, nondepolarizing neuromuscular blocking drugs should be used with caution supported by quantitative neuromuscular transmission monitoring. Immediately after successful intubation, a lung recruitment maneuver and the application of positive end-expiratory pressure for maintaining lung volume during surgery should be considered.[261,263]

Intraoperative Treatment. Impaired upper airway patency is of special concern whenever anesthetics are administered without a device that bypasses the collapsible upper airway—for example, during sedation for endoscopy.[264,265] While the overall rate of overt sedation-related complications for such procedures (e.g., endoscopy) appears low,[266] patients who are vulnerable to respiratory complications may suffer from sequelae of increased upper airway collapsibility beyond the immediately observable after intervention.

Opioids and GABAergic sedatives/hypnotics impair upper airway patency without any meaningful difference between compounds given at an equipotent dose of analgesics.[267-270] Of note, the impairing effects of GABAergic drugs on airway patency can be reversed by the respiratory stimulants (Fig. 10.14).[266] Thus it is recommended not to extubate patients at risk of postoperative airway collapse during hypocarbia but rather at mildly hypercarbic conditions.

Ketamine abolishes the impairment of upper airway patency during loss of consciousness and sleep,[271] and may be a viable adjunct to achieve postoperative pain therapy in patients at high risk of airway collapse.

Nondepolarizing neuromuscular blocking drugs should be titrated optimally by quantitative neuromuscular transmission monitoring to avoid residual neuromuscular blockade, which increases the risk of postoperative respiratory complications.[272-275] The effects of neuromuscular blockade should be reversed only when present, because inappropriate reversal can impair upper airway function in animals and humans.[274-276]

BOX 10.2 Special Sleep-Disordered Breathing Anesthesia Bundle: Special Procedures Performed During Anesthesia in Patients With Diagnosed Sleep-Disordered Breathing and Positive Airway Pressure or Noninvasive Ventilation Treatment

Preanesthesia Period

- Consider regional anesthetic techniques that minimize the chance of postoperative sedation.

Induction Strategy

- Monitoring: capnogram, tidal volume measurement
- Sniffing position
- Reverse Trendelenburg position
- Consider intubation without nondepolarizing NMBA; consider succinylcholine.
- Triple airway maneuver with two hands
- Utilize lung recruitment maneuvers immediately after intubation and apply PEEP for maintaining lung volume during surgery.
- PCV with PEEP
- Short-acting anesthetics and narcotics preferred
- Avoid high-dose steroidal NMBA.
- Use neuromuscular transmission monitoring.

Intraoperative Management

- Whenever possible, use of sedatives and narcotics should be reduced.
- Agents with reduced impairing effect on upper airway patency might be considered (e.g., ketamine, pentobarbital).
- Neuromuscular blockade should be monitored.
- Residual neuromuscular blockade should be reversed.

Extubation and Postanesthetic Care Unit

- Patient should be able to cooperate before extubation. Consider positioning of patients in PACU bed: upper body should be elevated by 45 degrees; lateral position preferred to minimize gravitational effects on the upper airway.
- In case of impaired respiratory function, a plan needs to be defined and documented for monitoring and treatment, including the consideration of noninvasive ventilation.
- Patients will be discharged to an unmonitored environment or home when they meet discharge criteria:
  - Vital signs within 20% from baseline
  - Adequate treatment of nausea
  - Pain score ≤40%
  - Aldrete-score ≥8
  - Passed room air challenge test

Pain Therapy

- Consider nonsteroidal antiinflammatory drugs to reduce opioid use whenever possible, if not contraindicated.
- Use caution when combining opioids with sedatives or hypnotics.

NMBA, Neuromuscular blocking agents; *PACU,* postanesthesia care unit; *PCV,* patient-controlled ventilation; *PEEP,* positive end-expiratory pressure.

Postoperative Care. OSA occurs during sleep and sedation;[277,278] therefore, tracheal extubation should be delayed until complete recovery of consciousness. Patients should be positioned with the upper body elevated by 45 degrees, which improves airway patency[261,262] and functional residual capacity. The lateral body position is an alternative for patients who do not tolerate an elevated upper body position. NIV is a viable treatment of postoperative respiratory failure and helps prevent deoxygenation and the development of postoperative negative pressure pulmonary edema; it can also prevent the respiratory depressant effects of opioids.[276,279]

Before discharge from the post anesthesia care unit, a room air-challenge test should be conducted. Several noninvasive monitoring devices have been developed for patients with and without risk for OSA. However, it is currently unclear if these devices can help prevent postoperative complications, and this requires further investigation.[280,281]

Pain Therapy. Pain treatment is of special concern during the postoperative period. Opioids dose-dependently reduce respiratory drive, and special caution is recommended when opioids are combined with sedatives or hypnotics. If not contraindicated, regional anesthesia and nonopioid analgesics should be considered to reduce opioid use whenever possible. If opioids are used, CPAP treatment throughout the early postoperative period may be beneficial in patients with high risk for OSA.[282] Pain intensity typically decreases over time following surgery. Decreasing opioid doses are typically required to maintain the balance of decreasing and increasing effects on respiratory drive.

Patients with SDB being treated with CPAP at home should proceed with these treatments throughout the perioperative period. Sufficient functioning of the treatment device needs to be checked preoperatively (see Box 10.2).

KNOWLEDGE GAPS AND FUTURE RESEARCH

Although a bold body of evidence on the effect of sleep-disordered breathing throughout the perioperative period has been published during the last decades, there are still large gaps of knowledge.[283,284] Respiratory, cardiovascular, and neuropsychological complications, as well as unfavorable clinical outcomes, may be more or less common in patients with OSA. However, there are many comorbidities that are potential confounders, such as obesity, diabetes, dyslipidemia, coronary artery disease, and increasing age. OSA is a heterogeneous disease, and detailed physiologic phenotyping could identify pathophysiologic mechanisms that increase or decrease risk of perioperative complications of OSA. Multiple mechanistic pathways that can lead to OSA (e.g., compromised anatomy, dilator muscle dysfunction, low arousal threshold, elevated loop gain, inadequate lung volume tethering, and vascular leak) are potentially relevant in a perioperative setting.[125] In-depth physiological studies are required until phenotyping can be accomplished with less time-intensive studies or through PSG. Noninvasive and readily available physiological studies or clinical prediction models that can characterize patients who have high-risk phenotypes of OSA are an important area of future research.

In this context, adequate screening tools for OSA during the perioperative period need to be identified. As stated

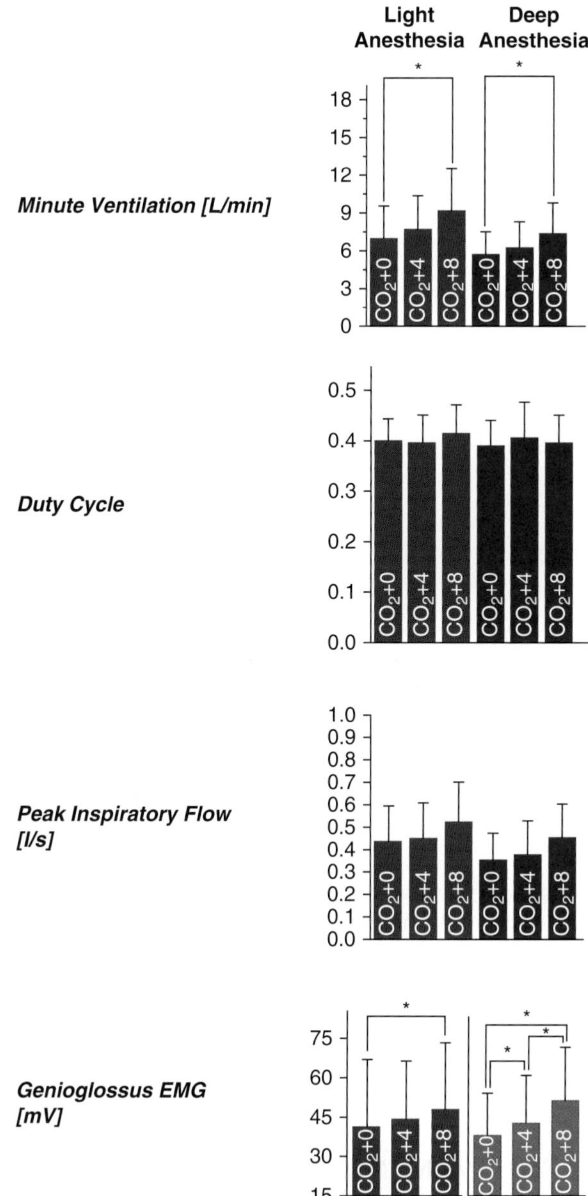

Fig. 10.14 Effect of carbon dioxide (CO2) level on genioglossus activity and respiratory function during anesthesia. Insufflation of CO2 to an increased pCO2 (+4 or +8 mm Hg) increases minute ventilation, peak inspiratory flow and upper airway dilating muscle activity (e.g. genioglossus muscle) in a dose-dependent fashion during deep (blue bars) and light (red bars) anesthesia. (Modified from Ruscic KJ, Bøgh Stokholm J, Patlak J, et al. Supplemental carbon dioxide stabilizes the upper airway in volunteers anesthetized with propofol. *Anesthesiology.* 2018;129(1):37–46.)

previously, PSG is often challenging to schedule before surgery, and ambulatory technologies may be more useful and should be studied. It might even be more important to identify patients at increased risk of postoperative complications due to specific type of surgery, required mode and depth of anesthesia and opioids, as well as other comorbidities, rather than the presence of SDB per se. It is currently unclear to which extent the risk for perioperative complications associated with SDB are due to or modulated by these coexisting factors. In addition, more severe OSA may be developed by some patients with no or mild OSA prior to anesthesia. Challenging factors are opioids, body position, or intravenous fluids. Some studies found early postoperative monitoring to detect patients with high risk for such aggravation of OSA severity. Additional research is needed to determine if and how postoperative monitoring is able to help stratify the risk for postoperative OSA. During the last few years, different approaches were made to improve postoperative management of patients with OSA (as discussed previously). However, open questions remain: What is the role of supplemental oxygen postoperatively? What are the barriers to CPAP adherence in the perioperative setting? Can patient adherence and positive airway pressure effectiveness be increased with educational resources? Should other respiratory support interventions be examined either in isolation or bundled with positive airway pressure? Is there a role for targeted positive airway pressure therapy, even with CPAP naive patients in very high risk groups? What are the medicolegal liability and patient safety factors to consider when starting CPAP in the hospital?[285]

Future research should aim to answer these questions to further improve the perioperative management of patients with sleep disordered breathing.[283] Testing a bundled approach to care (e.g., an algorithm of care including monitoring, positive airway pressure, education, and other respiratory supports) rather than each component individually might be more useful in initial clinical trials, as this may be more likely to be effective in improving outcomes.

The incidence of perioperative complications is low, and collaborative research networks are needed to identify a sufficient number of patients with OSA and answer the important research questions on perioperative outcomes. Patients with OHS might be at high risk. A minimal set of data elements required in prospective cohort studies should be identified to facilitate multisite collaboration and metaanalysis of independent studies. Case-control studies might also be nested within larger cohort studies. This would facilitate the choice of an appropriate control group. These studies may improve risk stratification and lead to novel targeted therapies. In addition, the identification of interventions that can optimize safety in this population is also important. Initial intervention trials should focus on patients at highest risk for sleep disordered breathing.[283]

Sleep and Sedation in the Intensive Care Unit

Impaired sleep is common in patients in the ICU,[286] with multiple contributing factors including noise, light, interruptions for medical procedures, and administration of fluids and nutrition, as well as endogenous factors such as pain, anxiety, and inflammation. Sleep duration in the ICU is variable depending on environmental conditions and the severity of the patient's disease.[287] Sleep fragmentation occurs consistently during sedation and mechanical ventilation.[288,289] The duration of deep NREM and REM sleep as well as circadian rhythms are severely reduced or abolished in ICU patients.[290-292] About 50% of sleep in these patients occurs during daytime hours.[286,287]. Altered EEG activity, not fitting into the standard criteria for sleep and wakefulness, was reported to occur in up to 70% of ICU patients who were receiving sedatives or being mechanically ventilated.[293] As a result, alternative classifications for sleep in the ICU have been developed;[294] however, these scoring classifications have not yet been validated.

TABLE 10.7 List of Studies Investigating Alteration of Circadian Rhythm and Sleep in Intensive Care Unit Patients

Measurement Method	Interactions	Reference
PSG studies	▪ Increased arousal during nighttime and disrupted sleep, due to: ▪ noise ▪ dim light ▪ medical intervention	292,296
	▪ Decrease N3- and REM-sleep ▪ Increase arousals and awakenings	302-304
	▪ Multiple discrete sleep episodes per 24 h ▪ Atypical EEG signal: ▪ disrupted sleep ▪ nonphysiologic sleep ▪ architecture, or evidence of coma	287,290,292,294
Melatonin blood levels and urinary 6-sulfatoxymelatonin urine levels	▪ Increasing chronodisruption with disease severity (rehabilitation patients, ICU patients, ICU patients with severe sepsis) ▪ Delayed melatonin peak at night	292,304-312
	▪ Reduced physiologic melatonin secretion at night, due to: ▪ sedation ▪ mechanical ventilation ▪ increased arousal	305,308,309
	▪ Increased melatonin levels during the day, due to: ▪ dim light ▪ severe sepsis	306,311
Blood pressure variation	▪ Reduced nocturnal blood pressure dip	305
Body temperature variation	▪ Reduced temperature variation ▪ Altered circadian rhythm with nadir dispersed widely across 24 h	23,305,313
Plasma cortisol level	▪ Abolished circadian rhythm ▪ Delayed peak of cortisol levels	305,310

EEG, Electroencephalography; *ICU*, intensive care unit; *N3*, sleep stage 3; *PSG*, polysomnography; *REM*, rapid eye movement.

NOISE AND LIGHT EXPOSURE

ICUs are among the most noisy areas in hospitals, with sound levels often exceeding those recommended by the World Health Organization (<45 dB).[289,295] Elbaz and associates[296] reported an increased incidence of arousals at sound levels above >77 dB in stable, mechanically ventilated ICU patients during the weaning phase. In the ICU setting, alarms from medical and monitoring devices were the most significant source of noise.

In addition to noise, changes in light exposure can alter sleep patterns and circadian rhythms. ICU patients are often exposed to dim light throughout the 24-hour cycle, resulting in increased light levels during the night and insufficient light exposure during the daytime.[297,298] This hinders the alignment (photoentrainment) of the internal circadian clock to the external 24-hour rhythm, potentially resulting in the disrupted sleep-wake pattern seen in many ICU patients.[299]

Impaired rhythmicity in melatonin secretion pattern in critically ill patients was reported in several studies (Table 10.7 for overview), and multiple factors influence melatonin rhythm in the ICU. Melatonin levels decrease with increasing age,[300] making older ICU patients more sensitive to circadian rhythm disruptions. Opioids increase melatonin levels throughout the 24-hour period.[301]

Similarly, β-agonists, including vasopressors, positive inotropes, and aerosolized albuterol, increase melatonin levels, whereas β-blockers decrease melatonin secretion. Also, endogenous production of catecholamines may induce periodic melatonin increases in patients with critical illness.[305] Benzodiazepines have inconsistent effects on melatonin.[314,315]

These interactive effects of critical illness and ICU treatment should be acknowledged while caring for ICU patients. Reduction of light and noise exposure during the night, and increased light levels during the day are recommended to improve sleep. In addition, earplugs and eye masks have been shown consistently to improve sleep quality in ICU patients and possibly reduce the risk of complications.[316-319]

MEDICATION AND MEDICAL PROCEDURES

Interruptions of sleep due to medical or nursing procedures are environmental factors in the ICU. Studies in different ICU settings found high numbers of interventions to be performed during the nighttime, ranging up to 60 interventions per night.[320-322]

Both NIV and ventilation via breathing tube impair sleep architecture and quality.[288,323] It is unclear how the issue of ICU-associated circadian disruption can be prevented or treated. Data suggest that weaning procedures during the daytime combined with assist control ventilation during the nighttime improve sleep, expressed as reduced numbers of arousal in patients requiring long-term ventilation.[291]

SLEEP AND SEDATION IN THE INTENSIVE CARE UNIT

Sedation is frequently required in the ICU to treat excessive agitation or to fulfill specific therapeutic needs; however, heavy sedation is associated with prolonged ICU and hospital stays.[324] GABA receptor agonists, such as propofol and benzodiazepines, may reduce REM sleep.[325,326]

Pain is a common experience for most patients in the ICU,[327] and failure to recognize pain can result in excessive administration of sedatives.[324] However, opioids have been shown to decrease REM-sleep and worsen sleep disorders, such as OSA in ICU patients.[131,328] Accordingly, an aggressive approach to managing pain while minimizing opioid utilization has been recommended.[329]

PHARMACOLOGICAL TREATMENT OF SLEEP DISTURBANCES IN INTENSIVE CARE UNIT PATIENTS

Medications currently used for the treatment of insomnia in the ICU interact with the GABA system. GABAergic neurotransmission has multiple functions throughout the brain, leading to daytime sedation, confusion, anterograde amnesia, and delirium.[330-332]

Melatonin has been selected as alternative sleep-promoting medication for critically ill patients in some countries. However, studies on the use of melatonin for the treatment of sleep disturbances and potential complications (e.g., delirium) in ICU patients have produced conflicting results. Administration of melatonin improved subjective and objective sleep quality in a small number of studies.[333-335] Melatonin may have side-effects such as dizziness, nausea, drowsiness, hypotension, and headache, potentially critical in the ICU setting. Recently melatonin receptor agonists have been developed and marketed for patients with circadian rhythm disorders.[336,337] These drugs may have fewer off-target effects than melatonin, but studies on their application in the ICU are very limited. It is therefore difficult to recommend treatment with melatonin agonists of any kind for ICU patients.[338]

The orexin receptor antagonist suvorexant has been approved by the FDA for the treatment of primary insomnia and might be another promising new approach for the treatment of insomnia in ICU patients. In a 4-week study in 254 patients with primary insomnia, suvorexant significantly improved sleep efficiency from the first night until the end of the study compared with placebo in a dose-dependent manner. In addition, suvorexant significantly improved wake after sleep onset and reduced sleep latency,[339] without an apparent delirium-promoting effect.[340] Additional research in the efficacy and safety of orexin receptor antagonists with critically ill patients is needed.

CONSEQUENCES OF SLEEP DISTURBANCE IN ICU PATIENTS

Compelling evidence links good sleep to proper metabolic, endocrine, immune, and neurobehavioral function.[341-345]

Regardless of controversies, the importance of a sufficient amount of good quality sleep for proper immunologic function, as well as the increased susceptibility for infection due to sleep loss, has gained increased acceptance.[346] Sleep deprivation during influenza vaccination delays the increase of antibody titers.[347,348] Sleep deprivation and insomnia is associated with decreased phagocytic activity of lymphocytes and natural killer T-cells, as well as lower levels of interleukin 2[349] and interleukin 7.[350] Interleukin 7 facilitates the transition of CD8þ effector to memory T-cells and lengthens survival of the T-cell memory cells.[351] Prolonged sleep deprivation, as may occur in long term ICU patients, may induce a persistent production of proinflammatory cytokines, producing a chronic low-grade inflammation, as well as immunodeficiency.[348]

Even short sleep deprivation in otherwise healthy young subjects has been shown to be associated with impaired glucose tolerance and insulin resistance, similar to levels usually seen in patients in the early course of diabetes mellitus.[352] In addition, sleep deprivation can induce the onset of a catabolic state: increased oxygen consumption, carbon dioxide production, and catecholamine levels, likely as signs of a stress response.[353] Changes in the activity of the hypothalamo-pituitary-adrenal axis with altered plasma levels of cortisol and thyrotropin,[354] as well as increased levels of inflammatory cytokines, are seen during sleep deprivation.[355]

It is likely that postoperative sleep deprivation also affects respiratory function, characterized as increased vulnerability to respiratory muscle fatigue,[356] decrease in ventilatory response to hypercapnia,[357] and greater upper airway collapsibility.[358]

Cognitive impairment after even short-term sleep deprived conditions is intuitive. Sleep deprivation causes bidirectional changes in brain activity and connectivity, thereby mainly affecting attention and working memory, and an increased vulnerability to delirium in critically ill patients.[359-361]

In addition, recent studies found beneficial effects of realignment of the sleep-wake cycles by pharmacologic and chronotherapeutic methods on the risk for delirium in these patients.[362-364] However, sleep-promoting agents per se can increase the vulnerability to delirium, and the optimal sleep-promoting agent that also minimizes the risk of delirium needs to be identified.

PERIOPERATIVE MANAGEMENT OF OTHER SLEEP DISORDERS

Narcolepsy

Narcolepsy is a neurologic sleep disorder with a prevalence of 0.05% to 0.8% in most ethnic groups.[365,366] It is characterized by excessive daytime sleepiness, involuntary daytime sleep episodes, disturbed nocturnal sleep, and sleep-associated muscular hypotension. Narcolepsy is divided into narcolepsy with or without cataplexy (sudden loss of muscle tone without loss of consciousness).[367]

An autoimmune pathology against hypothalamic orexin neurons may be involved in the pathogenesis of narcolepsy.[366] A mutation of the HCRT receptor 2 or loss of HCRT neurons have been shown to cause a narcolepsy-like state in animals,[368] and the deficiency of HCRT has been shown to be associated with narcolepsy in humans.[34] HCRT is involved in control of several biological functions such as feeding, cardiovascular regulation, upper airway stability, pain, locomotion, stress, and addiction.[369,370] Environmental factors play a key role in the pathogenesis of the disorder, as the disease concordance rate between monozygotic twins is only 20% to 35%.

Treatment of narcolepsy consists of behavioral treatment, as well as pharmacologic treatment for (1) daytime sleepiness and (2) cataplexies. Periodic and regular sleep times and scheduled daytime naps are recommended. Pharmaceutical treatments of daytime sleepiness include amphetamines, methylphenidate, modafinil, or selegiline (also effective for treatment of cataplexy), and cataplexies can be treated using tricyclic antidepressants, selective serotonin reuptake inhibitors, or γ-hydroxybutyrate/sodium oxybate. Medical treatment should always be accompanied by behavioral therapy.

Delayed emergence from anesthesia, postsurgical hypersomnia, and apneic episodes are in part related to an increased sensitivity to anesthetic drugs in narcolepsy patients.[371-373] Monitoring of anesthetic depth might be recommended in this patient population. Medical treatment of narcolepsy should be maintained during the preoperative period.[374,375] The most commonly used treatment of daytime sleepiness is modafinil, which acts via dopaminergic pathways and accelerates emergence from anesthesia.[376,377] Avoidance of sedative premedication and consideration of regional anesthesia may be indicated.[378] Of note, cataplectic events can also occur during regional anesthesia.[379]

Restless Legs Syndrome and Periodic Limb Movement Disorder

Restless legs syndrome, or Ekbom syndrome, is a neurologic disorder with a prevalence of 2% to 5% as defined by four cardinal features, including (1) the urge to move the limbs, usually associated with paresthesias or dysesthesias, (2) aggravating effects of rest, (3) ameliorating effects of physical activity, and (4) symptoms that worsen during the course of day, with a peak during the evening or at night. Patients with restless legs syndrome usually also complain about sensory symptoms in the legs.

Isolated periodic limb movement during sleep is a rare symptom, commonly referred to as *periodic limb movement disorder*. The characteristic periodic episodes of repetitive limb movements during sleep occur most often in the lower extremities, but occasionally in the upper extremities. These movements can be associated with frequent arousals leading to sleep disruption, causing excessive daytime sleepiness, which often is the only symptom reported by the patients themselves in most cases.[380]

Symptomatic restless legs syndrome can occur in patients with iron deficiency and uremia, during pregnancy,[381] or during the use of neurotropic medications (dopamine antagonists, neuroleptics, selective serotonin reuptake inhibitors, tricyclic antidepressants, antihistamines, caffeine, alcohol, nicotine). Although daytime symptoms of restless legs syndrome can be sufficiently diagnosed clinically (clinical examination in combination with standardized questionnaires), a PSG is recommended to rule out SDB, especially in patients complaining of daytime sleepiness or sleep fragmentation.

According to the most recent guidelines of the AASM, the first-line treatment of restless legs syndrome should consist of dopamine agonists (i.e., ropinirole and pramipexole) in the evening. Furthermore, gabapentin enacarbil, levodopa with dopa decarboxylase inhibitor, or opioids can be used. Medication impairing the dopaminergic system (dopamine antagonists, neuroleptics, selective serotonin reuptake inhibitors, and tricyclic antidepressants, antihistamines, caffeine, alcohol, and nicotine) should be avoided, if possible.

Exacerbation of restless legs syndrome may occur after general anesthesia,[382] and the urge to move the limbs may be misinterpreted as agitation or delirium.[383] The first manifestation of restless legs syndrome may occur after spinal anesthesia[384] or general anesthesia,[384] and the prevalence of restless legs syndrome after surgery seems to be higher than expected in this population.[382] To prevent perioperative exacerbation of symptoms, patients with restless legs syndrome should be scheduled for surgery early in the day. Restless legs syndrome medication should be continued until the day of surgery, whenever appropriate. Drugs that block the central dopamine transmission, such as neuroleptics, should be avoided. In contrast, ketamine might be the superior anesthetic drug for patients with restless legs syndrome.[385] In addition, intravenous or subcutaneous opioids and benzodiazepines during and after the surgery procedure might be beneficial in patients with restless legs syndrome. The best way to provide symptom relief in patients with restless legs syndrome might be early mobilization after surgery. In patients who are not eligible for mobilization, compression treatment[386] or intravenous administration of magnesium[387] and physiostigmine[388] have been shown to lead to relief of restless legs syndrome symptoms. Iron and ferritin blood levels should be monitored closely before, during, and after surgery, especially in surgical cases with iron loss (i.e., bleeding), to prevent symptomatic restless legs syndrome symptoms.

Acknowledgment

The editors, publisher, and Drs. Sebastian Zaremba and Matthias Eikermann would like to thank Dr. Nancy L. Chamberlin for her contribution to this chapter in the prior edition of this work. It has served as the foundation for the current chapter.

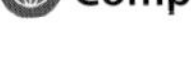

Complete references available online at expertconsult.com.

References

1. Rosner F, et al. *Anesth Analg.* 1971;50:298.
2. Rechtschaffen A, et al. *Perspect Biol Med.* 1998;41:359.
3. Mukherjee S, et al. *Am J Respir Crit Care Med.* 2015;191(12):1450.
4. Roesslein M, Chung F. *Eur J Anaesthesiol.* 2018;35(4):245.
5. Hobson JA. *Nature.* 2005;437(7063):1254.
6. Aserinsky E, Kleitman N. *Science.* 1953;118(3062):273.
7. Montgomery SM, et al. *J Neurosci.* 2008;28(26):6731.
8. Kronfeld-Schor N, Einat H. *Neuropharmacology.* 2012;62(1):101.
9. Kronfeld-Schor NaTD. *Biol Rhythm Res.* 2008;39(3):193.
10. Hastings MH, et al. *J Neuroendocrinol.* 2008;20(6):812.
11. Albrecht U. *Neuron.* 2012;74(2):246.
12. Lane JM, et al. *Nat Commun.* 2016;7:10889.
13. Danilenko KV, et al. *J Biol Rhythms.* 2003;18(2):170.
14. Borbely AA. *Hum Neurobiol.* 1982;1(3):195.
15. Dijk DJ, von Schantz M. *J Biol Rhythms.* 2005;20(4):279.
16. Hartse KM. *Handb Clin Neurol.* 2011;98:97.
17. Siegel JM. *Nature.* 2005;437(7063):1264.
18. Rial RV, et al. *Neurosci. Biobehav. Rev.* 2010;34(8):1144.
19. De Gennaro L, et al. *Neuroscience.* 2001;107(1):1.
20. Jahnke K, et al. *NeuroImage.* 2012;59(2):1631.
21. Kohsaka S, et al. *Neuroscience.* 2012;202:243.
22. Buckner RL, et al. *Ann N Y Acad Sci.* 2008;1124:1.
23. Alster J, et al. *Brain Inj.* 1993;7(3):191.

24. Lu J, et al. *J Neurosci.* 2006;26(1):193.
25. Pagel JF. *Curr Opin Pulm Med.* 2012;18(6):574.
26. Hallanger AE, et al. *J Comp Neurol.* 1987;262(1):105.
27. Satoh K, Fibiger HC. *J Comp Neurol.* 1986;253(3):277.
28. Lu J, et al. *Nature.* 2006;441(7093):589.
29. Fuller PM, et al. *J Comp Neurol.* 2011;519(5):933.
30. Aston-Jones G, Bloom FE. *J Neurosci.* 1981;1(8):876.
31. Kocsis B, et al. *Proc Nat Acad Sci U S A.* 2006;103(4):1059.
32. Peyron C, et al. *J Neurosci.* 1998;18(23):9996.
33. Kornum BR, et al. *Curr opin Neurobiol.* 2011;21(6):897.
34. Nishino S, et al. *Lancet.* 2000;355(9197):39.
35. Chemelli RM, et al. *Cell.* 1999;98(4):437.
36. Willie JT, et al. *Neuron.* 2003;38(5):715.
37. Fujiki N, et al. *Sleep.* 2003;26(8):953.
38. Adamantidis AR, et al. *Nature.* 2007;450(7168):420.
39. Trivedi P, et al. *FEBS Lett.* 1998;438(1-2):71.
40. Saper CB, et al. *Nature.* 2005;437(7063):1257.
41. Torrealba F, et al. *Neuroscience.* 2003;119(4):1033.
42. Mang GM, et al. *Sleep.* 2012;35(12):1625.
43. Dugovic C, et al. *J Pharmacol Exp Ther.* 2009;330(1):142.
44. Morairty SR, et al. *PLoS One.* 2012;7(7):e39131.
45. Gotter AL, et al. *Sci Rep.* 2016;6:27147.
46. von Economo C. *J Nerv Ment Dis.* 1930;71(3).
47. McGinty DJ, Sterman MB. *Science.* 1968;160(3833):1253.
48. Nauta WJ. *J Neurophysiol.* 1946;9:285.
49. Modirrousta M, et al. *Neuroscience.* 2004;129(3):803.
50. Hassani OK, et al. *Proc Natl Acad Sci U S A.* 2009;106(7):2418.
51. Takahashi K, et al. *Neuroscience.* 2009;161(1):269.
52. Sherin JE, et al. *Science.* 1996;271(5246):216.
53. Lu J, et al. *J Neurosci.* 2000;20(10):3830.
54. Saper CB, et al. *Neuron.* 2010;68(6):1023.
55. Anaclet C, et al. *J Neurosci.* 2012;32(50):17970.
56. Gerashchenko D, et al. *Proc Natl Acad Sci U S A.* 2008;105(29):10227.
57. Boissard R, et al. *Eur J Neurosci.* 2003;18(6):1627.
58. Lu J, et al. *Nature.* 2006;441(7093):589.
59. Johns MW. *Chest.* 1993;103(1):30.
60. Beaudreau SA, et al. *Sleep Med.* 2012;13(1):36.
61. Spira AP, et al. *J Gerontol A Biol Sci Med Sci.* 2012;67(4):433.
62. Sil A, Barr G. *J Laryngol Otol.* 2012;126(4):372.
63. Hesselbacher S, et al. *Open Respir Med J.* 2012;6:20.
64. Beaudreau SA, et al. *Sleep Med.* 2012;13(1):36.
65. Spira AP, et al. *J Gerontol A Biol Sci Med Sci.* 2012;67(4):433.
66. Chung F, et al. *J Clin Anesth.* 2007;19(2):130.
67. Aurora RN, et al. *Sleep.* 2012;35(8):1039.
68. Spruyt K, Gozal D. *Sleep Med Rev.* 2011;15(1):19.
69. Owens JA, et al. *Sleep.* 2000;23(8):1043.
70. Urfer-Maurer N, et al. *Sleep Med.* 2018;48:180.
71. Smarr BL. *J Biol Rhythms.* 2015;30(1):61.
72. Auger RR, et al. *Nat Sci Sleep.* 2013;5:125.
73. Kucharczyk E, et al. *Behav Sleep Med.* 2011;9(4):243.
74. Okun ML, et al. *J Clin Sleep Med.* 2009;5(1):41.
75. Chung F, et al. *Anesthesiology.* 2008;108(5):812.
76. Chung F, et al. *Br J Anaesth.* 2012;108(5):768.
77. Kessler RC, et al. *Sleep.* 2010;33(11):1539.
78. Walters AS, et al. *Sleep Med.* 2003;4(2):121.
79. Richards KC, et al. *J Nurs Meas.* 2000;8(2):131.
80. Wright JG, Feinstein AR. *J Clin Epidemiol.* 1992;45(11):1201.
81. Martin JL, Hakim AD. *Chest.* 2011;139(6):1514.
82. Paquet J, et al. *Sleep.* 2007;30(10):1362.
83. Ancoli-Israel S, et al. *Sleep.* 2003;26(3):342.
84. Henriksen A, et al. *J Med Internet Res.* 2018;20(3):e110.
85. Kushida CA, et al. *Sleep.* 2005;28(4):499.
86. Rechtschaffen A, et al. *A Manual of Standardized Terminology, Techniques and Scoring Systems for Sleep Stages of Human Subjects.* Washington, DC: National Health Institutes; 1977.
87. Berry RB, et al. *For the American Academy of Sleep Medicine. The AASM Manual for the Scoring of Sleep and Associated Events: Rules, Terminology and Technical Specifications.* Darien, IL: American Academy of Sleep Medicine; 2017. Version 2.4.
88. Epstein LJ, et al. *J Clin Sleep Med.* 2009;5(3):263.
89. Kuna ST, et al. *Proc Am Thorac Soc.* 2011;8(1):1.
90. Fleetham J, et al. *Can Respir J.* 2006;13(7):387.
91. Somers VK, et al. *J Am Coll Cardiol.* 2008;52(8):686.
92. Collop NA, et al. *J Clin Sleep Med.* 2007;3(7):737.
93. Kuna ST, et al. *Am J Respir Crit Care Med.* 2011;183(9):1238.
94. Finkel KJ, et al. *Sleep Med.* 2009;10(7):753.
95. Duce B, et al. *J Clin Sleep Med.* 2014;10(7):803.
96. Novelli L, et al. *J Sleep Res.* 2010;19(1 Pt 2):238.
97. White DP. *Am J Resp Crit Care Med.* 2005;172(11):1363.
98. Lindberg E. *Sleep Med Rev.* 2000;4(5):411.
99. Vozoris NT. *Sleep Med.* 2012;13(6):637.
100. Young T, et al. *WMJ.* 2009;108(5):246.
101. Schonbeck Y, et al. *PLoS ONE.* 2011;6(11):e27608.
102. Wang YC, et al. *Lancet.* 2011;378(9793):815.
103. Young T, et al. *N Engl J Med.* 1993;328(17):1230.
104. Kapur V, et al. *Sleep Breath.* 2002;6(2):49.
105. Bryson GL, et al. *Can J Anaesth.* 2012.
106. Stierer TL, et al. *J Clin Sleep Med.* 2010;6(5):467.
107. Weingarten TN, et al. *Br J Anaesth.* 2011;106(1):131.
108. Bamgbade OA, et al. *Int J Gynaecol Obstet.* 2017;138(1):69.
109. Young T, et al. *Am J Respir Crit Care Med.* 2002;165(9):1217.
110. Gottlieb DJ, et al. *Am J Respir Crit Care Med.* 1999;159(2):502.
111. Redline S, et al. *Am J Respir Crit Care Med.* 2010;182(2):269.
112. Carr GE, et al. *Chest.* 2012;141(3):798.
113. Selim B, et al. *Clin Chest Med.* 2010;31(2):203.
114. Tahrani AA, et al. *Am J Respir Crit Care Med.* 2012.
115. Yaffe K, et al. *JAMA.* 2011;306(6):613.
116. Torelli F, et al. *NeuroImage.* 2011;54(2):787.
117. Canessa N, et al. *Am J Respir Crit Care Med.* 2011;183(10):1419.
118. Lal C, et al. *Chest.* 2012;141(6):1601.
119. Balachandran JS, et al. *Am J Cardiol.* 2012;109(1):140.
120. Jennum P. *Kjellberg J. Thorax.* 2011;66(7):560.
121. Block AJ, et al. *N Engl J Med.* 1979;300(10):513.
122. Eikermann M, et al. *Chest.* 2007;131(6):1702.
123. Mak KK, et al. *Sleep Med.* 2010;11(3):268.
124. McNicholas WT, et al. *Am Rev Respir Dis.* 1982;126(4):625.
125. Subramani Y, et al. *Anesth Analg.* 2017;124(1):179.
126. Sasaki N, et al. *Anesthiology.* 2013.
127. Butler JE. *Respir Physiol Neurobiol.* 2007;159(2):115.
128. Pierce R, et al. *Eur Respir J.* 2007;30(2):345.
129. Chamberlin NL, et al. *J Physiol.* 2007;579(Pt 2):515.
130. Nicholas CL, et al. *Sleep.* 2012;35(5):699.
131. Timm FP, et al. *Sleep.* 2018;41(1).
132. Isono S, et al. *Anesthesiology.* 1997;87(5):1055.
133. Watanabe T, et al. *Am J Respir Crit Care Med.* 2002;165(2):260.
134. Isono S, et al. *Anesthesiology.* 2002;97(4):780.
135. Tagaito Y, et al. *Anesthesiology.* 2010;113(4):812.
136. Shiota S, et al. *Thorax.* 2007;62(10):868.
137. Su MC, et al. *Respir Physiol Neurobiol.* 2008;161(3):306.
138. Redolfi S, et al. *Am J Respir Crit Care Med.* 2011;184(9):1062.
139. Yumino D, et al. *Circulation.* 2010;121(14):1598.
140. Series F, Marc I. *J Appl Physiol.* 1994;77(2):840.
141. Hoffstein V. *Am Rev Respir Dis.* 1984;130(2):175.
142. Graaff Van de WB. *J Appl Physiol.* 1991;70(3):1328.
143. Graaff Van de WB. *J Appl Physiol.* 1988;65(5):2124.
144. Mead J, Loring SH. *J Appl Physiol.* 1982;53(3):750.
145. Schwartz AR, et al. *Am Rev Respir Dis.* 1991;144(3 Pt 1):494.
146. Isono S, et al. *J Appl Physiol.* 1997;82(4):1319.
147. Fogel RB, et al. *J Physiol.* 2003;550(Pt 3):899.
148. Jelev A, et al. *J Physiol.* 2001;532(Pt 2):467.
149. Jordan AS, White DP. *Respir Physiol Neurobiol.* 2008;160(1):1.
150. Gestreau C, et al. *Curr Opin Pulm Med.* 2008;14(6):512.
151. Fogel RB, et al. *J Physiol.* 2005;564(Pt 2):549.
152. Wilkinson V, et al. *Sleep.* 2008;31(4):525.
153. Lo YL, et al. *Thorax.* 2007;62(9):799.
154. Lan MC, et al. *Laryngoscope.* 2015;125(10):2408.
155. Isono S. *Eur Respir J.* 2017;50(3).
156. Safar P. *J Am Med Assoc.* 1958;167(3):335–341.
157. Sato S, et al. *Anesthesiology.* 2017;126(1):28.
158. Stanescu D, et al. *Eur Respir J.* 1996;9(10):2116.
159. Berry RB, Gleeson K. *Sleep.* 1997;20(8):654.
160. Pattinson KT. *Br J Anaesth.* 2008;100(6):747.
161. Szollosi I, et al. *Sleep.* 2006;29(8):1045.
162. Jordan AS, et al. *Am J Respir Crit Care Med.* 2011;184(10):1183.
163. Kushida CA, et al. *Sleep.* 2006;29(3):375.
164. Gay P, et al. *Sleep.* 2006;29(3):381.
165. Giles TL, et al. *Cochrane Database Syst Rev.* 2006;3:CD001106. 2006.

166. Schwab RJ, et al. *Am J Respir Crit Care Med*. 1996;154:1106.
167. McDaid C, et al. *Health Technol Assess*. 2009;13(4):143. iii, xi, 1.
168. Weaver TE, et al. *Am J Respir Crit Care Med*. 2012.
169. McEvoy RD, et al. *N Engl J Med*. 2016;375(10):919.
170. Morong S, et al. *Sleep Breath*. 2014;18(4):851.
171. Anandam A, et al. *Sleep Breath*. 2013;17(1):227.
172. Gunbey E, et al. *J Craniofac Surg*. 2015;26(4):1287.
173. Halle TR, et al. *Chest*. 2017;152(6):1214.
174. Lorenzi-Filho G, et al. *Respirology*. 2017;22(8):1500.
175. Kushida CA, et al. *Sleep*. 2006;29(2):240.
176. Corral J, et al. *Am J Respir Crit Care Med*. 2017;196(9):1181.
177. Malhotra A, et al. *Lancet Respir Med*. 2015;3(5):397.
178. Collop NA, et al. *J Clin Sleep Med*. 2011.
179. Randerath WJ, et al. *Eur Respir J*. 2011;37(5):1000.
180. Reckley LK. *Nat Sci Sleep*. 2018;10:105.
181. Kang KT, et al. *JAMA. Otolaygngol Head Neck Surg*. 2017;143(6):561.
182. Schwartz AR, et al. *Am J Respir Crit Care Med*. 2012;185(4):420.
183. Shelton KE, et al. *Am Rev Respir Dis*. 1993;148(2):462.
184. Oliven A, et al. *Eur Respir J*. 2008;32(5):1309.
185. Veasey SC, et al. *Sleep*. 2006;29(8):1036.
186. Morgenthaler TI, et al. *Sleep*. 2006;29(8):1031.
187. Roland PS, et al. *Otolaryngol Head Neck Surg*. 2011;145(suppl. 1):S1.
188. Malhotra A, Owens RL. *Respir Care*. 2010;55(9):1168.
189. Lanfranchi PA, et al. *Circulation*. 1999;99(11):1435.
190. Somers VK, et al. *Circulation*. 2008;118(10):1080.
191. Malhotra A, White DP. *Lancet*. 2002;360(9328):237.
192. Bixler EO, et al. *Am J Respir Crit Care Med*. 2001;163(3 Pt 1):608.
193. Young T, et al. *Arch Intern Med*. 2002;162(8):893.
194. Naughton MT, Lorenzi-Filho G. *Prog Cardiovasc Dis*. 2009;51(4):339.
195. MacDonald M, et al. *J Clin Sleep Med*. 2008;4(1):38.
196. Xie A, et al. *Am J Respir Crit Care Med*. 1950;152(6 Pt 1):1995.
197. Piper AJ. *Sleep Med Rev*. 2011;15(2):79.
198. Kessler R, et al. *Chest*. 2001;120(2):369.
199. Olson AL, Zwillich C. *Am J Med*. 2005;118(9):948.
200. Steier J, et al. *Thorax*. 2009;64(8):719.
201. Sampson MG, Grassino K. *Am J Med*. 1983;75(1):81.
202. Lopata M, Onal E. *Am Rev Respir Dis*. 1982;126(4):640.
203. Phipps PR, et al. *Thorax*. 2002;57(1):75.
204. Shimura R, et al. *Chest*. 2005;127(2):543.
205. Piper AJ, Grunstein RR. *Am J Respir Crit Care Med*. 2011;183(3):292.
206. Resta O, et al. *Respir Med*. 2000;94(3):240.
207. Zavorsky GS, Wilson B. *Respir Physiol Neurobiol*. 2010;170(1):120.
208. Ozsancak A, et al. *Chest*. 2008;133(5):1275.
209. Brown EN, et al. *N Engl J Med*. 2010;363(27):2638.
210. Kochs E, et al. *Anesthesiology*. 1994;80(5):1026.
211. Alkire MT, et al. *Science*. 2008;322(5903):876.
212. Hillman DR, et al. *Anesthesiol Clin*. 2010;28(3):443.
213. Lu J, et al. *J Comp Neurol*. 2008;508(4):648.
214. Tung A, Mendelson WB. *Sleep Med Rev*. 2004;8:213.
215. Nelson LE, et al. *Nat Neurosci*. 2002;5(10):979.
216. Moore JT, et al. *Curr Biol*. 2008;22(21):2012.
217. Harrison NL. *Nat Neurosci*. 2002;5(10):928.
218. Franks NP. *Nat Rev Neurosci*. 2008;9(5):370.
219. Eikermann M, et al. *Brain Res*. 2011;1426:30.
220. Tung A, et al. *Anesthesiology*. 2002;97(4):906.
221. Pal D, et al. *Anesthesiology*. 2011;114(2):302.
222. Brown EN, et al. *Annu Rev Neurosci*. 2011;34:601.
223. Leung LS, et al. *Prog Neurobiol*. 2014;122:24.
224. Guldenmund P, et al. *Br J Anaesth*. 2017;119(4):674.
225. Gogenur I, et al. *Br J Anaesth*. 2008;100(1):45.
226. Gogenur I, et al. *Surg Endosc*. 2009;23(5):1026.
227. Rosenberg J. *Sleep Med Rev*. 2001;5(2):129.
228. Rehberg S, et al. *Anesthesiology*. 2008;109(4):629.
229. Kjolhede P, et al. *J Clin Sleep Med*. 2012;8(4):395.
230. Krenk L, et al. *Br J Anaesth*. 2012.
231. Axelin A, et al. *Eur J Pain*. 2010;14(7):752.
232. Wang D, Teichtahl H. *Sleep Med Rev*. 2007;11(1):35.
233. Kondili E, et al. *Intensive Care Med*. 2012.
234. Gottschlich MM, et al. *J Burn Care Res*. 2011;32(5):535.
235. Mihara T, et al. *Anesth Analg*. 2012.
236. Cheeseman JF, et al. *Proc Natl Acad Sci U S A*. 2012;109(18):7061.
237. Poulsen RC, et al. *Sleep Med Rev*. 2018;37:35.
238. Lewczuk B, et al. *Neuro Endocrinol Lett*. 1999;20(3-4):171.
239. Sessler DI, et al. *Anesthesiology*. 1991;75(6):985.
240. Vandekerckhove M, Cluydts R. *Sleep Med Rev*. 2010;14(4):219.
241. Gupta RM, et al. *Mayo Clin Proc*. 2001;76(9):897.
242. Zaremba S, et al. *F1000Res*. 2016;5.
243. Benumof JL. *Curr Opin Anaesthesiol*. 2004;17(1):21.
244. Neligan PJ, et al. *Anesth Analg*. 2009;109(4):1182.
245. Eikermann M, et al. *Open Respir Med J*. 2010;4:58.
246. Kaw R, et al. *Br J Anaesth*. 2012.
247. Kaw R, et al. *Chest*. 2012;141(2):436.
248. Nagappa M, et al. *Anesth Analg*. 2017;125(6):2030.
249. Bateman BT, Eikermann M. *Anesthesiology*. 2012;116(4):753.
250. Mokhlesi B, et al. *Chest*. 2013;144(3):903.
251. Mokhlesi B, et al. *Obes Surg*. 2013;23(11):1842.
252. Berg G, et al. *Chest*. 2001;120(2):377.
253. Cullen A, Ferguson A. *Can J Anaesth*. 2012.
254. Lakdawala L. *J Perianesth Nurs*. 2011;26(1):15.
255. Nowbar S, et al. *Am J Med*. 2004;116(1):1.
256. Redline S, Strohl KP. *Clin Chest Med*. 1998;19(1):1.
257. Shin CH, et al. *BMC Anesthesiol*. 2017;17(1):71.
258. Memtsoudis SG, et al. *Anesth Analg*. 2018.
259. Mokhlesi B, et al. *Sleep Breath*. 2007;11(2):117.
260. Juvin P, et al. *Anesth Analg*. 2003;97(2):595; table of contents.
261. Corso RM, et al. *Minerva Anestesiol*. 2011;77(1):99.
262. Isono S, et al. *Anesthesiology*. 2005;103(3):489.
263. Myers TR. *Respir Care*. 2007;52(10):1308; discussion 1327.
264. Atkins JH, Mandel JE. *Curr Opin Anaesthesiol*. 2018;31(1):120.
265. Lo YL, et al. *J Clin Sleep Med*. 2015;11(9):1011.
266. Ruscic KJ, et al. *Anesthesiology*. 2018;129(1):37.
267. Simons JC, et al. *Anesthesiology*. 2016;125(3):525.
268. Overdyk FJ. *Anesthesiology*. 2010;113(1):259; author reply 260.
269. Hajiha M, et al. *J Physiol*. 2009;587(Pt 11):2677.
270. Eikermann M, et al. *Anesthesiology*. 2009;110(6):1327.
271. Eikermann M, et al. *Anesthesiology*. 2012;116(1):35.
272. Sundman E, et al. *Anesthesiology*. 2000;92(4):977.
273. Eikermann M, et al. *Am J Respir Crit Care Med*. 2007;175(1):9.
274. Sauer M, et al. *Eur J Anaesthesiol*. 2011;28(12):842.
275. Grosse-Sundrup M, et al. *BMJ*. 2012;345:e6329.
276. Eikermann M, et al. *Anesthesiology*. 2007;107(4):621.
277. Payne JP, et al. *Br J Anaesth*. 1980;52(1):69.
278. Fogel RB, et al. *Thorax*. 2004;59(2):159.
279. Zaremba S, et al. *Effects of CPAP treatment on respiratory function in the recovery room following weight loss-surgery: a cross-over design, randomized controlled trial*; 2013. ATS Abstract #43218 2013.
280. Zhang X, et al. *Front Med (Lausanne)*. 2017;4:26.
281. Rao Kadam V, Danesh M. *Sleep Sci*. 2016;9(3):142.
282. Zaremba S, et al. *Anesthesiology*. 2016;125(1):92.
283. Ayas NT, et al. *Ann Am Thorac Soc*. 2018;15(2):117.
284. Chung F, et al. *Anesth Analg*. 2016;123(2):452.
285. Gali B, et al. *Anesthesiology*. 2009;110(4):869.
286. Aurell J, Elmqvist D. *Br Med J (Clin Res Ed)*. 1985;290(6474):1029.
287. Freedman NS, et al. *Am J Respir Crit Care Med*. 2001;163(2):451.
288. Parthasarathy S, et al. *Am J Respir Crit Care Med*. 2002;166(11):1423.
289. Gabor JY, et al. *Am J Respir Crit Care Med*. 2003;167(5):708.
290. Cooper AB, et al. *Chest*. 2000;117(3):809.
291. Bosma K, et al. *Crit Care Med*. 2007;35(4):1048.
292. Gehlbach BK, et al. *Sleep*. 2012;35(8):1105.
293. Boyko Y, et al. *J Crit Care*. 2017;37:99.
294. Watson PL, et al. *Crit Care Med*. 2013;41(8):1958.
295. Tainter CR, et al. *Crit Care Med*. 2016;44(1):147.
296. Elbaz M, et al. *Ann Intensive Care*. 2017;7(1):25.
297. Fan EP, et al. *J Crit Care*. 2017;40:11.
298. Patel J, et al. *Anaesthesia*. 2014;69(6):540.
299. Oldham MA, et al. *Crit Care Med*. 2016;44(1):207.
300. Touitou Y. *Exp Gerontol*. 2001;36(7):1083.
301. Govitrapong P, et al. *J Pineal Res*. 1992;13(3):124.
302. Friese RS, et al. *J Trauma*. 2007;63(6):1210.
303. Hardin KA, et al. *Chest*. 2006;129(6):1468.
304. Elliott R, Nathaney A. *Aust Crit Care*. 2014;27(3):151.
305. Paul T, Lemmer B. *Chronobiol Int*. 2007;24(1):45.
306. Mundigler G, et al. *Crit Care Med*. 2002;30(3):536.
307. Olofsson K, et al. *Acta Anaesthesiol Scand*. 2004;48(6):679.
308. Frisk U, et al. *Clin Sci (Lond)*. 2004;107(1):47.
309. Perras B, et al. *Intensive Care Med*. 2007;33(11):1954.
310. Riutta A, et al. *Intensive Care Med*. 2009;35(10):1720.
311. Verceles AC, et al. *Intensive Care Med*. 2012;38(5):804.

312. Li CX, et al. *Mol Med Rep*. 2013;7(4):1117.
313. Gazendam JAC, et al. *Chest*. 2013;144(2):483.
314. Djeridane Y, Touitou Y. *Chronobiol Int*. 2003;20(2):285.
315. Morera AL, et al. *Prog Neuropsychopharmacol Biol Psychiatry*. 2009;33(6):1013.
316. Demoule A, et al. *Crit Care*. 2017;21(1):284.
317. Jones C, Dawson D. *Nurs Crit Care*. 2012;17(5):247.
318. Mills GH, Bourne RS. *Crit Care*. 2012;16(4):139.
319. Van Rompaey B, et al. *Crit Care*. 2012;16(3):R73.
320. Ugras GA, et al. *J Neurosci Nurs*. 2015;47(2):104.
321. Tamburri LM, et al. *Am J Crit Care*. 2004;13(2):102.
322. Celik S, et al. *J Clin Nurs*. 2005;14(1):102.
323. Ozsancak A, et al. *Crit Care Clin*. 2008;24(3):517. vi.
324. Kress JP, et al. *Am J Respir Crit Care Med*. 2002;166(8):1024.
325. Trompeo AC, et al. *Minerva Anestesiol*. 2011;77(6):604.
326. Kondili E, et al. *Intensive Care Med*. 2012;38(10):1640.
327. Turner JS, et al. *Crit Care Med*. 1990;18(9):966.
328. Bonafide CP, et al. *Anesthesiology*. 2008;108(4):627.
329. Shapiro BA, et al. *Crit Care Med*. 1995;23(9):1596.
330. Otmani S, et al. *Hum Psychopharmacol*. 2008;23(8):693.
331. Roth T. *J Clin Psychiatry*. 2007;68(suppl 5):13.
332. Hoque R, Chesson AL. *J Clin Sleep Med*. 2009;5(5):471.
333. Shilo L, et al. *Chronobiol Int*. 2000;17(1):71.
334. Ibrahim MG, et al. *Crit Care Resusc*. 2006;8(3):187.
335. Bourne RS, et al. *Crit Care*. 2008;12(2):R52.
336. Lockley SW, et al. *Lancet*. 2015;386(10005):1754.
337. Hatta K, et al. *Bellapart J, Boots R: Br J Anaesth*. 2012;108(4):572.
338. Bellapart J, Boots R. *Br J Anaesth*. 2012;108(4):572.
339. Herring WJ, et al. *Neurology*. 2012;79(23):2265.
340. Hatta K, et al. *J Clin Psychiatry*. 2017;78(8):e970.
341. Trinder J, et al. *Eur J Physiol*. 2012;463(1):161.
342. Imeri L. *Nat Rev Neurosci*. 2009;10(3):199.
343. Faraut B, et al. *Sleep Med Rev*. 2012;16(2):137.
344. Mullington JM, et al. *Prog Cardiovasc Dis*. 2009;51(4):294.
345. Lange T, et al. *Ann N Y Acad Sci*. 2010;1193:48.
346. Sareli AE, Schwab RJ. *Crit Care Clin*. 2008;24(3):613.
347. Spiegel K, et al. *JAMA*. 2002;288(12):1471.
348. Besedovsky L, et al. *Pflugers Arch*. 2012;463(1):121.
349. Irwin M, et al. *FASEB J*. 1996;10(5):643.
350. Benedict C, et al. *Brain Behav Immun*. 2007;21(8):1058.
351. Kaech SM, et al. *Nat Immunol*. 2003;4(12):1191.
352. Schmid SM, et al. *J Clin Endocrinol Metab*. 2007;92(8):3044.
353. Scrimshaw NS, et al. *Am J Clin Nutr*. 1966;19(5):313.
354. Spiegel K, et al. *Lancet*. 1999;354(9188):1435.
355. Sauvet F, et al. *J Appl Physiol (1985)*. 2010;108(1):68.
356. Chen HI, Tang YR. *Am Rev Respir Dis*. 1989;140(4):907.
357. White DP, et al. *Am Rev Respir Dis*. 1983;128(6):984.
358. Phillips B, et al. *South Med J*. 1987;80(1):16.
359. Krause AJ, et al. *Nat Rev Neurosci*. 2017;18(7):404.
360. Weinhouse GL, et al. *Crit Care*. 2009;13(6):234.
361. Ely EW, et al. *JAMA*. 2004;291(14):1753.
362. Potharajaroen S, et al. *Psychiatry Res*. 2018;261:21.
363. Burry L, et al. *BMJ Open*. 2017;7(3):e015420.
364. Luther R, McLeod A. *Nurs Crit Care*. 2017.
365. Longstreth WT, et al. *Sleep*. 2007;30(1):13.
366. Kornum BR, et al. *Curr Opin Neurobiol*. 2011;21(6):897.
367. Billiard M. *Sleep Med Rev*. 2007;11(5):377.
368. Lin L, et al. *Cell*. 1999;98(3):365.
369. Bonnavion P, de Lecea L. *Curr Neurol Neurosci Rep*. 2010;10(3):174.
370. Dauvilliers Y, et al. *Lancet*. 2007;369(9560):499.
371. Kelz MB, et al. *Proc Natl Acad Sci U S A*. 2008;105(4):1309.
372. Burrow B, et al. *J Clin Anesth*. 2005;17(1):21.
373. Mesa A, et al. *Anesthesiology*. 2000;92(4):1194.
374. Dahaba AA, et al. *Anesth Analg*. 2009;108(2):613.
375. Pelaez R, et al. *J Cardiothorac Vasc Anesth*. 2004;18(2):201.
376. Galvin E, et al. *Acta Anaesthesiol Scand*. 2010;54(2):154.
377. Larijani GE, et al. *Anesth Analg*. 2004;98(4):976.
378. Hu S, et al. *Anesth Analg*. 2018;126(1):233.
379. Soltanifar S, Russell R. *Int J Obstet Anesth*. 2010;19(4):440.
380. Aurora RN, et al. *Sleep*. 2012;35(8):1039.
381. Ohayon MM, O'Hara R. *Sleep Med Rev*. 2012;16(4):283.
382. Karroum EG, et al. *Ann Fr Anesth Reanim*. 2010;29(12):920.
383. Shin YK. *South Med J*. 1987;80(2):278.
384. Hogl B, et al. *Neurology*. 2002;59(11):1705.
385. Kapur N, Friedman R. *Anesth Analg*. 2002;94(6):1558.
386. Krishna M. *Anaesthesia*. 2007;62(9):973.
387. Bartell S, Zallek S. *J Clin Sleep Med*. 2006;2(2):187.
388. Alpert CC, et al. *Anesth Analg*. 2005;101(3):726; table of contents.

11 Cerebral Physiology and the Effects of Anesthetic Drugs

PIYUSH M. PATEL, JOHN C. DRUMMOND, and BRIAN P. LEMKUIL

KEY POINTS

- The brain has a high metabolic rate and receives approximately 12% to 15% of cardiac output. Under normal circumstances, cerebral blood flow (CBF) is approximately 50 mL/100 g/min. Gray matter receives 80% and white matter receives 20% of this blood flow.
- Approximately 60% of the brain's energy consumption supports electrophysiologic function. The remainder of the energy consumed by the brain is involved in cellular homeostatic activities.
- CBF is tightly coupled to local cerebral metabolism, a process called *neurovascular coupling.* When cerebral activity in a particular region of the brain increases, a corresponding increase in blood flow to that region takes place. Conversely, suppression of cerebral metabolism leads to a reduction in blood flow.
- CBF is autoregulated and remains constant over a mean arterial pressure (MAP) range estimated at 65 to 150 mm Hg, given normal venous pressure. CBF becomes pressure passive when MAP is either less than the lower limit or more than the upper limit of autoregulation. The lower and upper limits, as well as the range and slope of the plateau, manifest significant variability between individuals.
- CBF is also under chemical regulation. CBF varies directly with arterial carbon dioxide tension ($PaCO_2$) in the range of 25 to 70 mm Hg. When arterial partial pressure of oxygen (PaO_2) decreases to less than 60 mm Hg, CBF increases dramatically. Reductions in body temperature influence CBF primarily by the suppression of cerebral metabolism.
- Systemic vasodilators (e.g., nitroglycerin, nitroprusside, hydralazine, and calcium channel blockers) vasodilate the cerebral circulation and can, depending on the MAP, increase CBF. Vasopressors such as phenylephrine, norepinephrine, ephedrine, and dopamine do not have appreciable direct effects on the cerebral circulation. Their effect on CBF is via their effect on arterial blood pressure. When the MAP is less than the lower limit of autoregulation, vasopressors increase the MAP and thereby increase CBF. If the MAP is within the limits of autoregulation, then vasopressor-induced increases in systemic pressure have little effect on CBF.
- All volatile anesthetics suppress cerebral metabolic rate (CMR) and, with the exception of halothane, can produce burst suppression of the electroencephalogram. At that level, the CMR is reduced by approximately 60%. Volatile anesthetics have dose-dependent effects on CBF. In doses less than the minimum alveolar concentration (MAC), CBF is modestly decreased. In doses larger than 1 MAC, direct cerebral vasodilation results in an increase in CBF and cerebral blood volume (CBV).
- Barbiturates, etomidate, and propofol decrease the CMR and can produce burst suppression of the electroencephalogram. At that level, the CMR is reduced by approximately 60%. Because neurovascular coupling is preserved, CBF is decreased. Opiates and benzodiazepines effect minor decreases in CBF and CMR. In contrast, ketamine can increase CBF significantly, in association with a modest increase in CMR.
- Brain stores of oxygen and substrates are limited, and the brain is extremely sensitive to decreases in CBF. Severe decreases in CBF (<6-10 mL/100 g/min) lead to rapid neuronal death. Ischemic injury is characterized by early excitotoxicity and delayed apoptosis.
- Barbiturates, propofol, ketamine, volatile anesthetics, and xenon have neuroprotective efficacy and can reduce ischemic cerebral injury in experimental models. This anesthetic neuroprotection is sustained only when the severity of the ischemic insult is mild; with moderate-to-severe injury, long-term neuroprotection is not achieved. The neuroprotective efficacy of anesthetics in humans is limited. Administration of etomidate can decrease regional blood flow, which can exacerbate ischemic brain injury.

This chapter reviews the effects of anesthetic drugs and techniques on cerebral physiology—in particular, their effects on cerebral blood flow (CBF) and metabolism. The final section presents a brief discussion of pathophysiologic states, including cerebral ischemia and cerebral protection. Attention is directed to the rationale for selection and appropriate use of the anesthetic agents for neuroanesthetic management. Chapter 57 presents the clinical management of these patients in detail. Neurologic monitoring, including the effects of anesthetics on the electroencephalogram (EEG) and evoked responses, is reviewed in Chapter 39.

The Anatomy of the Cerebral Circulation

The arterial blood supply to the brain is composed of paired right and left internal carotid arteries, which give rise to the anterior circulation, and paired right and left vertebral arteries, which give rise to the posterior circulation. The connection of the two vertebral arteries forms the basilar artery. The internal carotid arteries and the basilar artery connect to form a vascular loop called the circle of Willis at the base of the brain that permits collateral circulation between both the right and left and the anterior and posterior perfusing arteries. Three paired arteries that originate from the circle of Willis perfuse the brain: anterior, middle, and posterior cerebral arteries. The posterior communicating arteries and the anterior communicating artery complete the loop. The anterior and the posterior circulations contribute equally to the circle of Willis.

Under normal circumstances, blood from the anterior and posterior circulations does not admix because the pressures in the two systems are equal. Similarly, side-to-side admixing of blood across the circle is limited. The vessels that originate from the circle provide blood flow to well-delineated regions of the brain. However, in pathologic circumstances during which occlusion of one of the arterial branches occurs, the circle of Willis can provide anterior-posterior or side-to-side collateralization to deliver flow to the region of the brain with reduced perfusion.

A complete circle of Willis is shown in Fig. 11.1*A*. However, substantial variability exists in the anatomy of the circle of Willis, and a significant proportion of individuals may have an incomplete circular loop.[1] The variations in the circle and their prevalence are shown in Fig. 11.1*B*.

Three sets of veins drain blood from the brain. The superficial cortical veins are within the pia mater on the brain's surface. Deep cortical veins drain the deeper structures of the brain. These veins drain into dural sinuses, of which the superior and inferior sagittal sinuses and the straight, transverse and sigmoid sinuses are the major dural sinuses. These ultimately drain into the right and left internal jugular veins.A schematic representation of the cerebral venous circulation is shown in Fig. 11.1*C*.

There is considerable asymmetry in the blood flow between the right and left internal jugular veins. In approximately 65% of patients, flow in the right IJV is greater than in the left; in the remainder, the left IJV is dominant.[2] The pattern of venous drainage may have implications for insertion of jugular venous catheters for the measurement of jugular venous oxygen saturation ($SjVO_2$). To ensure accurate measurement of $SjVO_2$, it has been advocated that the catheter be inserted into the dominant jugular vein. In most patients, the right IJV will be the dominant vein.

CEREBROSPINAL FLUID FORMATION AND CIRCULATION

Cerebrospinal fluid (CSF) is produced primarily by the choroid plexus in the lateral, third, and fourth ventricles; there are small contributions from the endothelial cells and from fluid that is produced as a consequence of metabolic activity. CSF production is the result of hydrostatic efflux from capillaries into the perivascular space, and then active transport into the ventricles. CSF reabsorption occurs primarily via the arachnoid granulations present in the dural sinuses. A smaller proportion of CSF, which tracks along cranial and peripheral nerves, perivascular routes, and along white matter tracts, gains access to the cerebral venous system by transependymal flow. The total CSF space is approximately 150 mL and total daily CSF production averages 450 mL. Therefore, there is a substantial daily turnover of CSF. CSF production is also under the influence of the circadian rhythm, with the peak production of CSF occurring during sleep.[3]

Recently, the concept of the glymphatic pathway as a means by which waste products are removed from the brain has been advanced. Conceptually, the glymphatic pathway can be visualized as a system akin to the lymphatic system in the systemic circulation (note, however, that the brain does not contain lymphatics other than those present in the meninges). Functionally, CSF enters the periarterial space, a space that is bounded by the vessels and the end-feet of astrocytes. Aquaporin channels on the end-feet facilitate this water exchange. From the periarterial space, CSF is transported to the brain parenchyma, and from there to the perivenous space and on to the ventricles. As such, the glymphatic system serves as a waste disposal system.[3] Of considerable interest is the observation that the periarterial space increases significantly during sleep and during general anesthesia; hence, glymphatic transport and waste clearance is increased during these states. Among anesthetic agents, glymphatic transport is reduced by volatile agents but is less affected by dexmedetomidine.[4]

REGULATION OF CEREBRAL BLOOD FLOW

Anesthetic drugs cause dose-related and reversible alterations in many aspects of cerebral physiology, including CBF, cerebral metabolic rate (CMR), and electrophysiologic function (EEG, evoked responses). The effects of anesthetic drugs and techniques have the potential to adversely affect the diseased brain and are thus of clinical importance in patients with neurosurgical disease. Conversely, the effects of general anesthesia on CBF and CMR can be altered to improve both the surgical course and the clinical outcome of patients with neurologic disorders.

The adult human brain weighs approximately 1350 g and therefore represents approximately 2% of total body weight. However, it receives 12% to 15% of cardiac output. This high flow rate is a reflection of the brain's high metabolic rate. At rest, the brain consumes oxygen at an average

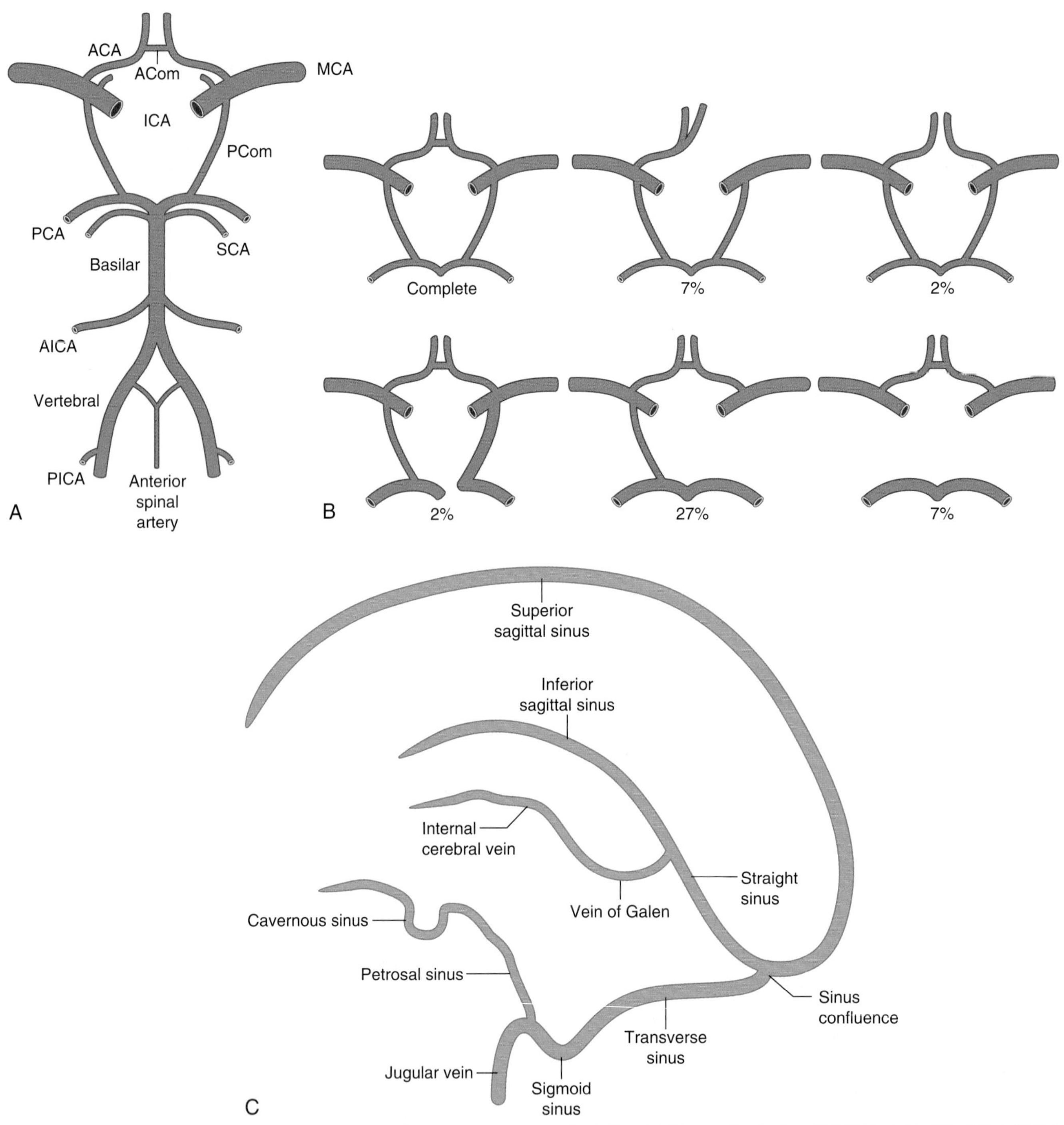

Fig. 11.1 Vascular anatomy of the blood supply to and drainage from the brain. (A) Arterial input into a complete circle of Willis. *ACA,* Anterior cerebral artery; *ACom,* anterior communicating artery; *AICA,* anterior inferior cerebellar artery; *ICA,* internal carotid artery; *MCA,* middle cerebral artery; *PCA,* posterior cerebral artery; *PCom,* posterior communicating artery; *PICA,* posterior inferior cerebellar artery; *SCA,* superior cerebellar artery. (B) Variations in the anatomy of the circle of Willis. The prevalence of each of the variations, expressed as percentage of adult patients, is provided for each variant. (C) Venous drainage of the brain.

rate of approximately 3.5 mL of oxygen per 100 g of brain tissue per minute. Whole-brain oxygen consumption (50 mL/min) represents approximately 20% of total body oxygen utilization. Normal values for CBF, CMR, and other physiologic variables are provided in Box 11.1.

Approximately 60% of the brain's energy consumption supports electrophysiologic function. The depolarization-repolarization activity that occurs, reflected in the EEG, requires expenditure of energy for the maintenance and restoration of ionic gradients and for the synthesis, transport, release, and reuptake of neurotransmitters. The remainder of the energy consumed by the brain is involved in cellular homeostatic activities (Fig. 11.2). Local CBF and CMR within the brain are very heterogeneous, and both are approximately four times greater in gray matter than in white matter. The cell population of the brain is also heterogeneous in its oxygen requirements. Glial cells make up approximately one half of the

BOX 11.1 Normal Cerebral Physiologic Values (Values Updated)

CBF	
Global	45-55 mL/100 g/min
Cortical (mostly gray matter)	75-80 mL/100 g/min
Subcortical (mostly white matter)	8-20 mL/100 g/min
$CMRO_2$	3-3.5 mL/100 g/min
CVR	1.5-2.1 mm Hg/100 g/min/mL
Cerebral venous Po_2	32-44 mm Hg
Cerebral venous So_2	55%-70%
rSO2	55%-80%
$SjVo_2$	60%-70%
ICP (supine)	8-12 mm Hg

CBF, Cerebral blood flow; *$CMRO_2$*, cerebral metabolic rate of oxygen; *CVR*, cerebral vascular resistance; *ICP*, intracranial pressure; *Po_2*, partial pressure of oxygen; *rSO_2*, regional oxygen saturation measured by near-infrared spectroscopy; *So_2*, oxygen saturation; *$SjVo_2$*, jugular venous oxygen saturation.

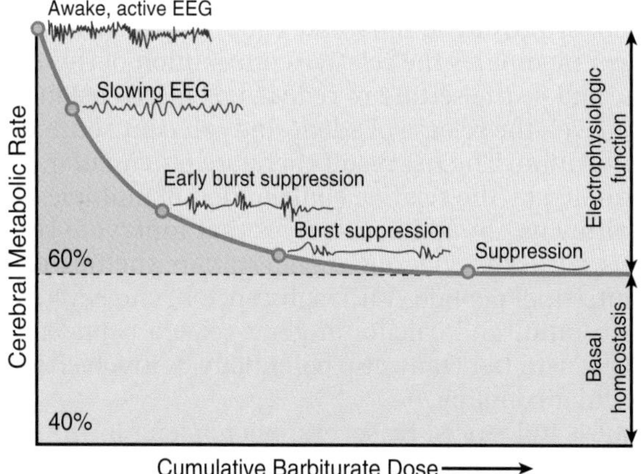

Fig. 11.2 Interdependency of cerebral electrophysiologic function and cerebral metabolic rate (CMR). Administration of various anesthetics, including barbiturates, results in a dose-related reduction in the CMR of oxygen ($CMRO_2$) and cerebral blood flow (CBF). The maximum reduction occurs with the dose that results in electrophysiologic silence. At this point, the energy utilization associated with electrophysiologic activity has been reduced to zero, but the energy utilization for cellular homeostasis persists unchanged. Additional barbiturates cause no further decrease in CBF or $CMRO_2$. *EEG*, Electroencephalogram.

brain's volume and require less energy than neurons. Besides providing a physically supportive latticework for the brain, glial cells are important in the reuptake of neurotransmitters, in the delivery and removal of metabolic substrates and wastes, and in blood-brain barrier (BBB) function.

Given the limited local storage of energy substrate, the brain's substantial demand for substrate must be met by adequate delivery of oxygen and glucose. However, the space constraints imposed by the noncompliant cranium and meninges require that blood flow not be excessive. Not surprisingly, elaborate mechanisms regulate CBF. These mechanisms, which include myogenic, chemical, and autonomic neural factors, are listed in Table 11.1.

TABLE 11.1 Factors Influencing Cerebral Blood Flow

Factor	Comment
CHEMICAL, METABOLIC, HUMORAL	
CMR	CMR influence assumes intact flow-metabolism coupling, the mechanism of which is not fully understood.
Anesthetics	
Temperature	
Arousal; seizures	
$Paco_2$	
Pao_2	
Cardiac output	
Vasoactive drugs	
Anesthetics	
Vasodilators	
Vasopressors	
MYOGENIC	
Autoregulation; MAP	The autoregulation mechanism is fragile; in many pathologic states, CBF is regionally pressure passive.
RHEOLOGIC	
Blood viscosity	
NEUROGENIC	
Extracranial sympathetic and parasympathetic pathways	Contribution and clinical significance are poorly defined.
Intraaxial pathways	

See text for discussion.

CBF, Cerebral blood flow; *CMR*, cerebral metabolic rate; *MAP*, mean arterial pressure; *$Paco_2$*, arterial partial pressure of carbon dioxide; *Pao_2*, arterial partial pressure of oxygen.

MYOGENIC REGULATION (AUTOREGULATION) OF CEREBRAL BLOOD FLOW

The conventional view of autoregulation is that the cerebral circulation adjusts its resistance to maintain CBF relatively constant over a wide range of mean arterial pressure (MAP) values. In normal human subjects, CBF is autoregulated between 70 mm Hg (lower limit of autoregulation, LLA) and 150 mm Hg (upper limit of autoregulation, ULA) (Fig. 11.3).[5] There is, however, considerable variation between subjects in the autoregulation limits. Cerebral perfusion pressure is the difference between the MAP and the intracranial pressure (ICP). Because ICP is not usually measured in normal subjects, cerebral perfusion pressure (CPP = MAP − ICP) is rarely available. Assuming a normal ICP of 5 to 10 mm Hg in a supine subject, an LLA of 70 mm Hg expressed as MAP corresponds to a LLA of approximately 60 to 65 mm Hg expressed as CPP. Above and below the autoregulatory plateau, CBF is pressure-dependent (pressure-passive) and linearly varies with CPP. Autoregulation is influenced by the time course over which the changes in CPP occur. Even within the range over which autoregulation normally occurs, a rapid change in arterial pressure will result in a transient (i.e., 3-4 minute) alteration in CBF.

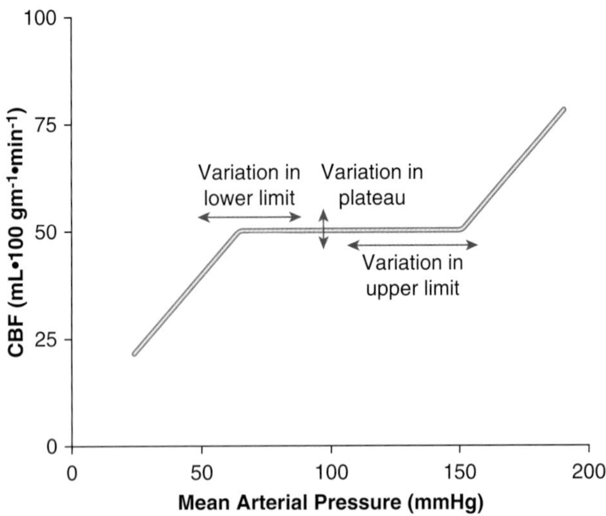

Fig. 11.3 The conventional view of cerebral autoregulation. Cerebral blood flow (CBF) is maintained within the normal range in the face of widely varying blood pressures. Below the lower limit of autoregulation, approximately 65 to 70 mm Hg in humans, and above the upper limit, approximately 150 mm Hg, the cerebral circulation is pressure passive and CBF decreases or increases, respectively, with corresponding changes in mean arterial pressure. Note that there is considerable intersubject variation in the limits of the autoregulatory plateau; the extent of this variation is depicted by the arrows. The autoregulatory curve should not be considered fixed and static but as a dynamically changing response to the cerebral circulation to changes in blood pressure.

The limits of autoregulation and the autoregulatory plateau are conceptual frameworks for the purpose of analysis. They do not represent physiologic "all-or-none" responses. There is considerable variability in the LLA and ULA as well as in the limits of the plateau (see the section on "An Integrated Contemporary View of Cerebral Autoregulation").

The precise mechanisms by which autoregulation is accomplished and its overlap with neurovascular coupling are not known. According to the myogenic hypothesis, changes in CPP lead to direct changes in the tone of vascular smooth muscle; this process appears to be passive. Nitric oxide (NO) and calcium channels may participate in the vasodilation associated with hypotension.

CHEMICAL REGULATION OF CEREBRAL BLOOD FLOW

Several factors, including changes in CMR, arterial partial pressure of carbon dioxide ($Paco_2$), and arterial partial pressure of oxygen (Pao_2) cause alterations in the cerebral biochemical environment that result in adjustments in CBF.

Cerebral Metabolic Rate

Regional CBF and metabolism are tightly coupled. They involve a complex physiologic process regulated, not by a single mechanism, but by a combination of metabolic, glial, neural, and vascular factors. Increased neuronal activity results in increased local brain metabolism, and this increase in the CMR is associated with a proportional change in CBF referred to as *neurovascular coupling*. The traditional view of neurovascular coupling is that it is a positive feedback mechanism wherein increased neuronal activity results in a demand for energy; this demand is met by an increase in CBF. More recent data indicate that coupling is based on a feed-forward mechanism wherein neuronal activity directly increases CBF, thereby increasing energy supply.[6] Although the precise mechanisms that mediate neurovascular coupling have not been defined, the data available implicate local by-products of metabolism (e.g., potassium ion [K^+], hydrogen ion [H^+], lactate, adenosine, and adenosine triphosphate [ATP]). Increased synaptic activity with the attendant release of glutamate leads to the downstream generation of a variety of mediators that affect vascular tone (Fig. 11.4). Glutamate, released with increased neuronal activity, results in the synthesis and release of NO, a potent cerebral vasodilator that plays an important role in neurovascular coupling. Glia also play an important role in neurovascular coupling. Their processes make contact with neurons, and these processes may serve as conduits for the coupling of increased neuronal activity to increases in blood flow. Glutamate activation of metabotropic glutamate receptors (mGluR) in astrocytes leads to arachidonic acid (AA) metabolism and the subsequent generation of prostaglandins and epoxyeicosatrienoic acids. Oxygen modulates the relative contribution of these pathways, and in the setting of reduced oxygen tension at the tissue level, the release of adenosine can contribute to vascular dilation. The net result therefore on vascular tone is determined by the relative contribution of multiple signaling pathways. In addition, nerves that innervate cerebral vessels release peptide neurotransmitters such as vasoactive intestinal peptide (VIP), substance P, cholecystokinin, somatostatin, and calcitonin gene–related peptide. These neurotransmitters may also potentially be involved in neurovascular coupling.

CMR is influenced by several phenomena in the neurosurgical environment, including the functional state of the nervous system, anesthetic drugs, and temperature.

Functional state. CMR decreases during sleep and increases during sensory stimulation, mental tasks, or arousal of any cause. During epileptic activity, increases in the CMR may be extreme, whereas regionally, after brain injury and globally with coma, the CMR may be substantially reduced.

Anesthetic drugs. The effect of individual anesthetic drugs on the CMR is presented in greater detail in the second section of this chapter. In general, anesthetic drugs suppress the CMR, with the exception of ketamine and nitrous oxide (N_2O). The component of the CMR on which they act is electrophysiologic function. With several anesthetics, including barbiturates, isoflurane, sevoflurane, desflurane, propofol, and etomidate, increasing plasma concentrations cause progressive suppression of EEG activity and a concomitant reduction in the CMR. However, increasing the plasma level beyond what is required to first achieve suppression of the EEG results in no further depression of the CMR. The component of the CMR required for the maintenance of cellular integrity, the "housekeeping" component, is unaltered by anesthetic drugs (see Fig. 11.2).

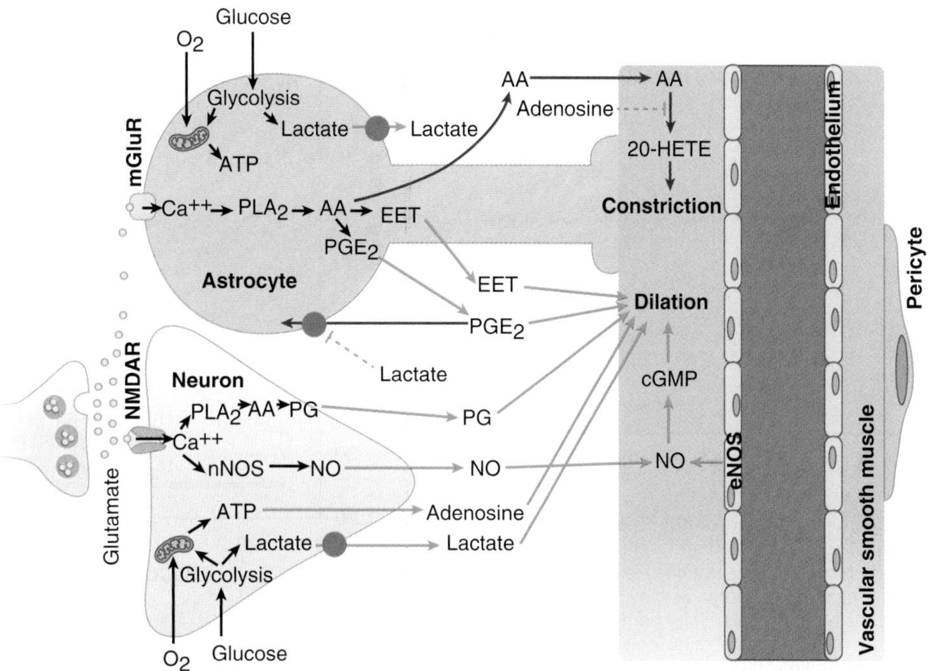

Fig. 11.4 Cerebral neurovascular coupling. Synaptic activity leads to glutamate release, activation of glutamatergic receptors, and calcium entry in neurons. This results in a release of arachidonic acid *(AA)*, prostaglandins *(PGs)*, and nitric oxide *(NO)*. Adenosine and lactate are generated from metabolic activity. These factors all lead to vascular dilation. Glutamate also activates metabotropic glutamate receptors *(mGluR)* in astrocytes, causing intracellular calcium entry, phospholipase A_2 *(PLA_2)* activation, release of AA and epoxyeicosatrienoic *(EET)* acid and prostaglandin E_2 *(PGE_2)*. The latter two AA metabolites contribute to dilation. By contrast, AA can also be metabolized to 20-hydroxyl-eicosatetraenoic acid *(20-HETE)* in vascular smooth muscle. 20-HETE is a potent vascular constrictor. *cGMP*, Cyclic guanosine monophosphate; *eNOS*, endothelial nitric oxide synthase; *NMDAR*, *N*-methyl D-aspartate (NMDA) glutamate receptor; *nNOS*, neuronal nitric oxide synthase. (Modified from Attwell D, Buchan AM, Charpak S, et al. Glial and neuronal control of brain blood flow. *Nature*. 2010;468(7321):232–243.)

When the complete suppression of EEG is achieved, the cerebral metabolic rate of oxygen ($CMRO_2$) is similar irrespective of the anesthetic agent used to achieve EEG suppression. Yet anesthetic-induced EEG suppression is not a single physiologic state and is influenced by the drug used to produce suppression. When barbiturates are administered to the point of EEG suppression, a uniform depression in the CBF and CMR occurs throughout the brain. When suppression occurs during the administration of isoflurane and sevoflurane, the relative reductions in the CMR and CBF are more intense in the neocortex than in other portions of the cerebrum. Electrophysiologic responsiveness also varies. Cortical somatosensory evoked responses to median nerve stimulation can be readily recorded at doses of thiopental far in excess of those required to cause complete suppression of the EEG but are difficult to elicit at concentrations of isoflurane associated with a burst-suppression pattern (~1.5 minimum alveolar concentration [MAC]). In addition, the EEG characteristics of the burst-suppression states that occur just before complete suppression differ among anesthetic drugs. These differences may be of some relevance to discussions of differences in the neuroprotective potential of drugs that can produce EEG suppression.

Temperature. The effects of hypothermia on the brain have been reviewed in detail.[7] The CMR decreases by 6% to 7% per degree Celsius of temperature reduction. In addition to anesthetic drugs, hypothermia can also cause complete suppression of the EEG (at approximately 18°C-20°C). However, in contrast to anesthetic drugs, temperature reduction beyond that at which EEG suppression first occurs *does* produce a further decrease in the CMR (Fig. 11.5). This decrease occurs because anesthetic drugs reduce only the component of the CMR associated with neuronal function, whereas hypothermia decreases the rate of energy utilization associated with both electrophysiologic function and the basal component related to the maintenance of cellular integrity. Mild hypothermia preferentially suppresses the basal component of the CMR. The $CMRO_2$ at 18°C is less than 10% of normothermic control values, which may explain the brain's tolerance for moderate periods of circulatory arrest at these and colder temperatures.

Hyperthermia has an opposite influence on cerebral physiologic function. Between 37°C and 42°C, CBF and CMR increase. However, above 42°C, a dramatic reduction in cerebral oxygen consumption occurs, an indication of a threshold for a toxic effect of hyperthermia that may occur as a result of protein (enzyme) denaturation.

$PaCO_2$. CBF varies directly with $Paco_2$ (Fig. 11.6*A*), especially within the range of physiologic variation of $Paco_2$. CBF changes 1 to 2 mL/100 g/min for each 1 mm Hg change in $Paco_2$ around normal $Paco_2$ values. This response is attenuated at a $Paco_2$ less than 25 mm Hg. Under normal circumstances, the sensitivity of CBF to changes in $Paco_2$ ($\Delta CBF/\Delta Paco_2$) is positively correlated with resting levels of CBF. Accordingly, anesthetic drugs that alter resting CBF cause changes in the response of the cerebral circulation

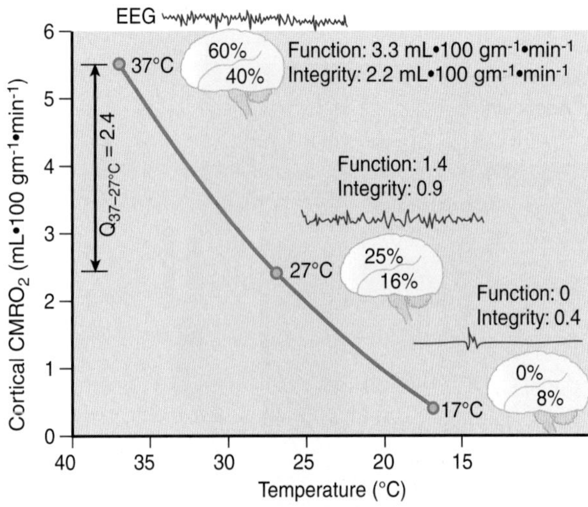

Fig. 11.5 Effect of temperature reduction on the cerebral metabolic rate of oxygen ($CMRO_2$) in the cortex. Hypothermia reduces both of the components of cerebral metabolic activity identified in Fig. 11.2—that associated with neuronal electrophysiologic activity (Function) and that associated with the maintenance of cellular homeostasis (Integrity). This is in contrast to anesthetics that alter only the functional component. The ratio of cerebral metabolic rate (CMR) at 37°C to that at 27°C, the Q10 ratio, is shown in the graph. Note that the $CMRO_2$ in the cortex (gray matter) is greater than global $CMRO_2$, considering the lower metabolic rate in white matter. *EEG*, Electroencephalogram. (Modified from Michenfelder JD. *Anesthesia and the brain: clinical, functional, metabolic, and vascular correlates*. New York: Churchill Livingstone; 1988.)

to CO_2. The magnitude of the reduction in CBF caused by hypocapnia is more intense when resting CBF is increased (as might occur during anesthesia with volatile agents). Conversely, when resting CBF is reduced, the magnitude of the hypocapnia-induced reduction in CBF is decreased slightly. It should be noted that CO_2 responsiveness has been observed in normal brain during anesthesia with all the anesthetic drugs that have been studied.

The role of MAP in the CO_2 responsiveness of the cerebral circulation is further highlighted by the impact of modest and severe hypotension.[8] With the former, the increase in CBF attendant upon hypercarbia is significantly reduced, whereas hypocapnia-induced vasoconstriction is only modestly affected. When hypotension is severe, a cerebrovascular response to changes in $Paco_2$ is not observed (Fig. 11.6*A*). The level of $Paco_2$ also modulates cerebral autoregulation. With hypercarbia, cerebral autoregulatory response to hypertension is attenuated. By contrast, with the induction of hypocapnia, CBF is autoregulated over a wider MAP range (Fig 11.6*B*).[9]

The changes in CBF caused by $Paco_2$ are dependent on pH alterations in the extracellular fluid of the brain. NO, in particular NO of neuronal origin, is an important although not exclusive mediator of CO_2-induced vasodilation.[10] The vasodilatory response to hypercapnia is also mediated in part by prostaglandins. The changes in extracellular pH and CBF rapidly occur after $Paco_2$ adjustments because CO_2 freely diffuses across the cerebrovascular endothelium and the BBB. In contrast with *respiratory* acidosis, acute systemic *metabolic* acidosis has little immediate effect on CBF because the BBB excludes H^+ from the perivascular space. The CBF changes in response to alterations in $Paco_2$

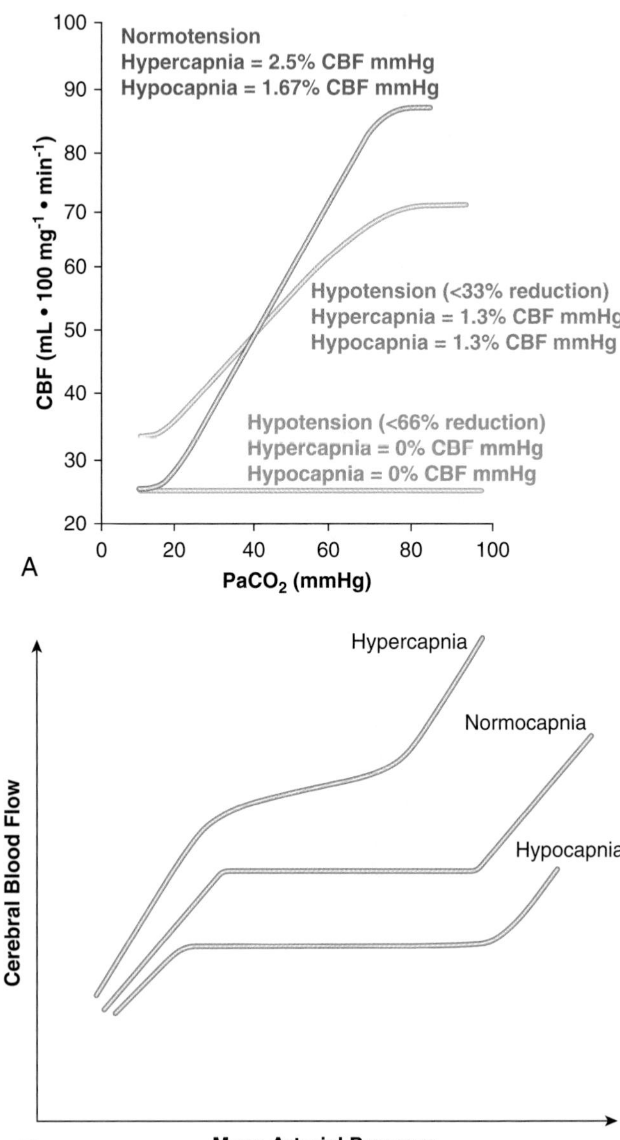

Fig. 11.6 *A*, Relationship between cerebral blood flow *(CBF)* and partial pressure of carbon dioxide *($Paco_2$)*. CBF increases linearly with increases in arterial $Paco_2$. Below a $Paco_2$ of 25 mm Hg, further reduction in CBF is limited. Similarly, the increase in CBF above a $Paco_2$ of approximately 75 to 80 mm Hg is also attenuated. The cerebrovascular responsiveness to $Paco_2$ is influenced significantly by blood pressure. With moderate hypotension (mean arterial pressure [MAP] reduction of <33%), the cerebrovascular responsiveness to changes in $Paco_2$ is attenuated significantly. With severe hypotension (MAP reduction of approximately 66%), CO_2 responsiveness is abolished. *B*, The effect of $Paco_2$ variation on cerebral autoregulation. Hypercarbia induces cerebral vasodilation and, consequently, the autoregulatory response to hypertension is less effective. By contrast, hypocapnia results in greater CBF autoregulation over a wider MAP variation. (Modified from Willie[8] and Rickards[9].)

rapidly occur, but they are not sustained. Despite the maintenance of an increased arterial pH, CBF returns toward normal over a period of 6 to 8 hours because the pH of CSF gradually returns to normal levels as a result of extrusion of bicarbonate (see Fig. 57.6). Consequently, a patient who has had a sustained period of hyperventilation or hypoventilation deserves special consideration. Acute restoration of a normal $Paco_2$ value will result in a significant CSF acidosis (after hypocapnia) or alkalosis (after hypercapnia). The

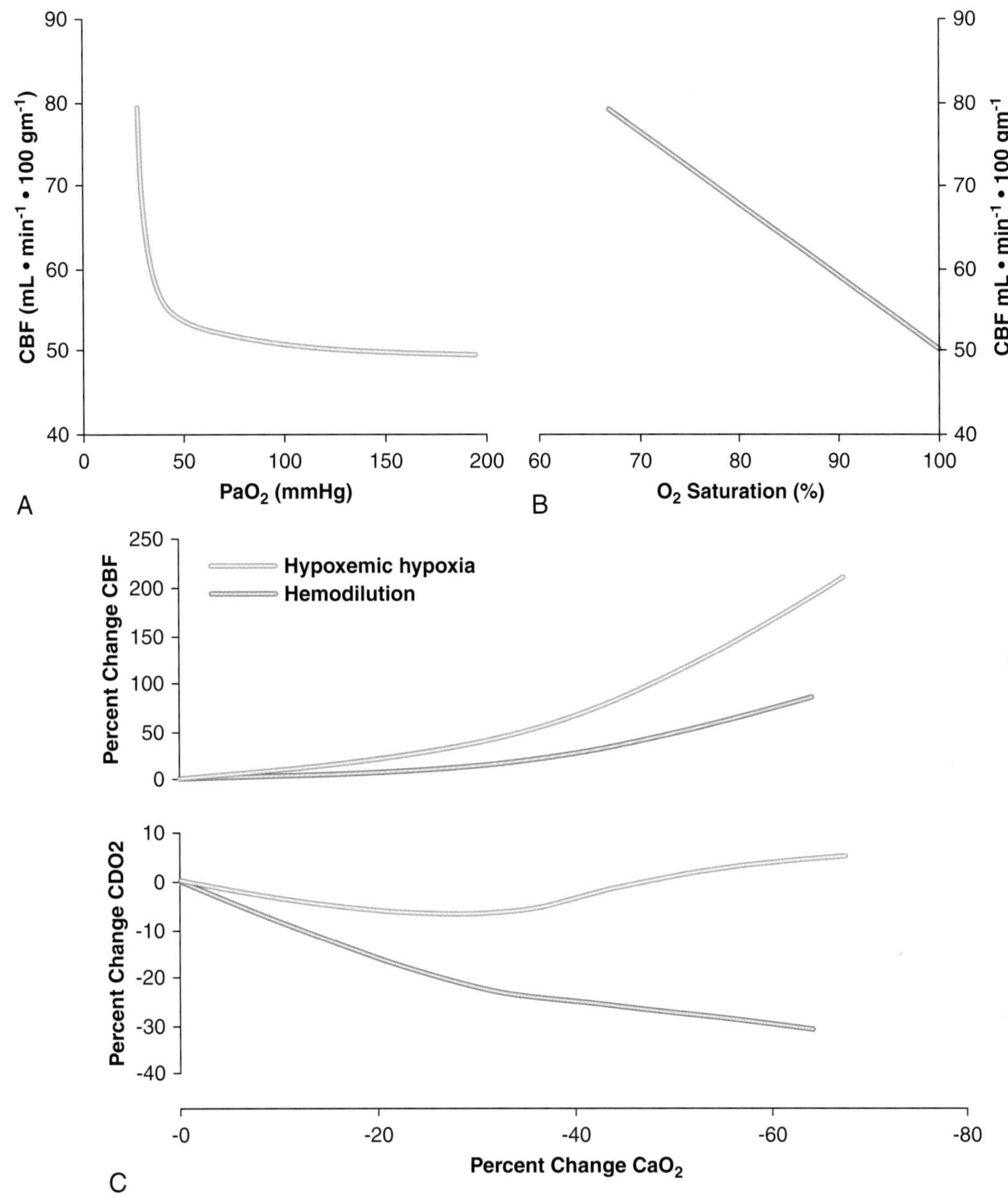

Fig. 11.7 (A) Relationship between cerebral blood flow *(CBF)* and partial pressure of oxygen *(Pao_2)*. Between the range of 60 and 200 mm Hg, Pao_2 has little impact on CBF. A reduction in Pao_2 to less than 60 mm Hg results in hemoglobin desaturation. There is significant cerebral vasodilation and a marked increase in CBF. (B) The relationship between hemoglobin saturation and CBF is inversely linear, with a gradual increase in CBF as saturation is decreased. (C) The impact of a reduction in cerebral oxygen delivery *(CDO_2)*, either by hypoxemic hypoxia or by hemodilution, is depicted. CBF increases significantly either with hypoxia or hemodilution; however, the CBF response is much greater with hypoxia *(upper panel)*. The total cerebral oxygen delivery is better maintained with hypoxia than hemodilution at a comparable level of arterial oxygen content *(CaO_2)* because of the greater CBF increase that occurs with the former. (Modified from Hoiland et al.[11] and Todd et al.[354,355].)

former results in increased CBF with a concomitant increase in ICP that depends on the prevailing intracranial compliance. The latter conveys a theoretic risk for ischemia.

Pao_2. Changes in Pao_2 from 60 to more than 300 mm Hg have little influence on CBF. A reduction in Pao_2 below 60 mm Hg rapidly increases CBF (Fig. 11.7*A*). Below a Pao_2 of 60 mm Hg, there is a rapid reduction in oxyhemoglobin saturation. The relationship between oxyhemoglobin saturation, as evaluated by pulse oximetry, and CBF is inversely linear (see Fig. 11.7*B*). The mechanisms mediating cerebral vasodilation during hypoxia may include neurogenic effects initiated by peripheral and neuraxial chemoreceptors, as well as local humoral influences. A reduction in arterial oxygen content, and therefore cerebral oxygen delivery, can be achieved either by a reduction in Pao_2 (hypoxemic hypoxia) or by a reduction in hemoglobin concentration (anemia, hemodilution). Both hemodilution and hypoxemic hypoxia lead to cerebral vasodilation and an increase in CBF. Of the two variables, however, hypoxemic hypoxia is a far more potent variable in CBF augmentation than hemodilution. Cerebral oxygen delivery is better maintained during hypoxia when arterial content is equivalently reduced by hypoxia or hemodilution (see Fig. 11.7*C*). Deoxyhemoglobin plays a central role in hypoxia-induced increases in CBF by causing the release of NO and its metabolites, as well as ATP.[11] Hypoxia-induced opening of ATP-dependent K^+ channels in vascular smooth muscle leads to hyperpolarization and vasodilation. The rostral ventrolateral medulla (RVLM) serves as an oxygen sensor within the brain. Stimulation of the RVM by hypoxia results in an increase in CBF (but not CMR), and lesions of the RVLM suppress the magnitude of the CBF response to hypoxia. The response to hypoxia is synergistic with the hyperemia produced by hypercapnia and acidosis. At high PaO_2 values, CBF modestly decreases. At 1 atmosphere of oxygen, CBF is reduced by approximately 12%.

NEUROGENIC REGULATION OF CEREBRAL BLOOD FLOW

The cerebral vasculature is extensively innervated.[12] The density of innervation declines with vessel size, and the greatest neurogenic influence appears to be exerted on larger cerebral arteries. This innervation includes cholinergic (parasympathetic and nonparasympathetic), adrenergic (sympathetic and nonsympathetic), serotoninergic, and VIPergic systems of extraaxial and intraaxial origin. An extracranial sympathetic influence via the superior cervical ganglion, as well as parasympathetic innervation via the sphenopalatine ganglion, certainly exists in animals. The intraaxial pathways likely result from innervation arising from several nuclei, including the locus coeruleus, the fastigial nucleus, the dorsal raphe nucleus, and the basal magnocellular nucleus of Meynert. Evidence of the functional significance of neurogenic influences has been derived from studies of CBF autoregulation and ischemic injury. Hemorrhagic shock, a state of high sympathetic tone, results in less CBF at a given MAP than occurs when hypotension is produced with sympatholytic drugs. During shock, a sympathetically mediated vasoconstrictive effect shifts the lower end of the autoregulatory curve to the right. It is not clear what the relative contributions of humoral and neural mechanisms are to this phenomenon; however, a neurogenic component certainly exists because sympathetic denervation increases CBF during hemorrhagic shock. Moreover, sympathetic denervation produced by a blockade of the stellate ganglion can increase CBF in humans.[13] Activation of cerebral sympathetic innervation also shifts the ULA to the right and offers some protection against hypertension-induced increases in CBF (which can in certain circumstances lead to a breakdown of the BBB).[8] Experimental interventions that alter these neurogenic control pathways influence outcome after standardized ischemic insults, presumably by influences on vascular tone and therefore CBF. The nature and influence of such pathways in humans are not known, and their manipulation for the purposes of clinical management remains to be systematically investigated.

EFFECTS OF BLOOD VISCOSITY ON CEREBRAL BLOOD FLOW

Blood viscosity can influence CBF. Hematocrit is the single most important determinant of blood viscosity.[14] In healthy humans, variation of the hematocrit within the normal range (33%-45%) probably results in only modest alterations in CBF. Beyond this range, changes are more substantial. In anemia, cerebral vascular resistance is reduced and CBF increases. However, this may result not only from a reduction in viscosity but also as a compensatory response to reduced oxygen delivery.[15] Although arterial oxygen content can be reduced by both hypoxia and by hemodilution, the increase in CBF that accompanies hypoxia is of a greater magnitude than that by hemodilution induced reduction in oxygen delivery.[11] The effect of a reduction in viscosity on CBF is more important with focal cerebral ischemia, a condition in which vasodilation in response to impaired oxygen delivery is probably already maximal. In this situation, reducing viscosity by hemodilution increases CBF in the ischemic territory. In patients with focal cerebral ischemia, a hematocrit of 30% to 34% will result in optimal delivery of oxygen. However, manipulation of viscosity in patients with acute ischemic stroke is not of benefit in reducing the extent of cerebral injury. Therefore, viscosity is not a target of manipulation in patients at risk as a result of cerebral ischemia, with the possible exception of those with hematocrit values higher than 55%.

CARDIAC OUTPUT

The conventional view of cerebral hemodynamics is that perfusion pressure (MAP or CPP) is the primary determinant of CBF and that the influence of cardiac output is limited. More recent data suggest that cardiac output impacts cerebral perfusion. In several investigations in which central blood volume was modulated, either reduced by application of lower body negative pressure, or increased by the infusion of fluid, a linear relationship between cardiac output and CBF, as measured as middle cerebral artery flow velocity (MCAfv) by transcranial Doppler, was clearly demonstrated.[8,16-20] An analysis of the pooled data from these investigations indicates that a reduction in cardiac output of approximately 30% leads to a decrease in CBF by about 10%.[21] In patients undergoing hip arthroplasty under hypotensive epidural anesthesia, the administration of epinephrine led to a maintenance of CBF even though the MAP was below the LLA.[22] Presumably, this maintenance of CBF was due to an epinephrine-induced increase in cardiac output. An association between CO and CBF has also been observed in acute stroke, subarachnoid hemorrhage-induced vasospasm, and sepsis. However, the CO–CBF relationship has not been demonstrated uniformly; in fact, augmentation of CO does not increase CBF in several disease states, including traumatic head injury, neurologic surgery, and cardiac surgery.[21] Collectively, the available data suggest that CO does influence CBF and that this effect may be of particular relevance in situations in which circulating volume is reduced and in shock states.

AN INTEGRATED CONTEMPORARY VIEW OF CEREBRAL AUTOREGULATION

The conventional view of cerebral autoregulation is that CBF is held constant as MAP increases between the lower limit and ULA. The currently available data, however, indicate that this view is now outmoded and is in need of revision. As discussed previously, CBF and the cerebral vasculature are influenced by a variety of variables. Clearly, MAP (perfusion pressure) is a major determinant of CBF. Cardiac output is increasingly being recognized as an important determinant of CBF. Cardiac output in turn is dependent on adequate circulatory volume, cardiac preload, contractility, afterload, and heart rate and rhythm. The presence of cardiovascular disease, in particular congestive heart failure, will limit the capacity of autoregulatory mechanisms to maintain CBF in response to hypotension. Arterial blood gas tensions affect vasomotor tone, and both hypercarbia and hypoxia attenuate autoregulation. The contribution of the sympathetic nervous system is of importance in the cerebrovascular response to hypertension. At the same time, sympathetic nerves reduce the vasodilatory capacity of the cerebral vessels during hypotension. A variety of medications can impact autoregulation, either through modulation of sympathetic nervous system activity (β-antagonists, α_2-agonists) or by direct reduction of vasomotor tone (calcium channel antagonists, nitrates, angiotensin receptor blockers, angiotensin converting enzyme [ACE] inhibitors). Anesthetics modulate autoregulation by a number of means, including suppression of metabolism, alteration of neurovascular coupling to a higher flow–metabolism ratio, suppression of autonomic neural activity, and by direct effect on cerebral vasomotor tone, and alteration of cardiac function and systemic circulatory tone.

Cerebrovascular tone and CBF are therefore under the control of a complex regulatory system (Fig. 11.8). Given the multitude of factors that determine the capacity of the cerebral circulation to respond to changes in perfusion pressure, the premise that cerebral autoregulation is static is now untenable. Rather, cerebral autoregulation should be viewed as a dynamic process and that the morphologic form of the autoregulatory curve is the result of the integration of all the variables that affect cerebrovascular tone in an interdependent manner.[8,23] Therefore, a continuum of vascular responsiveness in both the lower and upper limits and in the plateau probably exists as the ability of the cerebrovascular bed to dilate or constrict is exhausted. In a review of the available data from investigations in humans, the range of pressures that defined the LLA spanned from 33 mm Hg to as high as 108 mm Hg.[5]

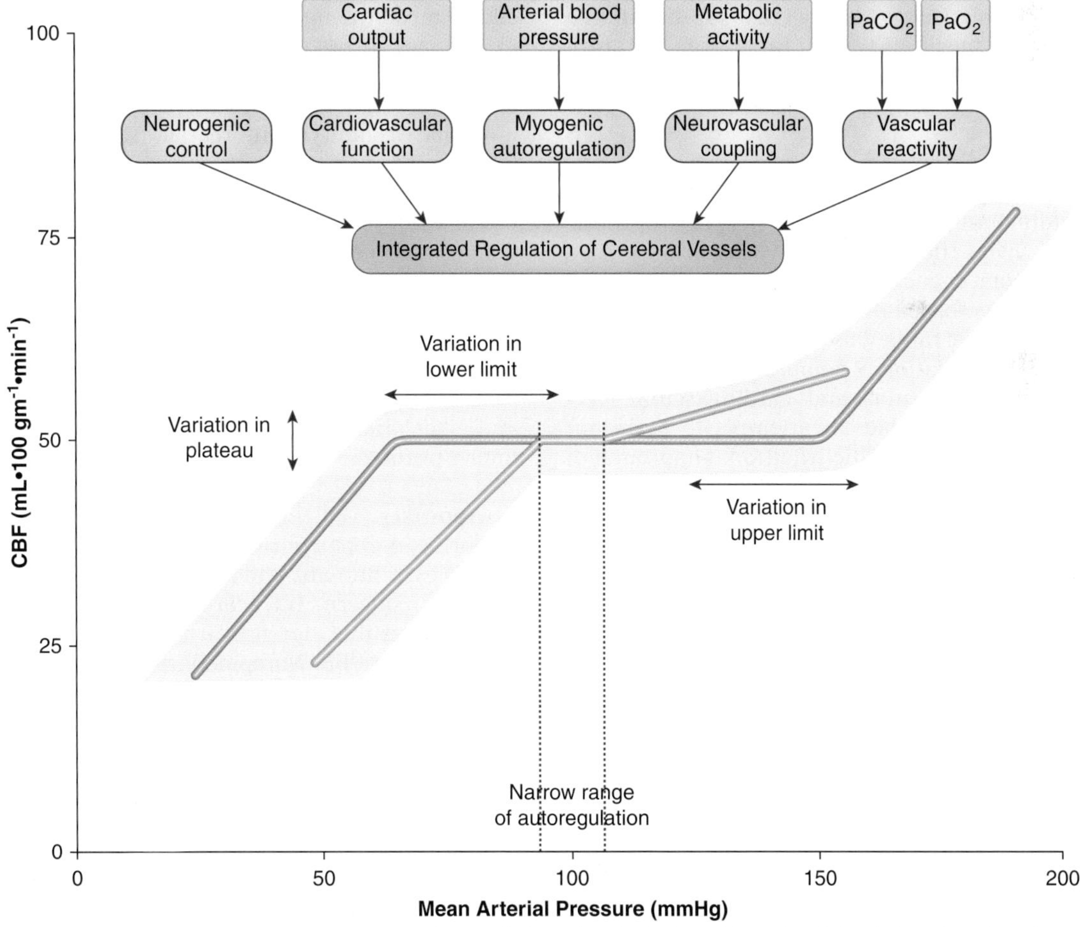

Fig. 11.8 Integrative regulation of cerebral blood flow *(CBF)*. The conventional view of cerebral autoregulation is that CBF is maintained constant with a variation in mean arterial pressure (MAP) of 65 to 150 mm Hg. A more contemporary view is that cerebral autoregulation is a dynamic process that is under the influence of a number of variables including myogenic autoregulation, neurovascular coupling, arterial CO_2 and O_2 tensions, autonomic (neurogenic) activity, and cardiovascular function. Anesthetic agents in particular affect autoregulation at multiple levels: suppression of metabolism, alteration in arterial blood gas tensions, direct cerebral vasodilation, suppression of autonomic activity, and modulation of cardiovascular function. Therefore, CBF at any given moment is a product of the composite of these variables. There is considerable variation in lower and upper limits as well as the plateau of the autoregulatory curve. The conventional autoregulatory curve is depicted in red. The red shaded area represents the range of variation in CBF. The autoregulatory curve depicted in blue was derived from 48 healthy human subjects. In that group, the lower limit of autoregulation was approximately 90 mm Hg and the range over which CBF remained relatively constant was only 10 mm Hg. *Paco₂*, Arterial partial pressure of carbon dioxide; *Pao₂*, arterial partial pressure of oxygen. (Modified from Tan et al.,[24] Willie et al.,[8] and Meng and Gelb.[23])

In healthy humans subjected to lower body negative pressure to reduce central blood volume and to reduce blood pressure, the autoregulatory plateau spanned a range of only 10 mm Hg (± 5 mm Hg from baseline)[24] as opposed to a range of 100 mm Hg in the once conventional representations of autoregulation. Above and below this narrow plateau, CBF was pressure passive. Even within this narrow plateau, a modest increase in CBF with increases in blood pressure is observable—that is, the plateau is not flat. The slope of the percentage change in MAP to percentage change in CBF relationship has been demonstrated to be 0.81 ± 0.77 with induction of hypotension and 0.21 ± 0.47 with the induction of hypertension. These data are consistent with the premise that the capacity of the cerebral circulation to adapt to increases in blood pressure is considerably greater than adaptation to hypotension.[8] Based on these more recent observations, the conventional view of autoregulation is probably not applicable to most subjects, and a revision of the framework of cerebral circulatory control along the lines of recent data is needed.[8,23] In this respect, it is the view of the authors that cerebral autoregulation should be accurately represented by a family of autoregulatory curves rather than a single static curve (see Fig. 11.8). In these dynamic autoregulatory curves, there is considerable heterogeneity in the LLA and ULA, as well as in the limits and slope of the plateau.

Clinical implications: Maintenance of cerebral perfusion is essential, and identification of a target range of MAP in individual patients is a key part of anesthetic management. Given the substantial variability in cerebral autoregulatory capacity, it may be difficult to identify the target range based on an LLA in most patients. Selection of the target range based on the baseline pressure, after due consideration of comorbid conditions that may impact cerebrovascular and cardiovascular performance, may be preferable. In attempts to maintain adequate perfusion pressure, the traditional approach of systemic vasoconstriction, for example with α_1-agonists, is reasonable. However, the adequate maintenance of circulatory volume and of cardiac output should also be considered; administration of agents that can also increase cardiac output may be of value. This may be of particular relevance in patients with compromised cardiac function.

VASOACTIVE DRUGS

Many drugs with intrinsic vascular effects are used in contemporary anesthetic practice, including both anesthetic drugs and numerous vasoactive drugs specifically used for hemodynamic manipulation. This section deals with the latter. The actions of anesthetics are discussed in the "Effects of Anesthetics on Cerebral Blood Flow and Cerebral Metabolic Rate" section.

Systemic Vasodilators

Most drugs used to induce hypotension, including sodium nitroprusside, nitroglycerin, hydralazine, adenosine, and calcium channel blockers (CCBs), also cause cerebral vasodilation. As a result, CBF either increases or is maintained at pre-hypotensive levels. In addition, when hypotension is induced with a cerebral vasodilator, CBF is maintained at lower MAP values than when induced by either hemorrhage or a noncerebral vasodilator. In contrast to direct vasodilators, the ACE inhibitor enalapril does not have any significant effect on CBF. Anesthetics that simultaneously vasodilate the cerebral circulation cause increases in cerebral blood volume (CBV) with the potential to increase ICP. The effects of these anesthetics on ICP are less dramatic when hypotension is slowly induced, which probably reflects the more effective interplay of compensatory mechanisms (i.e., shifts in CSF and venous blood) when changes occur more slowly.

Catecholamine Agonists and Antagonists

Numerous drugs with agonist and antagonist activity at catecholamine receptors (α_1, α_2, β_1, β_2, and dopamine) are in common use. The effects of these vasoactive drugs on cerebral physiology are dependent on basal arterial blood pressure, the magnitude of the drug-induced arterial blood pressure changes, the status of the autoregulation mechanism, and the status of the BBB. A drug may have direct effects on cerebral vascular smooth muscle or indirect effects mediated by the cerebral autoregulatory response to changes in systemic blood pressure (or both types of effects). When autoregulation is preserved, increases in systemic pressure should increase CBF if basal blood pressure is outside the limits of autoregulation. When basal pressure is within the normal autoregulatory range, an increase in systemic arterial pressure does not significantly affect CBF because the normal autoregulatory response to a rising MAP entails cerebral vasoconstriction (i.e., an increase in cerebral vascular resistance) to maintain a constant CBF. When autoregulation is defective, CBF will vary in direct relation to arterial pressure. The information in the following paragraphs and in Table 11.2 emphasizes data obtained from investigations of vasopressors in intact preparations, and gives priority to the results obtained in humans and higher primates.

α_1-Agonists. Will the administration of α_1-agonists (phenylephrine, norepinephrine) reduce CBF?

Studies in humans and nonhuman primates do not confirm this concern. Intracarotid infusions of norepinephrine in doses that significantly increase the MAP result in no change in CBF. Norepinephrine can increase CBF, but such increases might occur if autoregulation were defective or its limit exceeded. β-Mimetic drugs (norepinephrine has β_1 activity) may cause activation of cerebral metabolism[25] with a coupled increase in CBF. This effect is more apparent when these drugs can gain greater access to the brain parenchyma via a defective BBB (see Table 11.2). Administration of phenylephrine to patients undergoing cardiopulmonary bypass does not decrease CBF. In spinal cord–injured patients with relative hypotension, the administration of the α_1-agonist midodrine increased perfusion pressure and increased flow velocity in the middle cerebral artery (MCA) and the posterior cerebral artery.[26] In healthy patients,[27] and in those undergoing surgery in the beach chair position,[28] the administration of phenylephrine maintains or augments MCAfv. Collectively, these data suggest that norepinephrine and phenylephrine maintain cerebral perfusion.

TABLE 11.2 Best Estimates of the Influence of Pure Catecholamine Receptor Agonists and Specific Pressor Substances on Cerebral Blood Flow and Cerebral Metabolic Rate

Agonist	Cerebral Blood Flow	Cerebral Metabolic Rate
PURE		
α_1	0/–	0
α_2	–	–
β	+	+
β (BBB open)	+++	+++
Dopamine	++	0
Dopamine (high dose)	–	?0
Fenoldopam	–	?0
MIXED		
Norepinephrine	0/–	0/+
Norepinephrine (BBB open)	+	+
Epinephrine	+	+
Epinephrine (BBB open)	+++	+++

The number of symbols indicates the magnitude of the effect.
Where species differences occurred, data from primates were given preference. See text for complete discussion.
BBB, Blood-brain barrier; +, increase; –, decrease; 0, no effect.

The traditional view that CBF can be maintained by the administration of α_1-agonists without any adverse effect on cerebral oxygenation has been challenged. In anesthetized patients,[29-31] phenylephrine administration by bolus modestly reduced regional cerebral oxygen saturation (rSO_2), measured by near-infrared oximetry. Ephedrine, although increasing arterial blood pressure to a similar extent as phenylephrine, did not reduce rSO_2, presumably because of its ability to maintain cardiac output. In human volunteers, a norepinephrine-induced increase in arterial blood pressure slightly reduced MCAfv and cerebral oxygen saturation (Sco_2) and $SjVo_2$.[32] By contrast, although phenylephrine decreased rSO_2, MCAfv was increased and $SjVo_2$ was unchanged.[33] These data have led to the question of whether phenylephrine and norepinephrine administration negatively impact cerebral oxygenation. Several factors argue against this possibility.[34] The first concern is methodology. Near-infrared spectroscopy (NIRS) measures oxygenated and deoxygenated blood in a defined region of brain and is a composite of arterial, capillary, and venous blood. Vasopressors affect both arterial and venous tone. Even a minor change in the volume of arterial and venous volumes within the region of the brain can affect the rSO_2 measurement. Moreover, extracranial contamination is a significant component of the rSO_2 values reported by the currently available NIRS monitors.[35] This contamination is more important than the slight reduction in Sco_2 observed in these investigations. In the absence of direct measurement of brain tissue oxygenation, a modest reduction in Sco_2 in the face of increasing arterial blood pressure cannot be taken as evidence of impairment of cerebral oxygenation. In addition, phenylephrine did not decrease $SjVo_2$, a more global measurement of cerebral oxygenation. Although norepinephrine decreased $SjVo_2$ by approximately 3% (a mild reduction at best), its administration has been previously shown to increase the $CMRO_2$. Finally, the minor reduction in rSO_2 effected by phenylephrine is no longer apparent when an increase in the $CMRO_2$ is concurrent. Phenylephrine apparently does not prevent an increase in CBF when such an increase is warranted by increased brain metabolism.

These studies were conducted in patients with a normal central nervous system (CNS). Although unlikely, the concern is that α_1-agonists might reduce cerebral perfusion in the injured brain. In patients with a head injury, the administration of phenylephrine increased CPP and did not reduce regional CBF.[36] Transient changes may occur in CBF and rSO_2 (on the order of 2-5 minutes) in response to bolus doses of phenylephrine; however, with a continuous infusion, α_1-agonists have little direct influence on CBF and cerebral oxygenation in humans.[34] Thus maintenance of CPP with these vasopressors does not have an adverse effect on the brain.

α_2-Agonists. α_2-Agonists have both analgesic and sedative effects. This class of drugs includes dexmedetomidine and clonidine, with the latter being a significantly less specific and less potent α_2-agonist. Two investigations in human volunteers have confirmed the ability of dexmedetomidine to decrease CBF. Dexmedetomidine dose-dependently decreased MCAfv, with the maximum reduction being approximately 25%.[37] Dexmedetomidine (1 μg/kg loading dose and infusion at either 0.2 or 0.6 μg/kg/hr) decreased CBF by approximately 30%[38] in healthy human volunteers. In both these investigations, the CMR was not measured; whether the reduction in CBF was due to a direct vasoconstrictor activity of dexmedetomidine or to suppression of the CMR with a corresponding reduction in CBF is not clear. In a more recent study of dexmedetomidine during which both MCAfv and the CMR were measured in healthy humans, dexmedetomidine decreased MCAfv in parallel with a reduction in the CMR.[39] Similarly, in healthy patients[40] and those with traumatic brain injury[41] undergoing sedation with dexmedetomidine, the reduction in CBF was matched by a parallel reduction in CMR. Thus the effects of dexmedetomidine on CBF were primarily mediated by its ability to suppress the CMR; the reduction in CBF is commensurate with the reduction in CMR, and there is no evidence that dexmedetomidine causes cerebral ischemia. However, the well-known effect of dexmedetomidine in decreasing arterial blood pressure merits careful consideration if used in patients who are critically dependent on collateral perfusion pressure, especially in the recovery phase of an anesthetic.

β-Agonists. β-receptor agonists, in small doses, have little direct effect on the cerebral vasculature. In larger doses and in association with physiologic stress, they can cause an increase in the CMR with an accompanying increase in CBF. The β_1-receptor is probably the mediator of these effects. In doses that do not result in substantial changes in the MAP, intracarotid epinephrine does not change CBF in nonanesthetized humans. However, with larger doses that lead to an increase in the MAP, both CBF and $CMRO_2$ can increase by approximately 20%. A recent investigation has demonstrated that the administration of epinephrine in patients undergoing surgery under hypotensive epidural anesthesia can increase MCAfv, presumably by augmenting cardiac output (as discussed previously).[22]

Dobutamine can increase CBF and CMR by 20% and 30%, respectively. Dobutamine can increase CBF independent of its effect on blood pressure; the increase in CBF has been attributed to the augmentation of cardiac output by dobutamine.[36]

Evidence suggests that a defect in the BBB enhances the effect of β-agonists.[42] Intracarotid norepinephrine, which does not normally affect CBF and CMR, increases CBF and CMR when BBB permeability is increased with hypertonic drugs. Epinephrine caused an elevation in the $CMRO_2$, but only when the BBB was made permeable.[42] These observations beg the interpretation that β-agonists will increase CBF and CMR *only* when the BBB is injured. However, when epinephrine was given in doses that did not significantly increase the MAP, increases in CBF and CMR occurred. Accordingly, BBB injury may exaggerate but is not a necessary condition in humans for the occurrence of β-mediated increases in CBF and CMR.

β-Blockers. β-Adrenergic blockers either reduce or have no effect on CBF and CMR. In two investigations in humans, propranolol, 5 mg intravenously,[43] and labetalol, 0.75 mg/kg intravenously,[44] had no effect on CBF and cerebral blood flow velocity (CBFV), respectively. Modest reductions in CBF occur after the administration of labetalol to patients undergoing craniotomy who become hypertensive during emergence from anesthesia. Esmolol shortens seizures induced by electroconvulsive therapy (ECT), which suggests that esmolol does cross the normal BBB. Catecholamine levels at the time of β-blocker administration or the status of the BBB (or both) may influence the effect of these drugs. β-Adrenergic blockers are unlikely to have adverse effects on patients with intracranial pathology, other than effects secondary to changes in perfusion pressure.

Dopaminergic agents. Dopamine can be used for the treatment of hemodynamic dysfunction. It also augments the function of the normal cardiovascular system when an increase in the MAP is desired as an adjunct to the treatment of focal cerebral ischemia, especially in the setting of vasospasm. Nonetheless, its effects on CBF and CMR have not been defined with certainty. The likely predominant effect of dopamine in the normal cerebral vasculature, when administered in small doses, is probably slight vasodilation with a minimal change in the CMR.[45] Increased CMR in discrete regions of the brain, such as the choroid plexus and basal ganglia, can occur. However, overall cortical blood flow is not influenced. Vasoconstriction of the cerebral circulation is not observed even when dopamine is administered in doses of up to 100 μg/kg/min.[45] Fenoldopam is a dopamine agonist with activity at the DA_1-receptor and α_2-receptor. The administration of fenoldopam leads to systemic vasodilation and a decrease in arterial blood pressure. In humans, fenoldopam decreased systemic blood pressure to a level that was above the LLA; however, a modest (≈15%) reduction was observed in CBF that did not increase to normal levels when systemic blood pressure was supported.[46] The reason for the reduction of CBF is not clear.

Calcium channel blockers. CCBs are frequently used to treat acute hypertension in the neurologically injured patient population. Cerebral vessels are richly endowed with calcium channels, in particular the L-type calcium channel. CCBs therefore induce vasodilation of the pial and cerebral arteries. In healthy humans, intravenous administration of nimodipine does not change CBF; however, when the slight decrease in MAP and changes in $PaCO_2$ are taken into consideration, CBF increased by approximately 5% to 10%.[47] CMR and CO_2 reactivity are maintained. Nimodipine in human subjects does, however, blunt autoregulation moderately.[48] Intraarterial nimodipine for the treatment of cerebral vasospasm after subarachnoid hemorrhage increased regional CBF significantly provided MAP was maintained, indicating that nimodipine is a cerebral vasodilator.[49]

Nicardipine is perhaps the most commonly used CCB for perioperative blood pressure control because of its short half-life and easy titratability. Nicardipine is a modest cerebral vasodilator and has repeatedly been shown to increase CBF or CBFV while reducing systemic MAP. Cerebral CO_2 reactivity appears to be well preserved in the presence of nicardipine.[50,51]

Clevidipine is a third generation dihydropyridine CCB that has an ultrashort half-life because it undergoes rapid esterase-mediated metabolism. Its use in both the cardiac and neurologic patient populations has increased significantly given its rapid titratability. In healthy volunteers, clevidipine did not increase MCAfv. However, a substantial reduction in MAP of approximately 25% occurred.[52] The lack of increase in MCAfv in the face of hypotension suggests that clevidipine is a cerebral vasodilator and, like nicardipine, probably attenuates autoregulation to a moderate extent. CO_2 reactivity is preserved.

The available data indicate that CCBs are moderate cerebral vasodilators. Their net impact on CBF is therefore dependent on the extent of systemic vasodilation and MAP. When MAP is maintained, increases in CBF should be expected.

Angiotensin II, Angiotensin-Converting Enzyme Inhibitors, and Angiotensin Receptor Antagonists
There has been a renaissance of the use of angiotensin II (AII) for the treatment of vasodilatory shock that is refractory to conventional vasopressor agents. In these shock states, AII increased MAP and reduced the need for other vasopressors including norepinephrine and vasopressin. The acute effect of AII on the cerebral circulation has received only modest attention. Acute administration of AII increases cerebral microvascular constriction without affecting CBF; this effect precedes its impact on blood pressure. However, AII attenuates regional hyperemia that occurs with an increase in regional metabolism, thereby adversely impacting neurovascular coupling.[53] Given that CBF is maintained in the face of increased blood pressure, autoregulation and CO_2 responsivity appear to be maintained.[54]

Both ACE inhibitors and angiotensin-receptor blockers (ARBs) are commonly used to treat hypertension. In the surgical setting and in the neurocritical care unit, these drugs are administered to control arterial blood pressure acutely. ACE inhibitors and ARBs reduce arterial blood pressure when hypertension is present. However, they do not affect resting CBF, and autoregulation is maintained.[55] However, acute administration of ACE inhibitors and ARBs decreases the LLA (left shift of the autoregulatory curve in experimental animals);[56] the significance of this finding in humans is not clear. In patients with acute stroke, ACE inhibitors and ARBs reduce arterial blood pressure but do not acutely affect CBF.[57,58] Apparently, these drugs do not reduce CBF when arterial blood pressure is modestly decreased.

AGE

The loss of neurons is progressive in the normally aging brain from young adulthood to advanced age. There is approximately 10% neuronal loss in healthy aged brain.[59] The loss of myelinated fibers results in reduced white matter volume.[60] By contrast, the loss of synapses in the aged brain is considerably greater. The majority of excitatory synapses in the brain are on dendritic spines. Dendrite branching and volume decrease progressively, and the number of dendritic spines is reduced by approximately 25% to 35%.[60] Concomitant with the loss of neuropil, both CBF and $CMRO_2$ decrease by 15% to 20% at the age of 80 years.[61] Cerebral circulatory responsiveness to changes in $Paco_2$ and to hypoxia are slightly reduced in the healthy aged brain.[4,62]

Effects of Anesthetics on Cerebral Blood Flow and Cerebral Metabolic Rate

This section discusses the effects of anesthetic drugs on CBF and CMR. It includes limited mention of the influences on autoregulation, CO_2 responsiveness, and CBV. Effects on CSF dynamics, the BBB, and epileptogenesis are discussed later in the chapter.

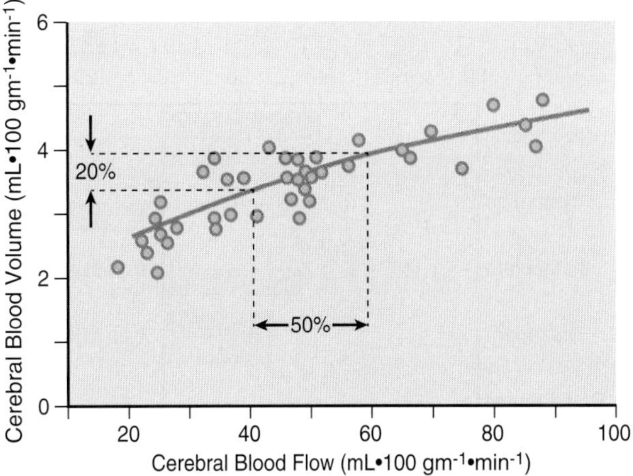

Fig. 11.9 Relationship between cerebral blood flow (CBF) and cerebral blood volume (CBV). Although a linear relationship exists between CBF and CBV, the magnitude of the change in CBV for a given change in CBF is considerably less. An increase in CBF of 50% results in a change in CBV of only 20%.

In the practice of neuroanesthesia, the manner in which anesthetic drugs and techniques influence CBF receives prime attention. The rationale is twofold. First, the delivery of energy substrates is dependent on CBF, and modest alterations in CBF can influence neuronal outcome substantially in the setting of ischemia. Second, control and manipulation of CBF are central to the management of ICP because as CBF varies in response to vasoconstrictor-vasodilator influences, CBV varies with it.[63] With respect to ICP, CBV is the more critical variable. In the normal brain, CBV is approximately 5 mL/100 g of brain, and over a $Paco_2$ range of approximately 25 to 70 mm Hg, CBV changes by approximately 0.049 mL/100 g for each 1 mm Hg change in $Paco_2$. In an adult brain weighing approximately 1400 g, this change can amount to 20 mL in total CBV for a $Paco_2$ range of 25 to 55 mm Hg. Because CBV is more difficult to measure than CBF few data exist, especially in humans.

Although CBV and CBF usually vary in parallel, the magnitude of change in CBV is less than the magnitude of change in CBF (Fig. 11.9). In addition, CBV and CBF vary independently under some circumstances. During cerebral ischemia, for example, CBV increases, whereas CBF is reduced significantly. Autoregulation normally serves to prevent MAP-related increases in CBV. In fact, as the cerebral circulation constricts to maintain a constant CBF in the face of an increasing MAP, CBV actually decreases. When autoregulation is impaired or its upper limit (≈150 mm Hg) is exceeded, CBF and CBV then increase in parallel as arterial blood pressure increases (see Fig. 11.8). A decreasing MAP results in a progressive increase in CBV as the cerebral circulation dilates to maintain constant flow, and exaggerated increases in CBV occur as the MAP decreases to less than the LLA. In normal subjects, the initial increases in CBV do not increase ICP because there is latitude for compensatory adjustments by other intracranial compartments (e.g., translocation of venous blood and CSF to extracerebral vessels and the spinal CSF space, respectively). When

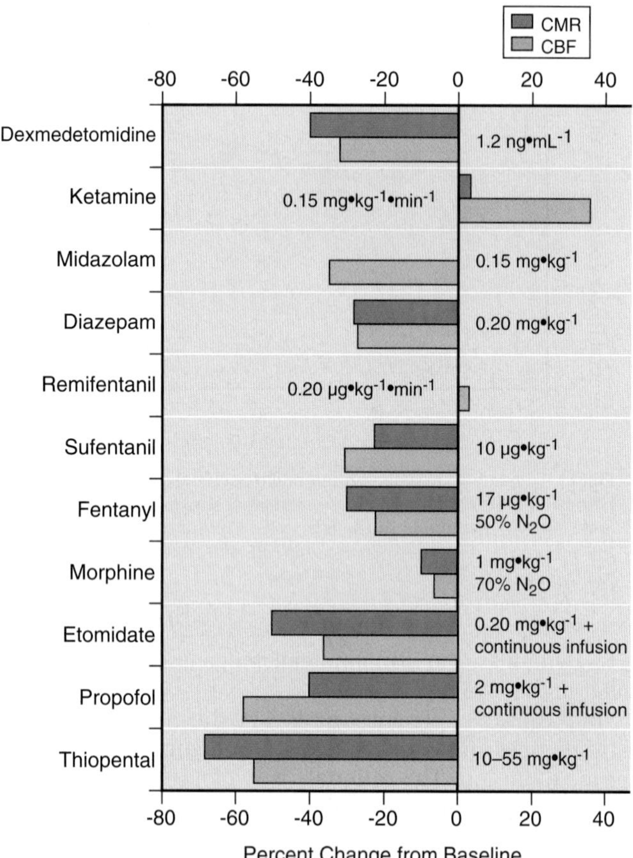

Fig. 11.10 Changes in cerebral blood flow *(CBF)* and the cerebral metabolic rate of oxygen ($CMRO_2$) caused by intravenous anesthetic drugs. The data are derived from human investigations and are presented as percent change from nonanesthetized control values. Dexmedetomidine CMR values were determined on a background of 0.5% isoflurane anesthesia (see the text for details). No data for the $CMRO_2$ effects of midazolam in humans are available. *CMR*, Cerebral metabolic rate. (Data from references 25, 47–59.)

intracranial compliance* is reduced, an increase in CBV can cause herniation or sufficiently reduce CPP to cause ischemia.

INTRAVENOUS ANESTHETIC DRUGS

The action of most intravenous anesthetics leads to parallel reductions in CMR and CBF. Ketamine, which causes an increase in the CMR and CBF, is the exception. The effects of selected intravenous anesthetic drugs on human CBF are compared in Fig. 11.10.[38,65-77]

Intravenous anesthetics maintain neurovascular coupling, and consequently changes in CBF induced by intravenous anesthetics are largely the result of the effects on the CMR with parallel (coupled) changes in CBF. Intravenous anesthetics have direct effects on vascular tone. Barbiturates, for example, cause relaxation of isolated cerebral vessels in vitro. However, *in vivo*, barbiturates suppress CMR, and the net effect at the point of EEG suppression is vasoconstriction and a substantial decrease in CBF.[78] In general, autoregulation and CO_2 responsiveness are preserved during the administration of intravenous anesthetic drugs.

Barbiturates

A dose-dependent reduction in CBF and CMR occurs with barbiturates. With the onset of anesthesia, both CBF and $CMRO_2$ are reduced by approximately 30%. When large doses of thiopental cause complete EEG suppression, CBF and CMR are reduced by approximately 50% to 60%.[78,79] Further increases in the barbiturate dose have no additional effect on the CMR.[78] These observations suggest that the major effect of nontoxic doses of depressant anesthetics is a reduction in the component of cerebral metabolism that is linked to electrical brain function (e.g., neurophysiologic activity) with only minimal effects on the second component, which is related to cellular homeostasis (see Fig. 11.2).

Tolerance to the CBF and CMR effects of barbiturates may quickly develop.[80] In patients with severe head injury in whom *barbiturate coma* was maintained for 72 hours, the blood concentration of thiamylal required to maintain EEG burst suppression was observed to be increased by the end of the first 24 hours and continued to increase over the next 48 hours.[81] During deep pentobarbital anesthesia, autoregulation and CO_2 responsiveness are maintained.

Propofol

The effects of propofol (2,6-diisopropylphenol) on CBF and CMR are similar to those of barbiturates. Both CBF and CMR decrease after the administration of propofol in humans.[82] In healthy volunteers, surgical levels of propofol reduced regional CBF by 53% to 79% in comparison with the awake state.[83,84] Cerebral glucose metabolism in volunteers was evaluated by positron-emission tomography (PET) before and during infusion of propofol to the point of unresponsiveness, and resulted in a decrease of the whole-brain metabolic rate of 48% to 58%, with limited regional heterogeneity.[85] When compared with isoflurane-fentanyl or sevoflurane-fentanyl anesthesia, a combination of propofol and fentanyl decreased subdural pressure in patients with intracranial tumors and decreased the arteriovenous oxygen content difference ($AVDO_2$).[86] Collectively, these investigations in human subjects indicate that propofol effects reductions in the CMR and secondarily decreases CBF, CBV, and ICP.

Both CO_2 responsiveness and autoregulation are preserved in humans during the administration of propofol,[87,88] even when administered in doses that produce burst suppression of the EEG.[89] The magnitude of the reduction in CBF during hypocapnia is decreased during propofol administration. This effect is probably due to the cerebral vasoconstriction induced by suppression of CMR, which limits further hypocapnia-mediated vasoconstriction.

Etomidate

The effects of etomidate on CBF and CMR are also similar to those of barbiturates. Roughly parallel reductions in CBF and CMR occur in humans,[65,90] and in general, they are accompanied by progressive suppression of the EEG.

*Note a well-entrenched misuse of terminology.[64] The "compliance" curve that is commonly drawn to describe the ICP-volume relationship (see Fig. 57-3) actually depicts the relationship $\Delta P/\Delta V$ (elastance) and not $\Delta V/\Delta P$ (compliance). References to "reduced compliance" in this text would more correctly be rendered as "increased elastance." However, because the existing literature most commonly uses the "compliance" terminology, the authors have left the misuse uncorrected herein.

Induction of anesthesia with either thiopental or etomidate resulted in a similar reduction in MCAfv by approximately 27%.[91] The changes in CBF and CMR are substantial. Etomidate, 0.2 mg/kg, reduced CBF and CMR by 34% and 45%, respectively, in adults.[65] As is the case with barbiturates, no further reduction in the CMR occurs when additional drug is administered beyond a dose sufficient to produce EEG suppression. Although this latter phenomenon has not been demonstrated in humans, etomidate has been demonstrated to reduce ICP only when EEG activity is well preserved; etomidate is ineffective in reducing ICP when EEG activity is suppressed in head injured patients.[92] The global CMR suppression attainable with etomidate is slightly less profound than that achieved with isoflurane and barbiturates. This finding is consistent with the observation that unlike barbiturates, which cause CMR suppression throughout the brain, the CMR suppression caused by etomidate is regionally variable and occurs predominantly in forebrain structures.

Etomidate is effective in reducing ICP without causing a reduction in CPP in patients with intracranial tumors[93] and patients with head injuries.[94] However, the administration of etomidate resulted in an exacerbation of brain tissue hypoxia and acidosis in patients in whom the MCA was temporarily occluded during surgery.[95] Additional concerns regarding the occurrence of adrenocortical suppression caused by enzyme inhibition and renal injury caused by the propylene glycol vehicle[96] will probably preclude more than episodic use.

Reactivity to CO_2 is preserved in humans during the administration of etomidate.[65,90] Autoregulation has not been evaluated. Myoclonus and epileptogenesis are discussed in the section, "Epileptogenesis."

Narcotics

Inconsistencies can be found in the available information, but narcotics likely have relatively little effect on CBF and CMR in the normal, unstimulated nervous system. When changes do occur, the general pattern is one of modest reductions in both CBF and CMR. The inconsistencies in the literature may largely arise because the control states entailed paralysis and nominal sedation in many studies, often with N_2O alone. In these studies, in which substantial reductions in CBF and CMR were frequently observed, the effect of the narcotic was probably a combination of the inherent effect of the drug plus a substantial component attributable to reduction of arousal. Comparable effects related to reduction of arousal may occur and can be clinically important. However, they should be viewed as nonspecific effects of sedation or pain control, or both, rather than specific properties of narcotics. The following discussion emphasizes investigations in which control measurements were unlikely to have been significantly influenced by arousal phenomena.

Morphine. When morphine (~1 mg/kg) was administered as the sole drug to humans, no effect on global CBF and a 41% decrease in the $CMRO_2$ were observed. The latter is a substantial reduction, and the absence of a simultaneous adjustment in CBF is surprising. No other investigations of morphine have been conducted in humans alone. Administration of morphine (1 mg/kg and 3 mg/kg) with 70% N_2O to patients did not significantly change CBF or CMR.[48] The N_2O that was used might be expected to have caused a tendency toward increases in CBF. The relative absence of *net* changes in these variables from awake control measurements suggests a small-to-moderate depressive effect of morphine on CBF and CMR at this large dose. However, morphine can cause a substantial release of histamine in individual patients. Histamine is a cerebral vasodilator that will cause an increase in CBV and a CBF effect that will vary, depending on the systemic blood pressure response.

Autoregulation was observed to be intact between MAP values of 60 and 120 mm Hg in human volunteers anesthetized with a combination of morphine, 2 mg/kg, and 70% N_2O.[97]

Fentanyl. Fentanyl, in a dose range of 12 to 30 (mean, 16) μg/kg, in combination with 50% N_2O, reduced CBF and CMR modestly, by 21% and 26%, respectively, in comparison to the awake control state. The data for fentanyl-N_2O presented in Fig. 11.10 are derived from these patients. In combination with 0.4 mg/kg of diazepam, high dose fentanyl (100 μg/kg) led to a reduction of CBF by 25%, although part of this effect may well have been a result of benzodiazepine (see later discussion in the section, "Benzodiazepine") rather than fentanyl *per se*. In sedative doses of 1.5 μg/kg, fentanyl increased CBF in the frontal, temporal, and cerebellar areas simultaneous with decreases in discrete areas associated with pain-related processing. CO_2 responsiveness and autoregulation are unaffected, and the hyperemic CBF response to hypoxia remains intact.

In conclusion, fentanyl will cause a moderate global reduction in CBF and CMR in the normal quiescent brain and will, similar to morphine, cause larger reductions when administered during arousal.

Alfentanil. Administration of alfentanil, 320 μg/kg, to pentobarbital-anesthetized dogs[98] did not affect CBF, CMR, CO_2 responsiveness, autoregulation, or CBF response to hypoxia. No studies of the effects of alfentanil on the CMR in humans have been conducted. In patients in whom anesthesia was induced with thiopental, administration of 25 to 50 μg/kg of alfentanil transiently decreased MCAfv, indicating a slight reduction in CBF.[99] By contrast,[100] no change in MCAfv was observed in response to 25 to 50 μg/kg of alfentanil given to patients during the maintenance of anesthesia with isoflurane-N_2O. An evaluation of the surgical field in patients undergoing craniotomy to whom alfentanil was administered did not reveal any adverse events.[101,102]

In general, alfentanil does not significantly impact the cerebral circulation, provided that alfentanil induced reduction in MAP is prevented.

Sufentanil. Studies in humans indicate that sufentanil causes, depending on the dose, either no change or a modest reduction in CBF and CMR. Induction of anesthesia with 10 μg/kg of sufentanil[68] resulted in a 29% reduction in CBF and a 22% reduction in $CMRO_2$. In healthy human volunteers, 0.5 μg/kg of sufentanil[103] does not affect CBF.

Sufentanil, at doses of 1.0 and 2.0 μg/kg, decreases MCAfv in head injured patients with increased ICP.

A logical conclusion is that no change and no reduction in ICP occur as a result of the administration of either sufentanil or alfentanil. However, in some investigations in humans, sufentanil was associated with modest increases in ICP. The increases in ICP associated with sufentanil are likely the consequence, in part, of a normal autoregulatory response to the sudden reduction in MAP that can occur as a consequence of sufentanil administration.[104] Therefore sufentanil and fentanyl should be administered in a manner that does not produce a sudden reduction of MAP. Such a decrease will reduce CPP and may increase ICP, each of which, in sufficient extreme, may be deleterious. However, ICP increases attributed to sufentanil are small. Furthermore, conditions in the surgical field, including pressure under brain retractors[101] and the state of brain relaxation, revealed no adverse influences attributable to sufentanil. Accordingly, sufentanil need not be viewed as contraindicated in any way, although its effect on MAP should be followed closely.

Remifentanil. Investigations of moderate doses of remifentanil in patients have revealed effects similar to those of other synthetic narcotics (with the exception of its substantially shorter duration of action). In patients undergoing craniotomy for supratentorial space-occupying lesions, 1 μg/kg of remifentanil caused no change in ICP.[105] In a second investigation in patients undergoing craniotomies, approximately 0.35 μg/kg/min of remifentanil resulted in CBF values comparable to those observed with moderately deep anesthesia with either isoflurane-N_2O or fentanyl-N_2O,[106] and CO_2 responsiveness was preserved. Greater doses of remifentanil may have more substantial effects. MCAfv decreased by 30% in response to 5 μg/kg, followed by 3 μg/kg/min of remifentanil at a constant MAP in patients being anesthetized for bypass surgery.[69] However, a lower dose of 2 μg/kg, followed by an infusion of 3 μg/kg/min, did not affect MCAfV. Quantitatively, the effects of remifentanil appear to be similar to those of sufentanil.

Remifentanil was administered with other drugs that might influence cerebral hemodynamics. More recent studies in human volunteers have demonstrated that the infusion of small (sedative) doses of remifentanil can increase CBF. A PET study in human subjects to whom remifentanil, 0.05 and 0.15 μg/kg/min, was administered revealed increases in CBF in the prefrontal, inferior parietal, and supplementary motor cortices; reductions in CBF were observed in the cerebellum, superior temporal lobe, and midbrain gray matter.[105] The relative increase in CBF was greater with the administration of the larger dose of remifentanil. Similar data were obtained by Lorenz and colleagues,[107] who used magnetic resonance imaging (MRI) to determine CBF.[107] In a PET investigation in human volunteers,[108] remifentanil-induced increases in regional CBF within the limbic system were observed. Although the underlying mechanisms of the increases in CBF are not clear, disinhibition produced by the small-dose remifentanil infusion, or perhaps the sensation of side effects (e.g., warmth, comfort, pruritus),[107] may have contributed. When combined with N_2O, CBF and CO_2 reactivity is similar in patients given remifentanil or fentanyl.[106] In conclusion, sedative doses of remifentanil alone can cause minor increases in CBF. With larger doses or with the concomitant administration of anesthetic adjuvants, CBF is either unaltered or modestly reduced.

Benzodiazepines

Benzodiazepines cause parallel reductions in CBF and CMR in humans. CBF and $CMRO_2$ decreased by 25% when 15 mg of diazepam was given to patients with head injuries. The effects of midazolam on CBF (but not on CMR) have also been studied in humans. Administration of 0.15 mg/kg of midazolam to awake healthy human volunteers resulted in a 30% to 34% reduction in CBF.[71,109] In an investigation using PET scanning, a similar dose of midazolam led to a global 12% reduction in CBF; the decreases occurred preferentially in the brain regions associated with arousal, attention, and memory.[110] CO_2 responsiveness was preserved.[111]

The available data indicate that benzodiazepines cause a moderate reduction in CBF in humans, which is coupled to metabolism. The extent of the maximal reductions of CBF and CMR produced by benzodiazepines is probably intermediate between the decreases caused by narcotics (modest) and barbiturates (substantial). It appears that benzodiazepines should be safe to administer to patients with intracranial hypertension, provided that respiratory depression (and an associated increase in $Paco_2$) or hypotension do not occur.

Flumazenil is a highly specific, competitive benzodiazepine receptor antagonist. It had no effect on CBF when administered to nonanesthetized human volunteers.[109,112] However, flumazenil reverses the CBF-, CMR-, and ICP-lowering effects of midazolam. When patients were aroused from midazolam anesthesia with flumazenil at the conclusion of craniotomy for brain tumor resection,[113] no change in either CBF or CMR was observed. By contrast, severe increases in ICP occurred when flumazenil was given to patients with severe head injury in whom ICP was not well controlled.[114] These latter observations are consistent with animal investigations during which flumazenil not only reversed the CBF and CMR effects of midazolam, but it also caused a substantial, although short-lived, overshoot above premidazolam levels in both CBF and ICP by 44% to 56% and 180% to 217%, respectively. The CMR did not rise above control levels, thus indicating that the increase in CBF was not metabolically coupled. The CBF overshoot effect is unexplained, but it may be a neurogenically mediated arousal phenomenon. Flumazenil should be used cautiously to reverse benzodiazepine sedation in patients with impaired intracranial compliance.

Droperidol

No human investigations of the CBF and CMR effects of droperidol have been conducted in isolation. However, the information available from animal investigations and combination drug administration in humans,[115] taken together, suggests that droperidol is not a cerebral vasodilator and probably has little effect on CBF and CMR in humans. The occasional increases in ICP that have been observed[115] probably reflect normal autoregulation-mediated vasodilation in response to an abrupt decrease in MAP.

Ketamine

Among the intravenous anesthetics, ketamine is unique in its ability to cause increases in both CBF and CMR.[116] Animal studies indicate that the changes in the CMR are regionally variable; substantial increases occur in limbic system structures with modest changes or small decreases in cortical structures.[117] PET studies in humans have demonstrated that subanesthetic doses of ketamine (0.2-0.3 mg/kg) can increase global CMR by approximately 25%.[118] The greatest increase in the CMR occurred in the frontal and anterior cingulate cortex. A relative reduction in the CMR in the cerebellum was also observed. Commercially available formulations of ketamine contain both the *(S)*- and *(R)*-ketamine enantiomers. The *(S)*-ketamine enantiomer substantially increases CMR, whereas the *(R)* enantiomer tends to decrease the CMR, particularly in the temporomedial cortex and in the cerebellum.[119] These changes in the CMR are accompanied by corresponding changes in CBF.[120] Global, as well as regional, increases in CBF in humans that were not accompanied by similar increases in the $CMRO_2$ after the administration of *(S)*-ketamine enantiomer have been observed. Both subanesthetic and anesthetic doses of ketamine increased global CBF by approximately 14% and 36%, respectively, without altering global $CMRO_2$. As expected, in the face of an unchanged CMR and increased CBF, the oxygen extraction ratio was reduced.[77] The majority of investigations indicate that autoregulation is maintained during ketamine anesthesia,[121] and CO_2 responsiveness is preserved. A recent metaanalysis concluded that, in humans, ketamine administration increases CBF, particularly in the anterior cingulate gyrus, medial prefrontal cortex, and occipital lobes. In aggregate, the available data indicate that ketamine does increase CBF, and the accompanying increase in CMR is at best modest. Ketamine does not increase CBV.[122]

The anticipated increase in ICP with an increase in CBF has not been confirmed to occur in humans. When examined in their entirety, the available data indicate that ketamine does not increase ICP in patients with nontraumatic neurologic illness[122] nor in patients with traumatic brain injury.[122] In fact, decreases in ICP occur when relatively large anesthetic doses of ketamine (1.5-5 mg/kg) are administered to patients with head injuries who are sedated with propofol.[123] However, it should be noted that, in most of the studies in which the ICP effects of ketamine have been evaluated, patients received sedative agents in addition to ketamine. It has been established that anesthetic drugs (diazepam, midazolam, isoflurane-N_2O, propofol, opioids, methohexital) blunt or eliminate the increases in ICP or CBF associated with ketamine.[116,124,125] Accordingly, although ketamine is probably best avoided as the sole anesthetic drug in patients with impaired intracranial compliance, it may be cautiously given to patients who are simultaneously receiving adjunctive sedative drugs.

Lidocaine

In nonanesthetized human volunteers, reductions in CBF and CMR of 24% and 20%, respectively, were observed after the administration of 5 mg/kg of lidocaine over a 30-minute period, followed by an infusion of 45 µg/kg/min.[126] When very large doses (160 mg/kg) were given to dogs maintained on cardiopulmonary bypass, the reduction in the $CMRO_2$ was apparently more than that observed with large-dose barbiturates.[127] The membrane-stabilizing effect of lidocaine probably reduces the energy required for the maintenance of membrane integrity.

The effectiveness of bolus doses of thiopental, 3 mg/kg, and lidocaine, 1.5 mg/kg, in controlling the acute increase in ICP that occurred after the application of a pin head holder or skin incision in patients undergoing craniotomies has been assessed.[128] The two regimens were equally effective in causing a reduction in ICP. However, the decrease in the MAP was greater with thiopental. Accordingly, a bolus dose of lidocaine is a reasonable adjunct to the prevention or treatment of acute increases in ICP and can prevent increases in ICP associated with endotracheal suctioning. Although large doses of lidocaine can produce seizures in humans, lidocaine-induced seizures have not been reported in anesthetized humans. Nonetheless, lidocaine doses should be adjusted to achieve serum levels less than the seizure threshold (>5-10 µg/mL) in awake humans. After a 2-mg/kg bolus, peak serum concentrations of 6.6 to 8.5 µg/mL are below the seizure threshold. Bolus doses of 1.5 to 2.0 mg/kg therefore seem appropriate.

INHALED ANESTHETICS

Volatile Anesthetics

The pattern of volatile anesthetic effects on cerebral physiology is quite different than that of intravenous anesthetics, which generally cause parallel reductions in CMR and CBF. All volatile anesthetics, in a manner similar to intravenous sedative-hypnotic drugs, suppress cerebral metabolism in a dose-related fashion.[129-132] Volatile anesthetics also possess intrinsic cerebral vasodilatory activity as a result of direct effects on vascular smooth muscle. The net effect of volatile anesthetics on CBF is therefore a balance between a reduction in CBF caused by CMR suppression and an augmentation of CBF caused by the direct cerebral vasodilation. When administered at a dose of 0.5 MAC, CMR suppression–induced reduction in CBF predominates, and net CBF decreases in comparison with the awake state. At 1 MAC, concentrations of isoflurane, sevoflurane, or desflurane, CBF remains unchanged; at this concentration, CMR suppression and vasodilatory effects are in balance. Beyond 1 MAC, the vasodilatory activity predominates, and CBF significantly increases, even though the CMR is substantially reduced (Fig. 11.11).[133] Vasodilation with increasing doses of volatile agents lead to an attenuation of cerebral autoregulation. With large doses, autoregulation is abolished and cerebral perfusion becomes pressure passive (Fig. 11.12).

The increase in CBF produced by volatile anesthetics at doses larger than 1 MAC has been referred to as reflecting a loss of neurovascular coupling. However, coupling (CBF adjustments paralleling changes in the CMR) persists during anesthesia with volatile anesthetics.[134-138] Accordingly, the conclusion should be that the CBF/CMR ratio is altered (increased) by volatile anesthetics. This alteration is dose related, and under steady-state conditions, increasing doses of volatile agents lead to greater CBF/$CMRO_2$ ratios[130,139]—that is, higher MAC levels cause greater luxury perfusion.

The important clinical consequences of the administration of volatile anesthetics are derived from the increases in

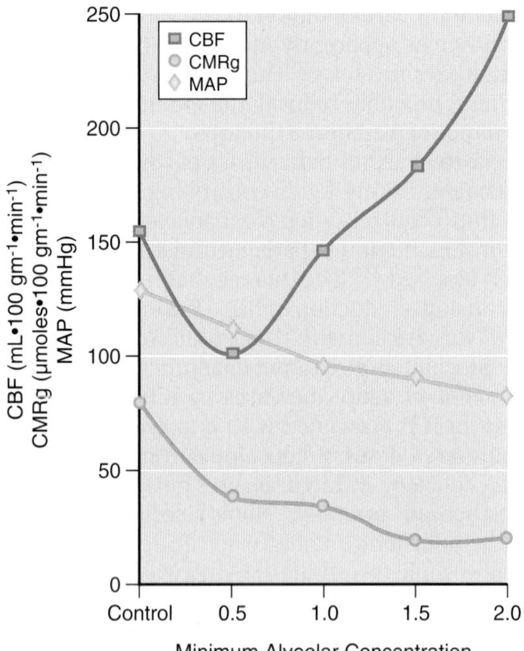

Fig. 11.11 Relationship between changes in the cerebral metabolic rate of glucose *(CMRg)* and cerebral blood flow *(CBF)* in the motor-sensory cortex in rats during isoflurane anesthesia. The majority of the suppression in the CMR caused by isoflurane has occurred by 1 minimum alveolar concentration; CBF is not increased in this concentration range. Thereafter, additional isoflurane causes little further reduction in the CMR, and cerebral vasodilation occurs. These data (± standard deviation) from Maekawa and colleagues[133] suggest the importance of metabolic coupling in determining the effects of isoflurane on CBF. *MAP,* Mean arterial pressure.

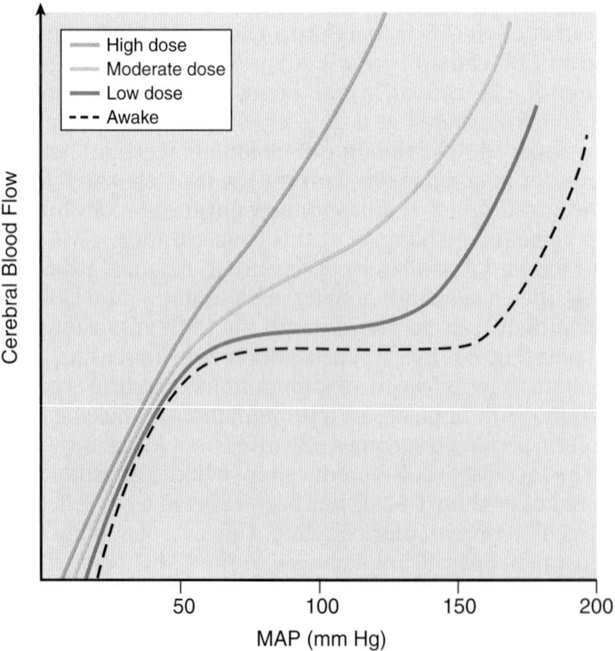

Fig. 11.12 Schematic representation of the effect of increasing concentrations of a typical volatile anesthetic drug on autoregulation of cerebral blood flow. Dose-dependent cerebral vasodilation results in attenuation of autoregulatory response to increasing mean arterial pressure *(MAP).* Both the upper and lower thresholds are shifted to the left.

CBF and CBV—and consequently ICP—that can occur. Of the commonly used volatile anesthetics, the order of vasodilating potency is approximately halothane ≫ enflurane > desflurane ≈ isoflurane > sevoflurane.

Effects on cerebral blood flow. Volatile anesthetics possess intrinsic vasodilatory activity, and they not only modify cerebral autoregulation, but they also produce a dose-dependent decrease in arterial blood pressure. Hence, their effects on CBF and CMR are best evaluated when arterial blood pressure is maintained at a constant level. In addition, the cerebrovascular effects of volatile anesthetics are modulated by the simultaneous administration of other CNS-active drugs. The control state—awake, sedated, or anesthetized—against which the CBF and CMR effects of volatile anesthetics are compared, is important to recognize. The best information concerning the cerebrovascular effects of volatile anesthetics is obtained in studies during which a nonanesthetized (awake) control state is used.

Data on the cerebrovascular effects of halothane and enflurane are limited. Initial studies in humans demonstrated that the administration of 1 MAC halothane significantly increases CBF, even when systemic blood pressure is substantially reduced, in comparison with preanesthetic CBF. When the MAP is maintained at 80 mm Hg, 1.1 MAC levels of halothane increase CBF by as much as 191% and decrease the CMR by approximately 10% (Fig. 11.13).[140,141] When compared with awake values, 1.2 MAC enflurane also increased CBF and decreased CMR by 45% and 15%, respectively.[142] The dramatic increases in CBF with a simultaneous modest reduction in the CMR attest to the cerebral vasodilatory properties of halothane and enflurane. Isoflurane, by contrast, does not increase CBF as much as halothane or enflurane. At concentrations of 1.1 MAC, isoflurane increases CBF by approximately 19% when arterial blood pressure is maintained within the normal range. The CMR is reduced by approximately 45%.[137]

Both sevoflurane and desflurane can reduce CBF significantly in humans when compared with CBF in awake, nonanesthetized patients. At 1 MAC concentrations, sevoflurane[143] and desflurane[142] decreased CBF by 38% and 22% and CMR by 39% and 35%, respectively. These results, which suggest that the cerebral vasodilation produced by isoflurane is greater than that produced by sevoflurane and desflurane, were obtained with CBF measured by the Kety-Schmidt technique. This technique primarily measures CBF within the cortex and therefore may have substantially underestimated global CBF. PET studies in healthy humans have shown that sevoflurane dose-dependently suppresses the $CMRO_2$ and CBF; at 1 MAC levels, the reduction in CBF and $CMRO_2$ is approximately 50% and 50% to 60%, respectively.[83,84] Even with a significant reduction in CBF, the administration of sevoflurane does not cause a decrease in CBV. Other investigations in humans, most using the measurement of MCAfv by transcranial Doppler, indicate that differences in the effects of isoflurane, desflurane (Fig. 11.14*A*), and sevoflurane are modest.[144-147] Unfortunately, a strictly quantitative comparison among these volatile anesthetics is not possible because of the variations in arterial blood pressure among study group patients. In addition, some discrepancy exists among studies in the

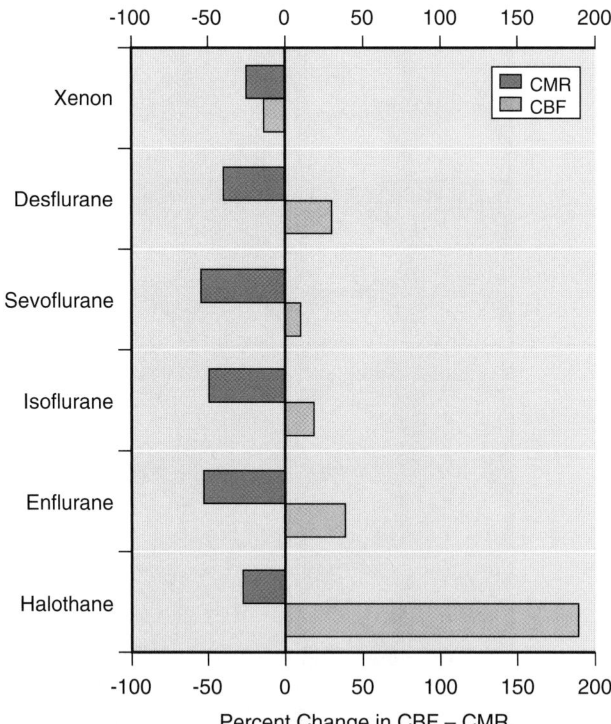

Fig. 11.13 Estimated changes in cerebral blood flow *(CBF)* and the cerebral metabolic rate of oxygen ($CMRO_2$) caused by volatile anesthetics. The CBF data for halothane, enflurane, and isoflurane were obtained during anesthesia (with blood pressure support) at 1.1 minimum alveolar concentration (MAC) in humans[356] and are expressed as percent change from awake control values. The $CMRO_2$ data for halothane, enflurane, and isoflurane were obtained in cats[130,140] and are expressed as percent change from N_2O-sedated control values. The data for sevoflurane were obtained during 1.1 MAC anesthesia in rabbits and are expressed as percent change from a morphine-N_2O–anesthetized control state.[132] CBF values were obtained in patients who received 1 MAC sevoflurane anesthesia.[143] Desflurane data were obtained in patients to whom 1 MAC desflurane was administered.[141] *CMR*, Cerebral metabolic rate.

literature regarding the magnitude of the effects of volatile anesthetics on CBF. Much of this inconsistency may occur as a result of the interaction of regionally selective CBF methods with the heterogeneity within the cerebrum of the CBF effects of volatile anesthetics. (See the later section, "Distribution of Changes in Cerebral Blood Flow/Cerebral Metabolic Rate.")

The anesthetic properties of xenon were recognized several decades ago, but this anesthetic is only now being evaluated for possible use in patients. The MAC of xenon has been estimated to be 63% to 71%, with female patients having significantly lower MAC values (51%).[147] Xenon exerts its anesthetic effect via noncompetitive antagonism of the *N*-methyl-D-aspartate receptor (NMDAR),[148] although activation of the TREK two-pore K^+ channel may also play a role.[149] In healthy humans, the administration of 1 MAC xenon resulted in a reduction in CBF by approximately 15% in the cortex and by 35% in the cerebellum. Interestingly, CBF in white matter increased by 22%.[150] This reduction in CBF is accompanied by a parallel reduction of the cerebral metabolic rate of glucose (CMRg) by 26%.[151] Cerebral autoregulation and CO_2 reactivity are preserved during xenon anesthesia in animals.[152] Under background pentobarbital anesthesia in an experimental model of increased ICP, the administration of xenon did not increase ICP, and the response to both hypocapnia and hypercapnia was preserved.[153] Diffusion of xenon into air-containing spaces such as the bowel does occur, although the magnitude of air expansion is considerably less than that with N_2O.[154] Nonetheless, caution will have to be exercised with the use of xenon in patients with intracranial air. These data indicate that xenon has a favorable profile for neuroanesthesia.

Effects on cerebral metabolic rate. All volatile anesthetics cause reductions in CMR. The degree of reduction in $CMRO_2$ that occurs at a given MAC is less with halothane

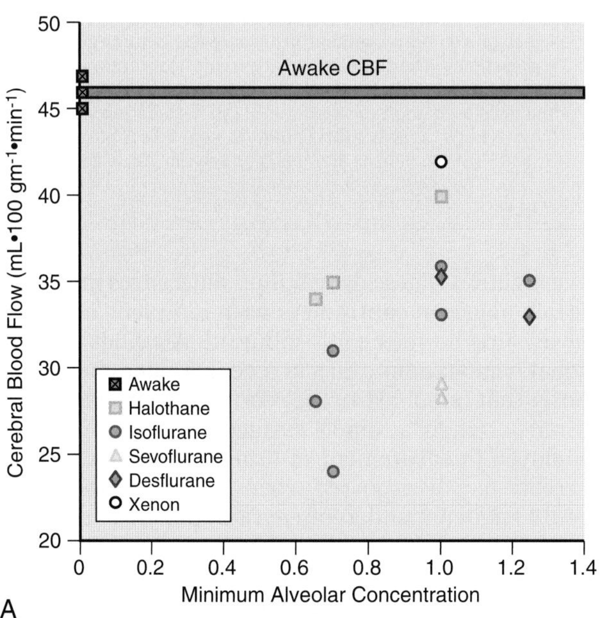

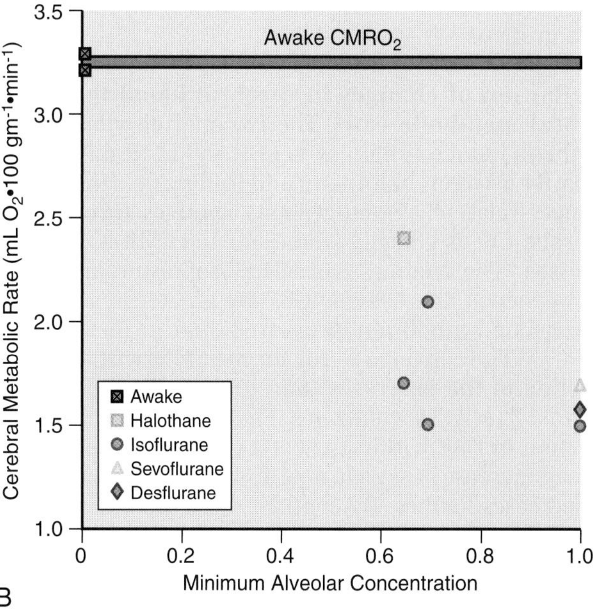

Fig. 11.14 Effect of volatile anesthetics on cerebral blood flow *(CBF)* (A) and the cerebral metabolic rate of oxygen *($CMRO_2$)* (B) in awake humans. The results are a composite of CBF and $CMRO_2$ values obtained from a number of separate investigations.[72,130,131,135-137,139-146,356-358] In these studies, arterial partial pressure of carbon dioxide ($PaCO_2$) was maintained in the normocapnic range (~35-40 mm Hg), and mean arterial pressure was supported. In most of the investigations, CBF was measured by a radioactive xenon washout technique; this technique primarily measures cortical CBF and, as such, may underestimate global CBF. This, in addition to species differences, probably account for the disparities between the data on the CBF effects attributed to volatile agents in this figure and Fig. 11.13.

than with the other four anesthetics. Sevoflurane's effect on the $CMRO_2$ is very similar to that of isoflurane. The available information, derived in separate investigations, suggests that desflurane causes slightly less suppression of the $CMRO_2$ than isoflurane, especially at concentrations above 1 MAC.[131] Although a direct comparison of the $CMRO_2$ effects of all of the volatile anesthetics has not been performed in humans, doses of 1 MAC isoflurane, sevoflurane, and desflurane clearly reduce the $CMRO_2$ by 25%,[155] 38%,[141] and 22%,[156] respectively. In PET studies, halothane (0.9 MAC) and isoflurane (0.5 MAC) can decrease the CMRg by 40% and 46%, respectively.[85,157] The decrease in the $CMRO_2$ is dose-related. With isoflurane (and almost certainly desflurane and sevoflurane as well), the maximal reduction is simultaneously attained with the occurrence of EEG suppression,[131] which occurs at clinically relevant concentrations, in the range of 1.5 to 2 MAC in humans. With additional isoflurane, 6% end-tidal concentration results in no further reduction in the CMR and no indication of metabolic toxicity. Halothane presents a contrast to this pattern. Halothane concentrations more than 4 MAC are required to achieve EEG suppression in animals, and additional halothane causes a further reduction in the $CMRO_2$ in concert with alterations in energy charge. The latter changes, which are reversible, suggest interference with oxidative phosphorylation by halothane.

Some nonlinearity exists in the CBF and CMR dose-response relationships for volatile anesthetics. The initial appearance of an EEG pattern associated with the onset of anesthesia with halothane, enflurane, and isoflurane is accompanied by a sharp decline in the $CMRO_2$.[131] Thereafter, the $CMRO_2$ declines in a slower dose-dependent manner. Such an effect has also been demonstrated for sevoflurane. In a dose escalation study in humans, the greatest reduction in entropy (i.e., a measure of anesthetic depth) was observed with 1 MAC sevoflurane anesthesia, with lesser reductions occurring at increasing concentrations.[158]

Distribution of changes in cerebral blood flow and cerebral metabolic rate. The regional distribution of anesthetic-induced changes in CBF and CMR differs significantly between halothane and isoflurane. Halothane produces relatively homogeneous changes throughout the brain. CBF is globally increased, and CMR is globally depressed. The changes caused by isoflurane are more heterogeneous. Increases in CBF are greater in subcortical areas and hindbrain structures than in the neocortex.[136,159] The converse is true for the CMR, with a larger reduction in the neocortex than in the subcortex.[133] In humans, 1 MAC sevoflurane (Fig. 11.15) results in a reduction in CBF within the cortex and the cerebellum. With an increase in sevoflurane dose, CBF within the cortex decreases further. By contrast, flow increases in the cerebellum with doses greater than 1.5 MAC.[83] These effects of sevoflurane are similar to those produced by isoflurane.[83,159] Desflurane has not been evaluated by local CBF studies. However, considering the similarity of its effects on the EEG (suggesting similar cortical CMR and CBF effects), an assumption of similar heterogeneity in CBF distribution seems reasonable, pending further

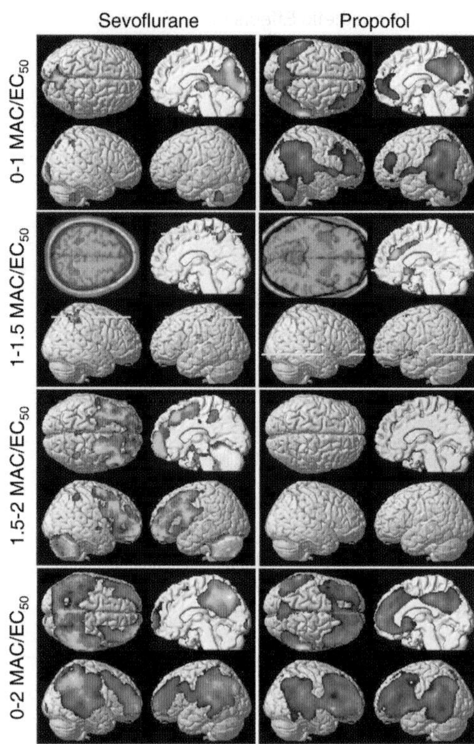

Fig. 11.15 Dose-dependent redistribution of cerebral blood flow (CBF) in humans. Positron-emission tomography (PET) scans demonstrate a dose-dependent reduction in CBF in both sevoflurane-anesthetized *(left)* and propofol-anesthetized *(right)* subjects. During sevoflurane anesthesia, there is a concentration dependent reduction in CBF within the cerebrum (indicated by blue color). An increase in concentration from 1.5 to 2 minimum alveolar concentration *(MAC)* leads to an increase in CBF within the cerebellum (indicated by the yellow-red color). A gradual reduction in the mean arterial pressure (MAP) occurred with increasing concentrations of sevoflurane, and the MAP was not supported. The CBF values would be expected to be considerably greater had blood pressure been maintained within the normal range. Therefore the CBF values represented in this figure probably *underestimate* true CBF during sevoflurane anesthesia. Propofol was administered in EC_{50} equivalents, defined as the plasma concentration that prevented movement in response to a surgical stimulus in 50% of patients. The target plasma propofol concentrations were 0, 6, 9, and 12 μg/mL. In propofol-anesthetized subjects, CBF was uniformly decreased and redistribution of CBF was not observed. (Modified from Kaisti K, Metsähonkala L, Teräs M, et al. Effects of surgical levels of propofol and sevoflurane anesthesia on cerebral blood flow in healthy subjects studied with positron emission tomography. *Anesthesiology.* 2002;96:1358–1370.)

investigation. These distribution differences may explain certain apparent contradictions in reported CBF effects in the existing literature for isoflurane. Methods that assess global hemodynamic effects reveal greater changes than those that emphasize the cortical compartment. For instance, when a xenon surface washout technique is employed (measurement of local cortical flow only), no increase in CBF occurred when isoflurane was administered to patients undergoing craniotomy.[160]

Time dependence of cerebral blood flow effects. The effects of volatile anesthetics on CBF are time-dependent in animal investigations. After an initial increase, CBF decreases and reaches a steady state near pre–volatile agent levels between 2.5 and 5 hours after exposure.[161-163] The mechanism of this effect is not

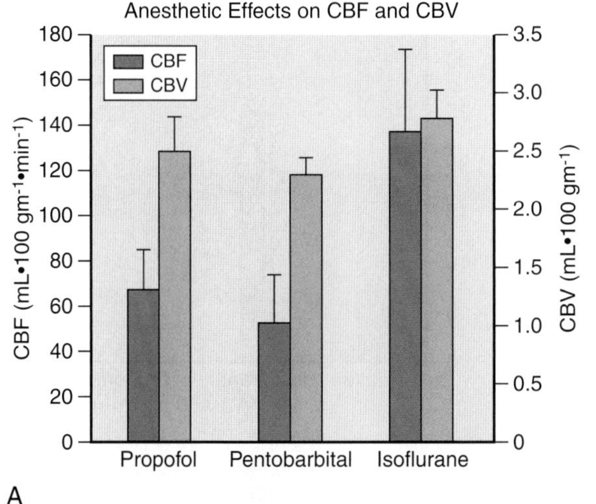

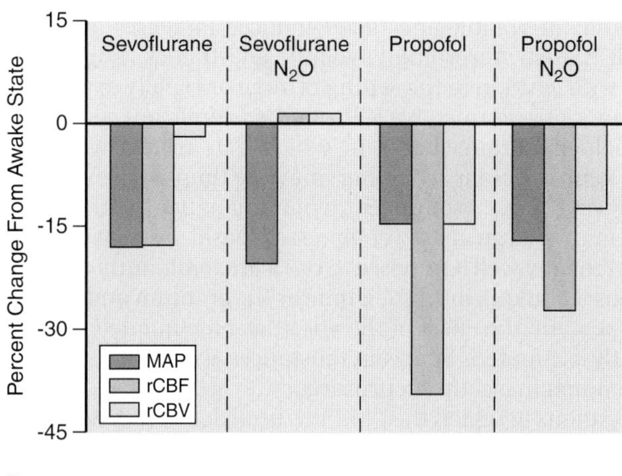

Fig. 11.16 Effect of anesthetic drugs on cerebral blood flow *(CBF)* and cerebral blood volume *(CBV)*. (A) When compared with isoflurane, propofol and pentobarbital effected substantial reductions in CBF. However, reductions in CBV were more modest.[151] (B) Although sevoflurane effected a significant reduction in regional CBF (rCBF), regional CBV (rCBV) was unchanged. Had blood pressure been supported to normal levels, rCBV may have been greater than the awake state. By contrast, propofol effected a significant reduction in both rCBF and rCBV. These data indicate that the magnitude of the effect of anesthetics on rCBF is substantially greater than on rCBV. Hence, decreases in rCBF may not lead to equivalent reductions in rCBV. *MAP,* Mean arterial pressure; *N_2O,* nitrous oxide.

understood, and the phenomenon was not evident in humans studied during a 3- or 6-hour exposure to halothane, isoflurane, desflurane, or sevoflurane.[146,164]

Cerebral blood volume. The extensive investigation of the influence of volatile anesthetics on CBF has been primarily based on the concern that the cerebral vasodilation produced by volatile anesthetics might increase ICP. However, it is CBV and not CBF, per se, that influences ICP. Most of the intracranial blood is within the cerebral venous circulation; although a reasonable correlation exists between vasodilation-induced increases in CBF and CBV, the magnitude of changes in CBF is considerably greater than that in CBV (see Fig. 11.9). Hence, changes in CBF do not reliably predict changes in CBV and, by extension, in ICP. CBV is considerably greater during isoflurane anesthesia than during propofol or pentobarbital anesthesia.[63] In human volunteers, 1 MAC sevoflurane reduced regional CBF but not regional CBV; by contrast, propofol reduced both regional CBF and regional CBV (Fig. 11.16).[84] In addition, CBV responds to changes in $Paco_2$ by a reduction in CBV with hypocapnia and an increase in CBV with hypercapnia. The magnitude of the change in CBV is, however, less than the change in CBF. In aggregate, although the effect of anesthetics and interventions on CBF may parallel the effect on CBV, substantial qualitative and quantitative differences may well be observed.

Carbon dioxide responsiveness and autoregulation. CO_2 responsiveness is well maintained during anesthesia with all volatile anesthetics.[145,165,166] As with all vasodilators, CBF is preserved up to lower MAP values during the administration of volatile anesthetics with no evidence of differences among the various anesthetics. Direct comparisons of CBF with isoflurane, desflurane, and sevoflurane anesthesia during hypotension are not available. By contrast, autoregulation of CBF in response to increasing arterial blood pressure is impaired, which is most apparent with the anesthetics that cause the most cerebral vasodilation and are dose related. Sevoflurane may cause less impairment of the autoregulatory response to increasing blood pressure than other volatile anesthetics. Recent studies surprisingly report no change in MCAfv in response to phenylephrine-induced increases in the MAP during anesthesia with 1.2 to 1.5 MAC sevoflurane[167,168] or in CBF during hemorrhagic hypotension.[169] The autoregulatory response to increasing blood pressure may be pertinent during acute episodes of hypertension, such as during laryngoscopy or mismatch of surgical stimulation to anesthetic depth.

Cerebral vasodilation by anesthetics—clinical implications. Isoflurane, desflurane, and sevoflurane may have a modest cerebral vasodilating effect in the human cortex when administered at doses of 1 MAC or less. In fact, the administration of volatile anesthetics may produce a net decrease in CBF (see Fig. 11.14*A*). These data, however, should be interpreted with the knowledge that the critical variable of interest in the clinical setting is CBV. Although a direct correlation exists between CBF and CBV, as noted earlier, the relationship is not strictly 1:1. The magnitude of the changes in CBV is significantly less than the magnitude of the changes in CBF, and modest reductions in CBF may not necessarily be accompanied by reductions in CBV. This finding is exemplified by clinical investigations in which a significant increase in ICP (and by extension, CBV) was observed in patients to whom isoflurane was administered at doses that should reduce CBF.[170,171] Although induction of hypocapnia mitigated the increase in ICP, hyperventilation may not be effective in blunting isoflurane-induced increases in ICP in patients with intracranial tumors.[172] In experimental investigations of cerebral injury, volatile anesthetics significantly increased ICP, which was not ameliorated by hypocapnia.[173] Collectively, these data suggest that volatile anesthetics have modest effects on cerebral hemodynamics in patients with normal intracranial compliance. However, in patients with abnormal intracranial compliance, the potential for volatile anesthetic–induced increases in CBV and ICP exist. Accordingly, volatile anesthetics should be used with caution in the setting of large or rapidly expanding mass lesions, unstable ICP, or other significant cerebral physiologic derangements in which CO_2 responsiveness and neurovascular coupling may be impaired. When they occur (e.g., a somnolent, vomiting patient with papilledema; a large mass; compressed basal cisterns), the clinician may well be advised to use a predominantly intravenous technique until such time as the cranium and dura are open and the effect of the anesthetic technique can be directly evaluated. Such circumstances will be relatively uncommon in elective neurosurgery.

Situations in which the CMR has been decreased by drug administration or disease processes should also justify caution in the use of volatile anesthetics. As previously noted, the vasodilation mediated increase in CBF induced by a volatile anesthetic is in part, and at low doses, offset by an opposing metabolically mediated vasoconstriction (see Fig. 11.11). In situations in which the CMR is already reduced, the vasodilatory activity will predominate and, therefore, the increase in CBF will be greater. For example, when CMR is only slightly reduced by morphine, isoflurane does not cause significant increase in CBF. However, under thiopental anesthesia, the introduction of isoflurane significantly increases CBF.[135] Similarly, prior propofol anesthesia produces near maximal suppression of CMR; in this situation, introduction of any of the volatile agents leads to significant increases in CBF.[89] In essence, antecedent CMR suppression unmasks the vasodilatory action of volatile anesthetics. These data also suggest that caution must be exercised in the administration of volatile anesthetics in pathologic conditions, such as traumatic brain injury, in which metabolism is already reduced.

The net vasodilating effects of equi-MAC concentrations of isoflurane, desflurane, and sevoflurane are less in humans than that of halothane, and the former are probably therefore preferable if a volatile anesthetic is to be used in the setting of impaired intracranial compliance. When hypocapnia is established before the introduction of halothane, the increases in ICP that might otherwise occur in a normocapnic patient with poor intracranial compliance can be prevented or greatly attenuated. Nonetheless, isoflurane, desflurane, or sevoflurane are preferred because the margin for error is probably wider than with halothane.

Nitrous Oxide

N_2O can cause increases in CBF, CMR, and ICP. At least a portion of the increases in CBF and CMR may be the result of a sympathoadrenal-stimulating effect of N_2O. The magnitude of the effect considerably varies according to the presence or absence of other anesthetic drugs (Fig. 11.17).[174,175] When N_2O is administered alone, substantial increases in CBF and ICP can occur. In sharp contrast, when N_2O is administered in combination with intravenous drugs, including barbiturates, benzodiazepines, narcotics, and propofol, its cerebral-vasodilating effect is attenuated or even completely inhibited. The addition of N_2O to anesthesia established with a volatile anesthetic will result in moderate increases in CBF.

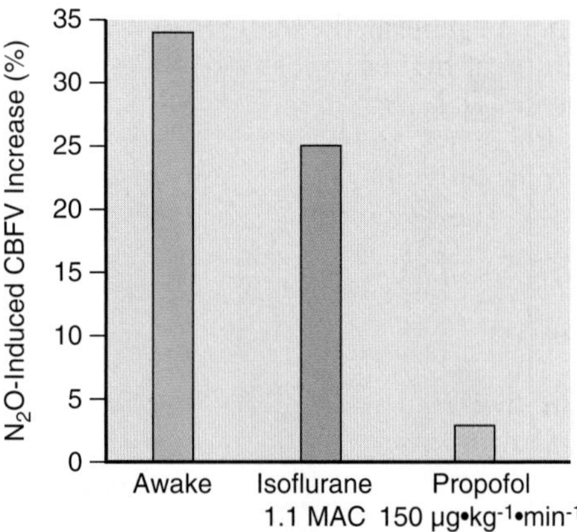

Fig. 11.17 Mean percent increases in cerebral blood flow velocity *(CBFV)* in the middle cerebral artery of normocapnic subjects exposed to 60% nitrous oxide (N_2O) after control recording in three conditions: awake;[174] 1.1 minimum alveolar concentration (MAC) of isoflurane;[179] and propofol, 150 μg/kg/min.[175]

The most dramatic increases in ICP or CBF in humans and experimental animals have occurred when N_2O was administered alone or with minimal background anesthesia. For instance, before and during spontaneous breathing of 66% N_2O by patients with intracranial tumors, mean ICP increased from 13 to 40 mm Hg.[176] The increases in CBF observed in humans are more modest than those observed in animals but are still substantial.[174] Whether these substantial increases represent the effects of N_2O, per se, or whether they reflect the nonspecific effects of a *second-stage* arousal phenomenon is not known.

When N_2O is administered in conjunction with certain intravenous anesthetics, its CBF effect may be considerably attenuated. In an investigation of patients with intracranial tumors and poor intracranial compliance (mean preinduction ICP, 27 mm Hg),[177] 50% N_2O introduced during barbiturate anesthesia and after the induction of hypocapnia had a negligible effect on ICP. Benzodiazepines administered alone have been shown to blunt the CBF response to N_2O in both animals and humans.[107] Narcotics appear to have a similar effect. Anesthesia with 1 mg/kg morphine and 70% N_2O resulted in no change in CBF from awake control values.[66] Because of the very minor effect of morphine on CBF, these data suggest that N_2O did not cause substantial cerebral vasodilation. Although the addition of N_2O to propofol anesthesia in children increased MCAfv in one study,[178] similar increases were not demonstrated by other investigators.[175]

In most investigations, including several in humans, during which N_2O has been added to a volatile anesthetic of 1 MAC or greater, substantial increases in CBF have been recorded.[179,180] A comparison of an approximately equi-MAC substitution of N_2O for isoflurane revealed that CBF was greater by 43% with 0.75 MAC isoflurane and 65% N_2O in comparison to 1.5 MAC isoflurane.[181] Several investigations have confirmed that CBF will be less with 1 MAC isoflurane than with a 1 MAC combination achieved with 50% to 65% N_2O and isoflurane.[179,181,182] These observations are consistent with a substantial additive vasodilating effect of N_2O in the presence of a volatile agent.

This vasodilating effect of N_2O may be positively correlated with the concentration of inhaled drug[180] and suggests that, in general, the increase in CBF caused by N_2O is exaggerated at higher concentrations of both halothane and isoflurane. Of importance, however, is the observation that the administration of 50% N_2O to healthy volunteers did not significantly alter CBV.[183] In support of this observation, N_2O did not have any effect on CBV when added to a background of 1 MAC sevoflurane anesthesia.[84] Although N_2O can increase CBF, these data indicate that its effect on CBV is modest.

Effects of nitrous oxide on cerebral metabolic rate. No uniform agreement has been reached concerning the effect of N_2O on the CMR. Parallel changes in CBF and CMR, increases in CBF without alteration of the CMR, and CMR alteration occurring without changes in CBF have all been reported. These findings are, doubtless, the product of differences in species, methods, depth of background anesthesia, and interactions with simultaneously administered anesthetics. In a recent investigation in humans, the administration of 70% N_2O on a background of either sevoflurane or propofol anesthesia resulted in modest increases in the $CMRO_2$, thus indicating that N_2O does indeed increase cerebral metabolism.[84]

The CBF response to CO_2 is preserved during the administration of N_2O.[184]

Clinical implications. Despite the inconsistencies that are evident, the vasodilatory action of N_2O can be clinically significant in neurosurgical patients with reduced intracranial compliance. However, N_2O-induced cerebral vasodilation can be considerably blunted by the simultaneous administration of intravenous anesthetics. By contrast, the addition of N_2O to a volatile drug–based anesthetic can modestly increase cerebral metabolism and blood flow. N_2O has been widely used in neurosurgery, and banishing it is inconsistent with the accumulated experience. Nonetheless, in circumstances wherein ICP is persistently elevated or the surgical field is persistently *tight*, N_2O should be viewed as a potential contributing factor. Because N_2O rapidly enters a closed gas space, it should be avoided or omitted when a closed intracranial gas space may exist or intravascular air is a concern.

MUSCLE RELAXANTS

Nondepolarizing Relaxants

The only recognized effect of nondepolarizing muscle relaxants on the cerebral vasculature occurs via the release of histamine. Histamine can result in a reduction in CPP because of the simultaneous increase in ICP (caused by cerebral vasodilation) and a decrease in the MAP. It is not entirely clear whether histamine directly causes cerebral vasodilation or whether it is a secondary (autoregulatory) response to a reduction in the MAP. *d*-Tubocurarine is the most potent histamine releaser among available muscle relaxants. Metocurine, atracurium, and mivacurium also release histamine in lesser quantities. This effect is likely to be clinically inconsequential unless these muscle relaxants are administered in the large doses necessary to achieve endotracheal intubation conditions rapidly. Of this group of drugs, cisatracurium has the least histamine-releasing effect. No evidence of histamine release was observed after the administration of 0.15 mg/kg of cisatracurium to neurosurgical patients in the intensive care unit.[185] Yet, cisatracurium's slow onset of action makes it less useful for a rapid sequence induction of anesthesia.

Vecuronium, in relatively large doses, does not have a significant effect on cerebral physiology in patients with brain tumors. The other aminosteroids, pipecuronium and rocuronium, should be similarly without direct effect, and no adverse events have been reported.

The indirect actions of relaxants may also have effects on cerebral physiology. Muscle relaxation may reduce ICP because coughing and straining are prevented, which decrease central venous pressure with a concomitant reduction in cerebral venous outflow impedance.

A metabolite of atracurium, laudanosine, may be epileptogenic. However, although large doses of atracurium caused an EEG arousal pattern in dogs, CBF, CMR, and ICP were unaltered.[186] In rabbits, the administration of laudanosine did not increase the severity of the epileptoid activity caused by the direct application of a cephalosporin to the cortical surface.[187] It appears highly unlikely that epileptogenesis will occur in humans with modest atracurium administration.[188]

In summary, vecuronium, pipecuronium, rocuronium, atracurium, mivacurium, cisatracurium, metocurine, and pancuronium (if acute MAP increases are prevented with the latter) are all reasonable muscle relaxants for use in patients with or at risk for intracranial hypertension. Doses of metocurine, atracurium, and mivacurium should be limited to ranges not associated with hypotension.

Rocuronium is increasingly being used for the induction of anesthesia, as well as for intraoperative relaxation. It has the most rapid onset time of any nondepolarizing muscle relaxant. With sugammadex, even a profound neuromuscular blockade can be rapidly reversed (see Chapters 27 and 28). The cerebrovascular effects of sugammadex have not yet been evaluated.

Succinylcholine

Succinylcholine can produce modest increases (~5 mm Hg) in ICP in lightly anesthetized humans. This effect appears to be the result of cerebral activation (as evidenced by EEG changes and increases in CBF) caused by afferent activity from the muscle spindle apparatus.[189] As might be expected with what appears to be an arousal phenomenon, deep anesthesia prevents succinylcholine-induced increases in ICP. The increase in ICP is also blocked by paralysis with vecuronium and by defasciculation with metocurine, 0.03 mg/kg.[190] The efficacy of other defasciculating anesthetics has not been examined in humans.

Although succinylcholine *can* produce increases in ICP, it can still be used for a rapid sequence induction of anesthesia. No change in ICP was observed after the administration of succinylcholine, 1 mg/kg, to 10 nonparalyzed, ventilated neurosurgical patients in the intensive care unit, 6 of whom had sustained a head injury.[191] Their observations are relevant because it is in precisely this population of patients that the issue of the use of succinylcholine arises most frequently. Considering that the ICP effects of succinylcholine may be an arousal phenomenon caused by increased afferent traffic from muscle spindles,[189] it is reasonable to assume that disease processes that substantially blunt the level of consciousness might similarly blunt this response. As with many anesthetics, the concern should

TABLE 11.3 Effects of Anesthetic Agents on the Rate of Cerebrospinal Fluid Secretion and Absorption

	Halothane	Enflurane	Isoflurane	Desflurane	Fentanyl	Etomidate
Secretion	↓	↑	—	↑	—	↓
Absorption	↓	↓	↑	—	↑	↑

Upward arrows indicate an increase in the rate of cerebrospinal fluid absorption or secretion, and downward arrows indicate a decrease. The information is presented nonquantitatively, and effects may vary with dose.

not be whether it is used but how it is used. When contraindications do not exist, with proper attention to the control of CO_2 tension, arterial blood pressure, and depth of anesthesia and after defasciculation, little hazard should attend succinylcholine administration.

Other Effects of Anesthetics on Cerebral Physiology

CEREBROSPINAL FLUID DYNAMICS

Anesthetics have been shown to influence both the rate of formation and the rate of reabsorption of CSF. Table 11.3 provides nonquantitative information about the direction of the influences of common anesthetic drugs. All the information has been derived from animals,[192-198] and these processes have not been examined in humans. Of the volatile anesthetics, halothane decreases the secretion of CSF, isoflurane has no effect, and enflurane and desflurane increase secretion. Absorption of CSF is reduced by halothane and enflurane, unchanged by desflurane, and increased by isoflurane. A theoretic concern might be in the setting of a prolonged closed-cranium procedure in a patient with poor intracranial compliance. The most deleterious potential combination of effects in a patient with poor intracranial compliance is increased CSF production and decreased reabsorption. This pattern occurs with enflurane in the dog, which is perhaps another reason (in addition to the potential for epileptogenesis in the presence of cerebral injury and hypocapnia) for omission of enflurane in this circumstance.

BLOOD-BRAIN BARRIER

In the majority of the body's capillary beds, fenestrations between endothelial cells are approximately 65 Å in diameter. In the brain, with the exception of the choroid plexus, in the pituitary, and in the area postrema, tight junctions reduce this pore size to approximately 8 Å. As a result, large molecules and most ions are prevented from entering the brain's interstitium (BBB). A limited number of studies of anesthetic effects on the BBB have been conducted. In experimental animals, 1% isoflurane leads to extravasation of albumin into the thalamus, indicating some compromise of the BBB integrity. At higher doses, isoflurane (3%) significantly increases protein extravasation, not only in the thalamus but also in the cortex.[199] This disruption of the BBB is quantitatively similar to that achieved by mannitol. In experimental models of brain injury, isoflurane has been reported to both exacerbate[200] and ameliorate[201] edema formation in the injured brain. Whether these effects are the result of isoflurane action at the BBB, *per se*, or to hemodynamic perturbations attendant upon anesthesia is not known. The clinical relevance of the potential BBB modulation by anesthetics is not clear. To the authors' knowledge, no peer-reviewed investigation has attempted a comparison of anesthetic effects on BBB function during anesthesia in normotensive humans.

EPILEPTOGENESIS

An extensive review of the pro- and anticonvulsant effects of anesthetics and adjuvants is available.[202,203] Several commonly used anesthetics have some epileptogenic potential, particularly in predisposed individuals. A concern is that seizure activity may go unrecognized in an anesthetized and paralyzed patient and may result in neuronal injury if substrate demand (CMR) exceeds supply for a prolonged period.[204] A second concern is that the epileptogenic effect will persist in the postanesthesia period when seizures may occur in less well-controlled circumstances than those that exist in the surgical unit. In practice, it appears that spontaneous seizures during or after anesthesia have been extremely rare events. Nonetheless, in patients with processes that might predispose them to seizures, the use of potentially epileptogenic drugs should be avoided in situations during which reasonable alternatives are available.

Volatile Anesthetics

Enflurane is potentially epileptogenic in clinical setting. Of particular relevance to neuroanesthesia is the observation that hypocapnia potentiates seizure-type discharges during enflurane anesthesia. A 50% decrease in the $CMRO_2$ was noted in human volunteers anesthetized with 3% enflurane; however, with the onset of seizure activity, the $CMRO_2$ returned to normal,[205] thus indicating preservation of neurovascular coupling. No evidence suggests that this type of EEG activity is deleterious when oxygen delivery is maintained during the event. However, because seizure activity can elevate brain metabolism by as much as 400%, the use of enflurane, especially at high doses and with hypocapnia, should probably be avoided in patients predisposed to seizures.

The EEG-activating property of enflurane has been used intraoperatively to activate and identify seizure foci that are to be surgically resected, and in this situation, spike activity not preoperatively present has been observed to persist after surgery.[206] However, adverse outcomes related to enflurane-induced seizures have not been reported.

Isoflurane can cause EEG spiking and myoclonus, but it has not been associated, in the experimental setting, with the frank epileptoid activity induced by enflurane. The clinical experience with isoflurane is extremely large, and unexplained seizure-like activity has been reported in only two patients. One occurrence was intraoperative,[207] and the other was immediately postoperative.[208] Therefore epileptogenesis does not appear to be a clinical concern with isoflurane. In fact, isoflurane has been successfully used to control EEG seizure activity in refractory status epilepticus.[209]

Seizures occur during the induction of anesthesia with high concentrations of sevoflurane in children, including those without a recognized seizure diathesis.[210] In two healthy humans, EEG burst suppression with 2 MAC sevoflurane was accompanied by epileptiform discharges that were observed during EEG monitoring.[211] These discharges were associated with a significant increase in CBF, thus demonstrating that neurovascular coupling was preserved. In patients with temporal lobe epilepsy, the administration of 1.5 MAC sevoflurane elicited widespread paroxysmal EEG activity. Of note was the observation that the paroxysmal activity was not restricted to the ictal focus and that the administration of sevoflurane did not provide any assistance in localizing the epileptogenic region of the brain.[212] The development of tonic-clonic movements suggestive of seizure activity has also been reported in otherwise healthy patients on emergence from sevoflurane anesthesia.[213,214] In all of the reported cases of seizure activity attributable to sevoflurane anesthesia, untoward sequelae have not been documented. These reports highlight sevoflurane's ability, albeit small, to evoke epileptiform activity; accordingly, the use of sevoflurane in patients with epilepsy should be undertaken with appropriate caution.

Methohexital

Myoclonic activity is sometimes observed with methohexital. Accordingly, this anesthetic has been used to activate seizure foci during cortical mapping.[211] In neurosurgical patients to whom larger doses of methohexital were administered to produce burst suppression of the EEG, refractory seizures have occurred.[215] Consequently, it appears that patients with seizures of temporal lobe origin, typically of the psychomotor variety or those to whom large doses are administered, are at risk for seizure activation by methohexital. However, prolonged seizure activity after single-dose methohexital administration has not been reported in patients who undergo ECT.

Ketamine

Ketamine can elicit seizures in patients with an epileptic diathesis.[216] Depth electrode recordings in epileptic patients have revealed the occurrence of isolated subcortical seizure activity originating in the limbic and thalamic areas during ketamine anesthesia and demonstrated that this subcortical activation may not be reflected in surface EEG recordings. On only two occasions, seizures have also been reported after ketamine anesthesia in subjects who were neurologically normal;[217,218] seizure thresholds may have been lowered by aminophylline in one of these instances. However, ketamine has also been employed for the purpose of controlling status epilepticus. Therefore, ketamine-induced seizure activity is not of significant concern.

Etomidate

Etomidate frequently produces myoclonus that is not associated with epileptiform activity on the EEG.[219] A single instance of severe, sustained myoclonus immediately after anesthesia with etomidate by infusion has been reported.[220] Etomidate has also been shown to precipitate generalized epileptic EEG activity in epileptic patients,[221] and its use in this population should probably be avoided. However, it has been electively used in low doses to activate seizure foci for the purposes of intraoperative EEG localization.[222] In the experience of the authors (unpublished), selective activation of a quiescent focus can be achieved with 0.1 mg/kg etomidate. Larger doses are more likely to lead to generalized activation.

Etomidate is also associated with longer seizures in response to ECT than seizures that occur after the administration of methohexital or propofol. Remarkably, etomidate, in the dose range of 0.15 to 0.3 mg/kg, does not cause dose-related seizure inhibition during ECT, as is readily demonstrated with methohexital or propofol.

The preceding information notwithstanding, no convincing reports indicate epileptogenesis in subjects who are neurologically normal, and the use of etomidate need not be restricted on this basis. In fact, etomidate has been used to control refractory status epilepticus.

Propofol

Abnormal body movements and opisthotonos can occur after propofol anesthesia. However, systematic studies in humans,[223] although identifying the occurrence of occasional dystonic and choreiform movements, have failed to confirm propofol as a proconvulsant. Furthermore, ECT seizures were shorter after induction with propofol than after induction with methohexital,[224] which is more consistent with an *anticonvulsant* effect. In addition, propofol sedation has been widely used during *awake* resection of seizure foci and other intracranial lesions. Although pronounced high-amplitude beta-frequency activity in the EEG has been observed,[225] unexpected incidences of seizures have not been reported.

Narcotics

Seizures or limbic system hypermetabolism (or both) can be readily elicited in some animal species with narcotics. Although an increase in CBF in deep brain structures associated with pain processing has been observed in human volunteers,[226] humans do not have a clinically apparent correlate of the hypermetabolism effect observed in animals. Several anecdotal accounts, unaccompanied by EEG recordings, have reported the occurrence of grand mal convulsions in patients who received both high and low doses of fentanyl. However, systematic investigations of EEG changes during the administration of relatively large doses of fentanyl, sufentanil, and alfentanil in humans have *not* documented neuroexcitatory activity,[227] and the seizures may have been an exaggerated rigidity phenomenon. There are exceptions. Partial complex seizures on the induction of anesthesia with fentanyl in patients undergoing anterior temporal lobectomy have been reported.[228] Eight of the nine patients displayed electrical seizure activity at a range of clinically relevant fentanyl doses (mean, 26 μg/kg).[228] Another study found that alfentanil, 50 μg/kg, augmented temporal lobe spike activity in patients with temporal lobe epilepsy.[229] Untreated rigidity may, itself, also have important CNS consequences. ICP elevation can occur during narcotic-induced rigidity, probably as a consequence of cerebral venous congestion.

NEONATAL ANESTHETIC NEUROTOXICITY

This subject is discussed in detail in Chapter 78.

Cerebral Physiology in Pathologic States

CEREBRAL ISCHEMIA—PATHOPHYSIOLOGIC CONSIDERATIONS

Critical Cerebral Blood Flow Thresholds

The brain has a high rate of energy utilization and very limited energy storage capacity. The brain is therefore extremely vulnerable in the event of interruption of substrate (e.g., oxygen, glucose) supply. Under normal circumstances, global CBF is maintained at approximately 50 mL/100 g/min. In the face of a declining CBF and therefore oxygen supply, neuronal function deteriorates in a progressive manner rather than in an all-or-none fashion (Fig. 11.18). There is substantial reserve below normal CBF levels, and not until EEG evidence of ischemia begins to appear is CBF decreased to approximately 20 mL/100 g/min. At a CBF level of approximately 15 mL/100 g/min, the cortical EEG is isoelectric. However, only when CBF is reduced to approximately 6 to 10 mL/100 g/min are indications of potentially irreversible membrane failure, such as increased extracellular potassium[230] and a loss of the direct cortical response, rapidly evident. As CBF decreases in the flow range between 15 and 10 mL/100 g/min, a progressive deterioration in energy supply occurs and eventually leads to membrane failure and neuronal death at a time course that may last hours rather than minutes. The brain regions falling within this CBF range (6-15 mL/100 g/min) encompass brain tissue in which neuronal dysfunction is temporarily reversible but within which neuronal death will occur if flow is not restored; such regions are referred to as the *ischemic penumbra*.[230,231] Studies defining progression to cerebral infarction within the penumbra have been performed principally in the cerebral cortex of primates, and the actual CBF levels at which the various decrements in function occur may vary with both anesthetic[232] and species. However, in humans anesthetized with halothane and N_2O, the CBF threshold for the initial EEG change[233] is similar to that observed in the animal investigations.

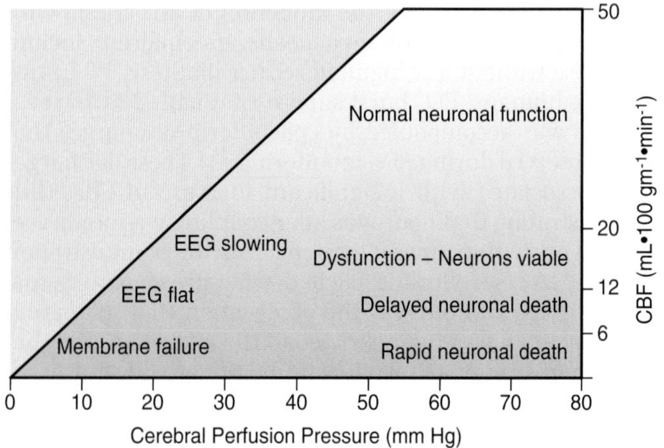

Fig. 11.18 Relationships between cerebral perfusion, cerebral blood flow *(CBF)*, the electroencephalogram *(EEG)*, and the functional status and viability of neurons. Note that in the approximate CBF range of 6 to 12 mL/100 g/min, the energy supply is insufficient to support electrophysiologic activity (i.e., flat EEG) but can prevent complete membrane failure and neuronal death for extended periods. These areas are referred to as the *ischemic penumbra*.[230] The data are derived from studies on the cerebral cortex of barbiturate-anesthetized baboons[230,359] and nonanesthetized monkeys.[360] The CBF and mean arterial pressure thresholds may vary with anesthetic and species.[232]

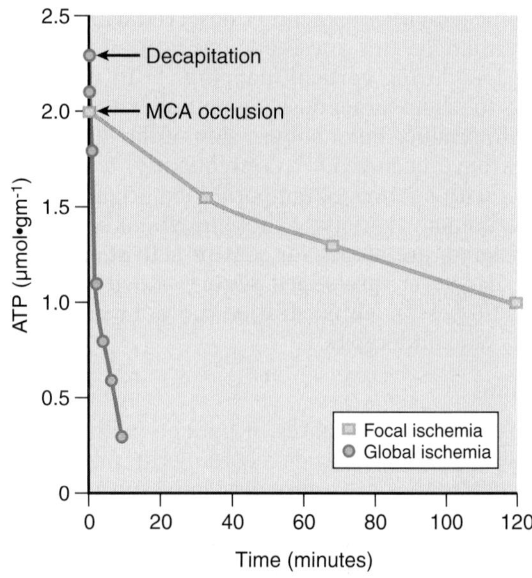

Fig. 11.19 Comparison of rates of failure of energy supply (adenosine triphosphate *[ATP]*) in complete global ischemia in dogs (produced by decapitation[235]) and in incomplete focal ischemia in monkeys (middle cerebral artery *[MCA]* occlusion[234]). In the presence of residual cerebral blood flow *(CBF)*, energy supply failure is substantially delayed.

Models of Cerebral Ischemia

How different is complete cerebral ischemia, as occurs during cardiac arrest, and incomplete cerebral ischemia, as may occur during occlusion of a major cerebral vessel or severe hypotension? From the clinician's vantage, the important difference is that the residual (i.e., collateral) blood flow during incomplete ischemia may result in enough delivery of oxygen to allow some generation of ATP and thereby stave off the catastrophic irreversible membrane failure that occurs within minutes during normothermic complete cerebral ischemia.[234] This difference in the rate of failure of the energy supply (Fig. 11.19)[234,235] can result in significantly greater apparent tolerance for focal or incomplete ischemia than for complete global ischemia (e.g., cardiac arrest).

Energy Failure and Excitotoxicity

Energy failure is the central event that occurs during cerebral ischemia.[236] ATP is required for the maintenance of the normal membrane ionic gradient, and energy failure is rapidly attended by membrane depolarization and influx of sodium (Na^+) and calcium (Ca^{2+}) into the neuron. Voltage-dependent Ca^{2+} channels are then activated, and Ca^{2+} gains entry into the cytosol. Depolarization of presynaptic terminals also results in the release of massive quantities of excitatory neurotransmitters, particularly glutamate, into the synaptic cleft. Activation of glutamatergic receptors, the NMDAR, and the α-amino-3-hydroxy-5-methyl-4-isoxazopropionic acid receptors (AMPARs), adds to the influx of Na^+ and Ca^{2+} (Fig. 11.20). Initiation of cellular signaling by the activation of the mGluR leads to the release of stored Ca^{2+} from the endoplasmic reticulum (ER) via

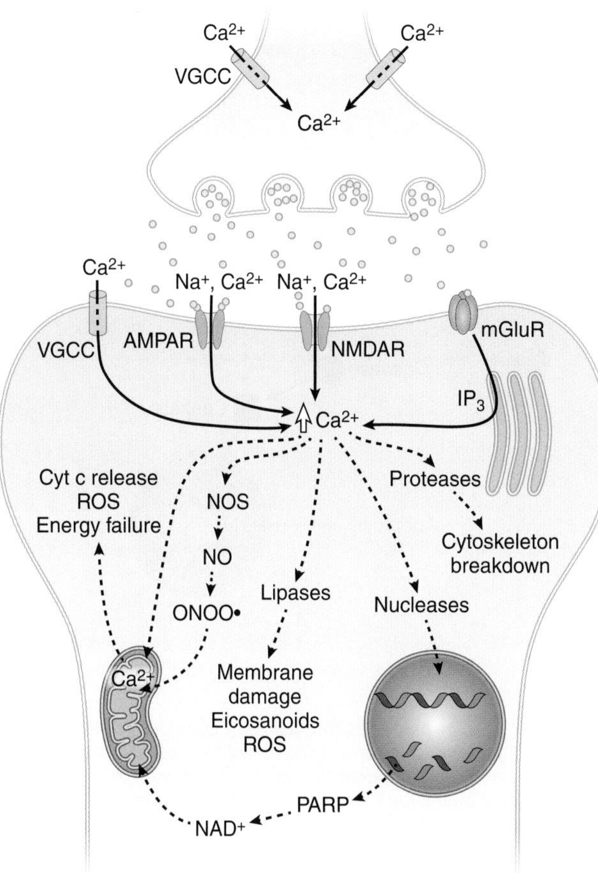

Fig. 11.20 During ischemia, depletion of adenosine triphosphate (ATP) leads to neuronal depolarization and the subsequent release of supranormal quantities of neurotransmitters, especially glutamate. Excessive stimulation of ligand-gated channels and the simultaneous opening of voltage-dependent calcium *(Ca^{2+})* channels permit rapid entry of Ca^{2+} into neurons. Stimulation of metabotropic glutamate receptors (mGluRs) generates inositol 1,4,5-triphosphate *(IP_3)*, which causes the release of Ca^{2+} from the endoplasmic reticulum (ER) and mitochondria. Activation of the α-amino-3-hydroxy-5-methyl-4-isoxazopropionic acid receptors *(AMPAR)*–gated subset of glutamate receptors also permits excessive entry of sodium *(Na^+)*. Excessive free Ca^{2+} results in the activation of numerous enzymes: protease activation causes the breakdown of the cytoskeleton of the neuron; lipases damage plasma membrane lipids and release arachidonic acid (AA), which is metabolized by cyclooxygenases and lipoxygenases to yield free radicals and other mediators of cell injury; activation of nitric oxide synthase *(NOS)* leads to the release of nitric oxide *(NO)* and, in turn, the generation of peroxynitrite *(ONOO)*, a highly reactive free radical; and activated endonucleases damage DNA, thereby rendering the neuron susceptible to apoptosis. Injury to the mitochondria leads to energy failure, generation of free radicals, and the release of cytochrome *c* *(cyt c)* from the mitochondria; the latter is one of the means by which neuronal apoptosis is initiated. *mGluR,* Metabotropic glutamate receptor; *NAD^+,* oxidized form of nicotinamide adenine dinucleotide; *NMDAR, N*-methyl-D-aspartate receptor; *PARP,* poly-ADP-ribose polymerase; *ROS,* reactive oxygen species; *VGCC,* voltage-gated calcium channel.

inositol 1,4,5-triphosphate (IP_3) receptors. Ionic influx is accompanied by an influx of water, and neuronal swelling rapidly occurs after membrane depolarization. The injury that is initiated by excessive glutamatergic activity is referred to as *excitotoxicity*.

Ca^{2+} is a ubiquitous second messenger in cells and is a cofactor required for the activation of a number of enzyme systems. The rapid, uncontrolled increase in cytosolic Ca^{2+} levels initiates the activation of a number of cellular processes that contribute to injury. Cytoskeletal proteins such as actin are cleaved by activated proteases. These enzymes also degrade a number of the protein constituents of the neuron. Lipases attack cellular lipids and produce membrane damage. An important lipase, phospholipase A_2, releases fatty acids such as AA from membranes. Metabolism of AA to prostaglandins and leukotrienes by cyclooxygenase and lipoxygenase is accompanied by the generation of superoxide free radicals. The latter, in combination with other free radicals generated in response to mitochondrial injury, can lead to lipid peroxidation and membrane injury. Prostaglandins and leukotrienes also evoke an inflammatory response and are powerful chemotactic drugs. Activation of platelets within cerebral microvessels, as well as an influx of white blood cells into damaged areas, aggravate the ischemic injury by occluding the vasculature.

Deoxyribonucleic acid (DNA) damage is also an important event during ischemic neuronal injury. Generation of free radicals from AA metabolism, from injured mitochondria, and from the production of peroxynitrite from NO leads to oxidative injury to DNA. Activation of endonucleases also produces DNA strand breaks. Under normal circumstances, DNA injury results in the activation of poly–adenosine diphosphate [ADP]–ribose polymerase (PARP), an enzyme that participates in DNA repair. With excessive DNA injury, PARP activity dramatically increases, which can lead to the depletion of nicotinamide adenine dinucleotide (NAD^+), a substrate of PARP. NAD^+ is also an important coenzyme in energy metabolism, and its depletion further exacerbates energy failure.

Lactate formation is an additional element of the pathophysiologic process. Lactic acid is formed as a result of the anaerobic glycolysis that takes place after failure of the supply of oxygen. The associated decrease in pH contributes to the deterioration of the intracellular environment. An increased preischemic serum glucose level may accelerate this process by providing additional substrate for anaerobic glycolysis.

NO, which has emerged as a probable mediator of CBF changes in many normal physiologic states (see the section "Cerebral Metabolic Rate"), is also of relevance to pathophysiologic ischemia. NO is, in fact, a weak free radical that in turn leads to the generation of a more reactive species (peroxynitrite), and it is the *killer substance* used by macrophages. In cerebral ischemia, NO is probably both friend and foe. During a period of focal ischemia, the vasodilating effect of NO (probably constitutively elaborated NO of endothelial origin) probably serves to augment collateral CBF. However, in the postischemic phase, NO (probably derived from neurons or macrophages) contributes to neuronal injury.

Collectively, the simultaneous and unregulated activation of a number of cellular pathways overwhelms the reparative and restorative processes within the neuron and ultimately leads to neuronal death.

The Nature of Neuronal Death

The neuronal death that occurs in response to these processes has been categorized as necrotic or apoptotic in nature. Necrotic death mediated by excitotoxic injury, is characterized by rapid cellular swelling, condensation and pyknosis of the nucleus, and swelling of the mitochondria and ER. A characteristic of these necrotic neurons is the presence of acidophilic cytoplasm.[237] Necrotic neuronal death results in local infiltration of the brain by inflammatory cells. A considerable amount of collateral damage is a consequence of this inflammation.

Neuronal apoptosis, a form of *cellular suicide*, has also been demonstrated in a variety of models of cerebral ischemia. Apoptosis is characterized by chromatin condensation, involution of the cell membrane, swelling of mitochondria, and cellular shrinkage. In the later stages of apoptosis, neurons fragment into several apoptotic bodies, which are then cleared from the brain.[237] The lack of a substantial inflammatory response to apoptotic death limits injury to surrounding neurons that have survived the initial ischemic insult.

A number of biochemical pathways that lead to apoptosis have been described. Initiation of apoptosis by the release of cytochrome *c* from injured mitochondria has been studied extensively (Fig. 11.21). Cytochrome *c* is restricted from the cytoplasm by the outer mitochondrial membrane.[238] When mitochondria are injured, pores within the outer membrane allow cytochrome *c* to be released into the cytoplasm, where it interacts with procaspase-9 and apoptosis-activating factor (APAF) to produce an apoptosome. Procaspase-9 undergoes activation by proteolytic cleavage. Activated caspase-9 then activates caspase-3. The latter serves as an executor of apoptosis by cleaving a number of protein substrates that are essential in DNA repair (such as PARP). Activation of caspase-3 can also occur by inflammatory signaling via tumor necrosis factor alpha (TNF-α) and the activation of caspase-8.[239] It should be noted that the neuronal injury that occurs in response to ischemia cannot be easily divided into necrosis or apoptosis. The nature of neuronal death probably encompasses a spectrum in which some neurons undergo either necrosis or apoptosis, whereas others undergo cell death that has features of both necrosis and apoptosis.

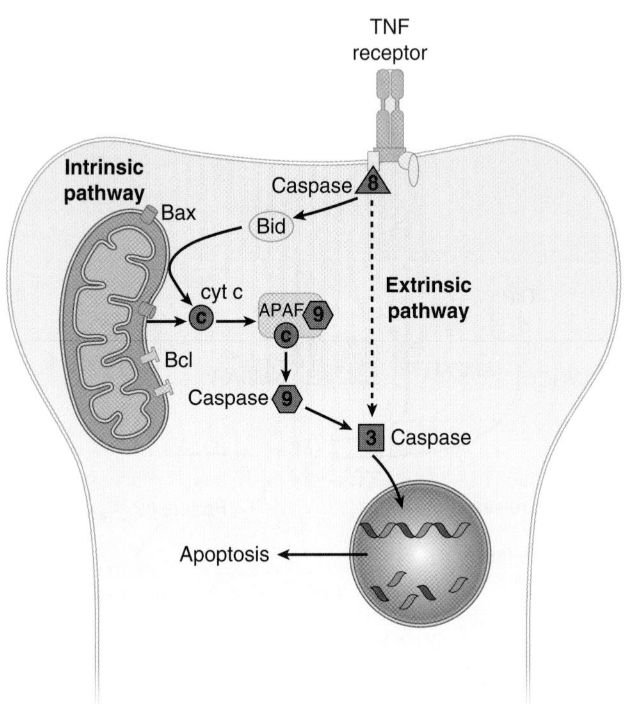

Fig. 11.21 Cellular processes that lead to neuronal apoptosis. Cytochrome *c (cyt c)*, which is normally restricted to the space between the inner and outer mitochondrial membranes, is released in response to mitochondrial injury. Cyt c, in combination with apoptosis-activating factor *(APAF)*, activates caspase-9 by proteolytic cleavage. Activated caspase-9 then leads to the activation of caspase-3. This enzyme cleaves a number of substrates, including those necessary for DNA repair. Within the mitochondria, Bax augments and Bcl prevents the release of cyt c. The release of cyt c can also be initiated by Bid, a substance that is activated by caspase-8 via tumor necrosis factor *(TNF)* signaling. In addition, caspase-8 can directly activate caspase-3. Excessive activation of poly-ADP-ribose polymerase, an enzyme integral to DNA repair, depletes cellular stores of oxidized nicotinamide adenine dinucleotide (NAD^+). Depletion of NAD^+ further exacerbates the energy failure because of its critical role in energy metabolism.

Timing of Neuronal Death

The traditional concept of ischemic injury was that neuronal death was restricted to the time of ischemia and during the early reperfusion period. However, more recent data indicate that postischemic neuronal injury is a dynamic process during which neurons continue to die for a long period after the initiating ischemic insult (Fig. 11.22).[240] This delayed neuronal death, which was first demonstrated in models of global cerebral ischemia, has been demonstrated during focal ischemia as well. The extent of delayed neuronal death depends on the severity of the ischemic insult. With severe ischemia, most neurons undergo rapid death. With more moderate insults, neurons that survive the initial insult undergo delayed death. This ongoing neuronal loss contributes to the gradual expansion of cerebral infarction after focal ischemia. In experimental studies, evidence of cerebral inflammation, which can theoretically contribute to further injury, has been demonstrated even 6 to 8 months after the primary ischemia.

The occurrence of delayed neuronal death has important implications for the evaluation of studies in which neuroprotective strategies are being investigated. A wide variety of interventions have shown neuroprotective efficacy in studies in which the extent of injury is evaluated within 3 to 4 days after ischemia. However, this neuroprotective efficacy may not be sustained. Recent data indicate that cerebral infarction undergoes gradual expansion and that a reduction in injury attributed to a particular therapeutic intervention is no longer apparent when the injury is evaluated after a long postischemic recovery period.[240] Long-term (>1 month) evaluation of the efficacy of a particular intervention is therefore important.

Much of the literature on the pathophysiologic process of cerebral ischemia has primarily been focused on neuronal injury. However, recent work has highlighted the importance of the contribution of astrocytes, microglia, vascular cells (e.g., endothelium, smooth muscle cells, pericytes), basement membranes, and extracellular matrix to stroke. These individual components in aggregate form the neurovascular unit. A detailed understanding of the contribution of each component of the neurovascular unit is a prerequisite, not only for the protection of the brain against ischemic and traumatic injury, but also for therapeutic approaches for the regeneration of the CNS.

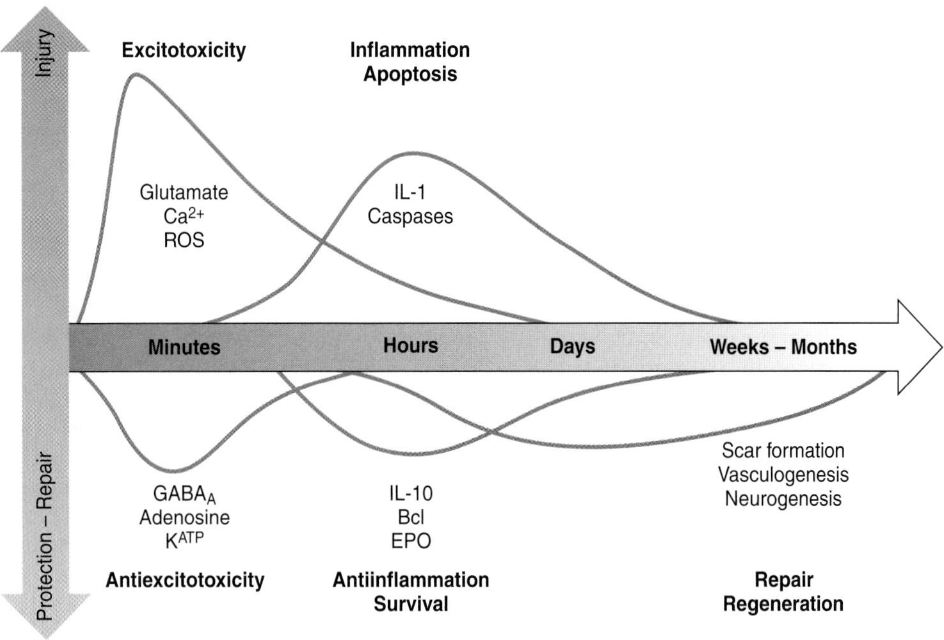

Fig. 11.22 Time course of neuronal death. Excitotoxic (glutamate-mediated) injury results in neuronal death within the first few hours after the onset of ischemia. Brain tissue injury elicits an inflammatory response—an important process in the removal of injured tissue and in healing—that leads to a substantial amount of collateral damage. Inflammation-mediated neuronal death can continue for several days. Neuronal apoptosis can occur in injured neurons that survived the initial insult. Apoptotic neuronal death has been demonstrated to occur for many days after the initiating ischemic insult. It is now apparent that ischemic neuronal death is a dynamic process during which neurons continue to die for a long period. *Ca^{2+}*, Calcium; *EPO*, erythropoietin; *GABAA*, gamma-aminobutyric acid A; *K^{ATP}*, adenosine triphosphate–regulated potassium; *IL-1*, interleukin 1; *IL-10*, interleukin 10; *ROS*, reactive oxygen species. (Adapted from Dirnagl U, Iadecola C, Moskowitz M. Pathobiology of ischaemic stroke: an integrated view. *Trends Neurosci.* 1999;22:391–397.)

BRAIN PROTECTION

Despite intense investigative efforts, pharmacologic agents that can protect the brain against ischemic injury have not been identified. The mainstay in the reduction of brain injury in the setting of acute ischemic stroke is thrombolysis. Management of thrombolysis has been reviewed in guidelines for the early management of patients with acute ischemic stroke.[241] Intravenous alteplase is recommended for patients in whom the time from onset of symptoms to treatment is less than 3 hours. Contraindications to thrombolysis include inability to identify onset of symptoms, intracranial hemorrhage, previous stroke or head trauma within 3 months, recent intracranial or spinal surgery, gastrointestinal malignancy, or bleeding and coagulopathy.[241] The window of thrombolysis may be extended to 4.5 hours in selected patients.

The narrow window for thrombolysis has limited the number of patients who may benefit from clot removal. Mechanical thrombectomy has recently considerably expanded this window. Previously, endovascular treatment of acute ischemic stroke with large clot in large vessels was restricted to a time period of no more than 6 hours from the time that the patients were last known to be well. Two recent trials demonstrated improved neurologic outcome following internal carotid or proximal MCA thrombectomy in patients up to 16 and 24 hours from the time they were last known well. A key enrollment requirement was the presence of a substantial volume of ischemic, but not yet infarcted, tissue that might be amenable to salvage (substantial mismatch between ischemic and infarcted tissue, indicating that noninfarcted tissue could be salvageable).

The DAWN trial used strictly defined mismatch criteria based upon discrepancy between the clinical neurologic deficit (National Institutes of Health Stroke Scale score) and the volume of infarcted tissue.[242] The DEFUSE 3 trial utilized imaging (computed tomography perfusion or MRI diffusion–perfusion) to identify mismatch between ischemic and infarcted tissue.[243] In both studies, the outcome was more favorable in patients who underwent thrombectomy. These studies will increase the number of patients that are eligible for endovascular treatment following acute ischemic stroke. Consequently, the frequency of involvement of the anesthesiologist in the care of these patients will increase significantly.

The literature on cerebral ischemia and brain protection is vast, and a detailed discourse on this topic is beyond the scope of the present discussion. A number of excellent recent reviews on the subject are available.[244-253]

Considerations Relevant to Complete Global Ischemia (Cardiac Arrest)

Maintaining adequate perfusion pressure after cardiac arrest is of considerable importance. Hypotension developing after resuscitation from cardiac arrest may aggravate the microcirculatory and vasospastic processes occurring at this time and may increase brain damage. A late phase of intracranial hypertension may occur and is due to the development of extensive cerebral edema (probably both vasogenic and cytotoxic edema) associated with brain necrosis. Attempts to control this type of intracranial hypertension with osmotherapy are particularly effective.

Both barbiturates and CCBs have been administered after cardiac arrest. The former are ineffective. In a small cohort (51 patients) of patients after cardiac arrest, nimodipine was shown to improve CBF but not neurologic outcome.[254] In a second trial with approximately 150 patients after cardiac arrest, no overall benefit in neurologic outcome was observed.[255] However, a subset of patients in whom the initiation of advanced life support was delayed for longer than 10 minutes demonstrated improved survival. This single study cannot serve as justification for the administration of nimodipine after cardiac arrest, especially in the face of the unequivocally negative results of the multicenter lidoflazine cardiac arrest study.[256] Once again, the important therapeutic objectives are the maintenance of normocapnia and normotension, normalization of systemic pH, avoidance of hyperoxia,[257] avoidance of hyperthermia, and prevention and treatment of seizures.

Induced mild hypothermia is effective in reducing mortality and morbidity in patients who sustain a cardiac arrest that is followed by altered mental status with a Glasgow Coma Scale score of 7 or less.[258] Induction of mild hypothermia in the range of 32°C to 34°C for a period of approximately 24 hours improved neurologic outcome and survival 6 months after cardiac arrest in comparison with a normothermic group. Mild hypothermia was induced without difficulty. Passive rewarming of patients was slowly accomplished over a period of 8 hours. The incidence of complications was similar to that in the control normothermic group. This important study is one of the first to demonstrate the feasibility and efficacy of induced hypothermia as a treatment to reduce injury from global ischemia. In neonates who sustained hypoxic-ischemic encephalopathy, induction of whole body hypothermia (33.5°C) for 72 hours resulted in a reduced incidence of mortality.[259] Long-term follow-up of patients enrolled in the study confirmed the potentially beneficial effects of mild hypothermia.[260] In many institutions, induced hypothermia has been added to the armamentarium for the treatment of cerebral complications of cardiac arrest or global neonatal hypoxic-ischemic encephalopathy.

Considerations Relevant to Focal (Incomplete) Ischemia

Before discussing individual anesthetics, it should be noted that anesthesia, *per se*, is protective. For undefined reasons, reducing the level of systemic stress associated with a standardized experimental insult results in an improved outcome.[261,262] In reviewing the protection-by-anesthetics literature, readers should be conscious of the possibility that the protective benefit ascribed to an intervention with an anesthetic drug may, in fact, be the product of exaggeration of the injury in a high-stress control state, such as N_2O sedation.

Barbiturates. Numerous demonstrations have revealed the protective efficacy of barbiturates in focal cerebral ischemia in animals,[263-265] and a single demonstration confirmed the effectiveness in humans.[266] The effect has been attributed principally to suppression of CMR. However, the effects of CBF redistribution and free radical scavenging[267] may contribute, and evidence indicates that CMR suppression is not the sole mechanism.[268] Suppression of CMR might logically be expected to be of benefit to brain regions in which oxygen delivery is inadequate to meet normal demands but is sufficient to allow energy consumption by some ongoing electrophysiologic activity (i.e., in which the EEG was abnormal but not flat). Such regions are likely to be limited in size in the setting of focal ischemia, yet several of the animal investigations suggest a very substantial protective effect.[263,264] Review of these experiments reveals that the methods used to monitor and maintain temperature, although accepted at the time, were below the standards that have evolved from a more recent understanding of the effects of both deliberate[269,270] and inadvertent hypothermia. Unrecognized cerebral hypothermia may well have been a factor in some of the cited investigations, and it is therefore possible that the protective efficacy of barbiturates may have been overestimated. Although more recent publications involving suitable temperature control methods do, in fact, indicate a protective effect of barbiturates,[268,271,272] the magnitude of that effect was modest when compared with the results of earlier studies. Barbiturate-induced EEG suppression in an already anesthetized patient may still be logical therapy when it can be applied before or early in the course of a period of temporary focal ischemia (e.g., temporary occlusion during aneurysm surgery). However, the decision to institute such therapy should be made only after considering the risk of the occlusive event, the patient's cardiovascular status, and the physician's willingness to accept the possibility of delayed emergence, together with an objective view of the probable magnitude of the protective effect.

Numerous investigations in animals and humans have failed to demonstrate any protective effect of barbiturates in the setting of global cerebral ischemia (e.g., cardiac arrest).

Because CMR suppression has been the presumed mechanism of effect, barbiturates have traditionally been administered to produce maximal reduction of the CMR (which is nearly complete when EEG burst suppression has been achieved). However, the same protective benefit (expressed as a reduction of infarct volume) was observed in an animal investigation with one third of the burst-suppression dose.[268] This raises a clinically important issue. The various barbiturates (e.g., thiopental, thiamylal, methohexital, pentobarbital) have similar effects on the CMR and have generally been assumed to have equal protective efficacy. However, if the mechanism of protection is a pharmacologic effect other than a reduction in the CMR, then is it reasonable to assume equivalence among the barbiturates? Recent data suggest that the neuroprotective efficacy of barbiturates is not similar. In a direct comparison of three clinically used barbiturates, methohexital and thiopental, but not pentobarbital, reduced injury in an animal model of focal ischemia.[273] These data suggest that mechanisms other than or at least in addition to metabolic suppression may contribute to the protective effect of barbiturates.

Volatile anesthetics. Isoflurane is also a potent suppressant of CMR in the cerebral cortex, and EEG evidence suggestive of a protective effect in humans has been reported.[232] In comparison with the awake or N_2O-fentanyl–anesthetized state, isoflurane is neuroprotective in models of hemispheric,[274] focal,[275] and nearly complete ischemia.[276,277] Of substantial clinical relevance is the observation in a preclinical investigation that isoflurane's neuroprotective efficacy is not sustained.[278] When injury was evaluated 2 days after ischemia, a robust reduction in injury was observed with isoflurane anesthesia. However, by 14 days, this reduction in injury was no longer apparent. These data indicate that neuronal injury continues well into the postischemic recovery period and that the neuroprotective benefit that is evident shortly after ischemia may not persist for the long term. More recent data have shown that isoflurane treatment can improve neuronal survival when the severity of ischemia is limited and the restoration of blood flow after ischemia is complete.[279] The neuroprotective effect of isoflurane is not substantially different from that of other volatile anesthetics. Sevoflurane reduces ischemic injury in animal models of focal[280] and hemispheric ischemia;[281] its efficacy is not different from that of halothane. Desflurane also reduces neuronal injury to the same extent that isoflurane does.[282] The available data therefore suggest that adequate anesthesia, *per se*, may have a protective effect[261,262] versus the awake state, but there does not appear to be any difference in neuroprotective efficacy among the volatile anesthetics.

Xenon. The inert gas xenon exerts its anesthetic action by noncompetitive blockade of NMDAR. As such, it is logical to suspect that it might provide neuroprotection against excitotoxic injury. The neuroprotective efficacy of xenon has been demonstrated against focal ischemia in vivo in mice,[283] and cardiopulmonary bypass–induced cognitive dysfunction in rats.[284] Of interest are observations that simultaneous administration of *subanesthetic* doses of xenon in combination with either hypothermia or isoflurane[285] significantly reduces neuronal injury and improves neurologic function in experimental models; this protective effect was apparent as late as 30 days after injury in a model of neonatal asphyxia. Note should be made, however, that long-term neuroprotection with xenon has not yet been demonstrated in experimental adult subjects. Currently, data are not available to support the specific use of xenon for the purpose of neuroprotection in humans.

Propofol. EEG suppression can also be achieved with clinically feasible doses of propofol. One case series and informal colleague communications indicate that it is being used to provide *protection* during both aneurysm surgery[286] and carotid endarterectomy (CEA). Cerebral infarction was significantly reduced in propofol-anesthetized animals in comparison with awake animals.[287] Direct comparison of propofol to pentobarbital has also demonstrated that cerebral injury after focal ischemia is similar in animals anesthetized with the two drugs.[288] Similar to the situation with volatile anesthetics, initial investigations revealed that propofol protection is not sustained.[289]

Etomidate. Etomidate was proposed as a potential protective anesthetic in the setting of aneurysm surgery.[290] It also produces CMR suppression to an extent equivalent to barbiturates, and similar to the barbiturates, etomidate is an agonist at the (inhibitory) $GABA_A$ receptor. Nonetheless, in an experimental model of focal ischemia, the volume of injury was not reduced by etomidate relative to a 1.2 MAC halothane-anesthetized control group. In fact, the volume of injury with etomidate was significantly larger than that in the control group. In patients subjected to temporary intracranial vessel occlusion, the administration of etomidate results in greater tissue hypoxia and acidosis than equivalent desflurane anesthesia. The aggravation of injury produced by etomidate (an imidazole) may be related to direct binding of NO as a consequence of etomidate-induced hemolysis[291] combined with direct inhibition of the NO synthase enzyme by etomidate. Therefore, no scientific studies support the current use of etomidate for cerebral protection and, in fact, suggest that it may actually be deleterious in the setting of focal ischemia.

Calcium channel antagonists. Orally administering nimodipine (the intravenous preparation is not approved for clinical use in North America) for 21 days beginning as soon as possible after subarachnoid hemorrhage (SAH) is now established clinical practice.[292] Other CCBs have reduced vasospasm after SAH but have not improved patient outcome, suggesting the benefit of nimodipine is a cellular rather than a vascular effect. However, by contrast with SAH, routinely administering nimodipine or any other CCB after neurologic stroke that has occurred in the surgical unit or in any other environment has not yet become standard practice. Despite favorable results in small trials, not all investigations of those who have sustained stroke have confirmed the benefits of nimodipine.[293] Although the administration of CCBs for the management of blood pressure is reasonable, their administration for the sole purpose of neuroprotection is not currently recommended.[241]

Other anesthetics. A remarkable number of anesthetics have shown neuroprotective efficacy in animal studies. However, to date, large-scale randomized trials of a variety of anesthetics in patients with stroke have not demonstrated neuroprotection for any drug. With the exception of tissue plasminogen activator (tPA) for thrombolysis, mechanical thrombectomy, and the CCBs nimodipine and nicardipine for the management of SAH, pharmacologic neuroprotective agents are not available for the treatment of patients with cerebral ischemia. Details about drugs that have undergone clinical trials and those that are currently being investigated in humans can be found at the Stroke Trials Registry (www.strokecenter.org/trials/clinicalstudies) of Washington University in St. Louis.

Cerebral Ischemia: Influence of Physiologic Variables

Cerebral perfusion pressure. Measures designed to augment CBF (an important determinant of energy supply) are also important. In the *ischemic penumbra* (described in the section "Critical Cerebral Blood Flow Thresholds"), small improvements in CBF have the potential to prolong neuronal survival substantially. Maintenance of high-normal CPP can augment collateral perfusion pressure and maintain CBF[294] and has been shown to result in improvement in neurologic function.[295] By contrast, hypotension can reduce CBF and exacerbate injury. In trials of nimodipine in patients with acute stroke, a reduction in blood pressure of 10% to 20% increased the probability of an adverse outcome (either death or dependency) fourfold,[296] thus emphasizing the adverse impact of blood pressure reduction on an injured brain. Therefore, in patients with cerebral ischemia, hypotension should be promptly treated and normotension restored. Although the target MAP should obviously be based on knowledge of a patient's preexisting blood pressure, data to provide specific guidelines are insufficient in humans.[241] In the majority of patients, maintenance of the MAP in the 70 to 80 mm Hg range should be adequate. The available data provide support for reducing blood pressure to less than 180/105 mm Hg in patients with stroke who have been treated with thrombolytic agents in the hope of reducing the incidence of hemorrhage into the ischemic brain.[241] In addition, blood pressure augmentation (after ensuring euvolemia) to a systolic pressure of approximately 180 mm Hg in patients with SAH-induced vasospasm[297] and to a CPP of 60 to 70 mm Hg in patients with traumatic brain injury[298] is reasonable.

Carbon dioxide tension. Hypercapnia has the potential to cause intracerebral steal and may worsen intracellular pH. Despite some support for the occurrence of a favorable so-called Robin Hood or inverse steal, hypocapnia has not generally proved effective in either laboratory or clinical settings. Pending further information and in the absence of a means of verifying the perfusion response to the manipulation of Pa_{CO_2}, normocapnia remains standard practice.[298]

Temperature. Hypothermia is the principal cerebral protective technique for circulatory arrest procedures. It unequivocally enhances cerebral tolerance for episodes of ischemia. For deep hypothermia, this effect is largely a function of the reduction in the CMR. Although barbiturates reduce only the component of the CMR associated with electrophysiologic work (approximately 60% of the $CMRO_2$ in the awake state), hypothermia causes a reduction in both electrophysiologic energy consumption and energy utilization related to the maintenance of cellular integrity; mild hypothermia may preferentially suppress the latter.[299] A substantial number of laboratory studies have demonstrated that mild degree of hypothermia (2°C-4°C) during an episode of ischemia can confer substantial protection as histologically measured.[269,270] In addition, hypothermia initiated in the immediate postischemic period confers a protective benefit.[300]

In light of this dramatic protective effect of mild hypothermia in the laboratory, its use in the surgical setting has been advocated. Proponents of its use argue that hypothermia is readily achieved and not accompanied by significant myocardial depression or arrhythmias. In addition, the patient can be easily rewarmed in the surgical unit after the risk of ischemia has subsided. Results of a pilot study clearly demonstrated a trend toward improved neurologic outcome in hypothermic patients undergoing intracranial aneurysm clipping.[301] Unfortunately, the subsequent definitive Intraoperative Hypothermia for Aneurysm Surgery Trial (IHAST) did not demonstrate any improvement in outcome that could be attributable to hypothermia.[302] However, the majority of the patients in that study had SAH of grades I, II, and III. In addition, the number of patients who had temporary clips applied in excess of 20 minutes was quite small (five to six patients). Consequently, an argument has been advanced that mild hypothermia may be of benefit in patients with high-grade aneurysms or in those in whom the complexity of the aneurysm clipping is such that prolonged temporary clipping may be required. Considering that temperature reduction takes time, the decision to induce hypothermia must be made in advance. It is therefore our view that the therapeutic use of hypothermia may be considered in such high-risk patients.[297]

The application of mild hypothermia after head injury reduced ICP[303] and improved neurologic outcome[304] in pilot trials. Complications attributable to hypothermia were not observed. Two subsequent multicenter trials of hypothermia in patients with head injuries, however, failed to confirm the findings of the pilot studies.[305,306] Induction of mild hypothermia did not improve long-term neurologic outcome.

A number of clinical trials of induced hypothermia in a limited number of patients with stroke have been conducted. To date, these trials have demonstrated the feasibility of inducing hypothermia in the range of 33°C to 35°C, even in patients who are not subjected to endotracheal intubation and mechanical ventilation.[307] Hypothermia was associated with improved ICP and CPP. However, complications, particularly thrombocytopenia, bradycardia, ventricular ectopy, hypotension, and infection, are frequent. In addition, an intractable increase in ICP can occur during rewarming, even if the elevation in temperature is gradual and accomplished over a period of several hours. These side effects attest to the need to conduct randomized trials to evaluate properly the efficacy of mild hypothermia in patients with stroke. At the current time, however, hypothermia for purposes of neuroprotection in the setting of acute ischemic stroke is not recommended.[241]

Data regarding the application of mild hypothermia in survivors of cardiac arrest are more positive. Two recent trials have demonstrated that the induction of hypothermia (32°C-34°C) after successful resuscitation from cardiac arrest resulted in a significantly better neurologic outcome 6 months after the arrest.[258,308] These studies demonstrate the clinical efficacy of hypothermia for the purposes of reducing ischemic cerebral injury and provide indirect support for the use of intraoperative hypothermia in patients who are considered to be at high risk.

By contrast, increases in brain temperature during and after ischemia aggravate injury dramatically.[309] An increase of as little as 1°C can increase injury. Ischemia that normally results in scattered neuronal necrosis produces cerebral infarction when body temperature is elevated. Therefore, avoiding hyperthermia in patients who have suffered an ischemic insult or in those who are at risk for cerebral ischemia seems prudent. In the surgical setting, hyperthermia is seldom a problem. In patients at risk of ischemic cerebral injury, treatment of hyperthermia with antipyretics is currently recommended.[241]

Glucose. Withholding glucose-containing solutions in situations during which cerebral ischemia may occur is now an established practice. The practice is based on numerous demonstrations in animal models of brain and spinal cord ischemia that elevation of plasma glucose before episodes of either complete or incomplete ischemia results in the aggravation of neurologic injury. However, the majority of investigations involved adult animals and that certainty concerning the adverse effects of hyperglycemia in immature subjects, such as neonates, is less.[310] Furthermore, only some[311,312] and not all[313] of the investigations in humans have provided confirmation of an independent effect of serum glucose on neurologic outcome. Nonetheless, in long-term outcome studies, diabetic and nondiabetic hyperglycemia has been shown to be an independent predictor of poor outcome.[312] In the National Institutes of Health–sponsored recombinant tPA stroke trial, hyperglycemia was associated with significantly lower odds for desirable clinical outcomes and a higher incidence of intracranial hemorrhage.[314] These data prompted a randomized clinical trial of the efficacy of insulin administration to patients with acute stroke. The results showed that the administration of insulin to control blood glucose levels in patients with stroke did not improve outcome 3 months after stroke.[315] A recurrent theme in the discussion of these studies is that glucose elevation may be the *result* of the stress associated with a severe insult, either ischemic or traumatic, rather than its *cause*. In addition, the inevitable questions of whether and how quickly immediate pretreatment of an elevated plasma glucose level with insulin reduces risk to normoglycemic levels have not been thoroughly examined. Based on the lack of the benefit of restoration of glucose within the normal range (referred to as "tight" control), the current recommendations, which call for the maintenance of blood glucose values in the 140 to 180 mg/dL range, represent reasonable clinical objectives.[241]

By contrast, hypoglycemia is also associated with cerebral injury. With a gradual reduction in blood glucose values to approximately 40 mg/dL, a shift in EEG frequencies occurs from alpha and beta toward delta and theta.[316] Below a blood glucose level of 20 mg/dL, suppression of the EEG (flat) is observed. Persistence of this level of hypoglycemia results in seizure activity and neuronal injury, particularly to the hippocampus.

Seizures. Seizures cause dramatic increases in CMR and CBF. Sustained seizure activity can significantly augment injury in the damaged brain. Accordingly, seizures should be promptly treated with appropriate antiepileptics in the setting of acute stroke (see the section "Coma and Epilepsy" later in the chapter).[241]

Intravascular volume and hematocrit manipulation. Hemodilution has not proved effective in studies of human stroke. Although hemodilution was often instituted in patients with ischemia associated with vasospasm in SAH with the goal of increasing CBF, current practice is focused more on the maintenance of euvolemia and induction of modest increases in blood pressure rather than on hemodilution. In addition, the data do not currently justify routine hemodilution (a hematocrit of 30%-35% is the theoretic optimum) in patients in whom focal ischemia *might* occur in the surgical unit.[317] An increased hematocrit, because of viscosity effects, reduces CBF.[14] In anticipation of a procedure wherein incomplete ischemia might occur, such as CEA, preoperative phlebotomy should be considered when hematocrit is in excess of 55%.

Hyperoxia. Hypoxia has repeatedly been shown to adversely affect outcome in patients with brain injury from a variety of causes. In an attempt to prevent hypoxia, administration of supplemental oxygen often leads to relative hyperoxia, with Pao_2 well in excess of normal values. Hyperoxia is associated with vasoconstriction and reduction in microvascular tissue flow, generation of reactive oxygen species, and augmentation of inflammation.[318] This has led to concerns about the potential adverse effects of excess oxygen in the injured brain.[319]

In patients who had sustained cardiac arrest and who were admitted to an intensive care unit after successful recovery of circulation, hyperoxia increased mortality.[320] The threshold Pao_2 that leads to this increase in mortality is greater than 300 mm Hg; Pao_2 in the range of 100 to 300 mm Hg was not associated with increased mortality.[321] By contrast, no adverse effect of hyperoxia on long-term outcome (12 months) was apparent among survivors of cardiac arrest.[322] In the setting of head injury, endothelial and tissue edema can reduce diffusion of oxygen to neurons. Hyperoxia improves cerebral metabolism but only in regions of the brain wherein metabolism has been significantly reduced.[323] Other investigations, however, have shown either worse outcomes in hyperoxic patients,[324] especially in those in whom Pao_2 was excessive (>487 mm Hg), or no effect on long-term outcome.[325] In acute stroke, oxygen administration by nasal cannula, oxygen mask, and endotracheal tube is not associated with adverse outcomes.[326] Similarly, supplemental oxygen administration to patients with SAH does not impact outcomes.[327]

With these conflicting data, it is difficult to draw firm conclusions that can inform clinical decisions. The available data do not allow for the determination of a target Pao_2, and this is not surprising, given the heterogeneous nature of cerebral injury. Consequently, oxygen administration should be customized in each patient, with the goal being the aggressive treatment of hypoxemia and avoidance of hyperoxia (>300 mm Hg) in patients in whom oxygenation is within normal limits.

Summary of Anesthetics and Neuroprotection

In comparison to the awake or lightly sedated state, the vulnerability of the brain to ischemic injury is reduced under anesthesia. Volatile anesthetics, barbiturates, propofol, xenon, and ketamine reduce injury in experimental models and may reduce injury in comparison with a pure N_2O-narcotic anesthetic. However, direct comparison has not demonstrated the superiority of any one anesthetic (or combination of anesthetics) over another. Therefore, based on the available data, the use of a specific anesthetic or anesthetic regimen for the purpose of brain protection in the clinical setting cannot be recommended.

There is a paucity of information about anesthetic neuroprotection in humans and the lack of clinical trials is understandable, considering the low frequency of stroke and ischemic injury in the perioperative setting. There are, however, a few clinical investigations from which inferences about anesthetic neuroprotection can be made. In the aforementioned IHAST aneurysm trial, a subset of patients received supplemental doses of thiopental, etomidate, or propofol for the purpose of neuroprotection. The neurologic outcome in these patients was no different than those who did not receive these anesthetics.[328] In the general anesthesia versus local anesthesia trial,[329] patients undergoing CEA were randomized to receive either general anesthesia or local anesthesia; in the latter group, patients were lightly sedated but were arousable during surgery. The outcome between the two groups was not different, indicating that the general anesthetic state did not provide any protective benefit.[329] Finally, in a recent retrospective trial of thrombolysis for acute stroke, patients who were anesthetized had a worse outcome than those who were only mildly sedated. Although the worse outcome with general anesthesia was attributed to a lower CPP in that group,[330] the results do not provide evidence of anesthetic neuroprotection. In aggregate, these data suggest that supplemental drugs that produce burst suppression of the EEG do not provide protection in anesthetized patients and that the state of general anesthesia does not improve neurologic outcome measurability.

The neuroprotective efficacy of anesthetic drugs in experimental studies is achieved only by rigorous maintenance of physiologic homeostasis; in fact, the potential for exacerbation of cerebral injury, either traumatic or ischemic, with physiologic mismanagement is significantly greater than the modest protection afforded by pharmacologic drugs—these are important observations. Accordingly, with respect to brain protection, efforts should be focused on the maintenance of physiologic parameters (e.g., perfusion pressure, oxygenation, normocapnia, temperature management, control of hyperglycemia, seizure prophylaxis) within the appropriate ranges and less on pharmacologic or anesthetic drugs to reduce cerebral injury.

Deferring Elective Procedures After Stroke

The risk of extension of cerebral infarction in the event of subsequent anesthesia and surgery has not been studied systematically. In patients who have suffered a stroke, CBF undergoes significant changes. Areas of both high and low CBF occur, and stabilization of regional CBF and CMR is apparent after approximately 2 weeks.[331] Loss of normal vasomotor responses (e.g., CO_2 responsiveness, autoregulation) in the early postinsult period is very common, and these changes persist beyond 2 weeks in a small percentage of patients with stroke. BBB abnormalities, as reflected by the accumulation of CT contrast material or brain scan isotopes, are still present 4 weeks after the insult,[332] and the histologic resolution of large infarcts is not complete for several months. Early CEA after stroke in patients with large strokes and neurologic disability was accompanied by an increased risk of intracerebral hemorrhage.[333] In a recent large cohort study, the occurrence of adverse cardiovascular events, including new stroke and myocardial infarction, was considerably greater in patients who underwent noncardiac surgery within 3 months of having a stroke; the complication rate stabilized 9 months after stroke.[334] Based on early experience with CEA, deferring CEA for at least 6 weeks after stroke is recommended.[333] A 6-week delay should give some assurance of the probable recovery of autoregulation, CO_2 responsiveness, and BBB integrity.

A delay in CEA after stroke, however, poses risks. In patients who have sustained a stroke, the incidence of a second stroke is approximately 12%.[335] The risk of a complete carotid occlusion is considerable with delayed surgery. In addition, early CEA can restore cerebral perfusion to the ischemic penumbra, possibly improving long-term functional recovery. However, the size and location of the infarction should be weighed. A small infarction in the silent cortex may offer wider latitudes than a large lesion that has resulted in a paresis that is still resolving. A small prospective study suggests that in patients with non-disabling stroke, early CEA can be performed safely within 2 weeks of the stroke.[336] Candidates for early CEA after stroke may include patients with relatively small cerebral infarctions, with complete or near complete resolution of neurologic symptoms, and those with ipsilateral carotid artery stenosis.[337] Delaying CEA in patients who have had large strokes with significant neurologic disability, reduced level of consciousness, and displaying a midline shift on the CT scan is generally preferable.

Outcome data to inform the decision about surgery for the patient after stroke, other than CEA, is lacking. With the extrapolation of the information from the CEA studies, pending other information, deferring elective surgery for at least 4 weeks after a cerebral vascular accident and preferably for 6 weeks from the point at which a stable postinsult neurologic state has been achieved seems reasonable.[334]

CHRONIC ARTERIAL HYPERTENSION

A recurrent concern is that of acceptable levels of arterial blood pressure reduction in patients who are chronically hypertensive. Firm guidelines have not been established. However, from the vantage of cerebral well-being, limiting elective MAP reduction 20% to 25% of resting mean levels seems appropriate for both hypertensive and normotensive patients. The same guidelines might apply in both populations, because in chronic hypertension, both the LLA and ULA are shifted to the right with apparently little distortion.[338]

The rationale for a limit of 20% to 25%% is as follows. MAP reductions of 50% in nonanesthetized patients, both normotensive and hypertensive, will commonly produce reversible symptoms of cerebral hypoperfusion.[338,339] Although even greater reductions will probably be tolerated provided that exposures are brief, the hematocrit is reasonable, and the cerebral vasculature is patent, the authors counsel against it. A reduction in the MAP of this magnitude will significantly increase the probability of CPP being close to or below the LLA, thereby reducing cerebrovascular reserve. It has been demonstrated that, on average, a 25% reduction in the MAP will bring both normotensive and hypertensive patients to the LLA.[338] As the reduction in the MAP exceeds 25% of baseline, CBF values will be below normal, albeit, in patients free of occlusive vascular disease, above the threshold for neurophysiologic dysfunction or injury (see Fig. 11.6). However, the physiologic reserve is being encroached upon, thereby leaving little margin for error or for other causes of impaired cerebral oxygen delivery such as low hematocrit or poor collateralization caused by congenital variation or unrecognized cerebrovascular disease.

In animals, treatment of chronic hypertension can restore the LLA to normal.[340, 341] A similar phenomenon has been observed in humans, although restoration was incomplete and had failed to occur after as long as 12 months of treatment in some patients.[338] It is an unexplored possibility that the extent of restoration of the LLA with antihypertensive therapy is agent dependent. Some may restore the LLA more effectively than others. In particular, ACE inhibitors have been shown to decrease the LLA acutely in both normotensive and hypertensive subjects.[342, 343]

Intracranial Hypertension

Control of intracranial hypertension is discussed in detail in Chapter 57.

BRAIN TUMORS

There are few data regarding the physiologic function of intracranial tumors. Measurement of CBF in cerebral tumors with laser Doppler technology revealed that tumors had lower CBF than the normal brain.[344] Autoregulation was occasionally apparent. Vascular responsiveness to changes in PaO_2[345] and $PaCO_2$[346] are generally preserved in patients with gliomas. Propofol reduces CBF in regions of the brain surrounding the tumor, and quantitatively, the reduction in CBF is similar to that in the contralateral normal hemisphere.[347] Measurement of regional CBF in the area of the tumor might also be a useful predictor of the grade of intracranial gliomas; both regional CBF and regional CBV are greater with high-grade gliomas.[348] Considerable edema is often associated with intracranial tumors, and the radiologic extent of the edema, which presumably represents the extent of abnormal vessel leakiness, correlates with the severity of the elevation in ICP that occurs in association with intubation-related hypertension.[349] Edema formation in the peritumoral region can be characterized as vasogenic with leakage of plasma proteins from the vascular space, hydrocephalic secondary to obstruction of CSF flow, or static as a result of venous obstruction by tumor.[350] Although the precise mechanisms by which edema formation occurs are not clear, the loss of integrity of the tight junctions of components of the BBB, an increased permeability induced by vascular endothelial growth factor expressed by tumors, and an increased expression of leukotriene C4 in peritumoral fluid probably play a role.[351] Osmotherapy with mannitol will effect a reduction in edema; however, with a permeable BBB, mannitol can diffuse into the peritumoral space and lead to rebound edema formation.[350] For acute reduction of ICP in the surgical unit, this concern is not significant. A reduction in osmotherapy-induced neuronal cell volume leads to the intraneuronal accumulation of "idiogenic" osmoles. The consequent increase in intraneuronal osmolarity leads to a reuptake of water into the cell in a compensatory attempt to restore cell volume. This process also contributes to the occurrence of rebound edema. The accumulation of idiogenic osmoles can be reduced significantly by loop diuretics such as bumetanide.[352] Dexamethasone remains the mainstay of treatment of tumor edema; it causes a reduction in edema formation with little effect on edema reabsorption. See Chapter 57 for a complete discussion.

COMA AND EPILEPSY

Regardless of its cause, coma reduces brain metabolism. In the case of lesions occurring in the reticular activating system, the reduction in the CMR probably represents a normal physiologic adjustment to reduced functional activity. During generalized seizure activity, CMR and CBF may increase dramatically.[187] The intensive motor and brain activity associated with generalized seizures leads to the development of systemic and cerebral acidosis, often accompanied by a reduction in arterial oxygenation, an increase in $PaCO_2$, and peripheral lactic acidosis. If generalized seizure activity continues unabated, then arterial hypotension ensues. With muscular relaxation and measures ensuring adequate oxygenation and ventilation, the systemic acidosis and hypotension can be avoided and the severity of the cerebral acidosis diminished. During relatively brief episodes of continuous seizures, the brain seems able to meet the high metabolic demands.[204] However, even with effective ventilation and maintenance of perfusion pressure, when seizures continue for a prolonged period, they can lead to the development of irreversible neuronal damage.[353] Therapy aimed at interrupting the seizure and restoring a normal balance between cerebral metabolic demand and blood flow is indicated. Barbiturates, benzodiazepines, or other potent anticonvulsants are appropriate. Adequate ventilation, oxygenation, and maintenance of arterial blood pressure are important adjunctive measures. Muscle relaxants must be viewed as purely symptomatic therapy because they do not alter the abnormal cerebral electrical activity. There is, in addition, the concern that muscle paralysis may mask seizure activity, especially when the EEG is not monitored.

The potentially injurious nature of seizures justifies attention to prevention. Practices vary. However, any patient in whom a substantial cortical incision is planned is at risk, and prophylactic anticonvulsants in the perioperative setting should be considered.

Complete references available online at expertconsult.com.

References

1. Hartkamp MJ, et al. *Stroke*. 1999;30(12):2671.
2. Beards SC, et al. *Anaesthesia*. 1998;53(7):627.
3. Benveniste H, et al. *Neuroscientist*. 2017. 1073858417691030.
4. Zhang N, et al. *Neurosci Biobehav Rev*. 2017;72:168.
5. Drummond JC. *Anesthesiology*. 1997;86(6):1431.
6. Attwell D, et al. *Nature*. 2010;468(7321):232.
7. Michenfelder JD. *Anesthesia and the Brain: Clinical, Functional, Metabolic, and Vascular Correlates*. New York: Churchill Livingstone; 1988.
8. Willie CK, et al. *J Physiol*. 2014;592(5):841.
9. Rickards CA. *Compr Physiol*. 2015;5(4):1585–1621.
10. Toda N, et al. *Can J Physiol Pharmacol*. 2009;87(8):581.
11. Hoiland RL, et al. *Am J Physiol Regul Integr Comp Physiol*. 2016;310(5):R398.
12. Branston NM. *Cerebrovasc Brain Metab Rev*. 1995;7(4):338.
13. Gupta MM, et al. *Br J Anaesth*. 2005;95(5):669.
14. Harrison MJ. *Cerebrovasc Brain Metab Rev*. 1989;1(1):55.
15. Cole DJ, et al. *J Neurol Sci*. 1994;124(1):15.
16. Brown CM, et al. *J Neurol Sci*. 2003;208(1-2):71.

17. Levine BD, et al. *Circulation*. 1994;90(1):298.
18. Ogawa Y, et al. *Anesth Analg*. 2007;105(5):1389.
19. Ogoh S, et al. *J Physiol*. 2005;569(Pt 2):697.
20. van Lieshout JJ, et al. *Stroke*. 2001;32(7):1546.
21. Meng L, et al. *Anesthesiology*. 2015;123(5):1198.
22. Bombardieri AM, et al. *Anesth Analg*. 2016;122(1):226.
23. Meng L, Gelb AW. *Anesthesiology*. 2015;122(1):196.
24. Tan CO. *J Appl Physiol. 1985*. 2012;113(8):1194.
25. Nemoto EM, et al. *Anesth Analg*. 1996;83(6):1262.
26. Phillips AA, et al. *J Cereb Blood Flow Metab*. 2014;34(5):794.
27. Ogoh S, et al. *Clin Physiol Funct Imaging. November*. 2011;31(6):445.
28. Soeding PF, et al. *Br J Anaesth*. 2013;111(2):229.
29. Meng L, et al. *Anesth Analg*. 2011;113(4):751.
30. Meng L, et al. *Br J Anaesth*. 2011;107(2):209.
31. Nissen P, et al. *Neurocrit Care*. 2010;12(1):17.
32. Brassard P, et al. *Br J Anaesth*. 2009;102(6):800.
33. Brassard P, et al. *J Appl Physiol*. 2010;108(6):1472.
34. Drummond JC. *Anesth Analg*. 2012;114(2):478.
35. Davie SN, Grocott HP. *Anesthesiology*. 2012;116(4):834.
36. Joseph M, et al. *Neurosurgery*. 2003;53(5):1044.
37. Zornow MH, et al. *J Cereb Blood Flow Metab*. 1993;13(2):350.
38. Prielipp RC, et al. *Anesth Analg*. 2002;95(4):1052.
39. Drummond JC, et al. *Anesthesiology*. 2008;108(2):225.
40. Farag E, et al. *Eur J Anaesthesiol*. 2017;34(11):732.
41. Wang X, et al. *Brain Inj*. 2013;27(13-14):1617.
42. Artru AA, et al. *J Neurochem*. 1981;36(6):1941.
43. Madsen PL, et al. *Eur J Clin Pharmacol*. 1990;39(3):295.
44. Schroeder T, et al. *Neurol Res*. 1991;13(1):10.
45. Bandres J, et al. *J Neurosurg Anesthesiol*. 1992;4(4):250.
46. Prielipp RC, et al. *Anesth Analg*. 2001;93(1):45.
47. Schmidt J, et al. *Acta Neurochirurgica*. 1991;111:49.
48. Tzeng YC, MacRae BA. *J Appl Physiol. 1985*. 2013;114(7):888.
49. Ott S, et al. *Biomed Res Int*. 2014;2014:970741.
50. Abe K, et al. *Anesth Analg*. 1993;76(6):1227.
51. Kawaguchi M, et al. *Stroke*. 1991;22(9):1170.
52. Lemkuil BP, et al. *J Neurosurg Anesthesiol*. 2016;28(4):337.
53. Capone C, et al. *Am J Physiol Heart Circ Physiol*. 2011;300(1):H397.
54. Kazama K, et al. *Am J Physiol Heart Circ Physiol*. 2003;285(5):H1890.
55. Estrup TM, et al. *J Renin Angiotensin Aldosterone Syst*. 2001;2(3):188.
56. Sigurdsson ST, et al. *J Cereb Blood Flow Metab*. 2014;34(3):467.
57. Nazir FS, et al. *Cerebrovasc Dis*. 2005;19(2):77.
58. Sare GM, et al. *J Hypertens*. 2008;26(6):1058.
59. Pakkenberg B, Gundersen HJ. *J Comp Neurol*. 1997;384(2):312.
60. Morrison JH, Baxter MG. *Nat Rev Neurosci*. 2012;13(4):240.
61. Aanerud J, et al. *J Cereb Blood Flow Metab*. 2012;32(7):1177.
62. Biagi L, et al. *J Magn Reson Imaging*. 2007;25(4):696.
63. Todd MM, Weeks J. *J Neurosurg Anesthesiol*. 1996;8(4):296.
64. Lanier WL, Warner DO. *Anesthesiology*. 1992;77(2):403.
65. Renou AM, et al. *Br J Anaesth*. 1978;50(10):1047.
66. Jobes DR, et al. *Anesthesiology*. 1977;47(1):16.
67. Vernhiet J, et al. *Ann Anesthesiol Fr*. 1977;18(10):803.
68. Stephan H, et al. *Anaesthesist*. 1991;40(3):153.
69. Paris A, et al. *Anesth Analg*. 1998;87(3):569.
70. Cotev S, Shalit MN. *Anesthesiology*. 1975;43(1):117.
71. Forster A, et al. *Anesthesiology*. 1982;56(6):453.
72. Pierce Jr EC, et al. *J Clin Invest*. 1962;41:1664.
73. Takeshita H, et al. *Anesthesiology*. 1972;36(1):69.
74. Stephan H, et al. *Anaesthesist*. 1987;36(2):60.
75. Kofke WA, et al. *Anesth Analg*. 2002;94(5):1229.
76. Zornow MH, et al. *Anesth Analg*. 1990;70(6):624.
77. Langsjo JW, et al. *Anesthesiology*. 2005;103(2):258.
78. Michenfelder JD, et al. *Anesthesiology*. 1974;41(3):231.
79. Astrup J, et al. *Acta Anaesthesiol Scand*. 1984;28(5):478.
80. Gronert GA, et al. *Anesthesiology*. 1981;55(2):110.
81. Sawada Y, et al. *Anesthesiology*. 1982;56(1):53.
82. Vandesteene A, et al. *Anaesthesia*. 1988;43(Suppl):42.
83. Kaisti K, et al. *Anesthesiology*. 2002;96:1358.
84. Kaisti KK, et al. *Anesthesiology*. 2003;99(3):603.
85. Alkire MT, et al. *Anesthesiology*. 1995;82(2):393.
86. Petersen KD, et al. *Anesthesiology*. 2003;98:329.
87. Fox J, et al. *Anesthesiology*. 1992;77(3):453.
88. Craen RA, et al. *J Neurosurg Anesthesiol*. 1992;4:298.
89. Matta BF, et al. *Anesthesiology*. 1995;83(5):980.
90. Cold GE, et al. *Acta Anaesthesiol Scand*. 1985;29(5):490.
91. Kofke WA, et al. *J Neurosurg Anesthesiol*. 1994;6(2):89.
92. Bingham RM, et al. *Br J Anaesth*. 1985;57(9):843.
93. Modica PA, Tempelhoff R. *Can J Anaesth*. 1992;39(3):236.
94. Dearden NM, McDowall DG. *Br J Anaesth*. 1985;57(4):361.
95. Hoffman WE, et al. *Anesthesiology*. 1998;88(5):1188.
96. Levy ML, et al. *Neurosurgery*. 1995;37(2):363.
97. Jobes DR, et al. *Anesthesiology*. 1975;42(1):30.
98. McPherson RW, et al. *Br J Anaesth*. 1985;57(12):1232.
99. Schregel W, et al. *Anaesthesist*. 1992;41(1):21.
100. Mayberg TS, et al. *Anesthesiology*. 1993;78(2):288.
101. Herrick IA, et al. *Anesth Analg*. 1991;72(3):359.
102. From RP, et al. *Anesthesiology*. 1990;73(5):896.
103. Mayer N, et al. *Anesthesiology*. 1990;73(2):240.
104. Werner C, et al. *J Neurosurg Anesthesiol*. 1992;4:313.
105. Wagner K, et al. *Anesthesiology*. 2001;94:732.
106. Ostapkovich ND, et al. *Anesthesiology*. 1998;89(2):358.
107. Lorenz IH, et al. *Neuroimage*. 2002;17(2):1056.
108. Kofke WA, et al. *Anesth Analg*. 2007;105(1):167.
109. Forster A, et al. *Anesth Analg*. 1987;66(4):309.
110. Veselis RA, et al. *Anesthesiology*. 1997;87(5):1106.
111. Forster A, et al. *J Cereb Blood Flow Metab*. 1983;3(2):246.
112. Wolf J, et al. *Br J Anaesth*. 1990;34(8):628.
113. Knudsen L, et al. *Br J Anaesth*. 1991;67(3):277.
114. Chiolero RL, et al. *Intensive Care Med*. 1988;14(3):196.
115. Misfeldt BB, et al. *Br J Anaesth*. 1976;48(10):963.
116. Strebel S, et al. *Anaesthesia*. 1995;50(3):223.
117. Cavazzuti M, et al. *J Cereb Blood Flow Metab*. 1987;7(6):806.
118. Vollenweider FX, et al. *Eur Neuropsychopharmacol*. 1997;7(1):25.
119. Vollenweider FX, et al. *Eur Neuropsychopharmacol*. 1997;7(1):9.
120. Holcomb HH, et al. *Neuropsychopharmacology*. 2001;25(2):165.
121. Schmidt A, et al. *Acta Anaesthesiol Scand*. 2003;47(5):569.
122. Zeiler FA, et al. *J Neurosurg Anesthesiol*. 2016;28(2):123.
123. Albanese J, et al. *Anesthesiology*. 1997;87(6):1328.
124. Mayberg TS, et al. *Anesth Analg*. 1995;81(1):84.
125. Sakai K, et al. *Anesth Analg*. 2000;90(2):377.
126. Lam AM, et al. *Anesthesiology*. 1993;79:A202.
127. Astrup J, et al. *Anesthesiology*. 1981;55(3):263.
128. Bedford RF, et al. *Anesth Analg*. 1980;59(6):435.
129. Michenfelder JD, Milde JH. *Stroke*. 1975;6:405.
130. Todd MM, Drummond JC. *Anesthesiology*. 1984;60(4):276.
131. Lutz LJ, et al. *Anesthesiology*. 1990;73(1):125.
132. Scheller MS, et al. *Anesthesiology*. 1988;68(4):548.
133. Maekawa T, et al. *Anesthesiology*. 1986;65(2):144.
134. Michenfelder JD, Cucchiara RF. *Anesthesiology*. 1974;40(6):575.
135. Drummond JC, et al. *Anesthesiology*. 1986;65(5):462.
136. Hansen TD, et al. *Anesthesiology*. 1988;69(3):332.
137. Lenz C, et al. *Anesthesiology*. 1998;89(6):1480.
138. Drummond JC. *Anesthesiology*. 2018;129(1):187.
139. Heath KJ, et al. *Anesth Analg*. 1997;85(6):1284.
140. Todd MM, et al. *Anesthesiology*. 1982;57:A332.
141. Mielck F, et al. *Br J Anaesth*. 1998;81:155.
142. Sakabe T. *Anesthesiology*. 1983;59(6):532.
143. Mielck F, et al. *Anesth Analg*. 1999;89:364.
144. Johnson J, et al. *Anesth Analg*. 1995;80:S214.
145. Ornstein E, et al. *Anesthesiology*. 1993;79(3):498.
146. Kuroda Y, et al. *Anesthesiology*. 1997;87(3):527.
147. Sanders RD, Maze M. *Curr Opin Anaesthesiol*. 2005;18(4):405.
148. Franks NP, et al. *Nature*. 1998;396(6709):324.
149. Gruss M, et al. *Mol Pharmacol*. 2004;65(2):443.
150. Laitio RM, et al. *Anesthesiology*. 2007;106(6):1128.
151. Rex S, et al. *Anesthesiology*. 2006;105(5):936.
152. Schmidt M, et al. *Anaesthesia*. 2002;57(10):960.
153. Schmidt M, et al. *Acta Anaesthesiol Scand*. 2005;49(4):494.
154. Reinelt H, et al. *Anesthesiology*. 2001;94(3):475.
155. Fraga M, et al. *Anesthesiology*. 2003;98:1085.
156. Milde LN, Milde JH. *Anesth Analg*. 1989;68:S196.
157. Alkire MT, et al. *Anesthesiology*. 1997;86(3):549.
158. Maksimow A, et al. *Anaesthesia*. 2005;60(9):862.
159. Reinstrup P, et al. *Anesthesiology*. 1995;82(2):359.
160. Eintrei C, et al. *Anesthesiology*. 1985;63(4):391.
161. Boarini DJ, et al. *Neurosurgery*. 1984;15(3):400.
162. Warner DS, et al. *Anesthesiology*. 1985;63(3):243.
163. Albrecht RF, et al. *Anesthesiology*. 1983;58(1):26.
164. Fleischer LH, et al. *Anesthesiology*. 1992;77:A167.
165. Madsen JB, et al. *Anesthesiology*. 1987;66(3):332.
166. Drummond JC, Todd MM. *Anesthesiology*. 1985;62(3):268.

167. Gupta S, et al. *Br J Anaesth*. 1997;79:469.
168. Vavilala MS, et al. *Br J Anaesth*. 2003;90(5):636.
169. Lu H, et al. *Anesth Analg*. 1998;87:854.
170. Adams RW, et al. *Anesthesiology*. 1981;54(2):97.
171. Campkin TV, Flinn RM. *Anaesthesia*. 1989;44(1):50.
172. Grosslight K, et al. *Anesthesiology*. 1985;63(5):533.
173. Scheller MS, et al. *Anesthesiology*. 1987;67:507.
174. Field LM, et al. *Br J Anaesth*. 1993;70(2):154.
175. Eng C, et al. *Anesthesiology*. 1992;77(5):872.
176. Henriksen HT, Jorgensen PB. *Br J Anaesth*. 1973;45(5):486.
177. Misfeldt BB, et al. *Br J Anaesth*. 1974;46(11):853.
178. Wilson-Smith E, et al. *Acta Anaesthesiol Scand*. 2003;47(3):307.
179. Lam AM, et al. *Anesth Analg*. 1994;78(3):462.
180. Strebel S, et al. *Acta Anaesthesiol Scand*. 1995;39(5):653.
181. Algotsson L, et al. *Acta Anaesthesiol Scand*. 1992;36(1):46.
182. Reinstrup P, et al. *Br J Anaesth*. 1997;78(4):407.
183. Reinstrup P, et al. *Anesthesiology*. 2001;95(5):1079.
184. Drummond JC, et al. *Anesth Analg*. 1987;66(11):1083.
185. Schramm WM, et al. *Anesth Analg*. 1998;86(1):123.
186. Lanier WL, et al. *Anesthesiology*. 1985;63(6):589.
187. Tateishi A, et al. *Stroke*. 1989;20(8):1044.
188. Standaert FG. *Anesthesiology*. 1985;63(6):577.
189. Lanier WL, et al. *Anesthesiology*. 1994;80(2):392.
190. Stirt JA, et al. *Anesthesiology*. 1987;67(1):50.
191. Kovarik WD, et al. *Anesth Analg*. 1994;78(3):469.
192. Artru AA. *Anesthesiology*. 1984;60(6):575.
193. Artru AA. *Anesthesiology*. 1983;58(6):533.
194. Artru AA. *Anesthesiology*. 1984;60(3):193.
195. Artru AA. *J Neurosurg*. 1984;60(2):252.
196. Artru AA, et al. *Anesthesiology*. 1982;57(4):255.
197. Maktabi MA, et al. *Anesthesiology*. 1993;78(1):72.
198. Artru AA. *J Neurosurg Anesthesiol*. 1993;5(3):178.
199. Tetrault S, et al. *Eur J Neurosci*. 2008;28(7):1330.
200. Thal SC, et al. *PLoS One*. 2012;7(12):e50752.
201. Altay O, et al. *Stroke*. 2012;43(9):2513.
202. Modica PA, et al. *Anesth Analg*. 1990;70(3):303.
203. Modica PA, et al. *Anesth Analg*. 1990;70(4):433.
204. Kreisman NR, et al. *J Cereb Blood Flow Metab*. 1991;11(1):77.
205. Wollman H, et al. *Fed Proc*. 1967;28:356.
206. Flemming DC, et al. *Anesthesiology*. 1980;52(5):431.
207. Hymes JA. *Anesth Analg*. 1985;64(3):367.
208. Harrison JL. *Anesth Analg*. 1986;65(11):1235.
209. Kofke WA, et al. *Anesthesiology*. 1989;71(5):653.
210. Komatsu H, et al. *Ann Acad Med Singapore*. 1994;23(suppl 6):130.
211. Kaisti K, et al. *Anesthesiology*. 1952;91(6):1999.
212. Hisada K, et al. *J Neurosurg Anesthesiol*. 2001;13:333.
213. Hilty CA, Drummond JC. *Anesthesiology*. 2000;93(5):1357.
214. Terasako K, et al. *Anesth Analg*. 2003;96(4):1239.
215. Todd MM, et al. *Anesthesiology*. 1984;61(5):495.
216. Bennett DR, et al. *Neurology*. 1973;23(5):449.
217. Steen PA, Michenfelder JD. *Anesthesiology*. 1979;50(5):437.
218. Hirshman CA, et al. *Anesthesiology*. 1982;56(6):464.
219. Ghoneim MM, Yamada T. *Anesth Analg*. 1977;56:479.
220. Laughlin TP, Newberg LA. *Anesth Analg*. 1985;64:80.
221. Ebrahim ZY, et al. *Anesth Analg*. 1986;65:1004.
222. Gancher S, et al. *Anesthesiology*. 1984;61:616.
223. Samra SK, et al. *Anesthesiology*. 1995;82(4):843.
224. Rampton AJ, et al. *Anesthesiology*. 1989;70(3):412.
225. Drummond JC, et al. *Anesthesiology*. 1992;76(4):652.
226. Firestone LL, et al. *Anesth Analg*. 1996;82(6):1247.
227. Smith NT, et al. *J Clin Monit*. 1985;1(4):236.
228. Tempelhoff R, et al. *J Neurosurg*. 1992;77(2):201.
229. Cascino GD, et al. *J Clin Neurophysiol*. 1993;10(4):520.
230. Astrup J, et al. *Stroke*. 1977;8(1):51.
231. Hossmann KA. *Ann Neurol*. 1994;36(4):557.
232. Michenfelder JD, et al. *Anesthesiology*. 1987;67(3):336.
233. Sundt Jr TM, et al. *Mayo Clin Proc*. 1981;56(9):533.
234. Michenfelder JD, Sundt Jr TM. *Stroke*. 1971;2(4):319.
235. Michenfelder JD, Theye RA. *Anesthesiology*. 1970;33(4):430.
236. Siesjo BK. *J Neurosurg*. 1992;77:169.
237. Lipton P. *Physiol Rev*. 1999;79(4):1431.
238. Fiskum G, et al. *J Cereb Blood Flow Metab*. 1999;19(4):351.
239. Velier JJ, et al. *J Neurosci*. 1999;19(14):5932.
240. Kawaguchi M, et al. *Anesthesiology*. 2000;92(5):1335.
241. Powers WJ, et al. *Stroke*. 2018;49(3):e46–e110.
242. Nogueira RG, et al. *N Engl J Med*. 2018;378(1):11.
243. Albers GW, et al. *N Engl J Med*. 2018;378(8):708.
244. Dirnagl U, et al. *Trends Neurosci*. 1999;22(9):391.
245. Del Zoppo GJ. *Stroke*. 2013;44(1):263.
246. Dirnagl U. *Ann NY Acad Sci*. 2012;1268:21.
247. Heiss WD. *Ann NY Acad Sci*. 2012;1268:26.
248. Hossmann KA. *J Cereb Blood Flow Metab*. 2012;32(7):1310.
249. van der Spuy WJ, et al. *Rev Neurosci*. 2012;23(3):269.
250. Kramer DR, et al. *J Clin Neurosci*. 2016;24:22.
251. Ma Y, et al. *Prog Neurobiol*. 2017;157:247.
252. Martin A, et al. *Ther Adv Neurol Disord*. 2018;11.1756286418774267.
253. Mayor D, Tymianski M. *Neuropharmacology*. 2018;134(Pt B):178.
254. Forsman M, et al. *Anesth Analg*. 1989;68(4):436.
255. Roine RO, et al. *JAMA*. 1990;264(24):3171.
256. No authors listed. *N Engl J Med*. 1991;324(18):1225.
257. Roberts BW, et al. *Circulation*. 2018;137(20):2114.
258. Hypothermia Group after Cardiac Arrest Study Group. *N Engl J Med*. 2002;346(8):549.
259. Shankaran S, et al. *N Engl J Med*. 2005;353(15):1574.
260. Shankaran S, et al. *N Engl J Med*. 2012;366(22):2085.
261. Hoffman WE, et al. *Anesth Analg*. 1991;73(4):460.
262. Hoffman WE, et al. *Anesth Analg*. 1993;76(2):279.
263. Smith AL, et al. *Stroke*. 1974;5(1):1.
264. Michenfelder JD, et al. *Arch Neurol*. 1976;33:345.
265. Nehls DG, et al. *Anesthesiology*. 1987;66:453.
266. Nussmeier NA, et al. *Anesthesiology*. 1986;64:165.
267. Shapiro HM. *Br J Anaesth*. 1985;57:82.
268. Warner DS, et al. *Anesthesiology*. 1996;84:1475.
269. Busto R, et al. *J Cereb Blood Flow Metab*. 1987;7(6):729.
270. Sano T, et al. *Anesthesiology*. 1992;76(2):221.
271. Warner DS, et al. *J Cereb Blood Flow Metab*. 1991;11(5):794.
272. Drummond JC, et al. *Neurosurgery*. 1995;37(4):742.
273. Cole DJ, et al. *Can J Anaesth*. 2001;48(8):807.
274. Baughman VL, et al. *Anesthesiology*. 1988;69:192.
275. Soonthan-Brant V, et al. *Anesth Analg*. 1999;88:49.
276. Mackensen GB, et al. *Anesthesiology*. 2000;93(4):1102.
277. Nellgard B, et al. *Anesthesiology*. 2000;93(2):431.
278. Kawaguchi M, et al. *J Neurosurg Anesthesiol*. 2000;12:385.
279. Sakai H, et al. *Anesthesiology*. 2007;106(1):92.
280. Warner DS, et al. *Anesthesiology*. 1993;79:985.
281. Werner C, et al. *Br J Anaesth*. 1995;75(6):756.
282. Engelhard K, et al. *Br J Anaesth*. 1999;83(3).
283. Homi HM, et al. *Anesthesiology*. 2003;99(4):876.
284. Ma D, et al. *Anesthesiology*. 2003;98(3):690.
285. Ma D, et al. *Ann Neurol*. 2005;58(2):182.
286. Ravussin P, de Tribolet N. *Neurosurgery*. 1993;32(2):236. discussion 240.
287. Gelb AW, et al. *Anesthesiology*. 2002;96(5):1183.
288. Pittman JE, et al. *Anesthesiology*. 1997;87(5):1139.
289. Bayona NA, et al. *Anesthesiology*. 2004;100(5):1151.
290. Batjer HH, et al. *J Neurosurg*. 1988;68:234.
291. Nebauer AE, et al. *Br J Anaesth*. 1992;69(1):58.
292. Pickard JD, et al. *BMJ*. 1989;298(6674):636.
293. No authors listed. *Lancet*. 1990;336(8725):1205.
294. Drummond JC, et al. *Stroke*. 1989;20(11):1538.
295. Young WL, et al. *Anesthesiology*. 1989;71:794.
296. Ahmed N, et al. *Stroke*. 2000;31(6):1250.
297. Connolly ES Jr, et al. *Stroke*. 2012;43(6):1711.
298. Carney N, et al. *Neurosurgery*. 2017;80(1):6.
299. Nemoto EM, et al. *J Neurosurg Anesthesiol*. 1996;8(1):52.
300. Buchan A, Pulsinelli WA. *J Neurosci*. 1990;10(1):311.
301. Hindman BJ, et al. *Neurosurgery*. 1999;44(1):23.
302. Todd MM, et al. *N Engl J Med*. 2005;352(2):135.
303. Shiozaki T, et al. *J Neurosurg*. 1993;79:363.
304. Clifton GL, et al. *J Neurotrauma*. 1993;10(3):263.
305. Clifton GL, et al. *Lancet Neurol*. 2011;10(2):131.
306. Clifton GL, et al. *N Engl J Med*. 2001;344(8):556.
307. Kammersgaard LP, et al. *Stroke*. 2000;31(9):2251.
308. Bernard SA, et al. *N Engl J Med*. 2002;346(8):557.
309. Wass CT, et al. *Anesthesiology*. 1995;83(2):325.
310. Vannucci RC, et al. *J Cereb Blood Flow Metab*. 1996;16(5):1026.
311. Mullner M, et al. *J Cereb Blood Flow Metab*. 1997;17(4):430.
312. Weir CJ, et al. *BMJ*. 1997;314(7090):1303.
313. Matchar DB, et al. *Ann Intern Med*. 1992;117(6):449.
314. Bruno A, et al. *Neurology*. 2002;59(5):669.
315. Gray CS, et al. *Lancet Neurol*. 2007;6(5):397.
316. Auer RN. *Forensic Sci Int*. 2004;146(2-3):105.

317. Archer DP, et al. *J Neurosurg Anesthesiol*. 1994;6(1):51.
318. Dell'Anna AM, et al. *Crit Care*. 2014;18(5):555.
319. de Jonge E, et al. *Crit Care*. 2008;12(6):R156.
320. Kilgannon JH, et al. *JAMA*. 2010;303(21):2165.
321. Elmer J, et al. *Intensive Care Med*. 2015;41(1):49.
322. Vaahersalo J, et al. *Crit Care Med*. 2014;42(6):1463.
323. Vilalta A, et al. *J Neurotrauma*. 2011;28(7):1139.
324. Davis DP, et al. *J Neurotrauma*. 2009;26(12):2217.
325. Brenner M, et al. *Arch Surg*. 2012;147(11):1042.
326. Roffe C, et al. *PLoS One*. 2011;6(5):e19113.
327. Lang M, et al. *Neurosurgery*. 2016;78(4):540.
328. Hindman BJ, et al. *Anesthesiology*. 2010;112(1):86.
329. Group GTC, et al. *Lancet*. 2008;372(9656):2132.
330. Davis MJ, et al. *Anesthesiology*. 2012;116(2):396.
331. Lenzi GL, et al. *J Cereb Blood Flow Metab*. 1982;2(3):321.
332. Olsen TS. *Acta Neurol Scand*. 1986;73(4):321.
333. Rockman CB, et al. *J Vasc Surg*. 2006;44(3):480.
334. Jorgensen ME, et al. Time elapsed after ischemic stroke and risk of adverse cardiovascular events and mortality following elective noncardiac surgery. *JAMA*. 2014;312(3):269.
335. Rantner B, et al. *Eur J Vasc Endovasc Surg*. 2005;30(1):36.
336. Ballotta E, et al. *Surgery*. 2002;131(3):287.
337. Keldahl ML, Eskandari MK. *Expert Rev Cardiovasc Ther*. 2010;8(10):1399.
338. Strandgaard S. *Circulation*. 1976;53(4):720.
339. Njemanze PC. *Stroke*. 1992;23(12):1743.
340. Vorstrup S, et al. *Stroke*. 1984;15(2):312.
341. Toyoda K, et al. *J Cereb Blood Flow Metab*. 1998;18(3):305.
342. Larsen FS, et al. *Stroke*. 1994;25(10):1985.
343. Waldemar G, et al. *J Hypertens*. 1989;7(3):229.
344. Arbit E, et al. *Neurosurgery*. 1989;24(2):166.
345. Julien C, et al. *Br J Cancer*. 2004;91(2):374.
346. Packard SD, et al. *Neoplasia*. 2003;5(4):330.
347. Rasmussen M, et al. *Anesthesiology*. 2010;112(1):50.
348. Shin JH, et al. *AJR Am J Roentgenol*. 2002;179(3):783.
349. Bedford RF, et al. *Anesth Analg*. 1982;61(5):430.
350. Kaal EC, Vecht CJ. *Curr Opin Oncol*. 2004;16(6):593.
351. Stummer W. *Neurosurg Focus*. 2007;22(5):E8.
352. McManus ML, Strange K. *Anesthesiology*. 1993;78(6):1132.
353. Wasterlain CG. *Epilepsia*. 1974;15(2):155.
354. Todd MM. *Adv Pharmacol*. 1994;31:595.
355. Todd MM, et al. *Am J Physiol*. 1994;267(5 Pt 2):H2025.
356. Murphy FL, et al. *Abstracts Annual Meeting Am Soc Anesthesiol*. 1974;1974:62.
357. Werner C, et al. *Anesth Analg*. 1991;72(2):177.
358. Wollman H, et al. *Anesthesiology*. 1964;25:180.
359. Branston NM, et al. *Exp Neurol*. 1974;45(2):195.
360. Jones TH, et al. *J Neurosurg*. 1981;54(6):773.

12 Neuromuscular Physiology and Pharmacology

J. A. JEEVENDRA MARTYN and MALIN JONSSON FAGERLUND

KEY POINTS

- The neuromuscular junction contains the distal nerve terminal, Schwann cell, synaptic cleft, and muscle end plate, which together provide an array of receptors and substrates for drug action. Neuromuscular transmission is predominantly dependent on acetylcholine as the natural transmitter. Acetylcholine, when released from the prejunctional nerve terminal, binds to acetylcholine receptors (AChRs) that are present either prejunctionally or postjunctionally within the neuromuscular junction (synapse) and, depending on their structural composition, are classified into the usual muscle subtype AChRs or a variety of neuronal subtype AChRs.
- Muscle relaxants have multiple sites of action. Although the major actions occur by mechanisms and at sites described as agonistic and antagonistic actions at postjunctional receptors for depolarizing and nondepolarizing muscle relaxants (NDMRs), this description of neuromuscular drug action is a simplistic one. Neuromuscular transmission is impeded by NDMRs because they prevent access of acetylcholine to its preferred recognition site on the postjunctional nicotinic AChRs.
- If the concentration of NDMR is increased, another, noncompetitive action—block of the ion channel—is superimposed. The postjunctional paralytic effects of muscle relaxants can be enhanced by the actions of the relaxant on prejunctional AChRs, which modulate the release of acetylcholine. The latter can be documented as *fade* that occurs with increased frequency of stimulation. Fade can also be seen when the postjunctional AChRs alone are functionally blocked (e.g., by bungarotoxin) or when the number of AChRs (e.g., myasthenia gravis) is decreased. Hence, the neuromuscular junction is a complex and dynamic system in which the phenomena produced by drugs are composites of actions that vary with the drug, dose, activity at the nerve terminal and muscle, time after administration, presence of anesthetics or other drugs, and age and condition of the patient.
- Inhibition of acetylcholinesterase enzyme by anticholinesterases (e.g., neostigmine) increases the concentration of acetylcholine in the synaptic cleft, which can compete with and displace the NDMRS and thus reverse the paralysis. These anticholinesterase drugs (e.g., neostigmine) also have other effects, including the nerve terminal and the receptor, by an allosteric mechanism. Acute bolus or prolonged administration of anticholinesterases can have deleterious effects on neuromuscular function in otherwise healthy patients. The modified cyclodextrin, sugammadex, is a novel and innovative class of compound that reverses paralysis of only steroidal muscle relaxants by encapsulation of this series of compounds.
- Depolarizing compounds (e.g., succinylcholine) initially react with the acetylcholine recognition site and, like the transmitter, open AChR ion channels during depolarization of the endplate membrane. Unlike the transmitter, they are not subject to hydrolysis by acetylcholinesterase and therefore remain in the junction. Soon after the administration of succinylcholine, some receptors are desensitized, and, although occupied by the agonist, they do not open to allow current to flow to depolarize the muscle membrane area.
- If the depolarizing relaxant is applied in higher-than-usual concentrations or is allowed to remain at the junction for a long time, then other neuromuscular effects occur; depolarizing relaxants in higher concentrations have effects on prejunctional structures, and the combination of prejunctional and postjunctional effects plus secondary ones on muscle and nerve homeostasis results in the complicated phenomenon known as *phase II block.* Some of the other drugs used clinically (e.g., Botox) have effects on the motor nerve and therefore indirectly on muscle. Systemic infection with clostridial toxins (*Clostridium botulinum*, gas gangrene) can lead to systemic paralysis as a result of decreased release of acetylcholine from the nerve terminal. NDMRs administered for 24 hours or longer can have effects on the postsynaptic receptor and simulate denervation state (chemical denervation) manifested by upregulated postsynaptic AChRs. Magnesium given to preeclamptic mothers decreases the release of acetylcholine with a potential for muscle weakness in the mother or newborn. In recognizing these sites and mechanisms, we begin to bring our theoretical knowledge closer to explaining the phenomena observed when these drugs are exposed to living humans.

Continued

- Contemporary research work has focused on the control of AChR expression on the postjunctional membrane in normal and diseased states. The presence or absence of the conventional mature and immature isoforms seems to complicate matters further. In certain pathologic states (e.g., denervation, stroke, sepsis, burns, immobilization, chronic use of NDMRs), AChRs are upregulated, with increased expression of the immature isoform and *de-novo* expression of the nicotinic α7 acetylcholine receptors (α7 AChRs). Altered functional and pharmacologic characteristics of the immature (fetal or γ-subunit–containing receptors) and α7 AChRs expressed in pathologic muscle wasting conditions result in increased sensitivity to succinylcholine with hyperkalemia and resistance (insensitivity) to NDMRs.
- An area of increasing attention is control of the expression of mature versus the other two receptor isoforms (immature γ- and α7 AChRs on the synapse). Re-expression of the immature γ- and α7 AChRs is probably related to aberrant growth factor signaling.
- Genetic mutations in the AChRs, that result in prolonged or fast open-channel time, can lead to a myasthenia-like state, even in the presence of normal receptor numbers. The weakness is usually related to ineffective depolarization or to the altered open-channel time, or to both.

Although cholinergic neurotransmission at the neuromuscular junction is the most widely studied synapse within the nervous system, complete knowledge of its workings has not yet been achieved. The physiology of neuromuscular transmission could be analyzed and understood at the simplest level by using the classic model of nerve signaling to muscle through the acetylcholine receptor (AChR). The mammalian neuromuscular junction and the nicotinic AChRs are the prototypical and most extensively studied synapse and receptor, respectively. Research has provided more detailed information on processes that, within the classic scheme, can modify neurotransmission and response to drugs. One example is the role of qualitative or quantitative changes in AChRs that modify neurotransmission and the response to drugs.[1-3] In myasthenia gravis, for example, the decrease in AChRs results in decreased efficiency of neurotransmission (and therefore muscle weakness)[4] and altered sensitivity to neuromuscular relaxants.[3] Another example is the importance of nerve-related (prejunctional) changes that alter neurotransmission and the response to muscle relaxants.[5-7] Yet, muscle relaxants act in ways that are not encompassed by the classic scheme of a unitary site of action. The observation that muscle relaxants can have prejunctional effects[5] or that some muscle relaxants can also have agonist-like stimulatory actions on the receptor,[8] whereas others have effects not explainable by purely postsynaptic actions on muscle,[9-11] has provided new insight into some previously unexplained observations. Although muscle relaxants are known to have effects on the presynaptic and postsynaptic receptors of the neuromuscular junction, recent evidence indicates that they can react with nicotinic and muscarinic AChRs other than those in muscle, including receptors on the carotid body, on the vagus to the heart, and on bronchial smooth muscle.[9-13] Although this multifaceted action-response scheme makes the physiologic and pharmacologic neurotransmission more complex, these added insights also bring experimentally derived knowledge much closer to clinical observations. This review dwells on the basic physiology and anesthesia-related pharmacology of the neuromuscular junction. Several reviews that provide more detailed insight into the physiological and pathological processes that alter function and pharmacology of the neuromuscular junction are available for the initiated reader.[14-19]

Neuromuscular Transmission

Neuromuscular transmission occurs by a fairly simple and straightforward mechanism. The nerve synthesizes acetylcholine and stores it in small, uniformly sized packages called *vesicles*. Stimulation of the nerve causes these vesicles to migrate to the surface of the nerve, rupture, and discharge acetylcholine into the cleft separating the nerve from muscle. AChRs in the end plate of the muscle respond by opening their channels for influx of sodium ions into the muscle to depolarize the muscle. The end-plate potential created is continued along the muscle membrane by the opening of sodium channels present throughout the muscle membrane to initiate a muscle contraction.[16,17] The acetylcholine immediately detaches from the receptor and is destroyed by the enzyme, acetylcholinesterase, which is also present in the cleft. Exogenous drugs that activate the nicotinic AChR, that is, agonists such as depolarizing muscle relaxants (e.g., succinylcholine or nicotine), can also act on these receptors and mimic the effect of acetylcholine and cause depolarization of the end plate. Nondepolarizing muscle relaxants (NDMRs) also act on the receptors, but they prevent acetylcholine from binding to the receptor and thus prevent depolarization by agonists. Because these NDMRs prevent the action of agonists (e.g., acetylcholine, carbachol, succinylcholine), they belong to the class of compounds known as *antagonists* at the muscle AChRs. Other compounds, frequently called *reversal drugs* or antagonists of neuromuscular paralysis (e.g., neostigmine, prostigmine), inhibit acetylcholinesterase and therefore impair the hydrolysis of acetylcholine. The increased accumulation of undegraded acetylcholine can effectively compete with NDMRs and thereby displace the latter from the receptor (i.e., law of mass action) and antagonize the effects of NDMRs.

MORPHOLOGY

The neuromuscular junction is specialized on both the nerve side and on the muscle side to transmit and receive chemical messages.[15-19] Each motor neuron runs without interruption from the ventral horn of the spinal cord or medulla to the neuromuscular junction as a large, myelinated axon (Fig. 12.1*A*). As the motor neuron approaches the muscle, the neuron repeatedly branches to contact many muscle

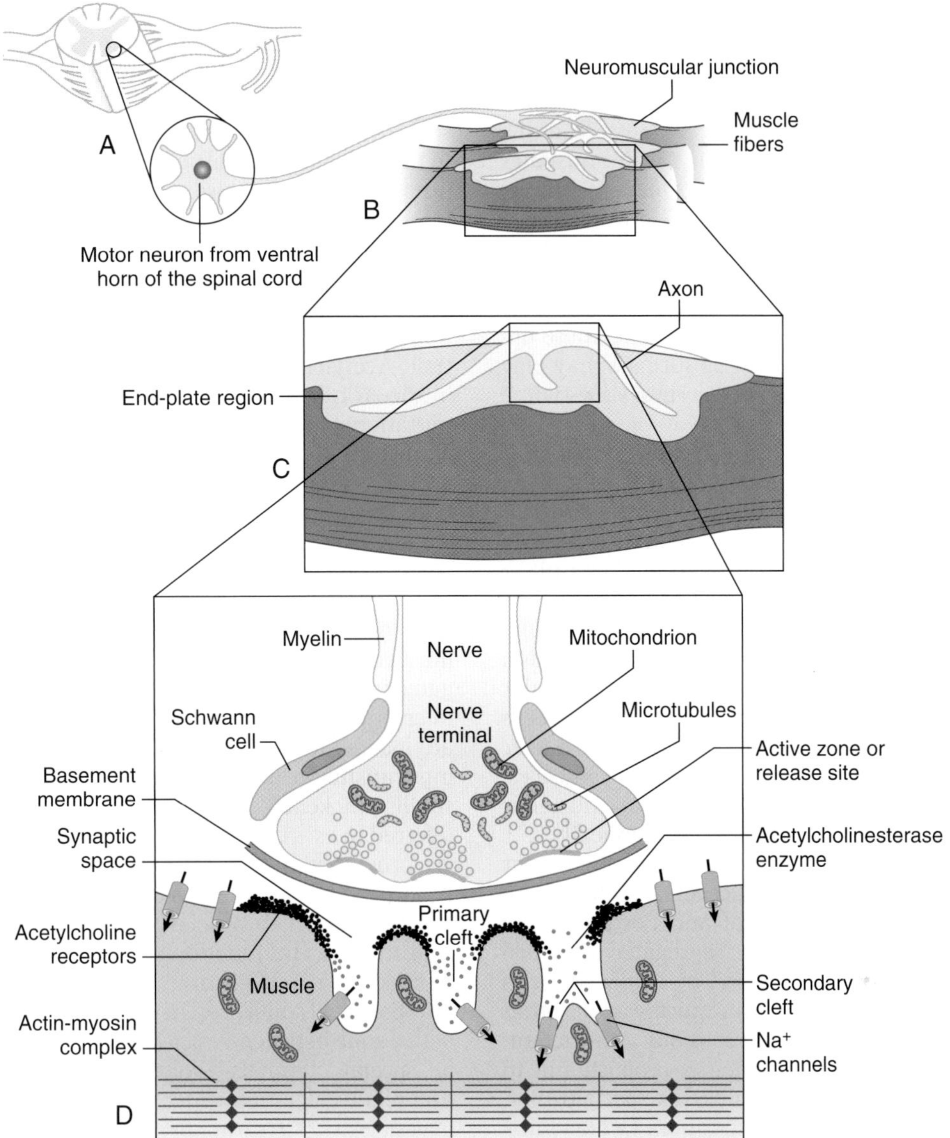

Fig. 12.1 Structure of the adult neuromuscular junction shows the three cells that constitute the synapse: the motor neuron (i.e., nerve terminal), muscle fiber, and Schwann cell. (A) The motor nerve originates in the ventral horn of the spinal cord or brainstem. (B) As the nerve approaches its muscle fibers and before attaching itself to the surface of the muscle fiber, the nerve divides into branches that innervate many individual muscle fibers. (C) Each muscle receives only one synapse. The motor nerve loses its myelin and further subdivides into many presynaptic boutons to terminate on the surface of the muscle fiber. (D) The nerve terminal, covered by Schwann cells, has vesicles clustered about the membrane thickenings, which are the active zones, toward its synaptic side and mitochondria and microtubules toward its other side. A synaptic gutter or cleft made up of a primary and many secondary clefts separate the nerve from the muscle. The muscle surface is corrugated, and dense areas on the shoulders of each fold contain acetylcholine receptors. Sodium (Na^+) channels are present at the bottom of the clefts and throughout the muscle membrane. The acetylcholinesterase and proteins and proteoglycans that stabilize the neuromuscular junction are present in the synaptic clefts.

cells and gather them into a functional group known as a *motor unit* (see Fig. 12.1*B*). The architecture of the nerve terminal is quite different from that of the rest of the axon. As the terminal reaches the muscle fiber, it loses its myelin, forms a spray of terminal branches against the muscle surface, and is covered by Schwann cells. This arrangement conforms to the architecture on the synaptic area of the muscle membrane (see Fig. 12.1*C*). The nerve is separated from the surface of the muscle by a gap of approximately 50 nm, called the *junctional cleft* or *synaptic cleft*. The nerve and muscle are held in tight alignment by protein filaments called *basal lamina* that span the cleft between the nerve and end plate. The muscle surface is heavily corrugated, with deep invaginations of the junctional cleft—the primary and secondary clefts—between the folds in the muscle membrane; thus, the end plate's total surface area is very large. The depths of the folds also vary between muscle types and species. Human neuromuscular junctions, relative to muscle size, are smaller than those of the mouse, although the junctions are located on muscle fibers that are much larger. Human junctions have longer junctional foldings and deeper gutters.[14,17] The sodium channels, which propagate the wave of depolarization, are located in the depths of the folds (see Fig. 12.1*D*). The shoulders of the folds are densely populated with AChRs, approximately 5 million of them in each junction. AChRs are sparse in the depths between the folds.

The trophic function of the nerve is vital for the development and maintenance of adequate neuromuscular function. Before birth, each muscle cell commonly has contacts with several nerves and has several neuromuscular junctions.[14,19] At birth, all but one of the nerves retract, and a single end plate remains (see section on "Neuromuscular Junction at the Extremes of Age"). Once formed, the nerve-muscle contact, especially the end plate, is durable. Even if the original nerve dies, the one replacing it innervates exactly the same region of the muscle. The nerve endings on fast muscles are larger and more complicated than those on slow muscles. The reason for this is unclear. These differences in the nerve endings on muscle surfaces may play a role in the difference in response of fast- and slow-twitch muscle fibers to muscle relaxants.

Because all the muscle cells in a unit are excited by a single neuron, stimulation of the nerve electrically or by an action potential originating from the ventral horn or by any agonist, including depolarizing relaxants (e.g., succinylcholine), causes all muscle cells in the motor unit to contract synchronously. Synchronous contraction of the cells in a motor unit is called *fasciculation* and is often vigorous enough to be observed through the skin. Although most adult human muscles have only one neuromuscular junction per cell, an important exception is some of the cells in extraocular muscles. The extraocular muscles are *tonic* muscles, and, unlike other mammalian striated muscles, they are multiply innervated with several neuromuscular junctions strung along the surface of each muscle fiber.[20-23] Quite in contrast to other muscles, even the adult ocular muscle contains mature and immature fetal receptors (see section on "Biology of Prejunctional and Postjunctional Nicotinic Acetylcholine Receptors") segregated into distinct synapses on different fibers.[20-22] The ocular muscles slowly contract and relax rather than quickly as do other striated muscles; they can maintain a steady contraction, or contracture, the strength of which is proportional to the stimulus received. Physiologically, this specialization apparently holds the eye steadily in position. Ocular muscles are important to an anesthesiologist because depolarizing muscle relaxants (e.g., succinylcholine) affect them differently than they do on most skeletal muscles. Instead of causing a brief contraction, followed by paralysis, the depolarizing drug causes a long-lasting contracture response that pulls the eye against the orbit and could contribute to an increase in intraocular fluid pressure.[22,23] The clinical significance of the succinylcholine-induced increase in intraocular pressure has been questioned. Although many textbooks invoke the reported extrusion of intraocular contents with succinylcholine, the basis for this effect seems to be anecdotal.[24] Clinical studies, however, have indicated that succinylcholine-induced contractions of the extraocular muscles can last as long as 1 to 2 minutes and isometric tensions larger than 12 g can develop for each extraocular muscle.[23] Thus, succinylcholine probably should not be given to patients with open eye injuries.

The perijunctional zone is the area of muscle immediately beyond the junctional area and is critical to the function of the neuromuscular junction. The perijunctional zone contains a mixture of receptors, including a smaller density of AChRs and a high density of sodium channels (see Fig. 12.1*D*). The admixture enhances the capacity of the perijunctional zone to respond to the depolarization (i.e., end-plate potential) produced by the AChRs and to transduce it into the wave of depolarization that travels along the muscle to initiate muscle contraction. The density of sodium channels in the perijunctional area is richer than in more distal parts of the muscle membrane.[25,26] The perijunctional zone is close enough to the nerve ending to be influenced by transmitter released from it. Moreover, special variants (i.e., isoforms) of receptors and sodium channels can appear in this area at different stages of life and in response to abnormal decreases in nerve activity (see section on "Biology of Prejunctional and Postjunctional Nicotinic Acetylcholine Receptors"). Congenital abnormalities in the AChRs or in the sodium and calcium channels (i.e., mutations) are also known.[25-27] These variabilities seem to contribute to the differences in response to relaxants that are observed in patients with different pathologic conditions and ages.[17,27]

QUANTAL THEORY

The contents of a nerve ending are not homogeneous. As illustrated in Figs. 12.1C and 12.2, vesicles are congregated in the portion toward the junctional surface, whereas microtubules, mitochondria, and other support structures are located toward the opposite side. The vesicles containing transmitter are ordered in repeating clusters alongside small, thickened, electron-dense patches of membrane referred to as *active zones* or *release sites*. This thickened area is a cross section of a band running across the width of the synaptic surface of the nerve ending that is believed to be the structure to which vesicles attach (active zones) before they rupture into the junctional cleft (see section on "Process of Exocytosis"). High-resolution scanning electron micrographs reveal small protein particles arranged alongside the active zone between vesicles. These particles are believed to be special channels—voltage-gated calcium channels—that allow calcium to enter the nerve and cause the release of vesicles.[28,29] The rapidity with which the neurotransmitter is released (200 μs) suggests that voltage-gated calcium channels are close to the release sites. Proteomic studies suggest that at least 26 genes encode presynaptic proteins, and mutations in 12 of them cause defects in presynaptic structure that can lead to decreased acetylcholine release and muscle weakness.[30] These defects can be related to exocytosis, endocytosis, formation of active and periactive zones, vesicle transport, and neuropeptide modulation.[30]

When observing the electrophysiologic activity of a skeletal muscle, small, spontaneous depolarizing potentials at neuromuscular junctions can be seen. These potentials have only one hundredth the amplitude of the evoked end-plate potential produced when the motor nerve is stimulated. Except for amplitude, these potentials resemble the end-plate potential in the time course and manner they are affected by drugs. These small-amplitude potentials are called *miniature end-plate potentials* (MEPPs). Statistical analysis led to the conclusion that they are unitary responses; that is, there is a minimum size for the MEPP, and the sizes of all MEPPs are equal to or multiples of this minimum size. Because MEPPs are too large to be produced by a single molecule of acetylcholine, it was deduced that they are produced by uniformly sized packages, or quanta, of transmitter released from the

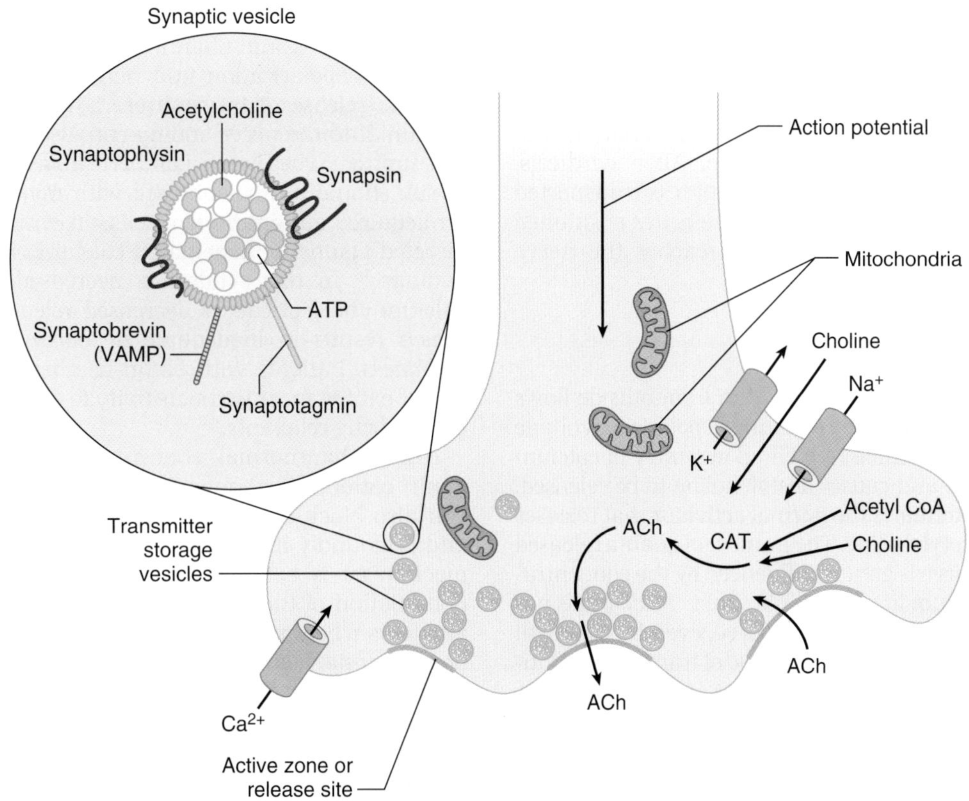

Fig. 12.2 The working of a chemical synapse, the motor nerve ending, including some of the apparatus for synthesis of transmitter, is illustrated. The large intracellular structures are mitochondria. Acetylcholine *(ACh)*, synthesized from choline and acetate by acetyl coenzyme A *(CoA)*, is transported into coated vesicles, which are moved to release sites. A presynaptic action potential that triggers the influx of calcium (Ca^{2+}) through specialized proteins (i.e., Ca^{2+} channels) causes the vesicles to fuse with the membrane and discharge transmitter. Membrane from the vesicle is retracted from the nerve membrane and recycled. Each vesicle can undergo various degrees of release of contents—from incomplete to complete. The transmitter is inactivated by diffusion, catabolism, or reuptake. The inset provides a magnified view of a synaptic vesicle. Quanta of ACh, together with adenosine triphosphate *(ATP)*, are stored in the vesicle and covered by vesicle membrane proteins. Synaptophysin is a glycoprotein component of the vesicle membrane. Synaptotagmin is the vesicle's calcium sensor. Phosphorylation of another membrane protein, synapsin, facilitates vesicular trafficking to the release site. Synaptobrevin (vesicle-associated membrane protein *[VAMP]*) is a SNARE protein involved in attaching the vesicle to the release-site proteins at the nerve terminal (see also Fig. 12.3). *CAT*, Choline acetyltransferase; K^+, potassium; Na^+, sodium.

nerve (in the absence of stimulation). The stimulus-evoked end-plate potential is the additive depolarization produced by the synchronous discharge of quanta from several hundred vesicles. The action potential that is propagated to the nerve ending allows the entry of calcium into the nerve through voltage-gated calcium channels, which causes vesicles to migrate to the active zone, fuse with the neural membrane at release sites, and discharge their acetylcholine into the junctional cleft.[28,29] Because the release sites are located immediately opposite the receptors on the postjunctional surface, little transmitter is wasted, and the response of the muscle is coupled directly with the signal from the nerve.[17,28]

Alignment of the presynaptic receptor site is achieved by adhesion molecules or specific cell-surface proteins located on both sides of the synapse that grip each other across the synaptic cleft and hold together the prejunctional and postjunctional synaptic apparatuses.[14,19,31] One such protein implicated in synapse adhesion is neurexin, which binds to neuroligins on the postsynaptic membrane. The amount of acetylcholine released by each nerve impulse is large, at least 200 quanta of approximately 5000 molecules each, and the number of AChRs activated by transmitter released by a nerve impulse is also large, approximately 500,000 molecules. The ions (mostly sodium and some calcium) that flow through the channels of activated (open) AChRs cause maximum depolarization of the end plate, which results in an end-plate potential that is greater than the threshold for stimulation of the muscle. This system is extremely vigorous. The signal is carried by more molecules of transmitter than are needed, and they evoke a response that is larger than needed. At the same time, only a small fraction of the available vesicles and receptors or channels are used to send each signal. Consequently, transmission has a substantial margin of safety, and, at the same time, the system has substantial capacity in reserve.[16-18,32]

Neuromuscular Junction

FORMATION OF NEUROTRANSMITTER AT MOTOR NERVE ENDINGS

The axon of the motor nerve carries electrical signals from the spinal cord to muscles and has all the biochemical apparatus needed to transform the electrical signal into a chemical one. All the ion channels, enzymes, other proteins, macromolecules, and membrane components needed by the nerve ending to synthesize, store, and release acetylcholine and other trophic factors are made in the cell body and transmitted to the nerve ending by axonal transport (see Fig. 12.2).[15,28,29] The simple molecules, choline and acetate, are obtained from the environment of the nerve ending, where choline is transported by a special system from extracellular fluid to the cytoplasm and acetate in the form of acetyl coenzyme A from mitochondria. The enzyme choline acetyltransferase brings about the reaction of choline and acetate to form acetylcholine. After synthesis, acetylcholine is stored in cytoplasm until it is transported and incorporated into vesicles, which are better positioned for release when an action potential reaches the nerve terminal.

NERVE ACTION POTENTIAL

During a nerve action potential, sodium from outside flows across the membrane, and the resulting depolarizing voltage opens the calcium channels, which allows entry of calcium ions into the nerve and causes acetylcholine to be released. A nerve action potential is the normal activator that releases the transmitter acetylcholine. The number of quanta released by a stimulated nerve is greatly influenced by the concentration of ionized calcium in extracellular fluid. If calcium is not present, then depolarization of the nerve, even by electrical stimulation, will not produce the release of transmitter. Doubling the extracellular calcium results in a 16-fold increase in the quantal content of an end-plate potential.[33] The calcium current persists until the membrane potential is returned to normal by outward fluxes of potassium from inside the nerve cell. Along with calcium channels on the nerve terminal are potassium channels, including the voltage-gated and calcium-activated potassium channels, whose function is to limit entry of calcium into the nerve and therefore depolarization.[26,32] The calcium current can be prolonged by potassium channel blockers (e.g., 4-aminopyridine, tetraethylammonium), which slow or prevent the efflux of potassium out of the nerve. The increase in quantal content produced in this way can reach astounding proportions.[17,34] An effect of increasing calcium in the nerve ending is also clinically observed as the so-called *posttetanic potentiation* (PTP), which occurs after a nerve of a patient paralyzed with an NDMR is stimulated at high, tetanic frequencies. Calcium enters the nerve with every stimulus, but it accumulates during the tetanic period because it cannot be excreted as quickly as the nerve is stimulated. Because the nerve ending contains more than the normal amount of calcium for some time after the tetanus, a stimulus applied to the nerve during this time causes the release of more than the normal amount of acetylcholine. The abnormally large amount of acetylcholine antagonizes the relaxant (temporarily) and causes the characteristic increase in the size of the twitch (i.e., post tetanic facilitation).

Calcium enters the nerve through specialized proteins called *calcium channels*.[15,35] Of the several types of calcium channels, two seem to be important for the release of transmitter: P channels and the slower L channels. P channels, probably the type responsible for the normal release of transmitter, are found only in nerve terminals.[13,35] In motor nerve endings, the calcium channels are located immediately adjacent to the active zones (see Fig 12.2). They are voltage-dependent and are opened and closed by changes in membrane voltage caused by the nerve action potential. In addition to calcium channels, several forms of potassium channels are present in the nerve terminal, including voltage-gated and calcium-activated potassium channels. Potassium channels limit the duration of nerve terminal depolarization and hence the entry of calcium and the release of transmitter.[26] Alterations in entry of calcium into the nerve ending can also alter the release of transmitter. The Eaton-Lambert myasthenic syndrome, which should not be confused with myasthenia gravis, is an acquired autoimmune disease in which antibodies are directed against voltage-gated calcium channels at nerve endings.[36] In this syndrome, decreased function of the calcium channel causes decreased release of transmitter, which results in inadequate depolarization and muscle weakness. Patients with Eaton-Lambert myasthenic syndrome exhibit increased sensitivity to depolarizing and nondepolarizing relaxants.[37]

Higher-than-normal concentrations of bivalent inorganic cations (e.g., magnesium, cadmium, manganese) can also block the entry of calcium through P channels and profoundly impair neuromuscular transmission. This mechanism is behind the typical muscle weakness and potentiation of the effect of muscle relaxants in a mother and fetus when magnesium sulfate is administered to treat preeclampsia. P channels, however, are not affected by calcium entry-blocking drugs such as verapamil, diltiazem, and nifedipine. These drugs have profound effects on the slower L channels present in the cardiovascular system. As a result, the L-type calcium channel blockers have no significant effect at therapeutic doses on the normal release of acetylcholine or on the strength of normal neuromuscular transmission. However, calcium entry-blocking drugs may increase the block in neuromuscular transmission induced by NDMRs. The effect is small, and not all investigators have been able to observe it. The explanation may lie in the fact that nerve endings also contain L-type calcium channels. The effects of calcium channels on depolarizing relaxants, if any, are unknown.

SYNAPTIC VESICLES AND RECYCLING

Two pools of vesicles seem to release acetylcholine, a readily releasable pool and a reserve pool, sometimes called VP1 and VP2, respectively.[38,39] Electron microscopic studies have demonstrated that the majority of synaptic vesicles (VP1) are sequestered in the reserve pool and tethered to the cytoskeleton in a filamentous network made up of primarily actin, synapsin (an actin-binding protein), synaptotagmin, and spectrin.[38,39] Vesicles in VP2 are a bit smaller and limited to an area very close to the nerve membrane, where they are bound to the active zones. These vesicles are the ones that ordinarily release transmitter. Release occurs when calcium ions enter the nerve through the P channels lined up on the sides of the active zones by soluble *N*-ethylmaleimide-sensitive attachment protein receptor (SNARE) proteins.[38,39] The SNARE proteins are involved in fusion, docking, and release of acetylcholine at the active zone. Calcium needs to move only a very short distance (i.e., a few atomic radii) to encounter a vesicle and activate the proteins in the vesicle wall involved in a process known as *docking* (see section on "Process of Exocytosis").[39] The activated proteins seem to react with the nerve membrane to form a pore through which the vesicle discharges its acetylcholine into the junctional cleft. Studies using fluorescent proteins

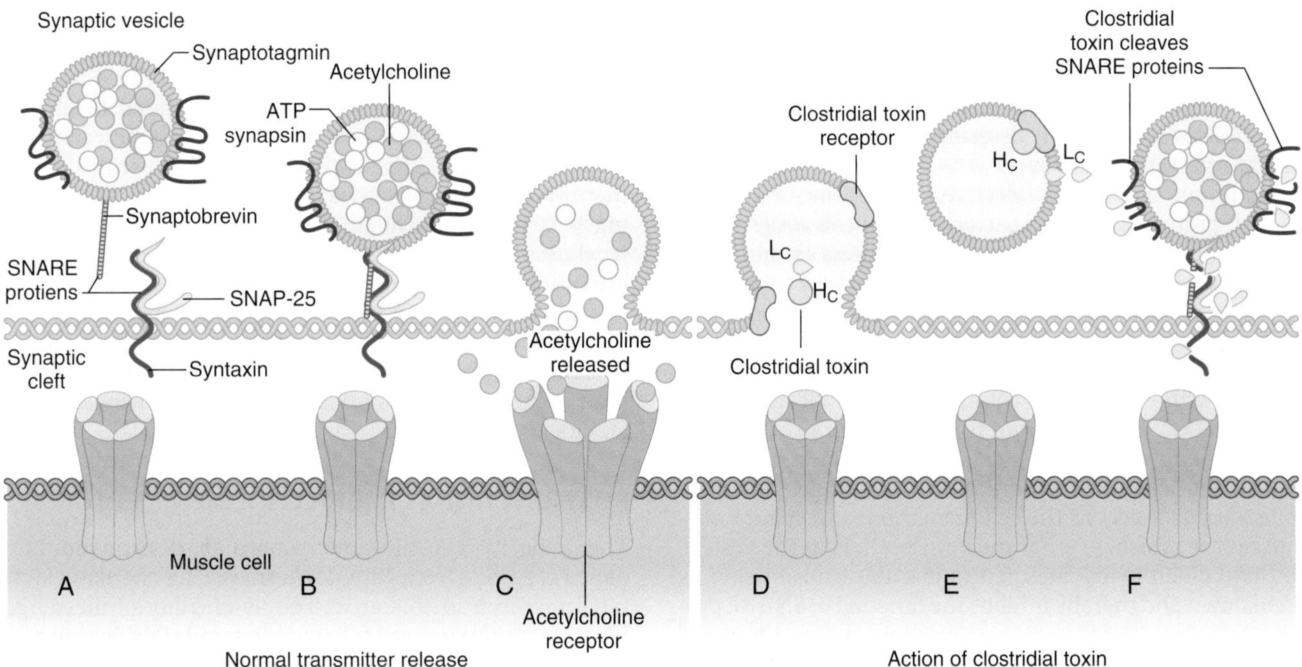

Fig. 12.3 Model of protein-mediated membrane fusion and exocytosis. (A) Release of acetylcholine from vesicles is mediated by a series of proteins collectively called *SNARE* proteins. Synaptotagmin is the neuronal calcium receptor that detects entry of calcium. Synaptobrevin (i.e., vesicle-associated membrane protein [VAMP]) is a filament-like protein on the vesicle. (B) During depolarization and entry of calcium, synapsin is also present on the vesicle membrane. Synaptobrevin on the vesicle unfolds and forms a ternary complex with syntaxin/SNAP-25 on the nerve terminal membrane. (C) Assembly of the ternary complex forces the vesicle in close apposition to the nerve membrane at the active zone with release of its contents, acetylcholine. The fusion is disassembled, and the vesicle is recycled. (D) Clostridial toxin, botulinum, inhibits the release of acetylcholine and causes paralysis of muscles. The toxin consists of a light chain *(L_c)* and a heavy chain *(H_c)*. The first stage in intoxication is the interaction of the toxin with a thus far unidentified receptor. (E) This interaction is followed by internalization of the toxin within the vesicle and the release of the L_c of toxin from the vesicle. (F) The liberated L_c cleaves a variety of SNARE proteins, depending on the type of toxin released, thereby preventing assembly of the fusion complex and thus blocking the release of acetylcholine. *ATP*, Adenosine triphosphate; *SNAP-25*, synaptosome-associated protein of 25-kd.

have visualized how synaptic vesicles fuse with release sites and release their contents, which are then retrieved. Some vesicles stay open briefly before retrieval and do not completely collapse into the surface membrane ("kiss and run"). Others stay open longer and probably do not completely collapse ("compensatory"). Still others completely collapse and are not retrieved until another stimulus is delivered ("stranded").[38,39]

The larger reserve (VP1) vesicles, from their position deep from the nerve ending and firmly tethered to the cytoskeleton by many proteins, including actin, synapsin (an actin-binding protein), synaptotagmin, and spectrin,[37,38] may be moved to the readily releasable store to replace worn-out vesicles or to participate in transmission when the nerve is called on to work especially hard (e.g., when it is stimulated at very high frequencies or for a very long time). Under such strenuous circumstances, calcium may penetrate more deeply than normal into the nerve or may enter through L channels to activate calcium-dependent enzymes that break the synapsin links holding the vesicles to the cytoskeleton, thereby allowing the vesicles to be moved to the release sites. Repeated stimulation requires the nerve ending to replenish its store of vesicles filled with transmitter, a process known as *mobilization*. The term is commonly applied to the aggregate of all steps involved in maintaining the nerve ending's capacity to release transmitter—everything from the acquisition of choline and the synthesis of acetate to the movement of filled vesicles to release sites. Uptake of choline and the activity of choline acetyltransferase, the enzyme that synthesizes acetylcholine, are probably the rate-limiting steps.[15,29]

PROCESS OF EXOCYTOSIS

The readily releasable pool of synaptic vesicles constitutes the vesicles directly available for release. During an action potential and calcium influx, neurotransmitter is released. Studies have shed some light on the inner workings by which the vesicle releases its contents. The whole process is called *exocytosis*. The SNARE proteins include (Fig. 12.3*A*) the synaptic-vesicle protein, synaptobrevin; the plasmalemma-associated protein, syntaxin; and the synaptosome-associated protein of 25-kd (SNAP-25).[38,39] The current model of protein-mediated membrane fusion in exocytosis is as follows. When there is an action potential and calcium ions enter, synapsin becomes phosphorylated, which frees the vesicle from its attachment to the cytoskeleton. Syntaxin and SNAP-25 are complexes attached to the plasma membrane. After the initial contact, the synaptobrevin on the vesicle forms a ternary complex with syntaxin and SNAP-25. Synaptotagmin is the protein on the vesicular membrane that acts as a calcium sensor, localizes the synaptic vesicles to synaptic zones rich in calcium channels, and stabilizes the vesicles in the docked state.[38] Assembly of the ternary complex forces the vesicle to move close to the underlying nerve terminal membrane (i.e., the active zone), and the vesicle is then ready for release (see Fig. 12.3*B*). The close proximity of release sites, calcium channels, and synaptic vesicles and the use of the calcium sensor lead to a burst of release of new transmitter synchronous with the stimulus (see Fig. 12.3*C*).[37-40] The vesicle can release part or all of its contents, some of which can be recycled to form new vesicles as previously described ("kiss and run," "compensatory," "stranded").[37-40]

Botulinum neurotoxin selectively digests one or all these SNARE proteins and blocks exocytosis of the vesicles,[41,42] which ultimately results in muscle weakness or more profound muscle paralysis. This toxin may produce a partial or complete chemical denervation. Botulinum toxin is therapeutically used to treat spasticity or spasm in several neurologic and surgical diseases, to prevent hyperhidrosis in patients with excessive sweating, and cosmetically to correct wrinkles.[43,44] Botulinum toxin consists of two protein segments known as heavy and light chains (see Fig. 12.3*D* and *E*). The heavy chain interacts with lipid molecules called *polysialogangliosides* in the cell membrane and synaptotagmin on the vesicle to enter the vesicle. Once in the vesicle, the light chain inactivates neuromuscular transmission by breakdown and thereby inhibits the function of SNARE proteins (see Fig. 12.3*F*). Some reports indicate an increased incidence of clostridial infections in both Canada and the United States, with *Clostridium botulinum* infection being particularly common after traumatic injuries, in drug abusers, and after musculoskeletal allografts.[6,7] Thus, systemic paralysis can occur after clostridial infection. Local injection for therapeutic purposes will usually result in localized paresis, although systemic effects have been reported.[7,45]

ACETYLCHOLINESTERASE

The acetylcholine released from the nerve diffuses across the junctional cleft and reacts with nicotinic AChRs in the end plate to initiate muscle contraction. Transmitter molecules that do not immediately react with a nicotinic AChR or those released after binding to the receptor are almost instantly destroyed by acetylcholinesterase in the junctional cleft. Acetylcholinesterase at the junction is the asymmetric or A12 form protein made in the muscle under the end plate. Acetylcholinesterase (enzyme classification 3.1.1.7) is type B carboxylesterase enzyme. A smaller concentration of the enzyme is found in the extrajunctional area. The enzyme is secreted from the muscle but remains attached to it by thin stalks of collagen fastened to the basement membrane.[15,37] Most of the molecules of acetylcholine released from the nerve initially pass between the enzymes to reach the postjunctional receptors; however, as they are released from the receptors, they invariably encounter acetylcholinesterase and are destroyed. Under normal circumstances, a molecule of acetylcholine reacts with only one receptor before it is hydrolyzed. Acetylcholine is a potent messenger, but its actions are very short lived because it is destroyed in less than 1 ms after it is released.

Some congenital and acquired diseases are caused by altered activity of acetylcholinesterase. The congenital absence of the secreted enzyme (in knock-out mice) leads to impaired maintenance of the motor neuronal system and organization of nerve terminal branches.[46] Many syndromes caused by congenital abnormalities in cholinesterase function have been described and result in neuromuscular disorders whose symptoms and signs usually resemble those of myasthenia gravis or myasthenic syndromes.[27,47] Denervation decreases acetylcholinesterase at the junctional and extrajunctional areas.[37] Other acquired diseases involving cholinesterases are related to chronic inhibition of acetylcholinesterase by organophosphate pesticides or nerve gas (e.g., sarin) or to chronic pyridostigmine therapy given as prophylaxis against nerve gas poisoning.[48,49] Symptoms ranging from chronic fatigue to muscle weakness have been attributed to chronic cholinesterase inhibition, thus underscoring the importance of acetylcholinesterase in normal and abnormal neuromuscular function. A rodent study confirms that the muscle weakness associated with chronic pyridostigmine therapy is related to both AChRs downregulation and to receptor-independent factors.[50]

POSTJUNCTIONAL ACETYLCHOLINE RECEPTORS

The similarity of AChRs among many species and the abundance of AChRs from *Torpedo electric fish* have greatly facilitated research in this area. The availability of messenger RNA from humans and other species and DNA has allowed the study of the receptor in artificial systems such as oocytes from frogs and in mammalian cells that do not express the receptor, such as COS or fibroblast cells. Receptors can also be mutated by molecular techniques to simulate pathologic states; the receptor function in these artificial systems can then be studied. By using these and related techniques, much has been learned about the synthesis, composition, and biologic function and mechanisms that underlie the physiologic and pharmacologic responses in AChRs.[51-53] Three isoforms of postjunctional nicotinic AChRs exist: a junctional or mature receptor, an extrajunctional or immature (fetal) receptor, and the more recently described neuronal $\alpha7$ nicotinic receptor (see section on "Biology of Prejunctional and Postjunctional Nicotinic Acetylcholine Receptors").[2,16,18] The differences between receptor subtypes, however, can be neglected in a general discussion of the role of receptors in neuromuscular transmission.

AChRs are synthesized in muscle cells and are anchored to the end-plate membrane by a special 43-kd protein known as *rapsyn*. This cytoplasmic protein is associated with the AChR in a 1:1 ratio.[16-19] The receptors, formed of five subunit proteins, are arranged like the staves of a barrel into a cylindrical receptor with a central pore for ion channeling (the key features are illustrated in Fig. 12.4). The receptor protein has a molecular mass of approximately 250,000 daltons. The mature receptor consists of $\alpha1$-, $\beta1$-, δ-, and ε-subunits, and the fetal (immature, extrajunctional) receptor consists of $\alpha1$-, $\beta1$-, δ-, and γ-subunits; there are two subunits of α and one each of the others. The neuronal $\alpha7$ AChR consists of five $\alpha7$-subunits.[16,18] Each of all receptor subunits consists of approximately 400 to 500 amino acids. The receptor-protein complex passes entirely through the membrane and protrudes beyond the extracellular surface of the membrane and into the cytoplasm. The binding site for acetylcholine is on each of the $\alpha1$- or $\alpha7$- subunits, is located on the extracellular component of the α-subunit protein, and these are the sites of competition between receptor agonists and antagonists. Agonists and antagonists are attracted to the binding site, and either may occupy the site, which is located near cysteine residues

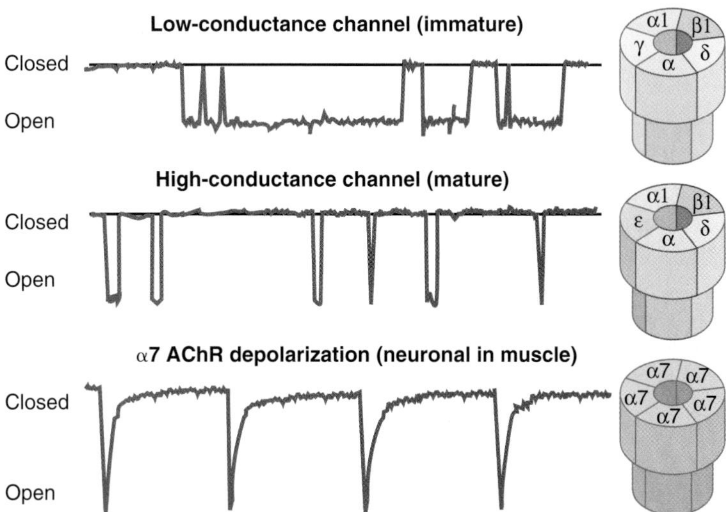

Fig. 12.4 Schematic illustration depicts acetylcholine receptor *(AChR)* channels *(right)* and tracings of cell-patch records of receptor channel openings *(left)*. The mature or junctional receptor consists of two α1-subunits and one each of β1-, δ-, and ε-subunits. The immature, extrajunctional, or fetal form consists of two α1-subunits and one each of β1-, δ-, and γ-subunits. The latter is thus called the γ-subunit receptor. Recently, a neuronal receptor consisting of five α7-subunits has been described in muscle. All the subunits are arranged around the central cation channel. The immature isoform containing the γ-subunit has long open times and low-amplitude channel currents. The mature isoform containing the ε-subunit has shorter open times and high-amplitude channel currents during depolarization. Substitution of the ε-subunit for the γ-subunit gives rise to the fast-gated, high-conductance channel type. As expected, application of acetylcholine to the α7 AChR also results in a fast, rapidly decaying inward current. All these depolarizing events are insensitive to treatment with muscarinic acetylcholine receptor antagonist, atropine, but sensitive to treatment with α-bungarotoxin or muscle relaxants, which block the flow of current. The affinity of the muscle relaxants to each of the three isoforms may be different, α7 AChR being the least sensitive to block.

(unique to the α-chain) at amino acid positions 192 to 193 of the α-subunit.[16-18] Radiolabeled α-bungarotoxin from the cobra, used to quantitate or fluorescent stain the receptor, binds to heptapeptide region 185 to 199 of the α-subunit.[54] Motor neuron-derived neuregulin-1β (NRβ-1), originally described as AChR-inducing activity (ARIA), induces AChR gene transcription in subsynaptic myonuclei by activating ErbB receptors.[16-19]

SYNTHESIS AND STABILIZATION OF POSTJUNCTIONAL RECEPTORS

Muscle tissue is formed from the mesoderm and initially appears as myoblasts. Myoblasts fuse to produce myotubes, which therefore have multiple nuclei. As the myotubes mature, the sarcomere, which is the contractile element of the muscle consisting of actin and myosin, develops.[55] The protein β-integrin seems to be essential for myoblast fusion and sarcomere assembly.[55] Shortly afterward, motor nerve axons grow into the developing muscle, and these axons bring in nerve-derived signals (i.e., growth factors), including agrin and neuregulins (NRβ-1 and NRβ-2), which are key to the maturation of myotubes to muscle.[19] Agrin is a protein from the nerve that stimulates postsynaptic differentiation by activating muscle-specific tyrosine kinase (MuSK), a tyrosine kinase expressed selectively in muscle. With signaling from agrin, the AChRs, which have been scattered throughout the muscle membrane, cluster at the area immediately beneath the nerve. Agrin, together with neuregulins and other growth factors, induce the clustering of other critical muscle-derived proteins, including MuSK, rapsyn, and ErbB proteins, all of which are necessary for maturation and stabilization of AChRs at the junction. In addition to the effects on postsynaptic differentiation, agrin and MuSK display effects on presynaptic differentiation as well. Agrin and MuSK induce retrograde signals that instruct axons to undergo neuron outgrowth and terminal differentiation.[19] Current understanding of presynaptic development of the neuromuscular junction, however, is significantly less advanced than the understanding of postsynaptic development. Just before and shortly after birth, the immature, γ-subunit-containing AChRs are replaced by the mature, ε-subunit-containing receptors. Although the mechanism of this change is unclear, a neuregulin, NRβ-1, also called *ARIA*, that binds to one of the ErbB receptors seems to play a role.[19,56]

BASIC ELECTROPHYSIOLOGY OF NEUROTRANSMISSION

Fig. 12.5 illustrates the results of the classic depolarizing action of acetylcholine on end-plate receptors. Normally, the pore of the channel is closed by approximation of the cylinders (i.e., subunits). When an agonist occupies both α-subunit sites, the protein molecule undergoes a conformational change with a twisting movement along the central axis of the receptor that results in the opening of the central channel through which ions can flow along a concentration gradient. When the central channel is open, sodium and calcium flow from the outside of the cell to the inside and potassium flows from the inside to the outside. The channel in the tube is large enough to accommodate many cations and electrically neutral molecules, but it excludes anions (e.g., chloride). The current transported by the ions depolarizes the adjacent membrane. The net current is depolarizing and creates the end-plate potential that stimulates the muscle to contract. In this instance, downward-going (i.e., depolarizing) current can be recorded by

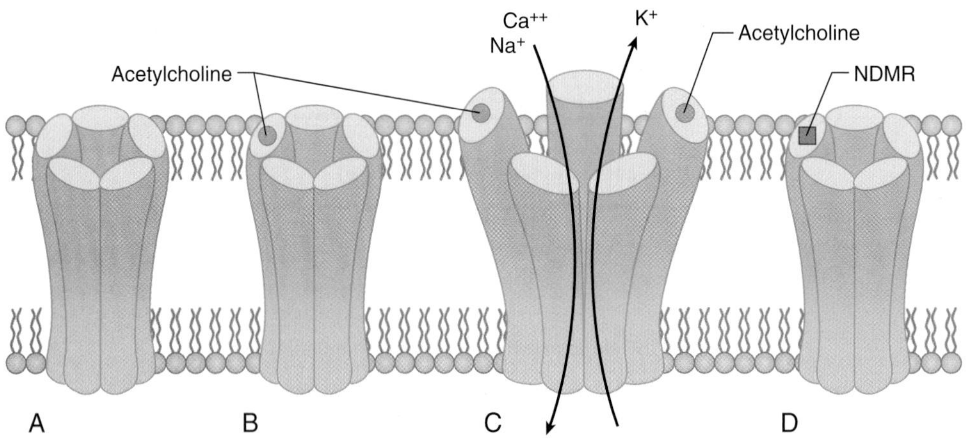

Fig. 12.5 Actions of acetylcholine or non-depolarizing muscle relaxant (NDMR) on end-plate receptors. (A) The ion channel is inactive and does not open in the absence of acetylcholine. (B) Although one acetylcholine molecule *(filled circle)* is binding to one of two binding sites, the central channel does not open. (C), When acetylcholine simultaneously binds to the recognition sites of both α-subunits *(filled circles)*, a conformation change is triggered that opens the channel and allows the cations to flow across the membrane. (D) Action of antagonists such as an NDMR *(filled square)*. Acetylcholine is in competition with NDMR for the receptor's recognition site but may also react with acetylcholinesterase. Inhibiting the acetylcholinesterase enzyme increases the lifetime of acetylcholine and the probability that it will react with a receptor. When one of the two binding (recognition) sites is occupied by an NDMR, the receptor will not open, even if the other binding site is occupied by acetylcholine. *Ca^{2++}*, Calcium ion; *K^+*, potassium ion; *Na^+*, sodium ion.

the patch-clamp electrophysiologic technique previously described (see Fig. 12.4).

The pulse stops when the channel closes by a reversed mechanical conformation (see earlier discussion), which is typically initiated when one or both agonist molecules detach from the receptor. In the activated, open state, the current that passes through each open channel is minuscule, only a few picoamperes (approximately 10^4 ions/ms). However, each burst of acetylcholine from the nerve normally opens approximately 500,000 channels simultaneously, and the total current is more than adequate to produce depolarization of the end plate and contraction of muscle. Opening of a channel causes conversion of chemical signals from a nerve to the flow of current on the muscle disease to cause end-plate potentials, thereby leading to muscle contraction. The end-plate potential has been viewed as a graded event that may be reduced in magnitude or extended in time by drugs, but, in reality, the end-plate potential is the summation of many all-or-nothing events simultaneously occurring at myriad ion channels. It is these tiny events that are affected by drugs.

Receptors that do not have two molecules of agonist (e.g., acetylcholine) bound remain closed. Both α-subunits must be simultaneously occupied by agonist; if only one of them is occupied, then the channel remains closed (see Fig. 12.5). This is the basis for preventing depolarization by antagonists. NDMRs act by binding to either or both α-subunits and thus preventing acetylcholine from binding and opening the channel. This interaction between agonists and antagonists is competitive, and the outcome—transmission or block—depends on the relative concentrations and binding characteristics of the drugs involved (see section on "Drug Effects on Postjunctional Receptors").

Individual channels are also capable of a wide variety of conformational states.[17,57] They may stay open or remain closed and thereby affect total current flow across the membrane, but they can do more. They may open for a longer or shorter time than normal, open or close more gradually than usual, open briefly and repeatedly (i.e., flickering), or pass fewer or more ions per opening than they usually do. Their function is also influenced by drugs, changes in fluidity of the membrane, temperature, electrolyte balance in the milieu, and other physical and chemical factors.[38,39] Receptor channels are dynamic structures that are capable of a wide variety of interactions with drugs and of entering a wide variety of current-passing states. All these influences on channel activity are ultimately reflected in the strength or weakness of neuromuscular transmission and contraction of a muscle.

Drug Effects on Postjunctional Receptors

CLASSIC ACTIONS OF NONDEPOLARIZING MUSCLE RELAXANTS

Neurotransmission occurs when acetylcholine released by the nerve action potential binds to nicotinic AChRs. All NDMRs impair or block neurotransmission by competitively preventing the binding of acetylcholine to the muscle AChR. The final outcome—block or transmission—depends on the relative concentrations of the chemicals and their comparative affinities for the receptor. Fig. 12.5 shows a system exposed to acetylcholine and the nondepolarizing neuromuscular blocking compound. One receptor has attracted two acetylcholine molecules and has opened its channel, where current will flow to depolarize that segment of membrane. Another has attracted one molecule of NDMR; its channel will not open, and no current will flow, even if one acetylcholine molecule binds to the other site. The third receptor has acetylcholine on one α-subunit and nothing on the other. What will happen depends on which of the molecules binds. If acetylcholine binds, then the channel will open and the membrane will be depolarized; if a NDMR binds, then the channel will remain closed and the membrane will not be depolarized. At other times, one or two molecules of NDMR may attach to the receptor, in which case the receptor is not available to agonists; no current flow is recorded. In the presence of moderate concentrations of NDMR, the amount of current flowing through the entire end plate at any instant is reduced from normal, which results in a smaller end-plate potential and, if carried far enough, a block in neurotransmission or the production of neuromuscular paralysis.

Normally, acetylcholinesterase destroys acetylcholine and removes it from competition for a receptor; therefore, an NDMR has a better chance of inhibiting transmission. If, however, an inhibitor of acetylcholinesterase such as neostigmine is added, then the cholinesterase cannot destroy acetylcholine. The concentration of agonist in the cleft remains high, and this high concentration shifts the competition between acetylcholine and a NDMR in favor of the former, thereby improving the chance of two acetylcholine molecules binding to a receptor even though NDMR is still in the environment. This mechanism causes the cholinesterase inhibitors to overcome the neuromuscular paralysis produced by NDMRs. The channel opens only when acetylcholine attaches to both recognition sites. A single molecule of antagonist, however, is adequate to prevent depolarization of that receptor. This modifies the competition by strongly biasing it in favor of the antagonist (relaxant). Mathematically, if the concentration of a NDMR is doubled, then the concentration of acetylcholine must be increased fourfold if acetylcholine is to remain competitive. Paralysis produced by high concentrations of muscle relaxants (antagonist) is more difficult to reverse with cholinesterase inhibitors than that produced by low concentrations. After large doses of NDMRs, cholinesterase inhibitors may be ineffective until the concentration of relaxant in the perijunctional area decreases to a lower level by the redistribution or elimination of the drug. This is the molecular basis for the recommendation to not administer anticholinesterases too early (i.e., at a deep block). In contrast to reversal with a cholinesterase inhibitor, cyclodextrin encapsulation takes place at any concentration of a steroid-based compound, such as vecuronium or rocuronium, and reversal by this novel mechanism can therefore be achieved at any level of neuromuscular block provided the amount of cyclodextrin (sugammadex) is large enough.

CLASSIC ACTIONS OF DEPOLARIZING MUSCLE RELAXANTS

Depolarizing relaxants (e.g., succinylcholine, decamethonium) initially simulate the effect of acetylcholine and can be considered agonists, despite the fact that they block neurotransmission after the initial stimulation. Structurally, succinylcholine is very similar to the natural ligand acetylcholine and consists of two molecules of acetylcholine bound together through their backbones. It is thus not surprising that succinylcholine can mimic the effects of acetylcholine.

Succinylcholine or decamethonium can bind to the receptor, open the channel, pass current, and depolarize the end plate. These agonists, similar to acetylcholine, attach only briefly; each opening of a channel is very short

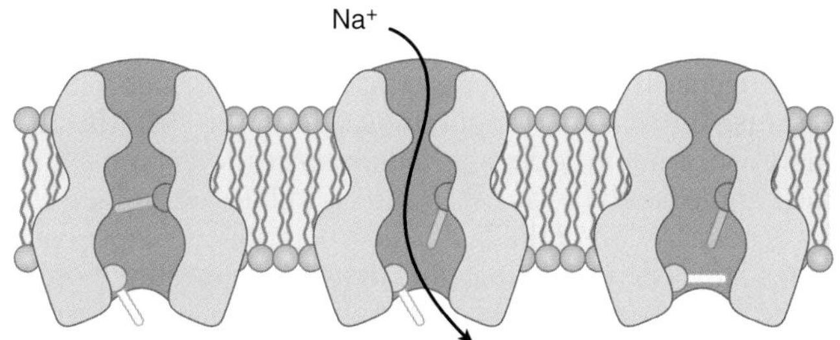

Fig. 12.6 Illustration of a sodium (Na^+) channel. The bars represent parts of the molecule that act as gates. The upper bar is voltage dependent; the lower bar is time dependent. The left side of the drawing represents the resting state. Once activated by a change in voltage, the molecule and its gates progress as illustrated *(left to right)*. See text for details.

in duration—1 ms or less. The response to acetylcholine, however, is over in milliseconds because of its rapid degradation by acetylcholinesterase, and the end plate resets to its resting state long before another nerve impulse arrives. In contrast, the depolarizing relaxants characteristically have a biphasic action on muscle—an initial contraction, followed by relaxation lasting from minutes to hours. Because they are not susceptible to hydrolysis by acetylcholinesterase, the depolarizing relaxants are not eliminated from the junctional cleft until after they are eliminated from plasma. The time required to clear the drug from the body is the principal determinant of how long the drug effect lasts. Whole-body clearance of the relaxant is very slow in comparison to acetylcholine, particularly when plasma (pseudo) cholinesterase is abnormal. Because the relaxant molecules are not quickly cleared from the cleft, compared with acetylcholine, they repeatedly react with receptors even with normal levels of plasma cholinesterase, almost immediately attaching to a receptor after separating from another, thereby repeatedly depolarizing the end plate and opening channels. For details on the effect of succinylcholine in patients with cholinesterase deficiency, also see Chapter 27.

The quick shift from excitation of muscle contraction to block of transmission by depolarizing relaxants occurs because the end plate is continuously depolarized. This comes about as a result of the juxtaposition of the edge of the end plate with a different kind of ion channel, the sodium channel that does not respond to chemicals but opens when exposed to a transmembrane voltage change. Just as the AChR, the sodium channel is also a cylindrical transmembrane protein through which sodium ions can flow. Two parts of its structure act as gates that allow or stop the flow of sodium ions.[58] Both gates must be open if sodium is to flow through the channel; closing of either cuts off the flow. Because these two gates act sequentially, a sodium channel has three functional conformational states and can progressively move from one state to another (Fig. 12.6). This whole process is short lived when depolarization occurs with acetylcholine.[58] The initial response of a depolarizing muscle relaxant resembles that of acetylcholine, but because the muscle relaxant is not rapidly hydrolyzed, depolarization of the end plate is not brief.

Depolarization of the end plate by the depolarizing relaxant initially causes the voltage gate in adjacent sodium channels to open, thereby producing a wave of depolarization that sweeps along the muscle and generates a muscle contraction. Shortly after the voltage-dependent gate opens, the time-dependent inactivation gate closes. Because the relaxant is not removed from the cleft, the end plate continues to be depolarized. Because the sodium channels immediately adjacent to the end plate are influenced by depolarization of the end plate, their voltage-dependent gates stay open and their inactivation gates stay closed. Since sodium cannot flow through a channel that has a closed inactivation gate, the perijunctional muscle membrane does not depolarize. When the flow of ions through sodium channels in the perijunctional zone stops because of a closure of the inactivation gates, the channels downstream (beyond the perijunctional zone) are freed of depolarizing influence. In effect, the perijunctional zone becomes a buffer that shields the rest of the muscle from events at the end plate. Consequently, the muscle membrane is separated into three zones: (1) the end plate, which is depolarized by succinylcholine; (2) the perijunctional muscle membrane, in which the sodium channels are frozen in an inactivated state; and (3) the rest of the muscle membrane, in which the sodium channels are in the resting state. Because a burst of acetylcholine from the nerve cannot overcome the inactivated sodium channels in the perijunctional zone, neuromuscular transmission is blocked. This phenomenon is also called *accommodation*. During accommodation, when the synapse is inexcitable through the nerve (transmitter), direct electrical stimulation of muscle causes muscle contraction because the sodium channels beyond the junctional area are in the resting excitable state.

The extraocular muscles are tonic muscles, which are multiply innervated and chemically excitable along most of their surfaces.[20-23] Despite their innervated state, the ocular muscles express both mature and immature receptors.[20,22] Accommodation does not occur, and these muscles can undergo a sustained contracture in the presence of succinylcholine. The tension that develops forces the eye against the orbit and accounts for part of the increase in intraocular pressure produced by depolarizing relaxants. The extraocular muscles contain a special type of receptor that does not become desensitized (see later discussion) during the continued presence of acetylcholine or other agonists.[21,23] A single dose of succinylcholine can cause contracture lasting several minutes.[23] Whether it is the immature γ-subunit AChR or the α7 AChR subunit that plays a role in this resistance to desensitization in the ocular muscles is unknown.

NONCLASSIC AND NONCOMPETITIVE ACTIONS OF NEUROMUSCULAR DRUGS

Several drugs can interfere with the receptor, directly or through its lipid environment, and can change transmission (Box 12.1). These drugs react with the neuromuscular receptor to change its function and impair transmission, but they do not act through the acetylcholine binding site. These reactions cause drug-induced changes in the dynamics of the receptor; instead of sharply opening and closing, the modified channels are sluggish. They open more slowly and stay open longer, or they close slowly and in several steps, or both. These effects on channels cause corresponding changes in the flow of ions and distortions of the end-plate potential. The clinical effect depends on the molecular events. For example, procaine, ketamine, inhaled anesthetics, or other drugs that dissolve in the membrane lipid may change the opening or closing characteristics of the channel.[57,59] If the channel is prevented from opening, then transmission is weakened. If, however, the channel is prevented from or slowed in closing, then transmission may be enhanced. These drugs do not fit the classic model, and the impaired neuromuscular function is not antagonized by increasing perijunctional acetylcholine concentrations with cholinesterase inhibitors. Such drugs can be involved in two clinically important reactions: receptor desensitization and channel block. The former occurs in the receptor molecule, whereas the latter occurs in the ion channel.

BOX 12.1 Drugs That Can Cause or Promote Desensitization of Muscle Nicotinic Receptors

- Volatile anesthetics
  - Halothane
  - Sevoflurane
  - Isoflurane
- Antibiotics
  - Polymyxin B
- Cocaine
- Alcohols
  - Ethanol
  - Butanol
  - Propanol
  - Octanol
- Barbiturates
  - Thiopental
  - Pentobarbital
- Agonists
  - Acetylcholine
  - Decamethonium
  - Carbachol
  - Succinylcholine
- Acetylcholinesterase inhibitors
  - Neostigmine
  - Pyridostigmine
  - Di-isopropyl-fluorophosphate
  - Edrophonium
- Local anesthetics
  - Dibucaine
  - Lidocaine
  - Prilocaine
  - Etidocaine
- Phenothiazines
  - Chlorpromazine
  - Trifluoperazine
  - Prochlorperazine
- Phencyclidine
- Calcium channel blockers
  - Verapamil

DESENSITIZATION BLOCK

The AChR, as a result of its flexibility and the fluidity of the lipid around it, is capable of existing in a number of conformational states.[57-61] Because the resting receptor is free of agonist, its channel is closed. The second state exists when two molecules of agonist are bound to the α-subunit of the receptor and the receptor has undergone the conformational change that opens the channel and allows ions to flow. These reactions are the bases of normal neuromuscular transmission. Some receptors that bind to agonists, however, do not undergo the conformational change to open the channel. Receptors in these states are called desensitized (i.e., they are not sensitive to the channel-opening actions of agonists). They bind agonists with exceptional avidity, but the binding does not result in the opening of the channel. The mechanisms by which desensitization occurs are not known. The receptor macromolecule, 1000 times larger by weight than most drugs or gases, provides many places at which the smaller molecules may act. The interface between lipid and receptor protein provides additional potential sites of reaction. Several different conformations of the protein are known, and because acetylcholine cannot cause the ion channel to open in any of them, they all are included in the functional term *desensitization*. Desensitization is accompanied by phosphorylation of a tyrosine unit in the receptor protein.[61,62]

Although agonists (e.g., succinylcholine) induce desensitization, the receptors are in a constant state of transition between resting and desensitized states, regardless of whether agonists are present. Agonists do promote transition to a desensitized state or, because they bind very tightly to desensitized receptors, trap a receptor in a desensitized state. NDMRs also tightly bind to desensitized receptors and can trap molecules in these states. This action of NDMRs is not competitive with that of acetylcholine; it may be augmented by acetylcholine if the latter promotes the change to a desensitized state. Desensitization can lead to significant misinterpretation of data. Superficially, the preparation seems to be normal, but its responsiveness to agonists or antagonists is altered. One variety occurs very rapidly, within a few milliseconds after application of an agonist, which may explain the increased sensitivity to nondepolarizing relaxant after the prior administration of succinylcholine. Desensitization may also be a part of the phenomenon known as *phase II block* (see section on "Phase II Block"), which is caused by a prolonged administration of depolarizing relaxants. Phase II block is frequently referred to as a desensitization block, but it should not be because desensitization of receptors is only one of many phenomena that contribute to the process.

Many other drugs used by anesthetists also promote the shift of receptors from a normal state to a desensitized state.[58-60] These drugs, some of which are listed in Box 12.1, can weaken neuromuscular transmission by reducing the margin of safety that normally exists at the neuromuscular junction, or they can cause an apparent increase in the capacity of NDMRs to block transmission. These actions are independent of the classic effects, based on competitive inhibition of acetylcholine. The presence of desensitized receptors means that fewer receptor channels than usual are available to carry transmembrane current. The production of desensitized receptors decreases the efficacy of neuromuscular transmission. If many receptors are desensitized, then insufficient normal ones are left to depolarize the motor end plate, and neuromuscular transmission will not occur. Even if only some receptors are desensitized, neuromuscular transmission will be impaired, and the system will be more susceptible to block by conventional antagonists such as atracurium or rocuronium.

CHANNEL BLOCK

Local anesthetics and calcium entry blockers prevent the flow of sodium or calcium through their respective channels, thus explaining the term *channel-blocking drugs*. Similarly, block of the flow of ions can occur at the AChR with concentrations of drugs used clinically and may contribute to some of the phenomena and drug interactions observed at the receptor. Two major types, closed-channel and open-channel block, can occur.[60,63,64] In a closed-channel block, certain drugs can occupy the mouth of the channel and prevent ions from passing through the channel to depolarize the end plate. The process can take place even when the channel is not open. In an open-channel block, a drug molecule enters a channel that has been opened by reaction with acetylcholine but does not necessarily penetrate all the way through. Open-channel block is a use-dependent block, which means that molecules can enter the channel only when it is open. In open- and closed-channel blocks, the normal flow of ions through the receptor is impaired, thereby resulting in the prevention of depolarization of the end plate and a weakened or blocked neuromuscular transmission. However, because the action is not at the acetylcholine recognition site, it is not a competitive antagonism of acetylcholine and is not relieved by anticholinesterases that increase concentrations of acetylcholine. Increasing the concentration of acetylcholine may cause the channels to open more often and, consequently, become more susceptible to block by use-dependent compounds. Evidence suggests that neostigmine and related cholinesterase inhibitors can act as channel-blocking drugs.[17,63]

Channel block may account for the antibiotic-, cocaine-, quinidine-, piperocaine-, tricyclic antidepressant-, naltrexone-, naloxone-, and histrionicotoxin-induced alterations in neuromuscular function. Muscle relaxants, in contrast, can bind to the acetylcholine recognition site of the receptor and occupy the channel. Pancuronium preferentially binds to the recognition site. Gallamine (not used clinically anymore) seems to act equally at the two sites (channel-blocking and acetylcholine-blocking sites). (Gallamine was synthesized by Daniel Bovet, a Swiss-born Italian pharmacologist and received the Nobel Prize in Physiology or Medicine in 1957 for his work on cardiovascular and neuromuscular pharmacology.) Tubocurarine, the first NDMR used clinically, is in between; at small doses that clinically produce minimal blockage of transmission, the drug is essentially a pure antagonist at the recognition site; at larger doses, it also enters and blocks channels. Decamethonium and succinylcholine, as agonists, can open channels and, as slender molecules, also enter and block them. Decamethonium and some other long, thin molecules can penetrate all the way through the open channel and enter the cytoplasm of muscle cells. Whether prolonged administration of NDMRs, as used in an intensive care unit, can result in the NDMR occupation of the channel, and even entry of drug into the cytosol, is unknown.

PHASE II BLOCK

A phase II block is a complex phenomenon associated with a typical fade in muscle during continuous exposure to depolarizing drugs. This fade phenomenon is likely due to the interaction of depolarizing action of succinylcholine on distinct neuronal (prejunctional) AChRs; these prejunctional receptors are blocked by higher-than-usual concentrations of succinylcholine. This fade after succinylcholine is at least partly dependent on a presynaptic interaction with cholinergic transmission of importance for neurotransmitter mobilization and release. However, fade in muscle during repetitive nerve stimulation can also be attributable to postjunctional AChR block.[65]

Other factors may also be involved. The repeated opening of channels allows a continuous efflux of potassium and influx of sodium, and the resulting abnormal electrolyte balance distorts the function of the junctional membrane. Calcium entering the muscle through the opened channels can cause disruption of receptors and the sub-end-plate elements themselves. The activity of the sodium-potassium adenosine triphosphatase pump in the membrane increases with increasing intracellular sodium and, by pumping sodium out of the cell and potassium into it, works to restore the ionic balance and membrane potential toward normal. As long as the depolarizing drug is present, the receptor channels remain open and ion flux through them remains frequent.[66]

Factors influencing the development of a phase II block include the duration of exposure to the drug, the particular drug used and its concentration, and even the type of muscle (i.e., fast or slow twitch). Interactions with anesthetics and other agents also affect the process. All these drugs may also have prejunctional effects on the rate and amount of transmitter released and mobilized. With so many variables involved in the interference with neuromuscular transmission, a phase II block is a complex and ever-changing phenomenon. The reversal response of a phase II block produced by a depolarizing muscle relaxant to the administration of cholinesterase inhibitors is difficult to predict. It is therefore best that reversal by cholinesterase inhibitors not be attempted, although the response to tetanus or train-of-four stimulation resembles that produced by NDMRs.

Biology of Prejunctional and Postjunctional Nicotinic Acetylcholine Receptors

POSTJUNCTIONAL CONVENTIONAL ACETYLCHOLINE RECEPTORS IN MUSCLE VERSUS NEURONAL ACETYLCHOLINE RECEPTORS IN MUSCLE

Currently, three variants of postjunctional AChRs have been identified. The AChR isoform present in the innervated, adult neuromuscular junction is referred to as the adult, mature, or junctional receptor. Another AChR isoform, also described more than 4 decades ago, is expressed when activity in muscle is decreased, as observed in the fetus before innervation or after chemically- or physically-induced immobilization; after lower or upper motor neuron injury, burns, or sepsis; or after other events that cause increased muscle protein catabolism, including sepsis or generalized inflammation.[1-3] In contrast with the mature or junctional receptors, the other isoform is referred to as the immature, extrajunctional, or fetal form of AChR. Some evidence suggests that the immature isoform is not observed in the muscle protein catabolism and wasting that occur with malnutrition.[67] Qualitative differences in the mature isoform can occur as a result of gene mutations, which therefore alters the subunit protein structure. These qualitative changes in AChR can also cause abnormalities in neurotransmission (e.g., slow- or fast-channel syndrome)[27,47] and therefore the response to muscle relaxants.

At the molecular level, the mature and immature receptors consist of five subunits (see Fig. 12.4).[1-3] The mature junctional receptor is a pentamer of two $\alpha1$-subunits and one each of the $\beta1$-, δ-, and ε-subunits. The immature receptor consists of two $\alpha1$-subunits and one each of the $\beta1$-, δ-, and γ-subunits; that is, in the immature receptor, the γ-subunit is present instead of the ε-subunit. The γ- and ε-subunits differ very little from each other in amino acid homology, but the differences are great enough to affect the physiologic function and pharmacologic characteristics of the receptor and its ion channel. Junctional receptors are always confined to the end-plate region of the muscle membrane. The immature, or extrajunctional, receptor may be expressed anywhere on the muscle membrane, although their junctional expression seems minimal.[16] During development and in certain pathologic states, junctional and extrajunctional receptors can coexist in the perijunctional area of the muscle membrane (Fig. 12.7).

Quite in contrast to the conventional muscle AChRs consisting of $\alpha1$-, $\beta1$-, δ-, and ε/γ-subunits described earlier, receptors formed of $\alpha7$ AChR subunits have recently been found in skeletal muscle during immobilization, sepsis, and denervation.[68,69] Two recent studies have evidenced the increased expression of $\alpha7$ AChR subunits in muscle by western blotting, ligand binding or genetic techniques after sepsis, and burn injury or immobilization, during which no overt denervation occurs.[16,70] These $\alpha7$ AChR subunits are homomeric (i.e., formed of the same subunits) channels arranged as pentameres (see Fig. 12.4). Ligand (drug)-binding pockets are thought to be formed at negative and positive faces of the $\alpha7$-subunit assembly interphases. As expected, the endogenous agonist, acetylcholine, binds to $\alpha7$ AChR subunits, and each of the five subunits has the potential to bind acetylcholine or succinylcholine molecules.[18,69] Other agonists, including nicotine and choline, and antagonists, including muscle relaxants, cobra toxin, and α-bungarotoxin, also bind to the $\alpha7$ AChR.[18,69-72]

The $\alpha7$ AChRs in muscle display unusual functional and pharmacologic characteristics when compared with conventional muscle ($\alpha1$, $\beta1$, δ, ε/γ) AChRs or neuronal $\alpha7$ AChRs in the brain. Choline, a precursor and metabolite of acetylcholine (and succinylcholine), is a weak agonist of conventional muscle AChRs but is a full agonist of muscle $\alpha7$ AChRs; that is, concentrations of choline that do not open conventional AChR channels will open $\alpha7$ AChR channels.[69] Furthermore, no desensitization of the $\alpha7$ AChRs occurs even during the continued presence of choline,[69] thus allowing a greater chance for potassium to efflux (approximately 145 mEq/L) from within the cell to the extracellular space, including plasma (approximately 4.5 mEq/L), down its concentration gradient. The chemical

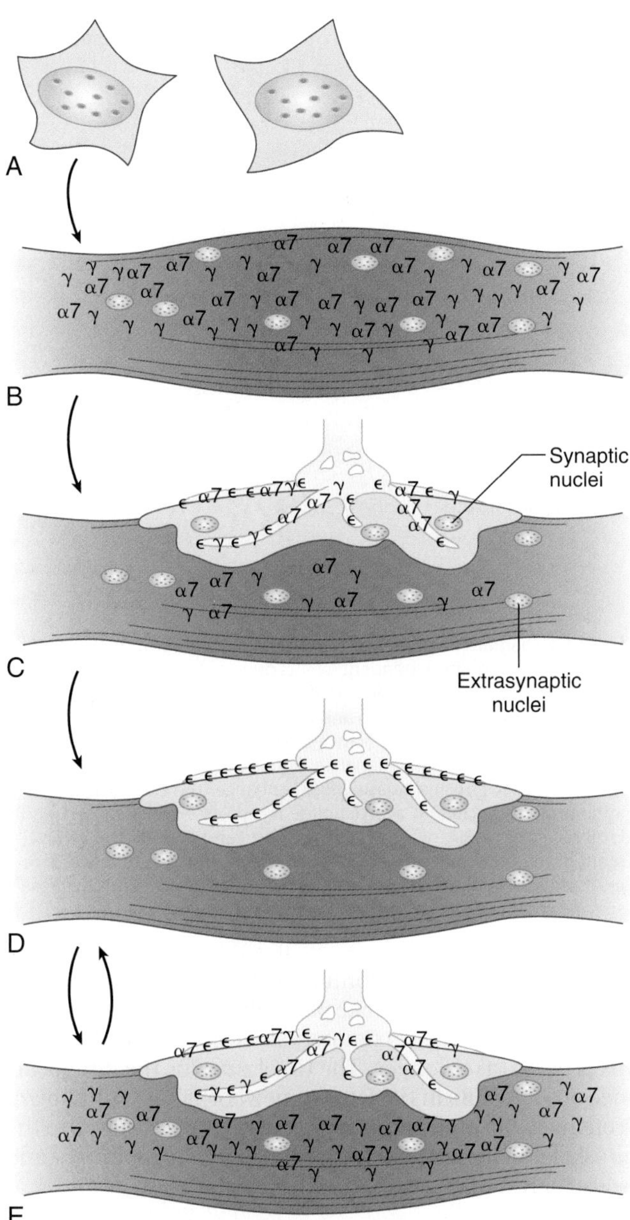

Fig. 12.7 Distribution of acetylcholine receptors in developing adult mature, denervated or immobilized muscle and in inflammation-induced catabolic muscle. (A and B) In the early fetal stage, mononucleated myoblasts, derived from the mesoderm, fuse with each other to form multinucleated myotubes. The γ-subunit-containing immature acetylcholine receptors (AChRs) and the neuronal α7-subunit AChRs are scattered throughout the muscle membrane before innervation. (C) As the nerve makes contact with muscle, clustering of the receptors occurs at the synapse and is associated with some loss of extrasynaptic receptors. (D) Maturation of the junction is said to occur when ε-subunit-containing receptors replace γ-subunit- and α7-subunit-containing AChRs at the neuromuscular junction. Even mature muscle is multinucleated, but it is devoid of extrasynaptic AChRs. (E) Denervation and some other pathologic states, even without anatomic denervation (e.g., burns, immobilization, chronic muscle relaxant therapy, stroke, sepsis), lead to the re-expression of the γ-subunit-containing AChRs mostly at the extrajunctional areas. The α7-subunit AChRs are expressed in the junctional areas and are also most likely in the extrajunctional areas. These receptor changes are potentially reversible if muscle immobilization, catabolism, and inflammation are restored to normal.

α-conotoxin GI from the snail specifically inhibits the conventional (mature and immature) AChRs in muscle but does not inhibit α7 AChRs. The important role of α7 AChRs in resistance to NDMRs is evidenced by the presence of immobilization-induced resistance in wild-type mice and the absence of resistance in α7 AChRs knockout mice.[73] The α7 AChRs expressed in neuronal tissue are also readily desensitized with choline, a feature that contrasts with muscle α7 AChRs, which do not desensitize with choline.[69] The α7 AChRs in muscle also have lower affinity for its antagonists, including pancuronium, rocuronium, atracurium, or α-bungarotoxin; higher concentrations of these drugs are therefore required to block agonist-induced depolarization in α7 AChRs in vitro or cause neuromuscular paralysis in vivo or ex vivo when α7 AChRs are upregulated.[69-72] In the conventional muscle AChRs, binding of even one of the α1-subunits by an antagonist results in inactivation of that receptor because acetylcholine needs both α1-subunits of the AChR for its activation. In α7 AChRs, however, even when three subunits are bound by an antagonist (e.g., muscle relaxant), two other subunits are still available for binding by agonist and cause depolarization. This feature may account for some of the resistance to muscle relaxants when α7 AChRs are expressed in muscle and other tissues in pathologic states.[69-73]

The clinical pharmacologic characteristics of the muscle α7 AChR have not yet been completely studied, but its basic composition also provides some insight into succinylcholine-related hyperkalemia. Chemical or physical denervation of muscle results in not only upregulation and qualitative (ε-subunit → γ-subunit) changes in AChRs, but it also results in upregulation of α7 AChRs in muscle. Succinylcholine, a synthetic analog of acetylcholine that consists of two molecules of acetylcholine joined together, is capable of depolarizing not only conventional AChRs but also α7 AChRs in muscle.[72] In addition, the metabolite of succinylcholine, choline, can depolarize α7 AChRs with little desensitization. The depolarizing effects of succinylcholine and choline on upregulated α7 AChRs can result in continued leakage of intracellular potassium and flooding of extracellular fluid, including plasma, thereby leading to hyperkalemia. Thus, differences in the subunit composition and increased numbers of the three isoforms junctionally and extrajunctionally expressed may account for aberrant responses to muscle relaxants clinically observed as resistant only to NDMRs and hyperkalemic response to succinylcholine.[2,72,73]

MAINTENANCE OF MATURE NEUROMUSCULAR JUNCTIONS

Quite unlike other cells, muscle cells are unusual in that they have many, usually hundreds, of nuclei per cell. Each nucleus has the genes to make all three isoform receptors. Multiple factors, including electrical activity, growth factor signaling (e.g., insulin, agrin, neuregulins), and the presence or absence of innervation, control the expression of the three types of receptor isoforms.[19,37] This control is most clearly observed in the developing embryo as the neuromuscular junction is formed. Before they are innervated, the muscle cells of a fetus synthesize only immature and α7 AChRs—hence the term *fetal isoform* for the former receptor. Synthesis is directed by nearly all of the nuclei in the cell, and the AChRs are expressed throughout the membrane of the muscle cell (see Fig. 12.7). As the fetus develops and the muscles become innervated, muscle cells begin to synthesize the mature isoform of receptors, which are exclusively inserted into the developing (future) endplate area.[14-19] The nerve releases several growth factors that influence the synthetic apparatus of the nearby nuclei. First, nerve-supplied factors induce the subsynaptic nuclei to increase synthesis of AChRs. Next, the nerve-induced electrical activity results in the repression of receptors in the extrajunctional area (see Fig. 12.7*B* and *C*). Nerve-derived growth factors, including agrin and ARIA/neuregulin, cause the receptors to cluster in the subsynaptic area and prompt the expression of the mature isoform.[19,37] Several lines of evidence indicate that clustering, expression, and stabilization of mature receptors are triggered by at least two growth factors: agrin, neuregulin/ARIA, and possibly calcitonin gene-related peptide.[56,74,75] Neuregulin and agrin are also released from muscle, but muscle-derived agrin is not as important in clustering and maturation of the receptor. ARIA is made in the nerve and plays a role in the maturation of vesicular arrangement and conversion of the γ-to-ε switch.[75] All of these growth factors interact with distinct membrane and cytosolic receptor proteins to cause phosphorylation and activation of nuclear (gene) transcriptional systems. Agrin signals through MuSK and neuregulins through ErbB receptors (Fig. 12.8). These receptors control qualitative and quantitative changes at the junction. Once begun, the process is very stable, and nuclei in the junctional area continue to express mature receptors. In certain pathologic state–induced insulin resistance, a concomitant proliferation of AChRs seems to occur beyond the junctional area. Conditions in which this form of insulin resistance (i.e., decreased growth factor signaling) has been observed include immobilization, burn injury, sepsis, and denervation[75-78]; in these conditions, not only does upregulation of total AChRs occur, but de novo upregulation of the immature and α7 AChR isoforms are also observed (see Fig. 12.7*D*).[1-3] This upregulation may be related to the lack of growth factor effects of agrin and possibly neuregulin, which signal via some of the same downstream signaling proteins as insulin (e.g., phosphoinositide 3-kinase).[56,76-79] Therefore, agrin and neuregulin signaling may be important for the suppression of α7 AChRs and immature AChRs in the normal neuromuscular junction.

Before innervation, as in the fetus, AChRs are present throughout the muscle membrane. After innervation, AChRs become more and more concentrated at the postsynaptic membrane and are virtually absent in the extrasynaptic area at birth. The innervation process progresses somewhat slowly during fetal life and matures during infancy and early childhood.[14-19] With time, the immature receptors diminish in concentration and disappear from the peripheral part of the muscle. In the active, adult, and normal innervated muscle, just the nuclei under and very near the end plate direct the synthesis of the receptor; only the genes for expressing mature receptors are active. Nuclei beyond the junctional area are not active, and therefore no receptors are expressed anywhere in the muscle cells beyond the perijunctional area. Conversion of all the

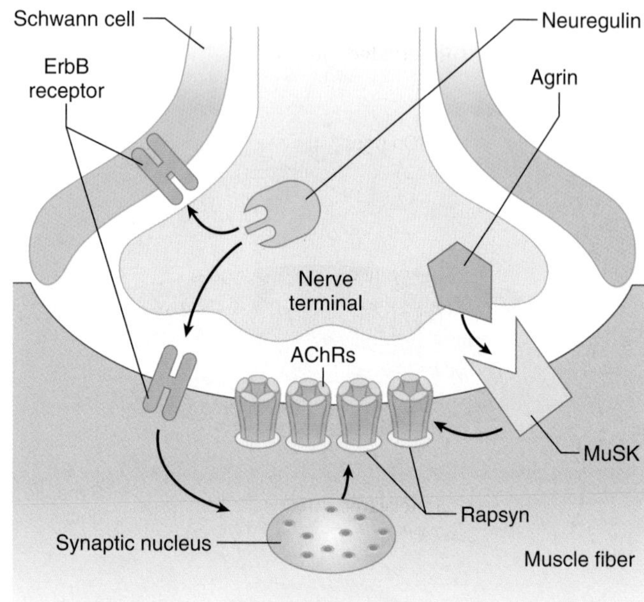

Fig. 12.8 Diagram of agrin- and acetylcholine receptor-inducing activity (ARIA)/neuregulin-dependent events during maturation of the neuromuscular junction. After the establishment of a nerve on the muscle, growth factors, including agrin and neuregulins, are released. Neuregulin signaling is essential for Schwann cell survival, and Schwann cells are essential for axonal maintenance. Agrin interacting with its receptor muscle-specific tyrosine kinase *(MuSK)* enhances the clustering of synaptic proteins, including acetylcholine receptors *(AChRs)*, rapsyn, and ErbB receptors. ARIA/neuregulin is the best candidate for the involvement in the conversion of γ-subunit-containing immature receptor to ε-subunit-containing mature (innervated) receptor, which is synapse specific and therefore not inserted in the extrajunctional area.

γ-subunit- to ε-subunit-containing AChRs in the perijunctional area continues to take place after birth. In the rodent, conversion takes approximately 2 weeks.[14-19] In humans, this process takes longer. The timeframe for the disappearance of α7 AChRs in the fetus or newborn is also unknown. Proteins implicated in the linking of mature receptors to the cytoskeleton include integrin, syntrophin, utrophin, α- and β-dystroglycan, and rapsyn, just to name a few.[14-19]

RE-EXPRESSION OF IMMATURE (FETAL) γ-SUBUNIT AND α7-SUBUNIT ACETYLCHOLINE RECEPTORS IN ADULT LIFE

The extrajunctional immature receptors can reappear soon after upper and lower motor denervation and in certain pathologic states (e.g., burns, sepsis, immobilization, chronic muscle relaxant therapy or botulism, loss of muscle electrical activity). Stimulation of a denervated muscle with an external electrical stimulus can prevent the appearance of immature receptors. It has been suggested that the calcium that enters the muscle during activity is important in the suppression process.[16,17] In the pathologic states previously enumerated, if the process is severe and prolonged, then extrajunctional receptors are inserted all over the surface of the muscle, including the perijunctional area (see Fig. 12.7*D*). The junctional nuclei also continue to make mature receptors. The synthesis of immature receptors is initiated within hours of inactivity, but it takes several

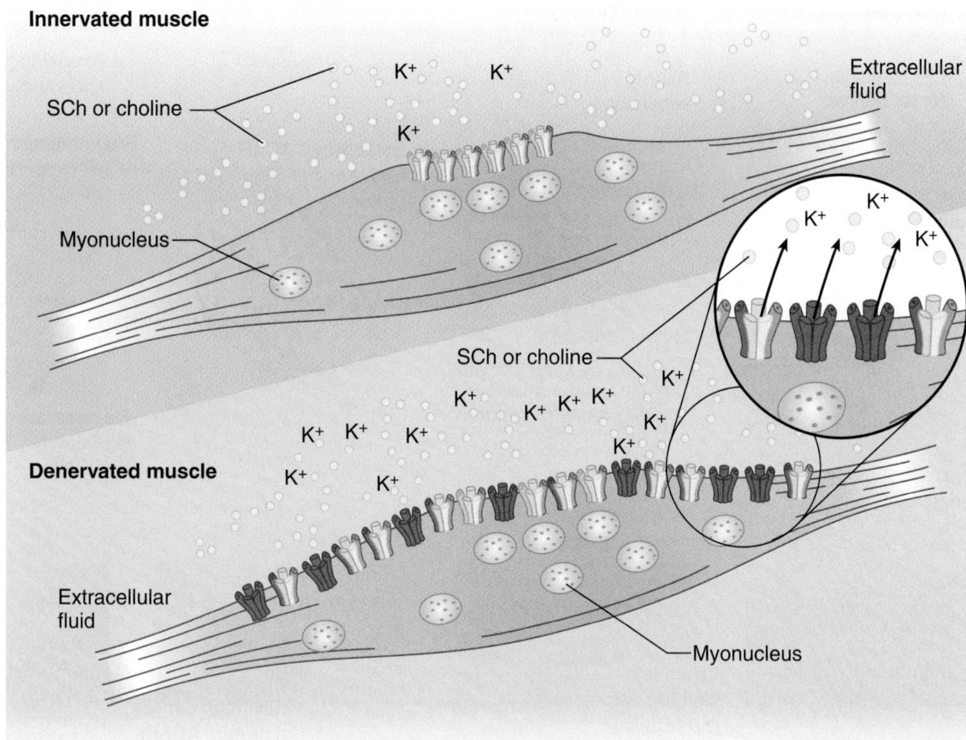

Fig. 12.9 Schematic of the succinylcholine (SCh)-induced potassium (K^+) release in an innervated *(top)* and denervated muscle *(bottom)*. In the innervated muscle, the systemically administered SCh reaches all the muscle membrane but depolarizes only the junctional ($\alpha1$, $\beta1$, δ/ε) receptors because acetylcholine receptors (AChRs) are located only in this area. With denervation, the muscle nuclei express not only extrajunctional ($\alpha1$, $\beta1$, δ/γ) AChRs but also $\alpha7$-nicotinic AChRs throughout the muscle membrane. Systemic SCh, in contrast to acetylcholine released locally, can depolarize all the upregulated AChRs, which leads to massive efflux of intracellular K^+ into the circulation, resulting in hyperkalemia. The metabolite of SCh, choline, and possibly succinylmonocholine, can maintain this depolarization via $\alpha7$-nicotinic AChRs, enhancing the K^+ release and maintaining the hyperkalemia. (From Martyn JAJ, Richtsfeld M. Succinylcholine-induced hyperkalemia in acquired pathologic states: etiologic factors and molecular mechanisms. *Anesthesiology*. 2006;104:158–169, 2006.)

days for the whole muscle membrane to be fully covered with receptors. This upregulation of receptors has implications for the use of depolarizing and possibly NDMRs. The changes in $\alpha7$ AChRs parallel the expression of immature receptors, although this has not been well studied.

The changes in subunit composition (γ vs. ε) in the receptor confer certain changes in electrophysiologic (functional), pharmacologic, and metabolic characteristics.[16-18] Mature receptors are metabolically stable, with a half-life approximating 2 weeks, whereas immature receptors have a metabolic half-life of less than 24 hours. Immature receptors have a smaller single-channel conductance and a twofold to tenfold longer mean channel open time than do mature receptors (see Fig. 12.4). The changes in subunit composition may also alter the sensitivity or affinity, or both, of the receptor for specific ligands. Depolarizing or agonist drugs such as succinylcholine and acetylcholine more easily depolarize immature receptors, thereby resulting in cation fluxes; doses one tenth to one hundredth of those needed for mature receptors can effect depolarization.[2] The potency of NDMRs is also reduced, as demonstrated by the resistance to their neuromuscular effects documented in patients with burns, denervation, sepsis, and immobilization.[1,3] In light of recent research, however, it seems that the resistance to nondepolarizers is more likely due to the junctional area expression of the $\alpha7$ AChRs, which has a decreased affinity to NDMRs.[16,69-73] Some NDMRs may also cause a partial agonist response in immature receptors, thus explaining the decreased potency in conditions in which upregulation of AChRs occurs.[8] The upregulation of immature AChRs in the perijunctional and extrajunctional areas may have a buffering effect for diffusion of relaxants, contributing to resistance to NDMRs.[80]

The altered sensitivity to muscle relaxants may occur in only certain parts of the body or certain muscles if only some muscles are affected by the diminution in nerve activity (e.g., after a stroke). Sensitivity to relaxants can begin to change beyond 72 hours after an injury or hospitalization. The most serious side effect with the use of succinylcholine in the presence of upregulated AChRs in one or more muscles is hyperkalemia.[1-3] In these subjects, the receptors can be scattered over a large surface of the muscle. The AChR channels opened by the agonist (succinylcholine) allow potassium to escape from the muscle and enter the blood (Fig. 12.9).[2,3] If a large part of the muscle surface consists of upregulated (immature) receptor channels, each of which stays open for a longer time, then the amount of potassium that moves from muscle to blood can be considerable. The resulting hyperkalemia can cause dangerous disturbances in cardiac rhythm, including ventricular fibrillation. Moreover, hyperkalemia probably cannot be prevented by prior administration of NDMRs because large doses required to

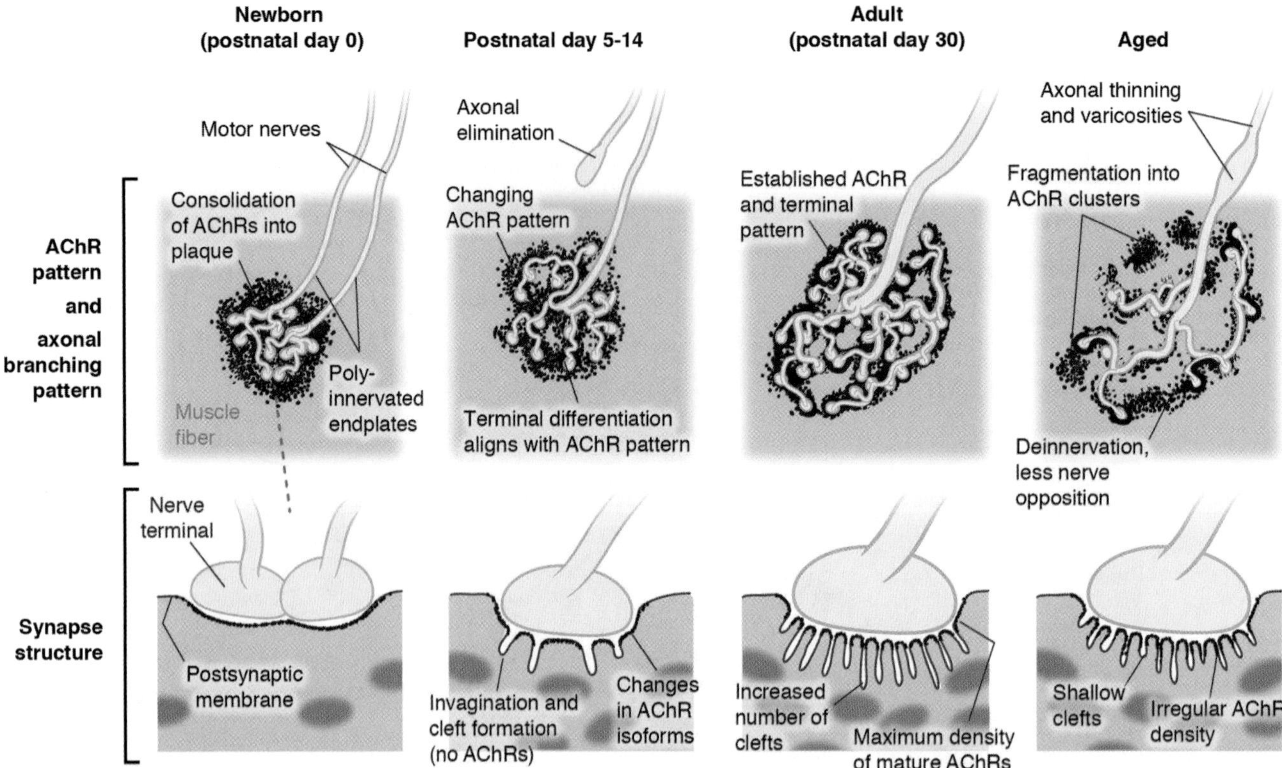

Fig. 12.10 Maturation of the postsynaptic apparatus. *Postnatal day 0 (Newborn)*: At the time of birth, the aggregates of acetylcholine receptors (AChRs) have consolidated to form an oval-like plaque with irregular borders. At this point, each junction may have more than one nerve terminal innervating it. *Postnatal day 5 to 14*: Approximately 5 to 14 days after birth, the postsynaptic membrane invaginates to form a gutter and small perforations develop on the plaque. These perforations reflect gaps due to the synaptic clefts (which do not have AChRs). During this time, the immature γ-subunit-containing AChRs are completely replaced by mature AChRs containing ε-subunit. The invaginations or clefts increase in numbers, resulting in more perforations in the synaptic AChRs giving it an almost pretzel-shaped junction. The perforations, as indicated, correspond to the synaptic clefts or folds. *Postnatal day 30*: The neuromuscular junction is completely developed (mature) at 30 days after birth with a larger pretzel-shaped appearance. The AChRs have maximal density. A distinct set of postsynaptic proteins and signaling molecules are selectively transcribed in the subsynaptic area, providing integrity to the neuromuscular junction and efficient neurotransmission. *Aged NMJ*: Examination of NMJ in the aged mice and humans reveal marked morphological changes. Some of the synapses undergo partial degeneration and synaptic staining becomes fainter. The synaptic folds are smaller in depth. The nerve terminals become thinner and appear swollen or bulbous with less apposition with the synapse. The Schwann cells seems to invade into the NMJ more (not shown). *NMJ*, neuromuscular junction.

block the AChRs, in and of itself, will cause paralysis, obviating the need for succinylcholine.[3] Larger-than-normal doses of NDMRs may attenuate the increase in blood potassium concentrations but cannot completely prevent it. In other words, no hyperkalemic response to succinylcholine has been seen earlier than 4 days after perturbations described previously.[50] However, hyperkalemia and cardiac arrest can occur after the administration of succinylcholine, even in the absence of denervation states. These effects are observed in certain congenital muscle dystrophies in which the muscle membrane is prone to damage by the depolarization produced by succinylcholine, resulting in potassium release via the membrane damage.[81]

PREJUNCTIONAL ACETYLCHOLINE RECEPTORS

Nicotinic AChRs exist in a variety of forms apart from that observed in muscle.[16,18] The classic muscle-type nicotinic AChR is postsynaptically present, whereas neuronal subtype receptors may be presynaptically and postsynaptically present. The neuronal subtype nicotinic AChRs expressed prejunctionally are usually heteromeric and built up by *only* α- and β-subunits. This family of nicotinic AChRs is widely expressed in the peripheral and central nervous systems, on autonomous nerves and ganglia on oxygen-sensing cells within the carotid bodies. There are also α7 AChRs in immune-competent cells, such as macrophages, microglia lymphocytes and granulocytes, and fibroblasts and chondrocytes.[16,18] Diverse genes encode the heterogeneous AChRs, and the ion channel is formed of multiple subunits (multimers). Seventeen AChR genes have been cloned from vertebrates. They include various combinations of α-subunits (α1 through α10) and β-subunits (β1 through β4) and one each of γ-, δ-, and ε-subunits. The γ-, δ-, and ε-subunits are found only in muscle.[16-18]

Prejunctional- or nerve terminal-associated cholinergic receptors have been demonstrated by morphologic pharmacologic and by molecular biologic techniques, but their form and functions are not as completely understood as those in the postjunctional area. Many drugs with an abundance of potential targets for drug action can affect the capacity of the nerve terminal to carry out its functions. The trophic function to maintain nerve-muscle contact involves the release and replenishment of acetylcholine together with other trophic factors that require signaling through many receptors, of which the prejunctional nicotinic AChR is just one. Succinylcholine produces fasciculations that can be prevented by NDMRs. Because a fasciculation is, by definition, the simultaneous contraction of the multitude of muscle cells in a single motor unit and because only the nerve can synchronize all the muscles in its motor unit, it became apparent that succinylcholine must also act on nerve endings. Because NDMRs prevent fasciculation, it was concluded that they acted on the same prejunctional receptor. Very small doses of cholinergic agonists (e.g., succinylcholine) and antagonists (e.g., NDMRs) affect nicotinic receptors on the nerve ending; the former by depolarizing the ending and sometimes inducing repetitive firing of the nerve and the latter by preventing the action of agonists.[5]

By the use of specific monoclonal antibodies, the presence of nicotinic α3-subunits has been demonstrated in the nerve terminal.[82] Another clue to the differences between prejunctional and postjunctional AChRs was the finding that some drugs (e.g., dihydro-β-erythroidine) bind only to prejunctional AChRs, whereas other drugs (e.g., α-bungarotoxin) bind only to postjunctional receptors.[65] Additional clues were found in the many demonstrations of quantitative differences in the reaction of prejunctional and postjunctional nicotinic receptors to other cholinergic agonists and antagonists.[65,82-84] For instance, it was known that tubocurarine, the first NDMR introduced to clinical practice in 1942 (not used in US or Europe), binds with lower affinity to the recognition sites of ganglionic nicotinic cholinoceptors and is not a competitive antagonist of acetylcholine at this site. Decamethonium (i.e., a depolarizing muscle relaxant no longer clinically used) is a selective inhibitor of the muscle receptor, and hexamethonium is a selective inhibitor of nicotinic receptors in the autonomic ganglia.[80-85] Instead, tubocurarine and hexamethonium can block the opened channels of these receptors and owe their ability to block ganglionic transmission to this property. The functional characteristics of prejunctional receptor channels may also be different. For example, the depolarization of motor nerve endings initiated by the administration of acetylcholine can be prevented by tetrodotoxin, a specific blocker of sodium flux with no effect on the end plate.

Specific information on the molecular organization of neuronal nicotinic receptors on the motor neuron terminal is still lacking. Some of the subunit composition is similar, but other subunits do not resemble those of the postjunctional receptor. Of the 16 different nicotinic AChR gene products identified, only 12 (α2 to α10 and β2 to β4) are thought to contribute nicotinic receptors expressed on neurons. Most strikingly, nervous tissue does not express γ-, δ-, or ε-receptor subunits; it contains genes only for the α- and β-subunits. The α- and β-subunit genes in nerve and muscle are not exactly the same; they are variants. To emphasize the distinction between neural and muscle nicotinic receptors, the former are sometimes designated *Nn* and the latter *Nm*. With so many different subunits available, possible combinations are many, and it is not known which combinations are found in motor nerves. Their physiologic roles have also not been completely characterized. Expression of neuronal nicotinic AChRs in *in vitro* systems has confirmed that muscle relaxants and their metabolites can bind to some of these neuronal AChRs.[53,83-85]

The nicotinic receptor on the junctional surface of the nerve (nerve terminal) senses transmitter in the cleft and, by means of a positive-feedback system, causes the release of more transmitter. In other parts of the nervous system, this positive feedback is complemented by a negative-feedback system that senses when the concentration of transmitter in the synaptic cleft has appropriately increased and shuts down the release system. It is believed that tetanic fade and train-of-four fade during neuromuscular block with NDMRs arise from presynaptic cholinergic autoreceptors at the motor nerved ending.[5,52]

The neuronal AChR subtype that is critically involved in acetylcholine release and subsequent fade phenomenon (as observed in tetanic or train-of-four stimulus patterns) has been identified as the α3β2-subtype nicotinic AChR.[10,84] When this prejunctional receptor is specifically blocked by a nondepolarizing relaxant such as tubocurarine, a reduction in neurotransmitter release occurs upon repeated stimulation with subsequent fade phenomenon. It should be noted, however, block of the prejunctional AChRs alone is not necessary and sufficient to induce fade; concomitant reduction in the safety of neurotransmission prejunctionally or postjunctionally must be present for it to be noticeable.[65] Although all clinically used nondepolarizing neuromuscular blocking drugs inhibit this prejunctional nicotinic AChR, as well as several other neuronal nicotinic AChRs, in the clinically relevant concentration range, succinylcholine neither activates nor inhibits the presynaptic α3β2 autoreceptor at clinically relevant concentrations.[53,85] However, the existence of the α3β2 autoreceptor at the prejunctional area has never been demonstrated by western blot or mRNA techniques. Thus, this prejunctional receptor has not been completely characterized.

This observation may be the reason for the typical lack of fade during succinylcholine-induced neuromuscular block. Succinylcholine, however, does not interact with α3β4 AChR found in autonomic ganglia.[53] It has also been shown that NDMRs reduce the hypoxic ventilatory response in partially paralyzed humans,[86] and the mechanism behind the depression might be related to inhibition of nicotine receptors on the carotid body.[11] Nicotinic α3, 7, and β2 AChRs have recently been documented in the human carotid body.[87] Whether the inhibition of these receptors plays a role in attenuated response to hypoxia drive needs further investigation. The motor nerve terminal is also known to bear several other receptors, such as opioid, adrenergic, dopamine, purine, and adenosine receptors, as well as receptors for endogenous hormones, neuropeptides, and a variety of proteins.[88,89] The physiologic roles of these receptors and the effects of anesthetics on them are unknown.

Neuromuscular Junction at Extremes of Age

NEWBORN

Just before birth, the AChRs are all clustered around the nerve in the junctional area, and minimal extrajunctional AChRs are present. The newborn postsynaptic membrane, itself, is not specialized, having almost no synaptic folds, a widened synaptic space, and a reduced number of AChRs.[14,19] The early postnatal AChR cluster appears as an oval plaque (Fig. 12.10). Within a few days, simplified folds appear. With continued maturation, the plaque is transformed to a multiperforated pretzel-like structure. The polyinnervated end plate is converted to a singly innervated junction because of a retraction of all but one terminal. In the adult, the terminals perfectly align with the AChR clusters. Morphologically, the postsynaptic membrane of the newborn and that from the patient with myasthenia gravis is not too different; the AChR number is decreased, and the postsynaptic folds are decreased. It is not surprising therefore that neurotransmission is not as efficient in the newborn and in patients with myasthenia gravis. For this reason, neonates and infants behave similar to patients with myasthenia gravis when NDMRs are administered to them.[90] In humans, maturation of the neuromuscular junction probably occurs at approximately 2 years of age.[90]

OLD AGE

With increasing life expectancy, typical changes associated with aging is a gradual loss of lean body mass and strength referred to as sarcopenia (Greek: sarco-flesh, penia- poverty), which has received increased attention recently.[91] These sarcopenic changes occur in association with denervation-like changes at the synapse and altered anabolic or growth factor signaling changes within muscle.[91-93] Old age-associated functional denervation, muscle wasting, and weakness is now well established.[91,92] Age-related morphologic changes include increase in length and area of the post-synaptic AChR, degenerating synaptic folds, and more invasion of synaptic folds by Schwann cells. The nerve terminals are thinned out and show terminal swelling with less apposition of the nerve to the synapse (see Fig. 12.10). Coupled with the morphologic changes in the neuromuscular junction that occur with aging, the functional changes that occur with it can include increased quantal content of neurotransmitter release and more rapid rundown of end-plate potential during stimulation of the preterminal neuron.[91-93] Regardless of these enumerated structured and functioned changes with aging, it appears that because of the superb margin of safety of neurotransmission, disability is not easily demonstrable by simple methods such as grip strength in most instances.[93] Despite the structural and functional changes associated with aging, the overall margin of safety is better in the older individual than in the neonate.[94] Even with these denervation-like changes in the elderly, there is no evidence that these patients are more prone to succinylcholine-induced hyperkalemia. There are also no studies confirming increased or decreased sensitivity to nondepolarizing blockers due to the neuromuscular junction changes. Some nondepolarizing neuromuscular blockers have prolonged effect in old age (e.g., vecuronium) due to pharmacokinetic causes.

Complete references available online at expertconsult.com.

References

1. Martyn JA, et al. *Anaesthesia*. 2009;64(suppl 1):1.
2. Martyn JA, Richtsfeld M. *Anesthesiology*. 2006;104:158.
3. Fagerlund MJ, Eriksson LI. *Br J Anaesth*. 2009;103(1):108.
4. Gilhus NE. *Curr Opin Neurol*. 2012;25:523.
5. Bowman WC, et al. *Ann N Y Acad Sci*. 1990;604:69.
6. Frick CG, et al. *Anesthesiology*. 2007;106:1139.
7. Frick CG, et al. *Anesth Analg*. 2012;114:102.
8. Lape R, et al. *Nature*. 2008;454:722.
9. Paul M, et al. *Eur J Pharmacol*. 2002;438:35.
10. Vizi ES, Lendvai B. *Pharmacol Ther*. 1997;73:75.
11. Jonsson M, et al. *Eur J Pharmacol*. 2004;497:173.
12. Sunaga H, et al. *Anesthesiology*. 2010;112:892.
13. Fryer AD, Maclagan J. *Naunyn Schmiedebergs Arch Pharmacol*. 1987;335:367.
14. Li L, et al. *Annu Rev Physiol*. 2018;80:159.
15. Tintignac LA, et al. *Physiol Rev*. 2015;95:809.
16. Lee S, et al. *Anesthesiology*. 2014;120(1):76–85.
17. Sine SM. *Physiol Rev*. 2012;92:1189.
18. Albuquerque EX, et al. *Physiol Rev*. 2009;89:73.
19. Shi L, et al. *Trends Neurosci*. 2012;35:441.
20. Fraterman S, et al. *Invest Ophthalmol Vis Sci*. 2006;47:3828.
21. Büttner-Ennever JA, Horn AK. *Mov Disord*. 2002;17(suppl 2):S2.
22. Kaminski HJ, et al. *Invest Ophthalmol Vis Sci*. 1996;37:345.
23. Lennerstrand G, et al. *Acta Ophthalmol*. 2010;88:872.
24. Vachon CA, et al. *Anesthesiology*. 2003;99:220.
25. Catterall WA. *J Physiol*. 2012;590:2577.
26. Catterall WA, et al. *J Biol Chem*. 2013;288:10742.
27. Engel AG, et al. *Ann N Y Acad Sci*. 2012;1275:54.
28. Heuser JE, Reese TS. *J Cell Biol*. 1981;88:564.
29. Rash JE, et al. *J Electron Microsc Tech*. 1988;10(153).
30. Sieburth D, et al. *Nature*. 2005;436:510.
31. Littleton JT, Sheng M. *Nature*. 2003;423:931.
32. Rich MM. *Neuroscientist*. 2006;12:134.
33. Wang X, et al. *J Neurosci*. 2004;24:10687.
34. Katz B, Miledi R. *Proc R Soc Lond B Biol Sci*. 1979;215:369.
35. Uchitel OD, et al. *Proc Natl Acad Sci U S A*. 1992;89:3330.
36. van Sonderen A, et al. *Curr Treat Options Neurol*. 2013;15:224–239.
37. Naguib M, et al. *Anesthesiology*. 2002;96:202.
38. Sudhof TC. *Neuron*. 2012;75:11.
39. Jahn R, Fasshauer D. *Nature*. 2012;490:201.
40. Heidelberger R. *Nature*. 2007;450:623.
41. Turton K, et al. *Trends Biochem Sci*. 2002;27:552.
42. Restani L, et al. *PLoS Pathog*. 2012;8:e1003087.
43. Schurch B. *Drugs Today (Barc)*. 2004;40:205.
44. Schiavo G. *Nature*. 2006;444:1019.
45. Lange DJ, et al. *Muscle Nerve*. 1991;14:672.
46. Heeroma JH, et al. *Neuroscience*. 2003;120:733.
47. Engel AG, Sine SM. *Curr Opin Pharmacol*. 2005;5:308.
48. Abraham RB, et al. *Anesthesiology*. 2002;97:989.
49. Karwa M, et al. *Crit Care Med*. 2005;33:S75.
50. Richtsfeld M, et al. *Anesthesiology*. 2013;119:412.
51. Kopta C, Steinbach JH. *J Neurosci*. 1994;14:3922.
52. Jonsson M, et al. *Anesthesiology*. 2006;105:521.
53. Jonsson M, et al. *Anesthesiology*. 2006;104:724.
54. Griesmann GE, et al. *J Neurochem*. 1990;54:1541.
55. Gullberg D. *Nature*. 2003;424:138.
56. Missias AC, et al. *Dev Biol*. 1996;179:223.
57. McCarthy MP, Stroud RM. *Biochemistry*. 1989;28:40.
58. Yamaoka K, et al. *Curr Pharm Des*. 2006;12:429.
59. Raines DE. *Anesthesiology*. 1996;84:663.
60. Gage PW. *Biophys Chem*. 1988;29:95.
61. Swope SL, et al. *Ann N Y Acad Sci*. 1995;757:197.
62. Plested CP, et al. *Neurology*. 2002;59:1682.
63. Albuquerque EX, et al. *J Pharmacol Exp Ther*. 1997;280:1117.
64. Maelicke A, et al. *J Recept Signal Transduct Res*. 1997;17:11.
65. Nagashima M, et al. *Anesth Analg*. 2013;116:994.
66. Creese R, et al. *J Physiol*. 1987;384:377.
67. Ibebunjo C, Martyn JAJ. *Anesth Analg*. 2000;91:1243.
68. Fischer U, et al. *Eur J Neurosci*. 1999;11:2856.
69. Tsuneki H, et al. *J Physiol*. 2003;54(7):169.
70. Liu L, et al. *Br J Anaesth*. 2014;112:159.
71. Lindstrom JM. *Ann N Y Acad Sci*. 2003;998:41.
72. Khan MA, et al. *Shock*. 2012;38:213.
73. Lee S, et al. *Alpha7 AChRs play a pivotal role in the immobilization-induced resistance to atracurium in mice*. Abstract A1007; Presented at the ASA Annual Meeting, 2012.
74. Placzek AN, et al. *Mol Pharmacol*. 2004;66:169.
75. Tansey MG, et al. *J Cell Biol*. 1996;134:465.
76. Hirose M, et al. *Am J Physiol*. 2000;279:E1235.

77. Sugita M, et al. *Metabolism*. 2012;61:127.
78. Hirose M, et al. *Metabolism*. 2001;50:216.
79. Samuel MA, et al. *PLoS One*. 2012;7:e456663.
80. Dilger JP. *Anesth Analg*. 2013;117:792.
81. Gronert GA. *Anesthesiology*. 2001;94:523.
82. Tsuneki H, et al. *Neurosci Lett*. 1995;196:13.
83. Chiodini F, et al. *Anesthesiology*. 2001;94:643.
84. Faria M, et al. *Synapse*. 2003;49:77.
85. Martyn J, Durieux ME. *Anesthesiology*. 2006;104:633.
86. Eriksson LI. *Acta Anaesthesiol Scand*. 1996;40:520.
87. Mkrtchian S, et al. *J Physiol*. 2012;590:3807.
88. Santafe MM, et al. *Eur J Neurosci*. 2003;17:119.
89. Wessler I. *Trends Pharmacol Sci*. 1989;10:110.
90. Goudsouzian NG, Standaert FG. *Anesth Analg*. 1986;65:1208.
91. Shafiee G, et al. *J Diabetes Metab Disord*. 2017;16:21.
92. Yang JC, Van Remmen H. *Exp Gerontol*. 2011;46(2-3):193.
93. Willadt, et al. *Ann NY Acad Sci*. 2018;1412:41–53.
94. Sanes JR, Lichtman JW. *Nat Rev Neurosci*. 2001;2:791.

13 Respiratory Physiology and Pathophysiology

BRIAN P. KAVANAGH† and GÖRAN HEDENSTIERNA

KEY POINTS

- Removal of carbon dioxide (CO_2) is determined by alveolar ventilation, not by total (minute) ventilation.
- Dead space ventilation can be dramatically increased in patients with chronic obstructive pulmonary disease and pulmonary embolism to more than 80% of minute ventilation.
- Breathing at small lung volumes increases airway resistance and promotes closure of airways.
- Hypoxemia can be caused by alveolar hypoventilation, diffusion impairment, ventilation-perfusion mismatch, and right-to-left shunt.
- Almost all anesthetics reduce skeletal muscle tone, which decreases functional residual capacity (FRC) to levels close to the awake residual volume.
- Atelectasis during anesthesia is caused by decreased FRC and the use of high inspired oxygen concentrations (FiO_2), including breathing oxygen before induction of anesthesia.
- General anesthesia causes ventilation-perfusion mismatch (airway closure) and shunts (atelectasis).
- Venous admixture is due to $\dot{V}_A/\dot{Q}$ mismatch (response to increased FiO_2) and shunts (unresponsive to increased FiO_2).
- Hypoxic pulmonary vasoconstriction is blunted by most anesthetics, and this results in increased ventilation-perfusion mismatching.
- Respiratory work is increased during anesthesia as a consequence of reduced respiratory compliance and increased airway resistance.

Respiratory Physiology Is Central to the Practice of Anesthesia

Respiratory function is inextricably linked to the practice of anesthesia. Adverse respiratory effects can occur during anesthesia,[1] and the most serious cases involve hypoxemia. These events range from intractable hypoxemia caused by loss of airway patency to postoperative respiratory depression from opioids or regional anesthesia.[2,3] In the absence of adverse outcomes, general anesthesia still has significant effects on respiratory function and lung physiology, documented by observations made in the operating and recovery rooms. Improved appreciation of anesthesia-induced physiologic alterations (e.g., mechanisms of bronchospasm,[4] impact of mechanical ventilation),[5] as well as pioneering developments in monitoring (e.g., pulse oximetry and capnography),[6] together are associated with the specialty of anesthesiology's emergence as a leader in patient safety.[7] Finally, integrative measures of respiratory function, ranging from exercise capacity,[8] spirometry to tissue oxygenation,[9] to global O_2 consumption,[8] may help predict outcomes following anesthesia and surgery.

Pulmonary Physiology in Health

The mechanisms by which anesthesia-associated respiratory dysfunction is caused can be determined with an examination of normal functions and mechanisms of respiration in health. We briefly review cellular respiration, whereby O_2 is consumed and CO_2 is produced, the transport of O_2 and CO_2 in the blood, and the principles by which the lung oxygenates blood and eliminates CO_2.

RESPIRATION IN THE CELL

The partial pressure of oxygen (PaO_2) in normal arterial blood is approximately 100 mm Hg, and decreases to 4 to 22 mm Hg in the mitochondrion, where it is consumed. Glucose ($C_6H_{12}O_6$) is converted into pyruvate (CH_3COCOO^-) and H^+ by glycolysis in the cytoplasm, and the pyruvate diffuses into the mitochondria and forms the initial substrate for Krebs cycle, which in turn produces nicotinamide adenine dinucleotide (NADH), as well as adenosine triphosphate (ATP), CO_2, and H_2O. The NADH is a key electron (and H^+) donor in the process of oxidative phosphorylation, wherein O_2 and adenosine diphosphate are consumed and ATP and H_2O are produced. Thus the net effect is oxidation of glucose to produce energy (ultimately as ATP), H_2O, and CO_2.[10]

TRANSPORT OF O_2 IN THE BLOOD

O_2 reaches the cells following transport by arterial blood, and the overall delivery of O_2 ($\dot{D}O_2$) is the product of the arterial blood O_2 content (CaO_2) and blood flow (cardiac output, $\dot{Q}$) as

†Deceased.

$$\dot{D}O_2 = CaO_2 \times \dot{Q}$$

Oxygen is carried in the blood in two forms: O_2 bound to hemoglobin (the vast bulk), and O_2 dissolved in the plasma, and the content is expressed as the sum of these components:

$$CaO_2 = \left[\begin{array}{l} (SaO_2 \times Hb \times O_2 \text{ combining capacity of } Hb) \\ + (O_2 \text{ solubility} \times PaO_2) \end{array} \right]$$

where CaO_2 (O_2 content) is the milliliters of O_2 per 100 mL of blood, SaO_2 is the fraction of hemoglobin (Hb) that is saturated with O_2, O_2-combining capacity of Hb is 1.34 mL of O_2 per gram of Hb, *Hb* is grams of Hb per 100 mL of blood, Pao_2 is the O_2 tension (i.e., dissolved O_2), and solubility of O_2 in plasma is 0.003 mL of O_2 per 100 mL plasma for each mm Hg Pao_2

The binding of O_2 to hemoglobin is a complex, allosteric mechanism. Important insights can be gained by understanding how characteristic abnormalities of blood O_2 carriage (e.g., carbon monoxide [CO] poisoning, methemoglobinemia) affect O_2 tension, content, and delivery.

Methemoglobin (MetHb), formed by the oxidation to Fe^{3+} (ferric) instead of the usual Fe^{2+} (ferrous) iron, is less able to bind O_2, resulting in diminished O_2 content and less O_2 delivery. Here, the Pao_2 (in the absence of lung disease) will be normal: if the O_2 content is calculated from the Pao_2, it will appear normal, but if directly measured, it will be low. In contrast, MetHb level will be elevated. In severe cases, lactic acidosis develops because of impaired O_2 delivery. In addition, because MetHb has a blue-brown color, the patient will appear blue, even if the fraction of MetHb is modest; specialized oximetry can separately measure MetHb levels.[11,12] The apparent cyanosis is not responsive to supplemental O_2, and therapy involves converting (i.e., reducing) the MetHb to Hb (e.g., by using methylene blue). Important medical causes of MetHb include benzocaine, dapsone, or in susceptible patients, inhaled nitric oxide (NO).

In CO poisoning, the CO binds to Hb, with far greater (over 200-fold) avidity than molecular O_2, tightly forming CO-Hb and resulting in two main effects.[13] First, formation of CO-Hb results in fewer sites available for O_2 binding, and this reduces the blood O_2 content. Second, the formation of CO-Hb causes conformational changes in the Hb molecule such that the tendency to release bound O_2 is reduced. This effect corresponds to a leftward shift of the Hb-O_2 dissociation curve, and although this aspect of CO binding does not reduce the O_2 content or "global" delivery of O_2, it does reduce the release of O_2 and its local delivery to the cells. Because the color of CO-Hb closely resembles that of O_2-Hb, the color of the blood (and the patient) is bright red; however, as with MetHb, the PaO_2 will be normal (assuming no pulmonary disease) as will be the calculated CaO_2; however, the measured CaO_2 will be low and if severe, a lactic acidosis will be present. Modern pulse oximeters can distinguish between Hb-O_2 and CO-Hb.[13]

Finally, the *Bohr effect* refers to a shift of the Hb-O_2 dissociation curve caused by changes in CO_2 or pH.[14] In the systemic capillaries, the Pco_2 is higher than in the arterial blood (and the pH correspondingly lower) because of local CO_2 production. These circumstances shift the Hb-O_2 dissociation curve to the right, which increases the offloading of O_2 to the tissues. The opposite occurs in the pulmonary capillaries; here, the Pco_2 is lower (and the pH correspondingly higher) because of CO_2 elimination, and the dissociation curve is shifted to the left to facilitate O_2 binding to Hb.

TRANSPORT OF CO_2 IN THE BLOOD

CO_2 is produced by metabolism in the mitochondria, where the CO_2 levels are highest. The transport path (involving progressively decreasing pressure gradients) is from mitochondria through cytoplasm, into venules, and finally, in mixed venous blood from where it is eliminated through the alveoli. In the blood, CO_2 is transported in three main forms: dissolved (reflected as $Paco_2$, partial pressure; accounts for approximately 5% of transported CO_2), bicarbonate ion (HCO_3–; almost 90%), and carbamino CO_2 (CO_2 bound to terminal amino groups in Hb molecules; approximately 5%).[10] The usual quantities of CO_2 in the arterial and (mixed) venous blood are approximately 21.5 and 23.3 mmol of CO_2 per liter of blood, respectively.

Breathing O_2 can sometimes induce hypercapnia, as occurs in patients with severe chronic lung disease who are breathing supplemental O_2. Although traditionally thought to occur because increased Pao_2 reduces ventilatory drive, this is now thought not to be the case,[15] resulting instead from the Haldane effect, as well as from impairment of hypoxic pulmonary vasoconstriction (HPV). The Haldane effect[16] is the difference in the amount of CO_2 carried in oxygenated versus deoxygenated blood, and two mechanisms explain this. First, increased Pao_2 decreases the ability to form carbamino compounds—reducing the amount of CO_2 bound to Hb—thereby raising the amount of dissolved CO_2 (i.e., elevated Pco_2). Second, the amino acid histidine, which has an imidazole group that is an effective H^+ buffer at physiologic pH, is an important linking molecule between heme groups and the Hb chains. Increasing the partial pressure of oxygen (PO_2) increases the amount of O_2 bound to Hb; this changes the conformation of the Hb molecule, which in turn alters the heme-linked histidine and reduces its H^+ buffering capacity. Therefore, more H^+ is free (not buffered) and binds to HCO_3–, releasing stored CO_2. Impairment of HPV by elevated O_2 allows increased perfusion to poorly ventilated regions; this has the effect of decreasing perfusion (and delivery of CO_2) to better ventilated regions, diminishing the efficiency of CO_2 exhalation. Patients with impaired ability to increase alveolar ventilation ($\dot{V}_A$) cannot compensate for the increased CO_2 availability, and therefore, in these patients, adding supplemental O_2 can result in elevated $Paco_2$.

OXYGENATION IN THE PULMONARY ARTERY

Systemic venous blood (central venous blood) enters the right ventricle via the right atrium. The O_2 saturation (SO_2) differs among the major veins: higher venous SO_2 reflects greater blood flow, less tissue oxygen uptake, or both.[17] SO_2 is usually higher in the inferior vena cava (IVC) than in the superior vena cava (SVC), possibly because of the high renal and hepatic flow relative to O_2 consumption. In the right ventricle, the central venous blood ($S_{cv}O_2$) from the SVC and IVC is joined by additional venous blood from the coronary circulation (via the coronary sinuses). In the right ventricle, an additional small amount of venous drainage from the myocardium enters through the thebesian veins, and as all this

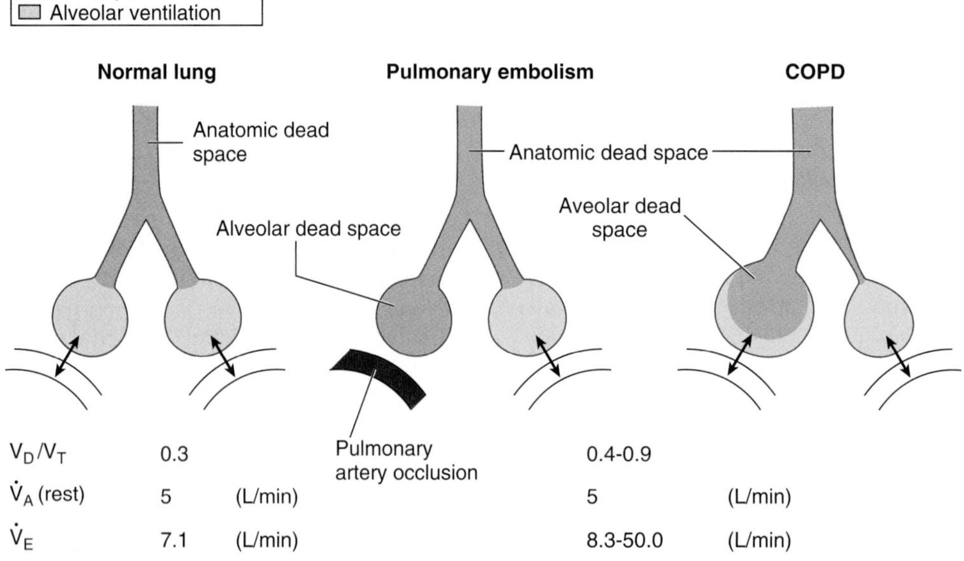

Fig. 13.1 Dead space and alveolar ventilation in normal and diseased lungs. Either cessation of blood flow or excessive alveolar ventilation relative to perfusion will cause an increase in dead space (V_D). If V_D is increased, a large compensatory increase in minute ventilation is required to preserve $\dot{V}_A$. V_D/V_T, dead space to tidal volume ratio; $\dot{V}_A$, alveolar ventilation; $\dot{V}_E$, minute ventilation. $\dot{V}_E = \dot{V}_A + f \times V_D$. *Double arrows* indicate normal CO_2 exchange. *COPD*, Chronic obstructive pulmonary disease. (From Hedenstierna G. *Respiratory measurement*. London: BMJ Books; 1998:184; see also book review of *Respiratory Measurement in Thorax* 1998;53:1096.)

venous blood enters the pulmonary artery, it is well mixed and is termed *mixed-venous blood* (S_vO_2); thus $S_vO_2 < S_{cv}O_2$, although the trends of each usually run in parallel.[18]

Ventilation

Ventilation refers to the movement of inspired gas into and exhaled gas out of the lungs.

ALVEOLAR VENTILATION

Fresh gas enters the lung by cyclic breathing at a rate and depth (tidal volume, V_T) determined by metabolic demand, usually 7 to 8 L/min.[19] While most inspired gas reaches the alveoli, some (100-150 mL) of each V_T remains in the airways and cannot participate in gas exchange. Such dead space (V_D) constitutes approximately one third of each V_T.[20] Anatomic V_D is the fraction of the V_T that remains in the "conducting" airways, and physiologic V_D is any part of a V_T that does not participate in gas exchange (Fig. 13.1).

For a single tidal volume (V_T, mL), the following is true:

$$V_T = V_A + V_D$$

The product of V_T (mL) times the respiratory rate (per minute) is the minute ventilation ($\dot{V}_E$). Aggregated over time, minute ventilation ($\dot{V}_E$, mL/min) is:

$$\dot{V}_E = \dot{V}_A + f \times V_D$$

The portion of the $\dot{V}_E$ that reaches the alveoli and respiratory bronchioles each minute and participates in gas exchange is called the *alveolar ventilation* ($\dot{V}_A$), and it is approximately 5 L/min. Because this is similar to the blood flow through the lungs (i.e., the cardiac output, also 5 L/min), the overall alveolar ventilation-perfusion ratio is approximately 1.

DEAD SPACE VENTILATION

Maintenance of $Paco_2$ is a balance between CO_2 production ($\dot{V}CO_2$, reflecting metabolic activity) and alveolar ventilation ($\dot{V}_A$). If $\dot{V}_E$ is constant but V_D is increased, $\dot{V}_A$ will naturally be reduced, and the $Paco_2$ will therefore rise. Therefore, if V_D is increased, $\dot{V}_E$ must also increase to prevent a rise in $Paco_2$. Such elevations in V_D occur when a mouthpiece or facemask is used, and in such cases, the additional V_D is termed "apparatus deadspace" (which can be up to 300 mL; anatomic V_D of the airways is 100-150 mL).[21]

Increases in the volume of the conducting airways (e.g., bronchiectasis) increase the overall V_D only slightly. Far more significant increases in V_D occur when perfusion to a large number of ventilated alveoli is interrupted, as occurs in a pulmonary embolus (see Fig. 13.1). Indeed, with multiple pulmonary emboli, V_D/V_T can exceed 0.8 (2.7-fold normal). In such a case, to maintain a normal $\dot{V}_A$ (5 L/min), the $\dot{V}_E$ would have to increase (also 2.7-fold) to almost 20 L/min. This effort would cause considerable dyspnea, in addition to the dyspnea induced by the lowered PaO_2.

Obstructive lung disease can result in diversion of inspired air into (nonobstructed) ventilated, but poorly perfused, regions of the lung. This results in local excesses of ventilation versus perfusion (high $\dot{V}_A/\dot{Q}$ ratio) in such regions,[22] which is equivalent to an increase in V_D/V_T (see Fig. 13.1). Patients with severe chronic obstructive pulmonary disease (COPD) may have a V_D/V_T ratio of up to 0.9, and would have to hyperventilate massively (30-50 L/min) to maintain normal $Paco_2$, which is not possible where ventilator reserve is diminished. Such patients demonstrate reduced $\dot{V}_A$ but often have an elevated $\dot{V}_E$. An important compensatory mechanism is that a lower level of $\dot{V}_A$ will maintain stable CO_2 excretion where the $Paco_2$ is increased (Box 13.1).

BOX 13.1 Alveolar Gas Equations

Alveolar Oxygen Tension (P_{AO_2})

$$P_{AO_2} = PIO_2 - \frac{P_{ACO_2}}{R} + \left[P_{ACO_2} \times FiO_2 \times \frac{1-R}{R}\right]$$

where PIO_2 is inspired oxygen tension, $PACO_2$ is alveolar CO_2 tension (assumed to equal arterial PCO_2), R is the respiratory exchange ratio (normally in the range of 0.8-1.0), and FiO_2 is the inspired oxygen fraction. The term within brackets compensates for the larger O_2 uptake than CO_2 elimination over the alveolar capillary membranes.

A simplified equation can be written without the compensation term:

$$P_{AO_2} = PIO_2 - \frac{P_{ACO_2}}{R}$$

Alveolar Ventilation

Alveolar ventilation ($\dot{V}_A$) can be expressed as

$$\dot{V}_A = f \times (V_T - V_{DS})$$

where f is breaths/min, V_T is tidal volume, and V_{DS} is physiologic dead space.

Alveolar ventilation can also be derived from:

$$\dot{V}_{CO_2} = c \times \dot{V}_A \times F_{ACO_2}$$

where $\dot{V}_{CO_2}$ is CO_2 elimination, c is a conversion constant, and $FACO_2$ is the alveolar CO_2 concentration.

If $\dot{V}_A$ is expressed in L/min, $\dot{V}_{CO_2}$ in mL/min, and $FACO_2$ is replaced by $PACO_2$ in mm Hg, $c = 0.863$. By rearranging:

$$\dot{V}_A = \frac{\dot{V}_{CO_2} \times 0.863}{P_{ACO_2}}$$

Static Lung Volumes—Functional Residual Capacity

The amount of air in the lungs after an ordinary expiration is called *functional residual capacity* (FRC; Fig. 13.2); it is usually 3 to 4 L and occurs because of the balance of inward (lung) forces and outward (chest wall) forces. The inward force is the "elastic recoil" of the lung and emanates from the elastic lung tissue fibers, contractile airway smooth muscle, and alveolar surface tension. The outward force is developed by passive recoil from the ribs, joints, and muscles of the chest wall. FRC is greater with increased height and age (loss of elastic lung tissue), and smaller in women and in obesity.[19,23]

There are two reasons why maintenance of gas in the lung at end-expiration (i.e., FRC) is important. First, inflating an already opened (inflated) lung is easier than when the lung is deflated. This is because complete collapse results in liquid-only surfaces interfacing in alveoli (high surface tension), whereas alveoli in partially inflated lung have air-liquid interfaces (lower surface tension). Second, although perfusion in the lung is phasic, the frequency is rapid and the oscillations in flow are low, resulting in nearly continuous flow. Ventilation is different: the frequency is far slower and the size of the oscillations far larger. If the lung (or large parts of it) completely deflate between breaths, the blood flowing from closed alveoli (that contain zero O_2) would have very low SO_2 (the same as mixed venous blood); this would mix into the overall blood flow from the lungs and cause a major O_2 desaturation after every exhalation.

Respiratory Mechanics

The study of respiratory mechanics tells us how inspired air is distributed within the lung and permits quantitation of the severity of lung disease. The components of overall impedance to breathing results from elastance (the reciprocal of compliance), resistance, and inertia.

COMPLIANCE OF THE RESPIRATORY SYSTEM

The lung is like a rubber balloon that can be distended by positive pressure (inside) or negative pressure (outside). Under normal circumstances, inflation of the lung is maintained because although the pressure inside (alveolar pressure) is zero, the outside pressure (i.e., the pleural pressure) is sufficiently negative. The net distending pressure, which is the difference of the (positive) airway pressure (P_{AW}) and the (negative) pleural pressure (P_{PL}) is termed the *transpulmonary pressure* (P_{TP}). Thus:

$$P_{TP} = P_{AW} - P_{PL}$$

Clearly, increasing the P_{AW} increases the P_{TP}. In addition, lowering the P_{PL} (which is usually negative and making it more negative) also increases the P_{TP}.

Compliance—the reciprocal of elastance—is the term that expresses how much distention (volume in liters) occurs for a given level of P_{TP} (pressure, cm H_2O); it is usually 0.2 to 0.3 L/cm H_2O.[24] However, although higher values of P_{TP} maintain greater levels of lung opening, the relationship—as with most elastic structures—between applied pressure and resultant volume is curvilinear (Fig. 13.3).[24] Lung compliance depends on the lung volume; it is lowest at an extremely low or high FRC (see Fig. 13.3). In lung diseases characterized by reduced compliance (e.g., ARDS, pulmonary fibrosis, or edema), the pressure-volume (PV) curve is flatter and shifted to the right (Fig. 13.4).[24] In contrast, although emphysema involves the loss of elastic tissue, the overall loss of lung tissue (as seen on computed tomography [CT] scanning)[25] means that the compliance is increased; the PV curve is therefore shifted to the left and is steeper (see Fig. 13.4).[24]

Chest wall impedance is not noticed during spontaneous breathing because the respiratory "pump" includes the chest wall. Chest wall mechanics can be measured only if complete relaxation of the respiratory muscles can be achieved[26]; however, during mechanical ventilation, the respiratory muscles can be completely relaxed. As the lung is inflated by P_{AW}, the properties of the chest wall will determine the resulting change in P_{PL}. Under these circumstances, the increase in lung volume per unit increase in P_{PL} is the chest wall compliance. Values of chest wall compliance are about the same as that of the lung and are reduced with obesity, chest wall edema, pleural effusions, and diseases of the costovertebral joints.[26]

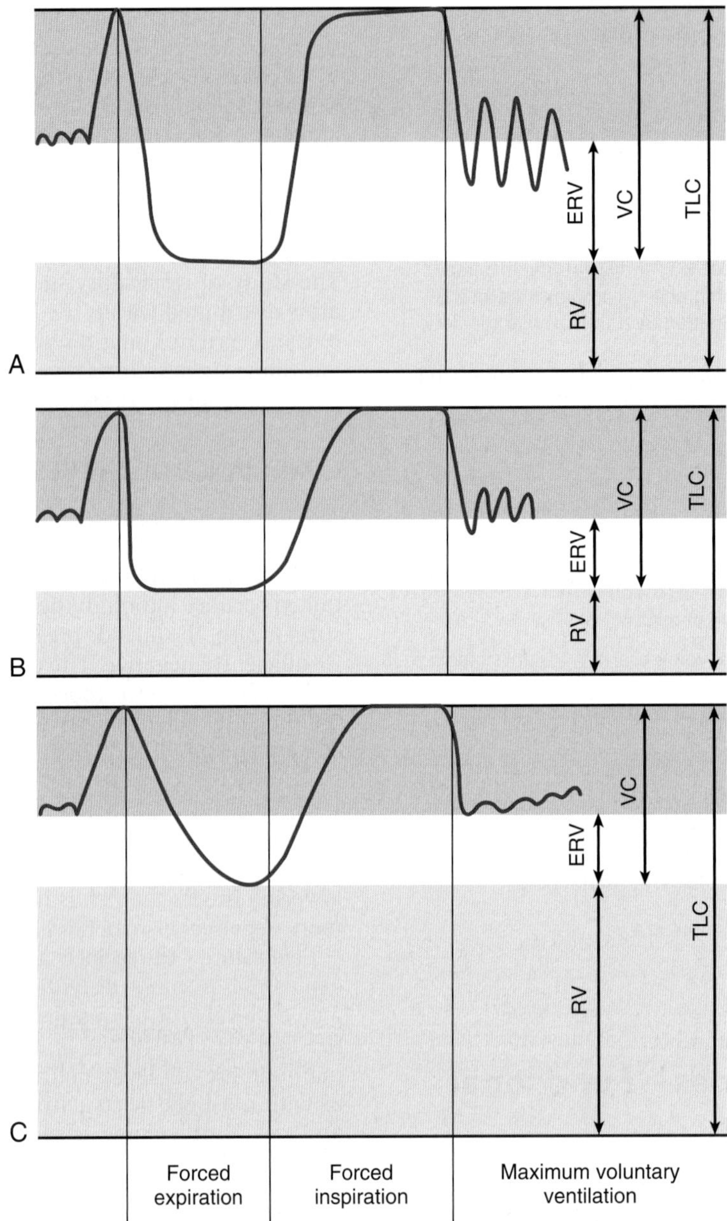

Fig. 13.2 (A) Ventilation and lung volumes in a healthy subject with normal lungs. (B) A patient with restrictive lung disease. (C) A patient with chronic obstructive pulmonary disease (COPD). In restrictive disease, the vital capacity *(VC)* is decreased and expiratory flow rate is increased (i.e., steeper than the normal slope of the forced expiratory curve). In COPD, the residual volume *(RV)* is increased, the VC is reduced, and forced expiration is slowed. *ERV*, Expiratory reserve volume; *TLC*, total lung capacity. (From Hedenstierna G. *Respiratory measurement*. London: BMJ Books; 1998:184; see also book review of *Respiratory Measurement in Thorax* 1998;53:1096.)

RESISTANCE OF THE RESPIRATORY SYSTEM

Airways

Resistance impedes airflow into (and out of) the lung. The major component of resistance is the resistance exerted by the airways (large and small), and a minor component is the sliding of lung and the chest wall tissue elements during inspiration (and expiration).[27] Resistance is overcome by (driving) pressure. In spontaneous breathing, driving pressure will be the P_{PL}; in positive pressure ventilation, the driving pressure will be the difference between the pressures applied to the endotracheal tube (P_{AW}; "source") and the alveolus (P_{ALV}; "destination"). Resistance (R) is calculated as driving pressure (ΔP) divided by the resultant gas flow (F):

$$R = \frac{\Delta P}{F}$$

The value of airway resistance is approximately 1 cm H_2O/L/sec, and is higher in obstructive lung disease (e.g., COPD, asthma); in severe asthma, it is elevated approximately tenfold.[28] The presence of an endotracheal tube adds a resistance of 5 (or 8) cm H_2O/L/min for a tube with internal diameter of size 8 (or 7) cm.[29] For any tube for which the airflow is laminar (smooth, streamlined), the resistance increases in direct proportion to the tube length and increases dramatically (to the fourth power) as the diameter of the tube is reduced.

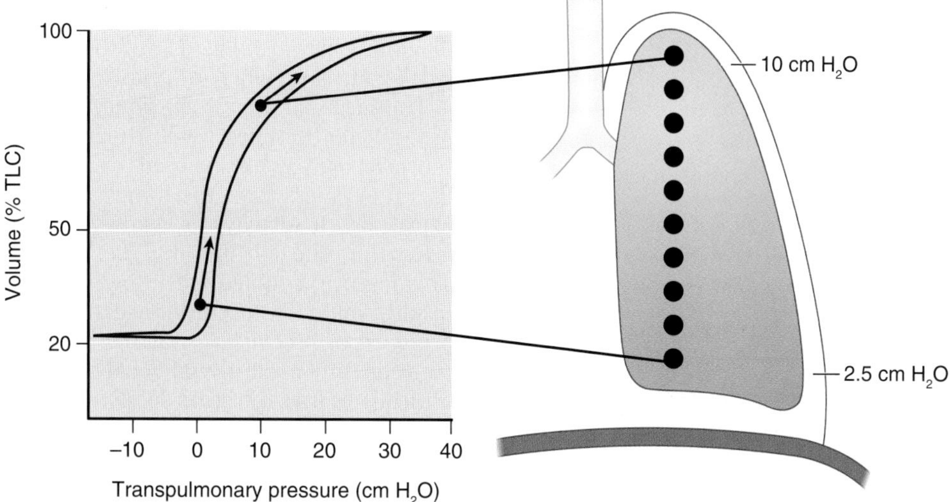

Fig. 13.3 The pressure-volume relationships of the lung. The relationship is curvilinear (typical for an elastic structure). The pleural pressure is lower (more subatmospheric) in the upper regions. In the upright subject, the transpulmonary pressure ($P_{TP} = P_{AW} - P_{PL}$) is higher in apical than in basal regions. This results in different positions on the pressure volume curve of the upper (flatter, less compliant) versus lower (steeper, more compliant) lung regions. Thus lower lung regions expand more (i.e., receive more ventilation) for a given increase in transpulmonary pressure than upper units. *TLC,* Total lung capacity.

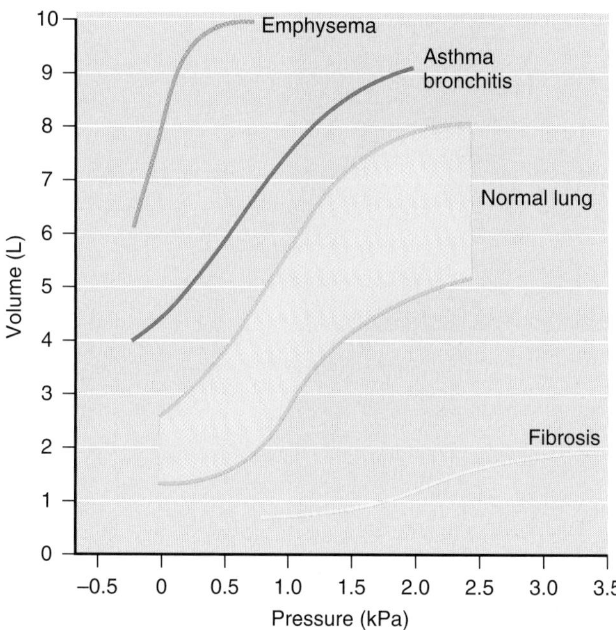

Fig. 13.4 Pressure-volume curves of the lung in healthy and lung-diseased patients. In fibrosis, the slope of the curve is flatter, reflecting considerable increases in pressure variation and in respiratory work. In asthma or bronchitis, there is a parallel *(upward)* shift of the pressure-volume curve, indicating an increase in lung volume but no change in compliance. In emphysema, the slope of the curve is steeper, reflecting tissue loss and possible increased compliance. However, in emphysema, asthma, or bronchitis, the airway resistance is increased; this increases work of breathing and overrides any benefit from increased compliance. (From Hedenstierna G. *Respiratory measurement*. London: BMJ Books; 1998:184; see also book review of *Respiratory Measurement in Thorax* 1998;53:1096.)

Two factors explain why most (approximately 80%) of the impedance to gas flow occurs in the large airways.[27] First, as bronchi progressively branch, the resistances are arranged in parallel and the total cross-sectional area at the level of the terminal bronchioles adds up to almost tenfold that at the trachea. Second, in tubes that are large, irregular or branched, the flow is often turbulent, not laminar. When flow is laminar:

$$F_{(lam)} = \frac{\Delta P}{R}$$

In contrast, when flow is turbulent:

$$F_{(turb)} = \frac{\Delta P}{R^2}$$

Therefore, for a given radius, far more pressure is required to achieve comparable flow where flow is turbulent; thus the effort required is greater and if prolonged or severe, respiratory failure is more likely.

Several factors can alter airflow resistance. First, resistance lessens as lung volume increases; this is intuitive, as increasing volume (positive pressure or spontaneous breathing) stretches the diameter of the airways. Because this is the key determinant of resistance, the resistance falls to a small extent. The opposite occurs with exhalation (Fig. 13.5). However, as lung volume approaches residual volume (RV)—as can happen during anesthesia—the airways are narrowed in parallel with the compressing lung tissue and the resistance rises exponentially. These effects are apparent with active or passive ventilation. Second, active ventilation has additional effects. Forced expiration can compress small airways (i.e., that do not contain cartilage).[27] In addition, forced expiration can cause turbulent flow in small airways in patients with COPD, precipitously dropping pressure in the lumen and thereby narrowing the bronchioles[30] and resulting in expiratory flow limitation and, after multiple breaths, eventual "dynamic hyperinflation."[31] Expiring against resistance (or pursed-lips breathing) is sometimes used by those with COPD to make breathing easier. This works by increasing expiratory resistance and slowing expiration. The slowed expiration reduces the pressure gradient driving expiration (i.e., pressure highest in the alveolus, lower toward the mouth). Therefore, the point along the airway tree at which pressure inside the airway has decreased to less than that outside the

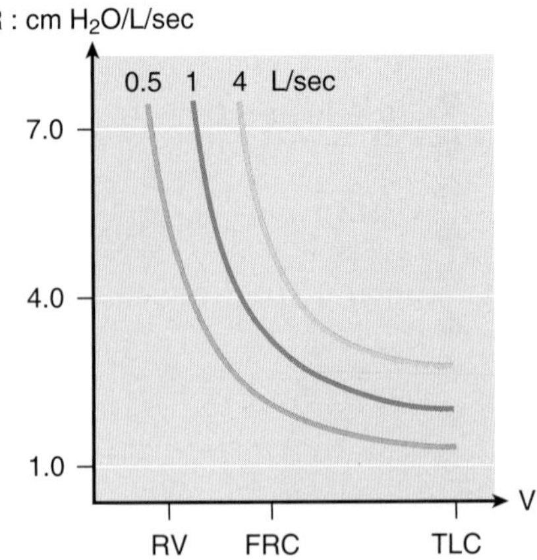

Fig. 13.5 Schematic drawing of airflow resistance against lung volume at different flow rates. As lung volume falls, the resistance to flow increases; the steepness of this increase is far greater at lung volumes below functional residual capacity *(FRC)*. In addition, higher airflow rates are associated with greater resistance. At extremely low lung volume, the resistance is comparable to values seen in moderate to severe asthma (6-8 cm $H_2O \times l^{-1} \times s$). *RV*, Residual volume; *TLC*, total lung capacity.

airway (equal to pleural pressure) is moved from smaller collapsible airways toward the mouth to noncollapsible, cartilaginous airways (Fig. 13.6); this prevents collapse of the smaller airways, which are vital for proper gas exchange.[32]

The large airways (i.e., pharynx, larynx, and trachea) are outside the chest wall. During inspiration, the intrathoracic airways are exposed to extraluminal pressure (i.e., P_{PL}) that is less than the lumen pressure; in contrast, the extrathoracic airways are exposed to lumen pressure that is less than the extraluminal (i.e., atmospheric) pressure.[27] This feature, coupled with downward stretch induced by inspiration, narrows the large extrathoracic airways; in the presence of preexisting narrowing (e.g., thyroid enlargement or tumor, paralyzed vocal cord, epiglottitis), this can critically reduce the cross-sectional area.

Tissue

Although not intuitively obvious, resistance of the lung tissue is the applied pressure on tissue divided by the resulting velocity of tissue movement. There are various approaches to determining this in humans, including separately

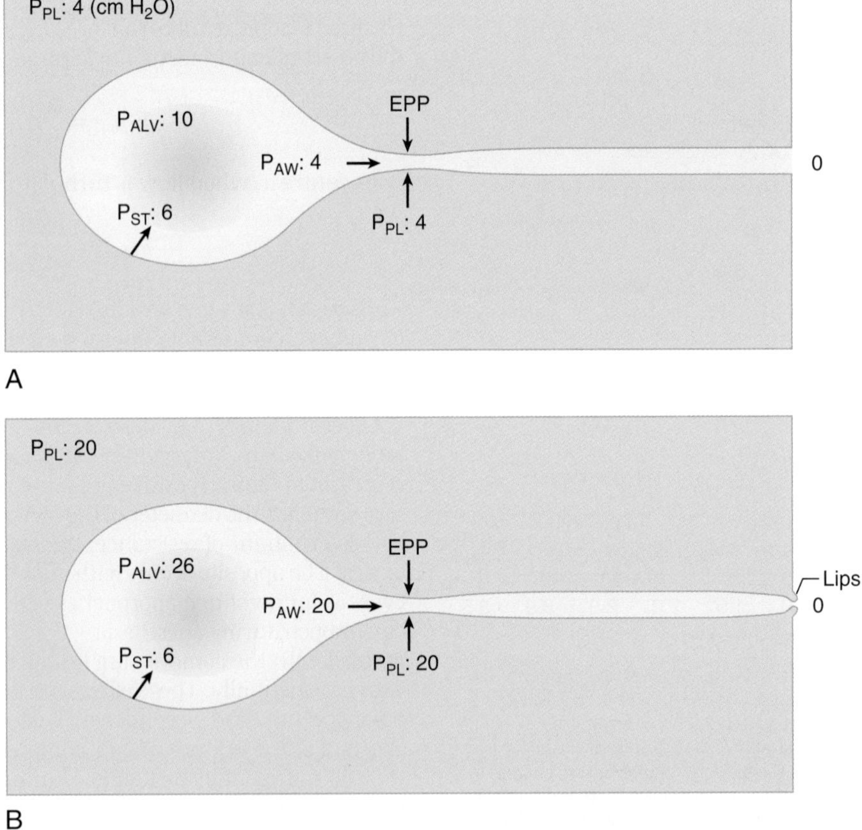

Fig. 13.6 Schematic drawings of the equal pressure point *(EPP)* concept and dynamic compression of airways. (A) Slightly forced expiration during otherwise normal conditions. With the application of some expiratory muscle effort, pleural pressure *(P_{PL})* is positive, 4 cm H_2O (0.4 kPa). The elastic recoil pressure *(P_{ST})* of the alveoli (6 cm H_2O) and the pleural pressure add together to yield intraalveolar pressure *(P_{ALV})* (10 cm H_2O). This causes expiratory flow. At some point downstream toward the airway opening, airway pressure *(P_{AW})* has dropped by 6 cm H_2O, so intraluminal pressure and pleural, extraluminal pressure are the same. This is the EPP. From this point to the mouth, intraluminal airway pressure is lower than the surrounding, extraluminal pressure and the airway may be compressed. (B) An attempt to stabilize the airway by so-called "pursed-lip" breathing. The increased resistance to expiratory flow requires increased expiratory effort to maintain gas flow. Thus pleural pressure is increased in comparison to the normal conditions (P_{PL} = 20 cm H_2O). Alveolar elastic recoil pressure (P_{ST}) is the same as in the earlier condition, provided that lung volume is the same. If expiratory flow is of the same magnitude as during normal breathing, pressure along the airway falls to the same extent as during normal breathing. Thus the EPP will have the same location as during normal breathing, and no stabilization of the airway has been achieved. The two ways of moving the EPP toward the mouth and to less collapsible airways is by raising alveolar recoil pressure (P_{ST}) by an increase in lung volume or by lowering the expiratory flow rate so that the pressure drop along the airway tree is slowed down.

considering the PV characteristics using plethysmography (where the area of the PV curve corresponds to work against total pulmonary resistance) and esophageal pressure (where the area of the PV curve corresponds to work against "tissue" resistance).[33] Alternative approaches mathematically model the lung responses to varying respiratory frequencies.[34] Lung tissue resistance amounts to 20% of the total resistance to breathing; it can be increased threefold or fourfold in chronic lung disease[35] and is reduced by panting respirations.[36] Finally, in adult respiratory distress syndrome (ARDS) the chest wall resistance is increased.[37]

INERTIA OR ACCELERATION OF GAS AND TISSUE

A final component of the total impedance to breathing is inertance, or the pressure required to accelerate air and tissue during inspiration and expiration. This component is minor, however, and can hardly be measured under normal breathing, regardless of whether the lungs are healthy. Nonetheless, tissue inertia is large during rapid ventilation,[38] and it could be important during the rapid, shallow breathing characteristic of weaning failure or during high-frequency oscillation.

Distribution of Inspired Gas

Inspired gas is not evenly distributed throughout the lung; naturally, more gas enters those lung units that expand most during inspiration. In the resting lung, the basal (dependent) regions are less aerated than the apical (nondependent) regions; therefore, they have the capacity to undergo greater expansion. During inspiration, most gas goes to the basal units (dorsal, when supine; lower right lung when in the right lateral position).[39] This distribution is because of the compliance properties of the lung and the effects of position on the distribution of the distending pleural pressure (i.e., the P_{PL} gradient). These changes are not related to the properties of the inspired gas.

In the upright position, the P_{PL} is less negative at the base of the lung than at the apex. Because the alveolus pressure (P_A) is uniform throughout the lung, the distending P_{TP} is greater at the apex; therefore, before inspiration commences, the apical lung is more open (and is less compliant) than the basal lung (Figs. 13.3 and 13.7). With inspiration, the contracting diaphragm lowers the P_{PL} by a comparable amount in all areas of the pleural surface (because of the fluid-like behavior of normal lung[39]) and distends the basal more than the apical regions (see Figs. 13.3 and 13.7). Because the pleural pressure gradient is oriented according to gravity, the distribution of ventilation changes with body position.

The P_{PL} gradient exists because lung density, gravity, and conformation of the lung to the shape of the thorax[40] result in crowding of the basal lung tissue, making the local P_{PL} less negative in the basal regions. Because the density of normal lung is approximately 0.3, P_{PL} will become more positive by 0.3 cm H_2O for each downward vertical

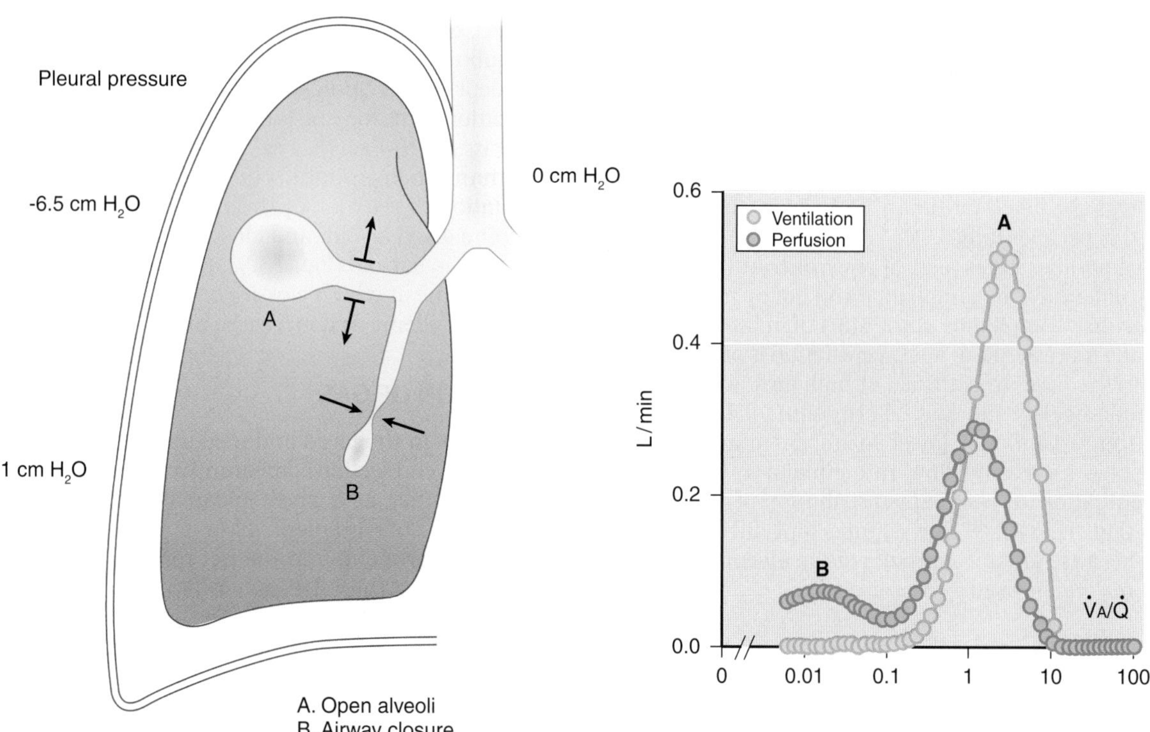

Fig. 13.7 Schematic of regional alveolar and airway volume at an upper *(A)* and a lower *(B)* lung level *(left panel)*. There is a vertical pleural pressure (P_{PL}) gradient between the uppermost and lowermost regions (−6.5 to 1 = −7.5 cm H_2O). Airway pressure (P_{AW}) is atmospheric, or 0 cm H_2O throughout; thus, in the upper regions, $P_{AW} > P_{PL}$ maintains airways open. In contrast, in the lower regions, $P_{PL} > P_{AW}$ causes airway closure—potentially exacerbated by subsequent alveolar gas absorption behind the occluded airway. The *right panel* shows the distribution of ventilation and perfusion ratios from the multiple inert gas elimination technique. A "normal" mode of ventilation and blood flow *(A)* can be seen corresponding to the open and ventilated alveoli in the upper parts of the lung. In addition, there is a range of low $\dot{V}_A/\dot{Q}$ ratios with more perfusion than ventilation *(B)*. This pattern is compatible with intermittent airway closure during breathing.

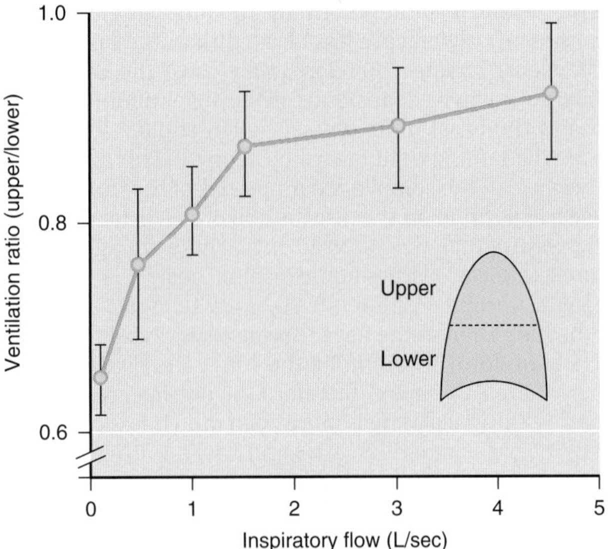

Fig. 13.8 Distribution of ventilation to upper versus lower lung regions as inspiratory flow is altered. At low flow, the bulk of the airflow goes to the lower regions. At higher flow rates (e.g., during exercise) the distribution is more even, ensuring more efficient use of all alveolar-capillary membranes for gas transfer (provided that pulmonary blood flow shows a similar distribution pattern).

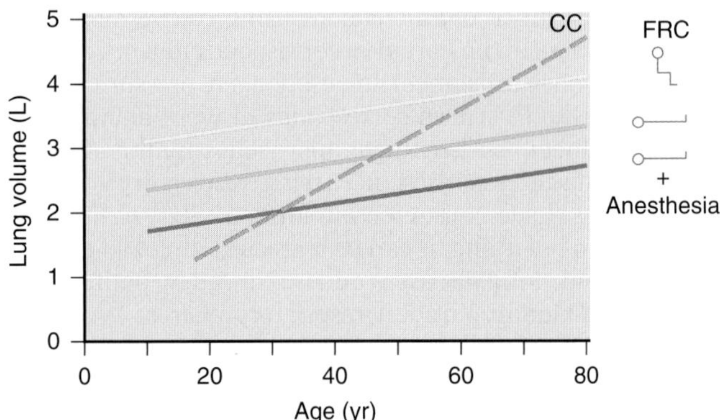

Fig. 13.9 Resting functional residual capacity *(FRC)* and closing capacity *(CC)*. FRC increases with age (because of loss of elastic tissue), and superimposed upon this is a step decrease in FRC with supine position (because of diaphragm elevation by abdominal contents), and a further decrease with anesthesia in the supine position. The CC is also increased with age, but far more steeply, causing airway closure above FRC in upright subjects (>65 yr) and in supine subjects (>45 yr). This relationship between CC and FRC explains decreasing oxygenation with age.

centimeter, and more so with injured or edematous lungs. Indeed, experimentally induced weightlessness decreases inhomogeneity in the distribution of ventilation,[41] but does not eliminate it; therefore, nongravitational (e.g., tissue, airway) factors also play a role.[42]

Although the vertical height of the lung is the same in the prone and supine positions, the vertical gradient P_{PL} is less when prone,[43] perhaps because the mediastinum compresses the dependent lung when supine but rests on the sternum when prone.[44] A more even distribution of inspired gas—with improved oxygenation—in the prone position was predicted by Bryan in 1974[44]; this has been confirmed experimentally.[45,46]

During low-flow states (e.g., at rest), distribution is determined by differences in compliance and not by airway resistance. Because compliance at the start of inflation is less in the (already more aerated) apex, ventilation is preferentially directed to the base. In contrast, at high airflow, resistance (not compliance) is the key determinant of distribution; because the resistance is lower in upper, more expanded lung regions, increasing flow rate equalizes the distribution of ventilation, as shown by distribution of ^{133}Xe gas in humans (Fig. 13.8).[47,48] This is important during exercise or stress because greater amounts of the alveolar-capillary surface area will be used.

AIRWAY CLOSURE

Expiration causes the airways to narrow, and deep expiration can cause them to close. The volume remaining above RV where expiration below FRC closes some airways is termed *closing volume* (CV), and this volume added to the RV is termed the *closing capacity* (CC; i.e., the total capacity of the lung at which closing can occur).[49] Closure of airways during expiration is normal and is potentiated by increasing P_{PL}, especially with active expiration. When P_{PL} exceeds the P_{AW}, the airway—if collapsible—will tend to close, and this usually commences at the bases because the basal P_{PL} is greatest (see Fig. 13.7).

Three applications of this important principle are of key relevance to anesthesia. First, airway closure depends on age: in youth, the closure does not occur until expiration is at or near RV, whereas with older age, it occurs earlier in expiration (i.e., at higher lung volumes). This occurs because P_{PL} is on average more "positive" (i.e., atmospheric, equal to P_{AW}) as age increases. Closing can occur at or above FRC in individuals aged 65 to 70 years,[50] such that dependent regions will undergo closure during normal expiration. This may be the major reason why oxygenation decreases with age. Second, in the supine position, FRC is less than when upright, but CC is unchanged; therefore, exhalation of a usual V_T (from FRC) encroaches on CC in a supine 45-year-old, and closure may be continuous in a supine 70-year-old (Fig. 13.9). Finally, COPD increases the lung volume at which closure occurs, possibly exacerbated by airway edema and increased bronchial tone.[49]

DIFFUSION OF GAS

Gas moves in the large and medium-sized airways by bulk flow (i.e., convection), meaning that the gas molecules travel together at a given mean velocity according to a driving pressure gradient. Flow is through multiple generations of bronchi, and the net resistance falls with each division. After the 14th generation, airways merge with alveoli and participate in gas exchange (respiratory bronchioles). The cross-sectional area expands massively (trachea, 2.5 cm^2; 23rd generation bronchi, 0.8 m^2; alveolar surface, 140 m^2),[51] resulting in a sharp drop in overall resistance. Because the number of gas molecules is constant, the velocity falls rapidly, which by the time the gas enters the alveoli is miniscule (0.001 mm/s); it is zero when it reaches the alveolar membrane. The velocity of the gas entering the alveolus is slower than the diffusion rates of O_2 and CO_2; therefore, diffusion—not convection—is necessary for transport in the distal airways and alveoli. Indeed,

CO_2 is detectable at the mouth after just seconds of breath-holding, because of rapid diffusion and because of cardiac oscillations (i.e., mixing).

Gas mixing is complete in the alveoli of a normal lung during normal breathing. However, if the alveolus expands (e.g., emphysema), the diffusion distance may be too great to allow complete mixing, potentially leaving a layer of CO_2-rich gas lining the alveolar membrane and a core of O_2-rich gas in the alveolus. This represents a "micro" version of inhomogeneous distribution of ventilation.[52]

Perfusion

The pulmonary circulation differs from the systemic circulation: it operates at a five to tenfold lower pressure, and the vessels are shorter and wider. There are two important consequences of the particularly low vascular resistance. First, the downstream blood flow in the pulmonary capillaries is pulsatile, in contrast to the more constant systemic capillary flow.[53] Second, the capillary and alveolar walls are protected from exposure to high hydrostatic pressures; therefore, they can be sufficiently thin to optimize diffusion (i.e., exchange) of gas but not permit leakage of plasma or blood into the airspace. Whereas an abrupt increase in the pulmonary arterial (or venous) pressure can cause breaks in the capillaries,[54] slower increases (i.e., months to years) stimulate vascular remodeling.[55] This remodeling might protect against pulmonary edema[56] (and possibly against lung injury[57]), but diffusion will be impaired.

DISTRIBUTION OF LUNG BLOOD FLOW

Pulmonary blood flow depends on driving pressure and vascular resistance; these factors (and flow) are not homogenous throughout the lung. The traditional thinking about lung perfusion emphasized the importance of gravity;[58] however, factors other than gravity are also important.

DISTRIBUTION OF BLOOD FLOW IN THE LUNG: THE EFFECT OF GRAVITY

Blood has weight and therefore blood pressure is affected by gravity. The height (base to apex) of an adult lung is approximately 25 cm; therefore, when a person is standing, the hydrostatic pressure at the base is 25 cm H_2O (i.e., approximately 18 mm Hg) higher than at the apex. The mean pulmonary arterial pressure is approximately 12 mm Hg at the level of the heart, and the pulmonary artery pressure at the lung apex can therefore approach zero. Thus less blood flow will occur at the apex (versus the base), and in the setting of positive pressure ventilation, the apical alveoli can compress the surrounding capillaries and prevent any local blood flow.

Based on such gravitational distribution of pulmonary artery pressure, as well as the effect of alveolar expansion, West and colleagues[59] divided the lung into zones I to III (Fig. 13.10). This system is based on the principle that perfusion to an alveolus depends on the pressures in the pulmonary artery (P_{PA}), pulmonary vein (P_{PV}), and alveolus (P_{ALV}). In the apex (zone I), the key issue is that pulmonary arterial pressure is less than alveolar pressure; therefore,

$$\text{Pulmonary vascular resistance (PVR)} = \frac{\bar{P}_{PA} - P_{LA}}{\dot{Q}_T}$$

(true only if lung is in zone III)

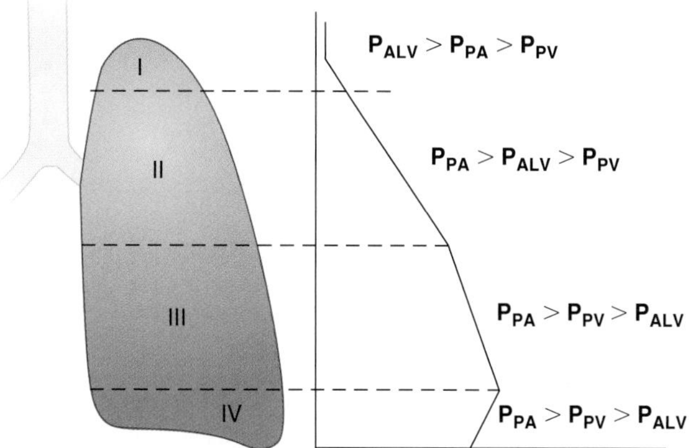

Fig. 13.10 Vertical distribution of lung blood flow. The so-called zones I, II, III, and IV are indicated. In zone I there is no perfusion, only ventilation. In zone II, pulmonary artery pressure exceeds alveolar pressure which in turn exceeds venous pressure; the driving pressure is $P_{PA}–P_{ALV}$. In zone III, arterial and venous pressures both exceed alveolar pressure, and here the driving pressure is $P_{PA}–P_{PV}$. In the lung base, blood flow is decreased possibly because of increased interstitial pressure that compresses extra alveolar vessels. P_{ALV}, intraalveolar pressure; P_{PV}, pulmonary vein pressure; P_{PA}, pulmonary artery pressure; Q_T, cardiac output.

no perfusion occurs. Zone I conditions can exist during mechanical ventilation and be exacerbated by low P_{PA}. Whenever zone I conditions exist, the nonperfused alveoli constitute additional dead space (V_D). Below the apex in zone II, P_{PV} is less than alveolar pressure, and the veins are collapsed except during flow, as in a "vascular waterfall." Although P_{ALV} is always greater than P_{PV}, perfusion occurs when P_{PA} exceeds P_{ALV} (i.e., intermittently, during systole). Below this zone is zone III, in which there are two important differences: P_{PA} and P_{PV} both always exceed P_{ALV}. As a result, there is perfusion throughout systole and diastole (and inspiration and expiration). Gravity results in equal increases in both P_{PA} and P_{PV} toward the lung base; therefore, gravity cannot affect flow throughout zone III by increasing the P_{PA} to P_{PV} pressure gradient alone. Nonetheless, it is possible that the greater weight of the blood nearer the base results in vessel dilatation, thereby lowering vascular resistance and increasing flow.[58] It was subsequently recognized that there is also a decrease in perfusion in the lung base, or zone IV, that is thought to occur because of the effects of gravity compressing the lung at the bases—and the blood vessels therein—and thereby increasing vascular resistance.[60]

Finally, additional evidence for the effect of gravity comes from volunteer experiments in which gravity was increased or abolished by altering the flight pattern of a jet aircraft.[61] In these experiments, zero gravity decreased cardiac oscillations of O_2 and CO_2 during a breath-hold, indicating development of more homogeneous perfusion. In contrast, more recent experiments of exhaled gas analysis (on the Mir space station) reported that the heterogeneity of lung perfusion was reduced, but not eliminated, in the presence of

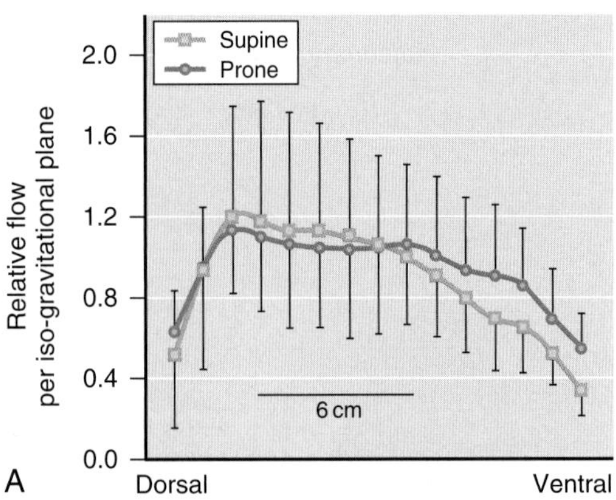

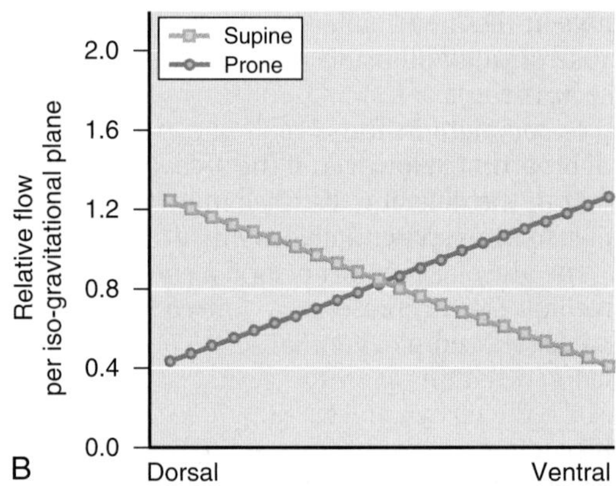

Fig. 13.11 Distribution of blood flow (ventral, dorsal) in supine versus prone position. The distributions from ventral to dorsal are similar, irrespective of position, suggesting that the anatomic features (and not simply gravity) determine the distribution of flow. The magnitude of the variability in either the prone (or in the supine) position (i.e., nongravitational inhomogeneity) is far greater than the differences in distribution between the prone and the supine positions (i.e., gravitational inhomogeneity). (From Glenny RW, Lamm WJ, Albert RK, Robertson HT. Gravity is a minor determinant of pulmonary blood flow distribution. *J Appl Physiol.* 1991;71:620–629.)

microgravity, indicating that gravity contributes to the heterogeneity of blood flow distribution but does not explain it entirely.[62] While the precise role of gravity is disputed, it is likely to play a smaller role when supine versus when upright.

DISTRIBUTION OF BLOOD FLOW IN THE LUNG: INFLUENCE OF FACTORS NOT RELATED TO GRAVITY

Key experiments have reconsidered the effects of gravity. Blood flow measured in the same gravitational plane was less per unit of lung tissue at the apex than at the base.[63] In addition, microsphere assessment demonstrated significant variability within iso-gravitational planes, and lung height appeared to account for less than 10% of the distribution of flow in either the prone or supine positions.[64] In addition, inhomogeneity in the horizontal planes can exceed that in the vertical direction (Fig. 13.11).[65] Other studies have reported a preponderance of perfusion to the central lung (versus peripheral) tissue,[66] which can be reversed by the application of positive end-expiratory pressure (PEEP).[67] Although greater length of radial blood vessels was considered to explain this central-peripheral difference, others have suggested that it is not significant.[64] Finally, differences have been reported among lung regions in local vascular resistance.[68]

Fractal distribution of blood flow may be more important than the influence of gravity.[69] A fractal pattern of perfusion means that in any given region, there will be "spatial correlation" (similarity) of the blood flow between neighboring regions.

Although the methods to study lung perfusion are complex—and there is a spectrum of opinion[70]—the aggregate data suggest that factors other than gravity contribute to the heterogeneity of the distribution of perfusion.

HYPOXIC PULMONARY VASOCONSTRICTION

HPV is a compensatory mechanism that diverts blood flow away from hypoxic lung regions toward better oxygenated regions.[71] The major stimulus for HPV is low alveolar oxygen tension (P_AO_2), whether caused by hypoventilation or by breathing gas with a low PO_2, and is more potent when affecting a smaller lung region. The stimulus of hypoxic mixed venous blood is weaker.[72,73] Whereas in humans older volatile anesthetics were thought to inhibit HPV more than intravenously based anesthesia, modern volatile anesthetics, including sevoflurane[74] and desflurane,[75] have little effect. During intravenously based anesthesia, exposure of one lung to an FiO_2 of 1.0 and the contralateral lung to a hypoxic gas mixture (FiO_2, 0.12 to 0.05) reduced perfusion to the hypoxic lung to 30% of the cardiac output.[76] Pulmonary hypertension, because of vascular remodeling owing to ongoing HPV, can develop in humans at high altitude[77] or in the presence of chronic hypoxemic lung disease.

Clinical Assessment of Lung Function

SPIROMETRY—TOTAL LUNG CAPACITY AND SUBDIVISIONS

The gas volume in the lung after a maximum inspiration is called the *total lung capacity* (TLC; usually 6 to 8 L). TLC can be increased in COPD either by overexpansion of alveoli or by destruction of the alveolar wall, resulting in loss of elastic tissue, as in emphysema (see Fig. 13.4).[78] In extreme cases, TLC can be increased to 10 to 12 L. In restrictive lung disease, TLC is reduced, reflecting the degree of fibrosis, and can be as low as 3 to 4 L (see Fig. 13.4).[78]

Following maximum expiratory effort, some air is left in the lung and constitutes the RV (approximately 2 L). However, usually no region develops collapse because distal airways (<2 mm) close before alveoli collapse,[79] trapping gas and preventing further alveolar emptying. In addition, there is a limit to how much the chest wall, rib cage, and diaphragm can be compressed. The importance of preventing collapse of lung tissue was presented earlier (see Fig. 13.6).

The maximum volume that can be inhaled and then exhaled is the vital capacity (VC; 4-6 L), and this is the difference between TLC and RV. VC is reduced in both restrictive and obstructive lung disease. In restriction, VC reduction reflects the loss of lung volume, such as from the constricting (i.e., shrinking) effects of fibrosis. In obstructive lung disease, long-term trapping of air increases the RV and can occur either by encroaching on (and reducing) the VC or in association with a (proportionally smaller) increase in FVC.[78]

Tidal volume (V_T, usually 0.5 L) is inspired from the resting lung volume reached at end-expiration (FRC, 2.0 L). With increased ventilation, as in exercise, V_T is increased and FRC may be reduced by approximately 0.5 L. However, in airway obstruction, exhalation is impeded such that inspiration commences before the usual resting lung volume is reached; thus end-expiratory volume is increased.[78] Such air trapping reduces the resistance to gas flow in the narrowed airways, but because the lung tissue is hyperinflated and mechanically disadvantaged, the work of breathing overall is increased.

FRC increases with age as elastic lung tissue is lost; this reduces the lung recoil force countering the outward chest wall force, and the lung assumes a higher volume. The rate of this aging process is accelerated in COPD because of the contributions of chronic air trapping and marked loss of elastic tissue.[19] FRC is reduced in fibrotic lung diseases,[78] sometimes to 1.5 L (see Fig. 13.4). Lung resection also reduces FRC, but the remaining lung will expand to fill the lung tissue void partially; this is called *compensatory emphysema* (see Chapter 53).

DIFFUSING CAPACITY (DL_{CO})—DIFFUSION ACROSS ALVEOLAR-CAPILLARY MEMBRANES

The diffusing capacity for carbon monoxide (DL_{CO}) test integrates many phenomena that are central to respiratory physiology. The test and the factors affecting its interpretation are described here. In the lungs, O_2 and CO_2 diffuse passively: O_2 from alveolar gas into plasma and red cells, where it binds to hemoglobin, and CO_2 in the opposite direction, from plasma to the alveoli. The amount that can diffuse across a membrane in a given period is the diffusing capacity, and it is determined with the following equation:

$$Diffusing\ capacity = \frac{(SA \times \Delta P \times Sol)}{\left(h \times \sqrt{MW}\right)}$$

where SA is the surface area of the membrane exposed to gas, ΔP is the gradient of partial pressure between administered gas versus blood tension, Sol is the solubility of the gas in the membrane, h is the thickness of the membrane, and MW is the molecular weight of the gas.

Assessment of diffusing capacity (sometimes called *transfer factor*) uses CO as the test gas; it is inhaled at a small concentration (0.3%) to TLC just after a maximal expiration, filling the lung as much as possible with the dilute CO. The breath is held and then deeply exhaled to RV. The difference between the quantity of CO exhaled versus inhaled will therefore either be taken up by the perfusing blood (i.e., hemoglobin) or remain in the lung (RV). The latter can be determined if the CO is coadministered with an insoluble gas (e.g., helium) that remains in the lung.

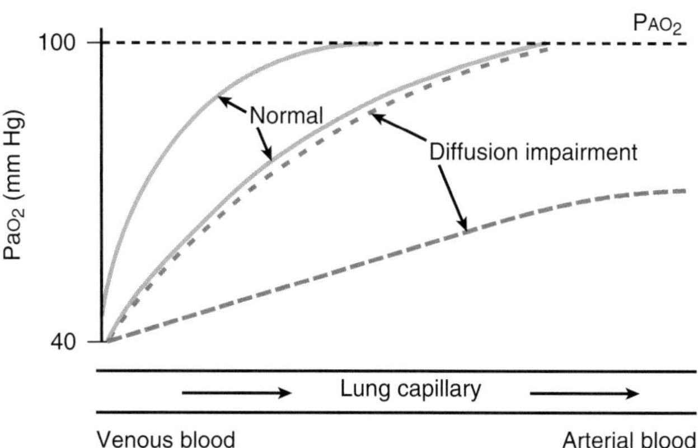

Fig. 13.12 Schematic of oxygenation of pulmonary capillary blood. In a healthy subject, there is a rapid equilibration (<30% capillary length) of the oxygen tension in capillary blood than that in alveolar gas; however, during exercise, the flow rate is greater (i.e., transit time shorter) and most of the capillary distance is used before equilibration is reached. This effect can be offset by distention and recruitment of pulmonary capillaries. If diffusion is impaired, equilibration takes longer, and it might not occur with exercise.

Surface Area

The surface area is taken as the area that is capable of exchanging gas on the alveolar and the capillary sides; thus it assumes a ventilated and perfused lung (i.e., not dead space). It will be lower in small lungs, lung fibrosis (restriction), after lung resection, or in cases of lung tissue destruction, such as emphysema.

Membrane Thickness

Thicker membranes reduce the CO transfer because the longer diffusion distance lowers the diffusion capacity, and the solubility of O_2 (and CO_2) is lower in fibrotic tissue than in plasma. Differentiating between effects of the volume of capillary blood and the membrane thickness can be difficult, but because oxygen and CO compete for binding to hemoglobin, distinguishing between these issues may be possible by measuring CO transfer with altered FiO_2 (see review by Hughes and colleagues).[80,81]

Pressure Gradient

The larger the O_2 or CO_2 tension difference (ΔP) between the gas phase (alveolus) and the plasma (capillary), the greater the rate of diffusion. The mixed venous blood entering the pulmonary capillary has a PO_2 of 40 mm Hg (5.3 kPa), and alveolar PO_2 is approximately 100 mm Hg (13.3 kPa); therefore, the driving pressure (ΔP) is 60 mm Hg (8 kPa).

When blood flows through the capillary, it takes up oxygen and delivers CO_2, but because oxygen pressure builds up in capillary blood, the diffusion rate slows down and becomes zero when pressure is equilibrated across the alveolar-capillary wall. At rest, equilibrium is usually reached within 25% to 30% of the capillary length, and almost no gas transfer occurs in the remaining capillary (Fig. 13.12). However, during exercise or stress (i.e., high cardiac output), blood flow through the capillary is faster, and a longer capillary distance is required before equilibrium is reached. Thickened alveolar-capillary membranes will also prolong the equilibration process and, if severe, can prevent equilibration occurring and increasing the propensity to hypoxemia. If the mixed venous PO_2 ($P_{mv}O_2$) is lower than normal, the driving pressure increases and partially compensates toward achieving equilibrium with alveolar O_2. The driving pressure is expressed:

$$\Delta P = (PaO_2 - P_{mv}O_2)\ mm\ Hg$$

Most of the oxygen that dissolves in plasma diffuses into the red cell and binds to hemoglobin; therefore, 1 L of blood (Hb 150 g/L) with a saturation of 98%—normal in arterial blood—carries 200 mL of Hb-bound O_2, compared with 3 mL that is dissolved (PaO_2 100 mm Hg). The Hb-bound oxygen creates no pressure in plasma, which is important because it allows much more oxygen to diffuse over the membranes before a pressure equilibration is reached. Anemia (or prior CO exposure) reduces—and polycythemia increases—diffusion capacity.

Molecular Weight and Solubility

The rate of diffusion of a gas is inversely related to the square root of its MW; the larger the molecule, the slower the diffusion. O_2 is a light gas (MW 32), and CO_2 is heavier (MW 44). However, diffusion is also directly proportional to solubility in tissue, and CO_2 is almost 30-fold more soluble than O_2. The aggregate effect is that CO_2 diffuses about 20-fold faster than O_2[82]; therefore, there is no lung disease compatible with life that measurably impairs CO_2 diffusion.

Intraoperative Respiratory Events

RESPIRATORY FUNCTION DURING ANESTHESIA

Anesthesia impairs pulmonary function, whether the patient is breathing spontaneously or is receiving mechanical ventilation. Impaired oxygenation of blood occurs in most subjects who are anesthetized,[83] and this is why supplemental O_2 (FiO_2 usually 0.3-0.5) is almost invariably used. Mild to moderate hypoxemia (SaO_2, 85% to 90%) is common and lasts from seconds to minutes; sometimes it is severe, and approximately 20% of patients may suffer from SaO_2 less than 81% for up to 5 minutes.[84] Indeed, greater than 50% of claims in anesthesia-related deaths relate to hypoxemia during anesthesia.[2] Beyond the operating room, the alterations in lung function acquired during anesthesia persist: clinically significant pulmonary complications can be seen in 1% to 2% of patients after minor surgery, and in up to 20% of patients after more major upper abdominal or thoracic surgery.[85] Such consequences of anesthesia place prime importance on ascertaining the causes of perioperative respiratory dysfunction and the clinical approaches to treatment.

In this section, we describe the effects of anesthesia and mechanical ventilation on lung function. The arrangement of this section parallels the sequence of events involved in oxygenating the blood and removing CO_2. Thus the first phenomenon that might be seen with anesthesia is loss of muscle tone with a subsequent change in the balance between outward forces (i.e., respiratory muscles) and inward forces (i.e., elastic tissue in the lung) leading to a fall in FRC. This causes or is paralleled by an increase in the elastic behavior of the lung (reduced compliance) and an increase in respiratory resistance. The decrease in FRC affects the patency of lung tissue with the formation of atelectasis (made worse with the use of high concentrations of inspired oxygen) and airway closure. This alters the distribution of ventilation and matching of ventilation and blood flow and impedes oxygenation of blood and removal of CO_2.

LUNG VOLUME AND RESPIRATORY MECHANICS DURING ANESTHESIA

Lung Volume

Resting lung volume (i.e., FRC) is reduced by almost 1 L by moving from upright to supine position; induction of anesthesia further decreases the FRC by approximately 0.5 L.[86] This reduces the FRC from approximately 3.5 to 2 L, a value close to RV. General anesthesia causes a fall in FRC (approximately 20%), whether breathing is controlled or spontaneous[87,88] and whether the anesthetic is inhalational or intravenous;[89] this is a major contributor to lowered oxygenation (discussed later). Muscle paralysis in the context of general anesthesia does not cause additional reduction in FRC.

The anatomic basis of the FRC reduction is not well understood. A landmark experiment on three volunteers using two-dimensional tomography suggested that a cephalad shift of the diaphragm, induced by anesthesia and paralysis, was responsible.[90] Recent studies using CT scanning also suggest cephalad diaphragm shift, as well as a decrease in the transverse chest area.[89,91] However, other data suggest little role for the diaphragm, with possible caudal (not cephalad) shift of its anterior aspect.[92] Simple CT suggests a cranial displacement, except in severe obstructive lung disease. Although the anatomic components of reduced FRC are debatable, the mechanism appears to be related to loss of respiratory muscle tone. FRC is maintained by a balance of the forces inward (lung recoil) versus forces outward (chest wall recoil, chest wall muscles, diaphragm). For example, maintenance of muscle tone using ketamine as the anesthetic does not reduce FRC.[89] Because patients are usually supine, the FRC will already have been reduced, and in elderly patients, this is particularly the case; in this context, the effects of anesthesia are more marked (see Fig. 13.9). As can be seen in the figure, FRC decreases with age assuming that weight does not change.

Compliance and Resistance of the Respiratory System

Static compliance of the total respiratory system (lungs and chest wall) is reduced on average from 95 to 60 mL/cm H_2O during anesthesia.[93] Most studies of lung compliance during anesthesia indicate a decrease compared with the awake state, and pooled data from several studies suggest that anesthesia is associated with a reduction in mean static compliance from almost 190 to approximately 150 mL/cm H_2O.[93] Data on changes in respiratory resistance are less clear. Although most studies suggest that anesthesia increases respiratory resistance, especially during mechanical ventilation,[93] no studies have corrected for lung volume and flow rates (both affect resistance considerably), and it is possible that changes in resistance occur merely because of volume (i.e., FRC) loss (Fig. 13.13).

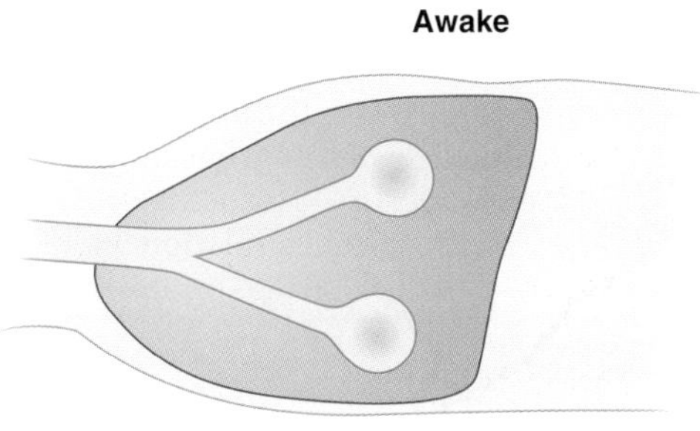

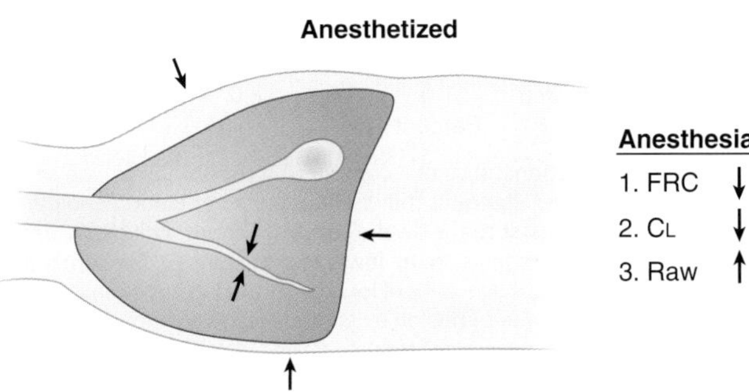

Fig. 13.13 Anesthesia induces cranial shift of the diaphragm and a decrease of transverse diameter of the thorax. These effects contribute to a lowered functional residual capacity *(FRC)*. The decreased ventilated volume (atelectasis and airway closure) can contribute to reduced compliance *(C_L)*. Decreased airway dimensions by the lowered FRC can contribute to increased airway resistance (Raw).

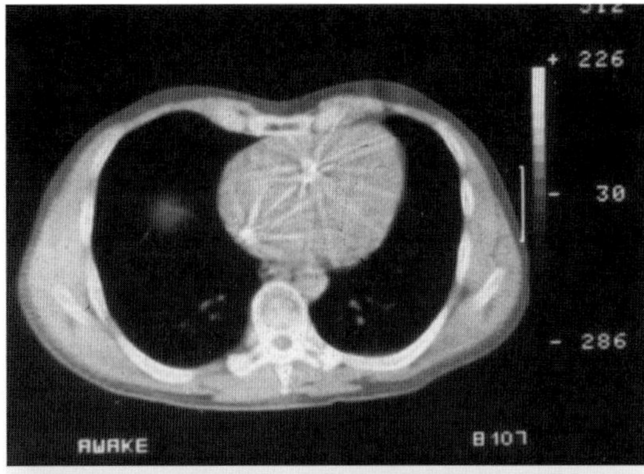

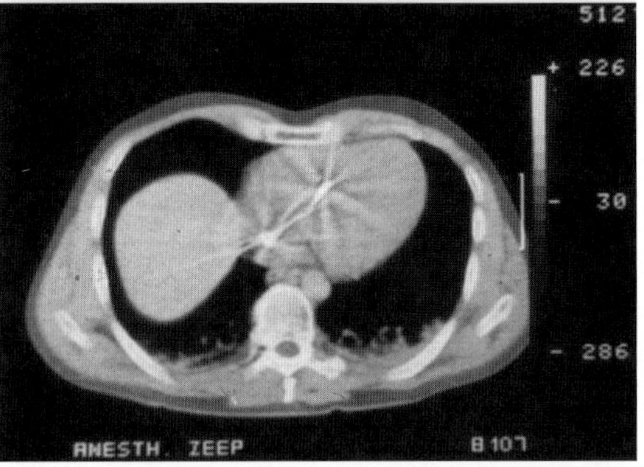

Fig. 13.14 Computed tomography with transverse exposures of the chest when the subject is awake *(upper panel)* and anesthetized *(lower panel)*. In the awake condition, the lung is well aerated (radiations from a pulmonary artery catheter are seen in the heart). During anesthesia, atelectasis has developed in the dependent regions *(grey/white irregular areas)*. The large grey/white area in the middle of the right lung field is caused by a cranial shift of the diaphragm and the underlying liver.

ATELECTASIS AND AIRWAY CLOSURE DURING ANESTHESIA

The classic article by Bendixen and colleagues[94] proposed "a concept of atelectasis" as a cause of impaired oxygenation and reduced respiratory compliance during anesthesia.[94] That study described a progressive decrease in compliance that paralleled decreases in oxygenation in both anesthetized humans and experimental animals, which was interpreted as progressive of atelectasis. However, others noticed an abrupt decrease in compliance and PaO_2 during induction of anesthesia, and yet atelectasis could not be shown on conventional chest radiography.

Since then, CT scanning has improved our knowledge of the nature of anesthesia-induced atelectasis, and the technique reveals prompt development of densities in the dependent regions of both lungs during anesthesia (data up to 1990 reviewed by Moller and associates).[84,95] Morphologic studies of these densities in various animals supported the diagnosis of atelectasis. An example of atelectasis as seen on a CT scan is shown in Fig. 13.14.

Atelectasis develops in approximately 90% of patients who are anesthetized, but it is unrelated to the choice of anesthesia.[96] It is seen during spontaneous breathing and after muscle paralysis, and with either intravenous or inhaled anesthetics.[89] The atelectatic area near the diaphragm is usually 5% to 6% of the total lung area, but can easily exceed 20%. The amount of lung tissue that is collapsed is larger, because the atelectatic area consists mostly of lung tissue, whereas normal aerated lung consists of 20% to 40% tissue (the rest being air). Thus 15% to 20% of the lung is atelectatic during uneventful anesthesia, before surgery has commenced; it decreases toward the apex, which usually remains aerated (Fig. 13.15). However, this degree of atelectasis is larger (upward of 50% of lung volume) after thoracic surgery or cardiopulmonary bypass, and can last for several hours.[97] Abdominal surgery adds little to the atelectasis, but after such surgery, it can persist for several days.[98]

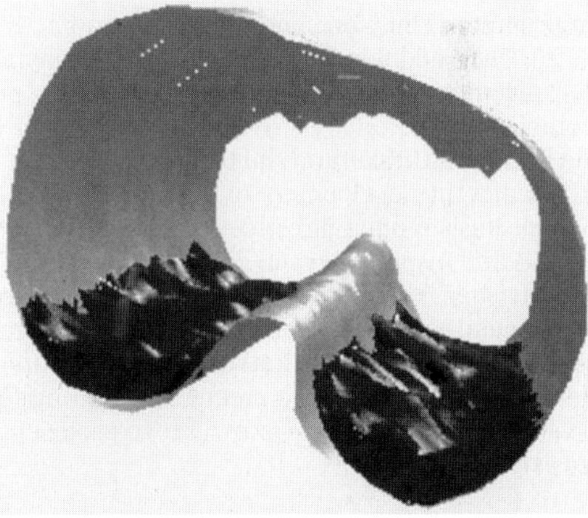

Fig. 13.15 A three-dimensional reconstruction of the thorax of an anesthetized patient with atelectasis in the dependent regions of both lungs. There is a slight decrease in the degree of atelectasis toward the apex (distal in this image). (Data from Reber A, Nylund U, Hedenstierna G. Position and shape of the diaphragm: implications for atelectasis formation. *Anaesthesia.* 1998;53:1054–1061.)

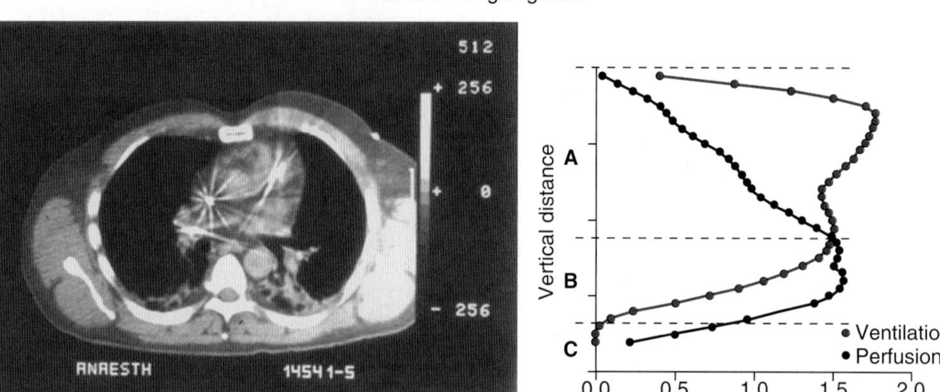

Fig. 13.16 Atelectasis and distribution of ventilation and blood flow. The *left panel* is a cross-sectional slice of a computed tomographic image of the chest of an anesthetized patient, illustrating atelectasis in the basal (dorsal) regions. The *right panel* illustrates the distribution of ventilation and perfusion throughout that slice. The bulk of the ventilation is to the upper lung region (zone *A*), in contrast to the awake subject without atelectasis, and it exceeds the level of local perfusion; this results in wasted ventilation (i.e., dead space) in the upper regions. In the lower region (zone *B*), the ventilation is less (probably because of intermittent airway closure) and is exceeded by the local perfusion, resulting in areas of low $\dot{V}_A/\dot{Q}$, causing hypoxemia. In the next lowest region (zone *C*), there is complete cessation of ventilation because of atelectasis, but some perfusion exists and causes a shunt. The farther from the top of the lung, the higher the perfusion; however, in the lowermost regions perfusion decreases (see text). (Data from Hedenstierna G. Alveolar collapse and closure of airways: regular effects of anaesthesia. *Clin Physiol Funct Imaging*. 2003;23:123–129.)

Atelectasis is an important cause of hypoxemia: there is a strong and significant correlation between the degree of atelectasis and the size of the pulmonary shunt (R = 0.81), where atelectasis is expressed as the percentage of lung area just above the diaphragm on CT scan and shunt is expressed as the percentage of cardiac output using the multiple inert gas elimination technique (MIGET).[96] The site of the increased shunt has been colocalized to the areas of atelectasis, using a technique that combines CT scanning and single photon emission computed tomography (SPECT; Fig. 13.16).[99] In addition to shunt, atelectasis may form a focus of infection and can certainly contribute to pulmonary complications.[100]

Aside from anesthesia (and the type of surgery), it is difficult to predict the development of atelectasis. The magnitude of atelectasis is often directly related to the body mass index (BMI) and inspired oxygen concentration.[87,89] Moreover, neither age[96] nor the presence of COPD[101] predicts the development or extent of atelectasis. In COPD, it may be that airway closure precedes (and therefore prevents) alveolar closure. Alternatively, the greater loss of lung (elastic recoil) versus chest wall tissue may serve to protect against atelectasis.

PREVENTION OF ATELECTASIS DURING ANESTHESIA

Several interventions can help prevent atelectasis[95] or even reopen collapsed tissue, as discussed in the following sections.

Positive End-Expiratory Pressure

The application of PEEP (10 cm H_2O) has been repeatedly demonstrated to reexpand atelectasis in part (Fig. 13.17). Some atelectasis may persist and might require higher PEEP and inspiratory airway pressure.[89] The application of larger levels of PEEP can have complex effects. Reversal of hypoxemia is not proportionally associated with applied PEEP, and a threshold exists in many cases. In addition, SaO_2 may decrease during the application of increased PEEP for two reasons. First, the increased P_{PL} owing to the PEEP can impair venous return, especially in the presence of hypovolemia, lowering the cardiac output and oxygen delivery (DO_2) and thereby reducing mixed venous O_2 content (C_vO_2). In the presence of an intrapulmonary shunt, such as with atelectasis, the mixed venous blood is shunted directly into pulmonary venous blood causing arterial desaturation. Second, increased PEEP can cause redistribution of blood flow away from the aerated, expanded regions (distended by PEEP) toward atelectatic areas (not distended by PEEP; Fig. 13.18).[102] In this context, persisting atelectasis in a dependent lung receives a larger proportion of the total pulmonary blood flow than without PEEP.[58] Finally, anesthesia-induced atelectasis rapidly reemerges after discontinuation of PEEP.[89] Indeed, Hewlett and coworkers[103] in 1974 cautioned against the "indiscriminate use of PEEP in routine anesthesia."

To avoid negative circulatory effects, the magnitude of PEEP should just be enough to open up a collapsed lung. A PEEP of 7 cm H_2O in normal-weight patients (BMI < 25 kg/m^2) without cardiopulmonary disease will recruit most of the lung, and keep it open with better oxygenation than in a comparable group without PEEP.[104] Thus a forceful dedicated recruit maneuver should not be needed. This effect was seen in nonabdominal surgery, and whether similar beneficial effect will be seen in abdominal surgery remains to be shown.

Recruitment Maneuvers

A sigh maneuver, or a large V_T, has been suggested for reversing atelectasis[10]; however, atelectasis is not uniformly reduced by a V_T increase or sigh up to P_{AW} of 20 cm H_2O.[105] Instead, a P_{AW} of 30 cm H_2O is required for initial opening, and 40 cm H_2O for more complete reversal (Fig. 13.19). In the presence of normal lungs, such inflation is equivalent to a VC and can therefore be called a *VC*

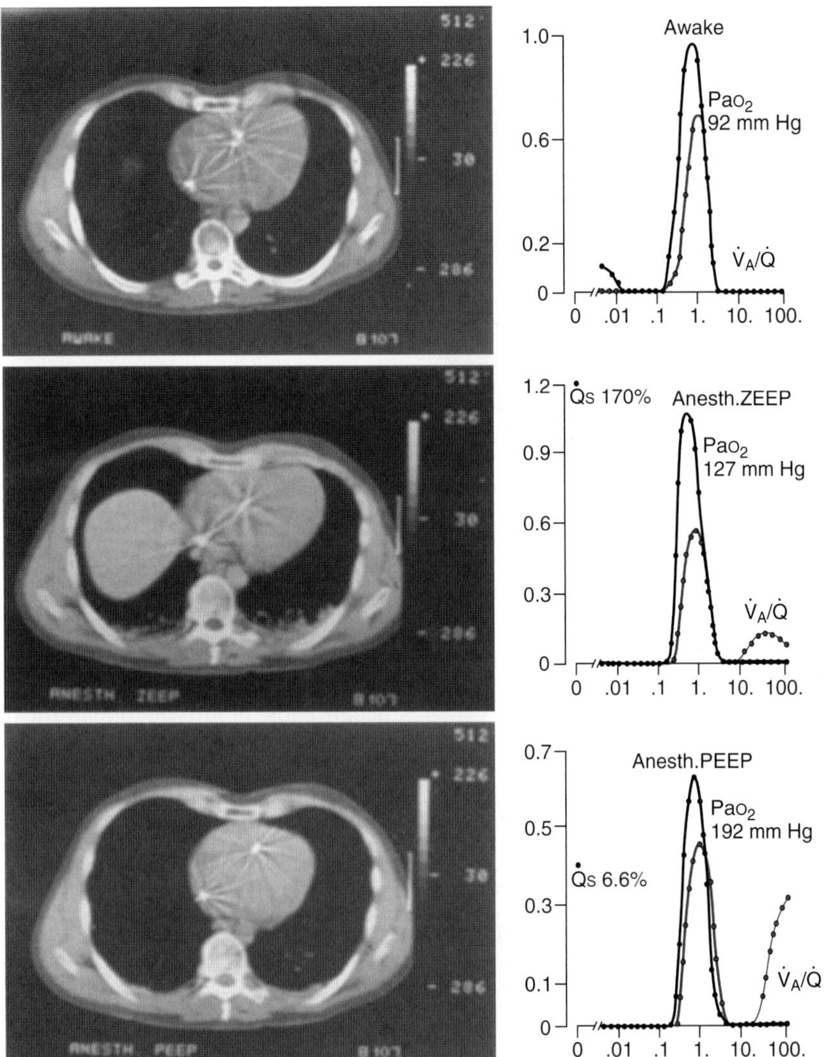

Fig. 13.17 Computed tomographic scans and $\dot{V}_A/\dot{Q}$ distributions in the lung of a healthy, awake subject during anesthesia (zero positive end-expiratory pressure *[ZEEP]*) and during anesthesia (10 cm H_2O positive end-expiratory pressure *[PEEP]*). In the awake state, there is no atelectasis and the corresponding minor low $\dot{V}_A/\dot{Q}$ distribution (*left side* of plot) may reflect intermittent airway closure. During anesthesia with ZEEP, atelectasis is apparent in the lung bases (and the diaphragm has been pushed cranially). The low $\dot{V}_A/\dot{Q}$ has been replaced by atelectasis and large shunt; in addition, a small "high" $\dot{V}_A/\dot{Q}$ mode (*right side* of plot) may reflect alveolar dead space in upper lung regions. With the addition of PEEP during anesthesia, the collapsed lung tissue has been recruited and the shunt has been reduced considerably. Moreover, the "high" $\dot{V}_A/\dot{Q}$ mode (*right side* of plot) has significantly increased; this may reflect additional inflation of nonperfused upper lung.

maneuver (albeit achieved with positive P_{AW}). In addition, a significant hemodynamic effect is likely if the VC maneuver is sustained; in fact, inflation with a P_{AW} of 40 cm H_2O for 7 to 8 seconds appears to successfully open almost all anesthesia-induced atelectasis.[106]

Minimizing Gas Resorption

Although recruitment of anesthesia-induced atelectasis is completely possible with either PEEP or a VC maneuver, continuous application of some level of PEEP is required to prevent rapid recurrence of the atelectasis.[107] However, nitrogen (N_2)—an insoluble gas that is not absorbed into the blood—can "splint" the alveolus if the alveolus is already opened. As a result, in anesthetized patients, a VC maneuver followed by ventilation with a gas mixture containing 60% N_2 (40% O_2) reduced the propensity for reaccumulation of atelectasis, with only 20% reappearing 40 minutes after recruitment.[107]

The same principles apply in the practice of preoxygenation of patients during induction of anesthesia. Here, the aim is to prevent O_2 desaturation (i.e., gain an O_2 safety margin) during induction before the airway has been secured when the anesthesiologist can better manage ventilation and oxygenation. Traditionally, the application of FiO_2 1.0 has been used. Although the SaO_2 is usually well maintained with this approach, atelectasis inevitably forms. The use of 30% versus 100% O_2 during induction was demonstrated in a clinical study to eliminate the formation of atelectasis.[108] Later, a comparison of breathing 100%, 80%, and 60% O_2 during induction demonstrated ubiquitous atelectasis with 100%, less with 80%, and even less with 60% O_2 (Fig. 13.20); however, the trade-off for less atelectasis was a shorter safety margin before occurrence of O_2 desaturation.[109]

An alternative approach may be continuous positive airway pressure (CPAP). Application of CPAP 10 cm

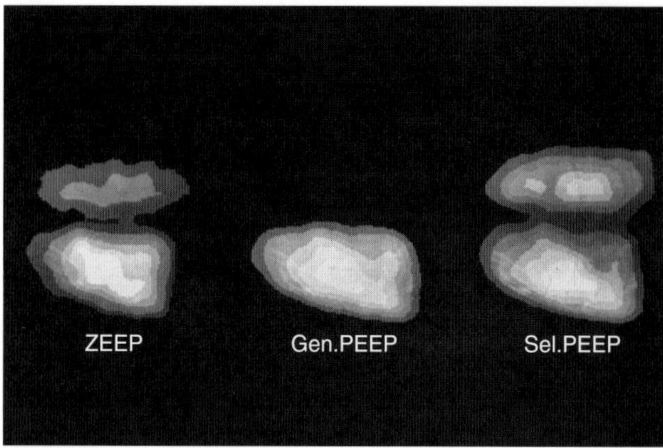

Fig. 13.18 Gamma camera images of lung blood flow in an anesthetized subject in the lateral position. During mechanical ventilation with zero end-expiratory pressure *(ZEEP)*, perfusion is predominantly (60%-70% of cardiac output) to the lower lung. Applying PEEP (10 cm H_2O) to both lungs forces more perfusion to the lower lung, leaving almost no perfusion to the upper lung (i.e., major increase in V_D). In contrast, selective application of PEEP to the lower lung causes redistribution of perfusion to the upper lung. Of course, the image presented is perfused tissue (not total anatomic lung tissue; in the right lateral position the upper-right lung would be larger). *PEEP*, Positive end-expiratory pressure. (From Hedenstierna G, Baehrendtz S, Klingstedt C, et al. Ventilation and perfusion of each lung during differential ventilation with selective PEEP. *Anesthesiology*. 1984;61:369–376.)

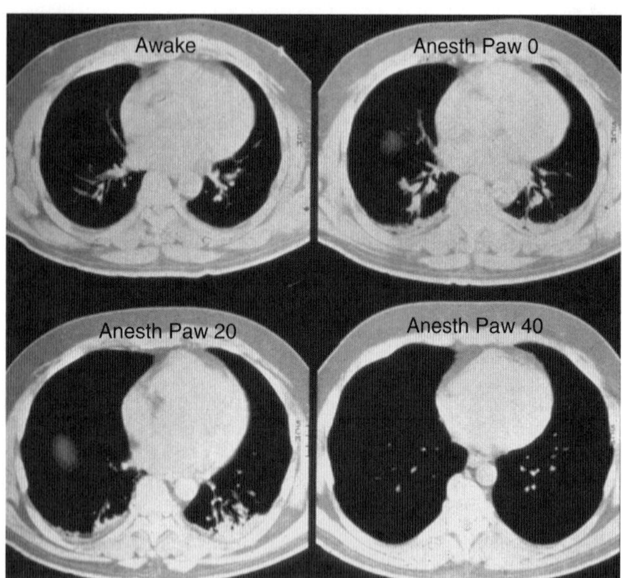

Fig. 13.19 Computed tomographic (CT) scans during awake and anesthetized states with altered airway pressure *(P_{AW})*. The CT scan in the awake subject *(upper left panel)* shows normal vasculature and no atelectasis. During anesthesia (P_{AW}, 0 cm H_2O; *upper right panel*), bilateral basal atelectasis is seen; the P_{AW} is increased in increments (20 cm H_2O shown), but the atelectasis is not reversed until a P_{AW} of 40 cm H_2O is applied (*lower right panel*). Thus a vital capacity maneuver was required to open the lung. (From Rothen HU, Sporre B, Engberg G, Wegenius G, Hedenstierna G. Re-expansion of atelectasis during general anaesthesia: a computed tomography study. *Br J Anaesth*. 1993;71:788–795.)

H_2O permitted the use of 100% inspired O_2 without formation of significant degrees of atelectasis.[110] This might provide an ideal combination of minimal risk of either O_2 desaturation or atelectasis, but it has not been repeatedly verified.

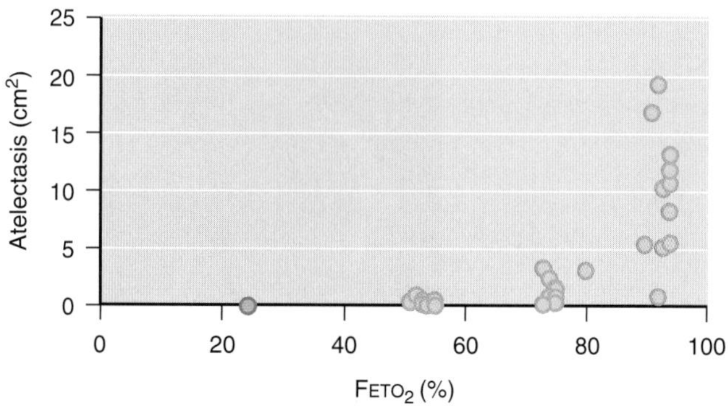

Fig. 13.20 Atelectasis formation in anesthetized subjects following preoxygenation with different inspired oxygen concentrations. Increasing the FiO_2 during preoxygenation increases the propensity to subsequent atelectasis (closed symbols), although there is much variability. The blue circle at around an expired oxygen concentration ($FETO_2$) of 25% represents data from anesthesia being induced while breathing 30% O_2. *$FETO_2$*, Expiratory oxygen fraction. (From Rothen HU, Sporre B, Engberg G, Wegenius G, Reber A, Hedenstierna G. Prevention of atelectasis during general anaesthesia. *Lancet*. 1995;345:1387–1391.)

Maintenance of Muscle Tone

Because loss of muscle tone in the diaphragm or chest wall appears to increase the risk of atelectasis, techniques that preserve muscle tone may have advantages. Intravenous ketamine does not impair muscle tone and is the only individual anesthetic that does not cause atelectasis. If neuromuscular blockade is added, atelectasis occurs as with other anesthetics.[90] Ketamine is an extremely useful anesthetic in special circumstances but has challenges with widespread use.

An experimental approach is restoration of respiratory muscle tone by diaphragm pacing. This approach is achieved with phrenic nerve stimulation, and it can modestly reduce the degree of atelectasis; however, the effect is minor and the approach is complicated.[111]

Atelectasis Following Surgery

Hypoxemia is common after anesthesia and surgery. It is enhanced by breathing oxygen before induction of anesthesia and suctioning of the airway (negative pressure) before extubation of the trachea. In addition, splinting and inhibition of coughing associated with pain can cause atelectasis postoperatively. Several approaches have been tried to address such atelectasis-associated hypoxemia following surgery. Administration of 100% O_2 coupled with a VC maneuver is not effective; this is probably because while the VC maneuver recruits the lung, the alveolar opening is not maintained (in fact closure is encouraged by the N_2-free O_2).[111] However, a VC maneuver followed by a lower O_2 concentration (40% O_2 in N_2) can maintain an open lung until the end of anesthesia.[106] Oxygenation is sustained for a longer period following ventilation with 50% O_2 in air (i.e., N_2) compared with 100%, following cardiopulmonary bypass.[113] In addition, use of 100% inspired oxygen before extubation increases the propensity to atelectasis[112] and treatment of postoperative hypoxemia, considered to be due to atelectasis, is associated with better outcomes when CPAP is used instead of 100% O_2.[114]

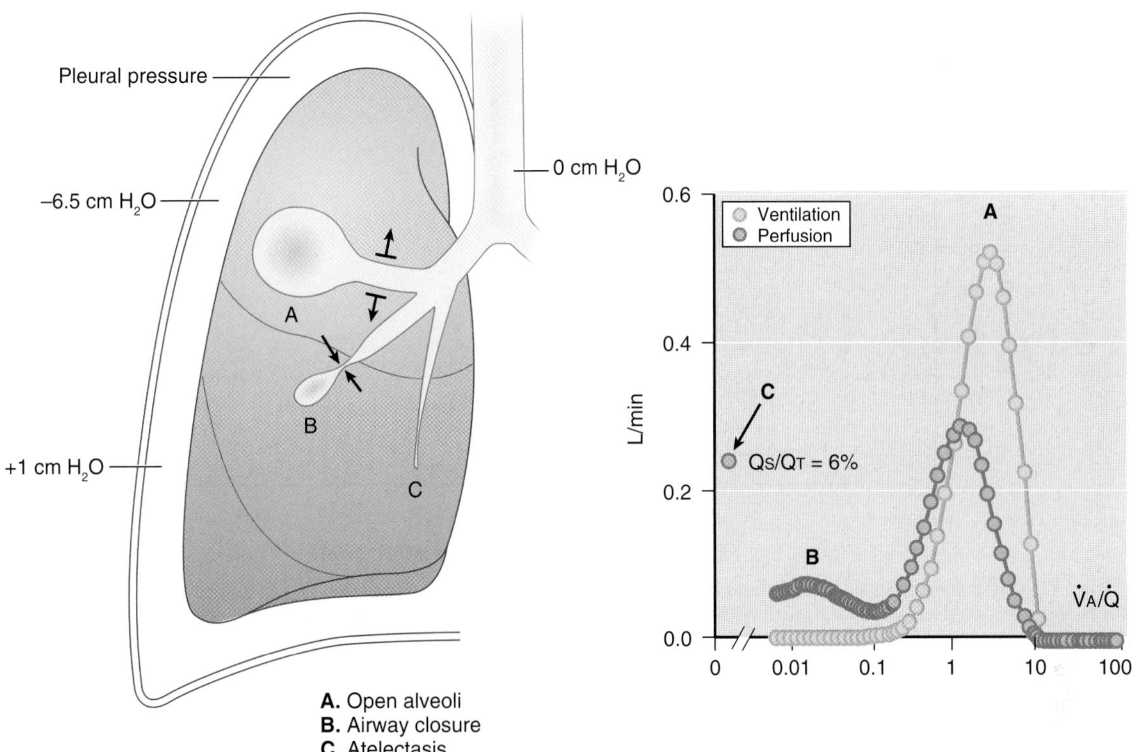

Fig. 13.21 A three-compartment model of ventilation and perfusion during anesthesia. In the upper regions, the alveoli and airways are open *(left panel, A)*. In the middle region, the airways are intermittently closed *(B)*, and atelectasis is present in the lower region *(C)*. The corresponding ventilation-perfusion distribution (multiple inert gas elimination technique) is illustrated in the *right panel*. Mode *A* reflects good ventilation and perfusion, whereas mode *B* reflects intermittent airway closure. In addition, there is a shunt in the atelectatic region (mode *C*). Q_S/Q_T, Venous admixture, or shunt equation.

AIRWAY CLOSURE

Intermittent airway closure reduces ventilation of the affected alveoli. Such lung regions can become regions of low $\dot{V}_A/\dot{Q}$ if perfusion is maintained or is not reduced to the same degree as ventilation. The propensity to airway closure increases with age (see Fig. 13.9),[49] as does perfusion to low $\dot{V}_A/\dot{Q}$ regions.[115] Anesthesia reduces FRC by about 0.5 L,[87] which increases airway closure during tidal ventilation.[116,117] In fact, the reduction in ventilation in the nonatelectatic lung (Fig. 13.21) is caused by airway closure. In addition, ventilation in these regions is less than perfusion (i.e., regions of low $\dot{V}_A/\dot{Q}$) and contributes to impaired oxygenation during anesthesia. Taken together, the combination of atelectasis and airway closure explain about 75% of the overall impairment in oxygenation.[88] In addition, where (CV–ERV) indicates the amount of airway closure occurring above FRC (and ERV is expiratory reserve volume), this value increased with induction of anesthesia, and there is good correlation between low $\dot{V}_A/\dot{Q}$ and the extent of airway closure.[88] In summary, a simple three-compartment lung model (normal $\dot{V}_A/\dot{Q}$ matching regions, region of airway closure, and atelectatic lung) describes well the components contributing to impairment of oxygenation during anesthesia (see Fig. 13.21).

DISTRIBUTION OF VENTILATION AND BLOOD FLOW DURING ANESTHESIA

Distribution of Ventilation

Redistribution of inspired gas away from dependent to nondependent lung regions has been demonstrated, using isotope techniques in anesthetized supine humans. Radiolabeled aerosol and SPECT demonstrate that ventilation is distributed mainly to the upper lung regions, with a successive decrease toward the lower lung regions, and an absence of ventilation in the lower-most regions, a finding consistent with the atelectasis demonstrable using CT (see Fig. 13.16).[100]

Recruitment maneuvers increase dependent lung ventilation in anesthetized subjects in the lateral[118] and supine[119] positions, restoring the distribution of ventilation to that in the awake state. Thus restoration of overall FRC toward the awake level returns gas distribution toward the awake pattern. The explanations are recruitment of atelectatic lung, reopening of closed airways, and further expansion of already expanded (upper) lung regions, decreasing regional compliance and lessening incremental ventilation.

Distribution of Lung Blood Flow

The distribution of lung blood flow has been studied by injection of radioactively labeled macroaggregated albumin and SPECT.[99] During anesthesia, a successive increase in perfusion occurs from upper toward lower regions, with a slight drop in perfusion in the lowermost portion of the lung, which is atelectatic on simultaneous CT (see Fig. 13.16). PEEP will impede venous return to the right heart and reduce cardiac output. It can also affect pulmonary vascular resistance, although this would have little effect on cardiac output. In addition, PEEP redistributes blood flow toward dependent lung regions,[59,119] reducing flow (and increasing dead space) in the upper lung; the increased dependent flow may increase shunt through atelectatic lung.[102]

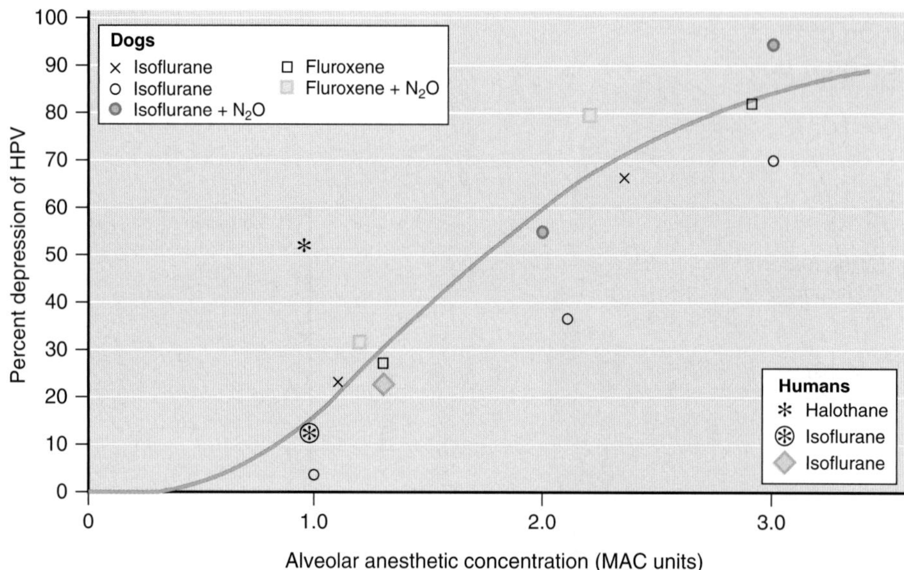

Fig. 13.22 Effect of inhaled anesthetics on hypoxic pulmonary vasoconstriction *(HPV)*. A concentration of 1 MAC causes a 20% to 30% depression of HPV, and the HPV depression decreases sharply with higher concentrations. The effect is that the shunt (i.e., perfusion through nonventilated regions) will be less reduced during inhalational anesthesia. *MAC*, Minimum alveolar concentration. (From Marshall BE. Hypoxic pulmonary vasoconstriction. *Acta Anaesthesiol Scand Suppl*. 1990;94:37–41.)

HYPOXIC PULMONARY VASOCONSTRICTION

Several inhaled—but not intravenous—anesthetics inhibit HPV in isolated lung preparations.[120] Human studies of HPV are complex with multiple parameters changing simultaneously, thereby confounding the HPV response with changes in cardiac output, myocardial contractility, vascular tone, blood volume distribution, pH, Pco_2, and lung mechanics. However, studies with no obvious changes in cardiac output indicated that isoflurane and halothane depress the HPV response by 50% at a minimum alveolar concentration (MAC) of 2 (Fig. 13.22).[121]

Ventilation-Perfusion Matching During Anesthesia

DEAD SPACE, SHUNT, AND VENTILATION-PERFUSION RELATIONSHIPS

CO_2 Elimination

Anesthesia impairs CO_2 elimination and oxygenation of blood. The explanation for reduced CO_2 elimination is reduced minute ventilation ($\dot{V}_E$) because of respiratory depression, or where this is preserved, because of an increase in the V_D/V_T. Single-breath wash out recordings demonstrate that "anatomic" dead space is unchanged, indicating that increased V_D/V_T is alveolar and confirmed by MIGET scan (Fig. 13.23).[10] Such high $\dot{V}_A/\dot{Q}$ can be explained by the perfusion of small corner vessels in interalveolar septa in the upper lung regions, where alveolar pressure can exceed pulmonary vascular pressure (zone I).[84] The impaired CO_2 elimination is most easily corrected by increasing the ventilation and is seldom a problem in routine anesthesia with mechanical ventilation.

Oxygenation

The impairment in arterial oxygenation during anesthesia is more marked with increased age, obesity, and

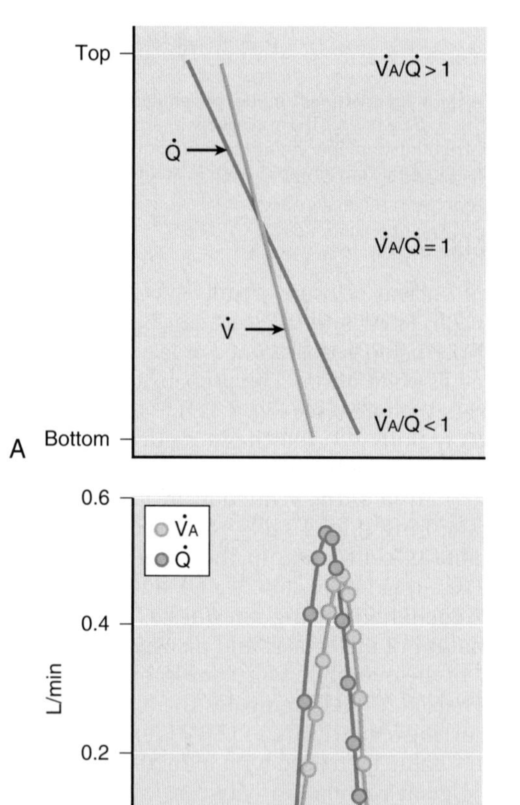

Fig. 13.23 A schematic drawing of (A) the vertical distributions of ventilation ($\dot{V}_A$) and blood flow through the lung ($\dot{Q}$) and (B) the resulting ventilation-perfusion distribution ($\dot{V}_A/\dot{Q}$). The $\dot{V}_A/\dot{Q}$ distribution is centered at a ratio of 1, corresponding to the intersection of the ventilation and perfusion distribution curves. The slightly larger ventilation than perfusion in upper lung regions contribute to the high $\dot{V}_A/\dot{Q}$ ratios greater than 1, whereas the larger perfusion than ventilation in the lower part of the lung is the cause of the lower $\dot{V}_A/\dot{Q}$ ratios, less than 1. Although there is a moderate increase in ventilation down the lung, the increase in perfusion is greater.

BOX 13.2 Derivation of the Venous Admixture (Shunt) Equation

$$Ca \times \dot{Q}_T = \left(Cc' \times \dot{Q}_C\right) + \left(C_{\bar{v}} \times \dot{Q}_S\right) \quad (1)$$

$$\dot{Q}_C = \dot{Q}_T - \dot{Q}_S \quad (2)$$

By inserting Equation (2) (accounts for all blood flow through the lungs) into Equation (1) (accounts for all oxygen carriage through the lungs),

$$Ca \times \dot{Q}_T = \left(C_c \times \left[\dot{Q}_T - \dot{Q}_S\right]\right) + \left(C_{\bar{v}} \times \dot{Q}_S\right)$$

Rearranging,

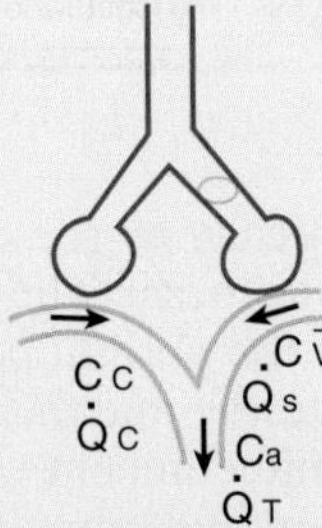

$$\frac{\dot{Q}_S}{\dot{Q}_T} = \frac{Cc' - Ca}{Cc' - C\bar{V}}$$

where Cc′, Ca, and Cv are oxygen content in pulmonary end-capillary, arterial, and mixed venous blood, respectively; $\dot{Q}_T$ is cardiac output; $\dot{Q}_C$ is capillary flow; and $\dot{Q}_S$ is shunt.

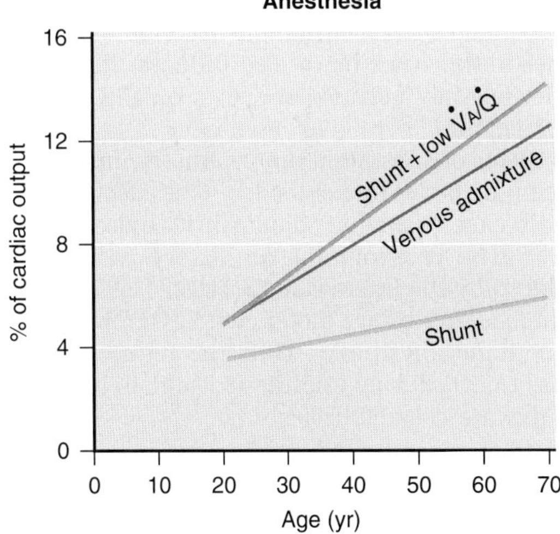

Fig. 13.24 **The effect of age on oxygenation during anesthesia. The combination of shunt with low $\dot{V}_A/\dot{Q}$ increases sharply with age (as does the degree of venous admixture). The increase in shunt with age, while significant, is less striking.** (From Gunnarsson L, Tokics L, Gustavsson H, Hedenstierna G. Influence of age on atelectasis formation and gas exchange impairment during general anaesthesia. *Br J Anaesth.* 1991;66:423–432.)

smoking.[122,123] Venous admixture, as calculated by the standard oxygen shunt equation, is also increased during anesthesia to approximately 10% of cardiac output. However, this is an averaged calculation that considers hypoxia caused by pure shunt only, when actually it is due to a combination of "true" shunt (i.e., perfusion of nonventilated lung), poor ventilation of some regions, and regions that are ventilated but are perfused in excess of their ventilation (low $\dot{V}_A/\dot{Q}$ regions). The combination of these effects is called *venous admixture*. The shunt equation (derived in Box 13.2) assumes that all blood flow through the lung goes to either of two compartments: in one (the non–shunt fraction), all the blood is oxygenated; and in the other (the shunt fraction), all blood is shunted.

The shunt equation (or venous admixture) can be written:[124]

$$\frac{\dot{Q}_S}{\dot{Q}_T} = \frac{(C_cO_2 - C_aO_2)}{(C_cO_2 - C_{\bar{v}}O_2)}$$

Because pulmonary end-capillary blood is assumed to be maximally saturated (therefore, $S_cO_2 = 1$), the quantity of dissolved O_2 can be ignored, and it can be the difference between $C_{\bar{v}}O_2$, and $C_{\bar{v}}O_2$ can be assumed to be small ($C_vO_2 = C_{\bar{v}}O_2$):

$$\frac{\dot{Q}_S}{\dot{Q}_T} = \frac{(1 - S_ao_2)}{(1 - S_vo_2)}$$

Thus the effect of interventions on estimated shunt can be calculated easily from the changes in SaO_2 and SvO_2.

The extent of venous admixture depends on the inspired oxygen fraction (FiO_2). The higher the inspired oxygen fraction, the less there are of the low $\dot{V}_A/\dot{Q}$ regions. However, with high FiO_2, regions with low $\dot{V}_A/\dot{Q}$ may collapse because of gas adsorption and be transformed to shunt regions.[125] A good correlation between venous admixture versus the sum of "true" shunt and perfusion of low $\dot{V}_A/\dot{Q}$ regions was seen in a study involving 45 anesthetized subjects (Fig. 13.24).[97] Derivation of the "oxygen shunt" or venous admixture is shown in Box 13.2.

In young healthy volunteers during anesthesia with thiopental and methoxyflurane, both ventilation and perfusion were distributed to wider ranges of $\dot{V}_A/\dot{Q}$ ratios, which can be expressed as an increase in the logarithmic standard deviation of the perfusion distribution (log SD$\dot{Q}$). In a similar group of patients studied during halothane anesthesia and muscle paralysis, log SD$\dot{Q}$ was almost doubled (0.43 awake, 0.80 during anesthesia). In addition, true shunt was increased to a mean of 8%. A similar increase in shunt from 1% awake to a mean of 9% during anesthesia was recorded in a study on middle-aged (37 to 64 years) surgical patients, and there was a widening of the distribution (log SD$\dot{Q}$: 0.47 awake, 1.01 during anesthesia). In older patients with more severe impairment of lung function, halothane anesthesia with muscle paralysis, with or without nitrous oxide, caused considerable widening of the $\dot{V}_A/\dot{Q}$ distribution (log SD$\dot{Q}$ 0.87 awake, 1.73 during anesthesia). In addition, shunt increased to a mean of 15%, with large variation among patients (0% to 30%). Thus the most consistent findings during anesthesia are an increased $\dot{V}_A/\dot{Q}$ mismatch, expressed as an increased log SDQ, and an increase in shunt. For review, see the article by Hedenstierna.[83]

Spontaneous ventilation is frequently reduced during anesthesia because inhaled anesthetics[126] or barbiturates[127] reduce sensitivity to CO_2. The response is dose-dependent and ventilation decreases with deepening anesthesia. Anesthesia also reduces the response to hypoxia, possibly because of effects on the carotid body chemoreceptors.[128]

The effects of anesthesia on respiratory muscle function are becoming better understood.[129] The effects are not uniform. Rib cage excursions diminish with deepening anesthesia.[130] The predominant ventilatory response to CO_2 is produced by the intercostal muscles,[131, 132] but with no clear increase in rib cage motion with CO_2 rebreathing during halothane anesthesia. Thus the reduced ventilatory response to CO_2 during anesthesia is due to impeded function of the intercostal muscles.

Factors that Influence Respiratory Function During Anesthesia

SPONTANEOUS BREATHING

Most studies of lung function have been performed on anesthetized, mechanically ventilated subjects or animals. Spontaneous breathing has been studied rarely. FRC decreases to the same extent during anesthesia, regardless of whether a muscle relaxant is used,[90,91] and atelectasis occurs to almost the same extent in anesthetized, spontaneously breathing subjects as during muscle paralysis.[133] Furthermore, the cranial shift of the diaphragm, as reported by Froese and Bryan,[90] was of the same magnitude both during general anesthesia with spontaneous breathing and with muscle paralysis, even though a difference in movement of the diaphragm from the resting position was noted. Thus, during spontaneous breathing, the lower, dependent portion of the diaphragm moved the most, whereas with muscle paralysis, the upper, nondependent part showed the largest displacement.

All these findings have raised the question of whether regional ventilation is different between spontaneous breathing and mechanical ventilation and whether mechanical ventilation worsens $\dot{V}_A/\dot{Q}$ as a consequence of poor ventilation of well-perfused, dependent lung regions. However, there is not much support for worsening of gas exchange by muscle paralysis if the lungs are normal (in contrast to injured lungs); there is also little support from the few studies of $\dot{V}_A/\dot{Q}$ distribution that have been performed. Dueck and colleagues[134] found the same increase in $\dot{V}_A/\dot{Q}$ mismatch in anesthetized sheep during anesthesia, regardless of whether they were spontaneously breathing or ventilated mechanically. The log SDQ, indicating the degree of mismatch, increased (0.66 [awake], 0.83 [inhaled anesthesia with spontaneous breathing], 0.89 [mechanical ventilation]). Shunt is also increased during anesthesia from 1% (awake) to 11% (anesthetized, spontaneous breathing) or 14% (anesthetized, mechanical ventilation). In a study of anesthetized human subjects, shunt and log SDQ increased from 1% and 0.47 while awake to 6% and 1.03 during anesthesia with spontaneous breathing and 8% and 1.01 during mechanical ventilation.[83] Thus most of the gas exchange effects of anesthesia occurs during spontaneous breathing, with little or no further derangement added by muscle paralysis and mechanical ventilation.

INCREASED OXYGEN FRACTION

In the studies cited thus far, an inspired oxygen fraction (FiO_2) of approximately 0.4 was used. Anjou-Lindskog and colleagues[135] induced anesthesia in subjects breathing air (FiO_2, 0.21) in middle-aged to older patients during intravenous anesthesia before elective lung surgery and found only small shunts of 1% to 2%, although log SDQ increased from 0.77 to 1.13. When FiO_2 was increased to 0.5, the shunt increased (by 3% to 4%). In another study of older patients during halothane anesthesia,[83] an increase in FiO_2 from 0.53 to 0.85 caused an increase in shunt from 7% to 10% of cardiac output. Thus increasing FiO_2 increases shunt, possibly because of attenuation of HPV by increasing FiO_2[121] or further development of atelectasis and shunt in lung units with low $\dot{V}_A/\dot{Q}$ ratios.[125]

BODY POSITION

FRC is reduced dramatically by the combined effect of the supine position and anesthesia. The effects on the FRC of inducing anesthesia in the upright position were tested by Heneghan and associates,[136] and there was no difference in oxygenation in the semirecumbent versus supine position. Decreased cardiac output and inhomogeneity of blood flow can outweigh any effects of posture. Fractional perfusion of the most dependent lung regions—likely poorly or not ventilated—may actually have been increased in the semirecumbent position. In the lateral position, differences in lung mechanics, resting lung volumes, and atelectasis formation between the dependent and nondependent portions of the lung have been demonstrated[137] and shown to result in further disturbance of the ventilation-perfusion match, with severe impairment in oxygenation. However, there are large and unpredictable inter-individual variations.[138] Using isotope techniques, an increase in $\dot{V}_A/\dot{Q}$ mismatch was also demonstrated in anesthetized, paralyzed patients in the lateral position,[139] and an improvement was noticed in the prone position.[140] In addition, the vertical inhomogeneity of perfusion distribution is less marked in the prone position,[68] possibly reflecting regional differences in vascular configuration that promote perfusion of dorsal lung regions, regardless of whether they are in a dependent or nondependent position. Finally, distribution of ventilation may be uniform in anesthetized subjects when prone.[141]

AGE

Oxygenation is less efficient in older patients.[10] However, the formation of atelectasis does not increase with age in adults, and the few CT studies of infants during anesthesia suggest greater degrees of atelectasis.[96] In addition, shunt is independent of age between 23 and 69 years. However, $\dot{V}_A/\dot{Q}$ mismatch increases with age, with enhanced perfusion of low $\dot{V}_A/\dot{Q}$ regions when awake and when anesthetized. The major cause of impaired gas exchange during anesthesia in those younger than 50 years is shunt, whereas beyond 50 years, $\dot{V}_A/\dot{Q}$ mismatch (i.e., increased log SDQ) becomes increasingly important (see Fig. 13.24). Because the correlation between log SDQ and age during anesthesia is almost parallel with that during the awake state, it can be said that anesthesia worsens $\dot{V}_A/\dot{Q}$ matching to the same extent as 20 years of aging.

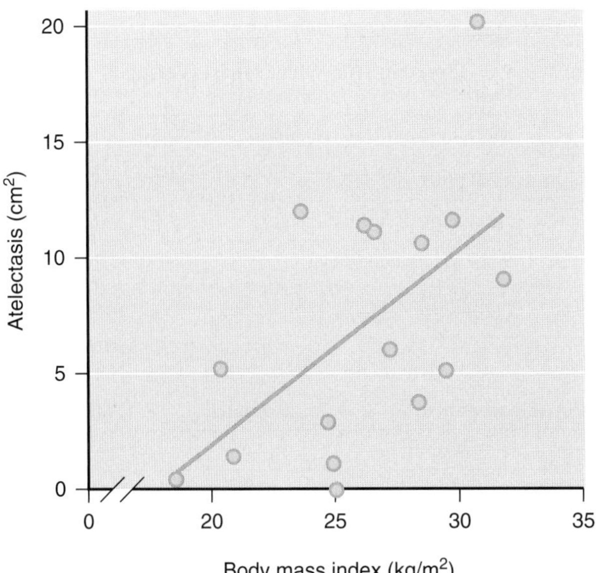

Fig. 13.25 Relationship between body mass index (BMI) and extent of atelectasis during general anesthesia. As BMI increases, so does the extent of atelectasis (although there is considerable variability). (From Rothen HU, Sporre B, Engberg G, Wegenius G, Hedenstierna G. Re-expansion of atelectasis during general anaesthesia: a computed tomography study. *Br J Anaesth.* 1993;71:788–795.)

OBESITY

Obesity worsens oxygenation[142,143] predominantly because of reduced FRC resulting in a greater propensity to airway closure.[144] In addition, the use of high inspired oxygen concentrations promotes rapid atelectasis formation in alveoli distal to closed airways,[87,109] and the atelectasis seems to be larger than in normal weight subjects (Fig. 13.25).[144,145]

Preventing a decrease in FRC by applying CPAP during induction of anesthesia probably reduces atelectasis formation, and thereby maintains oxygenation.[123,146,147] Indeed, the reduced "safety window" (the time taken to develop desaturation following breathing oxygen before induction of anesthesia) is much reduced in obese patients, and this may be prolonged by PEEP or CPAP[148] increasing lung volume and increasing the reservoir of O_2 available for diffusion into the capillary blood.

The use of high levels of inspired oxygen concentration, often almost 100%, to keep an acceptable level of oxygenation during anesthesia and surgery may be the simplest but not necessarily the best approach. It will promote further atelectasis formation,[108] and if the shunt is larger than 30%, which may be the case in these patients, additional oxygen will add little to arterial oxygenation.[149] The application of PEEP has been advocated, and it may reduce the atelectasis[122,144,146] but may also have adverse effects, such as propensity for aspiration, reduced cardiac output, and redistribution of blood flow toward residual collapsed lung regions. Ventilation with inflations close to VC to reopen collapsed tissue, followed by ventilation with added PEEP, is another option. Recruitment of the lung with inflation to 55 cm H_2O opened essentially all collapsed lung tissue in patients with a BMI of 40 kg/m^2 or more.[150] However, a recruitment alone did not keep the lung open for more than a few minutes. To keep the lung open, a PEEP of 10 cm H_2O after the recruitment was needed, and PEEP of 10 was not enough to open up the lung.[150] Body position can have a substantial effect on lung volume and should be considered to the extent that surgery allows.[151]

PREEXISTING LUNG DISEASE

Smokers and patients with chronic lung disease have impaired gas exchange in the awake state, and anesthesia-associated deterioration in oxygenation is greater than in healthy individuals.[10] Interestingly, smokers with moderate airflow limitation may have less shunt as measured by MIGET than in subjects with healthy lungs. Thus, in patients with mild to moderate bronchitis who were to undergo lung surgery or vascular reconstructive surgery in the leg, only a small shunt was noticed, but log SDQ was increased.[83] In patients with chronic bronchitis studied by MIGET and CT, no or limited atelectasis developed during anesthesia and no or only minor shunt;[101] however, a considerable mismatch was seen with a large perfusion fraction to low $\dot{V}_A/\dot{Q}$ regions. Consequently, arterial oxygenation was more impaired than in lung-healthy subjects, but the cause was different from that in healthy subjects. A possible reason for the absence of atelectasis and shunt in these patients is chronic hyperinflation, which changes the mechanical behavior of the lungs and their interaction with the chest wall such that the tendency to collapse is reduced. It should be kept in mind that a patient with obstructive lung disease may have large regions with low $\dot{V}_A/\dot{Q}$ ratios that can be converted over time to resorption atelectasis. Thus the protection against atelectasis formation during anesthesia by the obstructive lung disease might not last long. Regions with low $\dot{V}_A/\dot{Q}$ can be replaced by atelectasis as a result of slow absorption of gas behind occluded airways later during surgery and in the postoperative period.

REGIONAL ANESTHESIA

The ventilatory effects of regional anesthesia depend on the type and extension of motor blockade. With extensive blocks that include all the thoracic and lumbar segments, inspiratory capacity is reduced by 20% and expiratory reserve volume approaches zero.[152,153] Diaphragmatic function, however, is often spared, even in cases of inadvertent extension of subarachnoid or epidural sensory block up to the cervical segments.[152] Skillfully handled regional anesthesia affects pulmonary gas exchange only minimally. Arterial oxygenation and CO_2 elimination are well maintained during spinal and epidural anesthesia. This is in line with the findings of an unchanged relationship of CC and FRC,[154] and unaltered distributions of ventilation-perfusion ratios as assessed by MIGET during epidural anesthesia.[83]

CAUSES OF HYPOXEMIA AND HYPERCAPNIA

In the previous sections, we discussed ventilation, gas distribution, and the respiratory mechanics that govern distribution, diffusion, and pulmonary perfusion. All these components of lung function can affect the oxygenation of blood, and all except diffusion can also measurably affect CO_2 elimination. The different mechanisms behind hypoxemia and CO_2 retention, or hypercapnia or hypercarbia, have been mentioned previously but will be analyzed in more detail here.

TABLE 13.1 Causes of Hypoxemia

Disturbance	Pao_2 (Breathing Air) at Rest	Pao_2 (Breathing Oxygen) at Rest	Pao_2 (Breathing Air) With Exercise (Versus Rest)	$Paco_2$
Hypoventilation	Reduced	Normal	No change or further decrease	Increased
$\dot{V}_A/\dot{Q}$ mismatch	Reduced	Normal	No change or minor increase or decrease	Normal
Shunt	Reduced	Reduced	No change or further decrease	Normal
Diffusion impairment	Reduced	Normal	Small to large decrease	Normal

TABLE 13.2 Mechanisms of Hypoxemia in Different Lung Disorders

Disorder	Hypoventilation	Diffusion Impairment	$\dot{V}_A/\dot{Q}$ Mismatch	Shunt
Chronic bronchitis	(+)	–	++	–
Emphysema	+	++	+++	–
Asthma	–	–	++	–
Fibrosis	–	++	+	+
Pneumonia	–	–	+	++
Atelectasis	–	–	–	++
Pulmonary edema	–	+	+	++
Pulmonary emboli	–	–	++	+
Acute respiratory distress syndrome	–	–	+	+++

+++ Most Important; ++ Important; + Somewhat Important; – Unimportant.

Causes of hypoxemia include hypoventilation, $\dot{V}_A/\dot{Q}$ mismatch, impaired diffusion, and right-to-left shunt (Table 13.1). Hypercapnia is usually caused by hypoventilation, although it can be caused by $\dot{V}_A/\dot{Q}$ mismatch and shunt (Table 13.2). Increased $\dot{V}CO_2$ occurs in hypermetabolic conditions (e.g., fever, malignant hyperthermia, thyroid crisis) or with the use of CO_2-generating buffers such as sodium bicarbonate ($NaHCO_3$).

HYPOVENTILATION

If ventilation is low relative to metabolic demand, elimination of CO_2 will be inadequate, and CO_2 will accumulate in the alveoli, blood, and other body tissues. Hypoventilation is often defined as ventilation that results in a $Paco_2$ greater than 45 mm Hg (6 kPa). Thus hypoventilation could be present even when minute ventilation is high, provided the metabolic demand or dead space ventilation is increased to a greater extent.

The increased alveolar Pco_2 reduces the alveolar space available for oxygen. Alveolar PO_2 (PAO_2) can be estimated by the alveolar gas equation (see Box 13.1). The simplified equation is expressed:

$$PAO_2 = P_IO_2 - \left(\frac{PACO_2}{R}\right)$$

Assuming that the respiratory exchange ratio (R) is 0.8 (more or less true at rest), PAO_2 can be estimated. In the ideal lung, PaO_2 equals PAO_2. For example, if PiO_2 is 149 mm Hg (19.9 kPa) and $Paco_2$ is 40 mm Hg (5.3 kPa), then PaO_2 is 99 mm Hg (13.2 kPa). If hypoventilation develops and the $Paco_2$ rises to 60 mm Hg (8 kPa) and there is no other gas exchange impairment, the PaO_2 will fall to 74 mm Hg (9.9 kPa). Clearly, a decrease in PaO_2 caused by hypoventilation is easily overcome by increasing PiO_2 (i.e., by increasing FiO_2). If there is a gap between the PAO_2 (estimated from this equation) and the measured (actual) PaO_2, then a cause of hypoxemia in addition to hypoventilation is present. These causes are discussed in the following sections.

VENTILATION-PERFUSION MISMATCH

For optimal gas exchange, ventilation and perfusion must match each other in all lung regions. At rest, both ventilation and perfusion increase downward through the lung. However, perfusion increases more than ventilation, the difference between the uppermost and lowermost 5-cm segments being threefold for ventilation and tenfold for perfusion. This change results in a mean $\dot{V}_A/\dot{Q}$ ratio of approximately 1 somewhere in the middle of the lung and a range of $\dot{V}_A/\dot{Q}$ ratios (0.5 at the bottom, 5.0 in the apex; see Fig. 13.23, upper panel, the perfusion distribution being a simplified drawing of Fig. 13.11).

Another way of showing the matching between ventilation and blood flow is by illustrating a multicompartmental analysis of ventilation and distribution of blood flow against $\dot{V}_A/\dot{Q}$ ratios. This can be achieved with MIGET.[155] In short, MIGET is based on the constant intravenous infusion of a number of inert gases (usually six) with differing solubilities in blood. When passing through the lung capillaries, the different gases are eliminated via the alveoli and expired in indirect proportion to their solubility. A poorly

TABLE 13.3 Mean (SD) Ventilation-Perfusion Relationships With No Cardiopulmonary Disease (Normal, $N = 45$), Awake and During General Anesthesia and Muscle Paralysis

	$\dot{Q}$ mean	log SD$\dot{Q}$	$\dot{V}$ mean	log SD$\dot{V}$	Shunt (% Q_T)	Dead Space (% V_T)	PaO_2/FIO_2 (kPa)
Awake	0.76 (0-33)	0.68 (0.28)	1.11 (0.52)	0.52 (0.15)	0.5 (1.0)	34.8 (14.2)	59.5 (8.1)
Anesthetized	0.65 (0.34)	1.04 (0.36)	1.38 (0.76)	0.76 (0.31)	4.8 (4.1)	35.0 (9.9)	50.9 (15.2)

log SD$\dot{Q}$, Standard deviations of the logarithmic distribution of perfusion; log SD$\dot{V}$, standard deviations of the logarithmic distribution of ventilation; $\dot{Q}$ mean, mean $\dot{V}_A/\dot{Q}$ of the perfusion distribution; $\dot{V}$ mean, mean $\dot{V}_A/\dot{Q}$ of ventilation distribution. (Gunnarsson L, Tokics L, Gustavsson H, Hedenstierna G. Influence of age on atelectasis formation and gas exchange impairment during general anaesthesia. Br J Anaesth. 1991;66:423–432).

soluble gas will rapidly leave the bloodstream and be more or less completely eliminated and exhaled (e.g., sulfur hexafluoride); a gas with a high solubility in the blood will be almost completely retained in the blood and will not be exhaled (e.g., acetone); and a gas of intermediate solubility will be retained (and expired) to an intermediate extent (e.g., halothane).

As a result, the concentration of the different gases in arterial blood will differ, with higher concentrations of gases with high solubility. Retention can be calculated as the ratio between arterial and mixed venous blood concentrations. Similarly, the ratio of the concentrations (i.e., expired:mixed venous) can be calculated and gives the excretion for each gas. With knowledge of the retention, excretion, and solubility of each gas, an essentially continuous distribution of blood flow against $\dot{V}_A/\dot{Q}$ ratios can be constructed. The lower panel in Fig. 13.23 shows an example from a healthy subject. Note that ventilation and blood flow are well matched, being distributed to a limited number of compartments centered on a $\dot{V}_A/\dot{Q}$ ratio of 1. MIGET has a high discriminatory capacity of detecting different $\dot{V}_A/\dot{Q}$ disturbances, but does not provide topographic information. Several variables that reflect the degree of mismatch can be calculated and are shown in Table 13.3. In the following paragraphs, examples of $\dot{V}_A/\dot{Q}$ mismatch are discussed.

If ventilation and perfusion are not matched, gas exchange will be affected. The most common cause of impaired oxygenation is $\dot{V}_A/\dot{Q}$ mismatch. Low $\dot{V}_A/\dot{Q}$ will impede oxygenation because ventilation is insufficient to fully oxygenate the blood, and the degree of impairment is dependent on the degree of $\dot{V}_A/\dot{Q}$ mismatch; in fact, even normal lung regions $\dot{V}_A/\dot{Q}$ (0.5-1) cannot completely saturate the blood. Thus PaO_2 cannot equal alveolar PO_2, and a difference (PAO_2–PaO_2) of 3 to 5 mm Hg (0.4-0.7 kPa) is normal. With greater $\dot{V}_A/\dot{Q}$ mismatch, the PAO_2–PaO_2 difference is further increased. The $\dot{V}_A/\dot{Q}$ mismatch can account for all the hypoxemia seen in a patient with severe obstruction.[115] Shunt ($\dot{Q}$, but no $\dot{V}_A$), which is often claimed to exist in patients with COPD, is mostly absent when analyzed with a more sophisticated technique such as MIGET. Indeed, shunt in a patient with obstruction likely represents a complicating factor in the disease (Fig. 13.26).

In severe asthma, a distinct bimodal pattern of low ratios occurs when using MIGET (see Fig. 13.26).[156] The reason may be that alveoli behind airways obstructed by edema (or a mucous plug or spasm) can still be ventilated by collateral ventilation (i.e., alveolar pores, interbronchial communications); these regions would otherwise be shunt (no $\dot{V}_A$, some $\dot{Q}$), resulting in the additional peak in $\dot{V}_A/\dot{Q}$ explaining the bimodal distribution. Such collateral ventilation might be part of the reason that true shunt is not normally seen in COPD. Of course, if the standard shunt equation is used to explain hypoxemia, there is no capacity to distinguish between the contributions of low $\dot{V}_A/\dot{Q}$ versus shunt to hypoxemia (the net effect is best called *venous admixture*).

Airway obstruction is distributed unevenly, and a large variation in $\dot{V}_A/\dot{Q}$ ratios results. Indeed, ventilation is redistributed from regions with high airway resistance to other regions that can then become overventilated in proportion to their perfusion; this causes high $\dot{V}_A/\dot{Q}$ ratios. There are normally regions in the apex that have ratios of up to 5, but ratios of 100 or more exist in patients with obstruction, making the regions practically indistinguishable from true dead space; this is what causes the increase in physiologic dead space in obstructive lung disease. The effect of high $\dot{V}_A/\dot{Q}$ is also the same as for airway dead space—that is, ventilation that seems not to participate in gas exchange ("wasted ventilation"). Consequently, a patient with COPD has low $\dot{V}_A/\dot{Q}$ (impedes oxygenation) and high $\dot{V}_A/\dot{Q}$ (mimics dead space, impedes CO_2 elimination). However, MIGET is a complex, research-orientated tool, and the calculation of dead space for clinical purposes relies instead on expired CO_2. Derivation of the CO_2 dead space is shown in Box 13.3.

$\dot{V}_A/\dot{Q}$ mismatch exists to varying degrees in all patients with COPD, and it fully explains hypoxemia in most of them. Hypoventilation can also contribute, whereas impaired diffusion or shunt rarely contributes to hypoxemia. Diffusion capacity, or transfer test, can be reduced markedly in severe COPD, in particular in emphysema; in this case the decrease is not caused by thickened alveolar-capillary membranes but rather by reduced capillary blood volume and reduced area for diffusion.

Pulmonary vessels can be affected by lung disease and can cause $\dot{V}_A/\dot{Q}$ mismatch by impeding regional blood flow. Systemic diseases with vascular involvement can cause severe pulmonary dysfunction because of $\dot{V}_A/\dot{Q}$ mismatch, impaired diffusion, and shunt. $\dot{V}_A/\dot{Q}$ mismatch causes most of the hypoxemia in pulmonary fibrosis.[157] In addition, hypoxemia can be caused by impaired diffusion (in particular, during exercise, when it can dominate) and a varying degree of shunt (discussed later).

Pulmonary emboli cause $\dot{V}_A/\dot{Q}$ mismatch in three ways. First, vascular beds are occluded, causing extremely high $\dot{V}_A/\dot{Q}$ locally; this is manifest as increased dead space. Second, the occluded vascular bed diverts blood flow to other, already ventilated regions, thus converting these into low $\dot{V}_A/\dot{Q}$ regions. Finally, if P_{PA} (pulmonary artery pressure) is markedly increased, then any propensity to shunt will be increased.[158] In patients with acute pulmonary embolism,[159] hypoxemia appears to be principally caused by increased variability of $\dot{V}_A/\dot{Q}$, and this has been confirmed experimentally.[160]

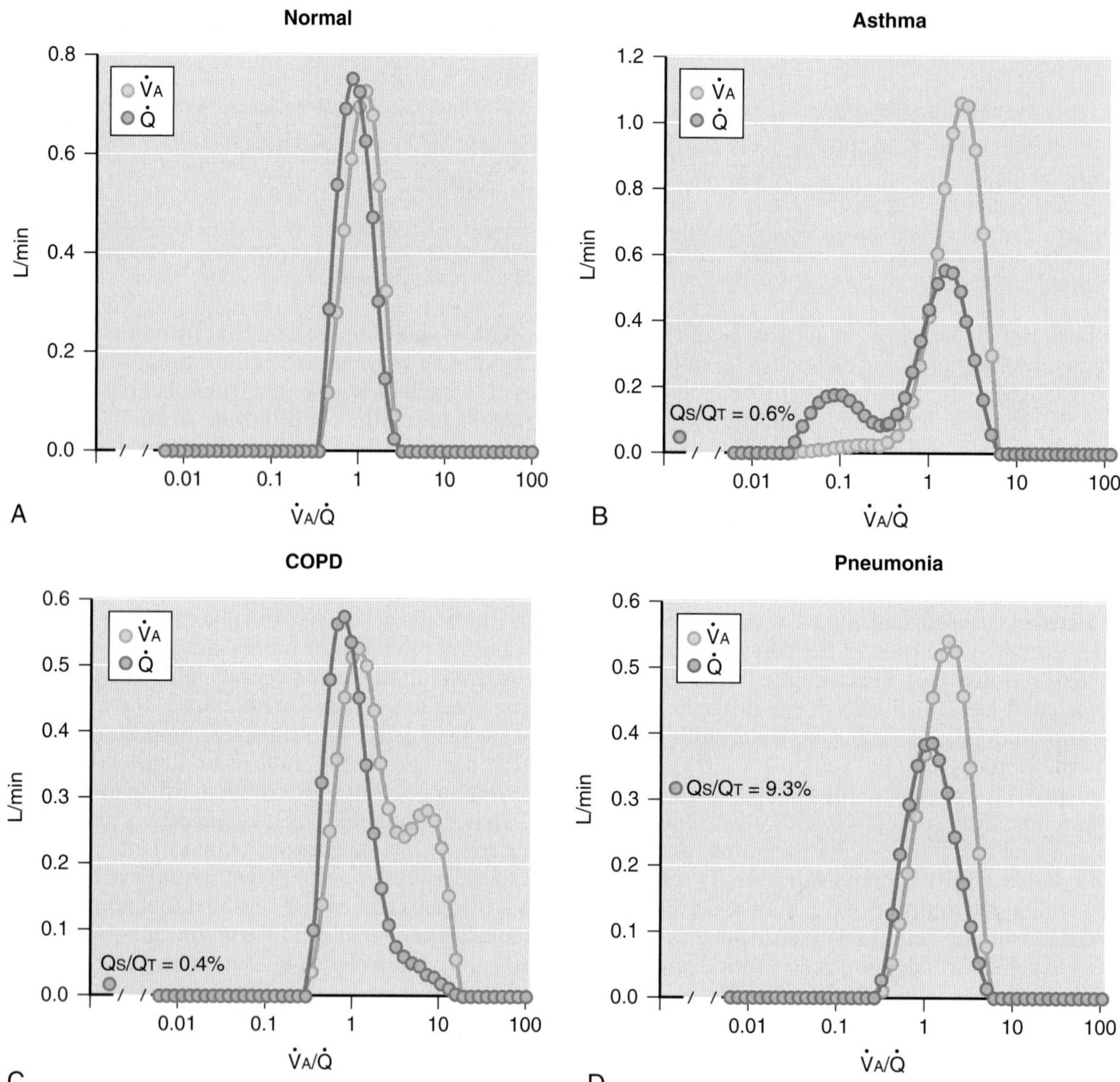

Fig. 13.26 Distribution of ventilation and perfusion in normal lungs, asthma, chronic obstructive pulmonary disease *(COPD)*, and pneumonia. In normal lungs (A) there is good matching between ventilation *(orange circle)* and perfusion *(blue circle)* with a mode centered around a $\dot{V}_A/\dot{Q}$ ratio of 1. This results in near optimal oxygenation of blood and CO_2 removal. In asthma (B) there is broader distribution of $\dot{V}_A/\dot{Q}$ with some regions being ventilated well in excess of perfusion ($\dot{V}_A/\dot{Q} = 10$ and greater), with another mode of low $\dot{V}_A/\dot{Q}$ centered around a ratio of 0.1. This mode can be explained by collateral ventilation maintaining gas exchange in alveoli behind occluded airways. There is no shunt seen in asthma. In COPD (C) the pattern is similar to asthma, but with an additional "high" $\dot{V}_A/\dot{Q}$ mode that adds to dead space such as ventilation. Shunt is not present, and the pattern of $\dot{V}_A/\dot{Q}$ distribution is not associated with significant hypoxemia. In lobar pneumonia (D) the major finding is pure shunt (consolidated, perfused, and poorly ventilated lobe); there is only minor widening of the $\dot{V}_A/\dot{Q}$ distribution.

Pneumonia involving large areas of consolidated, edematous, or atelectatic (i.e., all non-aerated) lung involves significant shunt, and areas of partial aeration contribute to $\dot{V}_A/\dot{Q}$ mismatch (see Fig. 13.26).[149] In bacterial pneumonia, HPV appears to be inhibited, which is an important mechanism that worsens hypoxemia.[161,162]

EFFECT OF $\dot{V}_A/\dot{Q}$ ON CO_2 ELIMINATION

A common misconception is that although $\dot{V}_A/\dot{Q}$ impedes oxygenation, it has little effect on CO_2 clearance. Actually, elimination of CO_2 is even more limited by $\dot{V}_A/\dot{Q}$ mismatch than is oxygenation of blood[82]; however, this seldom results in hypercapnia because minimal increases in $\dot{V}_A$ rapidly correct Pa_{CO_2}. If alveolar ventilation is already impaired and cannot be increased, the addition of $\dot{V}_A/\dot{Q}$ mismatch will increase Pa_{CO_2}.

IMPAIRED DIFFUSION

Hypoxemia can occur because of impaired diffusion in fibrosis or vascular diseases because of severely thickened alveolar-capillary membranes. Diffusion is slowed down and the entire length of capillary may be required before the capillary blood has been fully oxygenated, even in resting conditions. On the other hand, this means that a diffusion barrier is unlikely to cause hypoxemia provided the perfusion time and distance permits O_2 equilibration (see Fig. 13.12); however, when these reserves are spent, PaO_2 begins to fall. This decrease is particularly noticeable in patients with

BOX 13.3 Derivation of the Physiologic Dead Space Equation

FĒ
VT
FA
FI
VT−VD

The quantity of CO_2 expired in an exhaled tidal volume = $FECO_2 \times VT$

This comes from perfused lung and from nonperfused lung.

CO_2 exhaled from perfused lung = $FACO_2 \times VA = FACO_2 \times (VT - VD)$

CO_2 from nonperfused (dead space) lung is derived from inspired gas = $FICO_2 \times VD$

Thus, $FECO_2 \times VT = FACO_2(VT \cdot VD) + (FICO_2 \times VD)$

By rearranging,

$$\frac{V_{DS}}{V_T} = \frac{F_A - F_E}{F_A - F_I}$$

If FI = 0, F is replaced by P, and PA is replaced by Pa, for CO_2,

$$\frac{V_{DS}}{V_T} = \frac{PaCO_2 - PECO_2}{PaCO_2}$$

where FE, FA, and FI are mixed expired, alveolar, and inspired gas concentration, respectively, and VT, VDS, and VA are tidal volume, dead space, and part of the tidal volume to perfused alveoli, respectively.

pulmonary fibrosis, who might have normal PaO_2 at rest but show dramatic decreases during exercise.[82,115] Development of -or increasing- right-to-left shunting in the heart, such as with an atrial septal defect, can also cause this exercise-induced hypoxemia because the left-to-right shunt at rest becomes right-to-left (or a small right-to-left shunt increases) because of increased P_{PA}.

RIGHT-TO-LEFT SHUNT

If blood passes through the lung without contacting ventilated alveoli, then the blood will not oxygenate or release CO_2. This condition is called a *shunt*, and it lowers PaO_2 and can increase $PaCO_2$. Healthy people have a small shunt (2%-3% of cardiac output) that is caused by venous drainage of the heart muscle into the left atrium by the thebesian veins. In pathologic states, the shunt ranges from 2% to 50% of cardiac output.

Shunt is often confused with $\dot{V}_A/\dot{Q}$ mismatch. While a $\dot{V}_A/\dot{Q}$ of zero (some perfusion, no ventilation) constitutes a shunt, there are two clear and important differences between low $\dot{V}_A/\dot{Q}$ and shunt. First, the anatomy of a shunt differs from an area of low $\dot{V}_A/\dot{Q}$. Regions with low $\dot{V}_A/\dot{Q}$ are characterized by narrowing of the airways and vasculature, which reduces ventilation and blood flow in some regions and increases them in others. Examples are obstructive lung disease and vascular disorders. Shunt is caused by the complete cessation of ventilation in a region, usually as a result of collapse (atelectasis) or consolidation (e.g., pneumonia). Asthma or COPD does not involve the formation of a shunt[115]; if a shunt is present, it indicates a complication.

Second, supplemental O_2 improves the hypoxemia caused by low $\dot{V}_A/\dot{Q}$, but it has little effect on hypoxemia caused by shunt. Although aeration may be poor in regions of low $\dot{V}_A/\dot{Q}$, aeration does exist in these regions, and the concentration of O_2 in these alveoli can be enriched by increasing FiO_2. In contrast, supplemental O_2 cannot access the alveoli in a true (anatomic) shunt.

Anatomic shunt and low $\dot{V}_A/\dot{Q}$ usually coexist, and the net effect is sometimes referred to as *percent shunt* (per the standard shunt equation). In this situation, the low $\dot{V}_A/\dot{Q}$ component will contribute to the response from increasing FiO_2, and the regions of anatomic (true) shunt will not; therefore, shunt will always lower PaO_2 (at any FiO_2). When the calculated fraction increases to 25%, the response to increased FiO_2 will be small; when it increases to 30% or greater, the response will be negligible.[149] This varying response is the net effect of mixing blood with normal pulmonary end-capillary PO_2 and shunt blood, which has the same PO_2 as mixed venous blood. If shunt is a large enough fraction of total lung blood flow, the additional O_2 that can be physically dissolved by the raised FiO_2 is so small that it is almost immeasurable; such a shunt is said to be refractory.

RESPIRATORY FUNCTION DURING ONE-LUNG VENTILATION

Oxygenation can be a challenge during one-lung surgery. One lung is not ventilated but is still perfused, and in the postoperative period, restoration of lung integrity and ventilation–perfusion matching can take time.[163]

The technique of one-lung anesthesia and ventilation means that only one lung is ventilated and that the lung provides oxygenation of—and elimination of CO_2 from—the blood. Persisting perfusion through the nonventilated lung causes a shunt and decreases PaO_2 (Fig. 13.27); measures can be taken to reduce this blood flow.[164,165]

During one-lung anesthesia, there are two main contributors to impaired oxygenation: (1) the persisting blood flow through nonventilated lung and (2) development of atelectasis in the dependent lung, resulting in local shunt and low $\dot{V}_A/\dot{Q}$.[138] A recruitment maneuver can identify the influence of the dependent atelectasis;[166] serial increases in peak airway pressure and PEEP directed to the dependent, ventilated lung increased significantly the PaO_2, indicating that dependent atelectasis was an important cause of hypoxemia. In this situation, diversion of perfusion from the dependent (ventilated) to the nondependent (i.e., nonventilated) lung would have worsened oxygenation.

Recruitment can also affect V_D. Recruitment during one-lung anesthesia improved oxygenation, but also decreased V_D.[167] The slope of the CO_2 curve during a tidal expiration (phase III) was flatter, indicating a more even distribution of inspired gas throughout the lung and more synchronous alveolar emptying. Thus a secondary effect of recruiting collapsed lung tissue can be (presumably not when recruitment causes overinflation) more even distribution of ventilation and a decrease in the dead space fraction. This effect should facilitate the use of a smaller V_T. In contrast to an individual recruitment, the application of continuous elevated P_{AW} (PEEP titrated to optimal compliance in the ventilated lung) increased compliance by 10% but slightly worsened oxygenation, probably because of redistribution

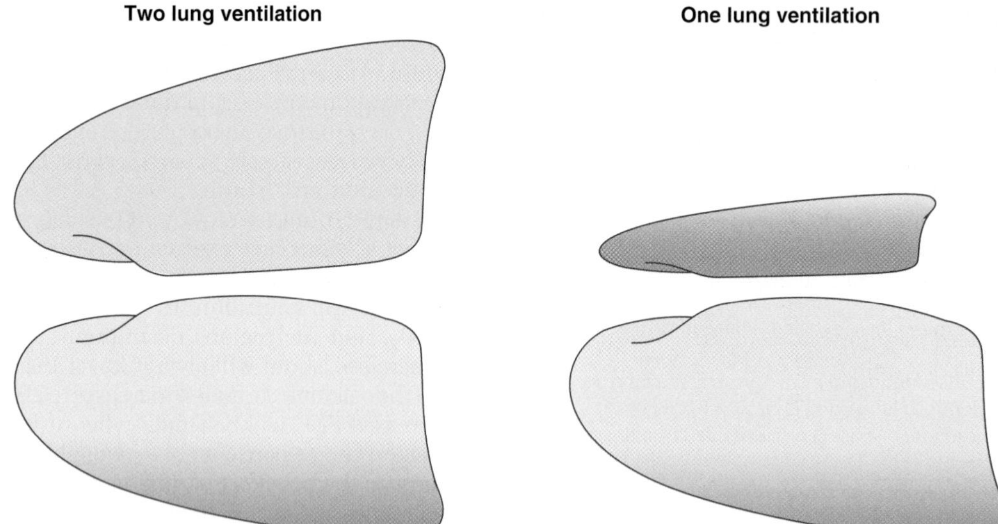

Fig. 13.27 Schematic drawing of the distribution of shunt during two-lung ventilation and one-lung ventilation during anesthesia. Shunt region is indicated by dark area in the lower lung during two-lung ventilation and in the lower lung—plus the entire upper lung—during one-lung ventilation.

of blood from the ventilated to the nonventilated (nondependent) lung.[168] The rationale for identifying and using optimal PEEP has also been reviewed.[169]

Maneuvers can also be applied to the nondependent lung. The effects of compressing the nondependent lung on oxygenation were examined using an intraarterial O_2 sensor, which provides instantaneous and continuous PaO_2.[170] Compression resulted in increased PaO_2, suggesting a shift of blood flow from the nondependent (nonventilated) to the dependent (ventilated) lung; development of complete absorption atelectasis in the nondependent lung may have similar effects.[171]

Inhaled NO (pulmonary vasodilator) and intravenous almitrine (pulmonary vasoconstrictor) have been studied alone and in combination. NO alone has little effect,[172] but oxygenation is improved when NO is combined with almitrine.[173,174] Almitrine alone also improves oxygenation[175] at a dose that does not alter P_{PA} or cardiac output. Although inhaled NO increases perfusion to already ventilated regions (increasing $\dot{V}_A/\dot{Q}$), almitrine potentiates HPV, decreasing perfusion to nonventilated (i.e., shunt) areas (reducing shunt) and potentially diverting blood flow to ventilated regions of the lung. Selective pulmonary vasodilation is reviewed.[176,177]

Careful analysis of the mechanical obstruction caused by kinking of pulmonary vessels and by HPV has shown that HPV is the important determinant of diversion of blood flow away from nonventilated lung (though not complete).[178] Moreover, positioning of the patient can affect the degree of shunting.[179]

PNEUMOPERITONEUM

Laparoscopic operations are usually performed by insufflation of CO_2 into the abdominal cavity. The effects are twofold. First, the consequences of hypercapnic acidosis[180,181] include depressed cardiac contractility, sensitization of the myocardium to the arrhythmogenic effects of catecholamines pulmonary vasoconstriction and systemic vasodilation.[182] There can also be long-lasting postoperative effects on breathing control.[183] In addition, the physical effects of pneumoperitoneum are important. These include decreased FRC and VC,[184] formation of atelectasis,[185] reduced respiratory compliance,[186] and increased peak airway pressure.[187] Nonetheless, shunt is reduced and arterial oxygenation is mostly improved during CO_2 pneumoperitoneum.[188] This paradox—more atelectasis and less shunt—suggests that efficient redistribution of blood flow away from collapsed lung regions is attributable to hypercapnic acidosis CO_2 potentiating hypoxic pulmonary vasoconstriction. Indeed, a recent experimental study showed that if the abdomen was inflated with air, a much larger shunt developed than if CO_2 had been used for inflation.[189]

Lung Function After Cardiac Surgery

Cardiac surgery produces the greatest degree of atelectasis in the postoperative period,[190] perhaps because both lungs are often collapsed. Spontaneous resolution of the atelectasis is gradual, leaving a residual shunt of up to 30% by day 1 or 2;[97,191] however, recruitment at the end of the case is possible. In some cases, 30 cm H_2O for 20 seconds is sufficient,[97] facilitated by the chest being open. A recruitment maneuver (with zero PEEP) causes transient increase in PaO_2 and end-expiratory lung volume (EELV), and with PEEP alone, EELV was increased but PaO_2 unchanged. However, a recruitment maneuver followed by PEEP resulted in a large and sustained increase in both PaO_2 and EELV.[192] The separation of effect whereby PEEP alone increases EELV to a greater extent than it increases oxygenation suggests further opening of an already opened lung rather than opening of atelectatic lung.

Head-to-head comparison of intermittent CPAP versus constant noninvasive pressure support ventilation reported intriguing findings. There was less radiographic evidence of atelectasis following pressure support, without differences in oxygenation of bedside pulmonary function testing.[193] Although the authors' conclusion was of no clinical benefit with noninvasive pressure support ventilation, differences in FiO_2 could cause differences in propensity to atelectasis. Recruitment maneuvers up to moderately high levels of airway pressure (46 cm H_2O) do not appear to affect the pulmonary vascular resistance or right ventricular afterload,[194] which is an issue of considerable importance following cardiac surgery. Nonetheless, it is prudent to consider RV loading and ejection in such circumstances, especially in the setting of diminished RV reserve or tricuspid regurgitation. Finally, many cardiac surgeries are now being performed "off pump," and the postoperative pulmonary effect is reduced, with less postoperative intrapulmonary shunt and correspondingly shorter hospital stays.[195]

Protective Ventilation

During the last few years, a concept of "protective ventilation" has appeared, based on three tools of ventilator support: (1) low tidal volume (assumed to reduce stress and strain of the lung), (2) recruitment maneuver (assumed to reopen any collapsed alveoli), and (3) PEEP (assumed to keep a recruited lung open during ongoing anesthesia and surgery).[196] These three tools have been adopted from intensive care, and one may ask whether they are equally useful in the mechanically ventilated, essentially lung healthy, anesthetized patient. As for (1) low tidal volume, a small tidal volume is reasonable, and a volume of 6 to 8 mL/kg/body weight, as is generally suggested, is the same size of what a normal subject is breathing spontaneously when awake. As for (2) recruitment maneuver and (3) PEEP, opening up and keeping the lung open is also reasonable and even important. Both a recruitment maneuver and PEEP will achieve this.

"Protective ventilation" has been claimed to reduce postoperative lung complications, although results vary between studies,[196,197] and which tool may be the most important remains also to be shown. Moreover, the protective ventilation concept covers the period from induction to emergence from anesthesia, and whether any positive effects remain in the postoperative period is unknown.[198] The atelectasis that develops intraoperatively may last for some days after surgery[199] and may be a cause of postoperative pulmonary complications. Further refinement of ventilatory support strategy may therefore rather be focused on the emergence from anesthesia and the postoperative period.

Postoperative Physiotherapy

Physiotherapy, much debated after surgery,[200] is associated with more effective lung recruitment (seen on thoracic CT) when involving deliberate approaches, such as flow bottles following exercise.[201] In effect, large and early inspiration following surgery may be key to preventing postoperative lung complications. Whether the deep inspiration needs to be accomplished with a specific forced breathing device is uncertain.

Intraoperative Hyperoxia

It has been suggested that ventilation with hyperoxic gas, 80% O_2, during anesthesia and for a couple of hours postoperatively will improve wound healing and reduce postoperative complications.[202] Based on a larger number of studies, the World Health Organization (WHO) presented guidelines in favor of perioperative hyperoxia.[203] However, the guidelines have met with criticism,[204] and large studies that have appeared after the publication of the guidelines do not support the use of hyperoxic gas.[205,206] Thus the potential advantage of elevating arterial oxygen tension may be offset by cellular responses with the formation of reactive oxygen species.[207]

Effect of Sleep on Respiration

Sleep has a major effect on many aspects of respiration, perhaps the most obvious being ventilation.[208] Sleep reduces V_T and inspiratory drive, and $\dot{V}_E$ falls by approximately 10%, depending on the sleep stage, with the most marked fall occurring during rapid-eye-movement (REM) sleep. Lung volume (i.e., FRC) is also reduced;[209] this commences almost immediately after the onset of sleep, and the lowest levels of FRC (down to 10% of resting levels) occur in REM sleep.[210] CT studies in healthy volunteers demonstrate that the sleep-induced decrease in FRC is accompanied by reduced aeration in the dependent lung.[211] Such loss in aeration was demonstrated in anesthetized patients when their FiO_2 was increased from 0.3 to 1.0; atelectasis developed rapidly. It is possible that during normal sleep, breathing with high levels of O_2 would also cause atelectasis.

 **Complete references available online at expertconsult.com.**

References

1. von Ungern-Sternberg BS, et al. *Lancet*. 2010;376:773.
2. Cook TM, et al. *Anaesthesia*. 2010;65:556.
3. Cheney FW, et al. *Anesthesiology*. 1991;75:932.
4. Woods BD, Sladen RN. *Br J Anaesth*. 2009;103(suppl 1):i57.
5. Pinsky MR. *Curr Opin Crit Care*. 2007;13:528. 2007.
6. Buhre W, Rossaint R. *Lancet*. 2003;362:1839.
7. Moonesinghe SR, et al. *Anesth Analg*. 2011;112:891.
8. Hennis PJ, et al. *Br J Anaesth*. 2012;109:566.
9. Poeze M, et al. *Intensive Care Med*. 2000;26:1272.
10. Nunn JF: *Nunn's Applied Respiratory Physiology*. 4th ed. London: Butterworth Heinemann; 1993.
11. Caboot JB, et al. *Pediatr Pulmonol*. 2012;47:808.
12. Shamir MY, et al. *Anesth Analg*. 2012;114:972.
13. Hampson NB, et al. *Am J Respir Crit Care Med*. 2012;186:1095.
14. Bohr C, et al. *Arch Physiol*. 1904;16:401.
15. Hanson CW, et al. *Crit Care Med*. 1996;24:23.
16. Jensen FB. *Acta Physiol Scand*. 2004;182:215.
17. Barratt-Boyes BG, Wood EH. *J Lab Clin Med*. 1957;50:93.
18. Chawla LS, Zia H, et al. *Chest*. 2004;126:1891.
19. Quanjer PH, et al. *Eur Respir J Suppl*. 1993;16:5.
20. Astrom E, et al. *Eur Respir J*. 2000;16:659.
21. Broughton SJ, et al. *Physiol Meas*. 2006;27:99.
22. Wilschut FA, et al. *Eur Respir J*. 1999;14:166.
23. Roca J, et al. *Respir Med*. 1998;92:454.
24. Grassino AE, Roussos C. Static properties of the lung and chest wall. In: Crystal RG, West JB, Weibel ER, Barnes PJ, eds. *The Lung: Scientific Foundations*. 2nd ed. Philadelphia: Lippincott-Raven; 1997:1187.
25. Goldin JG. *Radiol Clin North Am*. 2002;40:145.
26. Van Lith P, et al. *J Appl Physiol*. 1967;23:475.
27. Pedley TJ, Kamm RD. Dynamics of gas flow and pressure-flow relationships. In: Crystal RG, West JB, Weibel ER, Barnes PJ, eds. *The Lung: Scientific Foundations*. 2nd ed. Philadelphia, 1997, Lippincott Raven.
28. Slats AM, et al. *Am J Respir Crit Care Med*. 2007;176:121.

29. Holst M, et al. *Intensive Care Med.* 1990;16:384.
30. O'Donnell DE, et al. *Am Rev Respir Dis.* 1987;135:912.
31. Calverley PM, Koulouris NG. *Eur Respir J.* 2005;25:186.
32. Mead J, et al. *J Appl Physiol.* 1967;22:95.
33. Bachofen HJ. *Appl Physiol.* 1968;24:296.
34. Kaczka DW, et al. *J Appl Physiol.* 1997;82:1531.
35. Verbeken EK, et al. *J Appl Physiol.* 1992;72:2343.
36. Bachofen H, Scherrer M. *J Clin Invest.* 1967;46:133.
37. Tantucci C, et al. *Am Rev Respir Dis.* 1992;145:355.
38. Frostell C, et al. *J Appl Physiol.* 1983;55:1854.
39. Milic-Emili J. Ventilation distrbution. In: Hammid Q, Shannon J, Martin J, eds. *Physiologic Bases of Respiratory Disease.* BC Decker: Hamilton, Ontario; 2005.
40. Hubmayr RD. *Am J Respir Crit Care Med.* 2002;165:1647.
41. Guy HJ, et al. *J Appl Physiol.* 1994;76:1719.
42. Prisk GK. *J Appl Physiol.* 2000;89:385.
43. Ganesan S, et al. *Respir Physiol.* 1989;78:281.
44. Bryan AC. *Am Rev Respir Dis.* 1974;110:143.
45. Mayo JR, et al. *J Thorac Imaging.* 1995;10:73.
46. Petersson J, et al. *J Appl Physiol.* 2004;96:1127.
47. Bryan AC, et al. *J Appl Physiol.* 1964;19:395.
48. Bake B, et al. *J Appl Physiol.* 1974;37:8.
49. Milic-Emili J, et al. *Eur J Appl Physiol.* 2007;99:567.
50. Teculescu DB, et al. *Lung.* 1996;174(43).
51. Haefeli-Bleuer B, Weibel ER. *Anat Rec.* 1988;220:401.
52. Adaro F, Piiper J. *Respir Physiol.* 1976;26:195.
53. Dawson CA, Linehan JH. Dynamics of blood flow and pressure-flow relationships. In: Crystal RG, West JB, Weibel ER, Barnes PJ, eds. *The Lung: Scientific Foundations.* 2nd ed. Philadelphia: Lippincott-Raven; 1997:1503.
54. Bachofen H, et al. *Am Rev Respir Dis.* 1993;147:997.
55. Jeffery PK. *Proc Am Thorac Soc1.* 2004:176.
56. Townsley MI, et al. *Circ Res.* 1995;77:317.
57. Kornecki A, et al. *Anesthesiology.* 2008;108:1047.
58. Hughes JMB. In: Crystal RG, et al., ed. *The Lung: Scientific Foundations.* 2nd ed. Philadelphia: Lippincott-Raven; 1997:1523.
59. West JB, et al. *J Appl Physiol.* 1964;19:713.
60. Hughes JM, et al. *Respir Physiol.* 1968;4:58.
61. Michels DB, West JB. *J Appl Physiol.* 1978;45:987.
62. Verbandt Y, et al. *J Appl Physiol.* 2000;89:2407.
63. Reed JH Jr, Wood EH. *J Appl Physiol.* 1970;28:303.
64. Glenny RW, et al. *J Appl Physiol.* 1991;71:620.
65. Glenny RW, et al. *J Appl Physiol.* 1999;86:623.
66. Hakim TS, et al. *J Appl Physiol.* 1987;63:1114.
67. Hedenstierna G, et al. *J Appl Physiol.* 1979;47:938.
68. Hlastala MP, et al. *J Appl Physiol.* 1996;81:1051.
69. Glenny RW, Robertson HT. *J Appl Physiol.* 1991;70:1024.
70. Glenny R. Counterpoint. *J Appl Physiol.* 2008;104(1533);5–6; discussion.
71. Sylvester JT, et al. *Physiol Rev.* 2012;92:367.
72. Marshall BE, et al. *Intensive Care Med.* 1994;20:379.
73. Moudgil R, et al. *J Appl Physiol.* 2005;98:390.
74. Kerbaul F, et al. *Br J Anaesth.* 2000;85:440.
75. Kerbaul F, et al. *Can J Anaesth.* 2001;48:760.
76. Hambraeus-Jonzon K, et al. *Anesthesiology.* 1997;86:308.
77. Sartori C, et al. *Respir Physiol Neurobiol.* 2007;159:338.
78. Pellegrino R, et al. *Eur Respir J.* 1997;10:468.
79. Leith DE, Mead J. *J Appl Physiol.* 1967;23:221.
80. Hughes JM, Bates DV. *Respir Physiol Neurobiol.* 2003;138:115.
81. Aguilaniu B, et al. *Eur Respir J.* 2008;31:1091.
82. West JB. *Respiratory Physiology—The Essentials.* Baltimore: Williams & Watkins; 1990.
83. Hedenstierna G. *Thorax.* 1995;50:85.
84. Moller JT, et al. *Lancet.* 1998;351:857.
85. Kroenke K, et al. *Chest.* 1993;104:1445.
86. Wahba RW. *Can J Anaesth.* 1991;38:384.
87. Rothen HU, et al. *Br J Anaesth.* 1998;81:681.
88. Westbrook PR, et al. *J Appl Physiol.* 1973;34:81.
89. Hedenstierna G, Edmark L. *Intensive Care Med.* 2005;31:1327.
90. Froese AB, Bryan AC. *Anesthesiology.* 1974;41:242.
91. Reber A, et al. *Anaesthesia.* 1998;53:1054.
92. Warner DO, et al. *Anesthesiology.* 1996;85:49.
93. Don H. *Int Anesthesiol Clin.* 1977;15:113.
94. Bendixen HH, et al. *N Engl J Med.* 1963;269:991.
95. Duggan M, Kavanagh BP. *Anesthesiology.* 2005;102:838.
96. Gunnarsson L, et al. *Br J Anaesth.* 1991;66:423.
97. Tenling A, et al. *Anesthesiology.* 1998;89:371.
98. Lindberg P, et al. *Acta Anaesthesiol Scand.* 1992;36:546.
99. Tokics L, et al. *J Appl Physiol.* 1996;81:1822.
100. van Kaam AH, et al. *Am J Respir Crit Care Med.* 2004;169:1046.
101. Gunnarsson L, et al. *Eur Respir J.* 1991;4:1106.
102. Musch G, et al. *Anesthesiology.* 2004;100:323.
103. Hewlett AM, et al. *Br J Anaesth.* 1974;46:495.
104. Ostberg E, et al. *Anesthesiology.* 2018.
105. Rothen HU, et al. *Br J Anaesth.* 1993;71:788.
106. Rothen HU, et al. *Br J Anaesth.* 1999;82:551.
107. Rothen HU, et al. *Anesthesiology.* 1995;82:832.
108. Rothen HU, et al. *Lancet.* 1995;345:1387.
109. Edmark L, et al. *Anesthesiology.* 2003;98:28.
110. Rusca M, et al. *Anesth Analg.* 2003;97:1835.
111. Hedenstierna G, et al. *Anesthesiology.* 1994;80:751.
112. Benoit Z, et al. *Anesth Analg.* 2002;95:1777–1781.
113. Sinha PK, et al. *J Cardiothorac Vasc Anesth.* 2006;20:136.
114. Squadrone V, et al. *JAMA.* 2005;293:589.
115. Agusti AG, Barbera JA. *Thorax.* 1994;49:924.
116. Hedenstierna G. *Clin Physiol Funct Imaging.* 2003;23:123.
117. Dueck R, et al. *Anesthesiology.* 1988;69:854.
118. Hedenstierna G, et al. *Anesthesiology.* 1984;61:369.
119. Hulands GH, et al. *Clin Sci.* 1970;38:451.
120. Marshall BE. *Effects of Anesthetics on Gas Exchange.* London: Kluwer Academic; 1989.
121. Marshall BE. *Acta Anaesthesiol Scand.* 1990;94(suppl):37.
122. Pelosi P, et al. *Anesthesiology.* 1999;91:1221.
123. Coussa M, et al. *Anesth Analg.* 2004;98:1491; table of contents.
124. Walley KR. *Am J Respir Crit Care Med.* 2011;184:514.
125. Dantzker DR, et al. *J Physiol.* 1974;242:72P.
126. Sakai EM, et al. *Pharmacotherapy.* 2005;25:1773.
127. von Ungern-Sternberg BS, et al. *Br J Anaesth.* 2007;98:503.
128. Ide T, et al. *Anesthesiology.* 1999;90:1084.
129. Sasaki N, et al. *Anesthesiology.* 2013;118:961.
130. Morton CP, Drummond GB. *Br J Anaesth.* 1994;73:135.
131. Warner DO, Warner MA. *Anesthesiology.* 1995;82:20–31.
132. Warner DO, et al. *J Appl Physiol.* 1994;76:2802.
133. Strandberg A, et al. *Acta Anaesthesiol Scand.* 1986;30:154.
134. Dueck R, et al. *Anesthesiology.* 1984;61:55.
135. Anjou-Lindskog E, et al. *Anesthesiology.* 1985;62:485.
136. Heneghan CP, et al. *Br J Anaesth.* 1984;56:437.
137. Klingstedt C, et al. *Acta Anaesthesiol Scand.* 1990;34:315.
138. Klingstedt C, et al. *Acta Anaesthesiol Scand.* 1990;34:421.
139. Landmark SJ, et al. *J Appl Physiol.* 1977;43:993.
140. Mure M, et al. *Am J Respir Crit Care Med.* 1998;157:1785.
141. Nyren S, et al. *Anesthesiology.* 2010;112:682.
142. Yoshino J, et al. *Acta Anaesthesiol Scand.* 2003;47:742.
143. Brooks-Brunn JA. *Chest.* 1997;111:564.
144. Pelosi P, et al. *Anesth Analg.* 1998;87:654.
145. Eichenberger A, et al. *Anesth Analg.* 2002;95;1788; table of contents.
146. Cressey DM, et al. *Anaesthesia.* 2001;56:680.
147. Gander S, et al. *Anesth Analg.* 2005;100:580.
148. Berthoud MC, et al. *Br J Anaesth.* 1991;67:464.
149. Melot C. *Thorax.* 1994;49:1251.
150. Reinius H, et al. *Anesthesiology.* 2009;111:979.
151. Mynster T, et al. *Anaesthesia.* 1996;51:225.
152. Warner DO, et al. *Anesthesiology.* 1996;85:761.
153. Yamakage M, et al. *Acta Anaesthesiol Scand.* 1992;36:569.
154. McCarthy GS. *Br J Anaesth.* 1976;48:243.
155. Roca J, Wagner PD. *Thorax.* ;49. ; 1994:815.
156. Rodriguez-Roisin R, Roca J. *Thorax.* 1994;49:1027.
157. Agusti AG, et al. *Am Rev Respir Dis.* 1991;143:219.
158. Manier G, Castaing Y. *Thorax.* ;49. ; 1994:1169.
159. Santolicandro A, et al. *Am J Respir Crit Care Med.* 1995;152:336.
160. Altemeier WA, et al. *J Appl Physiol.* 1998;85:2337.
161. Light RB. *Semin Respir Infect.* 1999;14:218.
162. Light RB. *Am Rev Respir Dis.* 1986;134:520.
163. Benumof JL. *Anesth Analg.* 1985;64:821.
164. Karzai W, Schwarzkopf K. *Anesthesiology.* 2009;110:1402.
165. Hedenstierna G, Reber A. *Acta Anaesthesiol Scand.* 1996;40:2.
166. Tusman G, et al. *Ann Thorac Surg.* 2002;73:1204.
167. Tusman G, et al. *Analg.* 2004;98:1604; table of contents.
168. Mascotto G, et al. *Eur J Anaesthesiol.* 2003;20:704.
169. Slinger PD, et al. *Anesthesiology.* 2001;95:1096.
170. Ishikawa S, et al. *Br J Anaesth.* 2003;90:21.

171. Pfitzer J. *Br J Anaesth.* 2003;91:153; author reply -4.
172. Schwarzkopf K, et al. *Anesth Analg.* 2001;92:842.
173. Moutafis M, et al. *Anesth Analg.* 1997;85:1130.
174. Silva-Costa-Gomes T, et al. *Br J Anaesth.* 2005;95:410.
175. Moutafis M, et al. *Anesth Analg.* 2002;94:830; table of contents.
176. Dembinski R, et al. *Minerva Anestesiol.* 2004;70:239.
177. Schilling T, et al. *Anesth Analg.* 2005;101:957; table of contents.
178. Friedlander M, et al. *Can J Anaesth.* 1994;41:26.
179. Choi YS, et al. *J Thorac Cardiovasc Surg.* 2007;134:613.
180. McMahon AJ, et al. *Lancet.* 2000;356:1632.
181. Neudecker J, et al. *Surg Endosc.* 2002;16:1121.
182. Gutt CN, et al. *Dig Surg.* 2004;21:95.
183. Bablekos GD, et al. *Arch Surg.* 2006;141:16.
184. Hirvonen EA, et al. *Anesth Analg.* 1995;80:961.
185. Andersson LE, et al. *Anesthesiology.* 2005;102:293.
186. Makinen MT, et al. *Can J Anaesth.* 1998;45:865.
187. Sharma KC, et al. *Chest.* 1996;110:810.
188. Andersson L, et al. *Acta Anaesthesiol Scand.* 2002;46:552.
189. Strang CM, et al. *Minerva Anestesiol.* 2013;79(6):617.
190. Hachenberg T, et al. *Acta Anaesthesiol Scand.* 1992;36:800.
191. Hachenberg T, et al. *Anesthesiology.* 1997;86:809.
192. Dyhr T, et al. *Acta Anaesthesiol Scand.* 2004;48:187.
193. Pasquina P, et al. *Anesth Analg.* 2004;99:1001; table of contents.
194. Reis Miranda D, et al. *Br J Anaesth.* 2004;93:327.
195. Tschernko EM, et al. *J Thorac Cardiovasc Surg.* 2002;124:732.
196. Futier E, et al. *N Engl J Med.* 2013;369(5):428.
197. Las Vegas investigators. *Eur J Anaesthesiol.* 2017;34(8):492.
198. Hedenstierna G. *Anesthesiology.* 2015;123(3):501.
199. Lindberg P, et al. *Acta Anaesthesiol Scand.* 1992;36(6):546.
200. Pasquina P, et al. *BMJ.* 2003;327:1379.
201. Westerdahl E, et al. *Chest.* 2005;128:3482.
202. Greif R, et al. *N Engl J Med.* 2000;342(3):161.
203. Allegranzi B, et al. *Lancet Infect Dis.* 2016;16(12):e288.
204. Hedenstierna G, et al. *Anesthesiology.* 2017;126(5):771.
205. Staehr-Rye AK, et al. *Br J Anaesth.* 2017;119(1):140.
206. Kurz A, et al. *Br J Anaesth.* 2015;115(3):434.
207. Turrens JF. *J Physiol.* 2003;552(Pt 2):335.
208. Douglas NJ, et al. *Thorax.* 1982;37:840.
209. Hudgel DW, Devadatta P. *J Appl Physiol.* 1984;57:1319.
210. Ballard RD, et al. *J Appl Physiol.* 1990;68:2034.
211. Appelberg J, et al. *Chest.* 2007;131:122.

14 Cardiac Physiology

LENA S. SUN and NICHOLAS A. DAVIS

KEY POINTS

- The cardiac cycle is the sequence of electrical and mechanical events during a single heartbeat.
- Cardiac output is determined by the heart rate, myocardial contractility, and preload and afterload.
- The majority of cardiomyocytes consist of myofibrils, which are rod-like bundles that form the contractile elements within the cardiomyocyte.
- The basic working unit of contraction is the sarcomere.
- Gap junctions are responsible for the electrical coupling of small molecules between cells.
- Action potentials have four phases in the heart.
- The key player in cardiac excitation-contraction coupling is the ubiquitous second messenger calcium.
- Calcium-induced sparks are spatially and temporally patterned activations of localized calcium release that are important for excitation-contraction coupling and regulation of automaticity and contractility.
- β-Adrenoreceptors stimulate chronotropy, inotropy, lusitropy, and dromotropy.
- Hormones with cardiac action can be synthesized and secreted by cardiomyocytes or produced by other tissues and delivered to the heart.
- Cardiac reflexes are fast-acting reflex loops between the heart and central nervous system that contribute to the regulation of cardiac function and the maintenance of physiologic homeostasis.

"To err, to be deceived, is human." This was William Harvey's gentle repudiation to fellow physicians in his 1628 "Exercitatio Anatomica de Motu Cordis et Sanguinis in Animalibus," in which he advanced the concepts of circulation with the heart as the central pump, a major break from the centuries-old anatomic teaching of Galen.[1,2] Modern cardiac physiology includes this as well as concepts of cellular and molecular biology of the cardiomyocyte and regulation of cardiac function by neural and humoral factors. This chapter focuses on the physiology of the heart, beginning with the intact heart and advancing to cellular cardiac physiology. Finally, the various factors that regulate cardiac function are briefly discussed.

The basic anatomy of the heart consists of two atria and two ventricles that provide two separate circulations in series. The pulmonary circulation, a low-resistance and high-capacitance vascular bed, receives output from the right side of the heart, and its chief function is bidirectional gas exchange. The left side of the heart provides output for the systemic circulation. It functions to deliver oxygen (O_2) and nutrients and to remove carbon dioxide (CO_2) and metabolites from various tissue beds.

Physiology of the Intact Heart

Understanding the mechanical performance of the intact heart begins with the knowledge of the phases of the cardiac cycle and the determinants of ventricular function.

CARDIAC CYCLE

The cardiac cycle is the sequence of electrical and mechanical events during a single heartbeat. Fig. 14.1 illustrates the electrical events of a single cardiac cycle represented by the electrocardiogram (ECG) with corresponding mechanical events. Left atrial and left ventricular pressures are shown correlated in time with aortic flow and ventricular volume.[3]

Intrinsic to the specialized cardiac pacemaker tissues is automaticity and rhythmicity. The cardiac cycle begins at the sinoatrial (SA) node with the initiation of the heartbeat. Because the SA node can generate impulses at the greatest frequency, it is the natural pacemaker.

Electrical Events and the Electrocardiogram

Electrical events of the pacemaker and the specialized conduction system are represented by the ECG at the body surface. The ECG is the result of differences in electrical potential generated by the heart at sites of the surface recording. The action potential initiated at the SA node is propagated to both atria by specialized conduction tissue that leads to atrial systole (contraction) and the P wave of the ECG. At the junction of the interatrial and interventricular septa, specialized atrial conduction tissue converges at the atrioventricular (AV) node, which is distally connected to the His bundle. The AV node is an area of relatively slow conduction, and a delay between atrial and ventricular contraction normally occurs at this locus. The PR interval represents the delay between atrial and ventricular contraction at the level of the AV node. From the distal His

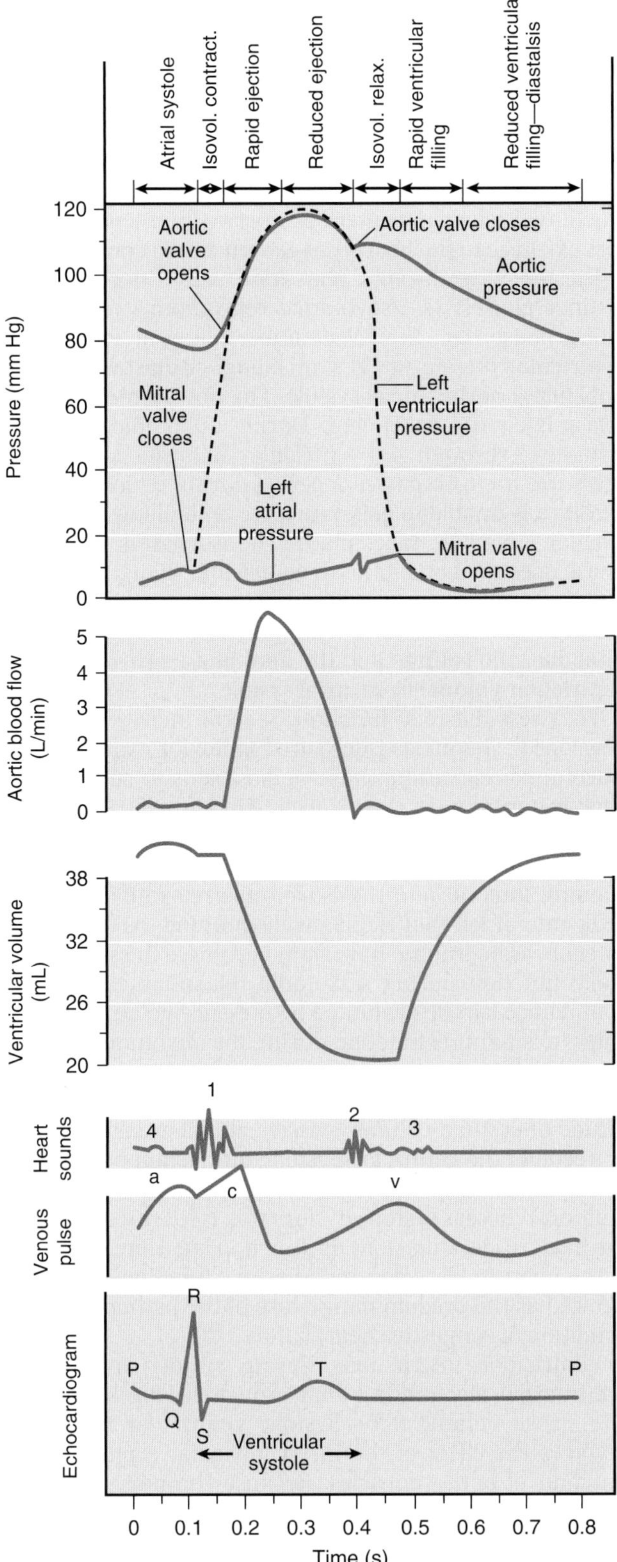

Fig. 14.1 Electrical and mechanical events during a single cardiac cycle. Aortic and atrial blood flow, ventricular volume, venous pulse, and the electrocardiogram are shown. (Berne RM, Levy MN: The cardiac pump. In *Cardiovascular physiology*, ed 8, St Louis, 2001, Mosby, pp 55-82.)

bundle, an electrical impulse is propagated through large left and right bundle branches and finally to the Purkinje system fibers, which are the smallest branches of the specialized conduction system. Finally, electrical signals are transmitted from the Purkinje system to individual ventricular cardiomyocytes. The spread of depolarization to the ventricular myocardium is exhibited as the QRS complex on the ECG. Depolarization is followed by ventricular repolarization and the appearance of the T wave on the ECG.[4]

Mechanical Events

The mechanical events of a cardiac cycle begin with the return of blood to the right and left atria from the systemic and pulmonary circulation, respectively. As blood accumulates in the atria, atrial pressure increases until it exceeds the pressure within the ventricle, and the AV valve opens. Blood passively flows first into the ventricular chambers, and such flow accounts for approximately 75% of the total ventricular filling.[5] The remainder of the blood flow is mediated by active atrial contraction or systole, known as the atrial "kick." The onset of atrial systole coincides with the depolarization of the SA node and the P wave. While the ventricles fill, the AV valves are displaced upward and ventricular contraction (systole) begins with closure of the tricuspid and mitral valves, which corresponds to the end of the R wave on the ECG. The first part of ventricular systole is known as isovolumic (or isometric) contraction. The electrical impulse traverses the AV region and passes through the right and left bundle branches into the Purkinje fibers, which leads to contraction of the ventricular myocardium and a progressive increase in intraventricular pressure. When intraventricular pressure exceeds pulmonary artery and aortic pressure, the pulmonic and aortic valves open and ventricular ejection occurs, which is the second part of ventricular systole.

Ventricular ejection is divided into the rapid ejection phase and the reduced ejection phase. During the rapid ejection phase, forward flow is maximal, and pulmonary artery and aortic pressure is maximally developed. In the reduced ejection phase, flow and great artery pressures taper with progression of systole. Pressures in both ventricular chambers decrease as blood is ejected from the heart, and ventricular diastole begins with closure of the pulmonic and aortic valves. The initial period of ventricular diastole consists of the isovolumic relaxation phase. This phase is concomitant with repolarization of the ventricular myocardium and corresponds to the end of the T wave on the ECG. The final portion of ventricular diastole involves a rapid decrease in intraventricular pressure until it decreases to less than that of the right and left atria, at which point the AV valve reopens, ventricular filling occurs, and the cycle repeats itself.

VENTRICULAR STRUCTURE AND FUNCTION

Ventricular Structure

The specific architectural order of the cardiac muscles provides the basis for the heart to function as a pump. The ellipsoid shape of the left ventricle (LV) is a result of the laminar layering of spiraling bundles of cardiac muscles (Fig. 14.2). The orientation of the muscle bundle is longitudinal in the subepicardial myocardium and circumferential

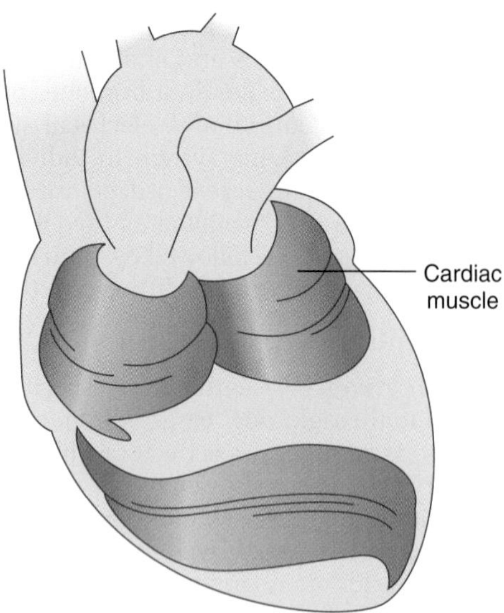

Fig. 14.2 Muscle bundles. (From Marieb EN. *Human Anatomy & Physiology.* 5th ed. San Francisco: Pearson Benjamin Cummings; 2001:684.)

in the middle segment and again becomes longitudinal in the subendocardial myocardium. Because of the ellipsoid shape of the LV, regional differences in wall thickness result in corresponding variations in the cross-sectional radius of the left ventricular chamber. These regional differences may serve to accommodate the variable loading conditions of the LV.[6] In addition, such anatomy allows the LV to eject blood in a corkscrew-type motion beginning from the base and ending at the apex. The architecturally complex structure of the LV thus allows maximal shortening of myocytes, which results in increased wall thickness and the generation of force during systole. Moreover, release of the twisted LV may provide a suction mechanism for filling of the LV during diastole. The left ventricular free wall and the septum have similar muscle bundle architecture. As a result, the septum moves inward during systole in a normal heart. Regional wall thickness is a commonly used index of myocardial performance that can be clinically assessed, such as by echocardiography or magnetic resonance imaging.

Unlike the LV, which needs to pump against the higher-pressure systemic circulation, the right ventricle (RV) pumps against a much lower pressure circuit in the pulmonary circulation. Consequently, wall thickness is considerably less in the RV. In contrast to the ellipsoidal form of the LV, the RV is crescent shaped; as a result, the mechanics of right ventricular contraction are more complex. Inflow and outflow contraction is not simultaneous, and much of the contractile force seems to be recruited from interventricular forces of the LV-based septum.

An intricate matrix of collagen fibers forms a scaffold of support for the heart and adjacent vessels. This matrix provides enough strength to resist tensile stretch. The collagen fibers are made up of mostly thick collagen type I fiber, which cross-links with the thin collagen type III fiber, the other major type of collagen.[7] Elastic fibers that contain elastin are in close proximity to the collagen fibers and account for the elasticity of the myocardium.[8]

Ventricular Function

The heart provides the driving force for delivering blood throughout the cardiovascular system to supply nutrients and to remove metabolic waste. Because of the anatomic complexity of the RV, the traditional description of systolic function is usually limited to the LV. Systolic performance of the heart is dependent on loading conditions and contractility. Preload and afterload are two interdependent factors extrinsic to the heart that govern cardiac performance.

Diastole is ventricular relaxation, and it occurs in four distinct phases: (1) isovolumic relaxation; (2) the rapid filling phase (i.e., the LV chamber filling at variable left ventricular pressure); (3) slow filling, or diastasis; and (4) final filling during atrial systole. The isovolumic relaxation phase is energy dependent. During auxotonic relaxation (phases 2 through 4), ventricular filling occurs against pressure. It encompasses a period during which the myocardium is unable to generate force, and filling of the ventricular chambers takes place. The isovolumic relaxation phase does not contribute to ventricular filling. The greatest amount of ventricular filling occurs in the second phase, whereas the third phase adds only approximately 5% of total diastolic volume and the final phase provides 15% of ventricular volume from atrial systole.

To assess diastolic function, several indices have been developed. The most widely used index for examining the isovolumic relaxation phase of diastole is to calculate the peak instantaneous rate of decline in left ventricular pressure ($-dP/dt$) or the time constant of isovolumic decline in left ventricular pressure (τ). The aortic closing-mitral opening interval and the isovolumic relaxation time and peak rate of left ventricular wall thinning, as determined by echocardiography, have both been used to estimate diastolic function during auxotonic relaxation. Ventricular compliance can be evaluated by pressure-volume relationships to determine function during the auxotonic phases of diastole.[9,10]

Many different factors influence diastolic function: magnitude of systolic volume, passive chamber stiffness, elastic recoil of the ventricle, diastolic interaction between the two ventricular chambers, atrial properties, and catecholamines. Whereas systolic dysfunction is a reduced ability of the heart to eject, diastolic dysfunction is a decreased ability of the heart to fill. Abnormal diastolic function is now recognized as the predominant cause of the pathophysiologic condition of congestive heart failure.[11]

Ventricular interactions during systole and diastole are internal mechanisms that provide feedback to modulate stroke volume (SV). Systolic ventricular interaction involves the effect of the interventricular septum on the function of both ventricles. Because the interventricular septum is anatomically linked to both ventricles, it is part of the load against which each ventricle has to work. Therefore, any changes in one ventricle will also be present in the other. In diastolic ventricular interaction, dilatation of either the LV or RV will have an impact on effective filling of the contralateral ventricle and thereby modify function.

Preload and Afterload. *Preload* is the ventricular load at the end of diastole, before contraction has started. First described by Starling, a linear relationship exists between

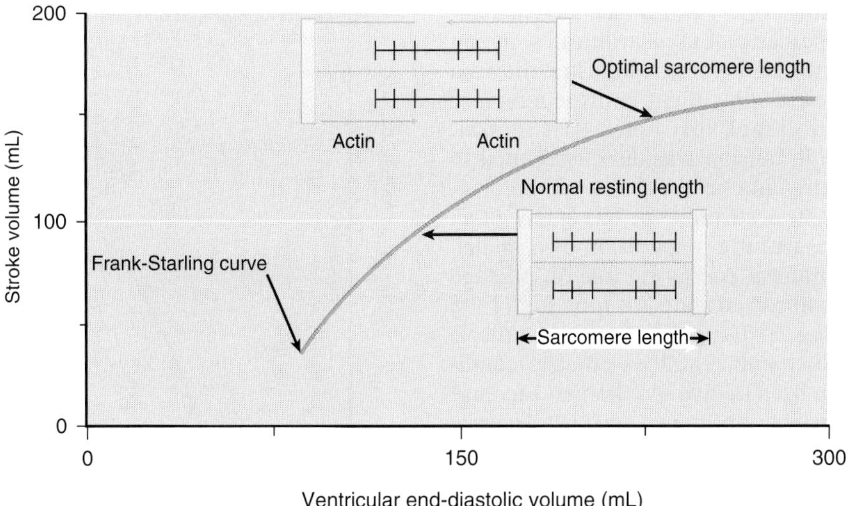

Fig. 14.3 Frank-Starling relationship. The relationship between sarcomere length and tension developed in cardiac muscles is shown. In the heart, an increase in end-diastolic volume is the equivalent of an increase in myocardial stretch; therefore, according to the Frank-Starling law, increased stroke volume is generated.

sarcomere length and myocardial force (Fig. 14.3). In clinical practice, surrogate representatives of left ventricular volume such as pulmonary wedge pressure or central venous pressure are used to estimate preload.[5] More direct measures of ventricular volumes can be made using echocardiography.

Afterload is the systolic load on the LV after contraction has begun. Aortic compliance is an additional determinant of afterload.[3] Aortic compliance is the ability of the aorta to give way to systolic forces from the ventricle. Changes in the aortic wall (dilation or stiffness) can alter aortic compliance and thus afterload. Examples of pathologic conditions that alter afterload are aortic stenosis and chronic hypertension. Both impede ventricular ejection, thereby increasing afterload. Aortic impedance, or aortic pressure divided by aortic flow at that instant, is an accurate means of gauging afterload. However, clinical measurement of aortic impedance is invasive. Echocardiography can noninvasively estimate aortic impedance by determining aortic blood flow at the time of its maximal increase. In clinical practice, the measurement of systolic blood pressure is adequate to approximate afterload, provided that aortic stenosis is not present.

Preload and afterload can be thought of as the wall stress that is present at the end of diastole and during left ventricular ejection, respectively. Wall stress is a useful concept because it includes preload, afterload, and the energy required to generate contraction. Wall stress and heart rate are probably the two most relevant indices that account for changes in myocardial O_2 demand. Laplace's law states that wall stress (σ) is the product of pressure (P) and radius (R) divided by wall thickness (h)[5]:

$$\sigma = P \times R / 2h$$

The ellipsoid shape of the LV allows the least amount of wall stress such that as the ventricle changes its shape from ellipsoid to spherical, wall stress is increased. By using the ratio of the long axis to the short axis as a measure of the ellipsoid shape, a decrease in this ratio would signify a transition from ellipsoid to spherical.

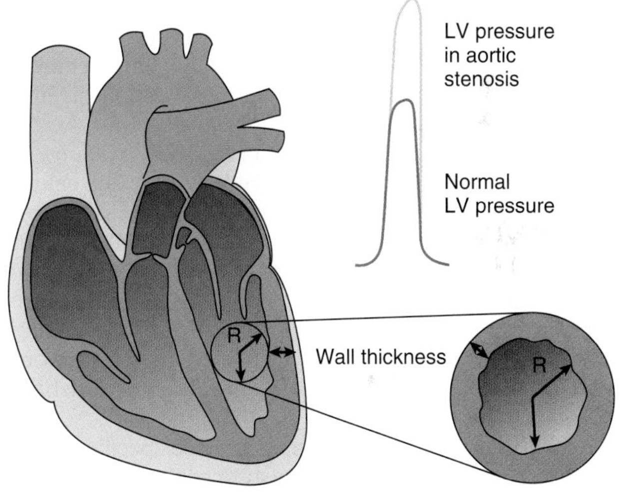

Fig. 14.4 In response to aortic stenosis, left ventricular *(LV)* pressure increases. To maintain wall stress at control levels, compensatory LV hypertrophy develops. According to Laplace's law, wall stress = pressure · radius *(R)* ÷ (2 × wall thickness). Therefore, the increase in wall thickness offsets the increased pressure, and wall stress is maintained at control levels. (From Opie LH. Ventricular function. In: *Heart Physiology From Cell to Circulation*. 4th ed. Philadelphia: Lippincott-Raven; 2004:355–401.)

Thickness of the left ventricular muscle is an important modifier of wall stress. For example, in aortic stenosis, afterload is increased. The ventricle must generate a much higher pressure to overcome the increased load opposing systolic ejection of blood. To generate such high performance, the ventricle increases its wall thickness (left ventricular hypertrophy). By applying Laplace's law, increased left ventricular wall thickness will decrease wall stress, despite the necessary increase in left ventricular pressure to overcome the aortic stenosis (Fig. 14.4).[12] In a failing heart, the radius of the LV increases, thus increasing wall stress.

Frank-Starling Relationship. The Frank-Starling relationship is an intrinsic property of myocardium by which stretching of the myocardial sarcomere results in enhanced myocardial performance for subsequent contractions (see Fig. 14.3). In 1895, Otto Frank first noted that in skeletal muscle, the change in tension was directly related to its length, and as pressure changed in the heart, a corresponding change in volume occurred.[13] In 1914, E.H. Starling, using an isolated heart-lung preparation as a model, observed that "the mechanical energy set free on passage from the resting to the contracted state is a function of the length of the muscle fiber."[14] If a strip of cardiac muscle is mounted in a muscle chamber under isometric conditions and stimulated at a fixed frequency, then an increase in sarcomere length results in an increase in twitch force. Starling concluded that the increased twitch force was the result of a greater interaction of muscle bundles.

Electron microscopy has demonstrated that sarcomere length (2-2.2 μm) is positively related to the amount of actin and myosin cross-bridging and that there is an optimal sarcomere length at which the interaction is maximal. This concept is based on the assumption that the increase in cross-bridging is equivalent to an increase in muscle performance. Although this theory continues to hold true for skeletal muscle, the force-length relationship in cardiac muscle is more complex. When comparing force-strength relationships between skeletal and cardiac muscle, it is noteworthy that the reduction in force is only 10%, even if cardiac muscle is at 80% sarcomere length.[13] The cellular basis of the Frank-Starling mechanism is still being investigated and is briefly discussed later in this chapter. A common clinical application of Starling's law is the relationship of left ventricular end-diastolic volume and SV. The Frank-Starling mechanism may remain intact even in a failing heart.[15] However, ventricular remodeling after injury or in heart failure may modify the Frank-Starling relationship.

Contractility. Each Frank-Starling curve specifies a level of contractility, or the inotropic state of the heart, which is defined as the work performed by cardiac muscle at any given end-diastolic fiber. Factors that modify contractility will create a family of Frank-Starling curves with different contractility (Fig. 14.5).[12] Factors that modify contractility are exercise, adrenergic stimulation, changes in pH, temperature, and drugs such as digitalis. The ability of the LV to develop, generate, and sustain the necessary pressure for the ejection of blood is the intrinsic inotropic state of the heart.

In isolated muscle, the maximal velocity of contraction (V_{max}) is defined as the maximal velocity of ejection at zero load. V_{max} is obtained by plotting the velocity of muscle shortening in isolated papillary muscle at varying degrees of force. Although this relationship can be replicated in isolated myocytes, V_{max} cannot be measured in an intact heart because complete unloading is impossible. To measure the intrinsic contractile activity of an intact heart, several strategies have been attempted with varying success. Pressure-volume loops, albeit requiring catheterization of the left side of the heart, are currently the best way to determine contractility in an intact heart (Fig. 14.6).[12] The pressure-volume loop represents an indirect measure of the Frank-Starling relationship between force (pressure) and muscle length (volume). Clinically, the most commonly used noninvasive index of ventricular contractile function is the ejection fraction, which is assessed by echocardiography, angiography, or radionuclide ventriculography.

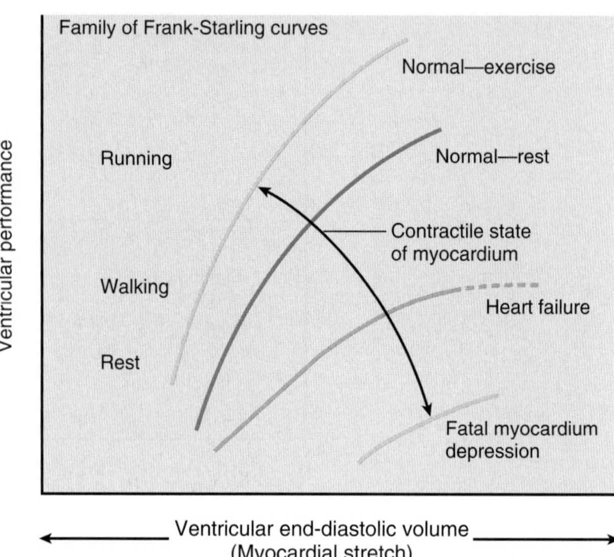

Fig. 14.5 A family of Frank-Starling curves is shown. A leftward shift of the curve denotes enhancement of the inotropic state, whereas a rightward shift denotes decreased inotropy. (From Opie LH. Ventricular function. In: *Heart Physiology From Cell to Circulation.* 4th ed. Philadelphia: Lippincott-Raven; 2004:355–401.)

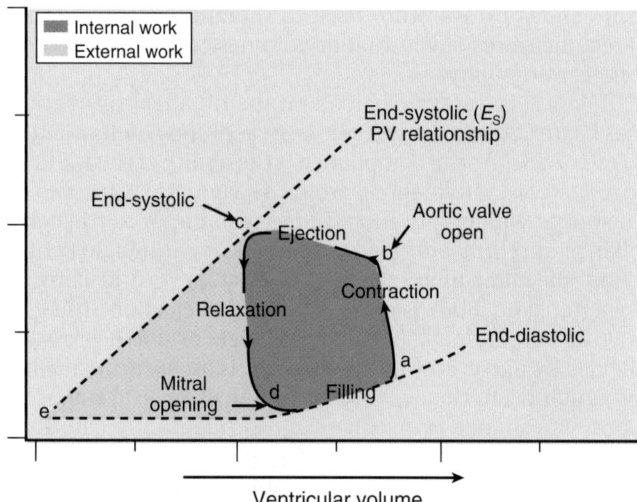

Fig. 14.6 Pressure-volume (PV) loop. Point *a* depicts the start of isovolumetric contraction. The aortic valve opens at point *b*, and ejection of blood follows *(points b→c)*. The mitral valve opens at point *d*, and ventricular filling ensues. External work is defined by points *a, b, c,* and *d,* and internal work is defined by points *e, d,* and *c.* The PV area is the sum of external and internal work. (From Opie LH. Ventricular function. In: *Heart Physiology From Cell to Circulation.* 4th ed. Philadelphia: Lippincott-Raven; 2004:355–401.)

$$\text{Ejection fraction} = (\text{LVEDV} - \text{LVESV})/\text{LVEDV}$$

where LVESV is left ventricular end-systolic volume.

Cardiac Work. The work of the heart can be divided into external and internal work. External work is expended to eject blood under pressure, whereas internal work is expended within the ventricle to change the shape of the heart and to prepare it for ejection. Internal work contributes to inefficiency in the performance of the heart. Wall stress is directly proportional to the internal work of the heart.[16]

External work, or stroke work, is a product of the SV and pressure (P) developed during ejection of the SV.

$$\text{Stroke work} = \text{SV} \times P \text{ or } (\text{LVEDV} - \text{LVESV}) \times P$$

The external work and internal work of the ventricle both consume O_2. The clinical significance of internal work is illustrated in the case of a poorly drained LV during cardiopulmonary bypass. Although external work is provided by the roller pump during bypass, myocardial ischemia can still occur because poor drainage of the LV creates tension on the left ventricular wall and increases internal work.

The efficiency of cardiac contraction is estimated by the following formula[10]:

$$\text{Cardiac efficiency} = \text{External work}/\text{Energy equivalent of } O_2 \text{consumption}$$

The corkscrew motion of the heart for the ejection of blood is the most favorable in terms of work efficiency, based on the architecture in a normal LV (with the cardiac muscle bundles arranged so that a circumferentially oriented middle layer is sandwiched by longitudinally oriented outer layers). In heart failure, ventricular dilation reduces cardiac efficiency because it increases wall stress, which in turn increases O_2 consumption.[13]

Heart Rate and Force-Frequency Relationship. In isolated cardiac muscle, an increase in the frequency of stimulation induces an increase in the force of contraction. This relationship is termed the *treppe*, which means *staircase* in German, and is the phenomenon of the force-frequency relationship.[10,17] At between 150 and 180 stimuli per minute, maximal contractile force is reached in an isolated heart muscle at a fixed muscle length. Thus, an increased frequency incrementally increases inotropy, whereas stimulation at a lower frequency decreases contractile force. However, when the stimulation becomes extremely rapid, the force of contraction decreases. In the clinical context, pacing-induced positive inotropic effects may be effective only up to a certain heart rate, based on the force-frequency relationship. In a failing heart, the force-frequency relationship may be less effective in producing a positive inotropic effect.[10]

CARDIAC OUTPUT

Cardiac output is the amount of blood pumped by the heart per unit of time ($\dot{Q}$) and is determined by four factors: two factors that are intrinsic to the heart—heart rate and myocardial contractility—and two factors that are extrinsic to the heart but functionally couple the heart and the vasculature—preload and afterload.

Heart rate is defined as the number of beats per minute and is mainly influenced by the autonomic nervous system. Increases in heart rate escalate cardiac output if ventricular filling is adequate during diastole. *Contractility* can be defined as the intrinsic level of contractile performance

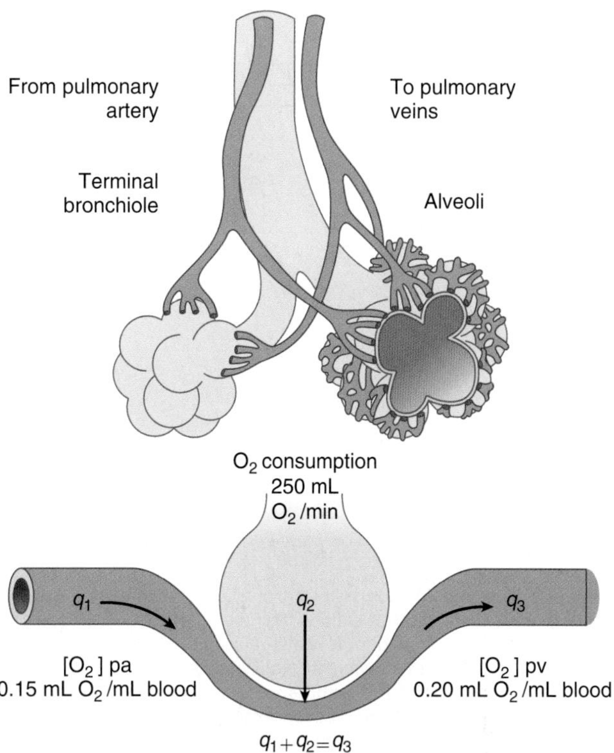

Fig. 14.7 Illustration demonstrates the principle of determination of cardiac output according to the Fick formula. If the oxygen (O_2) concentration in pulmonary arterial blood ($CpaO_2$), the O_2 concentration of the pulmonary vein ($CpvO_2$), and the O_2 consumption are known, then cardiac output can be calculated. *pa,* Pulmonary artery; *pv,* pulmonary vein. (Berne RM, Levy MN: The cardiac pump. In *Cardiovascular physiology*, ed 8, St Louis, 2001, Mosby, pp 55-82.)

that is independent of loading conditions. Contractility is difficult to define in an intact heart because it cannot be separated from loading conditions.[10,17] For example, the *Frank-Starling relationship* is defined as the change in intrinsic contractile performance, based on changes in preload. Cardiac output in a living organism can be measured with the Fick principle (a schematic depiction is illustrated in Fig. 14.7).[3]

The Fick principle is based on the concept of conservation of mass such that the O_2 delivered from pulmonary venous blood (q_3) is equal to the total O_2 delivered to pulmonary capillaries through the pulmonary artery (q_1) and the alveoli (q_2).

The amount of O_2 delivered to the pulmonary capillaries by way of the pulmonary arteries (q_1) equals total pulmonary arterial blood flow ($\dot{Q}$) times the O_2 concentration in pulmonary arterial blood ($CpaO_2$):

$$q_1 = \dot{Q} \times CpaO_2$$

The amount of O_2 carried away from pulmonary venous blood (q_3) is equal to total pulmonary venous blood flow ($\dot{Q}$) times the O_2 concentration in pulmonary venous blood ($CpvO_2$):

$$q_3 = \dot{Q} \times CpvO_2$$

The pulmonary arterial O_2 concentration is the mixed systemic venous O_2, and the pulmonary venous O_2

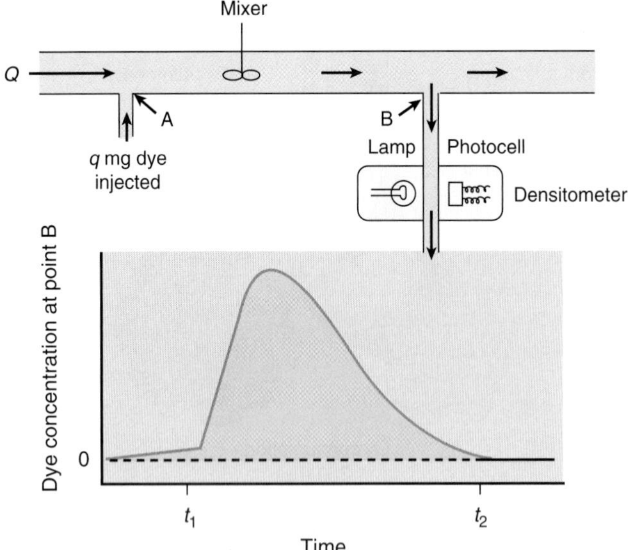

Fig. 14.8 Illustration demonstrates the principle of determining cardiac output with the indicator dilution technique. This model assumes that there is no recirculation. A known amount of dye *(q)* is injected at point *A* into a stream flowing at $\dot{Q}$ (mL/min). A mixed sample of the fluid flowing past point *B* is withdrawn at a constant rate through a densitometer. The change in dye concentration over time is depicted in a curve. Flow may be measured by dividing the amount of indicator injected upstream by the area under the downstream concentration curve. (Berne RM, Levy MN: The cardiac pump. In *Cardiovascular physiology*, ed 8, St Louis, 2001, Mosby, pp 55-82.)

concentration is the peripheral arterial O_2. O_2 consumption is the amount of O_2 delivered to the pulmonary capillaries from the alveoli (q_2). Because $q_1 + q_2 = q_3$,

$$\dot{Q}\,(CpaO_2) + q_2 = \dot{Q}\,(CpvO_2)$$

$$q_2 = \dot{Q}\,(CpvO_2) - \dot{Q}\,(CpaO_2)$$

$$q_2 = \dot{Q}\,(CpvO_2 - CpaO_2)$$

$$\dot{Q} = q_2 / (CpvO_2 - CpaO_2)$$

Thus, if the $CpaO_2$, $CpvO_2$, and O_2 consumption (q_2) are known, then the cardiac output can be determined.

The indicator dilution technique is another method for determining cardiac output also based on the law of conservation of mass. The two most commonly used indicator dilution techniques are the dye dilution and the thermodilution methods. Fig. 14.8 illustrates the principles of the dye dilution method.[3]

Cellular Cardiac Physiology

CELLULAR ANATOMY

At the cellular level, the heart consists of three major components: cardiac muscle tissue (contracting cardiomyocytes), conduction tissue (conducting cells), and extracellular connective tissue. A group of cardiomyocytes with its connective tissue support network or extracellular matrix make up a myofiber (Fig. 14.9). Adjacent myofibers are connected by strands of collagen. The extracellular matrix is the synthetic product of fibroblasts and is made up of collagen,

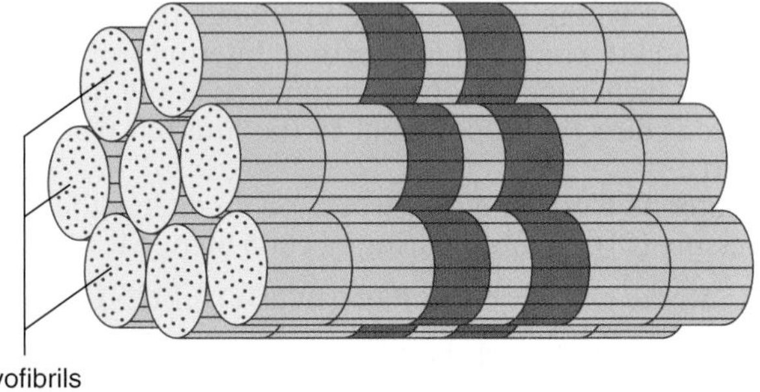

Fig. 14.9 Organization of cardiomyocytes. Fifty percent of cardiomyocyte volume is made up of myofibrils; the remainder consists of mitochondria, nucleus, sarcoplasmic reticulum, and cytosol.

which is the main determinant of myocardial stiffness, and other major matrix proteins. One of the matrix proteins, elastin, is the chief constituent of elastic fibers. The elastic fibers account for, in part, the elastic properties of the myocardium.[8] Other matrix proteins include the glycoproteins or proteoglycans and matrix metalloproteinases. Proteoglycans are proteins with short sugar chains, and they include heparan sulfate, chondroitin, fibronectin, and laminin. Matrix metalloproteins are enzymes that degrade collagen and other extracellular proteins. The balance between the accumulation of extracellular matrix proteins by synthesis and their breakdown by matrix metalloproteins contributes to the mechanical properties and function of the heart.[8]

CARDIOMYOCYTE STRUCTURE AND FUNCTION

Individual contracting cardiomyocytes are large cells between 20 μm (atrial cardiomyocytes) and 140 μm (ventricular cardiomyocytes) in length. Approximately 50% of the cell volume in a contracting cardiomyocyte is made up of myofibrils, and the remainder consists of mitochondria, nucleus, sarcoplasmic reticulum (SR), and cytosol. The myofibril is the rod-like bundle that forms the contractile elements within cardiomyocytes. Within each contractile element are contractile proteins, regulatory proteins, and structural proteins. Contractile proteins make up approximately 80% of the myofibrillar protein, with the remainder being regulatory and structural proteins.[18,19] The basic unit of contraction is the sarcomere (see discussion under Contractile Elements later in this chapter).

The sarcolemma, or the outer plasma membrane, separates the intracellular and extracellular space. It surrounds the cardiomyocyte and invaginates into the myofibrils through an extensive tubular network known as *transverse tubules* or *T tubules*, and it also forms specialized intercellular junctions between cells.[20,21]

Transverse or T tubules are in close proximity to an intramembranous system and the SR, which plays an important role in the calcium (Ca^{2+}) metabolism that is critical in the excitation-contraction coupling (ECC) of the cardiomyocyte. The SR can be further divided into the longitudinal (or network) SR and the junctional SR. The longitudinal SR is involved in the uptake of Ca^{2+} for the initiation of relaxation. The junctional SR contains large Ca^{2+}-release channels (ryanodine receptors [RyRs]) that release SR Ca^{2+} stores in response to depolarization-stimulated Ca^{2+} influx through the sarcolemmal Ca^{2+} channels. The RyRs are not only

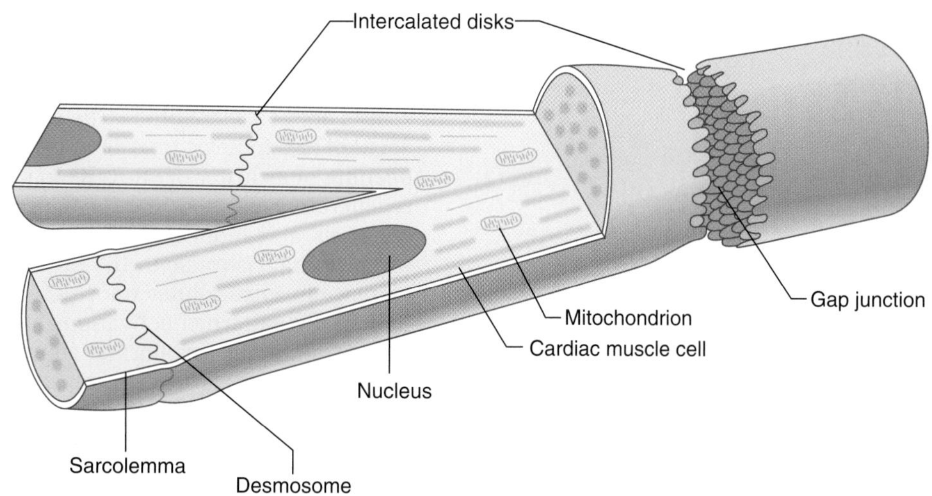

Fig. 14.10 The sarcolemma that envelops cardiomyocytes becomes highly specialized to form the intercalated disks where ends of neighboring cells are in contact. The intercalated disks consist of gap junctions and *spot* and *sheet* desmosomes.

Ca^{2+}-release channels, but they also form the scaffolding proteins that anchor many of the key regulatory proteins.[22]

Mitochondria are immediately found beneath the sarcolemma, wedged between myofibrils within the cell. They contain enzymes that promote the generation of adenosine triphosphate (ATP), and they are the energy powerhouse for the cardiomyocyte. In addition, mitochondria can also accumulate Ca^{2+} and thereby contribute to the regulation of the cytosolic Ca^{2+} concentration. Nearly all the genetic information is found within the centrally located nucleus. The cytosol is the fluid-filled microenvironment within the sarcolemma, exclusive of the organelles and the contractile apparatus and proteins.

Cardiac muscle cells contain three different types of intercellular junctions: gap junctions, *spot* desmosomes, and *sheet* desmosomes (or fasciae adherens) (Fig. 14.10).[20,23] Gap junctions are responsible for electrical coupling and the transfer of small molecules between cells, whereas desmosome-like junctions provide mechanical linkage. The adhesion sites formed by spot desmosomes anchor the intermediate filament cytoskeleton of the cell; those formed by the fasciae adherens anchor the contractile apparatus. Gap junctions consist of clusters of plasma membrane channels directly linking the cytoplasmic compartments of neighboring cells. Gap junction channels are constructed from connexins, a multigene family of conserved proteins. The principal connexin isoform of the mammalian heart is connexin 43; other connexins, notably connexins 40, 45, and 37, are also expressed but in smaller quantities.[22,23]

The conducting cardiomyocytes, or Purkinje cells, are cells specialized for conducting propagated action potentials. These cells have a low content of myofibrils and a prominent nucleus, and they contain an abundance of gap junctions. Cardiomyocytes can be functionally separated into (1) the excitation system, (2) the ECC system, and (3) the contractile system.

Excitation System

The cellular action potential originating in the specialized conduction tissue is propagated to individual cells where it initiates the intracellular event that leads to the contraction of the cell through the sarcolemmal excitation system.

Action Potential. Ion fluxes across plasma membranes result in depolarization (attaining a less negative membrane potential) and repolarization (attaining a more negative membrane potential). They are mediated by membrane proteins with ion-selective pores. Because these ion channel proteins open and close the pores in response to changes in membrane potential, the channels are voltage gated. In the heart, sodium (Na^+), potassium (K^+), Ca^{2+}, and chloride ($Cl-$) channels contribute to the action potential.

The types of action potential in the heart can be separated into two categories: (1) fast-response action potentials, which are found in the His-Purkinje system and atrial or ventricular cardiomyocytes; and (2) slow-response action potentials, which are found in the pacemaker cells in the SA and AV nodes. A typical tracing of an action potential in the His-Purkinje system is depicted in Fig. 14.11.[10] The electrochemical gradient for K^+ across the plasma membrane is the determinant for the resting membrane potential. Mostly as a result of the influx of Na^+, the membrane potential becomes depolarized, which leads to an extremely rapid upstroke (phase 0). As the membrane potential reaches a critical level (or threshold) during depolarization, the action potential is propagated. The rapid upstroke is followed by a transient repolarization (phase 1). Phase 1 is a period of brief and limited repolarization that is largely attributable to the activation of a transient outward K^+ current, i_{to}. The plateau phase (phase 2) occurs with a net influx of Ca^{2+} through L-type Ca^{2+} channels and the efflux of K^+ through several K^+ channels—the inwardly rectifying i_k, the delayed rectifier i_{k1}, and i_{to}. Repolarization (phase 3) is brought about when an efflux of K^+ from the three outward K^+ currents exceeds the influx of Ca^{2+}, thus returning the membrane to the resting potential. Very little ionic flux occurs during diastole (phase 4) in a fast-response action potential.

In contrast, during diastole (phase 4), pacemaker cells that show slow-response action potentials have the capability of spontaneous diastolic depolarization and generate the automatic cardiac rhythm. Pacemaker currents during phase 4 are the result of an increase in the three inward currents and a decrease in the two outward currents. The three

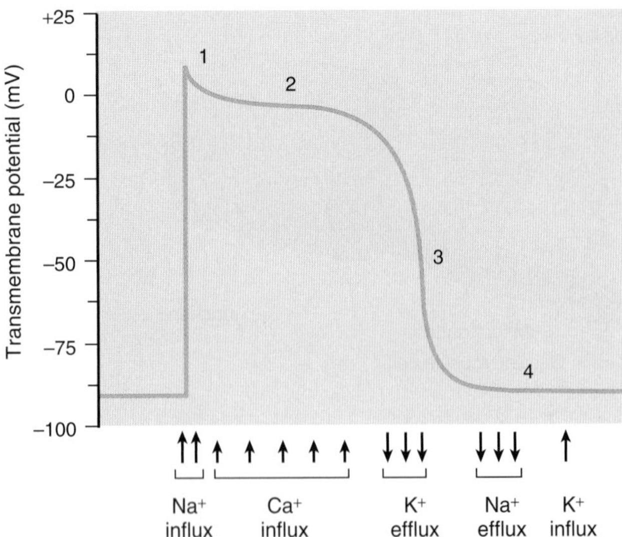

Fig. 14.11 Phases of cellular action potentials and major associated currents in ventricular myocytes. The initial phase (0) spike and overshoot (1) are caused by a rapid inward sodium (Na^+) current, the plateau phase (2) by a slow calcium (Ca^{2+}) current through L-type Ca channels, and repolarization (phase 3) by outward potassium (K^+) currents. Phase 4, the resting potential (Na^+ efflux, K^+ influx), is maintained by Na^+-K^+-adenosine triphosphatase (ATPase). The Na^+-Ca^{2+} exchanger is mainly responsible for extrusion of Ca^{2+}. In specialized conduction system tissue, spontaneous depolarization takes place during phase 4 until the voltage resulting in opening of the Na channel is reached. (From LeWinter MM, Osol G. Normal physiology of the cardiovascular system. In Fuster V, Alexander RW, O'Rourke RA, eds. *Hurst's the Heart*. 10th ed. New York: McGraw-Hill; 2001:63–94.)

inward currents that contribute to spontaneous pacemaker activity include two carried by Ca^{2+}, i_{CaL} and i_{CaT}, and one that is a mixed cation current, I_f.[24] The two outward currents are the delayed rectifier K^+ current, i_k, and the inward rectifying K^+ current, i_{k1}. When compared with the fast-response action potential, phase 0 is much less steep, phase 1 is absent, and phase 2 is indistinct from phase 3 in the slow-response action potential.[25] In SA node cells, the pacemaker I_f current is the principal determinant of duration diastolic depolarization, and it is encoded by four members of the hyperpolarization-activated cyclic nucleotide-gated gene (HCN1-4) family.[26]

During the cardiac action potential, movement of Ca^{2+} into the cell and Na^+ out of the cell creates an ionic imbalance. The Na^+-Ca^{2+} exchanger restores cellular ionic balance by actively transporting Ca^{2+} out of the cell against a concentration gradient while moving Na^+ into the cell in an energy-dependent manner.

Excitation-Contraction Coupling

Structures that participate in cardiac ECC include the sarcolemma, transverse tubules, SR, and myofilaments (Fig. 14.12A).[27] The process of ECC begins with depolarization of the plasma membrane and spread of electrical excitation along the sarcolemma of cardiomyocytes.

The ubiquitous second messenger Ca^{2+} is the key player in cardiac ECC (see Fig. 14.12B).[25] Cycling of Ca^{2+} within the structures that participate in ECC initiates and terminates contraction. Activation of the contractile system depends on an increase in free cytosolic Ca^{2+} and its subsequent binding to contractile proteins.

Ca^{2+} enters through plasma membrane channels concentrated at the T tubules, and such entry through L-type Ca^{2+} channels (dihydropyridine receptors) triggers the release of Ca^{2+} from the SR.[28] This evokes a *Ca^{2+} spark*. Ca^{2+} sparks are considered to be the elementary Ca^{2+} signaling event of ECC in heart muscle. A Ca^{2+} spark occurs with the opening of a cluster of SR RyRs to release Ca^{2+} in a locally regenerative manner. It, in turn, activates the Ca^{2+}-release channels and induces further release of Ca^{2+} from subsarcolemmal cisternae in the SR and thus leads to a large increase in intracellular Ca^{2+} (iCa^{2+}). These spatially and temporally patterned activations of localized Ca^{2+} release, in turn, stimulate myofibrillar contraction. The increase in iCa^{2+}, however, is transient, inasmuch as Ca^{2+} is removed by active uptake by the SR Ca^{2+} pump adenosine triphosphatase (ATPase), extrusion of Ca^{2+} from the cytosol by the Na^+-Ca^{2+} exchanger, and binding of Ca^{2+} to proteins.[29] Ca^{2+} sparks have also been implicated in pathophysiologic diseases such as hypertension, cardiac arrhythmias, heart failure, and muscular dystrophy.[30-32]

The SR provides the anatomic framework and is the major organelle for the cycling of Ca^{2+}. It is the depot for iCa^{2+} stores. The cyclic release plus reuptake of Ca^{2+} by the SR regulates the cytosolic Ca^{2+} concentration and couples excitation to contraction. The physical proximity between L-type Ca^{2+} channels and RyRs at the SR membrane makes Ca^{2+}-induced Ca^{2+} release occur easily. The *foot* region of the RyR is the part that extends from the SR membrane to the T tubules, where the L-type Ca^{2+} channels are located.[19,29,33]

The SR is also concerned with the reuptake of Ca^{2+} that initiates relaxation or terminates contraction. The sarcoplasmic/endoplasmic reticulum Ca^{2+}-ATPase (SERCA) pump is the ATP-dependent pump that actively pumps the majority of the Ca^{2+} back into the SR after its release. SERCA makes up close to 90% of all the SR proteins and is inhibited by the phosphoprotein, phospholamban, at rest. Phospholamban is an SR membrane protein that is active in the dephosphorylated form. Phosphorylation by a variety of kinases as a result of β-adrenergic stimulation or other stimuli inactivates phospholamban and releases its inhibitory action on SERCA. Positive feedback ensues and leads to further phospholamban phosphorylation and greater SERCA activity. Active reuptake of Ca^{2+} by SERCA then promotes relaxation.[19,29,33]

Once taken up into the SR, Ca^{2+} is stored until it is released during the next cycle. Calsequestrin and calreticulin are two storage proteins in the SR. Calsequestrin is a highly charged protein located in the cisternal component of the SR near the T tubules. Because it lies close to the Ca^{2+}-release channels, the stored Ca^{2+} can be quickly discharged for release once the Ca^{2+}-release channels are stimulated. Cytosolic Ca^{2+} can also be removed by extrusion through the sarcolemmal Ca^{2+} pump and the activity of the Na^+-Ca^{2+} exchanger. The protein, calmodulin, is an important *sensor* and regulator of iCa^{2+}.[21]

Errors in Ca^{2+} Handling. Because of the ubiquity of Ca^{2+} in cardiac signaling, changes in Ca^{2+} handling can be associated with numerous maladaptive outcomes. There is an increase in Ca^{2+} leak from the SR in the failing heart, which may be associated with removal of Ca^{2+} from the cytosole.

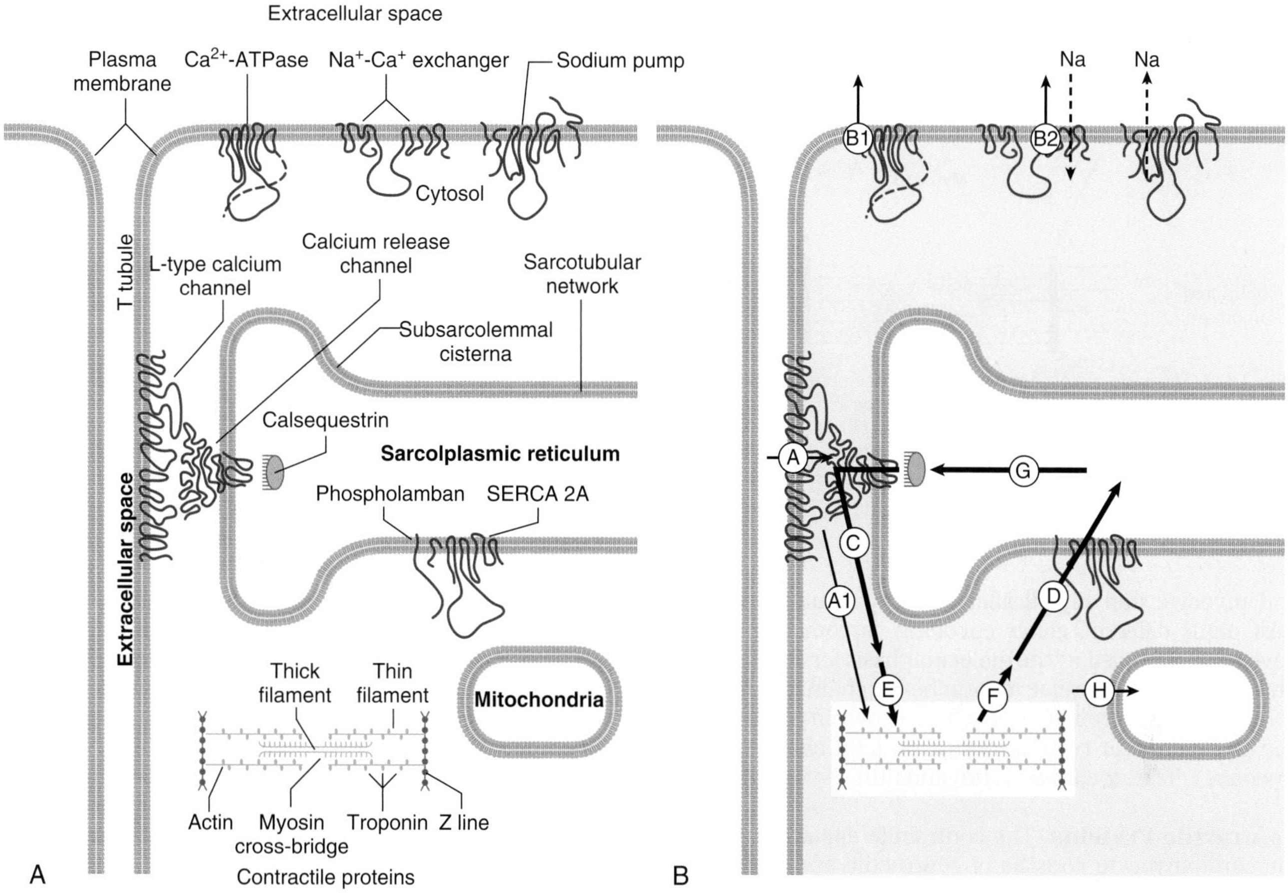

Fig. 14.12 (A) Diagram depicts the components of cardiac excitation-contraction coupling. Calcium pools are noted in **bold** letters. (B) Extracellular *(arrows A, B1, B2)* and intracellular calcium flux *(arrows C, D, E, F, G)* are shown. The thickness of the *arrows* indicates the magnitude of the calcium flux, and the vertical orientations describe their energetics: downward-pointing arrows represent passive calcium flux, whereas upward-pointing arrows represent energy-dependent calcium transport. Calcium entering the cell from extracellular fluid through L-type calcium channels triggers the release of calcium from the sarcoplasmic reticulum. Only a small portion directly activates the contractile proteins (*arrow A1*). Arrow B1 depicts active transport of calcium into extracellular fluid by means of the plasma membrane calcium adenosine triphosphatase (Ca^{2+}-ATPase) pump and the sodium-calcium (Na^+-Ca^{2+}) exchanger. Sodium that enters the cell in exchange for calcium *(dashed line)* is pumped out of the cytosol by the sodium pump. SR regulates calcium efflux from the subsarcolemmal cisternae *(arrow C)* and calcium uptake into the sarcotubular network *(arrow D)*. *Arrow G* represents calcium that diffuses within the SR. Calcium binding to *(arrow E)* and dissociation from *(arrow F)* high-affinity calcium-binding sites of troponin C activate and inhibit interactions of the contractile proteins. Arrow H depicts movement of calcium into and out of mitochondria to buffer the cytosolic calcium concentration. *SERCA 2A*, Sarcoplasmic/endoplasmic reticulum Ca^{2+}-ATPase. (From Katz AM. Calcium fluxes. In: *Physiology of the Heart*. 3rd ed. Philadelphia: Lippincott-Raven; 2001:232–233.)

This Ca^{2+} leak from the SR may significantly reduce contractile force in the heart and contributes to reduced inotropy in heart failure.[34,35] Uncoupling of β-AR activation of protein kinase A (PKA) and dysregulation of Ca^{2+} handling occurs in heart failure.[34] PKA, a cAMP-dependent protein kinase, is a key effector protein activated by β-AR agonists, which stimulates transsarcolemmal Ca^{2+} influx and its sequestration in the SR, leading to increased contractile function and lusitropy. Calcineurin, a Ca^{2+}-dependent signaling molecule, is consistently linked with myocardial hypertrophy via gene expression through a nuclear factor of activated T-cells pathway.[34,35] Calcium-calmodulin-dependent protein kinase II, in addition to calcineurin, is tightly coupled with Ca^{2+} homeostasis, and its prolonged activation can be proarrhythmic.

Contractile System

Contractile Elements. The basic working unit of contraction is the sarcomere. A *sarcomere* is defined as the distance between Z lines (Z is an abbreviation for the German word, *Zuckung*, meaning *contraction*), which join the sarcomeres in series. Each sarcomere consists of a central A band that is separated by one half of an I band from the Z lines on each side because the Z line bisects the I band. A schematic representation is depicted in Fig. 14.13.[10] Within each sarcomere are two principal contractile proteins (see the next section, Contractile Proteins) and one noncontractile protein, titin.[29] The two contractile proteins are actin, the thin filament, and myosin, the thick filament. Actin filaments and titin are both tethered to the Z line, but the thick myosin filaments do not actually reach the Z lines. Titin, the third filament protein, tethers the thick-filament myosin to the Z line. The Z lines at the two ends of the sarcomere are brought closer together during contraction as the thick-filament myosin heads interact with the thin actin filaments and slide over each other.[36,37]

Familial hypertrophic cardiomyopathy is an inherited autosomal dominant sarcomeric disease[38] that is the most common cause of sudden death in otherwise healthy individuals. Its clinical features are left ventricular hypertrophy

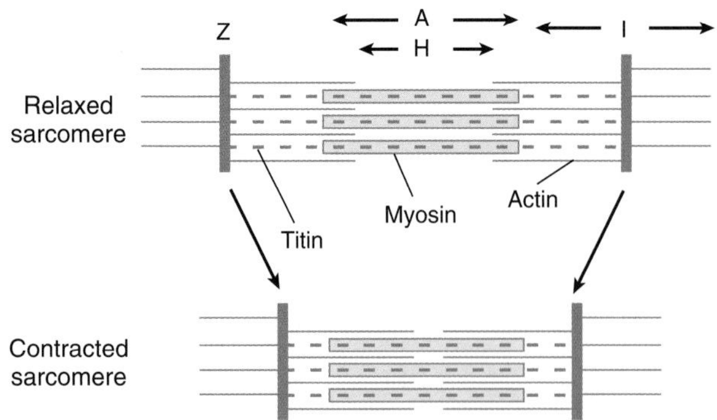

Fig. 14.13 The basic unit of contraction is the sarcomere. A contracted and relaxed sarcomere is depicted. Z lines are located at the ends of the sarcomere. The A band is the site of overlap between myosin and actin filaments. The I band is located on either side of the A band and contains only actin filament. The H zone is located in the center of the A band, and only myosin is present.

and myocyte and myofibrillar disarray. Mutations in at least eight different genes encoding sarcomere proteins have been identified as the molecular basis for the disorder. These genes are β-cardiac myosin heavy chain, cardiac troponin T (TnT), α-tropomyosin, cardiac myosin-binding protein C, essential or regulatory myosin light chain, cardiac troponin I (TnI), α-cardiac actin, and titin.[38]

Contractile Proteins. The contractile apparatus within the cardiomyocyte consists of contractile and regulatory proteins.[21,39,40] The thin-filament actin and the thick-filament myosin are the two principal contractile proteins. Actin contains two helical chains. Tropomyosin, a double-stranded α-helical regulatory protein, winds around the actin array and forms the backbone for the thin-filament actin. The thick-filament myosin is made up of 300 myosin molecules. Each myosin molecule has two functional domains: the body or filament and the bilobar myosin head. The myosin head is made up of one heavy chain and two light chains. The heavy head chain has two domains: the larger one interacts with actin at the actin cleft and has an ATP-binding pocket where myosin ATPase is located, and the other smaller one is flexible and attached to the two light chains. The regulatory troponin heterotrimer complex is found at regular intervals along tropomyosin. The heterotrimer troponins are made up of troponin C (TnC), the Ca^{2+} receptor; TnI, an inhibitor of actin-myosin interaction; and TnT, which links the troponin complex to tropomyosin. Tropomodulin is another regulatory protein. It is located at the end of the thin-filament actin and caps the end to prevent any excessive elongation of the thin filament.[36,37]

Myocyte Contraction and Relaxation. At rest, cross-bridge cycling and generation of force do not occur because either the myosin heads are blocked from physically reacting with the thin filament or they are only weakly bound to actin (Fig. 14.14).[18] Cross-bridge cycling is initiated on binding of Ca^{2+} to TnC, which increases TnC-TnI interaction and decreases the inhibitory TnI-actin interaction. These events, which ensue from the binding of Ca^{2+} to TnC, lead to conformational changes in tropomyosin and permit attachment of the myosin head to actin. Cross-bridging involves the detachment of the myosin head from actin and a reattachment of myosin to another actin on hydrolysis of ATP by myosin ATPase. Binding of ATP to the nucleotide pocket of the myosin head leads to the activation of myosin ATPase,[33,36,37] ATP hydrolysis, and changes in the configuration of the myosin head, all of which facilitate binding of the myosin head to actin and the generation of the power stroke of the myosin head. Based on this model, the rate of cross-bridge cycling is dependent on the activity of myosin ATPase.[40] Turnoff of cross-bridge cycling is largely initiated by the decrease in cytosolic Ca^{2+}.

Myocyte relaxation is an energy-dependent process because restoration of cytosolic Ca^{2+} to resting levels requires the expenditure of ATP. The decrease in cytosolic Ca^{2+} occurs through active reuptake of Ca^{2+} into the SR by SERCA and extrusion of Ca^{2+} by the Na^+-Ca^{2+} exchanger. This activity results in the release of Ca^{2+} binding to TnC and the separation of the myosin-actin cross-bridge. Myocyte relaxation is dependent on the kinetics of cross-bridge cycling, the affinity of Ca^{2+} for TnC, and the activity of the Ca^{2+}-reuptake mechanisms. Relaxation is enhanced by the increased kinetics of cross-bridge cycling, decreased Ca^{2+} affinity for TnC, and increased activity of Ca^{2+}-reuptake mechanisms.[29]

Titin is a giant string-like protein that acts as the third filament within the sarcomere. A single titin molecule spans one half of the sarcomere. Structurally, titin consists of an inextensible anchoring segment and an extensible elastic segment. Its two main functions involve muscle assembly and elasticity. Titin is the principal determinant of the passive properties of the myocardium at small ventricular volumes.[41]

The Frank-Starling relationship states that an increase in end-diastolic volume results in enhanced systolic function.[42,43] At the cellular level, the key component for the Frank-Starling relationship is a length-dependent shift in Ca^{2+} sensitivity.[44-46] Several possible mechanisms for this change in Ca^{2+} sensitivity have been implicated, including Ca^{2+} sensitivity: as a function of myofilament lattice spacing, involving positive cooperativity in cross-bridge binding to actin, and dependence on a strain of the elastic protein titin.[40,44]

Cytoskeleton Proteins. The cytoskeleton is the protein framework within the cytoplasm that links, anchors, or tethers structural components inside the cell.[18,21] Microfilaments (actin filaments), microtubules, and intermediate filaments are three classes of cytoskeleton proteins found in the cytoplasm. Microfilament proteins are actin filaments, either sarcomeric or cortical, depending on their location. Sarcomeric actin filaments are the thin filaments in the contractile machinery that have been previously described. Cortical actin filaments are found below the plasma membrane at the cell surface and are linked to several other microfilament proteins, including dystrophin, vinculin, and ankyrin. Microtubules assemble by polymerization of the α- and β-dimers of tubulin. They play a major role in intracellular transport and cell division.[47] Attachment of the ends of microtubules to cellular structures causes the microtubules to expand and contract, thereby pulling and pushing these structures around the cell. The intermediate filaments are relatively insoluble. They have been demonstrated to be important in normal mitochondrial function and behavior. The desmin intermediate filament in cardiomyocytes connects the nucleus to the plasma membrane and is important in the transmission of the stress and strain of contractile force between cells.[48]

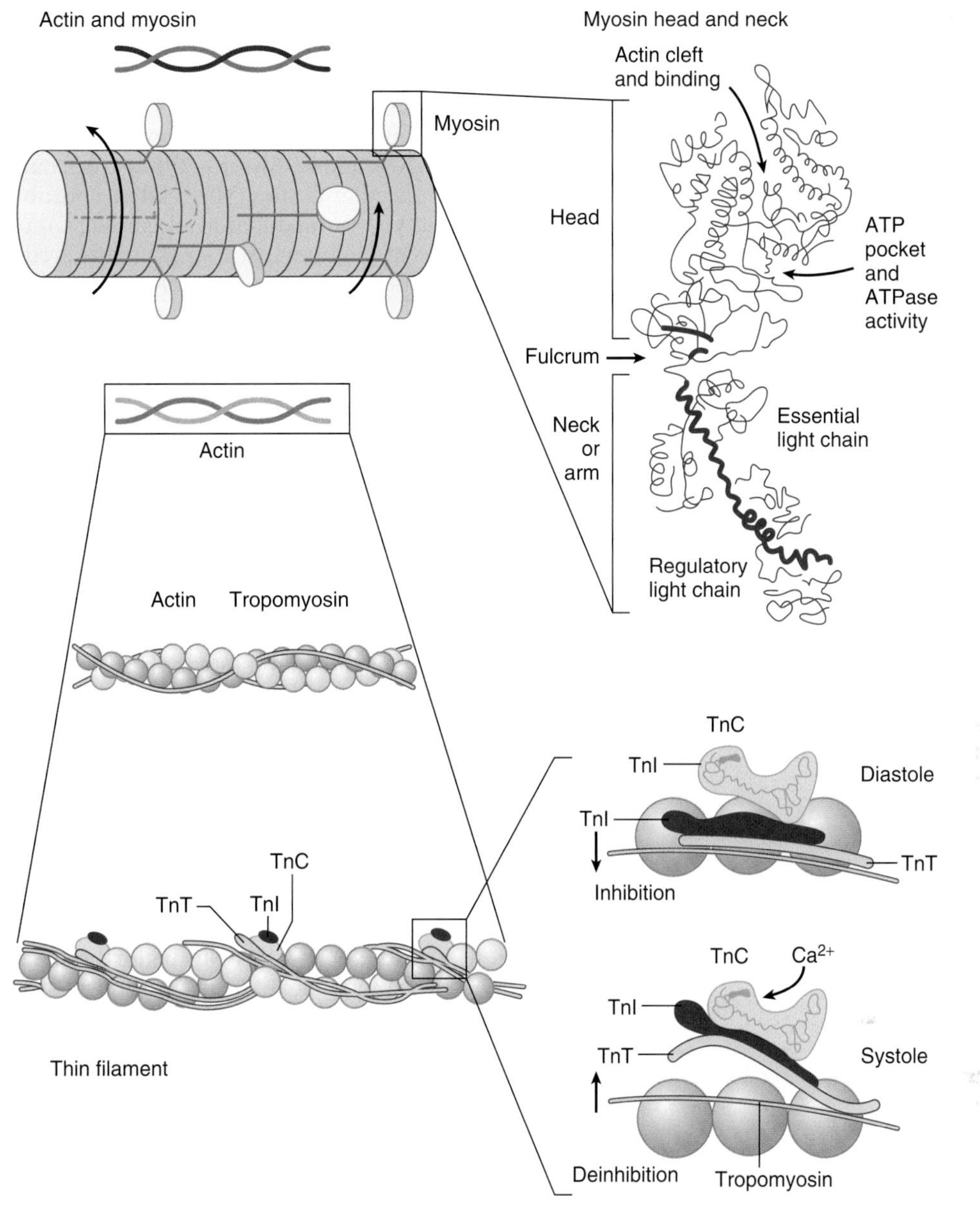

Fig. 14.14 Molecules of the contractile system, troponins C, I, and T (TnC, TnI, and TnT). *ATP*, Adenosine triphosphate; *ATPase*, adenosine triphosphatase. (From Opie LH. Ventricular function. In: *Heart Physiology From Cell to Circulation*. 4th ed. Philadelphia: Lippincott-Raven; 2004:209–231.)

The cytoskeleton provides the organization of microenvironments within the cell for enzyme and protein activity and interaction.

Whereas familial hypertrophic cardiomyopathy is a genetic sarcomeric disease, familial dilated cardiomyopathy (FDCM) is a disease of cytoskeleton proteins. The genetic basis of FDCM includes two genes for X-linked FDCM (dystrophin, G4.5) and four genes for the autosomal dominant form (actin, desmin, lamin A/C, and δ-sarcoglycan).[18]

Control of Cardiac Function

NEURAL REGULATION OF CARDIAC FUNCTION

The two limbs of the autonomic nervous system provide opposing input to regulate cardiac function.[49] The neurotransmitter of the sympathetic nervous system is norepinephrine, which provides positive chronotropic (heart rate), inotropic (contractility), and lusitropic (relaxation) effects. The parasympathetic nervous system has a more direct inhibitory effect in the atria and has a negative modulatory effect in the ventricles. The neurotransmitter of the parasympathetic nervous system is acetylcholine. Both norepinephrine and acetylcholine bind to seven-transmembrane-spanning G protein–coupled receptors (GPCRs) to transduce their intracellular signals and affect their functional responses (Fig. 14.15).[50] At rest, the heart has a tonic level of parasympathetic cardiac nerve firing and little, if any, sympathetic activity. Therefore, the major influence on the heart at rest is parasympathetic. During exercise or stress, however, the sympathetic neural influence becomes more prominent.

Parasympathetic innervation of the heart is through the vagal nerve. Supraventricular tissue receives significantly more intense vagal innervation than do the ventricles. The principal parasympathetic target neuroeffectors are the muscarinic receptors in the heart.[51,52] Activation of muscarinic receptors reduces pacemaker activity, slows AV conduction, directly decreases atrial contractile force, and exerts inhibitory modulation of ventricular contractile force. A total of five muscarinic receptors have been cloned.[53] M_2 receptors are the predominant subtype found in the mammalian heart. In the coronary circulation, M_3 receptors have been identified. Moreover, non-M_2 receptors have also been reported to exist in the heart. In general, for intracellular signaling, M_1, M_3, and M_5 receptors couple to $G_{q/11}$ protein and activate the phospholipase C-diacylglycerol-inositol phosphate system. On the other hand, the M_2 and M_4 receptors couple to the pertussis toxin-sensitive G protein, $G_{i/o}$, to inhibit adenylyl cyclase. M_2 receptors can couple to certain K^+ channels and influence the activity of Ca^{2+} channels, I_f current, phospholipase A_2, phospholipase D, and tyrosine kinases.

In contrast to vagal innervation, sympathetic innervation of the heart is more predominant in the ventricle than in the atrium. Norepinephrine released from sympathetic nerve terminals stimulates adrenergic receptors (adrenoreceptors [AdRs]) located in the heart. The two major classes of ARs are α and β, both of which are GPCRs that transduce their intracellular signals by means of specific signaling cascades (Fig. 14.16).

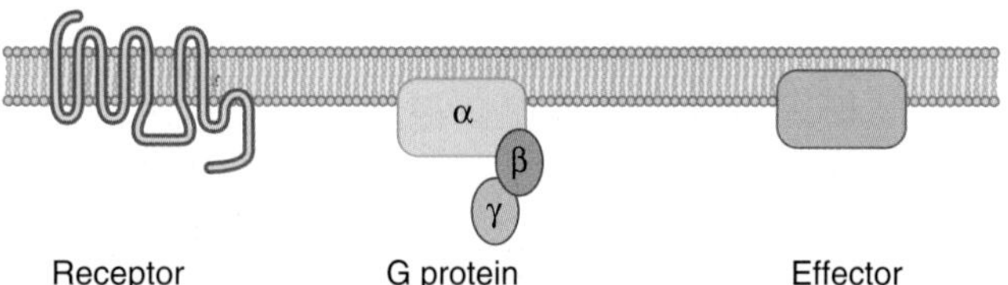

Fig. 14.15 General scheme for a G protein–coupled receptor consisting of receptor, the heterotrimeric G protein, and the effector unit. (Reprinted with permission from Bers DM. Cardiac excitation-contraction coupling. *Nature* 2002;415:198–205. Copyright MacMillan Magazines Ltd.)

β-ARs can be further divided into subpopulations of β_1, β_2, and β_3.[54] Although most mammalian hearts contain β1-ARs and β_2-ARs, β_3-ARs also exist in many mammalian ventricular tissues. The relative contribution of each β-AR subtype to modulation of cardiac function varies among species. In humans, β_1-ARs are the predominant subtype in both the atria and ventricles, but a substantial proportion of β_2-ARs are found in the atria, and approximately 20% of β_2-ARs are found in the LV. Much less is known about β_3-ARs, but they do exist in the human ventricle. Even though the β_1-AR population is more intense than the β_2-AR population, the cardiostimulant effect is not proportional to the relative densities of these two subpopulations, which is largely attributable to the tighter coupling of β_2-ARs than β_1-ARs to the cyclic adenosine monophosphate (cAMP) signaling pathway. Both β_1-ARs and β_2-ARs activate a pathway that involves the stimulatory G protein (Gs), activation of adenylyl cyclase, accumulation of cAMP, stimulation of cAMP-dependent PKA, and phosphorylation of key target proteins, including L-type Ca^{2+} channels, phospholamban, and TnI.

Both β_1-ARs and β_2-ARs are coupled to the G_s-cAMP pathway. Additionally, β_2-ARs can couple to G protein–independent pathways to modulate cardiac function, and also couple to the inhibitory G protein (Gi) to activate non–cAMP-dependent signaling pathways. β-AR stimulation increases both contraction and relaxation, as summarized in Fig. 14.17.

The two major subpopulations of α-ARs are α_1 and α_2. α_1-ARs and α_2-ARs can be further subdivided into different subtypes. α_1-ARs are GPCRs and include the α_{1A}, α_{1B}, and α_{1D} subtypes. The α_1-AR subtypes are products of separate genes and differ in structure, G protein coupling, tissue distribution, signaling, regulation, and function. Both

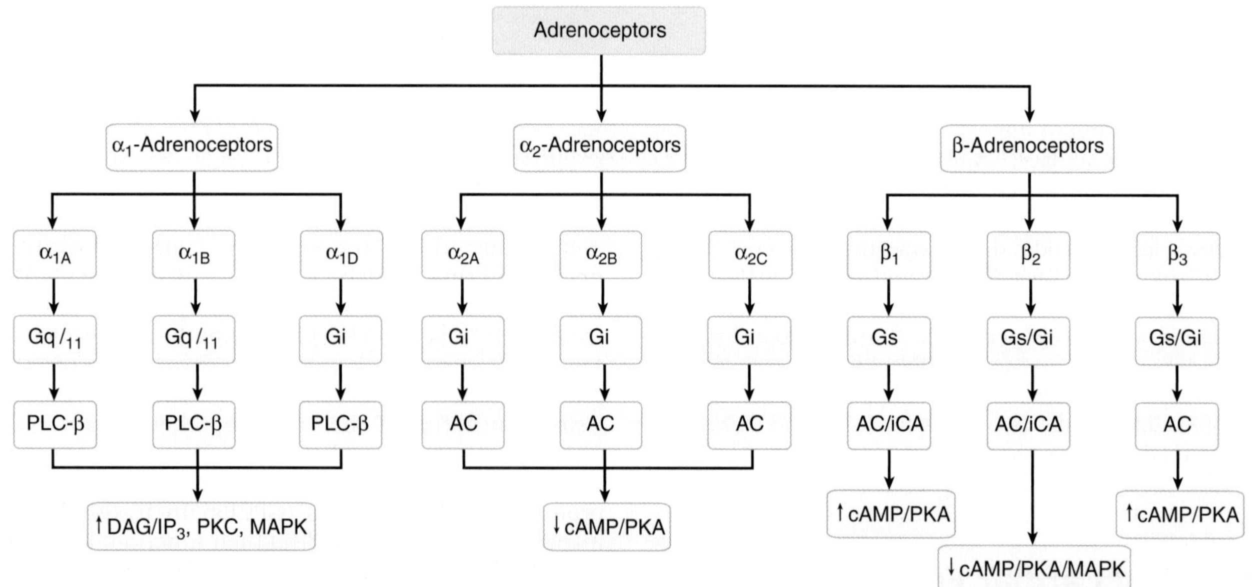

Fig. 14.16 Adrenoceptor signaling cascades involving G proteins and effectors are adenylyl cyclase *(AC)*, L-type calcium current *(iCA)*, and phospholipase β *(PLC-β)* in the heart. The intracellular signals are diacylglycerol *(DAG)*, inositol 1,4,5-triphosphate *(IP_3)*, protein kinase C *(PKC)*, cyclic adenosine monophosphate *(cAMP)*, protein kinase A *(PKA)*, and mitogen-activated protein kinase *(MAPK)*. *$Gq/_{11}$*, Heterotrimeric G protein; *Gi*, inhibitory G protein; *Gs*, stimulatory G protein.

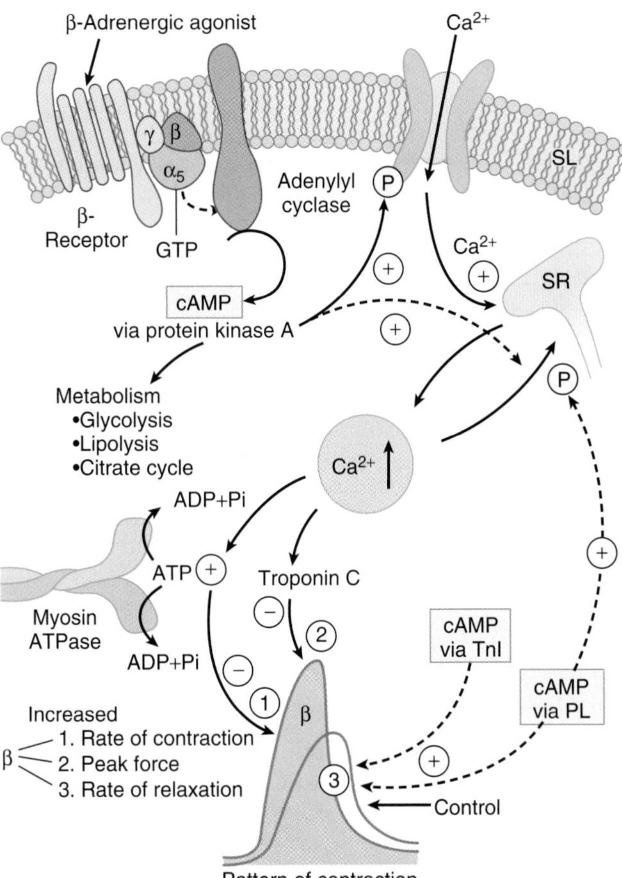

Fig. 14.17 The β-adrenoceptor signaling system leads to an increased rate and force of contraction and increased relaxation. *ADP*, Adenosine diphosphate; *ATP*, adenosine triphosphate; *ATPase*, adenosine triphosphatase; *cAMP*, cyclic adenosine monophosphate; *GTP*, guanosine triphosphate; *Pi*, phosphatidylinositol; *PL*, phospholipase; *SL*, sarcolemma; *SR*, sarcoplasmic reticulum; *TnI*, troponin I. (From Opie LH. Receptors and signal transduction. In: *Heart Physiology From Cell to Circulation*. 3rd ed. Philadelphia: Lippincott-Raven; 1998:195.)

α_{1A}-ARs and α_{1B}-ARs mediate positive inotropic responses. However, the positive inotropic effect mediated by α_1-ARs is believed to be of minor importance in the heart. α_1-ARs are coupled to phospholipase C, phospholipase D, and phospholipase A_2; they increase iCa^{2+} and myofibrillar sensitivity to Ca^{2+}.

Cardiac hypertrophy is primarily mediated by α_{1A}-ARs.[55,56] Cardiac hypertrophic responses to α_1-AR agonists involve activation of protein kinase C and mitogen-activated protein kinase through G_q-signaling mechanisms. Three subtypes of α_2-ARs are recognized: α_{2A}, α_{2B}, and α_{2C}. In the mammalian heart, α_2-ARs in the atrium play a role in the presynaptic inhibition of norepinephrine release. These prejunctional α_2-ARs are believed to belong to the α_{2C} subtype.

Neural regulation of cardiac function involves a complex interaction between the different classes and subpopulations of adrenoceptors and their signaling pathways. Targeted therapeutics in cardiovascular medicine involve the clinical application and manipulation of a basic understanding of adrenoceptor pharmacology.

HORMONES AFFECTING CARDIAC FUNCTION

Many hormones have direct and indirect actions on the heart (Table 14.1). Hormones with cardiac actions can be synthesized and secreted by cardiomyocytes or produced by other tissues and delivered to the heart. They act on specific receptors expressed in cardiomyocytes. Most of these hormone receptors are plasma membrane GPCRs. Non-GPCRs include the natriuretic peptide receptors, which are guanylyl cyclase-coupled receptors, and the glucocorticoid and mineralocorticoid receptors, which bind androgens and aldosterone and are nuclear zinc finger transcription factors. Hormones can have activity in normal cardiac physiologic function or are active only in pathophysiologic conditions, or both situations can apply. Most of the new information regarding the action of hormones in the heart has been derived from the endocrine changes associated with chronic heart failure.[57]

Cardiac hormones are polypeptides secreted by cardiac tissues into the circulation in the normal heart. Natriuretic peptides,[58,59] aldosterone,[60] and adrenomedullin[61] are hormones secreted by cardiomyocytes. Angiotensin II, the effector hormone in the renin-angiotensin system, is also produced by cardiomyocytes.[62,63] The renin-angiotensin system is one of the most important regulators of cardiovascular physiology. It is a key modulator of cardiac growth and function. Angiotensin II stimulates two separate receptor subtypes, AT_1 and AT_2, both of which are present in the heart. AT_1 receptors are the predominant subtype expressed in the normal adult human heart. Stimulation of AT_1 receptors induces a positive chronotropic and inotropic effect. Angiotensin II also mediates cell growth and proliferation in cardiomyocytes and fibroblasts, and induces the release of the growth factors aldosterone and catecholamines through the stimulation of AT_1 receptors. Activation of AT_1 receptors is directly involved in the development of cardiac hypertrophy and heart failure, as well as adverse remodeling of the myocardium. In contrast, AT_2 receptor activation is counterregulatory and generally antiproliferative. Expression of AT_2 receptors, however, is relatively scant in the adult heart because AT_2 receptors are most abundant in the fetal heart and decline with development. In response to injury and ischemia, AT_2 receptors become upregulated. The precise role of AT_2 receptors in the heart remains to be defined.

The beneficial effects of blockade of the renin-angiotensin system with angiotensin-converting enzyme inhibitors in the treatment of heart failure have been attributed to an inhibition of AT_1-receptor activity. In addition to the renin-angiotensin system, other cardiac hormones that have been shown to play pathogenic roles in the promotion of cardiomyocyte growth and cardiac fibrosis, development of cardiac hypertrophy, and progression of congestive heart failure include aldosterone,[60] adrenomedullin,[64-66] natriuretic peptides,[58,59] angiotensin,[67-69] endothelin,[70] and vasopressin.[71,72]

Increased stretch of the myocardium stimulates the release of atrial natriuretic protein (ANP) and B-type natriuretic protein (BNP) from the atria and ventricles, respectively. Both ANP and BNP bind to natriuretic peptide receptors to generate the second messenger cyclic guanosine monophosphate and represent part of the cardiac

TABLE 14.1 Actions of Hormones on Cardiac Function

Hormone	Receptor	Cardiac Action	Increase (+) or Decrease (−) With CHF
Adrenomedullin	GPCR	+ Inotropy/+ chronotropy	+
Aldosterone	Cytosolic or nuclear MR		+
Angiotensin	GPCR	+ Inotropy/+ chronotropy	+
Endothelin	GPCR		+
Natriuretic peptides	GCCR		
ANP (ANF)			+
BNP			+
Neuropeptide Y*	GPCR	− Inotropy	+
Vasopressin	GPCR	+ Inotropy/+ chronotropy	+
Vasoactive intestinal peptide†	GPCR	+ Inotropy	No
Estrogen	ERα/ERβ	Indirect	No
Testosterone	AR	Indirect	No
Progesterone	PR	Indirect	No
Thyroid hormones	NR	+ Inotropy/+ chronotropy	−
Growth hormones	IGF-1	+ Inotropy/+ chronotropy	−

ANF, Atrial natriuretic factor; *ANP,* atrial natriuretic peptide; *AR,* androgen receptor; *BNP,* B-type natriuretic peptide; *CHF,* congestive heart failure; *ER,* estrogen receptor; *GCCR,* guanylyl cyclase-coupled receptor; *GPCR,* G protein-coupled receptor; *IGF-1,* insulin growth factor 1; *MR,* mineralocorticoid receptor; *NR,* nuclear receptor; *PR,* progesterone receptor.

*Data from Grundemar L, Hakanson R. Multiple neuropeptide Y receptors are involved in cardiovascular regulation. Peripheral and central mechanisms. *Gen Pharmacol.* 1993;24:785–796; and Maisel AS, Scott NA, Motulsky HJ, et al. Elevation of plasma neuropeptide Y levels in congestive heart failure. *Am J Med.* 1989;86:43–48.

†Data from Henning RJ, Sawmiller DR. Vasoactive intestinal peptide: cardiovascular effects. *Cardiovasc Res.* 2001;49:27–37.

endocrine response to hemodynamic changes caused by pressure or volume overload. They also participate in organogenesis of the embryonic heart and cardiovascular system.[58,59] In patients with chronic heart failure, increases of serum ANP and BNP levels are a predictor of mortality.[73]

Adrenomedullin is a recently discovered cardiac hormone that was originally isolated from pheochromocytoma tissue. It increases the accumulation of cAMP and has direct positive chronotropic and inotropic effects.[61,64,65] Adrenomedullin, with interspecies and regional variations, has also been shown to increase nitric oxide production, and it functions as a potent vasodilator.

Aldosterone is one of the cardiac-generated steroids, although its physiologic significance remains to be defined. It binds to mineralocorticoid receptors and can increase the expression or activity (or both) of cardiac proteins involved in ionic homeostasis or the regulation of pH, such as cardiac Na^+/K^+-ATPase, the Na^+-K^+ cotransporter, Cl^--bicarbonate (HCO_3^{2+}), and the Na^+-hydrogen (H^+) antiporter.[60] Aldosterone modifies cardiac structure by inducing cardiac fibrosis in both ventricular chambers and thereby leads to impairment of cardiac contractile function.

Other hormones such as the growth hormone,[74] thyroid hormones,[75] and sex steroid hormones (see the following text) can also have cardiac effects through direct actions of nuclear receptors or indirect effects.

Sex Steroid Hormones and the Heart

Cardiac contractility is more intense in premenopausal women than in age-matched men, and withdrawal of hormone replacement therapy in postmenopausal women leads to a reduction in cardiac contractile function. The gender dimorphism in heart function and its adaptive responses to injury and disease states are partly mediated by sex steroid hormones. Indeed, healthy premenopausal women exhibit a lower cardiovascular risk compared to men, which suggests a mechanism for sex hormones in the modulation of cardiac function.[76]

The most extensively studied sex steroid hormones are estradiol-17β (E2) and its bioactive metabolites. They bind and act on the two subtypes of estrogen receptors (ERs) in the heart: ERα and ERβ. Progesterone and testosterone (two other sex steroid hormones) and the enzyme aromatase, which converts testosterone to estrogen, are much less well investigated. Progesterone and testosterone bind and act on their respective progesterone receptors and androgen receptors in the heart. Sex steroid hormones interact with their receptors to affect postsynaptic target cell responses and to influence presynaptic sympathoadrenergic function. Cardiomyocytes are not only targets for the action of sex steroid hormones, but they are also the source of synthesis and the site of metabolism of these hormones.[77]

E2 is derived from testosterone and is primarily metabolized in the liver to form hydroxyestradiols, catecholestradiols, and methoxyestradiols. Estradiol metabolism also takes place in vascular smooth muscle cells, cardiac fibroblasts, endothelial cells, and cardiomyocytes. Cardiomyocytes express nuclear steroid hormone receptors that modulate gene expression and nonnuclear receptors for the nongenomic effects of sex steroid hormones. They interact with

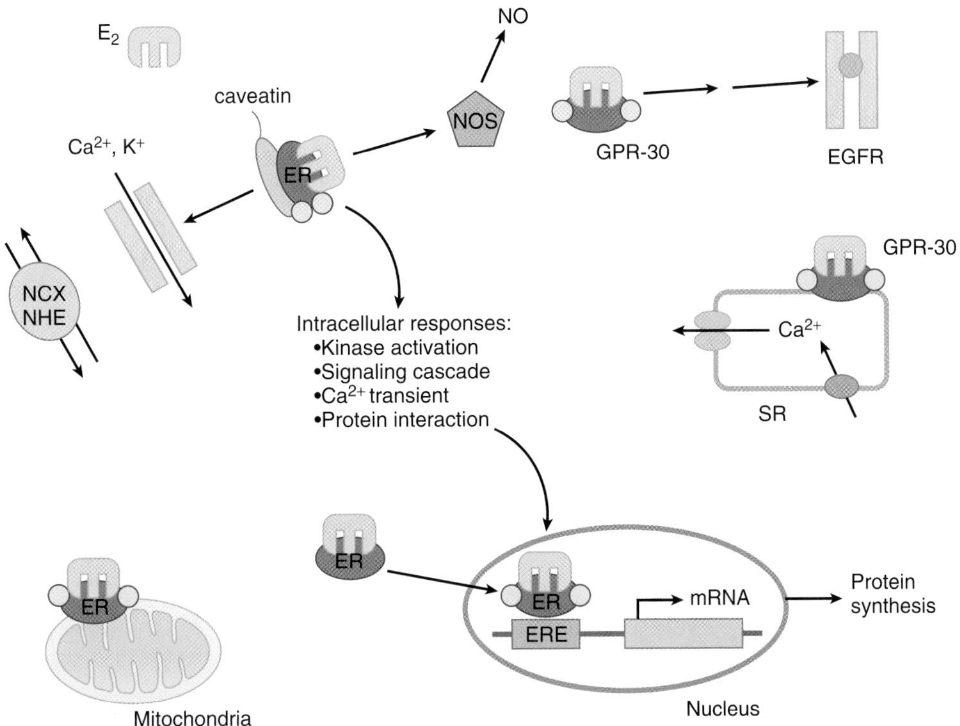

Fig. 14.18 Signaling mechanism of nuclear and nonnuclear localized estrogen receptor *(ER)* and the estrogen-binding receptor, GPR-30. Nuclear ER influences the transcription of target genes by binding to an ER-response element *(ERE)* within the promotor region of target genes. *E_2*, Estrogen; *EGFR*, epidermal growth factor receptor; *GFR*, growth factor receptor; *NCX*, Na^+-Ca^{2+} exchanger; *NHE*, Na^+-H^+ exchanger; *NO*, nitric oxide; *NOS*, nitric oxide synthase, *SR*, sarcoplasmic reticulum. (From Du XJ, Fang L, Kiriazis H. Sex dimorphism in cardiac pathophysiology: experimental findings, hormonal mechanisms, and molecular mechanisms. *Pharmacol Ther*. 2006;111:434–475.)

many different coregulators to confer tissue and temporal specificity in their transcriptional actions. These cell-specific coactivator and corepressor proteins are known as estrogen-related receptors.[78] Sex steroid hormones can activate rapid signaling pathways without changing gene expression (Fig. 14.18). One such example is stimulation of vascular endothelial nitric oxide synthase to mediate vascular dilation. Estrogen's vasodilatory effect might explain the lower systolic blood pressures of premenopausal women when compared with age-matched men. In men, aromatase-mediated conversion of testosterone to estrogen maintains normal vascular tone. In addition to sex steroid hormone stimulation of nuclear or nonnuclear receptors, sex steroid hormone receptors could also induce rapid signaling of growth factor pathways in the absence of ligands.

Gender differences exist in cardiac electrophysiologic function. The modulatory actions of estrogen on Ca^{2+} channels might be responsible for sex-based differences in repolarization of the heart, such as the faster resting heart rate of women, as well as the increased propensity of women to have prolonged QT syndrome.[79] Estrogen, through the activation of ERβ, confers protection after ischemia and reperfusion in murine models of myocardial infarction. In contrast, testosterone, in the same model, has the opposite effect. Aromatase also has protective effects, probably through its action to increase estrogen and to decrease testosterone.

Gender differences in cardiac physiology should include consideration of the cellular physiology of sex steroid hormones in males and females; intrinsic differences in the physiology of cardiomyocytes, vascular smooth muscle cells, and endothelial cells between males and females; and gender-based differences in the autonomic modulation of cardiac physiology.

CARDIAC REFLEXES

Cardiac reflexes are fast-acting reflex loops between the heart and the central nervous system (CNS) that contribute to regulation of cardiac function and the maintenance of physiologic homeostasis. Specific cardiac receptors elicit their physiologic responses by various pathways. Cardiac receptors are linked to the CNS by myelinated or unmyelinated afferent fibers that travel along the vagus nerve. Cardiac receptors are in the atria, ventricles, pericardium, and coronary arteries. Extracardiac receptors are located in the great vessels and carotid artery. Sympathetic and parasympathetic nerve input is processed in the CNS. After central processing, efferent fibers to the heart or the systemic circulation will provoke a specific reaction. The response of the cardiovascular system to efferent stimulation varies with age and duration of the underlying condition that elicited the reflex in the first instance.

Baroreceptor Reflex (Carotid Sinus Reflex)

The baroreceptor reflex is responsible for the maintenance of arterial blood pressure. This reflex regulates arterial pressure around a preset value through a negative-feedback loop (Fig. 14.19).[80,81] In addition, the baroreceptor reflex is capable of establishing a prevailing set point for arterial blood pressure when the preset value has been reset because of chronic hypertension. Changes in arterial blood pressure are monitored by circumferential and longitudinal stretch

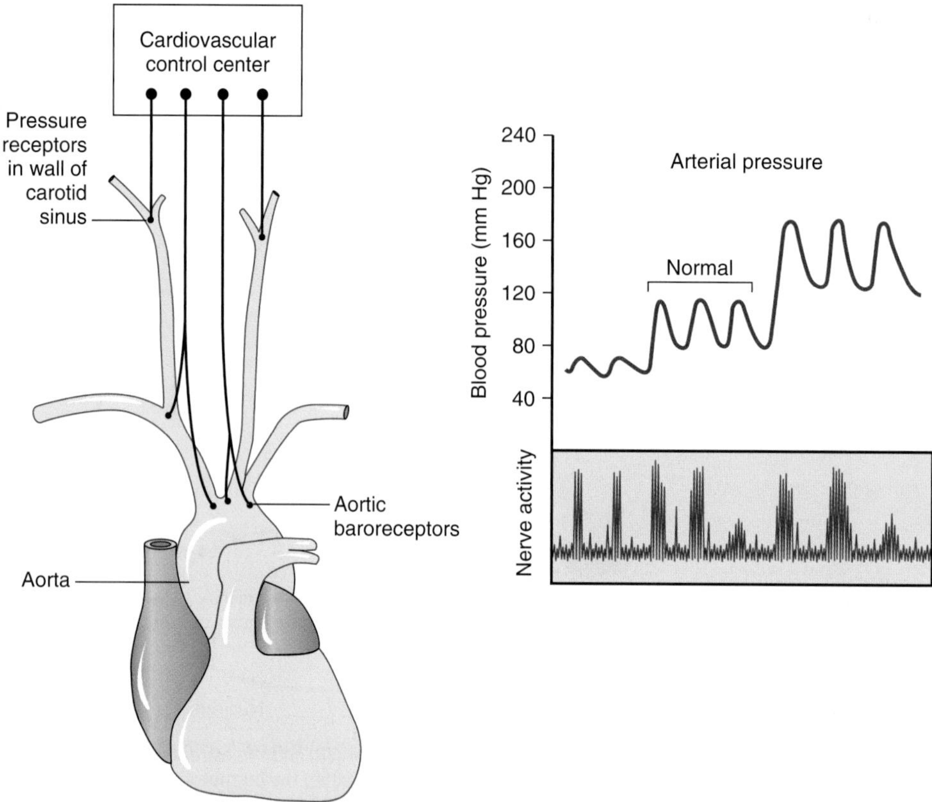

Fig. 14.19 Anatomic configuration of the baroreceptor reflex. Pressure receptors in the wall of the carotid sinuses and aorta detect changes in arterial pressure in the circulation. These signals are conveyed to afferent receptive regions of the medulla through the Hering and vagus nerves. Output from effector portions of the medulla modulates peripheral tone and heart rate. The increase in blood pressure results in increased activation of the reflex *(right)*, which affects a decrease in blood pressure. (From Campagna JA, Carter C. Clinical relevance of the Bezold-Jarisch reflex. *Anesthesiology.* 2003;98:1250–1260.)

receptors located in the carotid sinus and aortic arch. The nucleus solitarius, located in the cardiovascular center of the medulla, receives impulses from these stretch receptors through afferents of the glossopharyngeal and vagus nerves. The cardiovascular center in the medulla consists of two functionally different areas; the area responsible for increasing blood pressure is laterally and rostrally located, whereas the area responsible for lowering arterial blood pressure is centrally and caudally located. The latter area also integrates impulses from the hypothalamus and the limbic system. Typically, stretch receptors are activated if systemic blood pressure is greater than 170 mm Hg. The response of the depressor system includes decreased sympathetic activity, leading to a decrease in cardiac contractility, heart rate, and vascular tone. In addition, activation of the parasympathetic system further decreases the heart rate and myocardial contractility. Reverse effects are elicited with the onset of hypotension.

The baroreceptor reflex plays an important beneficial role during acute blood loss and shock. However, the reflex arch loses its functional capacity when arterial blood pressure is less than 50 mm Hg. Hormonal status and therefore sex differences may alter baroreceptor responses.[82] Furthermore, volatile anesthetics (particularly halothane) inhibit the heart rate component of this reflex.[83] Concomitant use of Ca^{2+}-channel blockers, angiotensin-converting enzyme inhibitors, or phosphodiesterase inhibitors will lessen the cardiovascular response of raising blood pressure through the baroreceptor reflex. This lessened response is achieved by either their direct effects on the peripheral vasculature or, more importantly, their interference with CNS signaling pathways (Ca^{2+}, angiotensin).[84] Patients with chronic hypertension often exhibit perioperative circulatory instability as a result of a decrease in their baroreceptor reflex response.

Chemoreceptor Reflex

Chemosensitive cells are located in the carotid bodies and the aortic body. These cells respond to changes in pH status and blood O_2 tension. At an arterial partial O_2 pressure (PaO_2) of less than 50 mm Hg or in conditions of acidosis, the chemoreceptors send their impulses along the sinus nerve of Hering (a branch of the glossopharyngeal nerve) and the tenth cranial nerve to the chemosensitive area of the medulla. This area responds by stimulating the respiratory centers and thereby increasing ventilatory drive. In addition, activation of the parasympathetic system ensues and leads to a reduction in heart rate and myocardial contractility. In the case of persistent hypoxia, the CNS will be directly stimulated, with a resultant increase in sympathetic activity.

Bainbridge Reflex

The Bainbridge reflex[85-87] is elicited by stretch receptors located in the right atrial wall and the cavoatrial junction. An increase in right-sided filling pressure sends vagal afferent signals to the cardiovascular center in the medulla. These afferent signals inhibit parasympathetic activity, thereby increasing the heart rate. Acceleration of the heart rate also results from a direct effect on the SA node by stretching the atrium. The changes in heart rate are dependent on the underlying heart rate before stimulation.

Bezold-Jarisch Reflex

The Bezold-Jarisch reflex responds to noxious ventricular stimuli sensed by chemoreceptors and mechanoreceptors within the left ventricular wall by inducing the triad of hypotension, bradycardia, and coronary artery dilatation.[80] The activated receptors communicate along unmyelinated vagal afferent type C fibers. These fibers reflexively increase parasympathetic tone. Because it invokes bradycardia, the Bezold-Jarisch reflex is thought of as a cardioprotective reflex. This reflex has been implicated in the physiologic response to a range of cardiovascular conditions such as myocardial ischemia or infarction, thrombolysis, or revascularization and syncope. Natriuretic peptide receptors stimulated by endogenous ANP or BNP may modulate the Bezold-Jarisch reflex. Thus, the Bezold-Jarisch reflex may be less pronounced in patients with cardiac hypertrophy or atrial fibrillation.[88]

Valsalva Maneuver

Forced expiration against a closed glottis produces increased intrathoracic pressure, increased central venous pressure, and decreased venous return. Cardiac output and blood pressure will be decreased after the Valsalva maneuver. This decrease will be sensed by baroreceptors and will reflexively result in an increase in heart rate and myocardial contractility through sympathetic stimulation. When the glottis opens, venous return increases and causes the heart to respond by vigorous contraction and an increase in blood pressure. This increase in arterial blood pressure will, in turn, be sensed by baroreceptors, thereby stimulating the parasympathetic efferent pathways to the heart.

Cushing Reflex

The Cushing reflex is a result of cerebral ischemia caused by increased intracranial pressure. Cerebral ischemia at the medullary vasomotor center induces initial activation of the sympathetic nervous system. Such activation will lead to an increase in heart rate, arterial blood pressure, and myocardial contractility in an effort to improve cerebral perfusion. As a result of the high vascular tone, reflex bradycardia mediated by baroreceptors will ensue.

Oculocardiac Reflex

The oculocardiac reflex is provoked by pressure applied to the globe of the eye or traction on the surrounding structures. Stretch receptors are located in the extraocular muscles. Once activated, stretch receptors will send afferent signals through the short- and long-ciliary nerves. The ciliary nerves will merge with the ophthalmic division of the trigeminal nerve at the ciliary ganglion. The trigeminal nerve will carry these impulses to the gasserian ganglion, thereby resulting in increased parasympathetic tone and subsequent bradycardia. The incidence of this reflex during ophthalmic surgery ranges from 30% to 90%. Administration of an antimuscarinic drug such as glycopyrrolate or atropine reduces the incidence of bradycardia during eye surgery.

Acknowledgment

The editors, publisher, and Dr. Lena Sun would like to thank Drs. Johanna Schwarzenberger and Radhika Dinavahi for their contribution to this chapter in the prior edition of this work. It has served as the foundation for the current chapter.

Complete references available online at expertconsult.com.

References

1. Harvey W. *On the Motion of the Heart and Blood in Animals* [Willis R, Trans]. *Scientific Papers: Physiology, Medicine, Surgery, Geology*, vol. 38. P. F. Collier & Son; 1910.
2. Shultz SG. *News Physiol Sci.* 2002:17:175–180.
3. Berne RM, Levy MN. The cardiac pump. In: *Cardiovascular Physiology.* St. Louis: Mosby; 2001:55–82.
4. Berne RM, Levy MN. Electrical activity of the heart. In: *Cardiovascular Physiology*. St. Louis: Mosby; 2001:7–32.
5. Katz AM. The heart as a muscular pump. In: *Physiology of the Heart.* Philadelphia: Lippincott-Raven; 2001:408–417.
6. Takayma Y, Costa KD, Covell JW. *Am J Physiol Heart Circ Physiol.* 2002;282:H1510.
7. Katz AM. Structure of the heart. In: *Physiology of the Heart.* Philadelphia: Lippincott-Raven; 2001:1.
8. Opie LH. Heart cells and organelles. In: *Heart Physiology From Cell to Circulation.* Philadelphia: Lippincott-Raven; 2004:42.
9. Little WC. Assessment of normal and abnormal cardiac function. In: Braunwald E, ed. *Heart Disease.* 6th ed. Philadelphia: Saunders; 2001:479.
10. LeWinter MM, Osol G. Normal physiology of the cardiovascular system. In: Fuster V, Alexander RW, O'Rourke RA, eds. *Hurst's the heart.* 10th ed. New York: McGraw-Hill; 2001:63.
11. Zile MR, Brutsaert DL. *Circulation.* 2002;105:1387.
12. Opie LH. Ventricular function. In: *Heart Physiology From Cell to Circulation.* Philadelphia: Lippincott-Raven; 2004:355.
13. Frank O. *Z Biol.* 1895;32:370.
14. Starling EH. *Linacre Lecture on the Law of the Heart.* London: Longmans Green; 1918.
15. Holubarsch CT, et al. *Circulation.* 1996;94:683.
16. Katz AM. The working heart. In: *Physiology of the Heart.* Philadelphia: Lippincott-Raven; 2001:418.
17. Opie LH. Mechanisms of cardiac contraction and relaxation. In: Braunwald E, ed. *Heart Disease.* 6th ed. Philadelphia: Saunders; 2001:443.
18. Roberts R. Principles of molecular cardiology. In: Alexander RW, O'Rourke RA, eds. *Hurst's the heart.* 10th ed. New York: McGraw-Hill; 2001:95.
19. Opie LH. Myocardial contraction and relaxation. In: *Heart Physiology From Cell to Circulation.* Philadelphia: Lippincott-Raven; 2004:221.
20. Severs NJ. *Bioessays.* 2000;22:188.
21. Katz AM. Contractile proteins and cytoskeleton. In: *Physiology of the Heart.* Philadelphia: Lippincott-Raven; 2001:123.
22. Yeager M. *J Struct Biol.* 1998;121:231.
23. Severs NJ. *Adv Myocardiol.* 1985;5:223.
24. DiFrancesco D. *Circ Res.* 2010;106:434.
25. Fill M, Copella JA. *Physiol Rev.* 2002;82:893.
26. Baruscotti M, Difrancesco D. *Ann N Y Acad Sci.* 2004;1015:111.
27. Kumar NM, Gilula NB. *Cell.* 1996;84:381.
28. Katz AM. The cardiac action potential. In: *Physiology of the Heart.* Philadelphia: Lippincott-Raven; 2001:478.
29. Katz AM. Calcium fluxes. In: *Physiology of the Heart.* Philadelphia: Lippincott-Raven; 2001:478.
30. Katz AM, Lorell BH. *Circulation.* 2000;102:69–74.
31. Cheng H, Lederer WJ. *Physiol Rev.* 2008;88:1491.
32. Cheng H, et al. *Cell Calcium.* 1996;20:129.
33. Bers DM. *Nature.* 2002;415:198.
34. Luo M, Anderson ME. *Circ Res.* 2013;113:690–708.

35. Hajjar RJ, Ishikawa K, Thum T. Molecular and cellular biology of the heart. In: Fuster V, Harrington RA, Narula J, Eapen ZJ. eds. Hurst's The Heart, 14e New York, NY: McGraw-Hill.
36. Opie LH. Excitation-contraction coupling. In: *Heart Physiology From Cell to Circulation*. Philadelphia: Lippincott-Raven; 2004:159.
37. de Tombe PP. *J Biomech*. 2003;36:721.
38. Bonne GL, et al. *Circ Res*. 1998;83:580.
39. Solaro RJ, Rarick HM. *Circ Res*. 1998;83:417.
40. Fuchs F, Smith SH. *News Physiol Sci*. 2001;16:5.
41. Trinick J, Tskhovrebova L. *Trends Cell Biol*. 1999;9:377.
42. Moss RL, Fitzsimons DP. *Circ Res*. 2002;90:11.
43. Alvarez BV, et al. *Circ Res*. 1999;85:716.
44. Konhilas JP, et al. *Circ Res*. 2002;90:59.
45. Konhilas JP, et al. *J Physiol*. 2002;544:225.
46. Fukuda N, et al. *Circulation*. 2001;104:1639.
47. Capetanaki Y. *Trends Cardiovasc Med*. 2002;12:339.
48. Howard J, Hyman AA. *Nature*. 2003;422:753.
49. Opie LH. Receptors and signal transduction. In: *Heart Physiology From Cell to Circulation*. Philadelphia: Lippincott-Raven; 2004:187.
50. Rockman HA, et al. *Nature*. 2002;415:206.
51. Mendelowitz D. *News Physiol Sci*. 1999;14:155.
52. Brodde OE, Michel MC. *Pharmacol Rev*. 1999;51:651.
53. Dhein S, et al. *Pharmacol Res*. 2001;44:161.
54. Kaumann AJ, Molenaar P. *Naunyn Schmiedebergs Arch Pharmacol*. 1997;355:667.
55. Endoh M. *Neurochem Res*. 1996;21:217.
56. Arteaga GMT, et al. *Ann Med*. 2002;34:248.
57. van der Horst IC, et al. *Neth Heart J*. 2010;18:190.
58. Cameron VA, Ellmers LJ. *Endocrinology*. 2003;144:2191.
59. de Bold AJ, et al. *Cardiovasc Res*. 1996;31:7.
60. Delcayre C, Silvestre JS. *Cardiovasc Res*. 1999;42:7.
61. Martinez A. *Microsc Res Tech*. 2002;57:1.
62. Dinh DT, et al. *Clin Sci*. 2001;100:481.
63. Schuijt MP, Jan Danser AH. *Am J Hypertens*. 2002;15:1109.
64. Kitamura K, et al. *Microsc Res Tech*. 2002;57:3.
65. Minamino N, et al. *Microsc Res Tech*. 2002;57:28.
66. Smith DM, et al. *Biochem Soc Trans*. 2002;30:432.
67. Mello De WC. *J Mol Med*. 2001;79:103.
68. Opie LH, Sack MN. *Circ Res*. 2001;88:654.
69. Scicchitano P, et al. *Molecules*. 2012;17:4225.
70. Kramer BK, et al. *J Mol Med*. 1997;75:886.
71. Chandrashekhar Y, et al. *J Mol Cell Cardiol*. 2003;35:495.
72. Walker BR, et al. *Am J Physiol*. 1988;255:H261.
73. Giannakoulas G, et al. *Am J Cardiol*. 2010;105:869.
74. Palmeiro CR, et al. *Cardiol Rev*. 2012;20:197.
75. Danzi S, Klein I. *Med Clin North Am*. 2012;96:257.
76. Clerico A, et al. *Am J Physiol Heart Circ Physiol*. 2011;301:H12–H20.
77. Mendelsohn ME. *Science*. 2005;308:1583.
78. Du XJ, et al. *Pharmacol Ther*. 2006;111:434.
79. Pham TV, Rosen MR. *Cardiovasc Res*. 2002;53:740.
80. Campagna JA, Carter C. *Anesthesiology*. 2003;98:1250.
81. Parlow JL, et al. *Anesthesiology*. 1999;90:681.
82. Huikuri HV, et al. *Circulation*. 1996;94:122.
83. Keyl C, et al. *Anesth Analg*. 2002;95:1629.
84. Devlin MG, et al. *Clin Exp Pharmacol Physiol*. 2002;29:372.
85. Crystal GJ, Salem MR. *Anesth Analg*. 2012;114:520.
86. Hakumaki MO. *Acta Physiol Scand*. 1987;130:177.
87. Ludbrook J. *Annu Rev Physiol*. 1983;45:155.
88. Thomas CJ, Woods RL. *Hypertension*. 2003;41:279.

15 Gastrointestinal Physiology and Pathophysiology

LAURIE O. MARK and A. SASSAN SABOURI

KEY POINTS

- The gastrointestinal (GI) tract forms a long tube from mouth to anus and its main functions are motility, digestion, absorption, excretion, and circulation. Each component of the GI tract has specific functions.
- The layers of the GI tract wall are (outermost to innermost): serosa, longitudinal muscle, circular muscle, submucosa, and mucosa. Within the mucosa is (outermost to innermost): muscularis mucosae, lamina propria, and epithelium.
- The GI tract is innervated by the autonomic nervous system. The extrinsic nervous system consists of the sympathetic, which is primarily inhibitory, and parasympathetic, which is primarily excitatory on GI tract motility. The enteric nervous system controls motility, secretion, and blood flow.
- Mixing movements and propulsive movements are the two primary movements within and along the GI tract. The mechanisms for each are altered significantly in the diseased state and there are multiple modalities for evaluating these alterations.
- The effect of general anesthesia on the GI tract is multifaceted and everything from the medications administered to the hemodynamic side effects can alter GI tract function. Opioids, in particular, have an adverse effect on the bowel and there are many efforts underway to decrease the use of opioids in GI surgery.
- Hemodynamic changes, bowel manipulation, and open abdominal surgeries can produce major effects on the anatomy and function of the GI tract including postoperative ileus, inflammatory states, mesenteric ischemia, and partial or total disruption of myogenic continuity.
- The innervation of the GI organs up to the proximal transverse colon is supplied by the celiac plexus, whereas the innervation of the descending colon and distal GI tract comes from the inferior hypogastric plexus.
- The celiac plexus can be blocked via different approaches, including: transcrural, intraoperative, endoscopic ultrasound-guided, and peritoneal lavage.
- Epidural anesthesia can suppress sympathetic mediated GI reflexes and reduce the incidence of postoperative ileus.
- Pain management strategies that use regional anesthetic techniques and avoid the use of systemic opioids help reduce the incidence of postoperative nausea and vomiting.
- The Enhanced Recovery after GI Surgery (ERAS) protocol and evidence-based practices helps to preserve natural GI physiology and is associated with shorter hospitalizations.
- The ERAS protocol focuses on: optimal perioperative pain control; nutrition; avoidance of unnecessary tubes, lines, and drains; temperature; fluid management; and early ambulation.

Introduction

The purpose of this chapter is to gain an understanding of the various components of gastrointestinal (GI) anatomy and their respective functions. This understanding of the GI system in the healthy state will pave the way for an understanding of how it is affected in different and common disease states. The chapter then transitions into a discussion of perioperative considerations for the anesthetist, including the effects of various anesthetic medications and surgical conditions on bowel function and physiology. The remainder of the chapter will focus on gastrointestinal innervation and how various regional anesthesia and pain management strategies are used when dealing with GI conditions and surgeries.

Gastrointestinal Anatomy and Function

The GI tract constitutes approximately 5% of the total human body mass. Its main functions are motility, digestion, absorption, excretion, and circulation. This section is composed of two parts. In the first part, the basic anatomy and innervation common to all parts of the GI tract are discussed. In the second part the specific anatomy and function of the esophagus, stomach, small bowel, and large bowel are discussed. The pancreas, liver, and biliary tract are covered in Chapter 16.

Common to all parts of the GI tract are the layers of the wall, but the functions of each layer differ from organ to organ.

From outermost to innermost these layers are the serosa, longitudinal muscle layer, circular muscle layer, submucosa, and mucosa. Within the mucosa is (outermost to innermost) the muscularis mucosae, lamina propria, and epithelium. The serosa is a smooth membrane of thin connective tissue and cells that secrete serous fluid that serves to enclose the cavity and reduce friction between muscle movements. The longitudinal muscle layer contracts in order to shorten the length of the intestinal segment whereas the circular muscle layer contracts to decrease the diameter of the intestinal lumen. These two layers work together to allow for gut motility. Between these smooth muscle layers is the myenteric (Auerbach) plexus, which regulates the gut smooth muscle. The submucosa contains the submucosal (Meissner) plexus, which transmits information from the epithelium to the enteric and central nervous systems (CNS). The mucosa is composed of a thin layer of smooth muscle called the muscularis mucosa, which functions to move the villi; the lamina propria, which contains blood vessels, nerve endings, and immune and inflammatory cells; and the epithelium, which is where the GI contents are sensed and where secretion of enzymes, absorption of nutrients, and excretion of waste products occur.

The GI tract is innervated by the autonomic nervous system. This is composed of the extrinsic nervous system, which has sympathetic and parasympathetic components, and the enteric nervous system. The extrinsic sympathetic nervous system is primarily inhibitory as stimulation can decrease or cease GI motility. The preganglionic fibers originate at the T5 to L2 segments of the spinal cord. They travel to the sympathetic chain of ganglia and synapse with postganglionic neurons. Then they travel to the gut where they terminate at the enteric nervous system. The primary neurotransmitter is norepinephrine. Vasoactive intestinal polypeptide (VIP) also transmits sympathetic signals. The extrinsic parasympathetic nervous system is primarily excitatory as it activates GI motility and function. Parasympathetic preganglionic fibers originate in the medulla and sacral region of the spinal cord. Vagus nerve fibers innervate the esophagus, stomach, pancreas, small intestine, and the first half of the large intestine. Pelvic nerve fibers innervate the second half of the large intestine, sigmoid, rectal, and anal regions. The primary neurotransmitter is acetylcholine.

The enteric nervous system is the independent nervous system of the GI tract, which controls motility, secretion, and blood flow. Two plexuses constitute the enteric nervous system: the myenteric (Auerbach) plexus and the submucosal (Meissner) plexus. The myenteric plexus controls motility, which is carried out by enteric neurons, interstitial cells of Cajal (pacemaker cells that generate intrinsic electrical activity of the GI tract), and smooth muscle cells. The submucosal plexus controls absorption, secretion, and mucosal blood flow. Both of these plexuses respond to sympathetic and parasympathetic stimulation. Sympathetic stimulation is inhibitory so it will increase the tone of the intestinal wall whereas parasympathetic stimulation is excitatory and will induce intestinal contractions and movement. Additionally, there are a variety of reflexes in the enteric nervous system. For example, when there is sympathetic stimulation the tone of the wall increases, the sphincters contract, and, reflexively, the amount of excitatory acetylcholine released is reduced. The mechanism is via α-2 activation, which inhibits the release of acetylcholine and through β activation which contracts sphincter muscles and relaxes intestinal muscles. These two actions work together to slow the transit of contents through the GI tract.

This next section serves to briefly discuss the anatomy and function of the various components of the GI tract. Only the esophagus, stomach, small intestine, and large intestine are covered. See Table 15.1 for an overview of GI tract anatomy and function.

The esophagus is a muscular tube that connects the pharynx to the stomach. It is the first passageway for food entry into the digestive system. It is approximately 18 to 25 cm in length and extends from the level of the hypopharynx at the C6 vertebrae down to the gastroesophageal (GE) junction at the T11 level.[1] The esophagus has three regions: cervical, thoracic, and abdominal. The cervical esophagus is approximately 4 to 5 cm long and is surrounded by the trachea anteriorly, the vertebral column posteriorly, and the carotid sheaths and thyroid gland laterally. The thoracic esophagus spans from the suprasternal notch to the diaphragmatic hiatus and lies posterior to the trachea. At the level of the carina, it deviates right to allow room for the aortic arch and runs posteriorly and underneath the left mainstem bronchus. From T8 to the diaphragmatic hiatus (T10) the esophagus runs anterior to the aorta. The abdominal esophagus extends from the diaphragmatic hiatus to the cardia of the stomach. The upper one-third of the esophagus is composed of striated muscle and the remaining two-thirds is smooth muscle. There are two areas of high pressure: the upper esophageal sphincter (UES) and the lower esophageal sphincter (LES). The UES lies at the level of the cricoid cartilage and is made up of the cricopharyngeal, inferior constrictor, and circular esophageal muscles. Resting tone ranges from 30–200 mm Hg. Opening and closing of the UES is coordinated with the pharyngeal pushing of food downstream. The LES is formed intrinsically by circular esophageal muscle and extrinsically by the diaphragm muscle. It has both sympathetic and parasympathetic innervation. Resting tone is 10–45 mm Hg.[2]

The stomach is a J-shaped dilation of the alimentary tract. It is divided into four regions: the cardia, fundus, body or corpus, and antrum. The stomach has three main functions: store large quantities of food (up to 1.5–2 liters), mix food with gastric secretions to form chyme and break down particle size, and slow emptying into the small intestine. The proximal stomach is the reservoir for undigested food and produces smooth, tonic contractions. The distal stomach grinds, mixes, and sieves food particles via high-amplitude contractions. Notable cell types in the stomach that aid in digestion are the mucous cells, which protect against harsh hydrochloric acid; parietal cells, which secrete hydrochloric acid; chief cells, which secrete pepsin; and G cells, which secrete gastrin. Together these cells' secretions break down and partially digest the food into chyme as well as reduce particle dimension to an appropriate size (2 mm or less) before it enters the small intestine.[2]

TABLE 15.1 Table of Gastrointestinal Components, Locations, and Functions

Component	Location	Function
Esophagus	Extends from C6 to T11	Propels food from the pharynx to the stomach
Stomach	Left upper abdominal cavity. Diaphragm along the top, pancreas posteriorly, greater omentum laterally	Receives food from the esophagus and initiates digestion. Breaks down food into chyme through physical and chemical mechanisms
Duodenum	Inferior to stomach, approximately 25–30 cm long	Chemically digests chyme for absorption in the small intestine
Jejunum	Between duodenum and ileum	Absorption of nutrients from chyme
Ileum	Between jejunum and cecum	Further nutrient absorption
Cecum	Lower right quadrant of abdominal cavity, inferior and lateral to the ileum	A space for mixing of chyme with bacteria to form fecal matter
Ascending colon	Runs superiorly from the cecum to the right inferior border of the liver where it turns 90 degrees to become the transverse colon	Peristaltic waves move the feces superiorly where bacteria digest the waste and further nutrients, water, and vitamins are absorbed
Transverse colon	Crosses abdominal cavity right to left just below the stomach	Fecal formation
Descending colon	Runs inferiorly along the left side of the abdominal cavity	Stores fecal matter prior to elimination. Further absorbs water, nutrients, vitamins
Sigmoid colon	Lower left quadrant of the abdominal cavity	Stores fecal matter prior to elimination
Rectum	Posterior pelvic cavity. Along the anterior surface of the sacrum and coccyx	Stores fecal matter prior to elimination. Distention will activate stretch receptors allowing the internal anal sphincter to relax and allow for defecation.

The duodenum is the first and smallest section of the small intestine. It is between 25 and 30 cm long and it forms a C-shaped loop around the pancreas. Its main function is to chemically digest the chyme received from the stomach in preparation for absorption. The pancreas, liver, and gallbladder secrete digestive enzymes through the ampulla of Vater into the middle portion of the duodenum.[2]

The jejunum is the second section of the small intestine and its primary function is to absorb nutrients. The digested chyme from the duodenum enters the jejunum where it is mixed and circulated for exposure to the jejunal walls for nutrient absorption. The walls of the jejunum are folded many times over to increase its surface area and allow for maximal absorption of nutrients. By the time chyme enters the ileum, almost 90% of all available nutrients are absorbed.[2]

The ileum is the final section of the small intestine. It serves to absorb vitamin B12 and other products of digestion that were not previously absorbed in the jejunum. It ends at the ileocecal valve—a circular muscle that serves to prevent reflux of colonic contents into the small intestine. It contracts in response to colonic dilation and relaxes in response to ileal dilation.[2]

The large intestine is composed of the cecum, appendix, ascending colon, transverse colon, descending colon, sigmoid colon, and rectum. Briefly, the cecum is a pouch at the beginning of the large intestine that allows for mixing of the chyme from the small intestine with bacteria to form fecal matter. The ascending colon transports the fecal matter superiorly along the right side up to the transverse colon. Along the way the ascending colonic wall absorbs water, nutrients, and vitamins. The transverse colon, the longest portion of the large intestine, crosses the abdominal cavity. Its contractions serve to mix the feces and allow bacteria to ferment the waste. Further absorption of water and nutrients also take place. The feces then enter the descending colon, which stores the feces until it is ready for transport, inferiorly and along the left side of the abdominal cavity to the sigmoid colon. Again, the walls of the descending colon allow for further absorption of water and nutrients. The sigmoid colon is an S-shaped, curved region that stores then transports fecal matter from the descending colon to the rectum and anus for elimination. The final portion of the large intestine is the rectum where feces are stored until elimination. As fecal matter accumulates it exerts pressure on the walls of the rectum. This activates stretch receptors and leads to relaxation of the internal anal sphincter allowing for elimination.[2]

Transit Time in Health and Disease

This section serves to discuss motility in the esophagus, stomach, small intestine, and large intestine. Emphasis is placed on mechanism, how motility and transit are altered by various disease states, and methods for evaluating motility.

Mixing movements and propulsive movements are the two primary movements within and along the GI tract. Mixing movements keep the contents of the intestine appropriately and thoroughly mixed throughout, while the propulsive movements, consisting of periodic contractions of certain GI tract segments (peristalsis), move the contents of the intestine along the tract.

Transit through the esophagus starts with swallowing. Swallowing starts with the oropharynx pushing food backward and downward while the muscles of the nasopharynx prevent food from entering the nasal passages. When ready to be swallowed the food is squeezed and rolled into the posterior pharynx by the tongue. The epiglottis moves upward in a protective mechanism over the larynx and trachea to prevent aspiration. The act of swallowing inhibits the respiratory center to protect from aspiration but it is so short-lived it is unnoticeable. Food enters the esophagus through the UES, which then constricts to prevent reflux back into the pharynx. The UES produces pressures around 30–200 mm Hg. Two waves of peristalsis move the food into the stomach through the LES, which also produces pressures between 20 and 60 mm Hg. Afferent nerve fibers transmit to the dorsal vagal complex activating efferent fibers that terminate either on the striated muscle of the esophagus or on the nerves of the enteric nervous system. Release of acetylcholine contracts the muscle while VIP and nitric oxide (NO) relax it. The LES responds to esophageal distention via myogenic and neurohormonal mechanisms.

Diseases of the esophagus are varied. Etiologies can be grouped into anatomical, mechanical, and neurologic, although many disease states involve overlap between two or all three. Anatomical etiologies include the presence of diverticula, hiatal hernia, and changes associated with chronic acid reflux. These anatomical abnormalities interrupt the normal pathway of food as it travels to the stomach which, in turn, changes many of the pressure zones of the esophagus. This can have dangerous sequelae as the luminal pressures may increase enough to overcome the resting pressures of the UES and LES allowing for reflux. Mechanical etiologies include achalasia, diffuse esophageal spasm, and hypertensive LES. There is also a neurologic component to these diseases but the result is the same—the esophagus is unable to relax properly for food travel. In achalasia the smooth muscles are unable to relax and move food down and the increased tone of the LES does not allow for complete relaxation. This results in dysphagia, regurgitation, and significant pain. In diffuse esophageal spasm the muscle contractions are uncoordinated and, as a result, food does not properly move downward. A hypertensive LES is defined as an LES with a mean pressure of 45 mm Hg or higher leading to dysphagia and chest pain. Neurologic disorders such as stroke, vagotomy, or hormone deficiencies will alter the nerve pathways such that the appropriate sensing and feedback are disrupted. A common result of neurologic disorders in the esophagus is dysphagia.

In evaluating esophageal function, it is important to select a study with an appropriate clinical correlation—is it a problem with motility or is it an anatomical abnormality? If it is a questionable motility problem, then an esophageal manometry study is best. A special catheter detects changes in pressure in the esophagus at various levels. First the pressure of the LES is recorded. The catheter is then pulled back into the esophagus and pressure measurements are made at different levels. Esophageal motor function between swallows is also evaluated. Finally the motor function of the UES is recorded and then the catheter is pulled out. Questionable anatomical problems are best studied using an upper GI series and ingested barium. These evaluate the act of swallowing and visualize the lining of the esophagus for anatomic abnormalities.

Before discussing the transit of food through the stomach and small intestine it is important to understand their actions during the fasting state. The migrating motor complex (MMC) occurs only during fasting, and is composed of waves of electrical activity in regular cycles originating in the stomach and terminating in the distal ileum.[3] Vagal stimulation releases motilin, which triggers an MMC leading to peristaltic waves. They occur every 45 to 180 minutes and are composed of four phases. Phase I is a period of quiescence. Phase II is composed of increased action potentials and low-amplitude smooth muscle contractility. Phase III is the most active as it is the time of peak electrical and mechanical activity producing bursts of regular, high-amplitude contractions. Phase IV demonstrates declining activity and will merge into the following MMC's phase I. The MMC is significant because it moves residual undigested food through the GI tract and also moves bacteria from the small intestine to the large intestine. Feeding interrupts it, and this is discussed next.

As described previously, the stomach is a J-shaped sac that serves as a reservoir for large volumes of food, mixes and breaks down food to form chyme, and slows emptying into the small intestine. Solids must be broken down into 1 to 2 mm particles before entering the duodenum, and they take approximately 3 to 4 hours to empty from the stomach. Liquids empty faster than solids. The motility of the stomach is controlled by intrinsic and extrinsic neural regulation. Parasympathetic stimulation to the vagus nerve increases the number and force of contractions whereas sympathetic stimulation inhibits these contractions via the splanchnic nerve. The intrinsic nervous system provides the coordination for motility. Neurohormonal control is also at play in that gastrin and motilin will increase the strength and frequency of contractions and the gastric inhibitory peptide will inhibit them.

Emptying of the stomach is controlled by neural and hormonal mechanisms as well as the composition of ingested food. Gastric distention, gastrin, and NO will promote emptying. Duodenal distention decreases the gastric tone to slow emptying, and increased fat content triggers the release of cholecystokinin to further inhibit stomach motility.

Gastric motility disorders that slow its emptying can increase the incidence of GE reflux disease. These disorders can be drug-induced, neurologic, or a result of critical illness. Drug-induced conditions include the administration of opioids (to be discussed later in the chapter), and the use of vasoactive agents. Vasoactive drugs increase catecholamine concentrations leading to sympathetic stimulation and, therefore, decreased motility. These drugs are often given intraoperatively or to critically ill patients for blood pressure control. Neurologic disorders resulting in decreased gastric motility include vagal neuropathies and gastroparesis. Finally, conditions that are commonly present in severely compromised patients, such as those with hyperglycemia, increased intracranial pressure, and mechanical ventilation can decrease gastric motility. Efforts to increase motility using drugs like erythromycin and metoclopramide have been used with some success.

The most prevailing test to evaluate gastric motility is the gastric emptying study. The patient fasts for at least 4 hours prior to the study then consumes a meal with a tightly bound radiotracer, commonly egg albumin. Continuous or frequent imaging occurs for the next 60 to 120 minutes and the measurement of time for 50% of the ingested meal to empty is determined. It is important to note that while gastric emptying scintigraphy has long been the standard study, it is affected by multiple factors including meal composition and data acquisition parameters.[4] Gastric motility studies can also be paired with small intestinal motility studies such as the small bowel manometry test. This will be discussed later.

Small intestinal motility mixes the contents of the stomach with digestive enzymes, further reducing particle size and increasing solubility. However, the major function of the small intestine is to circulate the contents and expose them to the mucosal wall in order to maximize absorption of water, nutrients, and vitamins before entering the large intestine. Again, there are mixing contractions and propulsive contractions. The circular and longitudinal muscle layers work in a coordinated fashion to achieve segmentation. Segmentation occurs when two nearby areas contract and thereby isolate a segment of intestine. Then a contraction occurs in the middle of that isolated segment, further dividing it. Contractions in the middle of those segments continue to occur and the process ensues. Segmentation allows the contents to remain in the intestine long enough for the essential substances to be absorbed into the circulation. It is controlled mainly by the enteric nervous system with modulation of motility by the extrinsic nervous system.

When considering small bowel dysmotility it is helpful to distinguish etiologies based on reversible and nonreversible causes. For reversible causes, mechanical obstruction should be the first to come to mind. In this case, there is a physical obstruction the muscles of the intestine cannot overcome. Hernias, malignancy, adhesions, and volvuluses are all examples. Bacterial overgrowth should be another consideration. Although the large intestine is rich with bacteria, the small intestine usually has fewer than 100,000 organisms per milliliter. Disrupting this condition with bacterial overgrowth leads to alterations in absorptive function leading to diarrhea. It is treated with antibiotics. Other reversible causes include ileus, electrolyte abnormalities, and critical illness. Nonreversible causes can be classified as structural or neuropathic. In structural causes there may be abnormalities with the intestinal smooth muscle, in which it cannot produce proper contractions. This occurs in diseases such as scleroderma and connective tissue disorders. In patients with an inflammatory bowel disease (IBD), there is a structural abnormality in the mucosa leading to decreased absorption of nutrients. Short bowel syndrome can be considered a structural etiology in that a large portion of the small intestinal structure is simply not present. In patients who have had a section of their small bowel resected, the remaining portion may not provide sufficient functional compensation, resulting in diarrhea, malnutrition, and weight loss. Neuropathic etiologies can produce a pseudo-obstruction in which the intrinsic and extrinsic nervous systems are altered in such a way that the intestines can only produce weak or uncoordinated contractions. This leads to symptoms of bloating, nausea, vomiting, and abdominal pain. Regardless of etiology, small intestinal dysmotility adversely affects nutrient absorption leading to malnutrition.

The most common test used to evaluate small intestine motility is small bowel manometry. This test is useful in patients with unexplained nausea, vomiting, abdominal pain, and manifested signs of obstruction without a clear obstructive cause. Similar to esophageal manometry, this test uses a small catheter with pressure sensors to evaluate the contractions of the intestine. The study evaluates contractions during three periods: fasting, during a meal, and postprandial. Normally the recording time is four hours for fasting, followed by ingestion of a meal, and two hours postprandial. Abnormal results are grouped into myopathic and neuropathic causes. In myopathic results, the MMC is absent or phase III exhibits very low amplitudes (normal phase III amplitude is 40 mm Hg). In neuropathic results, the contraction amplitude is adequate but either the contractions are uncoordinated (enteric neuropathy) or there is an inappropriate postprandial response, meaning postprandial antral hypomotility is present (extrinsic neuropathy). This manometry test is reported to result in a change of diagnosis in 8% to 15% of patients with unexplained nausea, vomiting, and abdominal pain.[5]

The large intestine acts as a reservoir for waste and indigestible material before elimination and extracts any remaining electrolytes and water. It plays an essential role in regulating defecation and consistency of stools. Distention of the ileum will relax the ileocecal valve to allow intestinal contents to enter the colon and subsequent cecal distention will contract it. The contractions of the colon are different from the rest of the gut. While there are still mixing and propulsive movements by the circular and longitudinal muscles, respectively, the colon also exhibits giant migrating complexes. The giant migrating complexes serve to produce mass movements across the large intestine. In the healthy state, these complexes occur approximately 6 to 10 times within 24 hours with mean amplitude of 115 mm Hg at a distance of about 1 cm/s for approximately 20 seconds each.[6] These complexes, as well as the mixing and propulsive movements, serve to transfer contents to the rectum. The giant migrating complexes that originate in the sigmoid colon will produce the urge to defecate. Rectal distention as well as VIP and NO release will promote relaxation of the internal anal sphincter and allow for defecation.

Colonic dysmotility manifests with two primary symptoms: altered bowel habits and intermittent abdominal cramping. The most common diseases associated with colonic dysmotility are irritable bowel syndrome (IBS) and IBD, both of which are clinical diagnoses. Rome II criteria define IBS as having abdominal pain/discomfort along with at least two of the following three features: defecation relieves pain or discomfort, onset of pain is associated with an abnormal frequency of stools (more than three times per day or fewer than three times per week), and onset of pain is associated with a change in the form of the stool.[7] In IBS with predominantly diarrheal symptoms, there is an increase in the frequency and amplitude of spontaneous giant migrating complexes, and this increase is directly proportional to the severity of symptoms. In IBS with predominantly constipation, there is a decreased amplitude and frequency of giant migrating complexes. In severe cases the giant migrating complexes may be completely absent. In addition, there is a depression of overall contractile activity in the colon leading to colonic distention and the sensation of pain. This phenomenon is exacerbated by stress in which there is significant motor dysfunction and visceral hypersensitivity as well as an increase in plasma norepinephrine stimulating the sympathetic nervous system. In IBD the mixing and propulsive movements as well as the tonic contractions are suppressed due to colonic wall compression by the inflamed mucosa, but the giant migrating complexes remain. There is an increased frequency of the giant migrating complexes and their large pressure effect further compresses the inflamed mucosa, which can lead to hemorrhage, thick mucus secretion, and significant erosions.

Methods of Evaluating Colonic Motility

Studies evaluating giant migrating complexes in patients with IBS and IBD are not routine but are performed only on patients with known diagnoses to help understand the physiology and mechanism causing them. There are, however, tests to evaluate the function and anatomy of the large intestine. The lower GI series, for example, involves the administration of a barium enema to a patient. The barium outlines the intestine and it is visible on radiograph. This allows for detection of colon and rectal anatomical abnormalities.

The Effects of General Anesthesia on Bowel Function

GI effects of the anesthetics are multifaceted and encompass a wide array of hemodynamic and physiological changes. This section is broken down into the various components that make up a general anesthetic and the GI effects of each of these components. Emphasis is placed on the effects of preoperative sedation, induction of anesthesia, hypnotic agents, volatile agents, paralysis, and reversal. Opioids will be discussed in another section. Please note that this discussion applies to the healthy state.

In the preoperative setting patients are often nervous and sympathetic stimulation is high. Inhibition of GI tract activity is directly proportional to the amount of norepinephrine secreted from sympathetic stimulation, so the higher the anxiety the higher the inhibition. Even though a good bedside manner and the use of behavioral approaches are beneficial, these may not be sufficient and patients are often given premedication with a benzodiazepine, usually midazolam, to alleviate anxiety. Midazolam acts by enhancing the effect of neurotransmitter, GABA, on GABA-A receptors. A study by Castedal and associates looked at the effect of midazolam on small bowel motility using antroduodenojejunal manometry.[8] The vast majority of the studied variables were not affected by the use of midazolam, but one significant change was noted—an increased duration of phase III of the MMC in the proximal and distal parts of the duodenum, which shortened the MMC by 27%. A clear explanation for this is not evident but there are a couple of considerations. One, the sedative effect of midazolam may be the reason for the change in MMC activity because MMC activity differs between awake and sleep states. Another consideration is that the resultant reduced anxiety decreases sympathetic stimulation allowing for less inhibition and higher activity. However, when applied clinically, there was no real difference seen in small intestinal motility patterns. Of the premedications, midazolam is widely used and considered well tolerated.

General anesthesia causes a loss of all protective reflexes. This is achieved with a variety of medications including opioids, hypnotics, and neuromuscular blocking agents. As mentioned, the effect of opioids will be discussed in a later section. Volatile anesthetics affect bowel function through various mechanisms including depression of spontaneous activity and changes in intestinal tissue oxygenation. Volatile anesthetics depress the spontaneous, electrical, contractile, and propulsive activity in the stomach, small intestine, and colon as demonstrated in many animal and human studies. The small intestine is the first part of the GI tract to recover, followed by the stomach in approximately 24 hours and then the colon 30 to 40 hours postoperatively. Between the various volatile anesthetics there are minor differences. One difference worth noting is that rapid increases in the concentration of desflurane induces greater sympathetic activation, as compared to other volatile agents, which coupled with sympathetic nervous system hyperactivity during surgical procedures can inhibit GI function and motility. In a study comparing desflurane and isoflurane, rapid increases in desflurane caused significantly greater effects on sympathetic and renin-angiotensin system activity as well as increases in blood pressure and heart rate as compared to isoflurane. However, this effect is short-lived as it is only seen with rapid increases in concentration and the surge in sympathetic stimulation tapers off quickly. This transient phenomenon is unlikely to have a lasting effect on bowel function.[9] The volatile anesthetics also affect splanchnic circulation and oxygenation in a dose-dependent manner, which is known to have an effect on bowel function. In horses receiving isoflurane for maintenance of anesthesia, microperfusion and intestinal tissue oxygenation decreased when isoflurane reached 2%.[10] In a human study by Muller and associates, the effects of desflurane and isoflurane on intestinal tissue oxygenation during colorectal surgery were evaluated. It was found that desflurane and isoflurane had comparable effects on intestinal tissue oxygenation. However, during periods of ischemia for resection and anastomosis, reactive hyperemia was better preserved in the patients given isoflurane.[11] This may have important implications in regaining coordinated and appropriate bowel function postoperatively and may determine maintenance with volatile versus total intravenous anesthesia. Whereas the volatile anesthetics depress spontaneous activity and affect blood flow, there is no clear-cut relationship between adverse GI effects and the use of volatile anesthetics. Also, when considering their use in clinical practice, there is very little difference between desflurane, isoflurane, and sevoflurane's effects on bowel function.

An alternative to maintenance with volatile anesthetics is total intravenous anesthesia. Propofol is the most common drug used for this purpose. When used intraoperatively, propofol-remifentanil anesthetic produced increased intestinal motility as compared to sevoflurane-remifentanil.[12] No adverse GI effects were reported, but it did cause a higher degree of surgeon dissatisfaction. A study by Jensen and colleagues looked at bowel recovery after open procedures and did not find a difference in overall recovery and bowel function when comparing isoflurane/nitrous oxide, propofol/air, and propofol/nitrous oxide.[13] Even in colorectal cancer patients there was no difference in inflammatory response among patients receiving either total intravenous anesthesia with propofol and remifentanil or inhalational anesthesia with sevoflurane and fentanyl.[14,15] There are few data on the effect of propofol on GI smooth muscle and many of the established studies show various and conflicting results when it comes to the recovery of bowel functions.

Nitrous oxide is 30 times more soluble than nitrogen in the blood and as such will diffuse into gas-containing cavities from the blood faster than the nitrogen already present in those cavities can diffuse out. This is especially important in the bowels as gut distention is correlated with the amount of gas already present in the bowel, the duration of nitrous oxide administration, and the concentration of nitrous oxide administered. Although it has been established that nitrous oxide causes bowel distention and it is prudent to avoid nitrous oxide in lengthy abdominal surgeries or when the bowel is already distended, the most recent ENIGMA trial did not relate the use of nitrous oxide to any significant adverse outcomes.[16]

Paralysis to achieve favorable surgical conditions is produced by administration of neuromuscular blocking agents. Neuromuscular blocking drugs only affect skeletal muscle so GI motility remains intact. However, special mention of the depolarizing neuromuscular blocker succinylcholine should be made. Succinylcholine mimics acetylcholine in that it produces an initial muscle contraction, which is visible as fasciculations. This contraction increases intragastric pressure, which may be so strong as to overcome the tone of the LES and allow reflux of gastric contents. Aspiration is certainly a concern, but this should not necessarily preclude the use of succinylcholine. Patient condition, including body habitus, technical difficulty of intubation, nothing by mouth (NPO) status, and comorbidities should be the determining factors in assessing the risk of aspiration.

Reversal of paralysis using the anticholinesterase, neostigmine, will increase parasympathetic activity and bowel peristalsis by increasing the frequency and intensity of contractions. In cases of fresh bowel anastomoses, this can be of concern as the increase in activity could result in dehiscence. This is partially offset by simultaneous administration of the anticholinergic medications, glycopyrrolate or atropine, which are used to attenuate the bradycardia from neostigmine. This effect is not seen with sugammadex, which may be a more prudent choice for reversal in situations of tenuous bowel anastomoses. There is some data to support the use of neostigmine in treating postoperative ileus but the adverse effects of bradycardia, vomiting, and abdominal cramps may preclude its use.

Surgical procedures on the GI tract produce an exaggerated stress response that may predispose to postoperative bowel dysfunction. Goals of anesthetic care should be to attenuate the stress response, optimize hemodynamic and fluid status, and maintain normothermia.[17,18] At present there is no evidence for recommendations on specific anesthetic and analgesic agents to avoid adverse GI effects.

Effect of Opioids on Bowel Function

Much attention has been given to the use and effects (beneficial and adverse) of opioid administration. There is a desire to only use adjunct techniques and nonopioid medications; however, opioids are often necessary to control perioperative pain. A major adverse effect, and one that is not associated with the development of opioid tolerance, is reduced GI motility and constipation. Opioids exert their function on both central and peripheral receptors, namely mu, delta, and kappa. It is the central effects that primarily mediate analgesia and produce the favorable effects. The peripheral effects are the adverse effects. There is a high density of peripheral mu-opioid receptors in the myenteric and submucosal plexuses. Activation of these mu-opioid receptors in the myenteric plexus has a dual effect on the neural pathways controlling motility—it inhibits excitatory pathways that depress peristaltic contraction and it also inhibits inhibitory pathways. These inhibitions increase GI muscular activity and increase resting muscle tone including tone in the ileocecal valve and internal anal sphincters. This produces spasm and nonrhythmic or propulsive motility. Activation of these receptors is also linked to the inhibition of acetylcholine release and promotion of nitrous oxide release that inhibits propulsive motility.[19] Together these effects will delay gastric emptying and slow transit through the intestine. Activation of these receptors in the submucosal plexus decreases nutrient secretion and increases fluid absorption. Coupled with reduced motility the stool will remain in the gut for a longer period of time and as more water is absorbed the stool becomes hard and dry leading to constipation.[20] Other adverse sequelae include nausea, anorexia, delayed digestion, abdominal pain, excessive straining during bowel movements, and incomplete evacuation.

Many efforts have been made and are currently underway to attenuate or avoid opioid-induced bowel dysfunction. The use of laxatives, stool softeners, and prokinetic agents, such as metoclopramide and neostigmine, have shown some success in alleviating opioid-induced constipation. Potentially switching to a different opioid is also offered as a treatment option. Tassinari and associates performed a meta-analysis demonstrating strong evidence supporting opioid switch in alleviating constipation, most strongly for morphine to transdermal fentanyl.[21] Another option is combining opioids with enteral opioid receptor antagonists. Naloxone was the first used. It is a nonselective, competitive opioid receptor antagonist. While its effect on the peripheral receptors in the gut produced favorable results of reversing gut motility inhibition, its nonselective profile meant it also worked on the central receptors and reversed the beneficial analgesic effect of opioids. Therefore, new attention is given to pure peripherally acting opioid receptor antagonists. Methylnaltrexone is a peripheral mu-opioid receptor antagonist and does not cross the blood-brain barrier. In healthy volunteers, the use of methylnaltrexone prevented delay in orocecal transit time after morphine administration.[22] Subsequent systematic reviews demonstrated that methylnaltrexone and alvimopan were better than placebo in reversing opioid-induced increased GI transit time and constipation.[23–25] However, long-term efficacy and safety have not been clearly established. Further studies are underway.

Effect of Open Abdominal Surgery, Ischemia, Stomas, and Bowel Anastomosis on Gastrointestinal Physiology and Function

The surgical procedure itself, even with purposes of correcting GI pathology, significantly affects GI physiology and function and predisposes to postoperative ileus. Recently, a standardized definition of postoperative ileus was established as "a transient cessation of coordinated bowel motility after surgical intervention, which prevents effective transit of intestinal contents and/or tolerance of oral intake."[26] Manipulation of the intestines is the main factor that initiates postoperative ileus. Additional contributors include immobility, electrolyte imbalance from fluid shifts and insensible losses, and intestinal wall swelling from excessive fluid administration. In open abdominal procedures, the surgical manipulation of the bowel induces a degree of trauma that sets in motion the whole process of postoperative ileus. There are two phases to uncomplicated postoperative ileus (i.e., in the absence of complications, such as perforation, bleeding, peritonitis). The first phase is an early neurogenic phase and the second is an inflammatory phase. In total, an uncomplicated postoperative ileus lasts about 3 to 4 days.[26]

The early neurogenic phase results when the intestine is manipulated, which is more extensive in open procedures than laparoscopic ones. This manipulation activates the sympathetic nervous system, increasing the inhibitory neural input that leads to decreased propulsive movements and almost complete cessation of GI motility. This lasts about 3 to 4 hours after surgery.

The late inflammatory phase also begins with surgical manipulation of the intestines. Surgical manipulation increases sympathetic stimulation of the myenteric plexus, which promotes the influx of leukocytes into the "traumatized" areas of the gut. Further release of cytokines, chemokines, and leukocytes as well as phagocytosis in the traumatized area occurs and eventually spreads through the entire GI tract. This inflammatory cascade increases permeability and allows for translocation of intraluminal bacteria, which further exacerbates the inflammatory process. However, peritonitis does not always develop because the mast cells and neutrophils are very effective in eliminating the translocated bacteria in the peritoneal cavity. This process occurs about 3 hours after intestinal manipulation and continues throughout the manipulated segment and the rest of the GI tract for the next 24 hours. It eventually subsides and within 3 to 4 days this uncomplicated ileus is usually resolved.[27,28]

Mesenteric ischemia, if left untreated, will lead to 100% mortality. This occurs when the supply of oxygen is insufficient to meet the oxygen demand of the intestines. It affects the small and large intestine and is classified as occlusive or nonocclusive. Etiologies of mesenteric ischemia include: strangulation, emboli (seen commonly in patients with atrial fibrillation), complications of aortic surgery or during cross-clamping, trauma, drug-induced, atherosclerosis, and inflammatory diseases. There are four stages of mesenteric ischemia. The first is the hyperactive stage when blood flow to the intestine is abruptly occluded. This produces severe pain and overactive peristalsis. There may be passage of loose stool with blood. The second stage is a paralytic stage that spreads diffusely across the intestines. The third stage involves leakage of fluid, proteins, and electrolytes through the bowel wall into the peritoneum. If the bowel becomes necrotic then peritonitis develops. The fourth stage is shock. End-organ damage is apparent and contributes to altered hemodynamics and critical illness. Treatment involves reperfusion of the occluded vessel through revascularization and possibly bowel resection.[29]

Bowel resections vary in terms of their effect on the remaining bowel. The degree of GI dysfunction depends on the portion of bowel resected. The colon primarily absorbs water and a full colonic resection is compatible with life. However, when the small intestine is resected the effect on the GI system is much more pronounced. The small intestine is responsible for absorbing vitamins and nutrients. This can be properly maintained if at least a third of the small bowel remains. The jejunum is the primary site for digestion and absorption of nutrients. After a jejunal resection, the ileum is usually able to adapt to fulfill its functions. The ileum absorbs vitamin B12 and bile salts. If the ileum is resected (especially more than 100 cm), the remaining small intestine cannot compensate for the loss of its function and severe malabsorption and diarrhea will result. The unabsorbed bile salts enter the colon and stimulate fat and water secretion. Small intestinal resection will increase gastric motility but this depends on the site and amount resected. If the terminal ileum and ileocecal valve are resected then intestinal content transit speeds up.[30]

Bowel anastomoses can significantly alter bowel function in that they disrupt normal motor activity. Partial transection usually preserves the wave of activity, though complete transection will interrupt it. There is a loss in myogenic continuity in that the intestine distal to the transection will no longer receive signals or respond to the pacemaker in the proximal duodenum. Now the part distal to transection has to rely on its own intrinsic slow-wave transmission. This can be attenuated by close approximation of the muscle layers. There is motor asynchrony across the anastomotic site but long-term studies report reasonable MMC activity is ultimately achieved with time. The mechanism explaining why this recovery occurs remains uncertain. The transection and anastomosis have little effect on intestinal homeostasis and are not associated with significant digestion or absorption side effects.[2]

Gastrointestinal System Nociception

Abdominal visceral pain and its associated symptoms are common in the GI perioperative period. For an understanding of GI nociception, a detailed knowledge of the anatomy and physiology of abdominal visceral innervation is essential.

ABDOMINAL VISCERA INNERVATION

Abdominal visceral pain signals are carried in both sympathetic and parasympathetic autonomic fibers.[31,32] Innervation of the parietal peritoneum, abdominal wall muscles, and skin is supplied by the ventral rami of thoracoabdominal nerves, which are part of the somatosensory system.

Sympathetic fibers for the upper abdomen, including the liver, stomach, pancreas, small bowel, and proximal part of the colon, originate from spinal cord segments T5 to L2. Those preganglionic fibers exit the cord as gray rami communicants to enter the sympathetic chain in the paravertebral region. These fibers terminate in the prevertebral (subdiaphragmatic) ganglia through splanchnic nerves and generate the celiac plexus, where they synapse with a large number of postganglionic, predominantly unmyelinated fibers. Postganglionic fibers will then innervate the

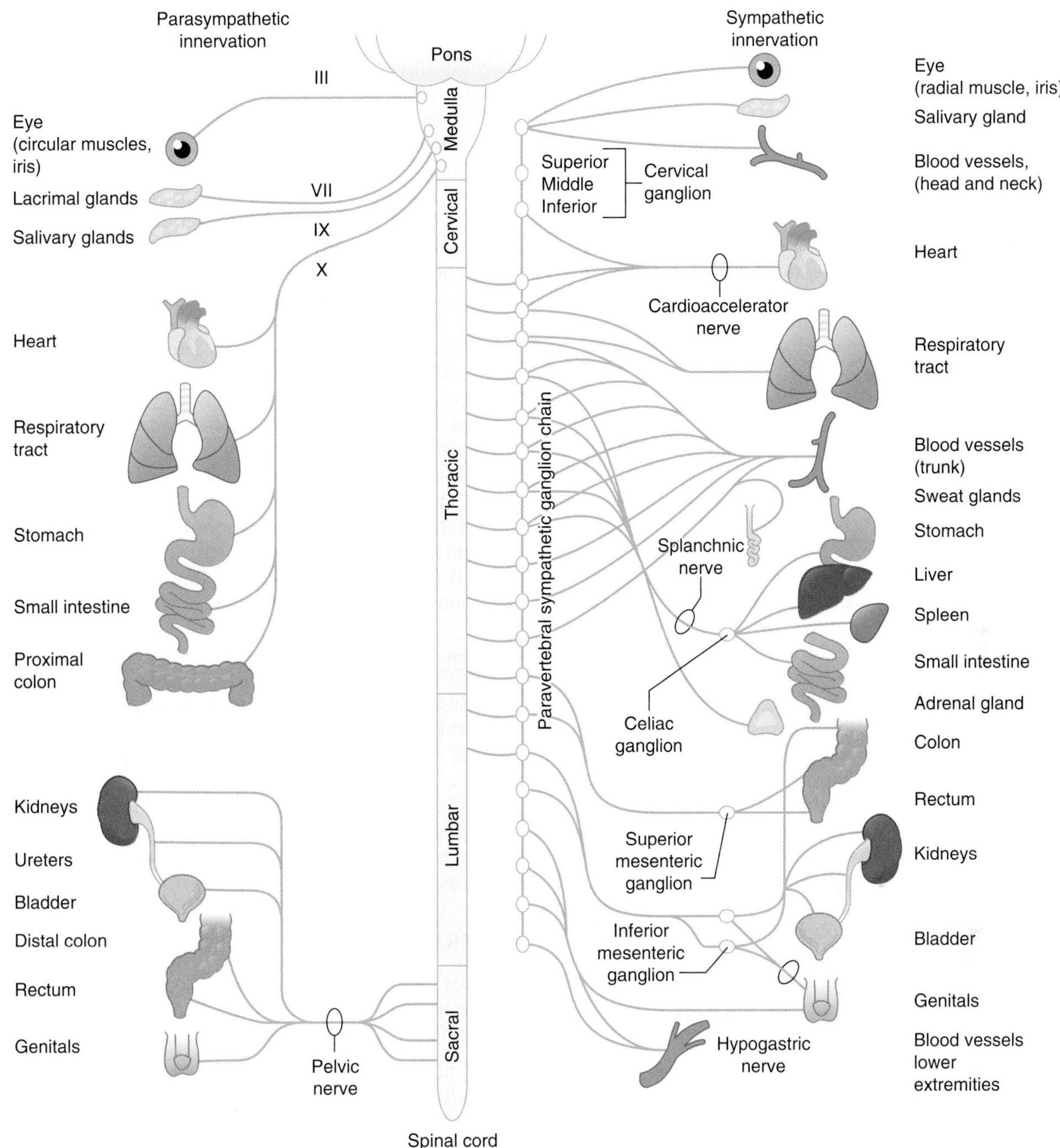

Fig. 15.1 Schematic diagram of sympathetic and parasympathetic innervation to the gastrointestinal (GI) tract. Sympathetic innervation of majority of the GI tract up to the rectum is supplied by the celiac plexus. (From Glick DB. The autonomic nervous system. In: Miller RD, ed. *Miller's Anesthesia*. 7th ed. Philadelphia: Elsevier; 2010.)

organs (see Fig. 15.5).[33] Innervation of the lower abdomen including the descending colon, sigmoid and rectum, bladder, and lower ureter originates from T9 to L3 and forms the inferior mesenteric and hypogastric ganglia and plexus.

Sympathetic afferent fibers transmit visceral pain, whereas sympathetic efferent nerves inhibit peristalsis and gastric distention as well as cause GI vasoconstriction.[33]

The parasympathetic nervous system supplies the abdominal viscera proximal to the splenic flexure of the colon via the vagus nerve. Some of the vagal fibers pass through the prevertebral fibers (celiac plexus). The parasympathetic postganglionic neurons are located in the myenteric and submucosal plexuses. Visceral afferent parasympathetic nerve fibers transmit the sensations of satiety, nausea, and distention, whereas efferent parasympathetic nerve fibers increase functions such as secretion, sphincter relaxation, and peristalsis.[34–36]

The colon, rectum, internal and external genitalia, and bladder are innervated by fibers from spinal cord segments S2 to S4, which run with the pelvic nerves (Fig. 15.1).[37–40]

Some of the characteristics of abdominal visceral innervation are: (1) they are almost exclusively myelinated A-delta and unmyelinated C fibers; (2) they have "dual-function" properties (sensory that carry sensory evoked potentials and afferent that regulate autonomic flow);[42]

(3) there are an abundance of connections between nerves, ganglia, and plexuses; (4) there is not a fine and distinct nerve; (5) considerable variation in anatomy can be found; (6) visceral innervation anatomy is affected by intraabdominal pathology; and (7) visceral innervation distribution is diffuse and capable of amplification. Once stimulated, it could be difficult to stop (self-aggravation).[41–46]

In summary, the innervation of the GI organs up to the proximal transverse colon is supplied by the celiac plexus, and innervation of the descending colon and distal GI tract comes from the inferior hypogastric plexus. Although each organ looks like it is innervated from specific cord segments, the fibers frequently communicate with each other (Table 15.2).

CELIAC PLEXUS ANATOMY

The celiac plexus is normally composed of two or three splanchnic nerves:

The greater (superior thoracic) splanchnic nerve comes from T5 to T9 (fibers can arise as high as T1 and as low as T11). The greater splanchnic nerve is usually anterolateral to the T12 vertebral body. It perforates the crura of the diaphragm and enters the retroperitoneal space where it joins the celiac plexus.

The lesser splanchnic nerve is formed from T9 to T11. In 30% of cases this nerve is not present. Two or more celiac ganglia are generated, which lie ventrolaterally to the aorta between the origin of the celiac arterial trunk and the renal arteries.

The celiac ganglia can vary considerably in size and number on each side. Usually they are oval shaped and can vary from 0.5 to 4.5 cm in width.

Fusion of these ganglia form a fine nerve plexus that may extend to the inferior border of the T12 vertebra and lower border of L2. They are mostly located close to the celiac artery trunk.[46]

The plexus and related nervous structures are contained in the prevertebral retroperitoneal space along with the aorta, inferior vena cava (IVC), veins of azygos system, lymph nodes, the cisterna chyli, and diaphragmatic crura (Fig. 15.2).

ABDOMINAL VISCERAL PAIN

Despite the fact that abdominal pain of visceral origin is a very common finding during the perioperative period, our knowledge and practice to control this pain are very limited.[47]

Visceral pain is different from somatic pain in many aspects; not all organs respond similarly to stimuli, some organs are more sensitive. For example, the pancreas is more sensitive than the stomach. Tissue destruction, ischemia, and inflammation will not always cause pain.[48] The most remarkable difference between visceral and superficial structures is the fact that visceral pain is poorly localized, produces strong affective responses, and refers to other locations with intense regional or muscle spasms and autonomic instability.[49–51]

The referral properties of visceral pain have been attributed to the conjunction of visceral and somatic inputs to the spinal cord and CNS. For the same reason, visceral pain can have somatic components. Merging of these inputs can modify pain sensation distal to the site of visceral inflammation, or pain from one intraabdominal organ can refer to another.[40]

Visceral pain is fervently associated with emotional fluctuation. IBS is thought to be related to gut-brain interaction and autonomic dysregulation.[52]

It was found that induced sadness was attenuated by fatty acid infusion, and increased neural activity in the part of the brain processing emotions was also observed.[53] Probiotic bacteria are beneficial in stress-related disorders, such as anxiety and depression, and during the course of common comorbidities and some bowel disorders.[54]

VISCERAL PAIN TREATMENT

Opioids are still the mainstay of visceral pain treatment, although their usage has been limited by many side effects such as decreased gut motility and constipation, sedation, nausea, and vomiting. In addition, prolonged usage of narcotics is associated with opioid-induced hyperalgesia and tolerance.[55] Usage of acetaminophen, nonsteroidal anti-inflammatory drugs, and serotonin components have been suggested, but the results are not specific.[56]

VISCERAL PAIN BLOCK TECHNIQUES

Noxious pain impulses originating from abdominal viscera can be blocked by the following regional anesthesia techniques (Fig. 15.3)

1. Spinal anesthesia extending to at least the level of T5
2. Epidural anesthesia covering T5 to Tl2 dermatomes
3. Paravertebral blocks comprising T5 to L2 spinal segments
4. Selective T5 to L2 sympathetic chain block
5. Celiac/splanchnic nerve block

TABLE 15.2 Summary of Visceral Innervation on Gastrointestinal Tract[47]

Organ	Sympathetic Sensory Supply	Parasympathetic Sensory Supply
Liver and biliary tract	T5-T10 via *Celiac plexus*	Vagus nerve
Stomach	T7-T9 via *Celiac plexus*	Vagus nerve
Pancreas	T6-T10 via *Celiac plexus*	Vagus nerve
Small bowel	T9-L1 via *Celiac plexus*	Vagus nerve
Cecum, ascending and transverse colon	T9-L1 via *Celiac plexus*	Vagus nerve
Descending colon	T9-T12 via *Celiac plexus*	S2-S4 via *Pelvic nerves*
Sigmoid, rectum	T11-L1 via *Inferior hypogastric plexus*	S2-S4 via *Pelvic nerves*

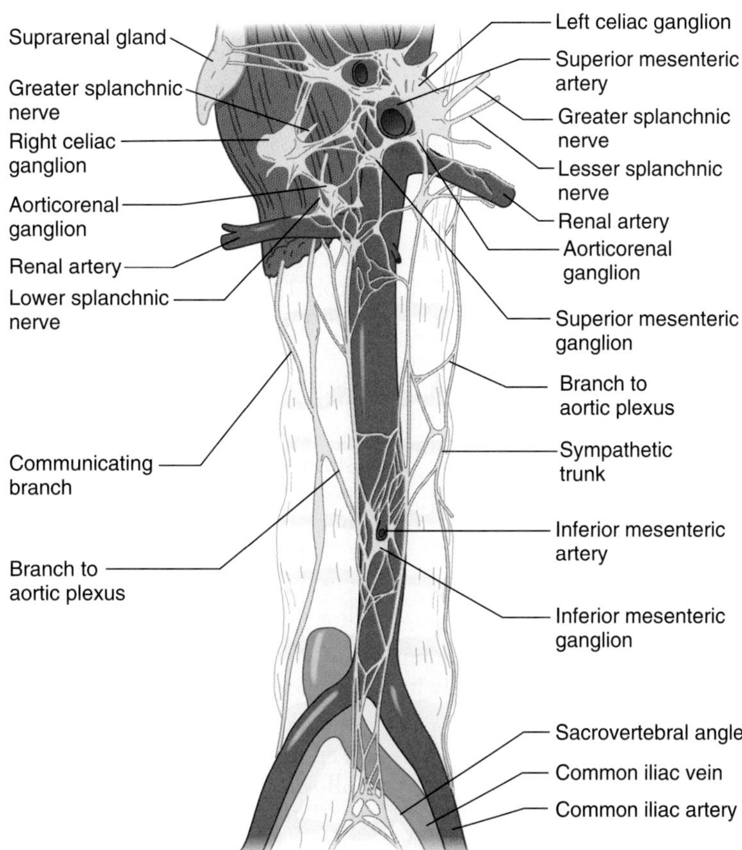

Fig. 15.2 Anatomy of the abdominal sympathetic trunk. (Redrawn from http://commons.wikimedia.org/wiki/File:Gray847.png#mediaviewer.)

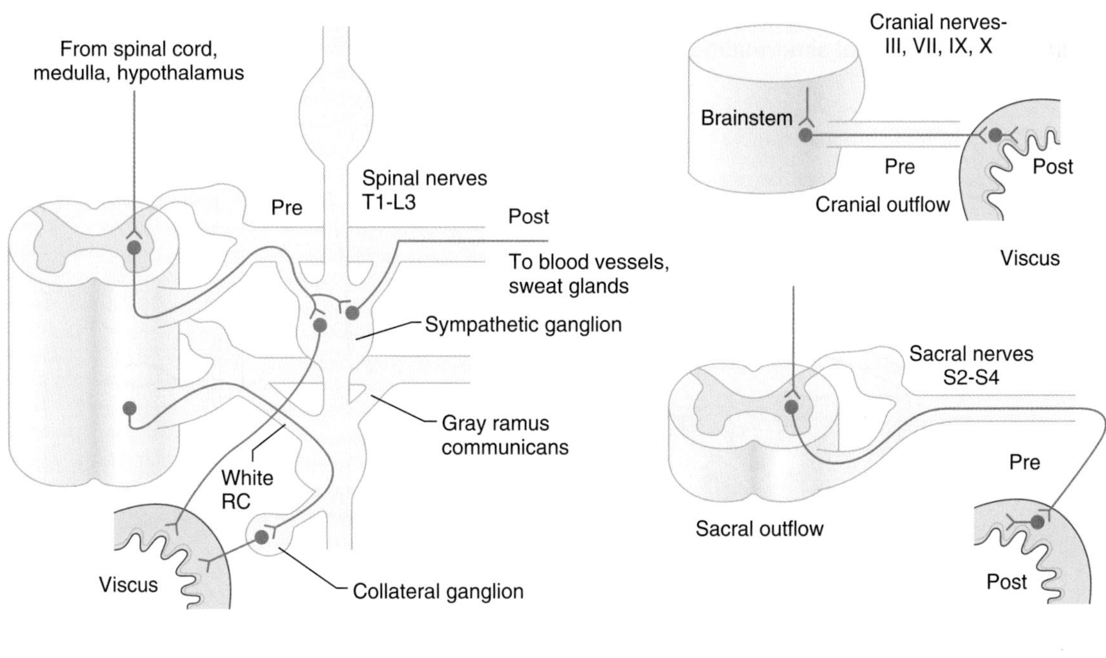

Fig. 15.3 Regional anesthetic techniques on gastrointestinal (GI) visceral sympathetic innervation: different regional techniques which can block sympathetic innervation of the GI tract at different levels. (From Glick DB. The autonomic nervous system. In: Miller RD, ed. *Miller's Anesthesia*. 7th ed. Philadelphia: Elsevier; 2010.)

Based on the type and extent of the regional technique, its effect on the GI physiology is different. Of note, the aforementioned regional anesthesia techniques are associated with the blockade of the sympathetic nervous system, whereas the parasympathetic system usually remains intact.

VISCERAL/CELIAC PLEXUS BLOCK

Blockage of the splanchnic/celiac plexus has been approached in many ways:

Intraperitoneal Regional Anesthesia or Peritoneal Lavage

Abdominal visceral pain can be blocked simply by instilling local anesthetic into the peritoneal cavity. A recent meta-analysis by Boddy and associates of intraperitoneal regional anesthesia in laparoscopic surgeries found an overall benefit, although there was no consistent analgesia, but also a remarkable absence of complications and side effects.[57]

Celiac Plexus Block—Posterior and Trans-Crural Approach

Radiography, fluoroscopy, or computed tomography scan is usually needed to perform this block safely, especially in lytic blocks.

This approach requires a special needle, usually a 15-cm, 20- or 22-G Chiba needle. The patient is in the prone or lateral position and the needle is inserted below the tip of the 12th rib on the left side. The needle is aimed at a 45-degree angle to touch the lateral side of the L1 vertebral body at a depth of 7 to 9 cm. Subsequently, the needle is nearly fully redirected 5 to 10 degrees and advanced to a depth of 11 to 14 cm. In this situation the pulsation of the aorta on the needle can sometimes be felt (Fig. 15.4).

Determination of the correct vertebral level is imprecise in patients with absence of the 12th rib, a markedly downsloping of the rib, or in other congenital abnormalities.

Celiac Plexus Block—Anterior Approach

The abdomen is opened and the left lobe of the liver is retracted upward. The stomach is pulled gently downward and to the left thereby exposing and stretching the lesser omentum. The index finger of the operator is then inserted at the highest possible point of the incision, palpating the pulsating aorta through the lesser omentum. The aorta is pushed aside to the left by passing the tip of the finger to the vertebrae whereby it is separated from the vena cava. A fine 22-G spinal needle is inserted alongside the finger and in the loose, retroperitoneal, prevertebral tissue between the IVC and aorta. Diluted local anesthetic is injected in this area after careful aspiration. The tip of the needle should be close to the diaphragm, above the origin of the celiac trunk, in the midline. A similar approach was described by Lillemoe in 1992 for postoperative pain control in pancreatic cancer patients: after lesser omentum exposure, the left index and middle fingers are placed on either side of the aorta and pulled caudad until the upper border of the pancreas is identified and 20 mL of solution is injected on either side of the aorta (Fig. 15.5).[58]

Endoscopic Ultrasound-Guided Celiac Plexus Block

Recent recognition that the celiac ganglia can be visualized and accessed by endoscopic ultrasound (EUS) now allows for a direct injection into the celiac plexus. The patient is placed in the left lateral decubitus position and under conscious sedation. From the posterior side of the lesser curvature of the gastric fundus EUS can visualize the aorta in a longitudinal plane. The aorta is traced distally to the celiac trunk, and the injection delivered around the celiac trunk. Meta-analysis has shown that EUS-guided celiac plexus blocks are safe and efficient (Fig. 15.6).[59]

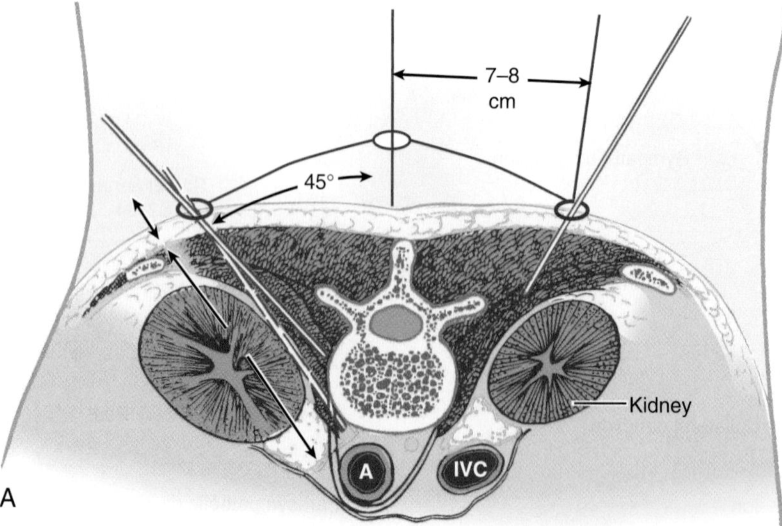

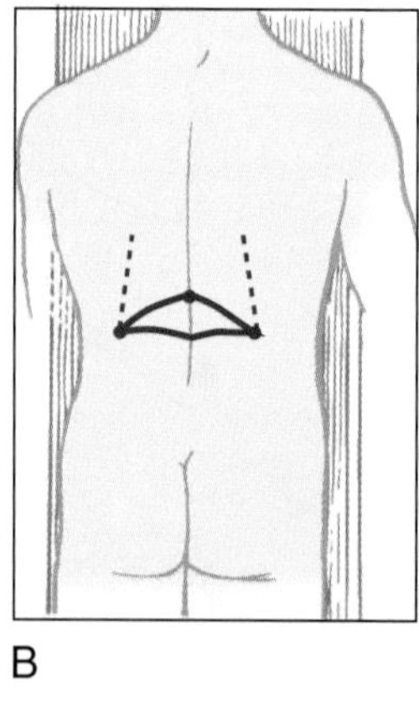

Fig. 15.4 (A) Schematic view of the posterior approach. Celiac plexus can be blocked by insertion of a 20- to 22-gauge 15-cm spinal needle (Chiba needle) at the level of T12. (B) Positioning and surface landmarks. (From Wedel DJ, Horlocker TT. Nerve blocks. In: Miller RD, ed. *Miller's Anesthesia*. 7th ed. Philadelphia: Elsevier; 2010.)

TECHNICAL ASPECTS OF VISCERAL PLEXUS BLOCKS

There is no established standard technique. It is important to completely disrupt all of the impulse traffic in the visceral innervation, as these impulses are widely spread and can be reinstated via very fine nerves.

Unfortunately, the success of splanchnic nerve and celiac plexus blocks cannot be verified by any objective signs. Hypotension is not a regular finding. If patients do have upper abdominal pain, analgesia typically results within a few minutes after the block. Failure of pain to subside is not only due to inappropriate technique but also due to the involvement of visceral plexuses, such as the hypogastric plexus.

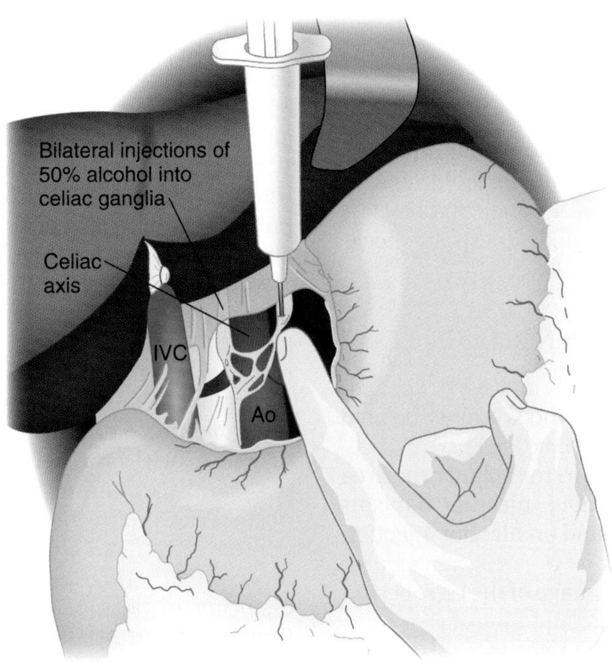

Fig. 15.5 Celiac plexus block (anterior approach): intraoperative celiac plexus block is performed using a 20- to 22-gauge spinal needle. Injection is performed at each side of the aorta and the level of celiac axis. (Redrawn from Lillemoe KD, Cameron JL, Kaufman HS, et al. Chemical splancnicectomy in patients with unresectable pancreatic cancer. A prospective randomized trial. *Ann Surg*. 1993;217:447–457.)

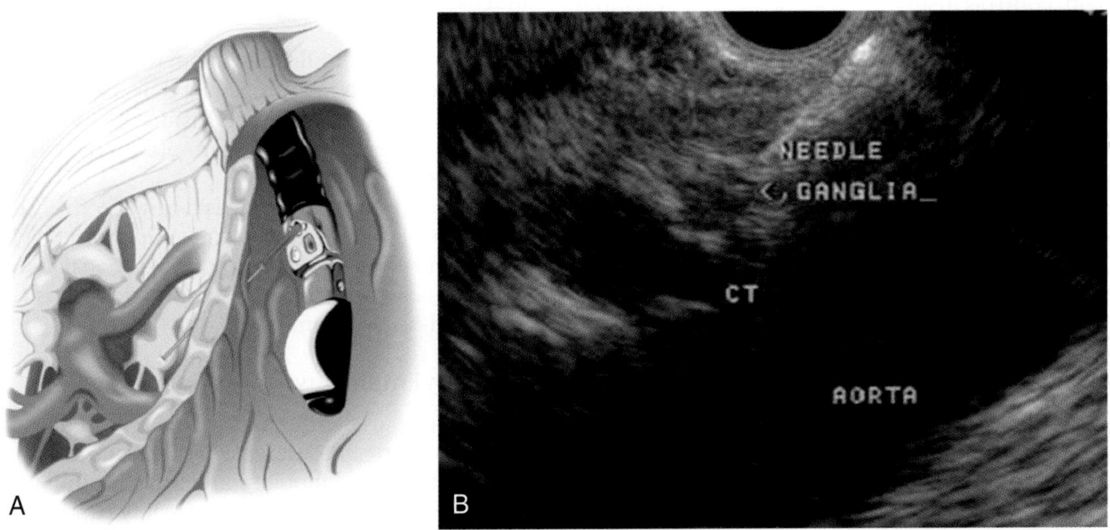

Fig. 15.6 Endoscopic ultrasound-guided celiac plexus block: (A) Ultrasound beams use lesser curvature of the gastric fundus as media to visualize the celiac trunk. (B) Ultrasonic image of celiac ganglia and needle during performance of endoscopic ultrasound-guided celiac plexus block. *CT*, Celiac trunk. (From Levy M, Wiersema M. EUS-guided celiac plexus neurolysis and celiac plexus block. *Gastrointest Endosc*. 2003;57(7):923–930.)

BOX 15.1 Complications of Celiac Plexus Blocks

Hypotension
Diarrhea
Intravascular injection and vascular trauma
Subarachnoid or epidural injection and paraplegia
Renal injury
Pneumothorax
Chylothorax
Damage to surrounding structures and retroperitoneal hematoma
Peritonitis and abscess

There is little information about the duration of a successful block induced by local anesthetics. Most of the blocks have been a combination of local anesthetic and lytic therapy for chronic pain. In order to avoid toxic side effects, local anesthetic doses must be reduced when the block is combined with another major regional anesthetic technique such as abdominal wall blocks.

COMPLICATIONS OF VISCERAL PAIN BLOCKS

The complication rate is between 0.5% and 32%, depending on the method, as radiologic methods are associated with a reduced rate of complications (Box 15.1).

Dilation of the capacitance vessels in the splanchnic area will cause hypotension. Subarachnoid injection happens mostly with a posterior approach, and an alcohol injection can cause paraplegia.

A chylothorax can result from damage of the retroperitoneal lymph nodes.

The most devastating complication occurs with vascular trauma, thrombosis, and retroperitoneal hematoma.[60]

INDICATIONS FOR A VISCERAL PAIN BLOCK

Post-Laparatomy Pain Relief

Visceral pain blocks are usually associated with somatosensory pain controls using central neuroaxial regional anesthesia techniques, such as epidural analgesia or paravertebral analgesia. A combination of a celiac plexus block with any other regional anesthesia technique is rarely used.

Cancer Pain

Splanchnic/celiac plexus blocks have been used for biliary and pancreatic cancers. The details of this indication of visceral pain control are discussed in the chronic pain management chapter (Chapter 51).

EFFECTS OF REGIONAL ANESTHESIA ON GASTROINTESTINAL PHYSIOLOGY

The degree to which the GI tract is affected by regional anesthesia depends on the type and extent of the block. Epidural analgesia, especially thoracic epidural analgesia (TEA), has been used extensively for a wide variety of GI surgeries. The clinical outcome of TEA after GI surgeries has been reviewed extensively in the literature; the focus of this chapter is its effect on GI physiology.

Effect on Gastrointestinal Motility and Postoperative Ileus

As described, postoperative ileus is a very common phenomenon in patients who undergo major abdominal surgery. Postoperative ileus is a temporary state of GI motor dysfunction that occurs after surgery in the abdominal cavity. This includes disruption of normal coordinated movements of the GI tract,[61] nonmechanical obstruction of the bowel, activation of the inhibitory reflexes, inflammatory mediators, bowel manipulation, electrolyte disturbances, opioid administration, sympathetic overactivity with surgical pain, and postoperative pain.[62–66] Transit time of the stomach may extend 24 to 48 hours and colon transfer time may increase 48 to 72 hours. Some of these effects may continue for up to 3 to 4 days after surgery.[67,68]

The main pathophysiologic event in postoperative ileus is neuroimmune interaction, which is based on the bidirectional communication between the immune system within and outside the GI tract and the autonomic nervous system.[69]

Manipulation of the intestines and the stress response associated with postoperative pain are the key factors initiating postoperative ileus. The surgical stress response is a multifaceted, neurohumoral response to a surgical stimulation and can be associated with considerable morbidity, including a systemic inflammatory response syndrome, which is associated with the release of systemic inflammatory response and adrenaline and noradrenaline hormones. This sympathetic overactivity will constrain mobility and directly inhibit gut smooth muscle via activation of α- and β-adrenergic receptors resulting in postoperative ileus.[70] Epidural administration of local anesthetic or opioids has been shown to suppress these responses.[71–73]

Epidural block with deposition of local anesthetic within the epidural space results in blockade of the afferent and efferent sympathetic-mediated GI reflexes, but parasympathetic innervation is left intact. The effect of an imbalanced sympathetic and parasympathetic nervous system has been associated with improved GI blood flow and anastomotic mucosal perfusion. This controls pain and decreases the need for opioids.[74–78]

However, it should be noted that severe hypotension (>50% reduction in systolic blood pressure) may be associated with worsened local perfusion.[79,80] Vasoactive drugs, such as norepinephrine, can attenuate this effect and improve colonic perfusion.[81]

In general, epidural analgesia can effectively decrease the incidence of postoperative ileus. A Cochrane review showed that epidural usage reduces postoperative ileus by 36 hours when a local anesthetic regimen was used as compared to an opioid-based regimen.[82]

Effect on Enteric Anastomosis Dehiscence

Unopposed parasympathetic activity with blockage of sympathetic fibers has increased concerns among clinicians that the increased mobility and intraluminal pressures will lead to anastomotic leaks and possibly rupture.[83] However, animal studies have failed to show any difference in anastomotic bursting pressure when epidural anesthesia is compared to general anesthesia.[84] In fact, it could be argued that with improvement of GI blood flow and tissue oxygenation the neuroaxial block can actually reduce the risk of anastomotic breakdown. However, the effect of neuroaxial blocks after GI procedures and laparotomies on enteric anastomotic leakage is not supported in the literature.[81,85]

Effect on Nutrition

The early postoperative period after GI surgery is characterized by a systemic stress response and catabolic activity. This effect, in conjunction with a lack of nutrition, results in postoperative weakness and muscle wasting. As discussed previously, epidural analgesia has been shown to decrease opioid requirements and reduce postoperative ileus. This, in turn, enhances enteral feeding.[86] Therefore, blockade of afferent stimuli and the endocrine metabolic responses, as well as the improvement in catabolism seen with epidural analgesia, are part of an enhanced recovery after surgery (ERAS) protocol for major GI surgeries to facilitate oral nutrition.[87]

Effect on Postoperative Nausea and Vomiting

Pain management plays a large role in postoperative nausea and vomiting therapy.[88] Avoiding systemic opioids and the use of epidural analgesia helps to reduce the incidence of nausea and vomiting. However, in the setting of regional anesthesia, attention should be paid to unopposed vagal activity, local anesthetic systemic toxicity, hypotension, and medication administration.

Spinal anesthesia poses the highest risk for the development of nausea and vomiting and is seen in 20% of patients. The effects of spinal anesthesia, especially with T6 to L1 blockade, include sympathetic innervation and unopposed vagal activity and result in GI hyperperistalsis, nausea, and vomiting.[89] In addition, TEA or spinal anesthesia that results in systemic hypotension severe enough to cause cerebral ischemia can cause nausea and vomiting.[90]

Effect on Gastrointestinal Blood Flow and Volume

The degree of arterial hypotension induced by spinal or epidural anesthesia is directly related to the extent of the blockade, the dose of local anesthetic used, and baseline hemodynamics.[91] Lumbar epidural anesthesia leads to arterial and venous dilation at the segments affected by the anesthetic. The constriction of the proximal part of the splanchnic vasculature shifts blood volume from the splanchnic system into the systemic circulation and usually results in preservation of stressed volume and blood pressure. TEA is associated with pronounced mesenteric vasodilation and arterial hypotension, while intestinal blood flow and oxygen consumption are maintained. A study using labeled red cells demonstrated that epidural anesthesia with sensory block at T4 to T5 increased blood volume in both the intrathoracic and splanchnic vasculature. The addition of a vasoconstrictor decreased volume within the splanchnic region, but increased volume within the thorax. The authors estimated that the use of a vasoconstrictor during TEA led to a shift of approximately 1 L of blood from the splanchnic area into the thoracic and systemic circulation.[92] Infusion of fluid or the use of adrenergic agonists apparently increases stressed volume. Infusion of fluid increases total (stressed and unstressed) blood volume, whereas adrenergic agonists move existing blood volume from unstressed to stressed.[93] In many situations, the use of α-adrenergic agonists might be more beneficial than infusion of fluid. Because veins are much more sensitive to adrenergic stimulation than arteries are, small doses of α-adrenergic agonists in normovolemic patients would constrict veins (increasing stressed volume) without affecting arteries or jeopardizing tissue perfusion.

ENHANCED RECOVERY AFTER SURGERY FOR GASTROINTESTINAL PROCEDURES—PHYSIOLOGIC BASIS

ERAS is an interdisciplinary, multimodal concept aimed at accelerating postoperative convalescence and reducing general morbidity by simultaneously applying several interventions. ERAS represents a paradigm shift in perioperative care. It reexamines traditional practice by replacing it with evidence-based practices.[94]

ERAS for GI procedures highlights a perioperative regimen with emphasis on[95,96]:

1. Regional anesthesia
2. Avoidance of opioids
3. Multimodal analgesia
4. Nutrition and preoperative carbohydrates
5. Selective bowel preparation
6. Fluid optimization
7. Temperature control
8. Early removal of drains and tubes
9. Early mobilization
10. Early oral intake

The use of ERAS protocols has been associated with shorter hospitalizations.[97]

PHYSIOLOGIC BASIS OF ERAS

Perioperative Pain Control

Many aspects of regional anesthesia, opioid-sparing anesthesia, and multimodal analgesia have already been discussed. The effect of pain control on postoperative outcomes has also been evaluated in multiple studies and is an inseparable part of ERAS protocols for many surgeries including GI procedures.[98–100] The favorable physiologic effects on the respiratory and cardiovascular systems by epidural analgesia may serve as yet another reason as to why epidural analgesia is a devoted part of ERAS protocols.[101–102]

Preoperative Carbohydrate Loading and Early Postoperative Feeding

There is strong evidence in animal studies demonstrating that fed animals tolerate stress much better than fasted animals. Perioperative oral carbohydrates raise insulin sensitivity by 50%. This means there is 50% less insulin resistance in the postoperative period, which also ameliorates ilium barrier failure. There is also less risk of development of hyperglycemic events and an improvement in retention of protein and lean body mass.[103,105] Enteric feeding is associated with prevention of bacterial translocation[104] or gut barrier failure.[105] Carbohydrate loading shifts the cellular metabolism to an anabolic state that will support postoperative nutrition.[106–108]

Most of the national and international societies now recommend a 6-hour preoperative fast for solids and a

2-hour fast for clear fluids, which includes carbohydrate drinks.[109–112]

In order to maintain metabolic and nutritional homoeostasis, early postoperative feeding has been suggested. A small study on patients after major colorectal surgery showed that immediate postoperative enteral feeding does not result in a net loss of body nitrogen.[113]

Temperature Control

In addition to the adverse effects of hypothermia (<35°C) on coagulation, cardiac, respiratory, and neurologic function, hypothermia triggers a whole-body thermoregulatory vasoconstriction response. Consequently, it reduces cutaneous flow and can result in tissue hypoxia and failure of the humoral immune defense system.[114–116] Hypothermia is associated with a threefold increase in the incidence of surgical site infection.[117]

Nasogastric Tubes

Regular use of nasogastric tubes following major intraabdominal surgery is for gastric decompression, thereby preventing anastomotic leakage and promoting early return of bowel function. However, routine use has been questioned as it is very uncomfortable for the patient and there is an associated risk of developing pulmonary complications, delays in the return of bowel function, and increasing the rate of wound infections.[118] In addition, the presence of gastric tubes is associated with increased gastric secretion and motility—a physiologic response to the presence of a foreign body.

Bowel Preparation

Bowel preparation for major GI procedures has been implemented in order to reduce postoperative complications related to infected bowel content,[119] with polyethylene glycol a most popular preparation. Adverse physiologic effects of this bowel preparation include decreased exercise capacity, lower weight, increased plasma osmolality, decreased urea and phosphate, and reduced plasma calcium and potassium.[120] These effects along with fasting can produce a very unpleasant experience for the patient.

The routine use of bowel preparation has been questioned repeatedly. In fact, recent studies have shown that mechanical bowel preparation can be safely omitted before elective colorectal surgery.[121,122]

Drains

Intraabdominal drains are placed to prevent accumulations of intraabdominal collections, to quickly discover postoperative bleeding, to diagnose anastomotic leakage, and to drain intraabdominal abscesses. However, routine use of drains simply placed prophylactically after major abdominal surgeries has recently been questioned. These drains are not innocuous as they can be associated with bacterial contamination, wound infection, incisional hernia, intestinal obstruction and fistula formation, and bleeding.[123] There is insufficient evidence to support the notion that routine use of drainage after colorectal anastomoses can prevent anastomotic leakage or any other related complications.[124]

Fluid Management

All patients having elective surgery undergo a preoperative starvation period that results in a fluid deficit. Typically, it is not enough to produce major fluid shifts, but it may stimulate the production of antidiuretic hormone, atrial natriuretic peptide, the renin-angiotensin-aldosterone system, and an increase in sympathetic activity. This relative hypovolemia is also more pronounced in patients who receive bowel preparation, experience diarrhea or vomiting, are exposed to high temperatures, or have high nasogastric tube output.

Recent NPO guidelines allow patients to have clear fluids up to 2 hours prior to surgery.[125] Intraoperative fluid management takes into account the preoperative fluid deficit, the presence of a regional anesthesia technique, hemorrhage, and third-space losses. However, prudent administration of intravenous fluids is necessary as free and rapid administration of salt and water will increase capillary hydrostatic pressure, cause tissue and bowel edema, and adversely affect anastomotic integrity. Optimizing fluid administration should focus on increasing tissue perfusion and oxygen delivery, and modulation of the hormonal and inflammatory response.[126]

Mobilization and Early Ambulation

Early postoperative ambulation is recommended for prevention and treatment of postoperative ileus.[127,128] It is believed that early ambulation helps with the restoration of normal bowel function. However, studies demonstrate that GI myoelectrical activity patterns are not always expedited by early postoperative ambulation; at least there is no correlation with the extent of ambulation.[129] Yet, early ambulation confers many other advantages, specifically prevention of postoperative thromboembolism and pulmonary complications.[130,131]

Acknowledgment

The editors and publisher would like to thank Drs. Matthias F. Stopfkuchen-Evans and Simon Gelman for contributing a chapter on this topic in the prior edition of this work. It has served as the foundation for the current chapter.

Complete references available online at expertconsult.com.

References

1. Agur A, et al. *Grant's Atlas of Anatomy*. Baltimore: Lippincott Williams & Wilkins; 2005.
2. Andreoli TE, Carpenter CCJ, Cecil RL. *Andreoli and Carpenter's Cecil Essentials of Medicine*. Philadelphia: Saunders; 2007. Print.
3. Quiqley EM, et al. *Braz J Med Biol Res*. 1998;31:889–900.
4. Seok JW. *J Neurogastroenterol Motil*. 2011;17(2):189–191.
5. Patcharatrakul T, Gonlachanvit S. *J Neurogastroenterol Motil*. 2013;19(3):395–404.
6. Sarna SK. *Colonic Motility: From Bench to Bedside*. San Rafael: Morgan & Claypool Life Sciences; 2010.
7. Thompson W, et al. *Gut*. 1999;45(suppl 2):1143–1147.
8. Castedal M, et al. *Aliment Pharmacol Ther*. 2000;14(5):571–577.
9. Weiskopf RB, et al. *Anesthesiology*. 1994;80(5):1035–1045.
10. Hopster K, et al. *Vet J*. 2015;205(1):62–68.
11. Muller M, et al. *Anaesthesia*. 2002;57(2):110–115.
12. Desmet M, et al. *Acta Anaesthesiologica Scandinavica*. 2016.
13. Jensen AG, et al. *Can J Anaesth*. 1992;39(9):938–943.

14. Tylman M, et al. *Minerva Anestesiol.* 2011;77:275–282.
15. Lee TL, et al. *Anesthesia & Analgesia.* 1999;89(5):1246–1249.
16. Leslie K, et al. *Anesth Analg.* 2011;112(2):387–393.
17. Patel S, et al. *J Anaesthesiol Clin Pharmacol.* 2012;28(2):162–171.
18. Woerlee GM. *Common Perioperative Problems and the Anaesthetist. Developments in Critical Care Medicine and Anaesthesiology.* Vol. 18. Springer Netherlands; 1988.
19. Galligan J, Akbarali H. *Am J Gastroenterol Suppl.* 2014;2(1):17–21.
20. Leppert W. *Contem Oncol (Pozn).* 2012;16(2):125–131.
21. Tassinari D, et al. *J Palliat Med.* 2008;11:492–502.
22. Yuan CS, et al. *Clin Pharmacol Ther.* 1997;61: 467–475.
23. McNicol E, et al. *Pain Med.* 2008;9:634–659.
24. McNicol E, et al. *Cochrane Database Syst Rev.* 2008;(2):CD006332.
25. Keller D, Stein SL. *Clin Colon Rectal Surg.* 2013;26(3):186–190.
26. Delaney C, et al. In: Bosker G, ed. *Clinical Consensus Update in General Surgery.* Roswell(GA): Pharmatecture, LLC; 2006.
27. Kumar C, Bellamy M. *Gastrointestinal and Colorectal Anesthesia.* New York: Taylor & Francis; 2006. Print.
28. Zeinali F, et al. *Can J Surg.* 2009;52:153–157.
29. Holzheimer RG, et al., eds. *Surgical Treatment: Evidence-Based and Problem-Oriented.* Munich: Zuckschwerdt; 2001.
30. Jeejeebhoy KN. *CMAJ.* 2002;166(10):1297–1302.
31. McSwiney BA. *Annu Rev Physiol.* 1944;(6):365–390.
32. Cervero F. *Physiol Rev. Jan.* 1994;74(1):95–138.
33. Scratchered T, Grundy D. *Br. J Anesth.* 1984;56:3–18.
34. Procacci P, et al. *Prog Brain Res.* 1986;67:21–28.
35. Paintal AS. *Prog Brain Res.* 1986;67:3–19.
36. Jänig W, Morrison JFB. *Prog Brain Res.* 1986;67:78–114.
37. Kuntz A. *The Autonomic Nervous System.* Philadelphia: Lea & Febiger; 1953.
38. Bornica JJ. *Anesthesiology.* 1968;29:793–813.
39. Gebhart GF. *Gut.* 2000;47(suppl 4):iv54–iv55; discussion iv8. PMID 11076915.
40. Altschuler SM, et al. *J Comp Neurol.* 1989;283(2):248–268.
41. Sengupta JN, Gebhart GF. Mechanosensitive afferent fibres in the gastrointestinal and lower urinary tracts. In: Gebhart GF, ed. *Visceral Pain.* Seattle: IASP Press; 1995:75–98.
42. Langley JN. *Brain.* 1903;(26):1–16.
43. Michell GAC. *Anatomy of the Autonomous Nervous System.* Livingstone: Edinburgh; 1953.
44. Sengupta JN, Gebhart GF. *J Neurophysiol.* 1994;71(6):2046–2060.
45. Al-Chaer ED, Traub RJ. *Pain.* 2002;96(3):221–225.
46. Renck H. Management of abdomino-visceral pain by nerve block techniques. *H Mediglobe.* 1992.
47. Sikandar S, Dickenson AH. *Curr Opin Support Palliat Care.* 2012;6(1):17–26.
48. Fields HL, Liebeskind JC. *Pharmacological Approaches to the Treatment of Chronic Pain: New Concepts and Critical Issues.* Seattle: 1994:11–30.
49. Procacci P, Zoppi M, Maresca M. Visceral sensation. In: Cervero F, Morrison JFB, eds. *Progress in Pain Research.* Amsterdam: Elsevier; 1986;39:21–28.
50. Hardy JD, et al. *J Clin Invest.* 1950;29(1):115–140.
51. Gebhart GF. *Visceral Pain, Progress in Pain Research and Management.* Seattle: IASP Press; 1995:3–23.
52. Mayer EA. *Am J Med.* 1999;107(5A). 12S–9S.
53. Van Oudenhove L, et al. *J Clin Invest.* 2011;121(8):3094–3099.
54. Mayer EA. *Nat Rev Neurosci.* 2011;12(8):453–466.
55. Chu LF, et al. *Clin J Pain.* 2008;24(6):479–496.
56. Castro-Lopes J, Raja SN, Schmelz M. *Pain 2008 Refresher Course Syllabus.* Seattle: IASP Press; 2008:381–389.
57. Boddy AP, et al. *Anesth Analg.* 2006;103(3):682–688.
58. Lillemoe KD, et al. *Ann Surg.* 1993;217:447–457.
59. Puli SR, et al. *Dig Dis Sci.* 2009;54(11):2330–2337.
60. Rana MV, et al. *Curr Pain Headache Rep.* 2014;18(2):394.
61. Liu SS, et al. *Anesthesiology.* 1995;83(4):757–765.
62. Leslie JB, et al. *Adv Prev Med.* 2011:1–10.
63. Yukioka H, et al. *Br J Anaesth.* 1987;59:581–584.
64. Wilder-Smith CH, et al. *Anesthesiology.* 1999;91:639–647.
65. Ingram DM, Sheiner HJ. *Br J Surg.* 1981;68:572–576.
66. Nimmo WS, et al. *Br J Clin Pharm.* 1975;2:509–513.
67. Desborough JP. *Br J Anaesth.* 2000;85(1):109–117.
68. Guha A, et al. *Eur J Anaesthesiol.* 2002;19(09):652.
69. Boeckxstaens GE, de Jonge WJ. *Gut.* 2009;58:1300.
70. Desborough JP. *Br J Anaesth.* 2000;85(1):109–117.
71. Kehlet H. *Br J Anaesth.* 1989;63:189–195.
72. Carli F, et al. *Br J Anaesth.* 1991;67:729–734.
73. Kouraklis G, et al. *Int Surg.* 2000;85:353–357.
74. Liu S, et al. *Anesthesiology.* 1995;82(6):1474–1506.
75. Holte K, Kehlet H. *Br J Surg.* 2000;87(11):1480–1493.
76. Shi WZ, et al. *Acta Anaesthesiol Scand.* 2014;58(8):923–932.
77. Steinbrook RA. *Anesth Analg.* 1998;86(4):837–844.
78. Guay J, et al. *Anesth Analg.* 2016;123(6):1591–1602.
79. Steinbrook RA. *Anesth Analg.* 1998;86:837–844.
80. Carpenter RL. *Reg Anesth.* 1996;21:13–17.
81. Michelet P, et al. *Chest.* 2005;128(5):3461–3466.
82. Jorgensen H, et al. *Cochrane Database Syst Rev.* 2000;4:CD001893.
83. Holte K, Kehlet H. *Reg Anesth Pain Med.* 2001;26:111–117.
84. Schnitzler M, et al. *Reg Anesth.* 1992;17:143–147.
85. Ryan P, et al. *Eur J Surg.* 1992;158:45–49.
86. Holte K, Kehlet H. *Clin Nutr.* 2002;21(3):199–206.
87. Lewis KS, et al. *Am J Hosp Pharm.* 1994;51(12):1539–1554.
88. Watcha MF, White PF. *Anesthesiology.* 1992;77(1):162–184.
89. Carpenter RL, et al. *Anesthesiology.* 1992;76(6):906–916.
90. Freise H, Fischer LG. *Curr Opin Anaesthesiol.* 2009;22(5):644–648.
91. Clemente A, Carli F. *Minerva Anestesiol.* 2008;74(10):549–563.
92. Stanton-Hicks M, et al. *Anesthesiology.* 1987;66(3):317–322.
93. Holte K, et al. *Anesthesiology.* 2004;100(2):281–286.
94. Ljungqvist O. *JPEN J Parenter Enteral Nutr.* 2014;38(5):559–566.
95. Varadhan KK, et al. *Clin Nutr.* 2010;29(4):434–440.
96. Ljungqvist O, et al. *JAMA Surg.* 2017;152(3):292–298.
97. Nygren J, et al. *Current Opinion in Clinical Nutrition and Metabolic Care.* 2003;6:593–597.
98. Pöpping DM, et al. *Ann Surg.* 2014;259(6):1056–1067.
99. Hughes MJ, et al. *JAMA Surg.* 2014;149(12):1224–12230.
100. Khan SA, et al. *Surg Endosc.* 2013;27(7):2581–2591.
101. Popping DM, et al. *Arch Surg.* 2008;143:990–999; discussion 1000.
102. Popping DM, et al. *Ann Surg.* 2014;259:1056–1067.
103. Soop M, et al. *Br J Surg.* 2004;91(9):1138–1145.
104. Wildhaber BE, et al. *J Surg Res.* 2005;123(1):8–16.
105. Mosenthal AC, et al. *Crit Care Med.* 2002;30(2):396–402.
106. Wang ZG, et al. *Br J Surg.* 2010;97:317–327.
107. Yuill KA, et al. *Clin Nutr.* 2005;24:32–37.
108. Bardram L, et al. *Lancet.* 1995;345(8952):763–764.
109. Smith MD, et al. *Cochrane Database Syst Rev.* 2014;8:CD009161.
110. American Society of Anesthesiologists Committee. *Anesthesiology.* 2011;114:495–511.
111. Soreide E, et al. *Acta Anaesthesiol Scand.* 2005;49:1041–1047.
112. Spies CD, et al. *Anaesthesist.* 2003;52:1039–4.
113. Soop M, et al. *Br J Surg.* 2004;91:1138–1145.
114. Hart SR, et al. *Ochsner J.* 2011;11(3):259–270.
115. van Oss CJ, et al. *J Reticuloendothel Soc.* 1980;27(6):561–565. PubMed.
116. Sheffield CW, et al. *Wound Repair Regen.* 1996;4(3):339–345.
117. Kurz A, et al. *N Engl J Med.* 1996;334(19):1209–1215.
118. Nelson R, et al. *Br J Surg.* 2005;92(6):673–680.
119. Nichols RL, Condon RE. *Surg Gynecol Obstet.* 1971;132(2):323–337.
120. Bucher P, et al. *Dis Colon Rectum.* 2004;47(8):1397–1402.
121. Slim K, et al. *Gastroenterol Clin Biol.* 2002;26:667–669. 8–9.
122. Guenaga KF, et al. *Cochrane Database Syst Rev.* 2005;1:CD001544.
123. Jesus EC, et al. *Cochrane Database Syst Rev.* 2004;4:CD002100.
124. Merad F, et al. *Surgery.* 1999;125(5):529–535.
125. Practice guidelines for preoperative fasting and the use of pharmacologic agents to reduce the risk of pulmonary aspiration: application to healthy patients undergoing elective procedures an updated report by the American Society of Anesthesiologists Task Force on Preoperative Fasting and the Use of Pharmacologic Agents to Reduce the Risk of Pulmonary Aspiration. *Anesthesiology.* 2017;126 (3):376–393.
126. Scott MJ, et al. *Acta Anaesthesiol Scand.* 2015;59(10):1212–1231.
127. Story SK. *Chamberlain RS Dig Surg.* 2009;26(4):265–275.
128. Brieger GH. *Ann Surg.* 1983;197:443–449.
129. Waldhausen JH, Schirmer BD. *Ann Surg.* 1990;212(6):671–677.
130. Wenger NK. *Cardiovascular Clinics.* 1978;9(3):107–115.
131. Parker HG, et al. *Surg Clin N Am.* 1976;56(3):667–672.

16 Hepatic Physiology, Pathophysiology, and Anesthetic Considerations

DOLORES B. NJOKU, HOVIG V. CHITILIAN, and KATE KRONISH

KEY POINTS

- The liver is the largest abdominal organ and carries out a number of vital functions including metabolism and detoxification.
- The liver receives approximately 25% of the resting cardiac output. The hepatic artery is responsible for 25% to 30% of the blood supply to the liver while the portal vein is responsible for 70% to 75%. They each deliver 50% of the total oxygen to the liver.
- For the purpose of hepatic resection, the liver can be divided into eight segments based on independent blood supply and drainage of blood and bile. A segment can be resected without compromising the blood flow and biliary drainage of other segments.
- The acinus is the basic functional unit of the liver. It is organized around the flow of blood from the portal triad to the central vein through the sinusoids. Hepatocytes in the acinus are organized into zones based on their proximity to the portal triad or central vein. Zone 1 or periportal hepatocytes are closer to the portal triads and receive oxygen and nutrient-rich blood. Zone 3 or perivenous hepatocytes are closer to the central veins and receive oxygen-poor blood. Hepatocytes in different zones serve different anatomic functions.
- The liver plays an integral role in carbohydrate, protein, lipid, and bile metabolism. It is also responsible for protein synthesis. Albumin is the most abundant plasma protein produced by the liver.
- Drug and toxin excretion is carried out by the hepatocytes by first polarizing the molecules then conjugating them to make them more hydrophilic. Drugs excreted in the bile may be reabsorbed through enterohepatic circulation leading to prolonged effects.
- Standard laboratory panels used to evaluate the hepatobiliary system help define broad categories of hepatobiliary pathology: hepatitis, hepatobiliary dysfunction, or insufficient protein synthesis. Specific diagnoses often require clinical context and radiologic studies.
- Cirrhosis is the result of chronic hepatic disease and can ultimately result in portal hypertension and liver failure. Liver failure can lead to significant dysfunction in all organ systems, giving rise to coagulopathy, thrombocytopenia, hyperdynamic circulation, esophageal varices, hepatic encephalopathy, hepatopulmonary syndrome, portopulmonary hypertension, and hepatorenal syndrome. The definitive treatment for hepatic failure is liver transplantation.
- Volatile anesthetics reduce mean arterial pressure and cardiac output, leading to a reduction in portal blood flow in a dose-dependent manner. The hepatic arterial buffer response is preserved with isoflurane, sevoflurane, and desflurane leading to the preservation total hepatic blood flow, but not with halothane.
- Advanced liver disease impairs the elimination of many drugs including vecuronium, rocuronium, morphine, meperidine, and benzodiazepines. Dosing should be adjusted in the setting of liver failure.
- Elective surgery is contraindicated in patients with acute hepatitis or liver failure. Patients with chronic hepatitis can safely undergo elective surgery. Hepatotoxic drugs should be avoided and hepatic perfusion maintained. Child-Turcotte-Pugh class and Model for End-Stage Liver Disease score can be used to predict risk of perioperative mortality.

Anatomy of the Liver

The liver is the second largest organ in the human body and is responsible for a host of functions to maintain homeostasis. The liver acts as the interface between the gastrointestinal tract and remainder of the body. It is responsible for metabolic, synthetic, immunologic, and hemodynamic functions. As a result, hepatic dysfunction has profound effects on all organ systems and introduces significant challenges to anesthetic management. It is therefore essential for the anesthesiologist to have a firm grasp of the anatomy, physiology, and pathophysiology of the liver.

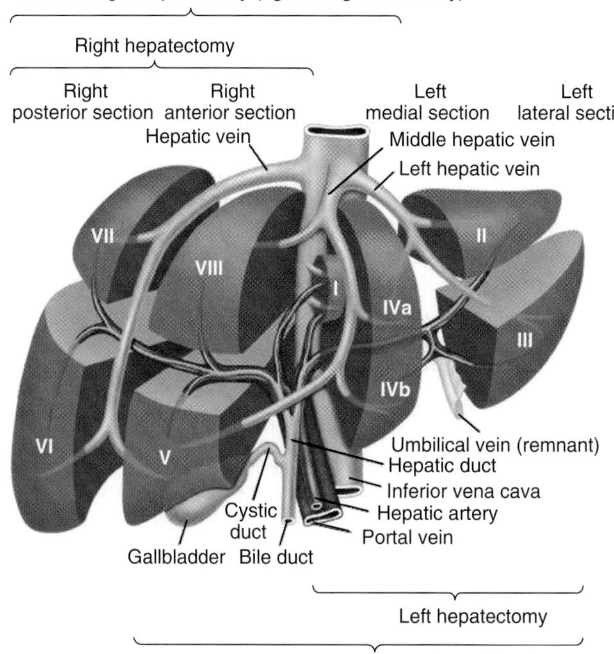

Fig. 16.1 Schematic depiction of Couinaud segmental liver anatomy and the normal portal venous structures. Bracketed text shows hepatic segments resected during partial hepatectomies. (Modified from Venook AP, Curley SA. Management of potentially resectable colorectal cancer liver metastases. http://www.uptodate.com/contents/management-of-potentially-resectable-colorectal-cancer-liver-metastases.)

SURGICAL ANATOMY, HEPATIC BLOOD FLOW, AND THE BILIARY TREE

The adult liver can range from around 600 to over 1800 g making the liver one of the heaviest organs in the body. In healthy females the liver ranges in size from 603 to 1767 g,[1] while in healthy males, the liver ranges in size from 968 to 1860 g.[2] In newborns, infants, and children, the liver is also one of the largest organs and the contribution of its weight to total body weight decreases with age. Thus the liver in a term 3 to 3.5 kg newborn can weigh 150 to 170 g,[3] which represents around 5% of the total body weight. In sharp contrast the adult liver represents 2% to 2.5% of the total body weight.

The liver receives approximately 25% of the resting cardiac output (CO).[4] The blood supply is through both the arterial and venous systems in the form of the hepatic artery and the portal vein (Fig. 16.1). The hepatic artery is responsible for 25% to 30% of the blood supply to the liver whereas the portal vein is responsible for 70% to 75%. The hepatic artery arises from the celiac trunk in 80% of the population. In the remainder, it arises from the superior mesenteric artery. After giving rise to the gastroduodenal artery, the common hepatic artery enters the hilum of the liver (porta hepatis) where it further branches into the right and left hepatic arteries, supplying the right and left sides of the liver, respectively. The right hepatic artery gives rise to the cystic artery that supplies the gallbladder.[4] The arteries continue to branch throughout the liver ultimately running through the portal tracts and terminating in the hepatic sinusoids (capillaries). Although part of the venous system, the portal vein is the primary source of oxygenated blood to the liver. The portal vein carries blood from the gastrointestinal tract, pancreas, and spleen to the liver. It drains the superior mesenteric, splenic, and inferior mesenteric veins. It also drains the gastric, cystic, and pancreaticoduodenal veins. The portal vein enters the hilum and, like the hepatic artery, branches into the right and left portal veins, supplying the respective sides of the liver.[4] The portal veins continue to branch throughout the liver in conjunction with the hepatic arteries. As with the arteries, they terminate in the hepatic sinusoids.

Venous drainage of the liver is through the hepatic veins directly into the inferior vena cava (IVC). The right and middle hepatic veins serve the right half and middle portions of the liver, respectively, while the left hepatic vein drains the left half of the liver. The biliary system removes bile from the liver and delivers it to the duodenum through the ampulla of Vater. The intrahepatic bile ducts typically travel with the portal veins, draining into right and left collections systems that ultimately form the common bile duct (CBD; see Fig. 16.1).[4]

From a historical perspective, the description of the gross anatomy of the liver has evolved from being rooted in the surface anatomy of the organ to its functional organization. Traditionally, the liver was divided into four lobes based on its surface features: right lobe, left lobe, quadrate, and caudate. The right and left lobes were divided by the falciform ligament, when viewed anteriorly. When viewed from below, the quadrate lobe was bounded by the porta hepatis posteriorly, the gallbladder fossa on the right, and the ligamentum teres on the left.[4] The caudate lobe was bounded by the porta hepatis anteriorly, the IVC on the right, and the ligamentum venosum fissure on the left. In the late 1800s, Sir James Cantlie demonstrated that the right and left hemilivers were defined by independent portal circulations and thus the functional midline of the liver was at the bifurcation of the portal vein, along a line connecting the gallbladder bed and the IVC ("Cantlie's line"), lateral to the falciform ligament. Cantlie recognized that the line defined a vascular watershed and described its implications for surgical resection of the liver.[5] With advances in hepatic surgery, anatomic descriptions of the liver were developed that further divided the hemilivers into segments based on the vascular distribution and biliary drainage. Each segment has its own independent vascular inflow and outflow, and biliary drainage. As a result, surgical resection of a segment does not compromise adjacent segments. The most commonly used organizational system was developed by Couinaud (see Fig. 16.1).[6] In the Couinaud model, the liver is divided into eight segments. The right and left hemilivers are divided at the bifurcation of the portal vein, along the middle hepatic vein. The right, middle, and left hepatic veins divide the liver vertically into four sectors: right posterior, right anterior, left medial, and left lateral sectors. The four sectors are divided in the horizontal plane by the branches of the portal vein, giving rise to the eight segments. In this system, the caudate lobe is referred to as segment 1 and the remainder of the segments are numbered in a clockwise fashion. Segments 2 and 3 are medial to the left hepatic vein, with segment 2 superior to segment 3. Segment 4 lies between the middle and left hepatic vein and is subdivided into 4a (superior) and 4b (inferior) subsegments. Segments 8 (superior) and 5 (inferior) are located between

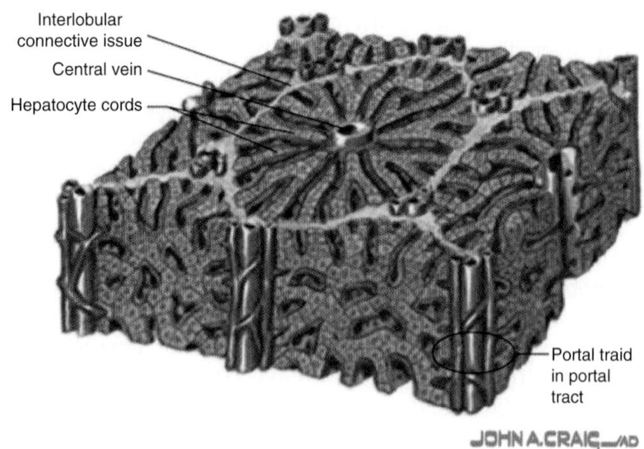

Fig. 16.2 Hepatic lobule. Liver arranged as a series of hexagonal lobules, each composed of a series of hepatocyte cords (plates) interspersed with sinusoids. Each lobule surrounds a central vein and is bounded by six peripheral portal triads (low magnification).

the middle and right hepatic veins. Segments 6 (inferior) and 7 (superior) are located between the right hepatic vein and the edge of the liver.[6] In clinical practice, contrast-enhanced computed tomography (CT) scanning and intraoperative ultrasound are used to define the anatomy unique to each individual and plan for the appropriate resection. To standardize the nomenclature used to describe hepatic resections, the International Hepatopancreatobiliary Association published consensus terminology in 2000 based on the Couinaud segments, known as the Brisbane 2000 terminology.[7] This system of terminology has gained traction but has not yet been uniformly adopted.[8,9]

CELLULAR ANATOMY

Liver Lobule and Acinus

The cellular architecture of the liver supports its functions of detoxifying the blood and metabolizing nutrients. Histologically, the liver parenchyma can be organized into anatomic units (liver lobules) or functional units (liver acinus). The liver lobule is the basic structural unit of the hepatic parenchyma (Fig. 16.2). The lobule typically appears hexagonal in shape with a portal canal at each corner and a hepatic venule (central vein) located in the center. Through each portal canal run the lymphatics, nerve fibers, and a portal triad. Each portal triad consists of a bile ductule, hepatic arteriole, and portal venule. From a functional standpoint, the acinus is the smallest unit of the liver (Fig. 16.3A). It is comprised of a portal tract at the center with central vein at the periphery. Oxygenated and nutrient-rich blood flows from the portal triads to the central hepatic veins through the hepatic sinusoids (see Fig. 16.3B). The walls of the sinusoids are composed of sinusoidal endothelial cells (SECs) that are separated by fenestrations of 50 to 150 nm in diameter. The fenestrations allow the passage of metabolites, plasma proteins, pharmaceutical molecules, lipoproteins, and other solutes into the space of Disse (SD) surrounding the sinusoids while retaining blood cells in the vessels. Larger macromolecules and potentially immunogenic peptides enter the SD by transcytosis through the SECs.[10] Once in the SD, the molecules are taken up by hepatocytes.

Hepatocytes

Hepatocytes make up 75% to 80% of the total cellular volume of the liver.[11] They are responsible for drug, protein, carbohydrate, lipid, and heme metabolism in addition to the synthesis of a variety of proteins necessary for the maintenance of homeostasis at baseline and in response to acute insults secondary to ischemia-reperfusion, viral and bacterial infections, and toxins. Hepatocytes are polarized with heterogenous plasma membranes to facilitate their varied functions. The basolateral (sinusoidal) portion of the membrane is in direct contact with the SD while the apical portion of the membrane makes up the bile canaliculus that drains bile to the ductules.[12] Hepatocytes are divided into different zones based on their proximity to the portal triad. Zone 1 is periportal, zone 3 is around the central vein (perivenous or pericentral), and zone 2 is in between (midzone). Zone 3 hepatocytes are furthest away from the portal tracts and thus receive blood with a lower oxygen tension and nutrient content.[13] The metabolic functions of the hepatocytes differ based on the zone in which they are located (see Fig. 16.3C). This metabolic zonation increases the efficiency of carbohydrate, amino acid, lipid, and xenobiotic metabolism. Periportal (zone 1) hepatocytes are the major sites of aerobic metabolism, and process such as glycogen synthesis and sulfation whereas perivenous (zone 3) hepatocytes are the major sites of anaerobic metabolism, glycolysis, and glucuronidation. By virtue of their location, zone 3 hepatocytes are most sensitive to hypoxia.[13]

Hepatic Stellate Cells

Hepatic stellate cells (HSCs) make up 8% to 10% of all resident liver cells.[14] These specialized cells reside in the SD between liver sinusoidal endothelial cells (LSECs) and the hepatocytes. In the normal liver, HSCs are believed to be in a quiescent state. In the setting of liver injury, these cells become activated in response to cytokines and chemokines generated by hepatocytes, LSECs, as well as leukocytes and Kupffer cells. The stellate cells proliferate and differentiate into myofibroblasts participating in hepatic inflammation and fibrosis.[15]

MYELOID CELLS

The myeloid cells that can be found in the liver consist primarily of Kupffer cells (20%-30%) also known as resident tissue macrophages, in addition to dendritic cells and myeloid-derived suppressor cells. At first glance, it may seem that these cells have a less important role than hepatocytes and LSEC. However, while Kupffer cells constitute around 20% to 30% of nonparenchymal cells, they constitute 80% to 90% of all tissue macrophages.[16] Kupffer cells reside in the portal and lobular liver sinusoids where they engulf both infectious and noninfectious particles by phagocytosis. Once phagocytosed, these particles are unable to induce proinflammatory responses in the liver. Thus by prevalence and location, these cells serve critical roles in innate and adaptive immunity by detoxification where they down-regulate potentially proinflammatory triggers that could disrupt hepatic homeostasis.[17]

Dendritic cells and myeloid-derived suppressor cells are the least abundant of myeloid cells. Hepatic dendritic cells are present in the normal liver and reside in the portal area and are believed to promote tolerance to phagocytosed

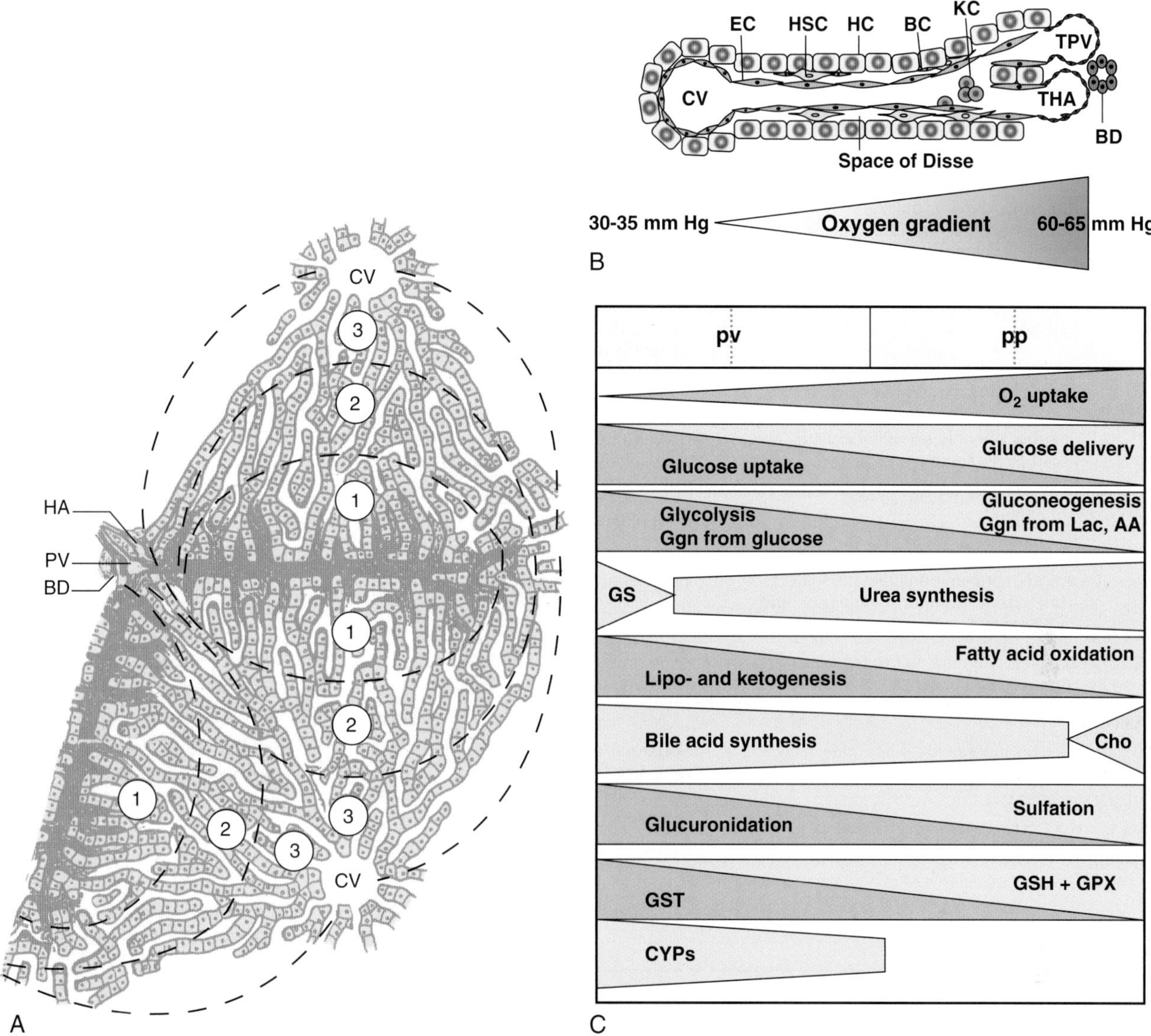

Fig. 16.3 (A) Blood supply of a liver acinus. Schematic representation of the acinus and hepatocyte zones. Hepatocytes can be divided into three zones based on their location along the sinusoid from the portal triad *(PT)* to the central vein *(CV)*. Zone 1—Periportal zone—hepatocytes are closest to the portal triad; Zone 3—perivenous, pericentral, or perilobular zone—hepatocytes are closest to the central vein. Zone 2 (intermediary) hepatocytes are in between. (B) Diagram of the sinusoid. The sinusoid is lined with sinusoidal epithelial cells *(EC)* separated by fenestrations that control the passage of solutes into the space of Disse. The space of Disse contains hepatic stellate cells *(HSC)* and is bound by the basolateral (sinusoidal) portion of the plasma membranes of the hepatocytes *(HC)*. The apical portion of the plasma membranes makes up the bile canaliculus *(BC)*. Oxygen and nutrient-rich blood flows from the terminal hepatic artery *(THA)* and portal vein *(TPV)* through the sinusoid to the central vein *(CV)*. There is an oxygen gradient along the length of the sinusoid. Kupffer cells *(KC)* are resident hepatic macrophages and found in the sinusoids. (C) Hepatocyte zonation. The major metabolic pathways in the hepatocytes along the sinusoid differ based on their proximity to the portal triad or the central vein. Predominant metabolic pathways are listed for the periportal *(pp)* hepatocytes and the perivenous *(pv)* hepatocytes. *AA,* Amino acid; *Cho,* cholesterol synthesis; *CYPs,* cytochrome P450 enzymes; *Ggn,* glycogen; *GPX,* glutathione peroxidase; *GS,* glutamine synthesis; *GST,* glutathione transferase; *Lac,* lactate. ([B and C] From Kietzmann T. Metabolic zonation of the liver: the oxygen gradient revisited. *Redox Biol.* 2017;11:622–630.)

particles.[18] Hepatic myeloid-derived supressor cells suppress immune response in the liver. In acute hepatitis they reduce inflammation and limit tissue injury. Their immune suppressive function has been associated with adverse effects in certain pathologic conditions. In chronic viral hepatitis, they may promote viral persistence. They have also been associated with suppression of immune response to hepatic tumors.[17]

LYMPHOCYTES

Cells of lymphatic origin that can be detected in the liver include natural killer (NK) cells, NK T cells (NKT), mucosal-associated invariant T cells, and γδ T cells in addition to major histocompatibility restricted CD4+ T cells, CD8+T cells, and B cells. These cells are distributed throughout the liver parenchyma and serve critical roles in the innate (NK, NKT, mucosal-associated invariant T cells, and γδ T cells) and adaptive (major histocompatibility restricted CD4+ T cells, CD8+T cells, and B cells) immune responses. These cells work primarily to maintain hepatic homeostasis by promoting tolerance to foreign substances. However, when necessary, these MHC-restricted cells can promote the clearance of foreign substances by expanding in response to them while recruiting additional cells from extrahepatic sources such as the lymph nodes and the spleen.[17]

TABLE 16.1 List of Well-Known Substrates, Inhibitors, and Inducers for Phase I, II, and III Metabolism Pathways

Enzymes	Substrates	Inhibitors	Inducers
PHASE I			
CYP3A	Midazolam, buspirone, felodipine, lovastatin, eletriptan, sildenafil, simvastatin, triazolam	Ketoconazole, clarithromycin, itraconazole, saquinavir, fluconazole, grapefruit juice, tipranavir/ritonavir	Phenytoin, rifampin, St. John's wort, efavirenz, etravirine, nafcillin, prednisone
1A2	Alosetron, caffeine, duloxetine, melatonin, ramelteon, tacrine, tizanidine	Ciprofloxacin, enoxacin, fluvoxamine, oral contraceptives, phenylpropanolamine,	Montelukast, phenytoin, smoking components of cigarettes
2C8	Repaglinide, paclitaxel	Gemfibrozil, fluvoxamine, ketoconazole, trimethoprim	Rifampin
2C9	Celecoxib, warfarin, phenytoin	Amiodarone, fluconazole, miconazole, oxandrolone, capecitabine, etravirine, fluvastatin, metronidazole, sulfinpyrazone, tigecycline	Carbamazepine, rifampin, aprepitant, bosentan, phenobarbital, St. John's wort
PHASE II			
UGTs	Bilirubin, phenols, estradiols, opiates, and carboxylic acids	Paclitaxel, midazolam, cyclosporine A, ketoconazole, phenobarbital, and phenytoin	Bilirubin, phenobarbitone, rifampin
SULTs	Phenols, alcohols, and amines	Flavonoids, mefenamic acids, salicylic acids, clomiphene, and danazol	Retinoic acid, methotrexate
NATs	Para-aminobenzoic acid, para-aminosalicylic acids, para-aminoglutamate, sulfamethazine, isoniazid, hydralazine, and sulfonamides	Caffeic acid, esculetin, quercetin, genistein, scopoletin, and coumarin	Androgens, aminophylline
GSTs	Epoxides, quinone, sulfoxides, esters, and peroxides	Phenols, quinone, vitamin C derivatives, dopamine, and *trans*retinoic acid	Extracts of broccoli, cabbage, Brussels sprouts, and grapefruit
PHASE III			
P-gp	Digoxin, loperamide, vinblastine, talinolol	Amiodarone, azithromycin, cyclosporine, diltiazem, dronedarone, erythromycin, itraconazole, ketoconazole, lopinavir/ritonavir, quinidine, verapamil	Avasimibe, carbamazepine, phenytoin, rifampin, St John's wort, tipranavir/ritonavir

From Almazroo OA, Miah MK, Venkataramanan R. Drug metabolism in the liver. *Clin Liver Dis.* 2017;21:1–20. Elsevier.

Hepatic Physiology

DRUG METABOLISM

The vast majority of drugs used in the conduct of anesthesia are metabolized in the liver. A variety of enzymes convert drug molecules into more water-soluble (hydrophilic) molecules or compounds to facilitate their excretion. These enzymes are designated as being either part of the Phase I pathway or Phase II pathway based on the types of reactions they mediate. Phase I enzymes consist of the cytochrome P450 family of enzymes that convert lipophilic drug molecules to hydrophilic molecules primarily through oxidation, reduction, or hydrolysis. Non-CYP450 enzymes include monoamine oxidases, alcohol dehydrogenases, and aldo-keto reductase. The phase II pathway consists of the conjugation of the products of the phase I pathway with hydrophilic endogenous moieties to make them more water-soluble. Polar molecules may undergo Phase II metabolism without having undergone Phase I metabolism. The most common Phase II reaction is glucuronidation, which is the conjugation of the drug compound to glucuronic acid. This reaction is carried out by a family of enzymes known as uridine 5′-diphospho-glucuronosyltransferases. Other Phase II enzymes include sulfotransferases (SULT), glutathione S-transferases (GST), and catechol O-methyltransferases.[19] The phase III pathway involves the excretion of compounds into the sinusoids or canalicular bile by molecular transporters that are transmembrane proteins which facilitate the movement of large or ionized molecules across cell membranes. The majority of these transmembrane proteins are part of a superfamily of ATP-binding cassette (ABC) transporters that use ATP to actively transport molecules. Common ABC-transporters include multidrug resistance protein (MDR), cystic fibrosis transmembrane conductance regulator, and multidrug resistance–related protein (MRP).

Some orally administered medications undergo extensive metabolism in the gut or liver prior to entering the systemic circulation. This metabolism is termed the first-pass effect and is responsible for the lower oral bioavailability of these medications.[20]

Drug metabolism is affected by a number of factors including genetic polymorphisms of metabolic enzymes, age, gender, pregnancy, liver disease, and concomitantly administered medications. The expression and function of Phase I and Phase II enzymes are reduced in neonates. The activities of some CYP450 enzymes are increased in women compared to men. Genetic polymorphisms in drug metabolizing enzymes and transporters can lead to wide variations in the pharmacokinetics of some drugs such as warfarin, with some patients having lower rates of metabolism based on the specific CYP450 polymorphism they carry. The concomitant administration of medications may also influence drug metabolism. A number of commonly encountered medications can serve as inducers or inhibitors of the enzymes involved in the different phases of drug metabolism.[20] Table 16.1 lists some of the commonly used drugs, which are metabolized and excreted by each of the three phases along with drugs that may serve as inhibitors or inducers for each phase.

See the pharmacokinetics chapter for further discussion of hepatic extraction ratio.

PROTEIN METABOLISM

The liver is responsible for the synthesis and catabolism of proteins, amino acids, and peptides. It is the site of synthesis for 80% to 90% of the circulating proteins including hormones, coagulant factors, cytokines, and chemokines. As such it plays a significant role in the functioning of the body. Albumin is the predominant protein produced by the liver, accounting for over 50% of total plasma protein. It functions to transport lipids and hormones and maintain blood volume. The liver plays a central role in protein degradation. Amino acids are catabolized through one of two reactions: deamination or transamination. Both reactions lead to the production of ammonia, which the liver converts to urea through the urea cycle. Urea is then excreted by the kidneys in the urine.[21]

CARBOHYDRATE METABOLISM

The liver is primarily responsible for storing and releasing glucose to meet the body's needs. In the postprandial state, the liver stores glucose through glycogenesis. Once the glycogen stores are complete, the liver converts excess glucose into fat through lipogenesis. In the fasting state, the liver provides the body with glucose by breaking down glycogen (glycogenolysis) or by generating glucose from carbohydrate precursors (gluconeogenesis).[22]

LIPID METABOLISM

The liver plays an important role in lipid metabolism. Nonesterified fatty acids can arise from the lipase-mediated breakdown of complex lipids, or from thioesterase-mediated hydrolysis of fatty acid-CoA.[23] These fatty acids can enter the liver following oral intake or they can enter the liver following the breakdown of adipose tissue. In the liver, fatty acid oxidation is regulated by two main factors: the supply of fatty acids to the liver (via lipolysis), and the amount of microsomal esterification that occurs.[23] Lipid metabolism is also influenced by the carbohydrate metabolism, as the acetyl-CoA formed during carbohydrate metabolism can be utilized to synthesize fatty acids. Fatty acids can undergo biotransformation to supply energy for the needs of the body. Alternatively, the liver can convert amino acids and intermediate products of carbohydrates into fats and transport them to the adipose tissues.

BOX 16.1 Drugs, Foreign Chemicals, and Their Metabolites That Are Excreted in the Bile

Amiodarone[114]	Estrone[115]	Phenol red[113]
Ampicillin[113,116]	Ezetimibe[110]	Phenolphthalein[117]
Benzylpenicillin[118]	2-Fluoro-β-alanine[119]	Phenytoin[117]
Bilirubin[120]	Gentamycin[118]	Pivampicillin[118]
Bromocresol green[121]	Glibenclamide (glyburide)[5]	Rifamide[113]
Bromosulfophthalein[122]	Gliclazide[123]	Rifamycin[113]
Cefixime[124]	Imipramine[125]	Roquinimex[126]
Ceftriaxone[127]	Indocyanine green[122]	Rose bengal[121]
Cefatzidime[128]	Indomethacin[125]	Spironolactone[125]
Cephaloridine[113]	Irinotecan[129]	Sulfamethoxazole[113]
Cephamandole[118]	Lanatoside C[118]	Sulindac[125]
Cephazolin[118]	Lorazepam[130]	Sulbactam[116]
Chenodeoxycholic acid[122,125]	Lomnetazepam[6]	Temafloxacin[131]
Chloramphenicol[118]	Methotrexate[113]	Testosterone[125]
Chlortetracycline[118]	Metronidazole[117]	Tetracycline[113,118]
Clindamycin[117]	Mezlocillin[132]	Thiamphenicol[113]
Demethylchlortetracycline[118]	Morphine[133]	Tolfenamic acid[134]
Diazepam[113]	Mycophenolic acid[135]	Toremifene[136]
Digitoxin[113]	Mycophenolate mofetil[137,138]	Troglitazone[139]
Digoxin[113]	Nortriptyline[131]	Trovafloxacin[7]
Doxycycline[118]	Novobiocin[131]	Ursodeoxycholic acid[122,125]
Erythromycin[113]	Oltiprazl[140]	Valproic acid[125]
Estradiol[125]	Pethidine (meperidine)[113]	Warfarin[133]

Roberts MS, Magnusson BM, Bruczynski FJ. Enterohepatic circulation. *Clin Pharmacokinet.* 2002;41:751–790, Table II, page 767.

BILE AND ENTEROHEPATIC CIRCULATION

The adult liver produces approximately 400 to 600 mL of bile each day. Bile facilitates the excretion of toxins as well as the absorption of dietary fats. It is the mechanism of excretion for compounds with molecular weights greater than 300 to 500 Daltons that are not readily excreted by the kidneys. It is used to excrete a host of endogenous and exogenous compounds, including bile acids, bilirubin, phospholipids, cholesterol, drugs, toxins, steroid hormones, and water-insoluble porphyrins. Box 16.1 lists drugs, chemicals, and their metabolites that are excreted in the bile. The other major function of bile is to assist in the digestion and absorption of dietary fats, cholesterol, and vitamins.[24] Bile is 95% water by volume, with the remainder consisting of bile acids, phospholipids, cholesterol, bilirubin, as well as other exogenous and endogenous substances. The two primary bile acids are cholic acid and chenodeoxycholic acid. Bile acids are synthesized by hepatocytes from cholesterol. They are then conjugated to reduce hepatotoxicity and increase solubility and secreted into the canaliculi. The canaliculi drain into the biliary ductules, which connect to form hepatic ducts. The walls of the intrahepatic bile ducts are made up of cholangiocytes that modify the volume and composition of the bile. The ducts ultimately form the left and right hepatic ducts, which join into the common hepatic duct. Bile is stored and concentrated in the gallbladder, which connects to the biliary tree through the cystic duct. The common hepatic duct and cystic duct join to form the CBD, which connects to the duodenum through the sphincter of Oddi (hepatopancreatic sphincter).[24] Following the ingestion of food, fatty acids in the duodenum stimulate the release of cholecystokinin (CCK) which causes the gallbladder to contract and the sphincter of Oddi to relax leading to the release of bile into the duodenum. The bile acids emulsify dietary fats and facilitate their absorption. The vast majority (95%) of the bile acids released into the duodenum are reabsorbed in the terminal ileum and returned to the liver to be reused. This pathway for recycling bile acids is known as the enterohepatic circulation (EHC).[25] Enterohepatic cycling can impact the pharmacokinetics and pharmacodynamics of drugs that undergo biliary excretion by increasing their bioavailability, reducing their elimination, as well as altering their plasma concentration curves. The effect of EHC on the properties of a drug depends on the physiologic activity of the excreted form of the drug (i.e., prodrug or activated form), the ease with which the excreted form is reabsorbed through the intestines, and whether it is recycled through the liver into the bile or the systemic circulation. In the case of some drugs, EHC can lead to secondary and tertiary peaks in plasma concentration as the drug is recycled into the system.[26]

ROLE OF THE LIVER IN COAGULATION

The liver plays a significant role in the coagulation system. It synthesizes all coagulation factors except factors III (thromboplastin), IV (calcium), and VIII (von Willebrand factor [vWF]). It also synthesizes proteins that regulate coagulation and fibrinolysis such as protein S, protein C, plasminogen activator inhibitor, and antithrombin III. Furthermore, it removes activated clotting and fibrinolysis products through the hepatic reticuloendothelial system. A number of factors require vitamin K to become active. Coagulation factors II, VII, IX, X, as well as protein C and protein S undergo posttranslational modification with vitamin K to become active. Briefly, glutamic acid in the amino terminus of these proteins is converted to gamma-carboxyglutamic acid. These gamma-carboxylated procoagulants can then bind calcium ions and form bridges to phospholipid surfaces that are essential for the formation of activation complexes.[27] Warfarin acts by inhibition gamma-carboxylation. In addition to these vitamin K–dependent factors, hepatocytes also synthesize factor V, XIII, fibrinogen, antithrombin, α_2 plasmin inhibitor, and plasminogen.[28] Thrombomodulin, tissue plasminogen activator, tissue factor plasma inhibitor, vWF, and urokinase are not synthesized in the liver. Instead these proteins are synthesized in endothelial cells, whereas urokinase is expressed by endothelial cells, macrophages, and renal epithelial cells. Tissue plasminogen activator is primarily removed from the bloodstream through the hepatic reticuloendothelial system.[29]

HEME METABOLISM, BILIRUBIN, AND PORPHYRIAS

The liver is involved in both heme synthesis and metabolism. Eighty to 90% of heme synthesis takes place in the bone marrow with the resultant heme used to produce hemoglobin. Most of the remainder of the heme is produced in the liver and used primarily to synthesize cytochrome P450 enzymes. Whereas the rate of heme synthesis in the bone marrow is a function of the availability of iron, the rate of synthesis in the liver is a function of the available free heme pool in the body.[30] Heme is synthesized through an eight-step enzymatic cascade known as the Shemin pathway. Synthesis begins with glycine and succinyl CoA and proceeds through porphyrinogen intermediaries. A deficiency in any of the enzymes involved in heme synthesis leads to the development of porphyria. The specific type of porphyria and its clinical manifestations depend on the specific enzyme that is deficient and the substrate that accumulates as a result. The most common porphyria is acute intermittent porphyria with an estimated incidence of 5 to 10 per 100,000. It is caused by a deficiency in porphobilinogen deaminase, which catalyzes the conversion of porphobilinogen to hydroxymethylbilane. Patients typically have adequate levels of the enzyme for heme homeostasis; however, in response to endogenous or exogenous triggers that induce the Shemin pathway, the capacity of the system is exceeded and they accumulate precursors leading to symptoms. Common triggers include erythromycin, trimethoprim, rifampicin, phenytoin, and barbiturates. Clinical symptoms of an attack include severe, poorly localized abdominal pain (in >90% of cases), nausea, vomiting, agitation, and confusion. Hyponatremia occurs in 40% of attacks. Change in urine color to dark red (especially on exposure to light) is a common finding. Treatment consists of discontinuing the triggering agent, administering pain medication, carbohydrates, and hematin.[30]

Bilirubin is a product of heme catabolism. The primary source is senescent erythrocytes that are phagocytosed by macrophages in the spleen, liver, and bone marrow. The released heme is metabolized by heme oxygenase into bilirubin, yielding carbon monoxide and iron in the process. Unconjugated bilirubin is water insoluble and thus tightly bound to albumin in the circulation. Hepatocytes convert bilirubin into a water-soluble form by conjugating it to glucuronic acid via the enzyme glucuronyl transferase. Conjugated bilirubin is then transported across bile canaliculi and excreted in the bile. In the colon, bilirubin is deconjugated, metabolized by bacteria, and converted into urobilinogen. Urobilinogens are either reabsorbed through the EHC or excreted in the urine and stool, giving urine and stool their characteristic colors.[31]

HEPATIC REGULATION OF HORMONES

The liver can participate in endocrine functions through hormone synthesis or hormone degradation. Hepatocytes synthesize hormones or prohormones such as hepcidin, insulin-like growth factor, and angiotensinogen, respectively. In addition to these hormones, thrombopoietin is also synthesized by hepatocytes and LSECs. These hormones and prohormones have specialized roles in the human body. Thus hepcidin is responsible for iron homeostasis and regulates intestinal iron absorption, plasma iron concentrations, and tissue iron distribution by inducing degradation of the hepcidin receptor, ferroportin.[32] Insulin-like growth factor promotes systemic growth, especially bone growth in children.[33] Angiotensinogen, the precursor of all angiotensin proteins, regulates the systemic blood pressure as well as the water and sodium composition of the body.[34] Thrombopoietin regulates platelet production by stimulating production and differentiation of megakaryocytes.[35] In addition to hormone synthesis, the liver participates in endocrine function by inactivating many hormones, including thyroxine, aldosterone, antidiuretic hormone, estrogens, androgens, and insulin.

TABLE 16.2 Liver Blood Tests and the Differential Diagnosis of Hepatobiliary Disorders

	PREDOMINANT ABNORMALITY		
Blood Test	**Bilirubin Overload (Hemolysis)**	**Hepatocellular Injury**	**Cholestasis**
Aminotransferases	Normal	Increased: May be normal or decreased in advanced stages	Normal: May be increased in advanced stages
Serum albumin	Normal	Decreased: May be normal in acute fulminant hepatic failure	Normal: May be decreased in advanced stages
Prothrombin time*	Normal	Prolonged	Normal: May be prolonged in advanced stages
Bilirubin (main form present)	Unconjugated (also mild increase in conjugates)	Conjugated	Conjugated
Alkaline phosphatase	Normal	Normal: May be increased by hepatic infiltrative disease	Increased
γ-Glutamyl transpeptidase 5′-nucleotidase	Normal	Normal	Increased
Blood urea nitrogen	Normal: May be increased by renal dysfunction	Normal: May be decreased by severe liver disease and normal kidney function	Normal
BSP/ICG (dye)	Normal	Retention of dye	Normal or retention of dye

*Used interchangeably with the international normalized ratio.
BSP/ICG, Bromsulphalein and indocyanine green.

Evaluation of the Liver

CLINICAL ASSESSMENT

There are often no signs or symptoms of liver disease until it is quite advanced. Even then, the only clues may be mild or nonspecific symptoms such as loss of appetite, fatigability, malaise, disrupted sleep patterns, or subtle cognitive changes. Major risk factors for liver disease include: alcohol use; illicit drug use; sexual promiscuity; blood transfusions; exposure to hepatotoxins; prior bouts of jaundice; and a family history of genetic diseases such as hemochromatosis, α_1-antitrypsin deficiency, and Wilson disease. Patients with advanced liver disease may have these nonspecific symptoms, as well as pruritus, easy bruising, and changes in urine or stool color. In advanced liver disease physical examination findings include jaundice, scleral icterus, ascites, spider angiomas, xanthelasma, asterixis, and palmar erythema.

STANDARD LABORATORY TESTS

Standard panels used to evaluate the hepatobiliary system are often called "liver function tests" (Table 16.2).[36] In fact, these tests do not measure specific liver functions. Instead, they help define broad categories of hepatobiliary pathology: hepatitis, hepatobiliary dysfunction, or insufficient protein synthesis.

DETECTION OF HEPATOCELLULAR INJURY

Aminotransferases

Serum alanine aminotransferase (ALT) and aspartate aminotransferase (AST), formerly named serum glutamic-pyruvic transaminase and serum glutamic-oxaloacetic transaminase, respectively, are most commonly elevated because of hepatocellular injury. Both are aminotransferases, enzymes involved in gluconeogenesis. ALT is mainly a cytoplasmic liver enzyme. In contrast, cytoplasmic and mitochondrial isozymes of AST are found in many extrahepatic tissues, including the heart, skeletal muscle, brain, kidney, pancreas, adipose, and blood. Therefore isolated elevations of AST likely represent non-liver sources, but concomitant elevations in AST and ALT usually represent liver injury. Rarely, elevations in AST and ALT levels may result from muscle injury.[37]

Practice guidelines provide recommendations for the evaluation of abnormal liver enzymes, based on the combination of clinical picture and degree of elevation of AST and ALT. Establishing normal reference ranges for AST and ALT have been complicated by studies with heterogeneous populations, since normal ranges differ with gender and body mass index (BMI). Nevertheless, multiple studies show that even mild elevations of AST and ALT above the upper limit of normal are associated with increased mortality. Some clinicians therefore argue that the normal limits should be lowered.[38]

Elevated ALT and AST levels are sometimes described in qualitative terms, ranging from mild (>100 IU/L), to extreme (>2000 IU/L). The extent of aminotransferase elevation can sometimes aid in the differential diagnosis. Mild elevations in AST and ALT can arise from any hepatocyte injury. Large elevations often reflect acute hepatocyte ischemia. Extreme elevations signify massive hepatic necrosis, such as from fulminant viral hepatitis, severe drug-induced liver injury, or shock liver.[51] However, aminotransferase levels do not reliably represent the extent of liver damage. Patients with so called "burnt out" livers, such as from chronic hepatitis, have insufficient functioning hepatocytes to bring about a transaminase increase.

The ratio of AST to ALT may help identify the cause of liver disease. Most causes of hepatic injury are associated with higher ALT than AST levels. However, Wilson disease and alcoholic liver disease are classically associated with an

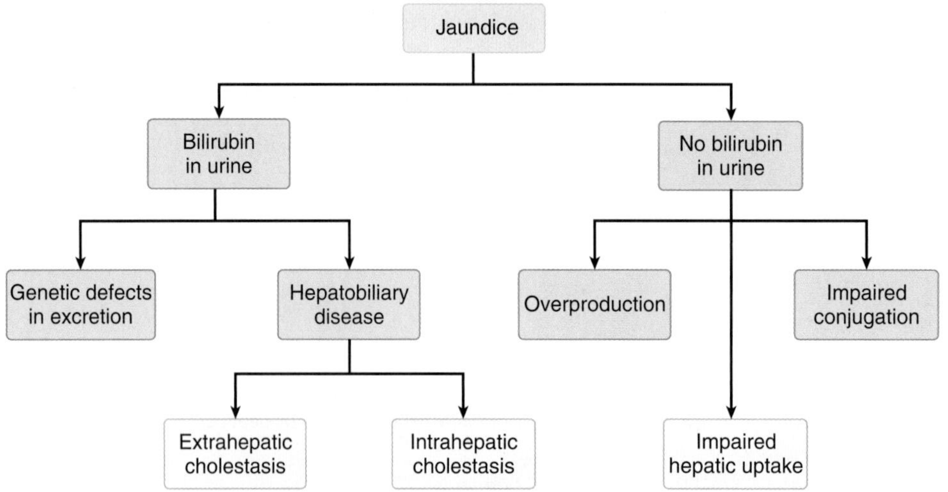

Fig. 16.4 Differential diagnosis of jaundice depending on whether bilirubin is or is not present in the urine.

AST-ALT ratio greater than 1; in some cases, a ratio of 4 has been documented. Chronic hepatitis with minimal fibrosis has a low AST-ALT ratio; however when cirrhosis develops the ratio is greater than 1. Although the AST-ALT ratio may have insufficient predictive value as a sole marker, it can be used in combination with other noninvasive tests to predict the degree of fibrosis in patients with chronic hepatitis.[39]

Lactate Dehydrogenase

Lactate dehydrogenase (LDH) is a nonspecific marker of hepatocellular injury. Extremely elevated LDH signifies massive hepatocyte damage, usually from ischemia or drug-induced hepatotoxicity (such as acetaminophen overdose). These patients will also have extreme elevations in AST and ALT. Elevated LDH concomitant with elevated alkaline phosphatase (AP) suggests malignant infiltration of the liver. Extrahepatic disorders that cause LDH elevation include hemolysis, rhabdomyolysis, tumor necrosis, renal infarction, acute stroke, and myocardial infarction.[37]

Glutathione-S-Transferase

GST is a sensitive test for liver injury, with a half-life (60-90 minutes) much shorter than AST or ALT. Following hepatocyte damage, serum GST rises quickly and serial GST measurements can help monitor for disease recovery.[40] The enzymes AST and ALT are found primarily in periportal hepatocytes (acinar zone 1), whereas GST is present in hepatocytes throughout the acinar zones.[41] Since centrilobular/perivenous hepatocytes are most susceptible to hypoxic injury and acetaminophen toxicity, GST is a useful marker particularly in early stages of injury.

DETECTION OF CHOLESTATIC DISORDERS

Alkaline Phosphatase

AP isoenzymes are present in many tissues, including liver, bone, intestine, and placenta. In the liver, AP is present in the canalicular membranes of the hepatocytes. Mild elevations in AP may be normal, as AP varies with gender, age, blood type, and smoking status.[42] Nonhepatic causes of AP elevation include bone disorders such as Paget disease, osteomalacia, and tumors of the bone; normal growth spurts in children; the third trimester of pregnancy; sepsis; renal failure; and some medications. Elevated AP from a hepatobiliary source is most commonly due to cholestatic disease and typically manifests as an increase to 2 to 4 times the upper limit of normal. Rarely, patients with cholestasis can have extreme elevations in AP (10 times the upper limit of normal).[51] AP will also be elevated to a lesser extent in hepatocellular disease such as hepatitis. The ALT to AP ratio helps differentiate hepatocellular injury (ALT:AP > 5) from cholestatic disease (ALT:AP < 2) from a mixed picture.[38]

AP elevation from cholestasis could be a result of either intrahepatic or extrahepatic biliary obstruction. Common causes include primary biliary cirrhosis, choledocholithiasis, and hepatic malignancy compressing small intrahepatic bile ducts. With a half-life of about 1 week, AP will be normal immediately after the onset of biliary obstruction, and it will remain elevated for days after resolution of obstruction.[37]

The source of AP isoenzyme elevation can be determined by electrophoresis, but this test is expensive and not routinely available. More commonly clinicians confirm the hepatic origin of the AP elevation with other tests that indicate cholestatic disease. The enzymes 5′-nucleotidase and gamma-glutamyl transpeptidase are also elevated in cholestatic disorders, coincident with AP. Simultaneous elevation of these enzymes help identify liver as the source of AP elevation.

Serum Bilirubin

Serum bilirubin is the most commonly used test to monitor for excretory dysfunction of the liver. Bilirubin is measured in serum assays as either direct or indirect bilirubin. Direct bilirubin measures the water-soluble form, which interacts directly with the assay's reagents. While direct bilirubin correlates with conjugated bilirubin levels, and indirect with unconjugated levels, the two terms are not synonymous. The level of unconjugated bilirubin is typically underestimated by the indirect bilirubin test. Distinguishing conjugated from unconjugated bilirubin is key to the differential diagnosis. The presence of bilirubin in the urine can also help differentiate the clinical cause. Bilirubinuria usually reflects conjugated hyperbilirubinemia, since only the water-soluble conjugated form is excreted by the kidney (Fig.16.4).[37]

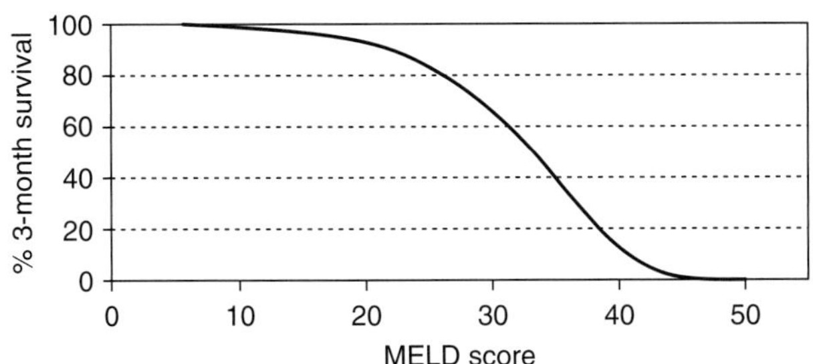

Fig. 16.5 Estimated 3-month survival as a function of the Model for End-Stage Liver Disease *(MELD)* score.

Elevation in the concentration of unconjugated bilirubin is either due to excessive heme breakdown, or the inability of the liver to conjugate bilirubin. One major cause is hemolysis, in which increased erythrocyte breakdown creates more unconjugated bilirubin than the liver is able to conjugate. Massive hemolysis will cause elevations in both forms of bilirubin, but with unconjugated predominance. Gilbert syndrome is a benign condition with genetically low levels of the hepatic enzyme glucuronyl transferase, associated with mild or intermittent elevation in unconjugated bilirubin. Various drugs may also produce unconjugated hyperbilirubinemia. High levels of unconjugated bilirubin are neurotoxic, particularly in infants.

Conjugated hyperbilirubinemia occurs due to either problems with the secretion of conjugated bilirubin from hepatocytes into canalicular bile or to the blockage of bile flow within the hepatobiliary tree. This can be due to a genetic defect in the excretion of bilirubin, or cholestasis (either intrahepatic or extrahepatic). Intrahepatic cholestasis is caused by an inflammatory or infiltrative process compressing small intrahepatic bile ducts, while extrahepatic cholestasis is due to biliary obstruction such as from stones or a pancreatic mass. Primary sclerosing cholangitis (PSC) can involve both intra- and extrahepatic bile ducts.[43]

ASSESSMENT OF HEPATIC PROTEIN SYNTHESIS

Serum Albumin

The serum albumin concentration is used to evaluate chronic liver disease and hepatocellular function (protein synthesis). However, it has poor specificity. Hypoalbuminemia has many other causes besides decreased protein synthesis, including increased catabolism, expansion of the plasma volume, renal losses, and maldistribution of total body albumin. The half-life of albumin in the serum is 20 days. As a result, changes in the synthetic function of the liver are not acutely reflected by the serum albumin concentration. Prealbumin is another protein synthesized in the liver that is also involved in transport and binding. It has a much shorter half-life than albumin. However, the level of prealbumin reflects the status of protein nutrition to a greater degree than liver synthetic function given its high percentage of essential amino acids.[37]

Prothrombin Time

Hepatic synthetic function can also be assessed by measuring the levels of liver-derived coagulation factors. The liver synthesizes coagulation factors in great excess, thus

TABLE 16.3 Interpretation of Hepatitis B Viral Serologies

Hepatitis B Virus Serologies	Interpretation
Hepatitis B surface antigen (HBsAg)	Acute or chronic infection
Antibody to hepatitis B surface antigen (Anti-HBs)	Immunity due to recovery from infection or vaccination
IgM antibody to hepatitis B core antigen (Anti-HBc IgM)	Previous or ongoing infection
IgG antibody to hepatitis B core antigen (Anti-HBc IgG)	Acute infection
INTERPRETATION OF CONSTELLATION OF RESULTS	
HBsAg NEG Anti-HBs POS Anti-HBc IgG POS	Immune due to recovery
HBsAg NEG Anti-HBs POS Anti-HBc IgG NEG	Immune by vaccination
HBsAg POS Anti-HBs NEG Anti-HBc IgM POS	Acute hepatitis B infection
HBsAg POS Anti-HBs NEG Anti-HBc IgG POS Anti-HBc IgM NEG	Chronic hepatitis B infection
HBsAg NEG Anti-HBs NEG Anti-HBc IgG NEG	Not immune, potentially susceptible

the prothrombin time (PT) will remain normal until significant hepatic impairment occurs. Coagulation factors have shorter half-lives than albumin, ranging from 4 hours for factor VII to 4 days for fibrinogen. Thus when severe liver dysfunction occurs, PT (or the international normalized ratio [INR]) can reflect acute liver failure more quickly than can albumin. It is also used to monitor for restoration of hepatic function, often improving before other clinical signs of improvement occur. However, prolonged PT/INR is not specific for liver disease. It may also represent vitamin K deficiency, warfarin effect, or a genetic factor deficiency.[37]

TESTING FOR DIAGNOSIS OF SPECIFIC DISEASES

In addition to the above standard laboratory tests, targeted testing can aid in the diagnosis of specific hepatobiliary diseases. Such testing includes serologic testing for viral and autoimmune diseases, genetic testing, and tumor marker assays. Viral markers, including antibodies, antigens, and genetic material, are used to diagnose hepatitis from hepatotropic viruses (A, B, C, D, and E) and herpesviruses such as cytomegalovirus and Epstein-Barr virus. Patients with acute or chronic hepatitis B infection and those with immunity due to resolved infection or vaccination can be distinguished based on measurements of hepatitis B surface antigens and surface and core antibodies (Table 16.3). HBV DNA testing has also emerged to monitor treatment effect and the development of chronic hepatitis B after resolution of acute hepatitis.[44]

Testing for hepatitis C is recommended for those with various risk behaviors and exposures (such as history of intravenous drug use, long term hemodialysis, or HIV infection) and as part of an evaluation for unexplained liver disease. American guidelines also recommend one-time screening for hepatitis C in all persons in the United States born between 1945 and 1965, as this birth cohort has the highest prevalence of hepatitis C. Screening entails testing for antibodies to HCV; a positive screen indicates exposure to the virus. Active infection can then be confirmed with nucleic acid testing for HCV RNA. Sustained viral response to treatment is defined as the absence of HCV RNA detected at least 12 weeks after the completion of therapy.[45] Currently, patients also receive HCV genotype testing prior to the initiation of treatment. New direct antiviral agents are highly effective in achieving sustained viral response for most genotypes and most clinical conditions. Therefore genotype testing may soon no longer be routinely required.[46]

Rapid HCV antibody testing and point of care RNA tests are useful in community-based settings serving high-risk populations and remote settings without access to centralized laboratories. The measurement of HCV core antigen (HCVcAg) can diagnose active hepatitis C infection with high sensitivity and specificity as a single test, although it is currently not the standard of care. HCVcAg measurement is particularly useful as a rapid, single test for diagnosis in populations who are at high risk of loss to follow-up. However, it is not yet available as a point of care test.[47]

Markers of hepatic malignancy include alpha fetoprotein (AFP) and protein induced by vitamin K absence or antagonist-II (PIVKA-II).[48-50] AFP is a glycoprotein synthesized in the liver, fetal yolk sac, and GI tract. The normal value of AFP is less than 20 ng/mL. A significantly elevated concentration of AFP, often greater than 1000 ng/mL, is common in patients with hepatocellular carcinoma (HCC). AFP is also elevated in testicular germ cell tumors, and less frequently in prostate and other gastrointestinal cancers. The concentration of AFP is used to monitor HCC disease progression and response to treatment. It is also widely used to screen for HCC in high-risk patients, along with ultrasound. However, AFP's role in HCC surveillance has recently been debated, as studies suggest that AFP has insufficient sensitivity as a screening tool for HCC, particularly for small and solitary tumors. AFP may be normal in 40% of HCC patients.[51,52] PIVKA-II, also known as des-γ-carboxylated prothrombin, is a biomarker for HCC with high specificity.[48,50] With a shorter half-life than AFP, PIVKA-II is useful in monitoring for treatment response and recurrence. PIVKA-II is also associated with worse survival. AFP and PIVKA-II combined can diagnose HCC with further increased sensitivity and specificity.[53]

TESTING IN MANAGEMENT AND PROGNOSIS OF LIVER DISEASE

Laboratory tests can help define the type of liver dysfunction, and even identify specific causes. In addition, some of these markers are used to assess disease severity, monitor disease progression and treatment, and predict mortality. Taken alone, thrombocytopenia is the earliest sign of cirrhosis among the routine serum tests, indicating both decreased hepatic function and splenic sequestration from portal hypertension.[54] Some markers are combined to create scoring systems, thereby improving the sensitivity and specificity of single tests. For example, the Model for End-Stage Liver Disease (MELD) score (a calculation that combines INR, bilirubin, and creatinine) was created to assess risk of mortality in cirrhotic patients undergoing transjugular intrahepatic portosystemic shunt (TIPS) procedures. The MELD score now is used for liver transplant listing, as it correlates with wait-list mortality. Standard tests such as INR, lactate and platelet count, as well as novel quantitative tests have been used to predict short-term outcome after liver transplantation.[55] The HCC-MELD score, which combines AFP, MELD, and tumor size, can predict survival after liver transplantation in HCC patients.[56] Elevated bilirubin predicts poor prognosis in acute or chronic liver disease, and AP and bilirubin together predict poor outcome in primary biliary cirrhosis.

Noninvasive Serum Testing for Fibrosis

Multiple models combining noninvasive measurements have been used to assess the severity of fibrosis. The goal of these models is to allow for disease staging (from mild fibrosis to cirrhosis) without requiring liver biopsy. Although liver biopsy remains the diagnostic gold standard, limitations include sampling error, subjectivity in interpretation, pain, bleeding, and cost.[54] These models include various combinations of standard tests such as aminotransferases, platelet count, and INR; as well serum markers of extracellular matrix turnover such as alpha-2-macroglobulin, apolipoprotein A1, and hyaluronic acid. New commercial panels test an array of direct markers of collagen turnover, which correlate with fibrosis.[39,57,58]

Quantitative Liver Tests

Quantitative liver function tests can estimate hepatocellular function by measuring the clearance of various substances metabolized by the liver. Two such substances are indocyanine green (ICG) and bromsulphalein. However, clearance techniques are imperfect tests, potentially influenced by extrahepatic uptake or clearance of the substance, changes in blood flow including portosystemic shunting, and other unknown factors. ICG is avidly extracted by the liver and undergoes minimal extrahepatic uptake and metabolism. Its elimination kinetics are expressed in the ICG plasma disappearance rate (PDR). It can be measured noninvasively by a transcutaneous method. The test is even sensitive to early changes in liver function, and it may be used to guide clinical management. By estimating functional hepatocellular mass, it may help predict outcomes after partial liver resections. It is also used as an early test of graft function following liver transplantation. However, like other highly extracted substances, ICG clearance is dependent on hepatic blood flow, and therefore reflects changes in both hepatic blood flow and hepatocyte function. In fact, ICG is also used specifically to test hepatic blood flow as discussed below. A drop in the ICG PDR may represent a reduction in hepatocellular function, a decrease in hepatic blood flow, or both. Bromsulphalein is another highly extracted substance that can be used to measure hepatic clearance. Bromsulphalein has been associated with severe systemic reactions, and therefore is largely no longer used.[59]

The capacity of the liver to metabolize drugs can also be measured by caffeine clearance, galactose elimination, aminopyrine breath test, and monoethylglycinexylidide (MEGX).[37,60-62] Caffeine clearance can be measured noninvasively through metabolites present in the saliva up to 24 hours after oral caffeine intake. MEGX is the primary metabolite of lidocaine and is measured in the serum after intravenous injection of lidocaine. MEGX concentration may be used to estimate liver function after partial hepatectomy and may have prognostic value in intensive care unit patients with liver dysfunction. MEGX was found to independently predict poor outcomes in patients with chronic hepatitis C, and it was more sensitive than standard liver tests in identifying these patients.[63] Expensive and time consuming, quantitative tests currently remain primarily research tools and require further validation.

MEASUREMENT OF HEPATIC BLOOD FLOW

Blood flow to the liver can be measured using clearance techniques, indicator dilution techniques, and direct measurements.

Clearance Techniques

Based upon the Fick principle, clearance techniques estimate the hepatic blood flow by measuring the rate of disappearance of substances that are exclusively and avidly cleared by the liver. Such substances with high extraction ratios include ICG, propranolol, lidocaine, and radiolabeled colloid particles. The primary limitation of clearance techniques is they assume normal hepatocyte function. Hepatic capacity to eliminate these substances can be variably or significantly diminished in liver disease. This is particularly problematic since liver dysfunction and altered hepatic flow are so often linked.[64]

The dual cholate test measures the clearance of cholate, a bile salt, given in both oral and intravenous form. The oral cholate undergoes a high first-pass extraction and allows for a calculation of portal circulation. Clearance from the systemic circulation is measured using the intravenous cholate. One can quantify the degree of portal-systemic shunting and calculate a disease severity index. This index correlates with degree of fibrosis on liver biopsy and can predict risk of cirrhosis and poor clinical outcomes.[63,65]

Indicator Dilution Techniques

Unlike clearance methods, indicator dilution techniques can measure hepatic blood flow even in the setting of liver dysfunction. A known quantity of a radiolabeled indicator (e.g., iodinated albumin) is injected into the portal system and hepatic artery. The concentration of that substance is then measured continuously from a hepatic vein. Hepatic blood flow can then be calculated by creating indicator dilution curves. The substance used should be resistant to hepatic clearance.[4] Indicator dilution techniques also presume uniform liver perfusion, and therefore results could be altered in patients with shunting. These techniques are invasive and are still primarily research tools as well.[64]

Direct Measurements

Blood flow through the portal vein or hepatic artery can be measured directly using electromagnetic or ultrasonic probes. These techniques are invasive and subject to significant error. The surgical procedures required to implant the probes can themselves alter hepatic blood flow. Once implanted, the probes are often left in place, and blood flow is then measured via telemetry. Implantable Doppler probes are sometimes used in patients immediately post-liver transplantation, and in patients who are at high risk for hepatic artery or portal vein thromboses.[64]

RADIOLOGIC METHODS

Radiologic techniques play important roles in diagnosing liver disease. Splenoportography evaluates the splenic and portal veins; it is useful in identifying varices and thromboses. Portal venography uses three-dimensional CT to create vascular maps of portosystemic collateral vessels. These noninvasive imaging techniques are particularly useful in surgical planning, such as before liver transplantation.[66]

Inexpensive and routinely available, ultrasound can help diagnose cirrhosis with high sensitivity and specificity. Ultrasonic signs of cirrhosis include surface nodularity, hepatomegaly, and hypertrophy of the caudate lobe, as well as signs of portal hypertension, such as ascites, splenomegaly, and increased portal vein diameter. Doppler ultrasonography can show diminished portal flow and portal venous flow reversal.[54,67,68] Fibrosis can also be estimated using elastography, a noninvasive measure of liver stiffness (LS). A shear wave is delivered across the liver via an ultrasound probe, and the wave propagation is then measured. Transient elastography is reproducible and easily performed in the office. Magnetic resonance elastography is especially useful in obese patients and those with ascites, where transient elastography is less accurate. Stiffness is a continuous measure which correlates with the histological stage of fibrosis, with high sensitivity and specificity.[67,69,70] The combination of serum tests along with elastography offers much improved accuracy in diagnosing fibrosis. These tests are now widely used in practice, although they have not yet supplanted the role of liver biopsy.

Patients with chronic liver disease and chronic hepatitis B virus carriers are at increased risk for developing HCC and require regular screening for the cancer. Ultrasound is the most widely used screening tool for HCC worldwide. Multiphasic, contrast-enhanced CT and MRI are used to evaluate focal liver lesions suspicious for HCC with high sensitivity and specificity. While normal liver parenchyma receives only 25% blood flow from the hepatic artery (the rest via the portal vein), HCC cells receive their blood supply primarily from the hepatic artery. Contrast-enhanced imaging reflects this fact with HCCs showing hyperintensity in the arterial phase and washout during the portal venous phase. The Liver Imaging Reporting and Data System (LI-RADS) is a standardized tool for the radiologic classification of liver lesions in patients with chronic liver disease. Use of the LI-RADS has improved radiologic diagnostic accuracy and reduced the need for biopsy in these patients. In fact, confirmatory biopsy is rarely used, even prior to liver transplantation for HCC.[54,71,72]

Hepatic Pathophysiology

CHOLESTATIC DISEASE

Cholestasis is the impairment of bile production or flow. Cholestatic disorders are characterized primarily by elevations of serum AP and gamma-glutamyl transferase (GGT), with or without elevations in bilirubin. Cholestasis can present as an acute or chronic condition and is thought to affect up to 20% of the population.[73] The impairment of flow leads to an increase in the concentration of bile salts in the serum and hepatocytes. As the bile salts accumulate in the liver, they dissolve hepatocyte cell membranes, leading to the release of AP and GGT, resulting in an increase in the serum concentrations of these enzymes.[74] Serum concentrations of AST and ALT, which are found in the cytoplasm of hepatocytes, are not increased to as great an extent. As the disease progresses, the serum concentration of conjugated bilirubin increases, giving rise to jaundice.[31] The majority of cases of cholestasis are benign; however, severe and prolonged cholestasis can lead to cirrhosis.

Signs and symptoms of cholestasis include fatigue, pruritus, dark urine, and pale stools. An elevation of AP on screening laboratory studies may be the first indication in asymptomatic patients. The evaluation consists of a history and physical exam followed by abdominal ultrasonography. Abdominal ultrasonography is used to distinguish between extrahepatic and intrahepatic cholestasis. Extrahepatic cholestasis results from mechanical obstruction of the extrahepatic bile ducts, typically by stones, strictures, or masses leading to ductal dilation. Definitive diagnosis and treatment is by endoscopic retrograde pancreatography (ERCP). If the etiology is unclear, further imaging can be conducted using endoscopic ultrasound or magnetic resonance cholangiopancreatography to identify the biliary lesion leading to obstruction.[75] Normal imaging results indicate intrahepatic cholestasis. Intrahepatic cholestasis can have several etiologies including immune-mediated, infectious, drug-induced, paraneoplastic, and ischemic. The first step in the evaluation is the measurement of antimitochondrial antibody (AMA) titers to rule out primary biliary cholangitis (PBC). Further evaluation may require ERCP and liver biopsy.

PRIMARY BILIARY CHOLANGITIS

Formerly known as primary biliary cirrhosis, PBC is an autoimmune disease that is characterized by the destruction of intrahepatic cholangiocytes and the presence of AMAs. It is one of the most common cholestatic liver disorders.[76] Reported prevalence rates vary from 20 to 490 cases per million inhabitants with the highest rates reported in the United States.[77] Over 90% of patients are female and the average age at diagnosis is typically in the sixth decade. The diagnosis is made based on an elevation of AP over 1.5 times the upper limit of normal for a duration greater than 24 weeks along with the presence of an AMA titer greater than 1:40.[76] A liver biopsy in these patients will reveal interlobular bile duct lesions. Up to 60% of patients may be asymptomatic at diagnosis. If present, the most common symptoms at presentation are fatigue and pruritus. A large number of patients may present with other autoimmune disorders such as keratoconjunctivitis sicca and Raynaud phenomenon. PBC may be associated with osteopenia as well as hyperlipidemia.[76] The disease develops as a result of the loss of tolerance to mitochondrial antigens, leading to autoimmune-mediated destruction of biliary epithelial cells (cholangiocytes). PBC can lead to cirrhosis and liver failure, ultimately requiring transplantation.

Treatment consists of ursodeoxycholic acid (UDCA) administration. UDCA, a bile acid, is thought to act by modifying the bile acid pool and reducing inflammation. Approximately 60% to 70% of patients with PBC respond to UDCA with improvement in serum AP and bilirubin levels and a delay in the progression to cirrhosis and liver transplantation. Patients who have a suboptimal response to UDCA have an increased risk of developing complications and liver failure. In these patients, the administration of obeticholic acid, a farnesoid-X receptor agonist, has been shown to reduce the serum levels of AP. Fibrates and corticosteroids have also shown benefit when combined with UDCA in patients who are unresponsive to UDCA alone.[78-83]

PRIMARY SCLEROSING CHOLANGITIS

PSC is a rare cholestatic, immune-mediated disease that occurs most frequently in men aged 30 to 40 years old. It is characterized by inflammation and fibrosis of the bile ducts. The majority of patients with PSC have ulcerative colitis as well. Approximately half of the patients are asymptomatic at diagnosis. The most common presenting symptoms are fatigue and pruritus. Blood tests demonstrate a cholestatic pattern. Patients may also have hypergammaglobulinemia and elevations in serum autoantibodies. Diagnosis is made based on the presence of multifocal strictures and segmental biliary dilations on cholangiography, and the exclusion of a number of other possible etiologies including bacterial cholangitis, choledocholithiasis, and surgical biliary trauma.[84] Patients have an increased risk of developing hepatobiliary carcinoma. The disease is progressive, with biliary fibrosis leading to cirrhosis and ultimately end-stage liver disease (ESLD). Liver transplantation is the only effective therapy.

CIRRHOSIS

Cirrhosis is the common pathologic endpoint of a variety of mechanisms of hepatic injury. In the United States, it is the 14th most common cause of death and has a prevalence of 0.3%.[85] The most common causes of cirrhosis in western countries are alcoholic liver disease, hepatitis C, and nonalcoholic steatohepatitis. In the Asia-Pacific region the most common cause is hepatitis B.[86] The morbidity and mortality associated with cirrhosis result mainly from portal hypertension. Chronic liver disease promotes apoptosis and regeneration of hepatocytes. The resultant inflammation leads to parenchymal injury and fibrosis, causing distortion and obstruction of the hepatic vascular architecture. These structural changes increase hepatic resistance to portal blood flow (PBF) and give rise to portal hypertension. Hepatic vascular resistance is further increased due to hepatic endothelial dysfunction, which results in a reduction of vasodilator (primarily nitric oxide [NO]) production and an increase in vasoconstrictor (i.e., thromboxane) production.[87] Portal hypertension and the release of angiogenic factors lead to the development of gastroesophageal varices as well as portosystemic shunts. As portal hypertension worsens, the locally released NO and prostaglandins cause the splanchnic circulation to vasodilate. This further increases portal inflow and exacerbates portal hypertension. Splanchnic vasodilation also leads to systemic hypotension that, in turn, increases sympathetic tone, activates the renin-angiotensin-aldosterone system, and increases antidiuretic hormone release, leading to the development of ascites and the hepatorenal syndrome (HRS). Other significant complications of cirrhosis and portal hypertension are spontaneous bacterial peritonitis, encephalopathy, HRS, portopulmonary hypertension (PoPH), cirrhotic cardiomyopathy, and HCC.[88]

Laboratory abnormalities in cirrhotic patients include elevations in ALT, AST, AP, GGT, as well as serum bilirubin. Hypoalbuminemia and elevations in the PT are indications of hepatic synthetic dysfunction. Although liver biopsy is the gold standard for diagnosing cirrhosis, it is often not necessary in the presence of an appropriate patient history, and laboratory and radiologic data. In patients who are suspected of having cirrhosis, abdominal ultrasonography is used to aid in the diagnosis and evaluation for HCC and portal hypertension. Serologic studies and ultrasound-based techniques for evaluating hepatic fibrosis are also available.[89]

The risk stratification of patients with cirrhosis is based on the presence and degree of portal hypertension, gastroesophageal varices, and synthetic dysfunction.[90] There are two stages of cirrhosis: compensated and decompensated. Decompensated cirrhosis is characterized by the presence of ascites, variceal hemorrhage, and/or hepatic encephalopathy (HE). Compensated cirrhosis is characterized by the absence of these clinical conditions. While the median survival in patients with compensated cirrhosis is greater than 12 years, in those with decompensated cirrhosis it is approximately 2 years.[91] Patients with compensated cirrhosis can be further stratified based on their degree of portal hypertension. Portal hypertension is defined as a hepatic venous pressure gradient (HVPG) greater than 5 mm Hg. Patients with an HVPG greater than 10 mm Hg are deemed to have clinically significant portal hypertension. They are at increased risk of developing varices, overt hepatic decompensation, postsurgical decompensation, and HCC compared to those with mild portal hypertension (HVPG between 5 mm Hg and 10 mm Hg).[92-94] Although HVPG is the gold standard for monitoring portal hypertension, its invasive nature precludes its routine use. A noninvasive measure of clinically significant portal hypertension is LS using transient elastography, an ultrasound-based approach. An LS value greater than 20 kPa has been shown to effectively discriminate mild from clinically significant portal hypertension.[95] Liver Doppler ultrasound may also aid in the diagnosis. The presence of portosystemic collaterals or reversal of portal venous flow on ultrasound imaging is also sufficient to diagnose clinically significant portal hypertension.[96] In patients with clinically significant portal hypertension, the presence of gastroesophageal varices portends a worse prognosis.[97]

The management of patients with compensated cirrhosis who don't have gastroesophageal varices focuses on preventing the advancement of the disease by treating the underlying etiology.[90] Patients with varices are treated with nonspecific beta-blockers (i.e., propranolol, timolol), carvedilol or endoscopic variceal ligation to prevent variceal hemorrhage. Nonspecific beta-blocker therapy reduces HVPG.[98-100]

Acute variceal hemorrhage is a medical emergency. Management consists of airway protection, volume resuscitation, and endoscopy with variceal ligation. The concomitant initiation of antibiotic prophylaxis (ceftriaxone 1 g/24 h) and vasopressor infusion (somatostatin, octreotide, or terlipressin) has been shown to improve outcome and is the standard of care. Once stabilized, preemptive TIPS may be performed in patients who are at high risk of rebleeding.[90]

ASCITES

The presence of ascites is a marker of decompensated cirrhosis. The 1-year mortality rate of patients who develop ascites is 20%.[100] Patients who develop ascites are at increased risk of developing further complications including spontaneous bacterial peritonitis and acute kidney injury (AKI). Management consists of dietary sodium restriction, nonspecific beta-blocker therapy to reduce portal pressure, and diuretic administration (spironolactone, furosemide). Midodrine can be added for refractory ascites. TIPS can improve transplant-free survival in certain patients with refractory ascites.[86]

Renal Failure and Hepatorenal Syndrome

Up to 40% of patients admitted to the hospital with ESLD develop renal failure. Renal failure is a sign of advanced disease and has a poor prognosis in liver failure. Seventy to 80% of cases are precipitated by hypovolemia or bacterial infections. HRS is less common and associated with a worse prognosis.[101,102] The diagnosis of HRS is one of exclusion. It is characterized by AKI in the absence of any apparent cause (shock, nephrotoxic drugs, obstruction, renal parenchymal disease) that is unresponsive to volume expansion and diuretic withdrawal. AKI is defined as a rise in creatinine greater than or equal to 0.3 mg/dL within 48 hours or a greater than 50% increase from baseline within 7 days.[103] HRS is subcategorized into Type 1 and Type 2 based on the rapidity of onset and degree of injury. Type 1 is rapidly progressive with a doubling of serum creatinine within 2 weeks. It is usually associated with a precipitating factor and has a worse prognosis. The treatment for HRS is aimed at increasing perfusion pressure to the kidneys. For critically ill patients, norepinephrine infusion with albumin boluses can be used. In more stable patients, terlipressin (if available) or midodrine with octreotide is administered along with albumin.[104] Dialysis may be used in the absence of response to medical therapy. Liver transplantation is the definitive treatment for HRS.[105]

HEPATIC ENCEPHALOPATHY

HE is brain dysfunction secondary to hepatic insufficiency or portosystemic shunting. It is a sign of decompensated cirrhosis. It occurs in 30% to 40% of patients with cirrhosis and 50% of patients with portosystemic shunts.[106] The clinical presentation is variable and can range from mild changes in personality to disorientation, somnolence, and coma. Asterixis is usually present in the early to middle stages.[107] The severity of HE is typically graded from I to IV using the West Haven criteria with Grade I indicating mild symptoms and Grade IV, coma (Table 16.4).[108] Common precipitating factors of HE include infections, variceal hemorrhage, and diuretic overdose. Diagnosis is based on the exclusion of other causes of brain dysfunction and the application of clinical criteria. Treatment consists of amelioration of

TABLE 16.4 West Haven Criteria for Grading Hepatic Encephalopathy

Grade	Description
I	Trivial lack of awareness; shortened attention span; disordered sleep
II	Lethargy; behavioral change; asterixis
III	Somnolence; confusion; gross disorientation; bizarre behavior
IV	Coma

Modified from Table 2, Page 719 in: Vilstrup H, Amodio P, Bajaj J, et al. Hepatic encephalopathy in chronic liver disease: 2014 practice guideline by the American Association for the Study of Liver Diseases and the European Association for the Study of the Liver. *Hepatol.* 2014;60:715–735.

precipitating factors and the administration of lactulose, a nonabsorbable disaccharide. Rifaximin can be added on to prevent recurrence.[108]

PULMONARY COMPLICATIONS

Hepatopulmonary syndrome (HPS), PoPH, and hepatic hydrothorax (HH) are pulmonary conditions that can develop in patients with cirrhosis and advanced liver disease. HPS has been reported in up to 30% of patients presenting for liver transplantation evaluation and is associated with increased mortality independent of the severity of liver disease.[109] It is defined as abnormal alveolar to arterial oxygen gradient (≥15 mm Hg) while breathing room air in sitting position. It is caused by intrapulmonary vascular dilation in the setting of cirrhosis. Its severity is determined by the PaO_2: greater than 80 mm Hg is mild, 60 to 80 mm Hg is moderate, 50 to 60 mm Hg is severe, and less than 50 mm Hg is very severe.[110] Patients may present with dyspnea at rest or on exertion. Approximately 25% of patients have platypnea (dyspnea when moving from supine to standing) or orthodeoxia (decrease in PaO_2 more than 5% or 4 mm Hg when moving from supine to standing). In advanced disease, patients may exhibit digital clubbing and cyanosis. Patients can be screened with pulse oximetry (SpO_2 < 96% on room air) and diagnosed based on PaO_2 values. Contrast-enhanced transthoracic echocardiography (TTE) may demonstrate intrapulmonary vascular dilation. No medical therapy has been shown to change outcome in patients with HPS. Supplemental oxygen is provided to maintain SpO_2 over 88%. Liver transplantation is the only effective treatment.[111] As such, MELD exception points are granted for patients with severe HPS (PaO_2 50-60 mm Hg). Patients with very severe HPS (PaO_2 < 50 mm Hg) have an increased risk for complications and mortality following liver transplantation although this risk may be lower in experienced centers.[111,112]

PoPH is pulmonary arterial hypertension in the setting of portal hypertension.[113] It is found in 5% of patients presenting for liver transplant evaluation and, in the absence of treatment, is associated with a 1-year survival of 46%.[114,115] The diagnosis is made by right heart catheterization showing a mean pulmonary artery pressure (mPAP) greater than 25 mm Hg, pulmonary vascular resistance (PVR) greater than 240 dynes/s/cm^5, and a pulmonary artery wedge pressure less than 15 mm Hg. PoPH is classified as mild (mPAP: 25-35 mm Hg), moderate (mPAP: 35-45 mm Hg), and severe (mPAP more than 45 mm Hg).[110] The pathophysiology of the disease remains to be elucidated. Patients are typically screened using TTE to measure right ventricular systolic pressure (RVSP). Those with RVSP greater than 50 mm Hg undergo right heart catheterization to confirm the diagnosis and determine the degree of PoPH. PoPH is treated with phosphodiesterase-5 inhibitors, prostacyclin analogs, and endothelin receptor antagonists to reduce PVR. mPAP greater than 45 mm Hg is an absolute contraindication to liver transplantation. MELD exception is considered for treatment-responsive PoPH.[110]

HH has a prevalence of 5% to 10% in cirrhotic patients.[116] It develops due to the passage of ascitic fluid from the peritoneal cavity into the pleural space through defects in the diaphragm, most often on the right side. Patients may present with dyspnea, cough, chest discomfort, and hypoxia. Chest radiography and thoracentesis are used for diagnosis. Medical therapy consists of sodium restriction and diuretic administration. Refractory HH is treated with TIPS placement. For patients who have failed TIPS, VATS with pleurodesis is an option.[117]

HEPATOCELLULAR CARCINOMA

HCC is the most common primary liver malignancy and the third most common cause of cancer death globally. It occurs with greater frequency in men than woman and with a higher incidence in Asia and Africa, although the incidence has been increasing in the United States.[118] Chronic liver disease is the most important risk factor for the development of HCC. Hepatitis B, hepatitis C, hemochromatosis, alcohol use, nonalcoholic fatty liver disease, diabetes mellitus, and obesity all increase the risk of developing HCC.[119] Screening is recommended for all patients with cirrhosis at 6-month intervals using ultrasound with or without serum AFP measurement. Masses over 1 cm should be imaged with dynamic MRI or four-phase multidetector CT to make the diagnosis noninvasively. A percutaneous biopsy is obtained for nodules that have nontypical appearance on imaging.[120] Staging is based on the size of the tumor, degree of extension into adjacent structures, presence of metastases, liver function, and the patient's physical status. There is no universally accepted system for staging. The tumor, node, metastasis and the Barcelona staging system (BCLC) are two of the more commonly used systems.[120]

Surgical resection of HCC is the definitive treatment for the disease. However, the diagnosis of HCC is typically made late in the course of the disease. In patients with preserved liver function and a solitary tumor confined to the liver, treatment with surgical resection carries a 5-year survival rate from 40% to 75%.[121] Transplantation may be an option for patients with hepatic dysfunction and tumors confined to the liver that meet certain size criteria.[122] Nonsurgical options for patients who are ineligible for resection or transplantation include radiofrequency ablation, transarterial chemoembolization, and systemic therapy.[120]

HEPATIC EFFECTS OF ANESTHETIC AGENTS

Inhalational Anesthetics

(See also chapter on pharmacokinetics/dynamics of volatile anesthetics.)

The hepatic effects of volatile anesthetics result primarily from alterations in liver perfusion. Total hepatic blood flow (THBF) is the sum of PBF and hepatic arterial blood flow (HABF). Reductions in PBF are matched by increases in HABF to maintain THBF through the hepatic arterial buffer response (HABR).[123] Volatile anesthetics reduce mean arterial pressure (MAP) and CO, leading to a reduction in PBF in a dose-dependent manner. The HABR is preserved with isoflurane, sevoflurane, and desflurane leading to preservation of THBF, but not with halothane.[124-126]

Xenon is an inert gas that can been used as an anesthetic.[127] It has favorable anesthetic properties including a low blood-gas partition coefficient (0.115) and a stable hemodynamic profile.[128,129] Hepatic perfusion during xenon anesthesia has been studied in pigs. In one study using radiolabeled microspheres, there was no difference in hepatic perfusion in pigs anesthetized with xenon when compared to propofol.[130] However, a second study using ICG reported a 17% reduction in portal venous blood flow in pigs anesthetized with a ketamine infusion that received a xenon anesthetic compared to controls. They reported no significant difference in hepatic arterial perfusion or hepatic function.[131] In a porcine model, the use of xenon anesthesia was associated with significantly higher hepatic venous oxygen content when compared with propofol.[132] It is not clear that there are relevant clinical consequences to these findings. The successful use of xenon anesthesia for the conduct of liver transplantation has been reported in a series of four cases.[133]

In general, intravenous anesthetics such as propofol, thiopental, etomidate, and methohexital do not adversely affect the liver. Furthermore, the pharmacokinetic properties of these agents are unchanged in patients with cirrhosis.[134-137] Cirrhotic patients may be more sensitive to their central nervous system depressant effects. Propofol has been found to increase hepatic blood flow and oxygen consumption in both animal and human studies that have measured flow using radiolabeled microspheres, Doppler, and electromagnetic flow meters.[138-141] Studies using ICG clearance to measure hepatic flow, however, have reported that propofol reduced hepatic flow.[142,143] These findings were confounded by the fact that propofol itself interferes with ICG clearance.[141,144] Clinically, propofol has no adverse effect on hepatic function. Midazolam elimination is impaired in liver dysfunction leading to prolongation of sedative effects.[145] Dexmedetomidine elimination is reduced in patients with hepatic impairment, necessitating dose reduction.[146]

In patients with significant cirrhosis, the metabolism of morphine, meperidine, and alfentanil is reduced and their durations of action are prolonged.[147-149] In patients with mild hepatic insufficiency, the pharmacokinetics of fentanyl, sufentanil, and remifentanil are unchanged when compared to normal controls.[150-152]

Reduced levels of pseudocholinesterase in patients with hepatic dysfunction may prolong the effects of succinylcholine and mivacurium.[153,154] The time to recovery from cisatracurium is unchanged as it is subject to Hoffman degradation.[155]

Aminosteroid neuromuscular blocking agents (vecuronium, rocuronium, pancuronium) have a larger volume of distribution in cirrhotic patients. They have a slower rate of onset and a longer duration of action, necessitating judicious dosing and close train-of-four monitoring.[156-158] Sugammadex has been shown to be effective for reversing rocuronium in patients with hepatic dysfunction.[159] The use of neostigmine for reversal is likewise unaffected by the presence of hepatic dysfunction.

Five studies have examined the effect of epidural anesthesia on hepatic blood flow. Four have shown a reduction in hepatic blood flow in response to lumbar or thoracic epidural anesthesia when measured using the PDR of ICG and transgastric hepatic vein Doppler. In one study, blood flow was restored with the infusion of colloid and dopamine.[160-162] Maintenance of MAP with ephedrine or norepinephrine further reduced hepatic blood flow. Unlike these studies, a study by Kortgen et al. found that thoracic epidural anesthesia increased hepatic blood flow when measured by PDR-ICG, whereas lumbar epidural anesthesia resulted in an overall reduction.[163] The clinical significance of these findings is uncertain.

Nonhepatic Surgery in Patients With Liver Disease

The preoperative evaluation of patients with liver disease should determine the severity of the disease and the presence of comorbid conditions associated with hepatic dysfunction. Given the mortality risk, elective surgery is contraindicated in patients with acute hepatitis or acute liver failure.[164] In the absence of cirrhosis and significant hepatic dysfunction, patients with chronic liver disease generally have no increased risk for undergoing elective surgery. Patients with cirrhosis who undergo nonhepatic surgery have a higher incidence of postoperative morbidity and mortality when compared to patients without cirrhosis.[165] A wide range of mortality rates has been reported in the literature (1%-50%), mostly in small, uncontrolled, institutional studies spanning 30 years. Mortality in these patients is a function of the severity of liver disease, its attendant comorbidities, and the type of surgical procedure.[165] The largest study of in-hospital mortality in patients with cirrhosis used data from the Nationwide Inpatient Sample. The outcomes of 22,569 cirrhotic patients undergoing one of four index operations (cholecystectomy, colectomy, coronary artery bypass grafting [CABG], and abdominal aortic aneurysm repair) from 1998 to 2005 were compared to those of 2.8 million control patients. It was found that 4214 of the cirrhotic patients had portal hypertension. Patients with cirrhosis had a three- to eight-fold increase in the risk of in-hospital mortality, depending on the operation, compared to control patients. Mortality risk worsened in those with more severe liver disease, ranging from 12- to 23-fold, depending on the specific operation. The greatest risk was seen in patients undergoing CABG.[166] A Taiwanese study comparing 24,282 cirrhotic patients undergoing major nonhepatic surgery with 97,128 matched control patients found an over two-fold increased risk of 30-day mortality in patients with cirrhosis (1.2% vs. 0.7%). Mortality was further increased in those cirrhotic patients with viral hepatitis, jaundice, ascites, gastrointestinal hemorrhage, and hepatic coma.[167]

In cirrhotic patients undergoing nonhepatic surgery, the Child-Turcotte-Pugh (CTP) and MELD scores have been shown to identify those who are at higher risk of morbidity and mortality.[168-172] The CTP score is calculated based on

TABLE 16.5 Child-Turcotte-Pugh (CTP) Score

	POINTS ASSIGNED		
	1	**2**	**3**
Ascites	Absent	Slight	Moderate
Bilirubin	<2 mg/dL	2-3 mg/dL	>3 mg/dL
Albumin	>3.5 g/dL	2.8-3.5 g/dL	<2.8 g/dL
PROTHROMBIN TIME			
Seconds over control	<4	4-6	>6
International normalized ratio	<1.7	1.7-2.3	>2.3
Encephalopathy	None	Grades 1-2	Grades 3-4
Point total	CTP class	Operative mortality	
5-6	A	2-10%	
7-9	B	12-31%	
10-15	C	12-82%	

The 30-day postoperative mortality predicted by the **Child-Turcotte-Pugh (CTP) score** is based on retrospective studies cited in text. Lower mortality rates have been reported in more recent studies.

From Pugh RN, Murray-Lyon IM, Dawson JL, et al. Transection of the oesophagus for bleeding oesophageal varices. *Br J Surg*. 1973;60(8):646–649. https://doi.org/10.1002/bjs.1800600817.

the values of five variables: degree of HE, degree of ascites, INR, serum albumin, and total bilirubin (Table 16.5). The score is then used to classify the patient into one of three groups: Class A (score of 5-6), Class B (score of 7-9), and Class C (score > 10).[173] A higher CTP class is associated with a greater risk of mortality. The mortality risk associated with each CTP class has decreased in more recent studies. In early retrospective series of cirrhotic patients undergoing abdominal surgery, the mortality risks associated with CTP Class A, B, and C were 10%, 30%, and 73% to 82%, respectively.[174,175] In a more recent series of 194 patients undergoing 212 general surgical procedures, 30-day mortality was reported to be 6%, 13%, and 53% for CTP Classes A, B, and C, respectively.[169] The risk has been found to be even lower in patients undergoing laparoscopic procedures (Class A: 2%; Class B: 12%; Class C: 12%), suggesting that improvements in perioperative care and surgical techniques have made surgery safer for patients with cirrhosis.[170] A disadvantage of the CTP score is that the grading of encephalopathy and ascites is subjective. Furthermore, the score doesn't take into account other predictors of operative risk such as the type of surgery or the etiology of the cirrhosis.[176]

As described above, the MELD score, calculated using the patient's INR, serum creatinine, serum bilirubin, and etiology of liver disease (Fig. 16.5) [177] is a validated measure of mortality risk in patients with ESLD and is the basis of the liver allocation system for transplantation.[178] A number of studies have validated the MELD score as a predictor of risk in cirrhotic patients undergoing abdominal, orthopedic, and cardiac surgery.[168,179-181] In a large, retrospective study of cirrhotic patients undergoing major abdominal, orthopedic, or cardiac surgery, MELD score was a predictor for mortality at 30 days, 90 days, 1 year, and 5 years. The 30-day mortality ranged from 5.8% in patients with a MELD under 8 to over 50% in patients with a MELD score greater than 20.[182] The incorporation of serum sodium into the MELD score (MELD-Na) as well as a combination of serum sodium and patient age (integrated MELD or iMELD) have been shown to improve the accuracy of predictions of survival over MELD.[183,184] The use of MELD-Na and iMELD may allow more accurate prediction of mortality following nonhepatic surgery; however more studies are needed.[169,185,186]

Studies comparing the predictive power of CTP to MELD have yielded conflicting results likely due to small sample sizes and differences in primary outcome measures and surgical procedures. Small studies in cardiac and general surgical patients have found the abilities of CTP and MELD to predict postoperative mortality to be comparable.[168,179] A study in cirrhotic patients undergoing extrahepatic abdominal surgery found MELD to be a better predictor than CTP for mortality or hepatic decompensation within 90 days of surgery.[180] A more recent study found neither to be a good predictor for death and hepatic decompensation in cirrhotic patients undergoing elective surgery requiring general anesthesia.[171] It has been suggested that both scores should be used in conjunction with other available patient data when attempting to risk-stratify cirrhotic patients for nonhepatic surgery.[187]

Apart from the severity of cirrhosis and the specific surgical procedure, risk factors associated with increased postoperative morbidity and mortality in cirrhotic patients include emergency surgery, American Society of Anesthesiologists (ASA) physical status classification, the presence of renal insufficiency, male gender, and advanced age.[168,170,188]

In addition to determining the severity of cirrhosis, the preoperative evaluation should determine the presence and severity of comorbidities associated with cirrhosis, including HE, pulmonary disease, cardiac disease, and renal dysfunction (see previous discussion). Preoperative laboratory evaluation should include a complete blood count to evaluate for anemia, thrombocytopenia, and leukocytosis. Additionally, INR, fibrinogen, serum electrolytes, creatinine, glucose, transaminases, bilirubin, and albumin should be measured.

Anesthetic Considerations for Procedures Involving the Liver

Transjugular Intrahepatic Portosystemic Shunt. TIPS placement is a catheter-based, endovascular procedure during which a shunt is created between the portal and hepatic venous systems through the parenchyma of the liver (Fig. 16.6). The goal of the procedure is to reduce portal hypertension.[189] The main indications for TIPS are the secondary prevention of variceal hemorrhage and the management of refractory ascites.[190] During acute variceal hemorrhage in high-risk patients (HVPG > 20), TIPS placement following endoscopic intervention has been shown to be reduce rebleeding.[191] Contraindications to the procedure include congestive heart failure, tricuspid regurgitation, and moderate to severe pulmonary hypertension. During the procedure, a catheter is typically inserted through the right internal jugular vein into a hepatic venous branch. A needle is then passed through the hepatic vein into the portal vein. The tract is dilated and a stent is placed across it. HVPG should be

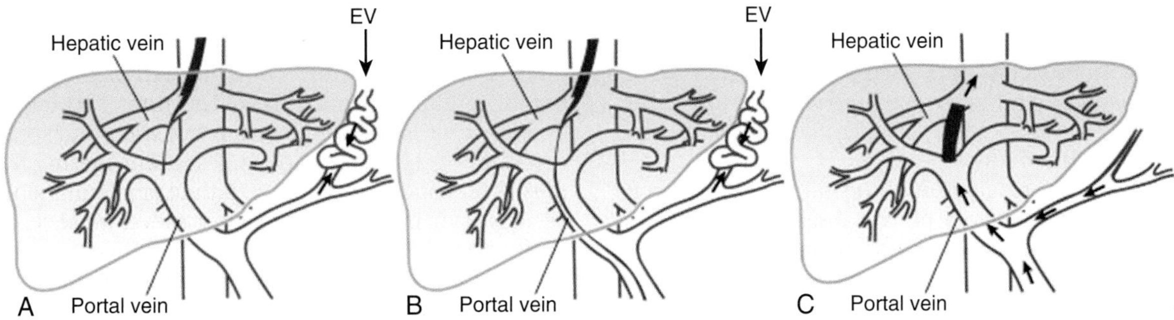

Fig. 16.6 Transjugular intrahepatic portosystemic shunt procedure. A stent (or stents) is passed through the internal jugular vein over a wire into the hepatic vein (A); dilated esophageal varices *(EV)* are apparent. The wire and stent or stents are then advanced into the portal vein (B), after which blood can pass through the portal vein into the hepatic vein and bypass and decompress dilated esophageal veins (C). (Reproduced with permission from University of Michigan Health System: www.med.umich.edu/1libr/topics/liver09.htm/ (not able to access/TG 9–21–18)

less than 12 mm Hg following the procedure. The incidence of major complications such as intra abdominal hemorrhage is on the order of 1% to 2%.[192]

TIPS may be carried out electively or emergently. The preoperative assessment should determine the extent of liver dysfunction and associated morbidity. Patients with advanced liver disease may be in a hyperdynamic state. They may have significant ascites with reductions in FRC as well as HH or HPS. Pulmonary function may be further compromised when the patient is in a supine position for the procedure. Patients may also have renal dysfunction, anemia, coagulopathy, and thrombocytopenia. Laboratory studies should screen for anemia, thrombocytopenia, and coagulopathy, as well as hyponatremia and elevations of creatinine and potassium. Patients should be transfused for a hemoglobin concentration less than 7 to 9 mg/dL, INR greater than 2, and a platelet count less than 50,000/μL.[193] The procedure can be conducted under local anesthesia, sedation, or general anesthesia. Consideration should be given to the acuity of the patient, their ability to tolerate supine positioning, and the anticipated length of the case. In patients with significant ascites or recent variceal hemorrhage, general anesthesia with rapid sequence induction for airway protection is preferred. Intraoperative pain may be experienced during the establishment of the intrahepatic shunt and the dilation of the stent. In a series of 150 patients undergoing TIPS with general anesthesia using TIVA, the authors reported a postoperative ICU admission rate of 6.6% primarily for intraoperative hemodynamic instability. They advocated for the use of general anesthesia for all TIPS procedures, given the concerns for airway protection, ability to maintain supine position, and pain associated with the procedure.[194] Postprocedure complications include heart failure due to increased venous return, HE, contrast-induced nephropathy, hemolytic anemia, and sepsis.[195,196]

Hepatic Resection. The most common indications for hepatic resection are for the treatment of secondary metastases (i.e., metastatic colon cancer), primary hepatic malignancies, biliary tract malignancies, and benign hepatic masses.[197] Hepatic resection is carried out along the functional segments of the liver. The liver is divided into eight functional segments based on the distribution of blood supply and biliary drainage. The left liver is comprised of segments II, III, and IV, while the right liver is comprised of segments V, VI, VII, and VIII. Segment I is the caudate lobe (see Fig.16.1). Right hepatectomy involves resection of segments V-VIII. Left hepatectomy involves resection of segments II-IV. Right lobectomy, also described as an extended right hepatectomy or right trisegmentectomy, involves resection of segments IV-VIII with or without segment I. An extended left hepatectomy (left trisegmentectomy) is the resection of segments II-V and VIII.[198] Mortality and morbidity rates are impacted by the extent of the resection. A review of the 4881 hepatic resections over a 5-year period in the American College of Surgeons – National Surgical Quality Improvement Program database reported 30-day mortality and morbidity rates of 1.9% and 13.1%, respectively, for patients undergoing partial hepatectomy. Those mortality and morbidity rates increased significantly for patients undergoing extended hepatectomies (lobectomies or trisegmentectomies) to 5.8% and 22.5%, respectively.[199,200] Other factors which have been shown to impact outcomes are the case volume of the performing center, patient age, history of cardiac, pulmonary or renal disease, blood loss, the presence of ascites, and reduced hepatic function.[199,200]

Laparoscopic hepatic resection is considered most appropriate for small (<5 cm), solitary lesions located in peripheral segments (II-VI), when performed in experienced institutions.[201,202] More extensive resections have been reported in experienced centers. A metaanalysis of 83 comparative case series (2900 patients) found a significantly lower rate of complications, transfusions, blood loss, and hospital stay in case-matched cohort of patients undergoing laparoscopic liver resection compared to open liver resection.[203] To date, the only randomized, controlled trial comparing laparoscopic to open liver resection found a significant reduction in postoperative complications in patients undergoing laparoscopic hepatic resection (19% vs. 31%; 95% confidence interval [CI], 1.67-21.8; P = .021) for colorectal cancer liver metastases requiring resection of fewer than three consecutive segments. Although the hospital length of stay was significantly shorter, there were no differences in blood loss or mortality.[204] Conversion from a laparoscopic to an open procedure is usually due to intraoperative hemorrhage and is reported to occur in 6% to 14% of cases. Risk factors for conversion include elevated BMI, increased age, diabetes mellitus, hypertension, and large tumor size.[205,206] A number of recent observational, retrospective studies have described the performance of robot-assisted hepatectomy for both minor and major resections.[207] A metaanalysis of seven studies published between 2010 and 2014, comparing laparoscopic to robotic hepatectomy, found that the laparoscopic approach is associated with significant reductions in blood loss and operative time without any difference in the conversion rate, postoperative morbidity, and the hospital length of stay.[208]

The preoperative evaluation of the patient should focus on determining the severity of liver disease and the presence of other comorbidities. Both cirrhosis and steatosis have been associated with increased mortality in patients undergoing liver resection. The decision to proceed is made based on the anticipated future liver remnant (FLR) that will remain following resection.[209,210] In patients with an anticipated FLR size that is considered unsafe, selective portal vein embolization (PVE) may be conducted in the weeks prior to the hepatic resection. Disruption of portal flow to the diseased portion of the liver leads to atrophy of the portion to be resected and hypertrophy of the FLR, allowing the patient to have adequate liver mass following resection. PVE is typically indicated for patients with an anticipated FLR less than 20% in the absence of cirrhosis, and less than 40% in the presence of cirrhosis.[120,211] Further preoperative evaluation and risk assessment should take place as outlined above. Laboratory investigations prior to hepatic resection should include a complete blood count, serum electrolytes, liver chemistries, albumin, coagulation studies, and a type and screen.

Strategies for Minimizing Blood Loss

Intraoperative blood loss during liver resection is associated with an increased risk of morbidity and mortality.[212-214] Several preoperative factors have been associated with an increased risk of transfusion. These include preoperative anemia, the need for an extrahepatic procedure, the need for caval exposure, major hepatectomy (>3 segments), tumor size, thrombocytopenia, cirrhosis, and a repeat operation.[215-217] For patients at increased risk of significant intraoperative hemorrhage, the use of techniques such as acute normovolemic hemodilution and intraoperative cell salvage have been shown to reduce the transfusion of allogeneic units.[218-221]

A number of strategies have been adopted to reduce blood loss in open hepatic resection and case series from high-volume centers routinely report losses less than 500 mL.[213,222,223] Such strategies include the use of temporary hepatic vascular occlusion and the intraoperative maintenance of low central venous pressure (CVP).[224,225]

Hepatic vascular occlusion techniques may be used by surgeons to limit blood loss by limiting blood flow to the liver. Although not routinely used in simple resections, familiarity with these techniques is important as they may be employed in more complex resections. The most commonly used vascular occlusion technique is occlusion of the hepatic artery and portal vein by clamping the hepatoduodenal ligament. Otherwise known as the Pringle maneuver, total hepatic inflow occlusion was first described in 1908 as a means of controlling hemorrhage in hepatic trauma (Fig.16.7A).[226] The drawback of this maneuver is the potential for hepatic ischemia and reperfusion injury.[227] To mitigate this effect, surgeons typically make use of intermittent clamping with 15- to 20-minute intervals of clamping interspersed with 5- to 10-minute intervals of unclamping for a total ischemic time of less than 120 minutes.[228] Tolerance of longer cumulative ischemic times has been reported.[229] The application of sevoflurane for 30 minutes of preconditioning prior to the Pringle maneuver has been shown in one single-center randomized, controlled trial to significantly reduce postoperative transaminitis and complications in cases with greater than 30 minutes of continuous inflow occlusion.[230] In a subsequent three-armed randomized controlled trial, the same group reported reductions in postoperative transaminitis and complications when sevoflurane was administered after the Pringle maneuver ("post-conditioning") or with the use of intermittent clamping.[231]

The utility of the Pringle maneuver for reducing blood loss in modern hepatic resection has been called into question. While two early randomized, controlled trials showed a significant reduction in blood loss with intermittent Pringle maneuver compared to no inflow occlusion, three, more recent, randomized controlled trials have reported no benefit.[232-236] The median blood loss values reported in these three more recent trials were much lower than those reported in the initial two studies. This finding suggests that in the context of current intraoperative approaches to hepatic resection, the routine use of the Pringle maneuver may not be necessary.[236,237]

An alternative technique that may be utilized is hemi-hepatic inflow occlusion. This maneuver involves exclusively clamping the branches of the portal vein and hepatic artery which supply the hemi-liver which is being resected in order to reduce ischemic injury to the remnant liver (see Fig. 16.7B and C).[238] Hemi-hepatic inflow occlusion hasn't been shown to reduce blood loss when compared to Pringle maneuver.[239-242] Total hepatic vascular exclusion (THVE) involves occlusion of the suprahepatic and infrahepatic IVC in addition to the portal vein and hepatic artery (see Fig. 16.7D)[243] THVE can result in significant hypotension due to the reduction in venous return as well as increased morbidity. It has not been shown to offer any benefit compared to the Pringle maneuver and its use is typically reserved for patients with tumor extension into the IVC. In such complex resections, it has been combined with hypothermic portal perfusion and venovenous bypass to mitigate the risks of hypotension and hepatic ischemia; however the reported mortality is high.[244,245] To avoid the hemodynamic effects of THVE, selective hepatic vascular exclusion (SHVE), which involves clamping the hepatic veins instead of the IVC, may be employed by the surgeon.[246] Some studies have shown that SHVE results in fewer complications than THVE; however it is technically demanding and has a limited role in uncomplicated hepatic resections.[247,248]

LOW CENTRAL VENOUS PRESSURE

While the Pringle maneuver occludes inflow to the liver, retrograde flow through the hepatic veins can still lead to substantial venous hemorrhage. The pressure in the hepatic veins is directly related to vena caval pressure, hence the strategy of maintaining a low CVP (<5 mm Hg) to minimize intraoperative blood loss.[249] Retrospective

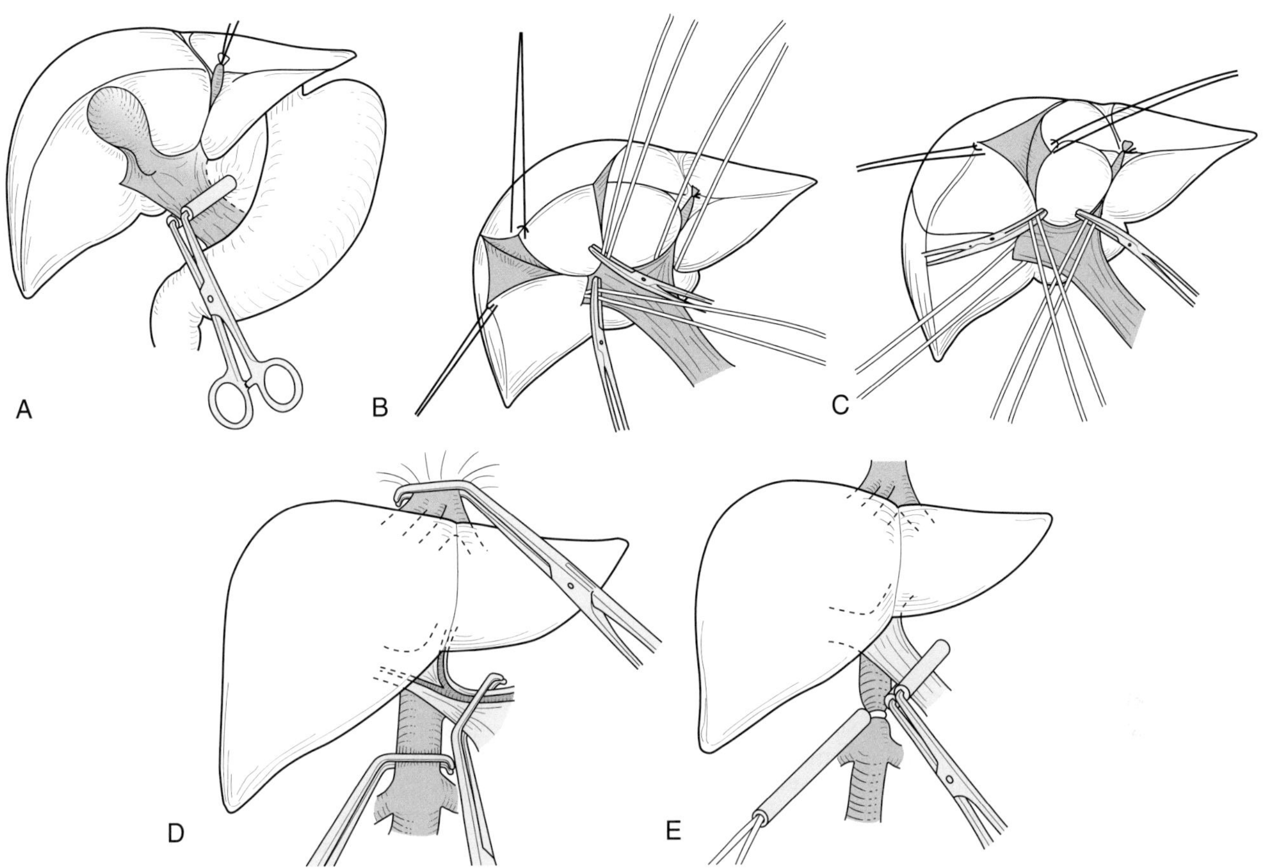

Fig. 16.7 (A–E) Vascular occlusion techniques in hepatic surgery. Surgical vascular occlusive techniques to reduce hemorrhage during hepatic resection include the Pringle maneuver (7A) during which a clamp is placed across the hepatoduodenal ligament to occlude hepatic arterial and portal venous inflow to the liver. Selective hepatic vascular exclusion (7B and C) involves clamping of the vessels perfusing the hemi-liver which is being resected. Total hepatic vascular exclusion (7D) is achieved by clamping the inferior vena cava above and below the liver along with the hepatoduodenal ligament. Another technique combines the application of a clamp across the infrahepatic IVC clamp with one across the hepatoduodenal ligament (7E). *IVC*, Inferior vena cava. (From Otsubo T. Control of the inflow and outflow system during liver resection. *J Hepatobiliary Pancreat Sci.* 2012;19:15–18.)

observational studies have reported reduced blood loss in patients managed with CVP less than 5 mm Hg without any significant adverse events.[250-253] Two randomized controlled trials comparing patients with CVP under 5 mm Hg with liberal volume administration have shown reductions in both intraoperative blood loss and the need for transfusion.[254,255] These studies have all been at risk for significant bias. Furthermore, in some of the trials the difference in estimated blood loss, though statistically significant, was clinically inconsequential.[256] Although standard practice in hepatic resections is to maintain low CVP, some studies have found no association between CVP and intraoperative blood loss. In retrospective studies of patients undergoing donor hepatectomies, no correlation was found between the CVP and intraoperative blood loss. This finding may be due to the fact that living liver donors are healthy patients with normal livers.[257,258] The largest of these studies consisted of over 900 patients. Although it found no correlation between CVP and estimated blood loss, nearly all of the patients were managed with CVPs less than 10 mm Hg, and the majority had CVPs in the 4 to 6 mm Hg range.[258]

A number of techniques have been described for reducing CVP during hepatic resection. The most commonly reported approach is the use of intraoperative fluid restriction with rates of 1 mL/kg/h. Vasopressors are used as needed to maintain SBP over 90 mm Hg and urine output more than 25 mL/h. Though seldom required, vasodilation using nitroglycerin or morphine, or forced diuresis with furosemide, can be instituted if fluid restriction is insufficient.[250,251,254,255,259] The use of milrinone, reverse Trendelenburg position, and epidural anesthesia have also been described, though there is insufficient data to recommend one particular approach.[256,260-262]

Clamping of the infrahepatic IVC (IIVC) has been described as a means of minimizing hemorrhage in the setting of an elevated CVP despite the interventions described earlier (see Fig. 16.7E).[263] A number of randomized controlled trials have demonstrated a significant reduction in blood loss and transfusion with the use of IIVC clamping in patients who tolerate the clamp or have a CVP greater than 5 mm Hg.[262,264-268] A metaanalysis of these trials, comprising of 714 patients, showed a significant reduction in intraoperative blood loss (mean difference −353 mL) with no difference in the rates of postoperative complications. Of note, in pooled analysis, there was no significant difference in reported CVP values between the two groups.[269]

OTHER APPROACHES TO REDUCE BLOOD LOSS

Two multicenter, randomized, placebo-controlled trials have examined the efficacy of prophylactic recombinant Factor VIIa (rFVIIa) administration to reduce transfusion patients undergoing hepatic resection. The studies found no benefit of prophylactic rFVIIa with respect to mortality, red blood cell transfusions, or adverse events.[270,271] A single randomized, controlled trial in 214 patients undergoing primarily minor hepatic resections (82% of cases) found that the administration of tranexamic acid (TXA) resulted in fewer transfusions and less blood loss compared to placebo. In the study group, 500 mg of TXA was administered intravenously prior to incision followed by 250 mg every 6 hours for 3 days.[272]

A recent Cochrane database analysis of 67 randomized clinical trials of methods to decrease blood loss during liver resection found a high risk of bias in all trials. Based on the outcomes that were available in more than one trial, there is low-quality evidence that the "clamp and crush" parenchymal resection technique may be associated with fewer adverse events than radiofrequency resection techniques. They reported very low quality evidence that blood loss, operating time, and total hospital stay were reduced with intraoperative low CVP management.[273]

ANESTHETIC MANAGEMENT

The anesthetic management of these cases should be tailored to the comorbidities of the patients, the surgical approach (open, laparoscopic), the anticipated extent of resection, and the need for vascular occlusive maneuvers. Adequate venous access should be obtained for the anticipated degree of hemorrhage. In cases where significant blood loss is anticipated, red blood cell salvage can be used and consideration should be given to the use of acute normovolemic hemodilution. In addition to standard ASA monitors, intra-arterial blood pressure monitoring should be used in cases during which significant hemorrhage or the need for vascular occlusion maneuvers is anticipated. Central venous catheters may be inserted for both vascular access and CVP monitoring, although some high-volume centers forgo the routine use of CVP monitoring.[274,275] Peripheral venous pressure monitoring may be considered as an alternative. Values are obtained through transduction of an antecubital vein and have been shown to correlate with the CVP in patients undergoing hepatic resection.[276,277] Stroke volume variation (SVV) has been investigated as an alternative to CVP for volume management in patients undergoing liver resection. A study of patients undergoing donor hepatectomy showed an SVV value ≤6% to be predictive of blood loss over 700 mL.[278] In two studies, targeting SVV values greater than 12% to 15% in patients undergoing open or laparoscopic hepatic resection yielded blood loss comparable to, or better than, maintaining low CVP.[279,280] In a study using milrinone to reduce CVP, SVV of 9% yielded a favorable surgical field. No correlation with CVP was noted in this study, possibly due to the lusitropic effects of milrinone.[281] The use of transesophageal echocardiography may be considered in patients with cardiac risk factors, although care must be taken in the presence of significant esophageal varices.

Hepatic resection may be associated with hemorrhage and, in extensive cases, the development of coagulopathy. There is insufficient data to recommend the routine use of viscoelastic hemostatic assays (rotational thromboelastography (TEG) or rotational thromboelastometry). A single randomized, controlled trial of TEG-guided transfusion in cirrhotic patients with coagulopathy (INR > 1.8 and/or platelet count <50 × 10^9/L) undergoing invasive procedures found a significant reduction in blood product administration with TEG compared to the standard lab value–based group. However, only half of the patients enrolled in the trial were undergoing procedures associated with greater than 3% risk of hemorrhage.[282]

With respect to pain management, thoracic epidural analgesia is a highly effective means of pain control for hepatic resection.[283,284] Although its use for this purpose has been described in a number of case series, it remains controversial due to the development of postoperative coagulopathy and thrombocytopenia following hepatic resection and the associated risk of epidural hematoma.[276,285-288] Postoperative coagulopathy and thrombocytopenia occur in 21% to 100% of patients undergoing liver resection, depending on the volume of tissue resected. The INR peaks around postoperative day (POD) one or two while the platelet count is lowest on POD three or four. The values typically return to baseline by POD four or five; however in some patients they may remain elevated for up to a week, leading to delays in epidural catheter removal or the decision to transfuse FFP to facilitate catheter removal.[276,285-289] An additional concern is the accidental dislodgment of the epidural catheter while the patient is coagulopathic which has been reported to occur in up to 7% of patients.[276,286] The degree of coagulopathy is influenced by the extent of the resection. In a review of 759 patients undergoing hepatic resection, the incidence of coagulopathy was 39.1% in patients who had undergone major hepatectomies (>2 segments) versus 21.3% in patients who had undergone minor hepatectomies (≤2 segments).[289] Other factors that are independently associated with postoperative coagulopathy included preexisting cirrhosis, preoperative INR ≥ 1.3, preoperative platelet count <150,000/μL, estimated blood loss ≥ 1000 mL, and the duration of surgery.[285,287,289] Although no case series has reported the complication of an epidural hematoma, epidural hematoma is quite rare and the numbers of published cases may have been inadequate to detect its occurrence.[290,291]

Rapid sequence induction should be considered in patients with significant ascites. Maintenance of general anesthesia has been described with both volatile anesthetics and intravenous anesthetics. There is no compelling clinical evidence for the benefit of one specific agent over another.[292-294] Regardless of the approach, anesthetic dosing should be titrated to the patient's requirements, taking into account the pharmacokinetics and pharmacodynamics of common anesthetic agents in patients with liver disease. The anesthesiologist should understand the vascular occlusion strategies that may be employed during the operation along with their hemodynamic effects. The Pringle maneuver, both during open and laparoscopic hepatic resections, leads to an increase in MAP and systemic vascular resistance and a decrease in CO.[295,296] During open hepatic resection, portal triad clamping leads to a decrease in left ventricular (LV) end-diastolic area (i.e., LV preload). During laparoscopic hepatic resection, in the presence of pneumoperitoneum, PTC also increases LV end-systolic wall stress (i.e., LV afterload).[297]

ENHANCED RECOVERY AFTER SURGERY AND LIVER RESECTION

A number of randomized controlled trials have been conducted comparing the use of enhanced recovery after surgery (ERAS) protocols with traditional management in patients undergoing both open and laparoscopic liver resections.[250,298-301] Although ERAS Society consensus guidelines exist, these trials differed with respect to the number and nature of ERAS elements.[302] Most incorporated preoperative education, early enteral nutrition, and early mobilization. The implementation of an ERAS protocol for liver resection surgery has been shown to reduce minor adverse events, hospital length of stay, hospital cost, and to improve patient quality of life. A metaanalysis published by the Cochrane group found that the use of ERAS protocols resulted in a reduction in mild adverse events, hospital length of stay, and cost. However, all studies were at high risk of bias and the quality of available evidence was determined to be low.[303]

Acknowledgment

The editors and publisher would like to thank Drs. Phillip S. Mushlin and Simon Gelman for contributing a chapter on this topic in the prior edition of this work. It has served as the foundation for the current chapter.

**Complete references available online at expertconsult.com.**

References

1. Molina DK, et al. *Am J Forensic Med Pathol.* 2015;36(3):182.
2. Molina DK, DiMaio VJM. *Am J Forensic Med Pathol.* 2012;33(4):368.
3. Pryce JW, et al. *BMC Clin Pathol.* 2014;14:(18).
4. Abdel-Misih SRZ, Bloomston M. *Surg Clin North Am.* 2010;90(4):643.
5. van Gulik TM, van den Esschert JW. *HPB (Oxford). England*; 2010;12:81.
6. Juza RM, Pauli EM. *Clin Anat.* 2014;27(5):764.
7. Strasberg SM. *J Hepatobiliary Pancreat.* 2005;12(5):351.
8. Strasberg SM, Phillips C. *Ann Surg.* 2013;257(3):377.
9. Bismuth H. Revisiting liver anatomy and terminology of hepatectomies. *Ann Surg.* 2013;257(3):383.
10. Poisson J, et al. *J Hepatol.* 2017;66(1):212.
11. Blouin A, et al. *J Cell Biol.* 1977;72(2):441.
12. Treyer A, Müsch A. *Physiol.* 2013;3(1):243.
13. T K. Metabolic Zonation of the Liver: The Oxygen Gradient Revisited; 2018. PubMed - NCBI. https://phstwlp2.partners.org:2052/pubmed/28126520.
14. Geerts A. *Semin Liver Dis.* 2001;21(3):311.
15. Tsuchida SL, Friedman T. Mechanisms of Hepatic Stellate Cell Activation; 2018. PubMed - NCBI. https://phstwlp2.partners.org:2052/pubmed/28487545.
16. Li P, et al. *Mol Immunol.* 2017;85:222.
17. Robinson MW, et al. *Cell Mol Immunol.* 2016;13(3):267.
18. Lau AH, Thomson AW. *Gut.* 2003;52(2):307.
19. Njoku DB. *Int J Mol Sci.* 2014;15(4):6990.
20. Almazroo OA, et al. *Clin Liver Dis.* 2017;21(1):1.
21. Trefts E, et al. *Curr Biol.* 2017;27(21):r1151.
22. Adeva-Andany MM, et al. *Biosci Rep.* 2016;36(6).
23. Nguyen P, et al. *J Anim Physiol Anim Nutr (Berl).* 2008;92(3):272.
24. Boyer JL. *Compr Physiol.* 2013;3(3):1035.
25. Roberts MS, et al. *Clin Pharmacokinet.* 2002;41(10):751.
26. Malik MY, et al. *Drug Metab Rev.* 2016;48(2):281.
27. Borowski M, et al. *J Biol Chem.* 1986;261(4):1624.
28. Dimova EY, Kietzmann T. *Thromb Haemost.* 2008;100(6):992.
29. Cesarman-Maus G, Hajjar KA. *Br J Haematol.* 2005;129(3):307.
30. Stein PE, et al. Update Review of the Acute Porphyrias; 2018.PubMed – NCBI. https://phstwlp2.partners.org:2052/pubmed/?term=27982422.
31. Sticova E, Jirsa M. *World J Gastroenterol.* 2013;19(38):6398–6407.
32. Ganz T, Nemeth E. *Biochim Biophys Acta.* 2012;1823(9):1434.
33. Yakar S, et al. *J Clin Invest.* 2002;110(6):771.
34. Lu H, et al. *Hypertens Res.* 2016;39(7):492.
35. Jelkmann W. *Eur J Gastroenterol Hepatol.* 2001;13(7):791.
36. Habib S, et al. Approach to jaundice and abnormal liver function test results. In: Sanyal AJ, et al., ed. *Zakim and Boyer's Hepatol: A Textbook of Liver Disease.* 7th ed. Philadelphia, PA: Elsevier; 2018:99–116.
37. Pratt DS. Liver chemistry and function tests. In: Feldman M, et al. ed. *Sleisenger and Fordtran's Gastrointestinal and Liver Disease: Pathophysiology, Diagnosis, Management.* 10th ed. Philadelphia: Saunders; 2016:1243–1253.
38. Kwo PY, et al. *Am J Gastroenterol.* 2017;112(1):18.
39. Eminler AT, Ayyildiz T, Irak K, et al. AST/ALT ratio is not useful in predicting the degree of fibrosis in chronic viral hepatitis patients. *Eur J Gastroenterol Hepatol.* 2015;27(12):1361.
40. Maina I, et al. *Jrnl App Lab Med.* 2016;1(2):119.
41. Redick JA, et al. *J Biol Chem.* 1982;257(24):15200.
42. Siddique A, Kowdley KV. *Clin Liver Dis.* 2012;16(2):199.
43. Fargo MV, et al. *Am Fam Physician.* 2017;95(3):164.
44. Liang TJ, Hepatitis B. The virus and disease. *Hepatology.* 2009; 49(suppl 5):13.
45. AASLD/IDSA HCV Guidance Panel. *Hepatology.* 2015;62(3):932.
46. Fourati S, et al. *J Int AIDS Soc.* 2018;21(suppl 2):e25058.
47. Freiman JM, et al. *Ann Intern Med.* 2016;165(5):345.
48. Ajisaka H, et al. *J Surg Oncol.* 2003;84(2):89.
49. Fujioka M, et al. *Hepatology.* 2001;34(6):1128.
50. Sugimoto H, et al. *Liver Int.* 2003;23(1):38.
51. Wong RJ, et al. *Clin Liver Dis.* 2015;19(2):309.
52. Song P, et al. *World J Gastroenterol.* 2016;22(1):262.
53. Yuen M, Lai C. *Best Pract Res Clin Gastroenterol.* 2005;19(1):91.
54. Tapper EB, Lok AS. *N Engl J Med.* 2017;377(23):2296.
55. Bolondi G, et al. *World J Gastroenterol.* 2016;22(26):5936.
56. Guerrini GP, et al. *Prog Transplant.* 2018;28(1):63.
57. Lin C, et al. *Intern Med.* 2008;47(7):569.
58. Younossi ZM, et al. *Hepatology.* 2018;68(1):349.
59. Sakka SG. *Curr Opin Crit Care.* 2007;13(2):207.
60. Denaro CP, et al. *Ther Drug Monit.* 1998;20(1):78.
61. Jover R, et al. *Am J Gastroenterol.* 1997;92(10):1905.
62. Wahlländer A, et al. *J Hepatol.* 1990;10(2):129.
63. Everson GT, et al. *Hepatology.* 2012;55(4):1019.
64. Chow PKH, et al. *J Surg Res.* 2003;112(1):1.
65. Helmke S, et al. *Curr Opin Gastroenterol.* 2015;31(3):199.
66. Kang HK, et al. *Radiographics.* 2002;22(5):1053.
67. Sharma S, et al. *World J Gastroenterol.* 2014;20(45).
68. Iranpour P, et al. *Ultrasonography.* 2016;35(1):3.
69. Barr RG, et al. *Radiology.* 2015;276(3):845.
70. Younossi ZM, et al. *Hepatology.* 2018;68(1):349.
71. Tang A, et al. *Radiology.* 2018;286(1):29.
72. Bialecki ES, Di Bisceglie AM. *HPB (Oxford).* 2005;7(1):26.
73. Pollock G, Minuk GY. *J Gastroenterol Hepatol.* 2017;32(7):1303.
74. Popper H, Schaffner F. Pathophysiology of cholestasis. *Hum Pathol.* 1970;1(1):1.
75. EASL. *J Hepatol.* 2009;51(2):237.
76. Lleo A, et al. *Hepatol Int.* 2017;11(6):485.
77. Boonstra K, et al. *J Hepatol.* 2012;56(5):1181.
78. Trivedi HD, et al. *Frontline Gastroenterol.* 2017;8(1):29.
79. Poupon RE, et al. *N Engl J Med.* 1991;324(22):1548.
80. Corpechot C, et al. *Hepatology.* 2008;48(3):871.
81. Hirschfield GM, et al. *Gastroenterol.* 2015;148(4):61.e8.
82. Lens S, et al. *Liver Int.* 2014;34(2):197.
83. Rautiainen H, et al. *Hepatology.* 2005;41(4):747.
84. Karlsen TH, et al. *J Hepatol.* 2017;67(6):1298.
85. Scaglione S, et al. *J Clin Gastroenterol.* 2015;49(8):690.
86. Tsochatzis EA, et al. *Lancet.* 2014;383(9930):1749.
87. Garcia-Pagan JC, et al. *J Hepatol.* 2012;57(2):458.
88. Runyon BA. *Hepatology.* 2013;57(4):1651.
89. De Robertis R, et al. *World J Gastroenterol.* 2014;20(23):7231.
90. Garcia-Tsao G, et al. *Hepatology.* 2017;65(1):310.
91. D'Amico G, et al. *J Hepatol.* 2018;68(3):563.
92. Ripoll C, et al. *Gastroenterology.* 2007;133(2):481.
93. Ripoll C, et al. *J Hepatology.* 2009;50(5):923.
94. Abraldes JG, et al. *Clin Liver Dis.* 2014;18(4):779.

95. Shi KQ, et al. *Liver Int.* 2013;33(1):62.
96. Vilgrain V, et al. *Gastrointest Radiol.* 1990;15(3):218.
97. Zipprich A, et al. *Liver Int.* 2012;32(9):1407.
98. Gluud LL, Krag A, et al. *Cochrane Database Syst Rev.* 2012;8:CD004544.
99. Shah HA, et al. *J Hepatol.* 2014;60(4):757.
100. D'Amico G, et al. *Gastroenterology.* 2006;131(5):1611.
101. Carvalho GC, et al. *Ann Hepatol.* 2012;11(1):90.
102. Martin–Llahi M, et al. *Gastroenterology.* 2011;140(2):496.e4.
103. Angeli P, et al. *J Hepatol.* 2015;62(4):968.
104. de Mattos AZ, et al. *Ann Hepatol.* 2016;15(4):474.
105. Boyer TD, et al. *Liver Transpl.* 2011;17(11):1328.
106. Nolte W, et al. *Hepatology.* 1998;28(5):1215.
107. Montagnese S, et al. *Metab Brain Dis.* 2004;19(3–4):281.
108. Vilstrup H, et al. *Hepatology.* 2014;60(2):715.
109. Swanson KL, et al. *Hepatology.* 2005;41(5):1122.
110. Krowka MJ, et al. *Transplantation.* 2016;100(7):1440.
111. Iyer VN, et al. *Hepatology.* 2013;57(6):2427.
112. Schiffer E, et al. *Am J Transplant.* 2006;6(6):1430.
113. Simonneau G, et al. *J Am Coll Cardiol.* 2013;62(suppl 25):34.
114. Krowka MJ, et al. Portopulmonary hypertension: Results from a 10–year screening algorithm. *Hepatology.* 2006;44(6):1502.
115. Swanson KL, et al. *Am J Transplant.* 2008;8(11):2445.
116. Malagari K, et al. *Hepatogastroenterology.* 2005;52(62):558.
117. Machicao VI, et al. *Hepatology.* 2014;59(4):1627.
118. GBD 2016 Risk Factors Collaborators. *Lancet.* 2017;390(10100): 1151.
119. Forner A, et al. *Lancet.* 2018;391(10127):1301.
120. Heimbach JK, et al. *Hepatology.* 2018;67(1):358.
121. Poon RT, et al. *Ann Surg.* 2002;235(3):373.
122. Mazzaferro V, et al. *N Engl J Med.* 1996;334(11):693.
123. Lautt WW. *Am J Physiol.* 1985;249(5 Pt 1):549.
124. Gelman S, et al. *Anesthesiology.* 1984;61(6):726.
125. Frink EJ Jr, et al. *Anesthesiology.* 1992;76(1):85.
126. Hartman JC, et al. *Can J Anaesth.* 1992;39(8):877.
127. Cullen SC, Gross EG. *Science.* 1951;113(2942):580.
128. Goto T, et al. *Br J Anaesth.* 1998;80(2):255.
129. Wappler F, et al. *Anesthesiology.* 2007;106(3):463.
130. Schmidt M, et al. *Anaesthesia.* 2001;56(12):1154.
131. Iber T, et al. *Minerva Anestesiol.* 2008;74(10):511.
132. Reinelt H, et al. *Acta Anaesthesiol Scand.* 2002;46(6):713.
133. Wilke HJ, et al. *Transplant Proc.* 2011;43(7):2683.
134. Servin F, et al. *Br J Anaesth.* 1990;65(2):177.
135. Pandele G, et al. *Anesthesiology.* 1983;59(2):123.
136. van Beem H, et al. *Anaesthesia.* 1983;38(Suppl):61.
137. Duvaldestin P, et al. *Acta Anaesthesiol Scand.* 1991;35(2):159.
138. Carmichael FJ, et al. *Anesthesiology.* 1993;79(5):1051.
139. Wouters PF, et al. *Anesth Analg.* 1995;81(1):125.
140. Zhu T, et al. *Can J Anaesth.* 2008;55(6):364.
141. Meierhenrich R, et al. *Anaesthesia.* 2010;65(11):1085.
142. Leslie K, et al. *Anesth Analg.* 1995;80(5):1007.
143. Runciman WB, et al. *Br J Anaesth.* 1990;65(3):353.
144. Sear JW, et al. *Br J Anaesth.* 1994;72(4):451.
145. MacGilchrist AJ, et al. *Gut.* 1986;27(2):190.
146. Weerink MAS, et al. *Clin Pharmacokinet.* 2017;56(8):893.
147. Mazoit JX, et al. *Anesth Analg.* 1987;66(4):293.
148. Klotz U, et al. *Clin Pharmacol Ther.* 1974;16(4):667.
149. Ferrier C, et al. *Anesthesiology.* 1985;62(4):480.
150. Haberer JP, et al. *Br J Anaesth.* 1982;54(12):1267.
151. Chauvin M, et al. *Anesth Analg.* 1989;68(1):1.
152. Dershwitz M, et al. *Anesthesiology.* 1996;84(4):812.
153. Devlin JC, et al. *Br J Anaesth.* 1993;71(2):227.
154. Viby–Mogensen J, Hanel HK. *Acta Anaesthesiol Scand.* 1978;22(4): 371.
155. De Wolf AM, et al. *Br J Anaesth.* 1996;76(5):624.
156. Lebrault C, et al. *Anesthesiology.* 1985;62(5):601.
157. Khalil M, et al. *Anesthesiology.* 1994;80(6):1241.
158. Duvaldestin P, et al. *Br J Anaesth.* 1978;50(11):1131.
159. Fujita A, et al. *Acta Anaesthesiol Taiwan.* 2014;52(2):54.
160. Tanaka N, et al. *Anesth Analg.* 1997;85(2):286.
161. Meierhenrich R, et al. *Anesth Analg.* 2009;108(4):1331.
162. Trepenaitis D, et al. *Medicina (Kaunas).* 2010;46(7):465.
163. Kortgen, et al. *Eur J Anaesthesiol.* 2009;26(2):111.
164. Friedman LS. *Trans Am Clin Climatol Assoc.* 2010;121:204. discussion 205.
165. de Goede B, et al. *Best Pract Res Clin Gastroenterol.* 2012;26(1):47.
166. Csikesz NG, et al. *J Am Coll Surg.* 2009;208(1):96.
167. Lin CS, et al. *Br J Surg.* 2013;100(13):1784.
168. Farnsworth N, et al. *Am J Surg.* 2004;188(5):580.
169. Neeff HP, et al. *Surgery.* 2014;155(4):623.
170. Telem DA, et al. *Clin Gastroenterol Hepatol.* 2010;8(5):7. quz e58.
171. Hoteit MA, et al. *World J Gastroenterol.* 2008;14(11):1774.
172. Pantel HJ, et al. *J Gastrointest Surg.* 2016;20(8):1511.
173. Pugh RN, et al. *Br J Surg.* 1973;60(8):646.
174. Garrison RN, et al. *Ann Surg.* 1984;199(6):648.
175. Mansour A, et al. *Surgery.* 1997;122(4):6.
176. Kiamanesh D, et al. *Br J Anaesth.* 2013;111(suppl 1):50.
177. Malinchoc M, et al. *Hepatology.* 2000;31(4):864.
178. Kamath PS, et al. *Hepatology.* 2001;33(2):464.
179. Suman A, et al. *Clin Gastroenterol Hepatol.* 2004;2(8):719.
180. Befeler AS, et al. *Arch Surg.* 2005;140(7):4. discussion 655.
181. Northup PG, et al. *Ann Surg.* 2005;242(2):244.
182. Teh SH, et al. *Gastroenterol.* 2007;132(4):1261.
183. Biggins SW, et al. *Gastroenterology.* 2006;130(6):1652.
184. Luca A, et al. *Liver Transpl.* 2007;13(8):1174.
185. Cho HC, et al. *Eur J Gastroenterol Hepatol.* 2011;23(1):51.
186. Kim DH, et al. *ANZ J Surg.* 2014;84(11):832.
187. Bhangui P, et al. *J Hepatol.* 2012;57(4):874.
188. Kim TH, et al. *Liver Int.* 2015;35(3):713.
189. Boyer TD, Haskal ZJ. *Hepatology.* 2010;51(1):306.
190. Parker R. *Clin Liver Dis.* 2014;18(2):319.
191. Monescillo A, et al. *Hepatology.* 2004;40(4):793.
192. Suhocki PV, et al. *Semin Intervent Radiol.* 2015;32(2):123.
193. Chana A, et al. *BJA Education.* 2016;16(12):405.
194. DeGasperi A, et al. *J Clin Monit Comput.* 2009;23(6):341.
195. Modha K, et al. *Cardiovasc Intervent Radiol.* 2018;41(4):564.
196. Suhocki PV, et al. *Semin Intervent Radiol.* 2015;32(2):123.
197. Dimick JB, et al. *Arch Surg.* 2003;138(2):185.
198. Aragon RJ, Solomon NL. *J Gastrointest Oncol.* 2012;3(1):28.
199. Kneuertz PJ, et al. *J Gastrointest Surg.* 2012;16(9):1727.
200. Chang CM, et al. *Medicine (Baltimore).* 2014;93(12):e59.
201. Wakabayashi G, et al. *Ann Surg.* 2015;261(4):619.
202. Abu Hilal M, et al. *Ann Surg.* 2018;268(1):11.
203. Ciria R, et al. *Ann Surg.* 2016;263(4):761.
204. Fretland AA, et al. *Ann Surg.* 2018;267(2):199.
205. Cauchy F, et al. *Br J Surg.* 2015;102(7):785.
206. Goh BK, et al. *Surg Endosc.* 2015;29(9):2636.
207. Nota CL, et al. *HPB (Oxford).* 2016;18(2):113.
208. Montalti R, et al. *World J Gastroenterol.* 2015;21(27):8441.
209. Capussotti L, et al. *Eur J Surg Oncol.* 2005;31(9):986.
210. Reddy SK, et al. *Hepatology.* 2012;56(6):2221.
211. van Lienden KP, et al. *Cardiovasc Intervent Radiology.* 2013;36(1):25.
212. Kamiyama T, et al. *J Am Coll Surg.* 2010;211(4):443.
213. Aramaki O, et al. *J Hepatobiliary Pancreat Sci.* 2014;21(8):585.
214. Katz SC, et al. *Ann Surg.* 2009;249(4):617.
215. McNally SJ, et al. *HPB (Oxford).* 2012;14(4):236.
216. Nanashima A, et al. *Surg Today.* 2013;43(5):485.
217. Janny S, et al. *HPB (Oxford).* 2015;17(4):357.
218. Fujimoto J, et al. *Arch Surg.* 1993;128(9):1065.
219. Matot I, et al. *Anesthesiol.* 2002;97(4):794.
220. Jarnagin WR, et al. *Ann Surg.* 2008;248(3):360.
221. Frankel TL, et al. *J Am Coll Surg.* 2013;217(2):210–220.
222. Imamura H, et al. *Arch Surg.* 2003;138(11):1206. discussion 1206.
223. Grazi GL, et al. *Ann Surg.* 2001;234(1):71.
224. Huntington JT, et al. *J Surg Oncol.* 2014;109(2):81.
225. Jiang B, et al. *Hepatol Res.* 2018;48(8):635.
226. Pringle JHV. *Ann Surg.* 1908;48(4):541.
227. Kim YI. *J Hepatobiliary Pancreat.* 2003;10(3):195.
228. Hoekstra LT, et al. *Dig Surg.* 2012;29(1):35.
229. Torzilli G, et al. *Ann Surg.* 2012;255(2):270.
230. Beck–Schimmer B, et al. *Ann Surg.* 2008;248(6):909.
231. Beck–Schimmer B, Breitenstein S, Bonvini JM, et al. *Ann Surg.* 2012;256(5):5.
232. Man K, et al. *Ann Surg.* 1997;226(6):3.
233. Man K, et al. *Br J Surg.* 2003;90(2):183.
234. Capussotti L, et al. *Br J Surg.* 2006;93(6):685.
235. Lee KF, et al. *Br J Surg.* 2012;99(9):1203.
236. Lee KF, et al. *World J Surg.* 2018.
237. Hanyong S, et al. *Eur J Surg Oncol.* 2015;41(2):243.
238. Makuuchi M, et al. *Surg Gynecol Obstet.* 1987;164(2):155.
239. Figueras J, et al. *Ann Surg.* 2005;241(4):582.

240. Liang G, et al. *HepatoGastroenterology*. 2009;56(91–92):745.
241. Fu SY, et al. *Am J Surg*. 2011;201(1):62.
242. Ni JS, et al. *J Gastrointest Surg*. 2013;17(8):1414.
243. Huguet C, et al. *Surg Gynecol Obstet*. 1978;147(5):689.
244. Belghiti J, et al. *Ann Surg*. 1996;224(2):155.
245. Azoulay D, et al. *Ann Surg*. 2015;262(1):93.
246. Elias D, et al. *Br J Surg*. 1995;82(11):1535.
247. Smyrniotis VE, et al. *Am J Surg*. 2002;183(2):173.
248. Smyrniotis VE, et al. *World J Surg*. 2003;27(7):765.
249. Melendez JA, et al. *J Am Coll Surg*. 1998;187(6):620.
250. Jones RM, et al. *Br J Surg*. 1998;85(8):1058.
251. Smyrniotis V, et al. *Am J Surg*. 2004;187(3):398.
252. Bui LL, et al. *HPB (Oxford)*. 2002;4(1):5.
253. Chen H, et al. *J Gastrointest Surg*. 2000;4(2):162.
254. Wang WD, et al. *World J Gastroenterol*. 2006;12(6):935.
255. Liu Y, et al. *Chin–Germ J Clin Oncol*. 2008;7:7.
256. Hughes MJ, et al. *HPB (Oxford)*. 2015;17(10):863.
257. Chhibber A, et al. *Liver Transpl*. 2007;13(4):537.
258. Kim YK, et al. *Acta Anaesthesiol Scand*. 2009;53(5):601.
259. Melendez JA, et al. *J Am Coll Surg*. 1998;187(6):620.
260. Ryu HG, et al. *Am J Transplant*. 2010;10(4):877.
261. Sand L, et al. *Acta Anaesthesiol Scand*. 2011;55(9):1106.
262. Rahbari NN, et al. *Ann Surg*. 2011;253(6):1102.
263. Otsubo T, et al. *Surgery*. 2004;135(1):67.
264. Chen XP, et al. *Langenbecks Arch Surg*. 2006;391(3):209.
265. Kato M, et al. *World J Surg*. 2008;32(6):1082.
266. Zhu P, et al. *Br J Surg*. 2012;99(6):781.
267. Zhou YM, et al. *Medicine (Baltimore)*. 2016;95(27):e4159.
268. Ueno M, et al. *Surgery*. 2017;161(6):1502.
269. Fancellu A, et al. *J Gastrointest Surg*.2018;22(5):941.
270. Lodge JP, Jonas S, Oussoultzoglou E, et al. *Anesthesiology*. 2005;102(2):269.
271. Shao YF, et al. *Am J Surg*. 2006;191(2):245.
272. Wu CC, et al. *Ann Surg*. 2006;243(2):173.
273. Moggia E, et al. *Cochrane Database Syst Rev*. 2016;10:CD010683.
274. Wax DB, et al. *Eur J Surg Oncol*. 2016;42(10):1608.
275. Niemann CU, et al. *Liver Transpl*. 2007;13(2):266.
276. Choi SJ, et al. *Liver Transpl*. 2007;13(10):1414.
277. Stephan F, et al. *Acta Anaesthesiol Scand*. 2008;52(3):388.
278. Kim YK, et al. *Transplant Proc*. 2011;43(5):1407.
279. Ratti F, et al. *HPB (Oxford)*. 2016;18(2):136.
280. Dunki–Jacobs EM, et al. *Ann Surg Oncol*. 2014;21(2):473.
281. Lee J, et al. *Anesth Analg*. 2017;125(2):423.
282. De Pietri L, et al. *Hepatol*. 2016;63(2):566.
283. Schreiber KL, et al. *Reg Anesth Pain Med*. 2016;41(4):460.
284. Ali M, et al. *Br J Anaesth*. 2010;104(3):292.
285. Matot I, et al. *Anesth Analg*. 2002;95(5):81.
286. Tsui SL, et al. *Anaesth Intensive Care*. 2004;32(5):630.
287. Yuan FS, et al. *J Clin Anesth*. 2012;24(5):398.
288. Elterman KG, Xiong Z. *J Anesth*. 2015;29(3):367.
289. Jacquenod P, et al. *Anesth Analg*. 2018;126(4):1142.
290. Christie IW, McCabe S. *Anaesthesia*. 2007;62(4):335.
291. Cook TM, et al. *Br J Anaesth*. 2009;102(2):179.
292. Ko JS, et al. *Transpl Int*. 2010;23(7):736.
293. Toprak HI, et al. *Transplant Proc*. 2012;44(6):1635.
294. Ko JS, et al. *Liver Transpl*. 2008;14(8):1150.
295. Decailliot F, et al. *Br J Anaesth*. 2001;87(3):493.
296. Delva E, et al. *Anesth Analg*. 1987;66(9):864.
297. Decailliot F, et al. *Anesth Analg*. 2005;100(3):864.
298. Ni CY, et al. *Eur J Surg Oncol*. 2013;39(6):542.
299. Qi S, et al. *J Clin Lab Anal*. 2018:e22434.
300. He F, et al. *Clin Transl Oncol*. 2015;17(9):694.
301. Liang X, et al. *Surg Endosc*. 2018;32(6):2746.
302. Melloul E, et al. *World J Surg*. 2016;40(10):2425.
303. Bond–Smith G, et al. *Cochrane Database Syst Rev*. 2016;2:CD011382.

17 Renal Anatomy, Physiology, Pharmacology, and Evaluation of Function

RICHARD M. PINO and ABRAHAM SONNY

KEY POINTS

- A molecule in the plasma must pass in succession through the endothelial fenestration, glomerular basement membrane (GBM), and epithelial slit diaphragm to cross the filtration barrier and enter the tubular fluid. The capillary endothelium restricts the passage of cells, while the GBM restricts albumin and larger molecules. The negatively charged glycoproteins of the GBM limit the passage of other negatively charged proteins. Thus, the filtration barrier is size selective and charge selective. The epithelial cells maintain the integrity of this capillary bed by producing several key signaling molecules and endocytosis of membrane receptors.
- A primary determinant of glomerular filtration rate (GFR) is glomerular filtration pressure, which depends on renal artery perfusion pressure and the balance between afferent and efferent arteriolar tone. With decreases in afferent arteriolar pressure or blood flow, mediators such as catecholamines, angiotensin II, and arginine vasopressin (AVP) constrict efferent arterioles to maintain glomerular filtration pressure. This is reflected by an increase in GFR.
- Tubuloglomerular feedback is a critical mechanism for renal autoregulation. When GFR is increased, distal tubular NaCl delivery is enhanced and the increase in chloride concentration is sensed by the macula densa to trigger the renin-angiotensin cascade. The result is afferent arteriolar vaso constriction as efferent arteriolar vasoconstriction increases GFR. Autoregulation enables the kidney to maintain solute and water regulation independently of wide fluctuations in arterial blood pressure. Tubular water reabsorption determines urinary flow rate and is closely related to the hydrostatic pressure in the peritubular capillaries. Hypotension of any cause results in decreased urinary flow rate that may be correctable only when arterial blood pressure is restored toward normal.
- The tubule has an enormous capacity for reabsorption of water and NaCl. Each day, 180 L of protein-free glomerular ultrafiltrate is formed, of which almost 99% of the water and 99% of the sodium is reabsorbed. The ability of the kidney to concentrate urine is dependent on the interaction of at least three processes: (1) generation of a hypertonic medullary interstitium by the countercurrent mechanism and urea recycling, (2) concentration and then dilution of tubular fluid in the loop of Henle, and (3) the action of AVP, also known as antidiuretic hormone, in increasing water permeability in the last part of the distal tubule and collecting ducts. The juxtaglomerular apparatus provides an important regulating system for arterial blood pressure, salt, and water homeostasis.
- The interactions of the sympathoadrenal axis, renin-angiotensin-aldosterone system, and AVP will respond to hypotension and hypovolemia by promoting vasoconstriction and the retention of salt and water. Prostaglandins and natriuretic peptides facilitate vasodilation and the excretion of salt and water excretion when there is hypertension and hypervolemia.
- Plasma osmolality is tightly controlled. The threshold for AVP secretion by the neurohypophysis between 280 and 290 mOsm/kg. Even mild dehydration results in rapid antidiuresis, and urine osmolality can increase from 300 to 1200 mOsm/kg. Decreases in intravascular volume stimulate AVP secretion.
- Serum creatinine reflects the balance between creatinine production from muscle and creatinine excretion by the kidney, which is dependent on GFR. Creatinine generation rate varies with muscle mass, physical activity, protein intake, and catabolism. However, when these processes are in equilibrium and renal function is stable, serum creatinine is a useful marker of GFR. The relationship between serum creatinine and GFR is inverse and exponential. A doubling of the serum creatinine implies a halving of GFR.

Introduction

The kidney exemplifies an exquisite structure-function relationship to regulate intravascular volume, osmolality, acid-base and electrolyte balance, and to excrete end products of metabolism and drugs. The kidney also produces hormones involved with fluid homeostasis (renin, prostaglandins, kinins), bone metabolism (1,25-dihydroxycholecalciferol) and hematopoiesis (erythropoietin).[1] In addition to these multiple roles in the healthy patient, almost every systemic disease will affect renal function. This chapter will describe the normal anatomy and physiology of the kidney and the basics for the clinical evaluation of renal function.

Organization of the Kidney

THE NEPHRON

The fundamental unit of the kidney is the nephron (Figs. 17.1 and 17.2). The nephron is composed of a vascular network close to a series of tubules with distinct physiologic functions that empty into collecting ducts to form urine. There are approximately 1 million nephrons in the normal kidney. The kidneys receive about 20% of the cardiac output and are responsible for 7% of total body oxygen consumption, although they account for only 0.5% of the total body weight.[2] Afferent arterioles from the renal arteries branch extensively to supply the renal and peritubular capillaries. Kidney disease can result from perturbations of these vascular, glomerular, and tubular components (see Chapter 42). Knowledge of these factors is important to the anesthesiologist to limit decrements in renal function during the perioperative period.

The kidney is divided into an outer layer, the cortex, which receives 85% to 90% of the renal blood flow (RBF), and an inner medulla (see Fig. 17.1). In the cortex are glomeruli (see Figs. 17.2 and 17.3), tufts of capillaries originating from afferent arterioles. The glomerular capillary endothelial cells have fenestrations that are barriers to red blood cells but allow the transit of plasma proteins and smaller molecules (Fig. 17.4). Their glycocalyx is an anionic barrier that repels large macromolecules and albumin. Knowledge of this is through experimental studies and diseases where albuminuria is seen after alteration of anionic sites in the glomerular basement membrane (GBM).[3,4] During development, these capillaries invaginate epithelial cells to form tufts of visceral epithelial cells with footlike morphologies called podocytes that are rich in actin cytoskeletons. These podocytes anchor to the GBM, closely interdigitate, and envelope the renal capillaries (Fig. 17.5). A thin membrane called the slit diaphragm has an ultrastructural zipper-like complex that spans the space between each of the foot processes of the podocytes.[5] Additional epithelial cells and their extravascular matrix make up the parietal

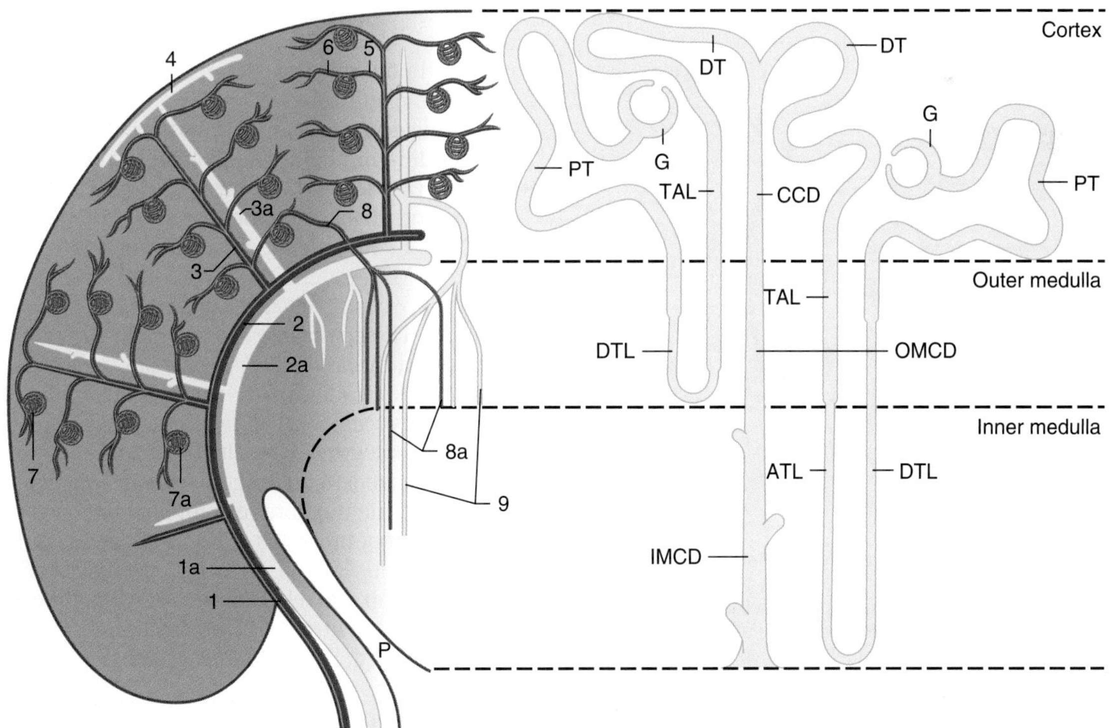

Fig. 17.1 Anatomic relationships of the nephron and the renal vasculature. The left side of the diagram represents the renal vasculature as distributed through the inner medulla, outer medulla, and cortex. Arteries are drawn as solid lines, veins as hollow tubes. The renal artery divides serially into interlobar arteries (1), arcuate arteries (2), and interlobular arteries (3). The afferent arterioles (5) branch off laterally and provide the capillary tufts of the renal glomeruli in the outer cortex (7a), whose efferent arterioles (6) supply the cortical capillary network (not shown). In the juxtamedullary zone (7b), the efferent arterioles become the vasa recta, which are closely applied to the long loops of Henle (8, 8a, 9). The venous drainage consists of stellate veins (4), interlobular veins (3a), arcuate veins (2a), and interlobar veins (1a). (Modified from Kriz W, Bankir L. A standard nomenclature for structures of the kidney. The Renal Commission of the International Union of Physiological Sciences (IUPS). *Kidney Int.* 1988;33[1]:1–7.)

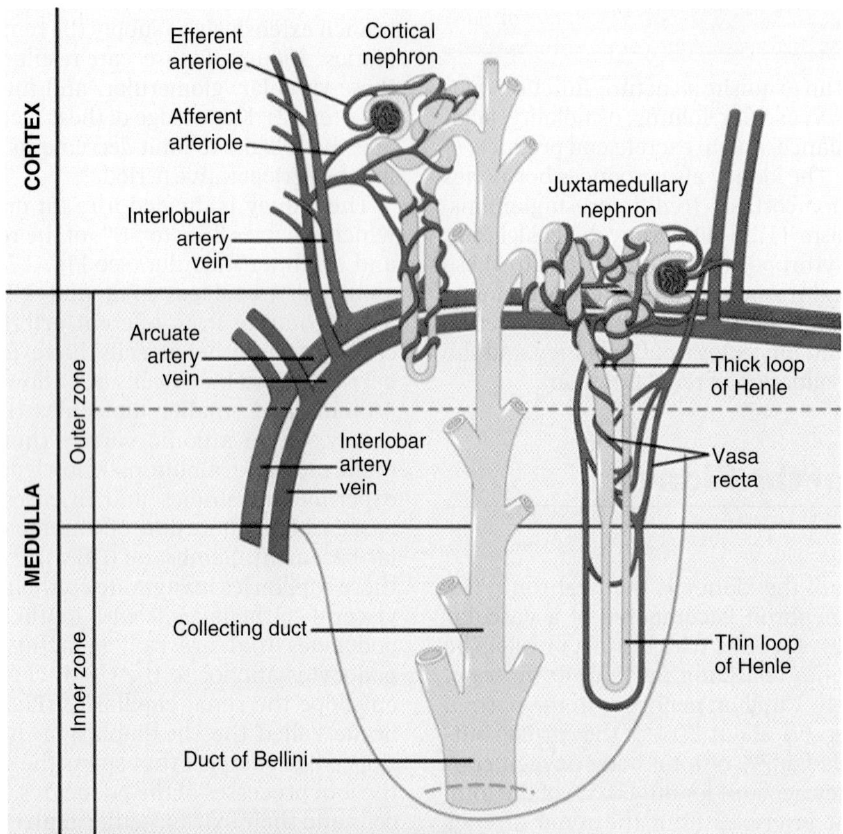

Fig. 17.2 Schematic of relations between blood vessels and tubular structures. (Redrawn from Hall JE. *Guyton and Hall Textbook of Medical Physiology*. 13th ed. Philadelphia: Elsevier; 2016.)

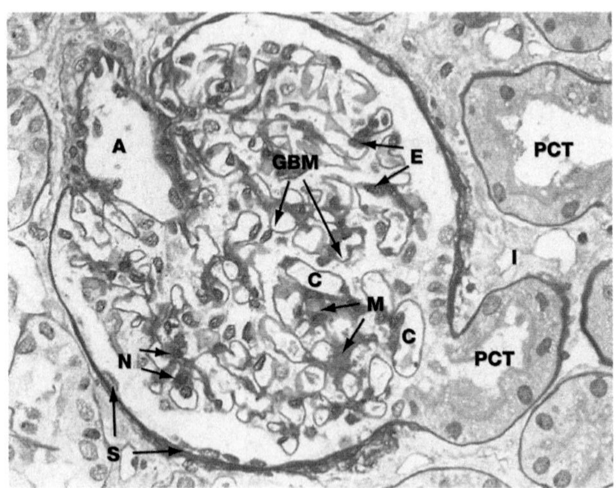

Fig. 17.3 Glomerulus. An afferent arteriole *(A)* enters the glomerulus and divides into numerous capillaries *(C)* adjacent to the glomerular basement membrane *(GBM)*. The squamous epithelial cells *(S)* lining Bowman space lead to the cuboidal proximal convoluted tubules *(PCT)* with brush borders. *E*, Nuclei of endothelial cells; *M*, mesangium; *N*, nuclei of mesangial cells. (From Young B, Woodford P, O'Dowd G. Urinary system. In: *Wheaton's Functional Histology. A Text and Colour Atlas*. 6th ed. Philadelphia: Elsevier Churchill Livingstone; 2014.)

epithelium that lines a pouch-like cistern, called Bowman space, which is the beginning of the renal tubular system.

The vasculature of the kidney is unique in that it has two capillary beds. Upon leaving the glomerulus, the glomerular capillary then forms the efferent artery that in turn leads to an anastomosing network of 10 to 25 long peritubular capillaries called vasa recta. The vasa recta are close around the ascending limb of the loop of Henle before anastomosis into veins that leave the kidney (see Fig. 17.2).

The endothelial and epithelial cells synthesize proteins that are essential components of the filtration barrier of the kidney, the GBM (see Fig. 17.5).[6] The GBM is rich in the anionic glycosaminoglycan heparin sulfate, Type IV collagen, and laminin.[6,7] The epithelial cells maintain the integrity of this capillary bed by producing several key molecules including vascular endothelial growth factor[8] and families of signaling proteins and receptors. The transmembrane protein nephrin supports the integrity of the slit pore diaphragms and its maintenance is dependent on the endocytosis of slit diaphragm proteins and plasma membrane components.[7,9,10] The interplay between the foot processes of the podocytes, slit diaphragms, and organization of the actin intracellular scaffolds is centered on nephrin and related proteins.[11] The functions of these numerous factors are often elucidated in experiential studies when found as etiologies of renal disease.[7,11]

THE RENAL TUBULES

The kidneys receive 20% of the total cardiac output but extract relatively little oxygen. The renal arteriovenous oxygen difference is only 1.5 mL/dL. However, there is marked dissimilarity between the renal cortex and medulla with regard to blood flow, oxygen delivery, and oxygen consumption (Table 17.1). The medulla receives only 6% of the

RBF and has an average oxygen tension (PO_2) of 8 mm Hg. Thus, severe hypoxia could develop in the medulla despite a relatively adequate total RBF; the metabolically active medullary thick ascending loop of Henle (mTAL) is particularly vulnerable.[12]

The terminology of the renal tubular system is based on morphology as seen with light microscopy. The system begins with the proximal convoluted tubule (PCT) that starts as a continuation of the parietal epithelium of the nephron (see Fig. 17.3). A high density of mitochondria and the extensive surface area of the apical (referred as the brush border) and basilar cell membranes mark the renal tubules and indicate high-energy requirements. In normal kidneys, 80% of the energy is required for Na^+/K^+-ATPase that maintains the osmotic gradient needed for the resorption of filtered molecules (Fig. 17.6).[2] In spite of this high-energy demand, the tubular system is supplied by only 10% to 15% of the RBF and is a key etiology for acute tubular necrosis after hypotension (see Chapter 42).

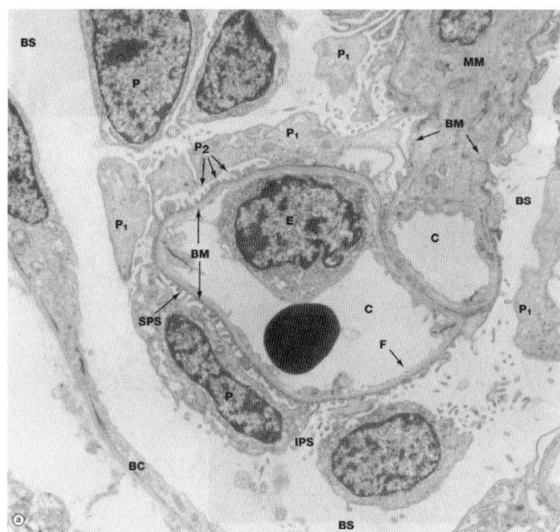

Fig. 17.4 Electron micrograph of glomerulus. The several glomerular capillaries *(C)* are lined by fenestrated endothelial cells. The podocytes *(P)* give rise to foot processes *(P_1, P_2)* that rest on the glomerular basement membrane *(BM)*. Mesangial cells *(M)* support the capillary loops. Bowman space *(BS)* is delineated by the podocyte bodies on one side and the parietal epithelial cells on the other. *E*, Nucleus of capillary; *IPS* interpodocyte space; *MM*, mesangial matrix; *SPS*, subpodocyte space. (From Young B, Woodford P, O'Dowd G. Urinary system. In: *Wheaton's Functional Histology. A Text and Colour Atlas*. 6th ed. Philadelphia: Elsevier Churchill Livingstone; 2014.)

A distal short straight length of the proximal tubule leads to the thinner epithelium of the descending thin limb of the loop of Henle. This makes a hairpin 180-degree turn to ascend toward the cortex and eventually becomes the medullary thick ascending limb of the loop of Henle (mTAL) and distal convoluted tube (see Fig. 17.2). Seventy to 80% of nephrons begin in the cortex and have short loops of Henle that enter only the outer margin of the medulla. The remaining juxtamedullary nephrons start at the corticomedullary junction and have elongated loops of Henle that descend into the most distal extent of the medulla. At the end of the distal tubule is the juxtaglomerular apparatus that is comprised of specialized epithelial cells, called the macula densa (by virtue of light microscopic image), cells of the afferent glomerular arteriole, and mesangial cells (Fig. 17.7). The juxtaglomerular apparatus is essential for the maintenance of blood pressure, as described later. The most distal end of the nephron is the collecting duct that empties the ultrafiltrate into the renal pelvis and then the ureters.

FORMATION OF URINE

Urine is formed by the interaction of three processes: glomerular filtration, tubular reabsorption, and tubular secretion.

Glomerular Filtration

The formation of the glomerular filtrate is dependent on the balance of Starling forces regulating fluid flux across the filtration barrier.[13] Central to this process is the pressure difference between the afferent and efferent arteries (Fig. 17.8). The hydrostatic pressure in the glomerular

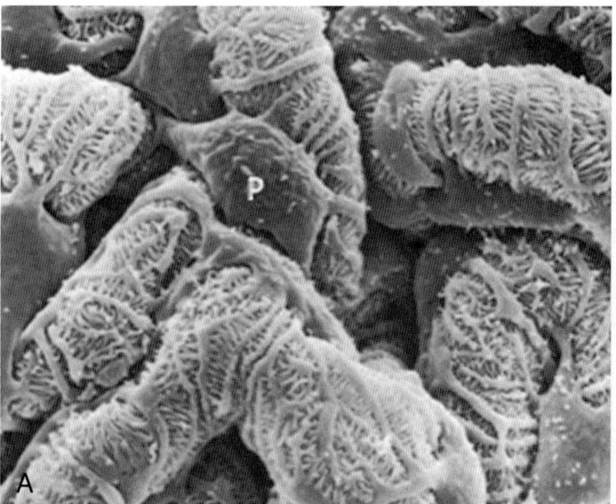

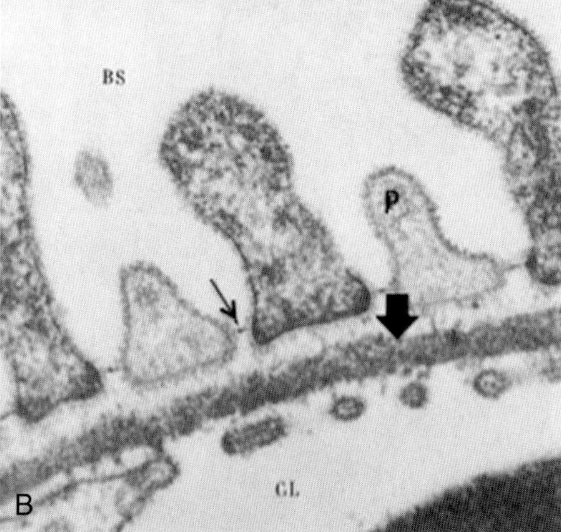

Fig. 17.5 (A) Scanning electron micrograph of podocytes *(P)* and their processes. (B) Electron micrograph of podocyte processes (P), the glomerular basement membrane, and glomerular capillaries. Slit diaphragms *(arrow)* span the podocyte processes. Large arrow points to the lamina densa of the glomerular basement membrane. *BS*, Bowman space; *CL*, glomerular capillary lumen. (Modified from Gartner LP. Urinary system. In: *Textbook of Histology*. 4th ed. Philadelphia: Elsevier; 2017.)

capillaries is 60 mm Hg, which is three times higher than in most capillary beds. This pressure difference drives plasma across the endothelial and epithelial filtration barriers (Table 17.2). A delicate balance in pressure maintenance is necessary because reduced pressures will decrease filtration, as increased pressures may cause renal damage. The glomerular filtration rate (GFR) depends upon the glomerular capillary pressure that is opposed by the hydrostatic pressure in Bowman space and the colloid osmotic pressure within the glomerular capillaries (Figs. 17.8 and 17.9). In healthy patients, the colloid osmotic pressure in Bowman

TABLE 17.1 Distribution of Renal Blood Flow Between Cortex and Medulla

	Cortex	Medulla*
Percentage of renal blood flow	94	6
Blood flow (mL/min/g)	5.0	0.03
PO2 (mm Hg)	50	8
O2 extraction ratio (VO2/DO2)	0.18	0.79

*The renal medulla receives only a small fraction of the total renal blood flow, and flow rates are extremely slow. As a result, the tissue oxygen tension is extremely low, and the medulla extracts almost 80% of the oxygen delivered to it. A very mild reduction in total and cortical renal blood flow may therefore induce ischemia and hypoxia in the renal medulla. *DO_2*, Oxygen delivery; *O_2*, oxygen; *PO_2*, oxygen tension; *VO_2*, oxygen consumption.
Data from Brezis M, Rosen S, Epstein F. The pathophysiological implications of medullary hypoxia. *Am J Kidney Dis*. 1989;13:253–258.

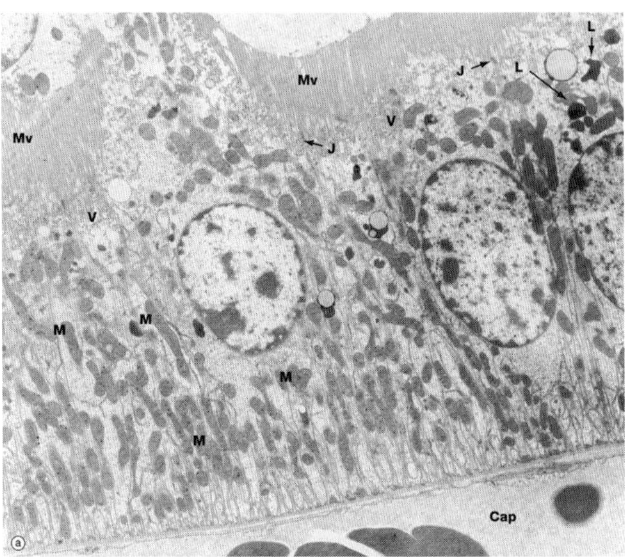

Fig. 17.6 Proximal convoluted tubule. The apical surface of the proximal convoluted tubule epithelium is marked by tall microvilli *(Mv)* that are seen as the brush border in light micrographs. The cytoplasm at the basal surface is filled with mitochondria *(M)* that are reflective of the high oxygen requirement needed for the maintenance of the basal lateral Na^+/K^+ ATPase. *Cap*, tubular capillary; *J*, tight intercellular junction; *L*, lysosome; *V*, vesicle. (From Young B, Woodford P, O'Dowd G. Urinary system. In: *Wheaton's Functional Histology. A Text and Colour Atlas*. 6th ed. Philadelphia: Elsevier Churchill Livingstone; 2014.)

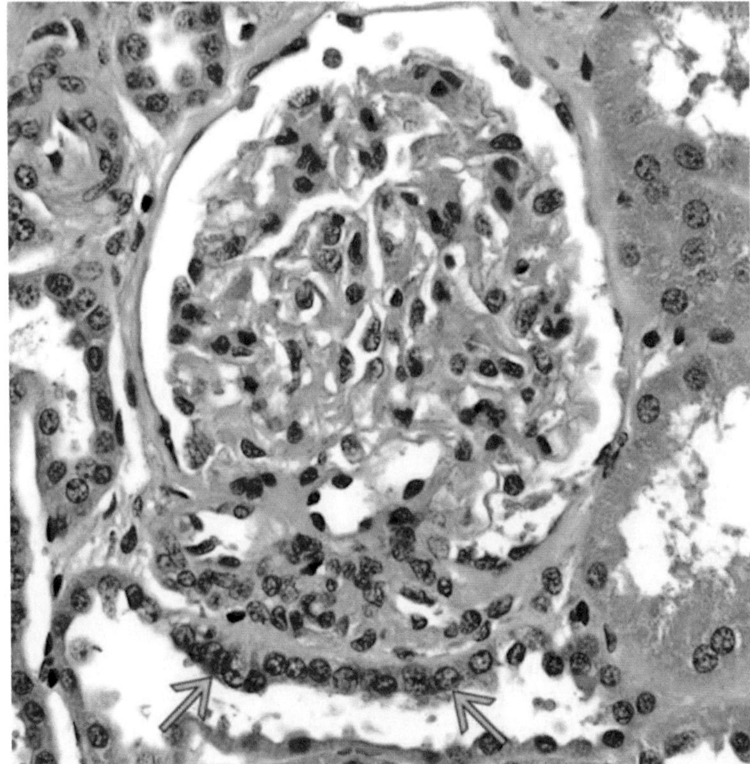

Fig. 17.7 The macula densa *(arrows)*. The cells of the macula densa represent a special portion of the distal tubule that is adjacent to the juxtaglomerular apparatus. (From Genitourinary and male genital tract. In: Lindberg MR, Lamps LW, eds. *Diagnostic Pathology: Normal Histology*. 2nd ed. Philadelphia: Elsevier; 2018.)

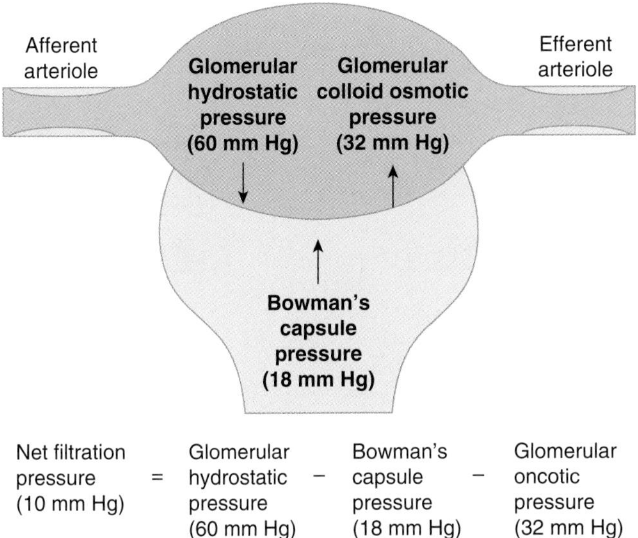

Fig. 17.8 Summary of forces causing filtration by the glomerular capillaries. (Redrawn from Hall JE. *Guyton and Hall Textbook of Medical Physiology*. 13th ed. Philadelphia: Elsevier; 2016.)

TABLE 17.2 Approximate Pressures and Vascular Resistances in the Circulation of a Normal Kidney

	PRESSURE IN VESSEL (MM HG)		Percent of Total Renal Vascular Resistance
Vessel	**Beginning**	**End**	
Renal artery	100	100	≈0
Interlobar, arcuate, and interlobular arteries	≈100	85	≈16
Afferent arteriole	85	60	≈26
Glomerular capillaries	60	59	≈1
Efferent arteriole	59	18	≈43
Peritubular capillaries	18	8	≈10
Interlobar, arcuate, and interlobular veins	8	4	≈4
Renal vein	4	≈4	≈0

From Hall JE. *Guyton and Hall Textbook of Medical Physiology*. 13th ed. Philadelphia: Elsevier; 2016.

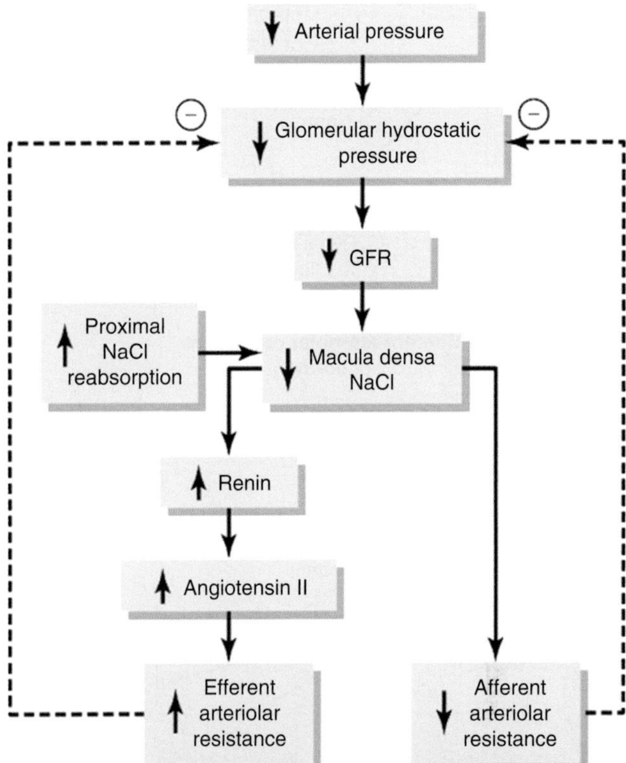

Fig. 17.9 Macula densa feedback mechanism for autoregulation of glomerular hydrostatic pressure and glomerular filtration rate *(GFR)* during decreased renal artery pressure. (Redrawn from Hall JE. *Guyton and Hall Textbook of Medical Physiology*. 13th ed. Philadelphia: Elsevier; 2016.)

Vasoconstrictor Systems	Vasodilator Systems
Sympathoadrenal system Renin-angiotensin system Aldosterone Antidiuretic hormone (ADH)	Prostaglandins Kinins Atrial natriuretic peptide (ANP)
↓ RBF ↓ GFR ↓ Urine flow ↓ Na excretion	↑ RBF ↑ GFR ↑ Urine flow ↑ Na excretion

Fig. 17.10 Neurohormonal renal regulatory systems. *GFR*, Glomerular filtration rate; *Na*, sodium; *RBF*, renal blood flow; ↓, decreased; ↑, increased. Modified from Sladen RN. Effect of anesthesia and surgery on renal function. *Crit Care Clin*. 1987;3(2):380–393.

space is negligible, since the GBM restricts the passage of proteins. The normal GFR is about 180 L/day.

Mediator Control of the Glomerular Filtration Rate

Control of this glomerular capillary pressure is exquisite. Hormones, peptides, and autacoids interact with receptors in the kidney to assure maintenance of RBF and GFR (Fig. 17.10).

α-Adrenergic Effect. The vascular myocytes of afferent and efferent arterioles have the pressure-dependent ability to contract or relax. This prevents increased diuresis, appropriately called pressure diuresis, when the blood pressure is elevated. Mild α-adrenergic stimulation constricts the efferent arteriole that preserves GFR (Fig. 17.11). Severe α-adrenergic activity decreases the filtration fraction by constricting the afferent and efferent arterioles to prevent a flow-induced decrease in GFR. This is the reason norepinephrine administration during sepsis may preserve diuresis. This is important to understand during shock, when the endogenous adrenergic response or the use of α agonists may worsen renal hypoperfusion and decrease the GFR. The kidney is relatively devoid of β2 receptors, so epinephrine release induces predominant vasoconstriction through α receptor or angiotensin activation.

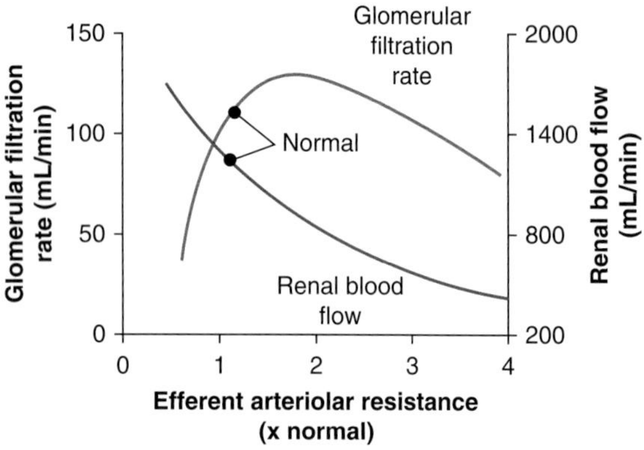

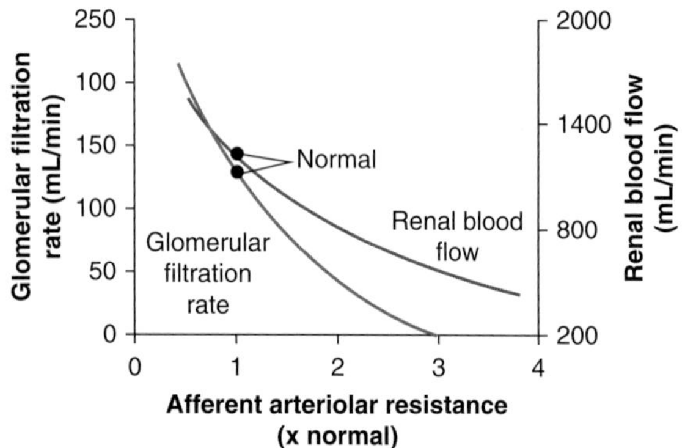

Fig. 17.11 Effect of change in afferent arteriolar resistance or efferent arteriolar resistance on glomerular filtration rate and renal blood flow. (Redrawn from Hall JE. *Guyton and Hall Textbook of Medical Physiology*. 13th ed. Philadelphia: Elsevier; 2016.)

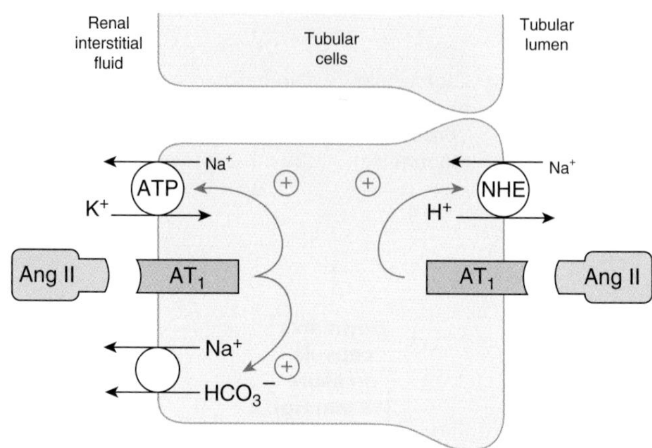

Fig. 17.12 Direct effects of angiotensin II *(Ang II)* to increase proximal tubular sodium reabsorption. Ang II stimulates sodium-hydrogen exchange *(NHE)* on the luminal membrane and the sodium-potassium ATPase transporter and sodium-bicarbonate co-transport on the basolateral membrane. *ATP*, Adenosine triphosphate. (Redrawn from Hall JE. *Guyton and Hall Textbook of Medical Physiology*. 13th ed. Philadelphia: Elsevier; 2016.)

Renin-Angiotensin. Adrenergic stimulation of the juxtaglomerular apparatus releases the enzyme renin from the cells of the macula densa and principal cells of the collecting ducts.[14] Renin, more appropriately called angiotensinogenase, converts the hepatic synthesized glycopeptide angiogensinogen to angiotensin I. Angiotensin-converting enzymes (ACEs) are present in diverse cell types,[12] including leukocytes and smooth muscle. The vascular endothelial cells of the kidney and lung are the major source of ACE that converts angiotensin I to angiotensin II.[12,15-17]

Angiotensin II stimulates two pathways that have opposing effects (Fig. 17.12). The principal receptor is AT_1 that is found on the luminal epithelial surface of the proximal tubular cell (PTC), mTAL, macula densa, distal tubules, and collecting ducts.[14,18] The angiotensin II-AT_1 interaction serves to maintain systemic blood pressure through vasoconstriction, and enhancement of tubular transport mechanisms to reabsorb sodium and water.[14,15,19] The binding of angiotensin II to "non-classical" receptors such as AT_7 opposes these actions and causes vasodilatation through nitric oxide (NO) and prostaglandin-mediated natriuresis, diuresis, and reduced oxidative stress.[19]

Angiotensin II is a potent vasoconstrictor of efferent arterioles, which increases the pressure difference and enhances filtration.[18] This maintains the glomerular filtration fraction in the face of mild to moderate decreases in RBF or perfusion pressure that may result from hypovolemia or systemic hypotension. Angiotensin II promotes systemic vasoconstriction at about one tenth of its renal effect. Renin secretion is stimulated by hypovolemia from hemorrhage, diuresis, or sodium loss/restriction and by reductions in perfusion as seen with positive pressure ventilation, congestive heart failure, sepsis, or cirrhosis with ascites. Angiotensin II feeds back to the juxtaglomerular apparatus to inhibit renin secretion. It also stimulates phospholipase A_2 to trigger the synthesis of vasodilatory prostaglandins.

Prostaglandins and Kinins. Intrarenal prostaglandins play an important role in endogenous renal protection by vasodilating juxtamedullary blood vessels and maintaining inner cortical blood flow.[20] Prostaglandins are called autacoids because, unlike true hormones, they are produced in minute amounts and have a local, evanescent action. Because their structure is based on a 20-carbon fatty acid, they are also referred to as eicosanoids, after *eicosa*, the Greek word for the number 20.

Phospholipase A_2 resides in the inner lipid layer of the cell membrane and controls prostaglandin production through its formation of the prime precursor, arachidonic acid. It is stimulated by ischemia, hypotension, norepinephrine, angiotensin II, and arginine vasopressin (AVP). Thus, the factors that induce and mediate the stress response simultaneously activate prostaglandins, which defend the kidney against their actions. Cyclooxygenase-1 acts on arachidonic acid to form the vasodilator prostaglandins that include PGD2, PGE2, and PGI2 (prostacyclin).[21] Vasodilation is through activation of cyclic adenosine monophosphate (cAMP) to oppose the action of catecholamines, angiotensin II, and AVP. Prostaglandins may be particularly important in decreasing the vasoconstrictor activity of angiotensin II on the afferent arteriole and mesangial cells. Drugs that inhibit prostaglandin synthesis, such as nonsteroidal anti-inflammatory agents, can upset this compensatory mechanism and result in medullary ischemia.

Kinins act directly as vasodilators, as well as stimulate phospholipase A_2, prostacyclin production, and endothelial cell NO formation.[22] Kinins are produced by cleavage of kininogen by the serine protease kallikrein. Over 90% of renal kallikrein is produced by the distal convoluted tubules

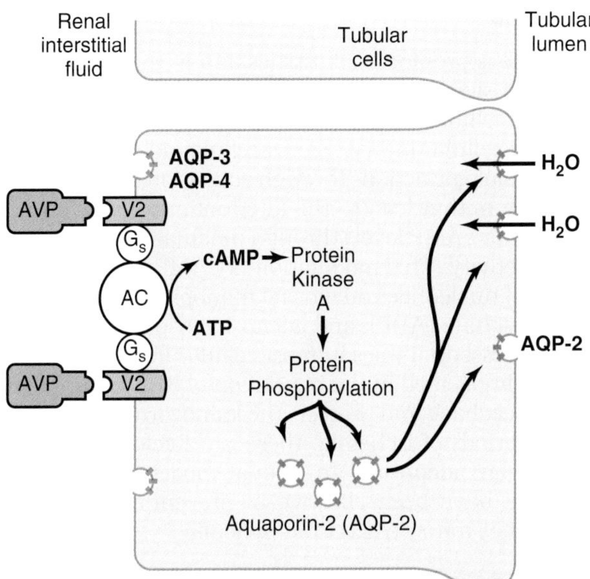

Fig. 17.13 Mechanism of action of arginine vasopressin. Arginine vasopressin *(AVP)* binds to receptors *(V_2)* that are coupled to G proteins *(G_s)* to activate adenylate cyclase *(AC)* and stimulate the formation of cyclic adenosine monophosphate *(cAMP)*. This will then activate protein kinase A to phosphorylate intracellular proteins and allow aquaporin-2 *(AQP-2)* to form water channels at the luminal side of the membrane. Other aquaporins *(AQP-3, AQP-4)* that are not controlled by AVP allow water to exit the cell at the basolateral cell membrane. *ATP*, Adenosine triphosphate. (Redrawn from Hall JE. *Guyton and Hall Textbook of Medical Physiology*. 13th ed. Philadelphia: Elsevier; 2016.)

in the cortex with decreased concentrations from outer to inner zones.[22] Renal kininase, which controls the level of bradykinin, is inhibited by ACE inhibitors and is the reason for angioedema.[23]

Arginine Vasopressin. AVP, also known as antidiuretic hormone (ADH), is produced by the posterior pituitary, and its release is stimulated by hyperosmolality or hypovolemia.[24] By far the most potent trigger for AVP release is systemic arterial hypotension, mediated by aortic and carotid baroreceptors. It overrides all other triggers, and plasma AVP may reach levels 10- to 1000-fold greater than normal. At these concentrations, AVP acts as a vasoconstrictor, especially in the outer renal cortex. It does so by stimulating the V_{1A} receptor that exists on vascular smooth muscle, glomerular mesangial cells, and the vasa recta and promotes vasoconstriction through the phosphatidylinositol pathway.[25] AVP maintains effective glomerular filtration pressure because it is an extremely potent constrictor of the efferent arteriole, and unlike catecholamines and angiotensin, it has little effect on the afferent arteriole, even at high plasma levels.[26] The binding to V_2 receptors on the medullary collecting ducts stimulates adenylate cyclase to form cAMP that enhances aquaporin-2 channels of the principal cells to increase water reabsorption (Fig. 17.13).[24,27] Anesthetics have little direct effect on AVP secretion, except via the changes that they induce in arterial blood pressure, venous volume, and serum osmolality. Surgical stimulation is a major stimulus to AVP secretion. This stress response, whether mediated by pain or by intravascular volume changes, is profound and lasts at least 2 to 3 days after the surgical procedure.

Natriuretic Peptides. Natriuretic peptides dilate vascular smooth muscle through activation of cyclic guanosine monophosphate by blocking the phospholipase C-linked receptors to the actions of norepinephrine and angiotensin II. Atrial natriuretic peptide (ANP)[28] is released from atrial myocytes in response to atrial wall stretch and increased atrial volume, brain (B-type) natriuretic peptide is released in response to cerebral ventricle stretch, and C-type is released from the endothelium of major blood vessels. Urodilatin is secreted by the epithelium of the distal tubules and collecting ducts in response to increases in mean arterial pressure and blood volume.

The natriuretic peptides cause prompt, sustained increases in GFR and glomerular filtration fractions even when RBF is not increased or when arterial pressure is decreased. They promote afferent arteriolar dilatation with or without efferent arteriolar constriction, antagonize endothelin (the endogenous vasoconstrictor peptide produced by vascular endothelial cells), inhibit renin secretion, and decrease angiotensin-stimulated aldosterone. These peptides also inhibit the release of aldosterone in the adrenal cortex and block its actions at the distal tubules and collecting ducts. Moreover, they inhibit the secretion of AVP through their effects on the brain and pituitary, which can lead to an enhanced diuresis. NaCl is resorbed, and diuresis is promoted.[29] These actions are important in oliguric patients (such as those with acute renal failure and chronic renal failure) to increase urine output.

Aldosterone. Aldosterone is a steroid hormone secreted by the zona glomerulosa of the adrenal cortex in response to hyperkalemia or hyponatremia.[30] Angiotensin II and adrenocorticotropic hormone also trigger its release. It acts at the thick ascending limb of the loop of Henle, the principal cells of the distal tubule, and the collecting duct to increase active absorption of sodium and passive absorption of water, culminating in an expanded blood volume. Sodium retention in vessel walls appears to enhance their response to vasoconstrictor agents. In contrast to the immediate sympathetic angiotensin II response to hypovolemia, there is a delay of about 1 to 2 hours from the secretion of aldosterone to its action on sodium reabsorption.

Aldosterone forms a complex with a receptor at the cell membrane in the principal cells of the distal tubule (Fig. 17.14). The aldosterone-receptor complex travels to the cell nucleus, where it induces cytoplasmic transcription of messenger ribonucleic acid. This fosters synthesis of proteins that form sodium channels in the apical cell membrane and enhance the Na^+/K^+/ATPase pump in the basolateral cell membrane.[31] Sodium is transported from the tubular fluid into the peritubular capillary in exchange for potassium. Long-standing stimulation of aldosterone secretion, characteristically induced by the intravascular volume depletion of chronic ascites, culminates in potassium depletion and hypokalemic alkalosis.

The Dopaminergic System

There are at least two subtypes of dopaminergic (DA) receptors.[32] DA1 receptors are present on the renal and splanchnic vasculature and also on the proximal tubule. Stimulation of the DA1 receptor activates cAMP and induces renal vasodilation, increased RBF and GFR, natriuresis, and diuresis. Dopamine inhibits the sodium-hydrogen antiporter system

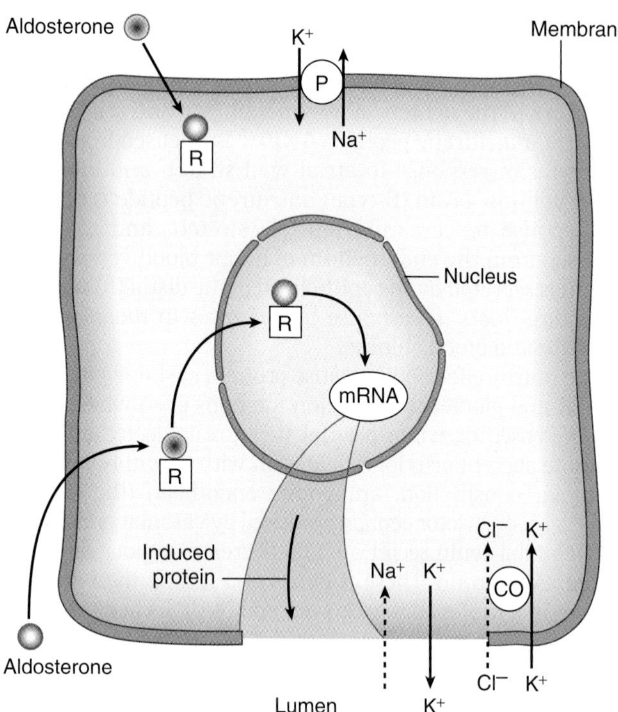

Fig. 17.14 Action of aldosterone. Aldosterone enters the distal tubular cytoplasm and attaches to a receptor, then migrates to the nucleus, where it induces the formation of messenger ribonucleic acid *(mRNA)*. The mRNA in turn induces the synthesis of a protein that enhances the permeability of the apical (luminal) membrane to sodium and potassium. The reabsorption of sodium stimulates the basolateral membrane Na-K-ATPase pump, the intracellular concentration of potassium rises, and it follows its concentration gradient out into the lumen. The net effect of aldosterone's action is sodium reabsorption and potassium loss. *Cl^-*, Chloride; *CO*, cotransporter (= symporter); *K^+*, potassium; *Na^+*, sodium; *P*, sodium-potassium ATPase pump; *R*, receptor. (From Wingard LB, Brody TM, Larner J, et al. Diuretics: drugs that increase excretion of water and electrolytes. In: Wingard LB, Brody TM, Larner J, et al., eds. *Human Pharmacology: Molecular-To-Clinical.* London: Wolfe Publishing Ltd; 1991:249, Fig. 19.4.)

at the brush-border membrane of the proximal tubule and the Na^+/K^+/ATPase pump at the basolateral membrane of the thick ascending limb of the loop of Henle to enhance NaCl reabsorption.

Stimulation of D2 receptors on the presynaptic terminal of postganglionic sympathetic nerves inhibits the release of norepinephrine from presynaptic vesicles to facilitate vasodilation. The DA system plays an integral role in the endogenous vasodilator-natriuresis system and the maintenance of normal blood pressure. Endogenous dopamine constitutively activates the DA2 receptor, which synergistically enhances the activation of the DA1 receptor and inhibits tubular Na^+/K^+-ATPase activity, especially when sodium intake is increased. It also opposes the anti-natriuretic effects of norepinephrine, angiotensin II, and aldosterone. Endogenous ANP acts via the renal dopamine system by recruiting "silent" DA1 receptors from the interior of the cell toward the plasma membrane and also enhances dopamine accumulation.[32,33]

Urinary dopamine excretion is increased with salt loading; decreased DA activity may contribute to the pathogenesis of idiopathic edema, which manifests as retention of salt and water in the upright position. There is evidence that the endogenous dopamine system is activated in compensated cirrhosis and helps to maintain renal sodium excretion.[32,33]

Adenosine

Adenosine is present in all tissues and in the extracellular space as a signaling molecule. It plays a role during conditions of cellular distress such as hypoxia, inflammation, and acute cellular injury.[34] Extracellular adenosine mainly exerts its biologic actions through activation of four adenosine receptors that lead to the attenuation or activation of intracellular cAMP levels through modulation of adenylate cyclase activity. This modulation of cAMP affects the production of nucleotides adenosine monophosphate, adenosine diphosphate (ADP), and adenosine triphosphate (ATP) that have essential roles in most cellular functions.[34] Adenosine is implicated in the regulation of RBF by tubuloglomerular feedback and protects the kidney from ischemia.[35] During periods of ischemia, there is a fivefold increase in extracellular adenosine. In animal models, receptors for adenosine have been effective in preventing or treating acute kidney injury (AKI) from ischemia.[35]

Nitric Oxide

Endogenous NO is a potent vasodilator of vascular smooth muscle. It is produced in many nephron segments including the cortical and medullary thick ascending limb of the loop of Henle (mTAL).[36] During oxidative stress, reactive oxygen species (ROS), including superoxide (O_2^-), hydrogen peroxide (H_2O_2), and the hydroxyl radical (OH), are produced. Under normal conditions, NO minimizes the influence of these ROS. NO acts at multiple points in the citric acid cycle and increases the efficiency of oxygen utilization within the kidney.[36] NO inhibits apical Na^+/H^+ cotransport and basolateral Na^+/K^+-ATPase activity in the proximal tubule, inhibits sodium reabsorption in the mTAL by blocking the $Na^+/K^+/2Cl^-$ cotransporter, and has a direct effect on apical sodium channels of the cortical collecting ducts to inhibit sodium transport.[36,37] NO produced in the epithelial cells of mTAL buffers the vasoconstriction in the medullary circulation in response to sympathetic stimulation and angiotensin II.[38] As for antagonism of O_2^- tubular activity, endogenous NO counteracts the vasoconstrictor effects of O_2^-.

Renal Tubular System Physiology

The renal tubular system compensates for the large glomerular filtration by resorption so that only 1.5 L/day of fluid is excreted as urine. The tubules also conserve and regulate molecules within appropriate physiologic ranges that are freely filtered such as ions, glucose, and amino acids (Table 17.3). Under most conditions, the kidneys excrete more than 95% of the ingested Na^+ at rates that match dietary Na^+ intake.[39] Approximately 65% of filtered sodium, chloride, and water is reabsorbed by the PCTs (Fig. 17.15). In the first segment of the PCT, sodium moves across the apical lumen by cotransport with amino acids, bicarbonate, and glucose and counter-transport mechanisms (Fig. 17.16). This reabsorption increases the concentration of chloride ions to 140 mEq/L from the initial filtrate concentration of 105 mEq/L and favors its diffusion through the intercellular junctions into the interstitial space. Organic acids and bases including waste products of metabolism, such as bile salts and urea, and multiple exogenous molecules are cleared by the PCT. This clearance has additional clinical importance since doses of drugs that are removed by the kidney, such as β-lactam antibiotics, will require dose

TABLE 17.3 Filtration, Reabsorption, and Excretion Rates of Different Substances by the Kidneys

	Amount Filtered	Amount Reabsorbed	Amount Excreted	Percent of Filtered Load Reabsorbed
Glucose (g/day)	180	180	0	100
Bicarbonate (mEq/day)	4,320	4,318	2	>99.9
Sodium (mEq/day)	25,560	25,410	150	99.4
Chloride (mEq/day)	19,440	19,260	180	99.1
Potassium (mEq/day)	756	664	92	87.8
Urea (g/day)	46.8	23.4	23.4	50
Creatinine (g/day)	1.8	0	1.8	0

From Hall JE. *Guyton and Hall Textbook of Medical Physiology*. 13th ed. Philadelphia: Elsevier; 2016.

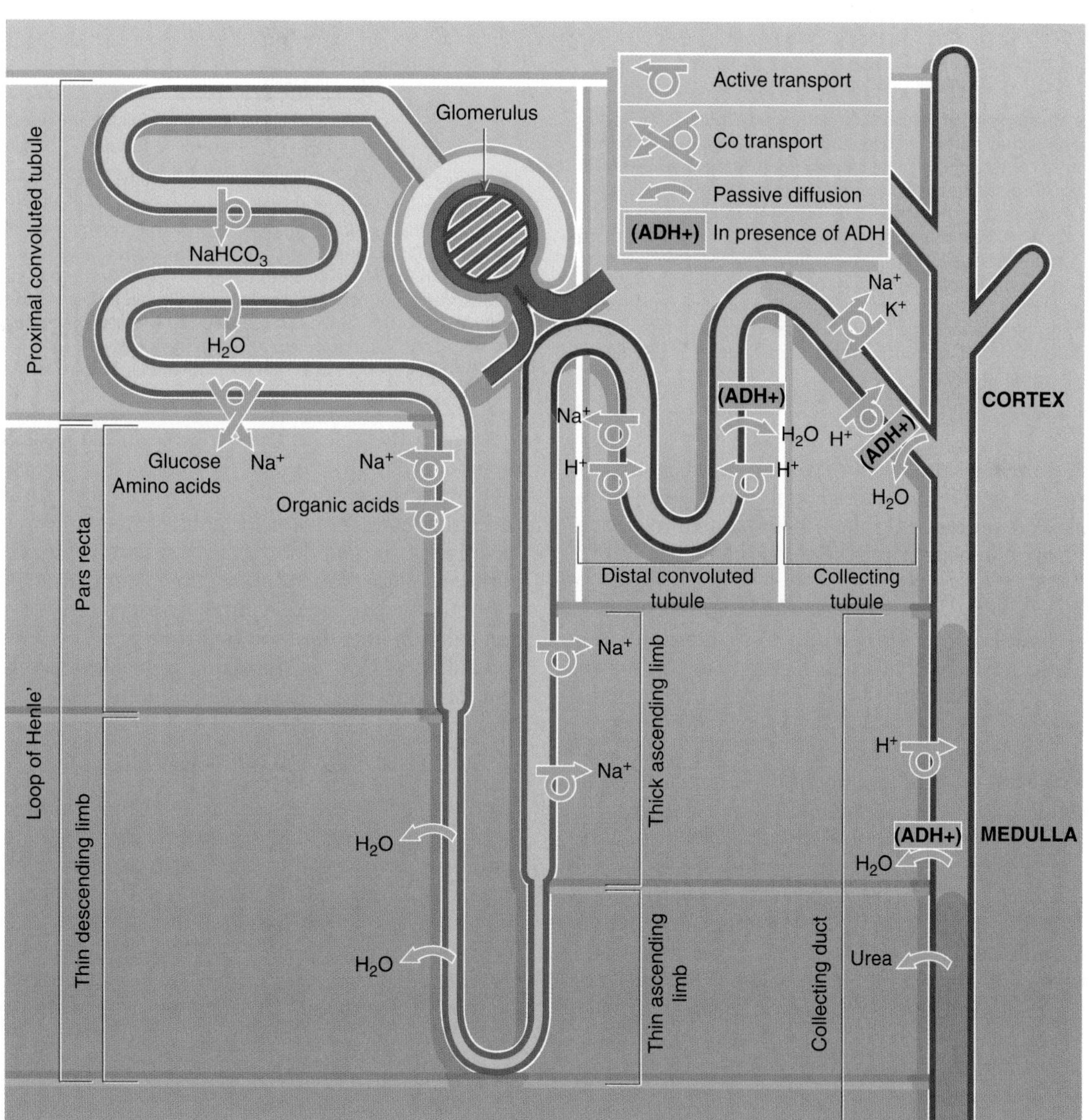

Fig. 17.15 Summary of major activities of different parts of the renal tubule. The ability of the tubule to produce concentrated urine is dependent on the high osmolality of the renal medulla created by the counter-current multiplier mechanism. This is dependent upon the active transport of NaCl in the water-impermeable thick ascending limb of the loop of Henle NaCl, the action of arginine vasopressin (antidiuretic hormone, *ADH*) on the collecting tubule and duct, the high concentration of urea created by passive diffusion, and the reabsorption of water reabsorbed into the hyperosmolar medulla by the vasa recta. (Redrawn from Young B, Woodford P, O'Dowd G. Urinary system. *Wheaton's Functional Histology. A Text and Colour Atlas*. 6th ed. Philadelphia: Elsevier Churchill Livingstone; 2014.)

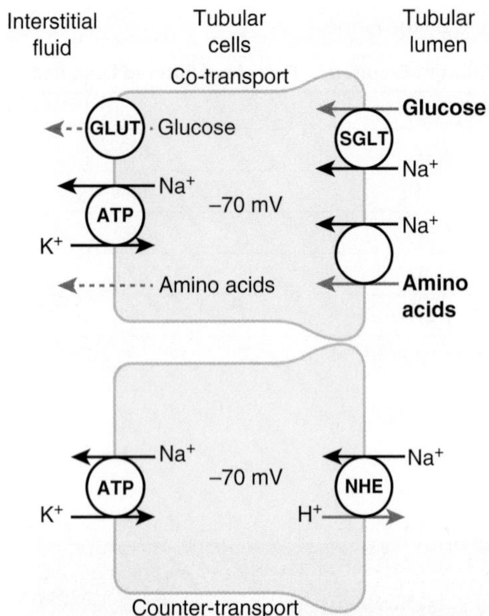

Fig. 17.16 Mechanism of secondary active transport. The upper cell shows the cotransport of glucose and amino acids along with Na^+ through the apical side of the tubular epithelial cells followed by facilitated diffusion through the basolateral membranes. The lower cell shows the counter-transport of hydrogen ions from the interior of the cell across the apical membrane and into the tubular lumen. The movement of sodium ions into the cell is down an electrochemical gradient established by the sodium-potassium pump at the basolateral membrane and provides the energy for transport of the hydrogen ions from the inside of the cell into the tubular lumen. *ATP*, Adenosine triphosphate; *GLUT*, glucose transporter; *NHE*, sodium hydrogen exchanger; *SGLT*, sodium-glucose co-transporter. (Redrawn from Hall JE. *Guyton and Hall Textbook of Medical Physiology*. 13th ed. Philadelphia: Elsevier; 2016.)

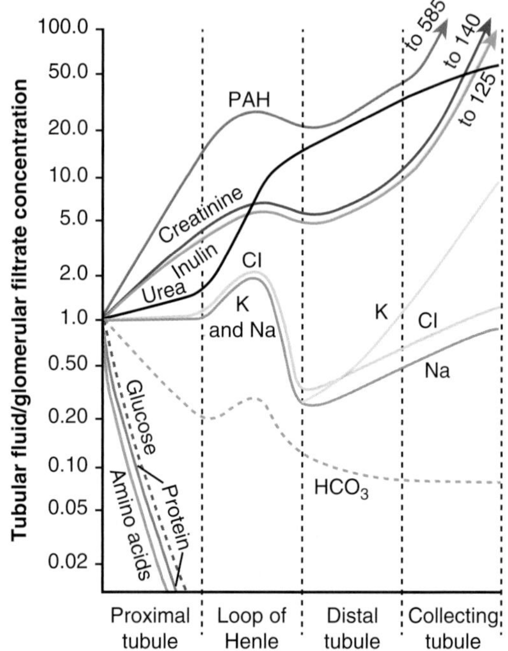

Fig. 17.17 Changes in the average concentrations of different substances at different points in the tubular system relative to the concentration of that substance in the plasma and in the glomerular filtrate. A value of 1.0 indicates that the concentration in the tubular fluid is the same as in the plasma, values below 1.0 indicate that the substance is reabsorbed more avidly than water, while values greater than 1.0 indicate that the substance is reabsorbed to a lesser extent than water or is secreted into the tubules. (Redrawn from Hall JE. *Guyton and Hall Textbook of Medical Physiology*. 13th ed. Philadelphia: Elsevier; 2016.)

adjustments to achieve therapeutic levels or to prevent toxicity in other organs. Fig. 17.17 outlines changes in the concentrations of different substances in the tubular system relative to the concentration in plasma and the glomerular filtrate.

The Loop of Henle

The loop of Henle is comprised of a thin descending limb, thin ascending limb, a medullary thick ascending limb (mTAL) as well as a cortical portion that leads to the distal convoluted tubule. The macula densa (see Fig. 17.1) is an area of closely packed cells lining the wall of the distal tubule at the point where it meets the thick ascending limb.The major function of the loop of Henle is the maintenance of an osmotic gradient in the interstitium by a countercurrent system to allow the resorption of 40% of the filtered sodium and 25% of filtered water (see later).[39] Differential permeability to water, transport of ions, and urea carriers provide the interstitial environment to concentrate urine (see Fig. 17.15). The tubules of the descending loop of Henle are freely permeable to water and allow for the reabsorption of about 20% of the filtered water. Both the medullary and cortical thick limbs are impermeable to water and function to concentrate urine. Urea, which comprises 90% of waste nitrogen, is passively absorbed in the tubules by osmosis and is facilitated by specific transporters. An increased concentration of urea in the tubular lumen favors its movement into the interstitium to create an extremely high interstitial osmolality at the tip that approaches 1200 mOsm/kg. Since the tubules are less permeable to urea than water, most of the urea is excreted into the urine.

As with the cells of the PCT, the mTAL cells have high metabolic activity. A $Na^+/K^+/2Cl^-$ cotransporter in this segment absorbs Na^+, Cl^-, and K^+ from the tubular lumen. Inhibition of this cotransporter is the mechanism of cationic (positively charged) loop diuretics such as furosemide. The positive charge of the tubular lumen compared to the interstitium allows the paracellular reabsorption of magnesium and calcium in addition to sodium and potassium. ATPase-dependent Na^+/K^+ pumps in the basilar membrane will reabsorb 25% of the filtered sodium and potassium.

DISTAL TUBULES AND MACULA DENSA

The first part of the distal tubule forms the macula densa of the juxtaglomerular apparatus. Approximately 5% of sodium is reabsorbed in the first part of the distal tubule by a sodium chloride cotransporter that moves ions from the tubular lumen into the cell and a Na^+/K^+ ATPase that moves Na^+ out of the cell.[39,40] Thiazide diuretics inhibit this cotransporter (see Fig. 17.16). The movement of chloride is passive. The permeability to water of the distal tubules, as well as the collecting tubules described later, is regulated by AVP (Fig. 17.18). With increased AVP, the tubules become more permeable and water is absorbed.

COLLECTING TUBULES

The collecting tubules are extensions of the distal tubules and have the same function of Na^+ resorption. The two cell types lining the collecting tubules are the principal

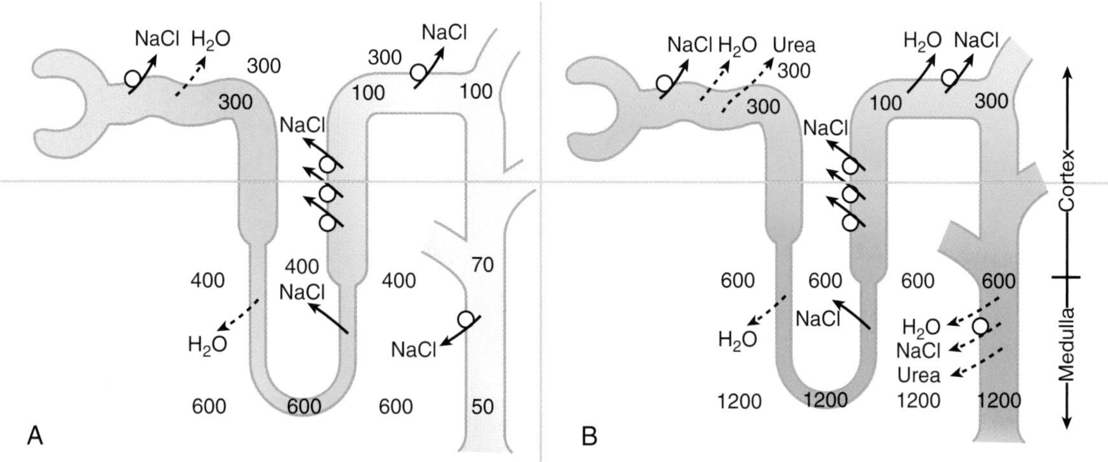

Fig. 17.18 Effect of arginine vasopressin on the formation of urine. (A) With low levels of arginine vasopressin (AVP), fluid in the ascending limb of the loop of Henle is dilute and becomes further diluted in the distal and collecting tubules by continued reabsorption of solutes (indicated as millimoles per liter) while water is not resorbed. (B) Urine is concentrated when AVP is high. Fluid leaving the loop of Henle becomes more concentrated as water is absorbed from the distal and collecting tubules. With high AVP levels, the osmolality of the urine (indicated as milliosmoles) is the same as in the renal medullary interstitial fluid. (Modified from Hall JE. *Guyton and Hall Textbook of Medical Physiology*. 13th ed. Philadelphia: Elsevier; 2016.)

cells and two types of intercalated cells. Principal cells use Na^+/K^+ ATPase to resorb Na^+ and K^+. These cells are the sites of action for the potassium-sparing diuretics such as spironolactone, a competitor of aldosterone. An additional mechanism is Na^+ channel blockade by diuretics such as amiloride.

Type A intercalated cells use H^+-ATPase and H^+/K^+-ATPase transporters to secrete hydrogen ions formed by carbonic anhydrase against a large concentration gradient. Bicarbonate ions are absorbed from the basolateral membrane. In contrast, the Type B intercalated cells transport hydrogen out of the cell on the basolateral side while bicarbonate is excreted into the tubular lumen. These cells are critical to the maintenance of acid-base balance, sodium reabsorption, and intravascular volume.[41]

COLLECTING DUCTS

The collecting ducts form as distal anastomoses of collecting tubules in the medulla and determine the final composition of urine. The principal cell of the collecting duct is a highly regulated epithelial cell. AVP controls water resorption. Urea is reabsorbed via transporters into the medullary interstitium, thereby raising the osmolality to assist in the concentration of urine. Hydrogen can also be secreted against a high concentration gradient to regulate acidosis.

RENAL AUTOREGULATION

The formation of urine is tightly controlled by complex autoregulation that maintains consistency of the RBF, GFR, and the resorption rate in tubules when there are changes in tubular flow. This autoregulation protects the kidney from injury secondary to elevated blood pressure by two mechanisms: autoregulation of RBF and tubuloglomerular feedback.[42]

Autoregulation of Renal Blood Flow

The smooth muscles of the afferent arterioles, as in other vascular beds, have the intrinsic ability to contract, called a myogenic response, to increases in blood pressure. The response can compensate for changes in pressure within 3 to 10 seconds over a mean arterial blood pressure range of 70 to 130 mm Hg.[43]

The Myogenic Mechanism of the Renal Blood Flow Autoregulation

Glomerulotubular balance compensates for increased GFR when blood pressure is elevated by preventing fluid loss through an augmented rate of tubular absorption in the PTC and loop of Henle. This process is more adaptable to slow changes in arterial pressure (>20 seconds) and more critical in maintaining GFR and RBF during sustained reductions in blood pressure (Fig. 17.19).[43] An increase in GFR provides enhanced NaCl delivery to the distal tubules. The increased chloride concentration is sensed by the macula densa and triggers the renin-angiotensin cascade to decrease the GFR through angiotensin II constriction of the afferent arteriole. This trigger is sent by the macula densa through the complex of mesangial cells to the smooth muscle of the vasculature by paracrine signaling. There are no intercellular connections between the macula densa, other components of the juxtaglomerular apparatus, and the blood vessels.[44] The increases in resorption proportionate to the GFR prevent distention of the distal tubular segments.

TUBULOGLOMERULAR FEEDBACK

The dynamic range of tubuloglomerular feedback is a NaCl concentration between 15 and 60 mmol/L with maximal responses at greater than 60 mmol/L.[44] In the tubules, more than 99% of water and most of the solutes are absorbed, pass through the interstitium, and enter the capillaries at a rate of 124 mL/min. As demonstrable for most capillary beds, the transit of fluids is dependent upon balance of hydrostatic and colloid forces (see Fig. 17.8). Intravascular pressure (13 mm Hg) and colloid osmotic pressure of the interstitium (15 mm Hg) oppose resorption, whereas the hydrostatic pressure in the interstitium (6 mm Hg), intravascular colloid osmotic pressure (32 mm Hg), and large surface area of the capillaries favor resorption.

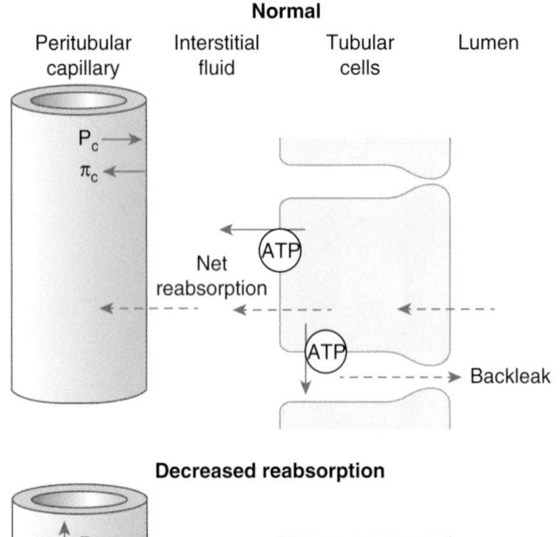

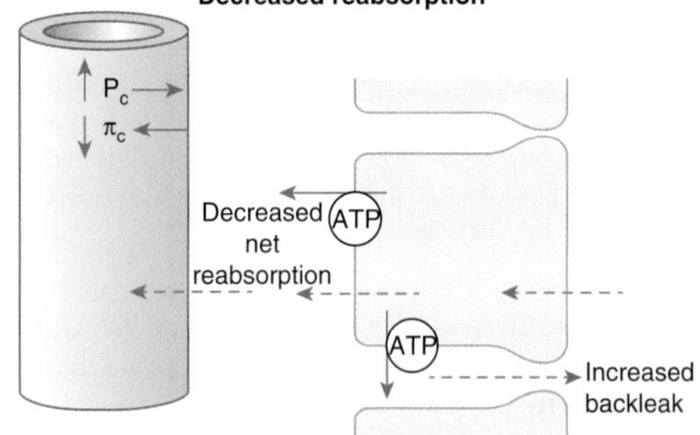

Fig. 17.19 Proximal and peritubular capillary reabsorption under normal conditions *(top)* and during decreased peritubular capillary reabsorption caused by increased hydrostatic pressure *(P_c)* or decreased colloid osmotic pressure *(π_c)*. As peritubular capillary reabsorption decreases, the net reabsorption of solutes and water is lowered by the increase in solutes and water that leak back into the tubular lumen through the tight junctions of the tubular epithelial cells. *ATP*, Adenosine triphosphate. (Redrawn from Hall JE. *Guyton and Hall Textbook of Medical Physiology.* 13th ed. Philadelphia: Elsevier; 2016.)

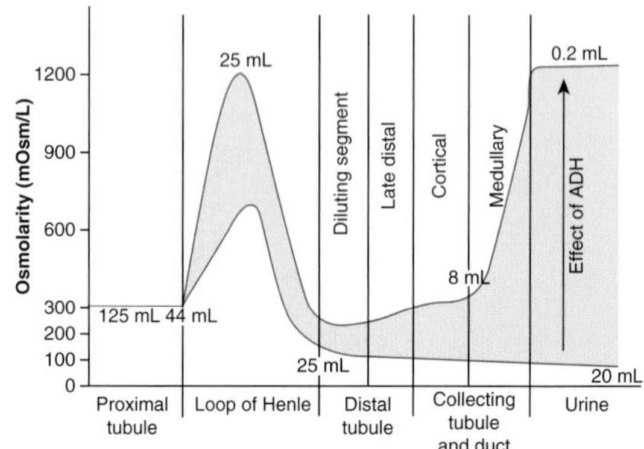

Fig. 17.20 Changes in osmolality of the tubular fluid as it passes through the different tubular segments (milliliters per minute) in the presence of high and low levels of arginine vasopressin (indicated here as the alternative term antidiuretic hormone *[ADH]*). (Redrawn from Hall JE. *Guyton and Hall Textbook of Medical Physiology.* 13th ed. Philadelphia: Elsevier; 2016.)

MAINTENANCE OF PLASMA OSMOLALITY

Definition

Prior to any description of this process, the definitions of osmolarity and osmolality should be reviewed. Osmolality is a measure of the osmoles (Osm) of solute per kilogram of solvent (Osm/kg) while osmolarity is defined as the number of osmoles of solute per liter of solution (Osm/L). Osmolarity is affected by changes in water content, temperature, and pressure. Osmolarity is slightly less than osmolality because the total solvent weight excludes any solutes. Clinically, the values for osmolarity and osmolality are very similar, and the terms are usually used interchangeably. The bedside calculation from laboratory data (2[Na^+ mmol/L] + 2[K^+ mmol/L] + BUN mg/dL/2.8 + glucose mg/dL/18) is in units of osmolarity. The clinical laboratory measurements determined with osmometers are reported as osmolality.

Regulation of Osmolality

Plasma osmolality is closely regulated between 275 and 300 mOsm/L. Acute alterations in osmolality, either hypoosmolality or hyperosmolality, can result in serious neurologic symptoms and death as the result of water movement in the brain. Normal patients can dilute and concentrate urine within the range of 40 to 1400 mOsm/L.[45] Maintenance of plasma osmolality is linked to the regulation of sodium concentration and water balance by the tubular system and the collecting ducts in concert with the vasa recta blood supply of the tubules through differences in tubular permeability to water and the control of sodium transport (Fig. 17.20). It is dependent on the interaction of at least three processes: the generation of a hypertonic medullary interstitium by the countercurrent mechanism and urea recycling, the concentration and then dilution of tubular fluid in the loop of Henle, and the action of AVP to increase water permeability in the last part of the distal tubule and collecting ducts.

ROLE OF PROXIMAL TUBULES AND LOOP OF HENLE

Osmosis, the spontaneous net movement of solvent molecules through a selectively permeable membrane into a region of higher solute concentration to equalize the solute concentrations on the two sides, takes place in the proximal tubule. Proximal tubule solutes and water are equally reabsorbed so that the fluid in the tubules is isosmotic with plasma. In contrast, the organization of the loop of Henle is designed to maintain hyperosmolality of the medullary interstitium that can approach 1200 mOsm/L. The major process for this is the active transport of Na^+ and co-transport of K^+ and Cl^- from the lumen of the thick limb of the loop of Henle that is impermeable to water to the interstitium. This allows for a concentration gradient of 200 mOsm/L.

Medullary Interstitium

The medullary interstitium becomes hypertonic by the countercurrent multiplier effect of the loop of Henle that is best understood diagrammatically (Fig. 17.21). The primary mechanism is by the combination of NaCl reabsorption and water impermeability in the ascending limb. The descending limb is freely permeable to water, which diffuses into the interstitium along the osmotic gradient, and the tubular fluid becomes progressively hyperosmotic at the bend of the loop.

Water entering the distal convoluted tubule after leaving the loop of Henle is dilute (about 100 mOsm/L).

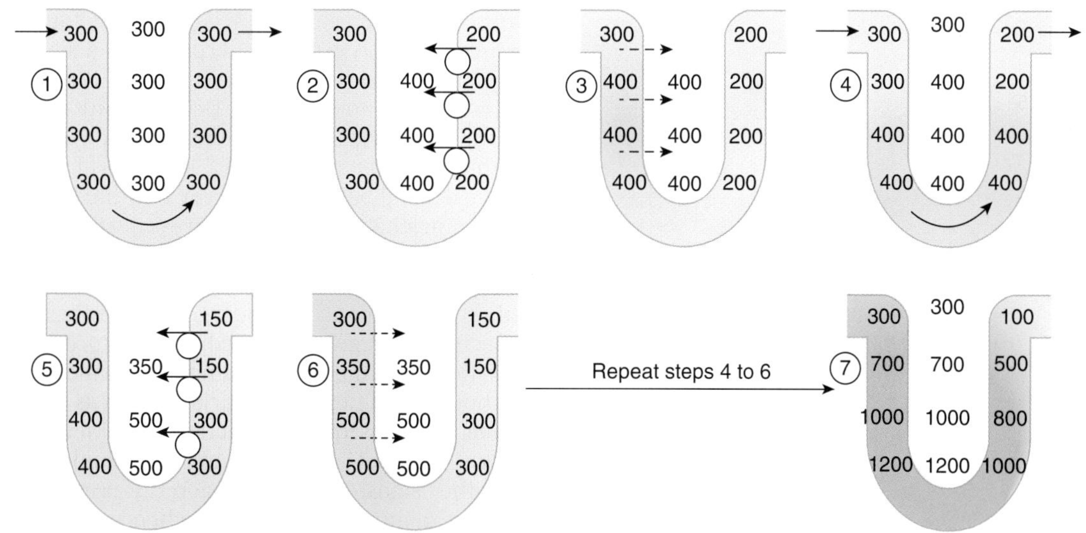

Fig. 17.21 Countercurrent multiplier system in the loop of Henle for producing a hyperosmotic (millimoles per liter) renal medulla. (Redrawn from Hall JE. *Guyton and Hall Textbook of Medical Physiology*. 13th ed. Philadelphia: Elsevier; 2016.)

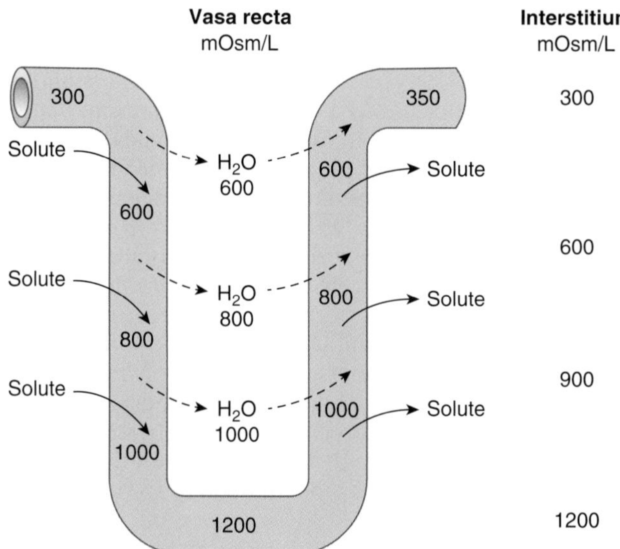

Fig. 17.22 Countercurrent exchange in the vasa recta. Plasma flowing down the descending limb of the loop of the vasa recta becomes more hyperosmotic (in millimoles per liter) as water diffuses out of the blood while solutes from the interstitial fluid flow into the blood. In the ascending limb, solutes diffuse back to the interstitial fluid and water diffuses back into the vasa recta. (Redrawn from Hall JE. *Guyton and Hall Textbook of Medical Physiology*. 13th ed. Philadelphia: Elsevier; 2016.)

This dilution is increased because of the active transport of NaCl and the impermeability of the epithelium. In the collecting tubule, resorption of water is dependent upon the action of AVP (ADH), since the epithelium is normally impermeable to water. With the action of AVP, large amounts of water are reabsorbed into the interstitium of the cortex and removed by the peritubular capillaries (see Fig. 17.18).

Vasa Recta

The vasa recta or straight arterioles of kidney are a series of straight capillaries that lie parallel to the loops of Henle of the juxtamedullary nephrons (Fig. 17.22). Only 5% of the RBF is through the vasa recta, creating a sluggish flow. As the capillaries descend into the medulla, the blood becomes more concentrated by solute entry from the interstitium. This high concentration in the ascending vasa recta in turn facilitates the entry of water from the ascending tubules. The combined interactions of tubular permeability and the vasa recta create the standing osmotic gradients in the cortex (300 mOsm/L), juxtamedullary zone (600 mOsm/L), and deep medulla (1200 mOsm/L).

The Role of Urea

A healthy person excretes 20% to 50% of the filtered load of urea. The concentration of urea entering the tubular system is related to the prerenal plasma concentration and the GFR. Urea contributes 40% to 50% of the osmolality of the medullary interstitium. The PCT are freely permeable whereas the loop of Henle, distal tubules, and the collecting ducts have little permeability to urea (Fig. 17.23). As water absorption increases with AVP action, the concentration of urea in the tubules progressively increases. With this high concentration, urea diffuses into the interstitial fluid facilitated by specific urea transporters that are activated by AVP. The simultaneous movement of urea and water out of the inner medullary collecting ducts maintains a high concentration of urea in the tubular fluid. As the concentration of urea increases in the medullary interstitium, it diffuses through the thin limb of the loop of Henle and transits through the ascending system again before it is excreted. This recirculation enhances the increased osmotic pressure in the medulla.

RENAL CONTROL OF INTRAVASCULAR VOLUME

Hypovolemia

Patients with hypovolemia, for example, from hemorrhage, gastrointestinal loss, or preoperative fasting, are commonly encountered in the perioperative period. Contraction of the extracellular volume by hypovolemia increases sympathetic outflow, activates the renin-angiotensin-aldosterone response, and releases AVP. Initially, the GFR and filtered load of sodium decrease. Sodium reabsorption in the proximal tubule is increased from about 66% to 80%

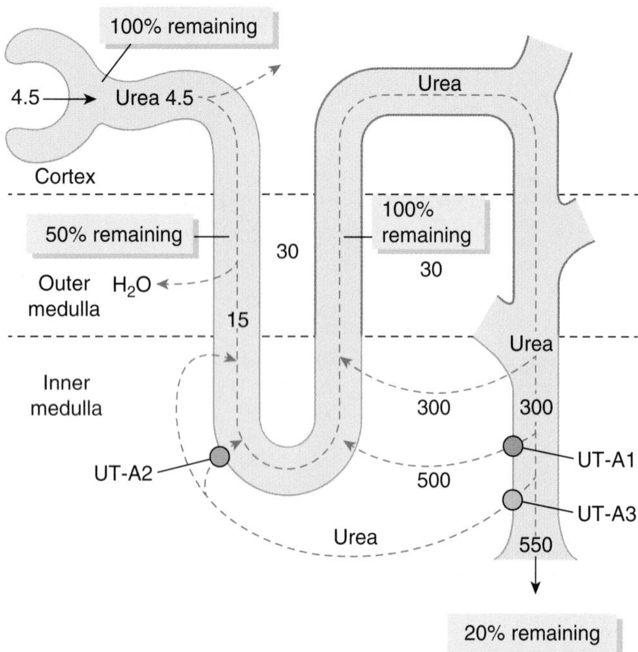

Fig. 17.23 Recirculation of urea absorbed from the medullary collecting duct into the interstitial fluid. Urea diffuses into the thin loop of Henle assisted by urea transporter UT-A2 through to the distal tubules and finally passes back to the collecting duct aided by urea transporters (*UT-A1* and *UT-A3*). This recirculation helps to trap urea in the renal medulla contributing to its hyperosmolality (millimoles per liter). Heavy lines indicate segments that are not very permeable to urea. (Redrawn from Hall JE. *Guyton and Hall Textbook of Medical Physiology*. 13th ed. Philadelphia: Elsevier; 2016.)

by sympathetic activity and angiotensin II, as well as by the decline in peritubular capillary pressure induced by renal vasoconstriction. Sodium delivery to the thick ascending loop of Henle, distal tubule, and collecting duct is decreased, but aldosterone promotes reabsorption of sodium at these sites. Under the influence of AVP, water is also avidly reabsorbed in the collecting duct so that the urine becomes highly concentrated (osmolality 600 mOsm/kg) but with virtually no sodium (10 mEq/L).

Hypervolemia

Expansion of the extracellular volume by hypervolemia is countered by an increase in the GFR and filtered sodium load due to a combination of reflex decreases in sympathetic and angiotensin II activity and the release of ANP. Together with the increase in peritubular capillary hydrostatic pressure, these responses cause sodium reabsorption in the proximal tubule to decrease from 67% to 50%. The decline in plasma aldosterone decreases sodium absorption from the thick ascending loop of Henle to the collecting duct. The presence of ANP and absence of AVP impairs water absorption at the collecting duct so that a dilute urine (osmolality 300 mOsm/kg) with abundant sodium (80 mEq/L) is produced.

CLINICAL TESTS FOR RENAL FUNCTION[46,47]

Urine Output

The measurement of urine output is simple and has been the traditional intraoperative and postoperative clinical evaluation of renal function in the absence of laboratory data. By consensus, oliguria is defined as a urine flow rate less than 0.5 mL/kg/h; it is often interpreted as a sign of renal dysfunction[48] and was first described by Galen and Ephesus between 100 and 200 AD. Urine output was listed as one of the most widely used indicators for volume expansion with intravenous fluids by 77% to 83% of anesthesiologists surveyed and based on a survey of United States and European anesthesiologists.[49] However, studies have shown that low urine output was not necessarily associated with renal failure.[50] Reduced intraoperative urinary output (<1 mL/kg/h) for patients undergoing anesthesia for thoracic resections was not associated with postoperative renal dysfunction regardless of the amount of fluid administered.[51] Although traditionally oliguria is taken as a sign of hypovolemia and subsequent reduction in kidney perfusion, perioperative oliguria is not always abnormal, especially when no other signs of hypoperfusion are present. Tolerance of modest oliguria is necessary when considering the relatively recent push for fluid limitations with enhanced recovery after surgery protocols.[52] Targeting urine output does not affect 30-day mortality, and oliguria is not a modifiable risk factor for mortality.[53] Oliguria has been correlated with AKI and may be a better threshold for the guidance of fluid administration.[54]

In the perioperative period, transient oliguria is almost inevitable, whether induced by hypotension, as an appropriate prerenal response to intravascular hypovolemia, or as a manifestation of the physiologic response to surgical stress.[55] It is a relative condition that depends on *expected* urine flow, and it may bear little, if any, relationship to GFR. When arterial blood pressure and intravascular volume are restored to normal levels, normal urinary flow should resume. Complete, often abrupt, cessation of urine flow (anuria) suggests postrenal obstruction. For patients with indwelling urinary catheters, obstruction of the catheter by malposition, blood, or kinking is the first diagnosis that must be ruled out and corrected immediately if confirmed. When the catheter is patent, obstruction from the surgical field must be considered dependent upon the procedure.

Creatinine

Creatine phosphate in muscle transfers high-energy phosphate to ADP, creating ATP necessary for contraction, and creatine. Creatinine results from the metabolism of creatine in the liver. Serum creatinine is a reasonable approximation of GFR since it is freely filtered by the glomerulus, is soluble, distributes through the total body water, and is not reabsorbed by the tubules. Creatinine varies with muscle mass, rate of catabolism, protein intake, and physical activity. Low GFR tends to overestimate renal function since little creatinine is secreted. The relationship between serum creatinine and GFR is inverse and exponential; that is, a doubling of serum creatinine implies a halving of GFR. The normal serum creatinine range is 0.5 to 1.2 mg/dL. Muscle mass must be taken into consideration since a normal creatinine in a malnourished, cachectic patient may reflect reduced GFR.

Blood Urea Nitrogen

Urea is formed in the liver by the deamination of amino acids and conversion to ammonia by the arginine cycle. It is not an indicator of GFR since it is rapidly reabsorbed by the tubules. Absorption of blood from the gastrointestinal tract, steroids, and sepsis may increase the blood urea nitrogen (BUN), whereas malnutrition or liver disease might result in its decrease. The normal ratio of BUN to serum creatinine ratio is between 10 and 15 to 1. The BUN to creatinine ratio may be useful in the diagnosis of renal failure from prerenal causes versus acute tubular necrosis (see Chapter 42).

RENAL CLEARANCE TECHNIQUES

Clearance is the pharmacokinetic measurement of the volume of plasma that is removed of a specific substance over a period of time. Classic renal physiology experiments used the plant polysaccharide that is freely filtered by the glomerulus and not secreted or reabsorbed by the tubules. ^{131}I-iothalamate has the same renal properties as inulin and is used in radiographic studies to assess clearance.[56]

In routine clinical practice, GFR [urine creatinine (mg/dL) × volume of urine (mL)/plasma creatinine (mg/dL)] has been employed. The traditional collection period is 24 hours but since the collection of urine can sometimes be impractical, shorter intervals can be used for estimations. A volume of urine is carefully collected over a defined time period and the creatinine concentration is measured. A comparison is then made with a blood sample that is taken during the midpoint of urine flow to determine the creatinine. The GFR may decrease significantly before serum creatinine increases above normal and can be inaccurate due to its variable tubular secretion, extrarenal elimination, and variable rates of generation. For these reasons, estimated GFR (eGFR) that is based on age, sex, and race is often calculated using either the Modification of Diet in Renal Disease (MDRD) or the Chronic Kidney Disease Epidemiology Collaboration (CKD-EPI) equation.[57]

Both methods normalize for sex, age, and race and are based on a stable steady-state production of creatinine and are not accurate with AKI when creatinine clearance is in flux. The MDRD formula is normalized to an average adult 1.73 m^2 body surface area. The CKD-EPI equation is more accurate for values less than 60 mL/min/1.73 m^2. Clinical laboratories will state which method is used when eGFR is reported. Extremes of muscle mass, pregnancy, dietary intake, and comorbidities are factors that will lead to errors in eGFR. Creatinine clearance is more accurate when drugs are dosed based on renal function.[58]

Measurement of Tubular Function

When oliguria is present, tests of renal tubular function may be useful to distinguish dehydration (prerenal azotemia) from acute tubular necrosis. In dehydration, the tubules function normally to retain Na^+ and water to maintain the blood volume. The osmolality of plasma is 280 to 300 mOs/kg but with dehydration, the urine osmolality can increase to greater than 450 mOs/kg. Acute tubular necrosis is a pathologic state (see Chapter 42) in which the concentrating ability of the tubules is defective. Sodium and water may be lost in the urine if nonoliguric.

The most common method of assessing for tubular concentration ability is the fractional excretion of sodium (FE_{Na}), which is a measure of sodium clearance as a percentage of creatine clearance. FE_{Na} is calculated by the following from simultaneous samples of blood and urine collection:

$$FE_{Na} = (\text{urine Na/plasma Na}) / (\text{urine creatinine/plasma creatinine}) \times 100$$

Effect of Anesthetics on Renal Function

All general anesthetics tend to decrease GFR and intraoperative urine flow as a consequence of decreased cardiac output and arterial blood pressure.[59] Some drugs also decrease RBF, but filtration fraction is usually increased, which implies that angiotensin-induced efferent arteriolar constriction limits the decrease in GFR that resolves after emergence from anesthesia. Any anesthetic technique that induces hypotension will result in decreased urine flow because of altered peritubular capillary hydrostatic gradients, even if renal autoregulation is preserved. Injury to kidneys seldom occurs unless there is preexisting kidney disease, nephrotoxic injury, hypovolemia, or a combination thereof, which will exacerbate renal dysfunction.[60] Volatile anesthetics induce mild to moderate reductions in RBF and GFR, primarily because of their myocardial depression and vasodilatory effects[61] that can be attenuated by prior intravenous hydration. Opioid-based anesthetics are considerably more effective than volatile anesthetics in suppressing the release of catecholamines, angiotensin II, aldosterone, and AVP. Ketamine increases RBF but decreases urine flow rate, possibly through sympathetic activation; it preserves RBF during hemorrhagic hypovolemia.[62]

The potential for AKI after the breakdown of volatile anesthetics to free fluoride ions causing tubular lesions is now of only historical interest.[63] The "older" volatile drug isoflurane produces minimal peak fluoride levels (<4 μm/L).[64] Initial studies of sevoflurane in rats reported nephrotoxicity through the formation of Compound A, a vinyl ether formed by degradation of sevoflurane at low flow through carbon dioxide absorbents.[65] Clinically significant renal injury has not been shown with desflurane, sevoflurane, or propofol in patients even with moderate preexisting renal dysfunction.[66]

There is growing evidence to support anesthetics as agents that ameliorate ischemia-reperfusion injury in the kidney and other organs.[67] The volatile anesthetics desflurane, sevoflurane, isoflurane, and halothane attenuated the increase in serum creatinine compared with pentobarbital or ketamine in animal models.[68] The mechanism is related to an induction of cytoprotective factors and suppression of proinflammatory cytokine and chemokine activation in response to ischemia-reperfusion. There is experimental evidence that propofol can prevent renal ischemia-reperfusion injury through inhibition of oxidative stress pathways.[69]

EFFECTS OF MECHANICAL VENTILATION ON RENAL FUNCTION

Mechanical ventilation and positive end-expiratory pressure (PEEP) may cause decreases in RBF, GFR, sodium excretion, and urine flow rate through changes in hemodynamics.[70] The increased airway and intrapleural pressures lead to decreased venous return, cardiac filling pressures, and cardiac output. Positive pressure ventilation increases inferior vena caval pressure and through increased renal venous pressure, may increase peritubular capillary pressure to increase tubular sodium reabsorption. The decrease in cardiac output and systemic arterial pressure results in a carotid and aortic baroreceptor-mediated increase in sympathetic nerve tone to the kidney, with renal vasoconstriction, antidiuresis, and anti-natriuresis. Volume receptors in the atria respond to decreased filling by decreased ANP secretion, resulting in increased sympathetic tone, renin activation, and AVP activity.

The renin-angiotensin-aldosterone system undoubtedly augments the renal responses to positive pressure ventilation. An increase in PEEP can depress cardiac output, RBF, GFR, and urine volume, and increase renin and aldosterone. Although the extent of depression of renal function depends on the mean airway pressure, there is no difference in creatinine clearance and FE_{Na} between volume-controlled and pressure support ventilation.[71] Permissive hypercapnia as employed during acute respiratory distress syndrome may promote renal vasoconstriction.[70]

Induced Hypotension

During anesthesia with induced hypotension, substantial reduction of GFR and urine flow rate is common. Although earlier studies suggested that hypotensive anesthesia can be well tolerated without permanent impairment of renal function, a more recent retrospective analysis suggests that mean arterial pressures less than 60 mmHg for 11 to 20 min or less than 55 mmHg for more than 10 min are associated with acute kidney injury.[72] Vasodilators used to induce hypotension differ in their effect on RBF. Administration of sodium nitroprusside decreases renal vascular resistance but tends to shunt blood flow away from the kidney. Moreover, its administration is associated with marked renin-angiotensin activation and catecholamine release, which results in rebound hypertension if the infusion is suddenly discontinued. Nitroglycerin decreases RBF less than sodium nitroprusside.[73] The selective DA1-dopaminergic agonist fenoldopam is capable of providing induced hypotension without any significant decrease in RBF.[74] Nicardipine increased creatinine clearance and attenuated the increase in FE_{Na} in patients undergoing spine surgery under deliberate hypotension[75] and improved renal function when given to patients with preexisting renal insufficiency who had robotic-assisted radical prostatectomy.[76]

Acknowledgment

The editors and publisher would like to thank Drs. David McIlroy and Robert N. Sladen for contributing a chapter on this topic in the prior edition of this work. It has served as the foundation for the current chapter.

 **Complete references available online at expertconsult.com.**

References

1. Jelkmann W. *J Physiol.* 2011;589:1251–1258.
2. Hansell P, et al. *Clin Exp Pharmacol Physiol.* 2014;40:123–137.
3. Washinzawa K, et al. *Pediatr Nephrol.* 1993;7:1–5.
4. Raats CJ, et al. *Kidney Int.* 2000;57:385–400.
5. Rodewald R, Karnovsky MJ. *J Cell Biol.* 1974;217:423–433.
6. Farquhar MG. *J Clin Invest.* 2006;116:2090–2093.
7. Neal CR. *Front Endocrinol.* 2015:6–9.
8. Schrijvers BF, et al. *Kidney Int.* 2004;65:2003–2017.
9. Inoue K, Ishibe S. *Am J Physiol Renal Physiol.* 2015;309:F398–F405.
10. Pulamen T, et al. *J Am Soc Nephrol.* 2002;13:1766–1772.
11. New LA, et al. *Curr Opin Nephrol Hypertens.* 2014;23:420–430.
12. Wu C-H, et al. *Arterioscler Thromb Vasc Biol.* 2018;38:e108–e116.
13. Koeppen BM, Stanton BA. Glomerular filtration and renal blood flow. In: Koeppen BM, Stanton BA, eds. *Renal Physiology.* 4th ed. Philadelphia: Mosby Elsevier; 2007:31.
14. Navar LG, et al. *Hypertension.* 2011;57:355–362.
15. Wilson BA, et al. *Am J Physiol Regul Integr Comp Physiol.* 2014;307:R487–R489.
16. Herichova I, Szantoova K. *Endocr Regul.* 2013;47:39–52.
17. Sparks MA, et al. *Compr Physiol.* 2014;4:1201–1228.
18. Li C, et al. *Am J Physiol Renal Physiol.* 2011;300:F1255–F1261.
19. Chappell MC. *Compr Physiol.* 2012;2:2733–2752.
20. Hao C-M, Breyer MD. *Ann Rev Physiol.* 2008;70:357–377.
21. Kim G-H. *Electrolyte and Blood Pressure.* 2008;6:35–41.
22. Scicli AG, Carretero OA. *Kidney Int.* 1986;29:120–130.
23. Baram M, et al. *J Allergy Clin Immunol Pract.* 2013;1:442–445.
24. Kortenoeven ML, et al. *Am J Physiol Renal Physiol.* 2015;15:F280–299.
25. Bayless PH. Posterior pituitary function in health and disease. *Clin Endocrin Metabolism.* 1983;12:747–770.
26. Edwards RM, et al. *Am J Physiol.* 1989;256:F526–F534.
27. Olesen ET, Fenton RA. *Am J Physiol Renal Physiol.* 2017;312:F744–F747.
28. de Bold AJ. *Can. J. Physiol. Pharmacol.* 2011;89:527–531.
29. Inoue T, et al. *Cardiovasc Res.* 2001;15:470–480.
30. Heras MM, et al. *J Diabetes Metab.* 2012:3:171.
31. Genuth SM. The adrenal glands. In: Berne RM, Levy EM, eds. *Physiology.* 4th ed. St Louis: Mosby; 1998:930–964.
32. Choi MR, et al. *Biomed Res Int.* 2014.
33. Sansoè G, et al. *Dig Dis Sci.* 2002;247:392–400.
34. Eltzschig HK. *Anesthesiology.* 2009;111:904–915.
35. Bauerle JD, et al. *J Am Soc Nephrol.* 2011;22:14–20.
36. Evans RG, Fitzgerald SM. *Curr Opin Nephrol Hypertens.* 2005;14:9–15.
37. Ortiz PA, Garvin JL. *Am J Physiol Renal Physiol.* 2002;282:F777–F784.
38. Cowley AW Jr, et al. *Am J Physiol Renal Physiol.* 2015;308:F179–F197.
39. Palmer LG, Schnermann J. *Clin J Am Soc Nephrol.* 2015;10:676–687.
40. McCormick JA, Ellison DH. *Compr Physiol.* 2015;5:45–98.
41. Roy A, et al. *Clin J Am Soc Nephrol.* 2015;10:305–324.
42. Carlström M, et al. *Physiol Rev.* 2015;95:405–511.
43. Burke M, et al. *Curr Vasc Pharmacol.* 2014;12:845–858.
44. Komlosi P, et al. *Acta Physiol Scand.* 2004;181:463–469.
45. Rose BD. Regulation of plasma osmolality. In: Rose BD, ed. *Clinical Physiology of Acid-Base and Electrolyte Disorders.* 4th ed. New York, NY: McGraw-Hill; 1994:261–273.
46. Winter WE. *The Kidney.* In: *Laposata's Laboratory Medicine Diagnosis of Disease in Clinical Laboratory.* 2nd ed. New York, NY: McGraw Hill; 2014:385–396.
47. Prowle JR, Forni LG. Functional biomarkers. In: Ronco C, Bellomo R, Kellum JA, Ricci Z, eds. *Critical Care Nephrology.* 3rd ed. Philadelphia: Elsevier, Inc; 2019:141–145.
48. Kunst G, Ostermann M. *Brit J Anaesth.* 2017;119:1075–1077.
49. Cannesson M, et al. *Critical Care.* 2011;15:R197.
50. Kheterpal S, et al. *Anesthesiology.* 2007;107:892–902.
51. Matot I, et al. *J Thorac Cardiovasc Surg.* 2013;146:461–466.
52. Makaryus R, et al. *Brit J Anaesth.* 2018;120:376–383.
53. van der Zee EN, et al. *BMC Anesthesiol.* 2017;17:22.
54. Matot I, et al. *Arch Surg.* 2012;147:228–234.
55. Sladen RN. *Anesthesiol Clin North America.* 2000;18:739–752. viii.
56. Seegmiller JC, et al. *Adv Chronic Kidney Dis.* 2018;25:84–92.
57. http://www.niddk.nih.gov/health-information/communication-programs/nkdep/laboratory-evaluation/glomerular-filtration-rate/estimating.
58. Hermsen ED, et al. *Pharmacotherapy.* 2009;29:649–655.
59. Priano LL. Effects of anesthetic agents on renal function. In: Barash PG, ed. *Refresher Courses in Anesthesiology.* Philadelphia: Lippincott; 1985:143–156.
60. Fukazawa K, Lee T. *J Am Soc Nephrol.* 2014;25:884–892.

61. Gelman S, et al. *Anesth Analg*. 1984;63:557–565.
62. Priano LL. *Anesth Analg*. 1982;61:853–862.
63. Mazze RI, et al. *Anesthesiology*. 1971;35:247.
64. Mazze RI, et al. *Anesthesiology*. 1974;40:536–542.
65. Higuchi H, et al. *Anesth Analg*. 2000;91:434–439.
66. Ebert TJ, Arain SR. *Anesthesiology*. 2000;93:1401–1406.
67. Motayagheni N, et al. *Am J Nephrol*. 2017;46:380–389.
68. Lee HT, et al. *Anesthesiology*. 2004;101:1313–1324.
69. Li Y, et al. *Cell Physiol Biochem*. 2015;37:14–26.
70. Kuiper JW, et al. *Crit Care Med*. 2005;33:1408–1415.
71. Botha J, et al. *Crit Care Resusc*. 2005;7:303–309.
72. Thompson GE, et al. *Anesthesiology*. 1978;48:91–96.
73. Colley PS, Silvarjan M. *Anesth Analg*. 1984;63:503–510.
74. Aronson S, et al. *J Cardiothorac Vasc Anesth*. 1991;5:29–32.
75. Park C, et al. *Clin Spine Surg*. 2017;30:E954–E958.
76. Huh H, et al. *J Int Med Res*. 2014;42:427–435.

18 Basic Principles of Pharmacology

TAE KYUN KIM, SHINJU OBARA, and KEN B. JOHNSON

KEY POINTS

- Pharmacokinetics describes the relationship between drug dose and drug concentration in plasma or at the site of drug effect over time. For anesthetic drugs, the processes of distribution and elimination (metabolism and excretion) govern this relationship.
- The time course of intravenously administered drugs is a function of distribution volume and clearance. Estimates of distribution volumes and clearances, pharmacokinetic parameters, are derived from mathematical formulas fit to measured blood or plasma concentrations over time following a known drug dose.
- Front-end kinetics refer to alterations in cardiac output that substantially influence the pharmacokinetic behavior of anesthetic drugs in terms of onset and duration of effect. Context-sensitive decrement time, which is defined as the time required to reach a certain plasma concentration after a termination of long infusion, characterizes the back-end kinetics.
- Hysteresis refers to the time delay between changes in plasma concentration and drug effect. Hysteresis accounts for the time required for drug to diffuse from the plasma to the site of action plus the time required, once drug is at the site of action, to elicit a drug effect.
- Pharmacodynamics describes what the drug does to the body. In particular, pharmacodynamics describes the relationship between drug concentration and pharmacologic effect.
- The effect-site concentration describes a mathematically derived virtual location where an anesthetic drug exerts its effect. This approach cannot describe a mechanism of drug action (e.g., drug-receptor interaction).
- A single anesthetic drug has multiple effects (i.e., analgesia, ventilatory depression, loss of response to laryngoscopy, and changes in the electroencephalogram) that typically occur at various effect-site concentrations.
- The concentration range where changes in drug effect occur is known as the dynamic range. Concentrations outside the dynamic range do not yield much change in drug effect. Levels below the dynamic range are ineffective and those above the dynamic range do not provide additional effect.
- Anesthesia is the practice of applied drug interactions. Anesthetics rarely consist of one drug, but rather a combination of drugs to achieve desired levels of hypnosis, analgesia, and muscle relaxation. Hypnotics, analgesics, and muscle relaxants all interact with one another such that rarely does one drug, when administered in the presence of other drugs, behave as if it were administered alone.
- Pharmacokinetic and pharmacodynamic principles characterize the magnitude and time course of drug effect, but because of complex mathematics, they have limited clinical utility. Advances in computer simulation have brought this capability to the point of real-time patient care in the form of drug displays.
- Special populations: many aspects of a patient's demographics and medical history are considered in finding the *correct dose*. Some of these include age; body habitus; gender; chronic exposure to opioids, benzodiazepines, or alcohol; presence of heart, lung, kidney, or liver disease; and the extent of blood loss or dehydration.
- Some patient characteristics (e.g., obesity and age) influence anesthetic drug behavior, while other patient characteristics (chronic opioid use, hepatic and renal failure) remain poorly described.

Introduction

The basic principles of pharmacology are fundamental to an anesthesia provider's knowledge base. The aim of this chapter is to provide an overview of key principles in clinical pharmacology used to describe anesthetic drug behavior. This chapter is divided into three major sections: pharmacokinetic principles, pharmacodynamic principles, and the importance of patient characteristics. Pharmacokinetics is the relationship between drug administration and drug concentration at the site of action. Core concepts include volumes of distribution, drug clearance, and transfer of drugs between plasma and tissues. The section on pharmacokinetics introduces both the physiologic processes that determine pharmacokinetics and the mathematical models used to relate dose to concentration.

Pharmacodynamics is the relationship between drug concentration and pharmacologic effect. An anesthetic rarely consists of only one drug. In fact, most anesthetics are a combination of several drugs with specific goals in analgesia, sedation, and muscle relaxation. This section reviews common pharmacodynamic interactions and how they influence anesthetic effect.

The last section briefly addresses patient demographics and how they influence anesthetic behavior. When formulating an anesthetic, the following factors need to be considered in determining the correct dose: age; body habitus; gender; chronic exposure to opioids, benzodiazepines, or alcohol; presence of heart, lung, kidney, or liver disease; and the extent of blood loss or dehydration. This section focuses on body habitus and age, both known to influence the pharmacology of many anesthetic drugs and both of which serve as excellent examples of altered pharmacokinetics and pharmacodynamics.

FUNDAMENTAL PHARMACOKINETIC CONCEPTS

Pharmacokinetics describes the relationship between drug dose and drug concentration in plasma or at the site of drug effect over time. The processes of absorption, distribution, and elimination (metabolism and excretion) govern this relationship. Absorption is not relevant to intravenously administered drugs but is relevant to all other routes of drug delivery. The time course of intravenously administered drugs is a function of distribution volume and clearance. Estimates of distribution volumes and clearances are described by pharmacokinetic parameters. Pharmacokinetic parameters are derived from mathematical formulas fit to measured blood or plasma concentrations over time following a known amount of drug dose.

Volume of Distribution

An over-simplified model of drug distribution throughout plasma and tissues is the dilution of a drug dose into a tank of water. The volume of distribution (Vd) is the apparent size of the tank in which a known amount of drug distributes to produce a measured drug concentration once the drug has had enough time to thoroughly mix within the tank (Fig 18.1). If an injected drug disperses and distributes instantaneously throughout the tank without any drug degradation, the distribution volume is estimated using the simple relationship between dose (e.g., mg) and measured concentration (e.g., mg/L) as presented in Eq. (18.1).

$$\text{Volume of distribution} = \frac{\text{Amount of dose}}{\text{Concentration}} \tag{18.1}$$

With an estimate of tank volume, drug concentration after any bolus dose can be calculated. Human bodies are not like water tanks. As soon as a drug is injected, it begins to be cleared from the body. To account for this in the schematic presented in Fig. 18.1, a faucet is added to the tank to mimic drug elimination from the body (Fig. 18.2). Considering the elimination of drug from the tank and the changes in concentration, the definition of distribution volume in Eq. (18.1) should be refined with the amount of drug and the concentration at a given time t.

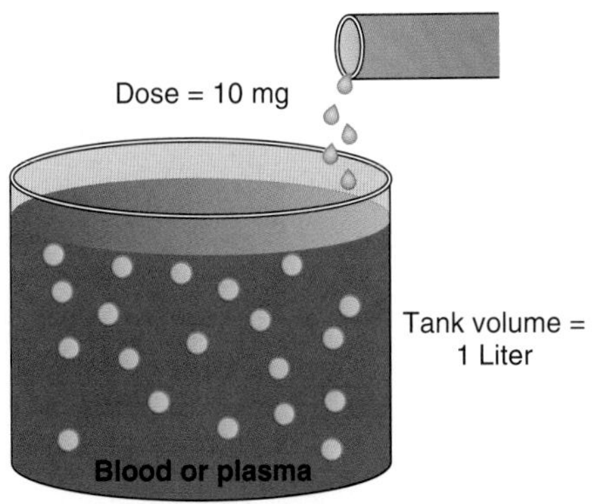

Fig. 18.1 Schematic of a single-tank model of distribution volume. The group of blue drops emerging from the pipe at the top right represent a bolus dose that, when administered to the tank of water, evenly distributes within the tank.

$$\text{Vd} = \frac{\text{Amount (t)}}{\text{Concentration (t)}} \tag{18.2}$$

If drug elimination occurs as a first-order process (i.e., elimination is proportional to the concentration at that time), in a tank model, the volume of distribution calculated by Eq. (18.2) will be constant (Fig. 18.3; see also Fig.18.2). When a drug is administered intravenously, some drug stays in the vascular volume, but most of the drug distributes to peripheral tissues. This distribution is often represented as additional tanks (peripheral distribution volumes) connected to a central tank (blood or plasma volume). Peripheral distribution volumes increase the total volume of distribution (Fig. 18.4). For the calculation of distribution volumes, peripheral tissue concentrations are difficult to measure whereas plasma concentrations are easily measured.

The schematic in Fig. 18.4 presents two tanks that represent plasma and peripheral tissue volumes. The peripheral tank represents the drug volume of distribution in peripheral tissues. There may be more than one peripheral tank (volume) to best describe the entire drug disposition in the body. The size of the peripheral volumes represents a drug's solubility in tissue relative to blood or plasma. The more soluble a drug is in peripheral tissue relative to blood or plasma, the larger the peripheral volumes of distribution.

An important point illustrated in Fig. 18.4 is that drug not only distributes to the peripheral tank and thus increases the volume of distribution, but it also binds to tissue in that tank. This process further lowers the measurable concentration in the central tank. Thus, the total volume of distribution may even be larger than the two tanks added together. In fact, some anesthetics have huge distribution volumes (e.g., fentanyl has an apparent distribution volume of 4 L/kg) that are substantially larger than an individual's vascular volume (0.07 L/kg) or extracellular volume (0.2 L/kg).

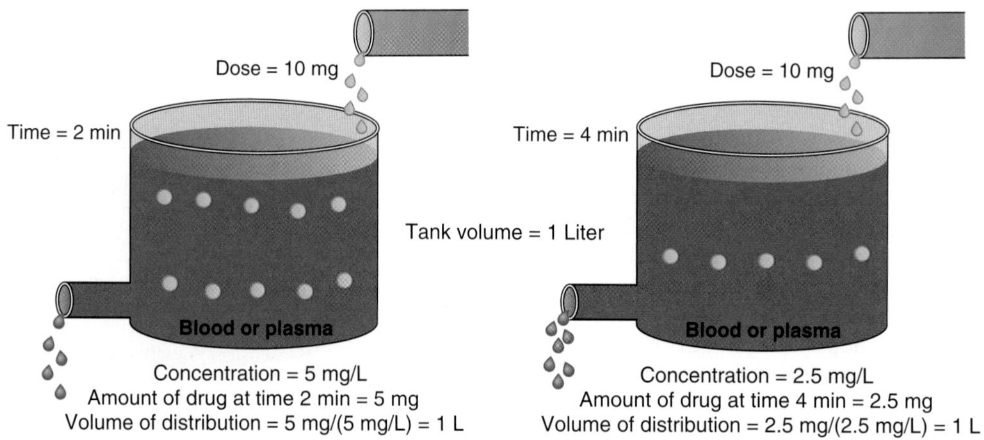

Fig. 18.2 Schematic of a single-tank model of elimination as a first-order process (eliminated at a rate of 50% to the amount of drug present at every two minutes). At 2 minutes *(left panel)* and 4 minutes *(right panel)* following a 10-mg drug bolus, tank concentrations are decreasing from 5 to 2.5 mg/mL. Accounting for elimination, estimates of the distribution volume at each time point are both 1 L.

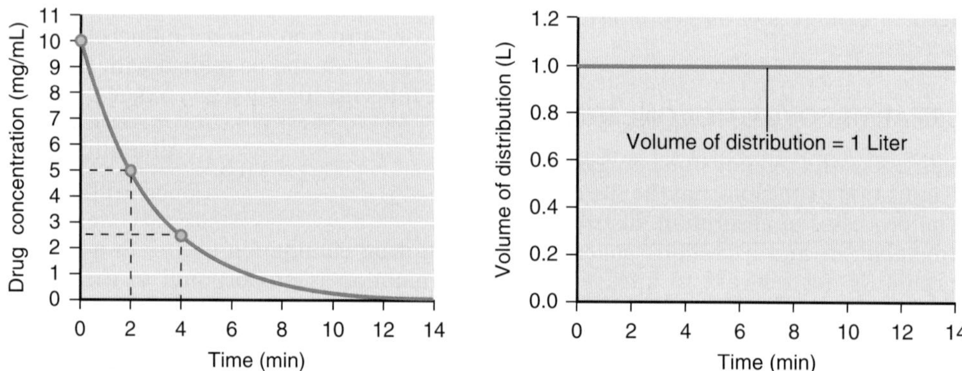

Fig. 18.3 Simulation of concentration *(left panel)* and distribution volume *(right panel)* changes over time following a bolus dose for a single-tank (one-compartment) model. The distribution volume remains constant throughout.

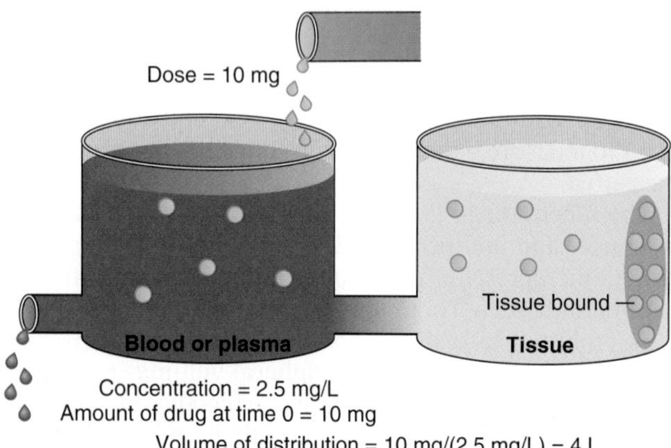

Fig. 18.4 Schematic of a two-tank model. The total volume of distribution consists of the sum of the two tanks. The brown ellipse in the peripheral volume represents tissue that binds up drugs. The measured concentration in the blood or plasma is 2.5 mg/mL just after a bolus dose of 10 mg. Using Fig. 18.1, this leads to a distribution volume of 4 L.

With additional distribution volumes, the overall volume of distribution can change over time and is a function of how drug is administered as well (e.g., as a bolus or a continuous infusion). For example, consider simulations of concentrations and distribution volumes over time following a bolus dose or a continuous infusion of an intravenous anesthetic as presented in Fig. 18.5. For a bolus dose, assume that the volume of distribution is 1 L at time = 0 and that it then increases to 14 L as the plasma concentration falls over the next 10 minutes. The increase of the distribution volume is due to the distribution of drug to peripheral tissue and a decrease in the plasma concentration. For a constant infusion, assume the volume of distribution is again 1 L at time = 0 and that it then increases to 5 L as the plasma concentrations also increase to a steady-state concentration over the next several hours. This is known as the steady-state volume of distribution. It is estimated as the sum of the central and peripheral apparent distribution volumes.

Clearance

Clearance describes the rate of drug removal from the plasma/blood. Two processes contribute to drug clearance: systemic (removal from the tank) and intercompartmental (between tanks) clearance (Fig. 18.6). Systemic clearance permanently removes drug from the body, either by eliminating the parent molecule or by transforming it into metabolites. Intercompartmental clearance moves drug between plasma and peripheral tissue tanks. By way of clarification, in this chapter, the words compartment and tank are interchangeable.

Clearance is defined in units of flow, that is, the volume completely cleared of drug per unit of time (e.g., L/min).

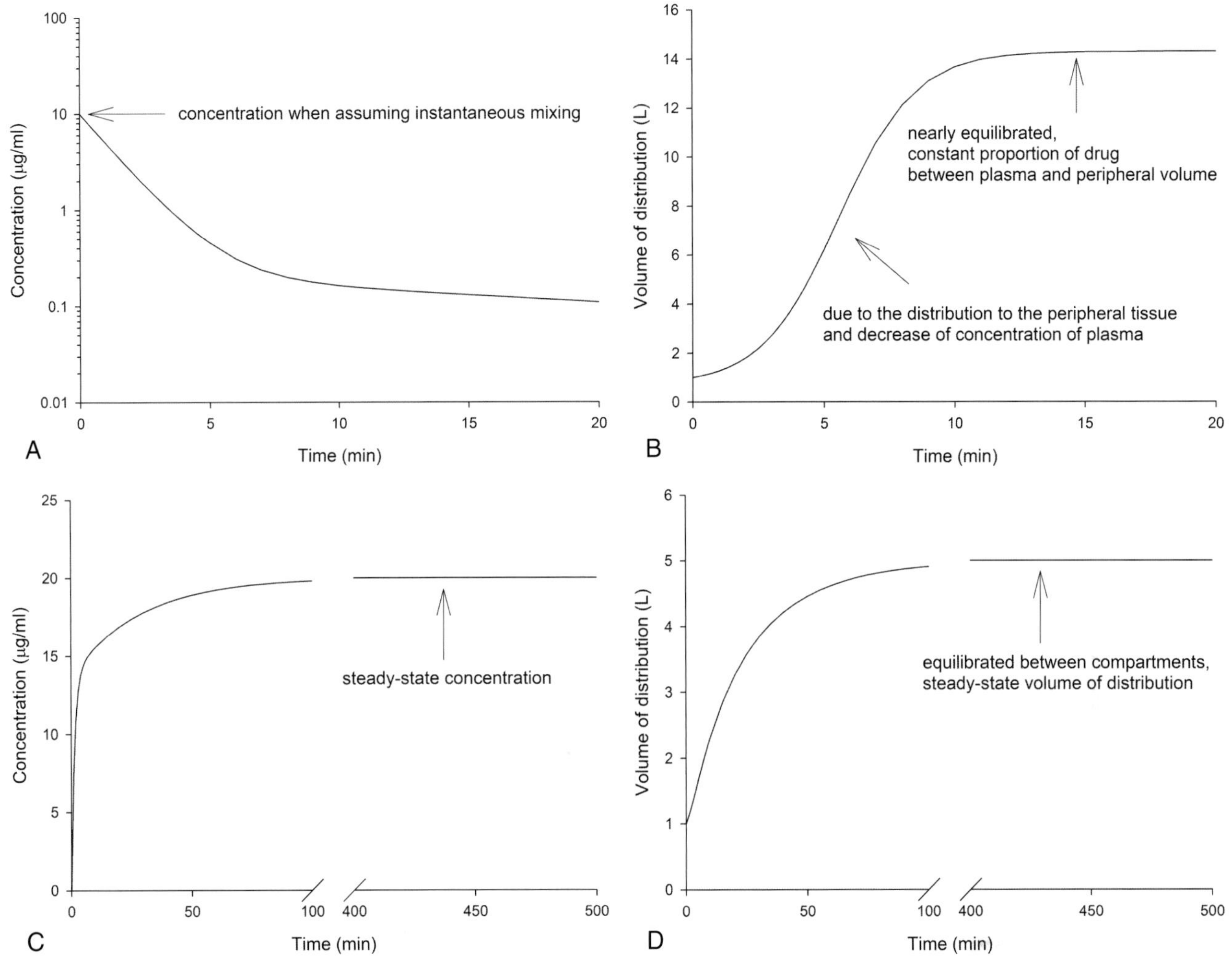

Fig. 18.5 Simulation of concentration and apparent distribution volume changes over time following a bolus dose for a two-tank (two-compartment) model. Panels A and C present drug concentrations over time. Panels B and D present the apparent distribution volume over time.

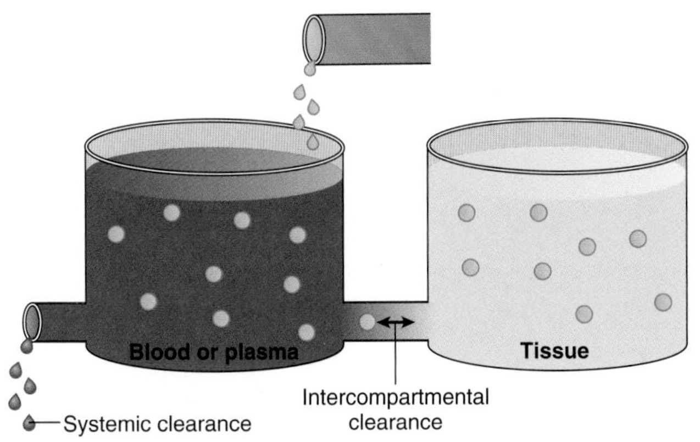

Fig. 18.6 Schematic of a two-tank model illustrating two sources of drug removal from the central tank (blood or plasma): systemic and intercompartmental clearance.

Clearance is not to be confused with elimination rate (e.g., mg/min). The elimination rate is not an accurate method of describing the mass of drug removed over time. For example, assuming a first-order process, when plasma concentrations are high, the rate of drug elimination is high. When low, the rate is also low. Clearance is a better descriptor as it is independent of drug concentration.

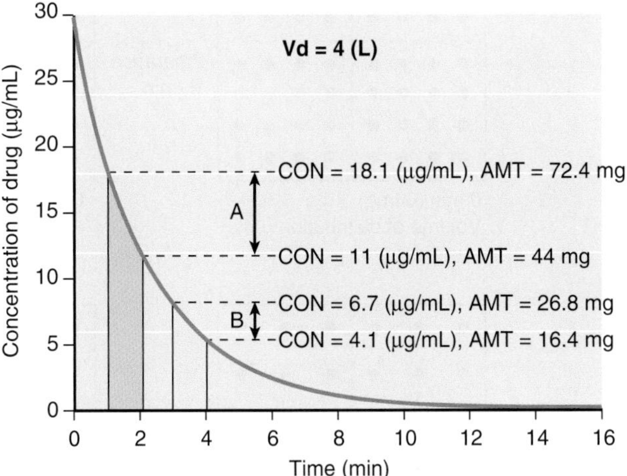

Fig.18.7 Simulation of drug concentration changes when a drug is administered to a single-tank model with first-order elimination (see Fig. 18.2). The concentration changes for two time windows are labeled with dashed lines from 1 to 2 minutes (time window *A*) and from 3 to 4 minutes (time window *B*), respectively. The concentrations *(CON)* at the beginning and end of each time window are used to calculate the amount *(AMT)* of drug that is eliminated (see text). *Vd*, Volume of distribution.

To illustrate this point, consider the simulation presented in Fig. 18.7. In this simulation, the total amount of drug at each time can be calculated from the known volume of distribution and measured concentration. The concentration change in time window A is larger than in time window B even though they are both 1 minute in duration. The elimination rates are 28.4 and 10.4 mg/min for time windows A and B, respectively. They are different, and neither can be used as a parameter to represent a measure of drug removal from the body. Because of this limitation with elimination rate, clearance was developed to provide a single number to describe the decay in drug concentration presented in Fig. 18.7.

For discussion purposes, assume that concentration is the power necessary to push drug out of the water tank. The higher the concentration, the larger the amount of drug eliminated. To standardize the elimination rate, the eliminated amount of drug is scaled to concentration. For example, when the elimination rate in time window A (28.4 mg/min) is scaled to the concentration at the middle of the time window (14.2 μg/mL), the clearance is 2 L/min. When the elimination rate in time window B (10.4 mg/min) is scaled to the concentration at the middle of the time window (5.2 μg/mL), the clearance is again 2 L/min. If the time interval is narrowed so that the time window approaches zero, the definition of clearance becomes:

$$\text{Clearance} = \frac{\frac{dA(t)}{dt}}{C(t)} \tag{18.3}$$

where dA(t)/dt is the rate of drug elimination at given time t, and C(t) is the corresponding concentration at that time. Rearranging Eq. (18.3) and integrating both numerator and denominator, the following relationship holds:

$$\text{Clearance} = \frac{\int_0^\infty dA(t)}{\int_0^\infty C(t)\,dt} \tag{18.4}$$

because the term $\int_0^\infty dA(t)$ is equal to the total amount of drug eliminated and $\int_0^\infty C(t)\,dt$ is the area under curve (AUC) in concentration versus time plot, then the following equation can be derived:

$$\text{Clearance} = \frac{\text{Dose}}{\text{AUC}} \tag{18.5}$$

With long infusions, drug concentrations reach a steady-state condition where the rate of drug elimination $\left(\frac{dA(t)}{dt}\right)$ is in equilibrium with the rate of drug administration (infusion rate). Clearance in a steady-state condition can be obtained using Eq. (18.3) as follows:

$$\text{Clearance} = \frac{\text{Infusion rate}}{\text{Css}} \tag{18.6}$$

where Css is the plasma concentration at steady state.

To illustrate the relationship between clearance and volume of distribution, consider the following simulation using a generic drug dosed in milligrams into a single compartment (tank) representing the distribution volume that has a clearance of 1 L/min. Assume that when drug is administered, the tank is well stirred and has instantaneous mixing throughout the entire volume. Assume the distribution volume is 4 L, the total dose of drug is 64 mg, and that drug elimination is proportional to the amount of drug present inside the tank at any given time. This rate of drug elimination is known as first-order elimination kinetics. When the drug is injected into the 4 L distribution volume, the drug will instantly evenly distribute throughout

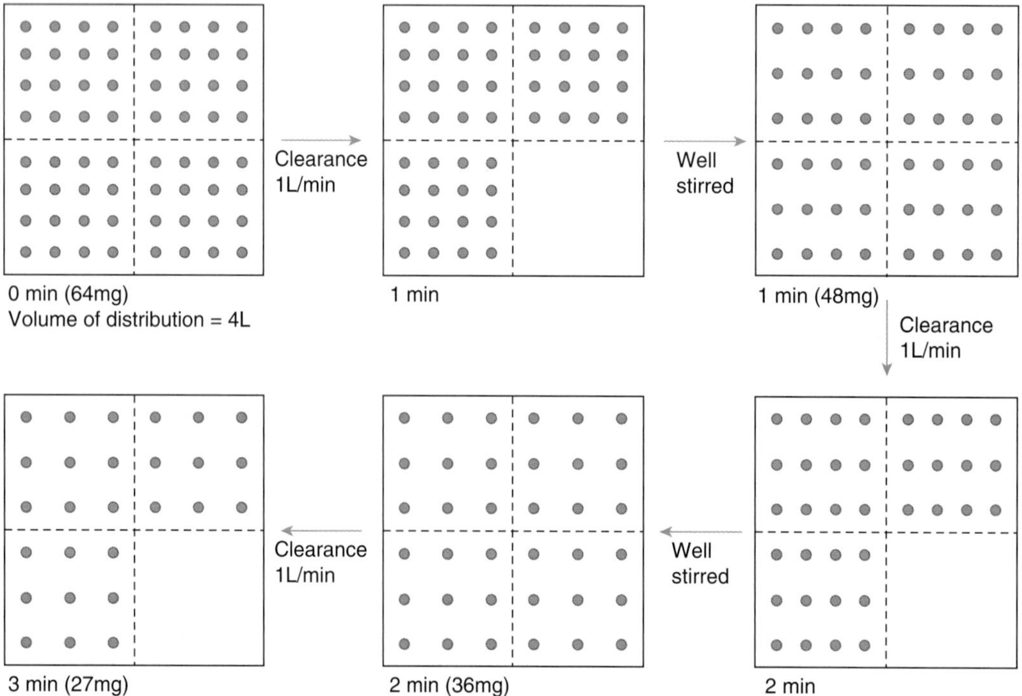

Fig. 18.8 Schematic representation of relationship among clearance, volume of distribution, and elimination rate constant. A generic drug dose of 64 mg is administered into a single compartment volume of 4 L that has a clearance of 1 L/min. Drug elimination is proportional to the amount of drug present inside the compartment at any given time, otherwise known as first-order elimination kinetics. At 1-minute intervals, one of the 4 L is cleared along with all drug contained in that liter. The drug amount decreases by 16, 12, and 9 mg at 1, 2, and 3 minutes.

the compartment (Fig. 18.8). With a clearance of 1 L/min, the amount of drug distributed to one fourth of compartment volume (1 L) will be cleared every minute. In the first minute, 16 mg drug is cleared. The remaining 48 mg will be redistributed evenly throughout the compartment. For the next minute, one fourth of the compartment volume (1 L) is again cleared. In the second minute, 12 mg of drug is cleared. This process repeats every minute. When assuming instantaneously mixing, the ratio of the amount of drug removed within the cleared portion of the distribution volume to the amount of drug within the total distribution volume will remain the same as illustrated in Eq. (18.7).

$$\frac{16\text{mg}}{64\text{mg}} = \frac{12\text{mg}}{48\text{mg}} = \frac{9\text{mg}}{36\text{mg}} = \frac{\text{cleared volume}}{\text{volume of distribution}} \qquad (18.7)$$

This ratio, known as the elimination rate constant (k), is described in Eq. (18.8).

$$\frac{\text{CL}}{\text{Vd}} = \text{k or CL} = \text{Vd} \times \text{k} \qquad (18.8)$$

Where CL is clearance with units of volume/time (L/min), Vd is the compartment distribution volume with units of liters (L), and k is the first-order elimination rate constant with units of inverse time (min^{-1}).

Physiologic Model for Clearance

Drug extraction by metabolic organs is illustrated in Fig. 18.9. This model contains a metabolic organ system responsible for drug elimination. According to mass balance, the rate at which drug flows *out* of metabolic organs is the rate at which drug flows *into* them minus the metabolic rate. The elimination rate (dA/dt) can be expressed as Q (C_{in} – C_{out}). Rearranging C(t) in Eq. (18.3) with C_{in}, clearance can be expressed as

$$\text{Clearance} = \frac{Q\,(C_{in} - C_{out})}{C_{in}} \qquad (18.9)$$

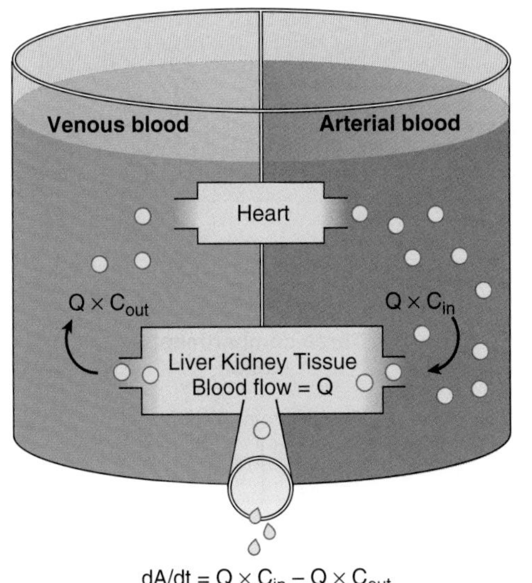

Fig. 18.9 Schematic of drug extraction. Q indicates blood flow. C_{in} and C_{out} indicate drug concentrations presented to and leaving metabolic organs. A indicates the amount of drug, and dA/dt is the drug elimination rate.

where Q is the blood flow to metabolic organs, C_{in} is the concentration of drug delivered to metabolic organs, and C_{out} is the concentration of drug leaving metabolic organs.

The fraction of inflowing drug extracted by the organ is $\frac{C_{in}-C_{out}}{C_{in}}$. This is called the extraction ratio (ER). Clearance can be estimated as organ blood flow multiplied by the ER. Eq. (18.9) can be simplified to

$$\text{Clearance} = \frac{Q\,(C_{in} - C_{out})}{C_{in}}$$

$$= Q \times \frac{C_{in} - C_{out}}{C_{in}} = Q \times \text{ER} \qquad (18.10)$$

The total clearance is the sum of each clearance by metabolic organs such as the liver, kidney, and other tissues.

Hepatic clearance has been well characterized. For example, the relationship among clearance, liver blood flow, and the ER is presented in Fig. 18.10.[1] For drugs with an ER of nearly 1 (e.g., propofol), a change in liver blood flow produces a nearly proportional change in clearance. For drugs with a low ER (e.g., alfentanil), clearance is nearly independent of the rate of liver blood flow. If nearly 100% of the drug is extracted by the liver, this implies that the liver has a very large metabolic capacity for the drug. In this case, the rate-limiting step in metabolism is the flow of drug to the liver, and such drugs are said to be "flow limited." As a consequence, any reduction in liver blood flow due to circulatory effects of anesthetic agents or changes in circulatory volumes in cases of perioperative bleeding or other situations of excessive fluid loss can be expected to reduce liver-dependent drug clearance. However, moderate changes in hepatic metabolic function per se will have little

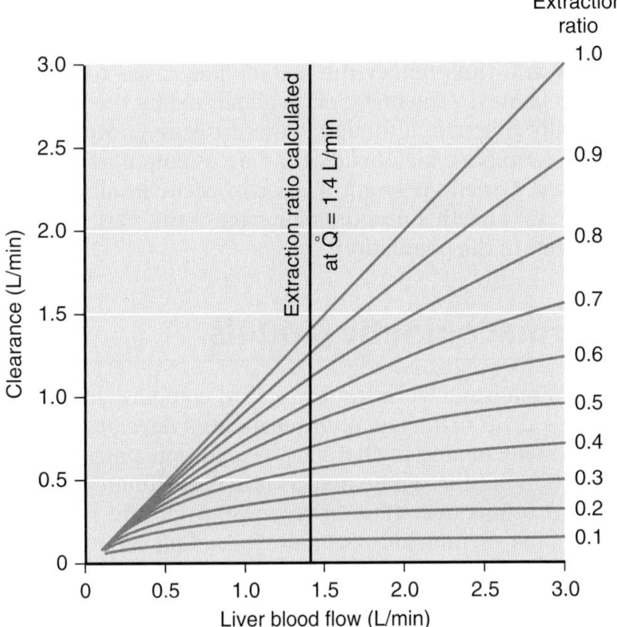

Fig. 18.10 Relationship among liver blood flow (Q), clearance, and extraction ratio. For drugs with a high extraction ratio, clearance is nearly identical to liver blood flow. For drugs with a low extraction ratio, changes in liver blood flow have almost no effect on clearance. (From Wilkinson GR, Shand DG. Commentary: a physiological approach to hepatic drug clearance. *Clin Pharmacol Ther.* 1975;18:377–390.)

impact on clearance because hepatic metabolic capacity is overwhelmingly in excess of demand.

For many drugs (e.g., alfentanil), the ER is considerably less than 1. For these drugs, clearance is limited by the capacity of the liver to take up and metabolize drug. These drugs are said to be "capacity limited." Clearance will change in response to any change in the capacity of the liver to metabolize such drugs, as might be caused by liver disease or enzymatic induction. However, changes in liver blood flow caused by the anesthetic regimen or other changes in splanchnic circulation usually have little influence on clearance because the liver handles only a fraction of the drug that it sees.

Although most anesthetic drugs are cleared by hepatic metabolism, remifentanil, succinylcholine, and esmolol are cleared in the plasma and tissues by ester hydrolysis, and pancuronium is cleared via the kidney. The relationship between metabolism and clearance is complex.

Hepatic Biotransformation

Most anesthetic drugs are cleared by hepatic biotransformation. The synthetic pathways for biotransformation are covered in detail in many biochemistry texts. Briefly, the liver metabolizes drugs through oxidation, reduction, hydrolysis, or conjugation. Oxidation and reduction occur in the cytochrome P450 system. These enzymes can be induced by exposure to certain drugs (e.g., the herbal remedy St. John's wort) and increase the liver's intrinsic metabolic capacity. Other drugs or hepatic disease can inhibit these enzymes (e.g., selected calcium channel blockers and selected antibiotics). Routes of oxidative metabolism include hydroxylation, dealkylation, deamination, desulfuration, epoxidation, and dehalogenation. Conjugation and hydrolysis often occur outside the P450 system, although glucuronidation involves the P450 system as well. The effect of conjugation is to transform hydrophobic molecules into water-soluble molecules through the addition of polar groups and thus render the metabolites easier to excrete via the kidneys. The metabolites generated by the liver are generally inactive, although some drugs (e.g., morphine, midazolam) have metabolites that are as potent as the parent drug. Genetic polymorphism can occur in all of these pathways, and this accounts for part of the variability in clearance in the population.

Pharmacokinetic Models

To create a framework from which to compare drugs and describe drug behavior, pharmacologists developed pharmacokinetic models to characterize drug concentrations as a function of time. These models provide estimates of drug concentrations over time in response to dosing regimens (e.g., bolus vs. infusion). Several types of pharmacokinetic models have been developed. Examples include complex physiologic models and the more common compartmental models.

Physiologic Models

Physiologic models are based on organ and tissue physiologic and anatomic data. Drug concentrations into and out of an organ, organ blood flow, and organ drug distribution volume are required. Capturing these metrics from all organs is nearly impossible in humans and very challenging in animal models. If obtained, this data is used to estimate volumes and clearances for each organ in the body. Individual organ models are assembled into a whole organism physiological model.[2] Once assembled, the combined models are complex and mathematically cumbersome. They may not offer a better prediction of plasma drug concentrations over time than simple compartmental models. If the intent of the model is to explore the ability of possible dosing regimens to achieve therapeutic plasma drug concentrations, compartmental models are usually adequate.

Compartmental Models

Compartmental models are built on the same basic concepts as physiologic models, but with significant simplifications. Compartment pharmacokinetic models are strictly empirical. They are based on fitting equations to measured plasma concentrations following a known dose. Kinetic models are transformed into models that characterize changes over time in terms of volumes and clearances. Part of the continuing popularity of pharmacokinetic models is that they can be transformed from an unintuitive exponential form to a more intuitive compartmental form as shown in Fig. 18.11.

Compartment models used to describe anesthetic drugs typically consist of one, two, or three compartments corresponding to the number of exponents in an equation needed to best fit the plasma versus concentration data (see Fig. 18.11). Exponents are difficult to work with and have little clinical meaning. Thus, they are converted into fictitious volumes and clearances. For example, in a three-compartment model, there is a central compartment and two peripheral compartments. The sum of the all volumes is the volume of distribution at steady state. Drug clearance

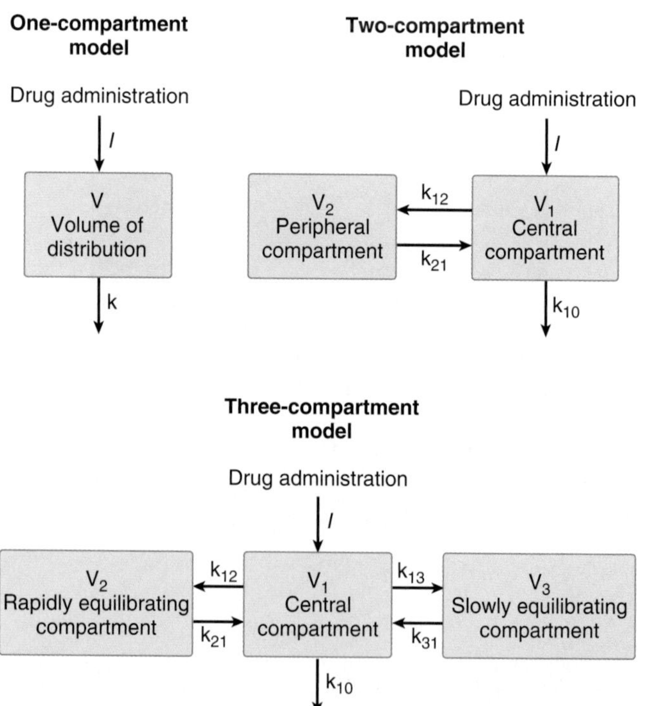

Fig. 18.11 One-, two-, and three-compartment mammillary models.

from the central compartment to the outside is the central clearance. Central clearance accounts for both metabolism and excretion. Clearances between the central and peripheral compartments is the "intercompartmental" clearance. Micro rate constants, expressed as k_{ij}, define the rate of drug transfer from compartment i to compartment j. For example, k_{10} is the micro rate constant describing drug transfer from central compartment to the outside. The intercompartmental micro rate constants (k_{12}, k_{21}, etc.) describe movement of drug between the central and peripheral compartments. Each peripheral compartment has at least two micro rate constants, one for drug entry and one for drug exit. The micro rate constants for the two- and three-compartment models are presented in Fig. 18.11.

Zero Versus First-Order Kinetics

Drug elimination can have one of two profiles, zero- and first-order kinetics. With zero-order kinetics, drug is eliminated at a constant rate. With first-order kinetics, drug is eliminated at a rate proportional to the amount of drug present at that time. These rates are expressed using the following equations.

$$\frac{dA(t)}{dt} = -k_0 \text{ for zero order kinetics} \tag{18.11}$$

$$\frac{dA(t)}{dt} = -k_1 E(t) \text{ for first-order kinetics} \tag{18.12}$$

where A(t) is the amount of drug at time t, dA(t) is the change in drug amount at time t. $-k_0$ is the zero-order elimination rate constant. Its units are mass/time (e.g., mg/min). $-k_1$ is the first-order elimination rate constant. Its units are the reciprocal time 1/time, (e.g., min^{-1}). Most anesthetic drugs have first-order kinetics. When the processes responsible for metabolism are saturated, the kinetics could change from first to zero order.

ONE-COMPARTMENT MODEL

For a one-compartment model with first-order kinetic elimination, the amount of drug at a given time t is described by Eq. (18.13).

$$A(t) = A_0 e^{-kt} \tag{18.13}$$

where A_0 is the initial drug amount (i.e., the initial dose), k is the first-order kinetic elimination rate constant. Note that k must be greater than 0. With this equation, there is an exponential decrease in drug amount.

The distribution volume (Vd) is a function of drug concentration and the total amount of drug in the compartment. Dividing Eq. (18.13) on both sides by Vd yields the following equation:

$$\frac{A(t)}{Vd} = \frac{A_0}{Vd} e^{-kt} \tag{18.14}$$

Drug concentration can be derived from this relationship with Eq. (18.15):

$$C(t) = C_0 \times e^{-kt} \tag{18.15}$$

where C(t) is the concentration at time t, C_0 is the initial concentration at time 0.

Taking the natural logarithm on both sides, the following expression is obtained:

$$\log C(t) = \log C_0 - kt \tag{18.16}$$

A plot of this equation shows a straight line with slope of –k and intercept of log C_0. To yield the time required for the concentration to decrease by half, replacing log C(t) in Eq. (18.16) to log $C_0/2$ and rearranging gives:

$$\log\frac{C_0}{2} = \log C_0 - kt \tag{18.17}$$

Solving this equation gives

$$t_{1/2} = \frac{0.693}{k} \tag{18.18}$$

where $t_{1/2}$ is the elimination half-life.

Multicompartment Models

Plasma concentrations over time after an intravenous bolus resemble the curve in Fig. 18.12. This curve has the characteristics common to most drugs when given by intravenous bolus. First, the concentrations continuously decrease over time. Second, the rate of decline is initially steep but continuously becomes less steep, until we get to a portion that is "log-linear." For many drugs, three distinct phases can be distinguished, as illustrated in Fig. 18.12. A "rapid-distribution" phase *(blue line)* begins immediately after bolus injection. Very rapid movement of the drug from plasma to the rapidly equilibrating tissues characterizes this phase. Frequently there is a second "slow-distribution" phase *(red line)*, which is characterized by movement of drug into more slowly equilibrating tissues and return of drug to plasma from the most rapidly equilibrating tissues. The terminal phase *(green line)* is a straight line when plotted on a semilogarithmic graph. The terminal phase is often called the "elimination phase" because the primary mechanism for decreasing drug concentration during the terminal phase is elimination of drug from the body. The distinguishing

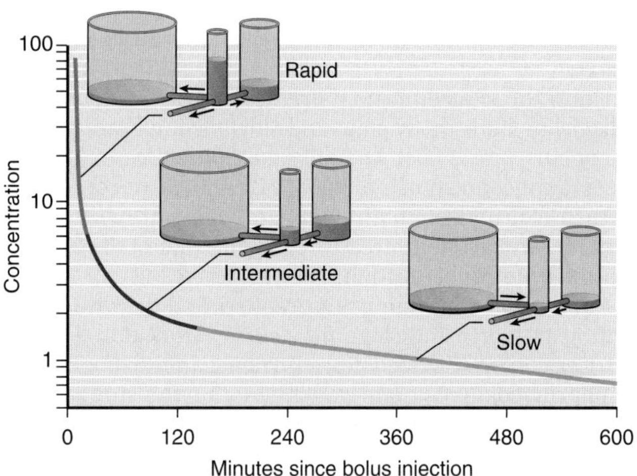

Fig. 18.12 Hydraulic model of fentanyl pharmacokinetics. Drug is administered into the central tank, from which it can distribute into two peripheral tanks, or it may be eliminated. The volume of the tanks is proportional to the volumes of distribution. The cross-sectional area of the pipes is proportional to clearance. (From Youngs EJ, Shafer SL. Basic pharmacokinetic and pharmacodynamic principles. In: White PF, ed. *Textbook of Intravenous Anesthesia*. Baltimore: Williams & Wilkins; 1997.)

characteristic of the terminal elimination phase is that the plasma concentration is lower than tissue concentrations and the relative proportion of drug in plasma and peripheral volumes of distribution remains constant. During this terminal phase, drug returns from the rapid- and slow-distribution volumes to plasma and is permanently removed from plasma by metabolism or excretion.

The presence of three distinct phases after bolus injection is a defining characteristic of a three-compartment model.[3] A useful metaphor in describing the features of this model is hydraulics. This model has three tanks corresponding (from left to right) to the slowly equilibrating peripheral compartment, the central compartment (the plasma, into which drug is injected), and the rapidly equilibrating peripheral compartment. The horizontal pipes represent intercompartmental clearance or (for the pipe draining onto the page) metabolic clearance. The volumes of each tank correspond to the volumes of each compartment. The cross-sectional areas of the pipes correlate with fentanyl systemic and intercompartmental clearance. The height of water in each tank corresponds to drug concentration.

By using this hydraulic model, we can follow the processes that decrease drug concentration over time after bolus injection. Initially, drug flows from the central compartment to both peripheral compartments via intercompartmental clearance and completely out of the model via metabolic clearance. Because there are three places for drug to go, the concentration in the central compartment decreases very rapidly. At the transition between the blue line and the red line, a change occurs in the role of the most rapidly equilibrating compartment. At this transition, the concentration in the central compartment falls below the concentration in the rapidly equilibrating compartment, and the direction of flow between them is reversed. After this transition *(red line)*, drug in plasma has only two places to go: into the slowly equilibrating compartment or out the drain pipe. These processes are partly offset by the return of drug to plasma from the rapidly equilibrating compartment. The net effect is that once the rapidly equilibrating compartment has come to equilibration, the concentration in the central compartment falls far more slowly than before.

Once the concentration in the central compartment falls below both the rapidly and slowly equilibrating compartments *(green line)*, the only method of decreasing the plasma concentration is metabolic clearance, the drainpipe. Return of drug from both peripheral compartments to the central compartment greatly slows the rate of decrease in plasma drug concentration.

Curves that continuously decrease over time, with a continuously increasing slope (i.e., curves that look like Fig. 18.12), can be described by a sum of negative exponentials. In pharmacokinetics, one way of denoting this sum of exponentials is to say that the plasma concentration over time is

$$C(t) = Ae^{-\alpha t} + Be^{-\beta t} + Ce^{-\gamma t} \quad (18.19)$$

where t is the time since the bolus, C(t) is the drug concentration after a bolus dose, and A, α, B, β, C, and γ are parameters of a pharmacokinetic model. A, B, and C are called coefficients, whereas α, β, and γ are called exponents. After a bolus injection, all six of the parameters in Eq. (18.19) will be greater than 0.

Special significance is often ascribed to the smallest exponent. This exponent determines the slope of the final log-linear portion of the curve. When the medical literature refers to the half-life of a drug, unless otherwise stated, the half-life will be the terminal half-life. Some literature occasionally refers to the half-life of the initial distribution phase as distribution half-life. The terminal half-life sets an upper limit on the time required for the concentrations to decrease by 50% after drug administration. Usually, the time needed for a 50% decrease will be much faster than that upper limit.

Special Interests in Anesthetic Pharmacokinetics

Front-End Kinetics

Front-end kinetics refers to the description of intravenous drug behavior immediately following administration. How a drug rapidly moves from the blood into peripheral tissues directly influences the peak plasma drug concentration. The amount of drug that moves to the peripheral tissue commonly surpasses the amount that is eliminated during the first few minutes after drug administration. As an example, consider a simulation of a propofol bolus that plots the accumulation of propofol in peripheral tissues and the amount eliminated over time (Fig. 18.13). During the first 4 minutes, the amount distributed to the peripheral tissue is larger than the amount eliminated out of the body. After 4 minutes, the amounts reverse.

With compartmental models, an important assumption is that an intravenous bolus instantly mixes in the central volume, with the peak concentration occurring at the moment of injection without elimination or distribution to peripheral tissues. For simulation purposes, the initial concentration and volume of distribution at time = 0 are extrapolated as if the circulation had been infinitely fast. This, of course, is not real. If drug is injected into an arm

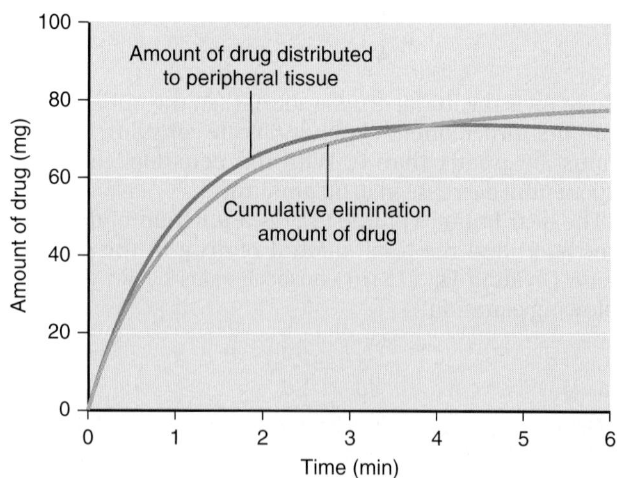

Fig.18.13 Simulation of propofol accumulation in the peripheral tissues *(blue line)* and the cumulative amount of propofol eliminated *(gold line)* following a 2-mg/kg propofol bolus to a 77-kg (170-lb), 53-year-old male who is 177 cm (5 ft 10 inch) tall, using published pharmacokinetic model parameters.[32] Drug indicates propofol.

vein and the initial concentration is measured in a radial artery, drug appears in the arterial circulation 30 to 40 seconds after injection. The delay likely represents the time required for drug to pass through the venous volume of the upper part of the arm, heart, great vessels, and peripheral arterial circulation. More sophisticated models (e.g., a recirculatory model)[4] account for this delay and are useful when characterizing the behavior of a drug immediately following bolus administration such as with induction agents where the speed of onset and duration of action are of interest (Fig. 18.14).

Back-End Kinetics

Using estimates of distribution volume and clearance, back-end kinetics is a useful tool that describes the behavior of intravenous agents when administered as continuous infusions. Back-end kinetics provides descriptors of how plasma drug concentrations decrease once a continuous infusion is terminated. An example is decrement time, which predicts the time required to reach a certain plasma concentration once an infusion is terminated. Decrement times are a function of infusion duration. Consider the example of decrement times for a set of continuous target- controlled infusions (TCIs; Fig. 18.15). In this simulation, TCI of propofol is set to maintain a concentration of 4 μg/mL for 30, 60, and 120 minutes. Once the infusion is stopped, the time to reach 0.5 μg/mL is estimated. As illustrated, the longer the infusion, the longer the time required to reach 0.5 μg/mL. This example demonstrates how drugs accumulate in peripheral tissues with prolonged infusions. This accumulation prolongs the decrement time.

Another use of decrement times is as a tool to compare drugs within a drug class (e.g., opioids). As a comparator, plots of decrement times are presented as a function of infusion duration. When used this way, decrement times are determined as the time required to reach a target percentage of the concentration just before the termination of a continuous infusion. Examples of 50% and 80% decrement times for selected opioids and sedatives are presented in Fig. 18.16. Of note, for shorter infusions, the decrement times are similar for both classes of anesthetic drugs. Once infusion duration exceeds 2 hours, the decrement times vary substantially. A popular decrement time is the 50% decrement time, also known as the context-sensitive half-time.[5] The term "context-sensitive" refers to infusion duration and the term "half-time" refers to the 50% decrement time.

Hysteresis

Hysteresis refers to the time delay between changes in plasma concentration and drug effect. Hysteresis accounts for the time required for drug to diffuse from the plasma to the site of action plus the time required, once drug is at the site of action, to elicit a drug effect. A simulation of various propofol bolus doses and their predicted effect on bispectral index are presented in Fig. 18.17. Of note, the time to peak effect for each dose is identical (approximately 1.5 minutes following the peak plasma concentration). The difference between each dose is the magnitude and duration of effect. A key principle here is that when drug concentrations are in flux (e.g., during induction and emergence), changes in drug effect will lag behind changes in plasma drug concentration. This lag between the plasma concentration and

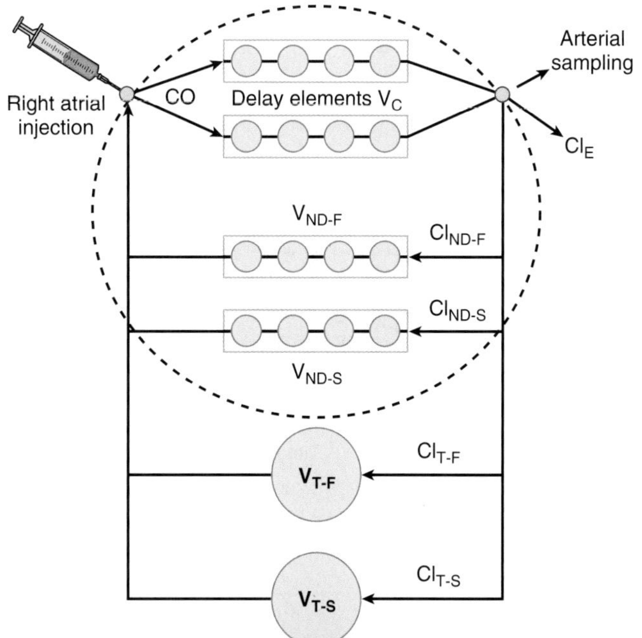

Fig. 18.14 A recirculatory model accounting for cardiac output *(CO)*, transit delays, pulmonary uptake (delay elements V and C), and nondistributive mixing pathways (V_{ND} and Cl_{ND}). All the components within the *dashed circle* are required to accurately model the central volume of distribution. In most situations, this complexity is not required, and the simpler approach of assuming instantaneous mixing within the central volume is an adequate approximation. Cl_{ND-F}, Fast nondistributive clearance; Cl_{ND-S}, slow nondistributive clearance; Cl_{T-F}, fast tissue clearance; Cl_{T-S}, slow tissue clearance; V_{ND-F}, fast nondistributive volume; V_{ND-S}, slow nondistributive volume; V_{T-F}, fast tissue volume; V_{T-S}, slow tissue volume. (From Krejcie TC, Avram MJ, Gentry WB. A recirculatory model of the pulmonary uptake and pharmacokinetics of lidocaine based on analysis or arterial and mixed venous data from dogs. J Pharmacokinet Biopharm. 1997;25:169–190.)

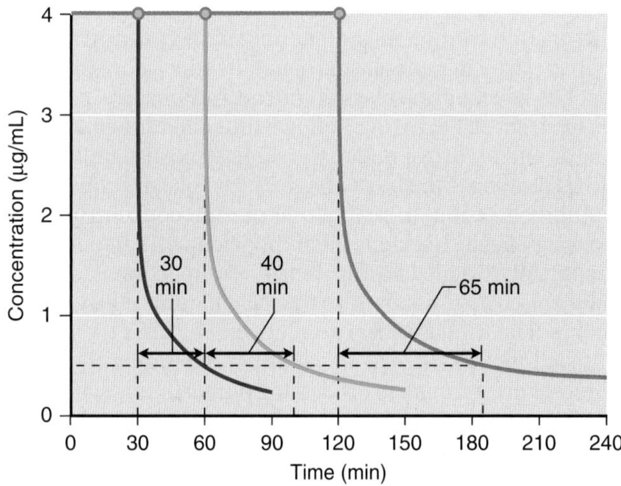

Fig. 18.15 Simulation of decrement times for a target-controlled infusion set to maintain a target propofol concentration of 4 μg/mL for 30, 60, and 120 minutes. Once terminated, the time required to reach 0.5 μg/mL was 30, 40, and 65 minutes for each infusion, respectively. Simulations of the decrement times used a published pharmacokinetic model. (From Schnider TW, Minto CF, Gambus PL, et al. The influence of method of administration and covariates on the pharmacokinetics of propofol in adult volunteers. *Anesthesiology*. 1998;88(5):1170–1182.)

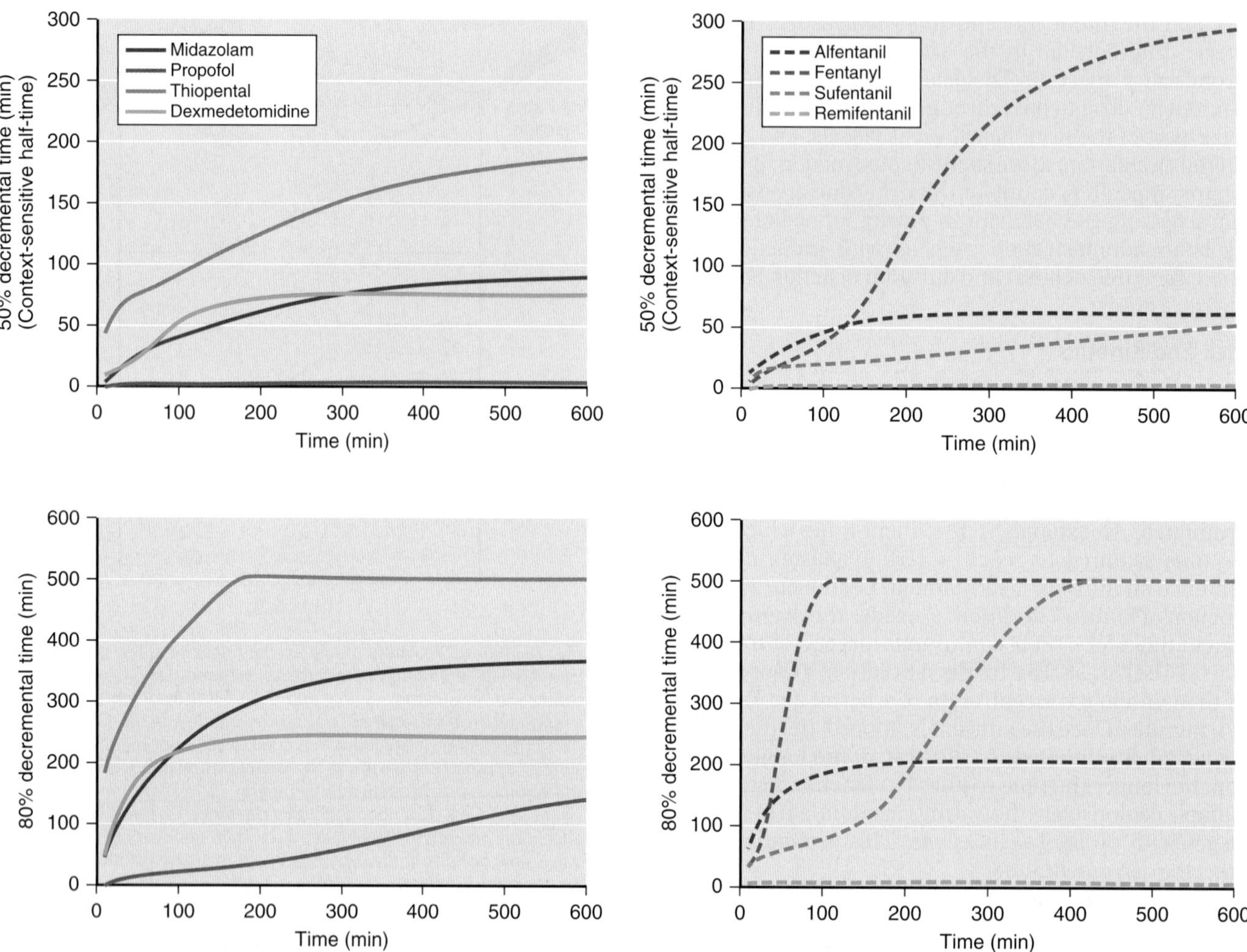

Fig. 18.16 Fifty percent and 80% decrement times for selected sedatives *(left side)* and opioids *(right side)*. The vertical axes refer to the time required to reach the desired decrement time. The horizontal axes refer to infusion duration. Simulations of the decrement times used published pharmacokinetic models for each sedative and analgesic. (Data from references 5, 43, 57, and 68-70.)

effect usually results in the phenomenon called hysteresis in which two different plasma concentrations correspond to one drug effect or one plasma concentration corresponds to two drug effects. Fig. 18.17 shows that different concentrations, C and c, correspond to the same bispectral index scale (BIS). To collapse the hysteresis between plasma concentration and effect and to match one plasma concentration to one drug effect, this lag is often modeled with an effect-site compartment added to the central compartment. Kinetic micro rate constants used to describe biophase include k_{1e} and k_{e0}. The k_{1e} describes drug movement from the central compartment to the effect site, and k_{e0} describe the elimination of drug from the effect-site compartment. There are two important assumptions with the effect-site compartment: (1) the amount of drug that moves from the central compartment to the effect-site compartment is negligible and vice versa, and (2) there is no "volume" estimate to the effect-site compartment.

Typically, the relationship between plasma and the site of drug effect is modeled with an "effect-site" compartment model, as shown in Fig. 18.18. The site of drug effect is connected to plasma by a first-order process. The equation that relates effect-site concentration to plasma concentration is

$$\frac{dCe}{dt} = k_{e0} \times (Cp - Ce) \qquad (18.20)$$

where Ce is the effect-site concentration, Cp is the plasma drug concentration, and k_{e0} is the rate constant for elimination of drug. The constant k_{e0} describes the rate of rise and offset of drug effect (Fig. 18.19).

In summary, although of interest to many clinicians, the conventional pharmacokinetic term *half-life* has limited meaning to anesthetic practice since the clinical behavior of drugs used in anesthesia is not well described by half-life. Instead, the pharmacokinetic principles discussed in this section (such as volume of distribution, clearance, elimination, front-end kinetics, back-end kinetics, context-sensitive half-time, and biophase) describe how drugs used in anesthesia will behave.

Pharmacodynamic Principles

Simply stated, pharmacokinetics describes what the body does to the drug, whereas pharmacodynamics describes what the drug does to the body. In particular, pharmacodynamics describes the relationship between drug concentration and pharmacologic effect.

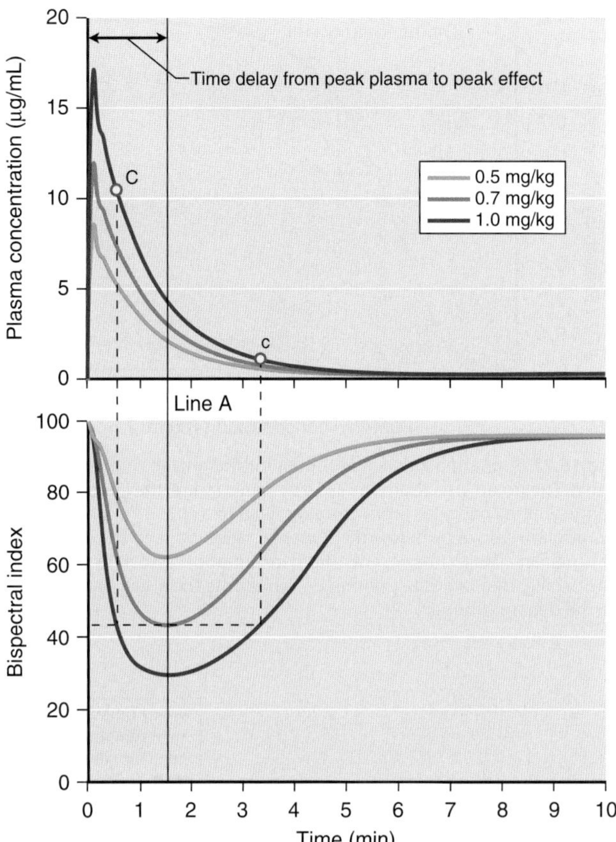

Fig. 18.17 Illustration of hysteresis. The top plot presents a simulation of three propofol doses and the resultant plasma concentrations. The bottom plot presents a simulation of the predicted effect on the bispectral index scale (BIS). These simulations assume linear kinetics: regardless of the dose, effects peak at the same time *(line A)* as do the plasma concentration. The time to peak effect is 1.5 minutes. Even the plasma concentrations of point *C* and *c* are different; the BIS of those two points are same. It shows the hysteresis between plasma concentration and BIS. Simulations used published pharmacokinetic and pharmacodynamic models. (Data from references 32 and 57.)

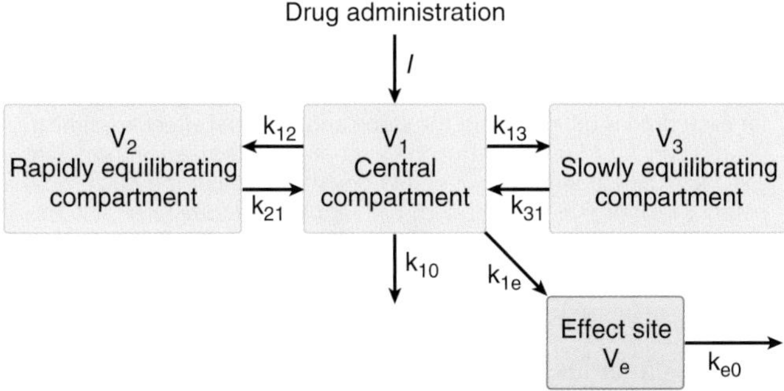

Fig. 18.18 A three-compartment model with an added effect site to account for the delay in equilibration between the rise and fall in arterial drug concentrations and the onset and offset of drug effect. The effect site is assumed to have a negligible volume.

Models used to describe the concentration-effect relationships are created in much the same way as pharmacokinetic models; they are based on observations and used to create a mathematical model. To create a pharmacodynamic model, plasma drug levels and a selected drug effect are measured simultaneously. For example, consider the measured plasma concentrations of a drug following a bolus dose and the associated changes in the spectral edge from one individual presented in Fig. 18.20. Spectral edge is an easily captured metric used to quantify the electroencephalogram (EEG). Shortly after the plasma concentration peaks, the spectral edge starts to drop, reaches a nadir, and then returns to baseline as the plasma concentrations drop to near 0.

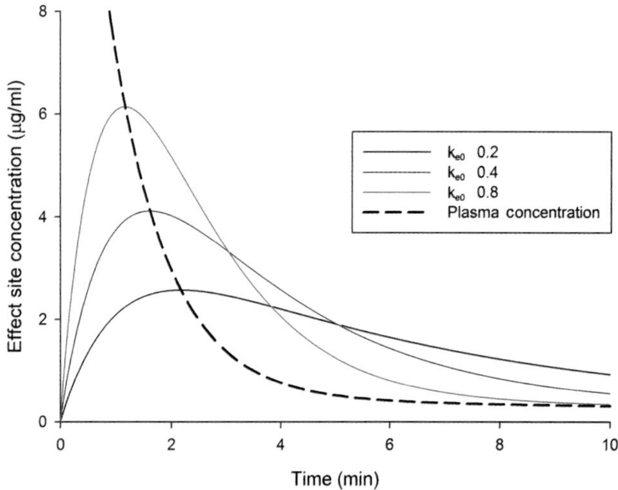

Fig. 18.19 Effect of the k_{eo} changes. As the k_{eo} decreases, the time to peak effect is prolonged. (Data from references 32, 57, 67.)

Combining data from several individuals and plotting the measured concentrations versus the observed effect (modified to be a percentage of the maximal effect across all individuals), the data create a hysteresis loop (Fig. 18.21). The ascending portion of the loop represents rising drug concentrations (see arrow). While rising, the increase in drug effect lags behind the increase in drug concentration. For the descending loop, the decrease in drug effect lags behind the decrease in drug concentration.

To create a pharmacodynamic model, the hysteresis loop is collapsed using modeling techniques that account for the lag time between plasma concentrations and the observed effect. These modeling techniques provide an estimate of the lag time, known as the $t_{1/2}k_{e0}$, and an estimate of the effect-site concentration (Ce) associated with a 50% probability of drug effect (C_{50}). Most concentration effect relationships in anesthesia are described with a sigmoid curve. The standard equation for this relationship is the "Hill Equation," also known as the "sigmoid E_{max} relationship" (Eq. 18.21),

$$\text{Effect} = E_0 + (E_{max} - E_0) * \left(C^g / \left(C_g^{50} + C^g\right)\right) \quad (18.21)$$

where E_0 is the baseline effect, E_{max} is the maximal effect, C is the drug concentration, and γ (gamma) represents the slope of the concentration-effect relationship. Gamma (γ) is also known as the "Hill coefficient." For values of $\gamma < 1$, the curve is hyperbolic; for values of $\gamma > 1$, the curve is sigmoid. Fig. 18.22 presents an example of this relationship: a fentanyl effect-site concentration-effect curve for analgesia. This example illustrates how C_{50} and γ characterize the concentration-effect relationship.

Potency and Efficacy

Two important concepts are relevant to this relationship: potency and efficacy. Potency describes the amount of drug

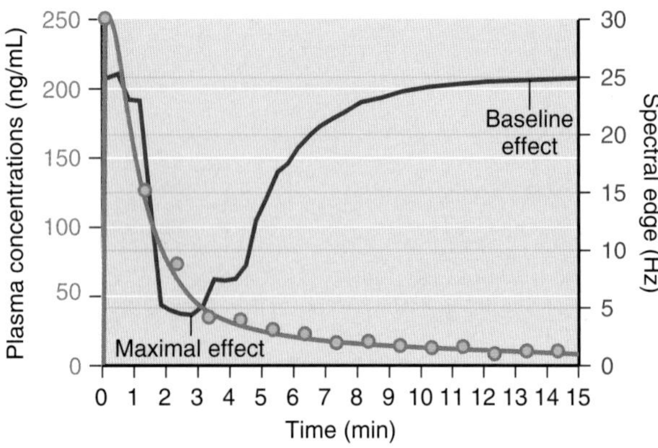

Fig. 18.20 Schematic representation of drug plasma concentrations *(blue circles)* following a bolus and the associated changes in the electroencephalogram's spectral edge *(red line)* measured in one individual. Note that changes in spectral edge lag behind changes in plasma concentrations.

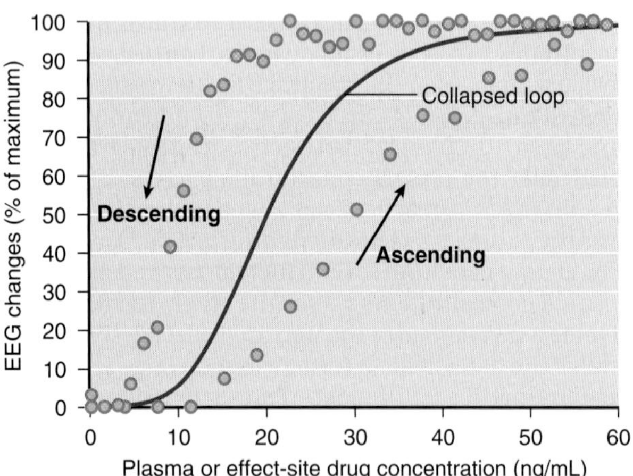

Fig.18.21 Schematic representation of plasma concentrations versus normalized spectral edge measurements (presented as a percentage of maximal effect) from several individuals *(blue circles)*. The black arrows indicate the ascending and descending arms of a hysteresis loop that coincide with increasing and decreasing drug concentrations. The red line represents the pharmacodynamic model developed from collapsing the hysteresis loop. *EEG*, Electroencephalogram.

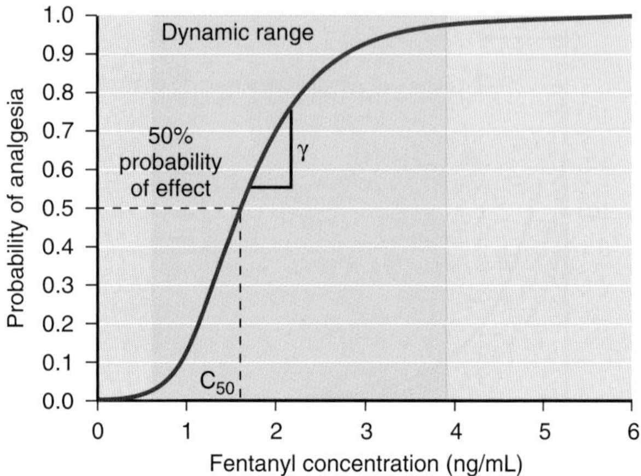

Fig.18.22 A pharmacodynamic model for the analgesic effect of fentanyl. The green area represents the dynamic range, the concentration range where changes in concentration lead to a change in effect. Concentrations above or below the dynamic range do lead to changes in drug effect. The C_{50} represents the concentration associate with 50% probability of analgesia. Gamma (γ) represents the slope of the curve in the dynamic range.

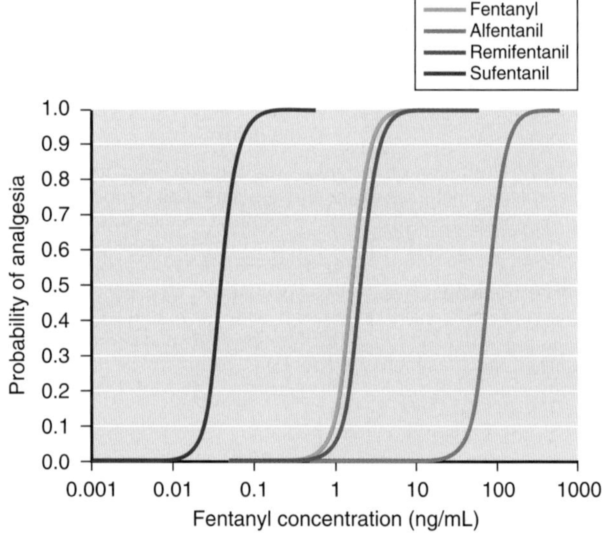

Fig. 18.23 Pharmacodynamic models for fentanyl congeners. The C_{50} for each drug is different, but the slope and maximal effect are similar. (From Egan TD, Muir KT, Hermann DJ, et al. The electroencephalogram (EEG) and clinical measures of opioid potency: defining the EEG-clinical potency relationship ("fingerprint") with application to remifentanil. *Int J Pharmaceut Med.* 2001;15(1):11–19.)

required to elicit an effect. The C_{50} is a common parameter used to describe potency. For drugs that have a concentration-versus-effect relationship that is shifted to the left (small C_{50}), the drug is considered to be more potent; the reverse is true for drugs that have a concentration-versus-effect relationship shifted to the right. For example, as illustrated in Fig. 18.23, the analgesia C_{50} for some of the fentanyl congeners ranges from small for sufentanil (0.04 ng/mL) to large for alfentanil (75 ng/mL). Thus, sufentanil is more potent than alfentanil.

Efficacy is a measure of drug effectiveness at producing an effect once it occupies a receptor. Similar drugs that work through the same receptor may have varying degrees of effect despite having the same receptor occupancy. For example, with G-protein coupled receptors, some drugs may bind the receptor in such a way as to produce a more pronounced activation of second messengers causing more of an effect than others. Drugs that achieve maximal effect are known as full agonists, and those that have an effect less than maximal effect are known as partial agonists.

Effective Versus Lethal Doses

A single drug can have multiple effects. The C_{50} concept is used to compare various drug effects for a single drug. For example, as illustrated in Fig. 18.24, fentanyl has a different C_{50} for analgesia (2 ng/mL), ventilatory depression (4 ng/mL), loss of response to laryngoscopy (15 ng/mL), and changes in the EEG (20 ng/mL).[6]

The concentration range where changes in drug effect occur is known as the *dynamic range*. In Fig. 18.22, the

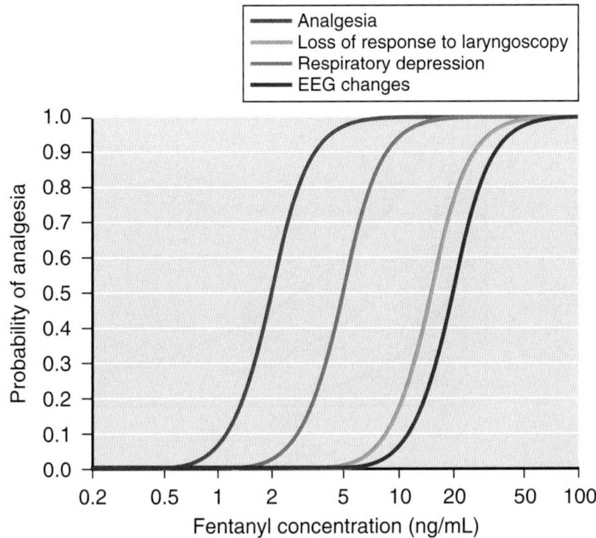

Fig. 18.24 Pharmacodynamic models for various fentanyl effects. *EEG*, Electroencephalogram. (From Egan TD, Muir KT, Hermann DJ, et al. The electroencephalogram (EEG) and clinical measures of opioid potency: defining the EEG-clinical potency relationship ("fingerprint") with application to remifentanil. *Int J Pharmaceut Med*. 2001;15(1):11–19.)

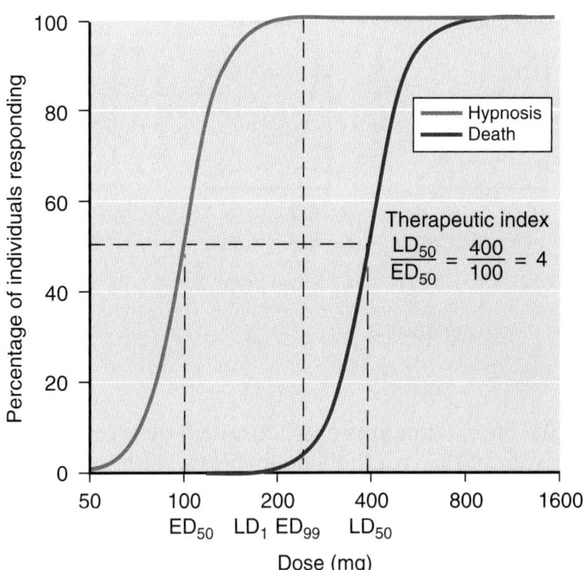

Fig. 18.25 Median effective dose (ED_{50}), median lethal dose (LD_{50}), and the therapeutic index. The blue curve represents the dose-effect relationship for a sedative hypnotic to achieve unresponsiveness. The red curve represents the dose-effect relationship for the same sedative hypnotic to achieve death. The therapeutic index is the ratio of the LD_{50}/ED_{50}, which in this example is 400. Also of interest are the ED_{99} and LD_1. The ED_{99} is the dose with a 99% probability of unresponsiveness, and the LD_1 is the dose with a 1% probability of death. In this example, the LD_1 is less than the ED_{99}, which is clinically unacceptable.

dynamic range is from 0.6 to 3.9 ng/mL to cover a probability of analgesia ranging from 2% to 97%. Concentrations outside the dynamic range do not yield much change in drug effect. Levels below the dynamic range are ineffective, and those above the dynamic range do not provide additional effect.

Like other effects, the concentration-relationship for death is also described with a sigmoid E_{max} curve. The relationship between drug and effect is expressed differently in that the horizontal axis uses dose in place of concentration. Similar to the C_{50}, the ED_{50} is the dose at which there is a 50% probability of effect, and the LD_{50} is the dose with a 50% probability of death. The therapeutic index of a drug is defined as the ratio between the LD_{50} and the ED_{50} (Fig. 18.25). The larger the ratio, the safer the drug is for clinical use.

Anesthetic Drug Interactions

Anesthetics rarely consist of one drug, but rather a combination of drugs to achieve desired levels of hypnosis, analgesia, and muscle relaxation. Hypnotics, analgesics, and muscle relaxants all interact with one another such that rarely does one drug, when administered in the presence of other drugs, behave as if it were administered alone. For example, when administering an analgesic in the presence of a hypnotic, analgesia is more profound with the hypnotic than by itself and hypnosis is more profound with the analgesic than by itself. Thus, anesthesia is the practice of applied drug interactions. This phenomenon is likely a function of each class of drug exerting an effect on different receptors.

Early work by McEwan and associates described interactions between two drugs and is illustrated in Fig. 18.26.[7] It presents the interaction between isoflurane, a likely GABA agonist, and fentanyl, an opioid receptor agonist. This plot illustrates two key points: First, with a relatively low fentanyl concentration (<2 ng/mL), there is a substantial decrease (>50%) in the end tidal isoflurane concentration necessary

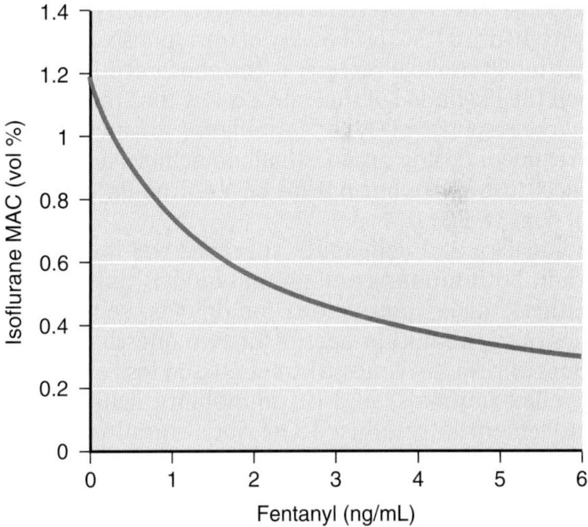

Fig. 18.26 The influence of fentanyl on the isoflurane minimal alveolar concentration *(MAC)* associated with a 50% probability of movement with skin incision. (Modified from McEwan AI, Smith C, Dyar O. Isoflurane minimum alveolar concentration reduction by fentanyl. *Anesthesiology*. 1993;78:864–869.)

to achieve minimal alveolar concentration (MAC) necessary to avoid movement with skin incision. Second, with fentanyl concentrations above 3 ng/mL, the end tidal concentration of isoflurane to maintain the MAC, although low, does not change much. Thus, there is a ceiling effect indicating that some isoflurane is necessary regardless of the fentanyl concentration to maintain a MAC of anesthesia.

A substantial body of work has been done to explore how anesthetic drugs interact with one another. As illustrated in Fig. 18.27, interactions have been characterized as antagonistic, additive, and synergistic. When drugs that have an

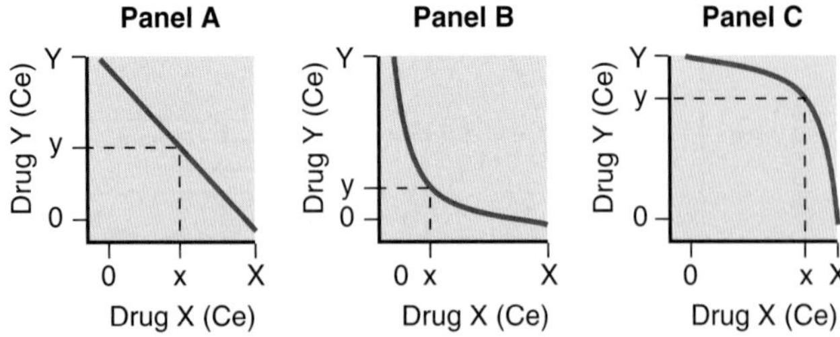

Fig. 18.27 Drug interactions. For two drugs, X and Y, Panel (A) represents additive, Panel (B) represents synergistic, and Panel (C) represents antagonistic interactions.

additive interaction are coadministered, their overall effect is the sum of the two individual effects. With antagonistic interactions, the overall effect is less than if the drug combination were additive; with synergistic interactions, the overall effect is greater than if the drug combination were additive.

A term used to characterize the continuum of drug concentrations across various combinations of drug pairs (X in combination with Y) is the isobole. The isobole is an isoeffect line for a selected probability of effect. A common isobole is the 50% isobole line. It represents all possible combinations of two-drug effect-site concentrations that would lead to a 50% probability of a given effect. Other isoboles are of more clinical interest. For example, the 95% isobole for loss of responsiveness represents the concentration pairs necessary to ensure a 95% probability of unresponsiveness. Similarly, the 5% isobole represents the concentration pairs in which the likelihood of that effect is low (i.e., most patients would be responsive). When formulating an anesthetic dosing regimen, dosing an anesthetic to achieve a probability of effect just above but not far beyond the 95% isobole is ideal (Fig. 18.28).

Hendrickx and colleagues surveyed the literature for work in both humans and animal models that described anesthetic drug interactions for opioids, sedative hypnotics, and inhalation agents for two anesthetic effects: (1) loss of responsiveness (humans) and loss of the righting reflex (animals) and (2) immobility defined as loss of movement in response to noxious stimulus in a nonparalyzed subject.[8] They found several interesting features of anesthetic drug combinations. First, inhalation agents when combined are strictly additive, suggesting a common mechanism of action, except for nitrous oxide, which has an infra-additive interaction with other inhalation agents. Second, interactions between various intravenous drugs and inhalation agents are synergistic except for nitrous oxide and GABA sedative hypnotics. Third, interactions between different classes of intravenous drugs (e.g., opioids and sedative hypnotics) are also primarily synergistic, except for ketamine and benzodiazepines (Fig. 18.29).

Several researchers have developed mathematical models that characterize anesthetic drug interactions in three dimensions. These models are known as response surface models and include effect-site concentrations for each drug, as well as a probability estimate of the overall effect. Fig. 18.30 presents the propofol–remifentanil interaction for loss of responsiveness as published by Bouillon and

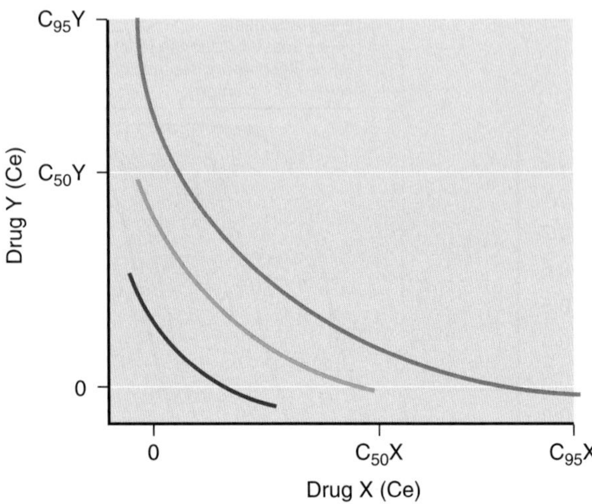

Fig. 18.28 Schematic illustration of iso-effect (isobole) lines. The red, green, and blue lines represent the 50% and 95% isoboles for a synergistic interaction between drugs X and Y. Isoboles represent concentration pairs with an equivalent effect. A set of 5%, 50%, and 95% isoboles can be used to describe the dynamic range of the concentrations for drugs X and Y for a given effect. As with single concentration effect curves, the ideal dosing leads to concentration pairs that are near the 95% isobole.

associates.[9] The response surface presents the full range of remifentanil-propofol isoboles (0%-100%) for loss of responsiveness. There are two common representations of the response surface model: the three-dimensional plot and the topographical plot. The topographical plot represents a top-down view of the response surface with drug concentrations on the vertical and horizontal axes. Drug effect is represented with selected isobole lines (i.e., 5%, 50%, and 95%).

Response surface models have been developed for a variety of anesthetic effects to include responses to verbal and tactile stimuli, painful stimuli, hemodynamic or respiratory effects, and changes in electrical brain activity. For example, with airway instrumentation, response surface models have been developed for loss of response to placing a laryngeal mask airway,[10] laryngoscopy,[11,12] tracheal intubation,[13] and esophageal instrumentation[14] for selected combinations of anesthetic drugs. Although many response surface models exist, there are several gaps in available models covering all common combinations of anesthetic drugs and various forms of stimuli encountered in the perioperative environment.

Recent work characterizing the interaction between sevoflurane and remifentanil has been done for a variety of drug effects to include loss of responsiveness, loss of response to several surrogates of surgical pain such as electrical tetany (up to 50 mA), pressure algometry (50 PSI pressure on the anterior tibial), loss of response to laryngoscopy, and temperature.[12] Using end tidal measures of sevoflurane was found to be inaccurate under non-steady state conditions (i.e., with a change in vaporizer settings). This was because end tidal concentrations did not account for the hysteresis (or time lag) between end tidal and effect-site concentrations. Improved model predictions were achieved when using estimated effect site concentrations.[15] Overall, for sevoflurane-opioid interactions, analgesic effects are

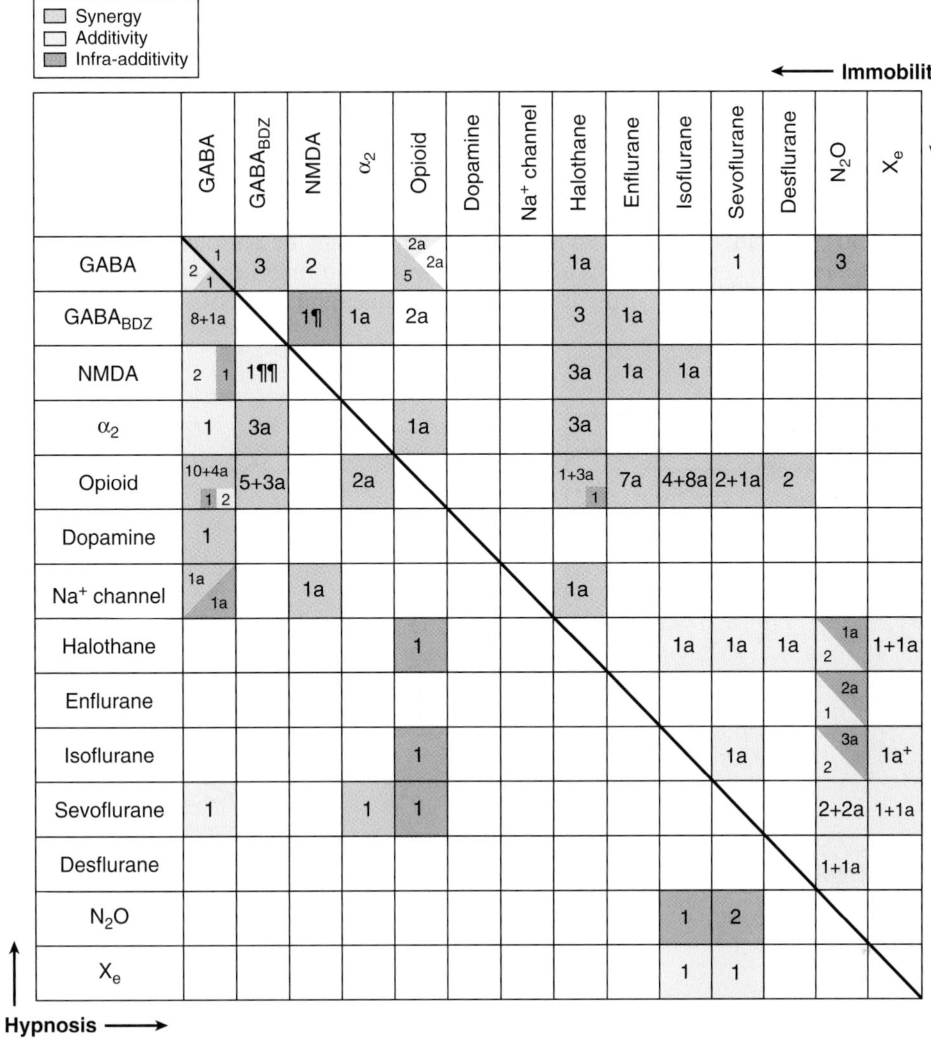

Fig. 18.29 Summary of drug interactions in humans and animals for hypnosis (loss of responsiveness in humans, loss of righting reflex in animals) and immobility (loss of movement in response to a noxious stimulus). The numbers in each cell refer to the number of papers supporting the finding. α_2 Agonists include dexmedetomidine and clonidine. Opioid agonists include morphine, remifentanil, fentanyl, sufentanil, and alfentanil. Dopamine agonists include droperidol and metoclopramide. Na+ (sodium) channel antagonists include lidocaine and bupivacaine. The letter "a" indicates the interaction was characterized in an animal model. The thick diagonal line separates studies characterizing drug-drug interactions of hypnosis *(bottom half)* and immobility *(top half)*. *GABA*, Gamma aminobutyric acid (GABA agonist drugs include propofol, thiopental, methohexital, and etomidate; GABA$_{BDZ}$ agonist drugs that work via benzodiazepine binding site include midazolam and diazepam); *NMDA*, N-methyl-D-aspartate (NMDA receptor antagonists include ketamine) (From Hendrickx J, Eger EI 2nd, Sonner JM, et al. Is synergy the rule? A review of anesthetic interactions producing hypnosis and immobility. *Anesth Analg*. 2008;107:494–506.)

markedly synergistic whereas sedative effects are somewhat synergistic.

Preliminary work has explored the adaptability of the sevoflurane-remifentanil interactions to other potent inhaled agent–opioid combinations using MAC and opioid equivalencies.[16] Predictions from sevoflurane-remifentanil models adapted to isoflurane-fentanyl correlated well with observed effects in patients undergoing elective general surgery procedures. Recent work has also explored the construction of models that characterize the interactions between three or more drugs.[17] For example, Vereecke and associates published a model that accounts for nitrous oxide, sevoflurane, and remifentanil.[18] This is of clinical relevance because most anesthetics consist of more than two anesthetic drugs.

Substantial work has explored interactions between sedative hypnotics and opioids, primarily propofol with alfentanil[19] or remifentanil[9,11,14,20,21] for a variety of effects. As with potent inhaled anesthetics and opioids, the interactions between sedative hypnotics and opioids for analgesic effects are markedly synergistic whereas sedative hypnotic effects are somewhat synergistic.

Some work has explored interactions between different types of sedative hypnotics. Two include midazolam combined with propofol[22,23] and propofol combined with a volatile anesthetic.[24–26] These interactions were found to be primarily additive.

Drug Displays

One major disadvantage to response surface models, as presented in the literature, is that they are complex and difficult to use in a clinical setting. Recent work has adapted these models to drug displays that allow clinicians to use them in real-time patient care settings.

These displays provide estimates of not only drug concentrations (both plasma and effect site) but various drug effects over time such as loss of responsiveness, analgesia, and reduction in response to peripheral train-of-four simulation (i.e., monitoring of muscle relaxant action), among others. With manual entry of patient demographics (age, gender, height, and weight) and drugs administered by syringe, either by bolus or continuous infusion along with automated data collection from an anesthesia machine (end tidal potent inhaled anesthetic concentrations and, in some instances, infusion pump information), drug displays provide predictions of drug concentration and effects. Drug displays are currently available from several anesthesia machine manufacturers (Navigator Suite from GE Healthcare, Wauwatosa, Wisconsin, USA, and SmartPilot View from Dräger, Lübeck, Germany). An example of a drug display is presented in Fig. 18.30. All drug display examples are based on response surface interaction models.

A unique feature of drug displays is that a given dosing regimen can be simulated prior to administration. This information may be useful in identifying the optimal dose in challenging patients, especially when more than one

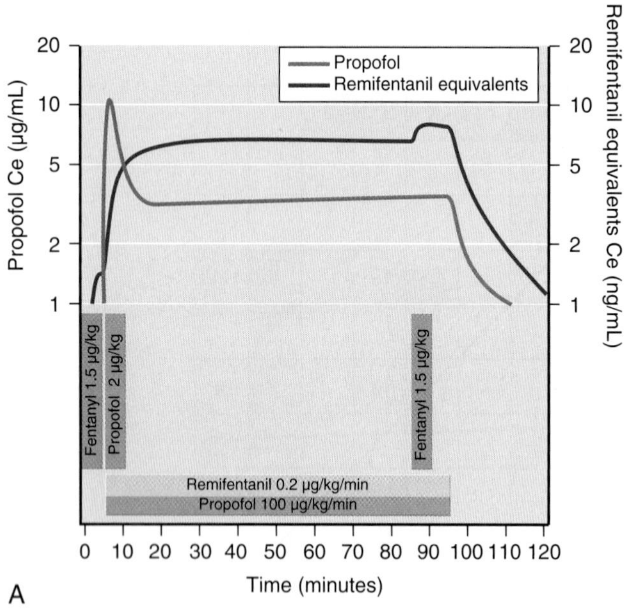

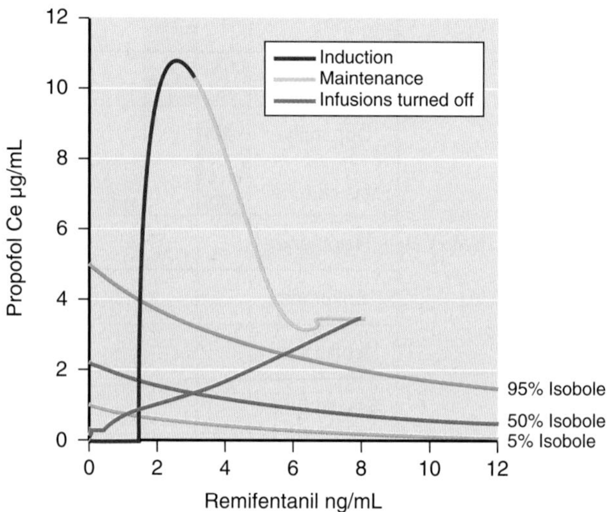

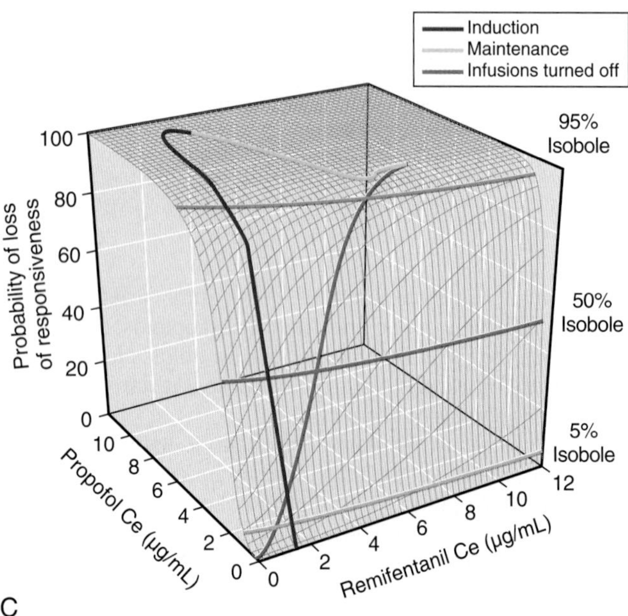

Fig. 18.30 (A–C) Simulation of a 90-minute total intravenous anesthetic consisting of propofol bolus (2 μg/kg) and infusion (100 μg/kg/min), remifentanil (0.2 μg/kg/min), and intermittent fentanyl boluses (1.5 μg/kg). (A) Resultant effect site concentrations (Ce) are presented. (B) Predictions of loss of responsiveness are presented on a topographical *(top-down)* view. (C) A three-dimensional response surface is shown. The light blue, purple, and green lines represent the 5%, 50%, and 95% isoboles. Each isobole presents the propofol-remifentanil pairs that yield the same effect. The inward bow of the isoboles indicates that the interaction is synergistic. The isoboles are in close proximity to one another indicating a steep transition from responsive to unresponsive.

drug is used. The drug displays use population models that, although generalizable, may not provide a good "fit" to every patient. For some drug display systems, observed patient responses are used to calibrate predictions of drug effect (Fig. 18.31). For example, with elderly or debilitated patients, smaller doses are often required to achieve a desired effect. Drug displays allow clinicians to identify concentrations that produce a desired response and can be used to titrate additional anesthetic.

There are several other advantages from using drug displays. When titrating an anesthetic, it is often difficult to appreciate when effect-site concentrations are near steady state. Clinicians may be tempted to administer additional drug assuming that drug concentrations have peaked (with bolus dosing) or are near steady-state conditions (with continuous infusions of potent inhaled anesthetics). Clinicians may also be impatient, assuming that drug concentrations are near zero when in fact they are still increased, even after terminating delivery (e.g., the end tidal potent inhaled agent concentration is 0 mm Hg but there is persistent unresponsiveness).

A second advantage is that drug displays provide a means of delivering passive TCI. Although widely used throughout the world, TCI is not used in the United States because of regulatory barriers.[27] TCI uses population pharmacokinetic models to drive infusion pumps. After entering the target plasma or effect-site concentration, a computer identifies the optimal infusion rate to achieve that concentration. With passive TCI, population models are used to display predicted effect-site concentrations and associated effects over time, but the models do not deliver information to drive infusion pumps as with TCI. With this approach,

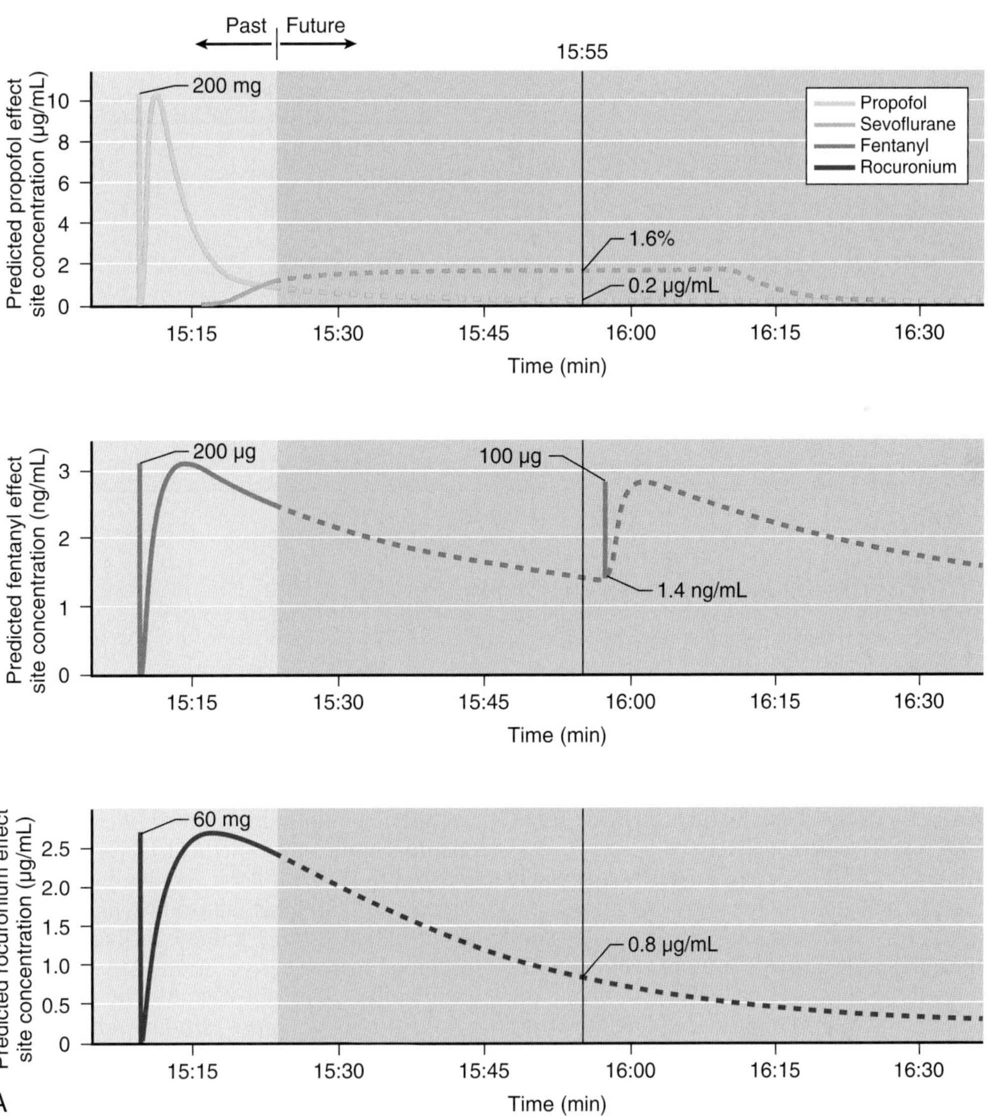

Fig. 18.31 (A) Example of a drug display. This example presents predictions of site effect concentrations (A) and drug effects (B) for a combined technique using fentanyl (2 µg/kg), propofol (2 mg/kg), and rocuronium (0.6 mg/kg) boluses and maintenance with sevoflurane (2%) and fentanyl bolus (1 µg/kg). This simulation assumes a 30-year-old, 100-kg male, 183 cm tall, with normal cardiac output and lung ventilation. (A) Predicted effect site concentrations for propofol *(bright yellow line)*, sevoflurane *(dark orange line)*, fentanyl *(blue line)*, and rocuronium *(red line)*. Bolus doses are represented as vertical lines, with the dose labeled adjacent to the line. Past predictions are solid lines and future predictions are dashed lines. The vertical black line represents a future prediction of effect site concentrations at 15:55 PM. Concentrations are reported.

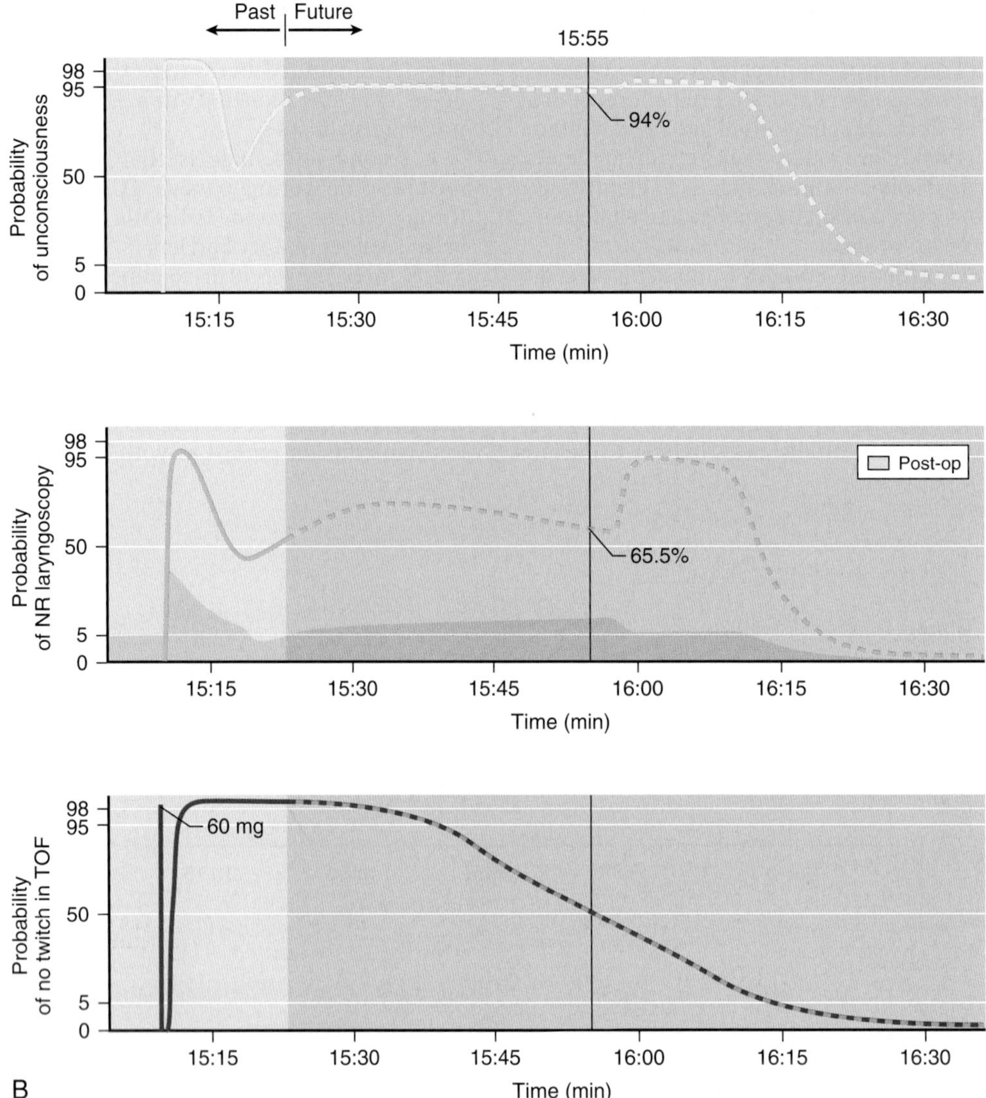

Fig. 18.31 Cont'd (B) Predicted drug effects. Probability of unresponsiveness *(yellow line)*, probability of no response to laryngoscopy *(blue line)*, and probability of loss of train-of-four *(red line)* from this combined technique. The white horizontal lines represent the 5%, 50%, 95%, and 98% probability of effect. The vertical black line represents a future prediction of drug effects at 15:55 PM. *NR*, No response to laryngoscopy; *TOF*, train-of-four. ([A] From Applied Medical Visualizations, Salt Lake City, Utah.)

clinicians can test out dosing regimens (bolus doses and infusion rates) before administering them to confirm they will achieve a desired effect. These features provide for a more consistent approach to drug delivery.

A third advantage is that they provide a better approach to dosing anesthetics. Instead of considering an anesthetic in terms of MAC, where 50% of patients may respond to surgical stimulus, drug displays provide a more refined characterization of anesthetic effect. Clinicians do not titrate an anesthetic to achieve a 50% probability of effect but rather aim for a 95% to 99% probability of effect. With response surfaces, anesthetic dosing regimens necessary to achieve this level of effect are easily visualized. Second, the concept of MAC does not fully embody the three elements of an anesthetic: analgesia, sedation and hypnosis, and muscle relaxation. Drug displays provide a means of visualizing all three effects simultaneously over a full 0% to 100% probability range.

Special Populations

When formulating an anesthetic, many aspects of patient demographics and medical history need to be considered to find the correct *dose*: age; body habitus; gender; chronic exposure to opioids, benzodiazepines, or alcohol; the presence of heart, lung, kidney, or liver disease; and the extent of blood loss or dehydration. Any of these factors can dramatically affect anesthetic drug kinetics and dynamics. Unfortunately, most studies characterizing anesthetic drug behavior have been conducted in healthy volunteers that rarely represent the general population presenting for surgery. Extensive work has explored how some patient characteristics (e.g., obesity) influence anesthetic drug behavior, whereas other patient characteristics remain difficult to assess (chronic opioid exposure). In addition, not all anesthetics have been studied. Most work has primarily focused on newer anesthetic drugs, such as propofol and remifentanil. This section will briefly summarize work that has been done to characterize the pharmacokinetics and pharmacodynamics in a few unique special populations.

Influence of Obesity on Anesthetic Drugs

Obesity is a worldwide epidemic, and overweight patients frequently undergo anesthesia and surgery. Furthermore, pharmacologic alterations of anesthetics occur in obese individuals. In general, manufacturer dosing recommendations are on a per-kg basis according to the actual total body weight (TBW). Anesthesia providers rarely use mg/kg dosing in obese patients for fear of administering an excessive dose (e.g., a 136-kg patient does not require twice as much drug as a patient of the same height who weighs 68 kg). To resolve this problem, several weight scalars were developed to avoid excessive dosing or under dosing in this patient population. Some of these include lean body mass (LBM), ideal body weight (IBW), corrected body weight (CBW), and fat-free mass (FFM). Table 18.1 presents the formulas used to estimate these weight scalars. Table 18.2 shows samples of the resultant scaled weight for lean and obese individuals. In general, the aim of weight scalars is to match dosing regimens for obese patients with what is required for normal-size patients. These scaled weights are usually smaller than TBW in obese patients and thus help prevent excessive drug dosing (Fig. 18.32). Scaled weights have been used in place of TBW for both bolus (mg/kg) and infusion (mg/kg/hr) dosing and also for TCI.

This section will discuss the pharmacologic (primarily pharmacokinetic) alterations of select intravenous anesthetic drugs (propofol, remifentanil, and fentanyl) in obese patients, review examples of weight scalars and their shortcomings when used in bolus and continuous infusion dosing, and when data are available, briefly describe pharmacologic models used to drive TCI.

Propofol

Dosing propofol in obese patients can be a challenge. For bolus dosing and continuous infusions, the choice of weight scalar is specific to the dosing technique being used (i.e., one is best for bolus dosing and another for continuous infusions). Furthermore, of the available propofol pharmacokinetic models, the one built from observations in obese patients may be best for TCI.

The influence of obesity on propofol pharmacokinetics is not entirely clear. Generally, in obese patients, the blood distributes more to nonadipose than to adipose tissues. This may result in higher plasma drug concentrations in obese patients with mg/kg dosing than in normal patients with less adipose mass. Furthermore, propofol clearance increases because of the increased liver volume and/or liver blood flow associated with obesity (and increased cardiac output). Distribution likely influences concentration peaks with bolus dosing, and clearance likely influences concentrations during and following infusions.

Dosing Scalars for Propofol. Simulations of an infusion using various weight scalars are presented in Fig. 18.33. The simulations predict propofol effect-site concentrations from a 60-minute infusion (167 μg/kg/min) in 176-cm (6-ft) males, obese (185 kg), and lean (68 kg). If dosed according to TBW, peak effect-site concentrations in a lean and obese individual are different; their respective peak propofol concentrations are approximately 5.2 and 7.1 μg/mL, respectively. If the obese individual is dosed to CBW, the peak concentration is near 4.5 μg/mL. The other weight scalars lead to much lower concentrations with the infusion.

Of the many available dosing scalars, authors recommend LBM[12] for bolus dosing (i.e., during induction) and TBW or CBW for infusions.[9,13] For continuous infusions, other weight scalars are likely inadequate (the most worrisome is LBM). When dosing to CBW, plasma concentrations may be lower than concentrations when dosed to TBW.

One concern with using TBW to dose continuous infusions is drug accumulation. Prior work, however, does not support this assumption. Servin and colleagues[28] performed pharmacokinetic analyses of propofol administration to normal and obese patients using TBW and CBW. The CBW was defined as the IBW + 0.4 × (TBW−IBW).[29] They found similar concentrations at eye opening in both groups

TABLE 18.1 Common Weight Scalars (Modified Added Modified Fat-Free Mass)

Name	Equations
Ideal body weight	Male: 50 kg + 2.3 kg for each 2.54 cm (1 inch) over 152 cm (5 ft) Female: 45.5 kg + 2.3 kg for each 2.54 cm (1 inch) over 152 cm (5 ft)
Corrected body weight	IBW + 0.4 × (TBW−IBW)
Lean body mass	Male: $1.1 \times TBW - 128 \times (TBW/Ht)^2$ Female: $1.07 \times TBW - 148 \times (TBW/Ht)^2$
Fat-free mass[66]	Male: $(9.27 \times 10^3 \times TBW)/(6.68 \times 10^3 + 216 \times BMI)$ Female: $(9.27 \times 10^3 \times TBW)/(8.78 \times 10^3 + 244 \times BMI)$
Pharmacokinetic mass[46,47]	$52/[1+(196.4 \cdot e^{-0.025\,TBW} - 53.66)/100]$ (fentanyl only)
Modified fat-free mass[28,36]	FFM + 0.4 × (TBW−FFM)

BMI, Body mass index; *FFM*, fat free mass; *Ht*, height in centimeters; *IBW*, ideal body weight; *LBM*, lean body mass; *TBW*, total body weight in kg.

TABLE 18.2 Dosing Weights Based on Various Dosing Scalars (Values Per K Johnson)

	176-cm (6 FT) Male	
	68 kg BMI = 22	185 kg BMI = 66
Dosing Scalar	**Dosing Weight (kg)**	**Dosing Weight (kg)**
Total body weight (TBW)	68	185
Ideal body weight (IBW)	72	72
Corrected body weight (CBW)	70	117
Lean body mass (LBM)	56	62
Fat-free mass (FFM)	55	88
Modified fat-free mass (MFFM)	60	127

BMI, Body mass index (kg/m²).

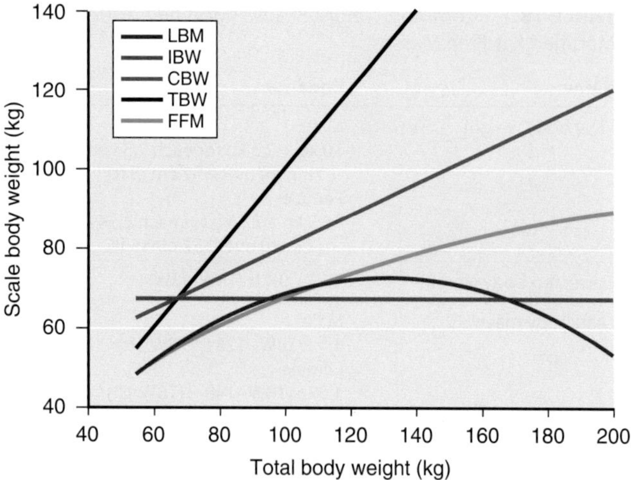

Fig. 18.32 Scaled weights as a function of total body weight *(TBW)*. Key points in this plot: IBW remains the same regardless of the TBW, and LBM starts to decline for weight increases above 127 kg. *CBW*, Corrected body weight; *FFM*, fat-free mass; *IBW*, Ideal body weight; *LBM*, lean body mass (for a 40-year-old male, 176 cm tall).

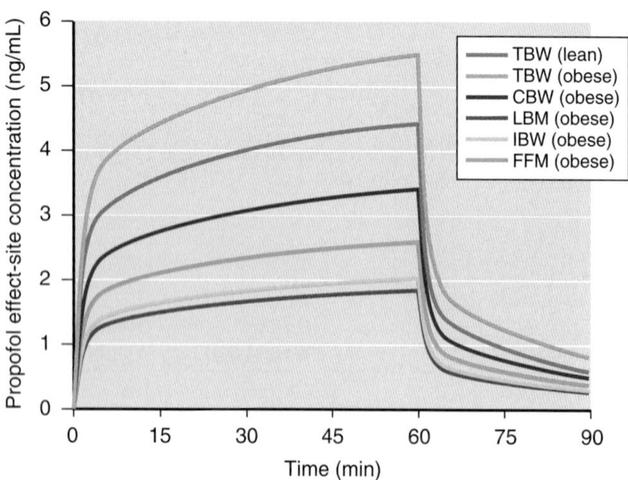

Fig. 18.33 Simulations of propofol effect site concentrations that result from a 60-minute infusion (10 mg/kg/h–167 µg/kg/min) to a 40-year-old male who is 176 cm tall. Simulations include the following dosing weights: total body weights *(TBW)* of 68 kg and 185 kg (body mass indices of 22 and 60, respectively) and scaled weights for the 185 kg weight to include Servin's corrected body weight *(CBW)*, lean body mass *(LBM)*, ideal body weight *(IBW)*, and fat-free mass *(FFM)*. Key points: At the 185-kg weight, when dosed to TBW, the infusion leads to high propofol concentrations, whereas when dosed to IBW or LBM, the infusion leads to low propofol concentrations. When the 185-kg individual is dosed using CBW, it best approximates the propofol concentrations that result from TBW in a lean individual. Predictions of propofol effect site concentrations were made using the Eleveld model.

and absence of propofol accumulation in obese patients; in fact, obese patients showed earlier awareness after the termination of propofol infusions than did the normal subjects. Data suggest that dosing infusions according to Servin's CBW may underdose obese patients.[30]

Propofol Kinetic Models Target-Controlled Infusions. Of the many available models, the two most widely used propofol kinetic models for TCI are those published by Marsh and associates and Schnider and associates.[31,32] In addition to model selection, as with bolus and continuous infusion dosing, identifying the ideal weight scalar to use is also important.

The Marsh model, although useful, was built from data collected in a pediatric population. Researchers have explored different dosing weights using this model in morbidly obese patients when coadministered with remifentanil with varied results. Albertin and colleagues[29] used CBW to dose a propofol TCI using the Marsh model. They found predicted substantially overestimated measured propofol concentrations and expressed concern for intraoperative awareness when using CBW with the Marsh TCI model. The same group[33] compared the predictive performance of the TCI using CBW versus TBW and found that CBW performed worse than TBW. They concluded that TBW, not CBW, should be used to administer propofol via TCI to morbidly obese patients. In contrast, recently, Cortinez and colleagues[34] evaluated the several pharmacokinetic models, and the use of CBW with the Marsh and Schnider models (described later) showed acceptable prediction performances. They stated that with both models using CBW is one of the best options for propofol TCI in obese patients, as their opinion. In any case, electroencephalographic monitoring is recommended to avoid the risk of awareness.

The Schnider model, although built from data collected in adults over a range of weights, heights, and ages, does not specifically include obese patients. This model uses the weight scalar LBM, which has limited application in morbidly obese patients.[32]

For comparison, the Marsh or the Schnider model has been applied on morbidly obese patients. Echevarria and colleagues[35] reported differences in effect-site propofol concentrations with a BIS of less than 60 between the two pharmacokinetic models when used for induction in morbidly obese patients. To achieve a 95% probability of effect, target concentrations of 4.2 and 5.5 µg/mL were required for the Marsh and Schnider models, respectively. This difference occurred because of the potential prediction errors in each pharmacokinetic model that was used (the actual drug concentrations in each patient are unknown).

Cortinez and colleagues used an international data repository called Open TCI (http://www.opentci.org) to build a model using propofol concentrations from a wide range of body weights.[36] They built a propofol kinetic model that scales normal-size to obese individuals using an empirically derived formula that uses allometric scaling. In this formula, TBW accounts for differences in distribution and clearances in obese patients. TBW is divided by a standard patient size (70 kg) and raised to the power of 1 for distribution volumes and by the power of 0.75 for clearances. Van Kralingen and colleagues[37] further modified this approach and reported better model performance with exponents of 0.71 for clearance. Eleveld and colleagues[38] constructed a general purpose allometric pharmacokinetic model for propofol using a large dataset containing data from young children, children, adults, elderly, and obese individuals (pharmacokinetic parameter estimates can be calculated by entering patient demographics at http://www.eurosiva.eu/tivatrainer/modeltranslate/calc_compartments.html; last accessed 2018/01/05). Cortinez and colleagues[34] evaluated the predictive performances of the five foregoing models (i.e., Marsh, Schnider, Cortinez, Van Kralingen, and Eleveld models) in data from obese patients and found that

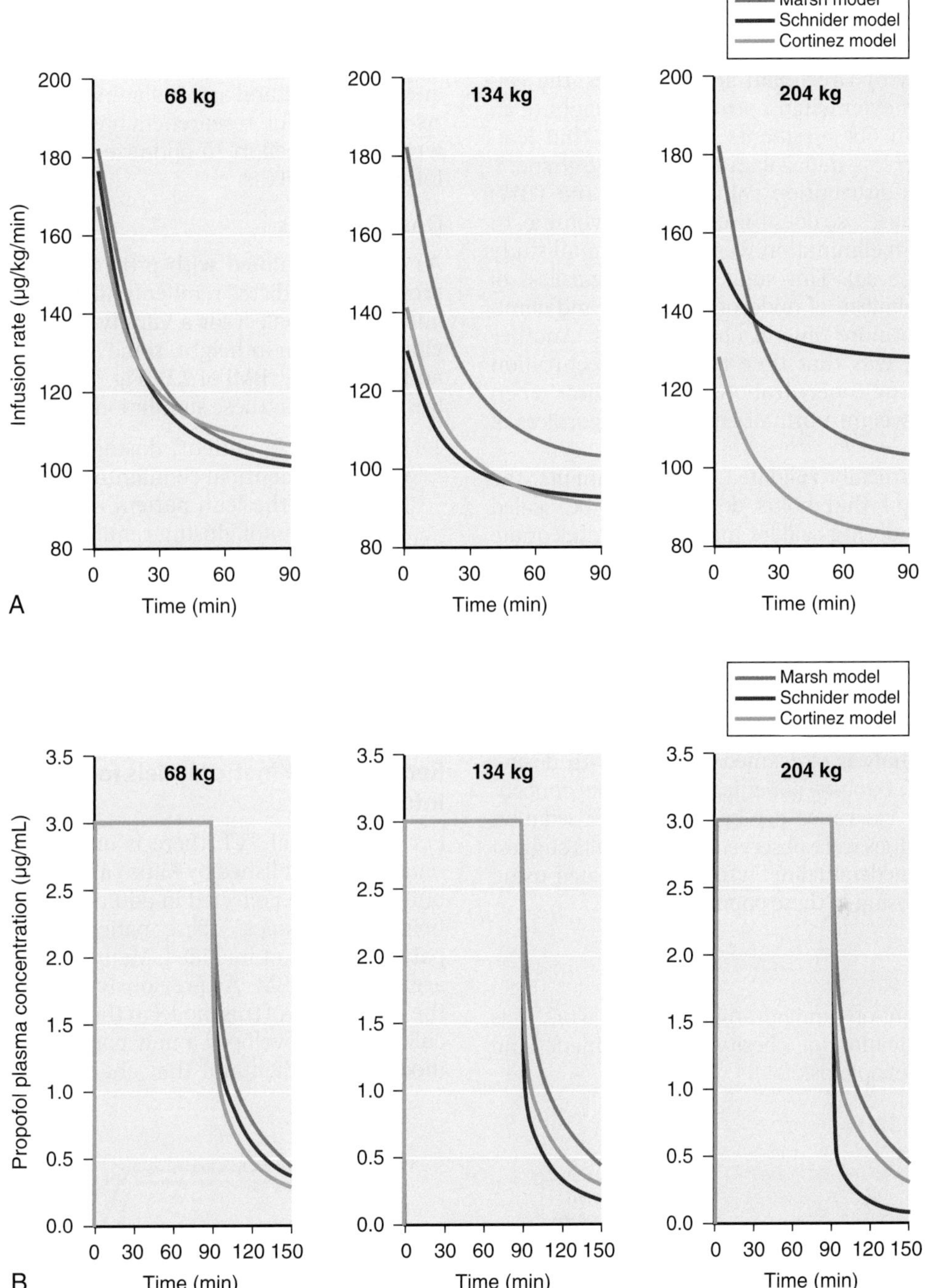

Fig.18.34 Simulations of a 90-minute propofol target-controlled infusion set to achieve and maintain a plasma concentration (Cp) of 3 µg/mL using four different published propofol pharmacokinetic models: Marsh and associates,[31] Schnider and associates,[32] Cortinez and associates,[36] and Eleveld and associates.[36,38] Simulations assumed 40-year-old males who are 176 cm tall and weigh 68, 134, or 204 kg. (A) Propofol infusion rates for each model at each weight. (B) Propofol plasma concentrations predicted by each model for each weight.

the Eleveld allometric pharmacokinetic model performed best. They stated that the Eleveld model using TBW is one of the best options for propofol TCI in obese patients.

Fig. 18.34 presents a simulation of propofol infusion rates and associated plasma concentrations using the Marsh, Schnider, Cortinez, and Eleveld models to drive a TCI to achieve a concentration of 3 µg/mL. Key points from this simulation include: TCI infusions based on the Marsh model are linear to TBW such that the infusion rates and plasma concentrations are identical across weights. With an increase in body weights, the degree of increase in total propofol amounts for TCI administrations is smaller with the Cortinez and Eleveld models than with the Marsh and Schnider models.

For propofol, the Eleveld model may be best suited for TCI in obese and morbidly obese patients. Unfortunately, this model is not yet available in many commercial TCI pumps. One caveat that is important to consider is that model differences are likely overshadowed by inter-individual variability. In sum, any one of the four models will likely yield similar clinical results if titrated to effect in conjunction with processed EEG monitoring.

Other Sedatives. Only limited information is available on the behavior of other sedatives (i.e., midazolam, ketamine, etomidate, dexmedetomidine, and barbiturates) in obese patients. In a study by Greenblatt and associates, the volume of distribution even when normalized to weight (e.g., L/kg) was larger in obese patients, suggesting that lean tissue may take up less midazolam than adipose tissue.[39] Thus, midazolam's distribution volume follows the TBW: as patient size increases, so does the distribution volume. In addition, midazolam elimination was the same in all study subjects (lean or obese). This suggests that regardless of dose, hepatic metabolism of midazolam is fixed and elimination will require more time in obese patients. Another interesting finding was that time to peak concentration and peak plasma drug concentrations were the same when administered in a weight-normalized fashion regardless of body habitus.

Although not clinically validated in obese patients, the authors recommend that bolus doses should be scaled to TBW and other dosing scalars may lead to inadequate effect. On the other hand, with a fixed elimination, continuous infusion rates should be dosed to IBW.[39]

Cortinez and colleagues[40] characterized the influence of obesity on pharmacokinetics of dexmedetomidine and found that fat mass is not related to a proportional increase in distribution volume and is associated with the impairment of clearance. Xu and colleagues[41] performed noncompartment pharmacokinetic analysis of dexmedetomidine with dosing calculated on TBW. In obese patients, higher initial concentrations and lower clearance per kg, and deeper sedation with lower SpO_2 values were observed. These results suggest that dosing of dexmedetomidine, which is calculated using TBW, can be overdosing in these populations.

OPIOIDS

With the exception of remifentanil, minimal work has explored the implication of obesity on the kinetic and dynamic behavior of opioids.

Remifentanil

In obese patients, largely due to its rapid metabolism by nonspecific esterases, the distribution volume and clearance of remifentanil are similar in lean and obese patients.[42] As with propofol, researchers have explored several scaled weights in an effort to optimize bolus dosing, continuous infusions, and TCIs.

Dosing Scalars

As previously noted with propofol, simulation is used to present the predicted remifentanil effect-site concentrations and analgesic effect for a variety of scaled weights in individuals 174 cm in height, some obese (185 kg, BMI of 60) and lean (68 kg, BMI of 22) (Fig. 18.35). Several key points are illustrated in these simulations:

1. For an obese patient, dosing scaled to FFM resulted in almost identical remifentanil effect-site concentrations as in the lean patient dosed according to TBW. Unlike propofol, dosing remifentanil to CBW *(red line)* leads to higher plasma concentrations compared with levels achieved when dosing to TBW in a lean individual.
2. Dosing scaled to LBM in the obese individual resulted in lower effect-site concentrations than those in a lean individual dosed according to TBW.

Remifentanil Kinetic Models for Target-Controlled Infusions

For remifentanil TCI, there is one available pharmacokinetic model published by Minto and associates.[43] Although built from data collected in adults over a range of weights, heights, and ages, obese patients and morbidly obese patients were not included. Many of the model parameters are scaled to LBM. As previously discussed, this may limit the application of this model in the morbidly obese. Kim and colleagues[44] developed a new population pharmacokinetic model for remifentanil that characterize the influence of

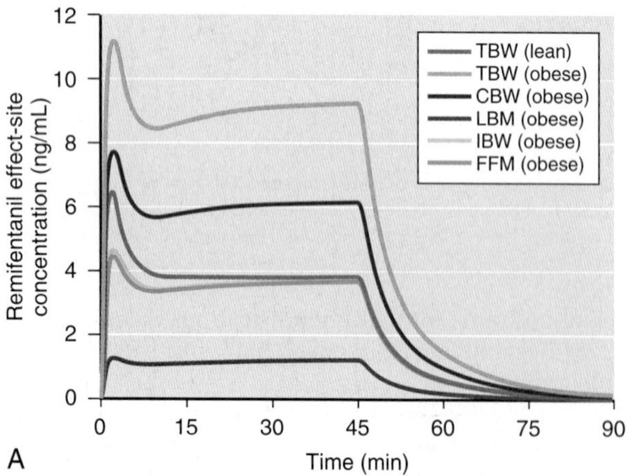

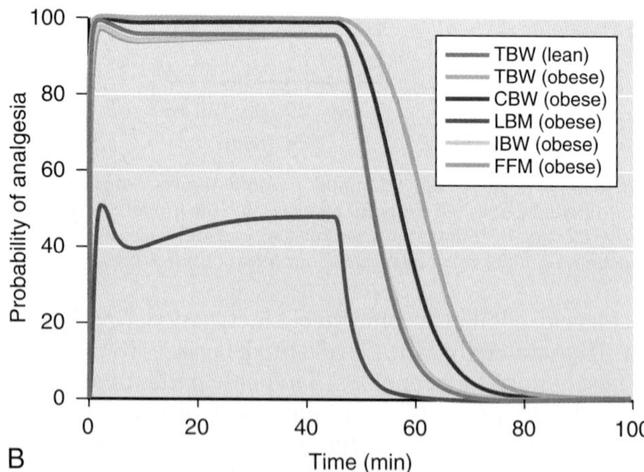

Fig. 18.35 (A and B) Simulations of remifentanil effect-site concentrations (A) and analgesic effect (B) that result from a 1 μg/kg bolus and a 60-minute infusion at a rate of 0.15 μg/kg/min to a 40-year-old male who is 176 cm tall. Simulations include the following dosing weights: total body weights *(TBW)* of 68 kg and 185 kg (body mass indices of 22 and 60, respectively) and scaled weights for the 185-kg weight to include Servin's corrected body weight *(CBW)*, lean body mass *(LBM)*, ideal body weight *(IBW)*, and fat free mass *(FFM)*. Remifentanil effect-site concentrations and estimates of analgesic effect were estimated using published pharmacokinetic models. (From Minto CF, Schnider TW, Egan TD, et al. Influence of age and gender on the pharmacokinetics and pharmacodynamics of remifentanil. I. Model development. *Anesthesiology*. 1997;86(1):10–23.)

body weight using allometric body mass scaling in the general adult population.

Fig. 18.36 presents a simulation of the predicted remifentanil plasma concentrations based on the Minto and Kim models. The Minto model overestimates remifentanil concentrations with increasing weight. This is likely due to the use of LBM when estimating pharmacokinetic parameters.

In summary, available models (Minto or Kim) are appropriate for TCI in this patient group but will administer different amounts of remifentanil and require titration to achieve desired yet avoid adverse clinical effects.

FENTANYL

Despite widespread use in the clinical arena, relatively little work has explored how obesity impacts fentanyl pharmacokinetics. Published fentanyl pharmacokinetic models[45] tend to overestimate fentanyl concentrations as TBW increases. A fentanyl kinetic model based on data collected in obese subjects has not (yet) been published. Shibutani and colleagues[46,47] explored ways to improve predictions using published models by modifying demographic data (e.g., either height or weight). They characterized a nonlinear relationship between fentanyl clearance and TBW and recommended the use of a modified weight, called the pharmacokinetic mass, to improve the predictive performance of one of the many available fentanyl kinetic models, a model published by Shafer and colleagues. They explored the use of pharmacokinetic mass when dosing obese patients with fentanyl in a postoperative setting. They found that dosing based on TBW may be excessive.[36]

Other Opioids

Even less information regarding the impact of obesity on drug behavior is available for opioids other than remifentanil and fentanyl. Sufentanil has been studied in obese patients, where its volume of distribution increases linearly with TBW[48] and clearance was similar between lean and obese individuals. It was recommended that bolus dosing use TBW and "prudently reduced" dosing for continuous infusions. For TCI, Slepchenko and colleagues found model estimates of sufentanil concentrations accurately predicted measured concentrations in morbidly obese patients[49] using a previously published mode of sufentanil kinetics by Gepts and associates.[50] This is likely due to the fact that the kinetic model was built from measured concentrations in patients with a weight range of 47 to 94 kg. de Hoogd and colleagues[51] performed a population pharmacokinetic analysis of intravenous morphine in morbidly obese individuals. They found that morphine pharmacokinetics were comparable to those of healthy volunteers. They concluded that no weight-based dosing adjustments were necessary. However, they also found that the elimination of pharmacologically active metabolite was decreased, resulting in an increased exposure to active metabolite with prolonged administrations. They concluded that the clinical relevance of this phenomenon was not clear.

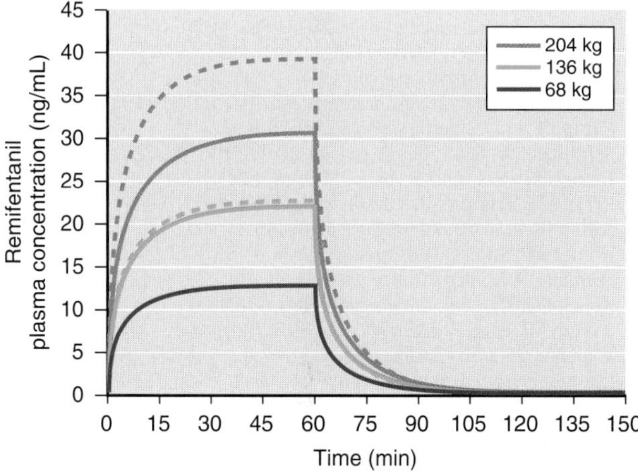

Fig. 18.36 Simulations of remifentanil plasma concentrations that result from a 60-minute infusion (0.5 µg/kg/min) in a 40-year-old male, 176 cm tall. The simulations include three total body weights: 68, 136, and 204 kg with body mass indices of 22, 44, and 66, respectively. Simulations were performed using pharmacokinetic parameters published by Minto and associates[43] *(dashed lines)* and Kim and colleagues[44] *(solid lines)*. In an extremely obese (204 kg) individual, Minto's model predicts very high remifentanil concentrations.

INHALED ANESTHETICS

The perception of volatile anesthetics is that they accumulate more in obese than in lean patients and that this leads to prolonged emergence. Studies on inhalation anesthetics in obese individuals, however, have not confirmed this perception.[52] Two phenomena contribute to this observation: first, blood flow to adipose tissue *decreases* with increasing obesity,[53] and second, the time required to fill adipose tissue with volatile anesthetics is long. The time required to achieve 63% of the final equilibrium within adipose tissue for desflurane and isoflurane are longer than 22 and 35 hours, respectively.[54,55]

INFLUENCE OF AGE ON ANESTHETIC DRUG PHARMACOLOGY

Clinicians are often faced with anesthetizing elderly adults and have long recognized that they usually require a smaller dosage of most anesthetics to produce the desired therapeutic effect while minimizing adverse effects. Age is one of the most valuable in covariates to consider when developing an anesthetic plan. The influence of age on pharmacokinetics and pharmacodynamics of many anesthetics has been well described. As with obesity, both remifentanil and propofol can serve as prototypes to understand how age influences anesthetic drug behavior. Studies specifically designed to assess the influence of age on remifentanil and propofol have characterized the influence of age in quantitative terms.[32,38,43,44,56,57]

With remifentanil, elderly patients require less drug to produce an opioid effect. Reduced doses are primarily a function of changes in pharmacodynamics, but may involve pharmacokinetic changes as well.[43] The concentration required to produce electroencephalographic changes is decreased. Based on previously published pharmacokinetic and pharmacodynamic models built from measurements over a wide age range,[32,43,56,57] simulations can be performed to explore how age may influence dosing. For example, to achieve equipotent doses in 20- and 80-year-olds, the dose for the 80-year-old should be reduced by 55%. A similar analysis for propofol recommends that the dose for an 80-year-old should be reduced by 65% compared to that of a 20-year-old.

The mechanisms for these changes are not clear, especially for pharmacodynamic changes. One possible source of change in pharmacokinetic behavior may be due to decreased cardiac output. Lower cardiac output in the elderly[58] results in slower circulation and subsequent changes in drug distribution and redistribution. This may lead to high peak concentrations[58,59] and decreased drug delivery to metabolic organs and reduced clearance. This is consistent with what has been reported for many intravenous anesthetics (propofol, thiopental, and etomidate), which have slower clearance and a smaller volume of distribution.[32,60–62] Beyond age-related changes in cardiac output, it is important to consider comorbidities that may reduce cardiovascular function.[63] Taking this into account, anesthesiologists often consider a patient's "physiologic" age instead of solely relying on actual age.[64,65] For some older adult patients, such as those with no significant coexisting disease, normal body habitus, and good exercise tolerance, a substantial reduction in dose may not be warranted.

Summary

This chapter reviewed basic principles of clinical pharmacology used to describe anesthetic drug behavior: pharmacokinetics, pharmacodynamics, and anesthetic drug interactions. These principles provide the information needed to make rational decisions about the selection and administration of anesthetics. From a practical aspect, these principles characterize the magnitude and time course of drug effect, but because of complex math requirements, they have limited clinical utility in everyday practice. Advances in computer simulation, however, have brought this capability to the point of real-time patient care. Perhaps one of the most important advances in our understanding of clinical pharmacology is the development of interaction models that describe how different classes of anesthetic drugs influence one another. This is especially relevant to anesthesiologists, given that they rarely use just one drug when providing anesthesia.

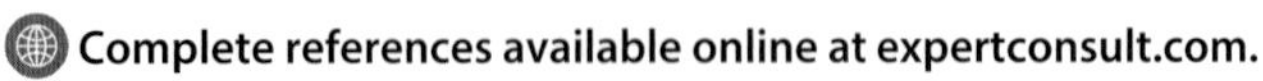

Complete references available online at expertconsult.com.

References

1. Wilkinson GR, Shand DG. *Clin Pharmacol Ther*. 1975;18:377.
2. Ebling WF, Wada DR, Stanski DR. *J Pharmacokinet Biopharm*. 1994;22:259.
3. Youngs EJ, Shafer SL. Basic pharmacokinetic and pharmacodynamic principles. In: White PF, ed. *Textbook of Intravenous Anesthesia*. Baltimore: William & Wilkins; 1997.
4. Krejcie TC, Avram MJ, Gentry WB. *J Pharmacokinet Biopharm*. 1997;25:169.
5. Hughes MA, et al. *Anesthesiology*. 1992;76(3):334.
6. Egan TD, et al. *Int J Pharm Med*. 2001;15(1):11.
7. McEwan AI, Smith C, Dyar O. *Anesthesiology*. 1993;78:864.
8. Hendrickx J, et al. *Anesth Analg*. 2008;107:494.
9. Bouillon TW, et al. *Anesthesiology*. 2004;100(6):1353.
10. Heyse B, et al. *Anesthesiology*. 2012;116(2):311.
11. Kern SE, et al. *Anesthesiology*. 2004;100(6):1373.
12. Manyam SC, et al. *Anesthesiology*. 2006;105(2):267.
13. Mertens MJ, et al. *Anesthesiology*. 2003;99(2):347.
14. LaPierre CD, et al. *Anesth Analg*. 2011;113(3):490.
15. Johnson KB, et al. *Anesth Analg*. 2010;111(2):387.
16. Syroid ND, et al. *Anesth Analg*. 2010;111(2):380.
17. Minto CF, Schnider TW. *Anesthesiology*. 2000;92:1603.
18. Vereecke HE, et al. *Anesthesiology*. 2013.
19. Vuyk J, Lim T, Engbers FH. *Anesthesiology*. 1995;83(8).
20. Johnson KB, et al. *Anesth Analg*. 2008;106(2):471.
21. Zanderigo E, et al. *Anesthesiology*. 2006;104(4):742.
22. Fidler M, Kern SE. *Anesthesiology*. 2006;105(2):286.
23. Vinik HR, et al. *Anesth Analg*. 1994;78(2):354.
24. Harris RS, et al. *Anesthesiology*. 2006;104(6):1170.
25. Schumacher PM, et al. *Anesthesiology*. 2009;111(4):790.
26. Sebel LE, et al. *Anesthesiology*. 2006;104(6):1176.
27. Egan TD, Shafer SL. *Anesthesiology*. 2003;99(5):1039.
28. Servin F, et al. *Anesthesiology*. 1993;78(4):657.
29. Albertin A, et al. *Br J Anaesth*. 2007;98(1):66.
30. Igarashi T, et al. *Masui*. 2002;51(11):1243.
31. Marsh B, et al. *Br J Anaesth*. 1991;67(1):41.
32. Schnider TW, et al. *Anesthesiology*. 1998;88(5):1170.
33. La Colla L, et al. *Eur J Anaesthesiol*. 2009;26(5):362.
34. Cortinez LI, et al. *Anesth Analg*. 2014;119(2):302.
35. Echevarria GC, et al. *Anesth Analg*. 2012;115(4):823.
36. Cortinez LI, et al. *Br J Anaesth*. 2010;105(4):448.
37. van Kralingen S, et al. *Br J Clin Pharmacol*. 2011;71(1):34.
38. Eleveld DJ, et al. *Anesth Analg*. 2014;118(6):1221.
39. Greenblatt DJ, et al. *Anesthesiology*. 1984;61(1):27.
40. Cortinez LI, et al. *Eur J Clin Pharmacol*. 2015;71(12):1501.
41. Xu B, et al. *J Anesth*. 2017;31(6):813.
42. Egan TD, et al. *Anesthesiology*. 1998;89:562–573.
43. Minto CF, et al. *Anesthesiology*. 1997;86(1):10.
44. Kim TK, et al. *Anesthesiology*. 2017;126(6):1019.
45. Shafer SL, et al. *Anesthesiology*. 1990;73:1091–1102.
46. Shibutani K, et al. *Anesthesiology*. 2004;101(3):603.
47. Shibutani K, et al. *Br J Anaesth*. 2005;95(3):377.
48. Schwartz AE, et al. *Anesth Analg*. 1991;73(6):790.
49. Slepchenko G, et al. *Anesthesiology*. 2003;98(1):65.
50. Gepts E, et al. *Anesthesiology*. 1995;83(6):1194.
51. de Hoogd S, et al. *Clin Pharmacokinet*. 2017;56(12):1577.
52. Cortinez LI, et al. *Anesth Analg*. 2011;113(1):70.
53. Lesser GT, Deutsch S. *J Appl Physiol*. 1967;23(5):621.
54. Eger EIn, et al. *Anesthesiology*. 1971;35(4):365.
55. Wahrenbrock EA, et al. *Anesthesiology*. 1974;40(1):19.
56. Minto CF, et al. *Anesthesiology*. 1997;86(1):24.
57. Schnider TW, et al. *Anesthesiology*. 1999;90(6):1502.
58. Upton RN, et al. *Anesth Analg*. 1999;89(3):545.
59. Krejcie TC, Avram MJ. *Anesth Analg*. 1999;89(3):541.
60. Arden JR, et al. *Anesthesiology*. 1986;65(1):19.
61. Homer TD, Stanski DR. *Anesthesiology*. 1985;62:714.
62. Stanski DR, Maitre PO. *Anesthesiology*. 1990;72(3):412.
63. Rodeheffer RJ, et al. *Circulation*. 1984;69(2):203.
64. Avram MJ, et al. *Anesthesiology*. 1990;72(3):403.
65. Williams TF. *Clin Pharmacol Ther*. 1987;42(6):663.
66. Janmahasatian S, et al. *Clin Pharmacokinet*. 2005;44(10):1051.
67. Doufas AG, et al. *Anesthesiology*. 2004;101:1112.
68. Lee S, et al. *J Clin Pharm Ther*. 2012;37:698.
69. Scott JC, Stanski DR. *J Pharmacol Exp Ther*. 1987;240:159.
70. Hudson RJ, et al. *Anesthesiology*. 1989;70:426.

19 Inhaled Anesthetics: Mechanisms of Action

MISHA PEROUANSKY, ROBERT A. PEARCE, HUGH C. HEMMINGS, and NICHOLAS P. FRANKS

KEY POINTS

- Anesthesia consists of separable and independent components, each of which involves distinct, but possibly overlapping, mechanisms at different sites in the central nervous system.
- The potencies of general anesthetics correlate with their solubility in oil, indicating the importance of interactions with predominantly hydrophobic targets.
- General anesthetics act by binding directly to amphiphilic cavities in proteins. Binding sites have been identified by a combination of site-directed mutagenesis and high-resolution structural analysis of anesthetic binding.
- Mutations made to render putative protein targets insensitive to inhaled anesthetics have been expressed in mice but have not generated breakthroughs analogous to the success of this strategy with intravenous anesthetics.
- The effects of inhaled anesthetics cannot be explained by a single molecular mechanism. Rather, several targets contribute to the component actions comprising the anesthetic effects of each anesthetic. However, these effects do converge on a limited number of states underlying the behavioral effects.
- The immobilizing effect of inhaled anesthetics involves actions in the spinal cord, whereas sedation/hypnosis and amnesia involve supraspinal mechanisms that interact with endogenous memory, sleep, and consciousness pathways and networks.
- Volatile inhaled anesthetics enhance inhibitory synaptic transmission postsynaptically by potentiating ligand-gated ion channels activated by γ-aminobutyric acid (GABA) and glycine, extrasynaptically by enhancing GABA receptors, and presynaptically by enhancing basal GABA release.
- Inhaled anesthetics suppress excitatory synaptic transmission presynaptically by reducing glutamate release (volatile anesthetics) and postsynaptically by inhibiting excitatory ionotropic receptors activated by glutamate (gaseous and to some extent volatile anesthetics).
- Inhaled anesthetics directly activate certain two-pore-domain potassium channels, which is likely to result in both pre- and post-synaptic effects.
- There is as yet no comprehensive theory of anesthesia that describes the sequence of events leading from the interaction between an anesthetic molecule and its targets to the behavioral effects.

Despite the widespread clinical use of general anesthetics, our current understanding of their molecular, cellular, and network mechanisms is incomplete. This critical gap in the pharmacology of one of medicine's most important drug classes not only impedes rational use of available anesthetics but also hinders the development of newer anesthetics that might selectively achieve the desirable end points of anesthesia with fewer adverse cardiovascular, respiratory, and possibly neuropathologic side effects. Although major progress has been made in understanding the pharmacology of the intravenous anesthetics by molecular genetic approaches, the actions of the inhaled anesthetics at the molecular and cellular levels are more enigmatic. It is still not possible to trace precisely the sequence of events that leads from inhaled anesthetic-target interactions, through ascending levels of biologic complexity, to the various behavioral effects that characterize the composite state of clinical anesthesia in humans. Nevertheless, investigations continue to reveal fundamental principles of action and have led to a framework for understanding anesthetic effects at different organizational levels.

The focus of this chapter is on the mechanisms involved in the principal therapeutic effects (anesthesia) and on the side effects of the inhaled anesthetics (Fig. 19.1), a chemically and pharmacologically diverse group that includes

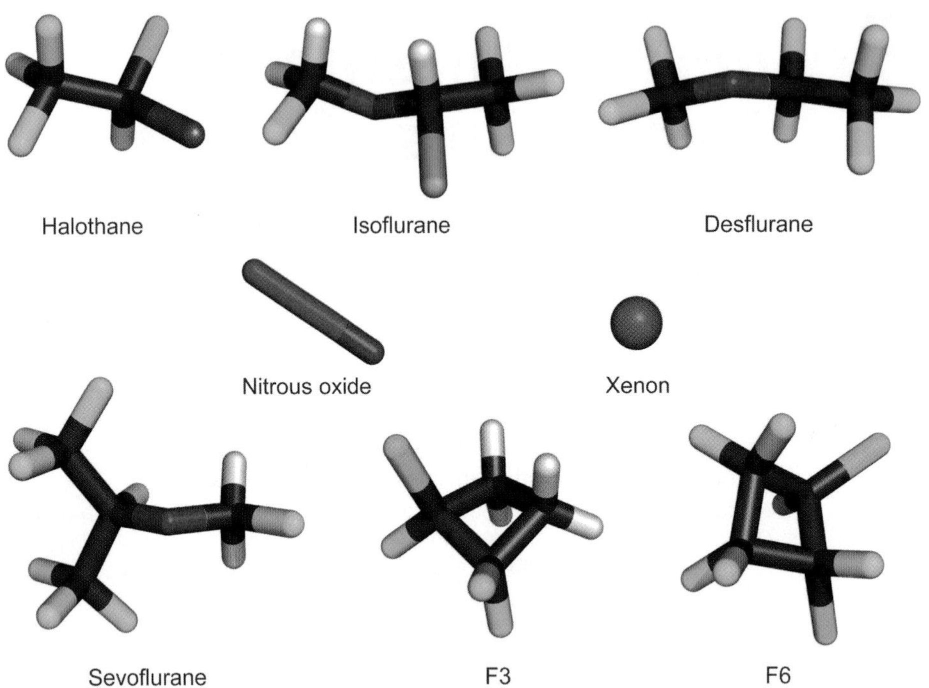

Fig. 19.1 Structures of some representative general anesthetics and a nonimmobilizer *(F6)*. The colors are bromine *(brown)*, carbon *(black)*, chlorine *(green)*, fluorine *(cyan)*, hydrogen *(gray)*, nitrogen *(blue)*, oxygen *(red)*, and xenon *(magenta)*. Note that halothane, isoflurane, desflurane, and *F3* all contain a chiral carbon; therefore each exists as two mirror-image enantiomers (only one enantiomer is shown). Also, the nonimmobilizer *F6* contains two chiral carbons and exists as two trans enantiomers and one cis stereoisomer (only one of the enantiomers is shown).

the potent halogenated ether (isoflurane, sevoflurane, desflurane, enflurane) and alkane (halothane) volatile anesthetics and the inorganic gaseous anesthetics (nitrous oxide and xenon). This critical summary of the current state of knowledge begins with an historical overview and a review of the behavioral end points of anesthesia. We then trace, where possible, inhaled anesthetic effects through ascending levels of organization from molecules, cells, circuits, networks, and organs to mammalian behavior. We also briefly address studies of anesthetic effects in very simple model organisms, with anesthetic end points being identified that as yet bear uncertain relationships to those in mammals.[1]

History

THE UNIFIED PARADIGM OF ANESTHETIC THEORIES

The first monograph reporting experimental work on anesthetic mechanisms, proposing a soon-to-be discredited lipid-elution theory of anesthetic action, was published only 6 months after Morton's public demonstration of ether anesthesia in Boston's Ether Dome. For decades thereafter, the phenomenon of anesthesia puzzled, inspired, and awed those who tried to understand it. An influential paradigm of anesthetic action formulated by Claude Bernard in the 1870s posited that anesthesia was a "unified" phenomenon—a unitary mechanism applicable to all forms of life. Although the anesthetized state could be brought about by a variety of agents, its essence was the same in all living creatures. In fact, Bernard thought that life itself was defined by susceptibility to anesthesia. Bernard also proposed a more specific theory of anesthesia, coagulation of protoplasm, which competed with a number of coexisting theories entertained by the scientific community. In a major work published in 1919, Hans Winterstein[2] summarized the perplexing diversity of anesthetic theories by listing more than 600 references, the majority to original laboratory work—a convincing testimony to the interest of the scientific world in this phenomenon. Of note, the work of Meyer and Overton at the end of the nineteenth century had only a limited effect on the trajectory of research until the 1960s. Only then was the striking simplicity of the Meyer-Overton correlation (Fig. 19.2*A*) of anesthetic potency with solubility in olive oil interpreted by the majority of researchers to indicate that lipids are likely to be the anesthetic target. This interpretation focused attention on anesthetic effects on the bulk physical properties of cell membranes, which were known to consist primarily of lipid molecules. Such nonspecific or "lipoid-based" anesthetic theories dominated the field from the 1960s to the 1980s.

MINIMUM ALVEOLAR CONCENTRATION—A BRIDGE BETWEEN PAST AND PRESENT

The potencies of inhaled anesthetics for immobilization were established in the classic studies in the 1960s of Eger and colleagues,[3,4] who defined the *minimum alveolar concentration* (MAC) as the inhaled anesthetic atmospheric pressure required to prevent movement in response to a defined noxious stimulus in 50% of subjects. The concept of MAC evolved within a unitary paradigm of anesthetic action and also reflected the priorities of clinical practice. As a result, prevention of movement (immobility) became a

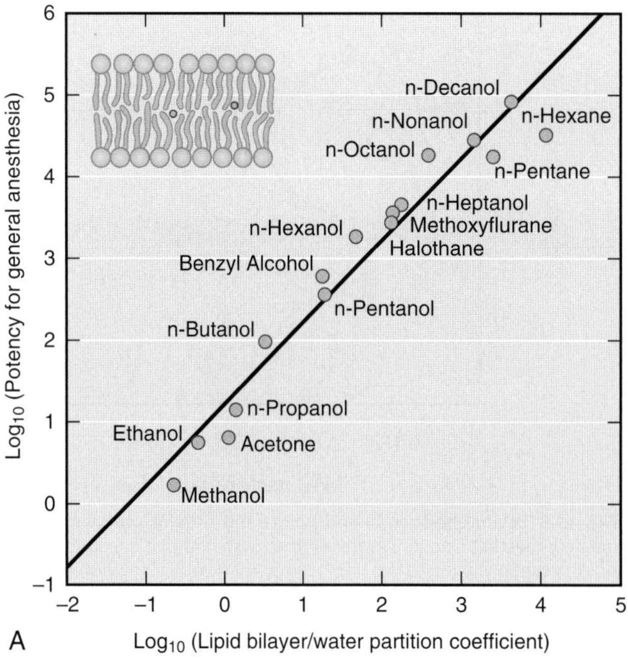

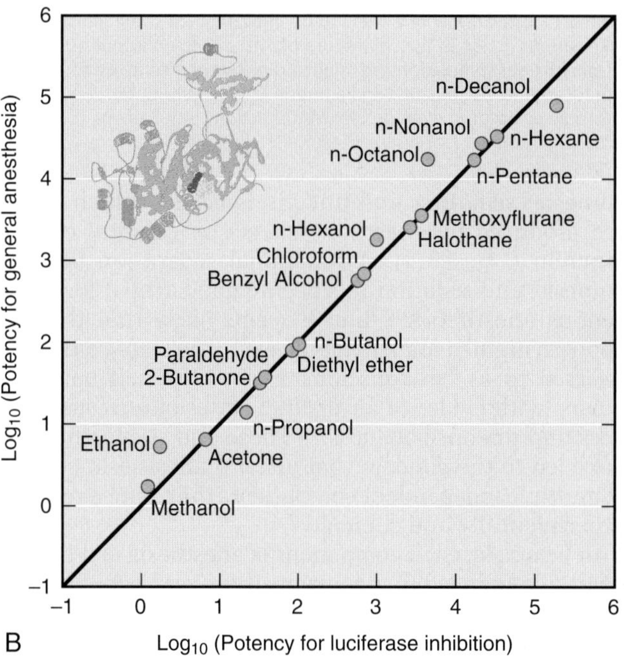

Fig. 19.2 General anesthetics act by binding directly to proteins. (A) The iconic Meyer-Overton correlation (c.1900) between anesthetic potency and the lipid-water partition coefficient was initially interpreted as evidence that lipids of nerve membranes were the principal anesthetic target sites. (B) Progress in the 20th century showed that general anesthetic potencies correlate equally well with their ability to inhibit activity of the soluble firefly enzyme luciferase, which is not a physiologically relevant anesthetic target itself but serves as a lipid-free model protein for anesthetic binding. *Inset*, The crystal structure of luciferase[110] with bound anesthetic *(red)*. (Reprinted with permission from Franks NP, Lieb WR. Molecular and cellular mechanisms of general anesthesia. *Nature*. 1994;367:607–614.)

universal yardstick for anesthetic effects, presumed to occur in the brain. Moreover, the simple elegance of the relationship between anesthetic potency and lipid solubility (see Fig. 19.2*A*) graphically illustrated Meyer and Overton's conclusion that "All chemically indifferent substances that are soluble in fat are anesthetics. Their relative potency as anesthetics will depend on their affinity to fat on the one hand and water on the other hand, that is, on the fat/water partition coefficient."[1] This was interpreted as favoring lipids as the primary targets of anesthetics and a single nonspecific theory to explain anesthesia. The appeal of a single unified mechanism to explain anesthesia was (and remains) intellectually appealing. This focused the bulk of research efforts on delineating how anesthetic interactions with lipid membranes might lead to the behavioral changes observed under anesthesia—the nonspecific lipoid theory.

Because inhaled anesthetic concentrations reflect concentrations in the tissues after equilibration, which is most rapidly achieved for well-perfused organs such as the brain and heart, MAC is analogous to the plasma concentration for 50% effect (EC_{50}) for intravenous anesthetics. In clinical applications, MAC is usually expressed as volume percent (vol%), which varies considerably with temperature owing to the large temperature dependence of partitioning between the gas phase and condensed phases (be they water, lipids, or proteins), whereas the equivalent condensed-phase molar concentrations are much less dependent on temperature.[5] The MAC concept provided researchers and clinicians with a universal standard whereby to measure a defined anesthetic end point (immobility), making meaningful comparisons of experimental results possible and accelerating clinical and laboratory research into anesthetic mechanisms. Today, a more nuanced understanding of MAC considers the structural and functional diversity of the physiologic targets for the different components of the anesthetic state.

SHIFT FROM LIPID- TO PROTEIN-CENTERED MECHANISMS

Lipid-centered mechanisms of anesthesia prevailed in the two decades after definition of the MAC concept. Alternative targets were occasionally proposed but largely neglected by the scientific mainstream. Experimental inconsistencies of lipid targets,[6-8] as well as evidence compatible with proteins as primary sites of action,[9,10] were largely ignored. A shift from lipid- to protein-centered mechanisms, however, began in the late 1970s, owing largely to the discoveries of Franks and Lieb,[11-15] who in an influential series of publications demonstrated that not only were lipids implausible targets but that protein targets were also compatible with the Meyer-Overton correlation (see Fig. 19.2*B*)—a proof of concept that, within a few years, redirected the bulk of research efforts toward proteins. As a corollary of this reorientation, evidence against lipid-based theories was recognized. Examples include the cutoff in anesthetic potency in homologous series of long-chain anesthetic alcohols[15,16] and the identification of hydrophobic drugs that do not obey the Meyer-Overton correlation.[1,17] The enantiomeric selectivity of several anesthetics further strengthened the case for specific binding sites on proteins because stereoselectivity is difficult to reconcile with lipid targets.[18-20] Today, there is widespread acceptance of the notion that lipid bilayers remain essentially unaffected by general anesthetics[11,21] and that critical signaling proteins (e.g., ion channels or ligand-gated receptors) are the relevant molecular targets of anesthetic action.[22] The exact identity of proteins contributing to specific anesthetic end points continues to be sought, with research addressing not only the "where" (target) but also the "how" (process) of anesthetic mechanisms.

DIVERSITY OF POTENTIAL ANESTHETIC TARGETS

At high concentrations in vitro, most inhaled anesthetics affect the functions of multiple proteins, several of which might be plausibly connected to the components of the anesthetic state or anesthetic side effects. However, when a specific anesthetic end point is considered, anesthetics are effective in vivo over a very narrow concentration range. This makes the concentration at which a relevant anesthetic effect is observed a critical consideration for deciding potential relevance. The mechanistic relevance of small effects observed in vitro at relevant concentrations is less clear; that is, what effect is too small to be considered relevant to anesthesia?[23-25]

Whether anesthesia results from the sum of minor perturbations at multiple sites or from substantial effects on a small number of targets remains to be determined. This should be resolved as more sophisticated molecular genetics experimental techniques are applied to test the relevance of putative targets. There are two reasons for believing that the number of relevant targets may be small. First, the extreme steepness of anesthetic concentration-response curves means that, for a given end point, substantial effects on two or three targets would be sufficient to account entirely for the in vivo effect. Second, the stereoselectivity observed in vivo[26] is comparable to the largest effects seen in putative targets in vitro,[18,20] suggesting that only a small number of targets are likely to be involved. Set against this logic is the experimental evidence that a rather large number of plausible target proteins are affected, albeit usually to small extents, and determining which of these are relevant to the various anesthetic end points remains a challenge.

ANESTHESIA: A COMPOSITE NEUROPHARMACOLOGIC STATE

Along with progress in identifying the molecular mechanisms of anesthesia, our understanding of the nature of the anesthetic state has evolved. Whereas a drug-induced coma-like state of general anesthesia can be induced by inhaled anesthetics administered at appropriate concentrations (approximately 1.3 times MAC, equivalent to the EC_{95} of an intravenous anesthetic), the use of such high concentrations can lead to short- and possibly long-term side effects. It is now clear that anesthesia consists of separable and at least partially independent components or substates, each of which involves distinct but possibly overlapping mechanisms in different regions of the central nervous system (CNS) and with variations in relative potencies between specific agents.[27] Immobilization, the core measure of MAC, is mediated largely at the level of the spinal cord by inhaled anesthetics[28,29] but not by barbiturates.[30] On the other hand, the spinal cord is clearly not the primary site of such phenomena as amnesia, sedation, and unconsciousness, which rather are produced by anesthetic effects on cerebral cortical function (Fig. 19.3). A functional separation between amnesia and sedation has been demonstrated for intravenous anesthetics,[31] and it seems likely that this will apply to inhaled anesthetics as well. The state commonly referred to as "unconsciousness" is in itself heterogeneous, with evidence for distinct states of unresponsiveness and unconsciousness.[32] These and similar findings have led to the concept that general anesthesia consists of multiple independent components that can be resolved experimentally and clinically.

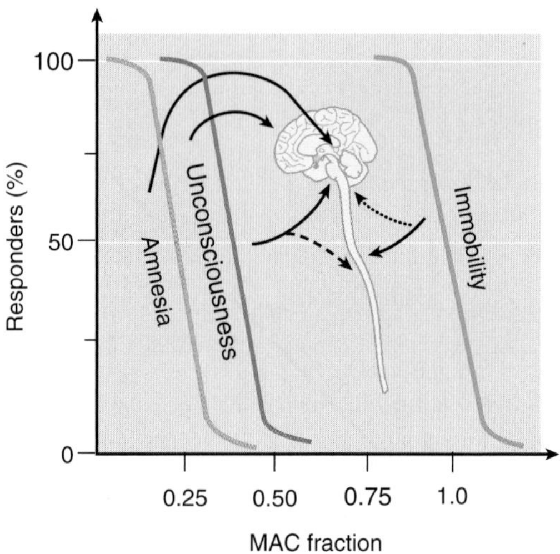

Fig. 19.3 Several behavioral end points and sites of action underlie inhaled anesthetic action. Amnesia, the most sensitive anesthetic end point, probably involves the hippocampus, amygdala, mediotemporal lobe, and other cortical structures. Unconsciousness likely involves the cerebral cortex, thalamus, and neuronal pathways of sleep and arousal. Sedation and hypnosis (loss of responsiveness) are part of the consciousness-unconsciousness continuum and are not shown. Immobility occurs by anesthetic action in the spinal cord, although supraspinal effects *(dotted arrow)* are likely to be important for some anesthetics. Anesthetic action in the spinal cord blunts ascending impulses arising from noxious stimulation and might indirectly contribute to anesthetic-induced unconsciousness and amnesia *(dashed arrow)*. Cardiovascular responses occur at even greater MAC fractions (not shown). (Courtesy Joseph Antognini, University of California, Davis, CA.)

In principle, each component of anesthesia can be preferentially induced in a concentration- and agent-specific manner using individual cellular/molecular pathways in various regions of the CNS. For example, injections of pentobarbital into discrete sites in the mesopontine tegmentum induce a comatose state,[33,34] whereas sedation induced by systemic administration of propofol can be reversed by microinjections of γ-aminobutyric acid $(GABA)_A$ receptor antagonists into the tuberomammillary nucleus, a sleep-regulating nucleus in the hypothalamus.[35] Thus general anesthetics produce separate identifiable anesthetic substates via agent-specific actions at discrete anatomic sites in the CNS through different molecular targets. An important consequence of this complexity is that MAC, which is based exclusively on a motor response, might not proportionately reflect other components of anesthesia. Although this heterogeneity of anesthetic actions complicates a mechanistic understanding, it does open the possibility of developing substate-specific drugs.

Integrated Effects on Central Nervous System Function

IMMOBILITY

Electroencephalography as a monitor of brain activity has been applied both to the study of anesthetic mechanisms and as a monitor of the anesthetic state. Failure to find a correlation between quantitative electroencephalographic activity and immobility in response to noxious stimulation led to the somewhat radical (at the time) hypothesis that immobility was not a cerebral cortex–mediated phenomenon.[36] Experimental demonstration that volatile anesthetics act on the spinal cord to suppress movement[28,29] supported this hypothesis and was a major factor leading to the contemporary separation of anesthetic substates, of which immobility requires the highest drug concentrations (see Fig. 19.3). Taking advantage of the atypical blood supply of goat CNS, which allows separate experimental perfusion of the brain and spinal cord, Antognini and colleagues[28,37] showed that immobility involves anesthetic effects at the spinal level because selective delivery of isoflurane or halothane only to the brain required 2.5-fold to 4-fold higher concentrations compared with delivery to the whole CNS. At the same time, experiments by Rampil and colleagues[29] that used surgical separation of the forebrain and midbrain from the spinal cord in rats led to the conclusion that immobilization involves primarily suppression of the nocifensive withdrawal reflex arc at the level of the spinal cord (Fig. 19.4).

In the 25 years since the identification of the spinal cord as the site of anesthetic-induced immobility, research has centered on pharmacologic, genetic, and complex network approaches. The conventional pharmacologic approach ("bulk" administration of agonists and antagonists into the CNS) to identify receptor-level contributions to isoflurane-induced immobility (isoflurane being the standard potent ether for experimental purposes) has severe limitations in the complex networks of the CNS. Nevertheless, it yielded at least one surprising insight—that actions at $GABA_A$ receptors appear not to be important for the end point of immobility, at least where inhalational agents are concerned.[38] Anesthetic-resistant transgenic mice confirmed that $GABA_A$ receptors containing α1- or α3-subunits do not contribute to the immobilizing action of isoflurane.[39,40] Perhaps less surprisingly, inhibition of central nicotinic acetylcholine receptors also plays no role in immobilization.[41] A role for voltage-gated sodium (Na^+) channels was suggested by the finding that intrathecal administration of a selective inhibitor of Na^+ channels potentiates anesthetic immobility (reduces MAC), whereas an enhancer of Na^+ channel activity does the opposite.[42]

In contrast, work in mutant mice suggests a potential role for tandem-pore domain potassium channels (K_{2P}) in anesthetic-induced immobility. Global knockout mice lacking the TASK-1, TASK-3, and TREK-1 K_{2P} channels are less sensitive to volatile but not intravenous anesthetics,[43-46] indicating a role for these channels possibly by a presynaptic mechanism.[47] An important limitation is that global knockout results almost invariably in wide-ranging compensatory changes in the molecular landscape of the organism with unpredictable consequences for the phenomenon under investigation.

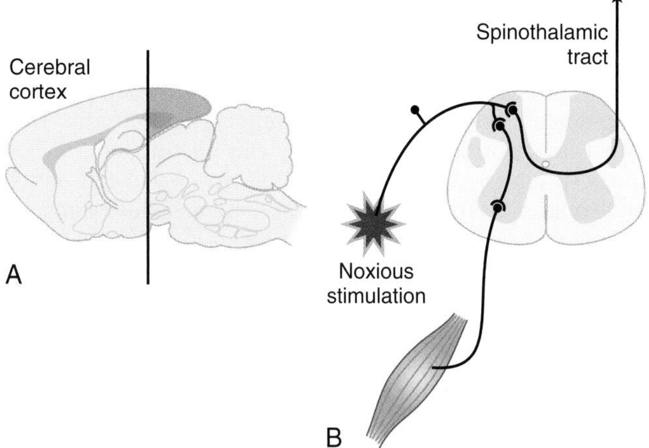

Fig. 19.4 Inhaled anesthetics produce immobility at the spinal level. (A) Decerebration by removal of the forebrain rostral to the *black line* does not alter the minimum alveolar concentration of isoflurane in rats, indicating that volatile anesthetic immobilization does not depend on the cerebral cortex.[28,29] (B) Anesthetics suppress the nocifensive withdrawal reflex response to noxious stimulation transmitted to the dorsal horn by sensory nerves at the spinal level. Current efforts are focused on identifying the molecular, cellular, and anatomic substrates for this effect.

Work with ex vivo preparations that attempt to preserve parts of the complex spinal cord circuitry suggests that anesthetic inhibition of afferent (noxious sensory) input to the dorsal horn plays a subordinate role to the suppression of the efferent (motor) output from the ventral horn, although this may vary by specific agent. This motor output is coordinated by neuronal networks organized in so-called central pattern generators that control the activity of cholinergic motoneurons.[48] Not unlike understanding the anesthetic effects on higher cognitive function, the key to understanding immobility will likely lie in resolving the effect of anesthetics on integrated spinal network activity after understanding the circuit physiology.

UNCONSCIOUSNESS

Compared with the other end points of anesthesia, research into the biologic basis of anesthetic-induced unconsciousness is relatively recent, but it has become an area of active investigation. Research is being conducted in animal models and human subjects and commercial interests are working to develop effective depth-of-anesthesia monitors. These efforts reflect increasing interest, and progress, in "consciousness science" in general.[49,50] Moreover, anesthetics are themselves being used as research tools to help unravel the neuronal underpinnings of consciousness.

Loss of consciousness (or hypnosis) is a hallmark of the onset of anesthesia. However, what is commonly referred to as *unconsciousness under anesthesia* might be more accurately described as *unresponsiveness*, a condition that could also encompass states of self-awareness without environmental awareness (as in dreaming) or environmental awareness without recall (e.g. conscious amnesia combined with neuromuscular paralysis during induction of anesthesia).[32,51]

Numerous theories have been advanced to explain anesthetic-induced unconsciousness. They can generally be divided into those that address "bottom-up" changes in the brain stem circuitry that controls arousal,[52,53] versus "top-down" changes in the thalamocortical circuits that integrate information.[54] Indeed, this distinction formed the basis for a recent suggestion that the *level* of consciousness reflects bottom-up processes whereas the *content* of consciousness reflects top-down processes—a notion with intuitive appeal.[55]

One of the most influential theories has been the "integrated information theory of consciousness (IITC)" of Tononi,[56] which emphasizes the need for simultaneous differentiation between brain states and their integration into a coherent whole.[57] Drugs or diseases that suppress consciousness could act through either process. Other information-based approaches use symbolic analysis,[58] transfer entropy,[59] chaos theory,[60] and more. The rich connectivity of the cerebral cortex and its hierarchical organization are especially suited to enable high levels of information integration in the human brain. Some brain areas present a "rich club" organization (i.e., highly connected nodes tend to be preferentially connected to other highly connected nodes), which has been suggested to be optimal for information integration.[61,62] These hubs are promising targets for the hypnotic action of general anesthetic drugs.

Anesthetics might act by interfering with the operational synchronicity and coherence of corticothalamic networks. Consequent disruption of functional and effective connectivity has been observed during natural slow-wave[63] and midazolam-induced loss of responsiveness.[64] This breakdown of cortical connectivity, rather than pharmacologic deafferentation from the environment, could underlie loss of consciousness.[65] Unconsciousness would then be characterized not by the absence but by the fragmentation of cortical processing.

Although the mechanism of "binding" (i.e., creating the unity of perception) is uncertain, synchronicity of neuronal activity in the 40- to 90-Hz range across functionally connected cortical areas (commonly referred to as 40-Hz- or γ-rhythm) is a viable candidate. Animal[66,67] and human[68] data implicate activity in the γ-band throughout the cortex as a network-level target of general anesthetics. Anesthetic actions on cortical information processing probably consist not merely of suppression of responses but of reduced complexity and variability reflected counterintuitively in the increased reliability and precision of evoked responses.[69,70]

A consistent and intriguing observation has been that anesthetics suppress descending more than ascending neural connectivity.[59,71] Within the framework of predictive coding,[72] this indicates that unconsciousness is associated with a reduction in internally generated predictions more than a suppression of incoming sensory information. The molecular and cellular mechanisms underlying this effect remain undefined, but the preferential suppression by isoflurane of cortico-cortical responses in brain slices in vitro[73,74] supports a top-down mechanism wherein the anesthetic acts directly on the thalamocortical circuitry.

By contrast, "bottom-up" theories attribute changes in consciousness to anesthetic modulation of subcortical arousal nuclei. An interesting theme has emerged from this line of research. There is substantial overlap between the centers whose activity is altered during natural slow-wave sleep and the state of general anesthesia.[35,75–77] That is, many anesthetics may induce unconsciousness, at least in part, by "hijacking" neural sleep[78,79] or arousal[80] pathways.

Thalamic theories of anesthetic-induced unconsciousness[81,82] incorporate aspects of both top-down and bottom-up mechanisms, reflecting not only the intermediate position of this structure in the hierarchical organization of the brain but also the different connection patterns of "sensory relay" versus higher-order "nonspecific" thalamic nuclei.[83]

LEARNING AND MEMORY

Anterograde amnesia, one of the core desirable anesthetic end points, is achieved at lower anesthetic concentrations (~0.25 MAC) than those required for unconsciousness (~0.5 MAC). Perhaps the closest analogue in rodents to explicit memory in humans is medial temporal lobe–dependent learning of temporal and spatial sequences known as *hippocampus-dependent spatial learning*. Other learning paradigms, such as fear conditioning to tone, are by contrast independent of the hippocampus. Spatial learning can be tested by a variety of experimental paradigms, including fear conditioning to context (Fig. 19.5). Isoflurane and the nonimmobilizer F6 both inhibit hippocampus-dependent learning at about half the concentration necessary for disrupting hippocampus-independent learning.[84] Similarly, anesthetic concentrations that inhibit explicit memory in humans (memory that can be explicitly recalled as opposed to motor learning, classical conditioning, and so on) are similarly lower than concentrations that impair implicit memory (not subject to willful recollection).[85] Taken together, these findings implicate effects on function of the medial temporal lobe, including the hippocampus, in the suppression of explicit memory by anesthetics. Effects on other structures, such as the amygdala, may be relevant to anesthetic impairment of implicit or other types of memory.[86]

Because inhaled anesthetics affect multiple cellular targets even at amnesic concentrations, it is likely that anesthetic-induced amnesia arises from multiple cellular-level changes. A quantitative comparison of the degree of change in synaptic inhibition in the hippocampus produced by equiamnestic concentrations of isoflurane versus etomidate indicated that the enhancement of GABAergic inhibition can account for a substantial portion of isoflurane's effect on memory.[87] Other contributing targets may include nAChRs,[88] HCN1 channels,[89] and excitatory glutamatergic synapses.[90] Conversely, it is also likely that suppression of learning and memory by drugs known to have different receptor affinities share common mechanisms at some level of integration. For example, θ-rhythms (4-12 Hz) are clearly important for hippocampus-dependent learning and memory.[91] Benzodiazepines[92] and cannabinoids[93] slow and suppress hippocampal θ-rhythms in proportion to their ability to impair hippocampus-dependent learning. Isoflurane and the nonimmobilizer F6 have comparable effects on θ-rhythms at amnesic concentrations while having different receptor-level profiles and opposite effects on sedation.[94] Thus alterations in neuronal synchrony may

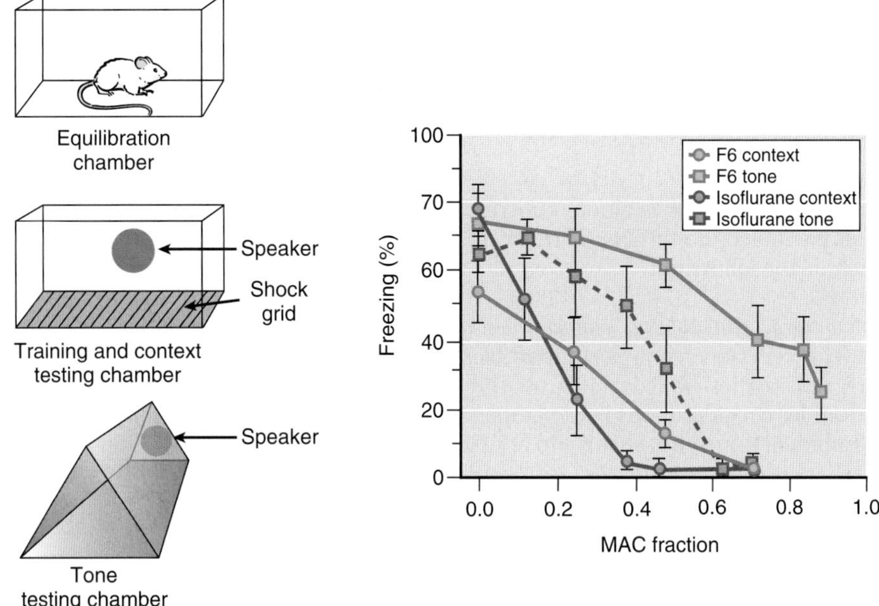

Fig. 19.5 Differential sensitivity of different types of learning to anesthetics and nonimmobilizers. Freezing in anticipation of a noxious stimulus is a measure of learning in rats; less freezing indicates less learning. *Left,* the learning protocol involves preequilibration of rats in the equilibration chamber to isoflurane or the nonimmobilizer *F6* at the desired concentration before placement into the training chamber. For testing of memory to context, the training and test chamber are identical. For testing of memory to tone, training and testing take place in different chambers. *Right,* hippocampus-dependent learning (fear conditioning to context, *closed symbols*) is inhibited by isoflurane *(purple circles)* at lower concentrations than hippocampus-independent learning (fear conditioning to tone, *purple squares*). This differential sensitivity is mirrored by the nonimmobilizer F6 (*blue circles* and *blue squares* for context and tone, respectively). (*Left panel* adapted with permission from Eger EI 2nd, Xing Y, Pearce R, et al. Isoflurane antagonizes the capacity of flurothyl or 1,2-dichlorohexafluorocyclobutane to impair fear conditioning to context and tone. *Anesth Analg.* 2003;96:1010–1018; *right panel* data points reconstructed from Dutton RC, Maurer AJ, Sonner JM, et al. Short-term memory resists the depressant effect of the nonimmobilizer 1-2-dichlorohexafluorocyclobutane (2N) more than long-term memory. *Anesth Analg.* 2002;94:631–639; and Dutton RC, Maurer AJ, Sonner JM, et al. The concentration of isoflurane required to suppress learning depends on the type of learning. *Anesthesiology.* 2001;94:514–519.)

provide a common network-level substrate for memory impairment. The synchronization between amygdalar and hippocampal θ-rhythms that occurs during fear memory retrieval indicates that this principle might also apply to other forms of memory and their impairment by anesthetics.[95] As with other components of the anesthetic state, the precise mechanisms of memory impairment by anesthetics and of memory itself remain to be fully elucidated.

SEDATION

Sedation (defined as a decrease in activity, alertness, arousal, and/or vigilance), which is on a behavioral continuum leading to hypnosis, is achieved at anesthetic doses similar to those that produce amnesia (<0.5 MAC). There is no clear mechanistic or clinical separation between sedation and hypnosis. By contrast, even though sedation can be difficult to separate from amnesia, for intravenous anesthetics there may be separate but overlapping substrates for these two end points.[31] The mechanisms involved in these behavioral effects are likely to resemble those of less promiscuous drugs, for which genetic approaches have been informative. An amino acid knockin mutation (H101R) in mice that renders the α_1 $GABA_A$ receptor subunit insensitive to modulation by benzodiazepines produces resistance to the sedative and amnesic effects of benzodiazepines while maintaining other behavioral effects, among them anxiolysis.[96] The α_1 subunit is abundantly expressed in the CNS, mainly in the cortical areas and thalamus. Volatile anesthetics have qualitatively similar effects on α_1-containing $GABA_A$ receptors (but also those containing other subunits) at low concentrations. The observation that the nonimmobilizer F6, which is devoid of sedative properties,[94] is amnesic[97] but does not modulate benzodiazepine-sensitive α_1-containing $GABA_A$ receptors,[98,99] is compatible with a role for α_1-containing receptors in volatile anesthetic-induced sedation, because few other targets are affected at purely sedative concentrations. Possible targets for the sedative effects of the gaseous anesthetics nitrous oxide and xenon, which do not affect $GABA_A$ receptors, include *N*-methyl-D-aspartate (NMDA) receptor antagonism[100] and K_{2P} channel activation.[101] Consistent with this distinct pharmacologic profile, nitrous oxide has strikingly different effects from those of benzodiazepines in behavioral tests aimed at evaluating sedation in mice.[102]

Recognizing that there may be more than a superficial similarity between natural sleep and anesthetic-induced sedation and hypnosis, the effects of some anesthetics apparently share natural sleep mechanisms by directly activating discrete sleep-promoting nuclei in the hypothalamus.[35] Indeed, the same neurons, or at least overlapping populations of neurons, that are activated by sleep deprivation are also activated during dexmedetomidine-induced sedation.[103] Electroencephalographic patterns during natural slow-wave sleep and anesthesia show similarities,[104] and recovery from sleep deprivation can occur under propofol[105,106] and inhalational anesthesia, supporting this concept. Anesthetic effects on other cortical[107] and subcortical structures[32] may also contribute to anesthetic-induced sedation and hypnosis.

Identification of Molecular Sites of Anesthetic Action

CRITERIA FOR IDENTIFYING SITES RELEVANT TO ANESTHESIA

Specific criteria have been proposed to evaluate the relevance of the many potential molecular targets of anesthetics.[108] These criteria include the following:

1. *Reversible alteration of target function at clinically relevant concentrations.* This criterion requires comparable in vivo and in vitro sensitivities and depends on the anesthetic end point under consideration. For example, targets involved in immobility must be sensitive to anesthetics near MAC, whereas targets mediating amnesia must be affected at a fraction of MAC. Recent evidence for persistent effects of inhaled anesthetics demonstrable in the absence of continued anesthetic exposure is challenging the notion of reversibility for certain effects.
2. *Expression of the target in appropriate anatomic locations to mediate the specific anesthetic end point.* For example, immobilization by inhaled agents appears to involve primarily actions in the spinal cord independent of actions in the brain.
3. *Concordant stereoselectivity of anesthetic effects in vivo and on the target in vitro.* Without a specific pharmacologic antagonist of anesthesia, correlation between the stereoselective actions of general anesthetics in vivo and in vitro is a useful test of pharmacologic relevance of putative molecular targets. Stereoselectivity data correlating in vivo potency and in vitro receptor actions implicate $GABA_A$ receptors as a target for the anesthetic actions of etomidate, pentobarbital, neurosteroid anesthetics, and isoflurane.
4. *Appropriate sensitivity or insensitivity to anesthetic and nonanesthetic compounds.* Anesthetic halogenated cyclobutanes together with structural analogs that do not produce anesthesia at concentrations predicted to be anesthetic by the Meyer-Overton correlation (nonimmobilizers) can be used to discriminate relevant volatile anesthetic targets in vitro. For example, the anesthetic F3 (1-chloro-1,2,2-trifluorocyclobutane), but not the structurally similar nonanesthetic F6 (1,2-dichlorohexa fluorocyclobutane), affect $GABA_A$, glycine, AMPA (α-amino-3-hydroxy-5-methyl-4-isoxazolepropionic acid), kainate, and 5-HT3 receptors; and Na^+ channels, consistent with possible roles in immobility, whereas both F3 and F6 affect neuronal nicotinic, M1 muscarinic, 5-HT2C, and mGluR5 receptors, indicating that these targets are not involved in immobility. F6 is interesting in that it lacks sedative and immobilizing effects but does possess amnesic effects, hence use of the more accurate term *nonimmobilizer*, making it a useful pharmacologic tool for discriminating targets for these actions.
5. *Predictable effects of genetic manipulations targeted to putative molecular targets.* The effects of targeted deletion of specific molecules implicated as anesthetic targets (knockout mutations) or genetic engineering to introduce specific mutations that modify anesthetic sensitivity (knockin mutations) in model organisms provide powerful approaches to test the roles of putative molecular targets of anesthetic action. This approach has been particularly successful in implicating specific $GABA_A$ receptor subtypes in the effects of the GABAergic intravenous anesthetics propofol and etomidate, where single amino acid substitutions in specific receptor subtypes eliminate anesthetic effects both in vitro and in vivo.[109] Targeted mutations of putative anesthetic targets provide a bridge between in vitro observations and whole-animal experiments essential for demonstrating anesthetic end points. The existence of multiple targets and redundancy among ion channel subtypes makes this a more challenging experimental approach for inhaled anesthetics compared with intravenous anesthetics (discussed later).

PHYSICOCHEMICAL PROPERTIES OF ANESTHETIC BINDING SITES

A convergence of x-ray crystallography, molecular modeling, and structure-function studies indicates that inhaled anesthetics bind in the hydrophobic cavities formed within proteins.[22] The lipophilic (or hydrophobic) nature of these binding sites explains their adherence to the Meyer-Overton correlation. An element of amphiphilicity (possessing both polar and nonpolar characteristics) is also required for effective interaction with these cavities, as indicated by improvements in the Meyer-Overton correlation with more amphipathic solvents (possessing both hydrophobic and hydrophilic properties).[7]

FROM MODEL PROTEINS TO RECEPTORS

Identifying inhaled anesthetic binding sites on plausible target proteins is difficult because of their low-affinity interactions, the paucity of atomic resolution structures of pharmacologically relevant target proteins, and the lack of specific antagonists. Consequently most anesthetic binding sites have been identified in well-characterized model proteins for which three-dimensional atomic resolution structures—such as luciferase[110] and serum albumin[111]—are available but are not themselves relevant to anesthesia. These studies indicate that anesthetics bind in pockets with both nonpolar and polar noncovalent chemical interactions.[23,112] Binding involves weak hydrogen bond interactions with polar amino acid residues and water molecules, nonpolar van der Waals interactions, and a polarizing effect of the amphiphilic binding cavity on the relatively hydrophobic anesthetic molecules. Occupation of a site, or sites, by an anesthetic provides a plausible mechanism for alteration of receptor and ion channel function by selectively binding to a particular conformation (e.g., an open or inactivated state of an ion channel).[22] Studies of glycine, $GABA_A$, and NMDA receptors provide convincing evidence for the existence of anesthetic binding sites in critical neuronal signaling proteins.[113] It is likely that before long, high-resolution crystal structures of these receptors will be determined with inhaled anesthetic bound. However, because anesthetics act by binding only to certain transient conformational states, the relevance of necessarily static crystal structures will have to be assessed with care.

Structural studies using the more accessible prokaryotic homologues of eukaryotic ion channels have provided a powerful tool for the study of anesthetic binding sites in biologically plausible proteins. For example, both propofol and desflurane have been cocrystalized with *Gloebacter violaceus*, a bacterial homologue of eukaryotic inhibitory ligand-gated ion channels (glycine and $GABA_A$ receptors). Both anesthetics bind to a common preexisting site in the upper part of the transmembrane domain between the transmembrane segments of a single subunit (Fig. 19.6).[114] Molecular modeling based on structurally homologous proteins has also been used to identify putative anesthetic binding sites in the transmembrane domains of vertebrate $GABA_A$ and glycine receptors (Fig. 19.7). These models

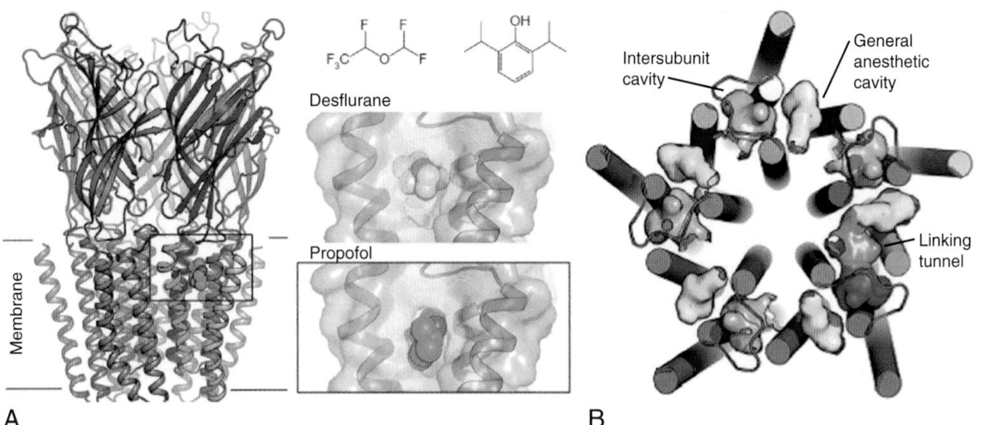

Fig. 19.6 X-ray structures of propofol and desflurane bound to a pentameric ligand-gated ion channel. (A) Cartoon of membrane-plane view of the bacterial homologue of mammalian pentameric ligand-gated ion channels *(Gloebacter violaceus)* with a bound general anesthetic molecule. (B) Molecular surface of the general anesthetic intrasubunit cavities *(yellow)* and neighboring intersubunit cavities *(pink)* of the whole pentameric channel. (Modified from Nury H, Van Renterghem C, Weng Y, et al. X-ray structure of general anaesthetics bound to a pentameric ligand-gated ion channel. *Nature.* 2011;469:428–433.)

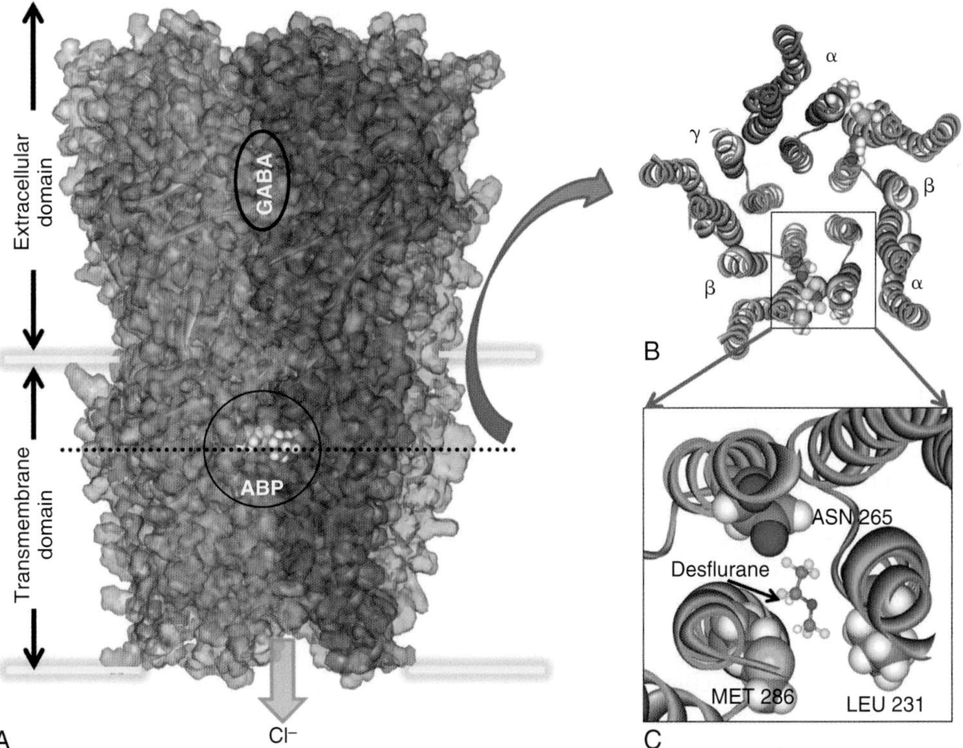

Fig. 19.7 Putative anesthetic binding sites on γ-aminobutyric acid (*$GABA_A$*) receptors identified by molecular modeling. (A) Molecular model of the mouse $GABA_A$ receptor built using homology modeling techniques with computational chemistry optimizations and molecular dockings. The amino acid backbone is displayed in ribbon format and outlined by the transparent solvent-accessible molecular surface. Each of the five subunits is colored uniquely. The *GABA* binding site is noted in the extracellular domain, whereas the putative anesthetic binding pocket *(ABP)* for potentiation is noted in the outer third of the transmembrane domain between the α and β subunits. Two binding sites are shown but only one has computationally docked desflurane. (B) A cross-section at the *dotted line* level in A showing orientation of subunits with pentameric symmetry about a central ion pore. (C) Magnified region of intersubunit anesthetic binding site derived from region in B showing relevant amino acid positions (in space-filling format) interacting with desflurane (in ball-and-stick format at the same scale). (Courtesy the Bertaccini laboratory, Stanford University, Stanford, CA.)

suggest that different drugs may either bind in different orientations within a single amphiphilic cavity or occupy different cavities within the protein, causing similar functional effects. Refinement of these molecular models will continue to provide new insights in the molecular basis for general anesthetic action that can be experimentally tested. For example, potential sites of interaction of xenon and isoflurane with the NMDA receptor have also been identified using this approach. One site, which can contain up to three xenon atoms or one molecule of isoflurane, overlaps the known binding site for the coagonist glycine in the NR1 subunit.[115] This suggests that two chemically dissimilar inhaled anesthetics inhibit NMDA receptors by direct competitive inhibition of coagonist binding.

Molecular Targets of Inhaled Anesthetics

Ion channels have emerged as the most promising molecular targets for inhaled anesthetics. Neurotransmitter-gated ion channels—in particular $GABA_A$, glycine, and NMDA-type glutamate receptors—are leading candidates owing to their appropriate CNS distributions, essential physiologic roles in inhibitory and excitatory synaptic transmission, and sensitivities to clinically relevant concentrations of anesthetics.[22,27,108,116] Other ion channels that are sensitive to inhaled anesthetics include the hyperpolarization-activated cyclic nucleotide (HCN)-gated family of channels that give rise to pacemaker currents[116] and regulate dendritic excitability, two-pore domain (K_{2P}) "leak" K^+ channels that maintain resting membrane potential in many cells,[117,118] and voltage-gated Na^+ and Ca^{2+} channels.[116]

LIGAND-GATED ION CHANNELS

Potentiation of Inhibitory $GABA_A$ and Glycine Receptors

The ether anesthetics (including isoflurane, sevoflurane, and desflurane), the alkane anesthetic halothane, most intravenous anesthetics (including propofol, etomidate, barbiturates), and the neurosteroid anesthetics enhance $GABA_A$ and glycine receptor (GlyR) function. $GABA_A$ and GlyRs are members of the same cys-loop ligand-gated ion channel superfamily that also includes the cation-permeable nicotinic acetylcholine and $5HT_3$ receptors. $GABA_A$ receptors are the principal transmitter-gated Cl^- channels in the neocortex and allocortex, whereas GlyRs fulfill this function in the spinal cord, with some overlap in the diencephalon and brain stem. Activated receptors conduct chloride ions, driving the membrane potential toward the Cl^- equilibrium potential. Both receptors are inhibitory (except in some cases during development) because the Cl^- equilibrium potential is usually more negative than the normal resting potential. Channel opening also reduces membrane resistance and "shunts" excitatory responses. Most functional $GABA_A$ and GlyRs are heteropentamers, typically consisting of three different $GABA_A$ subunits (e.g., two α, two β, and one γ or ∂)[119] or two different GlyR subunits (three α and two β).[120] The subunit composition of $GABA_A$ receptors determines their physiologic and pharmacologic properties and varies between and within brain areas as well as between different compartments of individual neurons. Examples are the preferential expression of the α_5 subunit in the dendritic field of the hippocampal CA1 area (a region important for memory formation), of the α_4 subunit in the thalamus, and of the α_6 subunit in the cerebellum. Presence of a γ subunit is required for benzodiazepine modulation of $GABA_A$ receptors and can also influence modulation by inhaled anesthetics. Although the molecular mechanisms of receptor modulation by inhaled anesthetics are not clear, these receptors have been key to our understanding of anesthetic-receptor interactions. Using chimeric receptor constructs between anesthetic-sensitive $GABA_A$ and insensitive GlyR subunits, specific amino acid residues in transmembrane domains 2 and 3 critical to the action of inhaled anesthetics have been identified.[121] This laid the groundwork for the construction of anesthetic-resistant $GABA_A$ receptors and the generation of transgenic mice with altered anesthetic sensitivity (discussed later).

The related cation-permeable 5-hydroxytryptamine (serotonin)-3 ($5HT_3$) receptors are similarly potentiated by volatile anesthetics.[122,123] $5HT_3$ receptors are involved with autonomic reflexes and also probably contribute to the emetogenic properties of volatile anesthetics.

Inhibition of Excitatory Acetylcholine and Glutamate Receptors

Neuronal nicotinic acetylcholine receptors (nnAChRs), like the other members of the cys-loop family, are heteropentameric ligand-gated ion channels but are cation-selective. They are composed of α and β subunits but functional homomeric receptors can be formed by certain α subunits. In the CNS, nnAChRs are localized primarily presynaptically.[124] Homomeric α_7 receptors have high permeability to Ca^{2+}, which can exceed that of NMDA receptors.[124] In contrast to $GABA_A$ and GlyRs, nnAChRs pass cations when activated and therefore depolarize the membrane potential. Receptors containing $\alpha_4\beta_2$ subunits are very sensitive to block by isoflurane.[125,126] Relevance of nnAChR block to immobilization, sedation, and unconsciousness by inhaled anesthetics is unlikely because nnAChRs are also blocked by nonimmobilizers, although it is possible that they do contribute to amnesia.

NMDA receptors are a major postsynaptic receptor subtype of inotropic receptors for glutamate, the principal excitatory neurotransmitter in the mammalian CNS.[127] Typical NMDA receptors, defined pharmacologically by their selective activation by the exogenous agonist NMDA, are heteromers consisting of an obligatory GluN1 subunit and modulatory GluN2 subunits. Channel opening requires glutamate (or another synthetic agonist such as NMDA) binding to the GluN2 subunit while the endogenous coagonist glycine binds to the GluN1 subunit. NMDA receptors also require membrane depolarization to relieve voltage-dependent block by Mg^{2+}. Depolarization is typically provided by the binding of glutamate to non-NMDA glutamate receptors (discussed later). Because of this requirement for both presynaptic transmitter release and postsynaptic depolarization, synaptic NMDA receptors function as coincidence detectors, and this characteristic is thought to be central to their role in learning and memory. NMDA receptors are also involved in the development of chronic pain, perhaps because of mechanisms similar to those underlying synaptic plasticity, and in ischemia-induced excitotoxicity by virtue of their capacity to allow entry of the ubiquitous intracellular signal Ca^{2+}. The nonhalogenated inhaled

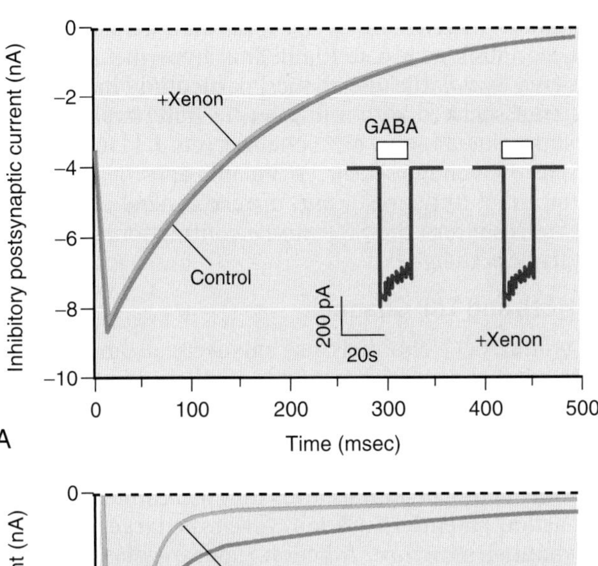

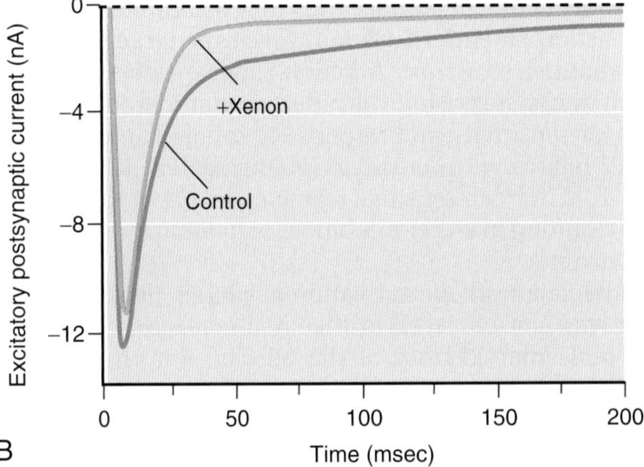

Fig. 19.8 The actions of xenon on inhibitory GABAergic and excitatory glutamatergic synapses in cultured rat hippocampal neurons. Xenon (3.4 mM, or 1 minimum alveolar concentration [MAC]) has no significant effect on the inhibitory postsynaptic current (A) but depresses the excitatory glutamatergic synaptic current, almost exclusively the slow *N*-methyl-D-aspartate receptor-mediated component of the current (B). In contrast, the principal effects of 1 MAC isoflurane are a prolongation in the inhibitory current decay and a reduction in excitatory current peak height, with little change in time course (not shown, see Fig. 19.10). (Reprinted in modified form by permission from de Sousa SLM, et al. Contrasting synaptic actions of the inhalational general anesthetics isoflurane and xenon. *Anesthesiology*. 2000;92:1055–1066.)

anesthetics xenon, nitrous oxide, and cyclopropane have minimal effects on $GABA_A$ receptors but depress excitatory glutamatergic synaptic transmission postsynaptically via NMDA glutamate receptor blockade (Fig. 19.8).[128,129] Volatile anesthetics can also inhibit isolated NMDA receptors at higher concentrations.[130] Along with presynaptic inhibition of glutamate release, this might contribute to their depression of NMDA receptor–mediated excitatory transmission.

A second class of inotropic glutamate receptors includes the non-NMDA receptors, which are subdivided into AMPA and kainate receptors based again on their sensitivities to selective exogenous agonists.[127] Inhaled anesthetics only weakly inhibit AMPA receptors; hence this action is unlikely to be important in their actions.[131] Interestingly, kainate receptors are enhanced by inhaled anesthetics, but this is unlikely to be involved in immobility because MAC is not altered in mice deficient in the GluR6 receptor subunit.[132] Most evidence suggests that the principal mechanism for depression of glutamatergic transmission by volatile anesthetics is presynaptic, with minor contributions from postsynaptic receptor blockade[133-135] (see section on "Cellular Mechanisms").

VOLTAGE-GATED AND OTHER ION CHANNELS

Volatile anesthetics have diverse effects on a wide variety of ion channels that are critically involved in their neurophysiologic, cardiovascular, and respiratory actions. A detailed understanding of these interactions is crucial to a pharmacologic description of this essential drug class.

Na^+ Channels

Voltage-gated Na^+ channels are critical to axonal conduction, synaptic integration, and neuronal excitability. In contrast to findings in invertebrate giant axons,[136] axonal conduction in small (0.1-0.2 μm) unmyelinated hippocampal axons is depressed by volatile anesthetics,[137,138] and small reductions in preterminal action potential amplitude significantly depress transmitter release and hence postsynaptic responses at a mammalian synapse.[139] Heterologously expressed mammalian voltage-gated Na^+ channels are sensitive to clinically relevant concentrations of volatile anesthetics. The Na^+ channel family consists of nine homologous pore-forming α subunits with distinct cellular and subcellular distributions.[140,141] Isoflurane and other volatile anesthetics inhibit the major mammalian Na^+ channel isoforms, including neuronal ($Na_v1.2$), skeletal muscle ($Na_v1.4$), cardiac ($Na_v1.5$), and peripheral ($Na_v1.8$) isoforms.[142] Volatile anesthetics but not nonimmobilizers also inhibit native neuronal and nerve terminal Na^+ channels,[141,143-146] lending support to the notion that Na^+ channel blockade contributes to the depression of synaptic neurotransmitter release.[147] In contrast, xenon has no detectable effect on Na^+, Ca^{2+}, or K^+ channels in isolated cardiomyocytes.[148] The demonstration that NaChBac, a prokaryotic homologue of voltage-gated Na^+ channels, is also inhibited by volatile anesthetics opens the way for structure-function studies of these channels.[145] These studies suggest that volatile anesthetics affect channel gating, probably via at least two drug binding sites.[149-151]

Ca^{2+} Channels

Multiple cellular functions depend on the tightly controlled concentration of intracellular free Ca^{2+} ($[Ca^{2+}]_i$), which is determined by the integrated activities of voltage-gated Ca^{2+} channels, capacitative Ca^{2+} channels, plasma membrane and sarcoplasmic/endoplasmic reticulum (ER) Ca^{2+}-adenosine triphosphatases (pumps), Na^+/Ca^{2+} exchangers, mitochondrial Ca^{2+} sequestration, and cytoplasmic Ca^{2+}-binding proteins. Alteration of any of these mechanisms can affect the many cellular processes regulated by the second-messenger actions of Ca^{2+}, including synaptic transmission, gene expression, cytotoxicity, and muscle excitation-contraction coupling. Excitable cells translate their electrical activity into action by Ca^{2+} fluxes mediated primarily by voltage-gated Ca^{2+} channels in the plasma membrane. Distinct Ca^{2+} channel subtypes are expressed in various cells and tissues, and are classified pharmacologically and functionally by the degree of depolarization required to gate the channel as low voltage–activated

(LVA; T-type) or high voltage–activated (HVA; L-, N-, R-, and P/Q-type) channels. Cloning and sequencing to identify their pore-forming α subunits has allowed molecular classification of these functionally identified channel subtypes.[141] Considerable evidence indicates that volatile anesthetics inhibit certain Ca^{2+} channel isoforms but not others.

Inhibition of presynaptic voltage-gated Ca^{2+} channels coupled to transmitter release has been proposed as a mechanism by which volatile anesthetics reduce excitatory transmission.[152,153] Indeed, N-type ($Ca_v2.2$) and P-type ($Ca_v2.1$) channels, which mediate Ca^{2+} entry coupled to neurotransmitter release, are modestly sensitive to volatile anesthetics[154,155] but not in all neuron types,[156] suggesting the importance of auxiliary subunits, posttranslational modification, or other potential modulators of anesthetic sensitivity. A modest contribution of R-type Ca^{2+} channels ($Ca_v2.3$) to anesthesia is suggested by their sensitivity to volatile anesthetics and a small increase in MAC produced by genetic deletion in mice.[157] T-type Ca^{2+} channels are particularly sensitive to volatile anesthetics[158] and nitrous oxide.[159] However, mutant mice lacking a major neuronal T-type Ca^{2+} channel isoform ($Ca_v3.1$) have normal volatile anesthetic sensitivity, although the onset of anesthesia is delayed.[160] Thus the role that inhibition of these or other Ca^{2+} channels plays in the CNS effects of inhaled anesthetics is unclear.

At higher doses, a role for Ca^{2+} channel inhibition in the negative inotropic effects of volatile anesthetics is well established. The force of myocardial contraction is determined by the magnitude of cytosolic Ca^{2+} increase after electrical excitation, the responsiveness of the contractile proteins to Ca^{2+}, and sarcomere length. Negative inotropic effects of volatile anesthetics are mediated by reductions in Ca^{2+} availability, Ca^{2+} sensitivity of the contractile proteins, and rate of cytosolic Ca^{2+} clearance. Volatile anesthetics reduce the Ca^{2+} transient and shorten action potential duration in cardiomyocytes primarily by inhibiting L-type ($Ca_v1.2$) Ca^{2+} currents, resulting in a negative inotropic effect and arrhythmogenicity.[161-163] In contrast, xenon does not depress myocardial function or inhibit L-type Ca^{2+}, Na^+, or K^+ currents in isolated cardiomyocytes.[164,165] Inhibition of trans-sarcolemmal Ca^{2+} influx through cardiac L-type Ca^{2+} channels plays a major role in the negative inotropic effects of volatile anesthetics—greatest for halothane—along with contributions from effects on myofilament Ca^{2+} sensitivity and sarcolemmal Ca^{2+} release.[162,166]

In contrast to voltage-gated Ca^{2+} channels that regulate the influx of extracellular Ca^{2+}, intracellular Ca^{2+} channels regulate Ca^{2+} release from intracellular stores, particularly the ER and sarcoplasmic reticulum (SR). These include 1,4,5-inositol triphosphate receptors (IP_3Rs), regulated by the second messenger IP_3, and ryanodine receptors (RyRs); the latter mediate the release of SR Ca^{2+}, which is critical to excitation-contraction coupling in muscle. Volatile anesthetic–induced Ca^{2+} leak occurs by effects on both IP_3R and RyR channels, which leads to depletion of intracellular Ca^{2+} stores from the SR and ER. In brain, volatile anesthetic activation of IP_3Rs has been proposed as a mechanism for anesthetic neurotoxicity.[167] This blunts changes in intracellular Ca^{2+} in response to stimulation and contributes to the smooth muscle–relaxing properties of volatile anesthetics that underlie bronchodilation and vasodilation.[168]

Malignant hyperthermia is a pharmacogenetic disorder that manifests as a potentially fatal hypermetabolic crisis triggered by volatile anesthetics, particularly halothane. It is often associated with mutations in RyR1 and the physically associated L-type Ca^{2+} channel ($Ca_v1.1$), which functions as the voltage sensor.[169] Volatile anesthetics activate the mutated RyRs, resulting in uncontrolled intracellular Ca^{2+} release from the SR, muscle contraction, and hypermetabolic activity.[170]

K^+, HCN, and TRP Channels

Potassium (K^+) channels are members of an extremely diverse ion channel family noted for their varied modes of activation. They regulate electrical excitability, muscle contractility, and neurotransmitter release. They are important in determining input resistance and in driving repolarization after action potentials; thus they determine excitability and action potential duration. Given the large diversity in K^+ channel structure, function, and anesthetic sensitivity, it is not surprising that there is considerable diversity in their sensitivity and response to inhaled anesthetics,[171] from relatively insensitive (voltage-gated K^+ channels $K_v1.1$, K_v3)[172] to sensitive (some members of the K_{2P} family), resulting in either inhibition, activation, or no effect on K^+ currents.

Volatile anesthetic activation of certain "leak" K^+ channels was first observed in the snail *Lymnaea*,[173] although the molecular identity of the affected ion channels was unknown. Activation of K_{2P} channels by volatile and gaseous anesthetics—including xenon, nitrous oxide, and cyclopropane—was subsequently observed in mammals.[118] Increased K^+ conductance can hyperpolarize neurons, reducing responsiveness to excitatory synaptic input and possibly altering network synchrony. Targeted deletion of the TASK-1, TASK-3, and TREK-1 K_{2P} channels in mice reduces sensitivity to immobilization by volatile anesthetics in an agent-specific manner, implicating these channels as contributory anesthetic targets in vivo.[44-47] The K^+ channel TREK-1 also contributes to the neuroprotective effects of xenon[174] and sevoflurane.[175]

Progress has recently been made in identifying anesthetic binding sites to K^+ channels using photoaffinity labeling, which has identified a sevoflurane binding site in the $K_v1.2$ channel; this is widely expressed in brain and positively modulated by volatile anesthetics.[176] Molecular modeling has also been used to identify likely binding sites in K_{2P} channels.[177]

The recognition that inherited channelopathies are arrhythmogenic and constitute an important contributor to sudden cardiac death,[178] particularly in young children,[179] highlights the importance of analyzing anesthetic modulation of cardiac ion channels. Recombinant hERG (human ether-a-go-go–related) channels are moderately inhibited by halothane, and their depression likely contributes to arrhythmogenic effects of volatile anesthetics[162,180]; they are also involved in acquired (drug-induced) and inherited long QT syndrome. Cardiac inward-rectifying (K_{IR}), voltage-gated (K_v), and Ca^{2+}-activated K^+ channels are generally relatively insensitive to clinical concentrations of volatile anesthetics and xenon.[162,164,181] In contrast, volatile anesthetics and xenon activate cardiac mitochondrial and sarcolemmal K_{ATP} channels,[182] which might contribute to anesthetic preconditioning to cardiac ischemia. Direct electrophysiologic effects of anesthetics with preconditioning properties have been demonstrated on both mitochondrial and sarcolemmal K_{ATP} channels, although the precise mechanisms remain to be clarified. The large conductance (BK) mitochondrial K^+ channel Slick of the *Slo2* gene family has been shown to be important for volatile anesthetic preconditioning in vivo.[183]

Volatile anesthetics also inhibit HCN pacemaker channels, reducing the rate of rise of pacemaker potentials and the bursting frequency of certain neurons that show autorhythmicity. They decrease the I_h conductance in neurons[184] and modulate recombinant HCN1 and HCN2 channel isoforms at clinically relevant concentrations.[185] Because HCN channels contribute to resting membrane potential, control action potential ring, dendritic integration, neuronal automaticity, and temporal summation, and also determine periodicity and synchronization of oscillations in many neuronal networks,[186] anesthetic modulation of these channels could play an important role in anesthetic effects on neuronal integrative functions. Selective knockout of HCN1 in mouse forebrain shows a role for these channels in the amnestic and hypnotic but not immobilizing effects of volatile anesthetics.[89]

INTRACELLULAR SIGNALING MECHANISMS

Cell signaling mechanisms are critical to all phases of organ and cellular function, which has made them attractive targets for producing the broad effects of general anesthetics on multiple organs. Anesthetics have complex actions on intracellular cell signaling pathways, which include processes downstream from cell surface receptors and ion channels, including effects on second messengers, protein phosphorylation pathways, and other regulatory mechanisms.[187]

G-Protein–Coupled Receptors

A variety of signals—including hormones, neurotransmitters, cytokines, pheromones, odorants, and photons—produce their intracellular actions by interactions with metabotropic receptors that activate heterotrimeric guanine nucleotide–binding proteins (G proteins). In contrast to inotropic receptors that directly couple to ion-selective channels, G proteins act as indirect molecular switches to relay information from activated plasma membrane receptors to appropriate intracellular targets.

Heterotrimeric G proteins consist of a large α-subunit and a smaller β/γ-subunit dimer, each expressed as multiple isoforms with distinct properties and downstream targets. G proteins regulate a plethora of downstream effectors to control the levels of cytosolic second messengers such as Ca^{2+}, cyclic adenosine monophosphate, and inositol triphosphate. These, in turn, regulate effector proteins such as ion channels and enzymes, either directly or via second messenger–regulated protein phosphorylation pathways. Ca^{2+} is a ubiquitous second messenger that regulates a number of downstream effectors, often mediated by the multifunctional Ca^{2+}-binding protein calmodulin. As volatile anesthetics have profound effects on intracellular Ca^{2+} concentrations via their effects on both plasma membrane and intracellular Ca^{2+} channels, transporters, and exchangers (see the section on ion channels earlier), many of the downstream effects of anesthetics are ultimately mediated by changes in the second-messenger actions of Ca^{2+}.

Drugs that act through G protein–coupled receptors (GPCRs) such as agonists for μ-opioid and α_2-adrenergic receptors can affect anesthetic sensitivity (reduce MAC). Inhaled anesthetics can also directly affect signaling via GPCRs.[188] For example, volatile anesthetics activate multiple olfactory GPCRs in the rat in vivo in a receptor- and agent-selective manner.[189] Analogous effects on related GPCRs more relevant to critical anesthetic end points are possible but remain to be demonstrated. The observation that both volatile anesthetics and nonimmobilizers inhibit mGluR5 glutamate receptors, 5-HT_{2A} serotonin receptors, and muscarinic acetylcholine receptors suggests that these GPCR effects do not contribute to anesthetic immobilization.[190-192]

Protein Phosphorylation

Phosphorylation of proteins on specific serine, threonine, or tyrosine hydroxyl groups, a posttranslational modification involved in the regulation of many anesthetic-sensitive receptors and ion channels, is pivotal to synaptic plasticity (e.g., long-term potentiation [LTP]). Phosphorylation is controlled by the balance of activity between protein kinases and phosphatases, several of which are plausible anesthetic targets. The protein kinase C (PKC) family of multifunctional protein kinases is activated by the lipid-signaling molecule diacylglycerol and is involved in the regulation of many ion channels and receptors. Halothane[193] and sevoflurane[194] enhance the activity of some PKC isoforms and stimulate phosphorylation of specific PKC substrates. Structural studies have identified a potential binding site in the diacylglycerol binding domain of PKCδ, consistent with the ability of certain anesthetics to mimic this natural regulator by binding to the activating site.[195] A specific role for a direct pharmacologically relevant effect related to general anesthesia mediated by anesthetic activation of PKC or of any other kinase has yet to be demonstrated. Intrathecal injection of isoform-specific inhibitors of PKC does not affect sensitivity to halothane in vivo.[196] Knockout mice lacking the PKCγ isoform show normal sensitivity to halothane and desflurane while isoflurane MAC was increased,[197] suggesting that PKC is not critical to volatile anesthetic immobilization.

An important role for effects of volatile anesthetics and xenon on cell signaling mechanisms has been discovered for anesthetic-induced preconditioning in the heart and brain against ischemic damage.[198-202] Anesthetic-induced and ischemic cardiac preconditioning share critical signaling mechanisms, including activation of multiple GPCRs (e.g., adenosine, opioid, adrenergic) and protein kinases (e.g., src kinase, PKCδ, PKCε, Akt, mitogen-activated protein kinases [MAPKs]), and their downstream targets, particularly sarcolemmal and/or mitochondrial K_{ATP} channels, possibly initiated by changes in reactive oxygen species as the critical second messenger.[203,204] Volatile anesthetics and xenon share cardioprotective and neuroprotective effects involving these signaling pathways.[202,205]

The effects of anesthetics on the phosphorylation of individual residues in specific substrates can be studied using phosphorylation state–specific antibodies that are able to detect the phosphorylated forms of kinase substrates. A comparison of the effects of three mechanistically diverse anesthetics (isoflurane, propofol, and ketamine) on critical intracellular protein phosphorylation signaling pathways that are known to integrate multiple second messenger systems reveals both shared and agent-specific actions in vivo.[206] All three anesthetics reduce phosphorylation of activating sites on NMDA and AMPA glutamate receptors and of the downstream extracellular signal-regulated kinase ERK2, all of which are known to be involved in synaptic plasticity, consistent with depression of normal glutamatergic synaptic transmission in the anesthetized mouse cerebral cortex. These effects are somewhat selective in that several other protein kinase A (PKA) substrates examined are not affected, indicating substrate-specific effects rather than a general inhibition of PKA activity.[207] Additional studies will be required to determine which anesthetic effects on kinase pathways represent direct effects, as occurs with PKC, and which are indirect because of anesthetic-induced alterations in signaling molecules known to regulate protein kinase and phosphatase activity such as Ca^{2+} and other second messengers.

Gene Expression

The ability of general anesthetics to alter gene expression in the brain was first observed for the highly reactive immediate early genes *c-fos* and *c-jun*.[208] Anesthetic effects on gene expression have since been observed for multiple anesthetics and organs.[209] In the hippocampus of aged rats, changes in gene expression persisted for up to 2 days in rats exposed to isoflurane and nitrous oxide,[210] and changes in protein expression have been observed 3 days after exposure to desflurane.[211] The significance of these changes in gene and protein expression persisting after recovery from the classic signs of anesthesia remains to be established (see review[212]). Recent findings suggest that certain anesthetic effects are mediated by epigenetic mechanisms involving specific posttranslational modifications of DNA-binding histone proteins by acetylase and deacetylase enzymes. For example, exposure of neonatal rats to general anesthesia led to reduced histone 3 acetylation and delayed cognitive deficits that could be reversed by a histone deacetylase inhibitor.[213]

Cellular Mechanisms

NEURONAL EXCITABILITY

Neuronal excitability is determined by resting membrane potential, threshold for action potential initiation, and input resistance (an indication of overall channel activity). Considerable diversity exists for each of these factors in different types of neurons, and membrane properties differ not only between neurons but also between compartments (e.g., soma versus dendrite). Moreover, anesthetic effects vary with the state of the individual neuron—that is, whether it is hyperpolarized or depolarized, stimulated by synaptic inputs, or quiescent. Therefore results obtained using model systems or reduced preparations (e.g. cultured neurons and brain slices) incompletely reflect anesthetic effects in vivo. Nevertheless much valuable information has been obtained using these approaches because they allow changes in neuronal activity to be attributed to specific cellular and molecular targets.

The intrinsic excitability of spinal motoneurons was reported to be little affected by halothane,[214] but changes in hippocampal pyramidal neuron excitability were shown to be substantial and complex. Threshold can be increased or decreased, and regional differences and dose-dependent effects on firing patterns have been observed.[215,216] Neurons in the ventral-posterior nucleus of the thalamus (possibly thalamic relay neurons) hyperpolarize in the presence of isoflurane and are less likely to fire action potentials because of a decrease in input resistance (increased shunting)—an effect that has been attributed to increased K^+ conductance.[217] Similar effects are observed in hypoglossal motoneurons and neurons from the locus coeruleus, where a TASK-type K_{2P} channel has been causally implicated.[218]

$GABA_A$ receptors located at extrasynaptic sites can also influence excitability by increasing membrane conductance and thereby "shunting" excitatory currents. These receptors have a high affinity for GABA; they are continually exposed to low ambient GABA concentrations and desensitize slowly.[219] Their importance to anesthesia, however, may hinge on exactly what these ambient concentrations are.[220] Tonic current in hippocampal pyramidal neurons arises primarily from α_5 subunit–containing $GABA_A$ receptors, which are highly sensitive to etomidate, propofol, midazolam, and isoflurane.[221-224] Thus they provide a potential substrate for the amnesic properties of anesthetics. These same receptors also contribute to slow phasic (synaptic) currents, which are produced by spillover of GABA from synapses.[225] Their slow time course and location, matching those of synaptic NMDA receptors, place them in an ideal position to modulate synaptic plasticity. Indeed, reducing or eliminating α_5-$GABA_A$ receptors by pharmacologic or genetic means attenuates the amnestic properties of the $GABA_A$ receptor-selective anesthetic etomidate. However, since elimination of α_5-$GABA_A$ receptors from pyramidal neurons does not reproduce this effect,[226] modulation of other cell types (interneurons or glia) may also play a role in anesthetic-induced amnesia and other anesthetic end points.

PRESYNAPTIC VERSUS POSTSYNAPTIC EFFECTS ON SYNAPTIC TRANSMISSION

General anesthetics have potent and specific effects on synaptic transmission, including presynaptic actions (by altering transmitter release) and postsynaptic actions (by altering the postsynaptic responses of neurons to specific transmitters). The relative contributions of presynaptic compared with postsynaptic anesthetic effects on synaptic transmission have been difficult to resolve, probably because the effects are transmitter- and synapse-specific. The net effect of anesthetics on synaptic transmission is determined by the relative magnitude and direction of both their presynaptic and postsynaptic effects. The general effects of inhaled anesthetics are to increase inhibitory synaptic transmission and to inhibit excitatory synaptic transmission (Fig. 19.9).

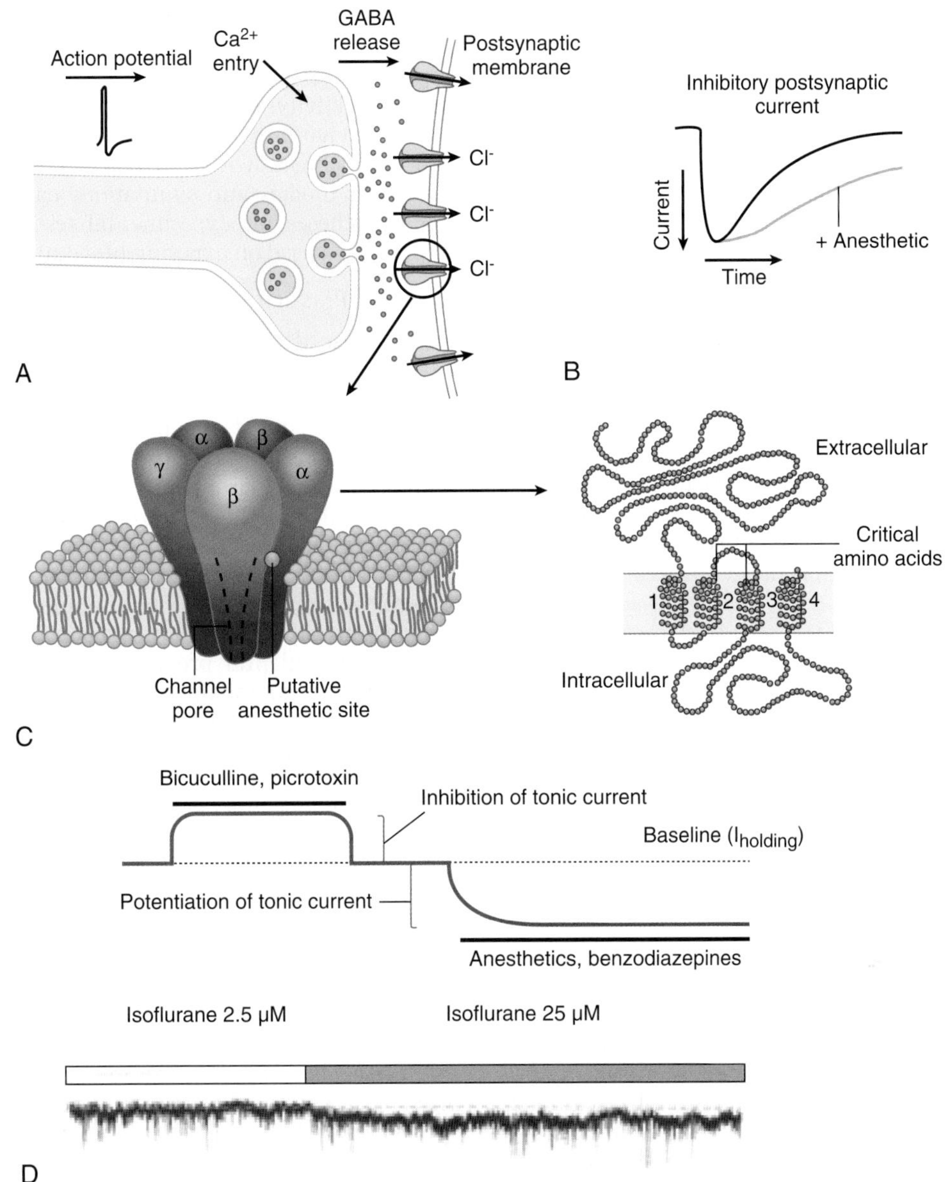

Fig. 19.9 Synaptic and extrasynaptic γ-aminobutyric acid (*GABA*$_A$) receptors are targets for inhaled anesthetics. (A) On binding of GABA to the GABA$_A$ receptor, its chloride-permeable channel opens, usually leading to hyperpolarization. Volatile anesthetics have a relatively low potency but high efficacy at synaptic GABA$_A$ receptors and a high potency and low efficacy at extrasynaptic GABA$_A$ receptors. (B) General anesthetics prolong channel opening and increase postsynaptic inhibition. The cartoon illustrates the prolongation of miniature inhibitory synaptic currents by the slowing of current decay. (C) A pentameric GABA$_A$ receptor complex in the lipid bilayer membrane *(left)*, with a blowup of a single subunit showing the location of residues critical to anesthetic efficacy in the second and third transmembrane domains *(right)*. (D) A tonic inhibitory conductance is revealed by the application of a GABA$_A$ receptor antagonist (bicuculline or picrotoxin), as shown by the upward shift in the baseline current. Anesthetics and benzodiazepines increase the tonic conductance, as indicated by the inward shift in the current. (Modified from Hemmings HC Jr, Akabas MH, Goldstein PA, et al. Emerging molecular mechanisms of general anesthetic action. *Trends Pharmacol Sci.* 2005;26:503–510.)

Excitatory synaptic excitation is generally decreased by volatile anesthetics (Fig. 19.10). Experiments in various slice preparations indicate that reduced excitation is primarily caused by presynaptic mechanisms.[87,133,214,227-229] A postsynaptic mechanism is also involved because the response to directly applied glutamate is reduced to some degree.[229-231] Volatile anesthetics have inconsistent effects on cloned AMPA or NMDA glutamate receptors, but they potentiate kainite receptors,[115,129,232,233] consistent with a predominantly presynaptic mechanism for glutamatergic synapses. By contrast, the effects of the nonhalogenated inhaled anesthetics (xenon, nitrous oxide, cyclopropane) appear to be mediated primarily by inhibition of postsynaptic NMDA receptors (discussed earlier). Under some circumstances, such as in patients with defects in mitochondrial complex 1[234] and in mice carrying mutations in mitochondrial complex 1,[235] inhaled agents suppress glutamate release by interfering with the energy-intensive glutamate recycling pathways,[236] thereby leading to extreme anesthetic sensitivity. Recent evidence from conditional knockout mice indicates this mechanism may contribute to various end points even in nonpathogenic states.[237]

Augmentation of GABAergic inhibition by most general anesthetics is mediated by both presynaptic and postsynaptic mechanisms. Enhancement of postsynaptic and extrasynaptic $GABA_A$ receptors is well recognized.[116] Volatile anesthetics increase spontaneous GABA release and inhibitory postsynaptic current (IPSC) frequency[238-242]—that is, their presynaptic effects at GABAergic terminals are distinct from those at glutamatergic synapses.

The mechanisms for the presynaptic effects of inhaled anesthetics, like those for their postsynaptic effects, are complex and involve multiple targets. Although a synapse-specific contribution of presynaptic Ca^{2+} channels is likely,[243] presynaptic Na^+ channels are more sensitive than the Ca^{2+} channels coupled to glutamate release. This finding is consistent with observations that the predominant Ca^{2+} channel coupled to neurotransmitter release at hippocampal glutamatergic synapses (P/Q-type) is insensitive to isoflurane.[156] Other presynaptic mechanisms have been proposed, including actions on the vesicle fusion process, as demonstrated in the model organism *Caenorhabditis elegans*.[244,245] However, isoflurane effects on exocytosis in rat hippocampal neurons occur primarily upstream of vesicle fusion.[139,246]

Simple Circuits and Complex Networks

SIMPLE CIRCUIT PHENOMENA

The development of a mechanistic understanding of phenomena involving complex circuits has been greatly facilitated by the study of anatomically reduced (in vitro) or physiologically simplified (in vivo) preparations complemented by computer simulations (in silico). These approaches are essential for integrating reductionist observations of the multiple molecular effects of anesthetics into functional models relevant to behavioral end points. Anesthetic effects have been studied in acute brain slice preparations from various regions of the CNS (hippocampus, amygdala, cortex, thalamus, brain stem, and spinal cord)—most often from rodents. Brain slices preserve native connections but usually lack natural inputs and outputs. Slices from developing mammalian brain can also be cultured in vitro. These "organotypic slice cultures" preserve a high degree of synaptic connectivity and display spontaneous network activity, typically absent from "acute slices." Simplified in vivo preparations involve phenomena (typically evoked responses) with *relatively* well-understood circuitry. Computer models and simulations can assist in generating hypotheses for experimental testing and developing hypotheses based on experimental data.

Synaptic Plasticity

Paired-pulse depression and paired-pulse facilitation are examples of short-term plasticity in response to external stimulation. Synaptic inhibition is prolonged by volatile anesthetics in vivo[247] and in vitro,[248] in general agreement with the notion that anesthetics enhance functional inhibition in the CNS. Enhancement of paired-pulse facilitation has been attributed to the presynaptic depressant effect of volatile agents (Fig. 19.11).[133,228]

LTP, a cellular model of learning and memory, is a use-dependent strengthening of glutamatergic excitatory synaptic connections. Volatile anesthetic effects on LTP depend on the experimental preparation. Halothane, enflurane, and isoflurane do not block LTP induction in vivo, whereas ketamine and the NMDA antagonist CPP do.[247,249] By contrast, isoflurane blocks LTP in the hippocampal slice by enhancing $GABA_A$ receptor–mediated inhibition (Fig. 19.12)[250] or blocking neuronal nicotinic receptors.[88] Long-term depression, a use-dependent weakening of excitatory connections that is effectively a homeostatic counterpart of LTP, is also blocked by isoflurane in vitro.[250] The discrepancy between findings in vivo and in vitro remains unexplained.

Spontaneously Active Circuits

Spontaneous neuronal activity is decreased by volatile anesthetics both in vivo and in cortical brain slices. This effect is largely $GABA_A$ receptor-dependent and marked even at low sedative concentrations.[107] Because the cortical brain slices lack subcortical input, these results suggest that volatile anesthetics can cause some effects (e.g., sedation)

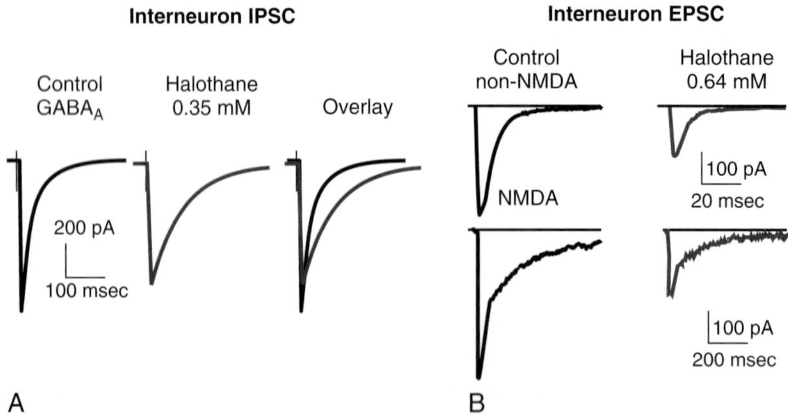

Fig. 19.10 Halogenated anesthetics enhance inhibitory and depress excitatory synaptic transmission. Halothane slows the decay of $GABA_A$ receptor–mediated inhibitory postsynaptic currents *(IPSCs)* (A) and depresses the amplitude of glutamatergic excitatory postsynaptic currents *(EPSCs)* without affecting the decay (B) in hippocampal interneurons. ([A] Redrawn with permission from Nishikawa K, MacIver MB. Membrane and synaptic actions of halothane on rat hippocampal pyramidal neurons and inhibitory interneurons. *J Neurosci.* 2000;20:5915–5923. [B] Redrawn with permission from Perouansky M, Baranov D, Salman M, Yaari Y. Effects of halothane on glutamate receptor-mediated excitatory postsynaptic currents. A patch-clamp study in adult mouse hippocampal slices. *Anesthesiology.* 1995;83:109–119.)

via direct cortical action. However, changes in raw neuronal firing rates do not provide a precise quantitative measure of higher cognitive function, which is better reflected by the relationship of firing patterns to the strength and phase of ongoing cortical rhythms (see next section). Anesthetic effects have also been tested on the circuitry underlying locomotion, a well-studied central pattern generator. Effects of isoflurane on in vitro lamprey and rat spinal cord preparations support the spinal cord as the primary target for volatile anesthetic–induced immobility.[251,252]

RHYTHMS AND SIMULATIONS

The brain perpetually generates complex electrical rhythms (oscillations in extracellular field potentials) that range in frequency from fractions to hundreds of Hertz (Hz; cycles per second), as recorded on the surface of the scalp as the electroencephalogram (EEG; the higher-frequency oscillations cannot be resolved in surface recordings). All oscillations are behavioral state–dependent and multiple oscillations coexist throughout the sleep-wake cycle. Lower-frequency rhythms allow for integration over longer time periods and typically engage larger areas of the brain. By contrast, higher-frequency rhythms allow for higher temporal resolution on local scales. Cross-frequency modulation allows for integration of both aspects of information processing. Although their physiologic roles are not clear, brain rhythms reflect, subserve, and/or constitute fundamental higher-order processing such that their modulation by anesthetics is of great interest. The current nomenclature of brain rhythms reflects historical conventions and is not based on underlying mechanisms.

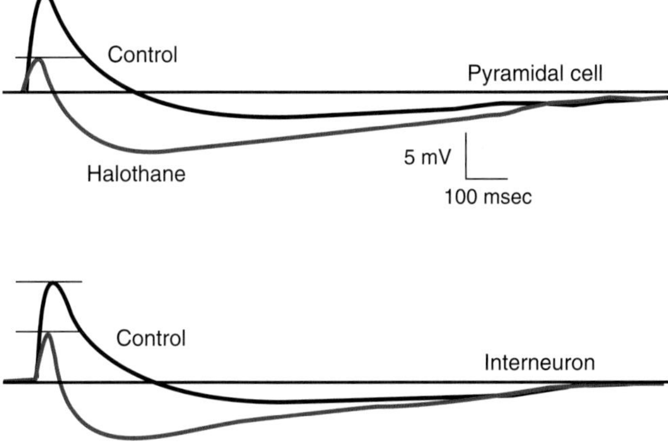

Fig. 19.11 Anesthetics affect excitation and inhibition simultaneously in opposite directions. Halothane depresses the excitatory depolarization and augments the inhibitory hyperpolarization in both hippocampal pyramidal cells and interneurons. The net result will depend on the underlying neuronal state as well as the neuronal network and its function. (Redrawn with permission form Nishikawa K, MacIver MB. Membrane and synaptic actions of halothane on rat hippocampal pyramidal neurons and inhibitory interneurons. *J Neurosci*. 2000;20:5915–5923.)

δ-Rhythms and Other Slow Rhythms

Oscillations with EEG frequencies from 1.5 to 4 Hz are generally referred to as δ-rhythms, and these oscillations are characteristic of deep sleep and are commonly observed under general anesthesia. Even slower rhythms (below 1 Hz) occur during non–rapid eye movement (NREM) sleep and appear at loss of consciousness induced by propofol[253] and sevoflurane.[254] During natural NREM sleep, δ-rhythms and sleep spindles are phase related to a slower oscillation, suggesting functional interaction.[255] Paroxysmal spindle-like waxing and waning oscillations overriding slower rhythms are also present in the cortical EEG under anesthesia. A change in δ-α phase relationships has been proposed as a "signature" of propofol-induced unconsciousness,[256] but how this comes about, whether similar changes occur for a wider range of anesthetics, and the underlying physiology and functional significance are unknown.

θ-Rhythms

θ-Rhythms, present in various cortical structures but most prominent in the hippocampus, are thought to signal the "online state." They are associated with sensorimotor and

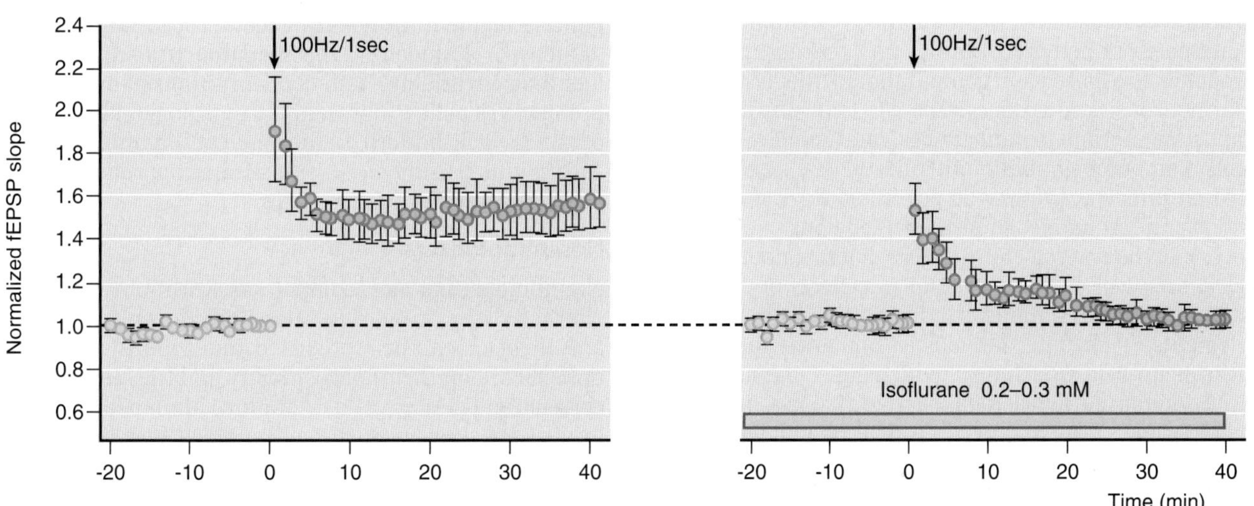

Fig. 19.12 Isoflurane blocks the induction of synaptic plasticity in vitro (a model of learning and memory). Long-term potentiation (an increase in synaptic strength), indicated by the increase in normalized excitatory postsynaptic potential *(EPSP)* slope, in hippocampal slices evoked by tetanic stimulation of excitatory synapses is blocked by 0.2 to 0.3 mM isoflurane. (Redrawn with permission from Simon W, Hapfelmeier G, Kochs E, et al. Isoflurane blocks synaptic plasticity in the mouse hippocampus. *Anesthesiology*. 2001;94:1058–1065.)

mnemonic functions during waking behavior.[257] One component of the θ-rhythm (type I or atropine-resistant) can be affected by amnestic concentrations of isoflurane as well as by the amnestic nonimmobilizer F6,[94] indicating a potential network-level signature effect for anesthetic-induced amnesia. Type II θ-rhythm (atropine-sensitive) can be evoked under anesthesia and is slowed and potentiated by halothane.[258] Interestingly, this halothane-induced oscillation disappears in TASK-3 knockout mice.[46]

γ-Rhythms

This designation includes an extremely broad and probably functionally and mechanistically heterogeneous spectrum of rhythms. It is frequently subdivided into slow γ (30-50 Hz; i.e., the spectrum above β-rhythms); γ (50-90 Hz), and fast-, ultra-γ, or ε-rhythms (>90 and up to hundreds of Hz). Fast $GABA_A$ ergic synaptic inhibition and the intrinsic resonant properties of neurons play important roles in γ-physiology, making these obvious candidates for anesthetic modulation. Isoflurane slows the frequency of evoked γ-oscillations (30-90 Hz, also known as "40-Hz rhythms") in humans.[259,260] Studies of γ-oscillations in vitro suggest that their frequency depends on the time constant of decay of $GABA_A$ receptor–mediated synaptic currents in inhibitory networks.[261] Isoflurane slows γ-rhythms in hippocampal[262] and neocortical slices[263] to a comparable degree as it does in humans,[259] providing a tentative link between receptor and circuit-level effects. However, the interaction between anesthetics and behaviorally relevant network effects is likely to be complex because flash-evoked γ-oscillations in the primary visual cortex are not affected by inhaled agents,[67] whereas feedback information transfer at γ-frequencies between the visual and frontal cortices is disrupted.[59,67] Moreover, many brain rhythms are interlinked (e.g., θ-rhythm modulates γ-oscillations (θ−γ nesting). The nature of their modulation by anesthetics as well as its relevance are far from clear.

Models and Simulations

On the macroscopic scale, computer simulations can provide an integrated picture of modulation of dynamic neuronal and network activity. "Bottom-up" neuron-by-neuron approaches are based on computational models of individual neurons, known *anesthetic effects* on intrinsic and synaptic membrane conductances, and simple network models. Computer simulations of anesthetic effects on integrated outputs can thereby be generated (e.g., the ring of pacemaker neurons).[264] These models obviously rely on the accuracy of the derived characteristics of real neurons and networks as well as knowledge of the effects of anesthetics; the scale of simulations is limited by the complexity of its elements.[265] An alternative is a "top-down" approach, such as mean-field modeling, in which molecular and cellular individual accuracy detail is sacrificed in favor of global dynamics. For example, global cortical phenomena, such as anesthetic-induced seizures, have been modeled as phase transitions based on mean interactions between populations of averaged neurons (analogous to the EEG signal that also averages the signals of neuronal populations).[266] This approach can be extended to other global cortical phenomena such as consciousness.[267] Neuronal modeling and computer simulations may gain importance in the future as bridges between theoretical and experimental studies of anesthesia.

Research Strategies for the Future

The search for anesthetic mechanisms is driven by advances in the basic sciences. Some strategies that should facilitate understanding of anesthetic mechanisms include use of agonists or antagonists in vivo, nonanesthetics or nonimmobilizers, high-resolution imaging of the functioning brain, transgenic animals, and the application of the latest techniques of molecular genetics.

PHARMACOLOGIC APPROACHES

Agonists, Antagonists, and Experimental Anesthetics

Use of receptor-specific agonists and antagonists provides a pharmacologic method for bridging in vitro with in vivo studies. In this approach, a receptor may be tested for its contribution to a specific end point (e.g., immobility) according to the criteria presented earlier. This approach was used to exclude an important role for NMDA receptor block in the immobilizing action of volatile anesthetics but did not yield conclusive results for the roles of $GABA_A$ and GlyR for immobilization,[267,268] probably owing to the intricacies of drug-receptor interactions on different levels of integration in complex networks like the spinal cord. A complementary pharmacologic approach using experimental anesthetics that inhibit NMDA receptors in vitro with different potencies supports the conclusion that NMDA receptor blockade does not contribute significantly to immobility by conventional volatile anesthetics.[269] Refinement of this strategy involves the anatomically discrete application of drugs to nuclei with known function. For example, the tuberomammillary nucleus (part of the endogenous sleep pathway) mediates the sedative component of anesthesia for some intravenous anesthetics (e.g., propofol).[35] A discrete site of general anesthetic action for GABAergic drugs in the mesopontine tegmentum has also been proposed based on this strategy.[33,34] However, these approaches suffer from the fact that, invariably, high concentrations of drugs have to be injected locally to observe pharmacologic effects (because of rapid redistribution), so that such observations need to be substantiated using more sophisticated approaches, such as genetic manipulations (see later).

Nonimmobilizers

Nonimmobilizers are compounds with physicochemical characteristics similar to those of conventional inhaled anesthetics, but their predicted anesthetizing concentrations (based on their lipid solubility and the Meyer-Overton correlation [MAC_{pred}]) do not induce immobility.[17] Initially termed *nonanesthetics*, the terminology was revised when it was discovered that at least some of them cause amnesia at similar MAC_{pred} fractions to classic volatile anesthetics.[98] If a molecular or cellular process is affected in similar ways by an anesthetic and a nonimmobilizer, that process is not relevant for the anesthetic state, with the notable exception of amnesia. Despite this elegant rationale, only a limited number of receptors have been excluded because, compared with volatile anesthetics, nonimmobilizers are relatively target selective. These compounds have the potential to provide insights beyond the initially envisaged receptor-level studies by allowing the separation of sedation from amnesia for the study of underlying network activity in vivo.[95]

Photoreactive Anesthetics

An approach that has proven to be very successful with intravenous drugs[270] is one in which an analog of an anesthetic is synthesized that bears a photoreactive group (often a tri-fluoro-diazirine) which, when irradiated at a wavelength of around 300 nm, reacts irreversibly with some amino acids in the anesthetic binding site. This approach, of course, requires that the pharmacologic profile of the analog is very similar to that of the parent compound, so that the relevant binding site is identified. Photoreactive analogs of inhaled anesthetics have been synthesized and four putative sites on $GABA_A$ receptors have been identified.[271]. One advantage of this approach over x-ray crystallography is that anesthetic binding to different conformational states of the receptor are, at least in principle, more accessible to analysis.

GENETIC APPROACHES

Whole-Organism Genetics

Genetic strategies on whole organisms take two forms: forward and reverse.[272] The reverse genetic approach focuses on a particular gene chosen because there are reasons to hypothesize that its product may be important to anesthesia. Examples of this strategy are targeted mutations that alter the sensitivity of specific neurotransmitter receptors to anesthetics.[121] Initially, these mutations were used to identify anesthetic binding sites. Subsequently, transgenic animals rendered resistant to anesthetics, either by deletion of a putative target protein from the genome or by expressing a target receptor engineered to be insensitive to an anesthetic, were used to test behavioral relevance of the altered gene product for the production of anesthesia. Forward genetics, by contrast, is a discovery process that involves the study of randomly generated mutations (either experimentally induced or naturally occurring polymorphisms) that affect the phenotype of interest (i.e., anesthetic end points) in a population. This approach, however, has not been widely used.

Molecular Genetics

A third genetic approach that is playing an increasing role in neuroscience is the selective modification of neuronal function using molecular genetics. Many different approaches are used, ranging from the selective knockdown of specific receptor populations using microRNA (a small noncoding piece of RNA that can selectively reduce protein expression), the block of neurotransmitter release from a population of neurons using tetanus toxin light chain, and the selective activation or inhibition of neuronal networks using optogenetics[273] or pharmacogenetics.[274] A powerful complement to these techniques is the ability to deliver artificial transgenes to defined neuronal populations using adeno-associated virus (AAV), and mouse lines that express Cre recombinase in particular cell types, which allow the selective expression of those genes in those specific cells. These approaches are only just beginning to be used to identify neuronal pathways that are involved in anesthetic action. For example, it has recently been shown that the sedative effects of propofol require the activation of the lateral habenula, an excitatory nucleus that lies close to the thalamus.[275] These approaches are likely to have an increasing impact on our understanding of the mechanisms of inhaled general anesthetics.

Knockout and Knockin Animals

In the knockout approach, expression of the gene encoding a protein of interest is disrupted by a specific deletion or insertion. Nearly all such studies have been carried out in mice. A well-recognized problem with the global knockout approach is that extensive compensatory changes can be induced, from anomalies that are lethal in utero to insidious (but experimentally confounding) influences that might be expressed only at maturity. A complementary strategy is the conditional knockout, in which the genetic deletion is restricted either anatomically (limited to certain brain regions) or temporally (at a known point in time). These strategies can minimize developmental anomalies and reduce the likelihood of compensatory changes. In the knockin approach, a mutation, usually of a single amino acid residue, is targeted to produce a protein with altered sensitivity to a drug of interest. Ideally, this mutation remains completely silent in the absence of the drug; that is, it does not perturb the normal expression and function of the protein of interest or alter the expression of other genes.

$GABA_A$ receptors. Results from transgenic animals illustrate both the utility and the difficulties of the genetic approach with respect to inhaled agents. The conditional forebrain-restricted $GABA_A$ receptor α_1-subunit knockout mouse was found to be less sensitive to isoflurane-induced amnesia than wild-type mice, which led to the conclusion that action at these receptors contributes to isoflurane's amnesic effects.[276] By contrast, a mouse harboring a mutation of the $GABA_A$ receptor α_1 subunit that renders the receptor insensitive to isoflurane in vitro did not show reduced sensitivity to either the amnesic or the immobilizing effects of isoflurane, leading to the conclusion that this subunit does not mediate the impairment of learning and memory by isoflurane.[40] Similar experiments indicate that action at the $GABA_A$ receptor β_3 subunit does not mediate immobility or amnesia by isoflurane.[39] This bottom-up genetic approach is a work-intensive but powerful tool that has yielded clear results with the receptor-specific intravenous anesthetics,[27] but it has proved challenging to apply it to the more promiscuous inhaled agents.

Glycine α1–containing receptors. Pharmacologic studies supported the notion that glycinergic neurotransmission might be the effector for the immobilizing action of inhaled anesthetics in the spinal cord, where glycine replaces GABA as the principal inhibitory transmitter. However, mice harboring mutations that render α_1 subunit–containing glycine receptors largely insensitive to alcohol and inhaled ether anesthetics did not demonstrate a concordant change in MAC values. Because α_1 is the most widely expressed subunit in adult animals, it is unlikely that action at glycine receptors plays an important part in the immobilizing action of inhaled anesthetics.[276]

Two-pore domain K^+ channels. Use of mice harboring knockout mutations of several two-pore domain K^+ channel (K_{2P}) family members (TASK-1, TASK-3, TREK-1) has demonstrated a role for these channels in volatile anesthesia.[44,45,47] For example, TREK-1 knockout mice are partially resistant to all volatile anesthetics tested with respect to both loss of righting reflex (a surrogate measure of consciousness) and immobility, but anesthesia can still be induced, albeit at higher anesthetic concentrations. Interestingly, responses to pentobarbital are unaffected, indicating that the mutation does not cause a generalized resistance to anesthesia.

FORWARD AND POPULATION GENETICS

The nematode *C. elegans* and the fruit fly *Drosophila melanogaster*, with 302 and 100,000 neurons, respectively, have also been used as model organisms in anesthesia research.[277] Mutations in a number of *C. elegans* genes affect sensitivity to volatile anesthetics,[278] most notably *unc-1*,[279] a close homologue of the mammalian protein stomatin.[280] Yeasts have also been used as model organisms, with even more obvious limitations with respect to identification of appropriate anesthetic end points.

Sensitivity to anesthetics is a quantitative trait (varying continuously in a population). Quantitative genetics is the study of the heritability of continuous traits. These traits are controlled by genes represented in quantitative trait loci (QTLs). A top-down population-based approach has been used to localize QTLs that govern susceptibility of individuals to anesthetics, in higher and lower organisms. Starting from the observation that inbred mouse strains vary in their sensitivity to isoflurane, microsatellite-based linkage analysis and, alternatively, single-nucleotide polymorphism–based analysis of genetic variation localized a QTL for isoflurane immobilization to the proximal part of mouse chromosome 7.[281] Genetic variability in the sensitivity of *D. melanogaster* to inhaled anesthetics has also been demonstrated.[282] This type of analysis promises to assist in defining the genetic basis for variability in the susceptibility to both primary anesthetic end points and side effects.

FUNCTIONAL IMAGING AND HIGH-DENSITY ELECTROENCEPHALOGRAPHY

Identification of the anatomic and functional substrates for anesthetic effects on consciousness, memory, and immobility is now approachable with improved imaging techniques. Imaging is based on mapping of either metabolic or hemodynamic changes as surrogate measures of neuronal activity, as in positron emission tomography (PET) and functional magnetic resonance imaging, or on mapping electrical activity with high-density EEG, magnetoencephalography, and low-resolution brain electromagnetic tomography. Properties of receptors can also be probed with radioactive ligands by PET. These techniques have the capacity to identify neuroanatomic substrates of drug action with method-specific limitations. Results from functional PET imaging suggest that propofol suppresses episodic memory by targeting the prefrontal and posterior parietal cortex as opposed to the medial temporal lobe[283] and that suppression of consciousness is caused by anesthetic action in the thalamus, parts of the medial and posterior parietal cortex, and/or the posterior cingulate and medial parietal cortex.[284] Although observations of regionally specific and global suppressive effects of anesthetics on metabolic activity are unlikely to provide a definitive mechanistic understanding, such information can facilitate hypotheses and experimentally testable predictions.

Advanced analytical approaches based on theories from mathematical and statistical sciences are being increasingly applied to enhance the power of existing technologies. Magnetic resonance images and high-density EEG recordings of the brain reveal strong interregional connections, but the considerable potential of this connectivity information to better understand the brain's response to anesthesia has only recently begun to be tapped. The growing use of invasive recording techniques (e.g., brain surface electrode grids and microelectrodes implanted deep into the brain for functional neurosurgical therapies) is also advancing the frontiers of neuroscience in general and the understanding of anesthetic mechanisms in particular.

Summary

The mechanisms of inhaled anesthetics have proved more difficult to explain than was envisaged a generation ago, when the paradigm shifted from lipids to amphiphilic cavities in proteins as targets for anesthetics. Despite a remarkable accumulation of information, a comprehensive theory of general anesthetic action has yet to be formulated. Progress toward this goal has been difficult for several reasons. Important pharmacologic characteristics of inhaled anesthetics that have impeded identification of their relevant molecular targets are their low potency (micromolar range), activity at multiple targets, lack of specific antagonists, and limitations in the neuroscience of memory and consciousness. This contrasts with the situation for intravenous anesthetics, which exhibit more conventional receptor pharmacology. Moreover, accumulating evidence indicates that no universal target exists to explain the actions of every general anesthetic or even of a single anesthetic agent. It is now clear that the composite state of anesthesia and its core components (amnesia, sedation/unconsciousness, immobility) are separable behavioral states in vivo. Resolution of these phenomena at the molecular and cellular levels represents the cutting edge of contemporary neuroscience. Of the multiple molecular and cellular anesthetic effects identified, it is unclear which are critical for the desired behavioral end points, which are harmless or beneficial side effects (e.g., preconditioning), and which, if any, could have long-lasting or delayed undesirable consequences (e.g., cell death, cognitive dysfunction). Progress in identifying the molecular targets of general anesthetics provides a foundation for identification of the network- and systems-level effects relevant to their behavioral and peripheral end points. As the biologic foundations of behaviors once thought to be exclusively the realm of psychology are unraveled, for which anesthetics provide a valuable investigative tool, a comprehensive theory of anesthesia will also develop.

Complete references available online at expertconsult.com.

References

1. Perouansky M. *Anesthesiology*. 2012;117:465.
2. Winterstein H. *Die Narkose in ihrer Bedeutung für die Allgemeine Physiologie*. Springer; 1919.
3. Eger EI. *Anesthesiology*. 2002;96:238–239.
4. Eger EI, et al. *Anesthesiology*. 1965;26:756–763.
5. Franks NP, Lieb WR. *Anesthesiology*. 1996;84:716–720.
6. Boggs JM, et al. *Mol Pharmacol*. 1976;12:127–135.
7. Franks NP, Lieb WR. *Nature*. 1978;274:339–342.
8. Franks NP, Lieb WR. *J Mol Biol*. 1979;133:469–500.
9. Featherstone RM, et al. *Anesthesiology*. 1961;22:977–981.
10. Ueda I, Kamaya H. *Anesthesiology*. 1973;38:425–436.
11. Franks NP, Lieb WR. *Nature*. 1982;300:487–493.
12. Franks NP, Lieb WR. *Nature*. 1984;310:599–601.
13. Franks NP, Lieb WR. *Anesthesiology*. 2004;101:235–237.
14. Franks NP, Lieb WR. *Nature*. 1981;292:248–251.
15. Franks NP, Lieb WR. *Nature*. 1985;316:349–351.
16. Franks NP, Lieb WR. *Proc Natl Acad Sci U S A*. 1986;83:5116–5120.
17. Koblin DD, et al. *Anesth Analg*. 1994;79:1043–1048.
18. Hall AC, et al. *Br J Pharmacol*. 1994;112:906–910.
19. Dickinson R, et al. *Biophys J*. 1994;66:2019–2023.
20. Franks NP, Lieb WR. *Science*. 1991;254:427–430.
21. Herold KF, et al. *Proc Natl Acad Sci U S A*. 2017;114:3109–3114.
22. Franks NP. *Nat Rev Neurosci*. 2008;9:370–386.
23. Eckenhoff RG. *Mol Interv*. 2001;1:258–268.
24. Eckenhoff RG, Johansson JS. *Anesthesiology*. 2001;95:1537–1539.
25. Eger 2nd EI, et al. *Anesthesiology*. 2001;94:915–921.
26. Dickinson R, et al. *Anesthesiology*. 2000;93:837–843.
27. Rudolph U, Antkowiak B. *Nat Rev Neurosci*. 2004;5:709–720.
28. Antognini JF, Schwartz K. *Anesthesiology*. 1993;79:1244–1249.
29. Rampil IJ, et al. *Anesthesiology*. 1993;78:707–712.
30. Stabernack C, et al. *Anesth Analg*. 2005;100:128–136.
31. Veselis RA, et al. *Anesthesiology*. 2001;95:896–907.
32. Sanders RD, et al. *Anesthesiology*. 2012;116:946–959.
33. Devor M, Zalkind V. *Pain*. 2001;94:101–112.
34. Minert A, et al. *J Neurosci*. 2017;37:9320–9331.
35. Nelson LE, et al. *Nat Neurosci*. 2002;5:979–984.
36. Rampil IJ, Laster MJ. *Anesthesiology*. 1992;77:920–925.
37. Antognini JF, et al. *Anesthesiology*. 2002;96:980–986.
38. Zhang Y, et al. *Anesth Analg*. 2004;99:85–90.
39. Liao M, et al. *Anesth Analg*. 2005;101:412–418.
40. Sonner JM, et al. *Anesthesiology*. 2007;106:107–113.
41. Raines DE, et al. *Anesth Analg*. 2002;95:573–577.
42. Zhang Y, et al. *Br J Pharmacol*. 2010;159:872–878.
43. Heurteaux C, et al. *EMBO J*. 2004;23:2684–2695.
44. Linden AM, et al. *J Pharmacol Exp Ther*. 2006;317:615–626.
45. Linden AM, et al. *J Pharmacol Exp Ther*. 2007;323:924–934.
46. Pang DS, et al. *Proc Natl Acad Sci U S A*. 2009;106:17546–17551.
47. Westphalen RI, et al. *Br J Pharmacol*. 2007;152:939–945.
48. Jinks SL, et al. *Anesthesiology*. 2008;108:1016–1024.
49. Koch C, et al. *Nat Rev Neurosci*. 2016;17:307–321.
50. Mashour GA, Hudetz AG. *Trends Neurosci*. 2018;41:150–160.
51. Sanders RD, et al. *Anesthesiology*. 2017;126:214–222.
52. Leung LS, et al. *Prog Neurobiol*. 2014;122:24–44.
53. Brown EN, et al. *Annu Rev Neurosci*. 2011;34:601–628.
54. Mashour GA. *Front Syst Neurosci*. 2014;8:115.
55. Mashour GA, Hudetz AG. *Front Neural Circuits*. 2017;11:44.
56. Tononi G. *Biol Bull*. 2008;215:216–242.
57. Tononi G, et al. *Nat Rev Neurosci*. 2016;17:450–461.
58. Lee U, et al. *Philos Trans A Math Phys Eng Sci*. 2015;373.
59. Imas OA, et al. *Neurosci Lett*. 2005;387:145–150.
60. MacIver MB, Bland BH. *Front Syst Neurosci*. 2014;8:203.
61. Bullmore E, Sporns O. *Nat Rev Neurosci*. 2012;13:336–349.
62. van den Heuvel MP, Sporns O. *J Neurosci*. 2011;31:15775–15786.
63. Massimini M, et al. *Science*. 2005;309:2228–2232.
64. Ferrarelli F, et al. *Proc Natl Acad Sci U S A*. 2010;107:2681–2686.
65. Alkire MT, et al. *Science*. 2008;322:876–880.
66. Imas OA, et al. *Anesthesiology*. 2005;102:937–947.
67. Imas OA, et al. *Neurosci Lett*. 2006;402:216–221.
68. John ER, et al. *Conscious Cogn*. 2001;10:165–183.
69. Burlingame RH, et al. *Anesthesiology*. 2007;106:754–762.
70. Ter-Mikaelian M, et al. *J Neurosci*. 2007;27:6091–6102.
71. Lee U, et al. *Anesthesiology*. 2013;118:1264–1275.
72. Wacongne C, et al. *Proc Natl Acad Sci U S A*. 2011;108:20754–20759.
73. Raz A, et al. *Front Syst Neurosci*. 2014;8:191.
74. Hentschke H, et al. *Br J Anaesth*. 2017;119:685–696.
75. Kelz MB, et al. *Proc Natl Acad Sci U S A*. 2008;105:1309–1314.
76. Moore JT, et al. *Curr Biol*. 2012;22:2008–2016.
77. McCarren HS, et al. *J Neurosci*. 2014;34:16385–16396.
78. Solt K. *Curr Biol*. 2012;22:R918–R919.
79. Scharf MT, Kelz MB. *Curr Anesthesiol Rep*. 2013;3:1–9.
80. Taylor NE, et al. *Proc Natl Acad Sci U S A*. 2016.
81. Alkire MT, et al. *Conscious Cogn*. 2000;9:370–386.
82. Baker R, et al. *J Neurosci*. 2014;34:13326–13335.
83. Saalmann YB. *Front Syst Neurosci*. 2014;8:83.
84. Dutton RC, et al. *Anesthesiology*. 2001;94:514–519.
85. Brown EN, et al. *N Engl J Med*. 2010;363:2638–2650.
86. Alkire MT, Nathan SV. *Anesthesiology*. 2005;102:754–760.
87. Dai S, et al. *Anesthesiology*. 2012;116:816–823.
88. Piao MH, et al. *Ann Fr Anesth Reanim*. 2013;32:e135–e141.
89. Zhou C, et al. *Anesth Analg*. 2015;121:661–666.
90. Kuo MC, Leung LS. *Anesthesiology*. 2017;127:838–851.
91. Vertes RP. *Hippocampus*. 2005;15:923–935.
92. Pan WX, McNaughton N. *Brain Res*. 1997;764:101–108.
93. Robbe D, et al. *Nat Neurosci*. 2006;9:1526–1533.
94. Perouansky M, et al. *Anesthesiology*. 2007;106:1168–1176.
95. Seidenbecher T, et al. *Science*. 2003;301:846–850.
96. Rudolph U, et al. *Nature*. 1999;401:796–800.
97. Kandel L, et al. *Anesth Analg*. 1996;82:321–326.
98. Mihic SJ, et al. *Mol Pharmacol*. 1994;46:851–857.
99. Zarnowska ED, et al. *Anesth Analg*. 2005;101:401–406.
100. Jevtovic-Todorovic V, et al. *Nat Med*. 1998;4:460–463.
101. Gruss M, et al. *Mol Pharmacol*. 2004;65:443–452.
102. Gries DA, et al. *Life Sci*. 2005;76:1667–1674.
103. Zhang Z, et al. *Nat Neurosci*. 2015;18:553–561.
104. Murphy M, et al. *Sleep*. 2011;34:283–291A.
105. Tung A, et al. *Anesthesiology*. 2004;100:1419–1426.
106. Nelson AB, et al. *Sleep*. 2010;33:1659–1667.
107. Hentschke H, et al. *Eur J Neurosci*. 2005;21:93–102.
108. Franks NP, Lieb WR. *Nature*. 1994;367:607–614.
109. Zeller A, et al. *Handb Exp Pharmacol*. 2008:31–51.
110. Franks NP, et al. *Biophys J*. 1998;75:2205–2211.
111. Bhattacharya AA, et al. *J Biol Chem*. 2000;275:38731–38738.
112. Bertaccini EJ, et al. *Anesth Analg*. 2007;104:318–324.
113. Howard RJ, et al. *Pharmacol Rev*. 2014;66:396–412.
114. Nury H, et al. *Nature*. 2011;469:428–431.
115. Dickinson R, et al. *Anesthesiology*. 2007;107:756–767.
116. Hemmings HC, et al. *Trends Pharmacol Sci*. 2005;26:503–510.
117. Patel AJ, et al. *Nat Neurosci*. 1999;2:422–426.
118. Franks NP, Honore E. *Trends Pharmacol Sci*. 2004;25:601–608.
119. Sieghart W. *Adv Pharmacol*. 2015;72:53–96.
120. Lynch JW. *Physiol Rev*. 2004;84:1051–1095.
121. Mihic SJ, et al. *Nature*. 1997;389:385–389.
122. Solt K, et al. *J Pharmacol Exp Ther*. 2005;315:771–776.
123. Jenkins A, et al. *Br J Pharmacol*. 1996;117:1507–1515.
124. Role LW, Berg DK. *Neuron*. 1996;16:1077–1085.
125. Flood P, et al. *Anesthesiology*. 1997;86:859–865.
126. Violet JM, et al. *Anesthesiology*. 1997;86:866–874.
127. Dingledine R, et al. *Pharmacol Rev*. 1999;51:7–61.
128. Franks NP, et al. *Nature*. 1998;396:324.
129. de Sousa SL, et al. *Anesthesiology*. 2000;92:1055–1066.
130. Solt K, et al. *Anesth Analg*. 2006;102:1407–1411.
131. Harris RA, et al. *FASEB J*. 1995;9:1454–1462.
132. Sonner JM, et al. *Anesth Analg*. 2005;101:143–148.
133. MacIver MB, et al. *Anesthesiology*. 1996;85:823–834.
134. Perouansky M, et al. *Anesthesiology*. 2004;100:470–472.
135. Winegar BD, MacIver MB. *BMC Neurosci*. 2006;7:5.
136. Haydon DA, Urban BW. *J Physiol*. 1983;341:429–439.
137. Berg-Johnsen J, Langmoen IA. *Acta Physiol Scand*. 1986;127:87–93.
138. Mikulec AA, et al. *Brain Res*. 1998;796:231–238.
139. Wu XS, et al. *Anesthesiology*. 2004;100:663–670.
140. Yu FH, Catterall WA. *Sci STKE*. 2004;2004:re15.
141. Catterall WA. *Annu Rev Cell Dev Biol*. 2000;16:521–555.

142. Herold KF, et al. *Anesthesiology*. 2009;111:591–599.
143. Ouyang W, Hemmings HC. *J Pharmacol Exp Ther*. 2005;312:801–808.
144. OuYang W, Hemmings HC. *Anesthesiology*. 2007;107:91–98.
145. Ouyang W, et al. *J Pharmacol Exp Ther*. 2007;322:1076–1083.
146. Ratnakumari L, et al. *Anesthesiology*. 2000;92:529–541.
147. Herold KF, Hemmings HC. *Front Pharmacol*. 2012;3:50.
148. Tang JX, et al. *Alzheimers Dement*. 2011;7:521–531.e521.
149. Barber AF, et al. *Proc Natl Acad Sci U S A*. 2014;111:6726–6731.
150. Kinde MN, et al. *Proc Natl Acad Sci U S A*. 2016;113:13762–13767.
151. Sand RM, et al. *J Gen Physiol*. 2017;149:623–638.
152. Miao N, et al. *Anesthesiology*. 1995;83:593–603.
153. Pocock G, Richards CD. *Br J Anaesth*. 1993;71:134–147.
154. Kameyama K, et al. *Br J Anaesth*. 1999;82:402–411.
155. Study RE. *Anesthesiology*. 1994;81:104–116.
156. Hall AC, et al. *Anesthesiology*. 1994;81:117–123.
157. Takei T, et al. *Neurosci Lett*. 2003;350:41–45.
158. Joksovic PM, et al. *Br J Pharmacol*. 2005;144:59–70.
159. Todorovic SM, et al. *Mol Pharmacol*. 2001;60:603–610.
160. Petrenko AB, et al. *Anesthesiology*. 2007;106:1177–1185.
161. Hanley PJ, et al. *Anesthesiology*. 2004;101:999–1014.
162. Huneke R, et al. *Acta Anaesthesiol Scand*. 2004;48:547–561.
163. Rithalia A, et al. *Anesth Analg*. 2004;99:1615–1622.
164. Huneke R, et al. *Anesthesiology*. 2001;95:999–1006.
165. Stowe DF, et al. *Anesthesiology*. 2000;92:516–522.
166. Davies LA, et al. *Anesthesiology*. 2000;93:1034–1044.
167. Joseph JD, et al. *Anesthesiology*. 2014;121:528–537.
168. Pabelick CM, et al. *Anesthesiology*. 2001;95:207–215.
169. Roberts MC, et al. *Anesthesiology*. 2001;95:716–725.
170. Mickelson JR, Louis CF. *Physiol Rev*. 1996;76:537–592.
171. Yost CS. *Anesthesiology*. 1999;90:1186–1203.
172. Friederich P, et al. *Anesthesiology*. 2001;95:954–958.
173. Franks NP, Lieb WR. *Nature*. 1988;333:662–664.
174. Dickinson R, Franks NP. *Critical care*. 2010;14:229.
175. Tong L, et al. *Br J Anaesth*. 2014;113:157–167.
176. Woll KA, et al. *ACS Chem Biol*. 2017;12:1353–1362.
177. Bertaccini EJ, et al. *ACS Chem Neurosci*. 2014;5:1246–1252.
178. Farwell D, Gollob MH. *Can J Cardiol*. 2007;23(suppl A):16A–22A.
179. Antzelevitch C. *J Electrocardiol*. 2001;34(suppl):177–181.
180. Li J, Correa AM. *Anesthesiology*. 2002;97:921–930.
181. Davies LA, et al. *Br J Pharmacol*. 2000;131:223–230.
182. Stadnicka A, et al. *J Anesth*. 2007;21:212–219.
183. Wojtovich AP, et al. *Anesthesiology*. 2016;124:1065–1076.
184. Sirois JE, et al. *J Physiol*. 2002;541:717–729.
185. Chen X, et al. *J Neurosci*. 2005;25:5803–5814.
186. Robinson RB, Siegelbaum SA. *Annu Rev Physiol*. 2003;65:453–480.
187. Girault JA, et al. In: Hemmings HC, et al, eds. *Foundations of Anesthesia*. Mosby; 2005:31.
188. Rebecchi MJ, Pentyala SN. *Br J Anaesth*. 2002;89:62–78.
189. Peterlin Z, et al. *Mol Cell Neurosci*. 2005;30:506–512.
190. Minami K, et al. *Mol Pharmacol*. 1998;53:148–156.
191. Minami K, et al. *J Pharmacol Exp Ther*. 1997;281:1136–1143.
192. Minami K, et al. *Eur J Pharmacol*. 1997;339:237–244.
193. Hemmings HC. *Toxicol Lett*. 1998;100–101:89–95.
194. Hasegawa J, et al. *Acta Histochem Cytochem*. 2006;39:163–172.
195. Das J, et al. *J Biol Chem*. 2004;279:37964–37972.
196. Shumilla JA, et al. *Anesth Analg*. 2004;99:82–84.
197. Sonner JM, et al. *Anesth Analg*. 1999;89:1030–1034.
198. Inoue S, et al. *Anesthesiology*. 2004;101:75–81.
199. Rasmussen LS, et al. *Acta Anaesthesiol Scand*. 2004;48:1137–1143.
200. Fukuda S, Warner DS. *Br J Anaesth*. 2007;99:10–17.
201. Turner CP, et al. *Neuroscience*. 2012;210:384–392.
202. Pratt PF, et al. *Curr Opin Anaesthesiol*. 2006;19:397–403.
203. Zaugg M, et al. *Br J Anaesth*. 2003;91:551–565.
204. Ludwig LM, et al. *Anesthesiology*. 2004;100:532–539.
205. Song IA, et al. *BMC Anesthesiol*. 2016;16:13.
206. Snyder GL, et al. *Neuropharmacology*. 2007;53:619–630.
207. Hemmings HC, Adamo AI. *Anesthesiology*. 1994;81:147–155.
208. Marota JJ, et al. *Anesthesiology*. 1992;77:365–371.
209. Hamaya Y, et al. *Anesth Analg*. 2000;90:1177–1183.
210. Culley DJ, et al. *Eur J Pharmacol*. 2006;549:71–78.
211. Futterer CD, et al. *Anesthesiology*. 2004;100:302–308.
212. Durieux M, Davis PJ. *Anesth Analg*. 2010;110:1265–1267.
213. Dalla Massara L, et al. *Anesthesiology*. 2016;124:1311–1327.
214. Kullmann DM, et al. *J Physiol*. 1989;412:277–296.
215. Fujiwara N, et al. *J Physiol*. 1988;402:155–175.
216. MacIver MB, Roth SH. *Br J Anaesth*. 1988;60:680–691.
217. Ries CR, Puil E. *J Neurophysiol*. 1999;81:1802–1809.
218. Sirois JE, et al. *J Neurosci*. 2000;20:6347–6354.
219. Semyanov A, et al. *Trends Neurosci*. 2004;27:262–269.
220. Houston CM, et al. *J Neurosci*. 2012;32:3887–3897.
221. Bai D, et al. *Mol Pharmacol*. 2001;59:814–824.
222. Bieda MC, MacIver MB. *J Neurophysiol*. 2004;92:1658–1667.
223. Caraiscos VB, et al. *Proc Natl Acad Sci U S A*. 2004;101:3662–3667.
224. Caraiscos VB, et al. *J Neurosci*. 2004;24:8454–8458.
225. Capogna M, Pearce RA. *Trends Neurosci*. 2011;34:101–112.
226. Rodgers FC, et al. *J Neurosci*. 2015;35:9707–9716.
227. Berg-Johnsen J, Langmoen IA. *Acta Anaesthesiol Scand*. 1992;36:350–355.
228. Kirson ED, et al. *Br J Pharmacol*. 1998;124:1607–1614.
229. Richards CD, Smaje JC. *Br J Pharmacol*. 1976;58:347–357.
230. Wakamori M, et al. *J Neurophysiol*. 1991;66:2014–2021.
231. Yang J, Zorumski CF. *Ann N Y Acad Sci*. 1991;625:287–289.
232. Dildy-Mayfield JE, et al. *J Pharmacol Exp Ther*. 1996;276:1058–1065.
233. Minami K, et al. *J Biol Chem*. 1998;273:8248–8255.
234. Morgan PG, et al. *Anesthesiology*. 2002;96:1268–1270.
235. Quintana A, et al. *PLoS One*. 2012;7:e42904.
236. Zimin PI, et al. *Curr Biol*. 2016;26:2194–2201.
237. Ramadasan-Nair R, et al. *PLoS One*. 2017;12:e0188087.
238. Banks MI, Pearce RA. *Anesthesiology*. 1999;90:120–134.
239. Murugaiah KD, Hemmings HC. *Anesthesiology*. 1998;89:919–928.
240. Nishikawa K, MacIver MB. *Anesthesiology*. 2001;94:340–347.
241. Westphalen RI, Hemmings HC. *J Pharmacol Exp Ther*. 2003;304:1188–1196.
242. Westphalen RI, Hemmings HC. *J Pharmacol Exp Ther*. 2006;316:216–223.
243. Baumgart JP, et al. *Proc Natl Acad Sci U S A*. 2015;112:11959–11964.
244. Nagele P, et al. *Anesthesiology*. 2005;103:768–778.
245. van Swinderen B, et al. *Proc Natl Acad Sci U S A*. 1999;96:2479–2484.
246. Hemmings HC, et al. *Mol Pharmacol*. 2005;67:1591–1599.
247. Pearce RA, et al. *Anesthesiology*. 1989;71:591–598.
248. Pearce RA. *J Physiol*. 1996;492(Pt 3):823–840.
249. Ballesteros KA, et al. *Int J Gen Med*. 2012;5:935–942.
250. Simon W, et al. *Anesthesiology*. 2001;94:1058–1065.
251. Jinks SL, et al. *Neuroreport*. 2011;22:655–659.
252. Jinks SL, et al. *Anesthesiology*. 2005;103:567–575.
253. Lewis LD, et al. *Proc Natl Acad Sci U S A*. 2012;109:E3377–E3386.
254. Guidera JA, et al. *Front Neural Circuits*. 2017;11:36.
255. Steriade M, et al. *J Neurosci*. 1993;13:3266–3283.
256. Purdon PL, et al. *Proc Natl Acad Sci U S A*. 2013;110:E1142–E1151.
257. Buzsaki G. *Neuron*. 2002;33:325–340.
258. Bland BH, et al. *Hippocampus*. 2003;13:38–47.
259. Munglani R, et al. *Br J Anaesth*. 1993;71:633–641.
260. Madler C, et al. *Br J Anaesth*. 1991;66:81–87.
261. Buzsaki G, Wang XJ. *Annu Rev Neurosci*. 2012;35:203–225.
262. Dickinson R, et al. *Neuropharmacology*. 2003;44:864–872.
263. Antkowiak B, Hentschke H. *Neurosci Lett*. 1997;231:87–90.
264. Gottschalk A, Haney P. *Anesthesiology*. 2003;98:548–564.
265. Storer KP, Reeke GN. *Anesthesiology*. 2012;117:780–790.
266. Wilson MT, et al. *Anesthesiology*. 2006;104:588–593.
267. Steyn-Ross ML, et al. *Prog Biophys Mol Biol*. 2004;85:369–385.
268. Zhang Y, et al. *Anesth Analg*. 2001;92:1585–1589.
269. Zhang Y, et al. *Anesth Analg*. 2001;92:123–127.
270. Forman SA, Miller KW. *Anesth Analg*. 2016;123:1263–1273.
271. Woll KA, et al. *FASEB J*. 2018: fj201701347R.
272. Nash HA. *Br J Anaesth*. 2002;89:143–155.
273. Kim CK, et al. *Nat Rev Neurosci*. 2017;18:222–235.
274. Roth BL. *Neuron*. 2016;89:683–694.
275. Gelegen C, et al. *Curr Biol*. 2018;28:580–587. e585.
276. Sonner JM, et al. *Mol Pharmacol*. 2005;68:61–68.
277. van Swinderen B, Kottler B. *Bioessays*. 2014;36:372–381.
278. Morgan PG, Sedensky MM. *Anesthesiology*. 1994;81:888–898.
279. Rajaram S, et al. *Proc Natl Acad Sci U S A*. 1998;95:8761–8766.
280. Sedensky MM, et al. *Am J Physiol Cell Physiol*. 2001;280:C1340–C1348.
281. Cascio M, et al. *Anesth Analg*. 2007;105:381–385.
282. Olufs ZPG, et al. *Sci Rep*. 2018;8:2348.
283. Veselis RA, et al. *Anesthesiology*. 2002;97:329–337.
284. Alkire MT, Miller J. *Prog Brain Res*. 2005;150:229–244.

20 Inhaled Anesthetic Uptake, Distribution, Metabolism, and Toxicity

STUART A. FORMAN and YUMIKO ISHIZAWA

KEY POINTS

- The alveolar anesthetic concentration (F_A) or partial pressure (P_{alv}) is important because it is the driving force determining anesthetic uptake into blood and target tissues in the central nervous system, and it can be monitored as a readout of anesthetic dosage. P_{alv} is influenced by both delivery and uptake of anesthetic gas.
- Inhaled anesthetic delivery to patients can be increased with larger fresh carrier gas flows, vaporizer output settings, and minute ventilation.
- Initial anesthetic uptake into blood increases with greater pulmonary blood flow (cardiac output) and high blood solubility of anesthetic gas. Increased uptake (as with a highly blood-soluble drug or high cardiac output) slows anesthetic induction because it slows the rate of rise of P_{alv}. Conversely, low anesthetic solubility in blood is associated with rapid onset and offset of anesthesia.
- Uptake of anesthetic into blood slows as blood and tissue partial pressures increase, resulting in higher anesthetic partial pressure in mixed venous blood.
- The higher the inspired anesthetic concentration, the less it diminishes because of uptake (the concentration effect). At 100% inspired concentration of a gas, uptake reduces the volume of gas in alveoli, but does reduce P_{alv}. During inhalation of anesthetic mixtures containing high nitrous oxide (N_2O) concentrations, the reduction of alveolar volume produced by rapid N_2O uptake sustains or increases the concentrations of other alveolar gases (the second gas effect).
- Factors that affect anesthetic uptake similarly affect pulmonary clearance of anesthetics. The rate of clearance is also context sensitive—that is, equivalent drops in alveolar and brain anesthetic concentrations are slower after a long exposure to inhaled anesthetic compared to a short exposure of equal depth.
- Toxicities of inhaled anesthetics that last beyond the exposure period are primarily associated with their biotransformation (metabolism). These toxic effects are usually produced in the tissues, such as liver and kidney, in which metabolism occurs. Modern inhaled anesthetics undergo less metabolism than older drugs, resulting in less hepatic and renal toxicity.
- Halothane hepatitis is a potentially fatal syndrome of fulminant liver damage after exposure to reactive metabolites produced by oxidation of volatile anesthetics. These metabolites covalently modify liver proteins, creating neohaptens that elicit an immune response against hepatocytes. The incidence of the syndrome varies with different anesthetics, paralleling the extent of drug metabolism: halothane >> enflurane > isoflurane > desflurane.
- Defluorination of inhaled anesthetics occurs in both the liver and kidney, producing high fluoride concentrations in blood. Renal toxicity characterized by high-output renal failure is almost exclusively associated with prolonged exposure to methoxyflurane. Sevoflurane metabolism also results in high fluoride levels in blood but does not damage kidneys. Factors that enhance the toxicity of methoxyflurane relative to sevoflurane include its higher tissue solubility, slower clearance, and higher degree of renal metabolism, resulting in high intrarenal fluoride levels for an extended time.
- In laboratory mammals, including nonhuman primates, all general anesthetics alter synapse and neural circuit formation during critical periods of brain development, resulting in abnormal memory and behavior. Clinical studies in children suggest that lengthy (>4 hours) anesthetic exposures at under 2 years of age are associated with detectable but quite small neurocognitive deficits, relative to unexposed controls (also see Chapter 77. Postoperative delirium and cognitive decline/dysfunction (POCD) in elderly patients is also a growing concern (see Chapter 83). Based on animal and clinical studies, both postsurgical neuroinflammation and exposure to general anesthesia may contribute to POCD.
- Anesthetics react with strong bases, particularly potassium hydroxide (KOH), in carbon dioxide (CO_2) absorbents, resulting in production of several potentially toxic substances. Sevoflurane

degrades to form compound A, which is associated with renal damage in rodents, but not in humans. This differential toxicity is associated with differential renal metabolism in rodents versus humans. Dry CO_2 absorbents in the breathing circuit react with inhaled anesthetics, releasing carbon monoxide and heat. New CO_2 absorbent materials that lack strong base chemicals prevent these reactions and subsequent potential harm to patients.

- N_2O is unique among anesthetics in its ability to inhibit methionine synthase by oxidizing a cofactor, vitamin B_{12}. In certain susceptible patients or with multiple frequent exposures to N_2O, methionine synthase inhibition can lead to hematologic and neurologic dysfunction. After prolonged N_2O exposure, methionine synthase inhibition also increases blood homocysteine, which is hypothesized to increase vascular inflammation and the risk of thrombosis. Large clinical trials show that N_2O exposure does not increase the risk of cardiovascular morbidity in most patients, but N_2O should be avoided in patients with deficiencies in dietary B_{12} intake or absorption or B_{12}-dependent metabolism.
- Inhaled anesthetics, when scavenged and ejected into the atmosphere, contribute to both global warming and ozone depletion. Minimizing the environmental impact of inhaled anesthetics requires reducing waste, through the routine use of low fresh gas flows and/or by use of new technologies that trap scavenged anesthetic gases. Reprocessing and reusing trapped anesthetic gases further reduce the environmental impact of drug production.

Introduction

Modern inhaled anesthetics are important pharmacologic tools for reversibly altering central nervous system (CNS) functions in patients. Because inhaled anesthetics are both taken up and eliminated through alveolar blood-gas exchange, drug dosage can be monitored in expired alveolar gases and tissue-dependent metabolism is unnecessary for drug clearance. Optimal delivery of systemic drugs via inhalation requires a full understanding of the factors influencing how gas-phase compounds move into and out of various body tissues and how they are metabolized (pharmacokinetics) together with knowledge of where and how these drugs and their metabolism affect tissue functions. Reversible anesthetic effects on the nervous, respiratory, and cardiovascular systems (pharmacodynamics) are covered elsewhere in this book (see Chapters 11, 14, 19, and 21).

Uptake and Distribution of Inhaled Anesthetics

In the first part of this chapter, we review and apply some of the basic principles of chemical equilibria to illuminate major factors influencing inhaled anesthetic uptake and distribution in patients. For this, we use a physiologic model that closely simulates clinical observations. The model, an elaboration of that introduced in 1973 by Mapleson,[1] is described both qualitatively and quantitatively (using mathematical expressions) to convey important concepts to readers with different learning styles.

BIOPHYSICAL PROPERTIES OF INHALED ANESTHETICS: PARTIAL PRESSURE, HYDROPHOBICITY, AND PARTITION COEFFICIENTS

Inhaled anesthetics are administered as a component of a gas mixture. Biophysical properties of inhaled anesthetics are summarized in Table 20.1.[2-11] ***Partial pressure*** is the portion of total pressure contributed by one component of a gas mixture, where each component contributes pressure in direct proportion to its molar fraction. For example, 1.5% isoflurane in air (21% O_2 and 79% N_2) at 1 standard atmosphere (atm) (760 mm Hg) is a mixture of O_2 at 157.2 mm Hg, N_2 at 591.4 mm Hg, and isoflurane at 11.4 mm Hg. The partial pressure of an anesthetic gas is a measure of its thermodynamic activity and determines its pharmacologic effect. The partial pressure of an anesthetic is usually reported as the percentage (or fraction) of the delivered gas mixture, where atmospheric pressure is near 1 atm (760 mm Hg). Correcting these values to absolute partial pressure is important under conditions when local atmospheric pressure differs significantly from standard, such as at high altitude, underwater, or in a hyperbaric chamber. The same inhaled concentration of an anesthetic gas results in a reduced pharmacologic effect at higher altitudes because the partial pressure of the anesthetic is lower. Because partial pressure is the thermodynamic force for gas transfer between compartments in a system, anesthetics move from regions of high partial pressure to low partial pressure, unaffected by the other components of the gas mixture, and equilibrium is achieved when the partial pressure of an anesthetic is equal in the different compartments.

The maximum partial pressure of a volatile compound is its ***vapor pressure***; this is the partial pressure of volatile anesthetic (VA) within the drug reservoir of a vaporizer. Vapor pressure is unique to each anesthetic and increases with increasing temperature. VAs are defined by a vapor pressure less than 1 atm at 20°C and a boiling point above 20°C (see Table 20.1). Gaseous anesthetics are defined by a vapor pressure above 1 atm at 20°C and a boiling point below 20°C (see Table 20.1). VAs typically compose a small fraction of the gas mixture delivered to patients. In contrast, gaseous anesthetics such as nitrous oxide (N_2O) and xenon, because of their relatively low anesthetic potencies, typically compose a large fraction of an inhaled gas mixture, and thus produce additional effects (e.g., concentration effect, second gas effect, and airspace expansion) that are negligible with VAs.

Hydrophobicity is a molecular property of certain chemicals, including most general anesthetics that do not

TABLE 20.1 Chemical Structures and Properties of Inhaled Anesthetics

Anesthetic	**Nitrous Oxide**	**Halothane**	**Methoxyflurane**	**Enflurane**	**Isoflurane**	**Desflurane**	**Sevoflurane**
Year Introduced into Clinic	**1840s**	**1956**	**1960**	**1966**	**1969**	**1990**	**1981**
Chemical structure	$N\equiv N^{+}-O^{-}$ ↕ $N^{-}=N^{+}=O$	F–C(F)(F)–C(Br)(Cl)–H	H–C(Cl)(Cl)–C(F)(F)–O–C(H)(H)–H	H–C(F)(Cl)–C(F)(F)–O–C(F)(F)–H	F–C(F)(F)–C(H)(Cl)–O–C(F)(F)–H	F–C(F)(F)–C(F)(H)–O–C(F)(F)–H	H–C(CF_3)(CF_3)–O–C(H)(H)–F
Molecular weight	44	197.4	165.0	184.5	184.5	168	200.1
Boiling point (°C)	−88.5	50.2	104.8	56.5	48.5	22.8	58.6
Density (g/ml)	1.84×10^{-3}	1.86	1.42	1.52	1.5	1.45	1.50
Vapor pressure (mm Hg)	43,880	243	22.5	175	238	664	157
Oil/gas partition coefficient at 37°C	1.3	197	950	98.5	90.8	19	47-54
Blood/gas partition coefficient at 37°C	0.47	2.5	12	1.9	1.4	0.45	0.65
MAC-immobility (% atm/mm Hg)*	104/800	0.75/5.7	0.2/1.52	1.58/12.0	1.28/9.7	6.0/45.6	2.05/15.6
MAC-awake*	71/540	0.41/3.21	0.081/0.62	0.51/3.88	0.43/3.27	2.4/19	0.63/4.79

*MAC is minimal alveolar concentration for subjects approximately age 40 years.
Partition coefficients are from the following references[2-6]:
MAC-immobility and MAC-awake values are from the following references[2,7-11]:
Properties are measured at standard temperature (20°C) and pressure (1 atm) unless otherwise specified.

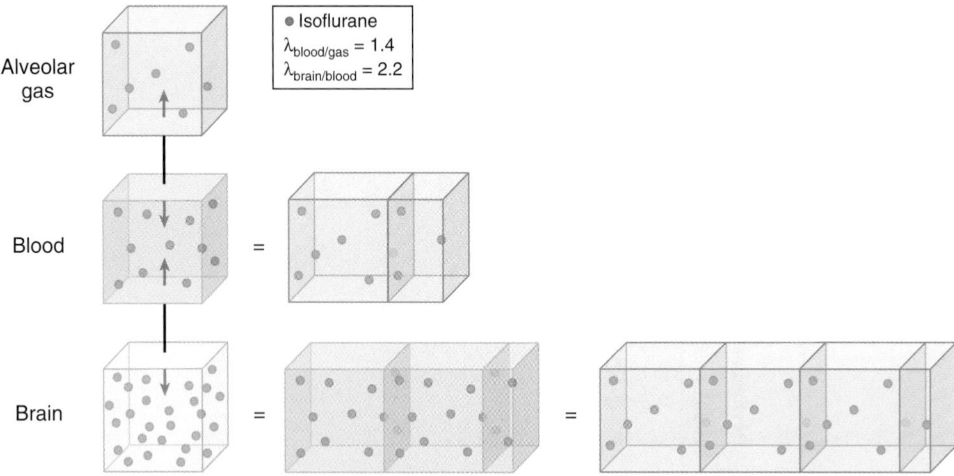

Fig. 20.1 Partitioning of anesthetic gases between different biophases. Left, Depicts the partitioning of isoflurane between gas phase *(blue)*, blood *(red)* and brain *(yellow)*. The blood:gas partition coefficient ($\lambda_{b/g}$) for isoflurane is 1.4 and the brain:blood partition coefficient ($\lambda_{CNS/blood}$) is 2.2 (see Table 20.2). At equilibrium, defined as equal isoflurane partial pressure in all compartments, a volume of blood contains 1.4-fold the quantity of isoflurane as the same volume of alveolar gas, whereas a volume of brain tissue contains 2.2-fold the quantity of isoflurane as the same volume of blood. Right, We also depict partition coefficients as effective (equivalent) volumes of another biophase. For example, 1 volume of blood contains the same amount of isoflurane as 1.4 volumes of alveolar gas, whereas 1 volume of brain contains the same amount of isoflurane as 2.2 volumes of blood or 3.1 volumes of gas.

readily form hydrogen bonds and therefore display low water solubility. Hydrophobic compounds are also usually *lipophilic*, demonstrating high solubility in low polarity solvents such as oils. Common measures of hydrophobicity are ***partition coefficients*** between water and olive oil (which is mostly oleic acid, an 18-carbon fatty acid) or between water and n-octanol. Usually represented by the Greek letter lambda (λ), a partition coefficient is the ratio of two solute concentrations *at* ***equilibrium*** (i.e., at equal partial pressure) in two separate but adjacent solvents or compartments such that the solute moves freely between the compartments (Fig. 20.1). Another useful way to conceptualize a partition coefficient is that it represents the *relative volume of two phases or compartments that contain an equal amount of the solute at equilibrium* (see Fig. 20.1).

Anesthetic partition coefficients between blood and gas ($\lambda_{b/g}$) and between tissue and blood ($\lambda_{t/b}$) are important factors in uptake and distribution of inhaled drugs as they move from pulmonary airspace to pulmonary blood and then from blood to various tissues (Tables 20.1 and 20.2).[6,12-15] The blood solubility of anesthetic gases (and other gases such as O_2, N_2, and CO_2) increases as temperature decreases.[16,17] Because most anesthetics are hydrophobic, they tend to display high solubility in tissues with high lipid content (e.g., fat), and also bind to many proteins that form hydrophobic or amphiphilic pockets.[13] Anesthetic partitioning into blood (blood solubility) increases after ingestion of fatty foods[18] and may decrease in anemic or malnourished patients. Methoxyflurane (no longer in clinical use) and halothane are notable for high blood solubility. N_2O, sevoflurane, and desflurane are characterized by low blood solubility.

ANESTHETIC DELIVERY, UPTAKE, AND DISTRIBUTION: A MULTICOMPARTMENTAL MODEL

Delivering an inhaled anesthetic agent to patients is analogous to an intravenous drug infusion with two major differences: (1) entry of drug into the body is via transalveolar exchange from gas to blood, and (2) clearance is mostly via the same route. Thus inhaled anesthetic delivery is dependent on pulmonary ventilation, whereas uptake and clearance of inhaled anesthetics are also dependent on pulmonary perfusion.

Upstream and Downstream Compartments and Anesthetic Transfer: Bulk Flow and Pressure Gradients

Uptake and distribution of inhaled anesthetic can be readily understood as a series of transfer steps from upstream compartments with high partial pressure to downstream compartments with low partial pressure as depicted in Fig. 20.2. First, drug is transferred from an anesthesia delivery device, typically an anesthesia machine with a vaporizer designed to deliver specified concentrations (in percent atm) of VA agent, into a fresh gas mixture flowing in a breathing circuit. Second, ventilation transfers gases from the circuit to the alveolar airspace in lung. Third, anesthetic moves by transcapillary diffusion into pulmonary venous blood. Fourth, arterial blood distributes anesthetic to various tissues including the primary target tissue, the CNS. Fifth, venous outflow from tissues converges in the pulmonary artery, and sixth, the mixed venous blood passes through alveolar capillaries where it again equilibrates with alveolar gases.

Gas flow from the anesthesia machine into the breathing circuit is unidirectional. Blood circulation is also largely unidirectional. In transfers from the anesthesia machine (the fresh gas outlet) to breathing circuit and then to alveolar airspace, anesthetic flow can simply be understood as exchange from upstream compartments into downstream compartments. In later steps, such as exchange between alveolar gases and pulmonary capillary blood, flow of anesthetic molecules occurs via diffusion between adjacent compartments separated by a permeable membrane. For simplicity, we have not treated blood as a separate compartment in our model. Distribution of anesthetic to and from various tissues involves both bulk transfer via blood flow

TABLE 20.2 Uptake and Distribution Model Parameters for Inhaled Anesthetics

Tissue	Blood		Heart			Kidney			Liver			CNS			Muscle			Fat			VPT		
	Blood Flow (L/min)	**Volume (L)**	**Blood Flow (L/min)**	**Volume (L)**		**Blood Flow (L/min)**	**Volume (L)**		**Blood Flow (L/min)**	**Volume (L)**		**Blood Flow (L/min)**	**Volume (L)**		**Blood Flow (L/min)**	**Volume (L)**		**Blood Flow (L/min)**	**Volume (L)**		**Blood Flow (L/min)**	**Volume (L)**	
	5	**5**	0.2	0.28		1.07	0.32		1.2	3.9		0.62	1.43		0.75	30		0.5	13		0.35	7	
Anesthetic Agent	V_{eff} (L)*		$\lambda_{tissue/blood}$	V_{eff} (L)	τ (min)	$\lambda_{tissue/blood}$	V_{eff} (L)	τ (min)	$\lambda_{tissue/blood}$	V_{eff} (L)	τ (min)	$\lambda_{tissue/blood}$	V_{eff} (L)	τ (min)	$\lambda_{tissue/blood}$	V_{eff} (L)	τ (min)	$\lambda_{tissue/blood}$	V_{eff} (L)	τ (min)	$\lambda_{tissue/blood}$	V_{eff} (L)	τ (min)
Nitrous oxide	2.35		0.87	0.24	1.2	0.93	0.3	0.3	1.1	4.1	3.4	1.1	1.6	2.6	1.2	36	48	2.3	30	60	1.4	9.9	29
Halothane	12.5		2.9	0.8	4.0	1.5	0.5	0.4	2.5	9.8	8.0	2.7	3.9	3.3	2.5	75	100	65	840	1700	2.3	16	47
Methoxyflurane	60		1.2	0.34	1.7	2.3	0.74	.69	2.5	9.8	8	2	2.9	4.7	1.6	48	64	76	980	1960	1.2	8.5	25
Enflurane	9		1.3	0.36	1.8	2.0	0.64	0.6	2.1	8.2	6.7	1.4	2.0	3.3	1.7	51	68	36	464	930	2	14	41
Isoflurane	7		1.3	0.36	1.8	2.3	0.74	0.69	2.4	9.4	7.6	1.5	2.1	3.5	2.9	87	116	45	580	1160	2	14	41
Desflurane	2.25		1.3	0.36	1.8	1.0	0.32	0.3	1.4	5.5	4.5	1.3	1.9	3.0	2.0	60	80	27	350	670	2	14	41
Sevoflurane	3.25		1.3	0.36	1.8	2.3	0.74	0.69	2.4	9.4	7.7	1.7	2.4	4.0	3.1	93	120	48	620	1240	2	14	41

Based on a 70 kg pt at rest. Blood and tissue partition coefficients are from references 6 and 12-14. Tissue volumes and blood flow values are approximate (Kennedy et al.[15] and Levitt[13]). Effective volumes are calculated as tissue volume × $\lambda_{tissue/blood}$ and exchange time constant (τ) for each compartment is V_{eff}/blood flow.

*Blood/gas partition coefficients for anesthetic agents are given in Table 20.1.

CNS, Central nervous system; *VPT*, vessel-poor tissues (e.g., skin, bone, and connective tissues).

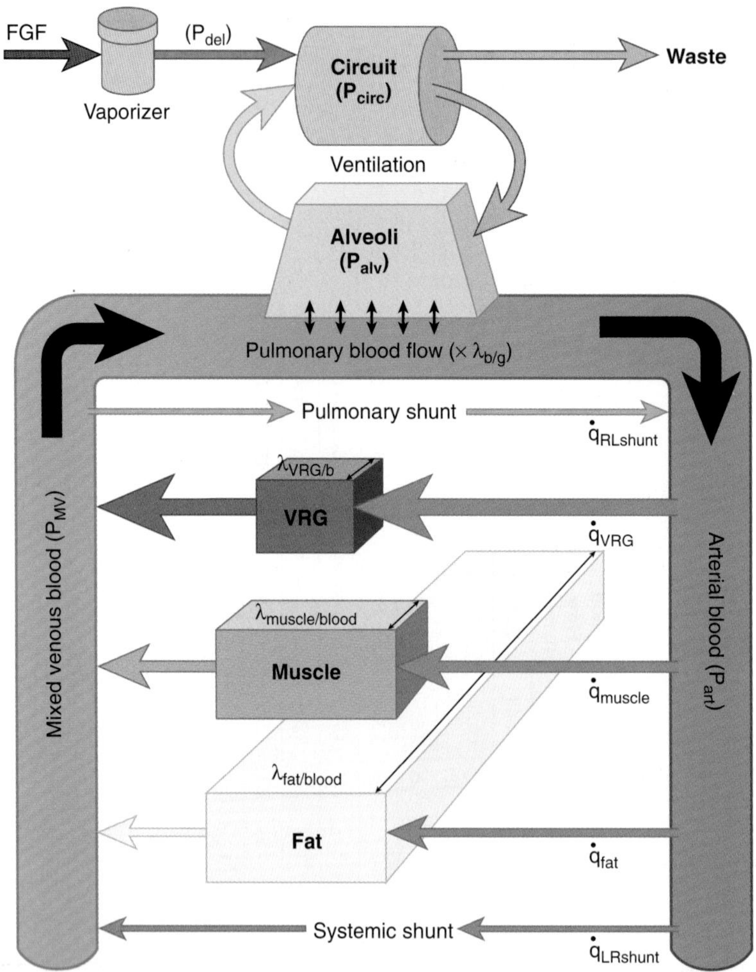

Fig. 20.2 Flow diagram for uptake and distribution of inhaled anesthetics. Major compartments for anesthetic flow are depicted, including the breathing circuit, alveolar gas space, and three major tissue compartments: vessel-rich group (VRG), muscle, and fat. The physiological volumes of the tissue compartments are approximately in proportion to the labeled face of the compartment, while the blood-tissue partition coefficients are depicted as the depth of the compartment. Thus the effective volume of the VRG is much smaller than that of muscle, which in turn is much smaller than that of fat. Carrier flows and exchange in different parts of the model are depicted by arrows: Fresh gas flow *(FGF)* moves anesthetic from the vaporizer to the circuit; ventilation drives exchange of anesthetic between the circuit and alveoli; pulmonary blood flow transfers anesthetic from alveoli into the circulation, which then distributes drug to different compartments depending on blood flow to various tissues. Relative blood flow is approximately proportional to the width of the arrows into and out of tissue compartments, as well as for shunts. The diagram depicts an early phase of anesthetic uptake when organs of the VRG, including the brain, are approaching equilibrium with alveolar and arterial anesthetic partial pressure, while anesthetic partial pressures in muscle and fat remain relatively low. Quantitative modeling of anesthetic gas movement in this system was performed using numerical integration of equations describing anesthetic flow into and out of each compartment (Eqs. 20.5, 20.8–20.11). Figs. 20.4–20.7, 26.9, 20.10, and 20.12 were all generated using this model. Standardized parameters used in the model are summarized in Table 20.2.

and diffusive equilibration across capillary membranes. Note that when anesthetic transfer occurs between gas and blood or between blood and tissue, the effective volume of the downstream compartment must be adjusted with the appropriate partition coefficient (see Table 20.2).

Rate of Wash-In of the Circuit: Equilibration Between Vaporizer and Circuit

Equipment for controlled delivery of inhaled anesthetic drugs are described elsewhere in this text (see Chapter 22). Wash-in of the ventilator breathing circuit represents an example of bulk transfer exchange, wherein the gas in circuit components is replaced by fresh gases emerging from the gas outlet of the anesthesia machine.

Anesthetic Delivery from the Vaporizer: VA delivery (in liters per minute of gaseous drug) from a vaporizer is closely approximated as the product of the delivered anesthetic concentration (fraction = F_{del} or partial pressure at 1 atm = P_{del}) of the anesthetic in a gas mixture and the fresh gas flow (FGF):

$$dVA_{del}/dt = P_{del} \times FGF. \tag{20.1}$$

Thus we can readily calculate the volume of delivered gas-phase anesthetic by simply integrating this function over time. In the simplest case where P_{del} and FGF remain constant,

$$VA_{del}(t) = P_{del} \times FGF \times t. \tag{20.2}$$

Fresh Gas Wash-In to the Breathing Circuit: The factors that affect the speed at which the gas mixture delivered from the anesthesia machine replaces gases in the breathing circuit (wash-in) are FGF and the breathing circuit volume (V_{circ}). Consider a typical situation where FGF at the beginning of an anesthetic is 6 L/min, and the gas volume inside the components of a breathing circuit is 6 L. If FGF is doubled to 12 L/min, then wash-in will proceed at twice the rate (halving the time). Conversely, if the V_{circ} doubles to 12 L, then wash-in will proceed at half the rate (doubling the time).

The gas exchange process is independent of the concentration of anesthetic in the circuit, because the exchange is simply through bulk flow and mixing. However, the *difference between the delivered concentration and that in the circuit determines the magnitude and direction of net anesthetic gas flow*. When the delivered anesthetic partial pressure (P_{del}) is greater than that in the circuit (P_{circ}), net anesthetic flow is into the circuit (and subsequently the patient). To remove anesthetic from the circuit, P_{del} must be less than P_{circ}. When there is no concentration gradient (i.e., equal partial pressures), bulk flow exchange may replace all the old anesthetic molecules with new ones, but there is no net flow and anesthetic concentrations in the circuit remain unchanged.

Mathematically, we can describe the breathing circuit exchange process as a differential equation that incorporates all of the above factors:

$$\frac{dP_{circ}}{dt} = \frac{FGF}{V_{circ}} \times (P_{del} - P_{circ}). \tag{20.3}$$

If P_{del} is constant, integrating this equation results in a single exponential function that defines P_{circ} at any given time following a change in P_{del} at t = 0:

$$P_{circ}(t) = P_{circ}(0) + (P_{del} - P_{circ}(0)) \times \left(1 - e^{-t/[V_{circ}/FGF]}\right) \tag{20.4}$$

P_{circ} approaches P_{del} following an exponential time course with a time constant of $\tau = V_{circ}/FGF$. Thus if V_{circ} = 6 L and FGF = 6 L/min, the exponential time constant will be 1 minute (Fig. 20.3). Each minute results in the fraction of old gas in the breathing circuit dropping by 63.1%, and after 4 minutes, less than 2% old gas remains. The half-life for the process (time for halving the vaporizer-circuit concentration difference) is $0.693 \times \tau$.

Breathing circuit components, such as CO_2 absorbents and the plastic or rubber of the circuit tubing and connectors, influence the rate of equilibration between vaporizer and circuit, because they absorb VAs, increasing the effective circuit volume.[19] The more hydrophobic VAs absorb more into circuit components, whereas absorption negligibly affects wash-in and wash-out of low-solubility anesthetics.

The clinical relevance of the wash-in process is readily appreciated. An example of the importance of FGF is "priming" the anesthetic circuit for a single-breath induction technique. The FGF setting and the circuit volume influence the required duration of priming. More generally, whenever the vaporizer settings are altered, the speed at which the new settings influence the wash-in or wash-out of the circuit (and subsequently the patient) will depend on FGF. Open (nonrebreathing) anesthetic breathing circuits are designed to have low exchange volumes and to be used with high fresh-gas flows. These features allow rapid changes in the delivered anesthetic concentration, while minimizing rebreathing of exhaled gases. The choice of an open versus

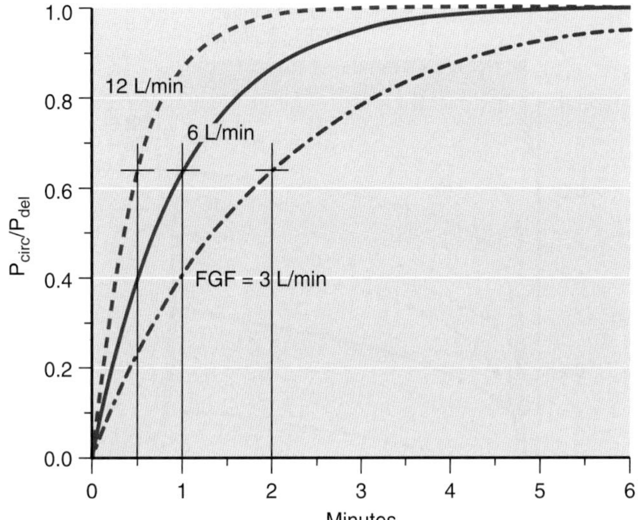

Fig. 20.3 Wash-in of the breathing circuit depends on fresh gas flow (FGF). The curves depict the rate of rise of anesthetic concentration (partial pressure) in a breathing circuit with 6 L gas volume, depending on FGF. Higher FGF results in more rapid exchange of circuit gases with fresh gas. The exponential time constant for the wash-in process is the circuit volume in liters divided by FGF flow in liters per minute (see Eq. 20.4). Cross marks overlaying the curves indicate time constants under different gas flow rates. Each time constant correlates with a 63.1% exchange.

rebreathing system influences the impact of various other factors that can affect uptake and distribution of inhaled anesthetics downstream from the breathing circuit. Some of the subsequent figures show models for both conditions.

Equilibration Between Circuit and Pulmonary Airspace

Transfer of anesthetic gases from the breathing circuit to the pulmonary airspace is another bulk exchange process similar to that from vaporizer to breathing circuit. In this case, gas flow via ventilation is cyclical and bidirectional, and the factors that determine the rate of anesthetic exchange are minute ventilation (MV) and total pulmonary airspace volume (V_{pulm}).[20] Because transfer from the circuit to the lungs represents anesthetic flow out of the circuit, we alter Eq. (20.3) to include both inflow to the circuit and outflow from the circuit,

$$\frac{dP_{circ}}{dt} = \frac{FGF}{V_{circ}} \times (P_{del} - P_{circ}) - \frac{MV}{V_{pulm}} \times (P_{circ} - P_{pulm}), \tag{20.5}$$

where P_{pulm} is a weighted average of the anesthetic partial pressure in dead space and alveolar space.

Eq. (20.5) describes how rebreathing affects the inhaled (breathing circuit) anesthetic concentration. Most inhaled anesthetics are delivered using a rebreathing circuit, which includes one-way flow valves and adsorbent material to chemically remove exhaled CO_2. Rebreathing depends primarily on the balance between fresh gas flow and MV. The anesthetic gas in the breathing circuit represents a mixture of fresh gas and exhaled gases. Increased fresh gas flow reduces rebreathing, whereas increased MV increases rebreathing.

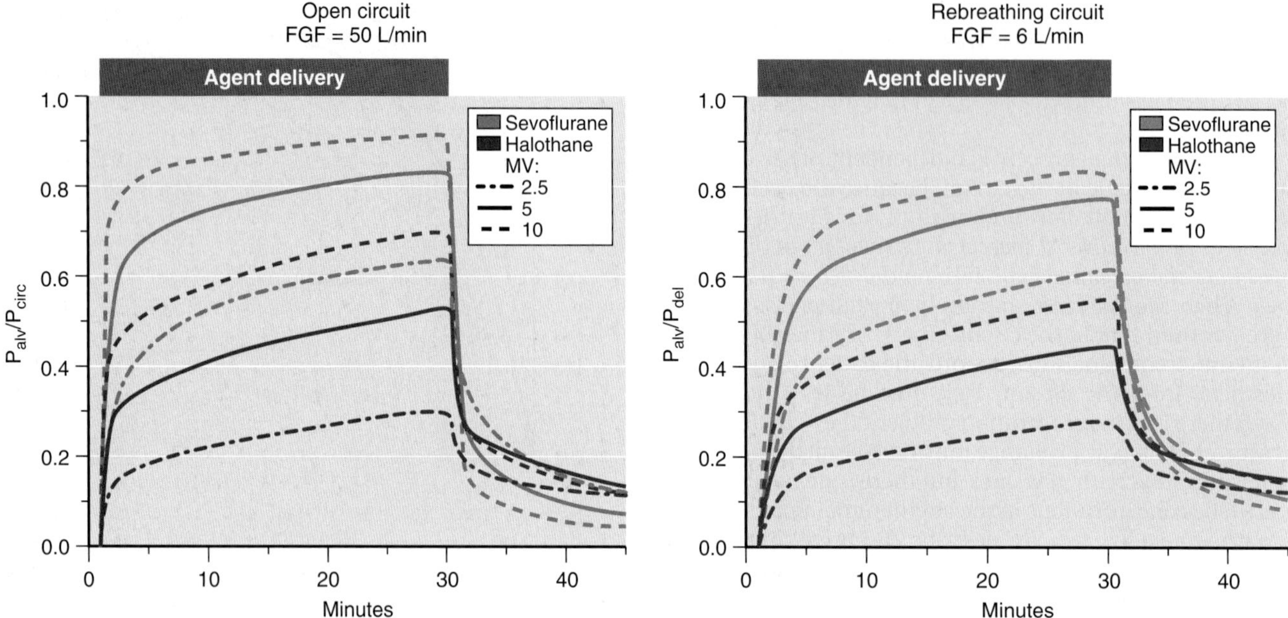

Fig. 20.4 Effect of ventilation on the rise of alveolar anesthetic partial pressure (P_{alv}). Left, A traditional open-circuit model with very high fresh gas flow *(FGF)* and therefore constant $P_{del} = P_{circ}$. Right, A more common clinical situation with constant vaporizer output (P_{del}) and partial rebreathing at a 6 L/min fresh gas flow rate. Raising minute ventilation accelerates the rise of P_{alv} by delivering more anesthetic to the lungs. The effect is seen whether anesthetic is highly soluble in blood (e.g., halothane) or relatively insoluble (e.g., sevoflurane). However, the relative size of the ventilation effect is greater for soluble agents. Increased ventilation also accelerates clearance of anesthetic agents after delivery ceases. *MV*, Minute ventilation; P_{circ}, Anesthetic partial pressure in the breathing circuit; P_{del}, delivered anesthetic partial pressure from the anesthesia machine gas outlet.

The Alveolar Anesthetic Concentration

The alveolar anesthetic concentration (P_{alv} or F_A) is a critically important factor in anesthetic uptake and distribution because (1) it is in rapid equilibrium with circulating blood and highly perfused tissues, including target tissues in the CNS, and (2) P_{alv} can be measured in exhaled end-tidal gases. Thus, except during periods of rapid change, P_{alv} in exhaled breath represents a useful estimate of the anesthetic concentration in the patient's CNS and other highly perfused organs.

Because only alveolar gas is relevant to transpulmonary exchange of anesthetic into and out of the body, *alveolar ventilation* ($\dot{V}_{alv}$) is the proper gas flow to calculate anesthetic exchange into this part of the pulmonary airspace,

$$\frac{dP_{alv}}{dt} = \frac{\dot{V}_{alv}}{V_{alv}} \times (P_{circ} - P_{alv}), \qquad (20.6)$$

where $\dot{V}_{alv}$ is MV corrected for dead space ventilation.

Alveolar Uptake of Anesthetic into Pulmonary Blood

During inhaled anesthetic induction, anesthetic flows from alveolar gas to pulmonary blood across the alveolar/capillary interface separating these compartments and is driven by the partial pressure gradient between alveolar gas (P_{alv}) and mixed venous blood (P_{MV}) entering the pulmonary arteries. The net flow of anesthetic reverses during anesthetic wash-out when P_{alv} drops below P_{MV}. Anesthetic uptake into blood also depends on the pulmonary blood flow (which is typically close to cardiac output, $\dot{Q}$) and the blood's capacity to solvate anesthetic from the gas state (the blood/gas partition coefficient, $\lambda_{b/g}$):

$$\text{uptake} = \dot{Q} \times \lambda_{b/g} \times (P_{alv} - P_{MV}). \qquad (20.7)$$

We therefore correct Eq. (20.6) to reflect both anesthetic inflow into alveolar airspace and its uptake into blood:

$$\frac{dP_{alv}}{dt} = \frac{\dot{V}_{alv}}{V_{alv}} \times (P_{circ} - P_{alv}) - \frac{\dot{Q} \times \lambda_{b/g}}{V_{alv}} \times (P_{alv} - P_{MV}). \qquad (20.8)$$

Thus, during an inhaled anesthetic induction, the rate of increase of P_{alv} relative to P_{circ} is governed by (1) alveolar ventilation, (2) cardiac output, and (3) anesthetic solubility in blood. Increased ventilation delivers more anesthetic from circuit to alveoli and increases P_{alv}/P_{circ} (Fig. 20.4). Importantly, increased pulmonary blood flow removes more anesthetic from alveoli, thereby decreasing the rate of increase in alveolar concentration of anesthetic (P_{alv}/P_{circ}) (Fig. 20.5). Indeed, significant decreases in cardiac output are suspected when end-tidal CO_2 ($ETCO_2$) decreases and end-tidal concentration of VA increases.[21] The more soluble an anesthetic is in blood (i.e., the higher its $\lambda_{b/g}$), the greater is the capacity for each volume of blood to take up anesthetic from alveolar gases (i.e., the larger the effective blood flow). Thus as $\lambda_{b/g}$ increases, P_{alv}/P_{circ} increases more slowly (Fig. 20.6).

Other Factors That Affect the Rate of Rise of P_{alv}

Other factors affecting alveolar uptake of anesthetic include ventilation-perfusion matching and the absolute concentration of anesthetic in alveolar gases.

Pulmonary Dead Space. Dead space (ventilated but not perfused pulmonary regions) reduces effective alveolar ventilation (see Eqs. 20.7 and 20.8), and thus slows anesthetic

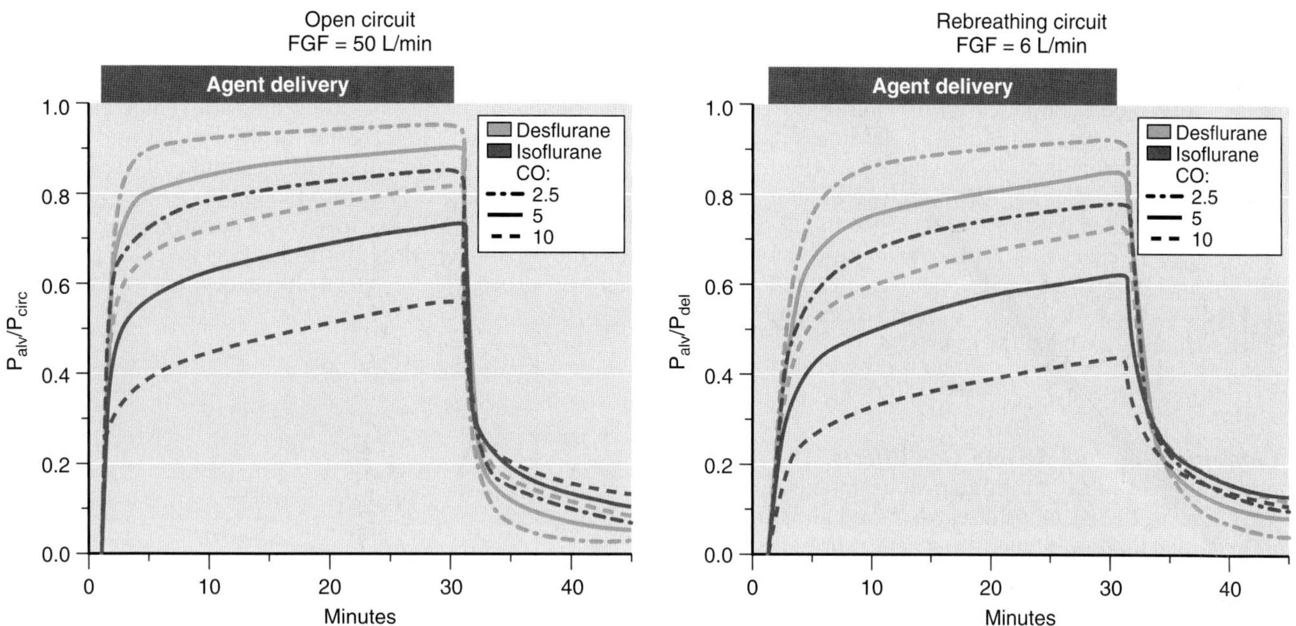

Fig. 20.5 Effect of cardiac output on the rise of alveolar anesthetic partial pressure (P_{alv}). Left, A traditional open-circuit model with very high fresh gas flows and therefore constant $P_{del} = P_{circ}$. Right, A more common clinical situation with constant vaporizer output (P_{del}) and partial rebreathing at a 6 L/min FGF. Increasing cardiac output slows the rise of P_{alv} by increasing anesthetic uptake into blood (removing anesthetic from alveolar gases). This effect is observed for both soluble (e.g., isoflurane) and relatively insoluble (e.g., desflurane) anesthetics, but the relative effect is greater for soluble agents. Cardiac output also affects clearance of anesthetics from the lungs in the same way it affects uptake (i.e., increased cardiac output slows anesthetic clearance rate). *CO*, Cardiac output; P_{circ}, anesthetic partial pressure in the breathing circuit; P_{del}, delivered anesthetic partial pressure from the anesthesia machine gas outlet.

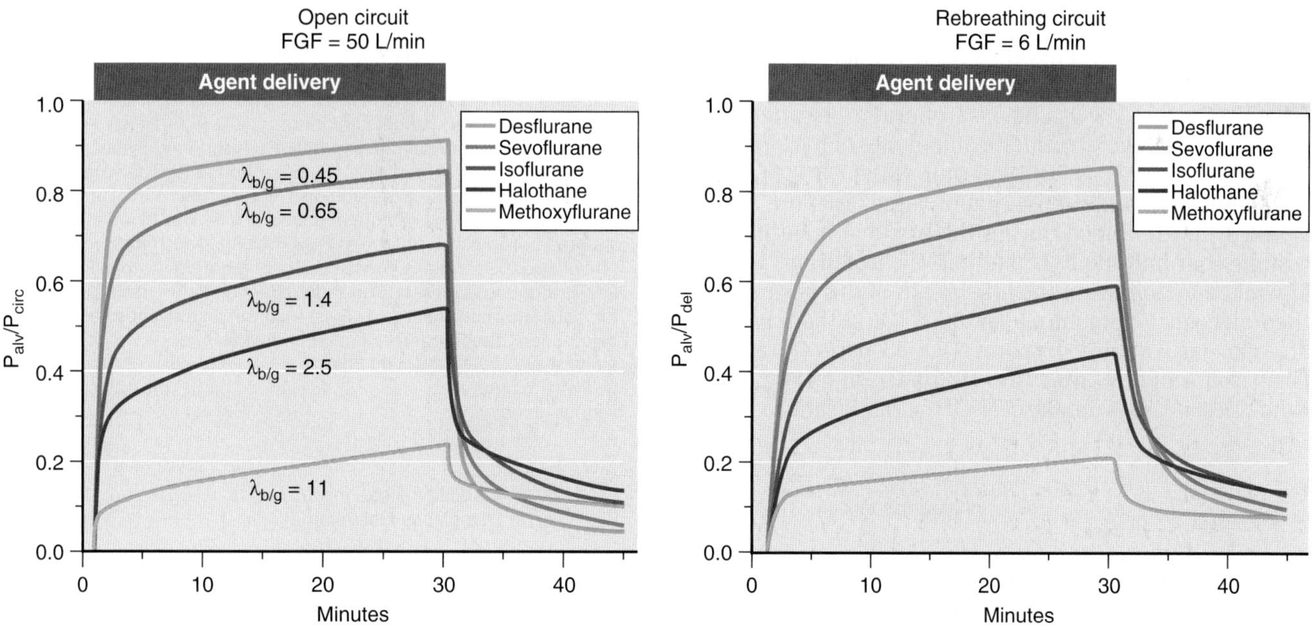

Fig. 20.6 Effect of blood solubility on the rise of alveolar anesthetic partial pressure (P_{alv}). Left, A traditional open-circuit model with very high fresh gas flow (FGF) and therefore constant $P_{del} = P_{circ}$. Right, A more common clinical situation with constant vaporizer output (P_{del}) and partial rebreathing at a 6 L/min FGF rate. As blood solubility ($\lambda_{b/g}$) increases, the rate of rise in P_{alv} slows, because uptake into blood is greater for high solubility agents. The major impact of blood solubility is the magnitude of the rapid initial rise in P_{alv}, which represents a balance between anesthetic delivery and uptake into pulmonary blood. Blood solubility similarly affects clearance from alveoli after anesthetic delivery ceases (i.e., increased blood solubility results in slower clearance from alveolar gas). P_{circ}, Anesthetic partial pressure in the breathing circuit; P_{del}, delivered anesthetic partial pressure from the anesthesia machine gas outlet.

uptake. This effect is strongest under conditions of high FGF and low blood-solubility agents, where alveolar ventilation is the limiting factor in uptake. Under conditions of low FGF and a highly blood-soluble agent, increased dead space, by reducing initial uptake, serves to maintain the inhaled anesthetic concentration (P_{circ}), which creates a compensatory increase in P_{alv} and subsequent uptake.

Pulmonary (Right to Left) Shunting. Pulmonary right to left shunting can be physiologic, pathologic, or iatrogenic, such as during one-lung ventilation. Right-to-left shunting results in a difference between P_{alv} and the partial pressure of anesthetic in arterial blood (P_{art}). This is because arterial blood represents a mixture of shunted mixed venous blood combined with blood that has equilibrated with alveolar gases (Eq. 20.9). Because such shunts also reduce transcapillary gas exchange in the lung and slow anesthetic uptake (Eqs. 20.7 and 20.8, after correcting pulmonary blood flow for shunt), right-to-left shunting sustains P_{circ}, an effect that is more pronounced for highly soluble drugs compared with insoluble anesthetics. Thus shunt reduces the ratio of P_{art}:P_{alv} more for insoluble anesthetics, such as N_2O (Fig. 20.7):[22,23]

$$P_{art} = P_{MV} \times \dot{q}_{RLshunt} + P_{alv} \times (\dot{Q} - \dot{q}_{RLshunt}). \quad (20.9)$$

Concentration and Second Gas Effects. The absolute concentration of anesthetic influences its uptake and that of other gases. In the previous discussion and illustrations, it was presumed that an inhaled anesthetic represents a small fraction of the inhaled gas mixture and that transalveolar uptake of the anesthetic results in a decrease in P_{alv} and negligible changes in alveolar gas volume. However, when the anesthetic represents a large fraction of the inhaled gas mixture, its rapid uptake results in a smaller relative alveolar anesthetic concentration drop, because the volume of alveolar gas also decreases. This is known as the ***concentration effect.***[24] In an imaginary situation where a patient is breathing 100% anesthetic, uptake into pulmonary blood reduces the volume of anesthetic gas in the alveoli without altering its concentration or partial pressure (oxygen-induced atelectasis occurs through a similar mechanism). A typical situation, illustrated in Fig. 20.8, is delivery of 66% N_2O with 33% O_2 and 1% isoflurane. Assuming cardiac output equals 5 L/min, the initial rate of N_2O uptake is given by Eq. (20.7) as 5000 mL/min × 0.47 × 0.66 atm = 1550 mL/min, indicating that a large fraction of N_2O is taken up into blood during the first few breaths. If we assume that half the N_2O and half the isoflurane are rapidly taken up following the first breath of this gas mixture, then alveolar volume drops by 33.5% and the remaining alveolar gas contains 33 parts N_2O, 33 parts O_2, and 0.5 parts isoflurane (49.6% N_2O, 49.6% O_2, and 0.8% isoflurane). Despite 50% uptake of N_2O, the significant reduction in alveolar gas volume results in a concentration of remaining alveolar N_2O that is only 24% less than its initial value.

The *second gas effect* is also evident in this example: the rapid uptake of N_2O and reduced alveolar gas volume sustains P_{iso} near its original inspired value and increases alveolar P_{O_2}, thereby augmenting uptake of these gases.[25] The rapid uptake of N_2O into blood also results in an effective increase in MV, because more gas from the breathing circuit is passively drawn into lung as alveolar gas is rapidly absorbed. These effects have been demonstrated in

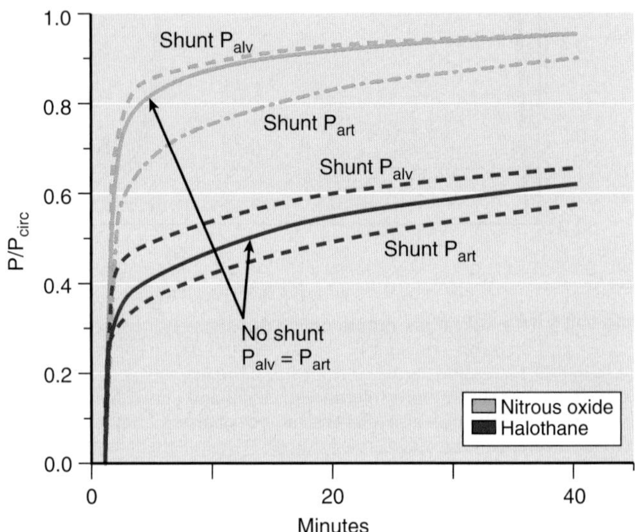

Fig. 20.7 Effect of right-to-left pulmonary shunt on the anesthetic partial pressure in alveolar gas and arterial blood. The curves represent anesthetic partial pressures in alveolar gases *(dashed lines)* and arterial blood *(dash-dot lines)* under conditions of 40% right-to-left shunt and no shunt *(solid lines)*. Pulmonary right-to-left shunting bypasses alveolar uptake, so less anesthetic is removed from pulmonary gases; this accelerates the rise in P_{alv}. In addition, the anesthetic partial pressure in arterial blood (P_{art}) is a mixture of pulmonary venous blood at P_{alv} and shunted mixed venous blood at P_{MV}. Thus P_{art}, which determines the rate of anesthetic uptake into tissues, rises more slowly than P_{alv} when R-to-L shunting is present. The shunt effect on P_{art} versus P_{alv} is larger for insoluble anesthetics (e.g., N_2O) than for soluble anesthetics (e.g., halothane). Other model parameters were set for open circuit delivery (constant P_{circ}) with MV = 6 L/min and CO = 5 L/min. *CO,* Cardiac output; *MV,* minute ventilation; *P_{MV},* anesthetic partial pressure in mixed venous blood; *P/P_{circ}*.

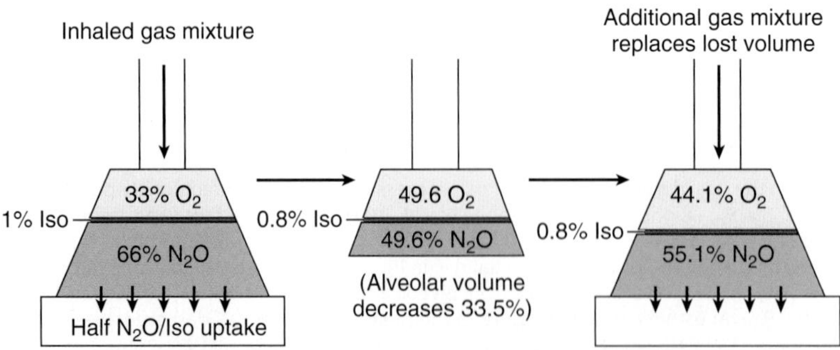

Fig. 20.8 Concentration and second gas effects. The figure depicts alveolar gases at the beginning of an anesthetic. After an initial inspiratory breath, alveoli are filled with the gas mixture in the circuit (66% N_2O, 33% O_2, 1% Isoflurane) at their normal end-inspiratory volume *(left panel)*. After half of the N_2O and isoflurane are absorbed into pulmonary blood, the alveolar gas volume is reduced by 33.5%. At this point, the volume of N_2O equals the volume of O_2 and the gas mixture is 49.6% N_2O, 49.6% O_2, 0.8% isoflurane. Inflow of additional inspired gas mixture returns alveolar volume to its original value, resulting in a gas mixture of 55.1% N_2O, 44.1% O_2, 0.8% isoflurane. The alveolar partial pressure of N_2O falls much less than the fractional uptake (the concentration effect). In addition, the partial pressure of O_2 *increases* relative to the inspired gas O_2 content, and the partial pressure of isoflurane is sustained close to the inspired value, increasing its rate of uptake (the second gas effect). *Iso,* Isoflurane; *N_2O,* nitrous oxide; *O_2,* oxygen.

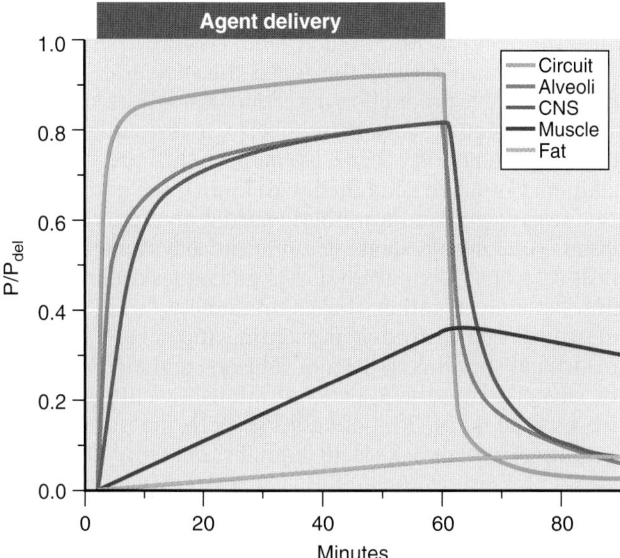

Fig. 20.9 The rate of anesthetic partial pressure rise in different tissue compartments. The curves represent model calculations for sevoflurane delivered at 6 L/min fresh gas flow, with 5 L/min ventilation and 5 L/min cardiac output. The anesthetic partial pressure in the central nervous system (*CNS; purple line*), part of the vessel rich group, equilibrates rapidly with P_{alv} *(blue line)*, although a lag-time of several minutes is evident when P_{alv} is rapidly rising or falling. The anesthetic partial pressures in both muscle *(red line)* and fat *(orange line)* rise and fall much more slowly, because muscle and fat compartments represent much larger effective volumes (see Fig. 20.2) and have lower blood flow than the vessel-rich group. Note that anesthetic partial pressure in fat continues to rise after anesthetic delivery stops, as long as partial pressure in alveolar gas (and arterial blood) is greater than that in the fat compartment.

humans[26] and lab animals.[25] Recent clinical studies and mathematical modeling indicate that, because of ventilation-perfusion heterogeneity, the second gas effect is greater in arterial blood than in expired gas, influenced by the blood solubility of VAs, and significantly affects anesthetic onset at relatively low rates of N_2O uptake.[27-29]

Distribution of Anesthetic into Tissues

Blood exiting the pulmonary capillaries enters the pulmonary vein and the left heart. Inhaled anesthetics are then distributed via arterial blood to various body tissues. The rate of increase of anesthetic partial pressure within each tissue is determined by tissue-specific arterial blood flow ($\dot{q}$), effective volume (the product of anatomic volume and tissue/blood partition coefficient, $\lambda_{t/b}$), and the anesthetic partial pressure gradient between arterial blood and the tissue,

$$\frac{dP_i}{dt} = \frac{\dot{q}_i}{V_i \times \lambda_{i/b}} \times (P_{art} - P_i), \qquad (20.10)$$

where i designates a particular organ or type of tissue. Values used in model calculations are summarized in Table 20.2. The time required for anesthetic partial pressure equilibration between arterial blood ($P_{art} = P_{alv}$) and a specified tissue is shorter if its blood flow is high, and longer if that tissue has a large effective volume (Figs. 20.2 and 20.9).

Traditionally, anesthetic distribution has been described for four distinct tissue groups. The ***vessel-rich group*** (VRG) includes the heart, brain, lungs, spinal cord, liver, and kidney. Together, these organs compose approximately 10% of the adult human body mass; however, they receive approximately 70% of cardiac output under normal resting conditions. As a result, time constants for anesthetic equilibration between blood and these organs are typically only a few minutes (see Table 20.2). Of particular interest is the equilibration time for the CNS, where anesthetic effects are mediated. After the highly perfused VRG tissues, ***skeletal muscle*** is the next compartment to equilibrate with inhaled anesthetics. Muscle composes approximately 40% of body mass in a healthy adult, making muscle the largest single compartment based on weight. Moreover, most inhaled anesthetics partition into muscle more than into brain, resulting in an increased effective volume for anesthetic uptake into this compartment. At rest, muscle receives about 10% to 15% of cardiac output (20 mL/kg/min), but this value can increase dramatically during exercise, stress, fever, or other states associated with high cardiac output.[30] Taken together, these factors generally result in slow equilibration between anesthetic in blood and muscle, with typical time constants of hours (see Table 20.2). The third tissue group is ***fat***, which in a healthy adult composes less than 25% of body mass and receives approximately 10% of cardiac output.[31] Potent VAs partition avidly into fat; therefore, fat represents the largest effective volume for uptake of these drugs (see Fig. 20.2, Table 20.2). The extremely large effective volume coupled with low blood flow results in very slow equilibration of anesthetics between blood and fat, with time constants approaching days. A fourth group, including skin, cortical bone, and connective tissue, is referred to as ***vessel poor tissues***. These tissues compose 10% to 15% of an average adult body while receiving less than 5% of cardiac output at rest. Induction of general anesthesia impairs normal sympathetic nervous function, resulting in increased blood flow to normally cool skin in the extremities.[32] The blood volume represents approximately 7% of body mass and may be considered another compartment for anesthetic uptake, while also conveying drug to other tissue compartments.

As stated previously, increased cardiac output results in increased anesthetic uptake and a slower rate of rise of P_{alv}. Clinical studies confirm that, other factors being equal, increasing cardiac output slows the induction of general anesthesia with inhaled anesthetics.[21,33] This result can seem counterintuitive when increasing cardiac output increases uptake of anesthetic into the patient's body and hastens its delivery to the tissues. However, during induction, the anesthetic partial pressure in blood and downstream tissue compartments cannot be higher than that in the upstream alveolar compartment. Increased cardiac output slows the rise of P_{alv} and thus also slows the rate of increase of the anesthetic partial pressure in blood (P_{art}), the CNS (P_{CNS}), and other highly perfused tissues. The extra anesthetic uptake is primarily into muscle, which is a large tissue compartment with a high capacity for anesthetic and is where much of the excess cardiac output flows. For example, a 50% increase in cardiac output can more than double muscle blood flow, diverting the majority of anesthetic to muscle, lowering P_{alv}, and thus slowing anesthetic uptake into target tissues in the CNS. If one could manipulate inhaled anesthetic delivery to maintain constant P_{alv}, which may be achievable with automated feedback control of vaporizer output and FGF,[34] then increased cardiac output might have a different effect. Model simulations where P_{alv} is maintained at a constant level show that uptake into VRG tissues, including brain tissue, increases more rapidly as cardiac output increases.[35]

In pediatric patients, the balance of cardiac output to various tissue beds differs from that in adults. Thus, although cardiac output per kilogram body weight is larger in children than in adults, anesthetic induction in young children is more rapid than in adults, because a disproportionate amount of perfusion goes to the vessel rich organs, such as the brain.[36]

The equilibrium distribution volumes for most inhaled anesthetics are extremely large, with the largest compartment by far being fat. However, equilibration with fat is so slow that this compartment usually plays a relatively minor role in the pharmacokinetics of inhaled anesthetics. During a typical general anesthetic lasting from 30 minutes to several hours, the blood, VRG organs, and muscle are the compartments into which inhaled anesthetics mostly distribute.

Although the model in Fig. 20.2 illustrates anesthetic distribution only via arterial blood flow, ***intertissue diffusion*** takes place between abutting tissues that have large interfacial surface areas. In particular, direct diffusion from organs with high anesthetic partial pressures to abutting tissues with low partial pressure and high capacity for anesthetic uptake may also contribute to drug distribution. Examples of this process include anesthetic diffusion from the heart, liver, and kidneys to surrounding fat in the pericardium and abdomen.[37,38]

The Mixed Venous Anesthetic Partial Pressure

The anesthetic partial pressure in mixed venous blood entering the pulmonary circulation is a weighted average of the venous outflows from all tissues and organs, which converge in the right ventricle:

$$P_{MV} = \sum_{i=1}^{n} \frac{\dot{q}_i}{\dot{Q}} \times P_i. \tag{20.11}$$

As P_{MV} rises, the gradient driving uptake of inhaled anesthetics from alveoli weakens. The difference between the delivered (inspired) and the alveolar (end-expiratory) anesthetic concentrations also shrinks, causing transpulmonary uptake to slow (Eq. 20.7). *Systemic (left to right) shunting* causes P_{MV} to increase more rapidly than it would in the absence of such shunts. When blood flow to other tissues remains normal and the left-to-right shunt simply represents excess cardiac output, the resulting increase in anesthetic uptake (Eq. 20.7) is offset by the increase in P_{MV}, resulting in a slight increase in the rate of anesthetic delivery or uptake into the brain, muscle, and other tissues. In cases where large left-to-right shunts result in reduced blood flow to other tissues, anesthetic equilibration in those tissues will be relatively slow.

Synthesis of the Model and Inhaled Anesthetic Induction: PK/PD

The earlier discussion emphasized the rate of equilibration (pharmacokinetics) of inhaled anesthetics among the various compartments involved in delivery to a patient: vaporizer, circuit, lung, blood, and various tissues. However, in a clinical setting, the goal of the anesthesia provider is the reversible production of certain desired effects (amnesia, unconsciousness, and immobility) in the patient within a reasonable period of time. To achieve this goal, pharmacokinetics must be combined with knowledge of the effects produced at different anesthetic partial pressures in target tissues (i.e., dose-response or pharmacodynamics).[39] The most relevant pharmacodynamic guidelines are minimum alveolar concentration (MAC)-immobility,[40] the alveolar anesthetic concentration preventing movement response to surgical stimulus in 50% of subjects, and MAC-awake,[7] the alveolar anesthetic concentration preventing perceptive awareness in 50% of subjects, both measured under conditions where P_{alv} is in equilibrium with anesthetic partial pressure in the CNS (P_{CNS}). MAC-awake for potent VAs is typically 0.34 × MAC-immobility,[41] whereas MAC-awake for N_2O is approximately 0.7 × MAC-immobility (see Table 20.1). During induction of anesthesia, the goal may be achieving a high probability of immobility following incision ($P_{CNS} \approx 1.2 \times$ MAC-immobility) within 15 minutes, while avoiding the deleterious effects of overly deep anesthesia. At the end of an anesthetic, return of consciousness is likely to occur when P_{CNS} decreases to less than MAC-awake. The targets used for this illustrative model patient are estimates. In clinical practice, the target for depth of general anesthesia should always minimize the risk of awareness (consciousness), but may vary, depending on patient factors, the presence of noxious stimuli, and other drugs that may be administered.

There are a variety of strategies to deliver inhaled anesthetics and to achieve the desired and reversible effects of anesthesia within a reasonable timeframe. The first important consideration is that P_{del} from the vaporizer must be higher than our target P_{alv} or P_{CNS} (***overpressure***). The more overpressure used, the more rapidly anesthetic is delivered. High fresh gas flows, large MV, and a low-solubility drug will also increase the rate of anesthetic delivery and the rate of rise of P_{alv} and P_{CNS}. These factors, and particularly overpressure, also increase the risk of delivering an overdose of anesthetic drug. A common strategy is to initiate inhaled anesthetic delivery with moderate to high fresh gas flows (≥ 6 L/min) and moderate overpressure (P_{del} = 2 × MAC-immobility), and reduce P_{del} after P_{alv} reaches or slightly exceeds the target level (Fig. 20.10, left). The need to maintain overpressure and slightly overshoot P_{alv} derives from the fact that distribution of drug to muscle maintains a high delivery requirement after the initial rapid phase of uptake. If P_{del} is decreased too quickly, then P_{alv} can decrease below the target. P_{del} or FGF is slowly adjusted downward as the anesthetic inspired-to-expired difference in anesthetic partial pressures ($P_{del}-P_{alv}$) decreases.

Closed-Circuit or Low-Flow Delivery of Anesthesia

The use of high or moderate fresh gas flows, while enabling use of less overpressure, results in far more anesthetic drug being delivered than being taken up into tissues. As illustrated in Fig. 20.10C, the amount of isoflurane delivered is 4.5-fold greater than that taken up, and delivered sevoflurane is 7.2-fold greater than absorbed drug. Thus more than 80% of delivered VA is waste using the moderately

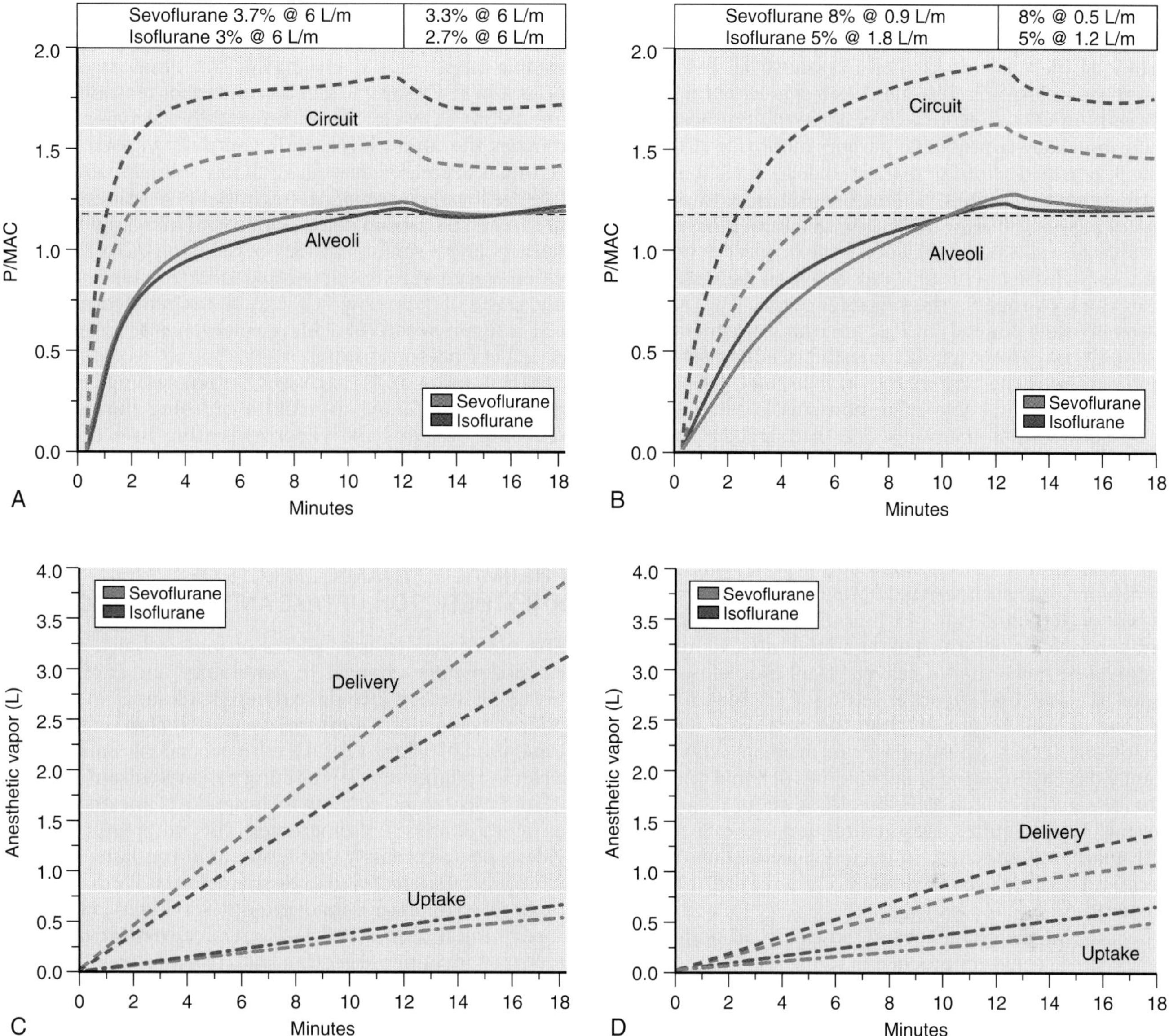

Fig. 20.10 Effect of induction technique on uptake and delivery of inhaled anesthetics. (A) Anesthetic partial pressures in both the circuit *(dashed lines)* and alveoli *(solid lines)* during inhalation induction with moderate (6 L/min) fresh gas flows and modest (twofold to threefold) overpressure for sevoflurane *(blue)* and isoflurane *(purple)*. P_{alv} reaches 1.2 × MAC in about 12 minutes, and approximately 10% downward adjustment of vaporizer settings results in maintenance of P_{alv} near this target level. Additional downward adjustments in vaporizer setting or fresh gas flows, or both, would be needed to further maintain this P_{alv} level. (B) Anesthetic partial pressures in both the circuit and alveoli during inhalation induction with low (<2 L/min) fresh gas flows and maximal (fourfold) overpressure for sevoflurane *(blue)* and isoflurane *(purple)*. P_{alv} reaches 1.2 × MAC in approximately 12 minutes, and a downward adjustment of fresh gas flow results in maintenance of P_{alv} near this target level. (C) The total anesthetic vapor delivered and taken up into the model patient from panel A. Note that delivery far exceeds uptake, more so for the low solubility anesthetic (sevoflurane). (D) The total amount of anesthetic vapor delivered and taken up into the model patient from panel B. Note that uptake is very similar to that in panel C, whereas delivery is much lower. The low fresh gas flow technique (panels B and D) reduces waste more so for anesthetics with low blood solubility (e.g., sevoflurane) than for soluble drugs (e.g., isoflurane). *MAC,* Minimum alveolar concentration; P_{alv}, alveolar anesthetic partial pressure.

high FGF approach illustrated in this example (settings are shown in Fig. 20.10*A*). Rebreathing circuits allow the use of fresh gas flows well below MV, which results in reduced anesthetic discharge into the waste-scavenging system. Less waste discharge translates into both reduced costs and reduced global environmental impact of anesthetic gases in the atmosphere, where they contribute to climate change (discussed later in this chapter). Additional benefits of low FGF and rebreathing include retention of expired heat and water vapor in rebreathed gas, improving airway epithelial health, and reducing accumulation of dried airway secretions.[42]

Closed-circuit anesthesia represents the ultimate limit of low gas flows, where fresh gases are delivered only in quantities sufficient to replace those taken up into tissues, metabolized (especially O_2), or otherwise lost to the environment, and the vast majority of gas in the breathing circuit undergoes rebreathing.[43] Achieving this goal requires a leak-free breathing circuit, complete removal of CO_2, and careful attention to the inspired-to-expired values of oxygen and anesthetic gases, and even to expired nitrogen that may slowly accumulate in the breathing circuit. Under these conditions, oxygen consumption in an anesthetized patient may be lower than 3 mL/kg/min, translating to

O_2 replacement of approximately 200 mL/min in a 70 kg patient. There are several significant limitations to this technique. Because all exhaled CO_2 must be removed by absorbents, closed-circuit anesthesia increases the risk of rebreathing CO_2 as absorbent capacity diminishes. Anesthetic breakdown products, carbon monoxide (CO), and slowly degassing nitrogen from blood can accumulate in the breathing circuit.[44] Clinicians must be aware that patient metabolism may deplete oxygen from the breathing circuit and result in delivery of a hypoxic gas mixture during use of closed circuit anesthesia. When using very low FGF values, changes in the vaporizer output (P_{del}) result in extremely slow changes in P_{circ} and the subsequent depth of anesthesia. Closed circuit anesthetic administration is often guided by the "square root of time rule," proposed by Severinghaus[45] and detailed in now classic descriptions.[46] This rule states that the rate of anesthetic uptake decreases approximately as the square root of delivery time. We can estimate the uptake of 1.2 MAC isoflurane during the first minute of anesthesia using Eq. (20.7). Thus cardiac output × $\lambda_{b/g}$ × 1.2 MAC = Initial uptake of isoflurane vapor (5000 mL/min × 1.4 × 0.0128 atm = 90 mL/min). Using the square-root of time rule, uptake at 4 minutes would be half of the initial rate (45 mL/min), and at 9 minutes, uptake would be one-third of the initial rate (30 mL/min). It should be noted that to deliver 90 mL/min of isoflurane vapor at a maximal vaporizer setting of 5% requires 1800 mL/min of FGF, far greater than the target FGF for closed circuit anesthesia. Anesthetists can overcome this limitation by directly injecting small volumes of liquid anesthetic into the expiratory limb of the breathing circuit;[47] however, this technique requires vigilant attention to the clock along with many other factors. In inexperienced hands, miscalculation or mistiming of anesthetic injection runs the risk of overdose.

Because of the challenges of closed-circuit administration, a more common practice is to use moderate to high fresh gas flows to achieve rapid changes during induction of anesthesia, reserving closed circuit anesthesia to periods where the $P_{circ}-P_{alv}$ difference is small. Even so, changes in a patient's metabolism because of temperature variation, degree of muscle relaxation, or surgical stimulation can result in the need for frequent adjustments to oxygen flow and anesthetic depth, making anesthesia delivery in a closed circuit system relatively unstable and difficult.

Low-flow anesthetic delivery, typically with fresh gas flows of 0.5 to 1.0 L/min during the maintenance phase of an anesthetic, is a compromise between closed-circuit conditions and the use of high fresh gas flows. Much of the waste and other problems associated with high fresh gas flows are avoided, while the instability associated with a strict closed-circuit technique is also moderated. As noted earlier (see section on "Equilibration Between Circuit and Pulmonary Airspace"), the inspired anesthetic concentration (P_{circ}) depends on both P_{del} and P_{pulm} when rebreathing occurs. Thus, as FGF diminishes, P_{del} must be adjusted upward to compensate for diminished delivery. Given that the maximal output setting on most vaporizers is about 4 × MAC-immobility, anesthetic delivery at 1 L/min and maximal P_{del} is still far less than the previous example with 6 L/min and P_{del} = 2 × MAC isoflurane. Higher FGF or a less soluble anesthetic drug, or both, is needed to achieve target P_{CNS} in less than 15 minutes, but as uptake diminishes, FGF can be gradually reduced (Fig. 20.10, right panels). With soluble anesthetics like isoflurane, maximal vaporizer settings and FGF near 2 L/min is required for reasonably rapid induction. FGF can be incrementally decreased as P_{alv} reaches the target level, and eventually vaporizer output setting is decreased as well. With low solubility anesthetics like desflurane or sevoflurane, initial FGF values near 1.0 L/min can be used in combination with maximal vaporizer settings and a similar strategy of reducing FGF. These conditions result in reasonably rapid induction while minimizing waste of VAs. Low FGF can be maintained until high FGF is again needed to achieve emergence at the end of the anesthetic administration.

When using high vaporizer output settings, diligence must be maintained to avoid overdosing the patient by reducing FGF and the vaporizer setting in a timely and deliberate manner. Use of significant overpressure should be avoided in situations when other clinical issues require the attention of the anesthesia provider.

PHARMACODYNAMIC EFFECTS OF ANESTHETICS ON UPTAKE AND DISTRIBUTION

The pharmacodynamic effects of most inhaled anesthetics also include changes in ventilatory and cardiac function that thereby introduce dynamic changes in the drug pharmacokinetics. ***Spontaneous ventilation*** is reduced by inhalation of potent VAs in a dose-dependent manner.[48] As a result, spontaneously breathing patients will autoregulate to some degree by reducing their uptake of anesthetic agent as depth of anesthesia increases. This autoregulation provides a degree of safety that is absent in ventilated patients, who may be subjected to excessive delivery of inhaled anesthetics if a vaporizer is inadvertently set to deliver overpressure.[49] Inhaled anesthetics also reduce ***cardiac output***, a pharmacodynamic effect that leads to a more rapid increase in P_{alv}/P_{circ} and consequently a more rapid increase in the anesthetic partial pressure in heart, brain, and other highly perfused tissues.[50] Halothane is the anesthetic associated with the greatest reduction in cardiac output. If anesthetic delivery continues in the face of a falling cardiac output, this can lead to a positive feedback loop of worsening cardiac depression and a rapid descent toward hemodynamic collapse. More details on the effects of inhaled anesthetics on respiratory and circulatory systems are provided in Chapter 21.

THE EFFECT OF NITROUS OXIDE ON GAS-FILLED SPACES

Because N_2O is often used at high partial pressures, it diffuses into and accumulates in spaces containing air or other immobile gases, with potentially deleterious physiologic consequences. Clinically relevant examples include intravascular air emboli,[51] pneumothorax,[52] air in the inner chamber of the ear,[53] intravitreal gas bubbles,[54] intrathecal air, pneumoencephalus,[55] and air in the gastrointestinal tract.[52] Air-filled spaces contain mostly nitrogen, a gas that composes 78% of air but is 30-fold less soluble in blood than N_2O ($\lambda_{b/g}$ for N_2 is 0.015). Thus N_2O diffuses down its pressure gradient from blood and surrounding tissues into

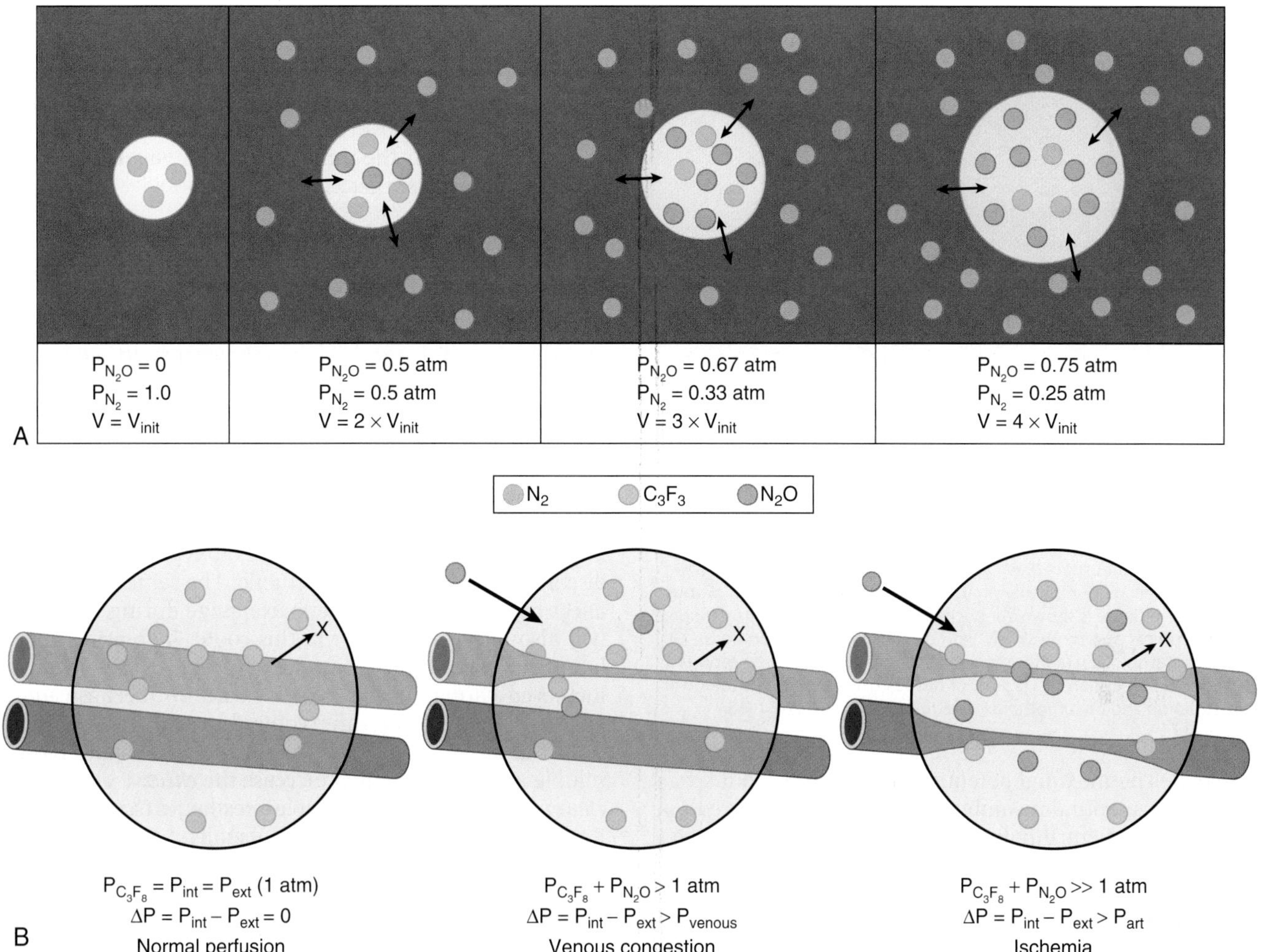

Fig. 20.11 Nitrous oxide accumulation in gas-filled spaces. A, Expansion of a compliant air-filled space (a small vascular air embolus) occurs as the partial pressure of nitrous oxide in surrounding blood increases. Each panel depicts the equilibrium condition with PN_2O inside the bubble equal to that in blood. Labels below each panel summarize the partial pressures of N_2O and N_2 in the bubble as well as the bubble volume relative to its initial value (Vinit). B, The increase in pressure inside a noncompliant, gas-filled compartment (e.g., an eye following perfluoropropane [C_3F_8] injection) with blood vessels passing through it. As N_2O accumulates, the pressure in the compartment increases, which can result in venous congestion (middle panel) or ischemia (right panel) in tissues that are perfused by the vessels in this compartment (e.g., the retina). *Atm*, Atmosphere; *ΔP*, difference between internal and external pressure; *N_2*, nitrogen; *N_2O*, nitrous oxide; *P_{art}*, arterial blood pressure; *PC_3F_8*, partial pressure of perfluoropropane; *P_{ext}*, pressure outside the compartment; *P_{int}*, internal compartment pressure; *PN_2*, partial pressure of nitrogen; *PN_2O*, partial pressure of N_2O; *P_{venous}*, venous blood pressure.

air-filled spaces, whereas N_2 elimination from these spaces is far slower, even with inspired $P_{N2} = 0$. As N_2O enters and the total number of gas molecules in an air space increases, it will expand in volume, increase in pressure, or both, depending on the compliance of the tissues surrounding the air-filled space.

In ***highly compliant air-filled spaces***, such as intravascular air bubbles or small pneumothoraces, N_2O accumulation increases the total volume of gas (Fig. 20.11*A*) with minimal changes in pressure. Air spaces expand as N_2O enters until the P_{N2O} within the air space matches that in surrounding blood, establishing equilibrium. The maximum potential gas volume expansion in a highly compliant space is

$$\frac{V}{V_{init}} = \frac{1}{1 - P_{N_2O}}. \qquad (20.12)$$

Thus administration of 50% N_2O can double air-space volume, whereas 67% can potentially triple air-space volume. N_2O can significantly worsen the cardiovascular or tissue consequences of intravascular air emboli, potentially making a nonlethal volume of venous air embolus become lethal.[51] Expansion of gastrointestinal gas volume by N_2O may impede surgical exposure or abdominal wound closure. Gas-space compartment compliance eventually decreases as volume expands, resulting in increased pressure. For example, N_2O may expand a small pneumothorax to a point where intrathoracic pressure rises, compressing lung, displacing the mediastinum, and reducing venous return (tension pneumothorax). N_2O is contraindicated in patients with intracranial air until after dural opening, in order to avoid intracranial hypertension.[56] The endotracheal tube cuff filled with air is also susceptible to expansion by N_2O. Increased tracheal cuff pressure may impair perfusion of surrounding mucosa.[57] Air-filled laryngeal mask airway cuffs[58] and the air-filled balloon of a Swan-Ganz catheter[59] may similarly expand during N_2O administration.

In ***noncompliant gas-filled spaces***, gas pressure rises as N_2O enters, until P_{N2O} within the air space matches that

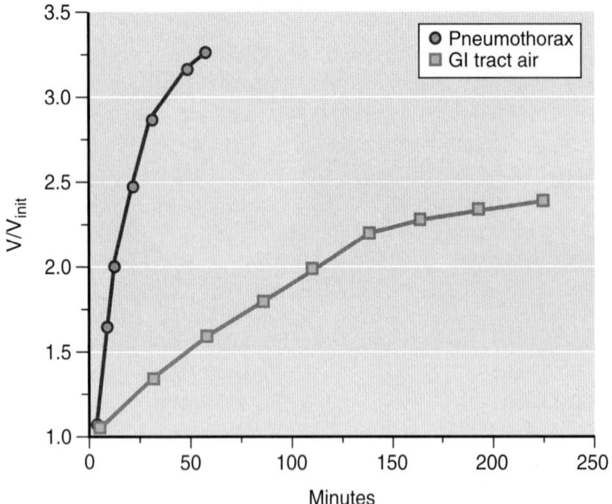

Fig. 20.12 The rate of air-space expansion during nitrous oxide administration. The rate and extent of expansion of air pockets injected into either the pleural space *(red circles)* or the gastrointestinal tract *(blue squares)* of dogs during the inhalation of a 25% oxygen/75% nitrous oxide gas mixture is shown. Air pockets in the stomach, small intestine, and colon expand more slowly than do those in a pneumothorax. *GI*, Gastrointestinal. (Data are approximations from the results reported in Eger EI II, Saidman LJ. Hazards of nitrous oxide anesthesia in bowel obstruction and pneumothorax. *Anesthesiology*. 1965;26:61–66.)

in blood. The maximal potential pressure in such a space, relative to surrounding ambient pressure, is therefore P_{N2O}. Thus, in a patient inhaling 50% N_2O, pressure in such a gas-filled compartment could approach 380 mm Hg, far greater than typical arterial perfusion pressures. A clinically important example is that of intravitreal sulfur hexafluoride (SF_6) or perfluoropropane (C_3F_8) bubbles, which are injected as the sclera is closed at the end of intraocular or retinal surgery (see Fig. 20.11*B*).[54] These gases persist even longer than N_2 does, because of their low blood solubility. If N_2O is administered to these patients at the time of intravitreal bubble injection, its diffusion into the bubble can rapidly increase intraocular pressure above that in retinal veins, producing retinal congestion. If the pressure in the eye further increases above systolic arterial pressure, retinal ischemia resulting in blindness may ensue.

The ***rate of N_2O diffusion into gas-filled spaces*** in the body depends on local blood flow and the surface to volume ratio of the space. Thus small air emboli expand within seconds, because they have high surface/volume ratios and are surrounded by a very high relative flow of blood containing dissolved N_2O. Larger air emboli expand more slowly, because their surface/volume ratios are smaller (spherical surface/volume is inversely proportional to radius). Small pneumothoraces typically have large surface/volume ratios and high local blood flow. Animal experiments show that inhalation of 75% N_2O approximately doubles pneumothorax volume in 10 minutes and triples it in 30 minutes (Fig. 20.12). Compared with a pneumothorax, gastrointestinal air pockets have lower surface/volume ratios and lower blood flow. Thus expansion of gas in the gastrointestinal tract is much slower than that in a pneumothorax. In animal studies (see Fig. 20.12), inhalation of 70% to 80% N_2O doubled intestinal gas volume after approximately 2 hours.[52]

N_2O use is contraindicated in patients with pneumothorax, pneumocephalus, and closed dura, or in those at high risk for vascular air embolus. Air-space expansion may impede surgery when substantial gastrointestinal air is present and N_2O exposure is prolonged, or it can be of little consequence when the initial volume of gas in the gut is small or when the surgery is brief.

RECOVERY FROM ANESTHESIA

Similarities and Differences to Induction

Clearance of inhaled anesthetics from target tissues (brain and spinal cord) is primarily via the same pathways used for anesthetic induction: anesthetic gases flow from tissue into venous blood and then to the lungs. If P_{alv} is less than P_{MV}, then the net flow of anesthetic will be out of the blood and into alveoli, where it is subsequently exhaled. To achieve the fastest clearance possible, P_{circ} must therefore be as low as possible, and this is achieved using high flows of nonanesthetic carrier gases (oxygen and air) after discontinuing delivery of anesthetic. The same factors that affect transalveolar anesthetic exchange during induction will also affect clearance via this route. Increasing ventilation will accelerate clearance (see Fig. 20.4), whereas increased cardiac output slows clearance, because more gas-exchange volumes are required to remove anesthetic from the larger blood flow (see Fig. 20.5). Highly blood-soluble anesthetics, which increase the *effective* blood flow, clear more slowly than insoluble anesthetics (see Fig. 20.6). Return-to-consciousness, which usually occurs after P_{CNS} decreases below MAC-awake, is faster following desflurane or sevoflurane anesthesia than after isoflurane anesthesia. N_2O, which is characterized by blood solubility similar to that of desflurane, provides an even faster return to consciousness, because of two additional advantages. First, the concentration effect works in reverse during clearance of N_2O, increasing effective alveolar ventilation and maintaining the gradient for flow from pulmonary blood to alveoli. Second, MAC-awake for N_2O (0.71 atm at 40 years old) is near typical inhaled concentrations during general anesthesia; therefore, elimination of only a small fraction of this drug is associated with return to consciousness. This is also why N_2O as the sole hypnotic drug is associated with a high risk of intraoperative awareness, which can be prevented by using a balanced gas mixture of N_2O together with end-tidal concentrations of about 1 × MAC-awake of a second potent inhaled anesthetic.

Body composition has an increasing impact as the length of anesthetic exposure increases, especially for highly soluble anesthetics. Compared with standard models, patients with increased muscle or fat will have larger volumes of anesthetic drug distribution over time, resulting in slower clearance rates.[60] One important difference between anesthetic uptake and clearance is that although overpressure can be utilized to hasten uptake and induction of anesthesia, the vaporizer setting cannot be set to less than zero. As a consequence, the most readily modifiable factors to affect the rate of anesthetic clearance are fresh gas flow and MV. Indeed, after prolonged (>4 hours) exposure to 1 × MAC inhaled anesthesia, maintenance of adequate ventilation should be a high priority, even after end-tidal anesthetic concentrations reach MAC-awake. Hypoventilation in this

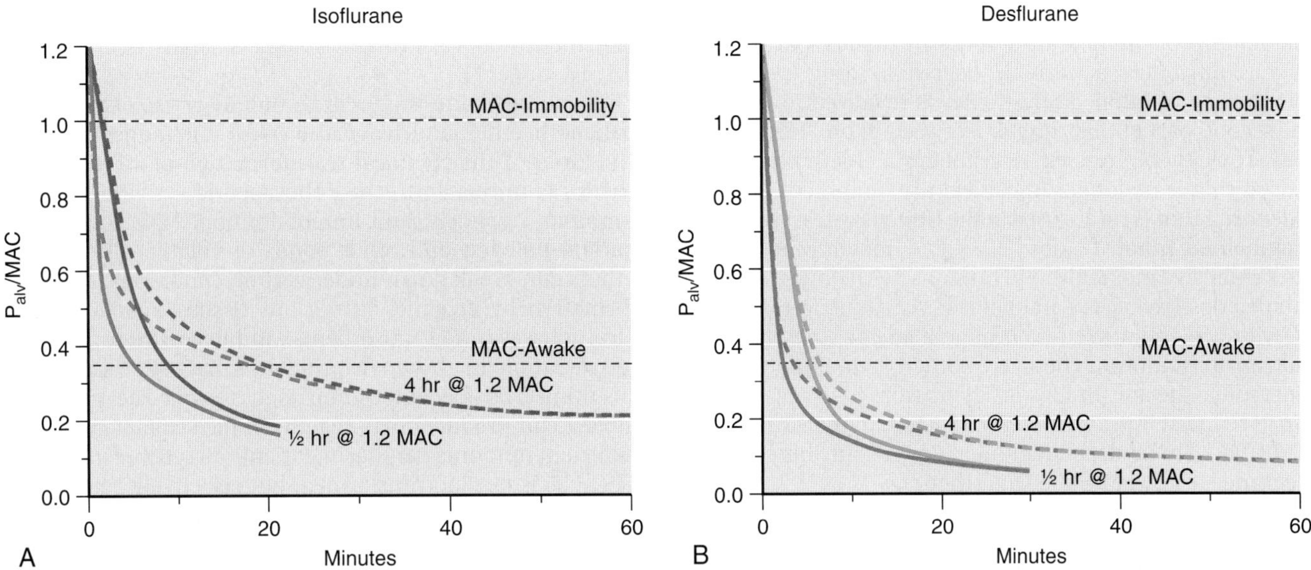

Fig. 20.13 Inhaled anesthetic wash-out and time to awakening depends on duration of anesthesia. The panels depict model calculations of P_{alv} and P_{CNS} normalized to MAC during wash-out at 10 L/min FGF and 5 L/min MV following anesthesia at approximately 1.2 × MAC-immobility for 30 minutes *(solid lines)* or 4 hours *(dashed lines)*. The MAC-awake (approximately 0.34 × MAC-immobility) is shown to indicate the threshold below which typical patients regain perceptive awareness after general anesthesia. Although P_{alv} drops earlier than P_{CNS}, the clinically relevant endpoint (return of consciousness) is predicted when P_{CNS} falls below MAC-awake. (A) Wash-out using a pharmacokinetic model for isoflurane (orange is P_{alv}, purple is P_{CNS}). The 30-minute isoflurane uptake was 990 mL of vapor, and the 4-hour isoflurane uptake was 3420 mL of vapor. Prolonged anesthesia with isoflurane dramatically increases the time required to wash-out sufficient drug to achieve awakening. After a 30-minute anesthetic, P_{CNS} (solid purple line) drops to MAC-awake in 9 minutes, whereas it takes more than 20 minutes of wash-out to reach the same P_{CNS} following a 4-hour anesthetic (dashed purple line). (B) Wash-out using a desflurane model (blue is P_{alv}, green is P_{CNS}). The 30-minute desflurane uptake was 1530 mL of vapor, and the 4-hour desflurane uptake was 4600 mL of vapor. The predicted times to awakening (solid versus dashed green lines reach MAC-awake at 5.2 and 6.3 minutes, respectively) are much closer following different durations of desflurane anesthesia, because of its low blood solubility. Clinical studies demonstrate that emergence and recovery (time to extubation) following isoflurane anesthesia nearly doubles when exposure increases from 20 to 75 minutes, whereas extubation is achieved in less than 10 minutes following desflurane anesthesia from 20 to 100 minutes' duration.[63] *FGF*, Fresh gas flow; *MAC*, minimum alveolar concentration; *MV*, minute ventilation; P_{alv}, Alveolar anesthetic partial pressure; P_{CNS}, anesthetic partial pressure in the central nervous system.

situation can result in reanesthetization caused by redistribution of anesthetic drug from muscle into blood and highly perfused tissues.[61]

Context Sensitive Recovery from Anesthesia

Although the concept of context sensitive half-time is typically applied to continuously infused anesthetics that distribute among multiple pharmacokinetic compartments, it also applies to inhaled anesthetics.[62] After a short period of inhalation and uptake, anesthetic clearance from blood is rapid through both exhalation and distribution to muscle and other tissues. As a result, P_{alv} decreases rapidly to a low value after discontinuing anesthetic delivery. After prolonged periods of inhalation and uptake, the anesthetic partial pressures in muscle and other compartments increase closer to that in blood, reducing the contribution of distributive clearance. Instead, clearance from the central blood compartment is slowed by the reverse flow of anesthetic from the high-capacity tissues. Thus, in comparison with a short period of inhalation, prolonged inhaled anesthesia is followed by a smaller initial decrease in P_{alv} and a more pronounced slow clearance phase, resulting in slower recovery from anesthesia (Fig. 20.13).[63] As with other factors, context sensitivity is exaggerated in highly soluble anesthetics, and it has less impact with anesthetics that display low blood and tissue solubilities.[63] The relative advantage of low blood solubility anesthetics increases with the duration of anesthesia. There is only a small (2.5 minutes) difference between predicted times to awakening after a short anesthetic with isoflurane versus desflurane, but significantly faster awakening can be achieved using the low-solubility drug for long cases.

Percutaneous and Visceral Anesthetic Loss

Aside from pulmonary exchange, some portion of inhaled anesthetics is lost by diffusion through other large area interfaces between the body and surrounding air. The skin surface area of an average human is about 2 m^2, and blood flow through skin during general anesthesia may be substantial because of inhibition of normal thermoregulatory vasoconstriction.[32] Nonetheless, transcutaneous losses of general anesthetics probably contribute negligibly to their clearance.[64,65] During open abdominal or thoracic surgery, visceral surfaces are also directly exposed to air, and under these circumstances, anesthetic losses via direct transfer and air movements are larger than those via skin, but still a small fraction of total clearance.[66]

Effect of the Anesthetic Circuit

As mentioned earlier, circuit components, including tubing, connectors, manual ventilation bag, and CO_2 absorbent material, absorb inhaled anesthetics, effectively creating another compartment that fills while anesthetic is flowing, and needs to be emptied during wash-out.[19] Low-level release of anesthetic gases from these components can continue for a considerable time.

Clearance via Metabolism of Anesthetics

Metabolism of inhaled anesthetics in tissues, particularly liver, contributes a variable degree to drug clearance. Metabolism of inhaled anesthetics is reviewed in detail in the second part of this chapter (see section on "Metabolism and Toxicity of Inhaled Anesthetics"). Methoxyflurane, a drug that is no longer in clinical use, and halothane, an older drug that is rarely used in the United States, are highly metabolized inhaled anesthetics. Methoxyflurane undergoes extensive metabolism in humans, with only 19% of an inhaled dose recovered in exhaled gases.[67] Approximately 20% to 25% of inhaled halothane is metabolized through biotransformation in the liver. A high rate of metabolism will reduce the anesthetic partial pressure in tissues, resulting in reduced P_{MV} and increased rates of overall anesthetic clearance. Tissue-dependent breakdown contributes less to clearance of newer inhaled anesthetics.

Additional Considerations and Possibilities

Modern inhaled anesthetics like sevoflurane and desflurane have low blood solubility, and therefore provide a distinct advantage for both anesthetic induction and recovery from anesthesia. However, they present no advantage over older drugs like isoflurane for maintenance of anesthesia during long cases and are far more expensive. What if anesthesia is induced with one drug, followed by a switch to isoflurane during the maintenance period, and then switched back to the more soluble drug, such as desflurane, for a period preceding emergence? This might allow for more rapid induction and wakeup than with isoflurane alone. Although a fast wakeup can be achieved by allowing sufficient time for near total washout of isoflurane and its replacement with desflurane, this type of crossover requires significant lead time and high fresh gas flows. As an illustration, Neumann and colleagues[68] compared 2-hour anesthetics at 1.25 × MAC (2 L/min FGF) with isoflurane alone, desflurane alone, or isoflurane with a crossover to desflurane during the last half hour. Although subjects awoke faster with desflurane alone, the crossover strategy did not result in acceleration of wakeup compared to isoflurane alone.

Diffusion Hypoxia

Diffusion hypoxia is another sequelae of rapid outgassing from the tissues of patients anesthetized with N_2O. During the initial 5 to 10 minutes after discontinuation of anesthesia, the flow of N_2O from blood into the alveoli can be several liters per minute, resulting in dilution of alveolar oxygen.[69] Another effect of rapid outgassing is reduction of alveolar P_{CO_2}, which may also reduce respiratory drive.[70] If the patient does not receive supplemental oxygen during this period, then the combined effects of respiratory depression from anesthesia, reduced alveolar P_{CO_2}, and reduced alveolar P_{O_2} can result in hypoventilation and oxyhemoglobin desaturation. This outcome is avoided by routinely providing supplemental O_2 for the first 5 to 10 minutes of recovery, together with vigilant attention to respiration and oxygenation.

Metabolism and Toxicity of Inhaled Anesthetics

This portion of the chapter focuses on adverse effects that are attributable to inhaled anesthetics, excluding most of the acutely reversible pharmacodynamic effects of inhaled anesthetics on various physiologic systems (see Chapters 11, 14, and 21).

The inhaled anesthetics are a unique group of drugs that can both enter and leave the body unchanged through the lungs. Thus chemical transformation of inhaled anesthetics is unrelated to their therapeutic activities such as amnesia, hypnosis, and immobilization. Nonetheless, the carbon-halogen and other bonds of volatile alkanes and ethers can break down under certain conditions: biotransformation by enzymes in various tissues, reactions with strong bases in CO_2 absorbents, and exposure to ultraviolet radiation in the environment. Anesthetic breakdown resulting from decomposition in tissues or the breathing circuit can produce toxic reactive intermediates, which in sufficient amounts can harm patients directly or indirectly. N_2O gas is not biotransformed, but selectively reacts with and inactivates vitamin B_{12} and perturbs B_{12}-dependent biochemical pathways. The breakdown of waste anesthetics in the atmosphere also has potential environmental and health consequences. There are potential long-term neurotoxic effects of anesthetic exposure in patients that are not associated with chemical breakdown. Potential neurotoxic properties of inhaled anesthetics are further described in Chapters 78 and 84.

BIOTRANSFORMATION OF INHALED ANESTHETICS

The extent and location of inhaled anesthetic metabolism depends on multiple chemical factors. Inhaled anesthetics undergo varying degrees of biotransformation (Table 20.3)[71] in various tissues. Methoxyflurane undergoes by far the greatest metabolism, estimated at 70%, and experiments indicate that only a small fraction of drug taken up into body tissues is exhaled.[67] Given the remarkable lipophilicity of methoxyflurane, respiratory clearance of this drug from muscle and fat extends over a period of days (see Tables 20.1 and 20.2). Halothane is the next most lipophilic drug and ranks second in metabolic clearance (see Table 20.3).[72-96] Thus prolonged residence in body tissues is an important factor in biotransformation of inhaled anesthetics. Chemical stability is another important factor. Isoflurane is an isomer of enflurane, and the two drugs display comparable respiratory uptake, distribution, and respiratory clearance. Nonetheless, isoflurane is metabolized only one tenth as much as enflurane. Although sevoflurane and desflurane represent another pair of anesthetics, both are characterized by rapid uptake, distribution, and respiratory clearance with 5% of sevoflurane biotransformed versus 0.02% of desflurane.

Of the major organs involved in anesthetic biotransformation, the liver and kidneys are exposed to the highest metabolite concentrations and thus are also most susceptible to damage from toxic metabolites. Clinically significant hepatotoxicity is primarily associated with exposure to halothane, and nephrotoxicity is associated with methoxyflurane.[71] Investigations into the mechanisms of these toxicities have influenced drug development and also provided important insights into human toxicology.[97]

TABLE 20.3 Metabolism of Halogenated Volatile Anesthetics

Anesthetic	Halothane	Methoxyflurane	Enflurane	Isoflurane	Desflurane	Sevoflurane
Extent of tissue metabolism (%)	25	70	2.5	0.2	0.02	5
Oxidizing enzymes	CYP2E1 CYP2A6	CYP2E1 CYP1A2, 2C9/10, 2D6	CYP2E1	CYP2E1	CYP2E1	CYP2E1
Oxidative metabolites	$F_3C\text{-}COOH$ HBr, HCl	$H_3C\text{-}O\text{-}CF_2\text{-}COOH$ $HCl_2C\text{-}COOH$ HOOC-COOH HF, HCl	$HF_2C\text{-}O\text{-}CF_2\text{-}COOH$ HCl, HF	$HF_2C\text{-}O\text{-}CO\text{-}CF_3$ $F_3C\text{-}COOH$ CF_2HOH HCl	$HF_2C\text{-}O\text{-}CO\text{-}CF_3$ $F_3C\text{-}COOH$ CF_2HOH HF	$HO\text{-}CH(CF_3)_2$ HF
Trifuoroacetylated hepatocellular proteins	+++++	n/a	++	+	+	none
Reducing enzymes	CYP2A6 CYP3A4	n/a	n/a	n/a	n/a	
Reductive metabolites	F^-, Br^- $F_2C{=}CHCl$ $F_3C\text{-}CH_2Cl$					
Tissue toxicities	Hepatic	Renal Hepatic	Renal Hepatic	Hepatic	Hepatic	Hepatic
Fulminant hepatitis incidence	1:20,000	Reported, incidence unknown	1:300,000	rare	rare	Few case reports
References	72-76	77-80	81-85	84,86-88	89-92	78,93-96

The plus signs indicate relative degree of protein modification. n/a, the specific enzymes are not identified in these cases. Kharasch ED. Adverse drug reactions with halogenated anesthetics. *Clin Pharmacol Ther.* 2008;84:158–162.

Biotransformation in the Liver

The liver is the major site of metabolism for most drugs, particularly lipophilic drugs, which typically are transformed into hydrophilic metabolites that are more readily excreted. The liver is large and contains high concentrations of many drug-metabolizing enzymes. Other organs that contribute to drug metabolism and clearance include the gastrointestinal tract, kidneys, and lungs.[98,99] Drug biotransformation reactions include oxidation, hydrolysis, and conjugation. A single drug may be transformed into several metabolites, depending on the relative rates of various enzyme reactions, the drug concentration in different tissues expressing relevant enzymes, competition at enzyme sites with other drugs or endogenous substances, and other factors. Oxidation and hydrolysis are also known as *phase 1 reactions*, and they result in the introduction or exposure of a polar group on the drug. The phase 1 enzymes that metabolize inhaled anesthetics in the liver are various cytochrome P450 (CYP) isoforms in the endoplasmic reticulum of hepatocytes. These catalyze oxidation reactions such as dehalogenation, N- and O-dealkylation, N- and S-oxidation, and deamination. These reactions require oxygen and NADPH-dependent cytochrome P450 reductase as cofactors. Under hypoxic conditions, some P450 enzymes can also catalyze reductive reactions. More than 50 CYP isoforms are active in humans, and CYP3A4 and CYP3A5 are the most abundant. Conjugations are also known as *phase 2 reactions*, and they often append highly polar groups such as glucuronic acid, sulfate, or glycine to polar groups on phase 1 metabolites. The resulting hydrophilic products are readily excreted in urine via the kidneys or in bile via the gastrointestinal tract. N-Acetylation reactions are an exception that result in metabolites that are less water-soluble than the parent drug.

Many factors affect hepatic drug metabolism, including concomitant drugs, disease, age, and genetics.[100] Induction and inhibition of enzymes are associated with exposure to certain drugs or other exogenous substances. Induction of specific CYP isoforms is a gene-mediated response to chronic exposure to substances that often are substrates of the enzyme, resulting in accelerated enzyme production or slowed turnover. For example, phenobarbital use results in increased production of CYP3A4 as well as NADPH-cytochrome P450 reductase, leading to dramatically increased metabolism of all CYP3A4 substrates. Enhanced metabolism can reduce drug efficacy (and therefore is one mechanism of drug tolerance) or, in cases of prodrug transformation to active metabolites, increased efficacy. If metabolites are toxic, as is the case with VAs, enhanced metabolism may increase toxicity. Conversely, CYP inhibition leads to enhanced activity of parent drugs and reduced metabolite effects. CYP enzyme inhibition is associated with hepatic disease and exposure to certain substances. An important example is CYP3A4 inhibition by grapefruit juice.[100] Regarding VAs, the major oxidative enzyme CYP2E1 is inducible by ethanol and isoniazid and is inhibited by disulfiram.[101] Diseases such as hepatitis, various cirrhotic diseases, and hepatocarcinoma can also reduce enzymatic activity, as can cardiac failure with reduced hepatic perfusion.

Neonates have different dominant CYP isoforms than adults. Impaired hepatic metabolism is common in premature and full-term infants, notably in bilirubin glucuronidation, leading to hyperbilirubinemia of the newborn.[102,103] Pharmacogenomics is a growing area of pharmacologic research that has linked variable drug metabolism to genetic variability. A well-established example in anesthesiology is homozygous inheritance of atypical butyrylcholinesterase,

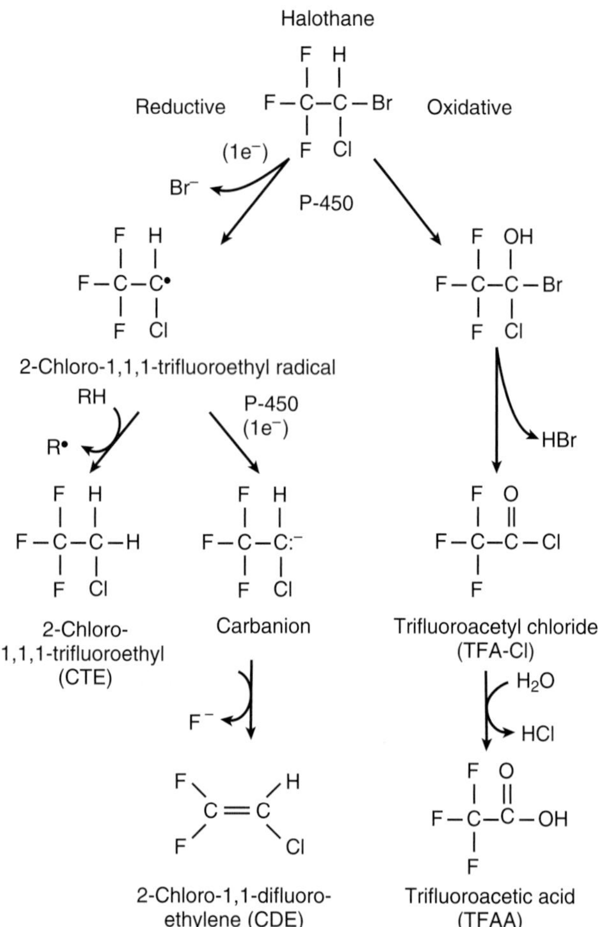

Fig. 20.14 Oxidative and reductive metabolism of halothane. Major products of hepatic CYP2E1 catalyzed halothane metabolism are shown. Under normal conditions, 24% of halothane undergoes oxidative metabolism, and 1% undergoes reductive metabolism.

resulting in slow hydrolysis of succinylcholine.[104] Genetic variations in CYP2D6 have clarified the basis for widely varying efficacies and toxicities of codeine (a prodrug), metoprolol, nortriptyline, dextromethorphan, and other substrate drugs.[105]

Hepatic CYP2E1 is particularly important in the oxidative metabolism of halogenated inhaled anesthetics (see Table 20.3). Under conditions of systemic hypoxia or decreased blood flow, or in liver regions of low P_{O_2}, CYP2A6 and CYP3A4 catalyze breakdown of VAs via reductive pathways. Halothane metabolism is primarily oxidative, and under normal conditions, about 1% of halothane undergoes reductive metabolism. Oxidative metabolism of halothane releases chloride and bromide ions, resulting in trifluoroacetyl chloride, which reacts with water to form trifluoroacetic acid (Fig. 20.14). Reductive metabolism of halothane results initially in loss of bromide, and the intermediate either reacts with a hydrogen donor to form 2-chloro-1,1,1-trifluoroethane or captures an electron, further reducing the carbon-carbon bond to form 2-chloro-1,1-difluoroethylene (see Fig. 20.14). Halothane reduces hepatic blood flow and can cause hepatocellular hypoxia in some regions in the liver, potentially leading to an increase in its reductive metabolism.[71] All of the ether anesthetics undergo similar oxidative metabolism catalyzed by CYP2E1 (see Table 20.3, Fig. 20.15). Oxidative metabolism of these drugs results in the release of fluoride (F^-) and chloride (Cl^-) ions and the formation of reactive intermediates that react with water to form carboxylic acids. Isoflurane and desflurane both produce trifluoroacetic acid, whereas enflurane forms 2-difluoromethoxy-2,2-difluoroacetic acid. Oxidative metabolism of methoxyflurane may follow several paths, releasing either Cl^- or F^- in sequential steps and producing methoxy-difluoroacetic acid, dichloroacetic acid, and acetic acid (see Table 20.3).

Halothane Hepatotoxicity

The first modern halogenated VA, halothane, was introduced in 1955. Clinical exposure to halothane is associated with two distinct types of hepatic injury.[76,106,107] Subclinical hepatotoxicity occurs in 20% of adults who receive halothane. It is characterized by mild postoperative elevations in alanine aminotransferase (ALT) and aspartate aminotransferase (AST), but is reversible and innocuous. Anaerobic halothane reduction by CYP2A6 to a 2-chloro-1,1,1-trifluoroethyl radical (see Fig. 20.14) is thought to mediate this mild hepatic injury.[72] The fulminant form of hepatotoxicity, commonly known as halothane hepatitis, is characterized by elevated ALT, AST, bilirubin, and alkaline phosphatase levels, and massive hepatic necrosis following the administration of halothane. Halothane hepatitis is rare (1 in 5000-35,000 administrations in adults) but is fatal in between 50% to 75% of cases. Because of the potential for fatal hepatitis, halothane is no longer used in adult patients in most countries.

Halothane hepatitis is caused by a hypersensitivity reaction associated with oxidative metabolism of halothane. The highly reactive trifluoroacetyl chloride metabolite of halothane oxidation can react with nearby liver proteins (see Table 20.3). In most patients who developed hepatic necrosis after halothane anesthesia, antibodies against trifluoroacetyl-modified proteins were detected, suggesting that the hepatic damage is linked to an immune response against the modified protein, which acts as a neoantigen (Fig. 20.16). Accordingly, patients who develop halothane hepatitis often have a history of prior exposures to halothane or other VAs, together with symptoms suggestive of immune reactivity, such as fever, rash, arthralgia, and eosinophilia.[75] It is hypothesized that trifluoroacetyl-protein adducts induce a cytotoxic T-cell reaction in sensitized individuals, which leads to liver damage.[76] However, definitive evidence that liver injury is immune-mediated in halothane hepatitis is lacking.

Hepatotoxicity and massive hepatic necrosis after halothane anesthesia also occurs in children. However, two large retrospective studies have demonstrated that the clinical syndrome of halothane hepatitis is even more rare in pediatric patients (1 in 80,000-200,000) than in adults.[108-110] Halothane is metabolized to a similar degree in adults and children, and children are immune competent from birth. Pediatric cases of halothane hepatitis are also associated with multiple anesthetic exposures, suggesting a mechanism similar to that in adults. Why the incidence of halothane hepatitis is significantly higher in the adult population remains unknown.

Other VAs including enflurane, isoflurane, and desflurane have also been associated with fulminant hepatic necrosis,[92,111-115] but compared with halothane, the incidence of

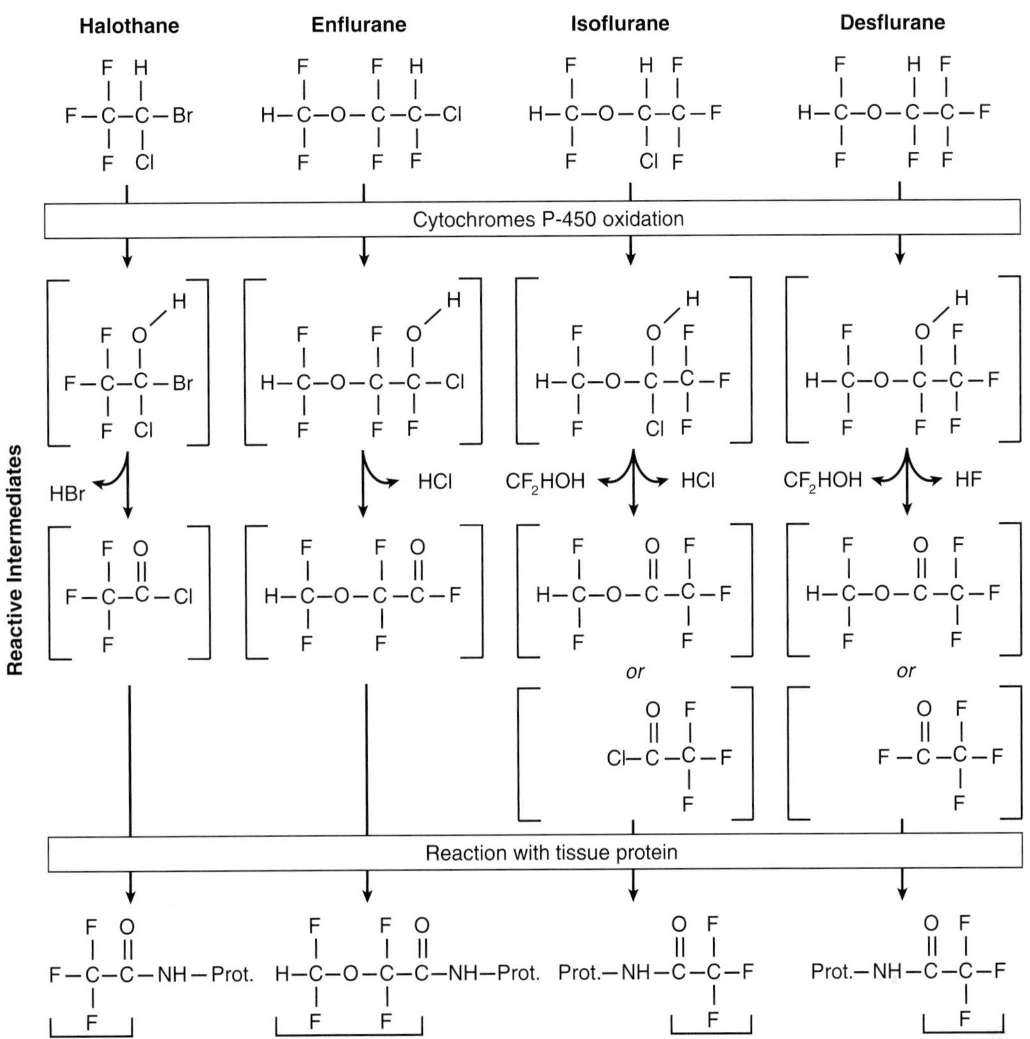

Fig. 20.15 Proposed pathways for inhaled anesthetic metabolism to reactive intermediates. CYP2E1 catalyzes oxidative metabolism of halothane, enflurane, isoflurane, and desflurane to a variety of reactive intermediates that can form adducts with hepatocellular proteins. Trifluoroacetylated proteins are identical after halothane, isoflurane, and desflurane, whereas adducts following enflurane are immunologically similar.

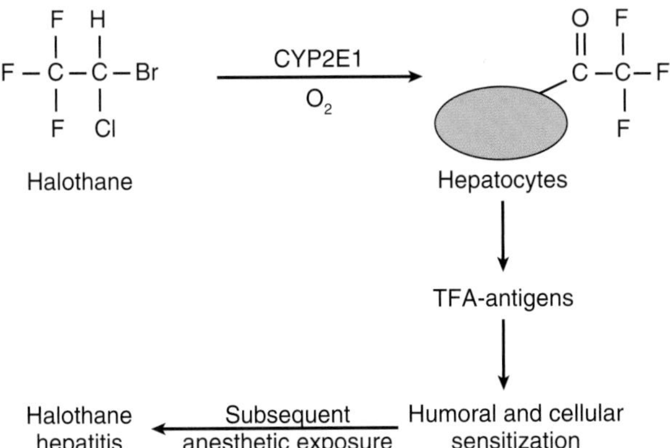

Fig. 20.16 Pathways generating the immune response after exposure to inhaled anesthetics. Halothane is metabolized to a reactive trifluoroacetyl intermediate that forms an amide bond with hepatocellular proteins. The altered protein triggers an immune response, which on subsequent exposure to anesthetic results in hepatocellular damage and necrosis. A similar process may ensue after exposure to other fluorinated drugs metabolized to similar halo-acyl intermediates. TFA, Trifluoroacetic acid. (Modified from Njoku D, Laster MJ, Gong DH, et al. Biotransformation of halothane, endflurane, isoflurane and desflurane to trifluoroacetylated liver proteins: association between protein acylation and liver injury. *Anesth Analg.* 1997;84:173–178.)

this potentially fatal toxicity is very rare after administration of these newer VAs. The mechanism of severe hepatitis following enflurane, isoflurane, and desflurane may be the same as for halothane, because all of these drugs are oxidatively metabolized to highly reactive intermediates that can covalently modify hepatic proteins (see Fig. 20.15). As with halothane, case investigations usually reveal that patients have had prior exposure to VAs, and antibodies to modified hepatic proteins can be detected. The extremely infrequent incidence of severe hepatitis for modern VAs is likely because of their lower degree of oxidative metabolism and subsequent immune sensitization. In fact, hepatitis was also commonly reported soon after introduction of methoxyflurane, another anesthetic that is mostly metabolized to highly reactive acidic intermediates.[77,116] Unlike all other VAs, sevoflurane is oxidized at the fluoromethoxy C-H bond and forms hexafluoroisopropanol and inorganic F^- (see Table 20.3; Fig. 20.17).[117,118] Hexafluoroisopropanol is relatively stable, and modified liver proteins are not formed after sevoflurane anesthesia. Cases of hepatitis and rapid death after sevoflurane anesthesia have been reported, but there was no evidence of an immune-mediated mechanism.[96]

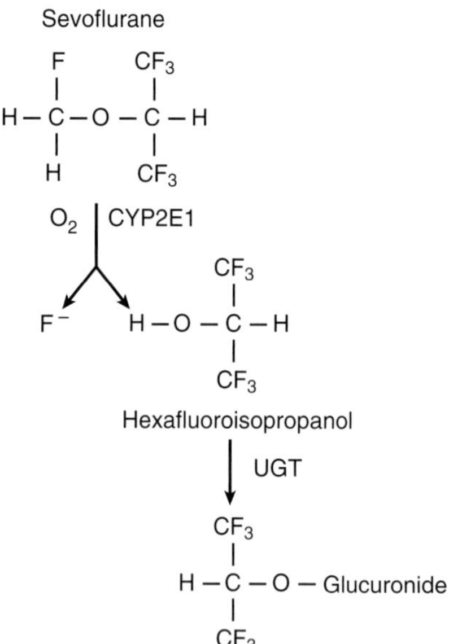

Fig. 20.17 Metabolic oxidation of Sevoflurane. CYP2E1 catalyzes phase 1 defluorination of sevoflurane, forming hexafluoroisopropanol. Phase 2 glucuronidation is catalyzed by uridine 5′-diphosphate glucuronosyltransferase (UGT).

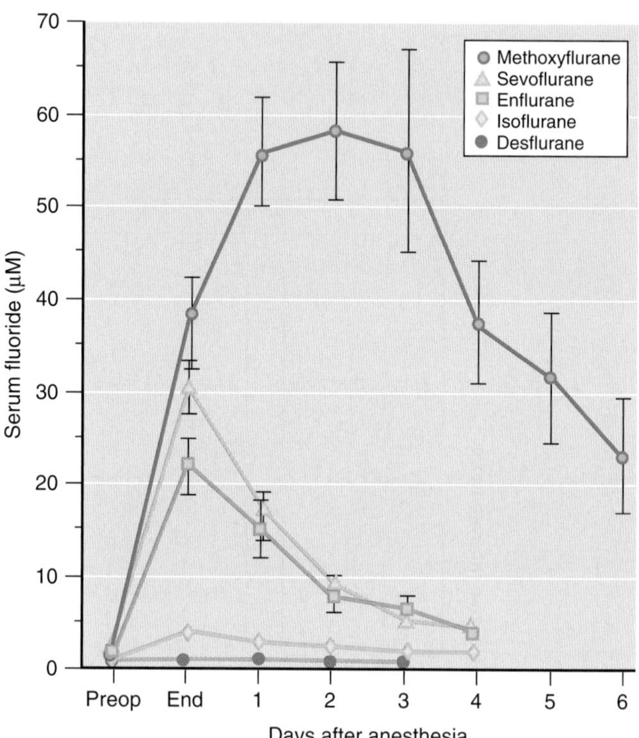

Fig. 20.18 Serum inorganic fluoride (F⁻) exposure during and after methoxyflurane anesthesia is much greater than with other anesthetics. Points represent serum F⁻ measurements (mean ± SD) from multiple subjects. After 2 to 3 MAC-hours of methoxyflurane anesthesia, F⁻ rises during and after drug administration ends, peaks above 60 μmol/L on postanesthesia days 2 and 3, then declines slowly, remaining elevated for more than 1 week. Sevoflurane anesthesia (3.7 MAC-hours) produces an early peak F⁻ concentration averaging 31 μmol/L, which declines over 3 to 4 days. Enflurane anesthesia (2.7 MAC-hours) results in an early average peak of 22 μmol/L that declines in 3 to 4 days. Isoflurane and desflurane result in small and negligible rises in serum F⁻ concentrations. Only methoxyflurane is associated with fluoride-associated renal toxicity. *MAC*, Minimum alveolar concentration (immobility).

Biotransformation in Kidneys

The kidneys are large organs that receive high blood flow. Renal physiologic activities include glomerular filtration of water-soluble metabolites, reabsorption of water and essential metabolites, urinary excretion of waste, and regulation of hormones involved in vascular tone (renin) and water balance (aldosterone). The kidneys clear most of the water-soluble metabolites resulting from biotransformation of inhaled anesthetics. Kidneys also contain CYP enzymes, including CYP2E1, that catalyze both phase 1 and phase 2 reactions and are therefore additional sites where inhaled anesthetic metabolism occurs. As in the liver, various CYPs in renal parenchyma may undergo induction or inhibition by exogenous substances.[119-122]

Fluoride-Associated Nephrotoxicity

The first modern halogenated ether anesthetic, methoxyflurane was introduced in 1959. Methoxyflurane causes polyuric renal insufficiency and is no longer used in clinical practice.[123] The nephrotoxic effect of methoxyflurane is attributed to inorganic fluoride (F^-) released during its metabolism. Investigations have provided significant insights into potential nephrotoxic mechanisms by fluorinated VAs and have influenced the development of subsequent halogenated anesthetic agents.

Absorbed methoxyflurane undergoes extensive biotransformation,[67] including cytochrome-catalyzed oxidation that releases inorganic fluoride ions (F^-) into blood. Animal studies provide clear evidence of the nephrotoxicity of methoxyflurane, which includes a strong relationship between methoxyflurane dose and renal injury,[124] increased nephrotoxicity with induction of CYP enzymes,[125,126] and decreased nephrotoxicity with inhibition of methoxyflurane metabolism.[84,127] Clinical data further indicate that severity of nephrotoxicity and mortality are associated with high plasma fluoride concentrations after methoxyflurane anesthesia.[128,129] Patients with serum inorganic fluoride levels below 50 μM had no evidence of renal injury, whereas patients with postmethoxyflurane serum F^- greater than 50 μM suffered high rates of renal dysfunction and increased mortality.[79,130] Moreover, serum F^- concentrations were significantly higher after the administration of methoxyflurane than with other halogenated VAs, which are not associated with nephrotoxicity (Fig. 20.18). Inorganic fluoride released during methoxyflurane metabolism probably causes renal injury, and the nephrotoxic threshold for plasma F^- is approximately 50 μM. Individual variability among patients in the degree of apparent renal injury after methoxyflurane exposure was observed. Genetic heterogeneity, drug interactions, and preexisting renal disease likely account for these differences.

Since the introduction of methoxyflurane, all prospective halogenated anesthetic agents have been extensively tested experimentally and clinically for their degree of defluorination and the resulting serum F^- concentrations. However, experience with newer drugs, particularly with sevoflurane, has caused investigators to reexamine the classical fluoride-induced nephrotoxicity hypothesis. Sevoflurane was initially synthesized in the 1970s, but because of its relatively large defluorination rate (2%-5%), its introduction into clinical practice was delayed. It was first widely used

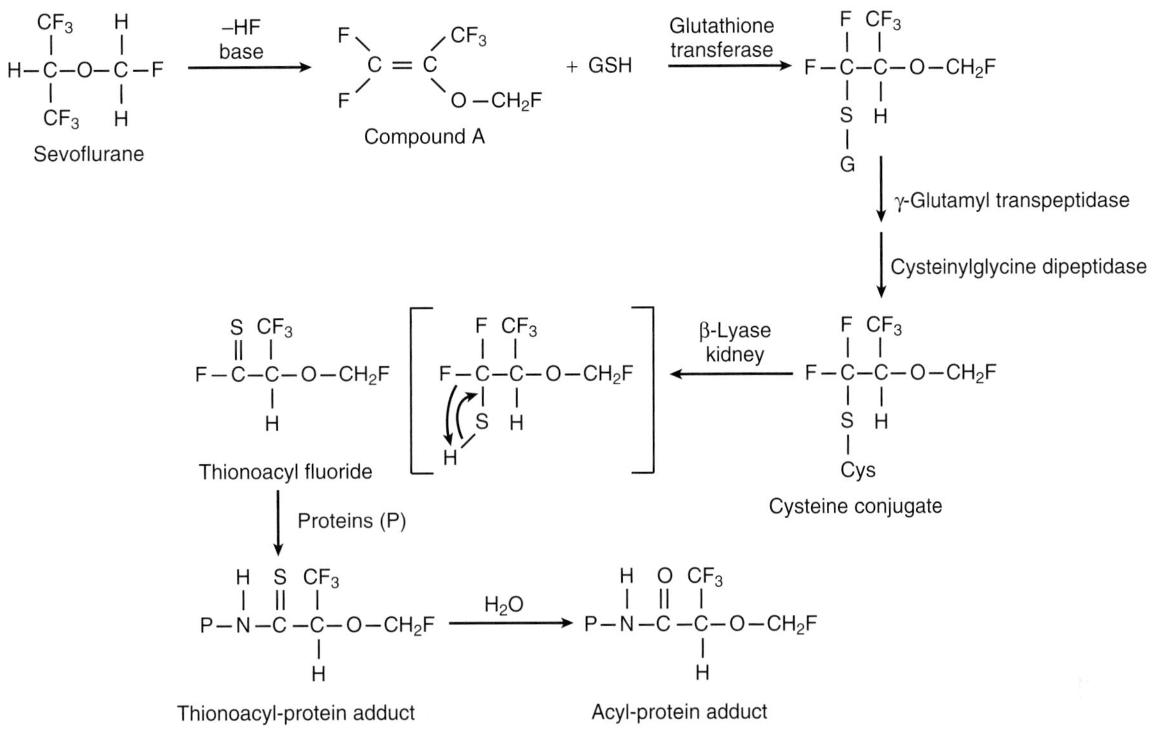

Fig. 20.19 Proposed pathway mediating nephrotoxic effects of compound A in rodents. Sevoflurane degrades to compound A in the presence of strong base in some CO_2 absorbent materials. Compound A itself is not nephrotoxic but undergoes hepatic S-conjugation with glutathione. In the kidney, additional metabolic steps produce a S-cysteine compound A conjugate, which is metabolized by β-lyase to a reactive thionoacyl fluoride that is proposed to damage proteins essential for kidney function. Humans have very low β-lyase activity, which is hypothetically the basis for the lack of reported nephrotoxicity in patients. *CO_2*, Carbon dioxide; *GSH*, glutathione; *HF*, hydrofluoric acid. (Adapted from Martin JL, Kandel L, Laster MJ, et al. Studies of the mechanism of nephrotoxicity of compound A in rats. *J Anesth.* 1997;11:32–37.)

in Japan in 1990. Subsequent clinical studies demonstrated no clinically significant nephrotoxicity after the administration of sevoflurane, even when the high peak blood F^- concentrations greater than 50 μM were confirmed.[117] Typical peak fluoride concentrations after 2 to 3 MAC-hours of sevoflurane anesthesia are 20 to 30 μM, and less than 5 μM after isoflurane and desflurane (see Fig. 20.18). Enflurane metabolism also often results in peak blood F^- concentrations greater than 20 μM. Isoflurane and desflurane are minimally metabolized and produce lower plasma fluoride concentrations. However, none of these anesthetics is associated with clinically significant renal toxicity, suggesting that methoxyflurane is unique in its ability to harm kidneys. One important difference between methoxyflurane and current VAs is its extreme lipophilicity and extremely long residence time in tissues. This results in prolonged elevated F^- concentrations in blood (see Fig. 20.18), suggesting that the length of F^- exposure is a key risk factor. However, prolonged moderate elevations of plasma fluoride (25-38 μM) during several days of isoflurane anesthesia without adverse renal effects have been documented.[131,132] Thus neither the peak level nor the duration of high plasma fluoride concentration entirely explains the nephrotoxic effects by the halogenated anesthetics. It is also not clear whether the integrated concentration multiplied by time exposure to inorganic F^- represents the key risk factor. However, methoxyflurane is metabolized to a large extent within kidney parenchyma, producing high intrarenal inorganic fluoride concentrations (likely much higher than those measured in blood), which are proposed to cause renal injury.[78,80] Thus, compared with methoxyflurane, the absence of renal toxicity with newer volatile halogenated agents likely derives from a combination of factors: (1) their lower tissue solubilities, particularly in kidney (see Table 20.2), resulting in lower intrarenal fluoride production; (2) lower overall degrees of biotransformation; and (3) more rapid respiratory clearance from the body.

ANESTHETIC DEGRADATION IN CARBON DIOXIDE ABSORBENTS

Sevoflurane, Compound A, and Renal Toxicity

Halogenated anesthetics can undergo chemical breakdown while interacting with carbon dioxide (CO_2) absorbents that contain strong bases such as sodium hydroxide (NaOH) and potassium hydroxide (KOH), which are present in soda lime and Baralyme.[133] Strong bases extract a proton from the isopropyl group of sevoflurane, primarily forming a haloalkene [fluoromethyl-2,2-difluoro-1-(trifluoromethyl) vinyl ether], known as *compound A* (Fig. 20.19). Compound A is volatile and can be absorbed via alveolar gas exchange. Compound A exposure is nephrotoxic in laboratory animals, causing proximal tubular necrosis and, with sufficient exposure, death. In rats, renal injury is observed with cumulative exposure to compound A above 150 parts per million (ppm)-hours (e.g., 50 ppm inhalation for 3 hours).[134,135] Moderately severe but reversible histopathologic damage was found in rats after 200 ppm-hour exposure, associated with increased blood and urea nitrogen (BUN), creatinine, and other measures of renal damage. Compound A exposure over 1000 ppm-hours is lethal in half of exposed rats.

Patients receiving sevoflurane anesthesia are routinely exposed to compound A in rebreathing circuits, and the inhaled concentration is dependent on the fresh gas flow rate and the type of CO_2 absorbent present. Fresh gas flows of 1 L/min result in maximal compound A concentrations around 20 ppm with soda lime and 30 ppm with Baralyme.[136] Higher FGF rates result in less compound A accumulation in the breathing circuit. However, compound A exposure is not associated with clinically significant nephrotoxicity in humans. There is no threshold exposure level known to cause more than subclinical renal damage. Numerous studies in which human subjects or patients were exposed to more than 200 ppm-hours of compound A have reported that clinical measures of renal function (BUN, creatinine, urinary protein or glucose, and urine concentrating ability) and laboratory tests for subtle renal damage (N-acetyl-β-glucoaminidase, alanine aminopeptidase, γ-GTP, and β2-microglobulin) remain unchanged.[81,86,137-139] Kharasch and colleagues[140] compared the effects of low-flow sevoflurane and isoflurane anesthesia in patients with stable renal insufficiency, and found no significant difference in postoperative renal function tests. Other studies have reported normal BUN and creatinine, but transient reversible abnormalities in other renal function test values following prolonged sevoflurane anesthesia at low FGF (>330 ppm-hour compound A exposure in one study).[141-144]

The evidence of nephrotoxicity in rats compared with the remarkably benign results in humans suggests that mechanisms of sevoflurane metabolism and toxicity differ between these species. The difference in the nephrotoxic effects of compound A between humans and rats may be attributed to the doses of compound A, interspecies differences in metabolic toxification, and sensitivity of the proximal tubular cells to compound A cytotoxicity.[71] Detailed studies show that in rats, compound A undergoes S-conjugation to cysteine, and that the resulting cysteine conjugate is metabolized by renal β-lyase to form a reactive thionoacyl fluoride intermediate that acylates proteins and has been proposed to mediate the nephrotoxic effect (see Fig. 20.19).[133,145] Human kidneys have far lower β-lyase activity than rat kidneys, accounting for the differential toxicity of compound A in the two species. Experiments testing whether inhibition of β-lyase with aminooxy-acetic acid (AOAA) protects rats from compound A nephrotoxicity have had mixed results.[146,147] Alternative mechanisms underlying compound A toxicity have been proposed, including formation of reactive sulfoxides catalyzed by CYP3A isozymes,[148] which are also more active in rat than human kidneys.

Although the mechanism underlying compound A toxicity in laboratory animals remains uncertain, the lack of significant sevoflurane nephrotoxicity in human clinical data is reassuring. Compound A exposure can be limited by careful selection of fresh gas flows, vaporizer output, and CO_2 absorbent materials. The use of 2 L/min fresh gas flows assures that for the vast majority of patients, exposure to compound A will be below the most conservative threshold for nephrotoxicity. Although clinical studies indicate that sevoflurane is most likely safe, even in patients with preexisting renal dysfunction, the drug should be administered in accordance with the approved package labeling guidelines.

Like sevoflurane, halothane degrades in the presence of CO_2 absorbents to form a reactive intermediate, bromochlorodifluoroethylene (BCDFE),[133] which has also been investigated as a possible nephrotoxin. Eger and colleagues[149] found that in comparison to compound A, BCDFE accumulates 20- to 40-fold less in breathing circuits and is 4-fold less reactive. Thus the risk of BCDFE nephrotoxicity is negligible.

TABLE 20.4 Composition of Base Chemicals and Water Content of Carbon Dioxide Absorbents

CO_2 absorbent	$Ca(OH)_2$ (%)	$Ba(OH)_2$ (%)	KOH (%)	NaOH (%)	LiOH (%)	H_2O (%)
Baralyme*	70	10	4.6	–	–	14
Soda lime I	80	–	2.6	1.3	–	15
Sodasorb	90	–	0.0005	3.8	–	16
Drägersorb 800 plus	82	–	0.003	2	–	16
Soda lime II/ Medisorb	81	–	0.003	2.6	–	16
Spherasorb	84.5	–	0.003	1.5	–	14
Amsorb	83.2	–	–	–	–	14.4
LofloSorb	84	–	–	–	–	16
Superia	79.5	–	–	–	–	17.5
Lithium hydroxide	–	–	–	–	99	1

*Baralyme was withdrawn from the market in 2004.

Various absorbents also contain other components, such as polyvinylpyrrolidine, calcium chloride, calcium sulfate, magnesium chloride, and aluminosilicate.

Data from Keijzer C, Perez RS, de Lange JJ. Compound A and carbon monoxide production from sevoflurane and seven different types of carbon dioxide absorbent in a patient model. *Acta Anaesthesiol Scand*. 2007;51:31–37, and Kharasch ED, Powers KM, Artru AA. Comparison of Amsorb, sodalime, and Baralyme degradation of volatile anesthetics and formation of carbon monoxide and compound A in swine in vivo. *Anesthesiology*. 2002;96:173–182.

Carbon Monoxide and Heat

In the presence of strong bases in dry CO_2 absorbents (water content <5%), some halogenated VAs undergo degradation, resulting in the formation of CO, trifluoromethane (CF_3H), and hydrogen fluoride (HF).[133] The factors that determine the amount of CO produced include the chemical makeup of CO_2 absorbent (KOH > NaOH >> $Ba(OH)_2$, $Ca(OH)_2$), dryness of the absorbent material, the concentration of volatile agent, and its chemical structure.[150] Baralyme contains 4.6% KOH, whereas soda lime contains 2.5% KOH and 1.3% NaOH, and reacts less vigorously with halogenated anesthetics. The relatively weak bases $Ba(OH)_2$ and $Ca(OH)_2$ are other major constituents in CO_2 absorbents, and do not catalyze CO formation (Table 20.4).[136,151] The anesthetics that contain a difluoromethyl group (difluoromethyl-ethyl ethers) are most susceptible to this degradation, and for these drugs CO production correlates with anesthetic concentration in the breathing circuit (desflurane > enflurane > isoflurane)[152] (Fig. 20.20).[152] Sevoflurane, methoxyflurane, and halothane also degrade in the presence of strong bases, but do not produce CO. Production of CO appears to require nearly complete desiccation (i.e., removal of moisture) of the CO_2 absorbent, and typically occurs after high-flow "flushing" of the breathing circuit for 1 to 2 days. Soda

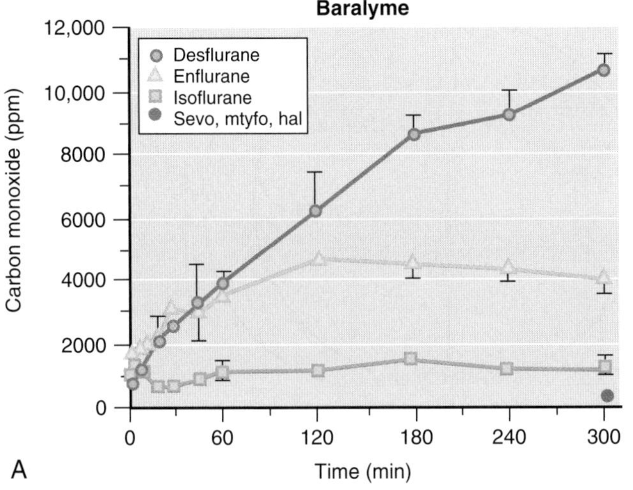

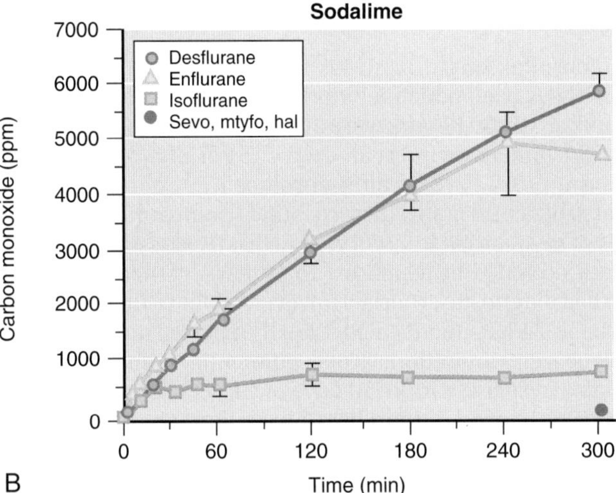

Fig. 20.20 Inhaled anesthetic degradation and carbon monoxide production. Points represent mean ± SD of three measurements with equivalent anesthetic doses (1.5 × MAC) in the presence of dry CO_2 absorbents at identical fresh gas flows. (A) Degradation and CO production with Baralyme. (B) Degradation and CO production with soda lime. Degradation and CO production was observed with anesthetics containing difluoromethoxy groups (desflurane, enflurane, and isoflurane), but not halothane *(hal)* or those with monofluoromethoxy groups such as sevoflurane *(sevo)* and methoxyflurane *(mtyfo)*. *CO*, Carbon monoxide; *MAC*, minimum alveolar concentration. (Adapted from Baxter PJ, Garton K, Kharasch ED. Mechanistic aspects of carbon monoxide formation from volatile anesthetics. *Anesthesiology*. 1998;89:929–941.)

lime contains 15% water by weight, and Baralyme contains 13% water by weight (see Table 20.4). CO production is observed when the water content of soda lime or Baralyme falls below 1.4% and 5%, respectively.[153] High ambient temperatures also accelerate desiccation of CO_2 absorbent materials and may increase the rate of CO producing reactions. As noted with compound A, CO accumulation in the breathing circuit is inversely related to the fresh gas flow.

Anesthetic degradation in the breathing circuit has resulted in CO poisoning during clinical anesthesia.[154,155] CO has 250-fold greater affinity for hemoglobin than O_2 does; therefore, the formation of carboxyhemoglobin reduces blood oxygen carrying capacity and tissue oxygen delivery, and is difficult to reverse. The detrimental effects and signs of CO toxicity are well known. However, during general anesthesia, signs of patient exposure to CO are masked and hypoxia may be difficult to detect because most pulse oximetry equipment cannot distinguish between carboxyhemoglobin and oxyhemoglobin.

The degradation of VAs by bases in CO_2 absorbents is an exothermic reaction that results in the production of heat. Sevoflurane produces the most heat when it is used with desiccated CO_2 absorbent. The absorbent canister and anesthetic circuit can reach extremely high temperatures, which can lead to explosion or fire, or both.[156,157]

Current recommendations to minimize anesthetic degradation to CO and heat include machine maintenance measures to avoid desiccation of CO_2 absorbents and the use of absorbents that contain less KOH and NaOH. Newer CO_2 absorbents (see Table 20.4) contain little or no strong base and do not degrade VAs, regardless of hydration status.[136,158,159] The use of the newer CO2 absorbents also reduces the production of compound A during sevoflurane anesthesia.[160–162]

NITROUS OXIDE, VITAMIN B12, AND HOMOCYSTEINE

N_2O is unique among anesthetics in irreversibly inhibiting cobalamins (vitamin B12) by oxidizing the Co (I) ligand. Cobalamins are ingested or produced by bacteria in the gut and are critical cofactors together with 5-methyltetrahydrofolate in the activity of methionine synthase (Fig. 20.21). Methionine synthase catalyzes methylation of homocysteine to methionine, while demethylating 5-methlytetrahydrofolate to tetrahydrofolate. Methionine, converted to S-adenosylmethionine, is the major substrate for methylation in biochemical pathways involved in the synthesis of DNA, RNA, myelin, and catecholamines[163] Chronic vitamin B12 deficiency (as in pernicious anemia) results in hematologic and neurologic dysfunction. Long-term N_2O exposure, typically among individuals who frequently inhale it as a recreational drug, can also cause megaloblastic anemia, myelopathy (subacute combined degeneration), neuropathy, and encephalopathy, sometimes presenting as psychosis.[164–167] N_2O is the eighth most commonly used recreational substance in the United Kingdom.[168] Risk factors that increase susceptibility to N_2O toxicity include pernicious anemia or other gastrointestinal malabsorption syndromes, extremes of age, alcoholism, malnutrition, a strict vegetarian diet, and inborn deficiencies in cobalamin or tetrahydrofolate metabolism.[164] Inhibitors of folate metabolism, such as methotrexate, may also enhance sensitivity to N_2O toxicity.[169]

In healthy surgical patients, megaloblastic changes in the bone marrow are rare, and reported only after a prolonged period of exposure (>12 hours) to N_2O. Healthy pediatric patients exposed to N_2O for up to 8 hours during spine surgery do not develop evidence of megaloblastic anemia.[170] However, in seriously ill patients or those with risk factors noted earlier, shorter (or repetitive) periods of N_2O exposure may lead to significant subacute pathology. Megaloblastic bone marrow changes can be induced after a short period (2-6 hours) of N_2O exposure.[171] Vitamin B12 deficiency or reduced methionine synthase activity can also lead to subacute myelopathy and neuropathy.[172-175] A case highlighting the potential importance of inborn

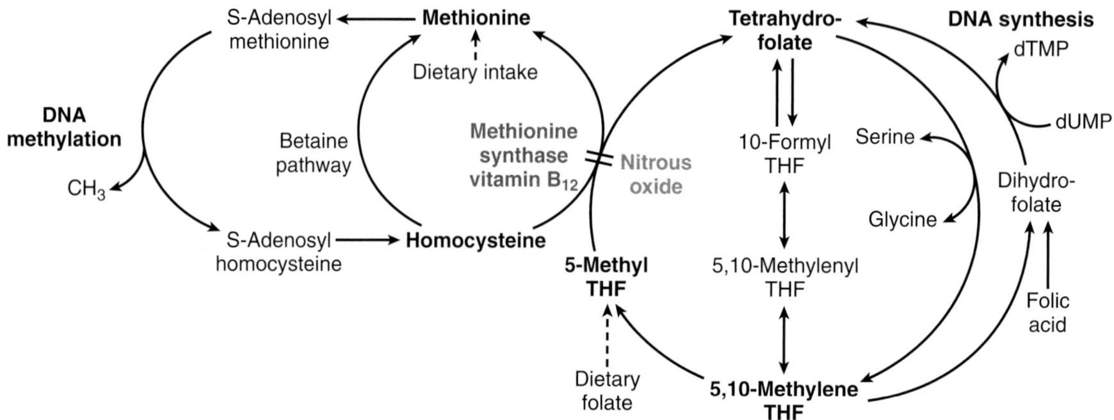

Fig. 20.21 Nitrous oxide inhibition of methionine synthase. Biochemical cycles involved in methylation reactions are shown. Methionine synthase *(red)* catalyzes methylation of homocysteine with 5-methyl tetrahydrofolate as the donor, producing methionine and tetrahydrofolate *(THF)*. Both vitamin B12 and folate are essential cofactors for methionine synthase. Nitrous oxide *(blue)* inhibits methionine synthase by oxidizing the cobalt of cobalamin (vitamin B_{12}). Methyl transfer pathways are important in synthesis of protein and DNA. *dTMP*, Deoxythymidine; *dUMP*, 2′-Deoxyuridine 5″-Monophosphate.

metabolism was reported by Selzer and colleagues.[176] In this case, a 4-month-old child developed an irreversibly and ultimately fatal seizure disorder several weeks after receiving N_2O during anesthesia. Autopsy revealed widespread brain atrophy and demyelination, and biochemical investigations revealed reduced methyltetrahydrofolate reductase (MTHFR) activity, which eventually were linked to several mutations in the gene encoding MTHFR.

Another consequence of reduced methionine synthase activity is accumulation of its substrate: homocysteine (see Fig. 20.21). Homocystinuria caused by severe inborn deficiency of methionine synthase activity is associated with extremely elevated blood homocysteine levels, early atherosclerosis of coronary and cerebral arteries, and premature death.[177] These observations led to the "homocysteine hypothesis," which postulates that homocysteine stimulates inflammation and atherosclerosis, and is a key modifiable factor in vascular morbidity and mortality. Despite some evidence that increased homocysteine levels are an independent risk factor for cardiac and cerebrovascular morbidity,[178,179] the association between homocysteine levels and atherothrombotic disease is weak, as some large prospective studies have found.[180] Moreover, studies in which diet and vitamin supplementation was used to reduce homocysteine levels demonstrate improvement in some markers of vascular risk, but do not reduce the rate of myocardial infarction and atherosclerotic stroke.[180,181] Thus it appears that the importance of chronic *moderate* elevation in homocysteine to cardiovascular outcomes is tenuous, or perhaps only pertinent to limited patient populations.

Does the rapid increase of homocysteine levels during N_2O anesthesia influence the risk of cardiovascular and neurovascular morbidity following surgery and anesthesia? Badner and colleagues[182] reported that N_2O administration significantly increased homocysteine levels and increased myocardial risk in carotid endarterectomy patients. The Evaluation of Nitrous Oxide in a Gas Mixture for Anaesthesia (ENIGMA) trial in more than 2000 patients reported that avoidance of N_2O combined with increased inspired oxygen concentration during anesthesia decreased the incidence of a variety of complications after major surgery, but found no reduction in death, myocardial infarction, stroke, or hospital length of stay.[183] In a follow-up study of the ENIGMA trial, patients reported that those exposed to N_2O for more than 2 hours were at increased risk (odds ratio 1.6; 95% confidence interval, 1.01-2.5) of myocardial infarction up to 5.7 years after enrollment.[184] No difference in rates of death or stroke were found. Unfortunately, diagnosis of myocardial infarction in ENIGMA was often based on data obtained in telephone interviews, rather than established diagnostic criteria. However, a follow-up randomized trial in 7112 patients (ENIGMA-II) reported no difference in myocardial infarction, stroke, pulmonary embolism, or cardiac arrest risk within 30 days of surgery.[185] A recent post hoc study of 5133 enrollees in the Perioperative Ischemic Evaluation (POISE) trial[186] also found no increase in rates of death, myocardial infarction, or stroke in approximately 1500 patients who received N_2O.

Anecdotally, N_2O use is thought to contribute to myocardial infarction in patients with elevated homocysteine levels at baseline.[187] Homocysteine elevation following N_2O inhalation is a useful marker for assessing the sensitivity of methionine synthase and related biochemical pathways to N_2O inhibition. Nagele and colleagues[188] studied a small group of surgical patients with common mutations in the gene encoding MTHFR, and found that those with 667C→T and 1298A→C mutations were at risk of developing abnormally high homocysteine levels after N_2O exposures of at least 2 hours. However, a common gene variant (66A→G) associated with reduced methionine synthase reductase activity did not result in abnormally high homocysteine levels after anesthesia with N_2O[189] Preoperative infusions of vitamin B12 and folate do not prevent the normal elevation in homocysteine observed following anesthesia with N_2O.[190]

The continued value of N_2O, first used as an anesthetic in the early 19th century, has been questioned by some who view its known and potential toxicities as outweighing benefits such as rapid onset and offset and relative cardiovascular stability during anesthesia.[191,192] Currently available data indicate that N_2O does not alter the risk of cardiovascular morbidity in the vast majority of patients. The authors recommend careful screening of patients to identify the few most likely to suffer N_2O toxicity, and to avoid the drug in these cases.

TABLE 20.5 Atmospheric Lifetimes and Environmental Effects of Inhaled Anesthetics

Compound		Lifetime (years)	Ozone-Depleting Potential	Global Warming Potential (20 years)	Global Warming Potential (100 years)
CFC-12	CCl_2F_2	100	1	11,000	10,900
Carbon dioxide	CO_2	5-200	–[§]	1	1
Nitrous oxide	N_2O	114	0.017[212]	289	298
Halothane	$CF_3CHBrCl$	7[213]	0.36	–	218
Isoflurane	$CHF_2OCHClCF_3$	2.6-3.6[214]	0.01	1230-1401[214]	350
Sevoflurane	$CH_2FOCH(CF_3)_2$	1.2-5.2[214]	0	349-1980[214]	575
Desflurane	$CHF_2OCHFCF_3$	10[214]	0	3714[214]	–

Ozone depleting potential (ODP) is the ratio of integrated perturbations to total ozone relative to an equal emission of CFC-12. Global warming potential (GWP) is defined as the cumulative radiative retention integrated over a period of time from the emission of gas relative to reference gas (Carbon Dioxide). The data are based on the Intergovernmental Panel on Climate Change (IPCC) Fourth Assessment Report[215] unless otherwise indicated. § CO_2 unlikely reacts and depletes ozone. However, CO_2 producing the greenhouse effect in the troposphere is predicted to reduce stratospheric temperatures and cause further ozone depletion.[216] Computed value for halothane relative to GWP for CFC-12.

INHALED ANESTHETICS AND NEUROTOXICITY

For a comprehensive description of potential neurotoxic properties of inhaled anesthetics, see Chapter 78.

The ability of general anesthetics to reversibly ablate consciousness has benefitted millions of patients and enabled dramatic advances in health care. While inhaled agents were the first class of anesthetics and continue to be used in the vast majority of cases, accumulating evidence suggests potential long-lasting neurotoxic effects of inhaled and other general anesthetics in patients of extreme ages (see Chapter 78).[193,194] The greatest concern surrounds the impact of general anesthetics in the youngest patients during periods of rapid brain development. In a seminal study, Jevtovic-Todorovic and coworkers[195] demonstrated widespread neuronal death (apoptosis) in the brains of 7-day-old rats after exposure to midazolam, isoflurane, and N_2O, associated with long-lasting (up to 4.5 months) changes in neurophysiological correlates of learning and memory, and performance deficits in spatial learning tests. Other animal studies in various species, including nonhuman primates, demonstrate that during sensitive periods of early brain development, exposure to most general anesthetics is associated with accelerated neuronal apoptosis and degeneration.[196-200] Neonatal primate studies suggest that exposure to anesthetics for as little as 3 hours leads to neuro-apoptosis and neurocognitive problems.[197,199,201] Other studies suggest that low nonapoptotic concentrations of general anesthetics may inhibit normal synapse formation and damage developing neuronal networks.[202] Mechanisms underlying neurodevelopmental toxicity are potentially linked to the same ion channels hypothesized to mediate general anesthesia. General anesthetic actions are attributed in part to both antagonism of N-methyl-D-aspartate (NMDA) receptor and potentiation of $GABA_A$ receptor signal transduction, and drugs with either or both of these activities damage developing brains.[194,203,204]

Based on preclinical studies showing that anesthetic exposure consistently impairs neurodevelopment, the US Food and Drug Administration (FDA) issued a safety announcement that repeated or lengthy exposures to general anesthetics and sedative drugs before the age of three have the potential to harm the development of children's brains (http://www.fda.gov/drugs/drugsafety/ucm532356.htm). Emerging clinical data, however, indicate either no or very modest associations between exposure to surgical procedures requiring general anesthesia and neurodevelopmental outcomes.[205–208] The Pediatric Anesthesia NeuroDevelopment Assessment (PANDA) trial compared a cohort of children who received general anesthesia for hernia repair before age 3 with siblings.[209] The neuropsychological outcomes showed no difference between groups. A randomized clinical study, the General Anesthesia Compared to Spinal Anesthesia (GAS) trial, compared infants who underwent hernia repair with awake-spinal versus inhaled general anesthesia. At age 2, cognitive scores in the two groups were equivalent,[210] whereas the primary outcome at age 5 has not been reported. Related clinical studies exploring a variety of long-term outcomes in children are underway, adding uncertainty to clinical decision making. A comprehensive examination of this topic is provided elsewhere in this textbook ("Pediatric Anesthesia," Chapter 78). For updated recommendations to healthcare providers and parents regarding exposure to anesthesia and surgery in early life, please consult https://smarttots.org/about/consensus-statement/. For a comprehensive description of long-term cognitive effects of surgery and anesthesia in adults, see Chapter 84.

INHALED ANESTHETICS AND ENVIRONMENTAL EFFECTS

Anesthetic gases in the workplace and in the outdoor environment have the potential to cause harm. An American Society of Anesthesiologists (ASA) Task Force released a comprehensive document on environmentally sustainable anesthesia practice, including the choice of anesthetic gases and reduction of waste: https://www.asahq.org/resources/resources-from-asa-committees/environmental-sustainability/greening-the-operating-room.[211] Three potential sequelae have been investigated: global warming, ozone depletion, and health effects from workplace exposure (Table 20.5).[212–216]

Global Warming Effects

Atmospheric trapping of thermal radiation from the Earth's surface is known as the *greenhouse effect*, which the

Intergovernmental Panel on Climate Change[217] deems a major contributor to global warming. Inhaled anesthetics are recognized greenhouse gases.[218,219] Isoflurane, sevoflurane, and desflurane, the most widely used current inhaled anesthetics, are minimally metabolized in the body and are substantially eliminated through exhalation. Most anesthesia waste scavenging systems transfer these gases directly and unchanged into the atmosphere, which has drawn attention to the ecotoxicologic properties of inhaled anesthetics. The global warming potential (GWP) takes into account the heat-trapping efficiency and life-span of atmospheric gases (i.e., the time for removal by chemical reaction with radicals, photolysis, and deposition). The GWP of halogenated anesthetics is reported to range from 1230-fold (isoflurane) to 3714-fold (desflurane)—that of an equal mass of CO_2. Ryan and Nielsen[214] suggested that the most common VAs can significantly influence global warming, with the greatest impact produced by atmospheric desflurane.[214]

The GWP of N_2O is approximately 300-fold greater than that of an equal mass of CO_2.[220,221] N_2O is administered to patients in much larger quantities relative to VA gases and is remarkably stable, with an atmospheric life-span of approximately 120 years.[222] Atmospheric N_2O is produced by natural sources in soil and water, as well as human sources, including agriculture (nitrogen-based fertilizers) and combustion of fossil fuels. Sherman and Cullen[223] first reported that N_2O could contribute to global warming and estimated that approximately 1% of man-made N_2O production was for anesthesia. Anesthetic use may contribute 3.0% of total N_2O emissions in the United States.[219] Although the use of N_2O is declining in many countries, data on the worldwide medical use of N_2O are not available.

Ozone Depletion

The ozone layer of the Earth's atmosphere, which has been declining 4% per decade since the 1970s, absorbs damaging ultraviolet B light (UVB; wavelengths 280-315 nm). The biologic consequences of increasing UVB radiation include increases in skin cancer, cataracts, damage to plants, and reduction of oceanic plankton populations. Halogenated VAs are similar to chlorofluorocarbons (CFCs), which are major ozone depleting pollutants. Ozone depletion by halocarbons depends on molecular weight, number and type of halogen atoms, and atmospheric life-span.[224] The atmospheric life-span of halogenated anesthetics is much shorter (4.0-21.4 years)[225] than that of many CFCs (up to 100 years). Fluorination is associated with longer atmospheric life-span because of the stability of carbon-fluorine (C-F) bonds. Chemicals with a lifetime of more than 2 years are believed to reach the stratosphere in significant quantities. There they are exposed to intense ultraviolet radiation that can break carbon-halogen bonds, creating halogen radicals that catalytically destroy ozone. Chlorine-containing anesthetics such as halothane, isoflurane, and enflurane may be more destructive to the ozone layer than sevoflurane and desflurane, which contain only C-F bonds. Carbon-hydrogen bonds are susceptible to attack by hydroxyl radicals (OH) in the troposphere,[226] making them less likely to reach the stratosphere. However, even compounds with a lifetime of a few months may potentially contribute to ozone destruction.[227] Contributions to total stratospheric ozone depletion were estimated as 1% for halothane and 0.02% for enflurane and isoflurane.[225]

N_2O is the primary source of stratospheric nitrogen oxides, NO and NO_2, and both destroy ozone. Because only 10% of N_2O is converted to NO_X, its ozone depleting potential is lower than that of an equal mass of CFCs. However, N_2O emission is reported to be the single largest ozone depleting human emission, and is expected to remain so for the rest of this century. [212] The use of N_2O could actually contribute additional environmental harm when used with halogenated anesthetics.

The environmental impact of all inhaled anesthetics could be reduced by 80% to 90% if closed circuit anesthesia is widely employed, and to a lesser degree if low carrier gas flow rates are routinely used (see Fig. 20.13). Technologies that trap anesthetics in waste gas flows have the potential to reduce emissions into the environment, and can reduce drug costs by reusing (after redistillation) the trapped drugs.[228] Physician education warning that the medical use of N_2O can significantly contribute to both the greenhouse effect and ozone depletion should be maintained. Avoiding N_2O when it provides no clinical advantage is suggested for a more environmentally sound anesthetic practice.[218]

Exposure to Waste Anesthetic Gases

Healthcare personnel can be exposed to waste anesthetic gases both in and out of the operating room environment. Possible adverse health effects by chronic exposure to trace concentrations of inhaled anesthetics has concerned healthcare professionals for many years.[229,230] Laboratory studies suggest reproductive abnormalities in animals exposed to high concentrations of N_2O (1000 ppm or greater).[231,232] Long-term occupational exposure to anesthetic gases may be associated with genomic alterations.[233] However, a long-term prospective study found no causal relationship between adverse health effects and exposure to waste anesthetic gases with or without a scavenging system.[234]

All inhaled anesthetics cross the placental-fetal exchange barrier. Teratogenicity, which has been demonstrated in animal fetuses chronically exposed to N_2O,[235,236] is of particular concern in pregnant healthcare workers, but there is no evidence of harm in humans. Furthermore, there is no definitive evidence of harm to fetuses of women anesthetized while pregnant,[237] although studies are underway addressing the possibility that anesthetics cause harm during critical phases of fetal brain development (see earlier section, "Inhaled Anesthetics and Neurotoxicity," and Chapter 78).[238] The US Occupational Safety and Health Administration (OSHA) recommends that no worker should be exposed to concentrations of halogenated anesthetic greater than 2 ppm for a period exceeding 1 hour during anesthesia administration (http://www.osha.gov/dts/osta/anestheticgases/index.html). OSHA also recommends that no worker should be exposed to 8-hour time-weighted average concentrations of N_2O greater than 25 ppm.

Potential postoperative exposure of healthcare workers to exhaled anesthetic gases in postanesthesia care units, intensive care units, and other patient care areas should also be recognized. Studies have documented excessive levels of waste anesthetic gases in poorly ventilated postanesthesia care areas.[239-241] However, no studies have documented significant adverse health effects.

Xenon and Other Noble Gases

Modern inhaled anesthetics represent vast improvements over earlier inhaled agents, with N_2O representing the longest surviving widely used anesthetic. The noble gas xenon was first shown to produce general anesthesia in 1951,[242] and subsequent studies have revealed that in comparison with other inhaled anesthetics, it approaches being the ideal agent.[243-245] It is most comparable to N_2O, but superior in a number of ways. Xenon is present as a minor constituent of air (50 parts per billion), and is isolated by distillation of liquefied air, along with liquefied nitrogen and oxygen. Xenon is entirely unreactive in the biosphere and is the only inhaled anesthetic that is not an environmental pollutant, although its distillation from air uses considerable energy and thus creates CO_2 and other pollutants as byproducts.[219] It is odorless, tasteless, nonflammable, and has a limitless shelf-life. Its solubility in blood ($\lambda_{b/g} = 0.14$) and body tissues is lower than that of any other inhaled anesthetic, including N_2O. As a result, it has extraordinarily rapid onset and respiratory clearance, with emergence times 2- to 3-fold faster when it replaces N_2O in clinical settings.[246-248] It undergoes no biotransformation or reactions with CO_2 absorbents or ultraviolet light. Moreover, xenon has favorable pharmacodynamic effects in comparison to most inhaled anesthetics. It produces minimal cardiovascular depression and is not arrhythmogenic.[248-251] As with N_2O, xenon has analgesic activity and reduces intraoperative opioid requirements.[252] It does not trigger malignant hyperthermia or produce any known toxicity.[253] In fact, xenon has been shown to have cardioprotective and neuroprotective activities in preclinical models.[243,245] Clinical trials in adult cardiac surgery patients,[254-256] partial nephrectomy patients,[257] and comatose survivors of cardiac arrest[258,259] have demonstrated that xenon reduces pressor requirements and modestly reduces the extent of organ damage, relative to other anesthetics. However, in these clinical settings and in others, xenon does not improve neurocognitive function or survival.[260-262]

Given all these advantages, why is xenon not a commonly used inhaled anesthetic? The main reason is its cost.[263] At more than $15/L in the gas form, xenon is greater than 100-fold more expensive than N_2O and far more expensive per patient than either desflurane or sevoflurane, which are currently the most expensive VAs. Xenon has a MAC-immobility of 0.61 atm, and even with a strict closed-circuit technique, greater than 10 L are needed to anesthetize a typical patient. To perform closed circuit anesthesia with xenon-oxygen also requires lengthy preanesthetic denitrogenation to prevent N_2 from accumulating in the rebreathing circuit.[264] Transitioning from 100% oxygen during denitrogenation to closed circuit xenon-oxygen anesthesia is another slow process because xenon is added to the circuit as oxygen is metabolized in the patient at 200 to 250 mL/min. High-flow xenon is otherwise necessary to make this transition short. To make xenon a more affordable anesthetic, specialized anesthesia machines have been designed to enable its efficient delivery,[265] and new waste-scavenging systems are being introduced with cryogenic traps that can condense xenon in a liquid form from waste gases.[266] This process allows relatively inexpensive recycling of xenon after it has been redistilled to a pure form.

In addition to cost, xenon presents a few other downsides. Xenon gas has a much higher density (5.9 g/L) than either N_2O (1.9 g/L) or air (1.2 g/L), resulting in increased flow resistance and work of breathing.[267] Thus it may be a poor choice for patients with compromised respiratory function. As with N_2O, high xenon partial pressures needed for anesthesia cause expansion of trapped air spaces and vascular air emboli.[268] Compared with propofol infusion or sevoflurane inhalation, xenon anesthesia results in a higher incidence of nausea and vomiting.[269,270]

Currently, xenon remains an experimental anesthetic, with clinical research focusing on its potential as an organ protectant, and the development of technologies to reduce its cost. Shifting the cost-benefit balance toward more xenon use in patients will depend on whether clinical studies end up supporting xenon's beneficial efficacy. Other noble gases also share some of xenon's neuroprotective actions in experimental model systems and are also under investigation as potential clinical anesthetics.[271]

Complete references available online at expertconsult.com.

References

1. Mapleson WW. *Br J Anaesth.* 1973;45:319.
2. Bovill JG. *Handb Exp Pharmacol.* 2008;182:121.
3. Eger 2nd EI. *Anesth Analg.* 1987;66:971.
4. Eger 2nd EI, Shargel R. *Anesthesiology.* 1963;24:625.
5. Cromwell TH, et al. *Anesthesiology.* 1971;35:401.
6. Yasuda N, et al. *Anesth Analg.* 1989;69:370.
7. Stoelting RK, et al. *Anesthesiology.* 1970;33(5).
8. Dwyer R, et al. *Anesthesiology.* 1992;77:888.
9. Gion H, Saidman LJ. *Anesthesiology.* 1971;35:361.
10. Rampil IJ, et al. *Anesthesiology.* 1991;74:429.
11. Katoh T, et al. *Anesth Analg.* 1993;77:1012.
12. Steward A, et al. *Br J Anaesth.* 1973;45:282.
13. Levitt DG. *BMC Anesthesiol.* 2002;2:5.
14. Wissing H, et al. *Br J Anaesth.* 2000;84:443.
15. Kennedy RR, et al. *Anesth Analg.* 2002;95:1616.
16. Munson ES, Eger 2nd EI. *Anesthesiology.* 1970;33:515.
17. Allott PR, et al. *Br J Anaesth.* 1973;45:294.
18. Munson ES, et al. *Anesth Analg.* 1978;57:224.
19. Eger 2nd EI, et al. *Anesth Analg.* 1998;86:1070.
20. Yamamura H, et al. *Anaesthesia.* 1963;18:427.
21. Kennedy RR, Baker AB. *Anaesth Intensive Care.* 2001;29:535.
22. Eger 2nd EI, Severinghaus JW. *Anesthesiology.* 1964;25:620.
23. Stoelting RK, Longnecker DE. *Anesthesiology.* 1972;36:352.
24. Stoelting RK, Eger 2nd EI. *Anesthesiology.* 1969;30:273.
25. Epstein RM, et al. *Anesthesiology.* 1964;25:364.
26. Taheri S, Eger 2nd EI. *Anesth Analg.* 1999;89:774.
27. Hendrickx JF, et al. *Br J Anaesth.* 2006;96:391.
28. Peyton PJ, Horriat M, Robinson GJ, Pierce R, Thompson BR. Magnitude of the second gas effect on arterial sevoflurane partial pressure. *Anesthesiology.* 2008;108:381–387.
29. Korman B, et al. *Anesthesiology.* 2018;129.
30. Barrett EJ, Rattigan S: Diabetes 61:2661
31. Larsen OA, et al. *Acta Physiol Scand.* 1966;66:337.
32. Matsukawa T, et al. *Anesthesiology.* 1995;82:662.
33. Watt SJ, et al. *Anaesthesia.* 1996;51:24.
34. Westenskow DR, et al. *Br J Anaesth.* 1986;58:555.
35. Van Zundert T, et al: Anaesth Intensive Care 38:76
36. Gallagher TM, Black GW. *Anaesthesia.* 1985;40:1073.
37. Carpenter RL, et al. *Anesth Analg.* 1986;65:575.
38. Yasuda N, et al. *Anesthesiology.* 1991;74:489.
39. Hendrickx J, et al. *Eur J Anaesthesiol.* 2016;33:611.
40. Eger EI, Brandstater B. *Anesthesiology.* 1965;26:756.
41. Eger 2nd EI. *Anesth Analg.* 2001;93:947.
42. Hunter T, et al. *Paediatr Anaesth.* 2005;15:750.
43. Baum JA. *Low flow anaesthesia: the theory and practice of low flow, minimal flow and closed system anaesthesia.* 3nd ed. Boston, Mass: Butterworth-Heinemann; 2001.

44. Levy RJ, et al. *Anesth Analg*. 2010;110:747.
45. Severinghaus JW. *J Clin Invest*. 1954;33:1183.
46. Lowe H, Ernst E. *The quantitative practice of anesthesia: use of closed circuit*. Baltimore, MD: Williams & Wilkins; 1981.
47. Lerou JG, et al. *Anesthesiology*. 1991;75:230.
48. Munson ES, et al. *Anesthesiology*. 1973;38:251.
49. Gibbons RT, et al. *Anesth Analg*. 1977;56:32.
50. Eger 2nd EI, et al. *Anesthesiology*. 1970;32:396.
51. Munson ES, Merrick HC. *Anesthesiology*. 1966;27:783.
52. Eger 2nd EI, Saidman LJ. *Anesthesiology*. 1965;26:61.
53. Perreault L, et al. *Anesthesiology*. 1982;57:325.
54. Wolf GL, et al. *Anesthesiology*. 1983;59:547.
55. Miller CF, Furman WR. *Anesthesiology*. 1983;58:281.
56. Singh M, et al. *J Surg Tech Case Rep*. 2015;7:20–22.
57. Stanley TH, et al. *Anesthesiology*. 1974;41:256.
58. Algren JT, et al. *Paediatr Anaesth*. 1998;8:31.
59. Kaplan R, et al. *Anesthesiology*. 1981;55:71.
60. Lemmens HJ, et al. *Anesth Analg*. 2008;107:1864.
61. Leeson S, et al. *Anesth Analg*. 2014;119:829.
62. Hendrickx JF, et al. *BMC Anesthesiol*. 2006;6:7.
63. Nordmann GR, et al. *Br J Anaesth*. 2006;96:779.
64. Cullen BF, Eger 2nd EI. *Anesthesiology*. 1972;36:168.
65. Fassoulaki A, et al. *Anesthesiology*. 1991;74:479.
66. Laster MJ, et al. *Anesth Analg*. 1991;73:209.
67. Yoshimura N, et al. *Anesthesiology*. 1976;44:372.
68. Neumann MA, et al. *Anesthesiology*. 1998;88:914.
69. Fink BR. *Anesthesiology*. 1955;16:511.
70. Rackow H, et al. *J Appl Physiol*. 1961;16:723.
71. Kharasch ED, et al. *Eur J Clin Pharmacol*. 2000;55:853.
72. Kenna JG. *J Hepatol*. 1997;26(suppl 1):5.
73. Kharasch ED, et al. *Lancet*. 1996;347:1367.
74. Garton KJ, et al. *Drug Metab Dispos*. 1995;23:1426.
75. Kenna JG. *J Hepatol*. 1997;26(suppl 1):5.
76. Gut J, et al. *Pharmacol Ther*. 1993;58(133).
77. Joshi PH, Conn HO. *Ann Int Med*. 1974;80:395.
78. Kharasch ED, et al. *Anesthesiology*. 1995;82:689.
79. Cousins MJ, Mazze RI. *JAMA*. 1973;225:1611.
80. Kharasch ED, et al. *Anesthesiology*. 2006;105:726.
81. Kharasch ED, et al. *Anesth Analg*. 2001;93:1511.
82. Christ DD, et al. *Drug Metab Dispos*. 1988;16:135.
83. Mazze RI, et al. *Anesthesiology*. 1982;57:5.
84. Kharasch ED, Thummel KE. *Anesthesiology*. 1993;79:795.
85. Christ DD, et al. *Anesthesiology*. 1988;69:833.
86. Mazze RI, et al. *Anesth Analg*. 2000;90:683.
87. Brunt EM, et al. *Hepatology*. 1991;13:1017.
88. Mazze RI, et al. *Anesthesiology*. 1974;40:536.
89. Sutton TS, et al. *Anesth Analg*. 1991;73:180.
90. Martin JL, et al. *Anesthesiology*. 1995;83:1125.
91. Jones RM, et al. *Br J Anaesth*. 1990;64:482.
92. Anderson JS, et al. *Anesth Analg*. 2007;104:1452.
93. Holaday DA, Smith FR. *Anesthesiology*. 1981;54:100.
94. Kharasch ED, et al. *Anesthesiology*. 1995;82:1379.
95. Kobayashi Y, et al. *Anesth Analg*. 1992;74:753.
96. Turillazzi E, et al. *Toxicol Pathol*. 2007;35:840.
97. Terrell RC. *Anesthesiology*. 2008;108:531.
98. Krishna DR, Klotz U. *Clin Pharmacokinet*. 1994;26:144.
99. Lohr JW, et al. *Pharmacol Rev*. 1998;50:107.
100. Wilkinson GR. *N Engl J Med*. 2005;352:2211.
101. Kharasch ED. *Acta Anaesthesiol Belg*. 1996;47:7.
102. Weiss CF, et al. *N Engl J Med*. 1960;262:787.
103. Young WS, Lietman PS. *J Pharmacol Exp Therap*. 1978;204:203.
104. Kalow W. *Hum Genomics*. 2004;1:375.
105. Ingelman-Sundberg M, et al. *Trends Pharmacol Sci*. 1999;20:342.
106. Summary of the national Halothane Study. Possible association between halothane anesthesia and postoperative hepatic necrosis. *JAMA*. 1966:197.
107. Ray DC, Drummond GB. *Br J Anaesth*. 1991;67:84.
108. Warner LO, et al. *Anesth Analg*. 1984;63:838.
109. Wark HJ. *Anaesthesia*. 1983;38:237.
110. Wark H, et al. *Br J Anaesth*. 1986;58:1224.
111. Tung D, et al. *Can J Anaesth*. 2005;52:133.
112. Ihtiyar E, et al. *Ind J Gastroenterol*. 2006;25:41.
113. Peiris LJ, et al. *J Clin Anesth*. 2012;24:477.
114. Turner GB, et al. *Eur J Gastroenterol Hepatol*. 2000;12:955.
115. Lewis JH, et al. *Ann Int Med*. 1983;98:984.
116. Lischner MW, et al. *Arch Int Med*. 1967;120:725.
117. Kharasch ED. *Anesth Analg*. 1995;81:S27.
118. Kharasch ED, et al. *Anesthesiology*. 1995;82:1369.
119. Ronis MJ, et al. *Biochem Pharmacol*. 1998;55:123.
120. Hotchkiss JA, et al. *Toxicol Lett*. 1995;78:1.
121. Chen TL, et al. *Can J Anaesth*. 2000;47:680.
122. Knights KM, et al. *Br J Clin Pharmacol*. 2013;76:587.
123. Mazze RI. *Anesthesiology*. 2006;105:843.
124. Mazze RI, et al. *Anesthesiology*. 1972;36:571.
125. Baden JM, et al. *Anesthesiology*. 1982;56:203.
126. Mazze RI, et al. *J Pharmacol Exp Therap*. 1974;190:523.
127. Cousins MJ, et al. *J Pharmacol Exp Therap*. 1974;190:530.
128. Taves DR, et al. *JAMA*. 1970;214:91.
129. Mazze RI, et al. *JAMA*. 1971;216:278.
130. Mazze RI, et al. *Anesthesiology*. 1971;35:247.
131. Murray JM, Trinick TR. *Anesth Analg*. 1992;74:236.
132. Spencer EM, et al. *Anesth Analg*. 1991;73:731.
133. Anders MW. *Annu Rev Pharmacol Toxicol*. 2005;45:147.
134. Keller KA, et al. *Anesthesiology*. 1995;83:1220.
135. Gonsowski CT, et al. *Anesthesiology*. 1994;80:566.
136. Kharasch ED, et al. *Anesthesiology*. 2002;96:173.
137. Bito H, Ikeda K. *Anesthesia Analg*. 1996;82:173.
138. Kharasch ED, et al. *Anesthesiology*. 1997;86:1238.
139. Bito H, et al. *Anesthesiology*. 1997;86:1231.
140. Conzen PF, et al. *Anesthesiology*. 2002;97:578.
141. Eger 2nd EI, et al. *Anesthesia Analg*. 1997;85:1154.
142. Ebert TJ, et al. *Anesthesiology*. 1998;88:601.
143. Higuchi H, et al. *Anesthesiology*. 1998;89:307.
144. Higuchi H, et al. *Anesth Analg*. 2001;92:650.
145. Kharasch ED, et al. *Anesthesiology*. 2005;103:1183.
146. Kharasch ED, et al. *Anesthesiology*. 1997;86:160.
147. Kharasch ED, et al. *Anesthesiology*. 1998;88:1624.
148. Altuntas TG, et al. *Chem Res Toxicol*. 2004;17:435.
149. Eger 2nd EI, et al. *Anesth Analg*. 1997;85:1164.
150. Wissing H, et al. *Anesthesiology*. 2001;95:1205.
151. Keijzer C, et al. *Acta Anaesthesiol Scand*. 2005;49:815.
152. Baxter PJ, et al. *Anesthesiology*. 1998;89:929.
153. Fang ZX, et al. *Anesthesia Analg*. 1995;80:1187.
154. Woehlck HJ, et al. *Anesthesiology*. 1997;87:228.
155. Berry PD, et al. *Anesthesiology*. 1999;90:613.
156. Wu J, et al. *Anesthesiology*. 2004;101:534.
157. Laster M, et al. *Anesth Analg*. 2004;99:769.
158. Baum J, van Aken H. *Eur J Anaesthesiol*. 2000;17:597.
159. Murray JM, et al. *Anesthesiology*. 1999;91:1342.
160. Kobayashi S, et al. *J Anesth*. 2004;18:277.
161. Struys MM, et al. *Anaesthesia*. 2004;59:584.
162. Kobayashi S, et al. *J Clin Anesth*. 2003;15:33.
163. Sanders RD, et al. *Anesthesiology*. 2008;109:707.
164. Reynolds E. *Lancet neurology*. 2006;5:949.
165. Doran M, et al. *BMJ*. 2004;328:1364.
166. Keddie S, et al. *J Neurol*. 2018.
167. Garakani A, et al. *Am J Addict*. 2016;25:358.
168. Kaar SJ, et al. *J Psychopharmacol*. 2016;30:395.
169. Fiskerstrand T, et al. *J Pharmacol Exp Therap*. 1997;282:1305.
170. Duma A, et al. *Anesth Analg*. 2015;120:1325.
171. Amos RJ, et al. *Lancet*. 1982;2:835.
172. Sesso RM, et al. *Neuroradiology*. 1999;41:588.
173. Hadzic A, et al. *Anesthesiology*. 1995;83:863.
174. McNeely JK, et al. *Anesthesiology*. 2000;93:1549.
175. Ilniczky S, et al. *Eur J Neurol*. 2002;9:101.
176. Selzer RR, et al. *N Engl J Med*. 2003;349:45.
177. McCully KS. *Am J Pathology*. 1969;56:111.
178. Nygard O, et al. *N Engl J Med*. 1997;337:230.
179. Mayer EL, et al. *J Am Coll Cardiol*. 1996;27:517.
180. Kaul S, et al. *J Am Coll Cardiol*. 2006;48:914.
181. Ntaios G, et al. *Arch Cardiovasc Dis*. 2009;102:847.
182. Badner NH, et al. *Anesth Analg*. 2000;91:1073.
183. Myles PS, et al. *Anesthesiology*. 2007;107:221.
184. Leslie K, et al. *Anesth Analg*. 2011;112:387.
185. Myles PS, et al. *Lancet*. 2014;384:1446.
186. Leslie K, et al. *Anesth Analg*. 2013.
187. Indraratna P, et al. *Heart Lung Circ*. 2017;26:e41.
188. Nagele P, et al. *Anesthesiology*. 2008;109:36.

189. Nagele P, et al. *Pharmacogenet Genomics*. 2009;19:325.
190. Rao LK, et al. *Anaesthesia*. 2010;65:710.
191. Nunn JF. *Br J Anaesth*. 1987;59:3.
192. Myles PS, et al. *Anaesth Intensive Care*. 2004;32:165.
193. Rappaport B, et al. *N Engl J Med*. 2011;364:1387.
194. Hudson AE, Hemmings Jr HC. *Br J Anaesth*. 2011;107:30.
195. Jevtovic-Todorovic V, et al. *J Neurosci*. 2003;23:876.
196. Loepke AW, Soriano SG. *Anesth Analg*. 2008;106:1681.
197. Slikker Jr W, et al. *Toxicol Sci*. 2007;98:145.
198. Zou X, et al. *Neurotoxicol Teratol*. 2011;33:592.
199. Brambrink AM, et al. *Anesthesiology*. 2010;112:834.
200. Brambrink AM, et al. *Anesthesiology*. 2012;116:372.
201. Schenning KJ, et al. *Neurotoxicol Teratol*. 2017;60:63.
202. Gascon E, et al. *Eur J Anaesthesiol*. 2007;24:213.
203. Mellon RD, et al. *Anesth Analg*. 2007;104:509.
204. Vutskits L, et al. *Paediatr Anaesth*. 2012;22:973.
205. Graham MR, et al. *Anesthesiology*. 2016;125:667.
206. Glatz P, et al. *JAMA Pediatr*. 2017;171:e163470.
207. Warner DO, et al. *Anesthesiology*. 2018;129(1):89.
208. Davidson AJ, Sun LS. *Anesthesiology*. 2018;128:840.
209. Schneuer FJ, et al. *Paediatr Anaesth*. 2018;28(6):528.
210. Davidson AJ, et al. *Lancet*. 2016;387:239.
211. Axelrod D, et al. *Greening the Operating Room and Perioperative Arena: Environmental Sustainability for Anesthesia Practice*. American Society of Anesthesiologists; 2014.
212. Ravishankara AR, et al. *Science*. 2009;326:123.
213. Langbein T, et al. *Br J Anaesth*. 1999;82:66.
214. Ryan SM, Nielsen CJ. *Anesth Analg*. 2010;111:92.
215. *Climate Change 2007: The Physical Science Basis*. New York: Cambridge University Press; 2007.
216. Austin J, et al. *Nature*. 1992;360:221.
217. Forster P, et al. In: Solomon S, Qin D, Manning M, eds. *Changes in Atmospheric Constituents and in Radiative Forcing, Climate Change 2007: The Physical Science Basis*. Cambridge: Contribution of Working Group I to the Fourth Assessment Report of the Intergovernmental Panel on Climate Change; 2007.
218. Ryan S, Sherman J. *Anesth Analg*. 2012;114:921.
219. Ishizawa Y. *Anesth Analg*. 2011;112:213.
220. Gutierrez MJF, et al. *Waste Manag Res*. 2005;23:133.
221. Maskell K, et al. *Lancet*. 1993;342:1027.
222. Schmeltekopf AL, et al. *Geophys Res Lett*. 1975;2:393.
223. Sherman SJ, Cullen BF. *Anesthesiology*. 1988;68:816.
224. Hammitt JK, et al. *Nature*. 1987;330:711.
225. Langbein T, et al. *Br J Anaesth*. 1999;82:66.
226. Brown AC, et al. *Nature*. 1989;341:635.
227. *Executive summary. scientific assessment of ozone depletion: 2002*. Geneva: World Meteorological Organization; 2002. Global Ozone Research and Monitoring Project Report No. 47.
228. Barwise JA, et al. *Anesth Analg*. 2011;113:1064.
229. McGregor DG. *Mayo Clinic*. 2000;75:273.
230. Burm AG. *Best Pract Res Clin Anaesthesiol*. 2003;17:147.
231. Vieira E, et al. *Anesth Analg*. 1980;59:175.
232. Fujinaga M, et al. *Anesthesiology*. 1988;69:401.
233. Yilmaz S, Calbayram NC. *J Clin Anesth*. 2016;35:326.
234. Spence AA. *Br J Anaesth*. 1987;59:96.
235. Szyfter K, et al. *J Appl Genet*. 2004;45:369.
236. Friedman JM. *Teratology*. 1988;37:69.
237. Kuczkowski KM. *Obstet Gynecol Surv*. 2004;59:52.
238. Reitman E, Flood P. *Br J Anaesth*. 2011;107(suppl 1):i72.
239. Sessler DI, Badgwell JM. *Anesth Analg*. 1998;87:1083.
240. McGregor DG, et al. *Anesth Analg*. 1999;89:472.
241. Krenzischek DA, et al. *J Perianesth Nurs*. 2002;17:227.
242. Cullen SC, Gross EG. *Science*. 1951;113:580.
243. Preckel B, et al. *Anesthesiology*. 2006;105:187.
244. Sanders RD, et al. *Br J Anaesth*. 2003;91:709.
245. Sanders RD, Maze M. *Curr Opin Anaesthesiol*. 2005;18:405.
246. Goto T, et al. *Anesthesiology*. 1997;86:1273.
247. Rossaint R, et al. *Anesthesiology*. 2003;98:6.
248. Law LS, Lo EA, Gan TJ. Xenon Anesthesia: A Systematic Review and Meta-Analysis of Randomized Controlled Trials. *Anesth Analg*. 2016;122:678–697.
249. Goto T, et al. *Anaesthesia*. 2004;59:1178.
250. Wappler F, et al. *Anesthesiology*. 2007;106:463.
251. Baumert JH, et al. *Br J Anaesth*. 2008;100:605.
252. Lachmann B, et al. *Lancet*. 1990;335(1413).
253. Wappler F. *Curr Opin Anaesthesiol*. 2010;23:417.
254. Al Tmimi L, et al. *Anesth Analg*. 2017;125:1118.
255. Al Tmimi L, et al. *Trials*. 2015;16:449.
256. Hofland J, et al. *Anesthesiology*. 2017;127:918.
258. Arola O, et al. *J Am Coll Cardiol*. 2017;70:2652.
259. Laitio R, et al. *JAMA*. 2016;315:1120.
260. Coburn M, et al. *Br J Anaesth*. 2007;98:756.
261. Coburn M, et al. *Eur J Anaesthesiol*. 2005;22:870.
262. Coburn M, et al. *Br J Anaesth*. 2018;120:127.
263. Nakata Y, et al. *J Clin Anesth*. 1999;11:477.
264. Rawat S, Dingley J. *Anesth Analg*. 2010;110:101.
265. Dingley J, et al. *Anesthesiology*. 2001;94:173.
266. Dingley J, Mason RS. *Anesth Analg*. 2007;105:1312.
267. Zhang P, et al. *Can J Anaesthesia = Journal canadien d'anesthesie*. 1995;42:547.
268. Lockwood G. *Br J Anaesth*. 2002;89:282.
269. Coburn M, et al. *Br J Anaesth*. 2008;100:787.
270. Fahlenkamp AV, et al. *PLoS One*. 2016;11:e0153807.
271. Dickinson R, Franks NP. *Crit Care*. 2010;14:229.

21 Pulmonary Pharmacology and Inhaled Anesthetics

OLEG V. EVGENOV, YAFEN LIANG, YANDONG JIANG, and JAMES L. BLAIR

KEY POINTS

- Inhaled anesthetics affect every part of physiology of the lungs and their pulmonary pharmacology is complex.
- Volatile anesthetics produce bronchodilation through decreases in cytoplasmic ionized calcium concentration and/or a reduction in calcium sensitivity of airway smooth muscle. Volatile anesthetics also attenuate an increase in pulmonary airway resistance induced by chemical and mechanical stimulation.
- Inhaled anesthetics reduce the rate of mucous clearance and affect function of type II alveolar cells; these effects can potentially contribute to postoperative pulmonary complications.
- Volatile anesthetics produce a biphasic response in pulmonary vascular smooth muscle. Although inhibition of hypoxic pulmonary vasoconstriction by volatile anesthetic is an overall small effect, it can contribute to worsening of hypoxemia in patients with underlying pulmonary disease.
- Volatile anesthetics depress respiratory function through a diminished respiratory drive and an increase in upper airway collapsibility. Following extubation, even at residual concentrations, volatile anesthetics can severely impair peripheral chemoreceptor inputs and hypoxic arousal reflexes.
- Volatile anesthetics produce dose-dependent reductions in tidal volume and minute ventilation, cause tachypnea, and blunt ventilatory response to hypercapnia and hypoxia.
- During anesthesia with volatile agents, diaphragmatic function remains relatively well preserved, whereas inspiratory rib cage muscles are significantly depressed resulting in insufficiency of breathing or paradoxical breathing.
- Volatile anesthetics can compromise upper airway patency. Even at low concentrations, upper airway obstruction can occur in susceptible patients, including elderly, obese, or critically ill patients.
- Volatile anesthetics vary in their ability to irritate airways and augment defensive airway reflexes. Sevoflurane causes the least amount of subjective airway irritation and is the anesthetic of choice for inhaled induction of anesthesia in infants and children.
- Preclinical and clinical evidence suggests therapeutic potential of isoflurane and sevoflurane in acute lung injury.
- Although concerns have been recently raised regarding the use of nitrous oxide, a lack of strong evidence does not justify abandoning it from clinical practice, especially considering its favorable cost-effectiveness.
- Xenon produces a fast on and off action and is a promising alternative for sedation in the critical care setting.

Introduction

Pulmonary pharmacology of inhaled anesthetics is complex. This chapter focuses in depth on pulmonary pharmacology of isoflurane, sevoflurane, desflurane, nitrous oxide, and xenon. The older anesthetics (including halothane, enflurane, and ether) are no longer in use in the developed countries, and are discussed here only for comparison. The lungs are unique in their exposure to a wide variety of physical forces including ventilation, blood flow, and surface tension as well as derangements of function caused by disease and environmental factors. The effects of inhaled anesthetics on ventilatory control, airway tone, mucociliary function, surfactant production, pulmonary vascular resistance (PVR), and acute lung injury (ALI) are examined in detail in this chapter.

The physical properties of commonly used inhalational anesthetics and clinical concerns are presented in Table 21.1.

Inhaled Anesthetics

ASTHMA AND BRONCHOSPASM OVERVIEW

Asthma is a chronic airway disease with an estimated worldwide annual death rate of 250,000. Asymptomatic asthma patients have relatively infrequent perioperative respiratory complications; however, bronchospasm

TABLE 21.1 The Physical Properties of Commonly Used Inhalational Anesthetics and Their Clinical Concerns

Property	Halothane	Isoflurane	Sevoflurane	Desflurane	Nitrous oxide	Xenon
Boiling point (°C)	50.2	49	59	24	−88	−108
Vapor pressure (mm Hg) at 20°C	241	238	157	669	38,770	–
Blood:gas partition coefficient	2.5	1.46	0.65	0.42	0.46	0.115
Oil:gas partition coefficient	224	91	47	19	1.4	1.9
Minimal alveolar concentration (MAC)	0.74	1.17	1.8	6.6	104	63-71
Metabolized in the body (%)	25	0.2	2-4	0.02	0	0
Clinical concerns	Hepatotoxicity		Compound A	Airway irritation	Gas expansion	Apnea

develops in about 9% of asthmatics in the perioperative period.[1] Twenty-five percent of asthmatics may present with wheezing after induction of anesthesia,[2] and 1.7% of asthma patients sustain a poor respiratory outcome.[3] In addition, acute bronchospasm can occur at induction, intubation, or during maintenance of anesthesia without prior history of asthma or COPD. According to the ASA Closed Claims Project[4] 40 cases of bronchospasm resulted in settled malpractice claims, with 88% involving brain damage or death. Importantly, only half of the patients had preexisting asthma or COPD. Adverse respiratory events accounted for 28% of claims related to anesthesia-related brain damage and death in the United States; they were associated with the highest mean cost per closed claim. In France, 7% of anesthesia-related deaths were also attributed to bronchospasm.[5] A nonallergic mechanism was involved in nearly 80% of cases. Although bronchospasm caused by airway irritation occurred more frequently in patients who had one or more predisposing factors including asthma, heavy tobacco smoking, or bronchitis, only 50% and 60% of patients with nonallergic and allergic bronchospasm, respectively, had history of asthma.

PHYSIOLOGY OF BRONCHIAL SMOOTH MUSCLE

Airway resistance is increased, at least in part, by an increase in bronchiolar smooth muscle (BSM) tone. BSM extends down to the terminal bronchioles and is controlled primarily by autonomic nervous system activity. Nonadrenergic, noncholinergic mechanisms, activated by the stimulation of the afferent bronchopulmonary sensory C fibers, play a role in BSM constriction to tachykinins, vasoactive intestinal peptide (VIP), adenosine, and calcitonin gene-related peptides.

Asthmatic bronchiolar constriction involves complex interactions of airway nerves, smooth muscle, epithelium, and inflammatory cells. In contrast, reflex bronchoconstriction caused by airway irritation is mediated by sensory afferents in the nucleus of the solitary tract (NTS), projecting to vagal preganglionic neurons (VPN). Glutamate modulates stimulation of NTS and VPN, whereas γ aminobutyric acid (GABA) is inhibitory from NTS projecting to VPN. VPN projections to the airways release acetylcholine (ACh) predominantly onto M3 receptors, inducing bronchoconstriction. Baseline airway tone is also mediated by the vagus nerve. The muscarinic acetylcholine receptors (mAChRs, M1-M5) on BSM are G protein-coupled receptors, three of which (M1, M2, and M3) are expressed in the lungs of humans and of most mammals.[6] Belmonte and colleagues[7] reviewed the essentials of muscarinic control of mAChRs in the lungs. Neuronal inhibitory M2 muscarinic ACh receptors on parasympathetic nerves are responsible for limiting ACh release from these nerves (Fig. 21.1).

ROLE OF CALCIUM

Alterations in cytoplasmic ionized calcium concentration (ICa^{+2}) and calcium (Ca^{+2}) influx result from the interplay of cyclic nucleotides in BSM that alters myosin light chain (MLC) and MLC kinase activity. Ca^{+2}/calmodulin-dependent MLC kinase is critical for tonic smooth muscle contraction.[8] Agonist activation of BSM also involves a second messenger, cADP ribose, resulting in inositol triphosphate (IP_3)-mediated release of Ca^{+2} from sarcoplasmic reticulum via activated ryanodine channels.[9] This release is followed by an increase in sodium (Na^+) influx across the cell membrane. This localized increase in Na^+ may switch the Na^+/Ca^{2+} exchanger into reverse mode, leading to even more Ca^{2+} influx and greater bronchial constriction. Several different cyclic adenosine monophosphate (cAMP) signaling compartments exist in airway smooth muscle that are responsive to different hormones and neurotransmitters.[10] The mechanical stretch of human BSM cells also causes contraction via an influx of Ca^{2+} through unique stretch-activated nonselective cation channels.[11] Adenosine indirectly enhances contraction of airway smooth muscle via the activation of mast cells and via nerves by directly stimulating adenosine type I receptors on airway smooth muscle, thereby rapidly mobilizing ICa^{2+} stores through G proteins and IP_3 signaling. Agonist-induced stimulation of *particulate* guanylyl cyclase relaxes bronchial smooth muscle by attenuating inward Ca^{2+} current, whereas stimulation of *soluble* guanylyl cyclase by substances such as nitric oxide (NO) reduces ICa^{2+} concentration and Ca^{2+} sensitivity.[12]

HISTAMINE

Release of histamine in the airway produces reflex bronchoconstriction from actions on H1 receptors on BSM, eliciting activation of phospholipase C and protein kinase C (PKC) downstream mediators, leading to release of Ca^{2+} from intracellular stores. This leads to calcium ion entry through calcium channels, cation channels of the transient receptor potential (TRP1) channel type, and stimulation of a Na^+/

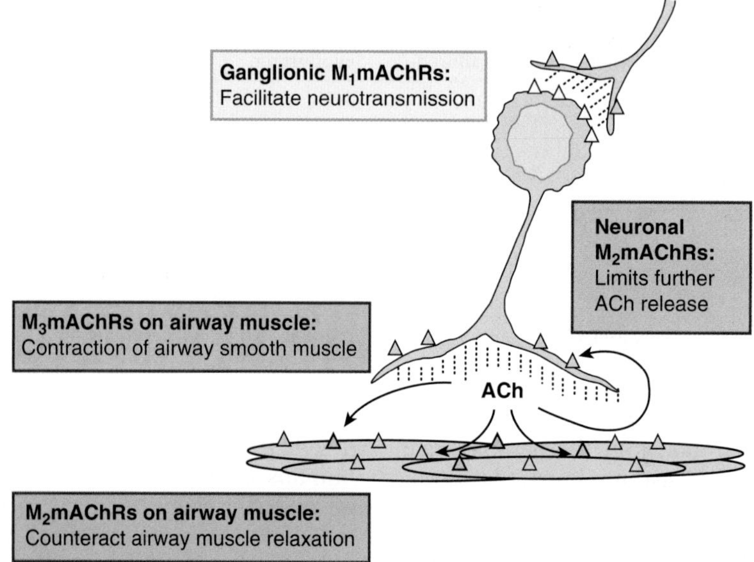

Fig. 21.1 Muscarinic acetylcholine receptors *(mAChRs)* on pulmonary parasympathetic nerves (PSN) and airway smooth muscle (ASM). Acetylcholine (ACh) released by PSN stimulates M2 mAChRs on ASM resulting in contraction. M2 mAChRs on ASM facilitate M3 mAChR-mediated contraction by counteracting the cyclic adenosine monophosphate relaxant pathway. Release of ACh by nerves is tightly controlled by M2 mAChRs found on PSN endings. M1 mAChRs found within parasympathetic ganglia are thought to facilitate cholinergic neurotransmission that is mediated primarily by nicotinic Ach receptors.[7] (Redrawn from Belmonte KE. Cholinergic pathways in the lungs and anticholinergic therapy for chronic obstructive pulmonary disease. *Proc Am Thorac Soc.* 2005;2(4):297–304. Used with permission.)

Ca^{2+} exchanger. Nicotinic acid adenine dinucleotide phosphate has also been suggested as a potential second messenger in histamine-induced Ca^{2+} release from lysosome-like acidic compartments, functionally coupled to the endoplasmic reticulum via H1 receptor in endothelial cells.[13] This increase in bronchomotor tone is attenuated by the cholinergic antagonist atropine. The histamine-degrading enzyme, histamine N-methyltransferase, has been localized to human airway epithelium and may play a protective role against histamine-mediated bronchoconstriction.[14] Histamine-induced bronchoconstriction, measured as altered pulmonary resistance (RL) and dynamic pulmonary compliance (C_{dyn}) in response to intravenous (IV) histamine was studied in dogs to determine the bronchodilatory effects of halothane, sevoflurane, isoflurane, and enflurane. All the volatile anesthetics demonstrated an inhibitory effect on increases in RL and decreases in C_{dyn} caused by histamine.[15]

ADRENERGIC RECEPTORS

Adrenergic receptors in BSM are classified into α and β_2 types. The α2 agonists clonidine and dexmedetomidine have been shown to produce bronchodilation in central airways,[16] which may be mediated through α2 central vagolytic effects. Clinically, the β_2-receptor subtypes play an important role in BSM responsiveness. Stimulation of β_2 adrenoceptors causes cAMP-mediated relaxation via activation of protein kinase A and subsequent Ca^{2+} efflux out of the cell and into the SR. Interestingly, asthma, as well as allergy- and methacholine-induced bronchospasm, do not appear to be genetically linked to a dominant β_2-adrenoceptor gene.[17]

Respiratory epithelium releases substances that modulate BSM tone. Removal of the epithelium enhances contractile responses to ACh, histamine, or serotonin in large airways and decreases relaxation responses to isoproterenol in small airways. These responses are similar to the effect of endothelial damage on vascular smooth muscle tone. Notably, cardiopulmonary bypass does significantly affect porcine bronchiolar epithelium-mediated bronchomotor activity, in contrast to vascular endothelium-mediated smooth muscle dysfunction.[18] While endogenous epithelial factors have been identified, endogenous NO produced in respiratory epithelium likely plays a bronchodilatory role similar to that of vascular endothelium. Endothelin-1 is a potent constrictor of vascular smooth muscle and BSM that activates the IP_3 pathway and produces greater pulmonary effects compared to the systemic circulation.[19] Clinically, evaluation of the effects of the inhalational agents may be framed against a background of the major physiologic mechanisms governing normal and pathophysiologic BSM activity. These include airway disease (asthma and COPD), the overarching complex chemistry of calcium release as the BSM stimulus-contraction coupler, intrinsic factors (afferent and efferent ACh signaling, α2 receptor signaling, NO and endothelin-1, allergy and histamine release), and extrinsic factors (physical and chemical irritants, e.g., endotracheal tubes), capable of promoting reflex bronchoconstriction.

Effects of Inhaled Anesthetics

In general, all volatile anesthetics are bronchodilators, making them a good choice for patients with increased airway resistance. Using computed tomography (CT), Brown and colleagues demonstrated that halothane causes dose-dependent bronchodilation in a dog (Fig. 21.2).[20]

Eliminating indirect effects of arterial carbon dioxide (CO_2) tension is important when examining the actions of volatile anesthetics on bronchial tone, especially during spontaneous ventilation. This is because hypercapnia-induced bronchodilation and hypocapnia-induced bronchoconstriction are both attenuated by isoflurane.[21] Thus a concentration-dependent bronchodilator effect

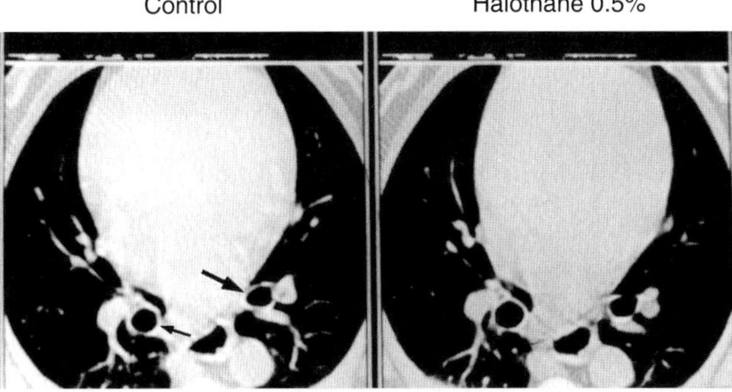

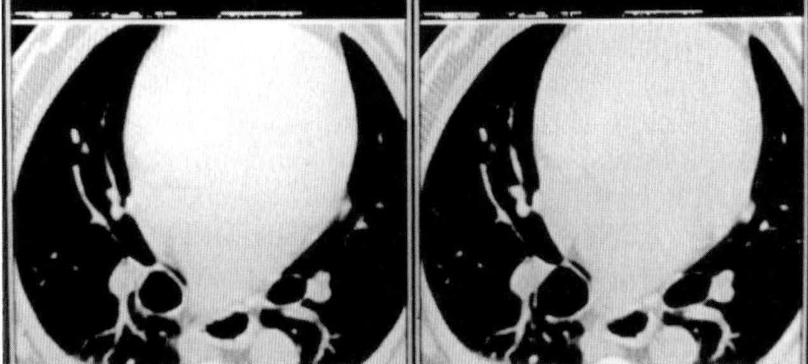

Fig. 21.2 High-resolution computed tomography scans from one dog. *Upper left:* Control. *Upper right:* During 0.5% halothane. *Lower left:* During 1.0% halothane. *Lower right:* During 1.5% halothane. Note the progressive dilation of the airways as indicated by the *arrows*. (Reproduced from Brown RH, Mitzner W, Zerhouni E, et al. Direct in vivo visualization of bronchodilation induced by inhalational anesthesia using high-resolution computed tomography. *Anesthesiology*. 1993;78:295. Used with permission.)

of volatile anesthetics may be indirectly attributable to increase in CO_2 tension. The structure of the respiratory epithelium changes from pseudostratified columnar cells of the large airways to thinner, cuboidal cells of the bronchioles, and thus a relatively large amount of histologic heterogeneity exists between these regions. The specific effects of volatile anesthetics on the bronchioles depend on the location in and the structure of the respiratory tree. In vitro, isoflurane preferentially relaxes the bronchioles rather than the bronchi.[22] Isoflurane and halothane dilate fourth order bronchi at equivalent minimum alveolar concentration (MAC) values.[23] Similarly, at up to 1 MAC, isoflurane, sevoflurane, and desflurane attenuate methacholine-induced bronchoconstriction in open-chest, pentobarbital-anesthetized rats.[24] Isoflurane and sevoflurane also appear to have greater inhibitory effects on bronchial contraction as compared with tracheal smooth muscle contraction.[25] Furthermore, halothane, desflurane, and isoflurane relax distal airways (e.g., bronchioles) to a greater extent than proximal airways (e.g., bronchi).[26] These differential effects appear to be related to the type of voltage-dependent Ca^{2+} (VDC) channels that are present in these regions.

Inhalation of 1 or 2 MAC halothane, enflurane, sevoflurane, and isoflurane did not alter baseline pulmonary resistance and dynamic pulmonary compliance, but these anesthetics significantly attenuated increases in airway resistance and decreases in dynamic respiratory compliance in response to intravenous histamine. Halothane was the most effective bronchodilator, whereas responses to isoflurane, enflurane, and sevoflurane were similar.[15] In an isolated lung model, desflurane produced bronchodilation at 1 MAC but increased airway resistance at 2 MAC,[27] presumably resulting in part from significant increases in inspired gas density at higher MAC. Isoflurane, sevoflurane, and desflurane at 1.0, 1.5, and 2.0 MAC in 25% O_2 were all examined in a two-chamber test lung model with fixed resistance. All anesthetics demonstrated increased density and calculated resistance at higher MAC, with desflurane producing the highest increase in resistance at 2.0 MAC.[28] In a randomized clinical trial evaluating the same agents at 1.0 and 1.5 MAC, total inspiratory resistance (R[rs]), minimal resistance (R[min]), and effective resistance (D[Rrs]) were calculated using the end-inspiratory occlusion technique. No significant differences of those parameters were observed during administration of the three agents at 1 MAC for 30 min. At 1.5 MAC, desflurane caused a maximum increase in R(rs) by 26% and in R(min) by 30% above baseline, in contrast to isoflurane and sevoflurane, which did not have a significant effect on R(rs) and R(min).[29] Presumably, this increased resistance is due at least in part to the greater net viscosity of the higher absolute concentration of desflurane at 1.5 MAC. Other factors may also cause the reduction in the bronchodilation of desflurane at higher concentrations, especially in smokers.[30] Halothane, enflurane, and sevoflurane are equivalent at dilating third- or fourth-generation bronchi as directly measured with a fiberoptic bronchoscope in vivo.[31]

It appears that desflurane can both augment or inhibit bronchoconstriction (see below). At 1 MAC desflurane and sevoflurane blocked, to a similar degree, the increase in central airway resistance after a cholinergic challenge in rabbits. Both anesthetics reduced basal bronchial tone by 30% to 40%. This effect was consistently observed in the presence or absence of allergic airway inflammation and bronchial hyperresponsiveness.[32] When the mechanism of constriction is centrally mediated, such as with a cholinergic challenge,[22,24,33,34] desflurane appears to play a beneficial role in attenuating bronchoconstriction. However, when the mechanism of airway constriction is due to nonadrenergic, noncholinergic activation with tachykinins, desflurane may augment and worsen constriction.[35,36] Thus clinicians tend to avoid using desflurane in patients with reactive airway disease.

EFFECTS OF INHALED ANESTHETICS ON BRONCHOMOTOR TONE IN HUMANS AND THE WORK OF BREATHING

Sevoflurane (1 MAC) reduced respiratory system resistance by 15% in patients undergoing elective surgery, whereas desflurane had no effect.[30] Rooke and associates[37] compared the bronchodilating effects of halothane, isoflurane, sevoflurane, desflurane, and thiopental–nitrous oxide in healthy patients undergoing induction of anesthesia and tracheal intubation. In contrast to thiopental–nitrous oxide, all volatile agents with the exception of desflurane significantly reduced respiratory resistance (Fig. 21.3).

The work of breathing is defined as pressure or force multiplied by the tidal volume during inspiration. Respiratory work is further divided into elastic work (required to overcome the recoil of the lung) and resistive work (required

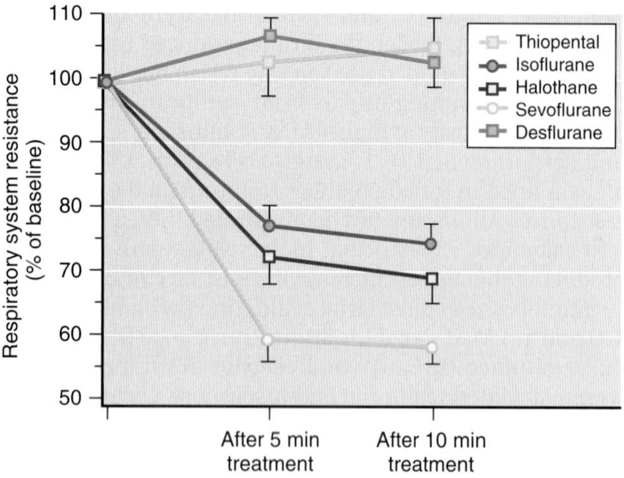

Fig. 21.3 Percent change in respiratory system resistance in patients after 5 and 10 minutes of maintenance anesthesia with either 0.25 mg/kg/min thiopental plus 50% nitrous oxide or 1.1 minimum alveolar concentration (MAC) sevoflurane, halothane, or isoflurane, or approximately 1 MAC desflurane. All volatile anesthetics except desflurane decreased resistance. Sevoflurane decreased resistance more than isoflurane. (Modified from Rooke GA, Choi JH, Bishop MJ. The effect of isoflurane, halothane, sevoflurane, and thiopental/nitrous oxide on respiratory system resistance after tracheal intubation. *Anesthesiology.* 1997;86:1294; and Goff MJ, Arain SR, Ficke DJ, et al. Absence of bronchodilation during desflurane anesthesia: a comparison to sevoflurane and thiopental. *Anesthesiology.* 2000;93:404. Used with permission.)

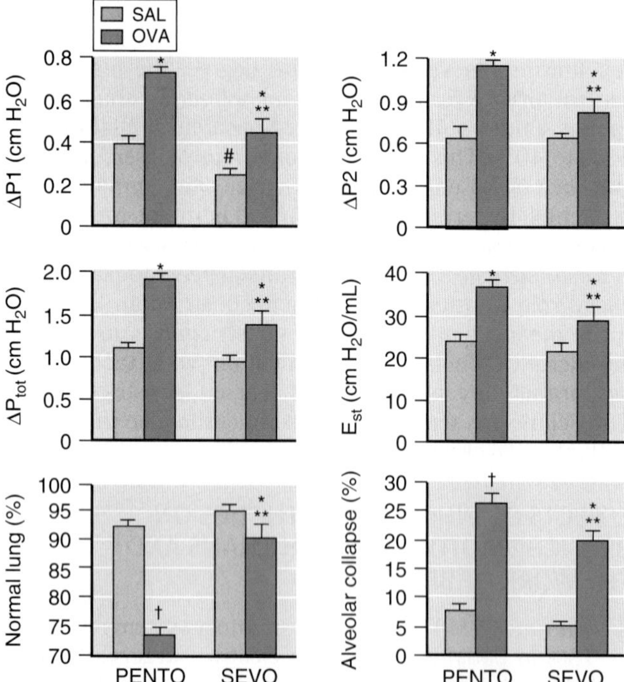

Fig. 21.4 Mean ± standard error of the mean for pressure to overcome airway resistance (ΔP1), viscoelastic lung properties (ΔP2), total of ΔP1 and ΔP2 (ΔP_{tot}), and static lung elastance (E_{st}). Also shown are the percent of normal area and the percent of alveolar collapse in mice repeatedly challenged with intratracheal instillation of saline *(SAL)* or ovalbumin *(OVA)*. Animals were anesthetized with pentobarbital sodium *(PENTO)* or sevoflurane *(SEVO)*, 1 minimum alveolar concentration (MAC). *$P < .05$ versus corresponding SAL group; **$P < .001$ versus OVA-PENTO group; #$P < .05$ versus SAL-PENTO group; †$P < .01$ versus the SAL-PENTO group. (Modified from Burburan SM, Xisto DG, Ferreira HC, et al. Lung mechanics and histology during sevoflurane anesthesia in a model of chronic allergic rhinitis. *Anesth Analg.* 2007;104:631. Used with permission.)

to overcome airway flow resistance and viscoelastic resistance of pulmonary tissues). The work of breathing is usually derived from transpulmonary pressure volume curves. Volatile anesthetics increase the work of breathing in adults and children. In rats, sevoflurane reduced pulmonary compliance at the lung periphery rather than at the airway level, thereby increasing viscoelastic and elastic pressures in the lung.[38] In addition, in a murine model of chronic asthma, sevoflurane significantly decreased resistance in central and distal airways and also lowered resistance in the lung periphery. These data suggest that sevoflurane exerts a beneficial effect in the presence of chronic airway obstruction and indicate that sevoflurane might reduce the work of breathing in comparison to other drugs (Fig. 21.4).[39]

Studies in humans demonstrate a ceiling effect where low concentrations of volatile anesthetics significantly reduce *upper airway resistance*, reflecting changes in airway smooth muscle tone in the major airways. In contrast, distal airways and lung parenchyma lack a smooth muscle component (with *lower airway and alveolar resistance* being more a measure of viscoelastic changes in the lung). Increasing concentrations of inhalational agents have diminished effect on these more distal pulmonary components and thus do not further reduce total lung resistance (Fig. 21.5).[40]

Expiration is passively affected by the recoil characteristics of the lung during normal breathing. In anesthetized patients, the ventilatory response to expiratory resistance is reduced to a greater extent than the response to inspiratory resistance. Conscious and anesthetized humans exhibit decreases in respiratory rate when expiratory resistive loads are applied, but only anesthetized subjects develop rib cage–abdominal wall motion dyssynchrony that causes less effective ventilation and reduction in minute alveolar ventilation. This concept may be particularly important in spontaneously breathing anesthetized patients who demonstrate expiratory obstruction, such as in cases of asthma, COPD, airway secretions, or during hypopharyngeal obstruction or partial breathing circuit occlusion.

Experimental studies demonstrating the equal potency of sevoflurane and isoflurane and the higher potency of halothane for bronchodilation must be extrapolated with caution because histamine-mediated experimental bronchospasm may not closely mimic tracheal intubation–induced bronchospasm in humans. Indeed, Arakawa and colleagues[41] showed that similar inspired concentrations of halothane, isoflurane, and sevoflurane produced nearly identical reductions in airway resistance in a patient with status asthmaticus. Volatile anesthetics may thus be an effective therapeutic modality in status asthmaticus when conventional therapy has failed.[42,43]

β-Adrenoceptor agonists may be beneficial for treating acute bronchospasm in patients anesthetized with halothane,[44,45] but their use may not be beneficial with other volatile anesthetics. For example, the β_2-adrenergic agonist fenoterol reduced respiratory system resistance after endotracheal intubation but did not further decrease resistance when administered in the presence of 1.3% isoflurane.[46] These findings should be interpreted with caution because the technique used to determine respiratory system resistance incorporates alterations in lung and chest wall resistance, as well as tissue viscosity. The most important functional change that occurs in the presence of lung disease is increased resistance. Resistance to airflow is

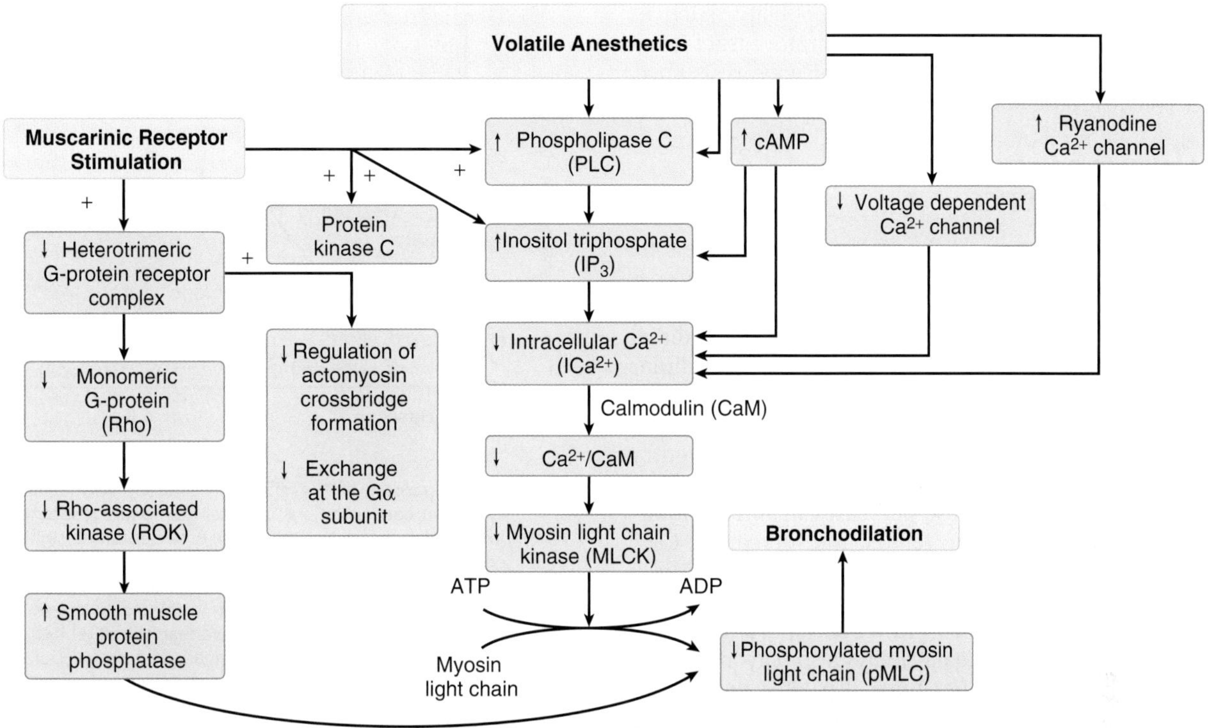

Fig. 21.5 Isoflurane (ISO) at 0.6% reduced respiratory system elastance (E in cm H_2O/L) and resistance (R in cm H_2O/L/s). *Total* represents the total respiratory system (lung and chest wall). Values are mean ± standard deviation (SD). No further reductions with increasing concentrations of isoflurane were observed. *$P < .05$ versus baseline; *ADP*, adenosine diphosphate; *ATP*, adenosine triphosphate; *cAMP*, cyclic adenosine monophosphate. (Modified from Ruiz P, Chartrand D. The effect of isoflurane 0.6% on respiratory mechanics in anesthetized-paralyzed humans is not increased at concentrations of 0.9% and 1.2%. *Can J Anaesth*. 2003;50:67. Used with permission.)

typically thought of as being determined by the flow rate and airway smooth muscle tension. However, nonmuscle elements, such as lung inflammation, airway thickening, altered lung volumes, lung recoil, airway wall remodeling, mucous hypersecretion, and loss of lung elastance, also play a clinically significant role in the amount of airway narrowing. The role of volatile anesthetics in altering many of these non–smooth-muscle elements responsible for airway resistance needs further elucidation.

The effects of volatile anesthetics on bronchomotor tone are also dependent on the substance used to produce contraction in vitro.[47] Relaxation of tracheal smooth muscle by halothane and isoflurane is greatest in the presence of the endogenous mediator serotonin (resulting from anaphylactoid or immunologic reactions) compared with ACh (representing the neutrally derived mediator of reflex bronchospasm). Thus inhaled anesthetics may remain effective bronchodilators, even in the presence of severe serotonin- or histamine-induced bronchospasm that is refractory to β_2-adrenoceptor therapy. It is important to note that in anesthetized patients, volatile anesthetic–induced decreases in bronchomotor tone and neurally mediated airway reflexes may be partially opposed by a simultaneous reduction in functional residual capacity (FRC). The well-known increased risk for morbidity and mortality in patients with asthma may be at least partially attributed to these FRC-mediated increases in airway resistance. Low temperature abolished the inhibitory effects of volatile anesthetics on carbachol-induced contraction of airway smooth muscle in dogs,[48] suggesting that intraoperative hypothermia may also attenuate volatile anesthetic–induced bronchodilation.

Bronchospasm may occur in conditions and with respiratory diseases other than asthma. For example, healthy patients undergoing surgical stimulation of lung parenchyma or airways including tracheal stimulation by an endotracheal tube are at risk of developing bronchospasm. Preoperative medications, sedatives, neuromuscular blockers, and volatile anesthetics are all important factors that may trigger or attenuate bronchospasms. Regardless of the airway sensitivity prior to induction, the different pathways involved in an individual patient may yield different responses to the volatile anesthetics. Iwasaki and colleagues[49] demonstrated that sevoflurane-induced relaxation of airway smooth muscle and VDC channels were dependent on the type of hyperreactive airway model. Sevoflurane had smaller effects in a model of chronic tobacco smoking (enlarged alveolar ducts and less muscarinic hyperreactivity), compared with an antigen-acute asthmatic (ovalbumin-sensitized) model. The morphologic changes in the peripheral airway may be responsible to some degree for a decrease in the efficacy of volatile anesthetics as bronchodilators in tobacco smokers, but sevoflurane and isoflurane still decrease respiratory system resistance in patients with COPD.[50]

In children undergoing elective imaging studies, sevoflurane produced progressive reductions in the cross-sectional area of upper airway, resulting in pharyngeal airway collapse[51] (also see Chapter 93). As observed with isoflurane in animal models, the effects of sevoflurane were not uniformly distributed along the upper airway. In healthy children, sevoflurane slightly decreased airway resistance, but desflurane had the opposite effect, presumably via reduced airway size.[52]

Children with documented airway susceptibility, such as those with asthma or a recent upper respiratory tract infection, exhibit significant increases in airway resistance. In these pediatric patients, desflurane should be avoided.

MECHANISMS OF ACTION OF VOLATILE ANESTHETICS

Volatile anesthetics attenuate airway smooth muscle tone by reducing smooth muscle contractility. This action is the result of the direct effects on bronchial epithelium and airway smooth muscle cells, combined with the indirect inhibition of reflex neural pathways. Several intracellular mediators responsible for Ca^{2+} mobilization are potential sites for the action for volatile anesthetics. Inhibition of cell membrane-associated VDC channels reduces Ca^{2+} entry into the cytosol.[53] Volatile anesthetic–induced increases in cAMP concentrations cause decreases in intracellular-free Ca^{2+} by stimulating Ca^{2+} efflux and increasing Ca^{2+} uptake into the sarcoplasmic reticular (SR). In addition, a decrease in Ca^{2+} sensitivity attributable to inhibition of PKC activity, inhibition of G-protein function, and attenuation of Rho/Rho-kinase signaling pathways also play important roles.[53,54] Volatile anesthetics may also alter pulmonary resistance by affecting the density of the gas mixture.[28] In an experimental lung model of fixed pulmonary resistance, high concentrations of volatile anesthetics increased the density of the gas mixture and the calculated resistance, with desflurane producing the largest increase (Fig. 21.6).[28] Such an effect is particularly profound for [55]xenon which has a molecular weight of 131.2 Daltons, making it four times as dense as room air.[55]

The effects of volatile anesthetics on proximal, compared with distal, airways may be related to the differential effects on VDC channels and the relative distribution of these channels. Long-lasting (L-type) VDC channels appear to be the predominant mechanism for Ca^{2+} entry in tracheal smooth muscle, whereas both transient (T-type) and L-type VDC channels are present in bronchial smooth muscle.[25,56] Isoflurane and sevoflurane inhibit both types of VDC channels in a dose-dependent fashion, and their effects on T-type VDC channels in bronchial smooth muscle are even more pronounced (Fig. 21.7).[25]

The differential effects of volatile anesthetics on tracheal smooth muscle, compared with bronchial smooth muscle, may also be related to actions on Ca^{2+}-activated chloride channel activity[57,58] or differential sensitivities of K^+ channel subtypes.[57]

The proposed signaling pathways underlying volatile anesthetic–induced bronchodilation are depicted in Fig. 21.8.[59,60]

Volatile anesthetic–induced reductions in ICa^{2+} result from the inhibition of both VDC and receptor-gated Ca^{2+} channels. In addition, volatile anesthetics deplete Ca^{2+} stores in SR by increasing Ca^{2+} leakage. Ca^{2+} influx occurring in response to depleted SR Ca^{2+} stores is known as store-operated Ca^{2+} entry (SOCE). By depleting Ca^{2+} stores in SR, volatile anesthetics may be expected to enhance SOCE. Nevertheless, at clinically relevant concentrations, volatile anesthetics (isoflurane more than sevoflurane) also inhibit SOCE in airway smooth muscle to further reduce available Ca^{2+}.[61]

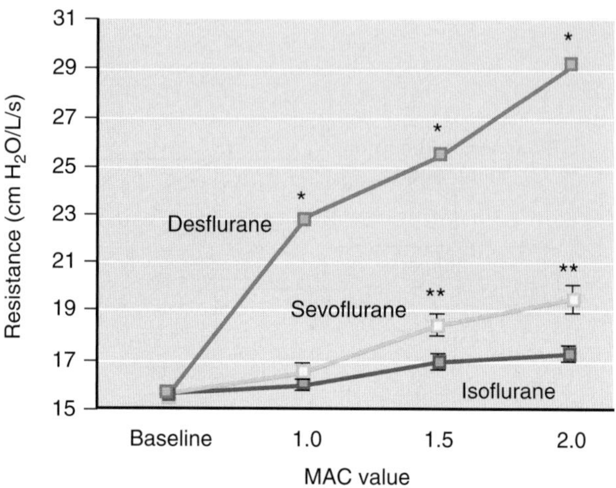

Fig. 21.6 Comparison of the effect of different volatile anesthetics at equivalent concentrations on total pulmonary resistance. At 1 minimum alveolar concentration (MAC), only desflurane significantly increased pulmonary resistance, compared with isoflurane and sevoflurane. At 1.5 and 2 MAC, sevoflurane significantly increased total pulmonary resistance compared with isoflurane, whereas desflurane caused a more pronounced increase than the other two agents. *Increased pulmonary resistance in comparison with sevoflurane and isoflurane; **increased pulmonary resistance in comparison with isoflurane. (Reproduced from Nyktari VG, Papaioannou AA, Prinianakis G, et al. Effect of the physical properties of isoflurane, sevoflurane, and desflurane on pulmonary resistance in a laboratory lung model. *Anesthesiology.* 2006;104:1202. Used with permission.)

Volatile anesthetic–induced reductions in SR Ca^{2+} appear to occur through enhancement of IP_3[62] and ryanodine-receptor channel activities.[59] Kai and coworkers[53] demonstrated that halothane attenuates ACh-induced Ca^{2+} sensitization in canine tracheal smooth muscle to a greater extent than does sevoflurane, whereas isoflurane has effect at concentrations equivalent to 2 MAC. This effect appears to be mediated, at least in part, by an increase in smooth muscle protein phosphatase,[60] modulation of G proteins (specifically G_q and G_I that exert actions on cyclic guanosine monophosphate [cGMP]),[53] or modulation of the Rho/Rho-kinase signaling pathways.[63,64] Volatile anesthetics interact with the muscarinic receptor–heterotrimeric G protein complex to prevent agonist-promoted nucleotide exchange at the Gα subunit of the G protein.[65,66] Halothane, sevoflurane, and, minimally, isoflurane exert direct effects on muscarinic receptor–mediated contraction of isolated airway smooth muscle.[67] The inhibitory effects of volatile agents on the biochemical coupling between the M_3 muscarinic receptor and the $G\alpha_q$ heterotrimeric G protein is completely reversible with time. Isoflurane-induced relaxation of precontracted bronchial smooth muscles is significantly augmented by pretreatment with a Rho-kinase inhibitor, whereas sevoflurane-inhibited guanosine-5′-triphosphate (GTP) γ S-stimulated contraction and membrane translocation of both Rho and Rho-kinase in a concentration-dependent manner. These latter actions play important roles in Ca^{2+} sensitization.[54] The final pathway in airway smooth muscle contraction is the generation of force and shortening of smooth muscles regulated by myosin cross-bridge number and kinetics. Isoflurane modulates both cross-bridge number and cycling rates of isolated rat airway smooth muscle.[67]

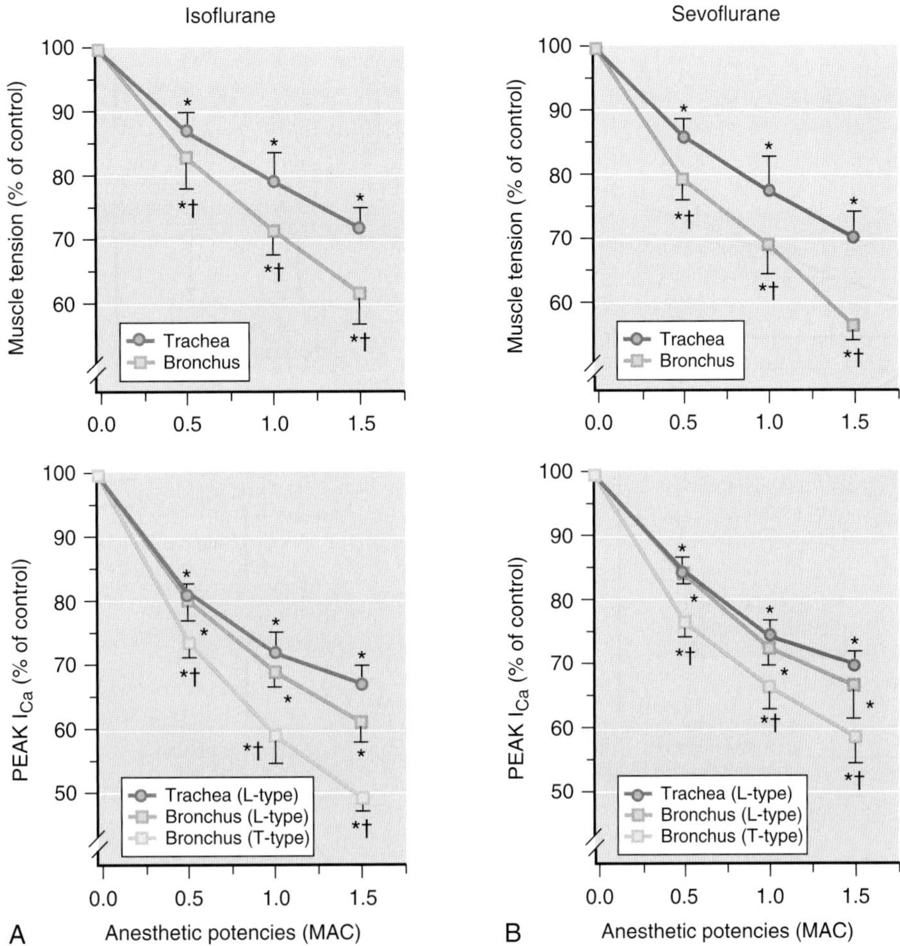

Fig. 21.7 Effect of isoflurane and sevoflurane on porcine tracheal versus bronchial smooth muscle tension or inward calcium (Ca^{2+}) current intercellular calcium (ICa^{2+}) through T- and L-type voltage-dependent Ca^{2+} (VDC) channels. No differences were observed in the inhibition of L-type VDC channels. Both anesthetics had greater inhibitory effects on T-type VDC channels in bronchial smooth muscle. Symbols represent mean ± standard deviation (SD). (A) *$P < .05$ versus 0 minimum alveolar concentration *(MAC)*. †$P < .05$ versus tracheal smooth muscle. (B) †$P < .05$ versus L-type VDC channels. (Reproduced from Yamakage M, Chen X, Tsujiguchi N, et al. Different inhibitory effects of volatile anesthetics on T- and L-type voltage dependent Ca^{2+} channels in porcine tracheal and bronchial smooth muscles. *Anesthesiology*. 2001;94:683. Used with permission.)

The bronchodilatory effect of volatile anesthetics is also mediated by GABA A ($GABA_A$) receptors in the brainstem or GABA B ($GABA_B$) receptors on preganglionic cholinergic nerves in the lung similar to the observations with propofol.[68] Indeed, $GABA_A$ and $GABA_B$ receptors, as well as glutamic decarboxylase (enzyme responsible for GABA synthesis), are located in airway epithelial and smooth muscle cells. GABA levels increase and localize to airway smooth muscle after contractile stimuli in upper airways. Furthermore, a GABA agonist reversed augmentation of cholinergic-induced tracheal ring contraction.[68,69]

Inhaled but not intravenous halothane attenuated bronchoconstricting effects of low inhaled concentrations of CO_2 in rat distal bronchi, suggesting that halothane exerts a direct action on airway muscle tone or local neural reflex arcs rather than centrally controlled reflex pathways. Consistent with this hypothesis, halothane-, isoflurane-, sevoflurane-, and desflurane-induced dilation of distal bronchial segments is partially dependent on the presence of bronchial epithelium.[23,70] Prostanoids (e.g., prostaglandin E_2 or I_2) or NO may be responsible for the bronchodilatory effects of volatile anesthetics under these conditions. Focal epithelial damage or inflammation may occur in small airways in patients with asthma or allergen exposure, resulting in a reduced bronchodilatory response to volatile anesthetics.[71] Nevertheless, the most pronounced bronchodilatory action of volatile anesthetics in patients with chronic reactive airway disease occurs primarily in the proximal rather than distal airways.

Direct stimulation of intrinsic airway nerves in vitro produces a contractile response that is inhibited by atropine. Volatile anesthetic–induced bronchodilation also occurs by modulation of this airway cholinergic neural transmission mediated through prejunctional and postjunctional mechanisms.[72,73] The combination of atropine and halothane did not increase airway caliber over that attained with either drug alone, suggesting that halothane dilates airways by blocking vagal tone during unstimulated conditions.[74] Potent tracheal constriction also occurs in response to the endogenously produced endothelin-1. Isoflurane attenuated the endothelin-1–induced airway smooth muscle contraction in rat tracheal rings, suggesting another potential mechanism for airway smooth muscle relaxation.[75]

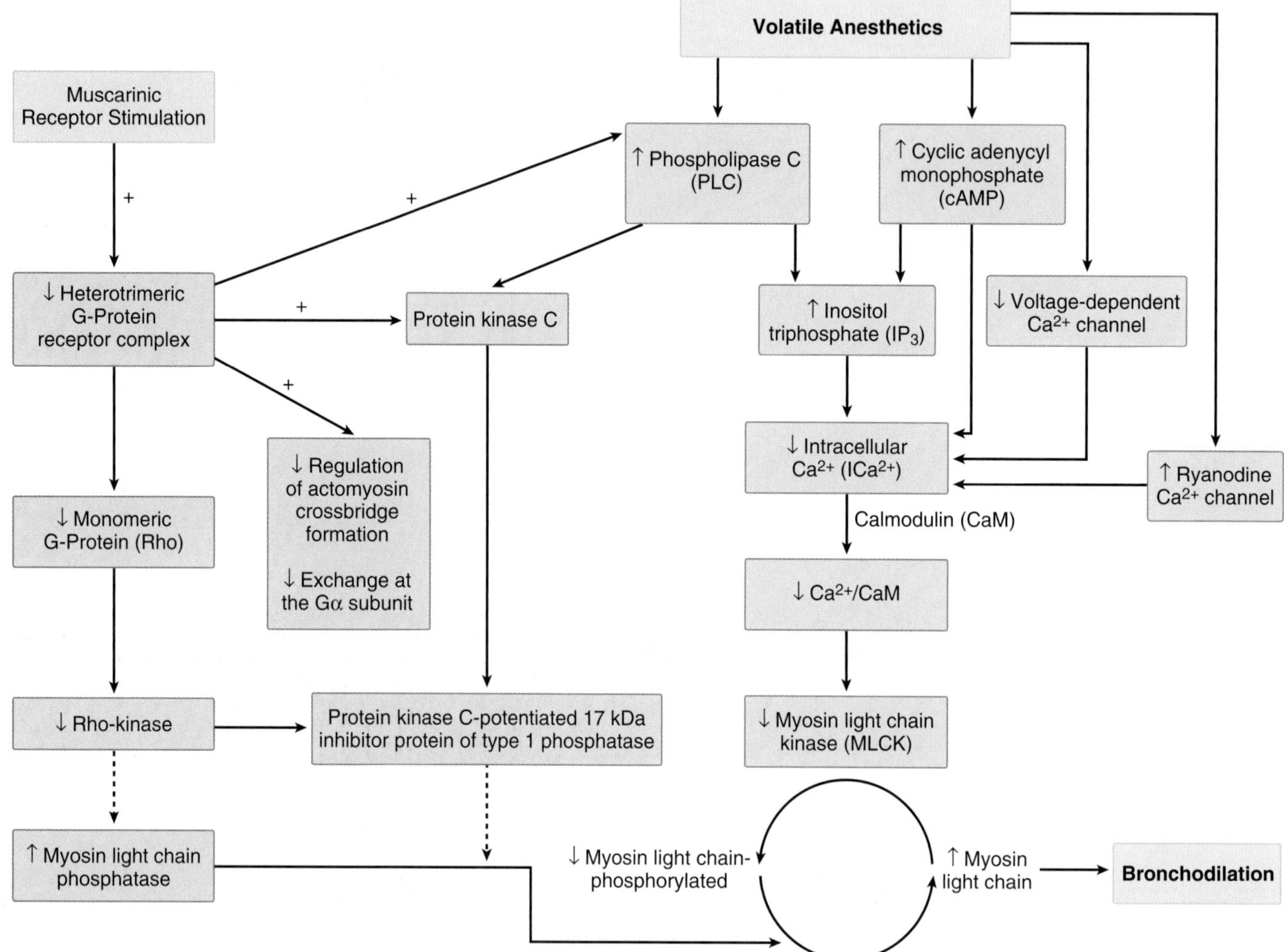

Fig. 21.8 Proposed signaling pathways underlying volatile anesthetic-induced bronchodilation and/or inhibition of muscarinic agonist–induced contraction of airway smooth muscle. +, Excitatory action of muscarinic-receptor agonist. ↑, Activation or increase attributable to the volatile anesthetic. ↓, Inhibition or decrease attributable to the volatile anesthetic. Volatile anesthetics play a role in decreasing intracellular calcium (ICa^{2+}) levels and decreasing calcium (Ca^{2+}) sensitivity.

Mucociliary Function and Surfactant

NORMAL MUCOCILIARY FUNCTION

The upward clearance of mucus from the tracheobronchial tree is responsible for removal of foreign particulate matter, microorganisms, and dead cells and is a primary pulmonary defense mechanism. Although ciliated respiratory epithelium cells are present throughout the respiratory tree, the density of ciliated respiratory epithelium progressively decreases from the trachea to the terminal bronchioles. Cilia are hair-like appendages, consisting of hundreds of proteins organized around a microtubular architecture. They are anchored to the apical cytoplasm by a basal body and extend from the cell surface into the extracellular space.[76,77] Cilia are classified as either motile or immotile (primary). Motile cilia were thought to be responsible for generating extracellular fluid movement or propelling individual cells, whereas primary cilia were believed to be vestigial. However, primary cilia are important environmental sensors. In human bronchial epithelium, they play a key role in sensing and transducing extracellular mechanochemical signals and are also capable of identifying smooth muscle injury.[78] Indeed, ciliopathies are responsible for a variety of pediatric disorders such as primary ciliary dyskinesia and autosomal recessive polycystic kidney disease.[76,79] Christopher et al. studied the effects of temperature (15°C-37°C) with varying combinations with fentanyl, dexmedetomidine, and isoflurane on the cilia of mouse tracheal epithelia. There was a linear correlation between cilia motility and temperature. Fentanyl exerted stimulatory effects on cilia, while dexmedetomidine and isoflurane both inhibited cilia function. When added together, fentanyl, dexmedetomidine, and isoflurane were all cilia inhibitory. In contrast, fentanyl plus dexmedetomidine did not significantly alter ciliary function, with results suggesting complex drug-drug and drug-temperature interactions not predicted by simple summation of effects.[80]

Ciliary motion consists of a rapid stroke in a cephalad direction, followed by a slower caudal recovery stroke. Movements of cilia are closely coordinated to move matter efficiently toward the trachea in a wave motion known as *metachronism*. Each motile cilium is organized in nine peripheral microtubule pairs surrounding a central pair (9+2). During a beat, dynein arms undergo an adenosine triphosphate (ATP)–dependent attachment, retraction, and release cycle with the adjacent doublet, which results in a sliding motion. The basal bodies of the motile cilia are anchored to the microtubules, nexin links, and radial spokes and are further restricted by the ciliary membrane. This anatomic constraint converts the sliding motion into a bend.

The quantity and physical properties of the mucous layer may also promote the coordination of ciliary beats. Mucus is a mixture of water, electrolytes, and macromolecules (e.g., lipids, mucins, enzymes) secreted by goblet cells and mucosal glands. Thicker layers of mucus slow the removal of surface particles from the airway, whereas low-viscosity mucus promotes more rapid ciliary transport. Impaired mucociliary function in the upper airways correlates with low levels of nasal NO, although the clinical significance of this finding is unclear.[81] Direct nervous system control of ciliary coordination has not been demonstrated in vertebrates, but mucociliary clearance is closely related to autonomic nervous system activity, most likely related to changes in physical characteristics of respiratory secretions (also see Chapter 103).[82]

Several factors affect mucociliary function in mechanically ventilated patients contributing to lung atelectasis and hypoxemia. For example, insufficiently humidified inspired gases reduce ciliary movement and desiccate mucus. In dogs, the flow rate of tracheal mucous was maintained within the basal range during a 40-minute exposure to inspired dry air at a temperature higher than 32°C. However, 3 hours of inhalation of dry air caused a complete cessation of the flow of tracheal mucus, which was restored by the subsequent use of inspired gases with 100% relative humidity at 38°C. Several anesthesia-related factors also reduce the rate of mucous movement, including high-inspired oxygen (O_2) concentrations, adjuvant medications (e.g., corticosteroids, atropine, β-adrenoreceptor antagonists) that affect bronchial tone, the presence of an endotracheal tube, and positive-pressure ventilation.[83]

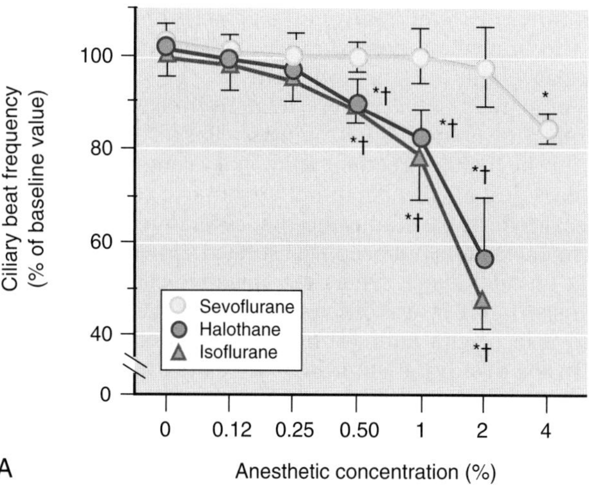

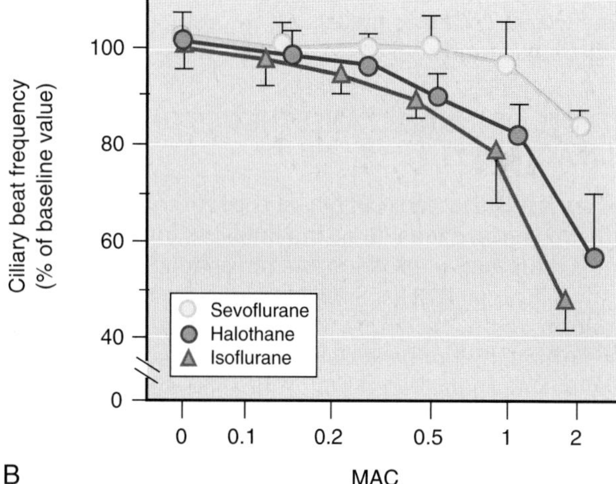

Fig. 21.9 Effects of sevoflurane, halothane, and isoflurane on ciliary beat frequency (CBF) in cultured rat tracheal epithelial cells. CBF was measured at baseline and 30 minutes after exposure to various anesthetic concentrations. Values represent mean ± standard deviation. (A) Plot of percent baseline CBF versus anesthetic concentration. $^*P < .05$ versus 0% vehicle. $^†P < .05$ versus sevoflurane at the same concentration. (B) Percent baseline CBF versus minimum alveolar concentration *(MAC)*. (Modified from Matsuura S, Shirakami G, Iida H, et al. The effect of sevoflurane on ciliary motility in rat cultured tracheal epithelial cells: a comparison with isoflurane and halothane. *Anesth Analg.* 2006;102:1703. Used with permission.)

EFFECTS OF INHALED ANESTHETICS ON MUCOCILIARY FUNCTION

Volatile anesthetics and nitrous oxide diminish the rates of mucous clearance by decreasing ciliary beat frequency, disrupting metachronism, and altering the physical characteristics or quantity of mucus. In contrast to many intravenous anesthetics,[84,85] halothane, enflurane, isoflurane, and sevoflurane all reduce ciliary movement and beat frequency in vitro.[84-87] Among the volatile anesthetics, sevoflurane exhibited the weakest cilioinhibitory effects in rat cultured tracheal epithelial cells in vitro (Fig. 21.9).[87]

Gamsu and colleagues[88] measured the rate of tantalum (a powder that adheres to airway mucus) clearance from the lungs of postoperative patients who received general anesthesia for intraabdominal or lower extremity surgeries. Tantalum retention was closely correlated with the retention of mucus and shown for as long as 6 days after intraabdominal surgery. The administration of halothane (1%-2%) and nitrous oxide (60%) rapidly decreased the rate of mucous movement in females undergoing gynecologic surgery. Little or no mucous motion was observed after 90 minutes of halothane–nitrous oxide inhalation.[89] Bronchial mucosal transport velocity was also determined using radiolabeled albumin microspheres distally deposited in the mainstem bronchi using a fiberoptic bronchoscope in healthy patients. In contrast to the findings of the study with halothane, mucous velocity was unchanged during the administration of 1.5 MAC isoflurane.[90]

Impairment of ciliary beat frequency, mucociliary clearance, and bronchial mucous transport contribute to pulmonary complications, including retention of secretions, atelectasis, and lower respiratory tract infection. A reduction in bronchial mucous transport of as little as 3.5 mm/min (normally 10 mm/min) was associated with an increase in pulmonary complications in patients who were mechanically ventilated for 4 days in the intensive care unit (ICU).[91] Thus pulmonary therapy directed at enhancing clearance of secretions from the airways may be beneficial in the immediate postoperative period, regardless of the type of volatile anesthetic chosen.

Compared to nonsmokers, tobacco smokers have significantly slower bronchial mucous transport velocities and are prone to more frequent pulmonary complications when undergoing major abdominal or thoracic surgeries.[92] The specific effects of volatile anesthetics on mucous movement in smokers have not been well studied. However, it is likely that an additive or synergistic negative effect on mucous transport may be present. Impairment of mucociliary function also occurs after lung transplantation. The mechanism for this dysfunction may be related to alterations in the surface properties of mucus and significant impairment of mucociliary transport distal to bronchial transection and re-anastomosis.[93] The effects of volatile anesthetics on mucous transport in lung transplant patients have not been described, but the baseline reductions in mucociliary movement would certainly predispose to postoperative respiratory complications.

EFFECTS OF INHALED ANESTHETICS ON SURFACTANT

Pulmonary surfactant decreases the work of breathing by reducing surface tension at the fluid-gas interface. Surfactant is a mixture of proteins and phospholipids synthesized by alveolar type II cells. Similar to mucus, surfactant plays a role in removing foreign particles from airways while also enhancing the bactericidal actions of alveolar macrophages. Halothane[94] and isoflurane[95] produced a transient dose-dependent reduction in phosphatidylcholine (a major component of surfactant) synthesis by alveolar cells during a 4-hour exposure. High concentrations of halothane also disrupted the energy metabolism of cultured alveolar cells as indicated by reduced ATP content and enhanced glycolytic metabolism. Halothane and isoflurane potentiated a hydrogen peroxide–induced reduction of phosphatidylcholine content in alveolar type II cells[95,96] by affecting cell energetics. Halothane decreased the Na^+/K^+–adenosine triphosphatase (Na^+/K^+-ATPase), and Na^+ channel activity in alveolar type II cells, probably related to alterations in ICa^{2+} or ATP depletion. A similar decrease in type II alveolar cell Na^+/K^+-ATPase occurs after the administration of isoflurane.[97] Transepithelial Na^+ transport helps regulate alveolar fluid balance, and, as a result, impairment of this transport system may contribute to alveolar edema. This observation may be especially relevant in surgical patients because volatile anesthetics decrease alveolar epithelial fluid clearance.[98]

The phospholipid composition of surfactant is critical to its functional integrity. Another crucial component of surfactant is the hydrophobic surfactant-associated protein C synthesized by alveolar type II cells. This protein facilitates the adsorption and spreading of phospholipids to form the surfactant monolayer and enhances the lipid uptake into alveolar type II cells. Exogenous surfactants that contain surfactant-associated protein C are effective at decreasing barotrauma and mortality in vivo. Clinically relevant concentrations of halothane increase surfactant-associated protein C messenger ribonucleic acid (mRNA) in vitro but cause the opposite effect in mechanically ventilated rats.[99] Extrapolation of these findings to patients should be approached with caution, but halothane and mechanical ventilation may play a potentially additive and deleterious role on surfactant production and homeostasis of the alveolar space, particularly in the presence of ALI. In a rat model, sevoflurane produced deterioration in surfactant composition and viscosity with impaired lung mechanics promoting alveolar collapse[100]; again, caution is warranted in extrapolating these findings to humans. Bilgi and colleagues compared the effects of low-flow and high-flow inhalational anesthesia with nitrous oxide and desflurane on mucociliary activity and pulmonary function tests in humans. The forced vital capacity and forced expiratory volume and mucociliary clearance of saccharin powder were better preserved with low-flow rather than a high-flow technique, suggesting that heated and humidified gases may have a greater impact than the inhaled anesthetics themselves.[101]

Prolonged administration of volatile anesthetics may produce mucous pooling and impair alveolar cell surfactant metabolism. These actions may result in adverse effects on pulmonary function including development of atelectasis and infections. Patients with excessive or abnormal mucous or surfactant production and patients with ALI, chronic bronchitis, asthma, cystic fibrosis, and chronic mechanical ventilation are at the greatest risk. Clinical studies of the effects of volatile anesthetics on mucociliary function, surfactant metabolism, and immunomodulation in patients with compromised pulmonary function are still sparse.

PULMONARY VASCULAR RESISTANCE

Regulation of Pulmonary Vascular Tone

The pulmonary vascular bed is a low-pressure, high-flow system. Normal pulmonary arterial (PA) pressure is approximately one-fifth of the systemic arterial pressure. Correspondingly, PVR is lower than systemic vascular resistance. The main pulmonary artery and its major branches have a thinner media and less vascular smooth muscle than the aorta and major proximal arterial vessels. Changes in pulmonary vascular smooth muscle tone alter PVR by affecting the slope of pressure-flow relation. Such direct changes may be produced by a rapid rise in cytoplasmic ICa^{2+} of the pulmonary vascular smooth muscle cell or by alterations in sympathetic nervous system activity, arterial O_2 and CO_2 tension, acid-base balance, or plasma catecholamine concentrations. Hypercapnia at constant pH (i.e., isohydria) does not alter tone in isolated pulmonary arteries, but normocapnic acidosis relaxes isolated pulmonary arteries by an endothelium-independent mechanism.[102] However, pulmonary endothelial dysfunction potentiates hypercapnia-induced vasoconstriction.[103] Changes in PA pressure and PVR exert important effects on pulmonary gas or fluid exchange. An increase in PVR occurring in conjunction with a corresponding increase in PA pressure promotes interstitial fluid transudation. An acute increase in PVR can be caused by large tidal volumes, high positive end-expiratory pressure, alveolar hypoxia, hypercarbia, acidosis, and critical closing pressure. Hypoxia and acidosis have a synergistic effect increasing PVR. In contrast to acute pulmonary hypertension, the development of chronic pulmonary hypertension involves endothelial dysfunction with persistent vasoconstriction due to imbalance between endogenous vasoconstrictors (including thromboxane A_2, angiotensin 2, and endothelin 1) and vasodilators (including NO and prostacyclin), smooth muscle proliferation, platelet aggregation, vascular remodeling and thrombosis, and formation of plexiform lesions that irreversibly obliterate pulmonary arterioles. Clinically, the use of positive inotropic medications (e.g., milrinone) or expanded blood volume can passively decrease PVR by increasing cardiac output. Volatile anesthetics may also have indirect effects on PVR through a reduction in lung volumes during spontaneous ventilation. To assess the total effect of the volatile anesthesia, the volume status and mechanical ventilation on the pulmonary pressures, and right heart function, either transthoracic or transesophageal echocardiography should be considered.

Endogenously produced NO plays an important role in the regulation of PVR both in the healthy, normoxic lung and during hypoxia. NO is generated via oxidation of a terminal guanidinium nitrogen on the amino acid L-arginine. The reaction utilizes molecular O_2 and NADPH as substrates, requires the presence of tetrahydrobiopterin, flavoproteins, calmodulin, and thiols as cofactors, and yields NO in addition to the co-product L-citrullin.[104] This oxidation is catalyzed by a single enzyme protein, NO synthase (NOS), which exists in three distinct isoforms. Constitutive calcium-dependent isoforms of the enzyme were originally purified from neuronal tissue (nNOS) and vascular endothelium (eNOS).[105,106] When stimulated by bacterial endotoxin and proinflammatory cytokines, a third calcium-independent isoform (iNOS) is induced in various cell types including endothelial and vascular smooth muscle cells, macrophages, and fibroblasts. Once expressed, iNOS is independent of calcium, and NO production continues at a maximum rate. All three NOS isoforms are widely distributed in the lung, extensively involved in vascular homeostasis, and intimately linked to the pulmonary O_2 environment.[107]

NO diffuses away from its point of synthesis and interacts with various intracellular molecular sites both within the generating cells and the target cells. The best-characterized target for NO is iron, bound within certain proteins, either as a heme group or as an iron-sulfur complex. The interaction of NO with the heme component of soluble guanylate cyclase stimulates enzymatic conversion of guanosine triphosphate to cGMP.[104] In turn, increased intracellular levels of cGMP cause relaxation of systemic and pulmonary vascular and nonvascular smooth muscles by several mechanisms. Besides lowering free intracellular calcium and attenuating calcium transients, cGMP causes hyperpolarization of muscle cells through activation of potassium channels.

Inhalation of gaseous NO produces selective pulmonary vasodilation in well-ventilated lung areas and may be beneficial in the treatment of neonatal pulmonary hypertension resulting from a variety of congenital heart diseases, hypoplastic lung, and meconium aspiration. Inhaled NO has also some benefits in the treatment of acute pulmonary hypertension in adults, provided that the PVR is not fixed by remodeling and hypertrophy of pulmonary vasculature. Additionally, the use of inhaled NO to reduce PVR in pediatric and adult patients during cardiac surgeries has become common (also see Chapters 67, 94, and 104).[108]

Prostacyclin is another endogenous vasodilator produced by the endothelium that causes smooth muscle relaxation through adenylyl cyclase stimulation and production of cAMP. Prostacyclin is used in inhaled or injected formulations to produce pulmonary vasodilation in patients with chronic PA hypertension. Another group of pulmonary vasodilators, including sildenafil and tadalafil, acts by inhibiting cGMP-specific phosphodiesterase type 5 (an enzyme that is responsible for cGMP degradation) and is used for therapy of refractory PA hypertension. Finally, riociguat, a novel drug that directly stimulates soluble guanylate cyclase independently of NO, has been recently approved for treating patients with chronic pulmonary hypertension and chronic thromboembolic pulmonary hypertension.[109]

MECHANISMS OF HYPOXIC PULMONARY VASOCONSTRICTION

Changes in PVR affect the regional distribution of blood flow within the lung and produce changes in ventilation-perfusion matching and gas exchange. The distribution of PA blood flow and ventilation in the lung is mainly a gravity-dependent phenomenon that is primarily mediated by the asymmetric branching of airways and blood vessels, thereby establishing regional heterogeneity.[110] An increase in PVR occurring within an area of atelectasis optimizes gas exchange by shifting blood flow away from the atelectatic segment to well-ventilated regions of the lung. This phenomenon, termed hypoxic pulmonary vasoconstriction (HPV), is unique to the pulmonary circulation because other vascular beds (e.g., coronary and cerebral) dilate in response to hypoxia. Thus HPV maintains oxygenation, while medications (including volatile anesthetics) that interfere with HPV may adversely affect gas exchange. HPV plays an especially important role in the presence of atelectasis, pneumonia, reactive airway disease, acute respiratory distress syndrome (ARDS), or one-lung ventilation (OLV). It usually does not contribute to pulmonary blood flow heterogeneity under normal conditions in supine humans.[111]

HPV is a locally mediated phenomenon that occurs when alveolar O_2 tension falls below approximately 60 mm Hg and is maximal when O_2 tension is approximately 30 mm Hg. HPV was first identified in 1894, and the precise mechanism is only now becoming clear. Specialized O_2-sensing cells modulate respiratory and circulatory function to maintain a normal O_2 supply. Hypercapnia-induced acidosis increases PVR in intact animals and in isolated, perfused lungs. Acidosis-induced increases in PVR are relatively small at normal alveolar O_2 tensions but are dramatically enhanced during alveolar hypoxia. Local acidosis and increases in alveolar CO_2 tension augment HPV and further improve arterial oxygenation in healthy lungs. High CO_2 concentrations reduce NO levels,[112] but whether this action plays a part in hypercarbia-induced improvements in the ventilation-perfusion ratio is unclear.[113]

Although the hypoxia-mediated endothelial-derived vasoconstrictor has yet to be identified,[114] hypoxia releases Ca^{2+} from smooth muscle SR via ryanodine receptors,[115] enhances Ca^{2+} sensitization,[114-116] and modulates voltage-gated K^+ channels in smooth muscles.[117] Other mediators of the hypoxic-response coupling have been identified.[116,118]

Wang and colleagues[119] have recently demonstrated that both connexin 40-mediated retrograde endothelial signal conduction for O_2 sensing, as well as Ca^{2+} influx at TRP1 channel V4 on pulmonary arterioles[120] are required for HPV. Ultimately, there are a number of contenders for the role of HPV oxygen sensor, yet there is still no consensus on how this happens in vivo, with most of the proposed mechanisms interlinked, depending on the phase of HPV, the degree of hypoxia, involvement of anesthetic or other agents.[121]

INHALED ANESTHETICS AND HYPOXIC PULMONARY VASOCONSTRICTION

All volatile anesthetics dilate the pulmonary vascular bed. In a thorough review, Akata[122] discussed the mechanisms by which inhaled anesthetics produce this vasodilation, including a reduction in free cytosolic Ca^{2+} and inhibition of myofilament Ca^{2+} sensitivity. However, the vasodilator effect of volatile anesthetics is modest in normal lungs, and the small attenuation of PVR is usually offset by a concomitant reduction in cardiac output. The net effect of these hemodynamic changes results in minor, if any, changes in PA pressure concomitant with a small decrease in total pulmonary blood flow. In contrast to their action as direct pulmonary vasodilators, volatile anesthetics also attenuate K_{ATP} channel-mediated and endothelium-dependent pulmonary vasodilation in chronically instrumented dogs.[123-125] This inhibition of pulmonary vasodilation is not a uniform observation under all experimental conditions. For example, isoflurane and halothane, but not enflurane, enhance isoproterenol-mediated vasodilation.[126,127] Unlike the findings with other volatile anesthetics, K_{ATP} channel–mediated pulmonary vasodilation in response to a K^+ channel agonist (lemakalim) is preserved during sevoflurane anesthesia.[125] Indeed, evidence suggests that halothane, enflurane, and isoflurane, but not sevoflurane, differentially modulate pulmonary vascular tension through Ca^{2+}-activated or voltage-sensitive K^+ channels, at least in isolated rabbit lungs.[128] Halothane- and enflurane-induced constriction of pulmonary vessels was potentiated by voltage-gated potassium (Kv) channel inhibition in this isolated rabbit lung preparation. In contrast, isoflurane did not affect pulmonary vessels when Kv channels were inhibited. Further, sevoflurane dilated pulmonary vessels and this dilation was unaffected by K^+ channel subtype inhibitors (Fig. 21.10).[128]

Smooth muscle TASK-1 channels also appear to contribute to volatile anesthetic–induced PA dilation.[129] Rather than causing immediate vasodilation, volatile anesthetics produce a paradoxical initial dose-dependent increase in force in isolated PA strips as a result of Ca^{2+} release from intracellular stores (Fig. 21.11).[122,130,131] Subsequently, a decrease in force, associated with a Ca^{2+}/calmodulin–dependent protein kinase II activation, occurs.[130,131] Extrapolation of these results to humans must be approached with caution, but these studies suggest that vasodilatory responses of volatile anesthetics may be more profound in patients with reduced SR Ca^{2+} stores (e.g., neonates) or those with depressed protein kinase activity (e.g., primary pulmonary hypertension).

In general, all volatile anesthetics attenuate HPV in isolated perfused lungs or in an in situ preparation with constant perfusion (Fig. 21.12),[121,132] whereas most intravenous anesthetics do not have such an effect.[118] The combined administration of a Ca^{2+}-channel blocker and a volatile anesthetic further reduces HPV by up to 40%, compared with either drug alone, suggesting that these drugs inhibit HPV through differing mechanisms. The mechanisms of HPV inhibition by volatile anesthetics are unclear but may be related to arachidonic acid metabolites[133]

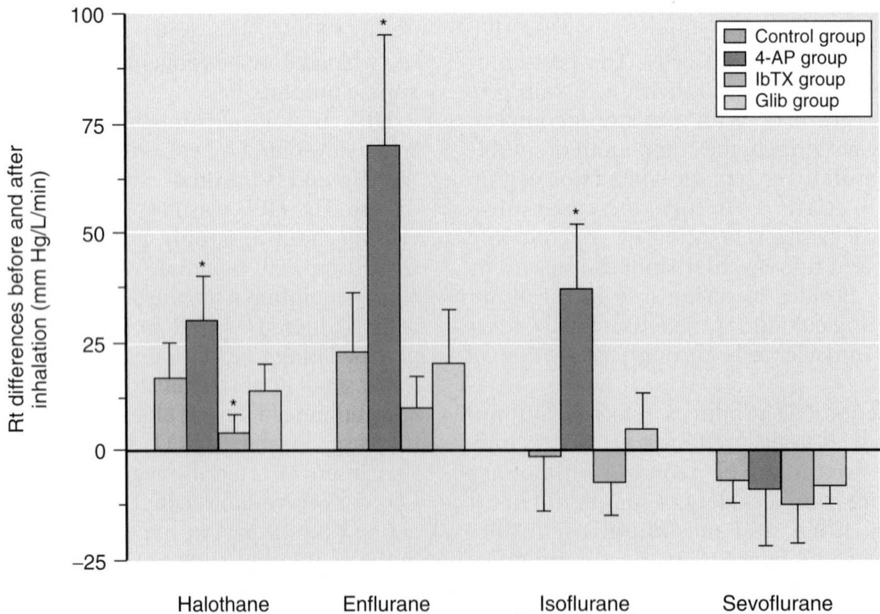

Fig. 21.10 Total pulmonary vascular resistance *(Rt)* before and after anesthetic inhalation. Data are mean ± standard deviation. $*P < .01$ versus control group. *4AP,* voltage-sensitive K^+ channel inhibitor; *Glib,* glibenclamide, an adenosine triphosphate–sensitive K^+ channel inhibitor; *IbTX,* calcium-activated K+ channel inhibitor; *Rt difference,* resistance after the administration of anesthetic minus resistance before administering the anesthetic. (Modified from Liu R, Ishibe Y, Okazaki N, et al. Volatile anesthetics regulate pulmonary vascular tensions through different potassium channel subtypes in isolated rabbit lungs. *Can J Anaesth.* 2003;50:301. Used with permission.)

or endothelial-derived vasodilating factors.[134] However, other evidence suggests that anesthetic-induced inhibition of HPV may occur independent of pulmonary vascular endothelium, NO, or guanylate cyclase.[135,136] Volatile anesthetics also disrupt Ca^{2+} homeostasis in vascular smooth muscle and thereby interfere with pulmonary vasoconstriction. Halothane and isoflurane attenuated endothelium-dependent vasodilation by inhibiting cGMP accumulation[137] and a K_{ATP} channel-mediated interaction between NO and prostacyclin in isolated canine PA rings.[138] In contrast, isoflurane modulated the HPV response, at least in part, through Ca^{2+}-activated and voltage-sensitive K^+ channels. Attenuation of HPV by sevoflurane occurred independent of K^+-channel function.[139]

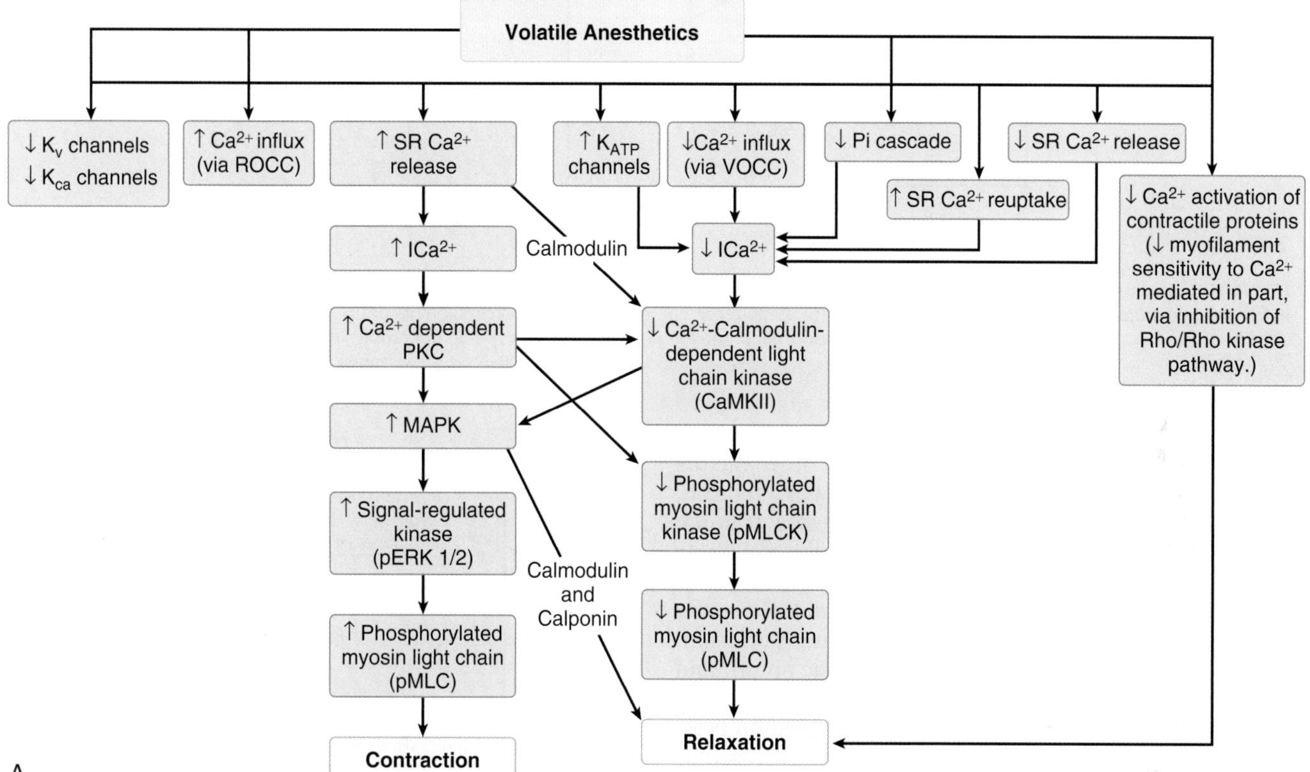

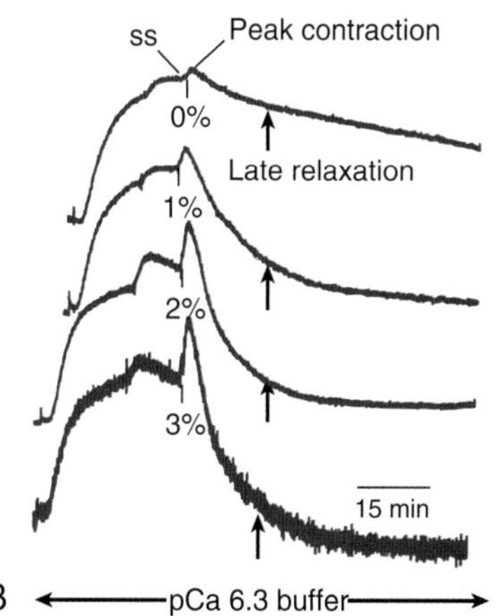

Fig. 21.11 (A) Proposed signaling pathways underlying volatile anesthetic-induced contraction and relaxation in pulmonary artery smooth muscle. Intracellular calcium (*ICa²⁺*) may be increased by release from the sarcoplasmic reticulum (*SR*), by the inhibition of voltage-sensitive potassium (*K_v*) or calcium-activated potassium (*K_{ca}*) channels, or by receptor-operated Ca^{2+} channels (*ROCC*). Increased ICa^{2+} results in an initial dose-dependent increase in force (associated with activation of protein kinase C *[PKC]* and increased mitogen-activated protein kinase *[MAPK]*). Volatile anesthetics also decrease ICa^{2+} by activating adenosine triphosphate–regulated potassium (*K_{ATP}*) channels, thereby inhibiting Ca^{2+} influx via voltage-operated Ca^{2+} channels (*VOCC*), decreasing SR-induced release of Ca^{2+}, inhibiting the phosphatidylinositol (*Pi*) cascade, and enhancing SR-mediated reuptake of Ca^{2+}. The resultant decrease in force is associated with activation of Ca^{2+}-calmodulin-dependent protein kinase II (*CaMKII*). It is important to note that there are many agent-specific effects of volatile anesthetics on each component of these pathways. *pERK,* Phosphorylated extracellular signal-regulated kinase. (B) Example of a biphasic (contraction/relaxation) effect of halothane on pulmonary arterial smooth muscle. *0%, 1%, 2%,* and *3%,* Halothane concentrations; *ss,* control force at steady state before halothane. Halothane dose dependently enhanced Ca^{2+}-activated peak force and late relaxation. (Data from Akata,[122] Su and Vo,[130] and Zhong and Su.[131])

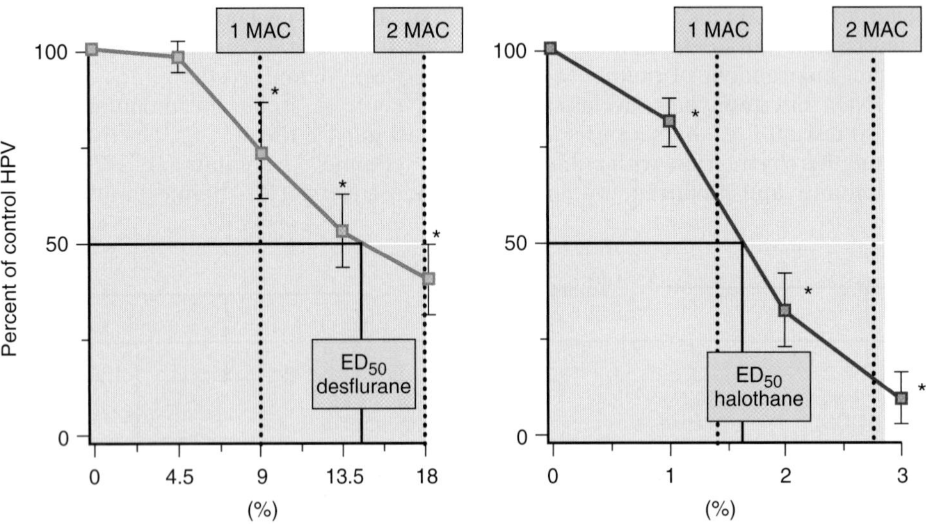

Fig. 21.12 Concentration-dependent inhibition of hypoxic pulmonary vasoconstriction *(HPV)* in isolated rabbit lungs by desflurane *(blue squares)* and halothane *(red squares)*. Values are mean ± standard error of the mean and expressed as a percentage of control. *$P < .05$ versus control HPV. The 50% effective dose (ED_{50}) values were within the range of 1 and 2 minimum alveolar concentrations *(MAC)* (for rabbits) for both agents. (Reproduced from Loer SA, Scheeren T, Tarnow J. Desflurane inhibits hypoxic pulmonary vasoconstriction in isolated rabbit lungs. *Anesthesiology.* 1995;83:552. Used with permission.)

The relative efficacy of volatile anesthetics on HPV in vivo is difficult to assess because several other factors impair HPV, including temperature, pH, CO_2 tension, degree of hypoxia, size of the hypoxic area, surgical trauma, and medications. During OLV, the direct inhibitory effects of volatile anesthetics on HPV may increase perfusion in the nonventilated lung and worsen hypoxemia. However, volatile anesthetics may also affect HPV, lung perfusion, and oxygenation by indirect actions on cardiac output and mixed venous O_2 saturation.[140] Baseline PA blood flow and pressure also modulate the effects of HPV. Elevated PA pressures may cause passive distension of constricted vascular beds and thereby reverse HPV. Alternatively, reflex pulmonary and systemic vasoconstriction in response to hypotension may increase PVR in healthy lung segments, leading to a shift of pulmonary blood flow to hypoxic areas of lung.[121]

Early studies suggested that nitrous oxide attenuates HPV in animal models in vivo. As opposed to the findings with isoflurane,[133] sevoflurane or desflurane did not inhibit HPV in chronically instrumented dogs subjected to gradual occlusion of the right main PA (Fig. 21.13).[141] Nitrous oxide,[142] desflurane, and isoflurane,[143] but not xenon,[142] reduced the mixed venous O_2 saturation, cardiac output, and arterial oxygenation during OLV in pigs. However, nitrous oxide,[142] xenon,[142] desflurane,[143,144] and isoflurane[143,145] did not alter perfusion of the nonventilated lung or reduce the shunt fraction during OLV. In animals with a preexisting impairment of gas exchange attributable to a pneumoperitoneum, sevoflurane, but not isoflurane, caused more profound abnormalities in gas exchange than did propofol.[146] Thus although reductions in HPV by volatile anesthetics have been relatively small in vivo, preexisting pulmonary disease may worsen anesthetic-induced gas exchange abnormalities.

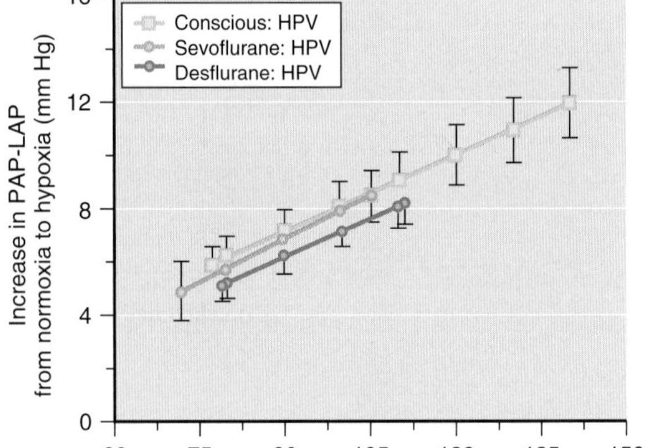

Fig. 21.13 Composite hypoxic pulmonary vasoconstriction *(HPV)* responses (increase in pulmonary artery pressure *[PAP]* minus left atrial pressure *[LAP]* as a function of left pulmonary flow in the same seven chronically instrumented dogs in the conscious state and during sevoflurane and desflurane anesthesia. Neither anesthetic affected the magnitude of HPV when compared with the response in the conscious state. (From Lesitsky MA, Davis S, Murray PA. Preservation of hypoxic pulmonary vasoconstriction during sevoflurane and desflurane anesthesia compared to the conscious state in chronically instrumented dogs. *Anesthesiology.* 1998;89:1501. Used with permission.)

EFFECTS OF VOLATILE ANESTHETICS ON PULMONARY VASCULATURE IN HUMANS

General anesthesia often impairs pulmonary gas exchange. In addition to specific effects of volatile anesthetics, many other factors including gravity, posture, atelectasis, differences in vessel conductance between lung regions, intrathoracic pressure, and HPV may all affect the distribution of pulmonary blood flow and ventilation during the administration of volatile anesthetics. Alterations in regional ventilation are related to variations in alveolar compliance, inspiratory rate, flow rate, pleural pressures, and ventilatory modes.[147] In spontaneously breathing healthy volunteers, sevoflurane (1 MAC for 20 minutes) administered via a facemask did not alter the relative distribution of either ventilation or perfusion in a ventral to dorsal direction measured by single photon–emission CT.[147] Similarly, no change in the distribution of ventilation, as measured by using electrical impedance tomography, occurred in spontaneously breathing adults receiving 0.7 MAC of sevoflurane via a laryngeal mask airway (LMA).[145] Interestingly, sevoflurane reduced regional heterogeneity of the perfusion distribution and increased regional heterogeneity of the ventilation/perfusion ($\dot{V}/\dot{Q}$) ratio with a tendency toward lower ratios in spontaneously breathing volunteers.[147] This alteration may contribute to less effective pulmonary gas exchange, but these effects were relatively small compared with alterations in $\dot{V}/\dot{Q}$ distribution that occur during mechanical ventilation.[148,149] Either pressure-controlled or pressure-supported ventilation with sevoflurane caused similar ventral redistributions of ventilation.[148]

Isoflurane produces no clinically significant effects on pulmonary shunt in healthy patients even at concentrations that cause systemic hypotension.[150] Thoracic surgeries are usually performed in the lateral position with an open chest and dramatically affect the relative distribution of ventilation and perfusion. Under these conditions, a diseased, nondependent lung may affect the pulmonary vascular response to hypoxia, as may surgical manipulation of the lung itself. Most studies in animal models or patients undergoing OLV did not demonstrate clinically significant attenuation of HPV by volatile anesthetics. Differences in shunt fraction, PVR, or oxygenation between isoflurane and sevoflurane anesthesia in patients undergoing OLV for lobectomy for lung cancer do not appear to be significant.[151] Some studies also demonstrated that shunt fraction is similar in patients receiving propofol or either isoflurane[152] or sevoflurane[153,154] during OLV. No significant differences in shunt fraction or arterial O_2 tension were observed during intravenous infusions of ketamine, which does not inhibit HPV, and inhalation of enflurane. In contrast, isoflurane[155,156] and sevoflurane[156] impaired oxygenation and increased shunt fraction more than an intravenous infusion of propofol during OLV. However, the differences in oxygenation observed in these studies were small and clinically insignificant. The relative depth of anesthesia may affect interpretation of the differences in oxygenation between intravenous and volatile anesthetics in these studies. When doses of propofol and sevoflurane were chosen based on a similar depth of anesthesia, assessed by a bispectral index monitor, similar reductions in arterial oxygenation were observed in patients undergoing OLV.[154] Similar changes in shunt fraction and oxygenation were shown to occur with halothane,[157] isoflurane,[151,157,158] desflurane,[158] and sevoflurane in patients undergoing thoracotomy and OLV (Fig. 21.14).[151,156-158]

Convincing evidence suggests that all volatile anesthetics may be safely used in patients undergoing thoracotomy and OLV. The increase in shunt and the decrease in oxygenation caused by halothane or isoflurane[157] were consistent with an approximately 20% inhibition of HPV at 1 MAC. Instead of the expected 50% reduction in pulmonary blood flow in a hypoxic lung in the absence of a volatile anesthetic, blood flow decreases by 40% during hypoxia in the presence of 1 MAC isoflurane. This change in flow corresponds to an increase in pulmonary shunt by approximately 4% of the cardiac output. Carlsson and colleagues[159] applied multiple inert gas elimination techniques to measure the true shunt fraction in humans

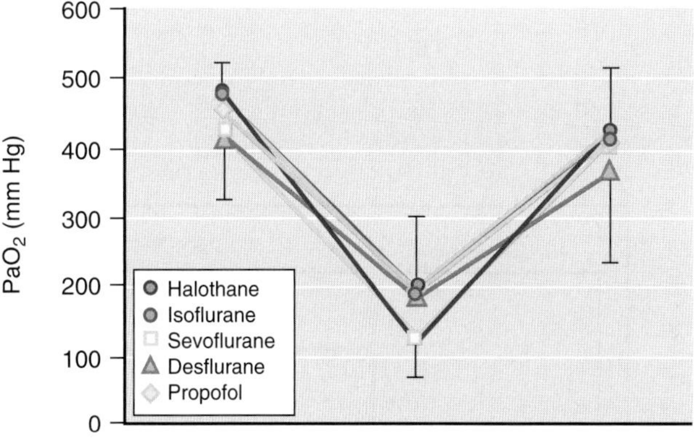

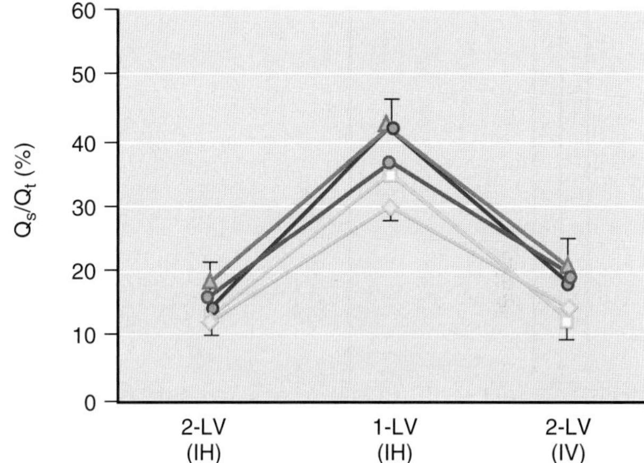

Fig. 21.14 Partial arterial pressure of oxygen *(PaO_2)* and intrapulmonary shunt fraction *(Q_s/Q_t)* in patients with both lungs ventilated *(2-LV)* or with one lung ventilated *(1-LV)*. Patients received an inhaled agent *(IH)* halothane, isoflurane, sevoflurane, or desflurane or the intravenous *(IV)* anesthetic propofol. Note the minimal effect on PaO_2 and shunt fraction that occurs in changing from a volatile anesthetic to an IV agent. (Data modified from Abe and colleagues,[148,153] Benumof and colleagues,[154] and Pagel and colleagues.[155])

anesthetized with volatile anesthetics and demonstrated a 2% to 3% increase in shunt fraction corresponding to approximately 20% HPV inhibition at 1.5% isoflurane. In addition, no significant effects on arterial oxygenation occurred with clinically relevant concentrations of isoflurane or enflurane. Indeed, the use of total intravenous anesthesia with propofol and alfentanil did not reduce the occurrence of hypoxemia during OLV, compared with a volatile anesthetic.[152]

Functionally, volatile anesthetics exert only mild, if any, inhibitory effects on HPV and oxygenation.[160,161] The relatively small inhibition of HPV should not significantly influence clinical decision making, especially considering the efficacy of drugs such as the peripheral chemoreceptor agonist, almitrine[162] (which enhances HPV), or inhaled NO (which selectively increases perfusion to adequately ventilated pulmonary regions). In addition, ventilatory strategies (e.g., nondependent lung continuous positive airway pressure, permissive hypercapnia) and fiberoptic bronchoscopy to ensure proper positioning of a double-lumen endotracheal tube help alleviate hypoxemia. The net effect of volatile anesthetics on HPV is multifactorial and depends on the direct effects of these agents not only on pulmonary vasomotor tone, but also by indirect actions that occur during anesthesia and surgery.

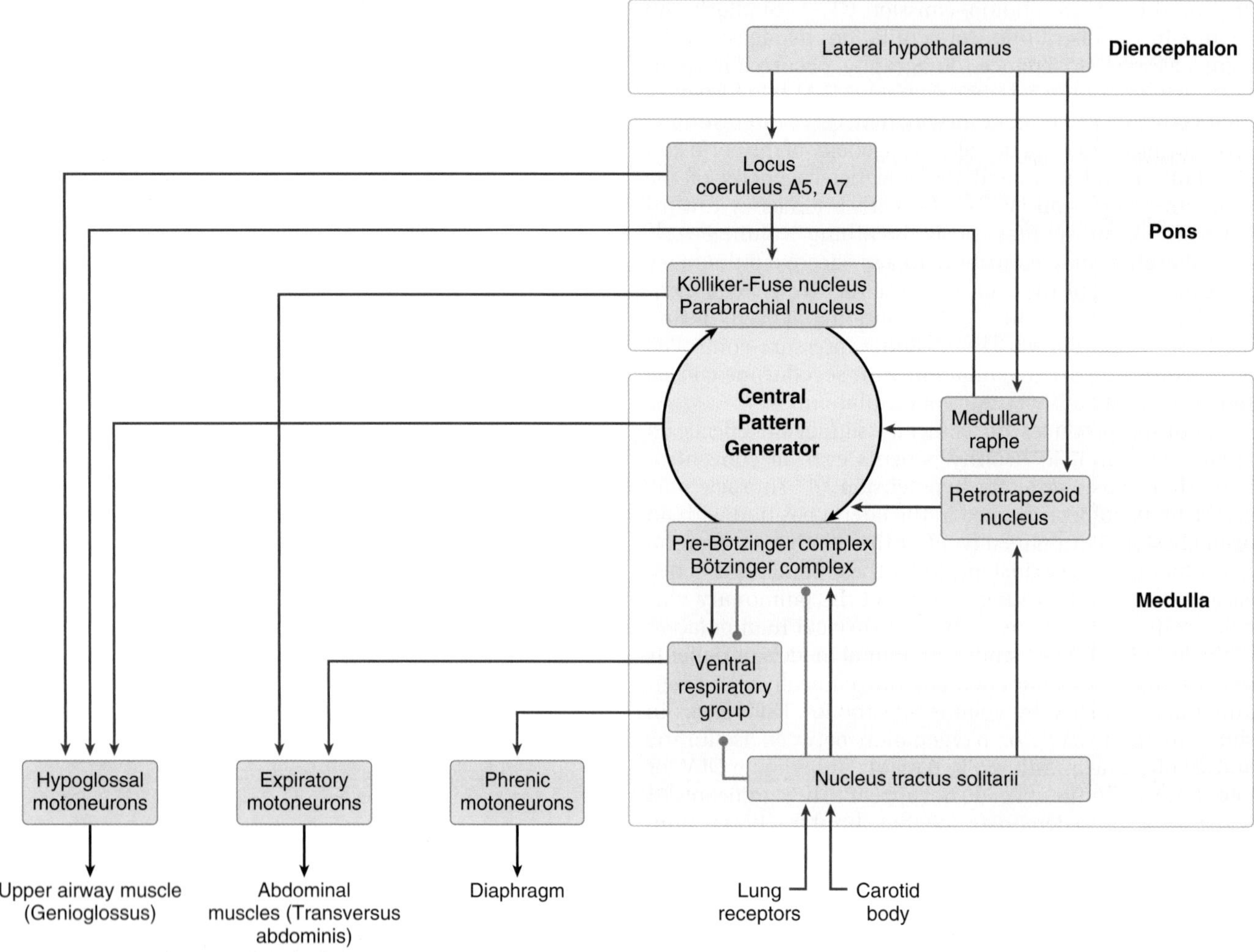

Fig. 21.15 Anatomic components of the respiratory system and the main nuclei involved in the generation of respiration from chemoreception to motoneuron activation (see text for details). Wakefulness drive is derived from the lateral hypothalamus. The *central pattern generator,* where respiratory drive is converted into a respiratory pattern, is thought to consist of several nuclei in the medulla and pons. Potential sites of central chemoreception are the locus coeruleus, areas A5 and A7, in the pons, and the medullary raphé and retrotrapezoid nucleus in the medulla. Expiratory and inspiratory excitatory drive is relayed to premotor neurons (ventral respiratory group), which project to expiratory motoneurons and inspiratory motoneurons (e.g., phrenic nerve) in the spinal cord. These motor nerves innervate abdominal muscles (expiratory) and diaphragm (inspiratory). Respiratory pattern and chemoreception are influenced by afferents from the lungs and carotid bodies. Excitatory inputs *(red arrows)*; inhibitory inputs *(blue buttons).*

CONTROL OF RESPIRATION

Components of the Respiratory Regulatory System

The regulation of respiratory function is very complex, occurs both on unconscious and conscious levels, and is precisely controlled by neuronal circuits, which are mainly located in the brainstem and include the medulla oblongata, pons, and midbrain (Fig. 21.15).

The neuronal networks in these areas are sufficient to generate involuntary, automatic breathing, which may be superseded by cortical centers for voluntary efforts such as speech, swallowing, laughing, sneezing, and coughing. Respiration per se is to ensure adequate gas exchange in order to meet metabolic demand during various levels of activity. Reflex inputs from the upper airways, lungs, and carotid bodies modulate respiration when inadequacy of gas exchange is sensed. Connections to the lateral hypothalamus also convey wakefulness drive to the respiratory center. Physiological status like sleep and pregnancy alter the respiratory function; so does nonphysiological status such as sedation. This chapter is not intended to discuss respiratory physiology in detail. Rather, its focus is on the major regulatory components of the respiratory system and how they are affected by inhalational anesthetics (Fig. 21.16).

Readers are referred to Chapters 13 and 41 for a detailed discussion of respiratory physiology and monitoring.

In general, respiratory drive is suppressed by all inhalational anesthetics except nitrous oxide.[163,164] Volatile anesthetics decrease glutamatergic excitatory drive to bulbospinal respiratory neurons and increase $GABA_A$ergic inhibitory mechanisms at the postsynaptic neuronal membrane.[165] In hypoglossal upper airway motor neurons, volatile anesthetics hyperpolarize neuronal membrane resting potential by activating K^+ channels that are linked to serotonin or norepinephrine receptors.[166,167] The magnitude of respiratory depression by volatile anesthetics may also depend on the position of the neuron in the neuronal hierarchy, which extends from the neurons generating excitatory respiratory drive to the respiratory pattern generator

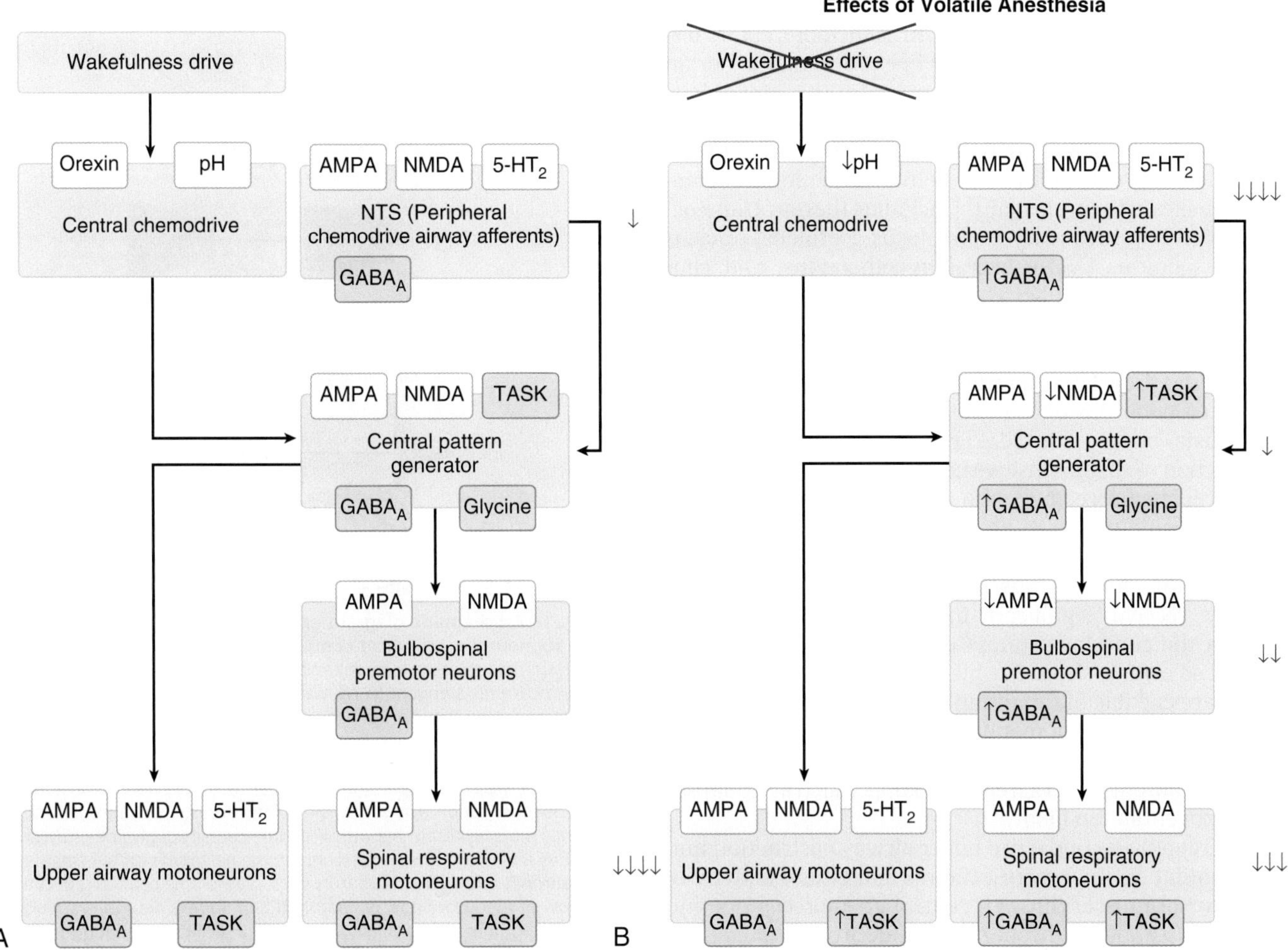

Fig. 21.16 (A) Ligand-gated receptors and ion channels on respiratory-related neurons. Excitatory receptors and channels are marked in *yellow*, inhibitory in *blue*. Opening of pH sensitive channels excites the neuron, whereas the opening of two-pore domain, acid-sensitive potassium (K^+) *(TASK)* channels causes membrane hyperpolarization and inhibition of neuronal discharge. (B) Effects of volatile anesthetics on respiratory-related neurons. Volatile anesthetics eliminate wakefulness drive to the respiratory system *(red cross out)*. *Black arrows* indicate changes in receptor function (*up*, increase; *down*, decrease) that have been published in the literature. Volatile anesthetics reduce the presynaptic release of glutamate and γ-aminobutyric acid A *($GABA_A$)* in respiratory premotor neurons. The cumulative anesthetic effects on the respective neuron groups are depicted *(red arrows)*. The relative magnitude of the depressant effect is visualized *(number of arrows)*. In humans, peripheral chemodrive is significantly more depressed than central chemodrive. Upper airway motoneurons are significantly more depressed than inspiratory motoneurons. *$5\text{-}HT_2$*, 5-Hydroxytryptamine; *AMPA*, alpha-amino-3-hydroxy-5-methyl-4-isoxazolepropionate acid; *NMDA*, *N*-methyl-D-aspartate; *NTS*, nucleus of the solitary tract.

and down to the phrenic and hypoglossal respiratory output motor neurons (see Fig. 21.16). Consequently, volatile anesthetics, which strongly affect synaptic neurotransmission, have a greater depressant effect on polysynaptic neuronal circuits that include many synapses, compared with those comprised of only few neurons (paucisynaptic). Fortunately, most connections between the single components of the respiratory system seem to be paucisynaptic, which may explain a relative resistance of automatic breathing to the depressant effects of volatile anesthetics.

The depressant effect of inhalational anesthetics on respiratory system may be further demonstrated at the molecular and genetic levels. Heterozygous paired-like homeobox 2b (PHOX2B) gene mutations have been found in the majority of patients diagnosed with late-onset central hypoventilation syndrome and may increase sensitivity of those patients to anesthetic-induced depression of breathing.[168] A recent study demonstrated that isoflurane can potentiate aggregation and mislocalization of PHOX2B variants, alter protein folding, and induce endoplasmic reticulum stress, indicating a mechanism by which these agents may affect respiratory neuronal function after surgery and promote the onset of the neurologic respiratory disease.[169]

Importantly, most data on respiratory regulatory systems are derived from animal models and may not directly translate to humans, as summarized in a review by Forster and Smith.[170] This section will therefore cover important animal study results to help understand the basic respiratory structure and function, as well as present recent clinical studies demonstrating the correlation of those findings to clinical practice.

CENTRAL CHEMORECEPTION

For many years, the prevailing view was that CO_2/H^+ sensitivity was due exclusively to the central chemoreceptors. Recent studies showed that central chemoreceptors contribute about two thirds of the ventilatory response to CO_2/H^+, while peripheral chemoreceptors contribute about one third.[170] These excitatory chemodrive mechanisms ensure automatic breathing under normoxic, normocapnic conditions in healthy individuals.[170] Central chemoreceptors discharge in response to the decrease in extracellular pH or an increase in [H+]. In addition, they project to other areas of the respiratory system where they form excitatory synapses. This pathway is well recognized, but its exact location remains to be defined. Animal studies have pointed to multiple chemosensitive sites in the brainstem[171] including the retrotrapezoid nucleus (RTN), medullary raphé, locus coeruleus, nucleus tractus solitarius (NTS), lateral hypothalamus, and caudal ventrolateral medulla. The RTN is a particularly strong candidate as the absence of RTN likely causes severe central apneas in congenital central hypoventilation syndrome. Glial cells in these areas may also theoretically contribute to chemoreception through their effect on extracellular pH or by hypoxia- or CO_2-induced ATP release potentially altering the function of chemosensitive neurons.[172]

Central chemoreceptors also promote excitatory drive to neurons regulating upper airway patency and arousal from sleep.[171] The genioglossus muscle, considered a typical representative for the muscles maintaining upper airway patency, receives significant tonic and phasic excitatory drive in the conscious state. Genioglossal muscle activity is reduced during sleep, but high levels of inspiratory CO_2 (>5%) are capable of recruiting near-normal levels of phasic activity. This phenomenon does not occur during rapid eye movement (REM) sleep because genioglossal muscle activity is absent, and therefore the upper airway collapses and hypoventilation follows.

Hypercapnia secondary to upper airway obstruction and hypoventilation may recruit the normal phasic activity of genioglossal muscle through central chemoreceptors and function as another mechanism (aside from hypoxia) by which patients with obstructive sleep apnea (OSA) arouse from sleep and reestablish airway patency. Residual subanesthetic concentrations of volatile anesthetics, which may be present for hours in postoperative patients, inhibit both peripheral hypoxic[173] and CO_2 chemosensitivity[174] and may also substantially impair the spontaneous arousal and resolution of upper airway obstruction that would otherwise occur with severe hypoxia or hypercarbia. This is a particularly important issue to recognize for same-day surgery patients, especially with a history of OSA.[175]

CENTRAL PATTERN GENERATOR

The cyclic breathing pattern is controlled by the central pattern generator (CPG). A recent review by Abdala and colleagues nicely summarizes the progress in the field.[176] Even though several models of the CPG network have been proposed, many of the circuit interactions and their functionalities remain unknown. CPG is believed to be located in nuclei of the pontomedullary network (see Fig. 21.15).[177] In the related nuclei, the network consists of excitatory and inhibitory neurons that control the inspiratory and expiratory phase of breathing. The breathing cycle is complexly regulated, and the type of neurons and the related neurotransmitters have been well illustrated (Fig. 21.17). This neuronal circuit can be pharmacologically modulated by inhaled anesthetics, affecting respiratory rate, upper airway patency, and relative contributions of the chest wall versus the diaphragm to tidal volume and minute alveolar ventilation.

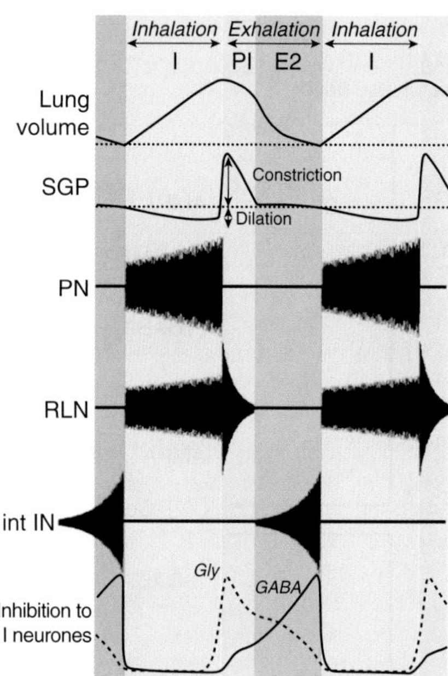

Fig. 21.17 Schematic diagram of a three–phase respiratory cycle and its neuro–mechanical components. Top schematic plots and neurograms represent lung volume, subglottal pressure *(SGP)*, phrenic *(PN)*, recurrent laryngeal *(RLN)*, and internal intercostal *(int IN)* nerve activities during the three phases of a respiratory cycle, i.e., inspiration *(I)*, postinspiration *(PI)*, and late expiration *(E2)*. Note that RLN conveys outputs from both abductor and adductor motoneurones, which fire respectively during inspiration (to dilate the glottis during inhalation) and postinspiration (to narrow the glottis during exhalation). Bottom overlay plots represent hypothetical time courses of glycine– *(Gly, dotted line)* and GABA–mediated *(continuous line)* inhibition to inspiratory (I) neurones during the respiratory cycle. These time courses reflect the activity of medullary postinspiratory (PI) inhibitory neurones, thought to be predominantly glycinergic, and GABAergic augmenting expiratory (E–AUG) inhibitory neurones active during E2 phase, both of which inhibit inspiratory neurones during expiration. Phasic inhibition of inspiratory neurones is minimal during inspiration, when active inspiratory neurones inhibit expiratory neurones, but rises abruptly during PI to orchestrate the inspiratory–expiratory phase transition and initiate exhalation. (Redrawn from Abdala AP, Paton JF, Smith JC. Defining inhibitory neurone function in respiratory circuits: opportunities with optogenetics? *J Physiol.* 2015;593[14]:3033–3046. Used with permission.)

INTEGRATION OF PERIPHERAL INPUTS

Afferent inputs from the periphery reach the brainstem respiratory center and influence respiratory drive. These inputs include the carotid body chemoreceptors, vagal inputs from the lungs and airways, and pulmonary baroreceptor inputs. The carotid body is the major peripheral chemoreceptor. It senses hypoxia or hypercapnia, which in turn increases carotid sinus nerve discharge. This information then reaches the RPG via NTS glutamatergic neurons, which also targets rostral ventrolateral medulla presympathetic neurons thereby raising sympathetic nerve activity (SNA). Chemoreceptors also regulate presympathetic neurons and cardio VPN indirectly via inputs from the RPG.[178] In essential hypertension, OSA, and congestive heart failure, chronically elevated carotid body afferent activity contributes to increasing SNA but breathing remains unchanged or becomes periodic.

The function of the carotid body was discovered nearly 80 years ago, and for a long time it was thought that the carotid body chemoreceptors function independently from central chemoreceptors.[179] However, more recent studies suggested that the peripheral and central chemoreceptors are not functionally separate but are interdependent. The sensitivity of the medullary chemoreceptors is critically determined by input from the peripheral chemoreceptors and possibly other breathing-related reflex afferents as well.[170] This effect might be mediated through interactions within the NTS and/or through NTS projections to parafacial respiratory group/RTN integrating neurons and/or through projections to neurons of a raphe-pontomedullary respiratory network.

Afferent vagal inputs from the lungs and airways are also relayed through the NTS. Pulmonary baroreceptor inputs project to second-order pump neurons in the NTS, which can provide both excitatory and inhibitory inputs to various parts of the medullary respiratory column. In general, pulmonary baroreceptor inputs promote the phase switch from inspiration to expiration. This vagal expiratory-facilitating reflex (Hering-Breuer reflex) is most prominent in immature mammals but also modulates respiratory phase-timing during resting ventilation in adult humans.[180] Although some of these inputs directly influence the CPG, others are integrated at the level of the bulbospinal or premotor neurons, which project to the motor neurons in the spinal cord.

RESPIRATORY MOTOR OUTPUT AND UPPER AIRWAY PATENCY

The pontomedullary respiratory network generates the respiratory pattern and then projects to and controls respiratory motor outputs in the brainstem and spinal cord. The phrenic motor neurons are the main inspiratory neurons in the spinal cord. They are located at the levels C_3 to C_5 of the spinal cord and innervate the diaphragm.[177] Phrenic motor neurons are also directly depressed by volatile anesthetics.[181] Expiratory motor neurons are located at approximately T_7-T_{12} of the spinal cord and innervate truncal abdominal muscles that aid with forceful expiration and with expiratory expulsive efforts such as coughing. Expiratory motor neurons receive inputs from expiratory bulbospinal neurons and the pons.[177] The spinal motor neurons are the final neurons in the respiratory neuronal hierarchy. Their activity tends to be reduced by the cumulative effect of anesthetics on all previous steps of chemoreception and neurotransmission.

To ensure effective ventilation, inspiratory muscle activity needs to be closely coordinated with upper airway muscles that maintain airway patency. Central respiratory motor output almost simultaneously engages both the phrenic motor neurons (serving chest wall pump muscles) and hypoglossal motor neurons (serving pharyngeal muscle dilators).[182,183] The hypoglossal motor nerve innervates upper airway muscles, particularly the genioglossal muscle. The strength of excitatory and inhibitory drive to hypoglossal motor neurons strongly depends on the level of consciousness and differs between the REM and non-REM sleep phases.

The onset of the sleeping state results in a reduced tonic activation of upper airway dilator musculature and enhances collapsibility. This effect is especially problematic for patients with OSA whose airway is narrower, longer, and more collapsible than that of those without OSA. Patients with OSA critically rely on compensatory activation of airway dilator muscles to maintain patency during wakefulness. The reduced lung volumes in obese recumbent patients during sleep also decrease caudal traction on the trachea, promoting pharyngeal collapse.[184,185] In addition, the loss of wakefulness removes an important vigilance component in the ventilatory control system, leaving the regulation of central respiratory motor output largely under chemoreceptor and mechanoreceptor feedback control.

The mechanisms of airway collapse during sleep and anesthesia are closely related. Hypoventilation and/or hypoxia secondary to upper airway collapse during anesthesia/sedation represent a significant challenge for anesthesia care providers, particularly in ambulatory surgery patients. The effect of inhalational anesthetics on pharyngeal airway collapsibility can best be illustrated by visualizing the changes as the depth of sedation increases.

EFFECTS OF INHALED ANESTHETICS ON RESTING VENTILATION

Volatile anesthetics suppress conscious control of breathing at concentrations of less than 1 MAC and completely abolish conscious breathing drive at higher concentrations. Breathing is then largely controlled by automatic brainstem mechanisms and chemoreflex inputs. All volatile anesthetics also cause a dose-dependent decrease in minute ventilation at concentrations greater than 1 MAC because of a decrease in tidal volume. However, in a pressure chamber, Hornbein and colleagues demonstrated that nitrous oxide does not significantly reduce minute ventilation within 1.5 MAC (well beyond an atmosphere).[186] The respiratory rate typically increases for all inhalational agents tested, except for xenon, which causes a significant reduction in respiratory rate (Fig. 21.18). Indeed, there are several reports indicating that xenon can cause hypopnea or apnea.[187,188]

Most volatile anesthetics cause an increase in respiratory rate by producing a decrease in both inspiratory and expiratory duration, whereas opioids cause a very prominent decrease in respiratory rate that primarily results from a large increase in expiratory duration. However, the observed modest decrease in minute ventilation with volatile anesthetics could underestimate the magnitude of the respiratory depressant effects of these agents. This is due to volatile anesthetic–induced hypoventilation increasing $PaCO_2$ in a closed central chemoreflex feedback loop. In turn, central chemoreceptors are stimulated, thereby increasing central chemodrive to the respiratory center and increasing minute ventilation.[199-202]

EFFECTS OF INHALED ANESTHETICS ON CHEMOREFLEXES

Volatile anesthetics impair peripheral chemoreceptor responses to hypoxia and hypercarbia in a dose dependent manner. In the presence of volatile anesthetic concentrations of 1 MAC or higher, breathing in humans is entirely dependent on the automatic control from the pontomedullary respiratory center and afferent excitatory inputs from the central chemoreceptors. These anesthetic concentrations lead to a complete depression of the peripheral chemoreflex loop with further respiratory depression rather than

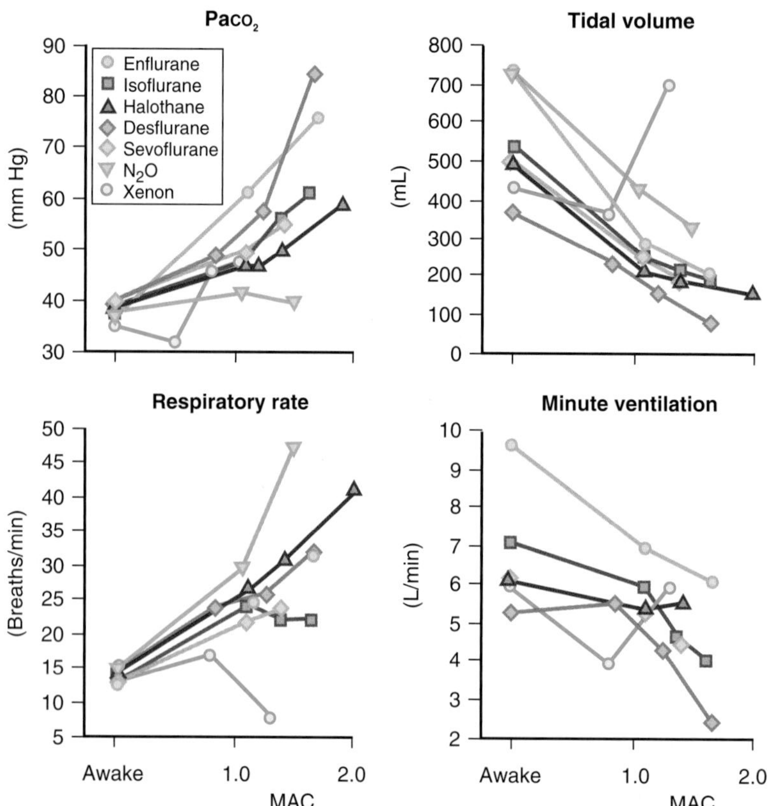

Fig. 21.18 Comparison of mean changes in resting partial arterial pressure of carbon dioxide ($PaCO_2$), tidal volume, respiratory rate, and minute ventilation in patients anesthetized with various inhaled agents. Most agents cause dose-dependent tachypnea, decreases in minute ventilation and tidal volume, and an increase in $Paco_2$. *MAC*, Minimum alveolar concentration, *N_2O*, nitrous oxide.[189-194] *Note: data for xenon has been extrapolated from references.*[195-198]

stimulation in response to hypoxia.[203] Even very low concentrations of the agent (0.1 MAC of isoflurane and sevoflurane) depress the peripheral chemoreflex loop, without affecting the central chemoreflex loop. Desflurane at the same MAC showed no effect on peripheral and central CO_2 sensitivity.[204] A loss of upper airway muscle tone and function accompanies this process, as does differential depression of neurotransmission at the level of the spinal cord.[205]

The effect of inhaled anesthetics on respiratory drive may not be clinically relevant in the patient undergoing controlled ventilation. However, it does matter in spontaneously breathing patients. Because the suppressive effect of inhaled anesthetics on respiratory drive is synergetic with narcotics and frequently these two drug classes are administered concurrently, the suppression on the hypoxic and hypercarbic drive can increase the risk of postoperative respiratory complications.

EFFECTS OF INHALED ANESTHETICS ON THE HYPERCAPNIC VENTILATORY RESPONSE

In awake humans, about one third of the CO_2-mediated respiratory drive is through peripheral chemoreceptors and other two thirds through the central chemoreceptors. The respiratory drive mediated by the peripheral chemoreceptors is augmented by hypoxia.[206] However, the hypoxia-mediated component is abolished by the majority of volatile anesthetics at concentration even under 1 MAC. When the anesthetic concentration increases above 1 MAC, the peripheral chemoreceptor-mediated portion of the CO_2 responsive respiratory drive are abolished, and only the central chemoreceptor loop remains functional.[173,207-209] Depression of the respiratory drive is often described in a quantitative manner by plotting the CO_2 response curve (an increase in $PaCO_2$ vs. an increase in minute alveolar ventilation). Volatile anesthetics also cause a rightward shift of the apneic threshold,[210] that is the minimum $PaCO_2$ required to initiate spontaneous respiration. Thus spontaneous breathing efforts do not occur if mechanical or assisted ventilation efforts drive the $PaCO_2$ levels below the CO_2 threshold during anesthesia.[211]

Patients under general anesthesia with volatile anesthetics become hypercarbic if they are spontaneously breathing without any ventilatory support. Pressure support ventilation is often used to counteract the suppression of the respiratory drive by the volatile anesthetics. However, it remains to be determined if an increase in pressure support would lead to a proportional increase in minute alveolar ventilation as the intrinsic CO_2 response curve at a given level of sedation is not altered. An increase in minute alveolar ventilation secondary to increased tidal volumes from pressure support may result in a decreased respiratory rate and therefore minute alveolar ventilation may not be increased as much as expected.

EFFECTS OF VOLATILE ANESTHETIC ON THE HYPOXIC VENTILATORY RESPONSE IN HUMANS

Hypoxic ventilatory response (HVR) is rarely encountered in conscious healthy humans at sea level. However, for

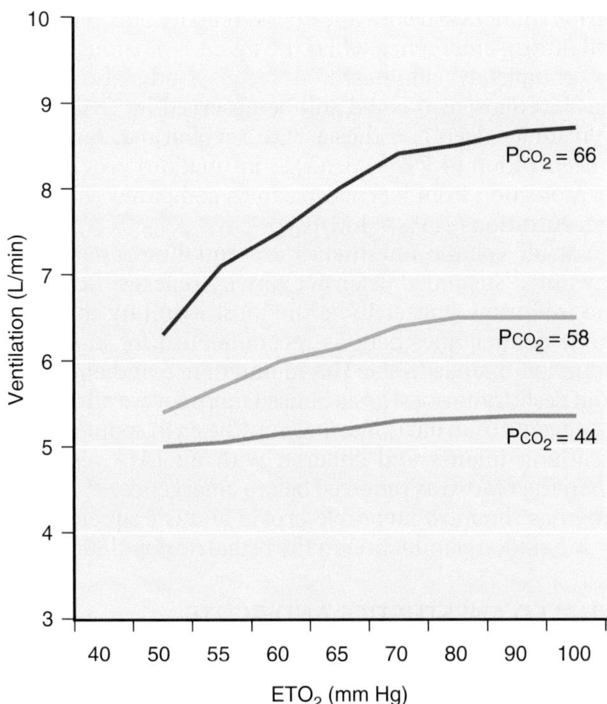

Fig. 21.19 Effects of halothane anesthesia on the hypoxic ventilatory response in humans at three steady-state levels of partial pressure of carbon dioxide (P_{CO_2}). Halothane anesthesia (1.1 minimum alveolar concentration) completely eliminates the hypoxic ventilatory response and the hypoxic hypercapnic interaction at the peripheral chemoreceptors. *ETO_2*, End-tidal oxygen. (Modified from Knill RL, Gelb AW. Ventilatory responses to hypoxia and hypercapnia during halothane sedation and anesthesia in man. *Anesthesiology*. 1978;49:244. Used with permission.)

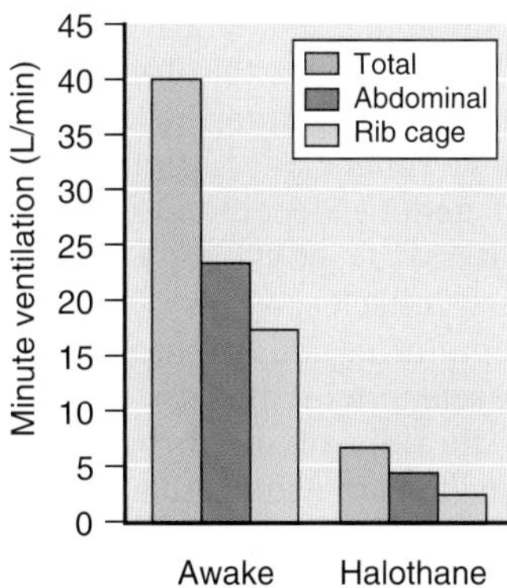

Fig. 21.20 Effects of halothane anesthesia on rib cage and abdominal ventilation during hypercapnia (calculated ventilation at partial arterial pressure of carbon dioxide [Pa_{CO_2}] of 55 mm Hg). Compared with being awake, halothane anesthesia strongly depresses minute ventilation. Halothane depresses the rib cage component to ventilation more than the abdominal component (diaphragmatic). Data are means. (Graph is based on data from Warner DO, Warner MA, Ritman EL. Mechanical significance of respiratory muscle activity in humans during halothane anesthesia. *Anesthesiology*. 1996;84:309.)

special occupations, such as tunnel workers at sea level, or mountain climbers staying at high attitude, hypoxia does occur and therefore the HVR becomes an important mechanism to compensate for low inspired O_2 concentrations. One example is humans living at high altitude. At the top of Mt. Everest (8848 m), the partial pressure of O_2 of ambient air is only about 50 mm Hg compared with 159.6 mm Hg at sea level. The corresponding arterial blood PaO_2 is only 37.6 mm Hg, which is lower than the partial pressure of O_2 in the mixed venous blood in healthy resting adults living at sea level. The estimated minute ventilation is approximately 166 L/min as a result of severe hypoxic hyperventilation.[212] However, this powerful compensation mechanism is significantly comprised under anesthesia with volatile anesthetics under 1 MAC and completely abolished at 1.1 MAC of halothane (Fig. 21.19). It is important to realize that even a subanesthetic concentration (0.1 MAC) of inhalational anesthetics profoundly diminishes hypoxic respiratory drive without concurrent use of narcotics.[213] The potency of the suppression of HVR has been proposed as the following order: halothane > enflurane > sevoflurane > isoflurane > desflurane.[173]

Certain patient populations are particularly vulnerable to the inhibition of hypoxic respiratory drive at subanesthetic concentrations, including premature infants and patients with OSA.[214,215] The depressant effect on the HVR is due to selective inhibition of the peripheral chemoreflex loop. The carotid body appears to be the most likely target. However, the mechanisms by which subanesthetic concentrations of volatile anesthetics attenuate hypoxic ventilatory drive are not completely understood. Interestingly, acute pain and central nervous system arousal do not restore impaired HVR during sevoflurane sedation. Thus compromise of the central nervous system arousal state per se does not contribute to the impairment of the acute HVR by sevoflurane.[216] Additionally, audiovisual stimulation does not prevent the blunting of acute HVR by low-dose halothane, but by isoflurane. This finding raises the possibility that volatile anesthetics might differently affect the hypoxic chemoreflex loop.[217]

EFFECTS OF INHALED ANESTHETICS ON RESPIRATORY MUSCLE ACTIVITY

Humans are bipeds and very different from the quadruped mammals in terms of contribution of various muscle groups, particularly the truncal muscles, to the normal respiratory effort, probably due to differences in posture. Thus the results of respiratory control studies in animals could not be directly extrapolated to humans, whether under normal resting conditions or under anesthesia. At quiet breathing in supine and conscious nonpregnant adult humans, scalene and parasternal inspiratory activity is universally present, but abdominal expiratory activity is absent.[218,219] This means that at quiet breathing, expiration is mostly passive and likely occurs via recoiling of chest wall and lungs. When breathing is stimulated by inhaling CO_2, the inspiratory activity is enhanced and expiratory muscles are recruited.

Volatile anesthetics, such as halothane, depress various respiratory muscles differently (Fig. 21.20). The diaphragm, as the main inspiratory muscle, is unique in that regard because it is relatively spared from the respiratory depression by volatile anesthetics, probably because of its low position in the hierarchy of the neurotransmission system. At 1 MAC of halothane, the tidal volume was reduced by 59%, respiratory rate was increased by 146%, and FRC was decreased by 335 ± 75 mL. The decrease in minute ventilation could be because of rib cage/chest wall activity but is not because of a reduction in abdominal breathing, and the contribution of the diaphragm is also substantially less affected.[220] Abdominal expiratory activity is routinely recruited during halothane anesthesia in male subjects.

The depressive effect of halothane on respiratory muscle is also gender dependent. Of note, pregnancy significantly alters the physiology and contribution of each respiratory muscle groups. The reduction in FRC is from both remaining activity of expiratory transverse abdominal muscles, which reduces thoracic volume, and cephalad motion of diaphragm. Paradoxical rib cage motion develops in some subjects during halothane anesthesia, such that the rib cage continues to expand during the first portion of expiration. Such paradoxical rib cage motion is exaggerated during a CO_2-stimulated rebreathing.[218,220]

EFFECTS OF INHALED ANESTHETICS ON THE UPPER AIRWAY

Inspiratory upper airway patency is maintained by the cortical wakefulness drive, fully preserved chemical chemoreceptor sensitivity and chemodrive transmission, and an optimal reflex feedback from upper airway receptors in the conscious state. These upper airway receptors are activated by the negative pressure and airflow[221,222] that are generated by the inspiratory muscles (e.g., diaphragm, respiratory chest wall muscles). During sleep or volatile anesthesia, the cortical wakefulness drive is absent, and the sensitivity of the chemoreceptors and upper airway receptors is decreased. Thus both phasic and tonic inspiratory excitatory drives to the upper airway muscles are decreased or entirely absent. The loss of tone in the upper airway muscles (genioglossus and other pharyngeal muscles) predisposes individuals with anatomic limitations to upper airway obstruction.[223,224] Even in the presence of subanesthetic concentrations of volatile anesthetics (frequently in immediate postoperative period), the cortical wakefulness drive, the drive from peripheral chemoreceptors, and excitatory inputs from upper airway mechanoreceptors are all significantly impaired. This may lead to partial or even complete upper airway obstruction, a situation that can be further complicated by inhibition of hypoxia-mediated arousal reflexes.[203]

EFFECTS OF INHALED ANESTHETICS ON DEFENSIVE AIRWAY REFLEXES

Humans have very effective protective mechanisms to prevent aspiration by closing glottis and coughing. Volatile anesthetics (≥1-1.3 MAC) progressively abolish defensive airway reflexes. The loss of airway protection against gastroesophageal reflux with consequent aspiration of orogastric content into the trachea can be catastrophic. However, lower concentrations of volatile anesthetics may paradoxically enhance and prolong the duration of protective defensive reflexes. Laryngospasm is the sustained and complete reflex glottic closure in response to foreign material (e.g., oral secretions) contacting the vocal cords, or to a poorly timed noxious stimulus (e.g., pain from incision, venipuncture) during the administration of inadequately low concentrations of a volatile anesthetic. This occurs during induction before anesthesia reaches adequate depth and during emergence when the agent is washing out but not completely eliminated. A recent study also showed that laryngospasm could still be observed in 18% of children under deep anesthesia with sevoflurane, but higher concentration (4.7% = MAC_{ED95} intubation) provided better protection from laryngospasm as compared with lower concentration (2.5% = 1 MAC).[225]

Not all volatile anesthetics are equally prone to elicit unwanted sustained defensive airway reflexes. Desflurane and isoflurane appear to be the most irritating to the airways; neither anesthetic is recommended for an inhaled induction of anesthesia. The maintenance and emergence from desflurane anesthesia caused more severe adverse airway events than did isoflurane anesthesia in spontaneously breathing infants and children with an LMA, especially when the LMA was removed before emergence.[226] Sevoflurane has the most favorable profile and is frequently used for inhalational induction in the pediatric population.

INHALED ANESTHETICS AND ACUTE LUNG INJURY

Pathophysiology of Sepsis-Induced Acute Lung Injury

ALI represents the pulmonary manifestation of a global inflammatory process that is commonly associated with gram-negative bacterial sepsis.[227-230] Derangements of pulmonary hemodynamics,[231] fluid filtration, and gas exchange are pathophysiological manifestations.[232] Bacterial endotoxin often triggers ALI.[233] In addition, other humoral and cellular cascades are involved, such as eicosanoids,[234] cytokines, O_2 free radicals, endothelin,[235] NO, as well as the coagulation, the NOTNOT complement,[236] the fibrinolytic, and the kinin/kallikrein systems,[237] as well as degradation fragments of NOT extracellular matrix.[238]

It is now well established that NO is involved in the pathogenesis of sepsis and sepsis-induced ALI. In hyperdynamic sepsis, increased iNOS-dependent formation of NO and, subsequently, cGMP is associated with myocardial depression, reduced contractile responses to vasoconstrictor agents, and circulatory shock.[239] In addition, NO may mediate cytotoxic effects following its reaction with the superoxide anion to yield the strong oxidant anion peroxynitrite and eventually its breakdown cytotoxic product OH•.[240] Large amounts of NO may also activate enzymes in the cyclooxygenase pathway and modify gene expression.[241] Interaction of NO with many molecular targets represents a pathway for its breakdown and inactivation. The most important is the reaction of NO with molecular O_2 to form nitrite, which in the presence of hemoproteins (i.e., hemoglobin) is oxidized further to nitrate.[242]

Moreover, NO may attenuate HPV, thereby contributing to derangement of gas exchange.[243] The latter changes may cause tissue hypoxia and microvascular damage that may result in multiple organ failure and death. However, in less extreme conditions, generation of minute amounts of NO by eNOS and/or iNOS might be protective. Vasodilatation may enhance tissue perfusion. NO inhibition of platelet adhesion and aggregation may produce antithrombotic effects. NO scavenging of superoxide anions and other free radicals and inhibition of leukocyte-endothelial cell adhesion may prevent crucial steps in the inflammatory reactions. Finally, stimulation of cGMP production may preserve the integrity of the microvascular barrier.[244,245]

EFFECTS OF INHALED ANESTHETICS ON EXPERIMENTAL SEPSIS-INDUCED ACUTE LUNG INJURY

There is a substantial debate surrounding the choice of anesthetic regimens for patients with ALI that require surgery. Animal studies suggest an important antiinflammatory role of volatile anesthetics in ALI. Pretreatment with sevoflurane significantly reduced the inflammatory response and attenuated LPS-induced chemotaxis of neutrophils from alveolar type II cells.[246] Compared with thiopental anesthesia, pigs anesthetized with sevoflurane exhibited decreased expression of TNFα and IL-1β in lung tissue.[247] Volatile anesthetics exert other antiinflammatory effects including reduction of proinflammatory cytokine production in alveolar type II cells, reduction of neutrophil migration into the lung interstitium and alveolar space, and decreased protein leakage and pulmonary edema.[248-250] In a rat model, LPS-induced ALI was markedly attenuated by sevoflurane compared with propofol anesthesia. Rats receiving sevoflurane demonstrated improved gas exchange, reduced amounts of albumin and total cell count in bronchoalveolar lavage fluid, and lower cytokine levels in bronchoalveolar lavage fluid and RNA levels in lung tissue compared with rats receiving propofol. Sevoflurane, but not propofol, also decreased the amount of pulmonary edema most likely through a reduction in edema formation rather than water reabsorption.[249] When administered after the onset of oleic acid–induced ALI in dogs, sevoflurane reduced the elevated PA pressure and PVR, attenuated pulmonary edema as evidenced by reduced extravascular lung water index, and decreased TNFα production and diffuse alveolar damage score compared with propofol. However, despite of these effects, sevoflurane worsened systemic oxygenation possibly via inhibition of HPV.[251] In a rat model of cecal ligation and puncture (CLP)–induced sepsis, both sevoflurane and isoflurane attenuated inflammatory response, lipid peroxidation, oxidative stress, and improved survival. Furthermore, sevoflurane was more effective in modulating sepsis-induced inflammatory response.[252] Induction of heme oxygenase-1 and suppression of iNOS expression provide cytoprotection in lung and vascular injury. In a rat model of ALI induced by CLP, the isoflurane posttreatment reduced pulmonary microvascular permeability, as well as lung injury as assessed by histological and immunohistochemical examinations. Furthermore, isoflurane decreased iNOS and increased heme oxygenase-1 expression in lung tissue. These findings suggest that the protective role of isoflurane postconditioning against CLP-induced ALI may be associated with its role in upregulating heme oxygenase-1.[253]

INHALED ANESTHETICS AND VENTILATOR-INDUCED LUNG INJURY

Mechanical ventilation is a life-saving clinical treatment, but it can also produce pulmonary inflammatory changes and injury known as ventilator-induced lung injury (VILI). Cyclic stretching of the lung during mechanical ventilation releases proinflammatory cytokines such as IL-1 and MIP-2 leading to pulmonary neutrophil accumulation; enhances activity of phospholipase A_2, which degrades surfactant; and results in pulmonary edema, hyaline membrane formation, and cellular infiltration.[254] Volatile anesthetics have been shown to attenuate lung injury due to mechanical ventilation. In mice, mechanical ventilation led to induction of lung injury, reactive O_2 species production, proinflammatory cytokine release, and neutrophil influx. Sevoflurane posttreatment reduced histological signs of VILI, as well as prevented increased production of reactive O_2 species, release of IL-1β and MIP-1β, and neutrophil transmigration.[255] Similarly, isoflurane reduced VILI in mice, as indicated by reduced inflammation, transmigration of neutrophils, and cytokine levels. Phosphorylation of Akt protein was significantly increased during mechanical ventilation with isoflurane. Inhibition of phosphoinositide 3-kinase/Akt signaling before mechanical ventilation completely reversed the lung-protective effects of isoflurane. These findings suggest that isoflurane-mediated pulmonary protection is mediated via phosphoinositide 3-kinase/Akt signaling.[256] Moreover, in a murine two-hit model of LPS-induced inflammation followed by VILI, isoflurane exposure before initiation of mechanical ventilation ameliorated VILI by improving both lung mechanics and vascular leakage. In addition, isoflurane prevented a decrease of a key tight junction protein (zona occludens 1) in lung tissue and lung epithelial cells.[257] In another study in murine VILI, animals anesthetized with isoflurane and sevoflurane showed thinner alveolar septa, lower VILI scores, lower polymorph neutrophil counts, lower IL-1β concentrations, less reactive O_2 species production, and higher glutathione contents compared to ketamine-anesthetized mice. Unexpectedly, desflurane-ventilated mice showed signs of lung injury similar to mice receiving ketamine anesthesia. Desflurane also failed to inhibit inflammatory responses and reactive O_2 species production in lung tissue.[258]

INHALED ANESTHETICS AND LUNG ISCHEMIA-REPERFUSION

Lung ischemia-reperfusion (IR) injury is a hallmark of many lung diseases, and it also occurs during surgical procedures such as lung transplantation. The re-establishment of blood flow and O_2 delivery into the previously ischemic lung exacerbates the ischemic injury and leads to increased microvascular permeability and PVR as well as activation of the immune response. These events trigger ALI with subsequent edema formation that can result in systemic hypoxemia and multiorgan failure. Reactive O_2 and nitrogen species have been suggested as crucial mediators of such responses during IR in the lung.[259] Isoflurane attenuated increases in PVR and the filtration coefficient and the wet-to-dry ratio in isolated rabbit lungs subjected to IR.[260] Isoflurane also protected against warm IR injury in an isolated, perfused rat lung model when it was administered after the onset of ischemia.[261] Moreover, reductions in inflammatory responses and oxidative stress were observed during sevoflurane compared with propofol anesthesia in a porcine model of IR injury.[262] In a rat lung transplantation model, preconditioning and postconditioning using sevoflurane significantly improved the oxygenation of lung grafts and decreased pulmonary edema. Sevoflurane treatment also reduced levels of

IL-1β, IL-6, and TNFα. In addition, sevoflurane significantly inhibited cell apoptosis by a decrease in cytochrome C release into cytosol and caspase-3 cleavage.[263] In contrast, pretreatment with desflurane exacerbated IR injury in isolated rabbit lungs perfused with saline by increasing pulmonary microvascular permeability and NO production.[264] Furthermore, postconditioning with xenon during prolonged ex vivo lung perfusion did not improve graft function in a porcine warm ischemic lung injury model.[265]

CLINICAL EVIDENCE

Clinical evidence supports potential beneficial effects of volatile anesthetics in ALI. For example, short-term positive pressure ventilation with high tidal volumes did not affect cytokine production in the lungs of healthy patients anesthetized with isoflurane.[266] Several studies investigated the effects of volatile anesthetics in patients undergoing thoracic surgery with OLV.[267-269] OLV is associated with hypoxia-reoxygenation injury in the deflated and subsequently reventilated lung. OLV increased the release of proinflammatory mediators in both the dependent and the nondependent lung.[268] Sevoflurane suppressed local alveolar inflammatory responses and cytokine release compared with propofol. Furthermore, the antiinflammatory effects of sevoflurane were greater in the dependent compared with the nondependent lung.[268,269] Patients receiving sevoflurane also had an improved postoperative course as indicated by a shorter ICU stay and fewer adverse events including pneumonia, pleural effusion, and bronchopleural fistula compared with those anesthetized with propofol.[267] In addition, a recent meta-analysis in cardiac surgical patients demonstrated that volatile as opposed to intravenous anesthesia is associated with a significant reduction in pulmonary complications and overall mortality.[270] However, in a randomized multicenter controlled trial in patients scheduled for surgery with OLV, the incidence of major complications during hospitalization and within 6 months from surgery was similar in propofol and desflurane groups.[271] This finding seems to be in agreement with an earlier study demonstrating that in healthy surgical patients desflurane increased lipid peroxidation as measured in BALF, indicating injury to the pulmonary alveolar membranes. Sevoflurane caused less pronounced effects, suggesting that it may exert a protective effect compared with desflurane.[272] Proinflammatory response and elevated levels of TNFα, IL-1β, and IL-6 in healthy patients undergoing tympanoplasty were also more evident following desflurane anesthesia compared with sevoflurane.[273]

In a recent parallel, open-label, single-center randomized controlled trial, adult patients with moderate-to-severe ARDS were randomized to receive either intravenous midazolam or inhaled sevoflurane for 48 hours. On day 2, PaO_2/FiO_2 ratio was significantly higher in the sevoflurane group than in the midazolam group. There was also a significant reduction in cytokines and the soluble form of the receptor for advanced glycation end-product levels in the sevoflurane group, compared with the midazolam group. No serious adverse events were observed with sevoflurane. This study suggests therapeutic utility of inhaled sevoflurane in patients with ARDS.[274] Moreover, the use of inhaled anesthetics in the ICU is conceptually appealing as they offer a safe, effective, and easily titratable method of sedation. A recent retrospective analysis of patients receiving inhaled sedation in the ICU suggests an association between its use and reductions in one-year and in-hospital mortality, perhaps related to a significant increase in ventilator-free days compared to sedation with intravenous agents.[275] Prospective randomized clinical trials are needed to further elucidate the therapeutic potential of inhaled anesthetics in intubated patients with ALI/ARDS and ICU patients requiring long term sedation.

Nonvolatile Inhaled Agents

The pharmacokinetics of all inhalational anesthetics follow the same principle. At initial uptake, the dynamic change of the ratio of the fraction of a gas in alveoli (FA) to its fraction in the inspiratory gas (FI) (FA/FI) is dependent on initial FI, solubility of the anesthetic, minute alveolar ventilation, and cardiac output. Fig. 21.21

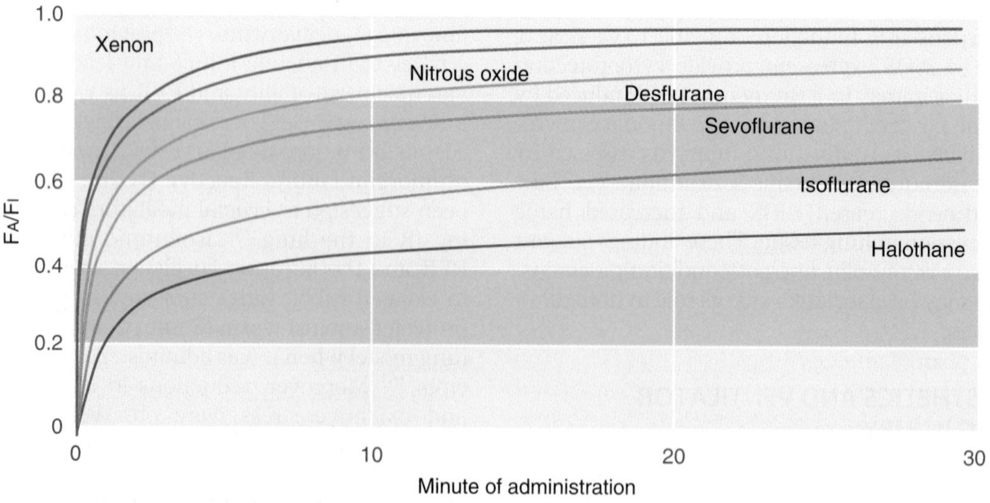

Fig. 21.21 Pharmacokinetics of the inhalational anesthetics. The rise in alveolar (FA) anesthetic concentration towards inspired (FI) is most rapid with the least soluble anesthetic, N2O, and slowest with the most soluble, methoxyflurane. All data from human studies (Data from Yashuda N, Lockhart SH, Eger EI II, et al. Kinetics of desflurane, isoflurane and halothane in humans. Anesthesiology 74:489-498, 1991; & Anesth Analg 72:316-24, 1991; Data for Xenon only recently available.

demonstrates the dynamic changes in FA/FI of inhalational anesthetics during the phase of uptake. Because xenon has the lowest solubility among the all inhalational anesthetics, it reaches equilibrium quickly, and even faster than nitrous oxide. The speed of washout of anesthetics also follows the same principle but in the reverse direction. Among the four factors affecting washout (solubility, fresh gas flow rate, minute alveolar ventilation, and cardiac output), fresh gas flow is the only one the provider can fully control besides partially controlling minute alveolar ventilation. Adequate fresh gas flow plays an important role in preventing rebreathing expired gas and affects the rate of its elimination. Fresh gas flow has to be higher than the peak inspiratory flow rate for the adult breathing circuit. If a tidal volume is 500 mL, respiratory rate is 10, and I:E ratio is 1:2, the inspiratory phase is 4 seconds. The mean inspiratory flow rate is 500 mL/4 seconds, 125 mL/s, or 7500 mL/min. Therefore maximal O_2 flow rate of 10 to 15 L/min for any given modern ventilator should be large enough to prevent rebreathing expired gas. For circuits used in pediatric patients, the minimal fresh gas flow rate for preventing rebreathing is dependent on the type of the circuit. In the following section, two commonly used nonvolatile gases, xenon and nitrous oxide, are discussed with focus on their clinically related aspects.

NITROUS OXIDE

Advantages of nitrous oxide (N_2O) are well established including the ability to quickly reach its target MAC value and quick washout. N_2O does not significantly interfere with respiratory drive and has no negative impact on bronchial mucosa or bronchial smooth muscle activity in healthy individuals. N_2O enhances catecholamine release and does not reduce systemic vascular resistance or cardiac output, maintaining hemodynamic stability. Because its MAC value is 104%, N_2O cannot be used as a sole anesthetic at 1 atmosphere pressure to achieve adequate sedation. However, because it is odorless, it is often used as an adjuvant at the beginning of inhalational induction, especially in pediatric patients, prior to administration of volatile anesthetics. It is also commonly used for analgesia and sedation for dental procedures.[276] Its use for labor pain has faded but it is still used for labor analgesia in some centers.[277]

Sedative and Analgesic Effects

Nitrous oxide has both sedative and analgesic effects. Because MAC is determined as the threshold of an individual's response to the painful stimulation of skin incision, and N_2O is analgesic, it is difficult to dissect its sedative from analgesic effects. Therefore the sedative potency of N_2O at equal MAC values is different from other inhalational anesthetics which do not possess analgesic effects. The MAC of N_2O and other inhalational anesthetics are additive relative to a subjects' movement in response to nociceptive stimulation, but not necessarily when it comes to the level of sedation. For most volatile anesthetics, MAC awake is approximately 0.3 MAC value.[278] However, the MAC awake of N_2O is 0.61 MAC (63.3%).[278] Even at 50% of N_2O or 0.48 MAC, the majority of adults may be conscious. Clinicians often use N_2O at the end anesthesia in order to facilitate washout of a volatile anesthetic. Even though the sum of the MAC values of the volatile anesthetic and that of N_2O is above the MAC awake value of the volatile anesthetic alone, this does not guarantee the unconsciousness of the patient. Awareness may occur even though it may not be associated with postoperative recall.[279]

In humans, the analgesic effect of 66% to 70% of N_2O is equal to that of an intravenous infusion of remifentanil at 0.085 to 0.17 mg/kg/min, or a whole-blood concentration of 2 ng/mL.[280,281] Analgesic potency of N_2O can be attenuated by sevoflurane (Fig. 21.22).[282] The detailed pathway of its analgesic action remains to be determined. However, animals tolerant to N_2O are cross-tolerant to morphine,[283] and the analgesic effect of N_2O can be reversed by naloxone.[284] This means that at least in part, the analgesic action of N_2O occurs via the mu opioid receptor. Small animals develop tolerance quickly (6-24 hours) following continuous administration of N_2O.[284] Humans can also develop acute tolerance to N_2O in only 40 minutes.[285] In clinical practice, N_2O is commonly administered for several hours. However, it is to be determined whether its sedative and/or analgesic effects remain during prolonged administration.

Gas Volume Expansion

Nitrous oxide has greater diffusibility across tissues than nitrogen. Therefore N_2O would diffuse into any closed air-containing space, more specifically any nitrogen-containing space, more quickly than nitrogen diffuses out, resulting in gas volume expansion. One of the major concerns related to this gas expansion effect is bowel dilatation.[286] However, this observation is based on surgical procedures lasting 3 hours. The increase in pressure and volume in a closed space due to accumulation of N_2O is dependent of the duration of exposure and pressure

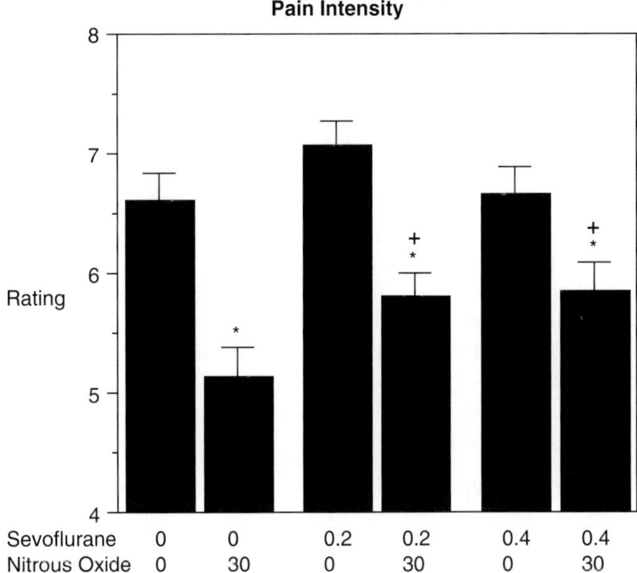

Fig. 21.22 Effects of sevoflurane and nitrous oxide on ratings of pain intensity to cold. Each bar is the mean across all subjects. *Brackets* represent SEM. *Significant decrease from placebo (0% sevoflurane/0% nitrous oxide) ratings. +Significant increase from the 0% sevoflurane/30% nitrous oxide ratings. (Redrawn from Janiszewski DJ, Galinkin JL, Klock PA, et al. The effects of subanesthetic concentrations of sevoflurane and nitrous oxide, alone and in combination, on analgesia, mood, and psychomotor performance in healthy volunteers. *Anesth Analg.* 1999;88(5):1149-1154. With permission.)

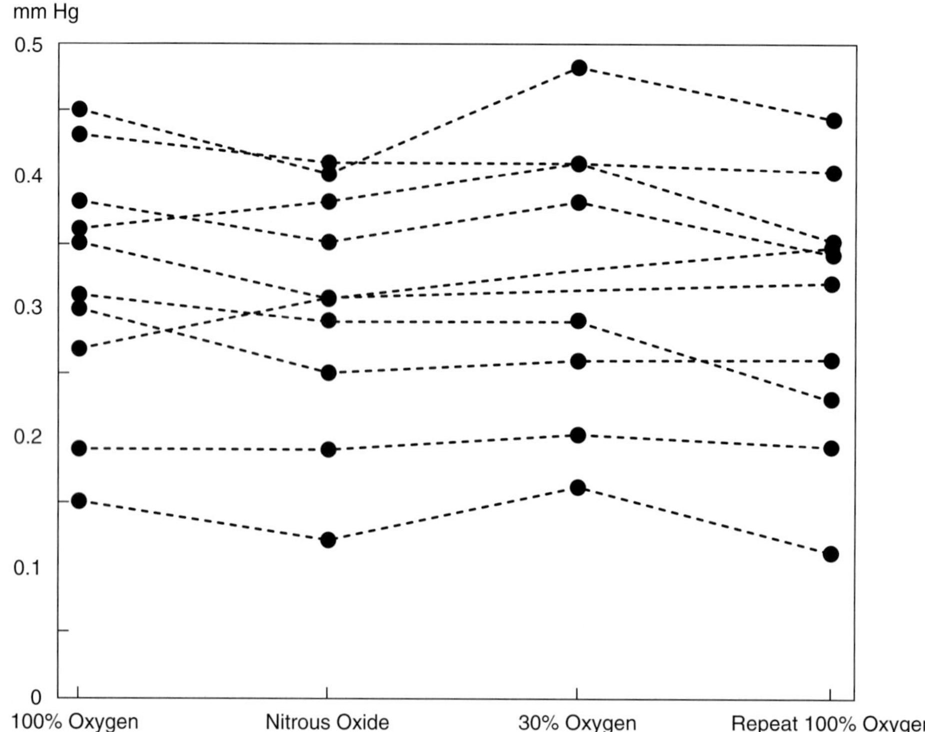

Fig. 21.23 **Individual patient responses in mean pulmonary arterial pressure (mm Hg) to nitrous oxide administration.** (Redrawn from Konstadt SN, Reich DL, Thys DM. Nitrous oxide does not exacerbate pulmonary hypertension or ventricular dysfunction in patients with mitral valvular disease. *Can J Anaesth.* 1990;37(6):613-617. With permission.)

gradient of N_2O. Briefly using N_2O for periods of 15 to 20 minutes during emergence enhances washout of volatile anesthetics and may not lead to clinically relevant bowel dilation.

Nausea And Vomiting

Postoperative nausea and vomiting (PONV) is a common complication of N_2O.[287] However, a recent meta-analysis demonstrated that N_2O–related PONV is clinically insignificant following a less than 1 hour exposure.[288] The authors suggested that a minor risk of PONV should not preclude N_2O use for a limited time period, such as for minor or ambulatory surgeries. Even though others questioned the methodology of the meta-analysis,[289,290] the trend consistently suggests that the incidence of PONV is associated primarily with the *duration* of N_2O exposure. Therefore clinicians can take advantage of the beneficial properties of N_2O, especially at the end of an anesthetic, to facilitate the washout of volatile agents and shorten the time of emergence.

Pulmonary Hypertension

Several studies were conducted to test whether N_2O worsens pulmonary hypertension with no consistent conclusions due to variation of the experimental protocols. In an earlier study, Konstadt and colleagues demonstrated no significant changes in PA pressure and cardiac output in patients with pulmonary hypertension when 70% N_2O versus 70% nitrogen was used (Fig. 21.23).[291] The authors concluded that N_2O does not have adverse effects on the pulmonary circulation or right ventricular function, and may be used with appropriate monitoring in patients with pulmonary hypertension. This conclusion should be interpreted with caution in patients with elevated PVR, particularly in the presence of right ventricular dysfunction and/or right coronary artery disease.[292] More recently, the ENIGMA II study, a large randomized clinical trial, demonstrated no difference in the risk of death or cardiovascular complications with N_2O.[293]

Potential Neurotoxicity of Nitrous Oxide

Prolonged use of N_2O can cause nitrous oxide–induced blockade of N-methyl-D-aspartate (NMDA) receptors and can manifest as swelling of neuronal organelles including mitochondria and endoplasmic reticulum,[294] presenting as neurotoxicity[295] with an acute neuropathy postoperatively.[296] Nitrous oxide also increases plasma homocysteine levels[297] caused by oxidation of methionine synthase.[298] As homocysteine can be easily measured in blood, it can be used as a biomarker of N_2O-induced modulation of methionine synthase activity. After an 8-hour exposure to N_2O, an eight-fold increase in blood homocysteine levels was detected.[299] Increased homocysteine may be prevented by continuous infusion of vitamin B_{12}, which is an enzyme cofactor of methionine synthase.[300]

XENON

Xenon has been suggested as an ideal inhalational anesthetic. It is stable, nonbiotransformable, nontoxic, nonflammable, nonirritant, and has a low blood–gas partition coefficient. Because of its specific molecular properties, xenon (Xe^{129}) can be hyperpolarized, with ventilation

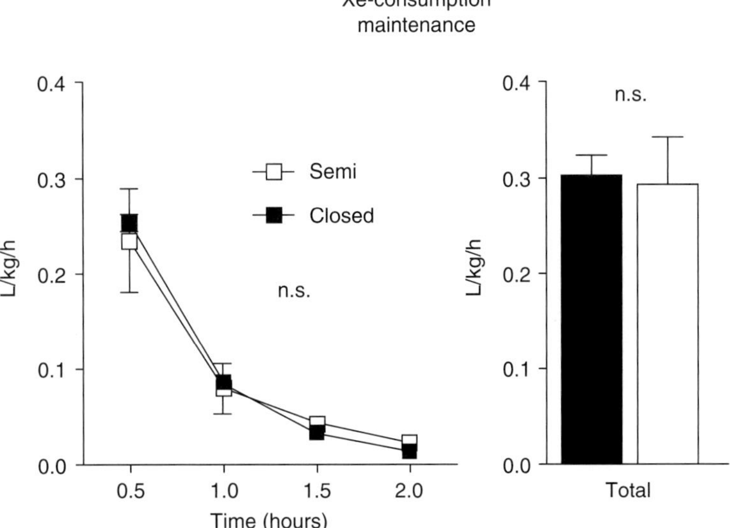

Fig. 21.24 **Xenon consumption during the maintenance phase in a semi-closed and closed circuit, shown for 30 minute intervals and in total for 2 hours. *n.s.*, not significant.** (Redrawn from Roehl AB, Goetzenich A, Rossaint R, et al. A practical rule for optimal flows for xenon anaesthesia in a semi-closed anaesthesia circuit. *Eur J Anaesthesiol.* 2010;27(7), 660–665. With permission.)

distribution and gas uptake yielding a highly selective tool for 3D MRI evaluation of lung disease.[301] Therefore xenon is used more frequently as an agent for imaging rather than as an inhalational anesthetic. However, its sedative effect is unique and mainly conferred by the inhibition of NMDA receptors in the central nervous system. In 1969, Cullen and colleagues determined the MAC of xenon to be 71% in O_2.[302] Using more modern measurements, Nakata and colleagues determined the MAC to be 63.1%.[303] A recent meta-analysis concluded that xenon anesthesia provides more stable intraoperative blood pressure, lower heart rate, and faster emergence from anesthesia than volatile agents and propofol, but xenon is associated with a higher risk of PONV (Fig. 21.24).[304]

Speed of Emergence and Postoperative Cognitive Dysfunction with Xenon

Compared with volatile anesthetics and propofol, anesthetic emergence is faster with xenon. It shortens time to extubation by approximately 4 minutes.[304] However, the shortening of emergence is not associated with the reduction in length of PACU or hospital stays. There is some evidence suggesting that, compared with other general anesthetic agents, xenon is associated with better neurological outcomes.[305] Therefore it might reduce the occurrence of postoperative cognitive dysfunction. A recent study did show that compared with sevoflurane, xenon was associated with faster emergence and with better early postoperative cognitive recovery.[306] However, such a benefit did not extend beyond 2 to 3 days post operation.[307] Xenon did not show benefits in postoperative cognitive dysfunction in elderly patients compared with desflurane[308] or propofol.[309] Therefore its neuro-protective potential remains debatable for patients undergoing general anesthesia.

Intraoperative Hemodynamics and Postoperative Outcome

Multiple studies have demonstrated that xenon produces a more stable intraoperative hemodynamic response. Xenon is a sympathetic stimulant and better maintains systolic, diastolic, and mean arterial blood pressures and reduces heart rate.[310] Such a favorable hemodynamic profile is very unique and beneficial in contrast to most volatile anesthetics that reduce systemic vascular resistance and perfusion pressure and increase heart rate. Hofland and colleagues recently demonstrated that compared with total intravenous anesthesia or anesthesia with sevoflurane, xenon reduces postoperative cardiac troponin I release and was noninferior to sevoflurane in low-risk, on-pump coronary artery bypass graft surgery patients.[311] However, the benefit of xenon as a cellular protectant observed in vitro[312] has not yet been demonstrated in human studies.

Use of Xenon in Critical Care

Sedation in the ICU usually lasts much longer than it does in anesthesia. Xenon could potentially be an ideal agent for sedation in the critical care setting, provided that its neuroprotective effect demonstrated in preclinical studies will be confirmed in humans.[313] However, there is currently a lack of clinical trials to determine the outcome of sedation with xenon compared to conventional sedation regimens in the ICU. A recent study by Bedi and colleagues[314] demonstrated the safety and feasibility of its use in critical care. Compared with a conventional propofol sedation regimen, similar sedation can be achieved at xenon concentrations of 28 ± 9.0% (range 9%-62%).[315]

Postoperative Nausea and Vomiting

Xenon is a potent antagonist at the 5-HT3 receptor,[316] and could theoretically exert intrinsic antiemetic properties. However, a previous study demonstrated that xenon causes an increase in risk of PONV by 72% (34.4% vs. 19.9%) when compared with volatile and propofol anesthesia.[304] In contrast, Schaefer and colleagues recently assessed the risk of nausea and vomiting among several anesthetic regimens and concluded that xenon causes nausea and vomiting no more frequently than other regimens.[317]

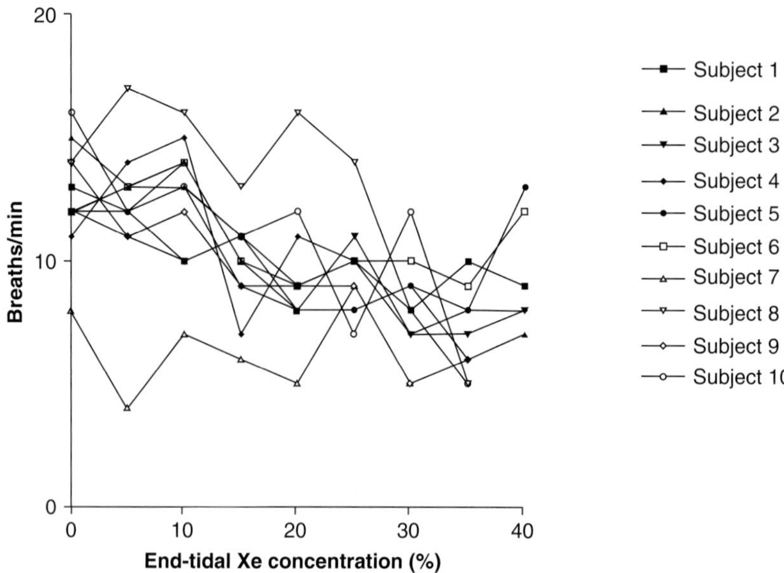

Fig. 21.25 The respiratory rate (breath/min) for individual subjects at increasing end-tidal concentration of xenon in oxygen. (Redrawn from Bedi A, McCarroll C, Murray JM, et al. The effects of subanaesthetic concentrations of xenon in volunteers. *Anaesthesia.* 2002;57(3):233–241. With permission.)

Airway Resistance

Xenon has a high density and viscosity. Therefore when using xenon, airway resistance is greater compared to other inhalational anesthetics at equivalent MAC values. The increase in airway resistance with 70% xenon mixed with 30% O_2 compared to 70% nitrogen mixed with 30% O_2 was minimal in healthy lungs in a pig model. However, the airway resistance was further increased in a bronchoconstriction model of asthma. Increased airway resistance is an intrinsic property of xenon and probably not a result of bronchoconstriction. The increase in airway resistance does not negatively affect oxygenation[318] and is not associated with decreased airway diameter.[319] Similar results were also reached in a dog model.[320] A human study with 33% xenon and 67% O_2 showed a significant increase in airway pressure but no alteration in oxygenation was reported.[321]

Apnea

Xenon is the only inhalational anesthetic that causes a decrease in respiratory rate(Fig. 21.25).[187] There are a few case reports describing prolonged apnea occurring in spontaneously breathing patients, even with subanesthetic concentrations of xenon.[188]

COMPARISON OF NITROUS OXIDE AND XENON

Both N_2O and xenon are nonvolatile inhaled anesthetics. Their pharmacodynamics are similar, although the solubility of N_2O is higher than that of xenon. The site of action of xenon[322,323] and N_2O[324,325] are believed to be the same: the NMDA receptor. However, imaging studies show that xenon and N_2O do not work on the same regions of the brain.[326,327] In addition, their sedative[328] and analgesic[329,330] properties, and their side effects[331,332] are not the same. Recently, concern has been raised for air pollution associated with the use of N_2O, and whether it should be routinely used in anesthesia. Since N_2O has not been shown to be associated with an increased rate of wound infections and its cost-effectiveness is favorable, there is no evidence to support abandoning N_2O for routine inhalational anesthetic use. On the other hand, since the superiority of xenon over the volatile anesthetics and N_2O remains to be determined and its cost is high, routine use of xenon as anesthetic is not recommended(Table 21.2).[333-335]

TABLE 21.2 Comparison of Xenon and Nitrous Oxide

	Nitrous oxide	Xenon
Pharmacodynamics	Comparable	Comparable
Sedation mechanism	NMDA	NMDA
Analgesic effect	Yes	Yes
Gas expansion	Yes	No
Nausea and vomiting	Yes	Yes
Increase in airway resistance	No	Yes
Increase in pulmonary vasculature resistance	Maybe	No
Diffusion hypoxia	Yes	No
MAC value	104%	63.1%-71%
MAC awake	63.3%	32.6%
Use as a sole anesthetic at ambient pressure at sea level	No	Yes
Respiratory rate	No effect	Decrease
Maintain hemodynamic stability	Yes	Yes
Acute tolerance	Yes	Unknown
Cost-efficiency	Favorable	Not favorable at present

MAC, Minimum alveolar concentration; *NMDA*, N-methyl-D-aspartate.

Summary

Even though the popularity of total intravenous anesthesia has been growing over the last two decades, inhalational anesthetics remain the most commonly used agents for general anesthesia. At least in part, this is due to our current thorough understanding of the pharmacology of these agents and their cost-efficiency. Measurement of the expiratory gas concentrations is readily available in any modern anesthesia machine and therefore the depth of sedation is much easier to determine and monitor, compared with intravenous anesthesia. Thus inhalational anesthesia will remain in the mainstream of anesthesia practice for the foreseeable future. Careful selection of a particular agent based on the mechanism of its action can improve quality of patient care. Such care will continue to be based on an individual's needs, with consideration of the pharmacokinetics and interactions of these agents with the respiratory system. Further research into the clinical utility of the inhalational agents is essential for advancing the goals of precision medicine in anesthesia.

Acknowledgment

This chapter is a consolidation of two chapters in the eighth edition, Chapter 27 Inhaled Anesthetics: Pulmonary Pharmacology and Chapter 28 Inhaled Anesthetics: Cardiovascular Pharmacology. The editors and publisher would like to thank the following authors: Neil E. Farber, Eckehard A.E. Stuth, Astrid G. Stucke, and Paul S. Pagel for their contributions to the prior edition of this work. It has served as the foundation for the current chapter.

Complete references available online at expertconsult.com.

References

1. Kumeta Y, et al. *Masui*. 1995;44:396.
2. Pizov R, et al. *Anesthesiology*. 1995;82:1111.
3. Forrest JB, et al. *Anesthesiology*. 1992;76:3.
4. Cheney FW, et al. *Anesthesiology*. 1991;75:932.
5. Auroy Y, et al. *Anaesthesia*. 2009;64:366.
6. Caulfield MP, Birdsall NJ. *Pharmacol Rev*. 1998;50(2):279.
7. Belmonte KE. *Proc Am Thorac Soc*. 2005;2(4):297. discussion 311.
8. Zhang WC, et al. *J Biol Chem*. 2010;285:5522.
9. Prakash YS, et al. *Am J Physiol Cell Physiol*. 1998;274:C1653.
10. Bogard AS, et al. *J Pharmacol Exp Ther*. 2011;337:209.
11. Ito S, et al. *Am J Resp Cell Mol Biol*. 2008;38:407.
12. Rho EH, et al. *J Appl Physiol*. 2002;92:257.
13. Panula P, et al. *Pharmacol Rev*. 2015;67(3):601.
14. Tamaoki J, et al. *Mediators Inflamm*. 1994;3:125.
15. Katoh T, Ikeda KCJA. *Can J Anaesth*. 1994;41:1214.
16. Yamakage M, et al. *Eur J Anaesthesiol*. 2008;25(1):67.
17. Emala CW, et al. *Chest*. 2002;121:722.
18. Park KW, et al. *Anesth Analg*. 2000;90:778.
19. Fehr JJ, et al. *Crit Care Med*. 2000;28:1884.
20. Brown RH, et al. *Anesthesiology*. 1993;78:1097.
21. D'Angelo E, et al. *Anesthesiology*. 2001;94:604.
22. Mazzeo AJ, et al. *Anesth Analg*. 1994;78:948.
23. Park KW, et al. *Anesthesiology*. 1997;86:1078.
24. Habre W, et al. *Anesthesiology*. 2001;94:348.
25. Yamakage M, et al. *Anesthesiology*. 2001;94:683.
26. Cheng EY, et al. *Anesth Analg*. 1996;83:162.
27. Dikmen Y, et al. *Anaesthesia*. 2003;58:745.
28. Nyktari VG, et al. *Anesthesiology*. 2006;104:1202.
29. Nyktari V, et al. *Br J Anaesth*. 2011;107(3):454.
30. Goff MJ, et al. *Anesthesiology*. 2000;93:404.
31. Hashimoto Y, et al. *J Cardiothorac Vasc Anesth*. 1996;10:213.
32. Myers CF, et al. *Can J Anaesth*. 2011;58:1007.
33. Lele E, et al. *Acta Anaesthesiol Scand*. 2006;50:1145.
34. Lele E, et al. *Anesth Analg*. 2013;116(6):1257.
35. Satoh J, Yamakage M. *J Anesth*. 2009;23:620.
36. Satoh JI, et al. *Br J Anaesth*. 2009;102:704.
37. Rooke GA, et al. *Anesthesiology*. 1997;86:1294.
38. Correa FCF, et al. *J Appl Physiol*. 2001;91:803.
39. Burburan SM, et al. *Anesth Analg*. 2007;104:631.
40. Ruiz P, Chartrand D. *Can J Anaesth*. 2003;50:67.
41. Arakawa H, et al. *J Asthma*. 2002;39:77.
42. Johnston RG, et al. *Chest*. 1990;97(3):698–701.
43. Koninckx M, et al. *Paediatr Respir Rev*. 2013;14(2):78.
44. Morimoto N, et al. *Anesth Analg*. 1994;78:328.
45. Tobias JD, Hirshman CA. *Anesthesiology*. 1990;72:105.
46. Wu RSC, et al. *Anesth Analg*. 1996;83:238.
47. Yamamoto K, et al. *Anesthesiology*. 1993;78:1102.
48. Yamakage M, et al. *Anesthesiology*. 2000;93:179.
49. Iwasaki S, et al. *Anesthesiology*. 2006;105:753.
50. Volta CA, et al. *Anesth Analg*. 2005;100:348.
51. Crawford MW, et al. *Anesthesiology*. 2006;105:1147.
52. von Ungern-Sternberg BS, et al. *Anesthesiology*. 2008;108:216.
53. Kai T, et al. *Anesthesiology*. 1998;89:1543.
54. Yu J, Ogawa K, et al. *Anesthesiology*. 2003;99:646.
55. Lynch C, et al. *Anesthesiology*. 2000;92(3):865.
56. Janssen LJ. *Am J Physiol Cell Physiol*. 1997;272:C1757.
57. Chen X, et al. *Anesthesiology*. 2002;96:458.
58. Yamakage M, et al. *Anesth Analg*. 2002;94:84.
59. Pabelick CM, et al. *Anesthesiology*. 2001;95:207.
60. Hanazaki M, et al. *Anesthesiology*. 2001;94:129.
61. Ay B, et al. *Am J Physiol Lung Cell Mol Physiol*. 2006;290(2):L278.
62. Jude JA, et al. *Proc Am Thorac Soc*. 2008;5(1):15.
63. Wettschureck N, Offermanns S, et al. *J Mol Med (Berl)*. 2002; 80(10):629.
64. Iizuka K, et al. *Eur J Pharmacol*. 2000;406(2):273.
65. Sakihara C, et al. *Anesthesiology*. 2004;101:120.
66. Nakayama T, et al. *Anesthesiology*. 2006;105:313.
67. Duracher C, et al. *Anesth Analg*. 2005;101:136.
68. Gallos G, et al. *Anesthesiology*. 2009;110:748.
69. Gallos G, et al. *Am J Physiol Lung Cell Moll Physiol*. 2011;302:L248.
70. Park KW, et al. *Anesth Analg*. 1998;86:646.
71. Mougdil GC. *Can J Anaesth*. 1997;44:R77.
72. Warner DO, et al. *Anesthesiology*. 1990;72:1057.
73. Wiklund CU, et al. *Br J Anaesth*. 1999;83:422.
74. Brown RH, et al. *Anesthesiology*. 1993;78:295.
75. Akhtar S, Brull SJ. *Pulm Pharmacol Ther*. 1998;11:227.
76. Berbari NF, et al. *Curr Biol*. 2009;19:R526.
77. Czarnecki PG, Shah JV. *Trends Cell Biol*. 2012;22:201.
78. Wu J, et al. *Chest*. 2009;136:561.
79. Ferkol TW, Leigh MW. *J Pediatr*. 2012;160:366.
80. Christopher AB, et al. *Front Pediatr*. 2014;2:111.
81. Lindberg S, et al. *Acta Otolaryngol*. 1997;117:728.
82. Lund VJ. *Allergy Asthma Proc*. 1996;17:179.
83. Keller C, Brimacombe J. *Anesth Analg*. 1998;86:1280.
84. Raphael JH, Butt MW. *Br J Anaesth*. 1997;79:473.
85. Iida H, et al. *Can J Anaesth*. 2006;53:242.
86. Raphael JH, et al. *Br J Anaesth*. 1996;76:116.
87. Matsuura S, et al. *Anesth Analg*. 2006;102:1703.
88. Gamsu G, et al. *Am Rev Respir Dis*. 1976;114:673.
89. Lichtiger M, et al. *Anesthesiology*. 1975;42:753.
90. Konrad F, et al. *Anaesthesist*. 1997;46:403.
91. Konrad F, et al. *Chest*. 1994;105:237.
92. Konrad FX, et al. *J Clin Anesth*. 1993;5:375.
93. Rivero DH, et al. *Chest*. 2001;119:1510.
94. Molliex S, et al. *Anesthesiology*. 1994;81:668.
95. Yang T, et al. *Drug Metabol Drug Interact*. 2001;18:243.
96. Patel AB, et al. *Anesth Analg*. 2002;94:943.
97. Li Y, et al. *Drug Metabol Drug Interact*. 2004;20:175.
98. Rezaiguai-Delclaux S, et al. *Anesthesiology*. 1998;88:751.
99. Paugam-Burtz C, et al. *Anesthesiology*. 2000;93:805.
100. Malacrida L, et al. *Pulm Pharmacol Ther*. 2014;28(2):122.
101. Bilgi M, et al. *Eur J Anaesthesiol*. 2011;28(4):279.
102. Sweeney M, et al. *J Appl Physiol*. 1998;85:2040.
103. Myers JL, et al. *Ann Thorac Surg*. 1996;62:1677.
104. Moncada S. *Pharmacol Rev*. 1991;43(2):109.
105. Bredt DS, et al. *Neuron*. 1991;7(4):615.
106. Lamas S, et al. *Proc Natl Acad Sci U S A*. 1992;89(14):6348.

107. Moncada S, Palmer RM. *Semin Perinatol.* 1991;15(1):16.
108. Ichinose F. *Circulation.* 2004;109(25):3106.
109. Lian TY. *Drug Des Devel Ther.* 2017;11:1195.
110. Galvin I, et al. *Br J Anaesth.* 2007;98:420.
111. Arai TJ, et al. *J Appl Physiol.* 2009;106:1057.
112. Adding LC, et al. *Acta Anaesthesiol Scand.* 1999;167:167.
113. Yamamoto Y, et al. *J Appl Physiol.* 2001;91:1121.
114. Robertson TP, et al. *Cardiovasc Res.* 2001;50:145.
115. Morio Y, McMurtry IF. *J Appl Physiol.* 2002;92:527.
116. Evans AM, et al. *Current Opinions Anesthesiology.* 2011;24:13.
117. Firth AL, et al. *Am J Physiol Lung Cell Mol Physiol.* 2008;295:L61.
118. Nagendran J, et al. *Current Opinions Anesthesiology.* 2006;19:34.
119. Wang L, et al. *J Clin Invest.* 2012;122(11):4218.
120. Goldenberg NM. *Anesthesiology.* 2015;122(6):1338–1348.
121. Lumb AB, Slinger P. *Anesthesiology.* 2015;122(4):932.
122. Akata T. *Anesthesiology.* 2007;106:365.
123. Gambone LM, et al. *Am J Physiol Heart Circ Physiol.* 1997;272:H290.
124. Seki S, et al. *Anesthesiology.* 1997;86:923.
125. Nakayama M, et al. *Anesthesiology.* 1998;88:1023.
126. Lennon PF, Murray PA. *Anesthesiology.* 1995;82:723.
127. Sato K, et al. *Anesthesiology.* 2002;97:478.
128. Liu R, et al. *Can J Anaesth.* 2003;50:301.
129. Olschewski A. *Adv Exp Med Biol.* 2010;661:459.
130. Su JY, Vo AC. *Anesthesiology.* 2002;97:207.
131. Zhong L, Su JY. *Anesthesiology.* 2002;96:148.
132. Loer SA, et al. *Anesthesiology.* 1995;83(3):552.
133. Lennon PF, Murray PA. *Anesthesiology.* 1996;84:404.
134. Johns RA. *Anesthesiology.* 1993;79:1381.
135. Marshall C, Marshall BE. *Anesthesiology.* 1993;79:A1238.
136. Marshall C, Marshall BE. *Anesthesiology.* 1990;73:441.
137. Jing M, et al. *Life Sci.* 1995;56(1):19.
138. Gambone LM, et al. *Anesthesiology.* 1997;86:936.
139. Liu R, et al. *Anesthesiology.* 2001;95:939.
140. Eisenkraft JB. *Br J Anaesth.* 1990;65:63.
141. Lesitsky MA, et al. *Anesthesiology.* 1998;89:1501.
142. Schwarzkopf K, et al. *Anesth Analg.* 2005;100:335.
143. Schwarzkopf K, et al. *J Cardiothorac Vasc Anesth.* 2003;17:73.
144. Karzai W, et al. *Anesth Analg.* 1999;89:215.
145. Schwarzkopf K, et al. *Anesth Analg.* 2001;93:1434.
146. Kleinsasser A, et al. *Anesthesiology.* 2001;95:1422.
147. Nyren S, et al. *Anesthesiology.* 2010;113:1370.
148. Radke OC, et al. *Anesthesiology.* 2012;116:1186.
149. Bindlsev L, et al. *Acta Anaesthesiol Scand.* 1981;25:360.
150. Nishiwaki K, et al. *Am J Physiol Heart Circ Physiol.* 1992;262:H1331.
151. Abe K, et al. *Anesth Analg.* 1998;86:266.
152. Reid CW, et al. *J Cardiothorac Vasc Anesth.* 1996;10:860.
153. Beck DH, et al. *Br J Anaesth.* 2001;86:38.
154. Pruszkowski O, et al. *Br J Anaesth.* 2007;98:539.
155. Kellow NH, et al. *Br J Anaesth.* 1995;75:578.
156. Abe K, et al. *Anesth Analg.* 1998;87:1164.
157. Benumof JL, et al. *Anesthesiology.* 1987;67:910.
158. Pagel P, et al. *Anesth Analg.* 1998;87:800.
159. Carlsson AJ, et al. *Anesthesiology.* 1987;66:312.
160. Ng A, Swanevelder J. *Br J Anaesth.* 2011;106:761.
161. Karzai W, Schwarzkopf K. *Anesthesiology.* 2009;110:1402.
162. Dalibon N, et al. *Anesth Analg.* 2004;98:590.
163. Teppema LJ, Baby S. *Respir Physiol Neurobiol.* 2011;177:80.
164. Stuth EAE, et al. Central Effects of General Anesthesia. In: Denham S, Ward ADLJT, eds. *Pharmacology and Pathophysiology of the Control of Breathing.* Boca Raton, FL: Tayor and Francis Group; 2005:571.
165. Stuth EA, et al. *Respir Physiol Neurobiol.* 2008;164:151.
166. Sirois JE, et al. *J Neurosci.* 2000;201:6347.
167. Sirois JE, et al. *J Physiol.* 2002;541:717.
168. Trochet D, et al. *Am J Respir Crit Care Med.* 2008;177:906–911.
169. Coghlan M, Richards E. *ER Trafficking.* 2018;8(1):5275.
170. Forster HV, Smith CA. *J Appl Physiol.* 2010;108:989.
171. Nattie E, et al. *J Appl Physiol.* 2011;110:1.
172. Erlichman JS, et al. *Respir Physiol Neurobiol.* 2010;173:305.
173. Pandit JJ. *Anaesthesia.* 2002;57:632.
174. Pandit JJ. *Anaesthesia.* 2005;60:461.
175. Baugh R, et al. *Otolaryngol Head Neck Surg.* 2013;148(5):867.
176. Abdala AP, et al. *J. Physiol.* 2015;593(14):3033.
177. Rybak IA, et al. *J Neurophysiol.* 2008;100:1770.
178. Smith CA, et al. *Respir Physiol Neurobiol.* 2010;173:288.
179. von Euler US LG, Zotterman Y. *Scand Arch Physiol.* 1939;83:132.
180. BuSha BF, et al. *J Appl Physiol.* 2002;93:903.
181. Lazarenko RM, et al. *J Neurosci.* 2010;30:7691.
182. Haxhiu MA, et al. *Respir Physiol.* 1987;70(2):183–193.
183. Horner RL. *Respir Physiol Neurobiol.* 2008;164:179.
184. Begle RL, et al. *Am Rev Respir Dis.* 1990;141(4 Pt 1):854.
185. Tagaito Y, et al. *J Appl Physiol (1985).* 2007;103(4):1379.
186. Hornbein TF, et al. *Anesth Analg.* 1982;61(7):553.
187. Bedi A, et al. *Anaesthesia.* 2002;57(3):233.
188. Cormack JR, Gott J, Kondogiannis S, et al. *A A Case Rep.* 2017;8(4):90.
189. Fourcade HE, et al. *Anesthesiology.* 1971;35(1):26.
190. Calverley RK, et al. *Anesth Analg.* 1978;57(6):610.
191. Lockhart SH, et al. *Anesthesiology.* 1991;74(3):484.
192. Doi M, Ikeda K, et al. *J Anesth.* 1987;1(2):137.
193. Hickey RF, Severinghaus JW. Regulation of breathing: drug effects. In: Hornbein TF, ed. *Regulation of Breathing - Pt. 2.* New York, NY: Marcel Dekker; 1981:1251–1312.
194. Eger EI. *Anesthesiology.* 1981;55(5):559.
195. Fujii Y, et al. *Int Anesthesiol Clin.* 2001;39(2):95.
196. Winkler SS, et al. *J Comput Assist Tomogr.* 1987;11(3):496.
197. Winkler STP, et al. Xenon effects on CNS control of respiratory rate and tidal volume-the danger of apnea. In: Hartmann AHS, ed. *Cerebral Blood Flow and Metabolism Measurement.* Berlin: Springer-Verlag; 1985:356–360.
198. Holl K, et al. *Acta Neurochir (Wien).* 1987;87(3-4):129.
199. Ballantyne D, Scheid P. *Adv Exp Med Biol.* 2001;499:17.
200. Ballantyne D, Scheid P. *Respir Physiol.* 2001;129:5.
201. Branco LG, et al. *J Appl Physiol.* 2009;106:1467.
202. Heeringa J, et al. *Respir Physiol.* 1979;37:365.
203. Knill RL, Gelb AW. *Anesthesiology.* 1978;49:244.
204. van den Elsen M. *Br J Anaesth.* 1998;80(2):174.
205. Kammer T, et al. *Anesthesiology.* 2002;97:1416.
206. Barnard P, et al. *J Appl Physiol.* 1987;63:685.
207. Dahan A, Teppema L. *Br J Anaesth.* 1999;83:199.
208. Sarton E, et al. *Anesthesiology.* 1999;90:1288.
209. van den Elsen MJLJ, et al. *Anesthesiology.* 1994;81:860.
210. Hickey RF, et al. *Anesthesiology.* 1971;35:32.
211. Nakayama H, et al. *Am J Respir Crit Care Med.* 2002;165:1251.
212. West JB. *Respiration physiology.* 1983;52(3):265.
213. Dahan A, et al. *Anesthesiology.* 1994;80:727.
214. Chung F, Liao P. *Anesthesiology.* 2014;120(2):287.
215. Chung F, et al. *Anesthesiology.* 2014;120(2):299–311.
216. Sarton E, et al. *Anesthesiology.* 1996;85:295.
217. Pandit JJ, et al. *Anesthesiology.* 2004;101(6):1409.
218. Warner DO. *Anesthesiology.* 1996;84(2):309.
219. Warner DO, et al. *Anesthesiology.* 1995;82:6.
220. Warner DO, Warner MA. *Anesthesiology.* 1995;82:20.
221. Gauda EB, et al. *J Appl Physiol.* 1994;76:2656.
222. Wheatley JR, et al. *J Appl Physiol.* 1991;70:2242.
223. Schwartz AR, et al. *Am J Respir Crit Care Med.* 1998;157(4 Pt 1):1051.
224. Kuna ST, et al. *Med Clin North Am.* 1985;69(6):1221.
225. Erb TO, et al. *Paediatric Anaesthesia.* 2017;27(3):282.
226. Lerman J, et al. *Paediatric Anaesth.* 2010;20:495.
227. Ulevitch RJ. *Adv Immunol.* 1993;53:267.
228. Chow JC, et al. *J Biol Chem.* 1999;274(16):10689.
229. Marini JJ, Evans TW. *Intensive Care Med.* 1998;24(8):878.
230. Meyrick B, et al. *Prog Clin Biol Res.* 1989;308:91.
231. Brigham KL. *Am Rev Respir Dis.* 1987;136(3):785.
232. Bulger EM, Maier RV. *Crit Care Med.* 2000;28(suppl 4):N27.
233. Ermert L, et al. *Am J Physiol Lung Cell Mol Physiol.* 2000;278(4):L744.
234. Quinn JV, Slotman GJ. *Crit Care Med.* 1999;27(11):2485.
235. Langleben D, et al. *Am Rev Respir Dis.* 1993;148(6 Pt 1):1646.
236. Suffredini AF, et al. *Am Rev Respir Dis.* 1992;145(6):1398.
237. O'Grady NP, et al. *Am J Respir Crit Care Med.* 2001;163(7):1591.
238. Bachofen M, Weibel ER. *Clin Chest Med.* 1982;3(1):35.
239. Kumar A, et al. *Am J Physiol.* 1999;276(1 Pt 2):R265.
240. McQuaid KE, Keenan AK. *Exp Physiol.* 1997;82(2):369.
241. Salvemini D. *Cell Mol Life Sci.* 1997;53(7):576.
242. Ignarro LJ, et al. *Proc Natl Acad Sci U S A.* 1993;90(17):8103.
243. Weissmann N, et al. *Am J Physiol Lung Cell Mol Physiol.* 2000;279(4):L683.
244. Singh S, Evans TW. *Eur Respir J.* 1997;10(3):699.
245. Westendorp RG, et al. *J Vasc Res.* 1994;31(1):42.
246. Suter D, et al. *Anesth Analg.* 2007;104(3):638.
247. Takala RS, et al. *Acta Anaesthesiol Scand.* 2006;50(2):163.

248. Giraud O, et al. *Anesthesiology*. 2003;98(1):74.
249. Voigtsberger S, et al. *Anesthesiology*. 2009;111(6):1238.
250. Schlapfer M, et al. *Clin Exp Immunol*. 2012;168(1):125.
251. Du G, et al. *Anesth Analg*. 2017;124(5):1555.
252. Bedirli N, et al. *J Surg Res*. 2012;178(1):e17.
253. Dong X, et al. *Exp Lung Res*. 2013;39(7):295.
254. Beitler JR, et al. *Clin Chest Med*. 2016;37(4):633.
255. Wagner J, et al. *PLoS One*. 2018;13(2):e0192896.
256. Faller S, et al. *Anesth Analg*. 2012;114(4):747.
257. Englert JA, et al. *Anesthesiology*. 2015;123(2):377.
258. Strosing KM, et al. *Anesth Analg*. 2016;123(1):143.
259. Pak O, et al. *Adv Exp Med Biol*. 2017;967:195.
260. Liu R, et al. *Anesth Analg*. 1999;89(3):561.
261. Fujinaga T, et al. *Transplantation*. 2006;82:1168.
262. Casanova J, et al. *Anesth Analg*. 2011;113:742.
263. Ohsumi A, et al. *Ann Thorac Surg*. 2017;103(5):1578.
264. Oshima Y, et al. *Springerplus*. 2016;5(1):2031.
265. Martens A, et al. *J Surg Res*. 2016;201(1):44.
266. Wrigge H, et al. *Anesthesiology*. 2000;93:1413.
267. De Conno E, et al. *Anesthesiology*. 2009;110:1316.
268. Schilling T, et al. *Anesthesiology*. 2011;115:65.
269. Sugasawa Y, et al. *J Anesth*. 2012;26:62.
270. Uhlig C, et al. *Anesthesiology*. 2016;124(6):1230.
271. Beck-Schimmer B, et al. *Anesthesiology*. 2016;125(2):313.
272. Koksal GM, et al. *Eur J Anaesthesiol*. 2004;21(3):217.
273. Koksal GM, et al. *Acta Anaesthesiol Scand*. 2005;49(6):835.
274. Jabaudon M, et al. *Am J Respir Crit Care Med*. 2017;195(6):792.
275. Bellgardt M, et al. *Eur J Anaesthesiol*. 2016;33(1):6.
276. Wilson KE. *Dent Update*. 2013;40(10):822, 826.
277. Likis FE, et al. *Anesth Analg*. 2014;118(1):153.
278. Goto T. *Anesthesiology*. 2000;93(5):1188.
279. Mashour GA, Avidan MS. *Br J Anaesth*. 2015;115(suppl 1):i20.
280. Mathews DM, et al. *Anesth Analg*. 2008;106(1).
281. Lee LH, et al. *Anesthesiology*. 2005;102(2):398.
282. Janiszewski DJ, et al. *Anesth Analg*. 1999;88(5):1149.
283. Berkowitz BA, et al. *Anesthesiology*. 1979;51(4):309.
284. Berkowitz BA, et al. *J Pharmacol Exp Ther*. 1977;203(3):539.
285. Ramsay DS, et al. *Pain*. 2005;114(1-2):19.
286. Akca O, et al. *Acta Anaesthesiol Scand*. 2004;48(7):894.
287. Fernandez-Guisasola J, et al. *Anaesthesia*. 2010;65(4):379–387.
288. Peyton PJ, Peyton PJ. *Anesthesiology*. 2014;120(5):1137.
289. Pace NL. *Anesthesiology*. 2014;121(6):1356.
290. Zhou L, Chen C, Yu H. *Anesthesiology*. 2014;121(6):1356.
291. Konstadt SN, et al. *Can J Anaesth*. 1990;37(6):613.
292. Schulte-Sasse U, et al. *Anesthesiology*. 1982;57(1):9.
293. Beattie WS, et al. *Anesth Analg*. 2018.
294. Jevtovic-Todorovic V, et al. *Br J Anaesth*. 2013;111(2):143.
295. Savage S, Ma D. *Brain Sci*. 2014;4(1):73.
296. Morris N, et al. *Muscle Nerve*. 2015;51(4):614.
297. Myles PS, et al. *Anesthesiology*. 2008;109(4):657.
298. Drummond JT, Matthews RG. *Biochemistry*. 1994;33(12):3742.
299. Nagele P, et al. *Anesth Analg*. 2011;113(4):843.
300. Kiasari AZ, et al. *Oman Med J*. 2014;29(3):194.
301. Mugler JP, et al. *Proc Natl Acad Sci U S A*. 2010;107(50):21707.
302. Cullen SC. *Anesthesiology*. 1969;31(4):305.
303. Nakata Y, et al. *Anesthesiology*. 2001;94(4):611.
304. Law LS. *Anesth Analg*. 2016;122(3):678.
305. Law LS, et al. *Can J Anaesth*. 2018;65(9):1041.
306. Bronco A, et al. *Eur J Anaesthesiol*. 2010;27(10):912.
307. Cremer J, et al. *Med Gas Res*. 2011;1(1):9.
308. Coburn M, et al. *Br J Anaesth*. 2007;98(6):756.
309. Hocker J, et al. *Anesthesiology*. 2009;110(5):1068.
310. Neukirchen M, et al. *Br J Anaesth*. 2012;109(6):887.
311. Hofland J, et al. *Anesthesiology*. 2017;127(6):918.
312. Petzelt C, et al. *BMC Neurosci*. 2004;5:55.
313. Sacchetti ML. *Stroke*. 2008;39(6):1659.
314. Bedi A, et al. *Crit Care Med*. 2003;31(10):2470.
315. Roehl AB, et al. *Eur J Anaesthesiol*. 2010;27(7):660.
316. Suzuki T, et al. *Anesthesiology*. 2002;96(3):699.
317. Schaefer MS, et al. *Br J Anaesth*. 2015;115(1):61.
318. Calzia E, et al. *Anesthesiology*. 1999;90(3):829.
319. Baumert JH, et al. *Br J Anaesth*. 2002;88(4):540.
320. Zhang P. *Can J Anaesth*. 1995;42(6):547.
321. Rueckoldt H, et al. *Acta Anaesthesiol Scand*. 1999;43(10):1060.
322. Dickinson R, et al. *Anesthesiology*. 2007;107(5):756.
323. Kratzer S, et al. *Anesthesiology*. 2012;116(3):673.
324. Nagele P, et al. *Proc Natl Acad Sci U S A*. 2004;101(23):8791.
325. Richardson KJ, et al. *J Pharmacol Exp Ther*. 2015;352(1):156.
326. Hagen T, et al. *J Comput Assist Tomogr*. 1999;23(2):257.
327. Reinstrup P, et al. *Anesthesiology*. 1994;81(2):396.
328. Yagi M, et al. *Br J Anaesth*. 1995;74(6):670.
329. Petersen-Felix S, et al. *Br J Anaesth*. 1998;81(5):742.
330. Utsumi J, et al. *Anesth Analg*. 1997;84(6):1372.
331. Yonas H. *J Comput Assist Tomogr*. 1981;5(4):591.
332. Kamp HD. *Klin Anasthesiol Intensivther*. 1993;42:17.
333. de Vasconcellos K, Sneyd JR. *Br J Anaesth*. 2013;111(6):877.
334. Imberger G, et al. *Br J Anaesth*. 2014;112(3):410.
335. Myles PS, et al. *Lancet*. 2014;384(9952):1446.

22 Inhaled Anesthetics: Delivery Systems

MICHAEL P. BOKOCH and STEPHEN D. WESTON

KEY POINTS

- The modern anesthesia workstation has evolved into a complex device with a number of safety features. However, if there is any possibility that the workstation or the breathing circuit is a potential cause of difficulty with ventilation or oxygenation, ventilating the patient using an oxygen cylinder and a manual ventilation bag is an appropriate decision. *When in doubt, ventilate and oxygenate the patient first via another method—troubleshoot later.*
- The most important part of the preanesthesia workstation checkout procedure is to verify the presence of a self-inflating resuscitation bag and that an alternative oxygen source (E-cylinder) is available.
- The Diameter Index Safety System (DISS) is designed to prevent the misconnection of hospital gas supply lines to the anesthesia workstation. The Pin Index Safety System (PISS) is designed to prevent incorrect gas cylinder connections in the anesthesia workstation. Quick coupling systems may be utilized to connect to the central gas supply. No system is immune to misconnection.
- In the event of hospital pipeline crossover or contamination, two actions must be taken: the backup oxygen cylinder valve must be opened, and the wall supply sources must be disconnected. Otherwise, the suspect hospital pipeline gas will continue to flow to the patient.
- The oxygen flush valve provides a high flow of 100% oxygen directly to the patient's breathing circuit, allowing the anesthesia provider to overcome circuit leaks or to rapidly increase inspired oxygen concentration. Improper use can be associated with barotrauma or patient awareness.
- When using nitrous oxide, there is a risk of delivering a hypoxic mixture to the patient. "Fail-safe" valves and nitrous oxide/oxygen proportioning systems help minimize this risk, but they are not truly fail-safe. Delivery of a hypoxic mixture to the fresh gas outlet can result from (1) the wrong supply gas, (2) a defective or broken safety device, (3) leaks downstream from these safety devices, (4) administration of a fourth inert gas (e.g., helium), and (5) dilution of the inspired oxygen concentration by high concentrations of inhaled anesthetic agents (e.g., desflurane).
- The low-pressure section (LPS) of the gas supply system includes the flow control valves, flowmeters or flow sensors, and the anesthetic vaporizers. This section of the anesthesia workstation is most vulnerable to leaks, which can cause delivery of a hypoxic gas mixture or an inadequate concentration of anesthetic agent to the patient. The workstation must be checked for leaks before delivery of an anesthetic.
- The oxygen analyzer is the only protection against a hypoxic mixture within the low-pressure section of the pneumatic system.
- Anesthesia workstations with a one-way check valve in the LPS require a manual negative-pressure leak test. On machines without a check valve in this location, manual positive-pressure testing or automated testing is used to test the LPS for leaks.
- On machines with manually controlled anesthetic vaporizers, internal vaporizer leaks can be detected only when the vaporizer is turned on. This is true even during automated machine self-tests. Machines with electronically controlled vaporizers (e.g., the GE/Datex-Ohmeda Aladin cassette vaporizer, Maquet FLOW-i anesthesia workstation vaporizer) can check the installed vaporizer during self-test.
- Variable bypass vaporizers route a portion of the fresh gas flow into a vaporizing chamber to create the desired anesthetic concentration. Injection-type vaporizers utilize microprocessor control to inject small amounts of anesthetic liquid into an evaporating chamber.
- Desflurane's low boiling point and high vapor pressure make it unsuitable for a variable bypass vaporizer. Misfilling a variable bypass vaporizer with desflurane could theoretically cause delivery of a hypoxic mixture and a massive overdose of inhaled desflurane.
- The major advantage of the *circle breathing system* is the capability to rebreathe exhaled gas, including volatile anesthetic. The major disadvantage is its complex design with multiple connections.
- Before an anesthetic agent is administered, the circle system must be checked both to rule out *leaks* and to verify *flow.* To test for leaks, a static test is performed: the circle system is pressurized and the airway pressure gauge is observed not to fall. An automated test may perform this

function on many modern machines. To rule out obstruction or faulty valves, a dynamic test is performed, ventilating a test lung (usually a breathing bag) using the anesthesia workstation's ventilator, and observing for appropriate "lung" motion.

- Increasing the fresh gas flow rate into the circle breathing system causes less rebreathing of volatile anesthetic gas and more waste gas. To avoid rebreathing of carbon dioxide, a carbon dioxide absorbent is essential to the circle system's function.
- Inhaled anesthetic agents can interact with carbon dioxide absorbents and produce potentially harmful degradation products. Sevoflurane can form compound A, especially at low fresh gas flows. Several volatile anesthetics, though especially desflurane, can lead to release of carbon monoxide when exposed to desiccated absorbents. Carbon dioxide absorbents without strong bases such as potassium hydroxide or sodium hydroxide decrease this risk.
- The Mapleson breathing circuits are simple, lightweight breathing systems that support both spontaneous and manual ventilation. The particular circuit design has implications on the required fresh gas flow to avoid rebreathing of exhaled gases. None are economical for volatile anesthetic use, as they do not support carbon dioxide absorbent use.
- Anesthesia ventilators differ from intensive care unit ventilators in that they must support the rebreathing of exhaled gases. Types of anesthesia ventilators include bellows, piston, volume reflector, and turbine. Each design has its own benefits and limitations. Contemporary anesthesia ventilators support a wide variety of ventilation modes similar to intensive care unit ventilators.
- For bellows-type anesthesia ventilators, ascending bellows (bellows that ascend during the expiratory phase) are safer than descending bellows (bellows that descend during the expiratory phase) because disconnections are readily manifested by failure of ascending bellows to refill.
- Piston ventilators can potentially draw room air into the breathing circuit if a leak is present. The Maquet FLOW-i volume reflector compensates for leaks with 100% oxygen. Both are susceptible to lower than expected levels of inhaled anesthetic.
- On older anesthesia machines, the portion of fresh gas flow that occurs during inspiration is added to the tidal volume. Therefore increased fresh gas flow leads to increased tidal volume and increased airway pressure during positive-pressure ventilation. Newer-generation anesthesia workstations either *decouple* the fresh gas flow from the inspired tidal volume, or *compensate* for the fresh gas flow in calculating the amount of gas to deliver as tidal volume. Anesthesia providers should know whether their machines compensate for changes in fresh gas flow.
- The anesthesia gas scavenging system protects the operating room from waste anesthesia gases. Active systems, which apply vacuum suction to the scavenge system, are most common in contemporary operating rooms. Obstruction of, or inadequate vacuum to, the scavenging system transfer tubing can result in increased breathing circuit pressure or discharge of waste anesthesia gases to the operating room, depending on design.
- The American Society of Anesthesiologists *Recommendations for Pre-Anesthesia Checkout Procedures (2008)* serves as an excellent template for the creation of machine-specific checkout procedures. However, it is not a one-size-fits-all checklist.

Although the modern anesthesia workstation bears little resemblance to the ether-soaked rags of the mid-1800s, it is at its heart a device for delivering inhaled anesthesia. Early inhaled anesthetics provided no certainty regarding the delivered concentration of anesthetic, relied on spontaneous breathing of room air, possessed little more than the vigilance of the anesthesia provider for safety systems, and exposed the operating room to the anesthetic vapor. The evolution of the anesthesia workstation has provided increasingly sophisticated solutions to each of these problems. Today, anesthesia workstations are designed to do all of the following:

- Deliver volatile anesthetic gas at precise concentrations.
- Individually meter oxygen and two or more other breathing gases, and continuously enrich the inhaled gas with anesthetic vapor.
- Allow the patient to be ventilated manually ("bag" ventilation) with adjustable breathing circuit pressure.
- Ventilate the patient mechanically, with sophisticated ventilator modes comparable to the intensive care unit (ICU).
- Allow rebreathing of the exhaled anesthetic gases after removing carbon dioxide.
- Eliminate ("scavenge") excess gas from the patient's breathing circuit and remove this gas from the room.
- Continuously measure and display the inspired oxygen concentration, as well as ventilatory parameters such as respiratory rate and tidal volume.
- Prevent hypoxic gas mixtures caused by operator error or gas supply failure.
- Provide a breathing circuit manual oxygen flush feature.
- Possess a backup supply of oxygen.
- Display gas pipeline and backup tank supply pressures.
- Provide an integrated platform for displaying anesthetic, hemodynamic, and respiratory parameters, and for collecting this data into an electronic medical record.

The sheer number of tasks and solutions for which the anesthesia workstation is designed explains its complexity. Newcomers to the specialty often find the anesthesia machine to be both mysterious and intimidating, even though they sometimes have had experience with other ventilation equipment, such as ICU ventilators. Understanding the anesthetic workstation is important because the workstation is one of the most essential pieces of equipment used by anesthesia care providers. Nevertheless, it is worth emphasizing that if there is any doubt about the correct functioning of an anesthesia workstation, and there is difficulty with ventilation or oxygenation, then ventilating the patient with an alternative source of oxygen such as an E-cylinder is of top priority. Troubleshooting the anesthesia machine can commence once the patient is safe.

While some of the design and engineering innovations in anesthesia workstations make the anesthesia provider's job easier or more efficient, many of the innovations aim to enhance patients' safety. Closed claims analysis of adverse anesthetic outcomes related to anesthetic gas delivery equipment shows that such claims now account for only approximately 1% of the claims in the American Society of Anesthesiologists (ASA) closed claims database.[1] Further, the severity of the events leading to the claims has tended to decrease compared with closed claims analysis of earlier decades, with more reports of awareness under anesthesia, and fewer reports of death or permanent brain injury.[1,2]

To prevent mishaps, anesthesia providers must be aware of the operational characteristics and functional anatomy of their anesthesia workstations. Many workstations and their components share very similar characteristics, but the variation among them is growing. Similarly, the operational and pre-use checkout procedures are becoming more divergent, thus mandating device-specific familiarity. Unfortunately, a lack of knowledge pertaining to the anesthesia workstation and a lack of understanding and application of a proper pre-use check are common.[3-7] Contemporary machines have automated pre-use checkout procedures, but performance adherence is uneven.[6] More importantly, machines can pass automated checkouts despite the presence of unsafe conditions.[8,9] Safe use requires a solid generic understanding of any anesthesia workstation, as well as machine-specific knowledge of features and checkout procedures.

Providing a detailed description of each gas system, subsystem component, and patient breathing circuit is not practical within the scope of a single chapter. However, because anesthesia workstations must adhere to basic standards, a generic approach to all machines will be presented. Although several subsystems are described in detail in this chapter, anesthesia providers must acquire a functional understanding of their own workstations and ensure that their local pre-use checkout procedures are suitable for their machines. This chapter will review guidelines for anesthesia workstations; functional anatomy including gas supply, vaporizers, breathing circuits, ventilators, and scavenging; and the anesthesia machine pre-use checkout.

Standards and Guidelines for Anesthesia Workstations

Standards for medical devices and anesthesia workstations provide guidelines for manufacturers regarding device minimum performance, design characteristics, and safety requirements. For the anesthesia workstation, many of these requirements are outlined in the standards of the International Organization for Standardization (ISO). The ISO is a developer of international voluntary consensus standards based on global expert opinion, including industry and academia, as well as governments, consumer organizations, and other nongovernmental organizations.[10] The current standards are defined within the *Particular Requirements for Basic Safety and Essential Performance of an Anesthetic Workstation*, ISO 80601-2-13, of 2011.[11] The ISO standards also reference a large number of other components such as: electrical standards, device construction and performance, and even software standards. The relevant standards promulgated by the ASTM International (formerly known as the American Society for Testing and Materials), were withdrawn in 2014 because they had not been updated. Additional key standards for machine subsystems arise from the Compressed Gas Association and the Institute of Electrical and Electronics Engineers.

The ISO standards for the anesthetic workstation—or "anesthesia workstation," or "anesthesia machine," all used interchangeably in this chapter—include standards for numerous aspects of the design and construction of the workstation, including the anesthetic gas delivery system and anesthetic breathing system, as well as for monitoring equipment, alarm systems, and protection devices. The focus of this chapter is on design and functional aspects of the anesthesia workstation relevant to the delivery of inhaled anesthesia.

The ASA publishes several guidelines pertaining to the anesthesia workstation.[11a] The *Recommendations for Pre-Anesthesia Checkout*, which was updated last in 2008, serves as a general guideline for individual departments and practitioners to design checkout procedures specific to their anesthetic delivery systems.[11b] The ASA *Guidelines for Determining Anesthesia Machine Obsolescence* helps assist anesthesia providers and other healthcare personnel, administrators, and regulatory bodies to determine when an anesthesia machine is obsolete by applying both absolute and relative criteria.[11c] Finally, the ASA publishes *Standards for Basic Anesthetic Monitoring*, which outlines minimal monitoring standards pertaining to oxygenation, ventilation, circulation, body temperature, and the requirements for the presence of anesthesia personnel.[11d] Standards and recommendations pertaining to the anesthesia workstation are published by several other international anesthesiology societies.[11e,11f]

Functional Anatomy of the Anesthesia Workstation

GAS SUPPLY SYSTEM

Modern anesthesia machines are often largely electronically controlled, such that the clinician's relationship with

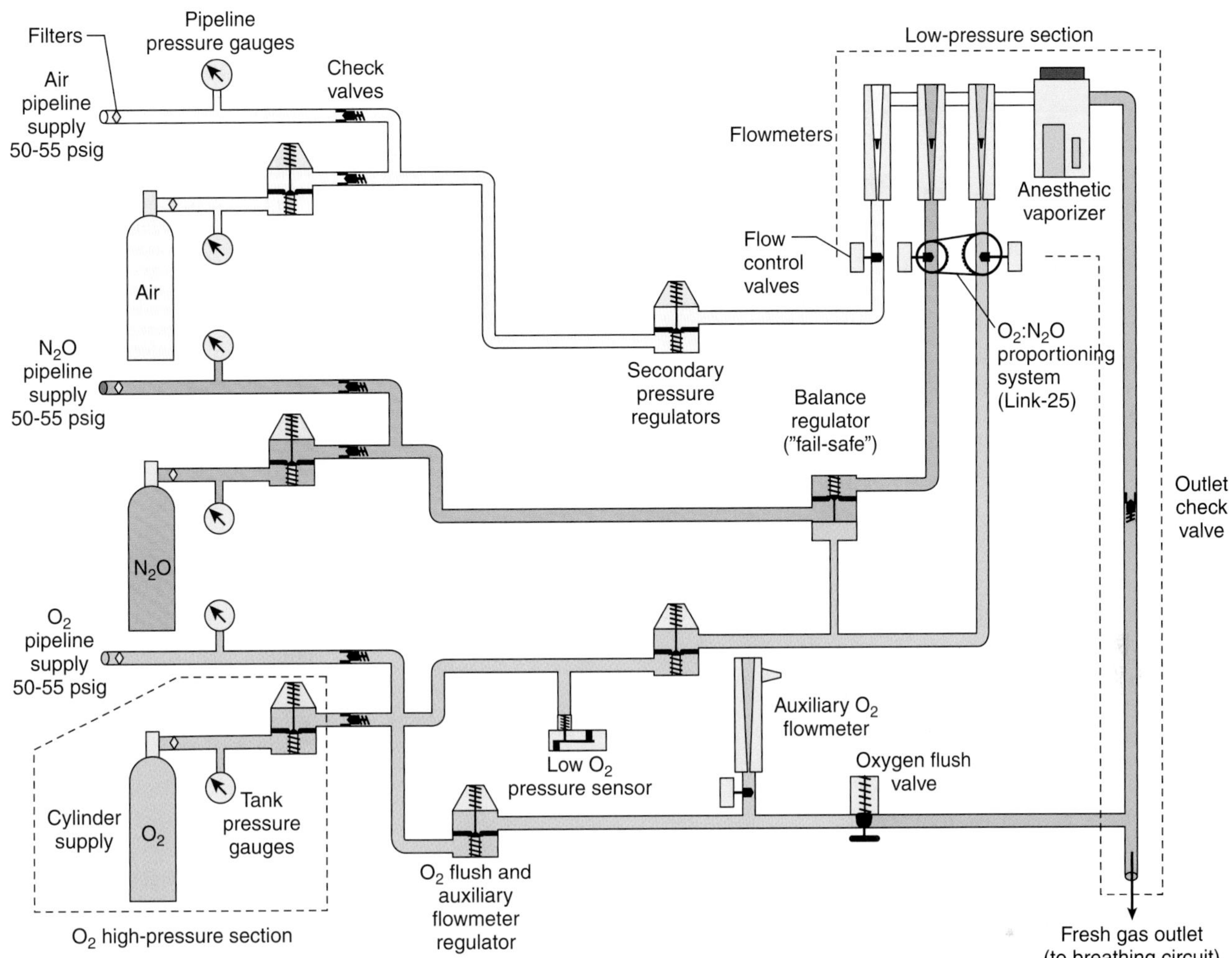

Fig. 22.1 The GE Healthcare Aespire anesthesia workstation gas supply system. The high-pressure system extends from the gas cylinders to the high-pressure regulators (*dashed lines* around O_2 high-pressure section only). The intermediate-pressure section extends from the high-pressure regulators to the flow control valves and also includes the tubing and components originating from the pipeline inlets. The low-pressure section *(dashed lines)* extends from the flow control valves to the breathing circuit. See text for additional details. (From Datex-Ohmeda. *S/5 Aespire Anesthesia Machine: Technical Reference Manual.* Madison, WI: Datex-Ohmeda; 2004.)

the pneumatic system is no longer mediated by a flowmeter, but rather by a touchscreen. However, the interior of the anesthesia machine remains a pneumatic system. It is where breathing gases are delivered from their supply sources, measured, mixed, passed through an anesthetic vaporizer, and delivered to the patient's breathing circuit. The details of this gas supply system may differ between the various manufacturers' anesthesia workstations, but their overall schematic is similar. Fig. 22.1 presents the gas supply system of a more traditional anesthesia machine, without electronic controls. Fig. 22.2 demonstrates a typical contemporary workstation with electronic controls.

The gas supply system consists of the following elements: oxygen, air, and nitrous oxide may enter the anesthesia machine from either the hospital gas pipeline system, or from E-cylinders mounted on the back of the anesthesia machine. The gases flow through pressure regulators to reach flow control valves before reaching flowmeters, anesthetic vaporizers, and the patient's breathing circuit via the fresh gas outlet. There are a number of safety mechanisms in place along this route to avoid delivering a hypoxic gas mixture at the fresh gas outlet. In addition, the system is designed to be able to rapidly fill the patient's breathing circuit with 100% oxygen (oxygen flush valve), and to provide 100% oxygen from a flowmeter; both of these features are active even when the machine is off or without power.

The gas supply system can be divided into three sections: high-pressure, intermediate-pressure, and low-pressure. The only high-pressure elements in the anesthesia machine are the auxiliary gas tanks (E-cylinders) on the back of the anesthesia machine. The pressure in these tanks (approximately 2000 pounds per square inch gauge [psig] for air and oxygen, 745 psig for nitrous oxide) is immediately stepped down to an intermediate pressure. The hospital's gas pipelines are themselves of intermediate pressure (50-55 psig), so the intermediate pressure section starts from the pipelines or from the stepped-down input from the E-cylinders, and extends up to the flowmeter control valves. The low-pressure section begins at the flowmeter control valves, includes the flowmeters and anesthetic vaporizer, and ends at the fresh gas outlet.

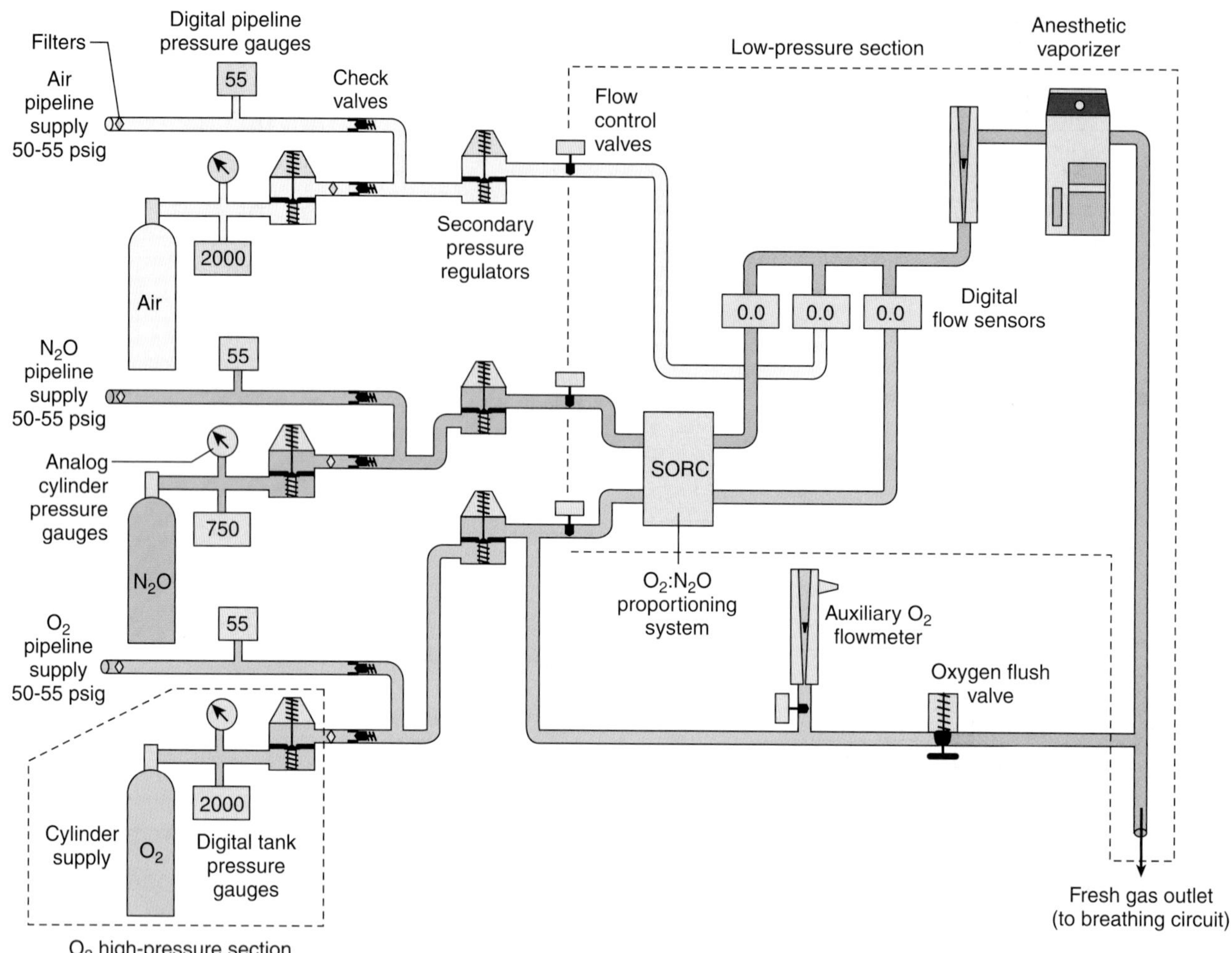

Fig. 22.2 Dräger Apollo anesthesia workstation gas supply system. The high-pressure system extends from the gas cylinders to the high-pressure regulators (*dashed lines* around O_2 high-pressure section only). The intermediate-pressure section extends from the high-pressure regulators to the flow control valves and also includes the tubing and components originating from the pipeline inlets. The low-pressure section *(dashed lines)* extends from the flow control valves to the breathing circuit. See text for additional details. (From Dräger Medical. *Instructions for Use: Apollo.* Telford, PA: Dräger Medical; 2012.)

High-Pressure Section

Auxiliary E-Cylinder Inlet. During normal operation, the high-pressure section of the anesthesia machine is not active, because the hospital's central gas supply system serves as the primary gas source for the machine. However, it is a requirement to have at least one attachment for an oxygen cylinder to serve as a backup oxygen source in case of failure of the hospital supply. Many machines have up to three and sometimes four E-cylinder attachment points to accommodate oxygen, air, and nitrous oxide. Some machines have attachments for two oxygen tanks, and some rare systems can accommodate carbon dioxide (CO_2) or helium tanks used for special applications. The cylinders are mounted to the anesthesia machine by the hanger yoke assembly, as seen in Fig. 22.3. The hanger yoke assembly orients and safely supports the cylinder, provides a gas-tight seal, and ensures unidirectional flow of gases into the machine.[12,13] Each yoke assembly must have a label designating which gas it is intended to accept. Each hanger yoke is also equipped with the Pin Index Safety System (PISS), which is a safeguard to reduce the risk of a medical gas error caused by interchanging cylinders. Two metal pins on the yoke assembly are arranged to project precisely into corresponding holes on the cylinder head–valve assembly of the tank. Each gas or combination of gases has a specific pin arrangement.[14] Although infrequent, failures of the PISS have been reported, and like all safety systems, the PISS should be considered partial protection. Conditions in which failure occurred have included the following: excessive seating (jamming) of the pins back into the hanger yoke; the presence of bent or broken pins; and an excessive use of washers between the cylinder and the yoke that can override pin alignment, yet allow for a gas-tight seal.[15-17] Medical gas cylinder errors can have tragic outcomes, so it is critical to ensure that the proper gas is being connected to the proper inlet by also checking the tank and yoke labels.[18]

Once a gas cylinder valve is opened by the operator, gas flows first through a filter to entrap any particulate matter from the tank inflow. The maximum pressure in full E-cylinders (approximately 750 psig for nitrous oxide, 2200 psig for air, and 2200 psig for oxygen) is much higher than the normal hospital pipeline supply pressure of 50 to 55 psig. A *high-pressure regulator* reduces the variable high pressure in the E-cylinder to a constant pressure slightly lower than

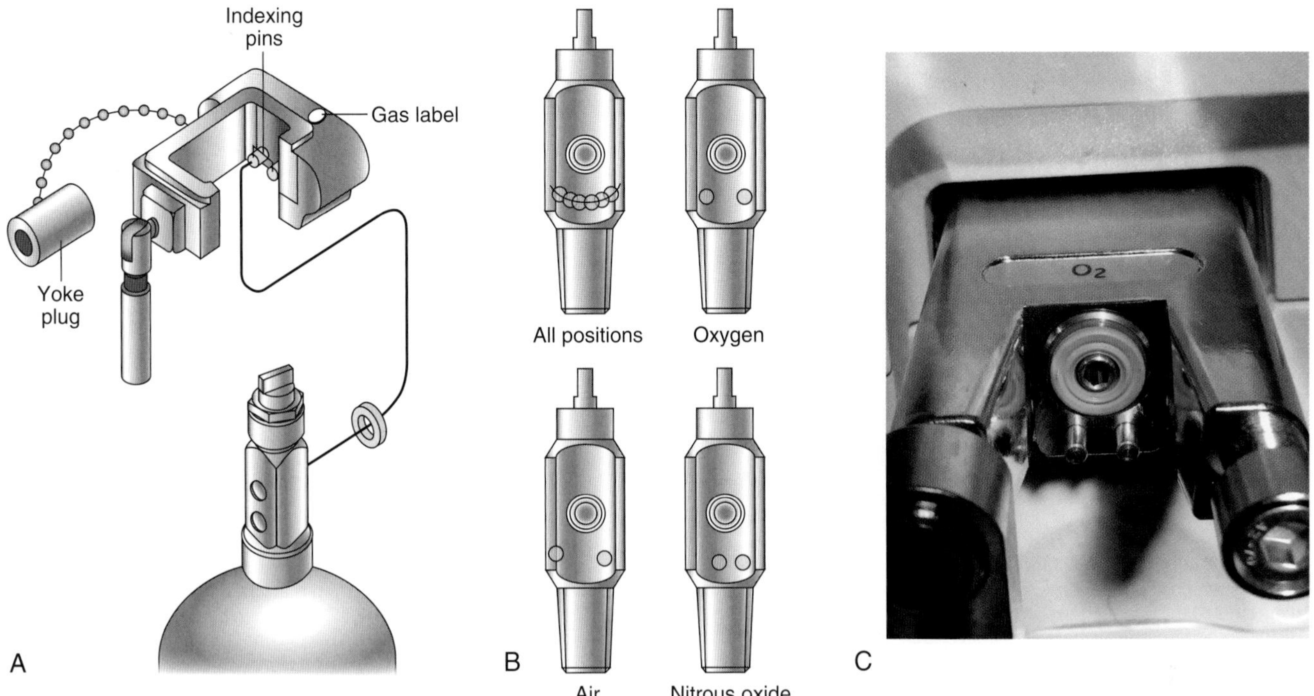

Fig. 22.3 E-cylinder hanger yoke assembly. (A) Standard E-cylinder hanger yoke assembly highlighting the gas-specific indexing pins, sealing gasket, and yoke plug. The yoke plug should be inserted when a tank is not in place. (B) Pin Index Safety System holes machined into the cylinder head–valve mechanism of the compressed gas cylinders. (C) Oxygen yoke with indexing pins. (A and B, From Yoder M. Gas supply systems. In: *Understanding Modern Anesthesia Systems*. Telford, PA: Dräger Medical; 2009.)

the normal pipeline supply pressure, approximately 40 to 45 psig (depending on the specific anesthesia machine)[13] (see the O_2 high-pressure section in Fig. 22.1). The lower pressure is a safety feature: if both the E-cylinder and the oxygen pipeline are connected and the E-cylinder is open, the anesthesia machine will draw its gas from the pipeline rather than the E-cylinder, thereby preserving the contents of the E-cylinder in case of pipeline failure. Fluctuations in the pipeline pressure below 40 to 45 psig could allow the E-cylinder to be drained, as could silent leaks in the high-pressure system, so E-cylinders should be closed during normal operation. One implication of this design warrants emphasis: in case of known or suspected pipeline contamination or crossover leading to delivery of a hypoxic gas mixture (as might be caused by nitrous oxide in the oxygen pipeline), backup oxygen from the E-cylinder will not flow unless the anesthesia machine is disconnected from the pipeline. Merely turning the backup tank on will not help, if the pipeline pressure remains higher than the high-pressure regulator's output.[13,18a]

After the high-pressure regulator, cylinder gas flows through a one-way valve called the cylinder check valve, which prevents any backflow of machine gas out through an empty yoke or back into a nearly empty cylinder (see Fig. 22.1). If the anesthesia machine allows two oxygen E-cylinders to be mounted on a common manifold, then each mount must have a check valve. On some machines, a single high pressure regulator is downstream from the two check valves; on others, each mount on the manifold has its own high pressure regulator and check valve. In either configuration, transfer of gas from a full tank to an empty tank is prevented, and the system allows for a cylinder to be exchanged while the other cylinder on the manifold continues to supply gas to the anesthesia machine.

As noted on Fig. 22.1, there are a number of pressure gauges in the system. The pressure in each of the gas pipelines and each of the auxiliary E-cylinder manifolds must be displayed on the front of the anesthesia machine. The E-cylinder pressures are accurate only when the tank is open; in the case of a two-tank manifold, the pressure of the open tank with higher pressure will be displayed. In systems with electronic pressure displays, the pipeline and tank pressures are visible only when the machine is on.

Two points about the safe use of the auxiliary E-cylinder system should be noted. First, checking the E-cylinders is *not* part of an automatic machine checkout. The practitioner must manually open each cylinder and check the pressure gauges on the front of the machine. In the case of a two-tank oxygen manifold, the tanks must be serially opened and checked. The oxygen flush valve may be used to vent the pressure from the system after closing the first tank, so the pressure in the second tank can be accurately assessed. Second, it is imperative to keep the auxiliary E-cylinders closed during normal operation using pipeline gases because of the possibility of small leaks in the high-pressure system, or fluctuations in pipeline pressures allowing flow from the cylinder to be activated. An open oxygen cylinder may allow the anesthesiologist to be unaware of catastrophic pipeline failure. When the oxygen cylinder is closed, the immediate result of oxygen pipeline failure is a low oxygen pressure alarm. The auxiliary E-cylinder can then be opened, ensuring continued flow of oxygen to the patient while troubleshooting occurs. If the oxygen tank is *already open* when pipeline failure occurs, there may be only a subtle indication from the anesthesia machine that the oxygen source has

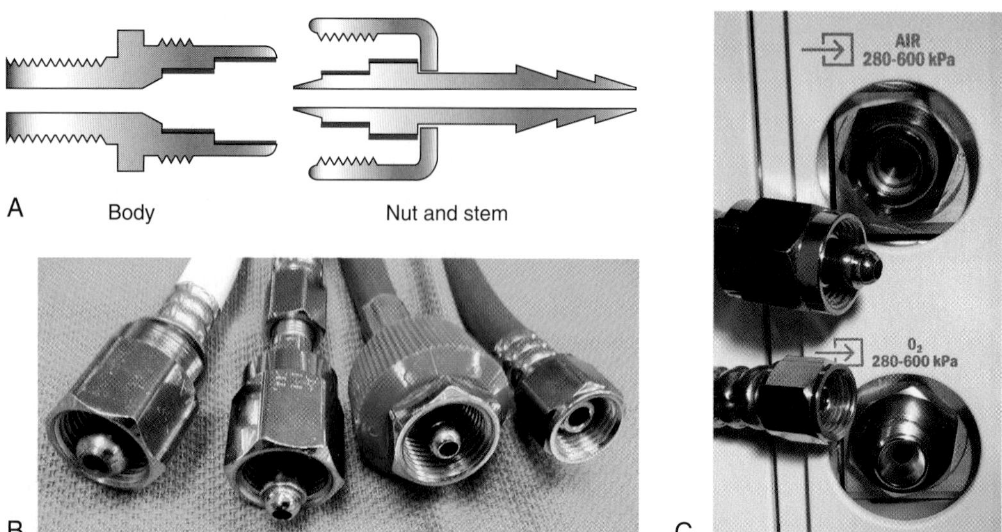

Fig. 22.4 Diameter Index Safety System. Diameter Index Safety System (DISS) connectors are used for noninterchangeable, removable medical gas connections at pressures less than 200 psig. They are also used for suction and waste gas connections. Indexing is accomplished through differing diameters of the connection components, resulting in key-like fitting when matched connectors come together. The oxygen connector is additionally distinguished from the other gas connectors by a unique threaded fitting diameter and a unique thread count. (A) DISS connector cross section. (B) Nut and stem connectors for (*left* to *right*) vacuum, air, nitrous oxide, and oxygen. (C) DISS connections at the back of an anesthesia workstation. (A, Modified from Yoder M. Gas supply systems. In: *Understanding Modern Anesthesia Systems*. Telford, PA: Dräger Medical; 2009.)

switched from pipeline to auxiliary tank. In this case, the low oxygen pressure alarm only occurs once the auxiliary tank has been depleted, nullifying the utility of the backup system.[12,19]

Intermediate-Pressure Section

Gas Pipeline Inlet: Central Gas Supply Source. Three gases are typically piped into the operating room by the hospital's central gas supply system: oxygen, air, and nitrous oxide. The main supply source of oxygen in a large hospital usually is a large cryogenic bulk oxygen storage system. These are refilled on site from a truck carrying liquid oxygen. Smaller hospitals may use liquid oxygen tanks that can be replaced rather than refilled on site, or even a bank of oxygen H-cylinders connected by a manifold. Oxygen storage systems must have backup supply and alarm systems in place.[14] Most hospitals use compressors to deliver cleaned, dried air to a pressurized reservoir for delivery to the pipeline system. Centrally supplied nitrous oxide arises either from a bank of H-type cylinders, or a bulk liquid storage system similar to that for oxygen.[14]

The gas pipeline terminates in patient care areas of the hospital with one of two types of connector: the Diameter Index Safety System (DISS) connector system, or the quick coupler system. Within each type, the connectors for oxygen, air, and nitrous oxide are mutually incompatible, which helps to minimize the potential for connecting to the wrong gas. DISS connectors (as seen in Fig. 22.4) rely on matching diameters in the male and female connections to properly seat and thread the connection.[14,20] The quick couplers (Fig. 22.5) utilize pins and corresponding slots on the male and female ends, respectively, in order to ensure correct connections. Because these connectors can be plugged together or released with a simple twisting motion, they are especially appealing for equipment that needs to be moved between locations. In addition, in both systems the wall plates and hoses are color-coded for ease of identification.

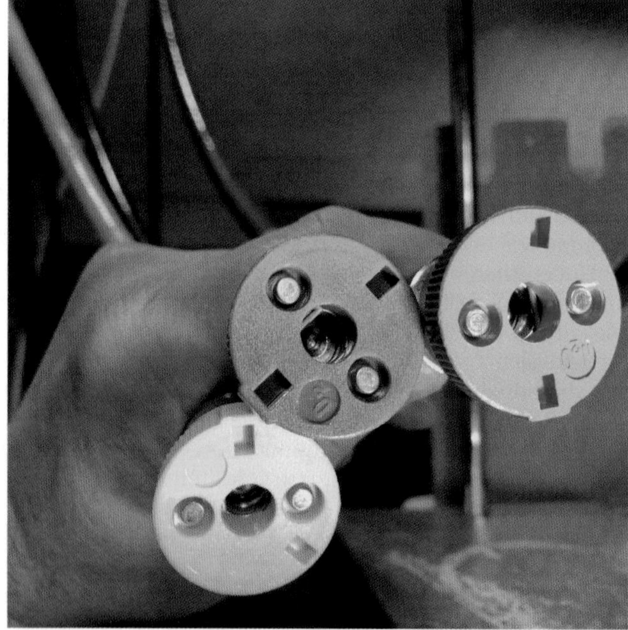

Fig. 22.5 Quick couplers. Quick couplers, like Diameter Index Safety System connectors, are used for noninterchangeable, removable medical gas, suction, and waste gas connections. Indexing is accomplished by the configuration of pins on one plate which match to recesses on the other plate (shown). The two plates lock together, allowing an airtight connection. A twist to the housing of the male plate allows the two plates to be disengaged.

The final medical gas pipeline connection to the anesthesia workstation is always through a DISS connector (Fig. 22.4C). Once the gas enters the machine, it encounters a filter followed by a pipeline check valve. This one-way valve prevents reverse flow of gas from the machine into the medical gas pipeline system or into the atmosphere from an open inlet. Interposed between the DISS inlet and the pipeline check valves is a sample port to measure pipeline oxygen pressure. The pipeline pressure must always be clearly visible on the front of the machine.

Oxygen Flush Valve. The oxygen flush valve is probably one of the oldest safety features on the machine and remains a machine standard today.[11,20,21] The oxygen flush valve allows manual delivery of a high flow rate of 100% oxygen directly to the patient's breathing circuit in order to overcome circuit leaks or to rapidly increase the inhaled oxygen concentration. Flow from the oxygen flush valve bypasses the anesthetic vaporizers (see Fig. 22.1). The intermediate-pressure segment of the gas supply system feeds the valve, which remains closed until the operator opens it. The feature is usually available even when the machine is not turned on because the valve is located upstream from the machine's pneumatic power switch. Flow from the oxygen flush valve enters the low-pressure circuit downstream from the vaporizers at a rate between 35 and 75 L/min, depending on the machine and operating pressure.[11,20,21]

Several hazards have been reported with the oxygen flush valve. A defective or damaged valve can stick in the fully open position and result in barotrauma.[22] Oxygen flow from a valve sticking in a partially open position or overzealous oxygen flushing can dilute the inhaled anesthetic agent concentration, potentially resulting in awareness under anesthesia.[23,24,24a] Oxygen flushing during the inspiratory phase of positive-pressure ventilation can produce barotrauma if the anesthesia machine does not incorporate a fresh gas decoupling feature or an appropriately adjusted inspiratory pressure controller. Fresh gas decoupling prevents the fresh gas inflow from either the flowmeters or the oxygen flush valve from increasing the delivered ventilator tidal volume presented to the patient's lungs (see section on fresh gas flow compensation and fresh gas decoupling). With most older anesthesia breathing circuits, excess volume could not be vented during the inspiratory phase of mechanical ventilation because the ventilator relief valve was closed and the breathing circuit adjustable pressure-limiting (APL) valve was either out of circuit or closed.[25]

Although the oxygen flush valve can potentially provide a high-pressure, high-flow oxygen source at the machine's fresh gas outlet suitable for jet ventilation, it has potential limitations. In some machines, the fresh gas outlet is no longer easy to access, and not all machines are capable of generating pressures at the outlet that are sufficient to deliver jet ventilation.[26,27] An alternate source of high-flow oxygen should be sought if jet ventilation is needed and cannot be supported by the machine's oxygen flush function.

Pneumatic Safety Systems. One of the primary safety goals of contemporary anesthesia machines is to guard against the potential of delivering an excessive concentration of nitrous oxide relative to oxygen (hypoxic mixture). ISO standards require delivery of a nonhypoxic gas mixture to the patient, or generation of an alarm condition.[11] Several safety devices discussed below have been introduced to prevent generating a hypoxic mixture.

OXYGEN SUPPLY FAILURE ALARM SENSOR. Within the oxygen circuit of the intermediate-pressure section of the machine is a sensor that provides an audible and visual warning to the clinician if the oxygen pressure drops below a manufacturer-specified minimum. The alarm is an ISO requirement[11]; under ASTM guidelines, it cannot be silenced until the pressure is restored to the minimum value.[20] The alarm is triggered by a loss of or significant decrease in pipeline pressure, or a nearly empty oxygen tank if the tank was the oxygen source. During normal operation this alarm signal serves as a prompt for the operator to open the oxygen E-cylinder on the machine and troubleshoot the oxygen pipeline source. The minimum threshold pressure for an alarm condition differs among manufacturers and models, because pipeline pressure standards vary significantly throughout the world. The conditions that trigger the alarm should be delineated in the manufacturer's instructions.[11] Numerous types of pneumatic-electrical switches serve as this sensor. Older machines had a purely pneumatic device that gave an audible signal when oxygen pressure dropped (the "Ritchie whistle").[27a] Current machines integrate the output from electronic pressure transducers to create an alarm if pressures drop below predetermined minimums.[21]

OXYGEN SUPPLY FAILURE PROTECTION DEVICES. In addition to generating an alarm condition, oxygen failure influences the flow of other gases within the gas supply system. Sometimes called "fail-safe valves," the oxygen supply failure protection devices are safeguards intended to link the flow of other gases in the gas supply system to the pressure of oxygen. They are an ISO standard.[11] In response to low oxygen pressure within the intermediate-pressure section of the anesthesia machine, the oxygen supply failure protection device either shuts off (binary valve), or reduces (proportional valve) the flow of other gases such as nitrous oxide or air. Unfortunately, the term *fail-safe* as it pertains to these valves is a misnomer and has led to the misconception that they can independently prevent the administration of a hypoxic mixture. If a gas other than oxygen pressurizes the oxygen circuit as a result of hospital pipeline contamination or crossover, the fail-safe valves will remain open. In such a case, only the inspired oxygen concentration monitor and clinical acumen would protect the patient.

Auxiliary Oxygen Flowmeter. Although auxiliary oxygen flowmeters are not mandatory, they are commonly encountered. During normal operation, the auxiliary flowmeter is a convenience feature that allows the use of low-flow oxygen for devices independent of the patient's breathing circuit. Similar to the oxygen flush feature, oxygen flow from the flowmeter is usually accessible even when the machine is not turned on, because the flowmeter is typically fed before the pneumatic power switch in the intermediate-pressure section. As long as oxygen is available from the pipeline inlet or from an attached E-cylinder, the auxiliary oxygen flowmeter can serve as a source of oxygen delivery for use with a manually powered resuscitation bag in the case of a system power failure. The auxiliary oxygen flowmeter may also potentially serve as gas source for a manual jet ventilator; however, not all machines can generate sufficient working pressure.[26,28] Some auxiliary oxygen flowmeters have a DISS connector that would be a better source for manual jet ventilation.[13]

The operator should be aware that the source of oxygen for the auxiliary flowmeter is the same as for the other oxygen flow control valves. This is an important consideration in cases of suspected hospital oxygen pipeline contamination or crossover. If the pipeline oxygen supply line is connected to the machine and the pressure is sufficient, the gas source will be the pipeline even if the auxiliary oxygen tank valve is opened. In a simulation experiment, a nitrous oxide–oxygen pipeline crossover situation was created whereby the inspired oxygen concentration became alarmingly low, and the "patient" became hypoxemic after turning the nitrous oxide flow off. Researchers noted that many study participants tried to make inappropriate use of the auxiliary oxygen flowmeter and oxygen E-cylinders on the machine as an external source of oxygen without disconnecting the pipeline source.[29] The participant's suboptimal management was attributed to a lack of knowledge of the anesthesia machine and its gas supply.

Second-Stage Pressure Regulators. Some machines have second-stage regulators located downstream from the gas supply sources in the intermediate-pressure circuit. These regulators supply constant pressure to the flow control valves and the proportioning system regardless of potential fluctuations in hospital pipeline pressures. They are adjusted to lower pressure levels than the pipeline supply, usually between 14 and 35 psig, depending on the workstation.[30,31,31a]

Low-Pressure Section

The purpose of the high- and intermediate-pressure sections of the anesthesia machine is to deliver a reliable source of breathing gases at a stable and known working pressure to the low-pressure section of the gas supply system. The low-pressure section of the gas supply system begins at the flow control valves and ends at the fresh gas outlet (see Figs. 22.1 and 22.2). The breathing circuit, including the circle system, breathing bag, and ventilator, will be treated separately. Key components include the flow control valves, the flowmeters or flow sensors, the vaporizer manifold, and the anesthetic vaporizers. The low-pressure section is the most vulnerable section to leaks within the gas supply system.

Flow Control Assemblies. The flow control valves on the anesthesia workstation allow the operator to select a *total fresh gas flow* of known composition that enters the low-pressure section of the anesthesia workstation. These valves separate the intermediate-pressure section from the low-pressure section. After leaving the flowmeters, the mixture of gases travels through a common manifold and may be directed through an anesthetic vaporizer if selected. The total fresh gas flow and the anesthetic vapor then travel toward the fresh gas outlet (see Figs. 22.1 and 22.2).[12,19]

ELECTRONIC FLOW SENSORS. Newer anesthesia workstations are increasingly equipped with electronic flow sensors instead of flow tubes. These systems may employ conventional control knobs or an entirely electronic interface to control gas flow. Flows can be displayed numerically or sometimes graphically in the form of a virtual, digitalized flowmeter. Numerous types of flow sensor technologies can be applied, such as hot-wire anemometers, a differential pressure transducer method, or mass flow sensors. An example of an electronic mass flow sensor is seen in Fig. 22.6. The illustrated device relies on the principle of specific heat to measure gas

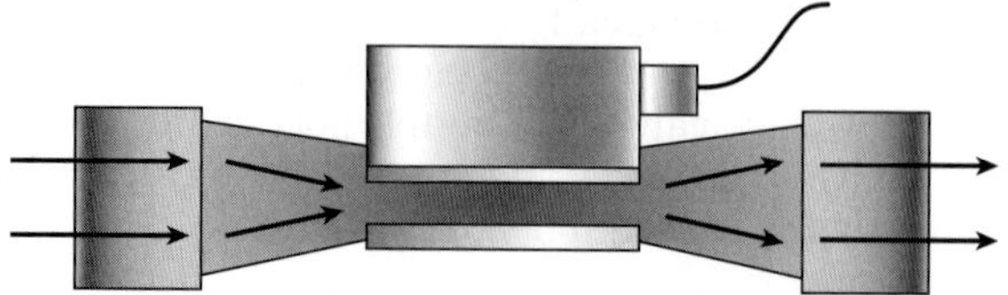

Fig. 22.6 Electronic mass flow sensor. Gas flows past a heated chamber of known volume. The amount of heat (electrical energy) that is required to maintain a set chamber temperature is proportional to the specific heat of the gas and its rate of flow through the chamber. Because the specific heat of the gas is relevant to the calculation, each gas must have its own mass flow sensor. Flow is accurately extrapolated from the energy required to keep the chamber at a constant temperature. (Modified from Yoder M. Gas supply systems. In: *Understanding Modern Anesthesia Systems*. Telford, PA: Dräger Medical; 2009.)

flow.[30] As gas flows through a heated chamber of known volume, a specific amount of electricity is required to maintain the chamber temperature. The amount of energy required to maintain the temperature is proportional to the flow and specific heat of the gas. Regardless of the mechanism of flow measurement, these systems depend on electrical power to provide a display of gas flow. When electrical power is totally interrupted, some backup mechanical means usually exists to control (mechanical flow control) and display (flow tube) oxygen gas flow.

MECHANICAL FLOWMETER ASSEMBLIES. Mechanical flow control and flow display still remain common, even on some newer workstations, either as primary or backup systems.[31a,31b]

FLOW CONTROL VALVES. The flow control valve assembly consists of a flow control knob, a tapered needle valve, a valve seat, and a pair of valve stops (Fig. 22.7).[12] The inlet pressure to the assembly is determined by the pressure characteristics of the machine's intermediate-pressure segment. The location of the needle valve in the valve seat changes to establish different orifices when the flow control valve is adjusted. Gas flow increases when the flow control valve is turned counterclockwise, and it decreases when the valve is turned clockwise. Because their use is frequent and the consequences of damage are significant, the controls must be constructed so extremes of rotation will not cause disassembly or disengagement.

Contemporary flow control valve assemblies have numerous safety features. The oxygen flow control knob is physically distinguishable from the other gas knobs. It is distinctively fluted, may project beyond the control knobs of the other gases, and is larger in diameter than the flow control knobs of other gases.[11] All knobs are color coded for the appropriate gas, and the chemical formula or name of the gas must be permanently marked on each knob. Flow control knobs are recessed or protected with a shield or barrier to minimize inadvertent change from a preset position. If a single gas has two flow tubes, the tubes are arranged in series and are controlled by a single flow control valve.[20]

FLOW TUBES. With a traditional flowmeter assembly, the flow control valve regulates the amount of flow that enters a tapered, transparent flow tube known as a *variable orifice flowmeter* or *Thorpe tube*. These glass tubes are narrowest at the bottom and widen at the top. A mobile indicator float inside the calibrated flow tube indicates the amount of flow passing through the associated flow control valve. The quantity of flow is indicated on a scale specific to the

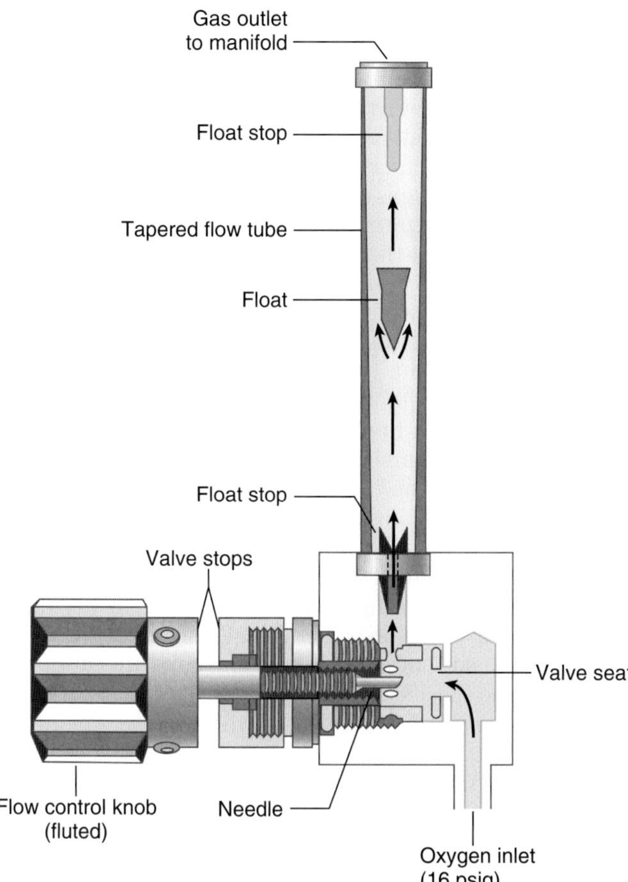

Fig. 22.7 Oxygen flowmeter assembly. The oxygen flowmeter assembly is composed of the flow control valve assembly and the flowmeter subassembly. (From Bowie E, Huffman LM. *The Anesthesia Machine: Essentials for Understanding.* Madison, WI: Ohmeda, BOC Group; 1985.)

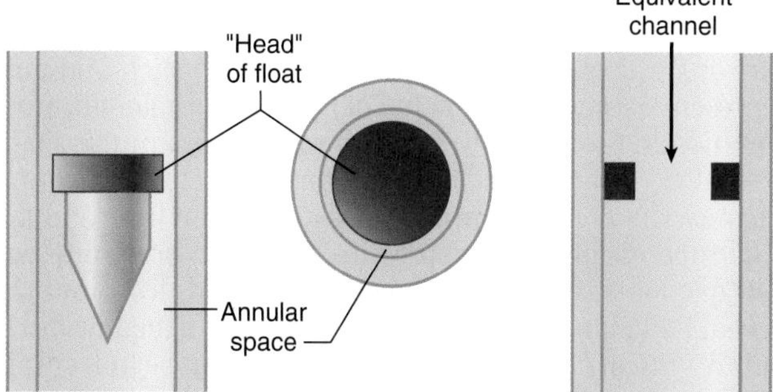

Fig. 22.8 The annular space. The clearance between the head of the float and the flow tube is known as the annular space. It can be considered equivalent to a circular channel of the same cross-sectional area. (Redrawn from Macintosh R, Mushin WW, Epstein HG, eds. *Physics for the Anaesthetist.* 3rd ed. Oxford: Blackwell Scientific; 1963.)

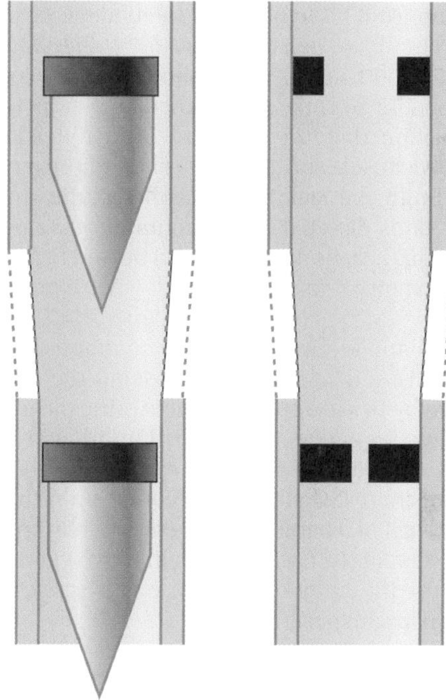

Fig. 22.9 Flow tube constriction. The *lower pair* of illustrations represents the lower portion of a flow tube. The clearance between the head of the float and the flow tube is narrow. The equivalent channel is tubular because its diameter is less than its length. Viscosity is dominant in determining the gas flow rate through this tubular constriction. The *upper pair* of illustrations represents the upper portion of a flow tube. The equivalent channel is orificial because its length is less than its diameter. Density is dominant in determining the gas flow rate through this orificial constriction. (Redrawn from Macintosh R, Mushin WW, Epstein HG, eds. *Physics for the Anaesthetist.* 3rd ed. Oxford: Blackwell Scientific; 1963.)

flow tube.[12,19] Opening the flow control valve allows gas to travel through the space between the float and the flow tube. This space is known as the *annular space*, and it varies in size depending on the position in the tube (Fig. 22.8). The indicator float hovers freely in an equilibrium position in the tube where the upward force resulting from gas flow equals the downward gravity force on the float at a given flow rate. The float moves to a new equilibrium position in the tube when flow is changed. These flowmeters are commonly referred to as *constant-pressure* flowmeters because the decrease in pressure across the float remains constant for all positions in the tube.[12,32,33]

Flow through the annular space can be laminar or turbulent, depending on the gas flow rate (Fig. 22.9). The characteristics of a gas that influence its flow rate through a given constriction are viscosity (laminar flow) and density (turbulent flow). Because the annular space behaves as a tube at low flow rates, laminar flow is present, and *viscosity* determines the gas flow rate. At high flow rates, the annular space behaves like an orifice. Turbulent gas flow is present and gas *density* predominantly influences the flow. Because the viscosity and density of the gas affect flow through annular space around the float, the calibrated flow tubes are gas specific. The tube, the float, and the scale are inseparable. Although temperature and barometric pressure can influence gas density and viscosity, under normal clinical circumstances, flow tube accuracy is not significantly affected by mild changes in temperature or pressure.

The float or bobbin within the flow tube is usually constructed so that it rotates to indicate that gas is flowing and that the indicator is not stuck in the tube. A stop at the top of the flowmeter tube prevents the float from occluding the outlet. Two flowmeter tubes are sometimes placed in series, with a fine flow tube displaying low flows and a coarse flow tube indicating higher flows.

Problems With Flowmeters. Flow measurement error can occur even when flowmeters are assembled properly. Dirt or static electricity can cause a float to stick and misrepresent actual flow. Sticking of the indicator float is more common in the low-flow ranges because the annular space is smaller. A damaged float can cause inaccurate readings because the precise relationship between the float and the flow tube is altered. Backpressure from the breathing circuit can cause a float to drop so that it reads less than the actual flow. Finally, if flowmeters are not aligned properly in the vertical position (plumb), readings can be inaccurate because tilting distorts the annular space.[12,34,35]

The flow tube has historically been a very fragile component of the anesthesia workstation. Subtle cracks and chips may be overlooked and can cause errors in delivered flow.[34] Leaks can also occur at the O-ring junctions between the glass flow tubes and the metal manifold. Flow tube leaks are a potential hazard because the flowmeters are located downstream from all hypoxemia safety devices, except the breathing circuit oxygen analyzer.[33,36,37] Fig. 22.10 shows an example where an unused air flow tube develops a large leak. When the nitrous oxide flowmeter is in the downstream position (Fig. 22.10*A* and *B*), a hypoxic mixture can occur because a substantial portion of the oxygen flow passes through the leak in the air flow tube, and mainly nitrous oxide is directed to the common gas outlet. Safer configurations are shown in Fig. 22.10*C* and *D*, in which the oxygen flowmeter is located in the downstream position. A portion of the nitrous oxide flow escapes through the leak, and the remainder goes toward the common gas outlet. A hypoxic mixture is less likely because all the oxygen flow is advanced by the nitrous oxide (this principle is known as the Eger flow sequence). It has been an industry standard that oxygen be delivered downstream of all other gases,[20] although current ISO standards require only that oxygen be at either end of a bank of flowmeters.[11] It is important to remember that in the case of a leak in the oxygen flow tube, a hypoxic mixture may result even when oxygen is located in the downstream position.[34]

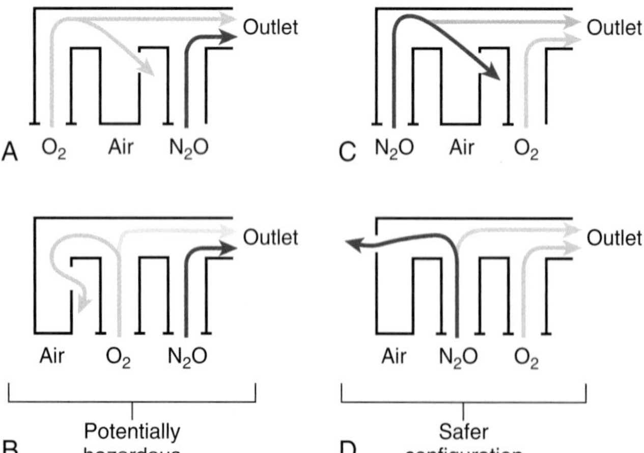

Fig. 22.10 The flowmeter sequence is a potential cause of hypoxia. In the event of a flowmeter leak, a potentially dangerous arrangement exists when nitrous oxide is located in the downstream position (A and B). A safer configuration exists when oxygen is located in the downstream position (C and D). See text for details. (Modified from Eger EI II, Hylton RR, Irwin RH, et al. Anesthetic flowmeter sequence: a cause for hypoxia. *Anesthesiology.* 1963;24:396.)

PROPORTIONING SYSTEMS. Anesthesia workstations are equipped with an oxygen failure protection device in the intermediate-pressure section that, in response to reduced oxygen pressure, either proportionally reduces or completely inhibits nitrous oxide. However, this system does not prevent the user from selecting a hypoxic gas mixture for delivery to the fresh gas outlet. On anesthesia workstations with electronically controlled gas flow, the machine is programmed to prevent the user from selecting a hypoxic gas mixture for delivery to the fresh gas outlet. For mechanically controlled flowmeters, the concern is that a user could mistakenly select oxygen and nitrous oxide flows that would result in a hypoxic mixture. According to the ISO, an alarm condition is insufficient and the machine must have a system to prevent delivery of a hypoxic mixture.[11] This is accomplished by a pneumatic-mechanical interface between the oxygen and nitrous oxide flows or by mechanically linking the oxygen and nitrous oxide flow control valves. This way, no matter how high the operator attempts to turn up the nitrous oxide, or how low the operator tries to turn down the oxygen flow, when nitrous oxide is running, the machine will automatically adjust the ratio of these flows so that a hypoxemic gas mixture cannot be delivered. The specific devices used to accomplish this control vary among manufacturers. Two examples are briefly discussed here.

The North American Dräger sensitive oxygen ratio controller system (SORC) is a pneumatic-mechanical, oxygen–nitrous oxide interlock system designed to maintain a ratio of no less than 25% oxygen to 75% nitrous oxide flow into the breathing circuit by limiting the nitrous oxide flow when necessary.[21] The SORC, located after the flow control valves, consists of an oxygen chamber with a diaphragm, a nitrous oxide chamber with a diaphragm, and a nitrous oxide proportioning valve (Fig. 22.11). All are interconnected by a mobile horizontal shaft. As oxygen flows out of the SORC, it encounters a resistor that creates backpressure in the oxygen chamber, which causes the diaphragm to move to the right, thereby opening the nitrous oxide proportioning valve. As the oxygen flow is increased, so too is the backpressure and the rightward motion of the shaft. If the nitrous oxide flow is now turned on, it will also flow into the SORC, through the proportioning valve, and past its resistor to create backpressure that will press on the diaphragm in its respective chamber. The counterbalance between the two gas flows (backpressures) determines the positioning of the nitrous oxide proportioning valve.[21] If the oxygen is turned down too low (<1/3 of the nitrous oxide flow), the shaft will move to the left and thus limit the nitrous oxide flow. If the operator tries to turn up the nitrous oxide too high relative to the oxygen flow, the SORC will limit the nitrous oxide flow because of the nitrous oxide backpressure and leftward movement of the valve. If the oxygen flow is decreased to less than 200 mL/min, the proportioning valve will close completely.[38]

A mechanical proportioning system that remains in use today on many anesthesia machines is the GE/Datex-Ohmeda Link-25 system. The system provides mechanical integration of the nitrous oxide and oxygen flow control valves to maintain a minimum oxygen concentration with a maximum nitrous oxide:oxygen flow ratio of 3:1. Independent adjustment of either valve is allowed as long as the minimum threshold is met. The Link-25 automatically increases oxygen flow when the nitrous oxide flow is increased above the 3:1 ratio. It also will lower nitrous oxide flow if oxygen flow is decreased below that ratio. Fig. 22.12 shows the Link-25 system. A 15-tooth sprocket is attached to the nitrous oxide flow control valve, a 29-tooth sprocket is attached to the oxygen flow control valve and a chain physically links the sprockets. When the nitrous oxide flow control valve is turned through two revolutions, the oxygen flow control valve will revolve once because of the 2:1 gear ratio. The final 3:1 flow ratio results because the flow control valve needle for nitrous oxide has a faster taper than does the oxygen valve needle. The Link-25 system uses a stop tab on each valve stem to allow for independent adjustment of oxygen or nitrous oxide as long as the mixture is at least 25% oxygen; attempting to turn the valve controller past that point will engage the chain and effect a change in the other gas. In addition, the system is designed so that nitrous oxide cannot flow unless the oxygen flow is at least 200 mL/min.[38a]

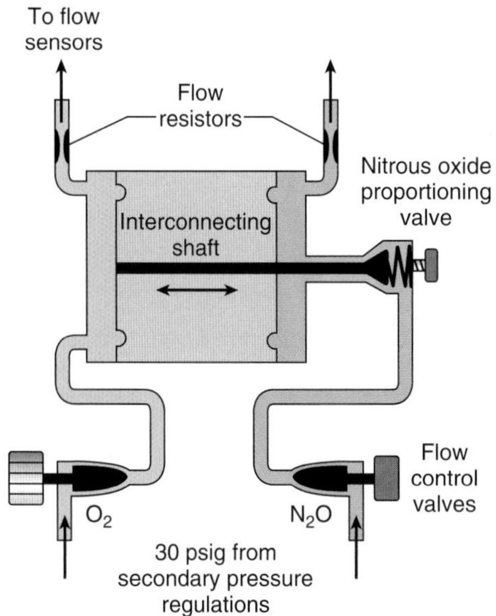

Fig. 22.11 North American Dräger sensitive oxygen ratio controller system (SORC) (Dräger Medical, Telford, PA). The SORC is a pneumatic-mechanical interlock system designed to maintain a ratio of no less than 25% oxygen/75% nitrous oxide regardless of operator input. Differential oxygen and nitrous oxide flows and the resultant chamber backpressures determine the position of the nitrous oxide proportioning valve. The SORC requires a minimum oxygen flow of 200 mL/min for the nitrous oxide proportioning valve to open. See text for details. (Modified from Yoder M. Gas supply systems. In: *Understanding Modern Anesthesia Systems*. Telford, PA: Dräger Medical; 2009.)

Although both proportioning systems are designed to prevent delivery of a hypoxic gas mixture to the common gas outlet, their effect on the output may be different. If the operator turns down oxygen flow below 25% oxygen, both the Link-25 and SORC systems will respond by decreasing the flow of nitrous oxide. If the operator subsequently increases the set oxygen flow, the nitrous oxide flow will remain at the new, lower value with the Link-25 system, because the mechanical linkage will have physically changed the nitrous oxide control valve setting. With the SORC system, on the other hand, the nitrous oxide flow will return to the higher, previously set value when adequate oxygen flow is restored. If the operator increases nitrous oxide flow beyond the set safe range, the Link-25 system will increase the oxygen flow by changing the setting on the oxygen control valve. The SORC system will instead prevent the increase in nitrous oxide flow from occurring. If the operator subsequently reduces the nitrous oxide flow setting, the oxygen flow will remain at the new, higher level with the Link-25, and will remain unchanged with the SORC.

PROPORTIONING SYSTEM MALFUNCTION. Proportioning systems are not immune from failure, and workstations equipped with proportioning systems can still deliver a hypoxic mixture under certain conditions. Many case reports have described proportioning system malfunction.[39-43] Other situations that may defeat the purpose of the proportioning system require operator vigilance. Both mechanical and pneumatic proportioning systems can be defeated if a gas other than oxygen is present in the oxygen pipeline. Proportioning systems such as the Link-25 function at the level of the flow control valves. A leak downstream from these devices, such as a broken

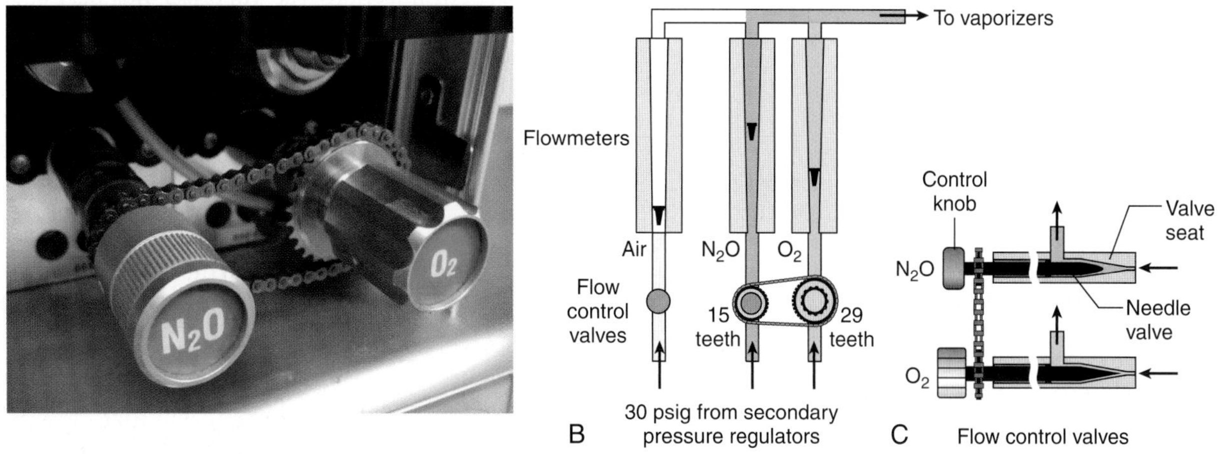

Fig. 22.12 GE/Datex-Ohmeda Link-25 nitrous oxide: oxygen proportioning system. The system prevents the operator from selecting more than a 75% nitrous oxide–25% oxygen (3:1) mixture by two separate but interdependent means. (A) Link-25 proportioning system on a GE Healthcare Aestiva anesthesia workstation with front panel removed. (B) Mechanical linkage of the control valves maintains no more than a 2:1 ratio. (C) A faster taper of the nitrous oxide valve needle allows more gas flow through the valve per turn relative to flow through the oxygen valve per turn, thus resulting in the maximal 3:1 ratio. A stable and equal pressure supply to the valves is provided by the secondary pressure regulator for oxygen and a balance regulator for nitrous oxide. See text for additional details. (Datex-Ohmeda: Aestiva anesthesia machine: technical reference manual, Madison, Wis: Datex-Ohmeda 2006.)

oxygen flow tube, could result in delivery of a hypoxic mixture to the common gas outlet. In this situation, oxygen escapes through the leak, and the predominant gas delivered is nitrous oxide. Finally, volatile inhaled anesthetic agents are added to the mixed gases downstream from both the flowmeters and the proportioning system. Concentrations of less potent inhaled anesthetic agents such as desflurane may account for a larger percentage of the total fresh gas composition than is the case with more potent agents. Because significant percentages of these inhaled anesthetic agents may be added downstream of the proportioning system, the resulting gas-vapor mixture may contain an inspired oxygen concentration less than 21% despite a functional proportioning system. The additional complexity of the circle system (discussed below) means that the oxygen concentration of the fresh gas flow delivered to the breathing circuit may be very different from the patient's actual fraction of inspired oxygen (FiO_2). In each case, the presence of a functioning oxygen analyzer in the patient's breathing circuit is the last protection against a hypoxic gas mixture.

Vaporizer Mount and Interlock System

VAPORIZER MOUNTING SYSTEMS. Removable modern vaporizer mounts allow for rapid replacement or exchange of anesthetic vaporizers. This allows for ease of maintenance, fewer required vaporizer positions on the workstation, and the ability to remove the vaporizer if malignant hyperthermia is suspected.[44] Detachable mounting systems can lead to problems such as low-pressure systems leaks or fresh gas flow obstruction as a result connection-related failures.[44-49] After adding or changing a vaporizer on the anesthesia machine, the operator should make sure it is seated properly and cannot be dislodged once locked. The operator should then perform a vaporizer leak test, if required by the manufacturer.

VAPORIZER INTERLOCK DEVICES. All anesthesia workstations must prevent fresh gas from flowing through more than one vaporizer at time.[11] The design of vaporizer interlock devices varies significantly. Operators should be aware that these devices are not immune from failure, and anesthetic overdose can be a potential consequence.[50-53]

Outlet Check Valve. Many older Datex-Ohmeda anesthesia machines and a few contemporary workstations (e.g., GE/Datex-Ohmeda Aestiva and Aespire) have a one-way check valve located between the vaporizer and the common gas outlet in the mixed-gas pipeline (see Fig. 22.1). The purpose of this valve is to prevent backflow into the vaporizer during positive-pressure ventilation, thereby minimizing the effects of intermittent fluctuations in downstream pressure on the concentration of inhaled anesthetics (see the discussion of intermittent backpressure in the section on anesthetic vaporizers). The presence or absence of this check valve historically influenced which *manual* leak test of the low-pressure system was indicated because it precluded positive-pressure tests to detect for leaks upstream of the valve (see the section on checking your anesthesia workstation).

ANESTHETIC VAPORIZERS

In 1846, William T. G. Morton performed the first public demonstration of ether anesthesia using an ingenious, yet simple inhaler (Fig. 22.13).[54-56] Although the device was effective in delivering anesthetic vapor, Morton's ether inhaler had no means of regulating output concentration or compensating for temperature changes caused by vaporization of the liquid anesthetic and the ambient environment. These two issues were central to the subsequent development and evolution of modern anesthetic vaporizers. Modern variable bypass–type vaporizers are temperature compensated and can maintain desired outputs accurately over a wide range of input gas flow rates. In 1993, with the introduction of desflurane to the clinical setting, an even more sophisticated vaporizer was introduced to handle the unique physical properties of this agent. Vaporizers blending both old technology and computer control have emerged as "cassette" vaporizer systems. An injection-type vaporizer has also been reintroduced. This vaporizer injects precise amounts of liquid anesthetic agent into the fresh gas stream. Before discussing these systems in detail, a brief review of physical/chemical principles is necessary to understand the operation, construction, and design of contemporary anesthetic vaporizers.

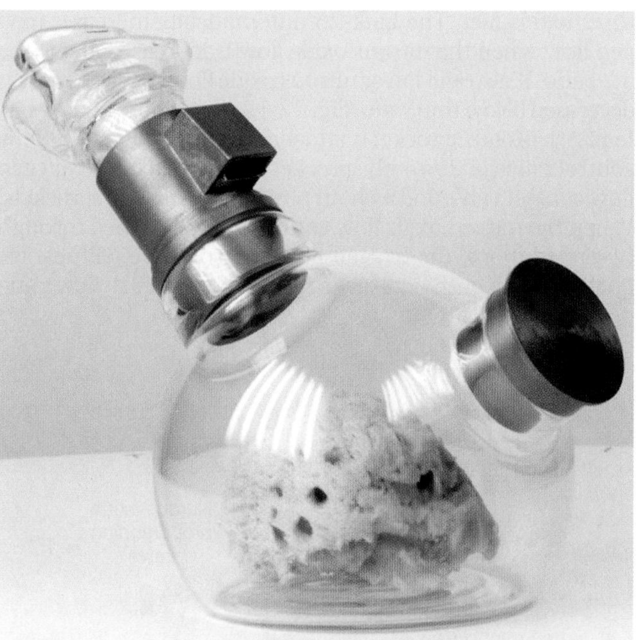

Fig. 22.13 Morton's ether inhaler: A replica of the inhaler used by William T. G. Morton during his public demonstration of ether anesthesia in October of 1846 at Massachusetts General Hospital in Boston. (Courtesy the Wood Library–Museum of Anesthesiology, Park Ridge, IL.)

Physics

The Ideal Gas Law. When sealed in a container, gas molecules collide with the walls and exert a force or pressure. This pressure is directly proportional to the number of molecules or moles *(n)* of gas present within the container and to the temperature *(T)* in degrees kelvin, and inversely proportional to the volume *(V)* that confines the gas. (One mole of a substance is equal to 6.022×10^{23} [Avogadro's number] molecules of that substance.) The ideal gas law is:

$$PV = nRT$$

R (the universal gas constant) = 8.314 L kPa/mol *K or 62.364 L mm Hg/mol*K

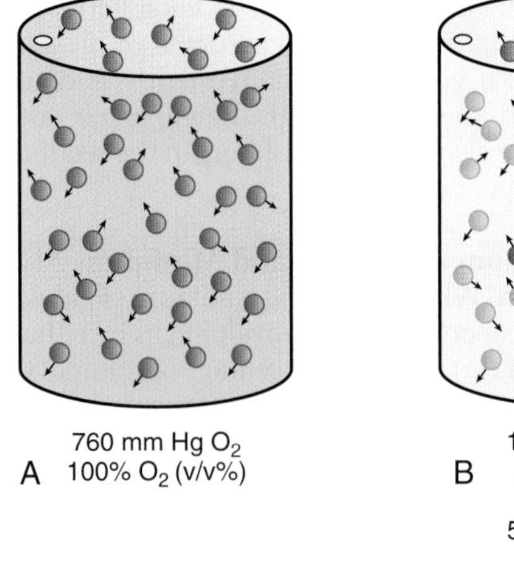
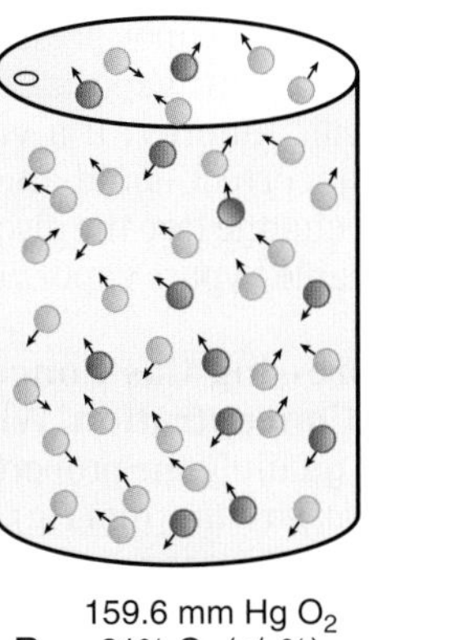

Fig. 22.14 Partial pressures. (A) Theoretical container filled with 100% oxygen at 1 atm pressure (760 mm Hg). The oxygen molecules account for the entirety of the pressure. $P_{total} = P_{oxygen} = 760$ mm Hg. (B) Pure oxygen is replaced with air, and now the nitrogen, oxygen, and other rare gases each contribute to the total pressure in proportion to their volume percent (v/v%). $P_{total} = P_{oxygen} + P_{nitrogen} + P_{other} = 760$ mm.

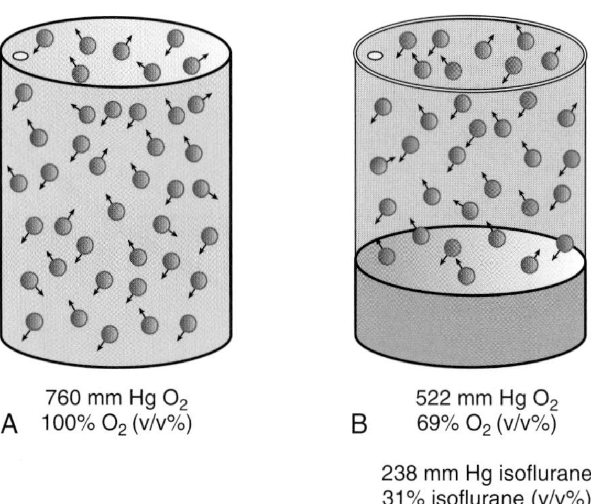

Fig. 22.15 Evaporation (vaporization) and vapor pressure. (A) Theoretical container with 100% oxygen. $P_{total} = P_{oxygen} = 760$ mm Hg, see Fig. 22.14. (B) Isoflurane is added to the container, and the temperature is maintained at 20°C (68°F). Evaporation commences, and isoflurane molecules begin to displace oxygen molecules out of the container. When the rate of vaporization is equal to the rate of condensation, the gas above the liquid is said to be "saturated" with isoflurane. The partial pressure of the isoflurane at this point is called the saturated vapor pressure (SVP), which at this temperature equals 238 mm Hg. $P_{total} = P_{oxygen} + P_{isoflurane} = 760$ mm.

The ideal gas law provides an important framework for understanding the behavior of anesthetic gases within vaporizers, anesthesia delivery equipment, and the pulmonary alveolus. Key assumptions of this law are that gas molecules (1) behave as points in space and (2) undergo perfectly elastic collisions without attracting or repelling one another or the walls of the container. These assumptions are valid for dilute anesthetic gases at normal operating conditions.

Dalton's Law of Partial Pressures. When a mixture of ideal gases exists in a container, each gas creates its own pressure, which is the same pressure as if the individual gas occupied the container alone. The total pressure may be calculated by simply adding together the pressures of each gas. This is known as Dalton's law of partial pressures, where the individual pressures (P_i) exerted by each of the constituent gases are referred to as *partial pressures*:[57,58]

$$P_{total} = P_1 + P_2 + P_3 + \ \ldots$$

Another useful expression, which can be derived by combining Dalton's law with the ideal gas law, is:

$$P_A = (n_A/n_{total})\,P_{total} = (v/v\%)\,P_{total}$$

which states that the partial pressure of gas A can be calculated by multiplying the total pressure of the mixture by the mole fraction (n_A/n_{total}), or the volume percent ($v/v\%$), of gas A. The volume percent tends to be more useful in day-to-day anesthesia practice (see below).

As a first step to understanding vaporizer function, it is useful to look at an example of Dalton's law of partial pressures. In Fig. 22.14*A*, pure oxygen fills a theoretical container that is open to the environment through a very small hole. The pressure in the container is equal to the ambient pressure, which at sea level is 760 mm Hg or 1 atm or 101.325 kPa, and generated entirely by the oxygen molecules. In Fig. 22.14*B*, the container is filled with air, and the total pressure is generated by the additive partial pressures of oxygen, nitrogen, and trace amounts of rare gases.

Evaporation and Vapor Pressure. Volatile liquids, such as inhaled anesthetic agents, are characterized by a high propensity to enter the gas phase, or *vaporize*. When a volatile liquid is exposed to air or other gases, molecules at the liquid surface with sufficient kinetic energy escape and enter the vapor phase. This process is known as *evaporation*, which is purely a surface phenomenon (in contrast to *boiling*, which occurs throughout the liquid). If liquid volatile anesthetic is placed within a contained space, such as a vaporizer, molecules will escape into the vapor phase until the rate of evaporation equals the rate of return to the liquid phase (a process known as *condensation*). When this equilibrium is reached, the gas above the liquid is said to be "saturated" with anesthetic (Fig. 22.15). The anesthetic molecules in the gas phase create a partial pressure known as the *saturated vapor pressure*, or simply *vapor pressure*. Liquids with a greater tendency to evaporate and generate higher vapor pressures are described as "more volatile."

Vapor pressure is an unique physical property of a substance at any given temperature (Fig. 22.16). Vapor pressure is *not* affected by changes in atmospheric pressure.[59] As illustrated in Fig. 22.17 for the isoflurane, evaporation is diminished at colder temperatures because fewer molecules possess sufficient kinetic energy to escape into the vapor phase. Conversely, at warmer temperatures, evaporation is enhanced and vapor pressure increases. Although

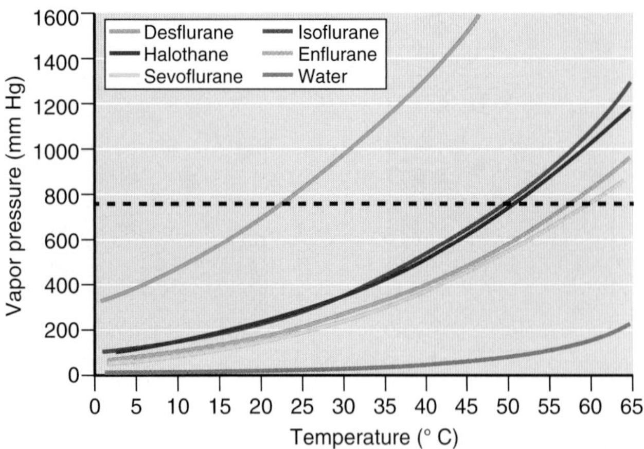

Fig. 22.16 Vapor pressure-versus-temperature curves for desflurane, isoflurane, halothane, enflurane, sevoflurane, and water. Note that the curve for desflurane differs dramatically from that of the other inhaled anesthetic agents. Also note that all inhaled agents are more volatile than water. Dashed line indicates 1 atm (760 mm Hg) of pressure, which illustrates the boiling point at sea level (normal boiling point). (From inhaled anesthetic package insert equations and Susay SR, Smith MA, Lockwood GG. The saturated vapor pressure of desflurane at various temperatures. *Anesth Analg.* 1996;83:864–866.)

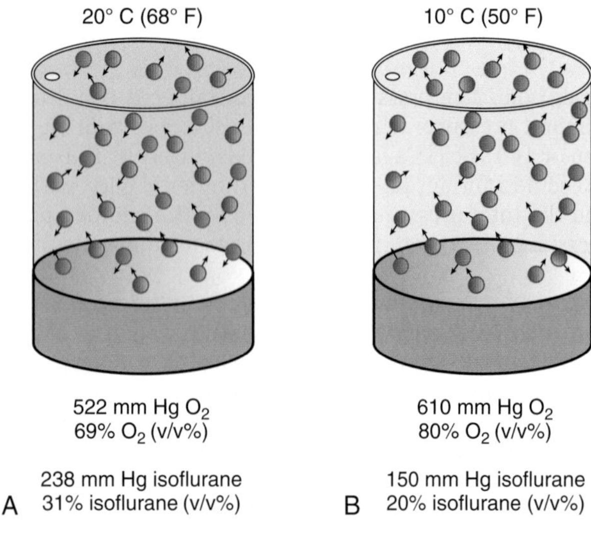

Fig. 22.17 The impact of temperature on vapor pressure. (A) Chamber containing oxygen and isoflurane at its saturated vapor pressure (SVP) at 20°C (68°F). At evaporative equilibrium, the SVP of isoflurane in the container represents 31% of the entire gas composition by volume (*v/v%*). (B) Decreasing the temperature to 10°C (50°F) substantially lowers the isoflurane vapor pressure to 150 mm Hg and causes isoflurane to represent only 20% of the entire gas volume (*v/v%*). This example assumes that some oxygen can enter the container through a tiny hole to replace the condensed isoflurane molecules.

operating room (ambient) temperature can raise or lower liquid anesthetic vapor pressure, the cooling influence of evaporation (the latent heat of vaporization, *see below*) has a far more pronounced and dynamic effect. The impact of evaporative temperature change on vaporizer and anesthetic inhaler output has been recognized since the mid-1800s, and addressing this phenomenon has been one of the principal factors influencing design of anesthetic vaporizers.

Because vapor pressures are unique to each liquid anesthetic agent, vaporizers must be constructed in an agent-specific manner. If a vaporizer is inadvertently filled with the incorrect liquid anesthetic agent, the vaporizer output will change (see the discussion of misfilling in the section on variable bypass vaporizers).[60,61]

Expressing Gas Concentrations and Minimum Alveolar Concentration. When describing a mixture of gases, we can quantify the proportion of an individual gas by either its *partial pressure* (mm Hg), or by the percentage of volume occupied by the gas relative to the sum of all gases present, which is known as *volume percent* or *volume-volume percent* (*v*/*v*%)[62]:

$$\text{Volume percent}(v/v\%) = (\text{volume of gas } x/\text{total gas volume}) * 100\%$$

The volume that an ideal gas occupies at a given temperature and pressure is related to the number of molecules of gas present, but not the size or identity of the molecules. This statement is known as the *Avogadro Hypothesis*. Using the ideal gas law, it is easy to calculate that at 1 atm (760 mm Hg) of pressure and 20°C (68°F or 293°K), conditions that might be found in a typical operating room, 1 mole of an ideal gas occupies a volume of about 24 L. The same is true for any mixture of ideal gases containing a total of 1 mole of gas molecules. Therefore, because partial pressure is directly proportional to the number of molecules of a gas present in the mixture, we can also use partial pressures to calculate the volume percent of any constituent gas[63]:

$$\text{Volume percent } (v/v\%) = (\text{partial pressure of gas } x/\text{total pressure}) * 100\% = (P_x/P_{\text{total}}) * 100\%$$

Using air at sea level ($P_{\text{total}} = P_{\text{atm}} = 760$ mm Hg) as an example:

Knowing the partial pressures of the constituent gases of air…

$$P_{\text{atm}} = P_{\text{oxygen}} + P_{\text{nitrogen}} + P_{\text{other}}$$

$$P_{\text{atm}} = 760\,\text{mm Hg} \approx (160 \text{ mm Hg oxygen}) + (592 \text{ mm Hg nitrogen}) + (8 \text{ mm Hg other gases})$$

… we can then calculate the volume percent (*v*/*v*%) of oxygen…

$$\text{Oxygen } (v/v\%) \sim P_{\text{oxygen}} / P_{\text{amt}} \sim 160 \text{ mm Hg} / 760 \text{ mm Hg} \sim 21\%$$

When anesthesiologists describe inhaled and exhaled anesthetic concentrations, they typically use volume percent. One percent isoflurane is equal to 7.6 mm Hg isoflurane at sea level. The amount of oxygen and nitrous oxide in the breathing gas is also typically described in terms of volume percent. However, CO_2 content (i.e., end-tidal carbon dioxide [$ETCO_2$]) is usually displayed as a partial pressure (mm Hg). This was probably adopted because of the relatively close correlation between $ETCO_2$ and arterial partial pressure of carbon dioxide ($PaCO_2$), and the latter's common expression as a partial pressure. Fig. 22.18 illustrates a typical composition of the breathing gases during anesthesia in terms of concentration (*v*/*v*%) and partial pressures.

The minimum alveolar concentration (MAC) is described in terms of volume percent. MAC is the concentration of anesthetic that prevents movement from surgical stimulus in 50% of individuals.[64] MAC is an age-dependent phenomenon,[65] and it can also be affected by other variables. MAC is a clinically useful value given that vaporizer control knobs are marked and calibrated in terms of anesthetic concentration. However, it is actually the anesthetic partial pressure (mm Hg) value in the brain that is responsible for anesthetic depth. The corresponding partial pressure for each MAC value is known as the minimal alveolar partial pressure (MAPP), as listed in Table 22.1.[66] When discussing anesthetic vaporizers, it is useful to think about their output in terms of partial pressure and how it relates to volume percent and MAC, especially when considering changes in ambient pressure.

Latent Heat of Vaporization. When a liquid such as a volatile anesthetic evaporates into the gas phase, energy is required to overcome the attractive intermolecular forces between molecules in the liquid phase (a property known as *cohesion*). The needed energy is absorbed from the surroundings in the form of *heat*, and is the reason why the human body is cooled by the evaporation of sweat. The amount of energy absorbed by a specific liquid during evaporation is referred to as the *latent heat of vaporization*. It is more precisely defined as the amount of energy in joules or calories (1 calorie = 4.184 joules) required to change 1 g of liquid into vapor at a constant temperature. In a well-insulated container, the energy for vaporization must come from the liquid itself. In the absence of an outside heat source, the remaining liquid cools as vaporization progresses. This leads to significant reductions in vapor pressure (see Fig. 22.16) and therefore the number of volatile anesthetic molecules in the gas phase (see Fig. 22.17).[44,59,67] If vaporizer design does not mitigate and compensate for evaporative cooling, output will decrease.

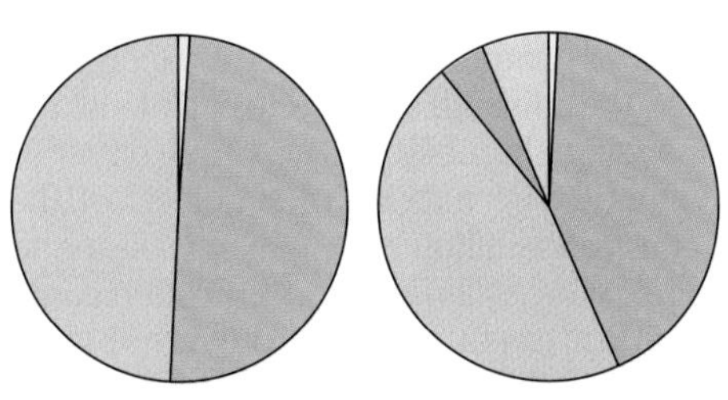

Gas	Inhalation mm Hg	Inhalation v/v%	Exhalation mm Hg	Exhalation v/v%
Sevoflurane	9	1.2	8	1.1
Oxygen	378	50	323	42
N_2O	373	49	347	46
CO_2	–	–	35	4.5
H_2O	–	–	47*	6.2
Total	760	100	760	100

*Saturated vapor pressure of water at body temperature.

Fig. 22.18 Common units of measure for breathing circuit gases: typical values for an oxygen-nitrous oxide-sevoflurane anesthetic. Anesthetic agent, oxygen, and nitrous oxide concentrations are typically expressed in volume percent (v/v%). Carbon dioxide is commonly described as a partial pressure (mm Hg).

Boiling Point. The *boiling point* of a liquid is defined as the temperature at which vapor pressure equals atmospheric pressure and the liquid begins to undergo rapid vaporization.[44,67] From the definition above, it is important to note that the boiling point changes depending on atmospheric pressure. Whereas evaporation is a surface phenomenon, boiling is a bulk phenomenon that occurs throughout the interior of the liquid. The boiling point of a liquid is inversely related to volatility. For example, water is not particularly volatile (see Fig. 22.16) and its boiling point of 100°C (212°F) at sea level is much higher than all of the inhaled anesthetic agents. Table 22.1 lists the *normal boiling point* (defined as the boiling point at a pressure of 1 atm) of the common volatile anesthetic agents. While most inhaled anesthetics boil in the range of 48° to 59°C (118°-138°F), desflurane has a normal boiling point close to room temperature (22.8°C or 73°F).

The boiling point of contemporary volatile anesthetic agents is not relevant to vaporizer design under most clinical situations. Desflurane, however, has a high saturated vapor pressure and boils at a temperature commonly encountered in clinical settings. These properties mandate a special vaporizer design to control agent delivery (see section on desflurane vaporizer). Isoflurane and halothane could theoretically boil at high altitudes and very high

TABLE 22.1 Physical Properties of Inhaled Volatile Anesthetic Agents

Property	Halothane	Isoflurane	Sevoflurane	Desflurane
SVP* @ 20°C (mm Hg)	243	238	157	669
SVC† @ 20°C at 1 atm‡ (v/v%)	32	31	21	88
MAC§ at age 40 year (v/v%)	0.75	1.2	1.9	6.0
MAPP¶ (mm Hg)	5.7	9.1	14.4	45.6
Boiling point @1 atm (°C)	50.2 (122.4°F)	48.5 (119.3°F)	58.6 (137.3°F)	22.8 (73°F)

**SVP*, Saturated vapor pressure. From anesthetic prescribing information.
†*SVC*, Saturated vapor concentration: the percentage of anesthetic agent relative to ambient pressure within an equilibrated (saturated) container (SVP/ambient pressure).
‡*1 atm*, 1 atmosphere = ambient pressure at sea level (760 mm Hg).
§*MAC*, Minimum alveolar concentration: the alveolar concentration that produces immobility in response to a noxious stimulus in 50% of subjects.[64] The denominator is approximately sea level pressure (760 mm Hg).
¶*MAPP*, Minimum alveolar partial pressure. The alveolar partial pressure that produces immobility in response to a noxious stimulus in 50% of subjects (the numerator in the MAC calculation).[66] Not affected by altitude. Calculated as MAC (fraction) × 760 mm Hg (i.e., for isoflurane = 0.012 × 760 mm Hg).
v/v%, Volume percent.

temperatures. At least one vaporizer manufacturer specifies a maximum safe operating temperature for these anesthetic agents.[68]

Specific Heat. The *specific heat* is the amount of energy required to increase the temperature of 1 g of a substance by 1°C.[44,67] Water, for example, has a specific heat of exactly 1 calorie g^{-1} deg^{-1}. The concept of specific heat is important to the design, operation, and construction of vaporizers in two ways. First, the specific heat of a liquid anesthetic determines how much heat must be supplied to maintain a constant temperature due to the latent heat of vaporization. Second, vaporizers are built from materials with a high specific heat in order to better resist temperature changes associated with evaporative cooling.

Thermal Conductivity. Thermal conductivity is a property that describes how well heat flows through a substance. The higher the thermal conductivity, the better a substance conducts heat.[44] Vaporizers are constructed of metals with relatively high thermal conductivity, which helps maintain a uniform internal temperature during evaporation by allowing efficient heat absorption from the environment. By contrast, coffee mugs should be made of materials with a low thermal conductivity to slow heat loss to the environment.

Modern Vaporizer Types

Vaporizer nomenclature can be somewhat confusing, especially if the historical context of vaporizer, workstation, and breathing circuit evolution is not considered (Table 22.2). Vaporizers are first designated as *in-circuit* or *out-of-circuit*, which describes their relationship to the patient's breathing circuit. Virtually all modern vaporizers are out-of-circuit, and their controlled output is introduced into the breathing circuit through a fresh gas line. In-circuit vaporizers are found mainly within the so-called *draw-over* anesthesia systems, which are of great historical significance in anesthesiology.

The second designation involves the specific types of vaporizers, and these currently include the variable bypass vaporizer (e.g., GE/Datex-Ohmeda Tec 7), the dual-circuit vaporizer (e.g., the classic GE/Datex-Ohmeda Tec 6 desflurane vaporizer), the cassette vaporizer (e.g., GE/Datex-Ohmeda Aladin cassette), the injection vaporizer (e.g., the Maquet vaporizer), and the now historical measured-flow vaporizer (e.g., Copper Kettle). Variable bypass vaporizers can be subcategorized as plenum type, which are out-of-circuit and have relatively high internal flow resistance (the term "plenum" refers to a chamber where gas flows under positive pressure), or draw-over type, which are in-circuit and have low internal resistance. Most modern variable bypass vaporizers are plenum type and are located out-of-circuit, like those seen in Figs. 22.1 and 22.2. Draw-over type vaporizers are uncommon today, but remain an option for providing anesthesia in resource-poor environments.[68a] Variable bypass vaporizers carry additional designations such as agent-specific, flow-over, temperature-compensated, and pressure-compensated, which are discussed later.

Variable Bypass Vaporizers. When volatile anesthetic agents evaporate, their resultant saturated gas concentrations greatly exceed those used clinically, so these concentrations must be diluted to safe ranges (see Table 22.1). *Variable bypass* refers to the method of diluting gas fully saturated with anesthetic agent with a more voluminous flow of gas. A diagram of a variable bypass vaporizer is shown in Fig. 22.19. Basic vaporizer components include a vaporizer inlet port (fresh gas inlet), the concentration control dial, the bypass chamber, the vaporizing chamber, the vaporizer outlet port, and the filling assembly. The maximum safe level of the vaporizer corresponds to the filling port, which is positioned to minimize the chance of overfilling. A concentration control dial determines the ratio of gas that flows through the bypass chamber and the vaporizing chamber, and a temperature-compensating device further adjusts that ratio. Vaporizer concentration control dials are labeled to set vaporizer output in terms of volume percent (*v*/*v*%), and the vaporizers are calibrated at sea level.

Fig. 22.20 illustrates volatile anesthetic equilibrium concentrations within a theoretical vaporizing chamber of a variable bypass vaporizer. As can be seen, the saturated vapor concentration of sevoflurane within the chamber (21%) far exceeds the clinical concentration. Fig. 22.20 also depicts the volume of anesthetic vapor that is added to the gas stream as it flows through the chamber. These properties are essential for a quantitative understanding of variable bypass vaporizer function (Box 22.1). Although this example and others in the chapter imply that the gas flowing through the vaporizing chamber becomes fully saturated with anesthetic vapor, this is actually not the case. There is insufficient time to reach evaporative equilibrium due to the constant inflow of fresh gas. As a result, the vaporizing chamber becomes only partially saturated with volatile anesthetic.[69] However, for the purposes of this discussion, it is useful to assume that full saturation occurs.

TABLE 22.2 Concise Summary of Modern Vaporizer Nomenclature

Type	Subtype(s)	Characteristics
Variable bypass vaporizers		
	Plenum type	Out-of-circuit, high resistance, gas flow under positive pressure
	Draw-over type	In-circuit, low resistance, gas flow under negative pressure; may be portable
Cassette vaporizer	GE Aladin and Aladin2	Computer-controlled variable bypass vaporizer
Dual-circuit (desflurane) vaporizer	GE Tec 6 and Dräger D-Vapor	Gas-vapor blender, heated & pressurized
Injection vaporizer	Maquet and Dräger DIVA	Direct injection of volatile anesthetic
Anesthetic reflector	AnaConDa, Mirus	Adsorption to and release from a carbon filter

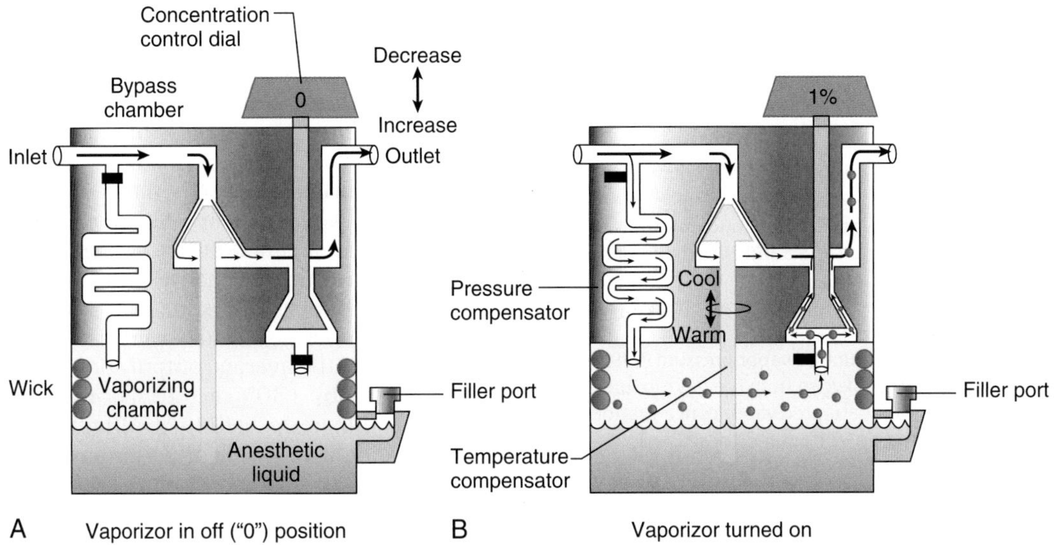

Fig. 22.19 Variable bypass vaporizer. (A) Basic components. Vaporizer in the off or "0" position. Fresh gas from the flowmeter assembly enters the vaporizer and then flows through the bypass chamber, around the temperature compensator, and out the vaporizer without passing through the vaporizing chamber. (B) Selecting a vaporizer output (turning the vaporizer "on") diverts an agent-specific ratio of gas through the pressure-compensating labyrinth, into the vaporizing chamber where it becomes saturated with anesthetic vapor, and then past the concentration cone where it reunites with the fresh gas stream. The temperature compensation device further adjusts the ratio of bypass to vaporizing chamber flow, to compensate for changes in anesthetic vapor pressure resulting from temperature changes. As the liquid anesthetic cools by evaporation, more gas is diverted to the vaporizing chamber to compensate for the decrease in vapor pressure. The labyrinth compensates for pressure fluctuations within the vaporizer from the gas supply side and the breathing circuit side to stabilize vaporizer output; it is *not* present to compensate for changes in atmospheric pressure. Please see text for additional details.

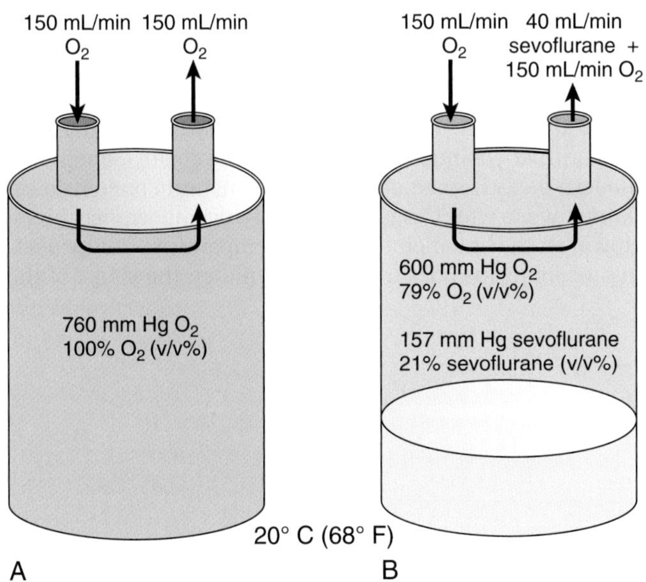

Fig. 22.20 Theoretical vaporizing chamber demonstrating the volume of anesthetic gas added to the gas flow stream as a result of evaporation: (A) Pure oxygen flows through the chamber. (B) Liquid sevoflurane is added to the chamber and evaporates to saturated vapor pressure (see Box 22.1 for details).

Fig. 22.21 illustrates a modern variable bypass vaporizer set to deliver 2% sevoflurane. Note how the majority of fresh gas flows straight through the bypass chamber. The bypass flow and vaporizing chamber output combine to create the desired output concentration. The fresh gas that is diverted to the vaporizing chamber becomes saturated with anesthetic gas by flowing through the wicks and over the liquid agent (hence the designation *flow-over*). The wicks and baffles serve to increase the surface area available for vaporization and promote mixing of the carrier gas with anesthetic vapor.[69a,69b] The specific ratio of fresh gas flow divided between the bypass chamber and the vaporizing chamber is determined by the concentration control dial setting and the temperature compensation device (see the later discussion of temperature compensation). Because the physical properties and clinical concentrations of each agent are unique, the diverting ratios are specific to each agent and dial setting (hence the designation *agent-specific*). The approximate variable bypass diverting or "splitting ratios" for the common anesthetic agents at 20°C are shown in Table 22.3. Variable bypass vaporizers cannot be used to deliver desflurane, because of this agent's unique physical properties (see section on the desflurane vaporizer).

Virtually all variable bypass vaporizers are equipped with a mechanism that helps maintain constant vaporizer output over a wide range of operating temperatures (hence the designation *temperature-compensated*). This mechanism automatically alters the ratio of gas flowing through the bypass and vaporizing chambers. Temperature compensation is accomplished by an expansion-contraction element, as seen in Fig. 22.19, or a bimetallic strip (Fig. 22.22). At cooler temperatures, the vapor pressure of liquid anesthetic decreases (Fig. 22.16), and it is necessary to reduce the splitting ratio to maintain output. In Fig. 22.19*B*, as the liquid anesthetic agent cools, the temperature-compensating cone moves upward, restricts bypass flow, and diverts more gas to the vaporizing chamber, thereby maintaining relatively stable vaporizer output. The inverse is also true: warmer temperatures cause the cone to move downward, increasing bypass flow, and diverting less gas to the vaporizing chamber. The most important function of temperature compensation devices is to correct for the effect of evaporative cooling on the liquid anesthetic.

BOX 22.1 Calculation of the Volume of Gas Added to a Fresh Gas Flow, and Proof of the Splitting Ratio

Step 1: Calculate the amount of volatile anesthetic added to the fresh gas stream that makes up a vaporizer chamber output.

- Assume that 150 mL/min of oxygen flows through a vaporizer chamber at 1 atm (760 mm Hg) pressure and 20°C (68°F) (Fig. 22.20*A*).
- Liquid sevoflurane is then added to the vaporizer chamber (Fig. 22.20*B*).
- Sevoflurane evaporates to its saturated vapor pressure (SVP) of 157 mm Hg, which displaces oxygen from the gas mixture. At this point, sevoflurane has a saturated vapor concentration (SVC) of 157 mm Hg/760 mm Hg ~21% (see Table 22.1).
- Sevoflurane makes up 21% of the gas flowing out of the vaporizer, and oxygen makes up 79%.
  - To calculate the amount of sevoflurane added to the fresh gas flow through the vaporizer, set up the simple proportion:
    - (*x* mL/min sevoflurane)/21% = (150 mL/min oxygen)/79%
  - Solve for *x*:
    - *x* = (150 mL/min) * 21%/79% ~ 40 mL/min sevoflurane
- Therefore 40 mL/min of sevoflurane is added to the vaporizer output, for a total of 190 mL/min (Fig. 22.20*B*).

Step 2: Prove the splitting ratio for a variable bypass vaporizer.

Building on the example in **Step 1**, consider a sevoflurane vaporizer with 2000 mL/min of fresh gas inflow. Prove that the splitting ratio must be ~12:1 in order to deliver 2% sevoflurane.

- A splitting ratio of 12:1 means that ~150 mL/min of fresh gas is diverted to the vaporizer chamber, and ~1850 mL/min flows through the bypass chamber (see Fig. 22.21).
- 40 mL/min of sevoflurane is added to the vaporizer output (see **Step 1**).
- The total vaporizer output is 2040 mL/min.
- Sevoflurane makes up (40 mL/min)/(2040 mL/min) ~2% of the total vaporizer output.

Variable bypass vaporizers are also constructed from materials with high specific heat, yielding temperature stability, and high thermal conductivity, which allows rapid transfer of ambient heat. Additionally, the vaporizer wick systems are located in contact with the metal walls to facilitate absorption of environmental heat.

FACTORS THAT INFLUENCE VARIABLE BYPASS VAPORIZER OUTPUT. An ideal variable bypass vaporizer would maintain a constant concentration output at a given setting regardless of variables such as the fresh gas flow rate, temperature, intermittent backpressure from the breathing circuit, carrier gas composition, and barometric pressure. ISO standards state that the average output should not deviate from the dial setting by +30% or −20% or more than +7.5% or −5% of the maximum setting.[11] Although modern vaporizers generally have excellent performance characteristics, it is important to understand how these challenges could potentially influence vaporizer output.

IMPACT OF GAS FLOW RATE. This factor is notable only at the extremes of flow rates and at higher concentration control dial settings. At low flow rates (<250 mL/min), the output tends to be slightly less than the dial setting due to the relatively high density of volatile anesthetic agents. Insufficient turbulence is generated in the vaporizing chamber to advance the vapor molecules upward. At high flow rates (such as 15 L/min), the output of most variable bypass vaporizers is somewhat less than the dial setting. This discrepancy is due to: cooling during rapid evaporation, incomplete mixing, and failure to saturate the carrier gas in the vaporizing chamber. In addition, the resistance characteristics of the bypass chamber and the vaporizing chamber can vary as flow increases.[68,70]

IMPACT OF TEMPERATURE CHANGE. Despite the impact of evaporative cooling and variation in ambient conditions, modern vaporizers maintain fairly constant concentration output over a wide range of common working temperatures. However, the linear change in the temperature-compensating mechanisms does not precisely match the shape of the

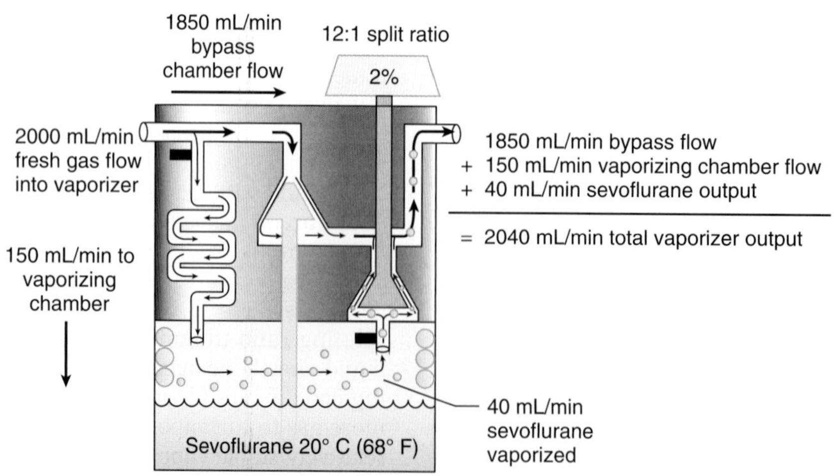

Fig. 22.21 Vaporizer set to deliver 2% sevoflurane at 1 atm (760 mm Hg): 2% sevoflurane requires a splitting ratio of 12:1 (see Table 22.3 and Box 22.1).

TABLE 22.3 Variable Bypass Vaporizer Splitting Ratios

Concentration Control Dial Setting (v/v%)	BYPASS CHAMBER–TO–VAPORIZING CHAMBER SPLITTING RATIOS AT 20°C (68°F)*		
	Halothane	**Isoflurane**	**Sevoflurane**
1	46:1	45:1	25:1
2	23:1	22:1	12:1
3	15:1	14:1	8:1

*Ratio of fresh gas flowing through the bypass chamber relative to the vaporizing chamber for the listed output concentrations. The temperature compensation device may alter the actual ratio. This applies to variable bypass vaporizers only. Calculated from: % volatile agent output = 100 × $P_V \times F_V/F_T\ (P_A - P_V)$ where P_A = atmospheric pressure, P_V = vapor pressure at 20°C, F_V = flow of fresh gas through vaporizing chamber (mL/min), and F_T = total fresh gas flow (mL/min).

From *Prescribing Information Forane [Isoflurane, USP]*. Deerfield, IL: Baxter Healthcare; 2009.

v/v%, Volume percent.

vapor pressure curves.[19,68] As a result, a slight correlation between vaporizer temperature and delivered concentration remains. This correlation is mainly apparent at higher temperatures and higher concentrations (Fig. 22.23). A dangerous but highly unlikely circumstance could occur if the boiling point of a volatile agent within a variable bypass vaporizer were reached. In this situation, the vaporizer output would be impossible to control by any compensatory mechanism. Although it would be rare to reach ambient temperatures around 50°C at sea level (see Table 22.1), at higher altitudes, where boiling points are lower, this is theoretically more likely. In fact, the Dräger Vapor 2000 user's manual decreases the high-altitude operating specification for the vaporizer from 9880 to 4800 feet if halothane or isoflurane is used at higher ambient temperatures. Manufacturers' published vaporizer operating temperatures range from 10°C to 40°C (50°F-104°F), although the specific ranges vary.[68,70-74]

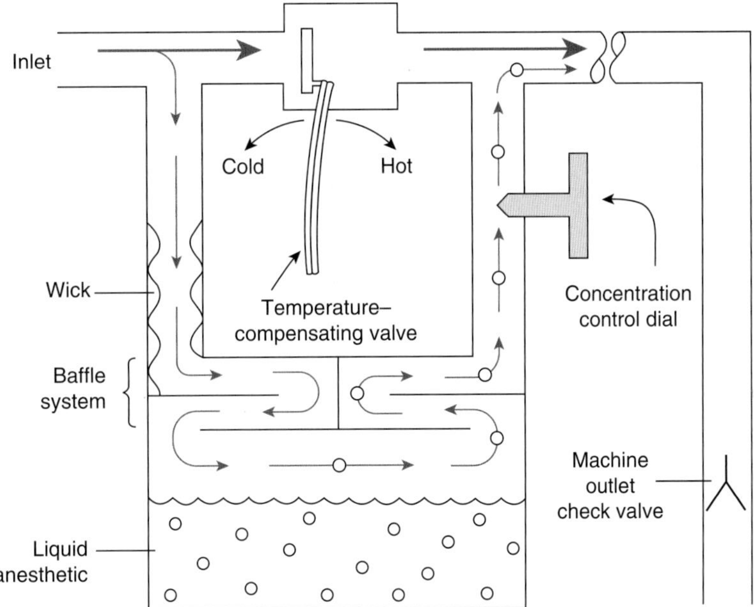

Fig. 22.22 Temperature compensation with a bimetallic strip. At cooler temperatures, the strip bends one way and diverts more flow through the vaporizing chamber. At warmer temperatures, the strip bends the opposite way and allows more flow through the bypass chamber. (From Chakravarti S, Basu S. Modern anaesthesia vapourisers. *Ind J Anaesth*. 2013;57[5]:464–471.)

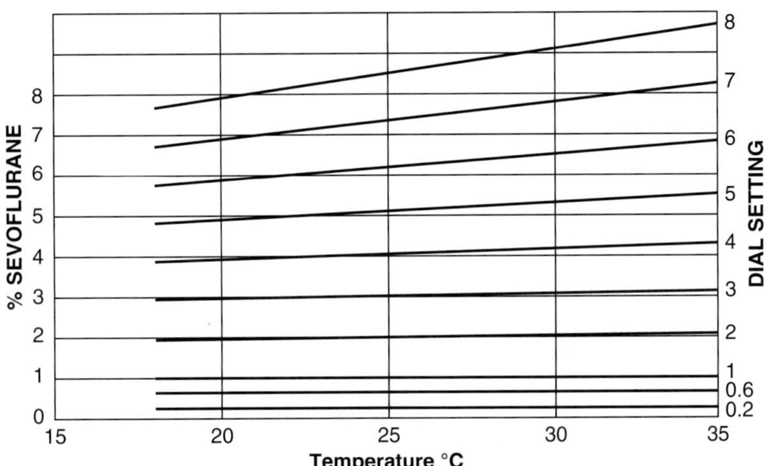

Fig. 22.23 Effect of ambient temperature on vaporizer output. See text for explanation. (Redrawn from Datex-Ohmeda. *Tec 7 Vaporizer: User's Reference Manual*. Madison, WI: Datex-Ohmeda; 2002.)

IMPACT OF INTERMITTENT BACKPRESSURE. The intermittent backpressure that results from either positive-pressure ventilation or use of the oxygen flush valve may lead to higher than expected vaporizer output. This phenomenon, known as the *pumping effect*, is more pronounced at low flow rates, low dial settings, and low levels of liquid anesthetic in the vaporizing chamber.[44,68,75-77] Additionally, the pumping effect is increased by rapid respiratory rates, high peak inspiratory pressures (PIPs), the use of anesthesia machines without fresh gas decoupling, and rapid drops in pressure during expiration.[44,59,67,68,78,79] Although contemporary variable bypass vaporizers are not highly vulnerable to the pumping effect, the proposed mechanism and preventative design features should be understood. The pumping effect is caused by retrograde transmission of pressure from the patient circuit to the vaporizer during the inspiratory phase of positive-pressure ventilation or use of the oxygen flush function. Gas molecules are compressed in both the bypass and vaporizing chambers. When the backpressure is suddenly released during the expiratory phase, vapor exits the vaporizing chamber both antegrade through the outlet and retrograde through the inlet. This occurs because the output resistance of the bypass chamber is lower than that of the vaporizing chamber, particularly at low dial settings. The enhanced output concentration results from the increment of vapor that travels in the retrograde direction to the bypass chamber.[68,76,77,80]

To decrease the pumping effect, modern vaporizing chambers are smaller than those of early variable bypass vaporizers so that only a small volume of vapor can be discharged retrograde into the bypass chamber.[77] Additionally, some vaporizers have a long spiral tube or labyrinth that serves as the inlet to the vaporizing chamber (see Fig. 22.19).[77] When the pressure in the vaporizing chamber is released, the vapor does not flow back into the bypass chamber because of tube length.[59] This serpentine passage also dampens pressure fluctuations and compensates for fluctuations in gas supply pressure. Other designs may also include an extensive baffle system in the vaporizing chamber. Finally, a one-way check valve can be inserted after the vaporizers and before the breathing circuit inlet to minimize the pumping effect (see the discussion of the gas supply system). This check valve can attenuate but does not eliminate the increase in pressure, because gas still flows from the flowmeters to the vaporizer during the inspiratory phase of positive-pressure ventilation.[44,81] Although intermittent backpressure can result in transient rises in anesthetic concentration at the common gas outlet, the effects are mitigated by dilution within the much larger anesthetic breathing circuit.[82] The goal of all these pressure-compensating mechanisms is to provide an even flow of gas through the vaporizing chamber despite changes in pressure, giving the vaporizers the additional designation *pressure-compensated*.

IMPACT OF CARRIER GAS COMPOSITION. Variable bypass vaporizer output can be influenced by fresh gas composition. This phenomenon is the result of differences in the solubility of carrier gases in volatile anesthetic liquids. This effect is most pronounced when nitrous oxide is introduced or removed as a carrier gas.[68,83-90] In the experimental example seen in Fig. 22.24, a change in carrier gas from 100% oxygen to 100% nitrous oxide results in a sudden decrease in halothane output (expressed as volume percent) followed by a slow increase to a new, lower, steady-state (see Fig. 22.24, label *B*).[88,89] Because nitrous oxide is more soluble than oxygen in the liquid anesthetic within the vaporizer sump, more of the carrier gas dissolves, and the volume output from the vaporizing chamber is transiently reduced.[88] Once the anesthetic liquid becomes saturated with nitrous oxide, the vaporizing chamber output increases and achieves a new steady state.

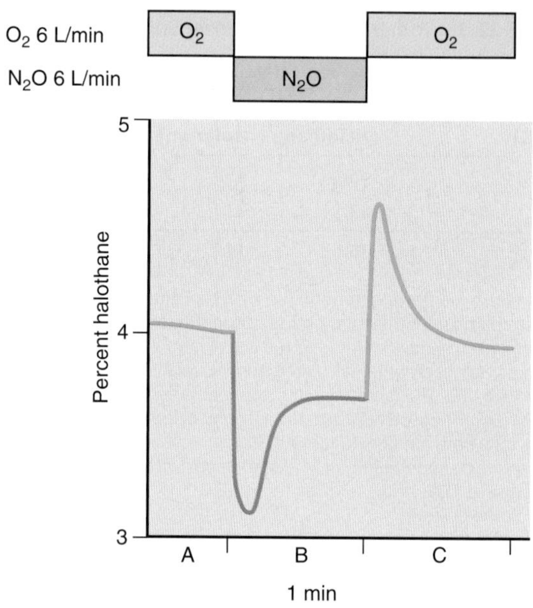

Fig. 22.24 Halothane output of a North American Dräger Vapor 19.n vaporizer (Dräger Medical, Telford, PA) with different carrier gases. The initial output concentration is approximately 4% halothane when oxygen is the carrier gas at flows of 6 L/min *(A)*. When the carrier gas is quickly switched to 100% nitrous oxide *(B)*, the halothane concentration decreases to 3% within 8 seconds. A new steady-state concentration of approximately 3.5% is then attained within about 1 minute. When O_2 flow is reestablished, halothane output increases abruptly and then settles back to baseline *(C)*. See text for details. (Modified from Gould DB, Lampert BA, MacKrell TN. Effect of nitrous oxide solubility on vaporizer aberrance. *Anesth Analg*. 1982;61:939.)

The explanation for the new steady-state output value is less well understood.[90] Differences in density and viscosity between oxygen and nitrous oxide are likely responsible[90a] because these physical properties affect the relative amount of gas flow through the bypass and vaporizing channels.[86,89,91] Helium, a gas with far lower density than either oxygen or nitrous oxide, has been shown to have variable effect on vaporizer output, depending on the vaporizer model and study design (although the changes tend to be minimal).[92,93]

Although the carrier gas composition can be demonstrated experimentally to affect vaporizer output, deviations are often within specified accuracy ranges. Vaporizer user's manuals usually specify the anticipated response to a change in carrier gas relative to the calibration gas, which may be air or oxygen, depending on the vaporizer model.[68,70,71,94]

IMPACT OF BAROMETRIC PRESSURE CHANGES. Understanding the influence of barometric pressure on variable bypass vaporizer output is probably more important for comprehending vaporizer function than for actual clinical reasons. With variable bypass vaporizers, the depth of anesthesia at a given dial setting is relatively independent of atmospheric pressure, and no adjustments need to be made (Table 22.4).[68]

TABLE 22.4 Comparative Performance of an Isoflurane Variable Bypass Vaporizer and the Tec 6 Desflurane Vaporizer During Changes in Barometric Pressure

		Isoflurane Variable Bypass Vaporizer With Dial Setting of 0.89% (v/v)			Tec 6 Desflurane Vaporizer With Dial Setting of 6%
Atm	**Ambient Pressure (mm Hg)**	**mL Isoflurane Vapor Entrained by 100 mL O_2**	**Vaporizer Isoflurane Output (v/v%)**	**Vaporizer Isoflurane Output (mm Hg)**	**Vaporizer Desflurane Output (mm Hg)**
0.66	500 (≈10,000 ft)	91	1.7	8.8	30
0.74	560 (≈8200 ft)	74	1.5	8	33.6
0.8	608 (≈6000 ft)	64	1.2	7.6	36.5
1.0	760 (sea level)	46	0.89	6.8	45.6
1.5*	1140	26	0.5	5.9	68.4
2*	1520	19	0.36	5.5	91.2
3*	2280	12	0.23	5.2	136

*ATA or *atmospheres absolute*. ATA = *atmospheric pressure + water pressure*. Hyperbaric oxygen chamber protocols apply ATA. Many protocols use depths from 2.0 to 2.5 ATA, but some conditions such as gas embolus or carbon monoxide poisoning may require depths to 3.0 ATA.[238] 2 ATA ≈ 33 feet of sea water (fsw) ≈ 1520 mm Hg *ambient pressure*.
atm, Atmospheres (1 atm = 760 mm Hg); *v/v%*, volume percent.
Modified from Ehrenwerth J, Eisenkraft J. Anesthesia vaporizers. In: Ehrenwerth J, Eisenkraft J, eds. *Anesthesia Equipment: Principles and Applications*. St. Louis: Mosby; 1993:69–71.

HIGHER ALTITUDE. As previously discussed, vapor pressure is independent of barometric pressure. Therefore as altitude increases and barometric pressure declines, the partial pressure of anesthetic agent in the vaporizing chamber remains constant despite decreases in the partial pressures of other constituent breathing gases and the total ambient pressure. This situation results in significantly increased volume percent concentration of anesthetic agent within the vaporizing chamber and at the outlet of the vaporizer (see Table 22.4). However, because anesthetic depth is determined by the *partial pressure* of volatile agent in the brain, the clinical impact is minor (see MAPP in Table 22.1).

Let us consider an example of moving a vaporizer from sea level to higher altitude. With a constant dial setting of 0.89%, at 1 atm, a well-calibrated isoflurane variable bypass vaporizer would deliver 0.89 *v/v%* isoflurane, and the partial pressure of isoflurane output would be 6.8 mm Hg. Assume that we maintain the same dial setting and lower the atmospheric pressure to 0.66 atm or 502 mm Hg (roughly equivalent to an elevation of 10,000 feet. This results result in an increase in the isoflurane concentration output to 1.75% (a 97% increase), but the partial pressure increases to only 8.8 mm Hg (a 29% increase). A similar change in output partial pressure at sea level, in terms of volume percent, would correspond to an isoflurane concentration increase of only 0.2%. So while the anesthetic concentration (*v/v%*) changes significantly in this example, it is the partial pressure of volatile agent in the brain that is ultimately responsible for anesthetic depth, and that change is minimal.

As described earlier, MAC values for contemporary inhalational anesthetic agents were determined at sea level. Similarly, anesthetic vaporizers are calibrated at sea level, thus ensuring that vaporizer output (*v/v%*) matches the dial setting. Using the isoflurane data shown in Table 22.4 as an example, one can see how confusion may arise when thinking of MAC in terms of volume percent and considering barometric change.

The MAPP at altitude is the same as at sea level because it is a partial pressure, whereas the MAC increases because it is a simple concentration. Table 22.4 shows that the *partial pressure output* of a variable bypass vaporizer changes proportionally less than the volume percent concentration as altitude increases. Because the partial pressure of volatile agent determines anesthetic depth, the operator *does not* need to adjust the dial to a higher setting to compensate for barometric pressure. This holds true for variable bypass vaporizers, but not for the desflurane Tec 6–style vaporizer (see later).

HYPERBARIC CONDITIONS. Although anesthesia is sometimes delivered in *hyperbaric conditions*, intravenous anesthesia is easier to deliver in this setting. Under hyperbaric conditions, the partial pressure of volatile anesthetic in the vaporizing chamber remains constant despite an increase in ambient pressure and the partial pressure of the other gases. The net theoretical effects on variable bypass vaporizers are a significant decrease in anesthetic concentration (*v/v%*) and a mild decrease in partial pressure output. However, the partial pressure of halothane was noted to increase slightly with increasing barometric pressure under experimental conditions.[95] Possible explanations for this finding include the effect of increased atmospheric gas density on the flow of gas through the vaporizer and the increased thermal conductivity of air at higher pressure. The clinical significance of these small changes in partial pressure output under hyperbaric conditions is unclear.

OTHER SAFETY FEATURES. Contemporary variable bypass vaporizers incorporate many other safety features. Agent-specific, keyed filling devices help prevent filling with the wrong agent. Overfilling is minimized by locating the filler port at the maximum safe liquid level. Modern vaporizers are firmly secured to a manifold on the anesthesia workstation to prevent tipping. Contemporary interlock systems prevent the administration of more than one inhaled anesthetic agent. However, virtually all safety systems have vulnerabilities, so it remains important to understand these potential hazards.

MISFILLING. Misfilling of anesthetic vaporizers with the wrong agent can result in an overdose or underdose of volatile anesthetic.[96,97] Vaporizer output in these circumstances depends on the erroneous agent's saturated vapor pressure and the splitting ratio of the misfilled vaporizer, since these key parameters must normally be matched to ensure accurate agent delivery (see earlier discussion). Similarly, mixtures of anesthetic agents can also result in harmful dosing.[60] Agent-specific filling devices have reduced, but not eliminated, misfilling. The potential for misfilling exists even in vaporizers equipped with keyed fillers,[98-100] and current standards do not mandate their use.[20] The use of breathing circuit gas analysis may alert the user to misfilling. If a variable bypass vaporizer for isoflurane or sevoflurane is misfilled with desflurane, a substantial overdose could occur because of the high vapor pressure of desflurane (see Fig. 22.16).

CONTAMINATION. Although rarely reported, contamination of anesthetic vaporizer contents has occurred. In one instance, organic contaminants (some volatile) in a bottle of isoflurane were detected because of an abnormal acrid odor emanating from the vaporizer.[101] In another report, water accumulation within sevoflurane vaporizers allowed bacteria *(Staphylococcus epidermidis)* to grow and metabolize liquid sevoflurane to volatile and potentially toxic compounds.[101a]

TIPPING. Tipping of a variable bypass vaporizer can occur when it is incorrectly removed, transported, or replaced. Excessive tipping can allow the liquid agent to enter the bypass chamber and cause an extremely high output.[102] Although some vaporizers are more sensitive than others, most should not be used after tipping until they have been flushed for a period of time at high flow rates. Manufacturers' instructions differ regarding their post-tipping procedures, so it is best to refer to each specific user manual.[68,70,71,94] A gas analyzer should be used to assess vaporizer output before replacing into clinical use. The Dräger Vapor and D-Vapor series vaporizers have a transport ("T") dial setting that isolates the vaporizer chamber from the bypass chamber to eliminate the possibility of internal overflow during transport.[68]

OVERFILLING. Improper filling procedures, combined with failure of the vaporizer sight glass, can cause patient overdose. If overfilled, liquid anesthetic may enter the bypass chamber, and a harmful dose of vapor could be delivered to the common gas outlet.[103] It is a requirement that contemporary vaporizers be designed so that they cannot be overfilled when they are used in a normal operating position.[20] Side-fill variable bypass vaporizers, as opposed to top-fill devices, largely prevent overfilling because the maximum safe level is predetermined by the position of the filler port (see Fig. 22.19). In addition, some vaporizers are equipped with an overflow hole as an additional safeguard.[68] Overfilling can still occur if the vaporizer is tipped or turned on while filling, or air enters at the bottle neck and filler adapter caused by a loose or faulty seal.[103-106]

LEAKS. Vaporizers and the vaporizer-machine interface are potential sources of gas leaks that can result in patient awareness during inhaled anesthesia. Loose filler caps, filler plugs, and drain valves are probably the most common sources of leaks. Such a leak may be obvious (e.g., an audible gas leak with spillage of anesthetic agent) or have a more subtle presentation (such as a lower than expected inhaled agent concentration, or the odor of anesthetic gas).[107,108] Another common source of gas leak occurs at the junction of the vaporizer and the mounting bracket or manifold, where broken mounting assemblies or foreign bodies can compromise the seal between the vaporizer and its point of attachment.[109-112] Gas leaks can also occur within the vaporizer itself as a result of mechanical failure.

ENVIRONMENTAL CONSIDERATIONS. Anesthesia delivery has become more common outside the operating rooms, and one challenging location is the magnetic resonance imaging (MRI) suite. The presence of a powerful magnetic field, significant noise pollution, and limited access to the patient during the procedure all complicate care in this setting. The anesthesia provider must appreciate the extremely powerful magnetic fields in these locations and know that only nonferrous (MRI-compatible) equipment can be used. Although some anesthesia vaporizers may appear nonferrous by testing with a horseshoe magnet, they may indeed contain substantial internal ferrous components. Inappropriate use of such devices in an MRI suite may turn them into dangerous missiles if left unsecured.[113]

Desflurane Vaporizer. Because of its unique physical characteristics, accurate delivery of desflurane required a different approach to vaporizer design. The Datex-Ohmeda Tec 6 vaporizer was released into clinical use in the early 1990s. The Tec 6 is an electrically heated, pressurized device specifically designed to deliver desflurane (Fig. 22.25).[114,115] Dräger Medical received approval from the U.S. Food and Drug Administration (FDA) for the D-Vapor, its version of the desflurane vaporizer in 2004. The operating principles apply to either system, although the discussion refers to the Tec 6 specifically. The Datex-Ohmeda Aladin cassette vaporizer and the Maquet vaporizers are discussed separately because their operating principles are different.

UNSUITABILITY OF CONTEMPORARY VARIABLE BYPASS VAPORIZERS FOR CONTROLLED VAPORIZATION OF DESFLURANE. Desflurane's high volatility and moderate potency (see Table 22.1) preclude its use with contemporary variable bypass vaporizers for three main reasons[114]:

1. *Desflurane's high rate of evaporation would require excessive diluting gas (bypass chamber) flow.* The vapor pressure of desflurane is 669 mm Hg at 20°C (68°F), which is significantly higher than other inhaled anesthetic agents (see Fig. 22.16).[116] At 1 atm and 20°C, 100 mL/min passing through the vaporizing chamber would entrain 735 mL/min of desflurane (as compared with 29, 46, and 47 mL/min of enflurane, isoflurane, and halothane, respectively).[114] To produce a 1% desflurane output, the amount of bypass flow required to dilute the large volume of desflurane-saturated anesthetic vapor would be approximately 73 L/min (in contrast to 5 L/min or less for the other three agents). Prohibitively high bypass chamber flow rates would be required to dilute the vaporizing chamber output to clinical concentrations.
2. *Desflurane's high rate of evaporation would cause substantial anesthetic cooling.* Variable bypass vaporizers require ambient heat to offset evaporative cooling. Although the latent heat of vaporization for desflurane

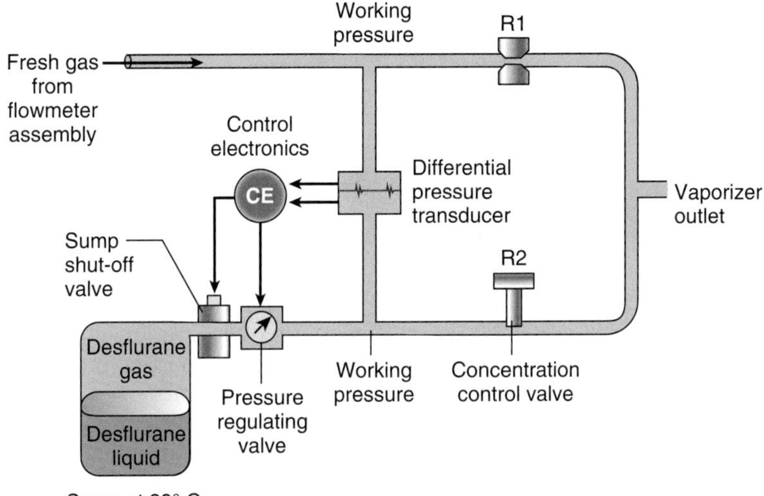

Fig. 22.25 Simplified schematic of the Tec 6 desflurane vaporizer (Datex-Ohmeda, Madison, WI). See text for details. (From Andrews JJ. *Operating Principles of the Ohmeda Tec 6 Desflurane Vaporizer: A Collection of Twelve Color Illustrations.* Washington, DC: Library of Congress; 1996.)

is approximately equal to that of enflurane, isoflurane, and halothane, its MAC is much higher. The amount of desflurane required to be vaporized over a given period is considerably greater than that of the other inhaled anesthetics. Supplying desflurane in equivalent MAC concentrations would lead to excessive cooling of the vaporizer and reduced output without an external heat source. Because of the broad range of temperatures seen in the clinical setting and desflurane's steep vapor pressure–versus-temperature curve (see Fig. 22.16), desflurane delivery would not be stable in a conventional variable bypass vaporizer.[114]

3. *Desflurane is more likely to boil.* The boiling point of desflurane is 22.8°C (73°F) at 1 atm. This temperature is at the higher end of normal operating room temperatures. If the anesthetic agent were to boil within a variable bypass–type vaporizer, the output would be uncontrollable. The amount of vapor produced would be limited only by heat transfer to the desflurane liquid, which depends upon the specific heat and thermal conductivity of the vaporizer (see discussion above).[114]

OPERATING PRINCIPLES OF THE TEC 6 AND TEC 6 PLUS. The Tec 6 desflurane vaporizer was the first clinically available vaporizer to be electrically heated and pressurized, making many aspects of the internal design and operating principles radically different from variable bypass vaporizers. The Tec 6 is probably more accurately described as a dual-gas blender than as a vaporizer. A simplified schematic of the Tec 6 is shown in Fig. 22.25. The vaporizer has two independent gas circuits arranged in parallel. The fresh gas circuit is shown in *orange*, and the vapor circuit is shown in *blue*. Fresh gas from the flowmeters enters at the fresh gas inlet, passes through a fixed restrictor (R1), and exits at the vaporizer gas outlet. The vapor circuit originates at the desflurane sump, which is a reservoir of desflurane vapor. It is electrically heated to 39°C, a temperature much higher than desflurane's boiling point. At 39°C, the vapor pressure in the sump is approximately 1300 mm Hg (~2 atm).[117] Just downstream from the sump is the shut-off valve. After the vaporizer warms up, the shut-off valve fully opens when the concentration control valve is turned to the "on" position.

TABLE 22.5 Fresh Gas Flow Rate Versus Working Pressure in the Tec 6 Desflurane Vaporizer

Fresh Gas Flow Rate (L/min)	Working Pressure at R1 and R2 (mm Hg)
1	7.4
5	37.0
10	74.0

From Andrews JJ, Johnston RV Jr. The new Tec 6 desflurane vaporizer. *Anesth Analg.* 1993;76:1338.

A pressure-regulating valve located downstream from the shut-off valve down regulates the pressure to the pressure of the background gas. The operator controls the output of desflurane by adjusting the concentration control valve (R2), which is a variable restrictor.[114]

The vapor flow through R2 joins the fresh gas flow through R1 at a point downstream from the restrictors. Until this point, the two circuits are physically separated. They are interfaced pneumatically and electronically, however, through differential pressure transducers, a control electronics system, and a pressure-regulating valve. When fresh gas flows past the fixed restrictor R1, a specific backpressure proportional to the flow rate pushes against the diaphragm of the differential pressure transducer. The transducer relays the pressure difference between the fresh gas circuit and the desflurane vapor circuit to the control electronics system. The control system tunes the pressure-regulating valve so that the pressure in the vapor circuit equals the pressure in the fresh gas circuit. This equalized pressure supplying R1 and R2 is the working pressure, which is constant at a fixed fresh gas flow rate. If the operator increases the fresh gas flow rate, more backpressure will be exerted on the diaphragm of the pressure transducer, and the working pressure of the vaporizer will increase.[114] Table 22.5 shows the linear relationship between fresh gas flow rate and working pressure for a typical Tec 6 vaporizer.

The following are two specific examples to demonstrate the operating principles of the Tec 6:[114]

TABLE 22.6 Dial Setting Versus Flow Through Restrictor R2 at 1 L/min Fresh Gas Flow in the Tec 6 Desflurane Vaporizer

Dial Setting (vol%)	Approximate Vapor Flow Rate Through R2 (mL/min)
1	10
6	64
12	136
18	220

From Andrews JJ, Johnston RV Jr. The new Tec 6 desflurane vaporizer. *Anesth Analg.* 1993;76:1338.

Example A: *Constant fresh gas flow rate of 1 L/min with an increase in the dial setting.* With a fresh gas flow rate of 1 L/min, the pressure supplying R1 and R2 is 7.4 mm Hg. As the operator increases the dial setting, the opening at R2 becomes larger, thereby allowing more vapor to pass through R2. Specific vapor flow values at different dial settings are shown in Table 22.6.

Example B: *Constant dial setting with an increase in fresh gas flow from 1 to 10 L/min.* At a fresh gas flow rate of 1 L/min, the working pressure is 7.4 mm Hg, and at a dial setting of 6%, the vapor flow rate through R2 is 64 mL/min (see Tables 22.5 and 22.6). With a 10-fold increase in the fresh gas flow rate, the working pressure increases to 74 mm Hg. Because R2 is supplied by 10 times more pressure, the vapor flow rate through R2 increases 10-fold to 640 mL/min. Both fresh gas flow and vapor flow increase proportionally, so vaporizer output is constant.

FACTORS THAT INFLUENCE TEC 6 DESFLURANE VAPORIZER OUTPUT. Barometric pressure and carrier gas composition influence the Tec 6 vaporizer output.

HIGHER ALTITUDE. Although ambient pressure changes affect the volume percent output of *variable bypass vaporizers* significantly, the effect on partial pressure output is minimal (and recall that the partial pressure of volatile agent in brain tissue is the main determinant of anesthetic depth). By contrast, the partial pressure output of Tec 6 style desflurane vaporizers is significantly affected by altitude, as can be seen in Table 22.4. One must remember that the Tec 6 device is more accurately described as a dual-gas blender than a vaporizer. Regardless of ambient pressure, the Tec 6 will maintain a constant volume percent output (v/v%), *not a constant partial pressure.* This means that at high altitudes, the partial pressure of desflurane will decrease in proportion to the reduction in atmospheric pressure divided by the calibration pressure (normally 760 mm Hg) per the following formula:

Required dial setting (%) = Normal dial setting × (760 mm Hg) / [Ambient pressure (mm Hg)]

For example, at an altitude of 2000 m, or 6564 feet, where the ambient pressure is 608 mm Hg, the operator must advance the concentration control dial from 10% to 12.5% to maintain the required anesthetic partial pressure. In hyperbaric settings, the operator must decrease the dial setting to prevent delivery of an overdose. At 2 atm or 1520 mm Hg of pressure, the desflurane output in mm Hg is twice that at sea level (91.2 vs. 45.6 mm Hg).

CARRIER GAS COMPOSITION. Vaporizer output most closely matches the dial setting when oxygen is the carrier gas because the Tec 6 vaporizer is calibrated with 100% oxygen. When a carrier gas other than 100% oxygen is used at low flow rates, a clear trend toward reduction in vaporizer output emerges. This reduction correlates with the decrease in viscosity of the carrier gas. Nitrous oxide is less viscous than oxygen, and generates lower backpressure upstream of resistor R1 (see Fig. 22.25). As a result, the working pressure is reduced. At low flow rates with nitrous oxide as the carrier gas, vaporizer output is approximately 20% less than the dial setting.

SAFETY FEATURES. Because desflurane's vapor pressure is nearly 1 atm, misfilling a variable bypass vaporizer with desflurane could theoretically result in both overdose and creation of a hypoxic gas mixture. Like most of its contemporaries, the desflurane vaporizer has a unique, anesthetic-specific filling system to minimize this potential hazard. Each desflurane bottle has a "SAF-T-FILL" adapter intended to prevent use with traditional vaporizers. The SAF-T-FILL is essentially a spring-loaded valve that seals the bottle until the bayonet fitment is fully engaged in the filler port of a desflurane vaporizer.[119] This mechanism also helps guard against evaporative loss of agent during storage. The adapter has an O-ring on the tip to minimize spillage during filling.[119a] Thus the SAF-T-FILL system helps prevent both misfilling of variable bypass vaporizers and leakage of desflurane to the atmosphere.[119b]

Major vaporizer faults cause the shut-off valve located just downstream from the desflurane sump (see Fig. 22.25) to close and terminate output. The valve closes, and a no-output alarm is activated, if any of the following conditions occur: (1) the anesthetic level decreases to less than 20 mL, (2) the vaporizer is tilted, (3) a power failure occurs, or (4) the pressure difference between the vapor and fresh gas circuits exceeds a specified tolerance. Although such automated safeguards can enhance patient safety, they may have unintended consequences. For example, a previous generation of Datex-Ohmeda D-Tec Plus vaporizer was reported to be incompatible with a certain model of Dräger anesthesia machine.[120] By design, this workstation interrupted fresh gas flow during the inspiratory phase of volume control ventilation as a means of fresh gas decoupling. These purposeful fresh gas flow interruptions caused an alarm and inappropriate termination of vaporizer output. Although the vaporizer was subsequently modified, this example serves as a reminder that new technology can bring about new problems.

SUMMARY. The Tec 6 and Dräger D-Vapor vaporizers are electrically heated, thermostatically controlled, constant-temperature, pressurized, electromechanically coupled dual-circuit, gas vapor blenders. The pressure in the vapor circuit is electronically regulated to equal the pressure in the fresh gas circuit. At a constant fresh gas flow rate, the operator regulates vapor flow with a conventional concentration control dial. When the fresh gas flow rate increases, the working pressure increases proportionally. For a given concentration setting, even when varying the fresh gas flow rate, the vaporizer output is constant because the amount of flow through each circuit remains proportional.[114]

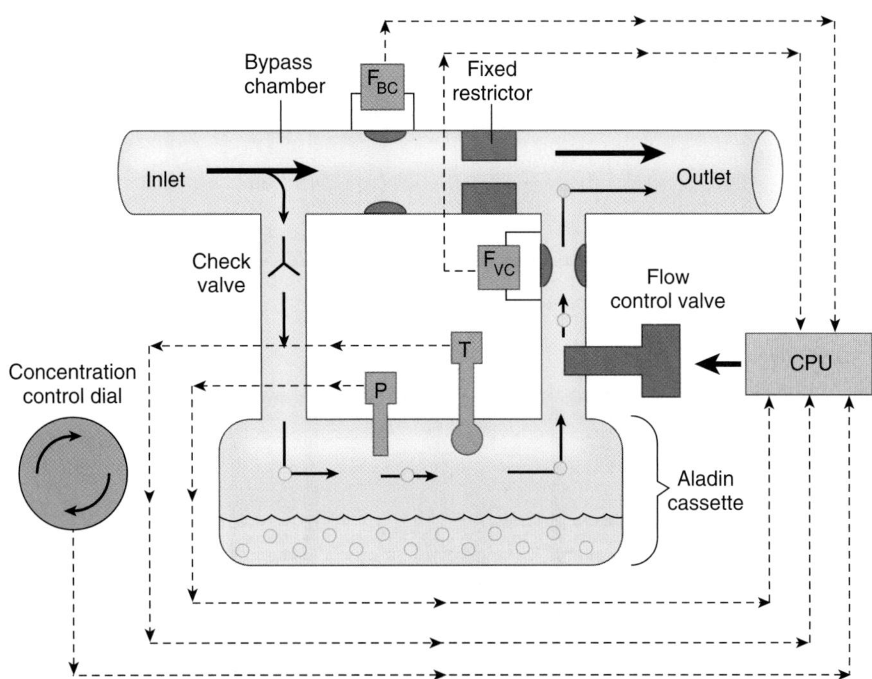

Fig. 22.26 Simplified schematic of Datex-Ohmeda Aladin cassette vaporizer (Datex-Ohmeda, Madison, WI). The black arrows inside the vaporizer represent flow from the flowmeters, and the yellow circles represent anesthetic vapor. The heart of the vaporizer is the electronically controlled flow control valve located in the outlet of the vaporizing chamber. *CPU,* Central processing unit; F_{BC}, flow measurement unit that measures flow through the bypass chamber; F_{VC}, flow measurement unit that measures flow through the vaporizing chamber; *P,* pressure sensor; *T,* temperature sensor. Please see text for additional details. (Modified from Andrews JJ. *Operating Principles of the Datex-Ohmeda Aladin Cassette Vaporizer: A Collection of Color Illustrations.* Washington, DC: Library of Congress; 2000.)

GE/Datex-Ohmeda Aladin and Aladin2 Cassette Vaporizers. The vaporizer system used in the GE Aisys anesthesia workstations (and some former Datex-Ohmeda models) is unique in that a single electronically controlled vaporizer is designed to deliver several different inhaled anesthetic agents. The vaporizer consists of a permanent internal control unit housed within the workstation and interchangeable cassettes that contain anesthetic liquid and serve as vaporizing chambers. The Aladin cassettes (now superseded by the Aladin2) are filled using agent-specific fillers and color-coded: red (halothane), orange (enflurane), purple (isoflurane), yellow (sevoflurane), and blue (desflurane). They are also magnetically coded to allow the anesthesia workstation to identify which cassette has been inserted.

Operationally, the Aladin cassette vaporizing system is best described, during most circumstances, as a computer-controlled variable bypass vaporizer (Fig. 22.26). It consists of a bypass section and vaporizing chamber, the latter of which is contained within the interchangeable cassette (Fig. 22.27). A fixed restrictor located in the bypass chamber causes gas flow from the inlet to split into two streams. One stream passes through the bypass chamber, and the other is diverted to the vaporizing chamber where it passes through a one-way check valve. This valve prevents retrograde flow of anesthetic vapor into the bypass chamber, and its presence is unique to the Aladin system. The one-way check valve is essential for precise delivery of desflurane (see below). Failure of the check valve to close can result in anesthetic overdose due to retrograde flow into the bypass chamber.

Within the cassette, anesthetic agent vaporizes freely to saturated vapor pressure. A flow control valve, modulated by a central processing unit (CPU), precisely meters the amount of gas flow through the vaporizing chamber, which then rejoins the bypass flow.[44] The CPU receives input from multiple sources: the concentration control dial, pressure and temperature sensors inside the vaporizing chamber, and flow sensors in the bypass and vaporizing chambers. The CPU also receives input from the flowmeters regarding the carrier gas composition, which can affect vaporizer output as described above. Using these data, the CPU precisely regulates fresh gas flow through the vaporizing chamber to obtain the desired vapor concentration output.[121]

As mentioned in the discussion of the Tec 6, controlled vaporization of desflurane presents a unique challenge, particularly when room temperature is higher than the boiling point (22.8°C [73°F]). If the desflurane were to boil, the pressure inside the vaporizing chamber would exceed ambient pressure. When vaporizing chamber pressure exceeds that in the bypass chamber, the one-way check valve closes and prevents carrier gas from entering the cassette. Carrier gas passes straight through the bypass chamber and its flow sensor. Under these conditions, the CPU adjusts the flow control valve to meter in the appropriate flow of pure desflurane vapor needed to achieve the desired final concentration. The vaporizer then begins functioning as an injector, as opposed to resembling a variable bypass unit.

During delivery of inhaled agents at high fresh gas flow rates and/or high dial settings, large quantities of anesthetic liquid are rapidly vaporized. As a result, the temperature of the vaporizer sump decreases due to evaporative

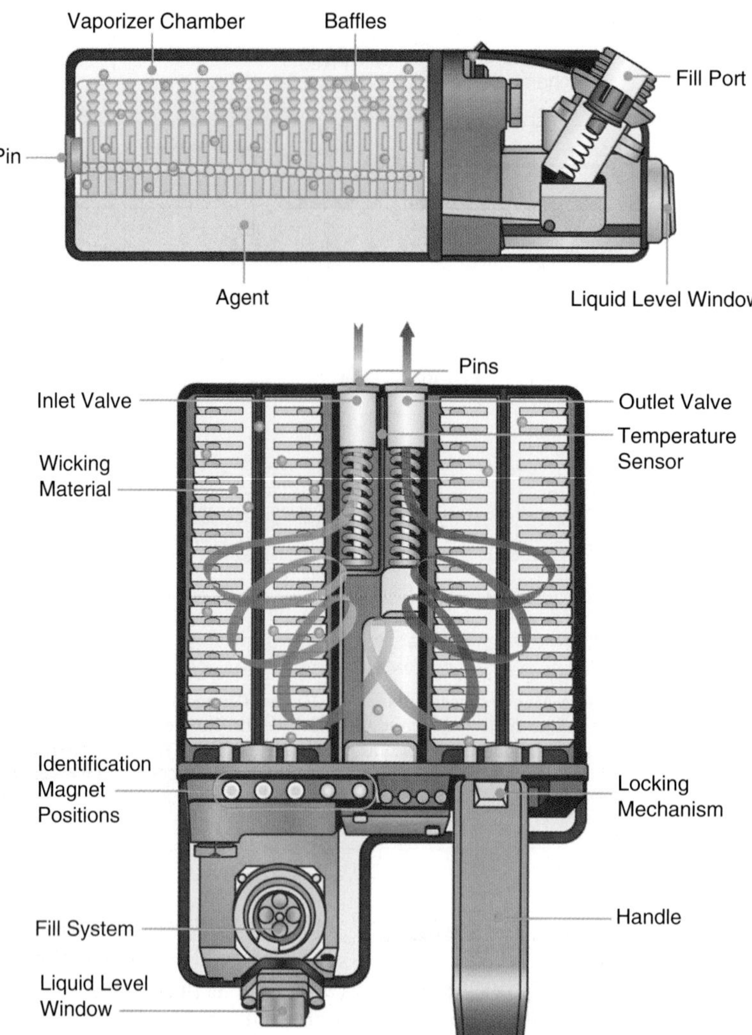

Fig. 22.27 Gas flow and safety features of the Aladin2 cassette. Top, side view illustrating filling system and baffles. Bottom, top view showing safety features, wicks, and gas flow during vapor uptake. (From GE HealthCare.)

cooling. To offset this cooling effect, some workstations are equipped with a fan that forces warmed air from a resistor across the cassette to raise its temperature when necessary. The fan is activated during two common clinical situations: (1) desflurane induction and maintenance and (2) sevoflurane induction.

The Aladin vaporizing system incorporates many important safety features. Electronic control of the carrier gas ratio guards against delivery of a hypoxic gas mixture. This ensures that no less than 25% oxygen is delivered at the common gas outlet regardless of carrier gas composition *and* concentration of anesthetic agent. This feature is unique, since conventional oxygen–nitrous oxide proportioning systems are not affected by the concentration of potent inhaled anesthetic agents. The system is also equipped with a safety relief valve that opens when cassette pressure exceeds 2.5 atm (1899 mm Hg). When the Aladin cassette is removed from the workstation, valves close to prevent loss of fresh gas. Another valve prevents liquid anesthetic from entering the fresh gas line. The system also has an overfilling protection mechanism.[121a] Finally, the Aladin cassette is immune to tipping and has no restrictions on orientation during handling or storage.[121]

Injection-Type Vaporizers: Maquet and Dräger Direct Injection of Volatile Anesthetic. The Maquet vaporizer is an electronically controlled, injection-type vaporizer that is used exclusively with Maquet FLOW-i anesthesia workstations. Because these vaporizers are located upstream from the patient's breathing circuit, they are designated as out-of-circuit vaporizers, similar to the desflurane vaporizers and most variable bypass vaporizers. The Maquet injection vaporizers are agent-specific and available for isoflurane, sevoflurane, and desflurane. Externally, the device has a lid, filling port, electronic level indicator, and alert indicators, but no concentration control dial. Vaporizer output adjustments are accomplished through an electronic interface on the workstation.

The Maquet vaporizer principle of operation is illustrated in Fig. 22.28. Gas from the anesthesia machine enters through the drive gas inlet and pressurizes a reservoir of liquid anesthetic. This pressure provides the force to drive

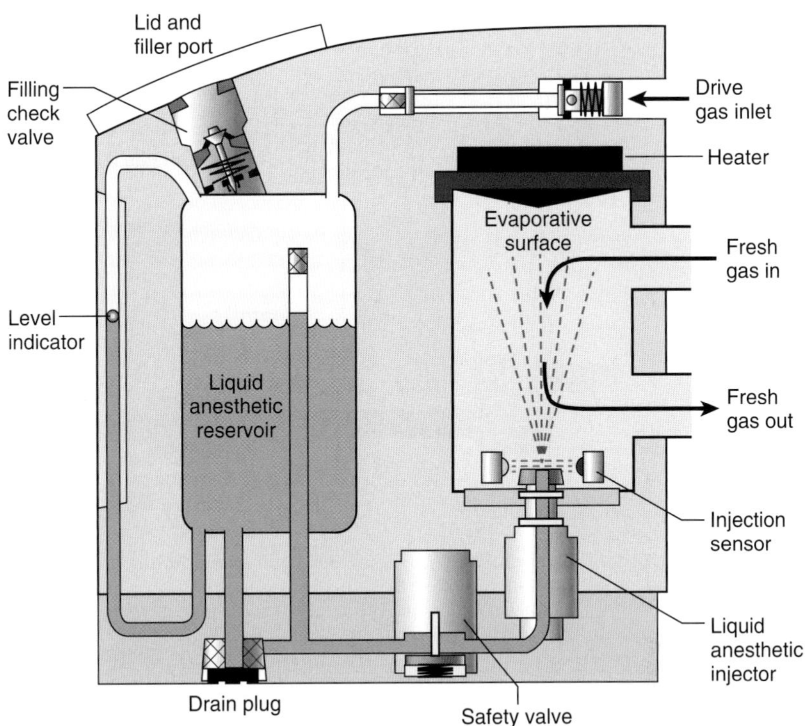

Fig. 22.28 The Maquet anesthetic vaporizer. Drive gas from the anesthesia machine is used to pressurize a liquid anesthetic reservoir. Under microprocessor control, liquid agent is injected into a vaporizing chamber. Injection is carefully monitored. A heated surface within the vaporizing chamber facilitates evaporation of the anesthetic agent. Fresh gas flows through the chamber and is enriched with anesthetic gas. A safety valve stops the flow of liquid agent in the case of vaporizer malfunction. (Personal communication, illustration adapted with permission from Maquet Critical Care, Solna, Sweden, January 14, 2013.)

liquid through the injector (and also minimizes evaporation within the reservoir chamber). Liquid anesthetic is injected into a heated vaporizing chamber in pulses that are under microprocessor control. Rapid evaporation occurs. Injection continues in small increments until the desired volume is obtained. The total amount injected in any given interval is based on the desired anesthetic concentration and the fresh gas flow through the vaporizer. A dedicated gas analysis line downstream from the vaporizer monitors the output. An optical sensor in the vaporizer monitors the integrity of the anesthetic injections (personal communication, Maquet Critical Care, January 14, 2013).

Fresh gas from the anesthesia workstation flows through the vaporizing chamber and is enriched with anesthetic agent. Although some of the injected liquid anesthetic evaporates while in flight within the vaporizing chamber, the remainder is deposited on a heated surface that ensures immediate evaporation. Heating of the evaporative surface is carefully regulated to compensate for evaporative cooling (personal communication, Maquet Critical Care, January 14, 2013).

During the daily workstation pre-use check, Maquet vaporizers are automatically tested with respect to functionality and leaks. A safety valve stops the flow of liquid agent in the event of vaporizer malfunction. The vaporizer is not vulnerable to tipping because it has no wicks to saturate, and agent cannot spill into the vaporizing chamber. The vaporizer can be filled during use, although no vaporizer output occurs during filling. An alarm triggers when the liquid anesthetic level is less than 10%, and a higher-priority alarm triggers when it reaches 5%. Limited data is available on the Maquet vaporizer's performance with different fresh gas flow rates,[121b] but the impact of changing barometric pressure, temperature, and fresh gas composition has not been reported.

Some Dräger anesthesia workstations are also equipped with vaporizers that function by the direct injection of volatile anesthetic (DIVA) principle (Fig. 22.29). Dräger DIVA vaporizers are agent specific. They consist of an interchangeable vaporizing module and a gas supply arrangement that is part of the workstation.[69a,121c] Liquid anesthetic agent is held in a reservoir. The liquid flows by gravity into a dosing chamber, where it is pressurized by gas supply from the workstation. The liquid passes through a dosing valve, and it is sprayed by a fuel injector into a heated vaporizing chamber. The anesthetic agent evaporates rapidly to its vapor pressure and is then conducted into the patient's breathing circuit under microprocessor control. The feedback control unit may be set to target a certain volatile agent concentration as a percentage of either the fresh gas stream or the patient's end-tidal gas.

Draw-Over Vaporizers in Contemporary Practice. As described above, most modern anesthesia workstations incorporate *plenum-type variable-bypass* vaporizers or other sophisticated units that require pressurized flow of carrier gases to drive vaporization and delivery. However, compressed medical gases (oxygen or air) are not available in many resource-constrained environments. *Draw-over* vaporizers remain a popular option for delivering anesthesia in such settings, including military field operations.[121d] They are characterized by (1) *in-circuit* location, (2)

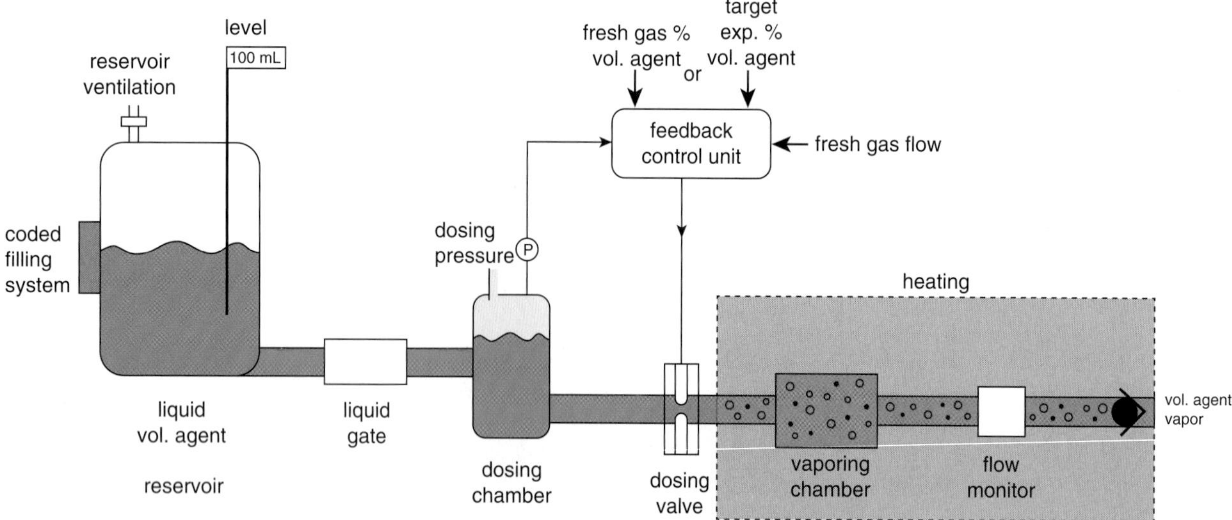

Fig. 22.29 Schematic of the Dräger DIVA vaporizer (Drägerwerk AG & Co. KGaA. Diagram reprinted with permission). The vaporizer consists of two modules: an interchangeable vaporizing module, and a gas supply module that is part of the anesthesia workstation. The vaporizing module includes a reservoir for liquid agent and a dosing chamber. The gas supply module consists of a feedback control unit that provides dosing pressure and control, as well as a system of valves. The valves may target vapor injection into either a mixing chamber (to mix with fresh gas flow) or directly into the breathing system (injection independent of fresh gas flow). See text for details.

low-resistance to gas flow, and (3) gas flow that is driven by negative downstream pressure (typically arising from the patient's respiratory effort, but potentially from a bellows or compressible bag). For a more thorough discussion of *draw-over* anesthesia technique in resource-limited settings, please see Chapter 2, Section 3. The basic design principles are worth a brief illustration.

The Oxford Miniature Vaporizer (OMV) is a stainless steel, variable-bypass, draw-over vaporizer that has been in use since 1968 and is particularly popular in the British Armed Forces.[121e] It has a robust, simple, and portable design and holds up to 50 mL of liquid anesthetic.[69b] A calibrated dial controls flow through an aperture between a slide valve and obturator located in the bypass chamber (Fig. 22.30).[121f] Closing the aperture directs more flow into the vaporizing chamber and increases output. Metal mesh wicks increase the surface area for vaporization yet add little resistance to gas flow. The OMV is not temperature compensated and output varies significantly with ambient temperature.[121g] It does feature a heat sink of water and ethylene glycol ("antifreeze") housed in the base to resist temperature swings. The OMV is not agent-specific, and different calibrated dials are available for halothane, isoflurane, and sevoflurane.[44] In order to deliver sufficient sevoflurane concentration for an inhaled induction, two OMVs must be used in series.[121h] Recently, the *Diamedica Draw-Over Vaporizer* (*DDV*) has been developed. Although similar in design to the OMV, the DDV tends to deliver more accurate results across a range of dial settings and ambient temperatures.[69a] It also has a larger reservoir (150 mL) for liquid agent and is available in two versions (halothane/isoflurane and sevoflurane).[121i]

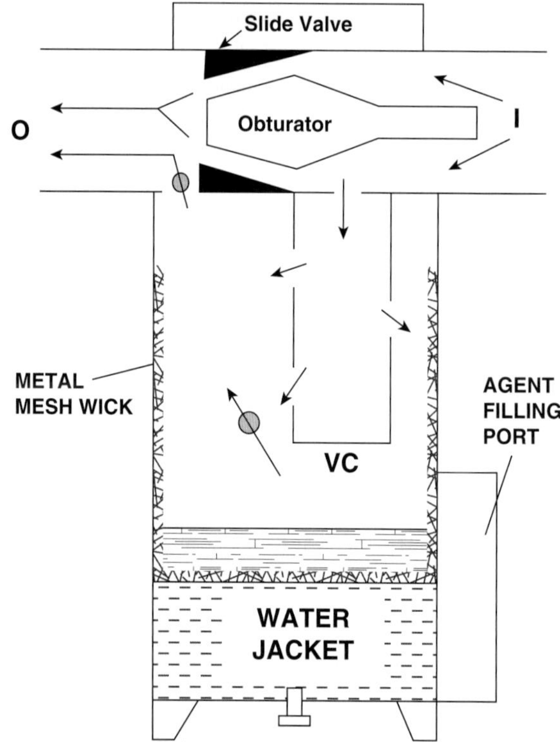

Fig. 22.30 Oxford miniature vaporizer. Gas flows from the inlet, *I*, through a slide valve and towards the outlet, *O*. A dial controls motion of an obturator that diverts flow to the vaporizing chamber, *VC*, and determines vaporizer output. (Redrawn from Dhulkhed V, Shetti A, Naik S, et al. Vapourisers: physical principles and classification. *Ind J Anaesth.* 2013;57[5]:455–419.)

Volatile Anesthetic Reflectors: AnaConDa and Similar Devices. There has been a resurgence of interest in providing inhaled volatile anesthetics to patients in locations outside of the operating room, such as the ICU, where commercial anesthesia workstations are not readily available.[121j] Indications for ICU delivery of volatile anesthetics include refractory bronchospasm and status epilepticus (see also Chapter 79), as well as a potential alternative to intravenous sedation.[121k] Barriers to providing volatile anesthesia in the intensive care setting include (1) rapid

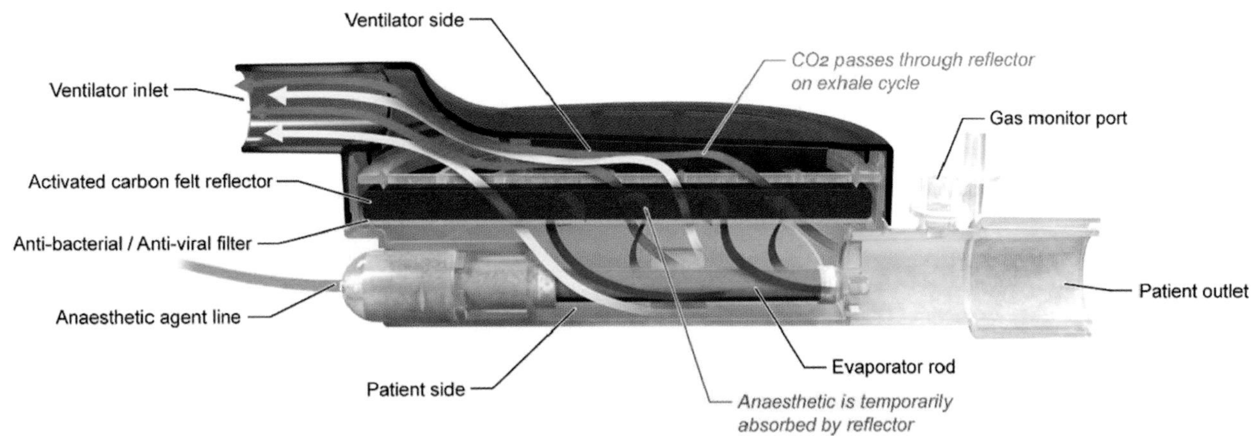

Fig. 22.31 **Anesthetic conserving device (AnaConDa) showing the flow of gas during exhalation.** (From Farrell R, Oomen G, Carey P. A technical review of the history, development and performance of the anaesthetic conserving device "AnaConDa" for delivering volatile anaesthetic in intensive and postoperative critical care. *J Clin Monitor Comput.* 2018;32[4]:595–604.)

consumption of volatile anesthetics due to the high gas flow rates of modern ICU ventilators, and (2) environmental safety and occupational health hazards due to atmospheric contamination and ineffective scavenging of waste gases.

One possible solution for ICU delivery of volatile anesthetics are *reflector*-style devices such as the *anesthetic conserving device* (AnaConDa) and *Mirus* device.[121l,121m] The AnaConDa is a single-use device based on a heat and moisture exchanger (HME) filter and does not require a power source or an anesthesia workstation (Fig. 22.31).[121n] Liquid volatile anesthetic (either isoflurane or sevoflurane) is injected into the device using a standard syringe pump and vaporized through a porous evaporator rod. The patient breathes in the anesthetic vapor normally. Upon exhalation, the breathing gases pass through several layers of filter. The first is an antimicrobial layer typical of HME filters. The second layer is activated carbon that rapidly adsorbs exhaled volatile anesthetic with high efficiency, while CO_2 and other exhaled gases pass through. Upon the next inspiratory cycle, the adsorbed volatile anesthetic molecules are released from the carbon filter and "reflected" towards the patient for re-breathing. The efficiency of the device is approximately 90%, with only 10% loss of vapor passing through the reflector to the ventilator waste gases. A gas sampling port allows for monitoring of end-tidal volatile agent concentration and titration of the syringe pump infusion rate. The Mirus device works on a similar concept, but is capable of delivering desflurane, and incorporates automatic control of end-tidal concentrations.[121l]

ANESTHETIC BREATHING CIRCUITS

Fresh gas departs from the supply system and enters the anesthetic breathing circuit through the fresh gas line. The functions of the breathing circuit are to deliver oxygen and other gases to the patient and to eliminate CO_2. The breathing system must contain a low-resistance conduit for gas flow, a reservoir that can meet the patient's inspiratory flow demand, and an expiratory port or valve to vent excess gas.[122] Beyond these fundamentals, circuits are categorized as those that use an absorber to eliminate CO_2 (the circle system) and those that do not (the Mapleson circuits).[123] Circle systems are the most common breathing circuits used for anesthetic delivery. However, certain Mapleson systems are used in anesthesia workstations, particularly in pediatrics, and they are often used by anesthesia providers during transport of patients, procedural sedation, liberation from tracheal intubation (the T-piece), and preoxygenation during out-of-the-operating-room airway management. Therefore both systems are discussed.

Leaks and obstruction represent the two most important hazards associated with the breathing circuit. Most of the time, these problems can be detected during the pre-use checkout of the workstation. However, a firm understanding of the components and function of the breathing system is critical if one is to perform a proper checkout and troubleshoot acute problems. The operator should also be aware of the various standards and alarms associated with this critical part of the anesthesia workstation.

Circle Breathing Systems

The circle breathing system is so named because it allows circular, unidirectional flow of gas facilitated by one-way valves. For many years, the overall design of the classic circle system changed little. Most anesthesia workstations had circle systems with similar schematics and components (Figs. 22.32–22.34). More recently, however, circle breathing systems have evolved along with the technological complexity of workstations. These changes have resulted from efforts to improve patient safety with features such as integrated fresh gas decoupling during positive-pressure ventilation.

The circle system consists of several essential components, including (1) a fresh gas inflow source, (2) inspiratory and expiratory unidirectional valves, (3) inspiratory and expiratory corrugated tubes, (4) a Y-piece that connects to the patient, (5) an overflow or APL or "pop-off" valve, (6) a reservoir or breathing bag, and (7) a canister containing a CO_2 absorbent (see Fig. 22.32). Several additional components are added to enhance patient safety, including a circuit pressure sensor, a pressure gauge, an expiratory (and possibly an inspiratory) flow sensor, and an inspired oxygen concentration sensor. A separate positive end-expiratory pressure (PEEP) valve may be present. Circle

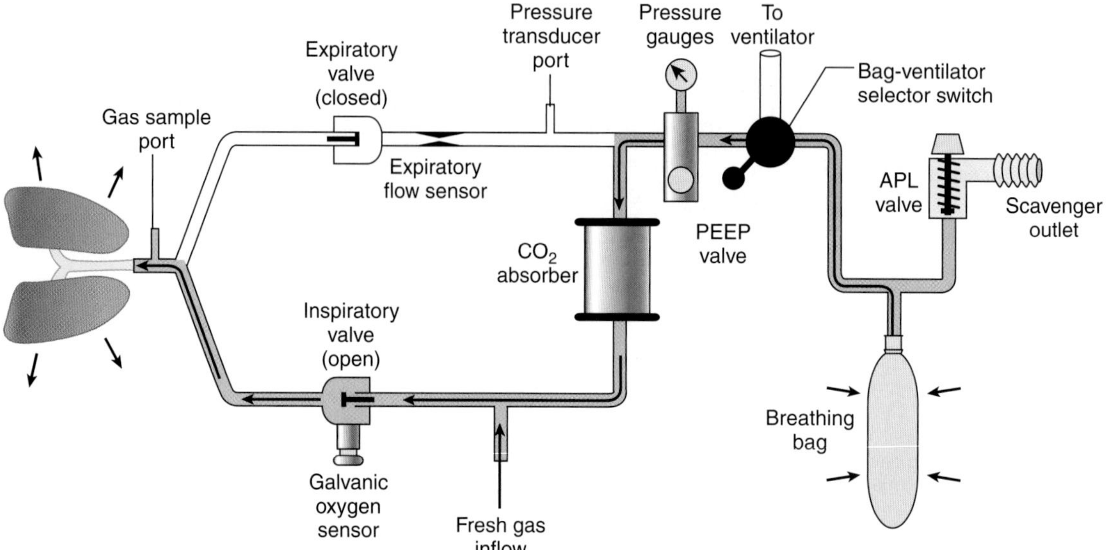

Fig. 22.32 Classic circle breathing system. Spontaneous breathing-inspiratory phase (ventilator not shown). Gas is drawn by the patient from the breathing bag and through the carbon dioxide *(CO_2)* absorber. It is then mixed with the fresh gas inflow from the gas supply system, traverses the inspiratory valve, and flows to the patient. The expiratory valve prevents rebreathing by not allowing flow to bypass the CO_2 absorber. *APL,* Adjustable pressure-limiting; *PEEP,* positive end-expiratory pressure. (Courtesy Dr. Michael A. Olympio; modified with his permission.)

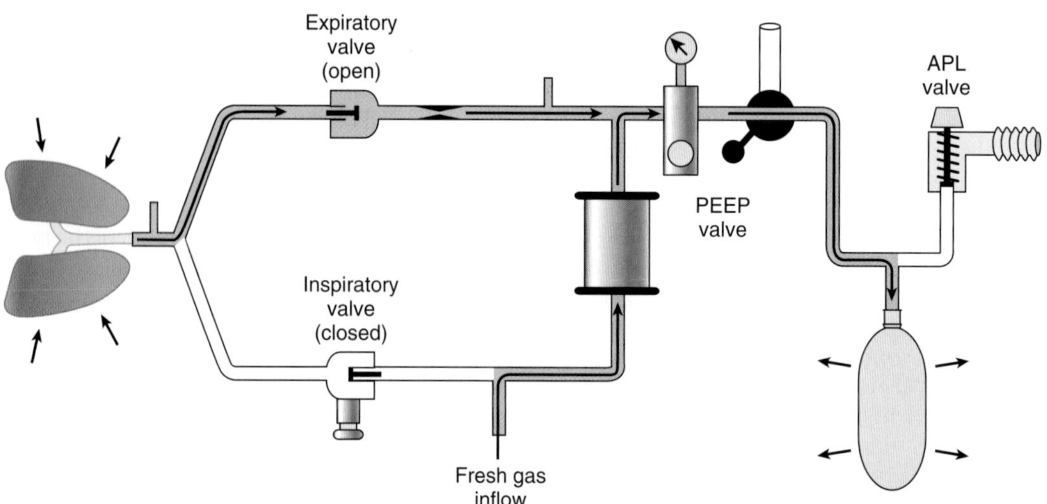

Fig. 22.33 Spontaneous breathing: early expiratory phase. The inspiratory unidirectional valve ensures that all exhaled carbon dioxide (CO_2)–containing gas flows toward the breathing bag and adjustable pressure-limiting *(APL)* valve before being scrubbed of CO_2. Fresh gas continues to flow, but now in retrograde fashion, and combines with the exhaled breath. The APL valve remains closed in this example because circuit pressure is still lower than the practitioner-set APL valve pressure threshold (i.e., 10 cm H_2O). *PEEP,* Positive end-expiratory pressure. (Courtesy Dr. Michael A. Olympio; modified with his permission.)

systems must allow for spontaneous ventilation, manual ventilation, and positive-pressure mechanical ventilation, and therefore must function with both the anesthesia reservoir bag and ventilator. The fresh gas inflow enters the circle by a connection from the common gas outlet of the anesthesia machine.

Some of the main advantages of the circle system include (1) maintenance of relatively stable inspired gas concentrations; (2) conservation of respiratory heat and moisture, and anesthetic gases; (3) elimination of CO_2; and (4) prevention of operating room pollution. The capability to rebreathe exhaled gases is a unique aspect of circle systems as compared with ICU ventilators. Carbon dioxide is efficiently removed to allow safe rebreathing of exhaled gases. Waste gas, which is composed of excess carrier gas, anesthetic agent, and CO_2, is scavenged and eliminated.

Circle breathing systems have several disadvantages. First, they have a complex design that may consist of ten or more individual connections. These multiple links set the stage for misconnections, disconnections, obstructions, and leaks. In a closed-claim analysis of adverse anesthetic outcomes arising from gas delivery equipment, 39% of malpractice claims resulted from breathing circuit misconnections or disconnection.[124] Malfunction of unidirectional valves can be life-threatening. The circle breathing system is large and compliant when compared with the Mapleson systems, and this property may compromise tidal volume

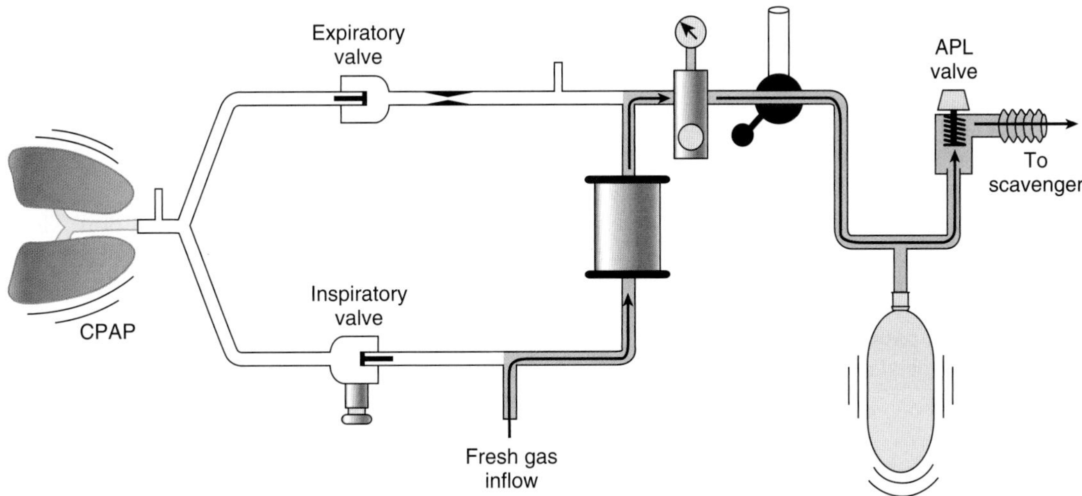

Fig. 22.34 Spontaneous breathing: end-expiratory phase with continuous positive airway pressure *(CPAP)*. Fresh gas continues to flow into the circuit generating pressure that maintains distention of the lungs (CPAP) and the breathing bag. Once the circuit pressure exceeds the adjustable pressure-limiting *(APL)* valve's set threshold (i.e., 10 cm H_2O), the valve opens, and excess gas flow is vented to the scavenger. (Courtesy Dr. Michael A. Olympio; modified with his permission.)

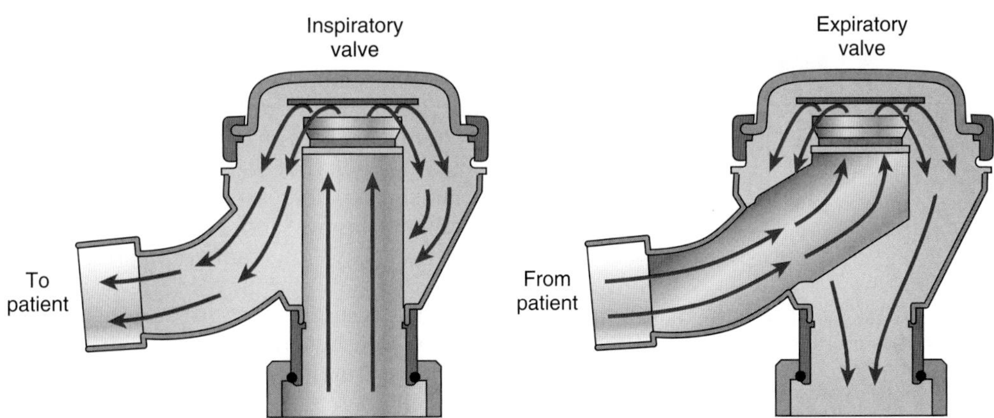

Fig. 22.35 Circle breathing system unidirectional valves. (Modified from Yoder M. Absorbers and breathing systems. In: *Understanding Modern Anesthesia Systems*. Telford, PA: Dräger Medical; 2009:83–126.)

delivery during controlled ventilation. Finally, because circle breathing systems use a CO_2 absorber, anesthetic degradation can occur (see section on Carbon Dioxide Absorbers).[125] Specific perils associated with each component of the circle system are discussed in detail in the sections to follow.

Mechanical Components of the Circle Breathing System

Unidirectional Valves. The one-way valves are essential elements of the circle breathing system (Fig. 22.35). They are constructed to resist the humidity that sometimes accumulates in the breathing system. However, these usually reliable valves can occasionally fail during use. The expiratory valve seems to be more vulnerable because it is subject to greater moisture exposure. If a unidirectional valve sticks in the open position, inappropriate rebreathing of CO_2 may occur.[125a] Capnography may help with diagnosis, as each valve demonstrates a characteristic CO_2 waveform when incompetent.[126,126a] If the valves are stuck shut, total occlusion of the circuit can result. An expiratory valve stuck in the closed position can lead to barotrauma. Assessing for proper unidirectional valve function should be part of the anesthesia workstation pre-use check out procedure. Anesthesia machines are constructed so that valve function and motion can either be visibly assessed, or malfunction is indicated by the workstation.[11]

Adjustable Pressure-Limiting Valve. The APL valve is an operator-adjustable relief valve that vents excess breathing circuit gas to the scavenging system and provides control of the breathing system pressure during spontaneous and manual modes of ventilation. Switching the workstation to a ventilator mode excludes or closes the valve.[127] Several other common names exist for these devices, including "pop-off" valve and pressure relief valve.[122] The two basic types of APL valves are the variable-orifice (or variable-resistor) type and the pressure-regulating type. The variable-orifice type functions as a needle valve, much like a flow control valve (Fig. 22.36). The operator adjusts the outlet orifice size, so the resultant breathing system pressure at any given adjustment is directly related to the fresh gas flow rate. Modern machines now mostly use pressure-regulating type APL valves (Fig. 22.37). This type of APL valve has an adjustable internal spring and an external scale indicating the approximate opening pressure. When the pressure in the system exceeds spring tension, a disk opens and gas is vented (see Fig. 22.37*B*). Waste gas is prevented from returning from the scavenging system by a downstream check valve. By adjusting spring tension, the operator can choose the desired maximal circuit pressure in manual mode.[38,122] Unlike variable-orifice type valves, the pressure-regulating APL valves are designed to maintain stable circuit pressure even as fresh gas flow is increased. This type of valve usually has a fully open (to atmosphere) position for spontaneous breathing (see Fig. 22.37*C*). Continuous positive airway pressure (CPAP) can be more reliably controlled using this type of APL valve.

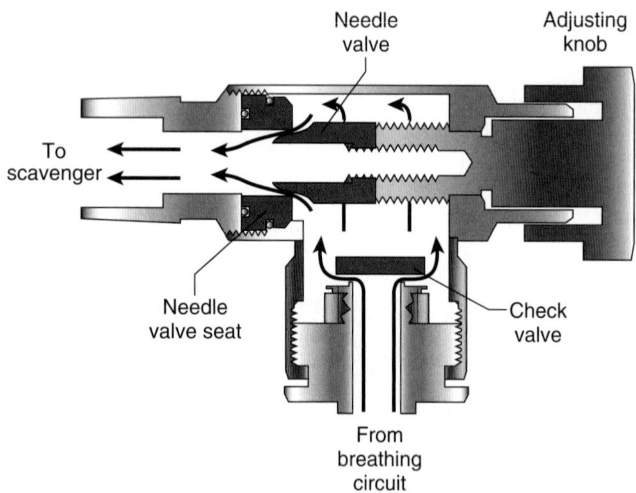

Fig. 22.36 Adjustable pressure-limiting valve: variable orifice type. A weighted check valve prevents gas from flowing backward after being sent to the scavenger. A variable orifice needle valve controls rate of gas egress from the breathing circuit, thereby controlling the circuit pressure. At any given adjusted valve orifice, the pressure in the circuit will depend on the fresh gas flow rate. (Modified from Yoder M. Absorbers and breathing systems. In: *Understanding Modern Anesthesia Systems*. Telford, PA: Dräger Medical; 2009:83–126.)

While APL valves are designed as a safety feature to allow precise control of circuit pressures during manual ventilation, problems do occur. A comparison of two modern anesthesia machines demonstrated that not all APL valves have equivalent linear behavior, and with certain valves the PIPs may routinely exceed set values.[127a] This serves as a reminder that the operator must vigilantly monitor circuit pressure during manual ventilation. Mechanical failures of APL valves have been reported due to breakage or trapping of gas sampling lines under the edge of the control knob.[127b,127c]

Anesthesia Reservoir Bag or "Breathing Bag." The anesthesia reservoir bag, or "breathing bag," provides several important functions, including (1) serving as a reservoir for exhaled gas and excess fresh gas, (2) providing a means of delivering manual ventilation or assisting spontaneous breathing, (3) serving as a visual or tactile means of monitoring a patient's spontaneous breathing efforts, and (4) partially protecting the patient from excessive positive pressure in the breathing system, such as in the case of inadvertent closure of the APL valve or an obstruction of the scavenge line [Fig. 22.38*A*]). Standard adult breathing bags have a nominal volume of 3 L; pediatric bags are available as small as 0.5 L. The reservoir bag is the most compliant part of the breathing system. The pressure-volume characteristics of standard bags are such that they inflate to a maximal pressure, and then slightly decrease to a plateau as filling continues to higher volumes (Fig. 22.38*B*).[122,128,129,129a] Anesthesia reservoir bags must adhere to pressure standards, which mandate a minimum pressure of approximately 30 cm H_2O and a maximum pressure of approximately 60 cm H_2O when the bag is filled to four times its stated capacity.[130] Although most bags adhere to these standards, some latex-free bags have exceeded the upper pressure limit.[129] Classically, the reservoir bag was excluded from the breathing circuit when the ventilator was in use. However, on most contemporary Dräger workstations,

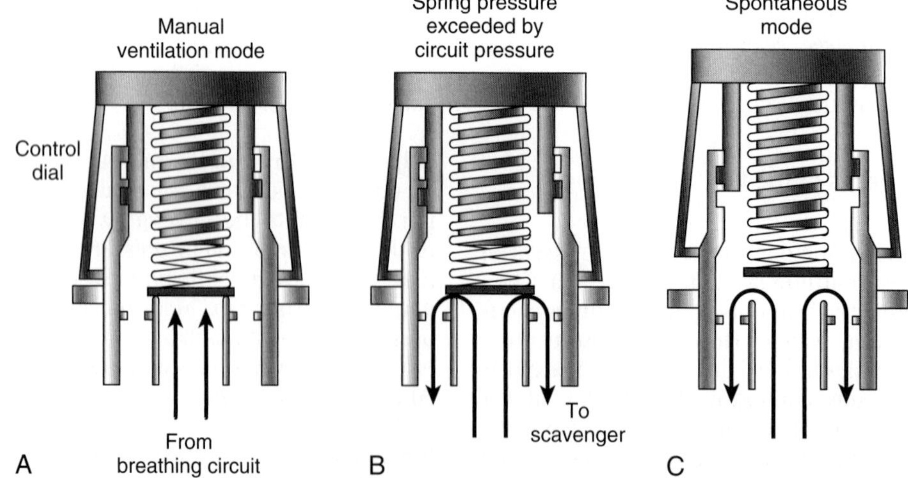

Fig. 22.37 Adjustable pressure-limiting valve: pressure-regulating type. (A) In the "manual" setting, the operator adjusts spring tension, thereby adjusting valve opening pressure. In this image the breathing circuit pressure has not yet exceeded spring tension. (B) Breathing circuit pressure has exceeded the set pressure (spring tension), and gas is vented to the scavenger. With the pressure regulating type of adjustable pressure-limiting valve, circuit pressure is independent of the fresh gas flow rate. (C) When the valve is placed in the spontaneous mode, the disk is lifted off the valve seat, and gas flows freely to the scavenger. A check valve downstream prevents waste gas from returning to the breathing circuit.

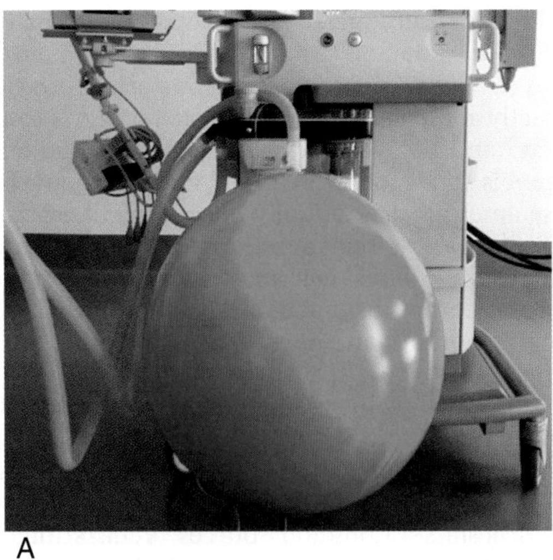
A

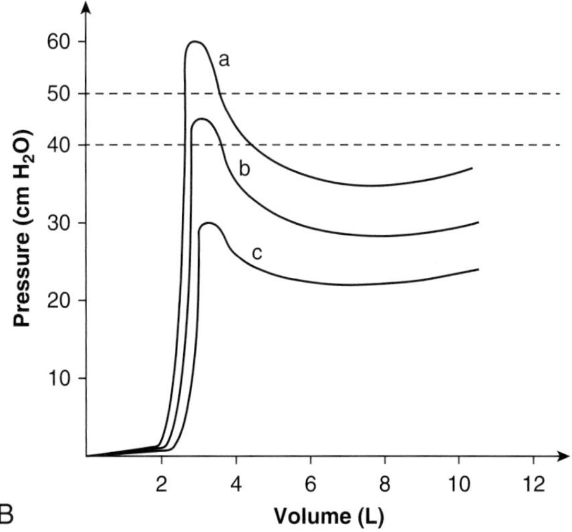

B

Fig. 22.38 Safety function of the breathing circuit reservoir bag when overdistended. The standard for reservoir bags is that the maximum pressure should not exceed approximately 60 cm H_2O at four times the stated capacity.[130] However, the pressure inside many reservoir bags peaks at a lower volume, and all should maintain a plateau pressure with further expansion.[128] (A) A breathing bag distended to a diameter of ~66 cm and volume of ~150 L. The pressure inside the bag is 34 cm H_2O. (B) Pressure versus volume filling curves for three different reservoir bags demonstrating a peak and plateau pressure. Vigilance should prevent overfilling from occurring because the continuing positive pressure alarm should be sounding while the bag is inflating. (From Křižmarić M. Functions of anesthesia reservoir bag in a breathing system. *Slov Med J.* 2017;86:226–235.)

the reservoir bag is integral to circuit function during mechanical ventilation, where it serves as an exhaled and fresh gas reservoir.[31b,38,131,131a]

Corrugated Breathing Circuit Tubing. The breathing circuit tubing, which accounts for most of the volume within the circle system, has certain vulnerabilities. First, these circuits are compliant, and some of the volume intended for delivery to the patient during positive-pressure ventilation is lost to distention of the tubing. Many modern anesthesia workstations perform a compliance test to compensate for this effect. Alternatively, the workstation may compensate for discrepancies in the set versus delivered tidal volume. It is important that these tests be performed with the actual circuit that is to be used for anesthesia delivery. For instance, if a circuit extension is to be used to facilitate turning the operating room table 180 degrees, the compliance, leak, and flow tests should be performed with the extension in place. Circuit tubing may also be a source of leaks or obstruction (see below).

Y-Piece. The Y-piece is the distal (nearest the patient) part of the circuit that merges the inspiratory and expiratory limbs. It has a 15-mm inner diameter to connect to an endotracheal tube or elbow connector, and a 22-mm outer diameter to connect to a face mask. The dead space in the circle breathing system begins at the Y-piece and continues to the patient (i.e., the portions of the circuit with bidirectional gas flow, compare Figs. 22.32 and 22.33).[131b] On modern anesthesia machines, the gas sampling port is located at or near the Y-piece to allow monitoring of both inspiratory and expiratory gases.

Filters and Heat and Moisture Exchangers. The use of HMEs and filters within the anesthesia breathing circuit is common. HMEs help replace the normal warming and humidifying function of the upper airway, which is often bypassed by an artificial airway during anesthesia.[132] Filters are used to prevent the transmission of microbes from the patient to the machine and hence potentially to other patients. No consensus agreement pertaining to their use exists. Current ASA recommendations endorse the use of filters only in the context of patients with tuberculosis.[133] If a filter is to be used for this purpose, it should have an efficiency rating higher than 95% for particle sizes larger than 0.3 μm. The filter should be placed between the endotracheal tube and the Y-piece.[134]

Sensors

Inspired Oxygen Concentration Monitor. The ASTM standards state that the workstation must be equipped with a sensor to monitor the oxygen concentration in the inspiratory limb or at the Y-piece of the breathing circuit. A low oxygen concentration alarm must sound within 30 seconds if the fraction of inspired oxygen (FiO_2) drops below a set limit, which cannot be adjustable to less than 18% v/v%.[20] The oxygen sensor is truly the patient's last line of defense from receiving a hypoxemic gas mixture. *Galvanic cell oxygen analyzers* are often used for this purpose, but they have a finite life span and are prone to drift.[134a] They therefore require daily calibration during the workstation pre-use check. A common location for galvanic sensors is in the housing of the inspiratory unidirectional valve (see Fig. 22.32). Modern anesthesia workstations (e.g., Dräger Apollo) increasingly use *side-stream multigas analyzers at the Y-piece* as the exclusive inspiratory oxygen monitor.[131a,134c] *Paramagnetic oxygen analyzers*, which require less frequent calibration, are typically used in these monitors.

Flow Sensors. Flow sensors are used on the anesthesia machine primarily to measure tidal volume. The workstation must have a device that monitors the patient's exhaled tidal volume, minute ventilation, or both.[11] These sensors may also be used to display flow waveforms and/or flow-volume loops. Finally, some workstations use flow sensor measurements as a feedback signal to maintain stable tidal volume delivery at varying fresh gas flow rates. Although early flow sensors were usually mechanical respirometers, contemporary machines may use differential pressure sensors, heated-wire anemometers, ultrasonic flow sensors, or variable-orifice flow sensors. The location of the flow sensor can vary, but a sensor for exhaled gas flow is required at a minimum.

Breathing Circuit Pressure Sensors. The continuous measurement of airway pressure in the breathing circuit is critical to patient safety. Several requirements must be met. First, anesthesia workstations must continuously display pressure in the breathing system. Second, operator-adjustable alarms must be present for *high pressure* as well as for *continuous positive pressure* lasting 15 seconds or longer. Excessive high pressure or prolonged positive airway pressure can compromise venous return, decrease cardiac output, interfere with ventilation, or cause barotrauma. An alarm must also sound if *negative pressure below −10 cm* H_2O occurs in the breathing circuit for more than 1 second. Finally, when automatic ventilation is in use, the machine must alarm whenever the breathing pressure falls below a preset or adjustable *threshold pressure* for more than 20 seconds. This alarm may serve as a disconnection alarm, but low-volume or exhaled CO_2 monitoring may also be used (see below).[11] The location of pressure sensors in the breathing system varies. They are often located in the nondisposable portion of either the inspiratory or expiratory limb near one of the unidirectional valves.[134b] Dräger machines transduce pressure from the CO_2 absorber system.[131a] It is important to remember that the breathing circuit pressure may not accurately represent the patient's airway pressure, especially if the pressure sensor is located far from the Y-piece.[134b] Older machines have a mechanical pressure gauge, while newer models may display a digital representation of this gauge.

Circle System Function—Semiclosed, Semiopen, and Closed Systems. Circle system function is illustrated in Figs. 22.32–22.34. The extent of rebreathing, and therefore the conservation of exhaled gases, depends on the fresh gas flow rate. Higher fresh gas flow rates result in less rebreathing and greater waste gas. Contemporary circle systems are usually operated in a *semiclosed* manner, meaning that some rebreathing occurs, but some waste flow is vented through the APL or waste gas valve of the ventilator. The delivery of *low-flow* anesthesia (≤1.0 L/min fresh gas flow) with a circle system exemplifies a *semiclosed* system. *Low-flow* anesthesia generally refers to a technique where fresh gas flow is less than minute ventilation, and at least 50% of expired gas is rebreathed after carbon dioxide removal.[131b]

A circle system operated in a *semiopen* manner implies a higher fresh gas flow rate with minimal rebreathing and more venting of waste gas. The advantages of conducting *low-flow* or *minimal-flow* (≤0.5 L/min) anesthesia include the decreased use of volatile anesthetic agents, improved temperature and humidity control, and reduced environmental pollution. The disadvantages include difficulty in rapidly adjusting anesthetic depth and the theoretical possibility of accumulating unwanted exhaled gases (e.g., carbon monoxide, acetone, methane) or volatile anesthetic degradation products (e.g., compound A, carbon monoxide—see section on carbon dioxide absorbers later).[135]

A *closed* system is one in which the rate of oxygen inflow exactly matches metabolic demand, rebreathing is complete, and no waste gas is vented. A volatile anesthetic agent is added to the breathing circuit in liquid form in precise amounts or is initially introduced through the vaporizer.[136] Closed-circuit anesthesia maximizes the advantages of *low-* and *minimal-flow* anesthesia. However, the vigilance demanded by this technique make it impractical for routine use with contemporary equipment; thus it is rarely employed.[137]

Potential Circle System Problems

LEAKS AND DISCONNECTIONS. Breathing circuit leaks and disconnections continue to cause critical incidents in anesthesia.[140] Common sources of leaks include disposable tubing and components, as well as points of connection within the breathing circuit and at the CO_2 absorber canister.[141] Although leaks can develop during the course of anesthesia, such as a partial disconnection, most can be detected during a thorough workstation pre-use checkout. Leaks can be small, and easily overcome by increasing fresh gas flow to compensate for lost volume, or they can be very large and render ventilation impossible. No matter the size, *all leaks should be investigated.* Several monitors can assist the anesthesia provider in detecting a leak or circuit disconnection during the course of anesthetic care (Table 22.7).

Breathing circuit pressure monitoring is an extremely important aid in diagnosing leaks and disconnections. As discussed earlier, breathing circuit pressure monitoring is a required feature of anesthesia workstations. The *threshold pressure* (or *low peak inspiratory pressure*) alarm is useful for detecting leaks and disconnections. When using a controlled ventilation mode, an audible and visual alarm is generated if the breathing system pressure drops below the threshold limit for more than 20 seconds (Fig. 22.39*A*). Visual alarm examples include "Apnea Pressure," "Check Breathing Circuit," and "Low Pressure."[38,141a,141b] The specific times required before sounding the alarm may vary slightly between machines. The *threshold pressure alarm* limit is operator-adjustable on some machines, and may also have an "autoset" feature that applies an algorithm to set an appropriate limit based on current airway pressures.[131,141c] As can be seen in Fig. 22.39*B*, setting the threshold limit too low may allow a partial disconnection (leak) to go unrecognized. Conversely, setting the threshold limit too high can result in an erroneous alarm.

Respiratory volume monitors (flow sensors) are useful in detecting leaks or disconnections. Low exhaled tidal volume and/or low minute ventilation alarms may first alert the operator to these problems. The user should bracket the minute ventilation alarms slightly higher and lower than the patient's requirements. An autoset feature may be available for minute ventilation monitoring as well.[131] Some workstations will alarm if a significant disparity exists between inhaled and exhaled tidal volumes, or when the measured tidal volume does not achieve the set tidal volume.[142]

Finally, all modern workstations have integrated gas monitoring with alarms for *exhaled* CO_2. Total loss of the

TABLE 22.7 Methods of Detecting Leaks and Disconnections During the Course of Anesthesia

Method	Leak Indications
Breathing circuit pressure sensors	*Threshold pressure alarm** Pressure waveform evaluation Trend of peak pressures
Workstation tidal volume sensors	Low minute ventilation or low tidal volume alarm Failure to deliver set tidal volume Disparity between inhaled and exhaled tidal volumes Decreasing trend of tidal volume and minute ventilation
Exhaled gas analysis	Exhaled carbon dioxide automated monitoring Abnormal appearance and trend of capnography tracing
Physiologic sensors (e.g., SpO_2, HR, BP)	*Late detection* of significant leaks and disconnections because the patient is already decompensating
A vigilant practitioner	Assesses breath sounds and chest wall excursion Pays close attention to alarms and responds promptly Observes workstation and physiologic monitors Notes that ventilator bellows is not refilling completely and tidal volumes are decreasing Notes that flow rate requirements are increasing to refill an ascending bellows Senses that breathing bag motion and feel are not normal Detects the odor of anesthetic gas Follows his or her instinct that something is not right

*ISO standard.
BP, Blood pressure; *HR*, heart rate; *SpO_2*, saturation of peripheral oxygen.

capnogram should alert the operator to a loss of ventilation and possible circuit disconnect. More subtle changes in capnogram amplitude or waveform may indicate a leak.

MISCONNECTIONS. Unfortunately, misconnections of the breathing system are not rare. Anesthesia workstations, breathing systems, ventilators, and scavenging systems incorporate many diameter-specific connections. Despite the efforts of standards committees to assign different diameters to various circuit connections, misconnections continue to occur. The ingenuity of some individuals in outwitting these "foolproof" systems has led to various hoses being adapted or forcefully fitted to inappropriate terminals, and even to various other solid cylindrical protrusions of the anesthesia machine.[143,144] Operators and technicians should be properly trained on their respective workstations and modifications should be discouraged.

OBSTRUCTION. Occlusion (obstruction) of the breathing circuit may occur and can have severe consequences. Tracheal tubes may kink. Breathing circuit valves or other components can malfunction. Hoses throughout the breathing circuit are subject to occlusion by internal obstruction or external mechanical forces that can impinge on flow. Blockage of HMEs by secretions can also cause significant obstruction.[145] Case reports describe bilateral tension pneumothorax caused by blockage of a bacterial filter in the expiratory limb,[146] or a misplaced disk in an expiratory valve.[147] Because retained CO_2 absorber canister wrappings have caused circuit obstruction, ASTM standards now require that absorbers be packaged in a way that immediately identifies the presence of a wrapper.[127,148,149] Defects associated with disposable circuit components or the tubing itself have caused severe circuit obstruction and sometimes injury to the patient.[150-154] Misplaced Luer caps have made their way into the elbow connector of the circuit because of packaging or processing and have caused obstruction.[155,156] Incorrect insertion of flow direction-sensitive components

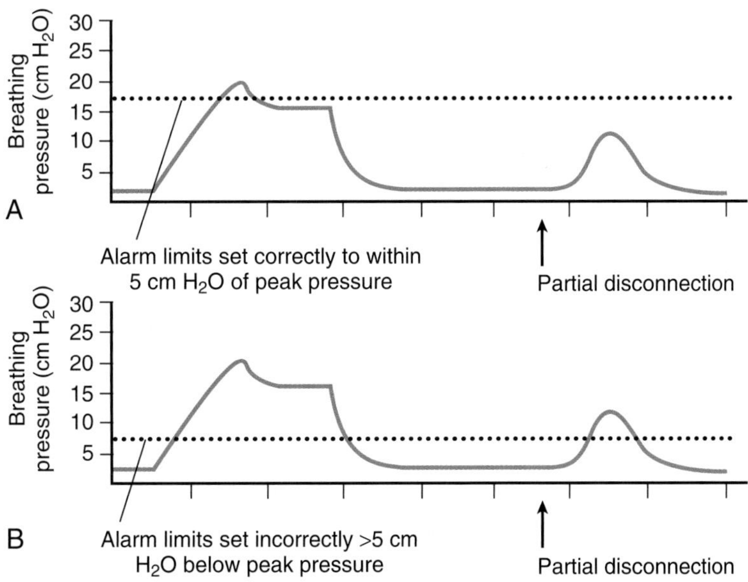

Fig. 22.39 Threshold pressure alarm limit. (A) The threshold pressure alarm limit *(dotted line)* has been set appropriately. An alarm is actuated when partial disconnection occurs *(arrow)* because the threshold pressure alarm limit is not exceeded by the breathing circuit pressure. (B) Partial disconnection is unrecognized by the pressure monitor because the threshold pressure alarm limit has been set too low. (Redrawn from North American Dräger. *Baromed Breathing Pressure Monitor: Operator's Instruction Manual.* Telford, PA: North American Dräger; 1986.)

can result in a no-flow state. Examples of these components include some older PEEP valves and cascade humidifiers. Only the performance of a manual circuit flow test, or a similar automated test, during the pre-use checkout will reliably detect an obstruction. *If you are struggling to ventilate a patient and are unsure why, do not delay in switching to a self-inflating resuscitation bag.* Ventilate the patient first, troubleshoot later.

Variations in Circle Breathing System Design. Numerous variations of the circle system are possible, depending on the relative positions of the unidirectional valves, the APL valve, the reservoir bag, the CO_2 absorber, and the site of fresh gas entry. However, to prevent rebreathing of CO_2 in a traditional circle system, three rules must be followed: (1) a unidirectional valve must be located between the patient and the reservoir bag on both the inspiratory and expiratory limbs, (2) the fresh gas inflow cannot enter the circuit between the expiratory valve and the patient, and (3) the APL valve cannot be located between the patient and the inspiratory valve. If these rules are followed, any arrangement of the other components will prevent rebreathing of CO_2.[125] Design departures from the traditional circle breathing system are becoming more common as workstations evolve. Some of these designs are driven by strategies to eliminate the impact of varying fresh gas flow rates or oxygen flush on inspiratory tidal volume and airway pressure during mechanical ventilations (fresh gas decoupling or compensation). These variations are addressed later, in section on anesthesia ventilators.

Carbon Dioxide Absorbers

Circle breathing systems require a means of CO_2 removal from the exhaled gases to avoid rebreathing and hypercapnia. Although increasing the fresh gas inflow to high levels can dilute out most CO_2 in the circle system, this is a very inefficient way to conduct an anesthetic. Because typical gas flows through the anesthesia machine are less than minute ventilation (*semiclosed* system), absorption of CO_2 is essential. If one could design an ideal CO_2 absorbent, its characteristics would include a lack of reactivity with common anesthetics, an absence of toxicity, low resistance to airflow, minimal dust production, low cost, ease of handling, and high efficiency. It should also be easy to assess for absorbent depletion (i.e., a diminished ability to remove CO_2). Finally, the container that houses the absorbent should be easy to remove and replace, should maintain breathing circuit integrity if quickly replaced during use, and should impose minimal risk of causing breathing system leaks or obstruction. Carbon dioxide absorbers are not unique to anesthesiology. They are also used in certain military and commercial diving equipment, submarines, space operations, mining and rescue operations, and hyperbaric facilities. In these environments, CO_2 absorbers are often referred to as *CO_2 scrubbers*.

Absorber Canister. Although CO_2 absorber canister configurations vary, they must be visible to the operator and transparent to monitor for absorbent presence and color. On traditional anesthesia machines, the absorber consists of a single clear plastic canister (or two canisters arranged in series). Opening a traditional canister assembly abolishes the integrity of the breathing circuit. If the absorbent needs to be changed in the course of anesthesia, and apnea cannot be tolerated, it is necessary to ventilate by other means. These older canisters are a common source of leaks due to their multiple components and compression assembly method.[141] The canisters are filled either with loose bulk absorbent or with factory-supplied disposable cartridges called *prepacks*. Loose granules from bulk absorbent may lodge between the canister and the O-ring gasket of the absorber and create a clinically significant leak. Leaks have also been caused by defective prepacks or those that were larger than factory specifications.[154,157] Prepacks can also cause total obstruction of the circle system if the clear plastic shipping wrapper is not removed before use.[148] Problems with rebreathing CO_2 have been caused by canister apparatus reassembly issues.[158-160]

Many modern workstations now use single canister absorbers that are disposable and easily replaceable. Increasingly, workstation design allows the canister to be replaced during anesthesia without interfering with breathing system integrity, sometimes referred to as a *bypass* feature.[141a] A potential risk imposed by this feature is that the machine may pass an automated or manual leak test *without* the absorber attached.

Chemistry of Absorbents. Carbon dioxide is removed from the breathing circuit through absorption by chemicals within the absorber canister. Through a series of reactions, CO_2 is transformed into water, heat, and other byproducts through a chemical process that neutralizes an acid (CO_2 or carbonic acid) with one or more basic compounds. Most absorbents use calcium hydroxide [$Ca(OH)_2$] to react with the expired CO_2, producing insoluble calcium carbonate ($CaCO_3$) (Box 22.2). However, because CO_2 does not react quickly with $Ca(OH)_2$, water and small amounts of stronger base catalysts are required to speed up the reaction. Calcium hydroxide-based absorbents vary in content of water, strong base

BOX 22.2 Carbon Dioxide Absorber Reactions (Net and Sequential)

Carbon Dioxide Reaction With Soda Lime

Net Reaction

$$CO_2 + Ca(OH)_2 \rightarrow CaCO_3 + H_2O + heat$$

Sequential Reactions

1. $CO_{2\,(gas)} + H_2O_{(liquid)} \rightleftharpoons H_2CO_{3\,(aqueous)}$
2. $H_2CO_3 + 2NaOH$ (or KOH) $\rightarrow Na_2CO_3$ (or K_2CO_3) $+ 2H_2O +$ heat
3. Na_2CO_3 (or K_2CO_3) $+ Ca(OH)_2 \rightarrow CaCO_3 + 2NaOH$* (or KOH*) + heat

Carbon Dioxide Reaction With Lithium Hydroxide Monohydrate

$$2\,LiOH{\bullet}H_2O + CO_2 + heat \rightarrow Li_2CO_3 + 3H_2O$$

*Note: Sodium hydroxide (NaOH) and potassium hydroxide (KOH) are catalysts in this reaction mechanism (they are neither created nor destroyed). *LiOH*, Lithium hydroxide.

catalysts (e.g., sodium hydroxide or potassium hydroxide), humectants (e.g., calcium chloride), and hardening agents such as silica. Newer absorbents only have trace amounts of potassium hydroxide (KOH) or sodium hydroxide (NaOH) because these bases have been associated with anesthetic degradation. One absorbent brand replaces $Ca(OH)_2$ entirely with lithium hydroxide (LiOH), which does not require any additional catalysts to react with CO_2. Key differences in absorbents include their capacity for CO_2 and their propensity to react with volatile anesthetics and produce potentially harmful degradation products (e.g., carbon monoxide and compound A). The composition of several absorbents is shown in Table 22.8.[161-166]

Soda lime is a mixture of chemicals that contains about 80% $Ca(OH)_2$, also known as *slaked lime*, along with water and small amounts of strong base (see Box 22.2). First, CO_2 reacts with liquid water present on and within the absorbent granules to yield carbonic acid (H_2CO_3). This step requires water and explains why all $Ca(OH)_2$-based absorbents contain approximately 15% H_2O by mass. Second, the strong base additives NaOH and KOH react quickly with H_2CO_3 to yield the soluble salts sodium carbonate (Na_2CO_3) and potassium carbonate (K_2CO_3). All available active strong base is quickly depleted. Third, the carbonates react with $Ca(OH)_2$ to yield insoluble $CaCO_3$. Note that NaOH and KOH are regenerated in this step and therefore meet the definition of catalysts. Since additional CO_2 cannot dissolve in water until H_2CO_3 is consumed by strong base (step 2), the rate of NaOH and KOH regeneration (step 3) is the rate-limiting step.[166a] Some CO_2 may react directly with $Ca(OH)_2$, but as mentioned, this reaction is slower. Byproducts of the entire process are water and heat.[167,168]

Unlike soda lime and the $Ca(OH)_2$-based absorbents, LiOH-based absorbents do not require catalysts. LiOH is a strong base and reacts quickly with CO_2. Although liquid water is not required to generate carbonic acid as in the classic $Ca(OH)_2$ reaction, some water molecules are still required for the CO_2 reaction with LiOH. These water molecules are supplied by humidity in the exhaled breathing gases and combine with the crystal lattice of LiOH in a 1:1 ratio through a process called "hydration."[168a] LiOH that does not contain water is referred to as *lithium hydroxide anhydrous*. LiOH chemically bound to water is called *lithium hydroxide monohydrate* (LiOH•H_2O). Because the hydration reaction is *exothermic* (gives off heat), absorbents composed of *LiOH anhydrous* generate heat as they extract humidity during use. *LiOH monohydrate*-based absorbents are hydrated at the factory and therefore generate less heat when used in circle breathing systems. Once hydrated, LiOH removes CO_2 from the breathing circuit through an endothermic reaction (absorbs heat) that produces insoluble lithium carbonate (see Box 22.2).

Interactions of Inhaled Anesthetics With Absorbents

FORMATION OF POTENTIALLY HARMFUL DEGRADATION PRODUCTS. Volatile anesthetic agents have long been known to interact with the strong bases (KOH and NaOH) found in $Ca(OH)_2$-based absorbents to form degradation products. For historical perspective, trichloroethylene, a volatile anesthetic introduced to clinical use in 1940, was found to be associated with neurologic toxicity (particularly cranial nerve neuropathies and encephalitis).[169,170] Experimental investigation determined that dichloroacetylene, a toxin, was being formed by a base-catalyzed reaction with prior formulations of soda lime. This reaction was more likely to occur if the soda lime had a high content of strong base and was dry. Today, the main degradation products of concern are compound A, associated with the use of sevoflurane, and carbon monoxide (CO), mainly associated with the use of desflurane, enflurane, and isoflurane.[171] Other degradation products include formaldehyde and methanol, but these are not discussed here.[165]

TABLE 22.8 Carbon Dioxide Absorber Comparisons

Absorbent (Reference)	$Ca(OH)_2$ (%)	LiOH (%)	H_2O (%)	NaOH (%)	KOH (%)	Other (%)
Classic soda lime (165)	80	0	16	3	2	–
Baralyme (164)*	73	0	11-16	0.0	5	11 $Ba(OH)_2$
Sodasorb (161)*	76.5	0	18.9	2.25	2.25	–
Dragersorb 800 Plus (162, 166)*	82	0	16	2	0.003	–
Medisorb (166)*	81	0	18	1-2	0.003	–
New soda lime*	73	0	<19	<4	0	–
Sodasorb LF (163)	>80	0	15-17	<1	0	–
Dragersorb Free (161, 164)	74-82	0	14-18	0.5-2	0	3-5 $CaCl_2$
Sofnolime*	>75	0	12-19	<3	0	–
Amsorb Plus (161, 165)	>75	0	14.5	0	0	<1 $CaCl_2$ and $CaSO_4$
Litholyme*	>75	0	12-19	0	0	<3 LiCl
SpiraLith*	0	≈95	0[†]	0	0	≤5 PE

*Materials Safety Data Sheets, Occupational Safety and Health Administration, U.S. Department of Labor.
[†]Up to 60% of LiOH is chemically bound 1:1 with H_2O as lithium hydroxide monohydrate (see text for details).
$Ba(OH)_2$, Barium hydroxide; *$CaCl_2$*, calcium chloride; *$Ca(OH)_2$*, calcium hydroxide; *$CaSO_4$*, calcium sulfate; *KOH*, potassium hydroxide; *LiCL*, lithium chloride; *LiOH*, lithium hydroxide; *NaOH*, sodium hydroxide; *PE*, polyethylene.

COMPOUND A PRODUCTION. Sevoflurane can undergo a base-catalyzed degradation into fluoromethyl-2,2-difluoro-1-(trifluoromethyl) vinyl ether, known as *compound A*. Compound A is nephrotoxic to rats at concentrations that can occur in the breathing circuit during clinical conditions.[169,172] Moreover, in a limited number of volunteer studies, sevoflurane was associated with transient albuminuria and glucosuria.[173,174] To date, however, mounting data show no relationship between sevoflurane use and postoperative renal dysfunction in humans (including patients with preoperative renal insufficiency).[169,175-180] The sevoflurane package insert states that patient exposure should not exceed 2 MAC-hours at flow rates between 1 and 2 L/min in order to minimize risk from compound A. Flow rates less than 1 L/min are not officially recommended, although these recommendations predate several studies demonstrating safety at lower flow rates.

Several physical factors may predispose to higher concentrations of compound A in the breathing circuit, including the following:

- Low-flow or closed-circuit anesthetic techniques
- Higher concentrations of sevoflurane
- Type of absorbent (KOH or NaOH-containing)
- Higher absorbent temperatures
- Fresh absorbent[171,172,175,181]

The type and ratio of strong bases within the CO_2 absorbent affects the degree of sevoflurane degradation. KOH seems to cause more breakdown than NaOH.[164,166] For example, classic soda lime and Baralyme (which was voluntarily withdrawn from the market) both contain significant amounts of KOH and have a greater propensity to generate compound A than newer absorbents (see Table 22.8).[166] LiOH-based absorbents and newer $Ca(OH)_2$-based absorbents that are free of KOH and NaOH generate zero or negligible amounts of compound A.[162,163,166,182,182a,182b] Given the safe track record of sevoflurane and ongoing improvements in CO_2 absorbents, it may be concluded that compound A poses minimal risk to patients during routine clinical practice.

CARBON MONOXIDE PRODUCTION. Strong-base containing absorbents that are extremely dry (desiccated) can also degrade inhaled anesthetics to clinically significant concentrations of CO.[164] Under certain conditions, this process can produce blood carboxyhemoglobin levels of 35% or greater in an exposed patient.[184] A typical scenario involving a dangerous CO exposure would be the first case on a Monday morning, after high continuous gas flows had accidentally been left on throughout the weekend and desiccated the absorbent.[185,186] Machines in remote locations are more frequently found with desiccated absorbent.[186] Prolonged fresh gas flow rates of 5 L/min or greater are sufficient to cause critical drying of the absorbent, especially when the breathing bag is left off the circle system. Because the inspiratory valve leaflet produces some resistance to flow, fresh gas tends to flow retrograde through the absorber and out the breathing bag mount (the path of least resistance). The presence of a breathing bag allows slight pressure build-up that resists this flow (see the classic circle breathing system in Fig. 22.32).[184] Desiccation of absorbent is unlikely to occur during anesthesia delivery since CO_2 absorption produces water (and patients exhale humidified gas).

Several factors increase the production of CO and risk of carboxyhemoglobinemia:

- Inhaled anesthetic used (for a given MAC multiple, the magnitude of carbon monoxide production is desflurane ≥ enflurane > isoflurane >> halothane = sevoflurane)
- Degree of desiccation of the absorbent
- Type of absorbent (KOH or NaOH-containing)
- Higher temperature
- Higher concentrations of anesthetic[187]
- Low fresh gas flow rates
- Smaller patient size[188,189]

As with compound A production, the presence of strong bases (KOH and NaOH) in the desiccated absorbent correlates with the propensity to degrade certain anesthetics and liberate CO. Therefore Baralyme (now withdrawn) and to a lesser extent soda lime were more likely to produce CO when desiccated than newer-generation absorbents (see Table 22.8).[190] Omission of NaOH and KOH from the $Ca(OH)_2$-based absorbents reduces or eliminates the potential to produce CO or compound A without significant impact on the capacity for CO_2 absorption.[182,191] LiOH absorbent produces essentially no CO and maintains excellent CO_2 absorption.[162,182b,191a]

ABSORBENT HEAT PRODUCTION. One extremely rare but potentially life-threatening complication related to CO_2 absorbent is the development of extreme exothermic reactions that lead to fires and explosions.[192-194] Specifically, this seems to occur when desiccated strong base absorbents (particularly Baralyme) interact with sevoflurane. Under experimental conditions, desiccated Baralyme absorbers exceeded 200°C (392°F) and higher, and fire was noted in some of the breathing circuits.[195] The buildup of very high temperatures, flammable degradation products (formaldehyde, methanol, and formic acid), and oxygen- or nitrous oxide-rich gases within the absorber provide all the ingredients necessary for combustion.[196] Avoiding the use of sevoflurane with strong base-rich absorbents (e.g., the now discontinued Baralyme), especially when desiccated, is the best way to prevent such complications. Anhydrous LiOH may also generate high temperatures by reacting with moisture from expired gas, but formulations of LiOH monohydrate do not.

A consensus statement established by the Anesthesia Patient Safety Foundation provides recommendations to reduce the risk of volatile anesthetic degradation by desiccated CO_2 absorbents[164]:

- Turn off all gas flow when the machine is not in use
- Change the absorbent regularly
- Change the absorbent if color change indicates exhaustion
- Change all absorbent (not just one canister in a two-canister system)
- Change the absorbent when uncertain about the state of hydration (e.g., if fresh gas flow is left on for an extensive or indeterminate period of time)
- If compact canisters are used, change them more frequently

Given the improvements in absorbent chemistry detailed above, it seems prudent to select an absorbent that minimizes risk of adverse reactions whenever possible. Finally, educating anesthesia personnel about these hazards and preventive measures may also reduce the likelihood of adverse events.

Indicators. Conventional absorbents contain an indicator dye, *ethyl violet*, that allows anesthesia personnel to visually assess the functional integrity of the absorbent. Ethyl violet is a substituted triphenylmethane dye that undergoes a color change around pH 10.3.[168] When the absorbent is fresh, the pH exceeds 10.3 and the dye is colorless. As the absorbent becomes exhausted, the pH drops below 10.3 and the dye becomes purple. The color change indicates that the absorptive capacity of the material has been depleted. Unfortunately, ethyl violet may not always be a reliable indicator. For example, prolonged exposure of ethyl violet to fluorescent light can photodeactivate the dye. When this occurs, the absorbent will remain white even when exhausted.[197] Similarly, color reversion (purple back to white) can occur with some absorbents due to the strongly alkaline nature of NaOH. Many newer indicators are resistant to color reversion, and several now endorse permanent color change. At least one absorbent contains no indicator and relies upon the detection of inspired CO_2 by the gas analyzer and/or a time schedule to trigger replacement.

Absorbent desiccation is impossible to detect by visual inspection. Therefore some newer generation $Ca(OH)_2$ absorbents also include desiccation indicators. Users should refer to the product manufacturer's literature to determine whether their absorbent uses this type of indicator.

Carbon Dioxide Removal Capacity and Absorber Resistance. The ability of the workstation's absorber to remove CO_2 is related to three main factors: (1) the amount of absorbent surface area exposed to the exhaled gas, (2) the intrinsic capacity of the absorbent to remove CO_2, and (3) the amount of nonexhausted absorbent remaining. The size and shape of the absorptive granules are intended to maximize surface area while minimizing resistance to airflow.[198] The smaller the granule size, the greater the surface area that is available for absorption. However, as particle size decreases, airflow resistance increases. The size and shape of the granules is proprietary, but most absorbents have a granule size between 4 and 8 mesh-a size at which surface area and resistance are optimized. (Mesh size refers to the number of openings per linear inch in a sieve through which the granular particles can pass. For example, a 4-mesh screen means that there are four quarter-inch openings per linear inch.[167]) The presence of excess liquid water within the canister can decrease the exposed granule surface area and therefore the efficiency of CO_2 absorption.

As the absorbent granules stack up in canisters, small passageways inevitably form. These passages allow gas to flow preferentially through low-resistance areas. This phenomenon, known as *channeling*, may substantially decrease the functional absorptive capacity.[199] Recently, a nongranular polymer matrix product was released that binds particles together in a solid sheet of absorbent that has molded airflow channels, eliminating the phenomenon of channeling (personal communication, Micropore, Inc., Elkton, MD, June 3, 2014).

If completely reacted, a pound of $Ca(OH)_2$ has the capacity to absorb 0.59 lb of CO_2. LiOH has a higher capacity of 0.91 lb of CO_2 per pound.[199a] Consequently, LiOH absorbents typically neutralize or "scrub" more CO_2 per unit weight (which is of great importance when planning submarine missions or space travel).[199a,199b]

Mapleson Breathing Systems

In 1954, Mapleson described and analyzed five different breathing circuits, designated A through E (Fig. 22.40).[200] In 1975, Willis and coauthors described the F system, which was added to the original five.[201] The Mapleson systems share certain features with the circle breathing system: they accept fresh gas flow, supply the patient with gas from a reservoir to meet inspiratory flow and volume requirements, and eliminate CO_2. They differ from the circle system by having bidirectional gas flow and lacking an absorber. To eliminate CO_2 and prevent rebreathing, these systems depend on a higher rate of fresh gas inflow. The Mapleson systems consist of several common components, including a connection point to a facemask or endotracheal tube, reservoir tubing, fresh gas inflow tubing, and an expiratory pop-off valve or port. All the circuits except for Mapleson E use a bag as an additional reservoir. The Mapleson A, B, and C systems are rarely used today, but the D, E, and F systems are commonly used. In the United States, the most popular representatives from the DEF group are the Bain circuit and the Jackson-Rees circuit.

Three distinct functional groups can be seen: A, BC, and DEF groups. The Mapleson A, also known as the "Magill circuit," has a spring-loaded pop-off valve located near the facemask. It is the only Mapleson circuit where fresh gas flow enters from the end of the circuit opposite the patient (in this case, near the reservoir bag). The Mapleson A is functionally quite different from the other circuits, and has drastically different performance when used for spontaneous versus controlled ventilation (see later). In the B and C systems, both the pop-off valve and fresh gas inlet tubing are located near the patient. The Mapleson C is known as the "Waters to-and-fro" circuit and lacks a corrugated tube. The reservoir tubing and breathing bag serve as a blind limb where fresh gas, dead space gas, and alveolar gas can collect. Finally, in the Mapleson D, E, and F, or "T-piece" group, fresh gas enters near the patient, and excess gas is vented off at the opposite end of the circuit. The Mapleson F circuit is known as the "Jackson-Rees" modification of the Mapleson E (also known as "Ayre's T-piece").

Even though the components and their arrangement are simple, functional analysis of the Mapleson systems is complex.[202,203] The amount of CO_2 rebreathing with each system is multifactorial and affected by: (1) the fresh gas inflow rate, (2) minute ventilation, (3) ventilation mode (spontaneous or controlled), (4) tidal volume, (5) respiratory rate, (6) the inspiratory-to-expiratory ratio, (7) the duration of the expiratory pause, (8) peak inspiratory flow rate, (9) the volume of reservoir tubing, (10) the volume of the breathing bag, (11) the airway device being used (mask or endotracheal tube), and (12) the CO_2 sampling site.

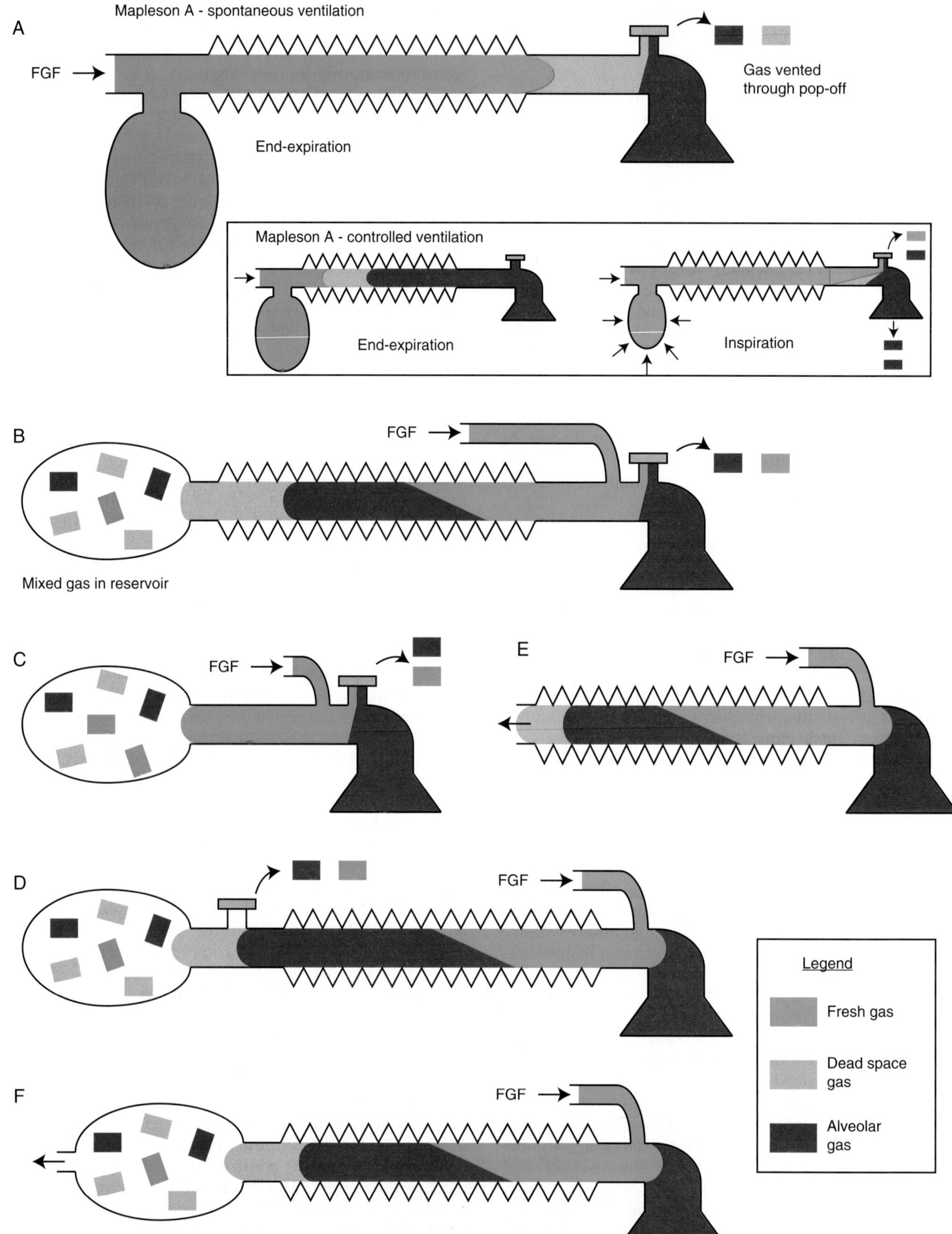

Fig. 22.40 Mapleson breathing systems. (A) Mapleson A system during spontaneous ventilation with gas distribution at end-expiration. A, *Inset,* Mapleson A system during controlled ventilation. (B–F) Mapleson systems B through F with gas distribution at end-expiration. *FGF,* Fresh gas flow. (Redrawn after Sykes MK. Rebreathing circuits. *Br J Anaesth.* 1968;40[9]:666–674; and Kaul TK, Mittal G. Mapleson's breathing systems. *Ind J Anaesth.* 2013;57[5]:507–519.)

Analysis of Gas Flow in the Mapleson A System. The performance of the Mapleson systems is best understood by studying the expiratory phase of the respiratory cycle.[204] Illustrations of the gas distribution at end-expiration is shown for each system (see Fig. 22.40).[204,204a] Of all the circuits, only the Mapleson A has markedly different performance when used for spontaneous versus controlled ventilation. During spontaneous ventilation, exhaled alveolar gas is vented through the pop-off during the expiratory phase (Fig. 22.40*A*). With the next inspiration, the patient primarily draws in fresh gas (and a small amount of dead space gas). Thus the Mapleson A has the best efficiency of the six systems for spontaneous breathing. A fresh gas inflow rate of greater than or equal to minute ventilation is sufficient to prevent rebreathing of CO_2.[205]

However, the Mapleson A has the worst efficiency during controlled ventilation. As the reservoir bag is squeezed to initiate inspiration, exhaled alveolar gas first flows into the patient (Fig. 22.40*A, inset*). The pop-off valve then opens and vents significant amounts of the fresh gas stream away from the patient during the inspiratory phase.[204a,205a] Significant rebreathing of CO_2 occurs unless minute ventilation is very high (>20 L/min). The key factor determining Mapleson A performance is the timing when the pop-off valve opens: during expiration for spontaneous ventilation, and during inspiration for controlled ventilation.[206] Due to the location of the fresh gas inflow near the patient, the gas flow patterns of the other Mapleson systems (Fig. 22.40*B–F*) do not differ as markedly between spontaneous and controlled ventilation as that of the Mapleson A.

Relative Efficiencies. The "T-piece" systems DEF are slightly more efficient than systems BC. To prevent rebreathing CO_2, the DEF systems require a fresh gas inflow rate of approximately 2 to 2.5 times minute ventilation, whereas the fresh gas inflow rates required for BC systems are somewhat higher.[203] The reason for this improved efficiency is the location of the pop-off valve relative to the fresh gas inflow. With the BC systems, significant fresh gas is vented through the pop-off at end-expiration (Fig. 22.40*B* and *C*). With the DEF systems, fresh gas flow drives exhaled alveolar gas away from the patient to minimize rebreathing (Fig. 22.40*E* and *F*).[204,205] The relative efficiency of different Mapleson systems with respect to prevention of rebreathing are: A > DFE > CB during spontaneous ventilation, and DFE > BC > A during controlled ventilation.[200,203]

Advantages and Disadvantages. Mapleson systems have low resistance to gas flow, they are small and contain few parts, and changes in the fresh gas flow composition result in rapid changes in the breathing circuit. In addition, the volatile anesthetic agents within a Mapleson breathing circuit have no chance of degradation because of the absence of a CO_2 absorber. However, given their need for higher gas flows to prevent rebreathing, they are not as economical with regards to carrier gas and volatile anesthetic usage as the circle system. Conservation of heat and humidity is less efficient. Finally, scavenging of waste gas can be challenging, with the exception of the Mapleson D, which has the pressure-limiting valve located away from the patient.[205]

Bain Circuit

The Bain circuit is a coaxial circuit and a modification of the Mapleson D system (Fig. 22.41). Fresh gas flows through a narrow inner tube nested within the outer corrugated hose.[207] The central fresh gas tubing enters the corrugated hose near the reservoir bag, but the fresh gas actually empties into the circuit at the patient's end. Exhaled gases pass down the corrugated hose, around the central tubing, and are vented through the pop-off valve near the reservoir bag.[205] Exhaled gases passing down the outer corrugated hose add warmth to the inspired fresh gases by countercurrent heat exchange.

The main hazards related to use of the Bain circuit are an unrecognized disconnection or kinking of the inner fresh gas hose. These problems can cause hypercapnia as a result of inadequate gas flow or increased respiratory resistance. The outer corrugated tube should be transparent to allow ongoing inspection of the inner tube. The integrity of the inner tube can be assessed by sending high-flow oxygen into the circuit while the patient's end is occluded until the reservoir bag is filled.[208] The patient's end is then opened, while oxygen is flushed into the circuit. If the inner tube is intact, the Venturi effect at the patient's end causes a decrease in

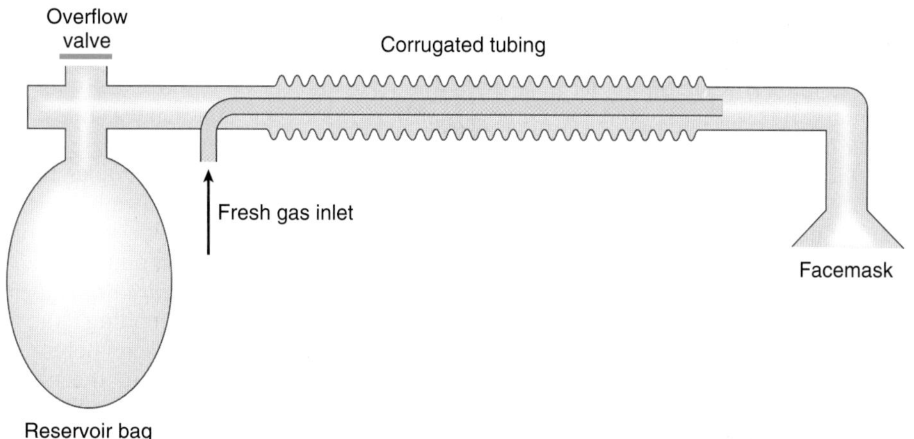

Fig. 22.41 The Bain circuit. (Redrawn from Bain JA, Spoerel WE. A streamlined anaesthetic system. *Can Anaesth Soc J*. 1972;19:426.)

pressure within the circuit, and the reservoir bag deflates. A leak in the inner tube allows fresh gas to escape into the expiratory limb, and the reservoir bag remains inflated. This test is recommended as part of the preanesthesia check if a Bain circuit is used.

Jackson-Rees Circuit. The Mapleson F circuit, also known as the "Jackson-Rees modification of the T-piece," has function similar to the Mapleson D. It incorporates a hole in the end of the reservoir bag distal to the patient for venting of gases (Fig. 22.40*F*). The hole may be occluded by the operator's hand to control bag distension and pressure, or fitted with a pop-off or PEEP valve for more precise control. The Jackson-Rees circuit is convenient for patient transport and preoxygenation during ICU or out-of-the-operating room procedures. The reservoir bag allows for easy tactile and visual monitoring of the patient's respiratory effort. This circuit may be used for spontaneous (with the venting hole open), or assisted/controlled ventilation (with the venting hole partially or totally occluded). The Jackson-Rees is effective when connected to a face mask, endotracheal tube, laryngeal mask airway, or tracheostomy tube.

Like the Bain circuit, the Jackson-Rees has many advantages. It is lightweight, convenient, and potentially reusable (if sterilized). Being a Mapleson system, it has low resistance work of breathing. Fresh gas flows required to prevent rebreathing are approximately 2.5 to 3 times minute volume for spontaneous breathing, and 1.5 to 2 times minute volume for controlled ventilation.[204a] Scavenging of gases from the expiratory valve is possible because the hole or valve is located away from the patient. Caution is advised when using HME filters between these Mapleson circuits and an endotracheal tube. Filters increase resistance and direct fresh gas flow away from the patient. An obstructed antimicrobial filter may produce hypoventilation and hypoxemia and mimic the signs and symptoms of severe bronchospasm.[209]

Self-Inflating Manual Resuscitators

While rarely used for delivery of inhaled anesthetics in modern practice, the manual resuscitation bag (e.g., Ambu bag, Laerdal resuscitator, or simply bag-valve-mask device) is an essential part of every anesthesia workstation. The key feature of this device is a compressible reservoir, typically made of silicone, that automatically expands upon release. Unlike the Mapleson circuits, the self-inflating manual resuscitator may be used for hand ventilation in the absence of an oxygen or air source. These devices are ubiquitous for patient transport, cardiopulmonary resuscitation, and for emergency back-up should the anesthesia machine ventilator or oxygen supply fail (see section on Checking Your Anesthesia Workstation).

In addition to the self-inflating reservoir bag, the manual resuscitator has several key components.[134b] (1) A T-shaped *nonrebreathing valve* is located between the bag and the patient in order to direct gas flow throughout the respiratory cycle. During inspiration, the valve opens to allow flow from the reservoir bag to the patient, and the expiratory port is blocked (see Fig. 22.42). During exhalation, the inspiratory port (to the bag) is blocked, and the expiratory port opens to vent alveolar gas to atmosphere. A variety of valve types exist (e.g., spring-disc, fishmouth). (2) An *inlet valve* permits refilling of the bag with reservoir gas or room air. (3) A *pop-off* valve may be present to limit the PIP, which can easily reach high levels with these devices.[209a] ISO standards require that manual resuscitators designed for infants or children have a valve to limit PIP to 45 cm H_2O.[209b] An override feature must be present should higher pressures be required (in case of poor lung compliance or high endotracheal tube resistance), and use of a manometer is recommended.

While manual resuscitators are extremely useful, portable, and convenient, they do have potential hazards.[134b] Dangerously high inspiratory pressures may be generated if the operator is untrained, uncareful, or if valve failure occurs.[209c] High pressures may lead to barotrauma or gastric insufflation. Similar to Mapleson circuits, significant variation of tidal volume, PIP, and PEEP is likely to occur when manual resuscitators are compared with mechanical ventilators.[209d] Finally, the nonrebreathing valves generate resistance and may significantly increase the work of breathing during spontaneous ventilation.

ANESTHESIA VENTILATORS

Automatic ventilation began to be added to anesthesia machines after the Second World War.[209e] Historical draw-over systems relied only on spontaneous breathing by the patient. Later, breathing bags were added to anesthetic delivery devices to allow positive-pressure ventilation. Today's anesthesia workstation ventilators incorporate ICU-like capabilities, including a variety of ventilation modes and the ability to allow for patient triggering. While ICU ventilators are simply open circuit, using entirely fresh gas for each breath, and venting all exhaled gas into the atmosphere, the anesthesia workstation must incorporate a means of collecting and redelivering the patient's exhaled gas in the semi-closed circle system. This requirement presents unique engineering challenges in the design and control of the anesthesia ventilator. Historically the most common solution to this challenge has been the inclusion of a bellow in the anesthesia workstation. Alternative engineering solutions to allow rebreathing include piston-type ventilators, the Maquet volume reflector, or the Draeger Perseus' turbine ventilator. The following discussion focuses on the classification, operating principles, and hazards associated with contemporary anesthesia ventilators.

Classification

Modern anesthesia ventilators can be best classified as either bellows or nonbellows. In bellows ventilators, the bellows serves as a volume reservoir for breathing gas, and the ventilator uses a double-circuit "bag in a bottle" design to deliver breaths. The bellows are typically driven pneumatically. Bellows-type ventilators can be subclassified as ascending or descending. The direction of bellows movement during the *expiratory phase* determines the bellows classification. An ascending (standing) bellows *ascends* during the expiratory phase, whereas a descending (hanging) bellows *descends* during the expiratory phase. Both types of bellows ventilators are illustrated in Fig. 22.43*A* and *B*. In nonbellows machines, the reservoir function may be served by the breathing bag itself (as in Draeger piston

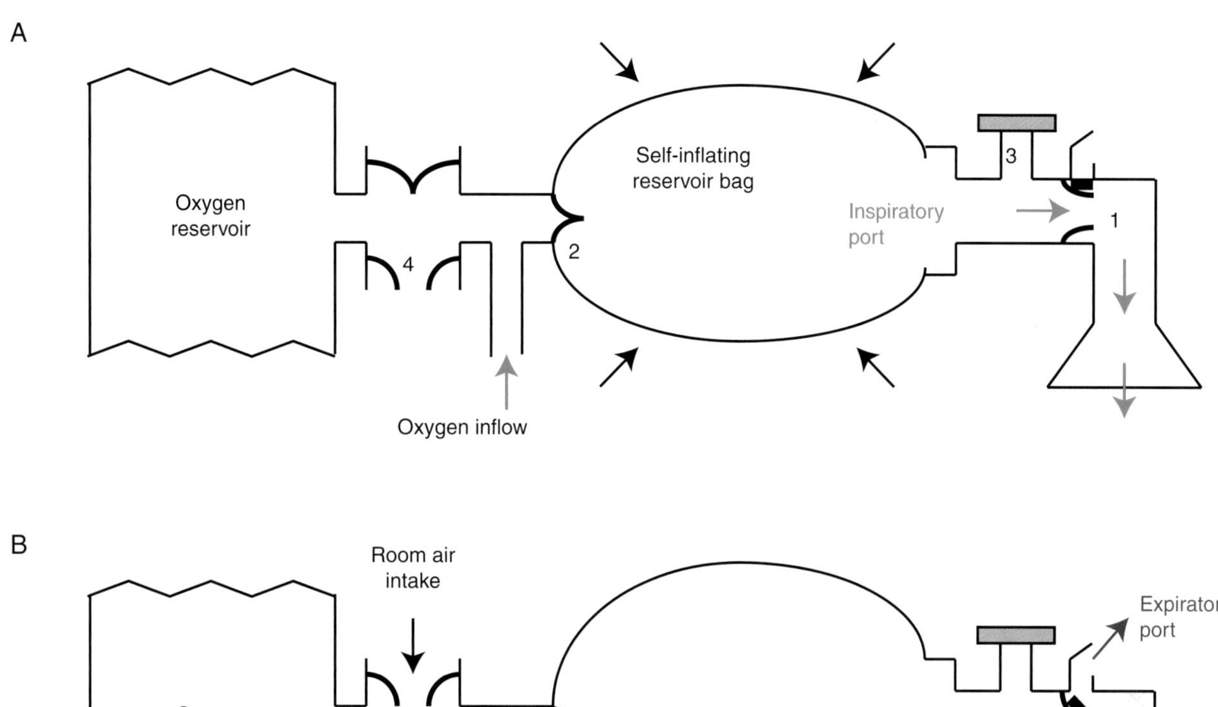

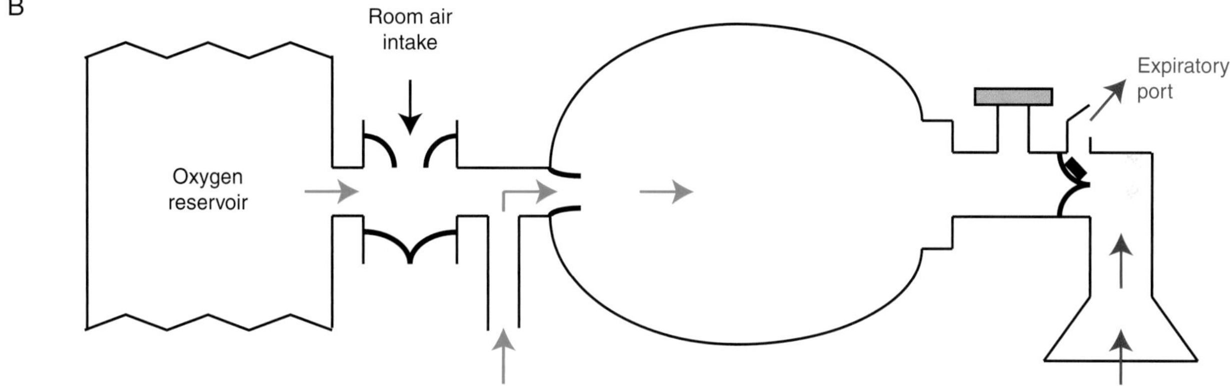

Fig. 22.42 Self-inflating manual resuscitator. (A) Flow of gas during inspiration. (1) Nonrebreathing valve, (2) bag inlet valve, (3) pop-off or pressure limiting valve (standard for pediatric and infant devices), and (4) outflow or excess-oxygen venting valve. (B) Flow of gas during expiration. See text for details. (Redrawn after Dorsch JA, Dorsch SE. The anesthesia machine. In Dorsch JA, Dorsch SE, eds. *Understanding Anesthesia Equipment*. 5th ed. Baltimore: Williams & Wilkins; 2008:83, Chapter 10 Manual Resuscitators; and Lien S, Verreault DJ, Alston TA. Sustained airway pressure after transient occlusion of a valve venting a self-inflating manual resuscitator. *J Clin Anesth*. 2013;25[5]:424–425.)

[see Fig. 22.43C] or turbine ventilators) or by the "volume reflector," in the Maquet Flow-i anesthesia workstation. The drive mechanism of piston and turbine ventilators is mechanical, while the Maquet ventilator is pneumatically driven.

Additional classifications involve the modes of ventilation that are available. Older anesthesia machine ventilators operated only in a time-cycled manner, or as "controller ventilators," without the ability to respond to a patient's spontaneous breathing efforts. Modern machines that offer synchronized intermittent mandatory ventilation (SIMV), assist/control (A/C), and pressure support ventilation (PSV) must offer the ability for the patient to trigger breaths, and are referred to as "controller/noncontroller" ventilators. In contemporary anesthesia workstations, the responsiveness to patient triggering efforts is comparable to ICU ventilators, but the clinician should be on the lookout for evidence of asynchrony in modes that allow triggering.[209f,209g] Contemporary anesthesia ventilators can function in volume-controlled or pressure-controlled modes. Finally, even though some ventilators may be pneumatically driven, all modern ventilators are under electronic control. The design of different anesthesia ventilators, with an emphasis on the integration between the ventilator and the circle breathing system, using specific workstations as examples are discussed below.

Pneumatically Driven Bellows Ventilator

The operating principle of the bellows ventilator is that it functions in a rigid airtight housing and serves as a reservoir for the patient's breathing gas. The driving force used to move gas from the bellows back to the patient is pressurized gas that flows into the bellows' housing under electropneumatic control. The bellows fills with the patient's exhalation and fresh gas flow. Once the bellows is refilled, excess circuit gas is vented to the scavenging system during the expiratory pause. The mechanisms that vent breathing circuit waste gas during mechanical ventilation with bellows ventilators differ among manufacturers and models. The bellows ventilator is traditionally designated as a *double circuit*, meaning that the ventilator drive gas and the breathing gas exist in two separate circuits. The bellows serves as the interface between the breathing gas and the drive gas, much like the reservoir bag serves as the interface between the breathing gas and the anesthesia care provider's hands.[209h] Figs. 22.44 and 22.45 illustrate the inspiratory and expiratory phases of mechanical ventilation with an ascending bellows ventilator on the GE Aisys workstation. Note that the bellows ventilator uses pressurized gas from the intermediate-pressure section of the anesthesia machine to drive the bellows. On older bellows ventilators,

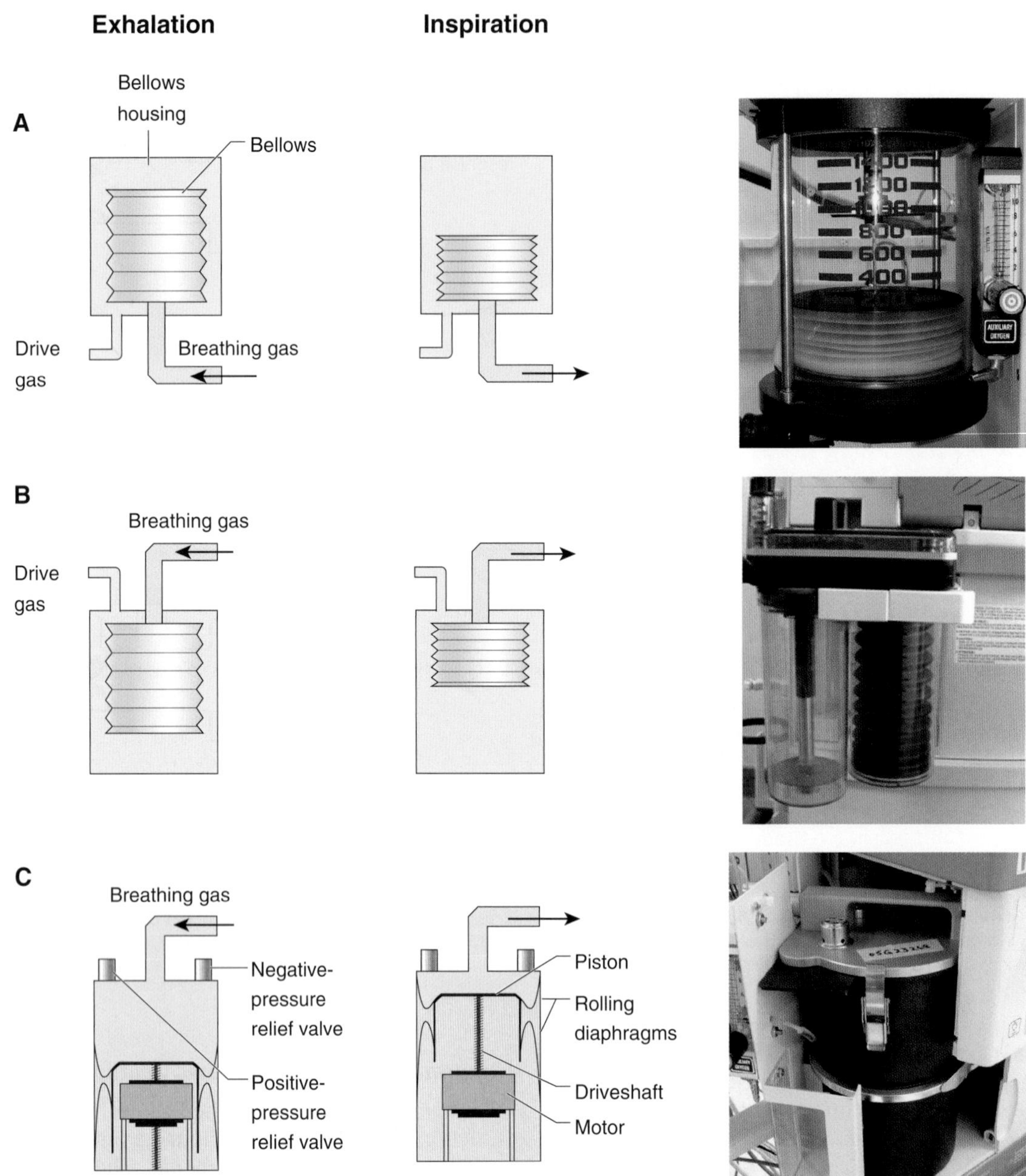

Fig. 22.43 Three types of anesthesia ventilators during exhalation *(left)* and inhalation *(middle)*, with photo *(right)*. To allow rebreathing and conservation of anesthetic gases, the anesthesia workstation ventilator must have a reservoir for the patient's exhaled breathing gas, just as the breathing bag does in manual and spontaneous modes of ventilation. This is a unique requirement of ventilators in anesthesia workstations. Intensive care unit ventilators, conversely, can simply vent exhaled gases into the environment. In the diagrams, breathing gas is green and ventilator drive gas is yellow. (A) Ascending bellows. (B) Descending (hanging) bellows. (C) Piston ventilator. See text for additional details. (Piston ventilator diagram modified from Yoder M. Ventilators. In: *Understanding Modern Anesthesia Systems*. Telford, PA: Dräger Medical; 2009.)

the user selected a tidal volume by setting a physical stop that restricted the bellows' filling (return stroke) to that point, making it a volume control ventilator.[131a] The modern bellows ventilator has primary control over the pressure applied to the bellows, and uses data integrated from the flow sensors to create volume control breaths.

The source of the drive gas for the bellows is either oxygen or air, which is obtained from the gas supply section of the workstation. Some workstations allow for the selection of either oxygen or air as the ventilator drive gas, and some can entrain room air through a Venturi effect into the oxygen drive gas flow, thereby decreasing the oxygen gas requirement. Knowing the type of gas used to drive the bellows ventilator can be important in oxygen failure emergencies. If oxygen is used as the drive gas, then the amount of oxygen consumed by the anesthesia machine will equal the amount of oxygen selected for fresh gas flow *plus* an amount approximately equal to the minute ventilation being delivered by the ventilator. Whereas a full E-cylinder can provide 10 hours of use with oxygen fresh gas flow of 1 L/min and manual ventilation through the circle system, that same E-cylinder will provide less than 2 hours' supply in an adult patient when oxygen is used as the ventilator drive gas.

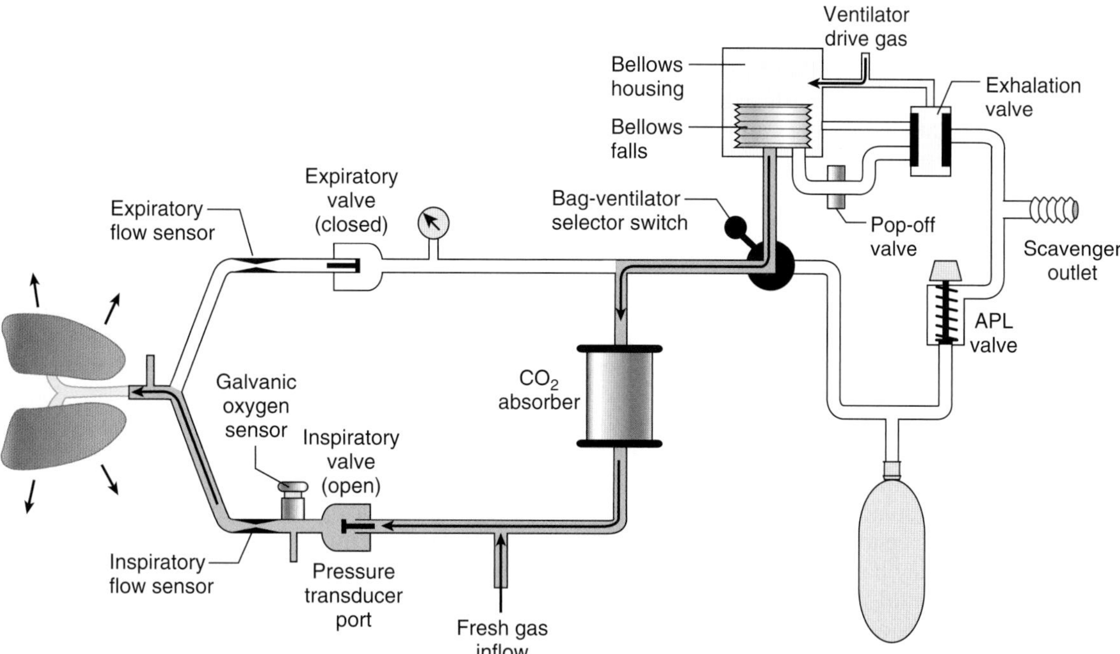

Fig. 22.44 Inspiratory phases of ventilation with an ascending bellows ventilator represented by GE Aisys anesthesia workstation. The ventilator drive gas circuit is located outside the bellows, and the patient's breathing circuit is inside the bellows. During the inspiratory phase the electronically controlled ventilator driving gas enters the bellows chamber and causes the pressure to increase, thereby compressing the bellows, which delivers gas to the patient's lungs. The drive gas also closes the exhalation valve and prevents the breathing gas from escaping into the scavenging system. Compensation for the impact of fresh gas flow on tidal volume accuracy is accomplished by monitoring the inhaled tidal volumes and adjusting ventilator drive gas volumes accordingly. *APL,* Adjustable pressure-limiting; *CO_2,* carbon dioxide. (Image courtesy Dr. Michael A. Olympio; modified with his permission. Adapted from Datex-Ohmeda. *Aisys Anesthesia Machine: Technical Reference.* Madison, WI: Datex-Ohmeda; 2005.)

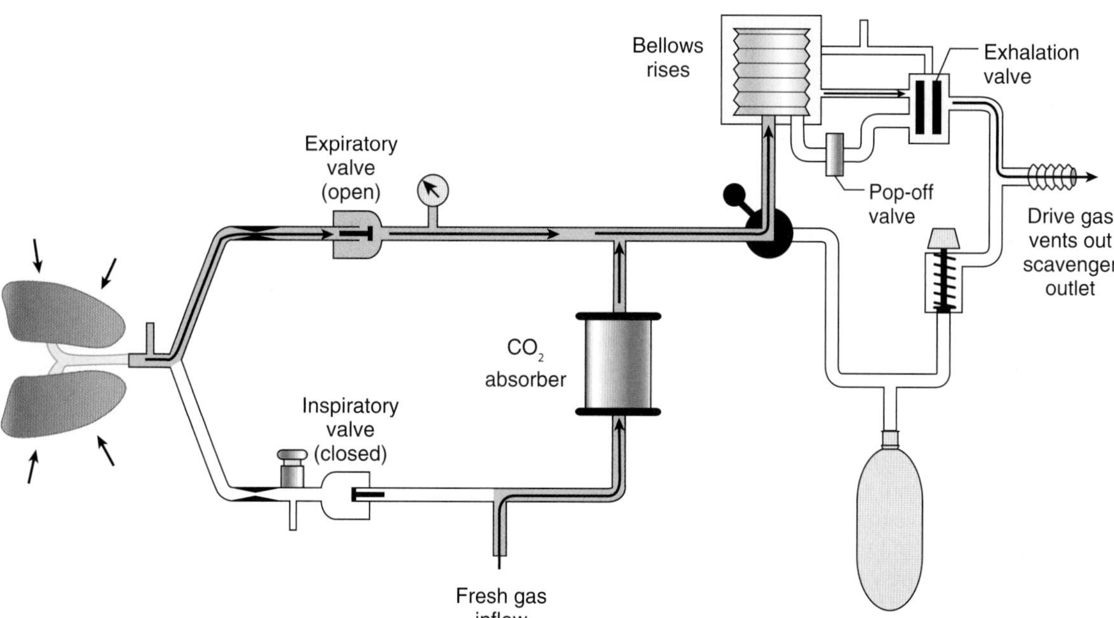

Fig. 22.45 During the early expiratory phase, the patient is able to exhale into the bellows because the ventilator exhalation valve is now open, thus allowing the drive gas in the bellows housing to vent through the scavenger outlet. The pop-off or ventilator relief valve prevents bellows gas from escaping at this point so the bellows can fill. In the late expiratory phase, positive end-expiratory pressure (PEEP) is provided by pressurization of the bellows housing and pressure modulation of the expiratory valve. (Courtesy Dr. Michael A. Olympio; modified with his permission. Adapted with permission from Datex-Ohmeda. *Aisys Anesthesia Machine: Technical Reference.* Madison, WI: Datex-Ohmeda; 2005.)

As described earlier, bellows-type ventilators can be classified according to the direction that they move during patient exhalation. Ascending bellows rise with exhalation, and descending bellows fall with exhalation (see Fig. 22.43). Older pneumatic ventilators and some newer anesthesia workstations use weighted descending bellows, but most contemporary bellows ventilators employ an ascending bellows design. Of the two configurations, the ascending bellows is considered safer. An ascending bellows will not fill if total disconnection occurs, or it may only partially fill if a circuit leak exceeds the fresh gas flow rate, providing an important visual cue for a circuit disconnect or leak. The bellows of a descending bellows ventilator, on the other hand, will continue its regular upward and downward movement despite patient disconnection: the drive gas pushes the bellows upward during the inspiratory phase, and during the expiratory phase the bellows "fills" with entrained room air instead of the patient's exhaled gas, because of the weighted bellows. The pressure monitor and the volume monitor may be fooled even if disconnection is complete.[36] An essential safety feature of any anesthesia workstation that uses a descending bellows is an integrated CO_2 apnea alarm that cannot be disabled while the ventilator is in use.

Problems With Bellows Ventilators. Correct function of the bellows ventilator requires that both the bellows housing and the bellows itself be free of leaks. Improper seating of the plastic bellows housing can result in inadequate ventilation because a portion of the driving gas is vented to the atmosphere.[209i] A hole in the bellows can lead to alveolar hyperinflation and possibly barotrauma in some ventilators because high-pressure driving gas can enter the patient's circuit. The oxygen concentration of the patient's gas may increase when the driving gas is 100% oxygen, or it may decrease if the driving gas is composed of air or an air-oxygen mixture.[210]

The ventilator relief valve (sometimes called the "exhalation valve"; see Fig. 22.44) can potentially cause problems. The function of this valve is to open during exhalation once the bellows has refilled, venting excess gas to the scavenger outlet. Hypoventilation can occur if the valve becomes incompetent because anesthetic gas is delivered to the scavenging system instead of to the patient during the inspiratory phase. Ventilator relief valve incompetency can result from a disconnected pilot line, a ruptured valve, or a damaged flapper valve.[211,212] A ventilator relief valve stuck in the closed or partially closed position can cause either barotrauma or undesired PEEP.[213] Excessive suction from the scavenging system can draw the ventilator relief valve to its seat and close the valve during both the inspiratory and expiratory phases.[37] In this case, breathing circuit pressure escalates because the excess anesthetic gas cannot be vented. A number of manufacturers' bellows-style anesthesia workstations send the used ventilator drive gas to the anesthesia gas scavenging system during exhalation. Under certain conditions, notably high fresh gas flows combined with high minute ventilation, the scavenging system can be overwhelmed, causing inadvertent high PEEP levels and/or pollution of the operating room with waste anesthetic gases (see section on scavenging systems). Other mechanical problems that can occur include leaks within the system, faulty pressure regulators, and faulty valves.

Mechanically Driven Piston Ventilator

Mechanically driven, electronically controlled piston-type ventilators use a computer-controlled stepper motor instead of compressed drive gas to deliver tidal volume (see Fig. 22.43). These are *single-circuit* ventilators, because there is not a separate ventilator drive gas circuit. The piston operates much like the plunger of a syringe in a cylinder of essentially zero compliance.[131a] The ventilator has primary control over the volume displaced in the circuit and uses the data from pressure sensors to create pressure control breaths. The computerized controls can support a variety of ventilator modes, including pressure or volume limited breaths, in controlled, synchronized, or spontaneous modes.

Because the patient's mechanical breath is delivered without the use of compressed gas to actuate a bellows, these systems consume dramatically less compressed gas during ventilator operation than do traditional pneumatic ventilators. This improvement in efficiency may have clinical significance when the anesthesia workstation is used in a setting where no pipeline gas supply is available (e.g., remote locations or office-based anesthesia practices). Another advantage of the piston ventilator is the potential for very accurate tidal volume delivery, because of the low compliance of the piston chamber. This is in contrast to bellows-type ventilators, in which the drive gas can be subject to varying degrees of compression. With either piston or bellows ventilators, feedback mechanisms that help maintain stable tidal volume delivery include circuit compliance compensation and the use of inspired tidal volume measurement as a feedback signal.

Figs. 22.46 and 22.47 illustrate the inspiratory and expiratory phases of mechanical ventilation with a piston ventilator, the Dräger Fabius workstation. Note the location of the ventilator within the breathing circuit between the fresh gas inflow and the inspiratory valve. The breathing bag participates in the circuit during mechanical ventilation, acting as the reservoir for rebreathing. The circuit employs a *fresh gas decoupling valve* to exclude fresh gas from being added to the tidal volume during inspiration. Therefore during inspiration the fresh gas is added to the breathing bag. During the expiratory phase, the breathing bag initially fills with exhaled gas; then, as the piston returns to its starting position, the fresh gas decoupling valve opens, and fresh gas flow plus gas from the breathing bag refill the piston chamber.

The piston in a piston ventilator tends to be fully or partially concealed from view, unlike the bellows on a bellows ventilator. The piston ventilator therefore does not naturally provide the visual feedback of a circuit disconnect or leak that is provided by the ascending bellows. However, the breathing bag, which serves as the reservoir during mechanical ventilation, moves with patient ventilation and can visually alert the provider to disconnect.

Additional feedback mechanisms have been incorporated on particular machines. For example, the Dräger Fabius Tiro has a transparent piston housing so that the user can visualize the motion of the piston, and the Dräger Apollo can be programmed to emit a breathing sound with the movement of the piston to provide an auditory cue.

A potential hazard associated with piston ventilators is that, like descending bellows ventilators, they will refill

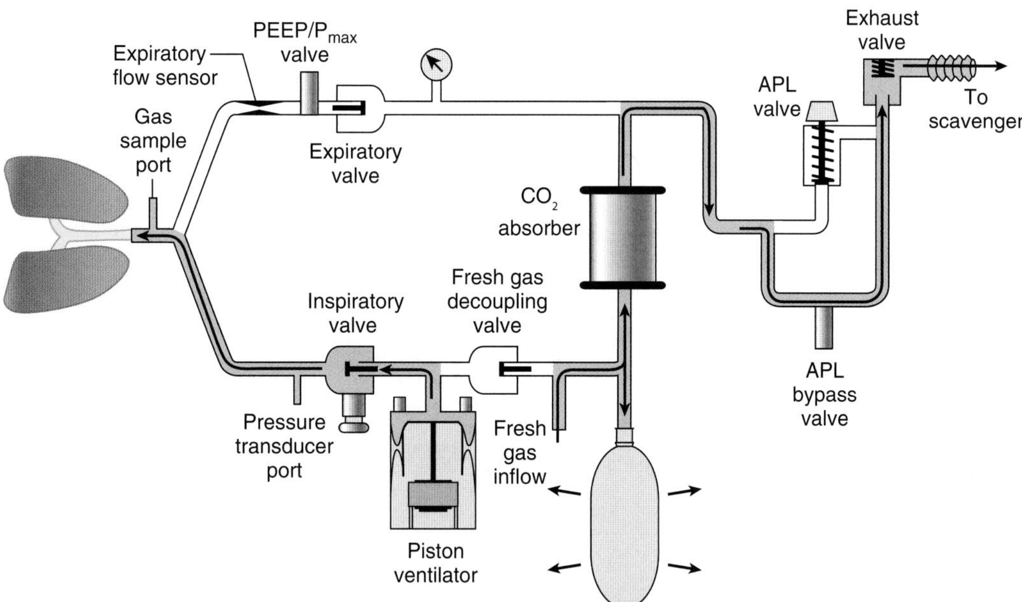

Fig. 22.46 Inspiratory phase of ventilation with a piston ventilator represented by Dräger Fabius anesthesia workstation. During inspiration, the positive end-expiratory pressure *(PEEP)*/maximum pressure *(P_{max})* valve is held closed. The pressure in the breathing circuit that is generated by the ventilator closes the fresh gas decoupling valve. This directs fresh gas flow toward the breathing bag during inspiration so it does not interfere with tidal volume accuracy. Excess fresh gas flows past the open adjustable pressure-limiting *(APL)* bypass valve, through the exhaust check valve, and to the scavenger. Note how the breathing bag is integral to circuit function during mechanical ventilation. In the manual and spontaneous modes of ventilation, the piston ventilator is held in the upward position, and the APL bypass valve closes, thus making the APL valve operable. (Courtesy Dr. Michael A. Olympio; modified with his permission. Adapted from Dräger Medical. *Dräger Technical Service Manual: Fabius GS Anesthesia System.* Telford, PA: Rev: E, Dräger Medical; 2002.)

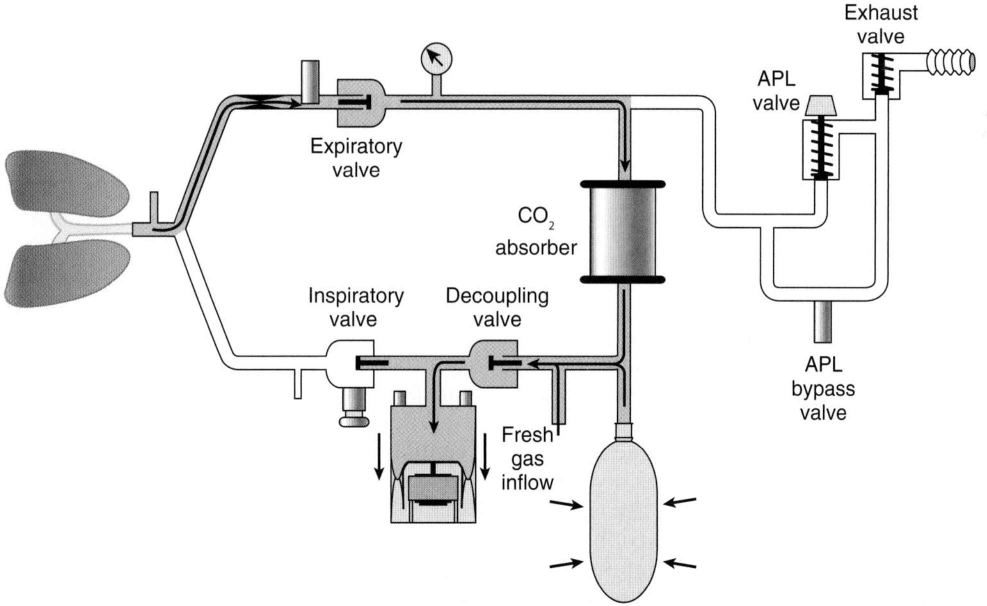

Fig. 22.47 During the initial phase of exhalation, before the piston begins moving back to starting position and the decoupling valve opens, the patient exhales into the breathing bag, and fresh gas continues to flow retrograde (not pictured). Once the decoupling valve opens, the piston's movement back to its starting position draws in gas stored within the breathing bag and fresh gas from the fresh gas inflow. Positive end-expiratory pressure (PEEP) is maintained by the PEEP/maximum pressure valve, which also prevents the ventilator from pulling in gas from the lungs. Once the piston reaches the bottom of its stroke, fresh gas flow reverses course and flows in retrograde fashion toward the breathing bag and the absorber (as in Fig. 22.46). Excess gas vents through the exhaust valve to the scavenger (Fig. 22.46). *APL,* Adjustable pressure-limiting. (Courtesy Dr. Michael A. Olympio; modified with his permission. Adapted from Dräger Medical. *Dräger Technical Service Manual: Fabius GS Anesthesia System.* Telford, PA: Rev: E, Dräger Medical; 2002.)

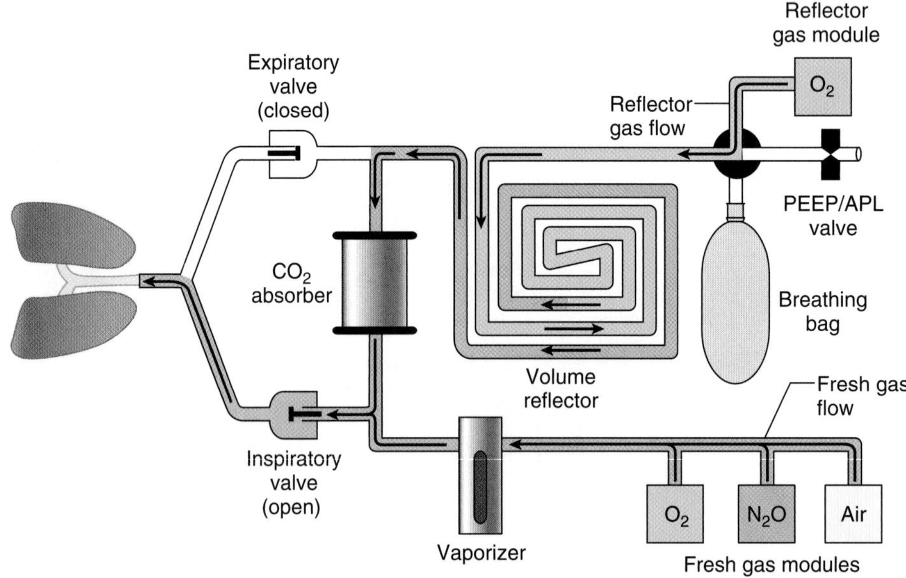

Fig. 22.48 Simplified schematic of the Maquet FLOW-i anesthesia workstation breathing circuit and gas supply system during inspiration in a controlled ventilation mode. The reflector gas module provides the driving force for ventilation by pushing gas out of the volume reflector to the patient. Volume reflector gas combines with the fresh gas flow downstream from the carbon dioxide *(CO_2)* absorber. *APL,* Adjustable pressure-limiting; *N_2O,* nitrous oxide; *O_2,* oxygen; *PEEP,* positive end-expiratory pressure. See text for additional details. (Adapted from Maquet Critical Care. *User's Manual: FLOW-i 1.2 Anesthesia System.* Solna, Sweden: Rev: 11, Maquet Critical Care; 2011.)

even if a circuit disconnection occurs. Similarly, if a circuit leak is present, piston ventilators may entrain room air through the leak, thereby diluting oxygen and anesthetic agent. The associated risks are hypoxemia and awareness. The Dräger Fabius series piston ventilator will entrain room air through an auxiliary air valve, seen in Fig. 22.43, to fill the piston chamber if the fresh gas flow fails or is inadequate (instead of causing negative pressure in the breathing circuit). However, if this occurs, an alarm will alert the operator. A positive-pressure relief valve on the ventilator prevents excessively high breathing circuit pressure (60-80 cm H_2O).[131a]

Maquet FLOW-i Anesthesia System With Volume Reflector

The Maquet FLOW-i anesthesia workstation uses a novel device called the *volume reflector* (Figs. 22.48 and 22.49) to act as the reservoir. The volume reflector is essentially a long plastic tube with a volume of 1.2 L, coiled compactly to fit in the anesthesia workstation. The volume reflector is functional and "in-circuit" during all modes of ventilation. It is interposed between the patient and the reflector gas module during positive-pressure ventilation or between the patient and the breathing bag during spontaneous or assisted ventilation. The volume reflector therefore acts as a volume reservoir while at the same time preventing mixing between the gas at the two ends of the tube.

Mechanical ventilation is powered by the *reflector gas module,* a solenoid-controlled oxygen flow source, which pushes gas out of the volume reflector through the CO_2 absorber and to the patient during inspiration, much like a piston (see Fig. 22.48). To understand the function of the volume reflector and reflector gas module, it is convenient to start with the expiratory phase (see Fig. 22.49), where exhaled patient gas fills the volume reflector's proximal end (nearest the patient), displacing reflector gas module gas out the PEEP valve and into the scavenging system. At the end of exhalation, the volume reflector is filled at the patient end with exhaled gas and is filled distally with a mixture of exhaled gases and reflector gas. The coiled design of the volume reflector prevents significant mixing between these gases of different compositions. The inspired tidal volume is generated by a combination of gas from the fresh gas modules and the reflector gas module, which work together in a coordinated manner to control gas flow and pressure in the breathing circuit so that operator-determined ventilation parameters are maintained. During mechanical ventilation on the FLOW-i, the fresh gas flow is not constant, but rather occurs primarily during inspiration. The inhaled anesthetic, if chosen, is injected into this flow (see earlier section on **Injection-Type Vaporizers**). All the gas modules use feedback loop–controlled, solenoid-actuated, pneumatic valves similar in function to those found in a servo-controlled ICU ventilator.[214]

When the workstation is in the spontaneous mode of ventilation, the breathing bag is enabled, and the reflector gas module is disabled. The patient breathes in and out of the volume reflector, and circuit pressure is controlled by the operator-adjustable APL valve. Excess gases in controlled and spontaneous modes of ventilation are vented to the scavenger through the dual-function PEEP-APL valve.

The FLOW-i system can compensate for breathing system leaks by increasing reflector gas module flow. The operator is informed if this occurs. Because the reflector gas module provides only 100% oxygen, dilution of anesthetic gas occurs in this circumstance. The machine is nearly entirely electronically interfaced; therefore an emergency manual ventilation backup mode is provided for cases of system failure. This emergency backup mode provides an oxygen flow meter and mechanical APL valve linked to the patient circuit.[214]

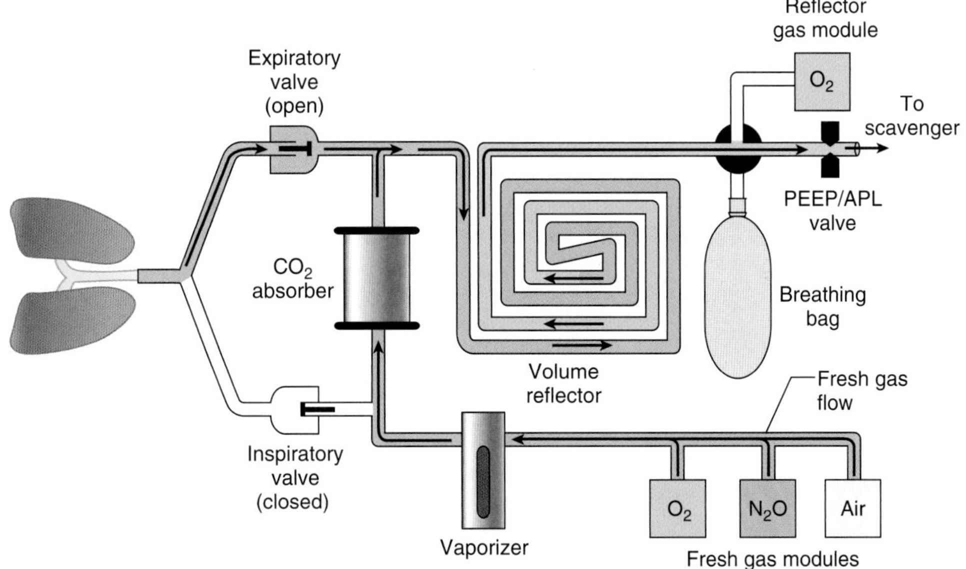

Fig. 22.49 Maquet FLOW-i breathing circuit and gas supply during exhalation in a controlled ventilation mode. The patient exhales into the volume reflector, which serves as an exhalation reservoir. The patient only partially fills the volume reflector. Fresh gas flows in retrograde fashion and combines with the exhaled gas. Excess gas is vented to the scavenger through the positive end-expiratory pressure *(PEEP)*/adjustable pressure-limiting *(APL)* valve, which also controls breathing circuit pressure (PEEP). When the machine is placed in the manual mode of ventilation, the breathing bag is enabled and the reflector gas module is disabled. In the manual mode, the patient breathes in and out of the volume reflector and can be assisted with the breathing bag. The PEEP/APL valve vents excess gas to the scavenger and controls breathing circuit pressure (continuous positive airway pressure). *CO_2*, Carbon dioxide, *N_2O*, nitrous oxide; *O_2*, oxygen. (Adapted from Maquet Critical Care. *User's Manual: FLOW-i 1.2 Anesthesia System.* Solna, Sweden: Rev: 11, Maquet Critical Care; 2011.)

Dräger Anesthesia Systems With Turbine Ventilators

A number of newer ventilators designed for the ICU utilize turbine technology to generate mechanical ventilation. Turbine ventilators use mechanical energy to spin a small turbine (fan) at very high speeds to create pressure and flow. Some possible functional advantages of turbine-based ventilators mentioned in bench testing include better responsiveness to patient triggering, more effective PSV, and, in some cases, more accurate tidal volume delivery under high ventilatory workload.[214a,214b,214c]

The Dräger Zeus and Perseus workstations incorporate turbine-type ventilators (Figs. 22.50 and 22.51). In constructing an anesthesia workstation, the major advantage of the turbine is that it can be placed directly within the circle system. Unlike the bellows or volume reflector, it does not require a separate quantity of gas to move the patient's tidal volume; and unlike a piston, it does not require refilling. During inspiration (see Fig. 22.50), the turbine blower generates flow and pressure directed into the inspiratory limb of the patient circuit, drawing gas from the breathing bag, which serves as a reservoir during mechanical ventilation. The fresh gas flow is incorporated as part of this inspiratory flow. During exhalation (see Fig. 22.51), exhaled gas fills the bag before escaping to the scavenge system, and that portion of the fresh gas flow that occurs during exhalation travels in the reverse direction toward the bag as well. As in the piston ventilators, the breathing bag is an integral part of the circuit during mechanical ventilation, continuing to serve a reservoir function. Unlike the piston ventilators, the turbine ventilator design implies that the breathing bag empties during inspiration and refills during expiration. The bag's motion may serve as a visual indicator of ventilation, and depending on set fresh gas flow, of circuit leak.

Unlike the piston, the turbine is primarily a pressure generator. The ventilator utilizes flow sensors and electronic controls to generate a number of modes of mechanical ventilation, including volume and pressure control, pressure support, and airway pressure release ventilation. In the spontaneous mode of ventilation, the operator may dial in a CPAP level.

Target-Controlled Inhalational Anesthesia

During traditional operation of the anesthetic workstation, the anesthesia provider controls the composition of the fresh gas flow that is added to the circle system every minute. Since this fresh gas mixes with the gases already in the circle breathing system, there may be a significant difference between the composition of the fresh gas flow and the final concentration of the inspired (or expired) gases. As the fresh gas flow is decreased, there may be a greater difference between the fresh gas composition and the actual inspired concentrations. If the oxygen in the fresh gas flow is less than the patient's metabolic oxygen requirement, then the amount of oxygen extracted from the circle breathing circuit every minute is more than the amount added, and the inspired gas will eventually become hypoxic.[214d] Reducing the fresh gas flow reduces the total amount of anesthetic agent used, which reduces cost and the environmental footprint. However, low-flow anesthesia can be challenging in practice, as it is easier to control the patient's actual inspired gas composition when the fresh gas flow is high.

On anesthesia workstations where the flow control valves and the anesthetic vaporizers are under electronic

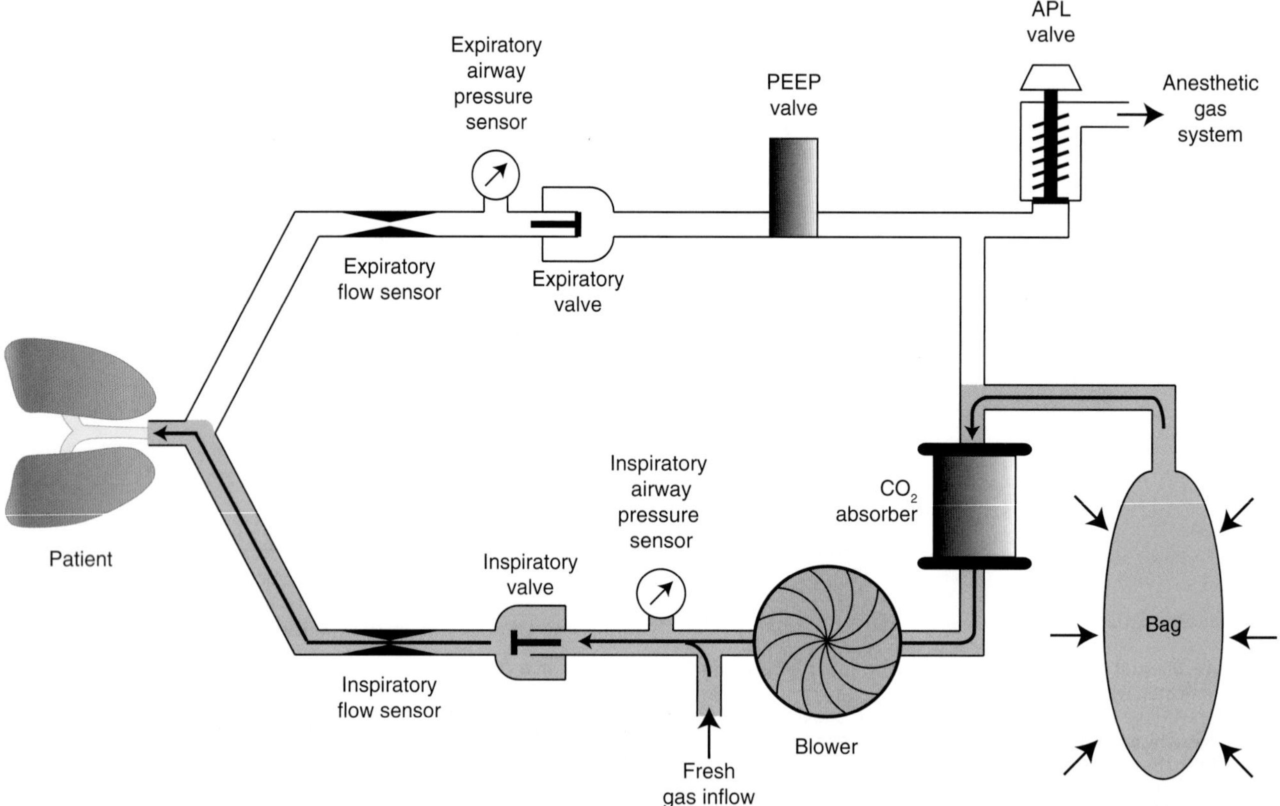

Fig. 22.50 Simplified schematic of the Dräger Perseus anesthesia workstation breathing circuit and gas supply system. During inspiration the positive end-expiratory pressure *(PEEP)* valve is held closed and pressure is generated by the turbine blower. There is no fresh gas decoupling valve. The flow generated by the blower draws gas from the breathing bag, which acts as a reservoir during mechanical ventilation, through the carbon dioxide *(CO_2)* absorber, and to the patient. In the manual and spontaneous modes of ventilation, the blower is passive, allowing the adjustable pressure-limiting *(APL)* valve to control the pressure in the breathing circuit. (Adapted from Drägerwerk AG & Co. *Technical Documentation IPM: Perseus A500 and Perseus A500 Ceiling*. Lübeck, Germany: Rev: 5.0; n.d.)

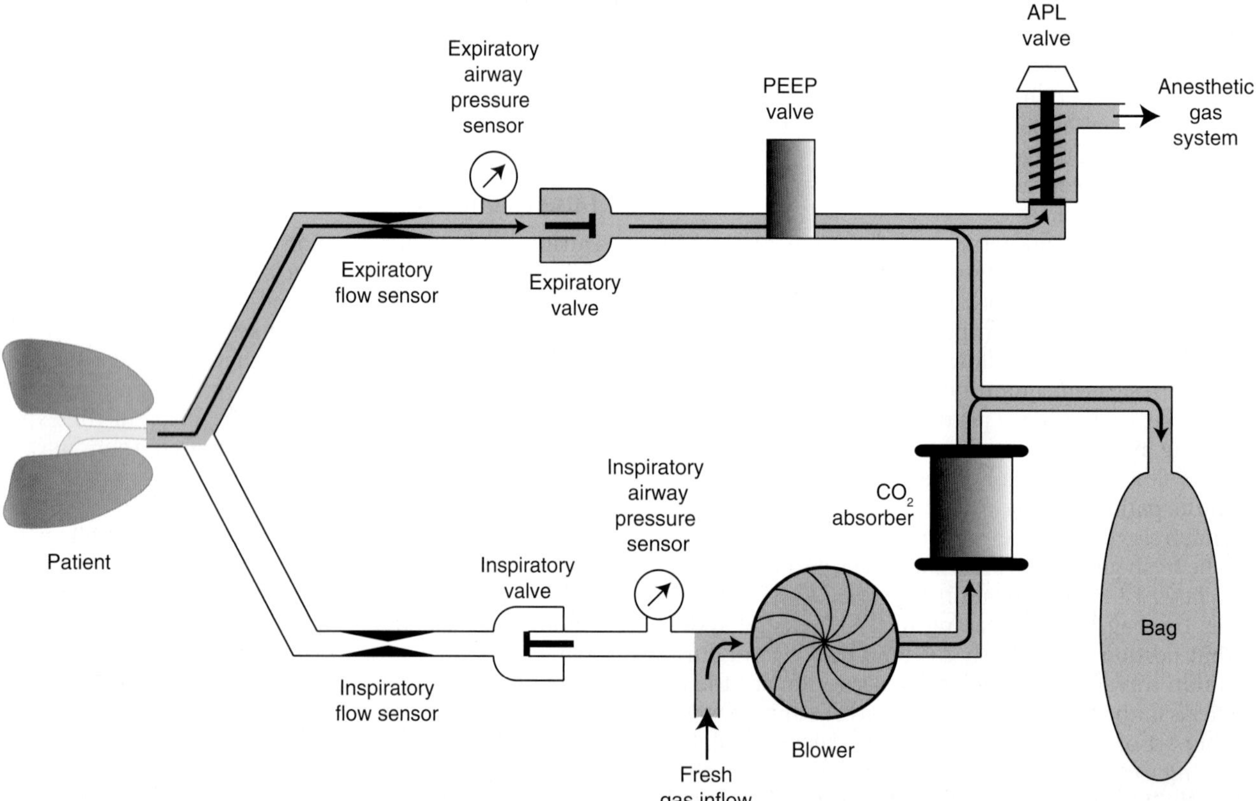

Fig. 22.51 Dräger Perseus anesthesia workstation breathing circuit and gas supply system during exhalation phase of controlled ventilation. The exhalation phase begins when the positive end-expiratory pressure *(PEEP)* valve opens and exhaled gas fills the breathing bag. The portion of fresh gas that flows during the exhalation phase also flows retrograde toward the breathing bag. Excess flow is vented to the anesthetic gas system (scavenge). Note that the adjustable pressure-limiting *(APL)* valve is not active during controlled ventilation. PEEP is maintained by a separate valve. ***CO2*, Carbon dioxide.** (Adapted from Drägerwerk AG & Co. *Technical Documentation IPM: Perseus A500 and Perseus A500 Ceiling*. Lübeck, Germany, n.d., Rev: 5.0.)

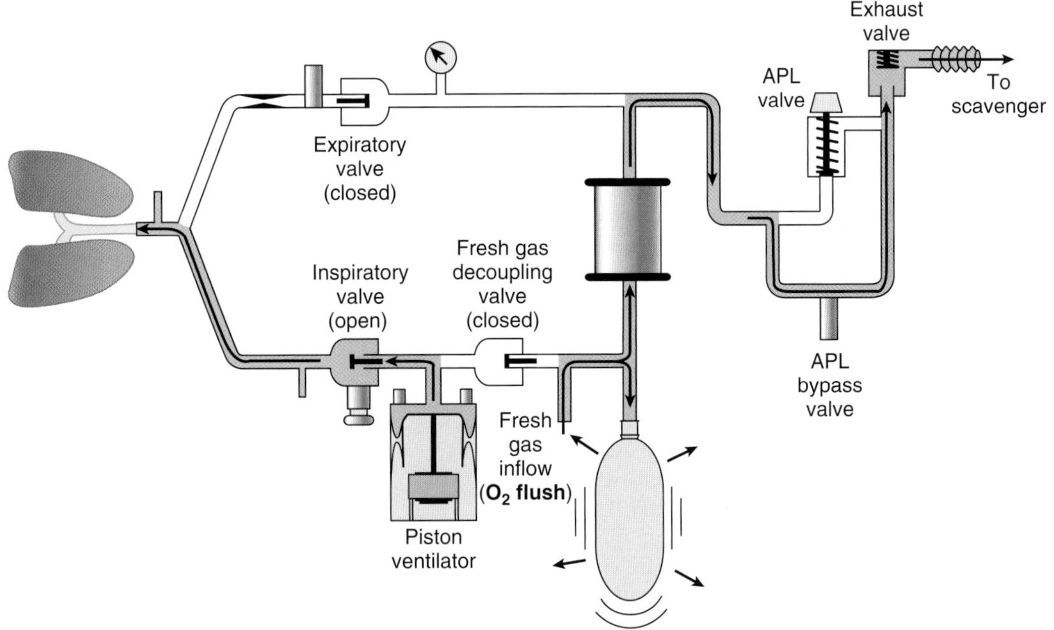

Fig. 22.52 Fresh gas decoupling during an oxygen *(O_2)* flush shown on the Dräger Fabius workstation. During inspiration the positive end-expiratory pressure/maximum pressure valve is held closed. The pressure in the breathing circuit that is generated by the ventilator closes the fresh gas decoupling valve. This directs the high-volume oxygen flush flow toward the breathing bag during inspiration so it does not contribute to inhaled tidal volume and breathing circuit pressure. The O_2 flush gas also flows past the open adjustable pressure-limiting *(APL)* bypass valve, through the exhaust check valve, and to the scavenger. (Modified image courtesy of Dr. Michael A. Olympio. Adapted from Dräger Medical: *Dräger Technical Service Manual: Fabius GS Anesthesia System.* Rev: E. Telford, PA: Dräger Medical; 2002.)

control, it is possible to implement *target-controlled inhalational anesthesia.* The targets subject to control are the end-tidal anesthetic agent and the end-tidal oxygen concentration. Currently, Dräger, GE, and Maquet all have target-controlled systems available. The major advantage of the target control is reduced consumption of anesthetic agent.[214f-214h] These systems rely on proprietary algorithms, and the actual savings may depend on how fast the algorithm tries to achieve the desired anesthetic depth. The target-controlled system might actually prioritize rapid achievement of set anesthetic agent (requiring high initial fresh gas flow) over reducing fresh gas flow and anesthetic agent consumption.[214i] The benefits of low-flow anesthesia could be realized by a vigilant anesthesia provider, but at the expense of significantly more key-strokes per case.[214h] Although the target-controlled modes of inhalational anesthesia seem likely to reduce anesthetic agent use, and to provide an additional layer of patient safety in low-flow anesthesia, none are currently approved by the FDA for use in the United States.

Fresh Gas Flow Compensation and Fresh Gas Decoupling

On older bellows-type anesthesia workstations, the portion of fresh gas flow that occurred during an inspiratory cycle was added to the set tidal volume, leading to variation in tidal volume depending on the set fresh gas flow. During the inspiratory phase of mechanical ventilation, the ventilator relief valve (also known as the ventilator pop-off valve) is typically closed, and the breathing system's APL valve is most commonly out of circuit. Therefore during positive-pressure ventilation, the patient's lungs received the volume from the bellows in addition to that from the flowmeters during the inspiratory phase. The amount of excess volume (and pressure) that the patient received was proportional to the direction and magnitude of the change in the fresh gas flow rate. As the practitioner turned up the fresh gas flow, the tidal volume increased. The opposite would occur if the flow rate were decreased from the baseline. It was therefore common knowledge that the operator needed to adjust the set tidal volume on the ventilator if the total fresh gas flow rate was changed to maintain stable tidal volumes and airway pressure.

Newer workstations have engineering features that provide compensation of fresh gas flow to maintain stable tidal volume delivery. Broadly speaking, the workstation will either exclude the fresh gas from the inspiratory limb of the circuit during inspiration, or it will use electronic controls to compensate for the fresh gas flow's contribution. The precise manner in which this is accomplished accounts for much of the variation in breathing system design. On the Dräger Fabius workstation, a principle called *fresh gas decoupling* is used to prevent changes in the fresh gas flow rate from altering positive-pressure tidal volumes and breathing circuit pressures. During the inspiratory phase of ventilation, a decoupling valve located upstream from the piston ventilator diverts the fresh gas stream toward the breathing bag and scavenge outlet during each positive-pressure breath (Fig. 22.52). The GE Aisys system, on the other hand, uses inspiratory tidal volume measurement as a feedback signal for the automatic adjustment of ventilator drive gas volume to compensate for changes in fresh gas flow and leaks.[214j]

On workstations without a fresh gas decoupling feature, inappropriate activation of the oxygen flush valve during the inspiratory phase of mechanical ventilation can add a substantial amount of volume to the circuit and can result in baro- and/or volutrauma because excess pressure and volume may not be able to be vented from the breathing circuit.[25] Although the circuit high-pressure alarm may provide warning, unless an adjustable inspiratory pressure limiter is set to a relatively low value, high pressures can be realized. On workstations equipped with adjustable inspiratory pressure limiters, maximal inspiratory pressure may be set by the user to a desired peak airway pressure. An adjustable pressure relief valve opens when the predetermined user-selected pressure is reached. This theoretically prevents the generation of excessive airway pressure. However, this feature depends on having preset the appropriate pop-off pressure. If the setting is too low, insufficient pressure for ventilation may be generated and can result in inadequate minute ventilation; if set too high, the excessive airway pressure may still occur and result in patient harm. Some machines may also include a factory-preset inspiratory pressure safety valve that opens at a preset airway pressure, such as 60 to 80 cm H_2O, to minimize the risk of barotrauma. Therefore modern workstations without fresh gas decoupling usually reach a maximum pressure limit and terminate ventilation, release pressure, or sustain at the pressure limit.[215] In machines with a fresh gas decoupling feature, the oxygen flush inflow is diverted away from the patient during positive-pressure ventilation, thereby maintaining stable volumes and pressures.

TABLE 22.9 National Institute for Occupational Safety and Health Recommendations for Trace Anesthetic Gas Levels

Anesthetic Gas	Maximum TWA Concentration (ppm)*
Halogenated agent alone	2
Nitrous oxide	25
Combination of halogenated agent plus nitrous oxide	
Halogenated agent	0.5
Nitrous oxide	25
Dental facilities (nitrous oxide alone)	50

*Time-weighted average sampling, also known as time-integrated sampling, is a sampling method that evaluates the average concentration of anesthetic gas over a prolonged period, such as 1 to 8 hours.
TWA, Time-weighted average.
From U.S. Department of Health, Education and Welfare. *Criteria for a Recommended Standard: Occupational Exposure to Waste Anesthetic Gases and Vapors.* Washington, DC: U.S. Department of Health, Education and Welfare; 1977.

SCAVENGING SYSTEMS

Scavenging is the collection and subsequent removal of waste anesthetic gases from both the anesthesia machine and the anesthetizing location. Scavenging is required because the fresh gas flow rates used during most anesthetic regimens deliver more anesthetic agent than necessary, as well as more oxygen than is being consumed. Without scavenging, operating room personnel could be exposed to anesthetic gases, and there could be an increased risk of an oxygen-rich environment supporting combustion.

In 1977, the National Institute for Occupational Safety and Health (NIOSH) prepared a document entitled *Criteria for a Recommended Standard: Occupational Exposure to Waste Anesthetic Gases and Vapors.*[216] Although it was maintained that a minimal safe level of exposure could not be defined, the NIOSH proceeded to issue the recommendations shown in Table 22.9. These same criteria remain in place today. Contemporary scavenging systems are governed by standards set forth by the ISO.[11,216a] In 1999, the ASA Task Force on Trace Anesthetic Gases developed a booklet entitled *Waste Anesthetic Gases: Information for Management in Anesthetizing Areas and the Postanesthesia Care Unit.* This publication describes the role of regulatory agencies, reviews scavenging and monitoring equipment, and provides recommendations.[217] Finally, the Occupational Safety and Health Administration (OSHA) publishes *Anesthetic Gases: Guidelines for Workplace Exposures* on its website; this document does not establish legal standards, but is a repository of information, guidelines, and references.[217a]

The two major causes of waste gas contamination in the operating room are the anesthetic technique used and equipment issues.[217,218] Regarding the anesthetic technique, causes of operating room contamination include: (1) failure to turn off the gas flow control valves or the vaporizer when the circuit is disconnected from the patient; (2) use of poorly fitting masks; (3) flushing of the circuit into the room; (4) filling of anesthetic vaporizers, particularly if spillage occurs; (5) use of uncuffed endotracheal tubes; and (6) use of breathing circuits other than the circle system. Equipment failure or lack of understanding of proper equipment use can also contribute to operating room contamination. Leaks can occur in the high-pressure hoses, the nitrous oxide tank mounting, the high- or low-pressure circuits of the anesthesia machine, or the circle system, particularly at the CO_2 absorber assembly. The anesthesia care provider must be certain that the room suction and scavenging system is operational and adjusted properly to ensure adequate scavenging. Waste flow from a side-stream gas analyzer (50-250 mL/min) must also be directed to the scavenging system or returned to the breathing system to prevent pollution of the operating room.[217,218]

Classifications and Components

Waste anesthesia gas scavenging systems can be classified as: *active* or *passive.* In active systems, the scavenging system is connected to a vacuum source, such as the hospital's suction system. Passive systems simply vent the waste gas into a heating, ventilation, and air conditioning (HVAC) system or through a hose to the building's exterior through a wall, ceiling, or floor. Passive systems rely only on the slight positive pressure of the gases leaving the gas-collecting assembly to provide the flow. If the passive system vents to an HVAC system, it is mandatory that it be a *nonrecirculating* system. Passive systems are less common in contemporary operating rooms.

Scavenging systems may also be *open* or *closed.* An open scavenging system allows for room air to be entrained into the flow of waste gas, whereas a closed system does not.[219] This distinction is discussed more thoroughly below.

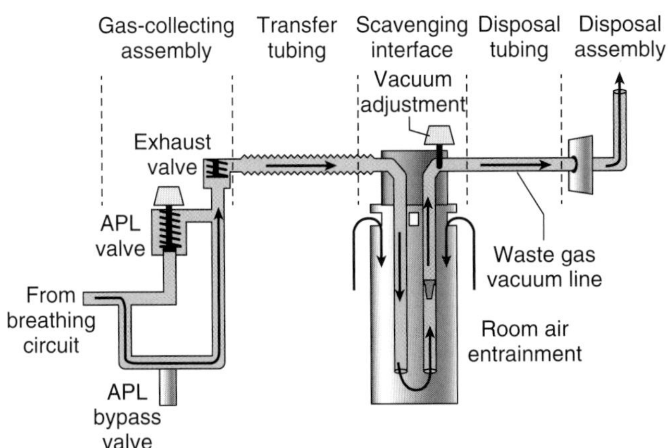

Fig. 22.53 Components of a scavenging system using the example of a Dräger Fabius system (Dräger Medical, Telford, PA) connected to an open, active scavenging system. The transfer tubing has a connector size distinct from the breathing circuit to prevent misconnections. Obstructions in the gas-collecting assembly or transfer tubing can cause high pressure in the breathing circuit. Leaks, inadequate suction, or failure of the scavenging interface can cause environmental contamination. *APL,* Adjustable pressure-limiting. See text for details. (From Brockwell RC. Delivery systems for inhaled anesthesia. In: Barash PG, ed. *Clinical Anesthesia.* 5th ed. Philadelphia: Lippincott Williams & Wilkins; 2006:589.)

Scavenging systems classically have five components (Fig. 22.53): (1) the gas-collecting assembly, (2) the transfer tubing, (3) the scavenging interface, (4) the gas disposal assembly tubing, and (5) an active or passive gas disposal assembly.[220]

Gas-Collecting Assembly. The gas-collecting assemblies are where waste gas exit from the breathing circuit and connect to the transfer tubing. Waste anesthetic gases are vented from the anesthesia system either through the APL valve or through some sort of ventilator relief valve. Excess patient exhaled gas must exit the breathing system through one of these valves or be shed into the room (e.g., poor face-mask fit, endotracheal tube leak, machine leak). Ventilator drive gas on contemporary bellows-type ventilators, as well as the flow from the reflector gas module on the Maquet FLOW-i, are vented via the scavenging system as well. This is significant because under conditions of high fresh gas flow and high minute ventilation, the gases flowing into the scavenging interface may overwhelm the evacuation system. If this occurs, waste anesthetic gases may overflow the system through the positive-pressure relief valve (closed systems) or through the atmospheric vents (open systems) and pollute the operating room. This scenario is less likely with pneumatically driven ventilators that exhaust their drive gas (100% oxygen or oxygen/air mixture) into the operating room through a small vent on the back of the ventilator control housing.

Transfer Tubing. The transfer tubing carries excess gas from the gas-collecting assembly to the scavenging interface. As specified by ISO standard 80601-2-13, the scavenging system must have 30-mm connectors, or some other proprietary connector that will prevent the scavenging system from connecting to other elements on the workstation.[11] Some manufacturers color-code the transfer tubing with yellow bands to distinguish it from 22-mm breathing system tubing. The tubing must be sufficiently rigid to prevent kinking to minimize the chance of occlusion, or it must contain some means of pressure relief in case of occlusion. Occlusion of the transfer tubing can be very problematic because it is upstream from the pressure-limiting features of the scavenging interface. If the transfer tubing is occluded by kinking or misconnection, breathing circuit pressure will increase and barotrauma can occur.[144,221-223] On machines that have separate transfer tubes for the APL valve and for the ventilator relief valve, the two tubes merge before or at the scavenging interface.

Scavenging Interface. The scavenging interface is the most important component of the system because it protects the breathing circuit or ventilator from excessive positive or negative pressure.[220] The interface should limit the pressure immediately downstream from the gas-collecting assembly to between −0.5 and +3.5 cm H_2O under normal working conditions.[11] Positive-pressure relief is mandatory irrespective of the type of disposal system used, so the system can vent excess gas in case of occlusion (or inadequate suction with active systems) downstream from the interface. If the disposal system is an active system, negative-pressure relief will also be necessary to protect the breathing circuit or ventilator from excessive subatmospheric pressure. Subatmospheric pressure in the scavenging system could induce gas flow from the patient's breathing system. A reservoir is highly desirable with active systems because it stores waste gases until the evacuation system can remove them.

OPEN INTERFACES. The open scavenge interface sets up a continual flow into the disposal tubing using an active interface. If the amount of waste gas being discharged from the anesthesia workstation is less than the continual flow in the scavenging system, then the balance of that flow is obtained from entrained room air. Because the anesthesia machine discharges waste gas intermittently in surges, peak flow may overwhelm the flow of the scavenging system, so open systems also require a reservoir canister (Fig. 22.54).[219] Waste gas enters the system at the top of the canister and travels to the bottom through an inner tube, where a vacuum line removes waste gases. When adjusted properly, the vacuum rate should exceed the rate of waste gas flow into the chamber, and some room air should also be drawn into the canister through the relief port. The vacuum flow rate is usually adjusted on the scavenging interface using a flow control valve and flowmeter. Adjusting the scavenger vacuum flow rate is an important part of the workstation daily pre-use checkout procedure. If vacuum flow is inadequate, waste gas can spill out into the room through the relief ports. The open system does not require positive- or negative-pressure relief valves because the canister is open to the atmosphere. Relief ports on the top of the canister provide positive- and negative-pressure relief. Some open scavenging systems can incorporate a reservoir bag instead of a canister.

CLOSED INTERFACES. Closed scavenging interfaces are isolated from the environment by pressure relief valves, so the relationship of waste gas flow, vacuum flow, and the size of the system's reservoir bag determines the effectiveness of the gas elimination. All closed interfaces must have a positive-pressure relief valve to vent excess system pressure in

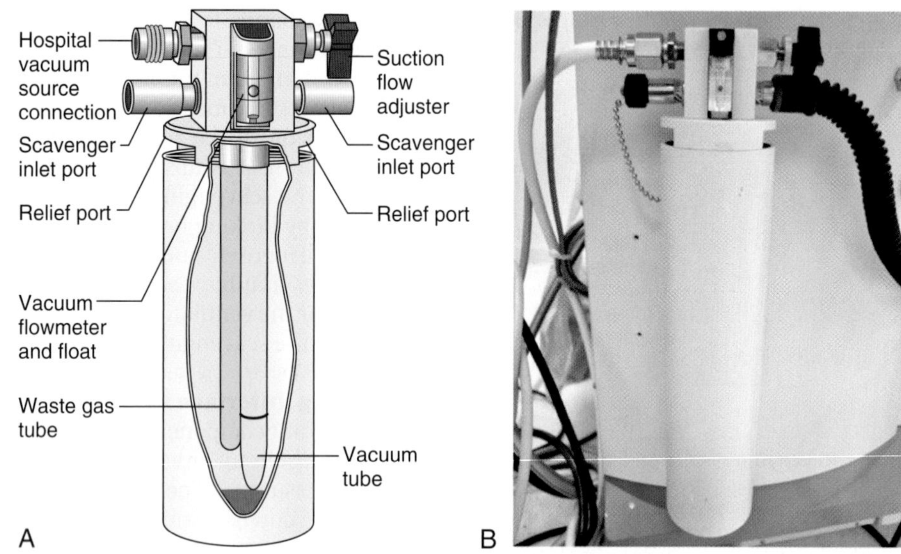

Fig. 22.54 (A and B) Open scavenge interface. When adjusted properly, room air is continually entrained via the relief port the top of the cannister. See text for details.

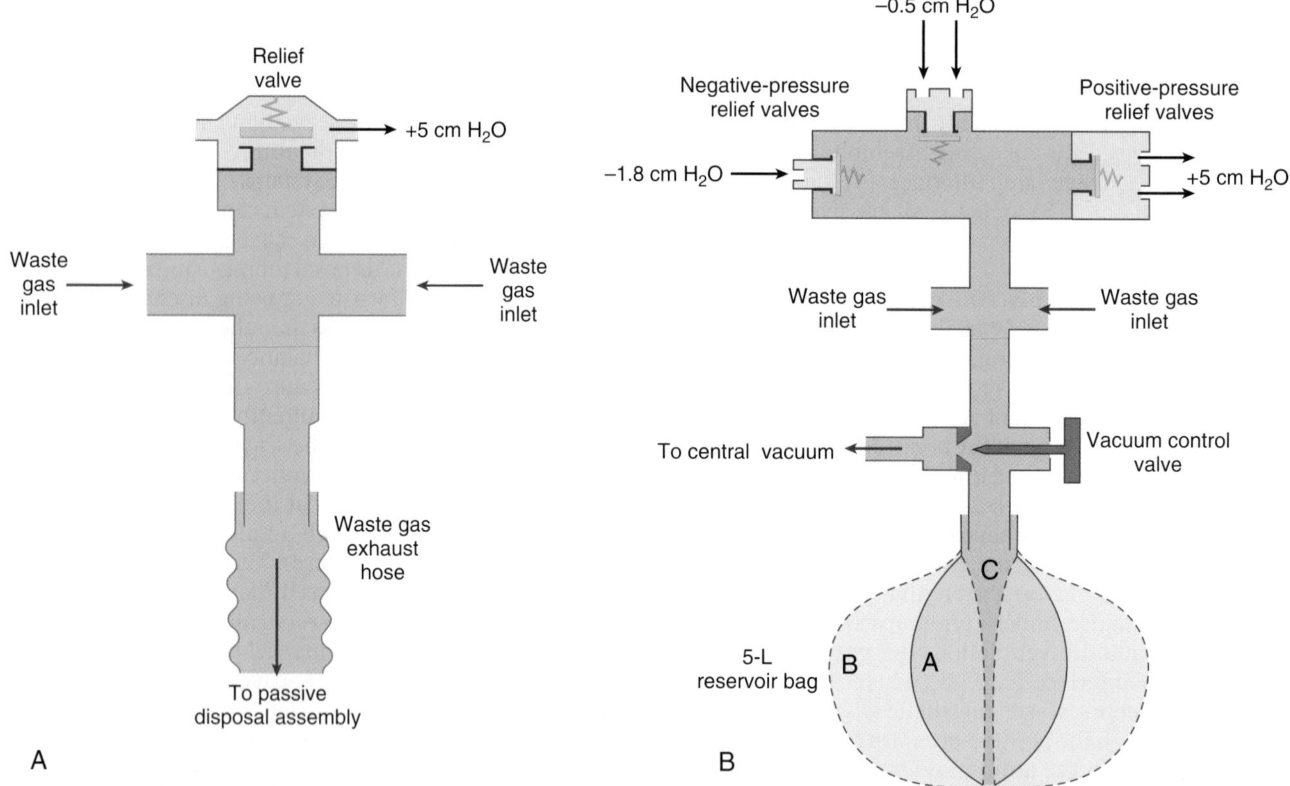

Fig. 22.55 Closed scavenging interfaces. (A) Interface used with a passive disposal system. (B) Interface used with an active system. In Panel B the labels on the 5-L reservoir bag refer to proper adjustment (A), over-distention (B), and completely deflated (C). See text for additional details. (A, Modified from North American Dräger. *Scavenger Interface for Air Conditioning: Instruction Manual.* Telford, PA: North American Dräger; 1984; B, From North American Dräger. *Narkomed 2A Anesthesia System: Technical Service Manual.* Telford, PA: North American Dräger; 1985.)

case of obstruction and a negative-pressure relief valve to protect the breathing system from subatmospheric pressure if an active disposal system is used.[220]

Two types of closed interfaces are used in clinical practice. One is used with passive scavenging systems and has positive-pressure relief only; the other is used with active scavenging systems and has both positive- and negative-pressure relief.

POSITIVE-PRESSURE RELIEF ONLY. A *closed, passive* scavenging system requires only a single positive-pressure relief valve (Fig. 22.55*A*). Waste gas enters the interface at the waste gas inlets. Transfer of the waste gas from the interface to the disposal system relies on the slight positive pressure of the gases leaving the patient's breathing system because a negative-pressure evacuation system is not used. Waste gases are then passively vented to a nonrecirculating HVAC system or to the outdoors. The positive-pressure relief valve opens at a preset value (such as 5 cm H_2O) if an obstruction between the interface and the disposal system occurs.[224] With this type of system, a reservoir bag is not required.

POSITIVE- AND NEGATIVE-PRESSURE RELIEF. A *closed, active* scavenging system requires a positive-pressure relief valve and at least one negative-pressure relief valve, in addition to a reservoir bag. Fig. 22.55*B*, is a schematic of Dräger Medical's closed scavenge interface for active suction systems. A variable volume of waste gas intermittently enters the interface through the waste gas inlets. The reservoir bag intermittently accumulates excess gas until the evacuation system eliminates it. The operator must adjust the vacuum control valve so that the reservoir bag remains properly inflated (see Fig. 22.55*B*, label *A*), and neither overdistended (label *B*) nor completely deflated (label *C*). Gas is vented to the operating room atmosphere through the positive-pressure relief valve if the system pressure exceeds a preset pressure (varies depending on manufacturer). Room air is entrained through the negative-pressure relief valve if the system pressure is more negative than that valve's opening pressure, approximately −0.5 cm H_2O. Some systems have a backup negative-pressure relief valve that opens at −1.8 cm H_2O if the primary negative-pressure relief valve becomes occluded by dust or other causes. The effectiveness of a closed system in preventing spillage depends on the rate of waste gas inflow, the evacuation flow rate, and the size of the reservoir. Leakage of waste gases into the atmosphere occurs only when the reservoir bag becomes fully inflated and the pressure increases sufficiently to open the positive-pressure relief valve. A "high PEEP" or sustained airway pressure alarm is often encountered in this circumstance.

Gas Disposal Assembly Conduit or Extract Flow. The gas disposal assembly conduit conducts waste gas from the scavenging interface to the receiving end of the gas disposal system (see Fig. 22.53). It should be collapse-proof and should run overhead, if possible, to minimize the chance of accidental occlusion. The connection to the scavenging interface can be a permanent or proprietary connector, but the connection to an active gas disposal system should be a DISS-type connector.[225]

Gas Disposal System. The gas disposal assembly ultimately eliminates excess waste gas (see Fig. 22.53). The two types of environmental disposal mechanisms, active and passive, have been described.

Hazards

Scavenging systems minimize operating room pollution, yet they add complexity to the anesthesia system. A scavenging system functionally extends the anesthesia circuit all the way from the anesthesia machine to the ultimate disposal site. This extension increases the potential for problems. Excessive vacuum applied to a scavenging system can cause undesirable negative pressures within the breathing system. Obstruction of scavenging pathways can cause excessive positive pressure in the breathing circuit. Even when the patient is protected from barotrauma by positive-pressure relief valves, alarm conditions can contribute to potentially unsafe conditions.[226] Inadequate vacuum to the interface can cause venting of waste gas into the operating room. An unusual report linked fires in engineering equipment rooms to design of some waste gas scavenging systems in which the waste gases were vented into machine rooms that have vents opening to the outside as opposed to directly outside.[21,230]

BOX 22.3 Requirements for Safe Delivery of Anesthesia Care

- Reliable delivery of oxygen at any appropriate concentration up to 100%.
- Reliable means of positive-pressure ventilation.
- Backup ventilation equipment available and functioning.
- Controlled release of positive pressure from the breathing circuit.
- Anesthesia vapor delivery (if intended as part of the anesthetic plan).
- Adequate suction.
- Means to conform to standards for patient monitoring.

From Sub-Committee of American Society of Anesthesiologists Committee on Equipment and Facilities: *Recommendations for Pre-Anesthesia Checkout Procedures* (2008).

Checking Your Anesthesia Workstation

A complete preanesthesia checkout procedure (PAC) must be performed each day before the anesthesia workstation is first used, and an abbreviated version should be performed before each subsequent case. Box 22.3 lists seven basic requirements for safe delivery of anesthesia care drawn from the ASA's *Recommendations for Pre-Anesthesia Checkout Procedures.*[11b] The anesthesia provider must have assurance prior to commencing any anesthetic that these requirements have been met. Institutions should develop and detail local procedures for meeting these basic safety requirements. These local procedures have taken on increased importance as increasing machine diversity make the applicability of a single, generic PAC remote.

Despite the fact that a PAC has been a mandatory part of anesthesia practice for over 30 years,[228] evidence suggests that anesthesia providers frequently do not perform a complete PAC,[6,229] and may miss faults even when explicitly looking for them on a sabotaged machine.[3] Furthermore, all contemporary anesthesia workstations have automated checkout procedures, none of which can assure that all the basic safety requirements for delivery of anesthetic care have been met.[8,231] In their 2008 *Recommendations*, the ASA suggests that many anesthesia providers are not fully aware of what elements are checked by the automated procedures.[11b] Even review of user's manuals does not always make it obvious.

The ASA's *Recommendations for Pre-Anesthesia Checkout Procedures*, summarized in Box 22.4, focus on ensuring the *availability* of key equipment, and assessing the *function* of that equipment. The *Recommendations* also give guidance as to which items may be carried out by a technician (such as an anesthesia technician or biomedical technician). When the party responsible is listed as "provider and technician," then the provider must perform that task; the task may *also* be assigned to the technician as an added layer of safety. Each institution should develop their own procedures in which the specific duties are delineated.

BOX 22.4 Summary Recommendations of the 2008 Preanesthesia Checkout Procedures

Items to Be Completed *Daily*

Item #	Task	Responsible Parties?
1	Verify that auxiliary oxygen cylinder and self-inflating manual ventilation device are available and functioning	Provider *and* technician
2	Verify that patient suction is adequate to clear the airway	Provider *and* technician
3	Turn on the anesthesia delivery system and confirm that AC power is available	Provider *or* technician
4	Verify the availability of required monitors, including alarms	Provider *or* technician
5	Verify that pressure is adequate on the spare oxygen cylinder mounted on the anesthesia machine	Provider *and* technician
6	Verify that the piped gas pressures are ≥50 psig	Provider *and* technician
7	Verify that vaporizers are adequately filled and, if applicable, that the filler ports are tightly closed	Provider *only*
8	Verify that the gas supply lines have no leaks between the flowmeters and the common gas outlet	Provider *or* technician
9	Test the scavenging system function	Provider *or* technician
10	Calibrate, or verify the calibration of, the oxygen monitor, and check the low-oxygen alarm	Provider *or* technician
11	Verify that carbon dioxide absorbent is not exhausted	Provider *or* technician
12	Perform breathing system pressure and leak testing	Provider *and* technician
13	Verify that gas flows properly through the breathing circuit during both inspiration and exhalation	Provider *and* technician
14	Document the completion of checkout procedures	Provider *and* technician
15	Confirm the ventilator settings, and evaluate readiness to deliver anesthesia care (Anesthesia Time Out)	Provider *only*

Items to Be Completed Before Each Procedure

Item #	Task	Responsible Parties?
1	Verify that patient suction is adequate to clear the airway	Provider *and* technician
2	Verify the availability of required monitors, including alarms	Provider *or* technician
3	Verify that vaporizers are adequately filled and, if applicable, that the filler ports are tightly closed	Provider only
4	Verify that carbon dioxide absorbent is not exhausted	Provider *or* technician
5	Perform breathing system pressure and leak testing	Provider *and* technician
6	Verify that gas flows properly through the breathing circuit during both inspiration and exhalation	Provider *and* technician
7	Document the completion of checkout procedures	Provider *and* technician
8	Confirm the ventilator settings, and evaluate readiness to deliver anesthesia care (Anesthesia Time Out)	Provider only

Modified from Sub-Committee of American Society of Anesthesiologists Committee on Equipment and Facilities: *Recommendations for Pre-Anesthesia Checkout Procedures* (2008).

2008 RECOMMENDATIONS FOR PRE-ANESTHESIA CHECKOUT PROCEDURES

The items in Box 22.4 are reviewed here. Fifteen items are required before commencing the day's anesthesia procedures. Eight items (see Box 22.4, items 2, 4, 7, 11-15) are required before each case.

Item 1: Verify Auxiliary Oxygen Cylinder and Self-Inflating Manual Ventilation Device Are Available and Functioning

Frequency: Daily
Responsible parties: Provider and technician

The anesthesia provider must always be prepared to keep the patient alive without the assistance of the anesthesia machine. The most important safety check in any anesthesia location prior to commencing the day's procedures is the presence of a self-inflating manual ventilation device and a source of oxygen that is separate from the anesthesia workstation and hospital pipeline oxygen supply. These items must be present at every anesthetizing location. The *Recommendations* advise checking the function of the self-inflating ventilation device; this can typically be done without opening the packaging. Note that the presence of a non–self-inflating Mapleson-type breathing circuit is *not* adequate to meet this item.

The auxiliary oxygen tank, typically an E-cylinder, should be checked to make sure it is full, and also for the presence of an attached flowmeter and a means to open the cylinder valve. After check, the valve should be closed to prevent inadvertent loss of the contents. Ensuring the presence of properly filled portable cylinders with attached flowmeters and cylinder wrenches benefits from the logistical support of support staff, but must ultimately be verified by the anesthesia provider.

Item 2: Verify Patient Suction Is Adequate to Clear the Airway

Frequency: Before each use
Responsible parties: Provider and technician

"Safe anesthetic care requires the immediate availability of suction to clear the airway if needed."[11b] Adequate suction with tubing of appropriate length and an oral suctioning tool (e.g., Yankauer suction tip) are necessary before the start of any case. Since these are normally changed with every case, this item is often shared between provider and technician. The provider must verify this item prior to commencing the anesthetic.

Item 3: Turn on Anesthesia Delivery System and Confirm That AC Power Is Available

Frequency: Daily
Responsible party: Provider or technician

Contemporary anesthesia workstations have backup battery power if wall power should fail. If a case is inadvertently started on battery backup power, the first obvious sign of power failure can be catastrophic system shutdown when the backup batteries are exhausted. Prior to commencing the day's anesthetic procedures, functioning AC power should be verified. The ASA also recommends verifying power supply to component subsystems such as desflurane vaporizers. This item may be completed by technician or provider.

Item 4: Verify Availability of Required Monitors and Check Alarms

Frequency: Before each use
Responsible party: Provider or technician

The ASA *Recommendations* include in this item both the presence of monitoring supplies (blood pressure cuffs of appropriate sizes, pulse oximetry probes, etc.), functional tests of critical monitoring equipment (pulse oximeter and capnography), and functional tests of alarm conditions. The importance of an audible alarm is emphasized.

Some elements of this item are straightforward, such as verifying the availability of the monitoring equipment and making sure that monitors are on and cables are properly plugged in. However, the process of checking alarm thresholds, and possibly resetting them, can be tedious. Monitor alarm settings may possibly vary within individual facilities as a result of provider manipulation of alarms for case requirements, a lack of standard default settings, and failure to reset alarm limits routinely. Departmental alarm default settings can be established and programmed into anesthesia workstation monitors. Alarm limit settings also include anesthesia machine alarms such as volume, pressure, and inspired oxygen concentration limits. The practitioner should ensure that critical alarm limits are set to values that permit these alarms to do what they were intended to do. Here, anesthesia technicians can improve the quality of the pre-use checkout by checking the function of standard monitors and confirming that critical alarm thresholds are set to established default values.

Item 5: Verify That Pressure Is Adequate on the Spare Oxygen Cylinder Mounted on the Anesthesia Machine

Frequency: Daily
Responsible parties: Provider and technician

In addition to verifying the presence of a separate source of cylinder oxygen (Item 1), the anesthesia provider should verify the presence of an adequately filled oxygen cylinder mounted on the anesthesia workstation. Verification of oxygen cylinder pressure is accomplished by opening the oxygen cylinder or cylinders on the back of the machine and evaluating the tank gauge pressure. The current recommendations do not provide a specific value that would prompt replacing the tank, but some manufacturer's manuals suggest changing the oxygen cylinder when the pressure is below 1000 psi.[31a]

The *Recommendations* affirm that other gas supply cylinders such as air, nitrous oxide, etc., need to be checked only if that gas is required for the anesthetic.

Item 6: Verify That Piped Gas Pressures Are 50 psig or Higher

Frequency: Daily
Responsible parties: Provider and technician

A daily check of adequate pipeline pressures is specified in the *Recommendations for Pre-Anesthesia Checkout Procedures*; this item should be performed by the provider even if it is part of the technician's workflow.

A more detailed daily pre-use check of the pipeline system may be part of institutional protocols. For example, a quick daily inspection of connections, supply hoses, gas pressures, and the presence of more than 90% oxygen in the inspiratory limb greatly minimizes risk. An important safety item on all machines is an audible and visual alarm that warns the operator of diminishing oxygen supply pressure. The only way to evaluate this safety device is to disconnect the wall oxygen supply and shut off the oxygen supply tank or tanks, in order to generate the alarm condition. The 2008 *Recommendations* do not mandate this maneuver.

Item 7: Verify That Vaporizers Are Adequately Filled and, If Applicable, That the Filler Ports Are Tightly Closed

Responsible parties: Provider (and technician if redundancy desired)

The anesthesia provider should verify that there is an adequate supply of anesthetic agent in the vaporizer if an inhaled anesthetic is planned. Because not every anesthetic utilizes an inhaled agent, alarm defaults may not include a low agent alarm. The risk of light anesthesia and recall can be mitigated by checking agent levels prior to proceeding.

Loose caps on vaporizer filler ports may be a source of leaks when the vaporizer is on. Because the breathing system pressure and leak test (see Item 12 below) is carried out with the vaporizer off, this source of leak may go otherwise undetected. Some vaporizers are designed to automatically close when the filling adapter is removed. Although not part of the 2008 PAC guidelines, some manufacturers recommend a check of their machine's vaporizer interlock system, which, if present, prevents more than one vaporizer from being activated simultaneously.

Item 8: Verify That No Leaks Are Present in the Gas Supply Lines Between the Flowmeters and the Common Gas Outlet

Frequency: Daily and whenever a vaporizer is changed
Responsible party: Provider or technician

As discussed above, the low-pressure section of the anesthesia workstation, from the flow control valves, through the vaporizers, and to the common gas outlet, is the most vulnerable to leaks. Leaks in this section of the machine can be associated with hypoxemia or patient awareness under anesthesia.[22,24]

Two areas of the low-pressure leak test deserve emphasis. First, some anesthesia workstations include an outlet check valve (see Fig. 22.1). The implication of this check valve is that positive pressure in the breathing circuit *cannot* be

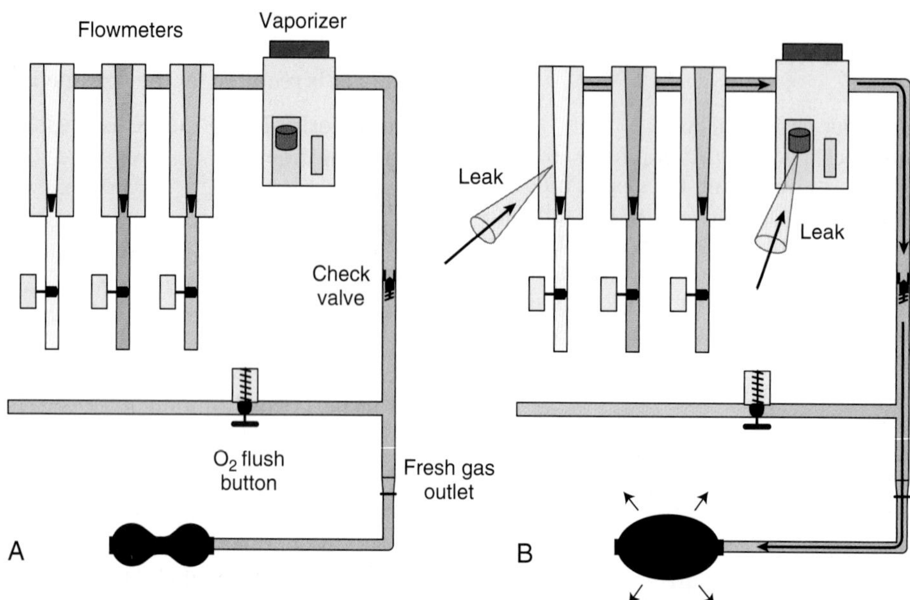

Fig. 22.56 The negative-pressure "universal" low-pressure system leak test. (A) A specially configured suction bulb is connected to the common (fresh) gas outlet and collapsed. Subatmospheric pressure is created in the low pressure circuit, thus opening the outlet check valve (if present) and exposing the vaporizers, tubing, and associated piping and connections to the vacuum. In a system without a leak, the bulb stays deflated. (B) Leaks in the system draw in ambient air and cause the suction bulb to inflate. *O_2*, Oxygen.

used to check for leaks upstream in the low-pressure system, because the pressure will not be transmitted past the check valve. On these machines, a negative pressure test must be performed. Second, most vaporizer leaks are not detected unless the vaporizer is on. Therefore a thorough low-pressure leak test can require testing multiple vaporizers, depending on machine configuration. Some workstations (Maquet anesthesia machines and GE Healthcare workstations) do perform automated vaporizer leak testing on their unique vaporizers (ADU vaporizer).

In machines with an outlet check valve, a negative-pressure test must be performed. The negative-pressure leak test is simple to perform and is highly sensitive, detecting leaks as small as 30 mL/min. This simple test requires that the flow control valves be fully closed to prevent any flow of gas into the low-pressure circuit. A specially configured suction bulb, which can either be constructed or obtained from the manufacturer, is then attached to the common gas outlet (Fig. 22.56). The bulb is then squeezed repeatedly until it is fully collapsed. If the bulb does not stay collapsed for a specified period of time, then air is being sucked by the bulb into the machine through a leak that will allow gas to escape when the machine is pressurized. The same maneuver is carried out with each vaporizer opened in turn to check for associated leaks.

The negative-pressure test *can* be performed on machines without a check valve. For this reason, the negative-pressure test is sometimes referred to as the "universal leak test." Several mishaps have resulted from application of the wrong leak test to the wrong machine.[231-234] When in doubt, the negative-pressure test is therefore preferred. However, many of the newer-generation anesthesia machines do not have an accessible common gas outlet; therefore negative-pressure low-pressure system testing cannot be performed. On these machines, either manual positive-pressure testing of the low-pressure system (and vaporizers) is performed during the pre-use checkout, or low-pressure testing is accomplished as part of an automated checkout feature. Note that the automated low-pressure test on some machines needs to be specifically selected.[214j]

Item 9: Test Scavenging System Function

Frequency: Daily
Responsible party: Provider or technician

Evaluation of the scavenging system is a manual maneuver. No automated checks are conducted. A test of the scavenging system begins by checking the proper assembly and integrity of each component and connection within the system including the gas transfer tubes leading from the APL valve and the ventilator relief valve to the scavenging interface. In the case of many modern machines, a single transfer tube may lead from a compact breathing system to the scavenge interface. The integrity of the vacuum tubing leading from the wall outlet to the scavenging interface should also be checked.

To test a closed, passive scavenger system (as seen in Fig. 22.55*A*), one creates high flow within the breathing system by occluding the patient "Y-piece" (or short-circuiting the inspiratory and expiratory limbs of the breathing circuit with breathing hose), occluding the exhaust hose outlet on the scavenging interface, and ensuring that the flow of gas exits the system through the positive-pressure safety relief valve so excess pressure does not build up in the breathing circuit (e.g., <10 cm H_2O). To test a closed, active scavenger system (as seen in Fig. 22.55*B*), two steps are required. A check of positive-pressure relief is conducted as just described for the passive, closed scavenger. Some manufacturers recommend that the suction needle valve be turned off for this step. A check of negative-pressure relief is conducted by setting scavenge interface suction to a routine setting, turning off all flow control valves on the anesthesia machine, and occluding inflow into the patient's breathing circuit at the patient's Y-piece (or short circuiting the inspiratory and expiratory limbs of the breathing circuit with breathing hose) and at the breathing bag mount. At this point, the breathing pressure gauge should indicate a negligible negative pressure (e.g., no lower than −1.0 cm H_2O). Generally speaking, the scavenging suction on active systems should be adjusted so the reservoir bag is never overinflated or underinflated, but it should remain slightly inflated during routine use. Because the volume of gas being passed into the scavenging system varies, it may be necessary to adjust the needle valve. Given the diversity of breathing systems, this check serves as another instance in which users must consider manufacturer-specified protocols when developing a local PAC.

Checking the function of an open, active system as seen in Fig. 22.54 is relatively simple compared with checking a closed, active system. After ensuring that all gas transfer tubes and the suction lines are properly connected, the scavenger suction needle valve is adjusted to place the flowmeter bobbin between the indicator lines. A positive-pressure test and a negative-pressure test are then conducted as described earlier.

Item 10: Calibrate, or Verify Calibration of, the Oxygen Monitor and Check the Low Oxygen Alarm

Frequency: Daily
Responsible party: Provider or technician

The oxygen concentration analyzer is one of the most important monitors on the anesthesia workstation. Older anesthesia workstations used a galvanic cell oxygen sensor located near the patient's breathing circuit inspiratory valve. These devices have a finite life span, which is inversely proportional to the amount of oxygen exposure.[234a] They are also vulnerable to drift. Therefore daily verification of calibration (and recalibration, if necessary) is recommended. Newer anesthesia workstations rely on side-stream multi-gas analyzers to measure the inspired oxygen concentration. The multi-gas analyzer is an irremovable and permanent component of the workstation. Thus it fulfills the requirement imposed on the manufacturer to provide inspired oxygen concentration monitoring. These monitors do not require daily calibration. Nevertheless, the function of the sensor should be checked in room air, to verify that the it reads 21%.

The function of the low-oxygen concentration alarm should be tested daily. This may be done by manually setting the low oxygen concentration alarm limit to more than 21% while exposing the analyzer to room air, generating the alarm condition. A prudent default setting would be somewhere between 25% and 30%, unless oxygen concentrations lower than this value are used routinely. In any case, it is wise to keep it set to at least 21%. These steps may be carried out by a technician, according to local protocols.

Item 11: Verify Carbon Dioxide Absorbent Is Not Exhausted

Frequency: Before each use
Responsible party: Provider or technician

In order to utilize rebreathed gas, the anesthesia circle system requires a CO_2 absorber. Prior to each anesthetic, the absorbent should be assessed for exhaustion. It is important for providers to know that absorbent color change is not as reliable as is the presence of *inspired* CO_2 on capnography in identifying exhausted absorbent. Capnometry should be used with every anesthetic that uses the circle system, and the provider should be vigilant for inspired CO_2 concentration greater than 0. A normal-appearing but nonfunctional absorbent is difficult to detect during the pre-use checkout procedure. It is no longer advised for providers to breathe in and breathe out of the breathing circuit manually to assess the functionality of the absorbent before a case.

Item 12: Breathing System Pressure and Leak Testing

Frequency: Before each use
Responsible parties: Provider and technician

This PAC item verifies that positive pressure can be developed and sustained in the breathing circuit, and that the APL ("pop-off") valve properly relieves pressure in the circuit. It is not rare for either the disposable breathing circuit components or the fixed anesthesia machine components to leak. Therefore a leak check of the breathing system is of paramount importance. Traditionally, this test has been performed manually after an inspection of the breathing circuit, removal of the gas sampling line, and capping of the gas sampling line port. With the machine set in the "bag" or the manual mode of ventilation, the gas flows are set to zero, the APL valve is closed, the patient's Y-piece is occluded, and breathing system is pressurized with the O_2 flush button to approximately 30 cm H_2O (Fig. 22.57). The circuit passes the leak test if it holds this pressure for at least 10 seconds. A decrease in pressure during the test should prompt a check of all plug-in, push-fit, and screw connectors, the seal of the absorber canister, and a careful inspection of the disposable tubing. One of the most common locations of a circuit leak is at the absorber canister, and it is particularly important for the anesthesia provider to apply this check rigorously immediately after the absorbent has been changed.

On many modern anesthesia machines, breathing circuit leak testing is an automated feature, although manual steps are still required for test preparation. Circuit compliance is often also automatically assessed on some machines during this phase to guide ventilator tidal volume delivery. Therefore the test should be performed with the circuit that is going to be used. The automated circuit leak test may be performed by a technician, but its completion should be verified by the provider. The importance of the leak test, on which depends the ability to deliver positive pressure ventilation, implies that it must be the provider's responsibility.

The APL valve should also be assessed at this time by opening it widely after the pressure test and ensuring that the breathing circuit pressure decreases rapidly to zero. A prompt pressure drop should occur regardless of APL valve design. The ability of the pressure-limiting type APL valve to maintain stable circuit pressure can be easily assessed, if required, by setting the APL valve to 30 cm H_2O, occluding the patient's Y-piece in a manual mode of ventilation, increasing gas flow to approximately 5 L/min, and ensuring the circuit pressure, once stable, remains within a range close to that set on the APL valve.

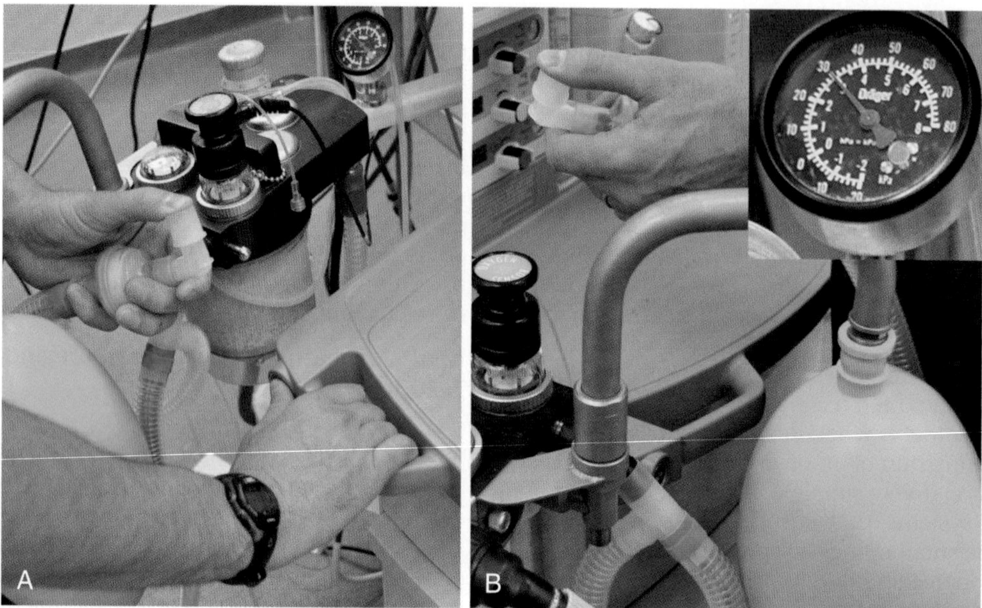

Fig. 22.57 Manual breathing system pressure and leak testing. Breathing system pressure and leak testing should be performed with the circuit configuration that will be used during anesthetic delivery. (A) The patient Y-piece or elbow is occluded, and the oxygen flush button is used to pressurize the breathing circuit to approximately 30 cm H_2O. (B) The circuit should hold pressure at this level for at least 10 seconds. It is important to ensure that the gas flows are set to zero (or their minimal values), the gas sample line is removed, and its circuit port is occluded.

Item 13: Verify That Gas Flows Properly Through the Breathing Circuit During Both Inspiration and Exhalation

Frequency: Before each use
Responsible parties: Provider and technician

This item assesses the circle breathing system for unobstructed flow and proper function of the unidirectional valves. This test of circuit flow is easily accomplished by placing a "test lung" or an extra breathing bag at the patient Y-piece. In the "bag" or a manual mode of ventilation, the operator ventilates the artificial "lung" with the breathing bag, then actively "exhales" (squeezes) the test lung back to the breathing bag in a to-and-fro motion (Fig. 22.58). This is the so-called *flow test*. The inspiratory valve should open and the expiratory valve should close during inspiration, and vice versa for exhalation. Obstruction to inspiratory flow during the flow test manifests as a "tight" breathing bag on "inspiration," whereas expiratory limb obstructions cause impeded "exhalation." Some form of flow test should be conducted because leak testing does not reliably identify circuit obstruction or unidirectional valve malfunction. Undetected circuit obstructions are particularly ominous and can manifest dramatically and sometimes immediately following induction.[147,148,150] Subtle circuit obstruction may not be appreciable except by capnometry.

Automated machine checks may not assess for (or detect) obstruction to flow within the breathing circuit. A number of complications and near-misses involving an obstructed breathing circuit have been reported despite the performance of the automated circuit check.[9,231,234b,234c] Although most user's manuals for machines that perform automated aspects of the pre-use checkout describe a leak test function, few specifically describe a flow test or an assessment of unidirectional valve function. In fact, some modern machines that incorporate automated checkout steps, including a leak test, recommend a manual assessment of the inspiratory and expiratory valves.[214,31a] In the experience of this chapter's authors, a full checkout procedure with test lung is uncommon in this era of automated machine checks. If this test is omitted, providers must be cognizant of the fact that unidirectional valve malfunction and breathing circuit obstruction have not been ruled out before starting the case.

Item 14: Document Completion of Checkout Procedures

Responsible parties: Provider and technician

Documentation of completion of the anesthetic checkout procedure by *providers* should occur within the anesthetic record. Currently, no guidance is available regarding where anesthesia or biomedical technician documentation of checkout procedures should occur. However, it would be prudent to maintain a detailed departmental log as a quality assurance tool.

Item 15: Confirm Ventilator Settings and Evaluate Readiness to Deliver Anesthesia Care (Anesthesia Time Out)

Frequency: Immediately before initiating the anesthetic regimen
Responsible parties: Provider

The authors of the 2008 *Recommendations* include as the last step in the PAC an "anesthesia time out." The time out asks the anesthesia provider to confirm 6 items:

- Monitors functional?
- Capnogram present?
- Oxygen saturation by pulse oximetry measured?
- Flowmeter and ventilator settings proper?
- Manual/ventilator switch set to manual?
- Vaporizer(s) adequately filled?[11b]

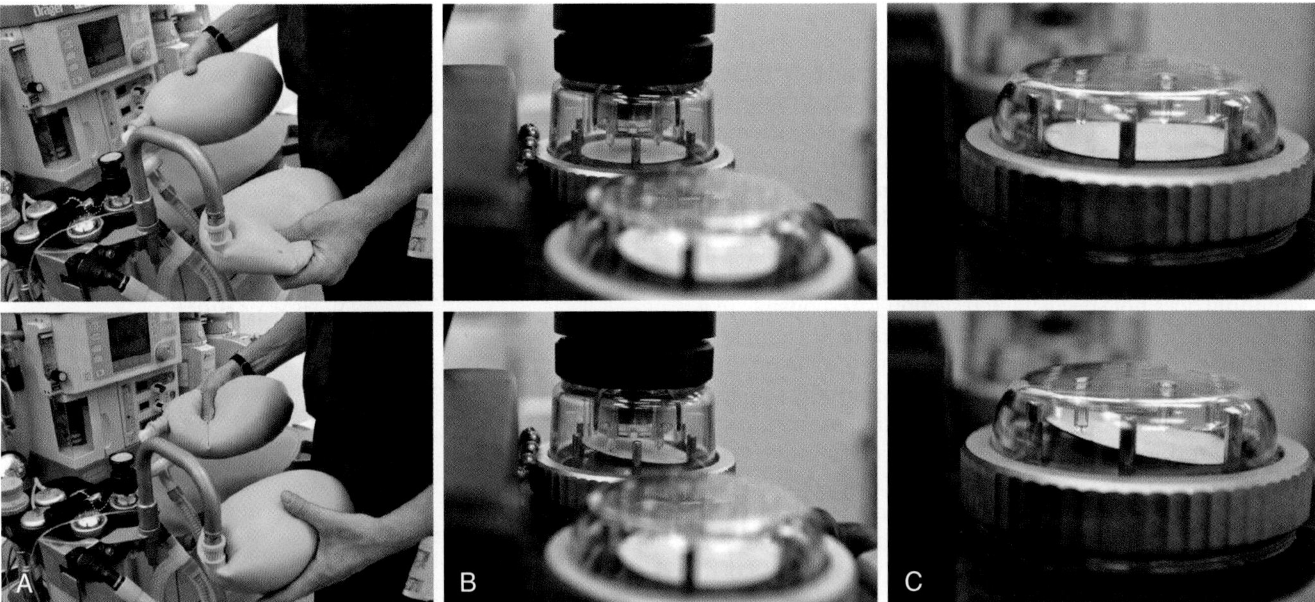

Fig. 22.58 (A–C) Verification that gas flows properly through the breathing circuit during both inspiration and exhalation with the to-and-fro "flow test." Top row, A test lung or second reservoir bag is placed on the patient elbow piece. A squeeze of the breathing bag should cause flow through the inspiratory limb, open the inspiratory valve, fill the test lung, and hold the expiratory valve closed. Bottom row, A reciprocal squeeze of the test lung should cause flow through the expiratory limb, open the expiratory valve, fill the breathing bag, and hold the inspiratory valve closed. Circuit flow during the test should be smooth and unimpeded.

This last step serves as a recommended final preinduction check list of the machine and other important items including the application of essential monitors. Verifying appropriate ventilator settings is an important safety check, especially in practices with mixed adult and pediatric cases. Many contemporary anesthesia workstations can be programmed to offer adult and pediatric "profiles" that adjust the anesthesia ventilator's default tidal volume and respiratory rate. Some older machines are more likely to retain the previous patient's settings, with the potential for under- or over-ventilation. Spending time adjusting ventilator settings in the immediate postinduction period can be distracting.

The checklist above focuses on the anesthesia workstation but does not include other key equipment such as medications, intubation supplies, monitoring transducers, etc. Some providers rely on final check mnemonic devices such as the MS MAIDS checklist (Box 22.5). Regardless of the specific steps, a final checklist that verifies the presence and function of key safety items is fundamental to the safe delivery of anesthesia.

BOX 22.5 The MS MAIDS Checklist*

- **Machine:** The machine checkout is complete; the vaporizers are filled, closed, and set to "0"; all gas flows knobs are set to zero flow; the ventilator and pressure settings are appropriate for the upcoming patient, with the machine in manual/spontaneous breathing mode, and the adjustable pressure-limiting valve is open.
- **Suction:** Patient suction is adequate to clear the airway.
- **Monitors:** All required standard monitors are present and ready to go.
- **Airway:** Primary airway equipment and appropriate backup equipment are ready to go.
- **Intravenous:** Intravenous lines, fluids, and associated equipment are ready to go.
- **Drugs:** All necessary medications are available and are properly labeled.
- **Special:** Any special or unique items (i.e., additional monitors) required for the case are available and ready.

*An example mnemonic for an "Anesthesia Time Out," which ensures that all appropriate checks have been completed, all essential equipment is available, and the machine is properly configured for the next patient.

Additional Comments Pertaining to the ASA's Pre-Anesthesia Checkout Procedure Recommendations (2008)

Although the 2008 PAC procedures are comprehensive, several steps that were part of the earlier PAC recommendations[228,235] did not appear in the current recommendations. Some of these are still found in machine user's manuals. The use of these steps should be based on local needs or requirements because the 2008 recommendations are not restrictive nor intended to be limiting. Some of these items are:

1. Disconnecting the central oxygen supply line to assess the low–oxygen supply pressure alarm and to purge the tank pressure gauges to zero
2. Inspecting the gas supply hoses for cracks or wear
3. Testing the flowmeters for smooth operation
4. Testing the proportioning system by attempting to create a hypoxic oxygen–nitrous oxide mixture

AUTOMATED ANESTHESIA MACHINE CHECKOUT PROCEDURES

Important points to consider regarding automated PAC features or "self-tests" are that (1) they differ between manufacturers and models; (2) it is sometimes difficult to determine precisely which segments or components are actually being checked by reading the user's manual, and (3) *no* machine automatically checks all the items on an effective PAC. At least some manual steps are required. Investigators have suggested that many providers do not understand exactly what is being checked by automated checks, or they make false assumptions regarding their respective machine's automated checkout procedure. It is easy to understand why the authors of the ASA's 2008 *Recommendations for Pre-Anesthesia Checkout Procedures* warned about an overreliance on the automated machine checkout. For example, one manufacturer's self-test screen reports a "leakage" amount, but the display or manual does not specify which section is responsible (e.g., the breathing circuit or the LPS). The operator must make an assumption that the low-pressure system is also being tested for leaks, and the manual does not state that any vaporizer should be turned "on" during leak testing. Finally, it was not clear in this manual whether the circuit is assessed for proper unidirectional flow or obstruction. When developing a local PAC procedure, providers should gain familiarity with their machine's automated checkout procedure through the user's manual. If an important item is not actually part of the described self-check or is not suggested in the user's manual, it should not be assumed that it can be neglected. Not requiring that conventional vaporizers be opened during a leak test of the low-pressure system is such an example.

MACHINE-EMBEDDED PREANESTHESIA MACHINE CHECKOUT CHECKLISTS

Some anesthesia machines have embedded PAC checklists, which are displayed during machine checkout. Like their paper counterparts, they help guide users through manual and self-test functions. If an embedded checklist provides a complete solution for a department, then it can be used exclusively. However, local requirements may exceed or depart from the embedded checklist. In these cases, the use of the embedded checklist (or a modification thereof) can become a line item within the local PAC checklist.

DEVELOPING A LOCAL PREANESTHESIA MACHINE CHECKOUT CHECKLIST

The goal of a PAC is to evaluate and configure the anesthesia workstation properly so it performs its functions safely and smoothly. The objectives of the PAC *checklist* are to guide the operator through an effective PAC and to promote compliance through ease of use. A PAC checklist can also serve as a quality control tool by codifying important items onto an organized list used by all providers.[236] The checkout procedure should be ergonomically ordered to minimize redundant movements and save time by placing procedures in a rational sequence.[237] Finally, the checklist should be as short as possible, yet be detailed enough so critical items are not omitted.

Acknowledgment

The editors and publisher would like to thank Drs. Steven G. Venticinque and J. Jeffrey Andrews for contributing a chapter on this topic in the prior edition of this work. It has served as the foundation for the current chapter.

 **Complete references available online at expertconsult.com.**

References

1. Mehta SP, et al. *Anesthesiology*. 2013;119:788.
2. Caplan R, et al. *Anesthesiology*. 1997;87:741.
3. Larson ER, et al. *Anesth Analg*. 2007;104:154.
4. Olympio MA, et al. *Anesth Analg*. 1996;83:618.
5. Armstrong-Brown A, et al. *Can J Anaesth*. 2000;47:974.
6. O'Shaughnessy SM, Mahon P. *Anaesthesia*. 2015;70:1005.
7. Mayor AH, Eaton JM. *Anaesthesia*. 1992;47:866.
8. Berry N, Mills P. *Anaesthesia*. 2012;67:927–927.
9. Yang KK, Lewis IH. *A A Case Rep*. 2014;2:143–146.
10. Organisation Internationale de Normalisation (ISO) n.d. Retrieved from https://www.iso.org/developing-standards.html Accessed 12/20/18.
11. International Organization for Standardization, 2011. ISO 80601-2-13:2011(en), https://www.iso.org/obp/ui/#iso:std:iso:80601:-2-13:ed-1:v1:en.

11a. American Society of Anesthesiologists. *Standards and Guidelines*. n.d. https://www.asahq.org/standards-and-guidelines.

11b. American Society of Anesthesiologists. *Recommendations for Pre-Anesthesia Checkout Procedures*; 2008.

11c. Dorsch JA. *ASA Monitor*. 2004;68:27–28.

11d. American Society of Anesthesiologists. *Standards for Basic Anesthetic Monitoring*. 1986.

11e. Association of Anesthetists of Great Britain and Ireland. *Checking Anesthetic Equipment 2012*; 2012.

11f. Australian and New Zealand College of Anesthetists. *Guidelines on Checking Anesthesia Delivery Systems*; 2014.

12. Dorsch JA, Dorsch SE. The anesthesia machine. In: Dorsch JA, Dorsch SE, eds. *Understanding Anesthesia Equipment*. 5th ed. Baltimore: Williams & Wilkins; 2008:83.
13. Eisenkraft JB. The Anesthesia Machine and Workstation. In: Ehrenwerth J, Eisenkraft JB, Berry JR, eds. *Anesthesia Equipment: Principles and Applications*. Philadelphia, PA: Saunders; 2013:25–63.
14. Malayaman SN, Mychaskiw G II, Ehrenwerth J. Medical Gases: Storage and Supply. In: Ehrenwerth J, Eisenkraft JB, Berry JR, eds. *Anesthesia Equipment: Principles and Applications*. Philadelphia, PA: Saunders; 2013:3–24.
15. Hogg CE. *Anesthesiology*. 1973;38:85.
16. Donaldson M, et al. *J Am Dent Assoc*. 2012;143:134–143.
17. Goebel WM. *Anesth Prog*. 1980;28:188–191.
18. Rose G, et al. *APSF Newsl*. 2010;25(16).

18a. Anderson WR, Brock-Utne JG. *J Clin. Monit*. 1991;7:39–41.

19. Bowie E, Huffman LM. *The Anesthesia Machine: Essentials for Understanding*. Madison, Wis: Ohmeda, BOC Group; 1985.
20. ASTM. Standard specification for particular requirements for anesthesia workstations and their components (ASTM F1850-00). In: *Medical Devices and Services*. vol. 13.01. Conshohocken, Pa: ASTM International; 2005:913.
21. Yoder M. Pneumatic safety system components. In: *Understanding Modern Anesthesia Systems*. Telford, Pa: Dräger Medical; 2009:23.
22. Anderson CE, Rendell-Baker L. *Anesthesiology*. 1982;56:328.
23. Mann D, et al. *Anesthesiology*. 2004;101(558).
24. Internal leakage from anesthesia unit flush valves. *Health Devices*. 1981;10(172).

24a. Mun SH, No MY. Internal leakage of oxygen flush valve. *Korean J Anesthesiol*. 2013;64:550–551.

25. Andrews JJ. Understanding your anesthesia machine and ventilator. In: *1989 Review Course Lectures*. Cleveland, Ohio: International Anesthesia Research Society; 1989:59.
26. Fassl J, et al. *Anesth Analg*. 2010;110(94).
27. Gaughan SD, et al. *Anesth Analg*. 1993;76:800.

27a. Loader J. *Anaesthesia*. 2009;64:574–574.

28. Doi T, et al. *BioMed Res. Int*. 2015:454807.
29. Mudumbai SC, et al. *Anesth Analg*. 2010;110:1292.
30. Yoder M. Gas supply systems. In: *Understanding Modern Anesthesia Systems*. Telford, Pa: Dräger Medical; 2009:1.
31. Datex-Ohmeda. *S/5 Aespire Anesthesia Machine: Technical Reference Manual*. Madison, Wis: Datex-Ohmeda; 2004.

31a. Mindray DS. *Operating Instructions: A7 Anesthesia System*. 2016. Mahwah, NJ; 2016.

31b. Draegerwerk AG & Co., n.d. *Perseus A500 and Perseus A500 Ceiling Technical Documentation IPM*. Lubeck, Germany: Draegerwerk AG & Co.: n.d.

32. Adriani J. Clinical application of physical principles concerning gases and vapor to anesthesiology. In: 2nd ed. Adriani J, ed. *The Chemistry and Physics of Anesthesia*. Springfield, Ill: Charles C Thomas; 1962:58.

33. Macintosh R, et al. Flowmeters. In: 3rd ed. Macintosh R, Mushin WW, Epstein HG, eds. *Physics for the Anaesthetist*. Oxford: Blackwell Scientific; 1963:196.
34. Eger II EI, Epstein RM. *Anesthesiology*. 1964;24:490.
35. Rendell-Baker L. *Int Anesthesiol Clin*. 1982;20(1).
36. Schreiber P. *Safety Guidelines for Anesthesia Systems*. Telford, Pa: North American Dräger; 1984.
37. Eger II EI, et al. *Anesthesiology*. 1963;24:396.
38. Dräger Medical. *Dräger technical Service manual: Fabius GS anesthesia system*, rev E. Telford, PA: Dräger Medical: 2002.
39. Gordon PC, et al. *Anesthesiology*. 1995;82:598.
40. Cheng CJ, Garewal DS. *Anesth Analg*. 2001;92:913.
41. Ishikawa S, et al. *Anesth Analg*. 2002;94:1672.
42. Paine GF, Kochan 3rd JJ. *Anesth Analg*. 2002;94:1374.
43. Richards C. *Anesthesiology*. 1989;71:997.
44. Dorsch JA, Dorsch SE. Vaporizers. In: Dorsch JA, Dorsch SE, eds. *Understanding Anesthesia Equipment*. 5th ed. Baltimore: Williams & Wilkins; 2008:121.
45. Kim HJ, Kim MW. *Korean J Anesthesiol*. 2010;59:270.
46. Liew WL, Jayamaha J. *Anaesthesia*. 2011;66:399.
47. Ong BC, et al. *Anesthesiology*. 2001;95:1038.
48. Lum ME, et al. *Anaesth Intensive Care*. 1992;20:501.
49. Aggarwal R, Kumar A. *J Anaesthesiol Clin Pharmacol*. 2018;34:135.
50. Webb C, et al. *Anaesthesia*. 2005;60:628.
51. Mitchell AM. *Anaesth Intensive Care*. 2007;35:804.
52. Jagannathan VK, Nortcliffe SA. *Eur J Anaesthesiol*. 2008;25:165.
53. Viney JP, Gartrell AD. *Anesthesiology*. 1994;81:781.
54. Haridas RP. *Anaesth Intensive Care*. 2009;37(suppl 1):30.
55. King AC. *Br Med J*. 1946;2:536.
56. Desbarax P. *Anaesthesia*. 2002;57:463.
57. Macintosh R, et al. Gas pressure: pressure in gaseous mixtures. In: Macintosh R, Mushin WW, Epstein HG, Jones PL, eds. *Physics for the Anaesthetist*. 4th ed. Oxford: Blackwell Scientific; 1987:73.
58. Ocasio I. *Principles of Chemistry*. John Wiley & Sons, Inc.
59. Macintosh R, et al. Gas pressure: pressure in gaseous mixtures. In: Macintosh R, Mushin WW, Epstein HG, Jones PL, eds. *Physics for the Anaesthetist*. 4th ed. Oxford: Blackwell Scientific; 1987:101.
60. Block Jr FE, Schulte GT. *J Clin Monit Comput*. 1999;15:57.
61. Korman B, Ritchie IM. *Anesthesiology*. 1985;63(152).
62. Eisenkraft JB. Anesthesia vaporizers. In: Ehrenwerth J, Eisenkraft JB, eds. *Anesthesia Equipment: Principles and Applications*. St. Louis: Mosby; 1993:57.
63. Middleton B, et al. *Physics in Anesthesia*. Banbury, United Kingdom: Scion; 2012.
64. Eger 2nd EI. *Anesth Analg*. 2001;93:947.
65. Nickalls RWD, Mapleson WW. *Br J Anaesth*. 2003;91:170.
66. James MF, White JF. *Anesth Analg*. 1984;63:1097.
67. Adriani J. Principles of physics and chemistry of solids and fluids applicable to anesthesiology. In: Adriani J, ed. *The Chemistry and Physics Of Anesthesia*. 2nd ed. Springfield, Ill: Charles C Thomas; 1962:7.
68. Dräger Medical: *Dräger Vapor 2000: anaesthetic vaporizer instructions for use*, ed 11. Lubeck, Germany: Dräger Medical; 2005.
68a. English WA, et al. *Anaesthesia*. 2009;64:84.
69. Yoder M, Vaporizers: In: *Understanding modern anesthesia systems*. Telford, PA: Dräger Medical; 2009:55.
69a. Chakravarti S, Basu S. *Indian J Anaesth*. 2013;57:464.
69b. Dhulkhed V, et al. *Indian J Anaesth*. 57: 455.
70. Datex-Ohmeda. *Tec 7 Vaporizer: User's Reference Manual*. Madison, Wis: Datex-Ohmeda; 2002.
71. Penlon. *Sigma Delta Vaporizer user Instruction Manual*. Abingdon, United Kingdom: Penlon; 2002.
72. Dräger Medical. *D-Vapor: desflurane vaporizer instructions for use*. Lubeck, Germany: Dräger Medical; 2004.
73. Datex-Ohmeda. *Anesthesia delivery unit: user's reference manual*. Bromma, Sweden: Datex-Ohmeda; 2003.
74. Maquet Critical Care. *Users manual: FLOW-i 1.2 anesthesia system*. rev 11. Solna, Sweden: Maquet Critical Care; 2011.
75. Schreiber P. *Anaesthetic equipment: performance, classification, and safety*. New York: Springer;1972.
76. Hill DW, Lowe HJ. *Anesthesiology*. 1962;23:291.
77. Hill DW. The design and calibration of vaporizers for volatile anaesthesia agents. In: Scurr C, Feldman S, eds. *Scientific Foundations of Anaesthesia*. 3rd ed. London: William Heineman; 1982:544.
78. Deleted in proofs.
79. Deleted in proofs.
80. Hill DW. *Br J Anaesth*. 1968;40:648.
81. Morris LE. *Int Anesthesiol Clin*. 1974;12:199.
82. Loeb RG. *Can J Anaesth*. 1992;39:888.
83. Stoelting RK. *Anesthesiology*. 1971;35:215.
84. Diaz PD. *Br J Anaesth*. 1976;48:387.
85. Nawaf K, Stoelting RK. *Anesth Analg*. 1979;58(30).
86. Prins L, et al. *Can Anaesth Soc J*. 1980;27:106.
87. Lin CY. *Anesth Analg*. 1980;59(359).
88. Gould DB, et al. *Anesth Analg*. 1982;61:938.
89. Palayiwa E, et al. *Br J Anaesth*. 1983;55:1025.
90. Scheller MS, Drummond JC. *Anesth Analg*. 1986;65(88).
90a. Habre, W., et al. *Br. J. Anaesth*. 87: 602.
91. Synnott A, Wren WS. *Br J Anaesth*. 1986;58:1055.
92. Deleted in proofs.
93. Carvalho B, Sanders D. *Br J Anaesth*. 2002;88:711.
94. Spacelabs Healthcare. *Blease Datum anesthesia vaporizers user's manual*. rev C. Issaquah, WA: Spacelabs Healthcare;1999.
95. Severinghaus J. *Anesthesia and Related drug Effects in Fundamentals of Hyperbaric Medicine*. Washington, DC: National Academy of Sciences; 1966:116.
96. Abel M, Eisenkraft JB. *J Clin Monit*. 1996;12:119.
97. Andrews JJ, et al. *Can J Anaesth*. 1993;40:71.
98. Riegle EV, Desertspring D. *Anesthesiology*. 1990;73:353–354.
99. Broka SM, et al. *Anesth Analg*. 1999;88:1194.
100. Keresztury MF, et al. *Anesth Analg*. 2006;103(124).
101. Lippmann M, et al. *Anesthesiology*. 1993;78:1175.
101a. Wallace AW. *A A Case Rep*. 2016;6:399.
102. Munson WM. *Anesthesiology*. 1965;26:235.
103. Craig DB. *Can J Anaesth*. 1993;40:1005.
104. Pratap JN, Harding L. *Eur J Anaesthesiol*. 2009;26:90.
105. Fernando PM, Peck DJ. *Anaesthesia*. 2001;56(1009).
106. Daniels D. *Anaesthesia*. 2002;57:288.
107. Vohra SB. *Anaesthesia*. 2000;55:606.
108. Lewis SE, et al. *Anesthesiology*. 1999;90:1221.
109. Terry L, da Silva EJ. *J Clin Anesth*. 2009;21:382.
110. Deleted in proofs.
111. Krishna KB, et al. *J Anaesthesiol Clin Pharmacol*. 2011;27:415.
112. Garstang JS. *Anaesthesia*. 2000;55:915.
113. Zimmer C, et al. *Anesthesiology*. 2004;100(1329).
114. Andrews JJ, Johnston Jr RV. *Anesth Analg*. 1993;76:1338.
115. Weiskopf RB, et al. *Br J Anaesth*. 1994;72:474.
116. Eger EI. *Anesthesiology*. 1994;80:906.
117. Susay SR, et al. *Anesth Analg*. 1996;83:864.
118. Deleted in proofs.
119. Jolly DT, Young J. *Anesth. Analg*. 2000;90:742.
119a. Jolly DT, Young J. *Can J Anesth*. 1999;46:709.
119b. Uncles DR, et al. *Anaesthesia*. 49: 547.
120. Kimatian SJ. *Anesthesiology*. 2002;96:1533.
121. Hendrickx JF, et al. *Anesth Analg*. 2001;93:391.
121a. Sansom GG. Arrangement for preventing overfill of anesthetic liquid. US6745800B1.
121b. Leijonhufvud F, et al. *F1000Research*. 2017;6:1997.
121c. Meyer JU, et al. *Handb Exp Pharmacol*. 2008;182:451–470.
121d. Gegel BT. *AANA J*. 2008;76(3):185–187.
121e. Eales M, Cooper R. *Anaesth Intensive Care Med*. 2007;8:111–115.
121f. Donovan A, Perndt H. *Anaesthesia*. 2007;62:609–614.
121g. Craig GR, et al. *Anaesthesia*. 50: 789–793.
121h. Brook PN, Perndt H. *Anaesth Intensive Care*. 2001;29:616–618.
121i. Payne T, et al. *Br J Anaesth*. 2012;108:763–767.
121j. Kim HY, et al. *Medicine (Baltimore)*. 2017;96:e8976.
121k. Marcos-Vidal JM, et al. *Heart Lung Vessels*. 2014;6:33–42.
121l. Bomberg H, et al. *Anaesthesia*. 2014;69:1241–1250.
121m. Farrell R, et al. *J Clin Monit Comput*. 2018;32:595–604.
121n. Enlund M, et al. *Anaesthesia*. 2001;56:429–432.
122. Dorsch JA, Dorsch SE. The breathing system: general principles, common components, and classifications. In: Dorsch JA, Dorsch SE, eds. *Understanding Anesthesia Equipment*. 5th ed. Baltimore: Williams & Wilkins; 2008:191.
123. Miller DM. *Anaesth Intensive Care*. 1995;23:281.
124. Metzner J, et al. *Clinical Anaesthesiology*. 2011;25:263.
125. Dorsch JA, Dorsch SE. The circle systems. In: Dorsch JA, Dorsch SE, eds. *Understanding Anesthesia Equipment*. 5th ed. Baltimore: Williams & Wilkins; 2008:223.
125a. Lee C, et al. *Korean J Anesthesiol*. 2013;65:337.

126. Eskaros SM, et al. Respiratory monitoring. In: Miller RD, Eriksson LI, Fleisher LA, et al., eds. *Miller's Anesthesia*. 7th ed. Philadelphia: Churchill Livingstone; 2010:1411.
126a. Kodali BS. *Anesthesiology*. 2013:118:192.
127. ASTM: Standard specification for minimum performance and safety requirements for anesthesia breathing systems (ASTM F1208-89), In: *Medical Devices and Services*, vol. 13.01. Conshohocken, PA: ASTM International;2005: 474.
127a. Thomas J, et al. *Anaesthesia*. 2017;72:28–34.
127b. Chaturvedi AU, Potdar MP. *Clin Pharmacol*. 2017;33:264.
127c. Oprea AD, et al. *J Clin Anesth*. 2011;23:58–60.
128. Johnstone RE, Smith TC. *Anesthesiology*. 1973;38:192.
129. Blanshard HJ, Milne MR. *Anaesthesia*. 2004;59(177).
129a. Križmarić M. *Slov Med J*. 2017;86:226.
130. International Standards Organization: ISO 5362:2006: Anesthetic reservoir bags ISO 5362. In: ISO 11.040.11: *Anaesthetic, respiratory and reanimation equipment*. http://www.iso.org/iso/home/store/catalogue_ics.htm/ Accessed 3/30/14.
131. Dräger Medical. *Operating instructions Apollo*. ed 2. Lubeck, Germany: Dräger Medical;2008.
131a. Yoder M, Ventilators: In *Understanding modern anesthesia systems*, Telford, Pa, 2009, Dräger Medical, p 145.
131b. Parthasarathy S. *Indian J Anaesth* 2013;57:516.
132. Wilkes AR. *Anaesthesia*. 2011;66:31.
133. American Society of Anesthesiologists. In: *Standards, guidelines, statements, and other documents*. <http://www.asahq.org/For-Members/Standards-Guidelines-and-Statements.aspx/> (Accessed 30.03.14).
134. Paulsen A, Klauss G. *APSF Newsl*. 2009;24(14).
134a. Dorsch JA, Dorsch SE. Gas Monitoring. In: Dorsch JA, Dorsch SE, eds. *Understanding Anesthesia Equipment*. 5th ed. Baltimore: Williams & Wilkins; 2008:685–727.
134b. Dorsch JA, Dorsch SE. *Understanding Anesthesia Equipment*. 5th ed. Philadelphia: Wolters Kluwer Health/Lippincott Williams & Wilkins; 2008.
134c. Yoder, JM. Draeger Medical. 2009;189.
135. Brattwall M, et al. *Can J Anaesth*. 2012;59:785.
136. Holzman R, Linter R. Principles and practice of closed circuit anesthesia. In: Sandberg W, Urman R, Ehrenfeld J, eds. *The MGH Textbook of Anesthetic Equipment*. Philadelphia: Saunders; 2011.
137. Baum J. *Acta Anaesthesiol Belg*. 1990;41:239.
138. Deleted in proofs.
139. Cassidy CJ, et al. *Anaesthesia*. 2011;66:879.
140. Dain S. *Can J Anaesth*. 2001;48:840.
141. Ianchulev SA, Comunale ME. *Anesth Analg*. 2005;101:774.
141a. Healthcare Spacelabs. *Arkon Anesthesia System User Manual, 070-241-00/rev A*. Issaquah, WA: Spacelabs Healthcare; 2012:212.
141b. Maquet Critical Care. *Users manual: FLOW-i 1.2 anesthesia system*, rev 11. Solna, Sweden: Maquet Critical Care;2011: 149.
142. Datex-Ohmeda. *Aisys user's reference manual*, software revision 7.x. Madison, WI: Datex-Ohmeda, p 7.
143. Hamad M, et al. *Anaesthesia*. 2003;58:719.
144. Khorasani A, et al. *Anesthesiology*. 2000;92:1501.
145. Wilkes AR. *Anaesthesia*. 2011;66(40).
146. McEwan AI, et al. *Anesth Analg*. 1993;76:440.
147. Dean HN, et al. *Anesth Analg*. 1971;50(195).
148. Norman PH, et al. *Anesth Analg*. 1996;83:425.
149. Ransom ES, Norfleet EA. *Anesth Analg*. 1997;84:703.
150. Monteiro JN, et al. *Eur J Anaesthesiol*. 2004;21:743.
151. Yang CH, et al. *Acta Anaesthesiol Taiwan*. 2012;50:35.
152. Smith CE, et al. *J Clin Anesth*. 1991;3:229.
153. Bajwa SJ, Singh A. *J Anaesthesiol Clin Pharmacol*. 2012;28:269.
154. Ramarapu S, Ramakrishnan U. *Anesth Analg*. 2012;115:477.
155. Nichols K, et al. *APSF Newsl*. 2004;19:35.
156. Krensavage TJ, Richards E. *Anesth Analg*. 1995;81:207.
157. Kshatri AM, Kingsley CP. *Anesthesiology*. 1996;84:475.
158. Agrawal P, et al. *J Anesth*. 2010;24:976.
159. Peters G, et al. *Anaesthesia*. 2007;62:860.
160. Phillips J, et al. *Anaesthesia*. 2007;62:300.
161. Kobayashi S, et al. *J Anesth*. 2004;18:277.
162. Keijzer C, et al. *Acta Anaesthesiol Scand*. 2007;51:31.
163. Yamakage M, et al. *Anaesthesia*. 2009;64:287.
164. Olympio MA. *APSF Newsl*. 2005;20(25).
165. Marini F, et al. *Acta Anaesthesiol Scand*. 2007;51:625.
166. Higuchi H, et al. *Anesth Analg*. 2000;91:434.
166a. The Sodasorb manual of CO_2 absorption. https://www.shearwater.com/?s=sodasorb+manual. Accessed 8-22-19 TG.
167. Adriani J. Carbon dioxide absorption. In: Adriani J, ed. *The Chemistry and Physics of Anesthesia*. 2nd ed. Springfield, Ill: Charles C Thomas; 1962:151.
168. Dewey & Almy Chemical Division. *The Sodasorb Manual of CO_2 Absorption*. New York: Grace; 1962.
168a. Wang TC, Bricker JL. *Environ. Int*. 1979; 2:425.
169. Anders MW. *Annu Rev Pharmacol Toxicol*. 2005;45:147.
170. Totonidis S. *Kathmandu Univ Med J (KUMJ)*. 2005;3(181).
171. Kharasch ED, et al. *Anesthesiology*. 2002;96:173.
172. Fang ZX, et al. *Anesth Analg*. 1996;82:775.
173. Eger 2nd EI, et al. *Anesth Analg*. 1997;85(1154).
174. Eger 2nd EI, et al. *Anesth Analg*. 1997;84(160).
175. Frink Jr EJ, et al. *Anesthesiology*. 1992;77:1064.
176. Conzen PF, et al. *Anesthesiology*. 2002;97:578.
177. Kharasch ED, et al. *Anesth Analg*. 2001;93:1511.
178. Higuchi H, et al. *Anesth Analg*. 2001;92:650.
179. Obata R, et al. *Anesth Analg*. 2000;91:1262.
180. Mazze RI, et al. *Anesth Analg*. 2000;90:683.
181. Morio M, et al. *Anesthesiology*. 1992;77:1155.
182. Versichelen LF, et al. *Anesthesiology*. 2001;95:750.
182a. Förster H, et al. *Anaesthesist*. 2000;49(106).
182b. Stabernack CR, et al. *Anesth Analg*. 2000;90(1428).
183. Deleted in proofs.
184. Berry PD, et al. *Anesthesiology*. 1999;90:613.
185. Baxter PJ, Kharasch ED. *Anesthesiology*. 1997;86:1061.
186. Woehlick HJ, et al. *Anesthesiology*. 1997;87:228.
187. Fang ZX, et al. *Anesth Analg*. 1995;80.
188. Holak E, et al. *Anesth Analg*. 2003;96:757.
189. Bonome C, et al. *Anesth Analg*. 1999;89:909.
190. Coppens MJ, et al. *Anaesthesia*. 2006;61:462.
191. Neumann MA, et al. *Anesth Analg*. 1999;89:768.
191a. Keijzer C1, et al. *Acta Anaesthesiol Scand*. 2005;49:815.
192. Fatheree RS, Leighton BL. *Anesthesiology*. 2004;101:531.
193. Wu J, et al. *Anesthesiology*. 2004;101:534.
194. Castro BA, et al. *Anesthesiology*. 2004;101(537).
195. Laster M, et al. *Anesth Analg*. 2004;99:769.
196. Holak E, et al. *Anesth Analg*. 2003;96:757.
197. Andrews JJ, et al. *Anesthesiology*. 1990;72(59).
198. Hunt HE. *Anesthesiology*. 1955;16(190).
199. Brown ES. *Anesthesiology*. 1959;20(41).
199a. Daley T. Submarine Air Monitoring and Atmosphere Purification Conference 2009, San Diego, CA.
199b. Wang TC. *Aviat Space Environ Med*. 1981;52:104.
200. Mapleson WW. *Br J Anaesth*. 1998;80:263.
201. Willis BA, et al. *Br J Anaesth*. 1975;47:1239.
202. Rose DK, Froese AB. *Can Anaesth Soc J*. 1979;26:104.
203. Froese AB, Rose DK. A detailed analysis of T-piece systems. In: Steward DJ, ed. *Some Aspects of Paediatric Anaesthesia*. Amsterdam: Elsevier North-Holland Biomedical Press; 1982:101.
204. Sykes MK. *Br J Anaesth*. 1968;40:666.
204a. Kaul T, Mittal G. *Indian J Anaesth*. 2013;57:507.
205. Dorsch JA, Dorsch SE. Mapleson breathing systems. In: Dorsch JA, Dorsch SE, eds. *Understanding Anesthesia Equipment*. 5th ed. Baltimore: Williams & Wilkins; 2008:209.
205a. Kain ML, Nunn JF. *Anesthesiology*. 1968;29:964–974.
206. Andersen PK, et al. *Acta Anaesthesiol Scand*. 1989;33:439.
207. Bain JA, Spoerel WE. *Can Anaesth Soc J*. 1972;19:426.
208. Pethick SL. *Can Anaesth Soc J*. 1975;22:115.
209. Aarhus D, et al. *Anaesthesia*. 1997;52:992.
209a. Hussey SG. *Arch Dis Child - Fetal Neonatal Ed*. 2004;89:F490–F493.
209b. ISO 10651-4:2002, Lung ventilators -- Part 4: Particular requirements for operator-powered resuscitators, 2002.
209c. Lien S, et al. *J Clin Anesth*. 2013;25:424–425.
209d. Lucy MJ, et al. *Pediatr Anesth*. 2018;28:788–794.
209e. Haupt J. *The History of Anesthesia at Draeger*. Lubeck, Germany: Draegerwerk AG; 1996.
209f. Jaber S, et al. *Anesthesiology*. 2006;105:944–952.
209g. Sáez JA. *Anesthesiology*. 2015;122:922.
209h. Modak RK, Olympio MA. Anesthesia Ventilaors. In: Ehrenwerth J, Eisenkraft JB, Berry JM, eds. *Anesthesia Equipment: Principles and Applications*. Philadelphia, PA: Elsevier Saunders; 2013.
209i. Saied N, et al. *Simul Healthc*. 2012;7:380–389.
210. Feeley TW, Bancroft ML. *Int Anesthesiol Clin*. 1982;20(83).
211. Khalil SN, et al. *Anaesth Analg*. 1987;66:1334.
212. Sommer RM, et al. *Anesth Analg*. 1988;67:999.
213. Bourke D, Tolentino D. *Anesth Analg*. 2003;97:492.

214. Maquet Critical Care. *FLOW-i 4.2 User's Manual.* Solna, Sweden: Maquet Critical Care;2015.
214a. Thille AW, et al. *Int Care Med.* 2009;35:1368.
214b. Boussen S, et al. *Respir Care.* 2013;58:1911–1922.
214c. Delgado C, et al. *Respir Care.* 2017;62:34–41.
214d. Walker SG, et al. Breathing Circuits. In: *Anesthesia Equipment: Principles and Applications.* Philadelphia, PA: Elsevier Saunders; 2013:95–124.
214e. Deleted in proofs.
214f. Carette R, et al. *J.Clin Monit Comput.* 2016;30:341–346.
214g. De Cooman S, et al. *BMC Anesthesiol.* 2008;8:4.
214h. Singaravelu S, Barclay P. *Br J Anaesth.* 2013;110:561–566.
214i. Wetz AJ, et al. *Acta Anaesthesiol Scand.* 2017;61:1262–1269.
214j. Datex-Ohmeda. *Aisys CS2 User's Reference Manual.* Madison, WI: Datex-Ohmeda; 2016.
215. Riutort KT, et al. The anesthesia workstation and delivery systems. In: 6th ed. Barash PG, Cullen BF, Stoelting RK, eds. *Clinical Anesthesia.* Philadelphia: Lippincott Williams & Wilkins; 2009:644.
216. U.S. Department of Health, Education and Welfare. *Criteria for a Recommended Standard: Occupational Exposure to Waste Anesthetic Gases and Vapors.* Washington, DC: U.S. Department of Health, Education and Welfare; 1977.
216a. International Standards Organization, 2007. ISO 7396-2.
217. McGregor DG. Waste anesthetic gases: information for management in anesthetizing areas and the postanesthesia care unit (PACU). ASA Task Force on Trace Anesthetic Gases. Park Ridge, IL: American Society of Anesthesiologists;1999: 3.
217a. Anesthetic Gases: Guidelines for Workplace Exposures | Occupational Safety and Health Administration https://www.osha.gov/dts/osta/anestheticgases/index.html (Accessed 12.20.18).
218. Kanmura Y, et al. *Anesthesiology.* 1999;90:693.
219. Eisenkraft JB, McGregor DG. Waste Anesthetic Gases and Scavenging Systems. In: Ehrenwerth J, Eisenkraft JB, Berry JM, eds. *Anesthesia Equipment: Principles and Applications.* Philadelphia, PA: Elsevier Saunders; 2013:125–147.
220. Dorsch JA, Dorsch SE. Controlling trace gas levels. In: Dorsch JA, Dorsch SE, eds. *Understanding Anesthesia Equipment.* 5th ed. Baltimore: Williams & Wilkins; 2008:373.
221. Carvalho B. *Br J Anaesth.* 1999;83:532.
222. Elakkumanan LB, et al. *J Anaesthesiol Clin Pharmacol.* 2012;28:270.
223. Joyal JJ, et al. *Anesthesiology.* 2012;116:1162.
224. North American Dräger. *Scavenger Interface for air Conditioning: Instruction Manual.* Telford, Pa: North American Dräger; 1984.
225. ASTM: Standard specification for anesthetic gas scavenging systems: transfer and receiving systems (ASTM F1343-02). In: *Medical devices and services.* vol. 13.01. Conshohocken, PA: ASTM International;2005: 554.
226. Saxena S, et al. *Anesth Patient Saf Found.* 2016;31:17.
227. Deleted in proofs.
228. Carstensen P. *APSF Newsl.* 1986;1:13–20.
229. Langford R, et al. *Eur J Anaesthesiol.* 2007;24:1050–1056.
230. Allen M, Lees DE. ASA Newsl. 2004;68:22.
231. Moreno-Duarte I, et al. *A A Case Rep.* 2017;8:192–196.
231a. Deleted in proofs.
232. March MG, Crowley JJ. *Anesthesiology.* 1991;75:724.
233. Lees DE. *APSF Newsl.* 1991;6(25).
234. Withiam-Wilson MJ. *APSF Newsl.* 1991;6(25).
234a. Eisenkraft JB, et al. Respiratory Gas Monitoring. In: *Anesthesia Equipment: Principles and Applications.* Philadelphia, PA: Elsevier Saunders; 2013:191–222.
234b. Cohen JB, Chaudhry T. *Anesth Patient Saf Found Newsl 27.* 2012.
234c. Huang J, et al. *J Anaesthesiol Clin Pharmacol.* 2012;28:230–231.
235. Anesthesia apparatus checkout recommendations. *Fed Regist.* 94–16618, 1994.
236. Degani A, Wiener EL. *Hum Factors.* 1993;35(345).
237. Federal Aviation Administration, Office of Integrated Safety Analysis, Human Factors Analysis Division: Human performance considerations in the use and design of aircraft checklists.
238. Tibbles PM, Edelsberg JS. *N Engl J Med.* 1996;3341642.

23 *Intravenous Anesthetics*

JAAP VUYK, ELSKE SITSEN, and MARIJE REEKERS

KEY POINTS

- The introduction of thiopental into clinical practice in 1934 marked the beginning of modern intravenous (IV) anesthesia. Today, IV anesthetics are used for induction and maintenance of anesthesia and sedation in a wide variety of circumstances.
- The most commonly used IV anesthetic is propofol, an alkylphenol presently formulated in a lipid emulsion. Propofol provides rapid onset and offset with context-sensitive decrement times of approximately 10 minutes when infused for less than 3 hours and less than 40 minutes when infused for up to 8 hours. Its mechanism of action is likely the enhancement of gamma-aminobutyric acid (GABA)-induced chloride currents. Propofol causes a dose-dependent decrease in arterial blood pressure predominantly through a decrease in systemic vascular resistance and causes moderate respiratory depression. A unique action of propofol is its antiemetic effect, even at concentrations less than those producing sedation. A growing body of evidence suggests propofol may have antitumor potential.
- Barbiturates were the most commonly used IV drugs administered to induce anesthesia prior to the introduction of propofol. Thiopental provides rapid onset and offset when used as a single dose, but it accumulates rapidly with repeated or prolonged administration thus postponing recovery from anesthesia. Methohexital has a rapid onset and offset similar to propofol for procedures lasting less than 2 hours. The barbiturates are administered as sodium salts diluted in a water base at an alkaline pH. Similar to propofol, the barbiturates provide their hypnotic effects largely through action on the GABAA receptor. Barbiturates provide cerebral protection and are, apart from induction of anesthesia, used primarily for this purpose. They cause a moderate dose-dependent decrease in arterial blood pressure (primarily as a result of peripheral vasodilation) and respiratory drive. The barbiturates are contraindicated in patients with porphyria.
- The benzodiazepines are used primarily for anxiolysis and amnesia or for conscious sedation. The water-soluble benzodiazepine midazolam is most frequently used intravenously because of its rapid onset and offset compared with other benzodiazepines (e.g., diazepam). The onset time of midazolam is slower than that of propofol and barbiturates, and its offset, especially with larger doses or a prolonged infusion, is considerably longer than that of propofol or methohexital and may be prolonged in hepatic and renal failure. The benzodiazepines act through the GABA receptor. Flumazenil is a specific benzodiazepine antagonist. It can be used to reverse the effects of benzodiazepines but should be used with caution because its antagonizing effect often lasts shorter than the benzodiazepine effect that it is supposed to antagonize. The benzodiazepines generally produce only a mild decrease in arterial blood pressure and mild-to-moderate respiratory depression. Remimazolam is the most recent benzodiazepine with an ultrashort duration of action due to its rapid clearance through plasma esterases.
- Ketamine is a phencyclidine derivative that acts primarily, but not entirely, as antagonist of the N-methyl-D-aspartate (NMDA) receptor. It produces a dissociative state of hypnosis and analgesia. It has been used for induction and maintenance of anesthesia. Ketamine is associated with significant adverse psychological effects from larger doses and has several other side effects. It is used now primarily for its analgesic properties. It has rapid onset and relatively rapid offset, even after an infusion of several hours. It has sympathomimetic effects that preserve cardiac function. Ketamine has minimal effect on respiration and tends to preserve autonomic reflexes. In addition, ongoing research suggests ketamine may play a role as an antidepressant.
- Etomidate is an imidazole derivative used primarily for induction of anesthesia, especially in elderly patients and patients who are cardiovascularly compromised. It has a rapid onset of effect and a rapid offset even after a continuous infusion. A dose used to induce anesthesia results in inhibition of adrenocortical synthesis and possible mortality in intensive care unit (ICU) patients. The major advantage of etomidate is its minimal effect on the cardiovascular and respiratory systems.
- Dexmedetomidine is the most recently released IV anesthetic. It is a highly selective α_2-adrenergic agonist that produces sedation, sympatholysis, hypnosis, and analgesia. Dexmedetomidine is approved for ICU sedation of initially intubated and mechanically ventilated patients, up to 24 hours. It may be advantageous for its ability to prevent delirium. Its second indication is procedural sedation of nonintubated patients. With increasing frequency dexmedetomine finds its use as a sedative during invasive or radiological procedures and as an adjunct in central or peripheral neural blockade. Its primary action is as an agonist on α_2-receptors in the locus caeruleus. It has minimal effect on respiration. Heart rate and cardiac output show a concentration-dependent decrease.

- Droperidol, a butyrophenone and major tranquilizer, was initially used to produce a state of neuroleptanesthesia. Its prolongation of the QT interval has resulted in its withdrawal in several countries and its limitation to the treatment of postoperative nausea and vomiting (PONV) with a black box warning in the United States. Because the use of low-dose droperidol (<1.25 mg) for PONV has not been approved by the US Food and Drug Administration (FDA), the black box warning does not relate to this use. Clinically significant prolongation of the QT interval by doses used for PONV (0.625 to 1.25 mg) has been challenged by several editorials, and this effect has not been substantiated by review of the reported cases or other literature. Low-dose droperidol remains an effective antiemetic therapy and is used as such in many European countries (also see Chapter 80).

Intravenous (IV) anesthesia can be traced back to 1656 with Percival Christopher Wren's and Daniel Johann Major's first experiments with the IV using a goose quill and bladder to inject wine and ale into a dog's vein. In 1665 German naturalist and physician Sigismund Elsholz made the first attempt at IV anesthesia in humans and investigated the possibilities of IV injection with opiates. IV anesthesia further evolved when Fedoroff started using hedonal in St. Petersburg in 1905 and entered the era of modern anesthesia with the release of thiopental in 1936.[1] Since these beginnings, and in particular during the past three decades, the pharmacokinetics and pharmacodynamics of IV anesthetics and their interactions have been described in increasingly greater detail. This body of knowledge and the availability of increasingly shorter-acting drugs now allow the anesthesia provider to administer anesthesia not on the basis of the needs of the population but to focus anesthesia on the individual needs of the patient. Today's anesthesia provider is supported by modern IV drug administration techniques like target-controlled infusion and central nervous system (CNS) monitoring devices to further optimize and individualize the application of IV anesthesia. This chapter describes the current status of the pharmacology of IV anesthetics and their place in modern anesthesia.

Propofol

HISTORY

Since its introduction in the 1970s, propofol has become the most used IV hypnotic today. Building on work on the sedative properties of phenol derivates in mice, propofol was developed in the United Kingdom by Imperial Chemical Industries as ICI 35868. The initial solution of propofol, as released in 1977 in Cremophor EL,[2] was withdrawn because of anaphylactic reactions, and replaced and reformulated as an emulsion of a soya oil/propofol mixture in water and relaunched in 1986. Propofol is used for induction and maintenance of anesthesia and for sedation in and outside the operating room.

PHYSICOCHEMICAL CHARACTERISTICS

Propofol (Fig. 23.1) is one of a group of alkylphenols that were explored for their hypnotic properties in animals.[3-5] The alkylphenols are highly lipid soluble and are insoluble in an aqueous solution.[6] Numerous formulations of propofol are marketed today. The formulation most used is that of 1% propofol, 10% soybean oil, and 1.2% purified egg phospholipid added as emulsifier, with 2.25% of glycerol as a tonicity-adjusting agent, and sodium hydroxide to change the pH. Following concerns regarding microbial growth in the emulsion, EDTA was added for its bacteriostatic activities. Propofol has a pH of 7 and appears as a slightly viscous, milky white substance, a result of small lipid droplets in solution. In Europe, a 2% formulation and a formulation in which the emulsion contains a mixture of medium-chain and long-chain triglycerides also are available. All formulations commercially available are stable at room temperature, are not light sensitive, and may be diluted with 5% dextrose in water. Propofol concentrations may be measured both in whole blood and in the exhaled air.[7-10]

In December 2008 the US Food and Drug Administration (FDA) approved fospropofol disodium (Lusedra) for monitored anesthesia care in adult patients undergoing diagnostic and therapeutic procedures. Fospropofol is a water-soluble prodrug of propofol that is metabolized by alkaline phosphatases in the liver to the active metabolite propofol. One millimole (mmol) of propofol is generated for each mmol of fospropofol sodium administered. About 1.86 mg of fospropofol sodium is the molar equivalent of 1 mg propofol. In April 2010, six studies on the pharmacokinetics and pharmacodynamics of fospropofol were retracted as a result of an analytical assay inaccuracy that was discovered after publication of these studies.[11,12] Since then, few data on the pharmacokinetics and pharmacodynamics of fospropofol have been published. Although fospropofol remains available for monitored anesthesia care, data now available are scarce and most pharmacokinetic-pharmacodynamic data that are available come from the United States as described in a recent review.[13] In contrast to propofol, fospropofol is not associated with pain on injection, although mild to moderate perineal paresthesias and pruritis minutes after a bolus injection of fospropofol have been reported and may be due to a phosphate metabolite.

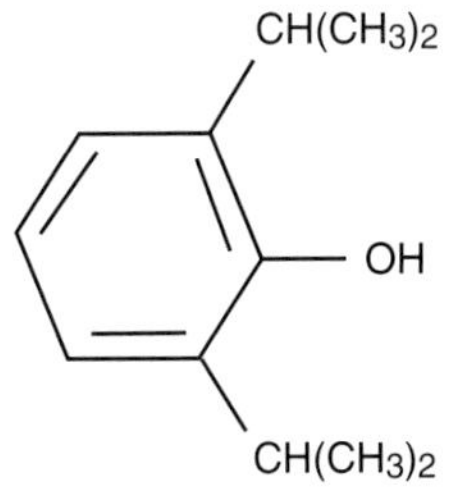

$CH(CH_3)_2$

OH

$CH(CH_3)_2$

Fig. 23.1 Structure of propofol, an alkylphenol derivative.

PHARMACOKINETICS

Propofol is oxidized to 1,4-diisopropyl quinol in the liver. Propofol and 1,4-diisopropyl quinol are conjugated with glucuronic acid to propofol-1-glucuronide, quinol-1-glucuronide, and quinol-4-glucuronide, which then may be excreted by the kidneys.[14,15] After a 2.5-hour anesthetic with propofol, patients excrete propofol and propofol metabolites for over 60 hours.[15] Less than 1% propofol is excreted unchanged in urine, and only 2% is excreted in feces. The metabolites of propofol are thought to be inactive. Because clearance of propofol (>1.5 L/min) exceeds hepatic blood flow, extrahepatic metabolism or extrarenal elimination may occur. Extrahepatic metabolism has been confirmed during the anhepatic phase of patients receiving a transplanted liver with the determination of propofol metabolites after propofol administration in the absence of liver tissue. The most important extrahepatic site for propofol metabolism is the kidney.[16,17] Renal metabolism of propofol accounts for up to 30% of propofol clearance, which explains the rapid clearance of propofol, which exceeds liver blood flow. The lungs also may play a role in the extrahepatic propofol metabolism.[18,19] In sheep, the lungs are responsible for approximately 30% of the uptake and first-pass elimination after a bolus dose. In humans, a 20% to 30% decrease in propofol concentration measured across the lung exists with a higher concentration of the metabolite 2,6-diisopropyl 1,4-quinol on the arterial side of the circulation.

Propofol is generally known for its hemodynamic depressant effects and may reduce hepatic blood flow. As such, it may reduce the clearance of other drugs metabolized by the liver, in particular those with a high extraction ratio.[20] In addition, propofol is known as a CYP3A4 inhibitor.[21] In contrast to enzyme induction that may take several days or weeks to develop, competitive inhibition of CYP activity may occur almost instantaneously due to the competition of two drugs (e.g., propofol and midazolam) for the enzyme's active site. A short-term exposure to propofol at a blood concentration of 3 μg/mL already reduces the CYP3A4 activity by about 37%.

Fospropofol[22-28,28a] is a water-soluble prodrug of propofol and is chemically described as phosphono-*O*-methyl-2, 6-diisopropylphenol, disodium salt ($C_{13}H_{19}O_5PNa_2$). Fospropofol is metabolized by alkaline phosphatases to propofol, formaldehyde, and phosphate. Formaldehyde is further metabolized to formate which is then eliminated, primarily by oxidation to carbon dioxide. Over 71% of fospropofol is recovered in the urine within 192 hours following a single 400 mg IV dose. Renal elimination is <0.02% and total body clearance in the order of 0.28 L/h/kg. The terminal elimination half-life of fospropofol is 0.88 hours. The pharmacokinetics of fospropofol and liberated propofol are not affected by race, sex, or mild to moderate renal impairment. Furthermore, fospropofol pharmacokinetics are not affected by age or alkaline phosphatase concentration. So far, no pharmacokinetic interactions have been found between fospropofol and fentanyl, midazolam, morphine, or with propofol. This is probably because fospropofol is not subject to cytochrome P450 enzyme mediated metabolism.[13]

The pharmacokinetics of propofol have been described by two-compartment and three-compartment models (Table 23.1).[28b] After a single bolus dose, whole blood propofol levels decrease rapidly as a result of redistribution and elimination (Fig. 23.2). The initial distribution half-life of propofol is 2 to 8 minutes. Studies in which the disposition of propofol is described by a three-compartment model give initial and slow distribution half-lives of 1 to 8 minutes and 30 to 70 minutes and an elimination half-life of 4 to 23.5 hours.[29-34] The context-sensitive half-time for propofol (Fig. 23.3) for infusions of up to 8 hours is less than 40 minutes.[35] Because the required decrease in concentration for awakening after anesthesia or sedation with propofol is generally less than 50%, recovery from propofol remains rapid even after prolonged infusion. The volume of distribution of the central compartment has been calculated between 6 and 40 L, and the volume of distribution at steady state has been calculated as 150 to 700 L. The

TABLE 23.1 Pharmacokinetic Variables for Commonly Used Intravenous Anesthetics

Elimination	Elimination Half-Life (h)	Clearance (mL/kg/min)	Vd_{SS} (L/kg)
Dexmedetomidine	2-3	10-30	2-3
Diazepam	20-50	0.2-0.5	0.7-1.7
Droperidol	1.7-2.2	14	2
Etomidate	2.9-5.3	18-25	2.5-4.5
Flumazenil	0.7-1.3	5-20	0.6-1.6
Ketamine	2.5-2.8	12-17	3.1
Lorazepam	11-22	0.8-1.8	0.8-1.3
Methohexital	2-6	10-15	1.5-3
Midazolam	1.7-2.6	6.4-11	1.1-1.7
Propofol	4-7	20-30	2-10
Thiopental	7-17	3-4	1.5-3

Vd_{SS}, Apparent volume of distribution at steady state.

From Reves JG, Glass P, Lubarsky DA, et al. Intravenous anesthetics. In: Miller RD, Eriksson LI, Fleischer LA, et al, eds. *Miller's Anesthesia,* 7th ed. Philadelphia: Churchill Livingstone; 2010: 719–768.

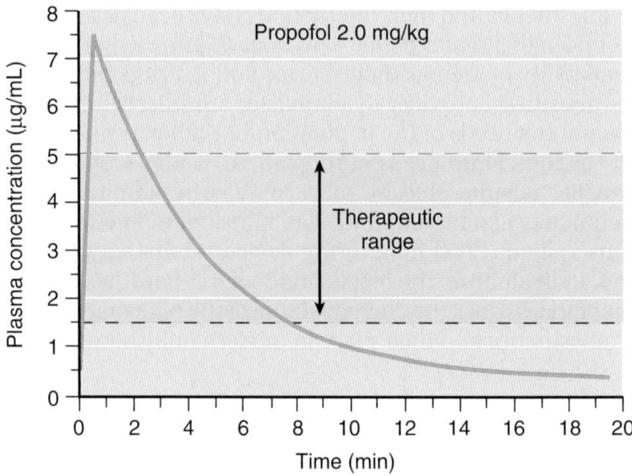

Fig. 23.2 Simulated time course of whole blood levels of propofol after an induction dose of 2 mg/kg. Blood levels required for anesthesia during surgery are 2 to 5 μg/mL, with awakening usually occurring at a blood level less than 1.5 μg/mL.

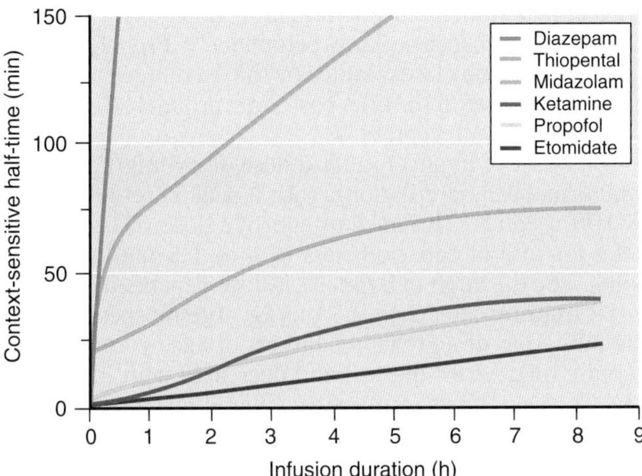

Fig. 23.3 The context-sensitive half-times for commonly used IV anesthetic drugs. The context-sensitive half-time is the time for the plasma level of the drug to decrease 50% after cessation of infusion. The duration of infusion is plotted on the horizontal axis. The rapidity with which the drug level decreases is directly related to the time of infusion (i.e., the longer the drug is infused, the longer the half-time). Etomidate, propofol, and ketamine have significantly shorter half-times than thiopental and diazepam, which makes them more suitable for prolonged infusion.

central compartment generally is smaller in the elderly as a result of the reduced cardiac output in these patients. A reduced cardiac output is associated with a higher peak plasma concentration, which is reflected by a smaller central compartment in the pharmacokinetic analysis. The clearance of propofol is extremely high—1.5 to 2.2 L/min. As discussed earlier, this exceeds hepatic blood flow, and extrahepatic metabolism has been shown.

The equilibrium constant for propofol based on suppression of the activity in the electroencephalogram (EEG) is about 0.3 min, and the half-life of equilibrium ($T^1\!/\!_2{}_{ke0}$) between plasma concentration and EEG effect is 2.5 minutes. The time to peak effect is 90 to 100 seconds. The onset of EEG effect with propofol seems to be independent of age. The onset of decreasing arterial blood pressure is much slower (double the time) and increases with age.[36] For EEG and blood pressure changes, elderly patients show a concentration dependent increasing sensitivity. The pharmacokinetics of propofol may be altered by various factors (e.g., gender, weight, preexisting disease, age, and concomitant medication).[37-39] Some studies suggest that propofol may exhibit nonlinear pharmacokinetics.[40] Because propofol has a high extraction ratio, this may impair its own clearance by decreasing cardiac output and thus hepatic blood flow.[41] As a result, a doubling of the dose of propofol may lead to a drug concentration that may be more than twice that initially experienced. In contrast, an increase in cardiac output induced by sympaticomimetic administration may lead to a decrease in the propofol plasma concentration. In a hemorrhagic shock model propofol concentrations increased 20% until uncompensated shock occurred, when there was a rapid and marked increase in propofol concentrations.[42]

In term and preterm neonates, variability of propofol clearance was accounted for largely by postmenstrual and postnatal age with very fast maturation of clearance in neonatal life. Dosing in these neonates needs to be calculated with extreme care.[43,44] Women have a larger volume of distribution and higher clearance rates, but the elimination half-life is similar for males and females. Elderly individuals have decreased clearance rates and a smaller central compartment volume.[45] Both may be the result of a reduced cardiac output. Because of this and because of an increased sensitivity to the propofol effect in the elderly, patients aged 80 years or older generally need 50% of the propofol dose of patients aged 20 years old to target the same level of sedation or hypnosis.[29,38,45,46] Children have a relatively larger central compartment volume (50%) and a more rapid clearance (25%).[31,47] In children older than 3 years, volumes and clearances should be weight adjusted (also see Chapter 77). Children younger than 3 years of age also show weight-proportional pharmacokinetic parameters, but with larger central compartment and systemic clearance values than in adults or older children. This finding explains the larger dose requirements in this age group.[48,49] Hepatic disease seems to result in larger steady state and central compartment volumes; clearance is unchanged, but the elimination half-life is slightly prolonged, as is time to recovery.[50,51] In clinical practice, no significant dose adjustment is required in case of hepatic disease. The extrahepatic clearance of propofol that may compensate for a reduced hepatic function may be responsible for this.

Midazolam affects the pharmacokinetics of propofol.[52] In the presence of a sedative midazolam concentration of 200 ng/mL, the blood propofol concentrations become elevated by about 25%. Midazolam reduces propofol metabolic clearance from 1.94 to 1.61 L/min, Cl_2 from 2.86 to 1.52 L/min, and Cl_3 from 0.95 to 0.73 L/min. The high extraction ratio of propofol of 0.79 to 0.92 suggests that the metabolic clearance of propofol may not be affected by enzyme inhibition but may be susceptible to changes in hepatic perfusion. The changes in the pharmacokinetics of propofol induced by midazolam thus may be the result of the hemodynamic alterations induced by the coadministration of midazolam.

Propofol in its turn affects midazolam pharmacokinetics as well.[20] In the presence of sedative concentrations of propofol, plasma midazolam concentrations increased by 27%. In the presence of propofol, midazolam is administered in a smaller central compartment from which midazolam is cleared and distributed less rapidly to peripheral tissues. For example, alfentanil[53] has been shown to increase blood propofol concentrations through a reduction in the elimination and distribution clearance of propofol. This is in line with other pharmacokinetic interactions between hypnotics and opioids when combined with propofol. Propofol has been shown to increase alfentanil concentrations by decreasing the elimination and the rapid and slow distribution clearances of alfentanil. Coadministration of propofol increased remifentanil concentrations via both a decrease in the central volume of distribution and distributional clearance of remifentanil by 41% and elimination clearance by 15%. Propofol kinetics is unaltered by renal disease.

As previously stated, pharmacokinetic data on the disposition of fospropofol are scarce. Phase I and phase II studies were conducted in Europe when a detection error became apparent resulting in the retraction of six published manuscripts. Currently, no further pharmacokinetic studies have been initiated. The pharmacokinetics of fospropofol in humans remains largely unknown.

Fospropofol protein binding is extensive (98%).[13] It has a small volume of distribution of 0.3 L/kg, a total body clearance of 0.36 L/kg/h with a terminal elimination half-life of 0.88 hours. After a bolus dose of 6 mg/kg of fospropofol, the parent drug peaks at 4 minutes and is rapidly metabolized to propofol with a peak plasma propofol concentration at 12 minutes after administration of fospropofol. With this fospropofol dose the highest plasma concentration reached (Cmax) of fospropofol was 78.7 μg/mL and the Cmax of propofol was 1.08 μg/mL. The total body clearance of fospropofol and propofol were 0.36 and 3.2 L/kg/h. The terminal half-lives were 0.88 and 1.13 hours, respectively.

Pharmacodynamics

EFFECTS ON THE CENTRAL NERVOUS SYSTEM

The hypnotic action of propofol is mostly mediated by enhancing γ-aminobutyric acid (GABA)-induced chloride current through its binding to the β-subunit of $GABA_A$ receptor. Sites on the β_1-subunit, β_2-subunit, and β_3-subunit of the transmembrane domains are crucial for the hypnotic action of propofol.[54,55] The α-subunit and γ_2-subunit subtypes also seem to contribute to modulating the effects of propofol on the GABA receptor. The effect of propofol has been described in two manners—indirect and direct. Propofol exhibits an indirect effect by potentiation of the ion channel activation by GABA, shifting the concentration-response relationship to the left. At higher propofol concentrations, propofol is also thought to directly activate $GABA_A$ receptor channels.[56-58] The exact mechanism and location of changes that are associated with the change from consciousness to the unconscious state are not yet fully understood. Some experts suggest that a proper functioning of the brain stem-thalamo-cortical arousal circuits are critical while others state that consciousness is more related to fronto-parietal association cortex activity. Propofol, through its action on $GABA_A$ receptors[59] in the hippocampus, inhibits acetylcholine release in the hippocampus and prefrontal cortex. The α_2-adrenoreceptor system also seems to play an indirect role in the sedative effects of propofol.[60] Resting state fMRI studies suggest that propofol's action may be related to a CNS that reduces its discriminable state and switches into stereotypic patterns of firing under propofol sedation.[61] The so called default mode network (DMN), including the posterior cingulated, the medial frontal cortex, and bilateral parietal cortices, is the anatomical substrate in which these stereotypical patterns become visible. Using positron emission tomography, propofol hypnosis is related with reduced activity in the thalamic and precuneus regions. These regions likely play an important role in propofol-induced unconsciousness.[62]

Propofol results also in widespread inhibition of the N-methyl-d-aspartate (NMDA) subtype of glutamate receptor through modulation of sodium channel gating, an action that also may contribute to the drug's CNS effects.[63,64] Propofol has a direct depressant effect on neurons of the spinal cord. In acutely dissociated spinal dorsal horn neurons, propofol acts on $GABA_A$ and glycine receptors.[65] The sense of well-being in patients with propofol is related to the increase in dopamine concentrations in the nucleus accumbens (a phenomenon noted with drugs of abuse and pleasure-seeking behavior).[66] Propofol's antiemetic action may be explained by the decrease in serotonin levels it produces in the area postrema, probably through its action on GABA receptors.[67]

The onset of hypnosis after a dose of 2.5 mg/kg is rapid (one arm–brain circulation), with a peak effect seen at 90 to 100 seconds. The median effective dose (ED_{50}) of propofol for loss of consciousness is 1 to 1.5 mg/kg after a bolus. The duration of hypnosis is dose-dependent, being 5 to 10 minutes after 2 to 2.5 mg/kg. Age markedly affects the induction dose, which is largest at ages younger than 2 years (ED_{95} 2.88 mg/kg) and decreases with increasing age. This is a direct result of the altered pharmacokinetics in children and elderly. Children exhibit a relatively larger central compartment and therefore need a higher dose to assure a similar blood-drug concentration.[68-70] In addition, the rapid clearance of propofol in children requires a larger maintenance dose as well. Increasing age decreases the propofol concentration required for loss of consciousness.

At subhypnotic doses, propofol provides sedation and amnesia. Propofol infusions of at least 2 mg/kg/h were necessary to provide amnesia in unstimulated volunteers. Awareness during surgery at higher infusion rates has been reported. During surgical procedures, extremely high infusion rates producing blood propofol concentrations in excess of 10 μg/mL may be necessary to prevent awareness if propofol is used as the sole anesthetic. Propofol also tends to produce a general state of well-being. Hallucinations, sexual fantasies, and opisthotonos occur after propofol administration.

The effect of propofol on the EEG, as assessed after 2.5 mg/kg followed by an infusion, shows an initial increase in alpha rhythm followed by a shift to gamma and theta frequency. Rapid infusion rates produce burst suppression at blood propofol concentrations higher than 8 μg/mL. Propofol causes a concentration-dependent decrease in the bispectral index (BIS), with 50% and 95% of patients unable to respond to a verbal command at a BIS of 63 and 51, respectively. The propofol concentration at which 50% of volunteers failed to respond to verbal command was 2.35 μg/mL. Lack of recall was observed in 95% of patients at a BIS value of 77.[71] Propofol effect site concentrations provide similar correlation with decreases in the spectral entropy variable derived from the EEG as it does with BIS, and a similar ability to titrate propofol anesthetic effect. The effect of propofol on epileptogenic EEG activity is controversial. Propofol may suppress seizure activity via GABA agonism, inhibition of NMDA receptors, and modulation of slow calcium ion channels. However, the same GABA agonism and glycine antagonism may also induce clinical seizures and EEG epileptiform changes.[72] This especially may occur during induction of and emergence from anesthesia. Propofol has a dose-dependent anticonvulsant. Propofol has even been used to treat epileptic seizures. Yet propofol can cause grand mal seizures and has been used for cortical mapping of epileptogenic foci.[73]

Unfortunately, propofol can be addictive. An important issue in the potential of abuse is the development of tolerance. Tolerance to a drug creates circumstances for abuse. Propofol is being used as a sedative in the intensive care unit (ICU); in 20% to 40% of patients, the propofol dosage regimen needs to be repeatedly adjusted upward in order to maintain the same effect.[74] Data on propofol abuse in the general public are unknown but the incidence of abuse is likely to be low compared to other substances. For healthcare workers, propofol is easy to access and case reports of lethal self-administration do occur. Some have suggested that there are more frequent incidences of propofol abuse by healthcare providers[75,76] and support stricter propofol regulation. In contrast to propofol, fospropofol was classified in 2009 by the US Drug Enforcement Administration (DEA) as a controlled substance.

Propofol decreases intracranial pressure (ICP) in patients with either normal or increased ICP (also see Chapter 57). The decrease in ICP (30% to 50%) is associated with significant decreases in cerebral perfusion pressure (CPP).[77] The use of propofol in head-injured patients should be restricted to doses providing mild-to-moderate sedation (i.e., blood concentration of 2 μg/mL, infusion of 25 to 75 μg/kg/min).[78] Anesthetics are neuroprotective because they reduce the metabolic oxygen use that is beneficial for the balance between energy supply and demand and because they increase the tolerance to hypoxia by the neuronal tissue. Propofol has no direct preconditioning effect but may attenuate glutamate-mediated excitotoxicity.[79-81] Propofol acutely reduces intraocular pressure by 30% to 40%. Compared with thiopental, propofol produces a larger decrease in intraocular pressure and is more effective in preventing an increase in intraocular pressure secondary to succinylcholine and endotracheal intubation. Normal cerebral reactivity to carbon dioxide and autoregulation are maintained during a propofol infusion.

The neuroprotective effects of propofol remain controversial.[82] In an incomplete ischemia model in rats, propofol administered to burst suppression results in significantly better neurologic outcome and less brain tissue injury compared with fentanyl. Propofol administered at sedative concentrations started either immediately after or at 1 hour after an ischemic insult significantly reduced infarct size compared with awake controls infused with intralipid.[83,84] Subanesthetic doses of propofol also induce neuroapoptosis in the infant mouse brain.[85] In addition, anesthetic doses of propofol in rats[86] induce complex changes that are accompanied by cell death in the cortex and thalamus of the developing rat brain. The neuronal protective effect of propofol may be due to the attenuation of changes in adenosine triphosphate, calcium, sodium, and potassium caused by hypoxic injury and its antioxidant action by inhibiting lipid peroxidation. Current evidence indicates that propofol can protect neurons against ischemic injury caused by excitotoxicity, but neuroprotection may be sustained only if the ischemic insult is relatively mild and is not sustained after a prolonged recovery period. Prolonged propofol sedation in children is associated with adverse neurologic sequelae.[87]

Many anesthetic-related drugs decrease the required dose or blood concentrations of propofol's pharmacologic action. The "required dose" is usually directly related to the required concentration for a given effect. The propofol Cp_{50} (blood concentration needed for 50% of subjects to not respond to a defined stimulus) for loss of response to verbal command in the absence of any other drug is 2.3 to 3.5 μg/mL.[88-90] The propofol Cp_{50} to prevent movement on skin incision is 16 μg/mL; this is markedly reduced by increasing concentrations (i.e., doses) of fentanyl or alfentanil. The propofol Cp_{50} for skin incision when combined with benzodiazepine premedication (lorazepam, 1 to 2 mg) and 66% nitrous oxide is 2.5 μg/mL (venous).[91] This concentration is reduced to 1.7 μg/mL when morphine (0.15 mg/kg) rather than lorazepam is used for premedication. The concentration of propofol (when combined with 66% nitrous oxide) required during minor surgery is 1.5 to 4.5 μg/mL, and the concentration for major surgery is 2.5 to 6 μg/mL.[92] Awakening usually occurs at concentrations less than 1.6 μg/mL and orientation occurs at concentrations less than 1.2 μg/mL when the propofol concentration is decreasing. Not surprisingly, awakening is postponed in the presence of high blood concentrations of opioids. Optimal propofol blood concentrations have been defined when combined with several opioids including remifentanil, alfentanil, sufentanil, and fentanyl that assure adequate anesthesia and the most rapid return to consciousness, postoperatively (Table 23.2). In the presence of remifentanil, a relatively large-dose opioid anesthetic is recommended. Yet, with fentanyl an accompanying large dose of propofol should be used to assure rapid return to recovery postoperatively (Fig. 23.4). When equilibration between blood and effect site is allowed, however, awakening concentrations (2.2 μg/mL) are similar to concentrations associated with loss of verbal command.[93]

EFFECTS ON THE RESPIRATORY SYSTEM

Apnea occurs after administration of an induction dose of propofol; the incidence and duration of apnea depend on dose, speed of injection, and concomitant premedication.[94] An induction dose of propofol results in a 25% to 30% incidence of apnea from the respiratory depressant effects of propofol and yet a normal partial pressure of carbon dioxide in the blood ($PaCO_2$) at induction in the absence of surgical stimulation. Metabolic depression further prevents the $PaCO_2$ to increase. Yet, the duration of apnea occurring with propofol may be prolonged to more than 30 seconds. The incidence of prolonged apnea (>30 seconds) is increased further by addition of an opiate, either as premedication or just before induction of anesthesia.[92,95] A maintenance infusion of propofol (100 μg/kg/min) results in a 40% decrease in tidal volume and a 20% increase in respiratory frequency, with an unpredictable change in minute ventilation. Doubling the infusion rate from 100 to 200 μg/kg/min causes a further moderate decrease in tidal volume but no change in respiratory frequency.[96] As with other hypnotic drugs, spontaneous ventilation is the result of the respiratory depressant effects of the hypnotic agents and the decrease in CO_2 production resulting from the metabolic depression versus the stimulatory effects of the increasing $PaCO_2$ resulting from apnea and the level of nociception. Propofol (50-120 μg/kg/min) also depresses the ventilatory response to hypoxia, presumably by a direct action on carotid body chemoreceptors.[97] Propofol induces bronchodilation in patients with chronic obstructive pulmonary disease. Propofol attenuates vagal (at low concentrations) and methacholine-induced (at high concentrations) bronchoconstriction and seems to have a direct action on muscarinic receptors. Propofol inhibits the receptor-coupled signal transduction pathway through inositol phosphate

TABLE 23.2 Infusion Schemes of Propofol and the Opioids Required to Maintain Effect-Site Concentrations of These Agents*

Opioid	**Alfentanil EC50-EC95 (90-130 ng/mL)**	**Fentanyl EC50-EC95 (1.1-1.6 ng/mL)**	**Sufentanil EC50-EC95 (0.14-0.20 ng/mL)**	**Remifentanil EC50-EC95 (4.7-8.0 ng/mL)**
Bolus	25-35 μg/kg in 30 sec	3 μg/kg in 30 sec	0.15-0.25 μg/kg in 30 sec	1.5-2 μg/kg in 30 sec
Infusion 1	50-75 μg/kg/h for 30 min	1.5-2.5 μg/kg/h for 30 min	0.15-0.22 μg/kg thereafter	13-22 μg/kg/h for 20 min
Infusion 2	30-42.5 μg/kg/h thereafter	1.3-2 μg/kg/h up to 150 min		11.5-19 μg/kg/h thereafter
Infusion 3		0.7-1.4 μg/kg/h thereafter		
Propofol	**Propofol EC_{50}-EC_{95} (3.2-4.4 μg/mL)**	**Propofol EC_{50}-EC_{95} (3.4-5.4 μg/mL)**	**Propofol EC_{50}-EC_{95} (3.3-4.5 μg/mL)**	**Propofol EC_{50}-EC_{95} (2.5-2.8 μg/mL)**
Bolus	2.0-2.8 mg/kg in 30 s	2.0-3.0 mg/kg in 30 s	2.0-2.8 mg/kg in 30 s	1.5 mg/kg in 30 s
Infusion 1	9-12 mg/kg/h for 40 min	9-15 mg/kg/h for 40 min	9-12 mg/kg/h for 40 min	7-8 mg/kg/h for 40 min
Infusion 2	7-10 mg/kg/h for 150 min	7-12 mg/kg/h for 150 min	7-10 mg/kg/h for 150 min	6-6.5 mg/kg/h for 150 min
Infusion 3	6.5-8 mg/kg/h thereafter	6.5-11 mg/kg/h thereafter	6.5-8 mg/kg/h thereafter	5-6 mg/kg/h thereafter

These optimal infusion schemes have been derived from data in female patients undergoing lower abdominal surgery. These should be used as guidelines and be adjusted to the individual needs of the patient.

Reproduced from Vuyk J, Mertens MJ, Olofsen E, et al. Propofol anesthesia and rational opioid selection: determination of optimal EC50-EC95 propofol-opioid concentrations that assure adequate anesthesia and a rapid return of consciousness. *Anesthesiology*. 1997;87:1549–1562, with permission from Lippincott Williams and Wilkins©, 1997; and Kataria BK, Ved SA, Nicodemus HF, et al. The pharmacokinetics of propofol in children using 3 different data-analysis approaches. *Anesthesiology*. 1994;80:104–122.

*When given in combination, within +/− 15% of the effect-site concentrations that are associated with a 50% and 95% probability of no response to surgical stimuli and the most rapid possible return of consciousness after termination of the infusions.

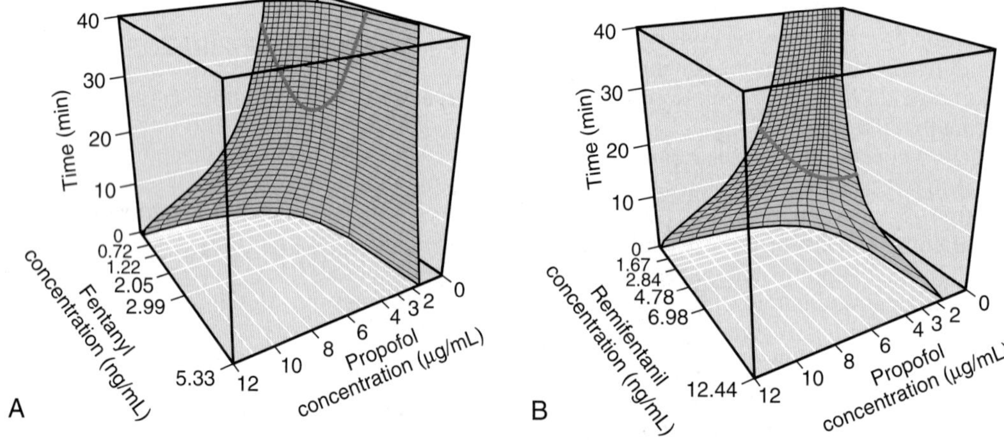

Fig. 23.4 Computer simulation of effect-site propofol and fentanyl (A) or remifentanil (B) concentrations vs. time during the first 40 min after termination of target-controlled infusions of propofol and fentanyl or remifentanil that had been maintained for 300 min at constant target blood or plasma concentration combinations associated with a 50% probability of no response to surgical stimuli. These concentration combinations are represented by the curved line on the bottom of the figure in the *x-y* plane. The decrease in concentrations following the intraoperative propofol-fentanyl and propofol-remifentanil combinations is represented by the curves running upward from the *x-y* plane. The curved lines in parallel to the *x-y* plane represent consecutive 1-min time intervals. The bold lines within the two figures represent the propofol-fentanyl-time and propofol-remifentanil-time relationships at which consciousness is regained in 50% of the patients. (Reproduced from Vuyk J, Mertens MJ, Olofsen E, et al. Propofol anesthesia and rational opioid selection: determination of optimal EC50-EC95 propofol-opioid concentrations that assure adequate anesthesia and a rapid return of consciousness. *Anesthesiology*. 1997;87:1549–1562, with permission from Lippincott Williams and Wilkins©, 1997.)

generation and inhibition of Ca^{2+} mobilization. The preservative used with propofol is important regarding its bronchodilator activity. Propofol with metabisulfite (compared with propofol without metabisulfite) does not inhibit vagal or methacholine-induced bronchoconstriction. Propofol potentiates hypoxic pulmonary vasoconstriction, an effect caused by inhibition of K(+) (ATP)-mediated pulmonary vasodilatation. Propofol has an impact on the pulmonary pathophysiology of adult respiratory distress syndrome. In an animal model of septic endotoxemia, propofol (10 mg/kg/h) significantly reduced free radical mediated and cyclooxygenase catalyzed lipid peroxidation. In addition, PaO_2 and hemodynamics were maintained closer to baseline. These benefits of propofol have not yet been confirmed in humans.

EFFECTS ON THE CARDIOVASCULAR SYSTEM

The cardiovascular effects of propofol for induction and maintenance of anesthesia have been evaluated (Table 23.3).[98] The most prominent effect of propofol is a decrease in arterial blood pressure during induction of

TABLE 23.3 Hemodynamic Changes % After Induction of Anesthesia With Nonbarbiturate Hypnotics

	Diazepam	Droperidol	Etomidate*	Ketamine	Lorazepam	Midazolam	Propofol
HR	−9 ± 13	Unchanged	−5 ± 10	0-59	Unchanged	−14 ± 12	−10 ± 10
MBP	0-19	0-10	0-17	0 ± 40	−7 to 20	−12 to 26	−10 to 40
SVR	−22 ± 13	−5 to 15	−10 ± 14	0 ± 33	−10 to 35	0-20	−15 to 25
PAP	0-10	Unchanged	−9 ± 8	+44 ± 47	—	Unchanged	0-10
PVR	0-19	Unchanged	−18 ± 6	0 ± 33	Unchanged	Unchanged	0-10
PAO	Unchanged	+25 ± 50	Unchanged	Unchanged	—	0-25	Unchanged
RAP	Unchanged	Unchanged	Unchanged	+15 ± 33	Unchanged	Unchanged	0-10
CI	Unchanged	Unchanged	−20 ± 14	0 ± 42	0 ± 16	0-25	−10 to 30
SV	0-8	0-10	0-20	0-21	Unchanged	0-18	−10 to 25
LVSWI	0-36	Unchanged	0-33	0 ± 27	—	−28 to 42	−10 to 20
dP/dt	Unchanged	—	0-18	Unchanged	—	0-12	Decreased

*The larger deviations are in patients with valvular disease.

CI, Cardiac index; *dP/dt*, first derivative of pressure measured over time; *HR*, heart rate; *LVSWI*, left ventricular stroke work index; *MBP*, mean blood pressure; *PAO*, pulmonary artery occluded pressure; *PAP*, pulmonary artery pressure; *PVR*, pulmonary vascular resistance; *RAP*, right atrial pressure; *SV*, stroke volume; *SVR*, systemic vascular resistance.

From Reves JG, Glass P, Lubarsky DA, et al. Intravenous anesthetics. In: Miller RD, Eriksson LI, Fleischer LA, et al, eds. *Miller's Anesthesia*, 7th ed. Philadelphia: Churchill Livingstone; 2010: 719–768.

anesthesia.[98a] Independent of the presence of cardiovascular disease, an induction dose of 2 to 2.5 mg/kg produces a 25% to 40% reduction of systolic blood pressure. Similar changes are seen in mean and diastolic blood pressure. The decrease in arterial blood pressure is associated with a decrease in cardiac output/cardiac index (±15%), stroke volume index (±20%), and systemic vascular resistance (15%-25%). Left ventricular stroke work index also is decreased (±30%). When looking specifically at right ventricular function, propofol produces a marked reduction in the slope of the right ventricular end-systolic pressure-volume relationship.

In patients with valvular heart disease, pulmonary artery and pulmonary capillary wedge pressure also are reduced, a finding that implies the resultant decrease in pressure is due to a decrease in preload and afterload. Although the decrease in systemic pressure after an induction dose of propofol is due to vasodilation, the direct myocardial depressant effects of propofol are more controversial. The decrease in cardiac output after propofol administration may be via its action on sympathetic drive to the heart. The hemodynamic response to propofol lags significantly behind that of the hypnotic effect. The effect-site equilibration half-life of propofol is in the order of 2 to 3 minutes for the hypnotic effect and about 7 minutes for the hemodynamic depressant effect.[36] This implies that hemodynamic depression increases in a few minutes after a patient has lost consciousness from an induction of anesthesia.

High concentrations of propofol abolish the inotropic effect of α- but not β-adrenoreceptor stimulation and enhance the lusitropic (relaxation) effect of β stimulation. Clinically, the myocardial depressant effect and the vasodilation are dose-dependent and plasma concentration-dependent.[99] Propofol is a vasodilator due to a reduction in sympathetic activity. The mechanism of this activity is a combination of a direct effect on intracellular smooth muscle calcium mobilization, inhibition of prostacyclin synthesis in endothelial cells, reduction in angiotensin II–elicited calcium entry,[100,101] activation of K adenosine triphosphate channels, and stimulation of nitric oxide. The stimulation of nitric oxide may be modulated by any intralipid rather than propofol itself.

Heart rate does not change significantly after an induction dose of propofol. Propofol either may reset or may inhibit the baroreflex, reducing the tachycardic response to hypotension. Propofol also decreases cardiac parasympathetic tone in a dose-dependent manner. Propofol has a minimal direct effect on sinoatrial node function or on normal atrioventricular and accessory pathway conduction. Propofol attenuates the heart rate response to atropine in a dose-dependent manner. Propofol suppresses atrial (supraventricular) tachycardias and probably should be avoided during electrophysiologic studies. The peak plasma concentrations obtained after a bolus dose are substantially higher than the concentrations seen with a continuous infusion and may reach concentrations up to 80 to 100 μg/mL. Because the vasodilatory and myocardial depressant effects are concentration-dependent, the decrease in arterial blood pressure from propofol during the infusion phase (maintenance of anesthesia) is much less than that seen after induction of anesthesia by an intravenous bolus administration of propofol. An infusion of propofol reduces myocardial blood flow and oxygen consumption. Thus, global myocardial oxygen supply-to-demand ratio is likely preserved. The cardioprotective effect of propofol versus volatile anesthetics in patients having cardiac surgery on- or off-cardiopulmonary bypass is less debatable. In two large studies comparing propofol with sevoflurane in patients undergoing cardiac surgery, postoperative troponin levels were lower and hemodynamic function better in patients receiving sevoflurane. A study comparing desflurane with propofol in patients undergoing off-pump coronary artery bypass showed similar results. In contrast, administration of a large-dose of propofol (120 μg/kg/min) or small-dose of propofol (60 μg/kg/min) during cardiopulmonary bypass, or titrating isoflurane throughout surgery, showed improved troponin levels and better hemodynamic function in the large-dose propofol group compared to the isoflurane or small-dose propofol group. This study suggests that cardio protection with propofol is dose-dependent.[102] Lastly, combinations of propofol with inhaled anesthetics may offer an optimal pre- and postconditioning strategy in patients scheduled for coronary bypass surgery. Isoflurane preconditioning combined with propofol postconditioning acts synergistically in attenuating postischemic myocardial reperfusion injury as determined by surrogate markers of myocardial injury and function.[103] Heart rate changes are variable when anesthesia is maintained with propofol. The extent of hypotension, the ability for the patient to compensate, and the use of any other concomitant drugs are likely the most important factors in determining what happens to the heart rate after propofol administration.

OTHER EFFECTS

Propofol, similar to thiopental, does not enhance neuromuscular blockade produced by neuromuscular blocking drugs. Propofol produces no effect on the evoked electromyogram or twitch tension; however, good or acceptable tracheal intubating conditions after propofol alone have been reported. Propofol does not trigger malignant hyperthermia and is an appropriate choice in patients with this condition.[104-106] Propofol after a single dose or a prolonged infusion does not affect corticosteroid synthesis or alter the normal response to adrenocorticotropic hormone (ACTH) stimulation. Propofol in the emulsion formulation does not alter hepatic, hematologic, or fibrinolytic function. Lipid emulsion per se reduces in vitro platelet aggregation, however. Anaphylactoid reactions to the present formulation of propofol have been reported. In at least some patients, the immune response was entirely due to propofol and not to the lipid emulsion. Most patients developing the anaphylactoid response to propofol had a previous history of allergic responses. Perhaps propofol should not be used in patients with multiple drug allergies.[107-109] Propofol alone in intralipid does not trigger histamine release. Fospropofol is metabolized to propofol and formate. Formate concentrations do not increase after fospropofol administration. Propofol also possesses significant antiemetic activity with small (subhypnotic) doses (i.e., 10 mg in adults). The median concentration of propofol with an antiemetic effect was 343 ng/mL, which also causes a mild sedative effect.[110] This concentration can be achieved by an initial dose of propofol infusion of 10 to 20 mg followed by 10 μg/kg/min. Propofol used as a maintenance anesthetic during breast surgery was more effective than 4 mg of ondansetron given as prophylaxis in preventing postoperative nausea and vomiting (PONV) (also see Chapter 80). Propofol as an infusion of 1 mg/kg/h (17 μg/kg/min) also has provided excellent antiemetic action after anticancer chemotherapy. At subhypnotic doses, propofol relieves cholestatic pruritus and is likely as effective as naloxone in treating pruritus induced by spinal opiates.

Propofol decreases polymorphonuclear leukocyte chemotaxis, but not adherence phagocytosis and killing. This action contrasts with the effect of thiopental, which inhibits all these chemotactic responses. However, propofol inhibits phagocytosis and killing of *Staphylococcus aureus* and *Escherichia coli*. There have been life-threatening systemic infections associated with the use of propofol.[111] In hospitals where these infections occurred, opened vials and syringes of propofol had positive cultures. The intralipid that acts as the solvent for propofol is an excellent culture medium. Disodium edetate or metabisulfite has been added to the formulation of propofol in an attempt to retard such bacterial growth. Strict aseptic technique still must be observed. The administration of propofol is associated with the development of pancreatitis,[112] which may be related to hypertriglyceridemia. Patients who developed hypertriglyceridemia tended to be older, had a longer ICU stay, and received propofol for a longer duration. If propofol is being used for prolonged sedation or at higher infusion rates (especially in elderly patients), serum triglyceride concentrations should be routinely monitored.

BOX 23.1 Uses and Doses of Intravenous Propofol

Induction of general anesthesia	1-2.5 mg/kg IV, dose reduced with increasing age
Maintenance of general anesthesia	50-150 μg/kg/min IV combined with N_2O or an opiate
Sedation	25-75 μg/kg/min IV
Antiemetic action	10-20 mg IV, can repeat every 5-10 min or start infusion of 10 μg/kg/min

IV, Intravenously; *N_2O*, nitrous oxide.

From Reves JG, Glass P, Lubarsky DA, et al. Intravenous anesthetics. In Miller RD, Eriksson LI, Fleischer LA, et al, eds. *Miller's Anesthesia*, 7th ed. Philadelphia: Churchill Livingstone; 2010: 719–768.

Uses

INDUCTION AND MAINTENANCE OF ANESTHESIA

Propofol is suitable for the induction and maintenance of anesthesia (Box 23.1). The intravenous induction dose is 1 to 2.5 mg/kg. Physiologic characteristics that best determine the appropriate dose to induce anesthesia are age, lean body mass, and central blood volume.[113] Propofol may be titrated on the basis of the BIS value for maintenance of anesthesia and to assure adequacy of anesthesia and prevention of overdosing. Premedication with an opiate or a benzodiazepine, or both, markedly reduces the necessary induction dose.[114-116] The induction dose needs to be reduced in elderly patients and a dose of 1 mg/kg (with premedication) to 1.75 mg/kg (without premedication) is recommended for inducing anesthesia in patients older than 60. Furthermore, older and sicker (ASA class III to IV) patients develop more profound hypotension, especially when propofol islcombined with an opiate (also see Chapter 65). To prevent hypotension in sicker patients or in patients presenting for cardiac surgery, intravenously administered fluids should be given as tolerated, and propofol titrated to achieve the desired anesthetic state. In general, for both pharmacokinetic and pharmacodynamic reasons elderly patients (>80 years old) require half the dose of young patients (<20 years)[117]. For induction in children, the ED_{95} (2-3 mg/kg) is increased, primarily because of pharmacokinetic differences. Children demonstrate a smaller central compartment, an increased metabolic clearance, and larger volumes of distribution of propofol relative to adult patients.[69] Propofol, when used for induction of anesthesia in short-lasting procedures, results in a significantly quicker recovery and an earlier return of psychomotor function compared with thiopental or methohexital, regardless of the anesthetic used for maintenance of anesthesia.

Several infusion schemes have been used to achieve adequate plasma concentrations of propofol. After an induction dose, an infusion of 100 to 200 μg/kg/min is usually needed. The infusion rate is titrated to individual requirements and the surgical stimulus. When combined with propofol, the required infusion rate and concentration of opiates, midazolam, clonidine, or ketamine should be reduced.[20,118] Because opioids alter the concentration of propofol required for adequate anesthesia, the time to awakening and recovery can be influenced by these drug combinations. Also, opioids affect both the pharmacokinetics and the pharmacodynamics of propofol. Alfentanil decreases the elimination clearance of propofol from 2.1 L/min to 1.9 L/min, the distribution clearance from 2.7 L/min to 2.0 L/min, and the peripheral volume of distribution from 179 L to 141 L. The pharmacokinetic parameters of propofol are affected by cardiac output, heart rate, and plasma alfentanil concentration.[39] Similarly, midazolam reduces propofol's metabolic clearance from 1.94 to 1.61 L/min, Cl_2 from 2.86 to 1.52 L/min, and Cl_3 from 0.95 to 0.73 L/min. Consequently, in the presence of both midazolam and alfentanil propofol concentrations become elevated by 20% to 30%.[53] The infusion rate required to achieve the combination with the shortest recovery is propofol, 1 to 1.5 mg/kg followed by 140 μg/kg/min for 10 minutes followed by 100 μg/kg/min, and alfentanil, 30 μg/kg followed by an infusion of 0.25 μg/kg/min, or fentanyl, 3 μg/kg followed by 0.02 μg/kg/min.

As indicated previously, increasing age is associated with a decrease in propofol infusion requirements, whereas these requirements are larger in children and infants. The blood levels of propofol alone for loss of consciousness are 2.5 to 4.5 μg/mL, and the blood concentrations (when combined with nitrous oxide) required for surgery are 2.5 to 8 μg/mL. Similar concentrations are necessary when propofol is combined with an opioid for a total IV technique. The knowledge of these levels and of the pharmacokinetics of propofol has enabled the use of pharmacokinetic model–driven infusion systems to deliver propofol as a continuous infusion for the maintenance of anesthesia. A meta-analysis of recovery data after either propofol for maintenance or the newer volatile anesthetics indicated only minor differences in times to reach recovery goals; however, the incidence of nausea and vomiting remained significantly less frequent in the patients given propofol for maintenance of anesthesia.

Propofol can be used as a maintenance of anesthesia infusion regimen for cardiac surgery. Using reduced and titrated doses of propofol for induction of anesthesia and titrated infusion rates of 50 to 200 μg/kg/min combined with an opioid for maintenance, propofol provides intraoperative hemodynamic control and ischemic episodes similar to those with either enflurane/opioid or a primary opioid technique.

Blood propofol concentrations increase in the presence of hemorrhagic shock. Shock affects the pharmacokinetics and pharmacodynamics of propofol. Shock results in slower intercompartmental clearances and shock shifts the concentration effect relationship to the left, demonstrating a 2.7-fold decrease in the effect-site concentration required to achieve 50% of the maximal effect in the BIS.[119] These pharmacokinetic changes may be reversed with intravenous fluid resuscitation. The propofol doses needed to reach a 50% decrease from baseline BIS, and no movement after noxious stimuli, are reduced by hemorrhagic shock by 54% and 38%, respectively. Hemorrhagic shock decreases the effect-site concentration that produced 50% of the maximal BIS effect from 11.6 ± 3.8 to 9.1 ± 1.7 μg/mL and that producing a 50% probability of movement from 26.8 ± 1.0 to 20.6 ± 1.0 μg/mL.[120]

SEDATION

Propofol has been evaluated for sedation during surgical procedures and for patients receiving mechanical ventilation in the ICU.[120a] As noted earlier, tolerance can occur with propofol. Increased propofol requirement occurs with repeated anesthetic administration in a limited time period in individual patients and an increased infusion requirement when propofol is infused for prolonged periods.[74] Infusion rates required for sedation to supplement regional anesthesia in healthy patients are half or less than the rates required for general anesthesia (i.e., 30-60 μg/kg/min). In elderly patients (>65 years old) and in sicker patients, the infusion rates that are necessary are markedly reduced up to 50% compared to 20-year-old patients. The infusion should be individually titrated to the desired effect. The pharmacokinetic profile of propofol makes it a suitable choice for long-term (days) sedation. This should always be weighed, though, against the hemodynamic side effects, tolerance, and rare occurrences of hypertriglyceridemia (and potential pancreatitis) or propofol infusion syndrome. Maintaining the smallest possible dose required for the desired level of sedation with potential "sedation holidays" should be considered as part of a long-term propofol sedation regimen. In addition, the FDA has specifically recommended against the use of propofol for the prolonged sedation of pediatric patients. The sedation guidelines of the American College of Critical Care Medicine also recommend "that patients receiving propofol for long-term sedation should be monitored for unexplained metabolic acidosis or arrhythmias. Drugs other than propofol should be considered for patients with escalating vasopressor or inotrope requirements or cardiac failure during large-dose propofol infusions." The recommended maximal dose of propofol infusion rate is 80 μg/kg/min (<5 mg/kg/h).[121] Generally, at propofol infusion rates more rapid than 30 μg/kg/min, patients are amnesic.

SIDE EFFECTS AND CONTRAINDICATIONS

In December 2016 the FDA issued a warning raising concerns about the potential risks to fetal brain development with general anesthetics, including propofol. Animal studies show that prolonged or repetitive propofol exposure to the developing fetal brain may be related to propofol neurotoxicity. Minimizing fetal exposure to propofol and other general anesthetics is therefore important and advisable.[121a,121b]

Next to its hypnotic effects, accumulating evidence suggests that propofol may affect cancer development through direct and indirect manners. Propofol exerts antitumor potential partly due to regulation of the expression and transfer of miRNAs. In addition, propofol impacts the degree of immunosuppression by modulating immune cells and cytokines. This results in reduced cancer cell mobility in some cancers and increased apoptosis of cancer cells in others. The clinical impact of the cancer-modulating effects of propofol needs further investigation.[121c] Induction of anesthesia with propofol is often associated with pain on injection, myoclonus, apnea, hypotension, and, rarely, thrombophlebitis of the vein into which propofol is injected.[122] Pain on injection is reduced by using a large vein, avoiding veins in the dorsum of the hand, and adding lidocaine to the propofol solution or changing the propofol formulation. Multiple other drugs and distraction techniques have been investigated to reduce the pain on injection of propofol. Pretreatment with a small dose of propofol, opiates, nonsteroidal anti-inflammatory drugs, ketamine, esmolol/metoprolol, magnesium, a flash of light, clonidine/ephedrine combination, dexamethasone, and metoclopramide all have been tested with variable efficacy.

Propofol infusion syndrome is a rare but lethal syndrome associated with infusion of propofol at 4 mg/kg/h or more for 48 hours or longer.[123] Yet, cases have been reported with smaller dosage schemes given for only 3 hours.[124] It was first described in children, but subsequently has been observed in critically ill adults.[125,126] The clinical features of propofol infusion syndrome are acute refractory bradycardia leading to asystole, in the presence of one or more of the following: metabolic acidosis (base deficit >10 mmol/L^{-1}), rhabdomyolysis, hyperlipidemia, and enlarged or fatty liver. Other features include cardiomyopathy with acute cardiac failure, skeletal myopathy, hyperkalemia, hepatomegaly, and lipemia. The symptoms and signs are the result of muscle injury and of the release of intracellular toxic contents. The major risk factors for its development are poor oxygen delivery, sepsis, serious cerebral injury, and large propofol dosage. Predisposing factors for the propofol infusion syndrome are likely genetic disorders impairing fatty acid metabolism, such as medium-chain acyl CoA (MCAD) deficiency and low carbohydrate supply. Because lipemia has been noted, a failure of hepatic lipid regulation, possibly related to poor oxygenation or a lack of glucose, may be the cause. In some cases, an increasing lipemia was the first indication of impending propofol infusion syndrome onset, so lipemia is a sign.

Barbiturates

HISTORY

Barbiturates were discovered in the early twentieth century. The first barbiturate to cause loss of consciousness within one arm-brain circulation time was hexobarbital. After the clinical introduction of thiopental by Waters and Lundy in 1934, thiopental became preferred clinically because of its rapid onset of action and short duration, without the excitatory effects of hexobarbital.[127] Although criticized after many casualties during the attack on Pearl Harbor as "the cause of more fatal casualties among the servicemen at Pearl Harbor than were the enemy bombs," the barbiturates continued to be widely used in clinical practice.[128] Many other barbiturate derivatives have been synthesized throughout the past decades, yet none have enjoyed the clinical success and popularity of thiopental.

Physicochemical Characteristics

CHEMISTRY AND FORMULATION

Barbiturates are hypnotically active drugs that are derivatives of barbituric acid (2,4,6-trioxohexahydropyrimidine), a hypnotically inactive pyrimidine nucleus that is formed by the condensation of malonic acid and urea (Fig. 23.5). The two major classes of barbiturates are the oxybarbiturates and thiobarbiturates with either an oxygen at position 2 or with a sulfur in position 2, respectively. Through keto-enol tautomerization, the oxygen or sulfur in position 2 becomes a reactive species in the enol form. This allows for the formation of water-soluble barbiturate salts in alkaline solutions and permits the IV use of barbiturates. Although tautomerization to the enol form allows for the creation of salts, the substitution of the hydrogen attached to the carbon atom in position 5 with aryl or alkyl groups gives the barbiturates their hypnotic activity. Only thiopental and thiamylal, thiobarbiturates, and methohexital, an oxybarbiturate, have been used for induction of anesthesia (Fig. 23.6). The formulation of barbiturates involves preparation as sodium

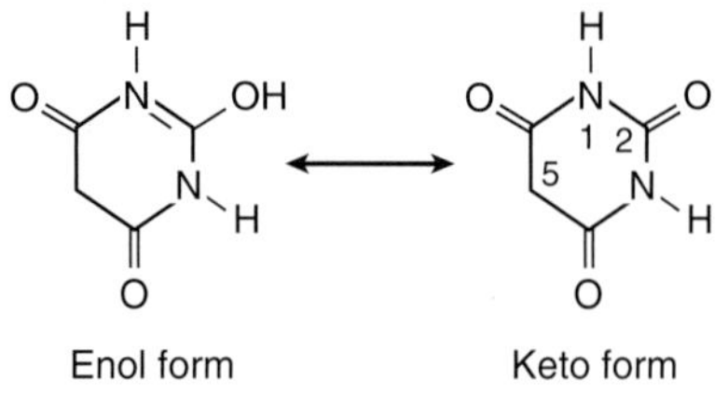

Enol form ⟷ Keto form

Fig. 23.5 The keto and enol tautomeric forms of barbituric acid with the sites of substitution in the hypnotically active barbiturates identified as 1, 2, and 5.

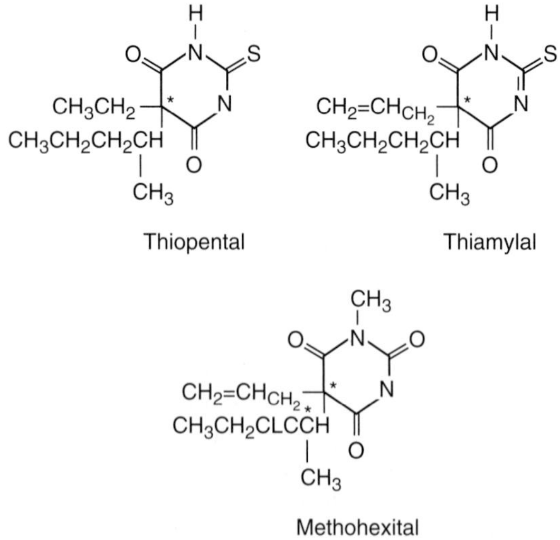

Thiopental

Thiamylal

Methohexital

Fig. 23.6 Hypnotically active barbiturates commonly used for induction, with their asymmetric centers indicated by an asterisk.

salts (mixed with 6% by weight anhydrous sodium carbonate) and then reconstitution with either water, glucose 5%, or normal saline to produce a 2.5% solution of thiopental, a 2% solution of thiamylal, or a 1% solution of methohexital. The thiobarbiturates are stable for 1 week if refrigerated after reconstitution, and methohexital remains available for use for 6 weeks after reconstitution. Barbiturates cannot be reconstituted with lactated Ringer solution or mixed with other acidic solutions, as a decrease in the alkalinity of the solution can result in precipitation of the barbiturates as free acids. Examples of drugs that are not to be coadministered or mixed in solution with the barbiturates are atracurium, vecuronium, rocuronium, suxamethonium, alfentanil, sufentanil, dobutamine, dopamine, esketamine, and midazolam. Mixing of thiopental with vecuronium or pancuronium results in the formation of precipitate that may occlude the IV line during a rapid sequence induction of anesthesia.[129]

Structure-Activity Relationships

As noted earlier, substitutions at the 5, 2, and 1 positions confer different pharmacologic activities to the barbiturate nucleus. Substitutions at position 5 with either aryl or alkyl groups produce hypnotic and sedative effects, whereas substitution at C5 with a phenyl group produces anticonvulsant activity. An increase in length of one or both side chains of an alkyl group at C5 increases hypnotic potency. Barbiturates used in clinical practice have either an oxygen or sulfur at C2. Substitution of a sulfur at position 2 produces a more rapid onset of action, as with thiopental. The addition of a methyl or ethyl group at position 1 also may produce a more rapid onset of action, as with methohexital. However, excitatory side effects, including tremor, hypertonus, and involuntary movement, may occur upon administration.

Pharmacokinetics

METABOLISM

The barbiturates (with the exception of phenobarbital) are metabolized hepatically. The metabolites are almost all inactive, water-soluble, and excreted in the urine. Barbiturates are biotransformed by four processes: (1) oxidation of the aryl, alkyl, or phenyl moiety at C5; (2) *N*-dealkylation; (3) desulfuration of the thiobarbiturates at C2; and (4) destruction of the barbituric acid ring.[130] Oxidation is the most important pathway, producing polar (charged) alcohols, ketones, phenols, or carboxylic acids. These metabolites are readily excreted in the urine or as glucuronic acid conjugates in the bile. Hydrolytic cleavage of the barbituratic acid ring forms a minimal contribution to the total metabolism of barbiturates, since the ring is stable in vivo. Drugs that induce oxidative microsomes or long-term administration enhance the metabolism of barbiturates. The hepatic enzyme induction by barbiturates is the reason that they are not recommended for administration to patients with acute intermittent porphyria. Barbiturates may precipitate an attack by stimulating γ-aminolevulinic acid synthetase, the enzyme responsible for the production of porphyrins.[131]

As mentioned earlier, hepatic metabolism accounts for the elimination of all of the barbiturates with the exception of phenobarbital. Renal excretion accounts for 60% to 90% of phenobarbital excretion in an unchanged form. The alkalinization of urine with bicarbonate enhances the renal excretion of phenobarbital. Other barbiturates are excreted unchanged by the kidney only in trivial amounts.

Methohexital is metabolized in the liver by oxidation to an alcohol and *N*-dealkylation. Methohexital exhibits similar distribution half-lives, volumes of distribution, and protein bindings as thiopental. A marked difference exists, however, in plasma disappearance and elimination half-lives (4 hours for methohexital and 12 hours for thiopental). This difference is due to the threefold more rapid rate of hepatic clearance of methohexital (mean 7.8-12.5 mL/kg/min).[132] The hepatic extraction ratio of methohexital (clearance to hepatic blood flow) is approximately 0.5, indicating that the liver extracts 50% of the drug presented to it. This ratio differs from the smaller hepatic extraction ratio of thiopental (0.15).

Barbiturate pharmacokinetics have been described in physiologic and compartmental models.[133] Both of these pharmacokinetic models describe rapid redistribution as the primary mechanism that terminates the action of a single induction dose. Physiologic models of barbiturates describe a rapid mixing of the drug within the central blood volume followed by a quick distribution of the drug to highly perfused, low-volume tissues (i.e., brain) with a slower redistribution of the drug to lean tissue (muscle), which terminates the effect of the initial (induction of anesthesia) dose. In these models, adipose tissue uptake and metabolic clearance (elimination) play only a minor role in the termination of the effects of the induction dose. This is a result of the minimal perfusion ratio of adipose tissue compared with other tissues and the slow rate of removal. Compartmental model values for thiopental and methohexital, the most commonly used barbiturates for induction of anesthesia, are given in Table 23.1. The compartmental model explains the delay of recovery when a continuous infusion of a barbiturate is used. This model describes how the termination of effect becomes increasingly dependent on the slower process of uptake into and redistribution from adipose tissue and elimination clearance through hepatic metabolism. After prolonged infusions, the pharmacokinetics of barbiturate metabolism is best approximated by nonlinear Michaelis-Menten metabolism. In usual doses (4-5 mg/kg), thiopental exhibits first-order kinetics (i.e., a constant *fraction* of drug is cleared from the body per unit time); however, at very high doses of thiopental (300-600 mg/kg) with receptor saturation, zero-order kinetics occur (i.e., a constant *amount* of drug is cleared per unit time). The volume of distribution is slightly larger in female patients, causing a longer elimination half-life.[134] Pregnancy also increases the volume of distribution of thiopental, prolonging the elimination half-life.[135] Even at advanced stages of liver cirrhosis, the clearance of thiopental is not altered. Because of its lipophilicity, relatively large volume of distribution, and low rate of hepatic clearance, thiopental can accumulate in tissues, especially if given in large doses over a prolonged period. The plasma drug level increases when repeated doses of drug are given. Although not used in routine clinical practice, appropriately designed infusion schemes ensure constant blood levels, maintaining the desired hypnotic effect.

Pharmacology

MECHANISM OF ACTION

The mechanisms of action of barbiturates on the CNS are largely unknown, with the exception of their action on the $GABA_A$ receptor.[136,137] Perhaps the NMDA receptors are involved with the effects of barbiturates.[138-140] The effects of barbiturates on the CNS have been grouped into two categories: (1) enhancement of the synaptic actions of *inhibitory* neurotransmitters, and (2) blockade of the synaptic actions of *excitatory* neurotransmitters.[141] GABA is the principal inhibitory neurotransmitter in the mammalian CNS, and the $GABA_A$ receptor is the only site proven to be involved in barbiturate-induced anesthesia.[137] The $GABA_A$ receptor is a chloride ion channel, composed of five subunits, with specific sites of action for GABA, barbiturates, benzodiazepines, and other molecules. The binding sites are at the interface of the specific subunits, where the combination of the adjacent subunits determine the affinity and selectivity for drugs like propofol, etomidate, or pentobarbital. Of each subunit multiple types exist, leading to various compositions of the $GABA_A$ receptor. Progressive insights in the composition of these binding sites may be useful in developing novel clinical anesthetics.[141a] Barbiturate binding to the $GABA_A$ receptor enhances and mimics the action of GABA by increasing chloride conductance through the ion channel. This causes hyperpolarization of the cell membrane and increases the threshold of excitability of the postsynaptic neuron. At low concentrations barbiturates enhance the effects of GABA, decreasing the rate of dissociation of GABA from its receptor and increasing the duration of GABA-activated chloride ion channel openings. This enhancement of the action of GABA is likely responsible for the sedative-hypnotic effects of the barbiturates. At larger concentrations, the barbiturates activate the chloride channels directly, without the binding of GABA, acting as the agonist itself. The GABA-mimetic effect at slightly higher concentrations may be responsible for what is termed barbiturate anesthesia.[137]

The second mechanism of action of barbiturates involves the inhibition of the synaptic transmission of excitatory neurotransmitters, such as glutamate and acetylcholine. The actions of the barbiturates to block excitatory CNS transmission are specific for synaptic ion channels. Thiopental, however, may exert GABA-independent effects on the glutaminergic-NMDA system. In two studies on effects in the rat prefrontal cortex, thiopental decreased extracellular glutamate levels in the CNS and decreased NMDA-gated currents in a concentration-dependent manner.[139,140]

Effects on Cerebral Metabolism (Also see Chapter 57)

Barbiturates, like other CNS depressants, have potent effects on cerebral metabolism. A dose-related depression of cerebral metabolic oxygen consumption rate ($CMRO_2$) progressively slows the EEG, reduces the rate of adenosine triphosphate consumption, and enhances protection from partial cerebral ischemia. The relationship between depressed metabolism and drug requirement was shown when thiopental was not eliminated (i.e., sustained with an extracorporeal circulation pump).[142] When the EEG became isoelectric, a point at which cerebral metabolic activity is roughly 50% of baseline,[143] no further decreases in $CMRO_2$ occurred. These findings support the hypothesis that metabolism and function of the brain are coupled. Barbiturates reduce the metabolic activity concerned with neuronal signaling and impulse traffic, not the metabolic activity corresponding to basal metabolic function. The only way to suppress baseline metabolic activity concerned with cellular activity is via hypothermia.[143] The effect of barbiturates on cerebral metabolism is maximized at a 50% depression of cerebral function, leaving all metabolic energy for the maintenance of cellular integrity. With the reduction in $CMRO_2$, there is a parallel reduction in cerebral perfusion, which is seen in decreased cerebral blood flow (CBF) and ICP. With reduced $CMRO_2$, cerebral vascular resistance increases, and CBF decreases.[144] The ratio of CBF to $CMRO_2$ remains unchanged. Even though the mean arterial pressure (MAP) decreases, barbiturates do not compromise the overall CPP because the CPP equals MAP minus ICP. In this relationship, ICP decreases more than MAP after barbiturate administration, preserving CPP.

Pharmacodynamics

Sufficient doses of barbiturates cause loss of consciousness, amnesia, and respiratory and cardiovascular depression, known as general anesthesia. The response to pain and other noxious stimulation during general anesthesia seems to be depressed. Pain studies reveal that barbiturates may decrease the pain threshold. This antianalgesic effect occurs only with low blood levels of barbiturates, which might be achieved with small doses of thiopental for induction of anesthesia or after emergence from thiopental. The amnesic effect of barbiturates is less pronounced than that produced by benzodiazepines.

Effects on the Central Nervous System

Drugs with high lipid solubility and a low degree of ionization cross the blood-brain barrier rapidly, producing a fast onset of action.[137] Most barbiturates exist in a nonionized form. Thiopental and methohexital are more lipid soluble than pentobarbital, which is clinically reflected by the more rapid onset of action of thiopental and methohexital compared to pentobarbital.[145] Only the nonionized form of a drug can directly traverse the cellular membranes. Thiopental has a pK_a of 7.6. Approximately 50% of thiopental is nonionized at physiologic pH, which accounts partly for the rapid accumulation of thiopental in the cerebrospinal fluid (CSF) after IV administration.[146] Methohexital is 75% nonionized at pH 7.4, which may explain the slightly more rapid effect of methohexital compared to thiopental. As pH decreases, with poor perfusion, barbiturates have a larger fraction of nonionized drug available to cross the blood-brain barrier.[146]

The onset of action in the CNS is affected by protein binding, because only unbound drug (free drug) can cross the blood-brain barrier.[147] Barbiturates are highly bound to albumin and other plasma proteins, where the thiobarbiturates are more highly protein bound than are the oxybarbiturates. The degree of protein binding of a drug is influenced by the physiologic pH and disease states, which alter the absolute amount of protein. Most barbiturates tend to experience peak protein binding at or around pH 7.5. The final factor governing the rapidity of drug penetration of the blood-brain barrier is the plasma drug concentration, causing a concentration gradient. The two primary determinants of the plasma concentration are the *dose* administered and the *rate* (speed) of administration. As the dose of thiopental over the same time is increased, an increased percentage of patients will be anesthetized.[148] Concerning absolute dose, 2 mg/kg produced anesthesia in 20% of patients, whereas a dose of 2.4 mg/kg produced anesthesia in 80% of patients. Similarly, the speed of injection influences the effect of thiopental. A smaller amount of drug is required to produce anesthesia when the dose rate of the administration is over 5 seconds as opposed to over 15 seconds.

Because of the equilibrium between brain concentration and plasma concentration, factors that determine the rate of onset of barbiturate effects also affect their termination. Lipid solubility, degree of ionization, and CSF drug concentration affect the movement of drug from the CSF to plasma. As plasma levels decrease, drug levels in the brain and CSF decrease. The most important factors in the termination of drug effect are those that govern plasma disappearance of the drug. These are generally divided into a rapid redistribution phase and a slow metabolic and second redistribution phase. In a classic pharmacologic study, Brodie and coworkers[149] showed that awakening from thiopental occurred because the plasma concentration rapidly declined. They further showed that the cause of the rapid plasma decay of thiopental was not metabolism of the drug but was rather due to a redistribution of the drug to other tissues throughout the body. The relationship of the plasma drug level and drug redistribution to the onset and termination of effect is illustrated in Fig. 23.7. Clinically, patients awake from a single dose of thiopental 5 to 10 minutes after administration, as the drug is redistributed from highly perfused CNS tissues to well-perfused lean tissues. The termination of effect after multiple drug administrations or constant infusion depends on the elimination of the drug from the blood, which becomes increasingly more dependent on first-order metabolism than redistribution and is a function of its context-sensitive decrement time (see Fig. 23.3). Awakening may be delayed in older patients because of increased CNS sensitivity, alterations in metabolism, or decreased central volume of distribution relative to younger adults.[150] The initial volume of distribution is less in elderly patients than in young patients, which explains a smaller dose requirement for the onset effect. Pediatric patients (<13 years old) seem to have a more rapid rate of total clearance and a shorter rate of plasma thiopental clearance than do adults, which theoretically might result in earlier awakening, especially after multiple doses of the drug.[151] There is little difference in distribution of thiopental and methohexital, which may explain the similar wakeup times. There is, however, a difference in the rate of total body clearance, being more rapid for methohexital. This disparity explains the difference found in the psychomotor skills of patients and the earlier full recovery after methohexital. Despite some residual effects, methohexital is cleared more rapidly than thiopental, which explains why methohexital is preferred for use by some clinicians when rapid awakening is desirable, such as in outpatient anesthesia. Prolongation of early and late recovery by the barbiturates is the primary reason behind the fact that they have been largely replaced by propofol.

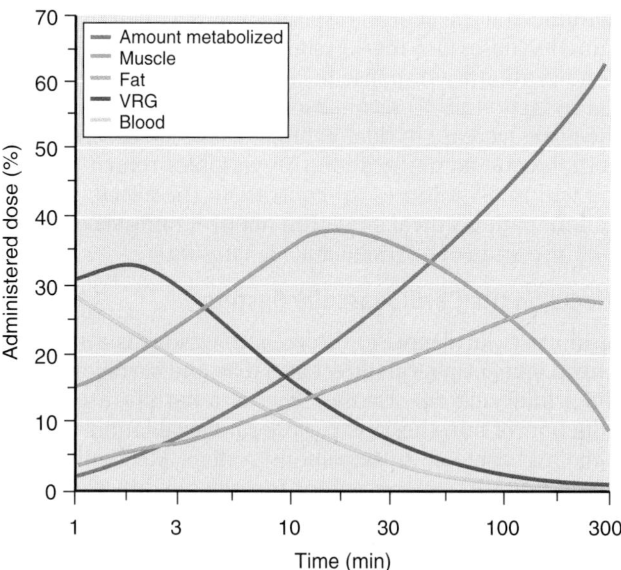

Fig. 23.7 After delivery of an IV bolus, the percentage of thiopental remaining in blood rapidly decreases as drug moves from blood to body tissues. The time to attainment of peak tissue levels is a direct function of tissue capacity for barbiturate relative to blood flow. A larger capacity or smaller blood flow is related to a longer time to a peak tissue level. Initially, most thiopental is taken up by the vessel-rich group *(VRG)* of tissues because of their high blood flow. Subsequently, drug is redistributed to muscle and to a lesser extent to fat. Throughout this period, small but substantial amounts of thiopental are removed and metabolized by the liver. In contrast to removal by tissues, this removal is cumulative. The rate of metabolism equals the early rate of removal by fat. The sum of this early removal by fat and metabolism is the same as the removal by muscle. (Redrawn from Saidman LJ. Uptake, distribution and elimination of barbiturates. In: Eger EI [ed]. *Anesthetic Uptake and Action*. Baltimore: Williams & Wilkins; 1974.)

Effects on the Respiratory System

Barbiturates produce dose-related central respiratory depression. The evidence for central depression is a correlation between EEG suppression and diminished minute ventilation. Peak respiratory depression (as measured by the slope of carbon dioxide concentration in the blood) and maximum depression of minute ventilation after delivery of thiopental (3.5 mg/kg) occurs 1 to 1.5 minutes after administration. These variables return to predrug levels rapidly, and within 15 minutes the drug effects are barely detectable.[152] Patients with chronic lung disease are slightly more susceptible to the respiratory depression of thiopental. The ventilatory pattern with thiopental induction has been described as "double apnea," that is an initial apnea of a few seconds occurring upon drug administration, succeeded by a few breaths of reasonably adequate tidal volume, which is followed by a more prolonged period of apnea, typically of approximately 25 seconds. This apnea occurs in at least 20% of cases. During the induction of anesthesia with thiopental, ventilation must be assisted or controlled to provide adequate respiratory exchange. Like thiopental, methohexital is a central respiratory system depressant.[152] Induction doses (1.5 mg/kg) significantly decrease the slope of the ventilatory response to carbon dioxide, with a maximal reduction at 30 seconds after drug administration.[153] The peak decrease in tidal volume occurs 60 seconds after methohexital administration. All variables return to baseline within 15 minutes. In contrast to the effects on ventilation, patients awaken within about 5 minutes after the administration of methohexital (1.5 mg/kg).

Effects on the Cardiovascular System

Cardiovascular depression from barbiturates is a result of central and peripheral (direct vascular and cardiac) effects. The primary cardiovascular effect of a barbiturate during induction of anesthesia is peripheral vasodilation causing a pooling of blood in the venous system. Mechanisms for the decrease in cardiac output include (1) direct negative inotropic action, due to a decrease of calcium influx into the cells, (2) decreased ventricular filling, due to increased capacitance, and (3) transiently decreased sympathetic outflow from the CNS.[154] The increase in heart rate (10% to 36%) that accompanies thiopental administration probably results from the baroreceptor-mediated sympathetic reflex stimulation of the heart in response to the decrease in output and pressure. The cardiac index, as well as the MAP, is unchanged or reduced. Hemodynamic changes are dependent on the infusion rate of thiopental. In the dose ranges hitherto studied, no relationship between plasma thiopental level and hemodynamic effect has been found. There is little difference in the responses after thiopental and methohexital administration in patients with heart disease. The increase in heart rate (11%-36%) encountered in patients with coronary artery disease anesthetized with thiopental (1-4 mg/kg) is potentially deleterious because of the obligatory increase in myocardial oxygen consumption that accompanies the increased heart rate. In a study in dogs, thiopental prolonged the QT interval, flattened T waves, and increased QT dispersion during and after induction.[150] Thiopental may not be the most appropriate choice for patients with a susceptibility to ventricular dysrhythmias or a prolonged QT interval, such as acidotic patients or conditions that prolong the QT interval, such as long-term dialysis or advanced cirrhosis. Patients who have normal coronary arteries have no difficulty in maintaining adequate coronary blood flow to meet the increased myocardial oxygen consumption.[155] Thiopental should be avoided in hypovolemic patients because there is a significant reduction in cardiac output (69%) and a significant decrease in arterial blood pressure.[156] Patients without adequate compensatory mechanisms may have serious hemodynamic depression with a thiopental induction of anesthesia.

Other Effects

The side effects of injecting barbiturates include a garlic or onion taste (40% of patients), allergic reactions, local tissue irritation, and rarely, tissue necrosis. A transient urticarial rash may develop on the head, neck, and trunk. More severe reactions such as facial edema, hives, bronchospasm, and anaphylaxis can occur. Treatment of anaphylaxis is symptomatic. Thiopental and thiamylal produce fewer excitatory symptoms with induction than methohexital, which produces cough, hiccups, tremors, and twitching approximately five times more often. Tissue irritation and local complications may occur more frequently with the use of thiopental and thiamylal than with methohexital.

The consequences of accidental arterial injection may be severe. The degree of injury is related to the concentration of the drug. Treatment consists of (1) dilution of the drug by the administration of saline into the artery, (2) heparinization to prevent thrombosis, and (3) brachial plexus block. Overall, the proper administration of thiopental intravenously is remarkably free of local toxicity.

Phenobarbital is used experimentally as an inducer of the cytochrome P450 (CYP) system in rodents, in particular of the CYP2B enzymes. In human hepatocyte culture, phenobarbital acts as an inducer of the CYP2B6, CYP2C9, CYP2C19, and CYP3A4 enzymes. This phenomenon may cause changes in the metabolism of drugs that are administered concomitantly.[157] On the other hand, the metabolism of thiopental can be influenced by concomitant drugs like selective serotonin reuptake inhibitors (SSRIs). These drugs are used frequently by patients who are treated by electroconvulsive therapy, in whom an induction with thiopental or thiamylal is performed.[158]

Uses

INDUCTION AND MAINTANANCE OF ANESTHESIA

Barbiturates are used clinically for induction and maintenance of anesthesia and premedication. Methohexital is the drug of choice for providing anesthesia during electroconvulsive therapy.[159] Other barbiturates used in this field are thiopental and thiamylal. Less frequently, barbiturates are used to provide cerebral protection in patients at risk of developing incomplete ischemia. The three barbiturates that are used most commonly for IV anesthesia induction and maintenance are thiopental, thiamylal, and methohexital. Thiopental is an excellent drug to use for induction of anesthesia. The prompt onset (15-30 seconds) of action and smooth induction are advantages for this drug. The rapid emergence, particularly after single use for induction, also was a reason for the widespread use of thiopental in this setting. Thiopental can be used to maintain general anesthesia because repeated doses reliably sustain unconsciousness and contribute to amnesia but should not be the drug of first choice as the hypnotic component in balanced anesthesia. A review of the role of anesthetics on the risk of awareness during surgery show that benzodiazepines reduce awareness compared to thiopental, ketamine, and placebo. Wakefulness is reduced by ketamine and etomidate, compared with thiopental. The evidence is not strong due to the risk of bias, the very small event rate, and the heterogeneity in definition of awareness.[160]

Methohexital is the only IV barbiturate used for induction of anesthesia that can compete with thiopental. With a dose of 1 to 2 mg/kg, induction and emergence from anesthesia is rapid. Methohexital also may be used as a hypnotic component to maintain anesthesia. Similar to thiopental, it is not an analgesic. Additional opioids or volatile anesthetics are required to provide a balanced technique satisfactory for general anesthesia during surgery. Because methohexital is

TABLE 23.4 Recommended Doses of Barbiturates for Anesthesia Induction and Maintenance

Drug	Induction Dose (mg/kg)*,†	Onset (s)	Intravenous Maintenance Infusion
Thiopental	3-4	10-30	50-100 mg every 10-12 min
Methohexital	1-1.5	10-30	20-40 mg every 4-7 min

*Adult and pediatric intravenous doses are roughly the same in milligrams per kilogram.
†Methohexital can be given rectally in pediatric patients as a 20 to 25 mg/kg/dose.
From Reves JG, Glass P, Lubarsky DA, et al. Intravenous anesthetics. In: Miller RD, Eriksson LI, Fleischer LA, et al, eds. *Miller's Anesthesia,* 7th ed. Philadelphia: Churchill Livingstone; 2010: 719–768.

cleared more rapidly than thiopental, it may be preferred to thiopental for the maintenance of anesthesia, as accumulation and saturation of peripheral sites takes longer. For brief infusion (<60 minutes), recovery from a methohexital infusion titrated to maintain hypnosis (50-150 μg/kg/min) is similar to that provided by propofol. There are probably upper limits of safe infusion doses yet to be defined, but seizures have occurred in neurosurgical patients after large doses of methohexital (24 mg/kg).[154] Methohexital may be given rectally and is absorbed rapidly, and can be used as a premedication drug in pediatric patients. The dose recommended for this use is 25 mg/kg rectal instillation (10% solution through a 14F catheter, 7 cm into rectum).[161] With this method of administration, sleep onset is rapid: mean peak plasma levels occur within 14 minutes.

Dosing

Dosing for the two most commonly used barbiturates is listed in Table 23.4. The usual doses of thiopental (3-4 mg/kg) and thiamylal (3-4 mg/kg) are about twice the dose of methohexital (1-2 mg/kg). In dose-response studies, the ED_{50} for thiopental ranged from 2.2 to 2.7 mg/kg, and the ED_{50} for methohexital was 1.1 mg/kg.[147] There is less interpatient variability in the dose response to barbiturates than to benzodiazepines when used for anesthesia induction, but there still is significant variability in the dose of thiopental required to induce anesthesia.[148] Interpatient dose variability is related to the presence of hemorrhagic shock, cardiac output, lean body mass, obesity, gender, and age. Hemorrhagic shock, lean body mass, age, and obesity explain variability of patient response owing to a decrease in the central volume of distribution. Finally, patients who have severe anemia, burns, malnutrition, widespread malignant disease, uremia, ulcerative colitis, or intestinal obstruction also require smaller induction doses of barbiturates.

Contraindications

The following conditions should be considered a contraindication for the use of IV barbiturates: (1) when there is respiratory obstruction or an inadequate airway, thiopental may worsen respiratory depression; (2) severe cardiovascular instability or shock contraindicate its use; (3) status asthmaticus is a condition in which airway control and ventilation may be worsened further by thiopental; (4) porphyria may be precipitated or acute attacks may be accentuated by the administration of thiopental; and (5) without proper induction equipment (IV instrumentation) and airway equipment (means of artificial ventilation), thiopental should not be administered.

Benzodiazepines

INTRODUCTION

The benzodiazepines have become a category of drugs widely used in anesthesia as anxiolytics, sedatives, and hypnotics. They exert their action through $GABA_A$ receptors, which are the key targets that mediate most of the clinically important effects of IV anesthetics.[162] In the clinical practice of daily anesthesia, midazolam is often used immediately before induction of anesthesia. The other agonists, diazepam, lorazepam, temazepam, and the antagonist flumazenil are sometimes used. Remimazolam, an ultrashort-acting $GABA_A$ receptor agonist, may be a useful new benzodiazepine in future anesthetic practice. Benzodiazepines are widely prescribed, and addiction to these drugs is a worldwide concern. Research is ongoing to elucidate the neural mechanism of the reward-related effects of benzodiazepines. Reynolds and associates conclude in their findings that α_2- and α_3-subunit–containing $GABA_A$ receptors are implicated as key mediators of the reward-related effects of benzodiazepines. This finding has important implications for the development of new drugs with less addictive properties.[163]

Surgical treatment of tumors is often the first line for several types of cancer. Several factors influence the metastatic spread of residual cancer cells. Midazolam is widely used during general anesthesia. Research in vitro and in vivo conclude that midazolam in contrast to dexmedetomidine has antitumorigenic properties in certain types of cancer in supraclinical dosage.[163a]

Benzodiazepines were discovered in 1954 by Sternbach and in 1959 chlordiazepoxide (Librium) was the first benzodiazepine patented. Diazepam was synthesized in 1963 in a search for a better compound and was used intravenously to induce anesthesia in 1965.[164] Oxazepam (Seresta), a metabolite of diazepam, was synthesized in 1961 by Bell. Lorazepam (Ativan), a 2′chloro-substitution product of oxazepam, was synthesized in 1971 in an attempt to produce a more potent benzodiazepine. The next major achievement was Fryer and Walser's synthesis in 1976 of midazolam (Versed, Dormicum), the first clinically used water-soluble benzodiazepine, produced primarily for use in anesthesia.[165] An ultrashort-acting benzodiazepine, remimazolam, is in its phase III trial and is promising.[166]

Physicochemical Characteristics

Four benzodiazepine receptor agonists are commonly used in anesthesia: midazolam, diazepam, lorazepam, and temazepam (Fig. 23.8). The physicochemical characteristics of the benzodiazepines used in anesthesia are listed in Table 23.5. These six molecules are relatively small and are lipid soluble at physiologic pH.

Of the clinically used benzodiazepines, midazolam is the most lipid soluble in vivo,[167] but because of its pH-dependent solubility, it is water soluble when formulated in a buffered acidic medium (pH 3.5). The imidazole ring of midazolam accounts for its stability in solution and its lipophilicity due

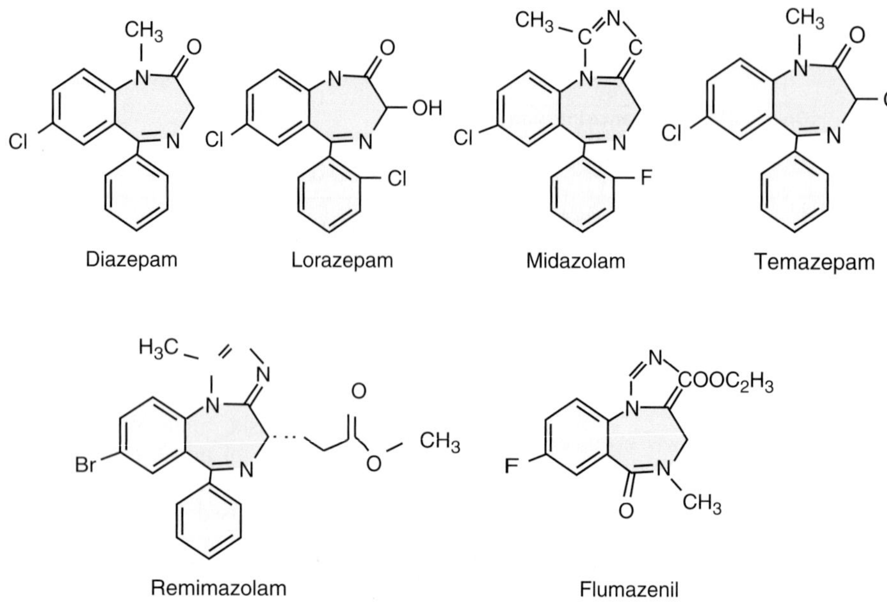

Fig. 23.8 **The structures of six benzodiazepines.**

TABLE 23.5 Physicochemical Characteristics of Benzodiazepines

	Molecular Weight	pK_a	Water Solubility	Lipid Solubility
	Da		g/L	Log P
Diazepam	284.7	3.4	0.051	2.801
Lorazepam	321.2	1.3	0.12	2.382
Temazepam	300.7	1.6, 11.7	0.28	2.188
Midazolam	325.8 (hydrochloride 362.2)	6.0	0.004 (2.0, pH 1)	3.798
Remimazolam	439.3 (besylate 597.5)	5.3	0.008 (7.5, pH 1)	3.724
Flumazenil	303.3	0.86	0.042	2.151

Water solubility values are in unbuffered water, maximal solubility at acidic pH in parenthesis. Data from http://scifinder.cas.org. pKa, dissociation constant. From Saari TI, Uusi-Oukari M, Ahonen J, Olkkola KT. Enhancement of GABAergic activity: neuropharmacological effects of benzodiazepines and therapeutic use in anesthesiology. *Pharmacol Rev*. 2011;63(1):243–267.

to rapid closing of the imidazole ring at physiological pH. The high lipophilicity of the compounds accounts for the rapid CNS effect and relatively large volumes of distribution.

Pharmacokinetics

The four benzodiazepines used in anesthesia are classified as short-acting (midazolam), intermediate-acting (lorazepam, temazepam), and long-acting (diazepam), according to their metabolism and plasma clearance (Table 23.6). The plasma disappearance curves of all benzodiazepines can be best described by a two- or three-compartment model.

Protein binding and volumes of distribution are not much different among these four benzodiazepines, but the clearance is significantly different. Factors that may influence the pharmacokinetics of benzodiazepines are age, gender, race, enzyme induction, and hepatic and renal disease. In addition, the pharmacokinetics of the benzodiazepines are affected by obesity. The volume of distribution is increased as drug diffuses from the plasma into the adipose tissue. Although clearance is not altered, elimination half-lives are prolonged, owing to the increased volume of distribution and delayed return of the drug to the plasma in obese patients.[168] Generally, sensitivity to benzodiazepines in some patient groups, such as elderly patients, is greater despite relatively modest pharmacokinetic changes; factors other than pharmacokinetics must be considered when these drugs are used.

Midazolam: After oral ingestion midazolam is absorbed completely and the peak plasma concentration is achieved in 30 to 80 minutes.[169] The bioavailability is less than 50% due to a significant first-pass metabolism in the intestinal wall and the liver.[169,170] After IV administration, midazolam is rapidly distributed, with a distribution half-life of 6 to 15 minutes.[170] The plasma protein binding is high: 94% to 98%.

The hepatic extraction ratio is low, ranging from 0.30 to 0.44, but is higher than the unbound free fraction of midazolam in plasma.[169] Thus, the protein binding is not a restrictive factor in drug extraction by the liver. With this intermediate hepatic extraction ratio, the metabolic clearance of midazolam may be susceptible both to changes in enzyme activity and to changes in hepatic blood flow.

The elimination half-life ranges from 1.7 to 3.5 hours.[170,171] The plasma clearance ranges from 5.8 to 9.0 mL/kg/min and is higher compared to that of the other benzodiazepines. This is due to the fused imidazole ring, which is rapidly oxidized in vivo—much more rapidly than the methylene group of the diazepine ring of other benzodiazepines.[172]

The pharmacokinetics of midazolam are affected by obesity, age, hepatic cirrhosis, and severity of critical illness. Because of its high lipophilicity (at physiological pH), midazolam distributes preferably to adipose tissue resulting in

TABLE 23.6 Pharmacokinetic Parameters of the Benzodiazepines

	Elimination half-life (h)	Clearance (mL/kg/min)	Vd (L/kg)	Plasma Protein Binding (%)	Reference
Midazolam	1.7-3.5	5.8-9.0	1.1-1.7	94-98	Dundee et al. (1984)
Diazepam	20-50	0.2-0.5	0.7-1.7	98-99	Greenblatt et al. (1980)
Lorazepam	11-22	0.8-1.5	0.8-1.3	88-92	Greenblatt et al. (1979)
Temazepam	6-8	1.0-1.2	1.3-1.5	96-98	Fraschini and Stankov (1993)
Remimazolam*	0.4	4521 mL/min	36.4 L	N.A.	Upton et al. (2010)
Flumazenil	0.7-1.3	13-17	0.9-1.9	40-50	Klotz and Kanto (1998)

*Noncompartmental analysis results from sheep.
N.A. is not available.
From Saari TI, Uusi-Oukari M, Ahonen J, Olkkola KT. Enhancement of GABAergic activity: neuropharmacological effects of benzodiazepines and therapeutic use in anesthesiology. *Pharmacol Rev.* 2011;63(1):243–267.

a prolonged elimination half-life in obese patients.[168] Liver cirrhosis reduces plasma clearance of midazolam due to decreased metabolism.[173]

Midazolam is metabolized by CYP3A4 and CYP3A5[174] to 1-hydroxymethylmidazolam (= α-hydroxymidazolam) and 4-hydroxymidazolam.[175] These metabolites possess similar sedative activities compared to the parent compound and, when given over a longer time, these metabolites may accumulate. These metabolites are rapidly conjugated and excreted in the urine and have, like midazolam, a marked increase in peripheral volume of distribution in obese/overweight adolescents.[175a] In comparison, 1-hydroxymethylmidazolam is less potent than its parent compound, the affinity to the receptor is about 60%, and weaker than that of midazolam. The metabolites are cleared more rapidly than midazolam itself, making them of little concern in patients with normal hepatic and renal function. In patients with renal impairment, though, they can cause profound sedation.[176]

Diazepam: After oral ingestion the bioavailability is about 94%.[177] Time to peak plasma concentrations after oral ingestion is approximately 60 minutes.[178] Diazepam is extensively bound to plasma proteins; the volume of distribution ranges from 0.7 to 4.7 L/kg. The plasma clearance of diazepam ranges from 0.2 to 0.5 mL/kg/min.[179]

The pharmacokinetics of diazepam are affected by obesity and liver dysfunction and particularly by age. Increasing age reduces the clearance of diazepam significantly.[180]

Metabolism occurs in the liver and is mediated mainly by CYP2C19 and CYP3A4. This accounts for 80% of the biotransformation of diazepam.[181-183] The metabolite N-desmethyldiazepam has pharmacodynamic characteristics similar to those of diazepam, but has a much slower elimination half-life extending to 200 hours. N-desmethyldiazepam is further metabolized to oxazepam, which is also pharmacologically active.

Temazepam, another metabolite of diazepam, is mainly conjugated to temazepam glucuronide and a smaller part is demethylated to oxazepam and thereafter conjugated to oxazepam-glucuronide.[184]

Lorazepam: The oral bioavailability is high, nearly 90%. Peak plasma concentrations are reached approximately 2 hours after oral ingestion, the mean elimination half-life is 15 hours, with a range of 8 to 25 hours.[185] Lorazepam has a large volume of distribution from 0.8 to 1.3 L/kg,[186] and it is highly bound to plasma proteins (>90%).

The clearance of lorazepam is 0.8 to 1.8 mL/kg/min. Lorazepam is conjugated in the liver to an inactive glucuronide and up to 70% is excreted in urine. The pharmacokinetics of lorazepam is little altered by age, and not altered by gender or renal disease, but clearance is decreased by hepatic dysfunction.[187]

Remimazolam (CNS 7056)

Remimazolam, a new short-acting $GABA_A$ receptor agonist with high affinity to the GABA receptor, is rapidly degraded in plasma by nonspecific esterases to its carboxylic acid metabolite CNS 7054. The incorporation of a carboxylic ester moiety into the benzodiazepine core of remimazolam renders it susceptible to nonspecific tissue esterases.[188] Preclinical studies in sheep showed a more rapid onset of action, greater depth of sedation, and more rapid recovery than midazolam. In sheep, remimazolam showed no dose-dependent depth of sedation like propofol.[189] In humans, remimazolam is eliminated by first-order pharmacokinetics, with no clear relationship registered between body weight and elimination clearance. Accumulation after prolonged infusion is unlikely. The clearance of remimazolam was rapid (overall mean clearance 70.3 ± 13.9 L/hr) and the volume of distribution moderately large (steady-state volume of distribution is 34.8 ± 9.4 L). No clear relation exists between body weight and systemic clearance. Level and duration of sedation are dose-dependent in humans.[190] Remimazolam trials conclude a safe administration for procedural sedation; it allows a faster recovery of neuropsychiatric function compared to midazolam. Possible benefit compared to propofol is the safe administration by endoscopists instead of healthcare providers trained in anesthesia.

Pharmacodynamics

Benzodiazepines act selectively at the $GABA_A$ receptor, which mediates fast inhibitory synaptic transmission in the CNS. Benzodiazepines enhance the response to GABA by facilitating the opening of the GABA-activated chloride channels resulting in hyperpolarization. A series of compounds are candidates as endogenous ligand of the $GABA_A$ receptor, such as diazepam binding inhibitor and other substances. This is an area of ongoing research.[191]

Translocator protein (TSPO, 18 kDa), first described as a peripheral binding site for benzodiazepines, which are not associated with GABA receptors, are expressed throughout the body and brain. While their precise function and pharmacologic significance remain only partly known, the TSPO role has many proposed functions depending on the tissue, like cholesterol transport, regulatory role in the heart, and immunomodulation related to inflammatory activation.[192]

EFFECTS ON THE CENTRAL NERVOUS SYSTEM

All benzodiazepines have hypnotic, sedative, anxiolytic, amnesic, anticonvulsant, and centrally produced muscle-relaxing properties. They may differ to some extent in their potency and efficacy with regard to some of these pharmacodynamic actions (e.g., anticonvulsive action). The neurotransmitter GABA is an inhibitory neurotransmitter and controls the state of a chloride ion channel. Activation of this chloride ion channel results in neuronal hyperpolarization (increased membrane potential in the direction away from the threshold potential) and accounts for the classification of the GABA system as "inhibitory." Benzodiazepines bind to their receptors with high affinity; the binding is stereospecific and saturable; the order of receptor affinity (potency) of three agonists is lorazepam > midazolam > diazepam. Midazolam is approximately 3 to 6 times, and lorazepam 5 to 10 times, as potent as diazepam.[193] As indicated previously, the mechanism of action of benzodiazepines is reasonably well understood.[194,195] The interaction of benzodiazepine ligands with the $GABA_A$ receptor is one of the few examples in which the complex systems of biochemistry, molecular pharmacology, genetic mutations, and clinical behavioral patterns can to some extent be explained. $GABA_A$ subtypes mediate the different effects (amnesic, anticonvulsant, anxiolytic, and sleep).[195] The $GABA_A$ receptor is a pentameric assembly built from 18 or more subunits (Fig. 23.9). Many different combinations of this pentameric assembly occur in different parts of the brain; linking this diversity to physiological function and pharmacologic specificity may be possible. The α-subunit of the pentameric complex occurs in six isoforms (α_1-α_6).[187] Sedation, anterograde amnesia, and anticonvulsant properties are mediated via α_1-subunits of the $GABA_A$ receptors,[195] and anxiolysis and muscle relaxation are mediated via the α_2-subunits. The "benzodiazepine receptors" are found in highest densities in the olfactory bulb, cerebral cortex, cerebellum, hippocampus, substantia nigra, and inferior colliculus, where lower densities in the striatum, lower brainstem, and spinal cord are found. Spinal cord benzodiazepine receptors can play an important role in analgesia; however, further elucidation of the mechanism of action of this drug class is required.[196] Intrathecal midazolam reduces excitatory GABA-mediated neurotransmission in interneurons, leading to a decrease in the excitability of spinal dorsal horn neurons.[196] A meta-analysis shows that intrathecal midazolam improves perioperative analgesia and reduces nausea and vomiting.[197]

The benzodiazepines reduce the $CMRO_2$ in a dose-related manner. Midazolam and diazepam maintain a relatively normal ratio of CBF to $CMRO_2$.[198] Midazolam, diazepam, and lorazepam all increase the seizure initiation threshold to local anesthetics and decrease the mortality rate in mice exposed to lethal doses of local anesthetics. Midazolam has neuroprotective effects by preventing lipid peroxidation and mitochondrial damage. There are indications in rats that the peripheral benzodiazepine receptor is involved in these actions.[199]

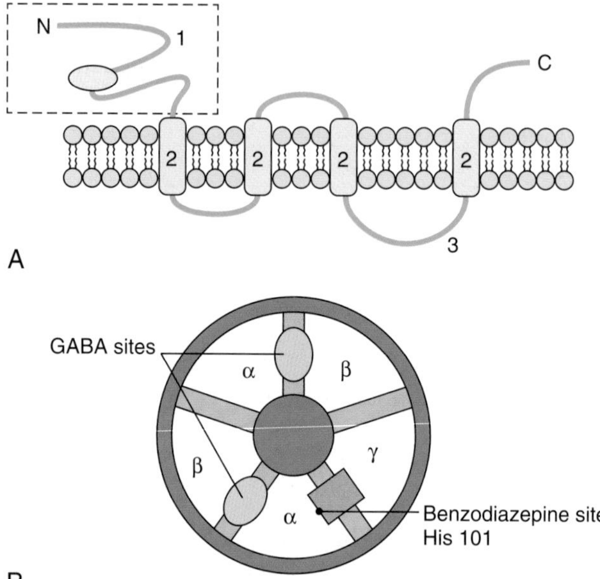

Fig. 23.9 Schematics of GABAA receptor structure and function. (A) topography of a GABAA receptor subunit partially embedded in the lipid bilayer. *1*, N-terminal extracellular domain responsible for transmitter and ligand binding and coupling of the binding sites with ion channel. This part is also important for the assembly of various receptor subunits into functional receptors. *2*, four transmembrane segments forming the anion channel are responsible for binding of hydrophobic ligands, ion selectivity, and channel binding sites. *3*, intracellular loop between transmembrane segments 3 and 4 forms the domain for regulatory phosphorylation sites and for the intracellular factors anchoring the receptors in appropriate locations. (B) hypothetical binding sites for GABA and benzodiazepines ligands in a pentameric receptor complex. (From Saari TI, Uusi-Oukari M, Ahonen J, Olkkola KT. Enhancement of GABAergic activity: neuropharmacological effects of benzodiazepines and therapeutic use in anesthesiology. *Pharmacol Rev.* 2011;63[1]:243–267.)

Effects on the Respiratory System

Benzodiazepines, similar to most IV anesthetics, produce dose-related central respiratory system depression. The benzodiazepines affect respiration in two different ways. First, they have an effect on the muscular tone leading to an increased risk of upper airway obstruction.[200] Second, they flatten the response of the respiratory curve to carbon dioxide.[201] In addition, sedative doses of midazolam depress the hypoxic ventilatory response in humans.[202]

Benzodiazepines and opioids produce additive or supra-additive (synergistic) respiratory depression, even though they act at different receptors.[203] Old age, debilitating disease, and other respiratory depressant drugs increase the incidence and degree of respiratory depression and apnea by benzodiazepines.

Effects on the Cardiovascular System

The hypothalamic paraventricular nucleus (PVN) is an important site for autonomic and endocrine homeostasis of the cardiovascular system. The PVN integrates afferent stimuli to regulate blood volume; the rostral ventrolateral medulla is the dominant brain region for tonic regulation of arterial blood pressure.[204] Under normal circumstances, the sympathetic nervous system is tonically inhibited. This inhibition is dependent on GABAergic signaling and nitric oxide.[205]

Benzodiazepines, when used alone, have modest hemodynamic effects. The predominant hemodynamic change is a modest decrease in arterial blood pressure, resulting from a decrease in systemic vascular resistance. The mechanism by which benzodiazepines maintain relatively stable hemodynamics involves the preservation of homeostatic reflex mechanisms. The hemodynamic effects of midazolam and diazepam are dose related, however, there is a plateau plasma drug effect above which little change in arterial blood pressure occurs. The plateau plasma level for midazolam is 100 ng/mL, and that for diazepam is about 900 ng/mL. Heart rate, ventricular filling pressures, and cardiac output are maintained after induction of anesthesia with benzodiazepines. More recent studies using heart rate variability variables as measurements to evaluate the effect of benzodiazepines on autonomic neurocardiac regulation conclude a biphasic effect. First, the vagal tone reduces and second, the cardiac pacemaker may decrease using intravenous premedication doses. In patients with increased left ventricular filling pressures, diazepam and midazolam produce a "nitroglycerin-like" effect by decreasing the filling pressure and increasing cardiac output. Notably, the stress of endotracheal intubation and surgery are not blocked by midazolam.

Drug Interactions

PHARMACOKINETIC DRUG INTERACTIONS

The pharmacokinetics of benzodiazepines may be altered by drug interactions. As cytochrome P450 is often involved in the metabolism of the benzodiazepines, drugs inducing or inhibiting CYP function often cause alterations in the pharmacokinetics of the benzodiazepines.

CYP-mediated drug interactions have extensively been examined utilizing midazolam, which is almost completely metabolized by CYP, particularly CYP3A4.

The inhibition of CYP3A by concomitantly administered drugs like—among many others—the azole antifungal agents, results in significant inhibition of the metabolism of midazolam.[206] Orally administered midazolam is especially affected by these inhibitors due to reduction of the first-pass metabolism elimination.[207]

Diazepam is primarily metabolized by CYP2C19 and CYP3A4. Different CYP2C19 alleles have varying activity, which results in ultra-rapid, extensive, intermediate, and poor metabolizer genotypes.[208,209] Pharmacokinetics and pharmacodynamics vary among these different metabolizers.[210,211] Strong inhibitors of CYP3A4 have a minor effect on the pharmacokinetics of diazepam.[212,213] Inhibitors of CYP2C19 like omeprazole, fluvoxamine, and ciprofloxacin consequently increase the plasma half-life of diazepam substantially.[214-216] The clearance of lorazepam is affected by probenecid and valproic acid, both of which decrease the formation clearance of lorazepam-glucuronide.[217,218] Remimazolam is not metabolized by CYP-dependent mechanisms, which decreases the chances of significant drug interactions occurring.

PHARMACODYNAMIC DRUG INTERACTION

All benzodiazepines act on the CNS and interact with other drugs targeting the CNS, in particular those causing CNS depression.

In anesthetic practice, opioids are often combined with benzodiazepines, which interact in a synergistic manner.[219] The interaction between midazolam and ketamine is additive,[220] while the interaction between the hypnotic effects of thiopental and midazolam and of propofol and midazolam are synergistic.[20,221]

Uses

PREMEDICATION

Benzodiazepines are the most commonly applied drugs for premedication. The goals of this application are anxiolysis, sedation, amnesia, vagolysis, and sympathicolysis, and reduction of PONV.[222] The amnestic effects are anterograde; retrograde memory is not affected.

Diazepam, lorazepam, and midazolam are given orally or intravenously for preoperative sedation. Midazolam is the most frequently used benzodiazepine for premedication in both adults and children.[223] The usual oral dose for adults ranges from 7.5 to 15 mg for midazolam, from 5 to 10 mg for diazepam, and from 10 to 20 mg for temazepam.[224] Many factors like age, ASA physical status, level of anxiety, and type and length of surgery determine the dose. Lorazepam is mostly used when a prolonged and intense anxiolysis is pursued, like in cardiac surgery. Typically, 2 to 4 mg lorazepam is administered orally 2 hours before anesthesia and surgery.[225]

For pediatric patients midazolam is available in several preparations (including a formulation for intranasal administration in some countries) and well tolerated. The dose is effective from 0.025 mg/kg and produces sedation and anxiolysis in 10 to 20 minutes.

Midazolam has minimal effects on respiration and oxygen saturation in adults, even in doses up to 1.0 mg/kg with a maximum of 20 mg.

Sedation

Relief of anxiety and lack of recall of unpleasant events during minor surgical and diagnostic procedures are the primary objectives of good sedation. Appropriately used sedation improves patient satisfaction.[222] Patients are seemingly conscious and coherent during sedation with benzodiazepines, yet they are amnesic for the procedure and events.[226] For this use drugs should be given by titration; end points of titration are adequate sedation or dysarthria (Table 23.7). The onset of action is rapid with midazolam, usually with a peak effect reached within 2 to 3 minutes of administration; time to peak effect is slightly longer with diazepam and even longer still with lorazepam. The duration of action of these drugs are dose-dependent. Although the onset is more rapid with midazolam than with diazepam after bolus administration, the recovery is similar, probably because both drugs have similar early plasma decay (redistribution) patterns.[227] (also see Fig. 23.10). With lorazepam, sedation and particularly amnesia are slower in onset and are longer lasting than with the other two benzodiazepines.[228] Lorazepam is particularly unpredictable with regard to duration of amnesia, and this is undesirable in patients who wish or need to have recall in the immediate postoperative period. The degree of sedation, the reliable amnesia, and the preservation of respiratory and hemodynamic function are better with benzodiazepines than with other sedative-hypnotic drugs used for conscious sedation. When midazolam is compared with propofol for sedation during procedures, the two are generally similar except that emergence or wake-up is more rapid with propofol. Sedation with propofol is safe in the hands of well-trained non-anesthetic professionals.[229,230]

There are studies showing that remimazolam has a favorable profile as a sedative for upper gastrointestinal endoscopy in patients as the time to recovery was shorter and more consistent than that observed after the use of midazolam.[188,190] The use of midazolam for sedation during regional and epidural anesthesia requires vigilance with regard to depth of sedation and respiratory function.[231]

Two studies report the use of midazolam during cesarean section either for sedation in preeclamptic parturients or prevention of nausea and vomiting; they showed that a single IV dose of midazolam was a safe practice, with no detriment in Apgar scores, neurobehavioral scores, continuous oxygen saturation, or the ability of the mother to recall the birth events.[232] Nitsun and associates found that 0.005% of the maternal dose of midazolam is transferred into the breast milk during a 24-hour milk collection.[233] Although verification of these findings is needed, they highlight an important clinical use of midazolam that may be safe for mother and infant.

Sedation for longer periods, such as in the ICU, can also be accomplished with benzodiazepines. Prolonged infusion may result in accumulation of drug and, in the case of midazolam, significant concentration of the active metabolite. Reviews have pointed out both concerns and advantages of benzodiazepine sedation.[234] The main advantages are the amnesia and hemodynamic stability, where the disadvantage is the potential lingering sedative effect after termination of the infusion when compared with propofol and a higher prevalence of delirium compared to dexmedetomidine. In 2013, the Society of Critical Care Medicine's (SCCM) American College of Critical Care Medicine (ACCM) published a revised version of its pain, agitation, and delirium (PAD) clinical practice guidelines for adult ICU patients. These guidelines suggest that sedation strategies using nonbenzodiazepine sedatives may be preferred over sedation with benzodiazepines, either midazolam or lorazepam, to improve clinical outcome in mechanically ventilated ICU patients.[235] To prevent overdosing and prolonged mechanical ventilation, evidence-based sedation algorithms have evolved. Daily interruption of sedation has not proven to decrease the time to extubation of the trachea or length of hospital stay.[236]

TABLE 23.7 Uses and Doses of Intravenous Benzodiazepines

	Midazolam	Diazepam	Lorazepam
Induction	0.05-0.15 mg/kg	0.3-0.5 mg/kg	0.1 mg/kg
Maintenance	0.05 mg/kg prn	0.1 mg/kg prn	0.02 mg/kg prn
	1 µg/kg/min		
Sedation*	0.5-1 mg repeated	2 mg repeated	0.25 mg repeated
	0.07 mg/kg IM		

*Incremental doses given until desired degree of sedation is obtained.
IM, Intramuscular; *prn*, as required to keep patient hypnotic and amnesic.
From Reves JG, Glass P, Lubarsky DA, et al. Intravenous anesthetics. In: Miller RD, Eriksson LI, Fleischer LA, et al, eds. *Miller's Anesthesia*, 7th ed. Philadelphia: Churchill Livingstone; 2010: 719–768.

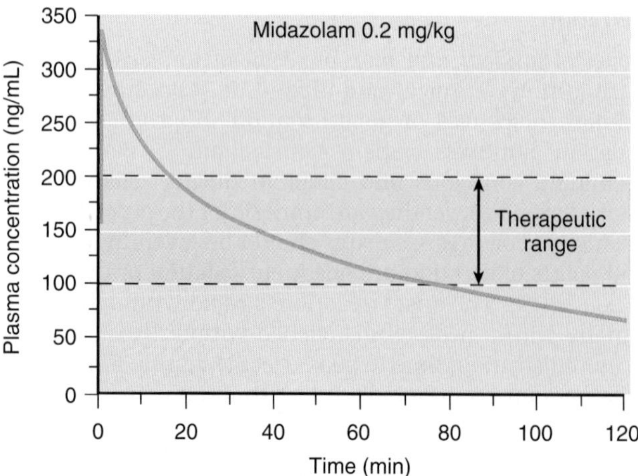

Fig. 23.10 Simulated time course of plasma levels of midazolam after an induction dose of 0.2 mg/kg. Plasma levels required for hypnosis and amnesia during surgery are 100 to 200 ng/mL, with awakening usually occurring at levels less than 50 ng/mL.

Induction and Maintenance of Anesthesia

Midazolam is the benzodiazepine of choice for induction of anesthesia. Numerous factors influence the rapidity of action of midazolam and the other benzodiazepines when used for induction of general anesthesia, including dose, speed of injection, degree of premedication, age, ASA physical status, and concurrent anesthetic drugs. The usual induction dose of midazolam is 0.1 to 0.2 mg/kg in premedicated patients, and up to 0.3 mg/kg in unpremedicated patients. The onset of anesthesia is within 30 to 60 seconds. The half-time of equilibrium between the plasma concentration and the EEG effects is about 2 to 3 minutes.[237]

Elderly patients require smaller doses of midazolam than younger patients (Fig. 23.11).[238]

When midazolam is combined with other anesthetic drugs (coinduction), often a synergistic interaction occurs, similar to that seen with propofol. This synergy is observed when midazolam is used with opioids or other hypnotics, similar to propofol in combination with opioids (Fig 23.12).[20,52,239]

Emergence time is related to the dose of midazolam and to the dose of adjuvant anesthetic drugs.

Benzodiazepines lack analgesic properties and must be used with other anesthetic drugs to provide sufficient analgesia; however, as maintenance anesthetic drugs during general anesthesia, benzodiazepines provide hypnosis and amnesia. The amnesic period after an anesthetic dose is about 1 to 2 hours.

A plasma level of more than 50 to 100 ng/mL occurs when used with adjuvant opioids (e.g., fentanyl) or inhaled anesthetics (e.g., nitrous oxide, volatile anesthetics) by a bolus initial dose of 0.05 to 0.15 mg/kg and a continuous infusion of 0.25 to 1 µg/kg/min.[240] This plasma level is sufficient to keep the patient asleep and amnesic but arousable at the end of surgery. Smaller infusion doses may be required in some patients or in combination with opioids. Midazolam, diazepam, and lorazepam accumulate in the blood after repeated bolus administrations or with continuous infusion. If the benzodiazepines do accumulate with repeated administration, prolonged arousal time can be anticipated. This is less of a problem with midazolam than with diazepam and lorazepam because of the shorter context-sensitive half-time and greater clearance of midazolam. Remimazolam might be a good alternative; it is rapidly metabolized and has a faster recovery profile than midazolam in sheep.[189,190]

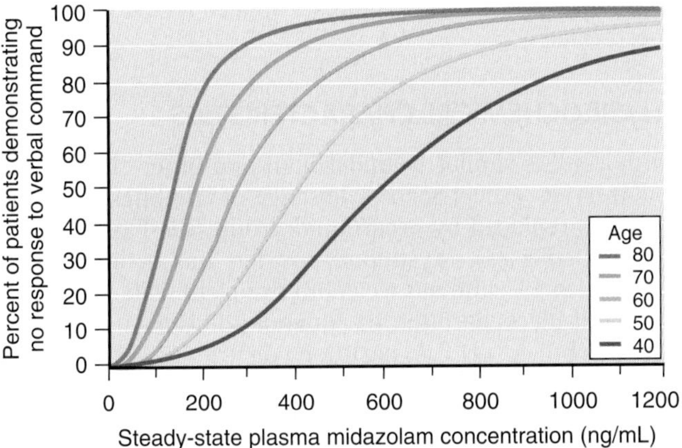

Fig. 23.11 Spectrum of the intrinsic activities of benzodiazepine receptor ligands, which range from agonists to inverse agonists. Structures of agonist, partial agonist, antagonist, partial inverse agonist, and inverse agonist compounds are shown. Intrinsic activity is greatest among agonists and is least among inverse agonists. Intrinsic activities are schematically indicated as positive by a plus sign and as negative by a minus sign, with 0 indicating a lack of intrinsic activity. *GABA*, γ-aminobutyric acid. (Redrawn with modification from Mohler H, Richards JG. The benzodiazepine receptor: a pharmacological control element of brain function. *Eur J Anaesthesiol.* 1988;Suppl 2:15–24.)

Nausea and Vomiting Prophylaxis

Numerous studies have highlighted the role that benzodiazepines, and specifically midazolam, may play in the prevention of PONV. A recent meta-analysis on the effect of intravenous midazolam on PONV concludes a significant decrease in overall PONV and rescue antiemetic drug. Jung and colleagues found that in women undergoing middle ear surgery, IV midazolam, 0.075 mg/kg after induction of anesthesia, reduced the incidence of PONV and the need for rescue antiemetics with no difference from placebo in pain intensity or drowsiness.[241] Furthermore, the combination of midazolam with dexamethasone proved more effective in preventing PONV than midazolam alone.[242] The incidence of PONV after minor gynecologic or urologic surgery was the same when comparing IV ondansetron, 4 mg, and IV midazolam, 2 mg.[243]

In children, IV midazolam, 0.05 mg/kg, reduced PONV significantly after pediatric (4-12 years old) strabismus surgery compared with placebo or IV dexamethasone 0.5 mg/kg. No child vomited with midazolam alone or with the midazolam dexamethasone combination.[244,245]

Finally, in a 2010 three-arm, placebo-controlled, double-blind clinical trial, Fuji and associates compared midazolam 0.050 mg/kg with 0.075 mg/kg in patients undergoing laparoscopic gynecologic surgery regarding PONV prophylaxis. The two doses of midazolam were not significantly different with regard to PONV (30% vs. 27% of patients experienced PONV) and both proved better than placebo (67%).[246]

Side Effects and Contraindications

Benzodiazepines have limited allergenic effects and do not suppress the adrenal gland. The most significant side effect with midazolam is respiratory depression. The major side effects of lorazepam and diazepam in addition to respiratory depression are venous irritation and thrombophlebitis, problems related to aqueous insolubility and requisite solvents.[165] When used as sedative or for induction and

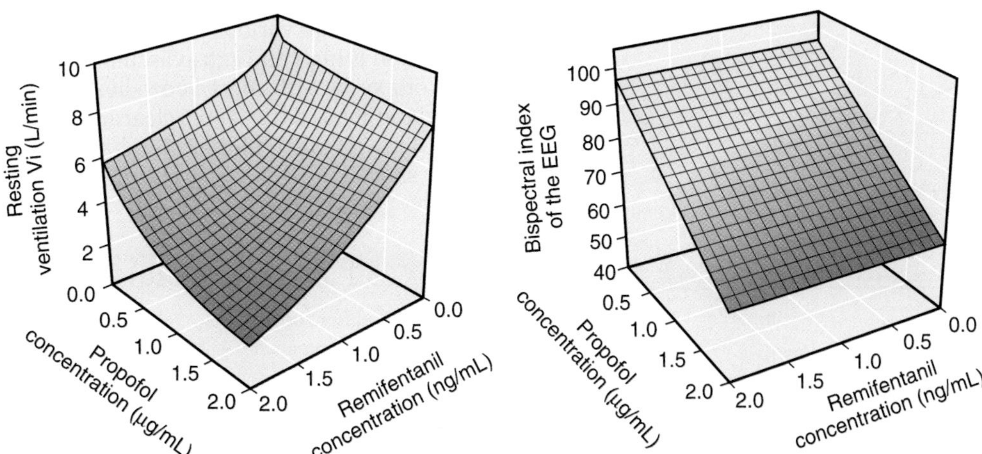

Fig. 23.12 Response surface modeling of the interaction of remifentanil and propofol on resting ventilation and the bispectral index of the electroencephalogram (BIS). Population response surface showing that the propofol–remifentanil interaction on respiration is synergistic and on BIS is inert since remifentanil had no effect on bispectral index irrespective of the propofol concentrations. Over this dose range, propofol causes a linear decrease in bispectral index with a 25% decrease occurring at 1.4 µg/mL. (From Nieuwenhuijs DJ, Olofsen E, Romberg RR, et al. Response surface modeling of remifentanil-propofol interaction on cardiorespiratory control and bispectral index. *Anesthesiology.* 2003; 98:312–322.)

maintenance of anesthesia, benzodiazepines may produce an undesirable degree or prolonged interval of postoperative amnesia, sedation, and, rarely, respiratory depression. These residual effects can be reversed with flumazenil.[247]

Flumazenil

Flumazenil (Anexate, Romazicon) is the first benzodiazepine antagonist approved for clinical use.[248] It is a benzodiazepine receptor ligand with high affinity, great specificity, and by definition minimal intrinsic effect. Flumazenil, similar to the agonists it replaces at the benzodiazepine receptor, interacts with the receptor in a concentration-dependent manner. It is a competitive antagonist at the benzodiazepine receptor and produces antagonism that is reversible and surmountable. In humans, flumazenil has minimal agonist activity, which means that its benzodiazepine receptor agonist effects are very weak, significantly less than those of clinical agonists.[249] Flumazenil, similar to all competitive antagonists at receptors, does not displace the agonist, but rather occupies the receptor when an agonist dissociates from the receptor. The half-time (or half-life) of a receptor-ligand bond is a few milliseconds to a few seconds, and new ligand receptor bonds are immediately formed. This dynamic situation accounts for the ability of either an agonist or an antagonist to readily occupy the receptor. The ratio of agonist to total receptors produces the effects of the agonist drug, but the antagonist can alter this ratio, depending on its concentration and dissociation constant. Flumazenil, which is an avid (high-affinity) ligand, replaces a relatively weak agonist, such as diazepam, as long as it is given in sufficient dose. Flumazenil is rapidly metabolically cleared, however, and the proportion of receptors occupied by the agonist then increases again, and the potential for rebound sedation and respiratory suppression exists (Fig. 23.13). This situation is less likely to occur when flumazenil is used to reverse midazolam, which has a more rapid clearance than other benzodiazepine agonists. Another important finding is that in the presence of extremely large doses of agonist (e.g., when a mistake in dosing has occurred, or suicide by means of an overdose is attempted), a small dose of flumazenil attenuates the deep CNS depression (loss of consciousness, respiratory depression) by reducing the fractional receptor occupancy by the agonist without decreasing the agonist effects that occur at low fractional receptor occupancy (drowsiness, amnesia).

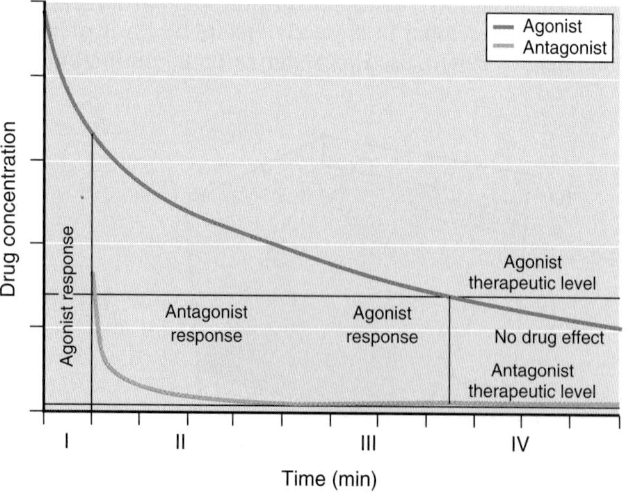

Fig. 23.13 Schematic representation of the interaction of a short-acting antagonist with a longer-acting agonist resulting in resedation. The upper curve shows disappearance of agonist from blood, and the lower curve shows disappearance of antagonist from plasma. Four conditions are represented: I, agonist response; II, antagonist response (the antagonist reverses the agonist effect); III, agonist response (resedation or resumption of agonist response with disappearance of short-lasting antagonist); and IV, no drug effect, with disappearance of agonist and antagonist (both drugs are below the therapeutic level).

Conversely, large doses of flumazenil in the presence of small doses of agonist completely reverse all the agonist effects. Flumazenil can precipitate withdrawal symptoms in animals or in humans physically dependent on a benzodiazepine receptor agonist.[250] However, this is not a problem when flumazenil is used to reverse clinical effects of benzodiazepine receptor agonists applied in the practice of anesthesia.

PHYSICOCHEMICAL CHARACTERISTICS

Flumazenil is similar to midazolam and other classic benzodiazepines except for the absence of the phenyl group, which is replaced by a carbonyl group (see Fig. 23.8). It forms a colorless, crystalline powder; has a dissociation constant of 1.7; and has weak but sufficient water solubility to permit its preparation in aqueous solution. Its octanol/aqueous buffer (pH 7.4) partition coefficient is 14, showing moderate lipid solubility at pH 7.4.[251]

PHARMACOKINETICS

Flumazenil, similar to the other benzodiazepines, is completely (99%) metabolized in the liver; is rapidly cleared from the plasma; and has three known metabolites: *N*-desmethylflumazenil, *N*-desmethylflumazenil acid, and flumazenil acid.[252] The metabolic end product, that is, flumazenil acid, has no pharmacologic activity. The major metabolites identified in urine are the de-ethylated free acid and its glucuronide conjugate. Flumazenil is a short-lived compound. Box 23.2 includes a summary of its pharmacokinetics, which are described in various clinical settings. The volume of distribution is high and extravascular distribution is rapid.

Compared with most benzodiazepine receptor agonists, flumazenil has a very rapid clearance and short elimination half-life.[253] Only remimazolam has a more rapid clearance and shorter half-life. The plasma half-life of flumazenil is

BOX 23.2 Uses and Doses of Flumazenil

Reversal of benzodiazepines	0.2 mg repeated up to 3 mg
Diagnosis in coma	0.5 mg repeated up to 1 mg

*The dose required to reverse each benzodiazepine (BZD) depends on residual BZD and the particular BZD (i.e., higher doses are required for more potent BZDs) (see text).

†The degree of reversal should be titrated by repeating 0.2-mg increments every 1 to 2 min until the desired level of reversal is achieved.

From Reves JG, Glass P, Lubarsky DA, et al. Intravenous anesthetics. In Miller RD, Eriksson LI, Fleischer LA, et al, eds. *Miller's Anesthesia,* 7th ed. Philadelphia: Churchill Livingstone; 2010: 719–768.

about 1 hour—it is the shortest lived of all benzodiazepines used in anesthetic practice. The rapid blood clearance of flumazenil approaches hepatic blood flow, a finding that indicates that liver clearance partially depends on hepatic blood flow. Compared with other benzodiazepines, flumazenil has a high proportion of unbound drug; plasma protein binding is about 40%. The potential exists for the antagonist to be cleared, leaving sufficient concentrations of agonist at the receptor site to cause resedation.[254] To maintain a constant therapeutic blood level over a prolonged time, either repeated administration or a continuous infusion is required. An infusion rate of 30 to 60 µg/min (0.5-1 µg/kg/min) has been used for this purpose.[255]

PHARMACODYNAMICS

When given in the absence of a benzodiazepine receptor agonist, flumazenil has little discernible CNS effect. When given to healthy subjects and patients in clinically relevant doses, flumazenil has no effect on the EEG or cerebral metabolism. Flumazenil is free of anticonvulsant properties, and reverses the anticonvulsant properties of benzodiazepines in local anesthetic-induced seizures.[256] When administered to patients who have benzodiazepine-induced CNS depression, flumazenil produces rapid and dependable reversal of unconsciousness, respiratory depression, sedation, amnesia, and psychomotor dysfunction.[257] Flumazenil can be given before, during, or after the agonist to block or reverse the CNS effects of the agonist.

Flumazenil has successfully reversed the effects of benzodiazepines like midazolam, diazepam, lorazepam, and flunitrazepam. It has also been used successfully to reverse the effects of chloralhydrate and cannabis intoxication in children, [258,259] carbamazepine and alcohol overdose,[260] and antihistamines overdose.[261] The onset is rapid, with peak effect occurring in 1 to 3 minutes, which coincides with the detection of C-flumazenil in the human brain.[257] Flumazenil reverses the agonist by replacing it at the benzodiazepine receptor, and its onset and duration are governed by the law of mass action. When flumazenil is given in the presence of agonists, there are significant respiratory effects because it reverses respiratory depression caused by the agonists (e.g., when given to volunteers made apneic with midazolam). For example, the reversal of midazolam-induced (0.13 mg/kg) respiratory depression with flumazenil (1 mg) lasts 3 to 30 minutes. Other agonists and other doses would have different durations of antagonism of respiratory depression.

Incremental doses up to 3 mg intravenously in patients with ischemic heart disease had no significant effect on cardiovascular variables.[257,262] Administration of flumazenil to patients given agonists is remarkably free of cardiovascular effects, in contrast to the experience of opioid reversal with naloxone.[263] Although flumazenil does reverse sedation, it does not increase blood concentrations of catecholamines. However, catecholamine levels may increase when arousal is more rapid after flumazenil.[264] The reversal of sedation by midazolam with flumazenil also restores the attenuated cardiac baroreflex function.[265]

In healthy subjects, flumazenil did not alter intraocular pressure but reversed the decrease in intraocular pressure observed after administration of midazolam (Romazicon package insert; www.fda.gov).

Uses and Doses

Application of a benzodiazepine antagonist (see Box 23.2) includes the diagnostic and therapeutic reversal of benzodiazepine receptor agonists. For diagnostic use in suspected benzodiazepine overdose, flumazenil may be given in incremental IV doses of 0.2 to 0.5 mg up to 3 mg. More commonly in anesthesia, flumazenil is used to reverse the residual sedation of a patient after administration of a benzodiazepine for premedication of a short surgical procedure, conscious sedation, or for general anesthesia. Flumazenil reliably reverses the sedation, respiratory depression, and amnesia caused by benzodiazepines. There are differential reversal effects on the different agonist actions. Flumazenil tends to reverse the hypnotic and respiratory effects more than the amnesic effects of the benzodiazepine agonist.[266,267]

The dose varies with the particular benzodiazepine being reversed, and the duration of reversal depends on the kinetics of the agonist and of flumazenil. Surveillance is recommended if a long-lasting benzodiazepine is reversed with a single administration of flumazenil because of the relatively short-lived effect. If a patient shows no signs of recurrent sedation within 2 hours after a 1-mg reversal dose of flumazenil, serious recurrent sedation at a later time is unlikely. Flumazenil may be administered by continuous infusion to prevent recurrent sedation by longer lasting benzodiazepine receptor agonists. The pharmacokinetic profile of flumazenil is unaltered in the presence of benzodiazepine agonists (diazepam, flunitrazepam, lormetazepam, midazolam) and vice versa.

Side Effects and Contraindications

Flumazenil has been given in large oral and IV doses with remarkably few toxic reactions.[257] It is free of local or tissue irritant properties, and there are no known organotoxicities. Similar to all benzodiazepines, it apparently has a high safety margin, probably higher than the safety margins of the agonists, because it does not produce prominent CNS depression. In patients using large doses of benzodiazepines over several weeks or longer, the administration of flumazenil may elicit symptoms of benzodiazepine withdrawal, including seizures.

Phencyclidines (Ketamine)

HISTORY

Ketamine (Ketalar) was synthesized in 1962 by Stevens and was first used in humans in 1965 by Corssen and Domino. Ketamine was released for clinical use in 1970 and is still used in various clinical settings. It produces dissociative anesthesia rather than generalized depression of the CNS through antagonistic actions at the phencyclidine (PCP) site of the N-methyl-D-aspartate receptor (NMDAR). Ketamine is a racemic mixture of the isomers R(-)-ketamine and S(+)-ketamine. It usually does not depress the cardiovascular and respiratory systems, but it does possess some of the adverse psychological effects found with the other phencyclidines.[268] The S(+)-isomer (Ketanest) is 3 to 4 times more potent as an analgesic with a faster clearance and recovery and with fewer psychomimetic side effects. Still, S-ketamine produces—besides analgesia—psychotropic effects, cognitive impairment, memory impairment, and a reduced

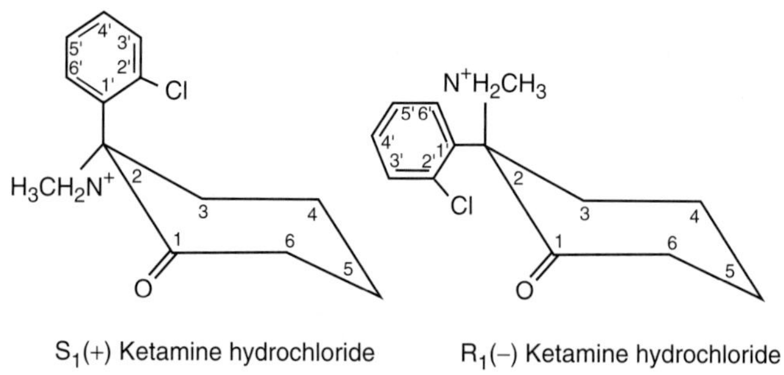

$S_1(+)$ Ketamine hydrochloride $R_1(-)$ Ketamine hydrochloride

Fig. 23.14 Stereoisomers of ketamine as it is formulated.

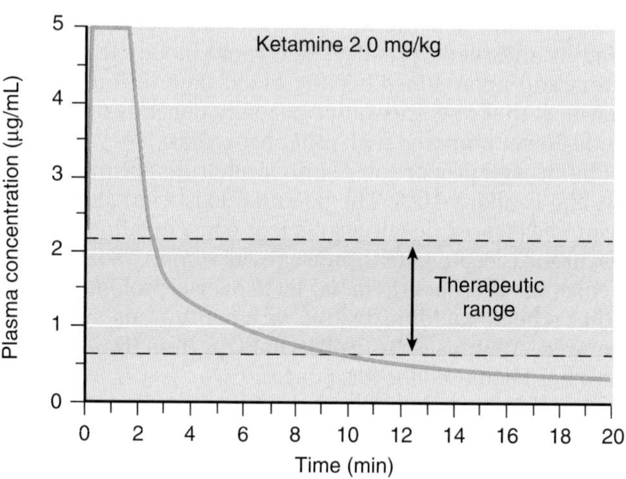

Fig. 23.15 Simulated time course of plasma levels of ketamine after an induction dose of 2 mg/kg. Plasma levels required for hypnosis and amnesia during surgery are 0.7 to 2.2 µg/mL, with awakening usually occurring at levels less than 0.5 µg/mL.

reaction time. Interest in ketamine has increased more recently because of its effects on hyperalgesia and opiate tolerance, use in chronic pain states, potential neuroprotective effects, increasing popularity of total IV anesthesia, and the availability in some countries of S(+) ketamine.[269] Lastly, ketamine receives growing interest because of its antidepressant effects.

PHYSICOCHEMICAL CHARACTERISTICS

Ketamine (Fig. 23.14) has a molecular weight of 238 kD, is partially water soluble, and forms a white crystalline salt with a pK_a of 7.5. It has a lipid solubility 5 to 10 times that of thiopental. Ketamine is only 12% bound to proteins. Its bioavailability is 93% after parenteral administration but only 20% after oral use, due to its high first-pass metabolism.[270]

PHARMACOKINETICS

Ketamine is metabolized by hepatic microsomal enzymes.[271,272] The major pathway involves *N*-demethylation to form norketamine (metabolite I), which is then hydroxylated to hydroxynorketamine, which is further conjugated to water-soluble glucuronide derivates and excreted in the urine. The activity of the principal metabolites of ketamine has not been well studied, but norketamine (metabolite I) has significantly less (20%-30%) activity than the parent compound. More recent modeling of norketamine suggests that it contributes in prolonging the analgesia provided by either a bolus or infusion of ketamine, although this conclusion is being questioned.[271,273,274] In contrast to previous reports, S-norketamine may have a negative contribution to S-ketamine-induced analgesia but shows absence of contribution to the cognitive impairment. This may explain the observation of ketamine-related excitatory phenomena (such as hyperalgesia and allodynia) upon the termination of ketamine infusions.[271,273,274]

Ketamine's pharmacokinetics have been examined after bolus administration of anesthetizing doses (2-2.5 mg/kg IV), after a subanesthetic dose (0.25 mg/kg IV), and after continuous infusion (steady-state plasma level 2000 ng/mL).

Regardless of the dose, ketamine plasma disappearance can be described by a two-compartment model. Table 23.1 contains the pharmacokinetic values from bolus administration studies. Of note is the rapid distribution reflected in the relatively brief distribution half-life of 11 to 16 minutes (Fig. 23.15). The high lipid solubility of ketamine is reflected in its large volume of distribution of nearly 3 L/kg.[272,275] Clearance also is high, 890 to 1227 mL/min, which accounts for the short elimination half-life of 2 to 3 hours. The mean total body clearance (1.4 L/min) is approximately equal to liver blood flow. Low-dose alfentanil increases the volume of distribution and clearance of ketamine. In addition, alfentanil increases the distribution of ketamine into the brain. The pharmacokinetic model of Clements provided the best accuracy when used to administer low-dose ketamine to volunteers using a target-controlled infusion device. The pharmacokinetics of the two isomers is different. S(+) ketamine has a larger elimination clearance and larger volume of distribution than R(−) ketamine. When the pharmacokinetics of S(+) ketamine were tested in a target-controlled infusion device for procedures of 1 hour and in combination with propofol, the authors found that the accuracy of the pharmacokinetic parameters was improved with a much smaller Vc* (167 mL/kg).[276] They also noted that ketamine clearance was not normally distributed, and this was not related to age. The S(+) enantiomer also seems to be more potent in suppressing the EEG than either R(−) or the racemic mixture. Ketamine is increasingly being given by alternative routes, especially orally and via an intranasal spray. Administration by either of these routes is subject to significant first-pass metabolism. The bioavailability via oral administration is 20% to 30%, and via the intranasal route is approximately 40% to 50%. In clinical and experimental studies hyperalgesic responses have been noted after the withdrawal of *S*(+)-ketamine.[273-275,277,278] Furthermore, no delay between concentration and effect has been observed for any of the antinociceptive end points. This indicates an almost immediate passage of S(+)-ketamine across the blood-brain barrier and rapid receptor kinetics.

Pharmacodynamics

EFFECTS ON THE CENTRAL NERVOUS SYSTEM

Ketamine produces dose-related unconsciousness and analgesia. Ketamine acts at multiple receptors including the NMDAR, opioid receptors, and monoaminergic receptors.

*Vc (central compartment volume of a three compartment model).

At high ketamine concentrations, sigma opioid receptors are also affected, muscarinic receptors are blocked, and GABAergic neurotransmission is facilitated. Its most important action is the inhibition of NMDAR-mediated glutamergic input to the GABAergic system leading to a changing excitatory activity in the cortex and limbic system that in the end results in unconsciousness. At the spinal cord level, ketamine has potent antinociceptive effects on NMDAR and inhibits acetylcholine release.[273-275] The anesthetized state has been termed *dissociative anesthesia* because patients who receive ketamine alone appear to be in a cataleptic state, in contrast with other states of anesthesia that resemble normal sleep. Patients anesthetized with ketamine have profound analgesia, but keep their eyes open and maintain many reflexes. Corneal, cough, and swallow reflexes all may be present, but should not be assumed to be protective. There is no recall of surgery or anesthesia, but amnesia is not as prominent with ketamine as with the benzodiazepines. Because ketamine has a low molecular weight, a pK_a near the physiologic pH, and relatively high lipid solubility, it crosses the blood-brain barrier rapidly and has an onset of action within 30 to 60 seconds of administration. The maximal effect occurs in about 1 minute.

After ketamine administration, pupils dilate moderately, and nystagmus occurs. Lacrimation and salivation are common, as is increased skeletal muscle tone, often with coordinated but seemingly purposeless movements of the arms, legs, trunk, and head. Although there is great inter-individual variability, plasma levels of 0.6 to 2 μg/mL are considered the minimum concentrations for general anesthesia; children may require slightly higher plasma levels (0.8-4 μg/mL). The duration of ketamine anesthesia after a single IV administration of a general anesthetic dose (2 mg/kg) is 10 to 15 minutes (see Fig. 23.15), and full orientation to person, place, and time occurs within 15 to 30 minutes. The S(+) enantiomer enables quicker recovery (by a couple of minutes) than the racemic mixture.[279,280] This is due to the smaller dose necessary to produce an equi-anesthetic effect and to the 10% faster hepatic biotransformation. Because there is a good correlation between blood concentration of ketamine and CNS effect, the relatively short duration of action of ketamine is probably due to its redistribution from the brain and blood to the other tissues in the body.

Concomitant administration of benzodiazepines, which is a common practice, may prolong the effect of ketamine. When used in combination with a benzodiazepine, the S(+) enantiomer was no different in terms of awareness at 30 minutes, but it was significantly better at 120 minutes than the racemic mixture. Analgesia occurs at considerably lower blood concentrations than loss of consciousness.

Ketamine provides important postoperative analgesia. The plasma level at which pain thresholds are elevated is 0.1 μg/mL or greater.[277,281,282] This means there is a considerable period of postoperative analgesia after ketamine general anesthesia, and subanesthetic doses can consequently be used to produce analgesia. Ketamine inhibits nociceptive central hypersensitization. Ketamine also attenuates acute tolerance after opiate administration. The NMDAR plays an important role in the induction of hyperalgesia and antinociceptive tolerance as induced by opioids. Preventive ketamine administration may thus prevent central sensitization and long-lasting enhancement in pain sensitivity as induced by opioids. Ketamine, just as other NMDAR antagonists, may thus prevent opioid-induced hyperalgesia.[283] The primary site of CNS action of ketamine seems to be the thalamoneocortical projection system. The drug selectively depresses neuronal function in parts of the cortex (especially association areas) and thalamus, while stimulating parts of the limbic system, including the hippocampus. This process creates what is termed a *functional disorganization* of nonspecific pathways in midbrain and thalamic areas. Ketamine acts via antagonism of the excitatory glutamatergic NMDA receptor. The NMDA receptor has a high expression in the temporal cortex, hippocampus, basal ganglia, cerebellum, and brainstem, all regions significantly affected by ketamine. There is also evidence that ketamine depresses transmission of impulses in the medial medullary reticular formation, which is important for transmission of the affective-emotional components of nociception from the spinal cord to higher brain centers. In volunteers experiencing heat pain, functional magnetic resonance imaging (MRI) studies showed ketamine produced a dose-dependent effect on pain processing by decreasing activation of the secondary somatosensory cortex (S2), insula, and anterior cingulate cortex. Ketamine occupies opiate receptors in the brain and spinal cord, and this property could account for some of the analgesic effects.[284,285] The S(+) enantiomer has some opioid μ-receptor activity, accounting for part of its analgesic effect. NMDA receptor interaction may mediate the general anesthetic effects and some analgesic actions of ketamine. The spinal cord analgesic effect of ketamine is postulated to be due to inhibition of dorsal horn wide dynamic range neuronal activity. In a resting state fMRI study, low-dose ketamine induced connectivity changes in brain areas involved in motor function, psychedelic effects, and pain processing. Ketamine's analgesic effect may arise from multiple pathways; a decreased connectivity in regions of the pain matrix responsible for the perception of pain (pain sensing) and the affective processing of pain. In addition, ketamine affected connectivity in brain areas involved in endogenous pain inhibition.[286,287]

Although some drugs have been used to antagonize ketamine, no specific receptor antagonist reverses all the CNS effects of ketamine.

Ketamine increases cerebral metabolism, CBF, and ICP. Because of its excitatory CNS effects, which can be detected by generalized EEG development of theta wave activity and by petit mal seizure-like activity in the hippocampus, ketamine increases $CMRO_2$. There is an increase in CBF, which appears higher than the increase in $CMRO_2$ would mandate. With the increase in CBF and the generalized increase in sympathetic nervous system response, there is an increase in ICP after ketamine. The increase in $CMRO_2$ and CBF can be blocked by the use of thiopental or diazepam. Cerebrovascular responsiveness to carbon dioxide seems to be preserved with ketamine; reducing $PaCO_2$ attenuates the increase in ICP after ketamine.

S(+) ketamine may influence the expression of apoptosis-regulating proteins in rat brains 4 hours after cerebral ischemia/reperfusion. The neuroprotection observed with ketamine may involve antiapoptotic mechanisms in addition to reducing necrotic cell death.

In contrast, ketamine and other anesthetics like propofol and volatile anesthetics, accentuate apoptosis in the brain of newborn animals and cause changes in the morphology of dendritic spines. This finding has sparked controversy over the use of ketamine in neonates. An editorial in the journal *Anesthesiology* and the Anesthetic and Life Support Drugs Advisory Committee of the FDA cautioned changing clinical practice based on present available data.

Ketamine, similar to other phencyclidines, produces undesirable psychological reactions, which occur during awakening from ketamine anesthesia and are termed *emergence reactions*. The common manifestations of these reactions, which vary in severity and classification, are vivid dreaming, extracorporeal experiences (sense of floating out of body), and illusions (misinterpretation of a real, external sensory experience). These incidents of dreaming and illusion are often associated with excitement, confusion, euphoria, and fear. They occur in the first hour of emergence and usually abate within 1 to several hours. The psychic emergence reactions occur secondary to ketamine-induced depression of auditory and visual relay nuclei, leading to misperception or misinterpretation of auditory and visual stimuli. The incidence of the psychic emergence reactions ranges from 3% to 100%. A clinically relevant range is probably 10% to 30% of adult patients who receive ketamine as a sole or major part of the anesthetic technique. Factors that affect the incidence of emergence reactions are age, dose, gender, psychological susceptibility, and concurrent drugs. Pediatric patients do not report as high an incidence of unpleasant emergence reactions as do adult patients; men also report a less frequent incidence compared with women. Larger doses and rapid administration of large doses seem to predispose patients to a frequent incidence of adverse effects. Finally, certain personality types seem prone to the development of emergence reactions. Patients who score high in psychotism on the Eysenck Personality Inventory are prone to develop emergence reactions, and individuals who commonly dream at home are more likely to have postoperative dreams in the hospital after ketamine. While numerous drugs have been used to reduce the incidence and severity of postoperative reactions to ketamine, the benzodiazepines seem to be the most effective group of drugs. Next to the undesirable psychological reactions, increasingly ketamine is described for its antidepressant effects. The dose often used for this indication is 0.5 mg/kg, given as a 40-minute infusion. This often results in a dramatic mood change within a day, often lasting for 3 to 12 days. A maintenance dose every 2 to 4 days may lengthen this effect.[288] The precise mechanism of action of the antidepressant effects of ketamine remain unknown.

EFFECTS ON THE RESPIRATORY SYSTEM

Ketamine has minimal effects on the central respiratory drive as reflected by an unaltered response to carbon dioxide. There can be a transient (1-3 minutes) decrease in minute ventilation after the bolus administration of an induction dose of ketamine (2 mg/kg intravenously). Unusually large doses can produce apnea, but this is seldom seen. In a μ-opioid knockout mouse model, though, at supraspinal sites S(+) ketamine interacts with the μ-opioid receptor system. This interaction contributes significantly to S(+) ketamine-induced respiratory depression and supraspinal antinociception.[289,290] With the use of adjuvant sedatives or anesthetic drugs, respiratory depression may become clinically significant. Ketamine depresses ventilatory control in children especially with bolus doses. Ketamine is a bronchial smooth muscle relaxant. When it is given to patients with reactive airway disease and bronchospasm, pulmonary compliance is improved.

Ketamine is as effective as halothane or enflurane in preventing experimentally induced bronchospasm. The mechanism for this effect is probably a result of the sympathomimetic response to ketamine, but there are isolated bronchial smooth muscle studies showing that ketamine can directly antagonize the spasmogenic effects of carbachol and histamine. Owing to its bronchodilating effect, administration of ketamine can treat status asthmaticus unresponsive to conventional therapy. A potential respiratory problem, especially in children, is the increased salivation that follows ketamine administration, which can be modulated by an anticholinergic drug such as atropine or glycopyrolate.

EFFECTS ON THE CARDIOVASCULAR SYSTEM

Ketamine increases arterial blood pressure, heart rate, and cardiac output in a biphasic manner. It produces a direct cardiodepressive, negative inotropic effect next to an indirect stimulatory effect due to activation of the sympathetic system. Ketamine causes the systemic release of catecholamines, inhibition of the vagal nerve, inhibition of norepinephrine reuptake at peripheral nerves and non-neuronal tissues such as the myocardium, and norepinephrine release from sympathetic ganglia.[291] Cardiodepression precedes stimulation after large-dose ketamine administration or occurs after repeated administrations when presynaptic catecholamine stores become depleted. Cardiovascular stimulation already occurs after small-dose ketamine infusion and is characterized by tachycardia, systemic and pulmonary hypertension, increases in cardiac output, and myocardial oxygen consumption. Whereas the cardiovascular stimulatory effects of ketamine generally are dominant, after termination of S-ketamine infusion, cardiovascular depression may become evident as cardiac output may decrease below pre-infusion values.[273] The cardiovascular stimulatory effects of S(+) ketamine are characterized by an increase in the cardiac output of 1 L/min in the presence of 243 ng/ml S(+) ketamine.[273] The cardiovascular stimulatory effect of S(+) ketamine is induced very rapidly with a half-life for onset/offset of the effect of ketamine on cardiac output of 1 to 2 minutes. The increase in hemodynamic variables is associated with increased work and myocardial oxygen consumption. The healthy heart increases oxygen supply by increased cardiac output and decreased coronary vascular resistance, so that coronary blood flow is appropriate for the increased oxygen consumption. In patients with congenital heart disease, there are no significant changes in shunt directions or fraction, or systemic oxygenation after ketamine induction of anesthesia. In patients who have increased pulmonary artery pressure (as with mitral valvular and some congenital lesions), ketamine causes a more pronounced increase in pulmonary than systemic vascular resistance. Ketamine injected directly into the CNS produces an immediate sympathetic nervous system hemodynamic response. Ketamine also causes the sympathoneuronal release of norepinephrine, which can be detected in venous blood. Blockade of this effect is possible with barbiturates, benzodiazepines, and droperidol. The centrally mediated sympathetic responses to ketamine usually override the direct depressant effects of ketamine. Some peripheral nervous system actions of ketamine play an undetermined role in the hemodynamic effects of the drug. Ketamine inhibits intraneuronal uptake of catecholamines in a cocaine-like effect and inhibits extraneuronal norepinephrine uptake.

Stimulation of the cardiovascular system is not always desirable, and certain pharmacologic methods have been used to block the ketamine-induced tachycardia and systemic hypertension. Probably the most fruitful approach has been prior administration of benzodiazepines. Modest doses of diazepam, flunitrazepam, and midazolam all attenuate the hemodynamic effects of ketamine. It also is possible to decrease the tachycardia and hypertension caused by ketamine by using a continuous infusion technique with or without a benzodiazepine. Inhalation anesthetics and propofol blunt the hemodynamic effect of ketamine.

Uses

The many unique features of ketamine pharmacology, especially its propensity to produce unwanted emergence reactions in 10% to 20% of patients, have limited its use for routine anesthesia. Nevertheless, ketamine has an important niche in the practice of anesthesiology when its unique sympathomimetic activity and bronchodilating capabilities are indicated during induction of anesthesia. It is used for premedication, sedation, induction, and maintenance of general anesthesia. There has been increased interest in the use of ketamine in small doses for preventive analgesia, for the treatment or prevention of opiate tolerance and hyperalgesia, and in treatment of acute and chronic pain.

Induction and Maintenance of Anesthesia

The cardiovascular stimulatory effects make ketamine a desirable drug for the induction of anesthesia in unstable cardiovascular patients suffering from hypovolemia, hemorrhagic shock, or cardiovascular depression in sepsis. Ketamine bronchodilation and profound analgesia allowing the use of high oxygen concentrations make ketamine an excellent choice for induction of anesthesia in patients with reactive airway disease. Trauma patients with extensive blood loss are typical candidates for rapid-sequence anesthesia induction with ketamine. Patients with septic shock also may benefit from ketamine. The intrinsic myocardial depressant effect of ketamine may manifest in this situation if trauma or sepsis has caused depletion of catecholamine stores before the patient's arrival in the operating room. Use of ketamine in these patients does not obviate the need for appropriate preoperative preparation, including restoration of intravascular blood volume. Other cardiac diseases that can be well managed with ketamine anesthesia are cardiac tamponade and restrictive pericarditis. The finding that ketamine preserves heart rate and right atrial pressure through its sympathetic stimulating effects makes ketamine an excellent anesthetic induction and maintenance drug in this setting. Ketamine also is often used in patients with congenital heart disease, especially patients in whom the propensity for right-to-left shunting exists. Ketamine has been successfully used in a patient susceptible to malignant hyperthermia. Ketamine combined with propofol or midazolam can be given by continuous infusion to produce satisfactory cardiac anesthesia for patients with valvular and ischemic heart disease. The combination of a benzodiazepine or of a benzodiazepine plus sufentanil with ketamine attenuates or eliminates the unwanted tachycardia and hypertension and postoperative psychological derangements. With this technique, there are minimal hemodynamic perturbations, profound analgesia, dependable amnesia, and an uneventful convalescence. The use of propofol plus small-dose ketamine also has gained increasing popularity as a total IV anesthesia technique for patients undergoing noncardiac surgery. The advantages of this combination are maintenance of stable hemodynamics and minimal ventilatory depression when allowing spontaneous ventilation.

Pain Management

Postoperative pain is a major concern of many patients and inadequately treated in as many as 30% to 50% of all postoperative patients. Multimodal analgesia combining various analgesic agents that act through different pathways is the way to manage postoperative pain. Ketamine is increasingly used as one of the constituents of this multimodal analgesia therapy. Over the years the ketamine dose used for perioperative analgesia has gradually been decreasing. Ketamine administered in small doses decreases postoperative analgesic consumption by 33%. Several meta-analyses of the use of small-dose ketamine (20 to 60 mg) perioperatively have been performed. These meta-analyses showed an overall decrease in opiate use or improved analgesia and a decrease in opiate-induced side effects, especially PONV. Side effects, especially psychomimetic effects, were minimal, especially if a benzodiazepine also was administered.

The epidural/caudal administration of ketamine (0.5 to 1 mg/kg) is effective. Although the efficacy of these doses of ketamine seems to be established, the safety of this technique has not yet received regulatory approval. The preservative of racemic mixture is potentially neurotoxic, whereas studies to date indicate preservative-free S(+) ketamine may be safe. Epidural preservative-free S(+) ketamine has been shown to be safe and of value in adjunct to corticosteroids in patients for the treatment of chronic low back pain secondary to radiculopathy.[292] The favorable hemodynamic effects and conservation of respiration makes intravenously and even intranasally administered ketamine useful for analgesia after extremity fractures.

The action of ketamine on opiate tolerance and hyperalgesia combined with its direct analgesic activity has led to its use in chronic pain states. Ketamine may be effective in the treatment of cancer pain, chronic peripheral and central neuropathic pain, phantom and ischemic limb pain, fibromyalgia, complex regional pain syndrome, visceral pain, and migraine. Multiple open-label studies conclude positively on the analgesic properties of ketamine in cancer pain. Randomized controlled trials, though, so far could not prove a clinical benefit of ketamine for this indication.[293] Thus, while ketamine is effective for relief of postoperative pain, causing reduced opioid consumption, ketamine for most other indications appears to have limited efficacy and results in no beneficial effects.

BOX 23.3 Uses and Doses of Ketamine

Induction of general anesthesia*	0.5-2 mg/kg IV 4-6 mg/kg IM
Maintenance of general anesthesia	0.5-1 mg/kg IV with N_2O 50% in O_2 15-45 μg/kg/min IV with N_2O 50%-70% in O_2 30-90 μg/kg/min IV without N_2O
Sedation and analgesia	0.2-0.8 mg/kg IV over 2-3 min 2-4 mg/kg IM
Preemptive or preventive analgesia	0.15-0.25 mg/kg IV

*Lower doses are used if adjuvant drugs such as midazolam or thiopental also are given. *IM*, Intramuscular; *IV*, intravenous; *N_2O*, nitrous oxide.
From Reves JG, Glass P, Lubarsky DA, et al. Intravenous anesthetics. In: Miller RD, Eriksson LI, Fleischer LA, et al, eds. *Miller's Anesthesia*, 7th ed. Philadelphia: Churchill Livingstone; 2010: 719–768.

Sedation

Often, ketamine is combined with premedication of a barbiturate or benzodiazepine and an antisialagogue (e.g., glycopyrrolate) to facilitate management. The premedications reduce the dose requirement for ketamine, and the antisialagogue reduces the sometimes troublesome salivation. In adults and children, ketamine can be used as a supplement or an adjunct to regional anesthesia, extending the usefulness of the primary (local anesthetic) form of anesthesia. Also, in the emergency department ketamine is increasingly used for short painful procedures. The dose used then is between 0.1 to 0.6 mg/kg. As previously described, ketamine also may be considered for sedation of patients in a critical care unit because of its combined sedative and analgesic properties and favorable effects on hemodynamics. Ketamine can even be used safely in head injury patients when they are adequately ventilated.[294,295]

Ketamine is particularly suitable for sedation of pediatric patients undergoing procedures outside of the operating room. Pediatric patients have fewer adverse emergence reactions than adults, and this feature makes the use of ketamine in pediatric patients more versatile.

Doses and Routes of Administration

Ketamine has been administered intravenously, intramuscularly, transcutaneously, orally, nasally, and rectally, and as a preservative-free solution epidurally or intrathecally. Most clinical use involves the IV and intramuscular (IM) routes, by which the drug rapidly achieves therapeutic concentrations. The dose depends on the desired therapeutic effect and on the route of administration. Box 23.3 contains general recommended doses for the IV and IM administration of ketamine for various therapeutic goals. Intranasal administration has an onset closer to IV administration; an oral dose of 3 to 10 mg/kg generates a sedative effect in 20 to 45 minutes. For sedation, ketamine may be given in an IM dose of 2 to 4 mg/kg. It also has been administered orally in doses of 3 to 10 mg/kg, with 6 mg/kg providing optimal conditions in 20 to 25 minutes in one study and 10 mg/kg providing sedation in 87% of children within 45 minutes in another study.

Side Effects and Contraindications

Contraindications to ketamine relate to specific pharmacologic actions and patient diseases. In patients with increased ICP and breathing spontaneously, ketamine should be used with caution because it can increase ICP and has been reported to cause apnea. There is increasing clinical use of ketamine in emergency airway management in brain injury patients with or without other body injuries. In this setting, the current knowledge on safe management of increased ICP is continuing to grow.[294,295]

In mechanically ventilated patients, ketamine retains the response of CBF to carbon dioxide, which makes it useful in head-injured patients because of its potential neuroprotective effect. Ketamine may be contraindicated in patients with an open eye injury or other ophthalmologic disorder, in which a ketamine induced increase in intraocular pressure would be detrimental. Because ketamine has a propensity to cause hypertension and tachycardia, with a commensurate increase in myocardial oxygen consumption, it may be contraindicated as the sole anesthetic in patients with ischemic heart disease. Likewise, it is unwise to give ketamine to patients with vascular aneurysms because of the possible sudden change in arterial blood pressure. Psychiatric disease, such as schizophrenia, and a history of adverse reaction to ketamine or one of its congeners also are contraindications. One also should consider carefully using ketamine when there is a possibility of postoperative delirium from other causes (e.g., delirium tremens, possibility of head trauma), and a ketamine-induced psychomimetic effect would confuse the differential diagnosis.

As mentioned earlier, ketamine or other NMDA receptor antagonists accentuate apoptosis in the newborn brain of animals, and the clinical implications of this are unknown. Finally, because ketamine's preservative—chlorobutanol—is neurotoxic, this formulation of ketamine for subarachnoid or epidural administration is contraindicated. S(+) ketamine is available in a preservative-free solution. The FDA has not approved the use of intrathecal or epidural ketamine. Caudal ketamine has been used for perioperative analgesia in children and neonates with 0.5 mg/kg as the optimal dose. Caudal analgesia, by combinations of ketamine and a local anesthetic, prolongs analgesia from 2.26 to 5.3 hours and reduces the need for nonopioid analgesics.[296-300]

Lastly, liver and renal toxicity occurs in the recreational abuse of ketamine. In addition, when ketamine is repeatedly administered in the treatment of chronic pain in patients with complex regional pain syndrome type 1 (CRPS), hepatotoxicity developed in patients that received two 100-hour infusions of S(+)-ketamine with a 16-day interval.[298,301,302]

Etomidate

HISTORY

The first report on etomidate was published in 1965.[303] Etomidate was introduced into clinical practice in 1972. The unique properties of etomidate include hemodynamic stability, minimal respiratory depression, cerebral protection, favorable toxicity profile, and pharmacokinetics enabling rapid recovery after either a single dose or a continuous infusion. In the 1970s, these beneficial properties led to widespread use of etomidate for induction, for maintenance of anesthesia, and for prolonged sedation in critically

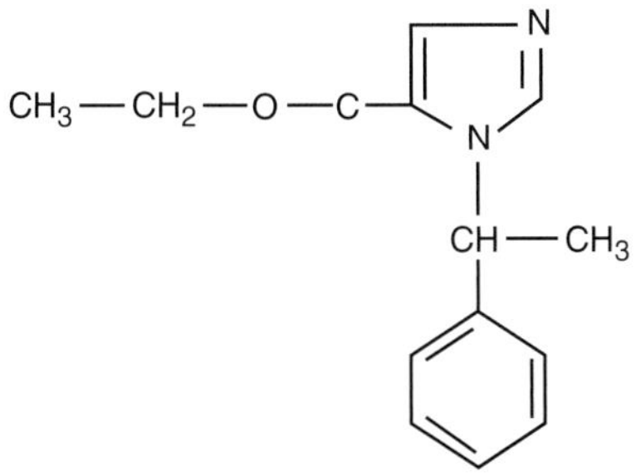

Fig. 23.16 **Structure of etomidate, an imidazole derivative.**

ill patients. The enthusiasm among clinicians for etomidate was tempered in the 1980s by reports that the drug can cause temporary inhibition of steroid synthesis after single doses and infusions.[304,305] This effect, combined with other minor disadvantages (e.g., pain on injection, superficial thrombophlebitis, myoclonus, and a frequent incidence of nausea and vomiting), led to several editorials questioning the role of etomidate in modern anesthetic practice.[306,307] Use of the drug decreased after those editorials, but its use has expanded again as a result of the rediscovery of etomidate's beneficial physiologic profile and a widening use in emergency departments and intensive care departments, combined with a lack of novel reports describing clinically significant adrenocortical suppression after induction or brief duration infusions.

PHYSICOCHEMICAL CHARACTERISTICS

Etomidate is an imidazole derivative (R-(+)-pentylethyl-1H-imidazole-5 carboxylate sulfate). Its chemical structure is illustrated in Fig. 23.16. Etomidate has a pK_a of 4.2 and is hydrophobic at physiologic pH. To increase its solubility it is formulated as a 0.2% solution either in 35% propylene glycol (Amidate; Hospira Inc., Lafe Forest, IL) or in a lipid emulsion (Etomidate-Lipuro; B. Braun, Melsungen, Germany).[308]

PHARMACOKINETICS

The pharmacokinetics of etomidate have been determined after single bolus doses and after continuous infusion. The time course of plasma disappearance after a 0.3 mg/kg bolus is shown in Fig. 23.17. The pharmacokinetics of etomidate are best described by an open three-compartment model.[309]

The drug has an initial distribution half-life of 2.7 minutes, a redistribution half-life of 29 minutes, and an elimination half-life of 2.9 to 5.3 hours.[310] Clearance of etomidate by the liver is high (18-25 mL/kg/min), with a hepatic extraction ratio of 0.5 ± 0.9.[309] Because redistribution is the mechanism whereby the effect after a bolus of etomidate is dissipated (Box 23.4), hepatic dysfunction should not appreciably alter recovery from a single induction dose. Etomidate is 75% protein bound.

A hemorrhagic shock model in pigs bled to a MAP of 50 mm Hg did not alter etomidate pharmacokinetics or pharmacodynamics.[311] This finding contrasts with the marked changes seen in this same model with other IV anesthetics. In patients with cirrhosis, the volume of distribution is doubled, whereas clearance is normal; the result is an elimination half-life that is twice normal.[312] The initial distribution

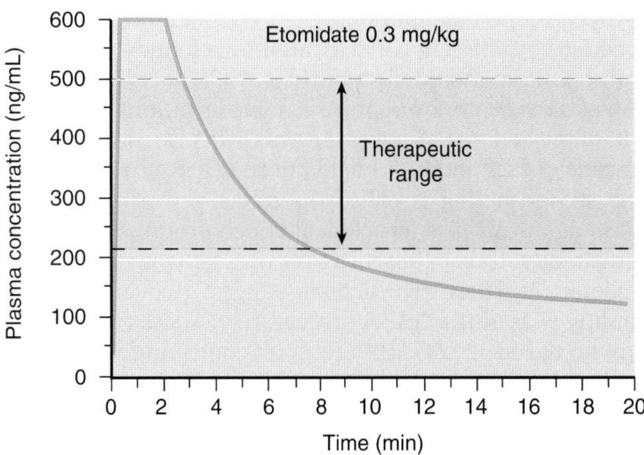

Fig. 23.17 Simulated time course of plasma levels of etomidate after an induction dose of 0.3 mg/kg. Plasma levels required for hypnosis during surgery are 300 to 500 ng/mL, with awakening usually occurring at levels less than 225 ng/mL.

BOX 23.4 Uses and Doses of Etomidate

Induction of general anesthesia	0.2-0.6 mg/kg IV
Sedation and analgesia	Limited to periods of brief sedation because of inhibition of corticosteroid synthesis

IV, Intravenous; *N_2O*, nitrous oxide.

From Reves JG, Glass P, Lubarsky DA, et al. Intravenous anesthetics. In Miller RD, Eriksson LI, Fleischer LA, et al, eds. *Miller's Anesthesia*, 7th ed. Philadelphia: Churchill Livingstone; 2010: 719–768.

half-life and clinical effect are likely unchanged. Increasing age is associated with a smaller initial volume of distribution and a decreased clearance of etomidate.[313]

The short elimination half-life and the rapid clearance of etomidate make it suitable for administration in a single dose, in multiple doses, or in a continuous infusion with its context sensitive half-time being shorter than that of propofol.[314] Continuous infusion was practiced in the first decade of its clinical availability, but the now widely recognized adrenal suppression limits this application. Etomidate is metabolized in the liver primarily by ester hydrolysis to the corresponding carboxylic acid of etomidate (major metabolite) and an ethanol leaving group.[315] The main metabolite is inactive. Only 2% of the drug is excreted unchanged, the remaining part being excreted as metabolites by the kidney (85%) and bile (13%). Pathologic conditions altering serum proteins (e.g., hepatic or renal disease) affect the amount of the free (unbound) fraction and may cause a dose to have an exaggerated pharmacodynamic effect.[316]

Pharmacodynamics

EFFECTS ON THE CENTRAL NERVOUS SYSTEM

The primary action of etomidate on the CNS is through the $GABA_A$ receptor and results in hypnosis,[317,318] which is achieved in one arm–brain circulation after a normal induction dose (0.3 mg/kg). The mechanism by which etomidate produces hypnosis is almost exclusively through

$GABA_A$ receptor facilitation.[318,319] This includes two effects produced by different concentrations of etomidate. The first is the positive modulation of the $GABA_A$ receptor: activation of the receptor by agonists at concentrations associated with clinical doses. A lower dose of GABA is required in the presence of etomidate to activate the $GABA_A$ receptor.[320] The second action is called the direct activation or allosteric agonism. In supraclinical concentrations etomidate can directly, thus in absence of GABA, activate the $GABA_A$ receptor.[321] These two actions suggest two independent binding sites at the $GABA_A$ receptor.[318] These two binding sites on the $\alpha1\beta2\gamma2$ $GABA_A$ receptor contribute equally and non-cooperatively to drug interaction and gating effects. At a dose of 0.2 to 0.3 mg/kg, etomidate reduces CBF by 34% and $CMRO_2$ by 45% without altering MAP. CPP is maintained or increased, and there is a beneficial net increase in the cerebral oxygen supply-to-demand ratio.[322] Etomidate, given in doses sufficient to produce EEG burst suppression, acutely decreases ICP by 50% in patients with already increased ICP, returning increased ICP to almost normal values.[323] The decrease in ICP is maintained in the period immediately after intubation. To maintain the effects of etomidate on ICP, high infusion rates (60 μg/kg/min) are necessary. Controversy remains on the neuroprotective qualities of etomidate. There is a dose-dependent increase in latency and a decreasing amplitude of the auditory evoked potentials.[324]

Preliminary animal experiments suggest that in a case of acute fetal distress and hypoxic injury propofol and midazolam may be preferred over etomidate to protect the fetal brain as the first choice anesthetic in cesarean delivery.[199,325,326] Etomidate has been associated with grand mal seizures and produces increased EEG activity in epileptogenic foci. This feature has proven useful for intraoperative mapping of seizure foci before surgical ablation.[327,328] BIS monitor values decrease after etomidate bolus administration and return to baseline during recovery.[329] During etomidate infusion, the BIS values reliably predict the depth of sedation and hypnosis.[330]

Effects on the Respiratory System

Etomidate has less effect on ventilation than other anesthetics used to induce anesthesia. It does not induce histamine release in healthy patients or in patients with reactive airway disease.[331] Ventilatory response to carbon dioxide is depressed by etomidate, but the ventilatory drive at any given carbon dioxide tension is greater than that following an equipotent dose of methohexital.[153] Induction with etomidate produces a brief period of hyperventilation, sometimes followed by a similarly brief period of apnea,[332] which results in a slight (±15%) increase in $PaCO_2$, but no change in the partial pressure of arterial oxygen (PaO_2).[333] Etomidate's action on pulmonary vascular tone is similar to the actions observed with ketamine and propofol; that is, they attenuate the vasorelaxant responses to acetylcholine and bradykinine.[334]

Effects on the Cardiovascular System

The hemodynamic stability seen with etomidate is due to its lack of effect on the sympathetic nervous system and on the function of the baroreceptor. The effect of etomidate on the $\alpha2$-adrenoceptors generates an increase in blood pressure in vivo; this may contribute to the cardiovascular stability after induction of anesthesia. The minimal effect of etomidate on cardiovascular function sets it apart from other rapid-onset anesthetics.[335,336] Etomidate has proven useful in patients with valvular or ischemic heart disease undergoing noncardiac surgery and in patients with poor cardiac function.[337,338] In patients receiving etomidate during induction of anesthesia, more hypertension and tachycardia occurs after etomidate compared to propofol.[339] The myocardial oxygen supply-to-demand ratio is well maintained.[340] Etomidate lacks analgesic efficacy, however, and needs to be combined with an opiate to prevent hemodynamic perturbations during laryngoscopy and intubation.

In the setting of a hemorrhagic shock, etomidate provides advantages for induction of anesthesia. In contrast to other drugs, in a pig model of hemorrhagic shock the pharmacodynamics and pharmacokinetics of etomidate were minimally altered.[311]

Endocrine Effects

In 1983 Ledingham and Watt reported retrospective data showing increased mortality among intensive care patients receiving long-term etomidate infusion compared to patients receiving benzodiazepines.[304] They postulated that adrenal cortical suppression could be the cause of this increased mortality.

Soon after this publication, clinical investigators confirmed the adrenocortical suppression by etomidate.[305,341]

The specific endocrine effects manifested by etomidate are a dose-dependent reversible inhibition of the enzyme 11β-hydroxylase, which results in decreased biosynthesis of cortisol. The blockade of the cytochrome P450-dependent enzyme 11β-hydroxylase also results in decreased mineralocorticoid production and an increased formation of intermediaries (11-deoxycorticosterone) (Fig. 23.18). Subsequent research showed that etomidate is far more potent as an inhibitor of steroid synthesis than as a sedative hypnotic agent.[341,342] The etomidate concentrations associated with adrenal cortical suppression are less than 10 ng/mL, which are much lower than the concentrations needed for hypnosis (more than 200 ng/mL). The disparate concentrations for hypnosis and adrenotoxicity may explain the dramatic difference in duration of these two actions.[57]

The concerns about the use of etomidate and etomidate-induced adrenal toxicity in critically ill patients is still a matter of strong debate in the critical care community. A Cochrane review in 2015 of single-dose etomidate versus other induction agents for endotracheal intubation in critically ill patients reveals no conclusive evidence that etomidate increases mortality.[343] As indicated earlier, etomidate is associated with suppression of adrenal steroidogenesis, which can last up to 72 hours. However, the clinical impact of this adrenal suppressive effect is not certain.[344]

The Corticosteroid Therapy of Septic Shock (CORTICUS) study followed 500 patients with septic shock, who were randomized to receive either low-dose corticosteroid therapy or placebo. Twenty percent of the patients received etomidate. The study concluded that there was no benefit of low-dose corticosteroid therapy to long-term outcome.[345] Retrospective analyses of the CORTICUS population suggest that patients receiving etomidate before enrollment

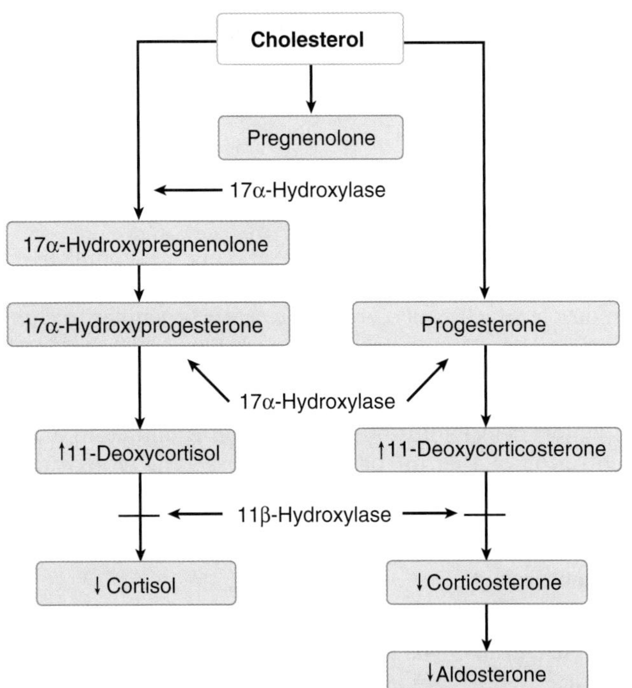

Fig. 23.18 Pathway for the biosynthesis of cortisol and aldosterone. The sites at which etomidate affects cortisol-aldosterone synthesis by its action on 11β-hydroxylase (major site) and 17α-hydroxylase (minor site) are illustrated.

had a 28-day mortality significantly higher and that steroid supplements provided no benefit.[346,347] Other studies designed to evaluate the effect of etomidate on morbidity and mortality and hospital and ICU length of stay are not conclusive.[348-351] In conclusion, the impact of the use of a single dose of etomidate in critically ill patients remains unclear.

Uses

INDUCTION OF ANESTHESIA

The induction dose of etomidate is 0.2 to 0.6 mg/kg.[352] The induction dose is reduced by premedication with an opiate, a benzodiazepine, or a barbiturate. Onset of anesthesia after a routine induction dose of 0.3 mg/kg of etomidate is rapid (one arm–brain circulation). Various infusion schemes have been devised to use etomidate as a maintenance anesthetic for the hypnotic component of anesthesia in the past. After the publications on the adrenocortical suppressive effects of etomidate, continuous infusion has been abandoned.

Etomidate is most appropriate in patients with cardiovascular disease, reactive airway disease, intracranial hypertension, or any combination of disorders indicating the need for an induction agent with limited or beneficial physiologic side effects. The hemodynamic stability of etomidate is unique among the rapid onset anesthetics used to induce anesthesia. In multiple studies, etomidate has been used for induction in patients with a compromised cardiovascular system who are undergoing coronary artery bypass surgery or valve surgery, and in patients requiring induction of general anesthesia for percutaneous transluminal coronary angioplasty, aortic aneurysm repair, and thoracic surgery. For cardioversion, the rapid onset, quick recovery, and maintenance of arterial blood pressure in these sometimes hemodynamically tenuous patients, combined with continued spontaneous respiration, make etomidate an acceptable choice.[353] Etomidate has been successfully used in neurosurgical procedures such as giant aneurysm clippings, making it a reasonable choice during neurosurgical induction.[354] In addition, etomidate should be considered as an anesthetic induction agent to reduce increased ICP when maintenance of cerebral or coronary perfusion pressure is also important.

Trauma patients with questionable intravascular volume status may be well served by an induction of anesthesia with etomidate. When using etomidate in trauma patients, loss of consciousness by itself can be associated with decreased adrenergic output, and controlled ventilation can exacerbate the cardiovascular effects of a decreased preload. Both of these factors may cause a significant decrease in arterial blood pressure during induction of anesthesia despite etomidate having no direct cardiovascular drug effect.

Short-term sedation with etomidate is useful in hemodynamically unstable patients, such as patients requiring cardioversion or patients requiring sedation after an acute myocardial infarction or with unstable angina for a minor operative procedure.[353] When used during electroconvulsive therapy, etomidate can produce longer seizures compared with other hypnotics.[355,356] Induction of anesthesia with etomidate is an independent risk factor in the development of an emergence delirium.[357]

Treatment in Hypercortisolemia

Etomidate has a special place in the treatment of endogenous hypercortisolemia. It is proven to be an effective parenteral treatment for this indication. In patients with unstable hemodynamics, patients with a sepsis, or patients with a psychosis, treatment should be performed under intensive care conditions.[358]

Side Effects

Although etomidate provides stable hemodynamics and minimal respiratory depression, it is associated with several adverse effects when used for induction, including PONV, pain on injection, myoclonic movement, and hiccups. More recently, etomidate in a lipid emulsion was associated with an equal or an increased incidence of postoperative nausea compared with propofol.[359-361]

The lipid formulation of etomidate is associated with a much less frequent incidence of pain on injection, thrombophlebitis, and histamine release.[362,363] Pain on injection may be reduced by injecting lidocaine, 20 to 40 mg immediately before injection of etomidate.

The incidence of muscle movement (myoclonus) and of hiccups is highly variable (0%-70%), but myoclonus is reduced by premedication with a hypnotic like midazolam or a small dose of magnesium 60 to 90 seconds before the induction dose of etomidate is given.[364,365]

Novel Etomidate Derivatives

Etomidate is a well-known and widely used anesthetic for induction of anesthesia. The limitations of etomidate are, as mentioned earlier, adrenocortical suppression, myoclonus, and PONV. Modifying etomidate could improve its clinical utility and produce etomidate derivatives with a better profile. Methoxycarbonyl etomidate (MOC) is an etomidate derivative and is rapidly metabolized to methoxycarbonyl etomidate carboxylic acid (MOC-ECA). MOC has almost equal hypnotic potency as etomidate, and the duration of the induced anesthesia is short due to rapid metabolization by nonspecific esterase enzymes. In preclinical studies MOC may not act as an inhibitor of adrenal steroid synthesis.[366] The accumulation of metabolites, leading to delayed recovery, makes it less than ideal for infusion.

Carboetomidate, another derivative, contains a five-membered pyrrole ring instead of an imidazole. In tadpoles and rats, carboetomidate reduces the adrenal suppression potency by three orders. Carboetomidate has potent hypnotic properties by activating $GABA_A$ receptors, which causes minimal hemodynamic changes.[367] Another potential benefit is its inhibition of the 5-HT3 receptor in a rat model; carboetomidate may have decreased emetogenic properties.

Another etomidate derivative, methoxycarbonyl-carboetomidate (MOC-carboetomidate), combines the favorable effects with no adrenal suppression and potency of the parent compound, but has a longer duration of action and makes it disadvantageous for longer infusions.

Cyclopropyl-methoxycarbonyl metomidate (CPMM) and dimethyl-methoxycarbonyl metomidate (DMMM) are the newest derivatives of etomidate. They have a higher potency and fast recovery time after infusion duration of 2 hours. So far, they are most promising in animal studies and inflammatory sepsis models.

Dexmedetomidine

HISTORY

The α_2-adrenergic receptor agonists have sedative, anxiolytic, hypnotic, analgesic, and sympatholytic effects. Its potential for use in anesthesia was recognized in patients who were treated with clonidine.[368] Soon a reduction of the minimum alveolar concentration (MAC) of halothane by clonidine was described.[369] Dexmedetomidine is a more selective α_2-agonist with a selectivity ratio for the α_2-receptor compared with the α_1-receptor of 1600:1, as compared to a ratio of 220:1 for clonidine. It was introduced in clinical practice in the United States in 1999 and approved by the FDA only as a short-term (<24 hours) sedative for mechanically ventilated adult ICU patients. Dexmedetomidine is used for prolonged sedation and anxiolysis in the ICU, as well as outside of the ICU in various settings, including sedation and adjunct analgesia in the operating room, sedation in diagnostic and procedure units, and for other applications such as withdrawal/detoxification amelioration in adult and pediatric patients.[370,371]

PHYSICOCHEMICAL CHARACTERISTICS

Dexmedetomidine is the S-enantiomer of medetomidine, a substance that has been used for sedation and analgesia in veterinary medicine for many years.[372] It shows a high ratio of specificity for the α_2-receptor ($\alpha_2/\alpha_1 = 1600:1$) compared with clonidine ($\alpha_2/\alpha_1 = 220:1$), making it a complete α_2-agonist.[373] The pK_a is 7.1. Dexmedetomidine belongs to the imidazole subclass of α_2-receptor agonists, similar to clonidine, and its structure is illustrated in Fig. 23.19. It is freely soluble in water and available as a clear isotonic solution containing 100 μg per mL and 9 mg sodium chloride per mL of water. Before infusion, this solution is diluted to a concentration of 4 μg/mL or 8 μg/mL by adding either saline, 5% glucose, mannitol, or Ringer lactate solution. It is not to be combined with amfoteracine B, amfoteracine B in liposomes, diazepam, phenytoin, gemtuzumab, irinotecan, or pantoprazole.

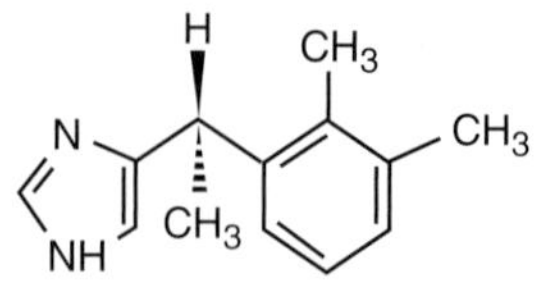

Fig. 23.19 Chemical structure of dexmedetomidine.

METABOLISM AND PHARMACOKINETICS

Dexmedetomidine undergoes almost complete biotransformation with very little unchanged dexmedetomidine excreted in urine and feces. Biotransformation involves both direct glucuronidation as well as cytochrome P450–mediated metabolism. The major metabolic pathways of dexmedetomidine are: direct N-glucuronidation to inactive metabolites, hydroxylation (mediated primarily by CYP2A6), and N-methylation. Polymorphism in CYP2A6 does not influence clinical dosing regimens.[374] Dexmedetomidine is 94% protein bound, and its concentration ratio between whole blood and plasma is 0.66. Dexmedetomidine has effects on cardiovascular variables, potentially causing bradycardia, transient hypertension or hypotension, and may alter its own pharmacokinetics. With large doses, there is marked vasoconstriction, which probably reduces the drug's volumes of distribution. The observed hypertension may be avoided by decreasing the loading dose or by increasing the time of administration.

In essence, dexmedetomidine displays nonlinear pharmacokinetics.[375] Its pharmacokinetics in volunteers are best described by a three-compartment model (see Table 23.1). Many subsequent studies in various patient populations have investigated the clinical pharmacokinetics and pharmacodynamics, the results of which are reviewed and summarized by Weerink and colleagues.[376] One of the findings is that the bodyweight adjustment dosing that is currently applied is only justified in a non-obese population. For obese patients, fat-free mass may be more appropriate, but this is still subject to investigation.

In subjects with varying degrees of hepatic impairment (Child-Pugh Class A, B, or C), clearance values for dexmedetomidine are slower than in healthy subjects. The mean clearance values for patients with mild, moderate, and severe hepatic impairment are 74%, 64%, and 53% of those observed in the normal healthy subjects, respectively.

The pharmacokinetics of dexemedetomidine are not influenced by renal impairment (creatinine clearance <30 mL/min) or age. In patients with severe renal disease, the sedative effect may be stronger, due to a lower

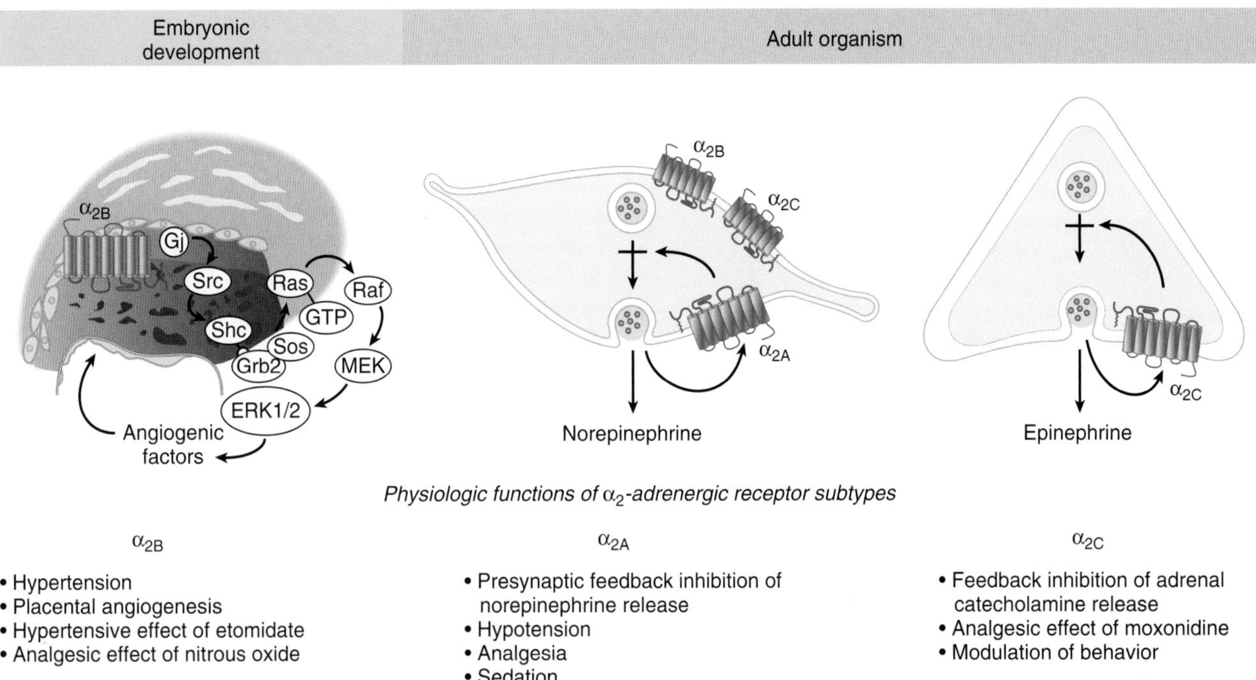

Fig. 23.20 The different physiologic functions of α2 adrenoreceptors. The top panel depicts the three α2 receptor subtypes acting as presynaptic inhibitory feedback receptors to control the release of norepinephrine and epinephrine from peripheral or central adult neurons. Also, a negative feedback loop has been seen in the adrenal gland. Alpha2B receptors have been involved in the development of the placental vascular system during prenatal development. The lower panel lists a series of physiologic effects with its associated α2 adrenoreceptors. (From Paris A, Tonner PH. Dexmedetomidine in anaesthesia. *Curr Opin Anaesthesiol.* 2005;18:412-418.)

degree of plasma protein binding. Clearance is a function of height.[375,377] The elimination half-life of dexmedetomidine is 2 to 3 hours, with a context-sensitive half-time ranging from 4 minutes after a 10-minute infusion to 250 minutes after an 8-hour infusion. Postoperative patients sedated with dexmedetomidine display similar pharmacokinetics to the pharmacokinetics seen in volunteers.[378] No clinically relevant cytochrome P450–mediated drug interaction has been found.

PHARMACOLOGY

Dexmedetomidine acts as a nonselective α_2-agonist on membrane bound G-protein coupled α_2-adrenoreceptors. Intracellular pathways include inhibition of adenylate cyclase and modulation of calcium and potassium ion channels. Three subtypes of α_2 adrenoreceptors have been described in humans: α_{2A}, α_{2B}, and α_{2C} (Fig. 23.20).[379] The α_{2A} adrenoreceptors are primarily distributed in the periphery, whereas α_{2B} and α_{2C} are in the brain and spinal cord. Postsynaptically located α_2 adrenoreceptors in peripheral blood vessels produce vasoconstriction, whereas presynaptic α_2 adrenoreceptors inhibit the release of norepinephrine, potentially attenuating the vasoconstriction. The overall response to α_2 adrenoreceptor agonists is related to the stimulation of α_2 adrenoreceptors located in the CNS and spinal cord. These receptors are involved in the sympatholysis, sedation, and antinociceptive effects of α_2 adrenoreceptors.[380] The α_2 agonists have the advantage that their effects are readily reversible by α_2-adrenergic antagonists (e.g., atipamezole).[381] Atipamezole is currently not approved for use in humans.

Effects on the Central Nervous System

SEDATION

The α_2 agonists produce their sedative-hypnotic effect by an action on α_2 receptors in the locus caeruleus and an analgesic action at α_2 receptors within the locus caeruleus and within the spinal cord.[382] Dexmedetomidine produces a decrease in activity of the projections of the locus caeruleus to the ventrolateral preoptic nucleus. As a result GABAergic and galanin release in the tuberomammillary nucleus is increased, producing a decrease in histamine release in cortical and subcortical projections.[383] The α_2 agonists inhibit ion conductance through L-type or P-type calcium channels and facilitate conductance through voltage-gated calcium-activated potassium channels. Dexmedetomidine induces sedation through different receptors than the sedative drugs propofol or benzodiazepines, which exert their action through the GABA system. The sedative effect of dexmedetomidine acts through the endogenous sleep-promoting pathways, generating natural sleep patterns (Fig. 23.21).[384] Patients have been described as being very easy to wake up and having the ability to follow commands and cooperate while being tracheally intubated. Undisturbed, patients were noted to fall asleep momentarily.[385] This characteristic allows for "daily wake up" tests to be done in a safe fashion. This critical test—when ventilated ICU patients are taken off all sedatives to assess their mental status and titrate sedation—shortens their ventilated and ICU length of stay.[386,387] The plasma concentration at which significant yet rousable sedation is achieved is about

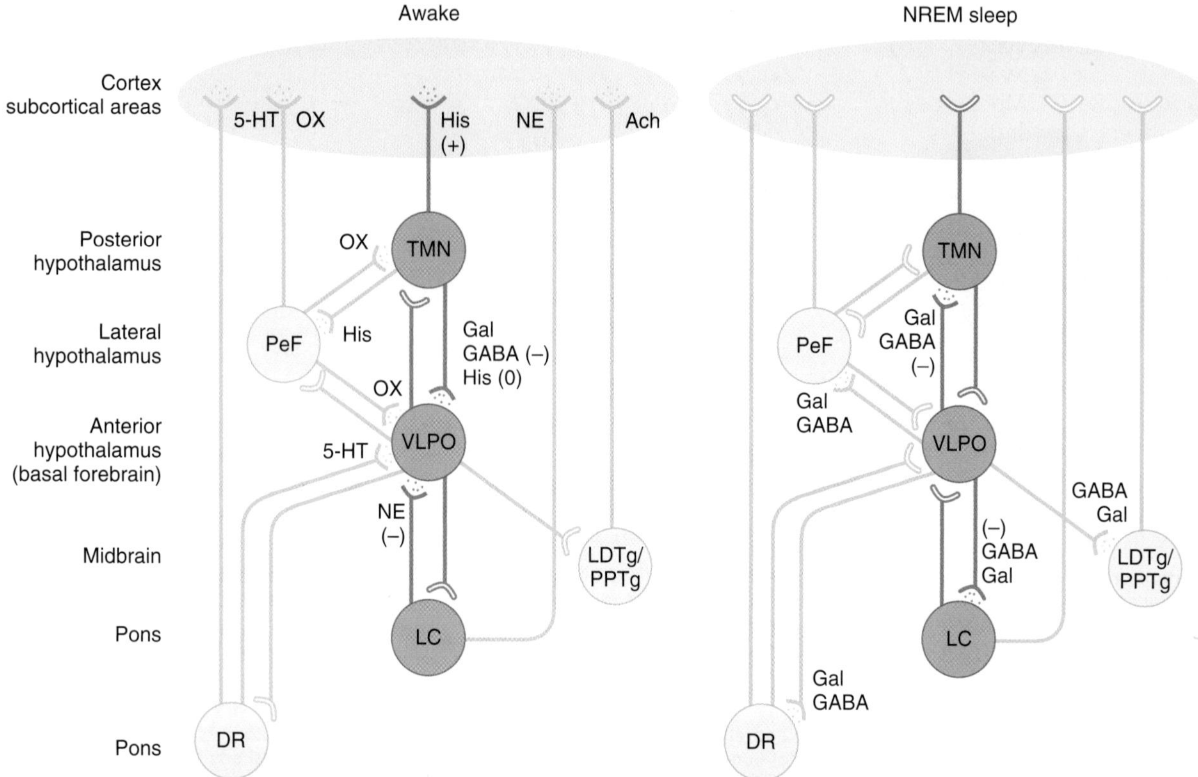

Fig. 23.21 Dexmedetomidine has been shown to induce a non–rapid eye movement sleeping pattern *(NREM)*. The stimulation of the locus caeruleus *(LC)* by dexmedetomidine (right diagram) releases the inhibition the LC has over the ventrolateral preoptic nucleus *(VLPO)*. The VLPO subsequently releases γ-aminobutyric acid *(GABA)* onto the tuberomammillary nucleus *(TMN)*. This inhibits the release of the arousal-promoting histamine on the cortex and forebrain, inducing the loss of consciousness. (From Ebert T, Maze M. Dexmedetomidine: another arrow for the clinician's quiver. *Anesthesiology*. 2004;101:569–570.)

0.2 to 0.3 ng/mL. Unarousable deep sedation is thought to occur at plasma concentrations above 1.9 ng/mL.[388]

The number of patients experiencing delirium in the ICU is significantly lower when sedated with dexmedetomidine, compared to propofol or lorazepam,[389] or midazolam.[390]

Although the precise mechanism by which dexmedetomidine preserves cognition is still unclear, there are data that suggest that the suppression of α5 γ-aminobutyric acid type A receptor expression after exposition to an anesthetic may play a role.[391]

ANALGESIA

The analgesic effect of the α_2 agonists is mediated through stimulation of the α_{2C} and α_{2A} receptor in the dorsal horn, directly suppressing pain transmission by reducing the release of pronociceptive transmitters, substance P and glutamate, and hyperpolarization of interneurons.[392] Systemic use of dexmedetomidine has an opioid sparing effect during surgery and postoperatively.[393] This is advantageous in patients who are prone to postoperative apnea or hypoventilation, as with patients undergoing bariatric surgery.[394] In the postoperative ICU setting, narcotic requirements are reduced by 50% when patients are receiving a dexmedetomidine drip compared with placebo.[385] During general anesthesia, it reduces the MAC of inhaled anesthetics.[395,396]

Like clonidine, dexmedetomidine is frequently used as an adjuvant in central or peripheral neural blockade. When administered caudally, 1 μg/kg as adjuvant to bupivacaine 0.25% 1 mL/kg, in children undergoing inguinal hernia repair, response to hernial sac traction is reduced and postoperative analgesia is prolonged.[397] Dexmedetomidine has been investigated in volunteers when administered as an adjuvant to ropivacaine in ulnar nerve block[398] and tibial nerve block.[399] Both studies showed intensification and foremost prolongation of the sensory blockade. This effect is likely elicited by prolonged hyperpolarization of the unmyelinated C-fibers (sensory), and to a lesser extent of the A-fibers (motor function).

Central Nervous System Protection and Other Central Nervous System Effects

The CNS protective effects are not well defined. Dexmedetomidine in animal models of incomplete cerebral ischemia and reperfusion reduces cerebral necrosis and improves neurologic outcome. The prevalent idea is that dexmedetomidine reduces the intracerebral catecholamine outflow during injury. The neuroprotection may be attributed to modulation of proapoptotic and antiapoptotic proteins.[400] Also, the reduction of the excitatory neurotransmitter glutamate during injury may explain some of the protective effects.[401]

In patients undergoing transsphenoidal hypophysectomy, dexmedetomidine has no effect on lumbar cerebral fluid pressure.[402] In other studies, CBF velocity at the middle cerebral artery, as measured by transcranial Doppler, decreased with increasing concentrations of dexmedetomidine but CO_2 responsiveness and autoregulation were preserved.[403,404] The decrease in CBF is not accompanied by a reduction in $CRMO_2$. More recently, in a study in six normal volunteers, the administration of dexmedetomidine to achieve serum levels of 0.6 ng/mL and 1.2 ng/mL (with and without hyperventilation) produced the predicted reduction of CBF with a concomitant reduction in $CRMO_2$.[405] This finding suggests that on the maintenance of the cerebral oxygen supply-to-demand relationship, further work in injured brains needs to be done.

Dexmedetomidine has been used in neurosurgical procedures involving neurophysiologic monitoring. Cortical evoked potentials, amplitudes, and latencies were minimally affected when using dexmedetomidine intraoperatively. It may also be suitable as an anesthetic adjunct during seizure surgery, since the epileptiform activity of seizure foci was not reduced by dexmedotomidine.[406]

EFFECTS ON THE RESPIRATORY SYSTEM

In spontaneous breathing volunteers, dexmedetomidine at concentrations producing significant sedation reduces minute ventilation, but results in no change in arterial oxygenation, pH, or the slope in the CO_2 ventilatory response curve. In a study comparing the effects of remifentanil and dexmedetomidine on respiratory parameters in normal volunteers, the hypercapnic ventilatory response was unaffected even at doses that produced unresponsiveness to vigorous stimulation.[407] Dexmedetomidine exhibited a hypercarbic arousal phenomenon, which has been described during normal sleep.

EFFECTS ON THE CARDIOVASCULAR SYSTEM

Ebert and colleagues performed a study in volunteers using a target-controlled infusion system to provide increasing concentrations (0.7 to 15 ng/mL) of dexmedetomidine (Fig. 23.22). The lowest two concentrations produced a decrease in MAP (13%) followed by progressive increase (12%). Increasing concentrations of dexmedetomidine also produce progressive decreases in heart rate (maximum 29%) and cardiac output (35%). The most commonly reported hemodynamic adverse reactions associated with dexmedetomidine in a phase III trial in 401 patients were hypotension (30%), hypertension (12%), and bradycardia (9%).[372] The initial increase in arterial blood pressure is probably due to the vasoconstrictive effects of dexmedetomidine

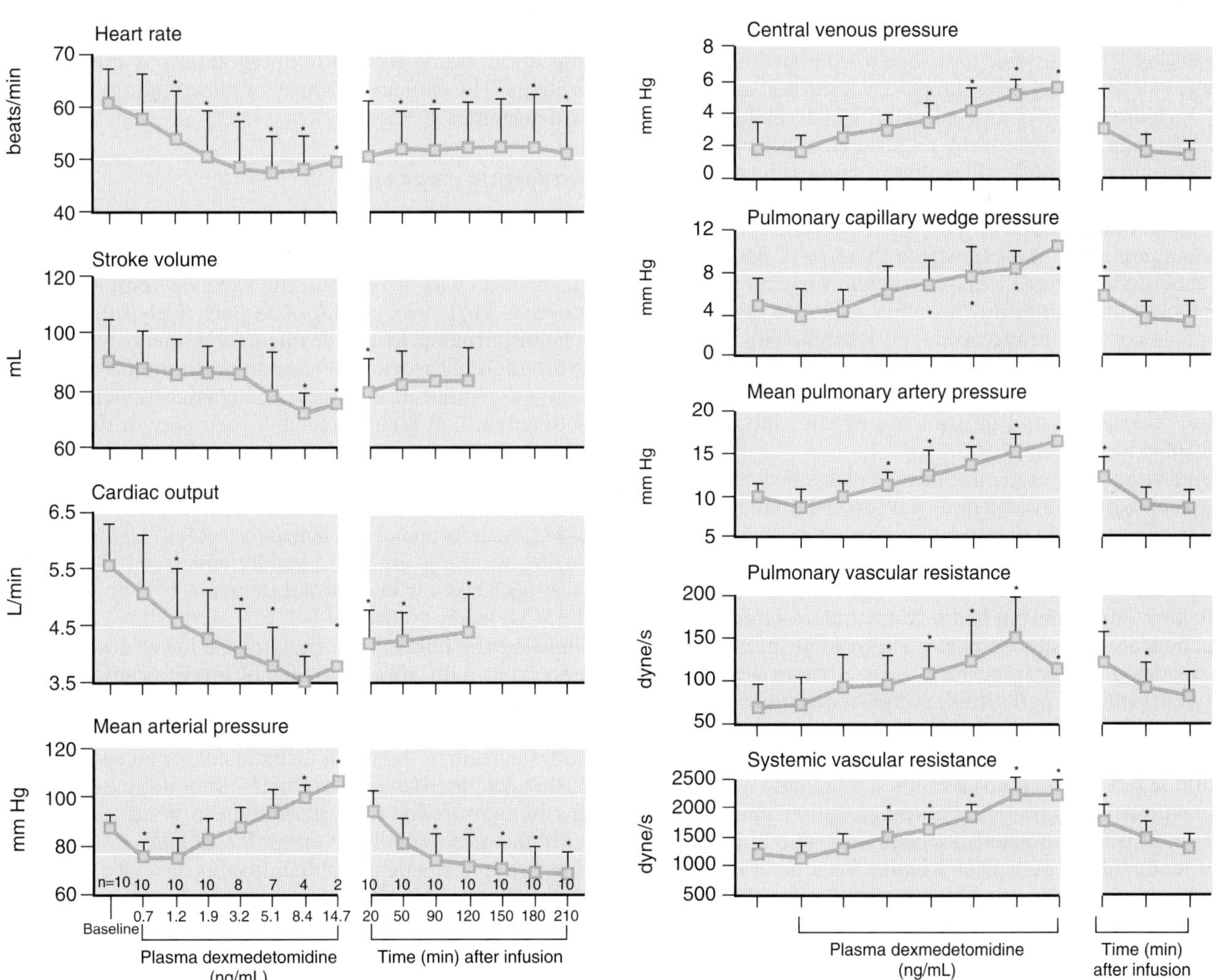

Fig. 23.22 Effects of increasing plasma concentrations of dexmedetomidine.

when stimulating peripheral α_2 receptors. The incidence of hypotension and bradycardia may be related to the administration of a large intravenous "loading" dose. Omitting the loading dose or not giving more than 0.4 μg/kg reduces the incidence of hypotension or makes it less pronounced. Giving the loading dose over 20 minutes also minimizes the transient hypertension.[408] In several studies after IM and IV administration, dexmedetomidine caused, in a small percentage of patients, profound bradycardia (<40 beats/min) and occasionally sinus arrest/pause. Generally, these episodes resolved spontaneously or were readily treated without adverse outcome by anticholinergics. No rebound effects have been found when discontinuing a dexmedetomidine infusion, even when it was given for more than 24 hours.[409] As clonidine and dexmedetomidine have shown to reduce perioperative oxygen consumption and blunt the sympathetic response to surgery, cardiac outcome may be improved.[410,411] However, more studies are needed to determine whether dexmedetomidine is beneficial in decreasing the risk of myocardial ischemia.

USES

Dexmedetomidine has been approved as a short-term sedative for adult intubated patients in the ICU. Given its well-documented beneficial effects of anxiolysis, sedation, analgesia, and sympatholysis with minimal respiratory depression, it also has been used in various other clinical scenarios. It is registered for use as a sedative during radiological or invasive procedures. Two studies, comprising 140 children 1 to 7 years old, reported successful sedation for MRI scans compared with midazolam or propofol.[412] For a thorough review of a wide range of studies on various procedures under sedation in different populations, we refer to Gerlach et al.[413]

As a premedicant, dexmedetomidine, at IV doses of 0.33 to 0.67 μg/kg given 15 minutes before surgery, seems efficacious, while minimizing the cardiovascular side effects of hypotension and bradycardia.[396] Dexmedetomidine has a high bioavailability when administered nasally or buccally. This improves compliance and absorption in younger children. A dose of 3 to 4 μg/kg 1 hour before surgery is safe and effective.

In a study comparing the efficacy of dexmedetomidine or propofol as a sedative agent in a group of 40 patients receiving local anesthesia or regional blocks, dexmedetomidine (1 μg/kg given over 10 minutes) when used for intraoperative sedation resulted in a slower onset than propofol (75 μg/kg/min for 10 minutes) but had similar cardiorespiratory effects when titrated to equal sedation. The average infusion rate of dexmedetomidine intraoperatively to maintain a BIS value of 70 to 80 was 0.7 μg/kg/min. Sedation was more prolonged after termination of the infusion, as was recovery of arterial blood pressure. Dexmedetomidine can also produce profound sedation, and it has been used as a total IV anesthetic when given at 10 times the normal sedation concentration range.[414] This characteristic, combined with the cooperative status of the patient at a lighter sedative level, and its analgesic effect with sparing of respiratory function, makes the drug suitable as a hypnotic during surgical procedures like awake craniotomy, deep brain stimulation, surgery near speech areas, or awake carotid endarterectomies, with fewer fluctuations from the desired sedation level and more stable hemodynamics.[403] A recent study shows that dexmedetomidine may be advantageous by improving the quality of emergence from general anaesthesia in avoiding coughing, agitation, hypertension, tachycardia, and shivering. This may be achieved by administration of dexmedetomidine 1 μg/kg intravenously at the end of surgery. Time to extubation is not prolonged.[415] The opioid-sparing effects are advantageous in the performance of bariatric surgery in patients who are prone to postoperative respiratory depression.[394]

Dexmedetomidine can be employed for addiction treatment; it has been described for use in rapid opioid detoxification, cocaine withdrawal, and iatrogenic-induced benzodiazepine and opioid tolerance after prolonged sedation.[416] The use in opioid/benzodiazepine withdrawal therapy in pediatric patients during mechanical ventilation in intensive care areas has been described as well.[417]

Dexmedetomidine may produce dry mouth due to a decrease in salivation. Combined with the sparing effect on respiratory function, this effect is beneficial for the facilitation of awake fiberoptic intubation, an application which is rapidly emerging.[418] Furthermore, dexmedetomidine decreases intraocular pressure and decreases the shivering threshold.[419]

The role of general anaesthesia in oncological surgery is still under debate. Studies of the in vitro and in vivo effects on lung carcinoma and neuroglioma cell lines have shown that dexmedetomidine enhanced cancer proliferation and migration, primarily by the upregulation of anti-apoptotic proteins. The clinical relevance of these findings remains to be determined.[163a]

INTENSIVE CARE UNIT

Dexmedetomidine may have advantages over propofol for sedation in mechanically ventilated postoperative patients. Heart rate was slower in the dexmedetomidine group, whereas MAP was similar. The PaO_2/FiO_2 ratio was significantly higher in the dexmedetomidine group. Time to extubation of the trachea after discontinuation of the infusion was similar at 28 minutes. Patients receiving dexmedetomidine had greater recall of their stay in the ICU, but all described this as pleasant overall.[421] Several other studies have confirmed the decreased requirement for opioids (>50%) when dexmedetomidine is used for sedation compared with propofol or benzodiazepines. Hemodynamics during weaning are more stable, which benefits patients with high risk for myocardial ischemia.[422] For sedation in the ICU, loading doses of 0.5 to 1 μg/kg have been used. Omitting the bolus dose or giving the lower dose has been associated with fewer episodes of severe bradycardia and other hemodynamic perturbations. Infusion rates of 0.1 to 1 μg/kg/h are generally needed to maintain adequate sedation. Delirium in the ICU is a risk factor for increased length of stay and increased mortality.[423] In a double-blind, randomized controlled trial of sedation in ventilated patients with dexmedetomidine versus lorazepam, it was found that using dexmedetomidine infusions provided more days alive without delirium or coma and a greater amount of time spent at the appropriate sedation level compared with lorazepam.[389] It also improved the patient's ability to communicate pain, compared to midazolam or propofol in two recent trials.[386] The unique characteristics of dexmedetomidine, that is providing adequate sedation with minimal respiratory depression, make this selective α_2-adrenoceptor agonist very useful when weaning patients from the ventilator.[424] While the FDA approved the use of dexmedetomidine infusions for 24 hours or less, multiple studies have shown the safety of using this agent for longer periods, even up to 30 days.[390]

Droperidol

HISTORY

Janssen[298,301] synthesized haloperidol, the first member of the butyrophenones, which became the primary neuroleptic component in neuroleptanesthesia. In 1959, DeCastro and Mundeleer combined haloperidol with phenoperidine (a meperidine derivative also synthesized by Janssen) in the forerunner to the practice of neuroleptanesthesia. Droperidol, a derivative of haloperidol, and fentanyl (a phenoperidine congener), both synthesized by Janssen, were used by DeCastro and Mundeleer in a combination they reported to be superior to haloperidol and phenoperidine. This neuroleptanesthesia combination produced more rapid onset of analgesia, less respiratory depression, and fewer extrapyramidal side effects. The fixed combination of droperidol and fentanyl, marketed as Innovar in the United States, was the drug primarily used for neuroleptanesthesia. The use of neuroleptanesthesia has largely disappeared in modern anesthetic practice. The primary use of droperidol in anesthesia has been as an antiemetic and to a lesser extent as a sedative and antipruritic. In addition, droperidol is used as an antipsychotic agent and to reduce agitation.[425]

In 2001, the FDA issued a black box warning regarding the use of droperidol and its potential for fatal arrhythmias and recommended that it be administered only during continuous electrocardiogram monitoring. With the withdrawal of droperidol in certain countries and more stringent labeling regarding potentially lethal dysrhythmias in others, the use of droperidol has decreased markedly. The validity of the risk of low-dose droperidol in causing QT prolongation, dysrhythmias, and death has been challenged by numerous editorials, articles, and letters reviewing the cases that prompted this action.[298,426-430] In Europe, 19 out of 25 countries with council members in the European Society of Anesthesiologists reported that droperidol is regularly used in a dosage of 0.5 to 2.5 mg for the prevention of PONV. Furthermore, in 2007, an international consensus panel recommended droperidol despite the FDA warning as a first-line antiemetic.[298,431]

Droperidol is a butyrophenone, a fluorinated derivative of phenothiazines (Fig. 23.23). Butyrophenones produce CNS depression, characterized by marked apparent tranquility and cataleptic immobility and are potent antiemetics. Droperidol is a potent butyrophenone, and, similar to the others, it produces its action centrally at sites where dopamine, norepinephrine, and serotonin act.[298,432] It has been postulated that butyrophenones may occupy GABA receptors on the postsynaptic membrane, reducing synaptic transmission and resulting in a build-up of dopamine in the synaptic cleft. In particular, droperidol results in a submaximal inhibition of the $GABA_A$ α_1, β_1, and γ_2 acetylcholine receptors and full inhibition of α_2 acetylcholine receptors. This submaximal inhibition of GABA receptors by droperidol may explain the anxiety, dysphoria, and restlessness that may occur with its administration.[298,433] An imbalance in dopamine and acetylcholine is thought to occur with subsequent alteration in normal transmission of signals in the CNS. The chemoreceptor trigger zone is the emetic center, and "red" astrocytes transport neurolept molecules from the capillary to dopaminergic synapses in the chemoreceptor trigger zone, where they occupy GABA receptors. This is thought to be the mechanism by which droperidol exerts its antiemetic effect.

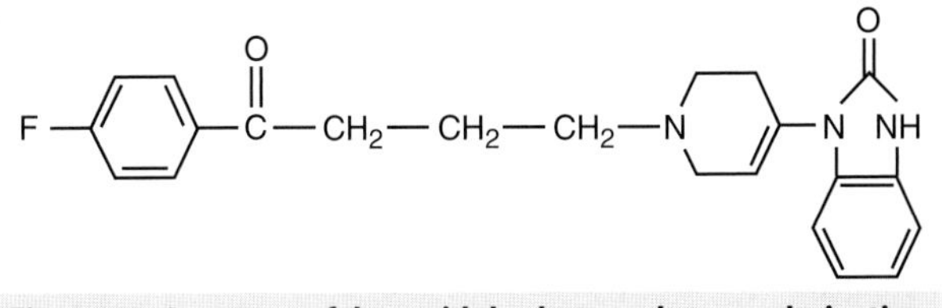

Fig. 23.23 Structure of droperidol, a butyrophenone derivative.

PHARMACOKINETICS

Droperidol is biotransformed in the liver into two primary metabolites. Its plasma decay can be described by a two-compartment model. The pharmacokinetics[298,434] is shown in Table 23.1.

Pharmacodynamics

EFFECTS ON THE CENTRAL NERVOUS SYSTEM

The effects of neurolept anesthetics on human CBF and $CMRO_2$ have not been studied. In dogs, droperidol causes potent cerebral vasoconstriction, producing a 40% reduction in CBF. No significant change in $CMRO_2$ occurs during droperidol administration. The EEG in conscious patients shows some reduction in frequency, with occasional slowing. Low-dose droperidol also has been shown to cause balance disturbances at the time of discharge after doses used for antiemetic prophylaxis. Droperidol may produce extrapyramidal signs and worsen symptoms of Parkinson disease, which is why the drug should be used with great caution in patients with this degenerative disorder. It also rarely may precipitate malignant neuroleptic syndrome.

EFFECTS ON THE RESPIRATORY SYSTEM

When used alone, droperidol has little effect on the respiratory system. Droperidol (0.044 mg/kg) given to surgical patients produced a slight reduction in respiratory rate, and IV droperidol (3 mg) had no significant effect on tidal volume in volunteers. More detailed respiratory studies are unavailable.

EFFECTS ON THE CARDIOVASCULAR SYSTEM

Similar to most antipsychotics, droperidol may prolong the QT interval by delaying myocardial repolarization and precipitating torsades de pointes.[298,435] This seems to be dose dependent and may be of clinical significance when other causes of QT prolongation also are present. Droperidol also may possess some antiarrhythmic effects that are similar to those of quinidine. Droperidol produces vasodilation with a decrease in blood pressure (see Table 23.3). This effect is considered to be a result of moderate α-adrenergic blockade. The dopamine-induced increase in renal blood flow (renal artery flowmeter methodology) is not significantly impaired by administration of droperidol. Droperidol has little effect on myocardial contractility.

USES

Use of droperidol today in the perioperative period is largely restricted to its antiemetic and sedative effects. It is an effective antiemetic; the dose for this use ranges from 10 to 20 μg/kg IV (typically 0.6-1.25 mg for a 70-kg individual).[298,436] Because droperidol in dosages below 1 mg produce antiemetic effects and because the cardiac side effects may be dose-dependent, an IV dose below 1 mg for prevention of PONV is advisable.[437] These doses of droperidol, given at the start of anesthesia for operations lasting 1 hour, reduce the incidence of nausea and vomiting by about 30%. These doses given at induction have little effect on wake-up time, but should they be given at the end of surgery, there could be some residual hypnotic effect. Overall, antiemetic efficacy of droperidol alone is equal to that of ondansetron and results in an equal number of side effects, but droperidol is more cost-effective. The efficacy of droperidol as an antiemetic is enhanced when used in combination with serotonin antagonists or dexamethasone, or both. Droperidol also has been shown to be effective in the treatment and prevention of pruritus secondary to opioid administration. It has been given intravenously and into the epidural space for this purpose. When used in this fashion, droperidol also effectively reduces nausea, but it increases sedation. The safety of droperidol administration into the epidural space has not been fully evaluated, however, and it is not approved for administration via this route.

Summary

Many different IV drugs are available for use in the care of patients requiring general anesthesia or sedation. The selection of a particular drug, but more often of a combination of drugs, must be based on the individual patient's need for hypnosis, amnesia, and analgesia. Drug selection must match the physiology and/or pathophysiology of the individual patient with the pharmacology of the particular drug(s). In addition, based on the pharmacokinetic and pharmacodynamic interactions now described, optimal dosage of hypnotic-analgesic combinations may be selected. A patient in shock who requires induction of anesthesia should receive the drug that produces rapid onset of effect without causing further hemodynamic compromise. The knowledge of the clinical pharmacology of each of the IV anesthetic drugs enables the clinician to induce and maintain sedation or general anesthesia safely and effectively. There is no single perfect drug for any particular patient, but rather the informed practitioner wisely employs the appropriate drug or drugs in the practice of good anesthesia care.

Acknowledgment

The editors and publisher would like to thank Drs. J.G. Reeves, Peter S.A. Glass, David A. Lubarsky, Matthew D. McEvoy, and Richardo Martinez-Ruiz for contributing a chapter on this topic in a previous edition of this work. It has served as the foundation for the current chapter.

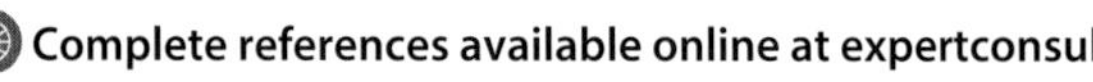
Complete references available online at expertconsult.com.

References

1. Jarman R. *Postgrad Med.* 1946;22:311.
2. Glen JB, et al. *Br J Anaesth.* 1982;54:231.
3. Adam HK, et al. *Br J Anaesth.* 1980;52:743.
4. Glen JB. *Br J Anaesth.* 1980;52:230.
5. Glen JB. *Br J Anaesth.* 1980;52:731.
6. James R, Glen JB. *J Med Chem.* 1980;23:1350.
7. Grossherr M, et al. *Br J Anaesth.* 2009;102:608.
8. Grossherr M, et al. *Xenobiotica.* 2009;39:782.
9. Liu B, et al. *J Clin Monit Comput.* 2012;26:29.
10. Cowley NJ, et al. *Anaesthesia.* 2012;67:870.
11. Struys MMRF, et al. *Eur J Anaesthesiol.* 2010;27:395.
12. Struys MMRF, et al. *Anesthesiology.* 2010;112:1056.
13. Garnock-Jones KP, Scott LJ. *Drugs.* 2010;70:469.
14. Vree TB, et al. *J Chromatogr B Biomed Sci Appl.* 1999;721:217.
15. Bleeker C, et al. *Br J Anaesth.* 2008;101:207.
16. Takizawa D, et al. *Clin Pharmacol Ther.* 2004;76:648.
17. Takizawa D, et al. *Anesthesiology.* 2005;102:327.
18. Kuipers JA, et al. *Anesthesiology.* 1999;91:1780.
19. Reekers M, et al. *Adv Exp Med Biol.* 2003;523:19.
20. Lichtenbelt BJ, et al. *Anesth Analg.* 2010;110:1597.
21. Chen TL, et al. *Br J Anaesth.* 1995;74:558.
22. Candiotti K, et al. *Crit Care Med.* 2010;38:U268.
23. Candiotti KA, et al. *Anesth Analg.* 2011;113:550.
24. Gan TJ, et al. *J Clin Anesth.* 2010;22:260.
25. Cohen LB, et al. *J Clin Gastroenterol.* 2010;44:345.
26. Abdelmalak B, et al. *Curr Pharm Des.* 2012;18:6241.
27. Patwardhan A, et al. *Anesth Analg.* 2012;115:837.
28. Sneyd JR, Rigby-Jones AE. *Br J Anaesth.* 2010;105:246.
28a. Feng AY, et al. *J Anaesthesiol Clin Pharmacol.* 2017;33(1):9.
28b. van den Berg JP, et al. *Br J Anaesth.* 2017;119(Issue 5):918.
29. Vuyk J, et al. *Br J Anaesth.* 2001;86:183.
30. Schnider TW, et al. *Anesthesiology.* 1999;90:1502.
31. Marsh B, et al. *Br J Anaesth.* 1991;67:41.
32. Marsh BJ, et al. *Can J Anaesth.* 1990;37:S97.
33. Gepts E, et al. *Anesth Analg.* 1987;66:1256.
34. Schuttler J, Ihmsen H. *Anesthesiology.* 2000;92:727.
35. Hughes MA, et al. *Anesthesiology.* 1992;76:334.
36. Kazama T, et al. *Anesthesiology.* 1999;90:1517.
37. Shafer A, et al. *Anesthesiology.* 1988;69:348.
38. Vuyk J, et al. *Anesthesiology.* 2000;93:1557.
39. Mertens MJ, et al. *Anesthesiology.* 2004;100:795.
40. Leslie K, et al. *Anesth Analg.* 1995;80:1007.
41. Upton RN, et al. *Anesth Analg.* 1999;89:545.
42. Kazama T, et al. *Anesthesiology.* 2002;97:1156.
43. Allegaert K, et al. *Br J Anaesth.* 2007;99:864.
44. Allegaert K, et al. *Neonatology.* 2007;92:291.
45. Kirkpatrick T, et al. *Br J Anaesth.* 1988;60:146.
46. Vuyk J. *Acta Anaesthesiol Belg.* 2001;52:445.
47. Kataria BK, et al. *Anesthesiology.* 1994;80:104.
48. Murat I, et al. *Anesthesiology.* 1995;83:A1131.
49. Murat I, et al. *Anesthesiology.* 1996;84:526.
50. Servin F, et al. *Anesthesiology.* 1988;69:887.
51. Servin F, et al. *Br J Anaesth.* 1990;65:177.
52. Vuyk J, et al. *Anesth Analg.* 2009;108:1522.
53. Mertens MJ, et al. *Anesthesiology.* 2001;94:949.
54. Krasowski MD, et al. *Mol Pharmacol.* 1998;53:530.
55. Krasowski MD, et al. *Neuropharmacology.* 2001;41:952.
56. Forman SA, Ruesch D. *Biophys J.* 2003;84:87A.
57. Forman SA. *Anesthesiology.* 2011;114:695.
58. Ruesch D, et al. *Anesthesiology.* 2012;116:47.
59. Franks NP. *Nat Rev Neurosci.* 2008;9:370.
60. Kushikata T, et al. *Anesth Analg.* 2002;94:1201.

61. Stamatakis EA, et al. *PLoS One*. 2010;5:e14224.
62. Xie G, et al. *Br J Anaesth*. 2011;106:548.
63. Lingamaneni R, et al. *Anesthesiology*. 2001;95:1460.
64. Lingamaneni R, Hemmings HC. *Br J Anaesth*. 2003;90:199.
65. Dong XP, Xu TL. *Anesth Analg*. 2002;95:907.
66. Pain L, et al. *Anesth Analg*. 2002;95:915.
67. Gelb AW, et al. *Anesthesiology*. 1995;83:A752.
68. Rigby-Jones AE, et al. *Anesthesiology*. 2002;97:1393.
69. Rigby-Jones AE, Sneyd JR. *Paediatr Anaesth*. 2011;21:247.
70. Murray DM, et al. *Br J Anaesth*. 2002;88:318P.
71. Glass PS, et al. *Anesthesiology*. 1997;86:836.
72. San-Juan D, et al. *Clin Neurophysiol*. 2010;121:998.
73. Hodkinson BP, et al. *Lancet*. 1987;2:1518.
74. Wilson C, et al. *Clin Toxicol*. 2010;48:165.
75. Kirby RR, et al. *Anesth Analg*. 2009;108:1182.
76. Wischmeyer PE, et al. *Anesth Analg*. 2007;105:1066.
77. Noterman J, et al. *Neurochirurgie*. 1988;34:161.
78. Steiner LA, et al. *Anesth Analg*. 2003;97:572.
79. Adembri C, et al. *Crit Care Med*. 2002;30:A24.
80. Adembri C, et al. *Anesthesiology*. 2006;104:80.
81. Adembri C, et al. *CNS Drug Rev*. 2007;13:333.
82. Kotani Y, et al. *J Cereb Blood Flow Metab*. 2008;28:354.
83. Gelb AW, et al. *Anesthesiology*. 2002;96:1183.
84. Gelb AW. *Anesth Analg*. 2003;96:33.
85. Cattano D, et al. *Anesth Analg*. 2008;106:1712.
86. Pesic V, et al. *Int J Dev Neurosci*. 2009;27:279.
87. Lanigan C, et al. *Anaesthesia*. 1992;47:810.
88. Vuyk J, et al. *Anesthesiology*. 1992;77:3.
89. Vuyk J, et al. *Anesthesiology*. 1996;84:288.
90. Vuyk J, et al. *Anesthesiology*. 1997;87:1549.
91. Spelina KR, et al. *Br J Anaesth*. 1986;58:1080.
92. Smith C, et al. *Anesthesiology*. 1994;81:820.
93. Kazama T, et al. *Anesth Analg*. 1998;86:872.
94. Dahan A, et al. *Adv Exp Med Biol*. 2003;523:81.
95. Nieuwenhuijs DJ, et al. *Anesthesiology*. 2003;98:312.
96. Goodman NW, et al. *Br J Anaesth*. 1987;59:1497.
97. Jonsson MM, et al. *Anesthesiology*. 2005;102:110.
98. Larsen R, et al. *Anaesthesia*. 1988;43(suppl):25.
98a. de Wit F, et al. *BJA: British Journal of Anaesthesia*. 2016;116(6):784.
99. Pagel PS, Warltier DC. *Anesthesiology*. 1993;78:100.
100. Samain E, et al. *Anesthesiology*. 2000;93:U169.
101. Samain E, et al. *Anesth Analg*. 2000;90:546.
102. Xia ZY, et al. *Anesth Analg*. 2006;103:527.
103. Huang ZY, et al. *Clin Sci*. 2011;121:57.
104. Denborough M, Hopkinson KC. *Lancet*. 1988;1:191.
105. Denborough MA. *Anesthesiology*. 2008;108:156.
106. Foster PS, et al. *Clin Exp Pharmacol Physiol*. 1992;19:183.
107. Mertes PM, Laxenaire MC. *Anaesthesia*. 2002;57:821.
108. Laxenaire MC, et al. *Anesthesiology*. 1992;77:275.
109. Laxenaire MC. *Ann Fr Anesth Reanim*. 1994;13:498.
110. Gan TJ, et al. *Anesthesiology*. 1997;87:779.
111. Bennett SN, et al. *N Engl J Med*. 1995;333:147.
112. Devlin JW, et al. *Pharmacotherapy*. 2005;25:1348.
113. Kazama T, et al. *Anesthesiology*. 2003;98:299.
114. Mertens MJ, et al. *Anesthesiology*. 2003;99:347.
115. Minto CF, et al. *Anesthesiology*. 2000;92:1603.
116. Short TG, et al. *Br J Anaesth*. 1992;69:162.
117. Reich DL, et al. *Anesth Analg*. 2005;101:622.
118. Lichtenbelt BJ, et al. *Clin Pharmacokinet*. 2004;43:577.
119. Johnson KB, et al. *Anesthesiology*. 2004;101:647.
120. Kurita T, et al. *Anesth Analg*. 2009;109:398.
120a. Reade MC, Finfer S. *N Engl J Med*. 2014;370:444.
121. Jacobi J, et al. *Crit Care Med*. 2002;30:119.
121a. Olutoyin OA, et al. *Am J Obstet Gynecol*. 2018;218:98.
121b. Malhotra A, et al. *Brain Sci*. 2017;7(8):107.
121c. Jiang S, et al. *Eur J Pharmacol*. 2018;831:1.
122. Jalota L, et al. *BMJ*. 2011;342:d1110.
123. Roberts R, et al. *Crit Care Med*. 2008;36:A180.
124. Fodale V, La Monaca E. *Drug Saf*. 2008;31:293.
125. Otterspoor LC, et al. *Curr Opin Anaesthesiol*. 2008;21:544.
126. Fudickar A, Bein B. *Minerva Anestesiol*. 2009;75:339.
127. Lundy JS. *J Am Assoc Nurse Anesth*. 1966;34:95.
128. Bennetts FE. *Br J Anaesth*. 1995;75:366.
129. Mahisekar UL, et al. *J Clin Anesth*. 1994;6:55.
130. Mark L. *Clin Pharmacol Ther*. 1963;4:504.
131. Granick S. *J Biol Chem*. 2012;238:PC2247.
132. Breimer DD. *Br J Anaesth*. 1976;48:643.
133. Henthorn TK, et al. *Clin Pharmacol Ther*. 1989;45:56.
134. Christensen JH, et al. *Br J Anaesth*. 1980;52:913.
135. Morgan DJ, et al. *Anesthesiology*. 1981;54:474.
136. Downie DL, et al. *Anesthesiology*. 2000;93:774.
137. Tomlin SL, et al. *Anesthesiology*. 1999;90:1714.
138. Fredriksson A, et al. *Anesthesiology*. 2007;107:427.
139. Liu H, Yao S. *Exp Brain Res*. 2005;167:666.
140. Liu H, et al. *Can J Anaesth*. 2006;53:442.
141. Judge SE. *Br J Anaesth*. 1983;55:191.
141a. Forman SA, Miller KW. *Anesth Analg*. 2016;123(5):1263.
142. Stullken EH, et al. *Anesthesiology*. 1977;46:28.
143. Baughman VL. *Anesthesiol Clin North Am*. 2002;20(vi):315.
144. Albrecht RF, et al. *Anesthesiology*. 1977;47:252.
145. Pancrazio JJ, et al. *J Pharmacol Exp Ther*. 1993;265:358.
146. Mark LC, et al. *J Pharmacol Exp Ther*. 1957;119:35.
147. Burch PG, Stanski DR. *Anesthesiology*. 1983;58:146.
148. Stella L, et al. *Br J Anaesth*. 1979;51:119.
149. Brodie BB, et al. *J Pharmacol Exp Ther*. 1960;130:20.
150. Homer TD, Stanski DR. *Anesthesiology*. 1985;62:714.
151. Sorbo S, et al. *Anesthesiology*. 1984;61:666.
152. Gross JB, et al. *Anesthesiology*. 1983;58:540.
153. Choi SD, et al. *Anesthesiology*. 1985;62:442.
154. Todd MM, et al. *Anesth Analg*. 1985;64:681.
155. Sonntag H, et al. *Acta Anaesthesiol Scand*. 1975;19:69.
156. Dundee JW, Moore J. *Anaesthesia*. 1961;16:50.
157. Touw DJ. *Drug Metabol Drug Interact*. 1997;14:55.
158. Bajwa SJ, et al. *J Anaesthesiol Clin Pharmacol*. 2011;27:440.
159. Ding Z, White PF. *Anesth Analg*. 2002;94:1351.
160. Messina AG, et al. *Cochrane Database Syst Rev*. 2016;10:CD007272.
161. Rodriguez E, Jordan R. *Emerg Med Clin North Am*. 2002;20:199.
162. Winsky-Sommerer R. *Eur J Neurosci*. 2009;29:1779.
163. Reynolds LM, et al. *Neuropsychopharmacology*. 2012;37(11):2531.
163a. Wang C, et al. *Anesthesiology*. 2018;129:1000–1014.
164. Stovner J, Endresen R. *Lancet*. 1965;2:1298.
165. Reves JG, et al. *Anesthesiology*. 1985;62:310.
166. Wesolowski AM, et al. *Pharmacotherapy*. 2016;36(9):1021–1027.
167. Greenblatt DJ, et al. *Clin Pharmacokinet*. 1983;8:233.
168. Greenblatt DJ, et al. *Anesthesiology*. 1984;61:27.
169. Thummel KE, et al. *Clin Pharmacol Ther*. 1996;59:491.
170. Allonen H, et al. *Clin Pharmacol Ther*. 1981;30:653.
171. Greenblatt DJ, et al. *Pharmacology*. 1983;27:70.
172. Dundee JW, et al. *Drugs*. 1984;28:519.
173. Pentikainen PJ, et al. *J Clin Pharmacol*. 1989;29:272.
174. Wandel C, et al. *Br J Anaesth*. 1994;73:658.
175. Heizmann P, et al. *Br J Clin Pharmacol*. 1983;16(suppl 1):43S–49S.
175a. van Rongen A, et al. *Br J Clin Pharnacol*. 2015;80:1185.
176. Bauer TM, et al. *Lancet*. 1995;346:145–147.
177. Divoll M, et al. *Anesth Analg*. 1983;62:1.
178. Gamble JA, et al. *Anaesthesia*. 1975;30:164.
179. Greenblatt DJ, et al. *Clin Pharmacol Ther*. 1980;27:301.
180. Klotz U, et al. *J Clin Invest*. 1975;55:347.
181. Andersson T, et al. *Br J Clin Pharmacol*. 1994;38:131.
182. Jung F, et al. *Drug Metab Dispos*. 1997;25:133.
183. Yang TJ, et al. *Drug Metab Dispos*. 1999;27:102.
184. Locniskar A, Greenblatt DJ. *Biopharm Drug Dispos*. 1990;11:499.
185. Greenblatt DJ, et al. *J Pharm Sci*. 1979;68:57.
186. Greenblatt DJ. *Clin Pharmacokinet*. 1981;6:89.
187. Saari TI, et al. *Pharmacol Rev*. 2011;63:243.
188. Rogers WK, McDowell TS. *IDrugs*. 2010;13:929.
189. Upton RN, et al. *Br J Anaesth*. 2009;103:848.
190. Antonik LJ, et al. *Anesth Analg*. 2012;115:274.
191. Tsukagoshi E, et al. *J Pharmacol Sci*. 2011;115:221.
192. Ostuni MA, et al. *Inflamm Bowel Dis*. 2010;16:1476.
193. Mould DR, et al. *Clin Pharmacol Ther*. 1995;58:35.
194. Mohler H, Richards JG. *Eur J Anaesthesiol Suppl*. 1988;2:15.
195. Mohler H, et al. *J Pharmacol Exp Ther*. 2002;300:2.
196. Kohno T, et al. *Anesthesiology*. 2006;104:338.
197. Ho KM, Ismail H. *Anaesth Intensive Care*. 2008;36:365.
198. Forster A, et al. *Anesthesiology*. 1982;56:453.
199. Harman F, et al. *Childs Nerv Syst*. 2012;28:1055.
200. Norton JR, et al. *Anesthesiology*. 2006;104:1155.
201. Sunzel M, et al. *Br J Clin Pharmacol*. 1988;25:561.
202. Alexander CM, Gross JB. *Anesth Analg*. 1988;67:377.

203. Tverskoy M, et al. *Anesth Analg.* 1989;68:282.
204. Coote JH. *Exp Physiol.* 2007;92:3.
205. Li YF, et al. *Am J Physiol.* 2006;291:H2847.
206. von Moltke LL, et al. *J Clin Pharmacol.* 1996;36:783.
207. Olkkola KT, et al. *Anesth Analg.* 1996;82:511.
208. Goldstein JA. *Br J Clin Pharmacol.* 2001;52:349.
209. Sim SC, et al. *Clin Pharmacol Ther.* 2006;79:103.
210. Ishizaki T, et al. *Clin Pharmacol Ther.* 1995;58:155.
211. Qin XP, et al. *Clin Pharmacol Ther.* 1999;66:642.
212. Ahonen J, et al. *Fundam Clin Pharmacol.* 1996;10:314.
213. Luurila H, et al. *Pharmacol Toxicol.* 1996;78:117.
214. Kamali F, et al. *Eur J Clin Pharmacol.* 1993;44:365.
215. Andersson T, et al. *Eur J Clin Pharmacol.* 1990;39:51.
216. Perucca E, et al. *Clin Pharmacol Ther.* 1994;56:471.
217. Abernethy DR, et al. *J Pharmacol Exp Ther.* 1985;234:345.
218. Samara EE, et al. *J Clin Pharmacol.* 1997;37:442.
219. Vinik HR, et al. *Anesth Analg.* 1989;69:213.
220. Hong W, et al. *Anesthesiology.* 1993;79:1227.
221. McClune S, et al. *Br J Anaesth.* 1992;69:240.
222. Bauer KP, et al. *J Clin Anesth.* 2004;16:177.
223. Kain ZN, et al. *Anesthesiology.* 1998;89:1147.
224. Hargreaves J. *Br J Anaesth.* 1988;61:611.
225. Pollock JS, Kenny GN. *Br J Anaesth.* 1993;70:219.
226. George KA, Dundee JW. *Br J Clin Pharmacol.* 1977;4:45.
227. Cole SG, et al. *Gastrointest Endosc.* 1983;29:219.
228. McNulty SE, et al. *Anesth Analg.* 1995;81:404.
229. Lee SH. *Dig Dis Sci.* 2012;57:2243.
230. Garewal D, et al. *Cochrane Database Syst Rev(6).* 2012:CD007274.
231. Tverskoy M, et al. *Reg Anesth.* 1996;21:209.
232. Frolich MA, et al. *Can J Anaesth.* 2006;53:79.
233. Nitsun M, et al. *Clin Pharmacol Ther.* 2006;79:549.
234. Walder B, et al. *Anesth Analg.* 2001;92:975.
235. Barr J, et al. *Crit Care Med.* 2013;41:263.
236. Mehta S, et al. *JAMA.* 1985;308:2012.
237. Breimer LT, et al. *Clin Pharmacokinet.* 1990;18:245.
238. Jacobs JR, et al. *Anesth Analg.* 1995;80:143.
239. Melvin MA, et al. *Anesthesiology.* 1982;57:238.
240. Theil DR, et al. *J Cardiothorac Vasc Anesth.* 1993;7:300.
241. Jung JS, et al. *Otolaryngol Head Neck Surg.* 2007;137:753.
242. Heidari SM, et al. *Adv Biomed Res.* 2012;1:9.
243. Lee Y, et al. *Anaesthesia.* 2007;62:18.
244. Riad W, et al. *Eur J Anaesthesiol.* 2007;24:697.
245. Riad W, Marouf H. *Middle East J Anesthesiol.* 2009;20:431.
246. Fujii Y, Itakura M. *Clin Ther.* 2010;32:1633.
247. Rinehart JB, et al. *Neurologist.* 2012;18:216.
248. Brogden RN, Goa KL. *Drugs.* 1991;42:1061.
249. File SE, Pellow S. *Psychopharmacology (Berl).* 1986;88:1.
250. Cumin R, et al. *Experientia.* 1982;38:833.
251. Haefely W, Hunkeler W. *Eur J Anaesthesiol Suppl.* 1988;2:3.
252. Klotz U, Kanto J. *Clin Pharmacokinet.* 1988;14:1.
253. Klotz U, et al. *Eur J Clin Pharmacol.* 1984;27:115.
254. Lauven PM, et al. *Anesthesiology.* 1985;63:61.
255. Kleinberger G, et al. *Lancet.* 1985;2:268.
256. Yokoyama M, et al. *Anesth Analg.* 1992;75:87.
257. Amrein R, et al. *Resuscitation.* 1988;16(suppl):S5.
258. Rubio F, et al. *Lancet.* 1993;341:1028.
259. Donovan KL, Fisher DJ. *BMJ.* 1989;298:1253.
260. Zuber M, et al. *Eur Neurol.* 1988;28:161.
261. Lassaletta A, et al. *Pediatr Emerg Care.* 2004;20:319.
262. Rouiller M, et al. *Ann Fr Anesth Reanim.* 1987;6:1.
263. Duka T, et al. *Psychopharmacology (Berl).* 1986;90:351.
264. Nilsson A. *Acta Anaesthesiol Scand Suppl.* 1990;92:51.
265. Ueda K, et al. *Acta Anaesthesiol Scand.* 2013;57:488.
266. Weinbrum A, Geller E. *Acta Anaesthesiol Scand Suppl.* 1990;92:65.
267. Ghoneim MM, et al. *Anesthesiology.* 1989;70:899.
268. White PF, et al. *Anesthesiology.* 1982;56:119.
269. Bovill JG. *Anesth Analg.* 2007;105:1186.
270. Bovill JG, et al. *Lancet.* 1971;1:1285.
271. Nimmo WS, Clements JA. *Br J Anaesth.* 1981;53:186.
272. Clements JA, Nimmo WS. *Br J Anaesth.* 1981;53:27.
273. Olofsen E, et al. *Anesth Analg.* 2012;115:536.
274. Olofsen E, et al. *Anesthesiology.* 2012;117:353.
275. Dahan A, et al. *Eur J Pain.* 2011;15:258.
276. White M, et al. *Br J Anaesth.* 2006;96:330.
277. Sigtermans M, et al. *Eur J Pain.* 2010;14:302.
278. Noppers I, et al. *Anesthesiology.* 2011;114:1435.
279. Kharasch ED, Labroo R. *Anesthesiology.* 1992;77:1201.
280. Kharasch ED, et al. *Anesthesiology.* 1992;77:1208.
281. Sigtermans M, et al. *Anesthesiology.* 2009;111:892.
282. Sigtermans MJ, et al. *Pain.* 2009;145:304.
283. Weinbroum AA. *Pharmacol Res.* 2012;65:411.
284. Niesters M, et al. *Anesthesiology.* 2011;115:1063.
285. Niesters M, et al. *Pain.* 2011;152:656.
286. Niesters M, et al. *Anesthesiology.* 2012;117:868.
287. Niesters M, Dahan A. *Expert Opin Drug Metab Toxicol.* 2012;8:1409.
288. Lee EE, et al. *Gen Hosp Psychiatry.* 2015;37(2):178.
289. Nieuwenhuijs D, et al. *Clin Exp Pharmacol Physiol.* 2002;29:A77.
290. Sarton E, et al. *Anesth Analg.* 2001;93:1495.
291. Timm C, et al. *Anaesthesist.* 2008;57:338.
292. Amr YM. *Pain Physician.* 2011;14:475.
293. Jonkman K, et al. *Curr Opin Support Palliat Care.* 2017;11(2):88.
294. Bar-Joseph G, et al. *Crit Care Med.* 2009;37:A402.
295. Bar-Joseph G, et al. *J Neurosurg Pediatr.* 2009;4:40.
296. Dahmani S, et al. *Paediatr Anaesth.* 2011;21:636.
297. Dahmani S. *Paediatr Anaesth.* 2011;21:1081.
298. Schnabel A, et al. *Br J Anaesth.* 2011;107:601.
299. Walker SM, Yaksh TL. *Anesth Analg.* 2012;115:638.
300. Walker SM, et al. *Anesth Analg.* 2012;115:450.
301. Janssen PA. *Int J Neuropsychiatry.* 1967;3(suppl 1):S10.
302. Noppers IM, et al. *Pain.* 2011;152:2173.
303. Godefroi EF, et al. *J Med Chem.* 1965;8:220.
304. Ledingham IM, Watt I. *Lancet.* 1983;1:1270.
305. Wagner RL, White PF. *Anesthesiology.* 1984;61:647.
306. Longnecker DE. *Anesthesiology.* 1984;61:643.
307. Owen H, Spence AA. *Br J Anaesth.* 1984;56:555.
308. Doenicke A, et al. *Br J Anaesth.* 1997;79:386.
309. Van Hamme MJ, et al. *Anesthesiology.* 1978;49:274.
310. Schuttler J, et al. *Eur J Anaesthesiol.* 1985;2:133.
311. Johnson KB, et al. *Anesth Analg.* 2003;96:1360.
312. van Beem H, et al. *Anaesthesia.* 1983;38(suppl):61.
313. Arden JR, et al. *Anesthesiology.* 1986;65:19.
314. Sear J. Total intravenous anesthesia. In: Longnecker DE, Brown DL, Newman MF, Zapol WM, eds. *Anesthesia.* New York: McGraw-Hill Medical; 2008:897.
315. Heykants JJ, et al. *Arch Int Pharmacodyn Ther.* 1975;216:113.
316. Meuldermans WE, Heykants JJ. *Arch Int Pharmacodyn Ther.* 1976;221:150.
317. Evans RH, Hill RG. *Experientia.* 1978;34:1325.
318. Guitchounts G, et al. *Anesthesiology.* 2012;116:1235.
319. Cheng VY, et al. *J Neurosci.* 2006;26:3713.
320. Carlson BX, et al. GABA-A receptors and anesthesia. In: Yaksh TL, Lynich C, Zapol WM, et al., eds. *Anesthesia: Biologic Foundations.* Philadelphia: Lippincott-Raven; 1998:259.
321. Rusch D, et al. *J Biol Chem.* 2004;279:20982.
322. Cold GE, et al. *Acta Anaesthesiol Scand.* 1986;30:159.
323. Modica PA, Tempelhoff R. *Can J Anaesth.* 1992;39:236.
324. Thornton C, et al. *Br J Anaesth.* 1985;57:554.
325. Drummond JC, et al. *Neurosurgery.* 1995;37:742.
326. Flower O, Hellings S. *Emerg Med Int.* 2012;2012:637171.
327. Ebrahim ZY, et al. *Anesth Analg.* 1986;65:1004.
328. Pastor J, et al. *Epilepsia.* 2010;51:602.
329. Lallemand MA, et al. *Br J Anaesth.* 2003;91:341.
330. Kaneda K, et al. *J Clin Pharmacol.* 2011;51:482.
331. Guldager H, et al. *Acta Anaesthesiol Scand.* 1985;29:352.
332. Morgan M, et al. *Br J Anaesth.* 1977;49:233.
333. Colvin MP, et al. *Br J Anaesth.* 1979;51:551.
334. Ogawa K, et al. *Anesthesiology.* 2001;94:668.
335. Gooding JM, Corssen G. *Anesth Analg.* 1977;56:717.
336. Gooding JM, et al. *Anesth Analg.* 1979;58:40.
337. Bovill JG. *Semin Cardiothorac Vasc Anesth.* 2006;10:43.
338. Sprung J, et al. *Anesth Analg.* 2000;91:68.
339. Möller PA, Kamenik M. *Br J Anaesth.* 2013;110:388.
340. Larsen R, et al. *Anaesthesist.* 1988;37:510.
341. Fragen RJ, et al. *Anesthesiology.* 1987;66:839.
342. Diago MC, et al. *Anaesthesia.* 1988;43:644.
343. Bruder EA, et al. *Cochrane Database Syst Rev.* 2015;1:CD010225.
344. Cherfan AJ, et al. *Pharmacotherapy.* 2012;32:475.
345. Sprung CL, et al. *N Engl J Med.* 2008;358:111.
346. Lipiner-Friedman D, et al. *Crit Care Med.* 2007;35:1012.
347. Cuthbertson BH, et al. *Intensive Care Med.* 2009;35:1868.

348. Hildreth AN, et al. *J Trauma*. 2008;65:573.
349. Tekwani KL, et al. *Acad Emerg Med*. 2009;16:11.
350. Ray DC, McKeown DW. *Crit Care*. 2007;11:R56.
351. Jung B, et al. *Crit Care*. 2012;16:R224.
352. Nimmo WS, Miller M. *Contemp Anesth Pract*. 1983;7:83.
353. Canessa R, et al. *J Cardiothorac Vasc Anesth*. 1991;5:566.
354. Kim TK, Park IS. *J Korean Neurosurg Soc*. 2011;50:497.
355. Wang N, et al. *J ECT*. 2011;27:281.
356. Avramov MN, et al. *Anesth Analg*. 1995;81:596.
357. Radtke FM, et al. *Minerva Anestesiol*. 2010;76:394.
358. Preda VA, et al. *Eur J Endocrinol*. 2012;167:137.
359. St Pierre M, et al. *Eur J Anaesthesiol*. 2000;17:634.
360. Mayer M, et al. *Anaesthesist*. 1996;45:1082.
361. Wu J, et al. *Contraception*. 2013;87:55.
362. Doenicke AW, et al. *Br J Anaesth*. 1999;83:464.
363. Nyman Y, et al. *Br J Anaesth*. 2006;97:536.
364. Huter L, et al. *Anesth Analg*. 2007;105:1298.
365. Un B, et al. *J Res Med Sci*. 2011;16:1490.
366. Cotten JF, et al. *Anesthesiology*. 2009;111:240.
367. Cotten JF, et al. *Anesthesiology*. 2010;112:637.
368. Maze M, Tranquilli W. *Anesthesiology*. 1991;74:581.
369. Bloor BC, Flacke WE. *Anesth Analg*. 1982;61:741.
370. Gerlach AT, Dasta JF. *Ann Pharmacother*. 2007;41:245.
371. Tobias JD. *Pediatr Crit Care Med*. 2007;8:115.
372. Bhana N, et al. *Drugs*. 2000;59:263.
373. Virtanen R, et al. *Eur J Pharmacol*. 1988;150:9.
374. Wang L, et al. *Expert Rev Clin Pharmacol*. 2018;11(9):917.
375. Dyck JB, et al. *Anesthesiology*. 1993;78:821.
376. Weerink MAS, et al. *Clin Pharmacokinet*. 2017;56(8):893.
377. De Wolf AM, et al. *Anesth Analg*. 2001;93:1205.
378. Venn RM, et al. *Br J Anaesth*. 2002;88:669.
379. Aantaa R, Jalonen J. *Eur J Anaesthesiol*. 2006;23:361.
380. Paris A, Tonner PH. *Curr Opin Anaesthesiol*. 2005;18:412.
381. Aho M, et al. *J Clin Anesth*. 1993;5:194.
382. Guo TZ, et al. *Anesthesiology*. 1996;84:873.
383. Nelson LE, et al. *Anesthesiology*. 2003;98:428.
384. Angst MS, et al. *Anesthesiology*. 2004;101:744.
385. Venn RM, et al. *Anaesthesia*. 1999;54:1136.
386. Jakob SM, et al. *JAMA*. 2012;307:1151.
387. Kress JP, et al. *N Engl J Med*. 2000;342:1471.
388. Ebert TJ, et al. *Anesthesiology*. 2000;93(2):382.
389. Pandharipande PP, et al. *JAMA*. 2007;298:2644.
390. Riker RR, et al. *JAMA*. 2009;301:489.
391. Wang D-S, et al. *Anesthesiology*. 2018;129:477.
392. Ishii H, et al. *Eur J Neurosci*. 2008;27:3182.
393. McCutcheon CA, et al. *Anesth Analg*. 2006;102:668.
394. Hofer RE, et al. *Can J Anaesth*. 2005;52:176.
395. Aho M, et al. *Anesthesiology*. 1991;74:997.
396. Aantaa R, et al. *Anesthesiology*. 1990;73:230.
397. Xiang Q, et al. *Br J Anaesth*. 2013;110:420.
398. Marhofer D, et al. *Br J Anaesth*. 2013;110:438.
399. Rancourt MP, et al. *Anesth Analg*. 2012;115:958.
400. Engelhard K, et al. *Anesth Analg*. 2003;96:524.
401. Talke P, Bickler PE. *Anesthesiology*. 1996;85:551.
402. Talke P, et al. *Anesth Analg*. 1997;85:358.
403. Bekker A, Sturaitis MK. *Neurosurgery*. 2005;57:1.
404. Zornow MH, et al. *J Cereb Blood Flow Metab*. 1993;13:350.
405. Drummond JC, et al. *Anesthesiology*. 2008;108:225.
406. Talke P, et al. *J Neurosurg Anesthesiol*. 2007;19:195.
407. Hsu YW, et al. *Anesthesiology*. 2004;101:1066.
408. Riker RR, Fraser GL. *Pharmacotherapy*. 2005;25:8S.
409. Venn M, et al. *Intensive Care Med*. 2003;29:201.
410. Jalonen J, et al. *Anesthesiology*. 1997;86:331.
411. Talke P, et al. *Anesthesiology*. 1995;82:620.
412. Koroglu A, et al. *Anesth Analg*. 2006;103:63.
413. Gerlach AT, et al. *Ann Pharmacother*. 2009;43(12):2064.
414. Ramsay MA, Luterman DL. *Anesthesiology*. 2004;101:787.
415. Aouad MT, et al. *Anesth Analg*. 2017.
416. Maccioli GA. *Anesthesiology*. 2003;98:575.
417. Phan H, Nahata MC. *Paediatr Drugs*. 2008;10:49.
418. Maroof M, et al. *Can J Anaesth*. 2005;52:776.
419. Yazbek-Karam VG, Aouad MM. *Middle East J Anesthesiol*. 2006;18:1043.
420. Deleted in proofs.
421. Venn RM, Grounds RM. *Br J Anaesth*. 2001;87:684.
422. Triltsch AE, et al. *Crit Care Med*. 2002;30:1007.
423. Ely EW, et al. *JAMA*. 2004;291:1753.
424. Siobal MS, et al. *Respir Care*. 2006;51:492.
425. Khokhar MA, Rathbone J. *Cochrane Database Syst Rev*. 2016;12:CD002830.
426. Dershwitz M. *J Clin Anesth*. 2002;14:598.
427. Gan TJ, et al. *Anesthesiology*. 2002;97:287.
428. Gan TJ. *Anesth Analg*. 2004;98:1809.
429. White PF, et al. *Anesthesiology*. 2005;102:1101.
430. White PF, Abrao J. *Anesthesiology*. 2006;104:386.
431. Gan TJ, et al. *Anesth Analg*. 2007;105:1615.
432. Gan TJ. *Anesth Analg*. 2006;47–51.
433. Flood P, Coates KM. *Anesthesiology*. 2002;96:987.
434. Fischler M, et al. *Anesthesiology*. 1986;64:486.
435. Wooltorton E. *CMAJ*. 2002;166:932.
436. Hill RP, et al. *Anesthesiology*. 2000;92:958.
437. Schaub I, et al. *Eur J Anesthesiol*. 2012;29:286.

24 Opioids

MARK SCHUMACHER and KAZUHIKO FUKUDA

KEY POINTS

- Opioids are a vital part of providing the analgesic component of anesthesia and often form the foundation for postoperative pain management.
- Opioids suppress pain by targeting multiple sites throughout the nervous system including action in brain, spinal cord, and peripheral nervous systems.
- An increased understanding of the molecular pharmacology of opioid receptors and opioid-induced cellular responses allows utilization of innovative techniques for analgesia.
- Opioids also affect multiple organ systems, including the respiratory and cardiovascular systems, and can cause a variety of adverse effects. Proper dosing and monitoring may allow these adverse effects to be minimized.
- Pharmacokinetic and pharmacodynamic properties of opioids are affected by a variety of factors, such as age, body weight, organ failure, shock, and drug interactions. To administer opioids, these factors should be taken into consideration.
- Although new opioid delivery systems such as transdermal patches provide certain clinical advantages, they can also pose additional risks such as respiratory depression.
- Opioid analgesics serve a critical role in acute pain management but their role in the long-term treatment of chronic noncancer pain has been called into question due to increased risks of overdose and addiction.

Introduction

The remarkable beneficial effects of opioids, as well as their toxic side effects and addictive potential, have been known for centuries. The term opioid refers broadly to all compounds related to opium. The word opium originates from *opos*, the Greek word for juice, the drug being derived from the juice of the opium poppy, *Papaver somniferum*. In contrast, the term opiate refers to natural products derived from the opium poppy and includes morphine, codeine, and thebaine.

The first undisputed reference to opium is found in the writings of Theophrastus in the third century B.C. During the Middle Ages, many of the uses of opium were appreciated. Opium contains more than 20 distinct alkaloids. In 1806, Sertürner reported the isolation of a pure substance in opium that he named morphine, after Morpheus, the Greek god of dreams. By the middle of the nineteenth century, the use of pure alkaloids rather than crude opium preparations began to spread throughout the medical world. Since then, there have been ongoing efforts to develop semisynthetic and synthetic opioid analgesics without the adverse side effects. Unfortunately, many of the synthetic opioids share side effects of natural opioids. The search for new opioid agonists led to the synthesis of opioid antagonists and compounds with mixed agonist/antagonist properties, which further expanded therapeutic options and provided important tools for exploring mechanisms of opioid actions. Although new methods of opioid administration, including patient-controlled analgesia (PCA) and computer-based infusion techniques, have been developed, opioids continue to act on common binding sites throughout the nervous system.

Pharmacology of Opioids

CLASSIFICATION OF OPIOID COMPOUNDS

Opioids can be classified as naturally occurring, semisynthetic, and synthetic (Box 24.1). The naturally occurring opioids can be divided into two chemical classes, phenanthrenes (morphine and codeine) and benzylisoquinolines (papaverine). The semisynthetic opioids are morphine derivatives in which one of several changes has been made. Synthetic opioids are classified into four groups, the morphinan derivatives (levorphanol), the diphenyl or methadone derivatives (methadone, *d*-propoxyphene), the benzomorphans (phenazocine, pentazocine), and the phenylpiperidine derivatives (meperidine, fentanyl, sufentanil, alfentanil, and remifentanil). Structures of opioid compounds are shown in Fig. 24.1[1] and Table 24.1.[1]

Opioids can be classified as agonists, partial agonists, mixed agonist-antagonist, and antagonists on the basis of their interaction with the opioid receptors.

BASIC STUDIES ON OPIOID RECEPTORS

In 1973, three independent teams of investigators described the presence of opioid binding sites in the nervous system from the radioligand binding assays. From pharmacologic experiments, three types of opioid receptors were postulated. They were named μ for morphine type, κ for the ketocyclazocine type, and σ for the SKF10047 (*N*-allylnormetazocine) type. In addition, a high-affinity receptor for enkephalins was found in the mouse vas deferens, and was named the δ-receptor. Furthermore, an ε-receptor was

BOX 24.1 Classification of Opioid Compounds

Naturally occurring
- Morphine
- Codeine
- Papaverine
- Thebaine

Semisynthetic
- Heroin
- Dihydromorphone, morphinone
- Thebaine derivatives (e.g., etorphine, buprenorphine)

Synthetic
- Morphinan derivatives (e.g., levorphanol, butorphanol)
- Diphenylpropylamine derivatives (e.g., methadone)
- Benzomorphan derivatives (e.g., pentazocine)
- Phenylpiperidine derivatives (e.g., meperidine, fentanyl, sufentanil, alfentanil, remifentanil)

From Bailey PL, Egan TD, Stanley TH. Intravenous opioid anesthetics. In: Miller RD, ed. *Anesthesia.* 8th ed. Philadelphia: Saunders; 2015. An imprint of Elsevier Inc., p. 865.

proposed as the binding site for β-endorphin in the rat vas deferens. Pharmacologic actions of opioids and the involved receptors have been analyzed (Table 24.2).

Since the early 1990s, molecular biologic studies have elucidated the molecular structures and signal transduction mechanisms of the opioid receptors. Four different complementary DNAs (cDNAs) have been isolated as members of the opioid receptor family.[2] Investigators demonstrated that three of them correspond to the pharmacologically defined μ-, δ-, and κ-opioid receptors. The fourth receptor did not bind with opioid ligands with high affinities. Later, a novel peptide, nociceptin/orphanin FQ, was identified as an endogenous agonist of the fourth member of the opioid receptor family.[3,4] The μ-, δ-, and κ-opioid receptors and the nociceptin receptor share approximately 50% amino acid sequence homology with each other. Characteristics of three opioid receptors and the nociceptin/orphanin FQ receptor are listed in Table 24.3. Hydropathy analysis of the primary structures of the opioid receptors predicted that the opioid receptors possess seven transmembrane domains (Fig. 24.2). This is a characteristic structural[5] feature of G-protein-coupled receptors. Crystallographic analysis revealed that the μ-, δ-, and κ-opioid receptors and the nociceptin receptor actually possess seven transmembrane domains and the agonist binds deeply within a large pocket (Fig. 24.3).[6] Furthermore, analysis of the crystal structure of the murine opioid receptor revealed agonist-induced conformational changes in detail, providing the basis for the development of new ligands.[7]

The σ (sigma) receptor, which was previously classified as a member of the opioid receptor, was shown to be an endoplasmic reticulum-resident protein, and has been implicated in many diseases, ranging from cocaine or alcohol addiction to the most recently reported familial adult or juvenile amyotrophic lateral sclerosis. The amino acid sequence of the σ-1 receptor does not resemble that of any other mammalian proteins.[8]

Further pharmacologic classification of the μ-receptor as the μ_1, μ_2, and μ_3 subtypes has been proposed, but the molecular identity of these receptor subtypes still remains to be clarified. Several possible molecular models of opioid receptor subtypes exist, including alternate splicing of a common gene product, receptor dimerization, and interaction of a common gene product with other receptor or signaling molecules.[9] Multiple μ-opioid receptor species can be produced from a gene product of the μ-opioid receptor gene by alternate splicing (Fig. 24.4).[10,11] Analysis of the alternate splicing products reveals differences in ligand binding and G-protein activation. However, their physiologic, pharmacologic, or clinical implications remain to be elucidated. Interestingly, it was recently reported that the analgesic action of 3-iodobenzoyl-6β-naltrexamide, a potent analgesic against thermal, inflammatory, and neuropathic pain, is mediated by its interaction with mMOR-1G, a truncated splice variant possessing only six transmembrane segments, in mice.[12]

G-protein-coupled receptors can form dimers, homodimers (same receptor), and heterodimers (different receptor types). The existence of these homodimers and heterodimers has been shown in cultured cells and *in vivo.* Among opioid receptors (μ, δ, κ, and nociception receptors), various combinations of the molecules have been shown to form dimers, and the dimer formation has been shown to affect the ligand binding properties and signal transduction mechanisms.[13] Physiologic and clinical implications of dimer formation of opioid receptors will be further clarified. For example, it is interesting that a bivalent ligand containing μ-agonist and δ-antagonist pharmacophores effectively bridges μ-δ opioid receptor heterodimers and exhibits enhanced efficacy and a reduced tendency for tolerance in mice.[14] However, in the peripheral nervous system, μ and δ receptors are apparently expressed in different sensory neuronal subpopulations.[15,16]

Taken together, the overwhelming evidence of opioid receptor diversity in structure, ligand binding, and distribution supports the concept they serve both essential and complex signaling roles throughout the nervous system.

GENETIC VARIATIONS WHICH INFLUENCE OPIOID EFFECTS

Several single nucleotide polymorphisms (SNPs) have been identified in the human μ-opioid receptor gene (Fig. 24.5).[17] The A118G mutation, the most common of these SNPs, leads to a change in the gene product in the human μ-opioid receptors, which is an A-to-G substitution in exon 1 that results in an amino acid exchange at position 40 from asparagine to aspartate (N40D). Patients with cancer who are homozygous for the A118G variant required higher doses of oral morphine for long-term treatment of their pain.[18] A118G mutation of the human μ-opioid receptor gene reduces analgesic responses to morphine-6-glucuronide (M6G), but it does not significantly affect the respiratory depression induced by M6G.[19] Furthermore, morphine consumption with intravenous PCA after total abdominal hysterectomy is significantly greater in women homozygous for the A118G variant than in other patients.[20] In a meta-analysis involving 18 studies and more than 4600 patients, carriers of A118G were observed to exhibit higher opioid analgesic requirements.[21] Another meta-analysis showed significant association between A118G polymorphism and susceptibility to opioid dependence or addiction in Asian populations.[22]

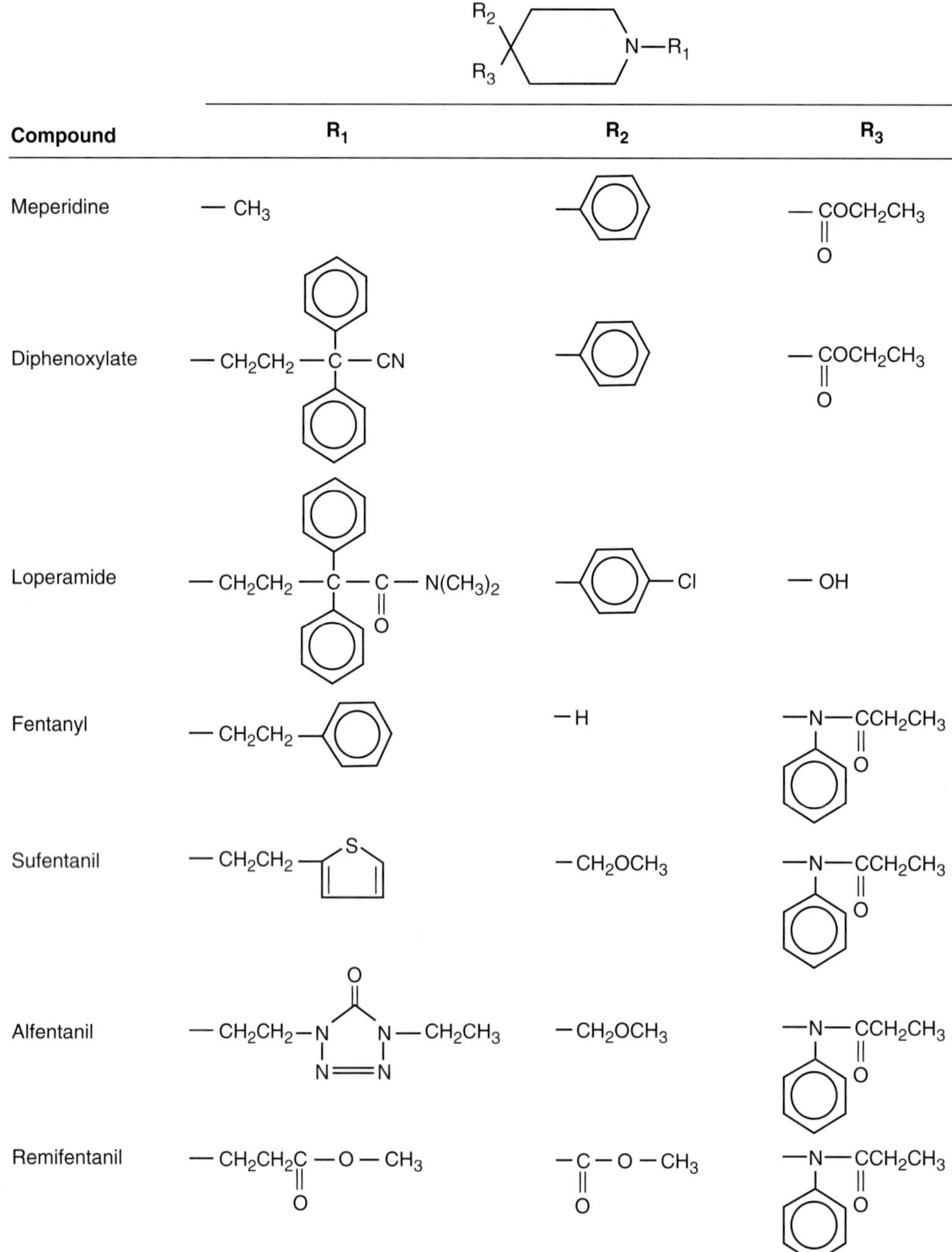

Fig. 24.1 **Chemical structures of piperidine and phenylpiperidine analgesics.** (From Gutstein HB, Akil H. Opioid analgesics. In: Hardman JG, Limbird LE, eds. *Goodman and Gilman's the Pharmacological Basis of Therapeutics*. 10th ed. New York: McGraw-Hill; 2001:569–619.)

In vitro experiments show that the variant receptors with A118G mutation are associated with higher binding affinity to and potency of β-endorphin, but lower potency of morphine.[23] Studies in mouse models with analogous substitution of human A118G showed reduced analgesic response to morphine in some regions of the mouse brain with the GG genotype when compared with the AA genotype.[24] A study also showed that 118A messenger RNA was 1.5- to 2.5-fold more abundant than the 118G messenger RNA in heterozygous brain autopsy tissues.[25]

Overall, these findings suggest that the 118G allele may result in changes in abundance and/or function of the μ-opioid receptor leading to differences in antinociceptive potency of opioid analgesics. This in turn could misdirect healthcare providers in providing the most effective and safe opioid-based analgesic plan.

The C17T mutation of the human μ-opioid receptor, located in exon 1, causes an amino acid exchange from alanine to valine at receptor protein position 6 of the extracellular receptor terminal. This mutation has been reported to occur in a higher overall proportion of opioid-dependent persons, but the effects of the C17T polymorphism on analgesic responses are unknown. A recent study using cultured cells reported that adenylate inhibition via the C17T polymorphism was decreased for many opioids, including the clinically significant drugs morphine, buprenorphine,

TABLE 24.1 Structures of Opioids and Opioid Antagonists Chemically Related to Morphine

Morphine

	CHEMICAL RADICALS AND POSITION*			
Nonproprietary Name	**3**	**6**	**17**	**Other Changes[†]**
Morphine	—OH	—OH	—CH_3	—
Heroin	—$OCOCH_3$	—$OCOCH_3$	—CH_3	—
Hydromorphone	—OH	=O	—CH_3	(1)
Oxymorphone	—OH	=O	—CH_3	(1), (2)
Levorphanol	—OH	—H	—CH_3	(1), (3)
Levallorphan	—OH	—H	—$CH_2CH{=}CH_2$	(1), (3)
Codeine	—OCH_3	—OH	—CH_3	—
Hydrocodone	—OCH_3	=O	—CH_3	(1)
Oxycodone	—OCH_3	=O	—CH_3	(1), (2)
Nalmefene	—OH	=CH_2	—CH_2—<	(1), (2)
Nalorphine	—OH	—OH	—CH_2CHKCH_2	—
Naloxone	—OH	=O	—$CH_2CH{=}CH_2$	(1), (2)
Naltrexone	—OH	=O	—CH_2—<	(1), (2)
Buprenorphine	—OH	—OCH_3	—CH_2—<	(1), (4)
Butorphanol	—OH	—H	—CH_2—◆	(1), (2), (3)
Nalbuphine	—OH	JOH	—CH_2—◆	(1),(2)

*The numbers 3, 6, and 17 refer to positions in the morphine molecule, as shown above.
[†]Other changes in the morphine molecule are as follows:
(1)Single instead of double bond between C7 and C8.
(2)OH added to C14.
(3)No oxygen between C4 and C5.
(4)Endoetheno bridge between C6 and C14; 1-hydroxy-1,2,2-trimethylpropyl substitution on C7.
From Gutstein HB, Akil H: Opioid analgesics. In: Hardman JG, Limbird LE, eds. *Goodman and Gilman's the Pharmacological Basis of Therapeutics*. 10th ed. New York: McGraw-Hill; 2001: 569–619.

and fentanyl, as well as endogenous opioids,[26] suggesting that this polymorphism may affect individual responses to opioid therapy, while the possible disruption of the endogenous opioid system may contribute to susceptibility to substance abuse.

It is known that genetic variation of genes other than opioid receptor genes can affect sensitivity to opioids. It has been demonstrated that the Val158Met polymorphism of the human catechol-*O*-methyltransferase (COMT) gene has contributed to differences in opioid consumption in patients treated for chronic cancer pain,[27] and is associated with variability in opioid consumption in postoperative nephrectomy patients.[28] COMT metabolizes biogenic amines including catecholamines such as dopamine, epinephrine, and norepinephrine, thereby acting as a key modulator of dopaminergic and adrenergic neurotransmission, and can affect the pharmacologic effects of opioids. Some studies have explored the relationship between gene-gene interactions and opioid responses. Kolesnikov and associates have demonstrated that the heterozygous patients with μ-opioid receptor A118G and COMT G1974A mutation consumed significantly less morphine compared with homozygous patients of A118.[29] As investigation into the clinical impact of genetic variability continues, it is revealing that even greater complexity exists between gene-gene interactions and postoperative morphine consumption.[30]

ENDOGENOUS OPIOID PEPTIDES

Enkephalin, β-endorphin, and dynorphin were identified as endogenous agonists for the δ-, μ-, and κ-opioid receptors, respectively. Following purification of these peptides from mammalian tissues, cDNAs for the precursors of these peptides were cloned. cDNA cloning and amino acid determination of preproopiomelanocortin demonstrated that the cleavage of this precursor protein produces not only β-endorphin but also several other neuropeptides including methionine-enkephalin, adrenocorticotropic hormone (ACTH), and α-melanocyte stimulating hormone. Amino acid sequence of preproenkephalin indicates that four methionine enkephalins and one leucine-enkephalin are cleaved from this precursor. Furthermore, the primary structure of preprodynorphin, the precursor of dynorphin, gives rise to dynorphin, leumorphin, and neoendorphin—ligands for the κ-opioid receptor.

Orphanin FQ or nociceptin, a novel endogenous opioid peptide with a significant sequence homology to dynorphin, was isolated in 1995[3,4] and so named because it lowered pain threshold under certain conditions in contrast to other endogenous opioid peptides. Pharmacologic and physiologic studies have demonstrated that orphanin FQ/nociceptin has behavioral and pain modulatory properties distinct from those of the three classic opioid peptides.[31] However, studies of the effect of orphanin FQ/nociceptin on pain sensitivity have produced conflicting results, which may suggest that the effects of orphanin FQ/nociceptin on pain sensitivity depend on the underlying behavioral state of the animal. Prepronociceptin, the precursor of orphanin FQ/nociceptin, was cloned, and its amino acid sequence suggested the existence of prepronociceptin-derived neuropeptides other than orphanin FQ/nociception.[32]

The search for endogenous ligand binding with the μ receptor with high affinity and high selectivity led to the discovery of a class of novel endogenous opioids termed endomorphin-1 and endomorphin-2.[33] These peptides are tetrapeptides with the sequence Tyr-Pro-Trp-Phe and Tyr-Pro-Phe-Phe, respectively. An endomorphin gene has yet to be cloned, and much remains to be learned about the anatomic distribution, mode of interaction with the opioid receptors, function in vivo, and potential existence of other related peptides that are highly selective for each of the opioid receptors. It was recently demonstrated that both endomorphin-1 and endomorphin-2 given centrally and peripherally produced potent antiallodynic activities in a mouse model of neuropathic pain,[34] and downregulation of endomorphin-2 correlates with mechanical allodynia in a rat bone cancer pain model.[35]

TABLE 24.2 Pharmacologic Actions of Opioids and Opioid Receptors in Animal Models

		ACTIONS OF	
	Receptor	**Agonists**	**Antagonists**
ANALGESIA			
Supraspinal	μ, δ, κ	Analgesic	No effect
Spinal	μ, δ, κ	Analgesic	No effect
Respiratory function	μ	Decrease	No effect
Gastrointestinal tract	μ, κ	Decrease transit	No effect
Psychotomimesis	κ	Increase	No effect
Feeding	μ, δ, κ	Increase feeding	Decrease feeding
Sedation	μ, κ	Increase	No effect
Diuresis	κ	Increase	
HORMONE SECRETION			
Prolactin	μ	Increase release	Decrease release
Growth hormone	μ and/ or δ	Increase release	Decrease release
NEUROTRANSMITTER RELEASE			
Acetylcholine	μ	Inhibit	
Dopamine	δ	Inhibit	

INTRACELLULAR SIGNAL TRANSDUCTION MECHANISM OF OPIOID RECEPTORS

The opioid receptors belong to the G-protein-coupled receptor family. It has been demonstrated that activation of the opioid receptors leads to activation of the pertussis toxin-sensitive G proteins (G_i or G_o or both). Expression of the cloned opioid receptors in cultured cells by transfection of the cloned cDNAs has facilitated analysis of the intracellular signal transduction mechanisms activated by the opioid receptors (Fig. 24.6).[2] Adenylate cyclase is inhibited by opioid receptor activation, with a resulting reduction of the cellular cyclic adenosine monophosphate (AMP) content. Electrophysiologically, the voltage-gated Ca^{2+}

TABLE 24.3 Characteristics of Opioid Receptors

	μ	**δ**	**κ**	**Nociceptin**
Tissue bioassay	Guinea pig ileum	Mouse vas deferens	Rabbit vas deferens	—
Endogenous ligand	β-Endorphin, Endomorphin	Leu-enkephalin, Met-enkephalin	Dynorphin	Nociceptin
Agonist	Morphine, Fentanyl, DAMGO	DPDPE, Deltorphin	Buprenorphine, Pentazocine, U50488H	—
Antagonist	Naloxone, Naltrexone	Naloxone, Naltrindole	Naloxone, NorBNI	—
Coupled G protein	$G_{i/o}$	$G_{i/o}$	$G_{i/o}$	$G_{i/o}$
Adenylate cyclase	Inhibition	Inhibition	Inhibition	Inhibition
Voltage-gated Ca^{2+} channels	Inhibition	Inhibition	Inhibition	Inhibition
Inward rectifier K^+ channels	Activation	Activation	Activation	Activation

DAMGO, [d-Ala^2, MePhe^4, Gly-ol^8]enkephalin; *DPDPE*, [D-penicillamine^2, D-penicillamine^5]enkephalin; *NorBNI*, norbinaltorphimine.

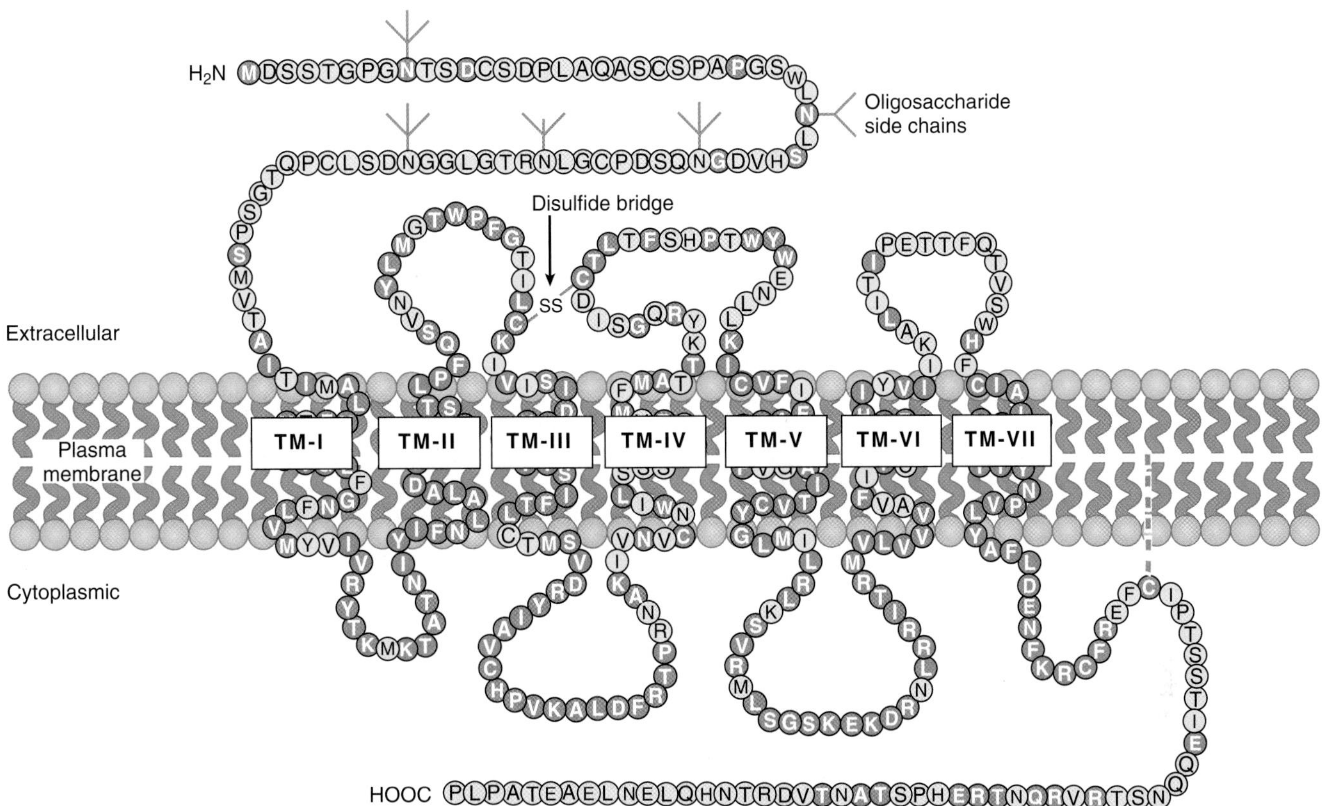

Fig. 24.2 Proposed structure of the μ-opioid receptor. *Black circles* indicate amino acid residues identical in the μ- and δ-opioid receptors. *TM-I* to *VII* show putative transmembrane segments composed of hydrophobic amino acid residues.

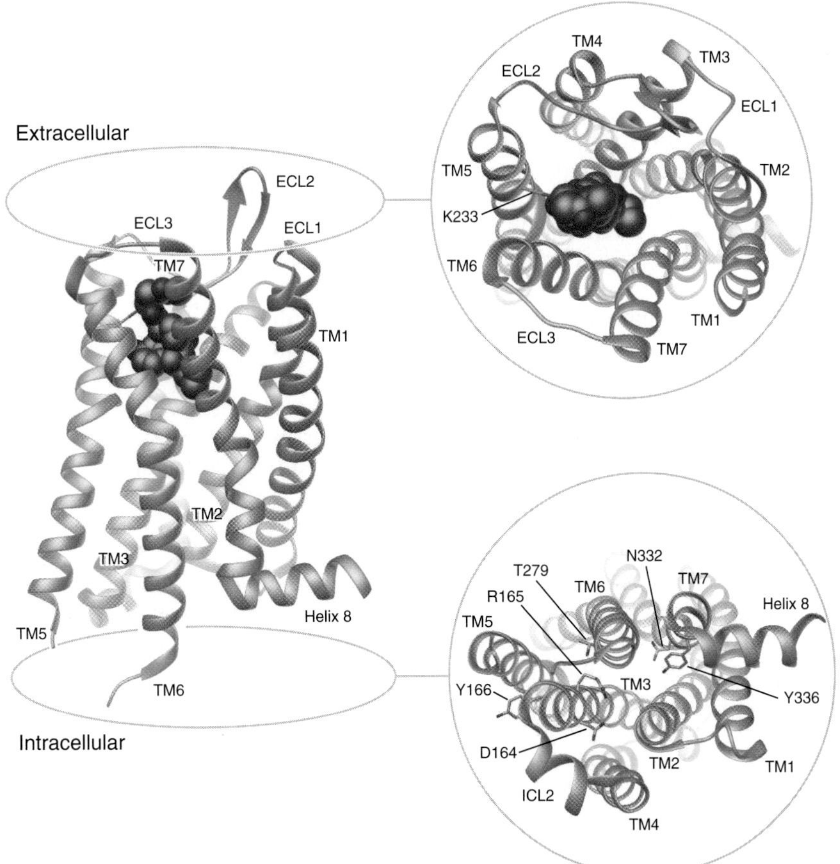

Fig. 24.3 Overall view of the μ-opioid receptor structure. Views from within the membrane plane *(left)*, extracellular side *(top)*, and intracellular side *(bottom)* show the typical 7-transmembrane G-protein-coupled receptor architecture of the μ-opioid receptor. β-FNA, a semisynthetic opioid antagonist derived from morphine, is shown in black spheres. (From Manglik A, Kruse AC, Kobilka TS, et al. Crystal structure of the μ-opioid receptor bound to a morphinan antagonist. *Nature*. 2012;485:321–326.)

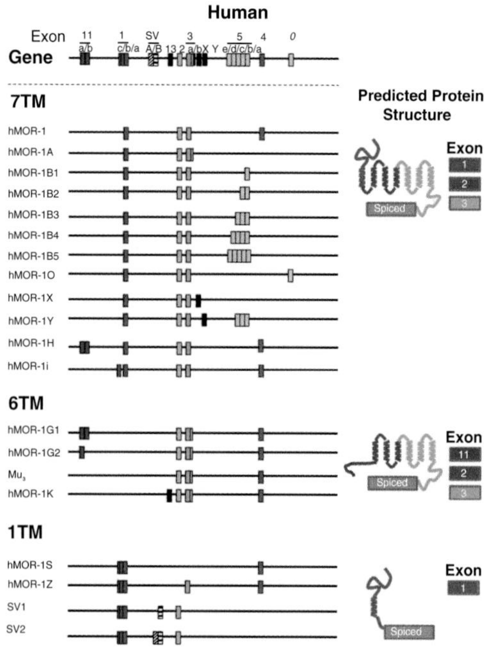

Fig. 24.4 μ-opioid receptor splicing in humans. Variants are grouped as full length, 7-transmembrane *(7TM)*, 6-transmembrane *(6TM)*, and 1-transmebrane *(1TM)* with the predicted structure shown to the right and the exons color-coded to match the splicing schematic. (From Pasternak GW, Pan YX. Mu opioids and their receptors: evolution of a concept. *Pharmacol Rev*. 2013;65:1257–1317.)

channel is inhibited and the inwardly rectifying potassium (K^+) channels are activated by the opioid receptors. As a result, neuronal excitability is reduced by activation of the opioid receptors. However, the role of adenylate cyclase in opioid receptor activation is complex. For example, long-term tolerance to opioids has been thought to be associated with superactivation of adenylyl cyclase activity, which is a counterregulatory response to the decrease in cyclic AMP levels seen after acute opioid administration.[36] That this effect is prevented by pretreatment of cells with pertussis toxin demonstrates involvement of G proteins (G_i or G_o or both).

Beyond adenylate cyclase, other regulatory components participate in the coupling of opioid receptor binding and a cellular response. It was shown that extracellular signal-related kinase, a class of mitogen-activated protein kinases, is activated by the opioid receptors.[37] Opioid-induced activation of extracellular signal-related kinase can lead to increase in arachidonate release[37] and expression of immediate early genes, c-fos and junB.[38]

Chronic exposure of the opioid receptors to agonists induces cellular adaptation mechanisms, which may be involved in opioid tolerance, dependence, and withdrawal symptoms. Several investigators have shown that short-term desensitization probably involves phosphorylation of the opioid receptors through protein kinase C.[39] A number of other kinases also have been implicated, including protein kinase A and β-adrenergic receptor kinase (BARK), a member of the G-protein-coupled receptor kinase (GRK).[40] BARKs selectively phosphorylate agonist-bound receptors and thereby promote interactions with β-arrestins, which interfere with G-protein coupling and promote receptor internalization. β-Arrestin 2 functions as a scaffolding protein that interacts with signal transducers, and the recruitment of β-arrestin 2 induced by opioid receptor activation is involved in the regulation of activity of c-Src, Akt, and mitogen-activated protein kinases (Fig. 24.7).[41] The c-Src inhibitor, dasatinib, attenuated and reversed morphine-induced tolerance in mice, suggesting that c-Src recruited by β-arrestin 2 is involved in the morphine-induced tolerance.[42] Acute morphine-induced analgesia was enhanced in mice lacking β-arrestin 2, suggesting that this protein contributes to regulation of responsivity to opioids *in vivo*.[43] Therefore, β-arrestin modification by associated kinases serves a critical role in the coupling between agonist binding to opioid receptors and their ability to develop and sustain an analgesic response.

Like other G-protein-coupled receptors, the opioid receptors can undergo rapid agonist-mediated internalization by a classic endocytic pathway.[44,45] These processes may be induced differentially as a function of the class of the ligand. For example, certain agonists, such as etorphine and enkephalins, cause rapid internalization of the μ receptor, whereas morphine, which decreases adenylyl cyclase activity equally well, does not cause μ receptor internalization in all cell types such as HEK293 cells.[46] Although these findings may suggest that different ligands induce different conformational changes in the receptor that lead to divergent intracellular events, they also have revealed that rapid morphine–dependent μ receptor endocytosis is still possible in subpopulations of central nervous system (CNS) neurons such as striatal neurons.[47] Taken together, they may help provide an explanation for differences in the efficacy and abuse potential of various opioids.[48]

BIASED AGONISM

Chemically distinct ligands binding to the same G-protein–coupled receptor can stabilize the receptor in multiple active conformations. In this way, differential activation of G-protein–coupled cell signaling pathways may produce divergent physiologic outcomes, a phenomenon known as biased agonism. Biased agonism can be exploited to design drugs that selectively activate desired signaling pathways, while minimizing other signaling pathways via the same receptor subtype and associated side effects.

Morphine binds to the μ-opioid receptor protein to form an active complex with signaling proteins, including $G_{i/o}$ and β-arrestin. The $G_{i/o}$ signaling pathway is thought to mediate analgesic action of morphine, whereas β-arrestin signaling results in unwanted side effects including euphoria, which can lead to addiction, respiratory depression, and gastrointestinal effects. Consistently, it was shown that the analgesic properties of morphine were enhanced but morphine-induced respiratory depression and constipation were attenuated in β-arrestin 2 knockout mice.[49] Emerging research in this evolving field includes a report by Manglik and associates, who computationally screened 3 million molecules, resulting in the compound PZM21, which showed high $G_{i/o}$-biased signaling and suppressed pain in mice without constipation, respiratory depression, hyperlocomotion, and addiction–related behaviors.[50] The clinical importance of these findings awaits further confirmation given other reports showing little difference in adverse effect profiles between morphine and PZM21 in

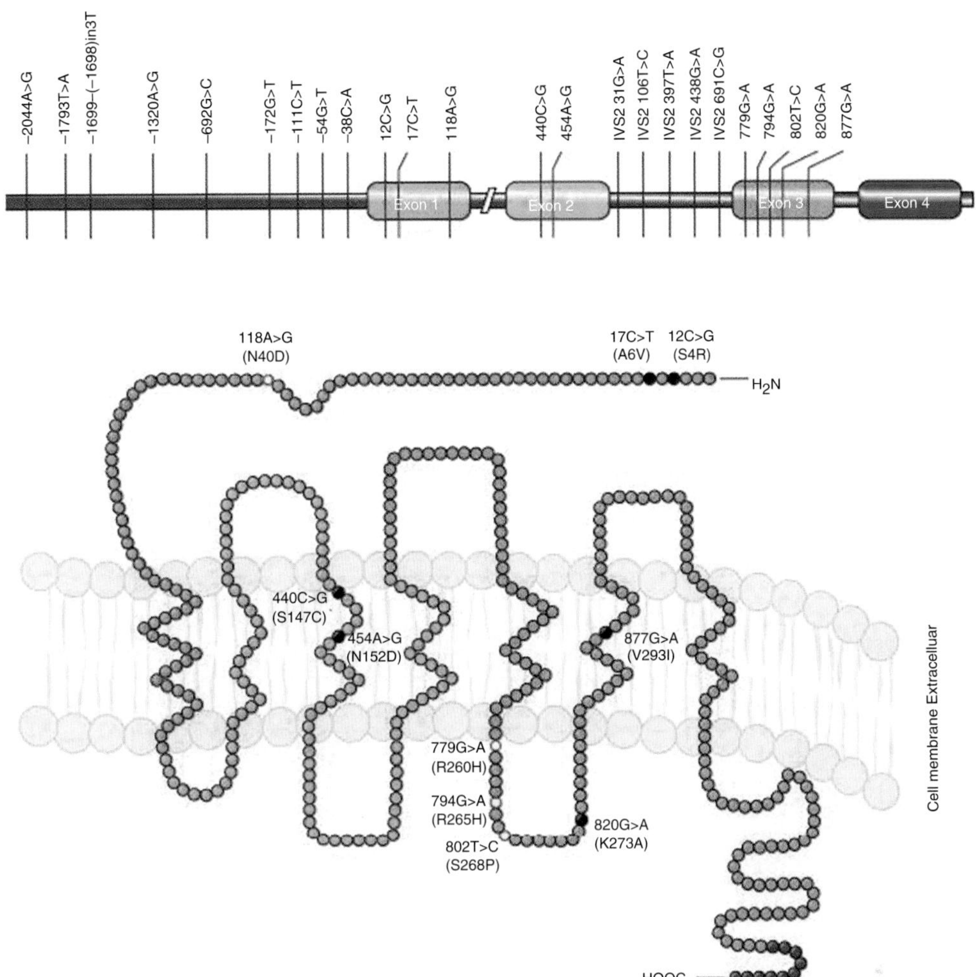

Fig. 24.5 Reported mutations in the μ-opioid receptor related to the exonic organization of the gene. Twenty-four mutations that produce an amino acid exchange and are frequently reportedly (>1%) or are proposed to have functional consequences are indicated in the gene. Amino acids are symbolized as circles, colored according to the exons by which they are coded. *Black circles* represent a naturally occurring mutation at the respective position, and *red circles* when functional consequences are shown at molecular level. Mutations are indicated by the nucleotide exchange and the resulting amino acid exchange. (From Lötsch J, Geisslinger G. Are μ-opioid receptor polymorphisms important for clinical opioid therapy? *Trends Mol Med.* 2005;11:82–89.)

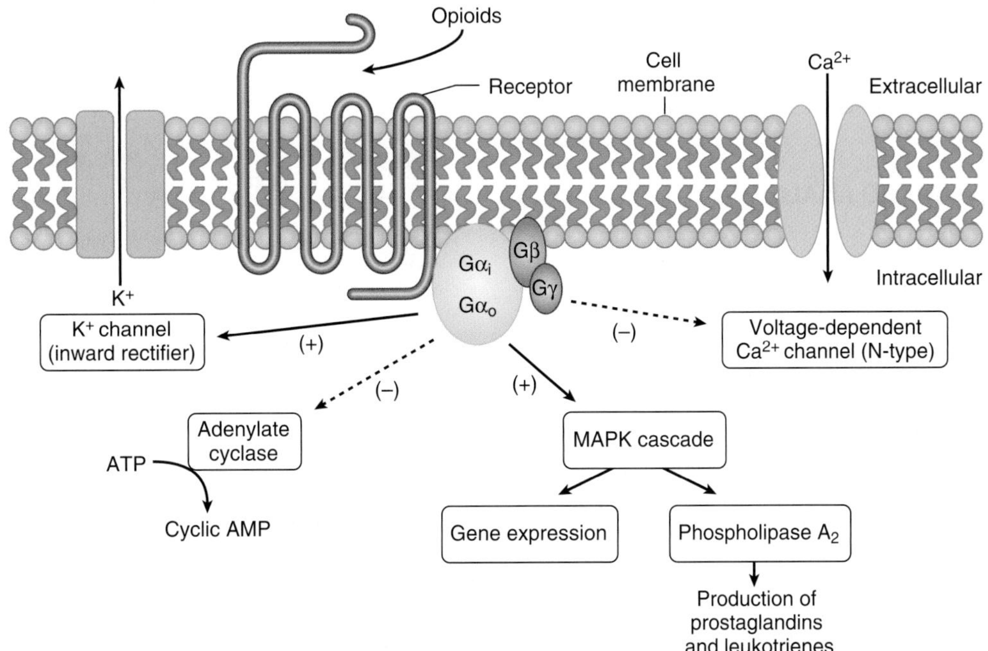

Fig. 24.6 Intracellular signal transduction mechanisms linked with the opioid receptors. Opioid agonists bind with the opioid receptors, leading to activation of the G protein. Activity of adenylate cyclase and the voltage-dependent calcium *(Ca^{2+})* channels is suppressed. On the other hand, inward rectifier potassium *(K^+)* channels and mitogen-activated protein kinase *(MAPK)* cascade are activated. *AMP*, Adenosine monophosphate; *ATP*, adenosine triphosphate.

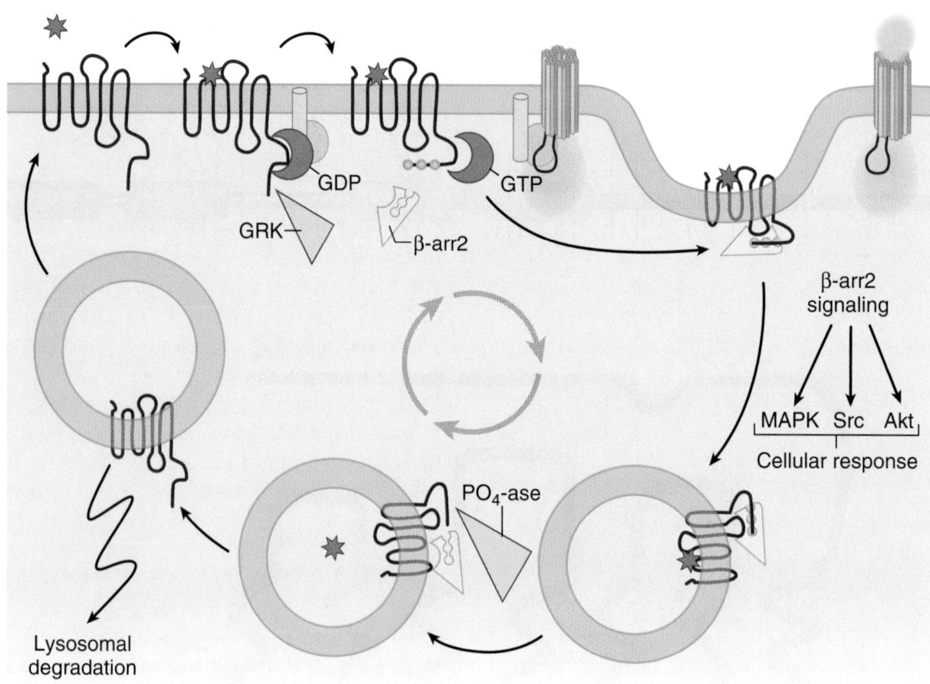

Fig. 24.7 β-Arrestin 2 and G protein in μ-opioid receptor recycling, signaling, and degradation. The *blue star* represents an opioid agonist and the trimeric membrane-associated complex in *brown, green,* and *blue* represents G protein α, β, and γ subunits, respectively. The α subunit is shown associated with guanosine diphosphate (*GDP*; resting state) or guanosine triphosphate (*GTP*; activated state). The βγ dimer interacts directly with the voltage-activated Ca^{2+} channel to inhibit calcium (Ca^{2+}) influx (indicated in *yellow*). β-arr2, β-arrestin 2; *GRK*, G-protein-coupled receptor kinase; *MAPK*, mitogen-activated protein kinase; *PO_4-ase*, phosphatase. (From Hales TG. Arresting the development of morphine tolerance and dependence. *Br J Anaesth*. 2011;107:653–655.)

mice.[51] However, TRV130, a "G protein-biased" μ-opioid ligand with G-protein–coupling efficacy similar to that of morphine, but markedly reduced receptor phosphorylation, recruitment of β-arrestin 2, and internalization, was tested in a randomized, double-blind, placebo-controlled crossover study in healthy volunteers.[52] TRV130 produced greater analgesia than morphine, but less respiratory depression and less severe nausea (Fig. 24.8). As additional biased-agonist candidates of the μ-opioid receptor emerge, so does the hope for a new generation of clinically effective analgesics with a reduced profile of harm.

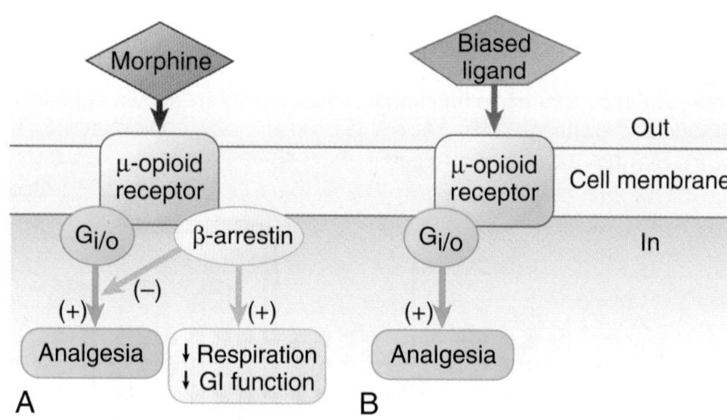

Fig. 24.8 Biased agonism. (A) Morphine binding to the μ-opioid receptor not only activates the G protein *($G_{i/o}$)* analgesic effect, but also recruits β-arrestins, which inhibits G protein coupling and promotes hypoventilation and gastrointestinal dysfunction. (B) *TRV130*, a G protein–biased agonist, engages G-protein coupling similarly to morphine but with less β-arrestin recruitment, resulting in analgesic effect similar to morphine and less effects on respiratory and gastrointestinal function.

MECHANISM OF OPIOID ANALGESIA

Brain

Pain control by opioids needs to be considered in the context of brain circuits modulating analgesia and the functions of the various types of receptors in these circuits.[53] It is well established that the analgesic effects of opioids arise from their ability to inhibit directly the ascending transmission of nociceptive information from the spinal cord dorsal horn and to activate pain control circuits that descend from the midbrain, through the rostral ventromedial medulla (RVM), to the spinal cord dorsal horn. Petrovic and colleagues used an experimental pain model and positron emission tomography (PET) to study mechanisms of action of the short-acting μ-opioid agonist remifentanil and found drug-induced activation of the rostral anterior cingulate cortex, insula, orbitofrontal cortex, and brainstem areas.[54] The activated brainstem regions overlapped with brain areas that have been implicated in pain modulation, such as the periaqueductal gray (PAG). Interestingly, placebo analgesia acts similarly on the activity of these brain areas, presumably via endogenous opioid release.[55]

Immunohistochemical studies and in situ hybridization analysis have demonstrated that opioid receptors are expressed in various areas in the CNS.[56] These areas include the amygdala, the mesencephalic reticular formation, the PAG, and the RVM. However, the role of the opioid receptors in all of these areas has not been completely clarified.

Microinjection of morphine into the PAG or direct electrical stimulation of this area produces analgesia that can be blocked by naloxone. Opioid actions at the PAG influence RVM, which in turn modulates nociceptive transmission in the dorsal horn of the spinal cord through the action of the descending inhibition pathway. Thus, opioids produce analgesia by direct actions on the spinal cord, as well as by neurally mediated action in the region separated from the site of opioid administration. Interestingly, a study by Dogrul and Seyrek reported that spinal serotonin 5-HT7 receptors play an important role on the antinociceptive effects of systemic morphine.[57]

It is well known that the actions of opioids in bulbospinal pathways are critical to their analgesic efficacy. It is clear that opioid actions in the forebrain contribute to analgesia, because decerebration prevents analgesia when rats are tested for pain sensitivity using the formalin test,[58] and microinjection of opioids into several forebrain regions are analgesic in this test.[59] Analgesia induced by systemic administration of morphine in both the tail-flick and formalin tests was disrupted either by lesioning or reversibly inactivating the central nucleus of the amygdala, thereby demonstrating that opioid actions in the forebrain contribute to analgesia after tissue damage, as well as after acute phasic nociception.[60]

The distribution of opioid receptors in descending pain control circuits indicates substantial overlap between μ and κ receptors. Interactions between the κ receptor and the μ receptor may be important for modulating nociceptive transmission from higher nociceptive centers, as well as in the spinal cord dorsal horn. The μ receptor produces analgesia within descending pain control circuits, at least in part, by the removal of γ-aminobutyric acidergic inhibition of RVM-projecting neurons in the PAG and spinally projecting neurons in the RVM.[53] The actions of μ-receptor agonists are invariably analgesic, whereas those of κ-receptor agonists can be either analgesic or antianalgesic. The pain-modulating effects of the κ-receptor agonists in the brainstem appear to oppose those of μ-receptor agonists.[61]

Spinal Cord

Analgesic actions of systemic morphine are in part mediated by a net inhibitory effect from the PAG and RVM on nociceptive processing in the spinal dorsal horn. It was demonstrated that morphine increased 5-HT release in the spinal dorsal horn by activation of serotonergic neurons in the RVM, and intrathecal pretreatment with ondansetron attenuated the analgesic effect of morphine in normal rats, suggesting the involvement of the 5-HT_3 serotonergic receptor in morphine analgesia.[62]

Local spinal mechanisms, in addition to descending inhibition, underlie the analgesic action of opioids. In the spinal cord, opioids act at synapses either presynaptically or postsynaptically. Opioid receptors are abundantly expressed in the substantia gelatinosa, where glutamate and substance P release from the primary sensory neuron is inhibited by opioids. Histamine receptors are known to participate in spinal cord nociceptive transmission, and previous studies have suggested that histaminergic receptors are also involved in the analgesic effects of morphine. An H_1 antagonist and H_3 agonist were found to potentiate the analgesic and antiedematogenic effects of morphine, suggesting that histaminergic and opioid spinal systems may be explored for means of improving analgesia, as well as peripheral antiinflammatory effects.[63]

Opioid-receptor ligand binding has been identified in both presynaptic and postsynaptic sites in the dorsal horn of the spinal cord. It is well known that opioids decrease the pain-evoked release of tachykinins from primary afferent nociceptors. However, the degree that opioids can suppress tachykinin signaling in response to noxious stimulation remains controversial.[64] These results suggest that although opioid administration may reduce tachykinin release from primary afferent nociceptors, the reduction may not be a major modulator on the actions of tachykinins on postsynaptic pain-transmitting neurons.

Peripheral Mechanism

Opioids may also produce analgesia through the peripheral mechanism.[65] Immune cells infiltrating the inflammation site may release endogenous opioid-like substances, which act on the opioid receptors located on the primary sensory neuron.[65] Interestingly, in cannabinoid receptor type 1 and type 2 knockout mice, the antinociceptive effect of morphine injected into the paw in the inflammatory phase of the formalin test was decreased by 87% and 76%, respectively.[66] This finding may suggest the possibility that the release of endogenous cannabinoids in structures along the pain pathway is involved in opioid analgesia by the peripheral mechanism.

Acupuncture

Acupuncture and electroacupuncture have been shown to block pain by activating a variety of bioactive chemicals through peripheral, spinal, and supraspinal mechanisms. Mechanistically, endogenous opioids and opioid receptors have been shown to be involved in acupuncture- and electroacupuncture-induced analgesia in various pain models.[67] Studies in carrageenan-induced inflammatory rat pain models show that an intraplantar injection of naloxone or selective antagonists against μ-, δ-, or κ-opioid receptors 1 hour before electroacupuncture treatment at acupoint *Zusanli* (ST36) dose-dependently blocked electroacupuncture-produced inhibition of mechanical hyperalgesia assessed through paw-pressure threshold.[68] In a capsaicin-induced inflammatory hind paw pain model, stimulation by 2 Hz of four-train pulses with 100 Hz of intratrain frequency at *Houxi* (SI3) and *San-yangluo* (TE8) on the forelimb significantly raised the mechanical pain threshold of the injected paw. This analgesic effect was blocked by intrathecal μ- or δ-opioid receptor antagonists but not by a κ-opioid receptor antagonist.[69] Precise mechanisms for acupuncture and electroacupuncture, including the involvement of physiologic systems other than the opioid receptors, remain to be elucidated.

MECHANISM OF MOOD ALTERATIONS AND REWARDING PROPERTIES

The mechanisms by which opioids produce euphoria, tranquility, and other alterations of mood (including rewarding properties) remain an area of active investigation, especially given the expanding scope of opioid diversion and misuse. Behavioral and pharmacologic evidence points to the role of dopaminergic pathways, particularly involving the nucleus accumbens (NAcc), in drug-induced reward. Functional magnetic resonance imaging studies demonstrated that a small intravenous dose (4 mg) of morphine induces positive signal changes in reward structures, including the NAcc, sublenticular extended amygdala, orbitofrontal cortex, and hippocampus, and decreases signal in cortical areas similar to the action of sedative-hypnotics such as propofol and midazolam.[70] These observations are consistent with results of pharmacologic studies.

The shell of the NAcc is the site that may be involved directly in the emotional and motivational aspects of drug-induced reward. All three opioid receptor types are present on the NAcc and are thought to mediate, at least in part, the motivational effects of opioid drugs.[56] Selective μ- and δ-receptor agonists are rewarding when defined by place preference and intracranial self-administration paradigms. Conversely, selective κ-receptor agonists produce aversive effects. Positive motivational effects of opioids are partially mediated by dopamine release at the level of the NAcc.

The locus ceruleus contains both noradrenergic neurons and high concentrations of opioid receptors and is postulated to play a critical role in feelings of alarm, panic, fear, and anxiety. Neural activity in the locus ceruleus is inhibited by both exogenous opioids and endogenous opioid peptides.

ANALYSIS OF KNOCKOUT MICE

The physiologic roles of the opioid receptors and endogenous opioid peptides have been investigated mainly by pharmacologic and physiologic methods. However, it has been difficult to analyze functional roles of these proteins. With analysis of knockout mice, in which a specific gene is inactivated by molecular biologic methods, additional insight into the physiologic role of the respective opioid receptors and/or endogenous opioid peptide precursors can be determined.[71]

In the μ-receptor knockout mice, analgesia, the reward effect, and the withdrawal effect of morphine were lost.[72] Morphine-induced respiratory depression was not observed in the μ-receptor knockout mice.[73] Therefore, the μ-receptor is a mandatory component of the opioid system for morphine action. In the μ-receptor knockout mice, ketamine-induced respiratory depression and antinociception are diminished,[74] a finding suggesting that ketamine interacts with the μ receptor to lead to these phenomena. Furthermore, minimum alveolar concentration (MAC) of sevoflurane was significantly higher in the μ-receptor knockout mice than wild-type mice, an observation suggesting the involvement of the μ receptor in the anesthetic potency of sevoflurane.[73] The δ-receptor knockout mice displayed a markedly reduced analgesic effect of opioids selective for δ-receptors at the spinal cord level.[75] However, at the supraspinal level, analgesia could be induced by δ-receptor agonists in δ-receptor knockout mice, a finding suggesting the existence of a second δ-like analgesic system. Disruption of the κ receptor abolished the analgesic, hypolocomotor, and aversive actions of the κ-receptor agonists and induced hyperreactivity in the abdominal constriction test; this finding indicates that the κ receptor is involved in the perception of visceral chemical pain.[76] Using gene knockout mice, a pharmacologic study demonstrated that the antinociceptive effect of N_2O may not be mediated by μ-receptor[77]; rather N_2O exerts its antinociceptive action and reduces MAC of volatile anesthetics in mice through complex mechanisms including activation of the κ receptor and the descending inhibitory pathway in the spinal cord, whereas its hypnotic potency is not dependent on κ-receptor activation.[78]

In the mice lacking β-endorphin, morphine induced normal analgesia, but naloxone-reversible stress-induced analgesia could not be observed.[79] The preproenkephalin knockout mice were more anxious than wild-type mice, and males displayed increased offensive aggressiveness.[80] The mutant mice showed marked difference from controls in supraspinal, but not in spinal, responses to painful stimuli.

Thus, the functional roles of individual components of the opioid system continue to be elucidated by analysis of knockout mice. The μ-opioid receptor continues to be recognized as a predominant signaling receptor for both the affective and antinociceptive action of opioid agonism.

ACTIONS OF OPIOIDS ON TARGETS OTHER THAN OPIOID RECEPTORS

Molecular pharmacologic analyses have shown that opioids can interact with molecules other than the opioid receptors. In cardiac myocytes, morphine can inhibit voltage-dependent sodium (Na^+) current in a naloxone-insensitive manner, a finding suggesting the existence of a signal transduction mechanism that is not dependent on the opioid receptors.[81] Buprenorphine, a partial μ-opioid receptor agonist, also has a local anesthetic property and blocks voltage-gated Na^+ channels through the local anesthetic binding site.[82] Meperidine is an agonist of both μ and κ receptors. In addition, meperidine can block voltage-dependent Na^+ channels in amphibian peripheral nerves,[83] as well as in the *Xenopus* oocyte expression system.[84] Furthermore, meperidine exerts agonist activity at the α_{2B}-adrenoreceptor subtype.[85] Yamakura and associates have shown that high concentrations of opioids, including meperidine, morphine, fentanyl, codeine, and naloxone, directly inhibit the *N*-methyl-D-aspartate (NMDA) receptor expressed in *Xenopus* oocytes.[86] Methadone is clinically used as a racemic mixture of the *l* and *d* isomers. The opioid-like activity of the racemate seems to be almost entirely the result of *l*-methadone, whereas *d*-methadone acts as an NMDA antagonist.[87] The commercially available remifentanil solution (Ultiva), which contains glycine, directly activates the NMDA receptor expressed in *Xenopus* oocytes.[88] Furthermore, an electrophysiologic study in rat spinal cord showed that remifentanil hydrochloride does not directly activate NMDA receptors, the NMDA current recorded after application of Ultiva is related to the presence of glycine, and the glycine-induced NMDA current is potentiated by application of remifentanil hydrochloride through a pathway involving the μ-opioid receptor.[89] The serotonin type 3A (5-HT_{3A}) receptor, which is directly and indirectly linked to gastrointestinal motility, visceral pain, nausea, and vomiting, is competitively inhibited by morphine and hydromorphone, as well as naloxone; however, fentanyl-like opioids did not significantly affect activity of the 5-HT_{3A} receptor.[90,91] The mechanism for tramadol analgesia is complex and appears to be composed of two actions that include reuptake inhibition of the noradrenergic serotonergic system and activation of the μ-opioid receptor. Tramadol's analgesic effect is only partially reversed by the μ-opioid receptor antagonist, naloxone. Furthermore, tramadol also acts as an agonist of transient receptor potential vanilloid-1 (TRPV1) heterologously expressed in cultured cells.[92] Tramadol may activate TRPV1 in sensory neurons, followed by local release of vasoactive neuropeptides and marked desensitization of the afferent fibers. Inhibition of the nicotinic acetylcholine receptor by tramadol has also been reported.[93] It remains to be clarified which of these "off-target" actions of opioids have physiologic or clinical implications.

PHYSIOLOGIC ROLE OF NOCICEPTIN/ORPHANIN FQ

Nociceptin or orphanin FQ is a 17-amino-acid peptide, the sequence of which resembles those of opioid peptides. Nociceptin or orphanin FQ precursor mRNA and peptide are present throughout the descending pain control circuits. In the spinal cord, nociceptin or orphanin FQ-receptor mRNA expression is stronger in the ventral horn than in the dorsal horn, but higher levels of ligand binding occur in the dorsal horn. Targeted disruption of the nociceptin or orphanin FQ receptor in mice had little effect on basal pain sensitivity in several measures, whereas targeted disruption of the N nociceptin or orphanin FQ precursor consistently elevated basal responses in the tail-flick test, findings suggesting an important role for nociceptin or orphanin FQ in regulating basal pain sensitivity.[94,95] Intrathecal injections of nociceptin or orphanin FQ have been shown to be analgesic[96]; however, supraspinal administration has produced hyperalgesia, antiopioid effects, or a biphasic hyperalgesic-analgesic response.[97] Nociceptin or orphanin FQ inhibits both pain-facilitating and analgesia-facilitating neurons in the RVM.[98] The effects of nociceptin or orphanin FQ on pain responses appear to depend on the preexisting state of pain in the animal. Involvement of nociceptin or orphanin FQ in physiologic functions such as regulation of feeding, body weight homeostasis, and stress response, and in psychiatric disorders such as depression, anxiety, and drug or alcohol dependence has also been reported.[99]

Systemic administration of nonpeptide nociceptin or orphanin FQ receptor agonists revealed that such compounds were effective analgesics in animal pain models. It was reported that a nociceptin or orphanin FQ receptor agonist, Ro64-6198, has antinociceptive and antiallodynic potency and efficacy without side effects of opioids such as itching, respiratory depression, and addiction in monkeys.[100] As nociceptin or orphanin FQ and opioid receptor agonists modulate pain by different targets, combining both mechanisms may constitute a novel approach for the development of innovative analgesics. Cebranopadol, a newly synthesized compound possessing nociceptin or orphanin FQ and opioid receptor agonist activity, exhibits highly potent and efficacious antinociceptive and antihyperalgesic effects in several rat models of acute and chronic pain (tail-flick, rheumatoid arthritis, bone cancer, spinal nerve ligation, diabetic neuropathy).[101] In a phase 1 clinical trial, it was shown that cebranopadol produced respiratory depression with a ceiling effect, in contrast to apnea produced by full μ-opioid receptor agonists.[102]

Expression of opioid receptors on peripheral blood mononuclear cells is controversial. Williams and associates reported that human peripheral blood mononuclear cells express the nociceptin receptor, but not μ-, δ-, or κ-opioid receptors.[103] Nociceptin, produced by the peripheral blood mononuclear cells, is involved in the control of immune functions.

Neurophysiologic Effects of Opioids

CHARACTERISTICS OF THE ANALGESIC ACTION OF OPIOIDS

In human beings, morphine-like drugs produce analgesia, drowsiness, changes in mood, and mental clouding. A significant feature of opioid analgesia is that it is not typically associated with loss of consciousness. When morphine in the same dose is given to a normal, pain-free individual, the experience may be unpleasant. The relief of pain by morphine-like opioids is relatively selective, in that other sensory modalities are not affected. Patients frequently report that the pain is still present, but that they feel more comfortable. It is also important to distinguish between pain caused by stimulation of nociceptive receptors and transmitted over intact neural pathways (nociceptive pain) and pain that is caused by damage to neural structures, often involving neural supersensitivity (neuropathic pain). Although nociceptive pain usually is responsive to opioid analgesics, neuropathic pain may respond poorly to opioid analgesics and require higher doses of drug.[104]

The analgesic effects, as well as side effects, of opioids vary greatly among individuals. A pharmacogenomic twin study has shown that the interindividual variations in opioid effects are likely the result of genetic and environmental factors.[105,106] Animal and human studies indicate the existence of sex-related differences in opioid-mediated behavior.[107] Sarton and associates examined the influence of morphine on experimentally induced pain in healthy volunteers, and demonstrated the gender differences in morphine analgesia, with greater morphine potency but slower speed of onset and offset in women.[108] In contrast, in a study examining interindividual variability in alfentanil analgesic sensitivity in experimental pain models in humans, no gender differences were detected.[109] In a study examining the effects of genetic factors on pain sensitivity, it was shown that males had higher pain thresholds in both thermal skin pain and muscle pressure pain than females.[110] The mechanism of the gender difference in pain sensitivity and opioid effects remains to be clarified.

The pharmacokinetic and pharmacodynamic characteristics of opioids often vary throughout the day, as demonstrated for oral morphine in chronic pain.[111] The duration of intrathecal sufentanil analgesia exhibited a temporal pattern, with 30% variation throughout the day in women in the first stage of labor.[112] Scavone and colleagues reported that the time of day of administration does not seem to influence duration of labor analgesia with spinal-epidural administration of fentanyl or with systemic hydromorphone administration.[113] The potential impact of chronobiology on clinical practice is not clear, and research on the influence of circadian rhythms on the actions of opioids is warranted.

Some controversy remains regarding analgesia produced by peripheral actions of opioids. One review concluded from meta-analysis that intraarticularly administered morphine has a definite but mild analgesic effect.[114] It may be dose dependent, and a systemic effect cannot be completely excluded. The addition of opioids in brachial plexus block improves the success rate and postoperative analgesia.[115] In contrast, the addition of sufentanil may not prolong the duration of brachial plexus block.[116]

Despite variations in effect ascribed to the type of pain stimuli, genetics, gender, time of administration, or site of action (central versus peripheral), opioids remain one of the most potent classes of analgesic drugs.

EFFECTS OF OPIOIDS ON CONSCIOUSNESS

Cortical acetylcholine originates in the basal forebrain and is essential for maintaining normal cognition and arousal. Injection of morphine to the substantia innominata or intravenous morphine administration significantly decreased acetylcholine release within the prefrontal cortex in the rat, and this effect may be the neurochemical basis of opioid-induced change in consciousness.[117] Although unconsciousness in humans can be produced with high doses of opioids alone, opioid-based anesthesia can be unpredictable and inconsistent.[118] Therefore, opioids are not suitable as sole intravenous induction agents.[119] The anesthetic potential of opioids was tested by measurement of MAC.[120] Fentanyl can reduce the MAC of isoflurane at skin incision in patients by at least 80%.[121] The relationship between the plasma fentanyl concentration and reduction in MAC is not linear, and fentanyl has a sub-MAC ceiling effect on reduction of the MAC of isoflurane. The MAC of sevoflurane was also dose dependently reduced by fentanyl, with 3 ng/mL resulting in a 61% reduction in MAC.[122] A ceiling effect was observed for MAC; 6 ng/mL fentanyl provided only an additional 13% reduction in the MAC of sevoflurane. Even potency ratios have been established for the "reduction of volatile anesthetic MAC" for most opioids such as sufentanil, fentanyl, remifentanil, and alfentanil. However, the MAC-reducing capabilities of the opioids are not complete; that is, these are not complete anesthetics. The opioids must be combined with other anesthetics to produce a "complete anesthetic."[121,123-125] Esmolol, a short-acting β_1-receptor antagonist, significantly decreased the MAC of isoflurane in the presence of alfentanil, although it did not significantly affect this parameter in the absence of alfentanil.[126] The mechanism of the interaction is unknown. Epidural fentanyl infusion reduces the awakening concentration of isoflurane more than does intravenous fentanyl infusion despite the lower plasma concentration, possibly by modulating the afferent nociceptive inputs in the spinal cord.[127]

The MAC that prevents movement in response to laryngoscopy and tracheal intubation in 50% of patients (MAC-TI) is higher than the MAC that prevents movement in response to surgical incision (MAC). The MAC-TI of sevoflurane was 3.55% and was reduced markedly to 2.07%, 1.45%, and 1.37% by the addition of fentanyl 1, 2, and 4 µg/kg, respectively, with no significant difference in the reduction between 2 and 4 µg/kg, thus showing a ceiling effect.[128] The MAC that prevents sympathetic responses to surgical incision in 50% of patients (MAC-BAR) decreased with increasing concentrations of fentanyl in plasma, and the initial steep reduction followed by a ceiling effect.[122]

The bispectral index (BIS) is often used to determine the level of consciousness under anesthesia. In the presence of fentanyl, alfentanil, remifentanil, or sufentanil, loss of consciousness occurred at a lower effect-site concentration of propofol and at a higher BIS value as compared with propofol alone.[129] Furthermore, Wang and associates reported that infusion of remifentanil (0.1-0.4 µg/kg/min) did not significantly change the median effective concentration (EC_{50}) of propofol necessary to lower the BIS value to 50 or less.[130] These results suggest that the hypnotic effect of propofol is enhanced by analgesic concentrations of opioids without changes in the BIS value. Conversely, infusion of remifentanil (effect-site target concentrations of 0.25, 2.5, and 10 ng/mL), combined with propofol infusion adjusted to a BIS of approximately 60, dose dependently decreased the BIS, thus suggesting a sedative or hypnotic effect of remifentanil.[131] Response surface analysis showed considerable synergy between opioids and hypnotics for sedation and suppression of responses to various noxious stimuli.[132] In contrast to the effect of opioids administered during anesthesia on the BIS, the impact of chronic opioid use on BIS is unknown. It was recently reported that the end-tidal concentration of sevoflurane necessary to maintain the BIS under 50 was 0.84% for chronic opioid users who received a stable dose of oral morphine of at least 60 mg/day according to the morphine equivalent daily dose for at least 4 weeks, which was lower than for opioid-naïve patients (1.18%).[133]

Opioids administered as a mainstay of postsurgical pain management can inhibit sleep on the first night after surgery. However, the effects of opioids on sleep and circadian rhythm are not clearly understood. A human study demonstrated that an overnight constant infusion of remifentanil inhibited rapid eye movement sleep without suppressing the nocturnal melatonin surge, findings that may suggest a minimal effect of opioids on the circadian pacemaker.[134]

Taken together, perioperative opioids have consistently been shown to dose dependently reduce the MAC and are well known to synergize with hypnotics to produce sedation; however, their ability to effect the BIS may vary depending on the context of opioid administration.

HALLUCINATION

Opioid-induced hallucination is an uncommon yet significant adverse effect of opioid treatment, frequently attributed to underlying psychiatric disease or personality disorder rather than a direct neurobiologic effect of opioids.[135] Hallucinations attributed to opioids have been typically described as auditory, visual, or rarely, tactile hallucinations. Although many reports have cited morphine as the causative agent, there is no evidence that across a population, one particular class of opioid is associated with a lower incidence of hallucinations. Moreover, there are reports of fentanyl, methadone, tramadol, hydromorphone, buprenorphine, pentazocine, and/or oxycodone–associated hallucinations and/or changes in mental status. Nevertheless, accumulation of morphine metabolites, particularly morphine-3-glucoronide, has been linked to the development of neurologic phenomena.[136] Many hypotheses have been advanced to explain the etiology of opioid-induced hallucinations. One common feature of these hypotheses involves opioid-induced dopamine dysregulation. Overactivation of the dopaminergic pathways is thought to result in auditory and visual hallucinations.[137] The simplest treatment for opioid-induced hallucination is discontinuing opioid therapy if practical. There are reports describing the successful use of naloxone and κ-selective opioid antagonists in the treatment of hallucinations associated with schizophrenia, although such κ-selective agents are known to be associated with hallucinations in subjects or patients without a diagnosis of mental illness.[138]

ELECTROENCEPHALOGRAPHY

Increasing concentrations of inhaled anesthetics produce a continuum of electroencephalogram (EEG) changes and eventually result in burst suppression and a flat EEG. In contrast, a ceiling effect is reached with opioids. Once this ceiling has been obtained, increasing opioid dosage does not further affect the EEG.[139]

Although the potency and rate of equilibrium between plasma and brain are different among opioids, the effects of fentanyl, alfentanil, sufentanil, and remifentanil are consistent (Fig. 24.9).[140] Small doses of fentanyl (2-5 μg/kg) produce minimal EEG changes, whereas higher doses (30-70 μg/kg) result in high-voltage slow (δ) waves suggesting a state consistent with anesthesia. Although transient isolated (usually frontotemporal) sharp wave activity can be observed after large doses of fentanyl and other opioids, it is not generalized. In a study examining the effect of morphine (3-10 mg) on EEG in patients (14.8 ± 2.8 years) who stayed overnight for pain relief after otologic surgery, it was

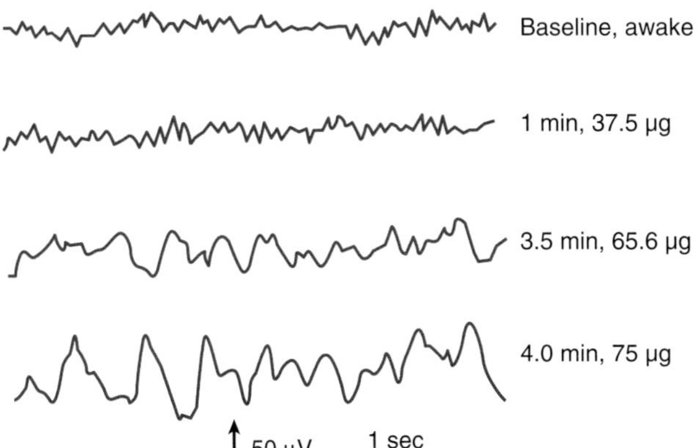

Fig. 24.9 Representative 4-s electroencephalogram (EEG) tracings during infusion of sufentanil (total dose shown in the right *column*). The awake baseline EEG consists of mixed β and α activity. At 1 minute, the EEG showed loss of β activity and the presence of primarily α waves (8-13 Hz). At 3.5 minutes, the EEG consisted of mixed θ (4-7 Hz) and δ (<4 Hz) waves, and at 4.0 min, it consisted of δ waves of high amplitude. (From Scott JC, Cooke JE, Stanski DR. Electroencephalographic quantitation of opioid effect: comparative pharmacodynamics of fentanyl and sufentanil. *Anesthesiology*. 1991;74:34–42.)

demonstrated that morphine reduced high-frequency β_1 (13.5-20 Hz) and β_2 (20-30 Hz) EEG powers and decreased coherence between frontal and occipital β_2 EEG activities compared to wakefulness and non–rapid eye movement sleep, indicating that morphine induced a deep sedative state (Fig. 24.10).[141] Khodayari-Rostamabad and associates studied the effect of remifentanil administration on resting EEG functional connectivity and its relationship to cognitive function and analgesia in healthy volunteers.[142] Remifentanil administration was associated with significant changes in functional cortical connectivity, which seem to disrupt the complex cortical network subserving normal brain function and can have the potential to be a biomarker for the sedative effects of opioids.

As an effect-site measure, EEG can be employed to assess onset of drug action and drug potency ratios. The spectral edge and serum concentration are closely parallel for remifentanil,[143] whereas a significant time lag is found for recovery of the spectral edge for fentanyl and sufentanil (Fig. 24.11).[144] In healthy volunteers, approximate entropy derived from a parietal montage showed significant correlation with remifentanil concentration, and it was shown to be appropriate for the assessment of the remifentanil effect on the EEG.[145] Potency ratios based on EEG studies are similar to those obtained from studies determining the plasma drug levels of each opioid necessary to reduce the MAC of isoflurane by 50%. Overall, opioids produce dose-dependent changes in the EEG that can mimic those of volatile anesthetics, however opioids show a ceiling effect at higher doses.

EVOKED RESPONSES

Because opioids do not appreciably alter sensory-evoked potentials elicited at the posterior tibial or median nerve, sensory-evoked potentials can be used for spinal cord function monitoring during anesthesia using opioids.[146] Although remifentanil produced dose-dependent reduction in auditory-evoked potentials,[147] it was also reported that remifentanil infusion (target plasma concentrations of 1, 2, and 3 ng/mL) did not affect evoked potential amplitudes and latencies.[148] In healthy human volunteers receiving 3 μg/kg fentanyl, amplitude and latency of motor-evoked responses to transcranial stimulation were not significantly affected.[149] This is consistent with the report by Kawaguchi and colleagues that intraoperative myogenic motor-evoked potential monitoring is feasible during isoflurane or sevoflurane anesthesia with fentanyl.[150]

Middle latency auditory-evoked potentials (MLAEPs) and their derivatives are increasingly used as a surrogate measure of the level of anesthesia. Changes in MLAEPs following the administration of opioids occur and may result from either a direct depressant effect of opioids on MLAEPs itself or an indirect effect reflecting the action of opioids in attenuating CNS arousal associated with noxious stimuli. Wright and associates examined the effect of remifentanil (1 or 3 μg/kg/min) on MLAEPs in tracheally intubated and nonintubated patients and showed that remifentanil has an effect on MLAEPs in attenuating the arousal associated with tracheal intubation but had no effect in the absence of a stimulus.[151] Similarly, Schraag and associates found no significant contribution of remifentanil alone on MLAEPs,

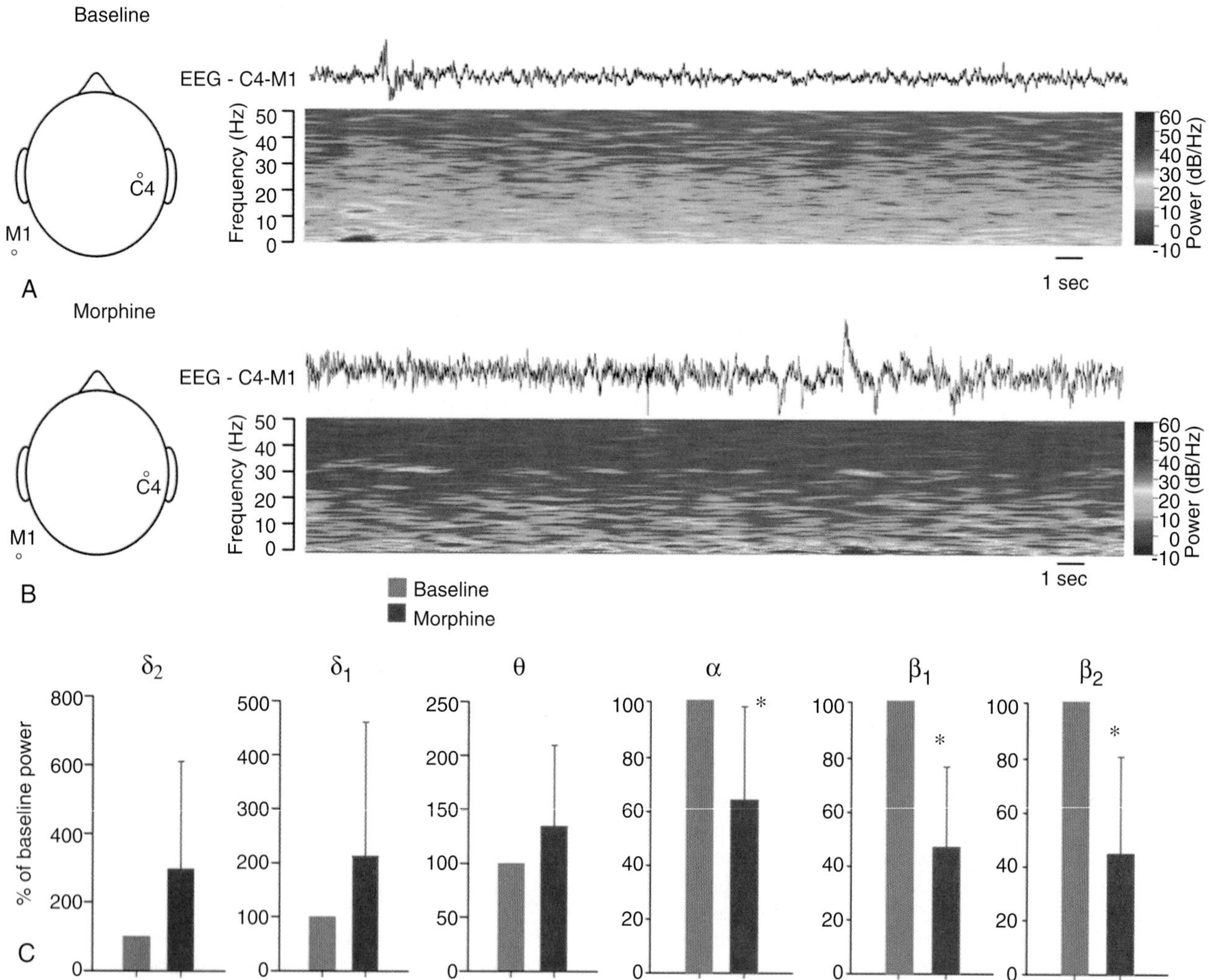

Fig. 24.10 Impacts of morphine on electroencephalography *(EEG)* spectral content. EEG activity of a representative 30-s epoch and power spectrograms of *C4-M1* (C4 = central electrode; M1 = mastoid electrode) derivation at baseline and after morphine administration. In a representative patient (A) and in the analyzed group data (B and C), high-frequency power (α, β_1, and β_2) was decreased by morphine. Mean data for 10 patients showed that morphine decreased α ($P = .039$, $n = 10$), β_1 ($P = .003$, $n = 10$), and β_2 ($P = .020$, $n = 10$) powers but did not change δ_2 ($P = .375$, $n = 10$), δ_1 ($P = .922$, $n = 10$), and θ ($P = .331$, $n = 10$) powers. Data are shown as mean ± 95% CI. *mean values significantly different from baseline with a $P < .05$. (From Montandon G, Cushing SL, Campbell F, et al. Distinct cortical signatures associated with sedation and respiratory rate depression by morphine in a pediatric population. *Anesthesiology*. 2016;125:889–903.)

whereas increasing the concentration of remifentanil led to a significant decrease of the calculated propofol effect-site concentrations necessary for unconsciousness.[152]

CEREBRAL BLOOD FLOW AND CEREBRAL METABOLIC RATE

Opioids generally produce modest decreases in cerebral metabolic rate and intracranial pressure (ICP), although the changes are influenced by the concomitant administration of other agents and anesthetic drugs, as well as by the patients' conditions. When vasodilation is produced by coadministered anesthetics, opioids are more likely to cause cerebral vasoconstriction. Opioids also decrease cerebral blood flow (CBF) when they are combined with nitrous oxide (N_2O). When opioids are administered alone or when the coadministered anesthetics cause cerebral vasoconstriction, opioids usually have no influence or result in a small increase in CBF.

Endogenous opioid activity is present in the cerebral arteries, although exogenously administered opioids were found to exert little effect on pial artery diameter in several animal models.[153] In the piglet, fentanyl, alfentanil, and sufentanil decreased arteriolar diameter in a dose-dependent naloxone-reversible manner.[154] In human volunteers, PET demonstrated that CBF changes induced by fentanyl are regionally heterogenous.[155]

In healthy volunteers, sufentanil (0.5 μg/kg intravenously [IV]) produces no significant effect on CBF.[156] Alfentanil (25-50 μg/kg IV), administered to patients receiving isoflurane (0.4%-0.6%)-N_2O anesthesia, produces minimal reductions in middle cerebral artery flow velocity.[157] A PET study in human volunteers showed that remifentanil induced dose-dependent changes in relative regional CBF in areas involved in pain processing, such as the lateral prefrontal cortex, inferior parietal cortex, and supplementary motor area.[158] In patients scheduled to undergo a supratentorial tumor surgical procedure and receiving N_2O,

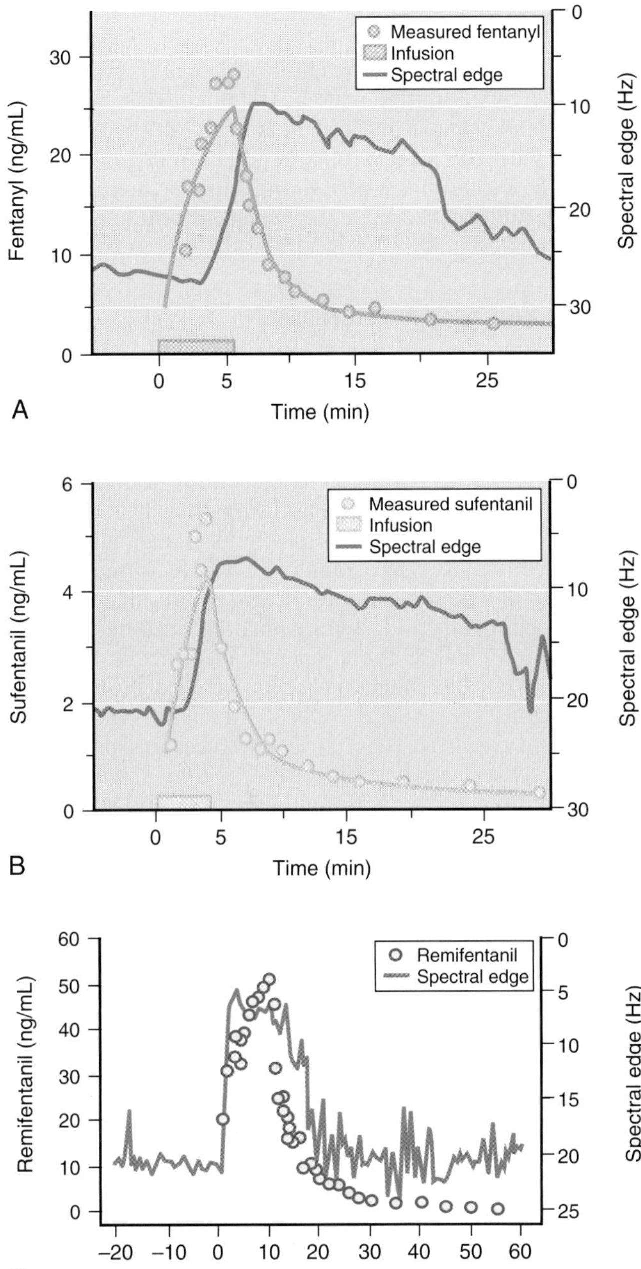

Fig. 24.11 Time course of spectral edge and serum opioid concentration. Fentanyl (A) and sufentanil (B) were infused at 150 μg/min and 18.75 μg/min, respectively. Remifentanil (C) was administered at 3 μg/kg/min for 10 minutes. The spectral edge changes lag behind the serum concentration changes in the case of fentanyl and sufentanil, whereas the spectral edge and serum concentration closely parallel in the cases of remifentanil. (From Scott JC, Ponganis KV, Stanski DR. EEG quantitation of narcotic effect: the comparative pharmacodynamics of fentanyl and alfentanil. *Anesthesiology*. 1985;62:234–241; and Egan TD, Minto CF, Hermann DJ, et al. Remifentanil versus alfentanil: comparative pharmacokinetics and pharmacodynamics in healthy adult male volunteers. *Anesthesiology*. 1996;84:821–833.)

remifentanil (1 μg/kg/min), similar to fentanyl (2 μg/kg/min), reduced CBF and did not significantly affect cerebrovascular carbon dioxide (CO_2) reactivity.[159]

Opioid-induced neuroexcitation and focal seizure activity can cause regional increases in brain metabolism. Regional increases in glucose use induced by high doses of alfentanil in the rat were associated not only with epileptiform activity but also with neuropathic lesions.[160] In humans, PET evaluation demonstrated that a 1 to 3 μg/kg/min infusion of remifentanil induces significant increase in the cerebral metabolic rate for glucose.[161] In summary, opioids, in general, do not significantly effect measures of CBF.

INTRACRANIAL PRESSURE

Opioids are generally thought to affect ICP minimally under conditions of controlled ventilation. When given with background anesthesia (isoflurane-N_2O), opioids do not cause significant increases in ICP undergoing craniotomy for supratentorial space-occupying lesions.[162,163] Opioid sedation does not alter ICP in patients with head injuries.[164] Light sedation with remifentanil (4.2 ± 1.8 μg/kg/h) does not result in higher ICP than that observed with propofol (4.3 ± 2.5 mg/kg/h) in patients undergoing stereotactic brain tumor biopsy, and cerebral perfusion pressure might be better preserved with remifentanil.[165]

Opioids may produce increases in ICP in patients undergoing craniotomy for excision of supratentorial space-occupying lesions, especially if intracranial compliance is compromised. In a study of patients with severe head injury who have preserved and impaired autoregulation, morphine (0.2 mg/kg) and fentanyl (2 μg/kg) moderately increased ICP, a finding suggesting that mechanisms other than vasodilation could be implicated in the opioid-induced ICP elevation.[166] Investigators also demonstrated no change in ICP in hydrocephalic children after administration of alfentanil (70 μg/kg).[167] Whether these discrepancies of the opioid effects on ICP reflect pressure assessment methods or the effects of other drugs is not clear. If opioids do increase ICP, whether cerebrovascular dilatation is directly induced by opioids or indirectly resulted from opioid-induced decrease in blood pressure is not known.

NEUROPROTECTION

Although certain early studies suggested potentially adverse effects of μ-opioid agonists on ischemic brain, other studies documented that certain opioid agents, such as the κ-agonists, can be neuroprotective in animal models of focal ischemia.[168] Investigators also showed that activation of δ-opioid receptors increases survival time of mice during lethal hypoxia.[169] An in vitro study using rat cerebellar brain slices demonstrated that pretreatment with morphine at clinically relevant concentrations induced acute neuroprotection mediated by activation of the δ_1-opioid receptors, activation of adenosine triphosphate (ATP)-sensitive K^+ channels, and free radical production in mitochondria.[170] In the rat focal ischemia model, fentanyl neither increased nor decreased brain injury compared with awake unanesthetized rats.[171] It was demonstrated that at a supraclinical concentration remifentanil had no pronecrotic effect but exerted ex vivo antiapoptotic action on the immature mouse brain, involving the opioid and NMDA receptors, and the mitochondrial-dependent apoptotic pathway.[172] A recent study reported that κ-opioid receptors were upregulated and played a critical role in brain ischemia and reperfusion in mice, and that κ-opioid receptor activation could potentially protect the brain and improve neurologic outcome via blood-brain barrier protection, apoptosis reduction, and inflammation inhibition.[173] Although there is contradicting evidence for a potential neuroprotection in animal models, there is no clear evidence for neuroprotective effects in humans.

MUSCLE RIGIDITY

Opioids can increase muscle tone and may cause muscle rigidity. The incidence of rigidity noted with opioid anesthetic techniques varies greatly because of differences in dose and speed of opioid administration, the concomitant use of N_2O, the presence or absence of muscle relaxants, and the patient's age. Opioid-induced rigidity is characterized by increased muscle tone that sometimes progresses to severe stiffness and associated clinical challenges (Table 24.4). Clinically significant opioid-induced rigidity usually begins just as, or after, a patient loses consciousness. Mild manifestations of rigidity, such as hoarseness, can occur in conscious patients. Vocal cord closure is primarily responsible for the difficult ventilation with bag and mask that follows the administration of opioids. Although opioids are generally thought to affect ICP minimally, it was demonstrated that alfentanil-induced rigidity can cause increase in ICP in rats.[174] Delayed or postoperative rigidity may be related to second peaks that can occur in plasma opioid concentrations, similar to the recurrence of respiratory depression.

The precise mechanism by which opioids cause muscle rigidity is not clearly understood. Muscle rigidity is not the result of a direct action on muscle fibers because it can be decreased or prevented by pretreatment with muscle relaxants. Mechanisms of opioid-induced muscle rigidity involving the CNS have been postulated. The nucleus raphe pontis within the reticular formation and the caudate nucleus within the basal ganglia have been implicated mechanistically.[175] Pharmacologic investigation using selective agonists and antagonists suggests that systemic opioid-induced muscle rigidity is primarily caused by the activation of central μ-receptors, whereas supraspinal δ_1 and κ_1 receptors may attenuate this effect.[176] Some aspects of opioid-induced catatonia and rigidity (increased incidence with age, muscle movements resembling extrapyramidal side effects) are similar to Parkinson disease and suggest similarities in neurochemical mechanisms. Patients with Parkinson disease, particularly if they are inadequately treated, may experience reactions such as dystonia following opioid administration.[177]

Pretreatment with or concomitant use of nondepolarizing muscle relaxants can decrease the incidence and severity of rigidity. Opioid-induced muscle rigidity can also be reversed with the μ-receptor antagonist naloxone. Induction doses of sodium thiopental and subanesthetic doses of diazepam and midazolam can prevent, attenuate, or successfully treat rigidity.

TABLE 24.4 Potential Problems Associated With Opioid-Induced Rigidity

System	Problem
Hemodynamic	↑CVP, ↑ PAP, ↑ PVR
Respiratory	↓ Compliance, ↓ FRC, ↓ ventilation Hypercarbia, Hypoxemia
Miscellaneous	↑ Oxygen consumption, ↑Intracranial pressure, ↑ Fentanyl plasma levels

CVP, Central venous pressure; *FRC*, functional residual capacity; *PAP*, pulmonary artery pressure; *PVR*, pulmonary vascular resistance.
Modified from Bailey PL, Egan TD, Stanley TH. Intravenous opioid anesthetics. In: Miller RD, ed. *Anesthesia*. 8th ed. Philadelphia: Saunders; 2015. An imprint of Elsevier Inc., p. 876.

NEUROEXCITATORY PHENOMENA

Fentanyl causes seizure activity seen on the EEG in animals, but EEG evidence of seizure activity after fentanyl, alfentanil, or sufentanil is generally lacking in humans. Remifentanil induced generalized tonic-clonic seizure-like activity in an otherwise healthy adult.[178] Morphine produces tonic-clonic activity after epidural and intrathecal administration.[179] Focal neuroexcitation on the EEG (e.g., sharp and spike wave activity) occasionally occurs in humans after large doses of fentanyl, sufentanil, and alfentanil.

The mechanisms underlying opioid-induced neuroexcitatory phenomena are not completely clear. Excitatory opioid actions may be related to coupling to mitogen-activated protein kinase cascades.[180] Local increases in CBF and metabolism are also of theoretic concern because prolonged seizure activity, even if focal, could lead to neuronal injury and/or cellular death. Fentanyl, alfentanil, and sufentanil in large doses also induced hypermetabolism and histopathologic alterations of the limbic system in rats.[181] Experimental study using excised mouse hippocampus showed that the proseizure effect of morphine is mediated by selective stimulation of the μ- and κ-opioid receptors but not the activation of the δ-opioid receptor.[182] In rats, midazolam, naloxone, and phenytoin prevented EEG seizure activity and histologically evident brain damage induced by large doses of fentanyl.[183]

Measurement of CBF by magnetic resonance imaging in human volunteers indicated that the cingulate cortex is the most susceptible to activation by remifentanil (0.05-0.2 μg/kg/min), and susceptibility is affected by the apolipoprotein E genotype.[184] These findings support the notion that neuroactivation of limbic areas by the perioperative use of opioids may have a role in the genesis of postoperative cognitive dysfunction.

PUPIL SIZE

Morphine and most μ− and κ−agonists cause constriction of the pupil by an excitatory action on the parasympathetic nerve innervating the pupil. Light induces excitation of the Edinger-Westphal nucleus leading to pupillary constriction, which is inhibited by hypercarbia, hypoxia, and nociception. Opioids release the effect of inhibitory neurons on the Edinger-Westphal nucleus, resulting in papillary constriction (Fig. 24.12).[185] After intravenous administration of morphine (0.125 mg/kg) in one report, a 26% decrease in pupil diameter occurred at 1 hour, and a period of more than 6 hours was necessary for complete recovery of pupil diameter.[186] The pupillary dilatation reflex has been successfully used to assess the analgesic component of a balanced anesthetic regimen. The pupillometer may be a valuable tool to

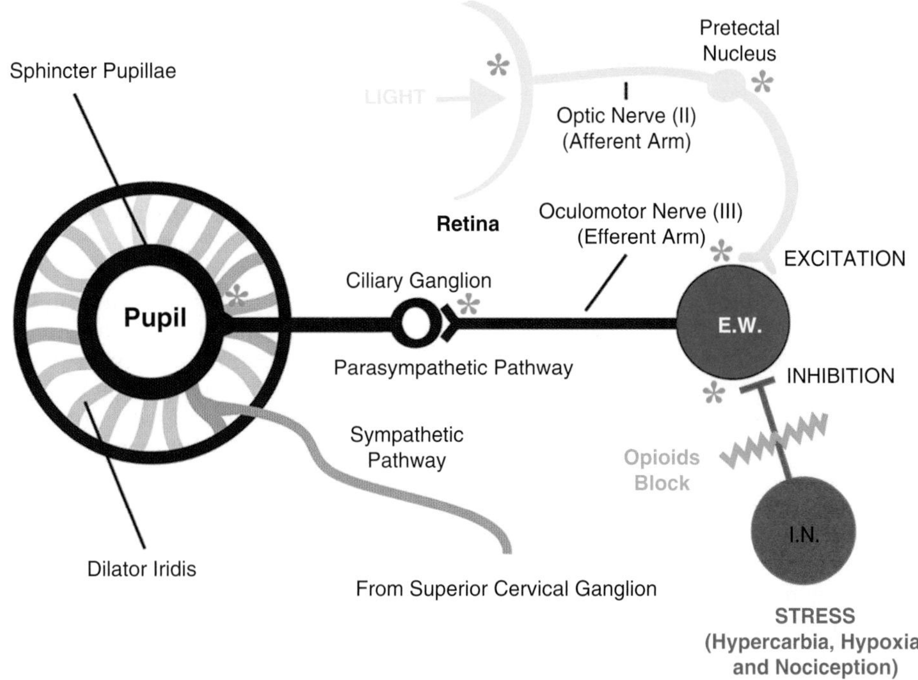

Fig. 24.12 Pathways and nerve centers that control pupil size and the pupillary light reflex in humans. *Colored* structures are the central nerve centers and pathways that modify the pupillary light reflex. Edinger-Westphal *(E.W.)* nucleus neurons are pacemaker cells that are modified by excitatory and inhibitory inputs. Opioids block the inhibition of the EW nucleus. Green asterisks (*) show locations where hypercarbia, hypoxia, and opioids might potentially interfere with the light reflex. * = locations where hypercarbia, hypoxia, and opioids might potentially interfere with the light reflex. *IN*, Inhibitory neuron. (From Rollins MD, Feiner JR, Lee JM, et al. Pupillary effects of high-dose opioid quantified with infrared pupillometry. *Anesthesiology.* 2014;84:1037–1044.)

guide morphine administration in the immediate postoperative period.[187] A prospective randomized study evaluated the impact of intraoperative pupillometry monitoring on perioperative opioid consumption in major gynecologic surgery. It was demonstrated that the use of pupillometry to guide intraoperative analgesia reduced intraoperative remifentanil consumption and postoperative morphine requirements.[188] Pupillary unrest is the fluctuation in pupil diameter, and pupillary unrest under ambient light (PUAL) is present even in well-rested individuals. Although the underlying mechanisms are unknown, PUAL is depressed by opioids. Administration of fentanyl to healthy volunteers diminishes PUAL, and the decrease is proportionally larger than the change in pupil diameter.[189] The pretreatment magnitude of PUAL is correlated with the analgesic response to opioid therapy, and patients who exhibit higher levels of PUAL change after opioid administration have a more beneficial analgesic effect from opioids.[190]

Pupillary constriction represents a well-known phenomenon following opioid administration and the use of pupillometry may help guide intraoperative opioid dosing to optimize analgesia.

THERMOREGULATION AND SHIVERING

Opioid-based anesthesia probably reduces thermoregulatory thresholds to a degree similar to that of the potent inhaled anesthetics.[191] However, meperidine is unique among opioids in its ability to effectively terminate or attenuate shivering. The antishivering effect of meperidine is primarily related to a reduction in the shivering threshold,[192] and seems to be mediated by meperidine's activity on the κ receptor.[193] However, the relatively specific κ-receptor agonist, nalbuphine, did not show significant antishivering activity.[194] Meperidine exerts agonist activity at the α_{2B}-adrenoreceptor subtype, a finding suggesting the involvement of this action in the antishivering action of meperidine.[85] Alfentanil, morphine, and fentanyl are not as effective as meperidine in the treatment of postoperative shivering. However, alfentanil and nefopam, a centrally acting analgesic, additively reduce the shivering threshold in humans.[195] Tramadol (0.5 mg/kg) suppressed postepidural anesthetic shivering in parturients as effectively as meperidine (0.5 mg/kg).[196] A quantitative systematic review of randomized controlled trials found that meperidine 12.5 to 35 mg and tramadol 35 to 220 mg were more effective than control for parenteral pharmacologic interventions for the prevention of postoperative shivering.[197]

Remifentanil is associated with an increased incidence of postanesthetic shivering, which is not related with intraoperative hypothermia. The higher incidence of postanesthetic shivering with higher doses of remifentanil probably reflects acute opioid tolerance and stimulation of the NMDA receptors.[198] A small dose of ketamine, 0.5 mg/kg at induction of anesthesia followed by infusion at 0.3 mg/kg/hour, can prevent remifentanil-induced postanesthetic shivering.

PRURITUS

Opioid-induced pruritis is one of several perpetual challenges associated with opioid-based analgesia. With the possible exception of morphine, histamine release, once thought to underlie this phenomenon, is not causative because non-histamine-releasing opioids also produce pruritus. Both central and peripheral nervous system mechanisms have been explored. Facial itching may not necessarily be a manifestation of direct opioid action at the level of the trigeminal nucleus, but rather, it may be a reflection of opioid-triggered neural transmission at a distant site. It is not known why the face is prone to pruritus even after spinal opioids. Interestingly, pruritus due to cholestasis is ameliorated by opioid antagonists.[199] Intrathecal morphine-induced itching in monkeys was suggested to be mediated by the μ receptor.[200] Activation of a μ-opioid receptor isoform MOR1D[11] by morphine induced activation of the gastrin-releasing peptide receptor that heterodimerized with MOR1D, thus resulting in activation of phospholipase β3 and intracellular Ca^{2+} increase in neurons leading to itch sensation in mice.[201]

Naloxone reverses opioid-induced itching, but opioid antagonists are not ideal therapeutic agents against pruritus because opioid analgesia is often reversed by these agents. A subcutaneous administration (12 mg) of methylnaltrexone bromide, a peripherally acting μ-opioid antagonist, did not reduce the overall severity or incidence of pruritus in women having elective cesarean section under spinal anesthesia with intrathecal morphine 100 μg, suggesting that peripheral mechanisms do not significantly contribute to spinal opioid-induced pruritus.[202] Ondansetron, a serotonin 5-HT_3 receptor antagonist has been proposed to treat spinal or epidural morphine-induced pruritus,[203] and a meta-analysis has demonstrated that prophylactic use of 5-HT_3 antagonists significantly reduced the severity and the need for treatment of pruritus.[204] Another meta-analysis showed that prophylactic intravenous administration of 8 mg ondansetron does not decrease the incidence of fentanyl- or sufentanil-induced pruritus but may decrease the need for pruritus rescue medication.[205] The application of mixed or partial opioid agonists, such as nalbuphine and butorphanol, are growing in popularity as antipruritics because they may partially antagonize μ receptor function with intact κ actions to maintain analgesia.[206] In fact, activation of the κ-opioid receptor inhibits pruritus evoked by subcutaneous and intrathecal morphine in animal models.[207]

Other agents that have been investigated include pentazocine (15 mg), an agonist of the κ-opioid receptor and partial agonist of the μ-opioid receptor. Pentazocine has been found to be superior to 4 mg of ondansetron for the treatment of pruritus induced by intrathecal morphine in parturients undergoing cesarean delivery.[208] It was recently reported that the antipruritic effect of κ-receptor agonists may not require interaction between the κ receptor and β-arrestins.[209] Tenoxicam, a nonsteroidal antiinflammatory drug (NSAID), was reported to be effective for pruritus induced by epidural fentanyl.[210] Other approaches include intravenous administration of droperidol (1.25 mg), propofol (20 mg), or alizapride (100 mg), which reduced the incidence of pruritus induced by the use of morphine 0.2 mg intrathecally in patients undergoing cesarean section under spinal anesthesia.[211] Preoperative gabapentin prevents pruritus induced by intrathecal morphine in patients undergoing lower limb surgery with spinal anesthesia.[212]

As opioid-induced pruritis continues to be a clinical challenge, current strategies have shifted away from the consequences of histamine release (morphine) and are focused on exploiting partial blockade/activation of the μ-opioid receptor, activation of the κ-receptor, and non-opioid receptor pathways.

OPIOID-INDUCED HYPERALGESIA

There is growing evidence that opioid-induced hyperalgesia (OIH) can represent a major adverse effect of opioid administration, especially when driven by potent formulations and escalating dosages. Experimentally, opioids have elicited hyperalgesia in animal models after repeated opioid administration or continuous delivery.[213] A systematic review to evaluate the clinical implication of OIH demonstrated that high intraoperative doses of remifentanil are associated with small but significant increases in acute pain after surgery as assessed by: pain intensity at rest 24 hours after surgery, 24-hour morphine use, pain intensity on movement, and hyperalgesia measured after an operation.[214] In a randomized, double-blind, crossover study with 24 healthy male volunteers, it was demonstrated that when compared with low-dose (1 μg/kg) fentanyl, high-dose fentanyl (10 μg/kg) increased the area of hyperalgesia from 4.5 to 6.5 hours after fentanyl administration. This result suggests that fentanyl can also produce OIH in humans.[215]

OIH was shown to be due to spinal sensitization to glutamate and substance P.[216] Activation of glycogen synthase kinase-3β (GSK-3β) contributes to remifentanil-induced hyperalgesia by regulating NMDA receptor plasticity in the spinal dorsal horn,[217] and further demonstrated that GSK-3β inhibition prevented remifentanil-induced postoperative hyperalgesia via regulating α-amino-3-hydroxy-5-methyl-4-isoxazolepropionic acid receptor (AMPAR) expression and function in the spinal dorsal horn.[218] Importantly, abrupt withdrawal of opioid administration may also contribute to induction of OIH, although its mechanism is not clear. In contrast to the high incidence of hyperalgesia induced after abrupt withdrawal of remifentanil (administered at 2.5 ng/mL for 30 minutes), no hyperalgesia was observed after gradual withdrawal by 0.6 ng/mL every 5 minutes.[219]

There have been reports that OIH and subsequent acute opioid tolerance can be prevented by ketamine, suggesting the involvement of the NMDA receptor.[220,221] Methadone is unique in possessing both μ-opioid receptor activating and NMDA antagonist properties. Opioid-induced hyperalgesia resulted from the presence in the racemate of the *l*-methadone (μ-opioid agonist) and was antagonized by the presence of the *d*-methadone (NMDA antagonist).[222] Low-dose buprenorphine (25 μg/h for 24 h), an opioid with NMDA antagonist activity, in patients receiving remifentanil infusion during major lung surgery prevented postoperative secondary hyperalgesia.[223] Butorphanol (0.2 μg/kg) was also effective for prevention of postoperative hyperalgesia after laparoscopic cholecystectomy performed with remifentanil (0.3 μg/kg/min).[224] N_2O, an inhalation anesthetic, is an effective NMDA antagonist. Intraoperative 70% N_2O administration significantly reduced postoperative opioid-induced hyperalgesia in patients receiving propofol (approximately 120 μg/kg/min) and remifentanil (0.3 μg/kg/min).[225] A randomized, double-blind, prospective study showed that a relatively high dose of remifentanil (0.2 μg/kg/min) enhances periincisional hyperalgesia in patients undergoing thyroidectomy, and intraoperative magnesium sulfate (30 mg/kg at induction followed by 10 mg/kg/h) can prevent remifentanil-induced hyperalgesia.[226]

Other strategies have focused on the upregulation of spinal cyclooxygenase-2 (COX-2) and increased prostaglandin E2 release in the spinal cord after morphine withdrawal in rats.[227] In humans, hyperalgesia after a 30-minute intravenous infusion of remifentanil (0.1 μg/kg/min) can be prevented by administration of parecoxib, a COX-2 inhibitor, before remifentanil infusion,[228] suggesting the involvement of COX-2 in OIH. Alternatively, it was reported that an ultra-low dose of naloxone blocked remifentanil-induced hyperalgesia but did not change opioid tolerance in rats under inhaled anesthesia, and that the MAC increase associated with hyperalgesia was also blocked by naloxone.[229] In patients undergoing elective thyroid surgery, intraoperative use of naloxone (0.05 μg/kg/h) reduced postoperative hyperalgesia after remifentanil infusion of 4 ng/mL.[230]

Genetic variants of the β_2-adrenergic receptor gene may explain some part of the differences between various strains of mice to develop OIH, and the selective β_2-adrenergic receptor antagonist butoxamine was shown to dose dependently reverse OIH.[231] In mice, systemic or intrathecal injection of the 5-HT_3 receptor antagonist, ondansetron, was shown to prevent or reverse opioid-induced tolerance or hyperalgesia.[232]

Interestingly, the occurrence of OIH might be affected by general anesthetics coadministered with opioids. When women undergoing breast cancer surgery were anesthetized with sevoflurane or propofol to keep BIS value at 40 to 50, postoperative hyperalgesia induced by intraoperative remifentanil infusion (effect-site target 4 ng/mL) was significant with sevoflurane anesthesia, but not apparent with propofol anesthesia.[233]

A follow-up study on the postoperative course of cardiac surgery demonstrated that intraoperative remifentanil was predictive for chronic thoracic pain 1 year after surgery in a dose-dependent manner.[234] It can be anticipated that hyperalgesia during the perioperative period is linked to peripheral and central pain sensitization and thereby correlates with the development of postoperative chronic pain.[235] This suggests that hyperalgesia due to remifentanil in the early postoperative period may explain the higher incidence of chronic pain.

Overall, human data generally support the existence of OIH in a few specific settings. Clinically relevant mechanisms of OIH include involvement of the NMDA receptor with ketamine as an appealing remedy. Although all potent opioids such as fentanyl are apparently capable of inducing OIH, ultrapotent opioid agonists such as remifentanil may pose even greater risks. The conditions under which OIH is expressed should be clarified and the extent of its clinical significance remains to be elucidated.[236]

Respiratory Effects of Opioids

The respiratory depressant actions of opioids represent their most serious adverse effect. Although some early studies indicated the involvement of both μ- and δ-opioid receptors, activation of the μ-opioid receptor in the caudal medullary raphe region, which is important for regulating pain and respiration, inhibits the ventilatory response to hypercapnia in anesthetized rats.[237] Furthermore, administration of morphine or M6G did not produce significant respiratory depression in the μ-opioid receptor knockout mice.[238] Polymorphism of the μ-opioid receptor at nucleotide position 118, which is known to affect M6G-induced analgesia, does not significantly change the susceptibility of respiratory depressive effect of M6G.[19] This result suggests that analgesia and respiratory depression may be mediated by different signal transduction mechanisms activated by the μ-opioid receptor.

EFFECTS ON AIRWAYS

The antitussive actions of opioids are well known and central in origin. Opioids blunt or eliminate somatic and autonomic responses to tracheal intubation. They allow patients to tolerate endotracheal tube placement without coughing or "bucking." Conversely, two successive doses of 1.5 μg/kg fentanyl did not effectively prevent laryngospasm in children aged 2 to 6 years old who were anesthetized with sevoflurane.[239] Opioids can also help avoid increases in bronchomotor tone in asthma. In addition, fentanyl also has antimuscarinic, antihistaminergic, and antiserotoninergic actions and may be more effective than morphine in patients with asthma or other bronchospastic diseases.

Nevertheless, several studies have reported a depressant effect of morphine on respiratory mucus transport, which is one of the most important defenses against respiratory tract infections. However, morphine had no effect on the beating frequency of nasal cilia in vitro.[240] Opioids can affect pharyngeal function, airway protection, and coordination of breathing and swallowing. A sedative dose of morphine (0.1 mg/kg) was associated with increased incidence of pharyngeal dysfunction and discoordinated breathing and swallowing, a combination impairing airway protection and potentially increasing the risk for pulmonary aspirations.[241]

More potent opioids such as remifentanil (effect-site concentration of 2 ng/mL) can suppress coughing induced by extubation after propofol or sevoflurane anesthesia.[242] In contrast, fentanyl, sufentanil, and alfentanil curiously elicit a brief cough in up to 50% of patients when the drug is injected by intravenous bolus. Fentanyl, administered through a peripheral intravenous cannula, provoked cough when it was injected rapidly, but the incidence of cough decreased significantly as the injection time was increased,[243] as well as by the administration of 1.5 mg/kg lidocaine 1 minute before fentanyl administration.[244] A meta-analysis showed that the lowest effective dose of lidocaine on the risk of opioid-induced cough was 0.5 mg/kg.[245] It was also reported that preemptive use of fentanyl 25 μg, administered 1 minute before bolus injection of fentanyl (125 or 150 μg), can effectively suppress fentanyl-induced cough.[246] Propofol, α_2 agonists (clonidine, dexmedetomidine), inhalation of β_2 agonists (terbutaline, salbutamol), and NMDA-receptor antagonists (ketamine, dextromethorphan) were also effective for suppression of fentanyl-induced cough.[247] A prospective randomized controlled study demonstrated that a huffing maneuver, consisting of a forced expiration against open glottis, just before intravenous fentanyl administration significantly reduced the incidence and severity of fentanyl-induced coughing in the majority of the patients.[248] Li and associates reported that nonsmoking women undergoing gynecological surgery who develop fentanyl-induced cough during induction of anesthesia have a higher incidence of postoperative nausea and vomiting (PONV).[249]

In summary, opioids engender potent antitussive properties that can help blunt airway responsiveness to endotracheal intubation. However, depending on the class of opioid and rate of administration, they may evoke a brief cough that can be subverted through the use of preadministered agents such as lidocaine. Ultimately, caution should be exercised in the administration of opioids as they can also interfere with protective aspects of airway physiology.

RESPIRATORY DEPRESSION

The lack of adequate pain relief can cause shallow respiration leading to postoperative respiratory dysfunction including atelectasis, and therefore opioids can serve as a foundational component of postoperative analgesia to prevent or correct respiratory impairment. However, opioids can also dose dependently depress respiration, representing the most feared adverse effect. The incidence of opioid-induced respiratory depression varies from 0.1% to 37%, depending on the route of opioid administration, the type of opioid, the definition and method of monitoring opioid-induced respiratory depression, and the prospective versus retrospective nature of the study, and is a significant cause of death and brain damage in the perioperative period.[250]

Opioids activating the μ receptor cause dose-dependent depression of respiration, primarily through a direct action on brainstem respiratory centers.[251] The stimulatory effect of CO_2 on ventilation is significantly reduced by opioids. Hypercapnic responses can be separated into central and peripheral components. In one report, morphine-induced changes in the central component were equal in men and women, whereas changes in the peripheral component were larger in women.[252] In addition, the apneic threshold and pressure of end-tidal carbon dioxide ($PETCO_2$) are increased by opioids (Fig. 24.13). Opioids also decrease hypoxic ventilatory drive.

Respiratory rate is usually drastically decreased in opioid overdose, although hypoxic CNS insult can counter this effect. The prolonged expiratory time in the respiratory cycle induced by opioids frequently results in greater reductions in respiratory rate than in tidal volume. Monitoring of breath intervals can sensitively detect fentanyl-induced respiratory depression and can be used as a measure of dynamic opioid effect.[253] High doses of opioids usually eliminate spontaneous respirations without necessarily producing unconsciousness. Patients receiving high doses of opioids may still be responsive to verbal command and often breathe when they are directed to do so.

Peak onset of respiratory depression after an analgesic dose of morphine is slower than after comparable doses of fentanyl, and respiratory depression induced by small doses of morphine usually lasts longer than after equipotent doses of fentanyl. Plasma fentanyl concentrations of 1.5 to 3.0 ng/mL are associated with significant decreases in CO_2 responsiveness. With higher doses of fentanyl (50-100 μg/kg), respiratory depression can persist for many hours. When moderately large doses (20-50 μg/kg or greater) of fentanyl are used, the potential need for postoperative mechanical ventilation should be anticipated. The effects of remifentanil are attenuated rapidly and completely within 5 to 15 minutes following termination of its administration. In healthy humans, the EC_{50} for depression of minute ventilation with remifentanil and alfentanil was 1.17 ng/mL and 49.4 ng/mL, respectively.[254] In healthy volunteers, fentanyl 1 μg/kg and remifentanil 0.5 μg/kg had similar maximum decreases in minute ventilation (~50%), but the onset of and recovery from ventilatory depression were faster with remifentanil.[255] Naloxone has been accepted as a standard therapy for opioid-induced respiratory depression. However, reports have noted naloxone-resistant respiratory depression after intrathecal morphine administration.[256]

A major component of the excitatory synaptic drive necessary for respiratory rhythmogenesis and activation of respiratory motoneurons is *via* the amino-3-hydroxy-5-methyl-4-isoxazolepropionate (AMPA) type of glutamate receptors.[257] This finding has led to investigations of ampakine (positive modulators of AMPA receptors) therapy to alleviate opioid-induced respiratory depression.[258] 5-HT released from the raphe nuclei potently alters the excitability of respiratory motoneurons, the preBötzinger complex (preBötC), and other brainstem respiratory nuclei. The activation of $5\text{-}HT_{1A}$ receptors with befiradol alleviates fentanyl-induced respiratory depression in rats.[259] PreBötC, the main region of respiratory rhythm–pattern generation, is the main target of opioid-induced respiratory depression.

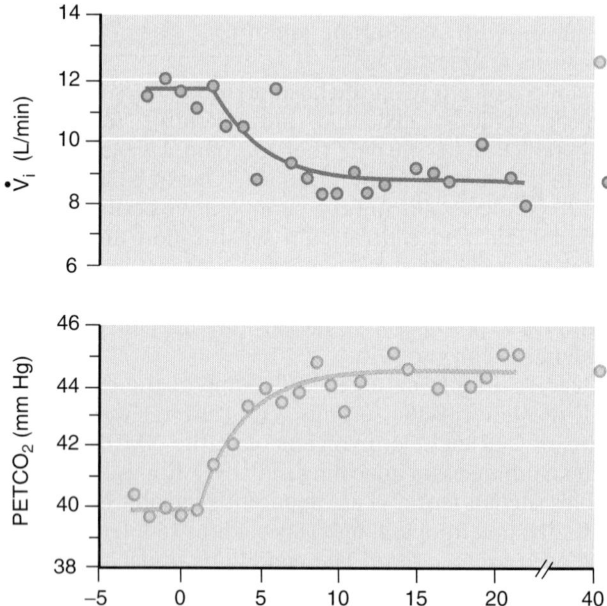

Fig. 24.13 Influence of morphine administration (bolus dose of 100 μg/kg given at the start of the infusion [0 minute], followed by a continuous infusion of 30 μg/kg/h) on resting inspired minute ventilation *(V_i)* and resting pressure of end-tidal carbon dioxide *($PETCO_2$)* in a single subject. A one-component exponential was fitted to the data. The estimated time constant for the V_i data is 3.0 minutes and for $PETCO_2$ data is 2.6 minutes. The time delays are between 1 and 2 minutes. (From Sarton E, Teppema L, Dahan A. Sex differences in morphine-induced ventilatory depression reside within the peripheral chemoreflex loop. *Anesthesiology*. 1999;90:1329–1338.)

However, it has been demonstrated that preBötC partially mediates opioid effects on respiratory phase timing, but does not mediate the opioid-induced depression of respiratory rate.[260] By the use of knockout mice and pharmacologic approaches, G-protein–gated inwardly rectifying κ channels were shown to contribute to respiratory depression by μ-opioid receptors and opioids.[261] In healthy humans, GAL021, a calcium-activated potassium (BKCa) channel blocker possessing a stimulatory effect on ventilation at the carotid bodies, was preliminarily shown to reverse alfentanil-induced respiratory depression.[262]

FACTORS AFFECTING OPIOID-INDUCED RESPIRATORY DEPRESSION

Many factors affect the magnitude and duration of opioid-induced respiratory depression (Box 24.2).

Older patients are more sensitive to the anesthetic and respiratory depressant effects of opioids and experience higher plasma concentrations of opioids administered on a weight basis. In addition, morphine can produce greater respiratory depression on a weight basis in neonates than adults, because morphine easily penetrates the brain of neonates and infants with incomplete blood-brain barriers.

The respiratory depressant effects of opioids are increased or prolonged (or both) when these drugs are administered with other CNS depressants, including potent inhaled anesthetics, alcohol, barbiturates, benzodiazepines, most intravenous sedatives, and hypnotics. However, droperidol, scopolamine, and clonidine do not enhance the respiratory depressant effects of fentanyl or other opioids. Curiously, Setnik and associates observed a decrease in end-tidal CO_2 when 0.7 g/kg ethanol was administered in addition to 80 mg oral morphine, suggesting a stimulatory effect of ethanol on opioid-induced respiratory depression.[263] However, it was reported that ethanol (1 g/L of breath ethanol concentration) caused a significant increase in the apneic events and increased end-tidal CO_2 induced by 20 mg oxycodone per os in opioid-naïve healthy volunteers.[264]

Although opioid action is usually dissipated by redistribution and hepatic metabolism, rather than by urinary excretion, the adequacy of renal function may influence the duration of opioid activity. In renal insufficiency, the respiratory depressant properties of morphine and hydromorphone, as well as of the morphine metabolite M6G, become evident as these accumulate.

Hypocapnic hyperventilation enhances and prolongs postoperative respiratory depression after fentanyl (10 and 25 μg/kg). Intraoperative hypercarbia produces the opposite effects. Possible explanations for these findings include increased brain opioid penetration (increased un-ionized fentanyl with hypocarbia) and removal (decreased CBF with hypocarbia). In patients who hyperventilate because of anxiety or pain, even small doses of intravenous opioids can result in transient apnea because of acute shifts in apneic thresholds. Respiratory depression by remifentanil (50 μg infused over 60 seconds) was more pronounced in hyperoxia (inhaling 50% O_2) than normoxia as determined by minute ventilation, end-tidal PCO_2, and respiratory rate.[265] During hyperoxia, respiratory depression may be masked when measuring SpO_2 as pulse oximetry remains in normal values during the first minutes of respiratory depression.

All opioid agonists with a longer plasma half-life than naloxone have a hypothetical potential to show renarcotization with time, especially when a bolus dose of naloxone is used to treat opioid-induced respiratory depression.

Overall, opioids exert their primary respiratory depressant effects through μ-receptor activation in the brainstem respiratory center, although other pathways have been defined. Dose-dependent opioid respiratory depression increases the apneic threshold, and reduces the respiratory stimulatory drive of CO_2 and hypoxia. Research efforts to block or reverse opioid-induced respiratory depression are ongoing and include a focus on AMPA, 5-HT_{1A}, and calcium-activated potassium channels. The μ-receptor antagonist, naloxone, continues to be the most commonly used clinical intervention to reverse opioid-induced respiratory depression, however its effectiveness may be limited if the administered opioid has a greater binding affinity and/or half-life than naloxone.

BOX 24.2 Factors Increasing the Magnitude and/or Duration of Opioid-Induced Respiratory Depression

- High dose
- Sleep
- Old age
- Central nervous system depressant
  - Inhaled anesthetics, alcohol, barbiturates, benzodiazepines
- Renal insufficiency
- Hyperventilation, hypocapnia
- Respiratory acidosis
- Decreased clearance
  - Reduction of hepatic blood flow
- Secondary peaks in plasma opioid levels
  - Reuptake of opioids from muscle, lung, fat, and intestine
- Pain

Cardiovascular Effects of Opioids

Numerous reports have demonstrated that large doses of opioid, administered as the sole or primary anesthetic, result in hemodynamic stability throughout the operative period. This remarkable physiologic state is a result of a number of complementary mechanisms.

NEUROLOGIC MECHANISMS

Key areas of the brainstem that integrate cardiovascular responses and maintain cardiovascular homeostasis are the nucleus solitarius, the dorsal vagal nucleus, the nucleus ambiguous, and the parabrachial nucleus. The nucleus solitarius and parabrachial nucleus play an important role in the hemodynamic control of vasopressin secretion. Enkephalin-containing neurons and opioid receptors are distributed in these regions. The direct administration of μ-agonists into the CNS of rats most commonly, but not always, produces hypotension and bradycardia.[266] The ventrolateral PAG region, a key central site mediating opioid analgesia, also affects hemodynamic control.[267] In addition, opioids can modulate the stress response through receptor-mediated actions on the hypothalamic-pituitary-adrenal axis. Most opioids reduce sympathetic and enhance vagal and parasympathetic tone. Patients who are volume depleted, or individuals depending on high sympathetic tone or exogenous catecholamines to maintain cardiovascular function, are predisposed to hypotension after opioid administration.

The predominant and usual effect of opioids on heart rate is bradycardia resulting from stimulation of the central vagal nucleus. Blockade of sympathetic actions may also play a role in opioid-induced bradycardia. Meperidine, in contrast to other opioids, rarely results in bradycardia, but it can cause tachycardia. Tachycardia after meperidine may be related to its structural similarity to atropine, to normeperidine, its principal metabolite, or to early manifestations of its toxic CNS effects.

CARDIAC MECHANISMS

The direct cardiac actions of opioids, in particular the effects on myocardial contractile mechanisms, are significantly less pronounced than are those of many other intravenous and inhaled anesthetics. However, opioid receptors exist in cardiac myocytes of several species.

Contractility

Morphine decreases Ca^{2+} transients but not cardiac contraction and enhances myofilament Ca^{2+} sensitivity through the action on the δ_1-opioid receptor expressed in the heart.[268] In rabbit ventricular myocytes, morphine prolonged action potential duration by increasing L-type Ca^{2+} current, an effect mediated by δ- and κ-opioid receptors, and hyperpolarized cardiac resting membrane potential by increasing the inwardly rectifying K^+ current, which is not mediated by opioid receptors.[269] Conversely, investigators demonstrated that morphine decreased the isometric force of contraction in atrial muscles from nonfailing and failing human hearts through a naloxone-insensitive mechanism.[270] Fentanyl produces little or no change in myocardial contractility.[271] Usually, most hemodynamic variables remain unchanged after large doses of fentanyl. Alfentanil, at concentrations achieved in clinical practice, increases contraction in ventricular cells by a mechanism involving an increase in the sensitivity of the contractile apparatus to Ca^{2+}.[272] The negative inotropic effect of tumor necrosis factor-α (TNF-α) and interleukin-1β (IL-1β) on ventricular myocytes caused by disruption of sarcoplasmic reticulum Ca^{2+} handling and Ca^{2+} transient was reported to be ameliorated by alfentanil, but this response may not be mediated by opioid receptors.[273] A study using transthoracic echocardiography demonstrated that continuous target-controlled infusion of remifentanil (target effect-site concentration 2 ng/mL, infusion rate 0.08-0.09 μg/kg/min) did not affect systolic and diastolic left ventricular function in young healthy subjects during spontaneous breathing.[274]

Cardiac Rhythm Conduction

Opioid-induced bradycardia is primarily mediated by the CNS. However, there have been reports on direct effects of opioids on cardiac pacemaker cells. Fentanyl may depress cardiac conduction by a mechanism mediated by direct membrane actions, as opposed to opioid receptor interactions.[275] During induction of anesthesia in patients undergoing coronary artery bypass graft surgery, the QT interval increased significantly after the injection of fentanyl.[276] However, pretreatment with fentanyl 2 μg/kg or remifentanil 1 μg/kg significantly attenuated QTc prolongation associated with laryngoscopy and tracheal intubation during propofol or sevoflurane induction.[277,278] Both sufentanil and alfentanil have been demonstrated to be devoid of electrophysiologic effects on the normal or accessory pathways in patients with Wolff-Parkinson-White syndrome.[279,280] Clinically, cardiac conduction disturbances attributable to opioids are rare, but they may be more likely to occur in the presence of Ca^{2+} channel or β-adrenergic blockers.

The overall effect of opioid anesthesia is antiarrhythmic. Naloxone, morphine, and levorphanol protected against arrhythmia induced by coronary artery occlusion in rats.[281] A direct effect on ionic currents in cardiac muscle was suggested as the mechanism of antiarrhythmic activity of opioids. It was also reported that opioid antagonists are more antiarrhythmogenic than agonists in rats.[282] Some of the electrophysiologic actions of opioids resemble those of class III antiarrhythmogenic drugs.

Myocardial Ischemia

Determining the effects and consequences of opioid action on myocardial ischemia is complex because results can depend on such factors as the species studied and experimental design. In an experimental model of myocardial ischemia in rabbits, fentanyl had antiarrhythmic and antiischemic action with central and peripheral opioid receptor involvement.[283] Opioids can mimic ischemic preconditioning. Opioid receptor stimulation results in a reduction in infarct size similar to that produced by ischemic preconditioning.[284] Although the preconditioning effect of opioids is mediated mainly by the cardiac κ- and δ-opioid receptors,[285] part of the protective effect of remifentanil may be produced by μ-agonist activity outside the heart.[286] Preconditioning with small doses of intrathecal morphine can provide comparable cardioprotection to myocardial ischemic preconditioning and preconditioning with intravenous morphine, and the effect seems to involve μ-, δ-, and κ-opioid receptors.[287] Late preconditioning, in which cardioprotective effects can be observed 24 hours after drug administration, was also produced by morphine-induced activation of the opioid receptor in rat hearts.[288]

It was found that remote preconditioning by brief ischemia of other distant organs, such as intestine, kidney, and limb, similarly provides cardioprotection that is as effective as classic ischemic preconditioning. The myocardial κ-opioid receptors were demonstrated to mediate cardioprotection by remote preconditioning.[289] Brief cycles of ischemia and reperfusion during the early phase of reperfusion protect the heart from infarction. This phenomenon, termed postconditioning, was shown to be induced by activation of the δ-opioid receptor in the heart.[290] Volatile anesthetics may also be capable of producing protection against ischemic injury when these drugs are administered solely on reperfusion. This anesthetic-induced postconditioning can be enhanced by morphine through the activation of phosphatidyl-3-kinase and opioid receptors.[291] It has been shown that brief exposure to exercise (1-3 days of moderate-intensity exercise) preconditions the heart against tissue injury and death resulting from myocardial ischemia–reperfusion. It was demonstrated that endogenous opioids produced in the heart mediate exercise-induced cardioprotection against ischemia–reperfusion injury through its action on the δ-opioid receptor in rats.[292] Stimulation of δ_1-opioid receptor also generates oxygen radicals through mitochondrial ATP-sensitive K^+ channels, with resulting attenuation of oxidant stress and cell death in cardiomyocytes.[293] Involvement of adenosine A1 receptor and protein kinase C in the cardioprotective effect of opioids was also suggested.[294,295] Whether the experimental results showing protective effects of opioid against myocardial ischemia will translate into reductions in morbidity and mortality in patients with coronary artery disease has yet to be established by clinical trials.[296] Clinically, high doses of opioids can maintain myocardial perfusion and the O_2 supply-demand ratio as well or better than can inhalation-based techniques.

Coronary Circulation

Opioids appear to have no significant effect on coronary vasomotion or myocardial metabolism, do not produce steal phenomena, nor diminish the ability of large coronary arterioles to respond to vasoactive agents.[297] Coronary conductance is regulated by arterial baroreflex control, and vasodilator response is induced by a rise in aortic pressure. This baroreflex control is enhanced by low plasma concentration of fentanyl (1-2 ng/mL), but appears to be depressed at increased concentrations of fentanyl.[298]

Circulatory Reflexes

In an experiment examining baroreceptor reflex responses induced by perfusion of the carotid sinus at predetermined levels, baroreceptor reflexes were well preserved by moderate doses of fentanyl while high doses of fentanyl depressed baroreceptor reflexes.[299] The oculocardiac reflex, which is caused by traction of extraocular muscles during strabismus surgery, was significantly augmented by fentanyl, sufentanil, and remifentanil.[300] Among pediatric patients undergoing strabismus surgery, anesthetized with propofol (12 mg/kg/h) and alfentanil (0.04 mg/kg/h), virtually all patients developed oculocardiac reflex and atrioventricular rhythm disorders were frequent.[301]

HISTAMINE RELEASE

It is well known that morphine causes histamine release and sympathoadrenal activation. Increases in plasma histamine after morphine cause dilation of terminal arterioles and direct positive cardiac chronotropic and inotropic actions. In patients pretreated with both H_1- and H_2-antagonists, the cardiovascular responses are significantly attenuated despite comparable increases in plasma histamine concentrations. Codeine and meperidine are examples of other opioids that can induce mast cell activation with the release of histamine, probably by a mechanism other than the μ-opioid receptors.[302] Unlike morphine or meperidine, the opioids fentanyl, alfentanil, sufentanil, and remifentanil do not produce increases in plasma histamine, subsequently hypotension is less frequent with their administration.

VASCULAR MECHANISMS

The pharmacologically defined opioid receptor subtype μ_3 is expressed in human endothelial cells and coupled to vasodilation via nitric oxide (NO) production. Although μ_3 is opiate alkaloid sensitive it is insensitive to opioid peptides including peptides previously shown to have affinities for the μ-opioid receptors. Morphine-induced vasodilation may be partially caused by activation of the μ_3 receptor.[303] Other pharmacologic studies evaluating alfentanil, fentanyl, and sufentanil in the dog also demonstrate direct peripheral vessel smooth muscle relaxation although exact mechanism(s) remains under study.[304,305] For example, measurement of forearm blood flow after infusion of sufentanil into the brachial artery indicated that sufentanil has a direct vasodilatory effect on human vascular tissue that is likely independent of a neurogenic or systemic mechanism.[306] A supraclinical dose of alfentanil attenuates the phenylephrine-induced contraction via an inhibitory effect on calcium influx by blocking the L-type calcium channels in the rat aortic vascular smooth muscle.[307] Remifentanil can cause transient instability in hemodynamic variables. However, this change may not be solely the result of autonomic or central nervous system inhibition or of centrally mediated vagal stimulation. A pharmacologic study using rat thoracic aortic rings indicated that remifentanil vasodilates by an endothelium-dependent mechanism, involving prostacyclin and NO released from the endothelium, and an endothelium-independent vasodilation probably mediated by the suppression of voltage-sensitive Ca^{2+} channels.[308] In patients with a total artificial heart in which cardiac output is preload-independent, remifentanil induces a dose-dependent and significant systemic vasodilation without significant effects on capacitance vessels.[309]

Opioids may affect the pulmonary vasculature as well as systemic circulation. It was shown that phenylephrine-induced contraction of canine pulmonary artery is primarily mediated by α_{1B}-adrenergic receptor activation, and is attenuated by fentanyl by binding to and directly inhibiting the α_{1B}-adrenergic receptor.[310] Pharmacologic studies in cats demonstrated that sufentanil and remifentanil have potent vasodepressor activity in the pulmonary vascular bed and these responses may be mediated by histamine and opioid receptor-sensitive pathway.[311,312]

OPIOIDS IN SHOCK

Opioids are often administered for patients requiring surgical intervention for the control of hemorrhage. An animal study demonstrated that pretreatment with morphine before inducing shock state decreases leukocyte adhesion and vascular permeability in the microcirculation of the mesenteric venule, suggesting the survival benefit for use of morphine during acute resuscitation.[313]

It has been shown that endogenous opioids contribute to the pathophysiology of hypovolemic shock through central and peripheral sympathetic inhibition and contributes to hypotension during severe hemorrhage. Liu et al. reported that the selective δ-opioid receptor antagonist (ICI 174,864) may be beneficial for the early management of traumatic hemorrhagic shock in rats, suggesting a pathophysiological role of the δ-opioid receptor in hemorrhagic shock.[314]

Endocrinologic Effects of Opioids

Opioids can induce a variety of endocrinological responses (Table 24.5).[315] In humans, opioids generally increase growth hormone, thyroid stimulating hormone, and prolactin, and decrease luteinizing hormone, testosterone, estradiol, and oxytocin. The effects of opioids on arginine vasopressin and ACTH are conflicting. The primary endocrine disorder that results from opioid misuse is hypogonadism, particularly in males.

Hormonal and metabolic responses to surgery are often extreme and are thought to contribute to operative mortality. Opioids are capable of reducing the stress response by modulating nociception at several levels of the neuraxis, as well as by influencing centrally mediated neuroendocrine responses. The main components of the neuroendocrine stress response are the corticotropin-releasing hormone brain centers (e.g., paraventricular hypothalamic nucleus) and the locus ceruleus-norepinephrine/autonomic nervous system. Increased levels of stress hormones are considered undesirable because they promote hemodynamic instability and intraoperative and postoperative metabolic catabolism. Opioids are potent inhibitors of the pituitary-adrenal axis.[316] Endogenous opioid peptides may serve as stress hormones themselves and not just as modulators of other hormones' secretion. This is suggested by the finding that β-endorphin and ACTH are derived from the same precursor preproopiomelanocortin and cosecreted during stress.

Morphine modifies hormonal responses to surgical trauma in a dose-related fashion through blockade of ACTH release, suppression of surgically induced increases in plasma cortisol, and attenuation of the pituitary-adrenal response to surgical stress. Morphine can increase some stress-responding hormones due to increases in plasma histamine release, adrenal medullary release mechanisms, and catecholamine release from sympathetic nerve endings.

TABLE 24.5 Summary of the Effects of Acute and Chronic Opioids on the Endocrine Systems of Animals and Humans

	ACUTE		CHRONIC	
Hormone	**Animals**	**Humans**	**Animals**	**Humans**
GH	↑	↑	=	?
PRL	↑	↑	↑	↑/=
TSH	↓	↑	?	?/=
ACTH	↑	↓	↓/↑	↓/=
LH	↓	↓↓	↓	↓↓
FSH	=	=	=	=
Estradiol	↓	↓↓	=	↓=
Testosterone	↓	↓↓	↓	↓↓
AVP	↑/↓	↑/↓	↑/↓	↑/↓
OT	↓	↓	↓/=	↓/=

↑, Stimulation; ↓, inhibition; ↑↓, conflicting; =, no change; ?, not studied.
ACTH, Adrenocorticotropic hormone; *AVP*, arginine vasopressin; FSH, follicle stimulating hormone; *GH*, growth hormone; *LH*, luteinizing hormone; *OT*, oxytocin; *PRL*, prolactin; *TSH*, thyroid stimulating hormone. https://www.ncbi.nlm.nih.gov/pmc/articles/PMC2852206/
From Vuong C, Van Uum SH, O'Dell LE, et al. The effects of opioids and opioid analogs on animal and human endocrine systems. *Endocr Rev.* 2010;31:98–132.

Fentanyl and its congeners are more effective than morphine in modifying hormonal responses to surgery. The efficacy of fentanyl in controlling the hormonal manifestations of the stress response can be dose-dependent. Fentanyl doses greater than or equal to 50 μg/kg can help to reduce the hyperglycemic response to cardiac surgery in pediatric patients to less than 200 mg/dL throughout operation.[317] In contrast, it has been demonstrated that neither fentanyl nor sufentanil alone can completely block sympathetic and hormonal stress responses and that perhaps no dose-response relationship exists for opioid-associated stress response control.[318] A randomized controlled trial showed that remifentanil (0.85 μg/kg/min), when compared with fentanyl (total doses of 15 and 28 μg/kg), blunts the hypertensive responses and cortisol excretion associated with cardiac surgery but is associated with more hypotension.[319]

STRESS REDUCTION AND OUTCOME

Anesthetic techniques or agents that minimize the stress response may reduce morbidity and mortality in a variety of circumstances. Anand and Hickey[320] evaluated the impact of sufentanil versus morphine-halothane anesthesia on hormonal and metabolic responses and morbidity and mortality in neonates undergoing cardiac surgery. Most strikingly, a difference in postoperative mortality was observed (0 of 30 given sufentanil versus 4 of 15 given halothane plus morphine). Mangano et al.[321] also reported that, after myocardial revascularization, patients receiving intense postoperative analgesia with sufentanil (1 μg/kg/h) experience a decrease in the incidence and severity of electrocardiographically documented ischemia compared with patients receiving intermittent IV morphine (2.2 ± 2.1 mg/h) for postoperative analgesia. It was also shown that large-dose opioids (remifentanil 0.85 μg/kg/min or fentanyl 28 μg/kg) were associated with a decreased rate of myocardial infarction after cardiac surgery.[319]

Many different hormonal changes induced by surgery have been described. However, the concomitant neural, cellular, immune, and biochemical changes have been less well defined, and little is understood or proven with regard to how modifying hormonal responses alters outcome.[322] Additional studies are necessary for complete elucidation of the relationship between control of the surgery-induced hormonal responses and outcome.

In summary, the mechanisms underlying the ability of opioids to provide perioperative cardiovascular stability include: a reduced sympathetic tone and enhanced parasympathetic activity often producing bradycardia; minimal changes in cardiac contractility; function generally as an antiarrhythmic; potentially function as cardioprotective agents to reduce the effect of ischemia by mimicking an endogenous opioid-peptide/preconditioning pathway; have no significant effect on the coronary circulation; produce modest vascular smooth muscle relaxation with the exception of a morphine-induced histaminergic mechanism; reduce the surgical stress response through the nervous system and adrenal-pituitary axis—depending on the opioid class.

OPIOID TOLERANCE

The precise mechanism(s) that drive opioid dependence and tolerance are not known, however they appear to encompass a range of factors including: genetic, molecular, cellular, physiologic, and functional. In the locus ceruleus, the major noradrenergic nucleus in the brain, long-term opioid exposure results in inhibition of adenylyl cyclase, reduced activity of protein kinase A, and upregulation of the cyclic AMP pathway.[323] Changes in μ-receptor density that occur prior to or during the development of tolerance do not appear to be essential for development of opioid tolerance.[324] Possible mechanisms involve protein kinase signal transduction cascades that link extracellular signals to cellular changes by regulating target gene expression. Central glucocorticoid receptors (GRs) have been implicated in the cellular mechanism of neuronal plasticity that has many cellular steps in common with the mechanism of opioid tolerance. It was shown that the development of tolerance to the antinociceptive effect of morphine was substantially attenuated when the GR antagonist was coadministered with morphine but the GR agonist dexamethasone facilitated the development of morphine tolerance, suggesting an important role of spinal GRs in the cellular mechanisms of morphine tolerance in rats.[325] Cholecystokinin and NMDA-NO system were also shown to be involved in development of acute tolerance to opioids,[326] which is also affected by spinal serotonin activity.[327] Neuroinflammation driven by chemokines may represent one of the major mechanisms underlying pathologic pain. A chemokine, CXCL1, was upregulated in both opioid-tolerant patients and rodents, and the onset and extent of opioid tolerance was affected by antagonizing intrathecal CXCL1/CXCR2 signaling.[328] A chemokine, CXCL12, was significantly upregulated in the cerebrospinal fluid of opioid-tolerant patients, and CXCL12 neutralizing antibody and antagonist for CXCR4, a receptor which interacts with CXCL12, attenuated morphine tolerance in rats.[329]

Morphine tolerance occurs more rapidly in younger rats than older rats and is unlikely to be the result of differences in drug metabolism or clearance, suggesting that aging may impact molecular processes involved in development of tolerance.[330] It has been suggested that activation of glial cells, including astrocytes and microglia, at the level of the spinal cord plays an important role in the development of opioid tolerance.[331,332] However, the mechanism for opioid-induced activation of glial cells is not completely understood.

Although the notion that opioid tolerance and dependence occur only after chronic administration has been widespread, it has now become recognized that tolerance can also develop rapidly after acute opioid exposure in animals and humans.[333,334] Intraoperative remifentanil infusion (0.3 μg/kg/min) in patients undergoing major abdominal surgery under desflurane anesthesia increased postoperative pain and morphine requirement compared with low-dose remifentanil (0.1 μg/kg/min), suggesting the development of acute remifentanil tolerance.[335] In contrast, there is a report that target-controlled infusion of alfentanil and remifentanil for postoperative analgesia does not lead to opioid tolerance.[336] In human volunteers, continuous infusion of remifentanil (0.08 μg/kg/min) for 3 hours did not decrease the pain threshold.[337] On the other hand, intraoperative use of 0.3 μg/kg/min remifentanil for approximately 3 hours did not induce acute tolerance, but the administration of 0.6 and 0.9 μg/kg/min remifentanil to young children resulted in acute tolerance for 24 hours after surgery revealed by increased use of postoperative fentanyl in an apparently dose-related manner.[338] Differences in these outcomes may reflect divergent methodologies and limited sample size and are an area of ongoing investigation.

Differential opioid tolerance, an important phenomenon in clinical opioid pharmacology, proposes that different targets of opioid drugs do not develop tolerance at the same rate and to the same degree.[339] In a study using rhesus monkeys, acute morphine administration predictably induced dose-dependent analgesia, and chronic morphine administration induced dose-dependent tolerance to the analgesic effect, while no tolerance development to the respiratory depressive effect could be demonstrated in the chronically opioid-treated animals (Fig. 24.14).[340] In humans, patients receiving chronic opioids for pain control, especially at high doses, most likely have developed opioid tolerance. However, there is little data to help predict the magnitude or clinical impact of an individual's loss of opioid-induced analgesia or potentially their resistance/vulnerability to the respiratory depressive effects of opioids. As discussed later, individuals chronically consuming opioids are dose dependently at increased risk for overdose and death.

MANAGEMENT OF OPIOID-DEPENDENT PATIENTS

A variety of problems should be taken into consideration for anesthetic management of opioid-dependent patients or patients suffering from opioid use disorder (OUD).[341] Complications in opioid-addicted patients include cardiopulmonary problems, renal problems, and anemia. Long-term morphine administration causes adrenal hypertrophy and impairs corticosteroid secretion. Viral and nonviral hepatitis, acquired immunodeficiency syndrome, osteomyelitis, muscle weakness, and neurologic complications may be found in patients suffering from OUD or poly substance use disorder. As it is common to underestimate and undertreat pain in opioid-dependent patients, it is important to identify the goals in their acute pain management (Box 24.3).[342] Anesthetic management for the opioid-dependent or patient with OUD should include adequate premedication with opioids, administration of supplemental intraoperative and postoperative opioids, and providing nonopioid analgesics and neural blockade. There is no ideal anesthetic agent or technique to employ in the patient with OUD or in the patient with an acute opioid overdose—with the possible exception of judicious use of an opioid antagonist as indicated. As mentioned previously, combined techniques utilizing regional anesthetic approaches, as well as concurrent use of low-dose ketamine and α2-agonists have been successful. Support of the circulatory system with fluids and monitoring of arterial blood gases and pulmonary function are essential.

Owing to the high risk of relapse, overdose, and death in individuals with OUD, medication-assisted treatment (MAT) in which opioids with different pharmacokinetic

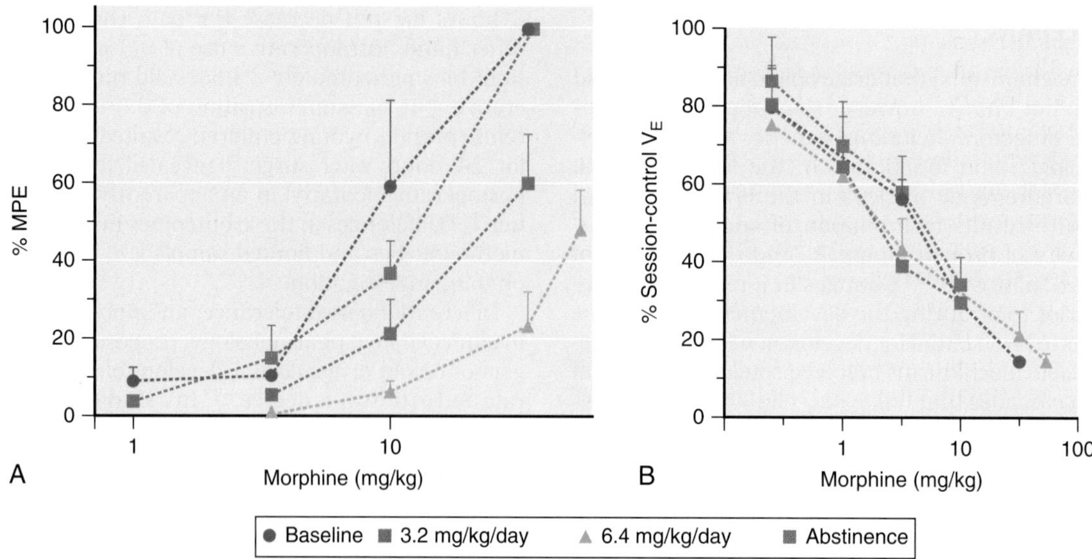

Fig. 24.14 The effects of chronic opioid administration on analgesia and respiratory response in rhesus monkeys. The animals were studied under baseline conditions, after receiving 3.2 or 6.4 mg/kg/day for 4 weeks, and after abstinence. After each treatment course, they were challenged with various doses of morphine, and analgesic and respiratory responses were assessed. Analgesic effects were assessed by tail withdrawal latency and shown as percentage of maximum possible effect *(MPE)*; respiratory depression was shown as decrease in minute ventilation *(V_E)*. The results show development of reversible tolerance to the analgesic effects of opioids (A), but no tolerance development to the respiratory depression (B). (From Paronis CA, Woods JH. Ventilation in morphine-maintained rhesus monkeys. ii: tolerance to the antinociceptive but not the ventilatory effects of morphine. *J Pharmacol Exp Ther.* 1997;282:355–362.)

BOX 24.3 Goals of Acute Pain Management in Opioid-Dependent Patients

1. Identification of the population of at-risk patients receiving long-term opioid therapy for various chronic pain situations (musculoskeletal disease, neuropathic conditions, sickle cell disease, HIV-related disease, palliative care), persons recovering in opioid maintenance programs
2. Prevention of withdrawal symptoms and complications
3. Symptomatic treatment of psychological affective disorders such as anxiety
4. Effective analgesic treatment in the acute phase
5. Rehabilitation to an acceptable and suitable maintenance opioid therapy

HIV, Human immunodeficiency virus.

and pharmacodynamic properties such as methadone or buprenorphine are commonly prescribed. Because of the injection-deterring potential of naloxone hydrochloride and a better safety profile compared with methadone, daily administration of combined buprenorphine and naloxone is becoming a first-line choice for MAT in a number of countries.[343] Other treatment approaches have emerged including rapid opioid detoxification with high-dose naloxone or naltrexone. For this treatment, general anesthesia is induced before the start of opioid antagonization and maintained for several hours to prevent perception of withdrawal symptoms by the patient.[344,345] Blockade of μ-opioid receptors by naloxone (total dose of 12.4 mg) in opioid-addicted patients induces sympathetic neural activation, including increase in plasma catecholamine concentration and cardiovascular stimulation, which can be managed in part by α_2-agonists.[346] Long-term opioid abstinence is not guaranteed, even with an ongoing program that includes MAT, given the neurobiology, societal factors involved in addiction, and potential for repeat exposure—often medically in the perioperative period.[347]

Renal and Urodynamic Effects of Opioids

Opioids can have significant effects on renal function. μ-receptor activation causes antidiuresis and decreases electrolyte excretion. κ-receptor stimulation predominantly produces diuresis with little change in electrolyte excretion. Indirect actions may involve inhibiting or altering the secretion of ADH and atrial natriuretic peptide. The absence of increases in plasma ADH, renin, and aldosterone indicate that fentanyl, sufentanil, alfentanil, and probably remifentanil most likely preserve or minimally alter renal function in humans. If renal function does change during opioid anesthesia and surgery, it is probably due to secondary changes in systemic and renal hemodynamics.

The mechanism by which opioids cause urinary retention is incompletely understood. Opioid effects on the lower urinary tract include disturbances of micturition characterized by urinary retention, especially after intrathecal opioid administration. Intrathecal administration of morphine and sufentanil caused dose-dependent suppression of detrusor contractility and decreased sensation of urge.[348] Mean times to recovery of normal lower urinary tract function were 5 and 8 hours after 10 or 30 μg sufentanil and 14 and 20 hours after 0.1 or 0.3 mg morphine, respectively. Not all opioid agonists behave similarly, and morphine appears to be particularly potent with regard to producing urodynamic problems. Malinovsky et al. compared urodynamic effects of intravenously administered morphine (10 mg), buprenorphine (0.3 mg), fentanyl (0.35 mg), and nalbuphine (20 mg).[349] It was shown that all of the opioids altered bladder sensations, but that detrusor contraction decreased only after administration of fentanyl and buprenorphine. Urinary retention induced by intravenous infusion of remifentanil, 0.15 μg/kg/min could be reversed by a single intravenous dose of methylnaltrexone 0.3 mg/kg or naloxone 0.01 mg/kg.[350] Reversal of urinary retention by methylnaltrexone indicates that peripheral mechanisms may play a role in opioid-induced bladder dysfunction.

A retrospective study for adult patients with chronic kidney disease undergoing orthopedic surgery estimated glomerular filtration rate during the postoperative period was significantly higher in the group in which remifentanil was used for anesthesia management than the group in which remifentanil was not used. This finding may suggest that anesthesia management using remifentanil may have a renal protective effect in adult patients with chronic kidney disease.[351]

Effects of Opioids on Digestive Organs

EFFECTS ON GASTROINTESTINAL TRACT

The adverse gastrointestinal effects of exogenous opioid treatment include nausea, vomiting, altered fluid dynamics, inhibited gastric emptying, inhibited intestinal coordinated propulsive activity, and increased transit time, all of which may contribute to postoperative ileus (Table 24.6).[352] Opioid-dependent mechanisms driving these effects are complex and those involving GI motility are believed to involve opioid receptors expressed throughout the myenteric plexus. Several opioid receptor types can be demonstrated on myenteric neurons, and both κ- and μ-receptor agonists regulate cholinergic transmission in the myenteric plexus. κ-Agonists appear to modulate acetylcholine release more potently than μ-agonists by inhibition of N-type voltage-sensitive Ca^{2+} channels via a pertussis toxin-sensitive G protein in guinea pig ileum.[353]

TABLE 24.6 Effects of Opioids on the Gastrointestinal Tract

Pharmacologic Action	Clinical Effect
Decreased gastric motility and emptying	Decreased appetite; increased gastroesophageal reflux
Decreased pyloric tone	Nausea and vomiting
Decreased enzymatic secretion	Delayed digestion; hard, dry stools
Inhibition of small and large bowel propulsion	Delayed absorption of medication; straining; incomplete evacuation; bloating; abdominal distension; constipation
Increased fluid and electrolyte absorption	Hard, dry stools
Increased nonpropulsive segmental contractions	Spasms; abdominal cramps; pain
Increased anal sphincter tone	Incomplete evacuation

From Viscusi ER, Gan TJ, Leslie JB, et al. Peripherally acting mu-opioid receptor antagonists and postoperative ileus: mechanisms of action and clinical applicability. *Anesth Analg*. 2009;108:1811–1822.

The effect of morphine on esophageal motility has been little explored. Morphine (80 μg/kg) increased the velocity but did not alter the amplitude or duration of primary peristalsis of the esophagus, and it decreased the duration and magnitude of swallow-induced lower esophageal sphincter relaxation.[354] Gastric emptying is delayed by opioids, via supraspinal (vagus nerve-mediated) and spinal, as well as peripheral, mechanisms. Intrathecal morphine (0.4 mg) significantly decreased the gastroduodenal propagation velocity and acetaminophen absorption, and intramuscular morphine (4 mg) gave additional effects.[355] Tramadol (1.25 mg/kg IV) has a measurable but smaller inhibitory effect on gastric emptying compared with codeine (1 mg/kg IV) or morphine (0.125 mg/kg IV).[356] Opioids administered epidurally as well as intrathecally reduce gastrointestinal motility.[355] It was reported that translocation of enteric microorganisms from the intestinal tract to extraintestinal sites is promoted by reduction of gut propulsion after morphine treatment in rats.[357] Propofol (0.3 mg/kg bolus and 1.0 mg/kg/h) abolished the decrease of gastric tone induced by morphine (0.1 mg/kg intravenously), but did not abolish morphine-induced delay of gastric emptying.[358]

Naloxone reverses opioid-induced delays in gastric emptying. Methylnaltrexone, a quaternary naloxone derivative that does not cross the blood-brain barrier, can attenuate morphine-induced delays in gastric emptying, suggesting that a peripheral mechanism is involved in the opioid effect on gastrointestinal tract.[359] Naloxone (0.7 mg/kg) significantly inhibited gastric emptying of saline and milk in rats.[360] This observation might suggest that opioids can affect the gastrointestinal tract by a mechanism independent from the opioid receptors. Intravenous, but not intramuscular, metoclopramide (10 mg) also can reverse morphine-induced delays in gastric emptying.[361]

Opioid effects on the intestine are complex. Transit time from mouth to ileum may not be significantly altered by morphine, because morphine enhances ileal propulsion before decreasing motility. Opioids increase tone and decrease propulsive activity in most of the intestine. Constipation is the frequent side effect in patients who are administered opioids. Naloxonazine attenuated the fentanyl-induced inhibition of gastrointestinal transit more potently than the inhibition induced by morphine or oxycodone. Naloxone methiodide suppressed the oxycodone-induced inhibition of gastrointestinal transit more potently than the inhibition induced by morphine.[362] Thus, μ-opioid receptor agonists induce the inhibition of gastrointestinal transit and drive constipation through different mechanisms.

BILIARY AND HEPATIC EFFECTS

Opioid agonists increase biliary duct pressure and sphincter of Oddi (choledochoduodenal sphincter) tone in a dose- and drug-dependent manner through opioid receptor-mediated mechanisms. However, the clinical consequences of opioid-induced biliary tract actions are usually minimal. Although traditional teaching dictates that morphine induces "spasm" in the sphincter of Oddi and should not be used in acute pancreatitis, no studies or evidence exist to indicate morphine is contraindicated for use in acute pancreatitis.[363] Increases in biliary pressure caused by opioids are, with the exception of meperidine, reversible with naloxone.

Oddi's sphincter manometry via choledochoscope demonstrated that the regular dose of morphine could increase common bile duct pressure, whereas pethidine had no effect on Oddi's sphincter motility and tramadol shows inhibited motility of the sphincter of Oddi.[364] Fragen et al. studied the effect of remifentanil (0.1 mg/kg/min) on the flow of dye from the gall bladder into the duodenum, and showed that remifentanil delays the drainage of dye from the gall bladder into the duodenum, but the delay is shorter than that reported after morphine or meperidine.[365]

Opioids produce minimal effects on liver function during anesthesia and surgery but can affect ischemia-reperfusion injury. Remifentanil pretreatment can attenuate liver injury induced by ischemia-reperfusion, which was shown to be mediated by inducible NO synthase expression and exhausting reactive oxygen species but does not involve opioid receptors.[366] Morphine administered either intravenously or intrathecally 10 minutes before 1 hour of ischemia protects against ischemia-reperfusion injury after 6 hours of reperfusion in both normal and cirrhotic rat liver by a mechanism involving the opioid receptor.[367] Remifentanil significantly attenuated increases in serum aminotransferase levels and the liver histological changes induced by ischemia-reperfusion injury of the liver in rats, by a mechanism possibly involving hepatic interleukin-18.[368] These reports might suggest the beneficial effects of opioids in anesthetic management of liver surgery.

NAUSEA AND VOMITING

Postoperative nausea and vomiting are serious problems which often embarrass anesthesiologists. Etiology, treatment, and prevention of PONV have been extensively investigated (Fig. 24.15).[369] Intraoperative use of opioids is a well-known risk factor for PONV .[370] Opioids stimulate the chemoreceptor trigger zone in the area postrema of the medulla possibly through δ-receptors, leading to nausea and vomiting. Alfentanil, compared with approximately equipotent doses of fentanyl and sufentanil, was found in one study to be associated with a lower incidence of PONV .[371]

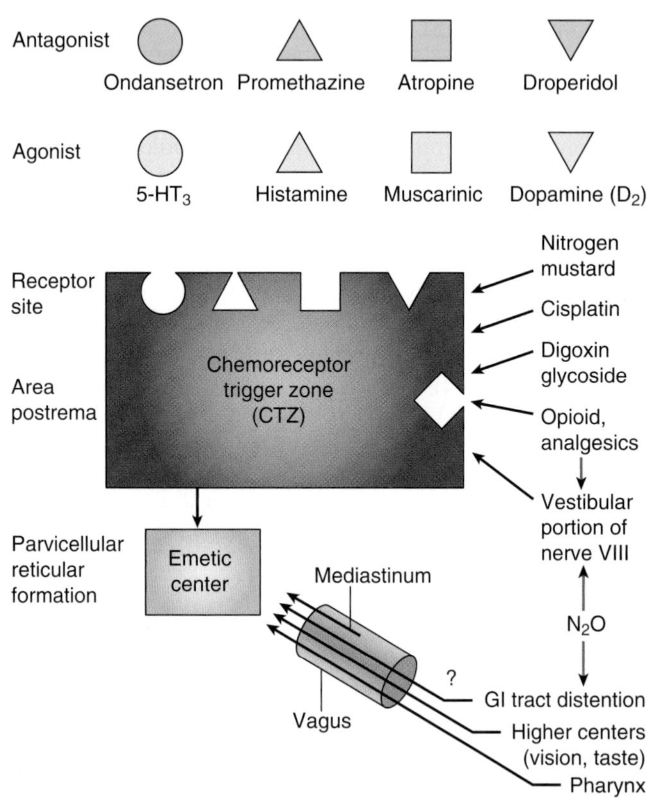

Fig. 24.15 The chemoreceptor trigger zone and the emetic center with the agonist and antagonist sites of action of various anesthetic-related agents and stimuli. *GI*, Gastrointestinal. (From Watcha MF, White PF. Postoperative nausea and vomiting: its etiology, treatment, and prevention. *Anesthesiology*. 1992;77:162–184.)

The use of propofol in balanced or total IV anesthesia (TIVA) significantly reduces the incidence of opioid-induced nausea and vomiting. When opioids are employed, antiemetic prophylaxis should be considered, which includes drugs with anticholinergic activity, butyrophenones, dopamine antagonists, serotonin antagonists and acupressure. Ondansetron, a serotonin type 3 (5-HT_3) receptor antagonist, was proved to be effective for postoperative opioid-induced nausea and vomiting.[372] A meta-analysis concluded that prophylactic use of 5-HT_3 receptor antagonists significantly reduced the incidence of PONV and the need of rescue antiemetic therapy in parturients who received intrathecal morphine for cesarean delivery.[204] Nausea and vomiting after epidural morphine (3 mg) for postcesarean section analgesia could be prevented by dexamethasone (8 mg IV) as efficiently as droperidol (1.25 mg IV).[373] Cannabinoid receptor agonists have been demonstrated to be effective antiemetics in some clinical settings. Animal experiments have shown that the cannabinoid agonist suppresses opioid-induced retching and vomiting by activation of the cannabinoid CB1 receptor.[374] A continuous low-dose naloxone infusion (0.25 μg/kg/h) ameliorates some of the opioid-induced side effects, including nausea, vomiting, and pruritus, in many but not all patients without adversely affecting analgesia.[375] Transdermal scopolamine was shown to be effective for prophylactic use in parturients receiving intrathecal morphine while undergoing cesarean delivery but was associated with higher incidence of side effects such as dry mouth and blurry vision.[376]

Taken together, the prevention and/or treatment of opioid-induced nausea and vomiting continues to be a clinical challenge. Strategies that include the administration of 5-HT_3 receptor antagonists and/or the steroid dexamethasone show efficacy in well controlled trials. However, such approaches require exposure to additional medications that, in themselves, may carry additional risks of side effects.

Other Opioid Effects

OBSTETRICS

The parenteral administration of opioids for oocyte retrieval and prior to delivery remains a commonly used method of analgesia.

Alfentanil and pethidine have been safely used as analgesics during the harvesting of human oocytes for subsequent *in vitro* fertilization.[377] Teratogenic actions of opioids, including fentanyl, sufentanil, and alfentanil, at least in animal models, appear to be minimal. Nociception due to uterine cervical distension could be suppressed by μ- and κ-agonists in rats,[378] but the analgesic effect of μ-agonist but not κ-agonist was reduced by estrogen.[379] Aortocaval compression and associated hypotension may be exacerbated by parenteral opioids, especially following morphine or meperidine. Fetal manifestations of maternal opioid administration include decreases in heart rate variability. Adverse neonatal effects can occur after either morphine or meperidine administration to mothers. Fetal acidosis increases opioid transfer from the mother. Attempts to minimize neonatal effects of opioids include restricting opioid administration to the first stage of labor. The short-acting opioid alfentanil administered before cesarean delivery attenuated the maternal stress response, but led to slightly reduced Apgar score.[380] In a randomized, double-blind, controlled study, it was shown that a single bolus of 1 μg/kg remifentanil administered to patients undergoing elective cesarean delivery effectively attenuated hemodynamic changes after induction and tracheal intubation, but remifentanil crosses the placenta and may cause mild neonatal depression.[381]

Because the fetus is capable of pain perception after the 26th week of gestation, adequate postoperative fetal pain management is essential after fetal surgery. It was shown that the sheep fetus absorbs sufentanil after intraamniotic instillation, and that significantly greater plasma concentrations were obtained in the fetal lamb as compared with the mother sheep.[382]

Morphine and meperidine have been found in the breast milk of mothers receiving intravenous opioid analgesia.[383,384] Although both fentanyl and morphine are concentrated in breast milk in milk-to-plasma ratios of 2 to 3:1, newborn exposure is reported to be insignificant. Newborns of mothers with OUD or taking prescription opioids can exhibit opioid withdrawal often referred to as neonatal abstinence syndrome (NAS) and require appropriate treatment and observation.[385,386]

ANAPHYLACTOID REACTIONS

True allergic reactions and systemic anaphylactoid reactions to opioids are rare. More commonly, local reactions caused by preservatives or histamine may occur. In 32% of heroin addicts dying suddenly after injection, the concentration of tryptase was elevated (>10 μg/L), but no correlation was found between the IgE levels and tryptase, supporting the hypothesis that mast cell degranulation was not mediated by allergic reaction.[387] This report suggests that heroin fatalities may be in part driven by anaphylactoid reaction.

OCULAR EFFECTS

The use of fentanyl, sufentanil, and alfentanil during induction of anesthesia can help to prevent increases in intraocular pressure. Fentanyl, alfentanil, and sufentanil doses as small as 2.5, 10, and 0.1 μg/kg, respectively, may be sufficient as long as appropriate anesthetic depth is achieved prior to tracheal intubation. Remifentanil (1 μg/kg) combined with propofol (2 mg/kg) or thiopental (5 mg/kg) was reported to be effective for prevention of intraocular pressure change after succinylcholine and tracheal intubation.[388,389]

IMMUNE EFFECTS

Opioids can affect immune function through adaptive immunity, innate immunity, and neuroendocrine system (Box 24.4).[390] The literature investigating the function of classical opioid receptors (μ, δ, and κ) present on immune cells suggest a complex relationship between clinically used opioids and immune function, including through indirect mechanisms. However, because the μ-opioid receptor knockout mice showed no immune modulatory effects after central administration of opioids, the central immune modulatory effect of opioids is mediated by μ-opioid receptors.[391]

It was shown that the maximal suppression of natural killer (NK) cell activity, proliferation of splenic T and B cells, and interferon-γ production are observed 0.5 to 1 hour after 15 mg/kg morphine injection in rats.[392] The time course

BOX 24.4 Opioid Effects on Immunity

Adaptive Immunity

↓ Splenic and thymic weight (rodents)
↓ T cell viability and proliferative response
↓ T-helper cell function
↓ CD4/CD8 population *in vivo*
↓ IL1β, IL-2, TNF-α, and IFN-γ (mouse splenocytes)
↓ Th1/Th2 ratio of T-helper cell population (PBMCs)
↓ NK cell activity
↓ Primary antibody response (B cells)
↓ B cells mitogenic response to bacterial LPS
↓ Macrophage activity
↓ TGF-β1 and IL-10 (antiinflammatory cytokines)
↑ T cell apoptosis (NF-κβ and AP-1/NFAT pathways)
Inhibition of CD3/28 mAb induced IL-2 transcripts

Innate Immunity

↓ Number of macrophages available to fight infections
↓ Leucocyte migration
↓ Peritoneal macrophages phagocytosis
↓ Respiratory burst activity and chemotaxis
Inhibition of Fc γ receptor mediated phagocytosis
↓ Superoxide production from neutrophils and macrophages
Alteration of IL-8 induced neutrophil chemotaxis
↓ Neutrophil cytokines involved in wound healing
↑ Apoptosis of macrophages impairing host defense barrier
↓ Leucocytes endothelial adhesion (intracellular adhesion molecules expression)

Neuroendocrine System

↑ Growth hormone, prolactin, and thyroid stimulating hormone secretion in humans
May affect the function of the HPA axis (ACTH and CRH) with risk of adrenal insufficiency
↓ Sex hormones [LH and testosterone (hypogonadism)], oxytocin, and estradiol

ACTH, Adrenocorticotropic hormone; *AP-1*, activator protein 1; *CRH*, corticotropin releasing hormone; *Fc*, fragment crystallizable region; *HPA*, hypothalamic pituitary adrenal axis; *IL*, interleukin; *IFN-γ*, interferon-gamma; *LH*, luteinizing hormone; *LPS*, lipopolysaccharides; *NF-κβ*, nuclear factor kappa beta; *NFAT*, nuclear factor of activated T-cells; *NK*, natural killer; *PBMC*, peripheral blood mononuclear cell; *TGF-β*, transforming growth factor beta; *TNF-α*, tumor necrosis factor-alpha.

From Al-Hashimi M, Scott SW, Thompson JP, Lambert DG. Opioids and immune modulation: more questions than answers. *Br J Anaesth.* 2013;111:80–88.

was nearly concordant with the antinociceptive effect of morphine. Postoperative administration of morphine (10 mg IM) did not significantly affect the NK cell activity, while tramadol (100 mg IM) enhanced NK cell activity.[393] It was reported that intravenously administered fentanyl causes a rapid increase in NK cell cytotoxicity, which was coincident with an increase in the percentage of $CD16^+$ and $CD8^+$ cells in peripheral blood.[394] Compared with fentanyl (1000 μg), administration of morphine (40 mg) as part of balanced anesthetic technique suppressed several components of the inflammatory response (IL-6, CD11b, CD18, postoperative hyperthermia) to cardiac surgery and cardiopulmonary bypass.[395]

As a potential mechanism for the immunosuppressive effects of morphine, it was demonstrated that NF-κβ activation induced by an inflammatory stimulus was inhibited by morphine-induced activation of μ_3-opioid receptors in a NO-dependent manner.[396] Several investigators have independently reported direct effects of morphine on apoptosis in cultured human peripheral blood lymphocytes, which may result in compromising immune functions.[397] However, there is also a report that morphine has no effect on apoptosis-related molecules and does not promote apoptosis of human peripheral blood lymphocytes.[398]

With respect to the effects of opioids on neutrophils, it was reported that remifentanil, but not sufentanil, alfentanil, or fentanyl, could attenuate activation of human neutrophils exposed to lipopolysaccharides, and decreased activation of intracellular signaling pathways, including p38 and ERK1/2, and expression of proinflammatory cytokines, including TNF-α, IL-6, and IL-8, through a mechanism involving the κ-opioid receptor.[399] It was also reported that remifentanil attenuates lipopolysaccharide-induced acute lung injury by inhibition of proinflammatory cytokine production by downregulating the NF-κβ pathway, suggesting a beneficial effect of remifentanil in acute lung injury or acute respiratory distress syndrome in sepsis.[400]

A prospective study for adult patients who underwent elective colorectal surgery demonstrated that the number of patients who developed surgical site infection was higher after remifentanil-based anesthesia (11.6%) compared with fentanyl-based anesthesia (3.4%).[401] A possible reason for this finding may be opioid-induced immunosuppression or opioid withdrawal-induced immunosuppression.

CANCER PROGRESSION

Epidemiological studies have suggested that patients who receive general anesthesia with opioids have a greater rate of cancer recurrence than patients who receive local or regional anesthetics,[402] although there is no direct evidence to support altering anesthetic technique in cancer patients. Opioids may directly stimulate proliferation and invasion of tumor cells and inhibit apoptosis of tumor cells, or indirectly affect cancer recurrence by immunosuppression.[403] Overexpression of the μ-opioid receptor in human non-small cell lung cancer was suggested to promote tumor growth and progression.[404] Furthermore, it was reported that women with A118G genotype of the μ-opioid receptor have decreased breast cancer-specific mortality, suggesting that opioid pathways may be involved in tumor growth.[405] Drawing from preclinical studies using animals or cultured cells opioids may promote tumor growth and metastasis through multiple mechanisms, whereas it is also reported that opioids can direct various anticarcinogenic pathways (Fig. 24.16).[406] Preclinical data have also suggested that μ-opioid receptor inhibition can reverse the adverse effect of μ-opioid receptor signaling on cancer progression, when a combination of methylnaltrexone, which blocks peripheral but not central μ-opioid receptor, and chemotherapy is tested.[407]

One of the mechanisms involved in the effects of opioids on cancer prognosis is their effects on angiogenesis. Morphine can stimulate angiogenesis by a variety of mechanisms involving NO, MAPK, VEGF, and Rho/Rho kinase.[408] Blebea et al. reported that activation of opioid receptors inhibited angiogenesis, via endogenous opioid ligands.[409] Although both pro- and anti-angiogenic actions of opioids have been reported, it is generally believed that the pro-angiogenic (or neo-vasculogenic) effects predominate.

The opioid growth factor receptor (OGFR) is localized in both the nucleus and the cytoplasm and functions as a receptor for OGF, also known as methionine-enkephalin. OGFR is distinguished from classic opioid receptors (μ, δ, and κ) as not having any role in analgesia but functions as a negative regulator of cell proliferation. Morphine can also interact with OGFR expressed in lung cancer tissues and cell lines and may suppress lung cancer progression.[410]

WOUND HEALING

Topical application of opioids has been explored as a strategy for reducing pain associated with cutaneous wounds. In addition to its analgesic functions, the peripheral opioid receptor system affects skin homeostasis by influencing cell differentiation, migration, and adhesion. Activation of peripheral opioid receptors on primary afferent neurons reduces the excitability of these neurons and suppresses the antidromic release of substance P and calcitonin gene-related peptide, which play an essential role in wound repair. It was shown that topical morphine application significantly reduced the number of myofibroblasts and macrophages in the closing wound.[411] These findings might limit the topical application of opioids as an analgesic therapeutic strategy in the treatment of painful cutaneous wounds. In contrast, it was shown that activation of the δ-opioid receptors destabilizes intercellular adhesion and promotes the migratory keratinocyte phenotype, which is required for fast wound closure.[412] If these divergent findings can be resolved in favor of wound healing and enhanced localized analgesia, there is great potential for opioid applications in wound healing. Most clinical studies have not focused on opioid effects on the wound healing process but substantial analgesic effects without delaying wound closure were found. Larger clinical trials are required to examine whether opioids interfere with wound healing by inhibition of proinflammatory cytokine release or by development of hypertrophic scars, as shown in animal studies.[413]

Pharmacokinetics and Pharmacodynamics of Opioids

With the advent of modern drug assay technology and the widespread availability of computers, it is now possible to

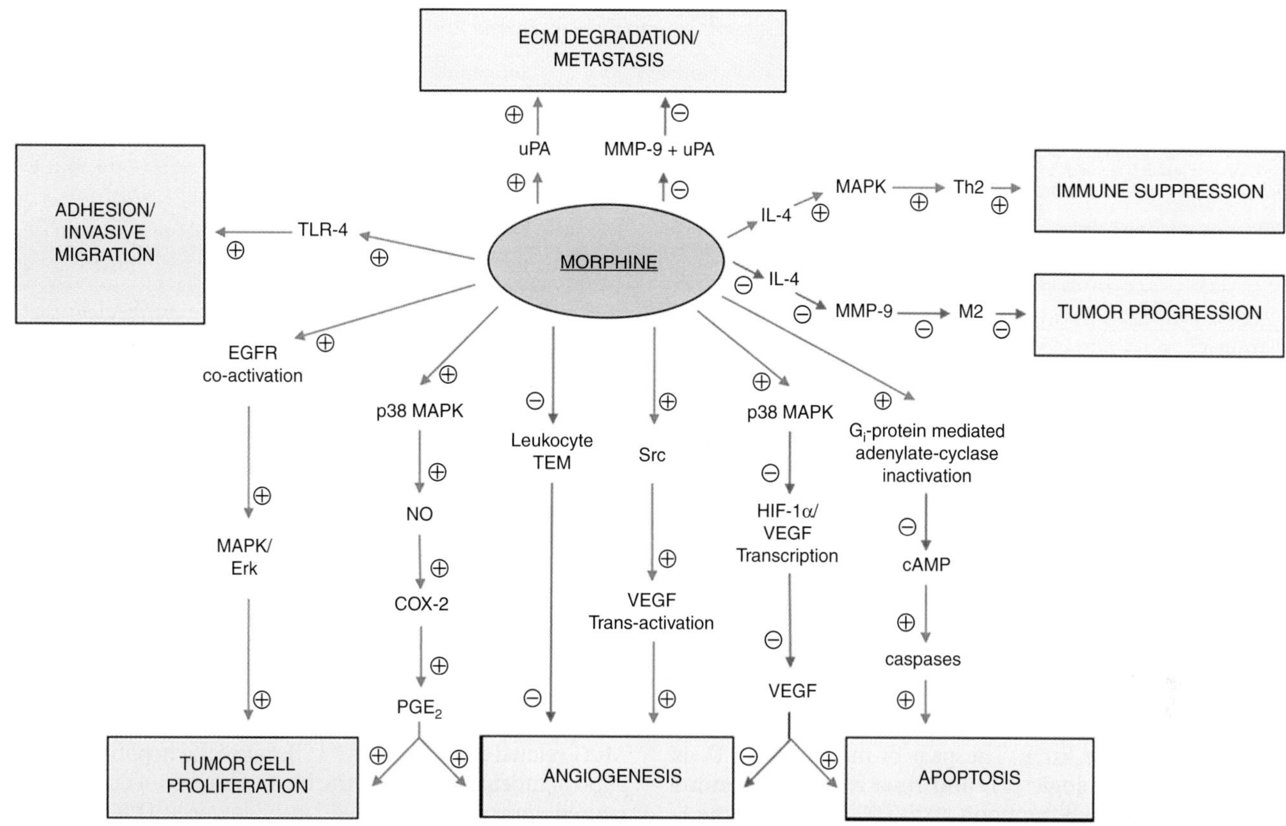

Fig. 24.16 Effects of morphine on cancer cells. It is important to note that the same pathway can have opposing end results, depending on the morphine doses, mode of administration, and animal models used. *cAMP*, Cyclic adenosine monophosphate; *COX-2*, cyclooxygenase-2; *ECM*, extracellular matrix; *EGFR*, epidermal growth factor receptor; *Erk*, extracellular-regulated kinase; *HIF-1α*, hypoxia inducible factor 1 alpha; *IL*, interleukin; *M2*, "alternative" activation of macrophages; *MAPK*, mitogen-activated protein kinase; *MMPs*, matrix metalloproteinases; *NO*, nitric oxide; *PGE₂*, Prostaglandin E_2; *Src*, non-receptor tyrosine kinase; *TLR-4*, toll-like receptor 4; *Th2*, T helper 2 cells; *uPA*, urokinase plasminogen activator; *VEGF*, vascular endothelial growth factor. (From Sekandarzad MW, van Zundert AAJ, Lirk PB, et al. Perioperative anesthesia care and tumor progression. *Anesth Analg*. 2017;124;1697–1708.)

analyze and model pharmacologic data which separates drug response into pharmacokinetic and pharmacodynamic components. Pharmacokinetic parameters govern the relationship between opioid dose and the opioid concentrations in the blood (or other body fluids). Pharmacodynamic parameters describe the relationship between opioid concentration in blood (or other fluids) and opioid effect.

Computer simulation techniques predict "context-sensitive half–times," the time necessary to achieve a 50% decrease in drug concentration after termination of a variable-length continuous infusion to a steady-state drug level (see Chapter 26). Such simulations are intended to provide more clinically relevant meaning to pharmacokinetic parameters. The context-sensitive half-time and computer simulations have helped clinicians to select opioids in a more rational fashion. After 1-hour continuous infusion, the context-sensitive half-time of fentanyl is nearly six times that of alfentanil or sufentanil. Remifentanil's context-sensitive half-time is independent of infusion duration.

PHYSICOCHEMICAL PROPERTIES

Opioids are weak bases. When dissolved in solution, they are dissociated into protonated and free-base fractions, with the relative proportions depending on the pH and pKa. The free-base fraction is more lipid-soluble than the protonated fraction. High lipid solubility facilitates opioid transport into the biophase or site of action. Therefore, highly lipid-soluble opioids have a more rapid onset of action. However, because the opioid receptor recognizes an opioid molecule in the protonated form, the intensity of opioid effects is closely related to the ionized concentration of drug in the biophase.

All opioids are to some extent bound to plasma proteins, including albumin and α_1-acid glycoprotein. It is only the un-ionized, unbound fraction that constitutes the diffusible fraction and provides the concentration gradient that promotes diffusion of opioid from the blood to the tissue of interest. Thus, the speed of onset of opioid effect is affected by both the lipid solubility and the protein binding.

PHARMACOKINETIC FEATURES OF INDIVIDUAL DRUGS

Representative pharmacokinetic parameters for the opioids commonly used in anesthesia are displayed in Table 24.7.

Morphine

Morphine pharmacokinetics is notably different from that of the fentanyl congeners. This difference is in large part due to morphine's comparatively low lipid solubility. There is relatively little transient first-pass uptake

TABLE 24.7 Physicochemical and Pharmacokinetic Data of Commonly Used Opioid Agonists

	Morphine	Fentanyl	Sufentanil	Alfentanil	Remifentanil
p*K*a	8.0	8.4	8.0	6.5	7.1
% Un-ionized at pH 7.4	23	<10	20	90	67?
Octanol/H_2O partition coefficient	1.4	813	1778	145	17.9
% Bound to plasma protein	20-40	84	93	92	80?
Diffusible fraction (%)	16.8	1.5	1.6	8.0	13.3?
$t_{1/2}\alpha$ (min)	1-2.5	1-2	1-2	1-3	0.5-1.5
$t_{1/2}\beta$ (min)	10-20	10-30	15-20	4-17	5-8
$t_{1/2\gamma}$ (h)	2-4	2-4	2-3	1-2	0.7-1.2
Vd_c (L/kg)	0.1-0.4	0.4-1.0	0.2	0.1-0.3	0.06-0.08
Vd_{ss} (L/kg)	3-5	3-5	2.5-3.0	0.4-1.0	0.2-0.3
Clearance (mL/min/kg)	15-30	10-20	10-15	4-9	30-40
Hepatic extraction ratio	0.6-0.8	0.8-1.0	0.7-0.9	0.3-0.5	NA

NA, Not applicable; pK_a, ion dissociation constant; $t_{1/2}$ α, β, γ, half-lives of a three-compartment model; Vd_c, volume of distribution of the central compartment; Vd_{ss}, volume of distribution at steady state.

From Bailey PL, Egan TD, Stanley TH. Intravenous opioid anesthetics. In: Miller RD, ed. *Anesthesia*. 8th ed. Philadelphia: Saunders; 2015. An imprint of Elsevier Inc., p. 887.

of morphine by the lung. The pKa of morphine (8.0) is greater than physiologic pH, and thus after intravenous injection only a small fraction (10%-20%) of morphine is un-ionized. Penetration of morphine into and out of the brain is presumably slower compared with that of other opioids. Approximately 20% to 40% of morphine is bound to plasma proteins, mostly albumin.

Morphine is principally metabolized by conjugation in the liver, but the kidney plays a key role in the extrahepatic metabolism of morphine. M3G is the major metabolite of morphine, but does not bind to opioid receptors and possesses little or no analgesic activity. M3G may actually antagonize morphine, and this effect may contribute to both variability in response and resistance to morphine analgesic therapy. M3G was reported to produce seizures in animals and cause allodynia in children.[414] M6G accounts for nearly 10% of morphine metabolite and is a more potent μ-receptor agonist than morphine with a similar duration of action. It was reported that M6G contributes substantially to morphine's analgesic effects even in patients with normal renal function.[415] A recent study reported that based on area under the concentration–time curve there was a major contribution of M6G to the overall analgesic effect; the mean contributions being estimated as 96.6%, 85.6%, 85.4%, and 91.3% after oral, subcutaneous, intravenous, and rectal administration of morphine, respectively.[416] In patients with renal insufficiency, 97.6% of the analgesic effect is caused by M6G when morphine is given orally. Especially in patients with renal dysfunction, the accumulation of M6G can lead to an increased incidence of adverse effects, including respiratory depression. Except for renal function, M6G accumulation was shown to be affected by transmembrane transporters inhibited by probenecid.[417] M6G can induce respiratory depression similarly as morphine, but the site of action in the ventilatory control system might be different between M6G and morphine.[418] It was suggested that SNP at the μ-opioid receptor affects the susceptibility to M6G-related opioid toxicity.[419] Because the hepatic extraction ratio of morphine is high, the bioavailability of orally administered morphine is significantly lower (20%-30%) than after intramuscular or subcutaneous injection. It appears that M6G is in fact the primary active compound when morphine is administered orally (Fig. 24.17).[420] In contrast to the reports suggesting the high potency of M6G, there have been reports showing that short-term intravenous administration of M6G does not provide effective analgesia.[421]

Fentanyl

A three-compartment model is typically used to describe plasma fentanyl concentration decay. The lungs exert a significant first-pass effect and transiently take up approximately 75% of an injected dose of fentanyl. Approximately 80% of fentanyl is bound to plasma proteins, and significant amounts (40%) are taken up by red blood cells. Fentanyl is relatively long acting, in large part because of this widespread distribution in body tissues.

Fentanyl is primarily metabolized in the liver by *N*-dealkylation and hydroxylation. Metabolites begin to appear in the plasma as early as 1.5 minutes after injection. Norfentanyl, the primary metabolite, is detectable in the urine for up to 48 hours after intravenous fentanyl in humans.

Alfentanil

Following IV injection, alfentanil plasma concentrations are described by either two-compartment or three-compartment model. Alfentanil is bound to plasma proteins (mostly glycoproteins) in higher proportions (92%) than fentanyl. At physiologic pH, it is mostly (90%) un-ionized because of its relatively low pKa (6.5). Thus, despite more intense protein binding, the diffusible fraction of alfentanil is higher than fentanyl. This explains, in part, its short latency to peak effect after intravenous injection.

The main metabolic pathways of alfentanil are similar to those of sufentanil and include oxidative *N*-dealkylation

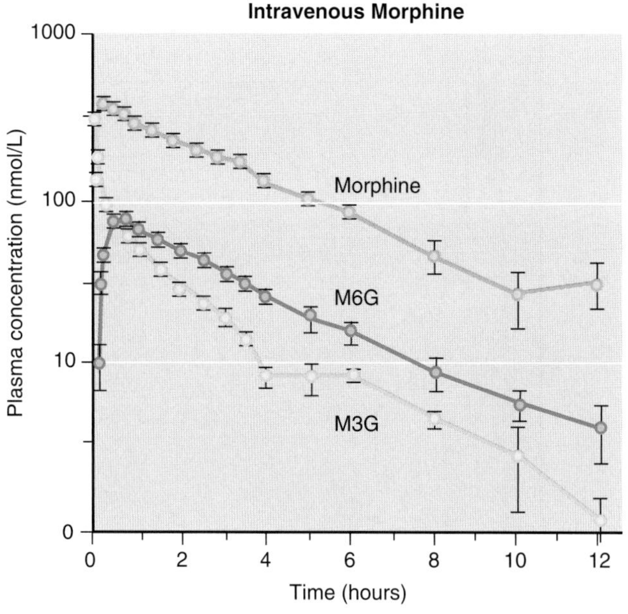

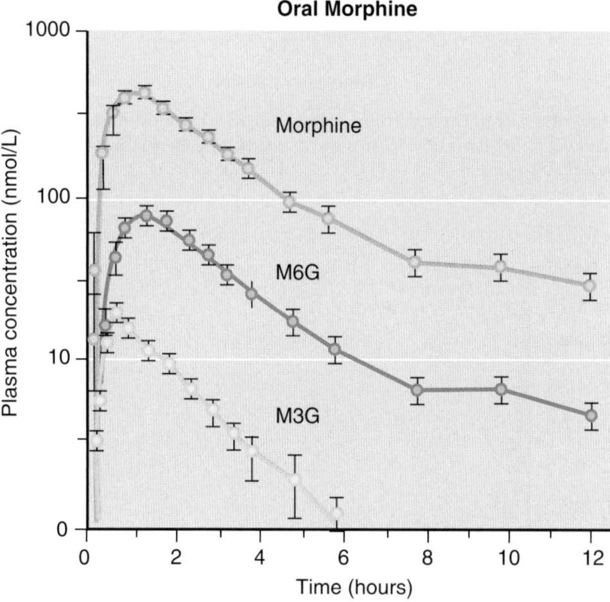

Fig. 24.17 Mean plasma concentrations (± standard error of means) of morphine, morphine-6-glucuronide *(M6G)*, and morphine-3-glucuronide *(M3G)* after intravenous and oral administration of morphine. (From Osborne R, Joel S, Trew D, et al. Morphine and metabolite behavior after different routes of morphine administration: demonstration of the importance of the active metabolite morphine-6-glucuronide. *Clin Pharmacol Ther*. 1990;47:12–19.)

and *O*-demethylation, aromatic hydroxylation, and ether glucuronide formation. The degradation products of alfentanil have little, if any, opioid activity. Human alfentanil metabolism may be predominantly, if not exclusively, by cytochrome P-450 3A3/4 (CYP3A3/4).[422] This enzyme is known to display at least 8-fold difference in activity in humans. Alfentanil is also metabolized by human liver microsomal CYP3A5, which shows more than 20-fold pharmacogenetic variability in expression level leading to significant differences in human liver alfentanil metabolism.[423] In vitro study demonstrated that propofol in clinically relevant concentrations interferes with oxidative metabolic degradation of alfentanil and sufentanil in the microsomal fraction of pig and human liver.[424]

Sufentanil

The pharmacokinetic property of sufentanil is adequately described by a three-compartment model. After intravenous injection, first-pass pulmonary extraction, retention, and release are similar to those of fentanyl.[425] The pKa of sufentanil at physiologic pH is the same as that of morphine (8.0), and, therefore, only a small amount (20%) exists in the un-ionized form. Sufentanil is twice as lipid-soluble as fentanyl and is highly bound (93%) to plasma proteins including α_1-acid glycoprotein.

The major metabolic pathways of sufentanil include *N*-dealkylation, oxidative *O*-demethylation, and aromatic hydroxylation. Major metabolites include *N*-phenylpropanamide.

Remifentanil

Although chemically related to the fentanyl congeners, remifentanil is structurally unique because of its ester linkages. Remifentanil's ester structure renders it susceptible to hydrolysis by blood- and tissue-nonspecific esterases, resulting in rapid metabolism and rapid reduction of blood concentration after an infusion has stopped (Fig. 24.18).[426] Remifentanil thus constitutes the first ultrashort-acting opioid for use as a supplement to general anesthesia.

Pharmacokinetic properties of remifentanil are best described by a three-compartment model. Its clearance is several times greater than normal hepatic blood flow, consistent with widespread extrahepatic metabolism. But, remifentanil is not significantly metabolized or sequestered in the lungs.[427] It is a weak base with a pKa of 7.07. It is highly lipid-soluble with an octanol/water partition coefficient of 19.9 at pH 7.4. Remifentanil is highly bound (= 70%) to plasma proteins (mostly α_1-acid glycoprotein). The remifentanil free base is formulated with glycine. Because glycine has been shown to act as an inhibitory neurotransmitter that causes a reversible motor weakness when injected intrathecally in rodents, remifentanil is not approved for spinal or epidural use.[428]

The primary metabolic pathway of remifentanil is de-esterification to form a carboxylic acid metabolite, GR-90291 (Fig. 24.19),[429] which is 0.003 to 0.001 times as potent as remifentanil. The low *in vivo* potency of GR90291 can be explained by its low affinity to the μ-receptor in combination with a poor brain penetration.[430] Excretion of GR-90291 is dependent on renal clearance mechanisms. Evidence from dogs suggests that the remifentanil metabolites are, for practical purposes, completely inactive, even in the face of renal failure. Its pharmacokinetics is not appreciably influenced by renal or hepatic failure. In blood, remifentanil is metabolized primarily by enzymes within erythrocytes. Remifentanil is not a good substrate for pseudocholinesterase and, therefore, is not influenced by pseudocholinesterase deficiency.[431]

SURROGATE MEASURES OF OPIOID POTENCY

Because a high-resolution measure of analgesia is not available, opioid potencies are usually estimated by some surrogate measures. Reduction of the MAC required to produce lack of movement to skin incision has been a

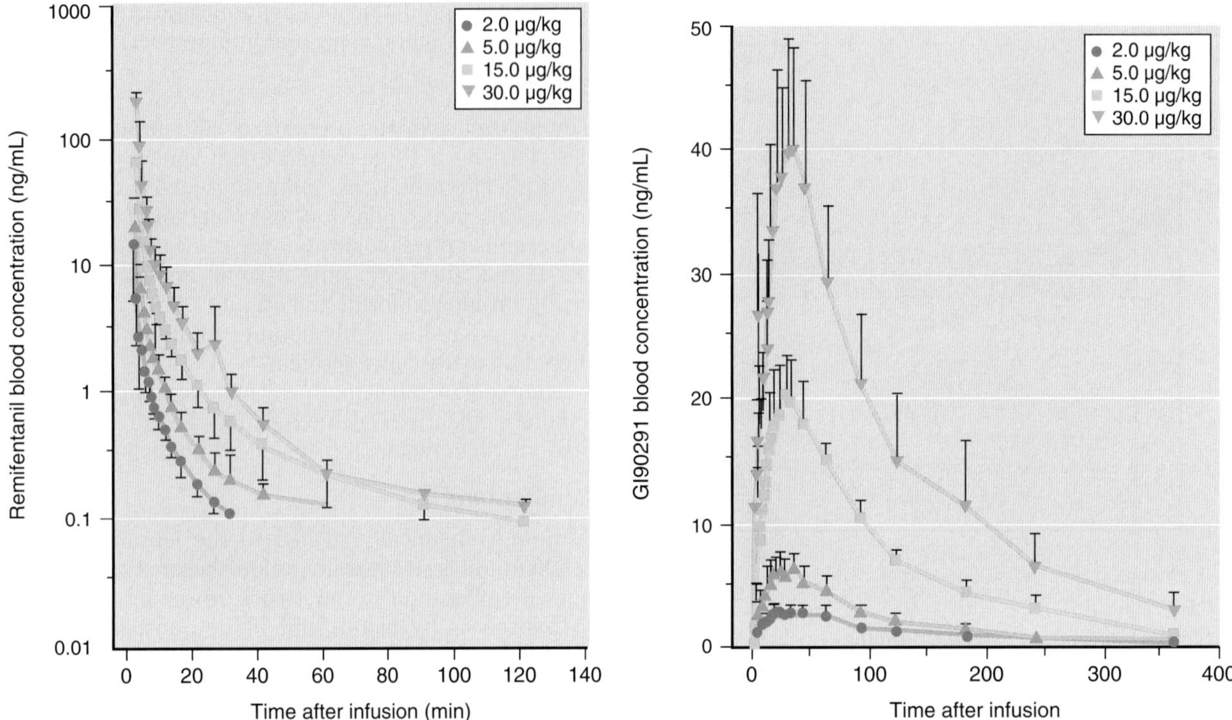

Fig. 24.18 Mean (± standard deviation) blood concentration-time curves of remifentanil and its metabolite GI90291 after a 1-minute transfusion of remifentanil of 2, 5, 15, and 30 μg/kg (*n* = 6 for each dose). (From Westmoreland CL, Hoke JF, Sebel PS, et al. Pharmacokinetics of remifentanil (GI87084B) and its major metabolite (GI90291) in patients undergoing elective inpatient surgery. *Anesthesiology*. 1993;79:893–903.)

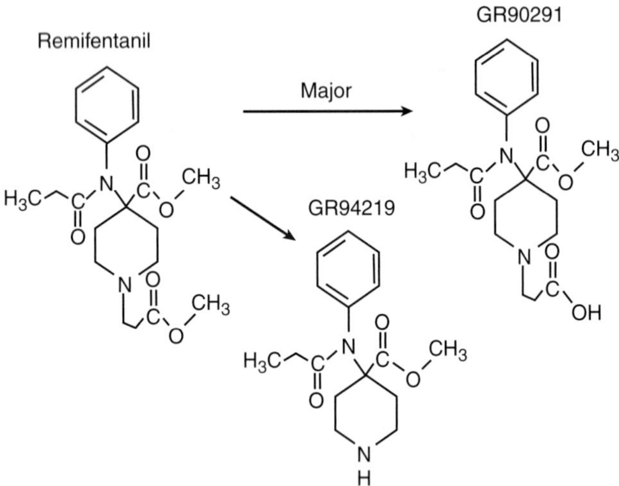

Fig. 24.19 Metabolic pathway of remifentanil. Deesterification by nonspecific plasma and tissue esterases to form a carboxylic acid metabolite *(GR90291)* that has only 1/300 to 1/1000 the potency of the parent compound is the primary metabolic pathway. *N*-dealkylation of remifentanil to *GR94219* is a minor metabolic pathway. (From Egan TD, Lemmens HJ, Fiset P, et al. The pharmacokinetics of the new short-acting opioid remifentanil (GI87084B) in healthy adult male volunteers. *Anesthesiology*. 1993;79:881–892.)

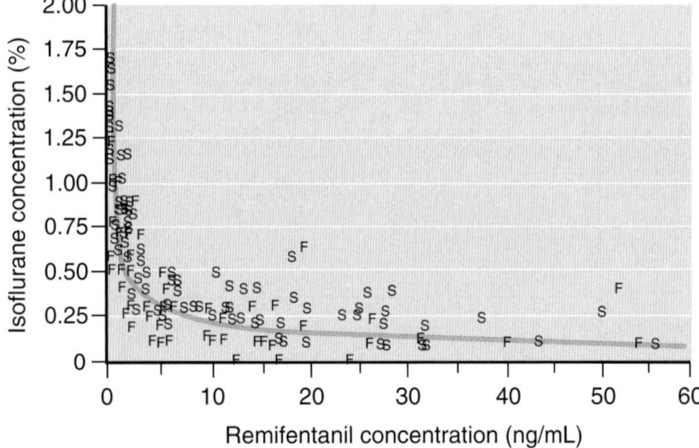

Fig. 24.20 The reduction in isoflurane concentration to prevent movement at skin incision in 50% of patients by increasing measured remifentanil whole blood concentrations. *F* represents a patient who moved and *S* represents a patient who did not move. The solid line is the logistic regression solution for a 40-year-old patient. (From Lang E, Kapila A, Shlugman D, et al. Reduction of isoflurane minimal alveolar concentration by remifentanil. *Anesthesiology*. 1995;85:721–728.)

frequently utilized surrogate measure in the estimation of opioid potency (Fig. 24.20).[125] However, MAC is not useful as a surrogate measure of opioid potencies outside the operation rooms.

To guide the administration of opioids in anesthetized patients, indirect parameters that reflect the patient's physiologic reaction to nociception like sweating, movement, heart rate, and blood pressure should be monitored. However, the low specificity of these signs can cause underdosage or overdosage of intraoperative analgesia. The Analgesia Nociception Index (ANI), derived from an electrocardiogram trace, has been proposed as a noninvasive guide to analgesia.[432] The ANI monitor calculates heart rate variation with respiration, a response mediated primarily by changes in the parasympathetic nervous system stimulation to the sinoatrial node of the heart. Patients receiving

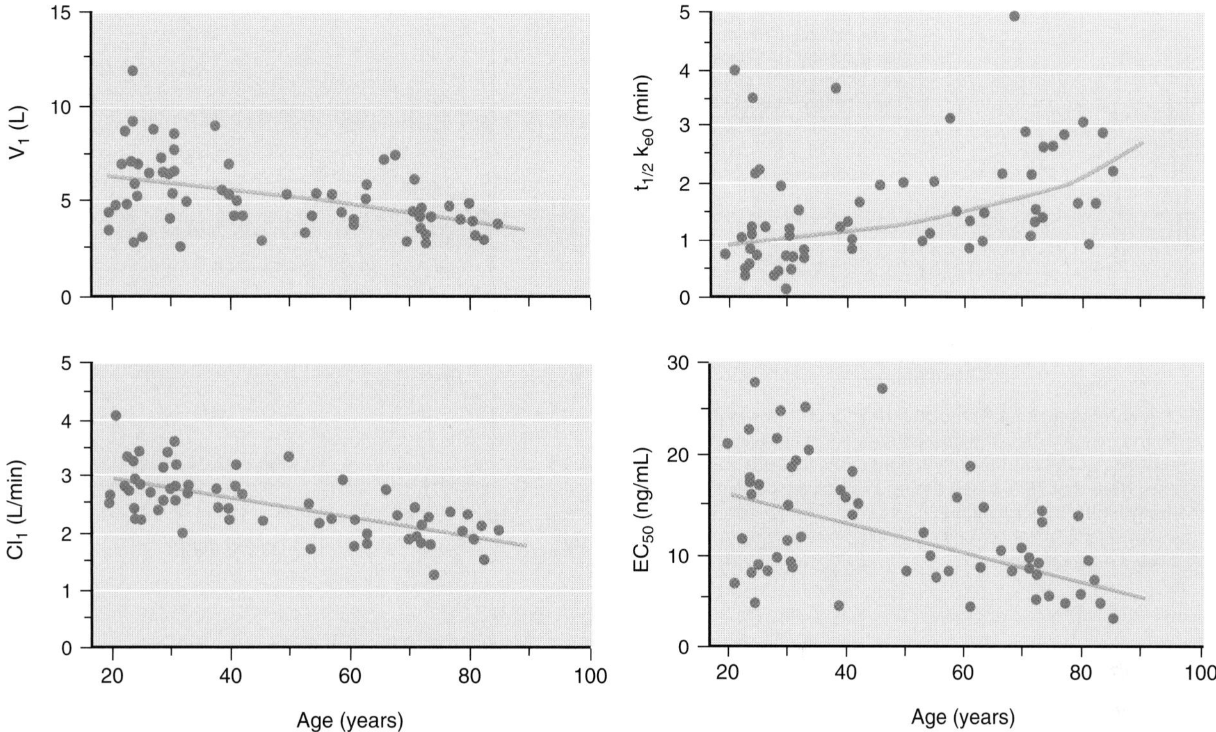

Fig. 24.21 Relationship between pharmacokinetic and pharmacodynamic parameters and age for remifentanil. Volume of distribution *(V_1)* and clearance *(Cl_1)* are estimated using a three-compartment model. $t_{1/2}k_{e0}$ is a half-life corresponding to k_{e0}, a first-order rate constant for elimination of drug from the effect compartment. (From Minto CF, Schnider TW, Shafer SL. Pharmacokinetics and pharmacodynamics of remifentanil. II. Model application. *Anesthesiology*. 1997;86:24–33.)

intraoperative ANI-guided fentanyl administration during sevoflurane anesthesia for lumbar discectomy and laminectomy demonstrated decreased pain in the recovery room, likely as a result of more objective intraoperative fentanyl administration.[433]

The EEG has been another widely utilized surrogate measure in estimating opioid potency. The EEG is advantageous, because it is noninvasive and can be used as an effect measure when an experimental subject is unconscious or apneic. When processed by Fourier spectral analysis, the raw EEG changes translate into a significant decrease in the value of the spectral edge, a parameter that quantitates the frequency below which a given percentage (usually 95%) of the power in the EEG signal is found. Although the clinical meaning of the EEG changes produced by opioids is unclear, the opioid potencies estimated using the EEG as a surrogate measure appear to be clinically reliable because they relate to clinically determined potencies in a proportional, reproducible fashion. However, because the surrogate measures do not always assess the drug effect of clinical interest (analgesia), estimations of potency based on surrogate measures must be interpreted with caution.

FACTORS AFFECTING PHARMACOKINETICS AND PHARMACODYNAMICS OF OPIOIDS

Age

Pharmacokinetics and pharmacodynamics of opioids can be influenced by age. It is clear that neonates exhibit a reduced rate of elimination of essentially all opioids.[434] This is presumably due to immature metabolic mechanisms, including the cytochrome P-450 system. The prolonged elimination of opioids observed in the neonatal period quickly normalizes toward adult values within the first year of life.[434]

Intraoperative requirements of opioids are different between adults and children. The infusion rate of remifentanil to block somatic and autonomic response to skin incision was almost 2-fold higher in children (2-11 years) than adults (20-60 years).[435,436] With advanced age, although pharmacokinetic changes may play a minor role, pharmacodynamic differences are primarily responsible for the decreased dose requirement in the elderly. Age was inversely correlated with central volume of distribution, clearance, and potency of remifentanil (Fig. 24.21).[437] These combined pharmacokinetic and pharmacodynamic changes mandate a reduction in remifentanil dosage by at least 50% or more in the elderly.

Body Weight

Many opioid pharmacokinetic parameters, especially clearance, appear to be more closely related to lean body mass. Total body weight-based dosing in an obese patient results in much higher remifentanil effect-site concentrations than does lean body mass-based dosing.[438] In contrast, for lean patients, the concentrations that result from total body weight-based dosing are not much greater than those based on body mass (Fig. 24.22). Clinically, context-sensitive half-times are not significantly different between obese and lean subjects (Fig. 24.23). There is mounting evidence to suggest that lean body mass is a better predictor of metabolic capacity than total body weight. Ideal body weight, a parameter closely related to lean body mass and one that

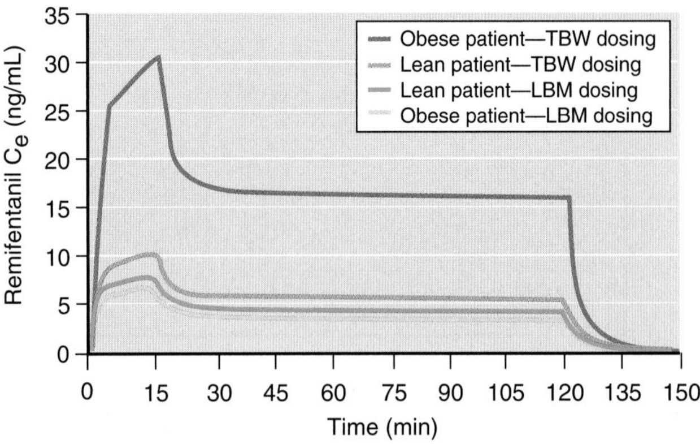

Fig. 24.22 A computer simulation of the time course of remifentanil concentration change, when the dosage regimen is calculated based on lean body mass *(LBM)* or total body weight *(TBW)* for both obese and lean patients. Note that TBW-based dosing in an obese patient results in dramatically higher concentrations. (From Egan TD, Huizinga B, Gupta SK, et al. Remifentanil pharmacokinetics in obese versus lean patients. *Anesthesiology*. 1998;89:562–573.)

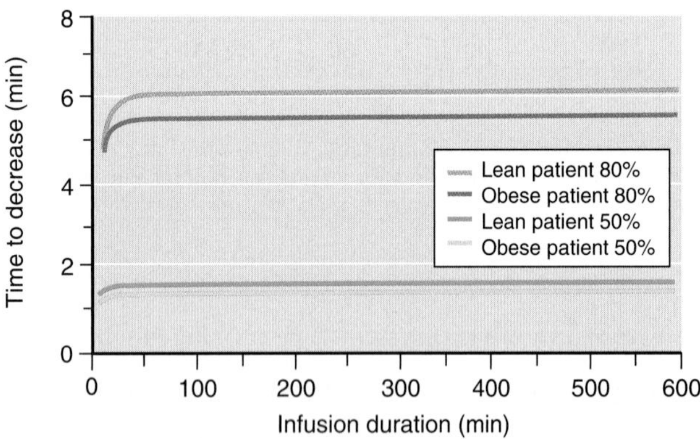

Fig. 24.23 A computer simulation of the context-sensitive half-times (50% decrement times) and 80% decrement times of remifentanil in obese vs. lean subjects. In clinical terms, the curves are not grossly different in obese and lean subjects. (From Egan TD, Huizinga B, Gupta SK, et al. Remifentanil pharmacokinetics in obese versus lean patients. *Anesthesiology*. 1998;89:562–573.)

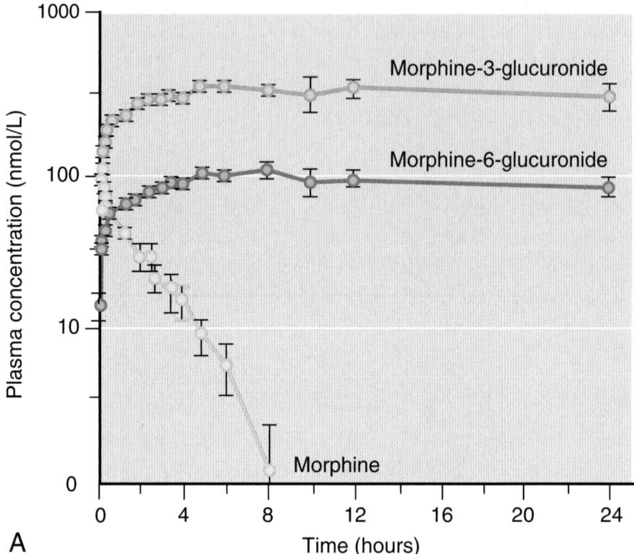

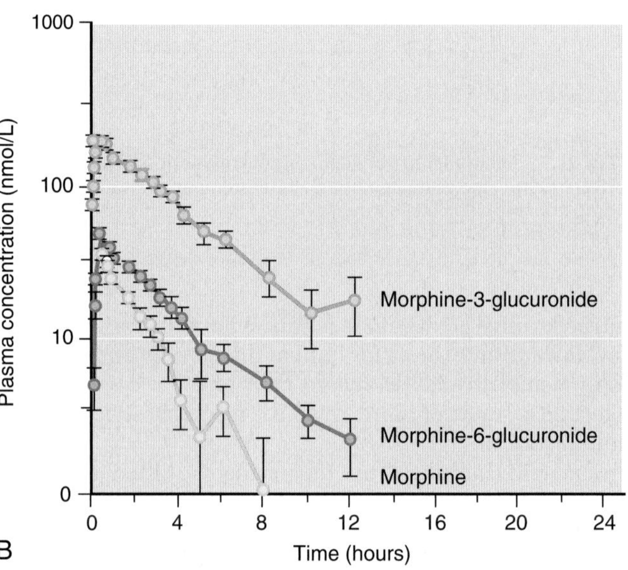

Fig. 24.24 Effect of renal failure on pharmacokinetics of morphine. The graphs show the time-dependent change of the serum concentration of morphine and its metabolite in patients of renal failure (A) and in patients with normal renal function (B) who received 0.1 mg/kg morphine intravenously. (From Osborne R, Joel S, Grebenik K, et al. The pharmacokinetics of morphine and morphine glucuronides in kidney failure. *Clin Pharmacol Ther*. 1993;54:158–167.)

is perhaps more easily estimated by the clinician, is probably an acceptable alternative of lean body mass. Because obesity and obesity-associated disease have increased and continue to do so, obese patients will frequently present for anesthesia and operations. Understanding the influence of obesity on the disposition of opioids is an important question in contemporary anesthesia practice. In response, new pharmacokinetic models incorporating the influence of body mass have been recently reported.[439,440]

Renal Failure

Renal failure has implications of major clinical importance with respect to morphine, hydromorphone, and meperidine. For the fentanyl congeners, the clinical importance of renal failure is less marked.

Morphine is an opioid with active metabolites that are dependent on renal clearance mechanisms for elimination. Morphine is principally metabolized by conjugation in the liver, and the water-soluble glucuronides (M3G and M6G) are excreted via kidney. The kidney also plays a role in the conjugation of morphine, accounting for nearly 40% of its metabolism.[441] Patients with renal failure can develop very high levels of M6G and life-threatening respiratory depression (Fig. 24.24).[442] In view of these changes induced by renal failure, morphine is not considered a good choice in patients with severely altered renal clearance mechanisms. There are similar concerns for the use of hydromorphone in the setting of renal dysfunction.

The clinical pharmacology of meperidine is also significantly altered by renal failure. Because normeperidine, the main metabolite of meperidine with analgesic and CNS excitatory effect, is subject to renal excretion, the potential CNS toxicity secondary to normeperidine accumulation is especially a concern in patients in renal failure.

In contrast, the clinical pharmacology of the fentanyl congeners is not grossly altered by renal failure, although a decrease in plasma protein binding may potentially alter the free fraction of the fentanyl class of opioids. In the presence of renal impairment, none of fentanyl, alfentanil, sufentanil, and remifentanil deliver a high active metabolite load, or suffer from significantly prolonged clearance.[443] Neither the pharmacokinetics nor the pharmacodynamics of remifentanil is altered by impaired renal function. Levels of GI-90291 that develop during a remifentanil infusion in patients in renal failure are not likely to produce any clinically significant effects.

HEPATIC FAILURE

Even though the liver is the metabolic organ primarily responsible for opioid biotransformation, the degree of liver failure typically observed in perioperative patients, with the exception of patients undergoing liver transplantation, does not have a major impact on the pharmacokinetics of most opioids. In addition to reduced metabolic capacity (i.e., cytochrome P-450 system and conjugation), liver disease may also lead to reductions in hepatic blood flow, hepatocellular mass, and plasma protein binding. The increase in total body water and the edema of advanced liver disease may alter the distribution characteristics of a drug. Enzyme induction such as observed in early alcoholism can actually increase metabolic capacity of the liver.

Morphine pharmacokinetics is relatively unchanged by developing liver disease, such as liver cirrhosis and hepatic carcinoma, because of the substantial compensatory extrahepatic metabolism of morphine. A reduction in hepatic blood flow would be expected to slow the decline of morphine plasma concentrations. After liver resection, M6G/morphine and M3G/morphine ratios were significantly reduced and circulating morphine concentration was increased mainly due to a lower morphine clearance.[444] In patients with cirrhosis, the metabolism of meperidine is decreased, leading to accumulation of the parent drug and possible CNS depressive effects similar to hepatic encephalopathy. Although the elimination of normeperidine is decreased as well in these patients, the ratio of normeperidine to meperidine is generally low, and the opioid effects of meperidine usually predominate.[445] The disposition of fentanyl and sufentanil appears to be unaffected in liver diseases.[446] Reductions in liver blood flow that result from either liver disease or some other disorder (e.g., shock) can affect the pharmacokinetic parameters of alfentanil, fentanyl, and sufentanil. It was demonstrated that there was a significant decrease in clearance of alfentanil in patients with mild to moderate cirrhosis compared with volunteers from the historical control group.[447] Remifentanil is an opioid whose pharmacokinetics is completely unchanged by liver disease (Fig. 24.25).[448] Its kinetics does not change during the anhepatic phase of orthotopic liver transplantation.[449] It was reported that 0.25 to 0.5 μg/kg/min remifentanil could provide perioperative analgesia without neurological deterioration in a patient suffering from chronic hepatic failure with mild encephalopathy.[450]

In summary, a reduction in renal function may have the greatest effects on morphine due to a decrease in capacity for extrahepatic glucuronidation and clearance. Therefore, fentanyl may be a safer choice in renal failure patients due to their lack of active metabolites. In contrast, only under conditions of severe hepatic failure does one observe clinically significant changes in morphine or fentanyl clearance.

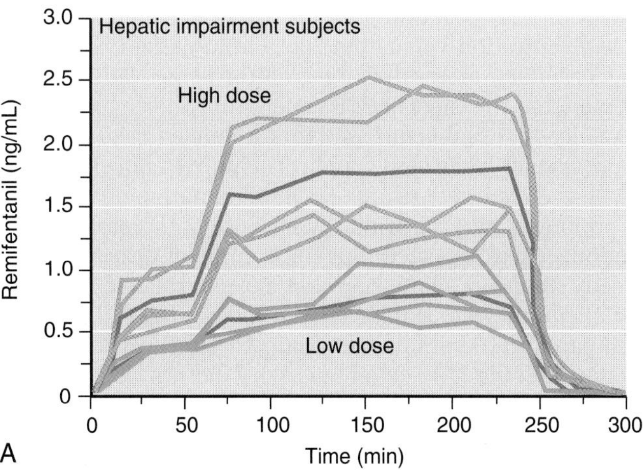

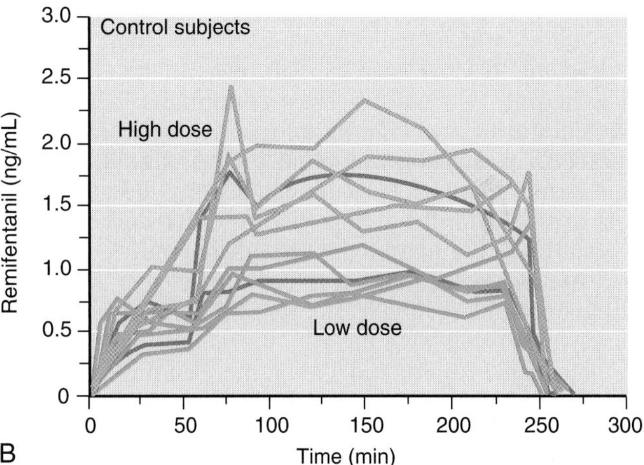

Fig. 24.25 Time-dependent changes of blood concentration of remifentanil in patients with liver disease (A) and in control subjects (B). In the low-dose group, remifentanil was infused at 0.0125 μg/kg/min for 1 hour and then 0.025 μg/kg/min for 3 hours. In the high-dose group, the infusion rate of remifentanil was 0.025 μg/kg/min for 1 hour and then 0.05 μg/kg/min for 3 hours. (From Dershwitz M, Hoke JF, Rosow CE, et al. Pharmacokinetics and pharmacodynamics of remifentanil in volunteer subjects with severe liver disease. *Anesthesiology*. 1996;84:812–820.)

Cardiopulmonary Bypass

CPB produces significant alterations in the pharmacokinetics of most opioids. These alterations are a result of CPB-induced modifications in distribution volumes (secondary to priming), changes in acid-base balance, organ blood flow, plasma protein concentrations, and body temperature. The binding of drugs to components of the bypass circuit can also alter opioid pharmacokinetics.

When morphine is given as a premedicant before cardiac anesthesia, its concentrations decline significantly on initiation of CPB. Miller et al. examined the effect of CPB on plasma fentanyl concentration and showed that total concentration of fentanyl in plasma was significantly decreased and the unbound fraction of fentanyl rose on initiation of CPB.[451] The total fentanyl concentration remained relatively stable during bypass until near the end of CPB when the mean total concentration increased, coinciding with rewarming. Population pharmacokinetic modeling applied to concentration-versus-time data from patients undergoing coronary artery bypass grafting using CPB demonstrated that the effect of CPB on fentanyl pharmacokinetics is clinically insignificant, and that a simple three-compartment model accurately predicts fentanyl concentrations throughout surgery using CPB.[452] Elimination of alfentanil is prolonged by CPB primarily because of increased distribution. It was reported that the volume of distribution in steady state (Vd_{ss}) and the volume of central compartment for alfentanil were significantly greater in the CPB groups, compared to the nonbypass group.[453] However, the elimination half-life (T1/2β) of alfentanil did not differ significantly between the normothermic CPB, hypothermic CPB, and nonbypass groups. Between the normothermic and hypothermic CPB groups no significant differences in Vd_{ss}, clearance, or T1/2β were found. The free fraction of alfentanil during CPB remains constant despite complex changes in binding protein concentrations.[454] In adult patients undergoing elective myocardial revascularization with hypothermic CPB who received continuous infusions of remifentanil 1.0 to 2.0 μg/kg/min, no evidence of accumulation or sequestration was found.[427] Russell et al. reported that normothermic CPB did not significantly affect the clearance of remifentanil, but hypothermic CPB reduced it by an average of 20%, and this was attributed to the effect of temperature on blood and tissue esterase activity.[455] In pediatric patients undergoing CPB for repair of atrial septal defect, there was no change in the Vd_{ss}, the volume of the central compartment, T1/2α, and T1/2β, but clearance values of remifentanil increased 20% in the postbypass period.[456] In patients undergoing coronary artery bypass graft surgery with hypothermic CPB receiving continuous infusion of remifentanil, the volume of distribution increased by 86% with institution of CPB and remained increased after CPB, and elimination clearance decreased by 6.37% for each degree from 37°C.[457] Thus, although clearance of remifentanil reduces during CPB, remifentanil remains a very short-acting drug even during CPB.

Acid-Base Changes

It was demonstrated that pH changes influence the protein binding of fentanyl, sufentanil, and alfentanil, resulting in an increase in protein binding with alkalosis and a decrease with acidosis. These effects are greater for fentanyl than sufentanil and sufentanil than alfentanil. Relative changes in the free-drug fraction with pH variation from 7.4 to 7.0 were much higher for fentanyl (52%) when compared with sufentanil (29%) and alfentanil (6%). The pH dependence of plasma protein binding of the opioids significantly correlates with their partition between an organic and aqueous phase, suggesting the hydrophobic character of the interaction between plasma proteins and opioids. Increased ionization decreases the amount of fentanyl available for hepatic metabolism or renal excretion. Intraoperative hyperventilation during surgical procedures can significantly influence the pharmacokinetics of sufentanil resulting in an increased distribution volume and a prolonged elimination half-time.

Thus, both intraoperative respiratory alkalosis and respiratory acidosis, especially in the immediate postoperative period, can prolong and exacerbate opioid-induced respiratory depression.

Hemorrhagic Shock

It is a common practice to administer reduced doses of opioids to patients suffering from hemorrhagic shock to minimize adverse hemodynamic consequences and to prevent prolonged opioid effect. This is at least partially attributable to a pharmacokinetic mechanism. Analysis with pigs receiving fentanyl suggested that central clearance and central- and second-compartment distribution volumes were significantly reduced in hemorrhagic shock, resulting in higher fentanyl concentrations for any given dosages and prolonged context-sensitive half-time (Fig. 24.26).[458] Hemorrhagic shock also altered pharmacokinetics of remifentanil, suggesting that less remifentanil would be required to maintain a target plasma concentration (Fig. 24.27).[459] However, because of its rapid metabolism, changes in context-sensitive half-time are small. In a stepwise hemorrhage model of pigs receiving total intravenous anesthesia with remifentanil (0.5 μg/kg/min) and propofol (6 mg/kg/h after 2 mg/kg bolus), the plasma remifentanil concentration showed a threefold greater increase than that of propofol.[460] Thus, the remifentanil dose should be reduced substantially compared with propofol during total intravenous anesthesia for patients with significant blood loss.

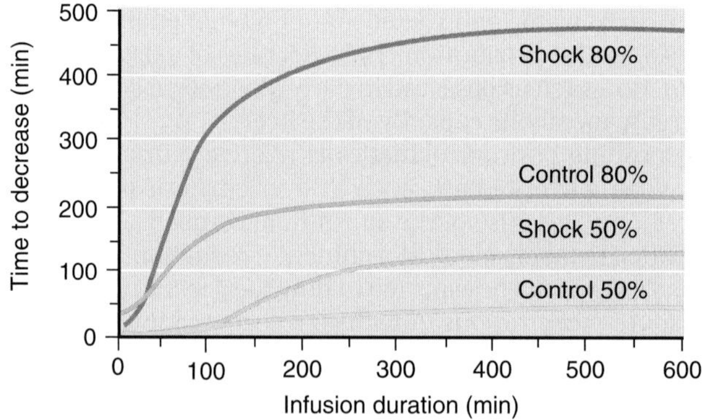

Fig. 24.26 A computer simulation of the context-sensitive half-times (50% decrement times) and 80% decrement times of fentanyl in shock versus control animals. (From Egan TD, Kuramkote S, Gong G, et al. Fentanyl pharmacokinetics in hemorrhagic shock: a porcine model. *Anesthesiology*. 1999;91:156–166.)

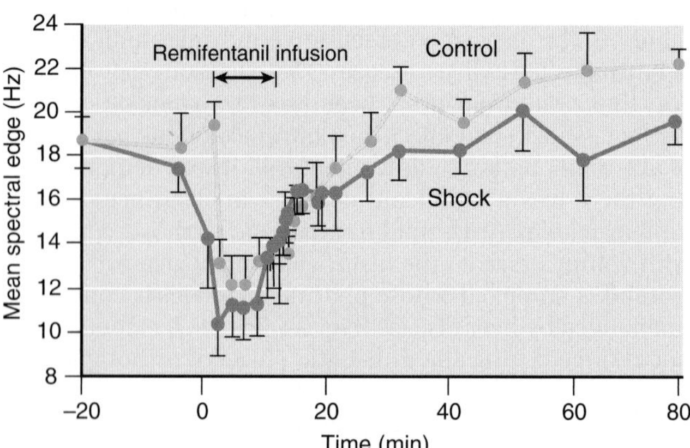

Fig. 24.27 Mean spectral edge changes versus time during remifentanil infusion. The graph indicates spectral edge measurements for control animals and for animals with hemorrhagic shock, respectively. (From Johnson KB, Kern SE, Hamber EA, et al. Influence of hemorrhagic shock on remifentanil: a pharmacokinetic and pharmacodynamic analysis. *Anesthesiology*. 2001;94:322–332.)

Genetic Variations in Opioid Metabolism

All opioid drugs are substantially metabolized mainly by cytochrome P450 (CYP) and to a lesser extent by UDP-glucuronosyltransferases (UGTs). Although CYP3A4 is involved in the metabolism of many of the opioids, it is the role of the highly polymorphic CYP2D6 that is of greater clinical interest with respect to the weaker opioids (codeine, dihydrocodeine, oxycodone, hydrocodone, and tramadol), because of the formation of their more potent hydroxyl metabolites (morphine, dihydromorphine, oxymorphone, and hydromorphone), which have about a 30-fold higher affinity for the μ-receptor. The CYP2D6 gene is highly polymorphic, with 100 allelic variants identified, and enzymatic activity of some alleles may be either significantly high or low. In the case of a variant more rapidly producing metabolites of higher affinity there exists the possibility of administering an unintended opioid overdose. This has been especially of concern for the use of codeine-containing products in pediatric populations resulting in changes in prescribing practice. Alternately, variants leading to low production of potent metabolites may result in subtherapeutic outcomes.[461] Finally, UGTs mediate mainly the formation of glucuronides from buprenorphine, codeine, dihydrocodeine, dihydromorphine, hydromorphone, morphine, naloxone, naltrexone, and oxymorphone. UGT2B7 gene is polymorphic, and less than 20 allelic variants have been identified. It is possible that differences in metabolic activity among UGT alleles affect pharmacokinetics of opioids.[461]

Anesthetic Techniques Using Opioids

ANALGESIA

Opioids are frequently used to relieve pain during monitored anesthesia care and regional anesthesia. A single bolus administration of opioids can provide significant pain relief. Morphine is slow in onset and does not allow rapid titration to effect. Meperidine (50-100 mg IV) produces variable degrees of pain relief and is not always effective in patients with severe pain. IV boluses of fentanyl (1-3 μg/kg), alfentanil (10-20 μg/kg), or sufentanil (0.1-0.3 μg/kg) can produce potent and short-lasting analgesia. Infusion rates range from 0.01 to 0.05 μg/kg/min for fentanyl, 0.0015 to 0.01 μg/kg/min for sufentanil, 0.25 to 0.75 μg/kg/min for alfentanil, and 0.05 to 0.25 μg/kg/min for remifentanil. Plasma concentrations of opioids necessary for various purposes are listed in Table 24.8.

Changes in the excitability of central neurons play an important role in establishment of pain. In rats, low doses of fentanyl block the synaptic form of central sensitization in the rat spinal cord in vivo, suggesting the possibility of preemptive analgesia by fentanyl, but higher doses do not have this effect.[462] In fact, dose escalation of fentanyl or other potent opioids may produce a hyperalgesic state—mentioned previously. Reductions in postoperative pain and improved recovery have been attributed to preemptive analgesia with either epidural fentanyl or bupivacaine after radical prostatectomy.[463] In contrast, in patients undergoing transperitoneal tumor nephrectomy, preoperative intravenous administration of a combination of morphine, ketamine, and clonidine failed to exert a clinically relevant effect on postoperative pain.[464] Aida et al. reported that the effectiveness of preemptive analgesia varies according to the type of surgery, and preemptive analgesia with epidural morphine was reliably effective in limb and breast surgeries but ineffective in abdominal surgery.[465] A meta-analysis demonstrated that the results of preemptive analgesia with systemic administration of opioids are equivocal.[466] Thus, whether or not preemptive analgesia can be effectively achieved clinically by the early administration of opioids remains uncertain and may be highly context specific.

Patient-controlled analgesia (PCA) with opioids has become a widely accepted technique in which to provide postoperative analgesia, but pharmacokinetic optimization of opioid treatment in acute pain is a complex matter. Without considering effect-site drug concentrations over time, the choice of opioid and the amount, method, and frequency of its administration cannot be optimal. Morphine and fentanyl are often used for PCA therapy, and piritramide is also frequently used for PCA in European countries. A double-blind randomized study demonstrated that effect-site target-controlled remifentanil PCA with a slow and progressive adapted algorithm is feasible in young women undergoing uterine artery embolization.[467] Combination of opioid with other drugs might be a method for improvement of PCA. For thoracic surgery, addition of ketamine to opioid for intravenous PCA was superior to intravenous PCA opioid alone, whereas the effect of added ketamine was not significant for orthopedic or abdominal surgery.[468] Despite the utility of an opioid-based PCA, critical considerations must also be made as to an individual patient's relative risk of opioid-induced respiratory depression with appropriate oversight and monitoring.

TABLE 24.8 Range of Approximate Plasma (or Whole Blood for Remifentanil) Opioid Concentration

	Fentanyl (ng/mL)	Sufentanil (ng/mL)	Alfentanil (ng/mL)	Remifentanil (ng/mL)
Predominant agent	15-30	5-10	400-800	—
Major surgery	4-10	1-3	200-400	2-4
Minor surgery	3-6	0.25-1	50-200	1-3
Spontaneous ventilation	1-3	<0.4	<200	0.3-0.6
Analgesia	1-2	0.2-0.4	50-150	0.2-0.4

From Bailey PL, Egan TD, Stanley TH. Intravenous opioid anesthetics. In: Miller RD, ed. *Anesthesia*. 8th ed. Philadelphia: Saunders; 2015. An imprint of Elsevier Inc,, p. 895.

SEDATION

Critically ill subjects in the intensive care unit (ICU) often experience anxiety and agitation while being exposed to numerous stressful or noxious stimuli. ICU patients generally require a combination of analgesia and sedation to relieve their state of anxiety, improve adaptation to the endotracheal tube, and aid compliance with mechanical ventilation. Morphine, fentanyl, and sufentanil are frequently used intravenous analgesic agents in the ICU. A randomized double-blind study indicated that remifentanil (0.15 μg/kg/min) and morphine (0.75 μg/kg/min) could provide comparable levels of sedation, and the remifentanil-based regimen allowed a more rapid emergence from sedation and facilitated earlier extubation.[469] However, use of ultrapotent opioid agents such as remifentanil may also drive tolerance development and OIH—as discussed previously.

BALANCED ANESTHESIA

Anesthesia with a single agent can often require doses that produce excessive hemodynamic depression. Alternately, "balanced anesthesia" with a balance of agents and techniques can be used to more selectively direct different components of anesthesia (i.e., analgesia, amnesia, muscle relaxation, and abolition of autonomic reflexes with maintenance of homeostasis). For example, inclusion of an opioid as a component of balanced anesthesia can reduce preoperative pain and anxiety, decrease somatic and autonomic responses to airway manipulations, improve hemodynamic stability, lower requirements for inhaled anesthetics, and provide immediate postoperative analgesia. Opioids interact synergistically and markedly reduce the dose of propofol and other sedative-hypnotics required for loss of consciousness and during noxious stimulation such as skin incision (Fig. 24.28).[470] Although the intent of combining opioids with sedative-hypnotics and/or volatile anesthetics is to produce anesthetic conditions with stable hemodynamics prior to as well as after noxious stimulation, this ideal is not always achieved.[471,472]

The timing, rate of administration, and dose of supplemental opioids should also be tailored to the specific condition of the patient and the expected duration of the operation in order to avoid problems. Giving a large dose of any opioid shortly before the end of surgery is very likely to result in postoperative respiratory depression. However, analgesic concentrations of opioids have little effect on the MAC awake of inhaled anesthetics.[473]

The ideal opioid would permit rapid titration, prevent unwanted responses to noxious stimuli, require little supplementation, not depress cardiovascular function, permit the return of adequate spontaneous ventilation in a timely manner, and produce effective postoperative analgesia with minimal side effects. Alfentanil and remifentanil provide the greatest ability to titrate opioids rapidly because of their extremely rapid time to onset (1-2 minutes) of peak effect. Sufentanil, alfentanil, and remifentanil are arguably superior to fentanyl in most respects. Antagonism of opioid action with naloxone for troublesome respiratory depression is required less frequently after alfentanil and sufentanil compared with fentanyl. Pharmacologic antagonism is not required after remifentanil administration because of its short half-life.

Fentanyl

Anesthetic induction is usually achieved by combining a loading dose of fentanyl (2-6 μg/kg) with a sedative-hypnotic, most commonly thiopental or propofol, and a muscle relaxant. Maintenance of anesthesia can be achieved with low concentrations of potent inhaled anesthetics, and additional fentanyl (intermittent boluses of 25-50 μg every 15-30 minutes or a constant infusion of 0.5-5.0 μg/kg/h).

The plasma concentration of fentanyl required for postoperative analgesia was approximately 1.5 ng/mL.[474] MAC of isoflurane at skin incision can be reduced by 50% and 63%

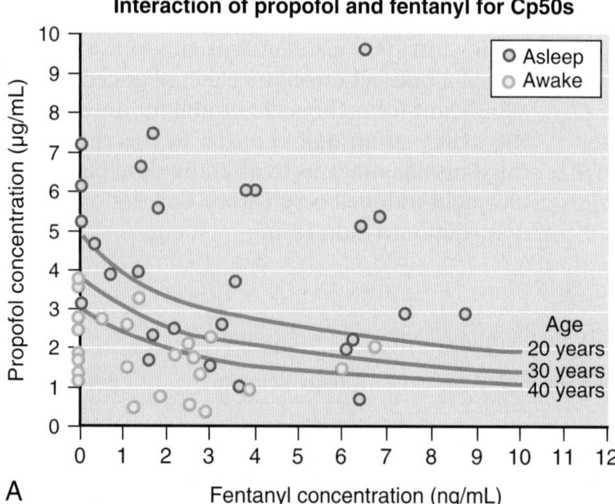

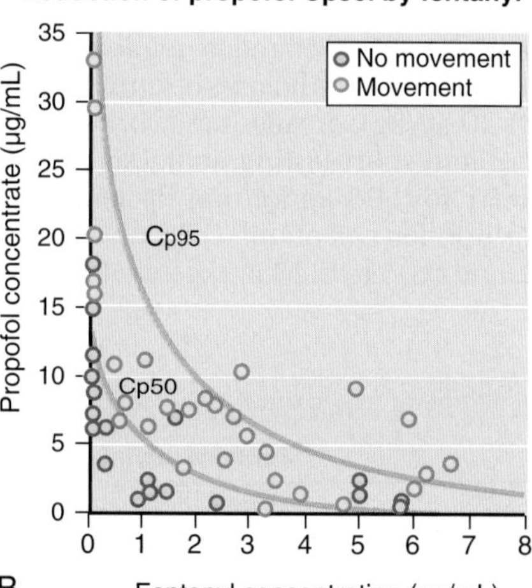

Fig. 24.28 (A) Measured arterial propofol and fentanyl concentrations at which patients did and did not respond to a verbal command at 10 minutes after the initiation of the infusion of these drugs. The *solid lines* represent the modeled concentration of propofol, according to decade of age when combined with the measured fentanyl concentrations, at which 50% of patients did not respond to verbal command (Cp50s). (B) Reduction by increasing concentration of fentanyl of propofol concentration at which 50% or 95% of patients did not move at skin incision (Cp50i and CP95i, respectively). The *solid lines* represent logistic regression solution. (From Smith C, McEwan AI, Jhaveri R, et al. The interaction of fentanyl on the Cp50 of propofol for loss of consciousness and skin incision. *Anesthesiology*. 1994;81:820–828.)

with plasma fentanyl concentrations of 1.67 and 3.0 ng/mL, respectively.[121] Increasing plasma fentanyl concentrations from 3.0 to 10 ng/mL only further reduced the MAC of isoflurane from 63% to 82%. Intraoperative requirement of propofol for hypnosis is also reduced by fentanyl. In patients undergoing spine fusion, to keep the mean arterial pressure within 15% of the control value when fentanyl was infused to keep the plasma concentration at 0, 1.5, 3.0, and 4.5 ng/mL, average propofol infusion rates were 10.1 ± 2.5 (mean ± SD), 7.5 ± 1.2, 5.7 ± 1.1, and 4.9 ± 1.2 mg/kg/h, respectively.[475]

Opioid pharmacokinetics and pharmacodynamics vary considerably among patients. It was reported that fentanyl dose based on total body weight may cause overdosing in obese patients.[474] As discussed previously, considerations for dosing based on lean body weight and/or ideal body weight may have merit in this context. Nevertheless, a balanced technique with fentanyl, titrating the opioid in anticipation of various stimuli and patient responses with pharmacokinetic guidelines in mind, will often result in a stable hemodynamic course and rapid awakening in a pain-free patient. Repeated doses or continuous infusions of fentanyl are most likely to result in significant depression of spontaneous ventilation.

Alfentanil

Because alfentanil penetrates the brain so rapidly, equilibration of alfentanil between plasma and CNS can be achieved while plasma alfentanil levels are relatively low compared with sufentanil and fentanyl. This property explains how low doses (10-30 μg/kg) of alfentanil, administered just before or simultaneously with a sedative-hypnotic, are effective.

Alfentanil (25-50 μg/kg IV), followed by small titrated sleep doses of any sedative-hyponic (e.g., 50-100 mg sodium thiopental), is usually successful in preventing significant hemodynamic stimulation from laryngoscopy and intubation. The optimum dose of alfentanil, coadministered with 2.5 mg/kg propofol, when inserting a classic laryngeal mask airway was 10 μg/kg.[476] Further opioid supplementation can be achieved with an alfentanil infusion (0.5-2.0 μg/kg/min) or intermittent boluses of alfentanil (5-10 μg/kg) for shorter procedures. In balanced anesthetic techniques in which potent inhaled anesthetics are also employed, relatively low plasma alfentanil concentrations (e.g., 29 ng/mL) can reduce the MAC of isoflurane by approximately 50%.[123] The EC50 of alfentanil during propofol anesthesia, in which plasma concentration of propofol was kept at target concentrations of 3 μg/mL, was 92 ng/mL for intubation, 55 ng/mL for skin incision, 84 ng/mL for the opening of the peritoneum, and 66 ± 38 ng/mL for the intraabdominal part of surgery.[477] It was reported that hemodynamic changes induced by propofol might have an important influence on the pharmacokinetics of alfentanil. Propofol (target concentration, 1.5 μg/mL) decreased the elimination clearance of alfentanil by 15%, rapid distribution clearance by 68%, slow distribution clearance by 51%, and lag time by 62%.[478] Alfentanil infusions or repeated doses should be minimized 15 to 30 minutes prior to the end of surgery in order to avoid problematic residual respiratory depression.

Sufentanil

CP_{50} for prevention of hemodynamic responses to laryngoscopy and tracheal intubation was 1.08 ng/mL with a range of 0.73 to 2.55 ng/mL. In combination with propofol for induction of anesthesia in children, bolus administration of sufentanil 0.3 μg/kg can completely abolish the cardiovascular response to tracheal intubation.[479] In healthy normotensive adult patients, a bolus sufentanil 0.1 μg/kg followed by a continuous infusion at 0.08 μg/kg/min for at least 5 minutes proved to be effective for blunting the cardiovascular response to intubation.[480] Maintenance of anesthesia can be achieved with sufentanil (intermittent boluses, 0.1-0.25 μg/kg, or constant infusion, 0.5-1.5 μg/kg/h). The CP_{50} for sufentanil during skin incision (2.08 ± 0.62 ng/mL) is twice as great as that for intubation in unpremedicated patients.[481] CP_{50} value ratios at skin incision for sufentanil, fentanyl, and alfentanil are approximately 1:2:150 and represent different, and probably more accurate, potency ratios than those traditionally published based on drug dose. In patients undergoing coronary artery bypass grafting, sufentanil greater than 1.25 ± 0.21 ng/mL reduced isoflurane requirements to less than 0.5% through the operation.[482]

Remifentanil

Very short duration of action of remifentanil mandates that an infusion (0.1-1.0 μg/kg/min) be started prior to or soon after a small bolus dose to ensure sustained opioid effect. Maintenance infusion rates of remifentanil range from 0.1 to 1.0 μg/kg/min for balanced anesthesia. Remifentanil can reliably suppress automatic, hemodynamic, and somatic responses to noxious stimulation and allows the most predictable and rapid trouble-free emergence from anesthesia without postoperative respiratory depression. Infusion rates of 0.1 ± 0.05 μg/kg/min should permit the return of spontaneous ventilation and responsiveness with maintenance of analgesia. A randomized, double-blind, placebo-controlled study demonstrated that combination of 0.05-0.1 μg/kg/min remifentanil and 2 mg midazolam provided effective sedation and analgesia during outpatient surgical procedures performed under local anesthesia.[483]

Associated with emergence from remifentanil anesthesia, the need for alternative analgesic therapies should be anticipated and administered in a timely fashion. Exposure to high doses of remifentanil may paradoxically reduce the pain threshold after its discontinuation, resulting in postoperative hyperalgesia, which is known to be associated with acute and persistent pain. It was reported that perioperative administration of morphine (0.15 or 0.25 mg/kg IV) or fentanyl (0.15 mg) did not provide entirely adequate immediate postoperative pain control after remifentanil-based anesthesia in major abdominal surgery.[484,485] Administration of ketamine (0.15 mg/kg followed by 2 μg/kg/min) decreased intraoperative remifentanil use during abdominal surgery and postoperative morphine consumption without increasing the incidence of side effects.[486] In children undergoing strabismus surgery, combination of sevoflurane (2.5%) and remifentanil (1 μg/kg followed by 0.1-0.2 μg/kg/min) showed less frequent postoperative vomiting but higher postoperative pain scores compared with fentanyl (2 μg/kg followed by 1 μg/kg every 45 minutes).[487]

Postoperative pain relief with low-dose remifentanil infusion was also reported. After general anesthesia with propofol (75 mg/kg/min) and remifentanil (0.5-1.0 mg/kg/min) for abdominal or thoracic surgery, continuous infusion of remifentanil (0.05 or 0.1 mg/kg/min) provided adequate analgesia.[488]

TOTAL INTRAVENOUS ANESTHESIA

Many different IV anesthetic and analgesic compounds can be employed in a number of combinations to provide TIVA. Most commonly, an opioid is combined with another drug more likely to provide hypnosis and amnesia. For example, combination of alfentanil and propofol can produce desirable TIVA. Alfentanil provides analgesia and hemodynamic stability while blunting responses to noxious stimuli. On the other hand, propofol provides hypnosis and amnesia and is antiemetic. Anesthetic induction with alfentanil (25-50 μg/kg) and propofol (0.5-1.5 mg/kg) followed by infusions of 0.5 to 1.5 μg/kg/min of alfentanil and 80 to 120 μg/kg/min of propofol will produce complete anesthesia for a variety of procedures. It is proposed that alfentanil concentrations as low as 85 ng/mL, when combined with a blood propofol concentration of 3.5 μg/mL, can produce both optimal anesthetic conditions and speed of recovery.[489] Stanski and Shafer suggested that bolus doses and initial infusion rates would be 30 μg/kg and 0.35 μg/kg/min for alfentanil and 0.7 mg/kg and 180 μg/kg/min for propofol.[490] Recognizing that these calculations were based on EC_{50} data in patients undergoing only moderately painful procedures, anesthesiologists should adjust these doses accordingly. In patients undergoing ear-nose-throat surgery, TIVA with remifentanil and propofol provided a more rapid respiratory recovery after brief surgical procedures, compared with TIVA with alfentanil and propofol.[491]

Maintenance infusions vary according to patient condition and surgical stimuli. Propofol (75-125 μg/kg/min) and alfentanil (1.0-2.0 μg/kg/min) were initially recommended. Propofol infusions should be terminated 5 to 10 minutes before anticipated patient awakening. Alfentanil infusion rates do not need to be less than 0.25 to 0.5 μg/kg/min until surgery is terminated. A multicenter evaluation demonstrated that in patients of elective inpatient surgery remifentanil 1 μg/kg IV followed by 1.0 μg/kg/min, when combined with propofol 75 μg/kg/min, effectively controlled responses to tracheal intubation.[492] Reduction of remifentanil infusion rate to 0.25-0.40 μg/kg/min after tracheal intubation was also recommended. Although midazolam-opioid combinations can also provide complete anesthesia, midazolam-alfentanil TIVA has not been found to compare favorably to propofol-alfentanil TIVA even with flumazenil reversal of benzodiazepine actions.[493]

TIVA techniques are especially useful when delivery of inhaled agents is compromised. By keeping the goals of balanced anesthesia in mind, combining modern opioids and other drugs, utilizing infusion pumps, and employing an increased understanding of pharmacokinetics, clinicians can successfully perform a variety of TIVA techniques. Approximate opioid doses and infusion rates for TIVA are listed in Table 24.9.

TABLE 24.9 Approximate Opioid Loading (Bolus) Doses, Maintenance Infusion Rates, and Additional Maintenance Doses for Total Intravenous Anesthesia

	Loading Dose (μg/kg)	Maintenance Infusion Rate	Additional Boluses
Alfentanil	25-100	0.5-2 μg/kg/min	5-10 μg/kg
Sufentanil	0.25-2	0.5-1.5 μg/kg/h	2.5-10 μg
Fentanyl	4-20	2-10 μg/kg/h	25-100 μg
Remifentanil	1-2	0.1-1.0 μg/kg/min	0.1-1.0 μg/kg

From Bailey PL, Egan TD, Stanley TH. Intravenous opioid anesthetics. In: Miller RD, ed. *Anesthesia*. 8th ed. Philadelphia: Saunders; 2015. An imprint of Elsevier Inc., p. 897.

OPIOID-BASED (HIGH-DOSE OPIOID) ANESTHESIA FOR CARDIAC SURGERY

Opioids can be administered as the primary anesthetic in opioid-based anesthetic techniques. High-dose opioid anesthesia was introduced as a stress-free anesthetic method for cardiac surgery. High-dose opioid anesthesia was first performed by the use of morphine, and fentanyl and sufentanil have been recommended later. However, several factors have diminished the popularity of high-dose opioid anesthesia, even in cardiac anesthesia. These include the lack of evidence substantiating any significant outcome benefit associated with the use of large doses of opioids, the added drug costs, and the trend toward "fast-track" approaches to the cardiac patient that can be impeded by large doses of opioids. However, opioids, particularly when administered by continuous infusion, are still among the most effective anesthetics for patients undergoing cardiac or other extensive operations.

In an attempt to decrease the costs of cardiac surgery, fast-track programs have become popular. Engoren et al. reported that the more expensive but shorter-acting opioids, sufentanil and remifentanil, produced equally rapid extubation, similar stays, and similar costs to fentanyl, indicating that any of these opioids can be recommended for fast-track cardiac surgery.[494]

Fentanyl

Many different techniques have been used to achieve anesthesia with fentanyl.[495,496] Rapid or slow bolus injections of fentanyl ranging from 5 to 75 μg/kg will establish plasma fentanyl concentrations (10-30 ng/mL) that are often sufficient to provide stable hemodynamics throughout the induction/intubation sequence. Continuous infusions of fentanyl for cardiac surgery range from 0.1 to 1.0 μg/kg/min up to or continuing through CPB. High-dose fentanyl anesthesia has also proved effective and safe for pediatric heart surgery. It was indicated that fentanyl 25 to 50 μg/kg combined with isoflurane 0.2% to 0.4% was sufficient to obtund hemodynamic and stress responses in the pre-CPB phase of open heart surgery in infants and young children (Fig. 24.29).[497] It was reported that 57 out of 59 eligible patients were successfully extubated at 34 ± 14 minutes after termination of fentanyl (total dose, 127 ± 64 μg/kg) with naloxone (total bolus, 3.4 ± 2.6 μg/kg), and recovered fully without ventilatory support under the naloxone infusion, which was terminated at 11 ± 7 hours.[498] These results suggest that naloxone infusion with individual dose titration can facilitate the use of high-dose opioid anesthesia, maintaining the advantage of this anesthesia. It was shown that high-dose fentanyl (50 μg/kg) is not associated

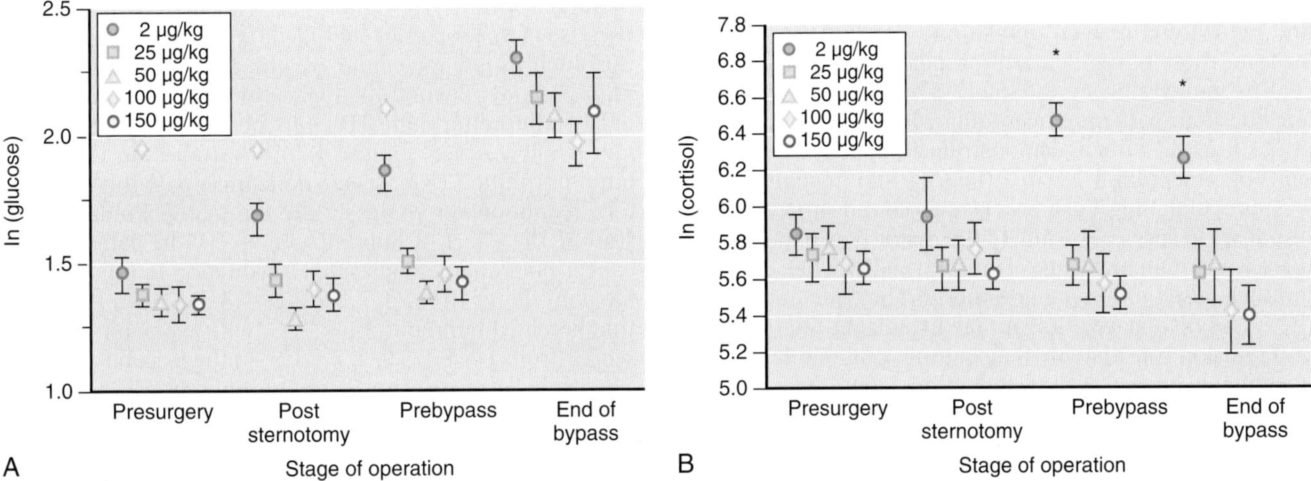

Fig. 24.29 Suppression of stress responses in the prebypass phase of open heart surgery in infants and young children by fentanyl combined with low concentration (0.2%-0.4%) of isoflurane. Mean (± SE) natural logarithm (ln) for glucose (A) or ln for cortisol (B) versus stage of surgery for each dose of fentanyl. The values for the 2 μg/kg group indicated by *asterisks* were significantly higher ($P < .01$) than in the other groups. (From Duncan HP, Cloote A, Weir PM, et al. Reducing stress responses in the pre-bypass phase of open heart surgery in infants and young children: a comparison of different fentanyl doses. *Br J Anaesth.* 2000;84:556–564.)

with a difference in the incidence of postoperative cognitive dysfunction at 3 or 12 months after coronary artery bypass surgery in the elderly, whereas low-dose fentanyl (10 μg/kg) leads to shorter postoperative ventilation times and may be associated with a greater incidence of postoperative cognitive dysfunction 1 week after surgery.[499]

Sufentanil

Advantages of high-dose sufentanil include more rapid induction, better blunting or elimination of hypertensive episodes, greater reduction in left ventricular stroke work, with higher cardiac outputs and more stable hemodynamics intraoperatively and/or postoperatively. Induction doses of sufentanil range from 2 to 20 μg/kg administered as a bolus or infused over 2 to 10 minutes. Total doses of sufentanil employed in high-dose techniques usually range from 15 to 30 μg/kg. However, no additional benefit could be demonstrated in terms of hemodynamic control or EEG signs by increasing the dose of sufentanil from 3 to 15 μg/kg for the induction of anesthesia in patients premedicated with lorazepam.[500] The amount of sufentanil required can be markedly influenced by the supplements employed concomitantly. For patients undergoing coronary artery surgery, induction (0.4 ± 0.2 μg/kg) and total maintenance (2.4 ± 0.8 μg/kg) doses of sufentanil were used in combination with propofol (1.5 ± 1 mg/kg for induction and 32 ± 12 mg/kg total). Interestingly, sufentanil requirements tripled when midazolam was employed instead of propofol.[501] Maintenance of anesthesia, utilizing infusion of sufentanil (1.0-2.0 μg/kg/h), in a balanced anesthetic technique, achieves the advantages of opioid-based anesthesia and avoids prolonged opioid action into the postoperative period.

Remifentanil

Remifentanil has been employed in cardiac anesthesia.[455] It was shown that induction with remifentanil 2 μg/kg with propofol and maintenance with remifentanil at 0.25 or 0.5 μg/kg/min provided appropriate anesthesia for

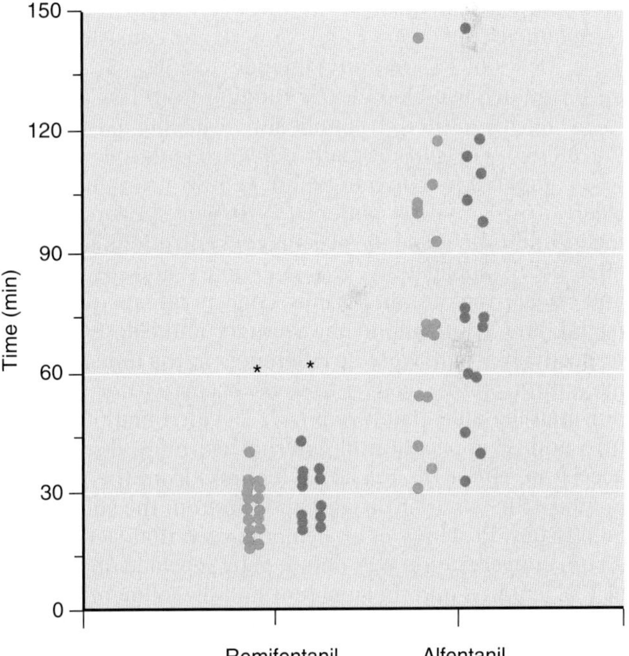

Fig. 24.30 Times to awakening *(green circles)* and tracheal extubation *(blue circles)* in patients who underwent minimally invasive direct coronary artery bypass surgery after intravenous anesthesia with remifentanil and propofol or alfentanil and propofol. (From Ahonen J, Olkkola KT, Verkkala K, et al. A comparison of remifentanil and alfentanil for use with propofol in patients undergoing minimally invasive coronary artery bypass surgery. *Anesth Analg.* 2000;90:1269–1274.)

minimally invasive coronary artery bypass surgery with rapid awakening and tracheal extubation (Fig. 24.30).[502] Kazmaier et al. compared high-dose remifentanil (2.0 μg/kg/min) and remifentanil 0.5 μg/kg/min combined with propofol (target-controlled infusion aiming at a plasma concentration of 2.0 μg/mL) in patients undergoing elective coronary artery bypass grafting.[503] It was demonstrated that high-dose remifentanil reduces stroke volume index, heart rate, mean arterial pressure, myocardial blood flow, and myocardial oxygen uptake and its effects do not differ from those of remifentanil/propofol anesthesia. Geisler et al. examined efficacy and safety of high-dose remifentanil anesthesia in patients undergoing coronary artery bypass graft surgery.[504] It was demonstrated that continuous infusions of remifentanil 1.0 to 2.0 µg/kg/min in combination with propofol 3 mg/kg/h provided profound suppression of responses to surgical stimuli in the majority of patients, but there was a high incidence of muscle rigidity when remifentanil was used to induce anesthesia. They concluded that there was no apparent advantage in starting the remifentanil infusion rate above 1.0 µg/kg/min and remifentanil is not suitable for use as a sole induction agent.

OTHER APPLICATIONS OF OPIOIDS

Transdermal Therapeutic System

Transdermal drug delivery generally requires high solubility in both water and oil, low molecular weight, high potency, and little or no skin irritation. Fentanyl is available in a transdermal therapeutic system (TTS). Potential advantages of delivering fentanyl transdermally include no first-pass drug metabolism by the liver, improved patient compliance, convenience and comfort, and consistent analgesia. Doses of TTS fentanyl include 25, 50, 75, and 100 µg/h and achieve blood levels ranging from less than 1.0 to 2.0 ng/mL, although significant variability exists. Pharmacokinetics of transdermally-delivered fentanyl (50 µg/h) was compared in 10 young adult (25-38 years) and eight elderly (64-82 years) patients.[505] It was shown that the mean half-time (time for plasma concentrations to double after patch application) was 4.2 hours and 11.1 hours and mean maximum plasma concentrations were 1.9 ng/mL and 1.5 n/mL, in the younger and elderly groups, respectively. There were no differences in the time at which maximum plasma concentrations occurred nor elimination half-life after patch removal. Elevated body temperature and/or application of external warming devices can accelerate either the release of fentanyl from the patch or increase the vascular bed distribution from the subcutaneous tissues. Portenoy et al. demonstrated that steady state serum concentration was obtained by repeated application of TTS fentanyl and the apparent half-life following system removal after repeated application was relatively long presumably due to ongoing absorption from a subcutaneous depot.[506]

Results of clinical trials utilizing TTS fentanyl for postoperative analgesia have demonstrated a high incidence of significant respiratory depression, and this application is not recommended and is contraindicated.[507] In cancer pain, TTS fentanyl offers an interesting alternative to oral morphine, and its effectiveness and tolerability in this indication has been demonstrated by a number of trials.[508] Its usefulness in chronic pain of nonmalignant origin remains to be confirmed in controlled trials just as there is a lack of evidence for the efficacy of chronic oral opioid administration in the treatment of nonmalignant pain. In general, TTS fentanyl produces the same adverse effects as other opioids, mainly sedation, nausea, vomiting, and constipation. In comparison with oral morphine, TTS fentanyl causes fewer gastrointestinal adverse events.

Buprenorphine is suitable for transdermal application because of its properties that facilitate transdermal absorption such as low molecular weight, high lipophilicity, and high potency. Beyond its application in the management of OUD, buprenorphine TDS may be effective for moderate and possibly severe cancer pain.[509] Studies on the use of buprenorphine TTS for severe noncancer pain that is refractory to nonopioid analgesia are emerging. Poulain et al. studied the effect of buprenorphine TDS in patients with cancer pain and demonstrated a reduction in mild–moderate pain scores (from 3.5 ± 2.2 to 1.5 ± 1.5) in the group that received buprenorphine TDS, with worsening of pain scores (from 1.5 ± 1.5 to 2.7 ± 1.9) in the placebo group.[510] The transdermal formulation of buprenorphine in the United States is currently available in 5 dosage strengths: 5, 7.5, 10, 15, and 20 µg/h, and the bioavailability decreases to 15% after a 7-day application.

Iontophoresis

Iontophoresis is a technique by which drug passage through the skin is augmented by an external electric current. Clinically significant doses of morphine and fentanyl can be delivered iontophoretically. The fentanyl hydrochloride iontophoretic transdermal system (fentanyl ITS) is a novel PCA system that has been approved in the USA and Europe for the management of acute, moderate-to-severe postoperative pain.[511] This system allows patients to self-administer preprogrammed doses of fentanyl noninvasively through the use of iontophoretic technology. To assess the efficacy and safety of patient-controlled ITS using fentanyl hydrochloride (40-µg infusion over 10 minutes) compared with a standard intravenous morphine PCA (1-mg bolus every 5 minutes; maximum of 10 mg/h), a prospective randomized controlled parallel-group trial was performed.[512] The results indicated that the fentanyl ITS can provide pain control equivalent to a standard morphine PCA, with a similar incidence of opioid-related adverse events. The fentanyl ITS may offer a number of clinical advantages over existing PCA modalities.[511] Its method of drug delivery avoids the risk of complications from needle-related injuries and infection, and its preprogrammed electronics eliminate the potential for manual programming errors and excessive dosing. In addition, the compact size of the system could enable greater patient mobility following surgery. The patient-controlled ITS with fentanyl has the potential to become a valuable option in the management of acute postoperative pain. Panchal and associates reported that fentanyl ITS was associated with a significantly lower incidence of analgesic gaps, which are defined as periods during which the patient does not have access to analgesia thus contributing to ineffective postoperative pain management, relative to morphine intravenous PCA.[513] Nevertheless, given potential variability in dose delivery and other factors, ITS systems may be restricted to monitored in-hospital facilities.

Transmucosal Drug Delivery

Similar to transdermal drug delivery, transmucosal delivery through the oropharynx and nasopharynx eliminates hepatic first-pass metabolism (drugs are absorbed directly into the systemic circulation) and improves patient comfort, convenience, and compliance.

Buprenorphine, a potent, synthetic morphine analogue with mixed opioid agonist-antagonist properties and a long half-time, is readily absorbed from sublingual mucosal tissues. The portion of the drug that is swallowed is almost completely metabolized by the liver, and only a small fraction can reach the systemic circulation when swallowed. Systemic bioavailability after sublingual buprenorphine is approximately 50% of that following intravenous administration. Sublingual buprenorphine (0.3 mg) was compared with transdermal buprenorphine (5, 10 and 20 μg/h) for osteoarthritis pain in the hips and/or knees and found to provide comparable analgesia.[514] Buccal buprenorphine was introduced and approved by the Food and Drug Administration in 2015 for the management of chronic pain. It is composed of flexible, water-soluble polymeric films that stick to the buccal mucosa and dissolve within a few minutes. The bioavailability of this formulation is 46%–65%, and it is useful in patients who are taking over 80 mg oral morphine sulfate equivalent per day for pain management.[515]

Initial experience with buccal morphine for postoperative analgesia had been promising. However, in female patients undergoing lower abdominal surgical procedures, buccal morphine did not significantly reduce postoperative pethidine consumption, compared with placebo, and all patients receiving buccal morphine reported a taste which reduced its acceptability.[516] Low lipid solubility of morphine makes it an unlikely candidate for effective transmucosal absorption. Opioids with high lipid solubility, such as buprenorphine, fentanyl, and methadone are more effectively absorbed sublingually than those with low lipid solubility such as morphine.

Oral transmucosal fentanyl citrate (OTFC) is a solid dosage form of fentanyl that consists of fentanyl incorporated into a sweetened lozenge on a stick. A portion of fentanyl is absorbed through the oral mucosa, and the rest is swallowed and absorbed through the gastrointestinal tract. The recommended doses range from 5 to 20 μg/kg.[517] OTFC should be administered approximately 30 minutes before surgery (or painful procedure) to obtain peak effect. Plasma concentrations after OTFC administration peak at 2.0 ± 0.5 ng/mL, 15 to 30 minutes after OTFC administration, then decline to less than 1 ng/mL an hour later.[518] Unlike transdermal fentanyl, OTFC leaves no significant depot in the mucosal tissues after it is removed. The systemic bioavailability of OTFC is 50% and reflects both buccal and gastrointestinal absorption. OTFC bioavailability is similar to that of buprenorphine (55%), but much greater than buccal morphine and other opioids with low lipid solubility. Egan et al. demonstrated that the pharmacokinetics of OTFC did not change with repeated dosing and the decline of plasma concentration was as rapid as when administered intravenously (Fig. 24.31).[519] Furthermore, Kharasch et al. reported that the pharmacokinetics of OTFC were not altered in older volunteers (67 ± 6 years), and no change in OTFC dosing in the elderly would appear necessary.[520] Peak fentanyl concentration and clinical effects after OTFC were minimally affected by hepatic/intestinal CYP3A induction by rifampicin and intestinal CYP3A inhibition by grapefruit juice, suggesting that first-pass metabolism minimally influences OTFC bioavailability.[521] Preoperative OTFC was reported to be effective for postoperative analgesia in pediatric tonsillectomy patients.[522] However, OTFC can induce perioperative emesis and respiratory depression. OTFC has also been introduced for treatment of breakthrough cancer pain.[523] OTFC may be ideally suited to treat breakthrough cancer pain because fentanyl is rapidly absorbed from OTFC and patients can easily self-administer OTFC.

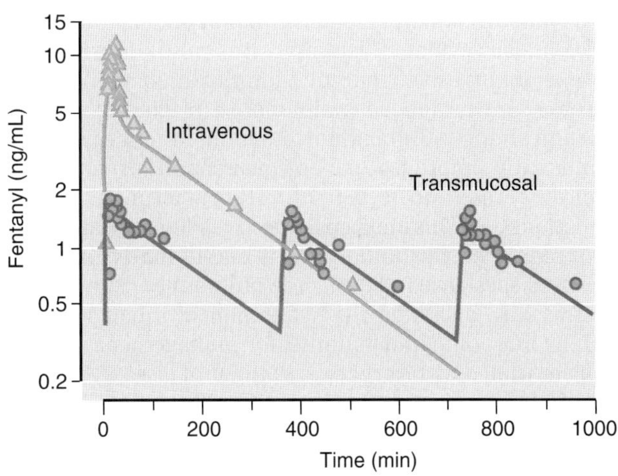

Fig. 24.31 A typical result of time-dependent change in plasma concentration of fentanyl after oral transmucosal fentanyl citrate (OTFC) application and intravenous administration. Three 800-μg doses of OTFC were administered with 6-hour intervals between doses, and fentanyl was infused at a constant rate of 50 μg/minute to a total of 15 μg/kg. (From Egan TD, Sharma A, Ashburn MA, et al. Multiple dose pharmacokinetics of oral transmucosal fentanyl citrate in healthy volunteers. *Anesthesiology*. 2000;92:665–673.)

Delivery of opioids through the nasal mucosa has also been investigated. Side effects of intranasal sufentanil in children include reduced ventilatory compliance (chest wall rigidity), hypoxemia, impaired manual ventilation, nausea, and vomiting.[524] Pharmacokinetic studies in volunteers are reported for fentanyl, alfentanil, sufentanil, butorphanol, oxycodone, and buprenorphine.[525] Mean times for achieving maximum serum concentrations vary from 5 to 50 minutes, while bioavailability varies from 46% to 71%. Fentanyl, pethidine, and butorphanol have been studied for postoperative pain. Mean onset times vary from 12 to 22 minutes and times to peak effect from 24 to 60 minutes. Transnasal butorphanol provides superior and more prolonged analgesia than similar doses given IV for postoperative pain after cesarean section. PCA with intranasal fentanyl was demonstrated to be effective for postoperative pain management.[526] There was no difference in the efficacy of intranasal fentanyl (2 μg/kg), intramuscular morphine (0.1 mg/kg), and intravenous morphine (0.1 mg/kg) in controlling postoperative pain and emergence delirium in children undergoing bilateral myringotomy and placement of ventilating tubes.[527] A novel intranasal morphine formulation composed of morphine monohydrate and chitosan, a nontoxic naturally occurring mucoadherent derived from shellfish, was shown to offer a noninvasive alternative to intravenous morphine for postoperative analgesia in patients after third molar extraction.[528] Intranasal administration of remifentanil (4 μg/kg) produces good intubating conditions in 2 to 3 minutes after induction of anesthesia with sevoflurane in children.[529]

Fentanyl (300 μg) inhalation produces low plasma drug level (0.1 ng/mL) after 15 minutes and analgesia that may be disproportionately greater than expected.[530] Inhaled liposome-encapsulated fentanyl was also demonstrated to be a noninvasive route of administration with a rapid increase and prolonged maintenance of plasma fentanyl concentration.[531] Inhalation of nebulized fentanyl citrate significantly improved patient perception of breathing, respiratory rate, and oxygen saturation in terminally ill cancer patients.[532] This inexpensive and readily available treatment may offer substantial relief of end-of-life dyspnea. The advent of specialized and efficient pulmonary drug delivery systems has facilitated the evaluation of inhaled opioids, such as morphine and fentanyl, for management of severe pain associated with surgery or malignant disease.[533] It was shown that remifentanil delivered by inhalation is rapidly absorbed, pharmacologically active, rapidly cleared, and noninjurious to respiratory tissues in rodents.[534]

The rectal mucosa is another site for transmucosal drug delivery. The bioavailability of 30-mg morphine sulfate controlled-release suppository formulation was significantly greater than that of 30-mg oral controlled-release morphine sulfate tablets, which may be the result of partial avoidance of hepatic biotransformation with rectal administration.[535] The hydrogel formulation of rectal morphine may also be useful for premedication and analgesia in pediatric patients.[536]

Oral Controlled-Release Medications

Despite the high first-pass metabolism of opioid analgesics, morphine has been formulated into an oral, sustained-release tablet (MST) and has been evaluated for premedication, postoperative analgesia, and as an analgesic for chronic cancer pain. MST provides unreliable preoperative anxiolysis and postoperative pain relief, possibly because of delayed time to onset of peak effects (3-5 hours), which can be increased by impaired gastric emptying and absorption from the small intestine. In addition, growing evidence has associated chronic use of sustained release formulation of opioids for noncancer pain to increase the risk of fatal overdose without significant benefit over other non-opioid modalities of analgesia. As an analgesic for chronic cancer pain, MST was shown to be an excellent formula.[537]

The relative analgesic potency of single doses of oral controlled-release oxycodone (20 or 40 mg) and oral controlled-release morphine (45 or 90 mg) was compared in a randomized, double-blind trial in women with moderate-to-severe pain following abdominal hysterectomy.[538] Controlled-release oxycodone at doses of 20 mg or 40 mg was comparable with controlled-release morphine at doses of 45 mg or 90 mg, respectively, for total and peak analgesic effects, indicating that oral controlled-release oxycodone was at least twice as potent as oral controlled-release morphine. A randomized, double-blind, crossover trial indicated that controlled-release oxycodone was as safe and effective as controlled-release morphine in the treatment of cancer pain.[539]

Extended-Release Epidural Morphine (DepoDur)

DepoDur is a novel drug that delivers morphine by using DepoFoam technology, a drug-delivery system composed of multivesicular lipid particles containing nonconcentric aqueous chambers that encapsulate the active drug. When the plasma morphine concentration after epidural administration of 5 mg of standard morphine was compared with those of 5 mg of DepoDur, the terminal half-life was comparable, but the peak concentration was significantly smaller and the peak systemic absorption occurs later with DepoDur. Randomized controlled studies demonstrated that 5-15 mg of DepoDur can be a potentially beneficial analgesic after elective cesarean delivery with no significant increases in adverse events for the period from 24 to 48 hours after surgery.[540,541] When compared to single-shot plain epidural morphine, DepoDur has been shown to provide a longer duration of postoperative pain control, and a decrease in the use of postoperative opioid in lower abdominal surgery,[542] total hip arthroplasty,[543] and total knee arthroplasty.[544] The adverse effect profile of DepoDur is similar to plain epidural morphine and includes nausea, vomiting, pruritus, and hypotension. It was reported that a large dose of epidural lidocaine before DepoDur administration alters the pharmacokinetics and drug effects of DepoDur.[545]

Other Opioid Agonists

CODEINE

Codeine (methylmorphine) is 6-7 fold less potent as morphine, has a high oral-parenteral potency ratio (2:3), and a plasma half-life of 2 to 3 hours. Codeine has mild to moderate analgesic but strong cough-suppressant properties after oral administration. Cytochrome P450 2D6 (CYP2D6) is the enzyme responsible for *O*-demethylation of codeine to morphine, and has genetic variants capable of rapid conversion of codeine to morphine in affected children and adults.[546] IV codeine produces profound hypotension and is neither approved nor recommended.

OXYCODONE

Although oxycodone has been widely used in pain management for more than 90 years, its pharmacokinetic properties are still poorly known. Oxycodone is extensively metabolized in humans mainly by hepatic cytochrome P450, and only 10% of oxycodone is excreted in unchanged form in urine. Rifampin, a strong inducer of several drug-metabolizing enzymes, induces cytochrome P450, reduces the plasma concentration of intravenous and oral oxycodone, and modestly attenuates pharmacologic effects of oxycodone.[547] The role of several metabolites in its analgesic activity is still not fully understood.[548] Oxycodone is a potent analgesic after systemic administration, but its analgesic potency is poor after intrathecal administration.[549] It was shown that oxycodone is more potent than morphine for visceral pain relief in intravenous patient-controlled postoperative analgesia after laparoscopic hysterectomy.[550] With respect to pharmacologic effects other than analgesic effects, it was reported that the extent and speed of onset of oxycodone-induced respiratory depression was dose-dependent and greater than an equivalent dose of morphine.[551]

MEPERIDINE (PETHIDINE)

Meperidine is predominantly a μ-opioid receptor agonist that produces pharmacologic effects similar, but not identical, to those of morphine. Meperidine sometimes causes excitation of the CNS, characterized by tremors, muscle twitches and seizures, that are largely due to accumulation of a metabolite, normeperidine. Meperidine has well-known local anesthetic properties.

Unlike morphine, after intravenous injection, first-pass uptake of meperidine by the lungs is approximately 65%. Meperidine is more highly bound to plasma proteins than is morphine, principally (70%) to α_1-acid glycoprotein. As with morphine, a relatively high hepatic extraction ratio results in biotransformation that depends on hepatic blood flow. The major metabolite normeperidine has analgesic activity and is roughly twice as potent as meperidine in producing seizures in animals. The elimination half-life of normeperidine is considerably greater than that of meperidine, and thus repeated doses can easily produce accumulation of this toxic metabolite in patients with renal disease, with the potential for inducing seizures.

Meperidine is frequently used for postoperative pain management. A comparative study demonstrated that morphine, meperidine, and tramadol resulted in equivalent pain scores in intravenous PCA after abdominal hysterectomy.[552] Meperidine is also used to relieve pain and distress in women in labor. Intravenous meperidine (50 mg) and butorphanol (1 mg) significantly reduced pain intensity 15 minutes after injection in women with moderate to severe labor pain, but the analgesia was often inadequate.[553] Meperidine can be administered as PCA in labor.[554] Meperidine (12.5 to 35 mg) is also effective for prevention and treatment of postoperative shivering.[197,555]

HYDROMORPHONE

Hydromorphone is structurally related to morphine but is approximately 5 to 10 times as potent. Because hydromorphone contains a keto-group in position 6 of the benzol ring, an active 6-glucuronate metabolite is not formed like morphine.[556] However, hydromorphone continues to represent an increased risk under conditions of renal insufficiency and failure due to a reduction in clearance and potential accumulation of hydromorphone-3-glucuronate. A bolus administration of hydromorphone reaches its peak effect in approximately 10-20 minutes, whereas an equivalent morphine bolus will require 20 minutes to reach peak. Analgesia after hydromorphone lasts 4 to 5 hours. Hydromorphone has been used for both acute and chronic pain conditions in adults and children.[557] It was reported that hydromorphone PCA provided adequate postoperative analgesia in gynecological surgery patients and there was no systematic difference between morphine and hydromorphone in opioid-related side effects.[558]

LEVORPHANOL

Levorphanol is the only available semisynthetic opioid agonist of the morphinan series with a long half-life. It is 5 times as potent as morphine with an IM/oral potency ratio of 1:2. Levorphanol may have particular utility in patients with chronic pain and who demonstrate morphine tolerance, perhaps because of differences in opioid receptor activity. Analgesia produced by levorphanol is mediated via its interactions with μ-, δ-, and κ-opioid receptors. Levorphanol is also an NMDA receptor antagonist. The long half-life of the drug increases the potential for drug accumulation.[559]

METHADONE

Methadone is a potent μ-opioid receptor agonist, with the longest half-life among the clinically used opioids. By virtue of one of methadone's isomers, it also exerts an inhibitory effect on NMDA receptors, which are implicated in the development of opioid tolerance, hyperalgesia, and chronic pain. Furthermore, methadone inhibits the reuptake of serotonin and norepinephrine, which may play a role in antinociception and mood elevation. Methadone itself is associated with less abuse potential than either morphine or heroin, and treatment with methadone has been considered to be the "gold standard" by which medication-assisted treatment (MAT) approaches are measured, as part of a comprehensive treatment program for OUD.

Methadone (IV) has an equivalent potency but longer duration of action than morphine. The plasma half-life of methadone is very long and variable (13-100 hours). Despite this property, many patients require dosing every 4 to 8 hours to maintain analgesic effects. Its major clinical applications are in the prevention of opioid withdrawal symptoms and in the treatment of chronic pain. It was shown that the same dose of IV methadone (20 mg) that is effective for postoperative pain is also suitable for the induction of anesthesia in combination with etomidate, and that methadone may have the potential for producing histamine release.[560] In patients undergoing posterior spinal fusion surgery, methadone 0.2 mg/kg at the start of surgery reduced postoperative opioid requirements, decreased pain scores, and improved patient satisfaction.[561] However, perioperative use of methadone represents a major clinical challenge, given the tremendous interpatient half-life variability which could contribute to unexpected postoperative respiratory depression.

OXYMORPHONE

Oxymorphone is a semisynthetic opioid agonist that is specific for the μ-opioid receptor and approved to treat both acute and chronic pain. Due to extensive liver metabolism, oral oxymorphone is contraindicated in patients with moderate-to-severe hepatic impairment.[562] Oxymorphone, structurally related to morphine, is almost 10 times as potent, but has a similar duration of action. It was shown that in patients with acute moderate-to-severe postsurgical pain, oral immediate-release oxymorphone 10, 20, or 30 mg provided significant dose-related pain relief compared with placebo, and this relief was maintained over several days with a safety profile comparable to that of immediate-release oxycodone.[563]

PIRITRAMIDE

Piritramide, a synthetic opioid structurally related to meperidine acting on the μ-opioid receptor, is often used for postoperative analgesia in several Eupropean[564] countries. Lack of hemodynamic effects and less side effects reported in early work made piritramide more suitable for postoperative pain control compared with other potent opioids.

Its relative analgesic potency compared with morphine is approximately 0.7. Intramuscular bolus injections of 7.5 to 15 mg were considered to be adequate for approximately 4 to 6 hours.[564] Pharmacokinetic analysis showed that piritramide is distributed extensively and eliminated slowly, and recommended for intermittent bolus administration.[565] A randomized controlled trial showed that intravenous PCA with piritramide can produce pain management as satisfactory as oral oxycodone after cesarean section.[566] It was also demonstrated that piritramide is at least as effective and as well tolerated as morphine for postoperative analgesia via a PCA system after hysterectomy.[567]

TRAMADOL

Tramadol is a prodrug that is metabolized by CYP2D6 and CYP3A4 to its more potent opioid analgesic metabolites, particularly the *O*-demethylation product M1. There is a significant variability in the efficiency and amount of CYP2D6 enzymes among individuals. Therefore, the large phenotypic variation affects the speed of metabolism and the rate of accumulation or elimination of tramadol.[568]

The action of tramadol to induce analgesia represents the combination of two predominant mechanisms, reuptake inhibition of the noradrenergic serotonergic system and activation of the μ-opioid receptor and to a lesser extent the δ- and κ-opioid receptors.[569] It was suggested that tramadol may also have a direct serotonin-releasing action.[570] Given the analgesic effect of tramadol is only partially reversed by naloxone, its serotonergic and noradrenergic effects likely represent its predominant analgesic action.

Tramadol is onefifth to onetenth as potent as morphine. In rats, tramadol could reduce MAC of isoflurane in a naloxone-sensitive manner.[571] It was shown that intravenously administered tramadol was effective for postthoracotomy pain relief.[572] Analgesic doses of tramadol may produce less respiratory depression in part because of its non-opioid receptor–mediated actions, and have minimal effects on gastrointestinal motor function.[573] Nevertheless, tramadol used as a sole drug cannot be considered the drug of choice after moderately severe painful surgery. The doses needed to relieve pain in 80% of patients are much larger than the usual dose of 50 to 100 mg.[574]

Tramadol added to lidocaine for intravenous regional anesthesia provided a shorter onset time of sensory block.[575] Tramadol added to 1.5% mepivacaine for brachial plexus block enhances the duration of analgesia in a dose-dependent manner with acceptable side effects.[576] Intraarticular tramadol was also used for management and prevention of pain after arthroscopic knee surgery. It was shown that the intraarticular admixture of tramadol 100 mg with 0.25% bupivacaine provides a pronounced prolongation of analgesia compared with either drug alone in patients undergoing arthroscopic knee surgery.[577]

Tramadol has dose- and time-dependent bactericidal activity against *Escherichia coli* and *Staphylococcus epidermidis*, as well as antibacterial activity against *Staphylococcus aureus* and *Pseudomonas aeruginosa*. The antibacterial properties of tramadol might be useful for reduction of bacterial infection after regional anesthesia.[578]

Coadministration of tramadol with proserotonergic medications can result in a hyperserotonergic state, serotonin syndrome, which can be subacute or chronic, and range from mild to severe. In mild cases, patients are afebrile and may report symptoms of diarrhea, tremor, tachycardia, shivering, diaphoresis, or mydriasis.[579] In severe cases, neuromuscular hyperactivity, autonomic hyperactivity, altered mental state, gastrointestinal symptoms, and even death have been reported. Serotonergic medications that can interact with tramadol include selective serotonin reuptake inhibitors, serotonin-norepinephrine reuptake inhibitors, tricyclic antidepressants, triptans (e.g., sumatriptan), antipsychotics, anticonvulsants, antiparkinsonian agents, cough and cold medications containing dextromethorphan, herbal products containing St. John's wort, and medications that inhibit the metabolism of serotonin, such as monoamine oxidase inhibitors. Because symptoms of serotonergic and norepinephrine withdrawal are possible upon abrupt cessation of tramadol, gradual tapering or symptomatic support are necessary when tramadol administration is stopped.[568]

MORPHINE-6-GLUCURONIDE

Morphine-6-glucuronide (M6G) is a potent metabolite of morphine. In contrast to morphine, M6G is not metabolized but excreted via the kidneys and exhibits enterohepatic cycling, as it is a substrate for multidrug resistance transporter proteins in the liver and intestines.[580] M6G exhibits a delay in its analgesic effect (blood–effect-site equilibration half-life 4-8 hours), which is partly related to slow passage through the blood-brain barrier and distribution within the brain compartment. M6G can be used as an analgesic in humans. Osborne et al. reported that 0.5 to 4 mg IV of M6G was effective for cancer pain for 2 to 24 hours without nausea and vomiting.[581] M6G 100 μg and 125 μg given intrathecally provided excellent analgesia after total hip replacement, as did intrathecal morphine sulfate 500 μg.[582] In a randomized double-blind study it was shown that M6G has an analgesic effect similar to that of morphine over the first 24 hours postoperatively. However, initial onset of M6G effect may be slower than morphine.[583] M6G has also paradoxically been observed to increase pain sensitivity in mice and humans. The pronociceptive effect of M6G can be shown in knockout mice lacking μ-, κ-, and δ-opioid receptors, and might be due to activation of the NMDA receptors.[584]

Agonist-Antagonist Opioid Compounds

Nalorphine, the first agonist-antagonist opioid, was successfully synthesized by Weijland and Erickson in 1942 and was found to be strongly antagonistic to almost all the properties of morphine. Although nalorphine was found to possess strong analgesic actions, it was unsuitable for clinical uses because of its psychotomimetic effects. Nalorphine was used in lower doses as an opioid antagonist.

Agonist-antagonist opioids are usually produced by alkylation of the piperidine nitrogen and addition of a three-carbon side chain such as a propyl, allyl, or methyl allyl to morphine. Buprenorphine is a partial agonist at the μ-receptor and an antagonist at the κ-receptor.

The other compounds are μ-antagonists and full or partial agonists at the κ-receptors. Agonist-antagonist opioids are less prone (but not immune) to abuse because they have analgesic ceiling effects, cause less euphoria, and are associated with less drug-seeking behavior and physical dependence.

Dosing data of these compounds are shown in Table 24.10. The agonist-antagonists compounds depress respiration similarly as morphine, but ceiling effects exist (Table 24.11). Effects on the cardiovascular system differ among these compounds (Table 24.12).

TABLE 24.10 Dosing Data for Agonist-Antagonist Opioids and Morphine

	Equianalgesic IM Dose (mg)	Duration of Analgesia (h)	Oral: IM Efficacy Ratio
Morphine	10	4-5	1:6
Buprenorphine	0.3-0.4	>6	1:2*
Butorphanol	2	3-4	—
Nalbuphine	10	3-6	1:4-5
Pentazocine	40	3	1:3

*Sublingual:IM ratio.
IM, Intramuscular.

TABLE 24.11 Respiratory Depressant Effects of Agonist-Antagonists Compared With Morphine*

Drug	Correlation of Respiratory Depression with Dose
Morphine	Increases proportionally with dose
Buprenorphine	Ceiling effect at 0.15-1.2 mg in adults
Butorphanol	Ceiling effect at 30-60 μg/kg
Nalbuphine	Ceiling effect at 30 mg in adults
Pentazocine	Ceiling effect suggested, but difficult to study because of psychotomimetic effects

*Low or moderate naloxone doses readily reverse the respiratory depressant effects produced by therapeutic doses of all drugs listed, except buprenorphine.
From Zola EM, McLeod DC. Comparative effects and analgesic efficacy of the agonist-antagonist opioids. *Drug Intell Clin Pharm*. 1983;17:411.

TABLE 24.12 Hemodynamic Effects of Agonist-Antagonist Compounds Compared With Morphine

Drug	Cardiac Workload	Blood Pressure	Heart Rate	Pulmonary Artery Pressure
Morphine	↓	↓	=↓	=↓
Buprenorphine	↓	↓	↓	?
Butorphanol	↑	=↑	=	↑
Nalbuphine	↓	=	=↓	=
Pentazocine	↑	↑	↑	↑

From Zola EM, McLeod DC. Comparative effects of analgesic efficacy of the agonist-antagonist opioids. *Drug Intell Clin Pharm*. 1983;17:411.

PENTAZOCINE

Analgesia produced by pentazocine is primarily related to κ-receptor stimulation. Pentazocine is onehalf to onefourth as potent as morphine. Ceilings to both analgesia and respiratory depression occur after 30 to 70 mg of pentazocine. Although the potential for abuse is less than with morphine, prolonged use of pentazocine can lead to physical dependence. Nalorphine-like dysphoric side effects are common, especially after high doses (>60 mg) of pentazocine in the elderly. The dysphoric effects of pentazocine can be reversed with naloxone. Pentazocine depresses myocardial contractility and increases arterial blood pressure, heart rate, systemic vascular resistance, pulmonary artery pressure, and left ventricular work index. Pentazocine also increases blood catecholamine levels. Pentazocine inhibits gastric emptying and gastrointestinal transit in rats, whereas U50488H, a pure κ-agonist, did not significantly inhibit either.[585] Therefore, it might be speculated that pentazocine affects gastrointestinal function through a mechanism other than the opioid receptors.

Pentazocine has been shown to be an effective treatment for pruritus after cesarean delivery under spinal anesthesia with opioids, the incidence of which is ranging from 50% to 100%. A single 15-mg dose of IV pentazocine after delivery was shown to reduce both the incidence and severity of pruritus in women who have received subarachnoid opioids during cesarean delivery.[586] Pentazocine has limited application, because it is associated with a high incidence of PONV, it provides limited analgesia, it partially antagonizes other opioids, and it can produce undesirable cardiovascular and psychotomimetic effects.

BUTORPHANOL

Butorphanol is an agonist at κ-receptors. Its activity at μ-receptors is either antagonistic or partially agonistic. It is 5 to 8 times as potent as morphine and is only available in parenteral form. After IM injection, onset of effect is rapid, and peak analgesia occurs within 1 hour. Whereas duration of action of butorphanol is similar to that of morphine, its plasma half-life is only 2 to 3 hours. Although butorphanol (10 mg IM) causes as much respiratory depression as the same dose of morphine, higher doses reach a ceiling. Side effects after butorphanol include drowsiness, sweating, nausea, and CNS stimulation. In healthy volunteers, butorphanol (0.03 or 0.06 mg/kg IV) produces no or minimal cardiovascular changes. However, in patients with cardiac disease, butorphanol causes significant increases in cardiac index, left ventricular end-diastolic pressure, and pulmonary artery pressure.

Because butorphanol decreases the MAC for enflurane by only a small fraction, it cannot serve like the fentanyl congeners as an anesthetic agent. Butorphanol is subject to less abuse and has less addictive potential than morphine or fentanyl. Acute biliary spasm can occur after butorphanol, but increases in biliary pressure are less than after equipotent doses of fentanyl or morphine. Transnasal butorphanol is effective in relieving migraine and postoperative pain.[587]

BUPRENORPHINE

Buprenorphine is a thebaine derivative, μ-receptor partial agonist, and similar in structure to morphine but approximately 33 times more potent. Whereas fentanyl dissociates rapidly from μ-receptors (half-life of 6.8 minutes), buprenorphine has a higher affinity and takes much longer (half-life of 166 minutes) to dissociate. Onset of action of buprenorphine is slow, its peak effect may not occur until 3 hours, and duration of effect is prolonged (<10 hours). Volume of distribution of buprenorphine is 2.8 L/kg and its clearance is 20 mL/kg/min. Plasma concentrations of the metabolites of buprenorphine, norbuprenorphine, buprenorphine-3-glucuronide, and norbuprenorphine-3-glucuronide may approximate or exceed those of the parent drug. Both glucuronide metabolites are biologically active and may contribute to the overall pharmacology of buprenorphine.[588]

Subjective effects (e.g., euphoria) of buprenorphine are similar to morphine. Buprenorphine produces depression of minute ventilation which leveled off at doses higher than 3.0 μg/kg to about 50% of baseline, in contrast to the case of fentanyl, in which dose-dependent respiratory depression results in apnea at doses higher than 2.9 μg/kg (Fig. 24.32).[589] Buprenorphine has been successfully used for premedication (0.3 mg IM), as the analgesic component in balanced anesthesia (4.5-12 μg/kg), and for postoperative pain control (0.3 mg IM). Buprenorphine, like the other agonist-antagonist compounds, is not acceptable as a sole anesthetic, and its receptor kinetic profile restricts its usefulness if other μ-agonists are used. Opioid withdrawal symptoms develop slowly (5-10 days) after buprenorphine is discontinued following long-term use.

A sublingual combination tablet composed of buprenorphine and naloxone in a fixed 4:1 ratio may provide pain relief in patients with chronic pain with OUD. However, the unique pharmacological profile of buprenorphine/naloxone confers it to be a weak analgesic relative to full μ-receptor agonists. Studies investigating the efficacy of buprenorphine/naloxone or buprenorphine alone for the management of non-malignant pain are ongoing. Possible mechanisms of pain relief by buprenorphine/naloxone therapy in opioid-dependent patients with chronic pain may include reversal of opioid-induced hyperalgesia and improvement in opioid tolerance and OUD.[590]

Acute administration of κ-opioid receptor agonists and antagonists has been shown to produce effects characterized as prodepressive or antidepressant, respectively, in rodent behavioral tests, encouraging further investigation of κ-opioid receptor antagonists as potential antidepressant treatments in humans.[591] In a preliminary clinical study, low doses of buprenorphine, which possess κ-receptor antagonist activity, produced impressive alleviation of depressive symptoms in patients that were considered treatment-resistant within 1 week of initiating administration.[592]

NALBUPHINE

Nalbuphine is an agonist-antagonist opioid that is structurally related to oxymorphone and naloxone, and binds to μ-receptors as well as to κ- and δ-receptors. Nalbuphine acts as an antagonist at the μ-receptor and an agonist at the κ-receptor. Activation of supraspinal and spinal κ-receptors results in limited analgesia, respiratory depression, and sedation. Nalbuphine, like other agonist-antagonist compounds, interferes with the analgesia produced by pure μ-agonists. In rats, coadministration of nalbuphine with morphine dose-dependently blocked the development of morphine tolerance and dependence, without attenuation of antinociceptive effect of morphine.[593] Nalbuphine is only available for parenteral use. Onset of effects is rapid (5-10 minutes), and duration is long (3-6 hours) because of a long plasma elimination half-life (5 hours).

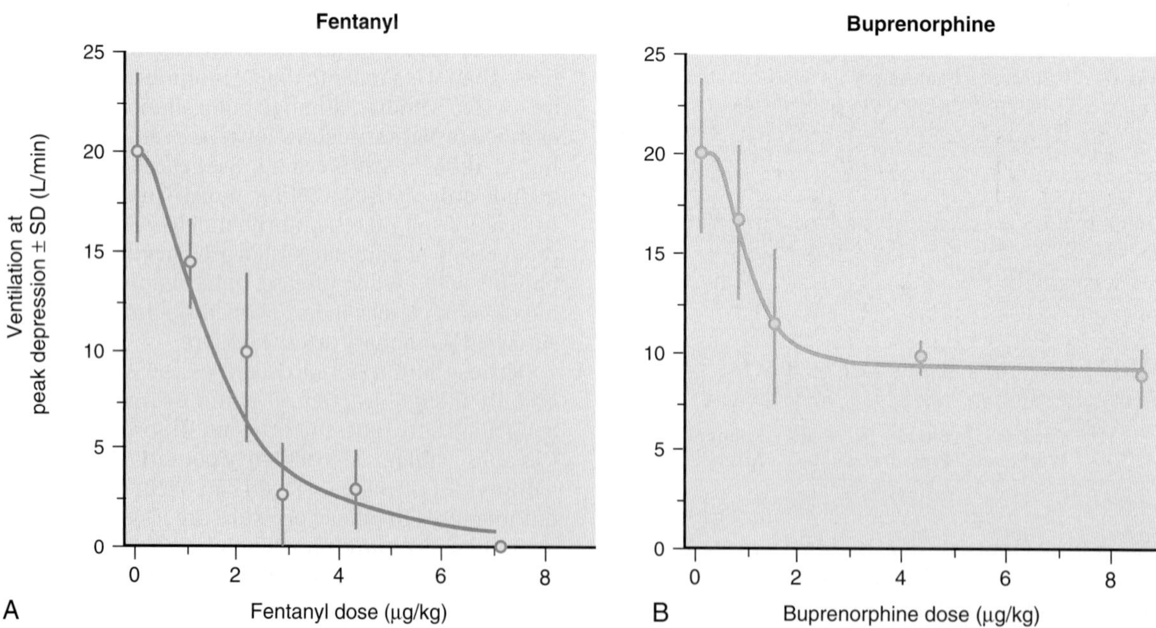

Fig. 24.32 Dose–response relationships for reduction of minute ventilation induced by fentanyl (A) and buprenorphine (B). The response is the peak ventilatory depression at each dose. The *line through the data* is the fit to the Hill equation. Placebo is 0 μg/kg. Data are mean ± standard deviation. (From Dahan A, Yassen A, Bijl H, et al. Comparison of the respiratory effects of intravenous buprenorphine and fentanyl in humans and rats. *Br J Anaesth.* 2005;94:825–834.)

Nalbuphine has been administered as an analgesic supplement for conscious sedation or balanced anesthesia, and as an analgesic for postoperative and chronic pain problems. In patients undergoing myocardial revascularization, continuous infusion of nalbuphine (0.05-0.1 mg/kg/min) and fentanyl (0.15-0.3 μg/kg/min) was compared.[594] It was shown that nalbuphine lacks the ability to attenuate cardiovascular and hormonal responses to tracheal intubation and surgical procedures, and was concluded that continuous infusion of nalbuphine cannot be recommended for anesthesia in patients undergoing myocardial revascularization. For postoperative patient-controlled epidural analgesia, the combination of hydromorphone 0.075 mg/mL and nalbuphine 0.04 mg/mL resulted in lower incidence of nausea and decreased need of bladder catheterization compared with hydromorphone alone.[595] A randomized double-blind controlled study in patients undergoing gynecological operations demonstrated that interaction between morphine and nalbuphine in intravenous PCA admixture is additive, and combination of the two drugs can decrease the incidence of pruritus.[596]

A prospective randomized double-blinded study demonstrated that nalbuphine (4 mg IV) was as effective as ondansetron (4-8 mg IV) for prevention of intrathecal morphine-induced pruritus after cesarean delivery.[597] Some reports showed that nalbuphine provides a rapid and potent antishivering effect similarly as meperidine.[598] However, a quantitative systematic review of randomized controlled trials did not support the conclusion.[197]

DEZOCINE

Dezocine is slightly more potent and acts faster than morphine, with a similar duration. Although no longer used clinically in Western countries, dezocine is gaining popularity in China as an alternative medication for perioperative pain management. A pharmacologic study showed the unique molecular pharmacologic profile of dezocine as a partial μ-receptor agonist, a κ-receptor antagonist, and a norepinephrine and serotonin reuptake inhibitor (*via* norepinephrine transporter and serotonin transporter).[368] Although dezocine was shown to be an effective alternative to fentanyl when administered during outpatient laparoscopy with propofol and N_2O, dezocine was associated with a high incidence of postoperative nausea and a delayed discharge time.[599] In adult patients who had arthroscopic surgery under general anesthesia, dezocine (5 mg IV) and morphine (5 mg IV) were similarly effective for postoperative analgesia and showed similar side effects.[600] A recent report showed that intravenous dezocine 0.1 mg/kg can effectively suppress cough induced by 5 μg/kg fentanyl.[601]

MEPTAZINOL

Meptazinol has been reported to cause minimal respiratory depression because of its selectivity for μ_1-receptors. In patients receiving meptazinol (2.5 mg/kg) with a barbiturate, no cardiovascular changes were observed at tracheal intubation, whereas blood pressure and heart rate were significantly increased in patients receiving fentanyl (5 μg/kg).[602] Side effects (nausea and vomiting) limit its use to relieve severe pain.

Opioid Antagonists

NALOXONE

Clinically, opioid antagonists are used to restore spontaneous ventilation in patients who breathe inadequately after opioid overdoses or opioid anesthesia. In addition, opioid antagonists can reduce or reverse opioid-induced nausea and vomiting, pruritus, urinary retention, rigidity, and biliary spasm associated with numerous therapies employing opioids, such as neuraxial analgesic techniques. It was reported that the potency ratio for naloxone:nalbuphine for antagonism of pruritic effects of epidural morphine was approximately 40:1.[603]

Morphine requirements were significantly less in patients receiving naloxone, suggesting that naloxone enhanced analgesia.[604] Proposed possible mechanisms for this apparent paradoxic effect of naloxone include enhanced release of endogenous opioids and opioid receptor upregulation.

Although naloxone is generally considered to be a pure opioid receptor antagonist, it delays gastric emptying of saline or milk, as does morphine in the rat.[360] Furthermore, high-dose naloxone possesses partial agonistic activity on the μ- and κ-opioid receptors in the cultured cells.[605]

Reversal of Respiratory Depression by Naloxone

In the early 1950s, nalorphine and levallorphan were evaluated as opioid antagonists. They were often found unacceptable because of a high incidence of side effects, as well as incomplete reversal. Naloxone was introduced into clinical practice in the late 1960s. There have been reports of side effects (increases in heart rate and blood pressure) and more serious complications (e.g., pulmonary edema). Initial naloxone dose recommendations ranged from 0.4 to 0.8 mg. Onset of action of IV naloxone is rapid (1-2 minutes), and half-life and duration of effect are short, approximately 30 to 60 minutes. If IV access is not available, naloxone, in doses similar to those given IV, is effectively absorbed after intratracheal administration. Reversal with naloxone is limited by high affinity for and slow dissociation from the μ-opioid receptor of buprenorphine, and depends on the buprenorphine dose and the correct naloxone dose window (Fig. 24.33).[606] Because respiratory depression from buprenorphine may outlast the effects of naloxone boluses or short infusions, a continuous infusion of naloxone may be required to maintain reversal of respiratory depression.[606]

Several mechanisms produce increases in arterial blood pressure, heart rate, and other significant hemodynamic alterations after naloxone reversal of opioids. These include pain, rapid awakening, and sympathetic activation not necessarily due to pain. When patients receiving naloxone for opioid agonist reversal are hypothermic due to intraoperative heat loss, O_2 consumption and minute ventilation can increase two- to threefold.[607] Such metabolic demands also stress the cardiovascular system, increasing cardiac output. In addition, greater degrees of hypercapnia at the time of opioid antagonism will result in greater degrees of cardiovascular stimulation because of associated sympathetic stimulation. Opioid reversal may be particularly hazardous in patients with pheochromocytoma or chromaffin tissue tumors. However, it was also reported that

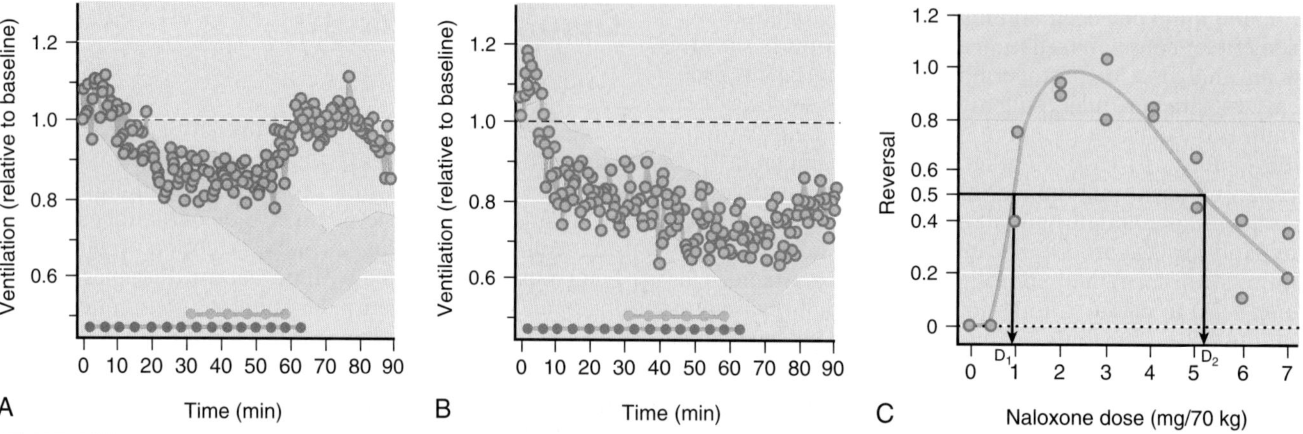

Fig. 24.33 Reversal of buprenorphine-induced respiratory depression with naloxone depends on the correct naloxone dose window. Respiratory depression induced by 0.2 mg buprenorphine was reversed by naloxone 2 mg (A) and 6 mg (B) given over 30 minutes in one subject. Gray field in the background is the result of the placebo group in which saline was infused instead of naloxone. Light gray dots and dark gray dots represent buprenorphine and naloxone infusion, respectively. (C) Influence of 0 (placebo) and 0.5-7 mg naloxone on 0.2 mg intravenous buprenorphine-induced respiratory depression. Reversal was calculated from the naloxone-induced change in ventilation, and it ranges from 0 (effect not different from placebo) to 1 (reversal to predrug baseline level). (From van Dorp E, Yassen A, Sarton E, et al. Naloxone reversal of buprenorphine-induced respiratory depression. *Anesthesiology*. 2006;105:51–57.)

IV administration of 10 mg naloxone did not significantly change plasma catecholamine concentration and blood pressure in pheochromocytoma patients.[608]

Recurrence of respiratory depression after naloxone is due to the short half-life of naloxone. "Renarcotization" occurs more frequently after the use of naloxone to reverse longer-acting opioids such as morphine. This is commonly not seen in clinical practice because opioid concentrations are often just above the threshold for respiratory depression, and treatment with a single or just a few effective bolus doses of naloxone is sufficient to reverse the respiratory depression induced by most opioids for the short time that the agonist concentration exceeds the respiratory depression threshold.[251] Short-acting opioids such as alfentanil rarely pose a danger of renarcotization, because of a rapid plasma decay curve and weak opioid receptor binding compared with fentanyl and sufentanil. Naloxone, although active at μ-, δ-, and κ-receptors, has greatest affinity for μ-receptors, which mediate most potent opioid effects, including respiratory depression and analgesia. Careful titration of naloxone often can restore adequate spontaneous ventilation without reversal of adequate analgesia.

Other Applications of Naloxone

Low-dose naloxone not only has been shown to block the development of acute opioid tolerance but also to ameliorate undesired opioid-induced side effects. Naloxone infusion 0.25 μg/kg/h prevented the acute opioid tolerance induced by a large dose of remifentanil at 0.30 μg/kg/min, provided a quicker recovery of bowel function, and reduced the length of hospital stay after open colorectal surgery.[609]

Reversal of effects of alcohol, barbiturates, and benzodiazepines by naloxone has been reported. However, it was also reported that naloxone potentiates anxiolytic-like action of benzodiazepines and barbiturates in the rat.[610] It is not advisable to try to reverse the effects of overdose of benzodiazepines and barbiturates by naloxone. Although it was suggested that the μ-opioid receptor is involved in the antinociceptive action of ketamine in mice,[74] naloxone did not affect the action of ketamine on secondary hyperalgesia induced by burn injury in humans.[611]

Evidence indicates that endogenous opioid peptides participate in the control of cardiovascular regulation during hemorrhagic shock. In patients with documented septic shock and resistance to a one-liter fluid challenge, administration of naloxone by initial bolus of 0.03 mg/kg followed by infusion at a rate of 0.2 mg/kg/h significantly increased mean arterial pressure, but did not affect survival.[612] This effect may be due to centrally mediated increases in sympathetic tone and decreases in parasympathetic output and/or antagonism of endogenous opioids. However, the clinical usefulness of naloxone to treat shock remains to be determined and additional randomized clinical trials are needed to assess its usefulness.[613]

One study indicated that opioids can elicit excitatory as well as inhibitory modulation of the action potentials of sensory neurons, and ultra-low doses of naloxone could selectively block the excitatory effect of opioids.[614] A prospective randomized double-blind study demonstrated that addition of an ultra-low dose of naloxone (100 ng) to 34 mL of 1.5% lidocaine solution with or without fentanyl in axillary brachial plexus block prolongs the time to first postoperative pain and motor blockade but also lengthens the onset time.[615]

It has been reported that naloxone may ameliorate the neurologic deficit following an ischemic or traumatic neurologic insult in animals.[616] In humans, a randomized controlled trial demonstrated that naloxone (a bolus of 5.4 mg/kg, followed by infusion at 4.0 mg/kg/h for 23 hours) does not improve neurologic recovery after acute spinal cord injury.[617] However, it was reported that combined use of cerebrospinal fluid drainage and naloxone reduces the risk of paraplegia in thoracoabdominal aneurysm repair.[618] Naloxone may also have a therapeutic role in heat stroke disorders[619] and cholestasis-induced pruritus.[620] Although intravenous naloxone has been claimed to produce pain relief in opioid-resistant central post-stroke pain, a double-blind trial concluded that intravenous naloxone was of no value in alleviating central post-stroke pain.[621]

NALTREXONE

Naltrexone is a μ-, δ-, and κ-opioid receptor antagonist. It is longer acting than naloxone (plasma half-life of 8-12 vs. 0.5-1.5 hours), and it is active when taken orally. A double-blind, placebo-controlled study for patients undergoing cesarean section indicated that naltrexone (6 mg) was an effective oral prophylactic against the pruritus and vomiting associated with intrathecal morphine, but was associated with shorter duration of analgesia.[622]

As a prescribed treatment for opioid dependence, extended-release naltrexone hydrochloride was compared directly with opioid medication treatment, which includes daily buprenorphine hydrochloride with naloxone hydrochloride. It was shown that extended-release naltrexone, administered 380 mg as monthly intramuscular injections, was as effective as buprenorphine-naloxone in maintaining short-term abstinence from heroin and other illicit substances and should be considered as a treatment option for opioid-dependent individuals.[343] Importantly, naltrexone induction requires individuals to be completely off opioids due to the likelihood of severe opioid withdrawal.

NALMEFENE

Nalmefene has a greater preference for μ- than δ- or κ-receptors. Nalmefene is equipotent to naloxone. Nalmefene is long-acting after oral (0.5-3.0 mg/kg) and parenteral (0.2-2.0 mg/kg) administration. Bioavailability after oral administration is 40% to 50%, and peak plasma concentrations are reached in 1 to 2 hours. The mean terminal elimination half-life of nalmefene is 8.5 hours, compared with 1 hour for naloxone. Prophylactic administration of nalmefene significantly decreased the need for antiemetics and antipruritic medications in patients receiving intravenous PCA with morphine.[623]

METHYLNALTREXONE

Methylnaltrexone is the first quaternary ammonium opioid receptor antagonist that does not cross the blood-brain barrier.[352] It can reverse adverse effects of opioid medications mediated by peripheral opioid receptors, while the opioid effects mediated by opioid receptors in the central nervous system, such as analgesia, are not affected. Delayed gastric emptying induced by 0.09 mg/kg morphine could be attenuated by 0.3 mg/kg methylnaltrexone in healthy volunteers.[359] Methylnaltrexone has been shown to be effective for management of opioid-induced constipation. It was reported that subcutaneous methylnaltrexone (0.15 mg/kg) rapidly induced laxation in patients who had received opioids for 2 or more weeks and who had received stable doses of opioids and laxatives for 3 or more days without relief of opioid-induced constipation.[624] It was also reported that methylnaltrexone (12 mg once daily) did not affect opioid-mediated analgesia in patients with chronic noncancer pain suffering from opioid-induced constipation who received more than 50 mg of oral morphine equivalents daily.[625] Because methylnaltrexone does not cross the dura, it might have potential to reverse peripherally mediated side effects of epidural opioids.[626] Randomized double-blind placebo-controlled studies have shown effectiveness of methylnaltrexone and alvimopan, another peripherally acting opioid receptor antagonist, in management of postoperative ileus, a transient cessation of coordinate bowel function after surgery.[352]

NALOXEGOL

Methylnaltrexone is restricted by the need for subcutaneous administration and is approved only for treatment of opioid-induced constipation in patients with advanced medical illness. Naloxegol, an oral peripherally acting μ-opioid antagonist, is a pegylated derivative of naloxone. Pegylation confers substrate properties for P-glycoprotein transporter and thus limits the ability of naloxegol to cross the blood–brain barrier. A double-blind study in outpatients with noncancer pain and opioid-induced constipation demonstrated that a daily dose of 12.5 mg or 25 mg naloxegol improved bowel movement, as compared with placebo, without changing pain scores and daily opioid dose.[627]

Drug Interactions With Opioids

GENERAL PRINCIPLES

Opioids are frequently combined with other anesthetic agents to produce optimal anesthetic conditions. Many drugs concomitantly administered for anesthesia can interact each other. Although some of these interactions are intentionally sought, others are unwanted and adverse. There are three general types of mechanisms of drug interactions—pharmaceutical, pharmacokinetic, and pharmacodynamic.[628]

Pharmaceutical interactions are chemical in nature, as illustrated when an alkaline solution of thiopental and an acidic solution of nondepolarizing muscle relaxants precipitate when simultaneously administered via IV.

Pharmacokinetic interactions occur when the administration of one agent alters the pharmacokinetics or disposition of another. Hemodynamic changes induced by one agent can affect pharmacokinetic behavior of the other agent. Sufentanil, which has a greater hepatic extraction ratio than alfentanil, is more likely to be affected by decreases in hepatic blood flow. Cimetidine can prolong opioid effects by decreasing hepatic blood flow and/or diminishing hepatic metabolism. Opioid plasma levels also increase in the presence of propofol.[629] Decreased opioid metabolism, by the CYP 3A4 isoform of the cytochrome P-450 enzyme responsible for the oxidative metabolism of more than 50 drugs, may also underlie pharmacokinetic interactions. A wide range of chemical compounds, including many drugs, can interact with the cytochrome P-450 system, causing either an increased activity (enzyme induction) or enzyme inhibition (Box 24.5).[628] Alfentanil, but not sufentanil, may have its action prolonged as a result of impaired metabolism in patients receiving erythromycin.[630,631]

Pharmacodynamic interaction between opioids and inhaled anesthetics were assessed with classic MAC reduction evaluations in animals and humans. Although marked synergism between opioids and inhaled anesthetics occurs with analgesic doses of opioids, there is a ceiling effect to MAC reduction by opioids. The pharmacodynamic

BOX 24.5 Drugs That Inhibit or Induce Cytochrome P-450 Enzymes

Inhibitors

- Antibiotics
  - Macrolides
  - Troleandomycin
  - Erythromycin
  - Fluoroquinolones
  - Isoniazid
- Azole antifungal drugs
  - Ketoconazole
  - Itraconazole
- Calcium entry blockers
  - Diltiazem
  - Verapamil
- Omeprazole
- Cimetidine
- Propofol
- Grapefruit juice

Inducers

- Barbiturates
- Antiepileptics
  - Carbamazepine
  - Phenytoin
  - Primidone
- Rifampicin
- Dichloralphenazone
- Ethanol
- Tobacco smoke

From Bovill JG. Adverse drug interactions in anesthesia. *J Clin Anesth.* 1997;9(Supp):3S.

synergism between opioids and sedative-hypnotics such as propofol is profound. Choosing an opioid with a short context-sensitive half-life allows greater doses of that opioid to be administered, along with reduced doses of propofol, without compromising the time for recovery from anesthesia. Thus, the optimal plasma level of propofol is estimated to be approximately 30% less when it is combined with remifentanil instead of alfentanil.[629]

Drug dosing regimens and plasma concentration of opioid and sedative-hypnotics to provide optimal hemodynamic control during a range of noxious stimuli are necessary. However, complicating our understanding of drug interactions is the observation that the same degree of interaction does not apply across different types of stimuli.

SEDATIVE-HYPNOTICS

Benzodiazepines

Alfentanil was found to reduce the midazolam ED50 value for the induction of anesthesia in a dose-dependent fashion. On the contrary, concerning the antinociceptive effect, interaction between these two types of drugs may be less than additive.[632] Midazolam enhanced opioid-induced antinociception at the spinal level but inhibited it at the supraspinal level.[633] Many studies reveal benzodiazepine-opioid interactions for many properties other than analgesia to be synergistic (supra-additive). Both the cardiovascular and respiratory actions of opioids can be significantly altered by the concomitant administration of benzodiazepines.[634] In anesthetized rabbits, fentanyl and midazolam synergistically caused depression of phrenic nerve activity.[635] Combinations of benzodiazepines and opioids, although occasionally preserving ventricular function, can cause significant and occasionally profound decreases in blood pressure, cardiac index, heart rates, and systemic vascular resistances. Fluid loading may attenuate circulatory depression that occurs when benzodiazepines and opioids are combined.

Barbiturates

Barbiturates can potentiate or produce hypotension if a large dose is administered with opioids. Hypotension after barbiturate-opioid combination is due to venodilatation, decreased cardiac filling, myocardial depression, and decreased sympathetic nervous system activity. Reducing induction doses of barbiturates administered concomitantly with opioids is recommended.

Propofol

Administration of propofol-opioid combinations provides unconsciousness and block responses to noxious stimuli. However, when given as an intravenous bolus for induction of anesthesia, propofol can create moderate to severe preintubation hypotension. Propofol-fentanyl and propofol-sufentanil anesthesia for coronary artery bypass surgery may provide acceptable conditions, but mean arterial pressure can decrease to levels that may jeopardize coronary perfusion, especially during the induction of anesthesia. In healthy volunteers, addition of alfentanil (effect-site concentration of 50 or 100 ng/mL) did not affect the changes in the BIS induced by propofol, but blocked BIS increase induced by painful stimuli.[636] In patients undergoing spine fusion, infusion of fentanyl (blood levels at 1.5-4.5 ng/mL) reduced the infusion rate of propofol necessary to keep mean arterial pressure, but delayed spontaneous eye opening and recovery of orientation.[475] In patients undergoing ambulatory gynecologic laparoscopy, administration of fentanyl (25-50 μg IV) at the time of anesthetic induction reduced maintenance propofol requirement, but failed to provide effective postoperative analgesia and increased the need of postoperative use of antiemetics.[637] Pharmacokinetic interaction as well as pharmacodynamic interaction between propofol and opioids has been reported. Target-controlled infusion of alfentanil (target concentration, 80 ng/ml) was shown to increase blood propofol concentration by 17%, and decrease the elimination clearance, the distribution clearance, and the peripheral volume of distribution of propofol.[638]

Etomidate

Etomidate can be combined in low doses with opioids with little loss of cardiovascular stability. In patients scheduled for coronary artery bypass grafting, etomidate (0.25 mg/kg) plus fentanyl (6 μg/kg) resulted in less hypotension after induction and intubation than propofol (1 mg/kg) plus fentanyl (6 μg/kg).[639]

Ketamine

Many studies on combinations of opioids and ketamine, an NMDA receptor antagonist, have been reported to optimize analgesic therapy to a variety of painful conditions. OIH and subsequent opioid tolerance can be prevented by ketamine in rats, suggesting the usefulness of combination of ketamine and opioids for postoperative analgesia. A pharmacologic study suggested that endogenous opioids and μ- and δ-opioid receptors are also involved in ketamine-induced central antinociception but the κ-opioid receptor is not involved in this effect.[640]

In the acute perioperative setting, results vary depending on the clinical context. Combination of ketamine (2.5 or 10 mg IV) and alfentanil (0.25 or 1 mg IV) provided no advantage over a larger dose of either drug alone in relieving pain caused by intradermal capsaicin injection in healthy volunteers.[641] Furthermore, combination of ketamine 1 mg/mL and morphine 1 mg/mL for PCA did not provide benefit to patients undergoing major abdominal surgery.[642] In contrast, Lauretti et al. reported that oral ketamine and transdermal nitroglycerine effectively reduced daily consumption of oral morphine in patients with cancer pain.[643] A prospective randomized double-blind controlled study demonstrated that intraoperative and postoperative administration of ketamine for the first 48 hours after surgery (2 μg/kg/min after a 0.5 mg/kg bolus) improved postoperative analgesia with a significant decrease of morphine consumption.[644] Furthermore, it was reported that a small dose of ketamine and memantine, a long-acting oral NMDA receptor antagonist, was effective in managing intractable pain in an opioid-tolerant patient.[645] Webb et al. reported that small-dose ketamine could be a useful addition to perioperative tramadol administration in patients undergoing abdominal surgery.[646]

INHALED ANESTHETICS

Volatile anesthetics are frequently combined with opioids in order to ensure amnesia and to promote immobility and hemodynamic stability. Clinical trials of opioids supplemented with volatile anesthetics for cardiac surgery demonstrate well-preserved cardiac output and minimal decreases in mean arterial blood pressure.[647] Myocardial ischemia may not, however, always be ameliorated by approaches that combine opioids with potent inhaled agents in spite of apparent "good" hemodynamic control. Some of the potent inhaled anesthetics can increase sympathetic nervous system activity and may increase the risk of myocardial ischemia in the cardiac patient.[648] Prior administration of fentanyl, in doses as low as 1.5 μg/kg, can markedly attenuate such responses. Alfentanil (10 μg/kg) is also effective in attenuating these effects.

MUSCLE RELAXANTS

Pancuronium bromide has been frequently used for muscle relaxation during high-dose opioid anesthesia. The vagolytic action of pancuronium can attenuate opioid-induced bradycardia and support blood pressure. In patients undergoing coronary artery bypass grafting administered with sufentanil (3-8 μg/kg), pancuronium (120 μg/kg) caused significant increase in mean arterial pressure, heart rate, and cardiac output but did not induce myocardial ischemia.[649] Pancuronium-induced tachycardia was easily and rapidly treated and caused no differences in ischemia or perioperative myocardial infarction. Many factors alter the impact of pancuronium and other muscle relaxants on hemodynamics when combined with opioids: the dose, timing, and rate of administration of each relaxant as well as the premedication, intravascular volume, left ventricular function, and presence of other drugs with autonomic nervous system actions.

Combinations of vecuronium and high doses of opioids may produce negative chronotropic and inotropic effects resulting in decreases in heart rate, cardiac output, and blood pressure, and increases in the need for vasopressor support. In patients scheduled for coronary artery surgery administered with 40 μg/kg sufentanil in combination with vecuronium (0.1 mg/kg), heart rate, mean arterial pressure, and systemic vascular resistance decreased from baseline values after tracheal intubation with neither significant change in cardiac output nor evidence of new myocardial ischemia.[650]

In patients anesthetized with fentanyl 50 μg/kg and scheduled to undergo elective coronary artery bypass grafting, rocuronium 0.6 mg/kg (approximately equivalent to 2 × ED_{95} dose) was associated with changes of only small magnitude in hemodynamic variables, including increases in stroke volume index (+15%) and cardiac index (+11%), and a decrease in pulmonary capillary wedge pressure (−25%).[651] In patients undergoing coronary artery bypass surgery under fentanyl anesthesia, mivacurium 0.15 or 0.2 mg/kg produced decreases in mean arterial pressure and systemic vascular resistance index possibly mediated by histamine release, whereas atracurium (0.5 mg/kg) produced no significant hemodynamic changes.[652]

MONOAMINE OXIDASE INHIBITORS

MAOI can underlie the most serious and potentially fatal drug interaction with opioids. Combination of meperidine and MAOI can induce the serotonin syndrome which is caused by excess serotonin availability in the CNS at the 5-HT_{1A} receptor and characterized by confusion, fever, shivering, diaphoresis, ataxia, hyperreflexia, myoclonus, or diarrhea. The phenylpiperidine series opioids, including meperidine, tramadol, and methadone, appear to be weak serotonin reuptake inhibitors and have all been involved in serotonin toxicity reactions with MAOIs, whereas morphine, codeine, oxycodone, and buprenorphine are known not to be serotonin reuptake inhibitors, and do not precipitate serotonin toxicity with MAOIs.[653] Alfentanil and remifentanil could be used with MAOIs without complications.[654,655]

CALCIUM CHANNEL BLOCKERS

Because opioids can inhibit voltage-dependent Ca^{2+} channel activity through the activation of G proteins, it may be possible that opioid action is potentiated by Ca^{2+} channel blockers. Numerous animal studies and a few clinical studies have documented that opioid-induced analgesia is potentiated by L-type Ca^{2+} channel blockers. However, there is also a report that L-type Ca^{2+} channel blockers do not potentiate morphine analgesia at clinically relevant doses.[656] N-type Ca^{2+} channels are involved in the release of neurotransmitters from sensory neurons in the spinal cord. It was reported that intrathecal administration of a blocker of this channel, ω-conotoxin GVIA, produced antinociception, and interacts synergistically with opioids at the spinal cord level.[657]

MAGNESIUM

Magnesium has been shown to have antinociceptive effects probably due to its antagonistic action on the NMDA receptor. Intravenous administration of magnesium sulfate 50 mg/kg preoperatively and 8 mg/kg/h intraoperatively significantly reduced intra- and postoperative fentanyl requirement.[658] However, passage of magnesium across the blood-brain barrier is limited. Intrathecal administration of fentanyl 25 μg plus magnesium sulfate 50 mg provided significantly prolonged analgesia compared with fentanyl alone, in patients requesting analgesia for labor.[659] It is likely that magnesium can potentiate opioid analgesia by both central and peripheral mechanisms.[660] A randomized, double-blind, prospective study showed that a relatively high dose of remifentanil (0.2 μg/kg/min) enhances periincisional hyperalgesia in patients undergoing thyroidectomy, and intraoperative magnesium sulfate (30 mg/kg at induction followed by 10 mg/kg/h) can prevent remifentanil-induced hyperalgesia.[226]

NONSTEROIDAL ANTIINFLAMMATORY DRUGS

NSAIDs such as ibuprofen, diclofenac, or ketorolac have been perioperatively administered to reduce opioid requirement. It was reported that perioperative administration of diclofenac (75 mg twice daily) reduced morphine consumption and the incidence of adverse effects such as sedation and nausea after total abdominal hysterectomy.[661] In a randomized double-blind trial, 0.1 mg/kg morphine was shown to be superior to 30 mg ketorolac as postoperative pain relief, but adding ketorolac to morphine reduces postoperative opioid requirement and opioid-related side effects in the early postoperative period.[662] Through the reduction of opioid requirements, NSAIDs are thought to help prevent opioid-induced hyperalgesia and/or the development of acute opioid tolerance although direct NSAID-dependent mechanisms are under investigation. A randomized double-blind placebo-controlled study has shown that 8 mg of lornoxicam prevented increase in postoperative morphine consumption induced by intraoperative fentanyl in female patients undergoing abdominal hysterectomy with spinal anesthesia.[663]

ACETAMINOPHEN

Acetaminophen has central analgesic and antipyretic effects that share similarity to those of NSAIDs, but has weak peripheral antiinflammatory action. Acetaminophen has been shown to have significant fentanyl-sparing effects and to reduce side effects when combined with fentanyl in intravenous parent- or nurse-controlled analgesia for postoperative pediatric pain management.[664] On the other hand, a randomized, placebo-controlled, double-blind study in children who received standard propofol-remifentanil anesthesia undergoing spine surgery showed that intravenously administered acetaminophen 90 mg/kg/day did improve analgesia, but did not diminish oxycodone consumption during 24 hours.[665]

GABAPENTINOIDS

Gabapentinoids, such as gabapentin and pregabalin, structural analogs of γ-aminobutyric acid, bind to the $\alpha_2\delta$ subunit of spinal voltage-gated calcium channel, and produce antihyperalgesic effects in neuropathic and other painful conditions. It was suggested that both pharmacodynamic and pharmacokinetic interaction between morphine and gabapentin leads to increased analgesic effects.[666] Furthermore, intrathecal administration of gabapentin was shown to prevent the development of opioid tolerance induced by repeated intrathecal injection of morphine.[667] It might be possible that systemic and intrathecal application of gabapentin prevents the development of OIH.[668] Preoperative administration of pregabalin is proposed as a promising way of enhancing postoperative pain control. A randomized, triple-blinded, placebo-controlled study demonstrated that preoperative administration of 300 mg pregabalin in patients undergoing transperitoneal nephrectomy reduces postoperative opioid consumption and decreases the area of mechanical hyperalgesia.[669]

ANTIDEPRESSANTS

Antidepressants are widely used to treat various chronic inflammatory and neuropathic pain conditions. Results in clinical studies were not consistent with respect to interactions between opioids and antidepressants. An isobolographic analysis demonstrated that systemic amitriptyline and morphine synergistically inhibit cutaneous orofacial inflammatory pain in rats.[670] Tricyclic antidepressants may cause respiratory depression in patients with chronic obstructive pulmonary diseases, and reduced CO_2 sensitivity has also been reported in patients receiving tricyclic antidepressants. An animal study demonstrated that pretreatment with amitriptyline increases morphine-induced hypercarbia through pharmacodynamic processes, suggesting that morphine doses should be reduced with careful titration, if patients are receiving concomitant treatment with tricyclic antidepressants.[671] It was demonstrated that perioperative administration of duloxetine, a potent selective serotonin and norepinephrine reuptake inhibitor, can reduce morphine requirement after knee replacement surgery.[672]

DIPHENHYDRAMINE

Diphenhydramine, a histamine H_1 receptor antagonist, is used as a sedative, an antipruritic, and an antiemetic agent. When administered alone, it modestly stimulates ventilation by augmenting the interaction of hypoxic and hypercarbic ventilatory drives. It was shown that diphenhydramine counteracts the alfentanil-induced decrease in the slope of the ventilatory response to CO_2.[673]

LOCAL ANESTHETICS

Systemic administration of local anesthetics can significantly reduce pain and perioperative systemic lidocaine can significantly reduce opioid requirements.[674] Curiously, previous evidence suggests that opioid-tolerant patients are less responsive to local anesthetics for postoperative pain management. In a study examining the effect of systemic morphine (seven daily subcutaneous injections of morphine 10 mg/kg) on the potency of lidocaine-induced block of the compound action potential in isolated rat sciatic nerves, it was shown that lidocaine potency was decreased due to the intrinsic changes in the peripheral nerve, and the loss of lidocaine potency remained 35 days after the last morphine injection.[675] Because there may be a decrease in potency of local anesthetics even in patients on moderate doses of opioids, additional study is necessary to better guide the perioperative use of systemic lidocaine.

Complete references available online at expertconsult.com.

References

1. Gutstein HB. Akil H. In: Hardman JG, Limbird LE, eds. *Goodman and Gilman's the Pharmacological Basis of Therapeutics*. 10th ed. New York: McGraw-Hill; 2001:569.
2. Minami M, Satoh M. *Neurosci Res*. 1995;23:121.
3. Reinscheid RK, et al. *Science*. 1995;270:792.
4. Meunier JC, et al. *Nature*. 1995;377:532.
5. Reuben SS, et al. *Anesth Analg*. 2002;94:55, table of contents.
6. Manglik A, et al. *Nature*. 2012;485:321.
7. Huang W, et al. *Nature*. 2015;524:315.
8. Kourrich S, et al. *Trends Neurosci*. 2012;35:762.
9. Dietis N, et al. *Br J Anaesth*. 2011;107:8.
10. Pasternak GW, et al. *Pharmacol Rev*. 2013;65:1257.
11. Pasternak GW. *Clin J Pain*. 2010;26(suppl 10):S3.
12. Lu Z, et al. *J Clin Invest*. 2015;125:2626.
13. Gomes I, et al. *Annu Rev Pharmacol Toxicol*. 2016;56:403.
14. Daniels DJ, et al. *Proc Natl Acad Sci*. 2005;102:19208.
15. Scherrer G, et al. *Cell*. 2009;137:1148.
16. Woolf CJ. *Cell*. 2009;137:987.
17. Lotsch J, et al. *Trends Mol Med*. 2005;11:82.
18. Klepstad P, et al. *Acta Anaesthesiol Scand*. 2004;48:1232.
19. Romberg RR, et al. *Anesthesiology*. 2005;102:522.
20. Chou WY, et al. *Anesthesiology*. 2006;105:334.
21. Hwang IC, et al. *Anesthesiol*. 2014;121:825.
22. Haerian BS, et al. *Pharmacogenomics*. 2013;14:813.
23. Kroslak T, et al. *J Neurochem*. 2007;103:77.
24. Mague SD, et al. *Proc Natl Acad Sci*. 2009;106:10847.
25. Zhang Y, et al. *J Biol Chem*. 2005;280:32618.
26. Knapman A, et al. *Br J Pharmacol*. 2015;172:2258.
27. Rakvag TT, et al. *Mol Pain*. 2008;4:64.
28. Candiotti KA, et al. *Anesth Analg*. 2014;119:1194.
29. Kolesnikov Y, et al. *Anesth Analg*. 2011;112:448.
30. De Gregori M, et al. *J Pain*. 2016;17:628.
31. Mogil JS, Pasternak GW. *Pharmacol Rev*. 2001;53:381.
32. Nothacker HP, et al. *Proc Natl Acad Sci U S A*. 1996;93:8677.
33. Zadina JE, et al. *Nature*. 1997;386:499.
34. Wang CL, et al. *Anesth Analg*. 2017;125:2123.
35. Chen L, et al. *Neuroscience*. 2015;286:151.
36. Avidor Reiss T, et al. *J Biol Chem*. 1996;271:21309.
37. Fukuda K, et al. *J Neurochem*. 1996;67:1309.
38. Shoda T, et al. *Anesthesiology*. 2001;95:983.
39. Mestek A, et al. *J Neurosci*. 1995;15:2396.
40. Pei G, et al. *Mol Pharmacol*. 1995;48:173.
41. Hales TG. *Br J Anaesth*. 2011;107:653.
42. Bull FA, et al. *Anesthesiology*. 2017;127:878.
43. Bohn LM, et al. *Science*. 1999;286:2495.
44. Trapaidze N, et al. *J Biol Chem*. 1996;271:29279.
45. Gaudriault G, et al. *J Biol Chem*. 1997;272:2880.
46. Keith DE, et al. *J Biol Chem*. 1996;271:19021.
47. Haberstock-Debic H, et al. *J Neurosci*. 2005;25:7847.
48. Hashimoto T, et al. *Anesthesiology*. 2006;105:574.
49. Raehal KM, et al. *J Pharmacol Exp Ther*. 2005;314:1195.
50. Manglik A, et al. *Nature*. 2016;537:185.
51. Hill R, et al. *Br J Pharmacol*. 2018;175:2653.
52. Soergel DG, et al. *Pain*. 2014;155:1829.
53. Fields HL, et al. *Annu Rev Neurosci*. 1991;14:219.
54. Petrovic P, et al. *Science*. 2002;295:1737.
55. Wager TD, et al. *Science*. 2004;303:1162.
56. Mansour A, et al. *Trends Neurosci*. 1995;18:22.
57. Dogrul A, Seyrek M. *Br J Pharmacol*. 2006;149:498.
58. Matthies BK, Franklin KB. *Pain*. 1992;51:199.
59. Manning BH, et al. *Neuroscience*. 1994;63:289.
60. Manning BH, Mayer DJ. *Pain*. 1995;63:141.
61. Pan ZZ, et al. *Nature*. 1997;389:382.
62. Kimura M, et al. *Anesthesiology*. 2014;121:362.
63. Stein T, et al. *Anesth Analg*. 2016;123:238.
64. Trafton JA, et al. *J Neurosci*. 1999;19:9642.
65. Stein C. *N Engl J Med*. 1995;332:1685.
66. Desroches J, et al. *Neuroscience*. 2014;261:23.
67. Zhang R, et al. *Anesthesiology*. 2014;120:482.
68. Taguchi R, et al. *Brain Res*. 2010;1355:97.
69. Kim HY, et al. *Pain*. 2009;145:332.
70. Becerra L, et al. *Anesth Analg*. 2006;103:208, table of contents.
71. Kieffer BL. *Trends Pharmacol Sci*. 1999;20:19.
72. Sora I, et al. *Proc Natl Acad Sci U S A*. 1997;94:1544.
73. Dahan A, et al. *Anesthesiology*. 2001;94:824.
74. Sarton E, et al. *Anesth Analg*. 2001;93:1495, table of contents.
75. Zhu Y, et al. *Neuron*. 1999;24:243.
76. Simonin F, et al. *EMBO J*. 1998;17:886.
77. Koyama T, et al. *Br J Anaesth*. 2009;103:744.
78. Fukagawa H, et al. *Br J Anaesth*. 2014;113:1032.
79. Rubinstein M, et al. *Proc Natl Acad Sci U S A*. 1996;93:3995.
80. Konig M, et al. *Nature*. 1996;383:535.
81. Hung CF, et al. *Br J Anaesth*. 1998;81:925.
82. Leffler A, et al. *Anesthesiology*. 2012;116:1335.
83. Brau ME, et al. *Anesthesiology*. 2000;92:147.
84. Wagner 2nd LE, et al. *Anesthesiology*. 1999;91:1481.
85. Takada K, et al. *Anesthesiology*. 2002;96:1420.
86. Yamakura T, et al. *Anesthesiology*. 1999;91:1053.
87. Davis AM, Inturrisi CE. *J Pharmacol Exp Ther*. 1999;289:1048.
88. Hahnenkamp K, et al. *Anesthesiology*. 2004;100:1531.
89. Guntz E, et al. *Anesthesiology*. 2005;102:1235.
90. Wittmann M, et al. *Anesth Analg*. 2006;103:747.
91. Wittmann M, et al. *Anesth Analg*. 2008;107:107.
92. Marincsak R, et al. *Anesth Analg*. 2008;106:1890.
93. Minami K, et al. *Arch Pharmacol*. 2015;388:999.
94. Nishi M, et al. *EMBO J*. 1997;16:1858.
95. Koster A, et al. *Proc Natl Acad Sci U S A*. 1999;96:10444.
96. Yamamoto T, Sakashita Y. *Anesth Analg*. 1999;89:1203.
97. Grisel JE, et al. *Neuroreport*. 1996;7:2125.
98. Pan Z, et al. *Neuron*. 2000;26:515.
99. Witkin JM, et al. *Pharmacol Ther*. 2014;141:283.
100. Ko MC, et al. *Neuropsychopharmacology*. 2009;34:2088.
101. Linz K, et al. *J Pharmacol Exp Ther*. 2014;349:535.
102. Dahan A, et al. *Anesthesiology*. 2017;126:697.
103. Williams JP, et al. *Anesth Analg*. 2007;105:998, table of contents.
104. Jadad AR, et al. *Lancet*. 1992;339:1367.
105. Angst MS, et al. *Anesthesiology*. 2012;117:22.
106. Angst MS, et al. *Pain*. 2012;153:1397.
107. Kest B, et al. *Anesthesiology*. 2000;93:539.
108. Sarton E, et al. *Anesthesiology*. 2000;93:1245; discussion, p 6A.
109. Olofsen E, et al. *Anesthesiology*. 2005;103:130.
110. Sato H, et al. *Mol Pain*. 2013;9:20.
111. Gourlay GK, et al. *Pain*. 1995;61:375.
112. Debon R, et al. *Anesthesiology*. 2004;101:978.
113. Scavone BM, et al. *Anesth Analg*. 2010;111:986.
114. Gupta A, et al. *Anesth Analg*. 2001;93:761.
115. Kapral S, et al. *Anesth Analg*. 1999;88:853.
116. Bouaziz H, et al. *Anesth Analg*. 2000;90:383.
117. Osman NI, et al. *Anesthesiology*. 2005;103:779.
118. Streisand JB, et al. *Anesthesiology*. 1993;78:629.
119. Jhaveri R, et al. *Anesthesiology*. 1997;87:253.
120. Michelsen LG, et al. *Anesthesiology*. 1996;84:865.
121. McEwan AI, et al. *Anesthesiology*. 1993;78:864.
122. Katoh T, et al. *Anesthesiology*. 1999;90:398.
123. Westmoreland CL, et al. *Anesth Analg*. 1994;78:23.
124. Brunner MD, et al. *Br J Anaesth*. 1994;72:42.
125. Lang E, et al. *Anesthesiology*. 1996;85:721.
126. Johansen JW, et al. *Anesth Analg*. 1998;87:671.
127. Inagaki Y, Tsuda Y. *Anesth Analg*. 1997;85:1387.
128. Katoh T, et al. *Br J Anaesth*. 1999;82:561.
129. Lysakowski C, et al. *Br J Anaesth*. 2001;86:523.

130. Wang LP, et al. *Anesth Analg.* 2007;104:325.
131. Koitabashi T, et al. *Anesth Analg.* 2002;94:1530.
132. Kern SE, et al. *Anesthesiology.* 2004;100:1373.
133. Oh TK, et al. *Anesth Analg.* 2017;125:156.
134. Bonafide CP, et al. *Anesthesiology.* 2008;108:627.
135. Sivanesan E, et al. *Anesth Analg.* 2016;123:836.
136. Smith MT. *Clin Exp Pharmacol Physiol.* 2000;27:524.
137. Johnson SW, et al. *J Neurosci.* 1992;12:483.
138. Welch EB, et al. *J Clin Pharm Ther.* 1994;19:279.
139. Chi OZ, et al. *Can J Anaesth.* 1991;38:275.
140. Gambus PL, et al. *Anesthesiology.* 1995;83:747.
141. Montandon G, et al. *Anesthesiology.* 2016;125:889.
142. Khodayari-Rostamabad A, et al. *Anesthesiology.* 2015;122:140.
143. Egan TD, et al. *Anesthesiology.* 1996;84:821.
144. Scott JC, et al. *Anesthesiology.* 1991;74:34.
145. Noh GJ, et al. *Anesthesiology.* 2006;104:921.
146. Langeron O, et al. *Br J Anaesth.* 1997;78:701.
147. Crabb I, et al. *Br J Anaesth.* 1996;76:795.
148. Haenggi M, et al. *Anesth Analg.* 2004;99:1728.
149. Kalkman CJ, et al. *Anesthesiology.* 1992;76:502.
150. Kawaguchi M, et al. *Anesth Analg.* 1996;82:593.
151. Wright DR, et al. *Eur J Anaesthesiol.* 2004;21:509.
152. Schraag S, et al. *Anesth Analg.* 2006;103:902.
153. Thorogood MC, Armstead WM. *Anesthesiology.* 1996;84:614.
154. Monitto CL, Kurth CD. *Anesth Analg.* 1993;76:985.
155. Adler LJ, et al. *Anesth Analg.* 1997;84:120.
156. Mayer N, et al. *Anesthesiology.* 1990;73:240.
157. Mayberg TS, et al. *Anesthesiology.* 1993;78:288.
158. Wagner KJ, et al. *Anesthesiology.* 2001;94:732.
159. Ostapkovich ND, et al. *Anesthesiology.* 1998;89:358.
160. Kofke WA, et al. *Anesth Analg.* 1992;75:953.
161. Kofke WA, et al. *Anesth Analg.* 2002;94:1229.
162. Warner DS, et al. *Anesth Analg.* 1996;83:348.
163. Jamali S, et al. *Anesth Analg.* 1996;82:600.
164. Lauer KK, et al. *Can J Anaesth.* 1997;44:929.
165. Girard F, et al. *Anesth Analg.* 2009;109:194.
166. de Nadal M, et al. *Anesthesiology.* 2000;92:11.
167. Markovitz BP, et al. *Anesthesiology.* 1992;76:71.
168. Takahashi H, et al. *Anesth Analg.* 1997;85:353.
169. Bofetiado DM, et al. *Anesth Analg.* 1996;82:1237.
170. Lim YJ, et al. *Anesthesiology.* 2004;100:562.
171. Soonthon Brant V, et al. *Anesth Analg.* 1999;88:49.
172. Tourrel F, et al. *Anesth Analg.* 2014;118:1041.
173. Chen C, et al. *Crit Care Med.* 2016;44:e1219.
174. Benthuysen JL, et al. *Anesthesiology.* 1988;68:438.
175. Coruh B, et al. *Chest.* 2013;143:1145.
176. Vankova ME, et al. *Anesthesiology.* 1996;85:574.
177. Mets B. *Anesth Analg.* 1991;72:557.
178. Haber GW, Litman RS. *Anesth Analg.* 2001;93:1532, table of contents.
179. Parkinson SK, et al. *Anesthesiology.* 1990;72:743.
180. Gutstein HB, et al. *Anesthesiology.* 1997;87:1118.
181. Kofke WA, et al. *Anesth Analg.* 1996;83:141.
182. Saboory E, et al. *Anesth Analg.* 2007;105:1729, table of contents.
183. Sinz EH, et al. *Anesth Analg.* 2000;91:1443.
184. Kofke WA, et al. *Anesth Analg.* 2007;105:167.
185. Rollins MD, et al. *Anesthesiology.* 2014;121:1037.
186. Knaggs RD, et al. *Anesth Analg.* 2004;99:108.
187. Aissou M, et al. *Anesthesiology.* 2012;116:1006.
188. Sabourdin N, et al. *Anesthesiology.* 2017;127:284.
189. Bokoch MP, et al. *Auton Neurosci.* 2015;189:68.
190. Neice AE, et al. *Anesth Analg.* 2017;124:915.
191. Kurz A, et al. *Anesthesiology.* 1995;83:293–299.
192. Ikeda T, et al. *Anesthesiology.* 1998;88:858.
193. Kurz M, et al. *Anesthesiology.* 1993;79:1193.
194. Greif R, et al. *Anesth Analg.* 2001;93:620.
195. Alfonsi P, et al. *Anesthesiology.* 2009;111:102.
196. Tsai YC, et al. *Anesth Analg.* 2001;93:1288.
197. Kranke Pet al. *Anesth Analg.* 2002;94:453, table of contents.
198. Nakasuji M, et al. *Br J Anaesth.* 2010;105:162.
199. Jones EA, Bergasa NV. *JAMA.* 1992;268:3359.
200. Ko MC, Naughton NN. *Anesthesiology.* 2000;92:795.
201. Liu XY, et al. *Cell.* 2011;147:447.
202. Paech M, et al. *Br J Anaesth.* 2015;114:469.
203. Borgeat A, Stirnemann HR. *Anesthesiology.* 1999;90:432.
204. George RB, et al. *Anesth Analg.* 2009;109:174.
205. Prin M, et al. *Anesth Analg.* 2016;122:402.
206. Dunteman E, et al. *J Pain Symptom Manage.* 1996;12:255.
207. Ko MC, et al. *J Pharmacol Exp Ther.* 2003;305:173.
208. Tamdee D, et al. *Anesth Analg.* 2009;109:1606.
209. Morgenweck J, et al. *Neuropharmacology.* 2015;99:600.
210. Colbert S, et al. *Anaesthesia.* 1999;54:76.
211. Horta ML, et al. *Br J Anaesth.* 2006;96:796.
212. Sheen MJ, et al. *Anesth Analg.* 2008;106:1868.
213. Celerier E, et al. *Anesthesiology.* 2000;92:465.
214. Fletcher D, Martinez V. *Br J Anaesth.* 2014;112:991.
215. Mauermann E, et al. *Anesthesiology.* 2016;124:453.
216. Li X, Clark JD. *Anesth Analg.* 2002;95:979, table of contents.
217. Yuan Y, et al. *Anesth Analg.* 2013;116:473.
218. Li YZ, et al. *Anesth Analg.* 2014;119:978.
219. Comelon M, et al. *Br J Anaesth.* 2016;116:524.
220. Laulin JP, et al. *Anesth Analg.* 2002;94:1263, table of contents.
221. Kissin I, et al. *Anesth Analg.* 2000;91:1483.
222. Holtman Jr JR, Wala EP. *Anesthesiology.* 2007;106:563.
223. Mercieri M, et al. *Br J Anaesth.* 2017;119:792.
224. Kong M, et al. *J Clin Anesth.* 2016;34:41.
225. Echevarria G, et al. *Br J Anaesth.* 2011;107:959.
226. Song JW, et al. *Anesth Analg.* 2011;113:390.
227. Dunbar SA, et al. *Anesthesiology.* 2006;105:154.
228. Troster A, et al. *Anesthesiology.* 2006;105:1016.
229. Aguado D, et al. *Anesthesiology.* 2013;118:1160.
230. Koo CH, et al. *Br J Anaesth.* 2017;119:1161.
231. Liang DY, et al. *Anesthesiology.* 2006;104:1054.
232. Liang DY, et al. *Anesthesiology.* 2011;114:1180.
233. Shin SW, et al. *Br J Anaesth.* 2010;105:661.
234. van Gulik L, et al. *Br J Anaesth.* 2012;109:616.
235. Voscopoulos C, Lema M. *Br J Anaesth.* 2010;105(suppl 1):i69.
236. Angst MS, Clark JD. *Anesthesiology.* 2006;104:570.
237. Zhang Z, et al. *Anesthesiology.* 2007;107:288.
238. Romberg R, et al. *Br J Anaesth.* 2003;91:862.
239. Erb TO, et al. *Anesthesiology.* 2010;113:41.
240. Selwyn DA, et al. *Br J Anaesth.* 1996;76:274.
241. Hardemark Cedborg AI, et al. *Anesthesiology.* 2015;122:1253.
242. Kim H, et al. *Anaesthesia.* 2012;67:765.
243. Lin JA, et al. *Anesth Analg.* 2005;101:670, table of contents.
244. Pandey CK, et al. *Anesth Analg.* 2004;99:1696, table of contents.
245. Sun L, et al. *Anesthesia.* 2014;28:325.
246. Hung KC, et al. *Anaesthesia.* 2010;65:4.
247. Kim JE, et al. *Anesthesia.* 2014;28:257.
248. Ambesh SP, et al. *Br J Anaesth.* 2010;104:40.
249. Li CC, et al. *Br J Anaesth.* 2015;115:444.
250. Lee LA, et al. *Anesthesiology.* 2015;122:659.
251. Dahan A, et al. *Anesthesiology.* 2010;112:226.
252. Sarton E, et al. *Anesthesiology.* 1999;90:1329.
253. Smart JA, et al. *Br J Anaesth.* 2000;84:735.
254. Glass PS, et al. *Anesthesiology.* 1999;90:1556.
255. Gelberg J, et al. *Br J Anaesth.* 2012;108:1028.
256. Krenn H, et al. *Anesth Analg.* 2000;91:432.
257. Funk GD, et al. *J Neurophysiol.* 1993;70:1497.
258. Ren J, et al. *Anesthesiology.* 2009;110:1364.
259. Ren J, et al. *Anesthesiology.* 2015;122:424.
260. Stucke AG, et al. *Anesthesiology.* 2015;122:1288.
261. Montandon G, et al. *Anesthesiology.* 2016;124:641.
262. Roozekrans M, et al. *Anesthesiology.* 2014;121:459.
263. Setnik B, et al. *Hum Psychopharmacol.* 2014;29:251.
264. van der Schrier R, et al. *Anesthesiology.* 2017;126:534.
265. Niesters M, et al. *Br J Anaesth.* 2013;110:837.
266. Feldman PD, et al. *Brain Res.* 1996;709:331.
267. Keay KA, et al. *Brain Res.* 1997;762:61.
268. Nakae Y, et al. *Anesth Analg.* 2001;92:602.
269. Xiao GS, et al. *Anesthesiology.* 2005;103:280.
270. Llobel F, Laorden ML. *Br J Anaesth.* 1996;76:106.
271. Kawakubo A, et al. *J Anesth.* 1999;13:77.
272. Graham MD, et al. *Anesth Analg.* 2004;98:1013, table of contents.
273. Duncan DJ, et al. *Br J Pharmacol.* 2007;150:720.
274. Bolliger D, et al. *Br J Anaesth.* 2011;106:573.
275. Weber G, et al. *Acta Anaesthesiol Scand.* 1995;39:1071.
276. Lischke V, et al. *Acta Anaesthesiol Scand.* 1994;38:144.
277. Chang DJ, et al. *Anaesthesia.* 2008;63:1056.
278. Kweon TD, et al. *Anaesthesia.* 2008;63:347.

279. Sharpe MD, et al. *Can J Anaesth*. 1992;39:816.
280. Sharpe MD, et al. *Anesthesiology*. 1994;80:63.
281. Sarne Y, et al. *Br J Pharmacol*. 1991;102:696.
282. McIntosh M, et al. *Eur J Pharmacol*. 1992;210:37.
283. Lessa MA, Tibirica E. *Anesth Analg*. 2006;103:815.
284. Schultz JE, et al. *Circ Res*. 1996;78:1100.
285. Zhang Y, et al. *Anesthesiology*. 2005;102:371.
286. Zhang Y, et al. *Anesthesiology*. 2004;101:918.
287. Li R, et al. *Anesth Analg*. 2009;108:23.
288. Frassdorf J, et al. *Anesth Analg*. 2005;101:934, table of contents.
289. Zhang SZ, et al. *Anesthesiology*. 2006;105:550.
290. Jang Y, et al. *Anesthesiology*. 2008;108:243.
291. Weihrauch D, et al. *Anesth Analg*. 2005;101:942, table of contents.
292. Miller LE, et al. *Exp Physiol*. 2015;100:410.
293. McPherson BC, Yao Z. *Anesthesiology*. 2001;94:1082.
294. Kato R, Foex P. *Br J Anaesth*. 2000;84:608.
295. Kato R, et al. *Br J Anaesth*. 2000;84:204.
296. Warltier DC, et al. *Anesthesiology*. 2000;92:253.
297. Blaise GA, et al. *Anesthesiology*. 1990;72:535.
298. Moore PG, et al. *Clin Exp Pharmacol Physiol*. 2000;27:1028.
299. Lennander O, et al. *Br J Anaesth*. 1996;77:399.
300. Arnold RW, et al. *Binocul Vis Strabismus Q*. 2004;19:215.
301. Hahnenkamp K, et al. *Paediatr Anaesth*. 2000;10:601.
302. Blunk JA, et al. *Anesth Analg*. 2004;98:364, table of contents.
303. Stefano GB. *J Neuroimmunol*. 1998;83:70.
304. White DA, et al. *Anesth Analg*. 1990;71:29.
305. Sohn JT, et al. *Anesthesiology*. 2004;101:89.
306. Ebert TJ, et al. *Anesth Analg*. 2005;101:1677.
307. Sohn JT, et al. *Eur J Anaesthesiol*. 2007;24:276.
308. Unlugenc H, et al. *Acta Anaesthesiol Scand*. 2003;47:65.
309. Ouattara A, et al. *Anesthesiology*. 2004;100:602.
310. Sohn JT, et al. *Anesthesiology*. 2005;103:327.
311. Kaye AD, et al. *Anesth Analg*. 2006;102:118.
312. Kaye AD, et al. *Eur J Pharmacol*. 2006;534:159.
313. Charleston C, et al. *Anesth Analg*. 2006;103:156, table of contents.
314. Liu L, et al. *Anesthesiology*. 2013;119:379.
315. Vuong C, et al. *Endocr Rev*. 2010;31:98.
316. Delitala G, et al. *J Endocrinol*. 1994;141:163.
317. Ellis DJ, Steward DJ. *Anesthesiology*. 1990;72:812.
318. Philbin DM, et al. *Anesthesiology*. 1990;73:5.
319. Myles PS, et al. *Anesth Analg*. 2002;95:805, table of contents.
320. Anand KJ, Hickey PR. *N Engl J Med*. 1992;326:1.
321. Mangano DT, et al. *Anesthesiology*. 1992;76:342.
322. Plunkett JJ, et al. *Anesthesiology*. 1997;86:785.
323. Nestler EJ, Aghajanian GK. *Science*. 1997;278:58.
324. Chan KW, et al. *Eur J Pharmacol*. 1997;319:225.
325. Lim G, et al. *Anesthesiology*. 2005;102:832.
326. Kissin I, et al. *Anesth Analg*. 2000;91:110.
327. Li JY, et al. *Anesth Analg*. 2001;92:1563.
328. Lin CP, et al. *Anesthesiology*. 2015;122:666.
329. Lin CP, et al. *Anesth Analg*. 2017;124:972.
330. Wang Y, et al. *Anesth Analg*. 2005;100:1733.
331. Narita M, et al. *Neuroscience*. 2006;138:609.
332. Mika J, et al. *Brain Behav Immun*. 2009;23:75.
333. Chia YY, et al. *Can J Anaesth*. 1999;46:872.
334. Vinik HR, Kissin I. *Anesth Analg*. 1998;86:1307.
335. Guignard B, et al. *Anesthesiology*. 2000;93:409.
336. Schraag S, et al. *Anesth Analg*. 1999;89:753.
337. Gustorff B, et al. *Anesth Analg*. 2002;94:1223, table of contents.
338. Kim SH, et al. *Anesthesiology*. 2013;118:337.
339. Hayhurst CJ, Durieux ME. *Anesthesiology*. 2016;124:483.
340. Paronis CA, Woods JH. *J Pharmacol Exp Ther*. 1997;282:355.
341. Mitra S, Sinatra RS. *Anesthesiology*. 2004;101:212.
342. Mehta V, Langford RM. *Anaesthesia*. 2006;61:269.
343. Tanum L, et al. *JAMA Psychiatry*. 2017;74:1197.
344. Kienbaum P, et al. *Anesthesiology*. 1998;88:1154.
345. Hensel M, et al. *Br J Anaesth*. 2000;84:236.
346. Kienbaum P, et al. *Anesthesiology*. 2002;96:346.
347. Clark DJ, Schumacher MA. *Anesth Analg*. 2017;125:1667.
348. Kuipers PW, et al. *Anesthesiology*. 2004;100:1497.
349. Malinovsky JM, et al. *Anesth Analg*. 1998;87:456.
350. Rosow CE, et al. *Clin Pharmacol Ther*. 2007;82:48.
351. Terashi T, et al. *Anesthesia*. 2013;27:340.
352. Viscusi ER, et al. *Anesth Analg*. 2009;108:1811.
353. Kojima Y, et al. *J Pharmacol Exp Ther*. 1994;268:965.
354. Penagini R, et al. *Am J Physiol*. 1996;271:G675.
355. Thorn SE, et al. *Acta Anaesthesiol Scand*. 1996;40:177.
356. Crighton IM, et al. *Anesth Analg*. 1998;87:445.
357. Runkel NS, et al. *Dig Dis Sci*. 1993;38:1530.
358. Hammas B, et al. *Acta Anaesthesiol Scand*. 2001;45:1023.
359. Murphy DB, et al. *Anesthesiology*. 1997;87:765.
360. Asai T, Power I. *Anesth Analg*. 1999;88:204.
361. McNeill MJ, et al. *Br J Anaesth*. 1990;64:450.
362. Mori T, et al. *J Pharmacol Exp Ther*. 2013;347:91.
363. Thompson DR. *Am J Gastroenterol*. 2001;96:1266.
364. Wu SD, et al. *World J Gastroenterol*. 2004;10:2901.
365. Fragen RJ, et al. *Anesth Analg*. 1999;89:1561.
366. Yang LQ, et al. *Anesthesiology*. 2011;114:1036.
367. Wang Y, et al. *Br J Anaesth*. 2012;109:529.
368. Liu R, et al. *Anesthesiology*. 2014;120:714.
369. Watcha MF, White PF. *Anesthesiology*. 1992;77:162.
370. Gan TJ. *Anesth Analg*. 2006;102:1884.
371. Langevin S, et al. *Anesthesiology*. 1999;91:1666.
372. Rung GW, et al. *Anesth Analg*. 1997;84:832.
373. Tzeng JI, et al. *Br J Anaesth*. 2000;85:865.
374. Simoneau II , et al. *Anesthesiology*. 2001;94:882.
375. Monitto CL, et al. *Anesth Analg*. 2011;113:834.
376. Harnett MJ, et al. *Anesth Analg*. 2007;105:764.
377. Lok IH, et al. *Hum Reprod*. 2002;17:2101.
378. Sandner-Kiesling A, Eisenach JC. *Anesthesiology*. 2002;97:966.
379. Sandner-Kiesling A, Eisenach JC. *Anesthesiology*. 2002;96:375.
380. Gin T, et al. *Anesth Analg*. 2000;90:1167.
381. Ngan Kee WD, et al. *Anesthesiology*. 2006;104:14.
382. Strumper D, et al. *Anesthesiology*. 2003;98:1400; discussion, p 5A.
383. Wittels B, et al. *Anesthesiology*. 1990;73:864.
384. Spigset O. *Acta Anaesthesiol Scand*. 1994;38:94.
385. Doberczak TM, et al. *J Pediatr*. 1991;118:933.
386. McQueen K, Murphy-Oikonen J. *N Engl J Med*. 2016;375:2468.
387. Edston E, van Hage-Hamsten M. *Allergy*. 1997;52:950.
388. Alexander R, et al. *Br J Anaesth*. 1998;81:606.
389. Ng HP, et al. *Br J Anaesth*. 2000;85:785.
390. Al-Hashimi M, et al. *Br J Anaesth*. 2013;111:80.
391. Gaveriaux-Ruff C, et al. *Proc Natl Acad Sci U S A*. 1998;95:6326.
392. Nelson CJ, et al. *Anesth Analg*. 1997;85:620.
393. Sacerdote P, et al. *Anesth Analg*. 2000;90:1411.
394. Yeager MP, et al. *Anesth Analg*. 2002;94:94.
395. Murphy GS, et al. *Anesth Analg*. 2007;104:1334, table of contents.
396. Welters ID, et al. *Anesthesiology*. 2000;92:1677.
397. Yin D, et al. *Nature*. 1999;397:218.
398. Ohara T, et al. *Anesth Analg*. 2005;101:1117, table of contents.
399. Hyejin J, et al. *Immunopharmacol Immunotoxicol*. 2013;35:264.
400. Zhang Y, et al. *Inflammation*. 2014;37:1654.
401. Inagi T, et al. *J Hosp Infect*. 2015;89:61.
402. Bovill JG. *Anesth Analg*. 2010;110:1524.
403. Lennon FE, et al. *Anesthesiology*. 2012;116:940.
404. Lennon FE, et al. *Anesthesiology*. 2012;116:857.
405. Bortsov AV, et al. *Anesthesiology*. 2012;116:896.
406. Sekandarzad MW, et al. *Anesth Analg*. 2017;124:1697.
407. Singleton PA, et al. *Cancer*. 2015;121:2681.
408. Mahbuba W, Lambert DG. *Br J Anaesth*. 2015;115:821.
409. Blebea J, et al. *J Vasc Surg*. 2000;32:364–373.
410. Kim JY, et al. *Anesth Analg*. 2016;123:1429.
411. Rook JM, et al. *Anesthesiology*. 2008;109:130.
412. Bigliardi PL, et al. *Br J Pharmacol*. 2015;172:501.
413. Stein C, Kuchler S. *Trends Pharmacol Sci*. 2013;34:303.
414. Lotsch J. *Anesthesiology*. 2009;110:1209.
415. Romberg R, et al. *Anesthesiology*. 2004;100:120.
416. Klimas R, Mikus G. *Br J Anaesth*. 2014;113:935.
417. Skarke C, et al. *Anesthesiology*. 2004;101:1394.
418. Teppema LJ, et al. *Anesthesiology*. 2008;109:689.
419. Lotsch J, et al. *Anesthesiology*. 2002;97:814.
420. Osborne R, et al. *Clin Pharmacol Ther*. 1990;47:12.
421. Motamed C, et al. *Anesthesiology*. 2000;92:355.
422. Kharasch ED, Thummel KE. *Anesth Analg*. 1993;76:1033.
423. Klees TM, et al. *Anesthesiology*. 2005;102:550.
424. Janicki PK, et al. *Br J Anaesth*. 1992;68:311.
425. Boer F, et al. *Br J Anaesth*. 1992;68:370.
426. Westmoreland CL, et al. *Anesthesiology*. 1993;79:893.
427. Duthie DJ, et al. *Anesth Analg*. 1997;84:740.
428. Buerkle H, Yaksh TL. *Anesthesiology*. 1996;84:926.

429. Egan TD. *Clin Pharmacokinet*. 1995;29:80.
430. Cox EH, et al. *Anesthesiology*. 1999;90:535.
431. Stiller RL, et al. *Anesthesiology*. 1995;83:A381.
432. Lang E, et al. *Anesthesiology*. 1996;85:721.
433. Upton HD, et al. *Anesth Analg*. 2017;125:81.
434. Olkkola KT, et al. *Clin Pharmacokinet*. 1995;28:385.
435. Munoz HR, et al. *Anesth Analg*. 2007;104:77.
436. Munoz HR, et al. *Anesthesiology*. 2002;97:1142.
437. Minto CF, et al. *Anesthesiology*. 1997;86:10.
438. Egan TD, et al. *Anesthesiology*. 1998;89:562.
439. Eleveld DJ, et al. *Anesthesiology*. 2017;126:1005.
440. Kim TK, et al. *Anesthesiology*. 2017;126:1019.
441. Mazoit JX, et al. *Clin Pharmacol Ther*. 1990;48:613.
442. Osborne R, et al. *Clin Pharmacol Ther*. 1993;54:158.
443. Murphy EJ. *Anaesth Intensive Care*. 2005;33:311.
444. Rudin A, et al. *Anesth Analg*. 2007;104:1409, table of contents.
445. Danziger LH, et al. *Pharmacotherapy*. 1994;14:235.
446. Tegeder I, et al. *Clin Pharmacokinet*. 1999;37:17.
447. Baririan N, et al. *Clin Pharmacokinet*. 2007;46:261.
448. Dershwitz M, et al. *Anesthesiology*. 1996;84:812.
449. Navapurkar VU, et al. *Anesthesiology*. 1995;83:A382.
450. Dumont L, et al. *Br J Anaesth*. 1998;81:265.
451. Miller RS, et al. *J Clin Pharm Ther*. 1997;22:197.
452. Hudson RJ, et al. *Anesthesiology*. 2003;99:847.
453. Petros A, et al. *Anesth Analg*. 1995;81:458.
454. Hynynen M, et al. *Br J Anaesth*. 1994;72:571.
455. Russell D, et al. *Br J Anaesth*. 1997;79:456.
456. Davis PJ, et al. *Anesth Analg*. 1999;89:904.
457. Michelsen LG, et al. *Anesth Analg*. 2001;93:1100.
458. Egan TD, et al. *Anesthesiology*. 1999;91:156.
459. Johnson KB, et al. *Anesthesiology*. 2001;94:322.
460. Kurita T, et al. *Br J Anaesth*. 2011;107:719.
461. Somogyi AA, et al. *Clin Pharmacol Ther*. 2007;81:429.
462. Benrath J, et al. *Anesthesiology*. 2004;100:1545.
463. Gottschalk A, et al. *JAMA*. 1998;279:1076.
464. Holthusen H, et al. *Reg Anesth Pain Med*. 2002;27:249.
465. Aida S, et al. *Anesth Analg*. 1999;89:711.
466. Ong CK, et al. *Anesth Analg*. 2005;100:757, table of contents.
467. Lipszyc M, et al. *Br J Anaesth*. 2011;106:724.
468. Carstensen M, Moller AM. *Br J Anaesth*. 2010;104:401.
469. Dahaba AA, et al. *Anesthesiology*. 2004;101:640.
470. Smith C, et al. *Anesthesiology*. 1994;81:820.
471. Vuyk J, et al. *Anesthesiology*. 1996;84:288.
472. Kazama T, et al. *Anesthesiology*. 1997;87:213.
473. Katoh T, et al. *Br J Anaesth*. 1994;73:322.
474. Shibutani K, et al. *Br J Anaesth*. 2005;95:377.
475. Han T, et al. *Anesth Analg*. 2000;90:1365.
476. Yu AL, et al. *Anesthesiology*. 2006;105:684.
477. Vuyk J, et al. *Anesthesiology*. 1993;78:1036; discussion, p 23A.
478. Mertens MJ, et al. *Anesthesiology*. 2001;94:949.
479. Xue FS, et al. *Br J Anaesth*. 2008;100:717.
480. Iannuzzi E, et al. *Minerva Anestesiol*. 2004;70:109.
481. Glass PS, et al. *Anesthesiology*. 1990;73:A378.
482. Thomson IR, et al. *Anesthesiology*. 1998;89:852.
483. Avramov MN, et al. *Anesthesiology*. 1996;85:1283.
484. Fletcher D, et al. *Anesth Analg*. 2000;90:666.
485. Kochs E, et al. *Br J Anaesth*. 2000;84:169.
486. Guignard B, et al. *Anesth Analg*. 2002;95:103, table of contents.
487. Eltzschig HK, et al. *Anesth Analg*. 2002;94:1173, table of contents.
488. Calderon E, et al. *Anesth Analg*. 2001;92:715.
489. Vuyk J, et al. *Anesthesiology*. 1995;83:8.
490. Stanski DR, Shafer SL. *Anesthesiology*. 1995;83:1.
491. Wuesten R, et al. *Anesthesiology*. 2001;94:211.
492. Hogue Jr CW, et al. *Anesth Analg*. 1996;83:279.
493. Vuyk J, et al. *Anesth Analg*. 1990;71:645.
494. Engoren M, et al. *Anesth Analg*. 2001;93:859.
495. Bell J, et al. *Br J Anaesth*. 1994;73:162.
496. Howie MB, et al. *Anesth Analg*. 1996;83:941.
497. Duncan HP, et al. *Br J Anaesth*. 2000;84:556.
498. Takahashi M, et al. *J Anesth*. 2004;18:1.
499. Silbert BS, et al. *Anesthesiology*. 2006;104:1137.
500. Sareen J, et al. *Can J Anaesth*. 1997;44:19.
501. Jain U, et al. *Anesthesiology*. 1996;85:522.
502. Ahonen J, et al. *Anesth Analg*. 2000;90:1269.
503. Kazmaier S, et al. *Br J Anaesth*. 2000;84:578.
504. Geisler FE, et al. *J Cardiothorac Vasc Anesth*. 2003;17:60.
505. Thompson JP, et al. *Br J Anaesth*. 1998;81:152.
506. Portenoy RK, et al. *Anesthesiology*. 1993;78:36.
507. Sandler AN, et al. *Anesthesiology*. 1994;81:1169.
508. Grond S, et al. *Clin Pharmacokinet*. 2000;38:59.
509. Schmidt-Hansen M, et al. *Cochrane Database Syst Rev*. 2015:CD009596.
510. Poulain P, et al. *J Pain Symptom Manage*. 2008;36:117.
511. Power I. *Br J Anaesth*. 2007;98:4.
512. Viscusi ER, et al. *JAMA*. 2004;291:1333.
513. Panchal SJ, et al. *Anesth Analg*. 2007;105:1437.
514. James IG, et al. *J Pain Symptom Manage*. 2010;40:266.
515. Aiyer R, et al. *Anesth Analg*. 2018;127:529.
516. Manara AR, et al. *Br J Anaesth*. 1990;64:551.
517. Friesen RH, Lockhart CH. *Anesthesiology*. 1992;76:46.
518. Streisand JB, et al. *Anesthesiology*. 1991;75:223.
519. Egan TD, et al. *Anesthesiology*. 2000;92:665.
520. Kharasch ED, et al. *Anesthesiology*. 2004;101:738.
521. Kharasch ED, et al. *Anesthesiology*. 2004;101:729.
522. Dsida RM, et al. *Anesth Analg*. 1998;86:66.
523. Mystakidou K, et al. *Drug Deliv*. 2006;13:269.
524. Zedie N, et al. *Clin Pharmacol Ther*. 1996;59:341.
525. Dale O, et al. *Acta Anaesthesiol Scand*. 2002;46:759.
526. Striebel HW, et al. *Anesth Analg*. 1996;83:548.
527. Hippard HK, et al. *Anesth Analg*. 2012;115:356.
528. Christensen KS, et al. *Anesth Analg*. 2008;107:2018.
529. Verghese ST, et al. *Anesth Analg*. 2008;107:1176.
530. Worsley MH, et al. *Anaesthesia*. 1990;45:449.
531. Hung OR, et al. *Anesthesiology*. 1995;83:277.
532. Coyne PJ, et al. *J Pain Symptom Manage*. 2002;23:157.
533. Farr SJ, Otulana BA. *Adv Drug Deliv Rev*. 2006;58:1076.
534. Bevans T, et al. *Anesth Analg*. 2016;122:1831.
535. Babul N, et al. *J Pain Symptom Manage*. 1992;7:400.
536. Lundeberg S, et al. *Acta Anaesthesiol Scand*. 1996;40:445.
537. Klepstad P, et al. *Pain*. 2003;101:193.
538. Curtis GB, et al. *Eur J Clin Pharmacol*. 1999;55:425.
539. Bruera E, et al. *J Clin Oncol*. 1998;16:3222.
540. Carvalho B, et al. *Anesth Analg*. 2005;100:1150.
541. Carvalho B, et al. *Anesth Analg*. 2007;105:176.
542. Gambling D, et al. *Anesth Analg*. 2005;100:1065.
543. Viscusi ER, et al. *Anesthesiology*. 2005;102:1014.
544. Hartrick CT, et al. *Bone Joint Surg Am*. 2006;88:273.
545. Atkinson Ralls L, et al. *Anesth Analg*. 2011;113:251.
546. Caraco Y, et al. *Drug Metab Dispos*. 1996;24:761.
547. Nieminen TH, et al. *Anesthesiology*. 2009;110:1371.
548. Lemberg KK, et al. *Anesth Analg*. 2008;106:463, table of contents.
549. Lemberg KK, et al. *Anesthesiology*. 2006;105:801.
550. Lenz H, et al. *Anesth Analg*. 2009;109:1279.
551. Chang SH, et al. *Anaesthesia*. 2010;65:1007.
552. Unlugenc H, et al. *Anesth Analg*. 2008;106:309, table of contents.
553. Nelson KE, Eisenach JC. *Anesthesiology*. 2005;102:1008.
554. Douma MR, et al. *Br J Anaesth*. 2010;104:209.
555. Kranke P, et al. *Anesth Analg*. 2004;99:718, table of contents.
556. Felden L, et al. *Br J Anaesth*. 2011;107:319.
557. Quigley C, Wiffen P. *J Pain Symptom Manage*. 2003;25:169.
558. Hong D, et al. *Anesth Analg*. 2008;107:1384.
559. Prommer E. *Support Care Cancer*. 2007;15:259.
560. Bowdle TA, et al. *Anesth Analg*. 2004;98:1692, table of contents.
561. Murphy GS, et al. *Anesthesiology*. 2017;126:822.
562. Chamberlin KW, et al. *Ann Pharmacother*. 2007;41:1144.
563. Gimbel J, Ahdieh H. *Anesth Analg*. 2004;99:1472, table of contents.
564. Morlion B, et al. *Br J Anaesth*. 1999;82:52.
565. Bouillon T, et al. *Anesthesiology*. 1999;90:7.
566. Dieterich M, et al. *Arch Gynecol Obstet*. 2012;286:859.
567. Dopfmer UR, et al. *Eur J Anaesthesiol*. 2001;18:389.
568. Miotto K, et al. *Anesth Analg*. 2017;124:44.
569. Halfpenny DM, et al. *Br J Anaesth*. 1999;83:909.
570. Bamigbade TA, et al. *Br J Anaesth*. 1997;79:352.
571. de Wolff MH, et al. *Br J Anaesth*. 1999;83:780.
572. James MF, et al. *Anesth Analg*. 1996;83:87.
573. Wilder Smith CH, Bettiga A. *Br J Clin Pharmacol*. 1997;43:71.
574. Thevenin A, et al. *Anesth Analg*. 2008;106:622, table of contents.
575. Acalovschi I, et al. *Anesth Analg*. 2001;92:209.
576. Robaux S, et al. *Anesth Analg*. 2004;98:1172, table of contents.
577. Zeidan A, et al. *Anesth Analg*. 2008;107:292.
578. Tamanai-Shacoori Z, et al. *Anesth Analg*. 2007;105:524.

579. Boyer EW, Shannon M. *N Engl J Med.* 2005;352:1112.
580. van Dorp EL, et al. *Anesth Analg.* 2006;102:1789.
581. Osborne R, et al. *Br J Clin Pharmacol.* 1992;34:130.
582. Grace D, Fee JP. *Anesth Analg.* 1996;83:1055.
583. Hanna MH, et al. *Anesthesiology.* 2005;102:815.
584. van Dorp EL, et al. *Anesthesiology.* 2009;110:1356.
585. Asai T, et al. *Br J Anaesth.* 1998;80:814.
586. Hirabayashi M, et al. *Anesth Analg.* 2017;124:1930.
587. Zacny JP, et al. *Anesth Analg.* 1996;82:931.
588. Brown SM, et al. *Anesthesiology.* 2011;115:1251.
589. Dahan A, et al. *Br J Anaesth.* 2005;94:825.
590. Chen KY, et al. *Anesthesiology.* 2014;120:1262.
591. Falcon E, et al. *Neuropsychopharmacology.* 2016;41:2344.
592. Nyhuis PW, et al. *J Clin Psychopharmacol.* 2008;28:593.
593. Lee SC, et al. *Anesth Analg.* 1997;84:810.
594. Weiss BM, et al. *Anesth Analg.* 1991;73:521.
595. Parker RK, et al. *Anesth Analg.* 1997;84:757.
596. Yeh YC, et al. *Br J Anaesth.* 2008;101:542.
597. Charuluxananan S, et al. *Anesth Analg.* 2003;96:1789, table of contents.
598. Wang JJ, et al. *Anesth Analg.* 1999;88:686.
599. Ding Y, White PF. *Anesth Analg.* 1992;75:566.
600. Cohen RI, et al. *Anesth Analg.* 1993;77:533.
601. Sun ZT, et al. *J Anesth.* 2011;25:860.
602. Freye E, Levy JV. *Eur J Anaesthesiol.* 2007;24:53.
603. Kendrick WD, et al. *Anesth Analg.* 1996;82:641.
604. Gan TJ, et al. *Anesthesiology.* 1997;87:1075.
605. Fukuda K, et al. *Anesth Analg.* 1998;87:450.
606. van Dorp E, et al. *Anesthesiology.* 2006;105:51.
607. Just B, et al. *Anesthesiology.* 1992;76:60.
608. Staessen J, et al. *J Cardiovasc Pharmacol.* 1990;15:386.
609. Xiao Y, et al. *Acta Anaesthesiol Scand.* 2015;59:1194.
610. Belzung C, et al. *Eur J f Pharma.* 2000;394:289.
611. Mikkelsen S, et al. *Anesthesiology.* 1999;90:1539.
612. Hackshaw KV, et al. *Crit Care Med.* 1990;18:47.
613. Boeuf B, et al. *Crit Care Med.* 1998;26:1910.
614. Crain SM, Shen KF. *Pain.* 2000;84:121.
615. Movafegh A, et al. *Anesth Analg.* 2009;109:1679.
616. Benzel EC, et al. *J Spinal Disord.* 1992;5:75.
617. Bracken MB, et al. *N Engl J Med.* 1990;322:1405.
618. Acher CW, et al. *J Vasc Surg.* 1994;19:236; discussion 247.
619. Romanovsky AA, Blatteis CM. *J Appl Physiol.* 1996;81:2565.
620. Bergasa NV. *Curr Treat Options Gastroenterol.* 2004;7:501.
621. Bainton T, et al. *Pain.* 1992;48:159.
622. Abboud TK, et al. *Anesth Analg.* 1990;71:367.
623. Joshi GP, et al. *Anesthesiology.* 1999;90:1007.
624. Thomas J, et al. *N Engl J Med.* 2008;358:2332.
625. Webster LR, et al. *J Pain Res.* 2015;8:771.
626. Murphy DB, et al. *Br J Anaesth.* 2001;86:120.
627. Chey WD, et al. *N Engl J Med.* 2014;370:2387.
628. Bovill JG. *J Clin Anesth.* 1997;9:3S.
629. Vuyk J. *J Clin Anesth.* 1997;9:23S.
630. Bartkowski RR, et al. *Anesthesiology.* 1993;78:260.
631. Bartkowski RR, McDonnell TE. *Anesthesiology.* 1990;73:566.
632. Schwieger IM, et al. *Anesthesiology.* 1991;74:1060.
633. Luger TJ, et al. *Eur J Pharmacol.* 1995;275:153.
634. Bailey PL, et al. *Anesthesiology.* 1990;73:826.
635. Ma D, et al. *Acta Anaesthesiol Scand.* 1998;42:670.
636. Iselin Chaves IA, et al. *Anesth Analg.* 1998;87:949.
637. Sukhani R, et al. *Anesth Analg.* 1996;83:975.
638. Mertens MJ, et al. *Anesthesiology.* 2004;100:795.
639. Haessler R, et al. *J Cardiothorac Vasc Anesth.* 1992;6:173.
640. Pacheco Dda F, et al. *Brain Res.* 2014;1562:69.
641. Sethna NF, et al. *Anesth Analg.* 1998;86:1250.
642. Reeves M, et al. *Anesth Analg.* 2001;93:116.
643. Lauretti GR, et al. *Anesthesiology.* 1999;90:1528.
644. Zakine J, et al. *Anesth Analg.* 2008;106:1856.
645. Grande LA, et al. *Anesth Analg.* 2008;107:1380.
646. Webb AR, et al. *Anesth Analg.* 2007;104:912.
647. Searle NR, et al. *Can J Anaesth.* 1996;43:890.
648. Weiskopf RB, et al. *Anesthesiology.* 1994;81:1350.
649. Shorten GD, et al. *Can J Anaesth.* 1995;42:695.
650. Cote D, et al. *Can J Anaesth.* 1991;38:324.
651. McCoy EP, et al. *Can J Anaesth.* 1993;40:703.
652. Loan PB, et al. *Br J Anaesth.* 1995;74:330.
653. Gillman PK. *Br J Anaesth.* 2005;95:434.
654. Ure DS, et al. *Br J Anaesth.* 2000;84:414.
655. Beresford BJ, et al. *J Ect.* 2004;20:120.
656. Hasegawa AE, Zacny JP. *Anesth Analg.* 1997;85:633.
657. Omote K, et al. *Anesthesiology.* 1996;84:636.
658. Koinig H, et al. *Anesth Analg.* 1998;87:206.
659. Buvanendran A, et al. *Anesth Analg.* 2002;95:661, table of contents.
660. Kroin JS, et al. *Anesth Analg.* 2000;90:913.
661. Ng A, et al. *Br J Anaesth.* 2002;88:714.
662. Cepeda MS, et al. *Anesthesiology.* 2005;103:1225.
663. Xuerong Y, et al. *Anesth Analg.* 2008;107:2032.
664. Hong JY, et al. *Anesthesiology.* 2010;113:672.
665. Hiller A, et al. *Spine.* 2012;37:E1225.
666. Eckhardt K, et al. *Anesth Analg.* 2000;91:185.
667. Hansen C, et al. *Anesth Analg.* 2004;99:1180, table of contents.
668. Van Elstraete AC, et al. *Anesthesiology.* 2008;108:484.
669. Bornemann-Cimenti H, et al. *Br J Anaesth.* 2012;108:845.
670. Luccarini P, et al. *Anesthesiology.* 2004;100:690.
671. Kozer E, et al. *Anesth Analg.* 2008;107:1216.
672. Ho KY, et al. *Br J Anaesth.* 2010;105:371.
673. Babenco HD, et al. *Anesthesiology.* 1998;89:642.
674. McKay A, et al. *Anesth Analg.* 2009;109:1805.
675. Liu Q, Gold MS. *Anesthesiology.* 2016;125:755.

25 Nonopioid Pain Medications

LUCY LIN CHEN and JIANREN MAO

KEY POINTS

- With a better understanding of pain pathways and mechanisms, it has been recognized that ion channels play an important role in the transduction, transmission, and modulation of nociceptive signals. This opens a new avenue of developing novel therapeutic agents for the treatment of acute or chronic pain, particularly neuropathic pain.
- Although the exact mechanism of action remains unclear for many drugs listed in this chapter, they often are a component of a multidrug treatment strategy that has been increasingly used for the management of chronic pain conditions.

Introduction

Recent advances in our understanding of pain mechanisms have enabled us to treat acute and chronic pain conditions with a variety of nonopioid pain medications. The option of using nonopioid pain medications is particularly meaningful given the growing global concern over prescription opioid abuse and overdose. Besides acetaminophen and nonsteroidal antiinflammatory drugs (NSAIDs), several new categories of nonopioid pain medications can be used for the management of acute or chronic pain and, in particular, neuropathic pain. Examples of these nonopioid pain medications include drugs that block voltage-sensitive sodium channels and voltage-sensitive calcium channels, facilitate opening of chloride channels, increase function of the endogenous γ-aminobutyric acid (GABA) system, and modulate the N-methyl-D-aspartate (NMDA) receptor activity. In particular, ion channel blockers possess the antihyperalgesic effect by targeting specific mechanisms of pathologic pain, although most analgesics in this category do not necessarily produce the typical analgesic effect (i.e., raising the pain threshold above the normal baseline).[1]

This chapter briefly discusses NSAIDs and acetaminophen and focuses on describing several ion channel blockers that are commonly used in the treatment of pain conditions, as listed in Box 25.1. They are grouped into two categories: calcium channel blockers and sodium channel blockers.

Nonsteroidal antiinflammatory drugs

NSAIDs include ibuprofen, naproxen, indomethacin, ketorolac, and diclofenac and are examples of a class of medication commonly used as analgesic to reduce myofascial pain, postoperative pain, and chronic pain conditions. In a recent Cochrane review of 16 randomized, controlled clinical trials (2144 patients), pain relief and function restoration were compared in patients with acute soft tissue injury treated with oral NSAIDs and other oral analgesics including acetaminophen with or without opioids. The analgesic effect was similar between NSAIDs and acetaminophen or opioid, and there were no differences in functional restoration at 7 days,[2] but the patients who were taking opioids reported more adverse side effects.[3] Although acetaminophen, indomethacin, or diclofenac produced similar pain reduction, the combination of acetaminophen and diclofenac showed slightly better pain reduction.[4] Intravenous ketorolac (15 or 30 mg) is a common medication of choice during the early postoperative period if there are no contraindications, such as renal insufficiency.[5] Ketorolac has also been successfully used in pediatric surgical patients.[6,7] A recent metaanalysis also found that NSAIDs were equivalent to opioids or paracetamol in the relief of acute renal colic pain.[8]

The cyclooxygenase-2 (COX-2) inhibitors are considered an alternative to NSAIDs (mixed COX-1/COX-2 inhibitors) while possessing reduced gastrointestinal side effects. However, COX-2 inhibition is associated with increased risk of adverse cardiovascular events, although recent clinical studies, including the data from the PRECISION trial that examined long-term cardiovascular safety issues, support the notion that both NSAIDs and COX-2 carry a certain degree of cardiovascular risk.[9]

Acetaminophen

For many decades, oral acetaminophen has been widely used as an analgesic to treat mild to moderate pain. Recently, intravenous acetaminophen has become available in the United States. Results of a randomized trial of patients who had colorectal surgery indicated that

BOX 25.1 Ion Channel Blockers as Pain Medications (Recommended Dosing)

Calcium Channel Blockers

Gabapentin: Starting dose 100–300 mg/day; titrating up to 1800–3600 mg/day
Pregabalin: Starting dose: 75–150 mg/day; titrating up to 450–600 mg/day
Zonisamide: Starting dose: 50–100 mg/day; titrating up to 450 mg/day
Ziconotide: Starting dose: 0.1 μg/h; titrating up to 0.4 μg/h
Levetiracetam: Starting dose: 250–500 mg/day; titrating up to 2000 mg/day

Sodium Channel Blockers

Lidocaine: Used in a lidocaine test: 1 mg/kg via slow intravenous push or drip
Mexiletine: Starting dose: 150–300 mg/day; titrating up to 600 mg/day
Carbamazepine: Starting dose: 100 mg/day; titrating up to 600 mg/day
Oxcarbazepine: Starting dose: 150 mg/day; titrating up to 900 mg/day
Lamotrigine: Starting dose: 25–50 mg/day; titrating up to 250–500 mg/day
Topiramate: Starting dose: 50–100 mg/day; titrating up to 300–400 mg/day.

intravenous acetaminophen decreased postoperative opioid consumption, reduced hospital stay, improved pain control, shortened time to return of bowel function, and lowered the rate of postoperative ileus.[10] Similar results were found after procedures for posterior spinal fusion,[11] craniotomy,[12] vitrectomy,[13] esophagectomy,[14,15] and total joint arthroplasty.[16]

Compared with an opioids-only option for postoperative pain management in adolescents with idiopathic scoliosis, patients treated with intravenous acetaminophen plus ketorolac consumed less opioids and had less severe constipation.[17] A retrospective analysis of the results of the Premier Database of 61,017 cholecystectomy patients showed that 31,133 (51%) of the patients who received intravenous acetaminophen had experienced a shorter length of hospital stay, a decrease in hospitalization costs, a reduced average daily morphine-equivalent dose, and lower rates of respiratory depression, nausea, and vomiting.[18] However, several studies have failed to show that intravenous acetaminophen achieved the positive results as described here.[19-21] The hepatic side effect is a significant concern for those with long-term acetaminophen use, particularly with alcohol. A recent analysis of nine prospective cohort studies has also linked long-term acetaminophen use with an increased risk of adverse neurodevelopmental outcomes following prenatal acetaminophen exposure.[22]

Calcium Channel Blockers

Opening of calcium channels is an important step of synaptic transmission because it facilitates release of neurotransmitters and neuromodulators from presynaptic sites. Changes in intracellular calcium concentration also modulate cell membrane excitability and initiate a cascade of intracellular responses. Therefore blocking calcium channels can play a significant role in modulating both nociceptive and antinociceptive processes. Drugs that reduce calcium influx into the intracellular compartment of neuronal or glial cells may be used as adjunctive or alternative medications for the treatment of various pain conditions, particularly chronic neuropathic pain conditions. Most calcium channel blockers used as antihypertensive drugs may be suitable for chronic pain management because of their side effects and site of action. Gabapentin, pregabalin, zonisamide, ziconotide, and levetiracetam are examples of drugs that block calcium channels as a part of their mechanisms of action and have been used in pain management.

GABAPENTIN

Gabapentin was initially approved by the U.S. Food and Drug Administration (FDA) as an anticonvulsant (partial seizure) and is currently extensively used for the treatment of neuropathic pain conditions. Although gabapentin's mechanism of action is unclear, it does block voltage-gated calcium channels by binding to the α_2-δ subunit,[23] thereby reducing calcium influx. By blocking calcium influx, gabapentin reduces the release of glutamate and substance P from primary nociceptive afferents, thereby modulating nociceptive transmission. Gabapentin has been used to treat painful diabetic neuropathy, postherpetic neuralgia, trigeminal neuralgia, complex regional pain syndrome, and painful peripheral neuropathies caused by human immunodeficiency virus (HIV), cancer, multiple sclerosis, and spinal cord injury.

Painful diabetic neuropathy is a debilitating condition commonly seen in patients with diabetes mellitus. Up to 25% of patients with diabetes may suffer from spontaneous pain, allodynia, hyperalgesia, paresthesias, and other pain symptoms.[24] Postherpetic neuralgia is another common neuropathic pain condition. The incidence of postherpetic neuralgia is estimated to be 9% to 34%, which increases significantly with age. Multiple classes of drugs have been tried to treat pain associated with painful diabetic neuralgia and postherpetic neuralgia, including tricyclic antidepressants (TCAs) such as amitriptyline, nortriptyline, imipramine, and desipramine. Because of the significant side effects of TCAs, gabapentin has been increasingly used in the treatment of these pain conditions.

Gabapentin is effective in reducing several salient symptoms of neuropathic pain such as burning and shooting pain, allodynia, and hyperalgesia.[25,26] The number needed to achieve at least 50% pain relief with antidepressants and gabapentin are 3.4 and 2.7, respectively.[27] Although both antidepressants and gabapentin may provide moderate pain relief, antidepressants may have more major side effects.

The recommended gabapentin dose range is 1800 to 3600 mg/day, starting at 100 to 300 mg/day and increasing 100 to 300 mg every 1 to 3 days. Adverse effects are usually mild to moderate and typically subside within 7 to 10 days after the treatment is started; however, serious side effects can occur including mood swing, edema, and suicidality. In general, a slow titration process can significantly reduce some otherwise intolerable side effects, such as dizziness. In addition to its use as a monotherapy, gabapentin has been extensively used in multimodal drug therapy in conjunction with TCAs and other anticonvulsants.[1] Multimodal drug therapy provides better pain control, requiring a smaller dose range for each drug included in the regimen. Gabapentin also can treat complex regional pain syndrome, phantom pain, trigeminal neuralgia, cancer-related neuropathic pain, multiple sclerosis, spinal cord injury, HIV-associated painful sensory neuropathy, and glossopharyngeal neuralgia.

The role of gabapentin in acute postoperative pain management remains unclear.

PREGABALIN

Pregabalin is an anticonvulsant that has a high affinity to the α_2-δ subunit of voltage-sensitive calcium channels. The mechanism of action of pregabalin is similar to that of gabapentin. Pregabalin decreases calcium influx, thereby reducing the release of excitatory neurotransmitters, including glutamate, substance P, and calcitonin gene–related peptide. Pregabalin has no activity on GABA or benzodiazepine receptors; therefore it has no significant drug-drug interactions with such agents.

Pregabalin has been used to treat painful diabetic neuropathy and postherpetic neuralgia, with a significant therapeutic effect.[28,29] It has a quick onset, and, in some cases, pain reduction can be expected on the first day of treatment with pregabalin (300 mg/day). Sustainable sleep improvement is also observed 1 week after the therapy is initiated. Common side effects are dizziness, somnolence, and mild to moderate peripheral edema.[30] Other concerns over pregabalin include behavioral changes such as mood swing and suicidality. Before starting pregabalin, it is recommended to check the baseline creatinine level. Moreover, pregabalin (at an average dose of 450 mg/day) is effective in patients with fibromyalgia, who often have clinical presentations including diffuse musculoskeletal pain, sleep disturbance, and fatigue.

ZONISAMIDE

Zonisamide blocks both voltage-sensitive sodium channels and N-type calcium channels. Studies suggest that zonisamide may be used to treat mania, Parkinson disease, and poststroke central pain or to provide migraine prophylaxis.[31,32] Its possible mechanisms of action include modulation of monoamine neurotransmitter release and free radical scavenging. Zonisamide is effective for the treatment of painful diabetic neuropathy (540 mg/day). The tolerability of zonisamide is difficult to assess because it is often used in multimodal drug therapy. Thus the data on the effectiveness and side effects of zonisamide remain limited.

ZICONOTIDE

Ziconotide is a synthetic peptide analogue of omega conotoxin derived from a marine snail, *Conus magus*. Ziconotide potently and selectively blocks N-type voltage-sensitive calcium channels. This drug is approved only for intrathecal use in patients with severe pain who are refractory to other treatment options, including intrathecal morphine. In early clinical trials, ziconotide exhibited severe central nervous system and psychiatric adverse effects with an initial intrathecal infusion rate of 0.4 μg/h and frequent dosing titration.[33] More recently, ziconotide has been shown to be effective for chronic pain conditions resulting from cancer, acquired immunodeficiency syndrome, and trigeminal neuralgia.[34,35] The role of ziconotide in postoperative pain management is less clear. Given ziconotide's significant side effects and restrictive delivery route, its routine use in acute postoperative pain management is not well justified.

The initial infusion rate of ziconotide should start at 0.1 μg/h intrathecally, with a slow titration of no more than 2 to 3 times the initial dose per week. An implanted intrathecal infusion system is required for the long-term use of this therapy if the initial ziconotide trial is effective.[36] Patients with severe psychiatric disorders may not be proper candidates for this therapy. On the other hand, ziconotide may be advantageous over intrathecal morphine because patients do not develop tolerance after a prolonged use of ziconotide. However, adverse neurologic effects associated with ziconotide therapy will require careful patient selection and monitoring. Using a smaller dose increment may help to avoid systemic toxicity.

LEVETIRACETAM

Levetiracetam is an anticonvulsant approved by the FDA for treatment of epilepsy.[37] Its mechanisms of action are less clear because it may have effects on several neurotransmitter systems, including dopaminergic, glutamatergic, and GABAergic systems. But at least one of its mechanisms of action is due to inhibition of N-type voltage-sensitive calcium channels. Levetiracetam improves neoplastic plexopathies, painful peripheral neuropathy, and postherpetic neuralgia. It also has been used in migraine headache prophylaxis. The dose range is 500 to 2000 mg/day. At this dose range, levetiracetam is well tolerated in clinical trials. Common adverse effects are dry eyes and dizziness.[38]

Sodium Channel Blockers

Sodium channels are primarily involved in nerve conduction. Sodium channels can be divided into two general categories based on their sensitivity to tetrodotoxin (TTX): TTX-sensitive (TTX-S) and TTX-resistant (TTX-R) sodium channels. TTX-S sodium channels are expressed mainly in large and medium dorsal root ganglion neurons, whereas TTX-R sodium channels are expressed mainly in small-diameter dorsal root ganglion neurons, including C-afferent neurons. Expression of both TTX-S and TTX-R sodium channels is likely to be altered when peripheral nerves are injured or severed (axotomy), producing aberrant high-frequency spontaneous ectopic discharges. Sodium channel blockers at a proper dose range are believed to suppress ectopic discharges without blocking normal nerve conduction, which forms the basis of using sodium channel blockers in the treatment of chronic pain conditions, particularly neuropathic pain. Selective Nav 1.7 and Nav 1.8 sodium channel blockers are being investigated for possible clinical applications. Currently, several representative sodium channel blockers include lidocaine, mexiletine, carbamazepine, oxcarbazepine, lamotrigine, and topiramate.[39]

LIDOCAINE

Lidocaine is a local anesthetic and cardiac antiarrhythmic. Since the 1980s, intravenous administration of lidocaine has been used as a diagnostic tool and, in some cases, a therapeutic tool for intractable neuropathic pain.[39] This treatment modality has been shown to improve chronic pain conditions induced by neurologic diseases, including stroke, neurogenic facial pain, and myofascial pain.[40,41] Up to 78% of cases are associated with a positive outcome when intravenous lidocaine is used.[42] A major pitfall of intravenous lidocaine treatment is its short duration, which requires frequent treatment sessions.

Topical 5% lidocaine patch and over-the-counter topical lidocaine gel or cream provide a local analgesic effect with a minimum systemic effect. Lidocaine patch has been used in patients with neuropathic pain conditions such as painful diabetic neuropathy, postherpetic neuralgia, and peripheral neuropathies. It reduces allodynia and hyperalgesia associated with such conditions.[43] Although the evidence remains weak and unclear, lidocaine patch has been used to treat chronic lower back pain. In some cases, lidocaine patch has become a part of multimodal drug therapy, such as a combination of topical lidocaine patch and gabapentin.[1]

MEXILETINE

Mexiletine is an oral lidocaine congener. It may be used to overcome the shortcoming of transient pain relief with intravenous lidocaine. In many cases, intravenous lidocaine is used as a test to determine whether the intended lidocaine treatment is effective. When a positive response is achieved, oral mexiletine is administered to maintain the therapeutic effect.[44,45] This treatment regimen reduces pain due to painful diabetic neuropathy refractory to other therapies.[46] Mexiletine alone has been used to treat phantom pain and pain after spinal cord injury.[46]

Fibromyalgia and myofascial pain are other clinical conditions that may be responsive to a lidocaine and mexiletine treatment regimen. In addition, anecdotal reports suggest that oral mexiletine may be used to treat primary erythromelalgia, metastasis bone pain, and headaches.

CARBAMAZEPINE

A primary mechanism of action of carbamazepine is sodium channel blockade, which decreases spontaneous firing of Aδ-fibers and C-fibers. Carbamazepine has been approved to treat trigeminal neuralgia, a neuropathic pain condition characterized by episodic lightning, lancinating, or shooting pain along the trigeminal nerve distribution.[47] Carbamazepine has been used for decades and was superior to placebo in a number of clinical trials. It was once considered a "gold standard" and remains a treatment of choice for trigeminal neuralgia, with a response rate of 89% within 5 to 14 days after the treatment is initiated. However, carbamazepine has significant drug-drug interactions and a long list of adverse effects, including central nervous system side effects. In the United States the FDA has issued black box warnings about this drug, including aplastic anemia and agranulocytosis. Therefore its clinical utility is rather limited considering that newer anticonvulsants are available with fewer and less severe side effects.

OXCARBAZEPINE

Oxcarbazepine is an analogue of carbamazepine, which acts as a sodium channel blocker and stabilizes neuronal membrane. In contrast to carbamazepine, oxcarbazepine has fewer drug-drug interactions and side effects, particularly severe blood dyscrasias. The most common side effects of oxcarbazepine are dizziness, drowsiness, hypotension, nausea, and asymptomatic mild hyponatremia. Oxcarbazepine has been used to treat intractable trigeminal neuralgia refractory to other anticonvulsants.[48] With a median dose of 750 mg/day, this novel drug appears to have the same efficacy as carbamazepine in the treatment of trigeminal neuralgia but a much lower incidence of side effects.

Oxcarbazepine also reduces pain associated with painful diabetic neuropathy and complex regional pain syndrome. For patients with postherpetic neuralgia that is unresponsive to carbamazepine and gabapentin, oxcarbazepine, starting at 150 mg/day and titrating up to a maintenance dose of 900 mg/day, may be a promising drug because it significantly reduces allodynia related to postherpetic neuralgia. Oxcarbazepine appears to be well tolerated and may serve as a reasonable alternative to other sodium channel blockers.

LAMOTRIGINE

Lamotrigine has multiple mechanisms of action, although it also blocks both sodium and calcium channels.[49] Lamotrigine is effective in the treatment of trigeminal neuralgia, neuralgia after nerve section, and pain related to HIV neuropathy. With a daily lamotrigine dose of 75 to 300 mg, the intensity of burning and shooting pain is relieved by 33% to 100%, and the frequency of shooting pain attack is reduced by 80% to 100%. In patients with spinal cord injury, lamotrigine decreases overall pain sensation to less than the level of injury in patients with incomplete spinal cord injury but has little effect on spontaneous and evoked pain in patients with complete spinal cord injury.

A typical starting dose for lamotrigine is 25 to 50 mg/day, which can be slowly titrated up over 2 to 3 weeks to 250 to 500 mg/day in divided doses. Tolerability is usually low at high doses (>300 mg/day). Up to 10% of patients may have rashes after taking this medication, with a 3 in 1000 incidence of Stevens-Johnson syndrome. Other side effects are mild dizziness, somnolence, nausea, and constipation.

TOPIRAMATE

Topiramate is another drug that has multiple mechanisms of action. However, at least one of its actions is to block voltage-sensitive sodium channels. It also may potentiate GABA inhibitory action, block voltage-sensitive calcium channels, and inhibit subtypes of glutamate receptors (non-NMDA receptors). Topiramate can cause significant weight loss (up to 7%), a side effect that could be beneficial for certain patient populations with chronic pain conditions. Topiramate, at a daily dose of 400 mg or greater, attenuates neuropathic pain, improves sleep quality, and reduces body weight.[48] When used to treat chronic lumbar radicular pain, the effect of topiramate is inconclusive because of a high dropout rate and frequent side effects in clinical trials. However, topiramate 30 to 80 mg/day is superior to placebo for the treatment of chronic tension, migraine, and cluster headaches with a substantial tolerability.[50]

 **Complete references available online at expertconsult.com.**

References

1. Vorobeychik Y, et al. *CNS Drugs*. 2011;25:1023.
2. Lyon C, et al. *J Fam Pract*. 2018;67(2):110.
3. Fathi M, et al. *Am J Emerg Med*. 2015;33(9):1205.
4. Woo WW, et al. *Ann Emerg Med*. 2005;46(4):352.
5. Duttchen KM, et al. *J Clin Anesth*. 2017;41:11.
6. Dorman RM, et al. *J Pediatr Surg*. 2017.
7. Marzuillo P. *Acta Paediatr*. 2017.
8. Pathan SA, et al. *Eur Urol*. 2017.
9. Walker C, et al. *Postgrad Med*. 2018;130(1):55–71.
10. Aryaie AH, et al. *Surg Endosc*. 2018.
11. Olbrecht VA, et al. *Clin J Pain*. 2017.
12. Artime CA, et al. *J Neurosurg Anesthesiol*. 2017.
13. Sadrolsadat SH, et al. *Anesth Pain Med*. 2017;7(3):e13639.
14. Ohkura Y, et al. *Medicine (Baltimore)*. 2016;95(44):e5352.
15. Ohkura Y, et al. *Surg Today*. 2017.
16. Sun L, et al. *Medicine (Baltimore)*. 2018;97(6):e9751.
17. Chidambaran V, et al. *Paediatr Anaesth*. 2018.
18. Hansen RN, et al. *Curr Med Res Opin*. 2018:1–7.
19. Sola R, et al. *Eur J Pediatr Surg*. 2018.
20. Towers CV, et al. *Am J Obstet Gynecol*. 2017.
21. Huang PS, et al. *J Arthroplasty*. 2017.
22. Bauer AZ, et al. *Horm Behav*. 2018.
23. Mao J, et al. *Anesth Analg*. 2000;91:680.
24. Backonja MM, et al. *JAMA*. 1831;280:1998.
25. Rauck RL, et al. *J Pain Symptom Manage*. 2013;46:219.
26. Beal B, et al. *Clin Interv Aging*. 2012;7:249.
27. Collins SL, et al. *J Pain Symptom Manage*. 2000;20:449.
28. Lesser H, et al. *Neurology*. 2004;63:2104.
29. Boyle J, et al. *Diabetes Care*. 2012;35:2451.
30. Jensen MP, et al. *Clin J Pain*. 2012;28:683.
31. Bialer M. *Adv Drug Deliv Rev*. 2012;64:887.
32. Kothare SV, et al. *Expert Opin Drug Metab Toxicol*. 2008;4:493.
33. Wermeling DP, et al. *Phamacotherapy*. 2005;25:1084.
34. Backonja MM. *Semin Neurol*. 2012;32:264.
35. Michiels WB, et al. *Clin J Pain*. 2011;27:352.
36. Rauck RL, et al. *Pain Pract*. 2009;9:327.
37. Lukyanetz EA, et al. *Epilepsia*. 2002;43:9.
38. Crepeau AZ, et al. *Expert Rev Neurother*. 2010;10:159.
39. Mao J, et al. *Pain*. 2000;87:7.
40. Nikolajsen L, et al. *Clin J Pain*. 2010;26:788.
41. Carroll I, et al. *Clin J Pain*. 2007;23:702.
42. Peterson P, et al. *Neurol Res*. 1986;8:189.
43. Argoff CE, et al. *Curr Med Res Opin*. 2004;20:S21.
44. Jungehulsing GJ, et al. *Eur J Neurol*. 2013;20:331.
45. Holbech JV, et al. *Eur J Pain*. 2011;15:608.
46. O'Connor AB, et al. *Am J Med*. 2009;122:S22.
47. Cruccu G, et al. *CNS Drugs*. 2013;27:91.
48. Wang QP, et al. *CNS Drugs*. 2011;25:847.
49. Wiffen PJ, et al. *Cochrane Database Syst Rev*. 2011;16(2):CD006044.
50. Hershey LA, et al. *Curr Treat Options Neurol*. 2013;15:56.

26 Intravenous Drug Delivery Systems

MICHEL MRF STRUYS, ANTHONY RAY ABSALOM, and
STEVEN L. SHAFER

KEY POINTS

- The pharmacokinetics of anesthetic drugs are described by multicompartment models. Accurate intravenous drug delivery requires adjusting the maintenance infusion rates to take into account the accumulation of the drug in the peripheral tissues.
- *Biophase* is the site of action of a drug. Initiation, maintenance, and titration of intravenous anesthetics must account for the delay in equilibration between plasma and the site of drug effect.
- Some drug effects directly reflect the concentration of the drug in the biophase (direct-effect models). Other drug effects reflect the alteration of feedback systems by anesthetics (indirect-effect models). The influence of opioids on ventilation reflects the dynamic influence of opioids on the feedback between ventilation and carbon dioxide and is thus an example of an indirect drug effect.
- The target concentration in the effect site is the same as the target concentration in plasma at steady state. Effect-site requirements are influenced by patient physiologic characteristics, surgical stimulation, and concurrent drug administration. Ideally, target concentrations should be set for the hypnotic (volatile anesthetic or propofol) and the analgesic (opioid) that properly accounts for the synergy between them.
- To achieve an effective target concentration, the conventional teaching of administering an initial dose as calculated by the product of target concentration and volume of distribution, followed by a maintenance rate as calculated as the product of target concentration and clearance, is inaccurate. The initial dose may be calculated as the product of target concentration and volume of distribution at peak effect. Maintenance rates must initially account for the distribution of drug in peripheral tissues and should only be reduced to the product of target concentration and clearance after equilibration of plasma and peripheral tissue concentrations.
- The terminal half-life does not reflect the clinical time course of drug plasma concentration. The context-sensitive decrement time is the time for a given decrement in drug concentration, as a function of the duration of infusion that maintains a steady plasma concentration. Context-sensitive decrement times properly incorporate the multicompartment behavior of intravenous anesthetics. The context-sensitive half-time is the time for a 50% decrement in concentration.
- Alfentanil, fentanyl, sufentanil, remifentanil, propofol, thiopental, methohexital, etomidate, ketamine, midazolam, and dexmedetomidine can all be administered as a continuous intravenous infusion. Specific caveats, infusion rates, and titration guidelines are presented in this text.
- Target-controlled infusions (TCIs) use pharmacokinetic models to determine intravenous anesthetic administration rates required to achieve specified plasma or effect-site drug concentrations. Various plasma and effect-site targeting TCI systems are commercially available worldwide (except within the United States) to administer hypnotics and opioids.
- Closed-loop drug delivery systems have used the median electroencephalographic frequency, bispectral index (BIS), or auditory-evoked potentials to control intravenous anesthetic delivery. Although these systems have generally performed well clinically, they remain under investigation.

Introduction

Drugs must reach their site of action to be effective. In 1628, William Harvey proved in Exercitatio Anatomica de Motu Cordis et Sanguinis in Animalibus that venous blood was transported to the arterial circulation and thus to body organs by the heart. That drugs injected into veins could be rapidly carried to the entire body was rapidly recognized. Consequently, for intravenous drug delivery to be successful, predictable intravenous access is essential.

The development of intravenous methods of anesthetic drug delivery has been made possible by technologic advances. In the middle of the 17th century, Christopher Wren and his Oxford contemporaries applied a feather quill and animal bladder to inject drugs into dogs and humans and rendered them unconscious. The hollow hypodermic needle and a functional syringe were developed by Frances Rynd (1801–1861) and Charles Pravaz (1791–1853), respectively. Contemporary needles, catheters, and syringes are descendants of these early devices. In the twentieth century, equipment began to be made of plastics, first polyvinyl chloride, then Teflon, and later, polyurethane. In 1950, Massa invented the Rochester needle (Fig. 26.1),[1] which led to the revolutionary concept of the "over-the-needle" catheter, which is still the gold standard for intravenous access for nearly all intravenous drug delivery today.[2]

Although fundamental principles of intravenously administering drugs were known in the 18th century, intravenous induction of anesthesia became common only in the 1930s after the discovery of barbiturates. Maintenance of anesthesia by intravenously administered anesthetics has become practical, safe, and popular in the past 2 decades. Intravenous drugs such as methohexitone and thiopental, although suitable for intravenous induction of anesthesia, are not suitable for use by infusion for the maintenance of anesthesia. In the case of thiopental, accumulation can lead to cardiovascular instability and delayed recovery, whereas methohexitone is associated with the excitatory phenomenon and epileptiform electroencephalographic (EEG) changes. Although the next generation of intravenous drugs, such as ketamine, althesin, and etomidate, possessed desirable pharmacokinetic characteristics, their use has been limited as a result of other side effects, including hallucinations, anaphylaxis, and adrenal suppression, respectively. The discovery of propofol in 1977 provided the anesthetic practice an intravenous drug suitable for both induction and maintenance of anesthesia; currently, propofol is still one of the most frequently used drugs for this purpose.[3] Other drugs suitable for continuous infusion used today are some of the opioids such as alfentanil and sufentanil and certainly the short-acting opioid remifentanil. In addition, some of the nondepolarizing neuromuscular blocking agents are used as continuous infusions in specific situations.

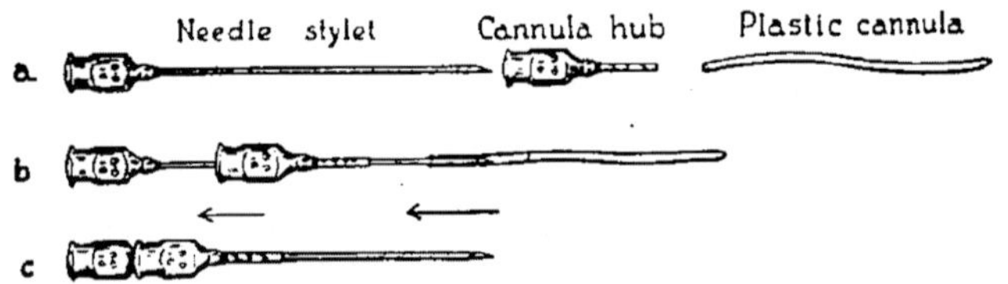

Fig. 26.1 Details of the assembly of the Massa plastic needle, sold by Rochester Products Company, Rochester, Minnesota. (From Massa DJ. A plastic needle. *Anesthesiology.* 1951;12:772–773. Used with permission.)

Drugs are still predominantly injected as a bolus or continuous infusion using standard dosing guidelines, thereby ignoring the large interindividual variability in the dose-response relationship.[4] In contrast to inhaled anesthetics, for which the inspired and end-tidal concentrations can be continuously measured in real time ("online"), the actual plasma or effect organ concentration of an intravenously administered drug is not immediately measurable in clinical practice. Therefore manually adjusting the intravenous drug injection regimens to maintain an online measured plasma concentration is impossible. It becomes even more complex if a specific effect-site concentration is the target. Optimal patient-individual dosing may be achieved by the application of pharmacokinetic-pharmacodynamic principles. Additionally, recent findings suggest that the pharmacokinetic and pharmacodynamic interactions during intravenous administration of various drugs are important and, as such, should be taken into account when optimizing drug administration.[5,6] Computer technology can be used to assist the clinician in titrating intravenous drug administration by using the therapeutic end point as the feedback signal for dosing (Fig. 26.2).

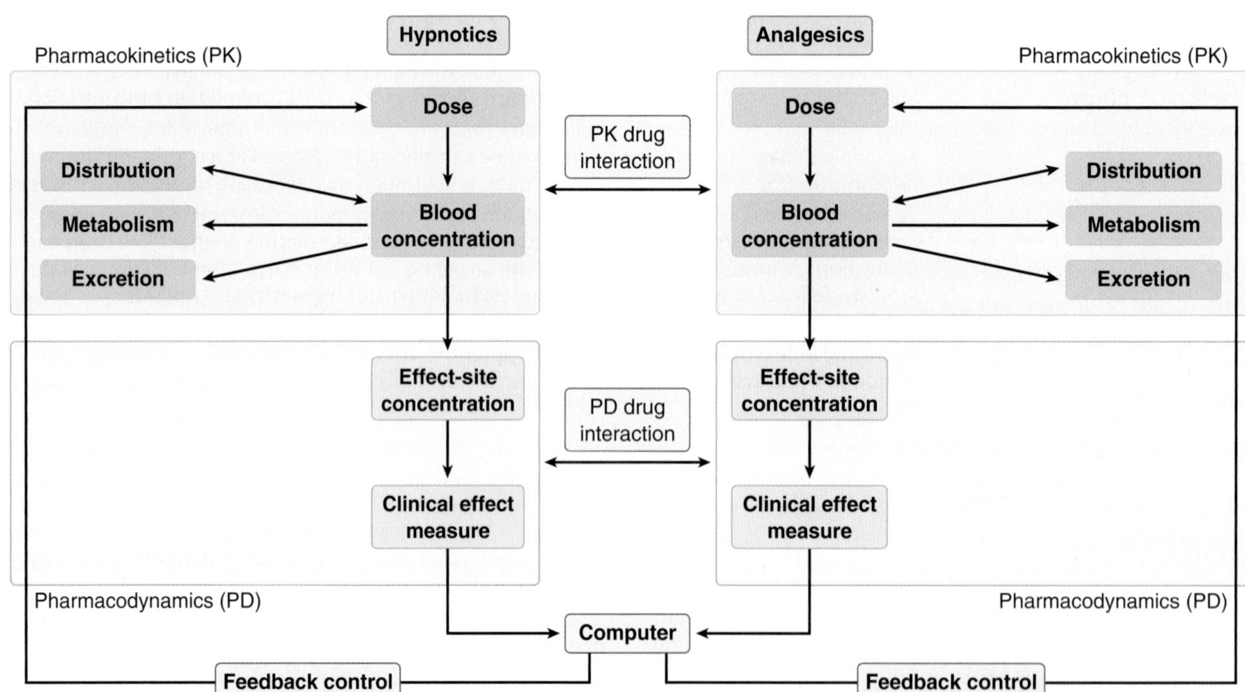

Fig. 26.2 Schematic representation of the dose-response relationship for both hypnotics and opioids. The pharmacokinetic *(PK) (green area)* and the pharmacodynamic *(PD) (yellow area)* parts of this relationship are shown. Closed-loop control of drug administration using the clinical measure is indicated as *feedback control.* PK and PD drug interactions are indicated. (From Sahinovic MM, Absalom AR, Struys MM. Administration and monitoring of intravenous anesthetics. *Curr Opin Anaesthesiol.* 2010;23:734–734. Used with permission.)

The development of the first mechanical syringe pumps in the 1950s improved the quality of intravenous drug administration. A more recent technologic development in intravenous anesthesia is the introduction of computerized pharmacokinetic model–driven continuous-infusion devices, enabling the attainment of desired plasma levels of an intravenous anesthetic drug by using a computer-controlled infusion pump operated in accordance with the published pharmacokinetics of the drug.[7] These efforts have resulted in the release of the first commercial target-controlled infusion (TCI) device in Europe, developed by Zeneca specifically for the administration of propofol. Since that time, several countries (with the exception of the United States) have approved the use of TCI devices for the delivery of anesthetic drugs.[8]

The ultimate development in anesthetic delivery systems will be devices for closed-loop administration of intravenous drugs during anesthesia. Systems have been developed for closed-loop administration of various drugs such as neuromuscular blocking agents, hypnotics, and opioids. The control variables for these systems have included various pharmacodynamic measures derived from techniques such as acceleromyography, automated blood pressure measurement, and electroencephalography.

The dose-response relationship can be divided into three parts (see Fig. 26.2): (1) the time course of the relationship between the given dose and the plasma concentration is defined as pharmacokinetics, (2) the relationship between the plasma concentration and/or effect-organ concentration and the clinical effect is defined as pharmacodynamics, and (3) the coupling between pharmacokinetics and pharmacodynamics is required when the blood is not the site of drug effect.

Before reviewing delivery techniques and devices for intravenous anesthesia, this chapter presents some pharmacokinetic and pharmacodynamic principles as background for understanding how to administer intravenous drugs to their best advantage. Further discussion of the principles of pharmacokinetics and pharmacodynamics can be found in Chapter 23.

Pharmacokinetic Considerations

The aim of optimal intravenous drug dosing is to reach and maintain a desired time course of therapeutic drug effect as accurately as possible, thereby preventing dose-related adverse drug effects. To be useful in anesthesia, this time course should include a rapid onset of clinical effects, smooth maintenance, and fast recovery after the termination of drug administration. The pharmacokinetics of many intravenous drugs can be described using mammillary multicompartment pharmacokinetic models. These models assume that the drug is directly given and mixed in the plasma, resulting in an immediate peak in its plasma concentration.

The easiest clinical technique is to administer a single dose, calculated to keep the plasma concentration above the therapeutic target concentration for the required time (Fig. 26.3). A constant concentration cannot be maintained, but it should not decrease to less than the therapeutic concentration. Unfortunately, when one single bolus is used, the initial dose must be large enough to maintain a concentration above the lowest therapeutic concentration even at the end of surgery. However, this sometimes very large dose of drug may cause numerous side effects attributable to the initially high concentrations in the body. It might be less harmful to keep the drug concentration above the lowest therapeutic level without very high initial concentrations by repeatedly injecting smaller doses; even with this technique, however, maintaining a stable plasma concentration is still impossible.

To produce a time course of drug effect that follows the time course of anesthetic requirement, a continuous infusion titrated to the perceived anesthetic requirement should be used. Typically, just enough amount of drug is given to achieve the therapeutic blood or plasma drug concentration. Drug administration thereafter should be continuously titrated throughout surgery. Although such a regimen does not overshoot the required concentration (and therefore avoids the risk of concentration-related side effects), yet another difficulty exists. Whereas, the large bolus approach produces an effective concentration (EC) from the onset, albeit with an excessive overshoot, a continuous infusion takes a long time to become effective because of the slow increase in concentration. Reaching steady state (see Fig. 26.3) takes a very long time during which the increase in concentration is rapid at first but then slows down as equilibrium is approached. For example, it will take longer than 1 hour for the propofol infusion to generate a plasma concentration that is at least 95% of the steady-state concentration. Consequently, although simple infusions are obviously very effective for maintaining constant blood concentrations once steady state is reached and for avoiding overshoot, infusions do not offer a clinically realistic approach. Therefore a combination of an initial bolus followed by a stepwise decreasing continuous infusion is more useful.[9,10]

Pharmacokinetic models can be used to calculate the required drug-dosing regimen to reach and maintain a therapeutic drug concentration as fast as possible without overshooting or accumulation. In this chapter, an explanation of how pharmacokinetic models can be used to calculate accurate dosing schemes for use with intravenous drug delivery systems is offered.

Pharmacokinetic models are mathematical descriptions of how the body *disposes* of drugs. The parameters describing this process are estimated by administering a known dose of the drug and measuring the resulting plasma concentrations. A mathematical model then relates the input over time, I(t), with the concentrations over time, C(t). These models can take many forms. Fig. 26.4 shows concentrations in plasma and effect site over time after a single intravenous bolus of drug at time 0. Drug concentrations continuously decrease after the bolus, and the rate of decrease is approximately proportional to the amount of drug in plasma. Typically, this behavior can be described with the use of exponential models. The curve might have a single exponent, in which case the plasma concentrations over time might be described by the function $C(t) = Ae^{-kt}$, where A is the concentration at time 0 and k is a constant that describes the rate of decrease in concentration. The relationship appears to be a straight line when graphed as the log of concentration versus time. The pharmacokinetics

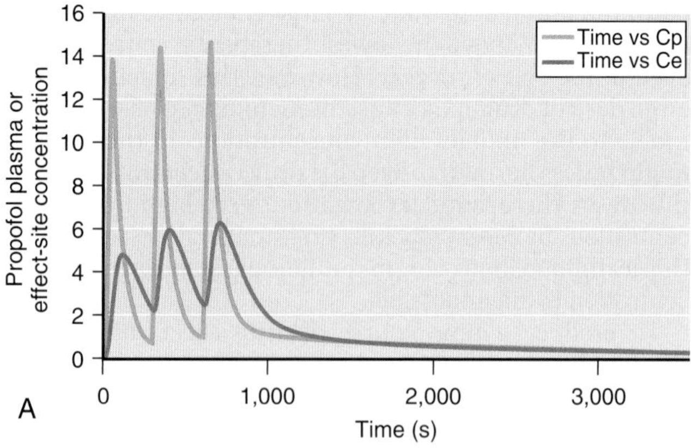

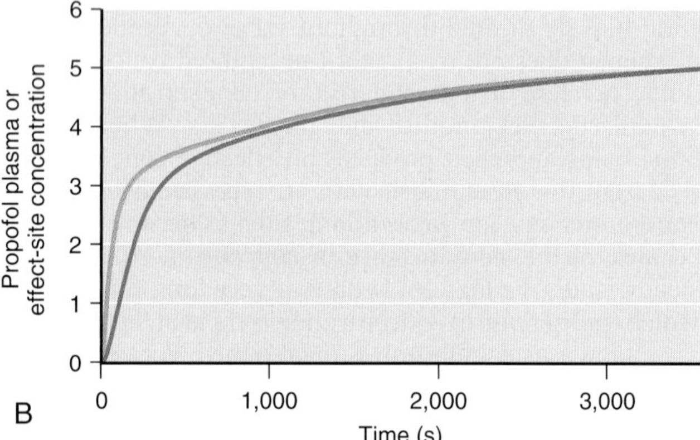

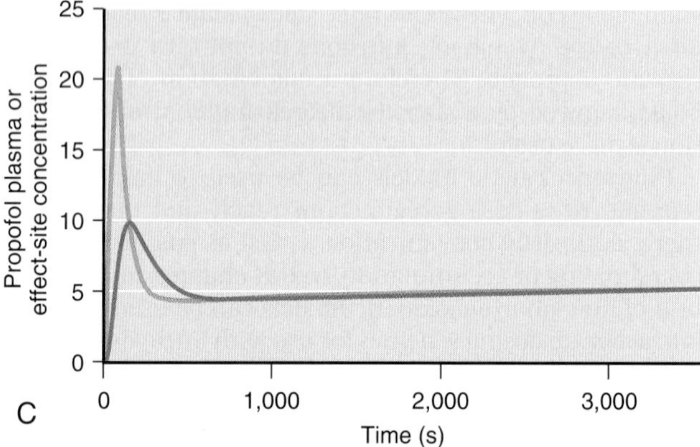

Fig. 26.3 Predicted propofol plasma concentration *(Cp)* and effect-site concentration *(Ce)* for a repeated bolus dose (1 mg/kg given at time 0 and after 5 and 10 minutes) (A), continuous infusion (10 mg/kg/h) (B), and a bolus (2 mg/kg) followed by a continuous infusion (10 mg/kg/h) (C). Simulated patient is a man, 45 years of age, 80 kg, 175 cm; Schnider model.

of intravenous anesthetic drugs is more complex because after the bolus, a period of rapid decline is observed before the terminal *log-linear* portion (i.e., the part that is a straight line when described as log concentration vs. time). This process can be modeled by taking several monoexponential curves and adding them together. The result is a polyexponential curve. For example, the concentrations after an intravenous bolus might be described by an equation with two exponents, $C(t) = Ae^{-}\alpha^{t} + Be^{-}\beta^{t}$, or an equation with three exponents, $C(t) = Ae^{-}\alpha^{t} + Be^{-}\beta^{t} + Ce^{-}\gamma^{t}$.

The aforementioned is applied to single bolus dosing, which is, of course, only one way of administering intravenous anesthetic drugs. A more general way to think of pharmacokinetics is to decompose the input into a series of small bits (boluses) and consider each bit of drug separately. The general pharmacokinetic model of drug disposition commonly used in anesthesia independently considers each bit of drug and analyzes its contribution by means of polyexponential decay over time. The formal mathematic description of each bit of drug in terms of polyexponential decay over time is the relationship (Eq. 26.1)

$$C(t) = I(t) * \sum_{i=1}^{n} A_i e^{-\lambda_i t} \tag{26.1}$$

where C(t) is the plasma concentration at time t and I(t) is drug input (i.e., a bolus or infusion). The summation after the asterisk (described later in this chapter) is the function describing how each bit of drug is disposed (hence the name, *disposition function*). Note that this is again a sum of *n* exponentials, as described in the previous paragraph.

Pharmacokinetic modeling is the process of estimating the parameters within this function. The integer *n* is the number of exponentials (i.e., compartments) and is usually two or three. Each exponential term is associated with a coefficient A_i and an exponent λ_i. The λ values are inversely proportional to the half-lives (half-life = ln 2/λ = 0.693/λ), with the smallest λ representing the longest (terminal) half-life. The A values are the relative contribution of each half-life to overall drug disposition. If a drug has a very long terminal half-life but a coefficient that is significantly smaller than the other coefficients, then the long half-life is likely to be clinically meaningless. Conversely, if a drug has a very long half-life with a relatively large coefficient, then the drug will be long lasting even after brief administration. The asterisk (*) operator is the mathematic process called *convolution*, which is simply the process of breaking the infusion into *bits* of drug and then adding up the results to observe the overall concentrations resulting from the disposition of the different bits up to a time point t.

The pharmacokinetic model shown has some useful characteristics that account for its enduring popularity in pharmacokinetic analysis. Most important, the model describes observations from studies reasonably well, the *sine qua non* for models. Second, these models have the useful characteristic of *linearity*. Simply stated, if the dose, I, is doubled (e.g., administering a bolus twice as large or an infusion twice as fast), then the resulting concentrations should be doubled.

More generally, linearity implies that the system (i.e., the body acting to produce a plasma drug concentration output from a drug dosage input) behaves in accordance with the principle of superposition. The superposition principle states that the response of a linear system with multiple inputs can be computed by determining the response to each individual input and then summing the individual responses. In other words, when the body treats each bit of drug by polyexponential decay over time, the *disposing* of each bit of drug does not influence the disposing of other bits of drug.

The third reason for the continuing popularity of these models is that they can be mathematically transformed from the admittedly nonintuitive exponential form shown

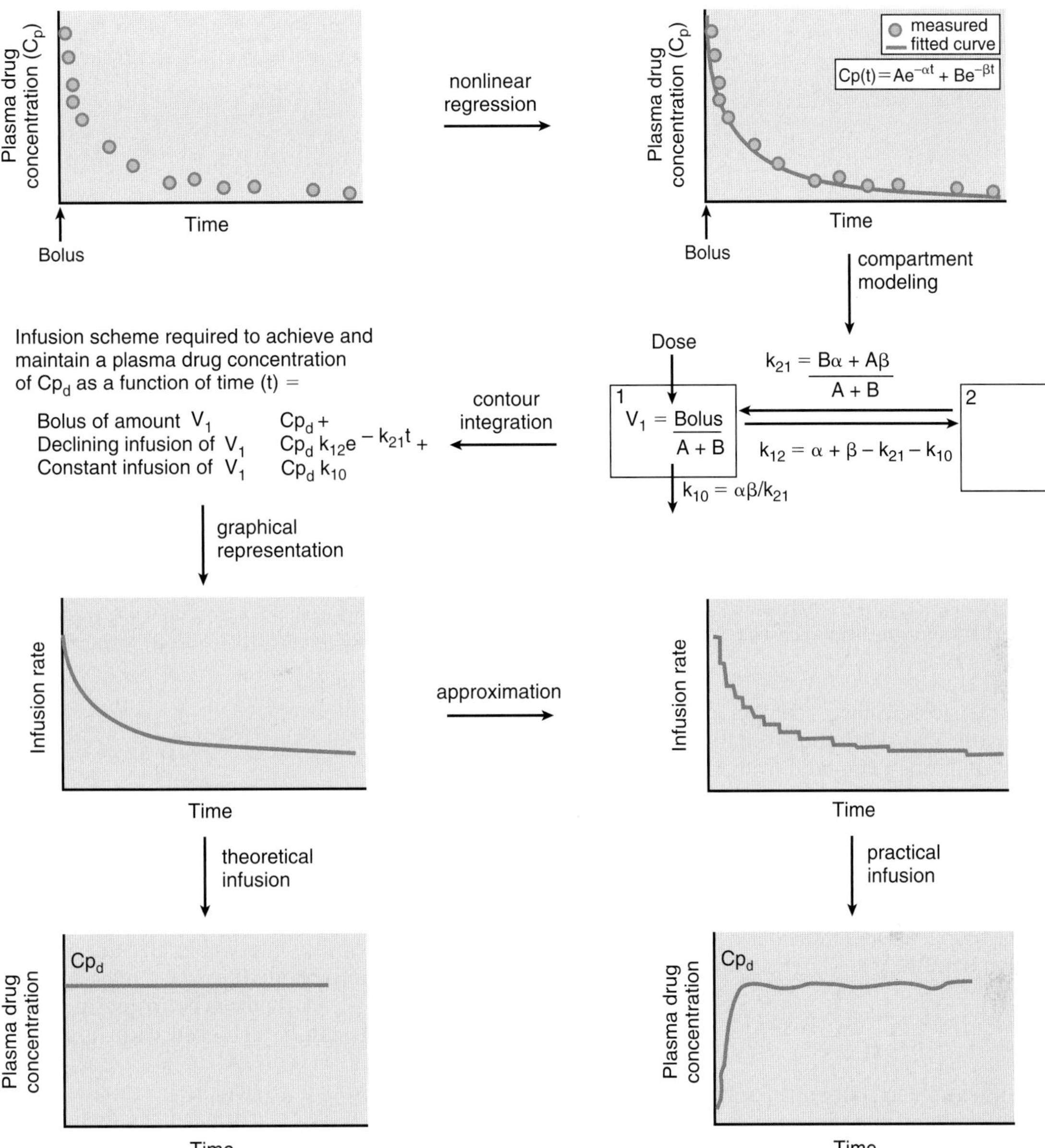

Fig. 26.4 Steps involved in pharmacokinetic model–driven infusion. Typically, pharmacokinetic models are derived from experiments in which plasma drug concentrations are measured at intervals after bolus administration of the drug. Nonlinear regression is used to fit a monoexponential, biexponential, or triexponential curve to the resulting concentration-versus-time data. An algebraic relationship exists between the exponential decay curves and a one-, two-, or three-compartment pharmacokinetic model. The bolus-elimination-transfer (BET) infusion scheme is developed and consists of a bolus, a continuous infusion to replace drug eliminated from the body, and an exponentially declining infusion to replace drug transferred out of plasma to other body compartments. BET infusion results in the maintenance of a constant specified plasma drug concentration. Practical implementation of the BET scheme with real infusion pumps and infusion rates that change only at discrete intervals of time results in a plasma drug concentration profile that approximates that resulting from a BET infusion.

earlier to a more intuitive compartment form (Fig. 26.5). The fundamental parameters of the compartment model are the volumes of distribution (central, rapidly equilibrating, and slowly equilibrating peripheral volumes) and clearances (systemic, rapid, and slow intercompartment). The central compartment (V_1) represents a distribution volume and includes the rapidly mixing portion of the blood and first-pass pulmonary uptake. The peripheral compartments are made up of tissues and organs that show a time course and extent of drug accumulation (or dissipation) different from that of the central compartment. In the three-compartment model, the two peripheral compartments may roughly correspond to splanchnic and muscle tissues (rapidly equilibrating) and fat stores (slowly equilibrating). The sum of the compartment volumes is the apparent volume of distribution at steady state (Vd_{ss}) and is the proportionality constant relating the plasma drug concentration at steady state to the total amount of drug in the body. The intercompartment rate constants (k_{12}, k_{21}, and so on) describe the movement of drug between the central and peripheral compartments. The elimination rate constant (k_{10}) encompasses processes acting through biotransformation or elimination that irreversibly removes drug from the central compartment.

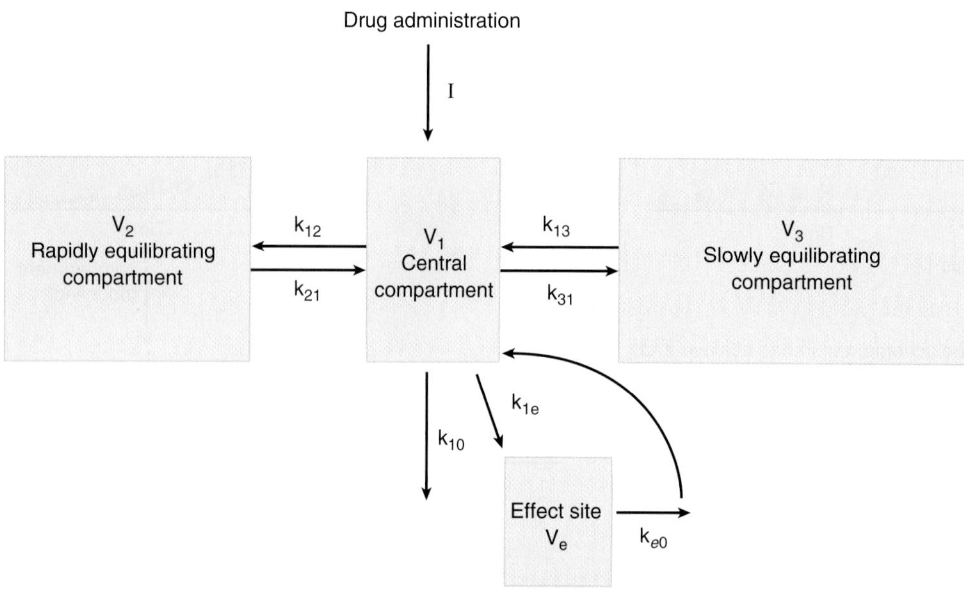

Fig. 26.5 Three-compartment model (including the biophase) illustrating the basic pharmacokinetic processes that occur after intravenous drug administration. *I*, Dosing scheme as a function of time; k_{10}, rate constant reflecting all processes acting to remove drug irreversibly from the central compartment; *k*, intercompartment rate constants; V_1, central compartment volume, usually expressed in liters or liters per kilogram.

Despite their physiologic flavor, compartment models are simply mathematic transformations of the polyexponential disposition functions computed from observed plasma concentrations. Thus physiologic interpretation of volumes and clearances (with the possible exception of systemic clearance and Vd_{ss} [the algebraic sum of the volumes]) is entirely speculative.

The last reason behind the popularity of these models is that they can be used to design infusion regimens. If the disposition function (Eq. 26.2)

$$\sum_{i=1}^{n} A_i e^{-\lambda_i t} \tag{26.2}$$

is abbreviated as simply D(t), then the relationship among concentration, dose, and the pharmacokinetic model D(t) can be rewritten as (Eq. 26.3)

$$C(t) = I(t) * D(t) \tag{26.3}$$

where * is the convolution operator, as noted earlier. In the usual pharmacokinetic study, I(t) is known, the dose that is given the patient, and C(t) is measured, the concentrations over time. The goal is to find D(t), the pharmacokinetic disposition function. Pharmacokinetic analysis can be thought of as a simple rearrangement of Eq. 26.3 to solve for D(t) (Eq. 26.4)

$$D(t) = \frac{C(t)}{I(t)} \tag{26.4}$$

where the symbol →← means *deconvolution*, the inverse operation of convolution. Deconvolution is similar to division, but of functions rather than simple numbers. When dosing regimens are designed from known pharmacokinetic models and a desired course for the plasma concentration over time, the known values are D(t) (the pharmacokinetics) and $C_T(t)$ (the desired target concentrations), and the drug dosing scheme is (Eq. 26.5)

$$I(t) = \frac{C_T(t)}{D(t)} \tag{26.5}$$

Thus the necessary infusion rates, I(t), can be calculated, given the desired target concentrations, $C_T(t)$, and the pharmacokinetics, D(t), by applying the same tools used to calculate the original pharmacokinetics. Unfortunately, such a solution might require some negative infusion rates, which are obviously impossible. Because a drug cannot be retracted from the body (i.e., give inverse infusions), clinicians must restrict themselves to plasma concentrations over time that can be achieved with noninverse infusion rates.

The standard pharmacokinetic model has one glaring shortcoming. It assumes that after a bolus injection there is complete mixing within the central compartment such that the peak concentration occurs precisely at time 0. It actually takes approximately 30 to 45 seconds for the drug to make its transit from the venous injection site to the arterial circulation. This model misspecification over the first minute or so may not seem significant, but it can cause problems in attempts to relate the drug effect after a bolus to drug concentrations in the body,[11] which becomes even more important when using effect-site TCI.[12] The standard polyexponential pharmacokinetic models are being modified to provide more accurate models of plasma drug concentration in the first minute after bolus injection, also taking into account infusion rate. Recently, Masui and associates[13] found that a pharmacokinetic model consisting of a two-compartment model with a LAG (the time shift of dosing as if the drug were, in fact, administered to the pharmacokinetic model at a later time) and presystemic compartments model accurately described the early pharmacologic phase of propofol during infusion rates between 10 and 160 mg/kg/h. The infusion rate has an influence on kinetics. Age was a covariate for LAG time (Fig. 26.6). Besides compartment models, various physiologically based

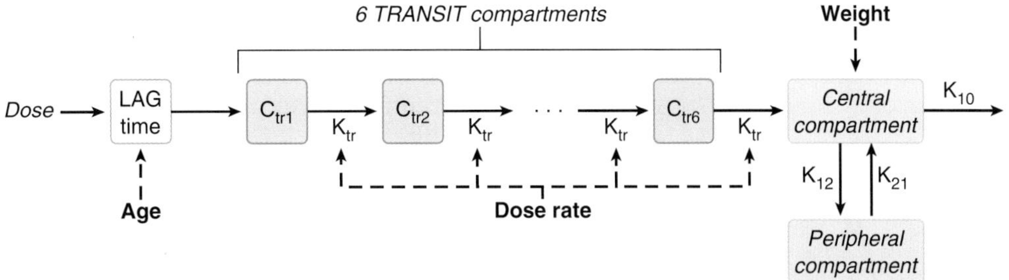

Fig. 26.6 Scheme of the final two-compartment pharmacokinetic model with a LAG time and six TRANSIT compartments (C_{tr} *n*). The equilibration rate constants between the central and peripheral compartments were calculated using the following equations: $k_{12} = C_{l2} \div V_1$, $k_{21} = Cl_2 \div V_2$. The elimination rate constant was calculated using the following equation: $k_{10} = Cl_1 \div V_1$. Cl_1, Clearance of central compartment; Cl_2, clearance of peripheral compartment; V_1, distribution volume of central compartment; V_2, distribution volume of peripheral compartment. LAG time represents the time shift of dosing as if the drug was, in fact, administered to the pharmacokinetic model at a later time. TRANSIT compartments depict a multiple-step process represented by a chain of presystemic compartments. (From Masui K, Kira M, Kazama T, et al. Early phase pharmacokinetics but not pharmacodynamics are influenced by propofol infusion rate. *Anesthesiology*. 2009;111:805–817. Used with permission.)

models have been developed to model the pharmacokinetic behavior of anesthetics.[14] So far, these models are not superior at predicting the time course of drug concentration.[13] None of these models have been used to control intravenous drug delivery devices.

Pharmacodynamic Considerations

THE BIOPHASE

The goal of drug titration during anesthesia is to reach and maintain a stable therapeutic drug concentration at the site of drug effect, also defined as the *effect site* or *biophase*. For most drugs used in anesthesia, the plasma is not the biophase and thus even after the drug has reached the arterial circulation, a further delay occurs before a therapeutic effect is observed. The reason is that additional time is required for the drug to be transported to the target organ, penetrate the tissue, bind to a receptor, and induce intercellular processes that ultimately lead to the onset of drug effect. This delay between peak plasma concentration and peak concentration at the effect site is called *hysteresis*. Fig. 26.7 illustrates an example of hysteresis revealed during an experiment published by Soehle and coworkers.[15] Two periods of continuous propofol infusions were given. The time course of the plasma concentration and effect-site concentration are simulated using pharmacokinetic and pharmacodynamic models. The cerebral drug effect was measured using the EEG-derived bispectral index (BIS). A clear delay between the time course of the plasma concentration and that of the BIS can be observed. The plasma concentration versus effect curve forms a counterclockwise hysteresis loop. This loop represents the plasma concentration, which is not the site of drug effect. Using nonlinear mixed-effect modeling, the hysteresis is minimized to reveal the effect-site concentration versus clinical effect relationship. The typical sigmoidal population model is also depicted in Fig. 26.7.

The concentration of drug in the biophase cannot be measured because it is usually inaccessible, at least in human subjects. The time course of drug effect can be calculated by using rapid measures of drug effect. Knowing the time course of drug effect, the rate of drug flow in and out of the biophase (or effect site) can be calculated with the use of mathematic models. As such, the time course of the plasma concentration and the measured effect can be linked using the concept of the *effect compartment*, developed by Hull[16] and Sheiner.[17] The effect-site concentration is not a real measurable concentration but rather a virtual concentration in a theoretic compartment without a volume and, as such, also without any significant amount of drug present. For any concentration in this virtual compartment, a corresponding assumed effect is observed. This relationship between the effect-site concentration and effect is usually nonlinear and static (i.e., does not explicitly depend on time). If the plasma concentration is maintained at a constant level, then the model assumes that, at equilibrium, the effect-compartment concentration equals the plasma concentration. The delay between the plasma and the effect compartment is mathematically described by a single parameter, defined as k_{e0}, the effect-site equilibration rate constant (see Fig. 26.5).[18]

Measures of drug effect used to characterize the time course of drug transfer between plasma and the biophase vary with the drug being evaluated. For some drugs, a direct measure of drug effect can be applied. For neuromuscular blocking agents, the response from peripheral nerve stimulation (i.e., the twitch) is an ideal measure of effect. Various authors have used the T1% (percentage change of the T1 response compared with baseline T1 response during supramaximal stimulus) derived from electromyogram to measure the drug effect of newer drugs such as rocuronium[19] and cisatracurium.[20] For other categories of drugs such as opioids and hypnotics, the real clinical effects (e.g., unconsciousness, amnesia, memory loss, antinociception) are not measurable. For these reasons, surrogate measures are used to quantify the time course of clinical effects. These surrogate measures can be categorical or continuous. For example, the Observer's Assessment of Alertness/Sedation (OAA/S) scale was used to measure quantal changes in hypnotic drug effects during propofol administration.[21] Egan and colleagues[22] applied a noxious pain stimulus and used an algometer to measure the balance between nociception and antinociception during remifentanil infusion. Various spontaneous and evoked EEG-derived and processed measures were used to measure cerebral drug effects for opioids and hypnotics.[15,23-27] Ludbrook and associates measured propofol concentrations in the carotid artery and

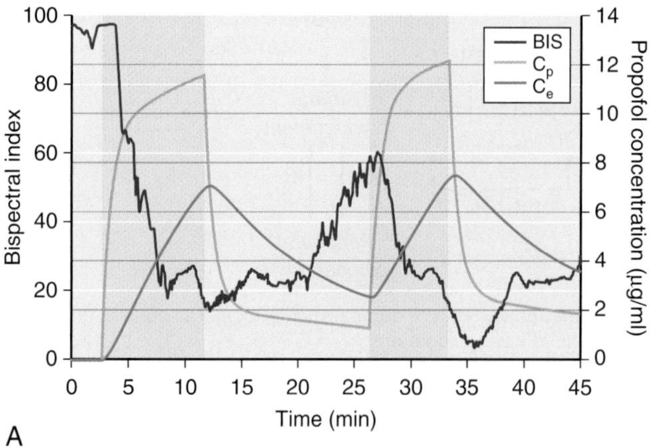

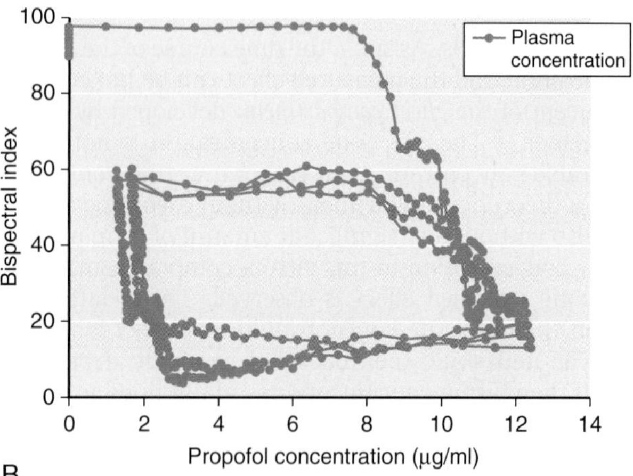

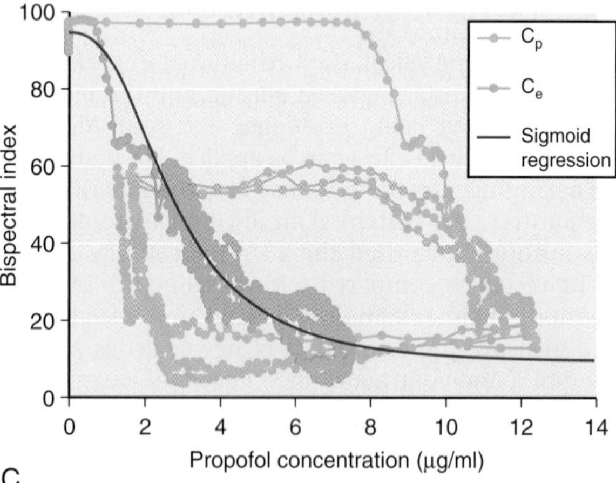

Fig. 26.7 (A) Time course of an experiment showing the hysteresis between plasma concentration *(C_p)* and hypnotic effect as measured by the electroencephalographic (EEG)-derived bispectral index (BIS). Propofol was given at a constant rate during the shaded periods, resulting in C_p *(orange line)* and effect-site concentration *(C_e) (blue line)*. The corresponding BIS values are shown as a *solid red line*. (B) Relation between C_p and BIS using data from the experiment reveals a hysteresis loop. (C) After modeling, this hysteresis is minimized as shown in the relation between the effect-site concentration and BIS. ([A] Modified from Soehle M, Kuech M, Grube M, et al. Patient state index vs bispectral index as measures of the electroencephalographic effects of propofol. *Br J Anaesth*. 2010;105:172–178. Used with permission; [B and C] Courtesy M. Soehle, Bonn, Germany.)

jugular bulb to establish movement of propofol into and equilibration with the brain. They simultaneously measured the BIS and found a close correlation between brain concentration (calculated by mass balance) and changes in the BIS.[28]

DIRECT-EFFECT MODELS

As with plasma pharmacokinetics, the biophase concentration is the convolution of an input function (in this case, the plasma drug concentration over time) and the disposition function of the biophase. This relationship can be expressed as (Eq. 26.6)

$$C_{biophase}(t) = C_{plasma}(t) * D_{biophase}(t) \qquad (26.6)$$

The disposition function of the biophase is typically modeled as a single exponential decay (Eq. 26.7)

$$D_{biophase}(t) = K_{e0}e^{-K_{e0}t} \qquad (26.7)$$

The monoexponential disposition function implies that the effect site is simply an additional compartment in the standard compartment model that is connected to the plasma compartment (see Fig. 26.5). The effect site is the hypothetical compartment that relates the time course of plasma drug concentration to the time course of drug effect, and k_{e0} is the rate constant of elimination of drug from the effect site. By convention, the effect compartment is assumed to receive such small amounts of drug from the central compartment that it has no influence on plasma pharmacokinetics.

Neither $C_{biophase}(t)$ nor $D_{biophase}(t)$ can be directly measured, but the drug effect can be measured. Knowing that the observed drug effect is a function of the drug concentration in the biophase, the drug effect can be predicted as (Eq. 26.8)

$$Effect = f_{PD}\left[C_{plasma}(t) * D_{biophase}(t),\ P_{PD},\ k_{e0}\right] \qquad (26.8)$$

where f_{PD} is a pharmacodynamic model (typically sigmoidal in shape), P_{PD} represents the parameters of the pharmacodynamic model, and k_{e0} is the rate constant for equilibration between plasma and the biophase. Nonlinear regression programs are used to find values of P_{PD} and k_{e0} that best predict the time course of drug effect. This method is called *loop-collapsing* (see Fig. 26.7). Knowledge of these parameters can then be incorporated into dosing regimens that produce the desired time course of drug effect.[29,30]

If a constant plasma concentration is maintained, then the time required for the biophase concentration to reach 50% of the plasma concentration ($t_{1/2}k_{e0}$) can be calculated as $0.693/k_{e0}$. After a bolus dose, the time to peak biophase concentration is a function of both plasma pharmacokinetics and k_{e0}. For drugs with a very rapid decline in plasma concentration after a bolus (e.g., adenosine with a half-life of several seconds), the effect-site concentration peaks within several seconds of the bolus, regardless of k_{e0}. For drugs with a rapid k_{e0} and a slow decrease in concentration after a bolus injection (e.g., pancuronium), the peak effect-site concentration is determined more by k_{e0} than by plasma pharmacokinetics.

An accurate estimation of k_{e0} demands an integrated pharmacokinetic-pharmacodynamic study combining rapid blood sampling with frequent measurements of drug effect, yielding an overall model for the dose-response behavior of the drug. Historically, the time constants of pharmacokinetic models and the k_{e0} of pharmacodynamic studies were sometimes naively merged, possibly leading to inaccurate predictions of the clinical drug effect. Coppens and colleagues proved that pharmacodynamic models of BIS in children developed by using estimates of plasma propofol concentrations from published pharmacokinetic models and estimating the pharmacodynamic model do not ensure good pharmacokinetic accuracy or provide informative estimates for pharmacodynamic parameters.[31] If no integrated pharmacokinetic-pharmacodynamic model exists, then the time to peak effect (t_{peak}) after a bolus injection can be used to recalculate k_{e0} using the pharmacokinetic model of interest to yield the correct time to peak effect. Under these circumstances, this alternative approach might lead to a more accurate prediction of the dose-response time course.[32,33] However, the correct covariates for t_{peak} should be estimated in a specific population.[34] A second caveat is that the time course of drug effect is specific for a given effect (e.g., cerebral drug effect as measured by a specific processed EEG). The time course of other side effects (e.g., hemodynamic effect for hypnotics) most frequently follows a different trajectory.[35,36] The time to peak effect and the $t_{1/2}$ k_{e0} for several intravenous anesthetics are listed in Table 26.1.

All methods discussed so far incorporate k_{e0} values calculated on the assumption that hysteresis between plasma concentration and clinical effect is explained by a delay in drug transfer between plasma and biophase and thus that anesthesia is a smooth, path- and state-independent, symmetric process. Although still commonly used, this assumption might be suboptimal. Data from animal experiments suggest that neural processes and pathways involved in anesthesia induction and recovery are different.[37,38] In an animal study, measured brain drug concentrations at loss of consciousness and at return of consciousness were significantly different.[39] If these data are confirmed, then a more complex model (e.g., one incorporating a second, serial effect-site model) might be required to depict the time course of drug effect. Several groups have investigated this hypothesis in humans, and so far the published findings are not consistent. One clinical study specifically designed to address this topic showed evidence supportive of the concept of neural inertia.[40] Two other studies involving secondary analyses of existing data, of which one indicated supportive evidence[41] and the other showed that neural inertia was not present in all subjects, and appeared to occur only with propofol (and not with sevoflurane), and to be present only with certain pharmacodynamic endpoints.[42]

TABLE 26.1 Time to Peak Effect and $t_{1/2}$ k_{e0} After a Bolus Dose

Drug	Time to Peak Drug Effect (min)*	$t_{1/2}$ k_{e0} (min)
Morphine	19	264
Fentanyl	3.6	4.7
Alfentanil	1.4	0.9
Sufentanil	5.6	3.0
Remifentanil	1.8	1.3
Ketamine	—	3.5
Propofol	1.6	1.7
Thiopental	1.6	1.5
Midazolam	2.8	4.0
Etomidate	2.0	1.5

*Measured by electroencephalography.

k_{e0} is the rate constant for transfer of drug from the site of drug effect to the environment.

$t_{1/2}$ k_{e0} = 0.693/k_{e0}

INDIRECT-EFFECT MODELS

Thus far, clinical effects that are an instantaneous function of drug concentration at the site of drug effect have been discussed, as implied by Eq. 26.8. For example, once a hypnotic drug reaches the brain or a neuromuscular-blocking drug reaches the muscles, drug action is almost immediately observed. On the other hand, some effects are significantly more complex. For example, consider the effect of opioids on ventilation. Initially, opioids depress ventilation, and arterial tension of carbon dioxide (CO_2) gradually accumulates. Yet, the accumulation of CO_2 at normal conditions is a strong stimulant for ventilation, thereby partly counteracting the ventilatory depressant effects of opioids. Ventilatory depression is an example in which direct and indirect drug effects are incorporated. The direct effect of the opioid is to depress ventilation, and the indirect effect is to increase arterial tension of CO_2. Modeling the time course of opioid-induced ventilatory depression requires consideration of both components. Bouillon and colleagues developed a model of ventilatory depression that incorporates both direct and indirect effects.[43-45] As is generally the case with indirect-effect models, characterizing drug-induced ventilatory depression requires a consideration of the entire time course of drug therapy, which is embodied by the following differential equation (Eq. 26.9):

$$\frac{d}{dt}PaCO_2 = k_{el} \bullet \left[1-\frac{Cp\,(t)\,\gamma}{C_{50}\gamma + C_p\,(t)\,\gamma}\right] \bullet \left[\frac{P_{biophase}\,CO_2\,(t)}{P_{biophase}\,CO_2\,(0)}\right]^F \bullet PaCO_2\,(t) \qquad (26.9)$$

where partial pressure of arterial carbon dioxide ($PaCO_2$) is arterial CO_2, $P_{biophase}CO_2$ is CO_2 in the biophase (i.e., brainstem respiratory control circuits), k_{el} is the rate constant for the elimination of CO_2, C_{50} is the effect-site opioid concentration associated with a 50% reduction in ventilatory drive, and F is the steepness or *gain* of the effect of CO_2 on ventilatory drive.

DOSE IMPLICATIONS OF THE BIOPHASE

The delay in onset of clinical effects has important clinical implications. After a bolus, the plasma concentration peaks nearly instantly and then steadily declines. The effect-site concentration starts at zero and increases over time until it equals the descending plasma concentration. The plasma concentration continues to decline. After the moment of identical concentrations, the gradient between plasma and the biophase favors removal of drug from the biophase, and the effect-site concentration decreases. The rate at which the effect-site concentration rises toward the peak after a bolus dictates how much drug must be injected into plasma to produce a given effect. For alfentanil, its rapid plasma effect-site equilibration (large k_{e0}) causes the effect-site concentration to rise rapidly, with a peak produced in approximately 90 seconds. At the time of the peak, approximately 60% of the alfentanil bolus has been distributed into peripheral tissues or eliminated from the body. For fentanyl, the effect-site concentration rises significantly more slowly and peaks 3 to 4 minutes after the bolus.[46] At the time of the peak, more than 80% of the initial bolus of fentanyl has been distributed into tissues or eliminated. As a result of slower equilibration with the biophase, relatively more fentanyl than alfentanil must be injected into plasma, which makes the rate of offset of drug effect after a fentanyl bolus slower than after an alfentanil bolus.

This difference in pharmacokinetics indicates that k_{e0} must be incorporated into dosing strategies on which rational drug selection is dependent. For rapid onset of effect, a drug with a large k_{e0} (short $t_{1/2}$ k_{e0}) should be chosen. For example, for rapid sequence induction of anesthesia, alfentanil or remifentanil may be the optimal opioid because its peak effect-site concentration coincides with the likely time of endotracheal intubation. However, for a slower induction of anesthesia in which a nondepolarizing neuromuscular blocking agent is used, an opioid with a slower onset of drug effect should be selected to coincide with the peak effect of the neuromuscular blocking agent. In this case, a bolus of fentanyl or sufentanil at the time of induction may be more appropriate. The time to peak effect for the commonly used opioids is shown in Fig. 26.8. Knowing k_{e0} (or time to peak effect) also improves titration of the drug by identifying the time at which the clinician should make an assessment of drug effect. For example, midazolam has a slow time to peak effect, and repeat bolus doses should be spaced at least 3 to 5 minutes apart to avoid inadvertent overdosing.

An accurate k_{e0} is also crucial during TCI titrating to a specific effect-site concentration because the initial bolus given to reach the targeted effect-site concentration depends on both the pharmacokinetics and the k_{e0}.[47]

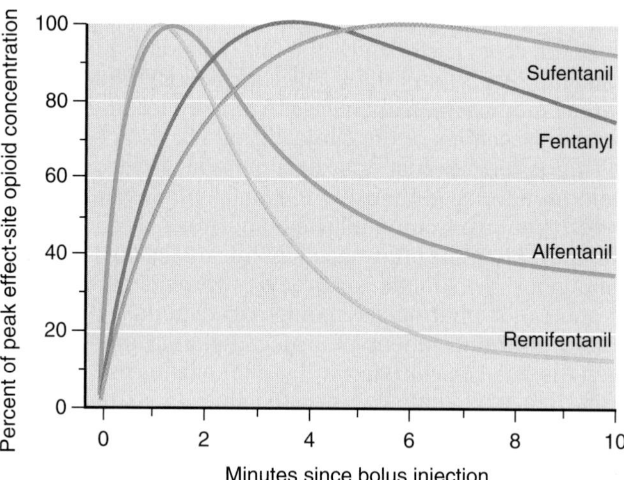

Fig. 26.8 Simulated onset and time to peak effect of commonly used opioids based on their k_{e0} and pharmacokinetic parameters. k_{e0}, Rate constant for the transfer of drug from the site of drug effect to the environment.

DRUG POTENCY

Single Drugs

Knowledge about adequate therapeutic drug concentration is crucial to achieve the aim of providing optimal anesthetic conditions. Therefore information on drug potency is essential. Analogous to the concept of minimum alveolar concentration (MAC), the concentration associated with a 50% likelihood of movement in response to skin incision for inhaled anesthetics[48] is the C_{50} for intravenous drugs, which provides a measure of relative potency between intravenous anesthetics.

There are many ways to look upon C_{50}, taking into consideration whether the clinical effect is a binary or continuous effect. When considering binary effects, the C_{50} might be the drug concentration that prevents response (e.g., movement, hypertension, release of catecholamines) to a particular stimulus (e.g., surgical incision, endotracheal intubation, spreading of the sternum) in 50% of patients. In this case, each combination of stimulus and response may have a unique C_{50}. When C_{50} is defined as the drug concentration that produces a given response in 50% of patients, a 50% probability of response is also likely in a given patient. Defining C_{50} as the concentration that produces a given drug effect in 50% of individuals implicitly assumes that the effect can be achieved in all individuals. Some drugs exhibit a ceiling effect. For example, a ceiling effect may exist on the ability of opioids to suppress response to noxious stimulation. When a ceiling in drug effect exists, some patients may not exhibit the drug effect even at infinitely large doses. In this case, C_{50} is not the concentration that causes the drug effect in 50% of patients but is the concentration associated with the drug effect in one half of whatever fraction of patients is able to respond.

Several studies have been performed to establish appropriate concentrations of intravenous anesthetics and opioids for various clinical endpoints and the effect of drug interactions (Table 26.2).[49-56]

Another interpretation of C_{50} is the concentration that produces 50% of the maximum possible physiologic response. For example, the C_{50} for an EEG response is the drug concentration that provides 50% depression of the maximal EEG effect. The C_{50} for EEG response has been measured for the opioids alfentanil,[57] fentanyl,[57] sufentanil,[58] and remifentanil.[59-61] It has also been determined for thiopental,[51,62,63] etomidate,[56] propofol,[24] and benzodiazepines (see Table 26.2).[57,64] Other measures such as pupillary dilation in response to a noxious stimulus[65] and pressure algometry[22] were used to measure opioid potency and revealed slightly different values for C_{50}, which indicates that observation of drug potency also depends on the applied measure of drug effect.

As mentioned, C_{50} can be used to compare potency among drugs. For example, Glass and colleagues[66] determined the potency of remifentanil compared with alfentanil using ventilatory depression as the measure of opioid effect. In their study, the C_{50} for depression of minute ventilation was 1.17 ng/mL and 49.4 ng/mL for remifentanil and alfentanil, respectively. Using this difference in C_{50},

TABLE 26.2 Steady-State Concentrations for Predefined Effects

Drug	C_{50} for EEG Depression*	C_{50} for Incision or Painful Stimulus†	C_{50} for Loss of Consciousness‡	C_{50} for Spontaneous Ventilation§	C_{50} for Isoflurane MAC Reduction	MEAC
Alfentanil (ng/mL)	500-600	200-300	—	170-230	50	10-30
Fentanyl (ng/mL)	6-10	4-6	—	2-3	1.7	0.5-1
Sufentanil (ng/mL)	0.5-0.75	(0.3-0.4)	—	(0.15-0.2)	0.15	0.025-0.05
Remifentanil (ng/mL)	10-15	4-6	—	2-3	1.2	0.5-1
Propofol (μg/mL)	3-4	4-8	2-3	1.33	—	—
Thiopental (μg/mL)	15-20	35-40	8-16	—	—	—
Etomidate (μg/mL)	0.53	—	0.55	—	—	—
Midazolam (ng/mL)	250-350	—	125-250	—	—	—

*C_{50} for depression of the EEG is the steady-state serum concentration that causes a 50% slowing of the maximal EEG, except for midazolam, in which the C_{50} is associated with 50% activation of the EEG.
†C_{50} for skin incision is the steady-state plasma concentration that prevents a somatic or autonomic response in 50% of patients.
‡C_{50} for loss of consciousness is the steady-state plasma concentration for absence of a response to a verbal command in 50% of patients.
§C_{50} for spontaneous ventilation is the steady-state plasma concentration associated with adequate spontaneous ventilation in 50% of patients.
Values in parentheses are estimated by scaling to the alfentanil C_{50} (see text for details).
EEG, Electroencephalography; *MAC*, minimum alveolar concentration; *MEAC*, minimum effective plasma concentration providing postoperative analgesia.

they concluded that remifentanil is approximately 40 times more potent than alfentanil.

To be entirely independent of dosing history, C_{50} must be determined at steady state, which is rarely possible because most anesthetic drugs do not reach steady state during a continuous infusion until many hours have passed. However, if the drug exhibits rapid equilibration between plasma and the effect site and the investigator waits long enough after starting the infusion, then this choice can be reasonably satisfactory. For example, Ausems and colleagues[67,68] used a continuous infusion of alfentanil in their experiments, which quickly equilibrated. They also recorded their measurements after the effect-site concentration had equilibrated with plasma.

A second alternative to performing a true steady-state experiment is to use mathematic modeling to calculate the effect-site concentrations of drug at the time of measurement, as proposed by Hull and colleagues[16] and Sheiner and colleagues.[17] The relationship between effect-site and plasma concentrations is graphically represented in Fig. 26.5 and mathematically in Eq. 26.6. Calculating effect-site concentrations is the same as attempting to determine the steady-state plasma concentrations that produce the observed drug effect. When the C_{50} reflects effect-site concentrations, it is represented as Ce_{50} to distinguish it from values of C_{50} that are based on plasma concentrations, which are then termed Cp_{50}. However, the distinction is artificial. In both cases, C_{50} is intended to represent the steady-state plasma drug concentration associated with a given drug effect.

A third alternative to performing a steady-state experiment is to establish a pseudo–steady state with the use of computer-controlled drug delivery. By this term we mean that a steady state is assumed to exist, because a varying rate drug infusion is being administered with the intent of achieving stable plasma concentrations. This method has become the state of the art for determining the C_{50} for anesthetic drugs, and many of the C_{50} values referenced earlier were determined at pseudo–steady state with the use of computer-controlled drug delivery. Commonly, two or more measurements of the plasma concentration during pseudo–steady state conditions are performed to verify whether this is indeed the case.[40-42] Typically, maintaining a constant plasma steady-state concentration for four to five plasma effect-site equilibration half-lives (e.g., 10-15 minutes for fentanyl) is required. Such a long delay is not necessarily needed when computer-controlled drug delivery is used.

Effect-compartment TCIs can be used to target the concentration at the effect site rather than the plasma concentration and thereby rapidly establishing plasma–effect site equilibration.[29,47] For example, Kodaka and associates reported predicted values of propofol effect-site concentration C_{50} between 3.1 μg/mL and 4.3 μg/mL for insertion of various laryngeal airway masks, depending on the type of laryngeal mask.[69] Cortinez and associates used TCI to determine the C_{50} of remifentanil and fentanyl for accurate pain relief during extracorporeal shock wave lithotripsy in relation with possible side effects and found that remifentanil and fentanyl C_{50} were 2.8 ng/mL and 2.9 ng/mL, respectively.[70] At C_{50}, the probability of having a respiratory rate less than 10 breaths per minute was 4% for remifentanil and 56% for fentanyl.

Likewise, TCI has been used to estimate the following C_{50} values for dexmedetomidine: the C_{50} for half-maximal effect on the BIS (BIS ~48) was 2.6 ng/mL, for half-maximal effect on the Modified Observer's Assessment of Alertness/Sedation (MOAA/S) scale was 0.438 ng/mL, for half-maximal hypotensive effect was 0.36 ng/mL, and the C_{50} for half-maximal hypertensive effects was 1.6 ng/mL.[71,72]

Thus there are several ways to establish C_{50} in terms of steady-state concentrations. C_{50} can be estimated through mathematic effect-site modeling or can be experimentally measured with the use of computer-controlled drug delivery to establish a pseudo–steady state quickly. Either way, when performing studies to define the concentration-effect relationship, equilibrium must exist or be modeled between the biophase (the site of effect) and plasma or blood (where the concentration is actually measured).

When C_{50} is defined in terms of the concentration associated with a response in one half of a population, that same C_{50} is the concentration associated with a 50% probability of response in a typical individual. However, individual patients are not typical individuals but rather will have their own value for C_{50}. Expressed in clinical terms, different patients have different anesthetic requirements for the same stimulus. For example, the minimal effective analgesic concentration of fentanyl is 0.6 ng/mL, but it varies among patients from 0.2 to 2.0 ng/mL.[73] The minimal effective analgesic concentrations of alfentanil[74] and sufentanil[75] similarly vary among patients by a factor of 5 to 10. This range encompasses both variability in the intensity of the stimulus and variability of the individual patient.

One factor known to be responsible for this interindividual pharmacodynamic variability is the patient age. Thus with the pharmacodynamic for propofol developed by Eleveld and colleagues, and based on pharmacokinetic-pharmacodynamic data from a large number of patients and volunteers, the estimated effect-site propofol concentrations required for a BIS of 47 for patients whose ages are 20, 40, and 70 years, are 3.5, 3.1, and 2.6 ug/mL, respectively.[76]

Although age has a strong effect on the C_{50}, it does not explain all the variability. This wide range reflects the clinical reality that must be accounted for when dosing regimens are designed. Because of this variability, intravenous anesthetics should be titrated to each patient's unique anesthetic requirement for the given stimulus.

Pharmacodynamic Drug Interactions

Drug interactions cause the potency of one drug (e.g., as measured by the C_{50}) to shift in response to the administration of a second drug. This drug interaction can be additive, supra-additive (synergistic), or infra-additive (antagonistic). As observed in the isobologram (Fig. 26.9), for additive drugs with equal potency, the cumulative effect resulting from doses a and b for substances A and B, respectively, equals the effect obtained with the injection of either drug A or B solely in a dose a + b. If the drugs interact synergistically, then the combination of A and B will generate a more pronounced effect than additive. For antagonistic drug interaction, the combination of A and B will result in a less pronounced effect than additive. In general, additive drug interactions occur when combining drugs acting by the same mechanism and synergistic or antagonistic interaction when combining drugs acting by a different mechanism.[77] Hendrickx and coworkers (Fig. 26.10) reviewed the available literature and summarized the available data on drug interactions in humans and animals for hypnosis and immobility.[77]

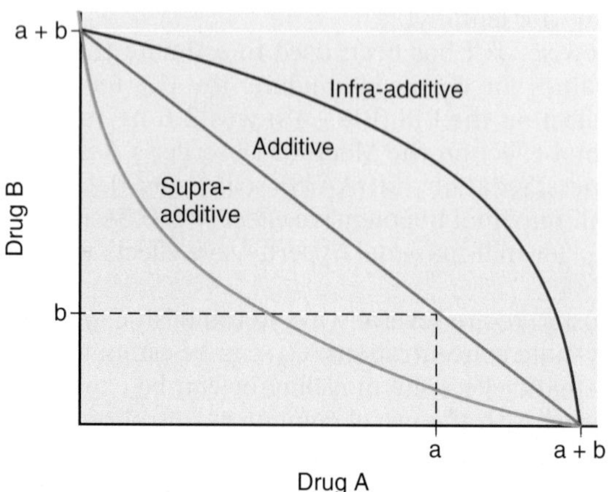

Fig. 26.9 Pharmacodynamic drug interactions.

Investigating only one isobole of the interaction spectrum (e.g., the 50% probability level of a specific drug response) provides a rudimentary insight into the interaction characteristics but reveals only limited information about other levels of drug effect (e.g., at the clinically more important level of 95% probability of drug response). As drug interactions may vary among drug effect levels (e.g., additive at the 50% level but synergistic at the 95% level), the ultimate aim is to characterize the response surface describing all levels of effect. Pharmacodynamic response surface models generate figures that are three- (or even higher) dimensional structures that have been developed to describe the relationship quantitatively between two or more drug concentrations and their combined clinical effect (Fig. 26.11). Response surface models are powerful representations of drug interactions as they combine information about the full range of isoboles resulting from the concentration response curves of all combinations of the drugs involved.[78,79] Using the mathematically defined response surface, the corresponding drug effect for any two or more drug concentrations of the interacting drugs can be predicted.[80,81] Various methodological approaches to response surface models are found in the literature.[82]

Intravenous opioids are frequently combined with volatile anesthetics during anesthesia. The reduction of the MAC for a given volatile by a given opioid dose can be applied to investigate the potency and efficacy of opioids.[83-85] These MAC reduction studies reveal a general pattern, irrespective of which opioid or volatile anesthetic has been used. Low concentrations of an opioid result in a substantial reduction of MAC (Fig. 26.12). With increasing concentrations of the opioid, MAC continues to decrease until a plateau is reached and, consequently, a further increase of the opioid dose is futile.[86]

The previously mentioned MAC reduction studies show the effect of a single opioid dose on a single point of a dose-response curve but, nonetheless, form the basis for more detailed surface interaction studies.[87] To characterize the interaction between sevoflurane and remifentanil in blunting responses to verbal (OAA/S scale) and painful stimuli (pressure algometry, electrical tetanic stimulus, and thermal stimulation), Manyam and coworkers constructed a response surface for each pharmacodynamic response using a Logit model approach and found synergy between sevoflurane and remifentanil for all responses. More specifically, a remifentanil effect-site concentration of 1.25 ng/mL was able to more than halve the sevoflurane requirements for preventing movement to pain.[88] Because this study suffered from nonsteady-state conditions at the moment of measurements, the authors improved their data using calculated effect-site sevoflurane concentrations and a Greco model instead of a Logit approach.[89] Accounting for the time lag between sevoflurane effect-site concentration and end-tidal concentration improved the predictions of responsiveness during anesthesia but had no effect on the accuracy of prediction of a response to a noxious stimulus in recovery. They concluded that models may be useful in predicting events of clinical interest, but large-scale evaluations with numerous patients are needed to better characterize model performance. Heyse and colleagues (Fig. 26.13) found that the pharmacodynamic interaction between sevoflurane and remifentanil for tolerance to shaking and shouting (TOSS), tetanic stimulation (TTET), laryngeal mask airway insertion (TLMA), and laryngoscopy (TLAR) using the Fixed $C50_O$ Hierarchical model was strongly synergistic for both the hypnotic and the analgesic components of anesthesia and showed the importance of exploring various surface model approaches when studying drug interactions.[82,90]

For total intravenous anesthesia, interactions associated with various drug combinations and concentrations have been described. The concept of *balanced* anesthesia is based on the assumption that drug combinations will be synergistic in anesthetic effect (however defined) but not in toxicity. Such synergism has been demonstrated for a variety of drug combinations but not for others (see Fig. 26.10).[77,91] Zanderigo and colleagues[92] developed the *well-being model*, a new interaction model to describe both positive and negative effects of drug combinations (Fig. 26.14).

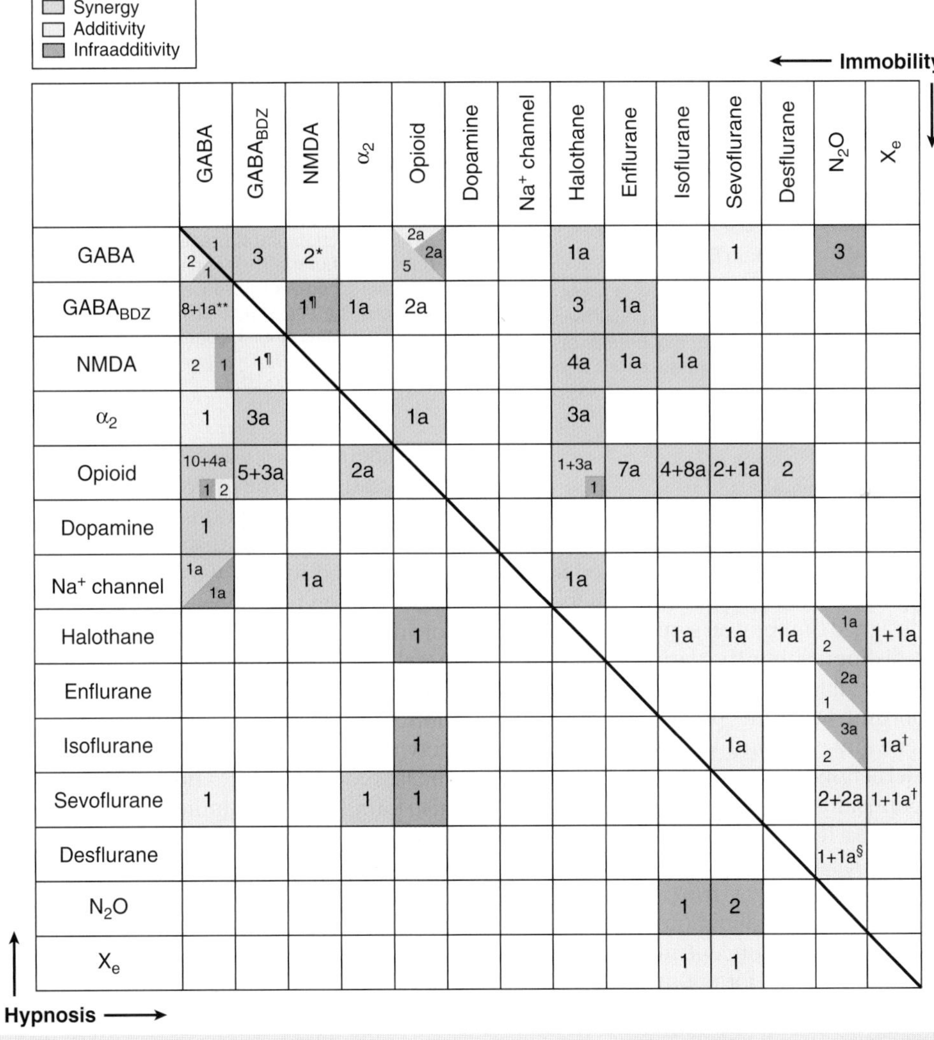

	GABA	$GABA_{BDZ}$	NMDA	α_2	Opioid	Dopamine	Na^+ channel	Halothane	Enflurane	Isoflurane	Sevoflurane	Desflurane	N_2O	X_e
GABA	1 2 1	3	2*		2a 2a 5			1a			1		3	
$GABA_{BDZ}$	8+1a**		1¶	1a	2a			3	1a					
NMDA	2 1	1¶						4a	1a	1a				
α_2	1	3a			1a			3a						
Opioid	10+4a 1 2	5+3a		2a				1+3a 1	7a	4+8a	2+1a	2		
Dopamine	1													
Na^+ channel	1a 1a		1a					1a						
Halothane					1					1a	1a	1a	1a 2	1+1a
Enflurane													2a 1	
Isoflurane					1						1a		3a 2	1a†
Sevoflurane	1			1	1								2+2a	1+1a†
Desflurane													1+1a§	
N_2O										1	2			
X_e										1	1			

Fig. 26.10 Interaction grid summarizing the available data on drug interactions in humans and animals for hypnosis and immobility. Drugs are organized by pharmacologic class: gamma-aminobutyric acid *(GABA)*–acting drugs (propofol, thiopental, methohexital, and etomidate); GABA agents acting at the benzodiazepine *($GABA_{BDZ}$)*-binding site (midazolam, diazepam); *N*-methyl-D-aspartate *(NMDA)*-receptor antagonist (ketamine); adrenergic agonists *(α_2)* (dexmedetomidine, clonidine); opioid-acting drugs at opioid receptor (morphine, alfentanil, fentanyl, sufentanil, and remifentanil); dopamine at dopamine antagonists (droperidol, metoclopramide); sodium (Na^+) channel blockers (lidocaine, bupivacaine); and anesthetic gases. The right upper half of the grid *(above the thick diagonal)* summarizes the interactions for the endpoint of immobility; the left lower half *(below the thick diagonal)* summarizes the interactions for the endpoint of hypnosis. Synergy is coded as *green*, additivity as *yellow*, and infra-additivity as *dark orange*. The number refers to the number of studies attesting to a particular interaction; if one study documents two interactions (e.g., isoflurane with both fentanyl and alfentanil), then they are counted separately. Animal data carry the suffix *a* after the number of studies, human data have no suffix. *Reanalysis: propofol-ketamine interaction in humans is infra-additive for immobility. **Reanalysis: thiopental-midazolam interaction in humans is additive for hypnosis. †Because the MAC of Xe in swine is uncertain, data in swine are not included. ¶Reanalysis: ketamine-midazolam interaction in humans is infra-additive for hypnosis and additive for immobility. §Infra-additivity between desflurane and nitrous oxide *(N_2O)* has been suggested in a small subgroup of 18- to 30-year-old patients. (From Hendrickx JF, Eger EI 2nd, Sonner JM, et al. Is synergy the rule? A review of anesthetic interactions producing hypnosis and immobility. Anesth *Analg*. 2008;107:494–506. Used with permission.)

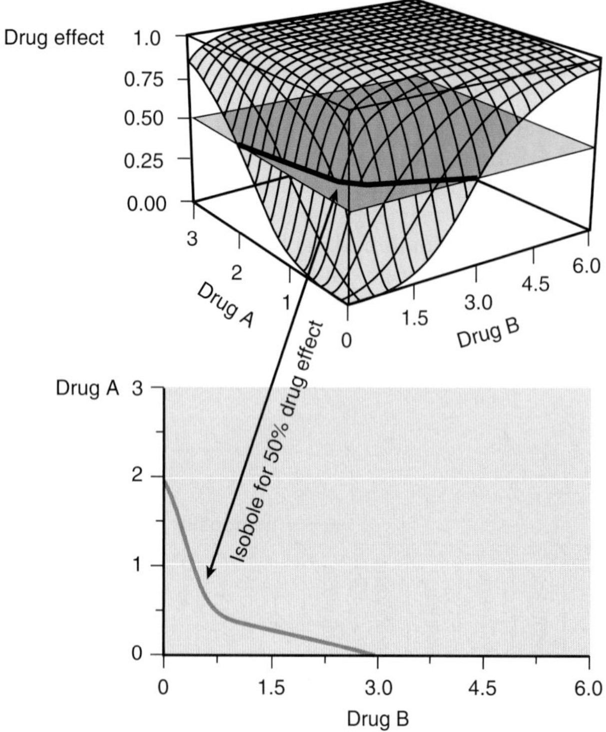

Fig. 26.11 Relationship between a response surface and a standard isobologram. Conventional isobolographic analysis, whether for doses or concentrations, describes only the concentration of both drugs that yields a 50% drug effect and thus fails to capture the entire response surface. (From Minto CF, Schnider TW, Short TG, et al. Response surface model for anesthetic drug interactions. *Anesthesiology*. 2000;92:1603–1616. Used with permission.)

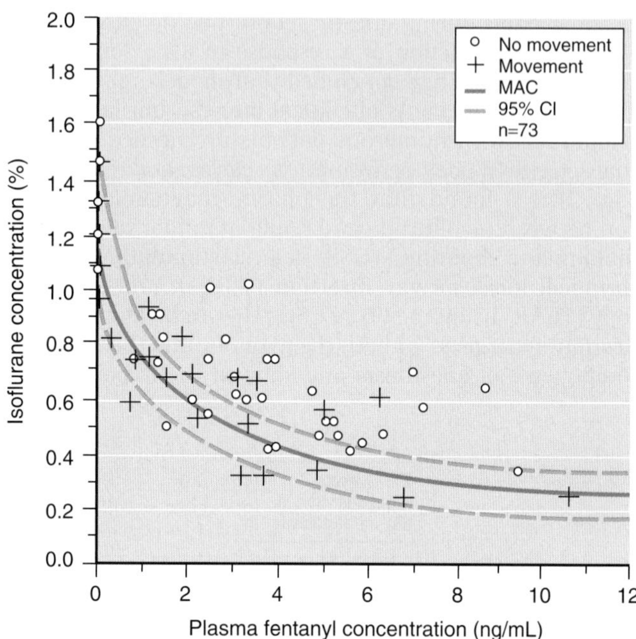

Fig. 26.12 Interaction of isoflurane and fentanyl in preventing a somatic response at skin incision (i.e., minimum alveolar concentration [MAC] reduction of isoflurane). The *blue line* represents the concentrations of isoflurane and fentanyl when administered together that are required to prevent purposeful movement in 50% of patients at skin incision. The *dotted gold lines* represent the 95% confidence interval (CI) of the MAC at each combination of fentanyl and isoflurane. (From McEwan AI, Smith C, Dyar O, et al. Isoflurane MAC reduction by fentanyl. *Anesthesiology*. 1993;78:864–869. Used with permission.)

More profound synergy for specific endpoints related to analgesia and hypnosis has also been demonstrated for the interaction between propofol and opioids. Thus when anesthetic regimens are designed that rely on synergy to produce the anesthetic state, distinguishing the desired endpoint—loss of consciousness or ablation of response to noxious stimulation—is important. Different combinations of drugs may be used to achieve any endpoint. Vuyk and colleagues characterized the interaction between propofol and alfentanil for several endpoints: loss of response to endotracheal intubation, loss of response to incision and retraction of the peritoneum, and emergence from anesthesia (Fig. 26.15).[93] The most profound stimulation was tracheal intubation, and when no opioid was used, the abolition of responses to that stimulus required a propofol concentration equal to or more than 12 μg/mL. More details for optimal drug combinations based on the findings from Vuyk and coworkers[93] are provided in Table 26.3.

Minto and colleagues published *response surfaces* for combinations of midazolam-alfentanil, propofol-alfentanil, and midazolam-propofol associated with the loss of response to verbal command (Fig. 26.16).[78] They also extended response surface methodology to describe the simultaneous interaction of three drugs. Rendering the full interaction surface for three drugs would require drawing the graph in four dimensions. If the graph is limited to the interaction at 50% drug effect, then it can be rendered in three dimensions (Fig. 26.17).

In addition to studies of quantal responses, various studies investigated the interaction between hypnotics and opioids as measured with continuous measures. The effect of combined drug administration on spontaneous and evoked EEG–derived indices was found to be important and existing but often in studies that did not provide sufficient data for full-response surface model development.[24,94,95] Fortunately, more accurately designed studies[81] using surface modeling techniques revealed the interaction between hypnotics and opioids. Bouillon and colleagues found synergy between propofol and remifentanil regarding hypnosis as measured by the BIS and EEG approximate entropy. They also found that both indices were more sensitive to propofol than remifentanil.[96] Others found conflicting results for the effect of opioids on the BIS.[97] More recently, Gambus and colleagues modeled the effect of propofol and remifentanil combinations for sedation-analgesia in endoscopic procedures using an adaptive neurofuzzy inference system.[98] Both spontaneous and evoked EEG–derived indices (e.g., BIS or autoregressive auditory-evoked potential index [AAI/2] and index of consciousness [IoC]) were used. They found, based on these models, that the propofol and remifentanil effect-site concentration pairs provide a Ramsay Sedation Score of 4 ranging from (1.8 μg/mL, 1.5 ng/mL) to (2.7 μg/mL, 0 ng/mL), associated with a BIS of 71 to 75, AAI/2 values of 25 to 30, and IoC of 72 to 76, respectively. The presence of noxious stimulation increases the requirements of propofol and remifentanil to achieve the same degree of sedative effects.[98]

Other effects of drug combinations were also studied. Bouillon and associates and Nieuwenhuijs and associates

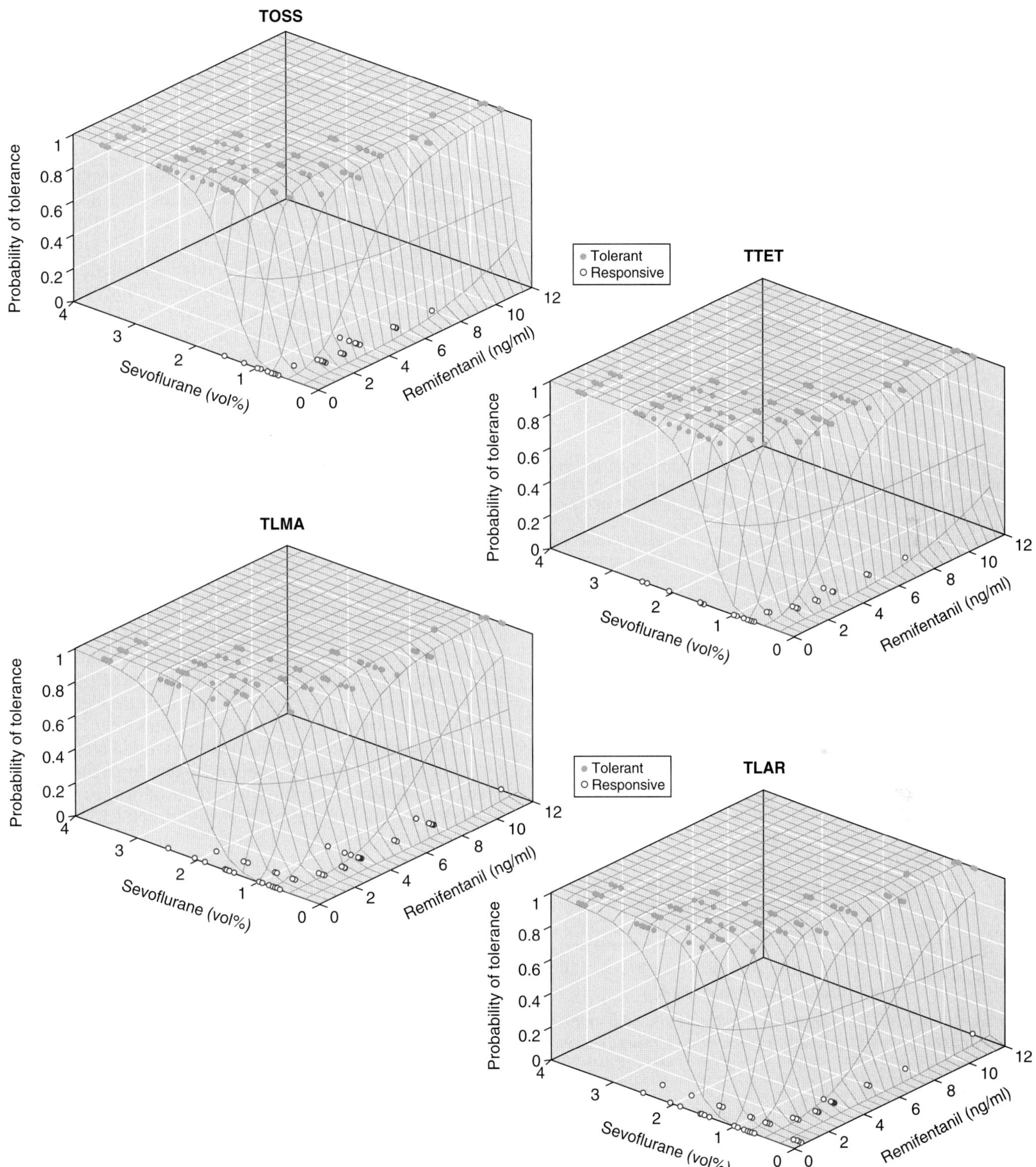

Fig. 26.13 Response surface for probability of tolerance to shaking and shouting *(TOSS)*, tetanic stimulation *(TTET)*, laryngeal mask airway insertion *(TLMA)*, and laryngoscopy *(TLAR)* for the Fixed C50(O) Hierarchical model. The solid lines at probability 0.5 represent the 50% isoboles. (From Heyse B, Proost JH, Schumacher PM, et al. Sevoflurane remifentanil interaction. comparison of different response surface models. *Anesthesiology*. 2012;116:311–323. Used with permission.)

investigated the effects of hypnotic-opioid combinations on cardiorespiratory control.[97,99] These data show dose-dependent effects on respiration at relatively low concentrations of propofol and remifentanil. When combined, their effect on respiration is strikingly synergistic, resulting in severe respiratory depression.

Surface models were also used to optimize drug administration in challenging situations such as short-duration

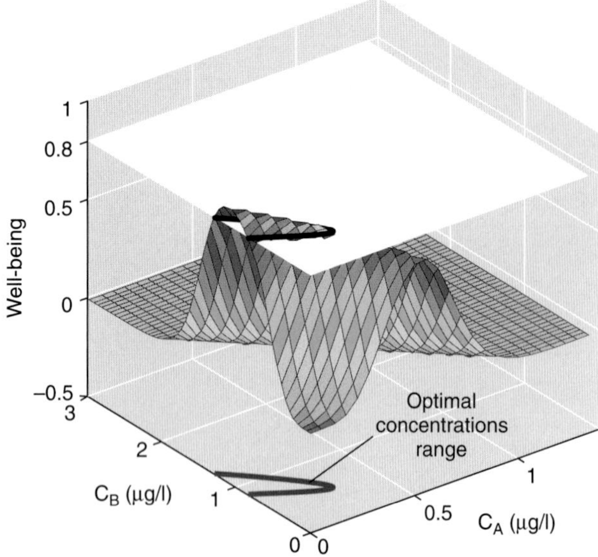

Fig. 26.14 Definition of the optimal concentrations range for the combined administration of drugs A and B, in the case of zero interactions. The optimal concentrations range results from the intersection between the well-being surface and the plane representing a well-being value of 0.8. (From Zanderigo E, Sartori V, Sveticic G, et al. The well-being model. A new drug interaction model for positive and negative effects. *Anesthesiology*. 2006;104:742–753. Used with permission.)

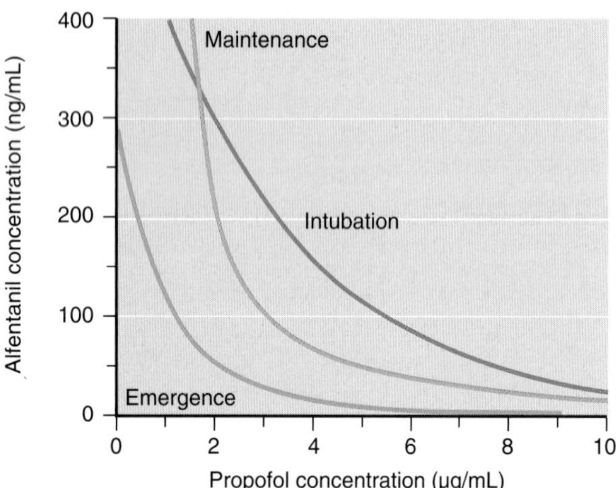

Fig. 26.15 Interaction between alfentanil and propofol on three different endpoints. Response to intubation *(blue line)*, maintenance of anesthesia *(gold line)*, and concentrations associated with emergence from anesthesia *(green line)*. The curve shows the concentrations associated with a 50% probability of the respective endpoint. (Modified from Vuyk J, Lim T, Engbers FH, et al. The pharmacodynamic interaction of propofol and alfentanil during lower abdominal surgery in women. *Anesthesiology*. 1995;83:8–22.)

procedures in spontaneous breathing patients. LaPierre and coworkers[100] explored remifentanil-propofol combinations that led to a loss of response to esophageal instrumentation, a loss of responsiveness, and/or an onset of ventilatory depression requiring intervention. They found that the combinations that allowed esophageal instrumentation and avoided intolerable ventilatory depression and/or loss of responsiveness primarily clustered around remifentanil-propofol effect-site concentrations ranging from 0.8 to 1.6 ng/mL and 1.5 to 2.7 µg/mL, respectively. However, blocking the response to esophageal instrumentation and avoiding both intolerable ventilatory depression and/or a loss of responsiveness is difficult. It may be necessary to accept some discomfort and blunt, rather than block, the response to esophageal instrumentation to consistently avoid intolerable ventilatory depression and/or loss of responsiveness.

In a previously mentioned study, using response surface modeling, Bouillon and colleagues also determined the interactions between propofol and remifentanil on the probability to tolerate laryngoscopy (PTOL).[96] Luginbuhl, working with a group that included Bouillon, normalized and calibrated PTOL, to produce an index called the noxious stimulus response index (NSRI).[101] The NSRI is a dimensionless integer number between 0 and 100, where 50 corresponds to a PTOL of 50% and 20 to a PTOL of 90%.

The interactions between hypnotics such as propofol and sevoflurane should also be understood, because these drugs are frequently used sequentially. Schumacher and colleagues[102] used response surface methodology to examine the influence of this interaction on the probability of TOSS and three noxious stimuli (TTET, TLMA, and TLAR). They found that for both EEG suppression and tolerance to stimulation, the interaction of propofol and sevoflurane were additive. Others found similar results on the C_{50} level.[103] Hammer and colleagues[104] determined the pharmacodynamic interaction of propofol and dexmedetomidine during pediatric esophagogastroduodenoscopy and concluded that the concentration of propofol at which 50% of patients are adequately anesthetized (EC_{50}) in children was unaffected by a concomitant intravenous infusion of dexmedetomidine 1 µg/kg body weight given over 10 minutes.

Hannivoort and colleagues took this work a step further by using response surface modeling to develop a model that predicts the effect of combinations of sevoflurane, propofol, and remifentanil in terms of PTOL and the NSRI.[105]

Although models of the pharmacokinetics and pharmacodynamics of drug, and models of drug interactions, are essentially just that—models that attempt to provide qualitative and quantitative representations of reality—they are based on many assumptions, and inherently involve many sources of error.[106] Nonetheless, the models provide information that is useful to clinicians to help guide rational practice. Information on drug interactions, including the NSRI, has been incorporated in commercially available anesthetic display monitors and are described by van den Berg and associates in a concise summary of current knowledge, and the ways that it has and can be incorporated into clinical practice.[107]

Designing Dosing Regimens

BOLUS DOSE CALCULATIONS

The definition of concentration is drug mass per unit of volume. The definition of concentration can be rearranged to find the amount of drug required to produce any desired concentration for a known volume (Eq. 26.10):

$$Amount = C_T \bullet Volume \qquad (26.10)$$

TABLE 26.3 Propofol/Opioid Combinations Associated with the Fastest Recovery from Anesthesia

Infusion Duration (min)		Propofol/Alfentanil (μg/mL; ng/mL)	Propofol/Sufentanil (μg/mL; ng/mL)	Propofol/Remifentanil (μg/mL; ng/mL)
15	$C_{optimal}$	3.25/99.3	3.57/0.17	2.57/4.70
	$C_{awakening}$	1.69/65.0	1.70/0.10	1.83/1.93
	Time to awakening (min)	8.2	9.4	5.1
60	$C_{optimal}$	3.38/89.7	3.34/0.14	2.51/4.78
	$C_{awakening}$	1.70/64.9	1.70/0.10	1.83/1.93
	Time to awakening (min)	12.2	11.9	6.1
300	$C_{optimal}$	3.40/88.9	3.37/0.14	2.51/4.78
	$C_{awakening}$	1.70/64.9	1.70/0.10	1.86/1.88
	Time to awakening (min)	16.0	15.6	6.7

$C_{optimal}$ represents combinations associated with a 50% probability of a response to surgical stimuli; $C_{awakening}$ concentrations represent the estimated concentrations at which consciousness will be regained; and Time to awakening represents the estimated time from termination of the infusion to return of consciousness in 50% of patients.

From Vuyk J, Mertens MJ, Olofsen E, et al. Propofol anesthesia and rational opioid selection. Determination of optimal EC_{50}-EC_{95} propofol-opioid concentrations that assure adequate anesthesia and a rapid return of consciousness. *Anesthesiology.* 1997;87:1549–1562; and modified from Absalom A, Struys MMRF. *An Overview of TCI and TIVA.* ed 2. Gent, Belgium: Academia Press; 2007. Used with permission.

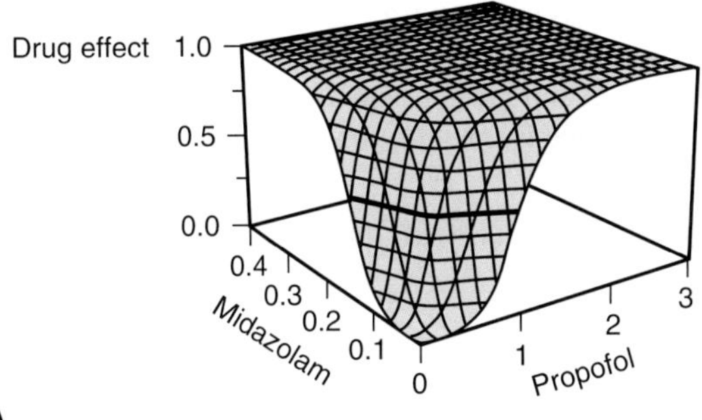

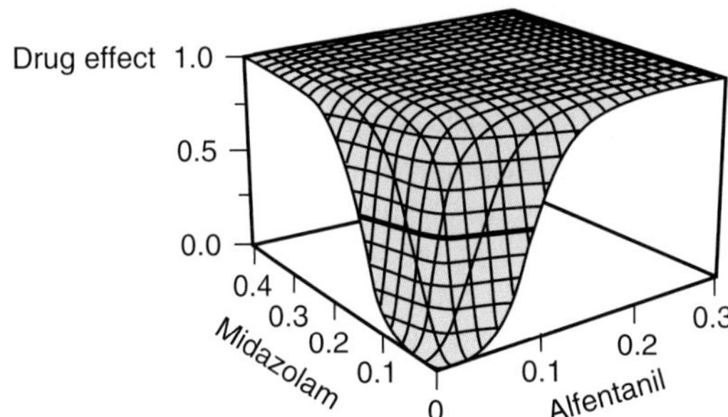

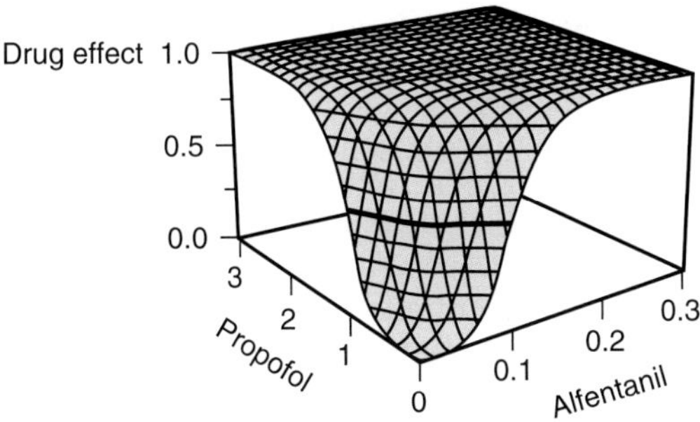

Fig. 26.16 Response surface for each of the paired interactions between propofol and midazolam (A), alfentanil and midazolam (B), and alfentanil and propofol (C) on the probability of opening eyes to a verbal command. The isoboles for a 10%, 20%, 30%, 40%, 50%, 60%, 70%, 80%, and 90% response are shown. (From Minto CF, Schnider TW, Short TG, et al. Response surface model for anesthetic drug interactions. *Anesthesiology.* 2000;92:1603–1616.)

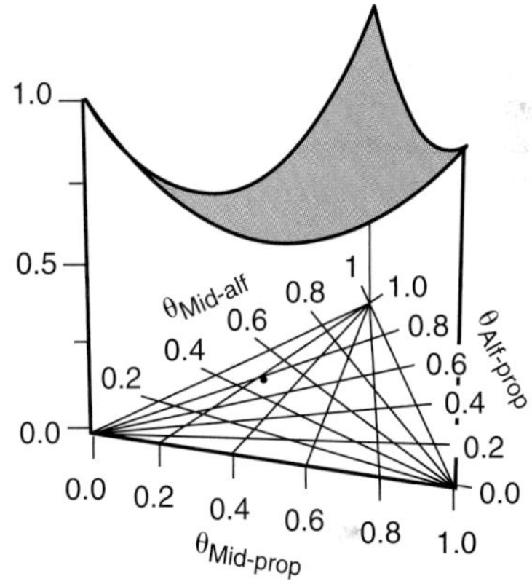

Fig. 26.17 Interaction at 50% drug effect (C_{50}) among propofol, midazolam, and alfentanil. Downward deflection of the surface represents synergy, in units of fractional reduction in C_{50}. The three edges represent relative amounts of propofol to midazolam ($\theta_{Mid\text{-}prop}$), alfentanil to midazolam ($\theta_{Mid\text{-}alf}$), and alfentanil to propofol ($\theta_{Alf\text{-}prop}$). The surface between the edges represents the relative synergy of all three drugs taken together. (From Minto CF, Schnider TW, Short TG, et al. Response surface model for anesthetic drug interactions. *Anesthesiology.* 2000;92:1603–1616.)

where C_T is the desired or *target* concentration. This formula is often used to calculate the initial (loading) bolus dose required to achieve a given concentration. The problem with applying this concept to anesthetic drugs is that there are several volumes of distribution: V_1 (central compartment), V_2 and V_3 (the peripheral compartments), and Vd_{ss} (the sum of the individual volumes). V_1 is usually significantly smaller than Vd_{ss}, and thus saying that the loading dose should be something between $C_T \times V_1$ and $C_T \times Vd_{ss}$ is tempting.

Consideration should be given to the dose of fentanyl required to attenuate the hemodynamic response to endotracheal intubation when combined with thiopental. The C_{50} for fentanyl, combined with thiopental for intubation, is approximately 3 ng/mL. The V_1 and Vd_{ss} for fentanyl are 13 L and 360 L, respectively. The aforementioned equations can thus be interpreted as suggesting that an appropriate dose of fentanyl to attenuate the hemodynamic response is between 39 μg (3 ng/mL × 13 L) and 1080 μg (3 ng/mL

× 360 L). A fentanyl bolus of 39 μg achieves the desired concentration in plasma for an initial instant, but plasma levels almost instantly decrease below the desired target. Levels at the effect site will never be close to the desired target concentration of 3 ng/mL. A fentanyl bolus of 1080 μg, not surprisingly, produces a significant overshoot in plasma levels that persists for hours (Fig. 26.18). Additionally, using equations to calculate the fentanyl dose if the resulting recommendation is to "use a fentanyl dose between 39 and 1080 μg" is absurd.

The usual dosing guidelines for a bolus dose, presented earlier, are designed to produce a specific plasma concentration. Because plasma is not the site of drug effect, calculating the initial bolus on the basis of a desired plasma concentration is irrational. By knowing the k_{e0} of an intravenous anesthetic, a dosing regimen can be designed that yields the desired concentration at the site of drug effect. To avoid an overdose for the patient, a bolus should be selected that produces the desired peak concentration at the effect site.

The decline in plasma concentration between the initial concentration after the bolus (amount/V_1) and the concentration at the time of peak effect can be thought of as dilution of the bolus into a larger anatomic volume than the volume of the central compartment. This introduces the concept of Vd_{pe}, the apparent volume of distribution at the time of peak effect,[28,94] or pseudoequilibration between plasma and the site of drug effect.[95] The size of this volume can be readily calculated from the observation that the plasma and effect-site concentrations are the same at the time of peak effect (Eq. 26.11):

$$Vd_{pe} = \frac{Bolus\ amount}{C_{pe}} \qquad (26.11)$$

where C_{pe} is the plasma concentration at the time of peak effect.

If the clinical goal is to select the dose required to achieve a certain drug effect without producing an overdose, then Eq. 26.11 can be rearranged by substituting C_T, the target concentration (which is the same in plasma and the effect site at the moment of peak effect), for C_{pe} to calculate the size of the initial bolus (Eq. 26.12)

$$Loading\ dose = C_T \times Vd_{pe} \qquad (26.12)$$

The Vd_{pe} for fentanyl is 75 L. To achieve a peak fentanyl effect-site concentration of 3.0 ng/mL requires 225 μg, which produces a peak effect in 3.6 minutes. This dosing guideline is more reasonable compared with the previous recommendation of a dose between 39 and 1080 μg. Table 26.4 lists V_1 and Vd_{pe} for fentanyl, alfentanil, sufentanil, remifentanil, propofol, thiopental, and midazolam. Table 26.1 lists the time to peak effect and the $t_{1/2}\ k_{e0}$ of the commonly used intravenous anesthetics.

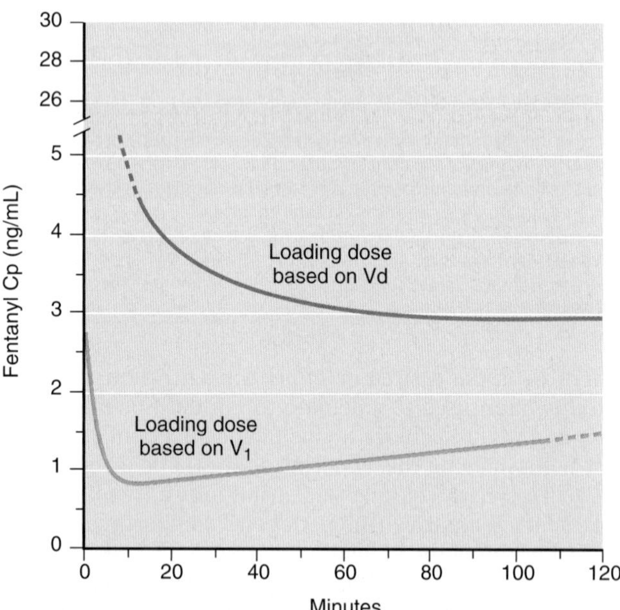

Fig. 26.18 Pharmacokinetic simulation demonstrating the limitations of infusion regimens based on simple pharmacokinetic parameters with fentanyl used as an example. These infusion schemes were designed to achieve a fentanyl plasma concentration *(Cp)* of 3 ng/mL. The *upper blue curve* shows that a regimen using a loading dose based on the volume of distribution followed by a constant infusion based on clearance results in a transient period of very high plasma concentrations. If the same maintenance infusion is given but the loading dose is based on the volume of the central compartment, then the distribution of drug to the peripheral compartments causes the plasma concentration to fall below the desired level until the compartments reach steady-state concentrations as shown in the *lower gold curve*.

MAINTENANCE INFUSION RATES

By definition, the rate at which active drug exits the body is systemic clearance (Cl_S) times the plasma concentration. To maintain a given target concentration (C_T), drug must be delivered at the same rate that it is exiting the body. Thus (Eq. 26.13),

$$Maintenance\ infusion\ rate = C_T \times Cl_S \qquad (26.13)$$

For drugs with multicompartment pharmacokinetics, which includes all of the intravenous drugs used in anesthetic practice, drug is distributed into the peripheral tissues, as well as cleared from the body. The rate of distribution into tissues changes over time as the tissues equilibrate with plasma. Eq. 26.13 is correct only after the peripheral tissues have fully equilibrated with plasma, which requires many hours. At all other times, this maintenance infusion rate underestimates the infusion rate necessary to maintain a target concentration.

Yet in some situations, this simple maintenance rate calculation may be acceptable. For example, if an infusion at this rate is used along with a bolus dose based on Vd_{pe} and the drug has a long delay between the bolus and peak effect, then most of the distribution of drug into tissues may have occurred by the time that the effect-site concentration reaches the target concentration. In this case, the maintenance infusion rate calculated as clearance times target concentration may be accurate because Vd_{pe} is sufficiently higher than V_1 to account for the distribution of drug into peripheral tissues. Unfortunately, most drugs used in anesthesia achieve sufficiently rapid equilibration between plasma and the effect site that Vd_{pe} does not adequately encompass the distribution process, thus making this approach unsuitable.

As such, approaches need to be used that are mathematically and clinically sound. Because the net flow of drug into peripheral tissues decreases over time, the infusion rate required to maintain any desired concentration must also decrease over time. If the initial bolus has been based on

Vd_{pe}, no infusion needs be administered until the effect-site concentration peaks. After the peak in effect-site concentration, the (nearly) correct equation to maintain the desired concentration is (Eq. 26.14)

Maintenance infusion rate

$$= C_T \times V_1 \times \left(k_{10} + k_{12}e^{-k_{21}t} + k_{13}e^{-k_{31}t}\right) \quad (26.14)$$

This equation indicates that a rapid infusion rate is initially required to maintain C_T. Over time, the infusion rate gradually decreases (see Fig. 26.14). At equilibrium (t = ∞), the infusion rate decreases to $C_T \times V_1 \times k_{10}$, which is the same as $C_T \times Cl_S$. Few clinicians would choose to solve such an equation during the administration of an anesthetic. Fortunately, simple techniques can be used in place of solving such a complex expression.

TABLE 26.4 Volume of Distribution at the Time of Peak Effect

Drug	V_1 (L)	Vd_{pe} (L)
Fentanyl	12.7	75
Alfentanil	2.19	5.9
Sufentanil	17.8	89
Remifentanil	5.0	17
Propofol	6.7	37
Thiopental	5.6	14.6
Midazolam	3.4	31

V_1, Volume of the central compartment; *Vd_{pe}*, apparent volume of distribution at the time of peak effect.

Fig. 26.19 is a nomogram in which Eq. 26.14 has been solved; the infusion rates at different times necessary to maintain any desired concentration of fentanyl, alfentanil, sufentanil, and propofol are shown. Because this nomogram is complex, the following review is provided:

The *y* axis represents the target concentration C_T. The *x* axis is the time since the beginning of the anesthetic (i.e., since the initial bolus). The suggested initial target concentrations (shown in gold) are based on the work of Vuyk and colleagues[93] with propofol and alfentanil (see Fig. 26.15) and are scaled to fentanyl and sufentanil according to their relative potencies.[108] The intersections of the target concentration line and the diagonal lines indicate the infusion rate appropriate at each point in time. For example, to maintain a sufentanil concentration of 0.16 ng/mL, the appropriate rates are approximately: 0.6 μg/kg/h at 5 minutes, 0.5 μg/kg/h at 10 minutes, 0.4 μg/kg/h at 20 minutes, and 0.3 μg/kg/h at 40 minutes. Of course, selecting target concentrations and different times of rate adjustment is possible, depending on the clinical circumstances and an assessment of how accurately the intravenous drug needs to be titrated.

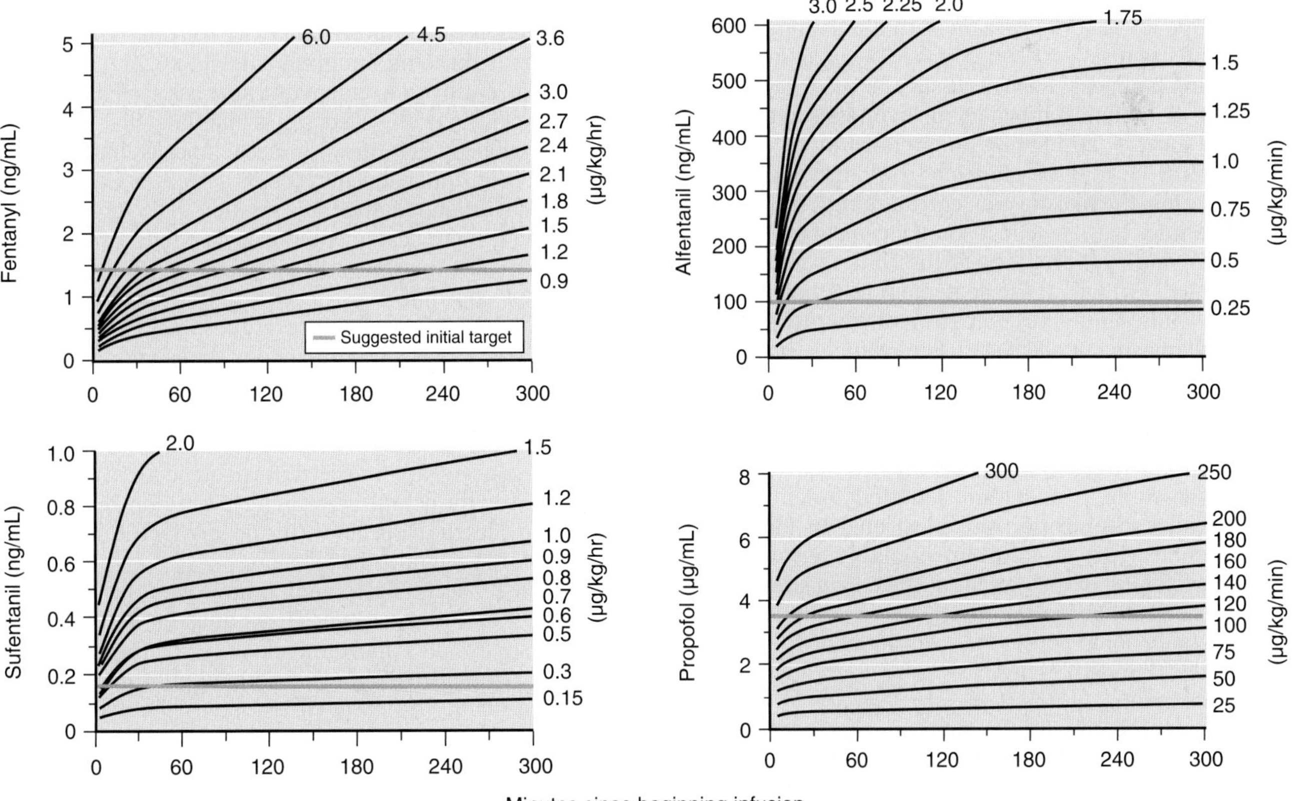

Fig. 26.19 Nomogram for calculating maintenance infusion rates to maintain a stable concentration of fentanyl, alfentanil, sufentanil, or propofol. The *y* axis is the desired concentration. The *x* axis is the time relative to the initial bolus. The *diagonal lines* show the infusion rates at different times required to maintain the desired concentration selected on the *y* axis.

RECOVERY FROM ANESTHESIA

Recovery from anesthesia is determined by the pharmacokinetic principles that govern the rate of decrease in drug from the effect compartment once drug administration is terminated, as well as by the pharmacodynamics of the drug. Although the terminal elimination half-life is often interpreted as a measure of how short- or long-lasting a drug is, the rate at which drug plasma concentration decreases is dependent on both elimination and redistribution of the drug from the central compartment. The contribution of redistribution and elimination toward the rate of decrease in drug concentration varies according to the duration for which the drug has been administered[108,109] and also the time since the infusion has stopped, because these processes have different rate constants.

In 1985, Schwilden[110] developed a mathematic model to relate the time course of offset of action of inhaled anesthetics to the duration of anesthetic drug delivery. Similarly, Fisher and Rosen[111] demonstrated how the accumulation of neuromuscular blocking agents in peripheral volumes of distribution results in slowed recovery with increasing duration of administration. They introduced two measures of the time course of recovery, the time for twitch tension to recover from 5% to 25% and the time for twitch tension to recover from 25% to 75%.

Since then, the time for the plasma concentration to decrease by 50% from an infusion that maintains a constant concentration (e.g., infusion given by (Eq. 26.14) has been termed the *context-sensitive half-time* (Fig. 26.20),[109] with the context being the duration of the infusion. The 50% decrease was chosen both for tradition (e.g., half-lives are the time for a 50% decrease with a one-compartment model) and because, very roughly, a 50% reduction in drug concentration appears to be necessary for recovery after the administration of most intravenous hypnotics at the termination of surgery. Depending on circumstances, decreases other than 50% may be clinically relevant. Additionally, sometimes it is the plasma concentration that is of interest, and sometimes it is the effect-site concentration that is of interest. A more general term is the context-sensitive *decrement time*,[112] in which the decrement in concentration is specifically noted, as is the compartment where the decrease is modeled (plasma or effect site). For example, the relationship between infusion duration and the time required for a 70% decrease in fentanyl effect-site concentration is the *context-sensitive 70% effect-site decrement time.*

Context-sensitive effect-site decrement times for varying percent decreases in alfentanil, fentanyl, sufentanil, and remifentanil concentration are illustrated in Fig. 26.21. To determine when an infusion should be terminated (to enable awakening of the patient at the end of surgery), the clinician needs to bear in mind the decrease in concentration necessary for recovery, the duration of the infusion (the context), and the context-sensitive, effect-site decrement time required for the necessary decrease.

Context-sensitive decrement times are fundamentally different from the elimination half-life. With monoexponential decay, each 50% decrease in concentration requires the same amount of time, and this time is independent of how the drug is given. This is not true for the context-sensitive half-time. First, as the name is intended to imply, the time needed for a 50% decrease is absolutely dependent on how long the drug was given, with infusion duration being the context to which the name refers. In addition, small changes in percent decrement can result in surprisingly large increases in the time required. The time required for a 60% decrease in drug concentration can be more than twice the time required for a 50% decrease in some situations (see Fig. 26.21).

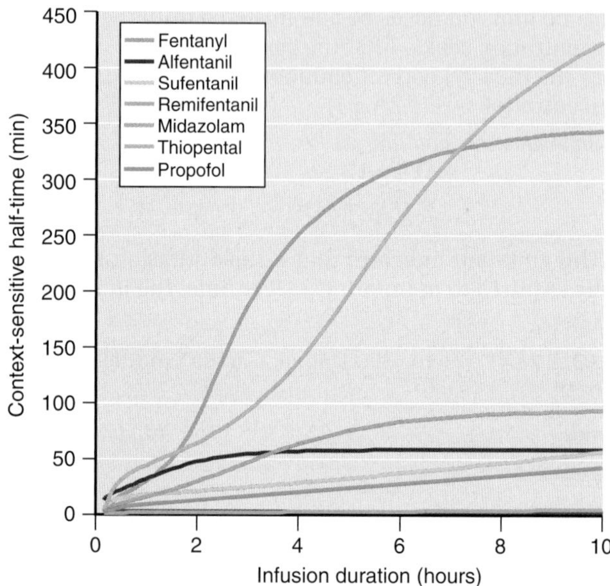

Fig. 26.20 Context-sensitive half-times as a function of infusion duration (context) derived from pharmacokinetic models of fentanyl, sufentanil, alfentanil, remifentanil, propofol, midazolam, and thiopental. (From Hughes MA, Glass PSA, Jacobs JR. Context-sensitive half-time in multicompartment pharmacokinetic models for intravenous anesthetic drugs. *Anesthesiology.* 1992;76:334–341.)

Context-sensitive decrement times are based on the assumption that plasma or the effect site is maintained at a constant concentration. Such is rarely the case clinically, but the maintenance of constant concentrations is a necessary assumption to provide a unique mathematic solution to the time required for a given percent decrement in plasma or effect-site concentration. Because plasma and effect-site concentrations are rarely kept constant, it is important that context-sensitive decrement times are used as *general* guidelines for interpreting the pharmacokinetics of intravenous drugs and not as *absolute* predictions for any given individual patient case or infusion regimen. Automated drug delivery systems can provide more precise predictions of the time required for the plasma or effect-site concentration to decrease to any desired concentration, based on the actual drug dosing in the individual patient, which provides the clinician with guidance for the most appropriate time to terminate the infusion.

Context-sensitive decrement times focus on the role of pharmacokinetics in recovery from anesthesia. Pharmacodynamics plays an important role in recovery as well. Bailey[113] used integrated pharmacokinetic-pharmacodynamic models to define the *mean effect time* as the average time to responsiveness after maintenance of anesthesia at the 90% probability of unresponsiveness. The mean effect time demonstrates that when drugs have a very shallow concentration-versus-response relationship, concentrations must decrease by a significant fraction to provide adequate emergence, which delays recovery from anesthesia. In contrast,

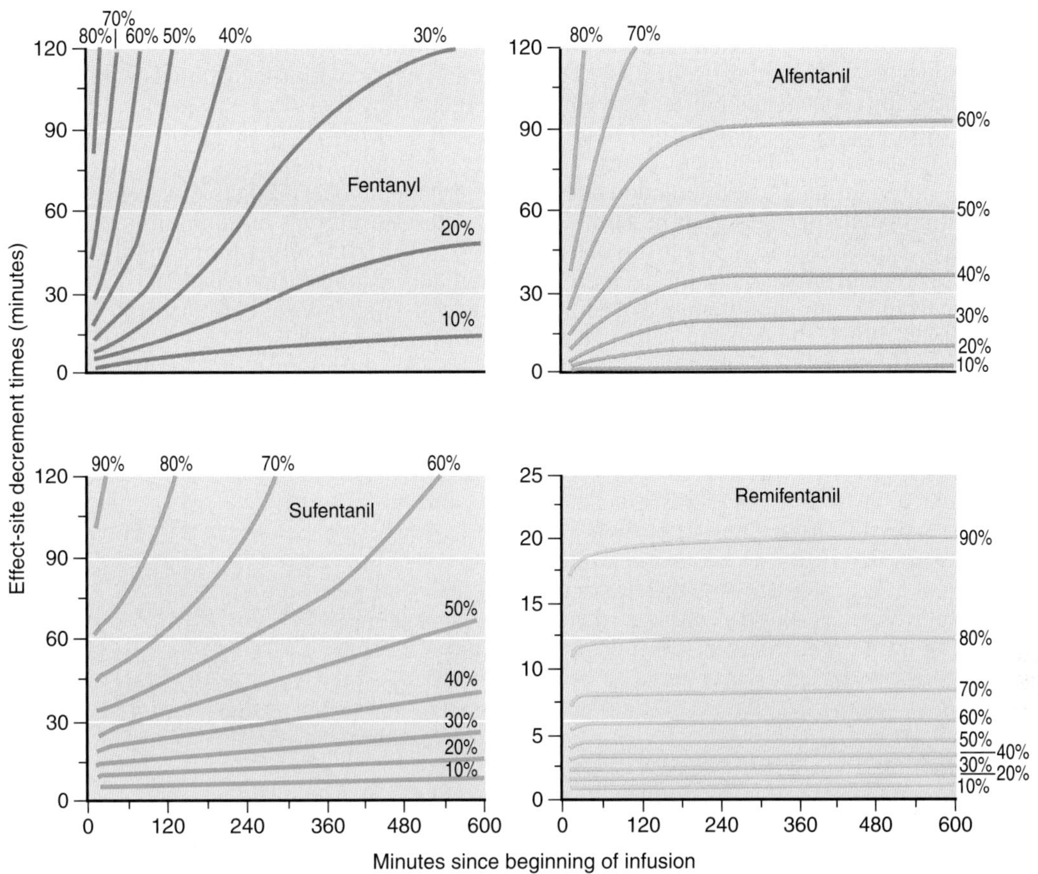

Fig. 26.21 Context-sensitive effect-site decrement times for alfentanil, fentanyl, sufentanil, and remifentanil showing the time required for decreases of a given percentage (labeled for each curve) from the maintained effect-site concentration after termination of the infusion.

recovery is hastened by a steep concentration-versus-response relationship, in which emergence from anesthesia occurs after a relatively small fractional decrease in concentration. Most intravenous hypnotics have a moderately steep concentration-versus-response relationship.

Pharmacodynamic drug interactions also play a role in recovery from anesthesia. Interaction relationships predict that the same anesthetic state can be achieved by different ratios of two drugs. One way of selecting the best ratio might be the combination that offers the most rapid recovery. For example, when an opioid is combined with a hypnotic, the rate of recovery from anesthesia depends on the opioid and hypnotic concentrations, the rate of decrease in both drug concentrations, and the relative synergy between them for loss of response to noxious stimulation (i.e., the state maintained during anesthesia) versus the relative synergy for loss of consciousness. Although the time course of decreases in opioid and hypnotic concentrations can be approximately described by their respective context-sensitive decrement times for both drugs (Fig. 26.22; see Fig. 26.15]), the influence of relative synergy for different endpoints must be captured by separate models of the interaction of the drugs for adequate anesthesia and emergence from anesthesia.

Vuyk and coworkers[54] modeled the predicted time to awakening from adequate anesthesia when propofol is combined with fentanyl, sufentanil, alfentanil, or remifentanil. Their calculations took into account the interaction between propofol and these opioids to provide adequate

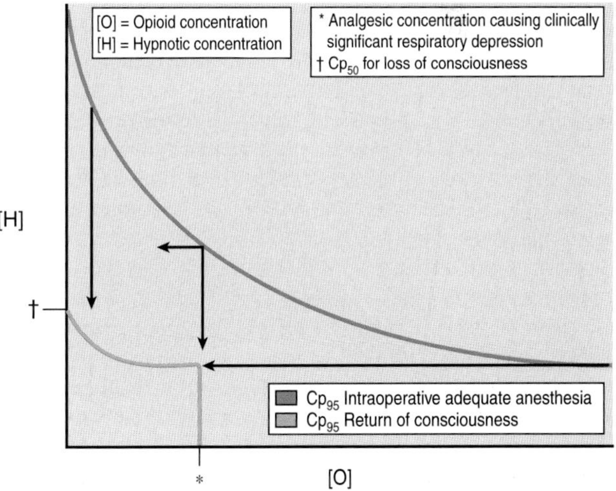

Fig. 26.22 Interaction between hypnotics and opioids for the prevention of movement after a noxious stimulus and for awakening and adequate spontaneous ventilation at the end of a surgical procedure. The time to recover at the end of a procedure is dependent on the concentration of both drugs used during surgery and the time for both to decrease below that required for consciousness and adequate spontaneous ventilation (i.e., their context-sensitive decrement times).

anesthesia and the interaction between propofol and opioids on consciousness levels on emergence from anesthesia (Figs. 26.23 and 26.24). Recovery times vary with the choice of opioid and the relative balance of opioid and propofol during maintenance of anesthesia. For example, the upper left of Fig. 26.23 simulates the emergence from a propofol-fentanyl anesthetic of 15-minute duration. The simulations assume a steady concentration of fentanyl and propofol throughout the anesthesia, similar to the underlying assumption of context-sensitive decrement times. The lowest curve on the response surface is the interaction curve between fentanyl and propofol; it ranges from no fentanyl and 12 μg/mL of propofol on the left to 5.33 ng/mL of fentanyl and 1.8 μg/mL of propofol on the right. In theory, any point along this curve would ensure maintenance of equivalent depth of anesthesia. When the infusion is turned off after 15 minutes of anesthesia, the concentrations of both drugs decrease. The decreasing concentrations of propofol and fentanyl when the infusion is turned off can be found by the upward lines drawn from different points on the interaction curve, with the distance away from the lower plane representing time. Taken together, these upward lines represent a *recovery surface*. The blue line drawn on the recovery surface shows the points at which the fentanyl-propofol interaction model predicts emergence.

After 15 minutes of maintaining 1.8 μg/mL of propofol and 5.33 ng/mL of fentanyl (right margin of the interaction curve), approximately 12 to 17 minutes is needed for the concentrations of both drugs to decrease sufficiently to permit emergence (see Fig. 26.23). However, if one maintains concentrations of 3.5 μg/mL of propofol and 1.5 ng/mL of fentanyl (toward the middle of the interaction curve),

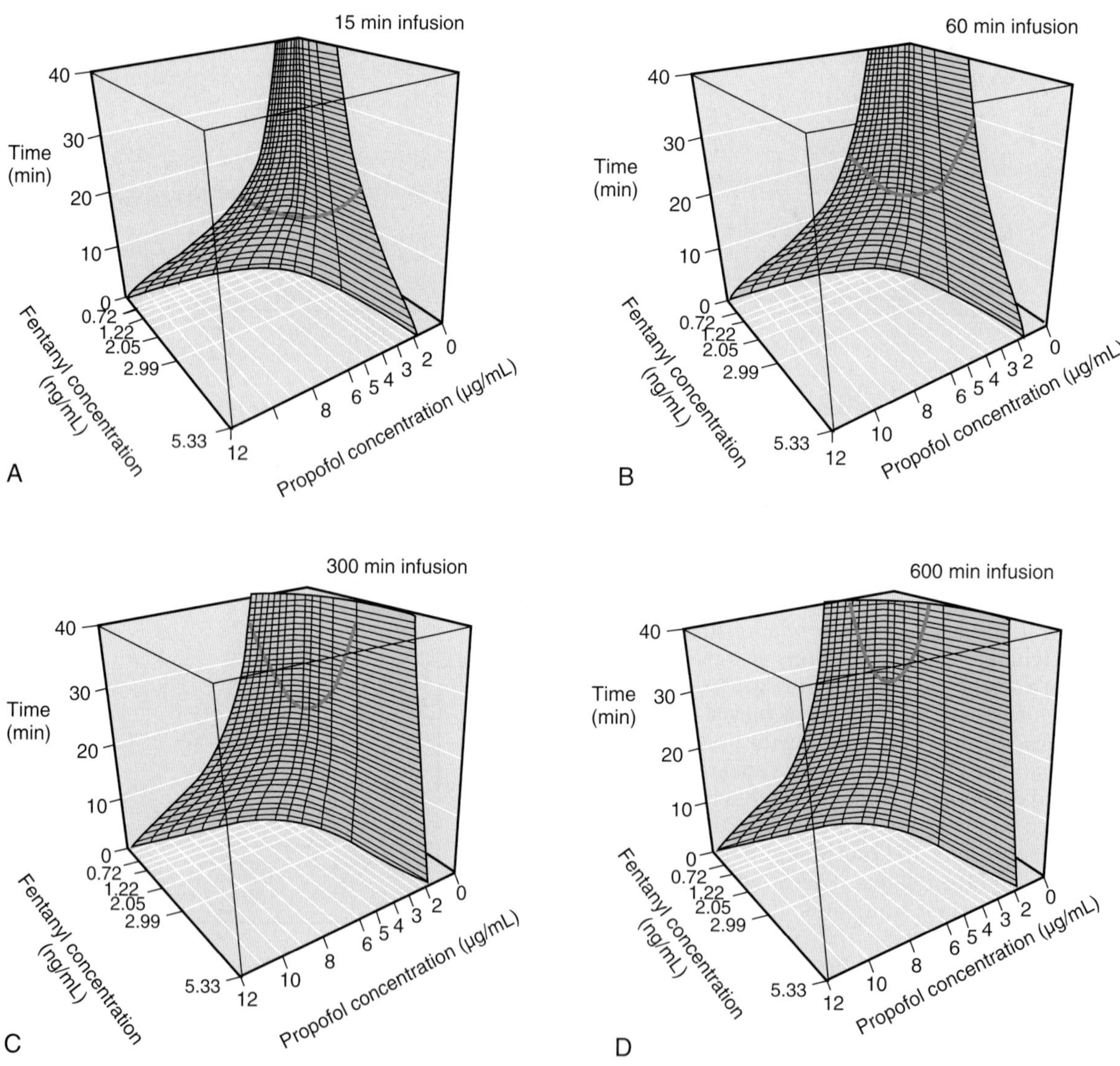

Fig. 26.23 Simulation of the interaction of propofol and fentanyl in preventing a somatic response at skin incision and time to recovery. On the *x* axis is the fentanyl concentration, and on the *y* axis is the propofol concentration. The *blue curve* in the lower plane shows the propofol-fentanyl interaction required to provide adequate anesthesia. When the infusion is turned off, the concentrations of each drug decrease, as shown on the *z* axis. The *blue curve* drawn on the recovery surface shows the time to emergence from anesthesia for combinations of fentanyl and propofol after an anesthetic of 15 minutes' (A), 60 minutes' (B), 300 minutes' (C), and 600 minutes' (D) duration. The optimal combination for the most rapid recovery is a propofol concentration of 3.0 to 3.5 μg/mL, combined with 1.5 ng/mL fentanyl. As the concentration of propofol or fentanyl increases, the time for recovery increases. In addition, the longer the duration of drug infusion, the longer recovery takes, especially if the optimal combination is not used. (Modified from Vuyk J, Mertens MJ, Olofsen E, et al. Propofol anesthesia and rational opioid selection. Determination of optimal EC50-EC95 propofol-opioid concentrations that assure adequate anesthesia and a rapid return of consciousness. *Anesthesiology*. 1997;87:1549–1562.)

then emergence can be expected only 8 minutes after the infusions are turned off. Examination of the curves for 60, 300, and 600 minutes of propofol-fentanyl anesthesia suggests that the fentanyl target concentration that provides the most rapid emergence is approximately 1.0 to 1.5 ng/mL, which requires a propofol concentration of approximately 3.0 to 3.5 μg/mL to maintain adequate anesthesia. In similar simulations, Vuyk and colleagues demonstrated that maintaining alfentanil and sufentanil concentrations in excess of the analgesic range (i.e., approximately 80 ng/mL for alfentanil and 0.15 ng/mL for sufentanil) is of little clinical benefit and can be expected to delay recovery from anesthesia. A second conclusion from these simulations is that if the patient demonstrates inadequate anesthesia, increasing the hypnotic concentration rather than increasing the opioid concentration beyond the analgesic range is preferable, so as to prevent prolongation of recovery.

The situation is different for remifentanil because of its unusual pharmacokinetic properties (see Fig. 26.24). When a remifentanil infusion is terminated, the extraordinarily fast clearance of remifentanil results in a very rapid offset of opioid drug effect. The lower plane again shows equivalent anesthetic states during maintenance with remifentanil and propofol (see Fig. 26.24). High doses of remifentanil permit a modest reduction in the dose of propofol needed for adequate anesthesia.[114] However, the recovery surfaces show that high doses of remifentanil, with a modest reduction in the propofol dose, permit considerably faster emergence

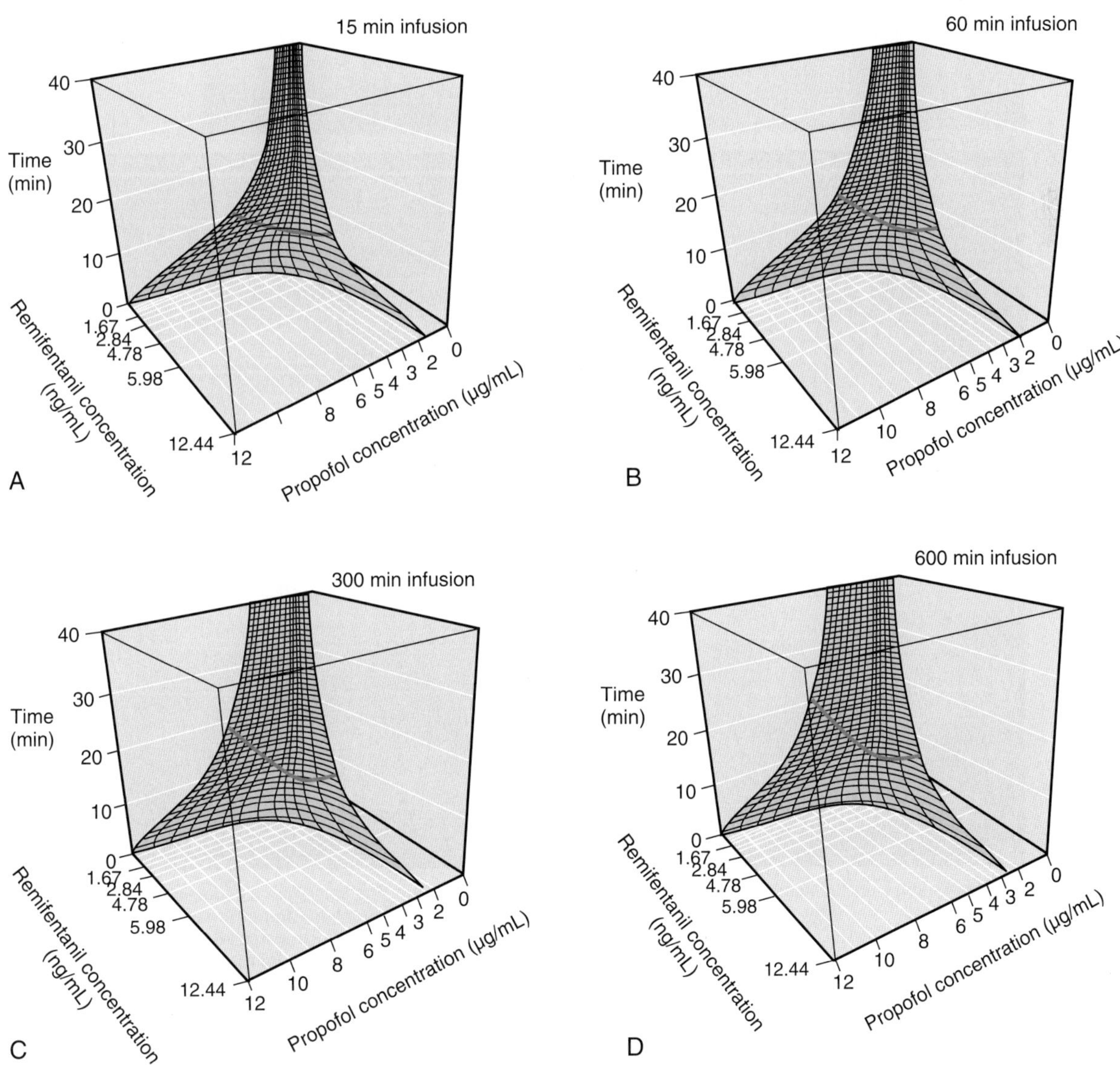

Fig. 26.24 Simulation of the interaction of propofol and remifentanil in preventing a somatic response at skin incision and time to recovery. The remifentanil concentration is on the *x* axis, and the propofol concentration is on the *y* axis. The *blue curve* in the lower plane shows the propofol-remifentanil interaction required to provide adequate anesthesia. When the infusion is turned off, the concentrations of each drug decrease, as shown on the *z* axis. The *blue line* drawn on the recovery surface shows the time to emergence from anesthesia for combinations of remifentanil and propofol after an anesthetic of 15 minutes' (A), 60 minutes' (B), 300 minutes' (C), and 600 minutes' (D) duration. With remifentanil, the optimal combination is a propofol concentration of 2.5 μg/mL and with remifentanil, 5 to 7 ng/mL. In addition, increasing the duration of the infusion has minimal impact on recovery time if the optimal dose of remifentanil is not used. However, if the propofol dose is increased, then recovery is prolonged. (Modified from Vuyk J, Mertens MJ, Olofsen E, et al. Propofol anesthesia and rational opioid selection. Determination of optimal EC50-EC95 propofol-opioid concentrations that assure adequate anesthesia and a rapid return of consciousness. *Anesthesiology*. 1997;87:1549–1562.)

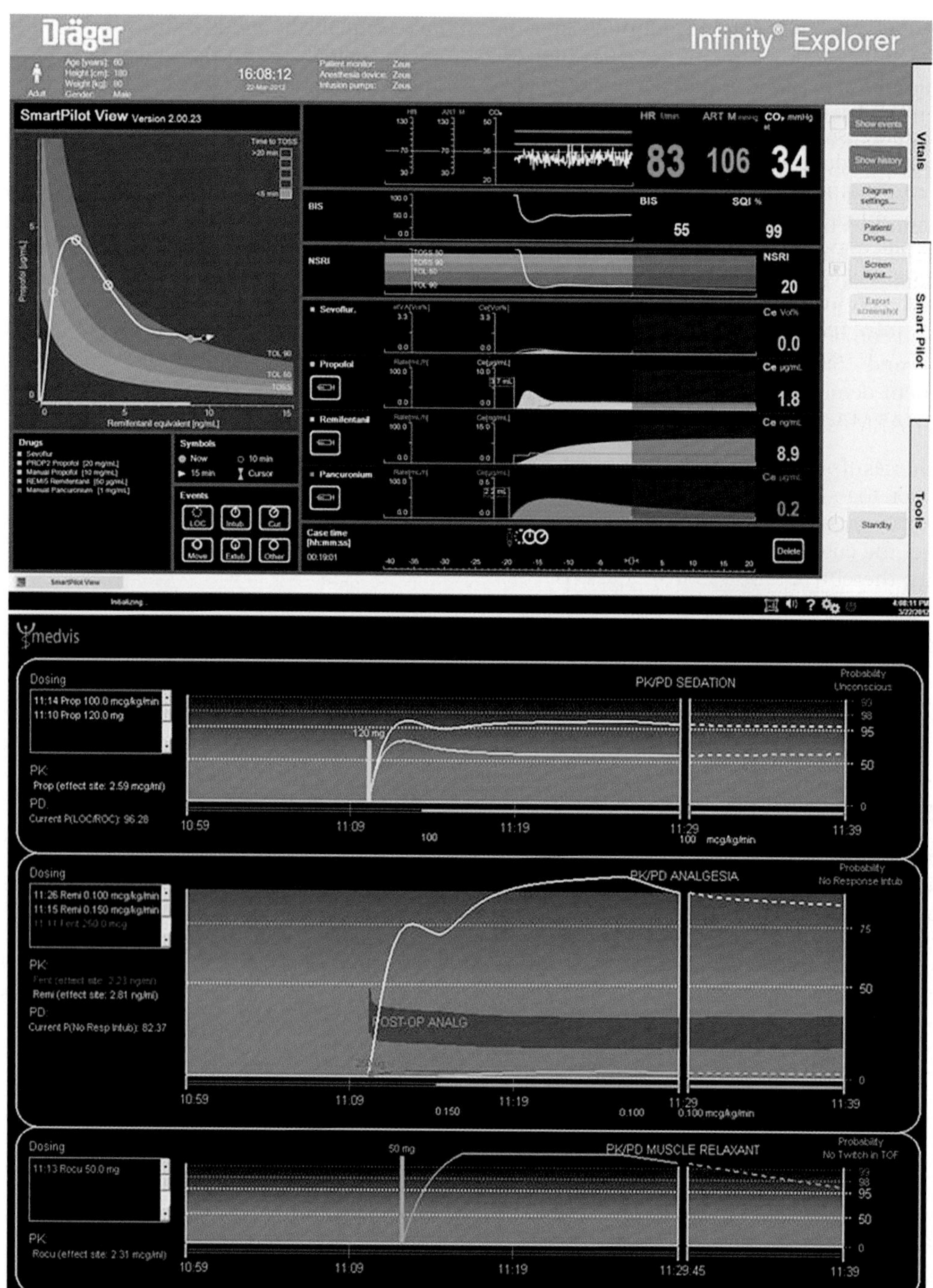

Fig. 26.25 On-line advisory displays including characteristics of drug behavior and interaction. The SmartPilot (Dräger, Lübeck, Germany) *(upper display)* is a two-dimensional display that shows the effect-site concentrations of combined drugs (opioids and intravenous or inhalation hypnotics), based on pharmacokinetic models and the resulting anesthetic effect and on pharmacodynamic models. Grey shaded areas indicate different levels of anesthesia. The *orange point* indicates the current combination of effect-site concentrations; the *white line* shows the retrospective concentrations; and a 10- and 15-minute prediction is marked by a *black point* and *arrow*—already calculated during presetting of delivery. Event markers may be set to show specific states of the patient related to the level of anesthesia. The time-based real-time curves, trends, and prediction of effect-site concentrations of individual drugs, resulting anesthetic effect (noxious stimulus response index [NSRI]), correlated bispectral index (BIS), vital signs, and event markers are shown as reference for interpretation. The Medvis display (Medvis, Salt Lake City, Utah) *(lower display)* shows a real-time visualization of anesthetic using pharmacokinetic and pharmacodynamic models to predict drug effect-site concentrations and drug effects in the past, current time, and 10 minutes into the future. Drug doses as boluses and infusions are administered via a separate data interface or user interface. Drugs are categorized according to sedation *(top plot)*, analgesia *(middle plot)*, and muscle relaxation *(bottom plot)*. Effects are depicted as a population-based probability of unconsciousness *(top plot)*, no response to tracheal intubation *(middle plot)*, and no twitch response to a train of four stimulus *(bottom plot)*. In addition, a second pharmacodynamic endpoint, POST-OP ANALG, represents a guideline therapeutic window for postoperative pain. Synergistic interactions of sedative-hypnotics and analgesics are shown by the *white curves* in the plot. For example, the top plot shows that with only propofol, the probability of unconsciousness is between 50% and 95% *(yellow curve)*, but because propofol interacts with the opioids, the probability of unconsciousness is greater than 95% *(white curve)*. Similarly, propofol potentiates the effect of the opioids in the middle plot.

from anesthesia. For example, it takes approximately 12 minutes to awaken from 600 minutes of anesthesia maintained with 3 μg/mL of propofol and 2.5 ng/mL of remifentanil (see Fig. 26.24*D*). On the other hand, if the remifentanil concentration is increased to 5 ng/mL, then the propofol concentration can be reduced to between 2 and 2.5 μg/mL, and emergence can be anticipated within 6 minutes of discontinuation of the infusions. One might be concerned that such a technique places patients at increased risk for awareness because a propofol concentration of 2 μg/mL is below the C_{50} value for wakefulness.[115] Therefore combining such a technique with intraoperative EEG monitoring to assess anesthetic adequacy is reasonable.[21,115]

DISPLAYING PHARMACOLOGIC INFORMATION

Integrating all sources of pharmacologic information including drug interaction together with measurements of patient response to a specific drug dose might offer a powerful advisory tool to depict the complete dose-response relationship of multiple drugs, thereby optimizing drug administration and improving patient care.[116,117] For example, Fig. 26.25 shows a drug interaction advisory display.

Intravenous Infusion Devices and Technologies

MANUAL INTRAVENOUS INFUSION

When an infusion of an intravenous anesthetic is administered, the infusion regimen can be controlled by a variety of mechanisms varying from the simple Cair clamp or Dial-a-Flo (Abbott Laboratories) to complex computer-controlled infusion pumps. Simplicity of mechanical design, however, is not necessarily correlated with ease of use, which has prompted ongoing advances in infusion device technology over the past decades.

Infusion devices can be classified as either controllers or positive displacement pumps. Explicit in their title, controllers contain mechanisms that control the rate of flow produced by gravity, whereas positive displacement pumps contain active pumping mechanisms.

The most commonly used pumps for administration of intravenous anesthetics are positive displacement syringe pumps that use a variety of mechanisms. These pumps have acceptable accuracy and have several features that make them particularly suitable for anesthetic delivery. An important advance has been the introduction of a calculator feature within the pump so that the clinician can input the weight of the patient, the drug concentration, and the infusion rate in dose/unit weight/unit time and the pump will then calculate the infusion in volume/unit time. These pumps also permit simple application of a staged infusion scheme by allowing an initial dose and a maintenance infusion rate to be programmed into the pump. Numerous syringe pumps also include automated recognition of syringe size. Further enhancements are drug libraries by class of drug, suggested dosing schemes, and maximal dosing alerts. These modest advances in pump technology and design enable intravenous anesthetics to be conveniently and safely delivered.

In addition to the pumps, the complete intravenous delivery systems' hardware must perform perfectly,[5] which means that the correct amount of drug should be delivered to the venous circulation in each unit of time. When the drug administration set has too large a *deadspace*, the actual delivery rate can be altered, depending on the flow rate of coadministered fluid.[118] The use of an antireflux valve is certainly advisable to prevent flow of the medication backward into the intravenous fluid bag rather than into the patient. Other factors include excessive compliance within the administration system (in the syringe plunger or in the administration lines) and the use of syringes with suboptimal lubrication, causing the plunger to advance in small jumps when infusion rates are slow; that is, with

TABLE 26.5 Manual Infusion Schemes

	ANESTHESIA		SEDATION OR ANALGESIA	
Drug	**Loading Dose (μg/kg)**	**Maintenance Infusion (μg/kg/min)**	**Loading Dose (μg/kg)**	**Maintenance Infusion (μg/kg/min)**
Alfentanil	50-150	0.5-3	10-25	0.25-1
Fentanyl	5-15	0.03-0.1	1-3	0.01-0.03
Sufentanil	0.5-5	0.01-0.05	0.1-0.5	0.005-0.01
Remifentanil	0.5-1.0	0.1-0.4	*	0.025-0.1
Ketamine	1500-2500	25-75	500-1000	10-20
Propofol	1000-2000	50-150	250-1000	10-50
Midazolam	50-150	0.25-1.5	25-100	0.25-1
Methohexital	1500-2500	50-150	250-1000	10-50
Dexmedetomidine			0.5-1 over 10 min	0.005-0.015

*For analgesia or during sedation, an initial loading dose of remifentanil should not be given because its very rapid onset may result in apnea or muscle rigidity.
After the loading dose, an initially high infusion rate to account for redistribution should be used and then titrated to the lowest infusion rate that will maintain adequate anesthesia or sedation. When using opiates as part of a nitrous-narcotic technique or for cardiac anesthesia, the dosing scheme listed under anesthesia is used. When the opiate is combined as part of balanced anesthesia, dosing listed for analgesia is needed.

small patients, low target concentrations, drug solutions of high concentration, or large-volume syringes.[5]

Manual intravenous drug delivery consists of a combination of a bolus dosage and a continuous infusion, as explained earlier when discussing the pharmacokinetic considerations. Table 26.5 offers recommendations for delivering intravenous anesthetics via conventional infusion pumps based on integrated pharmacokinetic-pharmacodynamic models. Ultimately, the adequate rate of drug administration is based on observation and examination. Individual patients vary significantly in their response to a given drug dose or concentration; therefore titrating to an adequate drug level for each individual patient is essential. Drug concentrations required to provide adequate anesthesia also vary according to the type of surgery (e.g., superficial surgery vs. intraabdominal surgery). Drug concentration requirements are often smaller during the end phase of surgery; therefore titration often involves judicious reduction of the infusion rate toward the end of surgery to facilitate rapid recovery.

If the infusion rate is insufficient to maintain adequate anesthesia, then both an additional loading (bolus) dose and an increase in infusion are required to increase the plasma (biophase) drug concentration rapidly. Various interventions also require larger drug concentrations, usually for brief periods (e.g., laryngoscopy, endotracheal intubation, skin incision). Consequently, the infusion scheme should be tailored to provide peak concentrations during these brief periods of intense stimulation. An adequate drug level for endotracheal intubation is often achieved with the initial loading dose; however, for procedures such as skin incision, an additional bolus dose may be necessary.

Infusion schemes (see Table 26.5) do not approach the convenience and precision of use associated with the delivery of an inhaled anesthetic via a calibrated vaporizer, particularly when the user is still required to calculate volume infusion rates (mL/hr) from the mass-based infusion rates given in the infusion schemes. The use of "calculator" pumps helps to simplify the task of the anesthesiologist. At start-up the user is required to input the weight of the patient and the drug concentration. Thereafter, the pumps are able to accept as input mass-based rates, from which they calculate and implement volume infusion rates. The level of convenience and precision of vaporizers can however be achieved by using TCI devices, such as the commercially available TCI pumps.

COMPUTER-CONTROLLED DRUG DELIVERY

As discussed in the introduction of this chapter, optimal patient-individual dosing may be achieved by the application of pharmacokinetic and pharmacodynamic principles. Using the dose-response relationship, drug titration should be performed as close as possible to the drug effect. Titrating to a specific effect or, if not possible, a specific effect-site concentration offers advantages. Because the effect-site or plasma concentrations are not continuously measurable online for most intravenous anesthetics (in contrast to inhaled anesthetics), a drug model using a computer that continuously updates the anesthetic administration rate to maintain an estimated drug effect or drug concentration is required (Fig. 26.26).

If a specific plasma or effect-site concentration is titrated, then this technique is called TCI. TCI is a *closed-loop control* system. The history of the development of TCI systems has recently been summarized.[119] In these systems the clinician serves as the *human controller* in the loop and, as a consequence, the control actions are intermittent and irregular in time.[120] Control theory is increasingly being applied in the development of computer-controlled drug delivery systems, among others in anesthetic closed-loop control applications. The aim of computer-controlled closed-loop systems is to formalize this process of observation and intervention to provide fine-tuned and more accurate control. Such systems use a near continuous signal of drug effect, calculate the error between the observed value and the set point value (selected by the user), and use this error figure in an algorithm to make frequent and regular adjustments to drug administration rates. Some computer-controlled drug delivery systems try to predict the future drug effect to make appropriate adjustments well in advance.[120]

TARGET-CONTROLLED INFUSION

Devices

The development of microprocessor-controlled syringe pumps and a better understanding of the dose-response relationship have enabled the development of TCI systems. A TCI is a computer- or microprocessor-controlled system that aims to achieve a user-defined estimated drug concentration in a body compartment or tissue. A clinician using a TCI system to administer an anesthetic drug is thus able to set and adjust a desired drug concentration, usually referred to as the *target concentration*, based on clinical observation of the patient or measurement of drug effect. Multicompartment pharmacokinetic-pharmacodynamic models are used by TCI systems to calculate the infusion rates required to achieve the target concentration (see Fig. 26.4). A computer or microprocessor is required to perform the complex calculations and to control the infusion pump. Typically, plasma or effect-site concentrations are targeted.[3]

TCI systems in use today still apply the theoretical approach described by Kruger-Thiemer[121] to achieve and maintain a steady-state blood concentration of a drug whose pharmacokinetic can be described by a multicompartment model. This approach was first clinically implemented by Schwilden.[7] The infusion schemes used, better known as bolus-elimination-transfer (BET) schemes (see Fig. 26.4), were initially designed for two-compartment models. Briefly, the infusion starts with an initial bolus of drug required to achieve the initial target concentration. Second, an infusion is administered to replace drug lost by elimination. Since the elimination rate constant is fixed, the amount of drug eliminated in each unit of time is proportional to the plasma concentration; accordingly, at steady-state plasma concentrations, drug removal by elimination can be compensated for by a constant rate infusion. Third, a second infusion is administered to replace drug distributed or transferred to peripheral tissues. The amount redistributed exponentially declines over time as the gradient between the central compartment and the peripheral compartment decreases. Replacing distributed drug requires an infusion at an exponentially declining rate to replace drug *lost* from the central compartment by distribution until steady state.[4]

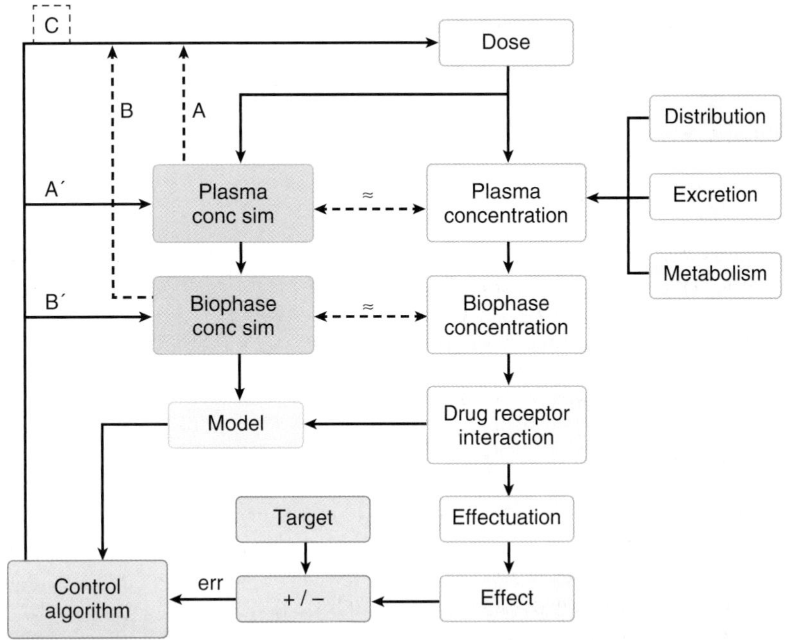

Fig. 26.26 Schematic representation of the pharmacokinetic and pharmacodynamic processes determining the relationship between administered doses and resulting effect intensity of a drug *(yellow)*. Pharmacokinetic factors such as distribution, metabolism, and/or excretion determine the relationship between drug dose and drug concentration in the biophase. In the biophase, the drug interacts with the receptor, and the pharmacologic effect is accomplished via effectuation processes. Target-controlled infusion (TCI) will use a model to estimate the plasma or biophase drug concentration *(red)*, and will calculate the dose needed to approach a target concentration in plasma *(A)* or biophase/effect-site *(B)*. Computer-controlled, closed-loop feedback measures the error between the effect and the target effect to control the dose administration *(blue)*. Better closed-loop performance can result if, rather than using the dose as a direct actuator, the *simulated* variable of a TCI system is used as actuated variable *(A/A´, B/B´)*. The TCI system then compensates for part of the complexity of the dose-interaction relationship. Advanced control algorithms may take into account a continuously updated model of the interaction *(light green)*. (Modified from Struys M, de Smet T. Principles of drug actions: target-controlled infusions and closed-loop administration. In: Evers AS, Maze M, Kharasch ED, eds. *Anesthetic Pharmacology: Basic Principles and Clinical Practice.* Cambridge: Cambridge University Press; 2011:103–122. Used with permission.)

BET schemes have some disadvantages such as the requirement of a no-drug status before infusion, which disables a change in the target concentration. In addition, more recent research concluded that the pharmacokinetics of most anesthetics is better described using a three- instead of a two-compartment model. Lastly, as previously discussed in this chapter, the plasma is not the site of drug effect. Consequently, effect compartment–controlled TCI algorithms were developed.[29] During the 1990s, various computer-based TCI prototypes were developed by researchers at Stanford (STANPUMP, California), Stellenbosch (STELPUMP, South Africa), Duke (computer-assisted continuous infusion [CACI], North Carolina), and Ghent (RUGLOOP, Belgium) universities. Groups in Erlangen, Germany, and Leiden, The Netherlands, produced software able to simulate pharmacokinetic trajectories (IVA-SIM and TIVA Trainer, respectively). Finally, the Diprifusor (AstraZeneca, London) became the first commercially available TCI pump. It was based on a prototype from the Kenny group[122] and was able to control a set plasma target concentration using specific prefilled syringes from AstraZeneca. Although the technology never became available in the United States,[8] this TCI pump was the first breakthrough in an attempt to optimize drug administration in daily clinical practice in many countries. More recently, various companies have commercialized more flexible *open TCI* pumps capable of administering multiple drugs in both plasma and effect compartment–control mode (Fig. 26.27).[8,119]

Effect compartment–control requires a rate constant that accurately describes the rate of equilibration between plasma (Fig. 26.28*A*) and effect-site concentrations (Fig. 26.28*B*). The benefits of effect compartment–controlled TCI were demonstrated for propofol by Wakeling and associates[123] and Struys and associates.[47] This mode is commonly used throughout Europe.

A detailed description of the history of the development of TCI and of the development and availability of TCI devices was published in 2016.[8,124]

Evaluation of Target-Controlled Infusion Delivery

Acceptance of target-controlled drug delivery of intravenous anesthetics requires evaluation of accuracy (defined as the difference between predicted and measured concentrations) and outcomes among patients in whom automated drug delivery has been used. The inaccuracies associated with pharmacokinetic model–driven devices are attributed to possible problems with the software and hardware, and more importantly to pharmacokinetic variability (Fig. 26.29).

Inaccuracy in the software results from incorrect mathematic implementation of the pharmacokinetic model. Computer simulations can be used to test the infusion rates as calculated by a software program, and thus software errors are fairly simple to identify and correct.[125] Inaccurate drug delivery from the infusion pump (i.e., failure to correctly infuse the amount intended by the system) infrequently

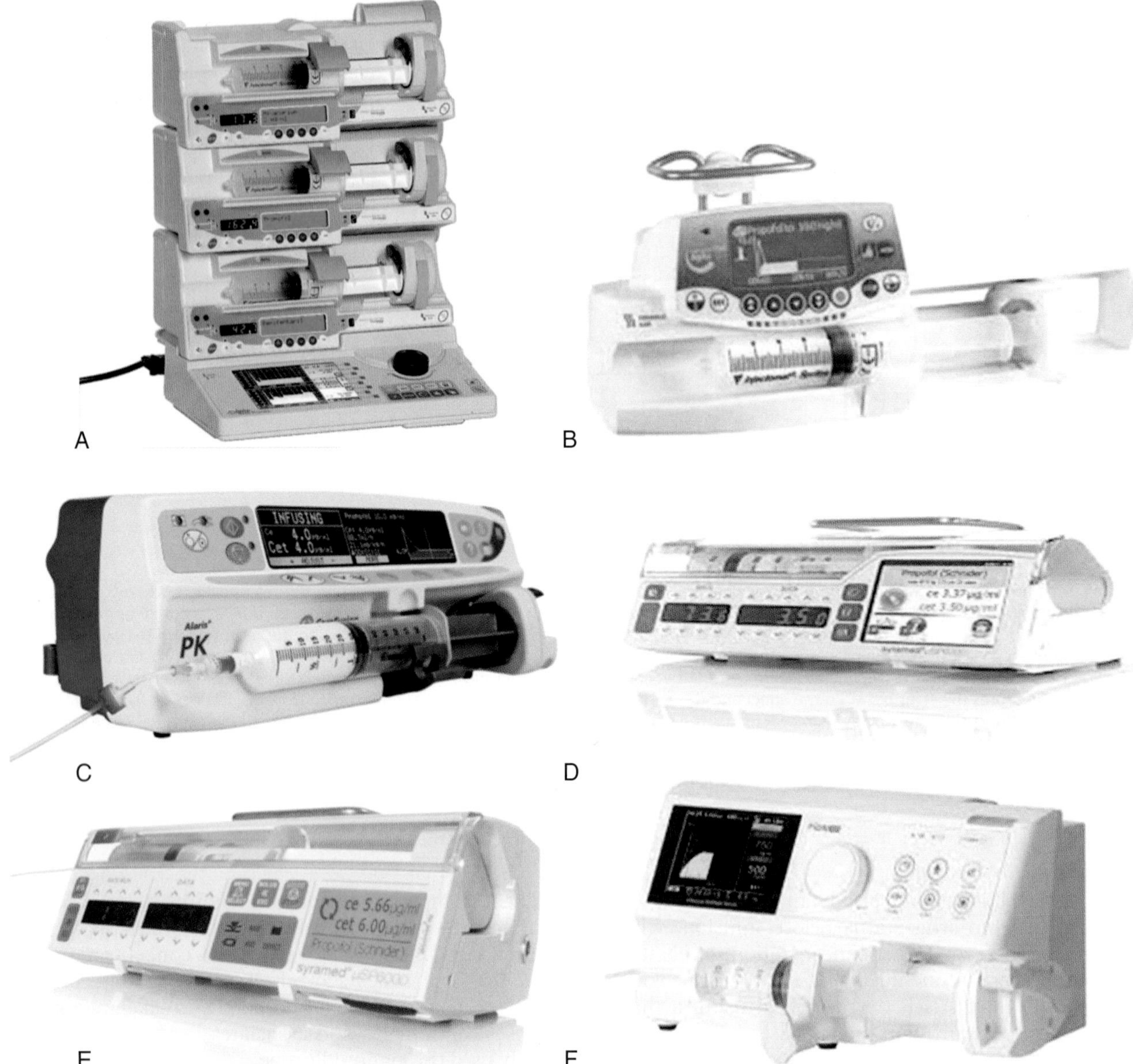

Fig. 26.27 Target-controlled infusion (TCI) pumps. (A) Fresenius Base Primea. (B) Fresenius Injectomat TIVA. (C) CareFusion Alaris PK. (D) Arcomed μSP 6000. (E) Arcomed μVP 7000. (F) Bionet PION TCI pump. (G) B. Braun Infusomat Space and Perfusor Space. (H) Veryark Concert-CL. (I) MedCaptain HP TCI. ([A and B] Courtesy Fresenius Kabi AG, Homburg, Germany; [C] Courtesy BD, Franklin Lakes, NJ; [D and E] Courtesy Arcomed, Zurich, Switzerland; [F] Courtesy Bionet, Seoul, Korea; [G] Courtesy B. Braun Medical Inc., Bethlehem PA; [H] Courtesy PRHOINSA, Madrid, Spain; [I] Courtesy Medcaptain, Shenzhen, P.R. China.)

occurs with present syringe-pump technology and contributes little to the overall inaccuracy of these devices.[126] The aforementioned safety review identified only two company reports of problems with TCI devices that were attributable to software programming errors, neither of which caused actual patient harm.[127]

The major cause of inaccuracy is biologic variability, of which there are two sources: (1) the pharmacokinetic model is always wrong,[106] and (2) the pharmacokinetics of the individual patient are not as programmed into the model. The pharmacokinetic model is always wrong because individuals are far more complex than implied by simple compartment models,[106] and no model can precisely predict the concentrations, even if the pharmacokinetic parameters in the individual were known with absolute precision. However, even if the pharmacokinetic model truly reflected the underlying biologic variables, the parameters of the model would be average parameters for the population and not the exact parameters of the patient. Even if the parameters were modified to reflect the influence of demographic factors such as age, gender, hypovolemia, and coadministration of other drugs, they would still deviate from the true pharmacokinetic parameters in the individual. Thus biologic variability fundamentally precludes the possibility of precisely achieving the desired target concentration when automated drug delivery devices are used. Realizing that biologic variability always exists, no matter how drugs are given, and that this same biologic variability affects all methods of drug delivery is important. Nonetheless, the variability with TCI devices will always be less than the variability observed after a single bolus injection.[128] The performance of computer-controlled drug administration

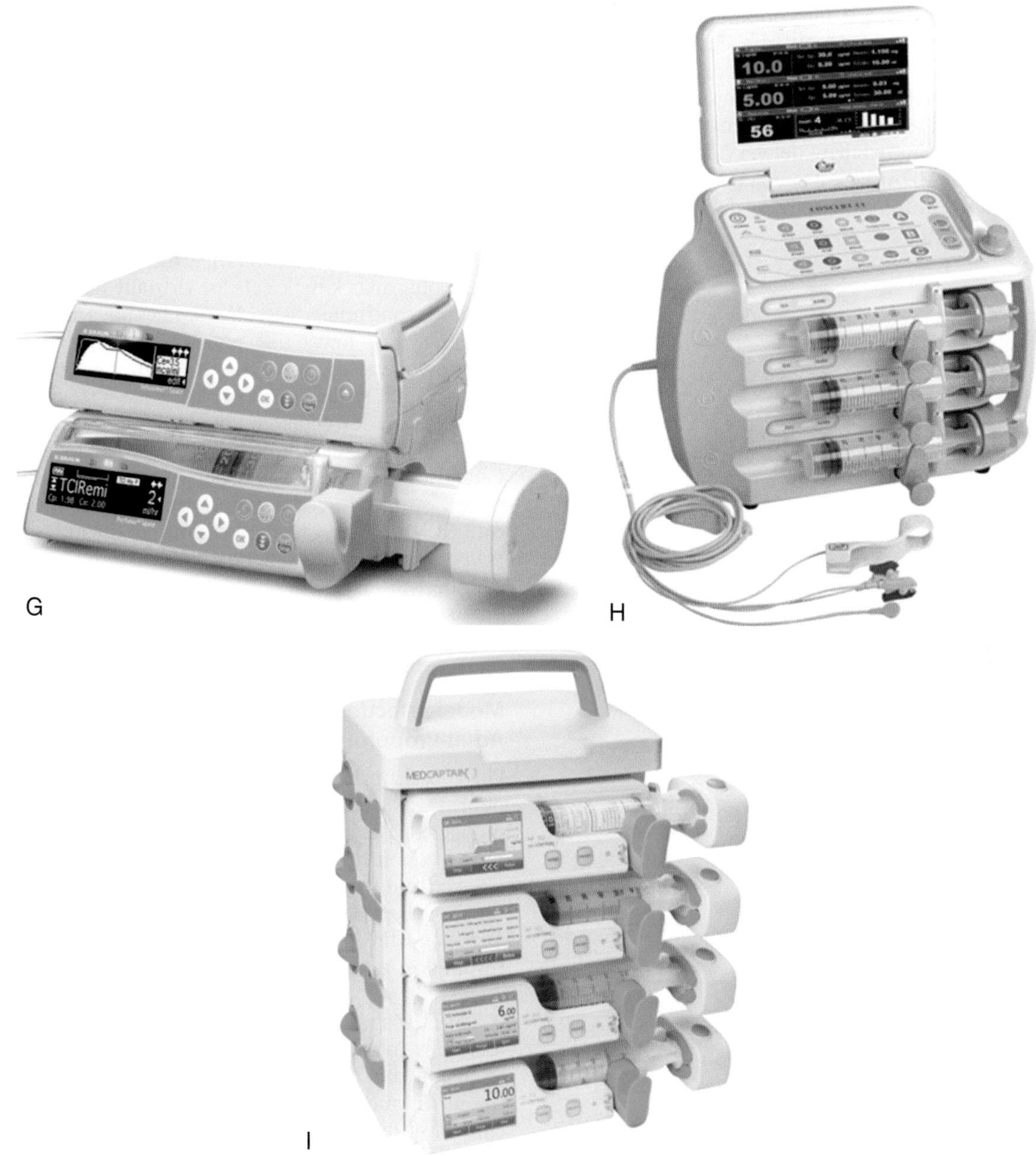

Fig. 26.27 cont'd

must be interpreted in terms of the therapeutic expectations of the clinician. Possible goals include accurately producing a desired concentration in plasma, precisely titrating the plasma drug concentration, achieving the desired drug effect, and producing the desired time course of drug effect. Over the past decade, investigators have addressed each of these goals and have refined the performance of automated drug delivery devices accordingly.

The ability of an automated drug delivery system to rapidly achieve and then maintain a selected target concentration is a logical measure of the performance of such a device. The difference between the measured and target concentrations can be expressed in several ways. Classic graphic representations are X-Y plots depicting predicted versus measured blood (plasma) drug concentrations (Fig. 26.30) or the relationship of the measured and predicted drug concentration versus time of administration (Fig. 26.31). Numerically, the primary concern is how far the measured concentration is from the predicted one; this relationship is now most frequently described in terms of performance errors, which is the difference between measured and target concentrations as a percentage of the desired target—for example, [(measured − target) ÷ target × 100%].[129] The median value of the performance error for a patient or population is referred to as the median performance error (MDPE) and represents the average overshoot or undershoot of the system. The median absolute performance error (MDAPE) is the median of the absolute values of all performance errors. The MDAPE is commonly used as a measure of the inaccuracy of an automated drug delivery device. An MDAPE of zero is perfect performance, and an MDAPE of 20% means that one half the plasma concentrations will be within 20% of the target and one half will be outside that range. A further assessment of accuracy is whether the system maintains a stable target concentration, which is best measured by the wobble of the system. Varvel and colleagues[129] asked a group of clinicians to evaluate the performance of automated drug delivery devices and demonstrated that the MDAPE best predicted the adequacy of performance of the automated delivery device, as judged by experienced clinicians.

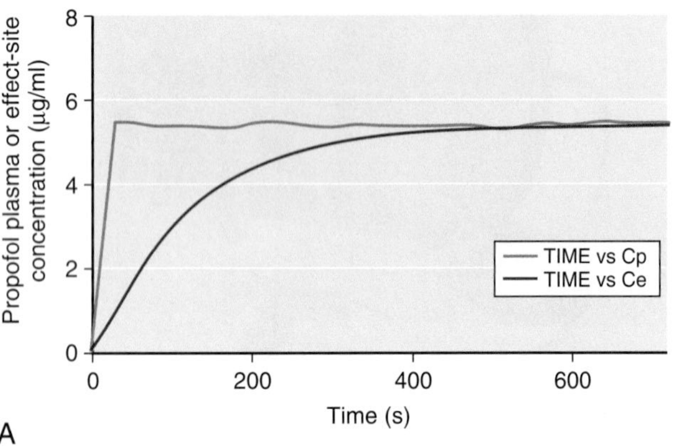

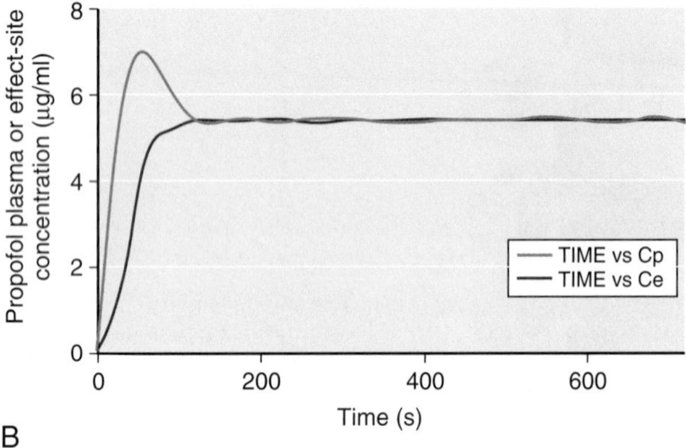

Fig. 26.28 Simulation of propofol plasma (A) versus effect compartment–controlled (B) target-controlled infusion.

As observed earlier, expecting all performance errors to be zero is not reasonable. However, it would be desirable if positive and negative errors offset each other so that the MDPE of an automated drug delivery device were 0%. The MDPE does not indicate the range of performance errors (because positive and negative performance errors offset each other), but it does indicate whether the plasma concentrations achieved with the device tend to overshoot (+MDPE) or undershoot (−MDPE) the desired target.

Many groups have evaluated the accuracy of many different pharmacokinetic sets for virtually all the intravenous hypnotics and analgesics. Most studies have involved healthy volunteers or lower-risk patients undergoing procedural sedation or anesthesia, and in these settings the authors have studied adult models for propofol,[13,31,130-137] midazolam,[138] ketamine,[139] dexmedetomidine,[140,141] fentanyl,[142-144] alfentanil,[67,145-147] sufentanil,[138,148,149] and remifentanil.[150,151] Pediatric models for propofol have also been evaluated.[152-155]

Few studies have been performed in the intensive care unit (ICU) setting. The performance of the Marsh model for propofol sedation in different adult populations has however been studied.[156,157]

Based on many of these studies, the expected predictive performance of such pharmacokinetic models, at best, tends to be around 20% to 30% MDAPE.

Model Selection for Target-Controlled Infusion: Adult Propofol Models

For most intravenous drugs, various multicompartment pharmacokinetic-pharmacodynamic models have been published. The pharmacokinetics of propofol have been the most frequently tested (see Fig. 26.6) of all anesthetic drugs. Coetzee and coworkers compared the accuracy of some of the models published before 1995 and found that propofol TCI using the model published by Marsh and coworkers resulted in acceptable performance (MDPE −7%; MDAPE 18%).[130]

The Marsh model was incorporated in the first commercially available TCI system (Diprifusor). Clinical studies using this plasma-controlled TCI system showed that the technique and model were clinically useful in various clinical situations.[158-162] The major drawback of the Marsh model is the lack of effect compartment information and

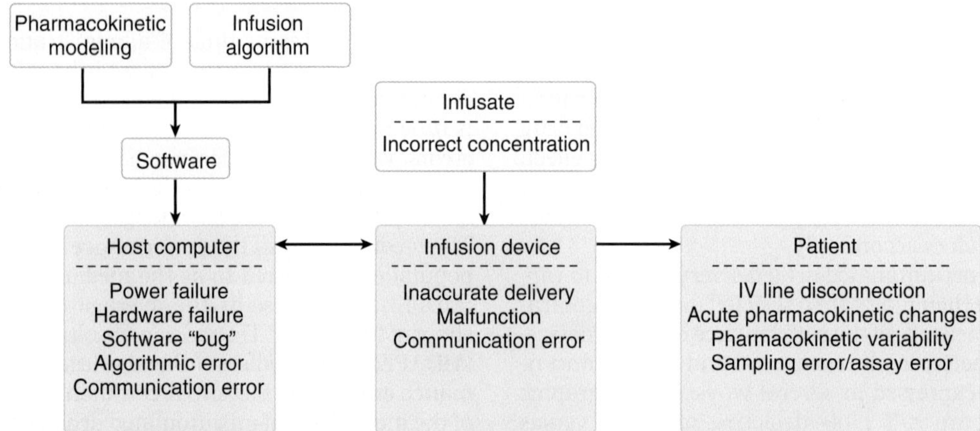

Fig. 26.29 Major sources of potential error in pharmacokinetic model–driven drug delivery. In a commercial device, the computer functions are incorporated into the infusion device. *IV*, Intravenous.

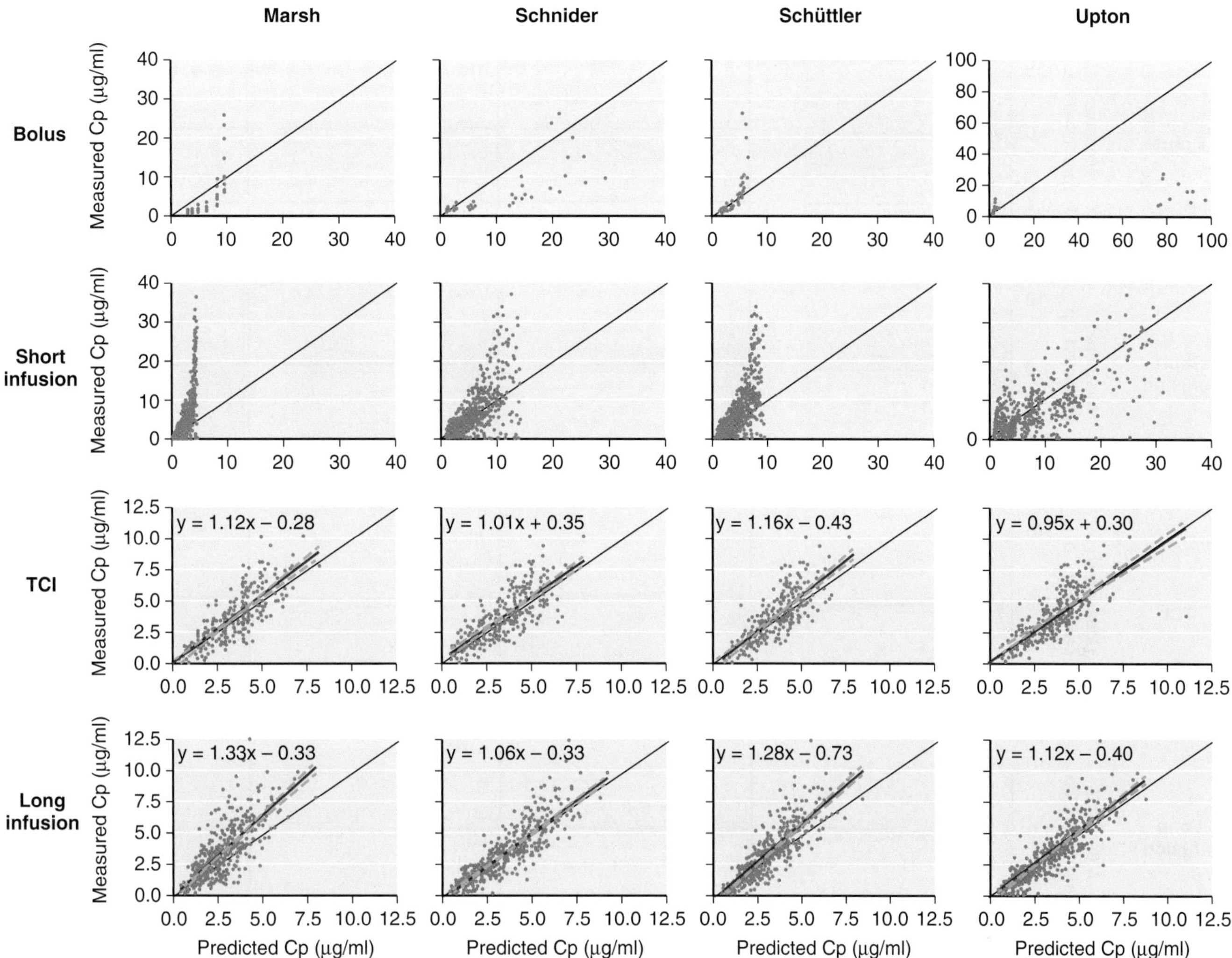

Fig. 26.30 Predicted versus measured propofol plasma concentration for the four pharmacokinetic models. Each point represents a single sample. *Thin black line* represents the line of identity. For target-controlled infusion *(TCI)* and long infusion conditions, the *bold red line* shows the regression line and the *bold dashed green line* indicates the 95% confidence interval for the regression line. The formula represents the equation from the linear regression. (From Masui K, Upton RN, Doufas AG, et al. The performance of compartmental and physiologically based recirculatory pharmacokinetic models for propofol. A comparison using bolus, continuous, and target-controlled infusion data. *Anesth Analg.* 2010;111:368–379. Used with permission.)

the fact that weight is the only covariate. Later, Schnider and coworkers[163,164] evaluated age, height, weight, and lean body mass as covariates in a new combined pharmacokinetic-pharmacodynamic three-compartment model. The large variability of the study population (age 18-81 years, weight 44-123 kg) provides a wide applicability of the model. Several validation studies rated this model accurate under various conditions. For example, Masui and colleagues[13] compared the measured propofol plasma concentrations with the predictions of four published models and revealed bias in all three compartment models during the bolus and short infusion regimens (see Figs. 26.30 and 26.31). During long infusions, a worse measured/predicted propofol plasma concentration at higher concentration was observed for the Marsh[152] and Schüttler[165] models than for the two other models. Less biased measured/predicted propofol plasma concentration was found for all models during TCI. In the bolus group, after 1 minute, a clear overprediction was observed for all three-compartment models for the entire 5-minute period; however, this initial error resolved after 4 minutes in the Schnider model. During the bolus and short infusion conditions, the Marsh model demonstrated worse MDPE and MDAPE when compared with the other models. During short infusion, MDAPE for the Schnider and Schüttler models was better. All models showed similar MDPE and MDAPE during TCI simulations. During long infusion, the Marsh and the Schüttler models underestimated the higher plasma concentrations. Interestingly, the physiologically based recirculatory model developed by Upton and coworkers[14] did not reveal a better description of the pharmacokinetic time course. The Schüttler model has a major practical drawback; it defined the infusion characteristics, being bolus or infusion, as a significant covariate, thereby discouraging TCI applicability.

An additional drawback of the Schnider model is the use of lean body mass as calculated using the equation developed by James.[12] The quadratic behavior of the lean body mass function makes it invalid (negative values!) when used in patients who are very obese. Therefore as changing population demographics such as obesity might influence the pharmacokinetics of propofol, models should ideally be applicable to a broad range of population demographics

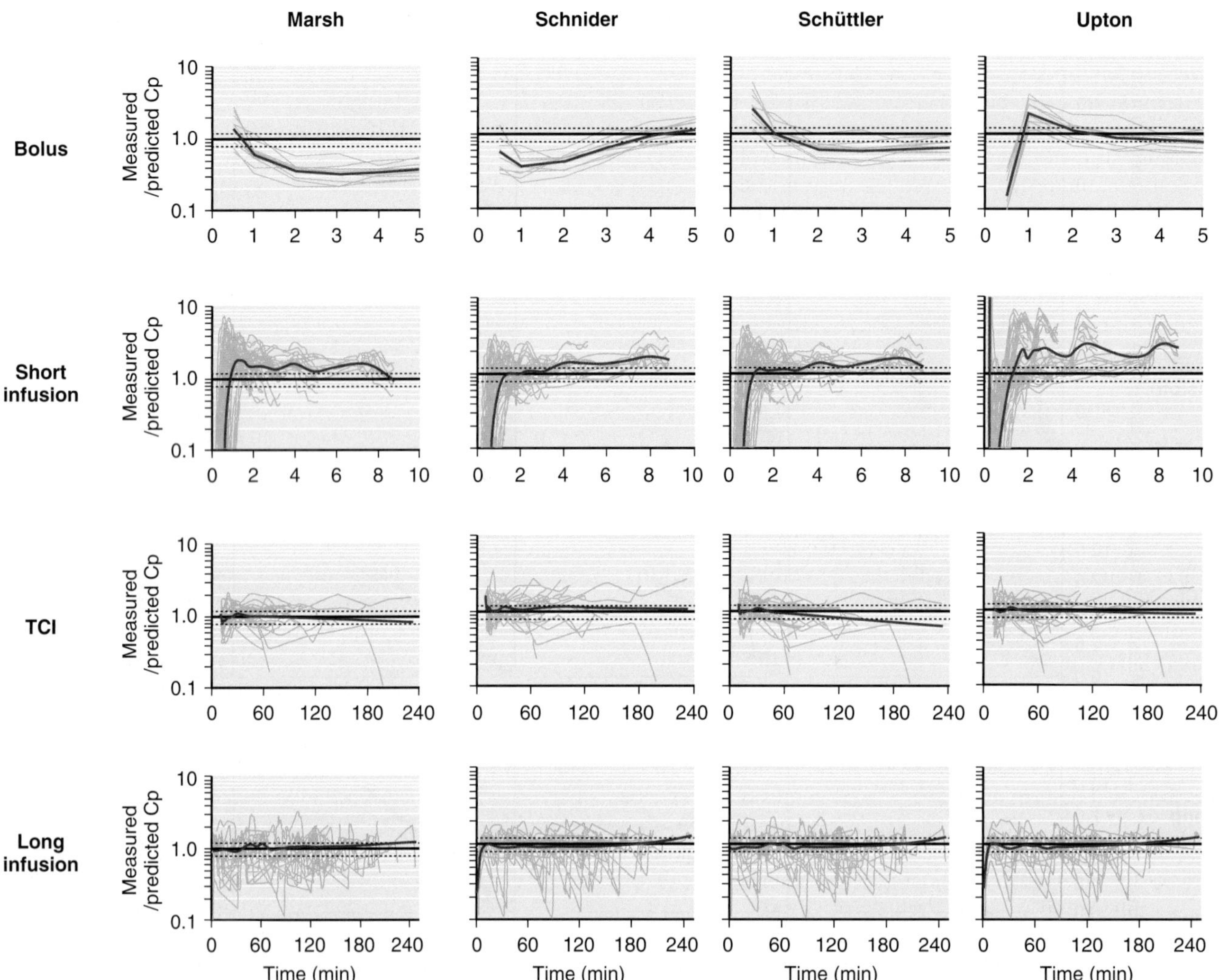

Fig. 26.31 Time course of the measured/predicted concentration relationship versus time of drug administration. The *dotted lines* indicate an acceptable range of measured/predicted plasma drug concentration *(Cp)*. The *red line* indicates the Friedman Super Smoother curve for the population data. (From Masui K, Upton RN, Doufas AG, et al. The performance of compartmental and physiologically based recirculatory pharmacokinetic models for propofol: a comparison using bolus, continuous, and target-controlled infusion data. *Anesth Analg*. 2010;111:368–379. Used with permission.)

before being used in clinical practice. One potential solution to the problem of scaling for size in obese patients is the application of allometric scaling. When using allometric scaling, growth and development can be studied using classic covariates (e.g., weight, age, sex). Size is the primary covariate and can be referenced to a 70-kg person with allometric scaling using a coefficient of 0.75 for clearance and 1 (one) for volume. Anderson and Holford[166] promote this approach because the use of these coefficients is supported by fractal geometric concepts and observations from biologically diverse areas.[167]

Cortinez and coworkers[168] derived a population pharmacokinetic model using obese and nonobese data to describe the pharmacokinetics of propofol over a wide range of body weights. A model using allometric scaling of total body weight as the size descriptor of volumes and clearances was better able to characterize propofol pharmacokinetics in obese patients than a model using size descriptors. The same model was later used to control TCI propofol administration in a new cohort of obese patients, and the predictive performance of this model was then compared with that of four other models (Marsh, Schnider, Eleveld, and van Kralingen).[133] While all models tended to underestimate measured concentrations in this study (i.e., measured concentrations were higher than those estimated), the Eleveld model provided the most accurate predictions. When, instead of using the total body weight with the Marsh and Schnider models, an adjusted body weight was used (adjusted weight = ideal weight + 40% × [total – ideal weight]), the predictive performance of these two models were then associated with the lowest MDPE and MDAPE of all models.[133]

Most recently, Cortinez and colleagues used the data from 47 patients enrolled in three previous studies to develop and prospectively evaluate a new pharmacokinetic-pharmacodynamic model for obese patients.[169] Interestingly, during the development phase, allometric scaling did not improve the fit of their new model, and thus their newest model uses linear scaling of compartmental volumes and clearances, with total body weight. When, in the second phase of their study, this newer model was tested prospectively in obese patients, the pharmacokinetic and pharmacodynamic components performed adequately; with regard to the pharmacokinetic component, the predictive performance of the Eleveld model was better than that of their older and newer models, and that of the Schnider model.

Attention has also been focused recently on the performance of propofol models in underweight patients. Lee and colleagues studied the predictive performance of the Marsh and Schnider model in underweight adults and showed that although predictive performance of both models was within limits considered clinically acceptable, the former tended to overestimate plasma concentrations, whereas the Schnider model tended to underestimate plasma concentrations.[135]

Interestingly, when the performance of the older Cortinez model, which uses allometric scaling of total body weight, was studied in volunteers of normal weight, the predictive performance was acceptable and similar to that of the Schnider model.[170] As mentioned earlier, the newer Cortinez model scales volumes and clearances linearly with total weight.[169] It may not extrapolate that well to patients of normal weight, and for this reason the authors do not recommend using it in patients of normal weight.

Different pharmacokinetic-pharmacodynamic models for propofol are associated with different k_{e0} values, which were sometimes derived in very different ways.[12] When effect-site targeting is used, not only is the accuracy of the pharmacokinetic model important for accurate drug administration, the validity of the k_{e0} is also important. First, the value of the k_{e0} will determine the degree of plasma concentration overshoot when the target concentration is increased, and second, it will determine the estimated values of the effect-site concentrations during periods when the plasma and effect-site are not in equilibrium. If one assumes that there is no hysteresis in the relationship between effect-site drug concentration and clinical effect, then it might be rational to evaluate the overall accuracy of propofol pharmacokinetic-pharmacodynamic models by experiments in which propofol is administered by effect-site TCI, by recording a measure of the clinical effect observed over a period of time and then comparing the time course of the estimated effect-site concentrations and clinical effect.

Barakat and colleagues compared the Marsh and Schnider models by observing BIS and MOAA/S scores after starting an effect-site targeted propofol TCI infusion at a fixed target concentration of 2 μg/mL.[171] Subsequently they compared the shapes of the curves of the time course of the estimated effect-site concentration and of measures of clinical effect (BIS and MOAA/S). They found that the shape of the effect-site concentration curve estimated by the Marsh model (with k_{e0} 0.26 min^{-1}) was more similar to the curves for clinical effect than the curve of the effect-site concentration estimated by the Schnider model.[171]

A more objective application of the preceding rationale is to observe clinical effect over a time period when a TCI system estimates that the effect-site concentration is stable. With this approach, one can reason that if the effect-site (target) concentration is kept constant, and there are no other changes (i.e., no other drugs are administered, and no new stimuli), then the most appropriate model will be the one for which a measure of clinical effect is most stable over time.

Using this approach to compare the Schnider and Marsh models, Coppens and coworkers[172] administered propofol by manual infusion until loss of consciousness. They then continued propofol administration in effect-site targeting TCI mode, using as target concentration the estimated effect-site concentration at the moment of loss of consciousness. They found that among 20 patients assigned to effect-site TCI propofol with the Marsh model, BIS values rose and all patients regained consciousness within the subsequent 20 minutes. On the other hand, among the 40 patients assigned to effect-site TCI propofol with the Schnider model (20 with a fixed k_{e0}, and 20 in whom an individual-specific k_{e0} was calculated using the Schnider pharmacokinetic parameters and a fixed time-to-peak effect of 1.6 minutes), only one regained consciousness and there was a general trend for the BIS to decline during the subsequent 20 minutes.

Thomson and colleagues applied the same rationale to a study in which they sought to determine the most suitable k_{e0} for use with the Marsh model when used in effect-site targeting mode for sedation.[173] Six sequential groups received sedation with the Marsh model with the k_{e0} set to 1.2, 0.8, 0.7, 0.6, 0.5, and 0.2 min^{-1}, respectively. In each patient, the initial target concentration was 0.5 μg/mL. Once the effect-site and plasma concentrations were calculated to have equilibrated, the effect-site target concentration was increased in increments of 0.2 μg/mL, until a MOAA/S score of 3 was reached. Thereafter the effect-site target concentration was fixed, and two-choice visual reaction times were recorded. Interestingly, while a k_{e0} of 0.6 min^{-1} seemed best overall, it should be noted that there was considerable interindividual variability. In every group there were patients where the sedation level (just by reaction times) remained stable, whereas in all groups except the 1.2 min^{-1} group there were patients where reaction times decreased (suggesting lightening of sedation depth) and in every group except the 0.2 min^{-1} group there were patients where reaction times increased (suggesting increasing sedation depth).

As mentioned previously, there is no strong consensus on which model is best for propofol administration. Clinician choices concerning which model to use and the mode of use (plasma versus effect-site targeting and method of implementation of effect-site targeting) are largely pragmatically made, based on geographical and historical issues, availability of equipment, and the choices made by the supplier of the equipment.[8,12] More fundamental research is required to better understand the mechanisms of anesthetic-induced loss of consciousness, to determine whether the aforementioned hysteresis occurs, and to subsequently fine-tune our understanding of the pharmacometric principles governing effect-site modeling.[120]

At present a variety of different adult and pediatric models for propofol are used in studies, but also in clinical use, having been implemented in commercially available TCI systems. This generates a potential source of confusion and error. A group in Groningen, The Netherlands, thus combined the data from a large number of pharmacokinetic-pharmacodynamic studies of propofol, involving subjects with a wide range of characteristics (age, weight, and patients vs. volunteers), and used nonlinear mixed effects modeling to generate a single model that applies to all patients. Initially, a pharmacokinetic-only model was produced.[174] This model is able to provide pharmacokinetic parameters for a wide range of patients, from small children to elderly patients, as well as for obese patients. Later a complete pharmacokinetic-pharmacodynamic model was produced, with the pharmacokinetic part involving the same structure as the previous model, but slightly updated parameters, and a sigmoidal Emax pharmacodynamic model.[76] Internal testing of the pharmacokinetic components of both models showed similar or better performance than that of specialist models designed for specific subpopulations (children, elderly, and obese).[76,174]

Model Selection for Target-Controlled Infusion: Pediatric Propofol Models

Two pharmacokinetic models for propofol in children are available in clinical TCI systems. Kataria and colleagues described the time course of propofol plasma concentration in a population of children between ages of 3 and 11 years using a three-compartment model with weight as the sole significant covariate. Weight-adjusting the volumes and clearances significantly improved the accuracy of the pharmacokinetics. Adjusting the pharmacokinetics for inclusion of additional patient covariates or using a mixed-effects model did not further improve the ability of the pharmacokinetic parameters to describe the observations.[175] An alternative propofol TCI model called *Paedfusor*,[153] developed by the Glasgow research group, incorporated a preliminary model published by Schüttler and coworkers[165] and was recently found to be more accurate than the Kataria model. Coppens and associates[31] were the first to publish a combined pharmacokinetic-pharmacodynamic model for propofol in children, revealing a k_{e0} of 0.79 min$-^{1}$ and a Ce_{50} of 3.85 μg/mL as measured using the BIS (Table 26.6). A recent study compared the predictive performance of 11 different models for propofol in children during long-duration anesthesia,[176] and found that in this setting, the Short[177] pediatric model performed best.

As can be seen in Table 26.6, several different models for children are available, and this can lead to errors. This problem, and the potential solution of the Eleveld general purpose model,[76,174] has been discussed previously.

Model Selection for Target-Controlled Infusion: Opioids

Table 26.7 shows the clinically used pharmacokinetic-pharmacodynamic models for remifentanil, fentanyl, sufentanil, and alfentanil. For sufentanil, the covariate model developed by Gepts and colleagues[178] is accurate with MDPE between −2.3% and 22.3% and MDAPE between 18.5% and 29%, even in patients who are obese.[138,148,149] Multiple pharmacokinetic models were developed for alfentanil. A combined analysis of these early study results using a true population analysis was used to develop a new alfentanil model.[179] A comparison showed a better performance for the Maitre alfentanil model (MDPE, 35%; MDAPE, 36%) than the Scott model (MDPE, 12%; MDAPE, 28%).[180] Other studies found contradictory results.[181]

A compartment fentanyl model without covariates specifically aiming for TCI was developed[143] and tested in both lean and obese patients.[144] A simulated plasma concentration required a specific correction in patients who were obese.[144] Various three-compartment combined pharmacokinetic-pharmacodynamic models for remifentanil were developed from studies with both volunteers and patients; however, only the model published by Minto and colleagues is applied in TCI.[61,182] Evaluation of this model showed an acceptable performance, with an MDPE of −15% and an MDAPE of 20%.[150] Because combined pharmacokinetic-pharmacodynamic models are lacking for some of the opioids, the times to peak effect after a bolus administration of alfentanil (1.4 minutes), fentanyl (3.6 minutes), and sufentanil (5.6 minutes) can be applied to calculate the effect-site concentration using the *tpeak algorithm*.[32]

Preliminary remifentanil models in children have been developed. For example, Rigby-Jones and colleagues[183] applied allometric scaling during a study of remifentanil pharmacokinetics in children and reported a single fixed allometric function scaled to a body mass of 10.5 kg that performed well across a broad range of patient weights. More recently, Eleveld and colleagues, using data from a variety of pharmacokinetic-pharmacodynamic studies of remifentanil, involving patients with a wide range of age, height, and weight characteristics, developed a model in which clearances are also allometrically scaled.[184] This model performed well on internal testing and is thought to be suitable for use in all patients, but now requires external prospective validation.

In addition to propofol and the opioids, compartment models have been published describing the time course of the plasma concentration and clinical effect of benzodiazepines, neuromuscular blocking agents, ketamine, and dexmedetomidine, although these drugs have not yet been included in the commercially available TCI pumps.

Rational Target Concentration Selection

No single regimen, concentration, or drug combination applies to all patients. While some sources of interindividual pharmacokinetic and pharmacodynamic variability are known, much of this variability remains unexplained.

Most of the previously mentioned pharmacokinetic-pharmacodynamic models have been derived from population pharmacologic studies. Interpatient variability limits the accuracy of the estimated drug concentration for the individual but can be counteracted if the model is built while exploring a wide variety of possible covariates using parametric modeling, optionally nonlinear mixed-effects modeling. Consequently, caution is needed when applying these models to patients who are obese, older, very young, diabetic, alcoholic, or unwell if similar participants were not part of the study population. The current commercial implementations of TCI, therefore, do not function well when used for patients with characteristics beyond the range of the model's development study population. As illustrated by Absalom and coworkers, the use of specific TCI algorithms outside the original studied population might result in dangerous drug infusion profiles.[12]

These investigators compared two currently used methods for calculating the effect-site concentration for propofol in patients who were obese, one using a fixed k_{e0} and the other using a fixed t_{peak} (see also "Direct-Effect Models" earlier in this chapter).

As the models in clinical use were not developed from data from obese patients, they should not be expected to perform accurately in obese patients. Tachibana and colleagues studied the influence of obesity on the predictive performance of the Marsh model, which scales compartment

TABLE 26.6 Commonly Applied Pharmacokinetic-Pharmacodynamic Models for Target-Controlled Infusion Systems for Hypnotics

Drug/Model	V_1	V_2	V_3	K_{10} (min^{-1})	K_{12} (min^{-1})	K_{13} (min^{-1})	K_{21} (min^{-1})	K_{31} (min^{-1})	k_{e0} (min^{-1})	TPPE (min)
Propofol/ Marsh[149]	0.228 L/kg	0.363 L/kg	2.893 L/kg	0.119	0.112	0.042	0.055	0.0033	0.26*	NA
Propofol/ Schnider[228,229]	4.27 L	18.9 − 0.391 (age 53) L	238 L	0.443 + 0.0107 × (weight − 77) − 0.0159 × (LBM − 59) + 0.0062 × (height − 177)	0.302 − 0.0056 (age 53)	0.196	(1.29 − 0.024 × [age − 53] ÷ (18.9 − 0.391 × [age − 53])	0.0035	0.456	1.69
Propofol/Paedfusor[230]	0.458 L/kg	1.34 L/kg	8.20 L/kg	70 × weight$^{-0.3}$ ÷ 458.3	0.12	0.034	0.041	0.0019	NA	NA
Propofol/Kataria[229]	0.52 L/kg	1.0 L/kg	8.2 L/kg	0.066	0.113	0.051	0.059	0.0032	NA	NA
Ketamine/Domino[232]	0.063 L/kg	0.207 L/kg	1.51 L/kg	0.4381	0.5921	0.59	0.2470	0.0146	NA	NA

LBM, Lean body mass; *TPPE,* time to peak effect.
*k_{e0} derived independently from the PK model by Schüttler and colleagues.[231]

TABLE 26.7 Commonly Applied Pharmacokinetic-Pharmacodynamic Models for Target-Controlled Infusion Systems for Analgesics

Drug	Remifentanil	Sufentanil	Fentanyl	Alfentani
Model	Minto[54,173]	Gepts[170]	Shafer[147]	Maitre[171]
V_1	(5.1 – 0.0201 [age – 40]) + 0.072 × (LBM – 55) L	14.3 L	6.09 L	♂ = 0.111 L/kg ♀ = 1.15 × 0.111 L/kg
V_2	(9.82 – 0.0811 [age – 40]) + 0.108 (LBM – 55) L	63.4 L	28.1 L	12.0 L
V_3	5.42 L	251.9 L	228 L	10.5 L
k_{10} (min^{-1})	(2.6 – 0.0162 [age – 40]) + 0.0191 (LBM – 55) ÷ V_1	0.0645	0.083	<40 year = 0.356/V_1 >40 year = 0.356 – (0.00269 [age – 40]) ÷ V_1
k_{12} (min^{-1})	(2.05 – 0.0301 [age – 40])/V_1	0.1086	0.4713	0.104
k_{13} (min^{-1})	(0.076 – 0.00113 [age – 40])/V_1	0.0229	0.22496	0.017
k_{21} (min^{-1})	$k_{12} \times V_1 \div V_2$	0.0245	0.1021	0.067
k_{31} (min^{-1})	$k_{13} \times V_1 \div V_2$	0.0013	0.00601	<40 year = 0.0126 >40 year = 0.0126-0.000113 (age – 40)
k_{e0} (min^{-1})	0.595 – 0.007(age-40)	NA	0.147*	0.77*

LBM, Lean body mass.
*k_{e0} is derived independently from the PK model by Scott and colleagues.[39]

volumes linearly with body weight.[134] In their study, they used a single target plasma propofol concentration (4 μg/mL) and found that whereas in nonobese patients the bias was reasonably low, in obese patients measured concentrations were consistently higher than those predicted, to the extent that they found that when they applied a correction factor involving the BMI to the predicted concentration, the bias was reduced.

Growing evidence suggests that gender, ethnic, and racial differences may be important sources of population pharmacokinetic-pharmacodynamic variability and should be considered when designing dosage regimens.[185]

The influence of different factors is often very complex. In one study involving the influence of age and gender on propofol clearance, clearance tended to be higher in females (and it declined with age), whereas age did not appear to have an influence in males.[186] Another study showed that different phases of the menstrual cycle were associated with significant differences in EC_{50} of propofol (predicted concentrations).[187] Xu and coworkers[55] confirmed that race can significantly influence propofol pharmacokinetics and pharmacodynamics. They evaluated the C_{50} for propofol-remifentanil TCI and the BIS at loss of consciousness and the response to noxious stimulus in patients of Chinese ethnicity and revealed that the predicted blood and effect-site concentrations at loss of consciousness were lower than those in previous publications involving Caucasian populations.

An additional caveat is required with the use of different formulations of a drug. For propofol, Calvo and colleagues[188] found that pharmacokinetics and pharmacodynamics were not equal for all formulations, which contributed to an increase in variability of the observed effect. Because of the aforementioned factors, no single regimen, concentration, or drug combination applies to all patients. Some guidance can be found in the ECs at which 50% and 95% of patients have accurate clinical effect (see Table 26.3). As with all drug administration in anesthesia, clinical judgment is always required, and the target concentration should be titrated according to the clinical response of the patient.

One of the major sources of variability in the clinical effect of propofol is interaction with concurrently administered drugs (see prior discussion). The interacting drugs may cause changes in the pharmacokinetics and/or pharmacodynamics of propofol. In this regard, the (mutual) interactions between hypnotics and opioids are currently best understood, but in fact, a wide array of drugs may interact with the hypnotics, including drugs that have been chronically administered during the preoperative phase.[107]

Finally, in individual cases, other obvious sources of reduced single-drug model accuracy are errors such as drug spills, excessive blood loss causing shock, or pharmacokinetic drug interaction.[189-191] The number of factors that can influence drug pharmacokinetics and pharmacodynamics is so large that it would not be practicable to develop models taking all the factors into account, and even less so to have different models to take into account factors such as race. Thus regardless of the accuracy and complexity of available models, it will probably always be necessary for clinicians to titrate anesthetic drug administration to clinical effect.

Benefits of Target-Controlled Infusion

The ability of TCI to rapidly achieve and maintain a steady concentration facilitates attainment of a desired drug effect, irrespective of the absolute achieved drug concentration in the target compartment. The application of TCI in most cases even reduces the variability of intersubject drug-response relationships.[128] As a result, clinical outcomes when comparing TCI versus manual infusion were found to be improved in various early studies, although contradictions exist in the literature.

In the 1980s, Ausems and coworkers[192] compared pharmacokinetic model–driven administration with intermittent bolus administration of alfentanil. Automated drug delivery produced fewer episodes of muscular rigidity, hypotension, and bradycardia on induction. Automated drug delivery during maintenance resulted in a significantly less frequent incidence of hemodynamic response, which resulted in a larger percentage of anesthesia time within

15% of the desired arterial blood pressure and heart rate. Recovery after TCI was associated with significantly less use of naloxone for adequate ventilation. Pharmacokinetic model–driven infusion of fentanyl during cardiac surgery resulted in better hemodynamic control with fewer additional drug interventions and significantly fewer episodes of either hypotension or hypertension than with bolus dose administration.[193]

Theil and colleagues[194] compared double-blind manual administration of fentanyl-midazolam with pharmacokinetic model–driven infusion of these two drugs in a small group of patients undergoing cardiac surgery. Both systems were simultaneously titrated (one containing placebo), with the aim of maintaining hemodynamics within 20% of baseline values. Both systems were equally effective in providing hemodynamic control as dictated by the protocol. The most significant difference between the two modes of delivery was the greater variability in drug plasma concentrations in the manual group, which suggested that pharmacokinetic model–driven infusion maintained patients within a more narrow therapeutic range.

TCI remifentanil provides improved hemodynamic control both intraoperatively and postoperatively with less remifentanil and similar propofol infusion rates.[195] Age dramatically influences the pharmacokinetics of remifentanil; consequently, a TCI model that includes age will result in a beneficial drug titration compared with a standard μg/kg/min infusion. For deep sedation in spontaneously breathing patients, Moerman and associates[196] found that the combination of remifentanil and propofol offered better conditions for colonoscopy than propofol alone; and that TCI remifentanil administration was associated with reduced propofol dosing and a less frequent incidence of apnea and respiratory depression, compared with manually controlled administration. Others have confirmed this finding.[192]

Using the first commercially available TCI system (Diprifusor), early studies administering propofol by plasma-targeted TCI showed some benefits.[159,197,198] These revealed a significant preference of clinicians for the TCI system, although this was their first use of the device.

Passot and coworkers[199] compared TCI and manual propofol infusion in high-risk older patients undergoing hip fracture surgery and concluded that TCI improved the time course of propofol-induced hemodynamic effects in these patients. Chen and colleagues found that similar induction and total doses of propofol were used when anesthesia was induced and maintained with either a manual or a TCI system, and the propofol administration was titrated to achieve a specific BIS value.[200]

Wang and colleagues compared the clinical conditions associated with TCI and manual propofol infusion during asleep-awake-asleep epilepsy surgery. TCI was associated with significantly improved awakening times and higher BIS values after the first asleep phase.[201] Chiang and associates found similar results when they compared TCI with manually controlled propofol infusions for combined upper and lower endoscopy.[202] Patients in the TCI group had better hemodynamic and respiratory stability and recovered more quickly from sedation than patients assigned to the manually controlled infusion group.

The Irwin group recently compared TCI and manual propofol administration in children.[203] Although they found that in children assigned to TCI propofol administration, higher total propofol doses were given, the amount of time the BIS was in an optimal range was greater and recovery times were similar. The authors concluded that TCI might facilitate easier titration of propofol to clinical effect.

TCI can theoretically facilitate rational drug administration for patients in the ICU, where drugs are commonly administered for prolonged periods. In this situation, by taking account of drug redistribution and eventually equilibration between compartments and thus reducing infusion rates, TCI systems have the potential to assist with maintenance of more stable sedation levels. McMurray and coworkers[156] studied TCI propofol in 122 adult ICU patients. Bias and median absolute performance error were within acceptable ranges at 4.3% and 19.6%, respectively. Acceptable sedation levels occurred for 84% of the sedation period. They proposed propofol plasma targets between 0.2 and 2.0 μg/mL for ICU sedation.

Overall, there is little high-quality evidence of improved outcome with the use of TCI as opposed to manual drug administration. Nonetheless, the popularity of TCI use has grown significantly since the introduction of the first commercially available devices. The systems are registered for use in at least 93 countries of the world, and we recently estimated that in Europe alone, more than 2 million patients per year received one or more drugs administered with a TCI system.[8]

Plasma Versus Effect-Site Targeting

Using experimental systems, Glass[123] and Struys[47] and their colleagues conducted similar studies in which they targeted either plasma or effect-site concentration of propofol and then observed the time and plasma versus effect-site concentration at loss of consciousness. In both studies, regardless of whether the effect-site or plasma concentration was targeted, loss of consciousness occurred when the appropriate *effect-site* concentration for loss of consciousness was achieved, thus validating the concept. Two other important observations were made during these studies. First, hemodynamic stability was not different for plasma or the effect-site targeting, although higher plasma concentrations were achieved in the effect-site group. This finding implies, at least for propofol, that the time course for its hemodynamic effects is similar or longer[204] to that for its anesthetic effects. Second, k_{e0} is dependent on the pharmacokinetic set from which it is derived.[32] A k_{e0} value cannot be taken from one pharmacokinetic set and used with another pharmacokinetic set.[31] Just as various demographics may alter the pharmacokinetics, they may also alter k_{e0}. Therefore using the k_{e0} best adapted for the clinical milieu is desirable. An ideal test of whether targeting plasma or the effect site is better is to compare their use in a closed-loop system in which a measure of effect (e.g., the BIS) is used as the target of control. In a small study of 10 patients per group, Absalom and Kenny showed that maintenance of the targeted BIS (as measured by MDPE, MDAPE, and wobble) was somewhat improved and induction times were significantly shorter when the pharmacokinetic model was for the effect site rather than for the plasma.[205] Effect compartment–controlled TCI systems are currently commercially available in many countries (not the United States).[8] They may offer better control of the dose-response relationship.[47,206,207]

Safety of Target-Controlled Infusion

In noncomparative studies, pharmacokinetic model–driven infusion has been used to administer most of the potent opioids, as well as the hypnotics. Different anesthetic techniques have also been tested with pharmacokinetic model–driven infusion devices, including nitrous oxide–opioid anesthesia, supplementation of volatile anesthetics, total intravenous anesthesia, sedation for monitored anesthesia care, and ICU sedation. In all these studies, outcome as measured by hemodynamics and recovery has been within the expectations of normal clinical care. Etomidate, methohexital, midazolam, propofol, thiopental, dexmedetomidine, alfentanil, fentanyl, remifentanil, and sufentanil have all been used with TCI. When these drugs were used with target-controlled drug delivery systems for total intravenous anesthesia or to supplement nitrous oxide or volatile anesthetics, hemodynamics were well maintained during induction and intubation, as well as during maintenance. Recovery milestones were reached at times comparable with those achieved with similar drug combinations used in manual infusion schemes. None of these studies have reported adverse outcomes resulting from target-controlled drug delivery.

A recent review shows that the safety and reliability of commercially available TCI systems has been exemplary, suggesting that the systems perform as intended and programmed.[127] Despite use of TCI systems in millions of patients around the world, a search of the medical literature, regulatory reports, and company safety statements revealed only a handful of possible problems specific to TCI device use, many of which were the result of user error and none of which resulted in product recalls or patient harm.

PATIENT-CONTROLLED ANALGESIA AND SEDATION

A particular method of intravenous drug administration is patient-controlled analgesia, mostly used for the postoperative administration of analgesics or for patient-controlled sedation (PCS) during therapeutic procedures. Although PCA can be considered as a method of computer-controlled or even closed-loop drug administration, most of these pumps currently do not include pharmacokinetic or pharmacodynamic algorithms. In some cases, the PCA or PCS pump is set to deliver a low, constant or *background* flow of medication. Additional doses of medication can be self-administered by the patient pressing a button as needed. Most commonly, no background infusion is provided, and the patient controls when he or she receives an analgesic bolus. To avoid overdosing, these pumps have built-in safety mechanisms such as lock-out times and limitations of the total amount of drug delivered per time unit. PCA is a common technique for delivery of postoperative pain medication such as morphine, piritramide, fentanyl, tramadol, and other drugs.[208-212] In a systematic review, Walder and colleagues showed that the literature presented some evidence that in the postoperative pain setting, PCA with opioids, compared with conventional opioid treatment, improved analgesia and decreased the risk of pulmonary complications; in general, patients preferred the technique.[213] Strict hospital guidelines may help avoid side effects such as oversedation and respiratory depression.[214] When epidural analgesia is contraindicated during labor, remifentanil PCA has been suggested as an alternative. Pilot trials suggested that this alternative is safe under strict observation.[215-220] However, a more recently published randomized-controlled trial showed that, in comparison with epidural analgesia, not only was remifentanil PCA associated with lower satisfaction scores, it was also associated with lower maternal oxygen saturation values.[221]

Although popular, PCA systems are imperfect, as they administer boluses that result in a time course of clinical effect that is unlikely to accurately match the time course of the painful stimulus the patient is suffering. The same applies to PCS systems, except that here the bolus will provide a time course of sedation or anxiolysis that does not match the experience of the patient. TCI technology has thus also been applied to PCA and PCS. With these patient-maintained analgesia and patient-maintained sedation systems, the system administers a TCI of analgesic or sedative, usually starting at a fixed low-target concentration, and after an initial period the patient is able to influence the target concentration. In some initial studies the target concentration was increased or decreased by a researcher using an algorithm,[70,74,180,211,222,223] but in others the patient was able to activate target concentration increases by pressing the button of a handset, once a lockout period had passed.[224]

Van den Nieuwenhuyzen and colleagues demonstrated the advantages of PCA-TCI with alfentanil over routine morphine PCA for postoperative analgesia.[74,180,222,223] Analgesia support using effect-site targeted TCI of remifentanil or fentanyl during extracorporeal shock-wave lithotripsy was tested by Cortinez and colleagues.[70] They found a remifentanil and fentanyl EC_{50} of 2.8 ng/mL and 2.9 ng/mL. At EC_{50}, the probability of having a respiratory rate less than 10 was 4% for remifentanil and 56% for fentanyl. Hypoxemia, vomiting, and sedation were more frequent in the fentanyl group, making this drug less suitable for this clinical application than remifentanil. Lipszyc and associates[211] used remifentanil effect-site PCA-TCI with a slow and progressive adapted algorithm for treatment of acute pain after uterine artery embolization and showed that it provided better care than PCA morphine in the first 4 hours of administration.

Schraag and colleagues studied the efficacy and safety of a remifentanil patient-maintained analgesic system for early analgesia after orthopedic surgery.[224] If the patient operated an activating handset then the target concentration was increased by 0.2 ng/mL; otherwise the system gradually reduced the target. The system was found to provide satisfactory analgesia, with little sedation and few respiratory adverse effects.

Jeleazcov and colleagues have developed and studied a TCI-PCA system for hydromorphone.[225] With this system the patient is also able to request higher target concentrations by means of a button push. The authors found that patients using this system after cardiac surgery had satisfactory pain control with only moderate adverse effects.

The initial developments of PCS systems enabled the patient to request bolus drug administration (propofol or midazolam), or occasionally an increase in drug infusion rate.[226-230] Studies on the quality and outcomes after PCS have shown that it reduces discomfort and fear by inducing sedation and amnesia during uncomfortable therapeutic procedures such as colonoscopy. Additionally, PCS facilitates the procedure by increasing the patient's tolerance. Although propofol offers no analgesic effect, several studies of patient control of propofol administration (bolus or short infusions) during procedures showed that it provided reasonably safe, light sedation, and that patients expressed a preference for being in control.[227,229,230] A recent study compared physician-controlled TCI propofol with PCS with boluses of propofol during endoscopic retrograde cholangiopancreatography. It showed that with PCS lower doses of propofol were used and recovery was more rapid.[231]

As bolus or even manual infusion regimens might produce fluctuating levels of sedation, Kenny and colleagues in Glasgow combined PCS with TCI of propofol to overcome this problem. Using a patient-maintained sedation system, the patient can set a specific propofol target concentration using an activating handset button. With the system, the patient was required to press twice within one second to request a target increase. If no validated presses occurred, the system initially kept the target propofol concentration unchanged, but if after 6 minutes no further presses occurred, then the target concentration was reduced by the incremental amount. A starting concentration and a lockout time is set by the clinician (commonly with the default being approximately the equilibration time between plasma and effect-site concentrations). In various applications requiring sedation, their experimental system was shown to be feasible[232-235]; however, even when using an effect-site controlled TCI system, some volunteers rendered themselves unconscious.[236] Whereas the system developed by Kenny and colleagues incorporated the Marsh model, Stonell and colleagues developed and tested a system enabling propofol effect-site targeted patient-maintained sedation with the Schnider model. They compared patient-maintained sedation with anesthetist-administered sedation and found that patient-maintained sedation was associated with fewer adverse events, higher sedation scores, and BIS values, but at the cost of slower induction times, while patient and operator satisfaction was similar.[237]

It is possible that safety can be improved further, particularly if a test or measure of responsiveness to a stimulus is added and if the control algorithm is incorporated to allow the facility to stop the infusion should the response become inadequate.[238-241]

Doufas and colleagues tested an automatic response test to optimize propofol administration for conscious sedation.[242,243] Although volunteers were required to push a delivery button in response to auditory and tactile stimuli, a TCI-like algorithm guided the propofol administration. The study showed that failure to respond to automated responsiveness monitoring precedes potentially serious adverse effects of sedation such as loss of responsiveness, and that the monitor was not susceptible to false-positive responses.[244]

An enlarged commercial version of this device, SEDASYS (Ethicon Endo-Surgery, Cincinnati, Ohio), was tested in two studies. It incorporated the automated responsiveness monitoring and built-in capnography and pulse oximetry. If the patient's responses to stimuli were inadequate, then the subsequent increases in infusion rates were limited. If apnea or hemoglobin oxygen desaturation were detected, then the infusion was stopped and additional oxygen given. After a successful feasibility study,[245] the system was then used in a large randomized study of sedation during upper gastrointestinal endoscopy and colonoscopy and was found to be associated with a reduced incidence of adverse events compared with standard care (5.8% vs. 8.7%, respectively).[246] Although the device was approved by the FDA in 2013 for the provision of moderate sedation during routine endoscopic procedures in ASA 1 and 2 patients, poor sales figures prompted a commercial decision by the vendor to cease marketing the device.[247,248]

Closed-Loop Controlled Intravenous Drug Delivery

The next step in computer-controlled drug delivery is to feed a continuous measure of drug effect directly back to the automated drug delivery device, thus providing a continuous closed-loop system. This system avoids the requirement of a clinician to titrate the target concentration manually, based on intermittent observations of the desired therapeutic effect. With manual control, attempts to achieve tight titration of hypnosis require high clinical expertise and a labor-intensive process and may divert the clinician's attention from critical actions resulting in a suboptimal therapy or even threatening the patient's safety. Applying closed-loop drug administration techniques could optimize this process of dose titration.[4] The application of closed-loop systems for drug administration is complex and requires a perfect balance for all the basic components of such a system: (1) a control variable representative for the targeted therapeutic effect; (2) a clinically relevant set-point or target value for this variable; (3) a control actuator which is, in this case, the infusion pump driving the drug; (4) a system, in this case a patient; and (5) an accurate, stable control algorithm.[249]

Control algorithms are all based on measuring the error between the target and the observed effect. Various control strategies are described in the literature to steer this closed-loop administration. Proportional-integral differential (PID) controllers are frequently used in engineering applications. This controller will adjust the infusion rates in a manner that is proportional to the magnitude of the error, the integral of the error over time, and the derivative of the error over time. The fine-tuning of a PID controller might be difficult in this particular setting because of the complexity of the system to control and the interindividual pharmacologic variability, and because directly counteracting the administration of excessive drug is not possible. A more appropriate approach could be to use a PID control system connected to a TCI system to decrease the order of complexity between dose and response (see Fig. 26.26).[250] An alternative control strategy is called *model-based adaptive control*. This controller has an internal model of the system, typically set up as an integrated pharmacokinetic-pharmacodynamic model that relates dose to concentration (pharmacokinetics) and concentration to drug effect (pharmacodynamics). The model is updated to explain the difference between the measured and predicted drug effect.

A reliable physiologic signal, which is a measure of the clinical drug effect, is the most important component of closed-loop technology. Vital signs such as arterial blood pressure or muscle activity have been used to guide intravenous closed-loop drug administration. For example, Kenny and coworkers[251] successfully evaluated closed-loop control of arterial blood pressure using a mixture of trimethaphan camsylate and sodium nitroprusside during controlled hypotensive anesthesia for local resection of intraocular melanoma. In the 1980s and the 1990s, various researchers investigated the accuracy of closed-loop controlled administration of atracurium[252,253] and vecuronium.[254] However, since the introduction of the novel reversal drug, sugammadex, interest in closed-loop administration of vecuronium or rocuronium has significantly declined.

The commercialization of various EEG-based *depth of anesthesia* monitors, such as the BIS, spectral entropy, and auditory-evoked potential, has renewed the interest of various research groups in closed-loop administration of intravenous hypnotics. Using an early version of the BIS as the control variable, Sakai and colleagues[255] concluded that their closed-loop system provided intraoperative hemodynamic stability and a prompt recovery from sedative-hypnotic effects of propofol. A similar propofol closed-loop system using the BIS and PID control of a plasma-controlled TCI system showed acceptable control during major orthopedic surgery[256] and during sedation.[257] Although these investigators improved the performance of their control system by switching toward effect-site targeted TCI, they also concluded that the PID controller might still face some stability problems. Similarly, Liu and colleagues used a closed-loop titration of TCI based on a proportional-differential algorithm guided by the BIS, allowing induction and maintenance of general anesthesia and compared this with manual propofol TCI. They found that closed-loop control resulted in less propofol consumption and longer induction times but with better hemodynamic stability, less excessive anesthetic levels (BIS <40), similar hemodynamic stability, and faster recovery.[250,258]

Liu and colleagues have developed a more advanced version of their initial system, now using full PID control, for closed-loop coadministration of both propofol and remifentanil, using the BIS as the controlled variable. A rule-based algorithm decides when to change the propofol or remifentanil targets. In a multicenter study, this system showed a better overall performance versus manual administration.[259] A similar approach was used with an alternative EEG-derived index, spectral entropy.[260] The same group has since used their system in various groups of patients in a variety of clinical settings, such as during sedation, pediatric surgery, and liver transplantation—and in a variety of applications in which it is used to provide an objective evaluation of the influence of pharmacological (e.g., use of dexmedetomidine) and nonpharmacological interventions (e.g., hypnosis) on anesthetic drug requirements for general anesthesia.[261-269]

Puri and colleagues in India developed a system that incorporates an adaptive PID algorithm to control propofol administration guided by the BIS. It has been extensively tested in a variety of circumstances, for general anesthesia and postoperative sedation, in adults and children, at high altitude, and in patients with pheochromocytoma and heart failure, and found to perform satisfactorily.[270-276] In a randomized controlled trial involving more than 200 patients, the system was shown to provide significantly more accurate control (defined as BIS within target range) than manually controlled anesthesia.[277]

A Canadian group lead by Dumont and Ansermino have also developed a PID-based closed-loop controller. For their system, they developed their own monitor (NeuroSENSE, NeuroWave Systems, Cleveland Heights, OH), which calculates the wavelet-based anesthetic value for central nervous system monitoring (WAV_{CNS}) and the burst suppression ratio.[278,279] The WAV_{CNS}, which has a range of 0 to 100, has also been used for monitoring sedation in the ICU.[280] A study comparing the performance of WAV_{CNS} with BIS and response entropy found that WAV_{CNS} performed well, and was particularly good at capturing rapidly occurring changes.[281] The system includes a PID algorithm, and initially was only used to control a propofol infusion.[282] It contains an infusion safety system to manage the infusion rate when the feedback variable (WAV_{CNS}) is unavailable or when the drug infusion exceeds predefined limits. Later, they developed and tested a so-called multi-input single-output system, in which the output remained the WAV_{CNS}, but the controller was able to control both a propofol and a remifentanil infusion.[282] The authors have shown that their system provides robust, stable, and safe control of anesthetic depth, even under challenging conditions such as significant bleeding,[283] and that the addition of automatic control of remifentanil administration improved the quality of control.[282]

Another group in Canada have gradually taken their closed-loop system (McSleepy) to the next level. Their initial version of McSleepy used a PID algorithm and the BIS to automatically control a propofol infusion and was shown to be able to provide more accurate and stable control of the BIS than an anesthesiologist manually controlling the propofol infusion rate.[284] They then developed McSleepy further to enable closed-loop control of three drugs: propofol and remifentanil infusions, and rocuronium boluses.[285] For propofol, a proportional integral algorithm is used with the BIS the control variable, whereas for remifentanil a rule-based proportional algorithm is used to control the Analgoscore (a nociception score based on heart rate and blood pressure),[286] and finally, rocuronium boluses are administered on the basis of simple rule set, to keep the train of four count less than 25%. This system has been shown to provide accurate control of all variables. The system has been adapted (the Analgoscore was adapted and the name changed to NociMap) and used for general anesthesia for cardiac surgery,[287] and more recently also adapted to provide propofol sedation[288] and used during transcatheter aortic valve implantation.[289]

Model-based adaptive control of BIS-guided propofol administration was previously used by Struys and colleagues for sedation during spinal anesthesia and for general anesthesia.[290,291] The control algorithm is based on a patient-specific pharmacodynamic profile estimated during induction. Compared with manually titrated propofol administration, patients in the closed-loop group reached the target BIS at a somewhat slower rate, but this resulted in less BIS overshoot and better hemodynamics after induction. During the maintenance phase, improved control of the BIS and systolic blood pressure was found in the closed-loop group and recovery was faster. Using simulations, these authors compared their model-based control system with a previously published PID controller

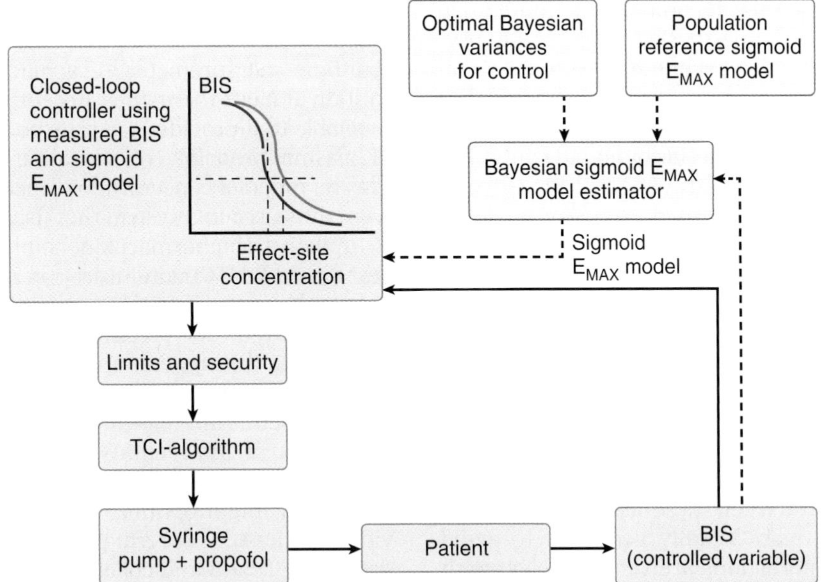

Fig. 26.32 Flow chart of the closed-loop system. The *solid lines* represent the closed-loop control system. Each time the required effect-site concentration is calculated by the controller this value is sent to an additional algorithm, taking the safety limits into account. The result of these calculations is the required effect-site concentration sent to the target-controlled infusion *(TCI)* algorithm, which steers a pump injecting propofol to the patient. The measured bispectral index *(BIS)* is used as the input of the closed-loop controller. The *dotted lines* represent the Bayesian sigmoid E_{MAX} model estimator. The estimator receives a priori information from the population sigmoid E_{MAX} model, the optimal Bayesian variances for control, and the patient-measured BIS values. (From De Smet T, Struys MM, Greenwald S, et al. Estimation of optimal modeling weights for a Bayesian-based closed-loop system for propofol administration using the bispectral index as a controlled variable: a simulation study. *Anesth Analg*. 2007;105:1629–1638. Used with permission.)

and found that the model-based controller outperformed, even under extreme control conditions such as low and high BIS levels and abrupt changes in the BIS levels.[292] De Smet and Struys later developed the adaptive part of the controller using Bayesian optimization (Fig. 26.32)[293] and compared the feasibility and accuracy of this system with manually controlled BIS-guided, effect compartment–controlled propofol TCI during ambulatory gynecologic procedures. They found that the closed-loop control system accurately titrated propofol administration resulting in BIS values close to the set point. The closed-loop control system was able to induce anesthesia in the patients within clinically accepted time limits and with less overshoot than the manual control group. Automated control resulted in beneficial recovery times. This closed-loop control group showed related acceptable clinical performance specified by similar hemodynamic respiratory stability, comparable movement rates, and quality scores as the manual control group.[294]

Alternative closed-loop systems have been developed for isoflurane administration using a controller with a cascade structure, originally described by Gentilini and associates.[295,296] More recently, Moore and Doufas designed a closed-loop system using an intelligent system technique called *reinforcement learning*, known as a mathematically robust method of achieving optimal control in systems challenged with noise, nonlinearity, time delay, and uncertainty.[297,298]

So far, closed-loop systems have only been used under strict experimental conditions. The challenge is now to prove their safety and utility when applied in clinical practice.[299,300] Liu and associates have shown improved stability of control of depth of anesthesia with their system in a large multicenter study.[259] More recently two meta-analyses have evaluated the available data concerning the performance of closed-loop systems for intravenous anesthesia and other applications.[301,302] Both found improved accuracy of control with closed-loop technology.

Liu and associates have also been able to show that the use of their system produces several secondary benefits, such as a reduction in the workload of the anesthesiologist.[303] Ultimately, clinicians will have to determine whether adaptive, intelligent computer systems with dual, interacting, closed-loop systems will facilitate better control and improve patient outcomes.[120]

Although closed-loop technology and automation are almost ubiquitous in our daily lives, closed-loop anesthesia is still only used within research settings. Recent editorials have discussed the relevance of closed-loop technology to anesthesia, and the likely time course over which applications will become a routine part of our daily work.[304-306] The theoretical benefits, however, are compelling, and so it is not surprising that the FDA recently held a workshop on the regulatory considerations for physiological closed-loop controlled medical for automation in critical care and anesthetic environments, and is currently formulating recommendations and regulatory proposals.[307]

Future Perspectives

For all existing drugs there is broad pharmacokinetic and pharmacodynamic variability. In anesthesia practice, inaccurate dosing can have serious consequences. Whereas overdosing might be associated with hemodynamic compromise and prolonged recovery, underdosing is particularly undesirable since it can result in unintended awareness during general anesthesia, with severe psychological consequences.[308] A recent study involving all hospitals in the United Kingdom and Ireland showed that accidental awareness during general anesthesia was more common with intravenous anesthesia compared with inhalational anesthesia.[309] Thus for intravenous drug delivery, there remains a strong need for methods to ensure accurate and individualized estimation and titration of dosing. Currently there exist several emerging techniques and technologies that might help realize this goal.

Hypnotic drugs used in anesthesia are known to have strong interaction reactions with other commonly used drugs. While pharmacokinetic interactions are common, pharmacodynamic interactions are much larger in magnitude, and thus clinically highly relevant. In the case of the hypnotics and opioid analgesics, the interactions are strongly synergistic, and so when these drugs are coadministered, dose adjustments are usually necessary to avoid adverse effects. These interactions are very complex, with the magnitude of the interaction effect dependent on the plasma and effect-site concentrations of all of the interacting drugs. Interactions between two drugs are best depicted on three-dimensional response surface plots.[80,96,99] As mentioned earlier, advisory displays have been developed to provide the anesthesiologist with real-time information on the likely magnitude of the clinical effect of drug combinations (see Fig. 26.25). Although seldom used in clinical practice, it is likely that these and similar systems will be more widely employed in the future, to help guide anesthesiologists to optimize anesthetic dosing.

A development that could potentially improve safety and accuracy is the broader implementation and clinical use of the new "universal" pharmacokinetic-pharmacodynamic models that have been developed for propofol[76] and remifentanil.[184] The models currently used to implement TCI were developed from studies of patients or volunteers with a rather narrow range of age, weight, and height characteristics; and so naturally these models are only applicable in patients of similar characteristics. On the other hand, the universal models were developed from a combined analysis of the data from a significant number of studies involving a large number of patients with different characteristics. The origin of the underlying data, along with the use of allometric scaling, should broaden the applicability of these models. Once these models have been prospectively validated, it is hoped that availability of a single, accurate model for propofol and remifentanil will enhance patient safety and encourage infusion system manufacturers to incorporate these models into their TCI pumps. This might also help reduce the likelihood of drug errors (e.g., those resulting from choice of an inappropriate model, or a lack of understanding of the model chosen), and this too might help improve the popularity and broaden the applications of TCI systems.

TCI systems contain population pharmacokinetic models, designed to provide the best estimate of the parameters of drug kinetics in a population, but not necessarily for an individual. Inevitably, there will be some degree of error when a pharmacokinetic-pharmacodynamic model is used to guide or determine drug infusion rates to a single patient. One possible solution to the inevitable problem of any mismatch between the pharmacokinetic behavior of a drug and the pharmacokinetic model used to guide administration is to perform real-time measurements of achieved concentrations, and to individualize the model. Recently, a system has become available that provides accurate point-of-care measurement of plasma propofol concentrations within 5 minutes.[310] Plasma propofol concentrations measured by this apparatus were thus used in a system that used Bayesian methodology to update the pharmacokinetic-pharmacodynamic model being used for TCI administration of propofol.[136] Although the results were somewhat disappointing—after adaptation bias improved, but precision did not—this was an initial effort using this system, and future research developments might show better results.

At present, no real-time plasma concentration measurements of intravenous drugs are routinely available for clinical use. Such measurements may improve drug delivery or might optimize TCI administration for the individual patient.[311] Several promising techniques have been described. Takita and colleagues found a strong and linear correlation between exhaled propofol concentrations measured by proton transfer mass spectrometry and estimated and measured arterial propofol concentrations.[312] Miekisch and coworkers[313] used headspace solid-phase microextraction coupled with gas chromatography mass spectrometry to measure alveolar (exhaled), arterial, central venous, and peripheral blood propofol concentrations, and found a good correlation between exhaled and arterial concentrations. Perl and colleagues[314] used an ion mobility spectrometer coupled to a multicapillary column for preseparation (multicapillary column–ion mobility spectrometer [MCC-IMS]), Hornuss and colleagues used ion molecule reaction mass spectrometry,[315,316] and Grossherr and colleagues used gas chromatography mass spectrometry.[317] The latter group also described the difference between blood/gas partition coefficient and pulmonary extraction ratio for propofol between species, which will be important when studying this technique in an animal setting.[318]

Varadajan,[319] Ziaian and colleagues,[320] and Kreuer and colleagues[321] have applied compartmental modeling to describe the kinetics of exhaled propofol. Colin et al. were able to show that standard compartmental models can easily be extended with an additional lung compartment (with a rate constant to model time delay) and a scaling factor (to convert units) to enable predictions of plasma propofol concentration, as well as online Bayesian model adaptation.[322] With this model it was also possible to estimate BIS values from exhaled propofol measurements.

Recently a system using MCC-IMS (Edmon, B. Braun, Germany) has become commercially available and is able to provide measurements every minute. Studies with a prototype system used a reference gas generator to confirm accuracy and precision over the clinical range of exhaled propofol measurements.[323]

Even with an online method for measurement of drug concentrations and/or of perfecting pharmacokinetic models, the clinician still faces the challenge of the broad variability in pharmacodynamic response to any given drug concentration. Automatic closed-loop control systems, which have been discussed extensively in this chapter, might provide a solution to this problem. A well-designed system with a robust measure of clinical effect should help to optimize drug administration and titration on an individual level by accurately titrating drug administration to clinical effect.

Finally, the use of nonlinear mixed effects modeling (NONMEM) techniques is currently considered to be the state-of-the-art for pharmacokinetic-pharmacodynamic analysis and for development of new models. Such development involves use of infusion rate, measured plasma concentration, and measures of clinical effect to generate mathematical models that are consistent with our knowledge of pharmacology.

This process produces the parameters for a structural model comprising two or more compartments, redistribution clearance, and metabolic clearance parameters that describe exponential processes. Artificial intelligence approaches using neural networks are providing powerful and effective solutions to modern problems, eliminating the need to start with models based on current knowledge.[324] This "deep learning" approach was recently applied to data from 231 patients to learn how to predict the BIS values associated with differing plasma and effect-site concentrations of propofol and remifentanil.[325] Remarkably the system was able to learn to predict BIS values more accurately than traditional pharmacokinetic-pharmacodynamic model-based approaches. Given the widespread ease of access of almost all anesthesiologists to web-based technology, it is reasonable to imagine a situation where the data from millions of patients around the world are fed into machine-learning systems that can learn to predict responses to different combinations of drugs, and, inversely, learn to accurately predict the doses required for given responses, without the need for complex models.

Complete references available online at expertconsult.com.

References

1. Massa DJ, et al. *Proc Staff Meet Mayo Clin*. 1950;25:413.
2. Rivera AM, et al. *Acta Anaesthesiol Belg*. 2005;56:271.
3. Absalom A, Struys MM. In: *An overview of TCI & TIVA*. Gent: Academia Press; 2007.
4. Struys M, de Smet T. In: Evers AS, et al., ed. *Anesthetic Pharmacology: Basic Principles and Clinical Practice*. Cambridge: Cambridge University Press; 2011:103.
5. Sahinovic MM, et al. *Curr Opin Anaesthesiol*. 2010;23:734.
6. Struys MM, et al. *Br J Anaesth*. 2011;107:38.
7. Schwilden H. *Eur J Clin Pharmacol*. 1981;20:379.
8. Absalom AR, et al. *Anesth Analg*. 2016;122(1):70.
9. Shafer SL. *J Clin Anesth*. 1993;5:14S.
10. Shafer SL. *Semin Anesth*. 1993;12:222.
11. Avram MJ, Krejcie TC. *Anesthesiology*. 2003;99:1078.
12. Absalom AR, et al. *Br J Anaesth*. 2009;103:26.
13. Masui K, et al. *Anesth Analg*. 2010;111:368.
14. Upton RN, Ludbrook G. *Anesthesiology*. 2005;103:344.
15. Soehle M, et al. *Br J Anaesth*. 2010;105:172.
16. Hull CJ, et al. *Br J Anaesth*. 1978;50:1113.
17. Sheiner LB, et al. *Clin Pharmacol Ther*. 1979;25:358.
18. Schnider TW, et al. In: Evers AS, et al., ed. *Anesthetic Pharmacology. Basic Principles and Clinical Practice*. Cambridge: Cambridge University Press; 2011:57.
19. Fernandez-Candil J, et al. *Eur J Clin Pharmacol*. 2008;64:795.
20. Chen C, et al. *Br J Anaesth*. 2008;101:788.
21. Struys MM, et al. *Anesthesiology*. 2003;99:802.
22. Egan TD, et al. *Br J Anaesth*. 2004;92:335.
23. Glass PS, et al. *Anesth Analg*. 1993;77:1031.
24. Vanluchene AL, et al. *Anesthesiology*. 2004;101:34.
25. Vereecke HE, et al. *Anesthesiology*. 2005;103:500.
26. Bruhn J, et al. *Br J Anaesth*. 2006;97:85.
27. Jospin M, et al. *IEEE Trans Biomed Eng*. 2007;54:840.
28. Ludbrook GL, et al. *Anesthesiology*. 2002;97:1363.
29. Shafer SL, Gregg KM. *J Pharmacokinet Biopharm*. 1992;20:147.
30. Jacobs JR, Williams EA. *IEEE Trans Biomed Eng*. 1993;40:993.
31. Coppens MJ, et al. *Anesthesiology*. 2011;115:83.
32. Minto CF, et al. *Anesthesiology*. 2003;99:324.
33. Cortinez LI, et al. *Br J Anaesth*. 2007;99:679.
34. Schnider T, Minto C. *Anaesthesia*. 2008;63:206.
35. Mourisse J, et al. *Br J Anaesth*. 2007;98:737.
36. Mourisse J, et al. *Br J Anaesth*. 2007;98:746.
37. McKay ID, et al. *Anesth Analg*. 2006;102:91.
38. Kelz MB, et al. *Proc Natl Acad Sci U S A*. 2008;105:1309.
39. Friedman EB, et al. *PLoS One*. 2010;5:e11903.
40. Sepulveda PO, et al. *Anaesthesia*. 2018;73(1):40.
41. Warnaby CE, et al. *Anesthesiology*. 2017;127(4):645–657.
42. Kuizenga MH, et al. *Br J Anaesth*. 2018;120(3):525–536.
43. Bouillon T, et al. *Anesthesiology*. 2003;99(4):779–787.
44. Bouillon T, et al. *Anesthesiology*. 2004;100(2):240–250.
45. Martinoni EP, et al. *Br J Anaesth*. 2004;92(6):800–807.
46. Scott JC, et al. *Anesthesiology*. 1985;62:234.
47. Struys MM, et al. *Anesthesiology*. 2000;92:399.
48. Eger 2nd EI, et al. *Anesthesiology*. 1965;26:756.
49. Telford RJ, et al. *Anesth Analg*. 1992;75:523.
50. Vuyk J, et al. *Anesthesiology*. 1992;77:3.
51. Hung OR, et al. *Anesthesiology*. 1992;77:237.
52. Glass PS, et al. *Anesthesiology*. 1993;78:842.
53. Jacobs JR, et al. *Anesth Analg*. 1995;80:143.
54. Vuyk J, et al. *Anesthesiology*. 1997;87:1549.
55. Xu Z, et al. *Anesth Analg*. 2009;108:478.
56. Kaneda K, et al. *J Clin Pharmacol*. 2011;51:482.
57. Scott JC, Stanski DR. *J Pharmacol Exp Ther*. 1987;240:159.
58. Scott JC, et al. *Anesthesiology*. 1991;74:34.
59. Egan TD, et al. *Anesthesiology*. 1993;79:881.
60. Egan TD, et al. *Anesthesiology*. 1996;84:821.
61. Minto CF, et al. *Anesthesiology*. 1997;86:10.
62. Homer TD, Stanski DR. *Anesthesiology*. 1985;62:714.
63. Stanski DR, Maitre PO. *Anesthesiology*. 1990;72:412.
64. Schnider TW, et al. *Anesthesiology*. 1996;84:510.
65. Barvais L, et al. *Br J Anaesth*. 2003;91:347.
66. Glass PS, et al. *Anesthesiology*. 1999;90:1556.
67. Ausems ME, et al. *Anesthesiology*. 1986;65:362.
68. Ausems ME, et al. *Br J Anaesth*. 1985;57:1217.
69. Kodaka M, et al. *Br J Anaesth*. 2004;92:242.
70. Cortinez LI, et al. *Eur J Anaesthesiol*. 2005;22:56.
71. Colin PJ, et al. *Br J Anaesth*. 2017;119(2):200–210.
72. Colin PJ, et al. *Br J Anaesth*. 2017;119(2):211–220.
73. Gourlay GK, et al. *Anesth Analg*. 1988;67:329.
74. van den Nieuwenhuyzen MC, et al. *Anesth Analg*. 1995;81:671.
75. Lehmann KA, et al. *Acta Anaesthesiol Scand*. 1991;35:221.
76. Eleveld DJ, et al. *Br J Anaesth*. 2018;120(5):942–959.
77. Hendrickx JF, et al. *Anesth Analg*. 2008;107:494.
78. Minto CF, et al. *Anesthesiology*. 2000;92:1603.
79. Bouillon TW. *Handb Exp Pharmacol*. 2008;182:471.
80. Minto CF, et al. *Anesthesiology*. 2000;92:1603.
81. Short TG, et al. *Anesthesiology*. 2002;96:400.
82. Heyse B, et al. *Anesthesiology*. 2012;116:311.
83. Sebel PS, et al. *Anesthesiology*. 1992;76:52.
84. McEwan AI, et al. *Anesthesiology*. 1993;78:864.
85. Lang E, et al. *Anesthesiology*. 1996;85:721.
86. Egan TD, Minto CF. In: Evers AS, et al., ed. *Anesthetic Pharmacology. Basic Principles and Clinical Practice*. Cambridge: Cambridge University Press; 2011:147.
87. Short TG. *Anesth Analg*. 2010;111:249.
88. Manyam SC, et al. *Anesthesiology*. 2006;105:267.
89. Johnson KB, et al. *Anesth Analg*. 2010;111:387.
90. Heyse B, et al. *Anesthesiology*. 2014;120(6):1390.
91. Kissin I. *Anesth Analg*. 1993;76:215.
92. Zanderigo E, et al. *Anesthesiology*. 2006;104:742.
93. Vuyk J, et al. *Anesthesiology*. 1995;83:8.
94. Bruhn J, et al. *Anesthesiology*. 2003;98:621.
95. Ropcke H, et al. *J Clin Anesth*. 2001;13:198.
96. Bouillon TW, et al. *Anesthesiology*. 2004;100:1353.
97. Nieuwenhuijs DJ, et al. *Anesthesiology*. 2003;98:312.
98. Gambus PL, et al. *Anesth Analg*. 2011;112:331.
99. Bouillon T, et al. *Anesthesiology*. 1999;91:144.
100. LaPierre CD, et al. *Anesth Analg*. 2011;113:490.

101. Luginbuhl M, et al. *Anesthesiology*. 2010;112(4):872–880.
102. Schumacher PM, et al. *Anesthesiology*. 2009;111:790.
103. Sebel LE, et al. *Anesthesiology*. 2006;104:1176.
104. Hammer GB, et al. *Paediatr Anaesth*. 2009;19:138.
105. Hannivoort LN, et al. *Br J Anaesth*. 2016;116(5):624.
106. Shafer SL. *Anesthesiology*. 2012;116(2):240.
107. van den Berg JP, et al. *Br J Anaesth*. 2017;118(1):44–57.
108. Shafer SL. *Varvel. JR. Anesthesiology*. 1991;74:53.
109. Hughes MA, et al. *Anesthesiology*. 1992;76:334.
110. Schwilden H. *Anasth Intensivther Notfallmed*. 1985;20:307.
111. Fisher DM, Rosen JI. *Anesthesiology*. 1986;65:286.
112. Youngs EJ, Shafer SL. *Anesthesiology*. 81:833.
113. Bailey JM. *Anesthesiology*. 1995;83:1095.
114. Milne SE, et al. *Br J Anaesth*. 2003;90:623.
115. Struys MM, et al. *Anesthesiology*. 2002;96:803.
116. Syroid ND, et al. *Anesthesiology*. 2002;96:565.
117. Drews FA, et al. *Hum Factors*. 2006;48:85.
118. Murphy RS, Wilcox SJ. *J Med Eng Technol*. 2009;33:470.
119. Struys MM, et al. *Anesth Analg*. 2016;122(1):56–69.
120. Absalom AR, et al. *Anesth Analg*. 2011;112(3):516–518.
121. Kruger-Thiemer E. *Eur J Pharmacol*. 1968;4(3):317–324.
122. White M, et al. *Anaesthesia*. 1990;45:204–209.
123. Wakeling HG, et al. *Anesthesiology*. 1999;90(1):92–97.
124. Struys MMRF, et al. *Anesth Analg*. 2016;122(1):56–69.
125. Shafer SL, et al. *Anesthesiology*. 1988;68(2):261–266.
126. Adapa RM, et al. *Anaesthesia*. 2012;67:33.
127. Schnider TW, et al. *Anesth Analg*. 2016;122(1):79–85.
128. Hu C, et al. *Anesthesiology*. 2005;102:639.
129. Varvel JR, et al. *J Pharmacokinet Biopharm*. 1992;20:63.
130. Coetzee JF, et al. *Anesthesiology*. 1995;82:1328.
131. Cowley NJ, et al. *Eur J Anaesthesiol*. 2013;30(10):627–632.
132. Glen JB, et al. *Anaesthesia*. 2014;69(6):550–557.
133. Cortinez LI, et al. *Anesth Analg*. 2014;119(2):302–310.
134. Tachibana N, et al. *Eur J Anaesthesiol*. 2014;31(12):701–707.
135. Lee YH, et al. *Br J Anaesth*. 2017;118(6):883–891.
136. van den Berg JP, et al. *Br J Anaesth*. 2017;119(5):918–927.
137. Lee AKY, et al. *J Cardiothorac Vasc Anesth*. 2018;32(2):723–730.
138. Barvais L, et al. *J Cardiothorac Vasc Anesth*. 2000;14:402.
139. Absalom AR, et al. *Br J Anaesth*. 2007;98(5):615–623.
140. Hannivoort LN, et al. *Anesthesiology*. 2015;123(2):357–367.
141. Obara S, et al. *J Anesth*. 2018;32(1):33–40.
142. Glass PS, et al. *Anesthesiology*. 1990;73(6):1082–1090.
143. Shafer SL, et al. *Anesthesiology*. 1990;73(6):1091–1102.
144. Shibutani K, et al. *Anesthesiology*. 2004;101:603.
145. Lemmens HJ, et al. *Clin Pharmacokinet*. 1990;19:416.
146. Crankshaw DP, et al. *Anesth Analg*. 1993;76:556.
147. Sigmond N, et al. *Br J Anaesth*. 2013;111(2):197–208.
148. Hudson RJ, et al. *J Cardiothorac Vasc Anesth*. 2001;15:693.
149. Slepchenko G, et al. *Anesthesiology*. 2003;98:65.
150. Mertens MJ, et al. *Br J Anaesth*. 2003;90:132.
151. Cho YJ, et al. *Anaesthesia*. 2017;72(10):1196–1205.
152. Marsh B, et al. *Br J Anaesth*. 1991;67:41–48.
153. Absalom A, et al. *Br J Anaesth*. 2003;91(4):507–513.
154. Sepulveda P, et al. *Br J Anaesth*. 2011;107(4):593–600.
155. Choi BM, et al. *J Pharmacokinet Pharmacodyn*. 2015;42(2):163–177.
156. McMurray TJ, et al. *Anaesthesia*. 2004;59(7):636–641.
157. Cortegiani A, et al. *J Clin Pharmacol*. 2018.
158. Struys M, et al. *Eur J Anaesthesiol*. 1995;10(suppl):85.
159. Struys M, et al. *Anaesthesia*. 1997;52:41.
160. Hoymork SC, et al. *Acta Anaesthesiol Scand*. 2000;44:1138.
161. Macquaire V, et al. *Acta Anaesthesiol Scand*. 2002;46:1010.
162. Fabregas N, et al. *Anesthesiology*. 2002;97:1378.
163. Schnider TW, et al. *Anesthesiology*. 1998;88(5):1170–1182.
164. Schnider TW, et al. *Anesthesiology*. 1999;90(6):1502–1516.
165. Schüttler J, Ihmsen H. *Anesthesiology*. 2000;92:727.
166. Anderson BJ, Holford NH. *Annu Rev Pharmacol Toxicol*. 2008;48:303.
167. Anderson BJ, Holford NH. *Paediatr Anaesth*. 2010;20:1.
168. Cortinez LI, et al. *Br J Anaesth*. 2010;105:448.
169. Cortinez LI, et al. *Anesth Analg*. 2018.
170. Frederico Avendano C, et al. *Rev Esp Anestesiol Reanim*. 2016;63(10): 556–563.
171. Barakat AR, et al. *Anaesthesia*. 2007;62:661.
172. Coppens M, et al. *Br J Anaesth*. 2010;104:452.
173. Thomson AJ, et al. *Anaesthesia*. 2014;69(5):420–428.
174. Eleveld DJ, et al. *Anesth Analg*. 2014;118(6):1221–1237.
175. Kataria BK, et al. *Anesthesiology*. 1994;80:104.
176. Hara M, et al. *Br J Anaesth*. 2017;118(3):415–423.
177. Short TG, et al. *Br J Anaesth*. 1994;72(3):302–306.
178. Gepts E, et al. *Anesthesiology*. 1995;83:1194.
179. Maitre PO, et al. *Anesthesiology*. 1987;66:3.
180. van den Nieuwenhuyzen MC, et al. *Anesthesiology*. 1993;79:481.
181. Raemer DB, et al. *Anesthesiology*. 1990;73:66.
182. Minto CF, et al. *Anesthesiology*. 1997;86:24.
183. Rigby-Jones AE, et al. *Br J Anaesth*. 2007;99:252–261.
184. Eleveld DJ, et al. *Anesthesiology*. 2017;126(6):1005–1018.
185. Chen L, Baker MD. *Pediatr Emerg Care*. 2006;22:485.
186. White M, et al. *Clin Pharmacokinet*. 2008;47(2):119–127.
187. Fu F, et al. *Br J Anaesth*. 2014;112(3):506–513.
188. Calvo R, et al. *Acta Anaesthesiol Scand*. 2004;48:1038.
189. Wietasch JK, et al. *Anesth Analg*. 2006;102:430.
190. Vuyk J, et al. *Anesth Analg*. 2009;108:1522.
191. Lichtenbelt BJ, et al. *Anesth Analg*. 2010;110:1597.
192. Ausems ME, et al. *Anesthesiology*. 1988;68:851.
193. Alvis JM, et al. *Anesthesiology*. 1985;63:41.
194. Theil DR, et al. *J Cardiothorac Vasc Anesth*. 1993;7:300.
195. De Castro V, et al. *Anesth Analg*. 2003;96:33.
196. Moerman AT, et al. *Anesth Analg*. 2009;108:828.
197. Kenny GN. *Eur J Anaesthesiol*. 1997;15(suppl):29.
198. Servin FS. *Anaesthesia*. 1998;53(suppl 1):82.
199. Passot S, et al. *Anesth Analg*. 2005;100:1338–1342.
200. Chen G, et al. *Eur J Anaesthesiol*. 2009;26:928.
201. Wang X, et al. *J Clin Anesth*. 2016;32:92–100.
202. Chiang MH, et al. *Endoscopy*. 2013;45(11):907–914.
203. Mu J, et al. *Br J Anaesth*. 2018;120(5):1049–1055.
204. Kazama T, et al. *Anesthesiology*. 1999;90:1517.
205. Absalom AR, Kenny GN. *Br J Anaesth*. 2003;90:737.
206. Raeder J. *Anesth Analg*. 2009;108:704.
207. Bejjani G, et al. *J Cardiothorac Vasc Anesth*. 2009;23:175.
208. Sveticic G, et al. *Anesthesiology*. 2003;98:1195.
209. Beilin B, et al. *Acta Anaesthesiol Scand*. 2005;49:78.
210. Ng KF, et al. *J Clin Anesth*. 2006;18:205.
211. Lipszyc M, et al. *Br J Anaesth*. 2011;106:724.
212. White I, et al. *Pharmacol Res*. 2012;66:185.
213. Walder B, et al. *Acta Anaesthesiol Scand*. 2001;45:795.
214. Cronrath P, et al. *Nurs Econ*. 2011;29:79.
215. Volmanen P, et al. *Acta Anaesthesiol Scand*. 2005;49:453.
216. Volmanen P, et al. *Acta Anaesthesiol Scand*. 2008;52:249.
217. Douma MR, et al. *Br J Anaesth*. 2010;104:209.
218. Volmanen P, et al. *Curr Opin Anaesthesiol*. 2011;24:235.
219. Volmanen PV, et al. *Acta Anaesthesiol Scand*. 2011;55:486.
220. Douma MR, et al. *Int J Obstet Anesth*. 2011;20:118.
221. Freeman LM, et al. *BMJ*. 2015;350:h846.
222. van den Nieuwenhuyzen MC, et al. *Br J Anaesth*. 1997;78:17.
223. van den Nieuwenhuyzen MC, et al. *Br J Anaesth*. 1999;82:580.
224. Schraag S, et al. *Br J Anaesth*. 1998;81(3):365–368.
225. Jeleazcov C, et al. *Anesthesiology*. 2016;124(1):56–68.
226. Loper KA, et al. *Anesth Analg*. 1988;67(11):1118–1119.
227. Osborne GA, et al. *Anaesthesia*. 1991;46:553–556.
228. Rudkin GE, et al. *Anaesthesia*. 1991;46:90–92.
229. Rudkin GE, et al. *Anaesthesia*. 1992;47:376–381.
230. Osborne GA, et al. *Anaesthesia*. 1994;49:287.
231. Mazanikov M, et al. *Endoscopy*. 2013;45(11):915–919.
232. Irwin MG, et al. *Anaesthesia*. 1997;52(6):525–530.
233. Murdoch JA, et al. *Br J Anaesth*. 1999;82(3):429–431.
234. Murdoch J, et al. *Br J Anaesth*. 2000;85(2):299–301.
235. Henderson F, et al. *Anaesthesia*. 2002;57(4):387–390.
236. Absalom AR, et al. *Anesthesiol* in press. 2000;93:A291.
237. Stonell CA, et al. *Anaesthesia*. 2006;61(3):240–247.
238. Chapman RM, et al. *Anaesthesia*. 2006;61(4):345–349.
239. O'Brien C, et al. *Anaesthesia*. 2013;68(7):760–764.
240. Anderson KJ, et al. *Anaesthesia*. 2013;68(2):148–153.
241. Allam S, et al. *Anaesthesia*. 2013;68(2):154–158.
242. Doufas AG, et al. *Anesthesiol*. 2001;94(4):585–592.
243. Doufas AG, et al. *Acta Anaesthesiol Scand*. 2003;47(8):944–950.
244. Doufas AG, et al. *Anesth Analg*. 2009;109(3):778–786.
245. Pambianco DJ, et al. *Gastrointest Endosc*. 2008;68(3):542–547.
246. Pambianco DJ, et al. *Gastrointest Endosc*. 2011;73(4):765–772.
247. Lin OS. *Intest Res*. 2017;15(4):456–466.
248. Goudra B, et al. *Anesth Analg*. 2017;124(2):686–688.
249. O'Hara DA, et al. *Anesthesiology*. 1992;77:563.
250. Liu N, et al. *Anesthesiology*. 2006;104:686.
251. Chaudhri S, et al. *Br J Anaesth*. 1992;69:607.

252. O'Hara DA, et al. *Anesthesiology*. 1991;74:258.
253. Edwards ND, et al. *Anaesthesia*. 1998;53:136.
254. Olkkola KT, et al. *Acta Anaesthesiol Scand*. 1991;35:420.
255. Sakai T, et al. *Acta Anaesthesiol Scand*. 2000;44:1007.
256. Absalom AR, et al. *Anesthesiology*. 2002;96:67.
257. Leslie K, et al. *Anaesthesia*. 2002;57:693.
258. Liu N, et al. *Eur J Anaesthesiol*. 2006;23:465.
259. Liu N, et al. *Anesth Analg*. 2011;112:546.
260. Liu N, et al. *Anesthesiology*. 2012;116:286.
261. Le Guen M, et al. *Intensive Care Med*. 2013;39(3):454–462.
262. Liu N, et al. *Can J Anaesth*. 2013;60(9):881–887.
263. Orliaguet GA, et al. *Anesthesiology*. 2015;122(4):759–767.
264. Restoux A, et al. *Br J Anaesth*. 2016;117(3):332–340.
265. Le Guen M, et al. *Anesth Analg*. 2014;118(5):946–955.
266. Liu N, et al. *Br J Anaesth*. 2014;112(5):842–851.
267. Le Guen M, et al. *Anesthesiology*. 2014;120(2):355–364.
268. Dumans-Nizard V, et al. *Anesth Analg*. 2017;125(2):635–642.
269. Bataille A, et al. *Eur J Anaesthesiol*. 2017.
270. Puri GD, et al. *Anaesth Intensive Care*. 2007;35(3):357–362.
271. Agarwal J, et al. *Acta Anaesthesiol Scand*. 2009;53(3):390–397.
272. Hegde HV, et al. *J Clin Monit Comput*. 2009;23(4):189–196.
273. Solanki A, et al. *Eur J Anaesthesiol*. 2010;27(8):708–713.
274. Puri GD, et al. *Indian J Aaesth*. 2012;56(3):238–242.
275. Biswas I, et al. *Paediatr Anaesth*. 2013;23(12):1145–1152.
276. Mahajan V, et al. *J Clin Anesth*. 2017;42:106–113.
277. Puri GD, et al. *Anesth Analg*. 2016;122(1):106–114.
278. Zikov T, et al. *IEEE Trans Biomed Eng*. 2006;53(4):617–632.
279. van Heusden K, et al. *IEEE Trans Biomed Eng*. 2013;60(9):2521–2529.
280. West N, et al. *J Clin Monit Comput*. 2018.
281. Bibian S, et al. *J Clin Monit Comput*. 2011;25(1):81–87.
282. West N, et al. *Anesth Analg*. 2017.
283. Brodie SM, et al. *A A Case Rep*. 2017;9(8):239–243.
284. Hemmerling TM, et al. *Can J Anaesth*. 2010;57(8):725–735.
285. Hemmerling TM, et al. *Br J Anaesth*. 2013;110(6):1031–1039.
286. Hemmerling TM, et al. *J Comput*. 2009;4:311–318.
287. Zaouter C, et al. *Anesth Analg*. 2016;123(4):885–893.
288. Zaouter C, et al. *J Clin Monit Comput*. 2017;31(2):309–317.
289. Zaouter C, et al. *Anesth Analg*. 2017;125(5):1505–1512.
290. Mortier E, et al. *Anaesthesia*. 1998;53(8):749–754.
291. Struys MM, et al. *Anesthesiology*. 2001;95(1):6–17.
292. Struys MM, et al. *Anesthesiology*. 2004;100(3):640–647.
293. De Smet T, et al. *Anesth Analg*. 2007;105(6):1629–1638.
294. De Smet T, et al. *Anesth Analg*. 2008;107(4):1200–1210.
295. Gentilini A, et al. *IEEE Trans Biomed Eng*. 2002;49(4):289–299.
296. Gentilini A, et al. *IEEE Trans Biomed Eng*. 2001;48(8):874–889.
297. Moore BL, et al. *Anesth Analg*. 2011;112(2):360–367.
298. Moore BL, et al. *Anesth Analg*. 2011;112(2):350–359.
299. Manberg PJ, et al. *Clin Pharmacol Ther*. 2008;84(1):166–169.
300. Liu N, et al. *Anesth Analg*. 2016;122(1):4–6.
301. Brogi E, et al. *Anesth Analg*. 2016;124(2):446–455.
302. Pasin L, et al. *Anesth Analg*. 2017;124(2):456–464.
303. Dussaussoy C, et al. *J Clin Monit Comput*. 2014;28(1):35–40.
304. Miller TE, et al. *Anesth Analg*. 2013;117(5):1039–1041.
305. Liu N, et al. *Anesth Analg*. 2016;122(1):4–6.
306. Loeb RG, et al. *Anesth Analg*. 2017;124(2):381–382.
307. Parvinian B, et al. *Anesth Analg*. 2017.
308. Tasbihgou SR, et al. *Anaesthesia*. 2018;73(1):112–122.
309. Pandit JJ, et al. *Br J Anaesth*. 2014;113(4):540–548.
310. Cowley NJ, et al. *Anaesthesia*. 2012;67(8):870–874.
311. Maitre PO, et al. *Anesthesiology*. 1988;69:652–659.
312. Takita A, et al. *Anesthesiology*. 2007;106(4):659–664.
313. Miekisch W, et al. *Clin Chim Acta*. 2008;395:32–37.
314. Perl T, et al. *Br J Anaesth*. 2009;103(6):822–827.
315. Hornuss C, et al. *Anesthesiology*. 2007;106(4):665–674.
316. Hornuss C, et al. *Anal Bioanal Chem*. 2012;403(2):555–561.
317. Grossherr M, et al. *Br J Anaesth*. 2009;102(5):608–613.
318. Grossherr M, et al. *Xenobiotica*. 2009;39(10):782–787.
319. Varadarajan BT. *Monitoring of Propofol in Breath; Pharmacokinetic Modeling and Design of a Control System*. Doctoral Thesis. Luebeck University; 2011.
320. Ziaian D, et al. *IEEE International Symposium on Medical Measurements and Applications*. MeMeA; 2014:1–5.
321. Kreuer S, et al. *Sci Rep*. 2014;4:5423.
322. Colin P, et al. *Clin Pharmacokinet*. 2016;55(7):849–859.
323. Maurer F, Walter L, Geiger M, et al. Calibration and validation of a MCC/IMS prototype for exhaled propofol online measurement. *J Pharm Biomed Anal*. 2017;145:293–297.
324. Gambus P, et al. *Anesthesiology*. 2018;128(3):431–433.
325. Lee HC, et al. *Anesthesiology*. 2018;128(3):492–501.

27 Pharmacology of Neuromuscular Blocking Drugs

SORIN J. BRULL and CLAUDE MEISTELMAN

KEY POINTS

- Two different populations of nicotinic acetylcholine receptors exist at the mammalian neuromuscular junction. In the adult, the nicotinic acetylcholine receptor at the postsynaptic (muscular) membrane is composed of $\alpha_2\beta\delta\varepsilon$ subunits, while the fetal (immature) receptor is composed of $\alpha_2\beta\gamma\delta$. The presynaptic (neuronal) nicotinic receptor is a pentameric complex composed of $\alpha_3\beta_2$ subunits. Each of the two α subunits of the postsynaptic receptors has a ligand (acetylcholine) binding site.
- Nondepolarizing muscle relaxants produce neuromuscular blockade by competing with acetylcholine for the postsynaptic α subunits. In contrast, succinylcholine acts directly with the recognition sites and produces prolonged depolarization that results in decreased sensitivity of the postsynaptic nicotinic acetylcholine receptor and inactivation of sodium channels so that propagation of the action potential across the muscle membrane is inhibited.
- Different patterns of stimulation examine neuromuscular blockade at different areas of the motor end plate. Depression of the response to single twitch stimulation is likely caused by blockade of postsynaptic nicotinic acetylcholine receptors, whereas fade in the response to tetanic and train-of-four stimuli results from blockade of presynaptic nicotinic receptors.
- Succinylcholine is the only available depolarizing neuromuscular blocking drug for clinical use. It is characterized by rapid onset of effect and ultrashort duration of action because of its rapid hydrolysis by butyrylcholinesterase.
- Available nondepolarizing neuromuscular blocking drugs can be classified according to chemical class (aminosteroid, benzylisoquinolinium, or other compounds) or by duration of action (long-, intermediate-, and short-acting drugs) of equipotent doses.
- The speed of onset is inversely proportional to the potency of nondepolarizing neuromuscular blocking drugs. With the exception of atracurium, molar potency is highly predictive of a drug's rate of onset of effect. Rocuronium has a molar potency that is approximately 13% that of vecuronium and 9% that of cisatracurium. Its onset of effect is more rapid than either of these muscle relaxants.
- Neuromuscular blockade develops faster, lasts a shorter time, and recovers faster in the more centrally located neuromuscular units (e.g., laryngeal adductors, diaphragm, and masseter muscle) than in the more peripherally located adductor pollicis muscle.
- Many long-acting neuromuscular blocking drugs undergo minimal or no metabolism, and they are primarily eliminated, largely unchanged, by renal excretion. Neuromuscular blocking drugs of intermediate duration of action have faster distribution and more rapid clearances than the long-acting drugs because of multiple pathways of degradation, metabolism, and elimination. Mivacurium, a short-acting neuromuscular blocking drug, is cleared rapidly and almost exclusively by metabolism by butyrylcholinesterase.
- After the administration of nondepolarizing neuromuscular blocking drugs, it is essential to ensure adequate return of normal neuromuscular function using objective (quantitative) means of monitoring. Residual neuromuscular paralysis decreases upper esophageal tone, coordination of the esophageal musculature during swallowing, and hypoxic ventilatory drive. Residual paralysis can increase healthcare costs and the patient hospital length of stay, morbidity, and mortality.

History and Clinical Use

In 1942, Griffith and Johnson described *d*-tubocurarine (dTc) as a safe drug to provide skeletal muscle relaxation during surgery.[1] One year later, Cullen described the use of this drug in 131 patients who had received general anesthesia for surgery.[2] In 1954, Beecher and Todd reported a six-fold increase in mortality in patients receiving dTc compared with patients who had not received a muscle relaxant.[3] The increased mortality resulted from a general lack of understanding of the clinical pharmacology and effects of neuromuscular blocking drugs (NMBDs). The effect of residual neuromuscular blockade postoperatively was not appreciated, guidelines for monitoring muscle strength had not been established, and the importance of pharmacologically antagonizing residual blockade was not understood.

Succinylcholine, introduced by Thesleff[4] and Foldes and associates[5] in 1952, rapidly gained widespread use and changed anesthetic practice drastically because the drug's rapid onset of effect and ultrashort duration of action allowed for both rapid endotracheal intubation and rapid recovery of neuromuscular strength.

In 1967, Baird and Reid reported on the clinical administration of the first synthetic aminosteroid, pancuronium.[6] The development of the intermediate-acting NMBDs was based on the compounds' metabolism and resulted in the introduction of vecuronium,[7] an aminosteroid, and atracurium,[8] a benzylisoquinolinium, into clinical practice in the 1980s. Vecuronium was the first muscle relaxant to have an intermediate duration of action and minimal cardiovascular actions. Mivacurium, the first short-acting nondepolarizing NMBD, was introduced into clinical practice in the 1990s,[9] as was rocuronium,[10] an intermediate-acting NMBD with a very rapid onset of neuromuscular blockade. Other NMBDs have been introduced into clinical practice since the use of dTc was first advocated. These include pipecuronium, doxacurium, cisatracurium, and rapacuronium. Although not all remain in clinical use today, each represented an advance or improvement in at least one aspect over its predecessors. Still other NMBDs, such as CW 002[11] and CW 1759-50[11a,11b] are undergoing investigation.

NMBDs should be administered only to anesthetized individuals to provide relaxation of skeletal muscles. Because this class of drugs lacks analgesic or amnestic properties, NMBDs should not be administered to prevent patient movement. Awareness during surgery[12] and in the intensive care unit (ICU)[13] has been described in multiple publications. As stated by Cullen and Larson, "muscle relaxants given inappropriately may provide the surgeon with optimal [operating] conditions in…a patient[14] [who] is paralyzed but not anesthetized—a state that [is] wholly unacceptable for the patient."[15] Additionally, "muscle relaxants used to cover up deficiencies in total anesthetic management…represent an…inappropriate use of the valuable adjuncts to anesthesia."[15] Administration of NMBDs intraoperatively to maintain neuromuscular block requires that the time course of block be monitored and the depth of anesthesia be assessed continuously.

NMBDs have been integrated into most anesthetic techniques for major surgery and have become key components in the continuous improvement of safe anesthetic practice and the development of advanced surgical techniques. As earlier stated by Foldes and colleagues,[5] "…[the] first use of…muscle relaxants…not only revolutionized the practice of anesthesia but also started the modern era of surgery and made possible the explosive development of cardiothoracic, neurologic, and organ transplant surgery." Certainly, NMBDs are now used routinely to facilitate endotracheal intubation and mechanical ventilation, and are commonly used to maintain neuromuscular blockade through any number of different surgical procedures. This chapter reviews the pharmacology and clinical use of NMBDs and anticholinesterases in anesthesia and intensive care settings.

Principles of Action of Neuromuscular Blocking Drugs at the Neuromuscular Junction

A brief description of the physiology of neuromuscular blockade is presented in this chapter. A more comprehensive overview is provided in Chapter 12.

POSTJUNCTIONAL EFFECTS

Nicotinic acetylcholine receptors (nAChRs) belong to a large pentameric family of ligand-gated ion channel receptors that include the 5-hydoxytryptamine$_3$ (5-HT$_3$), glycine, and γ-aminobutyric acid (GABA) receptors. They are synthetized in muscle cells and anchored to the end plate membrane by a special protein called rapsyn. Development of innervation in the first weeks of life leads to the replacement of the γ subunit by ε subunit. In adult mammalian skeletal muscle, the nAChR is a pentameric complex of two α subunits in association with single β, δ, and ε subunits (Fig. 27.1). Stoichiometrically, the receptor is represented as α2βεδ, while organizationally it is αεαδβ.

The subunits are organized to form a transmembrane pore, or channel, as well as extracellular binding pockets for acetylcholine and other agonists or antagonists.[16] The receptors are clustered on the crests of the junctional folds; the receptor density in this area is 10,000 to 30,000/μm^2. Each of the two α subunits has an acetylcholine-binding site. These sites are located in pockets within the receptor protein, approximately 3.0 nm above the surface membrane at the interfaces of the α_H-ε and α_L-δ subunits.[17] αH and αL indicate the high- and low-affinity binding sites for dTc; the difference in affinity probably results from the contribution of the different neighboring subunits.18 For instance, the binding affinity of dTc for the αH-ε site is approximately 100 to 500 times higher than that for the αL-δ site.[18] The fetal nAChR contains a γ subunit instead of an adult ε subunit. Once activated by acetylcholine, the mature nAChR has a shorter opening time and a higher conductance to sodium (Na^+), potassium (K^+), and calcium (Ca^{2+}) than the fetal nAChR, which has a smaller, single-channel conductance and a much longer open channel time.[16]

Functionally, the ion channel of the acetylcholine receptor is closed in the resting state. Simultaneous binding of two acetylcholine molecules to the α subunits is required to initiate conformational changes that open the channel. If one molecule of a nondepolarizer NMBD (i.e., a competitive antagonist) is bound to a subunit at the AChR, two agonist molecules of acetylcholine cannot bind simultaneously, and neuromuscular transmission is inhibited.[19]

Succinylcholine, a depolarizing NMBD, produces prolonged depolarization of the end plate region, which is similar to, but more persistent than, the depolarization induced by acetylcholine. This mechanism results in (1) desensitization of the nAChR, (2) inactivation of voltage-gated Na^+ channels at the neuromuscular junction, and (3) increases in K^+ permeability in the surrounding membrane.[19] The end results are failure of action potential generation and neuromuscular blockade.

The fetal nAChR is a low-conductance channel, in contrast to the high-conductance channel of the adult nAChR and upregulation of nAChRs found in states of functional

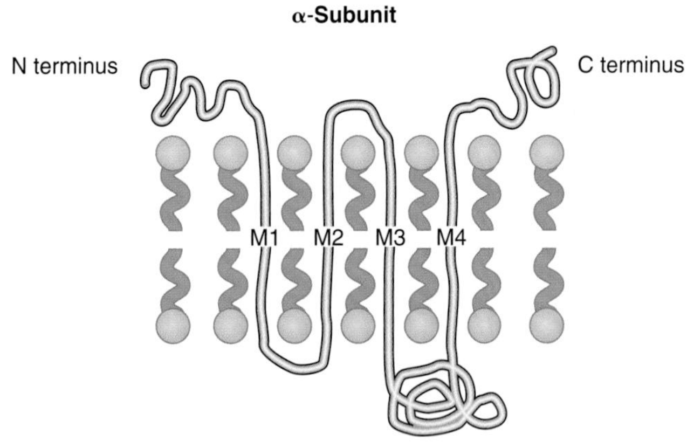

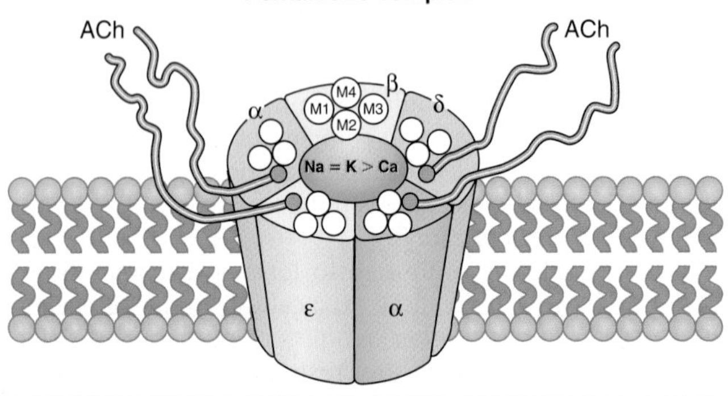

Fig. 27.1 Subunit composition of the nicotinic acetylcholine receptor (nAChR) in the end plate surface of adult mammalian muscle. The adult AChR is an intrinsic membrane protein with five distinct subunits *($\alpha_2\beta\delta\varepsilon$)*. Each subunit contains four helical domains, labeled M_1 to M_4. The M_2 domain forms the channel pore. The *upper panel* shows a single α subunit with its N and C termini on the extracellular surface of the membrane lipid bilayer. Between the N and C termini, the α subunit forms four helices (M_1, M_2, M_3, and M_4), which span the membrane bilayer. The *lower panel* shows the pentameric structure of the nAChR of adult mammalian muscle. The N termini of two subunits cooperate to form two distinct binding pockets for acetylcholine. These pockets occur at the ε-α and the δ-α subunit interface. The M_2 membrane-spanning domain of each subunit lines the ion channel. The doubly liganded ion channel has equal permeability to sodium *(Na)* and potassium *(K)*; calcium *(Ca)* contributes approximately 2.5% to the total permeability. (From Naguib M, Flood P, McArdle JJ, et al. Advances in neurobiology of the neuromuscular junction: implications for the anesthesiologist. *Anesthesiology*. 2002;96:202–231, with permission from *Anesthesiology*.)

CH_3–$N^+(CH_3)_2$–CH_2–CH_2–O–C(=O)–CH_3

Acetylcholine

CH_3–$N^+(CH_3)_2$–CH_2–CH_2–O–C(=O)–CH_2–CH_2–C(=O)–O–CH_2–CH_2–$N^+(CH_3)_2$–CH_3

Succinylcholine

Fig. 27.2 Structural relationship of succinylcholine, a depolarizing neuromuscular blocking drug, and acetylcholine. Succinylcholine consists of two acetylcholine molecules linked through the acetate methyl groups. Like acetylcholine, succinylcholine stimulates nicotinic receptors at the neuromuscular junction.

or surgical denervation is characterized by the spreading of predominantly fetal-type nAChRs. These receptors are resistant to nondepolarizing NMBDs and are more sensitive to succinylcholine.[20-22]

PREJUNCTIONAL EFFECTS

Prejunctional receptors are involved in the modulation of acetylcholine release in the neuromuscular junction. The existence of both nicotinic and muscarinic receptors on the motor nerve endings has been described. Prejunctional nicotinic receptors are activated by acetylcholine and function in a positive-feedback control system, which could mediate mobilization of the reserve store into the readily releasable store in case of high-frequency stimulation; this mobilization serves to maintain availability of acetylcholine when demand for it is high (e.g., during tetanic stimulation).[23] These presynaptic receptors are $\alpha_3\beta_2$ neuronal subtype receptors. Although most nondepolarizing NMBDs have a distinct affinity for the $\alpha_3\beta_2$ cholinergic receptor, succinylcholine lacks this affinity. The action of nondepolarizing versus depolarizing NMBDs at this neuronal cholinergic receptor explains the typical fade phenomenon after any nondepolarizing drugs, and the lack of such effect in the clinical dose range for succinylcholine. The G-protein–coupled muscarinic receptors also are involved in the feedback modulation of acetylcholine release.24 The prejunctional M1 and M2 receptors are involved in facilitation and inhibition of acetylcholine release, respectively, by modulating Ca2+ influx.[24] The prejunctional nicotinic receptors are involved with mobilization of acetylcholine but not directly with its release process.[25] Hence, blockade of the prejunctional nicotinic receptors by nondepolarizing NMBDs prevents acetylcholine from being made available fast enough to support tetanic or train-of-four (TOF) stimulation. In contrast, the prejunctional muscarinic receptors are involved with up-modulation or down-modulation of the release mechanism.

Pharmacology of Succinylcholine

STRUCTURE-ACTIVITY RELATIONSHIPS

All NMBDs contain quaternary ammonium compounds and as such are structurally closely related to acetylcholine. Positive charges at the quaternary ammonium sites of NMBDs mimic the quaternary nitrogen atom of acetylcholine and are the structural reason for the attraction of these drugs to muscle- and neuronal-type nAChRs at the neuromuscular junction. These receptors are also located at other sites throughout the body where acetylcholine is the transmitter. These sites include the neuronal-type nicotinic receptors in autonomic ganglia and as many as five different muscarinic receptors on both the parasympathetic and sympathetic sides of the autonomic nervous system. In addition, populations of neuronal nicotinic and muscarinic receptors are located prejunctionally at the neuromuscular junction.[19]

The depolarizing NMBD, succinylcholine, is composed of two molecules of acetylcholine linked through the acetate methyl groups (Fig. 27.2). As described by Bovet,[26] succinylcholine is a small, flexible molecule, and like the natural ligand acetylcholine, succinylcholine stimulates cholinergic receptors at the neuromuscular junction and muscarinic autonomic sites, thus opening the ionic channel in the acetylcholine receptor.

PHARMACOKINETICS AND PHARMACODYNAMICS

Succinylcholine is the only available NMBD with a rapid onset of effect and an ultrashort duration of action. The ED_{95} (the dose causing on average 95% suppression of neuromuscular response) of succinylcholine is 0.51 to 0.63 mg/kg.[27] Using cumulative dose-response techniques, Kopman and coworkers estimated that its potency is far greater,[28] and it has an ED_{95} of less than 0.3 mg/kg.

Administration of 1 mg/kg of succinylcholine results in complete suppression of response to neuromuscular stimulation in approximately 60 seconds.[29] In patients with genotypically normal butyrylcholinesterase (also known as plasma cholinesterase or pseudocholinesterase), recovery to 90% muscle strength following administration of 1 mg/kg succinylcholine requires 9 to 13 minutes.[30]

The ultrashort duration of action of succinylcholine results from its rapid hydrolysis by butyrylcholinesterase to succinylmonocholine and choline. Butyrylcholinesterase has a large enzymatic capacity to hydrolyze succinylcholine, and only 10% of the intravenously administered drug reaches the neuromuscular junction.[31] The initial metabolite, succinylmonocholine, is a much weaker NMBD than succinylcholine and is metabolized much more slowly to succinic acid and choline. The elimination half-life of succinylcholine is estimated to be 47 seconds.[32]

Because little or no butyrylcholinesterase is present at the neuromuscular junction, the neuromuscular blockade induced by succinylcholine is terminated by its diffusion away from the neuromuscular junction into the circulation. Butyrylcholinesterase therefore influences the onset and duration of action of succinylcholine by controlling the rate at which the drug is hydrolyzed before it reaches, and after it leaves, the neuromuscular junction.

BUTYRYLCHOLINESTERASE ACTIVITY

Butyrylcholinesterase is synthesized by the liver and found in the plasma. The neuromuscular blockade induced by succinylcholine is prolonged when the concentration or activity of the enzyme is decreased. The activity of the enzyme refers to the number of substrate molecules (μmol) hydrolyzed per unit of time, and it is often expressed in International Units. Because the normal range of butyrylcholinesterase activity is quite large,[30] significant decreases in activity result in only modest increases in the time required to return to 100% of baseline muscle strength (Fig. 27.3).

Factors that lower butyrylcholinesterase activity include liver disease,[33] advanced age,[34] malnutrition, pregnancy, burns, oral contraceptives, monoamine oxidase inhibitors, echothiophate, cytotoxic drugs, neoplastic disease, anticholinesterase drugs,[35] tetrahydroaminacrine,[36] hexafluorenium,[37] and metoclopramide.[38] Bambuterol, a prodrug of terbutaline, produces marked inhibition of butyrylcholinesterase activity and causes prolongation of succinylcholine-induced blockade.[39] The β-blocker esmolol inhibits butyrylcholinesterase but causes only a minor prolongation of succinylcholine-induced blockade.[40]

Decreased butyrylcholinesterase enzyme activity is not a major concern in clinical practice because even large decreases in butyrylcholinesterase activity result in only modest increases in the duration of action of succinylcholine.

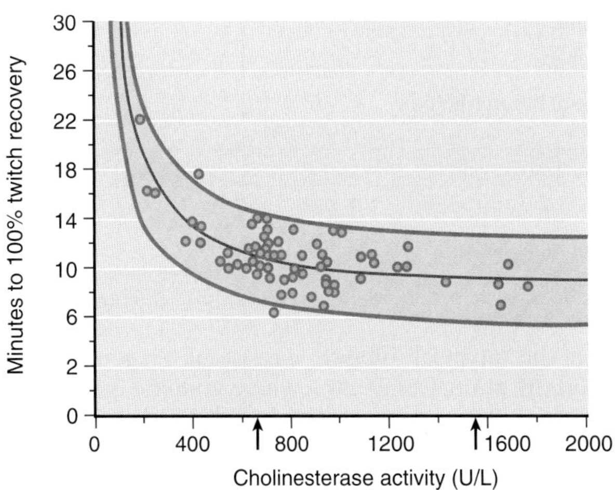

Fig. 27.3 Correlation between duration of succinylcholine neuromuscular blockade and butyrylcholinesterase activity. The normal range of activity lies between the *arrows*. (From Viby-Mogensen J. Correlation of succinylcholine duration of action with plasma cholinesterase activity in subjects with the genotypically normal enzyme. *Anesthesiology*. 1980;53:517–520.)

Even when butyrylcholinesterase activity is reduced to 20% of normal by severe liver disease, the duration of apnea after the administration of succinylcholine increases from a normal duration of 3 minutes to only 9 minutes. When glaucoma treatment with echothiophate decreased butyrylcholinesterase activity from 49% of control to no activity, the increase in the duration of neuromuscular blockade varied from 2 to 14 minutes. In no patient did the total duration of neuromuscular blockade exceed 23 minutes.[41]

DIBUCAINE NUMBER AND ATYPICAL BUTYRYLCHOLINESTERASE ACTIVITY

Succinylcholine-induced neuromuscular blockade can be significantly prolonged if a patient has an abnormal genetic variant of butyrylcholinesterase. Kalow and Genest discovered a variant that responded to dibucaine differently than it did to normal butyrylcholinesterase.[42] Dibucaine inhibits normal butyrylcholinesterase to a far greater extent than the abnormal enzyme. This observation led to the establishment of the dibucaine number. Under standardized test conditions, dibucaine inhibits the normal enzyme by approximately 80% and the abnormal enzyme by approximately 20% (Table 27.1). Many other genetic variants of butyrylcholinesterase have since been identified, although the dibucaine-resistant variants are the most important. A review by Jensen and Viby-Mogensen provides more detailed information on this topic.[43]

Although the dibucaine number indicates the genetic makeup of an individual with respect to butyrylcholinesterase, it does not measure the concentration of the enzyme in the plasma substrate. This is determined by measuring butyrylcholinesterase activity in plasma, and it may be influenced by comorbidities, medications, and genotype.

The molecular biology of butyrylcholinesterase is well understood. The amino acid sequence of the enzyme is known, and the coding errors responsible for most genetic variations have been identified.[43] Most variants result from a single amino acid substitution error or sequencing error at or near the active site of the enzyme. For example, in the

TABLE 27.1 Relationship Between Dibucaine Number and Duration of Succinylcholine or Mivacurium Neuromuscular Blockade

Type of Butyrylcholinesterase	Genotype	Incidence	Dibucaine Number*	Response to Succinylcholine or Mivacurium
Homozygous typical	$E_1^uE_1^u$	Normal	70-80	Normal
Heterozygous atypical	$E_1^uE_1^a$	1/480	50-60	Lengthened by 50%-100%
Homozygous atypical	$E_1^aE_1^a$	1/3200	20-30	Prolonged to 4-8 h

*The dibucaine number indicates the percentage of enzyme inhibited.

case of the "atypical" dibucaine-resistant (A) gene, a mutation occurs at nucleotide 209, where guanine is substituted for adenine. The resultant change in this codon causes substitution of glycine for aspartic acid at position 70 in the enzyme. In the case of the fluoride-resistant (F) gene, two amino acid substitutions are possible, namely, methionine for threonine at position 243, and valine for glycine at position 390. Table 27.1 summarizes many of the known genetic variants of butyrylcholinesterase: the amino acid substitution at position 70 is written as Asp ∅ Gly. New variants of butyrylcholinesterase genotypes continue to be discovered.[44]

SIDE EFFECTS

Cardiovascular Effects

Succinylcholine-induced cardiac dysrhythmias are many and varied. The drug stimulates cholinergic autonomic receptors on both sympathetic and parasympathetic ganglia[45] and muscarinic receptors in the sinus node of the heart. At low doses, both negative inotropic and chronotropic responses may occur. These responses can be attenuated by prior administration of atropine. With large doses of succinylcholine, these effects may become positive,[46] causing tachycardia. The clinical manifestation of generalized autonomic stimulation is the development of sinus bradycardia, junctional rhythms, and ventricular dysrhythmias. Clinical studies have described these dysrhythmias under various conditions in the presence of the intense autonomic stimulus of tracheal intubation. It is not entirely clear whether the cardiac irregularities are caused by the action of succinylcholine alone or by the added presence of extraneous autonomic stimulation. An in vitro study using ganglionic acetylcholine receptors subtype $\alpha_3\beta_4$ expressed in *Xenopus laevis* oocytes suggested that succinylcholine at clinically relevant concentrations had no effect on the expressed receptors.[47] Only high doses of succinylcholine caused inhibition of ganglionic acetylcholine receptors.[47] Whether or not these findings are applicable to clinical practice is unclear because the methodology (*X. laevis* oocytes expression model) has no clinical equivalent.

Sinus Bradycardia. Stimulation of cardiac muscarinic receptors in the cardiac sinus node causes sinus bradycardia. This side effect is particularly problematic in individuals with predominantly vagal tone, such as in children who have not received atropine. Sinus bradycardia can occur in adults and appears more commonly after a second dose of the drug administered approximately 5 minutes after the initial dose.[48] The bradycardia may be prevented by administration of atropine, ganglion-blocking drugs, and nondepolarizing NMBDs.[49] The ability of these drugs to prevent bradycardia implies that direct myocardial effects, increased muscarinic stimulation, and ganglionic stimulation may all be involved in the bradycardic response. The greater incidence of bradycardia after a second dose of succinylcholine suggests that the hydrolysis products of succinylcholine (succinylmonocholine and choline) may sensitize the heart to a subsequent dose.

Nodal (Junctional) Rhythms. Nodal rhythms occur commonly following administration of succinylcholine. The mechanism responsible for this likely involves relatively greater stimulation of muscarinic receptors in the sinus node, thus suppressing the sinus mechanism and allowing the emergence of the atrioventricular node as the pacemaker. The incidence of junctional rhythm is greater after a second dose of succinylcholine, and may be prevented by prior administration of dTc.[49]

Ventricular Dysrhythmias. Under stable anesthetic conditions, succinylcholine decreases the threshold of the ventricle to catecholamine-induced dysrhythmias in monkeys and dogs. Circulating catecholamine concentrations increase fourfold, and K^+ concentrations increase by one third, following succinylcholine administration in dogs.[50] Similar increases in catecholamine levels occur following administration of succinylcholine to humans.[51] Other autonomic stimuli, such as endotracheal intubation, hypoxia, hypercarbia, and surgery, may be additive to the effect of succinylcholine. The possible influence of drugs such as digitalis, tricyclic antidepressants, monoamine oxidase inhibitors, exogenous catecholamines, and anesthetic drugs such as halothane, which may lower the ventricular threshold for ectopic activity or increase the arrhythmogenic effect of the catecholamines, should also be considered. Ventricular escape beats may also occur as a result of severe sinus bradycardia and atrioventricular nodal slowing secondary to succinylcholine administration. The incidence of ventricular dysrhythmias is further increased by the release of K^+ from skeletal muscle as a consequence of the depolarizing action of the drug.

Hyperkalemia

The administration of succinylcholine to an otherwise healthy individual increases the plasma K^+ levels by approximately 0.5 mEq/dL. This slight increase in K^+ is well tolerated by most individuals and generally does not cause dysrhythmias. The increase in K^+ results from the depolarizing action of succinylcholine. With activation of the acetylcholine channels, movement of Na^+ into the cells is accompanied by movement of K^+ out of the cells.

Patients with renal failure are no more susceptible to an exaggerated response to succinylcholine than are those with normal renal function.[52] Patients who have uremic neuropathy may possibly be susceptible to succinylcholine-induced hyperkalemia, although the evidence supporting this view is scarce.[52,53,53a]

However, severe hyperkalemia may follow the administration of succinylcholine to patients with severe metabolic acidosis and hypovolemia.[54] In experimental animals (rabbit), the combination of metabolic acidosis and hypovolemia results in a high resting K^+ level and an exaggerated hyperkalemic response to succinylcholine.[55] In this situation, the K^+ originates from the gastrointestinal tract, rather than from muscle.[56] In patients with metabolic acidosis and hypovolemia, correction of the acidosis by hyperventilation and sodium bicarbonate administration should be attempted before succinylcholine administration. Should severe hyperkalemia occur, it can be treated with immediate hyperventilation, infusion of 500-1,000 mg calcium chloride or calcium gluconate over 3 minutes intravenously, and 10 units of regular insulin in 50 mL of 50% glucose for adults or, for children, 0.15 units/kg of regular insulin in 1.0 mL/kg of 50% glucose intravenously.

Kohlschütter and associates found that four of nine patients with severe abdominal infections had an increase in serum K^+ levels of as much as 3.1 mEq/L after succinylcholine administration.[57] The likelihood of a hyperkalemic response to succinylcholine increases in patients who have had intraabdominal infections for longer than 1 week.

Stevenson and Birch described a single, well-documented case of a marked hyperkalemic response to succinylcholine in a patient with a closed head injury without peripheral paralysis.[58]

Hyperkalemia after administration of succinylcholine is also a risk in patients who have had physical trauma.[59] The risk of hyperkalemia occurs 1 week after the injury, at which time a progressive increase in serum K^+ occurs during an infusion of succinylcholine. The risk of hyperkalemia can persist. Three weeks after injury, three of the patients studied in this series, who had especially severe injuries, became markedly hyperkalemic with an increase in serum K^+ of more than 3.6 mEq/L. Birch and coworkers also found that the prior administration of 6 mg of dTc prevented the hyperkalemic response to succinylcholine.[59] In the absence of infection or persistent degeneration of tissue, a patient is likely susceptible to the hyperkalemic response for at least 60 days after massive trauma or until adequate healing of damaged muscle has occurred.

Additionally, patients with conditions that result in the proliferation of extrajunctional acetylcholine receptors, such as upper or lower motor denervation, immobilization, burn injuries, and neuromuscular disease, are likely to have an exaggerated hyperkalemic response following the administration of succinylcholine. The response of patients with neuromuscular disease to NMBDs is reviewed in detail later in this chapter. Some of these disease states include cerebrovascular accident with resultant hemiplegia or paraplegia, muscular dystrophies, and Guillain-Barré syndrome. The hyperkalemia following administration of succinylcholine may be severe enough that cardiac arrest ensues. For a review of succinylcholine-induced hyperkalemia in acquired pathologic states, see Martyn and Richtsfeld.[22]

Increased Intraocular Pressure

Succinylcholine may cause an increase in intraocular pressure (IOP). The increased IOP develops within 1 minute of injection, peaks at 2 to 4 minutes, and subsides by 6 minutes.[60] The mechanism by which succinylcholine increases IOP has not been clearly defined, but it is known to involve contraction of tonic myofibrils and/or transient dilatation of choroidal blood vessels. Sublingual administration of nifedipine may attenuate the increase in IOP caused by succinylcholine, a finding suggesting a circulatory mechanism.[61] Despite this increase in IOP, the use of succinylcholine for eye operations is not contraindicated unless the anterior chamber is open. Although Meyers and colleagues were unable to confirm the efficacy of small (0.09 mg/kg) doses of dTc ("precurarization") in attenuating increases in IOP following succinylcholine,[62] numerous other investigators have found that prior administration of a small dose of nondepolarizing NMBD (e.g., 3 mg of dTc or 1 mg of pancuronium) prevents a succinylcholine-induced increase in IOP.[63] Furthermore, Libonati and associates described the anesthetic management of 73 patients with penetrating eye injuries who received succinylcholine.[64] Among these 73 patients, no extrusion of vitreous occurred. Thus, despite the potential concerns, the use of succinylcholine in patients with penetrating eye injuries, after pretreatment with a nondepolarizing NMBD and with a carefully controlled rapid-sequence induction of anesthesia, can be considered. Succinylcholine is only one of many factors that may increase IOP.[62] Other factors include endotracheal intubation and "bucking" on the endotracheal tube once it is positioned. Of prime importance in minimizing the chance of increasing IOP is ensuring that the patient is well anesthetized and is not straining or coughing. For instance, coughing, vomiting and maximal forced lid closure may induce increases in intraocular pressure that are 3-4 times greater (60-90 mm Hg) than those induced by succinylcholine administration.[63a] Because a nondepolarizing NMBD with a rapid onset of effect, rocuronium, is available, it is possible to perform a rapid sequence induction of anesthesia and endotracheal intubation without administering succinylcholine. Finally, should a patient become too lightly anesthetized during intraocular surgery, succinylcholine should not be given to immobilize the patient. Rather, the surgeon should be asked to pause while anesthesia is deepened. If necessary, the depth of neuromuscular blockade can also be increased with nondepolarizing NMBDs.

Increased Intragastric Pressure

Unlike the rather consistent increase in IOP following administration of succinylcholine, increases in intragastric pressure (IGP) are much more variable. The increase in IGP from succinylcholine is presumed to result from fasciculations of the abdominal skeletal muscle. This is not surprising because more coordinated abdominal skeletal muscle activity (e.g., straight-leg raising) may increase the IGP to values as high as 120 cm H_2O (88 mm Hg). In addition to skeletal muscle fasciculations, the acetylcholine-like effect of succinylcholine may be partly responsible for the observed increases in IGP. Greenan observed consistent increases in IGP of 4 to 7 cm H_2O (3-5 mm Hg) with direct vagal stimulation.[65]

Miller and Way found that 11 of 30 patients had essentially no increase in IGP after succinylcholine administration, yet 5 of the 30 had an increase in IGP of greater than 30 cm H_2O (22 mm Hg).[66] The increase in IGP from succinylcholine appeared to be related to the intensity of the fasciculations of the abdominal skeletal muscles. Accordingly, when fasciculations were prevented by prior administration of a nondepolarizing NMBD, no increase in IGP was observed.

Whether the increases in IGP following succinylcholine administration are sufficient to cause incompetence of the gastroesophageal junction are debatable. Generally, an IGP greater than 28 cm H_2O (21 mm Hg) is required to overcome the competence of the gastroesophageal junction. However, when the normal oblique angle of entry of the esophagus into the stomach is altered, as may occur with pregnancy or an abdomen distended by ascites, bowel obstruction, or a hiatus hernia, the IGP required to cause incompetence of the gastroesophageal junction is frequently less than 15 cm H_2O (11 mm Hg).[66] In these circumstances, regurgitation of stomach contents following succinylcholine administration is a distinct possibility, and precautionary measures should be taken to prevent fasciculations. Endotracheal intubation may be facilitated with administration of either a nondepolarizing NMBD or a defasciculating dose of nondepolarizing relaxant before succinylcholine use. Although the increase in IGP from succinylcholine is well documented, the evidence of clinical harm is not clear.

Succinylcholine does not increase IGP appreciably in infants and children. This may be related to the minimal or absent fasciculations from succinylcholine in these young patients.[67]

Increased Intracranial Pressure

Succinylcholine has the potential to increase intracranial pressure.[68] The mechanisms and clinical significance of this transient increase are unknown, but pretreatment with nondepolarizing NMBDs prevents intracranial pressure increases.[68]

Myalgia

The incidence of muscle pain following administration of succinylcholine varies widely, from 0.2% to 89%.[69] Muscle pain occurs more frequently after minor surgery, especially in women and in ambulatory, rather than bedridden, patients.[70] Waters and Mapleson postulated that pain is secondary to damage produced in muscle by the unsynchronized contractions of adjacent muscle fibers just before the onset of paralysis.[70] This concept has been substantiated by finding myoglobinemia and increases in serum creatine kinase following succinylcholine administration.[71] Prior administration of a small ("defasciculating") dose of a nondepolarizing NMBD clearly prevents fasciculations from succinylcholine.[71] The efficacy of this approach in preventing muscle pain is not clear; however, most investigators report that pretreatment with a nondepolarizing NMBD has minimal effect.[69] Pretreatment with a prostaglandin inhibitor (e.g., lysine acetyl salicylate) has been shown effective in decreasing the incidence of muscle pain after succinylcholine.[72] This finding suggests a possible role for prostaglandins and cyclooxygenases in succinylcholine-induced myalgias. Other investigators have found that myalgias following outpatient laparoscopic surgery (and atracurium administration) occur even in the absence of succinylcholine.[73] Other investigators reported a significant reduction in postoperative myalgia in elective oral surgery patients pretreated with rocuronium (20%) compared with vecuronium (42%) and placebo (70%).[73a]

Masseter Muscle Rigidity

An increase in tone of the masseter muscle is a frequent response to succinylcholine in adults[74] as well as in children.[75] Several studies have reported that an increase in masseter muscle tone of up to 500 g lasting 1 to 2 minutes is a normal finding in adults.[76] Most cases of the so-called masseter muscle rigidity (MMR) may represent simply the extreme of a spectrum of muscle tension changes that occur in response to succinylcholine. Meakin and associates suggested that the high incidence of spasm in children may result from inadequate dosage of succinylcholine.[75] In all likelihood, this increase in tone is an exaggerated contractile response at the neuromuscular junction and cannot be used to establish a diagnosis of malignant hyperthermia. Although an increase in tone of the masseter muscle may be an early indicator of malignant hyperthermia, this finding is not consistently associated with that syndrome.[76] Currently, no indication exists to change to a "nontriggering" anesthetic technique in instances of isolated MMR.[77]

Anaphylaxis

There is some controversy concerning the incidence of anaphylaxis following succinylcholine. The incidence of anaphylactic reactions may be close to 0.06%. Almost all cases of anaphylaxis have been reported in Europe or Australia. When the muscle relaxant cross-links with IgE, degranulation and release of histamine, neutrophil chemotactic factor, and platelet-activating factor occur. The release of these mediators can induce cardiovascular collapse, bronchospasm, and skin reaction.[77a] Patients with a history of anaphylactic reaction to succinylcholine may exhibit a cross-reaction, at least in vitro, with other NMBDs. The cross-reactivity is related to the common structural features of these drugs, all of which contain quaternary ammonium ions.

CLINICAL USES

In spite of its many adverse effects, succinylcholine remains in clinical use. Its popularity is likely the result of its rapid onset of effect, the profound depth of neuromuscular blockade it produces, and its short duration of action. Succinylcholine is not used as regularly as in the past for routine endotracheal intubation, but it is still a muscle relaxant frequently used for rapid-sequence induction of anesthesia and tracheal intubation. Although 1.0 mg/kg of succinylcholine is recommended to facilitate endotracheal intubation at 60 seconds, as little as 0.5 to 0.6 mg/kg may result in adequate intubating conditions 60 seconds after administration.[78] Reduction in the succinylcholine dose from 1.0 to 0.6 mg/kg decreases the incidence of hemoglobin desaturation but does not shorten the time to spontaneous diaphragmatic movements.[79] Decreasing the dose of succinylcholine is appealing as long as it does not interfere with provision of adequate conditions for endotracheal intubation and subsequent adequate ventilation.[79]

Typically, after administering succinylcholine for tracheal intubation, a nondepolarizing NMBD is given to maintain neuromuscular blockade. Prior administration of succinylcholine enhances the depth of blockade caused by a subsequent dose of nondepolarizing NMBD.[80,81] However, the effect on duration of action is variable. Succinylcholine has no effect on the duration of pancuronium,[82] but it increases the duration of atracurium and rocuronium.[80,83] The reasons for these differences are not clear.

With administration of large doses of succinylcholine, the nature of the block, as determined by a monitor of neuromuscular blockade, changes from that of a depolarizing drug (phase 1 block) to that of a nondepolarizing drug (phase 2 block). Clearly, both the dose and the duration of administration of succinylcholine contribute to this change. The relative contribution of each factor has not been established, however.

Posttetanic potentiation and fade in response to TOF and tetanic stimuli can be demonstrated after bolus administration of different doses of succinylcholine.[84] It seems that some characteristics of phase 2 blockade are evident from an initial dose (i.e., as small as 0.3 mg/kg) of succinylcholine.[84] Fade in response to TOF stimulation has been attributed to the presynaptic effects on NMBDs. The etiology of the appearance of fade phenomenon in the TOF response following excessive administration of succinylcholine has been suggested to be dependent on a concentration-dependent affinity for succinylcholine to the presynaptic $\alpha_3\beta_2$ neuronal subtype AChR in concentrations exceeding the normal clinical concentration range seen after routine doses.[47]

INTERACTIONS WITH ANTICHOLINESTERASES

Neostigmine and pyridostigmine inhibit butyrylcholinesterase, as well as acetylcholinesterase. If succinylcholine is administered after antagonism of residual neuromuscular block, as it may be with postextubation laryngospasm, the effect of succinylcholine will be pronounced and significantly prolonged. The effect of succinylcholine (1 mg/kg) was prolonged from 11 to 35 minutes when it was given 5 minutes after administration of neostigmine (5 mg).[35] Ninety minutes after neostigmine administration, butyrylcholinesterase activity will have returned to less than 50% of its baseline value.

Nondepolarizing Neuromuscular Blocking Drugs

The use of NMBDs in anesthesia has its origin in the arrow poisons or curares of South American Indians. Several nondepolarizing NMBDs were purified from naturally occurring sources. For example, dTc can be isolated from the Amazonian vine *Chondodendron tomentosum*. Similarly, the intermediates for the production of metocurine and alcuronium, which are semisynthetic, are obtained from *Chondodendron* and *Strychnos toxifera*. Malouetine, the first steroidal NMBD, was originally isolated from *Malouetia bequaertiana*, which grows in the jungles of the Democratic Republic of Congo in central Africa. The NMBDs pancuronium, vecuronium, pipecuronium, rocuronium, rapacuronium, atracurium, doxacurium, mivacurium, cisatracurium, gantacurium, and gallamine are all synthetic compounds.

Available nondepolarizing NMBDs can be classified according to chemical class, based on structure (steroids, benzylisoquinoliniums, fumarates, and other compounds), or, alternatively, according to onset or duration of action (long-, intermediate-, and short-acting drugs) of equipotent doses (Table 27.2).

STRUCTURE-ACTIVITY RELATIONSHIPS

Nondepolarizing NMBDs were originally classified by Bovet as pachycurares,[26] or bulky molecules having the amine functions incorporated into rigid ring structures. Two extensively studied chemical series of synthetic nondepolarizing NMBDs are the aminosteroids, in which the interonium distance is maintained by an androstane skeleton, and the benzylisoquinolinium series, in which the distance is maintained by linear diester-containing chains or, in the case of curare, by benzyl ethers. For a detailed account on structure-activity relationships, see Lee.[85]

Benzylisoquinolinium Compounds

dTc is an NMBD in which the amines are present in the form of two benzyl substituted tetrahydroisoquinoline structures (Fig. 27.4). Using nuclear magnetic resonance spectroscopy and methylation–demethylation studies, Everett and associates demonstrated that dTc contains three *N*-methyl groups.[86] One amine is quaternary (i.e., permanently charged with four nitrogen substituents), and the other is tertiary (i.e., pH-dependent charge with three nitrogen substituents). At physiologic pH, the tertiary nitrogen is protonated so that it is positively charged. The structure-activity relationships of the bis-benzylisoquinolines (see Fig. 27.4) have been described by Waser[87] and by Hill and associates,[88] and these relationships are as follows:

1. The nitrogen atoms are incorporated into isoquinoline ring systems. This bulky molecule favors a nondepolarizing rather than a depolarizing activity.

TABLE 27.2 Classification of Nondepolarizing Neuromuscular Blockers According to Duration of Action (Time to T1 = 25% of Control) after Twice the Dose Causing on Average 95% Suppression of Neuromuscular Response

	CLINICAL DURATION			
	Long-acting (>50 min)	**Intermediate-acting (20-50 min)**	**Short-acting (10-20 min)**	**Ultrashort-acting (<10 min)**
Steroidal compounds	Pancuronium	Vecuronium Rocuronium		
Benzylisoquinolinium compounds	*d*-Tubocurarine	Atracurium Cisatracurium	Mivacurium	
Asymmetric mixed-onium fumarates		CW 002		Gantacurium

Most nondepolarizing neuromuscular blockers are bisquaternary ammonium compounds. *d*-Tubocurarine, vecuronium, and rocuronium are monoquaternary compounds.

T1, First twitch of train-of-four.

2. The interonium distance (distance between charged amines) is approximately 1.4 nm.
3. Both the ganglion-blocking and the histamine-releasing properties of dTc probably result from the presence of the tertiary amine function.
4. When dTc is methylated at the tertiary amine and at the hydroxyl groups, the result is metocurine, a compound of greater potency (by a factor of two in humans) with much weaker ganglion-blocking and histamine-releasing properties than dTc (see Fig. 27.4). Metocurine contains three additional methyl groups, one of which quaternizes the tertiary nitrogen of dTc; the other two form methyl ethers at the phenolic hydroxyl groups.
5. Bisquaternary compounds are more potent than their monoquaternary analogues. The bisquaternary derivative of dTc, chondocurine, is more than twice as potent as dTc (see Fig. 27.4).

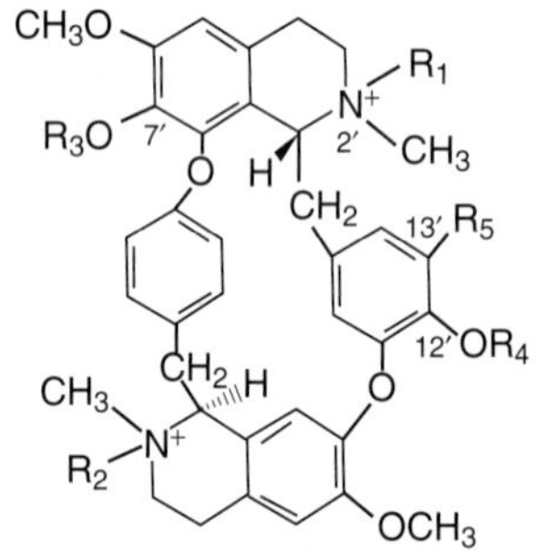

Cyclic benzylisoquinoline

Cyclic benzylisoquinoline derivatives

Name	R_1	R_2	R_3	R_4	R_5	1	1'
d-Tubocurarine	CH_3	H	H	H	H	*S*	*R*
Metocurine	CH_3	CH_3	CH_3	CH_3	H	*S*	*R*
Chondocurine	CH_3	CH_3	H	H	H	*S*	*R*

R and S represent the stereochemical configuration about the designated carbon

Fig. 27.4 Chemical structures of *d*-tubocurarine, metocurine, and chondocurine.

6. Substitution of the methyl groups on the quaternary nitrogen with bulkier groups causes a reduction in both potency and duration of action.

Atracurium is a bis-benzyltetrahydroisoquinolinium with isoquinolinium nitrogens connected by a diester-containing hydrocarbon chain (Fig. 27.5). The presence (in duplicate) of two-carbon separations between quaternary nitrogen and ester carbonyl renders it susceptible to the Hofmann elimination reaction.[89] The compound can also undergo ester hydrolysis. In a Hofmann elimination reaction, a quaternary ammonium group is converted into a tertiary amine through cleavage of a carbon-nitrogen bond. This is a pH- and temperature-dependent reaction in which higher pH and temperature favor elimination.

Atracurium has 4 chiral centers at each of the chiral carbons adjacent to the two amines. It is composed of 10 isomers.[89] These isomers have been separated into three geometric isomer groups that are designated *cis-cis, cis-trans,* and *trans-trans* according to their configuration about the tetrahydroisoquinoline ring system.[89] The ratio of the *cis-cis, cis-trans,* and *trans-trans* isomers is approximately 10:6:1, corresponding to 50% to 55% *cis-cis,* 35% to 38% *cis-trans,* and 6% to 7% *trans-trans* isomers.

Cisatracurium, the 1R *cis*–1′R *cis* isomer of atracurium, comprises approximately 15% of atracurium by weight but more than 50% in terms of neuromuscular blocking activity (see Fig. 27.5). R designates the absolute stereochemistry of the benzyl tetrahydroisoquinoline rings, and *cis* represents the relative geometry of the bulky dimethoxy and 2-alkyester groups at C(1) and N(1), respectively.[90,91] Like atracurium, cisatracurium undergoes Hofmann elimination. It is approximately four times as potent as atracurium, and in contrast to atracurium, it does not cause histamine release,[90,92] thus indicating that histamine release may be stereospecific.[90,93]

Mivacurium differs from atracurium by the presence of an additional methylated phenolic group (see Fig. 27.5). Compared with other isoquinolinium NMBDs, the interonium chain of mivacurium is longer (16 atoms).[88] Mivacurium consists of a mixture of three stereoisomers.[94] The two most active are the *trans-trans* and *cis-trans* isomers (57% and

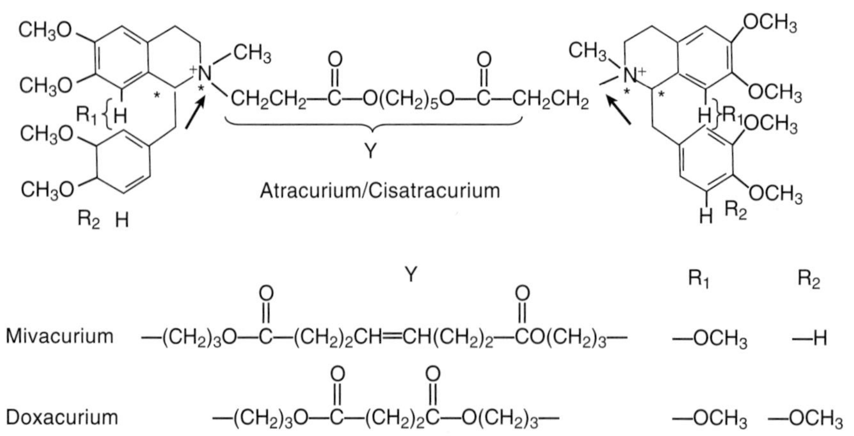

Atracurium/Cisatracurium

	Y	R_1	R_2
Mivacurium	$-(CH_2)_3O-C(=O)-(CH_2)_2CH=CH(CH_2)_2-C(=O)O(CH_2)_3-$	$-OCH_3$	$-H$
Doxacurium	$-(CH_2)_3O-C(=O)-(CH_2)_2C(=O)-O(CH_2)_3-$	$-OCH_3$	$-OCH_3$

Fig. 27.5 Chemical structures of atracurium, cisatracurium, mivacurium, and doxacurium. The *asterisk* indicates the chiral centers; *arrows* show cleavage sites for Hofmann elimination.

37% weight/weight, respectively), which are equipotent; the *cis-cis* isomer (6% weight/weight) has only one tenth the neuromuscular blocking activity of the more potent isomers in cats and monkeys.[94] Mivacurium is metabolized by butyrylcholinesterase to a monoester and a dicarboxylic acid at 70% to 88% the rate at which succinylcholine is metabolized by the same enzyme.[9]

Steroidal Neuromuscular Blockers

For the steroidal compounds to have neuromuscular blocking potential, it is likely that one of the compound's two nitrogen atoms be quaternized. The presence of an acetyl ester (acetylcholine-like moiety) facilitates their interaction with nAChRs at the postsynaptic muscle membrane.

Pancuronium is characterized by the presence of two acetyl ester groups on the A and D rings of the steroidal molecule. Pancuronium is a potent NMBD with vagolytic properties. It is also an inhibitor of butyrylcholinesterase (Fig. 27.6).[95] Deacetylation at the 3 or 17 positions decreases its potency.[96]

Vecuronium, in which the 2-piperidine substituent is not methylated, is the *N*-demethylated derivative of pancuronium (see Fig. 27.6).[7] At physiologic pH, the tertiary amine is largely protonated, as it is in dTc. The minor molecular modification results in the following: (1) a slight increase in the potency when compared with pancuronium; (2) a marked reduction in its vagolytic properties; (3) molecular instability in solution; and (4) increased lipid solubility, which results in a greater biliary elimination of vecuronium than pancuronium.[88]

Vecuronium is degraded by the hydrolysis of the acetyl esters at the C3 and the C17 positions. Hydrolysis at the C3 position is the primary degradation pathway because the acetate at the 3 position is more susceptible to hydrolysis in aqueous solutions than the acetate at the 17 position. This is because of the adjacent basic piperidine at the 2 position that facilitates hydrolysis of the 3-acetate. Therefore vecuronium cannot be prepared as a ready-to-use solution with a sufficient shelf life, even as a buffered solution. In contrast, the 2-piperidine of pancuronium is quaternized and no longer alkaline and therefore does not facilitate hydrolysis of the 3-acetate.

Rocuronium lacks the acetyl ester that is found in the A ring of the steroid nucleus of pancuronium and vecuronium (see Fig. 27.6). The introduction of cyclic substituents other than piperidine at the 2 and 16 positions results in a compound with a more rapid onset of effect than vecuronium or pancuronium.[97] The methyl group attached to the quaternary nitrogen of vecuronium and pancuronium is replaced by an allyl group in rocuronium. As a result of this change, rocuronium is approximately 6 and 10 times less potent than pancuronium and vecuronium, respectively.[97-99] The replacement of the acetyl ester attached to the A ring by a hydroxy group means that rocuronium is stable in solution. At room temperature, rocuronium is stable for 60 days. In contrast, pancuronium is stable for 6 months. The reason for this difference in shelf life is related to the fact that rocuronium is terminally sterilized in manufacturing, and pancuronium is not. Terminal sterilization causes some degree of degradation.

Asymmetric Mixed-Onium Fumarates and Analogues

These compounds share some structural properties with mivacurium. Gantacurium and CW 002 represent a new

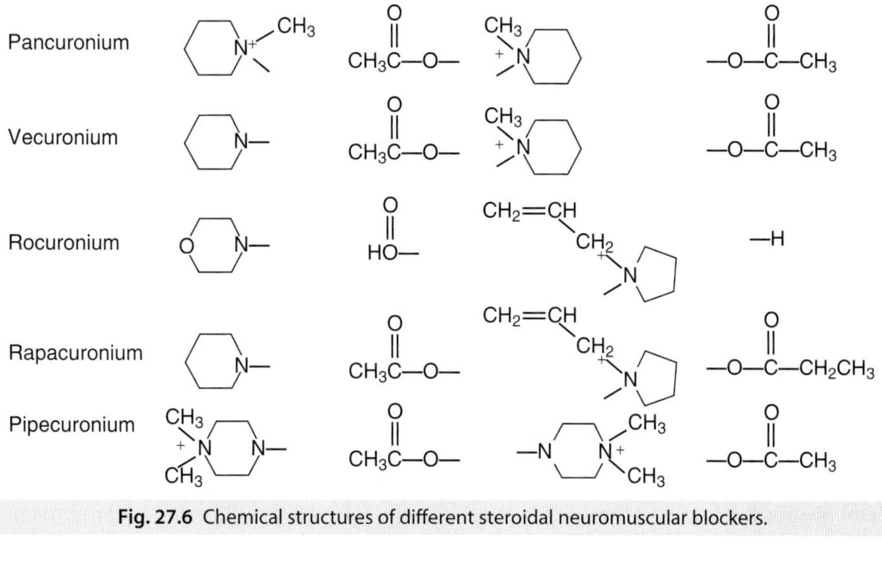

Fig. 27.6 Chemical structures of different steroidal neuromuscular blockers.

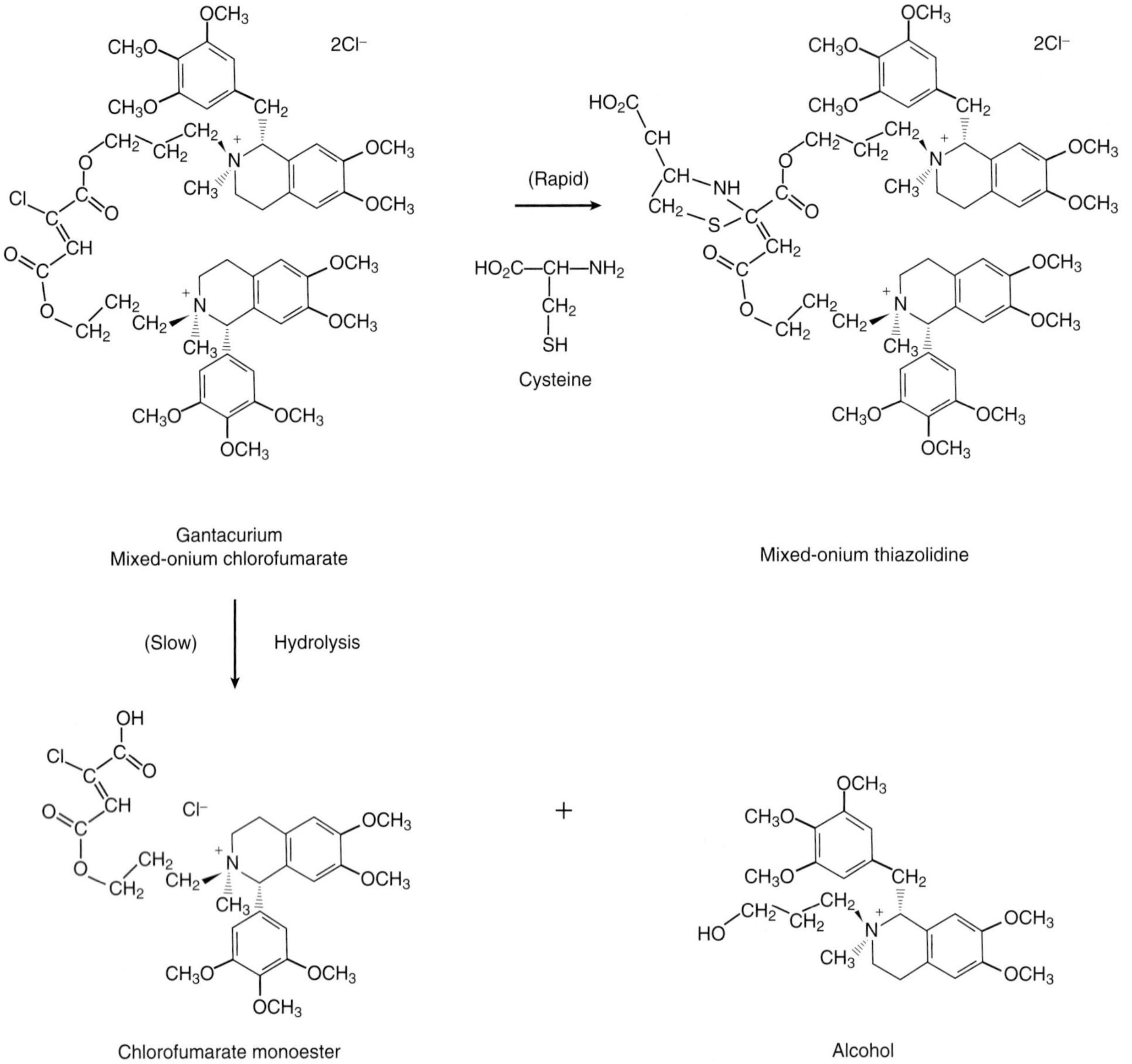

Gantacurium
Mixed-onium chlorofumarate

(Rapid) → Cysteine

Mixed-onium thiazolidine

(Slow) Hydrolysis

Chlorofumarate monoester + Alcohol

Fig. 27.7 Chemical structure of gantacurium (a mixed-onium chlorofumarate). In whole human blood, two pathways of deactivation occur, neither of which is enzymatic: (1) rapid formation of an apparently inactive cysteine adduction product, with cysteine replacing chlorine; and (2) slower hydrolysis of the ester bond adjacent to the chlorine substitution to chlorofumarate monoester and alcohol. (From Boros EE, Samano V, Ray JA, et al. Neuromuscular blocking activity and therapeutic potential of mixed-tetrahydroisoquinolinium halofumarates and halosuccinates in rhesus monkeys. *J Med Chem.* 2003;46:2502–2515.)

class of bisquaternary nondepolarizing NMBDs (Fig. 27.7). Gantacurium, an asymmetric mixed-onium chlorofumarate, is unique among nondepolarizing compounds in terms of its rapid onset of effect, its short duration of action, and its unique means of inactivation.[11,100] Because of the presence of three methyl groups between the quaternary nitrogen and oxygen atom at each end of the carbon chain, this compound does not undergo Hofmann elimination.[100]

Gantacurium has an ultrashort duration of action in human volunteers and in different animal species. In human volunteers receiving a nitrous oxide–opioid anesthetic, the ED_{95} of gantacurium is 0.19 mg/kg.[100] Onset of and recovery from block resemble those of succinylcholine. Following administration of approximately 2.5 times the ED_{95} dose, onset of maximal block occurs in 1.5 minutes. Spontaneous recovery to a TOF of 0.9 or greater occurs 10 minutes after administration of an ED_{95} dose, and complete spontaneous recovery occurs in 14 to 15 minutes after administration of doses ranging from 2 to 3.5 times the ED_{95}. Recovery is accelerated by administration of edrophonium at the beginning of spontaneous recovery. Transient hypotension and tachycardia occur following administration of doses three times the ED_{95} and greater, a finding suggesting that histamine release occurs with administration of these doses.[100]

Gantacurium appears to undergo two pathways of inactivation. One is a slower ester hydrolysis, and the second one, which occurs much more quickly, occurs through the adduction of cysteine, a nonessential amino acid, to create a new compound that can no longer bind to the nAChR of the neuromuscular junction.[101] This unique means of inactivation likely accounts for the drug's ultrashort duration of effect. It also provides a novel means of shortening recovery

TABLE 27.3 Dose-Response Relationships of Nondepolarizing Neuromuscular Blocking Drugs in Human Subjects

	ED_{50} (mg/kg)	ED_{90} (mg/kg)	ED_{95} (mg/kg)	References
LONG-ACTING				
Pancuronium	0.036 (0.022-0.042)	0.056 (0.044-0.070)	0.067 (0.059-0.080)	98, 103
d-Tubocurarine	0.23 (0.16-0.26)	0.41 (0.27-0.45)	0.48 (0.34-0.56)	103
INTERMEDIATE-ACTING				
Rocuronium	0.147 (0.069-0.220)	0.268 (0.200-0.419)	0.305 (0.257-0.521)	98, 104-106
Vecuronium	0.027 (0.015-0.031)	0.042 (0.023-0.055)	0.043 (0.037-0.059)	103
Atracurium	0.12 (0.08-0.15)	0.18 (0.19-0.24)	0.21 (0.13-0.28)	103
Cisatracurium	0.026 (0.015-0.031)	—	0.04 (0.032-0.05)	107-109, 371
SHORT-ACTING				
Mivacurium	0.039 (0.027-0.052)	—	0.067 (0.045-0.081)	9, 110-112
ULTRASHORT-ACTING				
Gantacurium	0.09		0.19	100

Data are the medians and ranges of reported values. ED_{50}, ED_{90}, and ED_{95} are the doses of each drug that produce, respectively, 50%, 90%, and 95% decrease in the force of contraction or amplitude of the electromyogram of the adductor pollicis muscle following ulnar nerve stimulation.

from gantacurium-induced neuromuscular block. Administration of L-cysteine (10 mg/kg) 1 minute after administration of gantacurium results in rapid return to complete neuromuscular function within 1 to 2 minutes.[102]

An analogue of the asymmetric fumarate gantacurium, CW 002 has been synthesized to undergo slower L-cysteine adduction. Because of its slower metabolism, it has an intermediate duration of action. In animals, it causes a nondepolarizing block that can be antagonized by neostigmine. Administration of L-cysteine 1 minute after administration of CW 002 effectively speeds recovery of neuromuscular function, whereas neostigmine does not.[22] Volunteer trials are required to determine whether onset, recovery, and ease of antagonism are improved over those using compounds that are currently available.

CW 011 (an asymmetrical maleate) is a nonhalogenated olefinic diester analogue of gantacurium[101] that can undergo L-cysteine adduction in animal models. Because this adduction reaction is slower than that of gantacurium, its duration of neuromuscular block is longer (approximately 21 minutes). Exogenous L-cysteine (50 mg/kg) administration can induce full recovery of neuromuscular block (after five times ED_{95} dose of CW 011) in 2 to 3 minutes.[101]

The clinical development of gantacurium was suspended in 2006, but since then, several other compounds similar to gantacurium have been tested. CW 1759-50 is a fast-onset, ultrashort-acting NMBA that is devoid of histaminoid side effects in animal testing.[11a,11b] CW 1759-50 is ultrashort acting because it is inactivated by plasma L-cysteine. Spontaneous recovery (5%-95% interval) from either bolus or infusion was similar (5-6 minutes), and reversal by L-cysteine required about 2 minutes.

POTENCY OF NONDEPOLARIZING NEUROMUSCULAR BLOCKING DRUGS

Drug potency is commonly expressed by the dose-response relationship. The dose of an NMBD required to produce an effect (e.g., 50%, 90%, or 95% depression of baseline

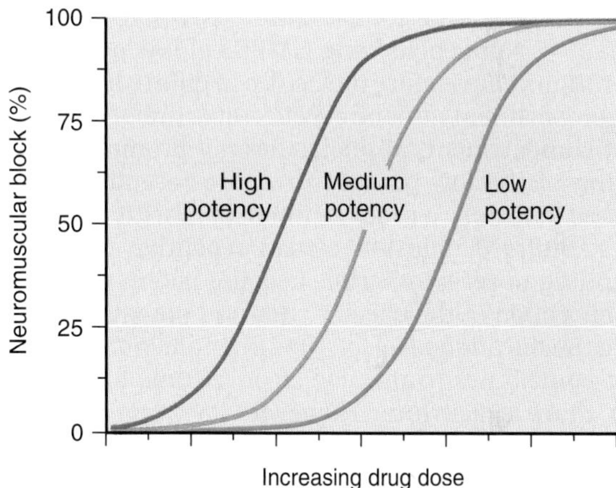

Fig. 27.8 Schematic representation of a semilogarithmic plot of a muscle-relaxant dose versus neuromuscular blockade. A drug of high potency is doxacurium, one of medium potency is atracurium, and one of low potency is gallamine. The graph illustrates that the relative potencies of the muscle relaxants span a range of approximately two orders of magnitude.

twitch height, commonly expressed as ED_{50}, ED_{90}, and ED_{95}, respectively) defines its potency.[9,98,103-114] The NMBDs have different potencies, as illustrated in Table 27.3 and Fig. 27.8. For factors affecting the potency of NMBDs, see the section on drug interactions later in this chapter. The dose-response relationship for nondepolarizing NMBDs is sigmoidal (see Fig. 27.8) and has been derived in various ways. The simplest method is to perform linear regression over the approximately linear portion of a semilogarithmic plot between 25% and 75% neuromuscular blockade. Alternatively, the curve can be subjected to probit or logit transformation to linearize it over its whole length, or the data can be subjected to nonlinear regression using the sigmoid E_{max} model of this form:

$$Effect\ (e) = F\left(dose_e^{\gamma},\ dose_e^{\gamma} + dose_{e50}^{\gamma}\right)$$

More complex models relating the concentration of NMBDs at the neuromuscular junction to their pharmacologic effect have been developed, and are discussed later.[115,116]

Factors that govern duration of action of NMBDs.

Onset

There is ample evidence that potent NMBDs have slower onset times than less potent drugs with similar physicochemical properties. These facts can be explained by the concept of the margin of safety. A critical number of receptors at the neuromuscular junction must be occupied before appearance of neuromuscular block, and at least 90% of the receptors must be occupied before block is complete at the adductor pollicis. When the drug reaches the synaptic cleft, most molecules will bind to receptors that are present with a high density. As the concentration of free drug decreases, more molecules are driven in and the process will continue until the concentrations of free drug within and outside the synaptic cleft are equal. When a potent drug is administered, fewer molecules are given than in a case of a less potent drug, and the onset will be slower compared to onset of lower potency NMBD.[116a] Nondepolarizing NMBDs of low potency (e.g., rocuronium) have more molecules to diffuse from the central compartment into the effect compartment. Once in the effect compartment, all molecules act promptly. Weaker binding of the low-potency drugs to receptors prevents buffered diffusion, a process that occurs with more potent drugs. Buffered diffusion causes repetitive binding and unbinding to receptors, thus keeping potent drugs in the neighborhood of the effector sites and potentially lengthening the duration of effect. This phenomenon is probably what contributes to the slower onset time for cisatracurium than atracurium. However, for very short-acting drugs, the ideal ED_{95} might be greater (0.5-1.0 mg/kg) because rapid metabolism in the plasma destroys some of the administered muscle relaxant before it reaches the neuromuscular junction. This phenomenon can explain the relatively slow onset time for mivacurium.

Plasma concentrations have only modest influence on onset time. Arterial plasma concentrations peak 25 to 35 seconds after administration, thus before onset of neuromuscular block. This paradox can be explained by assuming that the site of action, the neuromuscular junction, is represented by the effect compartment in which the concentration of the NMBD is directly related to the magnitude of neuromuscular blockade.[116b] The rate constant for transfer into the effect compartment is similar for most intermediate duration action NMBDs and corresponds approximately to neuromuscular junction blood flow divided by neuromuscular junction/plasma partition coefficient. Whatever muscle relaxant, the limiting factor appears to be the time required for the drug to reach the neuromuscular junction, which in turn depends on cardiac output, the distance of the muscle (and neuromuscular junction) from the central circulation, and muscle blood flow. Therefore in most cases, the onset time will be dependent on blood flow to muscle. Under normal circumstances, muscle blood flow increases when cardiac output increases, with a direct relationship between speed of onset and cardiac output. This may explain why infants and children have a faster onset of neuromuscular block, and elderly patients have a slower onset than younger individuals.

It is obvious that the intensity of maximum blockade is affected directly by the administered dose. However, when the dose increases in the subparalyzing range (that is, when maximum blockade is between 0% and 100%), time to reach maximum effect is dose-independent. This is because the time to peak concentration at the effect compartment is independent of the dose. When the administered dose, however, is sufficient to effect complete disappearance of neuromuscular response, time to maximum blockade becomes dose-dependent.

DURATION OF ACTION

Although it is commonly believed that the rate of decline of NMBD plasma concentrations during recovery from neuromuscular blockade determines the duration of action and the rate of recovery, further explanations are needed. It has been suggested that muscle blood flow is, to a certain extent, a limiting factor in the termination of action. For long-acting NMBDs, the dominant effect for the recovery from neuromuscular blockade is the rate of decrease of plasma concentration because there is pseudo-equilibrium between concentrations at the neuromuscular junction and plasma. Therefore changing blood flow will not affect the duration of action. For intermediate duration of action NMBD, after a single bolus dose, plasma concentrations decrease at a rate that differs slightly from the equilibrium half-life with muscle. It can induce a significant concentration gradient between neuromuscular junction and plasma during recovery, but provided that recovery rate is constant, the ratio of concentrations between the neuromuscular junction and plasma will remain relatively constant.

The most important factor is that the rate of decline of plasma concentration during recovery is not always related to the NMBD terminal half-life because after initial administration, plasma concentrations will decrease because of redistribution. It is only when redistribution will be complete that the decrease in plasma concentrations will be dependent on the terminal half-life and will decrease more slowly. For long-acting NMBD such as pancuronium, the recovery time will take place during the terminal half-life. In this situation the duration of action will be dependent on the rate of decrease of plasma concentrations. This is different for intermediate duration of action NMBDs. The terminal half-life of atracurium is around 20 minutes, whereas the elimination half-lives of both vecuronium and rocuronium are between 60 and 120 minutes. Although such differences can be observed, the duration of action and recovery from neuromuscular block of these three drugs are very similar. These apparent discrepancies can be explained by the fact that the distribution phase is the most important factor and extends for a much longer period than for long-acting NMBDs.[116c] If their duration of action and recovery rates are almost identical, it is due to the decrease of plasma concentrations to levels compatible with recovery during the redistribution phase.

CLINICAL MANAGEMENT

The main goal of neuromuscular blockade during induction of anesthesia includes paralysis of the vocal cords and muscles of the jaw to facilitate endotracheal intubation. Relaxation of the respiratory muscles, particularly the diaphragm, allows controlled ventilation. Paralysis of the abdominal muscles and the diaphragm is often required intraoperatively, particularly during abdominal, robotic, or laparoscopic surgery. During recovery from neuromuscular block, restoration of complete neuromuscular strength is essential to ensure adequate spontaneous ventilation with normal regulation of breathing during hypoxia and the patency of the musculature of the upper airway with maintained airway protection. The choice of the initial dose of NMBD, timing of readministration of NMBD, timing of administration of anticholinesterase, and interpretation of monitoring require an understanding of the varying sensitivities of different muscle groups to NMBDs.

Although the practice of administering an NMBD to facilitate tracheal intubation may be routine, it has been suggested that the combination of propofol with a rapid-acting opioid may provide good to excellent intubating conditions in most patients. However, relatively large doses of opioids are required to obtain satisfactory intubating conditions. Mencke and coworkers demonstrated that adding atracurium to a propofol-fentanyl induction regimen significantly improved the quality of intubating conditions and decreased the frequency of vocal cord lesions following intubation from 42% to 8%.[117] The rate of postoperative hoarseness was also significantly decreased to 16% from 44%.[117] Combes and associates confirmed that the use of NMBD for tracheal intubation decreased the incidence of adverse postoperative upper airway symptoms, resulted in better intubating conditions, and also reduced the rate of adverse hemodynamic effects caused by deeper levels of anesthesia.[118] Patients intubated without an NMBD had three to four times more Cormack scores of 3 to 4, and difficult intubation was more common (12% vs. 1%). In a cohort of more than 100,000 patients, Lundstrom and colleagues demonstrated that avoidance of NMBD was associated with more difficult tracheal intubation conditions compared with NMBD use, with an odds ratio of 1.5.[118a] A recent Cochrane review supported the use of an NMBD (vs. avoidance of NMBD) in order to create the best intubating conditions.[118b]

Several alternative approaches are available to enhance surgical relaxation when administration of additional NMBDs may be inappropriate. These options include increasing the depth of general anesthesia with a drug such as a volatile anesthetic or propofol, administering lidocaine, using regional anesthesia, positioning the patient properly on the operating table, and appropriately adjusting the depth of neuromuscular blockade. The choice of one or several of these options is determined by the estimated remaining duration of surgery, the anesthetic technique, and the surgical maneuver required. Importantly, the single best (and only) method to ensure appropriate dosing and timing of additional NMBD is assessment of the depth of neuromuscular block by objective (quantitative) means.[118c]

It is important to keep these options in mind to avoid relying on only neuromuscular blockade to achieve a desired degree of surgical relaxation.

Varying Sensitivities of Different Muscle Groups

The sensitivity of the neuromuscular junctions to the effects of neuromuscular relaxants among various muscle groups varies greatly. Paton and Zaimis[118d] demonstrated in 1951 that some of the muscles of respiration, such as the diaphragm, were more resistant to curare than others. The dose of nondepolarizing NMBDs needed to block the diaphragm is 1.5 to 2 times that of the adductor pollicis. Thus complete paralysis of the diaphragm is not expected with doses of NMBDs used to block neuromuscular transmission at the adductor pollicis.[119] Similarly, the laryngeal adductor muscles are more resistant to nondepolarizing NMBDs than the more peripheral muscles such as the adductor pollicis,[120] at which all dosing recommendations for NMBDs and their antagonists have been made. The sparing effect of NMBDs on the laryngeal adductor muscles has been documented with vecuronium, rocuronium, cisatracurium, and mivacurium.[120-122] Plaud and colleagues studied the pharmacokinetic-pharmacodynamic relationship of NMBDs at the adductor pollicis and the laryngeal adductors.[123] These investigators found that the concentration in the effect compartment producing 50% of the maximum block was significantly greater at the laryngeal adductor muscles (1.5 µg/mL) than that at the adductor pollicis muscle (0.8 µg/mL). Convincing evidence indicates that the EC_{50} for almost all drugs is 50% to 100% higher at the diaphragm or larynx than it is at the adductor pollicis. These differences may be caused by any of several factors. Waud and Waud found that following curare administration, neuromuscular transmission occurs when approximately 18% of the receptors are free at the diaphragm, whereas it does not occur at the peripheral muscles unless 29% of receptors are free.[124] The reason may be higher receptor density, greater release of acetylcholine, or less acetylcholinesterase activity. The lower density of acetylcholine receptors in slow muscle fibers, such as found in the peripheral muscles, explains, in part, the lower margin of safety for neuromuscular transmission when compared with that in the faster muscle fibers in the laryngeal adductors. Muscle sensitivity to succinylcholine is different from that of other NMBDs. Succinylcholine is the only muscle relaxant that, at equipotent doses, causes greater neuromuscular block at the vocal cords than at the adductor pollicis. Some data suggest that in contrast to nondepolarizing NMBDs, succinylcholine is more effective in blocking the muscles composed of primarily fast-contracting fibers.[125]

In spite of the relative resistance to NMBDs, the onset of neuromuscular block is significantly faster at the diaphragm and the laryngeal adductors than at the adductor pollicis. Fisher and associates postulated that more rapid equilibration (shorter effect site equilibration half-life [$t_{1/2}k_{e0}$]) of the NMBD between plasma[126] and the effect compartment at these more centrally located muscles was the explanation for this observation. The accelerated rate of equilibrium probably represents little more than differences in regional blood flow. Therefore muscle blood flow (i.e., the rate of drug delivery to the tissue), rather than a drug's intrinsic potency, may be more important in determining the onset and offset time of nondepolarizing NMBDs. Greater blood flow per gram of muscle at the diaphragm or larynx results in delivery of a higher peak plasma concentration of drug in the brief period of time

TABLE 27.4 Guide to Nondepolarizing Relaxant Dosage (mg/kg) Under Different Anesthetic Techniques

				DOSAGE FOR RELAXATION	
	ED_{95} Under N_2O/O_2	**Dose for Intubation**	**Supplemental Dose after Intubation**	**N_2O**	**Anesthetic Vapors***
LONG-ACTING					
Pancuronium	0.07	0.08-0.12	0.02	0.05	0.03
d-Tubocurarine	0.5	0.5-0.6	0.1	0.3	0.15
INTERMEDIATE-ACTING					
Vecuronium	0.05	0.1-0.2	0.02	0.05	0.03
Atracurium	0.23	0.5-0.6	0.1	0.3	0.15
Cisatracurium	0.05	0.15-0.2	0.02	0.05	0.04
Rocuronium	0.3	0.6-1.0	0.1	0.3	0.15
SHORT-ACTING					
Mivacurium	0.08	0.2-0.25	0.05	0.1	0.08
Continuous Infusion Dosage (µg/kg/min) Required to Maintain 90%-95% Twitch Inhibition Under N_2O/O_2 With Intravenous Agents					
Mivacurium	3-15				
Atracurium	4-12				
Cisatracurium	1-2				
Vecuronium	0.8-1.0				
Rocuronium	9-12				

*The potentiation of nondepolarizing relaxants by different anesthetic vapors has been reported to vary from 20% to 50%. More recent data suggest, however, that this variation may be much less, particularly in the case of the intermediate- and short-acting relaxants. Therefore for the sake of simplicity, this table assumes a potentiation of 40% in the case of all volatile anesthetics.

Suggested dosages provide good intubating conditions under light anesthesia. Satisfactory abdominal relaxation may be achieved at dosages listed after intubation without a relaxant or with succinylcholine. This table is intended as a general guide to dosage. Individual relaxant requirement should be confirmed with a neuromuscular monitor.

ED_{95}, Dose causing on average 95% suppression of neuromuscular response; *N_2O*, nitrous oxide; *O_2*, oxygen.

before rapid redistribution occurs. Plaud and colleagues confirmed this hypothesis by demonstrating a faster transfer rate constant (i.e., $t_{½}k_{e0}$) at the laryngeal adductors (2.7 minutes) than at the adductor pollicis (4.4 minutes).[123] Greater resistance to neuromuscular blockade accounts for the faster recovery of the respiratory muscles and the muscles of the abdominal wall than at the adductor pollicis muscle. Recovery occurs more rapidly because blood concentration of the NMBD must decrease more in the muscles of respiration than in the adductor pollicis for recovery of neuromuscular function to begin.

In contrast, the muscles of the upper airway are particularly sensitive to the effects of muscle relaxants. The masseter is 15% more sensitive to nondepolarizing NMBDs than is the adductor pollicis.[127] Significant weakness of the muscles of the upper airway may exist even when strength at the adductor pollicis has recovered almost to baseline values. A TOF ratio less than 0.9 at the adductor pollicis (with a calibrated neuromuscular monitor) is associated with impaired pharyngeal function, reduced resting tone in the upper esophageal sphincter muscle, and decreased coordination of the muscles involved in swallowing, all of which cause an increased incidence of misdirected swallows, or aspiration.[128] Because of the resistance of the diaphragm and laryngeal muscles to neuromuscular block, patients may be weak in pharyngeal muscle groups while being able to breathe as long as an endotracheal tube is in place. Once the trachea is extubated, however, patients may not be able to maintain a patent airway or protect their airway.[129] This is likely the reason that patients with a TOF less than 0.9 in the postanesthesia care unit (PACU) are more likely to develop critical respiratory events than those whose TOF ratio is 0.9 or greater.[129a] Some investigators[129b] have demonstrated that among patients who received NMBD, those who did not receive reversal were more than twice as likely to develop pneumonia after surgery.

The increase in ventilation during hypoxia is mainly governed by afferent neuronal input from peripheral chemoreceptors of the carotid body. Acetylcholine is involved in the transmission of afferent neuronal activity from the carotid body to the central nervous system (CNS). Eriksson and associates have shown that partial neuromuscular block (TOF ratio of 0.7) reduces specifically the ventilatory responses to isocapnic hypoxia without altering the response to hypercapnia. The ventilatory response to hypoxia returns to control values after recovery of a TOF ratio to above 0.9.[129c] The mechanism behind this interaction seems to be a spontaneous, reversible depression of carotid body chemoreceptor activity during hypoxia.[129d]

DOSAGE

General Dosage Guidelines

Proper selection of the dose of nondepolarizing NMBD and quantitative monitoring are required to ensure that the desired effect is achieved without overdose of the relaxant (Tables 27.4 and 27.5).

TABLE 27.5 Pharmacodynamic Effects of Succinylcholine and Nondepolarizing Neuromuscular Blockers

	Anesthesia	Intubating Dose (mg/kg)	Approximate ED_{95} Multiples	Maximum Block (%)	Time to Maximum Block (min)	Clinical Duration* (min)	References
Succinylcholine	Opioids or halothane	0.5	1.7	100	—	6.7	372
Succinylcholine	Desflurane	0.6	2	100	1.4	7.6	373
Succinylcholine	Opioids or halothane	1.0	2	100	—	11.3	372
Succinylcholine	Desflurane	1.0	3	100	1.2	9.3	373
Succinylcholine	Opioids	1.0	3	—	1.1	8	374
Succinylcholine	Opioids	1.0	3	—	1.1	9	375
Succinylcholine	Isoflurane	1.0	3	100	0.8	9	140
STEROIDAL COMPOUNDS							
Rocuronium	Opioids	0.6	2	100	1.7	36	142
Rocuronium	Isoflurane	0.6	2	100	1.5	37	140
Rocuronium	Isoflurane	0.9	3	100	1.3	53	140
Rocuronium	Isoflurane	1.2	4	100	0.9	73	140
Vecuronium	Isoflurane	0.1	2	100	2.4	41	140
Vecuronium	Opioids	0.1	2	100	2.4	44	376
Pancuronium	Opioids	0.08	1.3	100	2.9	86	148, 377
Pancuronium	Opioids	0.1	1.7	99	4	100	378
BENZYLISOQUINOLINIUM COMPOUNDS†							
Mivacurium	Opioids	0.15	2	100	3.3	16.8	9
Mivacurium	Opioids	0.15	2	100	3	14.5	142
Mivacurium	Halothane	0.15	2	100	2.8	18.6	379
Mivacurium	Opioids	0.2	2.6	100	2.5	19.7	9
Mivacurium	Opioids	0.25	3.3	100	2.3	20.3	9
Mivacurium	Opioids	0.25	3.3	—	2.1	21	375
Atracurium	Opioids	0.5	2	100	3.2	46	107
Cisatracurium	Opioids	0.1	2	99	7.7	46	323
Cisatracurium	Opioids	0.1	2	100	5.2	45	107
Cisatracurium	Opioids	0.2	4	100	2.7	68	107
Cisatracurium	Opioids	0.4	8	100	1.9	91	107
d-Tubocurarine	Opioids	0.6	1.2	97	5.7	81	378

*Time from injection of the intubating dose to recovery of twitch to 25% of control.
†For atracurium and mivacurium, slower injection (30 seconds) is recommended to minimize circulatory effects.
ED_{95}, Dose causing on average 95% suppression of neuromuscular response.

The intensity of maximum blockade is directly affected by dose. If a small dose of NMBD is administered, neuromuscular block may not occur because the amount administered is inadequate to overcome the margin of safety at the neuromuscular junction. When doses lower than those required to cause 100% neuromuscular blockade are administered, the time required to reach maximum effect is a function of the NMBD and blood flow to the muscles. It is independent of the dose administered. However, if the administered dose is high enough to cause 100% neuromuscular blockade, the time required for maximum block will depend on the dose of NMBD administered. Larger doses will, up to a certain point, produce a faster onset of effect.[130] Increasing the dose of NMBD beyond that point will not further decrease the time to onset of maximal effect, and may significantly prolong the total duration of neuromuscular blockade, contributing to residual postoperative paralysis.

In addition to a general knowledge of the pharmacodynamics and pharmacokinetics of NMBDs and understanding of the guidelines for dosing, optimal practice requires that dosing be adjusted to account for variability in individual patients' responses to NMBDs. This adjustment cannot be made without using a quantitative (objective) monitor of neuromuscular blockade any time that an NMBD is administered to a patient. Overdosage must be avoided for several

TABLE 27.6 Suggested Definitions of the Depth of Neuromuscular Block Based on Subjective and Objective Criteria

Depth of Block	Posttetanic Count	Train-of-Four Count	Subjective Train-of-Four Ratio	Measured Train-of-Four Ratio
Intense (profound) block	0	0	0	0
Deep block	≥1	0	0	0
Moderate block	NA	1-3	0	0
Light (shallow) block	NA	4	Fade present	0.1-0.4
Minimal block (near recovery)	NA	4	No fade	>0.4 but <0.90
Full recovery (normal function)	NA	4	No fade	≥0.90-1.0

NA, Not applicable.
From Brull SJ, Kopman AF. Current status of neuromuscular reversal and monitoring. Challenges and opportunities. *Anesthesiology.* 2017;126:173, see Table 1.

reasons: to limit the duration of drug effect so that it matches the anticipated length of surgery; to avoid unwanted cardiovascular side effects associated with large NMBD doses; and to minimize residual neuromuscular block postoperatively.

Initial and Maintenance Dosage

The initial dose of NMBD is determined by the reason for administration. Traditionally, doses used to facilitate tracheal intubation are twice the ED_{95} (see Table 27.4). If, however, the trachea has been intubated without the use of an NMBD and the purpose in administering an NMBD is to produce surgical relaxation, a dose that is slightly less than the ED_{95} (see Table 27.5) may be sufficient in most surgical settings. Administration of NMBDs solely for surgical relaxation does not prevent vocal cord injury and postoperative hoarseness caused by intubation without NMBD. Additionally, ensuring maximal neuromuscular block by using quantitative means (e.g., a TOF count of zero) rather than being guided by clinical judgment will result in less hemodynamic instability during laryngoscopy and better intubating conditions.[130a] Administering a smaller initial dose may be sufficient in the presence of any of the potent inhalational anesthetics (see the later section on drug interactions), but the dosing should always be guided by quantitative monitoring.

To avoid prolonged residual paralysis, inadequate antagonism of residual blockade, or both, the main goal in dosing NMBDs should be to use the lowest possible dose that provides adequate relaxation for surgery. Moreover, clinical management of individual patients should be guided by monitoring of the neuromuscular block, ideally with an objective neuromuscular monitoring technique, to allow safe intraoperative administration of the NMBD and its antagonism by neostigmine or sugammadex (see also Chapter 43, Neuromuscular Monitoring).

In an adequately anesthetized and monitored patient, little reason exists to abolish the TOF responses to peripheral nerve stimulation completely. However, if deep levels of block are required to maintain paralysis of the diaphragm and the abdominal wall muscles, response of the adductor pollicis to stimulation of the ulnar nerve may disappear. In this case, monitoring the depth of neuromuscular block can be accomplished using the posttetanic count (PTC) at the adductor pollicis or TOF ratio at the corrugator supercilii.[131,132] Supplemental (maintenance) doses of NMBDs should be approximately one tenth (in case of long-acting NMBDs) to one fourth (in the case of intermediate- and short-acting NMBDs) the initial dose and should not be given until quantitative evidence of beginning recovery from the previous dose is present.

Relaxation can be maintained by continuous infusion of intermediate- and short-acting drugs. This approach is useful in maintaining a stable depth of neuromuscular blockade and allows adjustment of the depth of relaxation according to surgical needs. The depth of neuromuscular blockade maintained is moderate, if possible, to ensure complete spontaneous recovery of neuromuscular function at the end of a surgical procedure or prompt antagonism of residual effects. Suggested definitions of the depth of neuromuscular block are listed in Table 27.6.[132a] Table 27.4 lists the approximate dose ranges that are typically required during infusions to maintain 90% to 95% blockade of the twitch (one twitch visible on TOF stimulation) during a nitrous oxide–oxygen anesthetic supplemented with intravenous anesthetics. Infusion dosage is usually decreased by 30% to 50% in the presence of potent volatile anesthetics.

NEUROMUSCULAR BLOCKING DRUGS AND TRACHEAL INTUBATION

Rapid onset of neuromuscular blockade is one of the requirements for securing an airway promptly. It is affected by several factors, including muscle blood flow, rate of delivery of the drug to the neuromuscular junction, receptor affinity, plasma clearance of the NMBD, and the mechanism of neuromuscular blockade (depolarizing vs. nondepolarizing)[96,116a,133](see Table 27.5 and Fig. 27.9). Onset time decreases as ED_{50} increases. When a potent NMBD is administered, fewer molecules are administered than in the case of an equipotent dose of a less potent drug. Because of this lower concentration gradient, more time is required for sufficient molecules of a potent drug to be delivered to the neuromuscular junction. Thus onset time is longer. This concept was verified by Kopman and colleagues, who demonstrated that, when giving equipotent doses of gallamine, dTc, and pancuronium, onset time was slower with the more potent pancuronium and faster with the less potent gallamine. Except for atracurium,[135] the molar potency (the ED_{50} or ED_{95} expressed as μM/kg) is highly predictive of a drug's initial rate of onset of effect (at the adductor pollicis muscle).[133] A drug's measured molar potency is the end result of many contributing factors: the drug's intrinsic potency (the CE_{50}, which is the biophase

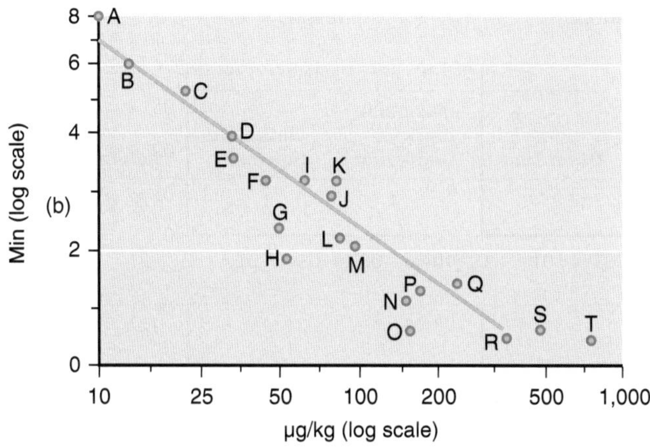

Fig. 27.9 Linear regression of onset of neuromuscular blockade (ordinate) versus potency of a series of steroidal relaxants studied in the cat model by Bowman and associates.[96] The data show that onset may be increased in compounds of low potency and encouraged the eventual development of rocuronium and rapacuronium (ORG 9487). *A*, Pipecuronium; *B*, ORG 8788; *C*, pancuronium; *D*, vecuronium; *E-M* and *O-T*, ORG 9274, 9360, 9273, 8715, 6502, 9216, 7931, 8730, 7617, 9275, 6368, 8764, 9382, and 7684 (respectively); *N*, RGH-4201. Data from Reference 96.

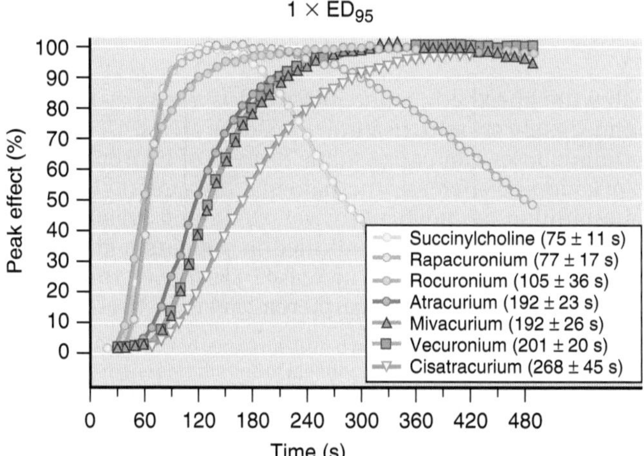

Fig. 27.10 Percentages of peak effect after a dose causing on average 95% suppression of neuromuscular response *(ED_{95})* of succinylcholine, rocuronium, rapacuronium, vecuronium, atracurium, mivacurium, and cisatracurium at the adductor pollicis muscle. Times (mean ± standard deviation) in seconds to 95% of peak effect are shown in parentheses. (Data from references 114, 133, and 135.)

concentration resulting in 50% twitch depression), the rate of equilibration between plasma and biophase (k_{e0}), the initial rate of plasma clearance, and probably other factors as well.[136] Notably, rocuronium has a molar potency (ED_{95}) of 0.54 μM/kg, which is approximately 13% that of vecuronium and only 9% that of cisatracurium; this finding illustrates the expected faster onset of rocuronium at the adductor pollicis muscle, as opposed to vecuronium and cisatracurium. Donati and Meistelman proposed a model to explain this inverse potency–onset relationship.[116a]

The times to 95% blockade at the adductor pollicis after administration of the ED_{95} dose of succinylcholine, rocuronium, vecuronium, atracurium, mivacurium, and cisatracurium are shown in Fig. 27.10.[114,133,135] The illustration shows that the most potent compound, cisatracurium,

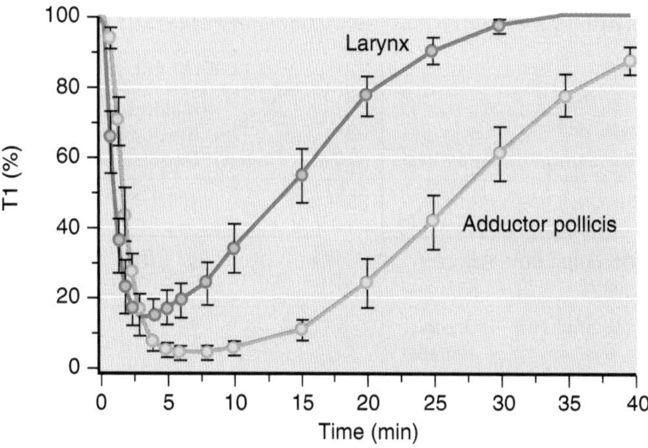

Fig. 27.11 Evolution of neuromuscular blockade in the larynx and thumb (adductor pollicis) after a 0.07 mg/kg dose of vecuronium. Onset and recovery from blockade occur more rapidly in the larynx. *T1*, First twitch of train-of-four. (From Donati F, Meistelman C, Plaud B. Vecuronium neuromuscular blockade at the adductor muscles of the larynx and adductor pollicis. *Anesthesiology.* 1991;74:833–837.)

has the slowest onset, and the least potent compound, rocuronium, has the most rapid onset.[114,133,135] Bevan also proposed that rapid plasma clearance is associated with a rapid onset of action.[137] The fast onset of succinylcholine's action is related to its rapid metabolism and plasma clearance.

The onset of neuromuscular blockade is much faster in the muscles that are relevant to obtaining optimal intubating conditions (laryngeal adductors, diaphragm, and masseter) than in the muscle that is typically monitored (adductor pollicis) (Fig. 27.11).[121] Thus neuromuscular blockade develops faster, has a shorter maximum depth and duration of effect, and recovers more quickly in these central muscles (Table 27.7).[120-122,138,139]

Paralysis following intravenous administration does not occur instantaneously even with large doses of muscle relaxants. Onset of blockade occurs 1 to 2 minutes earlier in the laryngeal muscles than at the adductor pollicis after administration of nondepolarizing NMBDs. The pattern of blockade (onset, depth, and speed of recovery) in the corrugator supercilii muscle is similar to that in the larynx,[119] the diaphragm, and the muscles of the abdominal wall. By monitoring the onset of neuromuscular blockade at the corrugator supercilii, one can predict the quality of tracheal intubating conditions. Good to excellent intubating conditions are observed in more than 90% of patients after disappearance of the TOF responses (a TOF count of zero) at the corrugator supercilii.[131] The onset of maximal blockade in the larynx also corresponds with the point at which the adductor pollicis muscle begins to show palpable evidence of weakening.

Rapid Tracheal Intubation

Rocuronium in high dose (0.9-1.2 mg/kg) or succinylcholine 1.5 mg/kg can be used interchangeably for rapid tracheal intubation because they provide adequate intubating conditions within 60 to 90 seconds. Hence if succinylcholine is considered undesirable or contraindicated, high doses of rocuronium can be administered.[140] The onset of action of other nondepolarizing NMBDs can be accelerated by administering a priming dose of the NMBD[141] or

TABLE 27.7 Time Course of Action and Peak Effect Data at the Laryngeal Adductors and Adductor Pollicis

		LARYNGEAL ADDUCTORS			ADDUCTOR POLLICIS			
Dose (mg/kg)	**Anesthesia**	**Onset Time (s)**	**Maximum Block (% Depression)**	**Clinical Duration (min)**	**Onset Time (s)**	**Maximum block (% Depression)**	**Clinical Duration (min)**	**Reference**
Succinylcholine, 1.0	Propofol-fentanyl	34 ± 12	100 ± 0	4.3 ± 1.6	56 ± 15	100 ± 0	8 ± 2	122
Rocuronium, 0.25	Propofol-fentanyl	96 ± 6	37 ± 8	—	180 ± 18	69 ± 8	—	121
Rocuronium, 0.4	Propofol-fentanyl	92 ± 29	70 ± 15	—	155 ± 40	99 ± 3	24 ± 7	122
Rocuronium, 0.5	Propofol-fentanyl	84 ± 6	77 ± 5	8 ± 3	144 ± 12	98 ± 1	22 ± 3	121
Vecuronium, 0.04	Propofol-fentanyl	198 ± 6	55 ± 8	—	342 ± 12	89 ± 3	11 ± 2	120
Vecuronium, 0.07	Propofol-fentanyl	198 ± 12	88 ± 4	9 ± 2	342 ± 18	98 ± 1	22 ± 2	120
Mivacurium, 0.14	Propofol-alfentanil	137 ± 20	90 ± 7	5.7 ± 2.1	201 ± 59	99 ± 1	16.2 ± 4.6	138
Mivacurium, 0.2	Propofol-alfentanil	89 ± 26	99 ± 4	10.4 ± 1.5	202 ± 45	99 ± 2	20.5 ± 3.9	139

Clinical duration is the time until the first twitch of train-of-four (T1) has recovered to 25% of its control value. Mean and standard deviation[122,138,139] or standard error of the mean.[120,121]

by using combinations of NMBDs.[142] Although combinations of mivacurium and rocuronium can achieve rapid onset without undue prolongation of action and without undesirable side effects,[142] combinations of compounds of different structures may result in a marked prolongation of neuromuscular blockade. Additionally, combining different NMBDs may not consistently result in a rapid onset of neuromuscular block.

Timing Technique. This technique entails administration of a single intubating dose (two times the ED_{95}) of a rapid-onset NMBD such as rocuronium to an awake patient, followed by the administration of the anesthetic induction agent at the onset of clinical signs of weakness such as ptosis or loss of ability to maintain the raised arm. Using this technique, 0.6 mg/kg rocuronium can provide good to excellent intubating conditions within 45 seconds after induction of anesthesia.[142a] Because of the potential for unpleasant symptoms and recall associated with neuromuscular paralysis in awake patients, this technique is no longer used clinically.

Priming Technique. Since the introduction of rocuronium into clinical practice, the use of priming technique has almost disappeared. When priming, a small, subparalyzing dose of the nondepolarizer (≈20% of the ED_{95} or ≈10% of the intubating dose) is administered 2 to 4 minutes before the intubating dose of the compound.[141] This procedure accelerates the onset of blockade for most nondepolarizing NMBDs only by 30 to 60 seconds, thereby indicating that intubation can be performed within 90 seconds of the second dose. However, the intubating conditions that occur after priming are only marginally improved and do not match those that occur after succinylcholine. The size of the priming dose is limited by its effects on the awake patient, since the anesthetic induction agent is administered only immediately prior to the intubating dose of NMBD. Further, priming doses can cause subtle degrees of neuromuscular blockade and increase the patient's discomfort, the risks of aspiration, and difficulty swallowing and breathing.[143] This technique is contraindicated in patients with abnormal airway anatomy or increased sensitivity to NMBDs such as patients with myasthenia gravis or those taking magnesium.

Large-Dose Regimen for Rapid Tracheal Intubation. Large doses of NMBDs are usually recommended when intubation must be accomplished in less than 90 seconds. High-dose regimens are associated with considerably prolonged duration of action and potentially increased cardiovascular side effects, however (see Table 27.5).[140,144] Increasing the dosage of rocuronium from 0.6 mg/kg (twice the ED_{95}) to 1.2 mg/kg (four times the ED_{95}) shortens the onset time of complete neuromuscular block from 89 to 55 seconds but essentially doubles the clinical duration of action of the compound (the recovery of the first twitch of TOF [T1] to 25% of baseline values) from 37 to 73 minutes.[140]

Small-Dose Relaxants for Tracheal Intubation. Small doses of NMBDs can be used for routine tracheal intubation. The use of smaller doses of NMBDs has the following two possible advantages: (1) it shortens the time to recovery from neuromuscular blockade, and (2) it reduces the requirement for anticholinesterase drugs. Rocuronium has the shortest onset time of all the nondepolarizing NMBDs currently available.[121,122] The maximal effect of either 0.25 or 0.5 mg/kg of rocuronium at the laryngeal muscles occurs after 1.5 minutes.[121] This interval is shorter than the 3.3 minutes reported after administration of equipotent

	Muscle X	Adductor pollicis
EC_{50} (μg/mL)	3.00	1.18
$t_{1/2}k_{e0}$ (min)	1.93	3.85
Hill coefficient	4.00	4.50

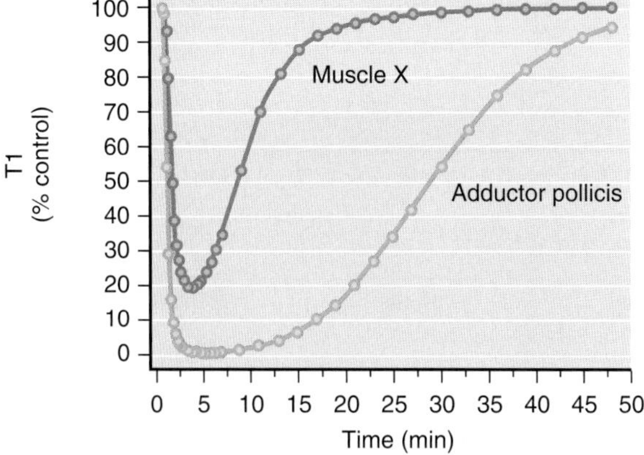

Fig. 27.12 A computer simulation based on Sheiner's model[115] and data reported by Wierda and colleagues. The dose causing on average 95% suppression of neuromuscular response (ED_{95}) of rocuronium at the adductor pollicis from this model is 0.33 mg/kg. Rocuronium, 0.45 mg/kg is given as a bolus at time zero. Muscle X represents a muscle (e.g., the diaphragm or the laryngeal adductors) that is less sensitive to the effects of nondepolarizing relaxants than the adductor pollicis but has greater blood flow. In this example, the concentration of rocuronium producing 50% block (EC_{50}) of muscle X is 2.5 times that of the adductor pollicis, but the half-life of transport between the plasma and effect compartment ($t_{½}k_{e0}$) of muscle X is only half as long. The rapid equilibration between plasma concentrations of rocuronium and muscle X results in the more rapid onset of blockade of muscle X than of the adductor pollicis. The greater EC_{50} at muscle X explains the faster recovery of this muscle than of the adductor pollicis from neuromuscular blockade. Lower blood concentrations of rocuronium must be achieved at the adductor pollicis than at muscle X before recovery begins. *T1,* First twitch of train-of-four. (From Naguib M, Kopman AF. Low dose rocuronium for tracheal intubation. *Middle East J Anesthesiol.* 2003;17:193–204, with permission from the *Middle East Journal of Anesthesiology.*)

doses of vecuronium (0.04 or 0.07 mg/kg),[120] and it is only slightly longer than the 0.9 minutes reported after 0.25 or 0.5 mg/kg of succinylcholine (see Table 27.7).[125]

With a better understanding of the multiple factors that contribute to satisfactory conditions for intubation, it is now possible to administer NMBDs thoughtfully in this fashion. Intubating conditions are related more closely to the degree of neuromuscular blockade of the laryngeal adductor muscles than to the degree of blockade typically monitored at the adductor pollicis. Fig. 27.12 demonstrates this principle.[136] In the presence of an adequate depth of anesthesia, complete blockade at the larynx or diaphragm, or both, may not be a prerequisite for satisfactory intubating conditions. Kopman and colleagues noted that 0.5 mg/kg of rocuronium (1.5 times the ED_{95}) provided satisfactory conditions for intubation in patients anesthetized with 12.5 μg/kg of alfentanil and 2.0 mg/kg of propofol if laryngoscopy was delayed for 75 seconds after drug administration.[145] It was furthermore estimated that 1.5 times the ED_{95} of rocuronium would produce at least 95% blockade in 98% of the population.[145] A similar or lower multiple of rocuronium's ED_{95} was shown to have a faster onset and shorter duration of action than those of atracurium[146] or cisatracurium.[109] In most patients receiving 15 μg/kg of alfentanil followed by 2.0 mg/kg of propofol and 0.45 mg/kg of rocuronium, good to excellent conditions for intubation are present 75 to 90 seconds after the completion of drug administration.

METABOLISM AND ELIMINATION

The specific pathways of the metabolism (biotransformation) and elimination of NMBDs are summarized in Table 27.8. Of the nondepolarizing NMBDs listed, pancuronium, pipecuronium, vecuronium, atracurium, cisatracurium, and mivacurium are the only drugs that are metabolized or degraded. Nearly all nondepolarizing NMBD molecules contain ester linkages, acetyl ester groups, and hydroxy or methoxy groups. These substitutions, especially the quaternary nitrogen groups, confer a high degree of water solubility with only slight lipid solubility. The hydrophilic nature of relaxant molecules enables easy elimination in the urine through glomerular filtration, with no tubular resorption or secretion. Therefore all nondepolarizing NMBDs show elimination of the parent molecule in the urine as the basic route of elimination; those with a long duration of action thus have a clearance rate that is limited by the glomerular filtration rate (1-2 mL/kg/min).

Steroidal Compounds

Long-Acting Neuromuscular Blocking Drugs. Pancuronium is cleared largely by the kidney[147] and, to a limited extent, by hepatic uptake and elimination. A small amount (15%-20%) is deacetylated at the 3 position in the liver, but this makes a minimal contribution to the total clearance. Deacetylation also occurs at the 17 position, but to such a small extent as to be clinically irrelevant. The three known metabolites have been individually studied in anesthetized humans.[148] The 3-OH metabolite is the most potent of the three, being approximately half as potent as pancuronium, and is the only one present in detectable concentrations in the plasma. This metabolite has pharmacokinetics and duration of action similar to those of pancuronium.[148] The 3-OH metabolite is most likely excreted largely by the kidney.[148] The parent compound and the 3-OH metabolite are also cleared in small amounts through a minor liver pathway. The total clearance is delayed, and the duration of action is significantly lengthened, by severe disorders of renal or hepatic function.[149-151]

Intermediate-Acting Neuromuscular Blockers. Vecuronium, the 2-desmethyl derivative of pancuronium, is more lipid soluble than pancuronium because of the absence of the quaternizing methyl group at the 2 position. It undergoes two to three times more metabolism than pancuronium. Vecuronium is taken up into the liver by a carrier-mediated transport system,[152] and it is then deacetylated at the 3 position by liver microsomes. Approximately 12% of vecuronium clearance is through conversion to 3-desacetylvecuronium,[153] and 30% to 40% of the drug is cleared in the bile as the parent compound.[154] Although the liver is the principal organ of elimination for vecuronium, the drug also undergoes significant (up to 25%) renal excretion, and this combined organ elimination gives it a clearance rate of 3 to 6 mL/kg/min.[153,155]

TABLE 27.8 Metabolism and Elimination of Neuromuscular Blocking Drugs

			ELIMINATION		
Drug	**Duration**	**Metabolism (%)**	**Kidney (%)**	**Liver (%)**	**Metabolites**
Succinylcholine	Ultrashort	Butyrylcholinesterase (98%-99%)	<2%	None	Monoester (succinyl monocholine) and choline; the monoester is metabolized much more slowly than succinylcholine
Gantacurium	Ultrashort	Cysteine (fast) and ester hydrolysis (slow)	?	?	Inactive cysteine adduction product, chloroformate monoester, and alcohol
Mivacurium	Short	Butyrylcholinesterase (95%-99%)	<5%	None	Monoester and quaternary alcohol; the metabolites are inactive and most likely are not metabolized any further
			(Metabolites eliminated in urine and bile)		
Atracurium	Intermediate	Hofmann elimination and nonspecific ester hydrolysis (60%-90%)	10%-40%	None	Laudanosine, acrylates, alcohols, and acids; although laudanosine has CNS-stimulating properties, the clinical relevance of this effect is negligible
			(Metabolites eliminated in urine and bile)		
Cisatracurium	Intermediate	Hofmann elimination (77%?)	Renal clearance is 16% of total		Laudanosine and acrylates; ester hydrolysis of the quaternary monoacrylate occurs secondarily; because of the greater potency of cisatracurium, laudanosine quantities produced by Hofmann elimination are 5-10 times lower than in the case of atracurium, thus making this a nonissue in practice
Vecuronium	Intermediate	Liver (30%-40%)	40%-50%	50%-60% ≈60%	The 3-OH metabolite accumulates, particularly in renal failure; it has ≈80% the potency of vecuronium and may be responsible for delayed recovery in ICU patients
			(Metabolites excreted in urine and bile) ≈40%		
Rocuronium	Intermediate	None	10%-25%	>70%	None
Pancuronium	Long	Liver (10%-20%)	85%	15%	The 3-OH metabolite may accumulate, particularly in renal failure; it is approximately two thirds as potent as the parent compound
d-Tubocurarine	Long	None	80% (?)	20%	None

3-OH, 3-hydroxy; *?*, unknown; *CNS*, central nervous system; *ICU*, intensive care unit.

The principal metabolite of vecuronium, 3-desacetylvecuronium, is a potent NMBD (≈80% of the potency of vecuronium). The metabolite, however, has slower plasma clearance and longer duration of action than vecuronium.[153] 3-Desacetylvecuronium has a clearance rate of 3.5 mL/kg/min, and renal clearance accounts for approximately one sixth of its elimination.[153] In patients with renal failure in the ICU, 3-desacetylvecuronium can accumulate and produce prolonged neuromuscular blockade.[156] Other putative metabolites are 17-desacetylvecuronium and 3,17-bisdesacetylvecuronium, neither of which occurs in clinically significant amounts.

Rocuronium is eliminated primarily by the liver, with a small fraction (≈10%) eliminated in the urine.[157] It is taken up into the liver by a carrier-mediated active transport system.[158] The putative metabolite, 17-desacetylrocuronium, has low (5%-10%) neuromuscular blocking activity of the parent drug and it has not been detected in significant quantities. The elimination of rocuronium occurs predominately through its biliary excretion. The organic anion transporting peptide 1A2 (OATP1A2) mediates the hepatocellular uptake of a variety of drugs, including rocuronium. The peptide is encoded by the *SLCO1A2* gene and is expressed in the bile duct cells (cholangiocytes) of the liver.[158a] Genetic polymorphism of the *SLCO1A2* gene has recently been reported, and was shown to reduce the clearance of rocuronium in patients undergoing elective surgeries.[158a] This reduction in the biliary excretion may partially explain the marked prolongation in the duration of action of rocuronium in some patients.[158b]

Benzylisoquinolinium Compounds

Short-Acting Neuromuscular Blocking Drugs. Mivacurium is hydrolyzed in the plasma by butyrylcholinesterase to a monoester and an amino alcohol,[9] which are excreted in urine and bile. They have less than 1% of the neuromuscular blocking activity of the parent compound. Less than 5% of mivacurium is excreted in the urine as the parent compound.

Mivacurium consists of three stereoisomers, and the clearances of the two most pharmacologically active isomers, the *cis-trans* and *trans-trans*, are approximately 100 and 50 to 70 mL/kg/min, respectively.[94,159,160] These two isomers show elimination half-lives of 2 to 3 minutes.[94] The third stereoisomer, the *cis-cis*, is present as only 4% to 8% of the mivacurium mixture and has less than 10% of the neuromuscular blocking potency of the other two isomers.[94] Consequently, even though it has a much longer elimination half-life (55 minutes) and lower clearance (≈4 mL/kg/min) than the two other isomers, it does not contribute significantly to the duration of action of mivacurium.[94] This rapid enzymatic clearance of mivacurium accounts for its short duration of action.[9,94] When butyrylcholinesterase activity is significantly decreased, however, as in the rare patient who is homozygous for genetically atypical enzymes, the duration of action of mivacurium is prolonged for up to several hours.[161-164]

CW 1759-50 is an ultrashort-acting nondepolarizing NMBD that was developed to minimize the histaminoid side effects associated with gantacurium. In laboratory animals, the ED_{95} of CW 1759-50 is 0.03 mg/kg (cat) and 0.069 mg/kg (rhesus monkey). Its total duration of action (spontaneous recovery) is approximately 8 minutes, and it is minimally prolonged (12 minutes) after administration of doses four times its ED_{95}.[11a,11b] It can be antagonized rapidly (2 minutes) by L-cysteine. Its development for clinical use is undergoing.

Intermediate-Acting Neuromuscular Blocking Drugs. Atracurium is metabolized through two pathways: Hofmann elimination and nonspecific ester hydrolysis. Hofmann elimination is a purely chemical process that results in loss of the positive charges by molecular fragmentation to laudanosine (a tertiary amine) and a monoquaternary acrylate, compounds that are thought to have no neuromuscular and little or no cardiovascular activity of clinical relevance.[165]

Because it undergoes Hofmann elimination, atracurium is relatively stable at pH 3.0 and 4°C and becomes unstable when it is injected into the bloodstream. Early observations of the breakdown of the drug in buffer and plasma showed faster degradation in plasma, a finding suggesting a possible enzymatic hydrolysis of the ester groups. Further evidence suggested that ester hydrolysis may be more important than originally realized in the breakdown of atracurium.[166] By using a pharmacokinetics analysis, Fisher and associates concluded that a significant amount of clearance of atracurium may be by routes other than ester hydrolysis and Hofmann elimination.[167] Thus it appears that atracurium's metabolism is complicated and may not be completely understood.[167]

Laudanosine, a metabolite of atracurium, has CNS-stimulating properties. Because it crosses the blood-brain barrier, laudanosine was thought to cause excitement and seizure activity. However, plasma concentrations of this metabolite are very low, and adverse effects are unlikely to occur with atracurium (or cisatracurium) use in either the operating room or the ICU.

Atracurium is a mixture of 10 optical isomers. Cisatracurium is the 1R *cis*–1′R *cis* isomer of atracurium.[90] Like atracurium, cisatracurium is metabolized by Hofmann elimination to laudanosine and a monoquaternary acrylate.[168,169] In contrast, however, no ester hydrolysis of the parent molecule occurs. Hofmann elimination accounts for 77% of the total clearance of 5 to 6 mL/kg/min. Twenty-three percent of the drug is cleared through organ-dependent means, and renal elimination accounts for 16% of this.[169] Because cisatracurium is approximately four or five times as potent as atracurium, approximately five times less laudanosine is produced, and, as with atracurium, accumulation of this metabolite is not thought to be of any consequence in clinical practice.

Long-Acting Neuromuscular Blocking Drugs. dTc has no active metabolism and the kidney is the major pathway of elimination, with approximately 50% of a dose eliminated through renal pathways. The liver is likely a secondary route of elimination.

Asymmetric Mixed-Onium Fumarates

Gantacurium and CW 002 are degraded by two chemical mechanisms, neither of which is enzymatic: (1) rapid formation of an apparently inactive cysteine adduction product and (2) slower hydrolysis of the ester

TABLE 27.9 Approximate Autonomic Margins of Safety of Nondepolarizing Neuromuscular Blockers

Drugs	Vagus*	Sympathetic Ganglia*	Histamine Release†
BENZYLISOQUINOLINIUM COMPOUNDS			
Mivacurium	>50	>100	3.0
Atracurium	16	40	2.5
Cisatracurium	>50	>50	None
d-Tubocurarine	0.6	2.0	0.6
STEROIDAL COMPOUNDS			
Vecuronium	20	>250	None
Rocuronium	3.0-5.0	>10	None
Pancuronium	3.0	>250	None

*In cats.
†In human subjects.
Definition: number of multiples of the dose causing on average 95% suppression of neuromuscular response (ED_{95}) for neuromuscular blockade required to produce the autonomic side effect (ED_{50}).

bond to presumably inactive hydrolysis products (see Fig. 27.7).[11,170] CW 1759-50 is degraded nonenzymatically by endogenous L-cysteine at physiological pH and temperature, which accounts for its ultrashort duration of action.

In summary, the only short-acting nondepolarizing NMBD, mivacurium, is cleared rapidly and almost exclusively by metabolism by butyrylcholinesterase, thus resulting in much greater plasma clearance than that of any other nondepolarizing NMBD.[9] NMBDs of intermediate duration, such as vecuronium, rocuronium, atracurium, and cisatracurium, have clearance rates in the range of 3 to 6 mL/kg/min because of multiple pathways of degradation, metabolism, and/or elimination. Atracurium is cleared two to three times more rapidly than the long-acting drugs.[171-174] Similar clearance values have been obtained for rocuronium[175-179] and cisatracurium.[168,169,180] The long-acting NMBDs undergo minimal or no metabolism, and they are eliminated largely unchanged, mostly by renal excretion. Hepatic pathways are less important in their metabolism.

ADVERSE EFFECTS OF NEUROMUSCULAR BLOCKING DRUGS

NMBDs seem to play a prominent role in the incidence of adverse reactions that occur during anesthesia. The Committee on Safety of Medicines in the United Kingdom reported that 10.8% (218 of 2014) of adverse drug reactions and 7.3% of deaths (21 of 286) were attributable to the NMBDs.[181]

Autonomic Effects

While NMBDs have little penetration through the blood-brain barrier, they may interact with nicotinic and muscarinic cholinergic receptors within the peripheral nervous system, in particular the sympathetic and parasympathetic nervous systems and at the nicotinic receptors of the neuromuscular junction.

Dose-response ratios comparing the neuromuscular blocking potencies of these drugs (the ED_{95}) with their potencies in blocking vagal (parasympathetic) or sympathetic ganglionic transmission (the ED_{50}) can be constructed (Table 27.9). These ratios are termed the autonomic margin of safety of the relaxant in question. The higher the dose ratio, the lower is the likelihood of, or the greater the safety ratio for, the occurrence of the particular autonomic effect. The side effect is considered absent (none) in clinical practice if the safety ratio is greater than 5; it is weak or slight if the safety ratio is 3 or 4, moderate if 2 or 3, and strong or prominent if the ratio is 1 or less.

These autonomic responses are not reduced by slower injection of the muscle relaxant. They are dose related and additive over time if divided doses are given. If identical to the original dose, subsequent doses will produce a similar response (i.e., no tachyphylaxis will occur). This is not the case, however, when the side effect of histamine release is in question. Cardiovascular responses secondary to histamine release are decreased by slowing the injection rate, and the response undergoes rapid tachyphylaxis. The autonomic effects of NMBDs are summarized in Table 27.10.

Histamine Release. Quaternary ammonium compounds (e.g., NMBDs) are generally weaker histamine-releasing substances than are tertiary amines such as morphine. Nevertheless, when large doses of certain NMBDs are administered rapidly, erythema of the face, neck, and upper torso may develop, as well as a brief decrease in arterial pressure and a slight to moderate increase in heart rate. Bronchospasm in this setting is very rare. The clinical effects of histamine are seen when plasma concentrations increase 200% to 300% of baseline values, and these effects involve chemical displacement of the contents of mast cell granules containing histamine, prostaglandin, and possibly other vasoactive substances.[182] The serosal mast cell, located in the skin and connective tissue and near blood vessels and nerves, is principally involved in the degranulation process.[182]

The side effect of histamine release is most often noted following administration of the benzylisoquinolinium class of muscle relaxants, although it has also been noted in steroidal relaxants of low potency. The effect is usually of short duration (1-5 minutes), is dose related, and is

TABLE 27.10 Clinical Autonomic Effects of Neuromuscular Blocking Drugs

Drug Type	Autonomic Ganglia	Cardiac Muscarinic Receptors	Histamine Release
DEPOLARIZING SUBSTANCE			
Succinylcholine	Stimulates	Stimulates	Slight
BENZYLISOQUINOLINIUM COMPOUNDS			
Mivacurium	None	None	Slight
Atracurium	None	None	Slight
Cisatracurium	None	None	None
d-Tubocurarine	Blocks	None	Moderate
STEROIDAL COMPOUNDS			
Vecuronium	None	None	None
Rocuronium	None	Blocks weakly	None
Pancuronium	None	Blocks moderately	None

clinically insignificant in healthy patients. The hypotensive cardiovascular response to 0.6 mg/kg of dTc in humans is prevented both by antihistamines and by nonsteroidal anti-inflammatory drugs (e.g., aspirin).[183] The final step in dTc-induced hypotension is modulated by prostaglandins that are vasodilators.[183] This side effect can be reduced considerably by using a slower injection rate that results in lower peak plasma concentrations of dTc. It is also prevented by prophylaxis with combinations of histamine_1 and histamine_2 blockers.[184] If a minor degree of histamine release such as described earlier occurs after an initial dose of an NMBD, subsequent doses will generally cause no response at all, as long as they are no larger than the original dose. This is clinical evidence of tachyphylaxis, an important characteristic of histamine release. A much more significant degree of histamine release occurs during anaphylactoid or anaphylactic reactions, but these are very rare.

Clinical Cardiovascular Manifestations of Autonomic Mechanisms

HYPOTENSION. The hypotension seen with the use of atracurium and mivacurium results from histamine release, whereas dTc causes hypotension by histamine release and ganglionic blockade.[185,186] The effects of dTc occur closer to the dose required to achieve neuromuscular blockade.[113] The safety margin for histamine release is approximately three times greater for atracurium and mivacurium than it is for dTc.[182,183,186] Rapid administration of atracurium in doses greater than 0.4 mg/kg and of mivacurium in doses greater than 0.15 mg/kg has been associated with transient hypotension secondary to histamine release (Fig. 27.13).

TACHYCARDIA. Pancuronium causes a moderate increase in heart rate and, to a lesser extent, in cardiac output, with little or no change in systemic vascular resistance.[187] Pancuronium-induced tachycardia has been attributed to the following: (1) vagolytic action,[187] probably from inhibition of M_2 receptors; and (2) sympathetic stimulation that involves both direct (blockade of neuronal uptake of norepinephrine) and indirect (release of norepinephrine from adrenergic nerve endings) mechanisms.[188] In humans a decrease in plasma norepinephrine levels was surprisingly found after administration of either pancuronium or atropine.[189] The investigators postulated that the increase in heart rate or rate-pressure product occurs because pancuronium (or atropine) acts through baroreceptors to reduce sympathetic outflow.[189] More specifically, the vagolytic effect of pancuronium increases heart rate and hence blood pressure and cardiac output, in turn influencing the baroreceptors to decrease sympathetic tone. Support for this concept is provided by the finding that prior administration of atropine attenuates or eliminates the cardiovascular effects of pancuronium.[187] However, a positive chronotropic effect that places emphasis on the vagolytic mechanism has not been found in humans.[190] The tachycardia seen with benzylisoquinolinium compounds is the result of histamine release.

DYSRHYTHMIAS. Succinylcholine and dTc actually reduce the incidence of epinephrine-induced dysrhythmias.[191] Possibly because of enhanced atrioventricular conduction,[192] the incidence of dysrhythmias caused by pancuronium appears to increase during halothane anesthesia.[187] There are reports of rapid tachycardia (>150 beats/min) that progressed to atrioventricular dissociation in two patients anesthetized with halothane who also received pancuronium.[193] The only other factor common to those two patients was that both were taking tricyclic antidepressant drugs.

BRADYCARDIA. Several case reports described the occurrence of severe bradycardia and even asystole after vecuronium or atracurium administration.[194,195] All these cases were also associated with opioid coadministration. Subsequent studies indicated that administration of vecuronium or atracurium alone does not cause bradycardia.[196] When combined with other drugs that do cause bradycardia (e.g., fentanyl), however, the nonvagolytic relaxants such as vecuronium, cisatracurium, and atracurium allow this mechanism to occur unopposed. Thus the moderate vagolytic effect of pancuronium is often used to counteract opioid-induced bradycardia.

Respiratory Effects. The muscarinic cholinergic system plays an important role in regulating airway function. Five muscarinic receptors have been cloned,[197] three of which (M_1 to M_3) exist in the airways.[198] M_1 receptors are under

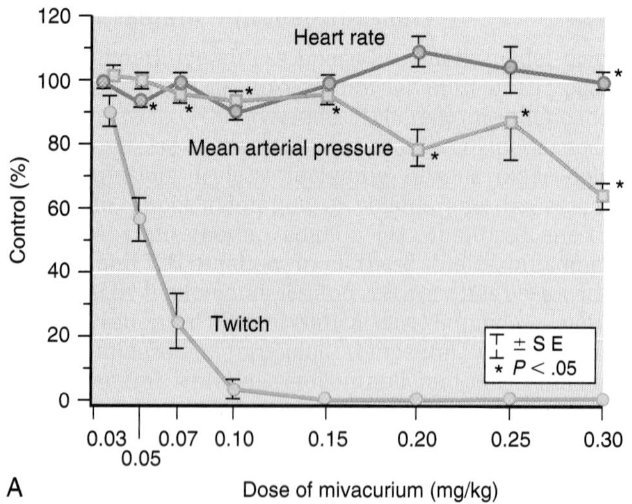

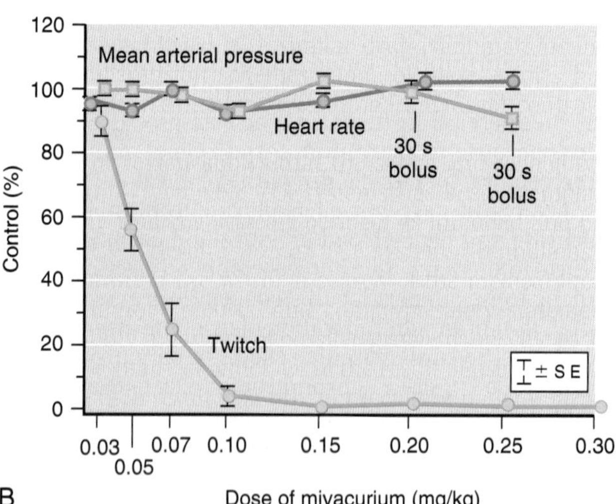

Fig. 27.13 Dose response to mivacurium in patients under nitrous oxide–oxygen-opioid anesthesia. Maximum changes at each dose are shown; $n = 9$ subjects per group. (A) With fast injection, a 15% to 20% decrease in arterial pressure occurred at 2.5 to 3 times the ED_{95} (0.20-0.25 mg/kg). (B) The changes were less than 10% when slower injection (30 seconds) was done. (From Savarese JJ, Ali HH, Basta SJ, et al. The cardiovascular effects of mivacurium chloride [BW B1090U] in patients receiving nitrous oxide–opiate-barbiturate anesthesia. *Anesthesiology.* 1989;70:386–394.)

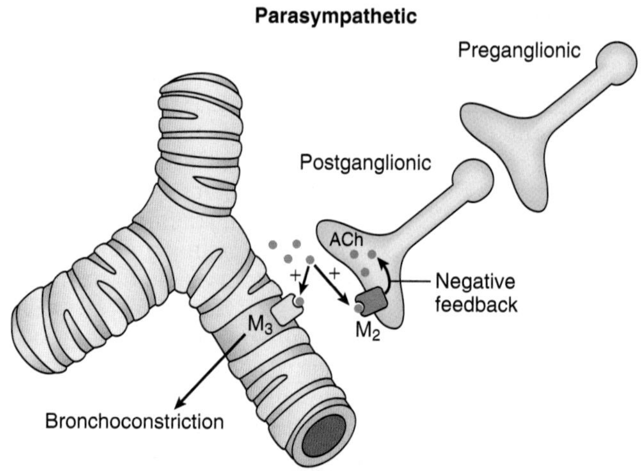

Fig. 27.14 The muscarinic *(M_3)* receptors are located postsynaptically on airway smooth muscle. Acetylcholine *(ACh)* stimulates M_3 receptors to cause contraction. M_2 muscarinic receptors are located presynaptically at the postganglionic parasympathetic nerve endings, and they function in a negative-feedback mechanism to limit the release of ACh.

sympathetic control, and they mediate bronchodilation.[199] M_2 receptors are located presynaptically (Fig. 27.14), at the postganglionic parasympathetic nerve endings, and they function in a negative-feedback mechanism to limit the release of acetylcholine. The M_3 receptors, which are located postsynaptically (see Fig. 27.14), mediate contraction of the airway smooth muscles (i.e., bronchoconstriction).[199] Nondepolarizing NMBDs have different antagonistic activities at both M_2 and M_3 receptors.[200] For example, blockade of M_3 receptors on airway smooth muscle inhibits vagally induced bronchoconstriction (i.e., causes bronchodilation), whereas blockade of M_2 receptors results in increased release of acetylcholine that acts on M_3 receptors, thus causing bronchoconstriction.

The affinity of the compound rapacuronium to block M_2 receptors is 15 times higher than its affinity to block M_3 receptors.[200] This explains the high incidence (>9%) of severe bronchospasm[201-203] reported with this drug that resulted in its withdrawal from the market. In laboratory animals (guinea pig), CW 1759-50 is reported to have five times greater safety at both M_2 and M_3 receptors than rapacuronium.[11b]

The administration of benzylisoquinolinium NMBDs (with the exception of cisatracurium) is associated with histamine release, which may result in increased airway resistance and bronchospasm in patients with hyperactive airway disease.

Allergic Reactions. The frequency of life-threatening anaphylactic (immune-mediated) or anaphylactoid reactions occurring during anesthesia has been estimated at 1 in 10,000 to 20,000 anesthetic procedures, whereas it is estimated at 1 in 6500 administrations of NMBDs in some countries.[204,205] In France, the most common causes of anaphylaxis in patients who experienced allergic reactions were reported to be NMBDs (60.6%), antibiotics (18.2%), dyes (5.4%), and latex (5.2%).[206,206a] Patients were sensitized to 2 or more NMBDS in approximately 50% of the cases and no cross-sensitivity could be predicted without skin testing. Anaphylactic reactions are mediated through immune responses involving immunoglobulin E (IgE) antibodies fixed to mast cells. Anaphylactoid reactions are not immune mediated and represent exaggerated pharmacologic responses in very rare and very sensitive individuals.

However, anaphylaxis to nondepolarizing NMBDs is not uncommon in patients without any previous exposure to any nondepolarizing NMBDs. Cross-reactivity occurs between NMBDs and food, cosmetics, disinfectants, and industrial materials.[207] Sensitization to nondepolarizing NMBDs may also be related to pholcodine, a cough-relieving medicine. Cross-reactivity is seen in 70% of patients with a history of anaphylaxis to an NMBD.[206] Six years after the withdrawal of pholcodine from the Norwegian market, the prevalence of IgE sensitization to NMBDs (succinylcholine) decreased significantly.[207a]

Steroidal compounds (e.g., rocuronium, vecuronium, or pancuronium) result in no significant histamine release.[186] For example, four times the ED_{95} of rocuronium (1.2

mg/kg) causes no significant histamine release.[208] Nevertheless, rocuronium and succinylcholine are reportedly associated with a 43.1% and 22.6% incidence, respectively, of anaphylaxis in France.[206] Rose and Fisher classified rocuronium and atracurium as having intermediate levels of risk for causing allergic reactions.[209] These investigators also noted that the increased number of reports of anaphylaxis with rocuronium is in line with the market share of that drug's usage. Watkins stated, "The much higher incidence of rocuronium reactions reported in France is currently inexplicable and is likely to remain so if investigators continue to seek a purely antibody-mediated response as an explanation of all anaphylactoid reaction presentations."[210] All nondepolarizing NMBDs may elicit anaphylaxis. More recent publications have highlighted the need for standardization of diagnostic procedures of anaphylactic reactions. Biochemical tests should be performed rapidly after occurrence of an anaphylactic reaction. An early increase in plasma histamine is observed 60 to 90 minutes after anaphylactic reactions. Serum tryptase concentration typically reaches a peak between 15 and 120 minutes, depending on the severity of the reaction, and is much more specific than histamine as a marker of anaphylactic reaction. It is highly suggestive of mast cell activation. Skin testing remains the gold standard for detection of the culprit agent.[77a] For many years, dilution thresholds have been debated. For instance, Laxenaire used a 1:10 dilution of rocuronium for interdermal skin testing,[212] whereas Rose and Fisher used a 1:1000 dilution.[209] Levy and associates showed that rocuronium in a 1:10 dilution can produce false-positive results in intradermal testing and suggested that rocuronium be diluted at least 100-fold to prevent such results.[213] The authors also reported that high concentrations ($\geq 10^{-4}$ M) of both rocuronium and cisatracurium were capable of producing a wheal-and-flare response to intradermal testing, which was associated with mild to moderate mast cell degranulation in the cisatracurium group only.[213] However, in contrast to control patients, skin tests with nondepolarizing NMBDs that were performed in patients who had an anaphylactic reaction were considered reliable. In the case of suspected anaphylactic reaction to any NMBD, it is mandatory to complete investigation for cross-reactivity with other commercially available NMBDs to identify safe alternative regimens.

All NMBDs can cause noncompetitive inhibition of histamine-N-methyltransferase, but the concentrations required for that inhibition greatly exceed those that would be used clinically, except in the case of vecuronium, with which the effect becomes manifest at 0.1 to 0.2 mg/kg.[214] This finding could explain the occurrence of occasional severe bronchospasm in patients after receiving vecuronium.[215] For goals of treatment of anaphylactic reactions, see Chapters 5 and 6.

DRUG INTERACTIONS AND OTHER FACTORS AFFECTING RESPONSE TO NEUROMUSCULAR BLOCKERS

A drug-drug interaction is an in vivo phenomenon that occurs when the administration of one drug alters the effects or kinetics of another drug. In vitro physical or chemical incompatibilities are *not* considered drug interactions.[216]

Many drugs interact with NMBDs or their antagonists, or both, and it is beyond the scope of this chapter to review them all.[216,217] Some of the more important drug interactions with NMBDs and their antagonists are discussed in the following sections.

Interactions Among Nondepolarizing Neuromuscular Blocking Drugs

Mixtures of two nondepolarizing NMBDs are considered to be either additive or synergistic. Antagonistic interactions have not been reported in this class of drugs. Additive interactions have been demonstrated after administration of chemically related drugs, such as atracurium and mivacurium,[218] or after coadministration of various pairs of steroidal NMBDs.[98] Conversely, combinations of structurally dissimilar (e.g., a steroidal with a benzylisoquinolinium) NMBDs, such as the combinations of pancuronium and dTc,[219] pancuronium and metocurine,[219] rocuronium and mivacurium,[142] or rocuronium and cisatracurium,[109] produce a synergistic response. An additional advantage (rapid onset and short duration) is noted for mivacurium-rocuronium combinations.[142] Although the precise mechanisms underlying a synergistic interaction are not known, hypotheses that have been put forward include the existence of multiple binding sites at the neuromuscular junction (presynaptic and postsynaptic receptors)[220] and the nonequivalence of binding affinities of the two α subunits (α_H and α_L). Further, inhibition of butyrylcholinesterase by pancuronium results in decreased plasma clearance of mivacurium and marked potentiation of the neuromuscular blockade.[221]

The pharmacodynamic response to the use of two different nondepolarizing NMBDs during the course of anesthesia depends not only on the specific drugs used but also on the sequence of their administration.[222,223] Approximately three half-lives are required for a clinical changeover (so that 95% of the first drug has been cleared) and for the duration of the blockade to begin to take on the characteristics of the second drug. After the administration of pancuronium, recovery from the first two maintenance doses of vecuronium is reportedly prolonged, although this effect becomes negligible by the third dose.[222] Similarly, Naguib and colleagues noted that the mean duration of the first maintenance dose of mivacurium to 10% recovery of the first twitch was significantly longer after atracurium (25 minutes) than after mivacurium (14.2 minutes).[218] However, the duration of the second maintenance dose of mivacurium after atracurium (18.3 minutes) was similar to that of mivacurium after mivacurium (14.6 minutes).

The apparent prolongation of action of the first maintenance dose of mivacurium administered after atracurium,[218] and of those reported with vecuronium after pancuronium,[222,223] is not related to synergism. Combinations of atracurium and mivacurium[218] and of vecuronium and pancuronium[98] are simply additive. However, this prolongation in the duration of action could be attributed to the relative concentrations of these drugs at the receptor site. Because most receptors remain occupied by the drug administered initially, the clinical profile depends on the kinetics or dynamics (or both) of the drug administered first, rather than on those of the second (maintenance)

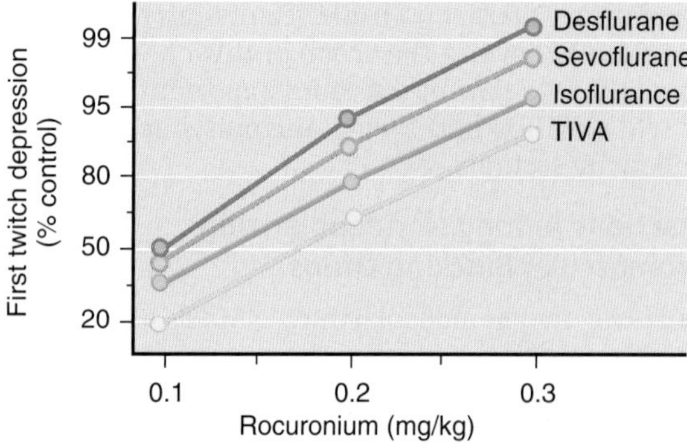

Fig. 27.15 Cumulative dose-response curves for rocuronium-induced neuromuscular blockade during 1.5 minimum alveolar concentration anesthesia with desflurane, sevoflurane, isoflurane, and total intravenous anesthesia *(TIVA)*. (From Wulf H, Ledowski T, Linstedt U, et al. Neuromuscular blocking effects of rocuronium during desflurane, isoflurane, and sevoflurane anaesthesia. *Can J Anaesth*. 1998;45:526–532, with permission from the *Canadian Journal of Anaesthesia*.)

drug. However, with further incremental doses of the second drug, a progressively larger proportion of the receptors is occupied by that second drug, and its clinical profile becomes evident.

Interactions Between Succinylcholine and Nondepolarizing Neuromuscular Blocking Drugs

The interaction between succinylcholine and nondepolarizing NMBDs depends on the order of administration and the doses used.[81,224,225] Small doses of different nondepolarizing NMBDs administered before succinylcholine to prevent fasciculations have an antagonistic effect on the development of subsequent depolarizing block produced by succinylcholine.[27,81] Therefore it is recommended that the dose of succinylcholine be increased after the administration of a defasciculating dose of a nondepolarizing NMBD.[27]

Studies of the effects of administering succinylcholine before nondepolarizing NMBDs have produced conflicting results. Several investigators reported potentiation of the effects of pancuronium,[224] vecuronium, and atracurium[225] by prior administration of succinylcholine. In contrast, other investigators found no significant influence of succinylcholine on subsequent administration of pancuronium, rocuronium, or mivacurium.[81,226,227]

Interactions With Inhaled Anesthetics

Deep anesthesia induced with potent volatile anesthetics (in the absence of neuromuscular blockade) may cause a slight reduction of neuromuscular transmission, as measured by depression of sensitive indicators of clinical neuromuscular function, such as tetanus and TOF ratio.[228] Inhaled anesthetics also enhance the neuromuscular blocking effects of nondepolarizing NMBDs. Inhaled anesthetics decrease the required dose of NMBDs, and prolong both the duration of action of the NMBD and recovery from neuromuscular block,[229] depending on the duration of anesthesia,[228,230,231] the specific inhaled anesthetic,[232] and the concentration (dose) given.[233] The rank order of potentiation is desflurane > sevoflurane > isoflurane > halothane > nitrous oxide/barbiturate/opioid or propofol anesthesia (Fig. 27.15).[234-236]

The greater clinical muscle-relaxing effect produced by less potent anesthetics is mainly caused by their larger aqueous concentrations.[237] Desflurane and sevoflurane have low blood-gas and tissue-gas solubility, so equilibrium between the end-tidal concentration and the neuromuscular junction is reached more rapidly with these anesthetics than with older inhaled anesthetics.

The interaction between volatile anesthetics and NMBDs is one of pharmacodynamics, not pharmacokinetics.[238] The proposed mechanisms behind this interaction include (1) a central effect on α motoneurons and interneuronal synapses,[239] (2) inhibition of postsynaptic nAChR,[240] and (3) augmentation of the antagonist's affinity at the receptor site.[237]

Interactions With Antibiotics

Most antibiotics can cause neuromuscular blockade in the absence of NMBDs. The aminoglycoside antibiotics, the polymyxins, and lincomycin and clindamycin primarily inhibit the prejunctional release of acetylcholine and also depress postjunctional nAChR sensitivity to acetylcholine.[241] The tetracyclines, in contrast, exhibit postjunctional activity only. When combined with NMBDs, the aforementioned antibiotics can potentiate neuromuscular blockade.[242] The cephalosporins and penicillins have not been reported to potentiate neuromuscular blockade. Because antagonism of neuromuscular blockade with neostigmine has been reported to be more difficult after the administration of aminoglycosides,[243] ventilation should be controlled until the neuromuscular blockade terminates spontaneously. Ca^{2+} should not be used to hasten the recovery of neuromuscular function for two reasons: the antagonism it produces is not sustained, and it may prevent the antibacterial effect of the antibiotics.

Temperature

Hypothermia prolongs the duration of action of nondepolarizing NMBDs.[244-246] The force of contraction of the adductor pollicis decreases by 10% to 16% per degree Celsius decrease in muscle temperature lower than 35.2°C.[247,248] To maintain the muscle temperature at or higher than 35.2°C, the central temperature must be maintained above 36.0°C.[244] The mechanical response recovery to 10% twitch height with 0.1 mg/kg of vecuronium increases from 28 minutes at a mean central temperature of 36.4°C to 64 minutes at 34.4°C.[244] The mechanism or mechanisms underlying this prolongation may be pharmacodynamic or pharmacokinetic, or both.[246] They include diminished renal and hepatic excretion, changing volumes of distribution, altered local diffusion receptor affinity, changes in pH at the neuromuscular junction, and the net effect of cooling on the various components of neuromuscular transmission.[244,249] Hypothermia decreases the plasma clearance and prolongs the duration of action of rocuronium and vecuronium.[246] Temperature-related differences in the pharmacodynamics of vecuronium have also been reported. The k_{e0} decreases (0.023/min/°C) with lower temperature, a finding suggesting slightly delayed equilibration of drug between the circulation and the neuromuscular junction during hypothermia.[246] The Hofmann elimination process of atracurium is slowed by a decrease in pH and especially by a decrease in temperature.[250] In fact, atracurium's duration of action is markedly prolonged by hypothermia.[245] For instance, the duration of action of a dose of 0.5 mg/kg atracurium is 44 minutes at 37°C but 68 minutes at 34.0°C when evoked mechanical responses are monitored.

Changes in temperature also affect the interpretation of the results of monitoring neuromuscular blockade. For example, the duration of action of vecuronium measured in an arm cooled to a skin temperature of 27°C is prolonged, and monitoring by PTC in that arm is unreliable.[251] In the same patient, TOF responses are different if the arms are at different temperatures, and the correlation of responses in the two arms becomes progressively poorer as the temperature difference between the arms increases.[252]

The efficacy of neostigmine is not altered by mild hypothermia.[253-255] Hypothermia does not change the clearance, maximum effect, or duration of action of neostigmine in volunteers.[255] Mild hypothermia prolonged sugammadex reversal of deep rocuronium block by 46 seconds, a prolongation considered clinically acceptable.[255a]

Interactions With Magnesium and Calcium

Magnesium sulfate, given for treatment of preeclampsia and eclamptic toxemia, potentiates the neuromuscular blockade induced by nondepolarizing NMBDs.[256,257] After a dose of 40 mg/kg of magnesium sulfate, the ED_{50} of vecuronium was reduced by 25%, the onset time was nearly halved, and the recovery time nearly doubled.[257] Neostigmine-induced recovery is also attenuated in patients treated with magnesium.[256] The mechanisms underlying the enhancement of nondepolarizing block by magnesium probably involve both prejunctional and postjunctional effects. High magnesium concentrations inhibit Ca^{2+} channels at the presynaptic nerve terminals that trigger the release of acetylcholine.[16] Further, magnesium ions have an inhibitory effect on postjunctional potentials and cause decreased excitability of muscle fiber membranes. In patients receiving magnesium, the dose of nondepolarizing NMBDs must be reduced and carefully titrated using an objective monitor to ensure adequate recovery of neuromuscular function prior to tracheal extubation.

The interaction between magnesium and succinylcholine is controversial, with some reports suggesting that magnesium antagonizes the block produced by succinylcholine.[258] Ca^{2+} triggers the release of acetylcholine from the motor nerve terminal and enhances excitation-contraction coupling in muscle.[16] Increasing Ca^{2+} concentrations decreased the sensitivity to dTc and pancuronium in a muscle-nerve model.[259] In hyperparathyroidism, hypercalcemia is associated with decreased sensitivity to atracurium and thus a shortened time course of neuromuscular blockade.[260]

Interactions With Lithium

Lithium is used for treatment of bipolar affective disorder (manic-depressive illness). The lithium ion resembles Na^+, K^+, magnesium, and Ca^{2+} ions, and therefore may affect the distribution and kinetics of all these electrolytes.[261] Lithium enters cells via Na^+ channels and tends to accumulate within the cells.

By its activation of K^+ channels, lithium inhibits neuromuscular transmission presynaptically and muscular contraction postsynaptically.[262] The combination of lithium and pipecuronium results in a synergistic inhibition of neuromuscular transmission, whereas the combination of lithium and succinylcholine results in additive inhibition.[262] Prolongation of neuromuscular blockade was reported in patients taking lithium carbonate and receiving both depolarizing and nondepolarizing NMBDs.[263] Only one report did not demonstrate prolongation of recovery from succinylcholine in patients receiving lithium.[264] In patients who are stabilized on lithium therapy and undergoing surgery, NMBDs should be administered in incremental and reduced doses and titrated to the degree of blockade required.

Interactions With Local Anesthetic and Antidysrhythmic Drugs

Local anesthetics act on the presynaptic and postsynaptic part of the neuromuscular junction. In large intravenous doses, most local anesthetics block neuromuscular transmission; in smaller doses, they enhance the neuromuscular blockade produced by both nondepolarizing and depolarizing NMBDs.[265] The ability of neostigmine to antagonize a combined local anesthetic–neuromuscular blockade has not been studied. Procaine also inhibits butyrylcholinesterase and may augment the effects of succinylcholine and mivacurium by decreasing their hydrolysis by the enzyme.

In small intravenous doses, local anesthetics depress posttetanic potentiation, and this is thought to be a neural prejunctional effect.[266] With larger doses, local anesthetics block acetylcholine-induced muscular contractions, a finding suggesting that local anesthetics have a stabilizing effect on the postjunctional membrane.[267] Procaine displaces Ca^{2+} from the sarcolemma and thus inhibits caffeine-induced contracture of skeletal muscle.[268] Most of these mechanisms of action probably apply to all local anesthetics.

Several drugs used for the treatment of dysrhythmias augment the blockade induced by NMBDs. Single-fiber electromyography found that verapamil and amlodipine impair neuromuscular transmission in subjects without neuromuscular disease.[269] Clinical reports suggested potentiation of neuromuscular block with verapamil[270] and impaired reversal of vecuronium in a patient receiving disopyramide.[271] However, the clinical significance of these interactions is probably minor.

Interactions With Antiepileptic Drugs

Anticonvulsants have a depressant action on acetylcholine release at the neuromuscular junction.[272,273] Patients receiving long-term anticonvulsant therapy demonstrated resistance to nondepolarizing NMBDs (except mivacurium[274] and probably atracurium as well[273]), as evidenced by accelerated recovery from neuromuscular blockade and the need for increased doses to achieve complete neuromuscular blockade. Vecuronium clearance is increased two-fold in patients receiving long-term carbamazepine therapy.[275] Other investigators, however, attribute this resistance to the increased binding (i.e., decreased free fraction) of the NMBDs to α_1-acid glycoproteins or to upregulation of neuromuscular acetylcholine receptors (or to both mechanisms).[276] The latter could also explain the hypersensitivity seen with succinylcholine.[277] The slight prolongation of succinylcholine's action in patients taking anticonvulsants has few clinical implications. Conversely, the potential hyperkalemic response to succinylcholine in the presence of receptor upregulation is of concern.

Interactions With Diuretics

Early results showed that in patients undergoing renal transplantation, the intensity and duration of dTc neuromuscular blockade was increased after a dose of furosemide (1 mg/kg intravenously).[278]

Furosemide reduced the concentration of dTc required to achieve 50% twitch tension depression in the indirectly stimulated rat diaphragm and intensified the neuromuscular blockade produced by dTc and succinylcholine.[279] Furosemide appears to inhibit the production of cyclic adenosine monophosphate. In addition, the breakdown of adenosine triphosphate is inhibited, resulting in reduced output of acetylcholine. Acetazolamide antagonized the effects of anticholinesterases in the rat phrenic-diaphragm preparation.[280] However, in one report, 1 mg/kg of furosemide facilitated recovery of the evoked twitch response after pancuronium.[281] Long-term furosemide treatment had no effect on either dTc- or pancuronium-induced neuromuscular blockade.[282]

In contrast, mannitol appears to have no effect on a nondepolarizing neuromuscular blockade. Increasing urine output by the administration of mannitol or other osmotic or tubular diuretics has no effect on the rate at which dTc and presumably other NMBDs are eliminated in the urine.[283]

Interactions With Other Drugs

Dantrolene, a drug used for the treatment of malignant hyperthermia, prevents Ca^{2+} release from the sarcoplasmic reticulum and blocks excitation-contraction coupling. Although dantrolene does not block neuromuscular transmission, the mechanical response to stimulation is depressed, resulting in potentiation of nondepolarizing neuromuscular blockade.[284]

Azathioprine, an immunodepressant drug that is used in patients undergoing renal transplantation, has a minor antagonistic action on muscle relaxant–induced neuromuscular blockade.[285]

Steroids antagonize the effects of nondepolarizing NMBDs in both humans[286] and animals.[287] Possible mechanisms for this interaction include facilitation of acetylcholine release because of the effect of steroids on the presynaptic motor nerve terminal.[288] Other reports, however, described a noncompetitive inhibition and channel blockade of the nAChR.[289] Endogenous steroids act noncompetitively on nAChRs.[290] Prolonged treatment with a combination of corticosteroids and NMBDs can result in prolonged weakness in patients receiving critical care (see the later section on NMBDs and weakness syndromes in critically ill patients).

Antiestrogenic drugs such as tamoxifen appear to potentiate the effects of nondepolarizing NMBDs.[291]

Special Populations

PEDIATRIC PATIENTS

The development of the neuromuscular junction is not complete at birth.[16] In humans, maturation of neuromuscular transmission occurs after the first 2 months of age, although immature junctions have been found up to 2 years of age. The main evolution during the first months of life is that the fetal receptors located outside the neuromuscular junction will disappear and will be replaced by mature receptors with ε subunits instead of γ subunits. These changes suggest that that the neonate's neuromuscular junction may exhibit evidence of its immaturity by changes in response to NMBDs, although NMBDs can be used safely in term and preterm infants.

The routine administration of succinylcholine to healthy children should be discontinued. In apparently healthy children, intractable cardiac arrest with hyperkalemia, rhabdomyolysis, and acidosis may develop after succinylcholine administration, particularly in patients with unsuspected muscular dystrophy of the Duchenne type[292] (see the section on complications of succinylcholine).

Significant age-related differences in the potency of nondepolarizing NMBDs exist in infants and children when compared with adults. Children require higher doses of nondepolarizing NMBDs than any other age group of patients. In infants less than 1 year old, the ED_{95} at the adductor pollicis is approximately 30% less than in older children. It is not apparent from older studies whether the neonate is more sensitive than adults to nondepolarizing NMBDs,[293] although most of the studies showed a wider range of dosage requirement in the neonate. These apparent discrepancies have been explained in studies by Fisher and associates on the pharmacokinetics and pharmacodynamics of NMBDs in infants, children, and adults.[294-296] Neonates and infants are more sensitive than adults to the neuromuscular blocking effects of dTc.[294] Plasma concentrations required to achieve a desired level of neuromuscular blockade are 57% and 32% lower in neonates and infants, respectively, when compared with children. However, the dosage should not be decreased as much because neonates and infants have a larger volume of distribution at steady state. This increased volume of distribution results from the increase in extracellular fluid volume during the first months of life. This increase, in association with a lower elimination clearance, contributes to a longer elimination half-life.[294,297] In infants, less frequent dosing (longer dosing intervals) of nondepolarizing NMBDs may be required than in older children.

Atracurium, vecuronium, cisatracurium, rocuronium, and mivacurium are commonly administered to children because many surgical procedures are of short duration in children and are compatible with the duration of action of a single intubating dose. Onset time of neuromuscular block is faster in infants (30%) and children (40%) when compared with adults. This age-related effect is probably caused by circulatory factors such as the relative decrease in cardiac output and increase in circulation time with age.

As for long-acting NMBDs, the sensitivity of infants to vecuronium is greater than that of children (ED_{95} 0.047 mg/kg vs. 0.081 mg/kg, respectively).[298,299] An increased duration of action in infants is most likely secondary to the increased volume of distribution of vecuronium because its clearance is unchanged.[295,297] An age-dependent prolongation of action has been demonstrated in infants. A dose of 0.1 mg/kg of vecuronium produces almost a complete neuromuscular block of approximately 60 minutes' duration in infants but of only 20 minutes' duration in children and adults. Vecuronium therefore acts as a long-acting muscle NMBD in the neonate.[295,297]

In contrast, the duration of action of atracurium is not significantly different in the pediatric patient from that in the adult.[300] As with vecuronium and dTc, the volume of distribution is increased in infants.[296] However, the clearance of atracurium is also more rapid.[296] Therefore the same dose (0.5-0.6 mg/kg) can be used in infants, children, and adults for tracheal intubation without any major differences among the three groups in the drug's duration of action. Atracurium recovery from neuromuscular blockade is little affected by age in pediatric patients more than 1 month old. Histamine release and the occurrence of untoward reactions caused by atracurium are less frequent in children than in adults. In children, a dose of 0.1 μg/kg of cisatracurium has an onset just longer than 2 minutes and a clinical duration of approximately 30 minutes during balanced or halothane anesthesia.[301] The calculated ED_{95} doses of cisatracurium in infants and children are 43 and 47 μg/kg, respectively.[302] The mean infusion rate necessary to maintain 90% to 99% neuromuscular blockade is also similar in infants and children.[302]

Rocuronium in adults is an intermediate-acting NMBD with a faster onset of action than other nondepolarizing NMBDs, and this is also true in infants and children.[303,304] The ED_{95} is approximately 0.4 mg/kg in children; it is approximately 20% to 30% greater than that in adults, but its onset is faster in adults.[304] In children, 0.6 mg/kg of rocuronium produces better conditions for rapid tracheal intubation (approximately 60 seconds) than does 0.1 mg/kg of vecuronium (approximately 100 seconds) or 0.5 mg/kg of atracurium (approximately 180 seconds).[303] Evidence indicates that, even during sevoflurane induction in infants, the addition of 0.3 mg/kg rocuronium significantly improves intubating conditions and significantly decreases the frequency of respiratory adverse events such as desaturation because of laryngospasm during induction.[305] As with adults, for rapid sequence induction and intubation (60 seconds) in the presence of a full stomach, a 1.2 mg/kg dose of rocuronium is suggested to provide rapid, excellent intubating conditions in pediatric patients.

The rate of recovery of intermediate- or short-acting NMBDs is faster than that of long-acting drugs in children. A neostigmine dose of 30 μg/kg in children is quite comparable to the usual dose of 40 μg/kg in adults and provides satisfactory antagonism of nondepolarizing NMBD. Neostigmine-assisted recovery is dependent on age and is more rapid in children than either infants or adults.[305a] Several studies have demonstrated that when children's tracheas were extubated using clinical criteria of recovery, the TOF ratio did not exceed 0.50 to 0.60, whereas a TOF ratio greater than 0.90 is required to guarantee full recovery from neuromuscular block. These results highlight the need for objective (quantitative) assessment of neuromuscular block, even in infants and children, because of their sensitivity and variability in their responsiveness to nondepolarizing NMBDs.

OLDER PATIENTS

The pharmacodynamics of NMBDs may be altered in older patients. Physiologic changes such as decreases in total body water and lean body mass, increases in total body fat, decreases in hepatic and renal blood flow and hepatic enzyme activity, and decreases in glomerular filtration rate (≈20%/year in adults) typically accompany the aging process. These changes may account for the altered responses of older adults to NMBDs. Some physiologic and anatomic changes at the neuromuscular junction also occur with aging. These include an increase in the distance between the junctional axon and the motor end plate, flattening of the folds of the motor end plate, decreased concentration of acetylcholine receptors at the motor end plate, decrease in the amount of acetylcholine in each vesicle in the prejunctional axon, and decreased release of acetylcholine from the preterminal axon in response to a neural impulse.[16]

Several studies found no differences in the initial dose requirement for nondepolarizing muscle relaxants in older adults. The dose-response curves of atracurium, pancuronium, and vecuronium were shifted slightly to the right of the curves for the younger adult subjects; however, no significant differences were noted. After a bolus dose of pancuronium, no significant difference was observed in any of the plasma concentrations corresponding to a fixed degree of neuromuscular block. Such results confirm that nondepolarizing muscle relaxants are as potent in older as in young adult patients. The onset of neuromuscular block can be delayed and can be correlated with age.[306] This age-related effect is probably caused by circulatory factors such as the decrease in cardiac output and increase in circulation time in older adults. These factors induce slower biophase equilibration with plasma. The onset of rocuronium neuromuscular block was prolonged to 3.7 from 3.1 minutes in older adults. Similarly, the onset of cisatracurium is delayed approximately 1 minute in this age group.

A prolongation of the duration of action of nondepolarizing muscle relaxants and a decrease in dose requirements for the maintenance of neuromuscular block have been observed with several currently available muscle relaxants in older adults. These results are explained by pharmacokinetic changes in this population. The distribution and elimination may be altered by any of the multitude of physiologic changes that accompany the aging process. The effect of aging alone, as opposed to disease states often associated with the aging process, may be difficult to distinguish in identifying mechanisms of altered NMBD action in older adults.

Pancuronium,[307] vecuronium,[295,308] and rocuronium[177] depend on the kidney or the liver (or both) for their metabolism and elimination. Therefore they all show altered pharmacodynamics and pharmacokinetics in older patients. Pancuronium has delayed recovery in older adults because of decreased plasma clearance secondary to delayed urinary excretion. Vecuronium dose requirements to maintain a constant neuromuscular block are decreased by approximately 36% in patients older than 60 years, and spontaneous recovery is significantly longer in older patients.[25] Plasma clearance is reduced by more than 50% and elimination half-life prolonged by 60% in older patients.[308] The prolongation of vecuronium action appears to be secondary to decreased drug elimination consistent with age-associated decreases in hepatic and renal blood flows. The duration of action of rocuronium and the recovery index are also increased in older adults. The prolongation of action can be explained by a 27% decrease in plasma clearance.

In the case of drugs whose elimination is independent of hepatic or renal blood flow, pharmacokinetics and pharmacodynamics should not be altered significantly by age. Atracurium has multiple routes of elimination. Degradation by Hofmann elimination and ester hydrolysis is independent of the liver and the kidney and is not affected by age. The only pharmacokinetic change is a slight increase of the volume of distribution at steady state leading to a modestly increased elimination half-life. Consequently, the duration of action, the recovery index, and the dose requirement during a continuous infusion are independent of age. Cisatracurium is mainly eliminated by Hofmann elimination, and unlike atracurium, cisatracurium does not undergo hydrolysis by specific esterases. It exhibits a slightly delayed onset of effect in older patients because of slower biophase equilibration. Clearances are not decreased in patients of advanced age. The slight prolongation of the elimination half-life of the drug in older adults is secondary to an increased volume of distribution at steady state (+10%). These minor pharmacokinetic changes are not associated with changes in the recovery profile in older patients.

Butyrylcholinesterase activity in older adults, although still in the normal range, is approximately 26% lower than that in young adults.[309] Because mivacurium is metabolized by butyrylcholinesterase, its clearance is likely to be slightly reduced in older patients, thus resulting in a 20% to 25% longer duration of action,[310] as well as a decreased infusion requirement to maintain a stable depth of block. Succinylcholine metabolism is unaffected by these changes.

In general, when maintaining neuromuscular blockade with nondepolarizing NMBDs in older patients, one can expect that, with the exception of atracurium and cisatracurium, the dosing interval will be increased to maintain the desired depth of neuromuscular blockade. The choice of drug and monitoring the depth of blockade are exceptionally important in this population because recovery of neuromuscular function is generally delayed in older patients. Inadequate or incomplete recovery of muscle strength after the use of pancuronium is associated with an increased incidence of perioperative pulmonary complications in this patient population.[129] The clear relationship between incomplete recovery from neuromuscular block and occurrence of critical respiratory events in the PACU highlights the need for objective monitoring to ensure recovery of neuromuscular block in older patients.

OBESE PATIENTS

The level of plasma pseudocholinesterase activity and the volume of extracellular fluid, which are the main determinants of the duration of action of succinylcholine, are increased in obese patients. For complete neuromuscular paralysis and predictable intubating conditions, a 1-mg/kg dose based on total-body weight (TBW) is recommended.[311]

Initial studies showed that obese subjects needed significantly more pancuronium than nonobese patients to maintain a constant 90% depression of twitch height. However, when corrected for body surface area (BSA), no significant difference was noted in dose requirement to maintain neuromuscular block.

The use of NMBDs with an intermediate duration of action should be preferred. Vecuronium doses based on TBW induce a prolonged duration of action in obese patients, although vecuronium pharmacokinetics is unaltered by obesity. The prolonged recovery in obese patients can be explained by the larger total dose of vecuronium administered to these patients. With larger doses, when administration is based on TBW, recovery occurs during the elimination phase when plasma concentration decreases more slowly than during the distribution phase.[312] The pharmacokinetics of rocuronium is not altered by obesity. In the same way, the duration of action of rocuronium is significantly prolonged when the dose is calculated according to TBW. In contrast, when rocuronium is dosed according to ideal body weight (IBW), the clinical duration is less than half.[313,314]

A correlation exists between the duration of action of atracurium and TBW when the dose is given as milligrams per kilogram of TBW. The clinical duration of action is doubled when the drug is given based on TBW versus IBW. There is little difference between obese and normal-weight patients in atracurium elimination half-life (19.8 vs. 19.7 minutes), volume of distribution at steady state (8.6 vs. 8.5 L), and total clearance (444 vs. 404 mL/min).[315] The finding that IBW avoids prolonged recovery of atracurium-induced blockade can be explained by an unchanged muscle mass and an unchanged volume of distribution in morbidly obese patients compared with normal-weight patients.[316] The duration of cisatracurium is also prolonged in obese patients when the drug is given on the basis of TBW versus IBW.

In summary, nondepolarizing NMBDs should be given to obese patients on the basis of IBW rather than on their actual body weight, to ensure that these patients are not receiving relative overdoses and to avoid prolonged recovery. When using maintenance doses, objective monitoring is strongly recommended to avoid accumulation.

SEVERE RENAL DISEASE

NMBDs contain quaternary ammonium groups that make them very hydrophilic. They are therefore usually completely ionized at a pH of 7.4 and are poorly bound to plasma proteins. The predominant pathway of elimination of steroidal muscle relaxants is ultrafiltration by the glomeruli before urinary excretion. Renal failure influences the pharmacologic characteristics of nondepolarizing NMBDs by producing either decreased renal elimination of the drug or its metabolites. Only atracurium, cisatracurium, and, to some extent, vecuronium are independent of renal function. Succinylcholine elimination is mainly independent of kidney function. However, succinylcholine is metabolized by plasma cholinesterases, and concentrations may be slightly decreased in patients with severe renal failure (Table 27.11). The decrease in plasma cholinesterase activity is always moderate (30%) and does not result in prolongation of succinylcholine-induced neuromuscular block. Succinylcholine induces a transient increase in plasma K^+ concentration (<0.5 mmol/L). Therefore succinylcholine is not contraindicated in severe renal failure when plasma K^+ concentrations are within the normal range. The duration of action of NMBDs may be prolonged in patients with renal failure.

Renal failure does not alter the sensitivity (dose response) of patients to the neuromuscular blocking action of pancuronium,[317] atracurium,[318] vecuronium,[319] or rocuronium.[320] All long-acting muscle relaxants are eliminated predominantly through the kidney, and renal failure is associated with reduced plasma clearance and increased elimination half-life for these drugs as well.[103] The elimination half-life of pancuronium is increased by 500% in patients with severe renal failure. As a consequence of these

TABLE 27.11 Pharmacokinetics of Neuromuscular Blocking Drugs in Patients With Normal Renal Function or Renal Failure

	PLASMA CLEARANCE (ML/KG/MIN)		VOLUME OF DISTRIBUTION (ML/KG)		ELIMINATION HALF-LIFE (MIN)		
	Normal Function	**Renal Failure**	**Normal Function**	**Renal Failure**	**Normal Function**	**Renal Failure**	**References**
SHORT-ACTING DRUGS							
Mivacurium isomers							160
Cis-trans	106	80	278	475	2.0	4.3	
Trans-trans	57	48	211	270	2.3	4.3	
Cis-cis	3.8	2.4*	227	244	68	80	
INTERMEDIATE-ACTING DRUGS							
Atracurium	6.1	6.7	182	224	21	24	172
	5.5	5.8	153	141	19	20	173*,†
	10.9	7.8	280	265	17.3	19.7	322
Cisatracurium	5.2	—	31	—	—	—	169
Vecuronium	3.0	2.5	194	239	78	97	324
	5.3	3.1*	199	241	53	83*	325
Rocuronium	2.9	2.9	207	264*	71	97*	175
LONG-ACTING DRUGS							
d-Tubocurarine	2.4	1.5	250	250	84	132	115
Pancuronium	74	20*	148	236*	97	475*	149†
	1.7	0.9	261	296*	132	257*	380

*Significant difference between normal renal function versus renal failure.
†Values expressed as mL/min, not weight adjusted.

pharmacokinetic changes, the duration of neuromuscular blockade produced by these drugs is longer and more variable than in patients with normal renal function. Because of the potential for prolonged blockade and the availability of intermediate- and short-acting NMBDs, long-acting NMBDs should not be used in patients with renal failure.

The pharmacokinetics and duration of action of atracurium are unaffected by renal failure.[321,322] This lack of effect is in part because Hofmann elimination and ester hydrolysis[173] account for 50% of its total clearance.[167] Laudanosine, the principal metabolite of atracurium, is eliminated unchanged by the kidney. The elimination half-life of laudanosine increases in renal failure.[322] Even during continuous administration of atracurium, laudanosine plasma concentrations are 10 times lower than concentrations associated with seizures in dogs.

In patients with chronic renal failure, the duration of action of cisatracurium is not prolonged.[323] Hofmann elimination accounts for 77% of the total clearance of cisatracurium,[169] and renal excretion accounts for 16% of its elimination.[169] The peak plasma laudanosine concentration is 10 times lower than after equipotent doses of atracurium. In patients with end-stage renal failure, the volume of distribution is unchanged, but there is a 13% reduction in clearance and an increase from 30 to 34 minutes in elimination half-life.

Vecuronium relies principally on hepatic mechanisms for its elimination. However, its clearance is reduced and its elimination half-life is increased in patients with renal failure.[324,325] In one study, the duration of action of 0.1 mg/kg of vecuronium was both longer and more variable in patients with renal failure than in those with normal renal function.[325] In three other studies, the duration of action of 0.05 to 0.14 mg/kg of vecuronium was not prolonged by renal failure, but this result was likely caused by the use of relatively small doses or inadequate sample sizes.[324] The principal metabolite of vecuronium, 3-desacetylvecuronium, has 80% of the neuromuscular blocking activity of vecuronium[153]; it may cause prolonged paralysis in patients with renal failure in the ICU.[156] In patients with renal failure, the duration of action and the rate of recovery from vecuronium- or atracurium-induced neuromuscular blockade during surgery are similar.[326]

The major routes of elimination of rocuronium are biliary and urinary excretion. Rocuronium is taken up by the liver and metabolized, excreted, or both, in bile and feces in high concentrations. After 0.6 mg/kg rocuronium, up to one fifth of the dose is recovered unchanged from the urine within 24 hours, and no active metabolites can be found in humans. Pharmacokinetic studies showed that the clearance of rocuronium was reduced by 33% to 39% in patients with renal failure.[326a] The distribution volume of this drug remained unchanged or slightly increased.[175] The elimination half-life was 70 and 57 minutes in patients with and without renal failure, respectively. The duration of action of single and repeated doses, however, was not affected significantly.[320]

In renal failure, there is no significant change in the volume of distribution of neostigmine. The clearance is decreased by two thirds and the elimination half-life is

TABLE 27.12 Pharmacokinetics of Neuromuscular Blocking Drugs in Patients With Normal Liver Function or Hepatobiliary Disease

	PLASMA CLEARANCE (ML/KG/MIN)		VOLUME OF DISTRIBUTION (ML/KG)		ELIMINATION HALF-LIFE (MIN)			
	Normal	**Disease**	**Normal**	**Disease**	**Normal**	**Disease**	**Hepatic Pathology**	**References**
SHORT-ACTING DRUGS								
Mivacurium isomers							Cirrhosis	159
Cis-trans	95	44*	210	188	1.53	2.48*		
Trans-trans	70	32*	200	199	2.32	11.1*		
Cis-cis	5.2	4.2	266	237	50.3	60.8		
INTERMEDIATE-ACTING DRUGS								
Atracurium	5.3	6.5	159	207*	21	22	Hepatorenal	318
	6.6	8.0*	202	282*	21	25	Cirrhosis	174
Cisatracurium	5.7	6.6*	161	195*	23.5	24.4	Transplantation	
Vecuronium	4.26	2.73*	246	253	58	84*	Cirrhosis	154
	4.30	2.36*	247	206	58	98*	Cholestasis	381
	4.5	4.4	180	220	58	51	Cirrhosis	155
Rocuronium	2.79	2.41	184	234	87.5	96.0	Cirrhosis	176
	217	217	16.4	23.4*	76.4	111.5*	Mixed	178†
	296	189	151	264*	56	98*	Cirrhosis	326c†
	3.70	2.66*	211	248	92	143*	Cirrhosis	179
LONG-ACTING DRUGS								
Pancuronium	123	59*	261	307*	133	267*	Cholestasis	151†
	1.86	1.45*	279	416*	114	208*	Cirrhosis	150
	1.76	1.47	284	425*	141	224*	Cholestasis	383

*Significant difference between normal hepatic function versus hepatobiliary disease.
†Values expressed as mL/min, or L, not weight adjusted.

prolonged from 80 to 183 minutes in patients with renal failure. The clearance of edrophonium is also significantly reduced and its elimination half-life significantly prolonged in patients with end-stage renal failure.

HEPATOBILIARY DISEASE

In comparison with renal elimination, liver function is a modest determinant of the pharmacokinetics of nondepolarizing muscle relaxants. The influence of hepatobiliary disease on the pharmacokinetics of NMBDs can be complex because of the different types of liver failure (Table 27.12). Cirrhosis is associated with an increased extracellular water compartment, edema, and, often, kidney dysfunction. Cholestasis induces decreased biliary excretion but is not associated with significant liver failure, contrary to acute hepatic failure.

A delayed onset of action and an apparent resistance to nondepolarizing muscle relaxants occur in patients with cirrhosis, although studies demonstrated that the sensitivity of the neuromuscular junction was unaltered. This is the consequence of the increased volume of distribution, which induces greater dilution of muscle relaxants in cirrhotic patients. The increase of terminal half-life can be secondary to either the increased volume of distribution or decreased biliary excretion for muscle relaxants dependent on hepatic function for elimination.[154] Following a single dose of nondepolarizing muscle relaxant, in most of the cases, no prolongation of the duration of action occurs because it is dependent on distribution. However, for muscle relaxants dependent on hepatic elimination, prolongation of neuromuscular block can be observed following repeated doses or continuous infusion.

Pancuronium is mainly eliminated through the kidney, although one third of the dose is metabolized and excreted through the liver. The elimination half-life increases from 114 to 208 minutes in cirrhotic patients.[150] This is the consequence of a 50% increase of the volume of distribution in conjunction with a 22% decrease in plasma clearance.[150] Cholestasis induces a 50% decrease in pancuronium clearance leading to a prolonged elimination half-life of 270 minutes. Severe acute hepatic failure also induces reduced plasma clearance and a prolonged elimination half-life.

Vecuronium elimination is mainly through the bile.[326b] Only a small fraction is metabolized to 3-hydroxyvecuronium, which still has 60-80% of the potency of vecuronium. This metabolic process is presumed to occur in the liver because 40% of the total dose of vecuronium is found in the liver and bile as both parent drug and metabolite.[147] The elimination half-life is increased in mildly decompensated cirrhotic patients as the result of a decreased clearance,[154] whereas the volume of distribution of the central compartment and the volume of distribution at steady state can be increased. In cirrhotic patients, the duration of action of vecuronium is related to the dose. A dose of 0.1 mg/kg has a slower onset of action and a shorter duration of action because the volume of distribution is increased. In contrast, after 0.2 mg/kg vecuronium, the duration of action is increased from 65 minutes to 91 minutes in cirrhotic patients because elimination is impaired. Cholestasis can increase plasma concentration of bile salts and thus reduce the hepatic uptake of vecuronium,[147] as well as pancuronium. This may explain the decreased clearance observed by some investigators. The duration of action of vecuronium is increased by 50% in patients with biliary obstruction.

Rocuronium is mainly excreted into the bile. The volume of both the central compartment (+33%) and the volume of distribution at steady state (+43%) are increased in cirrhotic patients, whereas clearance may be decreased.[326c] The duration of action is prolonged in patients with hepatic disease, and a correlation exists between the increased volume of distribution and the slower onset of action when compared with controls.[176]

Atracurium and cisatracurium share organ-independent modes of elimination.[165,168,169] As a consequence, their clearance should be little affected by hepatic disease. In fact, and in contrast to all other NMBDs, the plasma clearances of atracurium and cisatracurium are slightly increased in patients with liver disease (see Table 27.12).[174,180] Because elimination of atracurium and cisatracurium occurs outside of, as well as from within, the central compartment, investigators have suggested that a larger distribution volume should be associated with greater clearance.[169] In two studies,[174,180] volumes of distribution and clearances of the drugs increased with liver disease, thereby lending support to this hypothesis.[169] The increased clearance of the relaxant in patients with liver disease is not reflected in a decrease in the drug's duration of action.[174,180]

One concern raised about administering atracurium to patients with hepatic disease is the possible accumulation of laudanosine. Although laudanosine relies principally on hepatic mechanisms for its elimination, the concentrations encountered during liver transplantation are unlikely to be associated with clinical sequelae.[327]

Because of the wide interindividual variations seen in the response to nondepolarizing muscle relaxants in patients with hepatic disease, quantitative monitoring of neuromuscular block is required, with careful titration of doses.

In patients with severe liver disease, butyrylcholinesterase activity is decreased because of decreased synthesis of the hepatic enzymes. Consequently, the plasma clearance of the isomers of mivacurium is decreased by approximately 50% (see Table 27.12),[159] and the drug's duration of action is prolonged and may be almost tripled.[159]

TABLE 27.13 Conditions Associated With Upregulation and Downregulation of Acetylcholine Receptors

nAChR Upregulation	nAChR Downregulation
Spinal cord injury	Myasthenia gravis
Stroke	Anticholinesterase poisoning
Burns	Organophosphate poisoning
Prolonged immobility	
Prolonged exposure to neuromuscular blockers	
Multiple sclerosis	
Guillain-Barré syndrome	

nAChR, Nicotinic acetylcholine receptor.

BURNS

In patients with burn injuries, muscle relaxants can be used to facilitate mechanical ventilation, which can be associated with sustained improvement in oxygenation. After a period of immobilization, burn injury causes upregulation of both fetal ($\alpha_2\beta\gamma\delta$) and mature ($\alpha_2\beta\varepsilon\delta$) nAChRs.[328] This upregulation of nAChRs usually is associated with resistance to nondepolarizing NMBDs and increased sensitivity to succinylcholine.[329] Causes of upregulation of nAChRs are listed in Table 27.13. A significant increase in the quantal content of evoked acetylcholine release is typically noted by 72 hours after scald injury in rats.[330] This increase also contributes to the resistance to NMBDs in patients with burn injuries. In mice, thermal injury induces changes in diaphragm acetylcholinesterase with respect to total content and specific molecular forms.[331]

Resistance to the effects of nondepolarizing NMBDs is usually seen in patients with burns over at least 25% of their total BSA.[329,332,333] Recovery of neuromuscular function to preburn levels may take several months or even years after the burn injury.[334] The increase in serum K^+ concentration that normally follows succinylcholine administration is markedly exaggerated in burned patients and may be lethal.[335] K^+ concentrations as high as 13 mEq/L, resulting in ventricular tachycardia, fibrillation, and cardiac arrest, have been reported.[335] The magnitude of the hyperkalemic response does not appear to correlate closely with the magnitude of the burn injury. Potentially lethal hyperkalemia was seen in a patient with only an 8% total BSA burn.[336] Succinylcholine has been safely administered within 24 hours of a burn injury. It can be used for prehospital or emergency room intubation. After an initial 24-hour interval, however, sufficient alteration in muscle response may have occurred. Because of the unpredictability of occurrence of hyperkalemia, the use of succinylcholine is best avoided after 24 hours following a burn injury.

The time course of abnormal muscle membrane function corresponds with that of the healing process. Once normal skin has regrown and any infection subsides, the normal acetylcholine receptor populations appear to return.[334] Although normal responses to succinylcholine have been demonstrated in burned patients studied 3 years after injury,[334] the actual length of time during which a patient

BOX 27.1 Reported Indications for the Use of Muscle Relaxants in the Intensive Care Unit

Facilitation of mechanical ventilation
- Facilitation of endotracheal intubation
- Enabling patient to tolerate mechanical ventilation
- High pulmonary inflation pressures (e.g., acute respiratory distress syndrome)

Hyperventilation for increased intracranial pressure
Facilitation of therapeutic or diagnostic procedures
Tetanus
Status epilepticus
Reduction of oxygen consumption
- Abolishing shivering
- Reduction of work of breathing

BOX 27.2 Complications of Muscle Paralysis in the Intensive Care Unit

Short-term use
- Specific, known drug side effects
- Inadequate ventilation in the event of a ventilator failure or circuit disconnection
- Inadequate analgesia and/or sedation

Long-term use
- Complications of immobility
  - Deep vein thrombosis and pulmonary embolus
  - Peripheral nerve injuries
  - Decubitus ulcers

Inability to cough
- Retention of secretions and atelectasis
- Pulmonary infection

Dysregulation of nicotinic acetylcholine receptors
Prolonged paralysis after stopping relaxant
- Persistent neuromuscular blockade
- Critical illness myopathy
- Critical illness polyneuropathy
- Combination of the above

Unrecognized effects of drug or metabolites
- Succinylcholine and metabolic acidosis or hypovolemia
- 3-Desacetylvecuronium and neuromuscular blockade
- Laudanosine and cerebral excitation

with a burn injury may be at risk for the hyperkalemic response is not well defined. A conservative guideline therefore would be to avoid the use of succinylcholine in patients 24 hours after a thermal injury and for at least 1 or 2 years after the burned skin has healed.

USE OF NEUROMUSCULAR BLOCKING DRUGS AND WEAKNESS SYNDROMES IN CRITICALLY ILL PATIENTS

NMBDs are frequently used in conjunction with sedatives and analgesics in ICUs. The indications for the use of NMBDs in the ICU are outlined in Box 27.1. Few available data support their use, and evidence for a beneficial effect on pulmonary function or patient oxygenation is inconclusive.[337] However, a multicenter, double-blind trial showed that, in a subset of patients with acute respiratory distress syndrome, early and short-term administration of cisatracurium for 48 hours could be beneficial.[338] Half of the patients in the placebo group in that study received one or more doses of cisatracurium. The study was underpowered, and the effect on mortality was statistically borderline, with no between-group difference in crude mortality rate. Yet, nondepolarizing NMBDs are sometimes used in ICU patients. Of particular concern in intensive-care settings is the risk that paralyzed patients receive inadequate analgesia and sedation.[339] This reason for this concern may be that ICU nurses and physicians are unfamiliar with the pharmacology of the NMBDs.[339,340] For instance, pancuronium was thought to be an anxiolytic by 50% to 70% of ICU nurses and house staff, and 5% to 10% thought it was an analgesic.[339] In the United Kingdom, the erroneous use of NMBDs as sedatives in intensive care was not uncommon in the 1980s.[341] Approximately 96% of ICU patients received NMBDs to aid mechanical ventilation in 1980. By 1986, their use had decreased to 16% of ventilated patients.[341] Currently, intensivists are aware of the side effects and generally avoid administration of NMBDs to critically ill ICU patients. Clinical practice guidelines for management of critically ill adults who require neuromuscular paralysis have been published.[341a] Specific indications for the use of NMBDs in the ICU setting include severe, refractory hypoxemia; suppression of shivering during therapeutic hypothermia after cardiac arrest; elimination of unwanted movement in patients with status asthmaticus, high intracranial or intraabdominal pressure, massive hemoptysis, or to facilitate short procedures such as bronchoscopy or endoscopy; and acute respiratory failure in patients who require emergent tracheal intubation.[341a]

A prolonged ICU stay during critical illness is associated with disorders of neuromuscular function that contribute to morbidity, length of hospital stay, weaning difficulties, and prolonged rehabilitation.[342] The complications of long-term administration of NMBDs in the ICU are outlined in Box 27.2. In the ICU, duration of mechanical ventilation, sepsis, the dysfunction of two or more organs, female sex, administration of steroids, and hypercapnia are known risk factors for developing neuromuscular dysfunction. Syndromes of weakness in critically ill patients are relatively common and likely polymorphic in origin. In a retrospective study of 92 critically ill patients with clinically diagnosed weakness, electromyographic studies indicated that acute myopathy (critical illness myopathy [CIM]) is three times as common as acute axonal neuropathy (critical illness neuropathy): 43% versus 13%, respectively.[342] The additional healthcare cost of a single case of persistent weakness was estimated at approximately $67,000.[343] Conditions to consider when making a differential diagnosis of neuromuscular weakness in the ICU are listed in Box 27.3.

Critical Illness Myopathy

Lacomis and colleagues suggested using the term CIM,[344] instead of the current terms used in the literature, such as acute quadriplegic myopathy,[345] acute (necrotizing) myopathy of intensive care, thick filament myopathy, acute corticosteroid myopathy, and critical care myopathy.

Initial published reports of CIM in the ICU focused on patients with status asthmaticus[346] who typically had been treated with corticosteroids and nondepolarizing NMBDs.

BOX 27.3 Causes of Generalized Neuromuscular Weakness in the Intensive Care Unit

- Central nervous system
  - Septic or toxic-metabolic encephalopathy
  - Brainstem stroke
  - Central pontine myelinolysis
  - Anterior horn cell disorders (e.g., amyotrophic lateral sclerosis)
- Peripheral neuropathies
  - Critical illness polyneuropathy
  - Guillain-Barré syndrome
  - Porphyria
  - Paraneoplasia
  - Vasculitis
  - Nutritional and toxic neuropathies
- Neuromuscular junction disorders
  - Myasthenia gravis
  - Lambert-Eaton myasthenic syndrome
  - Botulism
  - Prolonged neuromuscular junction blockade
- Myopathies
  - Critical illness myopathy
  - Cachectic myopathy
  - Rhabdomyolysis
  - Inflammatory and infectious myopathies
  - Muscular dystrophies
  - Toxic myopathies
  - Acid maltase deficiency
  - Mitochondrial
  - Hypokalemia
  - Hypermetabolic syndromes with rhabdomyolysis (e.g., neuroleptic malignant syndrome)

From Lacomis D. Critical illness myopathy. *Curr Rheumatol Rep.* 2002;4:403–408.

Nevertheless, myopathy has also been documented in asthmatic patients and in patients with chronic lung disease without paralysis who received corticosteroids,[347] as well as in critically ill patients with sepsis who received neither corticosteroids nor nondepolarizing NMBDs.[348] The primary cause of this condition is a loss of myosin in myocytes with subsequent loss of contractile capacity. Animal studies also reveal that the number of cytosolic corticosteroid receptors is increased in immobilized muscles relative to that in contralateral controls.[349] It seems—at least in some patients—that prolonged immobility may be the key risk factor for myopathy in corticosteroid-treated patients,[350] and selective muscle atrophy is a result of changes in glucocorticoid sensitivity.[349]

Sepsis, immobility, and the catabolism associated with negative nitrogen balance may also result in myopathy.[16] Skeletal muscle hypoperfusion is noted in patients with severe sepsis despite normal or elevated whole blood oxygen delivery.[351] Antibodies to nAChRs were demonstrated in a rodent model of sepsis.[352] Thus myasthenia-like syndrome is also seen in critically ill patients. Evidence for local immune activation by cytokine expression in the skeletal muscle was reported in patients with CIM.[353]

The major feature of CIM is flaccid weakness that tends to be diffuse and sometimes also includes the facial muscles and diaphragm.[344] The clinical features of CIM overlap with those of critical illness polyneuropathy (CIP) and prolonged neuromuscular blockade.[344] Electrophysiologic studies and increases in serum creatine kinase concentrations may differentiate neuropathy from myopathy.[344] Lacomis and colleagues stated, "muscle biopsy should be considered if another myopathic process such as an inflammatory myopathy is suspected or if the histologic findings would affect management."[344]

Critical Illness Polyneuropathy

CIP is the polyneuropathy seen in critically ill patients. It affects both sensory and motor nerves and occurs in 50% to 70% of patients with multisystem organ failure and systemic inflammatory response syndrome.[354] Investigators have postulated that systemic inflammatory response syndrome contributes to CIP by releasing cytokines and free radicals that damage the microcirculation of the central and peripheral nervous systems.[353] Dysregulation of the microcirculation may render the peripheral nervous system susceptible to injury.

Although no pharmacologic treatment for muscle weakness syndromes in the critically ill patient currently exists, increasing evidence indicates the positive effects of early physical rehabilitation during ICU stay. Previously, intensive insulin therapy during critical illness was found to decrease the risk of CIP, and the maintenance of blood glucose at or below 110 mg/mL in critically ill patients may reduce the risk of CIP.

The outcomes from CIM and CIP appear to be similar. The reported mortality rate of patients with CIP syndrome is approximately 35%. In one study, 100% (13 of 13) of the patients who survived had abnormal clinical or neurophysiologic findings 1 to 2 years after the onset of the CIP syndrome, and quality of life was markedly impaired in all patients.[355]

Clinical Implications

Nondepolarizing NMBDs are the most common chemical agents producing immobilization and inducing a denervation-like state. In such circumstances, besides the mature or junctional nAChR formed of two α and one each of β, ε, and δ subunits, two other isoforms, the immature AChR or γAChR and the neuronal α7AChR, are expressed in the muscle. The immature AChR is also referred to as extrajunctional because it is expressed mostly in the extrajunctional part of the muscle. Upregulation of nAChRs was noted in the muscles of deceased critically ill adults who had received long-term infusions of vecuronium.[356] Upregulation refers to changes in the number of available receptors, but these changes usually do not involve a change in isoform configuration. These three types of receptors can coexist in the muscle.

Should Succinylcholine Be Used in Patients in the Intensive Care Unit?

It is likely that upregulation of nAChRs induced by immobilization and by prolonged administration of nondepolarizing NMBDs contributes to (1) the higher incidence of cardiac arrest associated with the use of succinylcholine in ICU patients[356] and (2) increased requirements for nondepolarizing NMBDs in ICU patients.[357] Even more important, succinylcholine more easily depolarizes immature nAChRs that may induce profound outward K^+ flux, with subsequent hyperkalemia. Moreover, the α7AChR can also be depolarized by succinylcholine, thus contributing to the K^+ efflux from the cell to the extracellular space. Therefore succinylcholine should be avoided in ICU patients in whom total body immobilization exceeds 24 hours.[16]

Should Nondepolarizing Neuromuscular Blocking Drugs Be Used in Patients in the Intensive Care Unit?

NMBD-associated persistent weakness appears to be a distinct pathologic entity and is not simply a manifestation of weakness syndromes in critically ill patients. In a prospective study, there was a 70% incidence of persistent weakness in ICU patients who received NMBDs for more than 2 days, compared with a 0% incidence in similar ICU patients who received no NMBD.[358] This is compelling evidence for the effects of nondepolarizing NMBDs in this complication.

Long-term weakness has been described after nondepolarizing NMBDs.[156,359,360] Approximately 20% of patients who received NMBDs for more than 6 days,[359] 15% to 40% of asthmatic patients who also received high-dose steroids,[346] and 50% of patients with renal failure who received vecuronium developed prolonged weakness.[156] Clinically, it appears that prolonged recovery from neuromuscular blockade occurs more frequently when steroidal NMBDs are used.[156,359]

However, prolonged weakness was also noted after the use of atracurium in ICU patients.[360] Further, the use of atracurium has raised concerns about its metabolite, laudanosine. Laudanosine, also detected in the cerebrospinal fluid (CSF) of ICU patients given atracurium,[361] is an analeptic and can trigger seizures in animals.[362] The toxic dose in humans is not known, but case reports have noted patients having seizures while receiving atracurium, and laudanosine has not been ruled out as a cause of these seizures.[363-365] Evidence also indicates that laudanosine can activate neuronal nicotinic receptors.[366] Cisatracurium is a single isomer of atracurium, and because it is four to five times more potent than atracurium, it is given in smaller total doses. Therefore the risk of laudanosine-related adverse effects should be minimal.[367]

Nondepolarizing NMBDs are polar molecules and do not readily cross the blood-brain barrier, but vecuronium and its long-acting active metabolite, 3-desacetylvecuronium, have been detected in the CSF of patients in the ICU. The CNS effects of NMBDs and their metabolites in humans have not been well studied, but in rats, atracurium, pancuronium, and vecuronium injected into the CSF caused dose-related cerebral excitation culminating in seizures.[362] Cerebral excitation with consequent increased cerebral oxygen demand is undesirable in ICU patients at risk of cerebral ischemia. Investigators have also suggested that nondepolarizing NMBDs can gain access to nerves during systemic inflammatory response syndrome, thus resulting in direct neurotoxicity.[362]

When nondepolarizing NMBDs are necessary, the use of an objective neuromuscular monitor is recommended, and periodic return of muscle function should be allowed. Adjusting the dosage of NMBDs by peripheral nerve stimulation versus standard "clinical dosing" in critically ill patients reduces drug requirements, produces faster recovery of neuromuscular function, and is cost-effective.[369] Daily interruption of sedative-drug infusions decreases the duration of mechanical ventilation and the length of stay in the ICU.[370] The effect of such an approach on the weakness syndromes in the ICU patient is unknown. When nondepolarizing NMBDs are used, the guidelines in Box 27.4 may help minimize the incidence of complications. As stated in the clinical practice guidelines for sustained neuromuscular blockade in the adult critically ill patient,[337] "*Independent of the reasons for using neuromuscular blockers, we emphasize that all other modalities to improve the clinical situation must be tried, using neuromuscular blockers only as a last resort.* To this admonition, we would add a plea that clinicians use objective monitors, whenever possible, to guide NMBD administration and assess readiness for tracheal extubation, whether in the operating room or ICU settings. The unquestionable benefits of quantitative neuromuscular monitoring are described in Chapter 43.

BOX 27.4 Recommendations for the Use of Neuromuscular Blockers in the Intensive Care Unit

- Avoid the use of neuromuscular blockers by
  - Maximal use of analgesics and sedatives
  - Manipulation of ventilatory parameters and modes
- Minimize the dose of neuromuscular blocker
  - Use a peripheral nerve stimulator with train-of-four monitoring
  - Do not administer for more than 2 days continuously
  - Administer by bolus rather than infusion
  - Administer only when required and to achieve a well-defined goal
  - Continually allow recovery from paralysis
  - Consider alternative therapies

Acknowledgment

The editors and publisher would like to thank Drs. Mohamed Naguib and Cynthia A. Lien for contributing a chapter on this topic in the prior edition of this work. It has served as the foundation for the current chapter.

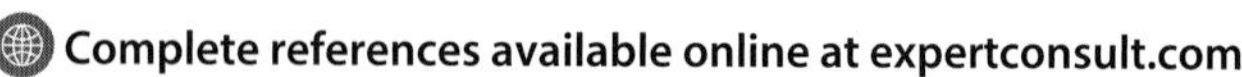
Complete references available online at expertconsult.com.

References

1. Griffith H, Johnson GE. *Anesthesiology*. 1942;3:418.
2. Cullen SC. *Surgery*. 1943;14:216.
3. Beecher HK, Todd DP. *Ann Surg*. 1954;140:2.
4. Thesleff S. *Nord Med*. 1951;46:1045.
5. Foldes FF, et al. *N Engl J Med*. 1952;247:596.
6. Baird WL, Reid AM. *Br J Anaesth*. 1967;39:775.
7. Savage DS, et al. *Br J Anaesth*. 1980;52(suppl 1):3S.
8. Stenlake JB, et al. *Eur J Med Chem*. 1981;16:515.
9. Savarese JJ, et al. *Anesthesiology*. 1988;68:723.
10. Wierda JM, et al. *Br J Anaesth*. 1990;64:521.
11. Lien CA, et al. *J Crit Care*. 2009;24:50.
11a. Savarese JJ. *Anesthesiology*. 2018;129:970.
11b. Deleted in proofs.
12. On being aware. *Br J Anaesth*. 1979;51:711.
13. Shovelton DS. *Br Med J*. 1979;1:737.
14. Poggesi I, et al. *Drug Metab Rev*. 2009;41:422.
15. Cullen SC, Larson CPJ. *Essentials of Anesthetic Practice*. Chicago: Year Book Medical; 1974.
16. Naguib M, et al. *Anesthesiology*. 2002;96:202.
17. Machold J, et al. *Eur J Biochem*. 1995;234:427.
18. Deleted in proofs.

19. Bowman WC. *Pharmacology of Neuromuscular Function*. 2nd ed. London: Wright; 1990.
20. Martyn JA. *Keio J Med*. 1995;44:1.
21. Kallen RG, et al. *Neuron*. 1990;4:233.
22. Martyn JA, Richtsfeld M. *Anesthesiology*. 2006;104:158.
23. Bowman WC. *Anesth Analg*. 1980;59:935.
24. Deleted in proofs.
25. Deleted in proofs.
26. Bovet D. *Ann NY Acad Sci*. 1951;54:407.
27. Szalados JE, et al. *Anesth Analg*. 1990;71:55.
28. Kopman AF, et al. *Anesth Analg*. 2000;90:1191.
29. Curran MJ, et al. *Br J Anaesth*. 1987;59:989.
30. Viby-Mogensen J. *Anesthesiology*. 1980;53:517.
31. Gissen AJ, et al. *Anesthesiology*. 1966;27:242.
32. Torda TA, et al. *Anaesth Intensive Care*. 1997;25:272.
33. Foldes FF, et al. *Anesth Analg*. 1956;35:609.
34. Lepage L, et al. *Clin Chem*. 1985;31:546.
35. Sunew KY, Hicks RG. *Anesthesiology*. 1978;49:188.
36. Lindsay PA, Lumley J. *Anaesthesia*. 1978;33:620.
37. Walts LF, et al. *Anesthesiology*. 1970;33:503.
38. Kao YJ, et al. *Br J Anaesth*. 1990;65:220.
39. Fisher DM, et al. *Anesthesiology*. 1988;69:757.
40. Barabas E, et al. *Can Anaesth Soc J*. 1986;33:332.
41. Pantuck EJ. *Br J Anaesth*. 1966;38:406.
42. Kalow W, Genest K. *Can J Biochem*. 1957;35:339.
43. Jensen FS, Viby-Mogensen J. *Acta Anaesthesiol Scand*. 1995;39:150.
44. Primo-Parmo SL, et al. *Pharmacogenetics*. 1997;7:27.
45. Galindo AHF, Davis TB. *Anesthesiology*. 1962;23:32.
46. Goat VA, Feldman SA. *Anaesthesia*. 1972;27:149.
47. Jonsson M, et al. *Anesthesiology*. 2006;104:724.
48. Stoelting RK, Peterson C. *Anesth Analg*. 1975;54:705.
49. Schoenstadt DA, Witcher CE. *Anesthesiology*. 1963;24:358.
50. Leiman BC, et al. *Anesth Analg*. 1987;66:1292.
51. Derbyshire DR. *Anesth Analg*. 1984;63:465.
52. Walton JD, Farman JV. *Anaesthesia*. 1973;28:666.
53. Powell JN, Golby M. *Br J Anaesth*. 1971;43:662.
53a. Thapa S, Brull SJ. *Anesth Analg*. 2000;91:237.
54. Schwartz DE, et al. *Anesth Analg*. 1992;75:291.
55. Antognini JF, Gronert GA. *Anesth Analg*. 1993;77:585.
56. Antognini JF. *Anesth Analg*. 1994;78:687.
57. Kohlschütter B, et al. *Br J Anaesth*. 1976;48:557.
58. Stevenson PH, Birch AA. *Anesthesiology*. 1979;51:89.
59. Birch Jr AA, et al. *JAMA*. 1969;210:490.
60. Pandey K, et al. *Br J Anaesth*. 1972;44:191.
61. Indu B, et al. *Can J Anaesth*. 1989;36:269.
62. Meyers EF, et al. *Anesthesiology*. 1978;48:149.
63. Miller RD, et al. *Anesthesiology*. 1968;29:123.
63a. Cunningham AJ, Barry P. *Can Anaesth Soc J*. 1986;33:195.
64. Deleted in proofs.
65. Greenan J. *Br J Anaesth*. 1961;33:432.
66. Miller RD, Way WL. *Anesthesiology*. 1971;34:185.
67. Salem MR, et al. *Br J Anaesth*. 1972;44:166.
68. Minton MD, et al. *Anesthesiology*. 1986;65:165.
69. Brodsky JB, et al. *Anesthesiology*. 1979;51:259.
70. Waters DJ, Mapleson WW. *Anaesthesia*. 1971;26:127.
71. McLoughlin C, et al. *Anaesthesia*. 1992;47:202.
72. Naguib M, et al. *Br J Anaesth*. 1987;59:606.
73. Smith I, et al. *Anesth Analg*. 1993;76:1181.
73a. Findlay GP, Spittal MJ. *Br J Anaesth*. 1996;76:526.
74. Leary NP, Ellis FR. *Br J Anaesth*. 1990;64:488.
75. Meakin G, et al. *Br J Anaesth*. 1990;65:816.
76. Van der Spek AF, et al. *Anesthesiology*. 1987;67:459.
77. Littleford JA, et al. *Anesth Analg*. 1991;72:151.
77a. Dewachter P, et al. *Anesthesiology*. 2009;111:1141.
78. Naguib M, et al. *Anesthesiology*. 2003;99:1045.
79. Naguib M, et al. *Anesthesiology*. 2005;102:35.
80. Donati F, et al. *Br J Anaesth*. 1991;66:557.
81. Naguib M, et al. *Br J Anaesth*. 1995;74:26.
82. Erkola O, et al. *Anesth Analg*. 1995;80:534.
83. Dubois MY, et al. *J Clin Anesth*. 1995;7:44.
84. Naguib M, et al. *Anesth Analg*. 2004;98:1686.
85. Lee C. *Br J Anaesth*. 2001;87:755.
86. Everett AJ, et al. *J Chem Soc D*. 1970:1020.
87. Waser PG. Chemistry and pharmacology of natural curare compounds. Neuromuscular blocking and stimulating agents. In: Cheymol J, ed. *International Encyclopedia of Pharmacology and Therapeutics*. Oxford: Pergamon Press; 1972:205.
88. Hill SA, et al. *Bailliere's Clin Anesthesiol*. 1994;8:317.
89. Stenlake JB, et al. *Eur J Med Chem*. 1984;19:441.
90. Wastila WB, et al. *Anesthesiology*. 1996;85:169.
91. Lien CA. *Curr Opin Anesthesiol*. 1996;9:348.
92. Lien CA, et al. *Anesthesiology*. 1995;82:1131.
93. Savarese JJ, Wastila WB. *Acta Anaesthesiol Scand Suppl*. 1995;106:91.
94. Lien CA, et al. *Anesthesiology*. 1994;80:1296.
95. Stovner J, et al. *Br J Anaesth*. 1975;47:949.
96. Bowman WC, et al. *Anesthesiology*. 1988;69:57.
97. Wierda JM, Proost JH. *Eur J Anaesthesiol Suppl*. 1995;11:45.
98. Naguib M, et al. *Br J Anaesth*. 1995;75:37.
99. Goulden MR, Hunter JM. *Br J Anaesth*. 1999;82:489.
100. Belmont MR, et al. *Anesthesiology*. 2004;100:768.
101. Savarese JJ, et al. *Anesthesiology*. 2010;113:58.
102. Heerdt PM, et al. *Anesthesiology*. 2010;112:910.
103. Shanks CA. *Anesthesiology*. 1986;64:72.
104. Booij LH, Knape HT. *Anaesthesia*. 1991;46:341.
105. Bartkowski RR, et al. *Anesth Analg*. 1993;77:574.
106. Bevan DR, et al. *Can J Anaesth*. 1993;40:127.
107. Belmont MR, et al. *Anesthesiology*. 1995;82:1139.
108. Savarese JJ, et al. *Anaesthesist*. 1997;46:840.
109. Naguib M, et al. *Anesthesiology*. 1998;89:1116.
110. Weber S, et al. *Anesth Analg*. 1988;67:495.
111. Caldwell JE, et al. *Anesthesiology*. 1989;70:31.
112. Diefenbach C, et al. *Anesth Analg*. 1992;74:420.
113. Wierda JM, et al. *Can J Anaesth*. 1994;41:213.
114. Kopman AF, et al. *Anesthesiology*. 2000;93:1017.
115. Sheiner LB, et al. *Clin Pharmacol Ther*. 1979;25:358.
116. Holford NH, Sheiner LB. *Pharmacol Ther*. 1982;16:143.
116a. Donati F, Meistelman C. *J Pharmacokinet Biopharm*. 1991;19:537.
116b. Ducharme J, et al. *Clin Pharmacokinet*. 1993;24:507.
116c. Donati F. *Semin Anesth*. 1994;13:310–320.
117. Mencke T, et al. *Anesthesiology*. 2003;98:1049.
118. Combes X, et al. *Br J Anaesth*. 2007;99:276.
118a. Lundstrøm LH, et al. *Br J Anaesth*. 2009;103:283.
118b. Lundstrøm LH, et al. *Cochrane Database Syst Rev*. 2017;5:CD009237.
118c. Naguib M, Brull SJ, et al. *Anesth Analg Nov*. 2017;30.
118d. Paton WD, et al. *J Physiol*. 1951;112:311.
119. Donati F, et al. *Anesthesiology*. 1990;73:870.
120. Donati F, et al. *Anesthesiology*. 1991;74:833.
121. Meistelman C, et al. *Can J Anaesth*. 1992;39:665.
122. Wright PM, et al. *Anesthesiology*. 1994;81:1110.
123. Plaud B, et al. *Clin Pharmacol Ther*. 1995;58:185.
124. Waud BE, Waud DR. *Anesthesiology*. 1972;37:417.
125. Meistelman C, et al. *Anesth Analg*. 1991;73:278.
126. Fisher DM, et al. *Anesthesiology*. 1997;86:558.
127. Smith CE, et al. *Anesthesiology*. 1989;71:57.
128. Sundman E, et al. *Anesthesiology*. 2000;92:977.
129. Berg H, et al. *Acta Anaesthesiol Scand*. 1997;41:1095.
129a. Murphy GS, Brull SJ. *Anesth Analg*. 2010;111:129.
129b. Bulka CM, et al. *Anesthesiology*. 2016;125:647.
129c. Eriksson LI, et al. *Anesthesiology*. 1993;78:693.
129d. Wyon N, et al. *Anesth Analg*. 1996;82:1252.
130. Chen BB, et al. *J Cardiothorac Vasc Anesth*. 1991;5:569.
130a. Nandi R, Basu SR, et al. *Indian J Anaesth*. 2017;61:910.
131. Plaud B, et al. *Anesthesiology*. 2001;95:96.
132. Lee HJ, et al. *Br J Anaesth*. 2009;102:869.
132a. Brull SJ, Kopman AF. *Anesthesiology*. 2017;126:173.
133. Kopman AF, et al. *Anesthesiology*. 1999;90:425.
134. Deleted in proofs.
135. Kopman AF, et al. *Anesth Analg*. 1999;89:1046.
136. Naguib M, Kopman AF. *Middle East J Anesthesiol*. 2003;17:193.
137. Bevan DR. *Can J Anaesth*. 1999;46:R88.
138. Plaud B, et al. *Anesthesiology*. 1996;85:77.
139. Hemmerling TM, et al. *Br J Anaesth*. 2000;85:856.
140. Magorian T, et al. *Anesthesiology*. 1993;79:913.
141. Mehta MP, et al. *Anesthesiology*. 1985;62:392.
142. Naguib M. *Anesthesiology*. 1994;81:388.
142a. Sieber TJ, Zbinden AM, et al. *Anesth Analg*. 1998;86:1137.
143. Engbaek J, et al. *Acta Anaesthesiol Scand*. 1985;29:117.
144. Savarese JJ, et al. *Anesthesiology*. 1989;70:386.
145. Kopman AF, et al. *Anesth Analg*. 2001;93:954.

146. Miguel RV, et al. *J Clin Anesth.* 2001;13:325.
147. Agoston S, et al. *Acta Anaesthesiol Scand.* 1973;17:267.
148. Miller RD, et al. *J Pharmacol Exp Ther.* 1978;207:539.
149. McLeod K, et al. *Br J Anaesth.* 1976;48:341.
150. Duvaldestin P, et al. *Br J Anaesth.* 1978;50:1131.
151. Somogyi AA, et al. *Br J Anaesth.* 1977;49:1103.
152. Mol WE, et al. *J Pharmacol Exp Ther.* 1988;244:268.
153. Caldwell JE, et al. *J Pharmacol Exp Ther.* 1994;270:1216.
154. Lebrault C, et al. *Anesthesiology.* 1985;62:601.
155. Arden JR, et al. *Anesthesiology.* 1988;68:771.
156. Segredo V, et al. *N Engl J Med.* 1992;327:524.
157. Khuenl-Brady K, et al. *Anesthesiology.* 1990;72:669.
158. Smit JW, et al. *Br J Pharmacol.* 1998;123:361.
158a. Costa ACC, et al. *Eur J Clin Pharmacol.* 2017;73:957–963.
158b. Leonard PA, Todd MM. *A A Case Rep.* 2017;9:190–192.
159. Head-Rapson AG, et al. *Br J Anaesth.* 1994;73:613.
160. Head-Rapson AG, et al. *Br J Anaesth.* 1995;75:31.
161. Goudsouzian NG, et al. *Anesth Analg.* 1993;77:183.
162. Maddineni VR, Mirakhur RK. *Anesthesiology.* 1993;78:1181.
163. Ostergaard D, et al. *Acta Anaesthesiol Scand.* 1993;37:314.
164. Naguib M, et al. *Anesthesiology.* 1995;82:1288.
165. Neill EA, et al. *Br J Anaesth.* 1983;55(Suppl 1):23S.
166. Stiller RL, et al. *Br J Anaesth.* 1985;57:1085.
167. Fisher DM, et al. *Anesthesiology.* 1986;65:6.
168. Lien CA, et al. *Anesthesiology.* 1996;84:300.
169. Kisor DF, et al. *Anesth Analg.* 1996;83:1065.
170. Boros EE, et al. *J Med Chem.* 2003;46:2502.
171. Fisher DM, et al. *Anesthesiology.* 1986;65:286.
172. Fahey MR, et al. *Anesthesiology.* 1984;61:699.
173. Ward S, et al. *Br J Anaesth.* 1987;59:697.
174. Parker CJ, Hunter JM. *Br J Anaesth.* 1989;62:177.
175. Szenohradszky J, et al. *Anesthesiology.* 1992;77:899.
176. Khalil M, et al. *Anesthesiology.* 1994;80:1241.
177. Matteo RS, et al. *Anesth Analg.* 1993;77:1193.
178. Magorian T, et al. *Anesth Analg.* 1995;80:754.
179. van Miert MM, et al. *Br J Clin Pharmacol.* 1997;44:139.
180. De Wolf AM, et al. *Br J Anaesth.* 1996;76:624.
181. Anaesthetists and the reporting of adverse drug reactions. *Br Med J (Clin Res Ed).* 1986;292:949.
182. Basta SJ. *Curr Opin Anaesthiol.* 1992;5:572.
183. Hatano Y, et al. *Anesthesiology.* 1990;72:28.
184. Scott RP, et al. *Br J Anaesth.* 1985;57:550.
185. Savarese JJ. *Anesthesiology.* 1979;50:40.
186. Naguib M, et al. *Br J Anaesth.* 1995;75:588.
187. Miller RD, et al. *Anesthesiology.* 1975;42:352.
188. Docherty JR, McGrath JC. *Br J Pharmacol.* 1978;64:589.
189. Roizen MF, et al. *J Pharmacol Exp Ther.* 1979;211:419.
190. Reitan JA, et al. *Anesth Analg.* 1973;52:974.
191. Wong KC, et al. *Anesthesiology.* 1971;34:458.
192. Geha DG, et al. *Anesthesiology.* 1977;46:342.
193. Edwards RP, et al. *Anesthesiology.* 1979;50:421.
194. Clayton D. *Br J Anaesth.* 1986;58:937.
195. Starr NJ, et al. *Anesthesiology.* 1986;64:521.
196. Cozanitis DA, Erkola O. *Anaesthesia.* 1989;44:648.
197. Bonner TI, et al. *Neuron.* 1988;1:403.
198. Mak JC, Barnes PJ. *Am Rev Respir Dis.* 1990;141:1559.
199. Coulson FR, Fryer AD. *Pharmacol Ther.* 2003;98:59.
200. Jooste E, et al. *Anesthesiology.* 2003;98:906.
201. Kron SS. *Anesthesiology.* 2001;94:923.
202. Naguib M. *Anesthesiology.* 2001;94:924.
203. Meakin GH, et al. *Anesthesiology.* 2001;94:926.
204. Laxenaire MC, et al. *Ann Fr Anesth Reanim.* 1990;9:501.
205. Fisher MM, More DG. *Anaesth Intensive Care.* 1981;9:226.
206. Mertes PM, et al. *Anesthesiology.* 2003;99:536.
206a. Tacquard C, et al. *Acta Anaesthesiol Scand.* 2017;61:290.
207. Baldo BA, Fisher MM. *Nature.* 1983;306:262.
207a. de Pater GH, Florvaag E, et al. *Allergy.* 2017;72:813.
208. Levy JH, et al. *Anesth Analg.* 1994;78:318.
209. Rose M, Fisher M. *Br J Anaesth.* 2001;86:678.
210. Watkins J. *Br J Anaesth.* 2001;87:522.
211. Deleted in proofs.
212. Laxenaire MC, Mertes PM. *Br J Anaesth.* 2001;87:549.
213. Levy JH, et al. *Br J Anaesth.* 2000;85:844.
214. Futo J, et al. *Anesthesiology.* 1988;69:92.
215. O'Callaghan AC, et al. *Anaesthesia.* 1986;41:940.
216. Naguib M, et al. *CNS Drugs.* 1997;8:51.
217. Miller RD. Factors affecting the action of muscle relaxants. In: Katz RL, ed. *Muscle relaxants.* Amsterdam: Excerpta Medica; 1975.
218. Naguib M, et al. *Br J Anaesth.* 1994;73:484.
219. Lebowitz PW, et al. *Anesth Analg.* 1981;60:12.
220. Paul M, et al. *Eur J Pharmacol.* 2002;438:35.
221. Motamed C, et al. *Anesthesiology.* 2003;98:1057.
222. Kay B, et al. *Anaesthesia.* 1987;42:277.
223. Rashkovsky OM, et al. *Br J Anaesth.* 1985;57:1063.
224. Katz RL. *Anesthesiology.* 1971;35:602.
225. Ono K, et al. *Br J Anaesth.* 1989;62:324.
226. Katz JA, et al. *Anesthesiology.* 1988;69:604.
227. Cooper R, et al. *Br J Anaesth.* 1992;69:269.
228. Kelly RE, et al. *Anesth Analg.* 1993;76:868.
229. Saitoh Y, et al. *Br J Anaesth.* 1993;70:402.
230. Miller RD, et al. *Anesthesiology.* 1972;37:573.
231. Miller RD, et al. *Anesthesiology.* 1976;44:206.
232. Rupp SM, et al. *Anesthesiology.* 1984;60:102.
233. Gencarelli PJ, et al. *Anesthesiology.* 1982;56:192.
234. Miller RD, et al. *Anesthesiology.* 1971;35:509.
235. Wulf H, et al. *Can J Anaesth.* 1998;45:526.
236. Bock M, et al. *Br J Anaesth.* 2000;84:43.
237. Paul M, et al. *Anesth Analg.* 2002;95:362.
238. Stanski DR, et al. *Anesth Analg.* 2002;95:362.
239. Pereon Y, et al. *Anesth Analg.* 1999;89:490.
240. Franks NP, Lieb WR. *Nature.* 1994;367:607.
241. Singh YN, et al. *Anesthesiology.* 1978;48:418.
242. Burkett L, et al. *Anesth Analg.* 1979;58:107.
243. Hasfurther D, Bailey P. *Can J Anaesth.* 1996;43:617.
244. Heier T, et al. *Anesthesiology.* 1991;74:815.
245. Leslie K, et al. *Anesth Analg.* 1995;80:1007.
246. Caldwell JE, et al. *Anesthesiology.* 2000;92:84.
247. Heier T, et al. *Anesthesiology.* 1989;71:381.
248. Heier T, et al. *Anesthesiology.* 1990;72:807.
249. Miller RD, et al. *J Pharmacol Exp Ther.* 1978;207:532.
250. Stenlake JB, Hughes R. *Br J Anaesth.* 1987;59:806.
251. Eriksson LI, et al. *Acta Anaesthesiol Scand.* 1991;35:387.
252. Thornberry EA, Mazumdar B. *Anaesthesia.* 1988;43:447.
253. Miller RD, et al. *J Pharmacol Exp Ther.* 1975;195:237.
254. Miller RD, Roderick LL. *Anesthesiology.* 1977;46:333.
255. Heier T, et al. *Anesthesiology.* 2002;97:90.
255a. Lee HJ, Kim KS, et al. *BMC Anesthesiol.* 2015;15:7.
256. Sinatra RS, et al. *Anesth Analg.* 1985;64:1220.
257. Fuchs-Buder T, et al. *Br J Anaesth.* 1995;74:405.
258. Tsai SK, et al. *Br J Anaesth.* 1994;72:674.
259. Waud BE, Waud DR. *Br J Anaesth.* 1980;52:863.
260. Al-Mohaya S, et al. *Anesthesiology.* 1986;65:554.
261. Price LH, Heninger GR. *N Engl J Med.* 1994;331:591.
262. Abdel-Zaher AO. *Pharmacol Res.* 2000;41:163.
263. Hill GE, et al. *Anesthesiology.* 1977;46:122.
264. Martin BA, Kramer PM. *Am J Psychiatry.* 1982;139:1326.
265. Usubiaga JE, et al. *Anesth Analg.* 1967;46:39.
266. Usubiaga JE, Standaert F. *J Pharmacol Exp Ther.* 1968;159:353.
267. Kordas M. *J Physiol.* 1970;209:689.
268. Thorpe WR, Seeman P. *J Pharmacol Exp Ther.* 1971;179:324.
269. Ozkul Y. *Clin Neurophysiol.* 2007;118:2005.
270. van Poorten JF, et al. *Anesth Analg.* 1984;63:155.
271. Baurain M, et al. *Anaesthesia.* 1989;44:34.
272. Selzer ME, et al. *Brain Res.* 1984;304:149.
273. Ornstein E, et al. *Anesthesiology.* 1987;67:191.
274. Spacek A, et al. *Br J Anaesth.* 1996;77:500.
275. Alloul K, et al. *Anesthesiology.* 1996;84:330.
276. Kim CS, et al. *Anesthesiology.* 1992;77:500.
277. Melton AT, et al. *Can J Anaesth.* 1993;40:939.
278. Miller RD, et al. *Anesthesiology.* 1976;45:442.
279. Deleted in proofs.
280. Deleted in proofs.
281. Deleted in proofs.
282. Hill GE, et al. *Anesth Analg.* 1978;57:417.
283. Matteo RS, et al. *Anesthesiology.* 1980;52:335.
284. Lee C, Katz RL. *Br J Anaesth.* 1980;52:173.
285. Glidden RS, et al. *Anesthesiology.* 1988;68:595.
286. Meyers EF. *Anesthesiology.* 1977;46:148.
287. Leeuwin RS, et al. *Eur J Pharmacol.* 1981;69:165.
288. Parr SM, et al. *Br J Anaesth.* 1991;67:447.

289. Bouzat C, Barrantes FJ. *J Biol Chem*. 1996;271:25835.
290. Valera S, et al. *Proc Natl Acad Sci U S A*. 1992;89:9949.
291. Naguib M, Gyasi HK. *Can Anaesth Soc J*. 1986;33:682.
292. Henderson WA. *Can Anaesth Soc J*. 1984;31:444.
293. Goudsouzian NG, et al. *Anesthesiology*. 1974;41:95.
294. Fisher DM, et al. *Anesthesiology*. 1982;57:203.
295. Fisher DM, et al. *Clin Pharmacol Ther*. 1985;37:402.
296. Fisher DM, et al. *Anesthesiology*. 1990;73:33.
297. Fisher DM, Miller RD. *Anesthesiology*. 1983;58:519.
298. Meretoja OA, et al. *Anesth Analg*. 1988;67:21.
299. Wierda JM, et al. *Br J Anaesth*. 1997;78:690.
300. Goudsouzian NG, et al. *Anesthesiology*. 1983;59:459.
301. Meretoja OA, et al. *Paediatr Anaesth*. 1996;6:373.
302. de Ruiter J, Crawford MW. *Anesthesiology*. 2001;94:790.
303. Scheiber G, et al. *Anesth Analg*. 1996;83:320.
304. Taivainen T, et al. *Paediatr Anaesth*. 1996;6:271.
305. Devys JM, et al. *Br J Anaesth*. 2011;106:225.
305a. Meakin G, et al. *Anesthesiology*. 1983;59:316.
306. Koscielniak-Nielsen ZJ, et al. *Anesthesiology*. 1993;79:229.
307. Duvaldestin P, et al. *Anesthesiology*. 1982;56:36.
308. Lien CA, et al. *Anesth Analg*. 1991;73:39.
309. Maddineni VR, et al. *Br J Anaesth*. 1994;72:497.
310. Maddineni VR, et al. *Br J Anaesth*. 1994;73:608.
311. Lemmens HJ, Brodsky JB. *Anesth Analg*. 2006;102:438.
312. Schwartz AE, et al. *Anesth Analg*. 1992;74:515.
313. Meyhoff CS, et al. *Anesth Analg*. 2009;109:787.
314. Leykin Y, et al. *Anesth Analg*. 2004;99:1086.
315. Varin F, et al. *Clin Pharmacol Ther*. 1990;48:18.
316. van Kralingen S, et al. *Br J Clin Pharmacol*. 2011;71:34.
317. Miller RD, et al. *J Pharmacol Exp Ther*. 1977;202:1.
318. Ward S, Neill EA. *Br J Anaesth*. 1983;55:1169.
319. Bevan DR, et al. *Can Anaesth Soc J*. 1984;31:491.
320. Khuenl-Brady KS, et al. *Anaesthesia*. 1993;48:873.
321. Hunter JM, et al. *Br J Anaesth*. 1982;54:1251.
322. Vandenbrom RH, et al. *Clin Pharmacokinet*. 1990;19:230.
323. Boyd AH, et al. *Br J Anaesth*. 1995;74:400.
324. Fahey MR, et al. *Br J Anaesth*. 1981;53:1049.
325. Lynam DP, et al. *Anesthesiology*. 1988;69:227.
326. Hunter JM, et al. *Br J Anaesth*. 1984;56:941.
326a. Robertson EN, et al. *Eur J Anaesthesiol*. 2005;22:4.
326b. Bencini AF, et al. *Br J Anaesth*. 1986;58:988.
326c. Servin FS, et al. *Anesthesiology*. 1996;84:1092.
327. Lawhead RG, et al. *Anesth Analg*. 1993;76:569.
328. Ward JM, et al. *J Burn Care Rehabil*. 1993;14:595.
329. Martyn JA, et al. *Anesthesiology*. 1980;52:352.
330. Edwards JP, et al. *Muscle Nerve*. 1999;22:1660.
331. Tomera JF, et al. *J Burn Care Rehabil*. 1993;14:406.
332. Marathe PH, et al. *Anesthesiology*. 1989;70:752.
333. Han T, et al. *Anesth Analg*. 2004;99:386.
334. Martyn JA, et al. *Anesthesiology*. 1992;76:822.
335. Schaner PJ, et al. *Anesth Analg*. 1969;48:764.
336. Viby-Mogensen J, et al. *Acta Anaesthesiol Scand*. 1975;19:169.
337. Murray MJ, et al. *Crit Care Med*. 2002;30:142.
338. Papazian L, et al. *N Engl J Med*. 2010;363:1107.
339. Loper KA, et al. *Pain*. 1989;37:315.
340. Hansen-Flaschen JH, et al. *JAMA*. 1991;266:2870.
341. Pollard BJ. *Br J Intens Care*. 1994;4:347.
341a. Murray MJ, et al. *Crit Care Med*. 2016;44:2079.
342. Lacomis D, et al. *Muscle Nerve*. 1998;21:610.
343. Rudis MI, et al. *Crit Care Med*. 1996;24:1749.
344. Lacomis D, et al. *Muscle Nerve*. 2000;23:1785.
345. Showalter CJ, Engel AG. *Muscle Nerve*. 1997;20:316.
346. Shee CD. *Respir Med*. 1990;84:229.
347. Hanson P, et al. *Muscle Nerve*. 1997;20:1371.
348. Deconinck N, et al. *Neuromuscul Disord*. 1998;8:186.
349. DuBois DC, Almon RR. *Endocrinology*. 1980;107:1649.
350. Hund E. *Crit Care Med*. 1999;27:2544.
351. Neviere R, et al. *Am J Respir Crit Care Med*. 1996;153:191.
352. Tsukagoshi H, et al. *Anesthesiology*. 1999;91:448.
353. De Letter MA, et al. *J Neuroimmunol*. 2000;106:206.
354. Tepper M, et al. *Neth J Med*. 2000;56:211.
355. Zifko UA. *Muscle Nerve Suppl*. 2000;9:S49.
356. Dodson BA, et al. *Crit Care Med*. 1995;23:815.
357. Coursin DB, et al. *Anesth Analg*. 69: 518.
358. Kupfer Y, et al. *Ann Intern Med*. 1992;117:484.
359. Op de Coul AA, et al. *Clin Neurol Neurosurg*. 1985;87:17.
360. Tousignant CP, et al. *Can J Anaesth*. 1995;42:224.
361. Gwinnutt CL, et al. *Br J Anaesth*. 1990;65:829.
362. Szenohradszky J, et al. *Anesth Analg*. 1993;76:1304.
363. Griffiths RB, et al. *Anaesthesia*. 1986;41:375.
364. Beemer GH, et al. *Anaesth Intensive Care*. 1989;17:504.
365. Eddleston JM, et al. *Br J Anaesth*. 1989;63:525.
366. Chiodini F, et al. *Anesthesiology*. 2001;94:643.
367. Chapple DJ, et al. *Br J Anaesth*. 1987;59:218.
368. Prielipp RC, et al. *Anesth Analg*. 1995;81:3.
369. Zarowitz BJ, et al. *Pharmacotherapy*. 1997;17:327.
370. Kress JP, et al. *N Engl J Med*. 2000;342:1471.
371. Kim KS, et al. *Br J Anaesth*. 1999;83:483.
372. Katz RL, Ryan JF. *Br J Anaesth*. 1969;41:381.
373. Kopman AF, et al. *Anesthesiology*. 2003;99:1050.
374. Wierda JM, et al. *Anesth Analg*. 1993;77:579.
375. Miguel R, et al. *Anesthesiology*. 1999;91:1648.
376. Agoston S, et al. *Br J Anaesth*. 1980;52(Suppl 1):53S.
377. Katz RL. *Anesthesiology*. 1971;34:550.
378. Savarese JJ, et al. *Anesthesiology*. 1977;47:277.
379. From RP, et al. *Br J Anaesth*. 1990;64:193.
380. Somogyi AA, et al. *Eur J Clin Pharmacol*. 1977;12:23.
381. Lebrault C, et al. *Br J Anaesth*. 1986;58:983.
382. Servin FS, et al. *Anesthesiology*. 1996;84:1092.
383. Westra P, et al. *Br J Anaesth*. 1981;53:331.

28 Reversal (Antagonism) of Neuromuscular Blockade

GLENN MURPHY, HANS D. DE BOER, LARS I. ERIKSSON, AND RONALD D. MILLER

KEY POINTS

- Appropriate reversal of a nondepolarizing neuromuscular blockade is essential to avoid adverse patient outcomes. Complete recovery of muscle strength should be present, and the residual effects of neuromuscular blocking drugs (NMBDs) should be fully pharmacologically reversed (or spontaneously recovered).
- Sufficient recovery from neuromuscular blockade for tracheal extubation can be confirmed by an adductor pollicis train-of-four (TOF) ratio of at least 0.90 (or 1.0 if acceleromyography [AMG] is used). Quantitative neuromuscular monitoring is the only method of assessing whether a safe level of recovery of muscular function has occurred.
- Residual neuromuscular blockade is not a rare event in the postanesthesia care unit (PACU). Approximately 30% to 50% of patients can have TOF ratios less than 0.90 following surgery.
- Patients with TOF ratios less than 0.90 in the PACU are at increased risk for hypoxemic events, impaired control of breathing during hypoxia, airway obstruction, postoperative pulmonary complications, symptoms of muscle weakness, and prolonged PACU admission times. Appropriate management of neuromuscular blockade can decrease the incidence of, or eliminate, residual blockade, which will reduce the risks of these adverse postoperative events.
- Neostigmine, pyridostigmine, and edrophonium inhibit the breakdown of acetylcholine, resulting in an increase in acetylcholine in the neuromuscular junction. However, there is a "ceiling" effect to the maximal concentration of acetylcholine that can be achieved with these drugs. Reversal of neuromuscular blockade with anticholinesterases should not be attempted until some evidence of spontaneous recovery is present. Neostigmine in the dose range of 30 to 70 μg/kg body weight antagonizes moderate to shallow levels of neuromuscular blockade. However, if these reversal drugs are given in the presence of full neuromuscular recovery, paradoxical muscle weakness theoretically may be induced.
- Sugammadex is a modified γ-cyclodextrin that shows a high affinity for the steroidal NMBDs rocuronium and vecuronium. Sugammadex is able to form a tight inclusion complex with either of these steroidal NMBDs, thereby inactivating the effects of rocuronium and vecuronium, resulting in rapid reversal of neuromuscular blockade.
- Sugammadex is able to reverse a moderate/shallow and a profound neuromuscular blockade with a dose of 2.0 mg/kg and 4.0 mg/kg, respectively. An immediate reversal of neuromuscular blockade induced by rocuronium is possible with a dose of sugammadex 16 mg/kg. Reversal of neuromuscular blockade by sugammadex is rapid and without many of the side effects encountered with anticholinesterase drugs.
- Fumarates (gantacurium [GW280430A, AV430A], CW002, and CW011) represent a new class of NMBDs in development that are inactivated primarily via adduction of cysteine to the double bond of the compounds, resulting in inactive breakdown products. Laboratory studies have shown that the administration of exogenous L-cysteine results in complete reversal of deep neuromuscular blockade within 2 to 3 minutes.

History

The paralytic effects of curare have been recognized since the time of Sir Walter Raleigh's voyage on the Amazon in 1595.[1] In 1935, the name *d*-tubocurarine was assigned to an alkaloid isolated from a South American vine *(Chondrodendron tomentosum)*. At approximately the same time, experiments from pharmacology and physiology laboratories in London suggested that acetylcholine was the chemical neurotransmitter at motor nerve endings.[2] Investigations from these same laboratories demonstrated that eserine (physostigmine)-like substances could reverse the effects of curare at the neuromuscular junction of frog nerve-muscle preparations.[2] In the clinical setting, Bennett (1940) described the use of curare in the prevention of traumatic complications during convulsive shock therapy.[3] In 1942, Griffith and colleagues reported on the effects of an extract of curare in 25 surgical patients; all patients appeared to recover fully without administration of an antagonist such as neostigmine.[4]

The importance of pharmacologic reversal of neuromuscular blockade was suggested in 1945. Specifically, use of neostigmine or physostigmine to antagonize curare was recognized and was recommended to be available whenever muscle relaxants were given in the operating room.[5] The first large case series examining the use of curare was published by Cecil Gray in 1946.[1] A crystalline extract, *d*-tubocurarine chloride, was administered in 1049 general anesthesia cases. No postoperative complications directly attributable to *d*-tubocurarine were noted, and physostigmine was administered to only two patients in the series. However, in a later review article (1959) from the same anesthesia department, the authors concluded that "it is safer to always use neostigmine when nondepolarizing relaxants have been administered."[6] By the mid-1960s, significant differences in neuromuscular management existed between the United States and Europe. As noted in an editorial from this time, "In Great Britain the majority of anesthetists have arbitrarily adopted the attitude that the dangers of reversal are far less than those of latent paresis, so that most patients receive at least some anticholinesterase drug at the end of anesthesia." In the United States, however, where smaller doses of curare were used, the emphasis was more on the mortality and morbidity associated with reversal drugs. Of greater importance was the use of muscle relaxants in smaller doses so that reversal drugs were not necessary.[7] In fact, in the senior author's training (Miller), the prevailing thinking was that emphasis in anesthesia should be on "properly anesthetizing rather than paralyzing" a patient; it was commonly said that "curare is not an anesthetic."

Despite more than seven decades of research, significant differences in opinion still exist regarding management of neuromuscular blockade at the conclusion of surgery and anesthesia. On a routine basis, some clinicians pharmacologically antagonize a nondepolarizing neuromuscular blocking drug (NMBD), whereas others antagonize neuromuscular blockade only when obvious clinical muscle weakness is present. The issue is whether clinically important weakness exists when it is not clinically apparent. Will monitoring of neuromuscular blockade improve patient care? The aim of this chapter is to review the consequences of incomplete neuromuscular recovery, the use of anticholinesterase drugs in clinical practice (benefits, risks, and limitations), and the recent developments in novel drugs to reverse/antagonize residual neuromuscular blockade.

Antagonism of Neuromuscular Blockade: Current Management Practices

A number of survey studies have been conducted to determine how clinicians evaluate and manage neuromuscular blockade in the perioperative period. In the late 1950s, a survey was sent to anesthetists in Great Britain and Ireland.[6] Forty-four percent of the respondents used neostigmine "always" or "almost always" when *d*-tubocurarine chloride or gallamine was used. Two thirds of respondents administered 1.25 to 2.5 mg when antagonizing these NMBDs.[6] Despite accumulating data demonstrating a continued frequent incidence of residual neuromuscular blockade, more-recent surveys indicate that attitudes toward reversal of neuromuscular blockade have changed little over the intervening decades. A questionnaire sent to German anesthesiologists in 2003 revealed routine reversal with neostigmine at the end of surgery was not practiced in 75% of anesthesia departments.[8] A similar survey of 1230 senior anesthetists in France reported that pharmacologic antagonism of neuromuscular blockade was "systematic" or "frequent" in only 6% and 26% of surgical cases, respectively.[9] In contrast, reversal of nondepolarizing NMBDs was routinely performed in Great Britain.[10]

A large-scale, comprehensive survey of neuromuscular management practices in the United States and Europe was conducted in order to better understand attitudes about doses of NMBDs, monitoring, and pharmacologic reversal.[11] Only 18% of European respondents and 34.2% of respondents from the United States "always" administered an anticholinesterase drug when a nondepolarizing relaxant was used. The findings from these surveys suggest that there is little agreement about best practices related to reversal of neuromuscular blockade. Despite perioperative guidelines from several international and national organizations, surveys from many countries reveal that most clinicians do not monitor or reverse a neuromuscular blockade in the operating room. Surprisingly, most anesthesiologists have not witnessed obvious adverse events directly attributable to incomplete recovery from neuromuscular blockade.[11] Therefore the potential hazards of reversal of neuromuscular blockade using an anticholinesterase drug (see later) are likely estimated to be more frequent than the risks of residual neuromuscular blockade. In the following sections, the definitions, incidence, and clinical implications of residual neuromuscular blockade are reviewed.

RESIDUAL NEUROMUSCULAR BLOCKADE

Assessment of Residual Neuromuscular Blockade

In order to optimize patient safety, tracheal extubation in the operating room should not occur until complete recovery of muscle strength is present and the residual effects of NMBDs have been fully reversed (or spontaneously recovered). Therefore methods to detect and treat residual muscle weakness are essential in improving postoperative outcomes. Three methods are commonly used in the operating room to determine the presence or absence of residual neuromuscular blockade: clinical evaluations for signs of muscle weakness, qualitative neuromuscular monitors (peripheral nerve stimulators), and quantitative (objective) neuromuscular monitors. A more detailed description of the types of neuromuscular monitors used perioperatively is provided in Chapter 43.

Clinical Evaluation for Signs of Muscle Weakness. Following the introduction of *d*-tubocurarine into clinical practice, residual paralysis and the need for neostigmine was determined primarily by the observation of "shallow, jerky movements of the diaphragm" at the end of surgery.[12] In the absence of any clinically observable respiratory impairment, neuromuscular function was assumed to be adequate, and no reversal drugs were administered. A peripheral nerve stimulator to assess neuromuscular

TABLE 28.1 Sensitivity, Specificity, Positive, and Negative Predictive Values of an Individual Clinical Test for a Train-of-Four <90% in 640 Surgical Patients

Variable	Sensitivity	Specificity	Positive Predictive Value	Negative Predictive Value
Inability to smile	0.29	0.80	0.47	0.64
Inability to swallow	0.21	0.85	0.47	0.63
Inability to speak	0.29	0.80	0.47	0.64
General weakness	0.35	0.78	0.51	0.66
Inability to lift head for 5 s	0.19	0.88	0.51	0.64
Inability to lift leg for 5 s	0.25	0.84	0.50	0.64
Inability to sustain hand grip for 5 s	0.18	0.89	0.51	0.63
Inability to perform sustained tongue depressor test	0.22	0.88	0.52	0.64

The sensitivity of a test is the number of true positives ÷ the sum of true positives + false negatives; the specificity is the number of true negatives ÷ the sum of true negatives + false positives. True positives are patients scoring positive for a test and having a train-of-four (TOF) <90%. False negatives are patients with a negative test result but a TOF <90%. True negatives have a negative test score and a TOF not <90%; false positives score positively but have a TOF not <90%. A *positive* test result means *inability* to smile, swallow and speak, general muscular weakness, and so on.

From Cammu G, De Witte J, De Veylder J, et al. Postoperative residual paralysis in outpatients versus inpatients. *Anesth Analg*. 2006;102:426–429.

blockade was first used in the 1960s by Harry Churchill-Davidson in the United Kingdom and later in the United States. However, routine use of a peripheral nerve stimulator did not occur. In fact, several decades later, the most commonly applied technique for evaluation of recovery of neuromuscular function continues to be the use of clinical tests for signs of apparent muscle weakness.[13] Furthermore, one of the primary factors that determines whether clinicians elect to administer a reversal drug at the end of surgery is the presence of signs of muscle weakness.[11] However, for decades an array of clinical studies from different countries have consistently shown that tests of muscle strength are not sensitive or reliable indices of adequate neuromuscular recovery. The most commonly applied criteria used to determine suitability for extubation of the trachea are a "normal" pattern of ventilation and a sustained head lift.[13] Unfortunately, the sensitivity of each test in detecting residual blockade is poor. At a level of neuromuscular recovery that allows for adequate ventilation in a patient whose trachea is intubated, the muscles responsible for maintaining airway patency and protection are significantly impaired.[14] Other investigators have observed that the majority of subjects could maintain a 5-second head lift at a train-of-four (TOF) ratio of 0.50 or less.[15,16] Additional clinical tests of muscle strength, such as sustained hand-grip, leg-lift, or eye opening, have been demonstrated to have a low sensitivity in predicting recovery of neuromuscular function (Table 28.1).[17,18]

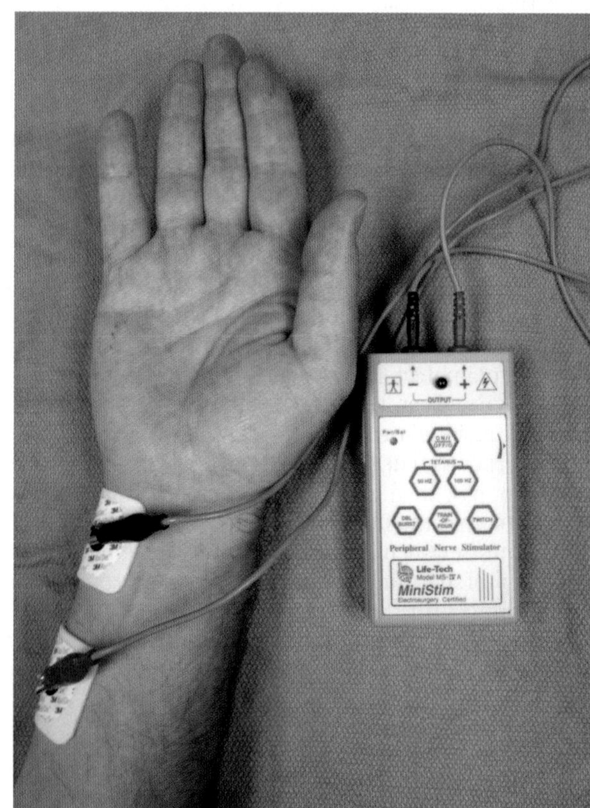

Fig. 28.1 Example of a qualitative neuromuscular monitor (or more appropriately, a peripheral nerve stimulator). (MiniStim, Halyard Health, Roswell, GA) A peripheral nerve is stimulated, and the response to nerve stimulation is subjectively (qualitatively) assessed using either visual or tactile (hand placed on the muscle) means. In this illustration, the ulnar nerve is stimulated, and movement of the thumb subjectively evaluated.

Qualitative Neuromuscular Monitoring. Qualitative neuromuscular monitors—or more accurately, peripheral nerve stimulators—deliver an electrical stimulus to a peripheral nerve, and the response to nerve stimulation is subjectively assessed by clinicians either visually or tactilely (i.e., placing a hand on the thumb to detect the muscle contraction after ulnar nerve stimulation) (Fig. 28.1). Three patterns of nerve stimulation are used in the clinical setting to assess patients for residual blockade: TOF, tetanic, and double-burst stimulation. TOF stimulation delivers four supramaximal stimuli every 0.5 seconds, tetanic stimulation consists of a series of extremely rapid (usually 50 or 100 Hz) stimuli typically applied over 5 seconds, and double-burst stimulation delivers two short bursts of 50-Hz tetanic stimuli separated by 750 ms. The presence of fade with these patterns of nerve stimulation indicates incomplete neuromuscular recovery. Although qualitative monitoring may guide management during early recovery from neuromuscular blockade, the sensitivity of these devices in detecting small degrees of

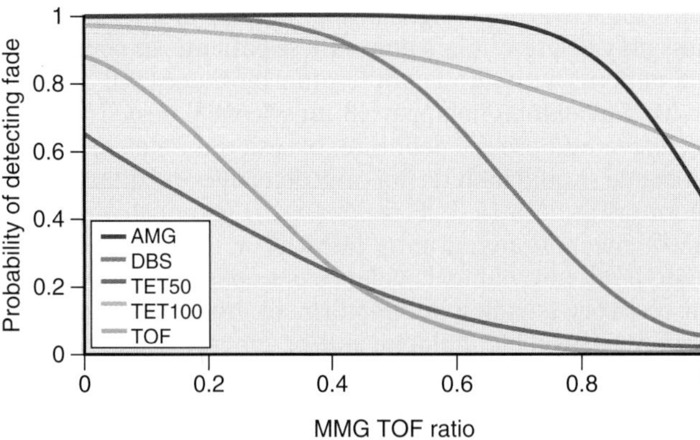

Fig. 28.2 Detection of fade with various neuromuscular monitoring techniques. Residual neuromuscular blockade was evaluated using acceleromyography *(AMG)*, tactile assessment of train-of-four *(TOF)*, double-burst stimulation *(DBS)*, 50-Hz tetanus *(TET50)*, or 100-Hz tetanus *(TET100)*. The mechanomyographic *(MMG)* adductor pollicis TOF ratio was measured at one extremity. During recovery, a blinded observer estimated tactile fade in the other extremity. Probability of detection of fade by logistic regression is presented. (From Capron F, Fortier LP, Racine S, Donati F. Tactile fade detection with hand or wrist stimulation using train-of-four, double-burst stimulation, 50-hertz tetanus, 100-hertz tetanus, and acceleromyography. *Anesth Analg*. 2006;102:1578–1584.)

residual paresis (TOF ratios between 0.50 and 1.0) is limited (Fig. 28.2). When using TOF stimulation, investigators have consistently observed that clinicians are unable to detect fade when TOF ratios exceed 0.30 to 0.40.[19-21] Similarly, the observation of fade during a 5-second, 50-Hz tetanic stimulation is difficult when TOF ratios are greater than 0.30.[21,22] The ability of clinicians to detect fade is improved with double-burst stimulation; the threshold for detection of fade is approximately 0.6 to 0.7 using this mode of stimulation.[20,21,23] However, regardless of the mode of nerve stimulation used, residual neuromuscular blockade cannot always be reliably excluded using qualitative monitoring.

Quantitative Neuromuscular Monitoring. Quantitative neuromuscular monitors are instruments that permit both stimulation of a peripheral nerve and the quantification and recording of the evoked response to nerve stimulation. Quantitative monitors allow an accurate assessment of the degree of muscle weakness using either TOF stimulation (TOF ratio displayed) or single-twitch stimulation (response compared with control "twitch" as a percentage). Although five different methods of quantifying neuromuscular function in the operating room have been developed, only one technology, acceleromyography (AMG, available as the Stimpod, Xavant Technology, Pretoria, South Africa), is commercially obtainable as a stand-alone monitor. The portable TOF-Watch AMG monitor (Bluestar Enterprises, San Antonio, Texas), which has been used in the majority of published clinical trials, is no longer sold in the United States (Fig. 28.3). In a study comparing AMG with standard qualitative tests (tactile fade to TOF, double-burst, 5-Hz tetanic, and 100-Hz tetanic stimulation), AMG was the most accurate technique in detecting residual paralysis (see Fig. 28.2).[21] In addition, the use of AMG in the operating room has been demonstrated to reduce the risk of residual neuromuscular blockade in the postanesthesia care unit (PACU)[24-27] and to decrease adverse respiratory events and

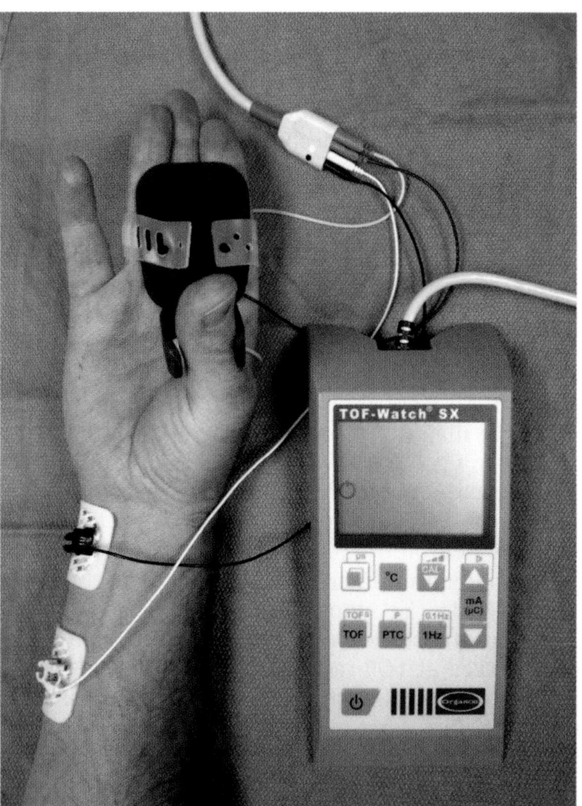

Fig. 28.3 Example of a quantitative neuromuscular monitor (acceleromyography). (TOF-Watch AMG, Bluestar Enterprises, San Antonio, TX) Ulnar nerve stimulation results in thumb movement, which is sensed by a piezoelectric sensor attached to the thumb. To improve the consistency of responses, a hand adapter applies a constant preload. Acceleration of the thumb is sensed by the piezoelectric sensor, and is proportional to the force of muscle contraction.

symptoms of muscle weakness associated with incomplete neuromuscular recovery.[26,27] In clinical practice, AMG is a valuable monitor in determining whether full recovery of neuromuscular function has occurred before tracheal extubation, and provides objective data to guide dosing of reversal drugs at the conclusion of surgery (see later).

A careful evaluation of the degree of residual blockade at the conclusion of a general anesthetic is essential in order to avoid the potential hazards of incomplete neuromuscular recovery following tracheal extubation. However, the methods used by most clinicians (ability to perform a head lift or maintain a stable pattern of ventilation; no fade observed to TOF or tetanic nerve stimulation) are insufficient in assuring safe recovery. At the present time, quantitative neuromuscular monitoring is the only method of determining whether full recovery of muscular function has occurred and reversal drugs safely avoided. In order to exclude with certainty the possibility of residual paresis, quantitative monitoring should be used. For a more comprehensive description of neuromuscular monitoring see Chapter 43.

Definitions of Residual Neuromuscular Blockade

QUANTITATIVE NEUROMUSCULAR MONITORING: TOF RATIO LESS THAN 0.70 AND LESS THAN 0.90 Traditionally, residual neuromuscular blockade has been defined using quantitative neuromuscular monitoring. Although peripheral nerve stimulation was used in the 1960s, Ali and colleagues first described the application of peripheral nerve stimulation for neuromuscular monitoring using the ulnar nerve–adductor pollicis unit as the site of monitoring in the early 1970s.[28,29] By comparing the amplitude of the fourth (T4) to the first (T1) evoked mechanical or electromyographic response (TOF response), the degree of neuromuscular recovery could be measured. Shortly thereafter, these same investigators performed several studies examining the association between the degree of residual blockade in the hand (defined using quantified T4/T1 ratio, i.e., TOF ratio) with symptoms of peripheral muscle weakness and spirometry measurements.[30-32] At adductor pollicis TOF ratios less than 0.60, signs of muscle weakness, tracheal tug, and ptosis were observed. When TOF ratios recovered to 0.70, the majority of patients were able to sustain head lift, eye opening, hand grasp, tongue protrusion, and a vital capacity exceeding 15 mL/kg. On the basis of these data, a TOF ratio of 0.70 was previously agreed on to represent acceptable neuromuscular recovery at the end of a general anesthetic that included administration of nondepolarizing NMBDs. Yet, more recently, clinically significant muscle weakness and impaired respiratory control have been observed at TOF ratios of up to 0.90. At TOF ratios less than 0.90, awake volunteers exhibit impaired pharyngeal function, airway obstruction, an increased risk of aspiration of gastric contents, an impaired hypoxic ventilatory control, and unpleasant symptoms of muscle weakness.[33-37] In surgical patients, an association between TOF ratios less than 0.90 and adverse respiratory events and prolonged PACU length of stay has been observed.[38,39] At the present time, it is generally agreed that adequate recovery of neuromuscular function is represented by an adductor pollicis TOF ratio of at least 0.90 (or even 1.0 when AMG is used).

Clinical Signs and Symptoms. A variety of clinical signs may be present in patients with residual neuromuscular blockade, including the following: inability to perform a head lift, hand grip, eye opening, or tongue protrusion; inability to clench a tongue depressor between the incisor teeth; inability to smile, swallow, speak, cough, track objects with eyes; or inability to perform a deep or vital capacity breath.[40] Symptoms of residual blockade that have been reported include subjective difficulty performing the aforementioned tests, as well as blurry vision, diplopia, facial weakness, facial numbness, and general weakness.[37,40] Although the majority of patients with TOF ratios of 0.90 to 1.0 will have recovered satisfactory strength in most muscle groups, signs and symptoms of muscle weakness may be present in some of these patients. In contrast, a few patients with significant residual blockade (TOF ratios < 0.70) may exhibit no apparent muscle weakness. The most inclusive and precise definition of residual neuromuscular blockade should include not only objective and quantifiable monitoring data (a TOF ratio < 0.90 demonstrated with AMG, mechanomyography [MMG], or electromyography [EMG]) but also clinical evidence of impaired neuromuscular recovery (swallowing impairment, inability to speak or perform a head lift, diplopia, and/or general weakness).

Incidence of Residual Neuromuscular Blockade

Residual neuromuscular blockade is not a rare event in the PACU. In 1979, Viby-Mogensen examined the efficacy of neostigmine in reversing *d*-tubocurarine, gallamine, or pancuronium blockade.[41] On arrival to the PACU, 42% of patients had a TOF ratio less than 0.70, and 24% were unable to perform a 5-second head lift (the majority of these subjects had TOF ratios <0.70). The authors concluded that the average dose of neostigmine given (2.5 mg) was insufficient for reversing neuromuscular blockade. Subsequent studies demonstrated a similarly frequent incidence of residual blockade in patients receiving long-acting NMBDs; 21% to 50% of patients in the early postoperative period had TOF ratios less than 0.70.[42-44] Subsequently, the risk of postoperative residual blockade was reduced if intermediate-acting NMBDs were used instead of long-acting drugs.[44-46] As the use of long-acting NMBDs began to decrease in clinical practices, many investigators hoped that residual blockade would become an uncommon occurrence in the PACU. However, incomplete neuromuscular recovery continues to be a common postoperative event. Large-scale studies (150–640 subjects) have demonstrated that approximately 31% to 50% of patients have clinically significant residual neuromuscular blockade with adductor pollicis TOF ratios less than 0.90 following surgery.[17,47,48] A recent multicenter investigation enrolling 1571 patients from 32 centers documented that 58% of patients had TOF ratios less than 0.90 at the time of tracheal extubation, despite the use of neostigmine reversal in 78% of subjects.[49]. In a metaanalysis of data from 24 clinical trials, Naguib and colleagues calculated the incidence of residual blockade by NMBD type and TOF ratio.[44] The pooled rate of residual blockade, defined as a TOF ratio less than 0.90, was 41% when studies using intermediate-acting NMBDs were analyzed (Table 28.2). In conclusion, a frequent incidence

TABLE 28.2 Pooled Estimated Incidence of Residual Neuromuscular Blockade by Muscle Relaxant Type and Train-of-Four Ratio

			HETEROGENEITY	
Sub-Population	**Pooled Rate of RNMB***	**Confidence Interval**	***P*-value**	**Inconsistency† (%)**
Long-acting MR (TOF <0.70)	0.351	(0.25-0.46)	<.001	86.7
Intermediate-acting MR (TOF <0.70)	0.115	(0.07-0.17)	<.001	85.9
Long-acting MR (TOF <0.90)	0.721	(0.59-0.84)	<.001	88.1
Intermediate-acting MR (TOF <0.90)	0.413	(0.25-0.58)	<.001	97.2

*Pooled rate of RNMB is the weighted average. The weight in the random-effect model takes into account both between and within studies variation.
†Inconsistency is the proportion of between studies variability that cannot be explained by chance.
MR, Muscle relaxant; *RNMB*, residual neuromuscular blockade; *TOF*, train-of-four.
From Naguib M, Kopman AF, Ensor JE. Neuromuscular monitoring and postoperative residual curarisation: a meta-analysis. *Br J Anaesth*. 2007;98:302–316.

of residual neuromuscular blockade still occurs worldwide in the immediate postoperative period; with current practice and inadequate monitoring, the incidence of this complication is not decreasing over time.

The observed incidence of postoperative residual blockade varies widely between studies, ranging from 5% to 93%.[44] A number of factors may influence the degree of neuromuscular recovery measured following tracheal extubation, accounting for the reported variability in the incidence of residual blockade (Box 28.1). The observed incidence of residual blockade is more frequent if a threshold definition of 0.90 is used (vs. the previous threshold of 0.70) (see Table 28.2). Similarly, a frequent incidence of residual paralysis is observed if there is a short time interval between reversal of NMBDs and quantification of TOF ratios (TOF ratios measured at the time of extubation vs. measurement in the PACU).[50] Furthermore, the technology used to quantify neuromuscular recovery may influence the percentage of patients with TOF ratios less than 0.90 following surgery. For example, when compared with MMG, AMG frequently overestimates the degree of neuromuscular recovery.[21] Additional factors influencing the degree of residual paralysis are discussed later.

Adverse Effects of Residual Blockade

Many investigations have demonstrated that approximately one half of patients will be admitted to the PACU with TOF ratios less than 0.90, as measured with AMG, MMG, or EMG.[44] The impact of this residual muscle weakness on clinical outcomes has been less well documented. Yet even minimal levels of neuromuscular blockade may have clinical consequences. The following section reviews the effects of residual blockade in both awake volunteer studies and in postoperative surgical patients.

Adverse Effects of Residual Blockade—Awake Volunteer Studies. Surgical patients receive a variety of anesthetics in the perioperative period, which complicates an assessment of the particular effect of residual neuromuscular blockade on clinical outcomes. Conducting awake volunteer trials allows investigators to more precisely quantify the impact of NMBDs and various degrees of neuromuscular blockade on physiologic systems in the absence of anesthetics. In general, these studies have titrated NMBDs to various TOF ratios in awake subjects and measured the effects on the respiratory system and on signs and symptoms of muscle weakness.

Early volunteer investigations concluded that respiratory impairment was minimal at TOF ratios of 0.60 to 0.70.[32] Respiratory frequency, tidal volume, vital capacity, and peak expiratory flow rates were not altered during the study, although vital capacity and inspiratory force were both significantly reduced compared with control values at a TOF ratio of 0.60.[32] The authors concluded that these changes were of minor clinical importance. Subsequent investigations have revealed that pharyngeal and respiratory function is impaired at TOF ratios as high as 0.90 to 1.0. Return of pharyngeal muscle function is essential for airway control following tracheal extubation. In series of human studies from the Karolinska Institutet, Sweden, a

BOX 28.1 Factors Influencing the Measured Incidence of Postoperative Residual Neuromuscular Blockade

Preoperative Factors

1. Definition of residual neuromuscular blockade
   - TOF ratio < 0.70 (before 1990)
   - TOF ratio < 0.90 (after 1990)
   - Presence of signs or symptoms of muscle weakness
2. Patient factors
   - Age (higher risk in older adults)
   - Gender
   - Preexisting medical conditions (renal or liver dysfunction, neuromuscular disorders)
   - Medications known to affect neuromuscular transmission (antiseizure medications)

Intraoperative Anesthetic Factors

1. Type of NMBD administered intraoperatively
   - Intermediate-acting NMBD (lower risk)
   - Long-acting NMBD (higher risk)
2. Dose of NMBD used intraoperatively
3. Use of neuromuscular monitoring
   - Qualitative monitoring (studies inconclusive)
   - Quantitative monitoring (lower risk)
4. Depth of neuromuscular blockade maintained
   - "Deeper blockade" (TOF count of 1-2) (higher risk)
   - "Lighter blockade" (TOF count of 2-3) (lower risk)
5. Type of anesthesia used intraoperatively
   - Inhalational agents (higher risk)
   - TIVA (lower risk)

Factors Related to Antagonism of Residual Blockade

1. Use of reversal agents (lower risk)
   - Neostigmine
   - Pyridostigmine
   - Edrophonium
   - Sugammadex
2. Dosage of reversal agent used
3. Time interval between reversal agent administration and quantification of residual blockade

Factors Related to Measurement of Residual Blockade

1. Method of objective measurement of residual neuromuscular blockade
   - Mechanomyography (MMG)
   - Electromyography (EMG)
   - Acceleromyography (AMG)
   - Kinemyography (KMG)
   - Phonomyography (PMG)
2. Time of measurement of residual neuromuscular blockade
   - Immediately

Postoperative Factors

1. Respiratory acidosis and metabolic alkalosis (higher risk)
2. Hypothermia (higher risk)
3. Drug administration in the PACU (antibiotics, opioids) (higher risk)

NMBD, Neuromuscular blocking drug; *PACU*, postanesthesia care unit; *TIVA*, total intravenous anesthetic; *TOF*, train-of-four.

functional assessment of the pharynx, upper esophageal muscles, and the integration of respiration with swallowing was performed during various levels of neuromuscular blockade.[33-34] At adductor pollicis TOF ratios less than 0.90, pharyngeal dysfunction was observed in 17% to 28% of young adult volunteers (Fig. 28.4),[33] increasing more than twofold in patients older than 60 years and associated with reduced upper esophageal sphincter resting tone and misdirected swallowing and aspiration (laryngeal penetration) of oral contrast material.[33,34,51] Eikermann and colleagues conducted a series of investigations examining the effect of residual paresis on respiratory muscle function in awake volunteers. Awake subjects were administered a rocuronium infusion, which was titrated to a TOF ratio 0.50 to 1.0. At a minimal level of residual blockade (approximately 0.80), the authors observed impaired inspiratory air flow and upper airway obstruction,[35] a marked decrease in upper airway volumes and upper airway dilator muscle function,[52] and increased upper airway closing pressure and collapsibility (Fig. 28.5).[53] In addition, evidence from human studies of respiratory control suggest that residual blockade inhibits hypoxic ventilatory control while leaving the ventilatory control during hypercapnia unaffected. In human volunteers, the hypoxic ventilatory response was attenuated by 30% after administration of either atracurium, vecuronium, or pancuronium at an adductor pollicis TOF ratio of 0.70, returning to normal after spontaneous recovery to a TOF ratio of greater than 0.90 (Fig. 28.6).[54] An increase in ventilatory drive during hypoxia is primarily mediated by afferent input from peripheral chemoreceptors in the carotid bodies located bilaterally at the carotid artery bifurcation, whereas ventilatory regulation during hypercapnia is mediated via CO_2 interaction with brainstem chemoreceptors. In experimental animals, the firing frequencies of carotid body chemoreceptors are almost abolished by the administration of a nondepolarizing NMBD via blockade of cholinergic neuronal subtype receptors within the carotid body oxygen signaling pathway.[55]

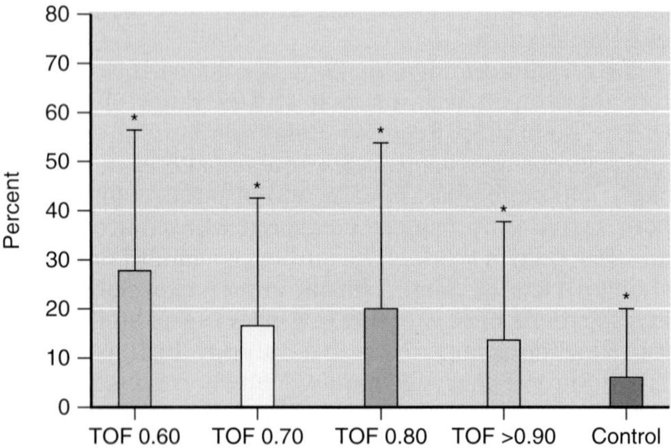

Fig. 28.4 Incidence of pharyngeal dysfunction during atracurium-induced partial neuromuscular blockade corresponding to steady-state adductor pollicis TOF ratio of 0.60, 0.70, 0.80, >0.90, and control in young volunteers. *TOF,* Train-of-four. (Modified from Sundman E, Witt H, Olsson R, et al. The incidence and mechanisms of pharyngeal and upper esophageal dysfunction in partially paralyzed humans. *Anesthesiology.* 2000;92:977–984.)

Awake volunteer studies have also revealed that unpleasant symptoms of muscle weakness are present in subjects with small degrees of residual neuromuscular blockade. Conscious subjects given a small "priming" dose of pancuronium noted blurred vision, difficulty swallowing, and keeping their eyes open, and jaw weakness at a TOF ratio of 0.81.[56] Symptoms of diplopia, dysarthria, and subjective difficulty swallowing were reported by subjects at TOF ratios of 0.60 and 0.70.[34] Reduced clarity of vision was described in all subjects receiving a mivacurium infusion at a TOF ratio of 0.81.[57] Kopman and associates examined 10 volunteers

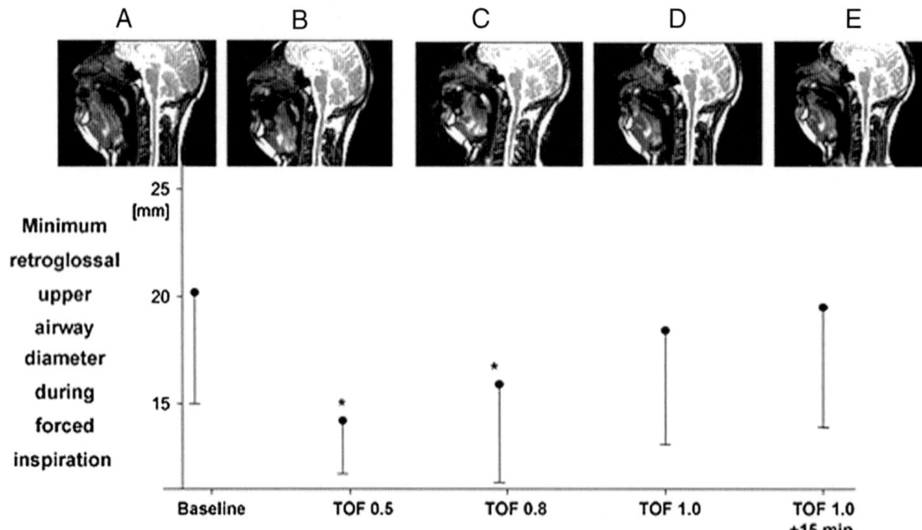

Fig. 28.5 An investigation examining the effect of residual neuromuscular blockade on respiratory muscle function in awake volunteers. Subjects were administered a rocuronium infusion, which was titrated to a train-of-four *(TOF)* ratio 0.5 to 1.0. Supraglottic airway diameter and volume was measured by respiratory-gated magnetic resonance imaging. Minimum retroglossal upper airway diameter during forced inspiration (A) before neuromuscular blockade (baseline), at a steady-state TOF ratio of (B) 0.50 and (C) 0.80, (D) after recovery of the TOF ratio to 1.0, and (E) 15 minutes later. Images from the volunteer show that a partial paralysis evokes an impairment of upper airway diameter increase during forced inspiration. $P < .05$ versus baseline. (From Eikermann M, Vogt FM, Herbstreit F, et al. The predisposition to inspiratory upper airway collapse during partial neuromuscular blockade. *Am J Respir Crit Care Med.* 2007;175:9–15.)

for symptoms and signs of residual paralysis at various TOF ratios.[37] Testing was performed at baseline (before an infusion of mivacurium), at a TOF ratio of 0.65 to 0.75, at 0.85 to 0.95, and at full recovery (1.0). All subjects had significant signs and symptoms at a TOF ratio of 0.70 (inability to maintain incisor teeth apposition, sit without assistance, drink from a straw, visual disturbances, facial numbness, difficulty speaking and swallowing, general weakness), and in seven subjects, visual symptoms persisted for up to 90 minutes after the TOF ratio had recovered to unity.

Adverse Effects of Residual Blockade—Postoperative Surgical Patients. Awake volunteers have impairment of respiratory function and a variety of symptoms of muscle weakness at TOF ratios of 0.50 to 0.90. Similar adverse events have been observed in postoperative surgical patients with TOF ratios less than 0.90 measured in the PACU. Incomplete neuromuscular recovery is a risk factor for hypoxemic events, airway obstruction, unpleasant symptoms of muscle weakness, delayed PACU length of stay, and pulmonary complications during the early postoperative period.

Clearly, an association exists between neuromuscular management characteristics and postoperative morbidity and mortality. Beecher and colleagues collected data from 10 university hospitals between the years 1948 to 1952 to determine anesthetic-related causes of mortality.[58] Risk of death related to anesthesia was six times more frequent in patients receiving NMBDs (primarily tubocurarine and decamethonium) compared with those administered no NMBDs (1:370 vs. 1:2100). Although the authors conclude that there is "an important increase in anesthesia death rate when muscle relaxants are added"[58] to an anesthetic, the use or omission of pharmacologic reversal in patients receiving NMBDs was not reported or analyzed. In another large-scale study, mortality data associated with anesthesia were collected over a 10-year period (1967-1976) at a single institution in South Africa.[59] An analysis of 240,483 anesthetics revealed that "respiratory inadequacy following myoneural blockade" was the second-most common cause of death. Again, data relating to the use of pharmacologic reversal drugs were not provided. A study from the Association of Anaesthetists of Great Britain and Ireland examined deaths that were judged "totally due to anesthesia" and reported that postoperative respiratory failure secondary to neuromuscular management was a primary cause of mortality.[60] Rose and associates examined patient, surgical, and anesthetic factors associated with critical respiratory events in the PACU.[61] Of the anesthetic management factors assessed, the most frequent rate of critical respiratory events was observed in patients receiving large doses of NMBDs (the use of reversal drugs was not analyzed). Two investigations of anesthetic complications resulting in admissions to the intensive care unit determined that "failure to reverse after muscle relaxants" and "ventilatory inadequacy after reversal of muscle relaxants" were the most common causes of admission.[62,63] Sprung and colleagues reviewed the medical records of patients who experienced a cardiac arrest over a 10-year period (223 of 518,284 anesthetics).[64] The most important category was the use of NMBDs, involving either hypoxia caused by inadequate pharmacologic reversal or asystole induced by anticholinesterase drugs. A large case-control investigation was performed of all patients undergoing anesthesia over a 3-year period (n = 869,483) in The Netherlands assessing the impact of anesthetic management characteristics on the risk of coma or death within 24 hours of surgery.[65] Reversal of the effects of NMBDs was associated with a significant reduction (odds ratio, 0.10; 95% confidence interval [CI], 0.03-0.31) in the risk of these complications. Two studies published in 2016 and 2017 examined the association between failure to reverse neuromuscular blockade and postoperative pneumonia.[66,67] In an investigation examining 13,100 surgical patients, Bulka and associates observed that the risk of postoperative pneumonia was 2.26 times more likely in patients that did not receive reversal with neostigmine.[66] Similarly, a retrospective study of 11,355 noncardiac patients revealed that the risk of respiratory complications (failure to wean from the ventilator, reintubation, or pneumonia) was significantly higher (odds ratio 1.75) in patients who were administered an NMBD without neostigmine compared to those given neostigmine.[66]

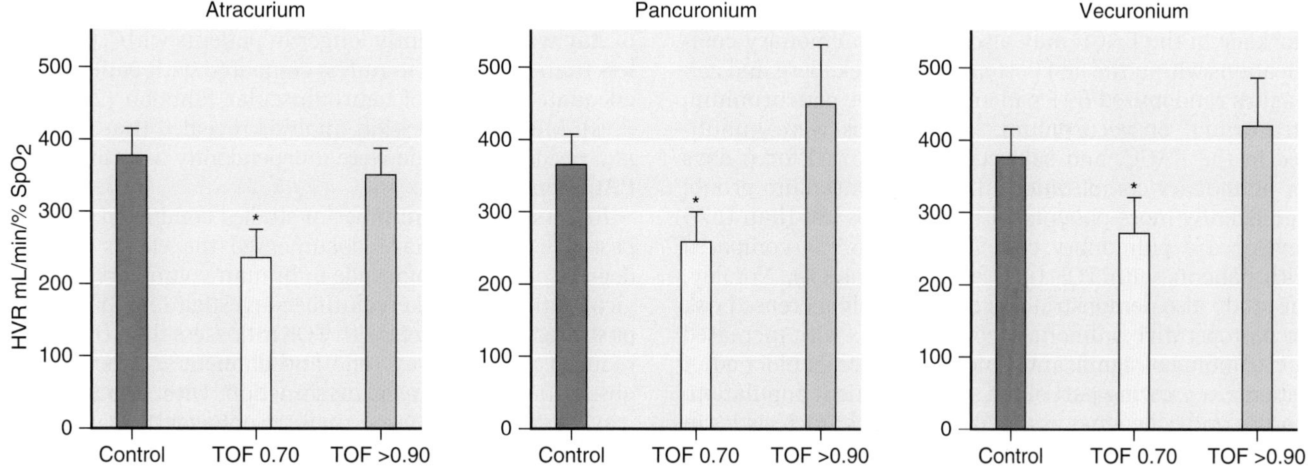

Fig. 28.6 Hypoxic ventilatory response *(HVR)* before (control); during steady-state infusion at train-of-four *(TOF)* ratio 0.70 of atracurium, pancuronium, and vecuronium; and after recovery (TOF ratio > 0.90). Data presented as means ± SD. * = P <.01. *SpO_2*, Saturation of arterial blood with oxygen. (From Eriksson LI. Reduced hypoxic chemosensitivity in partially paralysed man: a new property of muscle relaxants. *Acta Anaesthesiol Scand.* 1996;40:520–523.)

Epidemiologic studies thus suggest an association between incomplete neuromuscular recovery and adverse events in the early postoperative period. Notably, an important limitation of these outcome studies is that residual paresis was not quantified at the end of surgery. Therefore causality (residual blockade results in postoperative complications) can only be suggested but not proven.

In order to address these limitations, more recent studies have quantified TOF ratios in the PACU and documented a relationship between residual blockade and adverse outcomes. Several clinical investigations have documented an association between postoperative residual blockade and adverse respiratory events. In an observational study by Bissinger and colleagues, patients with TOF ratios less than 0.70 in the PACU had a more frequent incidence of hypoxemia (60%) compared with patients with TOF ratios 0.70 or greater (10%, $P < .05$).[68] Another small study of orthopedic surgical patients randomized to receive either pancuronium or rocuronium revealed that patients with TOF ratios less than 0.90 on arrival to the PACU were more likely to develop postoperative hypoxemia (24 of 39 patients) than those with TOF ratios greater than 0.90 (7 of 30 patients, $P = .003$).[69] Murphy and associates conducted a case-control study examining the incidence and severity of residual blockade in patients who developed critical respiratory events in the PACU.[38] Seventy-four percent of patients in the group with critical respiratory events had TOF ratios less than 0.70, compared with 0% in the matched control group (matched for age, sex, and surgical procedure). Because the two cohorts did not differ in any perioperative characteristics with the exception of neuromuscular recovery, these findings suggest that unrecognized residual paralysis is an important contributing factor to postoperative adverse respiratory events. Another investigation by this same group examined the effect of AMG monitoring on postoperative respiratory events.[26] Few patients randomized to AMG monitoring had postoperative TOF ratios less than 0.90, and a less frequent incidence of early hypoxemia and airway obstruction was observed in this group (compared with patients randomized to standard qualitative monitoring). A study of 114 patients randomized to neostigmine reversal or placebo (saline) documented a significantly more frequent incidence of both postoperative residual blockade and hypoxemia in the placebo group.[70] Residual blockade in the PACU may also result in pulmonary complications within the first postoperative week. Berg and colleagues randomized 691 patients to receive pancuronium, atracurium, or vecuronium.[71] TOF ratios were quantified in the PACU, and subjects were followed for 6 days for pulmonary complications. In the pancuronium group, significantly more patients with TOF ratios less than 0.70 developed a pulmonary complication (16.9%) compared with patients with TOF 0.70 or greater (4.8%). Notably, the study also demonstrated a continuously increased risk for postoperative pulmonary complications with increased age, a finding of significant clinical relevance for older adult patients, a growing part of the surgical patient population. Norton and colleagues assessed recovery characteristics in 202 consecutive patients arriving in the PACU. Thirty percent of patients had TOF ratios greater than 0.9; subjects with residual block had a significantly higher incidence of critical respiratory events, airway obstruction, hypoxemia, and respiratory failure.[72] An observational study enrolling 150 patients ages 18 to 50 and 150 patients more than 70 years old assessed the association between incomplete neuromuscular recovery (TOF < 0.9) and adverse events from the time of tracheal extubation until hospital discharge.[73] Elderly subjects had a higher risk of residual block (58% vs. 30%), and those elderly with TOF ratios less than 0.9 had a significantly higher incidence of airway obstruction episodes and hypoxemic events, as well as signs and symptoms of muscle weakness.[73] A multicenter study from Spain enrolling 763 patients from 26 centers reported that 27% of patients had TOF ratios less than 0.9 and that these subjects had a higher incidence of adverse respiratory events (odds ratio 2.57) and an increased risk of reintubation.[74] An additional study (340 patients) noted that patients with residual block had a greater than sixfold increase in postoperative adverse respiratory events.[75]

Residual blockade causes unpleasant symptoms of muscle weakness. This symptom of "general weakness" was the most sensitive "test" for determining whether patients had a TOF ratio of less than 0.90 in the PACU.[17] Orthopedic surgical patients given pancuronium had a more frequent risk of exhibiting both TOF ratios less than 0.90 and symptoms of blurry vision and general weakness during the PACU admission, compared with patients randomized to receive rocuronium.[69] Similar findings were observed in a cardiac surgical patient population not receiving anticholinesterase drugs.[76] The subjective experience of residual neuromuscular blockade after surgery was determined by examining 155 patients for 16 symptoms of muscle weakness during the PACU admission.[27] The presence of symptoms of muscle weakness was predictive of a TOF ratio less than 0.90 (good sensitivity and specificity).

The residual effects of NMBDs on postoperative muscle strength may impair clinical recovery and prolong PACU discharge times. In a small study of patients randomized to receive either pancuronium or rocuronium, the times required to meet and achieve discharge criteria were significantly longer in the pancuronium group, and patients in the cohort as a whole with postoperative TOF ratios less than 0.90 were more likely to have a prolonged PACU stay compared with those with TOF ratios greater than 0.90.[69] A larger investigation measured TOF ratios in 246 consecutive patients on arrival to the PACU.[39] The PACU length of stay was significantly longer in patients with TOF ratios less than 0.90 (323 minutes) compared with patients with adequate recovery of neuromuscular function (243 minutes). Multiple regression analysis revealed that only age and residual blockade were independently associated with PACU length of stay.

In conclusion, a number of studies conducted over the past five decades have documented the effects of small degrees of residual blockade in human volunteers and surgical patients. Awake volunteer investigations have demonstrated that subjects with TOF ratios less than 0.90 have reduced upper airway tone and diameters, upper airway obstruction, pharyngeal dysfunction with impaired airway integrity, decreased upper esophageal tone, and an increased risk of aspiration, impaired hypoxic ventilatory control, and unpleasant symptoms of muscle weakness. Epidemiologic outcome investigations have suggested an association between incomplete neuromuscular recovery and major morbidity and mortality. Prospective clinical trials have revealed that patients with TOF ratios less than 0.90 in the PACU are at increased risk for hypoxemic events, airway obstruction, postoperative pulmonary complications, symptoms of muscle weakness, and prolonged PACU admission times. These data suggest that residual blockade is an important patient safety issue in the early postoperative period. Therefore appropriate management of reversal of neuromuscular blockade and assessment of recovery from neuromuscular blockade are two essential clinical components to optimize patient outcomes.

Drugs Used to Antagonize (Reverse) Neuromuscular Blockade

Reversal of neuromuscular blockade is theoretically possible by three principal mechanisms: (1) an increase in presynaptic release of acetylcholine; (2) a decrease in enzymatic metabolism of acetylcholine by cholinesterase, thereby increasing receptor binding competition; and (3) a decrease in the concentration of the NMBD at the effect-site, freeing the postsynaptic receptors.

ANTICHOLINESTERASE REVERSAL OF NEUROMUSCULAR BLOCKADE

Nondepolarizing NMBDs inhibit neuromuscular transmission primarily by competitively antagonizing or blocking the effect of acetylcholine at the postjunctional nicotinic acetylcholine receptor (nAChR). Binding of nondepolarizing NMBDs to the nAChR occurs in a competitive fashion. If larger concentrations of acetylcholine are present at the neuromuscular junction, acetylcholine will attach to the postsynaptic receptor and facilitate neuromuscular transmission and muscle contraction. Conversely, if larger concentrations of a nondepolarizing NMBD are present at the neuromuscular junction, binding to α subunits of the receptor will preferentially occur, preventing central pore opening and muscle depolarization from occurring. A more detailed description of the neuromuscular junction is provided in Chapter 12.

One mechanism of reversing the effects of NMBDs is by an increase in the concentration of acetylcholine at the neuromuscular junction. This can be accomplished using an inhibitor of cholinesterase, which constrains the enzyme that breaks down acetylcholine at the neuromuscular junction (acetylcholinesterase). Three anticholinesterase drugs are commonly used in clinical practice: neostigmine, edrophonium, and pyridostigmine. Neostigmine is likely the most commonly administered drug. Over the prior six decades, anticholinesterases have been the only drugs used clinically to reverse neuromuscular blockade (until the recent introduction of sugammadex).

Mechanism of Action of Anticholinesterases

Acetylcholine is the primary neurotransmitter that is synthesized, stored, and released by exocytosis at the distal motor nerve terminal. Acetylcholinesterase is the enzyme responsible for the control of neurotransmission at the neuromuscular junction by hydrolyzing acetylcholine. Rapid hydrolysis of acetylcholine removes excess neurotransmitter from the synapse, preventing overstimulation and tetanic excitation of the postsynaptic muscle. Nearly half of the acetylcholine molecules released from the presynaptic nerve membrane are hydrolyzed by acetylcholinesterase before reaching the nAChR.[77] The action of acetylcholinesterase is quite rapid; acetylcholine molecules are hydrolyzed in approximately 80 to 100 μs (microseconds). Acetylcholinesterase is concentrated at the neuromuscular junction, and there are approximately 10 enzyme-binding sites for each molecule of acetylcholine released.[78] However, lower concentrations of acetylcholinesterase are present along the length of the muscle fiber. Each molecule of acetylcholinesterase has an active surface with two important binding sites, an anionic site and an esteratic site. The negatively charged anionic site on the acetylcholinesterase molecule is responsible for electrostatically binding the positively charged quaternary nitrogen group on the acetylcholine molecule. The esteratic site forms covalent bonds with the carbamate group at the opposite end of the acetylcholine molecule and is responsible for the hydrolytic process (Fig. 28.7).[78] In addition, a secondary or peripheral anionic site has been proposed. Binding of ligands to the peripheral anionic site results in inactivation of the enzyme.

The anticholinesterase drugs used by anesthesiologists interact with the anionic and esteratic sites of acetylcholinesterase. These drugs are characterized as either prosthetic inhibitors (edrophonium) or oxydiaphoretic (acid-transferring) inhibitors (neostigmine, pyridostigmine) of the enzyme. Edrophonium rapidly binds to the anionic site via electrostatic forces and to the esteratic site by hydrogen bonding.[77,78] Rapid binding may account for the short onset of action of edrophonium in clinical practice. During the time edrophonium is bound, the enzyme is inactive and edrophonium is not metabolized. However, the interaction between edrophonium and acetylcholinesterase is weak and short-lived. The dissociation half-life of this interaction is approximately 20 to 30 seconds, and the interaction between drug and enzyme is competitive and reversible. Because the nature of the binding is relatively brief, the efficacy of edrophonium in reversing neuromuscular blockade may be limited. Neostigmine and pyridostigmine are oxydiaphoretic inhibitors of acetylcholinesterase, which also

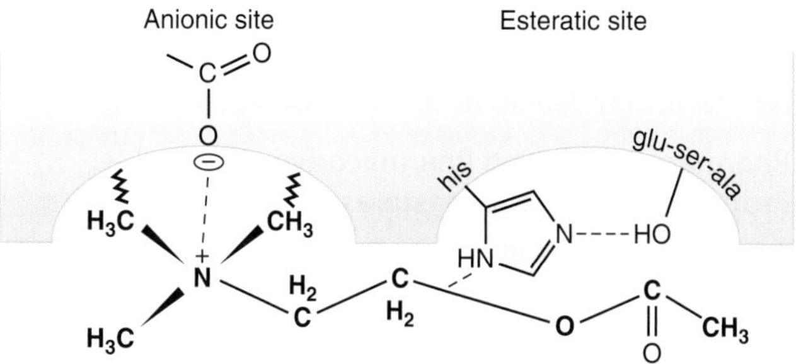

Fig. 28.7 Active binding sites on acetylcholinesterase. The positively charged quaternary nitrogen group on acetylcholine (Ach) binds by electrostatic forces to the negatively charged anionic site on the enzyme. The carbamate group at the opposite end of the Ach molecule forms covalent bonds with and is metabolized at the esteratic site. (From Caldwell JE. Clinical limitations of acetylcholinesterase antagonists. *J Crit Care.* 2009;24:21–28.)

bind to the anionic site. In addition, these drugs transfer a carbamate group to acetylcholinesterase, creating a covalent bond at the esteratic site.[77,78] This reaction results in an inactivation of the enzyme, as well as the hydrolysis of the drug. The stronger interaction between neostigmine and enzyme results in dissociation half-life of approximately 7 minutes.[78] Therefore the duration of enzyme inhibition is longer with neostigmine and pyridostigmine compared with edrophonium. These interactions at the molecular level likely have little impact on the duration of action in clinical practice. Duration of clinical effect is primarily determined by removal of anticholinesterase from the plasma.[79]

The administration of anticholinesterases has also been reported to produce presynaptic effects.[79] Laboratory investigations have demonstrated that these prejunctional effects may actually facilitate neuromuscular transmission. Anticholinesterases produce a reversible increase in the duration of the action potential and refractory period of the nerve terminal. Because the quantity of acetylcholine released is a function of the extent and duration of the depolarization of the terminal membrane, the period of acetylcholine release in response to nerve stimulation may be increased by anticholinesterase agents.[79] Excessive release of acetylcholine, coupled with decreased hydrolysis due to acetylcholinesterase inhibition, results in prolonged end-plate potentials and repetitive firing of muscle fibers. These prejunctional effects appear to account for the observations that spontaneous contractions of muscles can occur when anticholinesterases are given in the absence of NMBDs.[79]

Although neostigmine, pyridostigmine, and edrophonium inhibit the breakdown of acetylcholine, resulting in an increase in acetylcholine in the neuromuscular junction, there is a clinically relevant "ceiling" effect to the maximal concentration of acetylcholine. As concentrations of acetylcholine increase, some of the neurotransmitter diffuses away from the neuromuscular junction, while additional acetylcholine undergoes reuptake into motor nerve terminals. As the processes of diffusion and reuptake reach equilibrium with augmented release by enzyme inhibition, a "peak" level at the neuromuscular junction is reached.[78] Once the acetylcholinesterase enzyme is maximally inhibited by an anticholinesterase agent and peak concentrations of acetylcholine are present, the administration of additional drug will not further increase acetylcholine levels or enhance recovery of neuromuscular blockade. This "ceiling" effect of anticholinesterases is an important limitation of all clinically used agents; neuromuscular blockade cannot be adequately reversed if high concentrations of NMBDs are present at the neuromuscular junction.

Pharmacokinetic and Pharmacodynamic Properties of Anticholinesterases

A large number of clinical studies have examined the pharmacokinetic and pharmacodynamic characteristics of neostigmine, pyridostigmine, and edrophonium.

The pharmacokinetic profiles of neostigmine, pyridostigmine, and edrophonium are presented in Table 28.3. Most studies have used a two-compartment model to establish pharmacokinetic characteristics of each agent. Following a bolus administration, plasma concentrations peak rapidly and decline significantly within the first 5 to 10 minutes. This is followed by a slower decline in plasma concentrations due to the elimination phase.[79] In general, the pharmacokinetic profiles of all three anticholinesterases are similar. Early studies suggested that the duration of edrophonium was too short for clinical use. However, studies using larger doses (0.5 or 1.0 mg/kg) demonstrated that the elimination half-life of edrophonium was not significantly different from that of neostigmine or pyridostigmine and that edrophonium could produce prompt and sustained reversal of neuromuscular blockade.[80,81] The longer elimination half-life of pyridostigmine likely accounts for the longer duration of action compared with the other anticholinesterase drugs.[82]

TABLE 28.3 Pharmacokinetics of Neostigmine, Pyridostigmine, and Edrophonium in Patients Without and With Renal Failure

	WITHOUT RENAL FAILURE			WITH RENAL FAILURE		
	N	**P**	**E**	**N**	**P**	**E**
Distribution half-life ($T_{1/2}\alpha$, min)	3.4	6.7	7.2	2.5	3.9	7.0
Elimination half-life ($T_{1/2}\beta$, min)	77	113	110	181	379	304
Volume of central compartment (L/kg)	0.2	0.3	0.3	0.3	0.4	0.3
Total plasma clearance (mL/kg/min)	9.1	8.6	9.5	4.8	3.1	3.9

Data from references 73–76.
From Naguib M, Lien CA. Pharmacology of muscle relaxants and their antagonists. In: Miller RD, ed. *Miller's Anesthesia*. 7th ed. Philadelphia: Saunders; 2010.

The pharmacokinetics of anticholinesterases can be influenced by renal function, age, and body temperature. The elimination half-life of all three agents is altered by the presence of renal insufficiency or failure (see Table 28.3). Renal excretion accounts for approximately 50% of plasma clearance of neostigmine; elimination half-life is significantly prolonged and serum clearance decreased in anephric patients.[83] Similarly, renal function accounts for 70% to 75% of serum clearance of pyridostigmine and edrophonium.[82,84] The reduced plasma clearance of the anticholinesterases in renal failure patients provides a "margin of safety" against the risk of postoperative "recurarization" (the effects of the NMBD persist longer than that of the reversal agent, resulting in a worsening of residual paresis). The pharmacokinetics of edrophonium have been examined in older adult (age > 70 years) patients. When compared with a younger cohort, older adult patients exhibited a significant decrease in plasma clearance (5.9 ± 2 vs. 12.1 ± 4 mL/kg/min) and a prolonged elimination half-life (84.2 ± 17 vs. 56.6 ± 16 minutes).[85] Mild hypothermia (reduction in core temperature of 2°C) more than doubles the duration of action of intermediate-acting NMBDs.[86] In a study of human volunteers cooled to 34.5°C, the central volume of distribution of neostigmine decreased 38% and the onset time of maximal blockade increased from 4.6 to 5.6 minutes.[87] However, the clearance, maximal effect, and duration of action of neostigmine were not altered by a reduction in body temperature. Therefore if hypothermia influences the degree of neuromuscular recovery, it is likely

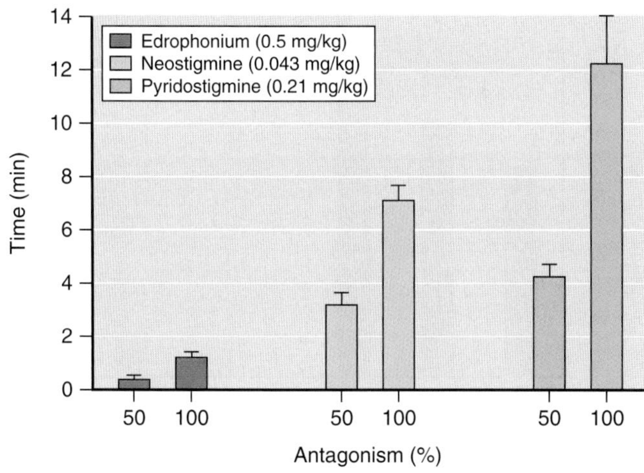

Fig. 28.8 Comparison of onset of action for edrophonium, neostigmine, and pyridostigmine. Values plotted are means ± SE. Edrophonium's onset was significantly faster than neostigmine or pyridostigmine. (From Cronnelly R, Morris RB, Miller RD. Edrophonium: duration of action and atropine requirement in humans during halothane anesthesia. *Anesthesiology*. 1982;57:261–266.)

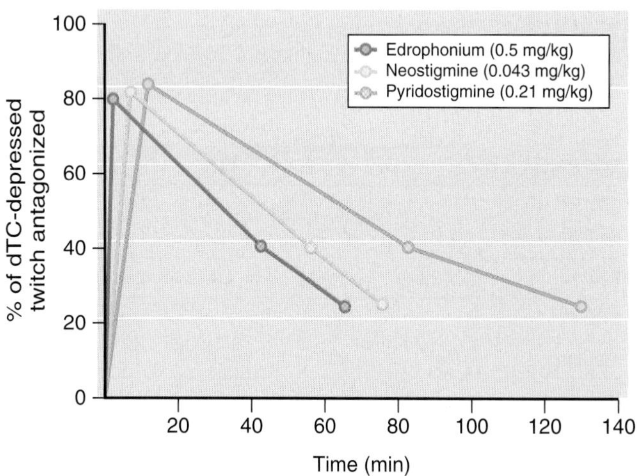

Fig. 28.9 Duration of antagonism compared at equipotent doses of neostigmine, pyridostigmine, and edrophonium. Values plotted are means. Edrophonium did not differ from neostigmine in duration; however, both were shorter than pyridostigmine. *dTC*, d-tubocurarine. (From Cronnelly R, Morris RB, Miller RD. Edrophonium: duration of action and atropine requirement in humans during halothane anesthesia. *Anesthesiology*. 1982;57:261–266.)

secondary to an effect on the pharmacology of NMBDs (not the anticholinesterase).

Onset of action may be more rapid with edrophonium than with either neostigmine or pyridostigmine. When *d*-tubocurarine neuromuscular blockade was reversed with approximately equipotent doses of the three clinically used anticholinesterases, the peak effect of antagonism was reached significantly faster with edrophonium (0.8-2.0 minutes) than with neostigmine (7-11 minutes) or pyridostigmine (12-16 minutes) (Fig. 28.8).[80] Similar findings have been observed in patients receiving other long- and intermediate-acting NMBDs. When larger doses (0.5-1.0 mg/kg) of edrophonium are administered during moderate levels of neuromuscular blockade (10% recovery of single-twitch height after pancuronium or atracurium), the onset time of edrophonium was faster than neostigmine.[88,89] During deeper levels of blockade (<10% recovery of single twitch), edrophonium 1.0 mg/kg and neostigmine 0.04 mg/kg had similar onset times when vecuronium was used (and both were faster than edrophonium 0.5 mg/kg).[90] When pancuronium was antagonized during deep blockade, edrophonium 1.0 mg/kg had a shorter onset time than neostigmine 0.04 mg/kg.[90] These findings suggest that onset time of antagonism is influenced by the type and dose of anticholinesterase used, the choice of NMBD administered intraoperatively, and the depth of neuromuscular blockade at the time of antagonism.

The duration of action of anticholinesterases is determined not only by the pharmacokinetic properties of the drugs, but also by the concentration of NMBD present at the neuromuscular junction at the time of reversal. Duration of neuromuscular blockade will naturally decrease over time as a result of metabolism and elimination of NMBDs. To accurately assess the duration of action of anticholinesterases during a stable, constant level of neuromuscular blockade, investigators have administered these agents to patients receiving an infusion of *d*-tubocurarine titrated to a 90% depression of single-twitch height.[80] The investigators observed that the duration of action of equipotent doses of neostigmine (0.043 mg/kg) and edrophonium (0.5 mg/kg) were similar (Fig. 28.9). The duration of both drugs, however, was significantly less than with pyridostigmine (0.21 mg/kg).

The comparative potencies of clinically used anticholinesterases have been calculated by constructing dose-response curves. In general, neostigmine is more potent than pyridostigmine, which is more potent than edrophonium. Neostigmine-to-pyridostigmine potency ratios of 4.4 to 6.7 have been reported (neostigmine is 4.4-6.7 times more potent than pyridostigmine).[80,91] Neostigmine is even more potent than edrophonium, with potency ratios of 5.7 to 19.5 estimated from dose-response curves.[80,91,92] The great variability in potency ratios described in the literature is related to several factors, which include the type of NMBD used in the studies, the endpoint selected to represent neuromuscular recovery, and the depth of blockade at the time of anticholinesterase administration.

In conclusion, pharmacokinetic and pharmacodynamic studies suggest that neostigmine, pyridostigmine, and edrophonium are all effective in reversing neuromuscular blockade when used in appropriate and equipotent doses. The following section will review factors that determine the efficacy of these agents in reversing neuromuscular blockade in the clinical setting.

Factors Determining the Adequacy of Recovery Following Administration of Anticholinesterases

Depth of Neuromuscular Blockade or Train-of-Four Count at the Time of Reversal. The primary anesthetic management variable determining the effectiveness of anticholinesterase agents in completely antagonizing neuromuscular blockade at the end of surgery is the depth of neuromuscular blockade at the time of reversal. As opposed to sugammadex (see later in this chapter), reversal of blockade by anticholinesterases should not be attempted until some evidence of spontaneous recovery is present. Kirkegaard-Nielsen and associates examined the optimal time for

TABLE 28.4 Time (min) from Neostigmine Administration to a Train-of-Four Ratio 0.70, 0.80, and 0.90 When Given at a Train-of-Four Count of 1-4

	GROUP*			
TOF Ratio	**I**	**II**	**III**	**IV**
0.70				
Median	10.3†	7.6‡	5.0	4.1
Range	5.9-23.4	3.2-14.1	2.0-18.4	2.4-11.0
0.80				
Median	16.6†	9.8‡	8.3	7.5
Range	8.9-30.7	5.3-25.0	3.8-27.1	3.0-74.5
0.90				
Median	22.2	20.2	17.1	16.5
Range	13.9-44.0	6.5-70.5	8.3-46.2	6.5-143.3

TOF, Train-of-four.
*Group I was reversed at a TOF count of 1, group II was reversed at a TOF count of 2, group III was reversed at a TOF count of 3, and group IV was reversed at a TOF count of 4.
†$P < .05$, group I > group II, III, and IV.
‡$P < .05$, group II > group IV.
From Kirkegaard H, Heier T, Caldwell JE. Efficacy of tactile-guided reversal from cisatracurium-induced neuromuscular block. *Anesthesiology*. 2002;96:45–50.

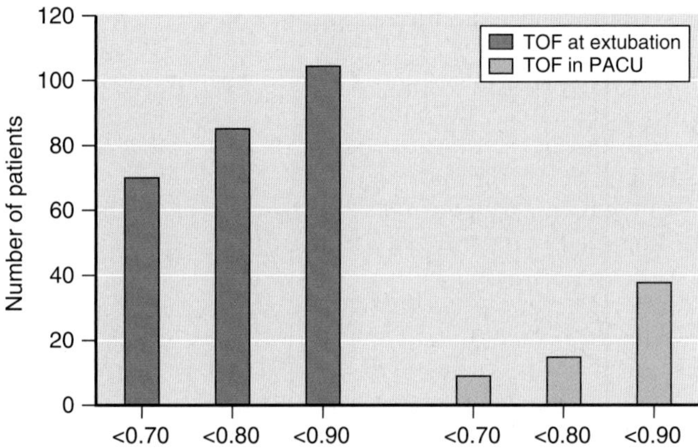

Fig. 28.10 Train-of-four (TOF) ratios measured immediately before tracheal extubation and again on admission to the postanesthesia care unit *(PACU)*. The graphs illustrate the number of patients (of a total of 120) with TOF ratios <0.70, <0.80, and <0.90 at each measurement interval. (From Murphy GS, Szokol JW, Marymont JH, et al. Residual paralysis at the time of tracheal extubation. *Anesth Analg*. 2005;100:1840–1845.)

neostigmine reversal of an atracurium blockade.[93] Administration of neostigmine 0.07 mg/kg during deep blockade (before the first twitch height reached 8%) resulted in significant prolongation of reversal times. In a similar investigation, atracurium was antagonized with neostigmine during intense blockade (posttetanic count [PTC] of 1 to >13).[94] Early administration of neostigmine did not shorten total recovery time and offered no clinical advantages. Similar findings have been observed during reversal of deep vecuronium blockade.[95] The total time to achieve a TOF ratio of 0.75 was the same whether neostigmine (0.07 mg/kg) was given 15 minutes after an intubating dose of vecuronium or whether single-twitch height had recovered to 10% of control.

The time required to achieve a TOF ratio of 0.90 after anticholinesterase administration is significantly shorter when a higher TOF count is present at reversal. Two studies have examined the efficacy of antagonizing residual blockade at varying TOF counts. Kirkegaard and colleagues randomized patients receiving cisatracurium to reversal with neostigmine (0.07 mg/kg) at the reappearance of the first, second, third, and fourth tactile TOF response (TOF count 1-4).[96] The median (range) time required to achieve a TOF ratio of 0.90 was 22.2 (13.9-44.0) minutes when reversal was attempted at a TOF count of 1. However, even when four responses were present, the time needed to attain a TOF ratio of 0.90 was 16.5 (6.5-143.3) minutes (Table 28.4). Kim and associates performed a similar study in which patients administered rocuronium were randomized to be reversed at the first through fourth tactile TOF responses.[97] In those patients receiving sevoflurane for anesthetic maintenance, the median (range) time required to achieve a TOF ratio of 0.90 was 28.6 (8.8-75.8) minutes when reversed at a TOF count of 1 and 9.7 (5.1-26.4) minutes when reversed at a TOF count of 4. In both investigations, a large interindividual variability in reversal times was observed.[96,97] This is likely a reflection of the individual response to the NMBD administered. The reason for marked prolongation of reversal times in some patients (up to 143 minutes) was not determined, but may be due to the "ceiling effect" with respect to the blockade (peak effect of the antagonist is followed by a plateau phase in which the balance between diminishing anticholinesterase activity and spontaneous recovery determines the slope of the recovery curve).[96] Both studies demonstrated that it was not possible to reliably achieve full neuromuscular recovery (TOF ratio of >0.90) in the majority of patients within 10 minutes of anticholinesterase administration. On the basis of data, expert opinion suggests that neostigmine should not be administered until the fourth "twitch" of the TOF count has returned.[98]

Time Interval Between Anticholinesterase Administration and Tracheal Extubation. Studies have suggested that if four responses to TOF nerve stimulation are present, approximately 15 minutes are needed to reach a TOF ratio of 0.90 in most patients.[96,97] Achieving a TOF ratio of 0.90 will require a significantly longer time (20–30 minutes) if a TOF count of 1 to 3 is observed at the time of reversal. To allow adequate neuromuscular recovery and ensure patient safety, anticholinesterase drugs should be given, on average, 15 to 30 minutes before clinicians anticipate removal of the endotracheal tube in the operating room. In many clinical situations, however, anticholinesterases are often administered at the conclusion of surgical closure, with tracheal extubation performed shortly thereafter. A survey of anesthesiologists from Europe and the United States revealed that approximately one half of respondents allowed only 5 minutes or less between anticholinesterase administration and tracheal extubation.[11] In a study of 120 surgical patients, TOF ratios were quantified at the time of tracheal extubation when clinicians had determined that full recovery of neuromuscular function had occurred using clinical criteria and qualitative neuromuscular monitoring (Fig. 28.10).[73] Mean TOF ratios of 0.67 were observed immediately before extubation, with

88% of patients exhibiting TOF less than 0.90. Of note, the median TOF count at reversal was 4, and the average time interval between neostigmine administration and tracheal extubation was only 8 minutes. The frequent incidence of residual blockade reported in multiple studies is likely attributable to the fact that anticholinesterases are not given early enough during the intraoperative anesthetic to ensure full neuromuscular recovery.

Type of Neuromuscular Blocking Drug Used Intraoperatively (Long-Acting Versus Intermediate-Acting). Two separate processes contribute to recovery of neuromuscular function following anticholinesterase administration. The first is the inhibition of acetylcholinesterase at the neuromuscular junction produced by neostigmine, pyridostigmine, or edrophonium. The second is the spontaneous process of decrease in the concentration of the NMBD at the neuromuscular junction over time due to redistribution and elimination. Therefore NMBDs that are redistributed and eliminated more rapidly from the plasma should be associated with more rapid recovery profiles after anticholinesterase use. Not surprisingly, the probability of satisfactorily antagonizing neuromuscular blockade is a function of the properties of the NMBD used to provide muscle relaxation. The ability of edrophonium (0.75 mg/kg) and neostigmine (0.05 mg/kg) to antagonize neuromuscular blockade produced by atracurium, vecuronium, and pancuronium following termination of steady-state infusions (single-twitch depression 10% of control) has been examined.[99] TOF ratios 20 minutes postreversal were 0.80 and 0.95 (atracurium with edrophonium or neostigmine), 0.76 and 0.89 (vecuronium with edrophonium or neostigmine), and 0.44 and 0.68 (pancuronium with edrophonium or neostigmine). Another clinical study investigated recovery of neuromuscular function in patients randomized to receive either intermediate-acting (rocuronium, vecuronium, atracurium) or long-acting (pancuronium) NMBDs.[100] Neostigmine (0.04 mg/kg) was given at 25% recovery of control twitch height, and TOF ratios were measured for 15 minutes. Mean TOF ratios had recovered to 0.88 to 0.92 in patients receiving intermediate-acting NMBDs, versus only 0.76 in the pancuronium group (Fig. 28.11).

A number of clinical investigations have examined the incidence of residual blockade in the PACU in patients receiving either intermediate- or long-acting NMBDs. These studies have consistently demonstrated that fewer patients given intermediate-acting NMBD have residual blockade compared with those receiving long-acting agents. A meta-analysis of 24 clinical trials examined the pooled estimated incidence of residual blockade (defined as a TOF ratio <0.90) by muscle relaxant type.[44] The risk of residual blockade was significantly less in patients given intermediate-acting NMBDs (41%) versus long-acting NMBDs (72%). In conclusion, the probability of incomplete neuromuscular recovery in the early postoperative period is decreased when shorter-acting NMBDs are used intraoperatively.

Type and Dose of Anticholinesterase. Complete recovery of neuromuscular function within 10 to 15 minutes with neostigmine, edrophonium, or pyridostigmine is difficult to achieve when profound neuromuscular blockade is present. Some investigations have suggested that edrophonium is less effective than neostigmine when reversing deep blockade; this may occur because the slopes of the dose-response relationships of neostigmine and edrophonium are not parallel (flatter dose-response curves are observed with edrophonium; Fig. 28.12).[90,92] In contrast, the recovery profile of edrophonium with larger doses (approximately 1.0 mg/kg) does not differ from neostigmine and pyridostigmine, and

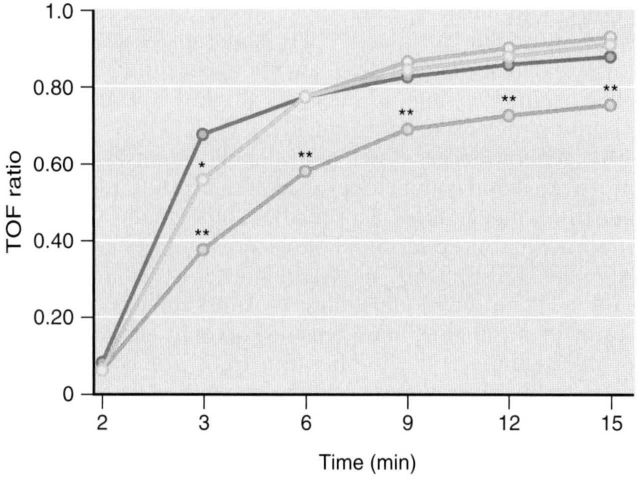

Fig. 28.11 Evolution of the train-of-four *(TOF)* ratio (mean) recorded at 3-minute intervals after administration of neostigmine 40 μg/kg when twitch height had returned to 25% of its initial value in groups of Roc *(green)*, Vec *(blue)*, Atr *(yellow)*, and Pan *(orange)*. **P* < .05, one-way analysis of variance and Duncan multiple classification range tests (group Vec vs. groups Roc and Atr). ***P* < .01, one-way analysis of variance and Duncan multiple classification range tests (group Pan versus groups Vec, Roc, Atr). (From Baurain MJ, Hoton F, D'Hollander AA, et al. Is recovery of neuromuscular transmission complete after the use of neostigmine to antagonize block produced by rocuronium, vecuronium, atracurium and pancuronium? *Br J Anaesth.* 1996;77:496–499.)

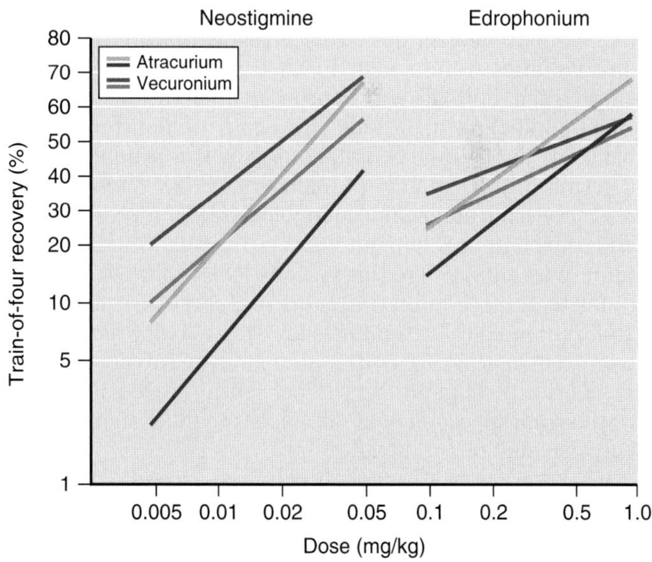

Fig. 28.12 Dose-response relationships of train-of-four assisted recovery evaluated 5 minutes (blue lines) or 10 minutes (purple lines) after administration of the antagonist as a function of the dose of neostigmine or edrophonium. The slopes of the curves obtained with edrophonium were usually flatter than the corresponding curves for neostigmine. (From Smith CE, Donati F, Bevan DR. Dose-response relationships for edrophonium and neostigmine as antagonists of atracurium and vecuronium neuromuscular blockade. *Anesthesiology.* 1989;71:37–43.)

edrophonium can produce rapid and sustained reversal of neuromuscular blockade.[88,90] At moderate levels of neuromuscular blockade all three agents appear to be similarly effective in reversing blockade, although the onset of edrophonium may occur more quickly.

In general, larger doses of anticholinesterases result in more rapid and complete reversal of neuromuscular blockade than smaller doses. This relationship remains true until the maximal dose of anticholinesterase has been administered. At this point, acetylcholinesterase is maximally inhibited, and additional amounts of anticholinesterase will result in no further antagonism. Maximal effective doses of neostigmine and edrophonium have not been clearly defined, but likely vary in relation to depth of blockade and type of NMBD used intraoperatively. Providing additional anticholinesterase beyond these maximum dose limits (neostigmine 60-80 μg/kg, edrophonium 1.0-1.5 mg/kg) provides no further benefit. When administered during deep neuromuscular blockade, a second dose of neostigmine (70 μg/kg) usually does not enhance recovery times beyond that observed with a single dose.[95]

AGE

INFANTS AND CHILDREN. The dose of neostigmine producing 50% antagonism of a *d*-tubocurarine neuromuscular blockade was slightly smaller in infants (13 μg/kg) and children (15 μg/kg) compared with adults (23 μg/kg).[101] The times to peak antagonism and duration of antagonism did not differ between infants, children, and adults. Pharmacokinetic modeling revealed that distribution half-lives and volumes were similar in all three cohorts, although elimination half-life was shorter in infants and children than adults. As in adults, the depth of neuromuscular blockade at the time of antagonism was a primary factor determining adequacy of recovery.[102,103] Spontaneous recovery from neuromuscular blockade is more rapid in children compared with adults.[103] However, when neostigmine was administered at various levels of blockade, the times to achieve neuromuscular recovery were similar in children and adults (the times to reach a TOF ratio of 0.90 were reduced by 30%–40% compared with spontaneous recovery).[103] Thus in the clinical setting, reversal of neuromuscular blockade does not appear to differ significantly between children and adults.

OLDER ADULTS. Physiologic changes occur during the aging process that result in alterations in the response of older patients to NMBDs. These changes include an increase in body fat, a decrease in total body water, and declines in cardiac, hepatic, and renal function. In addition, anatomic alterations occur at the neuromuscular junction in older adults, such as a decrease in the concentration of nAChRs at the motor end plate and a reduction in the release of acetylcholine from the preterminal axon. All of these factors contribute to a prolongation of effect of most NMBDs in older patients. In a study comparing older adults (age > 70) to younger controls, plasma clearance of edrophonium was decreased and elimination half-life prolonged in the aged cohort. Despite higher plasma concentrations of edrophonium, however, duration of antagonism was not increased. In contrast, Young and colleagues observed that the duration of action of both neostigmine and pyridostigmine was significantly longer in older adults (age > 60) compared with younger subjects.[104] These findings suggest that plasma concentrations and/or duration of action of both NMBDs and anticholinesterases (neostigmine and pyridostigmine) are prolonged in older patients, which should reduce the risk of recurarization. The risk of postoperative residual block in elderly patients (age > 70 years) who have received neostigmine is significantly higher than in a younger cohort receiving similar doses of this drug (ages 18–50, 58% vs. 30%, respectively).[73]

TYPE OF ANESTHESIA. Volatile anesthetics intensify the action of nondepolarizing NMBDs when compared with intravenous anesthetics. Furthermore, volatile anesthetics interfere with the antagonism of neuromuscular blockade.[105] Kim and colleagues randomized patients to receive a propofol or sevoflurane anesthetic (Table 28.5).[97] The times required to achieve a TOF ratio of 0.70, 0.80, and 0.90 were significantly longer in patients given the sevoflurane-based anesthetic compared with the propofol-based technique. Similar findings have been observed in patients randomized to receive either isoflurane or propofol (neuromuscular recovery was delayed when a volatile anesthetic was used).[105,106] These findings suggest that the probability of achieving a TOF ratio greater than 0.90 within 10 to 15 minutes of anticholinesterase administration is increased if a total intravenous anesthetic technique is administered as opposed to a volatile anesthetic.

CONTINUOUS INFUSION VERSUS BOLUS ADMINISTRATION OF NEUROMUSCULAR BLOCKING DRUGS. Recovery from neuromuscular blockade may also be influenced by mode of NMBD administration. Jellish and colleagues examined recovery characteristics of rocuronium and cisatracurium when given as either a bolus or continuous infusion.[106] The time required to reach a TOF ratio of 0.75 in the cisatracurium group was similar whether bolus or infusion techniques were used, whereas recovery was delayed when rocuronium was given as an infusion.[106] The authors conclude that cisatracurium may be the agent of choice for prolonged procedures since its recovery is not affected by length of infusion.

RENAL FUNCTION. As previously noted, renal excretion accounts for 50% to 75% of plasma clearance of neostigmine, pyridostigmine, and edrophonium. In anephric patients, elimination half-life of all three anticholinesterases is prolonged, and total plasma clearance of these agents is decreased (see Table 28.3). Similar changes in the pharmacokinetic characteristics of nondepolarizing NMBDs have been noted in patients with renal failure. Therefore management of anticholinesterase reversal should be similar in patients with normal and impaired renal function. Postoperative residual neuromuscular blockade in patients with renal failure is more likely secondary to improper titration of NMBDs intraoperatively rather than to inappropriate dosing of anticholinesterase agents.

ACID-BASE STATUS. The influence of metabolic status and respiratory acid-base balance on reversal of neuromuscular blockade has been investigated in the laboratory setting. Miller and associates noted that respiratory alkalosis and metabolic acidosis did not alter the dose of neostigmine needed to reverse a *d*-tubocurarine or pancuronium blockade. However, during respiratory acidosis and metabolic alkalosis, the dose of neostigmine needed to produce a comparable level of neuromuscular recovery was nearly twice

TABLE 28.5 Time (min) from Neostigmine Administration to a Train-of-Four Ratio of 0.70, 0.80, and 0.90 During Propofol- or Sevoflurane-Based Anesthesia

	GROUP*			
TOF Ratio	**I**	**II**	**III**	**IV**
PROPOFOL				
0.70	4.7 (2.5-7.8)†	4.0 (1.5-7.5)	3.4 (0.9-5.5)	2.1 (0.6-3.8)‡,§
0.80	6.4 (3.1-10.8)	5.5 (2.2-9.3)	4.4 (0.9-7.1)‡	3.3 (0.7-4.9)‡,§
0.90	8.6 (4.7-18.9)	7.5 (3.4-11.2)	5.4 (1.6-8.6)‡	4.7 (1.3-7.2)‡,§
SEVOFLURANE				
0.70	10.9 (3.6-28.9)¶	8.3 (2.5-22.3)¶	6.6 (2.4-18.5)‡,¶	5.4 (2.2-14.3)‡,§,¶
0.80	16.4 (5.9-47.5)¶	13.5 (5.1-37.2)¶	10.8 (4.2-29.2)‡,¶	7.8 (3.5-19.3)‡,§,¶
0.90	28.6 (8.8-75.8)¶	22.6 (8.3-57.4)¶	15.6 (7.3-43.9)‡,¶	9.7 (5.1-26.4)‡,§,¶

*Group I was reversed at a TOF count of 1, group II was reversed at a TOF count of 2, group III was reversed at a TOF count of 3, and group IV was reversed at a TOF count of 4.
†Values are median and (range).
‡$P < .05$ compared with group I.
§$P < .05$ compared with group II.
¶$P < .0001$ compared with propofol groups.
TOF, Train-of-four.
From Kim KS, Cheong MA, Lee HJ, Lee JM. Tactile assessment for the reversibility of rocuronium-induced neuromuscular blockade during propofol or sevoflurane anesthesia. *Anesth Analg*. 2004;99:1080–1085.

as large.[107,108] Although clinical studies have not been performed, the findings from laboratory investigations suggest that complete reversal of neuromuscular blockade may be difficult in the presence of respiratory acidosis and metabolic alkalosis. In particular, clinicians should be aware of the risk of residual blockade in the setting of respiratory acidosis. A number of anesthetics (opioids, benzodiazepines, volatile anesthetics) can potentially depress the ventilatory drive in the early postoperative period. This respiratory depression may result in respiratory acidosis, which limits the ability of anticholinesterases to reverse neuromuscular blockade. The resultant residual blockade may further depress the respiratory muscle strength and ventilatory drive and increase the risk of adverse postoperative events.

Neuromuscular Monitoring. Qualitative and quantitative neuromuscular monitoring should be used to guide dosing of both NMBDs and their reversal in the operating room. In general, if deeper levels of neuromuscular blockade are present at the end of surgery (1-2 responses to TOF stimulation), larger doses of anticholinesterases should be given. In these clinical scenarios, maximal doses of neostigmine (70 μg/kg), edrophonium (1.0-1.5 mg/kg), or pyridostigmine (350 μg/kg) should be considered. If three to four responses to TOF stimulation are present with observable fade of the fourth response, moderate doses of anticholinesterase should be administered (40-50 μg/kg of neostigmine, 0.5 mg/kg of edrophonium, 200 μg/kg pyridostigmine). If four responses are present with no fade, low doses of anticholinesterases can be considered (e.g., 20 μg/kg of neostigmine; see later).

Quantitative monitoring is also useful in guiding the dosing of anticholinesterases. Fuchs-Buder and colleagues investigated the dose-response relationship of neostigmine using AMG-based monitoring to guide neostigmine reversal (10, 20, or 30 μg/kg) given at TOF ratios of either 0.40 or 0.60 (Fig. 28.13).[109] All patients were able to achieve a TOF ratio of 0.90 within

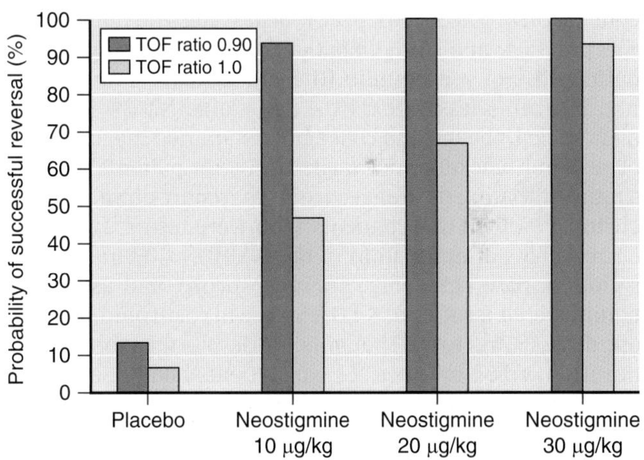

Fig. 28.13 Probability of successful reversal within 10 minutes after different doses of neostigmine or placebo. Neostigmine or placebo was given at a train-of-four ratio of 0.40. *TOF*, Train-of-four. (From Fuchs-Buder T, Meistelman C, Alla F, et al. Antagonism of low degrees of atracurium-induced neuromuscular blockade: dose-effect relationship for neostigmine. *Anesthesiology*. 2010;112:34–40.)

10 minutes of receiving 20 μg/kg of neostigmine. These findings demonstrate that small doses of neostigmine can be safely used if neuromuscular recovery is measured with quantitative monitoring. If muscle function is monitored manually with a peripheral nerve stimulator and no fade is detected manually with TOF stimulation, the TOF ratio is likely at least 0.40, but may be as high as 0.90 or 1.0. In the setting of full neuromuscular recovery, neostigmine administration may produce paradoxical muscle weakness (see later). This potential risk should be considered if neostigmine is used to reverse shallow blockade based on the results of qualitative neuromuscular monitoring.

In many clinical settings neuromuscular monitoring is unfortunately not used and decisions relating to the

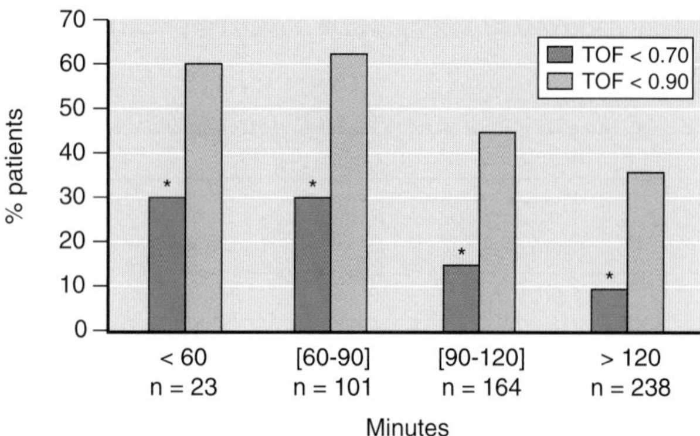

Fig. 28.14 The incidence of residual neuromuscular blockade after a single intubating dose of intermediate-duration nondepolarizing relaxant (rocuronium, vecuronium, or atracurium). Partial paralysis rate (percent) according to the delay between the administration of muscle relaxant and the arrival in the postanesthesia care unit. Partial paralysis was defined as a train-of-four *(TOF)* ratio less than 0.70 or less than 0.90. *n,* number of patients. *Significantly different from TOF < 0.90. (From Debaene B, Plaud B, Dilly MP, Donati F. Residual paralysis in the PACU after a single intubating dose of nondepolarizing muscle relaxant with an intermediate duration of action. *Anesthesiology.* 2003;98:1042–1048.)

administration of anticholinesterases are based on the time that has elapsed between the last dose of NMBD and the conclusion of the anesthetic. Clinical studies do not support this practice. In a study of patients receiving a single intubating dose of vecuronium (0.1 mg/kg), 8.4% of patients had TOF ratios less than 0.80 4 hours after NMBD administration.[110] Debaene and colleagues examined the incidence of residual blockade in a large cohort of patients given a single intubating dose of vecuronium, rocuronium, or atracurium.[47] Of the 239 patients who were tested 2 or more hours after administration of the NMBD, 37% had a TOF ratio less than 0.90 (Fig. 28.14). Murphy and associates administered a single 1 × ED 95 dose of rocuronium (average dose 25 mg) to 120 patients.[111] Despite an average case duration of 161 minutes, 21% of patients had not achieved a TOF ratio of 0.90 at the end of surgery. These investigations, as well as a number of pharmacokinetic and pharmacodynamic studies, demonstrate that the time course of spontaneous neuromuscular recovery is extremely variable from patient to patient. In order to detect and appropriately manage patients in whom delayed neuromuscular recovery may be present, quantitative neuromuscular monitoring is required.

Patients with Cholinesterase Deficiency. The duration of neuromuscular blockade following the administration of either succinylcholine or mivacurium is primarily determined by their rate of hydrolysis by plasma cholinesterase. Patients with abnormal plasma cholinesterase phenotypes and activity can demonstrate significant prolongation of clinical effect of these NMBDs. Mivacurium is four to five times more potent in patients phenotypically homozygous for the atypical plasma cholinesterase gene than in patients with normal cholinesterase activity.[112] Following standard intubating doses of mivacurium, recovery of neuromuscular function may require up to 4 to 8 hours in patients with cholinesterase deficiency.[113] Similar prolonged recovery times have been observed in patients administered succinylcholine who have atypical plasma cholinesterase genes.[114]

Human plasma cholinesterase has been used clinically to reverse neuromuscular blockade in patients with atypical serum cholinesterase. In 1977, Scholler and associates reported data on 15 patients with unexpected prolonged apnea lasting several hours after a dose of succinylcholine.[115] Adequate spontaneous ventilation was restored within an average time of 10 minutes in all subjects following the administration of human serum cholinesterase. Naguib and associates reported successful reversal of a profound mivacurium-induced neuromuscular blockade with three doses of a purified human plasma cholinesterase preparation and, in a subsequent study, established a dose-response relationship for plasma cholinesterase as a reversal agent for mivacurium in normal subjects.[113,116] The efficacy of exogenously administered plasma cholinesterase in antagonism of a mivacurium neuromuscular blockade was assessed in 11 patients phenotypically homozygous for atypical plasma cholinesterase.[117] A purified concentrate of cholinesterase (2.8-10 mg/kg) was administered 30 or 120 minutes after an intubating dose of mivacurium. Administration of cholinesterase restored plasma cholinesterase to normal levels, resulting in a 9- to 15-fold increased clearance and a shorter elimination half-life of mivacurium. The first response to TOF stimulation was observed in 13.5 minutes, and the time to achieve a TOF ratio of 0.80 ranged from 30 to 60 minutes. These data suggest that prolonged neuromuscular blockade secondary to low or abnormal plasma cholinesterase activity can be successfully managed with purified human plasma cholinesterase. Decisions relating to management of prolonged neuromuscular blockade in patients with atypical plasma cholinesterase should be based on the availability and cost of human plasma cholinesterase versus delaying tracheal extubation until spontaneous neuromuscular recovery has occurred.

Box 28.2 summarizes clinical management strategies that can be used by clinicians to reduce the risk of residual blockade when NMBDs are antagonized with anticholinesterases.

Complications Associated With Inhibitors of Acetylcholinesterase

Anticholinesterase-Associated Muscle Weakness. Anticholinesterases can antagonize moderate to shallow levels of neuromuscular blockade. However, if given when neuromuscular function is completely recovered, paradoxical muscle weakness theoretically may be induced. Large doses of neostigmine, pyridostigmine, and edrophonium may result in cholinergic hyperactivity and more intense fade in response to multiple nerve stimuli (decrease in TOF ratio) in an in vitro model.[118] The administration of a second dose of neostigmine (2.5 mg) to patients with small degrees of residual blockade resulted in a decrease in TOF ratios, tetanic height, and tetanic fade.[119,120] Caldwell examined neostigmine reversal (20 or 40 μg/kg) of residual neuromuscular blockade 1 to 4 hours after a single dose of vecuronium.[110] TOF ratios increased in 52 patients and decreased in 8 patients; TOF ratio decreases were only observed in patients with TOF ratios 0.90 or greater at the time of reversal (with 40 μg/kg doses of neostigmine but not 20 μg/kg dosing).

The clinical implications of administration of neostigmine after neuromuscular recovery has occurred have been

BOX 28.2 Clinical Management Strategies to Reduce the Risk of Residual Neuromuscular Blockade When Anticholinesterase Reversal Agents Are Used

Quantitative Monitoring Used (e.g., Acceleromyography)

1. TOF count of 1 or no TOF response—delay reversal until neuromuscular recovery is more complete (TOF count of 2 or greater).
2. TOF count of 2 or 3—administer doses of anticholinesterases (neostigmine [70 μg/kg], edrophonium [1.0–1.5 mg/kg], or pyridostigmine [350 μg/kg]). Extubate when the adductor pollicis TOF ratio has reached 0.90.
3. TOF ratio ≥ 0.40—administer moderate pharmacologic reversal doses of anticholinesterases (neostigmine [40–50 μg/kg], edrophonium [0.5 mg/kg], or pyridostigmine [200 μg/kg]). Extubate when the adductor pollicis TOF ratio has reached 0.90.
4. TOF ratio between 0.40 and 0.70—administer pharmacologic reversal, consider a low dose of neostigmine (20 μg/kg).
5. TOF ratio > 0.70—avoid anticholinesterase reversal; risk of anticholinesterase-induced muscle weakness if given.

Qualitative Monitoring Used (Peripheral Nerve Stimulator)

1. TOF count of 1 or no TOF response—delay reversal until neuromuscular recovery is detectable (TOF count of 2 or greater)
2. TOF count of 2 or 3 at the end of surgery—administer anticholinesterases (neostigmine [70 μg/kg], edrophonium [1.0–1.5 mg/kg], or pyridostigmine [350 μg/kg]). Allow at least 15-30 minutes before tracheal extubation is performed.
3. TOF count of 4 with observable fade at the end of surgery (likely adductor pollicis TOF ratio < 0.40)—administer anticholinesterases (neostigmine [40–50 μg/kg], edrophonium [0.5 mg/kg], or pyridostigmine [200 μg/kg]). Allow at least 10–15 minutes before tracheal extubation is performed.
4. TOF count of 4 with no perceived fade at the end of surgery (likely adductor pollicis TOF ratio ≥ 0.40)—administer pharmacologic reversal, consider a low dose of neostigmine (20 μg/kg).

No Neuromuscular Monitoring Used

1. Anticholinesterases should be considered. Spontaneous recovery of neuromuscular function may require several hours in a significant percentage of patients, even after a single intubating dose of an intermediate-acting NMBD.
2. Anticholinesterases should not be given until some evidence of recovery of muscle strength is observed since administration of an anticholinesterase during deep levels of paralysis may delay neuromuscular recovery.
3. Decisions relating to the use or avoidance of anticholinesterases should not be based upon clinical tests of muscle strength (5-second head lift). Many patients can perform these tests even in the presence of profound neuromuscular blockade (TOF ratio < 0.50). Other muscle groups may be significantly impaired (pharyngeal muscles) at the time when patients can successfully perform these tests.

NMBD, Neuromuscular blocking drug; *TOF*, train-of-four.
Modified from Brull SJ, Murphy GS. Residual neuromuscular block. Lessons unlearned. Part II: methods to reduce the risk of residual weakness. *Anesth Analg*. 2010;111:129–140.

examined in studies by Eikermann and colleagues. Rats were administered neostigmine after TOF ratios recovered to 1.0. Neostigmine administration resulted in decreases in upper airway dilator muscle tone and volume, impairment of diaphragmatic function, and reductions in minute ventilation.[121,122] In healthy volunteers given rocuronium, the administration of neostigmine after the recovery of the TOF to 1.0 induced genioglossus muscle impairment and increased upper airway collapsibility.[123] The adverse physiologic effects of neostigmine in the setting of complete neuromuscular recovery can potentially have negative respiratory consequences in postoperative surgical patients. The mechanisms proposed for this effect include sensitivity of the upper airway muscles to an overabundance of acetylcholine with desensitization of the ACh receptor, depolarizing blockade, or an open channel blockade. In contrast, Murphy and colleagues randomized 90 surgical patients to receive either 40 μg/kg of neostigmine or saline when TOF ratio of 0.90 to 1.0 was achieved at the end of surgery.[111] No decreases in TOF ratios were observed in any subjects given neostigmine, and no differences between groups were observed in the incidences of airway obstruction, hypoxemic events, or signs and symptoms of muscle weakness. Studies suggest that sugammadex does not appear to produce adverse effects on upper airway tone or normal breathing when given after neuromuscular recovery.[121]

Nausea and Vomiting. The impact of anticholinesterases on the incidence of postoperative nausea and vomiting remains controversial. Systemic anticholinesterases produce effects outside of the neuromuscular junction that may influence the risk of unwanted side effects following anesthesia and surgery. In addition to the action within the neuromuscular junction, anticholinesterase drugs result in muscarinic effects on the gastrointestinal tract, resulting in stimulation of secretion of gastric fluid and increases in gastric motility. The use of smaller doses of neostigmine in combination with atropine decreases lower esophageal sphincter tone.[124] Furthermore, neostigmine may produce nausea and vomiting via a central effect. Intrathecal neostigmine increases the incidence of nausea and vomiting, likely through a direct effect on the brainstem.

Anticholinergic drugs (e.g., atropine, glycopyrrolate) are routinely administered with anticholinesterases in order to attenuate the undesirable muscarinic effects of these reversal agents. Perhaps anticholinergic drugs have antiemetic properties.[125] When given to children receiving sedation (in the absence of anticholinesterases), atropine was associated with significantly less vomiting (5.3%) than either glycopyrrolate (10.7%) or no anticholinergic (11.4%).[126] Similarly, surgical patients who were randomized to receive atropine had significantly less nausea than those given glycopyrrolate.[127] Atropine is a tertiary amine that can readily cross the blood-brain barrier and produce central effects, whereas glycopyrrolate is a quaternary amine that does not penetrate the blood-brain barrier. The beneficial effects of atropine on nausea and vomiting are likely secondary to a central nervous system effect.

Several randomized clinical trials have been performed to determine whether anticholinesterase administration results in an increase in the incidence of postoperative nausea and vomiting. Unfortunately, most study populations were small (39-120 patients). Two systematic reviews have been conducted to address this limitation. Tramer

TABLE 28.6 Early and Delayed Postoperative Nausea and Vomiting With Neostigmine Versus Control—Results of a Metaanalysis

Outcome	Anticholinergics	Number of Studies	Number of Participants	Relative Risk (95% CI)
Early nausea (0-6 h)	Atropine and Glycopyrrolate	6	584	1.24 (0.86-1.80)
	Atropine	1	79	0.67 (0.36-1.26)
	Glycopyrrolate	5	505	1.39 (0.97-1.99)
Early vomiting (0-6 h)	Atropine and Glycopyrrolate	8	768	1.05 (0.72-1.55)
	Atropine	2	199	0.75 (0.52-1.08)
	Glycopyrrolate	6	568	1.35 (0.88-2.06)
Delayed nausea (6-24 h)	Glycopyrrolate	4	337	1.09 (0.76-1.57)
Delayed vomiting (6-24 h)	Glycopyrrolate	4	337	1.01 (0.58-1.78)

CI, Confidence interval.

From Cheng CR, Sessler DI, Apfel CC. Does neostigmine administration produce a clinically important increase in postoperative nausea and vomiting? *Anesth Analg*. 2005;101:1349–1355.

and Fuchs-Buder analyzed eight trials with data on 1134 patients that compared reversal with neostigmine or edrophonium with spontaneous recovery from long- or intermediate-acting NMBDs.[128] An analysis of the neostigmine data across all trials and doses revealed no evidence of an increased risk of early and late nausea and vomiting when neostigmine was administered. However, some evidence in adults suggested that antagonism with larger doses of neostigmine (2.5 mg) might increase the incidence of these events. No evidence was found for this effect with edrophonium. A later systematic review evaluated the effect of neostigmine on postoperative nausea and vomiting while considering the different anticholinergics as confounding variables.[125] Ten randomized trials (933 patients) that compared neostigmine to inactive control were included. The combination of neostigmine with either glycopyrrolate or atropine did not increase the incidence of nausea or vomiting, nor was there an increased risk when large doses of neostigmine were compared with smaller doses (Table 28.6). Atropine was associated with a reduction in the risk of vomiting, but glycopyrrolate was not. In conclusion, there is at present insufficient evidence to conclude that neostigmine or edrophonium is associated with an increased risk of postoperative nausea and vomiting.

Cardiovascular Effects. Pronounced vagal effects are observed following the administration of anticholinesterases—bradycardia and other bradyarrhythmias, such as junctional rhythms, ventricular escape beats, complete heart block, and asystole, have been reported. The time course of these bradyarrhythmias parallels the onset of action of the anticholinesterases, with the most rapid onset observed with edrophonium, slower for neostigmine, and slowest for pyridostigmine.[90] In order to counteract these cardiovascular effects, atropine and glycopyrrolate are administered concurrently with anticholinesterases. Atropine and glycopyrrolate have muscarinic (parasympathetic) blocking effects, but do not block nicotinic receptors. Atropine has a more rapid onset of action (approximately 1 minute) compared with glycopyrrolate (2-3 minutes), although the duration of action of both agents is similar (30–60 minutes). Despite the concurrent administration of anticholinergic drugs, a high incidence of bradyarrhythmias is observed following anticholinesterase reversal (up to 50%–60% of patients in some studies).[129] The risk of arrhythmias is influenced by the type of anticholinesterase and anticholinergic used, the dose of anticholinesterase and anticholinergic administered, and background anesthetic used (opioid-based vs. volatile anesthetic and type of NMBD).

Several investigations have examined the heart rate and rhythm responses to various anticholinesterase/anticholinergic combinations. In general, it is preferable to use atropine with edrophonium because the onset of action of both drugs is rapid. Edrophonium-atropine mixtures induced small increases in heart rate, whereas edrophonium-glycopyrrolate mixtures caused decreases in heart rate and occasionally severe bradycardia.[130] Similarly, the onset of cholinergic effects of neostigmine coincides with the onset of the anticholinergic effects of glycopyrrolate; glycopyrrolate is superior to atropine in protecting against neostigmine-induced bradyarrhythmias.[131] When atropine is given with edrophonium (0.5-1.0 mg/kg), doses of 5 to 7 μg/kg are recommended, although larger doses may be used in certain circumstances.[130,132] If glycopyrrolate is given with neostigmine, minimal changes in heart rate are observed if a dose equivalent of one fourth the dose of neostigmine is used (e.g., 1 mg glycopyrrolate with 4 mg of neostigmine).[131] Because the onset of action is slow with pyridostigmine, tachycardia may be observed when either atropine or glycopyrrolate is coadministered.

More recent investigations have examined the impact of atropine and glycopyrrolate, given with neostigmine, on autonomic control in the postoperative period. During physiologically stressful events, control of heart rate and arterial blood pressure is regulated by the sympathetic and parasympathetic nervous systems. Anticholinergic drugs attenuate the efferent parasympathetic regulation of heart rate and suppress cardiac baroreflex sensitivity and heart rate variability. This suppression of the parasympathetic system may predispose patients to cardiac arrhythmias following surgery. Marked decreases in baroreflex sensitivity and high-frequency heart rate variability have been observed in healthy volunteers given either atropine (20 μg/kg) or glycopyrrolate (7 μg/kg).[133] Although the times required to return to baseline values were prolonged in both groups, recovery times were significantly longer in the subjects given atropine (177-212 minutes) compared with those administered glycopyrrolate (82-111 minutes). Similar effects have been observed in healthy patients undergoing general anesthesia reversed with neostigmine and anticholinergics.[134] Neuromuscular blockade was antagonized with neostigmine 50 μg/kg and either atropine 20 μg/kg or glycopyrrolate 8 μg/kg. Two hours after giving neostigmine, patients given atropine had persistent impairment of baroreflex sensitivity and high-frequency heart rate variability, whereas these variables had returned to baseline values in patients receiving glycopyrrolate. These investigations demonstrate that the parasympathetic nervous system control of heart rate is less impaired by glycopyrrolate than by atropine.

Bronchoconstriction. Bronchospasm can occur after the administration of neostigmine in surgical patients.[135,136] Anticholinesterases (e.g., neostigmine) stimulate muscarinic receptors in airway smooth muscle; stimulation of these receptors can provoke bronchoconstriction. Neostigmine and pyridostigmine induce a phosphatidylinositol response (a reflection of smooth muscle contraction induced by a muscarinic agonist) in airway muscle, which can result in bronchoconstriction.[137] This response was inhibited in the presence of atropine, a direct bronchodilator. Edrophonium did not induce a phosphatidylinositol response. In patients with cervical spinal cord injuries, neostigmine alone caused bronchoconstriction, whereas neostigmine combined with glycopyrrolate caused bronchodilation.[138] The risk of perioperative bronchospasm appears low if anticholinesterases are administered concurrently with anticholinergics.

SUGAMMADEX REVERSAL OF NEUROMUSCULAR BLOCKADE

Sugammadex (Org 25969) is a modified γ-cyclodextrin and the first selective relaxant–binding agent based on an encapsulating principle for inactivation of a neuromuscular blocking drug (*su* refers to sugar, and *gammadex* refers to the structural molecule γ-cyclodextrin). This principle for reversal of rocuronium- and vecuronium-induced neuromuscular blockade was first introduced into clinical practice in 2008 and is now available for pediatric and adult anesthesia in most countries worldwide, including the United States and China. The complex formation of sugammadex and rocuronium or vecuronium occurs at all levels of neuromuscular blockade (profound through shallow) and results in a more fast-acting pharmacologic reversal when compared with anticholinesterase drugs. Consequently, sugammadex may markedly reduce postoperative residual neuromuscular blockade in the PACU.[139]

Structure-Activity Relationships and Mechanism of Action

The three natural unmodified cyclodextrins consist of six, seven, and eight cyclic oligosaccharides (i.e., dextrose units joined through one to four glycosyl bonds) and are called α-, β-, and γ-cyclodextrins, respectively.[140,141] Their three-dimensional structure resembles a hollow, truncated cone or a doughnut. The structure has a hydrophobic cavity and hydrophilic exterior because of the presence of polar hydroxyl groups. Hydrophobic interactions trap the lipophilic molecules in the cyclodextrin cavity, thereby resulting in the formation of a water-soluble guest-host complex. Sugammadex is built on this principle ring structure but is a modified γ-cyclodextrin. Although an unmodified γ-cyclodextrin possesses a larger lipophilic cavity (7.5-8.3 Å) than α- or β-cyclodextrins, it is still not deep enough to accommodate the larger rigid structure of the rocuronium molecule. Therefore the cavity is modified by adding eight side chains to extend it to 11 Å for better accommodation of the four hydrophobic steroidal rings of rocuronium. Furthermore, at the end of these side chains, negatively charged carboxyl groups are added to enhance electrostatic binding to the positively charged quaternary nitrogen of rocuronium (Fig. 28.15).[141,142] The stability of the rocuronium-sugammadex complex is a result of the combination of intermolecular forces (van der Waals forces), including thermodynamic (hydrogen bonds) and hydrophobic interactions.[141-143] Sugammadex forms a rigid complex in a 1:1 ratio with steroidal NMBDs (rocuronium and vecuronium) (Fig. 28.16).[141] There is some binding affinity with pancuronium, but this interaction is too low to have a significant clinical effect. The molecular mass of the sugammadex-rocuronium complex is 2532 g/mol (sugammadex 2002 g/mol and rocuronium 530 g/mol), and that of the sugammadex-vecuronium complex is 2640 g/mol (vecuronium 638 g/mol).[141] The rocuronium-sugammadex complex exists in an equilibrium with an association/dissociation rate of 1 molar concentration of sugammadex and rocuronium of 25,000,000:1, which means that sugammadex forms a very rigid complex and encapsulates rocuronium at 25 million times the rate that one molecule complex dissociates. The affinity of sugammadex toward vecuronium is 2.5 times smaller, but still high enough to form a tight complex.[141] Rapid binding of rocuronium and sugammadex results in removal of free rocuronium molecules from the plasma. This creates a

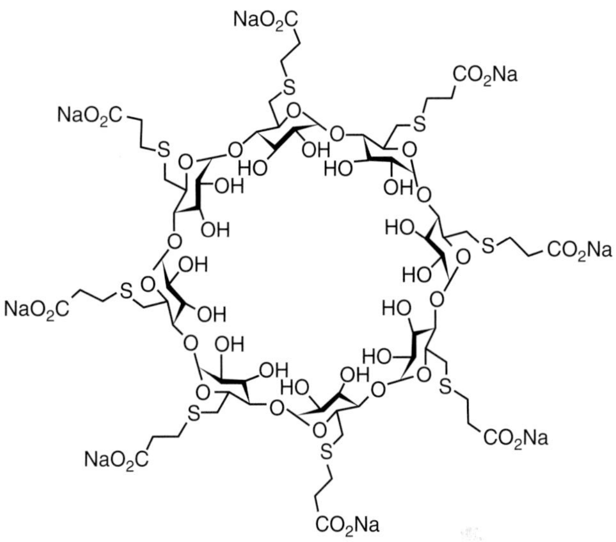

Fig. 28.15 Structure of the synthetic γ-cyclodextrin sugammadex (Org 25969). (From Bom A, Bradley M, Cameron K, et al. A novel concept of reversing neuromuscular block. Chemical encapsulating of rocuronium bromide by a cyclodextrin-based synthetic host. *Angew Chem*. 2002;41:266–270.)

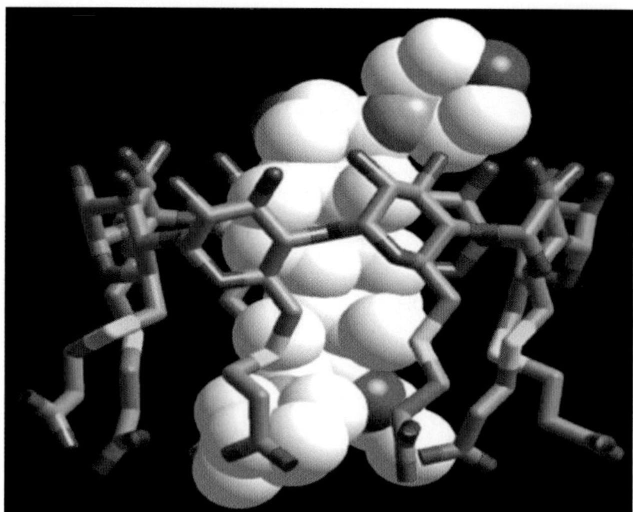

Fig. 28.16 **The sugammadex-rocuronium complex.** (From Bom A, Bradley M, Cameron K, et al. A novel concept of reversing neuromuscular block. Chemical encapsulating of rocuronium bromide by a cyclodextrin-based synthetic host. *Angew Chem.* 2002;41:266–270.)

concentration gradient favoring movement of the remaining rocuronium molecules from the effect site at the neuromuscular junction into plasma, where the drug is encapsulated by free sugammadex molecules. Neuromuscular blockade is quickly reversed as rocuronium is removed from the binding sites at the neuromuscular junction. Sugammadex administration results in an increase in the total plasma concentration of rocuronium (free and that bound to sugammadex).[144] Because sugammadex acts as a selective binding agent and has no direct or indirect action on the molecular components of cholinergic transmission (cholinesterase, nicotinic receptors, or muscarinic receptors), the need for coadministration of anticholinergic drugs is eliminated.[145]

Pharmacokinetics

The pharmacokinetic profile of sugammadex and rocuronium has been investigated in healthy volunteers and surgical patients.[146] Sugammadex, in a dose range of 0.1 to 8.0 mg/kg in healthy adult volunteers (without neuromuscular blockade), exhibited a dose-linear pharmacokinetic profile, a volume distribution of 18 L, an elimination half-life of 100 minutes, and a plasma clearance rate of 120 mL/min, with up to 80% of the dose being excreted in urine over 24 hours.[146] After encapsulation by sugammadex, rocuronium is less free to distribute to compartments other than those associated with the compartment in which sugammadex resides. During an infusion of rocuronium to maintain a stable depth of neuromuscular blockade, administration of sugammadex increased the measured plasma concentration of rocuronium; rocuronium redistributed from the effect compartment (including the neuromuscular junction) to the central compartment (mostly as the sugammadex complex) as it was encapsulated by sugammadex.[144] The volume of distribution of rocuronium decreases with increasing doses of sugammadex until the volume of distribution of rocuronium approaches the volume of distribution of sugammadex at higher doses.[144] Encapsulation changes the pharmacokinetics of rocuronium. In the absence of sugammadex, rocuronium is eliminated mainly by biliary excretion (>75%) and to a lesser degree by renal excretion (10%-25%).[147] The main difference in the pharmacokinetic profile of sugammadex and rocuronium is that the clearance of sugammadex is approximately three times slower than that of rocuronium.[146] The rate and amount of urinary excretion of rocuronium when administered alone is slow and small, but when sugammadex (a dose of 2.0 mg/kg or more) is administered, the plasma clearance of rocuronium is decreased by a factor of more than two.[146] This decreased clearance occurs because the biliary route of excretion becomes unavailable for the rocuronium-sugammadex complex as the large size of this complex prohibits additional renal excretion. The clearance of rocuronium after binding by sugammadex decreases to a value approaching the glomerular filtration rate (120 mL/min).[147] However, the renal excretion of rocuronium is increased by more than 100% after administration of 4.0 to 8.0 mg/kg of sugammadex.[147] Following the administration of sugammadex, encapsulation of rocuronium in the plasma results in a rapid decrease in free rocuronium in this compartment, although the total plasma concentration of rocuronium (both free and bound by sugammadex) increases. This results in a concentration gradient between the relatively high level of free rocuronium in the effect compartment (the neuromuscular junction) and the low level in the plasma compartment.[144] As a result, free rocuronium molecules rapidly diffuse towards the plasma compartment and are encapsulated by sugammadex. Thus the increase in plasma levels of rocuronium after sugammadex administration illustrates the mechanism responsible for the rapid reversal of neuromuscular blockade by sugammadex.

Because renal excretion is the primary route for the elimination of sugammadex and the rocuronium-sugammadex complex, studies on elimination by dialysis have considerable relevance in clinical practice. In a small subset of patients with severe renal impairment, an investigation on dialysis showed that the clearance of sugammadex and rocuronium in blood was 78 and 89 mL/min, respectively. Therefore hemodialysis using a high-flux dialysis method is effective in removing sugammadex and the sugammadex-rocuronium complex in patients with severe renal impairment.[148]

Pharmacodynamics

Clinical Use of Sugammadex in Healthy Patients

The first human exposure of sugammadex in male volunteers showed a large dose-dependent, more rapid recovery time from a rocuronium-induced neuromuscular blockade with sugammadex (0.1-8.0 mg/kg) as compared with placebo.[146] Administration of 8 mg/kg of sugammadex 3 minutes after a bolus dose of 0.6 mg/kg of rocuronium resulted in a recovery of the TOF ratio to 0.90 within 2 minutes compared with 52 minutes for placebo. Decreasing the dose of sugammadex to 4 mg/kg resulted in recovery of the TOF ratio to 0.90 in less than 4 minutes.[146] Similar recovery times were found in a study in which surgical patients received 0.6 mg/kg rocuronium, followed by different doses of sugammadex or placebo administered at a TOF count of 2.[149] Sugammadex reduced the median recovery time in a dose-dependent manner from 21 minutes in the placebo group to 1.1 minutes in the group receiving 4.0 mg/kg of sugammadex.[149] In another study, administration of sugammadex resulted in a more rapid and effective recovery from a rocuronium (0.6 mg/kg) or vecuronium

(0.1 mg/kg) neuromuscular blockade.[150] After a dose of 4.0 mg/kg of sugammadex, the mean recovery time to a TOF ratio of 0.90 was 1.1 minutes and 1.5 minutes after rocuronium and vecuronium, respectively (Figs. 28.17 and 28.18).[150] Reversal of neuromuscular blockade with larger doses of rocuronium (1.0–1.2 mg/kg) by different doses

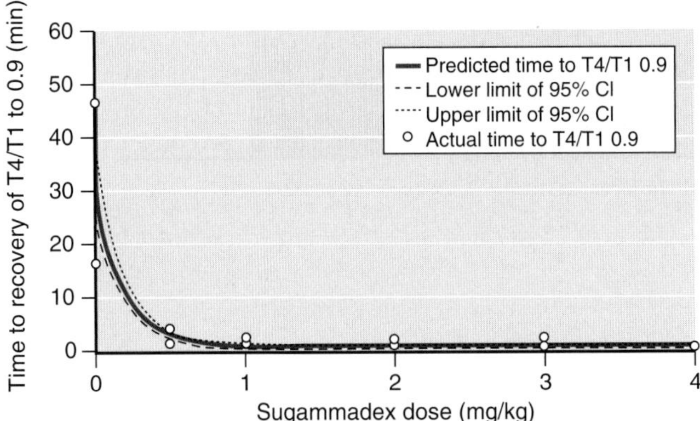

Fig. 28.17 The dose-response relation of sugammadex dose and time to recovery of the T4/T1 ratio to 0.9 with rocuronium 0.6 mg/kg. *T4/T1 ratio,* the degree of neuromuscular block. (From Suy K, Morias K, Cammu G, et al. Effective reversal of moderate rocuronium- or vecuronium-induced neuromuscular block with sugammadex, a selective relaxant binding agent. *Anesthesiology*. 2007;106:283–288.)

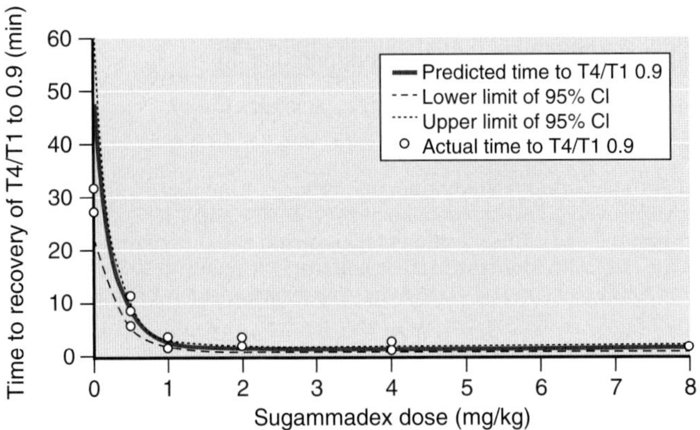

Fig. 28.18 The dose-response relation of sugammadex dose and time to recovery of the T4/T1 ratio to 0.9 with vecuronium 0.1 mg/kg. *T4/T1 ratio,* the degree of neuromuscular block. (From Suy K, Morias K, Cammu G, et al. Effective reversal of moderate rocuronium- or vecuronium-induced neuromuscular block with sugammadex, a selective relaxant binding agent. *Anesthesiology*. 2007;106:283–288.)

of sugammadex (2.0–16.0 mg/kg) at different time points (3–15 minutes after rocuronium) showed a dose-dependent, rapid, and effective reversal compared with placebo.[151-154]

Whereas anticholinesterase drugs, such as neostigmine, are unable to reverse deeper levels of neuromuscular blockade (e.g., posttetanic count of 1-2) because of a ceiling effect, sugammadex is effective in reversing profound neuromuscular blockade.[152,155] Optimal doses of sugammadex of 4.0 mg/kg produced prompt recovery of the TOF ratio to 0.90 within minutes (Table 28.7).[150-155] Therefore reversal of moderate and profound rocuronium and vecuronium neuromuscular blockades can be reliably achieved by administration of sugammadex, provided a dose of 2.0 and 4.0 mg/kg, respectively, is used. Because neostigmine has neuromuscular effects when given alone, some spontaneous recovery of the TOF should be evident before it is given. In contrast, sugammadex has no neuromuscular effects when given alone. Accordingly, sugammadex can be given even if there is no response to TOF stimulation. Sugammadex allows a profound neuromuscular blockade to continue until the end of surgery.

In contrast to the anticholinesterase drugs (e.g., neostigmine), intense neuromuscular blockade (no response to TOF and PTC stimulation) can be reversed by sugammadex immediately after the administration of rocuronium. In a multicenter investigation, patients were randomized to receive 1.2 mg/kg of rocuronium followed 3 minutes later by 16 mg/kg of sugammadex or a dose of 1.0 mg/kg of succinylcholine.[156] The mean time to 90% recovery of the first twitch (T1) from the start of sugammadex administration was 2.9 minutes and to a recovery of the TOF ratio to 0.90 was 2.2 minutes.[156] In contrast, the spontaneous recovery time from a succinylcholine neuromuscular blockade to 90% recovery of T1 was 10.9 minutes. Thus reversal of large doses of rocuronium with 16 mg/kg sugammadex was significantly faster than spontaneous recovery from succinylcholine (Fig. 28.19).[156] These findings were confirmed in a randomized trial that assessed how rapidly spontaneous ventilation could be reestablished after rapid sequence induction of anesthesia and intubation of the trachea, using either the combination of rocuronium (1.0 mg/kg)–sugammadex (16 mg/kg) or succinylcholine (1.0 mg/kg).[157] The median time from tracheal intubation to spontaneous ventilation was 406 seconds with succinylcholine and 216 seconds with rocuronium-sugammadex (Table 28.8).[157] These data demonstrated that sugammadex reversal of a large-dose rocuronium neuromuscular

TABLE 28.7 Recovery Times* of Reversal of a Rocuronium-Induced (1.2 mg/kg) Neuromuscular Blockade With Either Sugammadex or Placebo (NaCl 0.9%)

		SUGAMMADEX				
	Placebo (*n* = 4)	**2.0 mg/kg (*n* = 5)**	**4.0 mg/kg (*n* = 5)**	**8.0 mg/kg (*n* = 12)**	**12.0 mg/kg (*n* = 7)**	**16.0 mg/kg (*n* = 7)**
Mean (SD)	122.1 (18.1)	56.5 (5.4)	15.8 (17.8)	2.8 (0.6)	1.4 (0.3)	1.9 (2.2)
Median	126.1	55.3	12.3	2.5	1.3	1.3
Min-max	96.8-139.4	50.5-65.1	3.3-46.6	2.2-3.7	1.0-1.9	0.7-6.9

*Recovery times (minutes) from the start of administration of sugammadex or placebo to recovery of the train-of-four ratio to 0.90.
SD, Standard deviation.
From de Boer HD, Driessen JJ, Marcus MA, et al. Reversal of a rocuronium-induced (1.2 mg/kg) profound neuromuscular block by sugammadex: a multicenter, dose-finding and safety study. *Anesthesiology*. 2007;107:239–244.

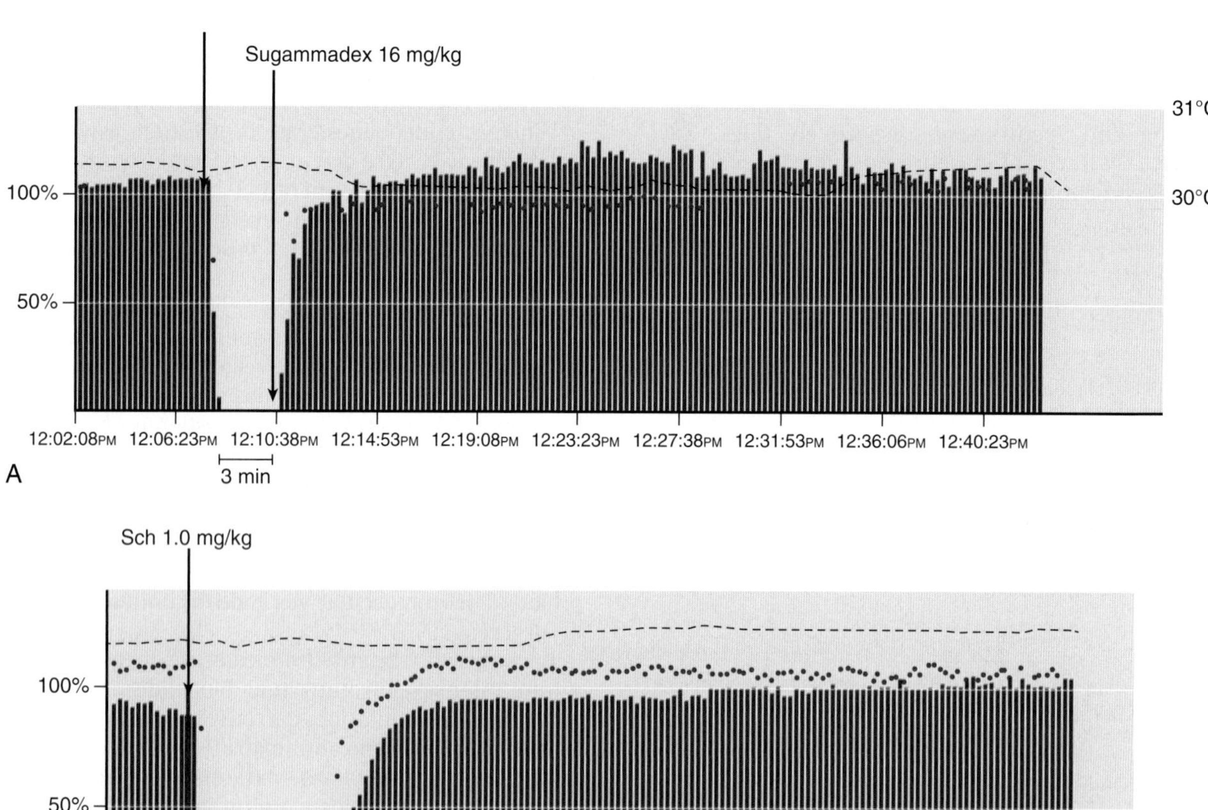

Fig. 28.19 (A) Recovery of T1 twitch height *(blue tracings)* and the train-of-four (TOF) ratio *(red dots)* after the administration of 1.2 mg/kg of rocuronium, followed 3 minutes later by 16 mg/kg of sugammadex, both given intravenously. Recovery to a first twitch height (T1) of 90% and a TOF ratio of 0.94 occurred 110 seconds later. The onset-offset time with this sequence (i.e., time from the end of the injection of rocuronium until T1 recovery to 90%) was 4 minutes, 47 seconds. (B) Effects of administering 1.0 mg/kg of succinylcholine *(Sch)* with spontaneous recovery to a T1 recovery to 90% occurring after 9 minutes, 23 seconds. *Black dashed line* represents hand skin temperature (°Celsius). (From Naguib M. Sugammadex: another milestone in clinical neuromuscular pharmacology. *Anesth Analg.* 2007;104:575–581.)

blockade was not only significantly faster than spontaneous recovery from succinylcholine, but that spontaneous ventilation could be restored more rapidly (i.e., this dose can be used to replace succinylcholine for endotracheal intubation). In clinical practice and during an unexpected difficult airway (cannot intubate, cannot ventilate scenario), a rocuronium neuromuscular blockade may be reversed by sugammadex immediately in order to restore spontaneous ventilation.

When sugammadex was compared with neostigmine or edrophonium, the time course of neuromuscular recovery was markedly different.[158-160] In a clinical study, patients received 0.6 mg/kg of rocuronium after which neuromuscular blockade was sustained with supplemental boluses of rocuronium given at the reappearance of the second twitch (second response to TOF stimulation or T2).[158] Fifteen minutes after the last dose of rocuronium either 70 µg/kg of neostigmine, 1 mg/kg of edrophonium, or 4.0 mg/kg sugammadex was administered. The average time to achieve a TOF ratio of 0.90 was 10 times longer after the administration of neostigmine than it was after sugammadex (1044 seconds vs. 107 seconds) and 3 times longer after the administration of edrophonium (331 seconds). In another study by Blobner and associates, similar differences were found when comparing reversal of rocuronium at the reappearance of the second twitch in the TOF response using 2 mg/kg sugammadex versus neostigmine 50 µg/kg.[159] This was also confirmed in an investigation that assessed the efficacy of sugammadex versus neostigmine for reversal of profound rocuronium-induced neuromuscular blockade.[160] More than 97% of patients reversed with sugammadex (4.0 mg/kg) at a PTC of 1 to 2 recovered to a TOF ratio of 0.90 within 5 minutes. In contrast, 73% of the patients administered neostigmine (70 µg/kg) recovered between 30 and 60 minutes after administration, with 23% requiring more than 60 minutes to recover to a TOF ratio of 0.90 (Fig. 28.20).

A randomized trial compared the efficacy of sugammadex reversal of a rocuronium (0.6 mg/kg) neuromuscular blockade with that of neostigmine reversal of a cisatracurium (0.15 mg/kg) neuromuscular blockade.[161] Time from the start of administration of reversal agent sugammadex 2.0 mg/kg or neostigmine 50 µg/kg) to recovery of the TOF

TABLE 28.8 How Rapidly Can Spontaneous Ventilation Be Reestablished After a Rapid Sequence Induction and Intubation of Anesthesia Using Either Succinylcholine- or Rocuronium-Sugammadex

	Succinylcholine (1 mg/kg) (*n* = 26)	Rocuronium (1 mg/kg) Sugammadex (16 mg/kg) (*n* = 29)	*P*-value
Time from start of procedure to tracheal intubation (seconds)	330 (313-351)	324 (312-343)	.45
Intubation conditions			.13
Excellent	20 (76%)	27 (93%)	
Good	6 (24%)	2 (7%)	
Poor	0 (0%)	0 (0%)	
Intubation difficulty score			.23
≤5	24 (92%)	28 (100%)	
>5	2 (8%)	0 (0%)	
Time from tracheal intubation to spontaneous ventilation (seconds)	406 (313-507)	216 (132-425)	.002
Time from tracheal intubation to T1 90% (seconds)	518 (451-671) (*n* = 17)	168 (122-201) (*n* = 27)	<.0001
Time from injection of NMBD to T1 90% (seconds)	719 (575-787) (*n* = 17)	282 (242-319) (*n* = 27)	<.0001

*These data include tracheal intubation conditions, time to reappearance of spontaneous ventilation, and recovery of neuromuscular function from either succinylcholine or the combination of rocuronium-sugammadex.

From Sørensen MK, Bretlau C, Gätke MR, et al. Rapid sequence induction and intubation with rocuronium-sugammadex compared with succinylcholine. A randomized trial. *Br J Anaesth*. 2012;108:682–689.

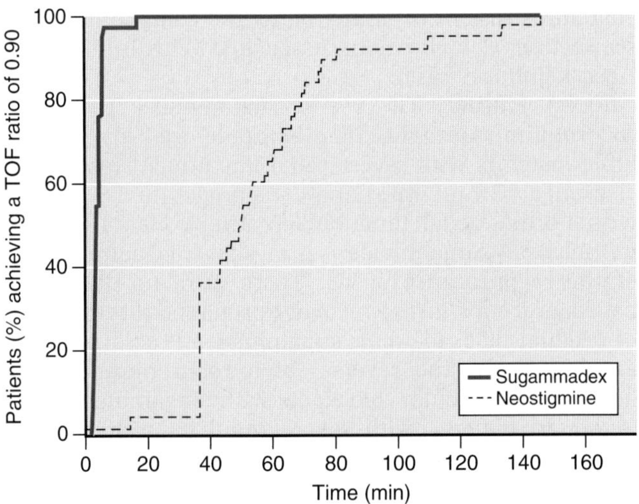

Fig. 28.20 Time to recovery of the train-of-four *(TOF)* ratio to 0.90 from profound rocuronium-induced neuromuscular blockade after administration of sugammadex 4 mg/kg or neostigmine 70 μg/kg. (From Jones RK, Caldwell JE, Brull SJ, et al. Reversal of profound rocuronium-induced blockade with sugammadex: a randomized comparison with neostigmine. *Anesthesiology*. 2008;109:816–824.)

ratio to 0.90 was 4.7 times faster with sugammadex than with neostigmine, 1.9 versus 9.0 minutes, respectively.

Unlike with neostigmine or edrophonium, the choice of anesthetic (e.g., propofol vs. sevoflurane) does not influence the ability of sugammadex to reverse rocuronium-induced neuromuscular blockade.[162,163] Provided that sugammadex is used in recommended dosages according to the level of neuromuscular blockade, a small risk exists of incomplete neuromuscular recovery or reoccurrence of neuromuscular blockade following surgery.

Clinical Use of Sugammadex in Pediatric and Older Adult Patients

Pediatrics. The use of sugammadex in pediatric patients was examined in a study enrolling 8 infants (28 days to 23 months), 24 children (2-11 years), and 31 adolescents (12-17 years).[164] Patients were anesthetized with propofol and opioids and received rocuronium 0.6 mg/kg. At the reappearance of T2 (second twitch), patients were given sugammadex 0.5, 1.0, 2.0, or 4.0 mg/kg or placebo. Recovery time to a TOF ratio of 0.90 decreased in a dose-dependent manner in all age groups. Residual neuromuscular blockade or recurarization was not observed, and no side effects were reported. In a more recent case report, sugammadex was used successfully in reversing a vecuronium-induced neuromuscular blockade in a 7-month-old infant.[165] Another case report described a 2-year-old patient who received readministration of rocuronium for reoperation after an initial successful reversal with sugammadex.[166] A recent systematic review showed that compared with neostigmine or placebo, sugammadex can reverse a rocuronium-induced neuromuscular blockade more rapidly with lower incidence of bradycardia.[167]

While sugammadex can be used safely in children and adolescents (2-17 years old), information on the use of sugammadex in pediatric patients less than 2 years old is still limited.

Older Adult Patients. Reversal of neuromuscular blockade by sugammadex has been assessed in older patients. One hundred and fifty patients were divided into three groups; an adult group (18–64 years old), an older adult group (65–75 years old), and an oldest adult group (75 years or older).[168] Patients received an intubating dose of rocuronium 0.6 mg/kg with maintenance doses of 0.15 mg/kg as required. Sugammadex 2.0 mg/kg was administered after the last dose of rocuronium at the

TABLE 28.9 Rocuronium Recovery Time (min) from the Administration of Sugammadex (2 mg/kg at Appearance of T2) Until the Recovery of Train-of-Four Ratios as Indicated in Patients With and Without Renal Failure

	PATIENT GROUP		
	CL_{CR} <30 mL/min (*n* = 15)	CL_{CR} ≥80 mL/min (*n* = 14)*	Anova
Recovery to TOF ratio 0.7, mean (SD)	1.45 (0.47)	1.17 (0.38)	NS
Recovery to TOF ratio 0.8, mean (SD)	1.60 (0.57)	1.32 (0.45)	NS
Recovery to TOF ratio 0.9, mean (SD)	2.00 (0.72)	1.65 (0.63)	NS

ANOVA, Analysis of variance; CL_{CR}, total plasma creatinine clearance; *NS*, not significant; *SD*, standard deviation; *TOF*, train-of-four.
*One patient was excluded from the control group (normal renal function) because of unreliable TOF traces.
From Staals LM, Snoeck MM, Driessen JJ, et al. Multicenter, parallel-group, comparative trial evaluating the efficacy and safety of sugammadex in patients with end-stage renal failure or normal renal function. *Br J Anaesth*. 2008;101:492–497.

reappearance of T2. Recovery of neuromuscular blockade by sugammadex was slightly (0.7 minutes) faster in patients younger than 65 years of age. In general, a prolonged circulation time secondary to a reduced cardiac output in older patients was anticipated to result in a longer recovery time from neuromuscular blockade after administration of sugammadex.[169,170] However, based on these results, no dose adjustments are needed in older patients.[168] Yet, if it is necessary to achieve a fast recovery in a short period of time, a higher dose of sugammadex might be considered.[171]

Clinical Use of Sugammadex in Special Patient Populations

Cardiac Disease. Studies evaluating the safety and efficacy of sugammadex in patients with underlying cardiovascular disease have not demonstrated an effect of sugammadex on electrocardiogram (no indication of a possible prolongation effect on the QTc interval).[172,173] A study designed to evaluate the effects of sugammadex on QTc prolongation in healthy subjects (in doses up to 32 mg/kg, alone or in combination with rocuronium or vecuronium) revealed that the administration of sugammadex was not associated with QTc prolongation.[173] In a case report of a patient with long QT syndrome, a vecuronium neuromuscular blockade was reversed with sugammadex 2 mg/kg without adversely affecting the QT interval.[174] Based on current data, sugammadex reversal is not associated with cardiovascular side effects in healthy patients or in those with cardiovascular comorbidities (also see earlier section Complications Associated With Inhibitors of Acetylcholinesterase).

Pulmonary Disease. Patients with a history of pulmonary disease have an increased risk of postoperative pulmonary complications such as pneumonia, respiratory failure, and exacerbation of the underlying pulmonary disease.[175] Sugammadex has been studied in patients with pulmonary disease.[175] Seventy-seven surgical patients with a diagnosis or known history of pulmonary disorders received sugammadex in doses up to 4 mg/kg in order to reverse a rocuronium neuromuscular blockade. As in other adult patient groups, reversal of a rocuronium-induced neuromuscular blockade was rapid, and there were no signs of residual neuromuscular blockade or recurarization.[176] Of the 77 patients treated with sugammadex, 2 patients developed bronchospasm, 1 minute and 55 minutes respectively, after the administration of sugammadex. Both patients were asthmatic, and there was no evidence that these symptoms were related to sugammadex. In other subsets of high-risk pulmonary patients (cystic fibrosis and end-stage lung disease), the successful use of sugammadex has been reported.[177] Reversal of a neuromuscular blockade with sugammadex has potential advantages compared with anticholinesterase drugs (e.g., neostigmine) in patients with pulmonary disease because sugammadex lacks interactions with the muscarinic cholinergic system, and there is no need for coadministration of anticholinergic compounds (also see section, Complications Associated With Inhibitors of Acetylcholinesterase).

Renal Failure. The use of sugammadex to reverse rocuronium neuromuscular blockade was investigated in 15 patients with severe renal impairment (creatinine clearance <30 mL/min) and compared with 15 patients with normal renal function (creatinine clearance >80 mL/min).[178] Sugammadex 2 mg/kg was administered at the reappearance of T2. There were no differences between groups in the recovery profile or the incidence of residual blockade after sugammadex (Table 28.9). In another study, the reversal of a rocuronium-induced deep neuromuscular blockade with sugammadex 4.0 mg/kg in patients with severe renal impairment (creatinine clearance <30 mL/min) showed a fast and stable reversal.[179] Sugammadex and sugammadex-rocuronium complex exposure is increased in patients with moderate and severe renal failure due to the decreased renal clearance.[180] The use of sugammadex in renal transplantation was described in two cases in which sugammadex was used for reversal of a rocuronium-induced neuromuscular block in pediatric patients and showed a fast and complete reversal without signs of residual neuromuscular blockade or recurarization.[181] More recently, the long-term efficacy and safety of rocuronium and sugammadex in patients undergoing renal transplantation were described in 57 patients diagnosed with severe renal failure.[182] Rocuronium and sugammadex appeared to be efficacious and safe in patients undergoing renal transplantation. Because complete elimination of the sugammadex-rocuronium complex remains poorly understood in renal impairment, sugammadex is at present not recommended for use in patients with severe renal failure. However, it can be used in patients with mild or moderate renal dysfunction as its safety profile is similar to that of healthy patients.[178] Theoretically, because of the molecular mass of the rocuronium/vecuronium-sugammadex complex, it is possible to decrease the plasma levels of this complex by dialysis. Hemodialysis using a high-flux dialysis method has been demonstrated to be effective in removing sugammadex and the sugammadex-rocuronium complex in patients with severe renal impairment.[148]

Hepatobiliary Disease. Sugammadex has not been studied in animal models or in patients with hepatic impairment. However, it is known that the biliary route of excretion becomes unavailable for either sugammadex or the rocuronium/vecuronium-sugammadex complex because the large size of this complex prohibits such excretion.[183] A population pharmacokinetic/pharmacodynamic (PK-PD) model was used to simulate the scenario of an immediate reversal, and reversal of a profound rocuronium-induced neuromuscular blockade in patients with hepatic impairment.[183] Under such study conditions, hepatic impairment had little effect on the reversal time when sugammadex (16 mg/kg) was administered 3 minutes after rocuronium (1.2 mg/kg). However, in other scenarios (sugammadex 2 mg/kg at reappearance of T2 and 4 mg/kg after 15 minutes), recovery from a rocuronium-induced (1.2 mg/kg) neuromuscular blockade was predicted to be longer than that seen in healthy patients.[183] In patients with hepatobiliary disease, the recovery of neuromuscular function after sugammadex administration will likely be faster than reversal with anticholinesterase drugs (but not be as rapid as patients without hepatobiliary disease). The explanation of the slower reversal is not yet fully understood and needs to be investigated in clinical studies. Based on limited available data, sugammadex should be used with caution in patients with hepatobiliary disease.

Obesity. Patients with obesity, particularly morbid obesity (body mass index [BMI] > 40 kg/m^2), are at risk for cardiovascular and respiratory complications perioperatively.[184] These patients are susceptible to critical respiratory events in the postoperative period, including hypoventilation, hypoxia, airway obstruction, and acute respiratory failure.[38,68] The presence of postoperative residual neuromuscular blockade may further increase the risk for postoperative complications in these patients by producing impairment of the integrity of the upper airway and upper airway collapse.[33,34] Therefore a rapid and complete reversal of neuromuscular blockade must be achieved before tracheal extubation is attempted. In this setting, sugammadex may have a more favorable recovery profile than traditional anticholinesterase drugs because it provides a more reliable recovery of neuromuscular functions and a less frequent risk of incomplete neuromuscular recovery.[184] A key issue is determining the appropriate dose of sugammadex to administer in a morbidly obese patient that is sufficient to capture remaining NMBD molecules. Whereas the dosing of NMBDs in obese patients should be based on lean/ideal body weight (because these drugs are hydrophilic and their volume of distribution is minimally affected by obesity), the dosing of sugammadex in obese patients is currently under debate. In order to ensure complete neuromuscular recovery, the dose of sugammadex must be sufficient to affect the gradient between the peripheral and central compartments and effectively encapsulate all rocuronium molecules. An inadequate dose of sugammadex may be incapable of sustaining this redistribution of rocuronium and lead to reoccurrence of the neuromuscular blockade.

The current product monograph recommends calculating the sugammadex dose based on the patient's actual body weight. However, because the low volume of distribution at steady state (estimated at 0.16 L/kg) restricts distribution to the intravascular space, it might be relevant to determine the dose of sugammadex based on the lean/ideal body weight and not on the actual body weight.[178] However, in a recently published pooled analysis (27 trials) on the use of sugammadex in patients with obesity (BMI > 30 kg/m^2), the authors concluded that the recommended dose on actual body weight provided rapid recovery from neuromuscular blockade in both obese and nonobese patients and that no dose adjustments should be undertaken in the obese patient.[185] Several studies have investigated the dosage of sugammadex based on lean or variations on the lean/ideal body weight.[186-189] In one investigation, a sugammadex dose of 4 mg/kg based on a lean/ideal body weight calculation was administered to morbidly obese patients during a profound rocuronium neuromuscular blockade.[188] Approximately 40% of these patients were inadequately reversed with a lean/ideal body weight–based dose of sugammadex. In these patients, an additional dose of sugammadex 2 mg/kg based on lean/ideal body weight was required to achieve a TOF ratio 0.90. The conclusion of the authors was that a sugammadex dose calculated according to lean/ideal body weight was insufficient for reversing both profound and moderate blockade in a considerable number of morbidly obese patients.[188]

In another study in morbidly obese patients, investigators examined reversal of a moderate level of a rocuronium neuromuscular blockade (at T1-T2) using a dose of sugammadex of 2.0 mg/kg.[187] Four different weight corrections were used: lean/ideal body weight, lean/ideal body weight +20%, lean/ideal body weight +40%, and actual body weight. This study demonstrated that a moderate rocuronium neuromuscular blockade could be effectively reversed with sugammadex 2.0 mg/kg using the calculation lean/ideal body weight + 40%.[187] In a more recent study, these findings were confirmed.[190] However, longer and larger interindividual variability of recovery times occur when dosing is based on lean/ideal body weight compared with dosing based on actual body weight.[187,188] Additionally, reoccurrence of neuromuscular blockade after suboptimal dosing of sugammadex has been reported in a morbidly obese patient.[189] Hence until more data are available, the dose of sugammadex should be based on the actual body weight.

Cesarean Section and Pregnant Patients. Induction of general anesthesia in late pregnancy and for patients undergoing cesarean section typically involves a rapid sequence induction of anesthesia with either thiopental or propofol and a rapid-onset NMBD. For decades, succinylcholine has been the prototypic NMBD used in these procedures to produce optimal endotracheal intubation conditions.[191] Rocuronium is an acceptable alternative to succinylcholine in rapid sequence induction of anesthesia procedures; rocuronium in doses larger than 1.0 mg/kg not only provides onset of action within 60 seconds, but also provides identical intubation conditions compared with succinylcholine.[192] However, the duration of action of rocuronium in dosages of 1.0 mg/kg or greater will result in a profound neuromuscular blockade of long duration (often more than 2 hours). Furthermore, the risk of failed intubation in the obstetric population is at least eight times higher compared with nonpregnant females.[193] In case of a failed endotracheal intubation scenario or a "cannot intubate, cannot ventilate" situation, rocuronium, even in dosages up to 1.2 mg/kg, can be immediately reversed with sugammadex 16 mg/kg.[156]

Preclinical animal data demonstrated that uteroplacental transfer of sugammadex is very small (<2% to 6%). Sugammadex does not have negative effects on pregnancy or on embryonic, fetal, or postnatal development.[191,194,195] Although no data are available about the excretion of sugammadex in human breast milk, excretion in breast milk is likely minimal, with insignificant clinical impact because oral absorption of cyclodextrins in general is small. Therefore sugammadex can be used in breastfeeding females. In two case series examining obstetric patients who received rocuronium and sugammadex (7 and 18 patients), no side effects were observed.[194,195] The efficacy and safety of sugammadex in obstetric anesthesia have not been determined; yet serious adverse events for the mother or the neonate have not been reported after sugammadex.

Neuromuscular Disorders. Neuromuscular disorders are frequently associated with an increased incidence of perioperative respiratory complications due to muscle weakness.[196,197] In these patient groups, administration of succinylcholine is often contraindicated and associated with potentially life-threatening side effects. The use of nondepolarizing NMBDs can on occasion be associated with prolonged spontaneous neuromuscular recovery, even after a single dose. Consequently, these patients have an increased risk for postoperative muscle weakness of multifactorial origin, one being residual neuromuscular blockade.[196,197] Prompt recovery of neuromuscular function is essential to optimize patient safety and reduce the risk of pulmonary complications. However, reversal with anticholinesterase (e.g., neostigmine), especially in neuromuscular disorders, can be associated with postoperative complications.[197]

Multiple case reports and case series describe the use of sugammadex in patients with various neuromuscular disorders such as myasthenia gravis, myotonic dystrophy, and spinal muscular atrophy (Fig. 28.21).[197-204] In general, dosing regimens for sugammadex were consistent with recommended doses adjusted to actual body weight and based on the level of neuromuscular blockade at the time of reversal. Sugammadex administration resulted in prompt reversal of neuromuscular blockade with a similar recovery profile as observed in normal patients. Although no studies have been performed in patients with neuromuscular disorders, the reported cases indicate that sugammadex should be considered as an alternative reversal drug (e.g., instead of neostigmine) in this patient population. These observations need to be confirmed in a larger series of patient studies.

Side Effects and Drug Interactions

Sugammadex is contraindicated in patients with known hypersensitivity to the drug. The potential for hypersensitivity is reported in several case reports. Hypersensitivity is a concern; however, this is difficult to study because hypersensitivity reactions occur rarely. In a recent retrospective analysis, the incidence of potential sugammadex-induced anaphylaxis at a single center over a period of 3 years was investigated. The overall incidence of intraoperative hypersensitivity was 0.22% (95% CI, 0.17%–0.29%), and the incidence of anaphylaxis was 0.059% (95% CI, 0.032%–0.10%). In total 15,479 patients were exposed to sugammadex in the study period and the incidence of anaphylaxis associated with sugammadex administration was 0.039% (n = 6; 95% CI, 0.014%–0.084%).[205] Prospective studies are needed to confirm the sugammadex anaphylaxis. Elevation of serum tryptase (positive predictive value of 93%, negative predictive value of 54%), skin testing (gold standard), and histamine levels in serum and urine are useful to confirm the diagnosis. Recently, a promising test, the basophil activation test, has been established to detect the causative compound of anaphylaxis with high specificity and sensitivity. However, more studies are needed to confirm this method to identify sugammadex-induced anaphylaxis.[206]

Other reported side effects include coughing, movement, parosmia (abnormal sense of smell), and elevated levels of *N*-acetyl-glucosaminidase in the urine.[183] Coughing and movement after the administration of sugammadex may have been due to the unmasking of inadequate anesthesia rather than a direct side effect of sugammadex. Initial studies showed a prolongation of activated partial thromboplastin and prothrombin time in healthy volunteers after sugammadex administration. However, in a more in-depth patient study that investigated the effect of sugammadex on postsurgical bleeding and coagulation variables, it was shown that sugammadex produced a limited, transient (<1 hour) increase in activated partial thromboplastin and

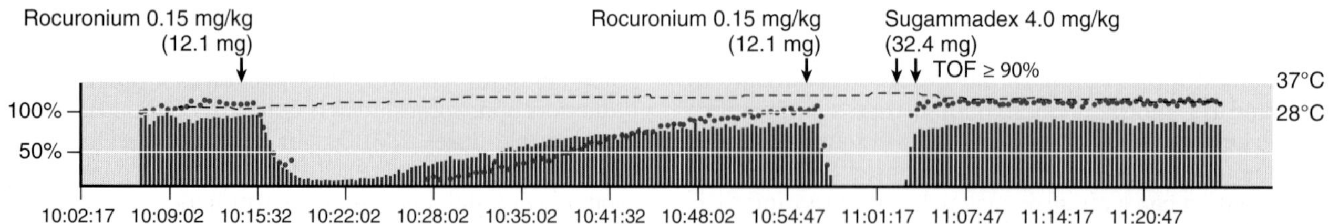

Fig. 28.21 Original tracing of sugammadex reversal in a patient with myasthenia gravis. The time to spontaneous recovery from the first profound rocuronium-induced neuromuscular blockade to a train-of-four *(TOF)* ratio was 36.5 minutes. The time from the start of the administration of sugammadex 4.0 mg/kg after the second dose of rocuronium to the recovery of the TOF ratio to 0.90 was 2.7 minutes. *Blue tracings* represent T1 recovery while *red dots* represent TOF ratio recovery. *Black dashed line* indicates hand skin temperature (degrees Celsius). (From de Boer HD, van Egmond J, Driessen JJ, et al. A new approach to anesthesia management in myasthenia gravis: reversal of neuromuscular blockade by sugammadex. *Rev Esp Anesthesiol Reanim*. 2010;57:81–84.)

prothrombin time but was not associated with increased risk of bleeding versus usual care.[207]

Cyclodextrins are a class of agents well known for their ability to form inclusion complexes with other compounds. Sugammadex forms a very tight complex with rocuronium or vecuronium in a 1:1 molecular ratio; however, because of its mechanism of action, it is possible that other relevant drug interactions may occur.[208] Theoretically, two important drug interactions can take place. First, sugammadex is capable of encapsulating endogenous or pharmaceutical molecules other than steroidal NMBDs, resulting in reduced efficacy of the encapsulated molecules. However, the ability to form complexes with steroidal or nonsteroidal molecules such as cortisone, atropine, and verapamil is clinically insignificant because the affinity for sugammadex is 120 to 700 times less than that of rocuronium.[208] In preclinical studies, an interaction of sugammadex with other steroidal compounds could be excluded up to a dose of sugammadex of 500 mg/kg/day.[209] Second, if the affinity of sugammadex for another molecule is very high, this molecule may displace rocuronium or vecuronium from the complex with sugammadex, resulting in reoccurrence of neuromuscular blockade. Both drug interactions may have potential clinical safety implications.[208] A modeling approach has been developed to evaluate 300 compounds (including the most commonly used drugs in the perioperative period) for possible displacement interactions with sugammadex.[208] In this screening, three compounds were identified as having possible displacement interactions: toremifene, fusidic acid, and flucloxacillin.[208] However, no clinically relevant reoccurrence of neuromuscular blockade was identified when sugammadex was used in combination with these drugs.[208] A clinical study reported that flucloxacillin did not cause reoccurrence of neuromuscular blockade after reversal with sugammadex; no clinically important displacement interaction was observed.[210]

Special Considerations

Reintubation of the Trachea After Initial Reversal of Neuromuscular Blockade With Sugammadex. Patients receiving sugammadex before extubation of the trachea who need reintubation require special consideration because the remaining circulating sugammadex molecules may potentially interfere with readministration of rocuronium or vecuronium. In this setting, two alternate strategies can reestablish a neuromuscular blockade. Within 24 hours of sugammadex administration, it is currently recommended that a nonsteroidal NMBD be used instead of rocuronium or vecuronium. This conservative approach is based on the maximum clearance time for sugammadex. However, preclinical and clinical studies have shown that it is possible to safely reestablish neuromuscular blockade with rocuronium earlier than 24 hours.[211] A modeling-based study in healthy volunteers revealed that high-dose rocuronium given 5 to 60 minutes after sugammadex reversal produced a complete neuromuscular blockade (T1 = 0%).[212] Rocuronium (1.2 mg/kg) administrated 5 minutes after sugammadex reversal produced a rapid onset of neuromuscular blockade (T1 = 0%), with a mean onset time of approximately 3 minutes. Thirty minutes after administration of sugammadex, an onset time of 1.5 minutes can be achieved with rocuronium (1.2 mg/kg). Hence an inverse relationship exists between the onset time and the time interval between sugammadex and the repeat dose of rocuronium, and a direct relationship exists between the duration of neuromuscular blockade and the time interval between sugammadex and the repeat dose of rocuronium.

Based on dose calculations using a model in which the equilibrium is described in the common volume of distribution of rocuronium and sugammadex, even a second reversal is possible using sugammadex with large doses between 8 and 20 mg/kg.[211]

Incomplete Reversal of Neuromuscular Blockade. Although sugammadex encapsulates rocuronium and vecuronium to form a rigid complex, case reports have described incomplete reversal of neuromuscular blockade.[151,213] In a dose-finding study, a case was described in which a temporary decrease in the TOF response was observed in a healthy patient after reversal with 0.5 mg/kg sugammadex.[213] The TOF ratio initially reached 0.70 before decreasing to 0.30 and then gradually increasing to 0.90 (Fig. 28.22). The authors hypothesized that the decrease in TOF ratio occurred because of redistribution of unbound rocuronium from the peripheral compartments, with insufficient sugammadex available for additional encapsulation of rocuronium. Similarly, incomplete reversal was reported in two healthy patients given suboptimal doses of sugammadex (0.5 mg/kg) during profound rocuronium-induced neuromuscular blockade.[151] In a study by Duvaldestin and associates, reversal of deep neuromuscular blockade with a low dose of sugammadex (0.5 and 1.0 mg/kg) found that five patients experienced recurrence of neuromuscular blockade.[163] In another study, both speed of reversal and effectiveness of sugammadex are dose-dependent; a single dose of 1.0 mg/kg of sugammadex (n = 15) administered at a deep neuromuscular blockade (PTC = 1) required

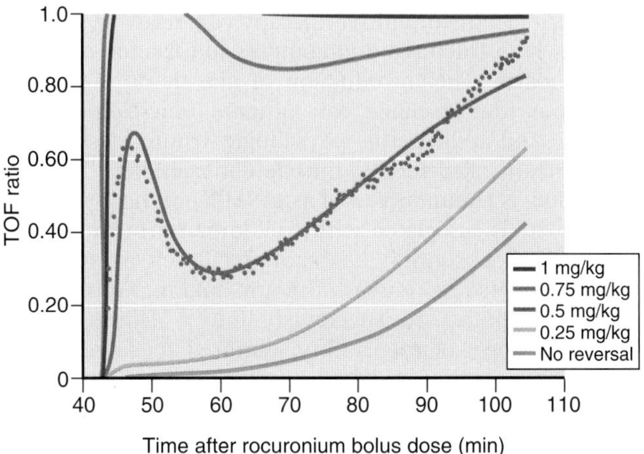

Fig. 28.22 The train-of-four data *(dots)* and the results of simulations *(solid lines)* of various sugammadex dosing amounts. Muscle relaxation rebound only occurs for sugammadex doses in a limited range. The simulations indicate that for this patient, doses larger than about 1 mg/kg are sufficient to achieve rapid muscle relaxation reversal and avoid muscle relaxation rebound. *TOF*, train-of-four. (From Eleveld DJ, Kuizenga K, Proost JH, et al. A temporary decrease in twitch response during reversal of rocuronium-induced muscle relaxation with a small dose of sugammadex. *Anesth Analg*. 2007;104:582–584.)

significantly longer time for reversal than a dose of 4.0 mg/kg (n = 60).[214] Interestingly, seven patients also exhibited residual (n = 3) and recurrence (n = 4) of neuromuscular blockade in the group of patients that received 1.0 mg/kg sugammadex. No patients who received the recommended dose of 4.0 mg/kg sugammadex had residual of recurarization of neuromuscular blockade. A similar pattern was observed with vecuronium-induced neuromuscular blockade. A longer reversal time and a higher incidence of residual and/or recurrence of neuromuscular blockade were noted in patients who received smaller (0.5 and 1.0 mg/kg) doses of sugammadex.[215] Therefore it is recommended that the dose be adjusted to the depth of neuromuscular blockade as underdosing of sugammadex is associated with an increased risk of residual neuromuscular blockade or recurrence of neuromuscular blockade.

Female Patients. Sugammadex may interact with hormonal contraceptive drugs. Possible capturing interactions, whereby unwanted encapsulation of a third drug by sugammadex reduces its clinical efficacy, have been investigated. In pharmacokinetic-pharmacodynamic simulations, it was predicted that 34% of (free) etonogestrel might be captured by 4 mg/kg sugammadex under very conservative modeling assumption conditions.[209] The interaction with this bolus dose of sugammadex resulted in a decrease in etonogestrel exposure, which was similar to the decrease seen after one missed daily dose of an oral contraceptive. Patients using hormonal contraceptives should be informed about the possible reduced effectiveness of hormonal contraceptive drugs after the administration of sugammadex. The use of an additional nonhormonal contraceptive method for the next 7 days should be considered in this patient population.

Electroconvulsive Therapy. Electroconvulsive therapy is the transcutaneous application of small electrical stimuli to the brain for treatment of selected psychiatric disorders like major depression. The tonic-clonic convulsions associated with electroconvulsive therapy can result in injuries such as limb fractures and compression fractures of vertebral bodies. The introduction of anesthesia, especially neuromuscular blockade, can mitigate tonic-clonic motor activity and reduce the physiologic trauma associated with uncontrolled tetanic muscle contractions.[216] Succinylcholine is commonly used as a NMBD in these patients, and its use is associated with well-known unwanted side effects.[216] Rocuronium has similar efficacy as succinylcholine in electroconvulsive therapy, making it an appropriate alternative to succinylcholine.[217] However, the increased doses of rocuronium required to decrease the onset time are associated with a prolonged duration of neuromuscular blockade. Several reports have evaluated the use of sugammadex in electroconvulsive therapy. These investigations demonstrated that sugammadex produced a complete and rapid reversal of neuromuscular blockade induced by rocuronium, without signs of residual blockade or other safety concerns.[217-220] Therefore the combination of rocuronium and sugammadex may be an alternative to succinylcholine for electroconvulsive therapy. However, the required dose of sugammadex in this clinical situation is not well established.

Historically, an important strategy in anesthesia has been to ensure that neuromuscular blockade is sufficiently recovered to achieve adequate antagonism by neostigmine. Having an intense neuromuscular blockade at the end of surgery would more likely result in residual blockade. With the availability of sugammadex, a profound, or deep, neuromuscular blockade has been recommended for the entire duration of laparoscopy. A profound neuromuscular blockade increases surgical space with smaller pressures for the pneumoperitoneum.[221] It is even possible that reducing insufflation pressures may improve patient outcomes.[221] Furthermore, Staehr-Rye and associates[222] have postulated that a deep or profound neuromuscular blockade is associated with more optimal surgical conditions, which leads to less postoperative pain and nausea and vomiting. A recent review and metaanalysis has shown that deep neuromuscular blockade during laparoscopic surgical procedures allows lower insufflation pressure, thereby improving surgical conditions and reducing postoperative pain.[223] Sugammadex, at doses of 2 to 8 mg/kg, was given to reverse the blockade when the TOF ratio was less than 0.90.

A recently published report describes the clinical experience in Japan.[224] Notably, although neuromuscular blockade was not routinely monitored intraoperatively, the TOF ratio was determined after tracheal extubation. A total of 249 patients were studied in three separate groups. Patients with spontaneous recovery (n = 23) were compared with patients being reversed with either neostigmine (n = 109) or sugammadex 2.7 mg/kg (n = 117). Although the sugammadex group had the least frequent incidence of residual neuromuscular blockade, all three groups had a surprisingly frequent incidence of residual neuromuscular blockade.[224]

A scholarly editorial written by Naguib and associates[225] placed prime emphasis on the dose of sugammadex used for reversal in combination with the lack of neuromuscular monitoring. Although proper monitoring is strongly advisable, an adequate dose of sugammadex is under current debate. Although the reversal effect of neostigmine is not improved by increasing the dose above the recommended dose interval, there are strong reasons to believe that sugammadex in doses larger than 2.7 mg/kg would be more effective for reversal. Others argue that a dose of sugammadex larger than 2.0 mg/kg would not be necessary if proper monitoring were used. Of course, another possibility exists. It would seem that a larger dose of sugammadex plus neuromuscular monitoring would be ideal.

In conclusion, sugammadex provides a novel concept in reversal of neuromuscular blockade. Although the expense of sugammadex continues to be an important factor that may limit its use, many institutions currently use sugammadex for routine reversal of neuromuscular blockade. We speculate whether, in the future, larger doses of sugammadex will likely be used and whether routine neuromuscular monitoring will finally be mandatory in anesthetic practice among countries worldwide.

CYSTEINE REVERSAL OF FUMARATE NEUROMUSCULAR BLOCKING DRUGS

A new class of nondepolarizing NMBDs called fumarates has been recently developed. These NMBDs are olefinic (double-bonded) isoquinolinium diester compounds that differ from symmetric benzylisoquinolines such as mivacurium in their unique method of inactivation. The developed drugs (gantacurium [GW280430A, AV430A], CW002, and CW011) bind to L-cysteine to form less active degradation products (Fig. 28.23). The administration of L-cysteine can rapidly inactivate fumarate compounds and reverse neuromuscular blockade.

Gantacurium is an asymmetric α-chlorofumarate that was developed to be a replacement for succinylcholine.[226] Gantacurium has a rapid onset and short duration of effect. The brief duration of gantacurium is primarily due to rapid reaction and subsequent inactivation of the drug with free cysteine in the plasma. The process of adduction of cysteine to gantacurium occurs at the central fumarate double bond. The adduction changes the stereochemistry of gantacurium so that it can no longer bind to the nAChR at the neuromuscular junction. Degradation also occurs through a slower secondary route (pH-sensitive ester hydrolysis) that yields two products without neuromuscular blocking properties.[226,227] CW 002 (a symmetrical fumarate) and CW 011 (an asymmetric maleate) are investigational NMBDs with no halogen (chlorine) substitution at the central double-bonded carbons. The absence of chlorine results in a slower adduction with cysteine; the inactivation of CW 002 and CW 011 is slower than gantacurium, resulting in a duration of action consistent with an intermediate-acting NMBD.

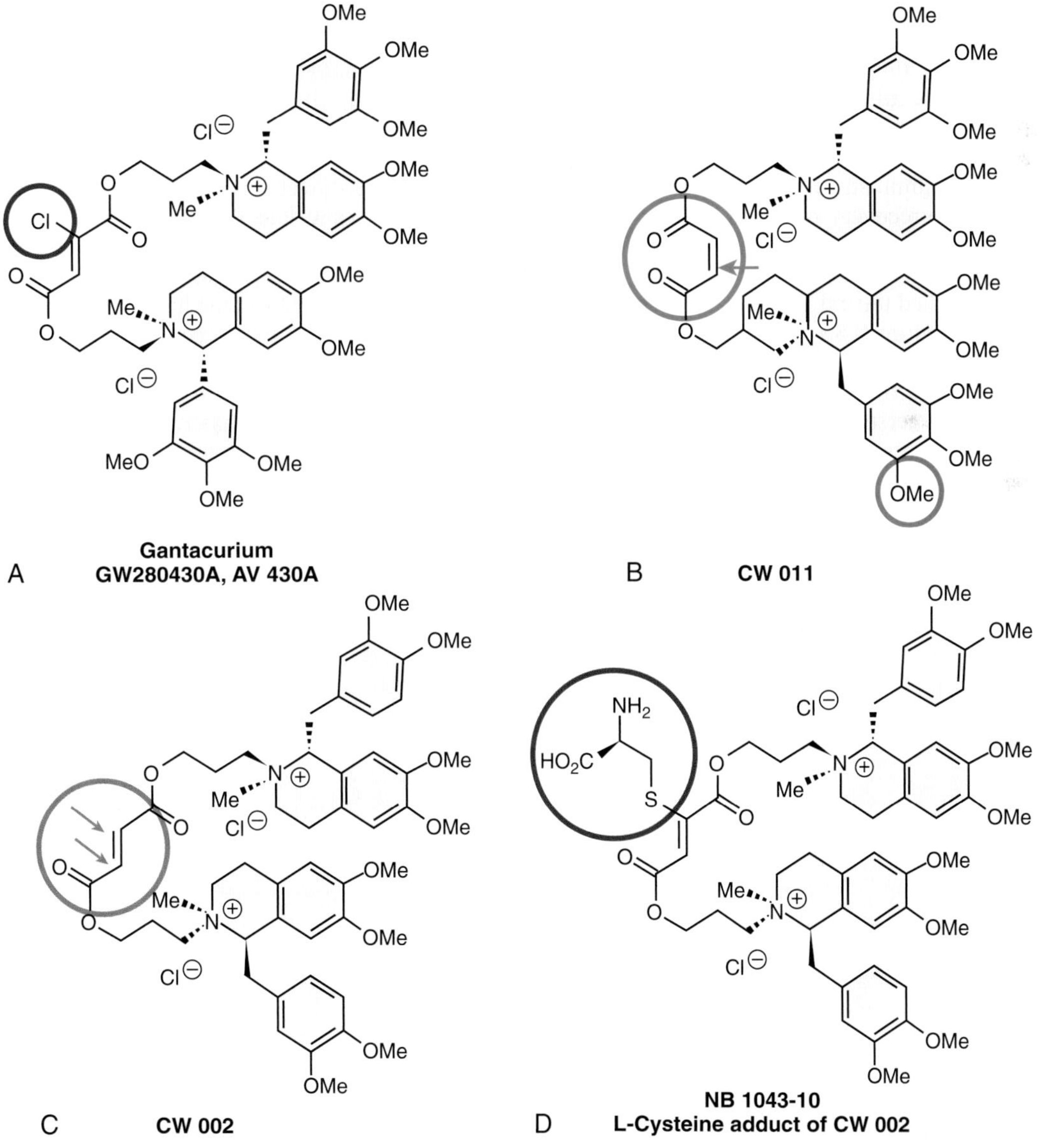

Fig. 28.23 The chemical formulas of gantacurium (A), CW 011 (B), and CW 002 (C). Chemical features are as follows. Chlorine substitution *(red circle)* on the olefinic double bond of gantacurium, a chlorofumarate, is designed to accelerate the L-cysteine adduction reaction. The fumarate CW 002 is symmetrical with no halogen (chlorine) substitutions and undergoes L-cysteine adduction more slowly than gantacurium, at either olefinic carbon *(blue arrows)*, enabled by the adjacent α-carboxyl (ester) groups. The maleate CW 011 is asymmetric in that one isoquinolinium group contains an extra methoxy substitution *(green circle)*. This may reduce access of L-cysteine to the olefin *(green arrow)* and may decrease the rate of the adduction reaction. The chemical formula of NB 1043-10, the L-cysteine adduct of CW 002, is also shown (D). The L-cysteine adduction is highlighted by the *red circle*. (From Savarese JJ, McGilvra JD, Sunaga H, et al. Rapid chemical antagonism of neuromuscular blockade by l-cysteine adduction to and inactivation of the olefinic (double-bonded) isoquinolinium diester compounds gantacurium (AV430A), CW 002, and CW 011. *Anesthesiology.* 2010;113:58–73.)

Cysteine is a nonessential endogenous amino acid derived from one molecule of serine and one molecule of methionine. It is composed of L- and D-enantiomers. L-Cysteine is a normal building block of protein and is a conditionally essential amino acid in infants.[228] Several therapeutic applications of cysteine in medicine are common. It is often added to total parenteral nutrition solutions for pediatric patients in doses of approximately 80 mg/kg/day. An acetylated derivative of cysteine (*N*-acetyl L-cysteine) is approved for use in the treatment of acute acetaminophen toxicity. In the doses used clinically for these applications, there does not appear to be obvious toxicity. L-Cysteine has also been studied for reversal of the neuromuscular blockade for fumarate NMBDs. Several laboratory investigations have attempted to define the L-cysteine dose necessary to effectively reverse gantacurium, CW 002, and CW 011 neuromuscular blockade.

The first of the fumarate NMBDs studied was gantacurium. In monkeys, the total duration of action was one half to one third that of mivacurium at equipotent doses; at three times the ED_{95} doses, the time until 95% twitch recovery was 8.5 ± 0.5 minutes versus 22.0 ± 2.6 minutes, respectively.[227] The administration of edrophonium 0.5 mg/kg accelerated the recovery of blockade. In a human volunteer trial, the time from administration of 0.40 mg/kg of gantacurium (2 × ED_{95}) until a TOF ratio 0.90 or greater was achieved was studied during spontaneous recovery or reversal with edrophonium 0.5 mg/kg.[229] Mean recovery time was significantly more rapid in the reversal group (3.8 minutes) compared with the spontaneous recovery group (14.3 minutes). The reversal of gantacurium with cysteine was investigated in monkeys.[228] A bolus of L-cysteine (10 mg/kg) given 1 minute after gantacurium reduced duration from 10.4 ± 3.1 minutes (spontaneous recovery) to 3.0 ± 1.0 minutes ($P < .001$). Antagonism of gantacurium was significantly faster at 1 minute with L-cysteine than edrophonium. These studies suggest that although gantacurium is a short-acting NMBD, recovery can be further enhanced by the administration of L-cysteine.

In contrast to gantacurium, CW 002 and CW 011 have a duration of action between a short-acting and intermediate-acting NMBD. In monkeys given four to five times the ED_{95} of CW 002 and CW 011, the duration of blockade was three times longer than gantacurium (28.1 and 33.3 minutes vs. 10.4 minutes), but only half the duration of cisatracurium.[228] The administration of neostigmine 1 minute after CW 002 did not accelerate neuromuscular recovery. Immediate reversal of CW 002 with cysteine (50 mg/kg), however, was highly effective in antagonizing neuromuscular blockade (95% of baseline twitch height within 2.2 ± 0.3 minutes and to a TOF ratio of 100% 1–2 minutes later) (Fig. 28.24).[228] Similar findings were observed with CW 011 using this model. Larger doses of L-cysteine were needed to optimally reverse CW 002 and CW 011 (50 mg/kg) compared with gantacurium (10 mg/kg); this is likely related to the slower rate of adduction of L-cysteine to these compounds, as well as the greater potency of CW 002 and CW 011. L-Cysteine reversal of CW 002 has also been investigated in a dog model given a dose of 9 × ED_{95}.[230] L-Cysteine (50 mg/kg) reduced the median duration of blockade from 70 minutes (spontaneous recovery) to less than 5 minutes. Doses of up to 200 mg/kg produced minimal hemodynamic changes and resulted in no anatomic, biochemical, or histologic evidence of organ toxicity.

In summary, fumarates are a new class of NMBDs that are inactivated primarily via adduction of cysteine to the double

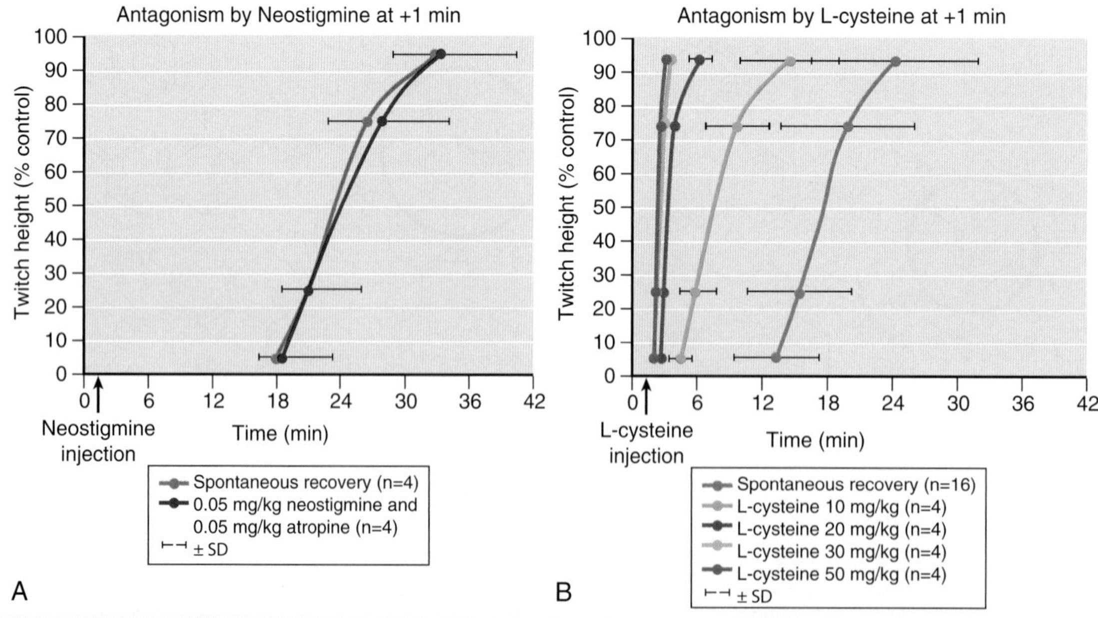

Fig. 28.24 Immediate antagonism of CW 002 blockade 1 minute after CW 002 dosage of 0.15 mg/kg, or ≈4 × ED_{95}, injected at $t = 0$. Neostigmine (0.05 mg/kg + atropine 0.05 mg/kg) or L-cysteine (10, 20, 30, or 50 mg/kg) was given at +1 min. Neostigmine did not shorten recovery (A), whereas L-cysteine produced a dose-related acceleration of recovery (B), peaking at 50 mg/kg. Data were taken from anesthetized rhesus monkeys. (From Savarese JJ, McGilvra JD, Sunaga H, et al. Rapid chemical antagonism of neuromuscular blockade by l-cysteine adduction to and inactivation of the olefinic (double-bonded) isoquinolinium diester compounds gantacurium (AV430A), CW 002, and CW 011. *Anesthesiology.* 2010;113:58–73.)

bond of the compounds, resulting in breakdown products that do not bind to the neuromuscular junction. Initial laboratory studies have shown that the administration of exogenous L-cysteine results in complete reversal of deep neuromuscular blockade within 2 to 3 minutes. These studies suggest that chemical antagonism of fumarate NMBDs will allow clinicians to rapidly and completely antagonize neuromuscular blockade, even when large doses of an NMBD have been recently administered. Early clinical trials in human volunteers have examined the pharmacology of gantacurium, and investigations of CW 002 in volunteers are currently ongoing. The optimal dose of L-cysteine is 50 mg/kg in an animal model. The dosing of L-cysteine needed to reverse the effects of gantacurium, CW 002, and CW 011 in humans has not been established. Additional investigations are also needed to determine whether large doses of cysteine produce adverse effects in humans. If future studies are consistent with these early findings, fumarate NMBDs may allow clinicians to maintain profound neuromuscular blockade throughout the surgical procedure with little risk of postoperative residual paralysis.

Complete references available online at expertconsult.com.

References

1. Gray TC, et al. JA. *Proc R Soc Med.* 1946;39:400.
2. Cowan SL. *J Physiol.* 1938;15:215.
3. Bennett AE. *JAMA.* 1940;114:322.
4. Griffith HR, Johnson GE. *Anesthesiology.* 1942;3:418.
5. Adams RC. *Surg Clin North Am.* 1945;25:735.
6. Gray TC, Wilson F. *Anesthesiology.* 1959;20:519.
7. Churchill-Davidson HC. *Anesthesiology.* 1965;26:132.
8. Fuchs-Buder T, et al. *Anaesthesist.* 2003;52:522.
9. Duvaldestin P, et al. *Ann Fr Anesth Reanim.* 2008;27:483.
10. Osmer C, et al. *Eur J Anaesthesiol.* 1996;13:389.
11. Naguib M, et al. *Anesth Analg.* 2010;111:110.
12. Cullen SC. *Anesthesiology.* 1944;5:166.
13. Grayling M, Sweeney BP. *Anaesthesia.* 2007;62:806.
14. Pavlin EG, et al. *Anesthesiology.* 1989;70:381.
15. Eikermann M, et al. *Anesthesiology.* 2003;98:1333.
16. Pedersen T, et al. *Anesthesiology.* 1990;73:835.
17. Cammu G, et al. *Anesth Analg.* 2006;102:426.
18. Hayes AH, et al. *Anaesthesia.* 2001;56:312.
19. Viby-Mogensen J, et al. *Anesthesiology.* 1985;63:440.
20. Brull SJ, Silverman DG. *Anesth Analg.* 1993;77:352.
21. Capron F, et al. *Anesth Analg.* 2006;102:1578.
22. Dupuis JY, et al. *Can J Anaesth.* 1990;37:397.
23. Brull SJ, Silverman DG. *Anesth Analg.* 1991;73:627.
24. Mortensen CR, et al. *Acta Anaesthesiol Scand.* 1995;39:797.
25. Gätke MR, et al. *Acta Anaesthesiol Scand.* 2002;46:207.
26. Murphy GS, et al. *Anesthesiology.* 2008;109:389.
27. Murphy GS, et al. *Anesthesiology.* 2011;115:946.
28. Ali HH, et al. *Br J Anaesth.* 1970;42:967.
29. Ali HH, et al. *Br J Anaesth.* 1971;43:473.
30. Ali HH, et al. *Br J Anaesth.* 1971;43:478.
31. Ali HH, Kitz RJ. *Anesth Analg.* 1973;52:740.
32. Ali HH, et al. *Br J Anaesth.* 1975;47:570.
33. Sundman E, et al. *Anesthesiology.* 2000;92:977.
34. Eriksson LI, et al. *Anesthesiology.* 1997;87:1035.
35. Eikermann M, et al. *Anesthesiology.* 2003;98:1333.
36. Eriksson LI, et al. *Anesthesiology.* 1993;78:693.
37. Kopman AF, et al. *Anesthesiology.* 1997;86:765.
38. Murphy GS, et al. *Anesth Analg.* 2008;107:130.
39. Butterly A, et al. *Br J Anaesth.* 2010;105:304.
40. Murphy GS, Brull SJ. *Anesth Analg.* 2010;111:120.
41. Viby-Mogensen J, et al. *Anesthesiology.* 1979;50:539.
42. Beemer GH, Rozental P. *Anaesth Intensive Care.* 1986;14:41.
43. Howardy-Hansen P, et al. *Acta Anaesthesiol Scand.* 1989;33:167.
44. Naguib M, et al. *Br J Anaesth.* 2007;98:302.
45. Andersen BN, et al. *Acta Anaesthesiol Scand.* 1988;32:79.
46. Bevan DR, et al. *Anesthesiology.* 1988;69:272.
47. Debaene B, et al. *Anesthesiology.* 2003;98:1042.
48. Hayes AH, et al. *Anaesthesia.* 2001;56:312.
49. Yu B, Ouyang B, Ge S. *Curr Med Res Opin.* 2016;32:1.
50. Murphy GS, et al. *Anesth Analg.* 2005;100:1840.
51. Cedborg AI, et al. *Anesthesiology.* 2014;120:312–325.
52. Eikermann M, et al. *Am J Respir Crit Care Med.* 2007;175:9.
53. Herbstreit F, et al. *Anesthesiology.* 2009;110:1253.
54. Eriksson LI. *Acta Anaesthesiol Scand.* 1996;40:520.
55. Eriksson LI. *Anesth Analg.* 1999;89:243.
56. Isono S, et al. *Anesthesiology.* 1991;75:980.
57. Heier T, et al. *Anesthesiology.* 2010;113:825.
58. Beecher HK, Todd DP. *Ann Surg.* 1954;140:2.
59. Harrison GG. *Br J Anaesth.* 1978;50:1041.
60. Cooper AL, et al. *Anaesthesia.* 1989;44:953.
61. Rose DK, et al. *Anesthesiology.* 1994;81:410.
62. Cooper AL, et al. *Anaesthesia.* 1989;44:953.
63. Barnes PJ, Havill JH. *Anaesth Intensive Care.* 1980;8:404.
64. Sprung J, et al. *Anesthesiology.* 2003;99:259.
65. Arbous MS, et al. *Anesthesiology.* 2005;102:257.
66. Bulka CM, et al. *Anesthesiology.* 2016;125:647.
67. Bronsert MR, et al. *Anesth Analg.* 2017;124:1476.
68. Bissinger U, et al. *Physiol Res.* 2000;49:455.
69. Murphy GS, et al. *Anesth Analg.* 2004;98:193.
70. Sauer M, et al. *Eur J Anaesthesiol.* 2011;28:842.
71. Berg H, et al. *Acta Anaesthesiol Scand.* 1997;41:1095.
72. Norton M, et al. *Rev Esp Anestesiol Reanim.* 2013;60:190.
73. Murphy GS, et al. *Anesth Analg.* 2003;96:1301.
74. Errando CL, et al. *Minerva Anestesiol.* 2016;82:1267.
75. Xará D, et al. *Arch Bronconeumol.* 2015;51:69.
76. Murphy GS, et al. *Anesth Analg.* 2003;96:1301.
77. Naguib M, et al. *Anesthesiology.* 2002;96:202.
78. Caldwell JE. *J Crit Care.* 2009;24:21.
79. Bevan DR, et al. *Anesthesiology.* 1992;77:785.
80. Cronnelly R, et al. *Anesthesiology.* 1982;57:261.
81. Morris RB, et al. *Anesthesiology.* 1981;54:399.
82. Cronnelly R, et al. *Clin Pharmacol Ther.* 1980;28:78.
83. Cronnelly R, et al. *Anesthesiology.* 1979;51:222.
84. Morris RB, et al. *Br J Anaesth.* 1981;53:1311.
85. Matteo RS, et al. *Anesth Analg.* 1990;71:334.
86. Heier T, Caldwell JE. *Anesthesiology.* 2006;104:1070.
87. Heier T, et al. *Anesthesiology.* 2002;97:90.
88. Ferguson A, et al. *Anesthesiology.* 1980;53:390.
89. Jones RM, et al. *Br J Anaesth.* 1984;56:453.
90. Rupp SM, et al. *Anesthesiology.* 1986;64:711.
91. Donati F, et al. *Anesthesiology.* 1987;66:471.
92. Smith CE, et al. *Anesthesiology.* 1989;71:37.
93. Kirkegaard-Nielsen H, et al. *Can J Anaesth.* 1996;43:932.
94. Engbaek J, et al. *Anesthesiology.* 1990;72:803.
95. Magorian TT, et al. *Anesthesiology.* 1990;73:410.
96. Kirkegaard H, et al. *Anesthesiology.* 2002;96:45.
97. Kim KS, et al. *Anesth Analg.* 2004;99:1080.
98. Hunter JM. *Br J Anaesth.* 2017;119(Suppl 1):i53.
99. Kopman AF. *Anesthesiology.* 1986;65:572.
100. Baurain MJ, et al. *Br J Anaesth.* 1996;77:496.
101. Fisher DM, et al. *Anesthesiology.* 1983;59:220.
102. Meistelman C, et al. *Anesthesiology.* 1988;69:97.
103. Bevan JC, et al. *Anesth Analg.* 1999;89:333.
104. Young WL, et al. *Anesth Analg.* 1988;67:775.
105. Reid JE, et al. *Can J Anaesth.* 2001;48:351.
106. Jellish WS, et al. *Anesth Analg.* 2000;91:1250.
107. Miller RD, et al. *Anesthesiology.* 1975;42:377.
108. Miller RD, Roderick LL. *Br J Anaesth.* 1978;50:317.
109. Fuchs-Buder T, et al. *Anesthesiology.* 2010;112:34.
110. Caldwell JE. *Anesth Analg.* 1995;80:1168.
111. Murphy G, et al. *Anesthesiology.* 2018;128:27.
112. Ostergaard D, et al. *Acta Anaesthesiol Scand.* 1995;39:1016.
113. Naguib M, et al. *Anesthesiology.* 1995;82:1288.
114. Levano S, et al. *Anesthesiology.* 2005;102:531.
115. Scholler KL, et al. *Can Anaesth Soc J.* 1977;24:396.
116. Naguib M, et al. *Anesthesiology.* 1995;83:694.
117. Østergaard D, et al. *Anesthesiology.* 2005;102:1124.
118. Bartkowski RR. *Anesth Analg.* 1987;66:594.
119. Goldhill DR, et al. *Anaesthesia.* 1989;44:293.

120. Astley BA, et al. *Br J Anaesth.* 1987;59:983.
121. Eikermann M, et al. *Br J Anaesth.* 2008;101:344.
122. Eikermann M, et al. *Anesthesiology.* 2007;107:621.
123. Herbstreit F, et al. *Anesthesiology.* 2010;113:1280.
124. Brock-Utne JG, et al. *Anesth Analg.* 1978;57:171.
125. Cheng CR, et al. *Anesth Analg.* 2005;101:1349.
126. Green SM, et al. *Acad Emerg Med.* 2010;17:157.
127. Salmenperä M, et al. *Acta Anaesthesiol Scand.* 1992;36:445.
128. Tramèr MR, Fuchs-Buder T. *Br J Anaesth.* 1999;82:379.
129. Urquhart ML, et al. *Anesthesiology.* 1987;67:561.
130. Azar I, et al. *Anesthesiology.* 1983;59:139.
131. Ostheimer GW. *Anesth Analg.* 1977;56:182.
132. Naguib M, et al. *Anesth Analg.* 1988;67:650.
133. Parlow JL, et al. *Anesth Analg.* 1997;84:155.
134. van Vlymen JM, Parlow JL. *Anesth Analg.* 1997;84:148.
135. Sun KO. *Anaesth Intensive Care.* 1993;21:457.
136. Pratt CI. *Anaesthesia.* 1988;43:248.
137. Shibata O, et al. *Anesth Analg.* 1996;82:1211.
138. Radulovic M, et al. *J Rehabil Res Dev.* 2004;41:53.
139. Miller RD. *Anesth Analg.* 2007;104:477.
140. Booij LHDJ, et al. *Semin Anesth Perioperat Med Pain.* 2002;21:92.
141. Bom A, et al. *Angew Chem.* 2002;41:266.
142. Adam JM, et al. *J Med Chem.* 2002;45:1806.
143. Baker MT, Naguib M. *Anesthesiology.* 2005;103:860.
144. Epemolu O, et al. *Anesthesiology.* 2003;99:632.
145. Caldwell JE, Miller RD. *Anaesthesia.* 2009;64(Suppl 1):66.
146. Gijsenbergh F, et al. *Anesthesiology.* 2005;103:695.
147. Sparr HJ, et al. *Anesthesiology.* 2007;106:935.
148. Cammu G, et al. *Br J Anaesth.* 2012;109:382.
149. Sorgenfrei IF, et al. *Anesthesiology.* 2006;104:667.
150. Suy K, et al. *Anesthesiology.* 2007;106:283.
151. Groudine SB, et al. *Anesth Analg.* 2007;104:555.
152. de Boer HD, et al. *Anesthesiology.* 2007;107:239.
153. Lemmens HJ, et al. *BMC Anesthesiol.* 2010;10:15.
154. Mosing M, et al. *Br J Anaesth.* 2010;105:480.
155. Shields M, et al. *Br J Anaesth.* 2006;96:36.
156. Lee C, et al. *Anesthesiology.* 2009;110:1020.
157. Sørensen MK, et al. *Br J Anaesth.* 2012;108:682.
158. Sacan O, et al. *Anesth Analg.* 2007;104:569.
159. Blobner M, et al. *Eur J Anaesthesiol.* 2010;27:874.
160. Jones RK, et al. *Anesthesiology.* 2008;109:816.
161. Flockton EA, et al. *Br J Anaesth.* 2008;100:622.
162. Vanacker BF, et al. *Anesth Analg.* 2007;104:563.
163. Duvaldestin P, et al. *Anesth Analg.* 2010;110:74.
164. Plaud B, et al. *Anesthesiology.* 2009;110:284.
165. Buchanan CC, O'Donnell AM. *Paediatr Anaesth.* 2011;21:1077.
166. Nishi M, et al. *Masui.* 2011;60:1189.
167. Liu G, et al. *Sci Rep.* 2017;7(1):5724.
168. McDonagh DL, et al. *Anesthesiology.* 2011;114:318.
169. Suzuki T, et al. *Br J Anaesth.* 2011;106:823.
170. Yoshida F, et al. *Acta Anaesthesiol Scand.* 2012;56:83.
171. Carron M, et al. *Clin Interv Aging.* 2018;13:13.
172. Dahl V, et al. *Eur J Anaesthesiol.* 2009;26:874.
173. de Kam PJ, et al. *Clin Drug Investig.* 2010;30:599.
174. Riley RH, et al. *Anaesth Intensive Care.* 2010;38:1138.
175. Craig RG, Hunter JM. *Anaesthesia.* 2009;64(Suppl 1):55.
176. Amao R, et al. *J Clin Anesth.* 2012;24:289.
177. Porter MV, Paleologos MS. *Anaesth Intensive Care.* 2011;39:299.
178. Staals LM, et al. *Br J Anaesth.* 2008;101:492.
179. Panhuizen IF, et al. *Br J Anaesth.* 2015;114(5):777.
180. Min KC, et al. *Int J Clin Pharmacol Ther.* 2017;55(9):746.
181. Carlos RV, et al. *Eur J Anaesthesiol.* 2016;33:383.
182. Ono Y, et al. *Eur J Anaesthesiol.* 34(e-suppl 55):397
183. Craig RG, Hunter JM. *Anaesthesia.* 2009;64(Suppl 1):55.
184. Ogunnaike BO, et al. *Anesth Analg.* 2002;95:1793.
185. Monk TG, et al. *Am J Ther.* 2017;24(5):e507–e516.
186. Gaszynski T, et al. *Br J Anaesth.* 2012;108:236.
187. Van Lancker P, et al. *Anaesthesia.* 2011;66:721.
188. Llauradó S, et al. *Anesthesiology.* 2012;117:93.
189. Le Corre F, et al. *Can J Anaesth.* 2011;58:944.
190. Duarte NMDC, et al. *Rev Bras Anestesiol.* 2018;68(3):219.
191. Sharp LM, Levy DM. *Curr Opin Anaesthesiol.* 2009;22:357.
192. Abrishami A, et al. *Cochrane Database Syst Rev.* 2009;(4):CD007362.
193. Dahl V, Spreng UJ. *Curr Opin Anaesthesiol.* 2009;22:352.
194. Pühringer FK, et al. *Br J Anaesth.* 2010;105:657.
195. Williamson RM, et al. *Acta Anaesthesiol Scand.* 2011;55:694.
196. Blichfeldt-Lauridsen L, Hansen BD. *Acta Anaesthesiol Scand.* 2012;56:17.
197. Baraka AS, Jalbout MI. *Curr Opin Anaesthesiol.* 2002;15:371.
198. Steward PA, et al. *Rev Esp Anestesiol Reanim.* 2012.
199. Vilela H, et al. *J Anesth.* 2012;26:306.
200. Unterbuchner C, et al. *Anaesthesia.* 2010;65:302.
201. de Boer HD, et al. *Rev Esp Anestesiol Reanim.* 2010;57:181.
202. Mavridou P, et al. *Acta Anaesthesiol Belg.* 2011;62:101.
203. de Boer HD, et al. *Eur J Anaesthesiol.* 2014;31(12):715.
204. Vymazal T, et al. *Ther Clin Risk Manag.* 2015;11:1593.
205. Miyazaki Y, et al. *Anesth Analg.* 2018;126(5):1505.
206. Horiuchi T, et al. *Anesth Analg.* 2018;126(5):1509.
207. Rahe-Meyer N, et al. *Anesthesiology.* 2014;121(5):969.
208. Zwiers A, et al. *Clin Drug Investig.* 2011;31:101.
209. US Food and Drug Administration. *Sugammadex, NDA 22-225, Anesthetic and Life Support Drugs Advisory Committee March.* ;11 ; 2008. http://wwwfdagov/ohrms/dockets/ac/08/slides/2008-4346s1-01-Schering-Plough-corebackuppdf>2008.
210. Kam PJ, et al. *Clin Drug Investig.* 2012;32:203.
211. de Boer HD, et al. *Can J Anaesth.* 2008;55:124.
212. Cammu G, et al. *Br J Anaesth.* 2010;105:487.
213. Eleveld DJ, et al. *Anesth Analg.* 2007;j104:582.
214. Drobnik L, et al. *Eur J Anaesthesiol.* 2010;27:866.
215. Asztalos L, et al. *Anesthesiology.* 2017;127:441.
216. Mirzakhani H, et al. *Acta Anaesthesiol Scand.* 2012;56:3.
217. Turkkal DC, et al. *J Clin Anesth.* 2008;20:589.
218. Hoshi H, et al. *J Anesth.* 2011;25:286.
219. Kadoi Y, et al. *J Anesth.* 2011;25:855.
220. Batistaki C, et al. *J ECT.* 2011;27:e47.
221. Lindekaer AL, et al. *J Vis Exp.* 2013;76:1.
222. Staehr-Rye AK, et al. *Dan Med J.* 2013;60:A4579.
223. Bruintjes MH, et al. *BJA.* 2017;118(6):834.
224. Kotake Y, et al. *Anesth Analg.* 2013;117:345.
225. Naguib M, et al. *Anesth Analg.* 2013;117:297.
226. Lien CA. *Br J Anaesth.* 2011;107(Suppl 1):i60.
227. Savarese JJ, et al. *Anesthesiology.* 2004;100:835.
228. Savarese JJ, et al. *Anesthesiology.* 2010;113:58.
229. Belmont MR, et al. *Anesthesiology.* 2004;100:768.
230. Sunaga H, et al. *Anesthesiology.* 2010;112:900.

29 Local Anesthetics

PHILIPP LIRK and CHARLES B. BERDE

KEY POINTS

- Local anesthetics block voltage-gated sodium channels and thereby interrupt initiation and propagation of impulses in axons, but they have a wide variety of other biologic actions, desirable and undesirable.
- Currently available local anesthetics are of two chemical classes: aminoesters and aminoamides.
- The low potency and lack of specificity of available local anesthetics are due in part to the very weak structural constraints at their binding site on the sodium channel. Most of their features derive from the requirement for high solubility, rapidly reversible protonation, and rapid diffusion in both aqueous environments and in the lipid phases of biologic membranes.
- Reversible protonation of the tertiary amine group tends to make local anesthetics less charged at more basic pH and more charged at neutral or acidic pH; the neutral base forms are more soluble in lipid environments, whereas the charged acid forms, the more potent species, are more soluble in aqueous environments.
- Aminoesters are metabolized primarily by plasma esterases, and aminoamides are metabolized primarily by hepatic cytochrome P450-linked enzymes.
- The principal systemic toxicities of local anesthetics involve the heart (including atrioventricular conduction block, arrhythmias, myocardial depression, and cardiac arrest) and the brain (including agitation, lethargy, seizures, and generalized central nervous system depression). Hypoxemia and acidosis exacerbate these toxicities. Resuscitation after bupivacaine overdose is particularly difficult. Therefore prevention of intravascular injection or overdose is crucial, and major nerve blockade should involve incremental, fractionated dosing. Ultrasound can reduce the incidence of systemic toxicity and Intralipid can help in the resuscitation.
- Local anesthetics are directly toxic to nerve at the concentrations supplied in commercial solutions. Intraneural concentrations during regional anesthesia are generally (but not always) below a threshold for toxicity because of spread of solutions through tissues and diffusion gradients from injection sites into nerve. Injection into a constrained tissue space increases the risk for local toxicity.
- Optimal use of local anesthetics in regional anesthesia requires an understanding of (1) the individual patient's clinical situation; (2) the location, intensity, and duration of regional anesthesia and analgesia required; (3) anatomic factors affecting deposition of drug near nerves; (4) proper drug selection and dosing; and (5) ongoing assessment of clinical effects after administration of a local anesthetic.
- Single-stereoisomer (as opposed to a racemic mixture) formulations have been developed in an effort to reduce systemic toxicity and improve sensory selectivity but true sensory selectivity has not been achieved with drugs currently available.
- The most important research avenues to improve local anesthetic action are slow release formulations, targeting of specific sodium channel subtypes, and targeting of nociceptive fibers.

Local anesthesia results from the blockade of nerve impulses to abolish sensation. All currently available, clinically useful agents are either aminoesters or aminoamides. These drugs, when applied in sufficient concentration at the site of action, prevent conduction of electrical impulses by the membranes of nerve and muscle. In addition to blockade of impulses, local anesthetics can inhibit various receptors, enhance release of glutamate, and depress the activity of certain intracellular signaling pathways. When local anesthetic agents are given systemically, the functions of cardiac, skeletal, and smooth muscle, as well as transmission of impulses in the central and peripheral nervous systems and within the specialized conducting system of the heart, may all be altered. Local anesthetics may abolish sensation in various parts of the body by topical application, injection near peripheral nerve endings and major nerve trunks, or instillation within the epidural or subarachnoid spaces. Toxicity may be local or systemic. The central nervous and cardiovascular systems are most commonly involved in acute clinical toxicity.

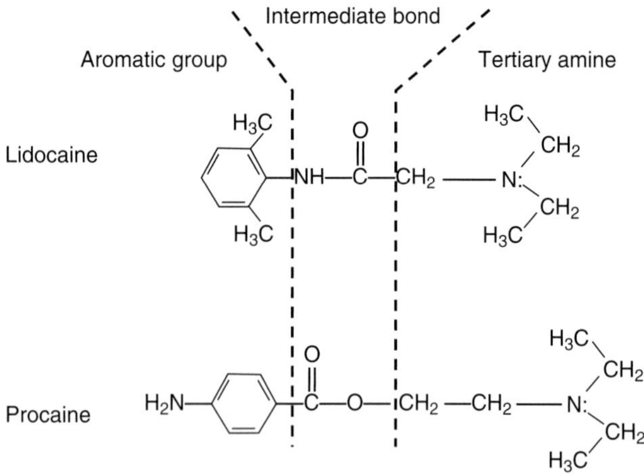

Fig. 29.1 Structures of two local anesthetics: the aminoamide lidocaine and the aminoester procaine. In both drugs, a hydrophobic aromatic group is joined to a more hydrophilic base, the tertiary amine, by an intermediate amide or ester bond.

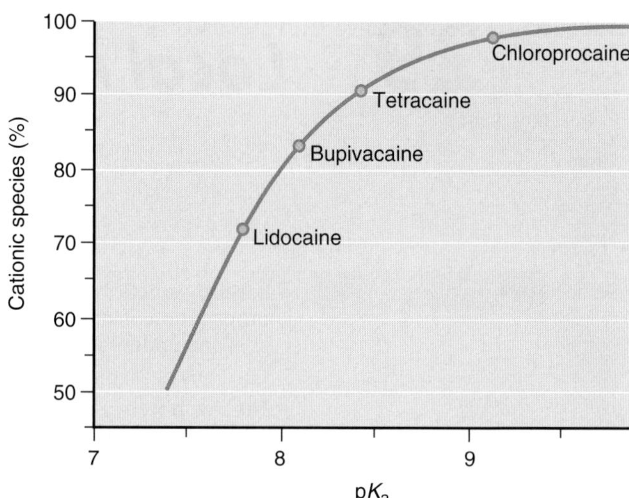

Fig. 29.2 Fraction of local anesthetic in the protonated, cationic form of an aqueous solution at physiologic pH (7.4) as a function of the pK_a of the drug. Lidocaine, the drug with the lowest pK_a, has the smallest fraction of its molecules protonated, the largest in the neutral form, and vice versa for chloroprocaine, the local anesthetic with the highest pK_a. Individual drug molecules become protonated and deprotonated in thousandths of a second in solution.

Basic Pharmacology

CHEMISTRY

The Local Anesthetic Molecule

The typical local anesthetic molecule, exemplified by lidocaine and procaine (Fig. 29.1), contains a tertiary amine attached to a substituted aromatic ring by an intermediate chain that almost always contains either an ester (see Fig. 29.1) or an amide linkage (Fig. 29.2).

Local anesthetics may therefore be classified as aminoester or aminoamide compounds. The aromatic ring system gives a lipophilic (membrane-liking) character to its portion of the molecule, whereas the tertiary amine end is relatively hydrophilic, particularly since it is partially protonated and thus bears some positive charge in the physiologic pH range (see Fig. 29.2). The structures of commonly administered local anesthetics are given in Table 29.1 and their physicochemical properties in Table 29.2.

STRUCTURE-ACTIVITY RELATIONSHIPS AND PHYSICOCHEMICAL PROPERTIES

The intrinsic potency and duration of action of local anesthetics are clearly dependent on certain features of the molecule.

Lipophilic-Hydrophilic Balance

The lipophilic versus hydrophilic character of a local anesthetic depends on the size of alkyl substituents on or near the tertiary amine and on the aromatic ring. "Lipophilicity" expresses the tendency of a compound to associate with membrane lipids, a property usually approximated by equilibrium partitioning into a hydrophobic solvent such as octanol.[1] Although octanol-buffer partition coefficients are comparable to membrane-buffer partition coefficients for the uncharged species of local anesthetics, they severely underestimate membrane partitioning for the charged, protonated species, octanol being a poor model for the polar regions near the membrane surface where local anesthetics are concentrated.[2] Here we use the term "hydrophobicity," expressed as octanol-buffer partitioning, to describe a physicochemical property of local anesthetics.

Compounds with a more hydrophobic nature are obtained by increasing the size of the alkyl substituents. These agents are more potent and produce longer-lasting blocks than their less hydrophobic congeners do.[3-5] For example, etidocaine, which has three more carbon atoms in the amine end of the molecule than lidocaine, is four times as potent and five times as long lasting when compared in the isolated sciatic nerve.

Hydrogen Ion Concentration

Local anesthetics in solution exist in a very rapid chemical equilibrium between the basic uncharged form (B) and the charged cationic form (BH^+). At a certain hydrogen ion concentration ($\log_{10}{}^{-1}$ [−pH]) specific for each drug, the concentration of local anesthetic base in solution is equal to the concentration of charged cation. The logarithm of this hydrogen ion concentration is called pK_a. The relationship is defined by

$$\frac{[BH^+]}{[B]} = 10\ pK_a - pH$$

pK_a values of local anesthetic agents in aqueous solution are listed in Table 29.2. The tendency to be protonated also depends on environmental factors, such as temperature and ionic strength, and on the medium surrounding the drug. In the relatively apolar milieu of a membrane, the average pK_a of local anesthetics is lower than in solution. This is chemically equivalent to saying that the membrane concentrates the base form of the local anesthetic

TABLE 29.1 Representative Local Anesthetics in Common Clinical Use

Generic* and Common Proprietary Names	Chemical Structure	Approximate Year of Initial Clinical Use	Main Anesthetic Use	Representative Commercial Preparation
Cocaine	CH_2—CH—$CHCOOCH_3$ NCH_3—$CHOOC_6H_5$ CH_2—CH—CH_2	1884	Topical	40-mg/mL solution
Benzocaine (Americaine)	H_2N—⟨ring⟩—C(=O)—OC_2H_5	1900	Topical	200 mg/mL
Procaine (Novocain)	H_2N—⟨ring⟩—$COOCH_2CH_2N(C_2H_5)_2$	1905	Topical Infiltration Spinal	200 mg/mL 10- and 20-mg/mL solutions 100-mg/mL solution
Dibucaine (Nupercaine)	⟨quinoline ring, N⟩—OC_4H_9 $CONHCH_2CH_2N(C_2H_5)_2$	1929	Spinal	0.667-, 2.5-, and 5-mg/mL solutions
Tetracaine (Pontocaine)	H_9C_4(H)N—⟨ring⟩—$COOCH_2CH_2N(CH_3)_2$	1930	Spinal	Niphanoid crystals—20- and 10-mg/mL solutions
Lidocaine (Xylocaine)	⟨ring with two CH_3⟩—$NHCOCH_2N(C_2H_5)_2$	1948	Infiltration Peripheral nerve blockade Epidural Spinal Topical Topical	5- and 10-mg/mL solutions 10-, 15-, and 20-mg/mL solutions 10-, 15-, and 20-mg/mL solutions 50-mg/mL solution 20-mg/mL jelly, viscous 25- and 50-mg/mL ointment
Chloroprocaine (Nesacaine)	H_2N—⟨ring with Cl⟩—$COOCH_2CH_2N(C_2H_5)_2$	1955	Infiltration Peripheral nerve blockade Epidural	10-mg/mL solution 10- and 20-mg/mL solutions 20- and 30-mg/mL solutions
Mepivacaine (Carbocaine)	⟨ring with two CH_3⟩—NHCO—⟨piperidine ring, N—CH_3⟩	1957	Infiltration Peripheral nerve blockade Epidural	10-mg/mL solution 10- and 20-mg/mL solutions 10-, 15-, and 20-mg/mL solutions
Prilocaine (Citanest)	⟨ring with CH_3⟩—NHCOCH(CH_3)—NH—C_3H_7	1960	Infiltration Peripheral nerve blockade Epidural	10- and 20-mg/mL solutions 10-, 20-, and 30-mg/mL solutions 10-, 20-, and 30-mg/mL solutions
Bupivacaine (Marcaine)	⟨ring with two CH_3⟩—NHCO—⟨piperidine ring, N—C_4H_9⟩	1963	Infiltration Peripheral nerve blockade Epidural Spinal	2.5-mg/mL solution 2.5- and 5-mg/mL solutions 2.5-, 5-, and 7.5-mg/mL solutions 5- and 7.5-mg/mL solutions
Ropivacaine (Naropin)	⟨ring with two CH_3⟩—NHCO—⟨piperidine ring, N—C_3H_7⟩	1992	Infiltration Peripheral nerve blockade Epidural	2.5- and 5-mg/mL solutions 5- and 10-mg/mL solutions 5- and 7.5-mg/mL solutions

*United States Pharmacopeia nomenclature.
From Covino B, Vassallo H. *Local Anesthetics: Mechanisms of Action and Clinical Use*. Orlando, FL: Grune and Stratton; 1976.

more than it concentrates the protonated cation form. The pH of the medium containing the local anesthetic influences drug activity by altering the relative percentage of the base and protonated forms. For example, in inflamed tissues the pH is lower than normal, and local anesthetics are more protonated than in normal tissue and thus penetrate the tissue relatively poorly (see later). The relationship between pK_a and the percentage of local anesthetic present in the cationic form is shown in Fig. 29.2. As described later, there are dual effects of pH on clinical effectiveness, depending on where the local anesthetic is injected and the importance of the base form for tissue penetration.

Anatomy of the Peripheral Nerve

Each peripheral nerve axon possesses its own cell membrane, the axolemma. Nonmyelinated nerves, such as autonomic postganglionic efferent and nociceptive afferent C fibers, contain many axons encased in a single Schwann cell sheath. In contrast, all large motor and sensory fibers are enclosed in many layers of myelin, which consists of the plasma membranes of specialized Schwann cells that wrap themselves around the axon during axonal outgrowth. Myelin greatly increases the speed of nerve conduction by insulating the axolemma from the surrounding conducting salt medium and forcing the "action current" generated by an impulse to flow through the axoplasm to the nodes of Ranvier, which are periodic interruptions in the myelin sheath where the active impulse is regenerated (Fig. 29.3). The Na^+ channels that serve generation and propagation of impulses are highly concentrated at the nodes of Ranvier of myelinated fibers[7a] but are distributed all along the axon of nonmyelinated fibers (see Fig. 29.3). A classification of peripheral nerves according to fiber size and physiologic properties is presented in Table 29.3. It is important to note that different fiber classes are not only distinguished by diameter and myelin thickness, but also by the structure of the neuronal membrane and ion channel composition.[6]

Each axon has its own connective tissue covering, the *endoneurium*. A typical peripheral nerve consists of several axon bundles, or fascicles. Each fascicle of many axons is encased by a second connective tissue layer, the epithelial-like *perineurium*, and the entire nerve is wrapped in a loose outer sheath called the *epineurium* (Fig. 29.4). To reach the nerve axon, a local anesthetic molecule must traverse any structures surrounding the nerve, such as the paraneurium of the distal sciatic nerve, the epineurium, the perineurium, and the endoneurium, as well as the neuronal plasma membrane. The main barrier to diffusion is the perineurium.[7a] Further, nerves are composed of both neuronal tissues and non-neuronal tissues, such as connective or fatty tissues, and blood vessels. When performing a popliteal sciatic nerve block for example, it should be kept in mind that here, approximately 60% of the nerve cross-section is non-neuronal tissue.[8]

STRUCTURE OF THE AXONAL MEMBRANE

Biologic membranes consist of a molecular lipid bilayer containing proteins adsorbed on the surfaces, as well as embedded in or spanning the hydrocarbon core (Fig. 29.5). The

TABLE 29.2 Relative In Vitro Conduction-Blocking Potency and Physicochemical Properties of Local Anesthetic Drugs

		PHYSIOCHEMICAL PROPERTIES	
Drug	**Relative Conduction-Blocking Potency***	**pK_a†**	**Hydrophobicity†**
LOW POTENCY			
Procaine	1	8.9	100
INTERMEDIATE POTENCY			
Mepivacaine	1.5	7.7	136
Prilocaine	1.8	8.0‡	129
Chloroprocaine	3	9.1	810
Lidocaine	2	7.8	366
HIGH POTENCY			
Tetracaine	8	8.4	5822
Bupivacaine	8	8.1	3420
Etidocaine	8	7.9	7320

*Data derived from C fibers of isolated rabbit vagus and sciatic nerve.
†pK_a and hydrophobicity at 36°C; hydrophobicity equals the octanol/buffer partition coefficient of the base. Values are ratios of concentrations.
‡Values at 25°C.
From Strichartz GR, Sanchez V, Arthur GR, et al. Fundamental properties of local anesthetics. II. Measured octanol: buffer partition coefficients and pK_a values of clinically used drugs. *Anesth Analg.* 1990;71:158–170.

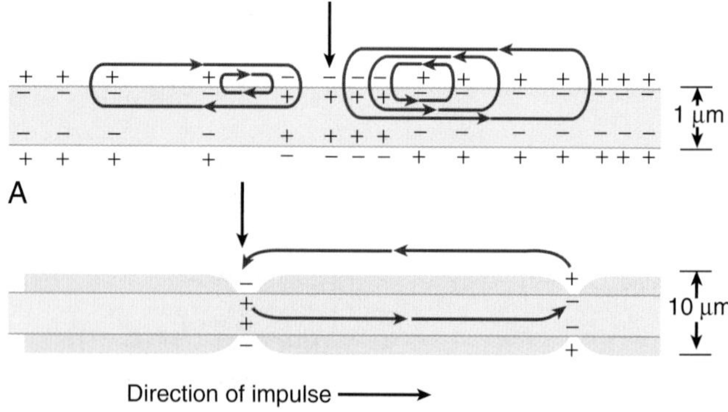

Fig. 29.3 Pattern of local circuit currents flowing during propagation of an impulse in a nonmyelinated C fiber's axon (A) and a myelinated axon (B). During propagation of impulses, from left to right, current entering the axon at the initial rising phase of the impulse *(large vertical arrows)* passes through the axoplasm (local circuit current) and depolarizes the adjacent membrane. Plus and minus signs adjacent to the axon membrane indicate the polarization state of the axon membrane: negative inside at rest, positive inside during active depolarization under the action potential, and less negative in regions where local circuit currents flow. This ionic current passes relatively uniformly across the nonmyelinated axon, but it is restricted in the myelinated axon to entry at the nodes of Ranvier, several of which are simultaneously depolarized during a single action potential.

character of the bilayer is determined by the phospholipids, which have long hydrophobic fatty acyl tails that lie in the center of the membrane, as well as by the polar hydrophilic head groups, which are usually composed of zwitterionic portions (containing positive and negative charges) that project into the cytoplasm or the extracellular fluid. Within the membrane there is both lateral and rotational diffusion, which allows lipids and certain proteins to migrate in a fluid mosaic, but most membrane proteins are fixed within specific regions of a membrane, anchored by connections to specific proteins of the cell's cytoskeleton.[9] A dynamic interaction exists between the cell's membrane and cytoplasm. Although we focus here on the channel-blocking actions of local anesthetics, it is noteworthy that many other cellular activities, including both metabolic and signal transduction pathways, are modulated by these drugs.

PHYSIOLOGY OF NERVE CONDUCTION

The neural membrane is able to maintain a voltage difference of −60 to −90 mV between the intracellular medium and the cell's outside, because at rest it is relatively impermeable to sodium ions (Na^+) but selectively permeable to potassium ions (K^+). The Na^+/K^+ pump, an

TABLE 29.3 Classification of Peripheral Nerves According to Anatomy, Physiology, and Function

Fiber Class	Subclass	Myelin	Diameter (μm)	Conduction Velocity (m/sec)	Location	Function	Susceptibility to Local Anesthetic Block
A	α	+	6-22	30-120	Efferent to muscles	Motor	++
	β	+	6-22	30-120	Afferent from skin and joints	Tactile, proprioception	++
	δ	+	3-6	15-35	Efferent to muscle spindles	Muscle tone	++++
		+	1-4	5-25	Afferent sensory nerves	Pain, cold temperature, touch	+++
B		+	<3	3-15	Preganglionic sympathetic	Various autonomic functions	++
C	sC	–	0.3-1.3	0.7-1.3	Postganglionic sympathetic	Various autonomic functions	++
	dC	–	0.4-1.2	0.1-2.0	Afferent sensory nerves	Various autonomic functions Pain, warm temperature, touch	+

From Bonica JJ. Principles and Practice of Obstetric Anesthesia and Analgesia. Philadelphia: FA Davis; 1967.

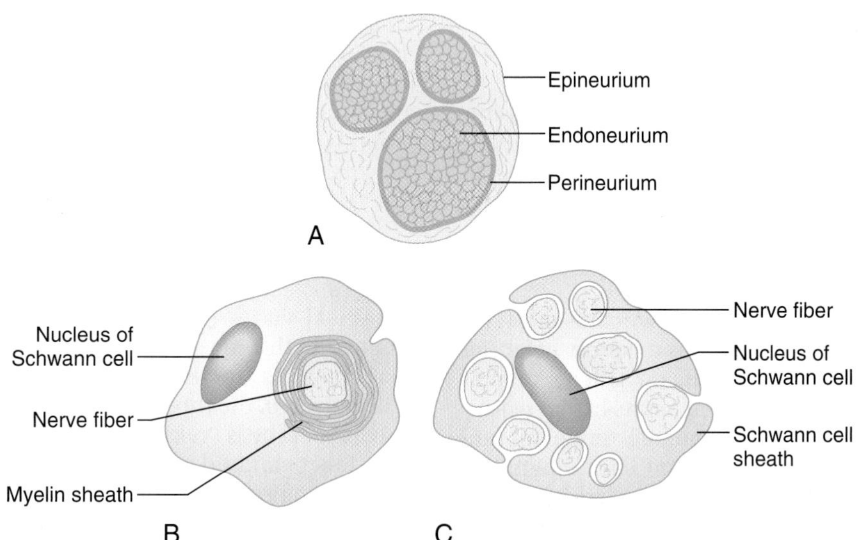

Fig. 29.4 (A) Transverse sections of a peripheral nerve showing the outermost epineurium; the inner perineurium, which collects nerve axons in fascicles; and the endoneurium, which surrounds each myelinated fiber. (B) Each myelinated axon is encased in the multiple membranous wrappings of myelin formed by one Schwann cell, each of which stretches longitudinally more than approximately 100 times the diameter of the axon. The narrow span of axon between these myelinated segments, the node of Ranvier, contains the ion channels that support action potentials. (C) Nonmyelinated fibers are enclosed in bundles of 5 to 10 axons by a chain of Schwann cells that tightly embrace each axon with but one layer of membrane.

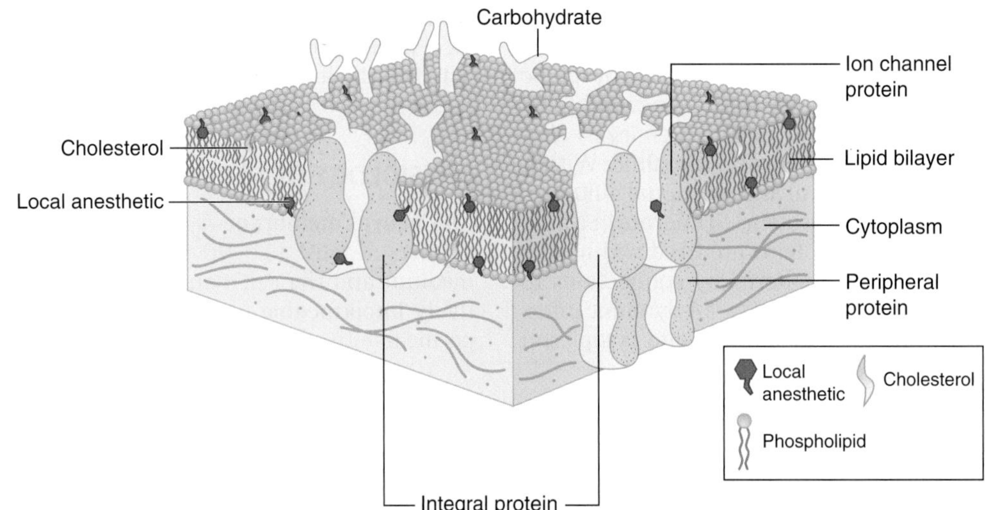

Fig. 29.5 A typical plasma membrane has at its core the lipid bilayer, composed of phospholipids and cholesterol molecules (in an approximately 5:1 ratio) embedding the membrane integral proteins, which are most often glycosylated by extracellular carbohydrates and include receptors and ion channels essential for intercellular communication. "Peripheral proteins" regulate the functions of membrane proteins, chaperone them to the plasma membrane, and stabilize them in the cell through interactions with both the cytoskeleton and the extracellular matrix. Probable membrane locations and protein sites for local anesthetics are also shown.

active, energy-dependent mechanism, sustains the ion gradients that drive this potential difference by constant extrusion of sodium from within the cell in exchange for a net uptake of potassium, with adenosine triphosphate used as an energy source. Although the membrane is relatively permeable to potassium ions, an intracellular-to-extracellular potassium ratio of 150 to 5 mM, or 30:1, is maintained by active removal of potassium as it leaks passively across the plasma membrane into the cell. The nerve at rest behaves largely as a "potassium electrode," according to the Nernst equation:

$$E_m \approx E_k = \left(\frac{-RT}{F}\right) \ln \left(\frac{[K^+]_i}{[K^+]_o}\right)$$

where E_m is the membrane potential, E_K is the potassium equilibrium potential, R is the gas constant, T is temperature (kelvin), F is Faraday's constant, and $[K^+]$ is the potassium ion concentration inside (i) and outside (o) the cell. For potassium, therefore,

$$E_k = -58 \log 30 \text{ or } -85.7 \text{ mV}$$

An opposite situation exists for Na^+, which is at higher concentration outside the cell and has a Nernst potential, E_{Na}, of approximately +60 mV. During an action potential, the nerve membrane transiently switches its higher permeability from K^+ to Na^+, thereby changing the membrane potential from negative to positive, and back again. The progress of this potential change and the underlying events are graphed in Fig. 29.6. They provide a basis for understanding local anesthetic conduction block.

Permeation of ions through membranes occurs via specialized proteins called ion channels.[10] The conformation of these channels is often sensitive to the membrane potential; both Na^+ and K^+ channels in nerve membranes are activated to an "open" conformation by membrane depolarization. Sodium channels, in addition, close to an "inactivated" conformation after their initial activation. A small membrane depolarization extending along an axon from a region of excited membrane, will begin to open both Na^+ and K^+ channels. The Na^+ channels open faster, and the inwardly directed Na^+ current (see Fig. 29.6) depolarizes the membrane further, thereby leading to opening of more Na^+ channels and increasing the inward Na^+ current even further (Fig. 29.7). This sequence of events continues during the *depolarizing phase* until some of the Na^+ channels have become inactivated and enough of the K^+ channels have opened to change the balance of current and result in a net outward current that produces membrane *repolarization* (see Fig. 29.7). After one action potential, the concentrations of Na^+ and K^+ have changed little for the large myelinated fibers but by as much as 10% for the small, nonmyelinated axons. The Na^+ ions entering and K^+ ions leaving the cell as a result of this process are restored by the Na^+/K^+ pump.

Depolarizations too weak to activate enough Na^+ channels to produce a net inward current are below the membrane's excitability *threshold*. The precise value of the threshold varies in different regions of the cell and can change with time. Directly after an impulse, when some Na^+ channels are still inactivated and some K^+ channels are still activated, the threshold is above its "resting" value and the membrane is "refractory" to stimulation. Over time, as Na^+ inactivation decays and K^+ channels return to their closed conformation, the original resting threshold value is restored. The action potential is a wave of depolarization that is propagated along the axon by continuous coupling between excited and nonexcited regions of membrane. Ionic current (the action current) enters the axon in the excited, depolarized region and then flows down the axoplasm and exits through the surrounding membrane, thereby passively depolarizing this adjacent region (see Fig. 29.3).

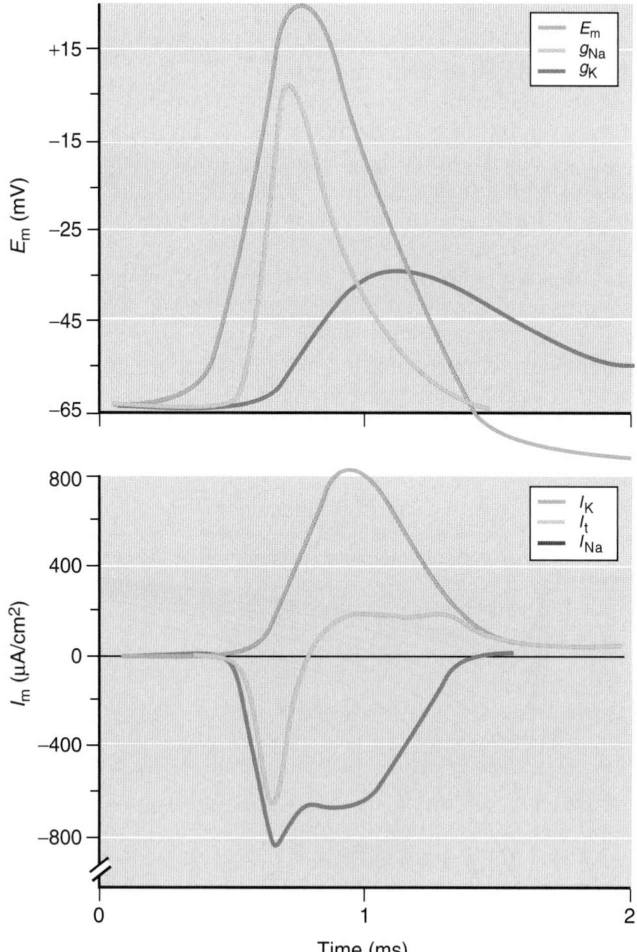

Fig. 29.6 Membrane potential *(E_m)* and the voltage-gated ionic conductance of sodium *(g_{Na})* and potassium *(g_K)*, which determine the corresponding membrane currents I_m (I_{Na} and I_K) during a propagated action potential. Modeled from the original studies of Hodgkin and Huxley on the squid giant axon (see Hodgkin[7b]), these relationships hold for almost all invertebrate and vertebrate nerve fibers. The direction of the total ionic current *(I_t)*, which is the sum of I_{Na} and I_K, is inward (negative values) for the depolarizing phase of the action potential and outward (positive values) for the repolarizing phase. (From Hodgkin A. *The Conduction of the Nervous Impulse*. Springfield, IL: Charles C. Thomas; 1964.)

Although this *local circuit current* spreads away from the excited zone in both directions, the region behind the impulse, having just been depolarized, is absolutely refractory, and propagation of impulses is thus unidirectional. The local circuit current spreads rapidly along a length of insulated internode in a myelinated axon (see Fig. 29.3), and many nodes of Ranvier in sequence are depolarized to threshold with little intervening delay. Single impulses do not jump from node to node as separate, discrete events; instead, active depolarization occurs simultaneously along several centimeters of the largest axons (see Fig. 29.3). Indeed, the local circuit current is so robust that it can skip past two completely nonexcitable nodes (e.g., blocked by local anesthetic) and successfully stimulate a third node. If excitability is partially reduced, such as by inhibition of some of the Na^+ channels, the amplitude of impulses in successive nodes falls accordingly, a process that can continue

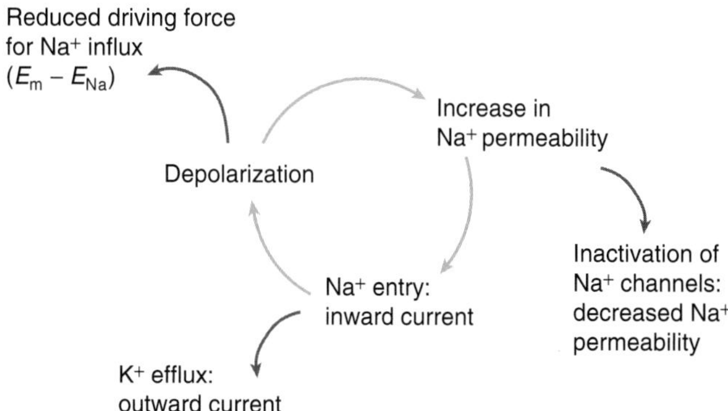

Fig. 29.7 The action potential can be understood in terms of the cyclic relationships between factors contributing to the regenerative, depolarizing phase and the passive, repolarizing phase. Positive factors *(yellow arrows)* increase the rate of depolarization in a positive-feedback loop, with each element in the cycle favoring the subsequent one. Negative factors *(gray arrows)* decrease the depolarization rate by reducing or opposing the related positive factor, with efflux of K^+ eventually dominating the ionic flow and repolarizing the membrane.

for many centimeters.[11] This situation probably occurs during certain phases of local anesthesia, as discussed later. When enough of the Na^+ channels are blocked, local circuit current fails to bring the adjacent resting region to threshold, and the impulse is fully extinguished.

Mechanism of Action of Local Anesthetics (Pharmacodynamics)

ACTIVE FORM

Local anesthetic bases are poorly to sparingly soluble in water but are quite soluble in relatively hydrophobic organic solvents. Therefore as a matter of chemistry (and to optimize shelf life), most of these drugs are formulated as hydrochloride salts. The pK_a of the drug and tissue pH determine the amount of drug that exists in solution as free base or as positively charged cation when injected into living tissue (see earlier). Furthermore, uptake of the drug by tissue, largely via lipophilic adsorption, will also alter its activity, both by shifting the effective pK_a downward, thereby favoring the neutral base form, and by limiting diffusion of the anesthetic away from the site of injection. Moderately hydrophobic local anesthetics block faster than either hydrophilic or highly hydrophobic ones, delivered at the same concentration, for the following reasons. Moderately hydrophilic local anesthetic block, such as lidocaine, are less bound to tissues than very hydrophobic drugs are (e.g., tetracaine) but are still more membrane permeant than very hydrophilic ones (e.g., 2-chloroprocaine). The highly hydrophobic local anesthetics, having higher intrinsic potencies (see Table 29.2), are therefore used in lower concentrations and their diffusion-controlled rate of onset is correspondingly reduced.

Which form of the local anesthetic, charged cation or neutral base, is actually responsible for blockade of impulses? More alkaline solutions of local anesthetics block nerve conduction more effectively. On sheath-free nerves, the rate of inhibition by tertiary amine anesthetics is greater at alkaline than at neutral external pH[12] because membrane permeation, favored by the base over the cationic species, determines the rate of access to the binding site. Direct control of axoplasmic pH (or internal perfusion with permanently charged quaternary amine homologs) shows that the dominant potency derives from the cationic species acting from the cytoplasmic surface.[13,14] The uncharged base also has intrinsic pharmacologic activity, however, which explains the effectiveness of benzocaine as a topical local anesthetic. The local anesthetic attaches to the binding site with its aromatic moiety, while the charged portion protrudes into the sodium channel's lumen.[15]

ELECTROPHYSIOLOGIC EFFECT OF LOCAL ANESTHETICS

The resting membrane potential of nerve is little affected by local anesthetics. As the concentration of local anesthetic applied to the nerve is increased, a decrease in the rate of depolarization and in the peak amplitude of the action potential occurs until the impulse is abolished. By using a "voltage-clamp" procedure, Na^+ currents and their inhibition by local anesthetics can be directly assayed (Fig. 29.8*A*). When the membrane of isolated neurons is rapidly depolarized to a constant value, the time course of ionic currents is observed. Sodium currents during one initial depolarization are reduced by subclinical doses of local anesthetic (e.g., 0.2 mM lidocaine) and totally abolished by clinical doses (e.g., 1% lidocaine ≈40 mM). If the test depolarization is applied repeatedly at frequencies higher than 5 Hz (five pulses per second), the partially depressed (*tonically* inhibited) Na^+ current is further reduced incrementally for each pulse until a new steady-state level of inhibition is reached.[13,16] This frequency-dependent inhibition, also called *phasic inhibition*, is reversed when stimulation is slowed or stopped, and currents return to the level of tonic inhibition observed in the resting nerve. Paralleling the phasic inhibition of Na^+ currents in voltage-clamped membranes is a "use-dependent" blockade of action potentials during normal physiologic function (see Fig. 29.8*B*).

Phasic actions are a manifestation of the selective affinity of local anesthetics for conformations of the Na^+ channel that result from depolarization. Both "open" and "inactivated" states of the channel bind local anesthetics more avidly than the resting state does. Repeated depolarization thus increases the fraction of drug-bound channels; dissociation of these bound drug molecules is usually a slower process than the normal recovery from inactivation (see earlier) and results in the use-dependent accumulation of channels in the blocked condition and the phenomenon of phasic block.

By its selective binding to a channel state, the local anesthetic stabilizes that state. During phasic block, therefore, more inactivated channels become drug bound, and reciprocally, less activation can occur. This relationship between state-dependent affinities and modification of transitions among states through drug binding is known as the "modulated receptor" model.[17] Overall binding of anesthetic is increased by membrane depolarization for two reasons: *more binding sites become accessible* during activation (the "guarded receptor" model) and drug *dissociation* from inactivated channels *is slower* than from resting channels (the modulated receptor model).

The potency of local anesthetics to produce tonic and phasic inhibition is similarly dependent on their structure, hydrophobicity, and pK_a. There appears to be a single, albeit complex, binding site for local anesthetics on the Na^+ channel, with a "tonic" affinity at rest and increased "phasic" affinity occurring as a result of depolarization. The sodium channel can be influenced by a number of drugs or toxins/venoms, and the different sites are numbered. The binding site for local anesthetics is referred to as Site 9, while the outer channel pore, binding site for tetrodotoxin (TTX) or saxitoxin (STX), is referred to as Site 1.

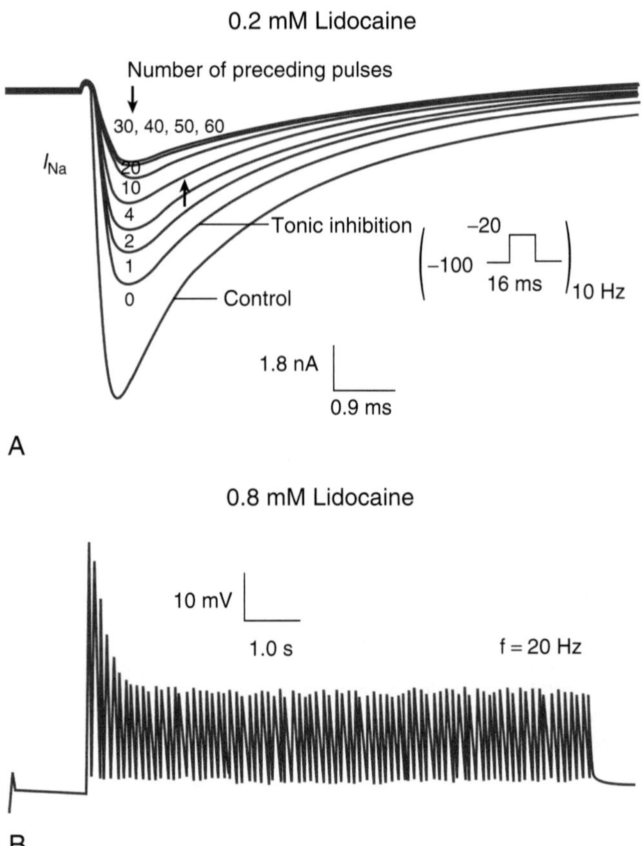

Fig. 29.8 Use-dependent actions of local anesthetics on excitable membrane properties. (A) Ionic Na^+ currents measured by a voltage-clamping technique are transiently activated by brief steps of depolarization applied infrequently (tonic test) or in a train at 10 times per second (phasic test, see E_m pattern in parentheses). After equilibration with 0.2 mM (0.005%) lidocaine, the currents measured tonically are reduced by approximately 30% from the control currents. Application of the phasic train of depolarizations results in a dynamic reduction of currents after each depolarization, with a steady-state value of phasic inhibition reached during the train of 75% of control currents. Recovery of currents to the tonic value occurs within a few seconds when phasic testing stops (not shown). (B) Action potentials are also inhibited in a phasic manner by local anesthetics. After equilibration with 0.8 mM lidocaine (0.02%), the action potential is tonically reduced by approximately 20% from its amplitude in drug-free solution (not shown). Stimulation by a train at 20 stimuli per second induces a phasic inhibition that further reduces the amplitude by about 70% from the control value. As with the ionic currents (A), phasic inhibition of the action potential recovers rapidly when high-frequency stimulation stops.

THE NATURE OF THE LOCAL ANESTHETIC

Binding Site

Intentional mutation of specific amino acids of the Na^+ channel has allowed definition of regions that interact directly with local anesthetics. The major functional protein of the Na^+ channel (the α-subunit) is composed of four homologous "domains" (D-1 to D-4), each of which contains six helical regions (S1 to S6) that span the core of the membrane (Fig. 29.9*A*). Each domain also has a loop, termed the "P region," that links the extracellular ends of its S5 and S6 transmembrane segments; the P regions extend inward between the transmembrane regions such that when the α-subunit folds together, each P loop contributes a quarter of the cylindrical ion "selectivity pore," the narrowest passage of an open channel (see Fig. 29.9*B*). Voltage sensitivity derives from the positive charges located on S4 segments, which slide or swing "outward" in response to membrane depolarization. By linkages still unknown, this movement of S4 results in a conformational rearrangement of the S6 segments, which form the inner, cytoplasmic entry to the channel. Closed-to-open channel gating results from movement of the S6 segments, whereas inactivation gating results from binding of the cytoplasmic loop located between D-3 and D-4 to the cytoplasmic opening of the channel.

Local anesthetics bind in the "inner vestibule" of the closed Na^+ channel (see Fig. 29.9*C*). Amino acid mutations in the S6 segments of D-1, D-3, and D-4 all modify local anesthetic action, thus suggesting either that these regions form a "pharmacophore" small enough to simultaneously contact the drug at three surfaces or that the local anesthetic molecule moves rapidly among these three segments. The rate constant for binding of local anesthetic to

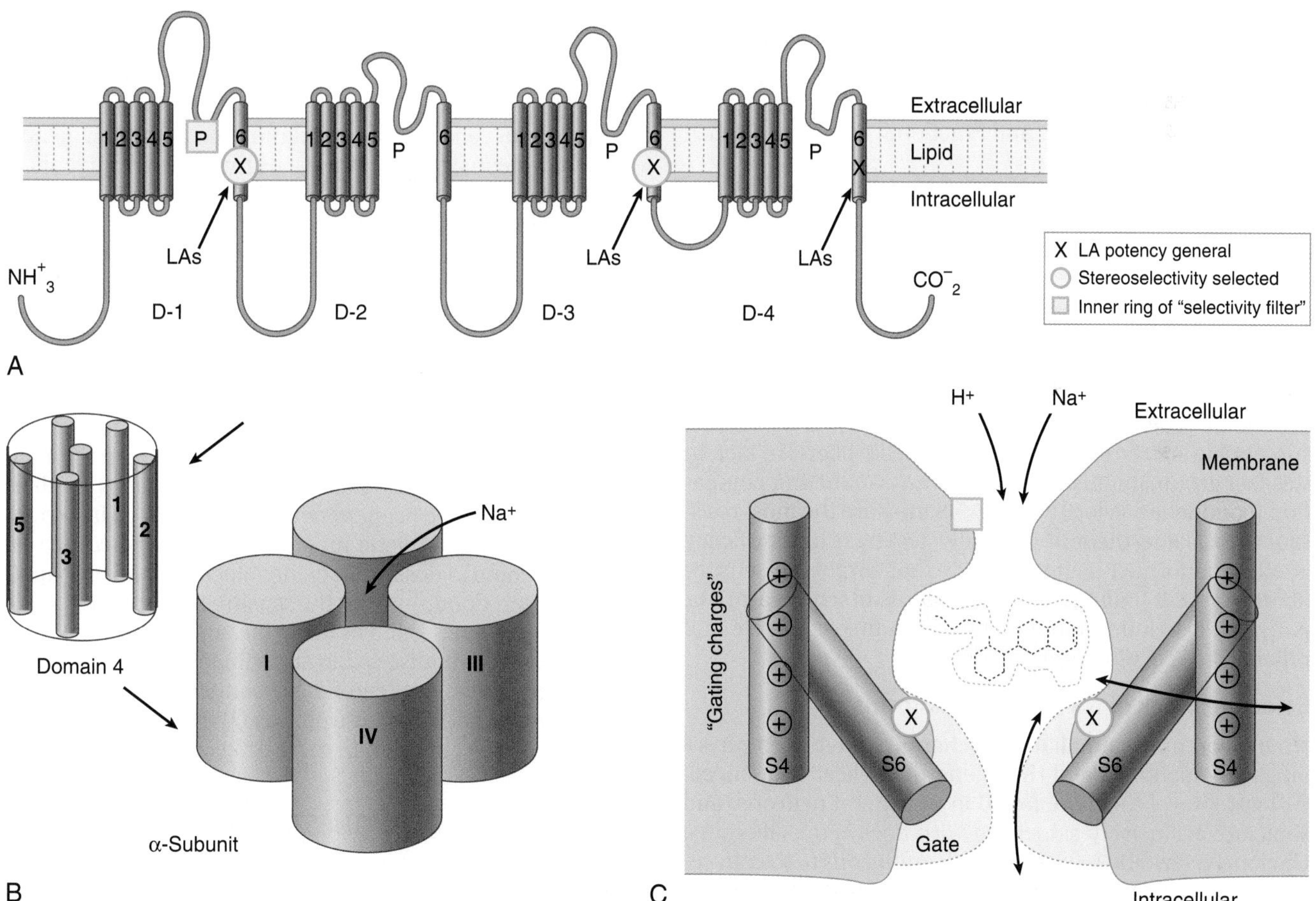

Fig. 29.9 Structural features of the Na^+ channel that determine local anesthetic *(LA)* interactions. (A) Consensus arrangement of the single peptide of the Na^+ channel α-subunit in a plasma membrane. Four domains with homologous sequences (D-1 through D-4) each contain six α-helical segments that span the membrane (S1 to S6). Each domain folds within itself to form one cylindrical bundle of segments, and these bundles converge to form the functional channel's quaternary structure (B). Activation gating leading to channel opening results from primary movement of the positively charged S4 segments in response to membrane depolarization (see panel C). Fast inactivation of the channel follows binding to the cytoplasmic end of the channel of part of the small loop that connects D-3 to D-4. Ions travel through an open channel along a pore defined at its narrowest dimension by the P region formed by partial membrane penetration of the four extracellular loops of protein connecting S5 and S6 in each domain. Intentional, directed mutations of different amino acids on the channel indicate residues that are involved in LA binding in the inner vestibule of the channel (X on S6 segments), at the interior regions of the ion-discriminating "selectivity filter" (*square* on the P region), and which are also known to influence stereoselectivity for phasic inhibition (*circle*, also on S6 segments). (C) Schematic cross section of the channel speculating on the manner in which S6 segments, forming a "gate," may realign during activation to open the channel and allow entry and departure of a bupivacaine molecule by the "hydrophilic" pathway. The closed (inactivated) channel has a more intimate association with the LA molecule, whose favored pathway for dissociation is no longer between S6 segments (the former pore) but now, much more slowly, laterally between segments and then through the membrane, the "hydrophobic" pathway. Na^+ ions entering the pore will compete with the LA for a site in the channel, and H^+ ions, which pass very slowly through the pore, can enter and leave from the extracellular opening, thereby protonating and deprotonating a bound LA molecule and thus regulating its rate of dissociation from the channel.

the closed Na^+ channel is larger for the more hydrophobic molecules, which suggest that drug molecules can reach the binding site (and depart from it) through a "hydrophobic" pathway. The charged species of local anesthetics dissociates much more slowly from closed and inactivated Na^+ channels than the neutral form does, which suggests that an ionic bond may be involved in drug binding or that the charged molecule moves only slowly along the hydrophobic pathway. In brief, hydrophobicity delivers the drug to the receptor and charge keeps it there.

NEUROPHYSIOLOGIC ASPECTS OF PHASIC INHIBITION

Different fiber types in the nerve are affected differently during local anesthesia. At least part of this difference arises from pharmacokinetic factors. At the onset of and during recovery from clinical block, in particular, longitudinal and radial diffusion of drug will produce concentration variations within and along the nerve. This variation is superimposed on the dynamic use-dependent inhibition to provide variable propagation, which depends on a fiber's geometry, position within the nerve, and functional as well as electrophysiologic properties.

Different fiber types are also differentially sensitive to local anesthetic blockade. In vivo experiments in which continuous superperfusion of peripheral nerve allows equilibration with drug, and experiments in which a drug bolus is delivered by percutaneous injection,[18] analogous to clinical peripheral nerve block, show that small myelinated axons (Aγ motor and Aδ sensory fibers) are the most susceptible to impulse suppression. Next in order of block are the large myelinated (Aα and Aβ) fibers, and the least susceptible are the small, nonmyelinated C fibers. In fact, in this last group, impulses in the slowest conducting population (conduction velocity of 0.5-0.8 m/s) are the most resistant to local anesthetic.[18] Clinically, testing of block efficacy is often performed using methods that target Aδ sensory fibers, so these findings suggest that loss of temperature or pin-prick discrimination does not guarantee complete and reliable block of all sensory modalities.

Selective Block of Na^+ Channel Isoforms

Nine different mammalian Na^+ channels have been physiologically identified and their genes have been sequenced. At least four of them are found in peripheral neurons, and some are exclusively associated with nociceptive afferents. Obviously, it would be clinically advantageous to selectively inhibit these channels and thus prevent or reduce pain while sparing other functions. Although selective channel blockade has been attained with naturally occurring small peptide toxins,[19] relatively little selective blockade by local anesthetics has been reported,[20] probably because the local anesthetic pharmacophore is too similar among the different channel isoforms and the local anesthetic molecules themselves have several rotational axes, which makes them poor structural templates for selecting among static binding pockets. Selectively blocking different sodium channel isoforms can lead to distinct effects because they are not evenly distributed across the nerve and react differently to activation. Specifically, one of the main functions of the Nav1.7 isoform is to act as an amplifier in the terminals of primary sensory neurons, while Nav1.8 is vital to the repetitive firing in these neurons, and Nav1.9 is able to generate persistent currents which can increase membrane excitability.[21] Some recent advances which hold promise to improve nerve block properties of local anesthetics are summarized toward the end of this chapter.

Sodium Channel Isoforms and Their Contribution to Human Diseases Characterized by Pain or Pain Insensitivity

We now know several mutations in the prototypical neuronal sodium channels (Nav1.7, 1.8, and 1.9) which can lead to states of either spontaneous pain[22,23] or profound and selective impairment of pain sensitivity.[24] This depends on the type of mutation and mode of inheritance. For example, mutations in Nav1.7 may lead to loss of channel function and, in the most extreme form, congenital insensitivity to pain. In contrast, activating mutations in the same channel can trigger erythromelalgia or paroxysmal extreme pain disorder.[21] Molecular studies reveal that these disorders involve several distinct types of mutations in NaV1.7 sodium channels.[22,23] When these channels are inserted into cells that lack sodium channels, they generate spontaneous, temperature-sensitive inward currents.[21] Another recent finding was that certain preclinical models of visceral pain (e.g., cystitis) are not responsive to therapies specifically targeting the NaV1.7 channels, while block of NaV1.9 channels was effective.[25] Lastly, it is important to note that mutations in nonneuronal sodium channels can have profound clinical consequences as well. For example, mutations of the Nav1.4 sodium channel isoform in skeletal muscle can produce myotonia, periodic paralysis, and congenital myasthenia.[26]

Aberrant impulses, which are often considered the hallmarks of various diseases of excitable membranes, such as abnormal repetitive firing in neuropathic pain or in certain types of inherited skeletal myotonia, are abolished by systemic lidocaine in doses that do not block normal propagating impulses. Conditions for the sensitivity of such impulses to local anesthetics, such as lidocaine, appear to result from the patterns of impulse spikes superimposed on slow membrane depolarizations caused by abnormal expression of Na^+ channels rather than from selective sensitivity of certain subtypes of channels to these drugs.[27]

SUMMARY OF LOCAL ANESTHETIC MECHANISMS

Impulse blockade by local anesthetics may be summarized by the following chronology:

1. Solutions of local anesthetic are deposited near the nerve. Removal of free drug molecules away from this locus is a function of tissue binding, removal by the circulation, and local hydrolysis of aminoester anesthetics. The net result is penetration of the nerve sheath by the remaining free drug molecules.
2. Local anesthetic molecules then permeate the nerve's axon membranes and reside there and in the axoplasm. The speed and extent of these processes depend on a particular drug's pK_a and on the lipophilicity of its base and cation species.

3. Binding of local anesthetic to sites on voltage-gated Na^+ channels prevents opening of the channels by inhibiting the conformational changes that underlie channel activation.
4. During onset of and recovery from local anesthesia, impulse blockade is incomplete and partially blocked fibers are further inhibited by repetitive stimulation, which produces an additional, use-dependent binding to Na^+ channels.
5. One local anesthetic binding site on the Na^+ channel may be sufficient to account for the drug's resting (tonic) and use-dependent (phasic) actions.
6. The clinically observed rates of onset and recovery from blockade are governed by the relatively slow diffusion of local anesthetic molecules into and out of the whole nerve, not by their much faster binding and dissociation from ion channels. A clinically effective block that may last for hours can be accomplished with local anesthetic drugs that dissociate from Na^+ channels in a few seconds.

Clinical Pharmacology

Successful use of regional anesthesia requires knowledge of the pharmacologic properties of the various local anesthetic drugs, as well as technical skill in performance of the nerve block. Local anesthetic requirements vary considerably, depending on factors such as the type of block, surgical procedure, and physiologic status of the patient.

Commonly used aminoester local anesthetics include procaine, chloroprocaine, tetracaine, and the first true local anesthetic, cocaine. Commonly used aminoamides include lidocaine, mepivacaine, prilocaine, bupivacaine (the racemic form and its levoenantiomer), ropivacaine, and etidocaine. The ester and amide local anesthetics differ in their chemical stability, locus of biotransformation, and allergic potential. Amides are extremely stable, whereas esters are relatively unstable in solution. Aminoesters are hydrolyzed in plasma by cholinesterase enzymes, but the amides undergo enzymatic degradation in the liver. Two exceptions to this trend include cocaine, an ester that is metabolized predominantly by hepatic carboxylesterase, and articaine, an amide local anesthetic widely used in dentistry that is inactivated by plasma carboxylesterase-induced cleavage of a methyl ester on the aromatic ring.

p-Aminobenzoic acid is one of the metabolites of ester-type compounds that can induce allergic-type reactions in a small percentage of patients. The aminoamides are not metabolized to *p*-aminobenzoic acid, and reports of allergic reactions to these agents are extremely rare.

GENERAL CONSIDERATIONS

Clinically important properties of the various local anesthetics include potency, speed of onset, duration of anesthetic action, and differential sensory/motor blockade. As previously indicated, the profile of individual drugs is determined by their physicochemical characteristics (see Table 29.2).

Anesthetic Potency

Hydrophobicity appears to be a primary determinant of intrinsic anesthetic potency[5] because the anesthetic molecule must penetrate into the nerve membrane and bind at a partially hydrophobic site on the Na^+ channel. Clinically, however, the correlation between hydrophobicity and anesthetic potency is not as precise as in an isolated nerve. Differences between in vitro and in vivo potency may be related to a number of factors, including local anesthetic charge and hydrophobicity (which influence partitioning into and transverse diffusion across biologic membranes) and vasodilator or vasoconstrictor properties (which influence the initial rate of vascular uptake from injection sites into the central circulation).

Onset of Action

The onset of conduction block in isolated nerves is related to the physicochemical properties of the individual agents. In vivo latency is also dependent on the dose or concentration of local anesthetic used. For example, 0.75% bupivacaine has more rapid onset than 0.25%. Chloroprocaine demonstrates a rapid onset of action in humans because its low systemic toxicity permits its use in high concentrations (3%).

Duration of Action

The duration of action of the various local anesthetics differs markedly. Procaine and chloroprocaine have a short duration of action. Lidocaine, mepivacaine, and prilocaine produce a moderate duration of anesthesia, whereas tetracaine, bupivacaine, ropivacaine, and etidocaine have the longest durations.

In humans, the duration of anesthesia is markedly influenced by the peripheral vascular effects of the local anesthetic drugs. Many local anesthetics have a biphasic effect on vascular smooth muscle; at low concentrations these agents tend to cause vasoconstriction, whereas at higher, clinically administered concentrations, they cause vasodilation.[28] However, differences exist in the degree of vasodilator activity of the various drugs. The effects of local anesthetics on vascular tone and regional blood flow are complex and vary according to concentration, time, and the particular vascular bed near the site of application. As a practical example, the topical local anesthetic formulation EMLA (eutectic mixture of the local anesthetics lidocaine and prilocaine) vasoconstricts cutaneous vessels initially and through most of the first hour of application, but vasodilation is observed after 2 or more hours of application.

Differential Sensory and Motor Blockade

Another important clinical consideration is the ability of local anesthetic agents to cause differential inhibition of sensory and motor activity. Bupivacaine became popular in the 1980s for epidural blocks because it was better than the previously available long-acting agents (e.g., etidocaine) in producing adequate antinociception without profound inhibition of motor activity, particularly when dilute solutions are used. Bupivacaine is widely used epidurally for obstetric analgesia and postoperative pain management because it can provide acceptable analgesia with only mild muscle weakness. Additional observations on the sensory selectivity of newer local anesthetics are detailed later in the section on chiral local anesthetics.

Traditional texts often state that small-diameter axons, such as C fibers, are more susceptible to local anesthetic block than larger-diameter fibers. However, when careful measurements are made of single-impulse annihilation in individual nerve fibers, exactly the opposite differential susceptibility is noted (see earlier).[29,30] Repetitive stimulation, such as occurs during propagation of trains of impulses, produces further, phasic inhibition of excitability, but it is not clear how this will affect a functionally selective failure of impulses. The length of drug-exposed nerve in the intrathecal space, imposed by anatomic restrictions, can perhaps explain clinically documented differential spinal or epidural blockade, with longer drug-exposed regions yielding block by lower concentrations of local anesthetic.[31] However, this reasoning does not explain the functionally differential loss from peripheral nerve block. Other factors may include actual spread of the drug along the nerve or its selective ability to inhibit Na^+ channels over K^+ channels,[32] which in itself can produce a differential block because these channels are present in very different proportions in different types of nerves. As a result of these confounding factors, conclusions about fiber-type involvement in chronic pain syndromes based on the dose or concentration requirement for pain relief in diagnostic nerve blockade should not be made.[33]

FACTORS INFLUENCING ANESTHETIC ACTIVITY IN HUMANS

Dosage of Local Anesthetic

As the dosage of local anesthetic is increased, the probability and duration of satisfactory anesthesia increases and the time to onset of block is shortened. The dosage of local anesthetic can be increased by administering either a larger volume or a more concentrated solution. For example, increasing the concentration of epidurally administered bupivacaine from 0.125% to 0.5% while maintaining the same volume of injectate (10 mL) resulted in shorter latency, an improved incidence of satisfactory analgesia, and a longer duration of sensory analgesia.[34] The volume per se of anesthetic solution probably influences the spread of anesthesia. For example, 30 mL of 1% lidocaine administered into the epidural space produced a level of anesthesia that was 4.3 dermatomes higher than that achieved when 10 mL of 3% lidocaine was given.

In selecting the volume and concentration for a specific block in a particular patient, clinicians must balance the risk of adverse effects from excessive dosing (e.g., systemic toxicity, excessive motor or autonomic blockade) against the increased risk of block failure if an inadequate volume or concentration is chosen. The degree to which additional volume can compensate for imprecise needle placement varies among different blocks. With the advent of very precise needle placement using ultrasound-guided blockade, it has become clear that the median effective volume for obtaining successful blockade can be achieved with smaller volumes than have been recommended from some previous clinical series based on traditional methods of needle localization. For example, in a recent dose-finding randomized trial for femoral nerve blockade, the median volumes for 50% or 95% success in obtaining dense sensory and motor block at 30 minutes under ultrasound guidance were 57% and 54% of the corresponding volumes with the use of nerve stimulation.[35] Interested readers will note the very wide confidence intervals found in this study and are encouraged to read recent work on some statistical design issues for dose-response studies involving all types of anesthetics.[36] As limited by toxicity considerations, the aim in most clinical situations should be to choose doses that provide high success rates; that is, an effective dose (ED) in 95% of patients (ED_{95}) is generally a more relevant guide to dose selection than an ED_{50} dose. These considerations are especially salient when performing regional anesthesia for patients with chronic pain, hyperalgesia, or a history of previous failed regional anesthesia. Also, decreasing the dose substantially may provide a satisfactory block after 30 minutes (a common endpoint for clinical studies), but at the same time, the block may have a decreased duration of action. Duration of action is important such that the block will cover the intensely painful period after surgery, and if this period is longer than could be achieved using plain local anesthetics, and in cases where continuous techniques are not feasible, adjuvants/additives may help in prolonging the block.

Addition of Additives

Epinephrine. Vasoconstrictors, usually epinephrine, are frequently included in local anesthetic solutions to decrease the rate of vascular absorption, thereby allowing more anesthetic molecules to reach the nerve membrane and thus improve the depth and duration of anesthesia. The use of epinephrine as a marker for inadvertent intravascular injection continues to be sensible, even though false negatives and false positives can occur, such as difficulty in interpretation for specific patient groups as with parturients and patients under anesthesia or on β-blockers.[37] Clinically used solutions typically contain 5 μg/mL or 1:200,000 of epinephrine, reflecting a balance between efficacy and vasoconstriction versus systemic side effects of epinephrine. The extent to which epinephrine prolongs the duration of anesthesia depends on the specific local anesthetic used and the site of injection. Epinephrine will significantly extend the duration of both infiltration anesthesia and peripheral nerve blockade with shorter-duration agents (e.g., lidocaine); epinephrine produces mild intensification of blockade but only most modest prolongation of epidural or peripheral blocks with bupivacaine.[36] Activation of α_2-adrenergic receptors in the spinal cord may contribute to the beneficial effect of epidural epinephrine.

Clonidine and Dexmedetomidine. The α-2 agonist clonidine prolongs the action of local anesthetics by about 2 hours with wide variation between studies[38], and its conjectured mechanisms of action include actions on α-2 receptors and on hyperpolarization-induced currents.[39] However, there is a large number of negative studies, and adverse systemic events are of concern, including hypotension, bradycardia, and sedation, such that limiting the clonidine dose to 0.5 to 1 μg/kg of ideal body weight has been proposed. Dexmedetomidine is a much more specific α-2 agonist, and prolongs both motor and sensory block by long-acting local anesthetics by approximately 4 hours.[40] Similar to clonidine, dexmedetomidine has also been shown to block the hyperpolarization-induced current.[41]

Nevertheless, risk of systemic adverse effects remains high, and optimal doses have not been determined. There seems to be no increased risk of neurotoxicity when clonidine or dexmedetomidine are used as nerve block adjuvants.

Buprenorphine. The partial μ-opiate receptor agonist, buprenorphine, intensifies blockade by two mechanisms, namely blockade of κ- and δ-opioid receptors, and blockade of voltage-gated sodium channel-blocking properties.[42] Blockade by long-acting local anesthetics is prolonged by about 6 hours, but at the price of a high incidence of nausea and vomiting, such that the use of buprenorphine has largely been abandoned.[43] Buprenorphine is considered safe in terms of neurotoxicity.

Dexamethasone. The most effective adjuvant for prolonging block duration with minimal side effects currently available is dexamethasone, able to prolong duration of medium-acting local anesthetics by 2 to 3 hours, and the block of long-acting local anesthetics by up to 10 hours on average.[44] Blocks can be prolonged by intravenous or perineural administration of dexamethasone. Despite the fact that perineural administration of dexamethasone seems to be more effective than systemic use, many providers use systemic dexamethasone to avoid mixing drugs which were not designed to be administered together, circumvent the problem of off-label perineural use, and profit from the antiemetic effects of systemic dexamethasone. Doses between 4 and 10 mg have typically been used in adults.[45] The precise mechanism of action of dexamethasone is not understood and the potential for neurotoxic side effects has not been adequately studied.

Site of Injection

The most rapid onset but the shortest duration of action occurs after intrathecal or subcutaneous administration of local anesthetics. The longest latencies and durations are observed after conventional non–ultrasound-guided large-volume brachial plexus blocks. For example, intrathecal bupivacaine will usually produce anesthesia within 5 minutes that will persist for 3 to 4 hours. However, when bupivacaine is administered for brachial plexus blockade, the onset time is approximately 20 to 30 minutes, and the duration of anesthesia (or at least analgesia) averages 10 hours.[46] These differences in the onset and duration of anesthesia and analgesia are due in part to the particular anatomy of the area of injection, which will influence the rate of diffusion and vascular absorption and, in turn, affect the amount of drug used for various types of regional anesthesia. In the subarachnoid space, for example, the lack of a nerve sheath around the spinal cord and deposition of the local anesthetic solution in the immediate vicinity of the spinal cord are responsible for the rapid onset of action, whereas the relatively small amount of drug used for spinal anesthesia probably accounts for the short duration of conduction block.

In contrast, the onset of brachial plexus blockade is slow because the anesthetic agent is usually deposited at some distance from the nerve and must diffuse through various tissue barriers before reaching the nerve membrane. The prolonged block with brachial plexus blockade may be related to several factors, including comparatively slow rates of vascular absorption from the brachial plexus sheath, larger doses of drug required for this regional anesthetic technique, and comparatively long segments of nerves exposed to local anesthetic.

Carbonation and pH Adjustment of Local Anesthetics

The addition of sodium bicarbonate to a solution of local anesthetic applied to an isolated nerve accelerates the onset and decreases the minimum concentration (C_m) required for conduction blockade by increasing pH and increasing the share of uncharged local anesthetic molecules that can more easily diffuse into the nerve cell.[47] Although the effect of carbon dioxide on local anesthetic activity is easily demonstrable in isolated nerve, controversy exists concerning the clinical utility of carbonated local anesthetic solutions[48] and the widespread introduction of ultrasound-guided nerve blockade with faster and more reliable block onset has decreased the relevance of carbonation, at least for peripheral nerve blockade.

Mixtures of Local Anesthetics

Mixtures of local anesthetics for regional anesthesia are sometimes used in an effort to compensate for the short duration of action of certain rapidly acting agents such as chloroprocaine and lidocaine, and the long latency of longer-acting agents such as tetracaine and bupivacaine. Mixtures of chloroprocaine and bupivacaine theoretically offer significant clinical advantages because of the rapid onset and low systemic toxicity of chloroprocaine and the long duration of action of bupivacaine; however, clinical results in studies of combinations have been mixed.[49] The use of catheter techniques for many forms of regional anesthesia makes it possible to begin with a rapid-onset local anesthetic such as lidocaine, mepivacaine, or chloroprocaine and then follow with an infusion of either a shorter-acting or longer-acting local anesthetic thereafter. Clinicians should be cautioned to not use maximum doses of two local anesthetics in combination in the mistaken belief that their toxicities are independent.[50] Toxicity in fact, is additive. Moreover, the use of ultrasound-guided nerve blockade has, in general, led to a decreased onset time and has made mixing local anesthetics less clinically relevant.

Pregnancy

The spread and depth of epidural and spinal anesthesia are greater in pregnant than in nonpregnant women. The effects of pregnancy on local anesthetic potency may reflect a combined effect of mechanical factors associated with pregnancy (i.e., dilated epidural veins decrease the volume of the epidural and subarachnoid spaces) and direct effects of hormones, especially progesterone, on the susceptibility of nerves to conduction blockade by local anesthetics.[51] Hormonal alterations are probably the more important of these two factors because greater spread of epidural anesthesia is already observed during the first trimester of pregnancy,[52] before any gross change in vascular dimensions within the epidural or subarachnoid spaces. The dosage of local anesthetics should probably be reduced in patients in all stages of pregnancy.

Choice of Local Anesthetic for Various Regional Anesthetic Procedures

On the basis of anatomic considerations, regional anesthesia may be divided into infiltration anesthesia, intravenous regional anesthesia (IVRA), peripheral nerve blockade (including plexus blockade), central neural blockade, and topical anesthesia. An additional method of local anesthetic injection, tumescent anesthesia, is included because it is widely used in office-based plastic surgery.

INFILTRATION ANESTHESIA

Any local anesthetic may be used for infiltration anesthesia. Onset of action is almost immediate for all agents after intradermal or subcutaneous administration; however, the duration of anesthesia varies (Table 29.4). Epinephrine will prolong the duration of infiltration anesthesia by all local anesthetic drugs, although this effect is most pronounced when epinephrine is added to lidocaine. The choice of a specific drug for infiltration anesthesia largely depends on the desired duration of action.

The dosage of local anesthetic required for adequate infiltration anesthesia depends on the extent of the area to be anesthetized and the expected duration of the surgical procedure. When large surface areas have to be anesthetized, large volumes of dilute anesthetic solutions should be used. These considerations are particularly important when performing infiltration anesthesia in infants and smaller children. As an example, consider a 4-kg infant receiving infiltration anesthesia with the maximum safe dose of lidocaine, 5 mg/kg. Dosing to 5 mg/kg permits 20 mg/4 kg, which is 1 mL of a 2% solution or 4 mL of a 0.5% solution. Lidocaine is effective for infiltration in concentrations as dilute as 0.3% to 0.5%, so the more dilute solution can be used more safely to anesthetize a larger area.

Patients frequently experience pain immediately after subcutaneous injection of local anesthetic solutions, in part because of the acidic nature of these solutions, and in part because lidocaine briefly activates transient receptor potential vanilloid-1 (TRPV-1) and transient receptor potential ankyrin-1 (TRPA-1) channels, causing pain, before sodium channel block subsequently silences the neuron.[53] Alkalinization of lidocaine solutions by the addition of sodium bicarbonate immediately before injection reduces pain on skin infiltration[54] and may improve onset (see earlier).

Infiltration analgesia and indwelling wound catheters are used increasingly as components of multimodal postoperative analgesia.[55-57] In particular, sustained-release formulations such as Exparel have been introduced into clinical practice (see the section Development of Prolonged-Duration and Sensory- or Nociceptive-Selective Local Anesthetics).

INTRAVENOUS REGIONAL ANESTHESIA

IVRA (Bier's block) involves the intravenous administration of a local anesthetic into a tourniquet-occluded limb. The local anesthetic diffuses from the peripheral vascular bed to nonvascular tissue such as axons and nerve endings. Both the safety and the efficacy of this regional anesthetic procedure depend on interruption of blood flow to the involved limb and gradual release of the occluding tourniquet.

Lidocaine and prilocaine have been the drugs used most frequently for IVRA. Drugs with a high cardiotoxic potential such as bupivacaine should not be used for IVRA. One might suppose a safety advantage with the aminoester-linked compounds because of their hydrolysis in blood; however, thrombophlebitis has been reported with chloroprocaine. In general, approximately 3 mg/kg (40 mL of a 0.5% solution) of preservative-free lidocaine without epinephrine is used for upper extremity procedures. For surgical procedures on the lower limbs, 50 to 100 mL of a 0.25% lidocaine solution have been used. Even though the safety profile of IVRA is considered very good, seizures have been reported with lidocaine doses as low as 1.4 mg/kg of lidocaine, and cardiovascular collapse (CC) can occur.[58]

TABLE 29.4 Infiltration Anesthesia

		PLAIN SOLUTION		EPINEPHRINE-CONTAINING SOLUTION	
Drug	**Concentration (%)**	**Maximum Dose (mg)**	**Duration (min)**	**Maximum Dose (mg)**	**Duration (min)**
SHORT DURATION					
Procaine	1-2	500	20-30	600	30-45
Chloroprocaine	1-2	800	15-30	1000	30
MODERATE DURATION					
Lidocaine	0.5-1	300	30-60	500	120
Mepivacaine	0.5-1	300	45-90	500	120
Prilocaine	0.5-1	350	30-90	550	120
LONG DURATION					
Bupivacaine	0.25-0.5	175	120-240	200	180-240
Ropivacaine	0.2-0.5	200	120-240	250	180-240

PERIPHERAL AND TRUNCAL NERVE BLOCKADE

Regional anesthetic procedures that inhibit conduction in fibers of the peripheral nervous system can be classified together under the general category of peripheral nerve blockade. This form of regional anesthesia has been arbitrarily subdivided into minor and major nerve blocks. Minor nerve blocks are defined as procedures involving single nerve entities such as the ulnar or radial nerve, whereas major nerve blocks involve the blockade of two or more distinct nerves or a nerve plexus or the blockade of very large nerves at more proximal sites (i.e., the femoral and sciatic nerves).

Most local anesthetic drugs can be used for minor nerve blocks. The onset of blockade is rapid with most drugs, and the choice of drug is determined primarily by the required duration of anesthesia. A classification of the various drugs according to their duration of action is shown in Table 29.5. It has become possible to define the minimum local anesthetic volume for ultrasound-guided peripheral nerve blockade and across several nerves; the volume was approximately 0.1 mL per mm^2 of nerve cross-sectional area.[59,60] However, as mentioned earlier, minimal volume to achieve sensory blockade 30 minutes after block may also mean decreased duration of the block as compared to "traditional" high volumes clinicians were accustomed to using during stimulator-guided regional anesthesia.

Brachial plexus blockade for upper limb surgery is the most common major peripheral nerve block technique, but many lower extremity procedures are now carried out under peripheral nerve blocks for anesthesia or postoperative analgesia. A significant difference exists between the onset times of various agents when these blocks are used (Table 29.6). In general, agents of intermediate potency exhibit a more rapid onset than the more potent compounds do.

Next to surgeries on the upper and lower extremities, peripheral nerve blocks have become popular for treating pain after thoracic and abdominal procedures. In the case of superficial thoracic surgery such as breast surgery, field blocks such as the PECS-1 and PECS-2 and Serratus plane block have been successfully used. Proximal intercostal nerve blocks and paravertebral blocks are also employed for mastectomies and reconstructions by some institutions, but more research is needed to define efficacy, precise indications, and procedure-specific details of technique.[61] Paravertebral and proximal intercostal techniques appear equally effective as epidural analgesia in treating pain after video-assisted thoracoscopic surgery (VATS) and thoracotomy and have fewer side effects.[62]

PERINEURAL AND PLEXUS INFUSIONS

Local anesthetics are being administered by continuous infusion for several days after surgery[56,63] or for periods of weeks to months for the treatment of chronic malignant and

TABLE 29.5 Minor Nerve Blocks

				AVERAGE DURATION (MIN)	
Drug	**Usual Concentration (%)**	**Usual Volume (mL)**	**Dose* (mg)**	**Plain Solutions**	**Epinephrine-Containing Solutions**
Procaine	2	5-20	100-400	15-30	30-60
Chloroprocaine	2	5-20	100-400	15-30	30-60
Lidocaine	1	5-20	50-200	60-120	120-180
Mepivacaine	1	5-20	50-200	60-120	120-180
Prilocaine	1	5-20	50-200	60-120	120-180
Bupivacaine	0.25-0.5	5-20	12.5-100	180-360	240-420
Ropivacaine	0.2-0.5	5-20	10-100	180-360	240-420

*Doses are for a 70-kg adult. For pediatric doses, see Chapter 76.

TABLE 29.6 Major Nerve Blocks

Drug	**Usual Concentration (%)**	**Usual Volume (mL)**	**Maximum Dose (mg) Without/With Epinephrine**	**Onset (min)**	**Duration (min)**
Lidocaine	1-2	30-50	350/500	10-20	120-240
Mepivacaine	1-1.5	30-50	350/500	10-20	180-300
Prilocaine	1-2	30-50	400/600	10-20	180-300
Bupivacaine	0.25-0.5	30-50	175/225	20-30	360-720
Levobupivacaine	0.25-0.5	30-50	200/225	20-30	360-720
Ropivacaine	0.2-0.5	30-50	200/250	20-30	360-720

See also Chapter 46. Doses are for a 70-kg adult receiving epinephrine-containing solutions. Doses should be reduced for children, for patients with specific risk factors, and for blocks in specific locations (e.g., interscalene). When two or more blocks are performed together, the sum of the doses for each of the individual blocks should not exceed the max dose listed here.

nonmalignant pain. However, because of the poor sensory selectivity of contemporary local anesthetics, prolonged use of catheters at times conflicts with the paradigm of fast mobilization, especially as neuraxial and lower extremity techniques are concerned. With prolonged infusions there is a theoretical potential for delayed systemic accumulation and toxicity. However, the activation of the acute-phase response after trauma or surgery also leads to an increase in α-1 acidic glycoprotein, which is potent at binding free local anesthetics and decreases the risk of cumulation of free local anesthetic.[64]

CENTRAL NEURAL BLOCKADE

Any of the local anesthetic drugs may be used for epidural anesthesia (Table 29.7), although procaine and tetracaine are rarely used because of their long onset times. Drugs of intermediate potency produce surgical anesthesia of 1 to 2 hours' duration, whereas long-acting drugs usually produce 3 to 4 hours of anesthesia. The duration of short- and intermediate-acting drugs is significantly prolonged by the addition of epinephrine (1:200,000), but the duration of long-acting drugs is only minimally affected by epinephrine. The onset of lumbar epidural anesthesia occurs within 5 to 15 minutes after the administration of chloroprocaine, lidocaine, mepivacaine, and prilocaine. Bupivacaine has a slower onset of action.

Bupivacaine epidural bolus doses at a concentration of 0.125% produce adequate postoperative analgesia in many clinical settings with only mild motor deficits.[65] Continuous epidural infusions of bupivacaine as dilute as 0.0625% to 0.1% are useful for labor epidural analgesia, especially when administered in combination with opioids and epinephrine. Bupivacaine 0.25% may be used for more intense analgesia (particularly during combined epidural-general anesthesia cases) with moderate degrees of motor block. Bupivacaine at concentrations of 0.5% to 0.75% is associated with a more profound degree of motor block, and surgical anesthesia. It should be emphasized that although high concentrations of local anesthetics may be appropriate for episodic bolus dosing for surgery, these concentrations (i.e., 0.25% for bupivacaine) should not be first choice for continuous epidural infusions. In some patients, increasing the local anesthetic dose or addition of adjuvants such as epinephrine and lipophilic opioids is necessary to achieve adequate block intensity. Bolus injections produce much more cephalocaudad spread than continuous infusions do. When concentrated bupivacaine solutions are used for infusions, they have the potential for excessive local effect with an associated risk for unwanted and very prolonged motor blockade. Drugs available for subarachnoid administration are shown in Table 29.8. Bupivacaine is widely used as a spinal anesthetic, either as a hyperbaric solution at a concentration of 0.75% with 8.25% dextrose or by using the nearly isobaric (though slightly hypobaric) 0.5% solution. Intrathecal bupivacaine possesses an anesthetic profile similar to that of tetracaine.[66]

The addition of vasoconstrictors may prolong the duration of spinal anesthesia; for example, the addition of 0.2 to 0.3 mg of epinephrine to lidocaine, tetracaine, or bupivacaine solutions will produce a 50% or greater increase in duration.[67,68] The duration of spinal anesthesia produced by tetracaine can also be increased to a similar extent by adding 1 to 5 μg of phenylephrine. The addition of epinephrine to bupivacaine or lidocaine may be more effective in prolonging the duration of spinal anesthesia in lumbosacral segments than in thoracic segments.

TOPICAL ANESTHESIA

A number of local anesthetic formulations are available for topical anesthesia (Table 29.9), lidocaine, dibucaine, tetracaine, and benzocaine being the drugs used most commonly. In general, these preparations provide effective but relatively short durations of analgesia when applied to mucous membranes or abraded skin. Their efficacy is determined by drug form, melting point, concentration, and skin permeability.[69] Lidocaine and tetracaine sprays are commonly used for endotracheal anesthesia before intubation or for mucosal analgesia for bronchoscopy or esophagoscopy.

A variety of topical local anesthetic formulations have been developed to penetrate intact skin. EMLA, which is a eutectic mixture of 2.5% lidocaine base and 2.5% prilocaine base, is widely used for venipuncture, intravenous cannulation, skin grafting, and a range of other uses, including circumcision.[70] This preparation must be applied under an occlusive bandage for 45 to 60 minutes to obtain effective

TABLE 29.7 Epidural Anesthesia

Drug With Epinephrine (1:200,000)	Usual Concentration (%)	Usual Volume (mL)	Maximum Dose (mg) Without/With Epinephrine	Usual Onset (min)	Usual Duration (min)
Chloroprocaine	2-3	15-30	700/900	5-15	30-90
Lidocaine	1-2	15-30	350/500	5-15	
Mepivacaine	1-2	15-30	350/500	5-15	60-180
Prilocaine	1-3	15-30	350/500	5-15	
Bupivacaine	0.25-0.5	15-30	175/225	15-20	180-350
Levobupivacaine	0.25-0.75	15-30	200/250	15-20	180-350
Ropivacaine	0.2-0.75	15-30	200/250	15-20	180-350

See also Chapter 45. Doses are for a 70-kg adult receiving epinephrine-containing solutions. Doses should be reduced for children, for patients with specific risk factors, and for specific catheter tip locations (e.g., upper thoracic).

TABLE 29.8 Spinal Anesthesia

Drug	Usual Concentration (%)	Usual Volume (mL)	Total Dose (mg)	Baricity	Glucose Concentration (%)	Usual Duration (min)
Procaine	10.0	1-2	100-200	Hyperbaric	5.0	30-60
Lidocaine	1.5, 5.0	1-2	30-100	Hyperbaric	7.5	30-90
Mepivacaine	4.0	1-2	40-80	Hyperbaric	9.0	30-90
Tetracaine	0.25-1.0	1-4	5-20	Hyperbaric	5.0	90-200
	0.25	2-6	5-20	Hypobaric		90-200
	1.0	1-2	5-20	Isobaric		90-200
Dibucaine	0.25	1-2	2.5-5.0	Hyperbaric	5.0	90-200
	0.5	1-2	5-10	Isobaric		90-200
	0.06	5-20	3-12	Hypobaric		90-200
Bupivacaine	0.5	3-4	15-20	Isobaric		90-200
	0.75	2-3	15-20	Hyperbaric	8.25	90-200
Levobupivacaine	0.5	3-4	15-20	Isobaric		90-200
	0.75	2-3	15-20	Hyperbaric		90-200
Ropivacaine	0.5	3-4	15-20	Isobaric		90-200
	0.75	2-3	15-20	Hyperbaric		90-200

Doses are for a 70-kg adult. Dosing may be reduced during pregnancy and with advancing age. Pediatric dosing is detailed in Chapter 76.

TABLE 29.9 Various Preparations Intended for Topical Anesthesia

Anesthetic Ingredient	Concentration (%)	Pharmaceutical Application Form	Intended Area of Use
Benzocaine	1-5	Cream	Skin and mucous membrane
	20	Ointment	Skin and mucous membrane
	20	Aerosol	Skin and mucous membrane
Cocaine	4	Solution	Ear, nose, throat
Dibucaine	0.25-1	Cream	Skin
	0.25-1	Ointment	Skin
	0.25-1	Aerosol	Skin
	0.25	Solution	Ear
	2.5	Suppositories	Rectum
Cyclomine	0.5-1	Solution	Skin, oropharynx, tracheobronchial tree, urethra, rectum
Lidocaine	2-4	Solution	Oropharynx, tracheobronchial tree, nose
	2	Jelly	Urethra
	2.5-5	Ointment	Skin, mucous membrane, rectum
	2	Viscous	Oropharynx
	10	Suppositories	Rectum
	10	Aerosol	Gingival mucosa
Tetracaine	0.5-1	Ointment	Skin, rectum, mucous membrane
	0.5-1	Cream	Skin, rectum, mucous membrane
	0.25-1	Solution	Nose, tracheobronchial tree
EMLA	Lidocaine, 2.5 Prilocaine, 2.5	Cream	Intact skin
TAC	Tetracaine, 0.5 Epinephrine, 1:200,000 Cocaine, 11.8	Solution	Cut skin
LET	Lidocaine, 4% Epinephrine, 1:20,000 Tetracaine, 0.5%	Solution	Cut skin

EMLA, Eutectic mixture of lidocaine and prilocaine; *LET*, lidocaine-epinephrine-tetracaine; *TAC*, tetracaine-epinephrine-cocaine.
From Covino B, Vassallo H. *Local Anesthetics: Mechanisms of Action and Clinical Use*. Orlando, FL: Grune and Stratton; 1976.

cutaneous anesthesia; longer application times increase the depth and reliability of skin analgesia. EMLA appears to be quite safe in neonates, and methemoglobinemia with the use of prilocaine is exceedingly uncommon. EMLA is more effective for newborn circumcision than placebo is but less effective than dorsal penile nerve block.[70,71] Several alternative topical local anesthetic formulations also are in use, including tetracaine gel[72] and liposomal lidocaine.[73] Physical methods to accelerate local anesthetic transit across skin, including iontophoresis, local heating, electroporation, and a variety of forms of needleless pressure injection, may lead to more rapid onset of cutaneous analgesia.[74] Synera (originally studied as S-Caine) is a formulation of lidocaine and tetracaine that was developed with a heating element (activated by opening the package to initiate an oxygen-dependent exothermic reaction). This formulation has a rapid onset and evokes vasodilatation.[75]

Topical anesthesia through cut skin is commonly used in pediatric emergency departments for liquid application into lacerations that require suturing. Historically, this had been provided by a mixture of tetracaine, epinephrine (adrenaline), and cocaine, known as TAC. TAC is ineffective through intact skin; in contrast, its rapid absorption from mucosal surfaces can lead to toxic, even fatal reactions. Another potential substance is ELA-max, a liposomal formulation of lidocaine which is useful for cuts or abrasions.[76] Lastly, Lidoderm patches have been in use for the topical treatment of postherpetic neuralgia.[77]

Because of concerns regarding cocaine toxicity and the potential for diversion and abuse, cocaine-free topical preparations are strongly recommended, and alternatives such as the combination of an α_1-adrenergic agonist (oxymetazoline or phenylephrine) and a local anesthetic such as 2% to 4% lidocaine should be used, with more dilute solutions being recommended for infants and children.

TUMESCENT ANESTHESIA

A technique of local anesthesia most commonly used by plastic surgeons during liposuction procedures involves the subcutaneous injection of large volumes of dilute local anesthetic in combination with epinephrine and other agents. Total doses of lidocaine ranging from 35 to 55 mg/kg have been reported to produce safe plasma concentrations around or below 5 μg/mL, but notably, these may only peak up to 20 hours after infusion, depending on the site of infiltration.[78] Despite these seemingly huge doses, very good safety outcomes have been reported in several case series.[79] Conversely, there have been several case series of cardiac arrest and death during plastic surgical procedures in patients with multiple risk factors. Here high local anesthetic concentrations and concomitant use of sedatives may have contributed to the patients' instability and deterioration.[80] Factors governing uptake and clearance from this method of local anesthetic delivery deserve further study.

SYSTEMIC LOCAL ANESTHETICS FOR POSTOPERATIVE PAIN AND NEUROPATHIC PAIN

Systemic lidocaine has been extensively investigated over the past 10 years for its potential to inhibit G protein-coupled receptors, especially those of the Gq11 subfamily. Systemic local anesthetics have a strong antiinflammatory effect, but their application has only been shown to be of clinical significance in visceral surgery where they decrease inflammation and pain, and speed recovery when compared to placebo.[81]

A broad variety of local anesthetics, antiarrhythmics, anticonvulsants, and other Na^+ channel blockers are administered intravenously, orally, or both, to relieve a number of forms of chronic neuropathic pain.[82] Clinical results are variable.[83] Although successful responses from intravenous lidocaine are often taken as a positive indication for oral mexiletine, some patients find mexiletine difficult to tolerate. When the signs of neuropathic pain are reversed by lidocaine infusion, normal nociception and other sensory modalities are unaffected, suggesting that the neurophysiologic correlate of the disease has an unusually high susceptibility to these drugs, present in plasma at concentrations 50 to 100 times lower than that required to block normal impulses in peripheral fibers. Laboratory studies suggest that ectopic impulse activity arising at a site of injury or elsewhere, such as the dorsal root ganglion, contributes to the neuropathic pain and that such impulses are particularly sensitive to use-dependent Na^+ channel blockers. It is noteworthy that relief of preexisting neuropathic pain, both clinically and in animal models,[84] can in some cases persist for days, weeks, or months after a single intravenous infusion of drug (e.g., lidocaine), far beyond the lifetime of the drug in vivo or any nerve block that it might affect. The mechanism of this remarkable action remains a mystery. Intuitively, this should be especially true for hereditary syndromes featuring gain-of-function mutations at the sodium channel, such as primary erythromelalgia and recent clinical experience and translational experiments have confirmed that mexiletine has the potential to normalize sodium currents in one specific mutation associated with erythromelalgia.[85]

Pharmacokinetics

The concentration of local anesthetics in blood is determined by the amount injected, the rate of absorption from the site of injection, the rate of tissue distribution, and the rate of biotransformation and excretion of the specific drug.[79,80] Patient-related factors such as age, cardiovascular status, and hepatic function influence the physiologic disposition and resultant blood concentration of local anesthetics.

ABSORPTION

The systemic absorption of local anesthetics is determined by the site of injection, dosage and volume, addition of a vasoconstrictor agent, and the pharmacologic profile of the agent itself.[86,87] Comparison of the blood concentration of local anesthetics after various routes of administration reveals that the anesthetic drug level is highest after intercostal nerve blockade, followed in order of decreasing concentration by injection into the caudal epidural space, lumbar epidural space, brachial plexus, and subcutaneous tissue. When a local anesthetic solution is exposed to an area of greater vascularity, a greater rate and degree of absorption occur. This relationship is of clinical significance because use of a fixed dose of a local anesthetic agent may be potentially toxic in one area of administration but not in others, and in one patient with specific physiology, but not in others. For example, the use of 400 mg of lidocaine without epinephrine for an intercostal nerve block results in an average peak venous plasma level of approximately 7 μg/mL, which is sufficiently high to cause symptoms of central nervous system (CNS) toxicity in some patients. By comparison, this same dose of lidocaine used for a brachial plexus block yields a mean maximum blood level of approximately 3 μg/mL, which is rarely associated with signs of toxicity.

The maximum blood concentration of local anesthetic drugs is related to the total dose of drug administered for any particular site of administration. For most drugs there is a proportionality between the amount of drug administered and the resultant peak anesthetic blood concentration. Epinephrine decreases the rate of vascular absorption of certain agents from various sites of administration and thus lowers their potential systemic toxicity. A 5-μg/mL concentration of epinephrine (1:200,000) significantly reduces the peak blood levels of lidocaine and mepivacaine irrespective of the site of administration. Resorption of local anesthetics follows a biphasic pattern, with an initial fast peak reflecting the fluid phase and later a slower second peak corresponding to resorption from the lipid compartment.[88] The addition of epinephrine to local anesthetic solutions slows the first phase.[89] The net clinical effect is a more profound block, and lower systemic levels.[90]

DISTRIBUTION

The systemic distribution of local anesthetics in many settings can be described sufficiently by a two-compartment model.[91] The rapid disappearance phase is believed to be related to uptake by rapidly equilibrating tissues (i.e., tissues that have high vascular perfusion). The slower phase of disappearance from blood is mainly a function of the particular compound.[86] Local anesthetic drugs are distributed throughout all body tissues, but the relative concentration in different tissues varies. In general, more highly perfused organs show higher concentrations of local anesthetic drug than less well perfused organs do. The primary extraction takes place in the liver, but local anesthetics are also rapidly extracted by lung tissue.[92,93]

BIOTRANSFORMATION AND EXCRETION

The pattern of metabolism of local anesthetic agents varies according to their chemical classification. The esters, or procaine-like drugs, undergo hydrolysis in plasma by the pseudocholinesterase enzymes; clearance of chloroprocaine is especially rapid.[94,95] The aminoamide drugs undergo enzymatic degradation primarily in the liver. Lidocaine is metabolized somewhat more rapidly than mepivacaine, which in turn is more rapidly metabolized than bupivacaine.[71,96,97] Excretion of the metabolites of amide-type local anesthetics occurs via the kidney. Less than 5% of the unchanged drug is excreted via the kidney into urine.

PHARMACOKINETIC ALTERATIONS BY PATIENT STATUS

Patient age may influence the physiologic disposition of local anesthetics. The half-life of lidocaine after intravenous administration averaged 80 minutes in human volunteers varying in age from 22 to 26 years, whereas volunteers 61 to 71 years of age demonstrated a significantly prolonged lidocaine half-life that averaged 138 minutes.[98]

Newborn infants have immature hepatic enzyme systems and hence prolonged elimination of lidocaine, bupivacaine, and ropivacaine.[99] Bupivacaine, for example, has a terminal elimination half-life in adults that averages around 3.5 hours. In neonates and some younger infants, terminal elimination half-lives may be as long as 8 to 12 hours. Prolonged elimination is particularly an issue for continuous infusions of local anesthetics in infants, and seizures have been associated with high bupivacaine infusion rates.[100] Based on analysis of these cases, a maximum infusion rate of 0.4 mg/kg/h for prolonged bupivacaine infusions has been proposed for children and adults, whereas prolonged infusion rates for neonates and young infants should not exceed 0.2 mg/kg/h.[101] Even at 0.2 mg/kg/h, plasma bupivacaine concentrations were found to be rising toward a toxic range in some younger infants after 48 hours.[102] Similarly, prolonged lidocaine infusions in neonates should not exceed 0.8 mg/kg/h. The potential for toxicity with lidocaine infusions in neonates is also increased by the accumulation of its principal metabolite, monoethylglycinexylidide (MEGX), which can cause seizures. Chloroprocaine may offer unique advantages for epidural infusion in neonates because it is rapidly cleared from plasma, even in preterm neonates.[103]

Decreased hepatic blood flow or impaired hepatic enzyme function can produce a substantial elevation of blood levels of the aminoamide local anesthetics. An average lidocaine half-life of 1.5 hours was reported in volunteers with normal hepatic function, whereas patients with liver disease demonstrated an average half-life of 5.0 hours. The rate of disappearance of lidocaine from blood has also been shown to be markedly prolonged in patients with congestive heart failure.[104]

In some patients CNS depression is seen without a preceding excitatory phase, particularly if other CNS depressant drugs had been administered.

Toxicity

Local anesthetic drugs are relatively safe if administered in an appropriate dosage and in the correct anatomic location. However, systemic and localized toxic reactions can occur, usually as a result of accidental intravascular or intrathecal injection or administration of an excessive dose. In addition, specific adverse effects are associated with the use of certain drugs, such as allergic reactions to the aminoester drugs and methemoglobinemia after the use of prilocaine.

SYSTEMIC TOXICITY

Systemic reactions to local anesthetics primarily involve the CNS and the cardiovascular system. In general, the CNS is more susceptible to the actions of systemic local anesthetics than the cardiovascular system, and thus the dose or blood level of local anesthetic required to produce CNS toxicity is usually lower than that resulting in circulatory collapse. However, a recent review of 93 cases showed that the symptoms encountered initially vary widely; and only 60% of patients actually exhibit the classic sequence of toxic events from minor CNS symptoms (e.g., perioral tingling, metallic taste, tinnitus), followed by major CNS symptoms (seizures) and cardiovascular collapse (CC).[105] Overall, the incidence of systemic toxicity following regional anesthesia is estimated at 1:1000 for nerve stimulator-guided blockade, and 1:1600 for ultrasound-guided regional anesthesia.[106]

Central Nervous System Toxicity

The initial symptoms of local anesthetic-induced CNS toxicity are feelings of lightheadedness and dizziness followed frequently by visual and auditory disturbances such as difficulty focusing and tinnitus. Other subjective CNS symptoms include disorientation and occasional feelings of drowsiness. Objective signs of initial CNS toxicity are usually excitatory in nature and include shivering, muscular twitching, and tremors initially involving muscles of the face and distal parts of the extremities. Ultimately, generalized convulsions of a tonic-clonic nature occur. If a sufficiently large dose or rapid intravenous injection of a local anesthetic is administered, the initial signs of CNS excitation are rapidly followed by a state of generalized CNS depression. Seizure activity ceases, and respiratory depression and ultimately respiratory arrest may occur. CNS excitation may be the result of an initial blockade of inhibitory pathways in the cerebral cortex by local anesthetic drugs but can also result from the net stimulation of release of glutamate, an excitatory amino acid neurotransmitter. Blockade of inhibitory pathways allows facilitatory neurons to function in an unopposed fashion, which results in an increase in excitatory activity leading to convulsions. A further increase in the dose of local anesthetic leads to inhibition of activity of both the inhibitory and facilitatory circuits, which results in a generalized state of CNS depression.

In general, a correlation exists between potency of the local anesthetic and intravenous CNS toxicity.[107] Convulsions caused by an inadvertent intravenous bolus of local anesthetic can generally be terminated by small intravenous doses of a benzodiazepine, such as midazolam, or by small intravenous doses of propofol. While propofol is faster acting, large doses should be avoided, especially in patients with hemodynamic instability.[108] Respiratory or metabolic acidosis increases the risks for CNS toxicity from local anesthetics.[109] Elevated $PaCO_2$ enhances cerebral blood flow and thus the anesthetic is delivered more rapidly to the brain. In addition, diffusion of carbon dioxide into neuronal cells decreases intracellular pH, which facilitates conversion of the base form of the drugs to the cationic form. The cationic form does not diffuse well across the nerve membrane, so ion trapping will occur, which will increase the apparent CNS toxicity of local anesthetics. Hypercapnia and acidosis also decrease the plasma protein binding of local anesthetic agents.[110] Accordingly, normocapnia should be targeted during episodes of local anesthetic systemic toxicity.

The clinical implication of this effect of hypercapnia and acidosis on toxicity deserves emphasis. Seizures produce hypoventilation and a combined respiratory and metabolic acidosis, which further exacerbates the CNS toxicity. In the setting of local anesthetic toxic reactions, it is essential to provide prompt assisted ventilation and circulatory support as needed to prevent or correct hypercapnia and acidosis and to prevent or correct hypoxemia, which also exacerbates CNS toxicity. Based on the preceding discussion, it should be apparent that clinicians performing major conduction blockade should make a routine practice of having the following ready at hand: monitoring equipment; an oxygen tank or wall oxygen outlet; rescue airway equipment; and drugs to terminate convulsions, such as midazolam, thiopental, or propofol.

Cardiovascular System Toxicity

Local anesthetics can exert direct actions on both the heart and peripheral blood vessels, as well as indirect actions on the circulation by blockade of sympathetic or parasympathetic efferent activity.

Direct Cardiac Effects. The main mechanisms of local anesthetic toxicity are blockades of cardiac sodium channels leading to negative inotropy and arrhythmia. Local anesthetics act directly by decreasing the conduction in Purkinje fibers and cardiomyocytes by prolonging the recovery time. Other facets of local anesthetic toxicity include inhibition of fatty acid metabolism, interference with calcium homeostasis, and disruption of the mitochondrial respiratory chain.[111] The primary cardiac electrophysiologic effect of local anesthetics is a decrease in the rate of depolarization in the fast conducting tissues of Purkinje fibers and ventricular muscle.[112] This reduction in rate is believed to be due to a decrease in the availability of fast sodium channels in cardiac membranes. Action potential duration and the effective refractory period are also decreased by local anesthetics. However, this effect is dose-dependent and substance-specific. Specifically, electrophysiologic studies have shown that high blood levels of local anesthetics will prolong conduction time through various parts of the heart, as indicated on the electrocardiogram (ECG) by an increase in the PR interval and duration of the QRS complex. Extremely high concentrations of local anesthetics depress spontaneous pacemaker activity in the sinus node, thereby resulting in sinus bradycardia and sinus arrest. Also, the electrophysiologic effects of various agents differ qualitatively. Bupivacaine depresses the rapid phase of depolarization (V_{max}) in Purkinje fibers and ventricular muscle to a greater extent than lidocaine does. In addition, the rate of recovery from a use-dependent block is slower in bupivacaine-treated papillary muscles than in lidocaine-treated muscles. This slow rate of recovery results in incomplete restoration of Na^+ channel availability between action potentials, particularly at high heart rates. These differential effects of lidocaine and bupivacaine have been advanced as explanations of the antiarrhythmic properties of lidocaine versus the arrhythmogenic potential of bupivacaine. All local anesthetics exert dose-dependent negative inotropic action on cardiac muscle; the depression of cardiac contractility is roughly proportional to conduction blocking potency. Thus bupivacaine and tetracaine are more potent cardio depressants than is lidocaine. Local anesthetics may depress myocardial contractility by affecting calcium influx and triggered release from the sarcoplasmic reticulum,[113] as well as by inhibiting cardiac sarcolemmal Ca^{2+} currents and Na^{+} currents. Lastly, mitochondrial metabolism is inhibited by bupivacaine, and, to a lesser extent, other long-acting local anesthetics such as ropivacaine,[114] while the effect of lidocaine is smaller.

Direct Peripheral Vascular Effects. Local anesthetics exert biphasic effects on peripheral vascular smooth muscle.[103] Low concentrations of lidocaine and bupivacaine produced vasoconstriction in the cremaster muscle of rats, whereas high concentrations produced vasodilation in both isolated tissue models and in vivo. Cocaine is the only local anesthetic that consistently causes vasoconstriction at all concentrations because of its ability to inhibit the uptake of norepinephrine by premotor neurons and thus to potentiate neurogenic vasoconstriction.

COMPARATIVE CARDIOVASCULAR TOXICITY

All local anesthetics, but especially bupivacaine, can cause rapid and profound cardiovascular depression. The cardiotoxicity of bupivacaine appears to differ from that of lidocaine in the following manner:

1. The ratio of the dosage required for irreversible CC and the dosage that will produce CNS toxicity (convulsions; i.e., the CC/CNS ratio) is lower for bupivacaine and etidocaine than for lidocaine.[115]
2. Ventricular arrhythmias and fatal ventricular fibrillation may occur more often after the rapid intravenous administration of a large dose of bupivacaine but far less frequently with lidocaine. The CNS effects of local anesthetics may contribute to the generation of arrhythmias.
3. A pregnant patient may be more sensitive to the cardiotoxic effects of bupivacaine than a nonpregnant animal or patient.[116] Consequently, the 0.75% solution of bupivacaine is no longer recommended for use in obstetric anesthesia in the United States.
4. Cardiac resuscitation is more difficult after bupivacaine-induced CC, and acidosis and hypoxia markedly potentiate the cardiotoxicity of bupivacaine.[117] Conversely, Intralipid is believed to be most effective in bupivacaine-induced toxicity. Despite the experimental or clinical anecdotal use of many different resuscitation drugs in the setting of bupivacaine overdose, current guidelines focus on standard cardiopulmonary resuscitation, albeit with titration rather than fixed doses of epinephrine, early administration of lipid emulsion, and avoidance of propofol in settings of hemodynamic instability.[108] Bupivacaine-induced ventricular arrhythmias should not be treated with vasopressin, calcium channel blockers, β-blockers, or other local anesthetics with antiarrhythmic potential (such as lidocaine).[118]

Pharmacokinetic studies have estimated that Intralipid decreases cardiac bupivacaine concentration by 11% within 3 minutes of administration, and cerebral bupivacaine content by 18% within 15 minutes.[119] Even though these findings are theoretical, they underline the notion that Intralipid should not be considered an antidote with full antagonistic properties. Rather, limited evidence suggests that it will considerably reduce the bupivacaine concentration in target organs, most likely improve metabolism, and potentially have direct beneficial effects at the sodium channel. Intralipid is a valuable contribution to, but not a substitute for, careful and meticulous conduct of regional anesthesia.[120]

The clinical implications for cardiac resuscitation after intravascular injection or overdose of local anesthetic are the following:

1. No medications are uniformly effective in facilitating resuscitation from bupivacaine-induced cardiac arrest or severe ventricular tachycardia (despite our recommendations regarding Intralipid later). Basic principles of cardiopulmonary resuscitation should be emphasized first, including attention to securing the airway, providing oxygenation and ventilation, and performing chest compressions as indicated.
2. Because resuscitation after local anesthetic-induced circulatory collapse is difficult, prevention of massive intravascular injection or excessive dosing is crucial.
3. Negative aspiration of the syringe does not always exclude intravascular placement. Incremental, fractionated dosing should be the rule for all patients undergoing major conduction blockade. Even though changes on the ECG are not present in all cases before circulatory collapse, they can often be seen, and continuous attention to the ECG (including changes in QRS and T-wave morphology, rate, rhythm, or ectopy) may be lifesaving by terminating injection before a cardiac arrest occurs.
4. Based on animal studies[121] and a growing number of human case reports, hospitals and clinics that perform major conduction blockade or large volume infiltration blockade should keep available for emergency use a supply of lipid emulsion such as Intralipid 20%. If a patient experiences profound cardiovascular depression or circulatory arrest after the administration of bupivacaine, ropivacaine, or by extrapolation, other local anesthetics, then along with initiation of basic life support and the ACLS protocol, a rapid bolus of Intralipid 20%, 1.5 mL/kg (approximately 100 mL in adults) is recommended, followed if necessary by an infusion of 0.25 mL/kg/min over the next 10 minutes.

Chiral Local Anesthetics: Ropivacaine and Levobupivacaine

Commercial bupivacaine is a racemic mixture of *(R)*- and *(S)*-stereoisomers. In response to the problem of cardiovascular toxicity as a result of accidental intravenous injection of bupivacaine, single enantiomers were developed in the hope that they would be potentially safer. Ropivacaine (Naropin)[122] and levo-*(S)*-bupivacaine (Chirocaine)[123] were formulated to exploit this stereoselectivity. Ropivacaine is a single *(S)*-stereoisomer that differs from levobupivacaine in the substitution of a propyl for the butyl group on the piperidine ring (see Fig. 29.2). With these designed changes in molecular structure, it was hoped that ropivacaine and levobupivacaine would be less intrinsically cardiotoxic. Conversely, it appears that the *(S)*-enantiomers of mepivacaine and bupivacaine are metabolized by the liver more slowly than the corresponding *(R)*-enantiomers, which would lead to somewhat greater systemic accumulation with prolonged infusions.

The very slow reversal of Na^+ channel blockade after a cardiac action potential, which is a hallmark of bupivacaine, is considerably faster with ropivacaine. In addition to these electrical differences, the negative inotropic potency of ropivacaine on isolated cardiac tissue appears to be considerably less than that of bupivacaine. Both electrical and mechanical differences in the toxic profiles may arise from the selective inhibition of Ca^{2+} currents by bupivacaine.

Do the data support the claim of a greater therapeutic index for ropivacaine than bupivacaine, particularly with regard to cardiotoxicity? In clinical studies comparing potencies of ropivacaine and bupivacaine administered for brachial plexus[124] or lumbar epidural block,[125] the anesthetic profiles of the drugs were almost identical. A third exemplary study comparing lumbar epidural 0.5% bupivacaine with 0.75% ropivacaine also found no significant differences in motor or sensory effects between the drugs at these different concentrations.[126] Overall, it appears that ropivacaine is slightly less potent than bupivacaine (1:1.3 to 1:1.5) for regional anesthesia. In some laboratory animal studies and in some human studies, ropivacaine also produced blocks of shorter duration than those induced by bupivacaine. Other studies in animals and humans have found equal durations of sensory and motor block for the two drugs.

At the projected equipotent doses for nerve block, are the drugs equally toxic? The overall impression is that ropivacaine is less cardiotoxic than bupivacaine. Studies in animals have generally found that bupivacaine more readily produces conduction disturbances, cardiac collapse, or ventricular fibrillation than ropivacaine does and that aggressive cardiac resuscitation after an intentional intravenous bolus in dogs leads to effective reversal of the toxic effects far more frequently with ropivacaine than with bupivacaine.[127]

The greater safety of ropivacaine than bupivacaine may be related both to the reduced toxicity of the single *(S)*-isomer and to the difference between the propyl- and butyl-*N*-piperidine substituent. In contrast to bupivacaine, the cardiotoxic profile of ropivacaine in pregnant ewes is the same as the corresponding profile in nonpregnant ewes.[128]

Levobupivacaine has been studied in a range of clinical settings and sites of administration. Although a number of publications have compared levobupivacaine with racemic bupivacaine and ropivacaine,[129,130] conclusions differ among studies regarding the relative potency and duration of block of these three drugs at different sites of administration with respect to sensory and motor end points. Clinicians should note that levobupivacaine is formulated as a weight percentage with regard to its free base content, whereas the weight percentage of most other local anesthetics is calculated on the basis of the hydrochloride salt.[131]

Acidosis and Hypoxia

As with CNS toxicity, hypercapnia, acidosis, and hypoxia potentiate the negative chronotropic and inotropic actions of lidocaine and bupivacaine in isolated cardiac tissue, and the combination of hypoxia and acidosis markedly potentiates the cardiodepressant effects of bupivacaine.[132] Hypoxia and acidosis also increased the frequency of cardiac arrhythmias and the mortality rate in sheep after the intravenous administration of bupivacaine. Hypercapnia, acidosis, and hypoxia occur very rapidly in some patients after seizure activity caused by the rapid accidental intravascular injection of local anesthetic agents.[133] Thus the cardiovascular depression observed in some patients after the accidental intravenous injection of bupivacaine may be related in part to the effect of seizures producing acidosis and hypoxia and thereby leading to an exacerbation of bupivacaine's intrinsic cardiotoxicity.

Indirect Cardiovascular Effects

High levels of spinal or epidural blockade can produce severe hypotension. A follow-up study of closed claims of patients who suffered perioperative cardiac arrest confirmed previous reports of a series of cardiac arrests involving generally healthy patients undergoing spinal or epidural anesthesia.[134] These events frequently occurred in conjunction with high dermatomal levels of blockade, liberal use of sedatives, and progression to cardiac arrest after a period of hypotension accompanied by bradycardia, often involving delays in recognition of the problem, delays in instituting airway support (particularly in sedated patients), and delays in administration of direct-acting combined α- and β-adrenergic agonists, such as epinephrine. Whereas mild to moderate degrees of hypotension generally respond well to indirect-acting sympathomimetics such as ephedrine or incremental dosing of phenylephrine, the combination of severe hypotension and severe bradycardia under spinal anesthesia should in most clinical settings be treated promptly with incremental dosing of epinephrine, initially at doses of 0.1 to 1 μg/kg.

METHEMOGLOBINEMIA

A unique systemic side effect associated with a specific local anesthetic is the development of methemoglobinemia after the administration of large doses of prilocaine.[135] In general, 600-mg doses are required for the development of clinically significant levels of methemoglobinemia in adults. Hepatic metabolism of prilocaine generates *O*-toluidine, which oxidizes hemoglobin to methemoglobin. Methemoglobinemia, if severe, may be treated by the intravenous administration of methylene blue. Standard dosing of the topical local anesthetic EMLA (a mixture of lidocaine and prilocaine) in term newborns produced minimal amounts of methemoglobin, and EMLA, if dosed appropriately, should be regarded as very safe in the great majority of newborns. Risk may be increased in newborns with rare metabolic disorders or after the concomitant administration of other drugs that impair reduction of methemoglobin.

ALLERGIES

Even though patients receiving local anesthetics may experience a range of local and systemic symptoms, prospective studies indicate that very few of these reactions are truly confirmed as allergic reactions.[136,137] Aminoester drugs such as procaine may produce allergic-type reactions more commonly than do the aminoamides, although even with aminoesters, the vast majority of reactions are not allergic. Aminoesters, unlike aminoamides, are derivatives of *p*-aminobenzoic acid, which is known to be allergenic. Some aminoamide solutions may contain a preservative, methylparaben, whose chemical structure is similar to that of *p*-aminobenzoic acid, but for most aminoamides, preservative-free solutions are available.[138] Contamination of vials with latex antigen has been suspected in some allergic reactions, although it has been difficult to confirm. In the very rare patient for whom confirmed allergy to both aminoamides and aminoesters precludes their use for spinal anesthesia, meperidine can be considered as an alternative.[128]

LOCAL TISSUE TOXICITY

All the clinically used aminoamide and aminoester local anesthetics can produce direct toxicity to nerves if they achieve sufficiently high intraneural concentrations.[139] Conversely, in the great majority of clinical applications, no damage to nerves occurs. Although local anesthetics are usually packaged and injected at concentrations well above their physiologically effective range, in the process of delivery they are generally diluted sufficiently that no harm is done. If such dilution does not occur, however, long-term or permanent neural deficits do result. Thus the application of 5% (200 mM) lidocaine in viscous, dense solutions through narrow intrathecal catheters had been associated with a high frequency of transient or longer-term radicular symptoms or even cauda equina syndrome.[140] Laboratory investigations have shown that such high concentrations of local anesthetics alone applied directly to bare nerve fibers produce an irreversible conduction block in less than 5 minutes.[141] Clinicians should be aware that the concentrations of formulated local anesthetic solutions are neurotoxic per se and that their "natural" dilution, which occurs in situ or in tissue, is essential for safe use.

If cauda equina syndrome was considered one catastrophic end of the spectrum, the opposite side would be transient neurologic syndrome, a temporary radicular irritation thought to be caused by local anesthetic application and influenced by patient positioning.[142] Single-shot spinal anesthesia with commonly recommended doses and concentrations of many different local anesthetics can produce more limited and transient neurologic symptoms (back pain, paresthesias, radicular pain, or hypesthesia).[143] Some studies and systematic reviews have found that mepivacaine and lidocaine at a range of dilutions cause more frequent symptoms than do bupivacaine and prilocaine.[144] The risk of transient neurologic symptoms after spinal anesthesia was not diminished by dilution of lidocaine from 5% to either 1% or 2%. Differences in study design, method of questioning, and criteria for inclusion may be partially responsible for differences in the prevalence of radicular sequelae in various studies. Despite these differences in study design, a meta-analysis concluded that the pooled relative risk for transient neurologic symptoms after spinal anesthesia with lidocaine was 6.7-fold higher than with bupivacaine and 5.5-fold higher than with prilocaine.[144] The addition of vasoconstrictors to local anesthetic solutions has been reported to potentially increase risk,[145] but within the limits of current dosing, neuraxial administration of vasoconstrictors as an adjuvant seems to be safe.[146] Neurotoxicity appears to be unrelated to conduction block per se, because STX, neosaxitoxin, and tetrodotoxin, highly potent blockers of sodium channels, can produce intense conduction blockade without histologic or behavioral signs of nerve injury.[147]

Skeletal muscle changes have been observed after the injection of local anesthetic agents such as lidocaine, mepivacaine, prilocaine, bupivacaine, and etidocaine.[148] In general, the more potent, longer-acting agents bupivacaine and etidocaine appear to cause more localized skeletal muscle damage than do the less potent, shorter-acting agents lidocaine and prilocaine. This effect on skeletal muscle, to the best of our current knowledge, is reversible due to the regenerative potential of skeletal muscle and the comparatively small area of the muscle affected, which is why it is often clinically inapparent.

Development of Prolonged-Duration and Sensory- or Nociceptive-Selective Local Anesthetics

Several methods for producing long-duration nerve blockade are under investigation. First, there have been efforts to use readily available drugs such as tricyclic antidepressants[149,150] or quaternary local anesthetic derivatives as novel local anesthetics,[151] but these efforts have consistently been hampered by concerns over neurotoxicity.

SLOW-RELEASE FORMULATIONS

Liposomal encapsulation can prolong nerve blockade, depending on the dose and the physical properties of the liposome (surface charge, size, lamellar structure).[141-143] This mode of action has been investigated for decades but the clinical introduction has only been recent. Liposomal bupivacaine (Exparel) has been licensed for infiltration analgesia[152] but its dose-response for blockade of peripheral nerves is less clear.[153] A recent study showed potential benefits when combining Exparel with bupivacaine for interscalene block,[154] and the Food and Drug Administration has moved to expand Exparel licensing to select nerve block indications. Despite strong basic science data, the clinical benefit of these formulations, especially for nerve blockade, and when compared to plain long-acting local anesthetics, is not as convincing as one would hope. Other modes of slow-release are embedding in bone wax, polylactic acid, polyglycolic acid, fatty-acid-based biodegradable polymers, and proliposomal formulations.[7] Finally, another variant of slow-release formulations is photo-triggered on-demand release.

SITE 1 BLOCKERS

Prolonged-duration local anesthesia also appears to be feasible with the use of site 1 sodium channel blockers.[148] The site 1 blocker neosaxitoxin has been used in humans in phase 1 and phase 2 clinical trials.[149-151] A combination of site 1 toxins with either local anesthetics or adrenergics results in prolongation of blockade and improvement in the therapeutic index.[155] Theoretically attractive features of site 1 toxins include their apparent lack of local tissue toxicity on nerves[137] or muscles[152] and their minimal cardiotoxicity.[153]

TARGETING OF SPECIFIC SODIUM CHANNEL ISOFORMS

Coming back to the nine different subtypes of sodium channels, research efforts have been directed at blocking specific isoforms thought to be of particular relevance for defined pain conditions. The Nav1.7 subtype, for example, has been linked to somatic pain, and to hereditary syndromes of hyperalgesia[156] or insensitivity to pain.[157] A monoclonal antibody has been described which is 1000 times more potent at blocking sodium currents through Nav1.7 than those of other isoforms.[158] Importantly, animal models of visceral pain suggest a substantial role of Nav1.9 in these syndromes.[25]

TARGETING OF NOCICEPTIVE FIBERS

High hopes had been raised by reports of sensory-selective blockade of peripheral nerves when a quaternary derivative of lidocaine was targeted into nociceptors using activation of TRPV-1 channels by lidocaine or capsaicin. TRPV channels are preferentially located in small sensory fibers.[159] After several promising studies, concerns over neurotoxicity[151] prevented this combination from entering clinical practice. Yet, the concept of targeting specific variants of local anesthetic drugs into specific fibers has been confirmed, and if a combination of drugs is found which can provide these effects with decreased neurotoxicity, the strategy as such may hold promise. Whether any quaternary derivatives of local anesthetics have less neurotoxicity than their parent compounds remains as of yet unanswered.

To summarize, several avenues of research may lead to new local anesthetics or new modes of application, but only liposomal bupivacaine has been introduced into clinical practice. Potentially, these new strategies may move us closer to the holy grail of regional anesthesia, where patients benefit from a tailored surgical block followed by prolonged periods of reliable sensory (or even nociceptive) block without impairment in motor function.

Biologic Mechanisms of Local Anesthetic Failure: Inflammation, Hyperalgesia, Tachyphylaxis, and Genetic Variants

Failure of local anesthesia is commonly ascribed to technical failure of delivery, insufficient volume or concentration of drug, or erroneous clinical decisions in selection of techniques. However, there are a number of clinical situations in which biologic processes contribute to failed local anesthesia, even with proper technique and drug selection.

For example, in patients going to the dentist with infections such as a tooth abscess or severe pulpitis, failure rates of standard doses of local anesthetic have been reported to be as high as 70%. Local anesthetic failure at a site of inflammation appears to reflect a combination of pharmacokinetic factors and pharmacodynamic factors. Pharmacokinetic factors include (1) increased local blood flow leading to accelerated removal of drug from perineural injection compartments; (2) local tissue acidosis leading to a greater proportion of the drug in the hydrochloride form, which diffuses more poorly across biologic membranes; and (3) local tissue edema, which increases diffusion distances for drug into nerves. Pharmacodynamic factors include the effects of inflammation on both peripheral sensitization of nerves and central sensitization.[120] It is noteworthy that in the setting of an infected mandibular tooth, inferior alveolar nerve block (performed proximally at a site presumably remote from the infected area) also has an unexpectedly high failure rate. Increasing the concentration of local anesthetic can still result in satisfactory, albeit shorter, blockade. In clinical practice, these patients require a higher local anesthetic dose to achieve sufficient analgesia. Inflamed tissue is more difficult, but not impossible, to anesthetize.

Apparent reductions in the effectiveness of local anesthetic infusions over time may be due to a number of causes unrelated to tolerance per se, including dislodgement of catheters and changes in the dermatomal origin or intensity of nociceptive input. In obstetric patients receiving epidural bolus injections, recurrence of pain before the next injection resulted in a reduction in the intensity and duration of blockade, whereas repeat injection before the return of pain prevented this rapidly occurring form of tolerance, or tachyphylaxis.[160] In postoperative patients, co-administration of systemic opioids prevented regression of segmental block in patients receiving thoracic epidural bupivacaine infusions.[161] Studies in rats suggest that both pharmacokinetic and pharmacodynamic mechanisms are involved. In a rat model, tachyphylaxis was linked to the development of hyperalgesia,[162] and drugs that inhibit hyperalgesia, including N-methyl-D-aspartate receptor antagonists and nitric oxide synthase inhibitors,[163] also prevented tachyphylaxis. Conversely, repeated sciatic injections of lidocaine resulted in reduced intraneural lidocaine content along with reduced duration of block.[164] The exact mechanism, however, has not been determined, and the clinical relevance with continuous use of long-acting local anesthetics is unclear.

Occasionally patients report that "local anesthetics don't work for me." Although this claim may reflect previous technical failures or a variety of other processes and patient- or procedure-specific factors, it is possible that in some cases these failures may involve genetic or acquired variation in local anesthetic responsiveness. Several mutations in the transmembrane segment IIIS6 of the rat brain α-subunit have been shown to decrease the affinity between sodium channels and local anesthetics and anticonvulsants[165] and similar investigations have also been carried out in sodium channel subtypes Nav1.7[166] or Nav1.5.[167] Of note, different mutations at specific points in the local anesthetic binding site led to differential response of these channels to sodium channel blockers, suggesting that the binding of local anesthetics to the "receptor" is a more dynamic, fluid, and structure-dependent process than commonly assumed. This is supported by a clinical study which showed that some percent of persons reporting inefficient regional anesthesia really did demonstrate partial resistance when tested in standardized manner, and some patients had selective resistance against specific local anesthetics.[168] While Clendenen and colleagues published the genetic workup of a family with inherited local anesthetic resistance,[167] there are preliminary hints that local anesthetic resistance may also be acquired. Interesting case reports suggest that repeated exposure to scorpion bites can elicit acquired resistance to local anesthetics.[169] Elements of scorpion toxin are known to interact with sodium channels, albeit at other sites (Site 3 and 4) than local anesthetics (which bind to Site 9),[170] and therefore the sustained modulation of sodium channel function by toxins is yet another fascinating potential facet of sodium channel and local anesthetic pharmacology.

Conclusions

Local anesthetics have been a central pillar in perioperative management of patients for more than a century, and continued research will assure that we know as much as possible about these drugs, and how we can use them as optimally as possible for the benefit of the patients whose care has been entrusted to us.

Acknowledgment

The editors, publisher, Dr. Charles B. Berde, and Dr. Philipp Lirk would like to thank Dr. Gary Strichartz for his contribution to this chapter in the prior edition of this work. It has served as the foundation for the current chapter.

Complete references available online at expertconsult.com.

References

1. Sanchez V, et al. *Anesth Analg*. 1987;66:159.
2. Zhang J, et al. *Biophys J*. 2007;92:3988.
3. Courtney KR. *J Pharmacol Exp Ther*. 1980;213:114.
4. Gissen AJ, et al. *Anesthesiology*. 1980;53:467.
5. Docherty RJ, Farmer CE. *Handb Exp Pharmacol*. 2009;194:519.
6. Lawson SN. *Exp Physiol*. 2002;87:239.

7a. Lirk P, et al. *Anesth Analg*. 2017.

7b. Hodgkin A, et al. *The Conduction of the Nervous Impulse*. Springfield, IL: Charles C. Thomas; 1964.

8. Moayeri N, Groen GJ. *Anesthesiology*. 2009;111:1128.
9. Ritchie JM, Rogart RB. *Proc Natl Acad Sci U S A*. 1977;74:211.
10. Savio-Galimberti E, et al. *Front Pharmacol*. 2012;3:124.
11. Ritchie JM, et al. *J Pharmacol Exp Ther*. 1965;150:160.
12. Hille B. *J Gen Physiol*. 1977;69:475.
13. Narahashi T, et al. *J Pharmacol Exp Ther*. 1970;171:32.
14. Strichartz GR. *J Gen Physiol*. 1973;62:37.
15. Haeseler G, et al. *Br J Pharmacol*. 2002;137:285–293.
16. Courtney KR, et al. *Anesthesiology*. 1978;48:111.
17. Hille B. *J Gen Physiol*. 1977;69:497.
18. Gokin AP, et al. *Anesthesiology*. 2001;95:1441.
19. Ekberg J, et al. *Proc Natl Acad Sci U S A*. 2006;103:17030.
20. Chevrier P, et al. *Br J Pharmacol*. 2004;142:576.
21. Bennett DL, Woods CG. *Lancet Neurol*. 2014;13:587–599.
22. Fertleman C, et al. *Neuron*. 2006;52:767.
23. Sheets PL, et al. *J Physiol*. 2007;581:1019.
24. Cox JJ, et al. *Nature*. 2006;444:894.
25. Hockley JR, et al. *J Physiol*. 2017;595:2661–2679.
26. Cannon SC. *Handb Exp Pharmacol*. 2017.
27. Persaud N, Strichartz G. *Pain*. 2002;99:333.
28. Johns RA, et al. *Anesthesiology*. 1985;62:141.
29. Fink BR. *Cairns AM: Anesthesiology*. 1984;60:111.
30. Fink BR, Cairns AM. *Anesth Analg*. 1987;66:948.
31. Raymond SA, et al. *Anesth Analg*. 1989;68:563.
32. Drachman D, Strichartz G. *Anesthesiology*. 1991;75:1051.
33. Hogan QH, Abram SE. *Anesthesiology*. 1997;86:216.
34. Littlewood DG, et al. *Br J Anaesth*. 1979;49:75.
35. Casati A, et al. *Br J Anaesth*. 2007;98:823.
36. Pace NL, Stylianou MP. *Anesthesiology*. 2007;107:144.
37. Tobias J. *Anesth Analg*. 2001;93:1156.
38. Popping DM, et al. *Anesthesiology*. 2009;111:406–415.
39. Kroin JS, et al. *Anesthesiology*. 2004;101:488–494.
40. Ping Y, et al. *Medicine (Baltimore)*. 2017;96:e5846.
41. Brummett CM, et al. *Anesthesiology*. 2011;115:836–843.
42. Kosel J, et al. *Expert Rev Clin Pharmacol*. 2016;9:375–383.
43. Kirksey MA, et al. *PLoS One*. 2015;10:e0137312.
44. Choi S, et al. *Br J Anaesth*. 2014;112:427–439.
45. Chong MA, et al. *Reg Anesth Pain Med*. 2017;42:319–326.
46. Klein SM, et al. *Anesth Analg*. 1998;87:1316–1319.
47. Wong K, et al. *Anesth Analg*. 1993;76:131.
48. DiFazio CA, et al. *Anesth Analg*. 1986;65:760.
49. Cohen SE, Thurlow A. *Anesthesiology*. 1979;51:288.
50. Kytta J, et al. *Reg Anesth*. 1991;16:89–94.
51. Popitz-Bergez FA, et al. *Reg Anesth*. 1997;22:363.
52. Fagraeus L, et al. *Anesthesiology*. 1983;58:184.
53. Leffler A, et al. *J Clin Invest*. 2008;118:763–776.
54. McKay W, et al. *Anesth Analg*. 1987;66:572.
55. Thornton PC, Buggy DJ. *Br J Anaesth*. 2011;107:656.
56. Gupta A, et al. *Acta Anaesthesiol Scand*. 2011;55:785.
57. Liu SS, et al. *J Am Coll Surg*. 2016;203:914–932.
58. Guay J. *J Clin Anesth*. 2009;21:585–594.
59. Eichenberger U, et al. *Reg Anesth Pain Med*. 2009;34:242–246.
60. Latzke D, et al. *Br J Anaesth*. 2010;104:239–244.
61. Abrahams M, et al. *Reg Anesth Pain Med*. 2016;41:275–288.
62. D'Ercole F, et al. *J Cardiothorac Vasc Anesth*. 2018;32:915–927.
63. Ilfeld BM. *Anesth Analg*. 2011;113:904.
64. Veering BT, et al. *Anesthesiology*. 2002;96:1062–1069.
65. Cohen SE, et al. *Anesthesiology*. 2000;92:387.
66. Brull SJ, Greene NM. *Anesth Analg*. 1989;69:342.
67. Yilmaz-Rastoder E, et al. *Reg Anesth Pain Med*. 2012;37:403.
68. Chambers WA, et al. *Anesth Analg*. 1981;60:417.
69. Kumar M, et al. *J Anaesthesiol Clin Pharmacol*. 2015;31:450–456.
70. Butler-O'Hara M, et al. *Pediatrics*. 1998;101:E5.
71. Arthur GR, et al. *Br J Anaesth*. 1979;51:481.
72. Browne J, et al. *Can J Anaesth*. 1999;46:1014.
73. Eichenfield LF, et al. *Pediatrics*. 2002;109:1093.
74. Galinkin JL, et al. *Anesth Analg*. 2002;94:1484.
75. Sethna NF, et al. *Anesthesiology*. 2005;102:403.
76. Friedman PM, et al. *Dermatol Surg*. 2001;27:1019–1026.
77. Davies PS, et al. *Drugs*. 2004;64:937–947.
78. Klein JA, Jeske DR. *Anesth Analg*. 2016;122:1350–1359.
79. Houseman TS, et al. *Dermatol Surg*. 2002;28:971.
80. Grazer FM, de Jong RH. *Plast Reconstr Surg*. 2000;105:436.
81. Kranke P, et al. *Cochrane Database Syst Rev*. 2015;7:CD009642.
82. Tremont-Lukats IW, et al. *Anesth Analg*. 2005;101:1738.
83. Carroll I, et al. *Clin J Pain*. 2007;23:702.
84. Araujo MC, et al. *Pain*. 2003;103:21.
85. Cregg R, Cox JJ, et al. *Br J Pharmacol*. 2014;171:4455–4463.
86. Tucker GT. *Br J Anaesth*. 1986;58:717–731.
87. Rosenberg PH, et al. *Reg Anesth Pain Med*. 2004;29:564.
88. Tucker GT, Mather LE. *Br J Anaesth*. 1975;47:213.
89. Lee BB, et al. *Anesth Analg*. 2002;95:1402–1407. Table of contents.
90. Hermanides J, et al. *Br J Anaesth*. 2012;109:144–154.
91. McCann ME, et al. *Anesth Analg*. 2001;93:893–897.
92. Lofstrom JB. *Int Anesthesiol Clin*. 1978;16:53.
93. Aoki M, et al. *Drug Metab Dispos*. 2010;38:1183–1188.
94. Kuhnert BR, et al. *Anesth Analg*. 1986;65:273.
95. Kuhnert BR, et al. *Anesthesiology*. 1980;53:21.
96. Scott DB, et al. *Br J Anaesth*. 1973;45:1010.
97. Katz JA, et al. *Anesth Analg*. 1990;70:16.
98. Nation RL, et al. *Br J Clin Pharmacol*. 1977;4:439.
99. Bösenberg AT, et al. *Paediatr Anaesth*. 2005;15:739.
100. Lonnqvist PA. *Paediatr Anaesth*. 2012;22:39–43.
101. Berde CB. *Anesth Analg*. 1992;75:164.
102. Larsson BA, et al. *Anesth Analg*. 1997;84:501.
103. Henderson K, et al. *J Clin Anesth*. 1993;5:129.
104. Thomson PD, et al. *Ann Intern Med*. 1973;78:499.
105. Di Gregorio G, et al. *Reg Anesth Pain Med*. 2010;35:181–187.
106. Barrington MJ, Kluger R. *Reg Anesth Pain Med*. 2013;38:289–297.
107. Scott DB. *Br J Anaesth*. 1975;47:328.
108. Neal JM, et al. *Reg Anesth Pain Med*. 2018;43:150–153.
109. Englesson S. *Acta Anaesthesiol Scand*. 1974;18:79.
110. Burney RG, et al. *Anesth Analg*. 1978;57:478.

111. Weinberg GL. *Anesthesiology*. 2012;117:180–187.
112. Clarkson CW, Hondeghem LM. *Anesthesiology*. 1985;62:396.
113. Chamberlain BK, et al. *J Biol Chem*. 1984;259:7547.
114. Sztark F, et al. *Anesthesiology*. 1998;88:1340–1349.
115. de Jong RH, et al. *Anesth Analg*. 1982;61:3.
116. Morishima HO, et al. *Anesthesiology*. 1985;63:134.
117. Rosen MA, et al. *Anesth Analg*. 1985;64:1089.
118. Neal JM, et al. *Reg Anesth Pain Med*. 2018;43:113–123.
119. Kuo I, Akpa BS. *Anesthesiology*. 2013;118:1350–1361.
120. Lirk P, et al. *Eur J Anaesthesiol*. 2014;31:575–585.
121. Weinberg GL, et al. *Anesthesiology*. 1998;88:1071.
122. Moller R, Covino BG. *Anesthesiology*. 1990;72:322.
123. Rutten AJ, et al. *Br J Anaesth*. 1991;67:247.
124. Hickey R, et al. *Anesthesiology*. 1991;74:639.
125. Brown DL, et al. *Anesthesiology*. 1990;72:633.
126. Katz JA, et al. *Reg Anesth*. 1990;15:250.
127. Feldman HS, et al. *Anesth Analg*. 1991;73:373.
128. Santos AC, et al. *Anesthesiology*. 1989;70:991.
129. Camorcia M, et al. *Anesthesiology*. 2005;102:646.
130. Benhamou D, et al. *Anesthesiology*. 2003;99:1383.
131. Rosenberg PH, Schug SA. *Br J Anaesth*. 2005;94:544.
132. Sage DJ, et al. *Anesth Analg*. 1984;63:1.
133. Moore DC, et al. *Anesthesiology*. 1980;53:259.
134. Lee LA, et al. *Anesthesiology*. 2004;101:143.
135. Lund P. *Cwik J: Anesthesiology*. 1980;53:259.
136. Ring J, et al. *Chem Immunol Allergy*. 2010;95:190–200.
137. Dewachter P, et al. *Anesthesiology*. 2009;111:1141–1150.
138. Eggleston ST, Lush LW. *Ann Pharmacother*. 1996;30:851–857.
139. Werdehausen R, et al. *Br J Anaesth*. 2009;103:711–718.
140. Rigler ML, et al. *Anesth Analg*. 1991;72:275–281.
141. Lambert LA, et al. *Anesthesiology*. 1994;80:1082–1093.
142. Kouri ME, Kopacz DJ. *Anesth Analg*. 2004;98:75–80. Table of contents.
143. Freedman JM, et al. *Anesthesiology*. 1998;89:633.
144. Eberhart LH, et al. *Anaesthetist*. 2002;51:539.
145. Sakura S, et al. *Anesthesiology*. 1997;87:771.
146. Neal JM. *Reg Anesth Pain Med*. 2003;28:124–134.
147. Sakura S, et al. *Anesth Analg*. 1995;81:338.
148. Brun A. *Acta Anaesthesiol Scand*. 1959;3:59–73.
149. Gerner P. *Reg Anesth Pain Med*. 2004;29:286–289.
150. Sudoh Y, et al. *Pain*. 2003;103:49–55.
151. Schwarz SK, et al. *Anesthesiology*. 2010;113:438–444.
152. Joshi GP, et al. *J Surg Orthop Adv*. 2015;24:27–35.
153. Ilfeld BM, et al. *Anesth Analg*. 2013;117:1248–1256.
154. Vandepitte C, et al. *Reg Anesth Pain Med*. 2017;42:334–341.
155. Lobo K, et al. *Anesthesiology*. 2015;123:873–885.
156. Yang Y, et al. *J Med Genet*. 2004;41:171–174.
157. Goldberg YP, et al. *Clin Genet*. 2007;71:311–319.
158. Lee JH, et al. *Cell*. 2014;157:1393–1404.
159. Binshtok AM, et al. *Anesthesiology*. 2009;111:127–137.
160. Bromage PR, et al. *J Clin Pharmacol*. 1969;9:30.
161. Lund C, et al. *Lancet*. 1985;2:1156.
162. Lee KC, et al. *Anesthesiology*. 1994;81:1284.
163. Wilder RT, et al. *Anesth Analg*. 1996;83:1251.
164. Choi RH, et al. *Life Sci*. 1997;61:PL177.
165. Yarov-Yarovoy V, et al. *J Biol Chem*. 2001;276:20–27.
166. Panigel J, Cook SP. *J Neurogenet*. 2011;25:134–139.
167. Clendenen N, et al. *Minerva Anestesiol*. 2016;82:1089–1097.
168. Trescot AM. *Pain Physician*. 2003;6:291–293.
169. Panditrao MM, et al. *Indian J Anaesth*. 2013;57:236–240.
170. Israel MR, et al. *Adv Pharmacol*. 2017;79:67–116.

SECTION III

ANESTHESIA MANAGEMENT

30 Risk of Anesthesia

RACHEL A. HADLER, MARK D. NEUMAN, and LEE A. FLEISHER

KEY POINTS

- Perioperative risk is multifactorial and may occur as a result of anesthesia-, surgery-, and/or patient-specific factors.
- Anesthesia-related (and surgery-related) risk is typically defined as morbidity and mortality occurring within 30 days of surgery, although events that occur at later points may still be related to anesthesia and/or surgery.
- The overall risk of anesthesia relates to both specific, organ-based complications and the rapidity with which they are managed (i.e., rescued).
- In the literature on anesthesia-related risk, the rates of morbidity and mortality reported across studies show a substantial variability in part attributable to the wide variety of definitions used in these studies.
- Historical studies of anesthesia-related risk identified anesthesia-related respiratory depression as the major cause of death and coma totally attributable to anesthesia. This finding prompted the creation of postanesthesia care units (PACUs).
- Research into anesthesia-related cardiac arrest has found it to be attributable to medication administration, airway management, and technical problems of central venous access.
- Multivariate modeling can be used to determine specific factors associated with an increased likelihood of adverse postoperative events, and it has been used to define a range of clinical risk indices to predict postoperative outcomes.
- Surveys of maternal mortality suggest that although the absolute rate of complications attributable to anesthesia has not decreased over time, the increased use of regional anesthesia may have led to improvements in outcome.
- Medication-related and cardiovascular events were the most common causes of cardiac arrest in the Pediatric Perioperative Cardiac Arrest (POCA) Registry.
- Growth in the number and variety of surgical procedures performed in hospital outpatient departments, ambulatory surgery centers, and physician offices creates novel challenges for assessing and managing perioperative risk.
- Initiatives established over time by the Anesthesia Patient Safety Foundation, the American Society of Anesthesiologists (ASA), and others have sought to decrease the potential risks of anesthesia through systems-level improvements, standardization of care processes, human-factors engineering, and simulation-based training.
- Emerging evidence suggests that the choice of anesthetic drugs, ventilator strategies, or technique may impact patient outcomes.

Introduction

Since the beginning of its modern history, the administration of anesthesia has been recognized as a hazardous enterprise,[1] with distinct risks to the patient and occupational risks to anesthesia providers. From the perspective of public health, understanding both the nature and the magnitude of these risks is important on multiple levels. For individual patients, receiving accurate information on the probability of specific perioperative complications is a prerequisite for informed decision making related to anesthesia and surgery. More broadly, understanding the extent to which rates of perioperative morbidity and mortality vary across patients, physicians, and hospitals provides an important opportunity for assessing and improving quality in healthcare.

Efforts to determine the risks of anesthesia are complicated by many potential perspectives from which such risks can be defined. The use of alternate periods of observation for morbidity and mortality—the intraoperative period alone, the first 48 hours after surgery, the duration of the hospital stay, or the first 30 days or longer after surgery—complicates simple conclusions about the risks faced by any individual patient undergoing anesthesia and surgery and at what point after surgery the likelihood of further adverse events has returned to baseline (Table 30.1). For example,

TABLE 30.1 Time Perspective of Anesthetic Morbidity and Mortality Studies

Study	Study Year	Time Perspective
Beecher and Todd	1954	All deaths on the surgical services
Dornette and Orth	1956	Deaths in the surgical unit or after failure to regain consciousness
Clifton and Hotten	1963	Any death under or attributable to anesthesia or without return of consciousness after anesthesia
Harrison	1978	Death within 24 h
Marx et al.	1973	Death within 5 days
Hovi-Viander	1980	Death within 3 days
Lunn and Mushin	1982	Death within 6 days
Tiret and Hatton	1986	Complications within 24 h
Mangano et al.	1992	Death within 2 years
Monk et al.	2005	Death within 1 year

Modified from Derrington MC, Smith G. A review of studies of anaesthetic risk, morbidity, and mortality. *Br J Anaesth*. 1987;59(7):815–833.

TABLE 30.2 Examples of Common Outcome Measures

Outcome	Example
Mortality Failure-to-rescue	Mortality after a postoperative complication
Morbidity Major	Myocardial infarction Pneumonia Pulmonary embolism Renal failure or insufficiency Postoperative cognitive dysfunction
Minor	Nausea Vomiting Readmission
Patient satisfaction Quality of life	

patients undergoing ambulatory surgery have the lowest risk of death the day of surgery as opposed to 1 month later.[2] At the opposite end of the spectrum, asymptomatic release of cardiac enzymes in the perioperative period can have implications for months to years.[3-5] Divergent conclusions would also be expected from studies that consider adverse events that are solely attributable to the administration of anesthesia versus those that examine the overall rates of morbidity and mortality after surgery, which anesthesia care may modify. Studies exclusively focusing on the intraoperative period have characterized contemporary anesthesia care as a patient safety "success story" as a result of the low rates of death directly attributable to anesthesia care. As a result, anesthesia has been hailed by the National Academy of Medicine as "an area in which very impressive improvements have been made" in terms of patient safety.[6]

Nonetheless, a broader perspective on perioperative outcomes presents a more complicated story. For example, in the case of a patient with established coronary artery disease who sustains a myocardial infarction after experiencing tachycardia during high-risk surgery, the cause of the patient's adverse outcome could arguably be attributed to both the patient's underlying coronary artery disease and to the absence of intraoperative heart rate control. In this situation, the decision to view the perioperative infarction primarily as a consequence of patient disease or as an event that could be prevented by anesthesia care carries vastly different implications for efforts to define and reduce the risks of anesthesia.

Finally, the diverse array of outcomes considered as hazards of anesthesia complicate the interpretation of the literature on the risks of anesthesia. Traditionally, investigators have focused on issues of death and major morbidity such as myocardial infarction, pneumonia, and renal failure. More recently, however, this view has been broadened to include economic outcomes, as well as patient-centered outcomes such as functional independence, quality of life, and satisfaction (Table 30.2). For example, unanticipated rehospitalization after ambulatory surgery or a delay in discharge as a result of postoperative nausea and vomiting are both potentially important from the perspectives of the patient's quality of life, as well as economics.

In this chapter, current theories regarding the underlying causes of adverse events in the perioperative period are reviewed, and the historical and contemporary literature regarding the nature and magnitude of risk related to both intraoperative anesthesia care and perioperative care are examined. Next, historical and recent efforts to characterize the patient-, provider-, and facility-level determinants of anesthetic and perioperative risk are reviewed through statistical risk indices, and clinically based approaches to patient classification, and available literature on the determinants of risk unique to the obstetric, pediatric, and geriatric populations are discussed. Finally, future directions in research and clinical care related to anesthetic risk are discussed, with a focus on the health policy implications of changing knowledge regarding the hazards of anesthesia.

Framework of Perioperative Risk

Perioperative risk is multifactorial and depends on the interaction of anesthesia-, patient-, and surgery-specific factors (Fig. 30.1). With respect to anesthesia, the selection and effects of medications, including volatile and intravenous anesthetic drugs, and the skills of the practitioner are important. Similarly, the surgeon's skills and the surgical procedure itself also affect perioperative risk. Further, practitioners may influence outcomes at multiple points in the postoperative course. Although the incidence of specific local or organ-based complications, such as perioperative myocardial infarction or central line–related bloodstream infection, may be modified by anesthetic or surgical care, variations in the adequacy of care delivered to patients who have already experienced a complication (i.e., failure to rescue) may largely explain hospital-to-hospital differences in surgical outcomes.[7-9] Notably, although past investigators have pointed to volume-outcome relationships as potentially mitigating these hospital-to-hospital outcome

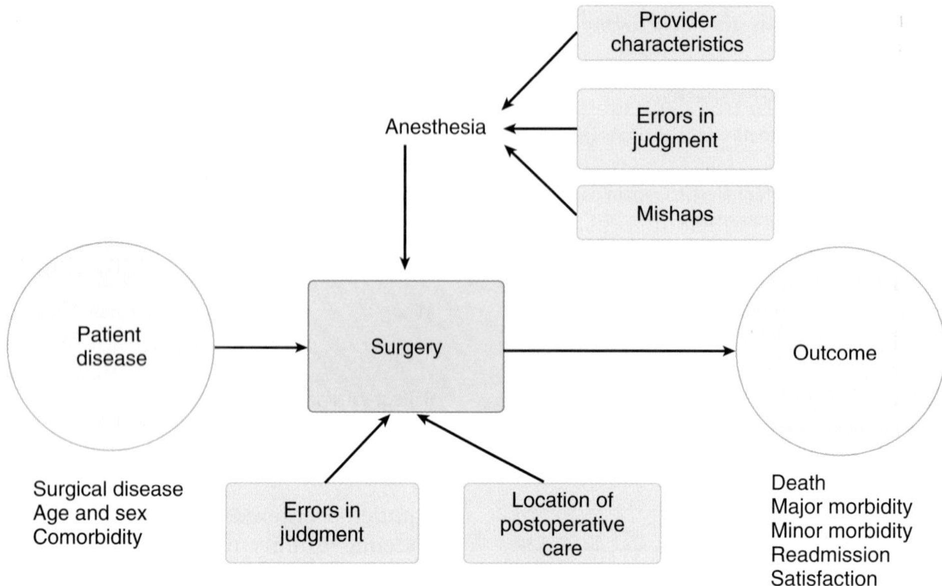

Fig. 30.1 Representation of the influences of various components on poor perioperative outcomes. Surgical, anesthetic, and patient characteristics all contribute to outcome. Anesthesia-related contributions can include issues of judgment and mishaps, as well as characteristics of the provider. The surgical procedure itself affects outcome, as does the location of intraoperative and postoperative care.

differences,[10,11] more recent data have suggested that local quality-improvement efforts, rather than large-scale efforts, at regionalization of care for elective surgeries hold the greatest potential to yield meaningful improvements in operative outcomes.[12]

The potential for anesthetic care to influence the overall hazard of surgery at multiple time points highlights both the complexity of measuring the risks of anesthesia and surgery, and the range of potential opportunities that may exist to reduce such risks. Given these challenges and opportunities, the goal of the next section is to summarize the current state of knowledge in this area, including the relative strengths and weaknesses of randomized and nonrandomized (i.e., observational) study designs used in efforts to understand patterns of outcomes after surgery and anesthesia.

Issues Related to Study Design

TYPES OF STUDIES

To interpret the literature related to anesthetic and perioperative risk, the strengths and limitations of various study designs must be understood. *Prospective cohort studies* involve the identification of a group of subjects who are monitored over time for the occurrence of an outcome of interest. The goal is to identify patients in whom the outcome develops. For studies of perioperative mortality, individual cases can be reviewed to determine the cause of mortality. Alternatively, data on all patients in the cohort study can be obtained, and discrete factors associated with the development of morbidity or mortality can be determined, often using multivariate regression techniques. An example of a prospective cohort study to identify factors associated with perioperative cardiac morbidity and mortality is that of Goldman and colleagues,[13] which led to development of the Cardiac Risk Index.

Although prospective cohort studies have important value in identifying risk factors for perioperative outcomes, they also have significant limitations. The range of patients enrolled in the cohort study, both in terms of baseline characteristics and the care they receive, may impact the generalizability of the study findings. Additional biases may be introduced by loss of patients to follow-up. Failure to anticipate the potential impact of some variables and collect data on them may limit the insights gained from a cohort study. Similarly, the inability to collect data on all potential confounders of the relationship between a putative risk factor and a given outcome limits the extent to which cohort studies can support causal inferences.

Randomized clinical trials offer stronger evidence of causality than do observational cohort studies. In a randomized trial, subjects are assigned by random allocation to one of two or more treatments (potentially including a placebo) and are observed for the development of a particular outcome. In the context of perioperative risk, randomized trials may be used to determine the efficacy of an intervention or anesthetic regimen intended to improve postoperative outcomes. For example, hypothermia in the perioperative period has been associated with an increased incidence of perioperative ischemia, a surrogate marker for morbidity.[14] In a randomized clinical trial, the use of forced-air warming to maintain normothermia was associated with a significantly less frequent incidence of perioperative morbid cardiac events.[15] Randomized clinical trials often build on hypotheses generated in cohort studies regarding the determinants of outcomes by testing interventions directed at a specific risk factor associated with adverse outcomes.

Randomized clinical trials derive their strength from their high degree of internal validity; the randomization scheme and the use of placebo (or accepted alternative treatments) provide strong evidence that the results are related to the intervention. Importantly, these trials may have a lower degree of external validity because the intervention tested in a particular trial may not work as well or in the same manner as when it is diffused into a more heterogeneous population. Further, as a result of sample size limitations, clinical trials may often be unable to detect subtle differences in outcomes among study groups or differences in rare events.

Retrospective studies involve the identification of patients who have sustained an outcome and definition of risk factors associated with the outcome. An example of a retrospective design is a case-control study. *Case-control studies* identify patients with the outcome of interest. Frequently, these patients are included as part of a prospective cohort study. The prevalence of a risk factor in patients with the outcome (i.e., cases) is compared with the prevalence of the risk factor in matched control participants to maximize the efficiency and power of the results. The ratio of cases to control participants can be varied to yield greater power with an increasing number of controls. An alternative retrospective design involves the systematic review of identifiable adverse events for patterns of error. For example, Cheney and colleagues[16] developed the American Society of Anesthesiologists' Closed Claims Project (ASA-CCP) to assess the risks associated with anesthesia care. By obtaining the records of major events that led to legal litigation, they were able to identify factors that contributed to bad outcomes. With this methodology, selected morbidities that led to litigation can be identified. The limitation of this methodology is that the actual rates of complications in the overall population are not known; only the number of closed legal claims is identified. Cases that do not result in litigation are not included in the database.

PROBLEMS INHERENT IN STUDYING ANESTHESIA-RELATED RISK

Studying anesthesia-related risk involves a range of methodologic challenges. On the most basic level, multiple definitions exist for key outcomes, such as perioperative mortality. In particular, the timeframe in which a death can be attributed to the surgery or the delivery of anesthesia or both varies. Notably, many events related to surgery may occur after discharge when monitoring of outcomes becomes more challenging. For this reason, the National Surgical Quality Improvement Program (NSQIP), a large, prospectively collected U.S. registry of surgical care and outcomes, requires 30-day follow-up on all patients to allow for consistent assessments of outcomes for all patients.

A second major challenge in any study of postoperative outcomes is the low observed rate of many key outcomes in the population of interest. Although some recent writers have called into question the safety of contemporary anesthesia care,[17] anesthesia-related death remains relatively uncommon in absolute terms. For example, the rate of anesthesia-related mortality described in the Confidential Enquiry into Perioperative Deaths (CEPOD) of 1987 was 1 in 185,000 patients as opposed to the 1 in 2680 cases reported by Beecher and Todd approximately 30 years earlier.[18,19] As a result, efforts to identify the range of factors that now contribute to anesthetic mortality are likely to require large patient cohort studies available either from administrative sources or collected over several years from multiple institutions. Several attempts have been made to establish large epidemiologic databases to address this challenge. One example of such an approach has been the work of Dennis Mangano and the Multicenter Study of Perioperative Ischemia Research Group with regard to cardiac surgery. This group used its database to evaluate issues such as the rate and importance of atrial fibrillation after cardiac surgery and the association of perioperative use of aspirin with cardiac surgical outcomes.[20,21] Other approaches include the development of cardiac surgery databases by the Society of Thoracic Surgeons, the U.S. Veterans Administration NSQIP, and the Northern New England Cardiovascular Disease Study Group.[22-25] These databases are used to define risk factors for poor outcome, to compare local with national complication rates, and as educational tools. In the United States, the Multicenter Perioperative Outcomes Group has undertaken such an enterprise by pooling electronically collected intraoperative and postoperative data.[26] Although these databases may provide extremely important information to improve care, the ability to generalize results to centers that do not have sufficient infrastructure to participate in such projects (e.g., smaller hospitals) is unknown.

Variations in care and outcomes across institutions may further complicate efforts to develop meaningful estimates of perioperative risk for use in clinical decision making by individual patients. Beyond the impact of patient illness, type of surgery, or anesthetic approach, hospital-level differences in postoperative care may have a profound impact on outcome. For example, the incidence of pulmonary embolism may be related to nursing care and the frequency of patient ambulation after surgery[27]; similarly, the presence of an intensivist who makes daily rounds and higher nurse staffing ratios may also affect outcome.[28]

Finally, issues of risk adjustment complicate efforts to determine changes in anesthesia risk over time. Common endpoints, such as mortality, are influenced by patient factors as well as by anesthesia and surgical care; as such, temporal trends in patient acuity may influence the apparent adverse outcomes associated with anesthesia and surgery in a given period. With appropriate risk adjustment, changes in mortality rates over short periods may provide some indication of changes in the quality of anesthesia or surgical care. When viewed over longer periods, however, it may be more difficult to reach firm conclusions regarding temporal changes in the safety of anesthesia or surgery based on differences in mortality rates over time. For example, if improvements in anesthetic technology have allowed for older and sicker patients to undergo surgery, then the safety of anesthesia may have improved without any apparent change in mortality rates because a sicker patient population is now offered surgery that, in the past, would have been avoided. Similarly, the rapid adoption of new but relatively high-risk procedures complicates simple comparisons of anesthesia-related complications over time.

STUDIES OF ANESTHESIA-RELATED MORTALITY

Efforts to understand the specific risks imposed by anesthesia care, above and beyond the surgical procedure itself, have represented an important dimension of research in anesthesia since the early 20th century. Although more recent trends in anesthesia research have emphasized a

TABLE 30.3 Estimates of the Incidence of Mortality Related to Anesthesia Before 1980

Study	Year	Number of Anesthetics	Primary Cause	Primary and Associated Causes
Beecher and Todd	1954	599,548	1:2680	1:1560
Dornette and Orth	1956	63,105	1:2427	1:1343
Schapira et al.	1960	22,177	1:1232	1:821
Phillips et al.	1960	—	1:7692	1:2500
Dripps et al.	1961	33,224	1:852	1:415
Clifton and Hotton	1963	205,640	1:6048	1:3955
Memery	1965	114,866	1:3145	1:1082
Gebbie	1966	129,336	—	1:6158
Minuck	1967	121,786	1:6766	1:3291
Marx et al.	1973	34,145	—	1:1265
Bodlander	1975	211,130	1:14,075	1:1703
Harrison	1978	240,483	—	1:4537
Hovi-Viander	1980	338,934	1:5059	1:1412

From Ross AF, Tinker JH. Anesthesia risk. In: Miller RD, ed. *Anesthesia*, ed 3. New York, NY: Churchill Livingstone; 1990;722.

broad view of perioperative outcomes not strictly limited to events primarily caused by anesthesia care,[30] the history of efforts to determine the safety of anesthesia management represents an important chapter in the development of modern perioperative medicine. This history also serves as important background for understanding current research and practice.

Research performed before 1980 demonstrated wide variation in reported rates of anesthesia-related mortality (Table 30.3). Beecher and Todd's 1954 report of anesthesia-related deaths at 10 institutions represents the earliest published major analysis of anesthesia outcomes.[18] Their study included 599,548 anesthesia procedures and found a rate of all-cause mortality of 1 per 75 cases (1.3%). In 1 out of every 2680 procedures, anesthesia represented the primary cause of mortality, and it was a primary or contributory cause of mortality in 1 of 1560 procedures. The work of Dornette and Orth[31] investigating perioperative deaths over a 12-year period at their institution corroborated these findings: they reported a mortality rate attributable to anesthesia in 1 in 2427 cases, and totally or partially attributable to anesthesia in 1 in 1343 cases. In contrast, Dripps and colleagues found the anesthesia-attributable mortality rate to be 1 in 852 in a similar single-institution longitudinal study.[32] These differences may be partially explained by Dripps' observation of 30-day, rather than intraoperative or 48-hour mortality, or differences in patient severity across studies.

Multiple additional studies on anesthetic mortality appeared between 1960 and 1980.[33] In the United States, these included the Baltimore Anesthesia Study Committee,[34] which reviewed 1024 deaths occurring on the day of or the day after a surgical procedure, and several single-institution studies.[35,36] Overall, the rate of anesthesia-related mortality in these studies varied

TABLE 30.4 Incidence of Complications Partially or Totally Related to Anesthesia

Complications	Partially Related	Totally Related	Total*
All complications	1:1887	1:1215	1:739
Death	1:3810	1:13,207	1:1957
Death and coma	1:3415	1:7924	1:2387

*Total number of anesthetics: 198,103. From Tiret L, Desmonts JM, Hatton F, Vourc'h G. Complications associated with anaesthesia—a prospective survey in France. *Can Anaesth Soc J*. 1986;33:336–344.

widely, ranging from 1 in 1232 cases in a study by Schapira et al[35] to 1 in 7692 cases in the Baltimore Anesthesia Study Committee report. Results from the international community during that period were similarly heterogeneous in methodology and findings.[37-40]

Studies of anesthetic risk published before 1980 varied widely in the definitions used for anesthesia-related mortality and in the mortality rates they reported; however, they suggested that death related solely to anesthesia was a relatively uncommon event. Moreover, an overall trend toward lower rates of anesthesia-related mortality across studies over time suggested potential improvements in anesthesia safety.

Studies since 1980 have generally been performed on a regional or national basis with a particular emphasis on documenting changes over time in anesthesia-related mortality. For example, Holland[41] reported deaths occurring within 24 hours after anesthesia in New South Wales, Australia. The incidence of anesthesia-attributable deaths decreased from 1 in 5500 procedures performed in 1960 to 1 in 26,000 in 1984. Based on these estimates, the investigators asserted that for all patients receiving surgery, it was more than five times safer to undergo anesthesia in 1984 than it was in 1960.[42]

Under the direction of the French Ministry of Health, Tiret and colleagues[43] carried out a prospective survey of complications associated with anesthesia in France between 1978 and 1982 from a representative sample of 198,103 anesthesia procedures from hospitals throughout the country. Death was solely related to anesthesia in 1 in 13,207 procedures and partially related in 1 in 3810 (Table 30.4). The French survey confirmed previous findings that major complications occur more frequently in older patients, those undergoing emergency surgical procedures, and those with more extensive comorbid conditions as measured by ASA physical status classification. More notably, the investigators found that postanesthesia respiratory depression was the leading principal cause among cases of death and coma that were solely attributable to anesthesia. Moreover, almost all the patients who had had respiratory depression leading to a major complication had received narcotics, as well as neuromuscular blocking drugs, but they had not received anticholinesterase medications for reversal of the agents.

Despite these observations, the low rates of anesthesia-attributable mortality documented in the French study offered compelling evidence of improvements in anesthesia safety. Such findings were reinforced by other, concurrent work in Finland[44] and in the United Kingdom,[45] resulting in the development of the United Kingdom CEPOD, which

TABLE 30.5 Death Totally Attributable to Each Component of Risk in the Confidential Enquiry into Perioperative Deaths

Component	Mortality Rate Contribution
Patient	1:870
Operation	1:2860
Anesthetic	1:185,056

Modified from Buck N, Devlin HB, Lunn JL. Report of a confidential enquiry into perioperative deaths. Nuffield Provincial Hospitals Trust, The King's Fund Publishing House, London, 1987.

TABLE 30.6 Most Common Clinical Causes of Death in the Confidential Enquiry into Perioperative Deaths

Cause of Death	Percent of Total
Bronchopneumonia	13.5
Congestive heart failure	10.8
Myocardial infarction	8.4
Pulmonary embolism	7.8
Respiratory failure	6.5

Modified from Buck N, Devlin HB, Lunn JL. Report of a confidential enquiry into perioperative deaths, Nuffield Provincial Hospitals Trust, The King's Fund Publishing House, London, 1987.

assessed almost 1 million anesthetics during a 1-year period in 1987 in three large regions of the United Kingdom.

Beyond confirming earlier work, CEPOD's findings suggested that anesthesia care was far safer than had been found in prior studies. Examining deaths within 30 days of surgery, CEPOD investigators observed 4034 deaths in an estimated 485,850 surgeries for a crude mortality rate of 0.7% to 0.8%. Anesthesia was considered the sole cause of death in only three individuals, for a rate of 1 in 185,000 cases, and anesthesia was contributory in 410 deaths, for a rate of 7 in 10,000 cases (Table 30.5).[19] The five most common causes of death in the CEPOD cohort study are shown in Table 30.6. Notably, of the 410 perioperative deaths, gastric aspiration was identified in 9 cases and cardiac arrest in 18 cases. Ultimately, CEPOD researchers concluded that avoidable factors were present in approximately 20% of the perioperative deaths. Contributing factors for anesthesiologists and surgeons tended to be failure to act appropriately with existing knowledge (rather than a lack of knowledge), equipment malfunction, fatigue, and inadequate supervision of trainees, particularly in off-hours shifts (Table 30.7).

Large national studies performed since the 1987 CEPOD report vary in the extent to which their findings agree with those of the CEPOD investigators. In a prospective study of 7306 anesthesia procedures in Denmark, Pedersen and colleagues[46] found complications attributable to anesthesia in 43 patients (1 in 170) and 3 deaths (1 in 2500), an incidence far higher than that documented by the CEPOD investigators. Complications in the 43 patients, in order of incidence, included cardiovascular collapse in 16 (37%), severe postoperative headache after regional anesthesia in 9 (21%), and awareness under anesthesia in 8 (19%).

TABLE 30.7 Grade of Physician According to Time of Surgery in the Confidential Enquiry into Perioperative Deaths

	ANESTHETIST		SURGEON	
Grade	**Day***	**Night†**	**Day***	**Night†**
Consultant	50	25	45	34
Others	50	75	55	66

*Represents Monday through Friday, 9 AM to 7 PM.
†Represents Monday through Friday, 7 PM to 9 AM, and Saturday and Sunday.
Modified from Buck N, Devlin HB, Lunn JL. Report of a confidential enquiry into perioperative deaths, Nuffield Provincial Hospitals Trust, The King's Fund Publishing House, London, 1987.

In the United States, Li and colleagues[47] conducted a population-level study to estimate epidemiologic patterns of anesthesia-related deaths, using International Classification of Diseases (ICD) codes listed in the United States multiple-cause-of-death data files for the years 1999 through 2005. Although the interpretation of Li's study is complicated by questions surrounding the sensitivity of ICD codes for anesthesia-related mortality,[48] their findings are in accord with those of the CEPOD report in presenting anesthesia-related mortality to be an extremely rare cause of death at the population level. The authors found anesthesia to be the underlying cause of death in 34 patients each year in the United States and a contributing factor in another 281 deaths annually, resulting in a 97% decrease in anesthesia-related death rates since the 1940s.

Recent European studies have taken a broader focus beyond anesthesia-related events to examine perioperative outcomes more generally, particularly among high-risk patients who Lagasse and others previously observed to account for the majority of postoperative deaths.[17] In a 2011 report, NCEPOD investigators prospectively collected data on all patients undergoing inpatient surgery, excluding obstetric, cardiac, transplant, or neurosurgery cases, in United Kingdom National Health Service facilities over a 1-week period.[49] In addition to prospectively collected patient-level data on clinical care and outcomes, the authors conducted a detailed institution-level survey of resources and practices. Although the authors observed an overall 30-day mortality rate of 1.6%, a subset of high-risk patients—approximately 20% of the full cohort—experienced a disproportionate share of adverse outcomes, accounting for 79% of all perioperative deaths. Notably, the authors identified important gaps in the perioperative management of these patients. A minority of the high-risk patients were monitored using an arterial line, a central line, or cardiac output monitoring; still more concerning was their observation that 48% of all high-risk patients who died were never admitted to a critical care unit for postoperative management. Similar findings were obtained in another study of surgical outcomes conducted across 28 European countries between April 4 and April 11, 2011.[50] Such patterns, which the authors describe as a "systematic failure in the process of allocation of critical care resources" in Europe, highlight the potential importance of "rescue"—the prevention of mortality among patients who experience postoperative complications—in determining the outcomes of surgical care. Further, to the extent that critical care use among patients who die after surgery is higher in the United States than in the United Kingdom,[51] such differences may offer insight into potential reasons for earlier observations of lower risk-adjusted postoperative mortality among American versus British surgical patients.[52]

In the United States, Whitlock and colleagues[52a] retrospectively analyzed 2,948,842 cases logged in the National Anesthesia Clinical Outcomes Registry between 2010 and 2014. They documented a mortality rate of 33 per 100,000. Increasing ASA physical status, emergency case status, time of day, and age less than 1 year or greater than 65 years were independently associated with perioperative mortality. After adjustment for confounding factors, mortality remained greater for cases started after 6 PM, suggesting that certain factors influencing perioperative mortality might be modifiable. The most common concurrent outcomes in patients who died within 48 hours of anesthesia were hemodynamic instability (35.0%) and respiratory complications (8.1%). Notably, due to data limitations, the authors did not comment on the number of deaths that were anesthesia associated.

In summary, research on anesthesia-related mortality offers a complex and still incomplete picture regarding the risks of anesthesia. Taken from the perspective of the 1987 CEPOD report or the findings of Li and colleagues, modern operative anesthesia could be characterized as an exceedingly safe enterprise with bad outcomes occurring as truly rare events; however, other studies have disputed these findings. More recent work has sought to go beyond efforts to quantify the contribution of anesthesia per se to overall operative risk to explore how anesthesia providers might be able to improve outcomes among high-risk patients—in essence asking not "how safe is anesthesia?" but instead "how can anesthesia providers help make surgery safer?" Ultimately, these studies' differing messages emphasize not only the dynamic nature of anesthesia risk over time, but also highlight important changes in how anesthetic risk has been defined across different periods and how alternate approaches to evaluating, describing, and mitigating such risk may be more or less relevant at a given moment in time.

TABLE 30.8 Selected Cardiac Arrest Series When the Denominator Is Greater Than 40,000 Anesthetics

Study	Years	Total Number of Anesthetics	Rate of Arrest
Hanks and Papper	1947-1950	49,728	1:2,162
Ehrenhaft et al.	1942-1951	71,000	1:2,840
Bonica	1945-1952	90,000	1:6,000
Blades	1948-1952	42,636	1:21,318
Hewlett et al.	1950-1954	56,033	1:2,061
Briggs et al.	1945-1954	103,777	1:1,038
Keenan and Boyan	1969-1978	107,257	1:6,704 (P)
Cohen et al.	1975-1983	112,721	1:1,427 (C)
Tiret et al.	1978-1982	198,103	1:3,358 (C)
Tiret et al.	1978-1982	198,103	1:11,653 (P)
Keenan and Boyan	1979-1988*	134,677	1:9,620 (P)
Newland et al.	1989-1999	72,959	1:14,493 (P)
Newland et al.	1989-1999	72,959	1:7,299 (C)
Olsson et al.	1967-1984	250,543	1:33,000
Biboulet et al.	1989-1995	101,769	1:7,828
Kawashima et al.	1994-1998	2,363,038	1:10,000 (P)
Sprung et al.	1990-2000	518,294	1:20,000 (P)
Braz et al.	1996-2005	53,718	1.9:10,000 (P)

*Since pulse oximetry was introduced in 1984, no preventable respiratory cardiac arrests have occurred.
C, Contributory cause; *P*, primary cause.
Modified from Brown DL. Anesthesia risk: a historical perspective. In: Brown DL, ed. *Risk and Outcome in Anesthesia*. 2nd ed. Philadelphia, PA: Lippincott; 1992:14.

ANALYSIS OF INTRAOPERATIVE CARDIAC ARREST

In an alternative approach to evaluating perioperative mortality specific to anesthesia, several studies have evaluated intraoperative fatal and nonfatal cardiac arrest. In contrast to efforts to estimate the mortality attributable to anesthesia per se, studies of intraoperative cardiac arrest may offer a broader picture of the potential hazards of anesthesia by examining an adverse outcome that is far more common than mortality yet remains highly consequential for long-term outcomes.

These studies offer a range of perspectives on the incidence of intraoperative cardiac arrest and the causes of such events. For example, Keenan and Boyan[53] studied the incidence and causes of cardiac arrest related to anesthesia at the Medical College of Virginia between 1969 and 1983. A total of 27 cardiac arrests occurred during 163,240 procedures, for an incidence of 1.7 per 10,000 cases. Fourteen patients died, for an incidence of 0.9 per 10,000 cases. Pediatric patients had a threefold higher risk of cardiac arrest than did adults, and emergency cases had a sixfold greater risk. Importantly, specific errors in anesthesia management could be identified in 75% of the cases; most common among these were inadequate ventilation and overdose of an inhaled anesthetic. Notably, the investigators identified progressive bradycardia preceding all but one arrest, suggesting that early identification and treatment may prevent complications.

Similar findings were reported by Olsson and Hallen,[54] who studied the incidence of intraoperative cardiac arrest at the Karolinska Hospital in Stockholm, Sweden, from 1967 to 1984. A total of 170 arrests occurred in 250,543 anesthesia procedures performed. Sixty patients died, for a mortality rate of 2.4 per 10,000 procedures. After eliminating cases of inevitable death (e.g., rupture of a cerebral aneurysm, trauma), the rate of mortality caused by anesthesia was 0.3 per 10,000 procedures. The most common causes of anesthesia-related cardiac arrest were inadequate ventilation (27 patients), asystole after succinylcholine (23 patients), and postinduction hypotension (14 patients). The incidence of cardiac arrest was highest in the patients with significant comorbid disease, as assessed by the ASA physical status classification. Notable is the finding that the incidence of cardiac arrest decreased over the study period. These findings were reproduced in other studies, including that of Biboulet and colleagues[55] and Newland and associates.[56]

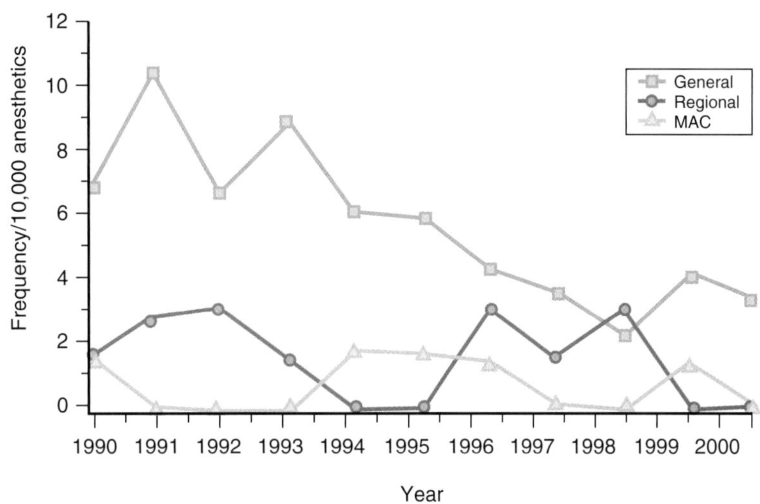

Fig. 30.2 Frequency of cardiac arrest by calendar year and type of anesthesia. *MAC*, Monitored anesthesia care. (From Sprung J, Warner ME, Contreras MG, et al. Predictors of survival following cardiac arrest in patients undergoing noncardiac surgery: a study of 518,294 patients at a tertiary referral center. *Anesthesiology*. 2003;99:259–269.)

TABLE 30.9 Cardiac Arrest Totally Attributable to Anesthesia During Anesthesia and Surgery and Its Outcomes, 1994 to 1998

		OUTCOMES				
	Number of Arrests	**Uneventful Recovery**	**Death in Surgical Unit**	**Death Within 7 Days**	**Vegetative State**	**Others**
5-year total	237	185	13	15	9	15
Incidence per 10,000	1.00	0.78	0.05	0.08	0.04	0.06
95% CI	0.88- ≈1.12	0.66- ≈0.89	0.2- ≈0.08	0.02- ≈0.13	0.03- ≈0.05	0.02- ≈0.10
Ratio	100%	78.1%	5.5%	6.3%	3.8%	6.3%
95% CI		55.3- ≈100	1.7- ≈9.3	3.0- ≈9.7	2.5- ≈5.3	1.7- ≈11.0

N = 2,363,038. *CI*, Confidence interval.
Reproduced with permission from Kawashima Y, Takahashi S, Suzuki M, et al. Anesthesia-related mortality and morbidity over a 5-year period in 2,363,038 patients in Japan. *Acta Anaesthesiol Scand*. 2003;47:809–817.

Sprung and colleagues[57] demonstrated similar findings with regard to incidence and outcome of cardiac arrest during 72,529 procedures between 1989 and 1999 in a teaching hospital in the United States. They also found that the frequency of arrest in patients receiving general anesthesia decreased over time (7.8 per 10,000 during 1990-1992; 3.2 per 10,000 during 1998-2000). The frequency of arrest during regional anesthesia (1.5 per 10,000) and monitored anesthesia care (MAC) (0.7 per 10,000) remained the same during the study period (Fig. 30.2). More recently, Ellis and group[57a] used an institutional quality improvement database to identify all instances of cardiac arrest occurring within a 24-hour perioperative period between 1999 and 2009. They identified 161 arrests in 217,365 anesthetics, 14 of which were found to be anesthesia-attributable (0.6 per 10,000 anesthetics) and 23 that were anesthesia-contributory (1.1 per 10,000). Of anesthesia-attributable events, the majority (64%) were caused by airway complications during induction or emergence. The mortality associated with these events was 29%.

Kawashima and colleagues identified even lower rates of cardiac arrest attributable to anesthesia in a survey-based study conducted in Japan from 1994 through 1998.[58] The average yearly incidence of cardiac arrest during surgery that was totally attributable to anesthesia was 1 per 10,000 cases (95% CI, 0.88-1.12). The average mortality per year in the surgical unit or within seven postoperative days that was totally attributable to anesthesia was 0.21 (0.15-0.27) per 10,000 cases. The two principal causes of cardiac arrest solely attributable to anesthesia were drug overdose or selection error (15.3%) and serious arrhythmia (13.9%). Preventable human errors caused 53.2% of cardiac arrests and 22.2% of deaths in the surgical unit that were totally attributable to anesthesia. The outcomes of cardiac arrests totally attributable to anesthesia are shown in Table 30.9.

Kheterpal and colleagues at the University of Michigan examined predictors of cardiac adverse events—including cardiac arrest, myocardial infarction, and clinically significant arrhythmia—among 7700 patients undergoing noncardiac surgery. Eighty-three patients (1.1%) experienced an adverse event. The authors identified nine independent predictors of an adverse event: (1) age 68 years or older, (2) body mass index of 30 or greater, (3) emergency surgery, (4) previous coronary intervention or cardiac surgery, (5) active congestive heart failure, (6) cerebrovascular disease, (7) hypertension, (8) operative time of 3.8 hours or longer, and (9) the intraoperative administration of one or more units of packed red blood cells.[60]

In summary, perioperative cardiac arrest is a relatively rare event whose incidence may be decreasing over time. Further, research in this area has highlighted the role of both patient factors and intraoperative care as contributing to the risk of intraoperative and postoperative cardiac arrest and emphasized the management of ventilation and the selection and dosing of anesthetic medications as key areas of focus for the prevention of such events.

PERIOPERATIVE MORTALITY AND MORBIDITY IN OUTPATIENT SURGERY

In the United States, an estimated 60% of all surgical procedures are performed on an outpatient basis, and this percentage is increasing annually. The type and extent of surgical procedures performed in an outpatient setting are constantly changing, and more complicated procedures associated with greater perioperative risk are increasingly being performed on an outpatient basis.

Notably, early research on the safety of two ambulatory surgical procedures—tonsillectomy and simple mastectomy—presented a negative view of the hazards of surgery in the outpatient setting. One of the first procedures advocated to be performed on an ambulatory basis was tonsillectomy. Although a 1968 case series of 40,000 outpatient tonsillectomies reported no deaths,[61] details on patient selection and length of postoperative monitoring were vague. Based on insurance company and state mandates, performance of tonsillectomy on an outpatient basis became routine.[62] Beginning in the mid-1980s and continuing in the 1990s, a number of articles evaluated outcomes with early discharge after tonsillectomy. For example, Carithers and colleagues[63] in 1987 at Ohio State University reported on 3000 tonsillectomies and argued that early discharge might be hazardous and economically unwarranted. The rate of readmission for active bleeding between 5 and 24 hours after surgery was reported to be between 0.2% and 0.5%.[64-67] More recently, Cote and his co-investigators in the Society for Pediatric Anesthesia[67a] used a survey instrument as well as analysis of the ASA-CCP to investigate adverse events associated with tonsillectomy in children. They identified a total of 111 events occurring between 1999 and 2010. Death was the most common outcome (66%), followed by neurologic injury (11%) and prolonged hospital stay (10%). Events in children at risk for obstructive sleep apnea (OSA) were more frequently attributed to apnea, whereas children not at risk for OSA were more likely to experience adverse events secondary to hemorrhage. Fifty percent of patients with postoperative events had received postoperative opioids, including 61% of those children who experienced apneic events in the next 24 hours. Events occurred in multiple locations (the operating room, postanesthesia care unit [PACU], and after discharge). In spite of the limitations in the largely self-reported data, these findings clearly suggest that tonsillectomy remains a procedure with significant associated risk, even in the ambulatory setting.

Mastectomy represents a second important case study in the development of surgery as an outpatient procedure. An analysis of Medicare claims demonstrated that the rate of outpatient mastectomy increased from a negligible proportion of all mastectomies in 1986 to 10.8% of all mastectomies performed among Medicare beneficiaries in 1995.[68] Within this population, simple mastectomies performed on an outpatient basis had a significantly higher rate of readmission than did those undergoing a 1-day hospital stay, with an adjusted odds ratio of 1.84. Additionally, rates of readmission after 1-day stays were significantly lower for infection (4.1 vs. 1.8 per 1000 cases), nausea and vomiting (1.1 vs. 0 per 1000 cases), and pulmonary embolism or deep venous thrombosis (1.1 vs. 0 per 1000 cases).

More recent research suggests that, for some procedures, mere exposure to anesthesia in the outpatient setting may present an increased risk for complications. In 2013, Cooper and colleagues[68a] reviewed outcomes for a sample of cancer-free Medicare beneficiaries in the Surveillance, Epidemiology, and End Results database undergoing outpatient colonoscopy without polypectomy, and compared outcomes including hospitalization and aspiration pneumonia for those undergoing procedures with or without deep sedation (anesthesia services). The researchers identified 35,128 (21.2%) procedures with anesthesia services in a total of 100,359 patients; overall complications were more common in patients who had received anesthesia (0.22% vs. 0.16%, $P < .001$). Aspiration was also more common in the anesthesia group (0.14% vs. 0.1%, $P = .02$). Multivariate analysis also demonstrated an increased risk of complications associated with use of anesthesia (odds ratio 1.46, 95% CI 1.09-1.94).

In contrast to these procedure-specific studies, the 1993 publication of Warner and colleagues[69] on major morbidity and mortality within 1 month of ambulatory surgery strongly argued for the safety and feasibility of surgery in the outpatient setting. Among the 38,598 patients included in Warner's study, four died. Of these four deaths, two were due to myocardial infarctions occurring more than 1 week after surgery; the other two deaths occurred in automobile accidents (Fig. 30.3). Partially as a result of these findings, the use of ambulatory surgery has dramatically grown between the early 1990s and the present, with a concurrent increase in the number and type of sites for ambulatory surgery. Such sites now include not only freestanding ambulatory surgery centers (ASCs) and physician's offices, but they also include interventional radiology units and other diagnostic and therapeutic sites not affiliated with any other healthcare facility.

In the context of such growth, investigators have sought to examine the relative safety of similar procedures performed across different outpatient settings. Fleisher and co-workers[2] performed a claims analysis of patients undergoing 16 different surgical procedures in a nationally representative (5%) sample of Medicare beneficiaries for the years 1994 through 1999. A total of 564,267 procedures were studied, with 360,780 in an outpatient hospital, 175,288 in an ASC, and 28,199 in a physician's office. On the day of surgery, no deaths occurred in the office, but four deaths occurred in the ASC (2.3 per 100,000) and nine deaths occurred in the outpatient hospital (2.5 per 100,000). The 7-day mortality rate was 35 per 100,000 in the office setting, 25 per 100,000 in the ASC, and 50 per 100,000 in the outpatient hospital. The rate of admission to an inpatient hospital within 7 days was 9.08 per 1000 in the office, 8.41 per 1000 in the ASC,

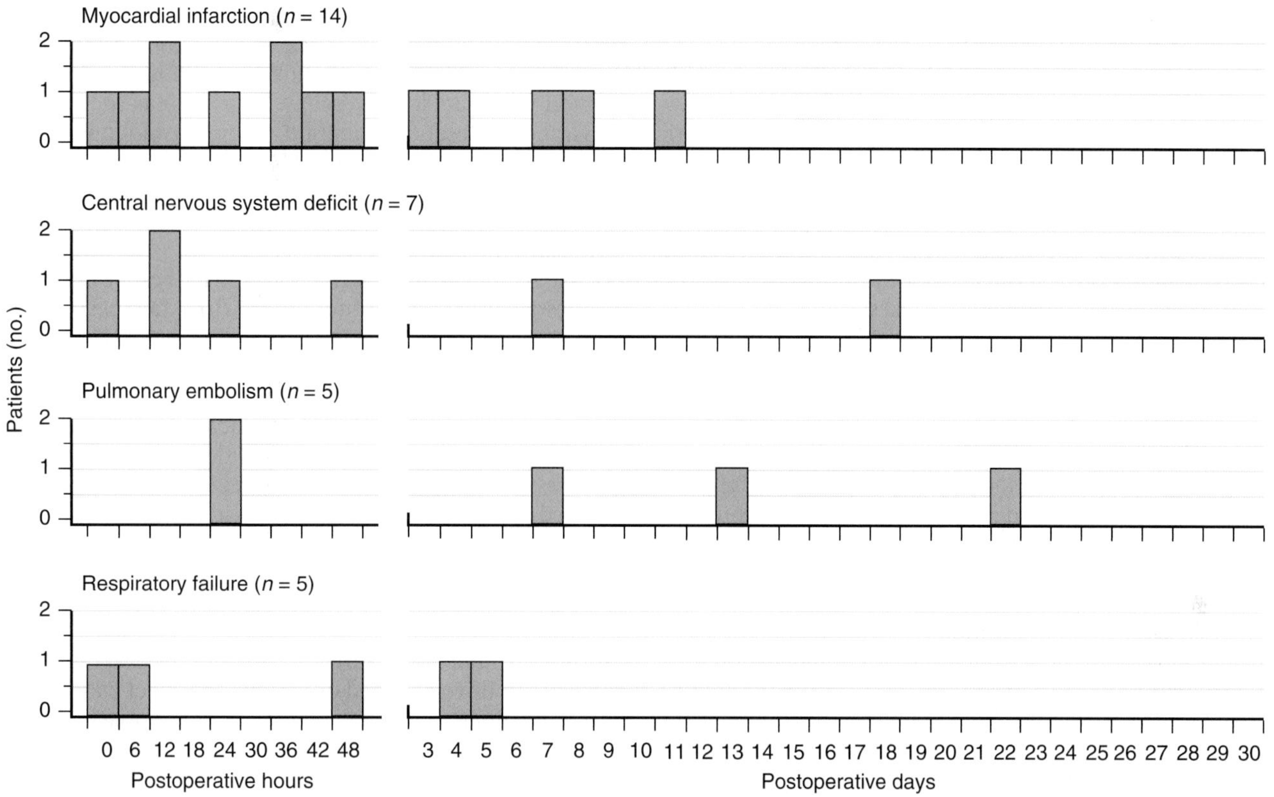

Fig. 30.3 Timing of perioperative events in patients undergoing ambulatory surgery. Many of the events occurring within the first 48 hours are probably related to the stress of surgery. A subset of events occurring after this period may be related to background event rates. The overall rate of morbidity was lower than expected for a similar cohort of age-matched nonsurgical patients. (From Warner MA, Shields SE, Chute CG. Major morbidity and mortality within 1 month of ambulatory surgery and anesthesia. *JAMA*. 1993;270(12):1437–1441.)

and 21 per 1000 in the outpatient hospital. Notably, the inferences of this study are limited by an inability to distinguish fully whether these differences in outcomes are related to the differences in the types of patients selected to have surgery in each setting versus the differences in the care patients received in each setting.

Subsequent work by Chukmaitov and colleagues compared quality outcomes between ASCs and hospital-based outpatient departments in the state of Florida between the years 1997 and 2004.[71] Although their conclusions were limited by differences in the data available for patients treated in each setting, they postulated that the difference in outcomes between the two locations may be related to variations in organizational structure, processes, and strategies.

In contrast to the growing literature on the safety of anesthesia and surgery in ASCs, limited information exists to quantify the incidence of complications in office-based settings. The American Association for Ambulatory Plastic Surgery Facilities mailed a survey to their members to determine the incidence of complications occurring in office facilities.[72] The overall response rate was 57%. The findings showed that 0.47% of patients had at least one complication, including bleeding, hypertension, infection, and hypotension, and 1 in 57,000 patients died. Although low in absolute terms, the observation of a rate of mortality after minor outpatient procedures that is three times the current estimate for anesthesia-related complications is concerning in this context.

Vila and colleagues reviewed all adverse incident reports to the Florida Board of Medicine for procedures dated April 1, 2000, to April 1, 2002.[73] Adverse incidents occurred at a rate of 66 and 5.3 per 100,000 procedures in offices and ASCs, respectively. The death rate per 100,000 procedures performed was 9.2 in offices and 0.78 in ASCs. The relative risk (RR) for injury and death for procedures performed in offices versus ASCs was 12.4 (95% CI, 9.5-16.2) and 11.8 (95% CI, 5.8-24.1), respectively. As a result, the authors concluded that if all office procedures had been performed in ASCs, approximately 43 injuries and 6 deaths per year could have been prevented. However, several other groups have also analyzed the Florida data and have been unable to document the increased risk in the office setting.[74-76]

In summary, although early research on ambulatory surgery placed an emphasis on the undue risks created by premature discharge, more recent analyses confirm that a range of surgeries can be safely performed in properly selected patients. Although some variations in outcomes have been observed across settings (i.e., hospital outpatient department vs. ASC), available literature suggests that, given proper patient selection, outpatient surgeries can be performed with a low rate of adverse events in multiple practice environments. Given the gradual expansion of outpatient surgery over time to include patients with greater burdens of comorbid disease and more extensive procedures, ongoing evaluations will be essential to characterize the dynamic, evolving nature of anesthetic risk in the ambulatory setting.

USE OF ANESTHESIA INFORMATION MANAGEMENT SYSTEMS

Over the past four decades, the use of computerized databases has enhanced the ability to assess perioperative risk and complications.

In one of the earliest computer analyses of postanesthesia deaths, Marx and associates[36] identified 645 individuals who died within 7 days after surgery out of a total cohort of 34,145 consecutive surgical patients. More recently, the growth of electronic anesthesia record systems has allowed for better insights into the causes of anesthesia-related events within the surgical unit, and, when used in combination with other data sources, on postoperative outcomes. An early example of such an analysis was that of Sanborn and colleagues,[77] who used a computer anesthesia record to identify intraoperative incidents. They were able to demonstrate that perioperative deaths occurred more frequently in patients who sustained an intraoperative incident of any type than in those who did not. Reich and colleagues similarly used computerized anesthesia records to evaluate hemodynamic variables and their relationship to risk.[78] They identified pulmonary hypertension, hypotension during cardiopulmonary bypass, and post–cardiopulmonary bypass pulmonary diastolic hypertension as independent predictors associated with mortality, stroke, and perioperative myocardial infarction over and above the effects of other preoperative risk factors.

More recently, data from the University of Michigan anesthesia information management system have been used to identify predictors of perioperative risk, including that of inadequate mask ventilation and of postoperative acute kidney injury. In the former evaluation of 22,660 patients,[79] limited or severely limited mandibular protrusion, abnormal neck anatomy, sleep apnea, snoring, and a body mass index of 30 kg/m^2 or greater were independent predictors of grade 3 or 4 mask ventilation and difficult intubation. Review of 15,102 patients who had a normal preoperative creatinine clearance and underwent noncardiac surgery[80] demonstrated that acute renal failure developed in 121 patients (0.8%), with 14 requiring renal replacement therapy (0.1%). Seven independent preoperative predictors were identified: age, emergency surgery, liver disease, body mass index, high-risk surgery, peripheral vascular occlusive disease, and chronic obstructive pulmonary disease necessitating chronic bronchodilator therapy. Acute renal failure was associated with increased mortality from any cause at 30 days, 60 days, and 1 year.

In an effort to expand upon the insights gained from single-institution studies, two major efforts have since been initiated to pool electronic data on anesthesia care from multiple sites as a means of more effectively comparing outcomes and defining risk factors related to outcomes after anesthesia. The first of these, the Multicenter Perioperative Outcomes Group, was initiated in 2008 under the leadership of investigators at the University of Michigan. This project currently collects electronic anesthesia data from over 50 participating anesthesia departments in two countries. To date, the group has released a series of observational studies, including a report on the risks and outcomes of epidural hematomas after perioperative and obstetric epidural catheterization[26] and a subsequent report evaluating the risk of epidural hematoma after neuraxial anesthesia in thrombocytopenic parturients.[80a] Other projects have evaluated predictors of difficult mask ventilation and intubation via direct laryngoscopy,[80b] as well as the success of a variety of rescue intubation techniques following direct laryngoscopy.[80c] The Multicenter Perioperative Outcomes Group recently established Initiative for Multicenter Perioperative Clinical Trials, an arm dedicated to clinical and translational research.

The second group, the National Anesthesia Clinical Outcomes Registry, is maintained by the Anesthesia Quality Institute, a nonprofit organization established by the ASA. This large-scale data warehouse collects paper and electronic anesthesia case data used to review anesthesia practices with the intent of optimizing local efforts to assess both the risk and the quality of care, and for research purposes for the specialty as a whole. The Registry has released data related to perioperative mortality (cited earlier).

OTHER APPROACHES TO DISCERN THE ROOT CAUSE OF MORBIDITY AND MORTALITY

Although mortality directly attributable to anesthesia appears to have declined over time, the exact causes of this decline remain unclear. Numerous factors have been implicated in the improved outcome, including new monitoring modalities, new anesthetic drugs, and changes in the anesthesia workforce. However, relating the reduced risk to any one factor on the basis of available epidemiologic data is difficult. Further, although the use of newer monitoring modalities, particularly pulse oximetry, would be expected to improve outcomes, no randomized trial has been able to document such a conclusion. This limitation supports the need for continued monitoring of complications and their root cause through a number of approaches.

Initiated by the Professional Liability Committee of the ASA, the ASA-CCP represents one important approach to understanding the root causes of important complications of anesthesia care. The ASA-CCP constitutes an ongoing, nationwide survey of closed insurance claims for major anesthesia-related adverse events. In an early publication based on data collected by the ASA-CCP, Caplan and colleagues reviewed both fatal and nonfatal outcomes resulting in claims against anesthesia providers. Among the fatal events, unexpected cardiac arrest during spinal anesthesia was observed in 14 healthy patients from the initial 900 claims.[81] These cases were analyzed in detail to identify patterns of care that might have led to the event. Two patterns were identified: oversedation leading to respiratory insufficiency and inappropriate resuscitation of high spinal sympathetic blockade.

Tinker and co-workers[82] queried the ASA-CCP to determine the role of monitoring devices in the prevention of anesthesia mishaps. They reviewed 1097 anesthesia-related claims and determined that 31.5% of the negative outcomes could have been prevented by the use of additional monitors, primarily pulse oximetry and capnography. Injuries that were deemed preventable with additional monitoring resulted in dramatically more severe injury and cost of settlement than did those judged to be nonpreventable with additional monitoring. These findings were reinforced by a subsequent study of intraoperative respiratory events by Caplan and colleagues (Table 30.10).[83] These claims represented the single largest class of injury (34%), with death or brain damage occurring in 85% of cases. They identified inadequate ventilation, esophageal intubation, and difficult tracheal intubation as the primary causes of respiratory events. The investigators believed most of the outcomes to be preventable with better monitoring, such as pulse oximetry or capnography (Fig. 30.4).[84] In more recent evaluations of MAC using the ASA-CCP, more than 40% of 121 claims associated with MAC involved death or permanent brain damage. Respiratory depression, after an absolute or relative overdose of sedative or opioid drugs, was the most common (21%, $n = 25$) of the complications.

A similar registry was developed by the Danish Patient Insurance Association.[85] For the years of 1996 through 2004, 1256 files were related to anesthesia, and 24 deaths were considered to be a result of the anesthetic procedure: 4 deaths were related to airway management, 2 to ventilation management, 4 to central venous catheter placement, 4 as a result of medication errors, 4 from infusion pump problems, and 4 after complications from regional blockade. Severe hemorrhage caused one death, and the cause was uncertain in one case.

TABLE 30.10 Distribution of Adverse Respiratory Events in the American Society of Anesthesiologists' Anesthesia Closed Claims Study

Event	Number of Cases	Percent of 522 Respiratory Claims
Inadequate ventilation	196	38
Esophageal intubation	94	18
Difficult tracheal intubation	87	17
Inadequate inspired oxygen concentration	11	2

From Caplan RA, Ward RJ, Posner K, Cheney FW. Unexpected cardiac arrest during spinal anesthesia: a closed claims analysis of predisposing factors. *Anesthesiology*. 1998;68(1):5–11.

Cooper and colleagues[86,87] took an alternate approach to examining perioperative mortality through the study of critical incidents, which were defined as those that were potentially preventable and could lead to undesirable outcomes. This definition included events that led to no harm or only transient effects. The investigation involved collecting data on anesthesia-related human errors and equipment failures from anesthesiologists, residents, and certified registered nurse anesthetists (CRNAs). In a series of reports, the authors identified frequent incidents, such as disconnections in breathing circuits, and causes of discovery of errors, such as intraoperative relief. They confirmed that equipment failure was a small cause of anesthesia mishaps (4%), whereas human error was a predominant factor. They suggested that future studies of anesthesia-related mortality and morbidity should classify events according to a strategy for prevention rather than outcome alone.

Other countries have developed similar databases, such as the Australian Incident Monitoring Study. Data from this database have been used to evaluate problems with ventilation, with vascular access, and in the PACU.[88,89]

ISSUES ASSOCIATED WITH ANESTHESIA-RELATED MORTALITY

The studies detailed in the preceding text focus on intraoperative or in-hospital deaths directly attributable to anesthesia care; nonetheless, perioperative complications may contribute to the risk of mortality beyond the immediate postoperative period. For example, a perioperative stroke or myocardial infarction may lead to death after the period of analysis. Notably, recent research has suggested that even small myocardial infarctions or unstable angina during the perioperative period have been associated with worsened long-term survival.[91] Should these *late* deaths be attributed to anesthesia complications for the purpose of such analyses? The answer depends on the outcome and its relationship to anesthesia management.

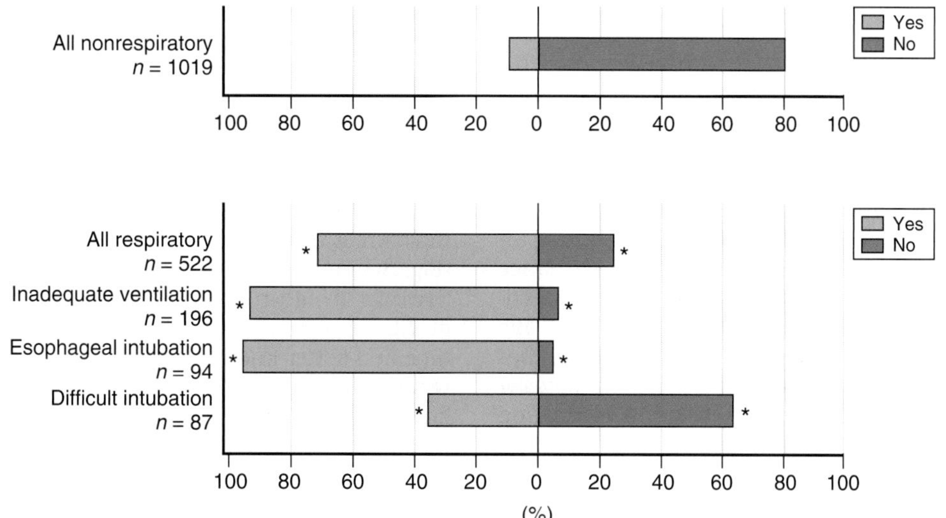

Fig. 30.4 Relationship between adverse events in the American Society of Anesthesiologists' Anesthesia Closed Claims Project and preventable complications. Preventable events related to respiratory complications were significantly more common than those related to all nonrespiratory complications. Of the respiratory complications, difficult intubation had the least number of preventable complications (*$P < .05$ vs. nonrespiratory claims). (From Caplan RA, Posner KL, Ward RJ, Cheney FW. Adverse respiratory events in anesthesia: a closed claims analysis. *Anesthesiology*. 1990;72(5):828–833.)

The potential effects of anesthesia on long-term survival were suggested by Monk and colleagues.[92] Using multivariate Cox proportional hazards models, these investigators identified three variables as significant independent predictors of mortality: patient comorbidity (RR, 16.116), cumulative deep hypnotic time (bispectral index < 45) (RR, 1.244/h), and intraoperative systolic hypotension (RR, 1.036/min). Further work is required to determine whether these results reflect a true pathophysiologic link between perioperative (anesthesia) management and long-term outcome or a simple statistical association. This study and others, however, emphasize the importance of evaluating all aspects of anesthesia care and short- and long-term outcomes to try to optimize both long- and short-term patient outcomes.

Risks Related to Patient Characteristics

Multiple studies have demonstrated that perioperative morbidity and mortality are increased in the presence of coexisting medical diseases. The ASA physical status classification system, originally proposed in 1941,[93] represents a widely used method of classifying the severity of coexisting disease among surgical patients. Since its introduction, this classification system has established a standardized terminology for anesthesia practice and has aided in developing valid statistical comparisons of outcomes among sites.[94]

The correlation between ASA physical status and mortality offers a simple illustration of the link between comorbidities and adverse operative outcomes. In 1961, Dripps and co-workers demonstrated that mortality increased as the severity of comorbid disease increased, as assessed by the ASA physical status classification.[32] Several investigators have reevaluated the relationship between operative mortality and ASA physical status and demonstrated similar findings.[43,46,95]

In Canada, Cohen and colleagues[96] analyzed 100,000 anesthesia procedures and determined mortality within 7 days of surgery by using governmental vital statistics mortality data between the years 1975 and 1984. For each patient, information was collected on age, preoperative conditions, ASA physical status, anesthetic technique, monitors, and other factors. The overall 7-day mortality rate was 71.04 deaths per 10,000 procedures. Risk markers for mortality are detailed in Table 30.11.

TABLE 30.11 Risk Factors Associated With Increased Odds of Dying Within 7 Days For All Cases

Variable	All Procedures: Relative Odds of Dying Within 7 Days	95% Confidence Limits
PATIENT RELATED		
Age (yr)		
60-79 vs. < 60	2.32	1.70-3.17
80+ vs. < 60	3.29	2.18-4.96
Sex (female vs. male)	0.77	0.59-1.00
ASA physical status classification (3-5 vs. 1-2)	10.65	7.59-14.85
SURGERY RELATED		
Major vs. minor	3.82	2.50-5.93
Intermediate vs. minor	1.76	1.24-2.5
Length of anesthesia (≤2 h vs. < 2 h)	1.08	0.77-1.50
	4.44	3.38-5.83
Emergency vs. elective		
OTHER FACTORS		
Year of surgery (1975-1979 vs. 1980-1984)	1.75	1.32-2.31
Complication in the surgical or recovery unit (yes vs. no)	1.42	1.06-1.89
ANESTHESIA RELATED*		
Experience of the anesthetist (>600 procedures for ≥ 8 years vs. <600 procedures for <8 years)	1.06	0.82-1.37
Inhalation with narcotic vs. inhalation alone	0.76	0.51-1.15
Narcotic alone vs. inhalation alone	1.41	1.01-2.00
Narcotic with inhalation vs. inhalation alone	0.79	0.47-1.32
Spinal vs. inhalation alone	0.53	0.29-0.98
Number of anesthetic drugs (1-2 vs. 3)	2.94	2.20-3.84

*All cases performed with the five most frequently used anesthetic techniques.

Modified from Cohen MM, Duncan PG, Tate RB. Does anesthesia contribute to operative mortality? *JAMA*. 1988;260(19):2859–2863.

One of the limitations of the ASA physical status classification system is that the ranking is determined by individual anesthesia providers; as such, there may be variance between providers, as demonstrated by Owens and co-workers.[97] In light of these limitations, other studies have attempted to define the specific patient characteristics that are most strongly associated with perioperative adverse events related to a particular organ system. In evaluating the risk directly related to the patient's condition, the limitations of the methodology must be understood. All such studies evaluate the predictive value of a clinical or laboratory risk factor for a defined perioperative complication. In this approach, a cohort of individuals of interest is defined. Ideally, the study is performed prospectively, and the outcome of interest is assessed in a rigorous, blinded fashion. Despite this, many available studies of perioperative risk factors focus on selected patients and include a retrospective design, methods that greatly limit their generalizability and validity. Many studies use multivariate modeling to determine the factors associated with increased risk. A major limitation in the use of multivariate modeling for this purpose is the assumption that the intraoperative period is a *black box* and that care is not modified by the knowledge of the risk factor (Fig. 30.5). However, anesthesiologists modify intraoperative care of high-risk patients in an attempt to minimize the likelihood of complications. Changes in medical care over time and better knowledge about high-risk patients should result in a reduction of the risk related to specified clinical factors. Such considerations make it difficult to design and complete formal investigations to validate individual management strategies in the context of current practice.

One common approach taken in past efforts to quantify operative risk has been to examine the relationship between a single risk factor and a broad range of adverse perioperative outcomes. For example, numerous studies have evaluated the importance of hypertension on perioperative risk. Goldman

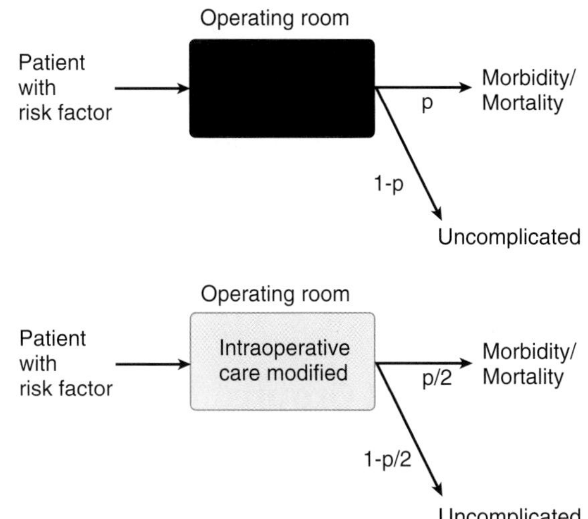

Fig. 30.5 The concept of the black box for risk indices. In developing a risk index, patients with a specific risk factor enter the operating room and have a complication at a rate *p*. If the anesthesiologist is aware of the importance of the risk factor and can modify care to reduce such risk (*p/2*), then the risk factor may no longer be significant. If the risk factor is ignored, then complications may again occur in such patients.

and Caldera[98] evaluated a cohort of patients undergoing noncardiac surgery under general anesthesia. Hypertension was not associated with increased perioperative risk, although the number of patients with diastolic blood pressure greater than 110 mm Hg was too small to draw any statistically significant conclusions. In contrast, Hollenberg and co-workers[99] identified hypertension and the presence of left ventricular hypertrophy as predictors of perioperative ischemia, but they did not consider their independent relationship to perioperative major morbidity. More recently, Baron and colleagues[99a] analyzed data from a prospective study examining perioperative care across 28 European countries to evaluate the impact of hemoglobin levels on in-hospital mortality. Patients with severe (hemoglobin < 8 g/dL) or moderate (8-11 g/dL) levels were found to have higher rates of in-hospital mortality as well as longer length of stay and a higher likelihood of postoperative admission to the intensive care unit.

An alternative to examining the impact of a single risk factor on perioperative outcomes involves a more general effort to identify multiple risk factors for one or more adverse perioperative outcomes. Multiple researchers have undertaken prospective and retrospective cohort studies with the goal of identifying patients at greatest risk for fatal and nonfatal myocardial infarction. One of the earliest attempts to define cardiac risk was performed by Goldman and colleagues at the Massachusetts General Hospital.[13] They studied 1001 patients older than 45 years of age who were undergoing noncardiac surgery. Using multivariate logistic regression, they demonstrated nine clinical factors associated with increased morbidity and mortality. Each risk factor was weighted in the logistic regression equation and converted into points in the index. An increasing number of points was associated with increasing perioperative cardiac morbidity or mortality.

Several attempts have been made to validate the Goldman Cardiac Risk Index in the surgical population.[100,101] The validity of the Cardiac Risk Index is more controversial for patients undergoing vascular surgery. Several groups[102-104] were able to demonstrate a similar, if not identical, pattern of increasing cardiac complication rate with increasing cardiac risk. Several other studies, however, were unable to demonstrate any relationship between the Cardiac Risk Index and perioperative cardiac complications, with a high incidence of complications found in patients with a Cardiac Risk Index of I or II.[105,106] When the ASA physical status classification system was compared with the Goldman Cardiac Risk Index in a cohort of 16,277 patients undergoing noncardiac surgery,[106] both indices demonstrated predictive value, although the objective Goldman Cardiac Risk Index provided little additional value over the more subjective ASA physical status classification.

Since the introduction of the Goldman Cardiac Risk Index, other investigators have put forward alternative risk indices for cardiac events after noncardiac surgery, such as the Detsky Modified Risk Index,[107] which confirms many of the factors identified by Goldman and allows calculation of a pretest probability of complications based on the type of surgery, after which the Detsky Modified Risk Index is applied with the use of a nomogram. The Detsky Modified Risk Index was advocated as the starting point for risk stratification in the American College of Physicians guidelines on preoperative evaluation.[108] Lee and colleagues[109] created a Revised Cardiac Risk Index (RCRI) incorporating six additional risk factors identified in a single-institution study: high-risk type of surgery, history of ischemic heart disease, history of congestive heart failure, history of cerebrovascular disease, preoperative treatment with insulin, and preoperative serum creatinine level higher than 2.0 mg/dL. The rate of major cardiac complications increased with the number of risk factors. The performance of the RCRI was examined in a metaanalysis conducted by Ford and colleagues,[110] who found that although the RCRI showed moderate discrimination for patients at low versus high risk for cardiac events after noncardiac surgery, it did not perform well at predicting death or at predicting cardiac events after vascular surgery.

Gupta and colleagues[111] used data collected by the NSQIP to evaluate the risk for cardiovascular events after noncardiac surgery. This model, which included five variables—type of surgery, dependent functional status, abnormal creatinine level, ASA physical status, and increasing age—demonstrated improved discrimination over the RCRI, which did not improve with the addition of the RCRI score to the model.

Vascular Events in Noncardiac Surgery Patients Cohort Evaluation Study (VISION) is a multinational cohort group actively investigating major perioperative vascular events and their impact on mortality. In a 2016 study of over 15,000 patients in 12 countries, Berwanger and colleagues[111a] noted a reduction in risk of a composite outcome of all-cause mortality, myocardial injury after noncardiac surgery (MINS), and stroke at 30 days (RR = 0.83, 95% CI 0.40-0.83, *P* = .007) associated with preoperative statin use. Perioperative statin use was also associated with a reduction in all-cause mortality, cardiovascular mortality, and MINS; however, there was no statistically significant difference in risk of myocardial infarction or stroke in statin users or non-users.

In a secondary analysis of the same patient cohort, Abbot and group[111b] investigated the association between elevated heart rate preoperatively and MINS within 30 days of surgery. Preoperative heart rate was stratified by deciles. The results showed that 7.9% of participants had sustained MINS, 2.8% myocardial infarction, and 2.0% died. After adjusting for confounders, the highest heart rate decile (preoperative heart rate more than 96 beats/min) was associated with increased risk of perioperative MINS (odds ratio 1.48, $P < .01$), MI (odds ratio 1.71, $P < .01$), and mortality (odds ratio 3.16, $P < .01$). Heart rates in the lowest decline (<60 beats/min) were independently associated with reduced mortality (odds ratio 0.05, $P = .02$). In a second subgroup analysis, preoperative hypercoagulability was associated with a higher risk of MINS.[111c]

Beyond the efforts at identifying those patients most at risk of postoperative cardiovascular events, recent research has sought to develop statistical models for a range of other organ-based preoperative outcomes. These have included risk models for acute kidney injury in cardiac[112] and noncardiac surgery patients,[60] postoperative respiratory failure,[113,114] and stroke after cardiac surgery[115] and carotid endarterectomy.[116]

In contrast to the efforts to determine risk factors for specific organ-based complications, other investigators have sought to develop risk-prediction models to identify those patients at risk of death from any cause in the immediate postoperative period. For example, Glance and colleagues from the University of Rochester used data from the NSQIP to derive and validate a predictive score for 30-day all-cause mortality for noncardiac surgery. They identified three factors that were highly predictive of death at 30 days after surgery: (1) ASA physical status, (2) emergency status, and (3) surgery type. Patients with ASA physical status I, II, III, IV, or V were assigned 0, 2, 4, 5, or 6 points, respectively; intermediate- or high-risk procedures were assigned 1 or 2 points, respectively; and emergency procedures were assigned 1 point. Patients with risk scores less than 5 had a predicted risk of mortality less than 0.5%, whereas patients with a risk score of 5 to 6 had a risk of mortality between 1.5% and 4%. Patients with a risk score greater than 6 had risk of mortality more than 10%.[117]

Beyond their clinical applicability, such risk indices have become important in the context of health policy by allowing for comparisons of risk-adjusted mortality rates across hospitals and physicians providing cardiac surgery. For example, the state of New York annually publishes data on mortality rates associated with coronary bypass grafting by surgeon and by hospital.[118-120] For comparison of rates across institutions, institutional mortality rates are typically risk-adjusted so that high-performing institutions that treat a high percentage of medically complex patients are not spuriously categorized as *poor performers* simply because of the features of their patient mix.

Beyond identifying clinical indicators of perioperative risk, historic and current research has focused on the role of genetics and genomics on the outcomes of major surgical procedures. Notably, the impact of genotype on perioperative risk has been well known since elucidation of the inheritance pattern of malignant hyperthermia. With malignant hyperthermia, a clear link exists between the autosomal dominant disease and an adverse outcome after administration of an anesthetic.[121] Interest in evaluating the impact of genetic polymorphism on overall perioperative outcome is increasing, even if the link to anesthesia is less well defined. For example, apolipoprotein E4 has been shown to modulate neurologic injury and recovery after a variety of acute ischemic insults, including coronary artery bypass grafting.[122] Polymorphism of the glycoprotein IIIa constituent of the platelet integrin receptor has also been correlated with postoperative cognitive decline.[123,124] Further research will be required to determine specific genetic profiles that will impact anesthetic management strategies, drug selection, and other aspects of care.

Special Patient Groups

OBSTETRICS

Anesthesia for the obstetric patient carries unique challenges, since both the mother and the fetus are potentially at risk for complications. Fortunately, maternal mortality is rare, and the anesthesia-related component of maternal delivery represents only a small fraction of all maternal deaths. As a result, studies of peripartum complications require a large number of patients from a diversity of clinical settings.

In parallel to the early efforts to determine the overall risk of anesthesia for surgery, a series of studies were performed between 1974 and 1985 that sought to determine the rate of obstetric complications in the United States and England, and to assess the contribution of anesthesia per se to the risk of adverse events in this group. Kaunitz and coauthors[125] reported an anesthesia-related death rate of 0.6 per 100,000 births with data from all 50 states. Endler and coworkers[126] studied births in Michigan between 1972 and 1984 and found a rate of 0.82 anesthesia-related deaths per 100,000 live births. Eleven of the 15 deaths were associated with cesarean section. Obesity and emergency surgery were risk factors in many patients. Complications related to regional anesthesia were identified as a problem in the earlier years of the study, whereas failure to secure a patent airway was the primary cause of mortality in the later years. No anesthesia-related maternal deaths occurred in the final 2 years of the study. Rochat and colleagues[127] studied 19 areas of the United States between 1980 and 1985 and reported 0.98 anesthesia-related deaths per 100,000 live births. They observed that maternal mortality did not decrease over the time of the study.

The Confidential Enquiry into Maternal Deaths in England and Wales has been assessing maternal deaths since 1952.[128] Morgan[128] reported the maternal deaths from anesthesia between 1952 and 1981 (Table 30.12). The total maternal mortality rate decreased over time, but the percentage of deaths related to anesthesia increased, although the absolute number of deaths associated with anesthesia decreased. Later reports identified technical difficulties with intubation as a major risk factor. The other major finding of this study was that the experience of the anesthesia provider in obstetric anesthesia was the most important factor in anesthesia-related maternal mortality.

More recent investigations have confirmed ongoing decreases over time in the hazards of obstetric anesthesia. Hawkins and associates[129] obtained data from the ongoing National Pregnancy Mortality Surveillance System of the

Centers for Disease Control and Prevention on births and fetal deaths from 1979 through 1990 to determine the possible risk related to anesthesia for obstetrics. They identified a total of 129 women who died of anesthesia-related causes during the study period. Most (82%) of the deaths occurred during cesarean section, and the incidence of anesthesia-related maternal mortality decreased over time (Table 30.13), possibly the result of a trend toward a greater use of neuraxial techniques. Importantly, among maternal deaths that occurred in the context of general anesthesia for cesarean delivery, 73% were related to airway problems.

In a subsequent study, Panchal and colleagues[130] conducted a retrospective case-control study using patients' records from a state-maintained anonymous database of deliveries between 1984 and 1997. Of the 822,591 hospital admissions for delivery during the 14-year study period, 135 maternal deaths occurred. The most common diagnoses associated with mortality during hospital admission for delivery were preeclampsia or eclampsia (22.2%), postpartum hemorrhage or obstetric shock (22.2%), pulmonary complications (14%), blood clot or amniotic embolism or both (8.1%), and anesthesia-related complications (5.2%). Notably, Panchal's study recorded differences by race in the rate of maternal death per 100,000 live births per year (Fig. 30.6). Although the potential causes of this difference remain to be elucidated, Panchal's findings also suggested potential improvements over time in both the overall risk of maternal mortality, as well as the degree to which such risk differed by race.

TABLE 30.12 Maternal Mortality Figures Obtained from the Confidential Enquiry into Maternal Deaths in England and Wales

Years	Maternal Mortality Per 1000 Total Births	Number of Deaths from Anesthesia	Percent of True Maternal Deaths from Anesthesia	Percent With Avoidable Factors
1952-1954	0.53	49	4.5	—
1955-1957	0.43	31	3.6	77
1958-1960	0.33	30	4.0	80
1961-1963	0.26	28	4.0	50
1964-1966	0.20	50	8.7	48
1967-1969	0.16	50	10.9	68
1970-1972	0.13	37	10.4	76
1973-1975	0.11	31	13.2	90
1976-1978	0.11	30	13.2	93
1979-1981	0.11	22	12.2	100

From Morgan M. Anaesthetic contribution to maternal mortality. *Br J Anaesth*. 1987;59(7):842–855.

More recent studies have continued to portray maternal mortality related to anesthesia as an important, although exceedingly rare event. Importantly, contemporary analyses of adverse maternal outcomes of anesthesia emphasize the particular risks associated with airway management in this population.[131,132] In 2004, the Society for Obstetric Anesthesia and Perinatology established the Serious Complication Repository Project to better capture the incidence of serious complications related to obstetric anesthesia. D'Angelo and colleagues[132A] collected outcomes of over 257,000 anesthetics at 30 institutions over a 5-year period. They identified a total of 157 serious complications, 85 of which were anesthesia-related (1 major complication per 3000 anesthetics). Maternal death occurred in 30 cases, but none were determined to be anesthesia-related. Complications frequently attributable to anesthesia included high neuraxial block, respiratory arrest, and unrecognized intrathecal catheter (Table 30.14).

In summary, extensive past research has indicated that the risks of major morbidity and mortality attributable to obstetric anesthesia care have decreased over time; nonetheless, recent research indicates that adverse outcomes continue to occur and may be of particular concern for patients receiving general anesthesia for cesarean delivery. As these risks are quantified with increasing precision using large databases, further research will be needed to validate these findings and identify the impact of variable care delivery (including the use of differing anesthetic techniques) and the maternal outcomes across institutions and practice environments.

PEDIATRICS

There are few studies of anesthesia-related risk in the pediatric population. Several themes emerge from these studies: very young infants are at increased risk of mortality, and anesthesia-related risk is reduced in centers with specialized pediatric anesthesia facilities. More recently, attempts have been made to define the neurocognitive risks presented by exposure to anesthesia at a young age.

In Beecher and Todd's classic 1954 study on anesthesia outcomes,[18] a "disproportionate number" of anesthesia-related deaths occurred in children younger than 10 years of age. Similarly, Graff and colleagues[133] from the Baltimore Anesthesia Study Committee reported 335 operative deaths

TABLE 30.13 Numbers, Case Fatality Rates, and Risk Ratios of Anesthesia-Related Deaths During Cesarean Section Delivery by Type of Anesthesia in the United States, 1979 to 1984 and 1985 to 1990

	NUMBER OF DEATHS		CASE-FATALITY RATE		RISK RATIO	
Population	**1979-1984**	**1985-1990**	**1979-1984**	**1985-1990**	**1979-1984**	**1985-1990**
General	33	32	20.0* (95% CI, 17.7-22.7)	32.3* (95% CI, 25.9-49.3)	2.3 (95% CI, 1.9-2.9)	16.7 (95% CI, 12.9-21.8)
Regional	19	9	8.6† (95% CI, 1.8-9.4)	1.9† (95% CI, 1.8-2)	Referent	Referent

*Per million general anesthetics for cesarean section.
†Per million regional anesthetics for cesarean section.
CI, Confidence interval.
Modified from Hawkins JL, Gibbs CP, Orleans M, et al. Obstetric anesthesia work force survey, 1981 versus 1992. *Anesthesiology*. 1997;87(1):135–143.

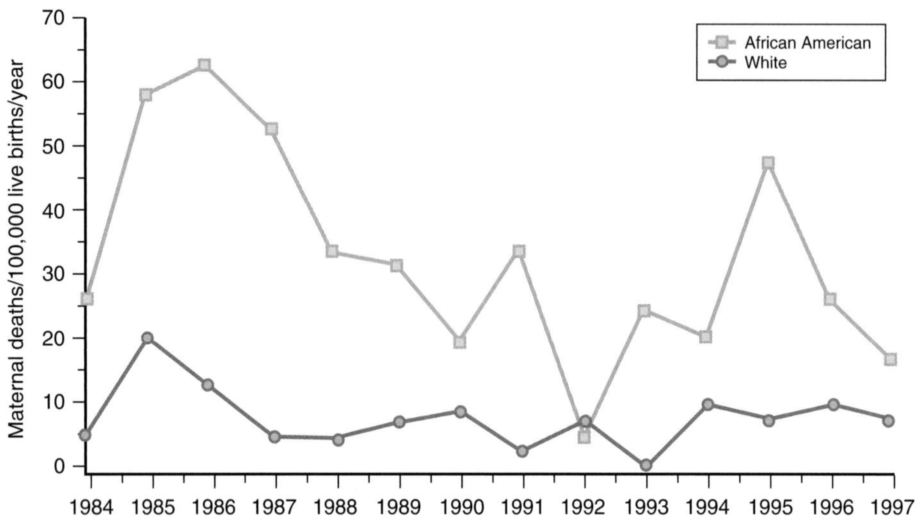

Fig. 30.6 Delivery mortality ratios by race in Maryland, from 1984 to 1997, according to discharge summaries. (From Panchal S, Arria AM, Labhsetwar SA. Maternal mortality during hospital admission for delivery: a retrospective analysis using a state-maintained database. *Anesth Analg.* 2001;93(1):134–141.)

TABLE 30.14 Incidence of Serious Complications Associated With Obstetric Anesthesia

Serious Complication	Totals	Incidence (95% CI)	Anesthesia Related	Incidence (95% CI)
Maternal death	30	1:10,250 (1:7,180-1:15,192)	0	
Cardiac arrest	43*	1:7,151 (1:5,319-1:9,615)	2	1:128,398 (1:35,544-1:1,060,218)
Myocardial infarction	2	1:153,758 (1:42,562-1:1,269,541)	2	1:128,398 (1:35,544-1:1,060,218)
Epidural abscess/meningitis	4		4	1:62,866 (1:25,074-1:235,620)
Epidural hematoma	1		1	1:251,463 (1:46,090-1:10,142,861)
Serious neurological injury	27	1:11,389 (1:7,828-1:17,281)	7	1:35,923 (1:17,805-1:91,244)
Aspiration	0		0	
Failed intubation	10		10	1:533 (1:290-1:971)
High neuraxial block	58		58†	1:4366 (1:3356-1:5587)
Anaphylaxis	5‡	1:61,499 (1:26,353-1:189-403)	0	
Respiratory arrest in labor suite	25	1:8,455 (1:5,714-1:12,500)	16	1:10,042 (1:6,172-1:16,131)
Unrecognized spinal catheter	14		14	1:15,435 (1:9,176-1:25,634)
Total	157§	1:1,959 (1:1,675-1:2,294)	85¶	1:3,021 (1:2,443-1:3,782)

*Fourteen cardiac arrests did not result in maternal death.
†Also includes high blocks on labor and delivery that resulted in respiratory arrest from local anesthetic administration.
‡The medications associated with anaphylaxis were administered by anesthesia personnel but were not anesthesia medications.
§There were 157 total serious complications; however, some complications are listed in more than one category.
¶There were 85 anesthesia-related complications; however, some complications are listed in more than one category.
Modified from D'Angelo R, Smiley RM, Riley ET, Segal S. Serious complications related to obstetric anesthesia: the serious complication repository project of the society for obstetric anesthesia and perinatology. *Anesthesiology.* 2014;120(6):1505–1512.

in the pediatric age group. Of these, 58 were thought to be primarily or partially attributable to anesthesia. The percentage of operative deaths attributable to anesthesia was relatively constant among age groups at 16.6% to 21.7%. The studies that followed those of Beecher and Todd and the Baltimore Anesthesia Study Committee provided further detail on the risks associated with pediatric anesthesia over time. Tiret and coauthors[134] prospectively studied major anesthesia-related complications in pediatric patients in 440 hospitals in France between 1978 and 1982. There were 27 major complications in 40,240 cases, which included 12 cardiac arrests and 1 death. The incidence of major complications and cardiac arrest was significantly higher in infants than in older children. Most complications in infants involved the respiratory system and predominantly consisted of airway problems and aspiration. Older children experienced respiratory and cardiac complications, which occurred most frequently during induction and recovery.

Cohen and colleagues[135] studied 29,220 anesthesia procedures at the Winnipeg Children's Hospital in the 1980s. Data on patients' coexisting medical conditions and postoperative follow-up were obtained within 72 hours. Complications included death, cardiac arrest, drug reactions, airway

TABLE 30.15 Summary of Perioperative Events by Age Group

	<1 Month (*n* = 361)	1-12 Months (*n* = 2,544)	1-5 Years (*n* = 13,484)	6-10 Years (*n* = 7,184)	11+ Years (*n* = 5,647)
Any intraoperative event	14.96	7.31	7.10	12.22	9.69
Any recovery room event	16.61	7.23	12.20	14.88	15.23
Any postoperative event	13.57	10.30	20.32	31.49	32.44
Minor event*	23.82	7.51	3.26	3.37	3.33
Major event†					
Any event‡	48.89	25.92	37.50	50.52	51.33
Among patients seen	41.55	23.47	33.16	45.04	45.78
Among all patients					

*Includes nausea and vomiting, sore throat, muscle pain, headache, dental conditions, positional conditions, conditions involving extremities, eye conditions, croup, temperature, behavioral problems, thrombophlebitis, arterial line problem, awareness, and "other" problems.
†Includes "other respiratory" conditions, cardiovascular disorders, nerve palsy, hepatic disorders, renal disorders, seizures, surgical complications, and death.
‡Percentage of total anesthetics in which at least one event occurred in the intraoperative unit, recovery unit, or later during the postoperative period.
All figures are given as the percentage of events per total anesthetics.
Modified from Cohen MM, Cameron CB, Duncan PG. Pediatric anesthesia morbidity and mortality in the perioperative period. *Anesth Analg*. 1990;70(2):160–167.

obstruction, and minor complications such as nausea and vomiting, arrhythmias, and sore throat. Neonates underwent a higher percentage of major vascular or cardiac and intraabdominal procedures, and older children had a higher incidence of extremity procedures. Intraoperative cardiac arrest occurred most frequently in patients younger than 1 year of age (4 in 2901 procedures). Postoperatively, minor events such as nausea and vomiting were more common in older children, whereas respiratory events were more common in infants and younger children (Table 30.15). When compared with adult patients, children experienced different complications, which frequently extended well into the postoperative period. In a comparison of 2-year periods between 1982 and 1987, rates of intraoperative events were found to be stable, and the rate of postoperative complications decreased.

More recently, van der Griend and colleagues reported on 24-hour and 30-day mortality associated with 101,885 anesthetics administered to 56,263 children at the Royal Children's Hospital in Melbourne, Australia. They noted a rate of all-cause 24-hour mortality of 13.4 per 10,000 anesthetics and a 30-day all-cause mortality of 34.5 per 10,000 anesthetics. The incidence of deaths related to anesthesia was far lower, occurring at a rate of 1 in 10,188 or 0.98 cases per 10,000 anesthetics performed. In all of the 10 anesthetic-related deaths that the authors observed, preexisting medical conditions were assessed to have been a significant contributing factor.[136]

In contrast to efforts to determine the incidence and predictors of mortality among pediatric surgical patients, a number of investigators have focused on cardiac arrest in the context of pediatric anesthesia. For example, Flick and associates[137] studied patients younger than 18 years of age who underwent surgery at the Mayo Clinic and experienced perioperative cardiac arrest between November 1, 1988 and June 30, 2005. A total of 92,881 anesthetics were administered during the study period, 4242 (5%) of which were for the repair of congenital heart malformations. The incidence of perioperative cardiac arrest during noncardiac procedures was 2.9 per 10,000, and the incidence during cardiac procedures was 127 per 10,000. The incidence of perioperative cardiac arrest attributable to anesthesia was 0.65 per 10,000 anesthetics. The incidence of cardiac arrest and mortality was highest in neonates (0 to 30 days of life) undergoing cardiac procedures (incidence, 435 per 10,000; mortality, 389 per 10,000).

Investigators at the Children's Hospital of Boston conducted a registry study to evaluate rates of arrest in patients undergoing surgery for congenital heart disease.[138] Over a 5-year period, 41 cardiac arrests occurred in 40 patients during 5213 anesthetics for an overall frequency of 0.79%. Eleven cardiac arrests (26.8%) were classified as either likely ($n = 6$) or possibly related ($n = 5$) to anesthesia (21.1 per 10,000 anesthetics) but with no mortality.

Efforts to understand the causes and outcomes of cardiac arrest in pediatric anesthesia patients have been aided by the development of large-scale clinical registries for research and quality improvement. In 1994, the Pediatric Perioperative Cardiac Arrest (POCA) Registry[139] was formed to determine the clinical factors and outcomes associated with cardiac arrest in anesthetized children. A total of 289 cardiac arrests occurred in the 63 institutions in the database during the first 4 years of the registry, 150 of which were judged to be related to anesthesia (1.4 per 10,000 anesthesia procedures), with a 26% mortality rate. Medication-related causes and cardiovascular causes of cardiac arrest were most common. Anesthesia-related cardiac arrest occurred most often in patients younger than age 1 year and in patients with severe underlying disease. In 2007, an update from the POCA registry was published.[140] From 1998 through 2004, 193 arrests (49%) were related to anesthesia. Cardiovascular causes of cardiac arrest (41%) were the most common, with hypovolemia from blood loss and hyperkalemia from transfusion of stored blood being the most common identifiable cardiovascular causes (Fig. 30.7). In contrast to the earlier study, medication-related arrests only accounted for 18% of all arrests.

In 2010, POCA investigators reported on anesthesia-related cardiac arrest in children with preexisting cardiac disease, comparing 245 cardiac arrests in children without heart disease with 127 cardiac arrests in children with cardiac conditions. Compared with children without cardiac disease, children with cardiac conditions were more often ASA physical status III, IV, or V and more often arrested from cardiovascular causes. Mortality was higher in children with heart disease than among children without heart

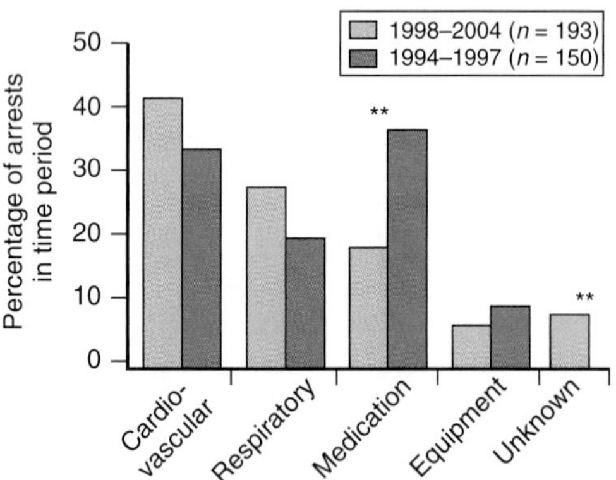

Fig. 30.7 Causes of anesthesia-related cardiac arrest in the Pediatric Perioperative Cardiac Arrest (POCA). Registry from 1998 to 2004 versus 1994 to 1997. (**$P < .01$ 1998-2004 vs 1994-1997 by Z test). (From Bhananker SM, Ramamoorthy C, Geiduschek JM, et al. Anesthesia-related cardiac arrest in children: update from the Pediatric Perioperative Cardiac Arrest Registry. *Anesth Analg.* 2007;105(2):344–350.)

disease (33% vs. 23%) but did not differ when adjusted for ASA physical status classification.[141]

In recent years, researchers have become increasingly interested in how anesthetic exposure in young children impacts neurocognitive development. In 2016, Sun and group[141a] published a sibling-matched cohort study conducted over 4 years at four university hospitals in the United States. They enrolled a total of 105 sibling pairs, one of whom had been exposed to inhalational anesthetics for an inguinal hernia repair before 36 months of age. Neurocognitive testing performed on both siblings did not demonstrate a statistically significant difference in intelligence quotient. Another group (Ing and colleagues)[141b] analyzed data from the Western Australia Pregnancy Cohort to evaluate the relationship between anesthetic exposure in children younger than 3 years of age and neuropsychological, academic, and behavioral outcomes in a cohort of 2868 children. They identified discrepancies in neuropsychological test and ICD-9 coded clinical outcomes, but did not identify any differences in academic achievement, and suggest that the unique attributes of specific tests may explain the variation in cognitive outcomes described in different studies. In another cohort study, Backeljauw and colleagues[141c] matched 5- to 18-year-old participants in a language development study who had undergone surgery with anesthesia before age 4 with unexposed peers. They found that exposed subjects had statistically significantly lower scores in listening comprehension and performance intelligence quotient, and that these changes were associated with lower gray matter density in key brain regions (occipital cortex and cerebellum). Given these conflicting results, further research is clearly needed to evaluate and quantify this impact in more detail.

OLDER ADULTS

The relationship of age to operative risk has been a subject of scientific and clinical debate since the early days of modern surgery. The nature of operative and anesthetic risk in older patients remains a vital area of inquiry particularly as the proportion of U.S. adults 65 years of age and older is anticipated to increase rapidly over the next three decades.

A key issue in research on the safety of surgery and anesthesia among older adults is the determination of what constitutes *old age* from the perspective of perioperative risk. Multiple definitions have been used for advanced age, including age older than 65, 70, 80, or 90 years. Denney and Denson[142] evaluated risk associated with surgery in patients older than 90 years of age. They reported 272 patients undergoing 301 operations at the University of Southern California Medical Center, finding a high perioperative mortality rate among older patients with serious bowel obstruction (63%). Taking a slightly different approach, Djokovic and Hedley-Whyte[143] studied outcome after surgery in 500 patients older than 80 years of age. They found that mortality was predicted by ASA physical status classification, with greater comorbid conditions associated with increasing risk. Myocardial infarction was the leading cause of postoperative death. Patients without significant comorbid diseases (ASA I classification) had a mortality rate of less than 1%.

Del Guercio and Cohn[144] investigated the value of preoperative invasive monitoring in obtaining hemodynamic and cardiopulmonary variables for predicting operative risk in the older adult. Among 148 consecutive patients older than 65 years of age who were treated in a surgical ICU, only 13.5% had normal physiologic measurements. Advanced and uncorrectable functional deficits were found in 63% of patients, and all in this group who underwent the planned surgery died.

Del Guerico and Cohn's work represented one of several studies that emphasized coexisting diseases, rather than aging itself, as the cause of apparently increased perioperative mortality among older adults. More recently, a growing body of literature has focused on the importance of functional disability and chronic geriatric syndromes, such as frailty and dementia, as determinants of postoperative outcomes among older individuals. Robinson and colleagues examined a cohort of 110 surgical patients with a mean age of 74 years, finding a 15% 6-month rate of mortality. Statistically significant predictors of 6-month mortality included impaired cognition, a recent fall, hypoalbuminemia, anemia, functional dependence, and comorbidity. Notably, functional dependence was the strongest predictor of 6-month mortality. Four or more markers in any one patient effectively predicted 6-month mortality (sensitivity, 81%; specificity, 86%).[145] Finlayson and colleagues observed high rates of mortality after major gastrointestinal surgery among older nursing home residents versus the overall Medicare population; the high rates of mortality were likely attributable to high rates of comorbidity and functional disability within this population.[146]

In this context, research on the risks of surgery and anesthesia in the older adult now focuses on broader definitions of *risk* that include functional outcomes and quality of life, in addition to traditional morbidity and mortality outcomes. Finlayson and colleagues examined 6822 older nursing home residents undergoing intestinal resections for colon cancer, noting a 53% 1-year mortality rate and a 24% rate of sustained decline in functional independence in activities of daily living among survivors. In multivariate regression, age older than 80 years, hospital readmission after surgical discharge, surgical complications, and functional decline before surgery all predicted functional decline at 1 year.[147]

As the older population continues to grow, researchers have recently begun to evaluate the neurocognitive impact of anesthesia on the elderly.

The measures of outcome relative to patient goals of care are becoming increasingly important in determining optimal strategies for perioperative management of the geriatric population. The ASA recently instituted a Perioperative Brain Health Initiative (Fleisher)[147a] dedicated to exploring the potential relationship between anesthetic exposure and postoperative cognitive function and delirium. This topic is discussed in more detail in Chapter 83.

Risks Directly Related to the Anesthetic Drug

Numerous studies have evaluated the influence of the choice of anesthetic on outcome, a question that is discussed throughout this book. From a global perspective, there does not appear to be a single best anesthesia technique for a particular surgery or group of surgeries, although emerging evidence begs for more research on this subject. In a multivariate analysis by Cohen and co-workers[96] of 100,000 anesthesia procedures performed in Canada, the choice of drug did not provide any additional prognostic information for predicting mortality beyond that of patient disease and the surgical procedure. In univariate analysis, MAC appeared to be associated with worse outcomes; however, this association was attributable to the use of MAC in sicker patients (see Table 30.11).

One question that has persisted within the anesthesia literature is the issue of whether anesthetic medications carry inherent toxicity. For example, numerous discussions have focused on the potential toxicity of halothane and sevoflurane. In the case of halothane, concern focused on the potential for fulminant, potentially fatal, hepatic necrosis with this medication. After several case reports of hepatic necrosis after halothane anesthesia, a large retrospective study of 856,500 anesthesia procedures at 34 institutions was undertaken.[148-150] In all but seven cases, hepatic necrosis could be explained by other causes. Halothane could be associated with hepatitis and hepatic failure, but the incidence was very low.

In the case of sevoflurane, concern has centered on the potential nephrotoxicity of its metabolite compound A. Although some laboratory studies have supported the contention that sevoflurane reacts with soda lime to form compound A and that this metabolite can lead to renal toxicity,[151,152] clinical studies have been unable to confirm this potentially detrimental effect[153,154] in the United States.

Some research groups have recently sought to identify and quantify other anesthesia-attributable effects. In 2016, Wigmore and colleagues[154a] published the results of a retrospective cohort study evaluating survival and recurrence outcomes in propensity-matched patients undergoing primary resection of malignancy with inhaled versus intravenous anesthetics in over 7000 patients in the United Kingdom. After adjusting for confounders, the investigators demonstrated a hazard ratio of 1.46 for death in patients receiving volatile anesthetic versus those receiving inhalational agents, a result which demands further prospective investigation.

In 2008, the GALA investigators[154b] published results of a randomized controlled trial comparing outcomes following carotid endarterectomy with local versus general anesthesia in 3526 patients with asymptomatic or symptomatic carotid stenosis. Primary outcomes included stroke, myocardial reinfarction, and 30-day mortality. Of the patients undergoing general anesthesia 4.8% experienced events, as compared to 4.5% of patients who were managed with local anesthetics (3 events preventable per 1000 treated). The investigators were not able to identify a statistically significant benefit to local or general anesthesia for individual primary outcomes, or for 30-day quality of life, hospital length of stay, or surgical duration. In a retrospective cohort study published in 2015, van den Berg and colleagues[154c] investigated outcomes of intraarterial treatment of patients with acute ischemic stroke with or without general anesthesia. Cases without general anesthesia were associated with good clinical outcome in a higher proportion than those treated with general anesthesia (26% vs. 14%), although there were notable distinctions between the two groups. They also found a nonsignificant mortality benefit in the non-general anesthesia group. The authors speculated that anesthetics might alter autoregulation of cerebral blood flow; however, their results were confounded by the determination that arterial recanalization was delayed by up to 20 minutes in patients undergoing interventions with general anesthesia.

Numerous studies have attempted to define the *safest* anesthetic for high-risk patients. In the late 1980s, there was concern that isoflurane caused coronary steal in patients with coronary stenosis and collaterals and that this could result in myocardial ischemia.[155,156] A series of studies were conducted to evaluate the rate of perioperative cardiac morbidity and mortality in patients undergoing coronary artery bypass grafting to determine the importance of the agent used for general anesthesia.[157-160] Taken together, these studies demonstrated negligible differences in outcome, thus supporting the contention that multiple safe approaches to general anesthesia may exist for an individual context. Other studies have focused on the relative safety of general anesthesia versus neuraxial or regional techniques (Basques et al.).[161,162,162a] For lower extremity and pelvic surgery, regional anesthesia was associated with a lower incidence of graft thrombosis and deep venous thrombosis, as well as decreased bleeding, decreased length of stay (Neuman et al.),[162b] reduced risk of surgical site infection, and risk of prolonged hospitalization (Helwani et al.).[162c] Regional anesthesia has also been specifically associated with lower major complication rates in patients with OSA (Memtsoudis et al.).[162d] In a more recent meta-analysis published by O'Donnell and colleagues,[162e] the findings were less favorable. Although they were able to determine a small difference in hospital length of stay attributable to regional anesthesia, the discrepancies in outcome reporting among the different studies were such that they were not able to identify definitively any other differences between the two approaches. The investigators of two randomized controlled trials currently underway, REGAIN (Neuman et al.)[162f] and RAGA-delirium, (Li et al.)[162g] are attempting to quantify the impact of anesthetic choice on morbidity, mortality, and cognitive outcomes in patients undergoing hip fracture surgery.

For patients undergoing vascular surgery, the primary finding favoring regional anesthesia was a lower incidence of graft thrombosis and the need for reoperation in patients undergoing infrainguinal bypass surgery; however, the largest of these studies was unable to demonstrate any difference in outcome based on anesthesia technique.[163-165] The rate of this complication was low in the total cohort in the largest trial, which made it impossible to detect any difference based on technique. Summarizing findings from several of these studies, Rodgers and co-workers[162] published an influential meta-analysis of regional versus general anesthesia. Neuraxial blockade was found to reduce postoperative mortality and other serious complications. As such, the magnitude of some of these benefits remained uncertain. Discussion of regional versus general anesthesia is presented in Chapters 45 and 46.

The impact of perioperative ventilation modality has also recently come under investigation: in 2015, Ladha's group[165a] published a hospital-based registry study examining outcomes of 69,239 patients undergoing noncardiac surgery requiring endotracheal intubation. Roughly 50% of patients received a protective ventilation strategy (reduced tidal volume and high positive end-expiratory pressure [PEEP]) versus standard care. Protective ventilation, defined as a PEEP of 5 cm H_2O and a plateau pressure of 16 cm H_2O or less, was associated with a reduced risk of postoperative respiratory complications. High driving pressure and plateau pressure were associated with an increased risk of respiratory complications. Severgnini and colleagues[165b] randomized 56 patients undergoing elective open abdominal surgery to a standard mechanical ventilation strategy (tidal volume of 9 mL/kg, ideal body weight [IBW], and zero PEEP), or "lung protective" ventilation (7 mL/kg, IBW, PEEP of 10 cm H_2O, recruitment maneuvers). Patients receiving protective ventilation demonstrated respiratory function and reduced Clinical Pulmonary Infection Score for several days postoperatively. Length of stay did not differ between groups.

Risks Related to Surgery

The surgical procedure itself significantly influences perioperative risk. In virtually every study performed, emergency surgery is associated with additional risk. [98] In some cases, the risk related to surgery is a function of the underlying disease processes and the stress related to the surgical procedure. As a category of surgical procedures, cardiovascular surgery has historically been associated with the highest risk of mortality and major morbidity. (The risks related to anesthesia for cardiac surgical procedures are reviewed in Chapter 54.) Vascular surgery is among the highest-risk group of noncardiac procedures. Although aortic reconstructive surgery has traditionally been considered the procedure with the highest risk, infrainguinal procedures have shown a similar rate of cardiac morbidity in several studies, possibly due to a higher burden of coronary artery disease in this population.[166,167] Other high-risk vascular procedures include amputation.[168] Intraabdominal, thoracic, and orthopedic procedures have also been associated with increased risk.[13,168]

Eagle and associates[170] evaluated perioperative cardiac morbidity and mortality among patients who had been treated for coronary artery disease and subsequently underwent major noncardiac surgery. Among these patients, major vascular surgery was associated with the highest risk of myocardial infarction or death, with a combined incidence of morbidity and mortality greater than 5%. Procedures associated with a combined complication rate of 1% to 5% included intraabdominal, thoracic, and head and neck surgical procedures. Low-risk procedures included breast, skin, urologic, and orthopedic surgeries. Ultimately, these groupings of surgical procedures came to form the basis for the definitions of surgical risk published in the American College of Cardiology/American Heart Association joint guidelines on perioperative cardiovascular evaluation for noncardiac surgery.[171] More recent statistical modeling efforts, such as those of Gupta[111] and Glance,[117] aimed at predicting postoperative outcomes have reinforced the important contribution of the type of surgical procedure to the overall operative risk.

Studies of the perioperative complication rate related to superficial procedures are generally reassuring. Backer and associates[172] evaluated the rate of perioperative myocardial reinfarction in patients who have a history of preexisting coronary artery disease and who underwent ophthalmologic surgery. They demonstrated that the rate of perioperative cardiac morbidity after ophthalmologic surgery was extremely low, even in patients with a recent myocardial infarction. Similar findings have been reported by multiple other investigators.[69,173]

More recent work suggests that surgical duration may also affect perioperative risk. Kim and group[173a] reviewed a cohort of over 1 million patients undergoing surgery under general anesthesia between 2005 and 2011 and demonstrated an association between surgery duration and the risk of development of venous thromboembolism. These results were preserved in analysis of individual procedures and classes of procedure by specialty.

Risks Related to the Location of Surgery and Postoperative Monitoring

Perioperative risk varies among hospitals for major procedures such as coronary artery bypass grafting and abdominal aortic aneurysm repair.[9,10,174] Multiple studies have documented a relationship between surgical volume and mortality. Although surgical skill most certainly plays a role in the rate of complications and mortality, local factors may also play an important role. For example, low surgical volume may lead to less skilled anesthesia and postoperative care. The influence of each of these factors on overall morbidity and mortality is unknown.

Although the value of postoperative monitoring and care in an ICU has never been documented in a randomized clinical trial, many investigators have suggested that such care is one of the primary reasons for the improved morbidity and mortality in recent years. For patients undergoing major vascular surgery, several investigators have suggested that more intense postoperative monitoring could obviate the need for preoperative cardiac testing and revascularization.[171] One potential value of risk assessment is the identification of patients who could benefit from referral to clinical centers with more extensive perioperative resources. Patients with a low probability of perioperative morbidity and mortality could have surgery performed locally, and individuals at higher risk could receive benefit from transfer to a center with high surgical volume.

Risks Related to the Anesthesia Provider

Over the past decade a great deal of attention has been paid to the role and skill of the anesthesia provider on patient outcome. Historically, anesthesia has been administered by a diverse group of providers with variable levels of supervision. The extent to which the skills and training of the individual anesthesia provider may affect outcomes has been assessed in a number of studies. In a now-classic paper, Slogoff and Keats[175] studied the association of perioperative myocardial ischemia and cardiac morbidity in patients undergoing coronary artery bypass grafting across multiple anesthesiologists working in a single practice. Notably, the rate of perioperative ischemia and infarction varied by anesthesiologist, and the authors concluded that operator technique and experience may affect risk. Subsequent work has moved beyond efforts to demonstrate variability in anesthesia outcomes at the level of the individual practitioner to examine whether outcomes might vary across different models of anesthesia care. Arbous and coauthors reported a case-control study over 1 year in the Netherlands,[176] in which they found that practice-level independent variables associated with a decreased risk for coma and death in 24 hours were (1) anesthesia equipment check performed with a checklist; (2) direct availability of an anesthesiologist by telephone, beeper, or walkie-talkie during maintenance anesthesia; (3) no change of anesthesiologist during the case; (4) presence of a full-time nurse anesthetist versus a part-time anesthetist during maintenance anesthesia; and (5) presence of two providers versus one person during emergence. This study was one of very few that attempted to identify practice characteristics rather than specific drugs or techniques that have an impact on anesthesia outcomes, and the results are striking, in spite of numerous issues with data reporting and matching. The finding that practitioner characteristics affect outcomes warrants further follow-up.

Attention has recently turned to the impact of handoffs of anesthesia care on patient outcomes. In 2018, Jones and colleagues[176a] published a retrospective cohort study evaluating outcomes including all-cause mortality, hospital readmission, and major postoperative complications in 313,066 patients undergoing major surgery. They identified an association between complete anesthesia handoffs (i.e., when one provider or team leaves the case permanently and is replaced by another) and increased incidence of primary outcomes, as well as with increased rates of ICU admission and hospital length of stay. The study design was limited by the inability to control for the career experience of the replacement anesthesiologist and surgeon as well as by the sole use of billing codes to determine exposure to a transition in anesthesia care.

Several studies have attempted to evaluate the complication rates and risks associated with various care provider models. Bechtoldt,[177] as a member of the North Carolina Anesthesia Study Committee, evaluated 900 perioperative deaths that occurred in an estimated 2 million anesthesia procedures performed in North Carolina between 1969 and 1976. The lowest rate of anesthesia-related deaths (1 per 28,166 procedures) occurred in patients who received anesthesia from an anesthesia care team (physician anesthesiologist and CRNA), and the highest rate (1 per 11,432 procedures) was associated with anesthesia administered by a dentist; the rate for the nurse anesthetist–only cohort was intermediate (1 per 20,723). A study by the Stanford Center for Health Care Research[178] demonstrated similar outcomes: the investigators reported that death plus severe morbidity was 11% higher than predicted in patients who received their care in a nurse anesthetist–only setting, 3% lower than predicted for physician-only care, and 20% lower than predicted for an anesthesia care team environment. Both studies demonstrated significant methodologic limitations.

The impact of specific provider types may be greatest in particular situations: for example, patients with significant comorbid diseases and those who sustain perioperative complications may benefit from providers with specific skill sets. One way to study such issues is to evaluate the rate of survival after complications. Silber and colleagues[7] at the University of Pennsylvania studied the medical records of 5972 surgical patients randomly selected from 531 hospitals. They evaluated patient and hospital characteristics, including the number and type of physicians, board certification status, and ratio of care providers. The 30-day mortality rate correlated with patient characteristics. Failure to rescue (i.e., failure to prevent death) after an adverse event was inversely associated with the proportion of board-certified anesthesiologists on staff in each facility. Improved perioperative survival was significantly associated with the presence of an increased number of board-certified anesthesiologists. These findings were corroborated in follow-up studies by the same group,[179,181] wherein analysis was again limited by database characteristics.[181] By contrast, Pine and co-workers evaluated mortality after eight specific surgical procedures[182] and used stepwise logistic regression to derive procedure-specific risk adjustment models. They found hospitals without anesthesiologists had results similar to those facilities in which anesthesiologists provided or directed anesthesia care. The authors did not evaluate failure to rescue or cause of mortality.

More recently, work by Needleman and Minnick compared obstetric outcomes in facilities with different obstetric anesthesia staffing patterns.[183] Although the authors observed consistent differences in maternal mortality and other quality indicators at facilities where nurse anesthetists practiced with minimal or no supervision by anesthesiologists versus anesthesiologist-only facilities, questions regarding risk adjustment and study design limit definitive interpretations of this work for policy making.[184] Similarly, a 2010 study by Dulisse and Cromwell suggested no changes in overall surgical patient outcomes in states that had enacted laws allowing nurse anesthetists to practice independently versus states that required anesthesiologist supervision.[185] However, as such new

BOX 30.1 Proposed Definitions from the 1984 International Symposium on Preventable Anesthesia Morbidity and Mortality

Outcome
- Normal
- Abandoned procedure
- Morbidity
- Death

Morbidity
- Unplanned, unwanted, undesirable consequence of anesthesia

Mortality
- Death that occurs before recovery from the effects of a drug or drugs given to facilitate a procedure
- Death that occurs during an attempt to relieve the pain of a condition
- Death that results from an incident that occurs while the drugs are effective

Modified from Pierce EC Jr. The 34th Rovenstine Lecture. 40 years behind the mask: safety revisited. *Anesthesiology.* 1996;84(4):965–975.

legislation was not associated with major changes in the number or types of surgery conducted without anesthesiologist supervision, Dulisse and Cromwell's work does not speak directly to the question of the gains or losses in safety associated with any specific provider type for a given type of surgery.

Ultimately, as concluded by Smith and associates[186] in a review of available published studies through 2004 on the influence of anesthesia providers, the relationship of patient outcomes to the type of anesthesia provider has not yet been conclusively demonstrated. Nurse anesthetists and other nonphysician providers are vital to the delivery of anesthesia care in the United States and elsewhere, and determining the optimal scope of practice for such providers remains an ongoing area of academic research and political debate.

Improving Anesthesia Safety

Over the past several decades, major improvements to the safety of anesthesia have been initiated. In 1984, Cooper, Kitz, and Pierce hosted a landmark International Symposium on Preventable Anesthesia Mortality and Morbidity in Boston. Approximately 50 anesthesiologists from around the world attended the meeting and, after much debate, established a series of definitions of outcome, morbidity, and mortality (Box 30.1). Beyond its specific conclusions, however, the symposium remains an event of major historical importance as a seminal early event in the movement to improve patient safety and as the context out of which the Anesthesia Patient Safety Foundation (APSF) was established. After its formal incorporation in October 1985, the APSF has since actively promoted a range of initiatives focused on fulfilling its mission to continually improve the safety of patients during anesthesia care by encouraging and conducting: (1) safety research and education, (2) patient safety programs and campaigns, and (3) national and international exchange of information and ideas. To this end, the APSF has focused on promoting research, practice improvement, and knowledge dissemination across a range of priority areas (Box 30.2). Overall, these efforts have stressed the potential for systems-level improvements, standardization of care processes, human-factors engineering, and simulation-based training to limit harms caused by preventable adverse events and errors in crisis management in the context of anesthesia care. Through this work, the APSF has come to serve as a leader in patient safety, not only in the context of anesthesia and perioperative care, but also more generally within medicine by establishing *patient safety* as a formal concept, discipline in medical care, and serving as a model for other organizations such as the U.S. National Patient Safety Foundation.[197]

BOX 30.2 Selected Areas of Focus of the Anesthesia Patient Safety Foundation, 1985 to 2012

- Use of anesthesia simulators for training and evaluation
- Improvement of standards for intraoperative monitoring
- Application of patient safety checklists to intraoperative care
- Promotion of standardized approaches to difficult airway management
- Prevention of medication-related adverse events
- Reuse and attempted resterilization of disposable anesthesia equipment
- Risks of outdated anesthesia machines without modern safety features
- Aiding the development of practice standards by the World Federated Societies of Anesthesiologists
- Surgery department crisis management, including teamwork, team training, and resource management
- *Production pressure*, causing dangerous omissions and cutting corners
- Intravenous procedural sedation by nonanesthesia personnel
- Contamination of medical gases and disruption of pipeline flow
- Contamination of intravenous medications
- Special risks of office-based anesthesia
- Patients with obstructive sleep apnea and their postoperative care
- Postoperative cognitive dysfunction (particularly in older adults)
- Possible long-term increase in morbidity and mortality after extensive general anesthesia
- Postoperative vision loss, especially in extensive prone spine surgery
- Wrong-site surgery
- Residual neuromuscular blockade and postoperative complications
- Protocols for assessing and managing adverse events
- Persistence of deaths from malignant hyperthermia
- Dangers and challenges in patients with coronary artery stents
- Maintenance of current protocols for the anesthesia machine checkout
- Possible impact of anesthesia management on cancer recurrence
- Persistence of surgical unit fires

Modified from Eichhorn JH. The Anesthesia Patient Safety Foundation at 25: a pioneering success in safety, 25th anniversary provokes reflection, anticipation. *Anesth Analg.* 2012;114(4):791–800.

Alongside the efforts of the APSF, other prominent organizations, such as the ASA, have sought to improve the safety of anesthesia care through the creation and dissemination of standards and guidelines for clinical practice.

In general, both standards and guidelines represent summations by clinicians of the available evidence about the benefits and risks of particular approaches to treatment. Typically, a practice standard implies that a therapy or practice should be performed for patients with a particular condition. Standards are approved only if an assessment of the probabilities and utilities of the group indicate that the decision to choose the treatment or a strategy would be virtually unanimous. At present, the ASA has established one set of practice standards for anesthesia care, which outline basic requirements for intraoperative monitoring.[198]

In contrast to practice standards, guidelines are intended to be more flexible than standards, but they should be followed in most cases. Depending on the patient, setting, and other factors, guidelines can and should be tailored to fit individual needs. Similar to standards, guidelines should be cost-effective methods. Specific guidelines have been created by the ASA for diverse issues such as a difficult airway,[199] the use of the pulmonary artery catheter,[200] and the use of blood components[201] with the goal of defining the evidence on which optimal practice can be based. In a similar vein, the World Health Organization has recently placed an emphasis on the potential for a simple preoperative checklist, modeled on the processes used in other high-risk industries such as aviation, to reduce the rates of adverse events in the perioperative period.[202] Driven in part by the findings of improved outcomes with checklist use in a multicenter, international study by Haynes and co-authors,[203] such expanding interest in the use of standardized safety checks offers new potential opportunities to decrease the risk of anesthesia further.

Applying further insights gained from the aviation industry to anesthesia care, the APSF and other organizations have focused on developing simulation-based approaches to train anesthesia providers and to evaluate their decision-making capabilities in crisis situations.[204-208] To date, an extensive array of standardized scenarios have been developed for making comparisons among individuals, and research is ongoing to examine how best to use this technology in anesthesia training and recertification. Ultimately, such efforts, combined with improved monitoring of adverse outcomes through large outcomes databases and those now being assembled by the Multicenter Perioperative Outcomes Group and the Anesthesia Quality Institute, hold potential to improve the safety of anesthesia care continually on both a national and an international level.

Summary

The risks related to anesthesia appear to have dramatically decreased over the past several decades. Clearly, death solely attributable to anesthesia is rare; rather, underlying patient disease and the nature and extent of surgery have a greater effect on overall outcome than do risks attributable to the anesthetic per se. Although these changes in the risk attributable to anesthesia could justifiably be considered a major achievement on the part of anesthesia providers over time, they also present a novel challenge to anesthesia providers to identify new opportunities to aid in more broadly decreasing both the morbidity and the mortality of surgical procedures and to aid in aligning the results of surgical interventions with individual patients' goals of care. At the same time, vigilance must be continued to maintain high standards of basic anesthesia care across both hospital- and nonhospital-based settings. Finally, anesthesia providers should play a role in systems-based thinking to improve perioperative care and the short- and long-term outcomes of patients undergoing surgery and anesthesia.

Complete references available online at expertconsult.com.

References

1. Snow SJ. *Blessed Days of Anesthesia: How Anaesthetics Changed the World*. Oxford: Oxford University Press; 2008.
2. Fleisher LA, et al. *Arch Surg*. 2004;139:67.
3. Devereaux PJ, et al. *JAMA*. 2012;307:2295.
4. Levy M, et al. *Anesthesiology*. 2011;114:796.
5. Mangano DT, et al. *JAMA*. 1992;268:233.
6. Institute of Medicine Committee on Quality of Health Care in America. *To Err Human: Building a Safer Health System*. The National Academies Press; 2000.
7. Silber JH, et al. *Med Care*. 1992;30:615.
8. Silber JH, et al. *Med Care*. 2007;45:918.
9. Ghaferi AA, et al. *Ann Surg*. 2009;250:1029.
10. Birkmeyer JD, et al. *N Engl J Med*. 2002;346:1128.
11. Birkmeyer JD, et al. *N Engl J Med*. 2003;349:2117.
12. Finks JF, et al. *N Engl J Med*. 2011;364:2128.
13. Goldman L, et al. *N Engl J Med*. 1977;297:845.
14. Frank SM, et al. *Anesthesiology*. 1993;78:468.
15. Frank SM, et al. *JAMA*. 1997;277:1127.
16. Cheney FW, et al. *JAMA*. 1989;261:1599.
17. Lagasse RS. *Anesthesiology*. 2002;97:1609.
18. Beecher HK, Todd DP. *Ann Surg*. 1954;140(2).
19. Buck N, et al. *Report of a Confidential Enquiry into Perioperative Deaths*. London: Nuffield Provincial Hospitals Trust; 1987.
20. Mangano DT. *N Engl J Med*. 2002;347:1309.
21. Mathew JP, et al. *JAMA*. 1996;276:300.
22. Clark RE. *Best Pract Benchmarking Healthc*. 1996;1:62.
23. Grover FL, et al. *Ann Thorac Surg*. 1996;62:1229.
24. Grover FL, et al. *Ann Thorac Surg*. 1996;62(S6).
25. Nugent WC. *Ann Thorac Surg*. 1997;64:S68.
26. Bateman BT, et al. *Anesth Analg*. 2013;116:1380.
27. Todd CJ, et al. *BMJ*. 1995;310:904.
28. Aiken LH, et al. *JAMA*. 2002;288:1987.
29. Memery HN. *JAMA*. 1965;194:1185.

29a. Minuck M. *Can Anaes Soc J*. 1967;14:197.

30. Takala J. *Anesth Analg*. 2011;112:745.
31. Dornette WH, Orth OS. *Curr Res Anesth Analg*. 1956;35:545.
32. Dripps RD, et al. *JAMA*. 1961;178:261.
33. Gebbie D. *Can Anaesth Soc J*. 1966;13:390.
34. Phillips OC, et al. *JAMA*. 1960;174:2015.
35. Schapira M, et al. *Anesth Analg*. 1960;39:149.
36. Marx GF, et al. *Anesthesiology*. 1973;39:54.
37. Clifton BS, Hotten WI. *Br J Anaesth*. 1963;35:250.
38. Dinnick OP. *Anaesthesia*. 1964;19:536.
39. Bodlander FM. *Br J Anaesth*. 1975;47:36.
40. Harrison GG. *Br J Anaesth*. 1978;50:1041.
41. Holland R. *Br J Anaesth*. 1987;59:834.
42. Warden JC, Horan BF. *Anaesth Intensive Care*. 1996;24:66.
43. Tiret L, et al. *Can Anaesth Soc J*. 1986;33:336.
44. Tikkanen J, Hovi-Viander M. *Acta Anaesthesiol Scand*. 1995;39:262.
45. Lunn JN. *Anaesthesia*. 1980;35:617.
46. Pedersen T, et al. *Acta Anaesthesiol Scand*. 1990;34:176.
47. Li G, Warner M, et al. *Anesthesiology*. 2009;110:759.
48. Lagasse RS. *Anesthesiology*. 2009;110:698.
49. Findlay G, et al. *Knowing the Risk: A Review of the Perioperative Care of Surgical Patients*. London: National Confidential Enquiry into Patient Outcome and Death; 2011.
50. Pearse R, et al. *Lancet*. 2012;380:1059.
51. Wunsch H, et al. *Am J Respir Crit Care Med*. 2009;180:875.
52. Bennett-Guerrero E, et al. *Br J Surg*. 2003;90:1593.

52a. Whitlock EL, et al. *Anesthesiology*. 2015;123(6):1312.

53. Keenan RL, Boyan CP. *JAMA*. 1985;253:2373.
54. Olsson GL, Hallen B. *Acta Anaesthesiol Scand*. 1988;32:653.

55. Biboulet P, et al. *Can J Anaesth*. 2001;48:326.
56. Newland MC, et al. *Anesthesiology*. 2002;97:108.
57. Sprung J, et al. *Anesthesiology*. 2003;99:259.
57a. Ellis SJ, et al. *Anesthesiology*. 2014;120(4):829–838.
58. Kawashima Y, et al. *Acta Anaesthesiol Scand*. 2003;47:809.
59. Deleted in proof.
60. Kheterpal S, et al. *Anesthesiology*. 2009;110:58.
61. Chiang TM, et al. *Arch Otolaryngol*. 1968;88:307.
62. Raymond CA. *JAMA*. 1986;256:311.
63. Carithers JS, et al. *Laryngoscope*. 1987;97:422.
64. Brigger MT, Brietzke SE. *Otolaryngol Head Neck Surg*. 2006;135:1.
65. Gabalski EC, et al. *Laryngoscope*. 1996;106:77.
66. Mitchell RB, et al. *Arch Otolaryngol Head Neck Surg*. 1997;123:681.
67. Schloss MD, et al. *Int J Pediatr Otorhinolaryngol*. 1994;30:115.
67a. Coté CJ, et al. *Anesth Analg*. 2014;118(6):1276–1283.
68. Warren JL, et al. *J Natl Cancer Inst*. 1998;90:833.
69. Warner MA, et al. *JAMA*. 1993;270:1437.
70. Deleted in proof.
71. Chukmaitov AS, et al. *Health Serv Res*. 2008;43:1485.
72. Morello DC, et al. *Plast Reconstr Surg*. 1997;99:1496.
73. Vila H Jr, et al. *Arch Surg*. 2003;138:991.
74. Coldiron B, et al. *Dermatol Surg*. 2004;30:1435.
75. Coldiron BM, et al. *Dermatol Surg*. 2008;34:285.
76. Clayman MA, Seagle BM. *Plast Reconstr Surg*. 2006;118:777.
77. Sanborn KV, et al. *Anesthesiology*. 1996;85:977.
78. Reich DL, et al. *Anesth Analg*. 1999;89:814.
79. Kheterpal S, et al. *Anesthesiology*. 2006;105:885.
80. Kheterpal S, et al. *Anesthesiology*. 2007;107:892.
80a. Lee LO, et al. *Anesthesiology*. 2017;126(6):1053.
80b. Kheterpal S, et al. *Anesthesiology*. 2013;119(6):1360.
80c. Aziz MF, et al. *Anesthesiology*. 2016;125(4):656.
81. Caplan RA, et al. *Anesthesiology*. 1988;68(5).
82. Tinker JH, et al. *Anesthesiology*. 1989;71:541.
83. Caplan RA, et al. *Anesthesiology*. 1990;72:828.
84. Bhananker SM, et al. *Anesthesiology*. 2006;104:228.
85. Hove LD, et al. *Anesthesiology*. 2007;106:675.
86. Cooper JB. *Int Anesthesiol Clin*. 1984;22:167.
87. Cooper JB, et al. *Anesthesiology*. 1984;60:34.
88. Singleton RJ, et al. *Anaesth Intensive Care*. 1993;21:664.
89. Van der Walt JH, et al. *Anaesth Intensive Care*. 1993;21:650.
90. Deleted in proof.
91. Lopez-Jimenez F, et al. *J Am Coll Cardiol*. 1997;29:1241.
92. Monk TG, et al. *Anesth Analg*. 2005;100:4.
93. Saklad M. *Anesthesiology*. 1941;2:281.
94. Keats AS. *Anesthesiology*. 1978;49:233.
95. Vacanti CJ, et al. *Anesth Analg*. 1970;49:564.
96. Cohen MM, et al. *JAMA*. 1988;260:2859.
97. Owens WD, et al. *Anesthesiology*. 1978;49:239.
98. Goldman L, Caldera DL. *Anesthesiology*. 1979;50:285.
99. Hollenberg M, et al. *JAMA*. 1992;268:205.
99a. Baron DM, et al. *Br J Anaesth*. 2014;113(3):416.
100. Zeldin RA. *Can J Surg*. 1984;27:402.
101. Larsen SF, et al. *Eur Heart J*. 1987;8:179.
102. Domaingue CM, et al. *Anaesth Intensive Care*. 1982;10:324.
103. Jeffrey CC, et al. *Anesthesiology*. 1983;58:462.
104. White GH, et al. *Am J Surg*. 1988;156:103.
105. Lette J, et al. *Ann Surg*. 1990;211:84.
106. McEnroe CS, et al. *J Vasc Surg*. 1990;11:497.
107. Detsky AS, et al. *J Gen Intern Med*. 1986;1:211.
108. Palda VA, Detsky AS. *Ann Intern Med*. 1997;127:313.
109. Lee TH, et al. *Circulation*. 1999;100:1043.
110. Ford MK, et al. *Ann Intern Med*. 2010;152:26.
111. Gupta PK, et al. *Circulation*. 2011;124:381.
111a. Berwanger O, et al. *Eur Heart J*. 2016;37(2):177.
111b. Abbott TE, et al. *Br J Anaesth*. 2016;117(2):172.
111c. Gorka J, et al. *Br J Anaesth*. 2017;118(5):713.
112. Wijeysundera DN, et al. *JAMA*. 2007;297:1801.
113. Arozullah AM, et al. *Ann Intern Med*. 2001;135:847.
114. Arozullah AM, et al. *Ann Surg*. 2000;232:242.
115. Hogue CW Jr, et al. *Circulation*. 1999;100:642.
116. McCrory DC, et al. *Stroke*. 1993;24:1285.
117. Glance LG, et al. *Ann Surg*. 2012;255:696.
118. Hannan EL, et al. *JAMA*. 1990;264:2768.
119. Hannan EL, et al. *Ann Thorac Surg*. 1994;58:1852.
120. Hannan EL, et al. *Am Heart J*. 1997;134:1120.
121. Hopkins PM. *Br J Anaesth*. 2000;85:118.
122. Tardiff BE, et al. *Ann Thorac Surg*. 1997;64:715.
123. Fox AA, et al. *Anesthesiology*. 2009;110:738.
124. Muehlschlegel JD, et al. *Circulation*. 2010;122:S60.
125. Kaunitz AM, et al. *Obstet Gynecol*. 1985;65:605.
126. Endler GC, et al. *Am J Obstet Gynecol*. 1988;159:187.
127. Rochat RW, et al. *Obstet Gynecol*. 1988;72:91.
128. Morgan M. *Br J Anaesth*. 1987;59:842.
129. Hawkins JL, et al. *Anesthesiology*. 1997;86:277.
130. Panchal S, et al. *Anesth Analg*. 2001;93:134.
131. Mhyre JM, et al. *Anesthesiology*. 2007;106:1096.
132. Bloom SL, et al. *Obstet Gynecol*. 2005;106:281.
132a. D'Angelo R, et al. *Anesthesiology*. 2014;120(6):1505.
133. Graff TD, et al. *Anesth Analg*. 1964;43:407.
134. Tiret L, et al. *Br J Anaesth*. 1988;61:263.
135. Cohen MM, et al. *Anesth Analg*. 1990;70:160.
136. van der Griend BF, et al. *Anesth Analg*. 2011;112:1440.
137. Flick RP, et al. *Anesthesiology*. 2007;106:226.
138. Odegard KC, et al. *Anesth Analg*. 2007;105:335.
139. Morray JP, et al. *Anesthesiology*. 2000;93(6).
140. Bhananker SM, et al. *Anesth Analg*. 2007;105:344.
141. Ramamoorthy C, et al. *Anesth Analg*. 2010;110:1376.
141a. Sun LS, et al. *JAMA*. 2016;315(21):2312.
141b. Ing CH, et al. *Anesthesiology*. 2014;120(6):1319.
141c. Backeljauw B, et al. *Pediatrics*. 2015;136(1):e1.
142. Denney JL, Denson JS. *Geriatrics*. 1972;27:115.
143. Djokovic JL, Hedley-Whyte J. *JAMA*. 1979;242:2301.
144. Del Guercio LR, Cohn JD. *JAMA*. 1980;243:1350.
145. Robinson TN, et al. *Ann Surg*. 2009;250:449.
146. Finlayson E, et al. *Ann Surg*. 2011;254:921.
147. Finlayson E, et al. *J Am Geriatr Soc*. 2012;60:967.
147a. Fleisher LA. *ASA Monitor*. 2016;80(6):10.
148. Subcommittee of the National Halothane Study of the Committee on Anesthesia NAoS, National Research Council. *JAMA*. 1966;197:775.
149. Aach R. *JAMA*. 1970;211:2145.
150. DeBacker LJ, Longnecker DS. *JAMA*. 1966;195:157.
151. Levine MF, et al. *Anesthesiology*. 1996;84:348.
152. Nishiyama T, et al. *Anesth Analg*. 1996;83:574.
153. Conzen PF, et al. *Anesth Analg*. 1995;81:569.
154. Rooke GA, et al. *Anesth Analg*. 1996;82:1159.
154a. Wigmore TJ, et al. *Anesthesiology*. 2016;124(1):69.
154b. Lewis SC, et al. *Lancet*. 2008;372(9656):2132.
154c. van den Berg LA, et al. *Stroke*. 2015;46(5):1257.
155. Becker LC. *Anesthesiology*. 1987;66:259.
156. Buffington CW, et al. *Anesthesiology*. 1987;66:280.
157. Leung JM, et al. *Anesthesiology*. 1991;74:838.
158. Leung JM, et al. *J Am Coll Cardiol*. 1992;20:1205.
159. Slogoff S, Keats AS. *Anesthesiology*. 1989;70:179.
160. Slogoff S, et al. *Anesth Analg*. 1991;72:22.
161. Neuman MD, et al. *Anesthesiology*. 2012;117:72.
162. Rodgers A, et al. *BMJ*. 2000;321:1493.
162a. Basques BA, et al. *J Bone Joint Surg Am*. 2015;97(6):455.
162b. Neuman MD, et al. *JAMA*. 2014;311(24):2508.
162c. Helwani MA, et al. *JBJS*. 2015;97(3):186.
162d. Memtsoudis SG, et al. *Reg Anesth Pain Med*. 2013;38(4):274.
162e. O'Donnell CM et al: *Br J Anaesth*.120(1):37.
162f. Neuman MD, et al. *BMJ Open*. 2016;6(11):e013473.
162g. Li T, et al. *BMJ Open*. 2017;7(10):e016937.
163. Christopherson R, et al. *Anesthesiology*. 1993;79:422.
164. Bode RH Jr, et al. *Anesthesiology*. 1996;84(3).
165. Tuman K, et al. *Anesth Analg*. 1990;70:S414.
165a. Ladha K, et al. *BMJ*. 2015:351.
165b. Severgnini P, et al. *Anesthesiology*. 2013;118(6):1307.
166. Krupski WC, et al. *J Vasc Surg*. 1992;15:354.
167. L'Italien GJ, et al. *J Vasc Surg*. 1995;21:935.
168. Ashton CM, et al. *Ann Intern Med*. 1993;118:504.
169. Deleted in proof.
170. Eagle KA, et al. *Circulation*. 1997;96:1882.
171. Fleisher LA, et al. *Circulation*. 2007;116:1971.
172. Backer CL, et al. *Anesth Analg*. 1980;59:257.
173. Schein OD, et al. *N Engl J Med*. 2000;342:168.
173a. Kim JS, et al. *JAMA surgery*. 2015;150(2):110.
174. Kantonen I, et al. *Eur J Vasc Endovasc Surg*. 1997;14:375.
175. Slogoff S, Keats AS. *Anesthesiology*. 1985;62:107.

176. Arbous MS, et al. *Anesthesiology*. 2005;102:257.
176a. Jones PM, et al. *JAMA*. 2018;319(2):143.
177. Bechtoldt AA Jr. *N C Med J*. 1981;42:253.
178. Forrest W. Outcome—the effect of the provider. In: Hirsch R, Forrest W, eds. *Health Care Delivery in Anesthesia*. Philadelphia: George F Stickley; 1980:137.
179. Silber JH. *LDI Issue Brief*. 2000;6:1.
180. Deleted in proof.
181. Silber JH, et al. *Anesthesiology*. 2002;96:1044.
182. Pine M, et al. *AANA J*. 2003;71:109.
183. Needleman J, Minnick AF. *Health Serv Res*. 2009;44:464.
184. Neuman MD, et al. *Health Serv Res*. 2010;45:1390.
185. Dulisse B, Cromwell J. *Health Aff (Millwood)*. 2010;29:1469.
186. Smith AF, et al. *Br J Anaesth*. 2004;93:540.
187. Deleted in proof.
188. Deleted in proof.
189. Deleted in proof.
190. Deleted in proof.
191. Deleted in proof.
192. Deleted in proof.
193. Deleted in proof.
194. Deleted in proof.
195. Deleted in proof.
196. Deleted in proof.
197. Eichhorn JH. *Anesth Analg*. 2012;114:791.
198. American Society of Anesthesiologists. *Standards for Basic Anesthesia Monitoring*. Park Ridge, Ill: American Society of Anesthesiologists; 2011.
199. American Society of Anesthesiologists. *Anesthesiology*. 2003;98:1269.
200. American Society of Anesthesiologists Task Force on Pulmonary Artery Catheterization. *Anesthesiology*. 2003;99:988.
201. American Society of Anesthesiologists. *Anesthesiology*. 2006;105:198.
202. *WHO Surgical Safety Checklist and Implementation Manual*. World Health Organization; 2008. http://www.who.int/patientsafety/safesurgery/ss_checklist/en/index.html.
203. Haynes AB, et al. *N Engl J Med*. 2009;360:491.
204. Gaba DM, et al. *Anesthesiology*. 1987;66:670.
205. Holzman RS, et al. *J Clin Anesth*. 1995;7:675.
206. Howard SK, et al. *Aviat Space Environ Med*. 1992;63:763.
207. Popp HJ, et al. *Int J Clin Monit Comput*. 1991;8:151.
208. Schwid HA, O'Donnell D. *Anesthesiology*. 1992;76:495.

31 Preoperative Evaluation

DUMINDA N. WIJEYSUNDERA and EMILY FINLAYSON

KEY POINTS

- The anesthesia preoperative evaluation, which is the clinical foundation for guiding perioperative patient management, reduces perioperative morbidity and enhances patient outcome.
- The fundamental purpose of preoperative evaluation is to obtain pertinent information regarding the patient's medical history, formulate an assessment of the patient's perioperative risk, and develop a plan for any requisite clinical optimization.
- The preanesthesia evaluation should include a focused clinical examination, documentation of comorbid illness, reduction of patients' anxiety through education, assurance that preexisting medical conditions are optimally managed, selective referrals to medical specialists, ordering of preoperative investigations, initiation of interventions intended to decrease risk, discussion of aspects of perioperative care, arrangements for appropriate postoperative care, and recommendations to delay or cancel the surgical procedure, if deemed appropriate.
- Comorbid medical diseases can influence anesthesia and perioperative management, thus requiring the anesthesiologist to be knowledgeable in many aspects of internal medicine.
- Patients require appropriate preoperative diagnostic and laboratory studies consistent with their medical history and the proposed surgical procedure. Routine preoperative testing cannot be justified because it is costly and often clinically inappropriate.
- The anesthesiologist-led preoperative evaluation outpatient clinic can enhance operating room efficiency, decrease day-of-surgery cancellations or delays, reduce hospital costs, and enhance the quality of patient care.
- New and updated preoperative evaluation consensus and evidence-based guidelines published by multiple medical specialties have important influences on the preparation of patients for anesthesia and surgery.
- Anesthesiologists must be aware of, and be compliant with, increasing regulatory and reporting requirements involving preoperative issues by healthcare agencies.
- The anesthesiologist is the perioperative medical specialist and thus is uniquely positioned to evaluate the risks associated with anesthesia or surgery, discuss these risks with the patient, and manage them perioperatively in collaboration with the surgical team, referring physician, and other medical specialists.

Preoperative evaluation is required prior to the administration of any anesthetic. Its practice and scope have changed dramatically. Initial changes were driven by a rapid transformation in practice from hospital admission of patients the night before surgical procedures to admission on the morning of surgery. More recently, preanesthesia evaluation has become integral to the Perioperative Surgical Home model that aims to develop an integrated model for managing the entire perioperative episode of care.[1] This evolution in practice has led to a new approach to preoperative evaluation, which is a vital role of the perioperative physician. Accordingly, many anesthesiologists have expanded their responsibilities from providers of intraoperative anesthesia care to *perioperative medical specialists* who use their unique knowledge and experience to manage medical complexities related to surgery.[2] This expanded role entails that anesthesiologists assume the leadership role in the assessment and optimization of patients who are scheduled for surgery.[3] This chapter provides a comprehensive discussion of the practice of preoperative evaluation, as well as a review of related concepts, current evidence, and consensus-based clinical practice guidelines.

Evolution of Preanesthesia Evaluation

All patients requiring anesthesia for surgery must undergo a preoperative evaluation by their anesthesia provider. The conduct of this evaluation has changed substantially. Historically, anesthesiologists assessed their patients for the first time either just before the surgical procedure or on the preceding day, with the remainder of preoperative evaluation and preparation being the responsibility of the surgeon, primary care provider, or other specialist. In some countries, this approach remains the usual clinical practice. Nonetheless, in many countries, anesthesiologists have increasingly taken on a leadership role in preoperative evaluation and preparation, well in advance of the scheduled procedure. This is particularly true for high-risk patients or those undergoing high-risk procedures.

Several factors explain this change. First, considerably fewer patients are admitted to the hospital prior to the day of surgery. In many countries, there is little financial justification for the previous model of admitting patients prior to the day of surgery. For example, most surgical procedures in the United States are performed on an outpatient or same-day admission basis, including major neurosurgical, cardiac, and cancer resection procedures. Second, surgical patients are increasingly likely to be older frail individuals with significant burdens of medical comorbidity.[4] For such patients, sufficient time is needed between the preanesthesia evaluation and the planned surgery to facilitate testing, interventions, and medical optimization. In the case of patients with very high-risk medical comorbidity, preoperative consultation by an anesthesiologist can help inform a shared decision-making process for proceeding with surgery (see section on "Frailty, Geriatric Conditions, and the Older Surgical Patient"). Third, anesthesia care increasingly extends beyond the operating room alone. Preoperative evaluation is an integral component of the anesthesiologists' role as perioperative physicians who are involved in integrated medical care before, during, and after surgery. The specialty is uniquely positioned for this role given its expertise in the management of medical complexities related to anesthesia and surgery. This view of preoperative evaluation as a key component of the integrated management of the entire perioperative episode of care is essential to the Perioperative Surgical Home model.[1]

Outpatient preoperative assessment clinics have been instrumental in facilitating greater involvement of anesthesiologists in preoperative evaluation. These clinics also impose new clinical and organizational challenges. In an institution where most surgical patients are evaluated in the preoperative assessment clinic, anesthesiologists may have less time to evaluate medically complex patients. Consequently, anesthesiologists must achieve a high level of efficiency and accuracy in the assessment of a patient's history, physical examination, and differential diagnosis, as well as in the planning of perioperative management. Conversely, in a hospital where only the highest-risk patients are referred for consultation at a preoperative assessment clinic, the anesthesia department must interact with surgical departments to establish general protocols that ensure capture of the information needed to perform anesthesia safely, as well as the appropriate selection of individuals who require preoperative anesthesia consultation. In addition to changes in the scope and timing of the preanesthesia evaluation, this assessment has increasingly been influenced and governed by practice guidelines. For example, in the United States, The Joint Commission mandates documentation of a history and physical examination for any surgical patient within 30 days before the planned procedure, as well as reassessment within the 48-hour period immediately preceding the surgical procedure. The American Society of Anesthesiologists (ASA) and European Society of Anaesthesiology (ESA) have published specific guidelines for preoperative anesthesia evaluation.[5,6] In addition, several other specialty societies published practice guidelines specifically relating to the preoperative management of medical issues in surgical patients.[7-12]

Goals and Benefits of Preanesthesia Evaluation

Preoperative evaluations help influence and improve perioperative care (Fig. 31.1). Indeed, inadequate preoperative evaluation was a contributing factor in 3% of perioperative adverse events in the Australian Incident Monitoring Study database.[13] The overarching goals of preanesthesia evaluation are to (1) ensure that the patient can safely tolerate anesthesia for the planned surgery; and (2) mitigate perioperative risks such as pulmonary or cardiovascular complications. In pursuit of these goals, preanesthesia evaluations offer opportunities to perform focused clinical examinations, better document comorbid illness, reduce the patient's (and family's) anxiety through education, optimize preexisting medical conditions, make selective referrals to medical specialists (e.g., cardiologists), order specialized investigations (e.g., cardiac stress tests), initiate interventions intended to decrease risk, discuss aspects of perioperative care (e.g., anticipated risks, fasting guidelines), and arrange appropriate levels of postoperative care (e.g., critical care unit). If a patient is deemed to be at very high risk for adverse perioperative outcomes, the anesthesiologist may also recommend consideration of a nonoperative or less invasive treatment. Such a recommendation helps inform shared decision making for surgery (see Clinical Examination During Preoperative Evaluation section). In some cases, preanesthesia evaluation can identify a previously unrecognized medical condition (e.g., hypertension) that may not significantly affect perioperative risks, but warrants longer-term follow-up by appropriate healthcare professionals.

Compared to preoperative evaluations performed by surgeons or primary care physicians alone, anesthesiologist-led preoperative evaluation is associated with more selective ordering of laboratory tests and referral to specialists, thereby leading to reduced healthcare costs.[14-17] Within the context of an anesthesiologist-led preoperative evaluation clinic, preanesthesia evaluations also associated with reduced anxiety,[18] improved acceptance of regional anesthesia,[19] fewer day-of-surgery case cancellations,[14,20-22] shorter hospital length-of-stay,[19,21,22] and lower hospital costs.[21]

Clinical Examination During Preoperative Evaluation

The *clinical examination*, consisting of the history and physical examination, is a fundamental component of preoperative evaluation by anesthesiologists. This information helps identify the underlying basis for the planned surgery, clarify the extent of comorbidities with specific perioperative relevance, identify opportunities for preoperative optimization, and select any appropriate preoperative testing. The consistency and quality of preoperative examinations are enhanced through standardization. Specifically, the baseline clinical examination of all surgical patients should include a consistent

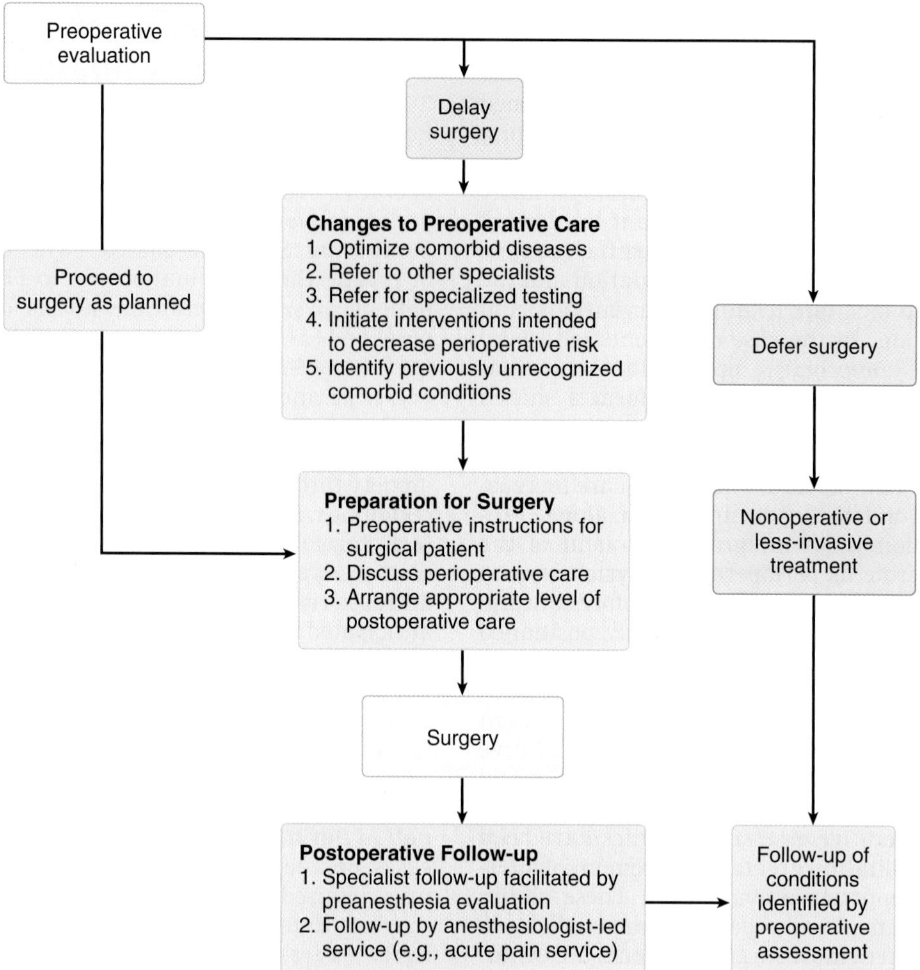

Fig. 31.1 Mechanisms by which preoperative evaluation can help influence and improve perioperative care.

set of components,[23] with opportunities for more detailed examination of one or more of these components (e.g., cardiovascular system) based on the findings from the standardized initial examination. Computer-based preoperative evaluation tools offer a mechanism for improving the standardization of high-quality preoperative assessments,[24,25] and are recommended in the 2018 ESA guidelines on preoperative evaluation.[6] The quality of the preoperative physical examination is further enhanced by appropriately considering evidence-based implications of different findings.[26]

COMPONENTS OF THE MEDICAL HISTORY

The important components of the anesthesia history are presented in the sample preoperative history form in Fig. 31.2. This information can be documented, either on paper or an electronic form, by anesthesia staff during an in-person or telephone interview with the patient. Alternatively, the patient can complete a form capturing the required information, either in person or remotely through a web-based program. The preanesthesia evaluation starts with the planned surgery and its indication. The development of the underlying condition necessitating surgery (e.g., cancer) and any prior related therapies need to be evident. Current known medical problems, past medical issues, previous surgeries, anesthesia types, and anesthesia-related complications must be noted. A simple notation of diseases or symptoms such as hypertension, diabetes mellitus, ischemic heart disease, shortness of breath, or chest pain is not sufficient. Rather, their associated severity, stability, associated activity limitations, exacerbations (current or recent), prior treatments, and planned interventions should be clearly documented. All related diagnostic test results, interventions, and names of treating physicians should be reviewed. The patient's responses to these initial questions may elicit further inquiry to establish a complete history.

Prescription and over-the-counter medications (including supplements and herbal medications) should be documented, along with their dosages and schedules. This information should include any recently interrupted medications with perioperative implications (e.g., recent corticosteroid therapy). The anesthesiologist should list any allergies to medications and other substances (e.g., latex, radiographic dye), with special emphasis on the patient's response to the exposure.

Patient's name__________ Age______ Sex______ Date of surgery______

Planned operation __________ Surgeon__________

Primary care doctor/phone #__________ Other physicians/phone #s__________

1. Please list **all operations** (and approximate dates)

a. __________ d. __________

b. __________ e. __________

c. __________ f. __________

2. Please list any **allergies** to medicines, latex, or other (and your reactions to them)

a. __________ c. __________

b. __________ d. __________

3. Please list **all medications** you have taken in the last month (include over-the-counter drugs, inhalers, herbals, dietary supplements, and aspirin)

Name of Drug	Dose and How Often	Name of Drug	Dose and How Often
a.		f.	
b.		g.	
c.		h.	
d.		i.	
e.		j.	

(Please check YES or NO and circle specific problems)	YES	NO
4. Have you taken steroids (prednisone or cortisone) in the last year?	☐	☐
5. Have you *ever* smoked? (Quantify in ______ packs/day for ______ years)	☐	☐
Do you still smoke?	☐	☐
Do you drink alcohol? (If so, how much?) __________	☐	☐
Do you use or have you ever used any illegal drugs? (we need to know for your safety)	☐	☐
6. Can you walk up one flight of stairs without stopping?	☐	☐
7. Have you had any problems with your heart? **(circle)** (chest pain or pressure, heart attack, abnormal ECG, skipped beats, heart murmur, palpitation, heart failure [fluid in the lungs], require antibiotics before routine dental care)	☐	☐
8. Do you have high blood pressure?	☐	☐
9. Have you had any problems with your lungs or your chest? **(circle)** (shortness of breath, emphysema, bronchitis, asthma, TB, abnormal chest x-ray)	☐	☐
10. Are you ill now or were you recently ill with a cold, fever, chills, flu or productive cough? Describe recent changes __________	☐	☐

A

Fig. 31.2 (A and B) Sample patient preoperative history form. (*ECG*, Electrocardiogram; *TB*, tuberculosis; *TMJ*, temporomandibular joint.)

Patients often claim an "allergy" to a substance when, in reality, the reaction was an expected side effect (e.g., nausea or vomiting with narcotics). Tobacco, alcohol, or illicit drug use must be documented. Tobacco exposure is best quantified using pack-years (number of packs of cigarettes smoked per day, multiplied by the number of years of smoking); as an example, an individual who smoked two packs of cigarettes daily for the prior 10 years is deemed to have a 20 pack-year history of tobacco use. A personal or family history of pseudocholinesterase deficiency and malignant hyperthermia (including a suggestive history such as hyperthermia or rigidity during anesthesia) must be clearly documented to facilitate appropriate planning before the day of surgery. Information from previous anesthetic records may clarify an uncertain history.

A standardized general review of all organ systems should then be performed. For example, patients should be asked whether they ever had problems with their heart, lungs, kidneys, liver, and nervous system. In addition, they should be asked about any history of cancer, anemia, bleeding problems, or prior hospitalization for any reason. The principal emphasis should be on airway abnormalities, anesthesia-related adverse events (personal or family history), as well as symptoms of cardiovascular, pulmonary, hepatic, renal, endocrine, or

(Please check YES or NO and circle specific problems)	YES	NO
11. Have you or anyone in your family had serious bleeding problems? **(circle)** (prolonged bleeding from nosebleed, gums, tooth extractions, or surgery)	☐	☐
12. Have you had any problems with your blood (anemia, leukemia, sickle cell disease, blood clots, transfusions)?	☐	☐
13. Have you ever had problems with your: **(circle)**	☐	☐
Liver (cirrhosis, hepatitis, jaundice)?	☐	☐
Kidney (stones, failure, dialysis)?	☐	☐
Digestive system (frequent heartburn, hiatus hernia, stomach ulcer)?	☐	☐
Back, neck or jaws (TMJ, rheumatoid arthritis)?	☐	☐
Thyroid gland (underactive or overactive)?	☐	☐
14. Have you ever had: **(circle)**	☐	☐
Seizures, epilepsy, or fits?	☐	☐
Stroke, facial, leg or arm weakness, difficulty speaking?	☐	☐
Cramping pain in your legs with walking?	☐	☐
Problems with hearing, vision or memory?	☐	☐
15. Have you ever been treated for cancer with chemotherapy or radiation therapy? **(circle)**	☐	☐
16. Women: Could you be pregnant? Last menstrual period began: ______________________	☐	☐
17. Have you ever had problems with anesthesia or surgery? **(circle)** (severe nausea or vomiting, malignant hyperthermia [in blood relatives or self], prolonged drowsiness, anxiety, breathing difficulties, or problems during placement of a breathing tube)	☐	☐
18. Do you have any chipped or loose teeth, dentures, caps, bridgework, braces, problems opening your mouth, swallowing or choking? **(circle)**	☐	☐
19. Do your physical abilities limit your daily activities?	☐	☐
20. Do you snore?	☐	☐
21. Please list any medical illnesses not noted above: ______________________		
22. Additional comments or questions for nurse or anesthesiologist? ______________________		

B

Fig. 31.2, cont'd.

neurologic disease. For example, a report of a patient who has experienced excessive sore throat, dental injuries, or "the need to have a small tube" with previous anesthetic cases may be an indication of previous difficulty with airway management. A history of snoring and daytime somnolence may suggest undiagnosed sleep apnea (see later section on "Obstructive Sleep Apnea"). Any history of chest discomfort (including its duration, precipitating factors, associated symptoms, and relieving factors) could be important. Similarly, a list of previous surgical procedures should be obtained and can help complete the medical history. Finally, records from primary care physicians, specialists, or inpatient admissions may reveal any issues the patient did not recall.

ASSESSMENT OF FUNCTIONAL CAPACITY

The assessment of the patient's cardiopulmonary fitness or functional capacity is an integral component of the preoperative clinical examination. This information is typically used to estimate a patient's risk for major postoperative morbidity or mortality, and to determine whether further preoperative testing is required.[7] Importantly, suboptimal functional capacity is common in many economically advanced countries. For example, only one-fifth of American adults meet federal guidelines for recommended levels of aerobic and strengthening activity.[27] Poor exercise capacity and cardiopulmonary disease have a bidirectional relationship. Specifically, lack of exercise may increase the risk of developing cardiopulmonary disease but preexisting cardiopulmonary disease can also prevent an individual from exercising. For example, patients with peripheral artery disease (PAD) may be limited by intermittent claudication, and patients with ischemic heart disease may be limited by exertional chest discomfort. There is a reasonable body of evidence demonstrating an association between poor preoperative functional capacity and increased perioperative risk. Most of these studies involved objective assessment of preoperative functional capacity using either exercise testing or cardiopulmonary exercise testing (CPET).[28-31] Several other large studies have demonstrated association between very significant preoperative functional impairment (i.e., difficulty or inability to perform activities of daily living) and increased risks of postoperative mortality,[32] cardiovascular complications,[33] and pulmonary complications.[34,35]

The challenge with assessment of preoperative functional capacity pertains to how best to assess it in usual clinical practice. Typically, the anesthesiologist will inquire about a patient's general activity levels during the preoperative interview, and on that basis, make a *subjective assessment* of the patient's functional capacity. Functional capacity is typically quantified in using the metabolic equivalent of task (MET), where one MET is approximately the rate of energy consumption at rest (3.5 mL/kg/min). A proposed scheme for estimating METs based on information from the preoperative interview is presented in Table 31.1. There are important limitations to the usual clinical approach for this integral component of the preoperative evaluation. First, subjective assessment does not accurately estimate the patient's true exercise capacity. In a multicenter prospective cohort study of 1401 patients undergoing major noncardiac surgery, anesthesiologists' subjective assessment had only 19% sensitivity and 95% specificity for identifying patients' inability to attain 4 or more METs during formal exercise testing.[36] In addition, subjective assessment has poor correlation with standardized questionnaires that have been validated for measuring functional capacity.[37,38] Second, subjective assessment has generally shown poor performance in predicting postoperative morbidity and mortality. In a single-center cohort study of 600 surgical patients, patients' self-reported poor exercise capacity (defined as inability to walk four blocks and climb two flights of stairs) was associated with increased risk of serious perioperative complications,[39] but the magnitude of the association was relatively weak (positive likelihood ratio of 1.3 and negative likelihood ratio of 0.6). For context, positive test results should have likelihood ratios greater than 2 to provide clinically meaningful information, whereas negative test results should have likelihood ratios of less than 0.5.[40] Furthermore, in both a multicenter prospective cohort study and single-center retrospective cohort study, subjective assessment was a poor predictor of postoperative mortality and morbidity.[36,41]

To improve preoperative evaluation of functional capacity, anesthesiologists should consider instead using structured questionnaires, such as the Duke Activity Status Index (DASI) (Table 31.2).[42] This 12-item self-administered questionnaire about activities of daily living has demonstrated correlation with gold-standard measures of functional capacity in surgical patients.[36,43] Furthermore, DASI scores have been shown to improve prediction of postoperative cardiac complications following noncardiac surgery.[36] While there is some varying opinion as to how DASI scores should be converted to METs, the original formula is presented below:

$$\text{Estimated METS} = \frac{(0.43 \times \text{DASI score}) + 9.6}{3.5}.$$

Other alternatives for estimating functional capacity include simple exercise tests (e.g., 6-minute walk test, incremental shuttle walk test),[44] exercise testing (e.g., electrocardiogram [ECG] exercise testing), or CPET. If using a standard exercise test (i.e., not CPET), extrapolation from the total treadmill time on a Bruce protocol exercise test results in overestimation of true exercise capacity. More importantly, resting left ventricular ejection fraction should not be used as a proxy measure of functional capacity.[45,46]

TABLE 31.1 Metabolic Equivalents* of Functional Capacity

METs	Equivalent Level of Exercise
1	Eating, working at computer, or dressing
2	Walking down stairs or in your house, or cooking
3	Walking 1 or 2 blocks on level ground
4	Raking leaves, gardening
5	Climbing 1 flight of stairs, dancing, or bicycling
6	Playing golf, or carrying clubs
7	Playing singles tennis
8	Rapidly climbing stairs, or jogging slowly
9	Jumping rope slowly, or moderate cycling
10	Swimming quickly, running or jogging briskly
11	Skiing cross country, or playing full-court basketball
12	Running rapidly for moderate to long distances

*One metabolic equivalent of task (MET) is the amount of oxygen consumed while sitting at rest, and is equivalent to an oxygen consumption of 3.5 mL/min/kg body weight.

Modified from Jette M, Sidney K, Blumchen G. Metabolic equivalents (METS) in exercise testing, exercise prescription, and evaluation of functional capacity. *Clin Cardiol.* 1990;13:555–565.

PHYSICAL EXAMINATION

At a minimum, the preanesthetic examination should include vital signs (i.e., arterial blood pressure, heart rate, respiratory rate, oxygen saturation), height, and

TABLE 31.2 Duke Activity Specific Index questionnaire

Can You	Points
1. Take care of yourself, that is, eat dress, bathe, or use the toilet?	2.75
2. Walk indoors, such as around your house?	1.75
3. Walk 200 yards on level ground?	2.75
4. Climb a flight of stairs or walk up a hill?	5.50
5. Run a short distance?	8.00
6. Do light work around the house like dusting or washing dishes?	2.70
7. Do moderate work around the house like vacuuming, sweeping floors, or carrying groceries?	3.50
8. Do heavy work around the house like scrubbing floors or lifting or moving heavy furniture?	8.00
9. Do yard work like raking leaves, weeding, or pushing a power mower?	4.50
10. Have sexual relations?	5.25
11. Participate in moderate recreational activities like golf, bowling, dancing, doubles tennis, or throwing a ball?	6.00
12. Participate in strenuous sports like swimming, singles tennis, football, basketball, or skiing?	7.50
Total score:	

From Hlatky MA, Boineau RE, Higginbotham MB, et al. A brief self-administered questionnaire to determine functional capacity (the Duke Activity Status Index). *Am J Cardiol.* 1989;64:651–654.

TABLE 31.3 Classification Scheme for Body Mass Index

Body Mass Index	Weight Status
ADULTS OVER 20 YEARS OLD	
BMI < 18.5	Underweight
BMI 18.5–24.9	Normal
BMI 25.0–29.9	Overweight
BMI 30.0 and above	Obese
FOR CHILDREN AND TEENS	
BMI-for-age < 5th percentile	Underweight
BMI-for-age 5th percentile to < 85th percentile	Normal
BMI-for-age 85th percentile to < 95th percentile	At risk of overweight
BMI-for-age ≥ 95th percentile	Overweight

BMI, Body mass index.
From Centers for Disease Control and Prevention. http://www.cdc.gov.

BOX 31.1 Components of the Airway Examination

Length of upper incisors (concerning if relatively long)
Condition of the teeth
Relationship of maxillary incisors to mandibular incisors (concerning if there is prominent overbite)
Ability to advance mandibular incisors in front of maxillary incisors (concerning if unable to do this)
Interincisor or intergum (if edentulous) distance (concerning if < 3 cm)
Visibility of the uvula (concerning if Mallampati class is 3 or more)
Shape of uvula (concerning if highly arched or very narrow)
Presence of heavy facial hair
Compliance of the mandibular space (concerning if it is stiff, indurated, occupied by mass, or nonresilient)
Thyromental distance (concerning if < 6 cm)
Length of the neck
Thickness or circumference of the neck
Range of motion of the head and neck (concerning if unable to touch tip of chin to chest or cannot extend neck)

From: Apfelbaum JL, Hagberg CA, Caplan RA, et al. Practice guidelines for management of the difficult airway: an updated report by the American Society of Anesthesiologists Task Force on Management of the Difficult Airway. *Anesthesiology.* 2013;118:251–270.

weight. Body mass index (BMI), which is calculated based on height and weight, is more informative than weight alone in establishing obesity. A scheme for classifying children and adults based on BMI is presented in Table 31.3. Information pertaining to BMI can help identify individuals at risk for difficulties with airway management, and some chronic diseases (e.g., heart disease, diabetes mellitus, obstructive sleep apnea [OSA]). An ideal body weight should also be calculated,[47] using available formulae such as the Devine equation.[48] Information on ideal body weight can better inform dose selection for some anesthesia-related medications, and settings for positive pressure ventilation. Readily available online calculators can be used to quickly determine both BMI and ideal body weight. Patients often have increased arterial blood pressure during the preoperative visit, even without a prior history of hypertension. This finding may be caused by anxiety, or patients having forgotten to take their usual dose of antihypertensive medication. Thus, a single reading during the preoperative evaluation may not reflect the patient's usual blood pressure control. Repeating the blood pressure measurement or obtaining previous readings, either by obtaining medical records (including prior ambulatory blood pressure testing) or asking patients about their "usual" blood pressure measurements are informative. Ideally, the referral documentation from the patient's primary care physician or surgeon should include information on the patient's usual blood pressure readings.[49]

From an anesthesiologist's perspective, inspection of the airway may be the most important component of the physical examination (see Chapter 44). The components of the airway examination are presented in Box 31.1.[50]

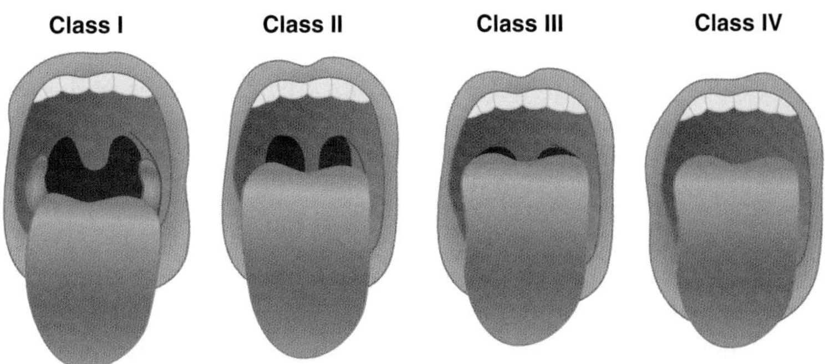

Fig. 31.3 Mallampati classification: class I, soft palate, fauces, entire uvula, pillars; class II, soft palate, fauces, portion of uvula; class III, soft palate, base of uvula; class IV, hard palate only. (From Bair AE, Caravelli R, Tyler K, et al. Feasibility of the preoperative Mallampati airway assessment in emergency department patients. *J Emerg Med.* 2010;38:677–680.)

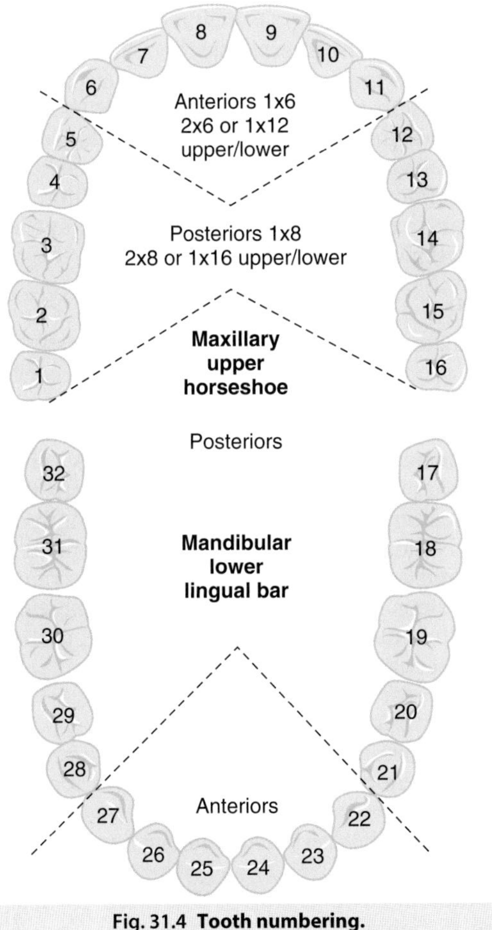

Fig. 31.4 Tooth numbering.

Documentation of an airway examination includes the Mallampati score (Fig. 31.3),[51] status of teeth, degree of neck mobility (especially extension), neck circumference (increased size predicts difficulty with laryngoscopy), thyromental distance, body habitus, and pertinent deformities. Because of the potential for dental injuries during anesthesia, any preexisting tooth abnormalities should be documented (Fig. 31.4). In a French prospective cohort study of 1501 patients, the following characteristics were identified as independent predictors of *difficult* bag-mask ventilation: age more than 55 years, BMI more than 26 kg/m^2, absence of teeth, presence of a beard, and a history of snoring.[52] These risk factors are largely consistent with those identified in an American retrospective cohort study of 22,660 patients: age 57 years or more, BMI 30 kg/m^2 or greater, presence of a beard, Mallampati classification III or IV, severely limited mandibular protrusion, and a history of snoring.[53] Other possible risk factors for difficult ventilation include an increased neck circumference, face and neck deformities (i.e., prior surgery, prior radiation, prior trauma, congenital abnormalities), rheumatoid arthritis, Trisomy 21 (Down syndrome), scleroderma, cervical spine disease, or previous cervical spine surgery. The physical examination must be supplemented by examination of previous anesthetic records, especially when there are indications of a potentially difficult airway. Patients with known difficult airways should be encouraged to obtain medical alert identification. When challenging airways are identified, advance planning ensures that necessary equipment and skilled personnel are available on the day of surgery. An evaluation of the heart, lungs, and skin is necessary, as well as further focus on organ systems involved with diseases reported by the patient. This evaluation should include cardiac auscultation, as well as inspection of arterial pulses, veins (peripheral and central), jugular venous distention, ascites, hepatomegaly, and peripheral edema. Inspection of peripheral veins can also help assess the ease of intravenous access. The auscultatory examination should assess for murmurs, abnormal heart sounds (e.g., third or fourth heart sounds), and pulmonary rales. If intravenous access sites are limited, possible central line placement can be discussed with the patient, or arrangements can be made for assistance from interventional radiology. Auscultation for carotid bruits is also important, especially in patients with a history of stroke, transient ischemic attacks (TIAs), or head and neck irradiation. The presence of a carotid bruit significantly increases the likelihood of an important lesion (i.e., 70%-99% stenosis) in both symptomatic or asymptomatic patients, but the absence of a bruit does not rule out carotid stenosis.[26] Examination of the pulmonary system should include both auscultation (i.e., wheezing, decreased breath sounds, abnormal breath sounds) and inspection (i.e., cyanosis, clubbing, accessory muscle use, respiratory effort). A basic screening neurologic examination should document deficits in mental status, speech, gait, cranial nerve function, motor nerve function, and sensory nerve function. For selected patients (e.g., those with deficits, or scheduled to undergo neurosurgery), a more extensive or focused neurologic examination should document preexisting abnormalities that may aid in diagnosis or interfere with positioning. In addition, the definition of a baseline preoperative neurologic state helps determine whether any postoperative deficits represent new deficits versus preexisting abnormalities.

Frailty, Geriatric Conditions, and the Older Surgical Patient

As patients age, the accumulation of comorbid conditions puts them at increased risk for adverse outcomes after surgery.[54] In addition, geriatric-specific risk factors such as functional and cognitive impairment are associated with poor postoperative outcomes.[54] These clinical conditions, which do not fit into discrete disease categories, are often overlooked in routine preoperative assessments. In order to (1) accurately inform patients of their surgical risk and (2) identify targets for preoperative optimization, assessment of geriatric vulnerabilities is essential before surgery. The American College of Surgeons (ACS) and the American Geriatrics Society (AGS) have established best practice guidelines to guide the preoperative assessment of older surgical patients.[55]

GERIATRIC-FOCUSED ASSESSMENT IN THE OLDER SURGICAL PATIENT

Function and Mobility

Preoperative functional decline is associated with morbidity, mortality, and loss of function after surgery.[54] Assessment of function prior to surgery is consequently essential for risk stratification and postdischarge planning in older surgical patients. Activities-of-daily-living (ADLs) assess the ability to perform basic tasks of selfcare, such as dressing, bathing, toileting, movement, continence, and eating. Instrumental ADLs determine an individual's ability to live independently by the ability to complete shopping, laundry, transportation, finances, medications, food preparation, and housekeeping. To determine additional functional vulnerabilities, determination of vision deficits, hearing deficits, and swallowing difficulties should be routine. Mobility impairment can be efficiently screened by enquiring about a history of falls, determining fall risk, and performing a Timed-Up-And-Go test.[56] The Timed-Up-And-Go test involves timing patients while they perform the following tasks in sequence:

1. Stand up from a chair (without using arm rests if possible)
2. Walk 10 feet
3. Turn around and walk back to chair
4. Sit down in chair

In a prospective cohort of older surgical patients, Timed-Up-And-Go test times were associated with risks of postoperative complications and 1-year mortality in a stepwise fashion.[57]

Cognition

Preoperative cognitive impairment is strongly linked to delirium, complications, functional decline, and death after surgery.[54] The Mini-Cog test (available at https://mini-cog.com), which consists of a three-item recall test and clock draw test, is an efficient tool to screen for preoperative cognitive impairment. Additional information about potential cognitive deficits should be elicited from someone who knows the patient well. Importantly, mild cognitive impairment that is not clinically apparent may have a critical impact on decision-making capacity. Patients should be able to describe, in their own words, the essential elements of the consent discussion—including the surgical condition, indications for surgery, risks, benefits, and alternatives to surgery. It is important to note the four legal criteria for medical decision-making capacity, namely that the patient can (1) clearly indicate his/her treatment choice; (2) understand the relevant information communicated by the physician; (3) acknowledge his/her medical condition, treatment options, and expected outcomes; and (4) engage in a rational discussion about treatment options.[55]

Nutrition

In general, most surgeons and anesthesiologists are keenly aware of the role nutritional status plays in recovery after surgery for all surgical patients. The most common adverse events related to poor nutritional status are infectious complications (i.e., surgical site infections, pneumonia, urinary tract infections), wound complications (i.e., dehiscence, anastomotic leaks), and increased length of stay. [54] The ACS National Surgical Quality Improvement Program (NSQIP) and AGS Best Practice Guidelines recommend the following steps to screen for poor nutritional status (older adults with limited material resources are at particular risk for food insecurity).[55]

1. *Document height, weight, and BMI*

A BMI value less than 18.5 kg/m^2 places an individual at elevated risk and should prompt referral for nutritional assessment.

2. *Measure baseline serum albumin and prealbumin concentrations*

Serum albumin concentration less than 30 g/L (in the absence of hepatic or renal dysfunction) should prompt referral for nutritional assessment.

3. *Inquire about unintentional weight loss in the last year*

Unintentional weight loss exceeding 10% to 15% of baseline weight within the prior 6 months is associated with severe nutritional risk and should prompt referral for nutritional assessment.

Frailty

Frailty, which is defined as a state of increased vulnerability to physiologic stressors, is associated with adverse health outcomes after medical and surgical interventions and

TABLE 31.4 Preoperative Assessment and Optimization in the Older Surgical Patient

Domain	Assessment	Preoperative Optimization
Cognition	▪ Mini-Cog Test ▪ Visual and hearing ▪ Impairment ▪ Alcohol abuse ▪ Medication review	▪ Formal assessment by geriatrician for patient identified to have cognitive impairment on screening ▪ Remind patient to bring all assistive devices (glasses, hearing aids) to hospital ▪ Limit use of sedating or psychotropic medications preoperatively
Function	▪ Evaluate ability to perform activities of daily living and instrumental activities of daily living ▪ Obtain history of falls ▪ Timed up and go test	▪ Refer patients with functional deficiencies or history of falls for formal evaluation by a physical therapist before surgery ▪ Exercise education ▪ Obtain assistive devices ▪ Plan for in-hospital and postdischarge rehabilitation therapy
Nutrition	▪ Document body mass index ▪ Measure albumin and prealbumin ▪ Query unintentional weight loss	▪ Patients at severe malnutritional deficit should be referred to dietician for formal assessment ▪ Preoperative nutritional supplementation and nutrition education

From Oresanya LB, Lyons WL, Finlayson E. Preoperative assessment of the older patient: a narrative review. *JAMA*. 2014;311:2110–2120.

limited life expectancy.[58] Numerous validated instruments measuring frailty are in current use in research and clinical practice. There are two primary models of frailty—the frailty phenotype and the deficit accumulation model. The frailty phenotype described by Fried and colleagues is based on the identification of traits associated with the occurrence of disease, hospitalization, falls, disability, and death in a large prospective cohort study.[59] This study defined the determinants of frailty as weight loss, exhaustion, physical activity, walk time, and grip strength. The deficit accumulation model of aging (based on data from the Canadian Study of Health and Aging) identified 92 signs, symptoms, functional impairments, and laboratory abnormalities that are proportionally weighted into a frailty index for predicting mortality.[60]

While numerous studies have demonstrated the association of patient frailty with adverse surgical outcomes,[54,61-64] the incorporation of a patient's level of frailty into routine clinical practice has not been broadly implemented. Many frailty instruments require special training, input of laboratory values or clinical data, and a fair amount of time to complete; hence, they are impractical in a busy clinical setting. A recent survey of surgical oncologists reported that although most surgeons expressed interest in preoperative optimization for older patients, only 6% currently perform geriatric assessments in their older patients.[65] Factors contributing to the low level of adoption include perceptions regarding the amount of time required to assess for vulnerabilities, and lack of specific programs designed to address them within typical clinical practices. To address this gap, several investigators have validated efficient strategies to measure frailty in clinical practice. Robinson and colleagues developed two alternative frailty assessment definitions for surgical patients,[66,67] which were

- Mini-Cog score of 3 or less, serum albumin concentration of 30 g/L or less, one or more falls in the prior 6 months, and hematocrit under 35%.
- Timed-Up-And-Go test 15 or more seconds, activity-of-daily-living dependence, and Charlson comorbidity index score 3 or greater.[68]

Frailty identified with the Edmonton Frail Scale (EFS) has been shown to be associated with adverse outcomes after surgery.[61] The EFS can be administered by an individual with no formal medical education, and has been validated in comparison to the geriatric specialist's comprehensive geriatric assessment.[69]

Additional Considerations

Anxiety, depression, substance abuse, and social isolation are common underdiagnosed conditions in older adults. Careful screening can identify these potential barriers to recovery, safe discharge after surgery, and maintenance of independence. Up to 11% of the population 71 years of age or more in the United States suffer from depression.[70] The Patient Health Questionnaire-2 is an efficient instrument to screen for depression that includes only two questions: "*In the past 12 months, have you ever had a time when you felt sad, blue, depressed, or down for most of the time for at least two weeks?*" and "*In the past 12 months, have you ever had a time, lasting at least two weeks, when you didn't care about the things that you usually care about or when you didn't enjoy the things that you usually enjoy?*" Among individuals aged 65 years or more, 13% of males and 8% of females consume at least two alcoholic drinks per day.[71] Alcohol and substance abuse are associated with increased rates of postoperative mortality and complications including pneumonia, sepsis, wound infection and disruption, and prolonged length of stay.[72] Consequently, the ACS NSQIP and AGS recommend screening for alcohol and substance abuse among older individuals with the modified CAGE (acronym of four clinical interview questions: cutting down, annoyance by criticism, guilty feeling, and eye-openers) questionnaire (see section on "Patients With a History of Substance Abuse").

PREOPERATIVE OPTIMIZATION FOR FRAIL GERIATRIC PATIENTS (TABLE 31.4)

One goal of the preoperative assessment of elderly surgical patients is to identify potentially modifiable risk factors—such as malnutrition, poor physical function, anxiety, and social isolation—in order to optimize surgical outcomes. Several recent geriatric *prehabilitation* models have emerged to help meet this need, with some demonstrating promising results. One of the first of such programs was the Proactive Care of Older People undergoing surgery (POPS) before-and-after study in United Kingdom.[73] The overarching aim of this project was to decrease complications and hospital length of stay among at-risk older adults undergoing elective surgery. The authors performed a structured geriatric team intervention that identified at-risk patients, and then facilitated coordinated multidisciplinary optimization of geriatric vulnerabilities. The interventions included preoperative home visits by occupational and physical therapists, social worker inputs, nutrition education, and relaxation techniques. In addition to preoperative optimization, interdisciplinary teams participated in daily inpatient rounds, weekly multidisciplinary meetings, and bi-weekly ward rounds led by a consultant or clinical nurse specialist. Compared to historical controls, surgical patients who received the POPS intervention experienced fewer postoperative complications (e.g., pneumonia, delirium), improved pain control, lower rates of delayed mobilization, lower rates of inappropriate urinary catheter use, and shorter hospital length of stay.

Similar findings were observed in the more recently reported Perioperative Optimization of Senior Health study, which was another before-and-after study.[74] This preoperative interdisciplinary clinic evaluated at-risk patients (either aged age ≥ 80 years, or aged ≥ 65 years with concurrent geriatric vulnerability) and designed targeted optimization. Compared to historical controls, the combination of geriatric prehabilitation and inpatient geriatric comanagement were associated with reduced hospital length of stay, reduced readmission rates, and increased rates of discharge to home with self-care. Another example of a promising prehabilitation program is the Michigan Surgical Home and Optimization Program,[75] which is a structured home-based preoperative training program with physical, nutritional, and psychological interventions. The intervention included (1) a home-based walking program with daily reminders and feedback; (2) incentive spirometry instructions starting 1 week prior to surgery; (3) education on nutrition, stress management, and care planning; and (4) resources for smoking cessation, when appropriate. Compared to matched historical controls, patients enrolled in the program experienced reductions in both hospital length of stay and healthcare costs. While promising, these studies do have methodological weakness as before-and-after studies, as opposed to methodologically more robust parallel arm randomized trials, cluster randomized trials, or stepped-wedge trials (see Chapter 90). Nonetheless, the consistency in findings across the studies is supportive of the notion that attention to preoperative and perioperative assessment in the older population can result in improved postoperative outcomes that benefit patients, hospitals, and healthcare systems.

DECISION MAKING FOR SURGERY IN OLDER ADULTS

The critical initial step in surgical decision making for the older patient is an assessment of the patient's decision-making capacity. Among older adults, only about 3% lack medical decision-making capacity. However, among older adults with mild cognitive impairment, this proportion is as high as 20%.[76] A Mini-Cog exam (see section on "Cognition") is an efficient way to screen for cognitive impairment in the surgical setting. If the patient does not have capacity, treatment goals and choices should be discussed with the patient's surrogate, with patient involvement as appropriate. Even cognitively intact patients may have difficulty grasping the risks and tradeoffs involved in decisions for surgery. The "teach-back" method (i.e., asking patients to communicate back information about their diagnosis, treatment plan, and potential risks of treatment) may be useful to confirm that the risks, expected benefits, and alternatives to surgery are fully understood. Various resources are available to aid in using the teach-back method (e.g., http://www.teachbacktraining.org).

Collaborative decision making is essential in older adults with limited life expectancy. Rather than a traditional conversation that focuses on the process of correcting the underlying surgical condition, the conversation should be driven by a focus on the older adult's overarching health goals. Using open-ended questions, physicians elicit the patient's global healthcare goals that may prioritize (1) life prolongation; (2) function and independence; (3) maintenance of cognition; or (4) comfort. Further discussion should be framed by the patient's most important health goal. A frank, realistic, and granular conversation about the ability of surgery to satisfy healthcare goals and priorities is essential. Invasive treatments should only be considered if there is a realistic possibility that overarching health goals can be achieved. These goals, however, are often dynamic and must be revisited as conditions change. Often, primary physicians who have longitudinal relationships with patients can provide important insight into their patient's health goals and should be included in this important deliberation. To assist in high-risk surgical decision making, preoperative palliative care consultation should be considered in individuals with poor prognoses who are electing to undergo surgery, particularly if they have a life expectancy of less than 6 months.

Preoperative Evaluation of Patients With Coexisting Disease

For some conditions commonly seen in the preanesthetic assessment clinic, preoperative optimization, testing, and intervention may be important (see also Chapter 32). Identification of these comorbid conditions might be an opportunity for the anesthesiologist to intervene to decrease perioperative risk. These conditions are best managed before the day of surgery, thus allowing ample time for thoughtful evaluation, consultation, and planning.

CARDIOVASCULAR DISEASE

Cardiovascular complications are serious perioperative adverse events that account for about 45% of all deaths within 30 days after major noncardiac surgery.[77] These events occur relatively frequently. For example, the multicenter Vascular Events in Noncardiac Surgery Patients Cohort Evaluation prospective cohort study found a 4% risk of myocardial infarction, 17% risk of prognostically important myocardial injury, and 0.7% risk of acute heart failure during the 30 days following major noncardiac surgery.[78] Evidence-based preoperative cardiovascular assessment guidelines have now been published in several countries, including the 2014 American College of Cardiology (ACC) and American Heart Association (AHA) guidelines,[7] 2014 European Society of Cardiology (ESC) and ESA guidelines,[9] 2017 Canadian Cardiovascular Society (CCS) guidelines,[8] 2017 Brazilian Society of Cardiology guidelines,[79] and 2014 Japanese Circulation Society guidelines.[80] While the guidelines provide generally similar guidance, there are some important differences that will be highlighted in the sections below.

Hypertension

Based on revised 2017 ACC/AHA guidelines, hypertension is defined as a blood pressure greater than 130/80 based on appropriately measured arterial blood pressure.[81] About 45% of adults in the United States have hypertension,[82] with a similar prevalence in other countries. While most individuals with hypertension have primary (or essential) hypertension, there are several important causes of secondary hypertension, including primary renal disease, OSA, pheochromocytoma, renovascular hypertension, Cushing syndrome, hyperthyroidism, and coarctation of the aorta. Hypertension leads to significantly increased risks of left ventricular hypertrophy (LVH), heart failure, ischemic heart disease, chronic kidney disease (CKD), ischemic stroke, intracerebral hemorrhage, and PAD. The duration and severity of hypertension are highly correlated with subsequent end-organ damage, morbidity, and mortality. These risks appear to increase once blood pressure exceeds 117/75, with each subsequent 20 mm Hg increase in systolic blood pressure and 10 mm Hg increase in diastolic blood pressure being associated with a two-fold increase in the risk of stroke and cardiovascular death.[83] In the perioperative setting, hypertension is associated with increased risks of postoperative death and myocardial infarction, but the magnitude of this association is relatively weak (odds ratio 1.35; 95% confidence limits, 1.17-1.56).[84]

In patients with hypertension, the goals of preoperative evaluation are to identify any secondary causes of hypertension, presence of other cardiovascular risk factors (e.g., smoking, diabetes mellitus), and evidence of end-organ damage. For example, paroxysmal hypertension or hypertension in young individuals should prompt a search for hyperthyroidism, illicit drug use (e.g., cocaine, anabolic steroids), and coarctation of the aorta. Similarly, a history of paroxysmal hypertension associated with episodic tachycardia and palpitations should raise suspicions about an underlying pheochromocytoma (see next section). The physical examination should focus on vital signs (including blood pressure measured in both arms), thyroid gland, peripheral pulses, and cardiovascular system (including bruits and signs of intravascular volume overload). Additional specialized testing is directed by the initial clinical evaluation. For example, patients with long-standing, severe, or poorly controlled hypertension should undergo an ECG and blood sampling to measure creatinine concentration. Individuals on diuretic antihypertensives (e.g., chlorthalidone, hydrochlorothiazide) may require evaluation of electrolytes. Patients with suspected hyperthyroidism will require thyroid function tests.

While preoperative hypertension is associated with an increased risk of cardiovascular complication,[84] this association is generally not evident for systolic blood pressure values less than 180 mm Hg or diastolic blood pressure values less than 110 mm Hg. Additionally, there is no compelling data that delaying surgery to optimize blood pressure control will result in improved outcomes. Accordingly, some international practice guidelines support proceeding with surgery if the systolic blood pressure is less than 180 mm Hg and diastolic blood pressure is less than 110 mm Hg.[9,49] Usual antihypertensive medication treatment should be continued in these patients during the perioperative period. For patients with severe hypertension (i.e., diastolic blood pressure > 110 mm Hg or systolic blood pressure > 180 mm Hg), anesthesiologists should weigh the potential benefits of delaying surgery to optimize antihypertensive treatment against the risks of delaying the procedure. In general, all long-term antihypertensive treatment should be continued up to the day of surgery, with the possible exception of angiotensin-converting enzyme inhibitors (ACEIs) and angiotensin receptor blockers (ARBs). Administration of these medications within 24 hours before surgery is consistently associated with increased risks of intraoperative hypotension,[85] and possibly associated with elevated risks of postoperative myocardial injury.[86] Accordingly, it is reasonable to withhold these medications for 24 hours before surgery, provided that they are restarted postoperatively once patients are hemodynamically stable. Importantly, failure to resume ACEI and ARB therapy postoperatively is itself associated with adverse outcomes.[87,88]

Even if surgery is not necessarily delayed to facilitate improved blood pressure control, the preanesthesia evaluation should also be viewed as an excellent opportunity to alter long-term consequences of diseases. Thus, appropriate postsurgery referrals should be made to facilitate improved long-term management of hypertension.

Ischemic Heart Disease

Ischemic heart disease (IHD) afflicts about 16.5 million adults in the United States, and 111 million people worldwide.[27] It also accounts for about 13% of all deaths, both in the United States and worldwide (http://www.who.int/mediacentre/factsheets/fs317/en/).[27] While death rates attributable to IHD are declining in many high-income countries,[89] other regions continue to experience high or increasing rates of IHD mortality. IHD mediates adverse effects because of its immediate impact (e.g., myocardial infarction, sudden cardiac death) and related diseases (e.g., heart failure, atrial fibrillation). Therapy for IHD includes antiplatelet therapy (e.g., aspirin, adenosine diphosphate receptor [$P2Y_{12}$] inhibitor), renin angiotensin system inhibitors (e.g., ACEI, ARB), β-adrenergic blockers, other antianginal therapies (e.g., calcium channel blocker, nitrates), lipid reducing agents (e.g., statins), and coronary revascularization with either coronary artery bypass grafting (CABG) or percutaneous coronary intervention (PCI). Based on recent randomized controlled trials, several newer types of medical therapy for IHD may be increasingly used, including novel antiinflammatory therapy (e.g., canakinumab),[90] low-dose direct oral anticoagulant (DOAC) therapy,[91] and antibody-based lipid-lowering agents.[92] Coronary revascularization—specifically with CABG—improves survival compared to medical therapy (pooled relative risk 0.80, 95% limits 0.70-0.91) in several high-risk IHD states,[93] namely left main coronary artery stenosis, triple-vessel coronary artery disease, and two-vessel coronary artery disease with proximal left anterior descending artery stenosis.[94] When PCI is used instead for these high-risk states, PCI with a newer generation drug eluting stent (DES) may also confer a survival benefit, albeit with marginal statistical significance.[93] In patients who meet indications for revascularization, CABG improves survival more than PCI in multivessel disease that is associated with either diabetes mellitus or higher coronary artery lesion complexity.[95] Notably, aside from these high-risk states (e.g., triple vessel coronary artery disease), PCI has not been shown to convincingly improve survival in stable IHD.[96]

In the perioperative setting, IHD is a risk factor for myocardial infarction and a prognostically important myocardial injury after surgery.[97,98] It is also associated with elevated risks of 30-day postoperative mortality,[99] especially if a patient had experienced a myocardial infarction, acute coronary syndrome, or severe angina (i.e., occurring at effort levels less than walking one to two blocks or climbing one flight of stairs) within the 6 months preceding surgery.[77,78] Surgical patients with IHD may also have important comorbidities with important perioperative implications, such as heart failure and atrial fibrillation (see sections of "Heart Failure" and "Atrial Fibrillation"). The goals of preoperative evaluation are to (1) ascertain whether the patient has previously undiagnosed significant IHD; (2) characterize any known IHD with respect to severity, functional limitations, therapy, and prior investigations; (3) determine whether additional preoperative specialized testing or consultations are warranted; and (4) identity opportunities for reducing perioperative risk related to IHD. In the case of patients without known IHD, evaluation of traditional risk factors for IHD (i.e., smoking, hypertension, increased age, male sex, hyperlipidemia, family history) is important when significance of suspicious symptoms (e.g., chest discomfort, dyspnea) or abnormal ECG. In patients with known IHD, the anesthesiologist should characterize any history of chest discomfort (i.e., pain, pressure, tightness) with respect to its duration, precipitating factors, associated symptoms, and relieving factors. Exertional dyspnea may represent an angina equivalent but is also a nonspecific finding that might be related to physical deconditioning, pulmonary disease, or heart failure. It is useful to classify any angina based on the CCS grading scale:

- CCS class I: Ordinary physical activity (e.g., walking, climbing stairs) does not cause angina. Angina with strenuous or rapid or prolonged exertion at work or recreation
- CCS class II: Slight limitation of ordinary activity. No angina is precipitated by walking more than two blocks on level ground or climbing more than one flight of stairs at a normal pace and in normal conditions. Angina is only precipitated by walking or climbing stairs rapidly, walking uphill, and walking or stair climbing under challenging conditions (e.g., after meals, in cold, in wind, under emotional stress, during the few hours after awakening).
- CCS class III: Marked limitation of ordinary physical activity. Angina precipitated by walking one or two blocks on level ground and climbing one flight of stairs in normal conditions and at normal pace.
- CCS class IV: Inability to carry on any physical activity without discomfort. Angina may be present at rest.

Patients with risk factors for IHD or suspicious symptoms may require an ECG, especially before intermediate-risk or high-risk surgical procedures.[9] Routine preoperative ECGs are not indicated (Box 31.2), especially in asymptomatic patients without known cardiovascular disease or risk factors.[7] While specific preoperative abnormalities are associated with increased perioperative cardiac risk (e.g., bundle branch blocks [BBBs]), these abnormalities do not enable clinicians to identify patients with increased perioperative cardiac risk more accurately when considered in combination with known clinical risk factors.[100] Establishing a baseline for postoperative comparison is often the most important reason to obtain a preoperative ECG; however, this decision should be based on the patient's likely risk of postoperative cardiovascular complications. Thus, a baseline ECG is unlikely to be helpful in an individual at very low risk for postoperative cardiac events. If a previous ECG is available from the previous 3 months and there has been no intervening change in clinical status, a repeat ECG is likely not needed.[7] Other typical preoperative laboratory tests that may be considered for patients with known or suspected IHD include creatinine and hemoglobin concentrations. Both chronic renal insufficiency and anemia are risk factors for perioperative cardiac complications.[97,101,102] In addition, anemia can modify the effects of β-adrenergic blockade in surgical patients, with evidence of increased harm when used in patients with perioperative anemia or significant bleeding.[103,104]

BOX 31.2 Recommendations for Preoperative Resting 12-Lead Electrocardiogram

Class IIa Recommendation: It Is Reasonable to Perform the Procedure

Preoperative resting 12-lead ECG is reasonable for patients with known IHD, significant arrhythmia, PAD, CVD, or other significant structural heart disease (except if undergoing low-risk surgical procedures).

Class IIb Recommendation: The Procedure May Be Considered

Preoperative resting 12-lead ECG may be considered for asymptomatic patients without known coronary heart disease, except for those undergoing low-risk surgical procedures.

Class III Recommendation: The Procedure Should *Not* Be Performed Because It Is Not Helpful

Routine preoperative resting 12-lead ECG is not useful for asymptomatic patients undergoing low-risk surgical procedures.

CVD, Cerebrovascular disease; *ECG*, electrocardiogram; *IHD*, ischemic heart disease; *PAD*, peripheral artery disease.

From Fleisher LA, Fleischmann KE, Auerbach AD, et al. 2014 ACC/AHA guideline on perioperative cardiovascular evaluation and management of patients undergoing noncardiac surgery: a report of the American College of Cardiology/American Heart Association Task Force on Practice Guidelines. *Circulation*. 2014;130:e278–e333.

Preoperative cardiac risk assessment algorithms have been proposed by several practice guidelines, including the ACC/AHA guidelines (Fig. 31.5)[7] and the CCS guidelines (Fig. 31.6).[8] These algorithms have somewhat differing target populations. The ACC/AHA algorithm encompasses patients with known IHD or associated risk factors who are having noncardiac surgery. The CCS guidelines focus on adults (≥18 years old) having inpatient surgery who are either 45 years or older, or who have significant cardiovascular disease (i.e., IHD, cerebrovascular disease [CVD], PAD, heart failure, severe pulmonary hypertension, severe obstructive cardiac valvular disease). While the algorithms have many fundamental similarities, they also have several key differences, which will be discussed below. Importantly, the algorithms should always be viewed as flexible guidance frameworks that should be tailored, as needed, to individual patients. The initial step in these risk assessment algorithms is consideration of the urgency of the planned surgery. The 2014 ACC/AHA guidelines define an *emergency* procedure as one where life or limb would be threatened if surgery did not proceed within 6 hours or less; an *urgent* procedure as one where life or limb would be threatened if surgery did not proceed within 6 to 24 hours; and a *time-sensitive* procedure as one where delays exceeding 1 to 6 weeks would adversely affect outcomes (e.g., most oncology surgery).[7] Based on this classification scheme, patients should proceed directly to any required emergency surgery without further preoperative cardiac assessment.[7,8] For these individuals, the focus should be on surveillance (e.g., serial cardiac enzymes, hemodynamic monitoring, serial ECGs) and early treatment of any postoperative cardiovascular complications.

In the second step, active cardiac conditions—such as acute coronary syndromes, decompensated heart failure, severe valvular disease (e.g., critical aortic stenosis), suspected significant pulmonary hypertension, or significant arrhythmias (e.g., atrial fibrillation with rapid ventricular rate, sustained ventricular tachycardia)—should be ruled

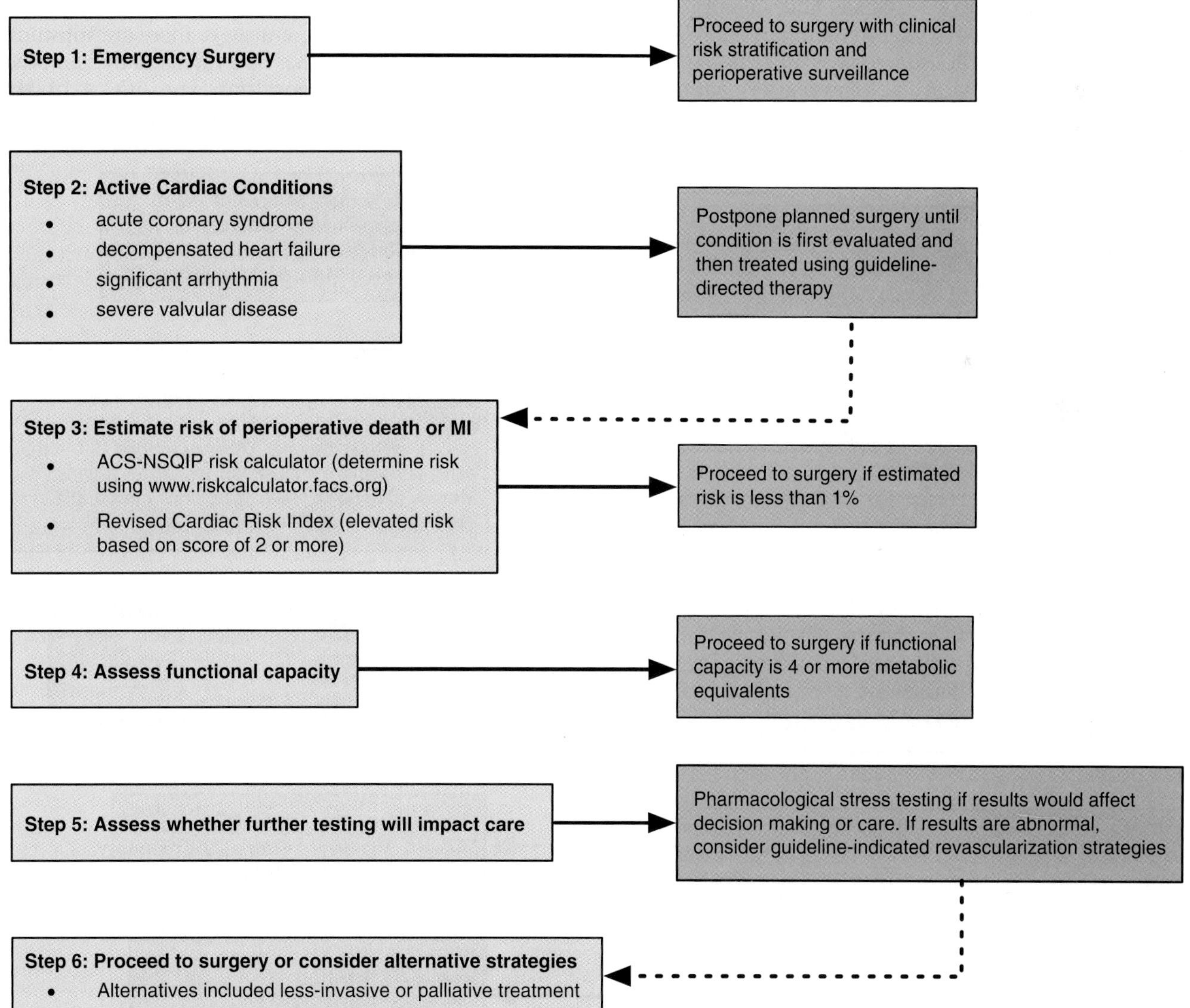

Fig. 31.5 Simplified cardiac evaluation algorithm for noncardiac surgery proposed by the 2014 American Heart Association and American College of Cardiology guidelines. *ACS-NSQIP*, American College of Surgeons National Surgical Quality Improvement Program; *MI*, myocardial infarction. (From Fleisher LA, Fleischmann KE, Auerbach AD, et al. 2014 ACC/AHA guideline on perioperative cardiovascular evaluation and management of patients undergoing noncardiac surgery: a report of the American College of Cardiology/American Heart Association Task Force on Practice Guidelines. *Circulation*. 2014;130:e278–e333.)

out in patients not requiring emergency surgery.[7] If any of these conditions are present, they must be initially treated, after which the original planned surgery can be reconsidered based on its risk-benefit balance. When assessing whether a patient has an active cardiac condition, the anesthesiologist should inquire about any recent myocardial infarction. In a study of about 560,000 patients who underwent major noncardiac surgery in the United States,[105] the risk of 30-day postoperative myocardial infarction or death was significantly elevated when surgery was performed within 60 days after a prior myocardial infarction. Thus, the 2014 ACC/AHA guidelines recommend deferring nonurgent surgery until 60 days after a recent myocardial infarction.[7]

In the third step, perioperative cardiac risk should be estimated based on readily available clinical information that encompasses both patient-level (e.g., comorbidities) and surgery-level (e.g., procedure type) characteristics. The 2014 ACC/AHA guidelines and 2014 ESC/ESA guidelines recommend using clinical risk indices, namely the Revised Cardiac Risk Index (RCRI) (Table 31.5),[97] ACS NSQIP surgical risk calculator (https://riskcalculator.facs.org/RiskCalculator),[32] or NSQIP Myocardial Infarction and Cardiac Arrest risk calculator.[33] If these indices find the estimated risk of postoperative myocardial infarction or death to be less than 1% (consistent with RCRI ≤ 1), the ACC/AHA guidelines recommend that patients simply proceed directly to surgery.[7] The 2017 CCS guidelines suggest using the RCRI, as opposed to the NSQIP risk calculators, largely because the NSQIP-risk models were developed using a database without routine postoperative troponin surveillance, implying that the predicted absolute myocardial infarction rate might underestimate the true rate by threefold,[98] and have not been externally validated.[8] In addition, the NSQIP risk calculators have largely not been externally validated. By comparison, the RCRI was derived in a cohort study with standardized cardiac biomarker surveillance,[97] and also has undergone extensive external validation.[106] Nonetheless, the RCRI has limitations, especially with respect to inadequate consideration of variations in cardiac risk across different surgical procedures.[107] The CCS guidelines recommend that patients proceed directly to surgery if they meet all the following criteria: age over 65 years, RCRI score of 1 or greater, and no history of significant cardiovascular disease (i.e., coronary artery disease, CVD, PAD, heart failure, pulmonary hypertension, or severe obstructive cardiac valvular disease).

In the fourth and subsequent steps, there are substantial differences between the American versus Canadian preoperative risk assessment algorithms. The ACC/AHA algorithm recommends that a patient with a functional capacity

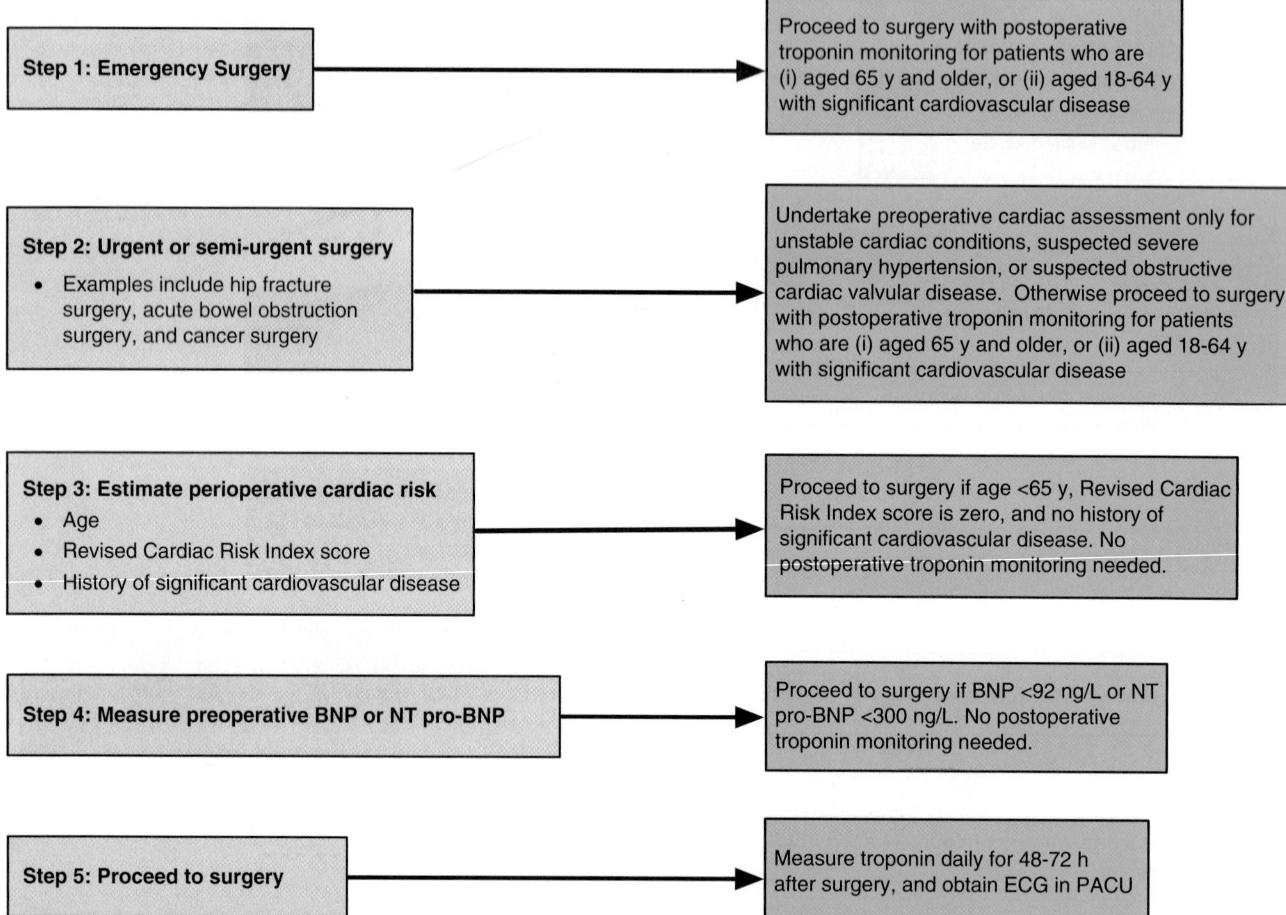

Fig. 31.6 Simplified cardiac evaluation algorithm for noncardiac surgery proposed by the 2017 Canadian Cardiovascular Society guidelines. *BNP,* Brain natriuretic peptide; *ECG,* electrocardiogram; *NT pro-BNP,* N-terminal-pro-BNP; *PACU,* postanesthesia care unit. (From Duceppe E, Parlow J, MacDonald P, et al. Canadian Cardiovascular Society guidelines on perioperative cardiac risk assessment and management for patients who undergo noncardiac surgery. *Can J Cardiol.* 2017;33:17–32.)

of 4 or more METs should proceed directly to surgery.[7] This guidance is largely based on older studies of preoperative exercise testing,[30,31] and more recent studies of preoperative CPET,[108,109] which found an association between poor functional capacity and elevated perioperative cardiac risk. The major clinical challenge with this recommendation pertains to how best to estimate patients' preoperative functional capacity in clinical practice (see earlier section on "Assessment of Functional Capacity"). Simple subjective assessment of functional capacity based on the usual preoperative history does not accurately estimate true exercise capacity,[36] and does not accurately predict postoperative cardiovascular complications.[36,41] Thus, in clinical practice, anesthesiologists should generally use a structured questionnaire, especially the DASI (see Table 31.2),[42] with consideration of formal exercise testing if the results would alter management. Notably, DASI scores improve the accuracy of prediction of cardiac complications following noncardiac surgery beyond that achieved with the RCRI alone.[36]

If a patient is deemed to have either low (i.e., < 4 METs) or uncertain functional capacity, the AHA/ACC guidelines recommend consideration of exercise or pharmacologic cardiac stress testing, if the results could plausibly inform decision making or clinical care. Patients with high-risk abnormal test results can be considered for subsequent coronary angiography, and possibly revascularization (if usual nonoperative indications for coronary revascularization are met). Importantly, the ACC/AHA guidelines emphasize the importance of considering alternative less invasive or nonsurgical treatment for the underlying condition, especially in patients found to be at very high cardiac risk.

As opposed to assessing functional capacity, the CCS guidelines recommend preoperative risk assessment with cardiac biomarkers,[8] specifically brain natriuretic peptide (BNP) or N-terminal-pro-BNP (NT pro-BNP). These neurohormones are secreted by the cardiac ventricles in response to stretch or ischemia of the atrial and ventricular walls. In the nonoperative setting, elevated natriuretic peptide concentrations are powerful markers of cardiovascular risk in individuals with IHD or associated risk factors, as well as in individuals with heart failure.[110] Interestingly, there is only slight-to-fair correlation between plasma levels of these biomarkers and measures of exercise capacity,[36] suggesting that natriuretic peptides measure a different patient characteristic. An individual patient data meta-analysis of 18 studies in noncardiac surgery found that preoperative natriuretic peptide concentrations can differentiate patients based on their perioperative cardiac risk (Table 31.6).[111] In general, BNP concentrations less than 100 ng/L or NT pro-BNP concentrations less than 300 ng/L are indicative of a patient at very low perioperative cardiac risk. Conversely, BNP concentrations above 300 ng/L or NT pro-BNP concentrations above 900 ng/L are indicative of a patient at high cardiac risk. Importantly, natriuretic peptides also improve the accuracy of risk estimation beyond that achieved with traditional clinical risk factors alone.[111] The CCS guidelines recommend that preoperative BNP or NT pro-BNP testing be used to inform the required level of postoperative surveillance. Specifically, they recommend

TABLE 31.5 Components of the Revised Cardiac Risk Index and Expected Cardiac Event Risk

Components of Revised Cardiac Risk Index*	Points Assigned
High-risk surgery (intraperitoneal, intrathoracic, or suprainguinal vascular procedure)	1
Ischemic heart disease (by any diagnostic criteria)	1
History of congestive heart failure	1
History of cerebrovascular disease	1
Diabetes mellitus requiring insulin	1
Creatinine > 2.0 mg/dL (176 μmol/L)	1
Revised Cardiac Risk Index Score	**Risk of Major Cardiac Events†,‡**
0	0.4%
1	1.0%
2	2.4%
≥3	5.4%

*Data from Lee TH, Marcantonio ER, Mangione CM, et al. Derivation and prospective validation of a simple index for prediction of cardiac risk of major noncardiac surgery. *Circulation*. 1999;100:1043–1049.

†Data from Devereaux OJ, Goldman L, Cook DJ, et al. Perioperative cardiac events in patients undergoing noncardiac surgery: a review of the magnitude of the problem, the pathophysiology of the events and methods to estimate and communicate risk. *CMAJ*. 2005;173:627–634.

‡Defined as cardiac death, nonfatal myocardial infarction, or nonfatal cardiac arrest.

TABLE 31.6 Risk of Death or Myocardial Infarction After Noncardiac Surgery Based on Preoperative Brain Natriuretic Peptide or N-Terminal-Pro-Brain Natriuretic Peptide Concentrations

Preoperative BNP Concentration (ng/L)	Likelihood Ratio* for Death or MI	Preoperative NT pro-BNP Concentration (ng/L)	Likelihood Ratio* for Death or MI
0–99	0.6	0–300	0.4
100–250	1.4	301–900	1.5
>250	3.9	901–3000	2.7
		>3000	5.0

*Positive test results should have likelihood ratios > 2 to provide clinically meaningful information, whereas negative test results should have likelihood ratios of < 0.5.

BNP, Brain natriuretic peptide; *MI*, myocardial infarction; *NT pro-BNP*, N-terminal-pro-BNP.

From Rodseth RN, Biccard BM, Le Manach Y, et al. The prognostic value of pre-operative and post-operative B-type natriuretic peptides in patients undergoing noncardiac surgery. B-type natriuretic peptide and N-terminal fragment of pro-B-type natriuretic peptide: a systematic review and individual patient data meta-analysis. *J Am Coll Cardiol*. 2014;63:170–180.

routine troponin surveillance for 48 to 72 hours after surgery in patients with elevated preoperative BNP (≥92 ng/L) or NT pro-BNP (≥300 ng/L) concentrations. No other preoperative testing or intervention is recommended based on the results of preoperative cardiac biomarker testing.

Although current evidence pertaining to risk assessment with preoperative natriuretic peptides is promising, there are also some important limitations. First, the event rate for death or myocardial infarction in this individual patient data meta-analysis was about 11%, which is considerably higher than would be expected in usual clinical practice. This high event rate is explained, in part, by the intermediate-to-high risk characteristics of the study sample, and by two large included studies that defined cardiovascular complications based on elevated troponin concentrations alone (as opposed to less frequent myocardial infarction events).[112,113] Therefore, further research remains needed to determine biomarker threshold levels and prognostic accuracy in generalizable study samples. Second, while elevated natriuretic peptide concentrations are indicative of elevated perioperative cardiac risk, they do not indicate underlying pathophysiological mechanism. Aside from ischemia and heart failure, other prognostically important conditions can cause elevated natriuretic peptide concentrations, including right ventricular dysfunction, cardiac valvular disease, and atrial fibrillation. Thus, further specialized testing (e.g., echocardiography) may be helpful in some patients with high preoperative BNP or NT pro-BNP concentrations, if the results might inform clinical care or decision making. Third, nonoperative data suggest natriuretic peptides have limitations as prognostic biomarkers in certain disease states, including obesity and chronic renal kidney.

The anesthesiologist has several other avenues for further investigating or optimizing known or suspected IHD before surgery—including consultations, biomarkers, stress testing, coronary angiography, coronary revascularization, and medical therapy. When considering the need for additional consultations before surgery, an initial phone call to the primary care physician or cardiologist often yields important information that obviates the need for further consultation. Any specialist consultation (e.g., cardiologist) initiated by the anesthesiologist should seek specific advice regarding the diagnosis, treatment, or further optimization of the patient's condition. It is preferable to ask specific questions, such as "*Does this patient have IHD?*" or "*Is this patient optimized for planned radical nephrectomy?*," to avoid unhelpful consultation reports that simply state that a patient is "*cleared for surgery.*"

Aside from BNP and NT pro-BNP, several other preoperative biomarkers have shown promise, with the most compelling data pertaining to high-sensitivity troponin assays. In the nonoperative setting, these high-sensitivity assays have demonstrated subtle resting elevations in cardiac troponin concentrations in an important segment of the population without any acute coronary syndrome. These individuals have significantly elevated risks of death, as well as progression to IHD or heart failure.[114,115] Perhaps unsurprisingly, many otherwise stable surgical patients may have elevated troponin concentrations even before surgery. For example, in a cohort study of 325 patients undergoing major inpatient noncardiac surgery, about 20% had a preoperative high-sensitivity troponin T concentration exceeding the 99th percentile for the assay.[116] Thus, especially in patients for whom postoperative troponin surveillance is planned, a preoperative troponin measurement is integral to determining whether any elevated postoperative concentration reflects acute injury versus chronic long-term elevation. Two large cohort studies have also shown that these preoperative troponin elevations may aid in risk stratification for noncardiac surgery.[117-119] Specifically, a preoperative high-sensitivity troponin T concentration above 14 ng/L is associated with increased risks of death and cardiovascular complications after major noncardiac surgery. Furthermore, addition of preoperative high-sensitivity troponin T appears to improve the accuracy of risk estimation beyond that achieved with traditional clinical risk factors and natriuretic peptides.[117,118] Further research remains needed to confirm these initial results, establish ideal screening thresholds, and replicate these analyses using other high-sensitivity troponin assays. Importantly, prognostically important conditions other than myocardial ischemia can cause elevated troponin concentrations, including right ventricular dysfunction, cardiac valvular disease, and atrial fibrillation.

When supplementing preoperative evaluation, cardiac stress testing can help diagnose IHD, assess its severity, and estimate perioperative cardiac risk. The tests therefore address both *diagnosis* and *prognosis*. Several stress tests are available that differ based on the stress modality (i.e., exercise, pharmacologic) and ischemia monitoring method (i.e., ECG, perfusion imaging, echocardiography). An exercise stress test is a preferred option for a patient who is capable of exercising and likely to achieve an adequate heart rate response during exercise. Exercise stress testing also allows for an objective measurement of functional capacity. An adequate test result is obtained when patients can exercise to 85% of their target heart rate (i.e., 220 minus age). Pharmacologic stress modalities (e.g., dobutamine, dipyridamole, adenosine, regadenoson) are indicated for an individual who cannot exercise or is unlikely to achieve an adequate heart rate response because of pacemakers, significant bradycardia, or high-dose negative chronotropic drugs (e.g., β-adrenergic blockers). The choice of pharmacologic stress modality is generally immaterial, but there are some exceptions. For example, since dobutamine uncovers ischemia by increasing contractility, heart rate, and blood pressure, it may not be the best choice in patients with pacemakers, significant bradycardia, aortic aneurysms, cerebral aneurysms, or poorly controlled hypertension. While adenosine and dipyridamole rely on their vasodilatory properties and do not depend on a heart rate response, they may exacerbate bronchospasm in patients taking theophylline. In addition, these drugs may cause dangerous reductions in preload in the presence of severe stenotic valvular heart disease.

An exercise ECG stress test is a reasonable option for a patient with a relatively normal baseline ECG who is capable of exercising with an adequate heart rate response. An imaging monitoring method (i.e., echocardiography, myocardial perfusion imaging) can be used instead if a patient has significant ECG abnormalities (e.g., left bundle branch block [LBBB], LVH with strain pattern) that may interfere with electrocardiographic detection of ischemia. Nonetheless, exercise myocardial perfusion imaging may still be problematic in patients with LBBB, because of false-positive results related to septal perfusion defects.[7] Stress echocardiography assesses for wall motion abnormalities both at rest and under stress conditions (i.e., exercise, dobutamine). Resting abnormalities indicate scar tissue from a prior infarction, while new abnormalities under stress conditions (i.e., inducible wall motion abnormalities) indicate limited blood due to stenotic coronary lesions. Nuclear myocardial perfusion imaging detects ischemia by comparing radioisotope uptake by viable myocardium under resting and stress conditions. Perfusion defects at rest are indicative of a prior infarction. Since normal coronary arteries vasodilate with exercise or specific pharmacologic stressors (i.e., adenosine, dipyridamole), normal myocardium maintains normal radioisotope uptake in stress conditions. By comparison, stenotic vessels are maximally vasodilated at rest, and unable to further vasodilate under stress conditions. Thus, myocardium with flow-limiting lesions has normal radioisotope update at rest, but decreased uptake under stress conditions (i.e., reversible perfusion defects). In general, the choice of test should be informed by patient factors (e.g., ability to exercise) and local expertise in cardiac stress testing.

Cardiac stress tests can also help predict whether patients are likely to experience perioperative cardiac complications. Since these events occur relatively infrequently, the prognostic performance of these tests should not be evaluated based on positive or negative predictive values. It is preferable to use positive likelihood ratio and negative likelihood ratio values, which can be readily calculated using sensitivity and specificity values.

$$\text{Positive likelihood ratio} = \frac{\text{sensitivity}}{1 - \text{specificity}}$$

$$\text{Negative likelihood ratio} = \frac{1 - \text{sensitivity}}{\text{specificity}}$$

There are relatively few data on the prognostic performance of preoperative exercise ECG stress testing. In a meta-analysis of studies in vascular surgery, exercise ECG stress testing had a positive likelihood ratio of 2.4 and negative likelihood ratio of 0.4 for predicting postoperative cardiac death or myocardial infarction.[120] Conversely, ECG stress testing had diminished predictive performance (positive likelihood ratio 1.8 and negative likelihood ratio 0.8) in a cohort study of 200 patients undergoing mixed noncardiac surgery.[30] Considerably more research has been published pertaining to the prognostic accuracy of preoperative stress testing based on myocardial perfusion imaging or echocardiography. In a meta-analysis in noncardiac surgery, stress echocardiography has a positive likelihood ratio of 4.1 and a negative likelihood ratio of 0.2 for predicting postoperative death or myocardial infarction. In the case of myocardial perfusion imaging, the positive likelihood ratio was 1.8 and negative likelihood ratio was 0.4.[121] The prognostic value of myocardial perfusion imaging might be further improved by considering the extent of reversible defects. In another meta-analysis in vascular surgery, reversible defects on preoperative myocardial perfusion imaging were associated with significantly increased cardiac risk only when the extent of reversibility exceeded 20% of the myocardium.[122] Notably, isolated fixed defects (i.e., no associated reversible defects) were not associated with elevated cardiac risk.[122] While available evidence does suggest that stress echocardiography has better prognostic accuracy, these data should be interpreted cautiously since they are older, heterogeneous, and do not account for varying local expertise in stress testing modalities. In addition, it remains unclear as to whether cardiac stress tests provide *incremental* prognostic information in patients who have already been assessed using clinical risk factors.

Some patients with high-risk findings on initial cardiac stress testing may require subsequent evaluation of coronary anatomy using either noninvasive computed tomography coronary angiography (CTCA) or invasive coronary angiography. These tests can diagnose IHD, assess its severity, and help assess perioperative cardiac risk. Using contemporary imaging technology, CTCA has reasonably high accuracy for detecting clinically significant coronary artery stenosis.[123,124] An initial retrospective cohort study found CTCA to improve prediction of cardiac complications after intermediate-risk noncardiac surgery, as compared to using the RCRI alone.[125] Conversely, a larger multicenter prospective cohort study found that the addition of CTCA to the RCRI was five times more likely to overestimate risk in low-risk individuals than correctly identify a previously misclassified high-risk individual.[126] Thus, CTCA does not appear to be an appropriate first-line test to supplement clinical risk stratification. Nonetheless, it may be a reasonable follow-up option in patients with high-risk cardiac stress test results.

Invasive coronary angiography is the gold standard for diagnosing IHD and may also be a follow-up option for patients with high-risk cardiac stress test results. Two Italian randomized trials in vascular surgery patients have suggested that routine preoperative invasive coronary angiography—followed by revascularization of any critical stenosis—reduces risks of postoperative myocardial ischemia,[127] and long-term mortality.[128,129] Although interesting, these findings still do not support a clinical shift to this invasive assessment strategy, largely because any patient-relevant benefits were seen over long-term follow-up, not the immediate postoperative period. Any merit for an invasive coronary artery assessment strategy is highly related to whether coronary revascularization before noncardiac surgery is beneficial. This issue remains controversial. The most relevant study is the Coronary Artery Revascularization Prophylaxis trial.[130] In the multicenter randomized controlled trial of 510 vascular surgery patients with known significant IHD, preoperative revascularization using CABG or PCI with bare metal stents (BMSs) did not reduce the risk of postoperative myocardial infarction or long-term mortality. Notably, the trial excluded patients with left main coronary artery stenosis, which is the only subgroup where revascularization was associated with improved survival in a related cohort study.[131] At present, both American and European guidelines only recommend consideration for revascularization in patients who meet usual nonoperative indications (e.g., left main coronary artery stenosis, triple-vessel coronary artery disease),[7,9] while the CCS guidelines recommend against preoperative revascularization in any patient with stable IHD.[8]

In general, randomized controlled trials have also *not* shown benefit from de novo medical therapy to decrease perioperative cardiac risk, including β-adrenergic blockers,[132,133] α_2-adrenergic agonists,[134,135] and low-dose aspirin.[136] Despite initial promising data on perioperative β-adrenergic blockade,[137] these benefits were not replicated in larger multicenter randomized trials, such as the Perioperative Ischemic Evaluation Study-1 (POISE-1) trial. Current randomized trial evidence shows that perioperative β-adrenergic blockade reduces the risk of postoperative myocardial infarction, but at the cost of increased risks of acute stroke, hypotension, and death.[133] Although it is possible that these risks are mitigated by starting β-adrenergic blockers several days before surgery,[138,139] and titrating therapy to a reasonable target heart rate without precipitating hypotension, there are no compelling data showing the efficacy and safety of this approach.[140] Caution should especially be exercised when using β-adrenergic blockers in individuals with known CVD because of the risks of perioperative stroke.[132,133]

Conversely, most *long-term* cardiovascular medications in patients with IHD should be continued up to surgery, including β-adrenergic blockers, statins, and most other antihypertensive medications. Nonetheless, there are some exceptions. Since ACEI and ARB administration within 24 hours before surgery is associated with increased risks of hypotension[85] and myocardial injury,[86] it is reasonable to withhold these medications for 24 hours before surgery, provided that they are restarted postoperatively (see section on "Hypertension").[87,88] Despite theoretical benefits,[141] randomized controlled trials to date have not shown benefits from routinely continuing aspirin before noncardiac surgery. For example, in the POISE-2 trial, continuing low-dose aspirin (100 mg/day) did not prevent cardiac complications but increased risks of major bleeding.[136] The lack of clear benefit may be explained, in part, by acute thrombosis being a relatively infrequent contributor to perioperative myocardial infarction.[142,143] Nonetheless, since only one third of participants in the POISE-2 trial had diagnosed vascular disease, it is possible that continuation of aspirin benefits some very high-risk subgroups. Consistent with this possibility, a relatively small post-hoc subgroup analysis from the POISE-2 trial found that perioperative aspirin reduced the risk of death or myocardial infarction in patients with prior PCI.[144] Based on these data, a reasonable strategy is to only continue aspirin *selectively* in patients where the risk of cardiac events is felt to exceed the risk of major bleeding. Other medications that should generally be withdrawn before surgery include $P2Y_{12}$ inhibitors (e.g., clopidogrel, ticagrelor, prasugrel) and DOACs (see sections on "Atrial Fibrillation" and "Preoperative Antiplatelet Therapy").

Coronary Stents

Following PCI with stent implantation, patients require an initial period of dual antiplatelet therapy (DAPT) with aspirin and a $P2Y_{12}$ inhibitor (e.g., clopidogrel, ticagrelor, prasugrel), after which they can be transitioned to aspirin monotherapy. The purpose of DAPT is to prevent potentially catastrophic stent thrombosis during the vulnerable period preceding stent reendothelialization. Temporary preoperative discontinuation of DAPT during this vulnerable period predisposes patients to cardiovascular complications, especially given the prothrombotic state triggered by surgical stress. Based on emerging evidence and improved DES technology, recommendations pertaining to minimum duration of DAPT before elective noncardiac surgery continue to evolve—as reflected in updated 2016 guidelines published by the ACC/AHA.[145] These guidelines recommend that elective noncardiac surgery should be delayed for 30 days or more after BMS implantation. In the case of DES, the ideal recommended minimum delay is 6 months, which is consistent with several cohort studies showing relatively low perioperative cardiac risk when elective noncardiac surgery was performed 6 months or more after DES implantation.[146,147] Based on expert opinion, the guidelines also indicate that elective noncardiac surgery can sometimes be performed from 3 to 6 months after DES implantation (particularly with new generation stents), if the risk of stent thrombosis is judged to be less than the risk of further delaying surgery.[145] When DAPT is temporarily interrupted before noncardiac surgery, the guidelines strongly recommend that aspirin be continued, and $P2Y_{12}$ inhibitor therapy be restarted as soon as possible after surgery.[145]

Although not explicitly indicated in the 2016 ACC/AHA guidelines, factors other than stent type and time interval since PCI should also inform judgments on the safety of performing elective noncardiac surgery in patients with coronary stents. For example, a large retrospective cohort study of about 26,600 patients found that the risks of noncardiac surgery early after stent implantation were increased when PCI had been performed for acute myocardial infarction, as opposed to unstable angina or non-acute coronary syndrome indications.[148] As a consequence, it may be particularly important to delay noncardiac surgery for 6 months when the indication for DES was treatment of an acute myocardial infarction.

During preoperative evaluation, the anesthesiologist should determine the presence, type (drug-eluting vs. bare-metal), location, and original indication of any coronary stent. Given the complex issues related to these patients, subsequent management should be performed in collaboration with a cardiologist and the responsible surgeon, especially for patients receiving DAPT.[145] Whenever possible, surgical procedures should be performed following critical time windows (i.e., 30 days after BMS, or 3-6 months after DES), aspirin should be continued throughout the perioperative period, and any $P2Y_{12}$ inhibitor therapy should be restarted as soon as possible after surgery. The importance of continuing aspirin perioperatively is supported by the substudy of the POISE-2 randomized trial.[144] In this subgroup analysis of 470 patients with prior PCI, aspirin reduced the risk of death or myocardial infarction (hazard ratio, 0.50; 95% confidence limits, 0.26-0.95) without any significantly increased bleeding risk. Unfractionated heparin and low-molecular-weight heparin (LMWH) should not be used to "bridge" patients who have been withdrawn from antiplatelet therapy, especially since heparin can paradoxically increase platelet aggregation.[149] Following surgery, close monitoring for myocardial injury (i.e., serial troponin measurement) should be strongly considered, with any suspected stent thrombosis treated using PCI. High-risk patients are thus ideally best managed in facilities with immediate access to interventional cardiology.

Heart Failure

Heart failure has been defined as a clinical syndrome resulting from impaired diastolic filling or systolic ejection of the cardiac ventricles.[150] Its major clinical manifestations are dyspnea, fatigue, and fluid retention. Although prevalence estimates are affected by differences in diagnostic criteria, recent estimates suggest that heart failure afflicts more than 6.5 million individuals in the United States,[27] and more than 23 million worldwide.[151] Heart failure is the sequelae of a broad array of underlying pathology, including ischemic heart disease (i.e., ischemic cardiomyopathy), hypertension, valvular heart disease, myocarditis, infiltrative disorder (e.g., sarcoidosis, amyloidosis), and peripartum cardiomyopathy. In addition, many affected individuals have no identifiable underlying cause (i.e., idiopathic dilated cardiomyopathy). Several approaches can be used to classify heart failure, including the presence versus absence of associated signs or symptoms (i.e., compensated vs. decompensated heart failure), and the extent of functional limitation. In heart failure patients, functional status is typically classified based on New York Heart Association (NYHA) categories:

- NYHA class I: no limitation of physical activity; ordinary activity not a cause of fatigue, palpitations, or syncope
- NYHA class II: slight limitation of physical activity; ordinary activity resulting in fatigue, palpitations, or syncope
- NYHA class III: marked limitation of physical activity; less than ordinary activity resulting in fatigue, palpitations, or syncope; comfort at rest
- NYHA class IV: inability to do any physical activity without discomfort; symptoms at rest

Heart failure can also be classified based on the severity of ventricular systolic dysfunction, namely as heart failure with reduced ejection fraction (HFrEF) versus heart failure with preserved ejection fraction (HFpEF).[152] Individuals with HFpEF (or diastolic heart failure) have normal left ventricular ejection fraction (≥50%), normal left ventricular end-diastolic volume, and abnormal diastolic function. By comparison, HFrEF (or systolic heart failure) is characterized by more significant left ventricular systolic dysfunction (i.e., ejection fraction ≤ 40%). Individuals with borderline left ventricular systolic function (i.e., ejection fraction 41%-49%) are classified as borderline HFpEF. They tend to have characteristics and outcomes similar to patients with HFpEF.[152] Among patients with heart failure, about half have HFpEF.[153] Although they have a high mortality risk (10%-20% at 1-year),[154,155] patients with HFpEF have lower adjusted risks of death (adjusted hazard ratio 0.68) over long-term follow-up than patients with HFrEF.[155] Most medical therapy for improving morbidity and mortality in heart failure (i.e., ACEI, ARB, aldosterone antagonist, β-adrenergic blocker, ivabradine) has only demonstrated efficacy in HFrEF.[156] In contrast, medical therapy for HFpEF is largely aimed at symptoms and underlying conditions (e.g., hypertension). Other heart failure-related treatments include diuretics (for volume overload), anticoagulants (for atrial fibrillation or left ventricular thrombus), implantable cardioverter-defibrillators (ICDs), or cardiac resynchronization therapy (CRT).

In the perioperative setting, heart failure is a recognized risk factor for mortality and morbidity after major surgery. *Symptomatic* heart failure has been consistently identified as a risk factor for adverse perioperative outcomes in multiple studies. For example, in a retrospective cohort study of about 159,000 Medicare beneficiaries in the United States, heart failure was associated with significantly higher risks of 30-day mortality (adjusted hazard ratio 1.63) after noncardiac surgery.[157] Similarly, a more recent matched cohort study using the NSQIP registry showed new or worsened heart failure within 30 days before surgery to be associated with increased risks of 30-day mortality (adjusted relative risk 2.08) or major morbidity (adjusted relative risk 1.54).[158] Symptomatic heart failure is also a component of the Revised Cardiac Index, which is commonly used for estimating perioperative cardiac risk cardiovascular complications. Among patients with heart failure, perioperative risk may be higher in patients with HFrEF versus HFpEF. Specifically, in a cohort study of 174 heart failure patients undergoing noncardiac surgery, an ejection fraction less than 30% was associated with much higher adjusted risks (adjusted odds ratio 4.88) of postoperative death, myocardial infarction, or heart failure exacerbation.[159] Nonetheless, HFpEF may still be prognostically important in the perioperative setting, as evidenced by a meta-analysis that found diastolic dysfunction to be associated with a doubling (pooled adjusted odds ratio 2.03) in the risk of postoperative adverse cardiac events.[160] Although symptomatic HF is a clear indicator of increased perioperative risk, the prognostic importance of *asymptomatic* systolic dysfunction is less clear. For example, in a cohort study of 339 individuals undergoing noncardiac surgery, a reduced ejection fraction was associated with increased cardiac morbidity, but this information did not improve risk prediction beyond that achieved with clinical risk factors.[161] Similarly, in another cohort study of 570 individuals undergoing noncardiac surgery, a reduced ejection only had prognostic importance within the subgroup with RCRI scores of 2 or greater.[162] Consistent with these data, the current ACC/AHA guidelines discourage routine preoperative assessment of ventricular function (Box 31.3).[7]

The clinical stability of heart failure symptoms prior to surgery is another important determinant of perioperative risk, as evidenced by a single-center retrospective cohort study from the United States.[163] After examination at a hospitalist-run preoperative evaluation clinic, clinically stable heart failure patients had relatively low risks of 30-day mortality (1.3%) after noncardiac surgery, albeit with longer hospital length of stay and higher readmission rates relative to matched controls. Consistent with these data, the ESC/ESA guidelines recommend that elective intermediate-risk and high-risk noncardiac procedures be deferred for at least 3 months after initiation of medical therapy in patients with newly diagnosed heart failure.[9]

The preoperative history pertaining to heart failure should clarify its type, etiology, severity, stability (including prior exacerbations), recent investigations (e.g., echocardiograms), and current therapy (medical and device-based). The anesthesiologist should inquire about recent weight gain, fatigue, shortness of breath, orthopnea, paroxysmal nocturnal dyspnea, nocturnal cough, peripheral edema, hospitalizations, and recent changes in medical management. The patient's functional status should be classified according to the NYHA categories. It is especially important to determine if the signs and symptoms of heart failure are

BOX 31.3 Recommendations for Preoperative Noninvasive Evaluation of Left Ventricular Function

Class IIa (Reasonable to Perform)

- It is reasonable for patients with dyspnea of unknown origin to undergo preoperative evaluation of LV function.
- It is reasonable for patients with heart failure with worsening dyspnea or other change in clinical status to undergo preoperative evaluation of LV function.

Class IIb (May Be Considered)

- Reassessment of LV function in clinically stable patients with previously documented LV dysfunction may be considered if there has been no assessment within a year.

Class III (Should Not Be Performed Since It Is Not Helpful)

- Routine preoperative evaluation of LV function is not recommended.

LV, Left ventricle.

From Fleisher LA, Fleischmann KE, Auerbach AD, et al. 2014 ACC/AHA guideline on perioperative cardiovascular evaluation and management of patients undergoing noncardiac surgery: a report of the American College of Cardiology/American Heart Association Task Force on Practice Guidelines. *Circulation*. 2014;130:e278–e333.

in their usual stable state (i.e., compensated heart failure) or have recently significantly worsened (i.e., decompensated heart failure). Decompensated heart failure is a very high-risk condition that warrants postponement of surgery for all except lifesaving emergency procedures.[7] No consensus exists on how long nonemergent surgery should be deferred after resolution of acute decompensated heart failure, although a reasonable approach is to delay elective procedures (including most time-sensitive procedures) for 1 month, and urgent procedures for 24 hours.

On physical examination, the findings of heart failure may be subtle. Furthermore, they can vary between HFrEF versus HFpEF, and between compensated versus decompensated states. More useful signs for determining heart failure include a third heart sound, jugular venous distension, pulmonary rales, and lower extremity edema.[26] A chest radiograph may provide further diagnostic guidance, especially in dyspneic patients, with pulmonary vascular redistribution and interstitial edema useful findings for supporting the presence of heart failure.[26] Natriuretic peptide measurement can further clarify whether a patient has heart failure. Both BNP and NT pro-BNP have excellent diagnostic performance, especially for ruling out heart failure, in the ambulatory setting (pooled negative likelihood ratio values 0.29-0.38 at manufacturers' recommended thresholds)[164] and emergency department setting (pooled negative likelihood ratio values 0.08-0.13 at manufacturers' recommended thresholds).[165] Preoperative natriuretic peptide concentrations also provide other potentially important information. Both BNP and NT pro-BNP concentrations are markers of perioperative cardiac risk (see section on "Ischemic Heart Disease"). In addition, for heart failure patients who have undergone prior natriuretic peptide measurement, preoperative BNP or NT pro-BNP testing provides insights into whether patients remained in their usual stable clinical state. Consistent with these data, the ESC/ESA guidelines recommend preoperative natriuretic peptide measurement in patients who have established or suspected heart failure, and are undergoing noncardiac intermediate or high-risk noncardiac surgery.[9] While routine preoperative echocardiography (or other noninvasive ventricular function measurement) is not useful, such specialized testing is helpful for assessment of dyspnea of unknown origin or recent altered clinical status in an individual with known heart failure. Furthermore, both American and European guidelines are supportive of selective preoperative echocardiography in clinically stable patients with known ventricular dysfunction,[9] especially in the absence of testing in the previous year (see Box 31.3).[7] Other tests for patients with heart failure include ECGs and blood sampling to measure electrolyte and creatinine concentration. Digoxin levels are not routinely determined unless toxicity, undertreatment, or noncompliance is suspected.

Consideration should be given for collaborative perioperative management with a cardiologist or heart failure specialist of severely affected heart failure patients (i.e., NYHA III or IV; decompensated heart failure) who will undergo intermediate-risk or high-risk procedures. Most medical therapy, including β-adrenergic blockers, hydralazine, nitrates, and digoxin, should be continued preoperatively. Loop diuretics (e.g., furosemide) can be continued on the day of surgery for most procedures since this strategy does not increase risks of intraoperative hypotension or adverse cardiac events.[166] The exception is lengthy high-risk procedures with projected significant blood loss or fluid requirements, in which potent diuretics should be held on the morning of surgery. Since ACEI and ARB administration within 24 hours before surgery is associated with increased risks of intraoperative hypotension,[85] and postoperative myocardial injury,[86] it is reasonable to withhold these medications for 24 hours before surgery, provided that they are restarted postoperatively once patients are hemodynamically stable (see section on "Hypertension").[87,88] Patients on anticoagulant therapy will likely need these medications temporarily discontinued before surgery (see later section on "Atrial Fibrillation"). In addition, patients with pacemakers, ICDs, and CRT devices have their own special perioperative considerations (see later section on "Cardiovascular Implantable Electronic Devices").

Murmurs and Valvular Abnormalities

When a cardiac murmur is identified during preoperative assessment, the subsequent goals are to identify any associated cardiovascular symptoms (e.g., dyspnea, chest discomfort, orthopnea, fatigue, syncope), determine the underlying cause of the murmur, and distinguish clinically significant murmurs from unimportant ones. For example, benign functional murmurs occur with turbulent flow across the aortic or pulmonic outflow tracts during high-flow states such as hyperthyroidism, pregnancy, or anemia. Murmurs can be graded according to loudness (Table 31.7), however, the loudness of a murmur does not necessarily indicate the severity of a lesion. In contrast, the location of the murmur, and changes in intensity associated with maneuvers can be informative (Table 31.8). A Valsalva maneuver decreases right- and left-heart filling, thereby reducing the intensity of most murmurs except those of mitral valve prolapse and hypertrophic cardiomyopathy. Standing also decreases preload, and thereby increases the intensity of murmurs of mitral valve prolapse and hypertrophic cardiomyopathy. Conversely, squatting increases venous return and afterload, thereby increasing most murmurs except those of mitral valve prolapse and hypertrophic cardiomyopathy. Having the patient repeatedly perform a hand grip increases heart rate and arterial blood pressure, thereby augmenting murmurs of mitral regurgitation and aortic insufficiency; conversely, this maneuver decreases murmurs of aortic stenosis and hypertrophic cardiomyopathy. The likelihood of a murmur being pathologic increases in the presence of increased age, cardiovascular risk factors, other abnormal heart sounds, cardiomegaly, abnormal ECG, evidence of excessive intravascular volume, and a history of rheumatic fever, pulmonary disease, or anorectic drug use. Diastolic or continuous murmurs are almost always pathologic and require further evaluation. Nonetheless, it is typically not easy to distinguish benign from pathologic murmurs based on history and physical examination alone. Thus, cardiovascular medicine guidelines now recommend transthoracic echocardiography for the initial evaluation of any patient with suspected valvular heart disease.[167] Additionally, perioperative guidelines recommend preoperative echocardiography for any patient who has clinically suspected moderate or severe valvular stenosis or regurgitation, and no echocardiogram within the previous year.[7,9] For patients with known valvular heart disease, repeat echocardiography is recommended if there has been a significant change in clinical status or physical examination since the last test.

TABLE 31.7 Grading the Intensity of Cardiac Murmurs

Grade	Description
I	Faintest that can be heard with difficulty
II	Faint but easily heard
III	Moderately loud without a thrill
IV	Loud with a palpable thrill
V	Very loud but still need stethoscope (thrill present)
VI	Heard without a stethoscope

Aortic Stenosis. Aortic valve stenosis is the leading cause of left ventricular outflow obstruction in adults. In high-income countries, aortic stenosis principally occurs because of the progressive calcific disease of a native trileaflet valve or a congenitally bicuspid valve. Stenosis of bicuspid valves typically occurs when individuals are in their fourth and fifth decades of life, whereas stenosis of native trileaflet valves occurs once individuals are age 60 years old or older. Aortic stenosis severity is classified based on the valve area and mean transvalvular pressure gradient (Table 31.9). A limitation of using the pressure gradient alone to assess severity is that the gradient may decrease if the left ventricle systolic function begins to decrease. In patients with known aortic stenosis, serial echocardiography is recommended every 6 to 12 months for patients with severe disease, every 1 to 2 years for moderate disease, and every 3 to 5 years for mild disease. After a prolonged asymptomatic phase, symptoms may develop in affected patients once stenosis becomes severe. The cardinal symptoms of severe aortic stenosis are angina, heart failure, and syncope, but patients are much more likely to complain of exertional dyspnea and decreased exercise tolerance.

Aortic stenosis causes a systolic ejection murmur (see Table 31.8), best heard in the right upper sternal border and often radiating to the neck. A similar murmur occurs with aortic *sclerosis*, which is defined as thickening of the aortic valve without associated stenosis. Aortic sclerosis is present in 25% of individuals age 65 years or older, and 50% of individuals age 80 years or older. Aortic sclerosis is associated with an increased risk of cardiovascular events, and a 2% annual risk of progression to aortic stenosis.[168] The radiating pattern of the systolic ejection murmur can help rule out aortic stenosis, with the absence of radiation to the right clavicle being associated with a negative likelihood ratio of 0.1 for aortic stenosis.[169] In addition to a systolic ejection murmur, aortic stenosis is associated with a delayed carotid upstroke and paradoxically split second heart sound. Any patient with a previously undiagnosed suspicious systolic murmur should have an echocardiogram, especially since noncardiologists have difficulty in distinguishing murmurs of aortic stenosis from those of aortic sclerosis. Typical ECG abnormalities associated with aortic stenosis include LVH (often with a strain pattern), left axis deviation, and LBBB.

TABLE 31.8 Descriptions of Murmurs Associated With Cardiac Abnormalities

Lesion	Location	Timing	Description
Aortic Stenosis	Second parasternal interspace	Midsystolic	Crescendo-decrescendo, radiates to the carotids; with or without S_3, S_4; Valsalva maneuver and sustained hand grip exercise decrease intensity
Aortic Insufficiency	Third and fourth parasternal interspaces	Holodiastolic	Decrescendo, blowing, high pitched, radiates to the carotids; Austin-Flint rumble at the apex; squatting, hand grip exercise, and leaning forward increase intensity
Mitral Stenosis	Apex	Middiastolic	Opening snap; low-pitched rumble radiates to the axilla; squatting and hand grip exercise increase intensity
Mitral Regurgitation	Apex	Holosystolic	High pitched, blowing, radiates to the axilla; loud S_3; standing decreases intensity; squatting and hand grip exercise increase intensity
Mitral Valve Prolapse	Apex	Late systolic	Crescendo, midsystolic click; Valsalva maneuver and standing increase intensity; squatting decreases intensity
Hypertrophic Cardiomyopathy	Apex, lower left sternal border	Midsystolic	S_4, Single S_2; Valsalva maneuver and standing increase intensity; squatting, passive leg raising, and hand grip exercise decrease intensity

Moderate to severe aortic stenosis is associated with increased risk of perioperative cardiovascular complications.[170,171] Nonetheless, contemporary studies suggest that noncardiac surgery can be performed with acceptable mortality risks in individuals with asymptomatic severe aortic stenosis[171] Thus, guidelines support proceeding with major elective noncardiac surgery in patients with asymptomatic severe aortic stenosis, provided that appropriate intraoperative and postoperative hemodynamic monitoring is available.[7,9] Conversely, for patients with symptomatic severe aortic stenosis, aortic valve replacement should be considered before their planned noncardiac surgery.[7,9] If a symptomatic patient is deemed high-risk or ineligible for surgical aortic valve replacement, alternative intervention options include transcatheter aortic valve replacement (TAVR) or percutaneous aortic balloon dilation.[7,9] Multidisciplinary collaboration with a cardiologist is invaluable for the perioperative management of these high-risk patients.

Patients with moderate to severe aortic stenosis also have an increased risk of bleeding from an *acquired* von Willebrand syndrome, which occurs in 67% to 92% of patients with severe stenosis.[172] The underlying pathophysiology is mechanical disruption of von Willebrand multimers during turbulent blood flow through the narrowed valve. Of note, prophylaxis for infective endocarditis is not recommended.[173]

Aortic Insufficiency. Aortic valve insufficiency occurs with valvular leaflet disease, aortic root dilation, or both. Causes of valvular disease include rheumatic heart disease, bicuspid valves, collagen vascular disease, and endocarditis. With respect to aortic root dilation, causes include ankylosing spondylitis, osteogenesis imperfecta, syphilis, hypertension, age-related degeneration, Marfan syndrome, and collagen vascular diseases. These causes generally lead to progressive chronic aortic insufficiency that remains asymptomatic for decades. In contrast, acute aortic insufficiency can result from trauma, infections, or aortic dissection; this is an emergent condition that results in cardiogenic shock.

On auscultation, aortic insufficiency is associated with a diastolic murmur (see Table 31.8), the intensity of which does not correlate well with the severity of regurgitation.[174] Patients typically have a widened pulse pressure, which manifests as Corrigan or water-hammer pulses (bounding carotid pulse with a rapid downstroke), de Musset sign (head bob with each heart beat), Duroziez sign (systolic and diastolic bruit heard over the femoral artery when it is partially compressed), and Quincke pulses (capillary pulsations in the fingertips or lips). Although auscultation by a cardiologist can help rule in or rule out aortic regurgitation (based on the presence or absence of an early diastolic murmur),[175] the accuracy of auscultation by noncardiologists is uncertain.[26] Thus, an echocardiogram is helpful for any patient suspected of having a diastolic murmur.

Limited prior research suggests that patients with moderate-to-severe aortic insufficiency experience increased risks of perioperative mortality and morbidity, especially in the presence of impaired left ventricular function (ejection fraction < 55%) or renal insufficiency.[176] Nonetheless, expert consensus from current guidelines is supportive of patients with asymptomatic severe aortic insufficiency to proceed with major noncardiac surgery accompanied by careful perioperative management, including hemodynamic monitoring, afterload control, and fluid balance.[7,9,167] Prophylaxis for infective endocarditis is not recommended.[173]

TABLE 31.9 Grading Severity of Aortic Stenosis

Grade	Transvalvular Jet Velocity (m/s)	Mean Pressure Gradient (mm Hg)	Valve Area (cm^2)
Mild	2.0–2.9	<20	≥1.5
Moderate	3–3.9	20–39	1.0–1.5
Severe	≥4	≥40	<1.0

Mitral Stenosis. Mitral stenosis is much rarer than aortic stenosis, and almost always related to rheumatic heart disease. Other less common causes include mitral annular calcification and radiation-associated valve disease. The normal mitral valve has a cross-sectional area of 4 to 6 cm^2. Mitral stenosis involves progressive reduction of this area, with shortness of breath with exertion occurring when the area falls below 2.5 cm^2, and symptoms at rest occurring once the area falls below 1.5 cm^2. Severe mitral stenosis is defined by a valve area less than 1 cm^2 and is typically associated with a pulmonary artery systolic pressure > 50 mm Hg, and a resting mean transvalvular gradient ≥ 10 mm Hg.

When mitral stenosis becomes symptomatic, patients experience dyspnea, fatigue, orthopnea, pulmonary edema, and hemoptysis because of increased left atrial pressures and decreased cardiac output. Atrial fibrillation can also develop, in turn causing heart failure in the short term and thrombosis in the long term. Patients with atrial fibrillation require long-term anticoagulation, with recent guidelines recommending vitamin K antagonist therapy (e.g., warfarin) as opposed to DOACs.[173] Pulmonary hypertension (see later section on "Pulmonary Hypertension") and right-sided heart failure can also occur in patients with significant stenosis. The physical examination should evaluate for rales and signs of right-sided heart failure such as jugular venous distention, peripheral edema, hepatomegaly, right ventricular heave, and ascites. On auscultation, mitral stenosis is associated with a diastolic murmur that should be evaluated with echocardiography.

Medical management includes β-adrenergic blockers for controlling heart rate, antiarrhythmic agents for preventing or controlling atrial fibrillation, and anticoagulants in patients with atrial fibrillation. Both β-adrenergic blockers and antiarrhythmic agents should be continued preoperatively, while anticoagulation should be managed in conjunction with the treating cardiologist and surgeon. Prophylaxis for infective endocarditis is not recommended.[173] If a patient with mitral stenosis meets guideline-based indications for valvular intervention (e.g., percutaneous mitral balloon commissurotomy),[167] consideration should be given to performing this intervention before major elective noncardiac surgery.[7,9] If an asymptomatic patient with severe mitral stenosis has valve morphology that is not favorable for a percutaneous intervention, it is still reasonable to proceed with major elective noncardiac surgery provided that appropriate intraoperative and postoperative hemodynamic monitoring is used.[7]

Mitral Regurgitation. Acute mitral regurgitation can occur in the setting of myocardial infarction, trauma, or infective endocarditis. Chronic mitral regurgitation is typically associated with degenerative mitral valve disease (including mitral valve prolapse), rheumatic heart disease, ischemic heart disease, and cardiomyopathies. Chronic mitral regurgitation progresses very gradually. Symptoms develop relatively late, and typically only after onset of left ventricular dysfunction. Associated symptoms are initially vague, but progress to fatigue, dyspnea, and atrial fibrillation with disease progression.

On auscultation, patients with mitral regurgitation usually have a holosystolic murmur heard best at the cardiac apex (see Table 31.8). The murmur grade is somewhat correlated with the severity of mitral regurgitation in primary mitral valve disease (e.g., degenerative mitral valve disease), but not in secondary functional regurgitation (e.g., ischemic heart disease, cardiomyopathies). Although auscultation by a cardiologist can help determine mitral regurgitation (based on the presence or absence of a late systolic or holosystolic murmur in the mid-left thorax), the accuracy of auscultation by noncardiologists is uncertain.[26] Thus, an echocardiogram is helpful for any patient with a suspicious systolic murmur. Chronic mitral regurgitation is generally well tolerated perioperatively, unless other valvular lesions (e.g., mitral stenosis) or left ventricular dysfunction coexist. Consistent with these observations, limited prior research suggests that patients with mitral regurgitation have increased risks of cardiovascular complications, but not mortality.[177] Current guidelines suggest that patients with asymptomatic severe mitral regurgitation can proceed to major elective noncardiac surgery provided that appropriate intraoperative and postoperative hemodynamic monitoring is available.[7] Prophylaxis for infective endocarditis is no longer recommended.[173]

Mitral Valve Prolapse. Mitral valve prolapse is characterized by the systolic billowing of an abnormally thickened mitral valve leaflet into the left atrium, with or without coexistent mitral regurgitation. Diagnostic criteria for mitral valve prolapse have evolved to the current definition based on echocardiography alone, namely ≥ 2 mm billowing of any portion of the mitral leaflets above the annular plane in the long axis view.[178] It is the common cause of isolated mitral regurgitation requiring surgical repair in high-income countries. Nonetheless, only 4% of patients with mitral valve prolapse have severe valvular regurgitation, with most affected individuals having mild, trace, or no mitral regurgitation.[179] The condition may be primary (i.e., myxomatous degeneration) or secondary (e.g., associated with Marfan syndrome, Ehlers-Danlos syndrome, and osteogenesis imperfecta). Nonspecific symptoms (e.g., atypical chest pain, palpitations, dyspnea, exercise intolerance, dizziness) have been attributed, albeit unreliably, to mitral valve prolapse—in what has been termed as the "mitral valve prolapse syndrome."

On auscultation, these patients may have a systolic click and a mid-systolic murmur at the cardiac apex (that intensifies with a Valsalva maneuver). Auscultation by a cardiologist can help diagnose mitral valve prolapse (based on the presence or absence of a systolic click and murmur); however, the accuracy of auscultation by noncardiologists is uncertain.[26] From the perioperative perspective, the key issue is to differentiate patients with clinically significant mitral valve regurgitation from those with an incidental finding of prolapse that does not warrant further evaluation. Thus, echocardiography may be helpful to further investigate murmurs suspected of representing significant mitral regurgitation. Prophylaxis for infective endocarditis is no longer recommended.[173]

Tricuspid Regurgitation. Tricuspid regurgitation is a common valvular abnormality, with 70% of normal adults exhibiting a small degree of tricuspid regurgitation on echocardiography. Since it is usually asymptomatic and not easily audible on physical examination, tricuspid regurgitation is most commonly noted as an incidental echocardiographic finding. Significant tricuspid regurgitation is most commonly caused by dilatation of the right ventricle and tricuspid annulus (i.e., secondary disease). Causes of secondary tricuspid regurgitation include left-sided heart failure, mitral valve disease (stenosis or regurgitation), primary pulmonary disease (e.g., pulmonary hypertension), left-to-right intracardiac shunts (e.g., atrial septal defect, ventricular septal defect), pulmonary artery stenosis, and right ventricle disease (e.g., arrhythmogenic right ventricular dysplasia). Tricuspid regurgitation is less commonly caused by processes directly affecting the tricuspid valve (i.e., primary disease), such as Ebstein anomaly, infective endocarditis (typically in intravenous drug users), rheumatic heart disease, carcinoid syndrome, connective tissue disorders (e.g., Marfan syndrome), myxomatous degeneration, or direct injury (e.g., permanent pacemaker or ICD lead). Certain drugs—namely anorectics (fenfluramine, phentermine) and pergolide (dopamine agonist)—have also been associated with primary tricuspid regurgitation.

Patients with mild or moderate tricuspid regurgitation are generally asymptomatic. Individuals with severe regurgitation may report pulsations in the neck (related to distended jugular veins), as well as symptoms of right-sided heart failure (e.g., ascites, peripheral edema) and underlying conditions (e.g., pulmonary hypertension). Relevant findings on physical examination include distended jugular veins, hepatomegaly, ascites, dependent edema, and a right ventricular heave on chest palpation. On auscultation, tricuspid regurgitation causes a holosystolic murmur that is heard best at the midsternal border or subxiphoid area. Nonetheless, the murmur is often absent or very soft, even with severe regurgitation. The intensity of the murmur can be increased using maneuvers that increase venous return (e.g., inspiration, abdominal pressure). Although auscultation by a cardiologist can help determine moderate-to-severe tricuspid regurgitation (based on the presence or absence of increased murmur intensity with inspiration or abdominal pressure), the accuracy of auscultation by noncardiologists is uncertain.[26] Thus, echocardiography may be helpful in a patient with a suspicious murmur, especially within the context of signs or symptoms of right-sided heart failure. The preoperative management of patients with severe tricuspid regurgitation should be guided by the presence of any underlying conditions, right-sided heart failure, and known or suspected pulmonary hypertension. Where indicated, perioperative management should be conducted collaboratively with a heart failure cardiologist or pulmonary hypertension specialist. Prophylaxis for infective endocarditis is no longer recommended.[173]

Hypertrophic Cardiomyopathy. Hypertrophic cardiomyopathy is a genetic disorder of the myocardium, which can result in dynamic left ventricular outflow tract obstruction, myocardial ischemia, diastolic dysfunction, and mitral regurgitation (related to systolic anterior motion of the mitral valve leaflets). Most affected individuals have a relatively normal lifespan; however others are at risk for progressive heart failure, sudden cardiac death, and atrial fibrillation. Most patients with hypertrophic cardiomyopathy are asymptomatic. When symptoms are present, they are quite variable, and not well correlated with the extent of LVH or outflow tract obstruction. Typical associated symptoms include fatigue, exertional dyspnea, atypical or angina chest pain, exertional presyncope or syncope, and palpitations. Symptomatic patients may be prescribed long-term medical therapy with negative inotropic agents (i.e., β-blockers, verapamil, disopyramide). Other symptomatic individuals with severe left ventricular outflow tract obstruction may require intervention with either surgical myectomy or alcohol septal ablation. Some patients may also undergo ICD insertion if they are deemed high-risk for sudden cardiac death.

Although the physical examination in a patient with hypertrophic cardiomyopathy may be normal, the classic finding on auscultation (see Table 31.8) is a mid-systolic murmur that increases with maneuvers to decrease ventricular size (e.g., Valsalva maneuver) and decreases with maneuvers to increase ventricular size (e.g., passive leg raise). Auscultation by a cardiologist can help rule in or rule out hypertrophic cardiomyopathy (based on decreased murmur intensity with passive leg elevation or increased murmur intensity with shifts from a squatting to standing position), however, the accuracy of auscultation by noncardiologists is uncertain.[26] Accordingly, an echocardiogram should be obtained if a patient has a personal (or family) history of exertional syncope or cardiac arrest; a suspicious murmur is found on auscultation; or concerning ECG findings (i.e., LVH, ST-segment abnormalities, T-wave abnormalities) are observed in an otherwise healthy nonhypertensive patient. In general, patients with hypertrophic cardiomyopathy can safely undergo most low-risk and intermediate-risk noncardiac surgical procedures, especially with close hemodynamic monitoring and management. Medical therapy (e.g., β-adrenergic blockers, verapamil) should be continued perioperatively, but prophylaxis for infective endocarditis is no longer recommended.[173] Appropriate perioperative management should be instituted for any patient who has an associated ICD.

Prosthetic Heart Valves. In patients with prosthetic heart valves, the preoperative evaluation should determine the underlying indication that led to valve replacement; type, age, and current status of the valve prosthesis; need for long-term anticoagulation entailed by the valve prosthesis; and planned perioperative anticoagulation management plan. The anesthesiologist should review the most recent echocardiogram, and order a repeat echocardiogram if there are any signs or symptoms suggestive of valve dysfunction (e.g., new onset heart failure).[167] In addition, a recent complete blood count may be helpful since these patients may have a valve-related hemolytic anemia.

Anticoagulation with a vitamin K antagonist (e.g., warfarin) is required for 3 to 6 months after open surgical bioprosthetic valve implantation, after which patients can be transitioned to aspirin therapy alone (75-100 mg daily).[167] Life-long aspirin therapy is recommended for patients who have undergone TAVR, as well as clopidogrel (75 mg daily) for the first 6 months in all patients and vitamin K antagonists for the first 3 months in select individuals.[173] Conversely, patients with mechanical prosthetic valves require life-long therapy with both aspirin and vitamin K antagonists.[167] Importantly, DOACs—such as dabigatran, rivaroxaban, edoxaban, or apixaban—should not be used for anticoagulation therapy in patients with mechanical heart valves.[167] In general, decisions about temporary preoperative discontinuation of anticoagulants, duration of anticoagulant discontinuation, need for "bridging" therapy with a shorter-acting drug, and type of bridging agent (intravenous heparin or LMWH) should be made in conjunction with the treating cardiologist and surgeon. Current guidelines make recommendations for bridging therapy largely based on the location of the mechanical heart valve and nature of planned surgery (Box 31.4).[173] Prophylaxis for infective endocarditis is recommended for

BOX 31.4 Recommendations for Preoperative Bridging Anticoagulation Therapy in Patients With Mechanical Heart Valves

Class I (Recommended)

- Continuation of vitamin K antagonist anticoagulation with a therapeutic INR is recommended in patients with mechanical heart valves undergoing minor procedures (e.g., dental extractions, cataract removal) where bleeding is easily controlled.
- Temporary interruption of vitamin K antagonist anticoagulation, without bridging agents while the INR is subtherapeutic, is recommended in patients with a bileaflet mechanical AVR and no other risk factors* for thrombosis who are undergoing invasive or surgical procedures.

Class IIa (Is Reasonable)

- Bridging anticoagulation therapy during the time interval when the INR is subtherapeutic preoperatively is reasonable on an individualized basis—with the risks of bleeding weighed against the benefits of thromboembolism prevention—for patients who are undergoing invasive or surgical procedures with a (i) mechanical AVR and any thromboembolic risk factor, (ii) older-generation mechanical AVR, or (iii) mechanical MVR.

*Risk factors include atrial fibrillation, previous thromboembolism, hypercoagulable condition, older-generation ball-cage or tilting disc mechanical valve, left ventricular systolic dysfunction, and ≥ 2 mechanical valves.

AVR, Aortic valve replacement; *INR,* international normalized ratio; *MVR,* mitral valve replacement.

From Nishimura RA, Otto CM, Bonow RO, et al. 2017 AHA/ACC Focused Update of the 2014 AHA/ACC Guideline for the Management of Patients With Valvular Heart Disease: A report of the American College of Cardiology/American Heart Association Task Force on Clinical Practice Guidelines. *Circulation.* 2017;135:e1159–e1195.

specific procedures (see section on "Infective Endocarditis Prophylaxis").[173]

Infective Endocarditis Prophylaxis

Patients at risk for infective endocarditis (e.g., valve replacement, complex congenital heart disease, previous endocarditis) and scheduled for procedures with the potential for transient bacteremia must be identified preoperatively. Current guidelines have dramatically scaled back the indications for prophylaxis. For example, current ACC/AHA guidelines recommended prophylaxis only for patients who are both at increased risk of developing infective endocarditis and also experiencing adverse outcomes from endocarditis (Box 31.5).[173] These target patient subgroups are also with those identified in the most recent ESC guidelines.[180] Prophylaxis is required when eligible patients undergo dental procedures that involve manipulation of gingival tissue, manipulation of the periapical region of teeth, or perforation of the oral mucosa. Prophylaxis is not required when these same individuals undergo nondental procedures (e.g., transesophageal echocardiography, gastroscopy, colonoscopy, cystoscopy, dermatological procedures), unless there is active infection at the procedure site.[173]

Rhythm Disturbances on the Preoperative Electrocardiogram

Arrhythmias and conduction disturbances are common during the perioperative period. Supraventricular and ventricular arrhythmias are associated with increased perioperative risk, both because of the arrhythmias themselves and because they are markers for cardiopulmonary disease. Uncontrolled atrial fibrillation (i.e., causing symptoms or hemodynamic compromise) and high-risk ventricular tachyarrhythmias (see section on "Ventricular Arrhythmias") are high-risk conditions that warrant postponement of elective surgery until evaluation and stabilization are complete. Rapid atrial fibrillation (rates > 100 beats/min), symptomatic bradycardia, or high-grade heart block (e.g., third-degree heart block) also warrants postponement of elective procedures to facilitate evaluation, stabilization, and possible cardiology evaluation.

First-degree atrioventricular (AV) block is defined as a PR interval exceeding 0.20 ms with an associated heart rate of 50 to 100 beats/min; it is considered generally benign. Second-degree heart block is defined by a PR interval exceeding 0.20 ms and the presence of some blocked atrial beats (resulting in a dropped or missing QRS complex after a P wave). There are two types of second-degree block. Mobitz type I block (also called Wenckebach block) is characterized by progressive lengthening of the PR interval until the dropped beat occurs. It is a more benign block that is related to AV nodal delay, easily responsive to atropine, and unlikely to progress to complete heart block. Mobitz type II block is characterized by a fixed and prolonged PR interval that does not change before the dropped QRS complex. It is related to an infranodal block, capable of progressing to complete heart block, and generally treated with a pacemaker (unless it is due to a reversible cause such as ischemia or drugs). Third-degree AV block or complete heart block, which is characterized by complete dissociation between the atrial and ventricular beats, requires pacemaker placement unless a reversible source is identified. A prolonged QT interval should prompt an evaluation of electrolytes (including magnesium and calcium), and search for any potentiating drugs. Syncope, presyncope, or a family history of sudden death in a patient with a prolonged QT interval mandates a cardiology consultation (see section on "Long QT Syndrome").

Three factors determine the need for permanent pacemaker treatment for an arrhythmia, namely whether the arrhythmia is associated with symptoms, where the conduction abnormality is located, and whether a reversible cause can be identified. Indications for perioperative pacemaker placement are the same as those in nonsurgical patients (common indications listed in Box 31.6).[181] In general, pacemaker placement is required for symptomatic bradycardia or conduction delays that lead to syncope or presyncope. Conduction disease below the AV node (i.e., in the His-Purkinje system) is also generally less stable and likely benefits from permanent pacemaker placement. The presence of such conduction disease is suggested by a normal or minimally prolonged PR interval, Mobitz type II block, and QRS complex abnormalities (BBB, fascicular block, or both).

BBBs can be classified as complete versus incomplete, and right bundle branch block (RBBB) versus LBBB. BBBs may be normal variants in some individuals, or the result of age-related fibrosis in the conduction system. Nonetheless, they can be associated with important underlying conditions. For example, LBBB may be related to structural heart disease (i.e., hypertensive heart disease, IHD, cardiomyopathies, valvular heart disease), while RBBB may be the result of elevated right ventricular pressures (i.e., pulmonary hypertension, cor pulmonale, pulmonary embolism), prior radiation exposure, myocarditis, and structural heart disease (i.e., IHD, cardiomyopathies, valvular heart disease, congenital heart disease). The presence of a BBB is not itself an indicator of increased perioperative cardiovascular risk,[182] especially after accounting for known clinical risk factors.[100] Nonetheless, data from the nonoperative

BOX 31.5 Cardiac Conditions for Which Endocarditis Prophylaxis Is Recommended

- Previous infective endocarditis
- Prosthetic cardiac valves, including transcatheter-implanted prostheses, and homografts
- Prosthetic material used for cardiac valve repair, such as annuloplasty rings and chords
- Unrepaired cyanotic congenital heart disease, including palliative shunts and conduits
- Repaired congenital heart disease, with residual shunts or valvular regurgitation at the site of or adjacent to the site of a prosthetic patch or prosthetic device
- Cardiac transplant with valve regurgitation due to a structurally abnormal valve

Prophylaxis is reasonable before dental procedures that involve manipulation of gingival tissue, manipulation of the periapical region of teeth, or perforation of the oral mucosa.

From Nishimura RA, Otto CM, Bonow RO, et al. 2017 AHA/ACC Focused Update of the 2014 AHA/ACC Guideline for the Management of Patients With Valvular Heart Disease: A Report of the American College of Cardiology/American Heart Association Task Force on Clinical Practice Guidelines. *Circulation.* 2017;135: e1159–e1195.

setting suggest that a recent onset or new diagnosis of a bundle branch should prompt a more extensive evaluation for undiagnosed cardiovascular disease. For example, LBBB is associated with increased risks of incident cardiovascular disease,[183] cardiovascular mortality,[183] and mortality in the nonoperative setting.[184] Additionally, RBBB is associated with increased risks of mortality in patients with suspected IHD, known IHD, and heart failure.[185,186] Based on this approach, if preoperative evaluation does not suggest significant pulmonary disease, IHD, structural heart disease, or Brugada syndrome (see section on "Brugada Syndrome"), no further preoperative evaluation of an isolated asymptomatic RBBB is warranted. Conversely, RBBB in a patient with known or suspected pulmonary disease (e.g., pulmonary hypertension) may suggest severe respiratory or vascular compromise; thus, consideration should be given to pulmonary evaluation and echocardiography if intermediate- or high-risk surgery is planned.

Atrial Fibrillation. Atrial fibrillation is a common arrhythmia characterized by a variable irregular ventricular response, and an absence of regular or organized atrial activity. The arrhythmia is classified as paroxysmal (i.e., terminates spontaneously or with intervention within 7 days of onset), persistent (i.e., fails to self-terminate within 7 days), long-standing persistent (i.e., lasts more than 12 months), or permanent (i.e., persistent atrial fibrillation where a joint decision has been made by the patient and clinician to no longer pursue a rhythm control strategy).[187] Atrial fibrillation can occur in the absence of any structural heart disease (previously termed "lone atrial fibrillation"), or in combination with underlying disorders. In high-income countries, hypertension and ischemic heart disease are the most common underlying disorders, while in low and middle-income countries, rheumatic heart disease is a very common associated condition. Other associated conditions include valvular heart disease, heart failure, hypertrophic cardiomyopathy, congenital heart disease, obesity, diabetes mellitus, CKD, and increased age. Potentially reversible acute triggers for atrial fibrillation are hyperthyroidism and recent surgery (especially cardiac or thoracic surgery).

Affected individuals are at elevated risk for death, heart failure, thromboembolic events (i.e., stroke), and hospitalization. In the nonoperative setting, treatment involves ventricular rate control, consideration of rhythm control to restore sinus rhythm, and prevention of systemic embolization. In large randomized trials, strategies that focused on heart rate control versus rhythm control have shown similar effects on the risks of stroke or death.[188,189] The CHA_2DS_2-VASc score (Table 31.10) can be used to estimate the long-term systematic embolization risk in patients with atrial fibrillation.[190] Based on this score, patients can be classified as low-risk (0 points: 0.2% annualized stroke rate), intermediate-risk (1 point: 0.6% annualized stroke rate), or high-risk (≥2 points: >2.2% annualized stroke rate).[191] Based on strong randomized controlled trial data,[192] current ACC/AHA guidelines recommend long-term oral anticoagulation for patients with nonvalvular atrial fibrillation (i.e.,

BOX 31.6 Common Indications for a Permanent Pacemaker

Class I Indications

- Sinus bradycardia with symptoms due to the bradycardia (typically seen with heart rates less than 40 bpm or with frequent sinus pauses)
- Symptomatic chronotropic incompetence (i.e., impaired heart rate response to exercise)
- Third-degree AV block
- Advanced second-degree AV block (block of ≥2 consecutive *P* waves)
- Symptomatic Mobitz I or II second-degree AV block
- Mobitz II second-degree AV block with a widened QRS or chronic bifascicular block, regardless of symptoms
- Exercise-induced second- or third-degree AV block

Class II Indications

- Sinus bradycardia (heart rate < 40 bpm) with symptoms suggestive (but not definitively so) of bradycardia
- Sinus node dysfunction with a history of unexplained syncope
- Chronic heart rates < 40 bpm in an awake but minimally symptomatic patient
- Asymptomatic Mobitz II second-degree AV block with a narrow QRS interval
- Bifascicular or trifascicular block associated with syncope possibly related to intermittent third-degree heart block
- First-degree AV block with a very long PR interval (which effectively leads to AV dissociation and hemodynamic compromise)

AV, Atrioventricular; *bpm,* beats per minute.
Class I Indications: *Permanent* pacing is definitely beneficial, useful, and effective.
Class II Indications: *Permanent* pacing may be indicated but there is conflicting evidence and/or divergence of opinion.
From Epstein AE, DiMarco JP, Ellenbogen KA, et al. 2012 ACCF/AHA/HRS focused update incorporated into the ACCF/AHA/HRS 2008 guidelines for device-based therapy of cardiac rhythm abnormalities: a report of the American College of Cardiology Foundation/American Heart Association Task Force on Practice Guidelines and the Heart Rhythm Society. *Circulation.* 2013;127:e283–e352.

TABLE 31.10 Scoring Scheme for the CHA_2DS_2-VASc Score

Risk Factor	Points
Heart Failure Associated signs and symptoms, or left ventricular systolic dysfunction	1
Hypertension	1
Age ≥ 75 years	2
Diabetes mellitus	1
Previous stroke, transient ischemic attack, or thromboembolism	2
Vascular Disease Myocardial infarction, peripheral artery disease, or aortic plaque	1
Age 65–74 years	1
Female sex	1

CHADS2, Congestive heart failure, hypertension, age > 75, diabetes, prior stroke/transient ischemic attack schema; CHA2DS2-VASc, Birmingham 2009 schema.
From Lip GY, Nieuwlaat R, Pisters R, et al. Refining clinical risk stratification for predicting stroke and thromboembolism in atrial fibrillation using a novel risk factor-based approach: the Euro heart survey on atrial fibrillation. *Chest.* 2010;137:263–272.

unrelated to mitral stenosis or prosthetic heart valves) and CHA_2DS_2-VASc scores of 2 or more, and support omitting anticoagulation in individuals with CHA_2DS_2-VASc scores of zero.[187] There is more uncertainty about the best treatment for individuals with CHA_2DS_2-VASc scores of 1. Consistent with this uncertainty, ACC/AHA guidelines indicate that (1) oral anticoagulant therapy, (2) aspirin therapy, or (3) omitting anticoagulation are all reasonable approaches in these intermediate-risk patients.[187] With respect to specific anticoagulant therapy, patients can be prescribed either a vitamin K antagonist (e.g., warfarin) or DOAC (e.g., dabigatran, rivaroxaban, edoxaban, apixaban) as reasonable options for patients with nonvalvular atrial fibrillation.

Although atrial fibrillation has typically been ignored during preoperative cardiac risk assessment, accumulating evidence challenges this approach in two main respects. Specifically, preexisting atrial fibrillation appears to be an indicator of increased perioperative risk. For example, in a large international multicenter prospective cohort study, preexisting atrial fibrillation was associated with an elevated risk of postoperative cardiovascular events (i.e., stroke, cardiovascular death, myocardial injury, heart failure, or cardiac arrest),[193] but not death.[77] In an American population-based retrospective cohort study, chronic atrial fibrillation was associated with a significantly higher risk of perioperative stroke.[194]

The preoperative evaluation of patients with atrial fibrillation focuses on underlying conditions (e.g., ischemic heart disease), complications (e.g., heart failure, stroke), rate or rhythm control strategies, and anticoagulation strategies. Patients with rapid ventricular rates (>100 beats/min) typically require rate control before any elective surgery. Patients with both atrial fibrillation and slow ventricular rate without rate-controlling medications may have sick sinus syndrome. They should be questioned regarding any previous episodes of syncope or presyncope. Any long-term β-adrenergic blockers, digoxin, calcium channel blockers, or antiarrhythmic medications should be continued.

The critical component for preoperative planning for most patients with atrial fibrillation is appropriate perioperative management of long-term anticoagulants. This management should ideally be conducted collaboratively with the treating physician and responsible surgeon. There are three overarching issues, namely (1) whether temporary preoperative discontinuation is needed, (2) when oral anticoagulants should be discontinued, and (3) whether bridging therapy with LMWH is required.[195] It is reasonable to continue vitamin K antagonist therapy if an individual does not have patient-related risk factors for bleeding (e.g., liver disease, abnormal renal function, prior bleeding complications), and is scheduled for a procedure without important bleeding risk (e.g., dental extraction, simple cutaneous procedures, pacemaker insertion). Otherwise, patients should have their anticoagulant medications temporarily discontinued before surgery, including all patients who are receiving DOACs or might need neuraxial anesthesia. If a decision to temporarily discontinue oral anticoagulants is made, vitamin K antagonists should be stopped 5 days before surgery. A longer discontinuation period may be needed for initial international normalized ratio (INR) values greater than 3.0. Ideally, the INR should be rechecked within 24 hours before surgery,[195] and a low dose of oral vitamin K administered for any INR result above 1.5. The timing of preoperative discontinuation of DOACs (Table 31.11) should be guided by the specific drug prescribed, expected procedural bleeding risk, renal function (based on estimated glomerular filtration rate [GFR]), and planned use of neuraxial anesthesia.[195,196] The ongoing multicenter Perioperative Anticoagulant Use for Surgery Evaluation prospective cohort study is expected to provide more high-quality data on the safety of a further simplified strategy for preoperative discontinuation of DOACs (Table 31.12).[197]

Accumulating evidence indicates that most patients with nonvalvular atrial fibrillation do not require bridging therapy if their anticoagulant therapy is temporarily discontinued before surgery. For example, in the multicenter Bridging Anticoagulation in Patients Who Require Temporary Interruption of Warfarin Therapy for an Elective Invasive Procedure and Surgery (BRIDGE) randomized trial, placebo was non-inferior to LMWH bridging therapy with respect to risks of arterial thromboembolism following perioperative interruption of vitamin K antagonist therapy.[198] In addition, bridging therapy led to increased risks of major bleeding. When interpreting the trial data, the challenge pertains to their generalizability to patients in clinical practice. For example, about 62% of the 1884

TABLE 31.11 Expert Consensus Recommendations on Preoperative Direct Oral Anticoagulant Discontinuation (Recommended Time Interval from Last Preoperative Dose)

Direct Thrombin Inhibitor (i.e., Dabigatran)	Direct Factor Xa Inhibitor (i.e., Rivaroxaban, Edoxaban, Apixaban)
LOW BLEEDING RISK PROCEDURES (ACC RECOMMENDATIONS)*	
eGFR ≥ 80 mL/min: ≥ 24 h eGFR 50–79 mL/min: ≥ 36 h eGFR 30–49 mL/min: ≥ 48 h eGFR 15–29 mL/min: ≥ 72 h eGFR < 15 mL/min: No data	eGFR ≥ 30 mL/min: ≥ 24 h eGFR 15–29 mL/min: ≥ 36 h eGFR < 15 mL/min: No data (consider ≥ 48 h)
UNCERTAIN, INTERMEDIATE, OR HIGH BLEEDING RISK PROCEDURES (ACC RECOMMENDATIONS)*	
eGFR ≥ 80 mL/min: ≥ 48 h eGFR 50–79 mL/min: ≥ 72 h eGFR 30–49 mL/min: ≥ 96 h eGFR 15–29 mL/min: ≥ 120 h eGFR < 15 mL/min: No data	eGFR ≥ 30 mL/min: ≥ 48 h eGFR < 30 mL/min: No data (consider ≥ 72 h)
PLANNED NEURAXIAL ANESTHESIA (ASRA RECOMMENDATIONS)†	
Uniform approach: 120 h Approach based on eGFR ▪ eGFR ≥ 80 mL/min: ≥ 72 h ▪ eGFR 50–79 mL/min: ≥ 96 h ▪ eGFR 30–49 mL/min: ≥ 120 h ▪ eGFR < 30 mL/min: Not recommended	72 h

ACC, American College of Cardiology; *ASRA*, American Society of Regional Anesthesiologists; *eGFR*, estimated glomerular filtration rate (Cockcroft-Gault equation).

*From Doherty JU, Gluckman TJ, Hucker WJ, et al. 2017 ACC Expert Consensus Decision Pathway for Periprocedural Management of Anticoagulation in Patients With Nonvalvular Atrial Fibrillation: A Report of the American College of Cardiology Clinical Expert Consensus Document Task Force. *J Am Coll Cardiol*. 2017;69:871–898.

†From Horlocker TT, Vandermeulen E, Kopp SL, et al. Regional anesthesia in the patient receiving antithrombotic or thrombolytic therapy: American Society of Regional Anesthesia and Pain Medicine Evidence-Based Guidelines (Fourth Edition). *Reg Anesth Pain Med*. 2018;43:263–309.

TABLE 31.12 Simplified Protocol for Preoperative Direct Oral Anticoagulant Discontinuation—as Assessed in the Perioperative Anticoagulant Use for Surgery Evaluation Study

Direct Thrombin Inhibitor (i.e., Dabigatran)	Direct Factor Xa Inhibitor (i.e., Rivaroxaban, Apixaban)
LOW BLEEDING RISK PROCEDURES (NO PLANNED NEURAXIAL ANESTHESIA)	
eGFR ≥ 50 mL/min: last dose 2 days before surgery eGFR 30–49 mL/min: last dose 4 days before surgery	eGFR ≥ 30 mL/min: last dose 2 days before surgery
HIGH BLEEDING RISK PROCEDURES (NO PLANNED NEURAXIAL ANESTHESIA)	
eGFR ≥ 50 mL/min: last dose 3 days before surgery eGFR 30–49 mL/min: last dose 5 days before surgery	eGFR ≥ 30 mL/min: last dose 3 days before surgery

eGFR, Estimated glomerular filtration rate*
*Should be calculated using the Cockcroft-Gault equation.
From Douketis JD, Spyropoulos AC, Anderson JM, et al. The Perioperative Anticoagulant Use for Surgery Evaluation (PAUSE) Study for patients on a direct oral anticoagulant who need an elective surgery or procedure: design and rationale. *Thromb Haemost.* 2017;117: 2415–2424.

participants in the BRIDGE trial had an expected 1-year stroke rate less than 5% (i.e., equivalent to CHA_2DS_2-VASc score ≤ 4), while about 14% had an expected 1-year stroke rate over 10% (equivalent to CHA_2DS_2-VASc score ≥ 7). To help clinicians better navigate clinical decision making, the ACC published a 2017 expert consensus report on perioperative anticoagulation management in nonvalvular atrial fibrillation.[195] In the case of vitamin K antagonist therapy, the recommended approach is to omit bridging therapy in low-risk patients who have CHA_2DS_2-VASc scores of 4 or less and no prior stroke, TIA, or systemic embolization. Conversely, bridging therapy should be considered for high-risk patients with CHA_2DS_2-VASc scores of 7 or more, recent (i.e., prior 3 months) stroke, TIA, or systemic embolization. For intermediate-risk patients (i.e., those not meeting either the low-risk or high-risk criteria), bridging therapy should be considered if there is no significant bleeding risk and a more remote time (more than 3 months) of stroke, TIA, or systemic embolization. Bridging therapy is generally not needed after preoperative interruption of DOACs because of their relatively short half-lives.

Supraventricular Arrhythmias. Supraventricular tachycardia can result from rapidly firing ectopic atrial foci with rapid conduction through the AV node, or from a reentry mechanism. Pathways for a reentry mechanism typically involve the AV node-Purkinje system and an accessory reentry pathway. In a reentry mechanism, the cycle self-perpetuates because conduction occurs down one pathway and up the other. Pharmacologic AV blockade (i.e., adenosine, verapamil, β-adrenergic blockers) can help slow the ventricular rate in most supraventricular tachycardias, with the exception of Wolff-Parkinson-White (WPW) syndrome. WPW syndrome is characterized by the presence of an accessory pathway (bundle of Kent) that permits *both* retrograde and antegrade conduction. Antegrade conduction over the accessory pathway results in a short PR interval (<0.12 ms) and a slurring of the upstroke of the QRS complex (termed a delta wave). Individuals with WPW syndrome are predisposed to supraventricular tachycardia. Additionally, treatment of supraventricular tachycardia in affected individuals with AV nodal blocking drugs can paradoxically increase conduction over the accessory pathway, thus potentially causing ventricular fibrillation. Thus, *acute* supraventricular tachycardia in these patients should be treated with electrical cardioversion (especially if hemodynamically unstable), ibutilide,[199] or procainamide. Long-term management of WPW syndrome typically involves catheter ablation of the recurrent accessory pathway. Long-term antiarrhythmic medications should be continued perioperatively in patients with known supraventricular tachycardia.[9]

Ventricular Arrhythmias. Ventricular ectopic beats can be differentiated from atrial ectopic beats by a wide QRS complex (>0.12 ms) and absence of an associated P-wave. To help predict the risk of sudden death, ventricular arrhythmias may be classified based on the type of rhythm disturbance and presence of underlying heart disease.

- *Benign* ventricular arrhythmias include isolated ventricular premature beats (VPBs) without associated heart disease. Affected individuals have no increased risk of sudden cardiac death, and do not need further cardiology evaluation.
- *Potentially lethal* arrhythmias include more than 30 VPBs per hour, or nonsustained ventricular tachycardia in association with underlying heart disease. Affected individuals are at moderately high risk of sudden cardiac arrest and may benefit from an ICD. They also require cardiology evaluation and echocardiography, along with the possible need for cardiac stress testing, coronary angiography, and electrophysiology testing.
- *Lethal* arrhythmias include sustained ventricular tachycardia, ventricular fibrillation, and VPBs associated with underlying heart disease, depressed cardiac function, and hemodynamic compromise. Affected individuals are at high risk for sudden cardiac arrest, and likely benefit from an ICD. They also require cardiology evaluation and echocardiography, along with possible cardiac stress testing, coronary angiography, and electrophysiology testing. In general, reversible causes of ventricular arrhythmias (e.g., hypokalemia, ischemia, acidosis, hypomagnesemia, drug toxicity, endocrine dysfunction) should be sought out and treated. Any long-term antiarrhythmic medications should be continued perioperatively.[9]

Long QT Syndrome. The long QT syndrome (LQTS) is a myocardial repolarization disorder associated with a prolonged QT interval. The QT interval is measured using a 12-lead ECG (preferably leads II and V5) from the onset of the QRS complex to the end of the T wave. Since the interval varies inversely with heart rate, a corrected QT interval (QT_c) can be calculated, with the most common formula being:

$$QT_c = \frac{\text{QT interval}}{\sqrt{\text{RR interval}}}$$

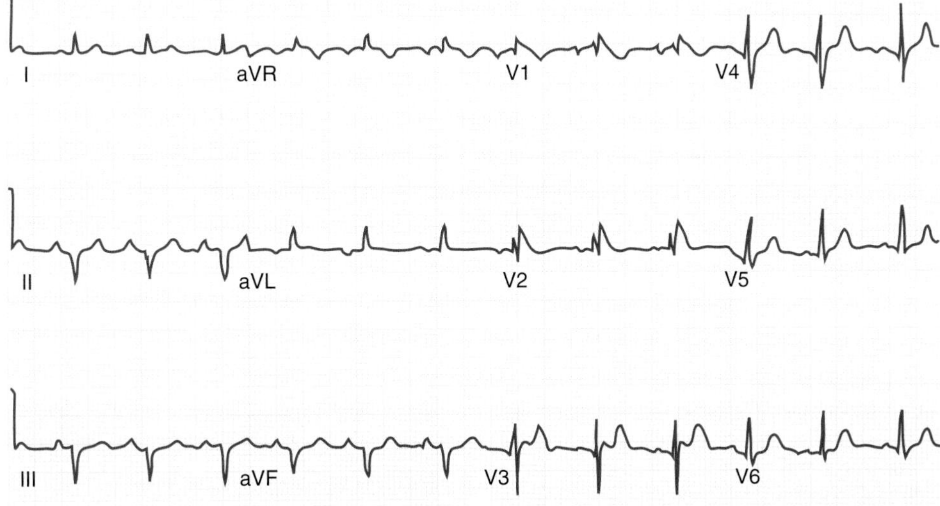

Fig. 31.7 Typical 12-lead electrocardiogram in a patient with Brugada syndrome.

In adults, an abnormally prolonged QTc is defined as a value exceeding the 99th percentile. The QTc is prolonged if exceeding 0.48 seconds in women and 0.47 seconds in men.[200] Individuals with LQTS are predisposed to developing *torsades de pointes*, a polymorphic ventricular tachycardia with frequent variations of the QRS axis or morphology. Affected patients are generally asymptomatic in the absence of arrhythmias. Conversely, after the onset of an arrhythmia, they may develop palpitations, syncope, seizures, and sudden cardiac death.

LQTS may be either congenital (i.e., genetic) or acquired. Causes of acquired LQTS include antiarrhythmic drugs (e.g., quinidine, sotalol, dofetilide, ibutilide), psychotropic medications (e.g., haloperidol, methadone), erythromycin, cisapride, and metabolic abnormalities (i.e., hypokalemia, hypomagnesemia, hypocalcemia). Notably, while amiodarone does markedly prolong the QT interval, it is rarely associated with *torsades de pointes* except in association with hypokalemia. The 2010 ACC/AHA scientific statement on the prevention of *torsades de pointes* suggests that QT_c be documented before initiation or after an increased dose of QT-prolonging drugs, and thereafter at least every 8 to 12 hours.[200] Other components of treatment for LQTS include β-adrenergic blockers (congenital LQTS), ICD implantation, and correction of underlying metabolic disorders.

Brugada Syndrome. Brugada syndrome is a rare cause of sudden cardiac arrest that occurs in the absence of structural heart disease. It is an autosomal dominant disorder that is more common in men, rarely diagnosed in children, and often affects individuals of Asian ethnicity. Patients usually have normal findings on echocardiography, stress testing, and cardiac magnetic resonance imaging (MRI). The most significant clinical manifestations are ventricular arrhythmias, syncope, and sudden death. Patients may also be at increased risk of atrial arrhythmias, especially atrial fibrillation. Brugada syndrome is characterized by an ECG with pseudo-RBBB and persistent ST-segment elevation in leads V_1 to V_3 (Fig. 31.7). Unlike usual RBBB, a widened S wave in the left lateral leads is usually absent in Brugada syndrome. In some patients, these ECG changes are transient and provoked by medications. Asymptomatic patients who have these typical ECG features but no other associated clinical criteria have been described as having "Brugada pattern." The website www.brugadadrugs.org lists drugs that are associated with adverse events in Brugada syndrome. These medications include some commonly used anesthetic drugs, such as propofol and bupivacaine. The syndrome has no proven pharmacologic treatment; indeed, class I antiarrhythmic medications (e.g., flecainide, procainamide) and β-adrenergic blockers can worsen the risk of lethal arrhythmias. ICD implantation is the standard of care for Brugada syndrome.

Cardiovascular Implantable Electronic Devices

Cardiovascular implantable electronic devices (CIEDs), which include both permanent pacemakers and ICDs, are very common. For example, in the United States alone, about 190,000 permanent pacemakers and 145,000 ICDs are implanted every year (see Chapter 38).[201,202] The preoperative evaluation should characterize the device with respect to type, age, manufacturer, model number, current settings, and timing of recent interrogation. Patients frequently carry a manufacturers' identification card with some of this relevant information. Permanent pacemaker capabilities are usually classified using a five-letter code (Table 31.13).[203] The anesthesiologist should also evaluate any coexisting cardiac disease because patients with CIEDs invariably have conditions such as heart failure, IHD, valvular heart disease, or potentially lethal arrhythmias—all of which have perioperative implications. It is especially important to note device features (e.g., rate modulation) that can malfunction with perioperative electromagnetic and other interferences. Sources of electromagnetic interference during the perioperative period include electrocautery (especially monopolar), radiofrequency ablation, lithotripsy devices, and radiation therapy, while direct mechanical interference can occur with guidewire movement during

TABLE 31.13 Pacemaker Nomenclature

Position I	Position II	Position III	Position IV	Position V
Chamber(s) Paced	Chamber(s) Sensed	Response to Sensing	Rate Modulation	Multisite Pacing
O = None	**O** = None	**O** = None	**O** = None	**O** = None
A = Atrium	**A** = Atrium	**I** = Inhibited	**R** = Rate modulation	**A** = Atrium
V = Ventricle	**V** = Ventricle	**T** = Triggered		**V** = Ventricle
D = Dual (A + V)	**D** = Dual (A + V)	**D** = Dual (T + I)		**D** = Dual (A + V)

From Bernstein AD, Daubert JC, Fletcher RD, et al. The revised NASPE/BPEG generic code for antibradycardia, adaptive-rate, and multisite pacing. North American Society of Pacing and Electrophysiology/British Pacing and Electrophysiology Group. *Pacing Clin Electrophysiol.* 2002;25:260–264.

central venous catheter insertion.[204] These sources of interference can result in CIED malfunction, such as inappropriate ICD discharge or inappropriate changes in pacing rates. Especially during delicate surgical procedures (e.g., intracranial, spinal, ocular), an unexpected ICD discharge with movement of the patient can have catastrophic results.

In general, the anesthesiologist conducting a preoperative evaluation of a patient with a CIED should collaboratively plan perioperative management with the relevant CIED care team (Box 31.7).[7,204] The CIED care team has been defined as the physicians and physician extenders who monitor the patient's CIED function. Ideally, patients with CIEDs should have these devices interrogated preoperatively, with recommendations that this be performed within the prior 6 months for an ICD, prior 12 months for a permanent pacemaker, and prior 3 to 6 months for any CRT device. Key issues for consideration when planning the perioperative care of a patient with a CIED include whether the patient has an ICD, whether the patient is pacemaker-dependent, and what happens with magnet placement over the CIED. In general, a magnet suspends antitachyarrhythmia therapy in most ICDs, and switch pacemakers (but not ICDs) to an asynchronous pacing mode. There is some disagreement among guidelines whether to place a magnet over the CIED during the intraoperative period,[204,205] versus arrange for temporary device reprogramming (i.e., switch pacemaker to asynchronous mode, and disable antitachyarrhythmia ICD).[206] Especially given the complexity of newer generation CIEDs, routine magnet use should not be viewed as an alternative for appropriate preoperative preparation. Collaboration with the CIED care team is the preferred approach for managing these patients in an individualized manner. Preoperative recommendations for CIEDs are presented in Box 31.8. In addition, these patients require a preoperative ECG. A chest radiograph is not mandatory before surgery but can reveal the device location and manufacturer's code.

BOX 31.7 **Proposed Principles for Cardiovascular Implantable Electronic Device Management**

The perioperative management of CIEDs must be individualized to the patient, type of CIED, and procedure being performed. A single recommendation for all CIED patients is not appropriate.

The CIED care team is defined as the physicians and physician extenders who monitor the CIED function of the patient.

The surgical or procedural team should communicate with the CIED care team to identify the type of procedure and likely risk of EMI.

The CIED care team should communicate with the procedure team to deliver a prescription for the perioperative management of patients with CIEDs.

For most patients, the prescription can be made from a review of the records of the CIED clinic. A small percentage of patients may require consultation from CIED specialists if the information is not available.

It is inappropriate to have industry-employed allied health professionals independently develop this prescription.

CIED, Cardiovascular implantable electronic devices; *EMI,* electromagnetic interference.

From Crossley GH, Poole JE, Rozner MA, et al. The Heart Rhythm Society (HRS)/American Society of Anesthesiologists (ASA) Expert Consensus Statement on the perioperative management of patients with implantable defibrillators, pacemakers and arrhythmia monitors: facilities and patient management: executive summary. *Heart Rhythm.* 2011;8:e1–e18.

Peripheral Artery Disease

PAD, which is defined as atherosclerosis of the large-sized and medium-sized noncardiac arterial vasculature, affects about 200 million people worldwide.[207] PAD is diagnosed based on an ankle-brachial index (ABI or ratio of ankle-to-arm systolic blood pressure) of less than 0.90.[208] The disease generally affects lower extremity vessels more than upper extremity vessels. PAD progresses variably across individuals, from an initially asymptomatic phase to intermittent claudication (i.e., extremity pain with activity) to critical limb ischemia. Risk factors for PAD include increased age, smoking, hypertension, diabetes mellitus, CKD, and known atherosclerosis in other sites (e.g., IHD). Conversely, patients with PAD likely have atherosclerosis in other sites (e.g., heart, brain). For example, a systematic review in the nonoperative setting found a prevalence of IHD in individuals with PAD ranged from 60% based on cardiac stress testing to 90% based on coronary angiography.[209] Individuals meeting diagnostic criteria for PAD (i.e., ABI < 0.90) have elevated risks for subsequent myocardial infarction, acute stroke, or cardiovascular death in the nonoperative setting.[210] PAD is also a marker of increased risk in surgical patients. An ABI less than 0.90 is independently associated with an increased risk of cardiovascular complications after noncardiac surgery.[211] Known PAD is also associated with elevated risks of mortality after major noncardiac surgery.[77,78] In addition, claudication related to PAD generally

BOX 31.8 Preoperative Recommendations for Cardiovascular Implantable Electronic Devices

- Inactivation of ICDs is not absolutely necessary for all procedures
- Not all pacemakers need to be altered to pace asynchronously in all patients or for all procedures
- Pacemakers can be reprogrammed or magnets can be used to force pacemakers to pace asynchronously to prevent inhibition
- ICDs can be reprogrammed or magnets can be used to inhibit ICD arrhythmia detection and tachyarrhythmia functions
- Magnets can/will *not* force pacemakers in ICDs to pace asynchronously
- Inactivation of ICDs is recommended for all procedures above the umbilicus involving electrocautery or radiofrequency ablation
- It is preferable to change to asynchronous pacing in pacemaker-dependent patients for procedures involving electrocautery or radiofrequency ablation above the umbilicus

The procedure team provides the following information to the CIED team:

- Type of procedure
- Anatomic site of procedure
- Patient position during procedure
- Will electrocautery (and type of cautery) be used?
- Are there other sources of EMI?
- Other issues such as likelihood of damage to leads (e.g., chest procedures), anticipated large blood loss, and surgery in close proximity to CIED

The CIED care team provides the following information to the procedure team:

- Type of device (e.g., pacemaker, ICD)
- Indication for device (e.g., sick sinus syndrome, primary or secondary prevention of lethal arrhythmias)
- Programming (e.g., pacing mode, rate, rate responsive, heart rates for shock delivery)
- Is the patient pacemaker-dependent, and what is the underlying heart rate/rhythm?
- Magnet response
  - Pacing rate
  - Is the device responsive to a magnet?
  - Will ICD functions resume automatically with magnet removal?
  - Does magnet need to be placed off-center?

CIED, Cardiovascular implantable electronic device; *EMI,* electromagnetic interference; *ICD,* implantable cardioverter-defibrillator.

Modified from Crossley GH, Poole JE, Rozner MA, et al. The Heart Rhythm Society (HRS)/American Society of Anesthesiologists (ASA) Expert Consensus Statement on the perioperative management of patients with implantable defibrillators, pacemakers and implantable monitors: facilities and patient management: executive summary. *Heart Rhythm.* 2011;8:e1–e18.

limits functional capacity and thereby masks the symptoms of underlying IHD or heart failure.

The preoperative evaluation of PAD should encompass related symptoms (e.g., intermittent claudication, rest pain), risk factors (e.g., hypertension, diabetes mellitus, smoking, CKD), and associated comorbidities (e.g., IHD, CVD). Arterial blood pressure should be measured in both upper extremities, along with the presence of peripheral arterial pulses. Auscultation for bruits over the abdomen and femoral arteries, as well as palpation for abdominal masses, should be part of the vascular examination. Typical preoperative laboratory testing includes an ECG and blood sampling for a complete blood count, creatinine concentration, and glucose concentration. These individuals may often need further specific workup for IHD with testing such as natriuretic peptides and cardiac stress testing (see section on "Ischemic Heart Disease"). Depending on concomitant risk factors and cardiovascular medications, patients may be on long-term therapy with aspirin, $P2Y_{12}$ inhibitors (e.g., clopidogrel), and DOACs. DOACs should be temporarily discontinued before surgery (see section on "Atrial Fibrillation"). In most cases, $P2Y_{12}$ inhibitor therapy should also be interrupted before surgery, with the possible exception of cases with very recent coronary stent implantation (see section on "Coronary Stents"). As a general strategy for patients undergoing noncardiac surgery, continuing aspirin perioperatively does not prevent cardiovascular complications except in those with drug-eluting coronary stents,[136] but leads to an increased risk of major bleeding (which is a risk factor for perioperative stroke).[132] Nonetheless, selective continuation of aspirin should be considered in patients undergoing vascular surgery (to mitigate risks of bypass graft occlusion), as well as those with high-risk IHD, prior PCI, or recent stroke (i.e., previous 9 months).[212]

PULMONARY DISORDERS

See Chapters 13 and 53.

Asthma

The Global Initiative for Asthma (http://ginasthma.org), describes asthma as a "*heterogeneous disease, usually characterized by chronic airway inflammation. It is defined by the history of respiratory symptoms such as wheeze, shortness of breath, chest tightness, and cough that vary over time and in intensity, together with variable expiratory airflow limitation.*" These episodes of airflow obstruction within the lung are often reversible, either spontaneously or with treatment. The airway obstruction can be precipitated by irritants (e.g., smoke), allergens, infections, medications, or airway instrumentation. Worldwide, it is estimated that asthma afflicts more than 300 million people, and is responsible for one in every 250 deaths.[213] Asthma is classified as intermittent, persistent mild, persistent moderate, and persistent severe, based on symptoms, nighttime awakenings, short-acting bronchodilator requirement, functional impairment, and pulmonary function test (PFT) abnormalities. Although spirometry is the preferred diagnostic test for asthma, a normal result does not exclude asthma. Typical findings on PFTs are a reduction in the ratio of the forced expiratory volume in 1 second (FEV_1) to forced vital capacity (FVC)—with a ratio below 0.7 being indicative of airflow obstruction. Importantly, normal initial PFT results do not necessarily exclude asthma. If results are normal but a diagnosis of asthma is still strongly suspected, a methacholine challenge test or a trial of bronchodilator therapy should be performed. Patients with mild well-controlled asthma have no greater perioperative risk than do individuals without asthma.[214] In addition, PFTs, while helping to establish the diagnosis of asthma, generally have no perioperative prognostic value in these patients.

In a patient with known asthma, the anesthesiologist should inquire about dyspnea, chest tightness, cough (especially nocturnal), recent exacerbations (with associated triggers), therapy (especially corticosteroids), prior hospitalizations, prior emergency department visits, prior critical care unit admissions, prior need for endotracheal intubation, and recent upper respiratory tract infections (see section on "Upper Respiratory Tract Infections"). It is helpful to ask patients to compare their current asthma symptoms to their "normal" or "best" status based on symptoms, exercise tolerance, and medication requirements. The physical examination should assess the quality of breath sounds, quantity of air movement, degree of wheezing, and oxygen saturation by pulse oximetry. The degree of wheezing does not always correlate with the severity of bronchoconstriction. With severe obstruction, airflow is dangerously restricted, and wheezing diminishes. Wheezing is common in asthma but it is not specific for the disease. For example, wheezing may be present in chronic obstructive pulmonary disease (COPD), gastroesophageal reflux disease, vocal cord dysfunction, tracheal stenosis, bronchial stenosis, cystic fibrosis, allergic bronchopulmonary aspergillosis, and heart failure. Observing the degree of accessory muscle use can also help gauge the severity of bronchoconstriction.

Arterial blood gases are not necessary unless the patient is having a severe acute exacerbation. Patients taking oral corticosteroids should have their blood glucose checked. Chest radiography is needed only if an infection or pneumothorax is suspected. Bronchodilators, corticosteroids (inhaled and oral), and any antibiotics must be continued on the day of surgery. β-adrenergic agonists are a useful prophylactic intervention to lower the risk of bronchospasm after induction of anesthesia. This therapy can be supplemented with a short preoperative course of oral corticosteroids (prednisone 20 mg-60 mg daily for 3-5 days) in any newly diagnosed or poorly controlled asthmatic patient.[215] Importantly, some asthmatics on chronic corticosteroid treatment may need perioperative "stress dose steroids" (see section on "Hypothalamic-Pituitary-Adrenal Disorders").

Chronic Obstructive Pulmonary Disease

COPD is a chronic respiratory disease that affects 175 million people worldwide, and causes 3 million deaths every year.[216] It is characterized by persistent airflow obstruction that occasionally is partially reversible (see Chapters 13 and 53). It may be the result of smoking, environmental pollutants (e.g., air pollution), α_1-antitrypsin deficiency, chronic infections, and long-standing asthma. The Global Initiative for Chronic Obstructive Lung Disease describes COPD as a "*common, preventable, and treatable disease that is characterized by persistent respiratory symptoms and airflow limitation that is due to airway and/or alveolar abnormalities usually caused by significant exposure to noxious particles or gases*" (http://www.goldcopd.org). COPD includes subtypes such as "chronic bronchitis" and "emphysema." Chronic bronchitis is defined as a chronic productive cough for 3 months in each of 2 successive years in a patient in whom other causes of chronic cough (e.g., bronchiectasis) have been excluded. Emphysema refers to pathologic structural changes in the lung that can occur with COPD, including enlargement of airspaces distal to the terminal bronchioles, as well as destruction of these airspace walls. The severity of COPD is classified based on both spirometry findings and symptoms. Once a patient has evidence of airway obstruction on spirometry (FEV_1/FVC ratio < 0.7), mild FEV_1 airflow limitation is at or greater than 80% of predicted, *moderate* limitation is FEV_1 between 50% and 79% of predicted, *severe* limitation is FEV_1 between 30% and 49% of predicted, and *very severe* limitation is FEV_1 is less than 30% of predicted. Symptom severity is classified separately using validated scales.[217] A COPD exacerbation is defined as "*an acute worsening of respiratory symptoms that result in additional therapy*" (http://www.goldcopd.org).

The preoperative evaluation of patients with COPD is similar to that of patients with asthma, with an additional emphasis on signs of recent infection (e.g., changes in sputum amount or color). A barrel chest and pursed-lip breathing also suggest advanced disease. COPD is a known risk factor for postoperative pulmonary complications (see section on "Postoperative Pulmonary Complications").[218] Nonetheless, there is no established threshold of COPD severity indicative of highly prohibitive perioperative risk. In general, PFTs are not useful for estimating perioperative risk in patients with COPD, with the exception of individuals undergoing lung resection surgery (see Chapter 53 and section on "Patients Scheduled for Lung Resection"). In general, preoperative PFTs are indicated when there is uncertainty as to whether the patient's lung function is optimized, or uncertainty as to the underlying basis for unexplained dyspnea. Patients who are hypoxic, or require supplemental oxygen, may benefit from further testing, including arterial blood gas measurement, in addition to routine measurement of oxygen saturation using pulse oximetry. A chest radiograph is useful only if infection or bullous disease is suspected. A key goal in the preoperative preparation of a patient with COPD is optimizing pulmonary function before any elective surgery. Accordingly, patients with a recent exacerbation may require more intensive bronchodilator treatment, brief courses of antibiotics or oral corticosteroids, and possible deferment of elective surgery. Smoking cessation should be encouraged for any ongoing smokers (see section on "Smokers and Second-Hand Smoke Exposure"). Additionally, consideration can be given to preoperative inspiratory muscle training and physiotherapy in high-risk patients, and discussion about the potential respiratory benefits of neuraxial anesthesia or analgesia (see section on "Postoperative Pulmonary Complications"). Inhalers and other long-term medications for COPD should be continued on the day of surgery, and individuals on chronic corticosteroid treatment may need "stress dose steroids" (see section on "Hypothalamic-Pituitary-Adrenal Disorders").

Restrictive Pulmonary Disorders

Restrictive lung disease is characterized by a reduced total lung capacity and may be related to both pulmonary or extrapulmonary conditions. Pulmonary causes include idiopathic interstitial pneumonia, prior lung resection, pulmonary fibrosis, and interstitial lung disease secondary to connective tissue disease. Extrapulmonary causes include chest wall limitations (e.g., kyphoscoliosis, obesity, ankylosing spondylitis), muscle dysfunction (e.g., muscular dystrophies, myasthenia gravis, diaphragm paralysis), and pleural disease (e.g., mesothelioma, effusion, pneumothorax). In a patient with suggestive symptoms or history of associated diseases, a chest radiograph and PFTs can help establish the diagnosis. Typically, the FEV_1 and the FVC are reduced proportionally such that the FEV_1/FVC ratio is normal (i.e., > 0.7). Preoperative PFTs can also help assess for acute or progressive worsening of known restrictive lung disease; however, routine testing is not necessary in the absence of clinical suspicion. These patients are also at risk of pulmonary hypertension that may not be recognized because of overlapping symptoms with restrictive lung disease. Thus, echocardiography may also be indicated to investigate causes of worsening symptoms in a patient with known restrictive lung disease.

Patients Scheduled for Lung Resection

Most patients scheduled for lung resection operations have underlying lung disease (this topic is covered in more detail in Chapter 53). Spirometry is useful in estimating risk and excluding patients who are highly likely to lack adequate pulmonary reserve after the planned resection (see Chapter 53). Current American College of Chest Physicians (ACCP) guidelines recommend measurement of both FEV_1 and diffusing capacity for carbon monoxide (D_{LCO}) in all patients being considered for lung resection surgery.[219] The amount of residual lung function after resection can be estimated by using a combination of spirometry and radionuclide quantitative lung scanning. The predicted postoperative FEV_1 (PPO FEV_1) is predicted by multiplying the preoperative FEV_1 by the percentage of perfusion to the nonoperative lung or lung region:

$$\text{PPO FEV}_1 = \text{Preoperative FEV}_1 \times \frac{\text{Perfusion to nonresected lung}}{\text{Total perfusion to lungs}}$$

The PPO D_{LCO} is calculated using an analogous equation for preoperative D_{LCO}. Patients with both PPO FEV_1 and PPO D_{LCO} values exceeding 60% of predicted are considered low-risk and can generally proceed directly to surgery. If either value is within the range of 30% to 60% of predicted, simple objective exercise testing with a shuttle walk test or symptom limited stair climbing test is recommended. For individuals with poor performance on these simple tests (i.e., < 400 m on shuttle walk test or < 22 m on stair climbing test), as well as for individuals with either PPO FEV_1 or PPO D_{LCO} values less than 30% predicted, the ACCP guidelines recommend CPET to measure peak oxygen consumption (VO_2 peak).[219] A preoperative VO_2 peak greater than 20 mL/kg/min is consistent with low perioperative risk, 10 to 20 mL/kg/min is consistent with moderate risk, and less than 10 mL/kg/min is consistent with high risk. Nonsurgical options should be considered in high-risk scenarios, while shared decision making should be incorporated in any intermediate-risk scenarios.

Obstructive Sleep Apnea

In North America, the prevalence of sleep-disordered breathing is 9% among females aged 30 to 60 years of age, and 24% among males in the same age group (see Chapter 10).[220] OSA is the most common type of sleep-disordered breathing, with varying prevalence across age groups, ethnicities, and countries. Recent North American estimates suggest that it afflicts about 9% of females aged 50 to 70 years, and 17% of males in this same age group.[221] OSA is characterized by recurrent upper airway collapse during sleep that leads to reduced or complete cessation of airflow, despite ongoing breathing efforts. Affected individuals develop intermittent hypercapnia, intermittent hypoxemia, and fragmented sleep. Risk factors for OSA include increased age, male sex, obesity, smoking, pregnancy, heart failure, end-stage renal disease, and craniofacial abnormalities. The diagnosis of OSA is based on the presence of symptoms, such as nonrestorative sleep, snoring, hypertension, and the frequency of sleep-related respiratory events during polysomnography or home sleep apnea testing. Once diagnosed, disease severity is typically characterized by the apnea-hypopnea index (AHI), which is the number of apneic and hypopneic episodes per hour of sleep. Mild OSA is defined by 5 to 15 episodes per hour, moderate disease by 16 to 30 episodes per hour, and severe disease by more than 30 episodes per hour. OSA is associated with an increased prevalence of systemic hypertension, pulmonary hypertension, IHD, heart failure, cardiac arrhythmias (i.e., atrial fibrillation, bradyarrhythmias, ventricular ectopy), stroke, type 2 diabetes mellitus, obesity hypoventilation syndrome, and nonalcoholic fatty liver disease. The main effective treatments for OSA in the nonoperative setting are continuous positive airway pressure (CPAP) and weight loss.[222-224]

Most cases of OSA in surgical patients remain undiagnosed at the time of surgery.[225] Screening questionnaires can help, in part, address this problem. For example, the eight-item STOP-Bang questionnaire is a straightforward validated tool to screen for OSA in preoperative evaluation clinics (Fig. 31.8).[226] Surgical patients with scores of 2 or less are at very low risk (negative likelihood ratio 0.24 for AHI ≥ 5), and those with scores of 5 or more are at increased risk (positive likelihood ratio 1.8 for AHI ≥ 5).[226] Since individuals with scores of 3 to 4 are in an indeterminate zone, additional screening criteria have been proposed for this subgroup, including serum bicarbonate concentration level at 28 mmol/L or greater,[227] and differentially weighting responses to the questionnaire.[228] There is some uncertainty as to the operational burden of screening all surgical patients for OSA, especially since the positive likelihood ratio for a higher STOP-Bang score is not particularly high. A reasonable option may be to apply screening in higher-risk populations, such as individuals with obesity, associated comorbidities, and known or suspected difficult intubation characteristics.

Patients with OSA are at increased perioperative risk because of the sleep disorder itself and associated comorbidities. Mask ventilation, direct laryngoscopy, endotracheal intubation, and fiberoptic visualization of the airway are more difficult in patients with OSA (see Chapter 44). In addition, these patients are also more sensitive to the respiratory depressant effects of opioids. In general, patients with OSA have elevated risks of perioperative airway obstruction, hypoxemia, atelectasis, pneumonia, cardiovascular complications, and prolonged hospitalizations.[229] There is uncertainty as to how much of this increased risk is explained by OSA itself, versus associated comorbidities (e.g., IHD, heart failure, diabetes mellitus, obesity). For example, some cohort studies that found that patients with known OSA, or patients screened as being high-risk for OSA, were not at elevated risk of mortality or postoperative hypoxemia, after accounting for coexisting comorbidities.[77,230,231]

STOP-Bang
Screening for Sleep Apnea

Have you been diagnosed with sleep apnea by a sleep study? Yes ☐ No ☐

Have you received treatment for sleep apnea, such as CPAP or Bi-PAP? Yes ☐ No ☐

Please answer the following four questions with a *yes* or *no* answer:

1) Do you snore loudly (louder than talking or loud enough to be heard through closed doors)?
   Yes ☐ No ☐

2) Do you often feel tired, fatigued, or sleepy during daytime?
   Yes ☐ No ☐

3) Has anyone observed you stop breathing during your sleep?
   Yes ☐ No ☐

4) Do you have or are you being treated for high blood pressure?
   Yes ☐ No ☐

FOR STAFF USE ONLY, DO NOT WRITE BELOW THIS LINE

---

5) Is the BMI ≥35 kg/m^2?
   Yes ☐ No ☐

6) Is the patient ≥50 years of age?
   Yes ☐ No ☐

7) Is the neck circumference greater than 15.7 inches (40 cm)?
   Yes ☐ No ☐

8) Is the patient male?
   Yes ☐ No ☐

Total number of questions answered YES: _____ Is the patient at high risk for OSA? Yes ☐ No ☐

High risk of OSA: Yes to >3 items

Fig. 31.8 Stop-Bang questionnaire to screen patients for obstructive sleep apnea. (From Chung F, Yegneswaran B, Liao P, et al. STOP Questionnaire: a tool to screen patients for obstructive sleep apnea. *Anesthesiology*. 2008;108:812–821.)

Preoperative evaluation focuses on characterizing all cases of known OSA, and selectively identifying patients at risk for undiagnosed OSA. In addition, associated comorbidities should be investigated and optimized as deemed clinically appropriate. For example, echocardiography may be indicated if undiagnosed heart failure or pulmonary hypertension is suspected. For patients with known OSA, the anesthesiologist should inquire about known disease severity, document current treatment, and instruct the patient to bring their CPAP equipment or oral appliances on the day of surgery (so that therapy can be restarted promptly after surgery).

Pulmonary Hypertension

Pulmonary hypertension is defined as a persistent mean pulmonary artery pressure of 25 mm Hg or more at rest. The condition may occur in isolation or with associated medical conditions. Based on the World Health Organization, pulmonary hypertension is classified into 5 groups (Box 31.9).[232] Idiopathic and heritable pulmonary arterial hypertension (formerly called primary pulmonary hypertension) are relatively rare. Other more common forms occur with a variety of diseases including cardiac, pulmonary, liver, thromboembolic, and collagen vascular diseases (e.g., scleroderma, systemic lupus erythematosus [SLE]). Pulmonary hypertension is also associated with human immunodeficiency virus (HIV) infection, anorectic drug exposure (e.g., fenfluramine), OSA, and chronic liver disease (especially with portal hypertension).

Patients with pulmonary hypertension have a high rate of perioperative morbidity and mortality.[233-235] Hypoxia, hypercarbia, hypothermia, vasoconstrictor use, and increased sympathetic tone (even from anxiety) during the perioperative period increase pulmonary vascular resistance, with the potential for acute decompensation with right-sided heart failure. Occult pulmonary hypertension is more problematic than the fully recognized disease because symptoms may be attributed to other diseases, and perioperative decompensation may occur unexpectedly. Current American and European guidelines recommend that affected patients be managed collaboratively with a pulmonary hypertension specialist team during the perioperative period, and that they undergo surgery at centers with requisite expertise.[7,9]

It may be challenging to detect pulmonary hypertension *de novo* during preoperative evaluation. The initial symptoms of pulmonary hypertension are usually nonspecific and insidious. Diagnosis is also typically delayed, with about 20% of patients having symptoms for more than 2 years prior to a formal diagnosis.[236] Typical initial symptoms

BOX 31.9 Classification Scheme for Pulmonary Hypertension

Pulmonary Arterial Hypertension

1. Idiopathic pulmonary arterial hypertension
2. Heritable pulmonary arterial hypertension
3. Drug-induced or toxin-induced pulmonary arterial hypertension
4. Associated with other conditions
   (a). Connective tissue disease
   (b). Congenital heart disease
   (c). Portal hypertension
   (d). Human immunodeficiency virus infection
   (e). Schistosomiasis
5. Pulmonary venoocclusive disease and/or pulmonary capillary hemangiomatosis
6. Persistent pulmonary hypertension of newborn

Pulmonary Hypertension Related to Left-heart Disease

1. Left ventricular systolic dysfunction
2. Left ventricular diastolic dysfunction
3. Valvular heart disease
4. Extrinsic compression of central pulmonary veins
5. Congenital or acquired obstruction of the left heart inflow or outflow tract, and congenital cardiomyopathies

Pulmonary Hypertension Related to Lung Disease or Hypoxemia

1. Chronic obstructive pulmonary disease
2. Interstitial lung disease
3. Other pulmonary diseases with mixed restrictive and obstructive pattern
4. Sleep disordered breathing
5. Alveolar hypoventilation disorders
6. Developmental lung disease
7. Chronic exposure to high altitude

Chronic Thromboembolic Pulmonary Hypertension

Pulmonary Hypertension with Unclear Multifactorial Etiology

1. Hematologic disorders (chronic hemolytic anemia, myeloproliferative disorders, splenectomy)
2. Systemic disorders (sarcoidosis, pulmonary histiocytosis, lymphangioleiomyomatosis)
3. Metabolic disorders (glycogen storage disease, Gaucher disease, thyroid disorders)
4. Other conditions (tumor obstruction, fibrosing mediastinitis, chronic kidney disease, segmental pulmonary hypertension

From: Simonneau G, Gatzoulis M, Adiata I, et al. Updated clinical classification of pulmonary hypertension. *J Am Coll Cardiol*. 2013;62: D34–D41.

are exertional dyspnea, lethargy, and fatigue. With disease progression, symptoms related to right ventricular overload develop—these symptoms include exertional chest pain, exertional syncope or presyncope, upper abdominal pain (i.e., liver congestion), and dependent edema. Physical examination may reveal a split S_2 with a loud second component, right ventricular heave, tricuspid regurgitation murmur, ascites, hepatomegaly, jugular venous distention, and peripheral edema. An ECG and echocardiogram are useful in patients with suspected pulmonary hypertension, and those with moderate-to-severe known disease. Typical ECG findings include right axis deviation, RBBB, right ventricular hypertrophy, and tall R waves in leads V_1 and V_2. Right atrial hypertrophy and "P-pulmonale" may be present in severe pulmonary hypertension, with peaked P waves, usually in leads II, III, aVF, and V_1. An echocardiogram is the initial screening test of choice for pulmonary hypertension. It can estimate pulmonary arterial pressures, assess right ventricular function, identify left-sided heart failure, and detect structural heart disease (e.g., valvular heart disease, congenital heart disease). Patients with significant echocardiographic findings may require subsequent right and left cardiac catheterizations, especially given the potential inaccuracy of estimating right-sided pressures by echocardiography alone. Other useful laboratory tests include complete blood count, electrolyte concentrations, creatinine concentrations, and liver function tests (i.e., liver congestion or drug-related side effects).

Patients with pulmonary hypertension may be receiving treatment with diuretics, calcium channel blockers, supplemental oxygen, phosphodiesterase type 5 inhibitors (e.g., sildenafil, tadalafil), endothelin receptor antagonists (e.g., bosentan, ambrisentan), and prostacyclin pathway agonists (e.g., iloprost, epoprostenol). Some drugs are given by continuous intravenous infusions, and even momentary interruption of therapy can be catastrophic. In general, all these medications should be continued perioperatively.[7,9] Some patients may be anticoagulated. The timing of any preoperative anticoagulant discontinuation, and assessment for bridging therapy, should be made collaboratively with a pulmonary hypertension specialist team.

Smokers and Second-Hand Smoke Exposure

Tobacco exposure, either directly or through "second-hand" smoke, increases the risk of many perioperative complications, including respiratory, cardiac, and infectious events. Current smokers have elevated risks for a range of postoperative complications, including mortality, cardiac complications, pulmonary complications, acute stroke, and surgical site infections.[237,238] Overall, about two thirds of smokers want to quit.[239] The U.S. Public Health Service recommends that "*all physicians should strongly advise every patient who smokes to quit because evidence shows that physician advice to quit smoking increases abstinence rates.*"[240] Even brief advice by a physician to quit smoking increases quit rates (relative risk 1.66; 95% CI, 1.42-1.94),[241] albeit from a very low baseline rate of 2% to 3%. Among intensive smoking cessation interventions, both behavioral counselling and medications have demonstrated efficacy, with evidence supporting further improvement in efficacy with combination therapy.[242] The main pharmacologic interventions for smoking cessation are nicotine replacement therapy (i.e., nicotine patches, gum, or lozenges), varenicline, and bupropion. Both bupropion and varenicline should be started at least 1 week before an attempt at quitting. Many hospitals, insurance companies, communities, and governmental agencies offer smoking cessation programs. Excellent advice and guidelines are available online (e.g., https://www.cdc.gov/tobacco/quit_smoking/index.htm and https://smokefree.gov) or via telephone (e.g., 1-800-QUIT-NOW in the United States).

Being scheduled for surgery is a "teachable moment" for promoting smoking cessation, with population-based survey data from the United States showing significant increases in smoking cessation rates after major surgery.[243] Within this context, interventions in the preoperative evaluation clinic result in higher rates of short-term smoking cessation (i.e., within 3-6 months after surgery).[244] Although there is uncertainty about the robustness of smoking cessation rates over the long term,[245] randomized controlled trials have demonstrated reduced nicotine dependence of up to 1 year postoperatively following perioperative smoking cessation interventions.[246,247]

The perioperative benefits of smoking abstinence are realized within the first year after cessation.[248] Nonetheless, there remains uncertainty regarding the minimum required period to accrue benefits. In previous systematic reviews, clinical benefits of preoperative smoking cessation were demonstrated only when it occurred at least 3 to 4 weeks before surgery.[249,250] These benefits include reduced risks for respiratory and wound healing complications. Despite an early study reporting an increased perioperative risk (this association was not statistically significant) in recent quitters,[251] a systematic review found no increased risk of adverse events with quitting smoking soon before surgical procedures (i.e., within 8 weeks).[252] Thus, motivated patients should be encouraged to quit smoking at any point before surgery. Quitting has many theoretical benefits, even within a few days before operation. Soon after a patient quits smoking, carbon monoxide levels decrease, thereby improving oxygen delivery and use. Cyanide levels decrease, which benefits mitochondrial oxidative metabolism. Other beneficial effects include lower nicotine levels (which improves vasodilatation) and clearance of many toxic substances that impair wound healing.

Upper Respiratory Tract Infections

Traditionally, elective surgical procedures were cancelled when patients, especially children, presented with current or recent upper respiratory tract infections. The concern pertains to associated airway hyperreactivity that predisposes patients to laryngospasm, bronchospasm, atelectasis, coughing, airway obstruction, hypoxia, stridor, and breath-holding.[253] Prior evidence suggests that this airway hyperreactivity lasts for 2 to 4 weeks after an upper respiratory tract infection.[253,254] Nonetheless, since most of these associated perioperative respiratory events are mild and easily managed with modern anesthesia care, cancellation is no longer routine. For patients with severe symptoms (e.g., high fever), especially in the presence of other health conditions (e.g., significant asthma, heart disease, immunosuppression), elective surgery should be postponed until 4 weeks after resolution of the infection. Conversely for mild or uncomplicated infections in otherwise healthy patients, it is reasonable to proceed with the planned surgery and avoid the inconvenience of a last-minute cancellation. The dilemma lies with patients between these two extremes, for whom decisions regarding the suitability to proceed should be made on an individualized basis.

Cystic Fibrosis

Cystic fibrosis is an autosomal recessive disease caused by altered chloride and water transport across epithelial cells. This genetic disorder can result in progressive chronic airway disease characterized by airway obstruction, destruction, and frequent pulmonary infections. Affected individuals can also develop exocrine pancreatic insufficiency (i.e., malnutrition, diabetes mellitus, pancreatitis), bowel obstruction, sinusitis, and liver disease (i.e., biliary cirrhosis, portal hypertension). The diagnosis is based on compatible clinical findings in at least one organ system (e.g., chronic airway disease, exocrine pancreatic insufficiency, chronic pansinusitis, cystic fibrosis) in a first-degree relative in combination with either biochemical (sweat chloride ≥ 60 mmol/L on two occasions) or genetic confirmation (presence of known disease-causing genetic mutations).[255]

The preoperative clinical evaluation should especially focus on respiratory, hepatic, and nutritional assessment. With respect to preoperative investigations, electrolyte levels, liver function tests, chest radiographs, and PFTs are useful. Collaborative perioperative management in conjunction with a pulmonologist or a cystic fibrosis specialist is ideal, with an important goal being optimization of pulmonary status (i.e., secretions, infections, bronchospasm) before surgery. Most medications for cystic fibrosis should be continued perioperatively.

Postoperative Pulmonary Complications

Postoperative pulmonary complications encompass several important clinical entities and these have been further defined in a recent systematic literature review and consensus-based process. Abbott and colleagues identified four standard outcome measures that are appropriate for widespread use in clinical trials of postoperative pulmonary complications, namely, pneumonia, atelectasis, acute respiratory distress syndrome, and aspiration.[256] In addition, the investigators proposed a new definition of postoperative pulmonary complications that incorporates the severity of the complication based on the degree of therapy required (e.g., supplemental oxygen, positive pressure ventilation).[256] There is considerable variation in how pulmonary outcome complications are defined and this is reflected in the inconsistent reporting of outcomes across studies and hinders interpretation of research findings. Despite the reporting inconsistencies, a reasonable estimate is that these complications develop in about 5% of patients undergoing nonthoracic surgery.[257,258]

Established risk factors for pulmonary complications pertain to two general domains: patient-level risk factors and procedure-related risk factors (Box 31.10).[218] Patient-level factors include general health status (e.g., ASA physical status [ASA-PS], functional dependency), smoking history, advanced age, COPD, preexisting pulmonary disease (e.g., recent infection, low oxygen saturation) pulmonary hypertension, anemia, heart failure, preexisting sepsis, poor nutritional status (e.g., albumin concentration), and obesity (BMI > 30 kg/m^2).[218,257,259,260] Notably absent from this list of patient-related factors are asthma, arterial blood gas results, or PFT results. The risk of complications is surprisingly low in patients who have well-controlled asthma or preoperative corticosteroid treatment.[214] The risk is higher in asthmatic patients with recent exacerbations, prior postoperative pulmonary complications, recent hospitalizations, or endotracheal intubations for asthma. Arterial blood gases are useful in predicting pulmonary function after lung resection operations, but do not estimate perioperative pulmonary risk. Findings on PFTs, such as the degree of FEV_1, are generally not predictive of pulmonary complications.[218] PFTs have clear roles in diagnosis ("*Is*

BOX 31.10 Selected Risk Factors for Postoperative Pulmonary Complications

Potential Patient-related Risk Factor

Advanced age
ASA-PS Class 2 or more
Congestive heart failure
Functionally dependent
Chronic obstructive pulmonary disease
Weight loss
Impaired sensorium
Cigarette use
Alcohol use
Abnormal findings on chest examination

Potential Procedure-related Risk Factor

Aortic aneurysm repair
Thoracic surgery
Abdominal surgery
Upper abdominal surgery
Neurosurgery
Head-and-neck surgery
Emergency surgery
Vascular surgery
General anesthesia
Perioperative transfusion

Potential Laboratory Test Risk Factor

Albumin concentration < 35 g/L
Chest radiograph abnormalities
BUN concentration > 7.5 mmol/L (> 21 mg/dL)

ASA-PS, American Society of Anesthesiologists Physical Status; *BUN*, blood urea nitrogen.
From Smetana GW, Lawrence VA, Cornell JE, et al. Preoperative pulmonary risk stratification for noncardiothoracic surgery: systematic review for the American College of Physicians. *Ann Intern Med.* 2006;144:581–595.

TABLE 31.14 Scoring Scheme for the ARISCAT* Perioperative Pulmonary Risk Index

Components of ARISCAT Score	Points Assigned
Age	
▪ ≤50 years	0
▪ 51–80 years	3
▪ >80 years	16
Preoperative oxygen saturation	
▪ ≥96%	0
▪ 91%–95%	8
▪ ≤91%	24
Respiratory infection in prior month	17
Preoperative anemia (<100 g/L)	11
Surgical incision location	
▪ Peripheral	0
▪ Upper abdominal	15
▪ Intrathoracic	24
Duration of surgery	
▪ ≤2 h	0
▪ >2–3 h	16
▪ >3 h	23
Emergency procedure	8
ARISCAT Score	**Risk of Pulmonary Complications†**
Low-risk: < 26 points	1.6%
Intermediate risk: 26–44 points	13.3%
High-risk: ≥ 45 points	42.1%

*Estimates risk of composite endpoint of respiratory infection, respiratory failure, pleural effusion, atelectasis, pneumothorax, bronchospasm, or aspiration pneumonitis.
ARISCAT, Assess Respiratory Risk in Surgical Patients in Catalonia group.
†Three patients were excluded because of a missing value in some variable.
From Canet J, Gallart L, Gomar C, et al. Prediction of postoperative pulmonary complications in a population-based surgical cohort. *Anesthesiology.* 2010;113:1338–1350.

dyspnea caused by lung disease or heart failure?") or informing management ("*Can dyspnea or wheezing be improved further?*"), but should not be used as a risk assessment tool or to deny a surgical procedure.[10,218] Procedure-related risk factors for pulmonary complications include the type of procedure (head-and-neck, thoracic, upper abdominal, aortic, neurosurgical), long-duration procedures, emergency procedures, general anesthesia, and residual neuromuscular blockade.[218,257]

Several preoperative clinical risk indices have been developed to estimate pulmonary risk.[34,35,257,259,260] Although these indices have reasonable predictive accuracy, they also have important limitations. Some only predict specific complication types (i.e., pneumonia vs. respiratory failure),[34,35,259,260] and others are too complex for easy clinical use.[34,35] The most straightforward, currently available index is likely the ARISCAT (Assess Respiratory Risk in Surgical Patients in Catalonia) score,[257] which has also been externally validated (Table 31.14).[261] The score classifies patients as low-risk, intermediate-risk, and high-risk strata.[257]

When high-risk patients are identified before surgery, the anesthesiologist has several available options to help decrease their perioperative pulmonary risk. These approaches include encouraging smoking cessation (see section on "Smokers and Second-Hand Smoke Exposure"), treatment of any recent asthma or COPD exacerbation, and treatment of any recent lower respiratory tract infection. These interventions may require medications (e.g., antibiotics, bronchodilators, corticosteroids), specialist referral (e.g., pulmonologists), or delay in the planned surgical procedure. There is accumulating evidence pointing to benefits from preoperative inspiratory muscle training and physiotherapy in high-risk patients undergoing cardiac or abdominal surgery.[262,263] The anesthesiologist can also use the preanesthesia evaluation to educate patients about the potential respiratory benefits of neuraxial anesthesia or analgesia,[19,264,265] and discuss options for less-invasive surgical procedures with the referring surgeon.

ENDOCRINE DISORDERS

Diabetes Mellitus

Diabetes mellitus afflicts about 420 million people worldwide.[266] The two main disease categories are type 1 diabetes (previously called "insulin-dependent diabetes" or "juvenile-onset diabetes") and type 2 diabetes (previously called "non–insulin dependent diabetes" or "adult-onset diabetes").[267] Type 1 diabetes, which accounts for about

5% to 10% of all cases of the disease, is the result of autoimmune destruction of pancreatic β-cells. Affected individuals have an absolute deficiency of insulin, but normal sensitivity to insulin. Since the disease has a typically early onset at a young age, and is often difficult to control, adults with type 1 diabetes are at risk of premature vascular disease, such as IHD, nephropathy, retinopathy, and peripheral neuropathy. They are also at risk of diabetic ketoacidosis. Type 2 diabetes is characterized by insulin resistance and a relative (but not absolute) deficiency in insulin. Most affected individuals are obese and seldom prone to ketoacidosis. Diabetes mellitus is associated with multiorgan dysfunction, including IHD, heart failure (independent of associated IHD), CVD, CKD, peripheral neuropathy, autonomic neuropathy (e.g., postural hypotension, gastroparesis), retinopathy, and reduced joint mobility (e.g., reduced cervical mobility affecting airway management). In the perioperative setting, diabetes mellitus is a risk factor for postoperative complications, including cardiac events,[97] acute kidney injury (AKI),[268,269] and surgical site infections.[270] Insulin therapy is the main treatment for type 1 diabetes mellitus, either as multiple daily injections or a continuous subcutaneous insulin infusion. In the case of type 2 diabetes, multiple treatment options are available, including nonpharmacologic therapy (i.e., diet, weight loss, exercise), metformin, sulfonylureas (e.g., glyburide, glipizide), repaglinide, glucagon-like peptide-1 (GLP-1) agonists (e.g., liraglutide), sodium-glucose cotransporter 2 (SGLT2) inhibitors (e.g., empagliflozin), dipeptidyl peptidase-4 (DPP-4) inhibitors (e.g., sitagliptin, saxagliptin, linagliptin, alogliptin), and insulin.

During the preoperative evaluation of a patient with diabetes mellitus, the anesthesiologist should document the disease type (i.e., type 1 vs. type 2), current usual glycemic control, history of hypoglycemic episodes, current therapy, and the severity of any end-organ complications. Given the effects of diabetes mellitus on other organ systems, the history and physical examination should especially focus on the cardiovascular, renal, and neurologic systems. Inquiries about postural dizziness, early satiety, and postprandial vomiting can help assess for any autonomic neuropathy. The physical examination should include an evaluation of pulses, skin breakdown, and joint (especially cervical spine) mobility. Informative preoperative laboratory tests include an ECG and blood sampling for electrolyte, creatinine, and blood glucose concentrations. To help better estimate renal function, an estimated GFR should be calculated (see section on "Kidney Disease"). Since patients are not typically fasting when they are evaluated in a preoperative evaluation clinic, glucose concentrations measured in the clinic cannot be used to evaluate general glycemic control. A diary of multiple glucose values (preprandial and postprandial) at varying times of the day is more informative for estimating the adequacy of therapy. Alternatively, a glycosylated hemoglobin (HbA_{1c}) concentration can help characterize the average plasma glucose concentration within the prior 3 months. Among surgical patients, preoperative HbA_{1C} is more informative than patients' self-reported history, fasting blood glucose concentrations, and random blood glucose concentrations in identifying preexisting poor glycemic control.[271] In the nonoperative setting, the American Diabetes Association recommends a target HbA_{1c} concentration under 7% for most diabetic patients. Although preoperative HbA_{1c} is correlated with postoperative glycemic control,[272] its role as a predictor of postoperative complications is largely restricted to diabetic patients undergoing orthopedic or vascular surgery.[273] Recently updated guidelines from the National Institute for Health and Care Excellence (NICE) in the United Kingdom[274] recommend offering HbA_{1c} testing to diabetic surgical patients who have not been tested in the prior 3 months, and ensuring the recent HbA_{1c} test results be included in referral materials from patients' primary care providers.

In the perioperative setting, the goals of glycemic management are to avoid hypoglycemia, prevent ketoacidosis, and avoid marked hyperglycemia. Tight perioperative glucose control in the immediate perioperative period is controversial. While aggressive management of hyperglycemia may theoretically help decrease postoperative complications, these theoretical clinical benefits of intraoperative intensive glucose control have not been observed in randomized trials of surgical patients.[275] Ideally, all diabetic patients should have their surgery as an early morning case to minimize any disruption of their diabetic management fasting. Normal treatment regimen for most non-insulin diabetic medications (metformin, sulfonylureas, repaglinide, GLP-1 agonists, DPP-4 inhibitors) should be continued until (and inclusive of) the day before surgery but held on the morning of surgery. The possible exception pertains to SGLT2 inhibitors, which have been associated with euglycemic diabetic ketoacidosis in the postoperative setting.[276] Thus, some guidelines recommend that the medications be discontinued at least 24 hours before elective surgery.[277] Diabetic patients should discontinue *short-acting* insulin while fasting. The exception pertains to patients with continuous subcutaneous insulin infusion pumps. These individuals should continue their infusion at the lowest basal rate, which is usually the nighttime fasting rate. With respect to management of *intermediate-acting* or *long-acting* insulin on the day of surgery, there is no uniform consensus on optimal perioperative protocols. A reasonable approach is for patients with type 1 diabetes mellitus to take a small amount (one third to one half) of their usual morning dose of intermediate-acting or long-acting insulin (e.g., lente, isophane) to avoid diabetic ketoacidosis. Patients with type 2 diabetes mellitus can either take no insulin or up to one half of their usual dose of intermediate-acting, long-acting, or combination (e.g., 70/30 preparations) insulin on the morning of surgery.

Thyroid Disease

Thyroid hormones are important for metabolism and its regulation. Mild to moderate thyroid dysfunction probably has minimal perioperative impact.[278,279] The major concern pertains to significant hyperthyroidism or hypothyroidism, which appears to increase perioperative risk. Symptoms and signs of hypothyroidism and hyperthyroidism can be subtle and nonspecific, especially with milder disease in older adults. Hyperthyroid individuals may manifest tachycardia, arrhythmias, palpitations, tremors, weight loss, and diarrhea. Patients with hypothyroidism may demonstrate hypotension, bradycardia, lethargy, weight gain, depressed cardiac function, pericardial effusions, and impaired ventilatory response to hypoxia or hypercarbia. Patients may also have goiters with related symptoms such as dysphagia, dyspnea, wheezing, and orthopnea. Individuals with hyperthyroidism due to Graves disease may also demonstrate proptosis.

The preoperative evaluation should clarify the patient's current medical therapy as well as any recent changes. In patients with known thyroid disease, additional preoperative thyroid function testing is not needed if the patient is on a stable medication dose and was assessed as being euthyroid within the previous 6 months. If additional preoperative testing is clinically indicated, thyroid-stimulating hormone (TSH) assays are best to evaluate for hypothyroidism, while free triiodothyronine (T_3), free thyroxine (T_4), and TSH levels are useful in hyperthyroid patients. Surgery, stress, or illness can precipitate myxedema or thyroid storm in patients with untreated or severe thyroid dysfunction. In general, if a patient has moderate or worse hypothyroidism (i.e., elevated TSH and low free T_4—with or without associated symptoms), elective surgery should be postponed until the individual is euthyroid. Similarly, elective *non-thyroid* surgery should also be delayed to facilitate treatment of patients with overt hyperthyroidism (i.e., suppressed TSH with elevated free T_4 or T_3 concentrations—with or without associated symptoms). Consultation with an endocrinologist is necessary if surgery is urgent in patients with thyroid dysfunction. If surgery is urgent, hyperthyroid patients can be treated with β-adrenergic blockers, antithyroid medications (e.g., methimazole, propylthiouracil, potassium iodide), and corticosteroids. Other potentially useful tests include chest radiography or computed tomography scans to evaluate tracheal or mediastinal involvement by a goiter. All thyroid replacement therapy and antithyroid drugs should be continued on the day of surgery.

Parathyroid Disease

Parathyroid hormone regulates calcium. Most cases of hyperparathyroidism are discovered based on an incidental elevated calcium level found during diagnostic testing. *Primary* hyperparathyroidism is caused by a primary disorder of the parathyroid glands (adenomas or hyperplasia). *Secondary* hyperparathyroidism is parathyroid gland hyperplasia induced by the hyperphosphatemia and hypocalcemia that occur during chronic renal failure. *Tertiary* hyperparathyroidism occurs when the parathyroid hyperplasia in secondary hyperparathyroidism functions autonomously. Hypercalcemia from parathyroid disease is associated with osteoporosis and bone loss. It is very unlikely that parathyroid glands become sufficiently enlarged to compromise the airway. Hypoparathyroidism is very uncommon, but it can be the consequence of a prior total parathyroidectomy.

Hypothalamic-Pituitary-Adrenal Disorders

The hypothalamus releases corticotropin-releasing hormone, which regulates adrenocorticotropic hormone (ACTH) release from the anterior pituitary gland. ACTH, in turn, regulates cortisol release from the adrenal cortex. Cortisol secretion varies with the circadian rhythm, with the highest release in the morning. Additionally, release increases with physical stress, psychological stress, fever, and hypoglycemia. Among physical stressors, surgery is one of the most potent activators of the hypothalamic-pituitary-adrenal axis. Although ACTH concentrations increase with surgical incision and through the surgical procedure, the greatest ACTH secretion occurs during termination of anesthesia and the immediate postoperative period.[280] The magnitude and duration of the cortisol response reflects the degree of physiological stress imposed by the surgical stress. In procedures with minimal associated stress (e.g., inguinal hernia repair), increased cortisol secretion lasts for about 24 hours.[280] In more complicated procedures (e.g., major abdominal surgery), the response is larger in magnitude and lasts for about 5 days after surgery.[280,281]

Excess adrenal hormones result from endogenous cortisol associated with pituitary or adrenal tumors, or exogenous glucocorticoids used to treat disorders such as asthma or inflammatory diseases. Cushing syndrome refers to the combinations and symptoms due to chronic excess glucocorticoid exposure (either endogenous or exogenous). Cushing disease is the specific situation when the excess glucocorticoids are related to an ACTH-producing pituitary tumor. Other causes of Cushing syndrome include exogenous corticosteroids, adrenal tumors, adrenal hyperplasia, and neoplasms that secrete ectopic ACTH. The major manifestations of Cushing syndrome are obesity (with characteristic patterns of fat deposition causing "moon facies" and a "buffalo hump"), diabetes mellitus, female virilization, OSA, hypertension, elevated cardiovascular risk, elevated venous thromboembolism (VTE) risk, osteoporosis, striae, skin atrophy, and easy bruising. Airway management can be challenging in affected patients due to obesity and OSA. In addition, peripheral intravenous access can be difficult because of skin atrophy and obesity. These patients may require an ECG and blood sampling for electrolytes and glucose. Despite easy bruising, they have normal coagulation profiles.

An important issue for patients with chronic corticosteroid exposure is whether perioperative "stress-dose steroids" are needed. Both endogenous and exogenous glucocorticoids exert important negative feedback suppression on the hypothalamic-pituitary-adrenal axis. Thus, chronic exogenous corticosteroid exposure suppresses the adrenals and may blunt the normal cortisol hypersecretion associated with surgery—even if the patient does not demonstrate Cushing syndrome. Perioperative corticosteroid supplementation is needed only when a patient is likely to have suppression of the hypothalamic-pituitary-adrenal axis. Thus, supplementation is not required for individuals who have received less than 5 mg prednisone (or its equivalent) daily,[282] or less than 3 weeks of corticosteroids (regardless of dose).[282] These individuals should simply continue their usual long-term corticosteroid regimen through the perioperative period. Conversely, patients taking prednisone (or its equivalent) in daily doses exceeding 20 mg/day for more than 3 weeks, and patients with Cushing syndrome should have perioperative corticosteroid supplementation. The need for supplementation is unclear for patients who have taken prednisone (or its equivalent) at a daily dose of 5 to 20 mg for more than 3 weeks. The options are to simply empirically provide perioperative corticosteroid supplementation or refer the patient to an endocrinologist for formal evaluation of their hypothalamic-pituitary-adrenal axis. There is no clear consensus on the optimal perioperative corticosteroid supplementation regimen.[284] A proposed regimen that accounts for contemporary evidence and different stress-response profiles across surgical procedures is presented in Table 31.15.[284]

TABLE 31.15 Recommendations for Perioperative Corticosteroid Coverage

Surgical Stress	Target Hydrocortisone Equivalent	Preoperative Corticosteroid Dose	Perioperative Corticosteroid Dose
Superficial procedure (e.g., biopsy, dental procedure)	8–10 mg/day	Usual daily dose	▪ Then usual daily dose
Minor (e.g., inguinal hernia repair, colonoscopy, hand surgery)	50 mg/day	Usual daily dose	▪ Hydrocortisone 50 mg IV before incision ▪ Hydrocortisone 25 mg IV every 8 h for 24 h ▪ Then usual daily dose
Moderate (e.g., colon resection, total joint replacement, lower extremity revascularization)	75–150 mg/day	Usual daily dose	▪ Hydrocortisone 50 mg IV before incision ▪ Hydrocortisone 25 mg IV every 8 h for 24 h ▪ Then usual daily dose
Major (e.g., esophagectomy, pancreatoduodenectomy, major cardiac, major vascular, trauma)	75–150 mg/day	Usual daily dose	▪ Hydrocortisone 100 mg IV before incision ▪ Continuous IV infusion of 200 mg of hydrocortisone over 24 h ▪ Then usual daily dose OR ▪ Hydrocortisone 50 mg IV every 8 h for 24 h ▪ Taper dose by 50% per day until usual daily dose is reached* ▪ Then usual daily dose

*Administer continuous IV fluids with 5% dextrose and 0.2% to 0.45% sodium chloride (based on degree of hypoglycemia).
IV, Intravenous.
From Liu MM, Reidy AB, Saatee S, et al. Perioperative steroid management: approaches based on current evidence. *Anesthesiology.* 2017;127:166–172.

Patients with adrenal insufficiency have weakness, weight loss, hypotension, orthostasis, hypovolemia, hyperpigmentation, and electrolyte abnormalities. Adrenal insufficiency results from destruction of the pituitary gland, destruction of the adrenal glands (e.g., autoimmune disease, tuberculosis, HIV infection), or long-term exogenous glucocorticoid administration (most common cause). To help establish the diagnosis and cause of adrenal insufficiency, patients require a morning cortisol concentration measurement, morning plasma ACTH concentration measurement, and often an ACTH stimulation test.[285,286] If the serum cortisol concentration is inappropriately low and a simultaneous plasma ACTH concentration is very high, primary adrenal insufficiency (i.e., primary adrenal disease) is the cause. Secondary (i.e., pituitary disease) or tertiary (i.e., hypothalamic disease) is the diagnosis if both serum cortisol and plasma ACTH concentrations are inappropriately low. Consultation with an endocrinologist is required if formal diagnostic testing for adrenal insufficiency is required, and to facilitate treatment of patients meeting the diagnostic criteria. Patients should continue their replacement corticosteroid therapy on the day of surgery and may need further supplementation based on the expected surgical stress response (see Table 31.15).

Importantly, aldosterone, although also produced by the adrenal cortex, is controlled instead by the renin-angiotensin system, not the hypothalamic-pituitary-adrenal axis. Aldosterone regulates volume and electrolytes (absorption of sodium and chloride; secretion of potassium and hydrogen ions).

BOX 31.11 Types of Multiple Endocrine Neoplasia Syndromes

Multiple Endocrine Neoplasia Type 1

1. Primary hyperparathyroidism
2. Entero-pancreatic tumor (e.g., gastrinoma, insulinoma, non-functioning)
3. Anterior pituitary tumor (e.g., prolactinoma)
4. Others
   (a). Foregut carcinoid tumor (e.g., thymus, gastric enterochromaffin-like tumor)
   (b). Adrenal cortical tumor (nonfunctioning)
   (c). Lipomas
   (d). Facial angiofibromas
   (e). Collagenomas

Multiple Endocrine Neoplasia Type 2A

1. MEN2A classical syndrome (i.e., medullary thyroid cancer, pheochromocytoma, primary hyperparathyroidism)
2. MEN2A with cutaneous lichen amyloidosis
3. MEN2A with Hirschsprung disease
4. Familial medullary thyroid cancer (no pheochromocytoma or parathyroid hyperplasia)

Multiple Endocrine Neoplasia Type 2B

1. Medullary thyroid cancer
2. Pheochromocytoma
3. Others
   (a). Mucosal neuromas
   (b). Intestinal ganglioneuromas
   (c). Marfanoid habitus

Multiple Endocrine Neoplasia Syndromes

Multiple endocrine neoplasia (MEN) syndromes are autosomal dominant inherited disorders. There are three types, namely MEN type 1, MEN type 2A, and MEN type 2B (Box 31.11). Although rare (2 in 100,000 for MEN type 1, and 3 in 100,000 for MEN type 2), recognition is important to facilitate treatment of the affected patient and evaluation of family members. MEN type 1 is characterized by the "3 Ps," namely tumors of the parathyroid glands, anterior pituitary, and pancreatic islet cells. Hyperparathyroidism is the most common manifestation of MEN type 1, with 90% penetrance by the age of 40 years. Affected individuals are also predisposed to other tumors, including gastrinomas (usually in the duodenum), carcinoid tumors (thymus or bronchi), enterochromaffin cell-like gastric tumors, adrenocortical adenomas, and lipomas. Individuals with gastrinomas can develop Zollinger-Ellison syndrome, which is characterized by multiple peptic ulcers due to gastrin hypersecretion. While testing for MEN type 1 gene mutations is possible,[287] there is little evidence that early detection improves the disease prognosis.

Within MEN type 2A, there are four subtypes, namely classical MEN type 2A, MEN type 2A with cutaneous lichen amyloidosis, MEN type 2A with Hirschsprung disease, and familial medullary thyroid cancer (see Box 31.11). Hyperparathyroidism in MEN type 2A is often mild or asymptomatic. Since pheochromocytoma (see section on "Pheochromocytoma") is present in about 50% of MEN type 2 cases, this diagnosis must be considered as a possible component of MEN type 2 syndrome. Furthermore, if a pheochromocytoma is present, it should be removed before any other tumor resections. Extraadrenal pheochromocytoma tumors are rare in MEN type 2, but bilateral adrenal disease is common. It is unusual for pheochromocytoma to precede a medullary thyroid carcinoma or be the initial manifestation of MEN type 2. In contrast to MEN type 1, early diagnosis of MEN type 2 through genetic screening is very important. This genetic testing predicts the clinical disease phenotype (e.g., age of onset, aggressiveness), guides surveillance for associated tumors, and informs timing of prophylactic thyroidectomy to prevent medullary thyroid carcinoma.

Pheochromocytoma

Pheochromocytomas are catecholamine-secreting tumors that arise from chromaffin cells of the adrenal medulla. Similar tumors arising from sympathetic ganglia are termed catecholamine-secreting paragangliomas or extraadrenal pheochromocytomas. Nonetheless, the term "pheochromocytoma" is often used to refer to either type of tumor. These rare tumors (incidence ~1 per 100,000 person-years)[288] occur most commonly between ages 40 and 60 years, with equal incidence in males and females. About 40% of cases occur as part of a familial disorder (i.e., von Hippel-Lindau syndrome, MEN type 2, neurofibromatosis type 1). These tumors tend to present at a younger age and are more likely to be bilateral adrenal pheochromocytomas or paragangliomas.

Pheochromocytomas are usually discovered when patients present with consistent symptoms, suggestive family history, or incidental adrenal mass. About half of patients have symptoms, which are typically paroxysmal. The classic triad of associated symptoms are episodic headaches (90% of symptomatic patients), sweating (60%-70% of symptomatic patients), and tachycardia. About half of patients have paroxysmal hypertension, 5% to 15% have normal blood pressure, and the remainder have what appears to be essential hypertension. Other manifestations include orthostatic hypotension, psychiatric disorders (i.e., panic attacks), pallor, blurred vision, weight loss, hyperglycemia, and cardiomyopathy. A diagnosis of pheochromocytoma should be considered if any of the following features is present.[289]

- Triad of episodic headaches, sweating, and tachycardia
- Hyperadrenergic spells (e.g., nonexertional palpitations, diaphoresis, headache, tremor)
- Hypertension that is difficult to control, or occurs at a young age
- Hypertension associated with new-onset or atypical diabetes mellitus
- Idiopathic dilated cardiomyopathy
- Family history of pheochromocytoma or suspicious familial syndrome (von Hippel-Lindau syndrome, MEN type 2, neurofibromatosis type 1)
- A history of gastric stromal tumors or pulmonary chondromas
- Incidentally discovered adrenal mass

Measurements of fractionated metanephrine and catecholamine concentrations in the urine and plasma generally establish the diagnosis of pheochromocytoma, with recent guidelines focusing on initial testing with either plasma-free metanephrines or urinary fractionated metanephrines.[290] Nonetheless, since testing algorithms vary considerably across hospitals and regions, a referral to an appropriate specialist (e.g., endocrinologist) should be made to facilitate a formal diagnosis in an individual with suspicious findings.

Patients scheduled for pheochromocytoma resection should undergo surgery at centers with experienced teams of anesthesiologists and surgeons. They also require about 10 to 14 days of medical preparation before surgery to mitigate perioperative risks. The overarching goals of this preparation are to control hypertension, control tachycardia, and normalization of intravascular volume status. The mainstay of medical therapy is preoperative α-adrenergic blockade started 7 to 14 days before surgery.[290] The preferred drug at many centers is phenoxybenzamine, which is an irreversible, long-acting, nonspecific α-adrenergic blocking drug. The initial dose is 10 mg once or twice daily, and the dose is increased by 10 to 20 mg every 2 to 3 days as needed. Most patients eventually need doses ranging from 20 to 100 mg daily. The arterial blood pressure target is less than 130/80 mm Hg in the seated position, with systolic pressure less than 90 mm Hg while standing. Typical side effects include orthostatic dizziness, fatigue, and nasal congestion. Given these side effects, as well as higher rates of postoperative hypotension after preoperative phenoxybenzamine treatment, some centers instead use selective α_1-adrenergic blocking drugs (e.g., prazosin, terazosin, doxazosin).[291] These agents are also preferable when long-term pharmacologic treatment is indicated (e.g., metastatic pheochromocytoma). The disadvantage of selective α_1-adrenergic blocking drugs is their incomplete degree of α-adrenergic blockade, thus resulting in more episodes of intraoperative hypertension.[291]

After adequate α-adrenergic blockade, β-adrenergic blockade may be started cautiously with short-acting drugs. As an example, 10 mg of propranolol every 6 hours can be used. After 24 to 48 hours, a long-acting preparation (e.g., metoprolol, atenolol) can be substituted, provided that the patient tolerates β-adrenergic blockade. The dose is then adjusted to achieve a heart rate between 60 and 80 beats/min. β-Adrenergic blockade should *never* be initiated before α-adrenergic blockade.[290] In the setting of unopposed α-adrenergic receptor stimulation, blockade of vasodilatory peripheral β-adrenergic receptors worsen hypertension, while acute depression of cardiac function can precipitate acute heart failure. In addition, initiation of β-adrenergic blockade may unmask a catecholamine-induced cardiomyopathy, with resulting acute pulmonary edema.

Alternatives to perioperative α-adrenergic blockade include calcium channel blockers and metyrosine.[290]

Nicardipine is the most commonly used calcium channel blocker for this indication, with a starting oral dose of 30 mg twice daily (sustained release preparation). The main role for calcium channel blockers is likely to supplement α- and β-adrenergic blockade when blood pressure control is inadequate, or to treat patients with intolerable side effects from usual therapy. Monotherapy with calcium channel blockers is not recommended.[290] Metyrosine, which inhibits catecholamine synthesis, has many side effects (e.g., sedation, diarrhea). As a consequence, it is also reserved for cases where conventional treatment is insufficient or not tolerated.

The preoperative evaluation of a patient with known pheochromocytoma should focus on the cardiovascular system (including orthostatic vital signs) and current medical treatment for pheochromocytoma (including adequacy of treatment). Laboratory testing includes an ECG, as well as blood sampling for a CBC, electrolyte concentrations, creatinine concentrations, and glucose concentrations. The patient may also warrant echocardiography or a cardiology consultation.

KIDNEY DISEASE

During preoperative evaluation, it is important to establish the severity, type, and underlying cause of preoperative renal impairment. Based on the Kidney Disease Improving Global Outcomes (KDIGO) guideline group, CKD is defined as a GFR less than 60 mL/min/1.73 m^2 for at least 3 months, regardless of the underlying cause.[292] Chronic kidney failure is defined as a GFR less than 15 mL/min/1.73 m^2 or the need for renal replacement therapy (i.e., dialysis). End-stage renal disease generally refers to chronic kidney failure that requires either dialysis or transplantation. GFR decreases with age; the renal reserve of a normal 80-year-old person is less than half that of a 40-year-old person. Thus, creatinine concentration is often not an accurate indicator of renal function, especially in older individuals.[293] The GFR can be reduced by 50% without a rise in creatinine concentration, while creatinine concentration does not exceed normal limits until GFR has fallen to less than 50 mL/min. Consequently, it is preferable to estimate renal function using an estimated GFR (eGFR) equation, such as the Cockcroft-Gault,[294] Modification of Diet in Renal Disease,[295] and current CKD-EPI equations.[296] Online calculators to estimate renal function are available (e.g., www.kidney.org/professionals/kdoqi/gfr_calculator). Calculating an eGFR is especially important in patients who are older, have elevated creatinine concentrations, or have other risk factors for CKD.[293] Given the inaccuracy of these equations at lower creatinine concentrations, values of eGFR that are greater than 60 mL/kg/min/1.73 m^2 should simply be reported as ">60 mL/kg/min/1.73 m^2." In the United States, the leading causes of end-stage renal disease are diabetes mellitus and hypertension.

AKI is a sudden decrease in renal function with the possible decrease in urine output. Episodes of AKI can occur in individuals with or without CKD. Several consensus-based criteria for classifying AKI have been developed, including the RIFLE classification scheme,[297] the Acute Kidney Injury Network classification scheme,[298] and the current KDIGO criteria.[299] AKI may be reversible if precipitating factors are identified and corrected. Classifying AKI into prerenal, renal, and postrenal causes allows for a systematic approach. Prerenal causes can often be differentiated by calculating the blood urea nitrogen-to-creatinine ratio. A ratio more than 20 suggests prerenal etiologies, with hypovolemia or hypotension the most common. A fractional excretion of sodium (FENa) less than 1% also suggests prerenal disease (in the absence of concomitant diuretic administration) and can be calculated using the following formula:

$$\text{FENa} = \frac{P_{Cr}/U_{Cr}}{P_{Na}/U_{Na}}$$

Obstruction, which results in dilated ureters and enlarged kidneys, should always be considered in the differential diagnosis of AKI. Prompt identification with ultrasound should lead to attempts to decompress the outflow tract.

Patients with CKD have many associated comorbidities, both related to the underlying diseases that led to CKD and its resulting end-organ complications. Cardiovascular issues include hypertension, IHD, ventricular dysfunction (diastolic and systolic), heart failure, CVD, PAD, pericarditis, pericardial effusions, and valvular heart disease (valvular calcification with resulting regurgitation or stenosis). Pulmonary hypertension and increased cardiac output occur in patients with arteriovenous fistulas. CKD is also associated with chronic anemia due to reduced erythropoietin production by the kidneys. While treatable with erythropoiesis stimulating agents, complete "normalization" of hemoglobin concentration (i.e., 135 g/L vs. 113 g/L) may actually increase morbidity and vascular events.[300] Hence, current KDIGO guidelines recommend using erythropoiesis stimulating agents to treat hemoglobin concentrations less than 90 g/L, but avoid increasing the concentration to above 130 g/L.[301] Other hematological abnormalities include platelet dysfunction and increased bleeding, despite normal platelet counts, prothrombin times, and activated partial thromboplastin time (aPTT). Once dialysis is begun, patients become more prone to hypercoagulable states. Patients with CKD can develop autonomic and peripheral (sensory and motor) neuropathies. Unsurprising, CKD is associated with many electrolyte disturbances. Chronic metabolic acidosis is common, but it is usually mild and compensated for by chronic hyperventilation. Hyperkalemia is the most serious electrolyte disturbance. Hypocalcemia is common in patients undergoing dialysis, although with long-term disease, secondary and tertiary hyperparathyroidism eventually develops. Chronically elevated troponin concentrations are common in end-stage renal disease, which does influence interpretation of any postoperative troponin elevations.[302] Since insulin is metabolized by the kidneys, worsening renal function should be suspected in diabetic patients with end-stage renal disease who develop improved glycemic control or unexpected hypoglycemia.

Preexisting CKD is a risk factor for increased postoperative complications, including cardiac complications,[97] AKI,[303,304] acute stroke,[305] and death.[99] Risk factors for *postoperative* AKI have also been identified. In cardiac surgery, several simple preoperative risk indices have been developed to predict postoperative AKI requiring dialysis.[268,269] Important risk factors in these indices include complex surgery, nonelective surgery, CKD, diabetes mellitus, heart failure, female sex, and COPD. In noncardiac surgery, identified risk factors for AKI include increased age, male sex, symptomatic heart failure, hypertension, liver disease (including ascites), CKD, PAD, COPD, nonelective surgery, and intraperitoneal surgery.[303,304] Preoperative identification of at-risk patients can facilitate care, such as preoperative hydration and avoidance of hypovolemia. Nonsteroidal antiinflammatory drugs (NSAIDs) and cyclooxygenase-2 (COX-2) inhibitors interfere with renal perfusion autoregulation and should be avoided or discontinued in patients with CKD. In contrast, these drugs do not increase the risk of postoperative AKI in patients with normal renal function.[306] Many drugs are also metabolized or cleared by the kidneys. Drugs with particular perioperative implications are the LMWHs since there is no easy method to monitor their anticoagulation effects. LMWHs are cleared by the kidneys and are not removed during dialysis; thus, they have a prolonged duration of action in patients with CKD. Similarly, dosing of DOACs have to be adjusted in CKD (see Table 31.11).

The preoperative evaluation of patients with CKD should emphasize the cardiovascular system, cerebrovascular system, intravascular volume status, and electrolyte status. The early stages of CKD typically cause no symptoms. The anesthesiologist should inquire about the cardiovascular systems (i.e., chest pain, orthopnea, paroxysmal nocturnal dyspnea), urine output, associated comorbidities, medications, dialysis schedules, and any hemodialysis catheter problems (e.g., infection, thrombosis). Information on the patient's target and current weight may be helpful for assessing volume status. Patients with CKD need an ECG and blood sampling to measure electrolyte, calcium, glucose, albumin, and creatinine concentrations. Further evaluation is needed if the ECG shows LVH (hypertension), peaked T waves (hyperkalemia), flattened T waves, a prolonged PR interval, or a prolonged QT interval (hypokalemia). A chest radiograph (infection, volume overload), echocardiogram (murmurs, heart failure), and cardiology evaluation may be necessary in some cases. Venous access sites or blood draws from the brachial, cephalic (antecubital), and central veins in the nondominant upper extremity should be avoided in patients who may eventually need fistulas in those locations for dialysis.

Preoperative renal replacement therapy (dialysis) schedules should be coordinated with the timing of the planned surgery. Dialysis is important for correct volume overload, hyperkalemia, and acidosis before planned surgery. Ideally, elective surgery should be performed about 24 hours after dialysis. Performance of surgery shortly after dialysis should be avoided, because of the risks of acute volume depletion and electrolyte alterations. Specifically, dialysis leads to fluid shifts and electrolyte (i.e., sodium, potassium, magnesium, phosphate) imbalance, especially related to shifting of electrolytes between intracellular and extracellular compartments.

Contrast-Induced Nephropathy

Contrast-induced nephropathy is defined as AKI that occurs after radiocontrast administration. Typically, the creatinine concentration increases within 24 to 48 hours after contrast exposure, after which it typically declines to baseline levels within 3 to 7 days. Recent (<24 hours) preoperative contrast exposure is also a risk factor for AKI following cardiac surgery.[307] Even when renal function returns to normal, patients with contrast-induced nephropathy experience elevated risks of short-term and long-term mortality.[308] Risk factors for contrast-induced nephropathy are CKD (especially diabetic nephropathy), heart failure, hypovolemia, and certain contrast exposure characteristics (i.e., high volume, ionic agents, hyperosmolal agents). Preventative strategies include avoiding volume depletion, discontinuing NSAIDs for 24 to 48 hours, using a low-risk contrast administration protocol (i.e., low volume of a low-osmolal or iso-osmolal agent), and periprocedure intravenous volume administration with normal saline. Despite initial promising results for N-acetylcysteine and sodium bicarbonate in relatively small randomized trials, a large trial with more than 5000 high-risk participants found that neither approach prevented contrast-induced nephropathy.[309]

HEPATIC DISORDERS

Liver disease can affect the hepatocytes and/or biliary system, thereby impacting protein synthesis (e.g., coagulation factors, albumin), bile regulation, and metabolism of drugs or toxins. Hepatocellular diseases, such as hepatitis (viral, alcoholic, autoimmune hepatitis) and hepatocellular carcinoma, affect hepatocytes and liver synthetic function. Obstructive disorders, including choledocholithiasis, bile duct tumors (extrahepatic), primary biliary cirrhosis (intrahepatic), and primary sclerosing cholangitis (extrahepatic and intrahepatic), cause bile stasis. Most drug-induced liver disease, as well as some forms of viral hepatitis, affect both hepatocytes and the biliary system.

The preoperative history typically reveals the underlying disease etiology, disease severity, therapies, and associated complications. Some patients with liver disease may be asymptomatic, whereas others may complain of fatigue, weight loss, dark urine, pale stools, pruritus, right upper quadrant pain, bloating, and jaundice. The physical examination should assess for weight, vital signs (including oxygen saturation), jaundice, bruising, ascites, pleural effusions, peripheral edema, hepatomegaly, splenomegaly, and altered mental status. The presence of encephalopathy, coagulopathy, ascites, volume overload, and infection should be determined before surgery. The bilirubin concentration generally must exceed 25 g/L before icterus is evident in mucous membranes and sclerae. If new-onset or worsening encephalopathy is identified, precipitating factors should be sought, such as infection, drug effects, bleeding, or electrolyte disturbances.

Baseline testing includes an ECG and blood sampling for CBC, electrolyte concentration, creatinine concentration, liver function tests, albumin concentration, and INR. Patients suspected of having hepatitis may require screening for the hepatitis A immunoglobulin M (IgM) antibody, the hepatitis B surface and core antigens, the hepatitis B surface antibody, and the hepatitis C antibody. A chest radiograph can help identify any suspected effusions. Coagulopathy can be a result of vitamin K deficiency (from cholestasis), factor deficiency (from loss of synthetic function), or thrombocytopenia (from splenomegaly and portal hypertension). Thus, therapy to correct coagulopathy should be directed at the cause. Vitamin K, fresh frozen plasma, or platelets may correct deficiencies. Vitamin K, taken at 1 to 5 mg orally or subcutaneously daily for 1 to 3 days, may correct a prolonged PT and carries minimal risk. The coagulopathy in patients with synthetic failure is not likely to correct, thus necessitating fresh frozen plasma transfusion aiming for an INR less than 1.5. Limited evidence suggests that lactulose (30 mL orally every 6 hours for 3 days preoperatively) with the last dose within 12 hours of surgery, or oral bile salts with intravenous hydration beginning the night before the operation, may reduce perioperative AKI in patients at risk.[310] Reduction of ascites preoperatively may decrease the risk of wound dehiscence and improve pulmonary function. Sodium restriction (in diet and intravenous solutions), diuretics (especially spironolactone), and paracentesis are useful for reducing ascites. If ascites fluid is aspirated, it should also be analyzed for infection. Encephalopathy is frequently precipitated by an additional acute insult such as infection, gastrointestinal bleeding, hypovolemia, or sedatives. It is therefore important to determine reversible factors and treat them accordingly. Lactulose (30 mL every 6 hours orally) is first-line therapy. Addressing nutritional deficiencies with enteral or parenteral supplementation may have benefits, especially in alcoholic patients. Patients who abuse alcohol may be at risk for neurologic deterioration (i.e., Wernicke-Korsakoff syndrome) if thiamine, folate, and vitamin B_{12} supplements are not provided, especially when these patients are given nutrition or glucose. These same patients are also at risk of alcohol withdrawal syndromes.

The perioperative risk of patients with chronic hepatitis or cirrhosis is predicted by histologic severity, portal hypertension, and impairment of liver function. Patients with severe liver disease have increased perioperative morbidity and mortality; common adverse events are bleeding, infection, liver failure, and hepatorenal syndrome. Predictors of poor perioperative outcome in patients with liver disease include the following:

- Child-Turcotte-Pugh class C cirrhosis, which is calculated using bilirubin concentration, albumin concentration, PT, ascites severity, and encephalopathy severity (Table 31.16)
- Model for end-stage liver disease (MELD)[311] score of 15 or more (the MELD score is calculated using serum bilirubin concentration, INR, and serum creatinine concentrations)
- Acute hepatitis (viral or alcoholic)
- Chronic active hepatitis with jaundice, encephalopathy, coagulopathy, or elevated liver enzymes
- Abdominal surgical procedures
- PT prolongation of 3 seconds or more that is refractive to vitamin K therapy

TABLE 31.16 Child-Turcotte-Pugh Classification

Parameter	1 point	2 points	3 points
Ascites	Absent	Slight	Moderate
Bilirubin (mg/dL)	<2	2–3	>3
Albumin (g/dL)	>3.5	2.8–2.5	<2.8
Prothrombin time (seconds over control)	<4	4–6	>6
Encephalopathy	None	Grade 1–2	Grade 3–4

Class A: <7 points.
Class B: 7-9 points.
Class C: >9 points.

The MELD score can be calculated as shown below (where creatinine and bilirubin concentrations are expressed in mg/dL):

$$\text{MELD} = 6.43 + [3.78 \times \log_e(\text{bilirubin})] + [11.2 \times \log_e(\text{INR})] + [9.57 \times \log_e(\text{creatinine})]$$

Online calculators are also available to calculate MELD scores readily (e.g., www.unos.org). In some cases, it may be appropriate to delay elective surgery until an acute episode of hepatitis (or exacerbation of chronic disease) has resolved, or until a diagnosis is established for newly discovered hepatic dysfunction. Elective surgery is contraindicated in patients with acute or fulminant liver disease. High-risk patients are best managed collaboratively with a liver specialist.

Hepatitis

Hepatitis, which is defined as hepatocyte inflammation, can be caused by drugs, alcohol, viruses (hepatitis A, B, C, D, and E), and autoimmune diseases (see also Chapter 16). These disorders generally have an initial acute phase, as well as a subsequent chronic phase that can progress to cirrhosis. Risk factors for hepatitis are alcohol use, sexual activity (i.e., multiple partners, sex industry workers, sex with sex industry workers, men who have sex with men), intravenous drug use, blood transfusions before 1992, obesity (i.e., nonalcoholic steatohepatitis [NASH]), tattoos, body piercing, and travel to developing countries. Hepatitis A is caused by contaminated food, contaminated water, or contact with an infected person. Since it rarely progresses beyond the acute illness, a remote history of hepatitis A has no perioperative significance. Hepatitis B is transmitted by sexual activity or contact with blood (rarely after implementation of screening in 1986). It varies in severity and can advance to cirrhosis; this has become much less common due to widespread hepatitis B vaccination. Additionally, antiviral therapy can treat the infection, albeit with variable efficacy. Hepatitis C is transmitted primarily through blood exposure (all blood has been screened since 1992), especially among intravenous drug users. Many patients are unaware of infection because the acute phase is often asymptomatic. While hepatitis C infection can advance to cirrhosis, currently available antiviral therapy can now eliminate infection in almost all patients. Hepatitis D occurs only in conjunction with hepatitis B infection, whereas hepatitis E is less common in high-income countries. Hepatitis D can progress to cirrhosis, while hepatitis E rarely progresses beyond the acute illness. Alcoholic hepatitis generally occurs after at least 20 years of moderate to heavy daily alcohol intake (>100 g/day) and may progress to cirrhosis. Autoimmune hepatitis primarily affects young females and has an as yet unknown etiology. Many different drugs (including herbal and over-the-counter preparations) can also cause hepatitis, with examples being statins, isoniazid, and acetaminophen.

Obstructive Jaundice

Extrahepatic bile duct obstruction may be caused by gallstones, tumors (e.g., pancreatic, gallbladder, bile duct, ampulla of Vater), or scarring. Patients can present with jaundice, pruritus, and abdominal pain. Risk factors for postoperative mortality in these patients include a hemoglobin concentration less than 100 g/L, serum bilirubin exceeding 20 mg/dL, and serum albumin lower than 25 g/L.[312] These patients are at elevated risk for postoperative AKI, which may be prevented using bile salts or lactulose.[310]

Miscellaneous Liver Diseases

Wilson disease, hemochromatosis, and α_1-antitrypsin deficiency are uncommon hereditary causes of liver disease. All three conditions can eventually lead to end-stage liver disease. In contrast, another hereditary liver disease, Gilbert disease, is characterized by a mildly elevated bilirubin level and no perioperative significance. NASH, also known as "fatty liver," progresses to liver fibrosis, cirrhosis, and end-stage liver disease (sometimes necessitating liver transplantation). The condition is associated with obesity, hypertension, dyslipidemia, and diabetes mellitus. Following a more than doubling in disease prevalence over the past two decades in the United States,[313] NASH is now the most common cause of chronic liver disease and the second most common indication for liver transplantation.[314,315] Primary biliary cirrhosis (or primary biliary cholangitis) is an autoimmune disorder characterized by intrahepatic biliary obstruction and antimitochondrial antibodies. Affected patients are predominantly female (>90%), may have other autoimmune disorders (e.g., Sjögren syndrome, autoimmune thyroid disease, limited cutaneous scleroderma, rheumatoid arthritis), and can progress to end-stage liver disease. Primary sclerosing cholangitis is characterized by bile duct destruction that can progress to cirrhosis and end-stage liver disease. The disease mainly affects males and may be idiopathic or associated with inflammatory bowel disease (i.e., ulcerative colitis, Crohn disease).

Unexpected Elevated Liver Function Tests

Elevated alanine aminotransferase (ALT) and aspartate aminotransferase (AST) concentration reflect hepatocyte damage. Bilirubin concentration measures the liver's ability to conjugate and excrete bile salts. Alkaline phosphatase (ALP) rises with impaired hepatic excretion, whereas albumin and INR measure the synthetic function of the liver. Routine preoperative laboratory screening may identify about 1 in 700 surgical patients as having unexpected liver diseases, most of which are not severe.[316] Nonetheless, if abnormal liver function test values are unexpectedly found, further testing or referral may be necessary in some cases. Elevated AST or ALT concentrations should prompt hepatitis screening with hepatitis A IgM antibody, hepatitis B antigens (surface and core), hepatitis B surface antibody, and hepatitis C antibody. Elevated concentrations of ALP or bilirubin, especially in association with normal or mild to moderate increased transaminase levels, may indicate obstruction in the biliary system. In these cases, abdominal ultrasound, computed tomography scans, or endoscopic retrograde cholangiopancreatography may establish a diagnosis.

Cirrhosis

Cirrhosis is defined as irreversible liver fibrosis and is the end result of most hepatotoxic conditions. This fibrosis leads to portal hypertension, impaired synthetic function (i.e., synthesis of proteins such as clotting factors), and impaired metabolic functions (i.e., clearance of toxins and drugs). Portal hypertension can lead to splenomegaly, esophageal varices, ascites, dependent edema, and pleural effusions. Patients with ascites may also develop spontaneous bacterial peritonitis, which is associated with increased perioperative mortality. Other complications include hepatic encephalopathy, bleeding, thrombocytopenia, low albumin concentrations, and prolonged INR. Hepatopulmonary syndrome may develop, resulting in hypoxemia and pulmonary hypertension because of pulmonary shunts. Jaundiced patients in particular are at risk for developing hepatorenal syndrome, which is renal insufficiency associated with hepatic disease but without any primary renal disease. The condition may be related to renal hypoperfusion. Patients with end-stage liver disease also develop a high–cardiac output state, characterized by decreased systemic vascular resistance. The Child-Turcotte-Pugh classification can predict perioperative morbidity and mortality, with especially high risks in patients assigned to class C (see Table 31.16). The MELD score also predicts perioperative risks, perhaps better than the Child-Turcotte-Pugh classification,[317] with scores exceeding 14 indicative of increased perioperative risk.

HEMATOLOGIC DISORDERS

Anemia

Anemia is a very common preoperative hematologic disorder with multifactorial etiology. It is strictly defined as a reduced number of circulating red blood cells (RBCs), however, more commonly it is defined based on the value of reduced hemoglobin concentration or reduced hematocrit. For example, the World Health Organization defines anemia as a hemoglobin level less than 130 g/L in adult men and less than 120 g/L in adult women. Anemia can be classified based on the underlying mechanisms as being related to decreased RBC production (e.g., bone marrow disorders, nutritional deficiencies), increased RBC destruction (e.g., hemolytic anemia, intravascular hemolysis), and blood loss (e.g., gastrointestinal blood loss). Anemia may also be classified morphologically based on the associated RBC size, which is itself characterized by the mean corpuscular volume (MCV). Based on this approach, anemia can be classified as microcytic (MCV < 80 femtoliter [fL]), macrocytic (MCV > 100 fL), or normocytic (MCV between 80 and 100 fL). Common causes of microcytic anemia are iron deficiency (including chronic blood loss), thalassemia minor, and anemia associated with inflammatory disease. Common causes of macrocytic anemia include alcoholism, liver disease, hypothyroidism, and vitamin B_{12} deficiency. Common causes of normocytic anemia are CKD, heart failure, and cancer.

Preexisting anemia is a consistently recognized risk factor for postoperative death and complications, including AKI, stroke, and infections.[318] Furthermore, this risk is proportional to the degree of anemia and independent of the patient's other comorbidities.[101,102,319] Nonetheless, there are some important caveats for consideration. First, it remains unclear whether anemia is the causal mechanism for these complications, or instead simply a marker of a high-risk patient. The limited available perioperative data generally suggest that anemia treatment strategies (e.g., erythropoiesis-stimulating agents) can improve hemoglobin concentrations and reduce transfusion requirements, but without convincing evidence for the prevention of death or complications.[320-322] These perioperative data are also generally consistent with findings in nonsurgical populations, such as patients with heart failure.[323-327] Second, there is no consistent hemoglobin concentration threshold that defines elevated perioperative risk. While data from noncardiac surgery performed in Jehovah's Witness patients suggest that risk increases substantially once preoperative hemoglobin concentrations fall below 100 g/L (especially in the presence of concomitant IHD),[328] simply increasing hemoglobin concentrations to this threshold with RBC transfusion is not consistently beneficial. Importantly, transfusion itself has also been associated with poor outcomes in observational studies.[329] In a multicenter randomized trial of 2016 patients undergoing hip fracture surgery, a strategy of transfusing in response to a 100 g/L threshold in hemoglobin concentration was not superior to a strategy of transfusing in response to a 80 g/L threshold or symptoms of anemia.[330] Similarly, in a multicenter randomized trial of 5243 patients undergoing cardiac surgery, a strategy of transfusing in response to a 75 g/L threshold was noninferior to a strategy of transfusing in response to a 95 g/L threshold.[331] These data suggest that the optimal perioperative hemoglobin concentration threshold varies between 75 g/L and 100 g/L across individuals, with interindividual differences largely explained by comorbid conditions (e.g., cardiopulmonary disease).

During the preoperative evaluation of known or suspected anemia, the overarching goals are to determine its etiology, duration, stability, related symptoms, and therapy. Thus, it is important to inquire about any history of anemia (including family history of anemia), colon cancer, gastrointestinal bleeding, genitourinary bleeding, menorrhagia, chronic infections, inflammatory diseases, nutritional deficiencies, and prior weight reduction procedures (e.g., bariatric surgery). The anesthesiologist should also consider the type of surgical procedure, anticipated blood loss, and comorbid conditions that may either affect oxygen delivery or be affected by decreased oxygen delivery (i.e., pulmonary, renal, hepatic, cerebrovascular, cardiovascular disease). In addition, an accurate determination of the patient's medications is helpful, especially because anemia has implications for the risk-to-benefit profile of some perioperative medications, such as β-adrenergic blockers.[103,104]

Patients with anemia or suspected anemia must have a CBC. In general, collaboration with a primary care physician or hematologist is helpful for further evaluation of newly diagnosed anemia. Usual initial studies include peripheral smear and MCV; subsequent studies, such as iron studies (i.e., ferritin, transferrin saturation), vitamin B_{12}, or folate levels, are guided by findings on the smear and the MCV.[332] The MCV is high and the vitamin B_{12} or folate levels are low in macrocytic anemia associated with these deficiencies. Low values in MCV, ferritin (<30 g/μL), and transferrin saturation (<20%) are indicative of iron deficiency anemia. In some cases of iron deficiency anemia, transferrin saturation may still be low (<20%) but ferritin concentrations are in an indeterminate zone (i.e., 30-100 g/μL). Conversely, ferritin and transferrin saturation are normal or high in anemia associated with chronic disease.

Blood type and screening may be necessary based on the level of preoperative anemia and anticipated degree of surgical blood loss. Elective procedures should be postponed in patients with significant anemia, regardless of the anticipated surgical blood loss. This delay allows for evaluation of the underlying cause, such as occult blood loss, vitamin deficiency, or undiagnosed chronic conditions (e.g., CKD). When delay in elective surgery is possible, updated 2015 guidelines from the ASA suggest preoperative treatment with an erythropoiesis-stimulating agent and iron in some patient subgroups (e.g., CKD, anemia of chronic disease, patient's refusal to receive blood transfusions), especially for anemic individuals scheduled for procedures with significant expected blood loss.[333] Similarly, preoperative iron therapy may be considered in patients with known iron deficiency anemia, when time permits.[333]

Sickle Cell Disease

Sickle cell disease is a hereditary hemoglobinopathy with associated vasoocclusive episodes that are responsible for most associated complications. Patients homozygous for hemoglobin S (HbS) have symptomatic disease; they are at risk for major morbidity and have a shortened life expectancy. Patients with SC disease, who have both HbS and HbC, have a much less severe clinical course with moderate anemia. Heterozygous patients (HbS and HbA) have sickle cell trait and rarely have any related consequences. Preoperative assessment should focus on evidence of organ dysfunction and recent patterns of acute exacerbations.[334] Patients may have CKD, loss of renal concentration ability (and therefore are prone to dehydration), splenomegaly, pulmonary hypertension, pulmonary infarctions, CVD, and heart failure. They are at risk for infections because of splenic infarctions. Predictors of perioperative vasoocclusive complications include recent increases in hospitalizations, advanced age, preexisting infections, and pulmonary disease.[334]

The preoperative examination focuses on the frequency, severity, and pattern of vasoocclusive crises. In addition, the anesthesiologist should evaluate the degree of pulmonary, cardiac, renal, and central nervous system damage. Useful tests include an ECG, chest radiograph, and blood sampling for CBC and creatinine concentration. Additional testing (e.g., echocardiogram, arterial blood gases) may be needed. Preoperative prophylactic transfusion is increasingly used in patients with sickle cell anemia who are undergoing any surgical procedure—other than short minor procedures (e.g., biopsy, myringotomy).[335] The objective of any red cell transfusion is to reduce the proportion of abnormal hemoglobin in the affected patient. A prior randomized trial found that prophylactic transfusion to a hemoglobin concentration greater than 100 g/L resulted in fewer adverse events following intermediate-risk surgery.[336] This simpler approach of transfusing to a hemoglobin concentration threshold (>100 g/L) is as effective as a more aggressive approach of transfusing to decrease

HbS concentration to under 30% (while also increasing hemoglobin concentration to ≥ 100 g/L)[337] in the setting of intermediate-risk surgery. It is likely that a more aggressive strategy (i.e., decreasing HbS concentration to < 30%) is preferable for high-risk surgery such as major cardiovascular or intracranial procedures. In general, the decision to transfuse preoperatively should be made only in concert with a hematologist familiar with the disease. Additionally, if the person with sickle cell is managed by a specialist sickle cell service, it is best to liaise with this team before surgery. The patient's surgical admission should be planned to minimize preoperative dehydration (e.g., minimize fasting period, schedule procedure as an early morning case).

Glucose-6-Phosphate Dehydrogenase Deficiency

Glucose-6-phosphate dehydrogenase deficiency is a hereditary Coombs-positive hemolytic anemia. Since it is an X-linked hereditary condition, affected individuals are typically males. Hemolysis may be triggered by drugs (e.g., antipyretics, nitrates, sulfonamides), food (e.g., fava beans), infection, hypoxia, hypothermia, or blood products. Lists of potentially triggering medications are available online (e.g., www.g6pd.org, www.g6pddeficiency.org). The severity of the hemolysis varies across individuals and the underlying genetic defects. Treatment involves avoidance of triggers, folic acid supplementation, and management of acute hemolytic episodes (i.e., hydration, red cell transfusion for severe anemia). The preoperative evaluation should focus on previous hemolysis episodes, predisposing factors, and current hematocrit.

Coagulopathies

Hypocoagulable states may be either inherited (e.g., hemophilia) or acquired (e.g., liver disease, malnutrition, drug exposure). To determine the diagnosis and associated bleeding risk, the anesthesiologist should inquire about known diagnoses, tests, treatments, previous bleeding episodes, and family history. A history of excessive bruising, prolonged bleeding after cuts, heavy menstrual cycles, and bleeding gums is sensitive but not specific. A *change* in these symptoms is likely more meaningful than a long-term history (because what one individual considers excessive may actually be normal). Excessive bleeding after previous procedures or childbirth (especially if transfusions were unexpectedly required) is more definitive but not diagnostic. Petechiae, multiple bruises, hematomas, jaundice, and frank bleeding are important findings. Diagnostic testing may include a CBC (including platelet count), INR, and aPTT; however, *routine* preoperative screening for coagulopathies is not indicated. Clinical indications include a known bleeding disorder, hepatic disease, and anticoagulant use.[5] National guidelines in the United Kingdom also recommend coagulation testing only in patients who are (1) ASA physical status class III or IV; (2) undergoing intermediate, major, or complex surgical procedures; and (3) known to take anticoagulant medications or have chronic liver disease.[274] If a specific cause of bleeding is suspected or known (e.g., liver disease, malnutrition), then additional targeted testing (e.g., liver function tests, protein, albumin) may be needed.

Patients may occasionally have abnormal INR or aPTT results on preoperative screening bloodwork. In patients without a history of vitamin K antagonist use, the most common causes of a prolonged INR are laboratory error, liver disease, and malnutrition. Consequently, the test should initially be repeated. If the repeat test result remains abnormal, both liver function tests and a hepatitis panel are warranted, with possible referral to a hematologist. A trial of oral vitamin K (1-5 mg daily for 3 days) can also be implemented. A prolonged aPTT can result from both hypocoagulable and hypercoagulable (e.g., factor V Leiden, anticardiolipin antibody, lupus anticoagulant, antiphospholipid antibody syndrome) conditions. The first steps are to repeat the test and ascertain possible exposure to heparin. Even small amounts of heparin in indwelling catheters can prolong the aPTT, especially if the blood is drawn from that site. Other than heparin exposure, other causes of a prolonged aPTT include von Willebrand disease (vWD; see section on von Willebrand Disease) and hemophilias (see section on "Hemophilias"). Mixing studies (in which normal blood is mixed with the subject's blood) allows for differentiation between factor deficiencies (aPTT will be corrected) versus inhibitors (no correction). Elective surgical procedures should be postponed until the etiology of abnormal tests is determined and corrections are made.

Hemophilias. Hemophilia A (factor VIII deficiency) and hemophilia B (factor IX deficiency) are X-linked recessive inherited disorders that almost exclusively manifest in males. Hemophilia B is also referred to as "Christmas disease." Hemophilia C is an autosomal recessive deficiency of factor XI (also called Rosenthal syndrome) that tends to affect individuals of Ashkenazi Jewish descent. Hemophilia A has a six-fold higher incidence than Hemophilia B (1 in 5000 male births vs. 1 in 30,000 male births). The severity of bleeding varies across individuals but is similar among relatives (who have the same underlying genetic mutation) and is directly related to the degree of factor deficiency. Severe hemophilia is characterized by less than 1% factor activity, moderate hemophilia by 1% to 5% activity, and mild hemophilia by more than 5% to under 40% activity. Increased disease severity is characterized by an early onset of bleeding episodes, as well as higher risks of both severe and spontaneous bleeding. About two thirds of hemophilia A cases are severe, while the proportion is 50% for hemophilia B. Patients with hemophilia have a prolonged aPTT, but a normal INR and platelet count.

A hematologist must be involved in the perioperative care of patients with hemophilia. A detailed plan to both measure and replace deficient factors is paramount. Current guidelines recommend that, in the setting of major surgery, factor replacement be used to increase preoperative levels to 80% to 100% for hemophilia A and 60% to 80% for hemophilia B.[338] After surgery, the target factor level is 50%, until the surgical wound is healed. The specific required dose of recombinant factor is informed by the targeted increase in factor levels, clinical expertise of the consulting hematologist, individual patient-level factors (e.g., history of previous bleeding episodes), and hospital protocols. The dose required to increase factor VIII levels is:

$$\text{Factor VIII dose} = \text{weight (kg)} \times 0.5 \times (\text{desired absolute \% increase in factor levels})$$

The typical required dose for factor IX replacement is:

$$\text{Factor IX dose} = \text{weight (kg)} \times (\text{desired absolute \% increase in factor levels})$$

To rapidly increase factor levels to close to 100%, the usual dose required is 50 units/kg for factor VIII and 100 to 120 units/kg for factor IX.[339] Intramuscular injections are to be avoided in these patients.

von Willebrand Disease. vWD is an inherited disorder of von Willebrand factor (vWF) that affects both sexes. It is the most common congenital coagulopathy, occurring in approximately 1% of individuals.[340] Several types (1, 2A, 2B, 2M, 2N) are autosomal dominant, while type 3 is autosomal recessive (Table 31.17). vWD can result from both quantitative and qualitative vWF deficiencies. Most affected patients have a normal INR and platelet count (although type 2B can have a mild thrombocytopenia), but typically elevated aPTT (although patients with mild disease may have normal aPTT). Indeed, vWD is the most common cause of a prolonged aPTT in patients not taking heparin. The condition is diagnosed by measuring plasma vWF functional activity (ristocetin cofactor, which causes platelet aggregation), plasma vWF antigen levels, and factor VIII levels. Most patients with vWD have a history of bleeding, but some do not receive a diagnosis until a challenge to coagulation occurs with major surgery or antiplatelet drug exposure (e.g., aspirin, NSAIDs).

A hematologist should be involved in the care of patients with vWD. Treatment options for vWD include desmopressin acetate (1-desamino-8-d-arginine vasopressin [DDAVP]) and vWF replacement therapy. DDAVP increases the release of factor VIII, vWF, and plasminogen activator from endothelial cells. It is contraindicated in patients with type 2B disease because it increases abnormal vWF release and may cause thrombocytopenia. In addition, it is not recommended in patients with type 3 disease (since there is minimal to no vWF available to be released from endothelial cells). In other cases, an intravenous dose of 0.3 μg/kg (given over 15-30 minutes to minimize hypotension, flushing, and tachycardia) typically raises vWF concentrations by three- to four-fold. Nonetheless, considerable variation in response exists among individuals. Hence, an initial test of DDAVP should be conducted prior to any bleeding episodes (e.g., surgery), while monitoring changes in vWF and factor VIII concentrations over the 4 hours after drug administration. DDAVP is also available as a nasal spray (150 μg for individuals under 50 kg, and 300 μg for individuals weighing 50 kg or more). For individuals who cannot be treated adequately with DDAVP, vWF preparations should be used instead. A variety of preparations are available, including vWF-containing factor VIII concentrates, purified vWF concentrates, and recombinant vWF products. These options, if available, are preferable to cryoprecipitate (which can be used nonetheless, but is associated with higher risks of viral transmission).

Thrombocytopenia. Thrombocytopenia is defined as a platelet count less than 150,000/mm^3. It may be the result of decreased production, increased destruction, or sequestration. Causes include malignant diseases, primary immune thrombocytopenia (ITP), drug-induced thrombocytopenia (e.g., quinine, sulfonamides, ampicillin), rheumatological autoimmune disorders (e.g., SLE, rheumatoid arthritis), pregnancy (i.e., gestational thrombocytopenia, preeclampsia), chronic liver disease (i.e., hypersplenism), alcohol, nutritional deficiencies, infection (e.g., hepatitis C, sepsis), hereditary disease, and disseminated intravascular coagulation. If a patient has an unexpectedly low platelet count, the initial steps are to repeat the test, examine the peripheral smear, and collect blood for the platelet count in a tube without ethylenediaminetetraacetic acid. This chemical is a chelating agent often used to prevent clotting in tubes used for determining CBC, but it can also cause clumping of platelets (termed pseudothrombocytopenia). ITP is a chronic autoimmune disorder characterized by autoantibodies that cause platelet destruction. Usual treatment includes corticosteroids, splenectomy (eliminates the major site of platelet removal), and intravenous immunoglobulin. Patients with ITP often have less bleeding than expected, even at very low platelet levels, likely because of increased platelet turnover with a resulting predominance of young platelets. A patient with newly discovered thrombocytopenia may require a hematology consultation before elective surgery.

Thrombocytopenia within the context of recent heparin exposure should raise a concern regarding potential heparin-induced thrombocytopenia (HIT), which generally occurs within 5 to 10 days after heparin exposure.[341] HIT is an immune-mediated disorder characterized by antibodies directed against platelet factor 4 complexed with heparin. While HIT is characterized by thrombocytopenia, affected patients are at risk for arterial thromboses,

TABLE 31.17 Classification of von Willebrand Disease

Type	Characteristics	Initial Treatment
1	80% of cases; quantitative defect	Desmopressin*
2A	Quantitative and qualitative defect	Desmopressin*
2B**	Rare; quantitative and qualitative defect, autosomal dominant	Cryoprecipitate or factor VIII concentrates with vWF
2M	Qualitative defect	Desmopressin*
2N	Qualitative defect; vWF levels normal; factor VIII reduced	Desmopressin* effect may be too short-lived
3	Rare; low to undetectable levels of vWF	Desmopressin* usually not effective

*Desmopressin acetate (DDAVP).
**With type 2B desmopressin acetate may cause thrombocytopenia. If desmopressin is not effective, factor VIII concentrates containing vWF may be used.
vWF, von Willebrand factor.

venous thromboses, stroke, skin necrosis, limb gangrene, and organ infarction. Since the results of definitive laboratory testing for HIT antibodies (i.e., immunoassay and/or functional assay for HIT antibodies) typically takes several days, the initial presumptive diagnosis is based on clinical presentation and available laboratory tests (e.g., decreasing platelet counts). This initial diagnosis can be aided with validated clinical prediction tools, such as the "4 Ts" score.[342] While waiting for the results of antibody testing in patients with suspected HIT, any heparin therapy (including LMWH) should be immediately discontinued and alternative anticoagulation therapy (e.g., danaparoid, argatroban, bivalirudin, fondaparinux, DOACs) instituted.

In otherwise healthy individuals (i.e., no other basis for elevated bleeding risks) neuraxial anesthesia is generally considered safe once the platelet count exceeds 50,000 to 80,000 per mm^3.[343-346] Surgery can be safely performed in patients with platelet counts higher than 50,000/mm^3.[346] The risk of bleeding increases progressively as the count falls further, to less than 50,000/mm^3. When platelet transfusions are used to treat thrombocytopenia, the platelet count generally rises by 10,000/mm^3 for every unit transfused.

Thrombocytosis. Thrombocytosis is a platelet count more than 450,000/mm^3. It may be physiologic (i.e., exercise, pregnancy), primary (e.g., myeloproliferative disorder), or secondary (e.g., iron deficiency, neoplasm, surgery, chronic inflammation). Increasing levels of thrombocytosis can increase risks for thrombotic events, such as strokes, myocardial infarction, pulmonary emboli, mesenteric emboli, and venous clots. Conversely, patients with primary thrombocytosis (also known as essential thrombocythemia) also have a tendency toward increased bleeding, which may be due to qualitative alterations in platelet function and an acquired von Willebrand syndrome associated with very high platelet counts (>1,000,000/mm^3). Treatments include medications (e.g., hydroxyurea, anagrelide, pegylated interferon) that decrease platelet production and thereby reduce platelet counts over 7 to 10 days. Plasmapheresis, which removes platelets from the circulation, can be used if an immediate lowering in platelet count is required. In cases of secondary thrombocytosis, treatment of the underlying disorder usually results in normalization of the platelet count.

Polycythemia. Polycythemia is characterized by an increased number of circulating RBCs and increased hemoglobin concentration. It can be defined based on hematocrit (>48% in females and >49% in males) and hemoglobin concentration (>160 g/L in females and > 165 g/L in males). Polycythemia can be a primary disorder (i.e., polycythemia vera) or secondary to conditions typically associated with chronic hypoxia (e.g., COPD, high altitude, cyanotic congenital heart disease). A steep increase in blood viscosity occurs once the hematocrit increases to more than 50%, resulting in an increased thrombogenic risk. High hematocrits are associated with increased atherosclerosis (e.g., carotid stenosis, stroke) and cardiac disease (e.g., heart failure, myocardial infarction). Reports on whether polycythemia increases perioperative risk are contradictory. For example, a hematocrit more than 51% was associated with increased postoperative mortality in a retrospective cohort study of more than 310,000 patients.[102] Conversely, a previous smaller study of 200 patients did not find an increased rate of perioperative complications in individuals with secondary polycythemia.[347]

The preoperative evaluation should focus on the pulmonary and cardiovascular systems. On physical examination, the anesthesiologist should examine for cyanosis, clubbing, wheezing, murmurs, and oxygen saturation (via pulse oximetry). Useful laboratory tests include an ECG, arterial blood gases, and chest radiograph. An unexpected finding of polycythemia should prompt an investigation for possible causes, which if not readily apparent, should raise the possibility of polycythemia vera. In such cases, elective surgery should be postponed pending a consultation by a hematologist.

Venous Thromboembolic Disorders. VTE is an important potential risk in hospitalized patients, including surgical patients.[348] Primary VTE prophylaxis is beyond the scope of this chapter and is covered extensively in specialty society practice guidelines.[11,12] Nonetheless, patients should be stratified preoperatively for their risks of perioperative VTE to inform the appropriate selection of prophylactic measures. The expected risk of postoperative VTE depends on both patient-related (e.g., inflammatory bowel disease, acute illness, smoking, malignant disease, obesity, increased age, prior VTE, estrogen use, hypercoagulable state, inherited thrombophilia) and procedure-related (e.g., invasiveness, trauma, immobilization) factors. A reasonable approach for estimating perioperative VTE risk is to use a validated clinical prediction index, a widely used example being the Modified Caprini Risk Assessment Model (Box 31.12).[11,349] A Caprini score of zero indicates very low VTE risk (0.5% risk in the absence of thromboprophylaxis), scores of 1 to 2 indicate low VTE risk (1.5% risk in the absence of thromboprophylaxis), scores of 3 to 4 indicate moderate VTE risk (3.0% risk in the absence of thromboprophylaxis), and scores of 5 or more indicate high VTE risk (6.0% risk in the absence of thromboprophylaxis).

Some subgroups of patients are at considerably higher risk for perioperative VTE, namely those with very recent VTE (i.e., within prior 3 months) and those with a history of VTE associated with a high-risk inherited thrombophilia.[350] For individuals with a very recent VTE episode, elective surgery should be delayed until 3 or more months have elapsed since the episode (during which time they should be anticoagulated).[351] Specifically, the risk of recurrent VTE is highest during the first 3 to 4 weeks after the initial episode; this risk then decreases over the next 2 months. Hereditary high-risk thrombophilias include Factor V Leiden, antithrombin III deficiency, protein C deficiency, protein S deficiency, prothrombin gene mutation, and antiphospholipid antibodies. Factor V Leiden and prothrombin gene mutations are the most common causes, together comprising up to 60% of cases.[352]

BOX 31.12 Modified Caprini Risk Assessment Model for Venous Thromboembolism

1 Point Each

Age 41–60 years
Minor surgery
BMI > 25 kg/m2
Swollen legs
Varicose veins
Pregnancy or postpartum
History of unexplained or recurrent spontaneous abortion
Oral contraceptives or hormone replacement
Sepsis (<1 month)
Serious lung disease, including pneumonia (<1 month)
Abnormal pulmonary function
Acute myocardial infarction
Heart failure (<1 month)
History of inflammatory bowel disease
Medical patient at bed rest

2 Points Each

Age 61–74 years
Arthroscopic surgery
Major open surgery (>45 min)
Laparoscopic surgery (>45 min)
Malignancy
Confined to bed (>72 h)
Immobilizing plaster cast
Central venous access

3 Points Each

Age ≥ 75 years
History of VTE
Family history of VTE
Factor V Leiden mutation
Prothrombin 20210A mutation
Lupus anticoagulant
Anticardiolipin antibodies
Elevated serum homocysteine
Heparin-induced thrombocytopenia
Other congenital or acquired thrombophilia

5 Points Each

Stroke (<1 month)
Elective arthroplasty
Hip, pelvis, or leg fracture
Acute spinal cord injury (<1 month)

BMI, Body mass index; *VTE*, venous thromboembolism.
From Gould MK, Garcia DA, Wren SM, et al. Prevention of VTE in nonorthopedic surgical patients: antithrombotic therapy and prevention of thrombosis, 9th ed: American College of Chest Physicians evidence-based clinical practical guidelines. *Chest.* 2012; 141: e227S–e277S.

Patients having minor procedures such as dental, endoscopic, cataract, or superficial operations usually do not require interruption of anticoagulant therapy. In other individuals, withholding warfarin for 5 days typically allows the INR to decrease to normal if the baseline INR is in the usual therapeutic target (2.0 and 3.0). A longer interval may be needed if the baseline INR is higher (see section on "Preoperative Anticoagulant Therapy"). During the time without warfarin, patients may be at risk for recurrent thromboembolism; however, the risk is relatively small in all but the highest-risk patients (i.e., VTE in prior 3 months, or VTE with high-risk inherited thrombophilia). The decision to bridge with intravenous unfractionated heparin or with LMWH subcutaneously in high-risk patients must be made collaboratively with the treating physician.

Preoperative Anticoagulant Therapy. Outpatient oral anticoagulant therapy includes vitamin K antagonists (e.g., warfarin) and DOACs. These agents increase perioperative bleeding, except in the case of very minor procedures. Thus, they should only be continued perioperatively if an individual does not have patient-related risk factors for bleeding (e.g., liver disease, abnormal renal function, prior bleeding complications), is scheduled for procedures without important bleeding risk (e.g., dental extraction, simple cutaneous procedures, cataract surgery without bulbar blocks), and is not being considered for neuraxial anesthesia. Otherwise, anticoagulant therapy must be temporarily discontinued before surgery.

Typically, vitamin K antagonists should be stopped 5 days before surgery, with consideration for a longer discontinuation period if the initial INR value is more than 3.0. Ideally, the INR should be rechecked within 24 hours before surgery,[195] and a low dose of oral vitamin K (1 to 5 mg administrated orally or subcutaneously) administered for any INR result greater than 1.5. Vitamin K has an effect within 6 to 10 hours after oral or subcutaneous administration (more predictable with oral administration), and it peaks within 24 hours to 48 hours.[353] Administration of higher doses may lead to warfarin resistance when therapy is initiated again. Some patients undergoing elective lower extremity joint replacement surgery may also receive an initial dose of warfarin before surgery for perioperative thromboprophylaxis. The 2018 American Society of Regional Anesthesiologists (ASRA) guidelines state that neuraxial anesthesia can still be performed in these patients when only a single dose of warfarin has been administered within a period of 24 hours or less before surgery.[196]

Patients are increasingly receiving DOACs for long-term anticoagulation, typically for nonvalvular atrial fibrillation, although some individuals may be prescribed low-dose DOAC therapy for IHD.[91] The timing of preoperative discontinuation of DOACs should be guided by the specific drug prescribed, expected procedural bleeding risk, renal function (based on estimated GFR), and planned use of neuraxial anesthesia. Some proposed approaches for preoperative DOAC discontinuation are outlined in Tables 31.11 and 31.12.[195-197]

Patients may require temporary bridging therapy during the intervening period between discontinuation of vitamin K antagonist therapy and the date of surgery. Such bridging therapy is generally not needed after interruption of DOACs because of their relatively short half-lives. *Most* patients with nonvalvular atrial fibrillation do not require bridging therapy if their anticoagulant therapy is temporarily discontinued before surgery (see section on "Atrial Fibrillation").[195,198] Conversely, many patients with mechanical heart valves will require bridging therapy, with the decision based on the location of the mechanical heart valve and nature of planned surgery (see Box 31.4).[173] Additionally, some patients who are at very high risk for recurrent VTE (e.g., VTE episode within prior 3 months) may also require bridging therapy. In general, decisions to use bridging therapy with intravenous unfractionated heparin or LMWH must be individualized, account for patients' risks of bleeding while on bridge therapy, and be made collaboratively with the treating physician.

If bridging is planned, either LMWH or intravenous unfractionated heparin can be started 2 or more days after the last administrated dose of vitamin K antagonist (e.g., warfarin). Bridging therapy should be started once the INR drops to under 2.0.[195] There are several available options for LMWH (e.g., enoxaparin, dalteparin). The specific choice and dose should be selected based on consultation with a hematologist or the patient's treating physician. For patients with impaired renal function (eGFR < 30 mL/min), intravenous heparin bridging is preferable, although some LMWH dosing adjustments remain possible if eGFR is in the range between 15 and 30 mL/min.[195] Intravenous unfractionated heparin is usually discontinued approximately 6 hours before the surgery to allow for normal intraoperative coagulation. The last dose of *bridging dose* LMWH should be given 24 hours preoperatively to allow normalization of coagulation by the time of surgery (based on an assumption of normal renal function). Both unfractionated heparin and LMWH are contraindicated in patients with an allergy to heparin or a history of HIT. Options for bridging therapy in such patients include argatroban (intravenous infusion), bivalirudin (intravenous infusion), fondaparinux (subcutaneous), or oral DOACs. The specific management strategy should be selected following consultation with a hematologist.

Based on the 2018 ASRA guidelines,[196] recommendations for management of preoperative anticoagulant therapy are more conservative if perioperative neuraxial techniques are being considered. These guidelines recommend that warfarin should be discontinued 5 or more days before surgery, and a repeat preoperative INR should confirm a normalized value before neuraxial blocks are performed.[196] The recommended intervals for timing of neuraxial blocks after discontinuing DOAC therapy are outlined in Table 31.11. The last *prophylactic* dose of LMWH should be 12 or more hours before any planned neuraxial block, whereas the last *therapeutic* dose (including bridging therapy) of LMWH should be 24 or more hours beforehand. Preoperative unfractionated intravenous heparin should be stopped 6 or more hours before planned spinal or epidural anesthesia.[196] In addition, return to normal coagulation can be monitored using aPTT or anti-factor Xa activity. Though the safety of performing neuraxial techniques in the presence of low-dose subcutaneous unfractionated heparin (i.e., 5000 units twice daily) has been described,[354] the 2018 ASRA guidelines include a Grade 2C recommendation for waiting 4 to 6 hours after subcutaneous injection before performing neuraxial blocks in patients receiving subcutaneous unfractionated heparin (i.e., 5000 units 2 or 3 times daily).[196] This Grade 2C rating indicates that the recommendation was relatively weaker ("*conflicting evidence or opinion on the usefulness*") and based entirely on case reports or expert opinion.[196] Any patients receiving fibrinolytic and thrombolytic drugs should not receive neuraxial anesthesia.

Preoperative Antiplatelet Therapy. Traditionally, aspirin has been discontinued before surgery (often 7-10 days before surgery) because of concern about increased bleeding. A withdrawal period of 7 to 10 days is likely excessive, especially because new platelets formed after aspirin discontinuation (half-life ≈15 minutes) are not inhibited. Since 10% of platelets are turned over every 24 hours, and about 50,000/mm^3 of normal functioning platelets are needed to control surgical bleeding, it is likely that aspirin need only be stopped 3 days before surgery to mitigate risks of increased bleeding. Continuation of aspirin until the time of surgery leads to increased bleeding during major noncardiac surgery,[136] but not during cardiac surgery.[355] *Withdrawing* aspirin itself has important theoretical risks with respect to a rebound hypercoagulable state and increased cardiac risk,[141,356] however, these theoretical risks have not been supported by data from large randomized trials.[136,355] Therefore, a reasonable standard approach for most surgical patients is to discontinue aspirin temporarily 3 days before surgery, with some notable exceptions. Specifically, aspirin should be continued in any patient with a prior PCI,[144] high-grade IHD, or high-risk CVD (e.g., stroke within prior 9 months).[212] Continuation of aspirin is not a contraindication to performance of neuraxial blocks.[196]

$P2Y_{12}$ inhibitors are the other relatively common type of antiplatelet medications that might be encountered during preoperative evaluation, especially among patients with known IHD or CVD. These medications include oral medications (clopidogrel, ticagrelor, prasugrel, ticlopidine) and an intravenous formulation (cangrelor). Aside from the case of patients with a recent PCI (see section on "Coronary Stents"), $P2Y_{12}$ inhibitor therapy should be temporarily discontinued before elective surgery. The usual recommended time interval for discontinuing these medications before surgery (including cases where neuraxial blocks are planned) is 5 to 7 days for clopidogrel, 5 to 7 days for ticagrelor, 7 to 10 days for prasugrel, 10 days for ticlopidine, and 3 hours for cangrelor.[196]

Some patients with either PAD or CVD may be on long-term therapy with dipyridamole, which causes vasodilation and impairment of platelet function. The drug is available as an immediate-release formulation, as well as an extended-release formulation combined with aspirin (i.e., Aggrenox). There are minimal data on the safety of continuing dipyridamole in patients undergoing surgery; current ASRA guidelines recommend discontinuing extended-release dipyridamole 24 hours before performing any neuraxial block.[196] Information on the perioperative safety of other antiplatelet therapies (e.g., glycoprotein IIb/IIIa inhibitors) is also limited. Platelet glycoprotein IIb/IIIa inhibitors (e.g., abciximab, eptifibatide, tirofiban) exert profound effects on platelet aggregation. Following administration, the time to restoration of normal platelet aggregation is 24 to 48 hours for abciximab, and 4 to 8 hours for eptifibatide and tirofiban. Neuraxial techniques should be avoided until platelet function has recovered after platelet glycoprotein IIb/IIIa inhibitor administration.[196]

NEUROLOGIC DISEASE

The preoperative history in a patient with neurologic disease should focus on recent exacerbations, prior investigations, and therapy (both current and prior). The basic neurologic examination should evaluate mental status, speech, cranial nerves, gait, motor function, and sensory function. This baseline determination also allows for comparison of any new postoperative deficits.

Cerebrovascular Disease

The major clinical manifestation of CVD is acute stroke with more than 10 million new strokes per year worldwide. In addition, about 6.5 million individuals die annually from stroke, making it the second leading cause of death globally.[357] The two main categories of stroke are hemorrhagic stroke and ischemic stroke. Hemorrhagic stroke is largely related to either intracerebral hemorrhage or subarachnoid hemorrhage. Common causes of intracerebral hemorrhage include hypertension, trauma, coagulopathies, illicit drug use (i.e., amphetamines, cocaine), and arteriovenous malformations (AVMs). Causes of subarachnoid hemorrhage are bleeding from aneurysms and AVMs (see section on "Aneurysms and Arteriovenous Malformations"). Ischemic stroke may be related to thrombosis of an artery through several different mechanisms (e.g., atherosclerosis, arterial dissection), embolism (e.g., related to atrial fibrillation), or systemic hypoperfusion (e.g., cardiac arrest). The other major manifestation of CVD is a TIA, which is a transient episode of neurologic dysfunction caused by focal ischemia in the brain, spinal cord, or retina, but without infarction.[358]

CVD has important perioperative implications. It is a risk factor for postoperative complications, including cardiac events,[97] stroke,[132,359,360] and death.[77] Furthermore, the risks of postoperative cardiac complications and recurrent stroke are particularly increased when elective noncardiac surgery is performed within 9 months after a prior stroke[212] or when surgical aortic valve replacement is performed within 3 months after a prior stroke.[212] Importantly, if emergency surgery needs to be performed after a stroke, it may be preferable to *not* delay surgery. Specifically, while the risks of postoperative cardiovascular complications are very high when emergency surgery is performed within 2 weeks after an ischemic stroke, these risks were reduced when surgery proceeded within 72 hours after the stroke.[361] This temporal pattern may be explained by progressively worsening cerebral autoregulation during the first 5 days after an ischemic stroke (which then recovers over the next 3 months).[362]

The preoperative evaluation should focus on the timing, presentation, etiology, and treatment of prior strokes or TIAs. It is important to document the etiology in order to distinguish carotid stenosis (i.e., atherosclerosis) from cardioembolic disease. Causes of cardiac emboli include stasis (i.e., atrial fibrillation, severe cardiomyopathy, ventricular aneurysm), thrombogenic (i.e., valvular heart disease, prosthetic heart valve), and paradoxical venous source (e.g., patent foramen ovale). The physical examination should include a brief neurologic exam to identify any preexisting deficits, auscultation for carotid bruits, and a precordial assessment to assess for murmurs or extra heart sounds. Depending on the underlying basis for CVD (i.e., atherosclerosis, atrial fibrillation), patients may be on long-term therapy with aspirin, $P2Y_{12}$ inhibitors (e.g., clopidogrel), vitamin K antagonists, and DOACs. Both vitamin K antagonists and DOACs should be temporarily discontinued before surgery (see section on "Atrial Fibrillation"). Similarly, $P2Y_{12}$ inhibitor therapy should be interrupted before surgery, with the possible exception of cases with very recent coronary stent implantation (see section on "Coronary Stents"). Continuing aspirin perioperatively does not prevent cardiovascular complications,[136] but leads to an increased risk of major bleeding (a risk factor for perioperative stroke).[132] Nonetheless, selective continuation of aspirin can be considered in patients with high-risk atherosclerotic CVD or recent stroke (i.e., previous 9 months).[212] In other cases, aspirin should be temporarily held 72 hours before surgery.[136] In addition, concomitant CVD should be carefully considered in any decision to initiate new β-adrenergic blocker therapy in a patient awaiting noncardiac surgery. Although β-blockade does decrease perioperative cardiac risk, it also significantly increases the risk for acute postoperative stroke.[132,133]

Asymptomatic Carotid Bruit

The presence of a carotid bruit significantly increases the likelihood of a significant lesion (i.e., 70%-99% stenosis) in both symptomatic or asymptomatic patients.[26] Thus, a newly discovered carotid bruit should prompt a careful search for any evidence of prior strokes or TIA, especially if the planned surgical procedure involves neck manipulation. At-risk individuals include those with risk factors for CVD (e.g., hypertension, smoker, diabetes mellitus, hyperlipidemia, IHD, PAD), as well as patients with prior head and neck radiation exposure. Patients may not volunteer pertinent symptoms until they are specifically probed, especially if the symptoms were transient. The anesthesiologist should specifically inquire about *amaurosis fugax*, dysphagia, dysarthria, and other symptoms of cerebrovascular insufficiency. Carotid Doppler ultrasound studies are simple, effective tools to evaluate suspicious carotid bruits. Significant abnormalities on Doppler studies may entail a referral to a neurologist or vascular surgeon. The risk of stroke in patients who have truly asymptomatic bruits is 1% to 2% per year, with most strokes preceded by transient symptoms.[363] No evidence indicates that truly asymptomatic bruits increase the risk of *perioperative* stroke.[364]

Seizure Disorder

The seizure type (e.g., *grand mal*, absence) and specific symptoms (e.g., staring, focal findings) are important to document in the preoperative evaluation. For example, absence (previously *petit mal*) seizures may be particularly difficult to recognize after surgery because they lack generalized motor signs. Hence, typical symptoms, such as staring and obtundation, may be misinterpreted as residual anesthetic effects in the postoperative period. It is important to determine the etiology of the seizure disorder because of possible associated morbidities, which include brain tumors, aneurysms, AVMs, classic epilepsy, drug toxicity, electrolyte disorders, infections, CVD, sickle cell disease, and SLE.

The anesthesiologist should document the anticonvulsant dosing regimen and adequacy of seizure control. Routine measurement of serum drug levels of anticonvulsants is not indicated unless there are concerns about drug toxicity or ongoing breakthrough seizures. Indeed, patients with good control of seizures may have levels outside the therapeutic range. Drug levels are highly influenced by when the blood draw occurs relative to the timing of drug administration. In general, trough levels should be measured. Anti-seizure medications have multiple side effects (e.g., bone marrow suppression, macrocytic anemia, leucopenia, hyponatremia), and testing may be needed based on suspected abnormalities. The most commonly ordered tests are CBC and electrolyte concentrations. All anticonvulsant therapy should be continued perioperatively. A patient with poorly controlled or new-onset seizures should be evaluated by a neurologist before any non-emergent surgery.

Multiple Sclerosis

Multiple sclerosis is believed to be an inflammatory immune disorder with two general clinical patterns: exacerbating-remitting and chronic progressive. Symptoms can include ataxia, motor weakness, sensory deficits, autonomic dysfunction, emotional lability, bladder or bowel dysfunction, and visual disturbances. Exacerbations of multiple sclerosis can be triggered by stress, infections, pregnancy, and elevated temperatures. Various treatments have been tried, including corticosteroids, immunosuppressants, monoclonal antibodies, plasmapheresis, benzodiazepines, and baclofen. The preoperative evaluation should document the history and pattern of disease, especially symptoms and physical deficits affecting the respiratory system (including oxygen saturation). Medications, previous triggers, and preexisting neurologic deficits should be documented. Testing is generally directed toward associated disturbances (e.g., chest radiography and CBC if pulmonary infection is suspected) and any medication side effects. For example, azathioprine can suppress bone marrow or affect liver function, cyclophosphamide may cause electrolyte abnormalities, and corticosteroids can cause hyperglycemia. Patients with stable minor disease require no special testing. Related medications should be continued on the day of surgery. No clear association has been shown between the type of anesthetic or a specific anesthetic drug and disease exacerbations. Nonetheless, regional anesthesia may offer theoretical advantages for patients with respiratory compromise or cognitive dysfunction.

Aneurysms and Arteriovenous Malformations

Aneurysms and AVMs can occur in the cerebral and spinal vascular beds. These lesions may be intact, ruptured, symptomatic, or incidental asymptomatic findings. Associated risk factors include polycystic kidney disease, fibromuscular dysplasia, type IV Ehlers-Danlos syndrome, and a family history. Some AVMs become large enough to exert a mass effect. The risk of aneurysmal bleeding, and possibly AVM bleeding, increases during pregnancy. Most patients have minimal symptoms before a rupture. A rupture can result in altered mental status, syncope, increased intracranial pressure, inappropriate antidiuretic hormone (ADH) secretion, and hemodynamic changes (i.e., bradycardia, tachycardia, ectopic beats). Typical testing includes an ECG and blood sampling to measure electrolyte, glucose, and creatinine concentrations. Chest radiography, echocardiography, and neurologic imaging (e.g., computed tomography scan) are also often needed. Importantly, the ECG changes seen following a rupture, which often include ST-segment and T-wave changes, mimic those seen with myocardial ischemia. In addition, troponin concentrations are often elevated, while echocardiography may reveal significant cardiac dysfunction with depressed contractility and wall motion abnormalities. Although the bleeding may be primarily responsible for these cardiovascular changes, concomitant IHD or preexisting cardiomyopathy should also be considered. Measures aimed at controlling increased intracranial pressure, arterial blood pressure, and blood glucose are important.

Parkinson Disease

Parkinson disease is a degenerative disorder of the basal ganglia characterized by failure of dopamine secretion and diminished inhibition of the extrapyramidal motor system. Patients typically have diminution of spontaneous movements, rigidity (cogwheel rigidity is classic), resting tremor, masked facies, difficulty speaking, difficulty walking, depression, and dementia. Autonomic dysfunction (including orthostatic hypotension), excessive salivation, and impaired thermoregulation may also occur. Patients are at risk of pulmonary complications resulting from difficulty swallowing, altered mental status, increased aspiration risk, and ventilatory muscle dysfunction. Pharmacologic treatments include levodopa, dopamine agonists (e.g., bromocriptine, pramipexole, ropinirole, rotigotine), monoamine oxidase type B inhibitors (e.g., selegiline, rasagiline, safinamide), anticholinergic agents (e.g., trihexyphenidyl, benztropine), amantadine, and catechol-O-methyl transferase inhibitors (tolcapone, entacapone). Levodopa can cause dyskinesias (i.e., dystonic and myoclonic involuntary movements). Some individuals also undergo implantation of deep brain stimulators to manage their symptoms.

Preoperative evaluation should assess the pulmonary system, signs of dysphagia, and degree of disability. Evidence of significant pulmonary symptoms or possible infection requires chest radiography, pulmonary consultation, and possible delay of the procedure for improvement. All associated medications should be continued. Abrupt withdrawal of levodopa may exacerbate symptoms (especially dysphagia and chest wall rigidity) or precipitate neuroleptic malignant syndrome. The latter disorder is characterized by autonomic instability, altered mental status, rigidity, and fever. Some medications encountered in the perioperative setting, such as metoclopramide and phenothiazines, may exacerbate symptoms of Parkinson disease by interfering with dopamine. Individuals with deep brain stimulators require deactivation of the devices before any procedures in which electrocautery will be used. The specific device should be identified, along with the severity of disease symptoms when the device is turned off. Perioperative management of the device ideally should be coordinated with the surgeon and the clinician managing the device.

Neuromuscular Junction Disorders

Myasthenia gravis is an autoimmune disorder of skeletal muscle neuromuscular junctions that is caused by antibodies against nicotinic acetylcholine receptors. The disease is characterized by skeletal muscle weakness that worsens with activity and improves with rest. Cardiac and smooth muscle function is unaffected. Weakness is exacerbated by stress, infections, hypokalemia, medications (e.g., aminoglycosides, propranolol, ciprofloxacin, clindamycin), and surgery. A classification system for severity of myasthenia gravis is presented in Box 31.13. Patients with myasthenia gravis commonly have other autoimmune diseases, such as rheumatoid arthritis, polymyositis, and thyroid disorders.

Ocular symptoms (i.e., diplopia, ptosis) are almost always present; often, they are the presenting complaint or sole complaint. Cranial nerve and bulbar involvement are common, with an associated aspiration risk related to pharyngeal and laryngeal muscle weakness. Affected individuals may have thymic hyperplasia and tumors. Since the thymus is located in the anterior mediastinum, thymic enlargement has potential implications for anesthesia care (see section on "Mediastinal Masses"). Patients are usually treated with thymectomy, acetylcholinesterase inhibitors (e.g., pyridostigmine, neostigmine), immunosuppressants (corticosteroids, azathioprine, mycophenolate, cyclosporine), plasmapheresis, and intravenous immunoglobulins. Worsening symptoms may reflect worsening disease (i.e., myasthenic crisis) or excessive acetylcholinesterase inhibitor treatment (i.e., cholinergic crisis). A short-acting anticholinesterase (edrophonium) can help distinguish the two states, since only a myasthenic crisis improves with more anticholinesterase. Plasmapheresis and intravenous immunoglobulins have been used to treat myasthenic crises and prepare patients for surgery, but still require several days to weeks to produce improvement.

All medications (with associated doses) should be documented and continued perioperatively. These drugs may also have implications themselves. For example, patients taking azathioprine require a CBC and liver function tests because of drug-induced bone marrow suppression and liver dysfunction. Patients treated with corticosteroids need measurement of blood glucose concentration, as well as possible perioperative corticosteroid supplementation. Since ventilatory function can be compromised, preoperative PFTs may also be indicated for selected patients, particularly those suspected of having severely affected ventilatory function. PFTs may be particularly helpful if patients are being considered for ambulatory surgery, especially in freestanding surgical centers. Drugs that can exacerbate myasthenic symptoms should also be avoided.

Lambert-Eaton syndrome is similar to myasthenia gravis, with muscle weakness including oculobulbar involvement and dysautonomia. It is caused by antibodies against voltage-gated calcium channels that result in decreased acetylcholine release. It is not associated with thymic abnormalities, but commonly occurs with malignant diseases, especially small cell lung cancer and gastrointestinal tumors. The other distinguishing feature of this disorder is that the muscle weakness classically improves with activity and is worse after inactivity. In addition to acetylcholinesterase inhibitors, typical treatments include 3,4-diaminopyridine, which is a selective potassium channel blocker. Preoperative evaluation and management are similar to those for myasthenia gravis. All related medications should be continued perioperatively.

BOX 31.13 Osserman Classification System for Myasthenia Gravis Clinical Classification System

Class I: Ocular myasthenia

Class IIA: Mild generalized myasthenia with slow progression: no crises, responsive to drugs

Class IIB: Moderately severe generalized myasthenia: severe skeletal and bulbar involvement but no crises; drug response less than satisfactory

Class III: Acute fulminating myasthenia: rapid progression of severe symptoms, with respiratory crises and poor drug response

Class IV: Late severe myasthenia, same as III but progression over 2 years from class I to II

Data from Osserman KE, Genkins G. Studies in myasthenia gravis: review of a twenty-year experience in over 1200 patients. *Mt Sinai J Med.* 1971;38:497–537.

Muscular Dystrophies and Myopathies

Muscular dystrophies and myopathies are inherited disorders that affect the neuromuscular junction. They share many similarities but do have a few differences. The hallmark of these disorders is progressive skeletal muscle weakness that commonly leads to respiratory failure. No effective therapy is available. Many individuals have associated cardiomyopathies and possible association with malignant hyperthermia.

Duchenne and Becker muscular dystrophies are X-linked recessive disorders that occur primarily in males. Affected individuals have elevated creatine phosphokinase levels, often preceding the onset of symptoms. Male patients with a family history of either Duchenne or Becker muscular dystrophy should be considered at risk (even when they have not been formally tested), and they require precautions similar to those in patients with diagnosed disease. Cardiomyopathy and respiratory failure are the usual causes of death. Female carriers of the abnormal gene may have dilated cardiomyopathy despite having no other manifestations of the disease. The preoperative evaluation should focus on the cardiovascular (e.g., palpitations, dyspnea, chest pain, syncope, orthopnea, dependent edema) and pulmonary (e.g., aspiration, pneumonia) systems. Potentially helpful additional preoperative tests include ECGs, PFTs, and echocardiography. Facioscapulohumeral muscular dystrophy (also known as faciohumeroscapular or Landouzy-Dejerine muscular dystrophy) is an autosomal dominant disorder that affects both sexes and causes a slow, progressive weakness of muscles in the shoulders and face. Cardiomyopathy occurs much less frequently than in other dystrophies, but arrhythmias have been reported. Limb-girdle dystrophies have a variable genetic inheritance pattern and primarily affect the muscles of the shoulders and pelvis. Conduction abnormalities are present in some patients, although frank cardiomyopathies are less frequent. The preoperative evaluation is largely similar to that described previously for Duchenne muscular dystrophy.

Myotonic Dystrophies. Myotonia is characterized by prolonged contraction and delayed relaxation of muscles. It is a common symptom of several dystrophies, including classic myotonic dystrophy, congenital myotonic dystrophy, myotonia congenital, and central core disease. Myotonic dystrophy, which is the most common of these conditions, is an autosomal dominant inherited disorder affecting both sexes. Congenital myotonic dystrophy is a severe form of this disease that manifests in infancy, often in the children of affected mothers. The classic findings are severe muscle wasting, typically involving the diaphragm, face, hands, pharynx, and larynx. Cold temperatures can often trigger myotonia. The disease severity is variable, with symptoms often not apparent until the second or third decade of life; hence, a family history is important. Cardiomyopathies, arrhythmias, and conduction abnormalities are common, while some patients also have cardiac valvular abnormalities. Cardiac involvement may not correlate with the degree of atrophy or weakness in skeletal muscle. Once an affected individual shows any evidence of second- or third-degree AV block, a pacemaker should be implanted (even if the patient is asymptomatic) because an unpredictably rapid progression of conduction disease may occur. Given this potential for rapid disease progression, pacemaker placement may be considered in patients with first-degree AV block, regardless of symptoms. Affected individuals are also at risk for aspiration, pneumonia, respiratory failure, and postoperative pulmonary complications. Central core disease is a rare disorder caused by deficiency of mitochondrial enzymes. The name derives from findings of muscle biopsies, which reveal "cores" of abnormalities. Affected individuals have proximal muscle weakness, scoliosis, and sometimes cardiomyopathies. As with myotonic dystrophy, patients are at risk for respiratory failure and aspiration. Myotonia congenita is a hereditary disorder that involves only skeletal muscles, causes less severe symptoms, and does not cause cardiac abnormalities.

Myotonia was historically thought to predispose patients to malignant hyperthermia, however, current evidence indicates that they are *not* at increased risk.[365] Nonetheless, succinylcholine should still be avoided in these patients because it may cause diffuse muscle contraction. Symptomatic treatments for myotonic contractions include corticosteroids, quinine, and procainamide; otherwise, these diseases have no cure. These treatments should be continued perioperatively. The preoperative evaluation focuses on the cardiopulmonary system, with special emphasis on evaluating for pulmonary infection, heart failure, syncope, conduction abnormalities, and valvular abnormalities. Preoperative testing includes an ECG, echocardiogram (except for myotonia congenita), and chest radiograph (if symptoms of pulmonary disease are present). Evidence of a conduction abnormality on ECG should trigger a cardiology consultation. Myotonia is not inhibited by regional anesthesia, but local anesthetic infiltration into muscle may provide symptomatic relief.

Central Nervous System Tumors

Pituitary tumors are classified as functioning (associated with endocrine abnormalities) versus nonfunctioning, as well as benign (adenomas are the most common pituitary lesion) versus malignant. The tumor can have mass effects that lead to associated symptoms, such as headaches, visual field defects, and increased intracranial pressure (with resulting gait disturbances, vomiting, cranial nerve deficits, bladder incontinence, bowel incontinence). Other symptoms may be related to pituitary insufficiency (e.g., hypoadrenalism, hypothyroidism, infertility) or overactivity. Manifestations of pituitary overactivity include Cushing syndrome from ACTH-secreting tumors; acromegaly from growth hormone secretion; hyperthyroidism from TSH production; and gynecomastia, lactation, and sex hormone-related changes from prolactin and gonadotropin (follicle stimulating and luteinizing hormones) secretion. These hormones are all produced by the anterior lobe of the pituitary and are controlled by a feedback loop from the hypothalamus. The posterior pituitary stores and secretes vasopressin and oxytocin, which are synthesized in the hypothalamus.

Acromegaly results in enlargement of connective tissue, bone, and visceral organs. Affected individuals have an enlarged jaw (i.e., macrognathia), nose, feet, hands, pharyngeal tissue, and laryngeal tissue (including macroglossia and enlarged epiglottis). Affected individuals have increased risks of sleep apnea (both central and obstructive), neuropathies (from nerve entrapment), hypertension, diastolic dysfunction, and cardiac valvular abnormalities. IHD, heart failure, diabetes mellitus, hypothyroidism, and difficult airway management (i.e., mask ventilation, laryngoscopy, intubation) may also occur. The preoperative evaluation should document any chest pain, dyspnea, snoring, numbness, polydipsia, headaches, and visual disturbances. The physical examination focuses on blood pressure, airway examination, murmurs, neurologic findings, and peripheral edema. It is important to plan for possible difficult airway management and inform the patient about the possible use of awake fiberoptic intubation. Preoperative testing may include an ECG and blood sampling for electrolyte concentration, glucose concentration, and thyroid function tests. TSH increases production of thyroid hormones (T_3 and T_4) by the thyroid gland (see section on "Thyroid Disease"). Prolactin- and gonadotropin-secreting tumors have little impact on anesthetic management, but their symptoms may alert clinicians to an undiagnosed pituitary tumor.

Posterior pituitary tumors result in failure to secrete vasopressin or ADH, which regulates renal water excretion. A deficiency results in diabetes insipidus, which is characterized by excessive urine output from a failure to reabsorb water. Unless treated with DDAVP, these patients may develop hypernatremia and volume depletion. The anesthesiologist should therefore carefully evaluate patients' intravascular volume status and conduct blood sampling for electrolyte concentrations and creatinine concentrations. Patients with pituitary tumors, pituitary apoplexy (hemorrhage into pituitary, which is associated with hypertension, trauma, or pregnancy), or previous pituitary tumor resection may require hormone replacement therapy (i.e., corticosteroids, thyroid replacement, DDAVP). These medications must not be interrupted during the perioperative period. The adequacy of replacement therapy can be determined based on the clinical evaluation, as well as blood sampling for electrolyte concentrations, creatinine concentrations, and thyroid function tests.

Other intracranial tumors include gliomas (45% of tumors), astrocytomas, ependymomas, medulloblastomas, oligodendrocytomas (malignant and highly lethal), benign meningiomas (15% of tumors), schwannomas, craniopharyngiomas, and dermoid tumors. Metastatic lesions (6% of intracranial tumors) can also occur with virtually all types of primary malignant diseases. Common sources of metastatic intracranial lesions include breast, colorectal, and lung cancers. Most intracranial tumors are detected either incidentally, or when patients develop seizures or symptoms related to mass effect. Symptoms of mass effect include headaches, strokelike symptoms, vomiting, visual disturbances, altered cognitive function, and ataxia. If the intracranial pressure becomes elevated, hypertension, bradycardia, arrhythmias, ECG abnormalities, and brainstem herniation may occur. Careful assessment of neurologic deficits is important. For patients with metastatic lesions, issues pertaining to the primary malignant disease and previous treatment (e.g., chemotherapy, radiation, corticosteroids, anticonvulsants) must be clarified. Continuation of preexisting corticosteroids (to treat cerebral edema) and anticonvulsant medications is important.

MUSCULOSKELETAL AND CONNECTIVE TISSUE DISEASES

These disorders are characterized by musculoskeletal deformities and chronic inflammation. Assessment of deformities is important because of their potential implications for airway management and regional anesthesia technique. Chronic inflammation—which occurs with rheumatoid arthritis, SLE, and systemic sclerosis—can cause vasculopathy and multiorgan dysfunction. Affected organ systems may include cardiovascular, pulmonary, renal, hematologic, integumentary, gastrointestinal, central nervous, and peripheral nervous systems.

Rheumatoid Arthritis

Rheumatoid arthritis is a chronic autoimmune disorder that primarily affects joints, but it often also affects multiple organ systems. The disease affects approximately 1% of the population, and women are 2 to 3 times more likely to be affected as are men.[366] Distal joints are involved more often than proximal, often in a symmetric pattern. Joint involvement is characterized by inflammation that can progress to severe deformity, although the disease course can vary dramatically. The temporomandibular joints and cricoarytenoid cartilage can be involved, resulting in limited mouth opening, hoarseness, and possible difficulties with airway management. Atlantodens subluxation and instability of the cervical spine can also occur. Subluxation, which is caused by ligamentous laxity, as opposed to joint disease, may also occur, although the prevalence appears to be decreasing with the advent of improved disease modifying agents. Cervical spine disease can be asymptomatic. IHD, pericardial effusions, aortic regurgitation, and conduction abnormalities may be present in affected individuals. Symptoms of myocardial ischemia may be masked in patients with rheumatoid arthritis because of impairment of functional status by concomitant joint disease. In addition, exertional dyspnea because of heart failure may be confused with pulmonary involvement. Pulmonary manifestations include restrictive lung disease secondary to decreased thoracic mobility, pulmonary fibrosis, and pleural effusions. Patients have an increased risk of renal dysfunction secondary to both vasculitis and long-term NSAID use. Peripheral neuropathy can result from vasculitis or entrapment. Anemia, leukocytosis, thrombocytosis (from chronic inflammation), and thrombocytopenia (from splenomegaly) may be present. Patients may also have rheumatoid nodules that occur subcutaneously (usually over extensor joints) or in the lungs.

The preoperative examination must document symptoms related to the many organ systems affected by rheumatoid arthritis. Special detail is directed to the neurologic, airway, pulmonary, and cardiovascular systems. Documentation of deformities and neurologic deficits is important to establish a baseline level of function. Significant hoarseness should prompt an evaluation by an otolaryngologist to assess the mobility of the vocal cords and the presence of cricoarytenoid arthritis. A careful history may elicit neurologic deficits, neck pain, upper extremity pain, or crunching sound with neck movement. Indications for preoperative cervical spine radiographs include neurologic findings, long-standing severely deforming disease, or procedures requiring prone positioning or manipulation of the cervical spine. The specific radiographs required are anteroposterior and lateral cervical spine films with flexion, extension, and open-mouth odontoid views.[367] Significant abnormalities (i.e., anterior atlas-dens interval >9 mm or posterior interval <14 mm) require consultation with a neurologist or neurosurgeon. Notably, disease duration, severity, and symptoms do not correlate with cervical spine subluxation. New or worsening pulmonary symptoms should prompt further evaluation with pulse oximetry, chest radiographs, PFTs, or possibly a pulmonary consultation. Muffled heart sounds, pericardial rubs, and low voltage on an ECG suggest a pericardial effusion, which necessitates an echocardiogram. Any suspicious murmur merits an echocardiogram in these patients. Because rheumatoid arthritis is associated with a very high prevalence of IHD, patients may require ECGs and possible cardiac stress testing (with subsequent cardiology referral as indicated). Other preoperative tests include blood sampling for CBC and creatinine concentrations.

Advanced planning for management of potential difficult airways is important, including discussion of regional anesthetic options and possible awake fiberoptic intubation. When possible, corticosteroids, analgesics, and nonbiological disease modifying agents (e.g., methotrexate, leflunomide, hydroxychloroquine, sulfasalazine) should be continued, although consideration can be given to stopping NSAIDs 2 to 3 days before surgery. There are more concerns regarding whether biological disease modifying agents (i.e., tumor necrosis factor alpha antagonists) should be stopped before surgery, especially since continued treatment may predispose patients to postoperative infections. Several guidelines recommend holding these agents before surgery,[368,369] although there is uncertainty regarding when treatment should be stopped relative to surgery. Especially since these drugs have different dosing cycles, patients with complex immunosuppressant therapy are best managed collaboratively with their rheumatologist, primary care physician, and surgeon. Stress-associated adrenal insufficiency may occur in patients taking preoperative corticosteroid therapy. Details on which patients warrant perioperative stress dose corticosteroids, as well as a suggested dosing regimen, are presented in the section on "Hypothalamic-Pituitary-Adrenal Disorders" and Table 31.15.

Ankylosing Spondylitis

Ankylosing spondylitis is a progressive inflammatory arthropathy that primarily affects the spine and sacroiliac joints, although peripheral joints may also be involved. It usually occurs in males. Ankylosing spondylitis can have important extraarticular manifestations, including uveitis, vasculitis, aortitis, and aortic insufficiency. Affected individuals may develop restrictive lung disease related to pulmonary fibrosis or chest wall movement restriction (joint fixation and kyphosis). Kyphosis can be so extreme that patients are unable to face forward, thereby making mask ventilation, direct laryngoscopy, and intubation very difficult. The patient's preoperative evaluation should focus on the cardiovascular, pulmonary, and musculoskeletal systems, with the physical examination including measurement of oxygen saturation on room air. The presence of a murmur on physical examination warrants an echocardiogram. If ventilatory compromise is suspected or present, a chest radiograph and PFTs are necessary. Most analgesic medications and non-biological disease modifying agents (e.g., sulfasalazine) can be continued preoperatively, although consideration can be given to stopping NSAIDs 2 to 3 days before surgery. Several guidelines recommend holding biological disease modifying agents (i.e., tumor necrosis factor alpha antagonists) before surgery,[368,369] although there is uncertainty regarding when treatment should be stopped relative to surgery. Especially since these drugs have different dosing cycles, patients with complex immunosuppressant therapy are best managed collaboratively with their rheumatologist, primary care physician, and surgeon. It is important to plan for perioperative airway management and inform the patient about the possibility of awake fiberoptic intubation. Peripheral nerve blocks are an option, but neuraxial anesthesia is often unsuccessful in the presence of severe spinal involvement.

Systemic Lupus Erythematosus

SLE is a systemic autoimmune disease that is predominantly caused by vasculitis. It has a variable course with flares and remission periods. SLE is more likely to affect females (i.e., seven-fold higher prevalence in adults), as well as individuals with East Asian or African-American ethnic backgrounds.[370] The multiorgan disease has musculoskeletal, cardiovascular, pulmonary, renal, neurological, dermatological, hematological, gastrointestinal, and constitutional manifestations. Common constitutional symptoms are fever and chronic fatigue. The fevers may be explained by disease activity itself, as well as frequent infections related to disease-induced immune dysfunction and immunosuppressant treatment. The musculoskeletal findings are typically a migratory arthritis of the small joints in the hands and feet. Many patients have dermatologic conditions including alopecia, photosensitivity, and a typical "butterfly rash" across the cheeks and nose. Vasospasm of the digits (i.e., Raynaud phenomenon), often associated with atrophy of nails and fingernails, can make it difficult to obtain pulse oximetry readings. Pulmonary manifestations include interstitial lung disease, pleural effusions, frequent respiratory infections, and pulmonary hypertension. Pulmonary hypertension, which can result from recurrent pulmonary emboli, pulmonary vasculopathy, and interstitial lung disease, carries a high risk of perioperative complications.[371] Cardiovascular involvement includes hypertension (often difficult to control), premature IHD, pericarditis, myocarditis, coronary artery vasculitis, cardiomyopathy, aseptic endocarditis, and pleural effusions. Neurologic disease includes cerebral vasculitis, stroke, CVD, cognitive dysfunction, seizures, peripheral neuropathy, headache, neuropsychiatric manifestations, and affective disorders. Lupus nephritis is a common end-organ complication that carries a poor prognosis and often results in ESRD. Patients with SLE may have anemia, leukopenia, thrombocytopenia, and antiphospholipid antibodies. Individuals with these antibodies typically have a prolonged aPTT, but are predisposed to pulmonary emboli, stroke, and recurrent venous or arterial thromboses.

The preoperative evaluation should assess all major organ systems and relevant medications. Patients with severe disease, infections, or exacerbations are best managed collaboratively with their rheumatologist or primary physician. The history should cover details on typical disease flairs (manifestations, timing, treatment), fevers, cardiovascular symptoms (e.g., dyspnea, chest pain, orthopnea), neurologic symptoms (e.g., stroke, seizures), renal disease, prior thromboembolic events, and fevers. Given the prevalence of IHD and CVD in these patients, the evaluation should include reviewing results of any previous relevant diagnostic studies (e.g., cardiac stress testing, echocardiography, computed tomography, MRI). The preoperative physical examination concentrates on the pulmonary (rales, decreased breath sounds), cardiac (pericardial rubs, murmurs, arrhythmias, jugular venous distention, peripheral edema), and nervous (motor deficits, sensory deficits, visual disturbances) systems. Helpful preoperative tests include an ECG and blood sampling for CBC, electrolyte concentrations, glucose concentrations, creatinine concentrations, and aPTT (unless the patient has a known antiphospholipid syndrome). Significant ECG abnormalities (e.g., conduction delays, arrhythmias, Q waves, low voltage) should prompt consideration for further testing, cardiology consultation, or pulmonology consultation. Other tests that may be considered include an INR (patients receiving warfarin), echocardiogram (murmurs, suspected heart failure, suspected effusion), chest radiograph (pulmonary symptoms or suspected heart failure), and PFTs (worsening or undiagnosed dyspnea). Patients with advanced cardiomyopathy, decompensated heart failure, pulmonary hypertension, systemic vasculitis, and recent or recurrent thromboembolism are considered to be at high risk, and they are best managed in concert with the appropriate specialists. Most medications, including corticosteroids and non-biological disease-modifying agents (e.g., hydroxychloroquine, cyclosporine, azathioprine, tacrolimus) should be continued. Patients on long-term corticosteroid therapy may need perioperative stress dose corticosteroids. Details on patient selection for such therapy, as well as a suggested dosing regimen, are presented in the section on "Hypothalamic-Pituitary-Adrenal Disorders" and Table 31.15. Medications that require temporary preoperative discontinuation include anticoagulant therapy; consultation with a hematologist may be necessary to plan perioperative anticoagulation management, including the possible need for bridging therapy. Similarly, patients with complex biological immunosuppressant therapy for SLE (e.g., belimumab) are best managed collaboratively with their rheumatologist.

Systemic Sclerosis

Systemic sclerosis (previously known as scleroderma) is an autoimmune multisystem disease that is characterized by excessive fibrosis. It occurs more commonly in females.[372] Aside from skin thickening, the most common skin manifestation is Raynaud phenomenon. Scleroderma has several variants, which are differentiated based on the extent of skin and internal organ involvement. *Localized scleroderma* involves just the skin, and no other organs. *Limited systemic sclerosis* has cutaneous manifestations "limited" to face and upper extremities, as well as systemic involvement in the gastrointestinal tract (e.g., dysphagia, reflux) and lungs (e.g., interstitial lung disease, pulmonary hypertension). *Diffuse systemic sclerosis* is characterized by generalized skin involvement and multiple end-organ damage. Manifestations include myocardial fibrosis, pericarditis, heart failure (right-sided and left-sided), coronary artery fibrosis, severe hypertension, ESRD, dysphagia, fatigue, weight loss, and gastroesophageal reflux. Pulmonary hypertension, which may result from interstitial lung disease or vasculopathy, is a leading cause of death in systemic sclerosis and is associated with increased perioperative risk.[371]

The preoperative evaluation focuses on the organ systems in the manner outlined previously in the section on SLE, with special attention to evidence of pulmonary hypertension (see section on "Pulmonary Hypertension"). The history should evaluate for any evidence of pulmonary disease (e.g., cough, dyspnea) or cardiac disease (e.g., dyspnea, orthopnea, chest pain). Patients may develop limited mouth opening, limited neck mobility, poor dentition, and oropharyngeal lesions secondary to skin involvement. Careful airway evaluation and planning for airway management are essential in such individuals, especially because they may also be at high risk for aspiration secondary to gastroesophageal reflux. Dermal involvement, edema, and contractures may also make venous access and regional anesthesia technically challenging. Thus, it is helpful to discuss central venous access and possible awake fiberoptic intubation during the preoperative assessment; in some cases, consideration should be given to arranging for interventional radiology to place intravenous lines.

Patients with systemic sclerosis usually need an ECG, and blood sampling for CBC (especially if receiving immunosuppressant therapy) and creatinine concentration. A chest radiograph and PFTs can be useful if interstitial lung disease or pulmonary fibrosis is suspected. Echocardiography (i.e., right ventricular size, right ventricular function, estimated right ventricular systolic pressure) may be useful to screen patients with suspected pulmonary hypertension. Antihypertensive agents (including calcium channel blockers for Raynaud phenomenon) and immunosuppressant therapy should be continued.

Raynaud Phenomenon

Raynaud phenomenon is an exaggerated vascular response to cold or emotional stress that results in color changes of the digits (typical sequence is pallor to cyanosis to rubor).[373] It is classified as primary (termed *Raynaud disease*) or secondary (termed *Raynaud phenomenon*). Raynaud phenomenon is associated with connective tissue diseases, autoimmune disorders, drugs, and use of vibrating tools. Connective tissue diseases associated with Raynaud phenomenon include systemic sclerosis, Sjögren disease, SLE, and possibly rheumatoid arthritis. Raynaud phenomenon most often affects the hands, typically resulting in a sudden onset of cold digits with sharply demarcated pallor or cyanosis. Cutaneous vasospasm is also common in other sites, such as the face and ears, where it causes pain and numbness. Criteria for the diagnosis of Raynaud disease include symmetric episodic attacks, absence of PAD, absence of tissue injury (or gangrene), normal nail fold capillary examination, normal erythrocyte sedimentation rate, and negative antinuclear antibody test. Raynaud disease requires no special additional preoperative evaluation. Secondary Raynaud phenomenon should prompt an assessment for associated disease states. It is also important to distinguish Raynaud phenomenon from PAD, especially given the difference in associated comorbidities. Calcium channel blockers are useful treatments in many patients and should be continued in the perioperative period.

Inherited Connective Tissue Disorders

Ehlers-Danlos syndrome is a disorder of collagen synthesis. It consists of several subtypes that have various manifestations but are almost all characterized by joint hypermobility. Type IV disease is more serious because affected individuals may have vascular fragility and skin fragility, as well as predisposition to vascular rupture, visceral rupture, and pneumothorax. Patients with type VI Ehlers-Danlos syndrome have muscle weakness, scoliosis, ocular fragility, skin fragility, and osteopenia.

Marfan syndrome is characterized by tall stature, arachnodactyly (i.e., long digits), scoliosis, pectus excavatum, valvular disease (e.g., aortic insufficiency, mitral valve prolapse, mitral regurgitation), arrhythmias, and ascending aortic dilatation. These patients are at risk for aortic dissection. Ocular (e.g., ectopia lentis, strabismus, glaucoma) and pulmonary (e.g., spontaneous pneumothorax) complications can also occur.[374] Other manifestations include retrognathia and high arched palates. Careful auscultation for the diastolic murmur of aortic insufficiency is important (see Table 31.8). If such a murmur is detected, subsequent tests should include an echocardiogram and chest radiograph. The most distinguishing feature of osteogenesis imperfecta is the propensity for fractures from extremely fragile bones.

These patients may have blue sclerae, short stature, scoliosis, joint hypermobility, hearing loss, muscle weakness, mitral valve prolapse, aortic insufficiency, and platelet dysfunction. An ECG and echocardiogram are necessary if physical examination reveals a murmur. Epidermolysis bullosa is distinguished by blistering, skin fragility, and scarring caused by abnormal epidermal-dermal anchoring. Even noninvasive blood pressure measurement may cause skin blistering and breakdown in an affected individual.

Kyphoscoliosis

Kyphoscoliosis is a curvature of the spine in both lateral and posterior directions. It can involve the thoracic region, the lumbar region, or both. Kyphoscoliosis may occur alone or as a manifestation of other diseases (e.g., collagen vascular disorders, Marfan syndrome, neurofibromatosis, muscular dystrophies, cerebral palsy). Therefore, the preoperative evaluation should also focus on identifying any coexisting abnormalities. Severe thoracic deformity may cause cardiopulmonary compromise as a consequence of restrictive lung disease, pulmonary hypertension, heart failure, tracheobronchial compression, or cardiac compression. The history should focus on assessing cardiopulmonary symptoms. The ability of the patient to lie supine (to facilitate airway access and management) must also be determined. The physical examination should evaluate vital signs (including oxygen saturation), pulmonary system (rales, decreased air entry), and cardiovascular system (murmurs, additional heart sounds, edema, jugular venous distention). A CBC, as well as a blood type and screen, is required in any patient scheduled to undergo spine correction surgery for kyphoscoliosis. Additionally, an ECG and chest radiograph may be useful. If heart failure is suspected based on clinical evaluation, a preoperative echocardiogram should be performed. Any reversible lung disease or heart failure must be optimized preoperatively.

CANCERS AND TUMORS IN PREOPERATIVE PATIENTS

Patients With Cancer

Patients with cancer may have complications related to both the disease itself and its treatment (e.g., chemotherapy, radiation therapy). Typically, patients are aware of the side effects of their cancer treatments. It is helpful to ask them whether any unexpected complications occurred during treatment, or whether chemotherapy or radiation therapy had to be interrupted because of adverse effects. A hypercoagulable state is also common in cancer, particularly advanced disease, primary brain tumors, ovarian adenocarcinoma, pancreatic cancer, colon cancer, gastric cancer, lung cancer, prostate cancer, and kidney tumors. The risk of thromboembolic events is increased six-fold in patients with cancer, with active cancer accounting for 20% of new cases of thromboembolism.

The preoperative evaluation focuses on cardiac, pulmonary, neurologic, and hematologic systems. Previous head and neck irradiation may cause carotid artery disease, hypothyroidism, or difficulty with airway management. Auscultation for bruits, thyroid function tests, and carotid Doppler studies are therefore recommended. Mediastinal, chest wall, or left breast irradiation can cause pericarditis, conduction abnormalities, cardiomyopathy, valvular heart disease, and premature IHD (even in the absence of traditional cardiovascular risk factors).[375] Thus, younger patients with a history of radiation therapy should be assessed for cardiac symptoms and undergo an ECG—even if they may not otherwise be at risk for heart disease. Based on these initial results, stress testing and echocardiography may be indicated. Previous irradiation to the lungs, breast, or mediastinum may also cause radiation pneumonitis. In such individuals, an oxygen saturation measurement and chest radiograph may be required, with consideration for PFTs if appropriate.

Other important chemotherapy-associated side effects include cardiomyopathy with trastuzumab and anthracyclines (e.g., doxorubicin); pulmonary toxicity with bleomycin; nephrotoxicity with cisplatin; hemorrhagic cystitis with cyclophosphamide; and peripheral neuropathy with vincristine or cisplatin. Many chemotherapeutic agents are toxic to the bone marrow, and patients commonly exhibit preoperative anemia. Patients who received corticosteroids as part of their cancer treatment may be at risk for adrenal insufficiency. These individuals may require supplemental perioperative corticosteroids; details on patient selection for such therapy, as well as a suggested dosing regimen, are presented in the section on "Hypothalamic-Pituitary-Adrenal Disorders" and Table 31.15. Other chemotherapy drugs result in impaired postsurgical wound healing, especially antiangiogenic agents (e.g., bevacizumab, sunitinib, sorafenib, pazopanib, vandetanib, cabozantinib, axitinib). Consequently, elective major surgery should be scheduled after temporary discontinuation of these agents, whenever feasible. The time interval for preoperative discontinuation varies across these agents from 28 days (bevacizumab) to 1 week (sunitinib, sorafenib, pazopanib, vandetanib, cabozantinib) to 48 hours (axitinib). Based on the type of chemotherapy, an ECG, chest radiograph, and blood sampling for CBC, electrolyte concentrations, creatinine concentration, and liver function tests may be needed. In some cases, consideration may be given to delaying the surgical procedure to allow resolution of neutropenia and thrombocytopenia. In general, advance planning of blood component replacement (including type and screening in the preoperative clinic) can avoid delays on the day of surgery.

The direct effects of cancers depend on the specific organ systems involved. Issues pertaining to intracranial tumors are discussed in the section on "Central Nervous System Tumors". Bone and liver involvement with metastases can commonly occur in patients with breast, colorectal, lung, and head and neck tumors. These bony lesions can in turn cause hypercalcemia or pancytopenia. Head and neck tumors, and their associated therapy (e.g., surgery, radiation), may cause thyroid dysfunction and difficulty with airway management. Lung cancer can cause airway problems, compromised pulmonary function, or mediastinal masses (see section on "Mediastinal Masses"). In these cases, computed tomography scans of the head, neck, or chest may be indicated. Paraneoplastic syndromes can complicate almost any type of malignant disease but are most commonly seen with lung cancer. Typical manifestations of these syndromes include hypercalcemia, inappropriate ADH secretion, Lambert-Eaton syndrome, Cushing syndrome, and neuropathies.

Patients who are receiving opioids on a long-term basis for cancer pain are likely to require larger than usual doses of medication for postoperative pain control (see the later section on "Planning for Postoperative Pain Management"). On the day of surgery, these patients typically take their usual analgesic medications, with the exception of NSAIDs (which, if possible, should be stopped 2-3 days before surgery).

Mediastinal Masses

Tumors that may occur in the anterior mediastinal space include lymphomas, thymomas, teratomas, thyroid goiters, and metastatic tumors. Anterior mediastinal masses can obstruct the great vessels (i.e., aorta, pulmonary arteries, pulmonary vein, superior vena cava), heart, trachea, and bronchi. Patients may complain of dyspnea, dysphagia, stridor, wheezing, coughing (especially when recumbent), and orthopnea. Compression of the superior vena cava can result in superior vena cava syndrome, which is characterized by jugular venous distention as well as edema in the face, neck, chest, and upper extremities. Affected individuals may also develop increased intracranial pressure and airway compromise. Imaging of the chest (with computed tomography or MRI) and echocardiography are needed if airway, cardiac, or vascular compression is suspected. Flow-volume loops may also be useful to assess the location (extrathoracic vs. intrathoracic) and degree of airway obstruction. Patients with tracheobronchial, cardiac, or major vessel compression require special anesthetic precautions, including possible awake fiberoptic intubation.

Von Hippel–Lindau disease

von Hippel–Lindau disease is an autosomal dominant inherited disorder characterized by a variety of benign and malignant tumors. Associated tumors include hemangioblastomas, retinal angiomas, clear cell renal cell carcinomas, pheochromocytomas, and neuroendocrine tumors of the pancreas. During preoperative evaluation, the anesthesiologist should assess for symptoms suggestive of a pheochromocytoma or neuroendocrine tumor (see relevant sections of this Chapter), as well as evaluate the patient's renal function. Any further testing (e.g., electrolytes, ECG, creatinine, glucose) should be guided by findings from the initial clinical evaluation.

Carcinoid Tumors

Carcinoid tumors are rare neuroendocrine tumors that release mediators. They are associated with MEN type 1. These tumors typically occur in the gastrointestinal tract and are the most common neoplasms of the appendix; in addition, they can also occur in the pancreas and bronchi. Carcinoid syndrome is caused by vasoactive amines (e.g., serotonin, norepinephrine, histamine, dopamine), polypeptides (e.g., bradykinin, somatostatin, vasoactive intestinal peptide, glucagon), and prostaglandins released by the tumors. Typical manifestations include flushing, tachycardia, arrhythmias, diarrhea, malnutrition, bronchospasm, and carcinoid heart disease. Nonetheless, most patients are asymptomatic because the liver inactivates the bioactive products of carcinoid tumors. Consequently, patients with gastrointestinal carcinoid tumors have manifestations of carcinoid syndrome only if they have hepatic metastases. Carcinoid heart disease is characterized by endocardial fibrosis of pulmonic and tricuspid valves. Affected individuals may then develop tricuspid regurgitation, pulmonic stenosis, pulmonic regurgitation, right-sided heart failure, peripheral edema, and hepatomegaly. They may also develop *carcinoid crisis*, which is associated with profound flushing, bronchospasm, tachycardia, and hemodynamic instability. These life-threatening episodes can occur with induction of anesthesia, intraoperative handling of a tumor, or other invasive procedure on a tumor (e.g., tumor embolization).[376]

The preoperative clinical evaluation should focus on dyspnea, orthopnea, wheezing, edema, arrhythmias, and murmurs; subsequent diagnostic tests are guided by the initial assessment. Patients with chronic diarrhea need measurement of electrolyte and creatinine concentrations. Patients with cardiac involvement must have an ECG and echocardiogram. Malnourished patients need an ECG, as well as measurement of electrolyte and albumin concentrations. Predictors of perioperative adverse events in these patients are carcinoid heart disease and elevated urinary 5-hydroxyindoleacetic acid concentrations.[377] The mainstay of pharmacologic treatment of carcinoid syndrome are somatostatin analogues, namely octreotide and lanreotide. Preoperative treatment with octreotide (300-500 μg intravenous or subcutaneously) helps mitigate the risks of intraoperative carcinoid crises.[378] An alternative approach for high-risk major procedures is to start a continuous intravenous 50 μg /hour infusion of octreotide 12 hours before surgery and continue it for at least 24 to 48 hours after surgery.[376]

Special Issues in Preoperative Evaluation

PSEUDOCHOLINESTERASE DEFICIENCY

A personal or family history of pseudocholinesterase, or butyrylcholinesterase, deficiency should be identified preoperatively (see Chapter 35). Pseudocholinesterase, which is found in the plasma, liver, pancreas, heart, and brain, is distinct from acetylcholinesterase, which is found in erythrocytes. Patients with an "allergy to succinylcholine" should be suspected of having either this disorder or malignant hyperthermia. Previous anesthetic records may help clarify an uncertain history. Additionally, inquiring whether the patient was intubated postoperatively, gravely ill, or in need of intensive care may be helpful.

Pseudocholinesterase activity may be permanently reduced because of abnormal genotypes, or transiently altered because of disease, drugs, pregnancy, or infancy. In patients with a history suggestive of pseudocholinesterase deficiency, recommended testing includes plasma cholinesterase activity, dibucaine number, and fluoride number. Plasma cholinesterase activity is a *quantitative* measure of enzyme activity, whereas the dibucaine number and fluoride number are *qualitative* measures. Plasma cholinesterase activity should not be confused with acetylcholinesterase activity, which is an assessment of erythrocyte cholinesterase. The *dibucaine number* represents the percentage inhibition of the enzyme by the local anesthetic dibucaine, and the fluoride number represents the percentage inhibition by fluoride. Normal individuals—who are homozygous for the wild-type gene—have a dibucaine number of 80 because their plasma cholinesterase is 80% inhibited by dibucaine. Individuals who are homozygous for the atypical genes have a dibucaine number of 20 (corresponding to 20% inhibition) and can be paralyzed for 4 to 8 hours after receiving succinylcholine. In heterozygous individuals who have a dibucaine number of 60 (corresponding to 60% inhibition), the duration of action of succinylcholine is prolonged by 50% to 100%. The combination of dibucaine number and plasma cholinesterase activity therefore differentiates genetic from acquired causes of prolonged apnea after succinylcholine administration. Patients with known or suspected pseudocholinesterase deficiency should be encouraged to obtain proper medical alert identification. Additionally, they should be educated that the enzyme also metabolizes ester-linked local anesthetics.

MALIGNANT HYPERTHERMIA

A known history or suggestive history (e.g., hyperthermia or rigidity during anesthesia) of malignant hyperthermia in a patient or family member must be clearly documented in the preoperative assessment. This information must also be communicated to the surgeon and eventual anesthesia provider—especially to ensure that appropriate arrangements are made preoperatively (see Chapter 35). Individuals who are genetically predisposed to malignant hyperthermia are asymptomatic until they are exposed to triggering agents. Certain neuromuscular diseases are also associated with elevated risks of malignant hyperthermia, including some muscular dystrophies (i.e., Duchenne, Becker, myotonic), King-Denborough syndrome, central core disease, periodic paralysis, osteogenesis imperfecta, myelomeningocele, and strabismus.

MORBIDLY OBESE PATIENTS

The morbidly obese patient presents special preoperative risks. Obesity is associated with several important comorbidities, including diabetes mellitus, hypertension, cardiovascular disease, CVD, cancer, OSA (see the earlier section on "Obstructive Sleep Apnea"), and poor functional capacity. Obese individuals are also at risk for NASH, which can result in abnormal liver function tests, liver fibrosis, and end-stage liver disease. In addition, patients with extreme obesity are at risk for right-sided heart failure and pulmonary hypertension. Such individuals can have obesity-hypoventilation syndrome (OHS), also known as Pickwickian syndrome. OHS is characterized by impaired central ventilatory drive and is distinct from OSA. It is associated with awake, chronic hypoxemia ($PaO_2 < 65$ mm Hg) without a diagnosis of COPD or primary lung disease. In the perioperative setting, obese patients experience higher rates of difficult bag-mask ventilation and difficult tracheal intubation.

The preoperative evaluation focuses on relevant coexisting diseases, airway, cardiopulmonary system, and vital signs (including pulse oximetry). When measuring blood pressure, the cuff should have a width that is approximately two thirds of the arm and a length that can adequately encircle the extremity. Assessment of neck circumference can also identify individuals at risk for difficulty with endotracheal intubation. It is also helpful to determine both actual body weight and ideal body weight. Determination of ideal body weight may be helpful in dose selection for certain medications (e.g., neuromuscular blockers),[379] and for determining optimal intraoperative mechanical ventilation settings. Treatments for obesity can have important perioperative implications. For example, drugs or other weight reduction methods (e.g., purging, diuretics, laxatives, gastric bypass procedures) may result in electrolyte abnormalities, vitamin deficiencies, malnutrition, anemia, and cardiopulmonary disorders. Two previously available antiobesity medications, fenfluramine and dexfenfluramine (both were withdrawn from the market in 1997), had significant cardiac side effects, including regurgitant valvular lesions and pulmonary hypertension. Any individual who was ever exposed to these drugs should undergo a cardiovascular evaluation, including an echocardiogram.

PATIENTS WITH TRANSPLANTED ORGANS

The number of patients with transplanted organs who require nontransplant surgical procedures increases yearly. During preoperative evaluation, these patients present special issues relating to transplant function, allograft denervation, immunosuppression, and other posttransplant physiologic and pharmacologic issues. Close interaction with the transplant team is one of the most important steps in the perioperative care of these patients. Clinicians performing the preoperative assessment should ensure that the transplant care providers are made aware of the upcoming procedure and are given an opportunity to make recommendations.

Some general preoperative considerations apply to all transplant recipients, as well as additional concerns based on the specific organ transplanted. In all transplant recipients, the level of function of the transplanted organ and the presence of any rejection should be evaluated. The dosage regimen of all immunosuppressant medications should be noted, and patients should be instructed to continue these medications perioperatively. However, these drugs can modify the pharmacology of many other agents administered during the perioperative period, as has been extensively summarized in the literature.[380,381] Patients should also be assessed for complications related to immunosuppressant therapy. These complications include the following: hyperglycemia and adrenal suppression (corticosteroids); increased risks of infection, hypertension, and renal insufficiency (corticosteroids, cyclosporine, tacrolimus); and myelosuppression causing anemia, thrombocytopenia, and leukopenia (azathioprine, sirolimus). Although transplant recipients are at increased risk for postoperative infections, no evidence indicates that higher doses of antibiotic prophylaxis provide added benefit. Instead, usual preoperative recommendations for antibiotic prophylaxis should be followed. Stress-associated adrenal insufficiency may occur in patients taking long-term corticosteroid therapy. Details on which patients warrant perioperative stress dose corticosteroids, as well as a suggested dosing regimen, are presented in the section on "Hypothalamic-Pituitary-Adrenal Disorders" and Table 31.15.

Cardiac evaluation is important in all transplant recipients because they are at increased risk for cardiovascular disease. The basis for this increased risk includes the underlying diseases that led to organ failure (e.g., diabetes mellitus, hypertension) and the potential for drug regimens, transplantation, and rejection episodes to create or worsen traditional cardiovascular risk factors. Preoperative renal function should also be assessed because long-term immunosuppressive regimens often lead to CKD. Although the effects of transplantation and immunosuppressive regimens on intravascular coagulation are controversial, thromboprophylaxis should be considered in all transplant recipients.

Kidney transplant recipients present some specific issues for preoperative evaluation. Despite the presence of a normal creatinine concentration, GFR in these individuals is generally decreased. This impairment in renal function predisposes these patients to electrolyte abnormalities and altered drug metabolism. Nephrotoxic drugs, such as NSAIDs and COX-2 inhibitors, should be avoided in all renal transplant recipients. In addition, their risk for cardiovascular disease is increased to approximately twice that of the general population. Careful preoperative cardiovascular evaluation is essential.

Successful liver transplantation usually resolves the hepatic and other end-organ effects of end-stage liver disease. Nonetheless, some pretransplant pulmonary problems may not resolve after transplantation, thus necessitating careful evaluation of pulmonary function. These disturbances can include hepatopulmonary syndrome, which involves hypoxemia from intrapulmonary vascular shunting. Other patients may continue to demonstrate ventilation-perfusion mismatch related to pulmonary effusions, ascites, or diaphragmatic dysfunction, as well as diffusion abnormalities resulting from interstitial pneumonitis or impaired hypoxic pulmonary vasoconstriction.

Following successful lung transplantation, recipients may require months to achieve peak pulmonary function. Compared with all other allografts, the transplanted lung is especially susceptible to infection and rejection as a result of its exposure to the external environment. Careful preoperative evaluation with PFTs should be considered in all lung transplant recipients, with postponement of elective surgery when allograft rejection or infection is suspected. Other perioperative considerations include airway hyperresponsiveness, loss of the cough reflex, and potential for injury to the airway anastomosis with intubation. These patients are also at increased risk for pulmonary edema, which has been attributed to disrupted lymphatic drainage in the transplanted lung.

Most issues relating to heart transplant recipients relate to the absence of autonomic innervation in the transplanted heart. This denervation has multiple physiologic effects, such as a higher than normal resting heart rate (from absence of vagal tone); the absence of cardiac baroreflexes; and the lack of response to carotid sinus massage, Valsalva maneuver, laryngoscopy, or tracheal intubation. Denervation also affects responses to medications; the allograft demonstrates a normal or augmented response to direct-acting drugs (e.g., epinephrine), a blunted response to indirect-acting agents (e.g., ephedrine), and no response to vagolytic agents. Chronic allograft rejection can manifest as accelerated IHD, and ventricular dysfunction (both systolic and diastolic). Because allograft denervation causes any myocardial ischemia to be silent, typical clinical manifestations include fatigue, ventricular dysrhythmias, heart failure, and ECG evidence of a silent myocardial infarction. Should preoperative evaluation raise clinical suspicions of worsening rejection, recent cardiac testing must be reviewed. Heart transplant recipients undergo routine periodic evaluation for IHD (cardiac stress testing or coronary angiography) and ventricular function (e.g., echocardiogram). The ECGs of these patients may reveal conduction abnormalities, and two P waves (a small nonconducted P wave from the native atria and a normal-sized conducted P wave from the donor atria). Many heart transplant recipients also require permanent pacemakers, and pacemaker function should be confirmed during the preoperative evaluation.

PATIENTS WITH ALLERGIES

The patient's preoperative evaluation record should carefully document any history of allergies and adverse drug reactions. True anaphylactic reactions should be distinguished from adverse side effects (e.g., nausea with opioid use), especially because a patient's definition of an allergy may differ significantly from the true clinical definition. In some cases, patients may incorrectly attribute previous perioperative difficulties to "allergies" to anesthetic or analgesic medications. The reported incidence of perioperative anaphylaxis is about 1 in 10,000 to procedures in large countrywide epidemiological studies, with consistent estimates based on studies from 2 different countries (France vs. United Kingdom) and time periods (2004 vs. 2016).[382,383] The overall incidence appears similar in these two epidemiological studies; however the common precipitating agents differ. In the older French study, the most common causes were neuromuscular blocking agents (58%), latex (20%), and antibiotics (13%).[383] Conversely, in the more recent United Kingdom study, the most common precipitating agents were antibiotics (53%), neuromuscular blocking agents (33%), and chlorhexidine (9%).[382] The mortality associated with an individual episode of anaphylaxis is about 4%,[384] but anaphylaxis accounts for up to 3% of perioperative deaths that are totally or partially related to anesthesia.[385] A careful history (including a review of records of prior allergic events and any associated laboratory tests) generally allows for avoidance of precipitating agents. In selected cases in which the clear diagnosis of a specific allergy is required to guide perioperative management, referral to an allergy specialist and possible skin testing (if the allergic reaction is believed to be immunoglobin E [IgE]-mediated) may be considered.

Allergic reactions to neuromuscular blocking drugs (NMBDs) are relatively more frequent in Europe as compared to North America. These differences have been attributed, in part, to the use of cough suppressants containing pholcodine in many European countries. Exposure to pholcodine is associated with development of IgE antibodies to NMBDs.[386] Confirmatory testing for an allergy to NMBDs can involve both skin testing and in-vitro assays for NMBD-specific IgE.

Although the rate of latex sensitization continues to increase, the development of better ways to identify at-risk patients has led to a decreased incidence of latex-induced anaphylaxis,[387] as evidenced by the absence of any latex-associated episodes in the recent epidemiological study from the United Kingdom.[382] The diagnosis of a latex allergy during preoperative evaluation is based on a careful history. Risk factors for latex allergy include a history of multiple surgeries, occupational exposure to latex (e.g., healthcare workers, food handlers), and an atopic history. This history may be supplemented with skin testing and latex-specific IgE antibody serology. When latex allergy is identified during the preoperative evaluation, the operative team should be notified in advance to ensure that all appropriate equipment is available. The ASA Task Force outlines detailed intraoperative considerations for these patients.[388] Among antibiotics, penicillins and cephalosporins are the most common causes of anaphylaxis. A small risk of cross-reactivity exists between penicillins and cephalosporins, but most of these reported reactions involve rashes, not anaphylaxis. Reported allergies to vancomycin should be distinguished from "red man syndrome." This histamine-induced side effect, which is associated with rapid injection of vancomycin, consists of flushing, pruritus, erythematous rash, and hypotension. With respect to other medications commonly encountered in the perioperative setting, anaphylactic reactions to amide local anesthetics are extremely rare. Most true anaphylactic reactions following exposure to ester local anesthetics do not involve an allergy to the local anesthetic, but rather to associated preservatives (e.g., *para*-aminobenzoic acid). Patients may incorrectly interpret adverse side effects from epinephrine in local anesthetic solutions as allergies, especially with dental procedures. Such reports should be carefully distinguished from true allergies. Similarly, true allergies to opioids are rare, with most reports of such "allergies" being simply opioid-related side effects, such as nausea and vomiting.

The scientific status of idiopathic environmental intolerance syndrome (formerly called multiple chemical sensitivity disorder) is very controversial. These individuals report chronic, diffuse, nonspecific symptoms with low levels of multiple chemical substances. Symptoms involve multiple organ systems and include fatigue, headache, memory loss, palpitations, and gastrointestinal symptoms. The symptoms are not generally accompanied by biologic test abnormalities or changes on physical examination, but they are frequently associated with psychiatric symptoms, notably depression and anxiety.[389] Preoperative evaluation of these patients can be extremely challenging because they have significant concerns about the multiple exposures involved during the perioperative period and the potential impact on their symptoms. No current recommendations are available on the perioperative care of these patients.

HUMAN IMMUNODEFICIENCY VIRUS INFECTION

Acute infection with HIV causes a mononucleosis-like illness, which then progresses to chronic lymphadenopathy (lasting 3-5 years). Infection can culminate in cell-mediated immune deficiency characterized by opportunistic infections, malignant diseases (e.g., Kaposi sarcoma, non-Hodgkin lymphoma), and death (usually secondary from infections, wasting, or cancer). The prognosis of untreated HIV infection and acquired immunodeficiency syndrome (AIDS) is very poor.[390] Nonetheless, outcomes have now improved substantially in individuals compliant with highly active antiretroviral therapy.[391] Risk factors for HIV infection include sexual contact with an infected individual, bloodborne contamination, men who have sex with men, sexual workers, and those having contact with sexual workers. Most infection transmitted by blood exposure occurs in intravenous drug users, whereas infection through blood product transfusion in the United States is very rare (1 per 1.5-2 million blood transfusions). Mothers can transmit the disease to infants, which occurs usually during breastfeeding or delivery.[392] Many patients infected with HIV are unaware of their status.

HIV infection is a multisystem disease.[393] Cardiac complications include myocarditis, dilated cardiomyopathy, valvular disease, pulmonary hypertension, pericardial effusions, and cardiac tamponade. Pulmonary effects include lymphoid interstitial pneumonitis, as well as drug-resistant infections with *Pneumocystis jiroveci*, *Mycobacterium avium*, or *Mycobacterium tuberculosis*, cytomegalovirus, and *Cryptococcus*. Nervous system manifestations include central nervous system tumors, infections, aseptic meningitis, and AIDS-related dementia. Malignant diseases can occur, such as lymphomas, Kaposi sarcoma, and cervical cancer. These tumors can also have direct consequences for anesthetic management. For example, supraglottic or intraoral Kaposi sarcoma may interfere with ventilation and intubation, whereas non-Hodgkin lymphoma can cause mediastinal masses. Gastrointestinal manifestations include dysphagia, diarrhea, and esophagitis, which can in turn cause malnutrition, dehydration, and electrolyte imbalance. Renal complications include acute tubular necrosis, glomerulonephritis, renovascular disease, and HIV-associated nephropathy with nephritic syndrome. Antiretroviral medications used to treat HIV infection also have important side effects. The major classes of antiretroviral medications include nucleoside reverse transcriptase inhibitors (e.g., lamivudine, zidovudine, tenofovir, abacavir), nonnucleoside reverse transcriptase inhibitors (e.g., nevirapine, efavirenz, rilpivirine), protease inhibitors (e.g., atazanavir, darunavir, lopinavir, fosamprenavir, saquinavir), attachment inhibitors (e.g., maraviroc), and integrase strand transfer inhibitors (e.g., raltegravir).[394] Side effects of relevance to anesthesiologists include lactic acidosis (nucleoside reverse transcriptase inhibitors), hepatotoxicity (nucleoside reverse transcriptase inhibitors, nonnucleoside reverse transcriptase inhibitors, protease inhibitors), hyperlipidemia (protease inhibitors), insulin resistance (protease inhibitors), premature IHD (protease inhibitors),[395] cardiac conduction abnormalities (protease inhibitors), and bone marrow suppression (all classes).

If the preoperative evaluation of a relatively young, otherwise healthy individual elicits a history of thrush, fever of unknown origin, chronic diarrhea, lymphadenopathy, or herpes zoster in more than one dermatome, these findings should raise concern of undiagnosed HIV infection. In these cases, the enzyme-linked immunosorbent assay (ELISA) is the primary initial screening test. It demonstrates very high sensitivity exceeding 99% but yields a high number of false-positive results. The Western blot technique is used as the confirmatory test following an initial positive ELISA result. Patients with known HIV infection frequently require further evaluation, including an ECG, a chest radiograph, and blood sampling for CBC, electrolyte concentration, creatinine concentration, and liver function tests. If the patient shows evidence of malnourishment or nephrotic syndrome, further blood tests for albumin, total protein, and magnesium concentrations may be beneficial. The patient's perioperative prognosis may be estimated based on the CD4 lymphocyte count and viral load, which reflect the patient's immunologic status during the previous 3 months. In general, rates of postoperative complications and mortality are higher among patients with CD4 counts lower than 200 cells/mm^3 and viral loads greater than 10,000 copies/mL.[396,397] Patients' antiretroviral therapy must be continued through the perioperative period.

PATIENTS WITH A HISTORY OF SUBSTANCE ABUSE

A patient with a history of current or previous alcohol or drug addiction presents special challenges for the perioperative team. The lifetime prevalence of these addictions is significant; for example, about 14% of the United States population suffers from alcohol addiction.[398] In a suggested classification system, abused drugs can be categorized as central nervous system depressants (e.g., opioids, alcohol, sedatives, hypnotics), stimulants (e.g., cocaine, amphetamines), and other psychotropic substances (e.g., cannabis).[399] Importantly, many addicts are polysubstance abusers. Thresholds for defining high-risk alcohol consumption are 5 or more standard drinks in a day (>14 drinks per week on average) for males under 65 years of age, and 4 or more standard drinks in a day (>7 drinks per week on average) for all females and males 65 or more years of age. Addictive disease should be considered *permanent* even in patients who have had long periods of abstinence. Some patients in the process of recovery from addiction may be receiving specific medications to maintain recovery. For example, previous opioid abusers may be receiving methadone (long-acting opioid agonist), buprenorphine (partial μ-agonist), or naltrexone (opioid antagonist).

Substance abuse disorders are risk factors for poor outcomes in the perioperative setting. For example, individuals with histories of alcohol misuse experience elevated rates of postoperative complications.[72,400-402] In addition, they are at risk for postoperative withdrawal, acute intoxication, and altered tolerance of anesthetic or opioid medications. Consequently, it is worthwhile to incorporate screening for substance abuse disorders into the preoperative evaluation. Several simple validated screening questionnaires for alcohol abuse disorders are available, including the four-item CAGE questionnaire,[403] the three-item AUDIT-C questionnaire,[404] and the U.S. National Institute on Alcohol Abuse and Alcoholism 2- and 4-question tests (NIAAA-2Q/4Q).[405] These screening tools appear to be more sensitive when administered through a computer-based self-assessment questionnaire than during an in-person interview with a nurse or anesthesiologist.[406] The accuracy of these questionnaires can be further augmented with additional screening laboratory tests, namely gamma gluteryl transferase and carbohydrate-deficient transferrin.[6,407] The preoperative evaluation is also an opportunity to obtain a detailed history of known addiction (drug type, routes of administration) and recovery (periods of abstinence, pharmacotherapy for addiction). The dosage of any pharmacotherapy should be documented and verified. Patients in recovery may also have heightened anxiety regarding upcoming surgical procedures because of concerns about relapse into addiction, and inadequate pain treatment (given their history of addiction). Such concerns may be appropriate. Patients receiving opioid substitution therapy do experience normal pain responses to nociceptive stimuli but require additional analgesia for control of post-procedural pain.[408] These patients should therefore be reassured that anxiety and pain will be adequately treated. The clinicians performing preoperative evaluation may have prejudicial attitudes and lack the educational background to formulate appropriate perioperative pain management plans. For example, pain medication may be under dosed and inappropriately restricted because of concerns about provoking relapses. Early involvement of the acute pain service and addiction specialists to assist in the management of these at-risk patients may be helpful.

The preoperative period should be used to develop appropriate management plans based on the types of abused drugs. All pertinent preoperative information and management plans should be transmitted to members of the perioperative team. Individuals addicted to alcohol, sedatives, or hypnotics may require stabilization with benzodiazepines, whereas heroin addicts may require substitution with methadone. It is important to document the dosage of opioids consumed by individuals abusing these drugs, especially to help guide postoperative pain management. To avoid inadequate analgesia (which could potentially activate addiction) in these patients, the preoperative evaluation should be used to discuss and plan the optimal use of nonopioid analgesics and regional techniques. Patients actively abusing cocaine and amphetamines are at especially high risk during anesthesia because of the potential for intraoperative hemodynamic instability. Urine testing may be helpful to rule out abused substances in such patients, but the results should be interpreted based on drug pharmacokinetics. For example, the half-life of cocaine is about 1.5 hours but its inactive metabolites may still be detectable in the urine for 14 days after consumption.[409] A history of intravenous drug use should prompt an evaluation for cardiovascular, pulmonary, neurologic, and infectious complications such as endocarditis, abscesses, osteomyelitis, hepatitis, and HIV infection. Opioid (including heroin) users have a tolerance to narcotics. Patients with alcoholism are at risk for delirium tremens, a potentially life-threatening form of withdrawal characterized by autonomic instability and hyperpyrexia. These patients may also have liver disease (alcoholic hepatitis, cirrhosis, portal hypertension, end-stage liver disease), alcohol-induced cardiomyopathy, arrhythmias, seizures, neuropathies, dementia, Wernicke-Korsakoff syndrome (ataxia and cognitive dysfunction secondary to thiamine deficiency), macrocytic anemia, and coagulopathies (from hepatic dysfunction or vitamin K deficiency). Cocaine and amphetamine addicts can develop cerebrovascular accidents, cardiomyopathy, and arrhythmias. Additionally, cocaine and amphetamines inhibit the uptake of sympathomimetic neurotransmitters, thereby increasing risks for hypertension, tachycardia, paranoia, anxiety, seizures, and myocardial ischemia. Long-term use can result in ventricular hypertrophy, myocardial infarction, and nasal septal perforation. Solvents can cause cardiac dysrhythmias, pulmonary edema, cerebral edema, diffuse cortical atrophy, and hepatic failure. Hallucinogens, such as lysergic acid diethylamide, can cause autonomic dysregulation and paranoia. Ecstasy, or more specifically 3,4-methylenedioxymethamphetamine, can cause excessive thirst that results in hyponatremia, pulmonary edema, or cerebral edema. Acute marijuana use can cause tachycardia, vasodilatation, and increased cardiac output. The risk of pulmonary complications in patients who smoke marijuana is similar to that of individuals who smoke tobacco.[410]

During the preoperative evaluation interview, patients who abuse alcohol or drugs may not give a reliable history. The subsequent physical examination should include careful measurement of vital signs, including temperature. For example, cocaine and amphetamines may cause hypertension and tachycardia, whereas acute opioid use may result in a slow respiratory rate. Acute opioid use may also manifest as lethargy and pinpoint pupils, and recent alcohol consumption can often be detected by smell. Especially in individuals suspected of being intravenous drug abusers, it is important to examine venous access sites for signs of abscesses and infections. In addition, careful auscultation for murmurs is essential because of the risk of bacterial endocarditis. Cocaine or alcohol abusers can also exhibit findings in their cardiovascular examination consistent with heart failure or arrhythmias. Long-term alcohol abuse may manifest with physical findings of chronic liver disease. In addition to identifying the presence of substance abuse and its related complications, clinicians should ascertain whether, and for how long, patients can stop consuming alcohol or addictive drugs. If patients do stop consumption occasionally, it is especially important to determine what complications, if any, occur. When an alcoholic patient reports previously interrupting drinking for several days, the interviewer should inquire whether agitation, seizures, delirium tremens, or other signs of withdrawal developed. Any testing is largely informed by findings on the preoperative clinical evaluation, as well as the specific drug being abused. For example, an ECG may be warranted to assess for previous myocardial infarction in an individual with a history of cocaine abuse or in an individual receiving methadone (which prolongs the QT interval).

Ideally, patients with drug or alcohol dependence should be drug free well before elective surgical procedures. The availability of randomized trial data is limited and suggest that preoperative alcohol cessation programs can help prevent postoperative complications.[411] Preanesthesia clinic staff should therefore be prepared to refer patients to addiction specialists or to prescribe medications to prevent withdrawal in the preoperative period if patients agree to abstinence. For example, benzodiazepines can be useful in preventing or treating alcohol withdrawal symptoms.

Some medications used to manage withdrawal or facilitate recovery have specific perioperative considerations.[412] Patients taking methadone should continue maintenance doses in the perioperative period. Patients who are taking disulfiram because of a history of alcohol abuse may have an altered response to sympathomimetic drugs; some authors therefore suggest that disulfiram be discontinued 10 days before the surgical procedure.[412] If disulfiram is continued, users can experience flushing, nausea, and tachycardia in response to small amounts of alcohol, such as amounts encountered in skin preparations or medications. For patients taking naltrexone for a history of alcohol abuse, consideration should be given to discontinuing it 3 days preoperatively.[412] Naltrexone alters responses to opioid analgesics and may make postoperative pain management very challenging. Buprenorphine-containing medications (i.e., Suboxone), which are used to treat opioid addiction (as well as chronic pain), also alter responses to opioid analgesics. In the case of relatively minor surgery with minimal levels of anticipated postoperative pain, it is reasonable to continue buprenorphine perioperatively and maximize the use of nonopioid analgesic approaches (e.g., regional anesthesia, NSAIDs). In other cases, the perioperative management of buprenorphine should be coordinated with the patient's addiction specialist.

BREASTFEEDING PATIENTS

Studies of milk levels and pharmacological properties of medications guide recommendations for the safety of anesthetics and medications in babies of breastfeeding mothers who receive these agents. For elective surgery, women may be advised to pump and store milk preoperatively to prepare for any missed feedings that occur in the postoperative period. With very few exceptions (e.g., codeine, tramadol, diazepam), most perioperative medications are likely compatible with lactation. Thus, when the mother is alert and able to breastfeed, she may do so. Recommending that lactating patients pump and discard milk after general anesthesia is no longer considered best practice. Mothers of very young or premature babies, especially those susceptible to apnea, may be advised to discuss the safety of breastfeeding while taking perioperative medications with their child's pediatrician.

PATIENTS WITH DO NOT RESUSCITATE ORDERS

Some patients scheduled for procedures have advance directives or a do-not-resuscitate (DNR) status.[413] The ASA adopted guidelines for the care of these patients and updated them in 2013 (Box 31.14).[414] Frequently, in circumstances with DNR orders, care providers are focused on a procedure-directed approach (i.e., do not intubate, do not administer resuscitative drugs). This approach is problematic in the perioperative period because much of anesthesia care involves such procedures. Within the context of anesthesia care, a better approach is to discuss DNR status in a goal-directed approach (i.e., from the perspective of the patient's values and objectives, such as quality-of-life concerns).[415] The ideal time to have this emotional and complex discussion is during the preoperative evaluation. Short discussions in the preoperative clinic have been shown to foster dialogue among patients, their proxies, and physicians regarding advance directives concerning end-of-life care, as demonstrated by a randomized trial of patients at a preoperative evaluation clinic.[416] In this trial, individuals who received the information session were significantly more likely to complete a durable power-of-attorney (27%

BOX 31.14 Do-Not-Resuscitate Orders in the Perioperative Period

Policies automatically suspending DNR orders or other directives that limit treatment before procedures involving anesthetic care may not sufficiently address a patient's rights to self-determination in a responsible and ethical manner. Such policies, if they exist, should be reviewed and revised, as necessary, to reflect the content of these guidelines.

1. *Full Attempt at Resuscitation*: The patient or designated surrogate may request the full suspension of existing directives during the anesthetic and immediate postoperative period, thereby consenting to the use of any resuscitation procedures that may be appropriate to treat clinical events that occur during this time.
2. *Limited Attempt at Resuscitation Defined With Regard to Specific Procedures*: The patient or designated surrogate may elect to continue to refuse certain specific resuscitation procedures (for example, chest compressions, defibrillation or tracheal intubation). The anesthesiologist should inform the patient or designated surrogate about which procedures are (1) essential to the success of the anesthesia and the proposed procedure, and (2) which procedures are not essential and may be refused.
3. *Limited Attempt at Resuscitation Defined With Regard to the Patient's Goals and Values*: The patient or designated surrogate may allow the anesthesiologist and surgical team to use clinical judgment in determining which resuscitation procedures are appropriate in the context of the situation and the patient's stated goals and values. For example, some patients may want full resuscitation procedures to be used to manage adverse clinical events that are believed to be quickly and easily reversible, but to refrain from treatment for conditions that are likely to result in permanent sequelae, such as neurologic impairment or unwanted dependence upon life-sustaining technology.

DNR, Do-not-resuscitate.

Modified from Committee on Ethics, American Society of Anesthesiologists: Ethical guidelines for the anesthesia care of patients with do-not-resuscitate orders or other directives that limit treatment, 2013. Available at http://www.asahq.org/For-Members/Standards-Guidelines-and-Statements.aspx.

vs. 10%) and discuss end-of-life care with their proxy decision makers (87% vs. 66%).

Preoperative Laboratory and Diagnostic Studies

The value of preoperative diagnostic testing is a central issue in delivering cost-effective health care to surgical patients. The role of preoperative testing to screen for disease and evaluate patients' fitness for surgery has been extensively studied. This research has largely concluded that routine preoperative testing in all surgical patients (i.e., without consideration for their demographics or comorbidities) cannot be justified. Routine preoperative testing in asymptomatic healthy patients has very poor diagnostic yield, provides little to no additional prognostic information, and has not shown any beneficial effect on outcomes.[274,417-420] Unnecessary testing is also expensive, and may lead to costly evaluation of borderline or false-positive test abnormalities. Aside from potentially causing operating room delays or cancellations, these unnecessary follow-up tests may pose risks to patients that are attributable to follow-up tests and any associated interventions. Therefore, the targeting of testing in appropriate patients has both clinical and economic benefits. At some hospitals where surgeons and primary care physicians order all preoperative tests, the common practice has been to order tests without any diagnostic focus, other than speculation that the anesthesiologist may "require them" for surgery to proceed without delay or cancellation. Other justifications offered for nonselective ordering of tests include routine screening for disease states, establishment of a diagnostic baseline, personal habit (e.g., "standard" testing checklist for all patients), physician reassurance, and a perceived medicolegal necessity "not to miss anything." This pattern of practice has led to a plethora of preoperative testing practices that are costly, highly variable across hospitals, and largely unrelated to patients' perioperative risk profiles.[421-423] For example, in 2011, almost half of Medicare beneficiaries (aged ≥ 65 years) in the United States underwent preoperative laboratory testing before cataract surgery, which is considered a very low-risk procedure.[423]

Preoperative diagnostic tests should be selectively ordered based on the patient's medical history, planned surgery, and expected degree of intraoperative blood loss. Testing should be for the detection of specific clinical indications that may increase perioperative risk. Randomized trials have demonstrated that such a shift in strategy from nonselective to selective preoperative testing in low-risk surgical procedures can reduce costs while preserving patients' safety.[418,419] As experts in perioperative medicine, anesthesiologists are in a unique position to appropriately select the preoperative laboratory tests needed to guide perioperative care. Indeed, anesthesiologist-led preoperative evaluation has been shown to result in more selective ordering of laboratory tests than evaluation led by surgeons or primary care physicians.[14-17] Thus, by educating and providing specific guidance to surgeons and other physician specialists on the appropriate ordering of preoperative tests, anesthesiologists can expedite patient care, reduce healthcare costs, and improve the delivery of perioperative medicine.

A framework for ordering preoperative diagnostic tests based on patients' medical history is presented in Table 31.18. These disease-specific recommendations are not intended as absolute, especially since many hospitals and regional jurisdictions (e.g., Ontario Pre-Operative Testing Grid)[424] have developed their own preoperative testing recommendations. In addition, the NICE in the United Kingdom published updated 2016 guidelines for preoperative testing following an extensive systematic review of the literature.[274] The NICE guidelines consider both patients' preoperative medical status and the extensiveness of the planned surgery to determine when preoperative testing is warranted. In these guidelines, surgical procedures are graded as minor (e.g., skin lesion excision), intermediate (e.g., inguinal hernia repair, varicose vein excision, tonsillectomy, knee arthroscopy), and major (e.g., total abdominal hysterectomy, transurethral prostate resection, lumbar spine discectomy, thyroidectomy, total joint replacement, lung operations, colon resection, radical neck dissection). Although the most recent 2012 ASA "Practice Advisory for Preanesthesia Evaluation" does recommend against routine preoperative testing,[5] it does

TABLE 31.18 Framework for Preoperative Diagnostic Testing Based on Patients' Medical History

Preoperative Diagnosis	ECG	CXR	CBC	Electrolytes	Creatinine	Glucose	Coagulation	LFTs	Drug Levels	Ca
Cardiac disease										
IHD	X		X	±						
HF	X	±								
HTN	X	±		X*	X					
Chronic atrial fibrillation	X								X†	
PAD	X									
Valvular heart disease	X	±								
Pulmonary disease										
COPD	X	±	X						X‡	
Asthma§										
Diabetes mellitus	X			±	X	X				
Liver disease										
Infectious hepatitis							X	X		
Alcohol/drug induced							X	X		
Tumor infiltration							X	X		
Renal disease			X	X	X					
Hematologic disorders			X							
Coagulopathies			X				X			
CNS Disorders										
Stroke	X		X	X					X	
Seizures	X		X	X		X			X	
Tumor	X		X							
Vascular/aneurysms	X		X							
Malignancy			X							
Hyperthyroidism	X		X	X						X
Hypothyroidism	X		X	X						
Cushing disease			X	X		X				
Addison disease			X	X		X				
Hyperparathyroidism	X		X	X						X
Hypoparathyroidism	X			X						X
Morbid obesity	X	±				X				
Malabsorption/poor nutrition	X		X	X	X	X				
Select Drug Therapies										
Digoxin	X			±					X	
Anticoagulants			X				X			
Phenytoin									X	
Phenobarbital									X	
Diuretics				X	X					
Corticosteroids			X			X				
Chemotherapy			X		±					
Aspirin/NSAID										
Theophylline									X	

*If the patient is taking diuretics.
†If the patient is taking digoxin.
‡If the patient is taking theophylline.
§Only test for consideration is pulmonary function testing if clinically indicated.
X, obtain; ±, consider.
Ca, Calcium; *CBC*, complete blood count; *HF*, heart failure; *CXR*, chest x-ray; *ECG*, electrocardiogram; *HTN*, hypertension; *IHD*, ischemic heart disease; *LFTs*, liver function tests; *NSAID*, nonsteroidal antiinflammatory drug; *PAD*, peripheral artery disease.

not make explicit recommendations about which tests should be ordered for specific clinical conditions. The practice advisory states that the indications for testing should be "*based on information obtained from medical records, patient interview, physical examination, and type and invasiveness of the planned procedure.*" In addition, it describes patient-related and surgery-related factors that anesthesiologists should consider when deciding whether to order a specific laboratory test.[5] Conversely, the updated 2018 ESA guidelines on preoperative evaluation do make some specific recommendations for when preoperative laboratory testing should be performed.[6]

The following subsections discuss specific preoperative laboratory tests. In general, testing does not have to be repeated during the preoperative evaluation of healthy patients (i.e., ASA-PS class 1 or 2) if similar testing has already been performed within the 2 months preceding surgery and there has been no major interval change in the patient's medical status (e.g., recent chemotherapy).[425]

COMPLETE BLOOD COUNT, HEMOGLOBIN, AND HEMATOCRIT

The proposed surgery, associated potential blood loss, and individualized patient-level clinical indications should determine the requirement for a preoperative CBC. Typical clinical indications include a history of increased bleeding, hematologic disorders, CKD, chronic liver disease, recent chemotherapy or radiation treatment, corticosteroid therapy, anticoagulant therapy, and poor nutritional status. The NICE guidelines recommend routine CBC testing only in ASA-PS class 3 or 4 patients undergoing intermediate grade procedures, and all patients undergoing major procedures.[274]

RENAL FUNCTION TESTING

Renal function tests assess renal tubular function and glomerular filtration. Primary clinical indications include diabetes mellitus, hypertension, cardiac disease, potential dehydration (e.g., vomiting, diarrhea), anorexia, bulimia, fluid overload states (e.g., heart rate, ascites), known renal disease, liver disease, relevant recent chemotherapy (e.g., cisplatin, carboplatin), and renal transplantation. The NICE guidelines recommend routine renal function testing in ASA-PS class 3 or 4 patients undergoing intermediate procedures, and ASA-PS class 2, 3, or 4 patients undergoing major procedures.[274] If patients are deemed to be at risk for perioperative AKI, testing may also be considered in ASA-PS class 3 or 4 patients undergoing minor procedures, and ASA-PS class 2 patients undergoing intermediate procedures.[274]

LIVER FUNCTION TESTING

The ordering of liver function tests should be based on a history of liver injury and physical examination findings. Primary clinical indications include a history of hepatitis (viral, alcohol, drug-induced, autoimmune), jaundice, cirrhosis, portal hypertension, biliary disease, gallbladder disease, hepatotoxic drug exposure, tumor involvement of the liver, and bleeding disorders.

COAGULATION TESTING

Routine preoperative coagulation testing is not indicated (even in patients undergoing regional procedures) unless a known or suspected coagulopathy is identified on preoperative evaluation. Primary clinical indications for testing include a known bleeding disorder, hepatic disease, and anticoagulant use.[5] The 2016 NICE guidelines state that coagulation testing should only be considered in patients who are (1) ASA-PS class 3 or 4; (2) undergoing intermediate, major, or complex surgical procedures; and (3) known to take anticoagulant medications or have chronic liver disease.[274]

URINALYSIS

There is no indication for routine preoperative urinalysis.[274] Primary clinical indications include a suspected urinary tract infection and unexplained fever or chills.

PREGNANCY TEST

Pregnancy testing is often determined by hospital-specific protocols. It can also be based on clinical indications such as sexual activity, birth control use, and date of the last menstrual period. Another important factor that should be considered is the potential for the planned surgical procedure harming a fetus, based on direct injury (e.g., uterine surgery), reduction in blood flow (e.g., major cardiac or vascular surgery), and exposure to teratogenic agents (e.g., x-rays). The 2012 ASA "Practice Advisory for Preanesthesia Evaluation" suggests offering pregnancy testing to female patients of childbearing age when the result would alter the patient's management. It also recommends that informed consent be obtained for such testing, or that there be a full discussion of the risks, benefits, and alternatives related to preoperative pregnancy testing. The NICE guidelines recommend that all women of childbearing potential be asked whether there is any possibility they could be pregnant, and that any women who could possibly be pregnant be made aware of the risks of anesthesia and surgery to a fetus. The guidelines also recommend documenting all discussions about whether or not to carry out pregnancy testing, and to conduct pregnancy testing with patient consent if there is any doubt about pregnancy status.[274]

SICKLE CELL TEST

Individuals at risk for sickle cell disease include those of African, Caribbean, Eastern Mediterranean, and Middle Eastern origin. Even in at-risk populations, routine preoperative screening for sickle cell disease has a very low yield,[426] especially in regions with newborn screening programs for sickle cell disease.[427] Consistent with this evidence, 2016 NICE guidelines recommend against routine preoperative testing for sickle cell disease or sickle cell trait.[274]

A reasonable approach is to consider testing in *previously untested* patients who have at-risk ethnic backgrounds and clinical indicators. These indicators include patient-related (e.g., family history of sickle cell disease, sickle cell symptoms) and surgery-related (e.g., deliberate hypothermia, cardiopulmonary bypass, intrathoracic procedures, intraabdominal procedures, orthopedic procedures with tourniquet use) factors.

ELECTROCARDIOGRAM

The ECG can help detect a prior myocardial infarction, cardiac rhythm disturbances, ischemia, chamber hypertrophy, and electrolyte disorders. Nonetheless, when combined with usual clinical examination, the preoperative ECG may not provide additional prognostic information to identify individuals at risk for postoperative cardiac complications.[100] Primary clinical indications for preoperative ECGs include a history of IHD, hypertension, diabetes mellitus, heart failure, chest pain, palpitations, abnormal valvular murmurs, peripheral edema, syncope, dizziness, dyspnea on exertion, orthopnea, paroxysmal nocturnal dyspnea, and CVD. The 2014 ESC/ESA guidelines suggest preoperative ECGs in patients with risk factors for IHD or suspicious symptoms, especially if they are undergoing intermediate-risk or high-risk surgery.[9] The 2014 ACC/AHA guidelines are fairly consistent in that they support preoperative ECGs for patients who are undergoing intermediate-risk or high-risk surgery, and who have known IHD, significant arrhythmia, PAD, CVD, or other significant structural heart disease.[7] The guidelines also recommend against routine preoperative ECGs (see Box 31.2), especially in asymptomatic patients without known cardiovascular disease or risk factors.[7] The NICE guidelines recommend routine preoperative ECGs in ASA-PS class 3 or 4 patients undergoing intermediate grade procedures, and ASA-PS class 2, 3, or 4 patients undergoing major procedures.[274] If patients have cardiovascular disease, CKD, or diabetes mellitus, testing may also be considered in ASA-PS class 2 patients undergoing intermediate procedures.[274]

CHEST RADIOGRAPH

Routine preoperative chest radiographs do not provide prognostically important information for assessing perioperative risk.[428] Preoperative chest radiographs should therefore not be ordered routinely,[274] but rather selectively based on abnormalities identified by preoperative evaluation. These indications include advanced COPD, bullous lung disease, suspected pulmonary edema, suspected pneumonia, suspected mediastinal masses, and suspicious findings on physical examination (e.g., rales, tracheal deviation).

Preoperative Risk Assessment

A critical component of the preanesthesia evaluation is assessment of a patient's risk for undergoing anesthesia and surgery. This assessment improves patients' understanding of the inherent perioperative risks and better informs healthcare providers' clinical decision making.

TABLE 31.19 American Society of Anesthesiologists Physical Status Classification

Category*	Definition
ASA-PS 1	A normal, healthy patient
ASA-PS 2	A patient with mild systemic disease
ASA-PS 3	A patient with severe systemic disease
ASA-PS 4	A patient with severe systemic disease that is a constant threat to life
ASA-PS 5	A moribund patient who is not expected to survive without the operation
ASA-PS 6	A declared brain-dead patient whose organs are being removed for donor purposes

*The addition of "E" to the classification category indicates emergency surgery.
ASA-PS, American Society of Anesthesiologists physical status.

For example, these risk assessments might help identify individuals who warrant enhanced levels of postoperative monitoring, consideration for alternative nonoperative or less invasive treatment options for their underlying condition, or initiation of interventions intended to decrease perioperative risk. An anesthesiologist's designation of a surgical patient as being high-risk is clinically important. Specifically, when the initial preanesthesia evaluation deems that a patient is at unacceptably high risk for anesthesia and surgery, adherence to the anesthesiologist's recommendations for further perioperative management is associated with lower postoperative complication rates.[429] In addition, accurate risk assessments facilitate fairer comparisons of perioperative outcomes; specifically, estimates of patients' risks are required by statistical methods that adjust for case-mix differences across providers and hospitals.

The most commonly used method by anesthesiologists to assess overall perioperative risk is the ASA-PS classification system (Table 31.19). This classification system, which was developed in 1941, was originally intended to facilitate collection and comparison of statistical data in anesthesia.[430] The ASA-PS classification system seeks to describe a patient's preoperative medical status, but it does not consider risks inherent to the planned surgical procedure. Although *not* intended to guide estimation of patients' risks for anesthesia and surgery, the ASA-PS is often used for this purpose, especially given its simplicity of use. Indeed, several studies have shown a correlation of ASA-PS scores with postoperative mortality and major complications.[97,218,431-433] An important limitation to the classification system is its inherent subjectivity; consequently, previous research has shown only fair to modest interrater agreement when different individuals attempt to assign an ASA-PS category to the same patient.[432,434-436]

In addition to patients' preoperative medical status, which is described by the ASA-PS system, the operative procedure is an important determinant of perioperative risk.[437-439] Overall perioperative risk is necessarily a function of both the risk associated with the specific operative procedure and the risk associated with a patient's underlying medical status. For example, ambulatory surgical procedures are very

TABLE 31.20 Johns Hopkins Surgery Risk Classification System

Category	Description
1	Minimal risk to the patient independent of anesthesia. Minimally invasive procedure with little or no blood loss. Procedures are often done in an office setting, with the operating room used principally for anesthesia and monitoring.
2	Minimal to moderately invasive procedure, with expected blood loss not exceeding 500 mL. Mild risk to patient independent of anesthesia.
3	Moderately to significantly invasive procedure, with expected blood loss of 500-1500 mL. Moderate risk to patient independent of anesthesia.
4	Highly invasive procedure, with expected blood loss exceeding 1500 mL. Major risk to patient independent of anesthesia.
5	Highly invasive procedure, with expected blood loss exceeding 1500 mL. Critical risk to patient independent of anesthesia. Usually requires postoperative critical care unit stay with invasive monitoring.

From Paternak LR, Johns A. Ambulatory gynaecological surgery: risk and assessment. *Best Pract Res Clin Obstet Gynaecol.* 2005;19:663–679.

safe with respect to risks of postoperative mortality and major adverse events,[440-442] as evidenced by a 7-day postoperative mortality rate of only 41 per 100,000 procedures in a large cohort of Medicare beneficiaries 65 years old or older.[440] Thus, although older patients with an increased burden of comorbidity do have increased relative risks of mortality and morbidity following ambulatory surgery, their *absolute* risks remain very low. Classification schemes have been proposed for assessing operative risk, such as the Johns Hopkins risk classification system (Table 31.20), elevated surgical risk category in the RCRI (see Table 31.5), and the strata employed by the ESA/ESC cardiovascular evaluation guidelines.[9,439] Importantly, individual operative procedures within broad categories (e.g., intraabdominal surgery) vary with respect to their perioperative risk.[107] As a consequence, there is a need to balance the desire to ensure that clinical prediction tools sufficiently capture the variability in operative risk across different procedures, against the need to ensure that these tools are sufficiently simple for straightforward clinical use.

Several commonly used and methodologically sound clinical indices can predict mortality and major morbidity after cardiac surgery with reasonable accuracy, such as the EuroSCORE,[443] Society of Thoracic Surgeons risk models,[444] and Cleveland Clinic AKI risk score.[269] A variety of prediction tools have also been developed for use in noncardiac surgery.[445] For example, the ACS NSQIP risk calculator is available on the Internet (http://riskcalculator.facs.org) and provides an estimate of risk based on patients' comorbidities and proposed surgical procedures.[32] High-quality validated indices have been developed for predicting specific major complications of noncardiac surgery, such as cardiovascular events (e.g., RCRI)[97,106] and respiratory complications (e.g., ARISCAT).[257,261] Other examples including the Surgical Risk Scale,[446] the Preoperative Score to Predict Postoperative Mortality (POSPOM),[99] and large multinational prospective epidemiologic studies of surgical patients (which included accurate capture of perioperative characteristics and outcomes),[77,78] will likely help lead to the development of other high-quality predictive indices.

ROLE OF SPECIALIZED TESTING IN PREOPERATIVE RISK ASSESSMENT

Based on an initial preoperative clinical evaluation, anesthesiologists may order subsequent specialized tests to help address diagnostic questions (e.g., "*Does this patient have aortic stenosis?*") or determine perioperative risk more accurately. Examples of such tests include noninvasive cardiac stress tests (see section on "Ischemic Heart Disease"), coronary angiography (see section on "Ischemic Heart Disease"), echocardiography, CPET, and PFTs (see section on "Pulmonary Disorders").

Resting echocardiography can provide information related to valvular lesions, pulmonary hypertension, fixed wall motion abnormalities, and ventricular function. Especially in cases of a suspicious murmur or other clinical indication, a preoperative echocardiogram can help diagnose prognostically important valvular or other cardiac lesions, such as aortic stenosis or pulmonary hypertension.[447,448] An echocardiogram can also identify fixed wall motion abnormalities consistent with a previous myocardial infarction. Although these findings can help support a diagnosis of IHD, fixed wall motion abnormalities are not themselves indicative of increased perioperative cardiac risk.[122] Similarly, while systolic ventricular dysfunction identified on echocardiography is associated with increased cardiac risk[161,162] this finding may not provide additional prognostic information when it is combined with routine preoperative clinical evaluation.[161] Thus, the overall role of echocardiography is to address focused *diagnostic* questions identified in usual clinical preoperative evaluation (e.g., suspicious systolic murmurs), not to provide important prognostic information pertaining to perioperative risk. Current guidelines therefore largely recommend preoperative echocardiography to assess dyspnea of unknown origin or recent altered clinical status in an individual with known heart failure (see Box 31.3).[7] In addition, repeat echocardiography is reasonable in clinically stable patients with known ventricular dysfunction who have not been tested in the previous year.[7] Conversely, routine preoperative echocardiography is discouraged.[7,8]

CPET is a noninvasive global assessment of exercise capacity; it involves a patient exercising on a bicycle or treadmill for 8 to 12 minutes while undergoing continuous measurement of respiratory gas exchange (i.e., oxygen uptake and carbon dioxide production).[449] Poor exercise capacity during CPET, based on either a low peak oxygen consumption or a low anaerobic threshold, is associated with increased risks of postoperative morbidity.[29,36,450] Thus, the test can help improve the accuracy of preoperative risk stratification. In some geographic settings,[451] CPET is a commonly used preoperative test. In these settings, it is used to aid preoperative risk assessment for major surgery, and to inform decisions on the appropriateness of planned major surgical procedures.

The role of PFTs for guiding preoperative assessment in the setting of specific comorbidities was discussed earlier in this chapter. These tests have an established and important role for assessing perioperative risk in lung resection surgery (see section on "Patients Scheduled for Lung Resection" and Chapter 53).[219] PFTs also play an important diagnostic role. For example, they help differentiate between pulmonary and cardiac causes of dyspnea of unknown origin. Aside from these specific circumstances, the *prognostic* value of preoperative PFTs is limited. Practice guidelines from the American College of Physicians recommend against routine preoperative spirometry for estimating risks for pulmonary complications after noncardiothoracic surgery.[10] Research has not found a consistent link between poor PFT results and increased risks for perioperative pulmonary complications, with older studies being generally limited by important methodologic flaws.[218] Furthermore, there does not seem to be a critical PFT threshold below which patients should not be offered surgery. For example, in a previous cohort study, individuals with severe obstructive findings (i.e., $FEV_1 < 50\%$ of predicted and FEV_1/FVC ratio < 0.7) had reasonably acceptable risks of postoperative death (5.6%) and respiratory failure (5.6%).[452]

Preoperative Medication Management

The patient's comorbidities and planned procedure must inform medication management during the perioperative period. Some medications have beneficial effects during surgical procedures, whereas others may be detrimental. In some cases, abrupt *withdrawal* of medications can have a negative effect. Management of specific preoperative medications has been discussed in the previous sections of this chapter. These recommendations are outlined again in Box 31.15. Although issues pertaining to many drugs are covered in other sections of this chapter, several issues merit special mention.

NSAIDs have *reversible* antiplatelet effects; hence, once the drugs have been eliminated, platelet function returns to normal. Concomitant NSAID use does not appear to increase the risk of spinal hematoma with neuraxial anesthesia.[196] Preoperative discontinuation of NSAIDs may be of value in patients at risk for perioperative AKI. Typically, NSAIDs are discontinued 24 to 72 hours preoperatively. Earlier discontinuation does not increase safety, and it may be burdensome to many patients with significant arthritis or chronic pain. COX-2 inhibitors (e.g., celecoxib) have minimal effect on platelet function and can usually be continued in the perioperative period. However, the long-term COX-2 inhibitor use in the nonoperative setting does increase the risk of cardiac events, in comparison with placebo or naproxen.[453] Conversely, COX-2 inhibitors have a cardiac risk profile similar to that of ibuprofen or diclofenac.[453] In general, no clear evidence indicates increased

BOX 31.15 Preoperative Management of Medications

Instruct patients to take these medications with a small sip of water, even if fasting.

1. **Antihypertensive medications**
   Continue on the day of surgery, except for ACEIs and ARBs
2. **Cardiac medications (e.g., β-blockers, digoxin)**
   Continue on the day of surgery.
3. **Antidepressants, anxiolytics, and other psychiatric medications**
   Continue on the day of surgery.
4. **Thyroid medications**
   Continue on the day of surgery.
5. **Oral contraceptive pills**
   Continue on the day of surgery.
6. **Eye drops**
   Continue on the day of surgery.
7. **Heartburn or reflux medications**
   Continue on the day of surgery.
8. **Opioid medications**
   Continue on the day of surgery.
9. **Anticonvulsant medications**
   Continue on the day of surgery.
10. **Asthma medications**
    Continue on the day of surgery.
11. **Corticosteroids (oral and inhaled)**
    Continue on the day of surgery.
12. **Statins**
    Continue on the day of surgery.
13. **Aspirin**
    Continue aspirin in patients with prior percutaneous coronary intervention, high-grade IHD, and significant CVD. Otherwise, discontinue aspirin 3 days before surgery.
14. **$P2Y_{12}$ inhibitors (e.g., clopidogrel, ticagrelor, prasugrel, ticlopidine)**
    Patients having cataract surgery with topical or general anesthesia do not need to stop taking thienopyridines. If reversal of platelet inhibition is necessary, the time interval for discontinuing these medications before surgery is 5–7 days for clopidogrel, 5–7 days for ticagrelor, 7–10 days for prasugrel, and 10 days for ticlopidine. Do not discontinue $P2Y_{12}$ inhibitors in patients who have drug-eluting stents until they have completed 6 mo of dual antiplatelet therapy, unless patients, surgeons, and cardiologists have discussed the risks of discontinuation. The same applies to patients with bare metal stents until they have completed 1 month of dual antiplatelet therapy.
15. **Insulin**
    For all patients, discontinue all short-acting (e.g., regular) insulin on the day of surgery (unless insulin is administered by continuous pump). Patients with type 2 diabetes should take none, or up to one half of their dose of long-acting or combination (e.g., 70/30 preparations) insulin, on the day of surgery. Patients with type 1 diabetes should take a small amount (usually one third) of their usual morning long-acting insulin dose on the day of surgery. Patients with an insulin pump should continue their basal rate only.
16. **Topical medications (e.g., creams and ointments)**
    Discontinue on the day of surgery.
17. **Non-insulin antidiabetic medications**
    Discontinue on the day of surgery (exception: SGLT2 inhibitors should be discontinued 24 hours before elective surgery)
18. **Diuretics**
    Discontinue on the day of surgery (exception: thiazide diuretics taken for hypertension, which should be continued on the day of surgery).
19. **Sildenafil (Viagra) or similar drugs**
    Discontinue 24 h before surgery.
20. **COX-2 inhibitors**
    Continue on the day of surgery unless the surgeon is concerned about bone healing.
21. **Nonsteroidal antiinflammatory drugs**
    Discontinue 48 hours before the day of surgery.
22. **Warfarin (Coumadin)**
    Discontinue 5 days before surgery, except for patients having cataract surgery without a bulbar block.
23. **Monoamine oxidase inhibitors**
    Continue these medications and adjust the anesthesia plan accordingly.

ACEI, Angiotensin converting enzyme inhibitors; *ARB*, angiotensin receptor blocker; *COX-2*, cyclooxygenase-2; *CVD*, cerebrovascular disease; *IHD*, ischemic heart disease; *P2Y12*, adenosine diphosphate receptor; *SGLT2*, sodium-glucose cotransporter 2 inhibitors.

cardiac risk from *short-term* perioperative administration of COX-2 inhibitors. The exception is valdecoxib (now withdrawn from the market), which caused an excess of cardiac events in patients undergoing cardiac surgery.[454]

Postmenopausal hormone replacement therapies that contain estrogen increase the risk of thromboembolic events.[455] It may therefore be reasonable to discontinue these medications before operations. Estrogens must be stopped approximately 4 weeks preoperatively for coagulation function to return to baseline. Most modern oral contraceptives contain low doses of estrogen. Nonetheless, these medications are still associated with some elevation in thrombotic risk.[456] Since the risk of unanticipated pregnancy may outweigh the benefits of discontinuing oral contraceptives preoperatively, it is reasonable to continue oral contraceptives in most patients during the perioperative period. In patients who are deemed to be a high risk for postoperative VTE (see section on "Venous Thromboembolic Disorders"), consideration may be given to stopping oral contraceptives 4 weeks before surgery (and temporarily switching to other forms of contraception). This decision should be made collaboratively with the patient and must balance the risk of VTE versus the risk of unwanted pregnancy.

Most medications for psychiatric and psychological problems should be continued into the preoperative period. Thus, most antidepressants, antipsychotics, and benzodiazepines are best maintained to avoid exacerbations of symptoms. Historically, monoamine oxidase inhibitor (MAOI) antidepressants were discontinued preoperatively; however, elimination of the risks associated with many of these drugs required drug discontinuation at least 3 weeks before surgery. This long withdrawal period is specifically applied to MAOIs that cause irreversible inhibition of MAO. Some newer agents, such as moclobemide, cause reversible enzyme inhibition and have effects lasting less than 24 hours. Preoperative withdrawal of these drugs has potential risks. Specifically, case reports of suicides or severe depression following discontinuation of MAOIs have been reported. Thus, the safest approach may be to continue these drugs and adjust the anesthetic plan accordingly (e.g., avoid meperidine and indirect-acting vasopressors such as ephedrine). If this approach is taken, it is critical that details of a patient's MAOI use must be clearly communicated to healthcare providers on the day of surgery. Patients receiving tricyclic antidepressants require a preoperative ECG, given the potential for a prolonged QT interval. Because tricyclic antidepressants block the reuptake of norepinephrine and serotonin, high doses may also result in augmented responses to vasopressor drugs, with the potential for exaggerated hemodynamic changes. Patients taking lithium require evaluation of electrolyte and creatinine concentrations. Discontinuation of lithium has also been associated with suicide. Continued perioperative use of selective serotonin reuptake inhibitors (SSRIs) are associated with increased surgical bleeding,[457,458] whereas abrupt discontinuation of SSRIs can also cause dizziness, chills, muscle aches, and anxiety. Overall, it is still reasonable to continue SSRI perioperatively in most patients, aside from those undergoing procedures where bleeding could have significant postoperative sequalae (e.g., intracranial surgery).

Complementary and alternative medications may interact with anesthetic drugs, alter effects of prescription medications, and increase bleeding. In addition, many patients do not consider these drugs "medications," and may not list them among their medications unless specifically asked. The perioperative management of complementary and alternative medications is discussed in further detail in Chapter 33.

Planning for Anesthesia

PREOPERATIVE FASTING STATUS

The overarching goal of preoperative fasting recommendations has been to reduce the risk of pulmonary aspiration. The ASA published practice guidelines pertaining to preoperative fasting in nonlaboring individuals undergoing elective procedures.[459] The recommended fasting period following clear fluids for all patients is 2 hours. In general, the volume of liquid ingested is less important than the type of liquid ingested. For neonates and infants, the recommended fasting period is 4 hours following breast milk, and 6 hours following formula, non-human milk, and solids. For patients other than infants, a fasting period of 6 hours after a light meal is recommended; this period may have to be increased to 8 or more hours if the meal includes fried or fatty foods. In addition to implementing these fasting intervals, the guidelines recommend that the preoperative evaluation include assessment of the potential for difficult airway management, as well as factors that may increase the risk for aspiration (e.g., gastrointestinal motility disorders, diabetes).

PLANNING FOR POSTOPERATIVE PAIN MANAGEMENT

A preoperative evaluation should always include baseline pain assessment. Standardization of pain measurement is difficult because of the subjective nature of the variable. It is therefore helpful to incorporate standardized pain measurement scales into the preoperative evaluation process. The scales may either be single-dimension scales, such as visual analog and numeric rating scales, or multidimensional scales such as the McGill pain questionnaire,[460] and Modified Brief Pain Inventory—Short Form.[461] Although multidimensional scales are longer, they capture a broader range of important details. For example, the 9-item Modified Brief Pain Inventory—Short Form captures details on the pain intensity, pain location, adequacy of analgesic treatment, and pain-related interference in activities. Consistent use of the same scale during the perioperative episode of care allows comparison when reassessments are performed after surgery.

The preoperative evaluation provides an important opportunity to discuss and plan for the management of acute postoperative pain, for several reasons. First, adequacy of perioperative pain control is a frequent concern for patients during preoperative evaluation.[462,463] Second, intensive preoperative pain instructions may help improve postoperative pain control in surgical patients.[464] Third, preoperative anesthesia consultation is associated with improved patient acceptance of perioperative regional techniques,[19] which can help improve the quality of postoperative analgesia.[465] Fourth, preoperative evaluation facilitates planning the perioperative care of patients with chronic pain conditions, who often present significant challenges with respect to managing postoperative analgesia. Specific issues include their tolerance to usual doses of opioid analgesics and the potential for acute withdrawal reactions if they receive insufficient doses of opioids postoperatively. The preoperative consultation should therefore be used to carefully document their usual baseline opioid requirements (to ensure adequate postoperative dosing), facilitate early involvement of an acute pain service or transitional pain specialist,[466] encourage regional analgesic techniques, and plan adjunct analgesic medications (e.g., NSAIDs, gabapentin, pregabalin, clonidine). Patients with preexisting chronic pain should be encouraged to develop reasonable goals for adequacy of postoperative pain control. They should be informed that although care providers will do everything possible to maintain comfort postoperatively, patients should not expect to have no pain at all.

In general, patients should not be weaned from pain medications before surgery. If instructed by their surgeons to temporarily discontinue NSAIDs or COX-2 analgesics, they may have to be transitioned to alternative analgesics before surgery. Patients should be instructed to take their usual morning dose of pain medication, including continued use of any transdermal medications.

Regulatory Issues

Providers must be aware of various governmental regulatory requirements, which often differ by individual municipalities and countries. These requirements may be driven by quality regulations, such as those developed by The Joint Commission or by payment requirements as set by the Centers for Medicare and Medicaid Services (CMS) in the United States. For example, the CMS has determined that a comprehensive anesthesia evaluation can be done within 30 days, and a focused update is required within 48 hours of a procedure requiring anesthesia services. The evaluation should be performed by a practitioner qualified to provide anesthesia. At a minimum, the preanesthesia evaluation must include the following:

- Notation of anesthesia risk (e.g., ASA-PS classification)
- Review of the medical, anesthesia, drug, and allergy history
- Interview and examination of the patient
- Potential anesthesia problems (e.g., difficult airway, limited intravascular access)
- Additional evaluation, if deemed necessary (e.g., stress tests, specialist consultation)
- Development of a plan for anesthesia, including the type of medications for induction, maintenance, and postoperative care
- Discussion of the risks and benefits of anesthesia with the patient or the patient's representative

Preoperative Evaluation Clinic

Many anesthesiology groups and medical centers have developed preoperative evaluation programs and outpatient clinics, with the objectives of improving patient care and operating room efficiency.[14,22,467] Although these programs may differ with respect to staffing, structure, financial support, and daily operations, they all share a common goal of preventing delays, last-minute cancellations, and adverse patient outcomes that could have been addressed before the day of surgery.

The decision to develop a preoperative evaluation clinic depends on several key factors. They include the anticipated daily volume of surgical patients, the predominant level of medical acuity among these patients, the availability of clinic facilities, relevant patient demographics (e.g., average travel distances from patients' homes to the clinic), and requisite support from the anesthesia department, perioperative staff, and hospital administration. If the decision to implement a preoperative evaluation program is made, anesthesiologists must play a key role in its leadership and management. When this role is instead undertaken by other specialties, such as internal medicine, anesthesiologists' expertise in perioperative patient management often becomes secondary. This shift to a secondary role can result in interdepartmental conflicts concerning patients' preoperative evaluation, risk stratification, and fitness to proceed with anesthesia and surgery. These conflicts can, in turn, result in unplanned delays or cancellations of planned surgical procedures, despite the completion of an assessment in an outpatient preoperative evaluation clinic.

Such conflicts often relate to surgeons' interpretation of a nonanesthesia specialist's judgment that a patient is "cleared for surgery" as evidence that the patient is fit for anesthesia. Unfortunately, this "clearance" is frequently made with limited knowledge of factors critical to the responsible anesthesiologist in the operating room, such as current anesthesia practice and intraoperative patient management. Indeed, previous research has shown that preoperative histories, physical examinations, and assessments performed by medical specialists often fail to address specific anesthesia-related concerns.[468] As the specialist who makes the final determination of whether a patient is fit to proceed with anesthesia and surgery, the responsible anesthesiologist is a critical "end-user" of any assessment performed in a preoperative evaluation clinic. Consequently, a reliance on nonanesthesia specialists can result in preoperative assessments that are deemed inadequate by the responsible anesthesia providers and that lead to potential last-minute surgical delays and cancellations, with associated significant frustration among both patients and surgeons. Conversely, preoperative-to-intraoperative communication is likely significantly improved when anesthesiologists are responsible for most outpatient preanesthesia evaluations, as confirmed by previous studies showing fewer last-minute case cancellations,[14,20,22,469] shorter durations of hospitalization,[22,469,470] lower hospital costs,[469] and possibly reduced postoperative mortality,[471] with institution of anesthesia-led preoperative evaluation programs.

Awareness of the local hospital context is critical if a preoperative evaluation program is to have good outcomes. In a hospital with limited resources that has mostly healthy outpatient and same-day-admission surgical patients, the anesthesia group may be unable to evaluate all patients preoperatively in a clinic before the day of surgery. In this situation, the preoperative program must develop a means for accurate screening and triage of patients based on their current health status. An accurate triage process helps target the use of preoperative clinic visits only among selected higher-risk patients without compromising patients' quality of care and outcomes.[24] An example of such a triage process may involve having patients initially complete an anesthesia screening questionnaire in their surgeons' office. This questionnaire can be a Web-based online document or even a paper version that would then be faxed to the anesthesia group before the date of surgery. The anesthesia group can develop local context-specific screening questionnaires, or adopt published instruments developed for this purpose.[472,473] In the case of a patient with a questionable medical history, a telephone call by the anesthesiologist could clarify any issues of concern. This opportunity to review a patient's medical history before the day of surgery helps reduce unresolved or unexpected medical concerns on the day of surgery. It also helps determine whether a patient requires formal preoperative consultation in advance of the surgical procedure, as opposed to evaluation on the day of surgery itself.

Conversely, anesthesia departments at hospitals with many medically complex surgical patients may benefit from the establishment of a formal preoperative evaluation facility with multiple examination rooms, dedicated staffing, and a full-time operational system. The establishment of a successful preoperative evaluation clinic requires commitment, collaboration, and support from several hospital disciplines.[14] At a minimum, the departments of anesthesia, surgery, nursing, and hospital administration must agree that such a clinic has value for the hospital, and they must commit to support its operational goals.

COLLABORATION, COMMITMENT, AND TEAMWORK

The preoperative evaluation clinic is a partnership among the departments of anesthesia, surgery, nursing, and hospital administration to achieve common goals. This collaboration conveys the important theme that the new clinical program is an integrated enterprise that requires shared obligation, endeavor, and financial responsibility. Although these clinics are best led by anesthesiologists,[14,20,22,469] collaborative engagement with medical specialists (e.g., cardiologists, geriatricians) and hospitalists remains important to the success of any preoperative program. These nonanesthesia specialties provide unique expertise in the preoperative management of selected medically complex patients; furthermore, they can facilitate enhanced postoperative monitoring of high-risk patients through, for example, the comanagement model of postoperative care (see section on "Role of the Medical Consultant in Preoperative Evaluation").

Surgeons may be initially reluctant to send their patients to a newly established anesthesia-led preoperative evaluation clinic. This reluctance often stems from an unclear understanding of the benefits of outpatient preoperative anesthesia evaluation. Consequently, the surgeons' hesitation can be reduced by clearly identifying the specific advantages of an integrated anesthesia-led preoperative evaluation program. First, the proven benefits of anesthesiology-led preoperative evaluation should be highlighted.[14,20,22,469-471] Second, anesthesiologists should emphasize the important practical advantages of an integrated assessment of medically complex surgical patients. Specifically, when relevant medical concerns are identified before the surgical procedure, the preoperative program can acquire all relevant prior medical data, coordinate any additional workup or consultation, prearrange any required specialized postoperative monitoring, and discuss the case beforehand with the surgeon and responsible anesthesiologist. This approach ensures that when such a patient presents for the operation, the responsible anesthesia provider is satisfied to proceed with the surgical procedure, and the perioperative team has all required medical information to manage the patient optimally during the hospitalization. This integration of the preoperative evaluation with the entire perioperative episode of care is an integral component of the Perioperative Surgical Home model.[1]

Third, informal assurances should be made to the surgical services that, if a patient is managed by the preoperative evaluation program, surgery will proceed without cancellation or delay by the assigned anesthesiologist unless an intervening illness or adverse medical event occurs between the outpatient evaluation and the scheduled operation. Because cancellations and delays on the day of surgery can be a prominent source of aggravation for surgeons and patients, these informal assurances would be viewed as a key strength of the newly developed preoperative program. Such assurances depend heavily on the anesthesia department's addressing relevant clinical practice variations. Specifically, issues that are subject to important interpractitioner differences, such as what fasting blood glucose level or degree of preoperative hypertension would merit cancelling a surgical case, must be discussed to achieve a departmental consensus standard. The absence of consensus standards can lead to situations in which half the anesthesia providers may proceed with a higher-risk surgical case, whereas the other half would cancel it instead. Wide inconsistency in practice will foster a lack of support among surgeons and will lead to reluctance to have their patients evaluated. Such a preoperative evaluation program is unlikely to be successful.

ROLE OF THE MEDICAL CONSULTANT IN PREOPERATIVE EVALUATION

Use of preoperative medical consultation varies across hospitals, likely depending on the expertise in perioperative medicine among the clinicians performing preanesthesia assessments. Since exposure to preoperative evaluation is inadequate at many anesthesia residency programs,[474] some anesthesia departments may prefer that medical specialists take primary responsibility for preoperative evaluations at their centers. Conversely, when anesthesiologists involved with preoperative evaluation develop improved comfort with interpreting ECGs, cardiac stress tests, or other specialized tests, rates of medical consultations can be substantially reduced.[17]

Medical consultants have a clear role in the preoperative care of selected surgical patients. For example, these consultations can help manage unstable medical conditions (e.g., unstable angina), optimize poorly controlled medical diseases (e.g., asthma exacerbation), or facilitate clinically indicated diagnostic workups (e.g., coronary angiography following high-risk cardiac stress test results).

Preoperative consultation by medical specialists or hospitalists can also help facilitate postoperative comanagement by these same individuals.[475] The comanagement model for postoperative care of surgical patients is increasingly common,[476] although its benefits with respect to clinical outcomes and healthcare costs remain uncertain.[477-482] Multidisciplinary collaboration with medical consultants can be especially helpful for perioperative management of complex or uncommon medical disorders. Indeed, some clinical practice guidelines recommend such multidisciplinary team management for patients with known cardiac disease undergoing high-risk noncardiac surgery,[9] as well as patients with significant pulmonary hypertension or adult congenital heart disease undergoing noncardiac surgery.[7]

Despite these theoretical benefits, preoperative medical consultation has shown a variable effect on postoperative outcomes. A randomized trial of outpatient preoperative evaluation demonstrated fewer last-minute surgical cancellations but no difference in hospital length of stay, as well as an increase in consultations.[483] In other nonrandomized studies, medical consultation was associated with increases in specialized testing, costs, hospital length of stay, and mortality.[484,485] Conversely, a transition from an anesthesiologist-led to a hospitalist-led preoperative assessment clinic was associated with reduced hospital length of stay in high-risk patients,[486] while preoperative geriatric consultation was associated with improved postoperative 90-day outcomes (i.e., survival, hospital length of stay, need for supported discharge, hospital readmission) in elderly patients (≥65 years) undergoing major elective noncardiac surgery.[487] Potential reasons for this variable effect may be the absence of recommendations or new interventions resulting from many medical consultations,[488,489] as well as disagreements among medical specialists, anesthesiologists, and surgeons on the intended purpose of these consultations.[468] In addition, increased burden of comorbidity is a very small determinant of whether patients are referred for preoperative medical consultations,[490-492] a finding suggesting poor patient selection during referral to medical specialists. Thus, during preoperative evaluation, the anesthesiologist should ensure that any referrals to medical specialists before surgery involve appropriate matching of patient profiles to specialist expertise. For example, patients with high-risk IHD should be referred to a cardiologist, while frail elderly patients should be referred to a geriatrician.

STRUCTURES AND ACTIVITIES OF THE PREOPERATIVE EVALUATION CLINIC

The daily operations of a preoperative evaluation clinic vary based on the patient volume, the general level of medical complexity among surgical patients, the type of available clinic facilities, and staffing resources. Nonetheless, a general operational structure can be proposed based on examination of several preoperative clinic models currently in practice.

Centers with large surgical case volumes should have their patients formally scheduled in the clinic before the day of evaluation, to allow for medical records and relevant outside information to be acquired and collated. The surgeon's office should schedule this clinic appointment at the same time that it books the operating room case. To ensure timely patient access and flow through the facility, these appointments should be booked using an efficient clinic scheduling system. Ideally, appointments should be scheduled to allow sufficient time between the clinic visit and the scheduled surgical procedure, to facilitate any additional preoperative testing, consultations, or interventions. Some degree of flexibility in the clinic schedule is also needed, especially to accommodate patients who have urgent indications for surgery. One approach for incorporating some flexibility is to include a few open appointment slots in the daily clinic schedule that can be used as needed for last-minute patient referrals. Such flexibility is required for individuals residing in rural and remote areas, who have been reported to have reduced rates of access to preoperative evaluation clinic facilities.[493] Anesthesiologists at some centers have also adopted telemedicine technology (defined as healthcare delivery and sharing of medical knowledge over a distance using telecommunications systems)[494] so that patients residing at remote locations can undergo preanesthesia consultations without traveling long distances to the clinic.[495]

At the clinic, a clinician interviews and examines the patient, obtains historical medical information and outside records, and determines whether (and which) additional laboratory tests, ECGs, radiographs, or other diagnostic tests are required. Phlebotomy, ECG, and hospital admitting and insurance registration services are typically available in the preoperative clinic facility. The ECGs are assessed during the clinic visit itself, whereas laboratory test results are evaluated at the end of each clinic day, with follow-up of abnormal findings as needed. In this manner, significant abnormalities can be addressed immediately; thus, any required delays or cancellations of surgical cases can occur well in advance of the scheduled day of surgery. This centralization of multiple services is also a significant convenience for patients, who no longer have to visit multiple hospital locations to complete their preoperative requirements. This arrangement should also centralize all medical data relevant to the scheduled hospital admission into a single chart, which remains in the preoperative evaluation clinic area until the date of surgery. In addition to addressing medical aspects relevant to the scheduled surgery, the preoperative evaluation program plays an important role in educating surgical patients. Typically, both the clinician performing the preoperative assessment and a specifically trained nurse educator discuss the forthcoming perioperative process with each patient and family members. By increasing patients' awareness of important components pertaining to their scheduled hospital admission (e.g., analgesic options, risks of anesthesia), this education process can decrease patients' anxiety,[18] as well as increase their willingness to receive regional analgesia.[19] The types of clinicians who perform the preanesthesia assessment include anesthesiologists and specially trained nurse practitioners. Some authors have questioned whether the responsible anesthesiologist in the operating room would be satisfied with preanesthesia assessments performed by another individual.[496] Patients themselves often report a preference for having the same anesthesiologist in both the preoperative clinic and the operating room.[497] Nonetheless, it is simply not feasible for all patients in the preoperative clinic to be evaluated by their eventual anesthesia providers. Furthermore, a large Dutch cohort study of about 21,000 surgical patients demonstrated that responsible anesthesia providers were satisfied with 95% of outpatient preanesthesia assessments performed by other anesthesiologists or trained nurses.[498]

Preoperative programs must adopt several strategies to ensure that anesthesia providers in the operating room will be satisfied with the quality of outpatient preoperative assessments. First, the anesthesia department must develop consensus standards for determining when patients should have scheduled surgery cancelled for medical reasons. Second, the documentation required for all preanesthesia assessments in the clinic should be standardized. This standardization helps prevent situations in which an assessment does not contain information needed by the anesthesia provider in the operating room to determine a patient's fitness for surgery or to develop an anesthetic management plan. Some national anesthesiology groups have initiated work on consensus-based documentation standards for all preanesthesia assessments.[23] Strategies for improving the consistency of documentation across preanesthesia assessments include the use of checklists, as well as structured electronic or paper-based forms for documenting preanesthesia assessments. Third, all nurse practitioners or other nonanesthesia clinicians assessing patients in the clinic should undergo an intensive and ongoing education in preoperative assessment. Anesthesiologists with strong interest and expertise in preoperative evaluation should lead this education program. Previous research has shown that well-trained nurses do perform effectively in both screening and evaluating patients in preoperative clinics.[499-501]

IMPACT ON OPERATING ROOM EFFICIENCY AND OUTCOMES

Anesthesia-led preoperative assessment clinics have had positive impact on operating room efficiency and outcomes (see the earlier section "Goals and Benefits of Preanesthesia Evaluation"). The demonstrated benefits of these clinics include fewer case cancellations on the day of surgery,[14,20,22,469] shorter duration of hospitalization,[22,469,470] and a possible reduction in postoperative mortality.[471] Other mechanisms whereby preoperative evaluation clinics reduce healthcare costs include more selective ordering of preoperative laboratory tests and specialist referrals.[14,16,17] Thus, although preoperative evaluation programs do incur costs (e.g., facility development costs, staff salaries), they can still lead to an overall reduction in hospital costs as a result of these associated cost savings.[469]

PATIENT SATISFACTION WITH PREOPERATIVE EVALUATION CLINICS

In addition to addressing perioperative efficiencies and clinical outcomes, preoperative programs should also consider the experience and satisfaction of patients attending their clinics. During development of strategies to improve patient satisfaction, the underlying determinants of improved satisfaction should be considered. They include being assessed by the same anesthesiologist who will administer anesthesia in the operating room, shorter wait times in the clinic, and good quality of communication from the clinic staff.[497,502,503] Because it is simply not feasible to have all patients in the clinic seen by their eventual anesthesia providers, the major focus should be on improving wait times and the quality of communication. Changes in appointment booking systems,[504] process flows, and clinic operations can decrease wait times,[499] which in turn can substantially improve patients' satisfaction.[499] In addition, preoperative programs can ensure that patients receive an accurate estimate of average waiting times before their scheduled clinic visit, and use any encountered wait times to conduct other clinic-related activities (e.g., physical therapy instructions, video-based preoperative education).

Conclusion

The practice of anesthesiology has changed. The expanding role of the anesthesiologist outside the operating room will redefine the specialty's contribution to high-quality patient care in the healthcare system. Within the context of preoperative evaluation, anesthesiologists must be knowledgeable and adept at assessing patients of highly varying medical complexity, whether in an outpatient preoperative evaluation clinic before the day of the surgical procedure or at the bedside immediately before induction of anesthesia. Anesthesiologists must be familiar with the impact of a broad range of chronic and acute medical conditions on patients' risks for anesthesia and surgery. In addition, this role entails awareness of multiple practice guidelines, regulatory requirements, and approaches for efficient management of outpatient clinics. Despite this evolving and expanding role of anesthesiologists in preoperative care, the primary purpose of preoperative evaluation will never change. It is the clinical foundation for guiding perioperative patient management, and it has the potential to reduce perioperative morbidity and enhance patient outcome.

Acknowledgment

The editors, publisher, and Dr. Duminda Wijeysundera would like to thank Dr. Bobbie-Jean Sweitzer for her contribution to this chapter in the prior edition of this work. It has served as the foundation for the current chapter.

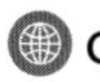 **Complete references available online at expertconsult.com.**

References

1. Kain ZN, et al. *Anesth Analg*. 2014;118(5):1126.
2. Saidman LJ. *Anesthesiology*. 1995;83:191.
3. Deutschman CS, Traber KB. *Anesthesiology*. 1996;85(1).
4. Etzioni DA, et al. *Am Surg*. 2003;69(11):961.
5. Apfelbaum JL, et al. *Anesthesiology*. 2012;116:522.
6. De Hert S, et al. *Eur J Anaesthesiol*. 2018;35(6):407.
7. Fleisher LA, et al. *Circulation*. 2009;120:e169.
8. Duceppe E, et al. *Can J Cardiol*. 2017;33(1):17.
9. Kristensen SD, et al. *Eur Heart J*. 2014;35(35):2383.
10. Qaseem A, et al. *Ann Intern Med*. 2006;144:575.
11. Gould MK, et al. *Chest*. 2012;141(suppl 2):e227S.
12. Falck-Ytter Y, et al. *Chest*. 2012;141(suppl 2):e278S.
13. Kluger MT, et al. *Anaesthesia*. 2000;55:1173.

14. Fischer SP. *Anesthesiology*. 1996;85:196.
15. Issa MRN, et al. *Rev Bras Anestesiol*. 2011;61:60.
16. Power LM, Thackray NM. *Anaesth Intensive Care*. 1999;27:481.
17. Tsen LC, et al. *Anesth Analg*. 2002;95:1563.
18. Klopfenstein CE, et al. *Can J Anaesth*. 2000;47:511.
19. Wijeysundera DN, et al. *Arch Intern Med*. 2009;169:595.
20. Ferschl MB, et al. *Anesthesiology*. 2005;103:855.
21. Pollard JB, et al. *Anesth Analg*. 1997;85:1307.
22. van Klei WA, et al. *Anesth Analg*. 2002;94:644.
23. Ahmadian L, et al. *Methods Inf Med*. 2009;48:155.
24. Grant C, et al. *Anaesth Intensive Care*. 2012;40(2):297.
25. Flamm M, et al. *J Am Med Inform Assoc*. 2013;20(e1):e91.
26. Simel DL, Rennie D. *The Rational Clinical Examination: Evidence-Based Clinical Diagnosis (Jama & Archives Journals)*. McGraw-Hill: Education / Medical; 2008.
27. Benjamin EJ, et al. *Circulation*. 2018;137(12):e67.
28. Hennis PJ, et al. *Postgrad Med J*. 2011;87(1030):550.
29. Moran J, et al. *Br J Anaesth*. 2016;116(2):177.
30. Carliner NH, et al. *Am J Cardiol*. 1985;56(1):51.
31. McPhail N, et al. *J Vasc Surg*. 1988;7(1):60–68.
32. Bilimoria KY, et al. *J Am Coll Surg*. 2013;217(5):833–842.e1.
33. Gupta PK, et al. *Circulation*. 2011;124(4):381–387.
34. Arozullah AM, et al. *Ann Intern Med*. 2001;135(10):847–857.
35. Arozullah AM, et al. *Ann Surg*. 2000;232(2):242–253.
36. Wijeysundera DN, et al. *Lancet*. 2018;39(10140):2631–2640.
37. Melon CC, et al. *JAMA Intern Med*. 2014;174(9):1507–1508.
38. Stokes JW, et al. *Perioper Med (Lond)*. 2016;5:18.
39. Reilly DF. *Arch Intern Med*. 1999;159:2185.
40. Jaeschke R, et al. *JAMA*. 1994;271(9):703–707.
41. Wiklund RA, et al. *Yale J Biol Med*. 2001;74:75.
42. Hlatky MA, et al. *Am J Cardiol*. 1989;64(10):651–654.
43. Struthers R, et al. *Br J Anaesth*. 2008;101(6):774–780.
44. Moran J, et al. *J Clin Anesth*. 2016:35446–35455.
45. Benge W, et al. *Circulation*. 1980;61(5):955–959.
46. Franciosa JA, et al. *Am J Cardiol*. 1981;47(1):33–39.
47. Pai MP, Paloucek FP. *Ann Pharmacother*. 2000;34(9):1066–1069.
48. Devine BJ. *Drug Intell Clin Pharm*. 1974:8650–8655.
49. Hartle A, et al. *Anaesthesia*. 2016;71(3):326–337.
50. Apfelbaum JL, et al. *Anesthesiology*. 2013;118(2):251–270.
51. Mallampati SR, et al. *Can Anaesth Soc J*. 1985;32:429.
52. Langeron O, et al. *Anesthesiology*. 2000;92(5):1229–1236.
53. Kheterpal S, et al. *Anesthesiology*. 2006;105(5):885–891.
54. Oresanya LB, et al. *JAMA*. 2014;311(20):2110–2120.
55. Chow WB, et al. *J Am Coll Surg*. 2012;215(4):453–466.
56. Podsiadlo D, Richardson S. *J Am Geriatr Soc*. 1991;39(2):142–148.
57. Robinson TN, et al. *Ann Surg*. 2013;258(4):582–588;discussion 588.
58. Fried LP. Chapter 24 - Frailty. In: Medina-Walpole A, Pacala JT, Potter JF, eds. *Geriatric Review Syllabus*. New York, NY, USA: American Geriatrics Society; 2016.
59. Fried LP, et al. *J Gerontol A Biol Sci Med Sci*. 2001;56(3):M146–M156.
60. Mitnitski AB, et al. *ScientificWorldJournal*. 2001:1323–1336.
61. Dasgupta M, et al. *Arch Gerontol Geriatr*. 2009;48(1):78–83.
62. McIsaac DI, et al. *JAMA Surg*. 2016;151(6):538–545.
63. McIsaac DI, et al. *Bone Joint J*. 2016;98-B(6):799–805.
64. McIsaac DI, et al. *Anesth Analg*. 2017;124(5):1653–1661.
65. Ghignone F, et al. *Eur J Surg Oncol*. 2016;42(2):297–302.
66. Robinson TN, et al. *Ann Surg*. 2009;250(3):449–455.
67. Robinson TN, et al. *J Am Coll Surg*. 2011;213(1):37–42;discussion 42.
68. Charlson ME, et al. *J Chronic Dis*. 1987;40(5):373–383.
69. Rolfson DB, et al. *Age Ageing*. 2006;35(5):526–529.
70. Steffens DC, et al. *Int Psychogeriatr*. 2009;21(5):879–888.
71. Blazer DG, Wu LT. *Am J Psychiatry*. 2009;166(10):1162–1169.
72. Nath B, et al. *J Gastrointest Surg*. 2010;14(11):1732–1741.
73. Harari D, et al. *Age Ageing*. 2007;36(2):190–196.
74. McDonald SR, et al. *JAMA Surg*. 2018.
75. Englesbe MJ, et al. *Surgery*. 2017;161(6):1659–1666.
76. Sessums LL, et al. *JAMA*. 2011;306(4):420–427.
77. Devereaux PJ, et al. *JAMA*. 2012;307(21):2295–2304.
78. Devereaux PJ, et al. *JAMA*. 2017;317(16):1642–1651.
79. Gualandro DM, et al. *Arq Bras Cardiol*. 2017;109(3 suppl 1):1–104.
80. Kyo S, et al. *Circ J*. 2017;81(2):245–267.
81. Whelton PK, et al. *Hypertension*. 2017.
82. Muntner P, et al. *Circulation*. 2018;137(2):109–118.
83. Lewington S, et al. *Lancet*. 2002;360(9349):1903–1913.
84. Howell SJ, et al. *Br J Anaesth*. 2004;92:570.
85. Rosenman DJ, et al. *J Hosp Med*. 2008;3:319.
86. Roshanov PS, et al. *Anesthesiology*. 2017;126(1):16–27.
87. Lee SM, et al. *Anesthesiology*. 2015;123(2):288–306.
88. Mudumbai SC, et al. *J Hosp Med*. 2014;9(5):289–296.
89. GBD Macodc. *Lancet*. 2015;385(9963):117–171.
90. Ridker PM, et al. *N Engl J Med*. 2017;377(12):1119–1131.
91. Eikelboom JW, et al. *N Engl J Med*. 2017;377(14):1319–1330.
92. Sabatine MS, et al. *N Engl J Med*. 2017;376(18):1713–1722.
93. Windecker S, et al. *BMJ*. 2014;348g:3859.
94. Yusuf S, et al. *Lancet*. 1994;344(8922):563–570.
95. Head SJ, et al. *Lancet*. 2018;391(10124):939–948.
96. Boden WE, et al. *N Engl J Med*. 2007;356(15):1503–1516.
97. Lee TH, et al. *Circulation*. 1999;100(10):1043–1049.
98. Botto F, et al. *Anesthesiology*. 2014;120(3):564–578.
99. Le Manach Y, et al. *Anesthesiology*. 2016;124(3):570–579.
100. van Klei WA, et al. *Ann Surg*. 2007;246(2):165–170.
101. Musallam KM, et al. *Lancet*. 2011;378:1396.
102. Wu WC, et al. *JAMA*. 2007;297:2481.
103. Beattie WS, et al. *Anesthesiology*. 2010;112:25.
104. Le Manach Y, et al. *Anesthesiology*. 2012;117:1203.
105. Livhits M, et al. *Ann Surg*. 2011;253(5):857–864.
106. Ford MK, et al. *Ann Intern Med*. 2010;152(1):26–35.
107. Liu JB, et al. *Anesthesiology*. 2018;128(2):283–292.
108. Forshaw MJ, et al. *Ann Thorac Surg*. 2008;85(1):294–299.
109. James S, et al. *Br J Anaesth*. 2014;112(3):491–497.
110. Balion C, et al. Rockville, MD: Agency for Healthcare Research and Quality; 2006.
111. Rodseth RN, et al. *J Am Coll Cardiol*. 2014;63(2):170–180.
112. Lurati Buse GA, et al. *Circulation*. 2012;126(23):2696–2704.
113. Rajagopalan S, et al. *Eur J Vasc Endovasc Surg*. 2011;41(5):657–662.
114. de Lemos JA, et al. *JAMA*. 2010;304(22):2503–2512.
115. deFilippi CR, et al. *JAMA*. 2010;304(22):2494–2502.
116. Kavsak PA, et al. *Clin Biochem*. 2011;44(12):1021–1024.
117. Weber M, et al. *Eur Heart J*. 2013;34(11):853–862.
118. Kopec M, et al. *Anesth Analg*. 2017;124(2):398–405.
119. Nagele P, et al. *Am Heart J*. 2013;166(2):325–332. e1.
120. Kertai MD, et al. *Heart*. 2003;89:1327.
121. Beattie WS, et al. *Anesth Analg*. 2006;102:8.
122. Etchells E, et al. *J Vasc Surg*. 2002;36:534.
123. Miller JM, et al. *N Engl J Med*. 2008;359(22):2324–2336.
124. Meijboom WB, et al. *J Am Coll Cardiol*. 2008;52(25):2135–2144.
125. Ahn JH, et al. *J Am Coll Cardiol*. 2013;61(6):661–668.
126. Sheth T, et al. *BMJ*. 2015;350:h1907.
127. Illuminati G, et al. *Eur J Vasc Endovasc Surg*. 2010;39(2):139–145.
128. Illuminati G, et al. *Eur J Vasc Endovasc Surg*. 2015;49(4):366–374.
129. Monaco M, et al. *J Am Coll Cardiol*. 2009;54:989.
130. McFalls EO, et al. *N Engl J Med*. 2004;351:2795.
131. Garcia S, et al. *Am J Cardiol*. 2008;102(7):809–813.
132. Devereaux PJ, et al. *Lancet*. 2008;371(9627):1839–1847.
133. Wijeysundera DN, et al. *Circulation*. 2014;130(24):2246–2264.
134. Devereaux PJ, et al. *N Engl J Med*. 2014;370(16):1504–1513.
135. Duncan D, et al. *Cochrane Database Syst Rev*. 2018;3:CD004126.
136. Devereaux PJ, et al. *N Engl J Med*. 2014;370(16):1494–1503.
137. Mangano DT, et al. *N Engl J Med*. 1996;335(23):1713–1720.
138. Ellenberger C, et al. *Anesthesiology*. 2011;114:817.
139. Wijeysundera DN, et al. *Can J Cardiol*. 2014;30(2):217–223.
140. Chen RJ, et al. *J Am Heart Assoc*. 2017;6:1.
141. Biondi-Zoccai GG, et al. *Eur Heart J*. 2006;27(22):2667–2674.
142. Sheth T, et al. *Br J Anaesth*. 2018;120(4):725–733.
143. Helwani MA, et al. *Anesthesiology*. 2018;128(6):1084–1091.
144. Graham MM, et al. *Ann Intern Med*. 2018;168(4):237–244.
145. Levine GN, et al. *Circulation*. 2016;134(10):e123–e155.
146. Hawn MT, et al. *JAMA*. 2013;310(14):1462–1472.
147. Wijeysundera DN, et al. *Circulation*. 2012;126:1355.
148. Holcomb CN, et al. *JAMA Surg*. 2016;151(5):462–469.
149. Webster SE, et al. *J Vasc Surg*. 2004;40:463.
150. Yancy CW, et al. *Circulation*. 2013;128(16):e240–e327.
151. McMurray JJ, et al. *Eur Heart J*. 1999;suppl 19:PP9-16.
152. Yancy CW, et al. *Circulation*. 2013;128(16):e240–e327.
153. Udelson JE. *Circulation*. 2011;124(21):e540–e543.
154. Bhatia RS, et al. *N Engl J Med*. 2006;355(3):260–269.
155. Meta-analysis Global Group in Chronic Heart Failure MAGGIC. *Eur Heart J*. 2012;33(14):1750–1757.

156. Yancy CW, et al. *Circulation*. 2017;136(6):e137–e161.
157. Hammill BG, et al. *Anesthesiology*. 2008;108:559.
158. Maile MD, et al. *Anesth Analg*. 2014;119(3):522–532.
159. Healy KO, et al. *Congest Heart Fail*. 2010;16(2):45–49.
160. Fayad A, et al. *Anesthesiology*. 2016;125(1):72–91.
161. Halm EA, et al. *Ann Intern Med*. 1996;125:433.
162. Rohde LE, et al. *Am J Cardiol*. 2001;87:505.
163. Xu-Cai YO, et al. *Mayo Clin Proc*. 2008;83(3):280–288.
164. Booth RA, et al. *Heart Fail Rev*. 2014;19(4):439–451.
165. Hill SA, et al. *Heart Fail Rev*. 2014;19(4):421–438.
166. Khan NA, et al. *Am J Med*. 2010;123(11):1059.e1–1059.e8.
167. Nishimura RA, et al. *Circulation*. 2014;129(23):e521–643.
168. Coffey S, et al. *J Am Coll Cardiol*. 2014;63(25 Pt A):2852–2861.
169. Etchells E, et al. *J Gen Intern Med*. 1998;13:699.
170. Agarwal S, et al. *Circ Cardiovasc Qual Outcomes*. 2013;6(2):193–200.
171. Tashiro T, et al. *Eur Heart J*. 2014;35:2372–2381.
172. Vincentelli A, et al. *N Engl J Med*. 2003;349:343.
173. Nishimura RA, et al. *Circulation*. 2017;135(25):e1159–e1195.
174. Desjardins VA, et al. *Am J Med*. 1996;100:149.
175. Choudhry NK, Etchells EE. *JAMA*. 1999;281(23):2231–2238.
176. Lai HC, et al. *Acta Anaesthesiol Scand*. 2010;54(5):580–588.
177. Bajaj NS, et al. *Am J Med*. 2013;126(6):529–535.
178. Bonow RO, et al. *Circulation*. 2008;118(15):e523–e661.
179. Freed LA, et al. *J Am Coll Cardiol*. 2002;40(7):1298–1304.
180. The 2015 ESC Guidelines for the management of infective endocarditis. *Eur Heart J*. 2015;36(44):3036–3037.
181. Epstein AE, et al. *Circulation*. 2013;127(3):e283–e352.
182. Dorman T, et al. *Arch Intern Med*. 2000;160(8):1149–1152.
183. Fahy GJ, et al. *Am J Cardiol*. 1996;77(14):1185–1190.
184. Eriksson P, et al. *Eur Heart J*. 2005;26:2300.
185. Hesse B, et al. *Am J Med*. 2001;110(4):253–259.
186. Zhang ZM, et al. *Am J Cardiol*. 2012;110(10):1489–1495.
187. January CT, et al. *Circulation*. 2014;130(23):e199–267.
188. Van Gelder IC, et al. *N Engl J Med*. 2002;347:1834.
189. Wyse DG, et al. *N Engl J Med*. 2002;347:1825.
190. Lip GY, et al. *Chest*. 2010;137(2):263–272.
191. Friberg L, et al. *Eur Heart J*. 2012;33(12):1500–1510.
192. Hart RG, et al. *Ann Intern Med*. 2007;146(12):857–867.
193. McAlister FA, et al. *J Thromb Haemost*. 2015;13(10):1768–1775.
194. Kaatz S, et al. *J Thromb Haemost*. 2010;8(5):884–890.
195. Doherty JU, et al. *J Am Coll Cardiol*. 2017;69(7):871–898.
196. Horlocker TT, et al. *Reg Anesth Pain Med*. 2018;43(3):263–309.
197. Douketis JD, et al. *Thromb Haemost*. 2017;117(12):2415–2424.
198. Douketis JD, et al. *N Engl J Med*. 2015;373(9):823–833.
199. Glatter KA, et al. *Circulation*. 2001;104(16):1933–1939.
200. Drew BJ, et al. *Circulation*. 2010;121:1047.
201. Greenspon AJ, et al. *J Am Coll Cardiol*. 2012;60(16):1540–1545.
202. Kremers MS, et al. *Heart Rhythm*. 2013;10(4):e59–65.
203. Bernstein AD, et al. *Pacing Clin Electrophysiol*. 2002;25:260.
204. Crossley GH, et al. *Heart Rhythm*. 2011;8:e1.
205. Healey JS, et al. *Can J Anaesth*. 2012;59(4):394–407.
206. American SOA. *Anesthesiology*. 2011;114(2):247–261.
207. Fowkes FG, et al. *Lancet*. 2013;382(9901):1329–1340.
208. Creager MA, et al. *J Am Coll Cardiol*. 2012;59(3):294–357.
209. Golomb BA, et al. *Circulation*. 2006;114(7):688–699.
210. Doobay AV, Anand SS. *Arterioscler Thromb Vasc Biol*. 2005;25(7): 1463–1469.
211. Fisher BW, et al. *Anesth Analg*. 2008;107(1):149–154.
212. Jørgensen ME, et al. *JAMA*. 2014;312(3):269–277.
213. Masoli M, et al. *Allergy*. 2004;59(5):469–478.
214. Warner DO, et al. *Anesthesiology*. 1996;85(3):460–467.
215. Silvanus MT, et al. *Anesthesiology*. 2004;100:1052.
216. GBD CRDC. *Lancet Respir Med*. 2017;5(9):691–706.
217. Gupta N, et al. *Eur Respir J*. 2014;44(4):873–884.
218. Smetana GW, et al. *Ann Intern Med*. 2006;144:581.
219. Brunelli A, et al. *Chest*. 2013;143(suppl 5):e166S–e190S.
220. Young T, et al. *N Engl J Med*. 1993;328(17):1230–1235.
221. Peppard PE, et al. *Am J Epidemiol*. 2013;177(9):1006–1014.
222. Gottlieb DJ, et al. *N Engl J Med*. 2014;370(24):2276–2285.
223. Chirinos JA, et al. *N Engl J Med*. 2014;370(24):2265–2275.
224. Araghi MH, et al. *Sleep*. 2013;36(10):1553–1562, 1562A.
225. Singh M, et al. *Br J Anaesth*. 2013.
226. Chung F, et al. *Br J Anaesth*. 2012;108(5):768–775.
227. Chung F, et al. *Chest*. 2013;143(5):1284–1293.
228. Chung F, et al. *J Clin Sleep Med*. 2014;10(9):951–958.
229. Opperer M, et al. *Anesth Analg*. 2016;122(5):1321–1334.
230. Lockhart EM, et al. *Sleep Med*. 2013;14(5):407–415.
231. Khanna AK, et al. *Br J Anaesth*. 2016;116(5):632–640.
232. Simonneau G, et al. *J Am Coll Cardiol*. 2013;62(25 suppl):D34–41.
233. Kaw R, et al. *Respir Med*. 2011;105(4):619–624.
234. Lai HC, et al. *Br J Anaesth*. 2007;99(2):184–190.
235. Ramakrishna G, et al. *J Am Coll Cardiol*. 2005;45(10):1691–1699.
236. Brown LM, et al. *Chest*. 2011;140(1):19–26.
237. Musallam KM, et al. *JAMA Surg*. 2013;148(8):755–762.
238. Turan A, et al. *Anesthesiology*. 2011;114(4):837–846.
239. Rigotti NA. *JAMA*. 2012;308(15):1573–1580.
240. A clinical practice guideline for treating tobacco use and dependence: 2008 update. A U.S. Public Health Service report. *Am J Prev Med*. 2008;35:158.
241. Stead LF, et al. *Cochrane Database Syst Rev*. 2013;(5):CD000165.
242. Stead LF, et al. *Cochrane Database Syst Rev*. 2016:3:CD008286.
243. Shi Y, Warner DO. *Anesthesiology*. 2010;112(1):102–107.
244. Zaki A, et al. *Can J Anaesth*. 2008;55:11.
245. Berlin NL, et al. *Am J Manag Care*. 2015;21(11):e623–e631.
246. Wong J, et al. *Anesthesiology*. 2012;117:755.
247. Lee SM, et al. *Anesth Analg*. 2015;120(3):582–587.
248. Turan A, et al. *Eur J Anaesthesiol*. 2018;35(4):256–265.
249. Mills E, et al. *Am J Med*. 2011;124(2):144–154.e8.
250. Wong J, et al. *Can J Anaesth*. 2012;59(3):268–279.
251. Warner MA, et al. *Mayo Clin Proc*. 1989;64:609.
252. Myers K, et al. *Arch Intern Med*. 2011;171:983.
253. von Ungern-Sternberg BS, et al. *Lancet*. 2010;376(9743):773–783.
254. Tait AR, et al. *Anesthesiology*. 2001;95(2):299–306.
255. Rosenstein BJ, Cutting GR. *J Pediatr*. 1998;132(4):589–595.
256. Abbott TEF, et al. *Br J Anaesth*. 2018;120(5):1066–1079.
257. Canet J, et al. *Anesthesiology*. 2010;113(6):1338–1350.
258. Yang CK, et al. *J Surg Res*. 2015;198(2):441–449.
259. Gupta H, et al. *Chest*. 2011;140(5):1207–1215.
260. Gupta H, et al. *Mayo Clin Proc*. 2013;88(11):1241–1249.
261. Mazo V, et al. *Anesthesiology*. 2014;121(2):219–231.
262. Katsura M, et al. *Cochrane Database Syst Rev*. 2015;(10):CD010356.
263. Boden I, et al. *BMJ*. 2018;360:j5916.
264. Guay J, et al. *Cochrane Database Syst Rev*. 2014;(1):CD010108.
265. Hausman MS, et al. *Anesth Analg*. 2015;120(6):1405–1412.
266. NCD Rfcncd-R. *Lancet*. 2016;387(10027):1513–1530.
267. American DA. *Diabetes Care*. 2014;37(suppl 1):S81–90.
268. Wijeysundera DN, et al. *JAMA*. 2007;297:1801.
269. Thakar CV, et al. *J Am Soc Nephrol*. 2005;16:162.
270. Martin ET, et al. *Infect Control Hosp Epidemiol*. 2016;37(1):88–99.
271. Koumpan Y, et al. *Can J Anaesth*. 2014;61(5):407–416.
272. Moitra VK, et al. *Can J Anaesth*. 2010;57:322.
273. Bock M, et al. *Eur J Anaesthesiol*. 2015;32(3):152–159.
274. Excellence Nifhac. Routine preoperative tests for elective surgery NICE guideline [NG45]. 2016
275. Buchleitner AM, et al. *Cochrane Database Syst Rev*. 2012;(9): CD007315.
276. Peacock SC, Lovshin JA. *Can J Anaesth*. 2018;65(2):143–147.
277. Handelsman Y, et al. *Endocr Pract*. 2016;22(6):753–762.
278. Weinberg AD, et al. *Arch Intern Med*. 1983;143:893.
279. Komatsu R, et al. *Anesth Analg*. 2015;121(3):716–726.
280. Chernow B, et al. *Arch Intern Med*. 1987;147(7):1273–1278.
281. Lamberts SW, et al. *N Engl J Med*. 1997;337(18):1285–1292.
282. Cooper MS, Stewart PM. *N Engl J Med*. 2003;348(8):727–734.
283. Deleted in proofs.
284. Liu MM, et al. *Anesthesiology*. 2017;127(1):166–172.
285. Oelkers W. *N Engl J Med*. 1996;335(16):1206–1212.
286. Bornstein SR, et al. *J Clin Endocrinol Metab*. 2016;101(2):364–389.
287. Thakker RV, et al. *J Clin Endocrinol Metab*. 2012;97(9):2990–3011.
288. Beard CM, et al. *Mayo Clin Proc*. 1983;58(12):802–804.
289. Young WF. Clinical presentation and diagnosis of pheochromocytoma. In: Nieman LK, Martin KA, eds. *UpToDate*. Waltham, MA: UpToDate; 2017
290. Lenders JW, et al. *J Clin Endocrinol Metab*. 2014;99(6):1915–1942.
291. Weingarten TN, et al. *Urology*. 2010;76:508.
292. Levey AS, et al. *Kidney Int*. 2005;67(6):2089–2100.
293. Wijeysundera DN, et al. *Anesthesiology*. 2006;104:65.
294. Cockcroft DW, Gault MH. *Nephron*. 1976;16(1):31–41.
295. Levey AS, et al. *Ann Intern Med*. 1999;130(6):461–470.
296. Levey AS, et al. *Ann Intern Med*. 2009;150:604.
297. Bellomo R, et al. *Crit Care*. 2004;8:R204.
298. Mehta RL, et al. *Crit Care*. 2007;11:R31.
299. Group KDIGOKDIGOAKIW. *Kidney Int Suppl*. 2012:21–138.

300. Singh AK, et al. *N Engl J Med.* 2006;355:2085.
301. Chapter 3: Use of ESAs and other agents to treat anemia in CKD. *Kidney Int Suppl (2011).* 2012;2(4):299–310.
302. Walsh M, et al. *J Am Soc Nephrol.* 2015;26(10):2571–2577.
303. Kheterpal S, et al. *Anesthesiology.* 2007;107:892.
304. Kheterpal S, et al. *Anesthesiology.* 2009;110:505.
305. Vlisides P, Mashour GA. *Can J Anaesth.* 2016;63(2):193–204.
306. Lee A, et al. *Cochrane Database Syst Rev.* 2007;(2):CD002765.
307. Mehta RH, et al. *Circulation.* 2011;124(suppl 11):S149–S155.
308. Giacoppo D, et al. *Circ Cardiovasc Interv.* 2015;8:e002475.
309. Weisbord SD, et al. *N Engl J Med.* 2018;378(7):603–614.
310. Pain JA, et al. *Br J Surg.* 1991;78:467.
311. Malinchoc M, et al. *Hepatology.* 2000;31:864.
312. Shirahatti RG, et al. *J R Coll Surg Edinb.* 1997;42:238.
313. Kabbany MN, et al. *Am J Gastroenterol.* 2017;112(4):581–587.
314. Younossi ZM, et al. *Clin Gastroenterol Hepatol.* 2011;9(6): 524–530.e1; quiz e60.
315. Cholankeril G, et al. *Dig Dis Sci.* 2017;62(10):2915–2922.
316. Schemel WH. *Anesth Analg.* 1976;55:810.
317. Befeler AS, et al. *Arch Surg.* 2005;140(7):650–654. discussion 655.
318. Fowler AJ, et al. *Br J Surg.* 2015;102(11):1314–1324.
319. Beattie WS, et al. *Anesthesiology.* 2009;110:574.
320. Voorn VM, et al. *Vox Sang.* 2016;111(3):219–225.
321. Froessler B, et al. *Ann Surg.* 2016;264(1):41–46.
322. Johansson PI, et al. *Vox Sang.* 2015;109(3):257–266.
323. Clevenger B, et al. *Eur J Heart Fail.* 2016;18(7):774–785.
324. Swedberg K, et al. *N Engl J Med.* 2013;368(13):1210–1219.
325. Pfeffer MA, et al. *N Engl J Med.* 2009;361(21):2019–2032.
326. Anker SD, et al. *N Engl J Med.* 2009;361(25):2436–2448.
327. Kansagara D, et al. *Ann Intern Med.* 2013;159(11):746–757.
328. Carson JL, et al. *Lancet.* 1996;348(9034):1055–1060.
329. Marik PE, Corwin HL. *Crit Care Med.* 2008;36:2667.
330. Carson JL, et al. *N Engl J Med.* 2011;365(26):2453–2462.
331. Mazer CD, et al. *N Engl J Med.* 2017;377(22):2133–2144.
332. Goodnough LT, et al. *Br J Anaesth.* 2011;106(1):13–22.
333. American Soatfopbm. *Anesthesiology.* 2015;122(2):241–275.
334. Firth PG, Head CA. *Anesthesiology.* 2004;101:766.
335. Koshy M, et al. *Blood.* 1995;86:3676.
336. Howard J, et al. *Lancet.* 2013;381(9870):930–938.
337. Vichinsky EP, et al. *N Engl J Med.* 1995;333:206.
338. Srivastava A, et al. *Haemophilia.* 2013;19(1):e1–47.
339. Hoots WK, Shapiro AD. Treatment of bleeding and perioperative management in hemophilia A and B. In: Mahoney DH, Leung LLK, Tirnauer JS, eds. *UpToDate.* Waltham, MA: UpToDate; 2017
340. Sadler JE, et al. *Thromb Haemost.* 2000;84(2):160–174.
341. Warkentin TE, Kelton JG. *N Engl J Med.* 2001;344:1286.
342. Cuker A, et al. *Blood.* 2012;120(20):4160–4167.
343. Bernstein J, et al. *Anesth Analg.* 2016;123(1):165–167.
344. Goodier CG, et al. *Anesth Analg.* 2015;121(4):988–991.
345. van Veen JJ, et al. *Br J Haematol.* 2010;148(1):15–25.
346. Kaufman RM, et al. *Ann Intern Med.* 2015;162(3):205–213.
347. Lubarsky DA, et al. *J Clin Anesth.* 1991;3:99.
348. Anderson FA, et al. *Am J Hematol.* 2007;82(9):777–782.
349. Caprini JA, et al. *Semin Thromb Hemost.* 1991;17(suppl): 3304–3312.
350. Douketis JD, et al. *Chest.* 2012;141(suppl 2): e326Se350S.
351. Douketis JD, et al. *Arch Intern Med.* 2000;160(22):3431–3436.
352. Dahlbäck B. *Blood.* 2008;112(1):19–27.
353. Kearon C, Hirsh J. *N Engl J Med.* 1997;336:1506.
354. Liu SS, Mulroy MF. *Reg Anesth Pain Med.* 1998;23(6 suppl 2): 157–163.
355. Myles PS, et al. *N Engl J Med.* 2016;374(8):728–737.
356. Beving H, et al. *Blood Coagul Fibrinolysis.* 1996;7(1):80–84.
357. Feigin VL, et al. *Neuroepidemiology.* 2015;45(3):161–176.
358. Easton JD, et al. *Stroke.* 2009;40(6):2276–2293.
359. Mashour GA, et al. *Anesthesiology.* 2011;114:1289.
360. Sharifpour M, et al. *Anesth Analg.* 2013;116(2):424–434.
361. Christiansen MN, et al. *Anesthesiology.* 2017;127(1):9–19.
362. Aries MJ, et al. *Stroke.* 2010;41(11):2697–2704.
363. Dodick DW, et al. *Mayo Clin Proc.* 2004;79:937.
364. Blacker DJ, et al. *Mayo Clin Proc.* 2004;79:223.
365. Walsh M, et al. *J Am Soc Nephrol.* 2015;26(10):2571–2577.
366. Spector TD. *Rheum Dis Clin North Am.* 1990;16(3):513–537.
367. Tokunaga D, et al. *Anesthesiology.* 2006;104(4):675–679.
368. Ledingham J, Deighton C. *Rheumatology (Oxford).* 2005;44(2): 157–163.
369. Saag KG, et al. *Arthritis Rheum.* 2008;59(6):762–784.
370. Petri M. *Best Pract Res Clin Rheumatol.* 2002;16(5):847–858.
371. Johnson SR, Granton JT. *Eur Respir Rev.* 2011;20(122):277–286.
372. Bernatsky S, et al. *Arthritis Rheum.* 2009;61(3):400–404.
373. Wigley FM. *N Engl J Med.* 2002;347(13):1001–1008.
374. Ho NC, et al. *Lancet.* 2005;366(9501):1978–1981.
375. Adams MJ, et al. *Crit Rev Oncol Hematol.* 2003;45(1):55–75.
376. Ramage JK, et al. *Gut.* 2012;61(1):6–32.
377. Kinney MA, et al. *Br J Anaesth.* 2001;87(3):447–452.
378. Boudreaux JP, et al. *Pancreas.* 2010;39(6):753–766.
379. Meyhoff CS, et al. *Anesth Analg.* 2009;109(3):787–792.
380. Kostopanagiotou G, et al. *Anesth Analg.* 1999;89:613.
381. Kostopanagiotou G, et al. *Paediatr Anaesth.* 2003;13:754.
382. Harper NJN, et al. *Br J Anaesth.* 2018.
383. Mertes PM, et al. *J Allergy Clin Immunol.* 2011;128(2):366–373.
384. Harper NJN, et al. *Br J Anaesth.* 2018.
385. Lienhart A, et al. *Anesthesiology.* 2006;105:1087.
386. Florvaag E, et al. *Acta Anaesthesiol Scand.* 2005;49(4):437–444.
387. Hepner DL, Castells MC. *Anesth Analg.* 2003;96:1219.
388. Holzman RS, Brown RH, Hamid R, et al. In *Natural Rubber Latex Allergy: Considerations for Anesthesiologists.* Park Ridge, Ill: American Society of Anesthesiologists; 2005.
389. Fisher MM, Rose M. *Br J Anaesth.* 2008;101:486.
390. Collaborative Group on AIDS Incubation and HIV Survival Including the CASCADE EU Concerted Action. *Lancet.* 2000;355:1131.
391. Egger M, et al. *Lancet.* 2002;360:119.
392. Mofenson LM. *Pediatr Infect Dis J.* 1995;14:169.
393. Evron S, et al. *Anesth Analg.* 2004;98:503.
394. Günthard HF, et al. *JAMA.* 2016;316(2):191–210.
395. Friis-Moller N, et al. *N Engl J Med.* 2007;356(17):1723–1735.
396. Albaran RG, et al. *Arch Surg.* 1998;133:626.
397. Tran HS, et al. *Am J Surg.* 2000;180:228.
398. Grant BF, et al. *JAMA Psychiatry.* 2015;72(8):757–766.
399. Jage J, Heid F. *Anaesthesist.* 2006;55:611.
400. Bradley KA, et al. *J Gen Intern Med.* 2011;26(2):162–169.
401. Harris AH, et al. *J Bone Joint Surg Am.* 2011;93(4):321–327.
402. Eliasen M, et al. *Ann Surg.* 2013;258(6):930–942.
403. Ewing JA. *JAMA.* 1984;252(14):1905–1907.
404. Bush K, et al. *Arch Intern Med.* 1998;158(16):1789–1795.
405. Agabio R, et al. *J Stud Alcohol Drugs.* 2012;73(1):126–133.
406. Kleinwächter R, et al. *Minerva Anestesiol.* 2010;76(1):29–37.
407. Conigrave KM, et al. *Alcohol Clin Exp Res.* 2002;26(3):332–339.
408. Savage SR. *J Pain Symptom Manage.* 1993;8:265.
409. Baxter JL, Alexandrov AW. *AANA J.* 2012;80(suppl 4):S33–S36.
410. Bryson EO, Frost EA. *Int Anesthesiol Clin.* 2011;49:103.
411. Oppedal K, et al. *Cochrane Database Syst Rev.* 2012;(7):CD008343.
412. May JA, et al. *Anesth Analg.* 2001;92(6):1601–1608.
413. Truog RD, et al. *Lancet.* 2005;365(9461):733–735.
414. Committee on Ethics ASOA. *Ethical Guidelines for the Anesthesia Care of Patients With Do-Not-Resuscitate Orders or Other Directives That Limit Treatment;* 2013.
415. Truog RD, et al. *Anesthesiology.* 1999;90:289.
416. Grimaldo DA, et al. *Anesthesiology.* 2001;95:43.
417. Benarroch-Gampel J, et al. *Ann Surg.* 2012;256:518.
418. Chung F, et al. *Anesth Analg.* 2009;108:467.
419. Schein OD, et al. *N Engl J Med.* 2000;342:168.
420. Johansson T, et al. *Br J Anaesth.* 2013;110(6):926–939.
421. Kirkham KR, et al. *CMAJ.* 2015;187(11):E349–E358.
422. Kirkham KR, et al. *Anesthesiology.* 2016;124(4):804–814.
423. Chen CL, et al. *N Engl J Med.* 2015;372(16):1530–1538.
424. Ontario Pre-Operative Task Force, Ontario Guidelines Advisory Committee: Ontario pre-operative testing grid. http://www.gacguidelines.ca/site/GAC_Guidelines/assets/docs/Projects_Preop_Grid.doc/. Accessed 24.02.14.
425. Ruetzler K, et al. *Anesth Analg.* 2018.
426. Crawford MW, et al. *Can J Anaesth.* 2005;52:1058.
427. O'Leary JD, et al. *Can J Anaesth.* 2013;60(1):54–59.
428. Joo HS, et al. *Can J Anaesth.* 2005;52:568.
429. Prause G, et al. *Acta Anaesthesiol Scand.* 1998;42:316.
430. Saklad M. *Anesthesiology.* 1941;2:281.
431. Pearse RM, et al. *Lancet.* 2012;380:1059.
432. Sankar A, et al. *Br J Anaesth.* 2014;113(3):424–432.
433. Koo CY, et al. *World J Surg.* 2015;39(1):88–103.
434. Cuvillon P, et al. *Eur J Anaesthesiol.* 2011;28:742.
435. Haynes SR, Lawler PG. *Anaesthesia.* 1995;50:195.
436. Owens WD, et al. *Anesthesiology.* 1978;49:239.

437. Dalton JE, et al. *Anesthesiology*. 2011;114:1336.
438. Noordzij PG, et al. *Anesthesiology*. 2010;112:1105.
439. Glance LG, et al. *Ann Surg*. 2012;255(4):696–702.
440. Fleisher LA, et al. *Arch Surg*. 2004;139:67.
441. Majholm B, et al. *Acta Anaesthesiol Scand*. 2012;56:323.
442. Warner MA, et al. *JAMA*. 1993;270:1437.
443. Nashef SA, et al. *Eur J Cardiothorac Surg*. 2012;41:734.
444. Shahian DM, et al. *Ann Thorac Surg*. 2018;105(5):1411–1418.
445. Moonesinghe SR, et al. *Anesthesiology*. 2013;119(4):959–981.
446. Sutton R, et al. *Br J Surg*. 2002;89(6):763–768.
447. Cowie B. *J Cardiothorac Vasc Anesth*. 2012;26:989.
448. Heiberg J, et al. *Anaesthesia*. 2016;71(9):1091–1100.
449. Guazzi M, et al. *Circulation*. 2016;133(24):e694–711.
450. Young EL, et al. *Eur J Vasc Endovasc Surg*. 2012;44(1):64–71.
451. Huddart S, et al. *Perioper Med (Lond)*. 2013;2(1):4.
452. Kroenke K, et al. *Arch Intern Med*. 1992;152:967.
453. Kearney PM, et al. *BMJ*. 2006;332:1302.
454. Nussmeier NA, et al. *N Engl J Med*. 2005;352:1081.
455. Grady D, et al. *Ann Intern Med*. 2000;132:689.
456. Vandenbroucke JP, et al. *N Engl J Med*. 2001;344(20):1527–1535.
457. Auerbach AD, et al. *JAMA Intern Med*. 2013;173(12):1075–1081.
458. Sajan F, et al. *Anesth Analg*. 2016;123(1):21–28.
459. Practice Guidelines for Preoperative Fasting and the Use of Pharmacologic Agents to Reduce the Risk of Pulmonary Aspiration: Application to Healthy Patients Undergoing Elective Procedures: An Updated Report by the American Society of Anesthesiologists Task Force on Preoperative Fasting and the Use of Pharmacologic Agents to Reduce the Risk of Pulmonary Aspiration. *Anesthesiology*. 2017;126(3):376–393.
460. Melzack R. *Pain*. 1975;1:277.
461. Gjeilo KH, et al. *J Pain Symptom Manage*. 2007;34(6):648–656.
462. Lam E, et al. *Can J Anaesth*. 2007;54:852.
463. Shafer A, et al. *Anesth Analg*. 1996;83:1285.
464. Egbert LD, et al. *N Engl J Med*. 1964;270:825.
465. Block BM, et al. *JAMA*. 2003;290:2455.
466. Katz J, et al. *J Pain Res*. 2015;8:695–702.
467. Starsnic MA, et al. *J Clin Anesth*. 1997;9:299.
468. Katz RI, et al. *Anesth Analg*. 1998;87(4):830–836.
469. Pollard JB, et al. *Anesth Analg*. 1997;85(6):1307–1311.
470. Wijeysundera DN, et al. *Cochrane Database Syst Rev*. 2009;(4): CD004126.
471. Blitz JD, et al. *Anesthesiology*. 2016;125(2):280–294.
472. Hilditch WG, et al. *Anaesthesia*. 2003;58(9):874–877.
473. Vetter TR, et al. *Anesth Analg*. 2016;123(6):1453–1457.
474. Tsen LC, et al. *Anesthesiology*. 2000;93:1134.
475. Salerno SM, et al. *Arch Intern Med*. 2007;167:271.
476. Sharma G, et al. *Arch Intern Med*. 2010;170:363.
477. Grigoryan KV, et al. *J Orthop Trauma*. 2014;28(3):e49–55.
478. Auerbach AD, et al. *Arch Intern Med*. 2004;170:2010.
479. Huddleston JM, et al. *Ann Intern Med*. 2004;141:28.
480. Kammerlander C, et al. *Osteoporos Int*. 2010;21(suppl 4):S637–S646.
481. Rohatgi N, et al. *Ann Surg*. 2016;264(2):275–282.
482. Batsis JA, et al. *J Hosp Med*. 2007;2(4):219–225.
483. Macpherson DS, Lofgren RP. *Med Care*. 1994;32:498.
484. Wijeysundera DN, et al. *Arch Intern Med*. 2010;170:1365.
485. Auerbach AD, et al. *Arch Intern Med*. 2007;167:2338.
486. Vazirani S, et al. *J Hosp Med*. 2012;7:697–701.
487. McIsaac DI, et al. *J Am Geriatr Soc*. 2017;65(12):2665–2672.
488. Katz RI, et al. *Can J Anesth*. 2005;52:697.
489. Groot MW, et al. *Neth Heart J*. 2017;25(11):629–633.
490. Wijeysundera DN, et al. *Anesthesiology*. 2012;116:25.
491. Thilen SR, et al. *JAMA Intern Med*. 2014;174(3):380–388.
492. Thilen SR, et al. *Anesthesiology*. 2013;118(5):1028–1037.
493. Seidel JE, et al. *BMC Health Serv Res*. 2006;6:13.
494. Strode SW, et al. *JAMA*. 1999;281:1066.
495. Wong DT, et al. *Anesthesiology*. 2004;100:1605.
496. Down MP, et al. *Can J Anesth*. 1998;45:802.
497. Soltner C, et al. *Br J Anaesth*. 2011;106:680.
498. van Klei WA, et al. *Br J Anaesth*. 2010;105:620.
499. Harnett MJ, et al. *Anesthesiology*. 2010;112:66.
500. Vaghadia H, Fowler C. *Can J Anesth*. 1999;46:1117.
501. van Klei WA, et al. *Anaesthesia*. 2004;59:971.
502. Edward GM, et al. *Br J Anaesth*. 2008;100:322.
503. Hepner DL, et al. *Anesth Analg*. 2004;98:1099.
504. Dexter F. *Anesth Analg*. 1999;89:925.

32 Anesthetic Implications of Concurrent Diseases

JESSE KIEFER, MONTY MYTHEN, MICHAEL F. ROIZEN, and
LEE A. FLEISHER

KEY POINTS

- The history and physical examination most accurately predict the risks of anesthesia and the likelihood of required changes in monitoring or therapy.
- For diabetic patients, end-organ dysfunction and the degree of glucose control in the perioperative and periprocedural periods are the critical issues with regard to risk.
- The keys to managing blood glucose levels in diabetic patients perioperatively are to set clear goals and then monitor blood glucose levels frequently enough to adjust therapy to achieve these goals.
- Obesity is associated with multiple comorbid conditions, including diabetes, hyperlipidemia, and cholelithiasis, but the primary concern is derangements of the cardiopulmonary system.
- Obstructive sleep apnea is important to recognize because of the increased sensitivity to and the consequence of the depressing effects of hypnotics and opioids on airway muscle tone and respiration, as well as the difficulty with laryngoscopy and mask ventilation.
- Although no controlled, randomized prospective clinical studies have been performed to evaluate the use of adrenergic receptor blocking drugs in patients undergoing resection of pheochromocytoma, the preoperative use of such drugs is generally recommended.
- For patients with hypertension, the routine administration of all drugs preoperatively is recommended, except angiotensin-converting enzyme inhibitors and angiotensin II antagonists.
- Evaluation of a patient with cardiovascular disease depends on clinical risk factors, the extent of surgery, and exercise tolerance.
- In patients with pulmonary disease, the following should be assessed: dyspnea, coughing and the production of sputum, recent respiratory infection, hemoptysis, wheezing, previous pulmonary complications, smoking history, and physical findings.
- In patients with pulmonary disease, several strategies have been suggested, including cessation of smoking 8 weeks or more preoperatively.
- Risk factors for perioperative renal dysfunction include advanced age, congestive heart failure, previous myocardial revascularization, diabetes, and increased baseline blood creatinine concentration.
- One of the primary objectives for a patient with renal disease is ensuring that the renal dysfunction is not augmented and thereby increasing the chance for renal failure, coma, and death.
- Mild perioperative anemia may be clinically significant only in patients with ischemic heart disease.
- Careful management of long-term drug administration should include questions about the effects and side effects of alternative as well as prescription drugs.

This chapter reviews many conditions requiring special preoperative and preprocedure evaluation, intraoperative or intraprocedure management, or postprocedure care. Patients undergoing surgical procedures move through a continuum of medical care to which a primary care physician, an internist or pediatrician, an anesthesiologist, and a surgeon, gastroenterologist, radiologist, or obstetrician-gynecologist contribute to ensure the best outcome possible. It may also involve comanagement with a hospitalist. No aspect of medical care requires greater cooperation among physicians than does performance of a surgical operation or a complex procedure involving multiple specialists and the perioperative care of a patient. Moreover, nowhere else can counseling make so huge a difference in so many lives. The preoperative evaluation also represents a time when education on tobacco cessation, physical inactivity, brain health, and poor food choices can be discussed. The importance of integrating physicians' expertise is even greater within the context of the increasing life-span of our population. As the number of older adults and very old adults (those >85 years old) grows, so does the need of surgical patients for preoperative consultation to help plan for comorbidity, frailty, and multiple drug regimens, the knowledge of which is crucial to successful patient management. At a time when medical information is encyclopedic, it is difficult, if not impossible, for even the most conscientious anesthesiologist to keep abreast of the medical issues relevant to every aspect of perioperative or periprocedure patient management. This chapter reviews such issues with primary emphasis on the anesthesiologist providing preoperative evaluation and care, rather than transferring these responsibilities to other providers.

As with "healthy" patients, the history and physical examination most accurately predict not only the associated risks but also the likelihood of whether a monitoring technique, change in therapy, or "prehabilitation" will be beneficial or necessary for survival. This chapter emphasizes instances in which specific information should be sought in history taking, physical examination, or laboratory evaluation. Although controlled studies designed to confirm that optimizing a patient's preoperative or preprocedure physical condition would result in a less frequent rate of morbidity have not been performed for most diseases, it is logical to assume that such is the case. That such preventive measures would cost less than treating the morbidity that would otherwise occur is an important consideration in a cost-conscious environment.

Minimally invasive procedures such as cataract extraction, magnetic resonance imaging (MRI), or diagnostic arthroscopy, performed in conjunction with the best current anesthetic practices, may pose no greater risk than daily living and thus may not be considered an opportunity for special evaluation. Nevertheless, the preoperative evaluation may identify conditions that could change perioperative management and that may improve both throughput of surgery and the speed of recovery. Examples include the following: ensuring the administration of long-term medications such as a β-adrenergic blocking drug, aspirin for patients with coronary stents, or a statin (or any combination); administering a histamine type 2 (H_2) antagonist 1 to 2 hours before entry into the operating room; ensuring the availability of equipment to measure blood glucose levels; obtaining a history of the patient's diabetic course and treatment from the primary care physician, as well as from the patient; and performing a fiberoptic laryngoscopic examination or procuring additional skilled attention.

The following conditions are discussed in this chapter:

1. Diseases involving the endocrine system and disorders of nutrition (discussed first because of its increasing importance to care)
2. Diseases involving the cardiovascular system
3. Disorders of the respiratory and immune system
4. Diseases of the central nervous system (CNS), neuromuscular diseases, and mental disorders
5. Diseases involving the kidney, infectious diseases, and disorders of electrolytes
6. Diseases involving the gastrointestinal (GI) tract or the liver
7. Diseases involving hematopoiesis and various forms of cancer
8. Diseases of aging or those that occur more commonly in older adults, as well as chronic and acute medical conditions requiring drug therapy

Role of the Primary Care Physician or Consultant

The roles of the primary care physician or consultant are not to select and suggest anesthetic or surgical methods but rather to optimize the patient's preoperative and preprocedure status regarding conditions that increase the morbidity and mortality associated with surgery and to alert the anesthesia care team about these conditions. Within the context of shared decision making, the primary care physician may also be involved in the decision to proceed with surgery.

Quotations and a box in a Medical Knowledge Self-Assessment Program published by the leading organization representing internists, the American College of Physicians, highlight this role for the consultant[1]:

Effective interaction with colleagues in other specialties requires a thorough grounding in the language and science of these other disciplines as well as an awareness of basic guidelines for consultation [Box 32.1]. The consulting internists' role in perioperative care is focused on the elucidation of medical factors that may increase the risks of anesthesia and surgery. Selecting the anesthetic technique for a given patient, procedure, surgeon, and anesthetist is highly individualized and remains the responsibility of the anesthesiologist rather than the internist.

BOX 32.1 Guidelines for Consultation Practice

- Complete a prompt, thorough, generalist-oriented evaluation.
- Respond specifically to the question or questions posed.
- Indicate clearly the perioperative importance of any observations and recommendations outside the area of initial concern.
- Provide focused, detailed, and precise diagnostic and therapeutic guidance.
- Emphasize verbal communication with the anesthesiologist and surgeon, particularly to resolve complex issues.
- Avoid chart notations that unnecessarily create or exacerbate regulatory or medicolegal risk.
- Use frequent follow-up visits in difficult cases to monitor clinical status and compliance with recommendations.

From American College of Physicians. Medical consultation. *Medical Knowledge Self-Assessment Program IX.* Part C. Book 4. Philadelphia: American College of Physicians; 1992: 939.

Optimizing a patient's preoperative and preprocedure condition and, in settings with a preoperative clinic, counseling a patient about needed future lifestyle changes such as exercise, food choices, and tobacco cessation are cooperative ventures between the anesthesiologist and the internist, pediatrician, surgeon, or family physician. If available, the primary care physician should affirm that the patient is in the very best physical state attainable (for that patient), or the anesthesiologist and primary care physician should do what is necessary to optimize that condition. Although not yet definitively proven, prehabilitation prior to surgery has been advocated by many groups.

Primary care physicians can prepare and treat a patient to provide optimal conditions for daily life. The preoperative clinic should collaborate with the primary care physician to start the process of preparing the patient for the needs of surgery or complex procedures. Although such education is more readily available and of better quality than in previous decades, and although cardiologic organizations have provided considerable data on the importance of this aspect of care,[2-4] the primary care physician's training, knowledge, and ability may not include an in-depth understanding of the perioperative evaluation. Without understanding the physiologic changes that occur perioperatively, appropriate therapy is difficult to prescribe. It is therefore part of the anesthesiologist's job to guide the patient's consultants about the type of information needed from the preoperative and preprocedure consultation.

Diseases Involving the Endocrine System and Disorders of Nutrition

PANCREATIC DISORDERS

Preoperative and Preprocedure Diabetes Mellitus

Diabetes mellitus is a heterogeneous group of disorders that have the common feature of a relative or absolute insulin deficiency. The disease is characterized by a multitude of hormone-induced metabolic abnormalities, diffuse microvascular lesions, and long-term end organ complications. The diagnosis of diabetes is made with a fasting blood glucose level greater than 110 mg/dL (6.1 mmol/L), and impaired glucose tolerance is diagnosed if the fasting glucose level is less than 110 mg/dL (6.1 mmol/L) but greater than 100 mg/dL (5.5 mmol/L). Diabetes can be divided into two very different diseases that share the same long-term end-organ complications. Type 1 diabetes is associated with autoimmune diseases and has a concordance rate of 40% to 50% (i.e., if one of a pair of monozygotic twins had diabetes, the likelihood that the other twin would have diabetes is 40%-50%). In type 1 diabetes, the patient is insulin deficient, principally from autoimmune destruction of the pancreatic β cells, and susceptible to ketoacidosis if insulin is withheld. Type 2 diabetes has a concordance rate approaching 80% (i.e., genetic material is both necessary and sufficient for the development of type 2 diabetes).[4a] How markedly the aging and end-organ effects of these genes are expressed is based on lifestyle choices of food and physical activity. These patients are not susceptible to the development of ketoacidosis in the absence of insulin, and they have peripheral insulin resistance through multiple defects with insulin action and secretion. Patients with non–insulin-dependent (type 2) diabetes account for the majority (>90%) of the diabetic patients in Europe and North America. These individuals tend to be overweight, relatively resistant to ketoacidosis, and susceptible to the development of a hyperglycemic-hyperosmolar nonketotic state. Plasma insulin levels are normal or increased in type 2 diabetes but are relatively low for the level of blood glucose. This hyperinsulinemia by itself is postulated to cause accelerated cardiovascular disease. Gestational diabetes develops in more than 3% of all pregnancies and increases the risk of developing type 2 diabetes by 17% to 63% within 15 years.

Type 1 and type 2 diabetes differ in other ways as well. Contrary to long-standing belief, a patient's age does not allow a firm distinction between type 1 and type 2 diabetes; type 1 diabetes can develop in an older person, and clearly, type 2 diabetes can develop in overweight children. Type 1 diabetes is associated with a 15% prevalence of other autoimmune diseases, including Graves disease, Hashimoto thyroiditis, Addison disease, and myasthenia gravis.

Over the next decade, the prevalence of diabetes is expected to increase by 50%. This growth is primarily the result of the increase in type 2 diabetes caused by excessive weight gain in adults and now also in the pediatric population. Large clinical studies show that long-term, strict control of blood glucose levels and arterial blood pressure, along with regular physical activity, results in a major delay in microvascular complications and perhaps indefinite postponement of type 2 diabetes in patients.[5,6]

The common administered drugs can be classified into eight major groups: acarbose, biguanides (e.g., metformin), dipeptidyl peptidase-4 inhibitors (e.g., sitagliptin, saxagliptin, vildagliptin), glucagon-like peptide-1 receptor agonists (e.g., albiglutide, dulagutide, or exenatide), meglitinide (e.g., repaglinide or nateglinide), sodium-glucose transport protein 2 inhibitors (e.g., canagliflozin or empagliflozin), sulfonylureas (e.g., glibenclamide, glipizide, glimepiride, gliquidone), and thiazolidinediones (e.g., pioglitazone or rosiglitazone).[6a]

Patients with insulin-dependent diabetes tend to be younger, nonobese, and susceptible to the development of ketoacidosis. Plasma insulin levels are low or un-measurable, and therapy requires insulin replacement. Patients with insulin-dependent diabetes experience an increase in their insulin requirements in the post-midnight hours, which may result in early morning hyperglycemia (dawn phenomenon). This accelerated glucose production and impaired glucose use reflect nocturnal surges in secretion of growth hormone (GH). Physiologically normal patients and diabetic patients taking insulin have steady-state levels of insulin in their blood. Absorption of insulin is highly variable and depends on the type and species of insulin, the site of administration, and subcutaneous blood flow. Nevertheless, attainment of a steady state depends on periodic administration of the preparations received by the patient. Thus it seems logical to continue the insulin combination perioperatively that the patient had been receiving after assessing previous blood glucose control.[6b]

The major risk factors for diabetic patients undergoing surgery are the end-organ diseases associated with diabetes: cardiovascular dysfunction, renal insufficiency, joint collagen tissue abnormalities (limitation in neck extension, poor wound healing), inadequate granulocyte production, neuropathies, and infectious complications.[7-15] Thus a major focus of the anesthesiologist should be the preoperative and preprocedure evaluation and treatment of these diseases to ensure optimal preoperative and preprocedure conditions. Poor preoperative glucose control, as measured by the hemoglobin A_{1C} (glycosylated hemoglobin) level, is an independent predictor of worse perioperative outcome.[16-18]

Glucotoxicity

Long-term tight control of blood glucose has been motivated by concern for three potential glucotoxicities, in addition to the results from major randomized outcome studies involving diabetic patients.[5-13]

1. Glucose itself may be toxic because high levels can promote nonenzymatic glycosylation reactions that lead to the formation of abnormal proteins. These proteins may weaken endothelial junctions and decrease elastance, which is responsible for the stiff joint syndrome (and difficult intubation secondary to fixation of the atlanto-occipital joint), as well as decrease wound-healing tensile strength.

2. Glycemia also disrupts autoregulation. Glucose-induced vasodilation prevents target organs from protecting against increases in systemic blood pressure. A glycosylated hemoglobin level of 8.1% is the threshold at which the risk for microalbuminuria increases logarithmically. A person with type 1 diabetes who has microalbuminuria of greater than 29 mg/day has an 80% chance of experiencing renal insufficiency. The threshold for glycemic toxicity differs for various vascular beds. For example, the threshold for retinopathy is a glycosylated hemoglobin value of 8.5% to 9.0% (12.5 mmol/L or 225 mg/dL), and that for cardiovascular disease is an average blood glucose value of 5.4 mmol/L (96 mg/dL). Thus different degrees of hyperglycemia may be required before different vascular beds are damaged. Another view is that perhaps severe hyperglycemia and microalbuminuria are simply concomitant effects of a common underlying cause. For instance, diabetic patients in whom microalbuminuria develops are more resistant to insulin, insulin resistance is associated with microalbuminuria in first-degree relatives of patients with type 2 diabetes, and persons who are normoglycemic but subsequently have clinical diabetes are at risk for atherogenesis before the onset of disease.

Diabetes itself may not be as important to perioperative outcome as are its end-organ effects. Epidemiologic studies segregated the effects of diabetes itself on the organ system from the effects of the complications of diabetes (e.g., cardiac, nervous system, renal, and vascular disease) and the effects of old age and the accelerated aging that diabetes causes. Even in patients requiring intensive care unit (ICU) management, long-standing diabetes does not appear to be as important an issue as the end-organ dysfunction that exists and the degree of glucose control in the perioperative or periprocedure and ICU periods.[6b,8-13]

The World Health Organization's surgical safety checklist bundle suggests control with a target perioperative blood glucose concentration of 6 to 10 mmol/L (acceptable range, 4-12 mmol/L) or 100 to 180 mg/dL.[19] Poor perioperative glycemic control has a significant impact on the risk of postoperative infection across a variety of surgical specialities.[20] Different regimens permit almost any degree of perioperative control of blood glucose levels, but the tighter the control desired, the greater the risk of hypoglycemia. Therefore, debate regarding optimal control during the perioperative period has been extensive. Tight control retards all these glucotoxicities and may have other benefits in retarding the severity of diabetes itself.[5-13,21] Management of intraoperative glucose may be influenced by specific situations, such as the following: the type of operation, pregnancy,[22] expected global CNS insult, the bias of the patient's primary care physician, or the type of diabetes.

Much of the research on perioperative control is derived from studies in the ICU, as opposed to the operating room. The first major trial demonstrating the benefit of tight glucose control was in medical ICU patients in Leuven, Belgium.[23] The most recent trial was from the NICE-SUGAR (Normoglycemia in Intensive Care Evaluation and Survival Using Glucose Algorithm Regulation) group.[24] In this randomized controlled trial, the investigators examined the associations between moderate and severe hypoglycemia (blood glucose, 41-70 mg/dL [2.3-3.9 mmol/L] and ≤40 mg/dL [2.2 mmol/L], respectively) and death among 6026 critically ill patients in ICUs. Intensive glucose control leads to moderate and severe hypoglycemia, both of which are associated with an increased risk of death. The association exhibits a dose-response relationship and is strongest for death from distributive shock. The optimal perioperative management has been reviewed elsewhere.[25] Guidelines have been developed on the use of insulin infusions in the critical care unit to achieve these goals (Table 32.1).[26]

Diabetes and Accelerated Physiologic Aging

Adverse perioperative outcomes have repeatedly and substantially correlated with the age of the patient,[2,3,27-30] and diabetes does cause physiologic aging. When one translates the results of the Diabetes Control and Complications Trials into age-induced physiologic changes, a patient with type 1 diabetes who has poor control of blood glucose ages approximately 1.75 years physiologically for every chronologic year of the disease and 1.25 years if blood glucose has been controlled tightly.[27-29] A patient with type 2 diabetes ages approximately 1.5 years for every chronologic year of the disease and approximately 1.06 years with tight control of blood glucose and blood pressure.[6,27-29,31] Thus when providing care for a diabetic patient, one must consider the associated risks to be those of a person who is much older physiologically; the physiologic age of a diabetic patient is considerably older than that person's calendar age just by virtue of having the disease.[1]

Obesity and lack of physical exercise seem to be major contributors to the increasing prevalence of type 2 diabetes. As with type 1 diabetes, tight control of blood glucose, increased physical activity, and reduction in weight appear to reduce the accelerated aging associated with type 2 diabetes, and possibly delay the appearance of the disease and aging from it substantially.[27-29,31] Although such a reduction in aging should reduce the perioperative risk for diabetic patients, no controlled trials have confirmed this theory.

The key to managing blood glucose levels perioperatively in diabetic patients is to set clear goals and then monitor blood glucose levels frequently enough to adjust therapy to achieve these goals.[31a]

Other Conditions Associated With Diabetes

Diabetes is associated with microangiopathy (in retinal and renal vessels), peripheral neuropathy, autonomic dysfunction, and infection. Diabetic patients are often treated with angiotensin-converting enzyme (ACE) inhibitors, even in the absence of gross hypertension, in an effort to prevent the effects of disordered autoregulation, including renal failure.[5,6,32]

Preoperatively, assessment and optimization of treatment of the potential and potent end-organ effects of diabetes are at least as important as assessment of the diabetic patient's current overall metabolic status. The preoperative evaluation of diabetic patients is also discussed in Chapter 31.

The presence of autonomic neuropathy likely makes the operative period more hazardous and the postoperative period crucial to survival. Evidence of autonomic neuropathy may be routinely sought before the surgical procedure. Patients with diabetic autonomic neuropathy are at increased risk for gastroparesis (and consequent aspiration

TABLE 32.1 Recommended Glucose Target Ranges for Intensive Care Patients and Related Subgroups

Society, Guideline	Patient Group	Trigger Blood Glucose Value to Start Insulin Infusion (mM [mg/dL])	Target range, (mM [mg/dL])	Rationale
Society of Critical Care Medicine's clinical practice guideline[26]	General recommendation	8.3 (150)	5.6-8.3 (100-150)	
	Cardiac surgical patients		<8.3 (150)	Decreased risk for deep sternal wound infection and death[73,118-121]
	Critically ill trauma patients	8.3 (150)	<10 (180)	
	Patients with traumatic brain injury	8.3 (150)	<10 (180)	
	Neurologic ICU patients Ischemic stroke Intraparenchymal hemorrhage Aneurysmal subarachnoid hemorrhage	8.3 (150)	<10 (180)	
American Diabetes Association guidelines[446]	General recommendation	10 (180)	7.8-10 (140-180)	
	Adaptation		6.1-7.8 (110-140)	Adjust to lower target range in documented low rate of severe hypoglycemia
American Association of Clinical Endocrinologists[447]	General recommendation		7.8-10 (140-180)	
	Surgical patients		Lower range	Only in units showing low rates of hypoglycemia
Surviving Sepsis Campaign[448]	General recommendation	10 (180)	<10 (180)	Based on the NICE-SUGAR study
Clinical Practical Guideline from the American College of Physicians[449]	General recommendation		7.8-11.1 (140-200)	If insulin infusion is applied; however, guideline does not recommend intensive insulin therapy
Spanish Society of Intensive Care Medicine and Coronary Units[450]	General recommendation		<8.3 (150)	
French Society of Anesthesia and Intensive Care[451]	General recommendation		10 (180)	
	Surgical patients		<6.1 (110)	
	Cardiac patients		<6.1 (110)	
Society of Thoracic Surgeons[452]	Cardiac surgical patients		<10 (180) except <8.3 (150) for those with devices in place	

ICU, Intensive care unit; *NICE-SUGAR*, normoglycemia in intensive care evaluation and survival using glucose algorithm regulation.
Data from Sebranek JJ, Lugli AK, Coursin DB. Glycaemic control in the perioperative period. *Br J Anaesth.* 2013;111(suppl 1):i18–i34; and Jacobi J, Bircher N, Krinsley J, et al. Guidelines for the use of an insulin infusion for the management of hyperglycemia in critically ill patients. *Crit Care Med.* 2012;40:3251–3276.

of gastric contents) and for perioperative cardiorespiratory arrest. Diabetic patients who exhibit signs of autonomic neuropathy, such as early satiety, lack of sweating, lack of pulse rate change with inspiration or orthostatic maneuvers, and impotence, have a very frequent incidence of painless myocardial ischemia.[15,33] Administration of metoclopramide, 10 mg preoperatively to facilitate gastric emptying of solids, may be helpful (Fig. 32.1). Interference with respiration or sinus automaticity by pneumonia or by anesthetic agents, pain medications, or sedative drugs is likely the precipitating cause in most cases of sudden cardiorespiratory arrest. Measuring the degree of sinus arrhythmia or beat-to-beat variability provides a simple, accurate test for significant autonomic neuropathy. The difference between the maximum and minimum heart rate on deep inspiration is normally 15 beats/min, but it is 5 beats/min or less in all patients who subsequently sustain cardiorespiratory arrest.[15,33]

Other characteristics of patients with autonomic neuropathy include postural hypotension with a decrease in arterial blood pressure of more than 30 mm Hg, resting tachycardia, nocturnal diarrhea, and dense peripheral neuropathy. Diabetic patients with significant autonomic neuropathy may have impaired respiratory responses to

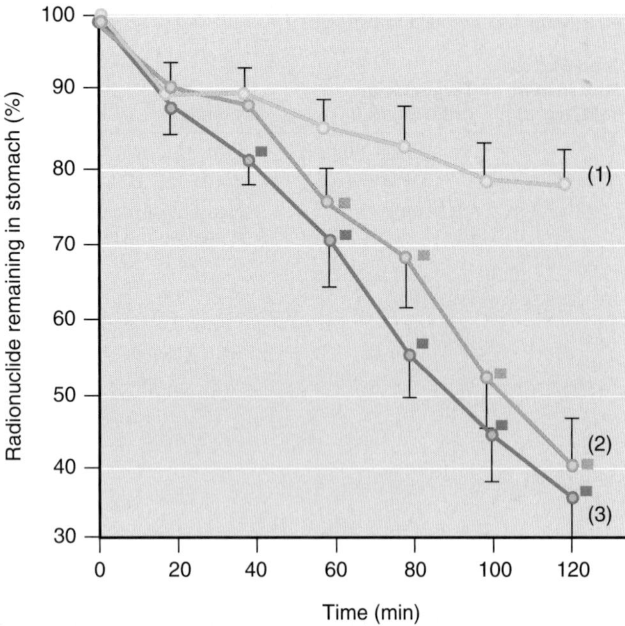

Fig. 32.1 Gastric emptying time (mean ± standard deviation) of a solid test meal in three groups of patients: diabetic patients *(line 1)*, diabetic patients given metoclopramide (10 mg intravenously) 1.5 hours before the test meal *(line 2)*, and nondiabetic patients *(line 3)*. (From Wright RA, Clemente R, Wathen R. Diabetic gastroparesis: an abnormality of gastric emptying of solids. *Am J Med Sci.* 1985;289:240–242.)

hypoxia and are particularly sensitive to the action of drugs that have depressant effects. These patients may warrant continuous cardiac and respiratory monitoring for 24 to 72 hours postoperatively, although this has not been tested in a rigorous, controlled trial.[15] In the absence of autonomic neuropathy, outpatient surgery is preferred for a diabetic patient if possible (see Table 32.1).[31a]

Emergency Surgery

Many diabetic patients requiring emergency surgery for trauma or infection have significant metabolic decompensation, including ketoacidosis. Frequently, little time is available to stabilize the patient, but even a few hours may be sufficient for correction of any fluid and electrolyte disturbances that are potentially life-threatening. It is futile to delay surgery in an attempt to eliminate ketoacidosis completely if the underlying surgical condition will lead to further metabolic deterioration. The likelihood of intraoperative cardiac arrhythmias and hypotension resulting from ketoacidosis will be reduced if intravascular volume depletion and hypokalemia are at least partially treated. During the initial resuscitation phase of ketoacidosis bicarbonate should initially be avoided with crystalloid fluids, potassium repletion, and intravenous insulin therapy favored.[33a]

Insulin therapy is initiated with a 10-unit intravenous bolus of regular insulin, followed by continuous insulin infusion. The rate of infusion is determined most easily by dividing the last serum glucose value by 150 (or 100 if the patient is receiving steroids, has an infection, or is considerably overweight [body mass index ≥35]). The actual amount of insulin administered is less important than is regular monitoring of glucose, potassium, and arterial pH. The maximum rate of glucose decline is fairly constant, averaging 75 to 100 mg/dL/h, regardless of the dose of insulin because the number of insulin binding sites is limited.[34] During the first 1 to 2 hours of fluid resuscitation, the glucose level may decrease more precipitously. When serum glucose reaches 250 mg/dL, the intravenous fluid should include 5% dextrose.

The volume of intravenously administered fluid required varies with the overall deficit; it ranges from 3 to 5 L and may be as large as 10 L. Despite losses of water in excess of losses of solute, sodium levels are generally normal or reduced. Factitious hyponatremia caused by hyperglycemia or hypertriglyceridemia may result in this seeming contradiction. The plasma sodium concentration decreases by approximately 1.6 mEq/L for every 100 mg/dL increase in plasma glucose greater than normal. Initially, balanced crystalloid solution is infused at a rate of 250 to 1000 mL/h, depending on the degree of intravascular volume depletion and cardiac status. Some measure of left ventricular volume should be monitored in diabetic patients who have a history of myocardial dysfunction. Approximately one third of the estimated fluid deficit is corrected during the first 6 to 8 hours and the remaining two thirds over the next 24 hours.[34a]

The degree of acidosis is determined by analysis of arterial blood gases and detection of an increased anion gap (see also Chapter 48). Acidosis with an increased anion gap (≥16 mEq/L) in an acutely ill diabetic patient may be caused by ketones in ketoacidosis, lactic acid in lactic acidosis, increased organic acids from renal insufficiency, or all three disorders. In ketoacidosis, plasma levels of acetoacetate, β-hydroxybutyrate, and acetone are increased. Plasma and urinary ketones can be measured semiquantitatively with Ketostix and Acetest tablets. The role of bicarbonate therapy in diabetic ketoacidosis is controversial, but could be considered in severe acidemia and hemodynamic instability as myocardial function and respiration are known to be depressed at a blood pH lower than 7.00 to 7.10.[34b] This careful consideration is because rapid correction of acidosis with bicarbonate therapy may result in alterations in CNS function and structure. These alterations may be caused by (1) paradoxical development of cerebrospinal fluid and CNS acidosis from rapid conversion of bicarbonate to carbon dioxide and diffusion of the acid across the blood-brain barrier, (2) altered CNS oxygenation with decreased cerebral blood flow, and (3) the development of unfavorable osmotic gradients. After treatment with fluids and insulin, β-hydroxybutyrate levels decrease rapidly, whereas acetoacetate levels may remain stable or even increase before declining. Plasma acetone levels remain elevated for 24 to 42 hours, long after blood glucose, β-hydroxybutyrate, and acetoacetate levels have returned to normal; the result is continuing ketonuria.[34] Persistent ketosis with a serum bicarbonate level less than 20 mEq/L in the presence of a normal glucose concentration is an indication of the continued need for intracellular glucose and insulin for reversal of lipolysis.

The most important electrolyte disturbance in diabetic ketoacidosis is depletion of total-body potassium. Deficits range from 3 to 10 mEq/kg body weight. Serum potassium levels decline rapidly and reach a nadir within 2 to 4 hours after the start of intravenous insulin administration. Aggressive replacement therapy is required. The potassium administered moves into the intracellular space with insulin as the acidosis is corrected. Potassium is also excreted in urine because of the increased delivery of sodium to the distal renal tubules that accompanies volume expansion. Phosphorus deficiency in ketoacidosis as a result of tissue catabolism, impaired cellular uptake, and increased urinary losses may give rise to significant muscular weakness and organ dysfunction. The average phosphorus deficit is approximately 1 mmol/kg body weight; no clear guidance for replacement exists, but replacement is appropriate in patients with cardiac dysfunction, anemia, respiratory depression, or if the plasma phosphate concentration is less than 1.0 mg/dL.[34]

Anticipated Newer Treatments of Diabetes

At least three major changes in the care of diabetic patients have made it to the clinical trial stage:

- Implanted (like a pacemaker) glucose analyzer with electronic transmission to a surface (watch) monitor
- New islet transplantation medication that makes islet cell transplants much more successful and rejection medication less hazardous
- Medications such as INGAP (islet neogenesis–associated protein) peptide, which may cause regrowth of normally functioning islet cells (without the need for transplantation)

Some of these treatments may radically change the therapies used in the perioperative period. If regrowth of islet cells becomes common, type 1 diabetes could all but disappear; if implanted minute-to-minute glucose reading is possible, tight control may be much easier and more expected.

Insulinoma and Other Causes of Hypoglycemia

Hypoglycemia in persons not treated for diabetes is rare. Hypoglycemia in nondiabetic patients can be caused by such diverse entities as pancreatic islet cell adenoma or carcinoma, large hepatoma, large sarcoma, alcohol ingestion, use of β-adrenergic receptor blocking drugs, haloperidol therapy, hypopituitarism, adrenal insufficiency, altered physiology after gastric or gastric bypass surgery, hereditary fructose intolerance, ingestion of antidiabetic drugs, galactosemia, or autoimmune hypoglycemia.[35] The last four entities cause postprandial reactive hypoglycemia. Because restriction of oral intake prevents severe hypoglycemia, the practice of keeping the patient NPO (nothing by mouth) and infusing small amounts of a solution containing 5% dextrose greatly lessens the possibility of perioperative postprandial reactive hypoglycemia. The other causes of hypoglycemia can cause serious problems during the perioperative period.[35]

Symptoms of hypoglycemia fall into one of two groups: adrenergic excess (tachycardia, palpitations, tremulousness, or diaphoresis) or neuroglycopenia (headache, confusion, mental sluggishness, seizures, or coma). All these symptoms may be masked by anesthesia, so blood glucose levels should be determined frequently in at-risk patients to ensure that hypoglycemia is not present. Because manipulation of an insulinoma can result in massive insulin release, this tumor should probably be operated on only at centers equipped with a mechanical pancreas. Perioperative use of the somatostatin analogue octreotide, which suppresses insulin release from such tumors, makes the perioperative period safer in anecdotal experience.

DISORDERS OF NUTRITION, INCLUDING OBESITY

Hyperlipoproteinemia, Hyperlipidemia, and Hypolipidemia

Hyperlipidemia may result from obesity, estrogen or corticoid therapy, uremia, diabetes, hypothyroidism, acromegaly, alcohol ingestion, liver disease, inborn errors of metabolism, or pregnancy. Hyperlipidemia may cause premature coronary, peripheral vascular disease, or pancreatitis.

Coronary events can be decreased by treating individuals with even normal levels of low-density lipoprotein (LDL) cholesterol with statins (3-hydroxy-3-methylglutaryl–coenzyme A [HMG-CoA] reductase inhibitors)—through an increase in high-density lipoprotein (HDL) and a decrease in LDL cholesterol levels. This approach has markedly decreased the rate of myocardial reinfarction in high-risk patients.[36-38] Secondary prevention efforts were successful when these high-risk patients stopped smoking, reduced their arterial blood pressure, controlled stress, increased physical activity, and used aspirin, folate, β-blocking drugs, angiotensin inhibitors, diet, and other drugs to reduce their levels of LDL and increase their levels of HDL.

Although controlling the diet remains a major treatment modality for all types of hyperlipidemia, the drugs fenofibrate and gemfibrozil, which are used to treat hypertriglyceridemia, can cause myopathy, especially in patients with hepatic or renal disease; clofibrate is also associated with an increased incidence of gallstones. Cholestyramine binds bile acids, as well as oral anticoagulants, digitalis drugs, and thyroid hormones. Nicotinic acid causes peripheral vasodilation and should probably not be continued through the morning of the surgical procedure. Probucol (Lorelco) decreases the synthesis of apoprotein A-1; its use is associated on rare occasion with fetid perspiration or prolongation of the QT interval, or both, and sudden death in animals.

The West of Scotland Coronary Prevention Study and its congeners produced convincing evidence that drugs in the statin class prevent the morbidity and mortality related to arterial aging and vascular disease, as well as their consequences, such as coronary artery disease (CAD), stroke, and peripheral vascular insufficiency.[37] Thus, the statins—lovastatin (Mevacor), pravastatin (Pravachol), simvastatin, fluvastatin, atorvastatin (Lipitor), and rosuvastatin (Crestor)—are mainstays of therapy, limited by patient tolerance most commonly secondary to musculoskeletal complaints.[38a]

However, the report of Downs and coworkers from the Air Force/Texas Coronary Atherosclerosis Prevention Study went further.[37] This report showed a 37% reduction in the risk for first acute major coronary events in patients who had no risk factors and normal (average) LDL cholesterol levels. In this study lovastatin did not alter mortality rates, but that had been true for many early short-term trials with the statins. Although much of the effect of the statins has been attributed to their lipid-lowering effects, statins also influence endothelial function, inflammatory responses, plaque stability, and thrombogenicity. In 2013, the American College of Cardiology (ACC) and the American Heart Association (AHA) released a new clinical practice guideline for the treatment of blood cholesterol in people at high risk for cardiovascular diseases.[39] They now advocate statin therapy for the following:

- Patients who have cardiovascular disease (coronary syndromes, previous myocardial infarction [MI], stable or unstable angina, previous stroke or transient ischemic attack, or peripheral artery disease)
- Patients with an LDL cholesterol level of 190 mg/dL or higher
- Patients with diabetes (type 1 or 2) who are between 40 and 75 years old
- Patients with an estimated 10-year risk of cardiovascular disease greater than 7.5% (the report provided formulas for calculating 10-year risk)

The 2014 National Lipid Association Recommendations for Patient-Centered Management of Dyslipidemia further emphasize the use of statins as a first-line therapy for dyslipidemia, but emphasize the inclusion of non-high density lipoprotein in addition to LDL as markers for risk. They further advocated for management of other atherosclerotic cardiovascular disease risk factors including high blood pressure, tobacco use, and diabetes mellitus.[39a]

Statins are drugs that block HMG-CoA reductase, the rate-limiting enzyme of cholesterol synthesis. Their use is occasionally accompanied by liver dysfunction, CNS dysfunction, and severe depression not related to the high cost of each drug and its congeners. Based on the available evidence, statin therapy should be continued in patients already taking these drugs.[40] Other drugs that reduce LDL and increase HDL cholesterol and decrease triglycerides are docosahexaenoic acid (an ω-3 fatty acid) and niacin. Statins also provide the substantial benefit of reversing inflammation in arteries, as evidenced by their ability to decrease highly specific C-reactive protein and pull cholesterol from plaque.[41]

Hypolipidemic conditions are rare diseases often associated with neuropathy, anemia, and renal failure. Although anesthetic experience with hypolipidemic conditions has been limited, some specific recommendations can be made: continuation of caloric intake and intravenous administration of protein hydrolysates and glucose should be continued throughout the perioperative period.

Obesity

Obesity is a risk factor for perioperative morbidity. In the study of Medicare claims in which obese patients were matched to non-obese patients undergoing surgery, the obese patients displayed increased odds of wound infection, renal dysfunction, urinary tract infection, hypotension, respiratory events, 30-day readmission, and a 12% longer length of stay.[41a] Although many conditions associated with obesity (diabetes, hyperlipidemia, cholelithiasis, gastroesophageal reflux disease, cirrhosis, degenerative joint and disk disease, venous stasis with thrombotic or embolic disease, sleep disorders, and emotional and altered body image disorders) contribute to chronic morbidity in these patients, the main concerns for the anesthesiologist have been the same since the 1970s—derangements of the cardiopulmonary system.

Morbid obesity with minimal or no coexisting pulmonary conditions (e.g., no obesity-hypoventilation syndrome or chronic obstructive pulmonary disease [COPD]) is referred to here as "simple" obesity. In simple obesity, the pathophysiology of mild alterations in daytime gas exchange and pulmonary function may also result from compression and restriction of the chest wall and diaphragm by excess adipose tissue.[42] Typically, in obese patients, the expiratory reserve volume and functional residual capacity are most affected and are reduced to 60% and 80% of normal, respectively. Care must be taken with medication choice and dosing, as simple obese patients may be more sensitive to sedative and narcotic agents leading to hypoventilation.[42a]

Other Eating Disorders: Anorexia Nervosa, Bulimia, and Starvation

Many endocrine and metabolic abnormalities occur in patients with anorexia nervosa, a condition characterized by starvation to the point of 40% loss of normal weight, hyperactivity, and a psychiatrically distorted body image. Many anorectic patients exhibit impulsive behavior, including suicide attempts, and intravenous drug use is much more common than in the general population. Acidosis, hypokalemia, hypocalcemia, hypomagnesemia, hypothermia, diabetes insipidus, and severe endocrine abnormalities mimicking panhypopituitarism may need attention before patients undergo anesthesia. Similar problems occur in bulimia (bulimorexia), a condition that may affect as many as 50% of female college students and is even unintentionally present in many older adults. As in severe protein deficiency, anorexia nervosa and bulimia may be accompanied by the following: alterations on the electrocardiogram (ECG), including a prolonged QT interval, atrioventricular (AV) block, and other arrhythmias; sensitivity to epinephrine; and cardiomyopathy.[43] Total depletion of body potassium makes the addition of potassium to glucose solutions useful; although, fluid administration can precipitate pulmonary edema in these patients and should be monitored judiciously. Esophagitis, pancreatitis, and aspiration pneumonia are more frequent in these patients, as is delayed gastric emptying. One review reported that in patients with severe anorexia, a body mass index less than 13 kg/m^2, marked hypoglycemia or leukocytopenia lower than $3.0 \times 10^9/L$, or both, potentially fatal complications frequently occur.[44] Intraoperatively, glucose or catecholamine administration may lead to disturbance of electrolytes or fatal arrhythmia. Intensive care and early nutritional support as soon as possible postoperatively are important to prevent surgical site infection with close monitoring for refeeding syndrome.

HYPERALIMENTATION (TOTAL PARENTERAL OR ENTERAL NUTRITION)

Hyperalimentation (i.e., total parenteral nutrition [TPN]) consists of concentrating hypertonic glucose calories in the normal daily fluid requirements. The solutions contain protein hydrolysates, soybean emulsions (i.e., Intralipid), or synthetic amino acids (or any combination of these ingredients). The major benefits of TPN or enteral nutrition have been fewer complications postoperatively and shorter hospital stays for patients scheduled to have no oral feeding for 7 days or who were malnourished preoperatively.[45,46] Starker and colleagues found that the response to TPN, as monitored by serum albumin levels, predicted the postoperative outcome.[47] The group of patients demonstrating

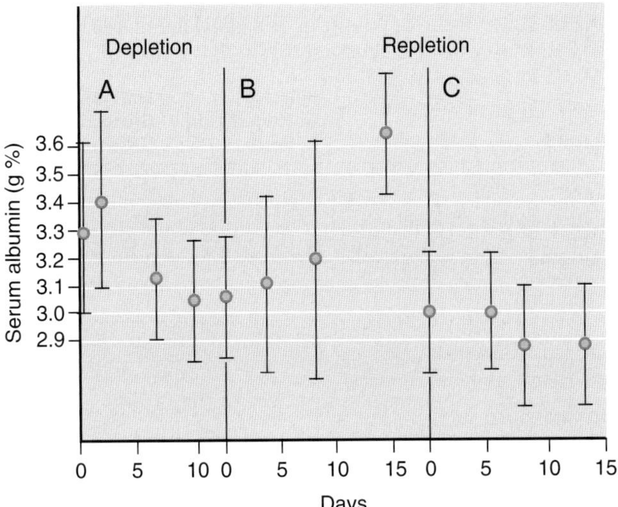

Fig. 32.2 The response to hyperalimentation (*A*, repletion), as measured by variation in serum albumin levels, predicted the outcome of surgery. Patients who responded *(B)* to nutritional support with increased albumin levels had a significantly better outcome than did those whose albumin level did not increase *(C)*. See the text for a more complete explanation. (Modified from Starker PM, Group FE, Askanazi J, et al. Serum albumin levels as an index of nutritional support. *Surgery*. 1982;91:194–199.)

an increase in serum albumin concentrations from TPN had diuresis, weight loss, and fewer complications (1 of 15 patients) than did the group that gained weight and had a decrease in serum albumin (8 of 16 patients had 15 complications; Fig. 32.2). The Veterans Administration (former name for Veterans Affairs [VA used for both]) studies also found that the serum albumin level was one of the most powerful predictors of perioperative outcome.[45]

The major complications of TPN are infection, metabolic abnormalities, and longer duration of ICU stay.[47a] The central lines used for TPN require an absolutely aseptic technique and should not be used as an intravenous access or as a route for drug administration during anesthesia and surgery. Major metabolic complications of TPN relate to electrolyte deficiencies, and the development of hyperosmolar states. Complications of hypertonic dextrose can develop if the patient has insufficient insulin (diabetes mellitus) to metabolize the sugar or if insulin resistance occurs (e.g., because of uremia, burns, or sepsis).

A gradual decrease in the infusion rate of TPN prevents the hypoglycemia that can occur on abrupt discontinuance. Thus the infusion rate of TPN should be decreased the night before anesthesia and surgery, or should be continued throughout the operation at its current rate. The main reason for slowing or discontinuing TPN before anesthesia is to avoid intraoperative hyperosmolarity secondary to accidental rapid infusion of the solution or hypoglycemia if the infusion is discontinued because of high levels of endogenous insulin and lower levels of glucose present in the usual crystalloid solutions.[45] Hypophosphatemia is a particularly serious complication that results from the administration of phosphate-free or phosphate-depleted solutions for hyperalimentation. The low serum phosphate level causes a shift of the oxygen dissociation curve to the left. The resulting low 2,3-diphosphoglycerate and adenosine triphosphatase levels mean that cardiac output must increase for oxygen delivery to remain the same. Hypophosphatemia of less than 1.0 mg/dL of blood may cause hemolytic anemia, cardiac failure, tachypnea, neurologic symptoms, seizures, and death. In addition, long-term TPN is associated with deficiencies in trace metals such as copper (refractory anemia), zinc (impaired wound healing), and magnesium.

ADRENOCORTICAL MALFUNCTION

Three major classes of hormones—androgens, glucocorticoids, and mineralocorticoids—are secreted by the adrenal cortex. For each class, an excess or a deficiency of hormone produces a characteristic clinical syndrome. The widespread use of steroids can also make the adrenal cortex unable to respond normally to the demands placed on it by surgical trauma and subsequent healing. The increase in computed tomography (CT) abdominal imaging procedures has meant that many adrenal masses have unfortunately been discovered incidentally. These adrenal "incidentalomas," as they are termed because they were initially thought a nuisance discovered by body scans, have proved more serious. As many as 30% are hormonally active; in one review of 2000 such masses, 82% were not hormonally active, 5.3% proved to be cortisone-secreting adenomas, 5.1% were pheochromocytomas, 4.7% were adrenal carcinomas, 2.5% were unsuspected metastatic disease, and 1% were aldosterone-secreting adenomas. "Incidentalomas" may therefore require serious pursuit; however, well accepted and utilized guidelines are absent, but caution should be taken during anesthesia.

Controlled comparisons of the perioperative management of patients who have disorders of adrenal function are lacking, although steroids are used more and more commonly, with the results of some controlled trials available for specific uses. However, a review of the possible pathophysiologic changes in the adrenal cortex and techniques for their management should enable physicians to improve the perioperative care of patients with adrenal abnormalities.

Physiologic Properties of Adrenocortical Hormones

Androgens. Androstenedione and dehydroepiandrosterone, weak androgens arising from the adrenal cortex, constitute major sources of androgen in women (and have gained prominence for their abuse among athletes). Excess secretion of androgen causes masculinization, pseudopuberty, or female pseudohermaphroditism. With some tumors, androgen is converted to an estrogenic substance, in which case feminization results. No special anesthetic evaluation is needed for such patients. Some congenital enzyme defects that cause androgen abnormalities also result in glucocorticoid and mineralocorticoid abnormalities that should be evaluated preoperatively. Most of these patients are treated with exogenous glucocorticoids and mineralocorticoids and may require supplementation of these hormones perioperatively.

Glucocorticoids. The principal glucocorticoid, cortisol, is an essential regulator of carbohydrate, protein, lipid, and nucleic acid metabolism. Cortisol exerts its biologic effects through a sequence of steps initiated by the binding of hormone to stereospecific intracellular cytoplasmic receptors.

This bound complex stimulates nuclear transcription of specific mRNA molecules. These molecules are then translated to give rise to proteins that mediate the ultimate effects of hormones.

Most cortisol is bound to corticosterone-binding globulin (CBG, transcortin). The relatively small amounts of unbound cortisol enter cells to induce actions or to be metabolized. Conditions that induce changes in the amount of CBG include liver disease and nephrotic syndrome, both of which result in decreased circulating levels of CBG, and estrogen administration and pregnancy, which result in increased CBG production. Total serum cortisol levels may become elevated or depressed under conditions that alter the amount of bound cortisol, and yet the unbound, active form of cortisol is present in normal amounts. The most accurate measure of cortisol activity is the level of urinary cortisol (i.e., the amount of unbound, active cortisol filtered by the kidney).

The serum half-life of cortisol is 80 to 110 minutes. However, because cortisol acts through intracellular receptors, pharmacokinetic data based on serum levels are not good indicators of cortisol activity. After a single dose of glucocorticoid, serum glucose is elevated for 12 to 24 hours; improvement in pulmonary function in patients with bronchial asthma can still be measured 24 hours after glucocorticoid administration. Treatment schedules for glucocorticoid replacement are therefore based not on the measured serum half-life but on the well-documented prolonged end-organ effect of these steroids. Hospitalized patients requiring long-term glucocorticoid replacement therapy are usually treated twice daily, with a slightly higher dose given in the morning than in the evening to simulate the normal diurnal variation in cortisol levels. For patients who require parenteral "steroid coverage" during and after surgery (see later paragraphs), administration of glucocorticoid every 6 to 12 hours is appropriate pending the type of surgery and expected stress response.[47b] The relative potencies of glucocorticoids are listed in Table 32.2. Cortisol is inactivated primarily in the liver and is excreted as 17-hydroxycorticosteroid. Cortisol is also filtered and excreted unchanged into urine.

The synthetic glucocorticoids vary in their binding specificity in a dose-related manner. When given in supraphysiologic doses (>30 mg/day), cortisol and cortisone bind to mineralocorticoid receptor sites, and cause salt and water retention and loss of potassium and hydrogen ions. When these steroids are administered in maintenance doses of 30 mg/day or less, patients require a specific mineralocorticoid for electrolyte and volume homeostasis. Many other steroids do not bind to mineralocorticoid receptors, even at high doses, and have no mineralocorticoid effect (see Table 32.2).[47b]

Secretion of glucocorticoids is regulated by pituitary adrenocorticotropic hormone (ACTH). ACTH is synthesized from a precursor molecule (pro-opiomelanocortin) that is metabolized to form an endorphin (β-lipotropin) and ACTH. Episodic secretion of ACTH has a diurnal rhythm that is normally greatest during the early morning hours in men and later in women and is regulated at least in part by light-dark cycles. Its secretion is stimulated by release of corticotropin-releasing factor (CRF) from the hypothalamus. (An abnormality in the diurnal rhythm of corticoid secretion has been implicated as a cause of so-called jet lag.) Cortisol and other glucocorticoids exert negative feedback at both the pituitary and hypothalamic levels to inhibit the secretion of ACTH and CRF. If the CRF- or ACTH-producing cells are destroyed, the adrenal gland takes more than 30 days to atrophy to the point at which short-term administration of exogenous ACTH will cause almost no adrenal responsiveness.[48]

TABLE 32.2 Relative Potencies and Equivalent Doses for Commonly Used Glucocorticoids

Steroids	Relative Glucocorticoid Potency	Equivalent Glucocorticoid Dose (mg)
SHORT ACTING		
Cortisol (hydrocortisone)	1.0	20.0
Cortisone	0.8	25.0
Prednisone	4.0	5.0
Prednisolone	4.0	5.0
Methylprednisolone	5.0	4.0
INTERMEDIATE ACTING		
Triamcinolone	5.0	4.0
LONG ACTING		
Betamethasone	25.0	0.60
Dexamethasone	30.0	0.75

Data from Axelrod L. Glucocorticoid therapy. *Medicine (Baltimore).* 1976;55:39–65.

Mineralocorticoids. Aldosterone, the major mineralocorticoid secreted in humans, comes from the zona glomerulosa of the adrenal cortex and causes reabsorption of sodium and secretion of potassium and hydrogen ions, thereby contributing to electrolyte and volume homeostasis. This action is most prominent in the distal renal tubule but also occurs in the salivary and sweat glands. The major regulator of aldosterone secretion is the renin-angiotensin system. Juxtaglomerular cells in the cuff of renal arterioles are sensitive to decreased renal perfusion pressure or volume and, consequently, secrete renin. Renin transforms the precursor angiotensinogen (from the liver) into angiotensin I, which is further converted by a converting enzyme, primarily in the lung, to angiotensin II. Angiotensin II binds to specific receptors to increase mineralocorticoid secretion, which is also stimulated by an increased potassium concentration and, to a lesser degree, by ACTH.

Adrenocortical Hormone Excess

Glucocorticoid Excess. Glucocorticoid excess (Cushing syndrome) resulting from either endogenous oversecretion or long-term treatment with glucocorticoids at higher than physiologic doses produces a moon-faced plethoric individual with a centripetal distribution of fat (truncal obesity and skinny extremities), thin skin, easy bruising, and striae. Skeletal muscle wasting is common, but the heart and diaphragm are usually spared. A test for this syndrome is to ask the patient to get up from a chair without using the hands with the inability to do so indicating proximal

TABLE 32.3 Clinical Features of Hyperadrenalism (Cushing Syndrome) and Hypoadrenalism

Cushing Syndrome	Hypoadrenalism
Central obesity	Weight loss
Proximal muscle weakness	Weakness, fatigue, lethargy
Osteopenia at a young age	Muscle, joint, and back pain
Hypertension	Postural hypotension and dizziness
Headache	Headache
Psychiatric disorders	Anorexia, nausea, abdominal pain, constipation, diarrhea
Purple striae	
Spontaneous ecchymoses	
Plethoric facies	
Hyperpigmentation	Hyperpigmentation
Hirsutism	
Acne	
Hypokalemic alkalosis	Hyperkalemia, hyponatremia
Glucose intolerance	Occasional hypoglycemia
Kidney stones	Hypercalcemia
Polyuria	Prerenal azotemia
Menstrual disorders	
Increased leukocyte count	

muscle weakness consistent with Cushing syndrome. These patients often have osteopenia as a result of decreased formation of bone matrix and impaired absorption of calcium. Fluid retention and hypertension (because of increases in renin substrate and vascular reactivity caused by glucocorticoid activity) are common. Such patients may also have hyperglycemia and even diabetes mellitus from inhibition of peripheral use of glucose, as well as anti-insulin action and concomitant stimulation of gluconeogenesis (Table 32.3).

The most common cause of Cushing syndrome is the administration of glucocorticoids for such conditions as arthritis, asthma, and allergies. In these conditions, the adrenal glands atrophy and cannot respond to stressful situations (e.g., the perioperative period) by secreting more steroid; therefore, additional glucocorticoids may be required perioperatively (see the later section "Patients Taking Steroids for Other Reasons"). Spontaneous Cushing syndrome may be caused by pituitary production of ACTH (65% to 75% of all spontaneous cases), which is usually associated with pituitary microadenoma, or by nonendocrine ectopic ACTH production (principally by tumors of the lung, pancreas, or thymus).[49] Ten percent to 20% of cases of spontaneous Cushing syndrome are caused by an ACTH-independent process, either an adrenal adenoma or carcinoma.[49]

Special preoperative and preprocedure considerations for patients with Cushing syndrome include regulating blood glucose control, managing hypertension, and ensuring intravascular volume and electrolyte concentrations are normal. Ectopic ACTH production may cause marked hypokalemic alkalosis. Treatment with the aldosterone antagonist spironolactone stops the potassium loss and helps mobilize excess fluid. Because of the incidence of severe osteopenia and the risk of fractures, meticulous attention must be paid to positioning of the patient. In addition, glucocorticoids are lympholytic and immunosuppressive, thus increasing the patient's susceptibility to infection. The tensile strength of healing wounds decreases in the presence of glucocorticoids, an effect that is at least partially reversed by the topical administration of vitamin A.

Ten percent to 15% of patients with Cushing syndrome exhibit adrenal overproduction of glucocorticoids from an adrenal adenoma or carcinoma. If either unilateral or bilateral adrenal resection is planned, the physician should begin administering glucocorticoids at the start of resection of the tumor. Despite the absence of definitive studies, 100 mg of hydrocortisone every 24 hours intravenously is reasonable. This amount can be reduced over a period of 3 to 6 days until a maintenance dose is reached. Beginning on day 3, the surgeons may also give a mineralocorticoid, 9α-fluorocortisol (0.05-0.1 mg/day). In certain patients, both steroids may require several adjustments. This therapy continues if the patient has undergone bilateral resection. For a patient who has undergone unilateral adrenal resection, therapy is individualized according to the status of the remaining adrenal gland. The incidence of pneumothorax in an open adrenal resection approach can be as high as 20%; the diagnosis of pneumothorax is sought and treatment is initiated before the wound is closed. The use of the laparoscopic technique has markedly decreased this complication.

Bilateral adrenalectomy (now performed laparoscopically) in patients with Cushing syndrome is associated with a perioperative morbidity rate up to 20% and a perioperative mortality rate up to 3%. This procedure often results in permanent mineralocorticoid and glucocorticoid deficiency.[49a] Ten percent of patients with Cushing syndrome who undergo adrenalectomy have an undiagnosed pituitary tumor. After cortisol concentrations are decreased by adrenalectomy, the pituitary tumor will likely enlarge. These pituitary tumors are potentially invasive and may produce large amounts of ACTH and melanocyte-stimulating hormone, thereby increasing pigmentation.

Approximately 85% of adrenal tumors are discovered incidentally during screening CT scans. Nonfunctioning adrenal adenomas are found in patients on autopsy, ranging from 1% to 32% in different series. Functioning adenomas are generally treated surgically; often, the contralateral gland resumes functioning after several months. Frequently, however, the effects of carcinomas are not cured surgically. In such cases, administration of inhibitors of steroid synthesis, such as metyrapone or mitotane (*o,p′*-DDD[2,2-bis(2-chlorophenyl4-chlorophenyl)-1,1-dichloroethane]), may ameliorate some symptoms, as these drugs and specific aldosterone antagonists may aid in reducing symptoms of ectopic ACTH secretion if the primary tumor is unresectable. Patients given these adrenal suppressants are also prescribed long-term glucocorticoid replacement therapy with the goal of therapy being complete adrenal suppression. Therefore, these patients should be considered to have suppressed adrenal function, and glucocorticoid replacement should be increased perioperatively.

Mineralocorticoid Excess. Excess mineralocorticoid activity (common with glucocorticoid excess because most glucocorticoids have some mineralocorticoid properties) leads to potassium depletion, sodium retention, muscle weakness, hypertension, tetany, polyuria, inability to concentrate urine, and hypokalemic alkalosis. These symptoms constitute primary hyperaldosteronism, or Conn syndrome (a cause of low-renin hypertension because renin secretion is inhibited by the effects of the high levels of aldosterone).

Primary hyperaldosteronism is present in 0.5% to 1% of hypertensive patients who have no other known cause of hypertension. Primary hyperaldosteronism most often results from unilateral adenoma, although 25% to 40% of patients have been found to have bilateral adrenal hyperplasia. Intravascular fluid volume, electrolyte concentrations, and renal function should be restored to within normal limits preoperatively by administering the aldosterone antagonist spironolactone. The effects of spironolactone are slow in onset and increase for 1 to 2 weeks. Frequently, a period of at least 24 hours is required to restore potassium equilibrium as the deficit can be up to 400 mEq; however, normal serum potassium level does not necessarily imply correction of a total-body deficit of potassium. In addition, patients with Conn syndrome have a high incidence of hypertension and ischemic heart disease; hemodynamic monitoring should be tailored to the individual patient.

A retrospective anecdotal study indicated that intraoperative hemodynamic status was more stable when arterial blood pressure and electrolytes were controlled preoperatively with spironolactone than when other antihypertensive agents were used. However, the efficacy of optimizing the perioperative status of patients who have disorders of glucocorticoid or mineralocorticoid secretion has not been clearly defined. Therefore, we have assumed that gradual restoration of physiologic norms is good medicine and expect that it would decrease perioperative morbidity and mortality.

Adrenocortical Hormone Deficiency

Glucocorticoid Deficiency. Withdrawal of steroids or suppression of synthesis by steroid therapy is the leading cause of underproduction of corticosteroids (its management is discussed in the later section "Patients Taking Steroids for Other Reasons"). Other causes of adrenocortical insufficiency include the following: defects in ACTH secretion and destruction of the adrenal gland by autoimmune disease, tuberculosis, hemorrhage (e.g., Sheehan syndrome), or cancer; some forms of congenital adrenal hyperplasia (see previous discussion); and administration of cytotoxic drugs.

Primary adrenal insufficiency (Addison disease) is associated with local destruction of all zones of the adrenal cortex and results in both glucocorticoid and mineralocorticoid deficiency if the insufficiency is bilateral; common symptoms and signs are listed in Table 32.3. Autoimmune disease is the most common cause of primary (nonexogenous) bilateral ACTH deficiency in the United States, whereas tuberculosis is the most common cause worldwide. Tuberculosis is associated not only with decreased adrenal function, but also large adrenal glands, which are a common finding in sarcoidosis, histoplasmosis, amyloidosis, metastatic malignant disease, heparin-induced thrombocytopenia, and adrenal hemorrhage. Further, destruction or injury by trauma, human immunodeficiency virus (HIV), and other infections (e.g., cytomegalovirus, mycobacteria, and fungi) is being recognized more frequently.

Autoimmune destruction of the adrenal glands may be associated with other autoimmune disorders, such as some forms of type 1 diabetes and Hashimoto thyroiditis. Enzymatic defects in cortisol synthesis cause glucocorticoid insufficiency, compensatory elevations in ACTH, and congenital adrenal hyperplasia. Because adrenal insufficiency usually develops slowly, such patients are subject to marked pigmentation (from excess ACTH trying to stimulate an unproductive adrenal gland) and cardiopenia (secondary to chronic hypotension).

Secondary adrenal insufficiency occurs when ACTH secretion is deficient, often because of a pituitary or hypothalamic tumor. Treatment of pituitary tumors by surgery or radiation therapy may result in hypopituitarism and subsequent adrenal failure.

If unstressed, glucocorticoid-deficient patients usually have no perioperative problems. However, acute adrenal crisis (addisonian crisis) can occur when even a minor stress is present (e.g., upper respiratory infection). Preparation of such a patient for anesthesia and surgery should include treatment of hypovolemia, hyperkalemia, and hyponatremia. Because these patients cannot respond to stressful situations, it was traditionally recommended that they be given a stress dose of glucocorticoids (≈200 mg hydrocortisone/day) perioperatively. However, Symreng and colleagues gave 25 mg of hydrocortisone phosphate intravenously to adults at the start of the operative procedure, followed by 100 mg intravenously over the next 24 hours.[50] Because using the minimum drug dose that would produce an appropriate effect is desirable, this latter regimen seems attractive. Such a regimen has proved to be as successful as a regimen using maximum doses (≈300 mg hydrocortisone/day). Thus we now recommend giving the patient's usual daily dose plus 50 to 100 mg of hydrocortisone before surgical incision and 25 to 50 mg of hydrocortisone every 8 hours for 24 to 48 hours, depending on the type and duration of surgery.[47b]

Mineralocorticoid Deficiency. Hypoaldosteronism, a less common condition, can be congenital, can occur after unilateral adrenalectomy, or be a consequence of prolonged heparin administration, long-standing diabetes, or renal failure. Nonsteroidal inhibitors of prostaglandin synthesis may also inhibit renin release and exacerbate this condition in patients with renal insufficiency. Plasma renin activity is lower than normal and fails to increase appropriately in response to sodium restriction or diuretic drugs. Most symptoms are caused by hyperkalemic acidosis rather than hypovolemia; in fact, some patients are hypertensive. These patients can have severe hyperkalemia, hyponatremia, and myocardial conduction defects. These defects can be treated successfully by administering mineralocorticoids (9α-fluorocortisol, 0.05-0.1 mg/day) preoperatively. Doses must be carefully titrated and monitored to avoid an increase in hypertension.

Patients Taking Steroids for Other Reasons

Perioperative Stress and the Need for Corticoid Supplementation. The adrenal responses of normal patients to the perioperative period, as well as the responses of patients taking steroids for other diseases, indicate the following:

1. Perioperative stress is related to the degree of trauma and the depth of anesthesia. Deep general or regional anesthesia delays the usual intraoperative glucocorticoid surge to the postoperative period.
2. A few patients with suppressed adrenal function will have perioperative cardiovascular problems if they do not receive supplemental steroids perioperatively.
3. Although a patient who takes steroids on a long-term basis may become hypotensive perioperatively; glucocorticoid or mineralocorticoid deficiency is seldom the cause. Longer duration and higher home steroid dose increase the likelihood of deficiency.[47b]
4. Acute adrenal insufficiency rarely occurs, but can be life-threatening.
5. Giving these patients steroid coverage equivalent to 100 mg of hydrocortisone perioperatively has little risk.[47b]

In a well-controlled study of glucocorticoid replacement in nonhuman primates, the investigators clearly defined the life-threatening events that can be associated with inadequate perioperative corticosteroid replacement.[48] In this study, adrenalectomized primates and sham-operated controls were given physiologic doses of steroids for 4 months. The animals were then randomly allocated to groups that received subphysiologic (one-tenth of the normal cortisol production), physiologic, or supraphysiologic (10 times the normal cortisol production) doses of cortisol for 4 days preceding abdominal surgery (cholecystectomy). The group given subphysiologic doses of steroid perioperatively had a significant increase in postoperative mortality. Death rates for the physiologic and supraphysiologic replacement groups were the same and did not differ from the rate for sham-operated controls. Death in the subphysiologic replacement group was related to severe hypotension associated with a significant decrease in systemic vascular resistance and a reduced left ventricular stroke work index. Filling pressures of the heart were unchanged when compared with those in control animals. No evidence of hypovolemia or severe congestive heart failure (CHF) was observed. Despite the low systemic vascular resistance, the animals did not become tachycardic. All these responses are compatible with the previously documented interaction of glucocorticoids and catecholamines, and thus suggest that glucocorticoids mediate catecholamine-induced increases in cardiac contractility and maintenance of vascular tone.

The investigators used a sensitive measure of wound healing involving accumulation of hydroxyproline. All treatment groups, including the group given supraphysiologic doses of glucocorticoids, had the same capacity for wound healing. Furthermore, perioperative administration of supraphysiologic doses of corticosteroids produced no adverse metabolic consequences.

This study confirmed long-standing intuitive impressions concerning patients who had inadequate adrenal function as a result of either underlying disease or administration of exogenous steroids—inadequate replacement of corticosteroids can lead to addisonian crisis and increased mortality, whereas the administration of supraphysiologic doses of steroids for a short time perioperatively can be safe. It is clear that inadequate corticosteroid coverage can cause death, but what is not so clear is what dose of steroid should be recommended for replacement therapy. Yong and colleagues reviewed the randomized controlled trials for a Cochrane Systemic Review and reported only two trials involving 37 patients that met the inclusion criteria.[51] These studies reported that supplemental perioperative steroids were not required during surgery for patients with adrenal insufficiency, but neither study reported any adverse effects or complications in the intervention or control groups. The authors concluded that they were unable to support or refute the use of supplemental perioperative steroids for patients with adrenal insufficiency during surgery. Because the risk is low and the benefit is high, physicians should consider providing supplementation for any patient who has received steroids within a year.[48,50]

How can one determine when adrenal responsiveness has returned to normal? The morning plasma cortisol level does not reveal whether the adrenal cortex has recovered sufficiently to ensure that cortisol secretion will increase adequately to meet the demands of stress. Inducing hypoglycemia with insulin has been advocated as a sensitive test of pituitary-adrenal competence, but it is impractical and is probably a more dangerous practice than simply administering glucocorticoids. If the plasma cortisol concentration is measured during acute stress, a value of greater than 25 μg/dL assuredly (and a value >15 μg/dL probably) indicates normal pituitary-adrenal responsiveness. In another test of pituitary-adrenal sufficiency, the baseline plasma cortisol level is determined. Then, 250 μg of synthetic ACTH (cosyntropin) is given, and plasma cortisol is measured 30 to 60 minutes later. An increase in plasma cortisol of 6 to 20 μg/dL or more is normal.[52,53] A normal response indicates recovery of pituitary-adrenal axis function. A lesser response usually indicates pituitary-adrenal insufficiency, possibly requiring perioperative supplementation with steroids.[53a]

Under perioperative conditions, the adrenal glands secrete 116 to 185 mg of cortisol daily. Under maximum stress, they may secrete 200 to 500 mg/day. Good correlation exists between the severity and duration of the operation and the response of the adrenal gland. "Major surgery" would be represented by procedures such as laparoscopic colectomy and "minor surgery" by procedures such as herniorrhaphy. In a study of 20 patients during major surgery, the mean maximal concentration of cortisol in plasma was 47 μg/dL (range, 22-75 μg/dL). Values remained higher than 26 μg/dL for a maximum of 72 hours postoperatively. During minor surgery, the mean maximal concentration of cortisol in plasma was 28 μg/dL (range, 10-44 μg/dL).

Although the precise amount required has not been established, we usually intravenously administer the maximum amount of glucocorticoid that the body manufactures in response to maximal stress (i.e., approximately 200 mg/day of hydrocortisone).[53b] For minor surgical procedures, we usually give hydrocortisone intravenously, 50 to 100 mg/day. Unless infection or some other perioperative complication develops, we decrease this dose by approximately 50%/day until the standard home dose is resumed. For major surgical procedures, we usually give 50 mg every 6 hours to 100 mg every 8 hours. Again unless a complication develops, this is decreased 50%/day until the standard home dose is resumed.[53b]

Risks of Supplementation. Rare complications of perioperative steroid supplementation include aggravation of hypertension, fluid retention, inducement of stress ulcers, and psychiatric disturbances. Two possible complications of short-term perioperative supplementation with glucocorticoids are abnormal wound healing and an increased rate of infections. This evidence is inconclusive, however, because it relates to short-term glucocorticoid administration and not to long-term administration of glucocorticoids with increased doses at times of stress. In contrast to a deleterious effect of perioperative glucocorticoid administration on wound healing in rats, a study involving primates suggested that large doses of glucocorticoids, administered perioperatively, do not impair sensitive measures of wound healing.[48] An overall assessment of these results suggests that short-term perioperative supplementation with steroids has a small but definite deleterious effect on wound healing that is perhaps partially reversed by topical administration of vitamin A.

Information on the risk of infection from perioperative glucocorticoid supplementation is also unclear as there are no controlled trials addressing these effects. In many studies of long-term use by patients and supplementation, no increased risk of serious infections was reported with long-term use of steroids alone. Data indicate that the risk of infection in a patient taking steroids on a long-term basis is real, but whether perioperative supplementation with steroids increases that risk is not clear.

Adrenal Cortex Function in Older Adults

Production of androgens by the adrenal gland progressively decreases with age; this change has no known implications for anesthesia. Plasma levels of cortisol are unaffected by increasing age. Levels of CBG are also unaffected by age, a finding suggesting that a normal fraction of free cortisol (1%-5%) is present in older patients. Older patients have a progressively impaired ability to metabolize and excrete glucocorticoids. In normal individuals, the quantity of 17-hydroxycorticosteroids excreted is reduced by half by the seventh decade. This decreased excretion undoubtedly reflects the reduced renal function that occurs with aging. When excretion of cortisol metabolites is expressed as a function of creatinine clearance, the age difference disappears. Further reductions in cortisol clearance may reflect impaired hepatic metabolism of circulating cortisol.

The rate of secretion of cortisol is 30% slower in older adults. This reduced secretion may be an appropriate compensatory mechanism for maintaining a normal cortisol level in the presence of decreased hepatic and renal clearance of cortisol. The reduced cortisol production can be overcome during periods of stress, and even extremely old patients (>100 years old) display an entirely normal adrenal response to the administration of ACTH and to stresses such as hypoglycemia.

Both underproduction and overproduction of glucocorticoids are generally considered diseases of younger individuals. The highest incidence of Cushing disease of either pituitary or adrenal origin occurs during the third decade of life. The most common cause of spontaneous Cushing disease is benign pituitary adenoma. However, in patients older than 60 years in whom Cushing disease develops, the most likely cause is adrenal carcinoma or ectopic ACTH production from tumors usually located in the lung, pancreas, or thymus.

ADRENAL MEDULLARY SYMPATHETIC HORMONE EXCESS: PHEOCHROMOCYTOMA

Less than 0.1% of all cases of hypertension are caused by pheochromocytomas, or catecholamine-producing tumors derived from chromaffin tissue.[54] Nevertheless, these tumors are clearly important to the anesthesiologist as previously 25% to 50% of hospital deaths in patients with pheochromocytoma occurred during induction of anesthesia or during operative procedures for other causes.[55] This high mortality has been reduced with the improvements in anesthesia management during our current era.[55a] Although usually found in the adrenal medulla, these vascular tumors can occur anywhere (referred to as paragangliomas), with a proportion of up to 20%.[55b] Malignant spread, which occurs in less than 15% of pheochromocytomas, usually proceeds to venous and lymphatic channels with a predisposition for the liver. This tumor is occasionally familial or part of the multiglandular-neoplastic syndrome known as multiple endocrine adenoma type IIa or type IIb, and is manifested as an autosomal dominant trait. Type IIa consists of medullary carcinoma of the thyroid, parathyroid adenoma or hyperplasia, and pheochromocytoma. What used to be called type IIb is now often called pheochromocytoma in association with phakomatoses such as von Recklinghausen neurofibromatosis and von Hippel–Lindau disease with cerebellar hemangioblastoma. Frequently, bilateral tumors are found in the familial form. Localization of tumors can be achieved by MRI or CT, metaiodobenzylguanidine nuclear scanning, ultrasonography, or intravenous pyelography (in decreasing order of combined sensitivity and specificity).

Symptoms and signs that may be solicited before surgery or procedures and are suggestive of pheochromocytoma are as follows: excessive sweating; headache; hypertension; orthostatic hypotension; previous hypertensive or arrhythmic response to induction of anesthesia or to abdominal examination; paroxysmal attacks of sweating, headache, tachycardia, and hypertension; glucose intolerance; polycythemia; weight loss; and psychological abnormalities. In fact, the occurrence of combined symptoms of paroxysmal headache, sweating, and hypertension is probably a more sensitive and specific indicator than any one biochemical test for pheochromocytoma (Table 32.4).

The value of preoperative and preprocedure adrenergic receptor blocking drugs probably justifies their use as these drugs may reduce the perioperative complications of hypertensive crisis, the wide arterial blood pressure fluctuations during tumor manipulation (especially until venous drainage is obliterated), and the myocardial dysfunction. Mortality is decreased with resection of pheochromocytoma (from 40% to 60% to the current 0% to 6%) when adrenergic receptor blockade is introduced as preoperative and preprocedure preparatory therapy for such patients.[56-60]

α-Adrenergic receptor blockade with prazosin or phenoxybenzamine restores intravascular plasma volume by counteracting the vasoconstrictive effects of high levels of catecholamines. This reexpansion of intravascular fluid volume is often followed by a decrease in hematocrit. Because some patients may be very sensitive to the effects of phenoxybenzamine, this drug should initially be

TABLE 32.4 Characteristics of Tests for Pheochromocytoma

Test/Symptoms	Sensitivity (%)	Specificity (%)	LIKELIHOOD RATIO Positive Result*	LIKELIHOOD RATIO Negative Result†
Vanillylmandelic acid excretion	81	97	27.0	0.20
Catecholamine excretion	82	95	16.4	0.19
Metanephrine excretion	83	95	16.6	0.18
Abdominal computed tomography	92	80	4.6	0.10
Concurrent paroxysmal hypertension, headache, sweating, and tachycardia‡	90	95	18.0	0.10

*The ratio representing the likelihood of a positive result is obtained by dividing the sensitivity by 1 and then subtracting the specificity.
†The ratio representing the likelihood of a negative result is obtained by subtracting the sensitivity from 1 and the dividing by the specificity.
‡Data for concurrent paroxysmal symptoms are best estimates from available data.
Modified from Pauker SG, Kopelman RI. Interpreting hoofbeats: can Bayes help clear the haze? *N Engl J Med.* 1992;327:1009–1013.

given in doses of 20 to 30 mg/70 kg orally once or twice a day. Most patients usually require 60 to 250 mg/day. The Endocrine Society Task Force guidelines from 2014 recommend α-adrenergic receptor blockade for all patients with active tumors.[60a] The efficacy of therapy should be judged by the reduction in symptoms and stabilization of arterial blood pressure. For patients who have carbohydrate intolerance because of inhibition of insulin release mediated by α-adrenergic receptor stimulation, α-adrenergic receptor blockade may reduce fasting blood glucose levels. For patients who exhibit ST-T changes on the ECG, long-term preoperative and preprocedure α-adrenergic receptor blockade (1-6 months) has produced ECG and clinical resolution of catecholamine-induced myocarditis.[56,57,59-63]

β-Adrenergic receptor blockade with propranolol is suggested for patients who have persistent arrhythmias or tachycardia,[56,57,59-63] the reason being that these conditions can be precipitated or aggravated by α-adrenergic receptor blockade. It is important to remember that β-adrenergic receptor blockade should not be used without concurrent α-adrenergic receptor blockade lest the vasoconstrictive effects of the latter go unopposed and thereby increasing the risk of malignant hypertension.

The optimal duration of preoperative therapy with α-adrenergic receptor blockade has not been well studied. The Endocrine Society Task Force guidelines from 2014 recommend α-adrenergic receptor blockade at least 7 to 14 days prior to surgery; however, most centers report a preoperative treatment duration of 2 to 6 weeks.[19] Most patients will require 10 to 14 days, as judged by the time needed to stabilize arterial blood pressure and ameliorate symptoms. The Endocrine Society Task Force guidelines further recommended a high sodium diet and fluid intake to reverse the catecholamine-induced volume contraction.[63a] Because the tumor spreads slowly, little is lost by waiting until medical therapy has optimized the patient's preoperative condition. The following criteria are reasonable for assessing the adequacy of treatment:

1. No in-hospital arterial blood pressure reading higher than 165/90 mm Hg should be evident for 48 hours preoperatively.
2. Orthostatic hypotension is acceptable as long as arterial blood pressure when the patient is standing is not less than 80/45 mm Hg.
3. The ECG should be free of ST-T changes that are not permanent.
4. No more than one premature ventricular contraction (PVC) should occur every 5 minutes.

Other drugs, including prazosin, calcium channel blocking drugs, clonidine, dexmedetomidine, and magnesium, have also been used to achieve suitable degrees of α-adrenergic blockade preoperatively. Multiple case series have confirmed the clinical utility of this approach in adults before tumor excision, including in a hemodynamic catecholamine crisis.[64] Magnesium therapy has shown efficacy for the resection of pheochromocytoma or paraganglioma during pregnancy. The dosing of magnesium for the management of pheochromocytoma has been reviewed elsewhere.[65]

The key clinical components of ideal patient care include optimal preoperative preparation, slow and controlled induction of anesthesia, and good communication among members of the perioperative team. Virtually all anesthetic drugs and techniques (including isoflurane, sevoflurane, sufentanil, remifentanil, fentanyl, and regional anesthesia) have been used with success, although all drugs studied were associated with a high rate of transient intraoperative arrhythmias.[59]

Because of ease of use, the preference is to give phenylephrine for hypotension and nitroprusside or nicardipine for hypertension. Phentolamine has too long an onset and duration of action. Painful or stressful events such as intubation often cause an exaggerated stress response in less than perfectly anesthetized patients who have pheochromocytoma. This response is caused by release of catecholamines from nerve endings that are "loaded" by the reuptake process. Such stresses may result in catecholamine levels of 200 to 2000 picograms (pg)/mL in normal patients. For a patient with pheochromocytoma, even simple stress can lead to blood catecholamine levels of ten times normal. However, infarction of a tumor, with release of products onto peritoneal surfaces, or surgical pressure causing release of products, can result in blood levels of 200,000 to 1,000,000 pg/mL—a situation that should be anticipated and avoided (if possible ask for a stay of surgery to increase vasodilator infusion). Once the venous supply is secured and if intravascular volume is normal, normal arterial blood pressure usually results. However, some patients may become hypotensive and occasionally require catecholamine infusions. Vasopressin has also been used for hemodynamic rescue in catecholamine-resistant vasoplegic shock after resection of a massive pheochromocytoma.[66] On rare occasion, patients remain hypertensive intraoperatively. Postoperatively, approximately 50% of patients remain hypertensive for 1 to 3 days and initially have markedly increased but declining plasma catecholamine levels—at which time all but 25% will become normotensive. Other family members should be advised to inform their future anesthesiologist about the potential for such familial disease.

HYPOFUNCTION OR ABERRATION IN FUNCTION OF THE SYMPATHETIC NERVOUS SYSTEM (DYSAUTONOMIA)

Disorders of the sympathetic nervous system include Shy-Drager syndrome, Riley-Day syndrome, Lesch-Nyhan syndrome, Gill familial dysautonomia, diabetic dysautonomia, and the dysautonomia of spinal cord transection.

Although individuals can function well without an adrenal medulla, a deficient peripheral sympathetic nervous system occurring late in life poses major problems; nevertheless, perioperative sympathectomy or its equivalent is often recommended.[67-73] A primary function of the sympathetic nervous system appears to be regulation of arterial blood pressure and intravascular fluid volume during changing of body position. Common features of all the syndromes with hypofunction of the sympathetic nervous system are orthostatic hypotension and decreased beat-to-beat variability in heart rate. These conditions can be caused by deficient intravascular volume, deficient baroreceptor function (as also occurs in carotid artery disease[74]), abnormalities in CNS function (as in Wernicke or Shy-Drager syndrome), deficient neuronal stores of norepinephrine (as in idiopathic orthostatic hypotension[75] and diabetes), or deficient release of norepinephrine (as in traumatic spinal cord injury[76]). These patients may have a compensatory upregulation of available adrenergic receptors causing an exaggerated response to sympathomimetic drugs. In addition to other abnormalities, such as retention of urine or feces and deficient heat exchange, hypofunction of the sympathetic nervous system is often accompanied by renal amyloidosis. Thus electrolyte and intravascular fluid volume status should be assessed preoperatively. Because many of these patients have cardiac abnormalities, cardiac function and intravascular volume status may require invasive assessment with echocardiography, central venous catheter, or a pulmonary artery catheter per the treating physician's discretion.

Because the functioning of the sympathetic nervous system is not predictable in these patients, slow and controlled induction of anesthesia and treatment of sympathetic excess or deficiency should be initiated through titratable direct-acting vasodilators (nicardipine/nitroprusside), vasoconstrictors (phenylephrine/norepinephrine), chronotropes (isoproterenol), or negative chronotropes (esmolol). A 20% perioperative mortality rate for 2600 patients after spinal cord transection has been reported, thus indicating that such patients are difficult to manage and deserve particularly close attention.

After reviewing 300 patients with spinal cord injuries, Kendrick and coworkers concluded that autonomic hyperreflexia syndrome does not develop if the lesion is below spinal dermatome T7.[77] If the lesion is above that level (splanchnic outflow), 60% to 70% of patients experience extreme vascular instability. The trigger to this instability, a mass reflex involving noradrenergic release and motor hypertonus, can be a cutaneous, proprioceptive, or visceral stimulus (a full bladder is a common initiator). The sensation enters the spinal cord and causes a spinal reflex, which in normal persons is inhibited from above. Sudden increases in arterial blood pressure are sensed in the pressure receptors of the aorta and carotid sinus. The resulting vagal hyperactivity produces bradycardia, ventricular ectopia, or various degrees of heart block. Reflex vasodilation may occur above the level of the lesion and result in flushing of the head and neck. In the acute injury period, modest therapeutic hypothermia may provide benefit but many note that further large randomized trials are needed; the anesthesiologist must be vigilant to avoid hyperthermia and maintain normothermia—hypothermia during procedures.[77a]

Depending on the length of time since spinal cord transection, other abnormalities may occur. In the short term (i.e., <3 weeks from the time of spinal injury), retention of urine and feces is common and, through elevation of the diaphragm, may affect respiration. Hyperesthesia is present above the lesion; reflexes and flaccid paralysis are present below the lesion. The intermediate period (3 days to 6 months) is marked by a hyperkalemic response to depolarizing drugs.[78] The chronic phase is characterized by return of muscle tone, Babinski sign, and, frequently, the occurrence of hyperreflexia syndromes (e.g., mass reflex [see earlier]).

Thus in addition to meticulous attention to perioperative intravascular volume and electrolyte status, the anesthesiologist should know—by history taking, physical examination, and laboratory data—the status of the patient's myocardial conduction (as revealed by the ECG), the status of renal functioning (by noting the ratio of creatinine to blood urea nitrogen [BUN]), and the condition of the respiratory muscles (by determining the ratio of forced expiratory volume in 1 second to forced vital capacity). The anesthesiologist may also obtain a chest radiograph if atelectasis or pneumonia is suspected on the basis of history taking or the physical examination. Temperature control, the presence of bone fractures or decubitus ulcers, and normal functioning of the urination and defecation systems must be assessed.

THYROID DYSFUNCTION

The major thyroid hormones are thyroxine (T_4), a prohormone product of the thyroid gland, and the more potent 3,5,3-triiodothyronine (T_3), a product of both the thyroid and extrathyroidal enzymatic deiodination of T_4. Under normal circumstances, approximately 85% of T_3 is produced outside the thyroid gland. Production of thyroid secretions is maintained by secretion of thyroid-stimulating hormone (TSH) in the pituitary, which in turn is regulated by secretion of thyrotropin-releasing hormone (TRH) in the hypothalamus. Secretion of TSH and TRH appears to be negatively regulated by T_4 and T_3. Many investigators believe that all effects of thyroid hormones are mediated by T_3 and that T_4 functions only as a prohormone.

TABLE 32.5 Biochemical Measurements of Thyroid Function That Account for Variation in Production of Thyroxine-Binding Globulin

	EXAMPLES OF NORMAL THYROID STATUS*						
	FT_4E	=	**T_4**	×	**THBR**	**TSH**
Normal	0.19 (0.12-0.25)	=	0.6 (0.4-0.9)	×	31% (25%-35%)	0.2 (0.2-0.8)
During use of oral contraceptives	0.19	=	1.3	×	15%	0.3
During use of corticosteroids	0.18	=	0.3	×	60%	0.3

*FT_4E is the free T_4 (thyroxine) estimate. It is usually obtained by multiplying the total T_4 concentration (the free amount and the amount bound to protein) by the thyroid hormone–binding ratio (THBR, formerly called the resin T_3 uptake). THBR is a measure of the bound thyroid hormone–binding protein. TSH is the thyroid-stimulating hormone secreted by the pituitary in the negative feedback loop. (TSH increases when FT_4E is low in hypothyroidism.)

BOX 32.2 Factors Influencing Serum Levels of Thyroxine-Binding Globulin

Conditions Increasing Serum Levels

- Use of oral contraceptives
- Pregnancy
- Use of estrogen
- Infectious hepatitis
- Chronic active hepatitis
- Neonatal state
- Acute intermittent porphyria
- Inherited conditions

Conditions Decreasing Serum Levels

- Testosterone
- Use of corticosteroids
- Severe illness
- Cirrhosis
- Nephrotic syndrome
- Inherited conditions

Because T_3 has greater biologic effect than does T_4, one would expect the diagnosis of thyroid disorders to be based on levels of T_3. However, this is not usually the case. The diagnosis of thyroid disease is confirmed by one of several biochemical measurements: levels of free T_4 or total serum concentrations of T_4 and the "free T_4 estimate." This estimate is obtained by multiplying total T_4 (free and bound) by the thyroid-binding ratio (formerly called resin T_3 uptake) (Table 32.5). Free T_4 can be accurately measured by many laboratories, this direct measurement of free T_4 obviates the need to account for changes in binding protein synthesis and affinity caused by other conditions. The T_3-binding ratio measures the extra quantity of serum protein-binding sites. This measurement is necessary because thyroxine-binding globulin (TBG) levels are abnormally high during pregnancy, hepatic disease, and estrogen therapy (all of which would elevate the total T_4 level; Box 32.2). Reliable interpretation of measurements of the total hormone concentration in serum necessitates data on the percentage of bound hormone. The thyroid hormone–binding ratio test provides this information. In this test, iodine-labeled T_3 is added to a patient's serum and is allowed to reach an equilibrium binding state. A resin is then added that binds the remaining radioactive T_3. Resin uptake is greater if the patient has fewer TBG-binding sites. In normal patients, resin T_3 uptake (the thyroid hormone–binding ratio) is 25% to 35%. When serum TBG is elevated, the thyroid hormone–binding ratio is diminished (see Table 32.5). When serum TBG is diminished, as in nephrotic syndrome, in conditions in which glucocorticoids are increased, or in chronic liver disease, the thyroid hormone–binding ratio is increased.

The free T_4 estimate and the free T_3 estimate are frequently used as measures of a patient's serum T_4 and T_3 hormone concentrations, respectively. To obtain these estimates, the concentration of total serum T_4 or total serum T_3 is multiplied by the measured thyroid hormone–binding ratio. Values of these two indices are normal in the event of a primary alteration in binding but not with an alteration in secretion of thyroid hormone.

Hyperthyroidism can be diagnosed by measuring levels of TSH after the administration of TRH. Although administering TRH normally increases TSH levels in blood, even a small increase in the T_4 or T_3 level in blood abolishes this response. Thus a subnormal or absent serum TSH response to TRH is a very sensitive indicator of hyperthyroidism. In one group of disorders involving hyperthyroidism, serum TSH levels are elevated in the presence of elevated levels of free thyroid hormone.

Measurement of the α-subunit of TSH has been helpful in identifying the rare patients who have a pituitary neoplasm and who usually have increased α-subunit concentrations. Some patients are clinically euthyroid in the presence of elevated levels of total T_4 in serum. Certain drugs, notably propranolol, glucocorticoids, and amiodarone, block the conversion of T_4 to T_3 and thereby elevate T_4 levels. Severe illness also slows this conversion, termed "sick thyroid" in a critical-illness setting. Levels of TSH are often high in situations in which the rate of conversion is decreased. In hyperthyroidism, cardiac function and responses to stress are abnormal; return of normal cardiac function parallels the return of TSH levels to normal.

Hyperthyroidism

Although hyperthyroidism is usually caused by the multinodular diffuse enlargement in Graves disease (also associated with disorders of the skin or eyes, or both), it can also occur with pregnancy, thyroiditis, thyroid adenoma, choriocarcinoma, or TSH-secreting pituitary adenoma. Five percent of women have thyrotoxic effects 3 to 6 months postpartum and tend to have recurrences with subsequent pregnancies. Major manifestations of hyperthyroidism are weight loss, diarrhea, warm and moist skin, weakness of large muscle groups, menstrual abnormalities, osteopenia, nervousness, jitteriness, intolerance to heat, tachycardia, cardiac arrhythmias, mitral valve prolapse, and heart failure. When the thyroid is functioning abnormally, the cardiovascular system is most at risk. When diarrhea is severe, the associated dehydration and electrolyte abnormalities should be corrected preoperatively. Mild anemia, thrombocytopenia, increased serum alkaline phosphatase, hypercalcemia, muscle wasting, and bone loss frequently occur in hyperthyroidism. Muscle disease usually involves the proximal large muscle groups; it has not been reported to cause respiratory muscle paralysis. In the apathetic form of hyperthyroidism (seen most commonly in persons >60 years old), cardiac effects predominate and include tachycardia, irregular heart rhythm, atrial fibrillation (in 10%), heart failure, and occasionally, papillary muscle dysfunction.

Although β-adrenergic receptor blockade can control the heart rate, its use is challenging in the setting of heart failure. However, a decreasing heart rate may improve heart-pumping function. Thus hyperthyroid patients who have fast ventricular rates and in heart failure, requiring emergency surgery, can be safely given short-acting β-blockers guided by clinical response. If slowing the heart rate with a small dose of esmolol (50 μg/kg) does not aggravate the heart failure, the physician should administer more esmolol, and titrate to effect. Antithyroid medications include propylthiouracil and methimazole, both of which decrease the synthesis of T_4 and may enhance remission by reducing TSH receptor antibody levels (the primary pathologic mechanism in Graves disease). Propylthiouracil also decreases the conversion of T_4 to the more potent T_3. However, the literature indicates a trend toward preoperative preparation with propranolol and iodides alone.[79] This approach is quicker (i.e., 7-14 days vs. 2-6 weeks); it shrinks the thyroid gland, as does the more traditional approach; it decreases conversion of the prohormone T_4 into the more potent T_3; and it treats symptoms but may not correct abnormalities in left ventricular function. Regardless of the approach, antithyroid drugs should be administered on a long-term basis and on the morning of the surgical procedure. If emergency surgery is necessary before the euthyroid state is achieved, if subclinical hyperthyroidism progresses without adequate treatment, or if hyperthyroidism is out of control intraoperatively, intravenous administration of esmolol, 50 to 500 μ/kg, could be titrated to restore a normal heart rate (assuming the absence of heart failure). In addition, intravascular fluid volume and electrolyte balance should be restored. However, administering propranolol or esmolol does not always prevent "thyroid storm." No specific anesthetic drug is preferred for surgical patients who have hyperthyroidism.

A patient with a large goiter and an obstructed airway can be managed in the same way as any other patient with a problematic airway. In this type of case, reviewing CT scans of the neck preoperatively may provide valuable information regarding the extent of compression. Maintenance of anesthesia usually presents little difficulty. Postoperatively, extubation of the trachea should be performed under optimal circumstances for reintubation in the event that tracheomalacia (the tracheal rings have been weakened and the trachea collapses) developed.

Of the many possible postoperative complications including: nerve injury, bleeding, metabolic abnormalities, and thyroid storm (discussed in the next section); bilateral recurrent laryngeal nerve trauma and hypocalcemic tetany are the most feared. Bilateral recurrent laryngeal nerve injury (secondary to trauma or edema) causes stridor and laryngeal obstruction as a result of unopposed adduction of the vocal cords and closure of the glottic aperture. Immediate endotracheal intubation is required, usually followed by tracheostomy to ensure an adequate airway. Fortunately, Lahey Clinic records indicate that this rare complication occurred only once in more than 30,000 thyroid operations. Unilateral recurrent nerve injury often goes unnoticed because of compensatory overadduction of the uninvolved cord. However, we often test vocal cord function before and after this operation by asking the patient to say "e" or "moon." Unilateral nerve injury is characterized by hoarseness, whereas aphonia characterizes bilateral nerve injury. Selective injury to the adductor fibers of both recurrent laryngeal nerves leaves the abductor muscles relatively unopposed, and pulmonary aspiration is a risk. Selective injury to the abductor fibers leaves the adductor muscles relatively unopposed, and airway obstruction can occur.

The intimate involvement of the parathyroid gland with the thyroid gland can result in inadvertent hypocalcemia during surgery for thyroid disease. Complications related to hypocalcemia are discussed in the later section on this disorder.

Because postoperative hematoma can compromise the airway, neck and wound dressings are placed in a crossing fashion (rather than vertically or horizontally) and should be examined for evidence of bleeding before a patient is discharged from the recovery room.

Thyroid Storm

Thyroid storm is the name for the clinical diagnosis of a life-threatening illness in a patient whose hyperthyroidism has been severely exacerbated by illness or surgery. Thyroid storm is characterized by hyperthermia or pyrexia, tachycardia, and striking alterations in consciousness. Its clinical appearance is similar to malignant hyperthermia, pheochromocytoma, and neuroleptic malignant syndrome, further complicating the differential.[79a] No laboratory tests are diagnostic of thyroid storm, and the precipitating (nonthyroidal) cause is the major determinant of survival. Therapy can include blocking the synthesis of thyroid hormones by administering antithyroid drugs and the release of preformed hormone with iodine. Blocking the sympathetic nervous system symptoms with reserpine, α- and β-receptor antagonists, or α_2 drugs may be exceedingly hazardous and requires skillful management with constant monitoring of the critically ill patient.

Thyroid dysfunction, either hyperthyroidism or hypothyroidism, develops in more than 10% of patients treated with the antiarrhythmic agent amiodarone.[80] Approximately 35% of the drug's weight is iodine, and a 200-mg tablet releases approximately 20 times the optimal daily dose of iodine. This iodine can lead to reduced synthesis of T_4 or increased synthesis. In addition, amiodarone inhibits the conversion of T_4 to the more potent T_3. These patients receiving amiodarone are in need of special attention preoperatively and intraoperatively, not just because of the arrhythmia that led to such therapy, but to ensure that no perioperative dysfunction or surprises result from unsuspected thyroid hyperfunction or hypofunction.[81]

Hypothyroidism

Hypothyroidism is a common disease that has been detected in 5% of a large population in Great Britain, in 3% to 6% of a healthy older population in Massachusetts, in 4.5% of a medical clinic population in Switzerland, and in 8.5% of a large Turkish population presenting to an anesthesiology preoperative clinic.[81a] The apathy and lethargy that often accompany hypothyroidism frequently delay its diagnosis, thus the perioperative period may be the first opportunity to spot many such hypothyroid patients. However, hypothyroidism is usually subclinical, serum concentrations of thyroid hormones are in the normal range, and only serum TSH levels are elevated. The normal range of TSH is 0.3 to 4.5 milliunits/L, and TSH values of 5 to 15 milliunits/L are characteristic of this entity. In such cases, hypothyroidism may have little or no perioperative significance. However, a retrospective study of 59 mildly hypothyroid patients found that more hypothyroid patients than control subjects required prolonged postoperative intubation (9 of 59 vs. 4 of 59), had significant electrolyte imbalances (3 of 59 vs. 1 of 59), and bleeding complications (4 of 59 vs. 0 of 59).[82] Because only a few charts were examined, these differences did not reach statistical significance. In another study, overt hypothyroidism later developed in a high percentage of patients with a history of subclinical hypothyroidism.[83,84]

Overt hypothyroidism is associated with slow mental functioning, slow movement, slow reflexes, dry skin, arthralgias, carpal tunnel syndrome, periorbital edema, intolerance to cold, depression of the ventilatory responses to hypoxia and hypercapnia, impaired clearance of free water with or without hyponatremia, slow gastric emptying, sleep apnea,[85] and bradycardia. In extreme cases, cardiomegaly, heart failure, pericardial and pleural effusions can develop, often presenting as orthopnea, dyspnea, or general fatigue. Hypothyroidism is often associated with amyloidosis, which may produce an enlarged tongue, cardiac conduction abnormalities, and renal disease. Hypothyroidism decreases the anesthetic requirement slightly. The tongue may be enlarged in a hypothyroid patient even in the absence of amyloidosis, and such enlargement may hamper endotracheal intubation.

An increasing TSH level is the most sensitive indicator of failing thyroid function. Ideal preoperative and preprocedure management of hypothyroidism consists of restoring normal thyroid status: the physicians should consider administering the normal dose of levothyroxine the morning of the surgical procedure, even though these drugs have long half-lives (1.4-10 days). Reduced GI absorption of levothyroxine may occur with the coadministration of cholestyramine or aluminum hydroxide, iron, a high-bran meal, or sucralfate or colestipol. For patients in myxedema coma who require emergency surgery, liothyronine (T3 hormone) can be given intravenously (with fear of precipitating myocardial ischemia, however) while supportive therapy is undertaken to restore normal intravascular fluid volume, body temperature, cardiac function, respiratory function, and electrolyte balance.[85a]

In hypothyroidism, respiratory control mechanisms and renal fluid balance do not function normally, however, the response to hypoxia and hypercapnia, and clearance of free water normalize with thyroid replacement therapy. Drug metabolism is anecdotally reported to be slowed, and awakening times from sedatives are reported to be prolonged by hypothyroidism. However, few formal studies, and none in humans, of the pharmacokinetics and pharmacodynamics of sedatives or anesthetic drugs in this population have been published. These concerns disappear when thyroid function is normalized preoperatively. Addison disease (with its relative steroid deficiency) is more common in hypothyroidism, and some endocrinologists routinely treat patients with noniatrogenic hypothyroidism with stress doses of steroids perioperatively because both conditions are commonly caused by autoimmune responses. The possibility that this steroid deficiency exists should be considered if the patient becomes hypotensive perioperatively. Body heat mechanisms are inadequate in hypothyroid patients, so temperature should be monitored and maintained, especially in patients requiring emergency surgery. Because of an increased incidence of myasthenia gravis in hypothyroid patients, a peripheral nerve stimulator is used to guide judicious administration of muscle relaxants.

Thyroid Nodules and Carcinoma

More than 90% of thyroid nodules are benign, yet identifying malignancy in a solitary thyroid nodule is a difficult and important procedure. Male patients and patients with previous radiation therapy to the head and neck have an increased likelihood of malignant disease in their nodules. Often, needle biopsy and scanning are sufficient for the diagnosis, but occasionally excisional biopsy is needed. Papillary carcinoma accounts for more than 70% of all thyroid carcinomas. Simple excision of lymph node metastases appears to be as efficacious as radical neck procedures for the patient's survival. Follicular carcinoma, which accounts for approximately 15% of thyroid carcinomas, is more aggressive, and has a less favorable prognosis.

Medullary carcinoma, the most aggressive form of thyroid carcinoma, is associated with a familial occurrence of pheochromocytoma, as are parathyroid adenomas. For this reason, a history should be obtained from patients with a surgical scar in the thyroid region so that the possibility of occult pheochromocytoma can be assessed and excluded.

DISORDERS OF CALCIUM METABOLISM

The three substances that regulate serum concentrations of calcium, phosphorus, and magnesium are parathyroid hormone (parathyrin, PTH), calcitonin, and vitamin D, which act on bone, kidney, gut, and their own receptors. Calcium excess in blood is caused by either malignant disease or hyperparathyroidism in more than 90% of patients.[86] PTH stimulates bone resorption, inhibits renal excretion of calcium, and increases conversion to active vitamin D, three conditions that lead to hypercalcemia. Calcitonin can be considered an antagonist to PTH. Through its metabolites, vitamin D aids in the absorption of calcium, phosphate, and magnesium from the gut and facilitates the bone resorptive effects of PTH. Secretion of PTH is modulated through the calcium-sensing receptor on the cell surface of parathyroid cells. An increase in ionized calcium stimulates this receptor and thus causes a decrease in PTH secretion. Recognition of this effect has led to reevaluation of the therapy for hyperparathyroidism inasmuch as a drug upregulating this receptor's sensitivity reduces PTH levels.[87]

Hyperparathyroidism and Hypercalcemia

Primary hyperparathyroidism occurs in approximately 0.1% of the population, most commonly begins in the third to fifth decades of life, and occurs two to three times more frequently in women than in men. Primary hyperparathyroidism usually results from enlargement of a single gland, commonly an adenoma and very rarely a carcinoma. Hypercalcemia almost always develops.

Calcium is the chief mineral component of the body; it provides structure to the skeleton and performs key roles in neural transmission, intracellular signaling, blood coagulation, and neuromuscular functioning. Ninety-nine percent of the 1000 g of calcium present in the average human body is stored in the bone mineral reservoir. Fifty percent to 60% is bound to plasma proteins or is complexed with phosphate or citrate. The normal total serum calcium level is 8.6 to 10.4 mg/dL, as measured in most laboratories; though this value depends on the albumin level, noting a decline of 0.8 mg/dL for each 1 g/dL drop in albumin. Binding of calcium to albumin depends on pH: binding decreases with acidic pH and increases with alkaline pH. Serum calcium, not ionized calcium, decreases with reductions in albumin levels. Although ionized calcium is the clinically significant fraction, the cost and technical difficulties of stabilizing the electrodes used for measurement have limited the available assays. Nevertheless, PTH and vitamin D_3 work to keep the level stable within 0.1 mg/dL in any individual.

Many of the prominent symptoms of hyperparathyroidism are a result of the hypercalcemia that accompanies it. Regardless of the cause, hypercalcemia can produce any of a number of symptoms, the most prominent of which involve the renal, skeletal, neuromuscular, and GI system, including anorexia, vomiting, constipation, polyuria, polydipsia, lethargy, confusion, renal calculi, pancreatitis, bone pain, and psychiatric abnormalities. Free intracellular calcium initiates or regulates muscle contraction, release of neurotransmitters, secretion of hormones, enzyme action, and energy metabolism.

Nephrolithiasis occurs in 60% to 70% of patients with hyperparathyroidism. Sustained hypercalcemia can result in tubular and glomerular disorders, including proximal (type II) renal tubular acidosis. Polyuria and polydipsia are common complaints.

Skeletal disorders related to hyperparathyroidism are osteitis fibrosa cystica, simple diffuse osteopenia, and osteoporosis. The rate of bone turnover is five times higher in patients with hyperparathyroidism than in normal controls. Patients may have a history of frequent fractures or may complain of bone pain, especially in the anterior margin of the tibia.

Because free intracellular calcium initiates or regulates muscle contraction, neurotransmitter signaling, hormone secretion, enzyme action, and energy metabolism, abnormalities in these end organs are often symptoms of hyperparathyroidism. Patients may experience profound muscle weakness, especially in proximal muscle groups, as well as muscle atrophy. Depression, psychomotor retardation, and memory impairment may occur. Lethargy and confusion are frequent complaints.

Peptic ulcer disease is more common in these patients than in the rest of the population. Production of gastrin and gastric acid is increased. Anorexia, vomiting, and constipation may also be present.

Approximately one third of all hypercalcemic patients are hypertensive, but the hypertension usually resolves with successful treatment of the primary disease. Neither hypertension nor minimally invasive surgery seems to alter the perioperative risk associated with surgery in such patients in comparison with the usual hypertensive patients.[88,89] Even octogenarians with asymptomatic hyperparathyroidism can be operated on without mortality and with morbidity no different from that in younger individuals, thus encouraging the use of parathyroidectomy as preventive therapy.[90] Long-standing hypercalcemia can lead to calcifications in the myocardium, blood vessels, brain, and kidneys. Cerebral calcifications may cause seizures, whereas renal calcifications lead to polyuria that is unresponsive to vasopressin.[90]

The most useful confirmatory test for hyperparathyroidism is radioimmunoassay for PTH. In fact, two changes have radically reduced anesthesia involvement in the care of patients with primary hyperparathyroidism. One change, the use of the calcimimetic drug class which modulates the calcium-sensitive PTH cell receptor and thereby decreases calcium levels, has been emphasized in older individuals. The other change is use of minimally invasive approaches after imaging procedures with just local anesthesia or a cervical plexus block—as with thyroidectomy.[91,92] Most surgeons now performing minimally invasive parathyroid removal monitor PTH levels intraoperatively to determine whether the causative adenoma has been resected. The baseline PTH level should be determined before induction of anesthesia because even monitored anesthesia care increases PTH levels.[93] In hyperparathyroid patients, hormone levels are abnormal for a given level of calcium. The level of inorganic phosphorus in serum is usually low, but it may be within normal limits. Alkaline phosphatase levels are elevated if considerable skeletal involvement is present.

Glucocorticoid administration reduces the level of calcium in blood in many other conditions that cause hypercalcemia, but not usually in primary hyperparathyroidism. In sarcoidosis, multiple myeloma, vitamin D intoxication, and some malignant diseases, all of which can cause hypercalcemia, administration of glucocorticoids may lower serum calcium levels through an effect on GI absorption. This effect occurs to a lesser degree in primary hyperparathyroidism.

Hypercalcemia may also occur as a consequence of secondary hyperparathyroidism in patients who have chronic renal disease. When phosphate excretion decreases as a result of decreased nephron mass, serum calcium levels fall because of deposition of calcium and phosphate in bone. Secretion of PTH subsequently increases, and this causes the fraction of phosphate excreted by each nephron to increase. Eventually, the chronic intermittent hypocalcemia of chronic renal failure leads to chronically high levels of serum PTH and hyperplasia of the parathyroid glands—one of the entities termed secondary hyperparathyroidism.

Symptomatic primary hyperparathyroidism in patients younger than 50 years or with serum calcium levels more than 1 mg/dL higher than the upper limit of normal, a 30% or greater reduction in the glomerular filtration rate (GFR), or severe bone demineralization is usually treated surgically. If the patient refuses surgery or if other illnesses render surgery inadvisable, medical management with the calcimimetic, cinacalcet, makes management much more feasible. The difficulty with such management is that the hyperfunctioning parathyroid glands secrete more hormone as the serum calcium concentration is lowered—as

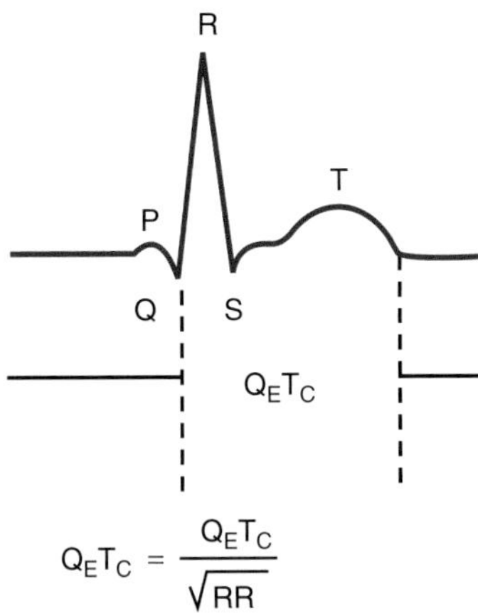

Fig. 32.3 Measurement of the QTc interval (properly termed Q_ET_C to indicate that it begins with the start of the Q wave, lasts throughout the QT interval, ends with the end of the T wave, and is corrected for heart rate). RR is the RR interval in seconds. (From Hensel P, Roizen MF. Patients with disorders of parathyroid function. *Anesthesiol Clin North Am.* 1987;5:287–291.)

though the calcium set point for feedback regulation of PTH secretion had been raised. Blanchard and colleagues demonstrated that patients with "asymptomatic" primary hyperparathyroidism have clinical improvement of their symptoms postoperatively even after 1 year, noting younger patients and those with higher preoperative calcium levels show the best improvement.[94]

Patients with moderate hypercalcemia who have normal renal and cardiovascular function present no special preoperative and preprocedure problems. The ECG can be examined preoperatively and intraoperatively for shortened PR or QT intervals (Fig. 32.3). Because severe hypercalcemia can result in substantial hypovolemia, normal intravascular volume and electrolyte status should be evaluated and then restored before anesthesia and surgery.

Management of hypercalcemia preoperatively should include (even in urgent or emergency situations) treatment of the underlying cause, a frequent strategy in surgical patients with malignancy-associated hypercalcemia. Therapy preoperatively for both malignant and nonmalignant causes of hypercalcemia include aggressive volume repletion, with the addition of diuresis only if volume overload develops. Intravenous fluid infusion rates of 250 to 500 mL/h preoperatively are commonly used to maintain urine output greater than 200 mL/h.[94a] Careful monitoring during this time is needed to avoid administration of an excessive amount of intravenous fluids, as many patients may have compromised cardiac function. In the setting of fluid overload, diuresis with furosemide can be warranted; however, evidence for benefit is limited and mainly theoreteical.[94a] Other complications of these interventions include hypomagnesemia and hypokalemia.

In emergency situations, vigorous expansion of intravascular volume usually reduces serum calcium to a safe level (<14 mg/dL). Phosphate should be given to correct hypophosphatemia because it decreases calcium uptake into bone, increases calcium excretion, and stimulates breakdown of bone. Hydration, accompanied by electrolyte repletion mainly phosphate, suffices in the management of most hypercalcemic patients. Other measures to decrease reabsorption of bone include the bisphosphonates pamidronate sodium (90 mg intravenously) and zoledronate (4 mg intravenously). Case reports note success in the setting of extreme hypercalcemia (>20 mg/dL) correction with a low calcium bath dialysate.[94b]

Calcitonin lowers serum calcium levels through direct inhibition of bone resorption. It can decrease serum calcium levels within minutes after intravenous administration. Side effects include urticaria and nausea. It is so rapid acting that it can be used to reduce calcium levels while waiting for hydration and a bisphosphonate to take effect.

It is especially important to know whether the hypercalcemia has been chronic because serious cardiac, renal, or CNS abnormalities may have resulted.

Hypocalcemia

Hypocalcemia (caused by hypoalbuminemia, hypoparathyroidism, hypomagnesemia, hypovitaminosis D, hungry bone syndrome after correction of hyperparathyroidism, anticonvulsant therapy, citrate infusion, or chronic renal disease) is not usually accompanied by a clinically evident cardiovascular disorder. The most common cause of hypocalcemia is hypoalbuminemia. In true hypocalcemia (i.e., when the free calcium concentration is low), myocardial contractility is affected, noting myocardial contractility varies directly with levels of blood ionized calcium. The clinical signs of hypocalcemia include clumsiness; convulsions; laryngeal stridor; depression; muscle stiffness; paresthesias; parkinsonism; tetany; Chvostek sign; dry and scaly skin, brittle nails, and coarse hair; low serum concentrations of calcium; prolonged QT intervals; soft tissue calcifications; and Trousseau sign.

Hypocalcemia delays ventricular repolarization, hence increasing the QTc interval (normal, 0.35-0.44 second). With electrical systole prolonged, the ventricles may fail to respond to the next electrical impulse from the sinoatrial node, with second-degree heart block resulting. Prolongation of the QT interval is a moderately reliable ECG sign of hypocalcemia, not for the population as a whole, but for the individual patient.[95] Thus monitoring the QT interval as corrected for the heart rate is a useful, but not always accurate means of monitoring hypocalcemia in any individual patient (see Fig. 32.3). Heart failure may also occur with hypocalcemia, but is rare. Because heart failure in patients with coexisting heart disease is reduced in severity when calcium and magnesium ion levels are restored to normal, these levels may be normalized preoperatively in a patient with impaired exercise tolerance or signs of cardiovascular dysfunction; normalization can be achieved intravenously over a 15-minute period if absolutely necessary. Sudden decreases in blood levels of ionized calcium (as with chelation therapy) can result in severe hypotension.

Patients with hypocalcemia may have seizures. They may be focal, petit mal, or grand mal in appearance, often indistinguishable from such seizures in the absence of hypocalcemia. Patients may also have a type of seizure called cerebral tetany, which consists of generalized tetany followed by tonic spasms. Therapy with standard anticonvulsants is ineffective and may even exacerbate these seizures (by an anti–vitamin D effect), calcium must be repleted for treatment. In long-standing hypoparathyroidism, calcifications may appear above the sella; these calcifications represent deposits of calcium in and around small blood vessels of the basal ganglia. They may be associated with a variety of extrapyramidal syndromes.

The most common cause of acquired hypoparathyroidism is surgery of the thyroid or parathyroid glands. Other causes include autoimmune disorders, therapy with iodine-131, hemosiderosis or hemochromatosis, neoplasia, and granulomatous disease. Idiopathic hypoparathyroidism has been divided into three categories: an isolated persistent neonatal form, branchial dysembryogenesis, and autoimmune candidiasis related to multiple endocrine deficiency.

Pseudohypoparathyroidism and pseudopseudohypoparathyroidism are rare hereditary disorders characterized by short stature, obesity, rounded face, and shortened metacarpals. Patients with pseudohypoparathyroidism have hypocalcemia and hyperphosphatemia despite high serum levels of PTH. These patients have a deficient end-organ response to PTH as a result of abnormalities in G-protein function.

Because treatment of hypoparathyroidism is not surgical, hypoparathyroid patients who come to the operating room are those who require surgery for unrelated conditions. Their calcium, phosphate, and magnesium levels should be measured both preoperatively and postoperatively. Patients with symptomatic hypocalcemia may be treated with intravenous calcium gluconate preoperatively. Initially, 10 to 20 mL of 10% calcium gluconate may be given at a rate of 5 mL/min. The effect on serum calcium levels is of short duration, but a continuous infusion with 10 mL/min of 10% calcium gluconate in 500 mL of solution over a period of 6 hours helps keep serum calcium at adequate levels. For severe symptoms in emergent settings, 10 mL of 10% calcium chloride may be given over 10 minutes, followed by a 10% calcium gluconate infusion. Magnesium and phosphate levels may also require normalization to normalize cardiovascular and nervous system function.

The objective of therapy is to bring the symptoms under control before the surgical procedure and anesthesia. For patients with chronic hypoparathyroidism, the objective is to keep the serum calcium level in the lower half of the normal range. A preoperative and preprocedure ECG is useful for maintaining the QTc interval. The preoperative and preprocedure QTc value may be used as a guide to the serum calcium level if rapid laboratory assessment is not possible. Changes in the calcium level may alter the duration of muscle relaxation; thus careful monitoring and titration of muscle relaxation with a twitch monitor is necessary.

The intimate involvement of the parathyroid gland with the thyroid gland can result in unintentional hypocalcemia during surgery for diseases of either organ. Because of the affinity of their bones for calcium, this relationship is crucial in patients with advanced osteitis. Internal redistribution of magnesium, calcium, or both ions may occur (into "hungry bones") after parathyroidectomy and may cause hypomagnesemia, hypocalcemia, or both. Because the tendency to tetany increases with alkalosis, hyperventilation should be avoided. The most prominent manifestations of acute hypocalcemia are distal paresthesias and muscle spasm (tetany). Potentially fatal complications of severe hypocalcemia include laryngeal spasm and hypocalcemic seizures. The clinical sequelae of magnesium deficiency include cardiac arrhythmias (principally ventricular tachyarrhythmias), hypocalcemic tetany, and neuromuscular irritability independent of hypocalcemia (tremors, twitching, asterixis, and seizures).

In addition to monitoring total serum calcium or ionized calcium postoperatively, one can test for the Chvostek and Trousseau signs. The Chvostek sign is a contracture of the facial muscles produced by tapping the ipsilateral facial nerve at the angle of the jaw, of note this sign can be elicited in up to 15% of patients who are not hypocalcemic, an attempt should be made to elicit this sign preoperatively to ensure that its appearance is meaningful. The Trousseau sign is elicited by applying a blood pressure cuff at a level slightly above the systolic level for a few minutes. The resulting carpopedal spasm, with contraction of the fingers and inability to open the hand, stems from the increased muscle irritability in hypocalcemic states, aggravated by ischemia produced by the blood pressure cuff.

Osteoporosis

Fifty percent of women who are older than 65 years sustain an osteoporotic fracture. (Because men are living longer, osteoporosis has become an increasing problem for them, too, and reports indicate a 15% per decade hip fracture rate for men >65 years old.)[95] Men with COPD (even without steroid treatment) are at high risk for vertebral fractures. Furthermore, in either gender, each vertebral fracture is associated with up to a 10% decrease in lung capacity. Diagnosis and treatment of these conditions have increased with routine use of dual-energy x-ray absorptiometry or quantitative ultrasonography. Because T-scores and Z-scores were developed to relate changes in white postmenopausal women to those at age 21 years, care must be used in interpreting the results. Known risk factors for osteoporosis include age, relative lifetime estrogen deficiency (late menarche, amenorrhea, early menopause, nulliparity), deficiency of dietary calcium, tobacco use, increased aerobic exercise in combination with decreased weight-bearing exercise, decreased weight-bearing exercise by itself, use of soft drinks, and Asian or white ancestry. Although therapy for osteoporosis (use of biphosphates, bone mineral depositors, weight-bearing exercises, calcium, vitamin D, estrogen, and now designer estrogens that may be useful for men, such as raloxifene [Evista]) does not have major known implications for anesthesia care.[96-98] Bone fractures in such patients have occurred on movement to and from an operating table, therefore these patients should be allowed to move and position themselves when possible. Recombinant PTH and calcitonin are also used, but again, no reports of perioperative interactions have been prominent.

PITUITARY ABNORMALITIES

Anterior Pituitary Hypersecretion

The anterior pituitary gland (or master endocrine gland) consists of five identifiable types of secretory cells and hormones produced: somatotrophs (GH), corticotrophs (ACTH), lactotrophs (prolactin), gonadotrophs (luteinizing hormone and follicle-stimulating hormone), and thyrotrophs (TSH). Secretion of these pituitary hormones is largely regulated by a negative-feedback loop by hypothalamic regulatory hormones and by signals that originate from the target site of pituitary action. Six hypothalamic hormones have been characterized: dopamine, the prolactin-inhibiting hormone; somatostatin, the GH release–inhibiting hormone; GH-releasing hormone; corticotropin-releasing hormone; gonadotropin-releasing hormone; and TRH. Most pituitary tumors (>60%) are hypersecretory and are classified according to the excess production of a specific anterior pituitary hormone.

The most common disorders of pituitary hypersecretion are those related to excesses of prolactin (amenorrhea, galactorrhea, and infertility), ACTH (Cushing syndrome), and GH (acromegaly). In addition to knowing the pathophysiologic processes of the disease involved, the anesthesiologist must determine whether the patient recently underwent air pneumoencephalography (almost obsolete, but still used rarely). If so, nitrous oxide should not be used to lessen the risk of intracranial hypertension from gas collection. CT or MRI of the sella has largely replaced neuroencephalography.

More than 99% of cases of acromegaly are attributable to pituitary adenoma (or use of recombinant human GH). Thus the primary treatment of acromegaly is transsphenoidal surgery (or withdrawal of drug) and symptomatic treatment of the carpal tunnel or other syndromes provoked. If the pituitary tumor is not totally removed, patients are often offered external pituitary irradiation. In the case of suprasellar extension, conventional transfrontal hypophysectomy is often performed. The dopaminergic agonist bromocriptine can lower GH levels, but the long-term follow-up with this drug is not favorable. Octreotide, a long-acting analogue of somatostatin, now given in depot form approximately once a month, produces effective palliation in 50% of patients. Other medical therapies such as pegvisomant or somatostatin analogues are also medications that have been tried before surgical intervention. In 2011, new guidelines were published with few changes to the available recommendations.[99] However, the new guidelines reported some evidence that medication taken preoperatively may result in a better postoperative outcome.

Difficulty with endotracheal intubation should be anticipated in a patient with acromegaly; lateral neck radiographs or CT scans of the neck and direct or indirect visualization can identify patients with subglottic stenosis or an enlarged tongue, mandible, epiglottis, or vocal cords. If placement of an arterial line is necessary, a brachial or femoral site may be preferable to a radial site.[100]

Anterior Pituitary Hypofunction

Anterior pituitary hypofunction results in deficiency of one or more of the following hormones: GH, TSH, ACTH, prolactin, or gonadotropin. No special preoperative and preprocedure preparation is required for a patient deficient in prolactin or gonadotropin; deficiency in GH, however, can result in atrophy of cardiac muscle, a condition that may necessitate preoperative and preprocedure cardiac evaluation. Nonetheless, anesthetic problems have not been documented in patients with isolated GH deficiency. Acute deficiencies are another matter.

Acute pituitary deficiency is often caused by bleeding into a pituitary tumor. In surgical specimens of resected adenomas, as many as 25% show evidence of hemorrhage. These patients often have acute headache, visual loss, nausea or vomiting, ocular palsy, disturbances of consciousness, fever, vertigo, or hemiparesis. In such patients, rapid transsphenoidal decompression should be accompanied by consideration of replacement therapy, including glucocorticoids and the treatment of increased intracranial pressure.

Obstetric anesthesiologists are often aware of these pituitary failure problems; Sheehan syndrome is the clinical manifestation of pituitary infarction associated with hypotension during or after obstetric hemorrhage. Conditions that strongly suggest this diagnosis are failure to start postpartum lactation, increasing fatigue, cold intolerance, and especially hypotension unresponsive to volume replacement and pressors; treatment is prompt hormone therapy.[100a]

Posterior Pituitary Hormone Excess and Deficiency

Secretion of vasopressin or antidiuretic hormone (ADH) is enhanced by increased serum osmolality or the presence of hypotension. Inappropriate secretion of vasopressin, without relation to serum osmolality, results in hyponatremia and fluid retention. This inappropriate secretion can result from the following: a variety of CNS lesions; drugs including nicotine, narcotics, tramadol, chlorpropamide, clofibrate, vincristine, vinblastine, and cyclophosphamide; and pulmonary infections, hypothyroidism, adrenal insufficiency, and ectopic production from tumors. Preoperative and preprocedure management of a surgical patient with inappropriate secretion of vasopressin includes appropriate treatment of the causative disorders and restriction of water. Occasionally, drugs that inhibit the renal response to ADH (e.g., lithium or demeclocycline) should be administered preoperatively to restore normal intravascular volume and electrolyte status.

Most of the clinical features associated with the syndrome of inappropriate secretion of antidiuretic hormone (SIADH) are related to hyponatremia and the resulting brain edema; such features include weight gain, weakness, lethargy, mental confusion, obtundation, and disordered reflexes and may culminate in convulsions and coma.

Investigators have recognized that up to 20% of long-distance runners have SIADH with increased vasopressin secretion. Because such people infrequently undergo surgical treatment of injuries, SIADH symptoms and laboratory evaluation may be routine for that group as well.

SIADH should be suspected in any patient with hyponatremia who excretes urine that is hypertonic relative to plasma. The following laboratory findings further support the diagnosis:

1. Urinary sodium greater than 20 mEq/L
2. Low serum levels of BUN, creatinine, uric acid, and albumin
3. Serum sodium lower than 130 mEq/L
4. Plasma osmolality lower than 270 mOsm/L
5. Urine hypertonic relative to plasma

Noting the response to water loading is a useful way of evaluating patients with hyponatremia. Patients with SIADH are unable to excrete dilute urine even after water loading. Assay of ADH in blood can confirm the diagnosis. Too vigorous treatment of chronic hyponatremia can result in disabling osmotic demyelination syndrome.[101,102] The increase in serum sodium should not be greater than 1 mEq/L/h.[101,102]

Patients with mild to moderate symptoms of water intoxication can be treated with restriction of fluid intake to approximately 500 to 1000 mL/day. Patients with severe water intoxication and CNS symptoms may need vigorous treatment consisting of intravenous administration of hypertonic saline solutions until symptoms resolve, followed by fluid restriction.

Treatment should be directed at the underlying problem. If SIADH is drug induced, use of the drug should be withdrawn. Inflammation should be treated with appropriate measures, and neoplasms should be managed by surgical resection, irradiation, or chemotherapy, whichever is indicated.

No drugs are available that can suppress release of ADH from the neurohypophysis or from a tumor. Phenytoin (Dilantin) and narcotic antagonists such as naloxone and butorphanol have some inhibiting effect on physiologic ADH release but are clinically ineffective in patients with SIADH. Drugs that block the effect of ADH on renal tubules include lithium, which is rarely used because its toxicity often outweighs its benefits, and demethylchlortetracycline in doses of 900 to 1200 mg/day. Demethylchlortetracycline interferes with the ability of the renal tubules to concentrate urine, thereby causing excretion of isotonic or hypotonic urine and lessening the hyponatremia. This drug can be used in ambulatory patients with SIADH when it is difficult to restrict fluids.

When a patient with SIADH comes to the operating room for any surgical procedure, fluids are managed by measuring volume status, when the clinical picture is unclear the use of arterial wave form analysis, central venous pressure, pulmonary artery pressure, or transthoracic and/or transesophageal echocardiography may be of value. Despite the common impression that SIADH is frequently seen in older patients in the postoperative period, studies have shown that the patient's age and the type of anesthetic used have no bearing on the postoperative development of SIADH. It is common to see several patients in the neurosurgical ICU suffering from this syndrome. The diagnosis is usually one of exclusion. Patients with SIADH generally require only restriction of intravenous fluids, very rarely is hypertonic saline needed.

Lack of ADH, which results in diabetes insipidus, is caused by pituitary disease, brain tumors, infiltrative diseases such as sarcoidosis, head trauma (including trauma after neurosurgery), or lack of a renal response to ADH. The last can result from such diverse conditions as hypokalemia, hypercalcemia, sickle cell anemia, obstructive uropathy, and renal insufficiency. Preoperative or preprocedure treatment of diabetes insipidus consists of restoring normal intravascular volume by replacing urinary losses, administering desmopressin acetate (DDAVP) nasally, and giving daily fluid requirements intravenously.

Perioperative management of patients with diabetes insipidus is based on the extent of the ADH deficiency. Management of a patient with complete diabetes insipidus and a total lack of ADH does not usually present any major problem as long as the side effects of the drug are avoided and the presence of the condition is known preoperatively. Just before the surgical procedure, the patient is given the usual dose of DDAVP intranasally or an intravenous bolus of 100 milliunits of aqueous vasopressin, followed by a constant infusion of 100 to 200 milliunits/h.[1] The dose is usually adjusted to permit the daily breakthrough polyuria that prevents the iatrogenic syndrome of SIADH. All the intravenous fluids given intraoperatively should be isotonic to reduce the risk of water depletion and hypernatremia. Plasma osmolality should be frequently measured, both intraoperatively and immediately postoperatively. If plasma osmolality rises much higher than 300 mOsm/L, hypotonic fluids can be administered; the rate of the intraoperative vasopressin infusion can be increased to greater than 200 milliunits/h.

For patients who have a partial deficiency of ADH, it is not necessary to use aqueous vasopressin perioperatively unless plasma osmolality rises to more than 300 mOsm/L. Nonosmotic stimuli (e.g., volume depletion) and the stress of surgery usually cause the release of large quantities of ADH perioperatively. Consequently, these patients require only frequent monitoring of plasma osmolality during this period.

Because of side effects, the dose of vasopressin should be limited to that necessary for control of diuresis. The oxytocic and coronary artery–constricting properties of vasopressin make this limit especially applicable to patients who are pregnant or have CAD.

Diseases Involving the Cardiovascular System

HYPERTENSION

Analysis of the perioperative treatment of hypertension is important because of the prevalence of the condition (33.5% of adults aged 20 and over in the United States), the great risk in perioperative care of a hypertensive patient, and the high cost of unnecessary delays in surgical treatment. Numerous studies over the years have evaluated the impact of hypertension as one of the risk factors for cardiac morbidity. However, the need to delay surgery because of poorly controlled hypertension has been questioned. Weksler and colleagues studied 989 hypertensive patients who were treated on a long-term basis and who underwent noncardiac surgery with diastolic blood pressure between 110 and 130 mm Hg and no previous MI, unstable or severe angina pectoris, renal failure, pregnancy-induced hypertension, left ventricular hypertrophy, previous coronary revascularization, aortic stenosis, preoperative dysrhythmias, conduction defects, or stroke.[103] The control group had their surgical procedures postponed and remained in the hospital for control of blood pressure, and the study patients received 10 mg of nifedipine intranasally. No statistically significant differences in postoperative complications were observed, thus suggesting that this subset of patients without significant cardiovascular comorbid conditions can proceed with surgery despite elevated blood pressure on the day of the operation.

Several studies have assessed the relationship between cardiovascular disease and preoperative hypertension. In a multicenter study of patients undergoing coronary artery bypass graft (CABG), the presence of isolated systolic hypertension was associated with a 30% increased incidence of perioperative cardiovascular complications when compared with normotensive individuals.[104] Kheterpal and colleagues integrated data from their anesthesia information system (AIMS) and the American College of Surgeons National Surgical Quality Improvement Project (NSQIP) and found hypertension to be one of the independent predictors of events.[105] Wax and colleagues used AIMS to identify independent predictors of troponin elevation or death, and independent predictors of adverse outcome included increased baseline systolic blood pressure (SBP), intraoperative diastolic blood pressure lower than 85 mm Hg, increased intraoperative heart rate, blood transfusion, and anesthetic technique, controlling for standard risk factors.[106] A delay of surgery did not result in interval normalization of blood pressure.

Although preoperative blood pressure (both systolic and diastolic) is a significant predictor of postoperative morbidity, no data definitively establish whether preoperative treatment of hypertension reduces perioperative risk. Until a definitive study is performed, we recommend letting the weight of evidence guide preoperative treatment of a patient with hypertension. Such treatment would be based on three general beliefs: (1) the patient should be educated regarding the importance of lifelong treatment of hypertension, even isolated systolic hypertension; (2) perioperative hemodynamic fluctuations occur less frequently in treated than in untreated hypertensive patients (as demonstrated by Prys-Roberts and colleagues[107] and confirmed by Goldman and Caldera[108] and Mangano and associates[109]); and (3) hemodynamic fluctuations have some relation to morbidity. Kheterpal and colleagues demonstrated that patients who sustained a cardiac adverse event were more likely to experience an episode of mean arterial pressure lower than 50 mm Hg, an episode of 40% decrease in mean arterial pressure, and an episode of heart rate higher than 100 beats/min.[105] The data of Pasternack and colleagues and Weksler and associates imply that rapid correction of blood pressure or prevention of increases in heart rate may be all that is needed.[103,110] Sessler and colleagues (2018) studied 9765 patients in the POISE-II trial to assess the relationship between perioperative hypotension and a composite of MI and death within 30-days of surgery.[110aa] Intraoperatively, the estimated average relative effect was 1.08 (98.3% confidence interval [CI], 1.03, 1.12; $P < .001$) per 10-minute increase in hypotension duration. The average relative effect odds ratio was 2.83 (98.3% CI, 1.26, 6.35; $P = .002$) in patients with hypotension during the subsequent 4 days of hospitalization. The Intraoperative Norepinephrine to Control Arterial Pressure (INPRESS) study was a multicenter, randomized, parallel-group clinical trial in adult patients ($n = 298$) at increased risk of postoperative complications of individualized management strategy aimed at achieving a SBP within 10% of the reference value (i.e., patient's resting SBP) or standard management strategy of treating SBP less than 80 mm Hg or lower than 40% from the reference value during and for 4 hours following surgery.[110a] Management targeting an individualized SBP, compared with standard management, reduced the risk of postoperative organ dysfunction. Taken together, these data suggest that maintenance of normal blood pressure is critical in patients with hypertension.

The INPRESS study demonstrated that preoperative data should be used to determine the individualized range of suitable arterial blood pressure values that are tolerable by a particular patient during and after a surgical procedure. Importantly, hypotension in patients at risk for a cerebrovascular event should be avoided. For example, the POISE (Perioperative Ischemic Evaluation) study demonstrated that short-term β-blocker administration resulted in an increased incidence of stroke and death that was associated with an increased rate of hypotension.[111]

Preoperative Administration of All Antihypertensive Drugs

Continuation of all antihypertensive drugs preoperatively should be considered, except ACE inhibitors or angiotensin II antagonists, for which no clear consensus exists. Coriat and colleagues found that ACE inhibitors were associated with hypotension in 100% of patients during induction versus approximately 20% in whom ACE inhibitors were withheld on the morning of the surgical procedure.[112] Bertrand and coworkers performed a prospective randomized study that demonstrated that more severe hypotensive episodes requiring vasoconstrictor treatment occurred after induction of general anesthesia in patients treated on a long-term basis with an angiotensin II antagonist and receiving the drug on the morning before the operation than in those in whom angiotensin II antagonists were discontinued on the day before the surgical procedure.[113] Kheterpal and colleagues performed a propensity-matched analysis of 12,381 noncardiac surgical cases.[114] Patients with long-term ACE inhibitor or angiotensin receptor blocker (ARB) and diuretic therapy showed more periods with a mean arterial blood pressure lower than 70 mm Hg, periods with a 40% decrease in SBP, periods with a 50% decrease in SBP, and vasopressor boluses than did patients receiving diuretic therapy alone. If these drugs are continued, vasopressin is the drug of choice for refractory hypotension. Investigators at the Cleveland Clinic evaluated 79,228 patients (9905 ACE inhibitor users [13%] and 66,620 [87%] non–ACE inhibitor users) who had noncardiac surgery between 2005 and 2009.[115] These investigators did not find any association between use of ACE inhibitors and intraoperative or postoperative upper airway complications. ACE inhibitor use was not associated with in-hospital complications or increased 30-day mortality. Investigators of the VISION trial studied the relationship between withholding ACE inhibitors/angiotensin II receptor blockers and a primary composite outcome of all-cause death, stroke, or myocardial injury after noncardiac surgery at 30 days. Withholding ACE inhibitors/angiotensin II receptor blockers before major noncardiac surgery was associated with a lower risk of death and postoperative vascular events (150/1245 [12.0%] vs. 459/3557 [12.9%]; adjusted relative risk, 0.82; 95% CI, 0.70-0.96). In an accompanying editorial, London suggested that the current study does provide strong impetus for a randomized trial but does not warrant changes in local practice until such a trial is completed.[116]

ISCHEMIC HEART DISEASE

Preoperative evaluation of a patient with ischemic heart disease and a discussion of the AHA/ACC guidelines can be found in Chapters 31 and 54.[117] New guidelines were published in 2014 by both the AHA/ACC and the European

Society of Cardiology as well as the Canadian Cardiovascular Society in 2017.[118] This chapter will focus on the AHA/ACC guideline approach.[119,120]

Role of Coronary Artery Bypass Graft or Percutaneous Coronary Interventions Before Noncardiac Surgical Procedures

Coronary revascularization may reduce the perioperative risk before noncardiac surgery, but the evidence suggests that it is limited to those with indications similar to the nonsurgical arena. The strongest retrospective evidence comes from the Coronary Artery Surgery Study registry, which enrolled patients from 1978 to 1981. Operative mortality in patients with CABG performed before noncardiac surgery was 0.9% but was significantly higher at 2.4% in patients without previous CABG. However, a 1.4% mortality rate was associated with the CABG procedure itself.

The benefit of percutaneous coronary intervention (PCI) before noncardiac surgery has also been examined in several cohort studies. Posner and colleagues used an administrative dataset of patients who underwent PCI and noncardiac surgery in Washington State.[121] These investigators matched patients with coronary disease who were undergoing noncardiac surgery with and without previous PCI and looked at cardiac complications. In this nonrandomized design, Posner and colleagues noted a significantly lower rate of 30-day cardiac complications in patients who underwent PCI at least 90 days before the noncardiac surgery. However, PCI within 90 days of noncardiac surgery did not improve outcome. Although the explanation for these results is unknown, they may support the notion that PCI performed "to get the patient through surgery" may not improve perioperative outcome because cardiac complications may not occur in patients with stable or asymptomatic coronary stenosis. PCI may actually destabilize coronary plaque, which becomes manifest in the days or weeks after noncardiac surgery.

Godet and associates studied a cohort of 1152 patients after abdominal aortic surgery in which 78 patients underwent PCI.[122] In the PCI group, the observed percentages of patients with a severe postoperative coronary event (9.0%; 95% CI, 4.4-17.4) or death (5.1% [95% CI, 2.0-12.5]) were not significantly different from the expected percentages (8.2% and 6.9%, respectively), which was confirmed by propensity analysis. PCI did not seem to significantly limit cardiac risk or death after aortic surgery.

Several randomized trials have addressed the value of testing and CABG or PCI, or both, in a subset of patients. McFalls and colleagues reported the results of a multicenter randomized trial in the VA Health System in which patients with documented CAD on coronary angiography, excluding those with left main CAD or a severely depressed ejection fraction (<20%), were randomized to CABG (59%), or percutaneous transluminal coronary angioplasty (PTCA; 41%) versus routine medical therapy.[123] At 2.7 years after randomization, mortality in the revascularization group was not significantly different (22%) from that in the no-revascularization group (23%; Fig. 32.4). Within 30 days after the vascular operation, postoperative MI, defined by elevated troponin levels, occurred in 12% of the revascularization group and in 14% of the no-revascularization group (P = .37). The authors suggested that coronary revascularization is not indicated in patients with stable CAD, and their results further support the lack of efficacy of PCI or CABG for single- or double-vessel disease before noncardiac surgery. However, in a follow-up analysis, Ward and coauthors reported improved outcome in the subset of patients who underwent CABG versus PCI.[124]

Poldermans and colleagues randomized 770 patients about to undergo major vascular surgery and considered to have intermediate cardiac risk, defined as the presence of 1 or 2 cardiac risk factors, to either undergo further risk stratification with stress imaging or proceed directly to surgery.[125] All patients received bisoprolol with a targeted heart rate of 60 to 65 beats/min initiated before and continued after the surgical procedure. The 30-day incidence of cardiac death and nonfatal MI was similar in both groups (1.8% in the no-testing group vs. 2.3% in the tested group). The conclusions of the authors were that further risk stratification in this group of patients considered to be at intermediate risk based on clinical history alone was unnecessary as long as perioperative β-blockers were used and that testing only delayed necessary vascular surgery. In a pilot study, Poldermans and associates tested patients with more than three risk factors; 101 (23%) showed extensive ischemia and were randomly assigned to revascularization (n = 49) or no revascularization.[126] Revascularization did not improve 30-day outcome; the incidence of the composite end-point was 43% versus 33% (odds ratio [OR], 1.4; 95% CI, 0.7-2.8; P = .30). In addition, no benefit during 1-year follow-up was observed after coronary revascularization (49% vs. 44%; OR, 1.2; 95% CI, 0.7-2.3; P = .48). Concern was expressed by Erasmus University (Rotterdam, the Netherlands) regarding the scientific integrity of studies led by Poldermans, as detailed in Erasmus MC Follow-up Investigation Committee: *Report on the 2012 follow-up investigation of possible breaches of academic integrity, September 30, 2012* (https://www.forbes.com/sites/larryhusten/2012/10/09/erasmus-medical-center-releases-final-report-on-cardiovascular-research-scandal/#675d592528ae). The articles have

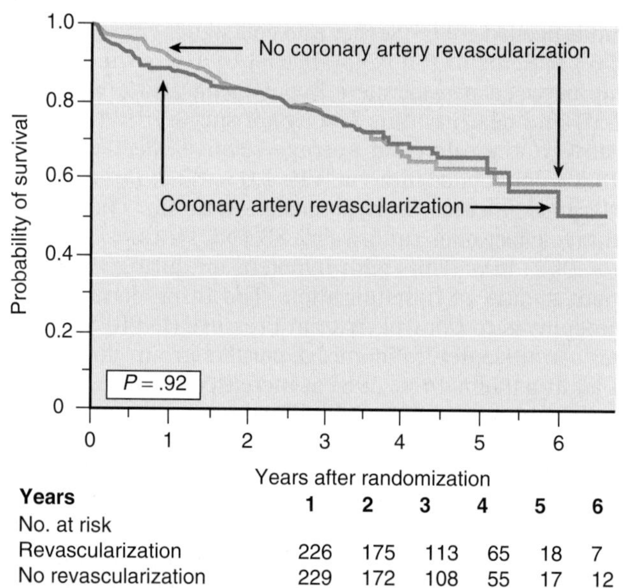

Years	1	2	3	4	5	6
No. at risk						
Revascularization	226	175	113	65	18	7
No revascularization	229	172	108	55	17	12

Fig. 32.4 Long-term survival in patients randomized to coronary revascularization or routine care in patients with coronary artery disease on angiography and undergoing major vascular surgical procedures in the Coronary Artery Revascularization Prophylaxis trial. (From McFalls EO, Ward HB, Moritz TE, et al. Coronary-artery revascularization before elective major vascular surgery. *N Engl J Med.* 2004;351:2795–2804.)

not been retracted, but these data should be viewed with some skepticism. The authors of the 2014 AHA/ACCF Guidelines decided that the nonretracted decrease publications and/or other derivative studies by Poldermans that are relevant to the topic can only be cited in the text with a comment about the finding compared with the current recommendation but did not form the basis of that recommendation.

One issue in interpreting the results is that the length of time between coronary revascularization and noncardiac surgery most likely has an impact on its protective effect and potential risks. Back and coworkers studied 425 consecutive patients undergoing 481 elective major vascular operations at an academic VA Medical Center.[127] Coronary revascularization was classified as recent (CABG < 1 year; PTCA < 6 months) in 35 cases (7%), prior (CABG >1 year and ≤5 years; PTCA >6 months and ≤2 years) in 45 cases (9%), and remote (CABG ≥ 5 years; PTCA ≥ 2 years) in 48 cases (10%). Outcomes in patients with previous PTCA were similar to those after CABG ($P = .7$). Significant differences in adverse cardiac events and mortality were found among patients with CABG performed within 5 years or PTCA within 2 years (6.3%, 1.3%, respectively), individuals with remote revascularization (10.4%, 6.3%), and nonrevascularized patients stratified at high risk (13.3%, 3.3%) or intermediate/low risk (2.8%, 0.9%). The authors concluded that previous coronary revascularization (CABG < 5 years; PTCA < 2 years) may provide only modest protection against adverse cardiac events and mortality after major arterial reconstruction.

PCI using coronary stenting poses several special issues. Kaluza and associates reported on the outcome of 40 patients who underwent prophylactic coronary stent placement less than 6 weeks before major noncardiac surgery requiring general anesthesia.[128] Among these patients, 7 MIs, 11 major bleeding episodes, and 8 deaths were noted. All deaths and MIs, as well as 8 of the 11 bleeding episodes, occurred in patients subjected to surgical procedures less than 14 days after stenting. Four patients died after undergoing surgical procedures 1 day after stenting. Wilson and colleagues reported on 207 patients who underwent noncardiac surgery within 2 months of stent placement.[129] Eight patients died or suffered an MI, all of whom were among the 168 patients who had surgical procedures 6 weeks after stent placement. Vicenzi and coworkers studied 103 patients and reported that the risk of suffering a perioperative cardiac event was 2.11-fold greater in patients with recent stents (<35 days before surgery) than in those who underwent PCI more than 90 days before surgical procedures.[130] Leibowitz and associates studied a total of 216 consecutive patients who underwent PCI within 3 months of noncardiac surgery (PTCA, 122; stent, 94).[131] A total of 26 patients (12%) died, 13 in the stent group (14%), and 13 in the PTCA group (11%), a nonsignificant difference. The incidence of acute MI and death within 6 months was not significantly different (7% and 14% in the stent group and 6% and 11% in the PTCA group, respectively). Significantly more events occurred in the two groups when noncardiac surgery was performed within 2 weeks of PCI. Based on the accumulating data, elective noncardiac surgery after PCI, with or without stent placement, should be delayed for 4 to 6 weeks.

Drug-eluting stents may represent an even greater problem during the perioperative period based on case reports. Nasser and coauthors described two patients with in-stent thrombosis occurring 4 and 21 months after the implantation of sirolimus-eluting stents.[132] Drug-eluting stents may represent an additional risk over a prolonged period (≤12 months), particularly if antiplatelet drugs are discontinued.[133] One study demonstrated that although the frequency of major noncardiac surgery in the year after drug-eluting stent placement was more than 4%, the overall risk of adverse outcomes was less than previously reported when surgical procedures were performed months after drug-eluting stent placement.[134] However, the risk was significantly increased in the week after major noncardiac surgery. A population-based study in Canada using administrative healthcare databases demonstrated that the earliest optimal time for elective surgery is 46 to 180 days after bare-metal stent implantation or more than 180 days after drug-eluting stent implantation.[135] Hawn and colleagues used a national, retrospective cohort study of 41,989 VA and non-VA operations occurring in the 24 months after coronary stent implantation between 2000 and 2010.[136] Among patients undergoing noncardiac surgery within 2 years of coronary stent placement, major adverse cardiac events were associated with emergency surgery and advanced cardiac disease but not stent type or timing of surgery beyond 6 months after stent implantation. The 2016 DAPT Guidelines (Fig. 32.5) suggest continuing aspirin therapy in all patients with a coronary stent and discontinuing clopidogrel for as short a time interval as possible for patients with bare-metal stents less than 30 days or drug-eluting stents less than 6 months; with DAPT it can be discontinued.[136a]

Based upon the non-perioperative literature, there is a suggestion that holding clopidogrel for the traditional 8 days may actually increase risk associated with a hypercoagulable rebound suggesting a shorter period of time may be optimal. A recent cohort study suggests that withdrawal of antiplatelet agents greater than 5 days is associated with increased major adverse cardiac events.[136b]

Perioperative Risk Factors for Cardiac Morbidity and Mortality

A thorough history should focus on cardiovascular risk factors and symptoms or signs of unstable cardiac disease states, such as myocardial ischemia with minimal exertion, active CHF, symptomatic valvular heart disease, and significant cardiac arrhythmias. The presence of unstable angina is associated with a 28% incidence of perioperative MI.[137] Such patients would benefit from delaying elective surgery to address their CAD. For those patients with chronic stable angina, exercise tolerance appears to be a good method of assessing perioperative risk.

In virtually all studies, the presence of active CHF has been associated with increased perioperative cardiac morbidity.[138] In addition, multiple studies have demonstrated that reduced ejection fraction is associated with an increased incidence of perioperative cardiac events.[139,140] Flu and colleagues performed echocardiography in patients undergoing vascular surgery and found that for open surgical procedures, asymptomatic systolic left ventricular dysfunction and asymptomatic diastolic left ventricular

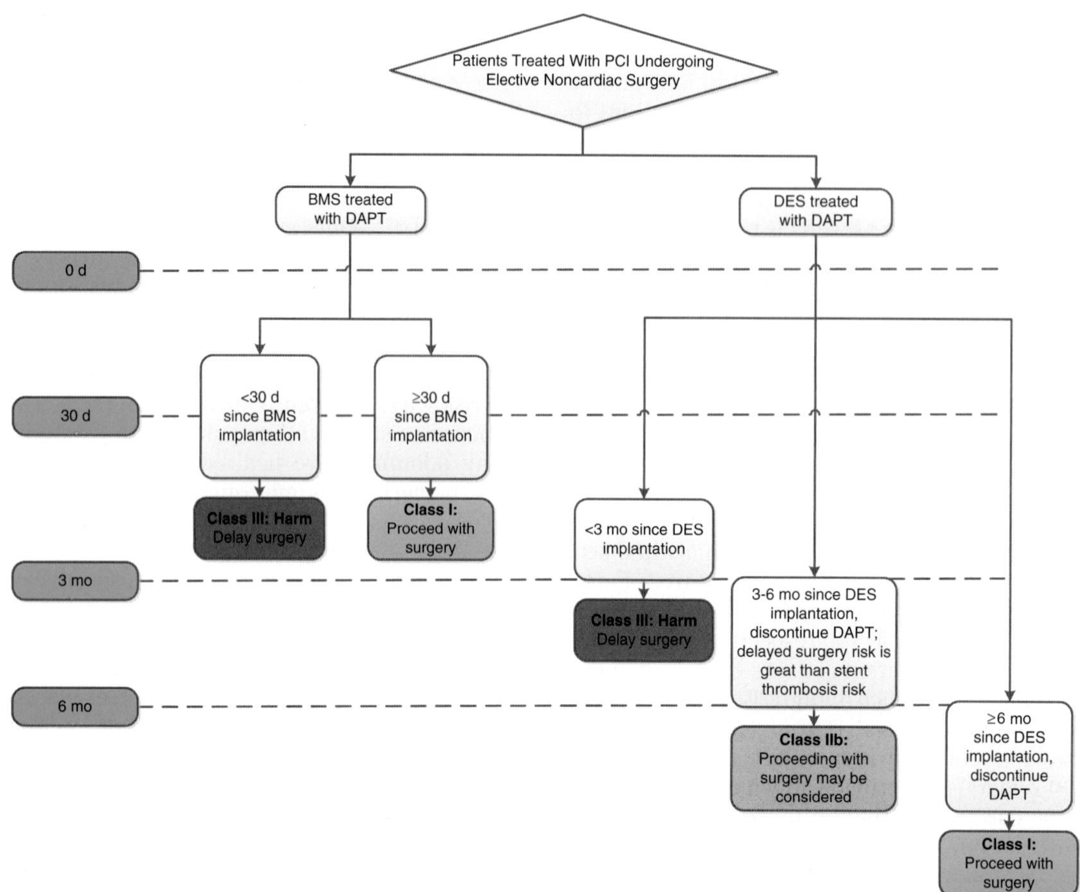

Fig. 32.5 Proposed algorithm for antiplatelet management in patients with percutaneous coronary intervention and noncardiac surgery. ***ASA,*** **Aspirin;** ***BMS,*** **bare metal stent;** ***DAPT,*** **dual antiplatelet therapy;** ***DES,*** **drug-eluting stent.** (From Fleisher LA, Fleischmann KE, Auerbach AD, et al. 2014 ACC/AHA guidelines on perioperative cardiovascular evaluation and management of patients undergoing noncardiac surgery: a report of the American College of Cardiology/American Heart Association Task Force on practice guidelines. *J Am Coll Cardiol.* 2014;64:e77–e137.)

dysfunction were both associated with increased 30-day cardiovascular event rates (OR, 2.3; 95% CI, 1.4-3.6; and OR, 1.8; 95% CI 1.1 to 2.9, respectively) and long-term cardiovascular mortality (hazard ratio, 4.6; 95% CI 2.4-8.5; and hazard ratio, 3.0; 95% CI 1.5 to 6.0, respectively).[141] In patients undergoing endovascular surgery (n = 356), only symptomatic heart failure was associated with an increase in 30-day cardiovascular events and long-term cardiovascular mortality. These results suggest that stabilization of ventricular function and treatment of pulmonary congestion is prudent before elective surgery.

A recent MI has traditionally been an important predictor of perioperative risk. The more recent the MI, particularly within 3 to 6 months, the greater is the perioperative risk. However, like the Goldman Cardiac Risk Index, medicine has changed and outcomes are improved. The 2014 AHA/ACC Foundation (AHA/ACCF) guidelines advocate the use of 60 days as being high risk.[119] After that time, further risk stratification depends on clinical symptoms.

For those patients without overt symptoms or a history of CAD, the probability of CAD varies with the type and number of atherosclerotic risk factors present. Diabetes accelerates the progression of atherosclerosis, which can frequently be silent, leading many clinicians to assume that diabetes is a CAD equivalent and treating patients as such. Diabetes is an independent risk factor for perioperative cardiac morbidity, and the preoperative treatment with insulin has been included in the Revised Cardiac Risk Index (RCRI). In attempting to determine the degree of the increased risk associated with diabetes, the treatment modality, duration of the disease, and other associated end-organ dysfunction should be taken into account.

Significant intraoperative factors that correlate with perioperative risk and that may be avoided or altered are (1) unnecessary use of vasopressors,[142,143] (2) unintentional hypotension[144-146] (this point is controversial, however, because some investigators have found that unintentional hypotension does not correlate with perioperative morbidity[143]), (3) hypothermia,[147] (4) too low or too high a hematocrit,[148,149] and (5) lengthy operations.[145]

Significant intraoperative factors that correlate with perioperative morbidity and probably cannot be avoided are (1) emergency surgery and (2) thoracic or intraperitoneal surgery or above-the-knee amputations.[145,150-164]

Several risk indices were developed in a prospective cohort study by Lee and associates.[164] They studied 4315 patients 50 years old or older who were undergoing elective major noncardiac procedures in a tertiary care teaching hospital. The six independent predictors of complications included in a RCRI were high-risk type of surgery, history of ischemic heart disease, history of CHF, history of cerebrovascular disease, preoperative treatment with insulin, and preoperative serum creatinine greater than 2.0 mg/dL; increasing cardiac complication rates were noted with an increasing number of risk factors.[164] The RCRI has become the standard tool in the literature for assessing perioperative cardiac risk in a given individual and has been used to direct the decision to perform cardiovascular testing and implement perioperative management protocols. It has been validated for both short-term and long-term cardiovascular outcomes.[165] It has also been shown to predict long-term quality of life.[165] Therefore, the RCRI can be used to help define both the short-term and long-term risks of cardiovascular disease in the surgical patient.

The American College of Surgeons NSQIP created a Surgical Risk Calculator from 525 participating hospitals and more than 1 million operations.[166] This risk calculator uses the specific current procedural terminology code of the procedure being performed to enable procedure-specific risk assessment and includes 21 patient-specific variables (e.g., age, sex, body mass index, dyspnea, previous MI). From this input, it calculates the percentage of risk of a major adverse cardiac event, death, and eight other outcomes. Use of this risk calculator may offer the best estimation for surgery-specific risk of a major adverse cardiac event and death.

The American College of Surgeons NSQIP Myocardial Infarction and Cardiac Arrest risk prediction rule is more specific for cardiac complications.[167] Using these definitions of outcome and chart-based data collection methods, the authors derived a risk index that was robust in the derivation and validation stages and appeared to outperform the RCRI (which was tested in the same dataset) in terms of discriminative power, particularly among patients undergoing vascular surgery.

A primary issue with all these indices is that a simple estimate of risk does not help in refining perioperative management for an individual patient. Therefore, the consultant must communicate the extent and stability of the patient's CAD, rather than make a simple statement of risk classification.

The goal in providing anesthesia to patients with ischemic heart disease is to achieve the best preoperative condition obtainable by treating conditions that correlate with perioperative risk. The next step is to intraoperatively monitor for conditions that correlate with perioperative risk and avoid circumstances that lead to perioperative risk.

Preoperative and Preprocedure Therapy

The only way known to increase oxygen supply to the myocardium of patients with coronary artery stenosis is to maintain adequate diastolic blood pressure, hemoglobin concentration, and oxygen saturation. The main goals of anesthesia practice for these patients have been to decrease the determinants of myocardial oxygen demand, heart rate, ventricular wall tension, and contractile performance, and to improve plaque stabilization. Thus medical management designed to preserve all viable myocardial tissue may include the following:

1. Multiple studies have demonstrated improved outcome in patients given perioperative β-blockers, especially if heart rate is controlled, acknowledging the previously discussed concerns regarding the quality of the studies from the Erasmus group.[167a,b] Subsequent studies demonstrated that β-blockers may not be effective if heart rate is not well controlled, or in lower risk patients.[167c-e] The POISE trial was published in which 8351 high-risk β-blocker-naïve patients were randomized to high-dose continuous-release metoprolol versus placebo.[167f]
2. There was a significant reduction in the primary outcome of cardiovascular events associated with a 30% reduction in MI rate, but with a significantly increased rate of 30-day all-cause mortality and stroke. Several recent cohort studies continue to support the fact that high-risk patients on β-blockers were associated with improved outcome. A Canadian administrative dataset suggested that the perioperative morbidity would be higher if β-blockers were started within 7 days as compared to 8 days or greater. As part of the update to the current ACC/AHA Guidelines, an Evidence Review Committee was formed to independently review the data on perioperative β-blockade. Perioperative β-blockade started within 1 day or less before noncardiac surgery prevents nonfatal MI but increases risks of stroke, death, hypotension, and bradycardia.[167g] Without the controversial DECREASE studies, there are insufficient data on β-blockade started two or more days prior to surgery. Wallace and associates reported that perioperative β-blockade administered according to the Perioperative Cardiac Risk Reduction protocol is associated with a reduction in 30-day and 1-year mortality.[167h] Perioperative withdrawal of β-blockers is associated with increased mortality. The current ACCF/AHA Guidelines on perioperative β-blockade advocate that perioperative β-blockade is a Class I indication and should be used in patients previously on β-blockers. The new recommendations changed the recommendation from a Class IIa to IIb for patients undergoing vascular surgery who are at high cardiac risk owing to CAD or the finding of cardiac ischemia on preoperative testing (Box 32.3).
2. Vasodilation (with nitroglycerin or its "long-acting" analogues nitroprusside, hydralazine, or prazosin) to decrease ventricular wall tension may be beneficial, although currently no randomized trials support the prophylactic use of these agents.[109,110,168] There are no data to support the routine use of pulmonary artery catheters and transesophageal echocardiography for this type of patient.[158,169] The intraoperative management of patients with ischemic heart disease is discussed in further detail in Chapters 31 and 54 and in published guidelines.[117]
3. Other medications. In POISE II, α-2 agonists were not shown to improve perioperative outcome.[169a] POISE II also evaluated the effectiveness of aspirin therapy in a cohort of patients without a recent stent. Administration of aspirin before surgery and throughout the early postsurgical period had no significant effect on the rate of a composite of death or nonfatal MI but increased the risk of major bleeding.[169b] Most recently, perioperative statins have been shown to improve cardiac outcome. Durazzo and colleagues published a randomized trial of 200 vascular surgery patients in which statins were started an average of 30 days prior to vascular surgery.[169c] A significant reduction in cardiovascular complications was demonstrated using this protocol. Le Manach and colleagues demonstrated that statin

BOX 32.3 2014 ACC/AHA Recommendations for Perioperative β-Blockade

Class I

- β-Blockers should be continued in patients undergoing surgery who have been on β-blockers chronically.[111-117] **(Level of Evidence: B)**

Class IIa

- It is reasonable for the management of β-blockers after surgery to be guided by clinical circumstances, independent of when the agent was started.[110,117,118] **(Level of Evidence: B)**

Class IIb

- In patients with intermediate- or high-risk myocardial ischemia noted in preoperative risk stratification tests, it may be reasonable to begin perioperative β-blockers.[119] **(Level of Evidence: C)**
- In patients with three or more RCRI risk factors (e.g., diabetes mellitus, heart failure, coronary artery disease, renal insufficiency, cerebrovascular accident), it may be reasonable to begin β-blockers before surgery.[117] **(Level of Evidence: B)**
- In patients with a compelling long-term indication for β-blocker therapy but no other RCRI risk factors, initiating β-blockers in the perioperative setting as an approach to reduce perioperative risk is of uncertain benefit.[111,117,120] **(Level of Evidence: B)**
- In patients in whom β-blocker therapy is initiated, it may be reasonable to begin perioperative β-blockers long enough in advance to assess safety and tolerability, preferably more than 1 day before surgery.[110,121-123] **(Level of Evidence: B)**

Class III: Harm

- β-Blocker therapy should not be started on the day of surgery.[110] **(Level of Evidence: B)**

RCRI, Revised cardiac risk index.

From Fleisher LA, Fleischmann KE, Auerbach AD, et al. 2014 ACC/AHA guideline on perioperative cardiovascular evaluation and management of patients undergoing noncardiac surgery: a report of the American College of Cardiology/American Heart Association Task Force on practice guidelines. *J Am Coll Cardiol*. 2014;64(22):e77–e137.

withdrawal greater than 4 days was associated with a 2.9 odds ratio of increased risk of cardiac morbidity in vascular surgery.[169d] The guidelines advocate continuing statin therapy in patients currently taking statins as a Class I indication. A multimodal approach to medical management should be taken in high-risk patients. There continues to be controversy regarding the optimal management of ACE inhibitors and ARBs. In the Veterans Administration, withholding ARB postoperatively is strongly associated with increased 30-day mortality, especially in younger patients, although residual confounding may be present.[169e] In the VISION trial, compared to patients who continued their ACE inhibitors/angiotensin II receptor blockers, the ACE/ARB users who withheld their agents in the 24 hours before surgery were less likely to suffer the primary composite outcome of all-cause death, stroke, or myocardial injury (adjusted relative risk, 0.82; 95% CI, 0.70 to 0.96; $P = .01$); and intraoperative hypotension (adjusted relative risk, 0.80; 95% CI, 0.72-0.93; $P < .001$).[169f] The current AHA/ACC Guidelines suggest that continuation of ACE inhibitors or angiotensin-receptor ARBs perioperatively is reasonable, but should be restarted as soon as reasonable. The new study questions this recommendation, but further randomized trials are needed.

4. Perioperative transfusion therapy is discussed in more detail in Chapter 49. The FOCUS (Functional Outcomes in Cardiovascular Patients Undergoing Surgical Repair of Hip Fracture) trial was unable to demonstrate benefit in high-risk patients with hip fracture between a high and low transfusion trigger.[170]

VALVULAR HEART DISEASE

Major alterations in the preoperative management of patients with valvular heart disease have been made regarding the use of anticoagulant therapy and are now based on the causes of the disease. Preoperative and intraoperative management of patients with valvular heart disease is discussed in Chapters 31 and 54.

The prognosis and the perioperative risk for patients with valvular heart disease depend on the stage of the disease. Although stenotic lesions typically progress faster than regurgitant lesions, regurgitant lesions from infective endocarditis, rupture of the chordae tendineae, or ischemic heart disease can be rapidly fatal. Left ventricular dysfunction is common in the late stage of valvular heart disease, both stenotic and regurgitant.

Preoperative maintenance of drug therapy can be crucial; for example, a patient with severe aortic stenosis can deteriorate rapidly with the onset of atrial fibrillation or flutter because the atrial contribution to left ventricular filling can be critical in maintaining cardiac output. One of the most serious complications of valvular heart surgery and of preoperative valvular heart disease is cardiac arrhythmia. Conduction disorders and long-term therapy with antiarrhythmic and inotropic drugs are discussed elsewhere in this chapter. The reader is referred to Chapter 78 and to other sources for discussion of the management of a child with congenital heart disease who is undergoing noncardiac surgery.[171]

Preoperative Antibiotic Prophylaxis for Endocarditis

Patients who have any form of valvular heart disease, as well as those with intracardiac (ventricular septal or atrial septal defects) or intravascular shunts, should be protected against endocarditis at the time of a known bacteremic event. Endocarditis has occurred in a sufficiently significant number of patients with hypertrophic cardiomyopathy (subvalvular aortic stenosis, asymmetric septal hypertrophy) and mitral valve prolapse to warrant the inclusion of these two conditions in the prophylaxis regimen.

Bacteremia occurs after the following events: dental extraction, 30% to 80%; brushing of teeth, 20% to 24%; use of oral irrigation devices, 20% to 24%; barium enema, 11%; transurethral resection of the prostate (TURP), 10% to 57%; upper GI endoscopy, 8%; nasotracheal intubation, 16% (4 of 25 patients); and orotracheal intubation, 0% (0 of 25 patients). The most recent guidelines from the AHA consisted of an update in 2008 from the AHA/ACC on endocarditis in patients with valvular heart disease, with changes from the 2006 document shown in Table 32.6.[172]

TABLE 32.6 Changes Related to Endocarditis Prophylaxis: American College of Cardiology/American Heart Association Guidelines on Valvular Heart Disease

2006 VHD Guideline Recommendations	2008 VHD Focused Update Recommendations	Comments
Class I	**Class IIa**	
Prophylaxis against infective endocarditis is recommended for the following patients: Patients with prosthetic heart valves and patients with a history of infective endocarditis *(level of evidence: C)* Patients who have complex cyanotic congenital heart disease (e.g., single-ventricle states, transposition of the great arteries, tetralogy of Fallot) *(level of evidence: C)* Patients with surgically constructed systemic pulmonary shunts or conduits *(level of evidence: C)* Patients with congenital cardiac valve malformations, particularly those with bicuspid aortic valves, and patients with acquired valvular dysfunction (e.g., rheumatic heart disease) *(level of evidence: C)* Patients who have undergone valve repair *(level of evidence: C)* Patients who have hypertrophic cardiomyopathy when there is latent or resting obstruction *(level of evidence: C)* Patients with MVP and auscultatory evidence of valvular regurgitation and/or thickened leaflets on echocardiography* *(level of evidence: C)*	Prophylaxis against infective endocarditis is reasonable for the following patients at highest risk for adverse outcomes from infective endocarditis who undergo dental procedures that involve manipulation of either gingival tissue or the periapical region of teeth or perforation of the oral mucosa: Patients with prosthetic cardiac valves or prosthetic material used for cardiac valve repair *(level of evidence: B)* Patients with previous infective endocarditis *(level of evidence: B)* Patients with CHD *(level of evidence: B)* Unrepaired cyanotic CHD, including palliative shunts and conduits *(level of evidence: B)* Completely repaired congenital heart defect repaired with prosthetic material or device, whether placed by surgery or by catheter intervention, during the first 6 months after the procedure *(level of evidence: B)* Repaired CHD with residual defects at the site or adjacent to the site of a prosthetic patch or prosthetic device (both of which inhibit endothelialization) *(level of evidence: B)* Cardiac transplant recipients with valve regurgitation as a result of a structurally abnormal valve *(level of evidence: C)*	Modified recommendation (changed class of recommendation from I to IIa, changed text); no class I recommendations exist for infective endocarditis prophylaxis

CHD, Congenital heart disease; *MVP,* mitral valve prolapse; *VHD,* valvular heart disease.

*This footnote is obsolete. Please see 2006 VHD Guideline 3 for footnote text, in Bonow RO, Carabello BA, Kanu C et al. ACC/AHA 2006 guidelines for the management of patients with valvular heart disease: a report of the American College of Cardiology/American Heart Association Task Force on practice guidelines (writing committee to revise the 1998 guidelines for the management of patients with valvular heart disease). Developed in collaboration with the Society of Cardiovascular Anesthesiologists: endorsed by the Society for Cardiovascular Angiography and Interventions and the Society of Thoracic Surgeons. *Circulation.* 2006;114:e84–e231.

From Nishimura RA, Carabello BA, Faxon DP, et al. ACC/AHA 2008 guideline update on valvular heart disease: focused update on infective endocarditis. A report of the American College of Cardiology/American Heart Association Task Force on practice guidelines: endorsed by the Society of Cardiovascular Anesthesiologists, Society for Cardiovascular Angiography and Interventions, and Society of Thoracic Surgeons. *Circulation.* 2008;118:887–896.

Cardiac Valve Prostheses and Anticoagulant Therapy and Prophylaxis for Deep Vein Thrombosis

In patients with prosthetic valves, the risk of increased bleeding during a procedure in a patient receiving antithrombotic therapy must be weighed against the increased risk of thromboembolism caused by stopping the therapy. Common practice in patients undergoing noncardiac surgery with a mechanical prosthetic valve in place is cessation of anticoagulant therapy 3 days preoperatively. This time frame allows the international normalized ratio to fall to less than 1.5 times normal. The oral anticoagulants can then be resumed on postoperative day 1. Using a similar protocol, Katholi and colleagues found no perioperative episodes of thromboembolism or hemorrhage in 25 patients.[173] An alternative approach in patients at high risk for thromboembolism is conversion to heparin during the perioperative period. The heparin can then be discontinued 4 to 6 hours preoperatively and resumed shortly thereafter. Current prosthetic valves may have a lower incidence of this complication, and the risk associated with heparin may outweigh its benefit in the perioperative setting. According to the AHA/ACC guidelines, heparin can usually be reserved for patients who have had a recent thrombus or embolus within 1 year, those with demonstrated thrombotic problems when previously off therapy, and those with more than three risk factors (atrial fibrillation, previous thromboembolism, hypercoagulable condition, and mechanical prosthesis).[174] A lower threshold for recommending heparin should be considered in patients with mechanical valves in the mitral position, in whom a single risk factor would be sufficient evidence of high risk. Subcutaneous low-molecular-weight heparin offers an alternative outpatient approach.[175] It is appropriate for the surgeon and cardiologist to discuss the optimal perioperative management for such a patient, including a review of the most recent guidelines.[176] A new guideline publication was published in 2014.[176a]

Regional anesthetic techniques may be avoided, although this issue is controversial as many practitioners will use regional anesthesia in patients who are receiving prophylaxis for deep vein thrombosis.[177-180] However, epidural hematoma has been associated with anticoagulant therapy in many reports. Large retrospective reviews of outcome after epidural or spinal anesthesia, or both, during or shortly before initiation of anticoagulant therapy with heparin have not reported neurologic dysfunction related to hematoma formation in any patient.[181,182] This paucity of damaging epidemiologic evidence, although reassuring, does not reduce the need for frequent evaluation of neurologic function and a search for back pain in the perioperative period after regional anesthesia in any patient receiving any anticoagulation or antiplatelet.[177,183-185] The risk of regional anesthesia concurrent with prophylaxis for deep vein thrombosis with heparin is greater with the use of low-molecular-weight heparin. Heparin-induced thrombocytopenia has been treated successfully with intravenous immunoglobulin.[179] The American Society of Regional

Anesthesia and Pain Management has issued a consensus statement on the use of regional anesthesia in anticoagulated patients.[186] They suggest that the decision to perform spinal or epidural anesthesia or analgesia, and the timing of catheter removal in a patient receiving antithrombotic therapy should be made on an individual basis, with the small but definite risk of spinal hematoma weighed against the benefits of regional anesthesia for a specific patient.

It was, previously, determined that venous thromboembolism is so common in postoperative patients that almost 1% of postsurgical patients die of fatal pulmonary embolism (Table 32.7).[187] More recently, it has been estimated that venous thromboembolism is responsible for up to 10% of all hospital-related deaths.[187a] Because of this high mortality risk, prophylaxis against deep vein thrombosis has attained widespread acceptance; thus prophylaxis begins with 5000 units of heparin given subcutaneously 2 hours preoperatively.[187-189] Other trials have shown equal effect with external pneumatic sequential compression devices.[188,190] The most current recommendations are available from the American College of Chest Physicians for prophylaxis against venous thromboembolism in 2012.[190a]

Another problem that can arise is managing a pregnant patient with a prosthetic valve during delivery. It is recommended that warfarin be replaced by subcutaneous heparin during the peripartum period. During labor and delivery, elective induction of labor is advocated with discontinuance of all anticoagulant therapy, as indicated for the particular valve prosthesis (discussed earlier).[191]

Auscultation of the prosthetic valve should be performed preoperatively to verify normal functioning. Abnormalities in such sounds warrant preoperative consultation and verification of functioning.

CARDIAC CONDUCTION DISTURBANCES: CARDIAC ARRHYTHMIAS

Bradyarrhythmias, especially if profound or associated with dizziness or syncope, are generally managed with pacemakers. However, chronic bifascicular block (right bundle branch block with a left anterior or posterior hemiblock or left bundle branch block with combined left anterior and posterior hemiblocks), even when only a first-degree heart block is present, can progress to complete heart block and sudden perioperative death on rare occasion. In six studies, less than 2% of the approximately 266 patients with bifascicular block progressed to complete heart block perioperatively.[192] Conversely, these patients have a high 5-year mortality rate (160 of 554 patients, or 29%). Most of the deaths were related to tachyarrhythmias or ischemic events not usually preventable by traditional pacemakers.[193] Thus the presence of a bifascicular block on the ECG should make the anesthesiologist worried about associated CAD or left ventricular dysfunction; an echocardiogram should be evaluated perioperatively. Nevertheless, these patients rarely have complete heart block perioperatively. Therefore, prophylactic preoperative insertion of temporary pacing wires for bifascicular block does not seem warranted; however, central access can be established in advance in the event that a temporary pacemaker needs to be inserted (most operating rooms do not rely on transthoracic pacing, although it may be attempted if available).[194] The actual pacemaker equipment and appropriate personnel should be immediately available, and the equipment should be tested regularly, because symptomatic heart block does occur perioperatively in more than 1% of patients. One study appears to have confirmed this rate of at least 1% for patients undergoing cardiac surgery.[195] One percent of patients in whom a pacing pulmonary artery catheter was not inserted preoperatively subsequently required pacing before cardiopulmonary bypass. By contrast, 19% of patients who had such a catheter in place underwent cardiac pacing before cardiopulmonary bypass. Predictors of the need for pacing included previous symptomatic bradyarrhythmia, a history of transient complete AV block, and aortic valve disease.

Older studies demonstrated that a rate of more than five PVCs per minute on preoperative examination correlates

TABLE 32.7 Incidence of Deep Vein Thrombosis and Fatal Pulmonary Embolism

	INCIDENCE OF		
Type of Surgery	**Deep Vein Thrombosis (%)**	**Proximal Deep Vein Thrombosis (%)**	**Fatal Pulmonary Embolism (%)**
GENERAL			
Age >40 years	10	<1	0.1
Age >60 years	10-40	3-15	0.8
Malignancy	50-60		
Thoracic	30		
VASCULAR			
Aortic repair	26		
Peripheral	12		
UROLOGIC			
Open prostatectomy	40		
TURP	10		
Other urologic	30-40		
MAJOR GYNECOLOGIC			
With malignancy	40		
Without malignancy	10-20		
NEUROSURGERY			
Craniotomy	20-80		
Laminectomy	4-25		1.5-3.0
ORTHOPEDIC			
Total hip replacement	40-80	10-20	1.0-5.0
Hip fracture	48-75		1.0-5.0
Tibial fracture	45		
Total knee replacement	60-70	20	1.0-5.0
Head, neck, chest wall	11		
MEDICAL			
Acute myocardial infarction	30	6	
Stroke	60-75		
Acute spine injury	60-100		
Other bed bound	26		

TURP, Transurethral resection of the prostate.

with perioperative cardiac morbidity.[144,151-153] To the classic criteria for treating PVCs (the presence of R-on-T couplets, the occurrence of more than three PVCs per minute, and multifocality of PVCs) must be added frequent (>10/h over a 24-hour period) and repetitive ventricular beats. Electrophysiologic and programmed ventricular stimulation studies are being used to indicate and guide treatment of patients with ischemic heart disease or recurrent arrhythmias and survivors of out-of-hospital cardiac arrest. Although such patients are often treated with antiarrhythmic therapy, attention to their underlying condition should be a focus of our preoperative management. Long-term antiarrhythmic therapy is discussed in the last section of this chapter, on drug therapy. Torsades de pointes is an arrhythmia characterized by episodes of alternating electrical polarity such that the major vector of the QRS complex seems to alternate around an isoelectric line. The hallmark enabling differential diagnosis from ventricular tachycardia is the unusual response of this arrhythmia to commonly used antiarrhythmic drugs. In other words, the use of drugs that prolong the QT interval (e.g., quinidine, procainamide, disopyramide, some of the antihistamines, and the antipsychotic phenothiazines) may well make the arrhythmia more frequent or of longer duration. Reports of the sudden occurrence of torsades de pointes during surgical procedures have been rare in the anesthesia literature. Immediate therapy consists of the administration of magnesium or electrical cardioversion, followed by overdrive cardiac pacing or the administration of β-adrenergic agonists and discontinuation of drugs that prolong the QT interval.

Premature atrial contractions and cardiac rhythms other than sinus also correlate with perioperative cardiac morbidity.[144,152] These arrhythmias may be more a marker of poor cardiovascular reserve than a specific cause of perioperative cardiac complications.

Preexcitation syndrome is the name for supraventricular tachycardias associated with AV bypass tracts.[196] Successful treatment, which is predicated on an understanding of the clinical and electrophysiologic manifestations of the syndrome, consists of either catheter ablation techniques or surgery using preoperative and intraoperative techniques that avoid release of sympathetic and other vasoactive substances and therefore tachyarrhythmias.[193,197,198] Anesthesia for electrophysiologic procedures is discussed in Chapter 55.

Disorders of the Respiratory and Immune Systems

GENERAL PREOPERATIVE AND PREPROCEDURE CONSIDERATIONS

Pulmonary complications after procedures requiring anesthesia are as common as cardiovascular complications—even more common if venous thromboembolism is included. It has, relatively recently, been estimated that postoperative respiratory complications can occur in up to 80% of surgical patients, noting obesity, preexisting pulmonary disease, and advanced age are among the chief risk factors.[198a] Thus pulmonary complications are equally as important or more important to the patient and the health system in terms of morbidity, mortality, length-of-stay extension, and cost. Today there is an even greater appreciation of the effects of smoking and sleep apnea on perioperative and long-term care has increased.[199-216] (Preoperative and preprocedure identification and perioperative care of patients with sleep apnea are discussed in the earlier section on obesity and in Chapter 58.)

The main purpose of preoperative testing is to identify patients at risk for perioperative complications so that appropriate perioperative therapy can be instituted to foster return to functional status. Preoperative assessment can also establish baseline function and the feasibility of surgical intervention. Whereas numerous investigators have used pulmonary function tests to define inoperability or high-risk versus low-risk groups for pulmonary complications, few have been able to demonstrate that the performance of any specific preoperative or intraoperative measure, except perhaps smoking cessation and physical activity such as a walking program, reliably decreases perioperative pulmonary morbidity or mortality and improves patient outcomes. Because routine preoperative pulmonary testing and care are discussed extensively in Chapter 41, the current discussion is limited to an assessment of the effectiveness of this type of care.

In fact, few randomized prospective studies indicate an outcome benefit of preoperative preparation. Stein and Cassara randomly allocated 48 patients to undergo preoperative therapy (cessation of smoking, administration of antibiotics for purulent sputum, and use of bronchodilating drugs, postural drainage, chest physiotherapy, and ultrasonic nebulizer) or no preoperative therapy.[212] The no-treatment group had a mortality of 16% and morbidity of 60%, as opposed to 0% and 20%, respectively, for the treatment group. In addition, the treatment group spent an average of 12 postoperative days in the hospital as compared with 24 days for the 21 survivors in the no-treatment group.[212]

Collins and colleagues prospectively examined the benefits of preoperative antibiotics, perioperative chest physiotherapy and therapy with bronchodilating drugs, and routine postoperative analgesia (morphine) on postoperative respiratory complications in patients with COPD.[217] Of these therapies, only preoperative treatment with antibiotics had a beneficial effect.

Hulzebos and colleagues performed a single-center randomized trial of intensive inspiratory muscle training.[218] Preoperative inspiratory muscle training reduced the incidence of postoperative pulmonary complications and the duration of postoperative hospitalization in patients at high risk of developing a pulmonary complication who were undergoing CABG surgery.

Warner and coworkers collected data retrospectively about smoking history and prospectively (concurrently) about pulmonary complications for 200 patients undergoing CABG.[219] These investigators documented that 8 weeks or more of smoking cessation was associated with a 66% reduction in postoperative pulmonary complications. Smokers who stopped for less than 8 weeks actually had an increase (from 33% for current smokers to 57.1% for recent quitters) in the rate of one or more of the six complications surveyed: purulent sputum with pyrexia; need for respiratory therapy care; bronchospasm requiring therapy; pleural effusion or pneumothorax (or both) necessitating drainage; segmental pulmonary collapse, as confirmed by radiography; or pneumonia necessitating antibiotic therapy. Other investigators have found that both shorter and longer periods of cessation of smoking were needed before achieving cardiovascular[220] and hematologic benefit.[221] Bluman and associates performed a retrospective chart review of 410 patients undergoing noncardiac surgery at a VA hospital.[222] Current smoking was associated with a nearly 6-fold increase in the risk of a postoperative pulmonary complication. Reduction in smoking within 1 month of surgery was not associated with a decreased risk for postoperative pulmonary complications. Nakagawa and coauthors also reported higher pulmonary complication rates in patients undergoing pulmonary surgery who quit within 4 weeks of surgery than in current smokers or those who had stopped smoking for more than 4 weeks.[223] Wong and colleagues performed a systematic review of 25 studies of smoking cessation.[224] At least 4 weeks of abstinence from smoking reduced respiratory complications, and abstinence of at least 3 to 4 weeks reduced wound healing complications. Short-term (<4 weeks) smoking cessation did not appear to affect the risk of postoperative respiratory complications.

Two randomized trials focused on smoking cessation. Wong and colleagues performed a prospective, multicenter, double-blind, placebo-controlled trial, in which 286 patients were randomized to receive varenicline or placebo.[225] A perioperative smoking cessation intervention with varenicline increased abstinence from smoking 3, 6, and 12 months after elective noncardiac surgery with no increase in serious adverse events. Lee and colleagues randomized patients to a group receiving no specific smoking cessation intervention or to an intervention group that received (1) brief counseling by the preadmission nurse, (2) brochures on smoking cessation, (3) referral to the Canadian Cancer Society's Smokers' Helpline, and (4) a free 6-week supply of transdermal nicotine replacement therapy.[226] All outcome assessors and caregivers on the operative day were blinded to group assignment. Smoking cessation occurred in 12 patients (14.3%) in the intervention group as compared with 3 patients (3.6%) in the control group (relative risk, 4.0; 95% CI, 1.2-13.7; $P = .03$). The overall rate of combined intraoperative and immediate postoperative complications was not significantly different between intervention and control groups. At follow-up 30 days postoperatively, smoking cessation was reported in 22 patients (28.6%) in the intervention group compared with 8 patients (11%) in controls (relative risk, 2.6; 95% CI, 1.2-5.5; $P = .008$).

When Skolnick and coworkers studied 602 children prospectively, exposure to passive smoking (as measured by urinary cotinine, the major metabolite of nicotine) correlated directly with airway complications. Children with the least exposure to passive smoke had the fewest complications.[210] Secondhand smoke may be a model for particulate air pollution, which can have immediate and long-term effects in increasing lung dysfunction and inflammatory stimuli throughout the body.[227,228]

Celli and associates performed a randomized prospective controlled trial of intermittent positive-pressure breathing (IPPB) versus incentive spirometry and deep-breathing exercises in 81 patients undergoing abdominal surgery.[229] The groups exposed to a respiratory therapist (regardless of the treatment given) had more than a 50% lower incidence of clinical complications (30%-33% vs. 88%) and shorter hospital stays than did the control group. Thus this demonstrates that the outcome improves when any concern about lung function is shown by someone knowledgeable in maneuvers designed to clear lung secretions.

Bartlett and coworkers randomly assigned 150 patients undergoing extensive laparotomy to 1 of 2 groups.[230] One group received preoperative instruction in and postoperative use of incentive spirometry (10 times/h). The other group received similar medical care but no incentive spirometry. Only 7 of 75 patients using incentive spirometry had postoperative pulmonary complications, as opposed to 19 of 75 in the control group. However, Lyager and colleagues randomly assigned 103 patients undergoing biliary or gastric surgery to receive either incentive spirometry with preoperative and postoperative chest physiotherapy or only preoperative and postoperative chest physiotherapy.[231] No difference in the postoperative course or pulmonary complications was found between the groups. Other studies have shown a specific benefit (i.e., greater than that provided by routine care) for chest physiotherapy and IPPB. These studies are usually poorly controlled, not randomized, or retrospective in design (or any combination); these deficiencies probably substantially bias the results toward finding a benefit in reducing postoperative pulmonary complications. Although randomized prospective studies showed no benefit or actual harm from chest physiotherapy and IPPB on the resolution of pneumonia or postoperative pulmonary complications, the studies cited earlier[212,217,229,230] and numerous retrospective studies strongly suggest that preoperative evaluation and treatment of patients with pulmonary disease actually decrease perioperative respiratory complications.

Meta-analyses have suggested a benefit of anesthetic and pain management with respect to respiratory outcomes. Rodgers and associates reviewed 141 trials involving 9559 patients who had been randomized to receive neuraxial blockade or general anesthesia. Overall mortality was significantly less frequent in the neuraxial blockade group (2.1% vs. 3.1%). The relative risk of pneumonia in the neuraxial blockade group was 0.61 (CI, 0.48-0.81), and the relative risk of respiratory depression was 0.41 (CI, 0.23-0.73).[211] Further, Neuman and colleagues examined a retrospective cohort of 18,158 patients undergoing surgery for hip fracture in 126 hospitals in New York in 2007 and 2008.[232] Patients receiving regional anesthesia experienced fewer pulmonary complications (359 [6.8%] vs. 1040 [8.1%]; $P < .005$). Regional anesthesia was associated with a lower adjusted odds of mortality (OR, 0.710; 95% CI, 0.541, 0.932; $P = .014$) and pulmonary complications (OR, 0.752; 95% CI, 0.637, 0.887; $P < .0001$) relative to general anesthesia. In subgroup analyses, regional anesthesia was associated with improved survival and fewer pulmonary complications among patients with intertrochanteric fractures but not among patients with femoral neck fractures.

Not all studies demonstrate beneficial effects of pharmacologic pretreatment. In afebrile outpatient American Society of Anesthesiologists (ASA) class I and II children with no lung disease or findings who underwent noncavitary, nonairway surgery lasting less than 3 hours, neither albuterol nor ipratropium premedication decreased adverse events.[233]

Evaluation of dyspnea is especially useful. Boushy and coworkers found that grades of preoperative dyspnea correlated with postoperative survival. (Grades of respiratory

TABLE 32.8 Grade of Dyspnea Caused by Respiratory Problems (Assessed in Terms of Walking on a Level Surface at a Normal Pace)

Category	Description
0	No dyspnea while walking on a level surface at a normal pace
I	"I am able to walk as far as I like, provided I take my time"
II	Specific (street) block limitation ("I have to stop for a while after one or two blocks")
III	Dyspnea on mild exertion ("I have to stop and rest while going from the kitchen to the bathroom")
IV	Dyspnea at rest

Modified from Boushy SF, Billing DM, North LB, et al. Clinical course related to preoperative pulmonary function in patients with bronchogenic carcinoma. *Chest.* 1971;59:383–391.

dyspnea are provided in Table 32.8.)[234] Mittman demonstrated an increased risk of death after thoracic surgery, from 8% in patients without dyspnea to 56% in patients with dyspnea.[235] Similarly, Reichel found that no patients died after pneumonectomy if they were able to complete a preoperative treadmill test for 4 minutes at the rate of 2 mph on level ground.[236] Other studies have found that the history and physical examination of an asthmatic subject can also predict the need for hospitalization.[201] Wong and colleagues found that the risk index correlated with postoperative pulmonary complications (Table 32.9).[237]

Arozullah and associates developed the first validated multifactorial risk index for postoperative respiratory failure, defined as mechanical ventilation for more than 48 hours after surgical procedures, or reintubation and mechanical ventilation after postoperative extubation.[238] In a prospective cohort study of 181,000 male veterans as part of the National Veterans Administration Surgical Quality Improvement Program, seven factors independently predicted risk (Table 32.10). With increasing numbers of risk factors present, the rate of complications increased from 0.5% (class 1) to 26.6% (class 4). Arozullah and colleagues subsequently developed a risk index for postoperative pneumonia by using data on 160,805 patients undergoing major noncardiac surgery and validated the index by using data on an additional 155,266 patients.[239] Patients were divided into five risk classes by using risk index scores (Table 32.11). Pneumonia rates were 0.2% in patients with 0 to 15 risk points, 1.2% in those with 16 to 25 risk points, 4.0% in those with 26 to 40 risk points, 9.4% in those with 41 to 55 risk points, and 15.3% in those with more than 55 risk points.

Gupta and colleagues used the American College of Surgeons NSQIP to develop a risk model for postoperative respiratory failure.[167] On multivariate logistic regression analysis, five preoperative predictors of postoperative respiratory failure were identified: type of surgery, emergency case, dependent functional status, preoperative sepsis, and higher ASA class (Table 32.12).

TABLE 32.9 Classification of Risk of Pulmonary Complications for Thoracic and Abdominal Procedures

Category	Points
I. EXPIRATORY SPIROGRAM	
A. Normal (% FVC + [% FEV_1/FVC] > 150)	0
B. % FVC + (% FEV_1/FVC) = 100-150	1
C. % FVC + (% FEV_1/FVC) <100	2
D. Preoperative FVC < 20 mL/kg	3
E. Post bronchodilator FEV_1/FVC <50%	3
II. CARDIOVASCULAR SYSTEM	
A. Normal	0
B. Controlled hypertension, myocardial infarction without sequelae for >2 years	0
C. Dyspnea on exertion, orthopnea, paroxysmal nocturnal dyspnea, dependent edema, congestive heart failure, angina	1
III. NERVOUS SYSTEM	
A. Normal	0
B. Confusion, obtundation, agitation, spasticity, discoordination, bulbar malfunction	1
C. Significant muscular weakness	1
IV. ARTERIAL BLOOD GASES	
A. Acceptable	0
B. $Paco_2$ >50 mm Hg or PaO_2 <60 mm Hg on room air	1
C. Metabolic pH abnormality >7.50 or <7.30	1
V. POSTOPERATIVE AMBULATION	
A. Expected ambulation (minimum, sitting at bedside) within 36 h	0
B. Expected complete bed confinement for ≥36 h	1

FEV_1, Forced expiratory volume in 1 second; *FVC*, forced vital capacity; *$Paco_2$*, arterial partial pressure of carbon dioxide; *PaO_2*, arterial partial pressure of oxygen.

Modified from Wong DH, Weber EC, Schell MJ, et al. Factors associated with postoperative pulmonary complications in patients with severe COPD. *Anesth Analg.* 1995;80:276–284.

SPECIFIC DISEASES

Pulmonary Vascular Diseases

Pulmonary vascular diseases include pulmonary hypertension secondary to heart disease (postcapillary disorders), parenchymal lung disease (pulmonary precapillary disorders), pulmonary embolism, and cor pulmonale from COPD.[240] Optimal preoperative management of these conditions requires treatment of the underlying disease and avoidance of worsening the process.[240-242] Because pulmonary embolism can be particularly difficult to diagnose as clinical findings of pulmonary emboli are not always present or specific for the diagnosis and include a history of tachypnea, dyspnea, palpitations, syncope, chest pain, or hemoptysis. Physical examination can reveal a pleural rub, wheezing, rales, a fixed and split second heart sound, right ventricular lift, or evidence of venous thrombosis. If the ECG shows an S_1Q_3 pattern, spiral CT or lung perfusion scans can be obtained to rule out the diagnosis of pulmonary emboli. A high degree of suspicion is necessary to warrant angiography and anticoagulation or fibrinolytic therapy. If possible, the reactivity of the pulmonary vasculature should be determined because it may be enhanced or decreased by such drugs as nifedipine, hydralazine, nitroglycerin, prazosin, tolazoline, phentolamine, sildenafil citrate, and nitric oxide.

TABLE 32.10 Preoperative Predictors of Postoperative Respiratory Failure

Variable	Odds Ratio (95% Confidence Interval)
TYPE OF SURGERY	
Abdominal aortic aneurysm	14.3 (12.0-16.9)
Thoracic	8.14 (7.17-9.25)
Neurosurgery, upper abdominal, or peripheral vascular	4.21 (3.80-4.67)
Neck	3.10 (2.40-4.01)
Other surgery*	1.00 (reference)
Emergency surgery	3.12 (2.83-3.43)
Albumin < 30 g/L	2.53 (2.28-2.80)
Blood urea nitrogen > 30 mg/dL	2.29 (2.04-2.56)
Partially or fully dependent status	1.92 (1.74-2.11)
History of COPD	1.81 (1.66-1.98)
AGE (YEARS)	
≥70	1.91 (1.71-2.13)
0-69	1.51 (1.36-1.69)
<60	1.00 (reference)

COPD, Chronic obstructive pulmonary disease.
*Other surgery includes ophthalmologic, ear, nose, mouth, lower abdominal, extremity, dermatologic, spine, and back surgery.
From Arozullah AM, Daley J, Henderson WG, et al. Multifactorial risk index for predicting postoperative respiratory failure in men after major noncardiac surgery: the National Veterans Administration Surgical Quality Improvement Program. *Ann Surg*. 2000;232:242–253.

TABLE 32.11 Postoperative Pneumonia Risk Index

Preoperative Risk Factor	Point Value
TYPE OF SURGERY	
Abdominal aortic aneurysm repair	15
Thoracic	14
Upper abdominal	10
Neck	8
Neurosurgery	8
Vascular	3
AGE	
80 years	17
70-79 years	13
60-69 years	9
50-59 years	4
FUNCTIONAL STATUS	
Totally dependent	10
Partially dependent	6
Weight loss >10% in past 6 months	7
History of COPD	5
General anesthesia	4
Impaired sensorium	4
History of cerebrovascular accident	4
BLOOD UREA NITROGEN LEVEL	
<2.86 mmol/L (0.8 mg/dL)	4
7.85-10.7 mmol/L (22-30 mg/dL)	2
≥10.7 mmol/L (≥30 mg/dL)	3
Transfusion >4 units	3
Emergency surgery	3
Steroid use for chronic condition	3
Current smoker within 1 year	3
Alcohol intake >2 drinks/day in past 2 weeks	2

COPD, Chronic obstructive pulmonary disease.
From Arozullah AM, Khuri SF, Henderson WG, et al. Development and validation of a multifactorial risk index for predicting postoperative pneumonia after major noncardiac surgery. *Ann Intern Med*. 2001;135:847–857.

Monitoring of pulmonary artery pressure is often required. Preoperative measures should be undertaken to ensure that the patient is not exposed to conditions that elevate pulmonary vascular resistance (e.g., hypoxia, hypercapnia, acidosis, lung hyperinflation, hypothermia)[243] or increased systemic vascular resistance, as this can precipitate acute or worsened right heart failure.

Infectious Diseases of the Lung

Preoperative evaluation and treatment should follow the basic guidelines outlined in the introduction to this section and in Chapter 31. Treatment of the underlying disease should be completed before all but emergency surgery is performed.

Even though elective surgery should be postponed whenever infectious diseases of the lung are present, patients undergoing emergency surgery can have nosocomial infections and immunocompromised systems. The predominant pathogens for nosocomial pneumonia are gram-negative bacilli, *Staphylococcus aureus*, *Haemophilus influenzae*, anaerobes, and pneumococci. Previously, the incidence of tuberculosis increased in the late 1980s and in the 1990s, probably because of reactivation in patients infected with HIV, through increased funding and directly observed antituberculosis treatment the incidence has steadily declined. Tuberculosis can lead to chronic pulmonary and systemic symptoms. Affected patients may have malaise, headache, fever, hemoptysis, and extrapulmonary diseases affecting the skin, cervical lymph nodes, kidneys, pericardium, and meninges. Active disease is treated with four-drug therapy: isoniazid, pyrazinamide, ethambutol or streptomycin, and rifampin for 9 months. Therapy should probably be started preoperatively.

Management of these emergency patients (many of whom have adult respiratory distress syndrome [ARDS]) before they are brought to the operating room may include initiation of antiinfective therapy, optimization of fluid status, facilitation of gas exchange, and therapy for the underlying pathophysiologic process.

Chronic Diseases of the Lung

Treatment of COPD may include the use of short and long acting β-adrenergic drugs, parasympatholytic agents (especially for exercise-induced asthma), systemic or inhaled corticosteroids, and leukotriene antagonists. An estimated

TABLE 32.12 Preoperative Variables Significantly Associated With an Increased Risk for Postoperative Respiratory Failure in 2007 Model from the American College of Surgeons National Surgical Quality Improvement Project*

Parameter	Adjusted OR	95% Wald CI
Totally dependent functional status†	4.07	3.68-4.51
Partially dependent functional status†	2.16	1.98-2.34
ASA class 1‡	0.03	0.02-0.05
ASA class 2‡	0.14	0.11-0.17
ASA class 3‡	0.54	0.44-0.67
ASA class 4‡	1.28	1.04-1.57
Preoperative sepsis (none)§	0.46	0.42-0.50
Preoperative sepsis§	1.32	1.16-1.49
Preoperative septic shock§	2.47	2.16-2.82
Emergency case (absence versus presence)	0.56	0.52-0.61
Anorectal¶	0.26	0.15-0.44
Aortic¶	2.94	2.35-3.68
Bariatric¶	0.36	0.27-0.49
Brain¶	2.08	1.15-3.78
Breast¶	0.07	0.04-0.12
Cardiac¶	1.32	0.92-1.88
Ear, nose, and throat¶	1.11	0.26-4.71
Foregut/hepatopancreatobiliary¶	2.64	2.13-3.27
Gallbladder, appendix, adrenals, and spleen¶	0.57	0.45-0.71
Intestinal¶	1.78	1.44-2.18
Neck¶	0.59	0.33-1.07
Obstetrics and gynecology¶	0.29	0.09-0.94
Orthopedic¶	0.42	0.33-0.55
Other abdominal¶	1.27	1.001-1.62
Peripheral vascular¶	0.79	0.63-0.98
Skin¶	0.73	0.55-0.95
Spine¶	0.593	0.25-1.39
Thoracic¶	1.96	1.43-2.68
Venous¶	0.134	0.05-0.37
Urologic¶	1.36	0.82-2.28

ASA, American Society of Anesthesiologists; *CI*, confidence interval; *OR*, odds ratio.
*The estimate and the standard error (SE) refer to the estimate of the logistic regression coefficient for the specific variable and its associated SE. C-statistic, 0.894.
†Reference group, independent functional status.
‡Reference group, ASA class 5.
§Reference group, preoperative systemic inflammatory response syndrome.
¶Reference group, hernia surgery.
From Gupta H, Gupta PK, Fang X, et al. Development and validation of a risk calculator predicting postoperative respiratory failure. *Chest.* 2011;140:1207–1215.

5% of this population has bronchospasm. Some investigators recommend using inhaled bronchodilators as first-line drugs and reducing the dose of inhaled steroids, such as beclomethasone dipropionate, budesonide, mometasone, and fluticasone, which are inactivated after absorption. However, in large doses, these "inhaled" steroids can suppress adrenal function, and supplemental systemic corticosteroids may be needed at times of stress (see the earlier discussion in the section on adrenocortical malfunction). Preoperative assessment must include gaining knowledge of drug regimens and their effects and education of the patient regarding proper use of an inhaler (Box 32.4), given that these drugs can interact dangerously with anesthetics (see the last section of this chapter) or can be used inappropriately and therefore produce side effects without maximum benefit.[199-209] No known interaction between the inhaled anticholinergic ipratropium bromide and muscle relaxants has been reported. An estimated 10% of asthmatic patients exhibit sensitivity to aspirin and may react not only to compounds containing aspirin but also to tartrazine, yellow dye

BOX 32.4 Procedures for Correct Use of a Metered-Dose Inhaler

Remove the cap and hold the inhaler upright.
Shake the inhaler.
Tilt the head back slightly and exhale steadily to functional residual capacity.
Position the inhaler by using a spacer between the actuator and the mouth.
Press down on the inhaler while taking a slow, deep breath (3-5 s).
Hold the full inspiration for at least 5 and up to 10 s, if possible, to allow the medication to reach deeply into the lungs.
Repeat inhalations as directed. Waiting 1 min after inhalation of the bronchodilator may permit subsequent inhalations to penetrate more deeply into the lungs and is necessary to ensure proper delivery of the dose. Rinse your mouth and expectorate after using the inhaler.

number five, indomethacin, other nonsteroidal antiinflammatory drugs, and aminopyrine.[244]

Cystic fibrosis is characterized by dilatation and hypertrophy of the bronchial glands, mucous plugging of the peripheral airways, and frequently, bronchitis, bronchiectasis, and bronchiolectasis. For all these conditions, the measures recommended earlier in this section, as well as appropriate hydration to allow mobilization of secretions, constitute optimal preprocedure therapy.

Surgical resection is the primary therapy for non–small cell carcinomas (e.g., adenocarcinoma, squamous cell carcinoma, and large cell carcinoma). These carcinomas account for 75% of all lung carcinomas, 12% of all malignant tumors, and 20% of all cancer deaths in the United States.[245] Success of surgery can be predicted by the stage of the tumor.

The combination of chemotherapy and radiation therapy is the current treatment of choice for small cell carcinomas of the lung.[246] Oat cell (small cell) carcinoma of the lung and bronchial adenomas are known for their secretion of endocrinologically active substances, such as ACTH-like hormones. Squamous cell cancers in the superior pulmonary sulcus produce Horner syndrome, as well as characteristic pain in areas served by the eighth cervical nerves and first and second thoracic nerves. These tumors are now treated with preoperative radiation; surgical resection leads to an almost 30% "cure" rate. For all these patients, their preoperative assessment should be viewed as a "three-legged stool," including lung mechanics, parenchymal function, and cardiopulmonary reserve.

Anaphylaxis, Anaphylactoid Responses, and Allergic Disorders Other than Those Related to Lung Diseases and Asthma

Anaphylactic and Anaphylactoid Reactions. Anaphylaxis is a severe life-threatening allergic reaction. Allergic applies to immunologically mediated reactions, as opposed to those caused by pharmacologic idiosyncrasy, direct toxicity or drug overdosage, or drug-drug interaction.[247-249] Anaphylaxis is the typical immediate hypersensitivity reaction (type I) produced by immunoglobulin E (IgE) mediated release of pharmacologically active substances. These mediators in turn produce specific end-organ responses in the skin (urticaria), the respiratory system (bronchospasm and upper airway edema), and the cardiovascular system (vasodilation, changes in inotropy, and increased capillary permeability). Vasodilation occurs at the level of the capillary and postcapillary venule and leads to erythema, edema, and smooth muscle contraction. This clinical syndrome is called *anaphylaxis*. By contrast, an *anaphylactoid reaction* denotes an identical or very similar clinical response that is not mediated by IgE or (usually) an antigen-antibody process.[248,249] A large perioperative database review found that hemodynamically significant anaphylaxis occurred in 1 of every 8400 cases.[249a] Further, a personal history of anaphylaxis was the best predictor of occurrence.

In anaphylactic reactions, an injected or inhaled (or ingested) substance—usually drugs, food, or insect venom—can serve as the allergen itself. Low-molecular-weight agents are believed to act as haptens that form immunologic conjugates with host proteins. The offending substance, regardless of whether it is a hapten, may be the parent compound, a nonenzymatically generated product, or a metabolic product formed in the patient's body. When an allergen binds immunospecific IgE antibodies on the surface of mast cells and basophils, histamine and eosinophilic chemotactic factors of anaphylaxis are released from storage granules in a calcium- and energy-dependent process.[248,249] Other chemical mediators are rapidly synthesized and are subsequently released in response to cellular activation. These mediators include the following: slow-reacting substance of anaphylaxis, which is a combination of three leukotrienes; other leukotrienes;[248,249] kinins; platelet-activating factors; adenosine; chemotactic factors; heparin; tryptase; chymase; and prostaglandins, including the potent bronchoconstrictor prostaglandin D_2; eosinophil growth and activating factors; mast cell growth factors; and proinflammatory and other factors that contribute to the IgE isotype switch.

The end-organ effects of the mediators produce the clinical syndrome of anaphylaxis. Usually, a first wave of symptoms, including those caused by vasodilation and a feeling of impending doom, is quickly followed by a second wave as the cascade of mediators amplifies the reactions. In a sensitized patient, onset of the signs and symptoms caused by these mediators is usually immediate but may be delayed 2 to 15 minutes or, in rare instances, as long as 2.5 hours after the parenteral injection of antigen.[250,251] After oral administration, manifestations may occur at unpredictable times.

Mast cell proliferation, together with severe progressive inflammation, contributes to the worsening of symptoms that occurs even after an allergen load is no longer present. The antigen present in cells and lymphocytes, as well as activated mast cells, starts to induce the production of cytokines. These proinflammatory cytokines recruit more inflammatory cells, a process that leads to tissue edema and mediates a second wave of mast cell degranulation. This second wave can promote the recurrence of severe symptoms 6 to 8 hours later and necessitates, some believe, at least 8 hours of continued ICU-like observation.

In addition, biologically active mediators can be generated by multiple effector processes to produce an anaphylactoid reaction. Activation of the blood coagulation and fibrinolytic systems, the kinin-generating sequence, or the complement cascade can produce the same inflammatory substances that result in an anaphylactic reaction. The two mechanisms known to activate the complement system are called classical and alternative. The classical pathway can be initiated through IgG or IgM (transfusion reactions) or plasmin. The alternative pathway can be activated by lipopolysaccharides (endotoxin), drugs (Althesin), radiographic contrast media,[252] membranes (nylon tricot membranes for bubble oxygenators), cellophane membranes of dialyzers, vascular graft material,[253] latex or latex-containing products,[254,255] and perfluorocarbon artificial blood.

Muscle relaxants were previously believed to be the most common drug associated with anaphylaxis, though recent evidence supports protamine and antibiotics with increased risk.[249a] However, this may change with the recent approval of sugammadex as one of the primary concerns regarding the delaying its approval in the United States was "hypersensitivity reactions," which includes anaphylaxis. Latex continues to account for a significant number of these reactions, and the incidence of intraoperative anaphylaxis caused by latex is increasing. In addition, histamine can be liberated independent of immunologic reactions.[256] Mast cells and basophils release histamine in response to chemicals or drugs. Most narcotics can release histamine,[256] and they can produce an anaphylactoid reaction, as can radiographic contrast media.[252] What makes some patients more susceptible to the release of histamine in response to drugs is unknown, but hereditary and environmental factors may play a role.

Intravenous contrast material is probably the most frequently used agent that causes anaphylactoid reactions. Because diagnostic (skin and other) tests are helpful only in IgE-mediated reactions, pretesting is not useful for contrast reactions. Pretreatment with diphenhydramine, cimetidine (or ranitidine), and corticosteroids has been reported to be useful in preventing or ameliorating anaphylactoid reactions to intravenous contrast material.[252,257] Unfortunately, very large doses of steroids (1 g of methylprednisolone intravenously) may be necessary to obtain a beneficial effect, though the efficacy of large-dose steroid therapy has not been confirmed.[258] Other common substances associated with anaphylactic or anaphylactoid reactions that may merit preoperative therapy include antibiotics, intravascular volume expanders, and blood products.[258] The anesthesiologist should always be prepared perioperatively to treat an anaphylactic or anaphylactoid response.

Minimizing Risks Preoperatively. Although virtually all evidence on this subject is merely anecdotal, enough consistent thought recurs through the literature to justify proposing an optimal approach to these problems. First, predisposing factors should be sought; patients with a history of atopy or allergic rhinitis should be suspected of being at risk. Other risk factors of note include multiple previous procedures, history of spina bifida, history of asthma, food allergies associated with latex allergy (including avocado, kiwi, banana, pineapple, papaya, chestnut, and buckwheat), systemic mastocytosis, and hereditary angioedema.[258a] Because anaphylactic and anaphylactoid reactions to contrast media occur 5 to 10 times more frequently in patients with a previously suspected reaction, consideration should be given to the administration of low-osmotic agents and both H_1- and H_2-receptor antagonists for 16 to 24 hours before exposing these patients to a suspected allergen. H_1-receptor antagonists appear to require this much time to act on the receptor. Volume status can be optimized,[248] and perhaps large doses of steroids (1 g of hydrocortisone) should also be administered before exposing patients to agents associated with a high incidence of anaphylactic or anaphylactoid reactions.[258] Older patients and patients taking β-adrenergic blocking drugs present special problems; they are at higher risk of having complications from both pretreatment (especially vigorous hydration) and therapy for anaphylactic reactions (glucagon is useful here to overcome epinephrine resistance) and are less responsive to treatment regimens.[259] One approach is to avoid drugs likely to trigger anaphylactic or anaphylactoid reactions or alter the treatment protocol for this group. Drawing blood for later analysis, especially of tryptase, can be useful in clarifying the diagnosis.[260]

With the increasing incidence of latex hypersensitivity, attempts have been made to make much of the operating room environment latex free; however, costs and preferences have resulted in the continued use of latex-containing gloves in many hospitals. Nonetheless, more hospitals are totally latex free. In allergic patients, care should be taken to ensure that no latex-containing products are present in the operating room.

Primary Immunodeficiency Diseases

Primary immunodeficiency diseases usually manifest early in life as recurrent infections. Along with survival achieved with antibiotic and antibody treatment have come new prominent features: cancer and allergic and autoimmune disorders.

Hereditary angioedema is an autosomal dominant genetic disease characterized by episodes of angioedema involving the subcutaneous tissues and submucosa of the GI tract and airway and often manifested as abdominal pain. These patients have a functionally impotent inhibitor or deficiency of an inhibitor to complement component C1 leading to an overproduction of bradykinin resulting in vascular permeability. The most feared complication for the anesthesiologist is airway edema resulting in an unexpected difficult airway.[260a] The mainstay of treatment of an acute attack is supportive because epinephrine, antihistamines, and corticosteroids often fail to work. The severity of attacks can be prevented or decreased by drugs that are either antifibrinolytics (e.g., ε-aminocaproic acid [EACA] and tranexamic acid) or attenuated androgens (e.g., danazol and stanozolol). Because trauma can precipitate acute attacks, prophylactic therapy with plasma derived C1-INH, attenuated androgens, antifibrinolytics, or all three is recommended before elective surgery; a repeat dose of C1-INH can be given if edema develops.[260a] Fresh frozen plasma has been used during acute attacks with success because it contains C1-INH, though FFP could theoretically worsen an attack, as it contains other complement components and should only be used if no other treatment is available.[260a]

Most of the 1 in 700 persons who have selective IgA deficiency (i.e., <5 mg/dL) have repeated serious infections or connective tissue disorders. These infections commonly involve the respiratory tract (e.g., sinusitis, otitis) or GI tract (manifested as diarrhea, malabsorption, or both). If the patient has rheumatoid arthritis, Sjögren syndrome, or systemic lupus erythematosus, the anesthetist should consider the possibility of an isolated IgA deficiency;

however, patients with this disorder can be otherwise healthy. Because antibodies to IgA may develop in these patients if they were previously exposed to IgA (as could occur from a previous blood transfusion), subsequent blood transfusions can cause anaphylaxis, even when they contain washed erythrocytes. Transfusions should therefore consist of blood donated by another IgA-deficient patient.

Many immunomodulators are now being given to augment cancer treatments[261]; no interactions among these modulators, no effects on the incidence of immune reactions during anesthesia, and no interactions with anesthetic effects have been reported except those regarding immunosuppressant drugs (see the last section of this chapter).

Immunonutrition is increasingly being used preprocedurally by patients and prescribed by providers to decrease inflammatory responses.[254] Whereas excellent data on the benefits of probiotics in changing the intestinal milieu to decrease inflammation can be found, data on probiotics' role in prevention of intestinal complications, improvement in wound healing, incidence of perioperative infections is under investigation, though benefits may outweigh the risks.[261a-c]

Diseases of the Central Nervous System, Neuromuscular Diseases, and Psychiatric Disorders

Evaluation of a patient with neurologic or psychiatric disease can be found in Chapter 31. Information gathered from the history that warrants further investigation includes a previous need for postoperative ventilation in a patient without inordinate lung disease, which indicates the possibility of metabolic neurologic disorders such as porphyria, myopathies, neuropathies, and neuromuscular disorders such as myasthenia gravis. Other historical information warranting further investigation includes the use of drugs such as the following: steroids; guanidine; anticonvulsant, anticoagulant, and antiplatelet drugs; lithium; tricyclic antidepressants; phenothiazines; and butyrophenones.

Although preoperative treatment of most neurologic disorders may not lessen perioperative morbidity, knowledge of the pathophysiologic characteristics of these disorders is important in planning intraoperative and postoperative management. Thus preoperative knowledge about these disorders and their associated conditions (e.g., cardiac arrhythmias with Duchenne muscular dystrophy, or respiratory and cardiac muscle weakness with dermatomyositis) may reduce perioperative morbidity. A primary goal of neurologic evaluation is to determine the site of the lesion in the nervous system. Such localization to one of four levels (supratentorial compartment, posterior fossa, spinal cord, peripheral nervous system) is essential for accurate diagnosis and appropriate management. (Disorders accompanied by increased intracranial pressure and cerebrovascular disorders are discussed in Chapters 11 and 57.)

COMA

Little is known about specific anesthetic, perioperative, or periprocedural choices that alter outcome for a comatose patient, but as for all other conditions, the cause of the coma should be known so that drugs can be avoided that may worsen the condition or that may not be metabolized because of organ dysfunction. First, the patient should be observed. Yawning, swallowing, or licking of the lips implies a "light" coma with major brainstem function intact. If consciousness is depressed but respiration, pupillary reactivity to light, and eye movements are normal and no focal motor signs are present, metabolic depression is likely. Abnormal pupillary responses may indicate hypoxia, hypothermia, local eye disease, or drug intoxication with belladonna alkaloids, narcotics, benzodiazepines, or glutethimide; pupillary responses may also be abnormal, however, after the use of eye drops. Other metabolic causes of coma include uremia, hypoglycemia, hepatic coma, alcohol ingestion, hypophosphatemia, myxedema, and hyperosmolar nonketotic coma. Except in extreme emergencies, such as uncontrolled bleeding or a perforated viscus, care should be taken to render the patient as metabolically normal as possible before the surgical procedure. This practice and documenting the findings on the chart preoperatively lessen any confusion regarding the cause of intraoperative and postoperative problems. However, too rapid correction of uremia or hyperosmolar nonketotic coma can lead to cerebral edema, a shift of water into the brain as a result of a reverse osmotic effect caused by dysequilibrium of the urea concentration.

The physical examination is extremely helpful preoperatively in assessing the prognosis. Arms flexed at the elbow (i.e., decorticate posture) imply bilateral hemisphere dysfunction but an intact brainstem, whereas extension of the legs and arms (bilateral decerebrate posture) implies bilateral damage to structures at the upper brainstem or deep hemisphere level. Seizures are often seen in patients with uremia and other metabolic encephalopathies. Hyperreflexia and upward-pointing toes suggest a structural CNS lesion or uremia, hypoglycemia, or hepatic coma; hyporeflexia and downward-pointing toes with no hemiplegia generally indicate the absence of a structural CNS lesion. It is important to compare preoperative physical examination with previous different providers' examinations, trending Glasgow Coma Scores can provide utility and standardization.

EPILEPTIC SEIZURES

A seizure is the term for the clinical event defined as a paroxysmal alteration in neurologic function caused by a synchronous, rhythmic depolarization of brain cortical neurons. Epilepsy is the condition manifested by recurrent, unprovoked seizures. Epileptic seizures result from paroxysmal neuronal discharges of abnormally excitable neurons. Six percent to 10% of individuals younger than 70 years old will experience a seizure at some time during their lifetime. Fifty percent to 70% of patients with one seizure will never have another. However, 70% of people with two seizures will have an epileptic focus, be candidates for antiseizure medications, and be subject to withdrawal seizures after anesthesia if such medications are not continued.[262] Overall, epilepsy has a prevalence of 0.5% to 1% of the population, with the highest incidence in extremes of age and in those with anatomic neurologic abnormalities.[262a]

Sometimes syncopal episodes can be mistaken for seizures, especially when interviews are compressed in the short time frame of a preoperative visit. Twenty-five percent of patients with a seizure have a normal electroencephalogram (EEG) when they are interictal; thus a negative EEG result does not indicate that someone with a seizure will not have a withdrawal seizure when emerging from anesthesia. Seizures can be generalized (arising from deep midline structures in the brainstem or thalamus, usually without an aura or focal features during the seizure), partial focal motor, or sensory (the initial discharge comes from a focal unilateral area of the brain, often preceded by an aura). As with cerebrovascular accidents and coma, knowing the origin may be crucial to understanding the pathophysiologic processes of the disease and to managing the patient's intraoperative and postoperative course.

Epileptic seizures can arise from discontinuation of sedative-hypnotic drugs or alcohol, use of narcotics, uremia, traumatic injury, neoplasms, infection, congenital malformation, birth injury, drug use (e.g., amphetamines, cocaine), hypercalcemia or hypocalcemia, blood in the ventricle or hypoxia, and vascular disease and vascular accidents. Up to 30% of patients with severe traumatic brain injury develop early seizures (within 7 days of injury).[262b] Thirty percent of epileptic seizures have no known cause. Most partial seizures are caused by structural brain abnormalities (secondary to tumor, trauma, stroke, infection, and other causes).

Most authorities believe that anticonvulsant medications should be given in the therapeutic range,[262-264] and they should be continued through the morning of the surgical procedure, even in pregnant women. They should also be given postoperatively, even in mothers who plan to breastfeed, according to guidelines published by the American Academy of Neurology. Many of the epileptic drugs, including phenytoin, carbamazepine, and phenobarbiturate, alter the hepatic metabolism of many drugs and induce cytochrome P450 enzyme activity. Drug-drug interactions are much less problematic with the newer epileptic drugs such as gabapentin and topirimate.[262] Appropriate treatment of status epilepticus refractory to antiepileptic drugs includes general anesthesia and carries high morbidity.[264] In one controlled trial, phenobarbital was more rapidly effective in controlling status epilepticus than was diazepam followed by phenytoin.[264] The frequency of side effects and of required tracheal intubation was similar for both regimens. Thus other than the use of current drug therapy and heeding precautions taken for the underlying disease, no known changes in perioperative management seem to be indicated, though many agents may possess both proconvulsant and anticonvulsant properties pending dose utilized; therefore knowledge of anesthetics agents is crucial.

INFECTIOUS DISEASES OF THE CENTRAL NERVOUS SYSTEM, DEGENERATIVE DISORDERS OF THE CENTRAL NERVOUS SYSTEM, AND HEADACHE

Many degenerative CNS disorders have been traced to slowly developing viral diseases or even the presence of certain proteins or viral particles ("prions"). No special perioperative anesthetic considerations appear to apply for infectious disorders of the CNS other than those for increased intracranial pressure and avoidance of occupational exposure and transmission of disease to healthcare workers. The appropriate prophylactic measures to take if one comes in contact with meningococcal disease or other infectious CNS diseases are still not well established. The use of *H. influenzae* type B vaccine has made meningitis an adult disease.[265]

Parkinson disease is a degenerative disorder of the CNS that may or may not be caused by a virus. Clinically, Parkinson disease, chronic manganese intoxication, phenothiazine or butyrophenone toxicity, Wilson disease, Huntington chorea, the effects of street drug toxins such as methylphenyltetrahydropyridine, and carbon monoxide encephalopathy all have similar initial features: bradykinesia, muscular rigidity, and tremor.

In Parkinson disease, therapy is directed at (1) increasing presence of dopamine, (2) increasing the neuronal release of dopamine or the receptor's response to dopamine, (3) stimulating the receptor directly with dopamine agonists (i.e., bromocriptine), (4) direct stimulation of dopaminergic tissue (i.e., deep brain stimulator), or (5) decreasing cholinergic activity. Anticholinergic agents have been the initial drugs of choice because they decrease tremor more than muscle rigidity. Dopamine does not pass the blood-brain barrier, so its precursor L-dopa (levodopa) is used. Unfortunately, L-dopa is decarboxylated to dopamine in the periphery and can cause nausea, vomiting, and arrhythmia. These side effects are diminished by the administration of α-methylhydrazine (carbidopa), a decarboxylase inhibitor that does not pass the blood-brain barrier. Refractoriness to L-dopa develops, and it is now debated whether the drug should be used only when symptoms cannot be controlled with other anticholinergic medications. "Drug holidays" have been suggested as one means of restoring the effectiveness of these compounds, but cessation of such therapy may result in marked deterioration of function and need for hospitalization. Therapy for Parkinson disease should be initiated preoperatively and be continued through the morning of the surgical procedure; such treatment seems to decrease drooling, the potential for aspiration, and ventilatory weakness.[266,267] Reinstituting therapy promptly after surgery is crucial,[263,266-270] as is avoiding drugs such as the phenothiazines and butyrophenones, which inhibit the release of dopamine or compete with dopamine at the receptor.[266] Carbidopa or levodopa in low doses (20-200 mg nightly vs. the usual 60-600 mg/day for Parkinson disease) is commonly used in the nonparkinsonian restless leg syndrome of older adults (present in 2%-5% of individuals >60 years old). This drug also should be given the night before and the night immediately after the surgical procedure. Clozapine does not appear to worsen the movement disorders of Parkinson disease and has been used postoperatively to stop levodopa-induced hallucinations. Patients with Parkinson disease may also undergo deep brain stimulation under monitored anesthesia care. Postoperatively patients with Parkinson disease benefit from early physical therapy, appropriate analgesia, pulmonary hygiene, and autonomic assessment with necessary intervention.[270a]

Dementia, a progressive decline in intellectual function, can be caused by treatable infections (e.g., syphilis, cryptococcosis, coccidioidomycosis, Lyme disease, tuberculosis), depression (a trial of antidepressants is indicated in most patients), side effects of medications (digitalis has slowed brain function more than the heart rate), myxedema, vitamin B_{12} deficiency, chronic drug or alcohol intoxication, metabolic causes (liver and renal failure), neoplasms, partially treatable infections (HIV), untreatable infections (Creutzfeldt-Jakob syndrome), or decreased acetylcholine in the cerebral cortex (Alzheimer disease). This last condition occurs in more than 0.5% of Americans.[271-274] As of 2013, some degree of Alzheimer disease affects approximately 11% of Americans aged 65 and older, and affects approximately 32% of Americans aged 85 and older.[274a] Although these patients are often given cholinergic agonists, controlled trials of these drugs have not as yet shown major significant benefit.[272,273,275] Gingko has improved subjective symptoms in 37% of patients versus 23% of those given placebo. Although further controlled trials failed to confirm its benefit in early Alzheimer disease or in healthy older individuals, gingko is still popular. Cholinergic medications improve functioning in patients with Alzheimer disease.[276] These families often desire surgery, but the interactions of these drugs and therapies with perioperative analgesic and anesthetic drug therapies are not well established. One case report noted intraoperative bradycardia in such patients with two cholinergic drugs.[277] A link may exist among Alzheimer disease, postoperative cognitive dysfunction, and inhaled anesthetics.[278,278a] Deposition of β-amyloid can occur in animals exposed to inhaled anesthetics.[279-281] Whether this link is clinically relevant in humans remains to be determined. Most reversible dementias represent either delirium (commonly infection, metabolic, or drug induced) or depression.[272,273,282] Creutzfeldt-Jakob disease (prion driven) has been transmitted inadvertently by surgical instruments and corneal transplants; the causative virus or protein particle is not inactivated by heat, disinfectants, or formaldehyde.

More than 90% of patients with chronic recurring headaches are categorized as having migraine, tension, or cluster headaches. The mechanism of tension or cluster headaches may not differ qualitatively from that of migraine headaches; all may be manifestations of labile vasomotor regulation.[283] A headache is said to be migraine if it is characterized by four of the following five "POUNDing" conditions: if it is Pulsating, if it lasts One day or more, if it is Unilateral, if Nausea occurs, and if it Disturbs daily activities.[284]

Treatment of cluster and migraine headaches centers on the use of serotonin drugs such as sumatriptan or ergotamine and its derivatives.[283-285] Other drugs that may be effective are propranolol, calcium channel inhibitors, cyproheptadine, prednisone, antihistamines, tricyclic antidepressants, phenytoin, and diuretic drugs, as well as biofeedback techniques. Giant cell arteritis, glaucoma, and all the meningitides, including Lyme disease, are other causes of headache that may benefit from preoperative treatment.[286] No other special treatment is indicated preoperatively for a patient who has a well-delineated cause for the headaches. Acute migraine attacks can sometimes be terminated by ergotamine tartrate aerosol or by injection of sumatriptan or dihydroergotamine mesylate intravenously; general anesthesia has also been used. We normally continue all prophylactic headache medicine, although the decision to continue aspirin through the morning of the surgical procedure is usually left to the surgeon.

BACK PAIN, NECK PAIN, AND SPINAL CANAL SYNDROMES

Acute spinal cord injury is discussed earlier in the section on autonomic dysfunction. Although it is a common problem, little is written about the anesthetic management of syndromes related to herniated disks, spondylosis (usually of advancing age), and the congenital narrowing of the cervical and lumbar spinal canal that gives rise to symptoms of nerve root compression. One report stresses the importance of the vascular component in the mechanism of damage to the spinal cord and hence the theoretic desirability of slight hypertension perioperatively.[287] Another report suggests the use of awake intubation, a fiberoptic bronchoscope, and monitoring of evoked potentials.[288] Patients with back pain may be receiving large doses of narcotics that may influence the anesthetic plan and necessitate the need for a perioperative multimodal analgesic approach, including the continuation of home analgesic regimens. A thoughtful preanesthetic discussion with the patient regarding analgesia following surgery is essential for a successful postsurgical regimen.

DEMYELINATING DISEASES

Demyelinating diseases constitute a diffuse group of diseases ranging from those with uncertain cause (e.g., multiple sclerosis, in which genetic, epidemiologic, and immunologic factors are probably all involved and interferon-β appears to be a promising treatment[289]) to those that follow infection, vaccination (e.g., Guillain-Barré syndrome), or antimetabolite treatment of cancer. Therefore, demyelinating diseases can have very diverse symptoms, with a risk of relapse of disease existing immediately after surgery. Because relapse may occur as a result of rapid electrolyte changes and hyperthermia in the perioperative period, such changes should be avoided and temperature tightly regulated.[289a] In addition, perioperative administration of steroids may be a protective measure.[100] Both spinal anesthesia and epidural anesthesia have been administered without problems.[290,291] Multiple sclerosis and demyelinating diseases in general are the most common causes of nontraumatic disability in young adults with a prevalence reported between 2 and 150/100,000 people.[289a] The age-adjusted survival rate is 80% of that of unaffected individuals (i.e., the average patient with multiple sclerosis ages 1.2 years for every year with the disease). No treatment alters most of these disease processes, although ACTH, steroids, interferon-β, glatiramer acetate (Copaxone), and plasmapheresis may ameliorate or abbreviate a relapse, or even alter disease progression, especially progression of multiple sclerosis and (if started within 2 weeks of onset) Guillain-Barré syndrome.[292] Such an effect is consonant with the hypothesis of an immunologic disorder as the cause of these diseases. Care should be taken to avoid succinylcholine in these patients because of the risk of hyperkalemia secondary to extrajunctional acetylcholine receptors.

METABOLIC DISEASES

Included in the category of metabolic diseases is nervous system dysfunction secondary to porphyrias, alcoholism, uremia, hepatic failure, and vitamin B_{12} deficiency. The periodic paralysis that can accompany thyroid disease is discussed in the later section on neuromuscular disorders.

Alcoholism or heavy alcohol intake is associated with the following: acute alcoholic hepatitis, the activity of

which declines as alcohol is withdrawn; myopathy and cardiomyopathy, which can be severe; and withdrawal syndromes. Within 6 to 8 hours of withdrawal, the patient may become tremulous, a state that usually subsides within days or weeks. Alcoholic hallucinosis and withdrawal seizures generally occur within 24 to 36 hours. These seizures are generalized grand mal attacks; when focal seizures occur, other causes should be sought. Delirium tremens usually appears within 72 hours of withdrawal and is often preceded by tremulousness, hallucinations, or seizures. These three symptoms, combined with perceptual distortions, insomnia, psychomotor disturbances, autonomic hyperactivity, and, in a large percentage of cases, another potentially fatal illness (e.g., bowel infarction or subdural hematoma), are components of delirium tremens. This syndrome is now treated with benzodiazepines. Nutritional disorders of alcoholism include alcoholic hypoglycemia and hypothermia, alcoholic polyneuropathy, Wernicke-Korsakoff syndrome, and cerebellar degeneration. In patients with alcoholism (i.e., those who drink at least two six packs of beer or one pint of hard alcohol/day or the equivalent), emergency surgery and anesthesia (despite alcoholic hepatitis), are not associated with worsening abnormalities in liver enzymes. In addition, approximately 20% of patients with alcoholism also have respiratory disease. Further, postoperatively these patients can have poor wound healing, altering levels of consciousness/delirium, and difficulty with analgesia.[292a] A patient who has a history of alcohol abuse therefore warrants careful examination of many systems for quantification of preoperative physical status.

Although hepatic failure can lead to coma with high-output cardiac failure, unlike uremia, it does not lead to chronic polyneuropathy. Uremic polyneuropathy is a distal symmetric sensorimotor polyneuropathy that may be improved by dialysis. The use of depolarizing muscle relaxants in patients with polyneuropathies has been questioned. We believe that patients who have neuropathy associated with uremia should not be given succinylcholine because of a possible exaggerated hyperkalemic response.

Pernicious anemia caused by vitamin B_{12} deficiency may result in subacute combined degeneration of the spinal cord; the signs are similar to those of chronic nitrous oxide toxicity. Both pernicious anemia and nitrous oxide toxicity are associated with peripheral neuropathy and disorders of the pyramidal tract and posterior column (which governs fine motor skills and the sense of body position). Combined-system disease can also occur without anemia, as can nitrous oxide toxicity in dentists and nitrous oxide abusers. Patients with vitamin B_{12} deficiency and anemia, if treated with folate, improve hematologically but progress to dementia and severe neuropathy. It may thus be prudent to give an intramuscular injection of 100 µg of vitamin B_{12} or 800 µg orally before giving folate to a patient who has signs of combined-system degeneration.[293]

The porphyrias are a constellation of metabolic diseases that result from an autosomally inherited lack of functional enzymes active in the synthesis of hemoglobin. Fig. 32.6 schematically depicts the abnormalities that result from these enzyme deficits. Type 1, 3, and 4 porphyrias can cause life-threatening neurologic abnormalities. These conditions are characterized by the presence of aminolevulinic

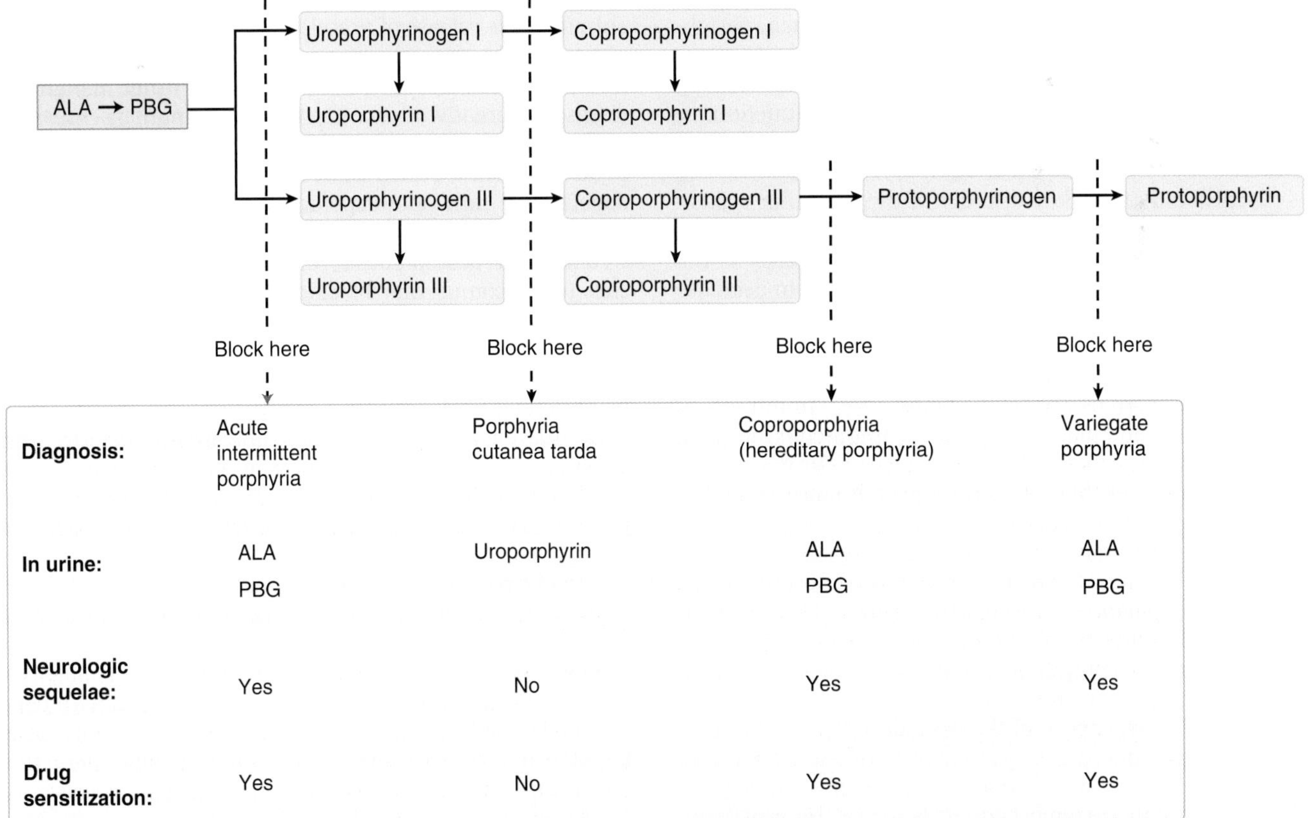

Fig. 32.6 Schematic depiction of the functional enzyme deficits that occur in some of the porphyrias. *ALA*, Aminolevulinic acid; *PBG*, porphobilinogen.

acid (ALA) or porphobilinogen, or both, in urine; these substances do not occur in porphyria cutanea tarda, a disease that does not incur neurologic sequelae.[294] In acute intermittent porphyria, the typical pattern consists of acute attacks of colicky pain, nausea, vomiting, severe constipation, psychiatric disorders, and lesions of the lower motoneuron that can progress to bulbar paralysis. Often, these patients will have had multiple previous surgeries. Certain drugs can induce the enzyme ALA synthetase and thereby exacerbate the disease process.[295-297] Drugs considered unsafe include barbiturates (all types), phenytoin, valproic acid, carbamazepine, primidone, oral contraceptives, progestins, carisoprodol, and sprinolactone.[297a] Clonazepam, ketamine, imipramine, sulfa antibiotics, erythromycin, fluconazole, nitrofurantoin, and rifampicin are considered possibly unsafe and should be used with caution.[297a] Patients can have attacks during infection, fasting, or menstruation. Administration of glucose suppresses ALA synthetase activity and prevents or ablates acute attacks. Drugs used in anesthetic management that are reported to be safe for patients with porphyria include neostigmine, atropine, succinylcholine, nitrous oxide, procaine, propofol, etomidate, meperidine, fentanyl, morphine, droperidol, promazine, promethazine, and chlorpromazine.[295-297] Although ketamine has previously been used, postoperative psychoses attributable to the disease may be difficult to distinguish from those possibly caused by ketamine. Propofol has been used without provoking porphyria in at least two susceptible patients.[295,296]

NEUROMUSCULAR DISORDERS

Neuromuscular disorders consist of conditions affecting any major component of the motor unit: motoneuron, peripheral nerve, neuromuscular junction, and muscle. Neuropathies may involve all components of the nerve, thereby producing sensory, motor, and autonomic dysfunction, or only one component. Myopathies may involve the proximal muscles, the distal muscles, or both.

Myasthenia gravis is a disorder of the muscular system caused by partial blockade or destruction of nicotinic acetylcholine receptors by IgG antibodies. The severity of the disease correlates with the ability of antibodies to decrease the number of available acetylcholine receptors.[298] Treatment of myasthenia is usually begun with anticholinesterase drugs, but in moderate and severe disease, treatment progresses to steroids and thymectomy.[298,299] Immunosuppressive drugs and plasmapheresis are initiated if the more conservative measures fail, and intravenous immunoglobulin, a rapid-onset therapy, is reserved for acute exacerbations and myasthenic crises.[298,299]

One major problem for the anesthesiologist involves the use of muscle relaxants and their reversal.[300] Because much of the care of patients with myasthenia gravis involves tailoring the amount of anticholinesterase medication to the maximal muscle strength of the patient, derangement of the course of the patient during the surgical procedure could necessitate reassessment of the drug dosage. For that reason, all anticholinergic drugs may be withheld for 6 hours preoperatively, and medication should be reinstituted postoperatively with extreme caution because the sensitivity of these patients to such drugs may have changed. Small doses of succinylcholine can be used to facilitate endotracheal intubation; extremely small doses of nondepolarizing drugs can be used for intraoperative relaxation not achieved by regional anesthesia or volatile anesthetics. Of prime importance is monitoring neuromuscular blockade as the guide for muscle relaxant administration and their reversal. Previously, controlled mechanical ventilation was frequently required for 24 to 48 hours postoperatively; however, immediate extubation has become more common.[299-301] Postoperative ventilation is especially important in patients with myasthenia gravis of more than 6 years' duration, COPD, a daily pyridostigmine requirement of 750 mg in association with significant bulbar weakness, and vital capacity of less than 40 mL/kg (PFTs are an important part of the preoperative workup).[301] One study in myasthenic patients found rapid recovery of neuromuscular function in patients receiving rocuronium when sugammadex was used for reversal.[302] This combination could be a rational alternative for myasthenic patients for whom neuromuscular blockade is mandatory during surgical procedures. Another study found that epidural analgesia intra- and postoperatively reduced the requirement of mechanical ventilation following thymectomy, though this was retrospective in nature.[302a] This technique may provide benefit and allow for minimal use of muscle relaxation.

Lambert-Eaton syndrome (myasthenic syndrome) is characterized by proximal limb muscle weakness and is associated with antibodies directed against the voltage-gated calcium channels in presynaptic nerve terminals. Strength or reflexes typically increase with repetitive effort, as affected patients exhibit decreased release of acetylcholine at the neuromuscular junction and repetitive use increases the available junctional acetylcholine. Guanidine therapy enhances the release of acetylcholine from nerve terminals and improves strength. Men with this syndrome generally have small cell carcinoma of the lung or other malignant disease, whereas women often have malignant disease, sarcoidosis, thyroiditis, or a collagen-related vascular disease. In addition, these patients have increased sensitivity to both depolarizing and nondepolarizing muscle relaxants.[303] These patients have an increased risk of prolonged muscle weakness or postoperative respiratory failure after exposure to neuromuscular blocking drugs, particularly when untreated preoperatively.[303a] Lambert-Eaton syndrome is also associated with an autonomic nervous system defect manifested by gastroparesis, orthostatic hypotension, and urinary retention.

Dermatomyositis and polymyositis are characterized by proximal limb muscle weakness with dysphagia. These conditions are associated with malignant disease or collagen-related vascular disease and often involve respiratory and cardiac muscle.

Periodic paralysis is another disease in which sensitivity to muscle relaxants increases. Periodic weakness starts in childhood or adolescence and is precipitated by rest after exercise, sleep, cold, surgery, or pregnancy. Hypokalemic and hyperkalemic forms exist and are associated with cardiac arrhythmias. Like thyrotoxic periodic paralysis, these hypokalemic and hyperkalemic forms usually spare the respiratory muscles. Anesthetic management consists of minimizing stress, maintaining normal fluid and electrolyte status, and controlling body temperature.[303-306]

Patients with muscular dystrophy now survive into their late 20s or early 30s. Because the disease involves the muscles themselves and not their innervation, conduction anesthesia cannot produce adequate relaxation of tonic muscles. Gastric dilation is also a problem. As with the other forms of muscular dystrophy, most problems in myotonic dystrophy arise from cardiac arrhythmias and inadequacy of the respiratory muscles.[307] The preoperative workup for all muscular dystrophies should include echocardiography and PFTs.[307a] For all the forms of muscular dystrophy, problems have been related to exaggerated release of serum potassium after the administration of depolarizing muscle relaxants. Volatile anesthetics are associated with anesthesia-induced rhabdomyolysis, hyperkalemia, and cardiac arrest; therefore, total intravenous anesthesia is the preferred method of general anesthesia. Of note, sugammadex has been used with success for muscle relaxation reversal.[307a]

Malignant hyperthermia in the patient or in a relative of the patient merits careful history taking and at least consideration of performing a test for susceptibility to the condition. Prophylaxis with intravenous dantrolene sodium may also be warranted with high risk patients. Through genotyping malignant hyperthermia has been associated with central core disease, multiminicore myopathy, congenital myopathy with cores and rods, centronuclear myopathy, congenital fiber type disproportion, King-Denborough syndrome, periodic paralysis, nemaline rod myopathy, Native American myopathy, and idiopathic hyperCKemia.[307b] Further genotyping has demonstrated that Duchene muscular dystrophy and Beck muscular dystrophy are better classified as a nonmalignant hyperthermia anesthetic-induced rhabdomyolysis, despite similar clinical appearances.[307b] Appropriate preparation for a patient with previous masseter spasm, or trismus, remains a matter of considerable debate. Malignant hyperthermia occurs most frequently in children and adolescents; the incidence is 1 in 14,000 administrations of anesthesia. The incidence increases to 1 in 2500 patients requiring strabismus surgery.

DOWN SYNDROME

Down syndrome (trisomy 21) occurs once in 1000 live births. It is associated with congenital cardiac lesions such as endocardial cushion defects (40%), ventricular septal defects (27%), patent ductus arteriosus (12%), and tetralogy of Fallot (8%). Prophylactic antibiotics should be used before predictable bacteremic events. Down syndrome is also associated with upper respiratory infections, with atlantooccipital instability (in approximately 15% of patients[308-311]) and laxity of other joints, with thyroid hypofunction (50%), with an increased incidence of subglottic stenosis, and with enlargement of the tongue (or a decreased oral cavity size for a normal-sized tongue).[310,312] Often, the atlantooccipital instability is asymptomatic and undiagnosed, so all patients should be treated as though they have atlantooccipital instability. No abnormal responses to anesthetic agents or anesthetic adjuvants have been substantiated. A reported sensitivity to atropine has been disproved, although administration of atropine to any patient receiving digoxin for atrial fibrillation should be done with care.[312] Examination for the conditions associated with Down syndrome should precede surgery.

PREOPERATIVE PREDICTION OF INCREASED INTRACRANIAL PRESSURE DURING NEUROSURGERY

Symptoms and signs of increased intracranial pressure include morning headache or headache made worse by coughing, nausea, vomiting, disturbances in consciousness, history of large tumors, tumors involving the brainstem, neck rigidity, and papilledema. Patients with these signs, large ventricles (as seen on radiography or images of the brain), or edema surrounding supratentorial tumors should be considered at risk for intraoperative intracranial hypertension. These patients may benefit from preoperative treatment or anesthetic management that assumes this possibility.[313]

MENTAL DISORDERS

Perhaps the most important preoperative consideration for patients with mental disorders, in addition to developing rapport, is understanding their specific drug therapy and its effects and side effects. Lithium, tricyclic antidepressants, selective serotonin reuptake inhibitors (SSRIs), other antidepressants that defy classification (e.g., bupropion), phenothiazines, butyrophenones, and MAOIs are used in these patients.[314] These drugs have potent effects and side effects that are discussed in the last section of this chapter, on drug therapy.

Renal Disease and Electrolyte Disorders

The anesthesiologist has an important role to play in preventing the onset and consequences of renal failure and its initiators. The linking of renal failure to electrolyte disorders is more obvious: the kidney is the primary organ for regulating body osmolality and fluid volume and has a major role in excretion of the end products of metabolism. In performing these functions, the kidney becomes intimately involved in the excretion of electrolytes.

A patient with renal insufficiency whose own kidneys are still functioning is distinct not only from a patient with end-stage renal disease whose renal functions are provided by dialysis but also from a patient who has a transplanted kidney. These three groups of patients require very different preoperative preparation. In addition, acute changes in renal function present quite a different problem than do chronic alterations in function. Certain renal diseases require different preoperative preparation than others, but generally, renal disease of any origin presents the same preoperative problems.

RENAL DISEASE

Causes and Systemic Effects of Renal Disorders

Nephrotic syndrome may develop in patients with glomerular diseases without disturbing tubular function. The soundness of tubular function is an important consideration because tubular dysfunction with attendant uremia presents problems quite different from those presented by glomerular disease with only nephrotic syndrome. This is not to minimize the adverse effects of glomerular disease; nephrotic syndrome consists of massive proteinuria and consequent hypoalbuminemia. The resulting reduction in plasma oncotic pressure diminishes plasma volume and calls forth compensatory mechanisms that result in retention of sodium and water. As a result, a common clinical finding in nephrotic syndrome is diffuse edema. Thus patients with nephrotic syndrome may have excess total-body water and decreased intravascular volume. In addition, diuretics are often given in an attempt to decrease edema. Although serum creatinine and creatinine clearance estimations have limitations as indices of the GFR (insulin clearance is the reference standard), these measurements are, for now, the most readily available to the anesthesiologist. Plasma creatinine levels reflect endogenous muscle catabolism and dietary intake, as well as urinary excretion. Urinary excretion depends on both filtration and secretion by the kidney. Drugs that are commonly used in the preoperative and perioperative periods can distort this measure of glomerular filtration. Moreover, the commonly used methods for measuring creatinine have a 95% confidence limit of greater than 20% for a GFR higher than 30 mL/min. Thus a normal creatinine level of 1.3 mg/dL may give a measured value ranging from 1.1 to 1.5 mg/dL.

Furthermore, in patients with nephrotic syndrome in whom renal tubular function has been preserved, hypovolemia appears to be a significant cause of deteriorating tubular renal function.[315-317] No randomized study has shown that close control of intravascular volume status in these groups of patients preserves renal tubular function (or any other measure of perioperative morbidity) to a greater degree than does less rigid control.

Uremia, the end result of renal tubular failure (i.e., failure of the concentrating, diluting, acidifying, and filtering functions) manifests in many ways. Changes occur in the cardiovascular, immunologic, hematologic, neuromuscular, pulmonary, and endocrine systems, as well as in bone. These alterations are ascribed either to the toxic end products of protein metabolism or to an imbalance in functioning of the kidney. As the number of functioning nephrons diminishes, the still-functioning nephrons attempt to increase some solute and body composition preservation functions at the expense of other functions, such as excretion of phosphate. The accumulation of phosphate increases PTH levels, which in turn produce osteodystrophy. Osteodystrophy can be managed by (1) restriction of dietary phosphate, (2) the use of binding agents (e.g., aluminum hydroxide or carbonate) that bind with intestinal phosphate, (3) calcium supplementation, or (4) parathyroidectomy.

Certain alterations in patients with uremia, such as neuropathy, are most logically attributed to an accumulation of toxic metabolites. Peripheral neuropathy is most often sensory and involves the lower extremities, but it may also be motor; peripheral neuropathies are frequently improved with hemodialysis and can be dramatically reversed with renal transplantation. Tubular function is commonly assessed by acidifying and concentrating capabilities.[318] Although such tests are crude, these capabilities are usually readily evaluated by measuring urine pH and specific gravity. Along with the altered volume status and cardiac complications in uremic patients, autonomic neuropathy may contribute to hypotension during anesthesia. Atherosclerosis is often accelerated in uremic patients; hypertension, with its attendant consequences, is very common.

Cardiac failure frequently occurs in uremic patients because of the presence of many adverse conditions: anemia with increasing myocardial work, hypertension, atherosclerosis, and altered volume status. Pericarditis can manifest by pericardial rub alone or by pain (with or without hemorrhage), the ECG will show diffuse ST changes in multiple coronary distributions—when available, these should be correlated to previous coronary catherization findings. Cardiac tamponade should be ruled out on the basis of clinical features and by echocardiography if this diagnosis is seriously suspected preoperatively. In addition, cardiac tamponade should be treated or planned for preoperatively.

If anemia is present, its severity generally parallels the degree of uremia; chronically uremic patients seem to adapt well to anemia. No hard data have substantiated the need to give a preoperative blood transfusion to a chronically uremic patient, even when the preoperative hemoglobin is approaching 7 g/dL. Even in nonuremic patients in an ICU and during cardiac surgery, randomized trials were unable to demonstrate improved outcomes with a liberal transfusion strategy,[319] and transfusions increase the risk for immune system compromise.[320,321a] In uremic patients, coagulation and platelet adhesiveness may be abnormal, and factor VIII and von Willebrand factor activity may be decreased; often, these patients may require DDAVP for enhancement of coagulation intraoperatively. However, DDAVP must be used with caution as it can lead to fluid retention and hypotension with rapid infusion.[321b]

Uremic patients exhibit a wide variety of metabolic and endocrinologic disorders in addition to hyperparathyroidism, including impaired carbohydrate tolerance, insulin resistance, type IV hyperlipoproteinemia, autonomic insufficiency, hyperkalemia, and anion-gap acidosis (caused by an inability of the kidneys to reabsorb filtered bicarbonate and excrete sufficient ammonium into urine). Furthermore, the excretion and pharmacokinetics of drugs are different in uremic patients than in normal patients. In addition, complications of hemodialysis include nutritional deficiencies, electrolyte and fluid imbalances, and mental disorders. Because these conditions can lead to serious perioperative morbidity, they should be evaluated preoperatively.

As with uremic patients, preoperative optimization of volume status is paramount in patients with kidney stones, and both are affected by carbohydrate intolerance.[321,322] Seventy-five percent of all kidney stones are composed of calcium oxalate. Patients with these stones frequently take diuretic drugs, consume calcium- and citrate-rich foods, and restrict salt intake. Prevention of dehydration by institution of intravenous fluid therapy along with restricted oral intake of protein may be as important for these patients as it is for patients with struvite or uric acid stones. Struvite stones often result from urinary infection. Uric acid stones can be prevented by treatment with allopurinol, by preoperative hydration, or by alkalinization of urine. Acidosis may contribute to stone formation. Again, optimal intravascular volume status is important in preventing stones and preserving renal function. More thorough discussion of renal function and physiology is provided in Chapter 17. Chapter 59 deals with the complexities of managing patients for renal surgery and other urologic procedures.

Creatinine clearance in conjunction with free water clearance appears to be the most accurate way of quantifying, for pharmacokinetic purposes, the degree of decreased renal function.[322] For a patient with stable renal function, creatinine clearance, which is a rough estimate of GFR, can be approximated by noting the serum creatinine level: a doubling of the creatinine level represents a halving of the GFR. Thus a patient with a stable serum creatinine level of 2 mg/dL would have a GFR of approximately 60 mL/min. A stable serum creatinine level of 4 mg/dL would accompany a GFR of approximately 30 mL/min, and a stable serum creatinine level of 8 mg/dL would accompany a GFR of 15 mL/min or less.

$$\text{Creatinine clearance} = \frac{(140 - \text{Age [yr]}) \times \text{Body weight (kg)}}{72 \times \text{serum creatinine}\left(\frac{\text{mg}}{\text{dL}}\right)}$$

$$\text{Free water clearance} = \text{Urine flow (mL/hour)}$$

$$\frac{\text{Urine osmolality}\left(\frac{\text{mOsm}}{\text{L}}\right) \times \text{Urine flow}\left(\frac{\text{mL}}{\text{hour}}\right)}{\text{Plasma osmolality}\left(\frac{\text{mOsm}}{\text{L}}\right)}$$

Free water clearance is a measure of renal concentrating ability, and it is normally −25 to +100 mL/h; it becomes more positive in renal insufficiency states. It may also become more positive in patients who have a head injury or high blood alcohol levels or in those undergoing aggressive fluid infusion or administration of diuretics.[323]

Patients With Insufficient but Functioning Kidneys

One of the greatest challenges for the anesthesiologist is presented by patients with insufficient renal function whose renal function must be preserved during surgical procedures. In addition, the presence of chronic renal failure is associated with higher rates of perioperative cardiac morbidity, which may warrant further evaluation for the presence of occult CAD.[324] The many uremic symptoms and great perioperative morbidity associated with uremia can probably be avoided by attention to detail in the preoperative and perioperative management of patients with insufficient but still functioning kidneys.[315-317]

First, studies demonstrate that acute postoperative renal failure is associated with an extremely high mortality rate.[325] The development of perioperative renal dysfunction has multiple risk factors, the most important of which include preexisting renal disease, heart surgery involving cardiopulmonary bypass or aortic surgery involving cross-clamping of the thoracic or abdominal aorta, and ongoing sepsis. Perioperative renal dysfunction accounts for upward of 40% of all in-hospital cases of acute kidney injury.[325a]

Moreover, acute perioperative renal failure is most likely to occur in patients who have renal insufficiency before the surgical procedure, are older than 60 years, and have preoperative left ventricular dysfunction.[323,325] Proper preoperative hydration probably decreases mortality after acute renal failure induced by radiocontrast agents.[317] Clues to the presence of hypovolemia or hypervolemia should be sought from the history and physical examination (e.g., weight loss or gain, thirst, edema, orthostatic hypotension and tachycardia, flat neck veins, dry mucous membranes, decreased skin turgor). Other causes of deterioration in function in chronic renal insufficiency are low cardiac output or low renal blood flow (in prerenal azotemia, whether because of cardiac failure or fluid depletion from diuretic drugs, BUN often increases disproportionately to increases in creatinine), urinary tract infection, use of nephrotoxic drugs, hypercalcemia, and hyperuricemia. These conditions and drugs should be avoided; if any of these conditions exist, they should be treated preoperatively.

Management of patients with renal disease is discussed in Chapter 59.

Patients Undergoing Dialysis

Patients with chronic (and at times acute) renal failure require renal replacement therapy, including conventional intermittent hemodialysis, peritoneal dialysis, and continuous renal replacement therapy (CRRT). CRRT includes a wide variety of techniques whose perioperative management has been reviewed (Table 32.13).[326] Although the primary indication for CRRT is acute renal failure, it can also be used for fluid clearance, correction of electrolyte abnormalities, management of metabolic acidosis, and removal of some toxins. It can be used in surgical patients without significant hemodynamic abnormalities. These patients may return to the operating room, and their assessment and management may be complicated by the underlying disease and the use of systemic anticoagulation to prevent filter and circuit clotting. In patients undergoing intermittent treatment with hemodialysis or peritoneal dialysis, the procedure is discontinued before entering the operating room. For patients on CRRT, the anesthesiologist must determine the appropriateness of discontinuing the therapy. With short procedures,

TABLE 32.13 Characteristics of Renal Replacement Therapy

Renal Replacement Therapy	Blood Pump	Replacement Fluid (RF)/Dialysate (D)	Intraoperative Use
Conventional intermittent hemodialysis	Yes	D	No
Peritoneal dialysis	No	D	No
Slow continuous ultrafiltration	Yes/no	None	Yes
Continuous arteriovenous hemodialysis	No	D	No
Continuous arteriovenous hemodiafiltration	No	RF/D	No
Continuous venovenous hemofiltration	Yes	RF	Yes
Continuous venovenous hemodialysis	Yes	D	Yes
Continuous venovenous hemodiafiltration	Yes	RF/D	Yes

From Petroni KC, Cohen NH. Continuous renal replacement therapy: anesthetic implications. *Anesth Analg.* 2002;94:1288–1297.

the therapy can usually be stopped safely provided the initial indication for therapy has improved (i.e., resolution of acidosis or hyperkalemia). If continued, CRRT can also be used to manage fluids during the surgical procedure by changing the dialysate, but the effect on drug dosing must be recognized. In addition to effects on renal elimination of drugs, CRRT has effects resulting from changes in protein binding and volume of distribution, as well as drug removal effects from membrane permeability, membrane surface area, the ultrafiltration rate, and the dialysate flow rate.

Because a patient undergoing conventional dialysis has already lost natural renal functioning, the emphasis in preoperative assessment shifts toward protecting other organ systems and optimally maintaining vascular access sites for cannulation. Usually, this does not require invasive monitoring. Emphasis is placed on intravascular fluid volume and electrolyte status, which can be ascertained by knowing when the patient last underwent dialysis, how much weight was normally gained or lost with dialysis, whether the fluid loss was peritoneal or intravascular, and what electrolyte composition the blood was dialyzed against. Although preoperative dialysis may benefit patients who have hyperkalemia, hypercalcemia, acidosis, neuropathy, and fluid overload, the resulting dysequilibrium between fluid and electrolytes can cause problems. Because hypovolemia induced by dialysis can lead to intraoperative hypotension, we try to avoid weight and fluid reduction in patients undergoing preoperative dialysis focusing on clearance of solutes and management of acid-base balance.

When renal transplant recipients have subsequent surgical procedures, the status of their renal function must be determined (i.e., whether they have normal renal function, insufficient but still functioning kidneys, or end-stage renal disease requiring hemodialysis). Descriptions of side effects of immunosuppressive drugs should also be sought. The drugs used preoperatively and intraoperatively to prevent acute rejection themselves have serious side effects that encourage close monitoring of blood glucose and cardiovascular function.[327] Because renal transplantation greatly increases the risk of infection, it is very important to consider invasive monitoring carefully and if indicated follow strict aseptic technique.

Drugs in Patients With Renal Failure

Patients with renal azotemia have a threefold or higher risk of having an adverse drug reaction than do patients with normal renal function.[328-330] The risk is increased by two conditions. First, excessive pharmacologic effects result from high levels of a drug or its metabolite (e.g., the metabolite of meperidine) in blood because of physiologic changes in target tissues induced by the uremic state. An example is excessive sedation in a uremic patient with standard blood levels of sedative-hypnotic drugs. Second, excessive administration of electrolytes with drugs also increases the risk of having an adverse drug reaction. Administration of standard doses of drugs that depend on renal excretion for their elimination can result in drug accumulation and enhanced pharmacologic effect. In one report, patients with end-stage renal disease required significantly higher propofol doses to achieve the clinical endpoint of hypnosis than did patients with normal renal function.[330]

INFECTIOUS DISEASE

Sepsis is a leading cause of postoperative morbidity,[317,331] probably through a decrease in systemic vascular resistance related to activation of the complement system and other mediators. Thus attention to the effects of antibiotic drugs must be supplemented by attention to intravascular volume status.[315-317,331-333] The degree of impairment of the infected organ and its effect on anesthesia should be assessed. Further, note that not all sepsis is the same, and often the source requires special consideration. For instance, endocarditis merits examination of the following: intravascular volume status; antibiotic and other drug therapy and side effects[334]; myocardial function; and renal, pulmonary, neurologic, and hepatic function—organ systems that can be affected by endocarditis.

Although all surgery except emergency or essential operations is proscribed when an acute infectious disease is present, many such diseases (e.g., influenza and pneumococcal pneumonia) and even inflammatory conditions are becoming less frequent because of successful immunization recommendations and programs.[335] Furthermore, even though acute infections are less common, surgery in patients with chronic viral diseases such as hepatitis and HIV infection is more frequent. Many of these patients may also harbor opportunistic infections such as tuberculosis or may have other systemic problems. Whether anesthesia or surgery, or both, exacerbates these infections or their systemic manifestations is not clear.

ELECTROLYTE DISORDERS

Disorders of calcium, magnesium, and phosphate balance are discussed in the earlier section on diseases involving the endocrine system and disorders of nutrition.

Hyponatremia and Hypernatremia

Electrolyte disorders are usually detected by determining the levels of electrolytes in serum. These concentrations reflect the balance between water and electrolytes. The osmolality of all body fluids is normally maintained within the narrow physiologic range of 285 to 295 mOsm/kg H_2O by integration of three key processes: thirst, release of ADH, and responsiveness of the medullary collecting ducts to ADH. Because of the permeability of biologic membranes, intracellular osmolality and extracellular osmolality are almost always equal.

$$2\left[\mathrm{Na}^{2+}\right](\mathrm{mEq/L}) + \frac{[\mathrm{Glucose}]\,(\mathrm{mg/dL})}{18} + \frac{[\mathrm{BUN}]\,(\mathrm{mg/dL})}{2.8} = \mathrm{mOsm/kg}$$

Hyponatremia is the most common electrolyte disorder in hospitalized patients, with a prevalence in ICUs patients as high as 40%, highlighting hyponatremia as a common and important clinical condition that adds complexity to the care.[335a] Hyponatremia can occur in isotonic, hypertonic, or hypotonic forms. For example, isotonic hyponatremia can develop in protein or liquid accumulation states such as myeloma. Hypertonic hyponatremia can be present with hyperglycemia or with infusions of glycine (as in the TURP syndrome). Hypotonic hyponatremia is the largest classification and is subdivided according to the status of the extracellular fluid into hypovolemic, isovolumic, or hypervolemic hypotonic hyponatremia. All three types require that excretion of renal water be impaired despite continued intake of dilute fluid. Common causes of hypovolemic

BOX 32.5 Types and Causes of Hypotonic Hyponatremia

Hypovolemic

- Gastrointestinal losses
  - Vomiting
  - Diarrhea
- Skin losses
- Third-space losses
- Lung losses
- Renal losses
  - Diuretics
  - Renal damage
  - Urinary tract obstruction
- Adrenal insufficiency

Isovolumic

- Syndrome of inappropriate secretion of antidiuretic hormone
- Renal failure
- Water intoxication
- Hypokalemia
- Dysfunctional osmostat

Hypervolemic

- Congestive heart failure
- Nephrosis
- Liver dysfunction

Serum osmolality less than 280 mOsm/L.

hypotonic hyponatremia are GI losses (vomiting, diarrhea), third-space losses (diuretics or salt-wasting nephropathy), and adrenal insufficiency (Box 32.5). Hypervolemic hypotonic hyponatremic states complicate severe cardiac failure, cirrhosis, nephrotic syndrome, and renal failure, and are characterized by retention of sodium with disproportionately larger amounts of water.

The most common isovolumic hypotonic hyponatremia is caused by retention of water without sodium, often edema is not usually clinically apparent. Edema is most often caused by SIADH, which in turn may be caused by CNS or pulmonary tumors or dysfunction. Secretion of ADH increases with age, thus rendering older adults more prone to hyponatremia. Drugs that potentiate the secretion of ADH (tricyclic antidepressants and vincristine) or its effects on the medullary collecting duct system in the kidney (nonsteroidal antiinflammatory drugs and thiazides) or that have similar effects (oxytocin and desmopressin) may be more likely to cause hyponatremia in older adults. To establish the diagnosis of SIADH, the physician should determine that the patient is free of renal and cardiac dysfunction, has normal adrenal and thyroid function, and is normovolemic—it is a diagnosis of exclusion. Urine osmolality would then be found to exceed 100 mOsm/kg, serum osmolality would be low, and urine sodium excretion would be higher than 20 mEq/L (20 mOsm/L).

Disturbances in serum sodium therefore may reflect alterations in glucose metabolism, renal function, or accumulation of body water. The last can be affected by disturbances in thirst, release of ADH, and renal function. Thus hyponatremia reflects a relative excess of free water and can occur when total-body sodium increases (as in edematous disorders), when total-body sodium is normal (as in excess of free water because of SIADH), or when total-body sodium decreases (as occurs with too aggressive use of diuretic drugs). Definition of the cause defines the treatment. For instance, water restriction is the mainstay of therapy for SIADH. Administration of demeclocycline is another option that corrects severe SIADH by inducing a reversible nephrogenic diabetes insipidus. The anesthesiologist is faced with the question of which levels of electrolytes require treatment before anesthesia. Although slowly developing hyponatremia usually produces few symptoms, the patient may be lethargic, apathetic, or unbalanced. Chronic hyponatremia is better tolerated than acute hyponatremia because of mechanisms regulating intracellular fluid volume that alleviate brain edema; the loss of other solutes from cells decreases the osmotic movement of water into cells. Nonetheless, severe chronic hyponatremia (i.e., serum sodium levels <123 mEq/L) can cause the development of brain edema.

By contrast, acute hyponatremia may be manifested by severe symptoms requiring emergency treatment: profound cerebral edema with obtundation, coma, convulsions, and disordered reflexes and thermoregulatory control.[100,101,336] Depending on the cause and relative total sodium and water content, treatment can range from the administration of hypertonic saline (with or without diuretic drugs) to restriction of fluids or administration of other drugs.[100,101,336] Because neurologic damage may develop if the serum sodium concentration is increased too rapidly, the rate of increase should not exceed 1 mEq/L/h.[100,101,336] After the serum sodium concentration has reached 125 mEq/L, therapy may consist of water restriction; more rapid correction may result in the osmotic demyelination syndrome.[335a] In hyponatremic patients who have excess total-body water secondary to SIADH, serum levels can be corrected by giving furosemide and saline to replace the loss of electrolytes in urine.[100,101,336] The diagnosis of SIADH is discussed earlier in this chapter (see the section on pituitary abnormalities).

Neither acute nor chronic hyponatremia necessitates restoration of serum sodium to normal levels, just until resolution of neurologic symptoms; brain swelling usually resolves at a serum sodium level of 130 mEq/L.

Hypernatremia occurs much less commonly than hyponatremia. It is often iatrogenic (e.g., it can be caused by failure to provide sufficient free water to a patient who is unconscious or who has had a recent stroke-induced deficit of the thirst mechanism) and can occur in the presence of low, normal, or excess total-body sodium. The primary symptoms of hypernatremia relate to brain cell shrinkage. Because too rapid correction of hypernatremia can lead to cerebral edema and possibly osmotic demyelination syndrome with convulsions, coma, and death; correction should be made gradually. Despite lack of data, there is general belief that all patients undergoing surgical procedures should have serum sodium concentrations of less than 150 mEq/L before anesthesia unless a therapeutic for hypernatremia exists (i.e., hypertonic therapy for cerebral edema in neurologic injury).

Hypokalemia and Hyperkalemia

Hypokalemia and hyperkalemia are also discussed in Chapters 31 and 47. The relationship between the measured potassium concentration in serum and total-body potassium stores can best be described with a scattergram. Only 2% of total-body potassium is stored in plasma (4200 mEq in cells and 60 mEq in extracellular fluid). In normal persons, 75% of the 50 to 60 mEq/L of total-body potassium is stored in skeletal muscle, 6% in red blood cells, and 5% in the liver. Thus a 20% to 25% change in potassium levels in plasma could represent a change in total-body potassium of 1000 mEq or more if the change were chronic or as little as 10 to 20 mEq if the change were acute.

As with serum sodium levels, acute changes in serum potassium levels are less well tolerated than chronic changes. Chronic changes are relatively well tolerated because of the equilibration of serum and intracellular stores that takes place over time to return the resting membrane potential of excitable cells to nearly normal levels.

Hyperkalemia can result from the following: factitious increase of potassium administration (as in red blood cell hemolysis); excessive exogenous potassium from sources such as salt substitutes; cellular shifts in potassium (as a result of metabolic acidosis, tissue and muscle damage after burns, use of depolarizing muscle relaxants, or intense catabolism of protein); and decreased renal excretion (as occurs in renal failure, renal insufficiency with trauma, and therapy with potassium-sparing diuretic drugs, especially when combined with ACE inhibitors or mineralocorticoid deficiency).[337-339] Factitious hyperkalemia can occur when a tourniquet is left on too long or even by simple fist clenching.[340]

The major danger in anesthetizing patients who have disorders of potassium balance appears to be abnormal cardiac function (i.e., both electrical disturbances and poor cardiac contractility).[337] Hyperkalemia lowers the resting membrane potential of excitable cardiac cells and decreases the duration of the myocardial action potential and upstroke velocity. This decreased rate of ventricular depolarization, in addition to the beginning of repolarization in some areas of the myocardium while other areas are still undergoing depolarization, produces a progressively widening QRS complex that merges with the T wave into a sine wave on the ECG.

At a potassium level greater than 6.7 mEq/L, the degree of hyperkalemia and the duration of the QRS complex correlate well.[337] This correlation is even better than the correlation between the serum potassium level and T-wave changes. Nevertheless, the earliest manifestations of hyperkalemia are narrowing and peaking of the T wave. Although not diagnostic of hyperkalemia, T waves are almost invariably peaked and narrow when serum potassium levels are 7 to 9 mEq/L. When serum potassium levels exceed 7 mEq/L, atrial conduction disturbances appear, as manifested by a decrease in P-wave amplitude and an increase in the PR interval. Supraventricular tachycardia, atrial fibrillation, PVCs, ventricular tachycardia, ventricular fibrillation, or sinus arrest may all occur.

The ECG and cardiac alterations associated with hyperkalemia are potentiated by low serum levels of calcium and sodium. Intravenous administration of bicarbonate, glucose with insulin (1 unit/2 g glucose), can reverse these changes temporarily by shifting extracellular potassium into the cells. Calcium is administered to stabilize the cardiac membrane; it has no effect on plasma concentrations of potassium. Furosemide should be given to start the removal process of excess potassium from the body and decrease serum potassium levels. Sodium polystyrene sulfonate (Kayexalate) enemas can be given to bind potassium in the gut in exchange for sodium, these should be used with caution in perioperative patients as there are reports of intestinal necrosis.[340a,340b] Dialysis against a hypokalemic solution also decreases serum potassium levels.

β-Adrenergic stimuli also cause redistribution of potassium into the cell. Indeed, the plasma potassium concentration measured in samples immediately before surgical procedures is usually 0.2 to 0.8 mEq/L lower than that measured during the less stressful period 1 to 3 days before surgery.[341] β-Adrenergic receptor blocking drugs can be used to prevent such an effect preoperatively. A β-adrenergic receptor stimulating agent (20 mg of nebulized albuterol for a 70-kg patient) can be used to treat hyperkalemia when it occurs; it decreases potassium levels 1.0 mEq/L within 30 minutes, and its effect lasts 2 hours.[342] Although nebulized β_2-agonists effectively lower plasma potassium concentrations by stimulating sodium- and potassium-dependent adenosine triphosphatase, this therapy should be used as an adjunct to rather than a substitute for more established measures.

In a hyperkalemic patient, hypoventilation can be dangerous during anesthesia because each 0.1 change in pH can produce a 0.4 to 1.5 mEq/L change in serum potassium levels in the opposite direction. For example, if pH decreases from 7.4 to 7.3, serum potassium levels could increase from 5.5 to 6.5 mEq/L.

Hypokalemia can be caused by inadequate intake of potassium, excessive GI loss (through diarrhea, vomiting, nasopharyngeal suctioning, long-term use of laxatives, or ingestion of cation exchange resins, as in certain wines), excessive renal loss (because of the use of diuretic drugs, renal tubular acidosis, chronic chloride deficiency, metabolic alkalosis, mineralocorticoid excess, excessive ingestion of licorice, use of antibiotics, ureterosigmoidostomy, and diabetic ketoacidosis), and shifts of potassium from extracellular to intracellular compartments (as occurs in alkalosis, insulin administration, administration of a β-adrenergic agonist, stress, barium poisoning, and periodic paralysis). As with hyperkalemia, knowledge of the cause of the potassium deficiency and appropriate preoperative evaluation and treatment of that cause may be as important as treatment of the deficiency itself. Also like hyperkalemia, hypokalemia may reflect small or vast changes in total-body potassium. Acute hypokalemia may be much less well tolerated than chronic hypokalemia. The major worrisome manifestations of hypokalemia pertain to the circulatory system, both the cardiac and peripheral components. In addition, chronic hypokalemia results in muscle weakness, hypoperistalsis, and nephropathy.

Cardiovascular manifestations of hypokalemia include the following: autonomic neuropathy, orthostatic hypotension, decreased sympathetic reserve, impaired myocardial contractility, and electrical conduction abnormalities. Conduction abnormalities can present as sinus tachycardia, atrial and ventricular arrhythmias, and intraventricular conduction disturbances that can progress to ventricular fibrillation. In addition to arrhythmias, the ECG shows widening of the QRS complex, ST-segment abnormalities, progressive diminution of the T-wave amplitude, and a progressive increase in the U-wave amplitude. Surawicz found these changes to be invariably present when serum potassium levels decreased to less than 2.3 mEq/L.[337] Although U waves are not specific for hypokalemia, they are sensitive indicators of the condition. Replenishing the total-body potassium deficit for a depletion reflected by a serum deficit of 1 mEq/L (e.g., from 3.3 to 4.3 mEq/L) may require 1000 mEq of potassium. Even if this amount could be given instantaneously (and it should not be replenished at a rate exceeding 250 mEq/day), it would take 24 to 48 hours to equilibrate in all tissues. Potassium-depleted myocardium is unusually sensitive to digoxin, calcium, and most important, potassium. Rapid potassium infusion in a hypokalemic patient can produce arrhythmias as severe as those produced by hypokalemia itself, again, slow correction is preferred.[343]

Thus the decision to proceed with surgery and anesthesia in the presence of acute or chronic depletions or excesses of potassium depends on many factors.[344-349] The cause and treatment of the underlying condition creating the electrolyte imbalance and the effect of that imbalance on perioperative risk and physiologic processes must be known. The urgency of the operation, the degree of electrolyte abnormality, the medications given, the acid-base balance, and the suddenness or persistence of the electrolyte disturbance are all considerations. For example, a small study of patients undergoing vascular access procedures with preoperative potassium levels of higher than 6 mmol/L demonstrated no adverse outcomes.[347] Similarly, in a cohort study in which 38 patients had a preoperative potassium level higher than 5.5 mEq/L, no dysrhythmias or major morbidity were associated with the use of succinylcholine.[348]

Retrospective epidemiologic studies attribute significant risk to the administration of potassium (even long-term oral administration).[344] In one study, 1910 of 16,048 consecutive hospitalized patients were given oral potassium supplements. Of these 1910 patients, hyperkalemia contributed to death in 7, and the incidence of complications of potassium therapy was 1 in 250.[350] Armed with such data, many internists do not prescribe oral potassium therapy for patients given diuretic drugs, yet these patients frequently become moderately hypokalemic.[350] Modest hypokalemia occurs in 10% to 50% of patients given diuretic drugs.

Three studies investigated whether modest hypokalemia was a problem by prospectively seeking arrhythmias on the ECGs of patients who had various preoperative levels of potassium.[345,346,349] No difference in the incidence of arrhythmias occurred in 25 normokalemic ($K^+ > 3.4$ mEq/L) patients, 25 moderately hypokalemic ($K^+ = 3\text{-}3.4$ mEq/L) patients, and 10 severely hypokalemic ($K^+ < 2.9$ mEq/L) patients.[345] Wahr and coauthors studied 2402 patients undergoing elective CABG and concluded that a serum potassium level less than 3.5 mmol/L was a predictor of perioperative arrhythmia (OR, 2.2; 95% CI, 1.2-4.0), intraoperative arrhythmia (OR, 2.0; 95% CI, 1.0-3.6), and postoperative atrial fibrillation/flutter (OR, 1.7; 95% CI, 1.0-2.7).[349]

Modest hypokalemia can have severe consequences.[350,351] Holland and coworkers treated 21 patients with 50 mg of hydrochlorothiazide twice a day for 4 weeks.[351] These patients had a history of becoming hypokalemic during diuretic therapy; no patients had cardiac disease or were taking other medications. Before and after diuretic therapy, 24-hour ambulatory ECGs were recorded. This study is also subject to the limitations of Holter monitoring. Ventricular ectopy, including complex ventricular ectopy (multifocal PVCs, ventricular couplets, ventricular tachycardia), developed in 7 of the 21 patients (33%). Potassium repletion decreased the number of ectopic ventricular beats per patient from 71.2 to 5.4/h. Apparently, some patients are sensitive to even minor potassium depletion. In the Multiple Risk Factor Intervention Trial involving 361,662 patients, more than 2000 of whom were treated for hypertension with diuretics, the reduction in serum potassium after diuretic therapy was greater in patients with PVCs.[350]

Gastrointestinal and Liver Diseases

GASTROINTESTINAL DISEASE

Preoperative Search for Diverse Associated Disorders in Gastrointestinal Disease

Although preoperative preparation of the GI tract is usually the responsibility of the surgeon, GI disease can and often does cause derangements in many or all other systems. Such disturbances can affect the safety of anesthesia for the patient. Preoperative preparation should include knowledge of disease processes and their effects to guide the patient smoothly through the perioperative period. The major advances of correcting fluid and electrolyte disorders and optimizing nutritional status preoperatively allow surgical procedures to be performed in patients with GI disease previously deemed to be at too great a risk and may have lessened the risk for others.[45-47,352] Nonetheless, in patients with GI disease, thorough assessment of intravascular fluid volume, electrolyte concentrations, and nutrition is essential, including an evaluation of the supervening side effects of these therapies (e.g., hypophosphatemia from parenteral nutrition, hyperkalemia or cardiac arrhythmias from too vigorous treatment of hypokalemia, and volume overload from too rapid or too vigorous treatment of hypovolemia).

In addition to the vast alterations in fluids, electrolytes, and nutrition that can occur with such diverse GI diseases as neoplasms and pancreatitis, patients with GI disorders can have gastroesophageal reflux disease,[353] bowel obstruction, vomiting, or hypersecretion of acid. These effects may merit rapid induction of anesthesia with the application of cricoid pressure or endotracheal intubation with the patient unanesthetized (awake), preoperative nasogastric suctioning, or preoperative use of histamine receptor blocking drugs. Clotting abnormalities may need to be corrected because fat-soluble vitamin K (often malabsorbed) is necessary for the synthesis of factors II, VII, IX, and X in the liver. Liver disease is often associated with GI disease and, if severe enough, can also result in a deficiency of clotting factors synthesized by the liver.

Other factors should be remembered in the perioperative management of any patient with GI disease. First, closed spaces containing gas expand by absorbing nitrous oxide, as such expansion can lead to ischemic injury, rupture of GI viscera, or both. Second, GI surgery predisposes the patient to blood stream contamination, which can lead to sepsis and decreased peripheral vascular resistance, massive fluid requirements, cardiac failure, and renal insufficiency. The surgical site infection rate has been declining. This decrease may be attributable to the use of better technique, more appropriate prophylactic timing and use of antibiotics, better nutrition, less invasive (laparoscopic and endoscopic) surgery, maintenance of normothermia, and surgical resection of even tumors.[354-358] Third, patients with GI disease may have many other associated disorders not directly related to the GI tract. For example, they may be anemic from deficiencies in iron, intrinsic factor, folate, or vitamin B_{12}.

They may also manifest neurologic changes from combined-system disease. Respiration may be impaired because of tobacco abuse, peritonitis, abscess, pulmonary obstruction, previous incisions, aspiration, or pulmonary embolism (as occurs with ulcerative colitis or with thrombophlebitis in bedridden patients). These patients may also have hepatitis, cholangitis, side effects from antibiotic drugs or other medications, massive bleeding with anemia and shock, or psychological derangements.

Because GI disease can be accompanied by so many diverse associated disorders, the clinician must clearly search for involvement of other systems and preoperatively assess and treat such disorders appropriately. Discussion of two specific diseases, ulcerative colitis and carcinoid tumor, highlights the importance of involvement of other systems in GI disease.

Ulcerative Colitis and Carcinoid Tumors as Examples of Gastrointestinal Disease Affecting Other Systems

Ulcerative colitis is a chronic inflammatory disease of the colonic mucosa, typically starting in the rectum and extending proximally through the colon. It is often marked with an unpredictable clinical course with periods of remission and exacerbation. Patients with ulcerative colitis may also have the following: phlebitis; deficiencies in iron, folate, or vitamin B_{12}; anemia; or clotting disorders caused by malabsorption. They can present as malnourished or dehydrated, or with electrolyte abnormalities. In addition, ulcerative colitis can be accompanied by massive bleeding, bowel obstruction, bowel perforation, toxic megacolon, hepatitis, arthritis, iritis, spondylitis, diabetes, or pancreatitis.

The site of origin of carcinoid tumors in more than 60% of patients is the GI tract.[358a] Within the GI tract, carcinoid tumors have been documented to occur from the esophagus to the rectum. Tumors arising in the ileocecal region have the highest incidence of metastases. Carcinoid tumors originating from sites other than the GI tract, such as the head and neck, lung, gonads, thymus, breast, and urinary tract, have also been reported. Cardiac involvement, although frequently reported, is usually limited to right-sided valvular and myocardial plaque formation.[359]

Not all patients with carcinoid tumors have symptoms attributable to secretion of hormone by the tumor. Some do, however, and unexpected carcinoid can manifest intraoperatively by hypersecretion of gastric fluid. The most comprehensive series in the literature indicates that only 7% of patients have carcinoid syndrome, which typically consists of flushing, diarrhea, and valvular heart disease. Of those patients with the syndrome, approximately 74% have cutaneous flushing, 68% have intestinal hypermotility, 41% have cardiac symptoms, and 18% have wheezing. Factors influencing symptoms include the location of the tumor and the specific hormones produced and secreted. Although it is generally believed that if patients do not exhibit carcinoid syndrome, the tumors are not producing serotonin (5-hydroxytryptamine [5-HT]), such may not be the case. Approximately 50% of patients with carcinoid tumors of the GI tract demonstrate evidence of 5-HT production as manifested by elevated urinary levels of 5-hydroxyindoleacetic acid (5-HIAA), a metabolic product of 5-HT. Carcinoid syndrome is usually associated with ileal carcinoid tumors that have metastasized to the liver. Presumably, the liver clears mediators released from the tumor. Impairment of this clearing ability by the metastatic tumor results in carcinoid syndrome.

Most patients with carcinoid tumors and increased urinary 5-HIAA levels have typical carcinoid tumors originating from the midgut (ileum or jejunum). These patients excrete only small amounts of 5-hydroxytryptophan (5-HTP). Patients with atypical carcinoid tumors that originate in the foregut (bronchus, stomach, and pancreas) excrete large amounts of 5-HT and 5-HTP, as well as moderately higher amounts of 5-HIAA.

Although it is generally agreed that 5-HT is responsible for the diarrhea experienced by patients with carcinoid tumors, other neurohumoral agents may contribute to the flushing and hypotension, including dopamine, histamine, and some of the neuropeptides such as substance P, neurotensin, vasoactive intestinal peptide, and somatostatin.

The net physiologic effect of circulating 5-HT represents a composite of both direct action (mediated by 5-HT receptors) and indirect action (mediated through modulation of adrenergic neurotransmission). The existence of several subtypes of 5-HT receptors may account for the different effects of 5-HT on various serotonin-sensitive tissue beds. Indirect actions are effected through alterations in catecholamine release and depend on the level of circulating 5-HT.

5-HT has little, if any, direct effect on the heart. With increased levels, however, positive chronotropic and inotropic myocardial effects may occur, mediated by the release of noradrenaline (norepinephrine). Effects of serotonin on the vasculature include both vasoconstriction and vasodilation.

Alterations in GI function attributed to 5-HT include increased motility and net intestinal secretion of water, sodium chloride, and potassium. 5-HT reportedly causes bronchoconstriction in many animals, but rarely in humans. Patients with asthma are a possible exception. Carcinoid tumors frequently manifest as diarrhea with fluid and electrolyte abnormalities. Because these tumors secrete vasoactive substances, patients can exhibit hypotension or hypertension along with the flush associated with release of vasoactive substances. Vasoactive substances can be released from the tumor by any number of substances, including catecholamines. The anesthesiologist needs to be ready and able to treat hypotension, decreased peripheral vascular resistance, bronchospasm, and hypertension. This difficulty in managing carcinoid syndrome seemed to change with the availability of a somatostatin analogue, octreotide, and lanreotide. In fact, somatostatin is such a powerful inhibitor of the release of peptides from carcinoid tumors and an inhibitor of the peptic effects on receptor cells that it is the therapy of choice for preoperative, intraoperative, and postoperative management of carcinoid symptoms and crises.[360,361] In cardiac surgical patients, mortality has declined over time, and vasopressors have been shown to be safe in conjunction with octreotide.[362] However, the ease of management of most patients[360,361,363-366] should not lull the anesthesiologist into being unprepared—in fact, somatostatin has caused problems of its own and has failed to prevent severe hypotension and bronchospasm.[367,368]

In patients with severe hypotension that is not treatable with somatostatin, the drug of choice is vasopressin; angiotensin has demonstrated benefit but only recently become available in the United States. However, the vasoactive substances released by carcinoid tumors cause fibrosis of the heart valves that often results in pulmonic stenosis or tricuspid insufficiency. To increase cardiac output in a patient with tricuspid insufficiency, the anesthesiologist should avoid drugs or situations that increase pulmonary vascular resistance. In addition, the production of large amounts of 5-HT (equal to 200 mg/day of 5-HIAA) can lead to the development of niacin deficiency with pellagra (as occurs with diarrhea, dermatitis, and dementia).

Steroids have been effective in treating the symptoms of bronchial carcinoid tumors. Although prophylactic preoperative administration and intraoperative therapeutic use have been described, controlled studies of beneficial effects are lacking. Aprotinin, like steroids, inhibits the kallikrein cascade by blocking the proteinase activity of kallikrein, and some reports have described a dramatic clinical response, though it is not available in the United States.

A subset of patients with symptoms of carcinoid syndrome excretes histamine at increased levels in their urine. Histamine causes vasodilation of small blood vessels, which leads to flushing and decreased total peripheral resistance. Histamine is known to cause bronchoconstriction, particularly in patients with bronchial asthma and other pulmonary diseases. Histamine receptor blocking drugs have been used with some success in alleviating the flushing associated with carcinoid syndrome. H_2 antagonism alone was found to be just as effective as combination therapy in preventing symptoms; pure H_1 antagonism, however, was ineffective. These therapies have been relegated to a second-line defense since the use of somatostatin.

Catecholamines aggravate the symptoms of carcinoid syndrome, presumably by stimulating release of hormone by the tumor. Adrenergic receptors have not been demonstrated in carcinoid tumors, nor do these tumors usually have neural innervation. Perhaps adrenergic stimuli work through their mechanical effects on the gut and vessels to stimulate the release of tumor products. Treatment of patients with carcinoid tumors by means of α- and β-adrenergic antagonists has been beneficial in ameliorating flushing in some instances but ineffective in others.

The results of prospective studies on somatostatin to ameliorate the symptoms of carcinoid syndrome have been dramatic. Somatostatin appears to have been a major advance in the treatment of carcinoid syndrome, it is now the mainstay of medical treatment perioperatively.

Bronchospasm with or without flushing also develops in many patients when vasoactive substances are released. Thus a patient with a carcinoid tumor may be well or may be severely incapacitated by pulmonary, neurologic, nutritional, fluid, electrolytic, or cardiovascular disturbances.

Therefore, although the GI system in itself may not require extensive preoperative preparation, GI disease can cause disturbances in any or all other systems that require extensive preoperative preparation to optimize the patient's condition in addition to preoperative knowledge of physiology and the effects of diseases to guide patients through the perioperative period smoothly. In addition, the anesthesiologist's understanding of the nature of the surgical procedure aids in determining the system involvement caused by the GI disorder.

Another perioperative consideration is that patients with GI diseases have had to endure the psychosocial trauma of having to live with their disease for long periods or the necessity of facing such a prospect.[369] They need emotional support, kindness, and empathy as much as, if not more than, other patients without sacrificing scientific rigor in the treatment of their condition. Obtaining relevant psychological data while gathering medical information, sitting while taking the history, and empathizing with the patient about how difficult it must be to accomplish tasks with this disease legitimize the physician's interests in and support of the patient's pain and other psychosocial issues. The time spent sitting and talking with the patient also allows the anesthesiologist to discuss options for pain therapy with the patient, and other issues that show the anesthesiologist to be both a competent physician and particularly concerned with that patient's well-being.

LIVER DISEASE

What are the risks of giving anesthesia to patients with acute liver disease who require emergency surgery? What are the risks of giving anesthesia to patients with chronic impairment of liver function? What can be done to minimize these risks? Although one may think that the experiences gained from providing anesthesia for liver transplantation would answer many of these questions, a substantial difference exists between optimizing cardiovascular function to meet the needs of a new liver (e.g., supply of nutrients) and maintaining liver function in a diseased liver. Hepatic physiology and pathology are discussed in Chapter 16.

Hematologic Disorders and Oncologic Disease

HEMATOLOGIC DISORDERS

Sickle Cell Anemia and Related Hemoglobinopathies

The sickle cell syndromes constitute a family of hemoglobinopathies caused by abnormal genetic transformation of amino acids in the heme portion of the hemoglobin molecule. The sickle cell syndromes arise from a mutation in the β-globin gene that changes the sixth amino acid from valine to glutamic acid. A major pathologic feature of sickle cell disease is the aggregation of irreversibly sickled cells in blood vessels. The molecular basis of sickling is the aggregation of deoxygenated hemoglobin B molecules along their longitudinal axis.[370] This abnormal aggregation distorts the cell membrane and thereby produces a sickle shape. Irreversibly sickled cells become dehydrated and rigid and can cause tissue infarcts by impeding blood flow and oxygen to tissues.[370-373] Several studies show enhanced adhesion of sickled erythrocytes to vascular endothelium, as well.[374] Some other abnormal hemoglobins interact with hemoglobin S to various degrees and give rise to symptomatic disease in patients heterozygous for hemoglobin S and one of the other hemoglobins such as the hemoglobin of thalassemia (hemoglobin C).

Three tenths of 1% of the African American population in the United States have sickle cell-thalassemia disease (hemoglobin SC); these patients also have end-organ disease and symptoms suggestive of organ infarction. For these patients, perioperative considerations should be similar to those for patients with sickle cell disease (hemoglobin SS).

Whereas 8% to 10% of African Americans have the sickle cell trait (hemoglobin AS), 0.2% are homozygous for sickle cell hemoglobin and have sickle cell anemia. Sickle cell trait is a heterozygous condition in which the individual has one βS globin gene and one βA globin gene, which results in the production of both hemoglobin S and hemoglobin A, with a predominance of hemoglobin A. Sickle cell trait is not clinically significant because hemoglobin AS cells begin to sickle only when the oxygen saturation of hemoglobin is less than 20%. Minimal difference has been found between physiologically normal persons (i.e., those with hemoglobin AA) and those with hemoglobin AS regarding survival rates, though there is one exception—patients with hemoglobin AS have a 50% increase in pulmonary infarction. However, single case reports of a perioperative death and a perioperative brain infarct in two patients with hemoglobin AS disease do exist, as does a report of death believed to be caused by aortocaval compression during general anesthesia that resulted in a sickling crisis.[375] Frequent measurement of oxygen saturation (pulse oximetry) in multiple areas of the body is recommended when caring these AS patients, including the ear and toe in pregnant patients.[375]

The pathologic end-organ damage that occurs in sickle cell states is attributable to three processes: the sickling or adhesion of cells in blood vessels, which causes infarcts and subsequent tissue destruction secondary to tissue ischemia; hemolytic crisis secondary to hemolysis; and aplastic crises that occur with bone marrow exhaustion, which can rapidly result in severe anemia. Patients currently in crisis should not undergo surgery except for emergencies, and then only after an exchange transfusion.[372,374-378]

Because sickling is increased with lowered oxygen tensions, acidosis, hypothermia, and the presence of more desaturated hemoglobin S; current therapy includes keeping the patient warm and well hydrated, giving supplemental oxygen, maintaining high cardiac output, and avoiding areas of stasis with pressure or tourniquets. Meticulous attention to these practices in periods when we do not usually pay most careful attention (i.e., waiting in the preinduction area) or when gas exchange may be most unmatched to the cardiovascular-metabolic demands (early postoperative period) may be important in lessening morbidity. Following these measures routinely succeeded in reducing mortality to 1% in several series of patients with sickle cell syndromes.[375,378,379] Retrospective review of patients' charts led the authors of those studies to conclude that, at most, a 0.5% mortality rate could be attributed to the interaction between sickle cell anemia and anesthesia.

Several investigators have advocated using partial exchange transfusions perioperatively. In children with sickle cell anemia and acute lung syndromes, partial exchange transfusion improved clinical symptoms and blood oxygenation. In addition, serum bilirubin levels decreased in patients with acute liver injury. Clinical improvement of pneumococcal meningitis and cessation of hematuria in papillary necrosis also accompanied exchange transfusion.[371] The goal of transfusion therapy is to lower the concentration of hemoglobin S to less than 30%, minimize splenic sequestration, treat severe anemia, and avoid acute chest syndrome due to low PaO_2.[379a] Exchange transfusion serves to lower the concentration of hemoglobin S, while red blood cell transfusions serve to correct anemia. To date only regular transfusion therapy has been associated with improved mortality in the extended period.[379b,c] Two studies demonstrated a possible decrease in perioperative morbidity after partial exchange transfusion when compared with the risks of exchange transfusion.[373,380] A retrospective review of 14 patients with sickle cell anemia who were undergoing total hip revision supported the decision to perform a simple transfusion preoperatively only if the patient's hemoglobin is significantly lower than their steady-state hemoglobin level.[381] Transfusion can be used intraoperatively according to hemoglobin level or blood loss volume. Other conditions are common in sickle cell syndromes: pulmonary dysfunction with increased shunting, renal insufficiency, gallstones, small MIs, priapism, stroke, aseptic necrosis of bones and joints, ischemic ulcers, retinal detachment as a result of neovascularization, and complications of repeated transfusions.

In thalassemia, globin structures are normal, but because of gene deletion, the rate of synthesis of either the α or β chains of hemoglobin (α- and β-thalassemia, respectively) decreases.[382-384] Two copies of the gene that codes for the α-globin chain are located on chromosome 16. Deletion of all four of these genes causes cell death in utero, and three deletions cause severe chronic hemolysis and a shortened life span. α-Thalassemia-1 (trait) occurs when two genes have been deleted and mild anemia results; α-thalassemia-2 (silent) occurs when the two genes have been deleted but no mild anemia or microcytosis results. In α-thalassemia trait, the hemoglobin A_2 level is normal. β-Thalassemia is associated with an excess of α chains, which denature developing erythrocytes, thereby leading to their premature death in marrow or to shortened survival in the circulation. An elevated hemoglobin A_2 level is the hallmark of β-thalassemia trait, a common cause of mild anemia and microcytosis. These syndromes are common in Southeast Asia, India, and the Middle East and in people of African descent.

In thalassemia, facial deformity from erythropoietin-stimulated ineffective erythropoiesis (ineffective because of a genetic inability to produce useful hemoglobin) was reported to make endotracheal intubation difficult.[382,383] The anemia associated with these syndromes often produces compensatory hyperplasia of the erythroid marrow, which in turn is associated with severe skeletal abnormalities.[382-384]

Cytoskeletal Anemias (Hereditary Spherocytosis and Elliptocytosis), Enzyme-Deficient Anemias, and Autoimmune Hemolytic Anemias

Congenital abnormalities of the erythrocyte membrane are becoming better understood. In elliptocytosis and hereditary spherocytosis, the membrane is more permeable to cations and is more susceptible to lipid loss when cell energy is depleted than is the membrane of a normal red blood cell. Both hereditary spherocytosis (present in 1 in 5000 people) and hereditary elliptocytosis are inherited as autosomal dominant traits. In both disorders, defects in the membrane are thought to result from a mutation of spectrin, a structural protein of the membrane cytoskeleton.[385] Although the therapeutic role of splenectomy in these diseases is not fully defined, in severe disease, splenectomy is known to improve the shortened life span of the red blood cell from 20-30 days to 40-70 days. Because splenectomy predisposes the patient to gram-positive septicemia (particularly pneumococcal), perhaps patients should be given pneumococcal vaccine preoperatively. No specific problems related to anesthesia have been reported for these disorders.

Glucose-6-phosphate dehydrogenase (G6PD) deficiency (a gender-linked recessive trait) has been recognized as the most common enzymopathy worldwide, most often expressed in males, and in patients of African, Asian, Mediterranean, or Middle Eastern descent.[385a] Young cells have normal activity, but older cells are grossly deficient when compared with normal cells. A deficiency in G6PD results in hemolysis of the erythrocyte and the formation of Heinz bodies. Red blood cell hemolysis can also occur with intercurrent infections or after the administration of drugs that produce substances requiring G6PD for detoxification (e.g., methemoglobin, glutathione, and hydrogen peroxide). Drugs to be avoided are sulfa drugs, quinidine, prilocaine, lidocaine, antimalarial drugs, antipyretic drugs, nonnarcotic analgesics, vitamin K analogues, and perhaps sodium nitroprusside.

The autoimmune hemolytic anemias include cold antibody anemia, warm antibody anemia (idiopathic), and drug-induced anemia and occur from antibody mediate destruction of red blood cells.[386-388] Cold antibody hemolytic anemia is mediated by IgM or IgG antibodies, which at room temperature and lower temperatures cause red blood cells to clump. When these patients are given blood transfusions, the cells and all fluid infusions must be warm, and body temperature must be meticulously maintained at 37°C if hemolysis is to be prevented. Warm antibody (or idiopathic) hemolytic anemia is mediated by IgG and is a difficult management problem characterized by chronic anemia, the presence of antibodies active against red blood cells, a positive Coombs test, and difficulty crossmatching blood. For patients undergoing elective surgery, autologous transfusions, predeposit of blood with or without erythropoietin stimulation,[389] and blood from rare Rh-negative red blood cell donors or the patient's first-degree relatives (or both) can be used. In emergency situations, the possibility of autotransfusion, splenectomy, corticosteroid treatment, rituximab, cyclophosphamide, or azathioprine should be discussed with a hematologist knowledgeable in this area.[389a]

Drug-induced anemias have three mechanisms. In receptor-type hemolysis, a drug (e.g., penicillin) binds to the membrane of the red blood cell, and the complex stimulates the formation of an antibody against the complex. In "innocent bystander" hemolysis, a drug (e.g., quinidine, sulfonamide) binds to a plasma protein, thereby stimulating an antibody (IgM) that cross-reacts with an erythrocyte. In autoimmune hemolysis, the drug stimulates the production of an antibody (IgG) that cross-reacts with the erythrocyte. Drug-induced hemolytic anemias generally cease when therapy with the drug ends.

Granulocytopenia

Granulocyte mechanisms have undergone experimental elaboration since 2000, partly because of the molecular biologic revolution: in addition to erythropoietin, more than 14 hemolymphopoietic growth factors or cytokines have been characterized biochemically and cloned genetically. These growth factors interact with cell-surface receptors to produce their major actions (Table 32.14).[390] Use of the colony-stimulating factors has permitted more intense oncologic treatment. The few reports related to their perioperative effects detail the unfavorable adverse consequences that such therapies can have on gas exchange when adverse immunologic effects occur.[391]

In patients who have fewer than 500 granulocytes/mL of blood and established sepsis, the use of growth factor and granulocyte transfusion has been shown to prolong life.[392-394] Although bone marrow transplantation is being used increasingly, complications usually occur after transplantation, not on harvesting of cells. Abnormal results on pulmonary function testing before bone marrow transplantation seem to predict complications after transplantation, but not so strongly as to preclude transplantation.[395]

Platelet Disorders

Although inherited platelet disorders are rare, acquired disorders are quite common and affect at least 20% of all patients in medical and surgical ICUs, with infections and drug therapies being the leading causes.[396] Both acquired and inherited platelet conditions cause skin and mucosal bleeding, whereas defects in plasma coagulation produce deep tissue bleeding or delayed bleeding. Perioperative treatment of inherited platelet disorders (e.g., Glanzmann thrombasthenia, Bernard-Soulier syndrome, Hermansky-Pudlak syndrome) consists of platelet transfusions. EACA has been used successfully to decrease perioperative bleeding in thrombocytopenic patients. The much more common acquired disorders may respond to one of several therapies. Immune thrombocytopenias, such as those associated with lupus erythematosus, idiopathic thrombocytopenic purpura, uremia, hemolytic-uremic syndrome, platelet transfusions, heparin, and thrombocytosis, may respond to steroids, splenectomy, plateletpheresis, eradication of *Helicobacter pylori*, or alkylating agents, or may require platelet transfusions, plasma exchange, whole blood exchange, or transfusion; sometimes these disorders do not respond to anything.[179,397,398] Traditionally, splenectomy is performed when steroid therapy fails or reaches a dosage that poses unacceptable risks of toxicity. Immunoglobulin infusions and rituximab may induce desirable remissions in idiopathic thrombocytopenic purpura without splenectomy.

Thrombotic thrombocytopenic purpura is a rare immune-mediated thrombotic microangiopathic disorder caused by antibodies to ADAMTS 13 (A Disintegrin AND Metalloproteinase with a Thrombospondin type 1 motif, member 13) that, despite various therapies, still carries a high mortality rate.[398a] The current therapies of plasma exchange, corticosteroids, and rituximab have improved survival rates, though new therapies are under investigation.[398b] One uncontrolled study implies that the benefit lies not only in improvement of the hematologic picture but also in prevention of ARDS, a leading cause of death in these patients.[398] In that study, early institution of plasmapheresis improved oxygenation.

By far the largest number of platelet abnormalities consists of drug-related defects in the aggregation and release of platelets. Aspirin irreversibly acetylates platelet cyclooxygenase, the enzyme that converts arachidonic acid to prostaglandin endoperoxidases. Because cyclooxygenase is not regenerated in the circulation within the life span of the platelet and because this enzyme is essential for the aggregation of platelets, one aspirin tablet may affect platelet function for a week. All other drugs that inhibit platelet function (e.g., vitamin E, indomethacin, sulfinpyrazone, dipyridamole, tricyclic antidepressant drugs, phenothiazines, furosemide, steroids) do not inhibit cyclooxygenase function irreversibly; these drugs disturb platelet function for only 24 to 48 hours. If emergency surgery is needed before the customary 8-day period for platelet regeneration after aspirin therapy or if the 2-day period for other drugs has not elapsed, administration of 2 to 5 units of platelet concentrate will return platelet function

TABLE 32.14 Major Effects of Hemolymphopoietic Growth Factors and Cytokines

Cytokine	Other Names	Biologic Effects
Erythropoietin		Erythrocyte production
Interleukin-3 (IL-3)	Multicolony-stimulating factor Stem cell–activating factor Persisting cell-stimulating factor Hemopoietin-2	Stimulates proliferation and differentiation of granulocyte, macrophage, eosinophil, mast cell, megakaryocyte, and T- and B-cell lineage and early myeloid stem cells Interacts with erythropoietin to stimulate erythroid colony formation, stimulates proliferation of AML blasts, and stimulates histamine release by mast cells
Granulocyte colony-stimulating factor (G-CSF)	Differentiation factor MGI-2	Stimulates granulocyte lineage proliferation and differentiation Acts on early myeloid stem cells, especially in association with other factors; synergizes with IL-3 to stimulate megakaryocyte colony formation Increases neutrophil phagocytes and antibody-dependent cell-mediated cytotoxicity Releases neutrophils from bone marrow and is chemotactic for neutrophils and monocytes Enhances phagocytosis and antibody-dependent cell-mediated cytotoxicity and oxidative metabolism of neutrophils Stimulates monocyte killing of *Mycobacterium avium-intracellulare* and *Candida* species, tumoricidal activity of monocytes, antibody-dependent cell-mediated cytotoxicity, and expression of cell-surface proteins
Granulocyte-macrophage colony-stimulating factor (GM-CSF)		Stimulates granulocyte, macrophage, and megakaryocyte proliferation and differentiation, early myeloid stem cells, and—in the presence of erythropoietin—erythropoiesis Enhances the cytotoxic and phagocytic colony-stimulating factor activity of neutrophils against bacteria, yeast, parasites, and antibody-coated tumor cells Increases surface expression of neutrophil adhesion proteins and enhances eosinophil cytotoxicity, macrophage phagocytosis, and basophil histamine release Amplifies IL-2–stimulated T-cell proliferation and stimulates B-cell lines to proliferate
Colony-stimulating factor-1	Macrophage colony-stimulating factor	Stimulates predominantly macrophage-monocyte proliferation and differentiation with lesser effects on granulocytes Acts synergistically with other factors on earlier myeloid stem cells Stimulates macrophage phagocytosis, killing, migration, antitumor activity, and metabolism Stimulates secretion of plasminogen activator, G-CSF, interferon, IL-3, or tumor necrosis factor by peritoneal macrophages
Interleukin-1 (α and β)	Endogenous pyrogen Hemopoietin-1 Osteoclast-activating factor Lymphocyte-activating factor	Induces synthesis of acute-phase proteins by hepatocytes Activates resting T cells, cofactor for T- and B-cell proliferation Chemotactic for monocytes and neutrophils Induces production of growth factors, including G-CSF, GM-CSF, IL-6, CSF-1, IL-3, and interferon by many cells Radioprotective in mice
Interleukin-2	T-cell growth factor	Growth factor for T cells, activates cytotoxic T lymphocytes, promotes synthesis of other cytokines, enhances natural killer cell function
Interleukin-4	B-cell–stimulating factor-1 (BSF-1) B-cell differentiation factor (BCDF) IgG induction factor	Enhances antibody production (IgG and IgE) and up-regulates class II MHC molecules and Fc receptors on B cells Costimulant with anti-IgM antibodies for induction of DNA synthesis in resting B cells Stimulates growth of activated T cells In the presence of IL-3, enhances mast cell growth; with G-CSF, enhances granulocytes of GM colony formation; and with erythropoietin and/or IL-1, stimulates erythroid and megakaryocyte colony formation
Interleukin-5	Eosinophil differentiation factor (EDF) T-cell–replacing factor (TRF) B-cell growth factor-II (BCGF-II) B-cell differentiation factor (BCDF)	Enhances antibody production (IgA) Promotes proliferation and IgG secretion by B-cell lines and induces hapten-specific IgG secretion in vitro by in vivo–primed B cells Promotes differentiation by normal B cells Stimulates eosinophil production and differentiation (GM-CSF and IL-3 act synergistically with IL-5 to stimulate eosinophil proliferation and differentiation) Enhances synthesis of IL-2 receptors
Interleukin-6	B-cell–stimulating factor-2 (BSF-2) Interferon-β_2 T-cell activation factor Hybridoma growth factor	B-cell differentiation and IgG secretion T cells activated to cytotoxicity Synergizes with IL-3 on early marrow myeloid stem cells and stimulates proliferation and differentiation of granulocytes, macrophages, eosinophils, mast cells, and megakaryocytes, as well as platelet production (may be a thrombopoietin)
Interleukin-7	Lymphopoietin-1	Stimulates pre–B-cell production Stimulates T-cell proliferation
Interleukin-8*	Neutrophil-activating factor T-cell chemotactic factor	Inflammatory mediator; stimulates activation of neutrophils
Interleukin-9		Stimulates erythroid colony formation and proliferation of a megakaryocyte cell line

TABLE 32.14 Major Effects of Hemolymphopoietic Growth Factors and Cytokines—cont'd

Cytokine	Other Names	Biologic Effects
Interleukin-10	Cytokine synthesis–inhibiting factor	Inhibits cytokine production by T_H1 cells
Interleukin-11		Stimulates B-cell, megakaryocyte, and mast cell lineages
C-kit ligand	Mast cell factor Stem cell factor Hemolymphopoietic growth factor-1	Acts on relatively early stem cells synergistically with other cytokines Stimulates pre-B cells

*Not considered a true growth factor but included here for completeness.
AML, Acute myeloblastic leukemia; *IgA*, immunoglobulin A; *IgG*, immunoglobulin G; *IgM*, immunoglobulin M; *MHC*, major histocompatibility complex; T_H1, first of the thymus-derived cells.

in a 70-kg adult to an adequate level and platelet-induced clotting dysfunction to normal. Only 30,000 to 50,000 normally functioning platelets per milliliter are needed for normal clotting. One platelet transfusion will increase the platelet count from 5,000 to 20,000/mL blood; the platelet half-life is approximately 8 hours.

Heparin-induced thrombocytopenia can develop within hours on reexposure to heparin in a previously sensitized patient; prevalence has been shown to be increasing, particularly in ICU populations.[398c] The diagnosis starts with a clinical assessment, most commonly the 4-T score (Thrombocytopenia, Timing of fall, presence of Thrombosis, and other causes for Thrombocytopenia), with enzymatic immunoassays for confirmation.[398d] Treatment can be initiated prior to confirmatory test results, if suspicion is high. Argatroban is a direct thrombin inhibitor effective as therapy for heparin-induced thrombocytopenia.[399]

Major risk factors for thrombosis include factor V Leiden and prothrombin 20210A mutations, elevated plasma homocysteine, and the antiphospholipid antibody syndrome.[400,401] Clinicians facing these challenging patients may seek expert local consultation for help with management. This issue is discussed more fully in Chapter 50.

Hemophilia and Related Clotting Disorders

Abnormalities in blood coagulation as a result of defects in plasma coagulation factors are either inherited or acquired. Inherited disorders include X-linked hemophilia A (a defect in factor VIII activity), von Willebrand disease (defect in the von Willebrand component of factor VIII), hemophilia B (a sex-linked deficiency of factor IX activity), and other less common disorders. The sex-linked origin of some of these disorders means that hemophilia occurs almost exclusively in the male children of female carriers; men do not transmit the disease to their male children.

In elective surgery, levels of the deficient coagulation factor should be assayed 48 hours preoperatively and the level restored to 40% of normal before the surgical procedure. One unit of factor concentrate per kilogram of body weight normally increases the factor concentration by 2%. Thus, in an individual essentially devoid of activity, administration of 20 units/kg body weight would be required as an initial dose. Because the half-life is 6 to 10 hours for factor VIII and 8 to 16 hours for factor IX, approximately 1.5 units/h/kg of factor VIII or 1.5 units/2 hours/kg of factor IX should be given. Additional administration of factors VIII and IX should be guided by the activity of the clotting factors for approximately 6 to 10 days postoperatively.[402-404]

An antibody that inactivates factor VIII or IX (fresh frozen plasma fails to increase clotting factor activity after incubation with the patient's plasma) develops in approximately 10% of patients with either hemophilia A or B. These acquired anticoagulants are usually composed of IgG, are poorly removed by plasmapheresis, and are variably responsive to immunosuppressive drugs. The use of prothrombin complex concentrates can be lifesaving to bypass the inhibitor.

Patients who come to the operating room after having received many units of blood (as in massive GI bleeding and trauma) may have deficient clotting caused by depletion of platelets and later coagulation factors, which occurs after administration of approximately 10 units of blood. Treatment of these deficiencies can be corrected with platelet concentrates and fresh frozen plasma. In settings of massive hemorrhage requiring large volume transfusion, the approximation of whole blood through a one to one to one ratio of packed red blood cells to plasma to platelets can be advantageous.

Urokinase, streptokinase, and tissue-type plasminogen activator (t-PA) have been used to treat pulmonary embolism, deep vein thrombosis, stroke, and arterial occlusive disease. These drugs accelerate the lysis of thrombi and emboli, in contrast to heparin, which may prevent and slow propagation, but will not dissolve a thrombus. Bleeding complications associated with these fibrinolytic agents are the result of dissolution of hemostatic plugs and can be quickly reversed by discontinuing the medication and replenishing plasma fibrinogen with cryoprecipitate or plasma. However, cryoprecipitate and plasma are seldom needed preoperatively because the fibrinolytic activity of urokinase and streptokinase usually dissipates within 1 hour of discontinuing their administration. Nonetheless, insufficient data have accumulated to prescribe the ideal preoperative preparation and intraoperative management of hemostasis in patients recently treated with urokinase, streptokinase, or t-PA. Postponing surgery for three half-lives of the drug (increases in plasmin activity in blood can be assayed for ≥4 to 8 hours) may not be possible, and meticulous observation of the operative field for hemostasis may not suffice.[405,406] The process may be even more complex in a patient with a vascular or cardiac condition who requires heparin administration intraoperatively. To correct the fibrinogen deficiency in these patients, some clinicians administer fibrinogen as cryoprecipitate preoperatively, and EACA at heparin administration.

DDAVP has been used in operations associated with high blood loss as a routine measure to decrease bleeding and transfusion requirements. DDAVP therapy began as treatment of platelet dysfunction in von Willebrand disease but has since expanded to routine use in patients undergoing cardiovascular surgery and to frequent use in other high-blood loss operations. A meta-analysis of cardiac surgery concluded that DDAVP was not associated with a clinically significant reduction in exposure to blood transfusion in unselected patients, and therefore the authors were unable to recommend the routine use of DDAVP in patients exposed to CPB.[407] However, DDAVP may reduce postoperative bleeding in patients who have received preoperative aspirin within 7 days of surgery, patients with CPB times in excess of 140 minutes, and patients with demonstrable platelet dysfunction. The authors suggested that DDAVP could be used selectively in these subgroups.

ONCOLOGIC DISEASE

Patients with malignant tumors may be otherwise healthy or may be chronically ill with nutritional, neurologic, metabolic, endocrinologic, electrolyte, cardiac, pulmonary, renal, hepatic, hematologic, or pharmacologic disabilities. Thus determining the other morbidities accompanying malignant tumors requires through evaluation of all systems. Abnormalities frequently accompanying such tumors include hypercalcemia either by direct bone invasion or by ectopic elaboration of PTH or other bone-dissolving substance, uric acid nephropathy, hyponatremia (especially with small cell, or oat cell, carcinoma of the lung), nausea, vomiting, anorexia and cachexia, fever, tumor-induced hypoglycemia, intracranial metastases (10%-20% of all cancers), peripheral nerve or spinal cord disorders, meningeal carcinomatosis, toxic neuropathies secondary to anticancer therapy, and paraneoplastic neurologic syndromes (dermatomyositis, Eaton-Lambert syndrome, myopathies, and distal neuropathies).

Many patients with malignant tumors are given large doses of analgesics and should be kept comfortable during the perioperative period, it is of particular importance in terminally ill patients.[408] Immunomodulators, stimulating factors or cytokines, gene identification,[409,410] and drugs for treating side effects (e.g., midazolam, ondansetron, and even marijuana) have given new hope for safer, more effective therapy with fewer limiting side effects. The effect of ondansetron in preventing vomiting and the effect of midazolam in preventing memory-stimulated vomiting have been important additions. The neurokinin-1 antagonists have also been approved for treatment in oncologic patients.

The toxicity of cancer chemotherapy is related to the drugs used and the dose. For radiation therapy, damage occurs when the following doses are exceeded: lungs, 1500 rad; kidneys, 2400 rad; heart, 3000 rad; spinal cord, 4000 rad; intestine, 5500 rad; brain, 6000 rad; and bone, 7500 rad. The toxicities of biologic and immunomodulating therapies are related to the change in immune function that they cause. Alkylating agents cause bone marrow depression, including thrombocytopenia, as well as alopecia, hemorrhagic cystitis, nausea, and vomiting. The alkylating agents, including cyclophosphamide and mechlorethamine, can act as an anticholinesterase and prolong neuromuscular blockade.[411] The antineoplastic alkaloid vincristine produces peripheral neuropathy and SIADH, and vinblastine produces myelotoxicity. Cisplatin is also associated with peripheral neuropathy and severe nausea. Nitrosoureas can produce severe hepatic and renal damage, as well as bone marrow toxicity, myalgia, and paresthesia. Folic acid analogues such as methotrexate have been linked to bone marrow depression, ulcerative stomatitis, pulmonary interstitial infiltrates, GI toxicity, and occasionally, severe liver dysfunction. Fluorouracil and floxuridine, both pyrimidine analogues, cause bone marrow toxicity, megaloblastic anemia, nervous system dysfunction, and hepatic and GI alterations. Purine analogues (mercaptopurine, thioguanine) have bone marrow depression as their primary toxic effect. Anthracycline antibiotics (doxorubicin, daunorubicin, mithramycin, mitomycin C, bleomycin) can all cause pulmonary infiltrates, cardiomyopathy (especially doxorubicin and daunorubicin), myelotoxicity, and GI, hepatic, and renal disturbances. Knowing these expected side effects and complications allow general anesthesia to be safely provided to this patient population with the appropriate preoperative plan.

Patients Given Drug Therapy for Chronic and Acute Medical Conditions

A steadily increasing number of potent drugs are being used to treat disease, and the average hospitalized patient receives more than 10 drugs. Many drugs have side effects that may make anesthesia challenging and patient management more difficult. Knowing the pharmacologic properties and potential side effects of commonly used drugs helps the anesthesiologist avoid pitfalls during anesthesia and surgery.

ANTIHYPERTENSIVE DRUGS

ACE inhibitors (e.g., captopril, enalapril, and lisinopril) and angiotensin II receptor blockers (e.g., valsartan, candesartan) are being used increasingly as first-line drugs and appear to improve the quality of life of patients taking antihypertensive drugs. ACE inhibitors and angiotensin II receptor blockers may be associated with more peripheral vasodilation and hypotension on induction of anesthesia than are sympatholytic agents. Both ACE inhibitors and angiotensin II receptor blocking agents are associated with such severe hypotension with standard anesthetic induction that we discontinue or at least consider discontinuing the use of these drugs preoperatively (see earlier).

Catecholamine or sympathetic receptor blocking drugs affect the three major types of catecholamine receptors: α-adrenergic, β-adrenergic, and dopaminergic. The existence of subdivisions (e.g., β_1 and β_2) suggested the possibility that some drugs would be found to affect only one set of receptors. For example, terbutaline is used more frequently than isoproterenol because terbutaline is said to exert a preferential effect on β-$_2$ receptors (i.e., dilation of bronchial smooth muscle), thereby avoiding the cardiac stimulation produced by drugs that stimulate β_1-receptors. In fact, the selectivity is dose related. At a certain dose, a direct β_2-receptor stimulating drug affects only those receptors but, at a higher dose, stimulates both β_1 and β_2 receptors. The effect of a given dose varies with each patient. A certain dose may stimulate β_1 and β_2 receptors in one patient but neither receptor in another patient. More and more selective blocking drugs are being developed in the hope of widening the margin among β_1-, β_2-, and α-adrenergic effects. Ultimately, however, even more selectivity is desired. It would be advantageous to be able to decrease the heart rate without changing myocardial contractility or to increase contractility without changing the heart rate.

Metoprolol, atenolol, propranolol, betaxolol, timolol, esmolol, pindolol, oxprenolol, acebutolol, carteolol, penbutolol, and nadolol are widely available β-adrenergic receptor blocking drugs used for therapy in the United States. Because nadolol has poor lipid solubility, it has a long elimination half-life

(17-24 hours) and does not cross the blood-brain barrier readily. Although selective β-adrenergic receptor blocking drugs should be more appropriate in patients with increased airway resistance or diabetes, this advantage is apparent only when low doses are used. The use of β-adrenergic receptor blocking drugs has become widespread because these drugs treat everything from angina and hypertension to priapism and stage fright. These drugs appear to decrease morbidity and mortality in patients who have initially survived MI, and they may increase perioperative survival in selected patients.[412,413]

When administration of β-adrenergic receptor blocking drugs is terminated, sympathetic stimulation often increases, as though the body had responded to the presence of these drugs by increasing sympathetic neuron activity. Thus propranolol and nadolol withdrawal can be accompanied by a hyper–β-adrenergic condition that increases myocardial oxygen demands. Administering propranolol or metoprolol can cause bradycardia, exacerbations of decompensated heart failure, fatigue, dizziness, depression, psychoses, bronchospasm, and Peyronie disease. The POISE study emphasized the concerns that inadequate titration of these agents can lead to stroke or increased mortality.[111] Side effects of dopaminergic receptor blocking drugs are discussed later.

Prazosin, terazosin, and oxazocine are α_1-adrenergic receptor blocking drugs used to treat hypertension, ischemic cardiomyopathy, receding hairlines, and benign prostatic hypertrophy because they dilate both veins and arteries and reduce sphincter tone. These drugs are associated with vertigo, palpitations, depression, dizziness, weakness, and anticholinergic effects.

Some sympathomimetic drugs stimulate α-adrenergic receptors in the brainstem. Clonidine, a drug with a half-life of 12 to 24 hours, dexmedetomidine, and guanfacine are α_2-adrenergic receptor stimulants. Presumably, α_2-adrenergic agonists, including clonidine, dexmedetomidine, and guanfacine, lower arterial blood pressure on a long-term basis through the central brainstem adrenergic stimulation referred to previously. They may also be used on a long-term basis to treat opiate, cocaine, food, and tobacco withdrawal. Occasionally, withdrawal from clonidine can precipitate a sudden rebound hypertensive crisis. Tricyclic antidepressant drugs and presumably phenothiazines and the butyrophenones interfere with the action of clonidine. Although administration of a butyrophenone (e.g., droperidol) to a patient taking clonidine, dexmedetomidine, or guanfacine on a long-term basis could theoretically precipitate a hypertensive crisis, this has not been reported. Clonidine administration can be accompanied by drowsiness, dry mouth, orthostatic hypotension, bradycardia, and impotence. Acute clonidine or dexmedetomidine administration decreases anesthetic requirements by at least 40% to 60%; long-term administration decreases requirements by 10% to 20%.[414,415] Because of the relative safety of these drugs and their ability to decrease anesthetic requirements, block narcotic-induced muscle rigidity, and provide pain relief, their popularity preoperatively, intraoperatively, and in ICU sedation is increasing dramatically.[414-418]

Three other classes of antihypertensive drugs affect the sympathetic nervous system indirectly: diuretics, arteriolar dilators, and calcium channel blocking agents. Thiazide diuretic drugs are associated with hypochloremic alkalosis, hypokalemia, hyperglycemia, hyperuricemia, and hypercalcemia. The potassium-sparing diuretic drug spironolactone is associated with hyperkalemia, hyponatremia, gynecomastia, and impotence. All diuretic drugs can cause dehydration. The thiazide diuretics and furosemide appear to prolong neuromuscular blockade.

The arteriolar dilator hydralazine can cause a lupus-like condition (usually with renal involvement), nasal congestion, headache, dizziness, CHF, angina, and GI disturbances. Such a syndrome is nonexistent with the other direct vasodilator on the U.S. market, minoxidil.

The calcium channel blocking drugs (slow-channel calcium ion antagonists) inhibit the transmembrane influx of calcium ions into cardiac and vascular smooth muscle. Such inhibition reduces the heart rate (negative chronotropy), depresses contractility (negative inotropy), decreases conduction velocity (negative dromotropy), and dilates coronary, cerebral, and systemic arterioles (Fig. 32.7).[419] Verapamil, diltiazem, and nifedipine all produce such effects, but to varying degrees and apparently by similar, but different mechanisms. These mechanisms relate to the three different classes of calcium channel antagonists that they represent: the phenylalkyl amines, the benzothiazepines, and the dihydropyridines, respectively. Nifedipine is the most potent of the three as a smooth muscle dilator, whereas verapamil and diltiazem have negative dromotropic and inotropic effects, and weak vasodilating properties. Diltiazem has weak vasodilating properties when compared with nifedipine and has less of an AV conduction effect than does verapamil. Thus verapamil and diltiazem can increase the PR interval and produce AV block. In fact, reflex activation of the sympathetic nervous system may be necessary during the administration of diltiazem, and especially during verapamil therapy, to maintain normal conduction. Clearly, verapamil and diltiazem must be titrated very carefully when a patient is already taking a β-adrenergic receptor blocking drug or when adding β-blocking drugs to a patient already taking verapamil or diltiazem.

The use of calcium channel blocking drugs has several important implications for anesthetic management.[419-421] First, the effects of inhaled and narcotic anesthetics and nifedipine in decreasing systemic vascular resistance, arterial blood pressure, and contractility may be additive. Similarly, verapamil and anesthetics (inhaled anesthetics, nitrous oxide, and narcotics) increase AV conduction times and additively decrease arterial blood pressure, systemic vascular resistance, and contractility. Second, verapamil and presumably the other calcium channel blocking drugs have been found to decrease anesthetic requirements by up to 25%. These drugs can produce neuromuscular blockade, and potentiate both depolarizing and nondepolarizing neuromuscular blocking drugs. Finally, because slow-channel activation of calcium is necessary to cause spasms of cerebral and coronary vessels, bronchoconstriction, and normal platelet aggregation, these drugs may have a role in treating cerebral vasospasm (nimodipine), coronary artery graft vasospasm (nicardipine), bronchoconstriction, and unwanted clotting disorders perioperatively. These drugs are highly protein bound and may displace or be displaced by other drugs that are also highly protein bound (e.g., lidocaine, bupivacaine, diazepam, disopyramide, and propranolol). Adverse consequences can be minimized by titrating the inhaled or narcotic drug to the hemodynamic and anesthetic effects. Hemodynamic, but not electrophysiologic, changes can usually be reversed by administering calcium. Reversal of the electrophysiologic effects may occur if high doses of β-adrenergic agonists are given.

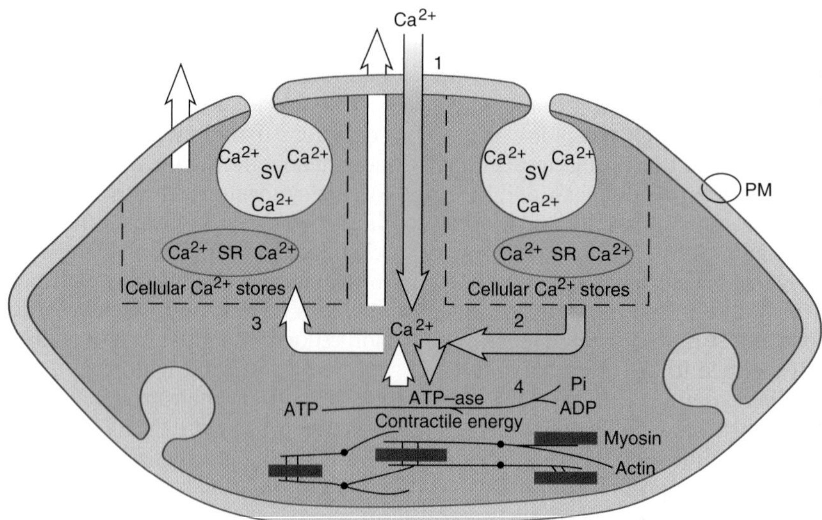

Fig. 32.7 Schematic drawing of a smooth muscle cell showing calcium *(Ca^{2+})* flux and possible sites of interference by halothane and nifedipine. The concentration of calcium in the cytoplasm increases *(green arrows)* because of entry through the plasma membrane *(PM)* and release from surface vesicles *(SV)* or the sarcoplasmic reticulum *(SR)*. When the concentration of cytoplasmic Ca^{2+} is sufficiently high, adenosine triphosphate *(ATP)* is activated. Splitting of ATP by adenosine triphosphatase *(ATPase)* into phosphatidylinositol *(Pi)* and adenosine diphosphate *(ADP)* provides the interaction and contraction of actin filaments and myosin particles constituting muscle fibers. The concentration of cytoplasmic Ca^{2+} decreases *(white arrows)* with the return of Ca^{2+} to cellular stores and the extracellular transport of Ca^{2+}. Both halothane and nifedipine probably (1) inhibit the entry of Ca^{2+} and (2) may also interfere with cytoplasmic Ca^{2+} flux by reducing the release of Ca^{2+} by the SR, by (3) reducing storage and reuptake, or by (4) blocking ATPase or the contractile mechanism (or both). (Redrawn from Tosone SR, Reves JG, Kissin I, et al. Hemodynamic responses to nifedipine in dogs anesthetized with halothane. *Anesth Analg.* 1983;62:903–908.)

MOOD-ALTERING DRUGS

Mood-altering drugs are the most frequently prescribed medications in the United States.[422,423] They include MAOIs, SSRIs, phenothiazines, tricyclic antidepressant drugs, other antidepressants that do not fall into previous drug category classifications such as bupropion, and drugs of abuse such as cocaine. MAOIs, which include isocarboxazid, phenelzine, pargyline, tranylcypromine, and deprenyl, bind irreversibly to the enzyme MAO, thereby increasing intraneuronal levels of amine neurotransmitters (serotonin, norepinephrine, dopamine, epinephrine). This increase is associated with an antidepressant effect, an antihypertensive effect, an antinarcoleptic effect, elevation of liver enzymes, and delayed onset of Parkinson disease. Because two forms of the enzyme (MAO-A and MAO-B) are selective in vitro for substrate (MAO-A is selective for serotonin, dopamine, and norepinephrine; MAO-B for tyramine and phenylethylamine), presumably MAOIs selective for MAO-A or MAO-B would have different effects.[424]

Interactions between MAOIs and a variety of foods and drugs containing indirect-acting sympathomimetic substances such as ephedrine or tyramine (found in aged hard cheeses) can occur for as long as 2 weeks after the last dose of MAOI is given. The most serious effects of this interaction are convulsions and hyperpyrexic coma (particularly after narcotics).

Anesthetic management of a patient given an MAOI can be challenging; for this reason it is widely accepted practice to discontinue MAOIs at least 2 to 3 weeks before any planned operation, further MAOIs are seen quite infrequently.[422-428] Severe reactions have occurred when too short an interval existed between the administration of MAOIs and tricyclic antidepressants. Emergency surgery in patients given MAOIs can be punctuated by hemodynamic instability. A regional block can be attempted as treatment of postoperative pain to avoid having to give narcotics. Cases of hyperpyrexic coma after the administration of most narcotics have been reported in humans, and animal studies document a 10% to 50% incidence of hyperpyrexic coma in animals pretreated with MAOIs and then given a variety of narcotics.[422-428] These reactions appear to be treated best by supportive care.

Alternative drugs for the treatment of severe depression include the tricyclic antidepressant drugs: amitriptyline, imipramine, desipramine, doxepin, nortriptyline, trazodone, and others.[422,423] Tricyclic antidepressant drugs also block the reuptake of neurotransmitters and cause their acute release. Given on a long-term basis, these drugs decrease stores of noradrenergic catecholamines. Tricyclic antidepressant drugs also produce side effects similar to those of atropine (dry mouth, tachycardia, delirium, urinary retention) and can cause changes on the ECG (changes in the T wave, prolongation of the QRS complex, bundle branch block or other conduction abnormalities, or PVCs). Although arrhythmias induced by tricyclic antidepressants have been treated successfully with physostigmine, bradycardia has sometimes occurred.[422,423] Drug interactions with tricyclic antidepressants include those related to blockade of the reuptake of norepinephrine. Such interactions, although predictable for a population of patients, may not alter a patient's threshold for arrhythmias. The selective serotonin reuptake inhibitors have gained popularity and include citalopram, escitalopram, fluoxetine, fluvoxamine, paroxetine, and sertraline, though these can also have serious side effects. For instance, fluoxetine causes nausea, vomiting, headaches, nervousness, and possibly paranoia and ideas of suicide more commonly than do the tricyclics[422,423]; however, it is less likely to cause systemic anticholinergic effects or orthostatic hypotension. Bupropion, which is fundamentally different than the SSRIs, may cause nausea, vomiting, seizures, agitation, tremor, excitement, and increased motor activity, but it only rarely causes anticholinergic effects or orthostatic hypotension. Discontinuing drugs can cause withdrawal symptoms or precipitate recurrence of psychiatric illness. Switching among drugs for depression can cause hyperpyrexia and coma; thus switching drugs preoperatively should not be requested casually.[422,423]

The effectiveness of phenothiazines and butyrophenones in schizophrenia suggests a dopamine receptor blocking action. In addition, these drugs possess varying degrees of parasympathetic stimulation and ability to block α-adrenergic receptors. The phenothiazines include chlorpromazine, promazine, triflupromazine, fluphenazine, trifluoperazine, prochlorperazine, and many others. The butyrophenones include droperidol and haloperidol. Both the phenothiazines and butyrophenones produce sedation, depression, and antihistaminic, antiemetic, and hypothermic responses. They are also associated with cholestatic jaundice, impotence, dystonia, and photosensitivity. Other side effects associated with phenothiazines include orthostatic hypotension (partly as a result of α-adrenergic blockade) and abnormalities on the ECG such as prolongation of the QT or PR intervals, blunting of T waves, depression of the ST segment, and on rare occasion, PVCs and torsades de pointes.[422,423,429,430]

Several important drug interactions are noteworthy for the phenothiazine derivatives. The effects of CNS depressants (especially narcotics and barbiturates) are enhanced by the concomitant administration of phenothiazines. In addition, the CNS seizure threshold is lowered by the administration of phenothiazines, which should be avoided in patients who are epileptic or withdrawing from any drug that depresses the CNS. Lithium carbonate is used to treat manic depression, but it is more effective in preventing mania than in relieving depression. In excitable cells, lithium mimics sodium and decreases the release of neurotransmitters both centrally and peripherally. Lithium prolongs neuromuscular blockade and may decrease anesthetic requirements because it blocks brainstem release of norepinephrine, epinephrine, and dopamine.

Psychoactive drugs such as the amphetamines (including methamphetamines, and crystal methamphetamine) and cocaine acutely release norepinephrine, epinephrine, and dopamine and block their reuptake. Taken on a long-term basis, they deplete nerve endings of these neurotransmitters.

Drugs that appear to increase central α-adrenergic release increase anesthetic requirements, whereas drugs that appear to decrease central α-adrenergic release decrease anesthetic requirements. (This may not be the mechanism by which they alter anesthetic requirements, but it is a convenient way of remembering the alteration.) Drugs that affect only the β-adrenergic receptors do not alter anesthetic requirements.

ANTIARRHYTHMIC DRUGS

Antiarrhythmic drugs include local anesthetics (lidocaine, procaine), anticonvulsant (phenytoin), β-adrenergic blocking agents, calcium channel blocking drugs, or primary antiarrhythmic drugs. These drugs are classified into five major categories: local anesthetics that alter phase 0 and phase 4 depolarization (quinidine, procainamide, and flecainide), local anesthetics that affect only phase 4 depolarization (lidocaine, mexiletine, tocainide, phenytoin, encainide), β-adrenergic receptor antagonists, antiadrenergic drugs (bretylium, disopyramide, amiodarone), and calcium entry blockers. A lack of adverse reports does not imply that all these drugs should be continued through the time of surgery.

The pharmacologic characteristics of the various antiarrhythmic drugs can affect anesthetic management. Disopyramide is similar to quinidine and procainamide in its antiarrhythmic effectiveness. Disopyramide is excreted mainly by the kidneys, but hepatic disease increases its half-life. This drug often produces anticholinergic effects, including tachycardia, urinary retention, and psychosis. Hepatitis has also been reported to have occurred after its use.[431] Little is known of the interaction of bretylium with anesthetic agents; however, since it blocks the release of catecholamines, long-term therapy with this drug has been associated with hypersensitivity to vasopressors.[431] Quinidine depends on the kidneys for excretion, can produce vagolytic effects that can decrease AV block, and is associated with blood dyscrasias and GI disturbances.[431] Most of the antiarrhythmic drugs enhance nondepolarizing neuromuscular blockade. Reports have confirmed this enhancement for quinidine, phenytoin, lidocaine, procainamide, and propranolol.[432-440] No data document such an effect for depolarizing muscle relaxants. Amiodarone, an antiadrenergic drug used to treat recurrent supraventricular and ventricular tachycardia, causes thyroid dysfunction as a result of the large amount of iodine in its structure, as well as peripheral neuropathy, and has been associated with hypertension, bradyarrhythmias, and reduced cardiac output during anesthesia.[441] The drug has a half-life of 29 days, and its pharmacologic effects persist for more than 45 days after discontinuance.[442]

ANTIBIOTICS

Many antibacterial drugs are nephrotoxic or neurotoxic, or both, and many prolong neuromuscular blockade.[434-443] The only antibiotics devoid of neuromuscular effects appear to be penicillin G and the cephalosporins.[439] Most enzyme-inducing drugs do not increase the metabolism of the volatile agents. Appropriate antibiotic prophylaxis for surgery requires a knowledge of the probability of infection for that type of surgical procedure and, if the incidence of infection warrants, the use of a drug regimen directed against the most likely infecting organisms.[443]

MEDICATIONS FOR GLAUCOMA

Medications for glaucoma include two organophosphates: echothiophate and isoflurophate. These drugs inhibit serum cholinesterase, which is responsible for the hydrolysis and inactivation of succinylcholine and ester-type local anesthetics such as procaine, chloroprocaine, and tetracaine.[444,445] These ester-type local anesthetics should be avoided in patients treated with eye drops containing organophosphate. Table 32.15 lists other medications related to anesthesia and their side effects (from the National Registry for Drug-Induced Ocular Side Effects, Oregon Health Sciences University, 3181 SW Sam Jackson Park Road, Portland, OR 97201; 503-279-8456).

TABLE 32.15 Common Ophthalmologic Drugs and Their Anesthetically Important Interactions

Drug (Trade Name)	Toxicities and Specific Treatments
GLAUCOMA: PRIMARY GOAL IS TO REDUCE IOP BY Miotics and epinephrine: increase outflow of aqueous humor β-Blockade and carbonic anhydrase inhibitors: reduce production of aqueous humor Osmotic drugs: transiently decrease volume	
MIOTICS Parasympathomimetics Pilocarpine (Adsorbocarpine, Isopto Carpine, Pilocar, Pilocel) Carbachol	
ACETYLCHOLINESTERASE INHIBITORS Physostigmine Demecarium Isoflurophate (Floropryl) Echothiophate (Echodide, Phospholine)	Tox: Hypersalivation, sweating, N/V, bradycardia, hypotension, bronchospasm, CNS effects, coma, respiratory arrest, death Rx: Atropine, pralidoxime (Protopam) Ix: Succinylcholine—prolonged apnea (drugs must be discontinued 4 weeks before)
EPINEPHRINE (EPITRATE, MUROCOLL, MYTRATE, EPIFRIN, GLAUCON, EPINAL, EPPY)	Tox: (rare) Tachycardia, PVCs, HTN, headache, tremors Ix: Avoid drugs that sensitize to catecholamines (e.g., halothane)
β-BLOCKERS Timolol (Timoptic) Betaxolol (Betoptic) Levobunolol (Betagan)	Tox: β-Blockade with bradycardia, exacerbation of asthma, CNS depression, lethargy, confusion Synergy noted with systemic drugs
CARBONIC ANHYDRASE INHIBITORS Acetazolamide (Diamox) Dichlorphenamide (Daranide, Oratrol) Ethoxzolamide (Cardrase, Ethamide) Methazolamide (Neptazane)	Tox: Anorexia, GI disturbances, "general miserable feeling" and malaise, paresthesias, diuresis, hypokalemia (transient), renal colic and calculi, hyperuricemia, thrombocytopenia, aplastic anemia, acute respiratory failure in patients with COPD
OSMOTIC DRUGS Glycerin (Glyrol, Osmoglyn) Isosorbide (Ismotic) Urea (Urevert, Ureaphil) Mannitol (Osmitrol) Intraocular acetylcholine (Miochol)	Tox: Dehydration, hyperglycemia, nonketotic hyperosmolar coma (rare); fatalities with mannitol secondary to CHF or intracranial bleeding; urea may cause thrombosis Tox: Hypotension, bradycardia Rx: Atropine
MYDRIATICS AND CYCLOPLEGICS: PROVIDE PUPILLARY DILATATION AND PARALYSIS OF ACCOMMODATION Anticholinergics block muscarinic receptors; paralyzing in iris α-Adrenergics contract the dilator of the iris	
ANTICHOLINERGICS Atropine (Atropisol, Bufopto, Isopto Atropine) Cyclopentolate, alone (Cyclogyl) or with phenylephrine-homatropine (Cyclomydril) Homatropine (Homatrocel, Isopto Homatropine) Scopolamine (Isopto Hyoscine, Murocoll 19) Tropicamide (Mydriacyl)	Tox: Dry mouth, flushing, thirst, tachycardia, seizure, hyperactivity, transient psychosis, rare coma, and death Rx: Physostigmine
β-ADRENERGICS Phenylephrine (Efricel, Mydfrin, Neo-Synephrine) Hydroxyamphetamine (Paredrine)	Tox: Tachycardia, HTN, PVCs, myocardial ischemia, agitation

CHF, Congestive heart failure; *CNS*, central nervous system; *COPD*, chronic obstructive pulmonary disease; *GI*, gastrointestinal; *HTN*, hypertension; *IOP*, intraocular pressure; *Ix*, interaction; *N/V*, nausea and vomiting; *PVCs*, premature ventricular contractions; *Rx*, treatment; *Tox*, toxicity.

Modified from the National Registry for Drug-Induced Ocular Side Effects, University of Oregon Health Sciences Center, Portland, OR.

Complete references available online at expertconsult.com.

References

1. Wei JY. *N Engl J Med*. 1992;327:1735.
2. Fleisher LA, Eagle KA. *N Engl J Med*. 2001;345:1677.
3. Goldman L, et al. *N Engl J Med*. 1977;297:845.
4. Fleisher LA, et al. *J Am Coll Cardiol*. 2007;50:159.

4a. van Tilburg J, et al. *J Med Genet*. 2001;38:569.

5. Diabetes Control and Complications Trial (DCCT)/Epidemiology of Diabetes Interventions and Complications Research Group. *N Engl J Med*. 2000;342:381.
6. U.K. Prospective. Diabetes Study Group. *BMJ*. 1998;317:703.

6a. Thrasher J. *Am J Cardiol*. 2017;120:S4.

6b. Iqbal A, et al. *Diabetes Metab J*. 2018;42:3.

7. Albacker T, et al. *Ann Thorac Surg*. 2008;86:20.
8. Krinsley JS. *Mayo Clin Proc*. 2004;79:992.
9. Advance Collaborative Group. *N Engl J Med*. 2008;358:2560.
10. Van den Berghe G, et al. *N Engl J Med*. 2001;345:1359.
11. Ingels C, et al. *Eur Heart J*. 2006;27:2716.
12. Finney SJ, et al. *JAMA*. 2003;290:2041.
13. Krinsley JS. *Mayo Clin Proc*. 2003;78:1471.
14. Freeman R. *Lancet*. 2005;365:1259.
15. Charlson ME, et al. *J Am Coll Surg*. 1994;179:1.
16. O'Sullivan CJ, et al. *Eur J Vasc Endovasc Surg*. 2006;32:188.
17. Halkos ME, et al. *Ann Thorac Surg*. 2008;86:1431.
18. Gustafsson UO, et al. *Br J Surg*. 2009;96:1358.
19. Bhadresha S, et al. *Anaesthesia*. 2009;64:1372.
20. Gandhi GY, et al. *Ann Intern Med*. 2007;146:233.
21. Diabetes Control and Complications Trial Research Group. *Ann Intern Med*. 1998;128:517.
22. Ramanathan S, et al. *Anesth Analg*. 1991;73:105.
23. Van den Berghe G, et al. *N Engl J Med*. 2006;354:449.
24. NICE-SUGAR Study Investigators, et al. *N Engl J Med*. 2012;367:1108.
25. Sebranek JJ, et al. *Br J Anaesth*. 2013;111(suppl 1):i18.
26. Jacobi J, et al. *Crit Care Med*. 2012;40:3251.
27. Roizen MF. *RealAge: Are You as Young as You Can be?*. New York: HarperCollins; 1999.
28. Roizen MF. *The RealAge Makeover: Take Years Off Your Looks and Add Them to Your Life!*. New York: HarperCollins; 2004.
29. Roizen MF, Oz MC. *YOU: the owner's manual*. New York, 2005.
30. Khuri SF, et al. *J Am Coll Surg*. 1997;185:315.
31. Tuomilehto J, et al. *N Engl J Med*. 2001;344:1343.

31a. Joshi GP, et al. *Anesth Analg*. 2010;111:1378.

32. Ravid M, et al. *Ann Intern Med*. 1998;128:982.
33. Page MM, Watkins PJ. *Lancet*. 1978;1:14.

33a. Tran TTT, et al. *Front Endocrinol (Lausanne)*. 2017;8:185.

34. Chiasson JL, et al. *CMAJ*. 2003;168:859.

34a. Fayfman M, et al. *Med Clin North Am*. 2017;101:587.

34b. Kamel KS, et al. *Am J Kidney Dis*. 2016;68:967.

35. Pasternak JJ, et al. *Mayo Clin Proc*. 2008;83:406.
36. Larsen ML, Illingworth DR. *Med Clin North Am*. 1994;78:225.
37. Downs JR, et al. *JAMA*. 1998;279:1615.
38. Fowkes FGR, et al. *BMJ*. 1998;316:1764.

38a. Rosenson RS, et al. *J Am Coll Cardiol*. 2017;70:1290.

39. Stone NJ, et al. *Circulation*. 2014;129(25 Suppl 2):S1.

39a. Jacobson TA, et al. *J Clin Lipidol*. 2014;8:473.

40. Fleisher LA, et al. *Circulation*. 2009;120:e169.
41. Nissen SE, et al. *JAMA*. 2004;291:1071.

41a. Silber JH, et al. *Ann Surg*. 2012;256:79.

42. Pelosi P, et al. *J Appl Physiol*. 1997;82:811.

42a. Bluth T, Pelosi P, de Abreu MG. *Opin Anaesthesiol*. 2016;29:421.

43. Daniels L. *Australian Prescriber*. 2003;26:136.
44. Hirose K, et al. *Br J Anaesth*. 2014;112:246.
45. Veterans Administration Total Parenteral Nutrition Cooperative Study Group. *N Engl J Med*. 1991;325:525.
46. Nicholas JM, et al. *Am J Surg*. 2003;186:583.
47. Starker PM, et al. *Ann Surg*. 1983;198:720.

47a. Elke G, et al. *Crit Care*. 2016;20:117.

47b. Liu MM, et al. *Anesthesiology*. 2017;127:166.

48. Udelsman R, et al. *J Clin Invest*. 1986;77:1377.
49. Ezzat S, et al. *Cancer*. 2004;101:613.

49a. Guerin C, et al. *Endocr Relat Cancer*. 2016;23:R131.

50. Symreng T, et al. *Br J Anaesth*. 1981;53:949.
51. Yong SL, et al. *Cochrane Database Syst Rev*. 2009;(4):CD005367.
52. Nieman LK, et al. *J Clin Endocrinol Metab*. 1993;77:1308.
53. Dorin RI, et al. *Ann Intern Med*. 2003;139:194.

53a. Bornstein SR, et al. *J Clin Endocrinol Metab*. 2016;101:364–389.

53b. Marik PE. *Varon J: Arch Surg*. 2008;143:1222.

54. Bravo EL. *Endocr Rev*. 1994;15:356.
55. St John Sutton MG, et al. *Mayo Clin Proc*. 1981;56:354.

55a. Naranjo J, et al. *J Cardiothorac Vasc Anesth*. 2017;31:1427.

55b. Lenders JW, et al. *Lancet*. 2005;366:665.

56. Prys-Roberts C. *Br J Anaesth*. 2000;85:44.
57. Witteles RM, et al. *Anesth Analg*. 2000;91:302.
58. Lucon AM, et al. *J Urol*. 1997;157:1208.
59. Roizen MF, et al. *Anesthesiology*. 1982;57:A43.
60. Roizen MF, et al. *Surgery*. 1983;94:941.

60a. Lenders JW, et al. *J Clin Endocrinol Metab*. 2014;99:1915.

61. Allen GC, Rosenberg H. *Can J Anaesth*. 1990;37:593.
62. Zakowski M, et al. *Anesthesiology*. 1989;70:875.
63. Roizen MF, et al. *Anesthesiol Clin North Am*. 1987;5:269.

63a. Esteve-Turrillas FA, et al. *Analyst*. 2014;139:3636.

64. Lord MS, Augoustides JG. *J Cardiothorac Vasc Anesth*. 2012;26:526.
65. Herroeder S, et al. *Anesthesiology*. 2011;114:971.
66. Augoustides JG, et al. *Anesthesiology*. 2004;101:1022.
67. Roizen MF. *Anesthesiology*. 1988;68:482.
68. Stone JG, et al. *Anesthesiology*. 1988;68:495.
69. Mangano DT, et al. *N Engl J Med*. 1996;335:1713.
70. Flacke JW, et al. *Anesthesiology*. 1987;67:11.
71. Yeager MP, et al. *Anesthesiology*. 1987;66:729.
72. Fleisher LA, et al. *Am Heart J*. 1991;122:980.
73. Levine JD, et al. *J Neurosci*. 1986;6:3423.
74. Wade JG, et al. *N Engl J Med*. 1970;282:823.
75. Ziegler MG, et al. *N Engl J Med*. 1977;296:293.
76. Goldstein DS, et al. *N Engl J Med*. 1997;336:696.
77. Kendrick WW, et al. *Treat Serv Bull (Ottawa)*. 1953;8:437.

77a. Martirosyan NL, et al. *Clin Neurol Neurosurg*. 2017;154:79.

78. Gronert GA, Theye RA. *Anesthesiology*. 1975;43:89.
79. Feek CM, et al. *N Engl J Med*. 1980;302:883.

79a. Strowd SM, et al. *A A Pract*. 2018;10:97.

80. Loh KC. *Postgrad Med J*. 2000;76:133.
81. Williams M, Lo Gerfo P. *Thyroid*. 2002;12:523.

81a. Saritas A, et al. *Turk J Anaesthesiol Reanim*. 2015;43:240–245.

82. Weinberg AD, et al. *Arch Intern Med*. 1983;143:893.
83. Surks MI, et al. *JAMA*. 2004;291:228.
84. Vanderpump MPJ, et al. *Clin Endocrinol*. 1995;43:55.
85. Hattori H, et al. *Acta Otolaryngol Suppl*. 2003;550:59.

85a. Mathew V, et al. *J Thyroid Res*. 2011;2011:462.

86. Stewart AF. *N Engl J Med*. 2005;352:373.
87. Peacock M, et al. *J Clin Endocrinol Metab*. 2005;90:135.
88. Lind L, Ljunghall S. *Exp Clin Endocrinol*. 1994;102:409.
89. Kebebew E, et al. *Arch Surg*. 2003;138:867.
90. Oltmann SC, et al. *Ann Surg Oncol*. 2013;20:4195.
91. Carling T, et al. *Arch Surg*. 2006;141:401.
92. Allain TJ, Dhesi J. *Gerontology*. 2003;49:273.
93. Hong JC, et al. *Surgery*. 2011;150:1069.
94. Blanchard C, et al. *Eur J Endocrinol*. 2013;169:665.

94a. Minisola S, et al. *BMJ*. 2015;350:h2723.

94b. Basok AB, et al. *BMJ Case Rep*. 2018;2018.

95. Rumancik WM, et al. *JAMA*. 1978;240:366.
96. Moyad MA. *Urol Clin North Am*. 2004;31:321.
97. Cauley JA, et al. *JAMA*. 2003;290:1729.
98. Keller MI. *Cleve Clin J Med*. 2004;71:829.
99. Katznelson L, et al. *Endocr Pract*. 2011;17:636.
100. Rojiani AM, et al. *J Neuropathol Exp Neurol*. 1987;46:495.

100a. Matsuzaki S, et al. *BMC Pregnancy Childbirth*. 2017;17:188.

101. Ayus JC, et al. *Ann Intern Med*. 1992;117:891.
102. Robertson GL. *Endocrinol Metab Clin North Am*. 1995;24:549.
103. Weksler N, et al. *J Clin Anesth*. 2003;15:179.
104. Aronson S, et al. *Anesth Analg*. 2002;94:1079.
105. Kheterpal S, et al. *Anesthesiology*. 2009;110:58.
106. Wax DB, et al. *J Cardiothorac Vasc Anesth*. 2010;24:927.
107. Prys-Roberts C, et al. *Br J Anaesth*. 1971;43:122.
108. Goldman L, Caldera DL. *Anesthesiology*. 1979;50:285.
109. Mangano DT, et al. *N Engl J Med*. 1990;323:1781.
110. Pasternack PF, et al. *Am J Surg*. 1989;158:113.

110a. Futier E, et al. *JAMA*. 2017;318:1346.

110aa. Sessler DI, et al. *Anesthesiology*. 2018;128:317–327.

111. POISE Study Group, et al. *Lancet*. 2008;371:1839.
112. Coriat P, et al. *Anesthesiology*. 1994;81:299.
113. Bertrand M, et al. *Anesth Analg*. 2001;92:26.
114. Kheterpal S, et al. *J Cardiothorac Vasc Anesth*. 2008;22:180.
115. Turan A, et al. *Anesth Analg*. 2012;114:552.

116. London MJ. *Anesthesiology*. 2017;126:1.
117. Fleisher LA, et al. *Circulation*. 2007;116:e418.
118. Duceppe E, et al. *Can J Cardiol*. 2017;33:17.
119. Fleisher LA, et al. *J Am Coll Cardiol*. 2014.
120. Kristensen SD, et al. *Eur Heart J*. 2014.
121. Posner KL, et al. *Anesth Analg*. 1999;89:553.
122. Godet G, et al. *Anesthesiology*. 2005;102:739.
123. McFalls EO, et al. *N Engl J Med*. 2004;351:2795.
124. Ward HB, et al. *Ann Thorac Surg*. 2006;82:795; discussion 800.
125. Poldermans D, et al. *J Am Coll Cardiol*. 2006;48:964.
126. Poldermans D, et al. *J Am Coll Cardiol*. 2007;49:1763.
127. Back MR, et al. *J Vasc Surg*. 2002;36:526.
128. Kaluza GL, et al. *J Am Coll Cardiol*. 2000;35:1288.
129. Wilson SH, et al. *J Am Coll Cardiol*. 2003;42:234.
130. Vicenzi MN, et al. *Br J Anaesth*. 2006;96:686.
131. Leibowitz D, et al. *Am J Cardiol*. 2006;97:1188.
132. Nasser M, et al. *Catheter Cardiovasc Interv*. 2005;65:516.
133. Schouten O, et al. *J Am Coll Cardiol*. 2007;49:122.
134. Berger PB, et al. *JACC Cardiovasc Interv*. 2010;3:920.
135. Wijeysundera DN, et al. *Circulation*. 2012;126:1355.
136. Hawn MT, et al. *JAMA*. 2013;310:1462.
136a. Levine GN, et al. *Circulation*. 2016;134:e123.
136b. Albaladejo P, et al. *Heart*. 2011;97:1566.
137. Shah KB, et al. *Anesth Analg*. 1990;70:240.
138. Hammill BG, et al. *Anesthesiology*. 2008;108:559.
139. McEnroe CS, et al. *J Vasc Surg*. 1990;11:497.
140. Mantha S, et al. *Anesth Analg*. 1994;79:422.
141. Flu WJ, et al. *Anesthesiology*. 2010;112:1316.
142. Smith JS, et al. *Anesthesiology*. 1988;69:846.
143. Riles TS, et al. *Surgery*. 1979;85:249.
144. Materson BJ, et al. *N Engl J Med*. 1993;328:914.
145. Goldman L, et al. *Medicine (Baltimore)*. 1978;57:357.
146. Charlson ME, et al. *Ann Surg*. 1990;212:66.
147. Frank SM, et al. *JAMA*. 1997;277:1127.
148. Eriksson G, et al. *J Intern Med*. 1993;234:493.
149. Nelson AH, et al. *Crit Care Med*. 1993;21:860.
150. Eagle KA, Boucher CA. *N Engl J Med*. 1989;321:1330.
151. Lette J, et al. *Am J Cardiol*. 1989;64:276.
152. Kennedy JW, et al. *Circulation*. 1981;63:793.
153. Detsky AS, et al. *J Gen Intern Med*. 1986;1:211.
154. Gerson MC, et al. *Ann Intern Med*. 1985;103:832.
155. Higgins TL, et al. *JAMA*. 1992;267:2344.
156. Rivers SP, et al. *J Vasc Surg*. 1990;11:70; discussion 76.
157. Berlauk JF, et al. *Ann Surg*. 1991;214:289.
158. American Society of Anesthesiologists Task Force on Pulmonary Artery Catheterization. *Anesthesiology*. 1993;78:380.
159. Eagle KA, et al. *Ann Intern Med*. 1989;110:859.
160. Boucher CA, et al. *N Engl J Med*. 1985;312:389.
161. Santos AL, Gelperin A. *J Am Geriatr Soc*. 1975;23:42.
162. Raby KE, et al. *N Engl J Med*. 1989;321:1296.
163. Fletcher JP, et al. *J Cardiovasc Surg*. 1988;29:666.
164. Lee TH, et al. *Circulation*. 1999;100:1043.
165. Hoeks SE, et al. *Am J Med*. 2009;122:559.
166. Cohen ME, et al. *J Am Coll Surg*. 2013;217:336.
167. Gupta PK, et al. *Circulation*. 2011;124:381.
167a. Mangano DT, et al. *N Engl J Med*. 1996;335:1713.
167b. Poldermans D, et al. *N Engl J Med*. 1999;341:1789.
167c. Juul AB, et al. *BMJ*. 2006;332:1482.
167d. Lindenauer PK, et al. *N Engl J Med*. 2005;353:349–361.
167e. Yang H, et al. *Am Heart J*. 2006;152:983–990.
167f. Devereaux PJ, et al. *Lancet*. 2008;371:1839.
167g. Wijeysundera DN, et al. *J Am Coll Cardiol*. 2014.
167h. Wallace AW, et al. *Anesthesiology*. 2010;113:794.
168. Ellis JE, et al. *Anesth Analg*. 1992;74:S85.
169. Naylor CD, et al. *JAMA*. 1993;269:2407.
169a. Devereaux PJ, et al. *N Engl J Med*. 2014.
169b. Devereaux PJ, et al. *N Engl J Med*. 2014.
169c. Durazzo AE, et al. *J Vasc Surg*. 2004;39:967.
169d. Le Manach Y, et al. *Anesth Analg*. 2007;104:1326; table of contents.
169e. Lee SM, et al. *Anesthesiology*. 2015;123:288–306.
169f. Roshanov PS, et al. *Anesthesiology*. 2017;126:16.
170. Carson JL, et al. *N Engl J Med*. 2011;365:2453.
171. Hollinger I. In: Katz R, Steward D, eds. *Anesthesia and Uncommon Pediatric Diseases*. Philadelphia: Saunders; 1993:93.
172. Nishimura RA, et al. *Circulation*. 2008;118:887.
173. Katholi RE, et al. *Am Heart J*. 1976;92:162.
174. Bonow RO, et al. *Circulation*. 1998;98:1949.
175. Ezekowitz MD. *J Heart Valve Dis*. 2002;11(suppl 1):S56.
176. Bonow RO, et al. *Circulation*. 2006;114:e84.
176a. Nishimura RA, et al. *Circulation*. 2014;129:2440.
177. Vandermeulen EP, et al. *Anesth Analg*. 1994;79:1165.
178. Rao TLK, El-Etr AA. *Anesthesiology*. 1981;55:618.
179. Frame JN, et al. *Ann Intern Med*. 1989;111:946.
180. Waldman SD, et al. *Anesth Analg*. 1987;66:267.
181. Bargon HC, et al. *J Vasc Surg*. 1987;6:144.
182. Onishchuk JL, Carlsson C. *Anesthesiology*. 1992;77:1221.
183. Horlocker TT, et al. *Anesth Analg*. 1990;70:631.
184. Macdonald R. *Br J Anaesth*. 1991;66(1).
185. Amrein PC, et al. *JAMA*. 1981;245:1825.
186. Horlocker TT, et al. *Reg Anesth Pain Med*. 2003;28:172.
187. International Multicentre Trial. *Lancet*. 1975;2:45.
187a. Gordon RJ, Lombard FW, et al. *Anesth Analg*. 2017;125:403.
188. Consensus Conference. *JAMA*. 1988;256:744.
189. Collins R, et al. *N Engl J Med*. 1988;318:1162.
190. Gallus A, et al. *Br J Surg*. 1983;70:17.
190a. MacLean S. *Chest*. 2012;141:e1S.
191. Lutz DJ, et al. *Am J Obstet Gynecol*. 1978;131:460.
192. Gauss A, et al. *Anesthesiology*. 1998;88:679.
193. Ruskin JN. *N Engl J Med*. 1991;324:1660.
194. Kelly JS, Royster RL. *Anesth Analg*. 1989;69:229.
195. Risk SC, et al. *J Cardiothorac Vasc Anesth*. 1992;6:275.
196. Prystowsky EN. *Curr Probl Cardiol*. 1988;13:225.
197. McAnulty JH, et al. *N Engl J Med*. 1982;307:137.
198. Rose MR, Koski G. *Anesthesiology*. 1988;69:A146.
198a. Fisher BW, et al. *Am J Med*. 2002;112:219.
199. Anthonisen NR, et al. *JAMA*. 1994;272:1497.
200. European Respiratory Society. *Eur Respir J*. 1995;8:1398.
201. Holleman Jr DR, Simel DL. *JAMA*. 1995;273:313.
202. Lacasse Y, et al. *Chest*. 1997;111:1077.
203. Saint S, et al. *JAMA*. 1995;273:957.
204. Thompson WH, et al. *Am J Respir Crit Care Med*. 1996;154:407.
205. NAEP Expert Panel Report 2. *Guidelines for the Diagnosis and Management of Asthma*. Public Health Service. U.S. Department of Health and Human Services publication no. 97-4051A; 1997. http://www.nhlbi.nih.gov/nhlbi/nhlbi.htm/. (Accessed 12.06.14.).
206. Sin DD, et al. *JAMA*. 2004;292:367.
207. Tilles SA. *Med Clin North Am*. 2006;90:61.
208. Dompeling E, et al. *Ann Intern Med*. 1993;118:770.
209. Calligaro KD, et al. *J Vasc Surg*. 1993;18:914.
210. Skolnick ET, et al. *Anesthesiology*. 1998;88:1144.
211. Rodgers A, et al. *BMJ*. 2000;321:1493.
212. Stein M, Cassara EL. *JAMA*. 1970;211:787.
213. Khan MA, Hussain SF. *J Ayub Med Coll Abbottabad*. 2005;17:82.
214. Rock P, Passannante A. *Anesthesiol Clin North Am*. 2004;22:77.
215. Qaseem A, et al. *Ann Intern Med*. 2006;144:575.
216. Smetana GW, et al. *Ann Intern Med*. 2006;144:581.
217. Collins CD, et al. *BMJ*. 1968;1:401.
218. Hulzebos EH, et al. *JAMA*. 2006;296:1851.
219. Warner MA, et al. *Mayo Clin Proc*. 1989;64:609.
220. Robinson K, et al. *Br Heart J*. 1989;62:16.
221. Ernst E, Matrai A. *Atherosclerosis*. 1987;64:75.
222. Bluman LG, et al. *Chest*. 1998;113:883.
223. Nakagawa M, et al. *Chest*. 2001;120:705.
224. Wong J, et al. *Can J Anaesth*. 2012;59:268.
225. Wong J, et al. *Anesthesiology*. 2012;117:755.
226. Lee SM, et al. *Anesth Analg*. 2013;117:605.
227. McCreanor J, et al. *N Engl J Med*. 2007;357:2348.
228. Downs SH, et al. *N Engl J Med*. 2007;357:2338.
229. Celli BR, et al. *Am Rev Respir Dis*. 1984;130:12.
230. Bartlett RH, et al. *Surg Gynecol Obstet*. 1973;137:925.
231. Lyager S, et al. *Acta Anaesthesiol Scand*. 1979;23:312.
232. Neuman MD, et al. *Anesthesiology*. 2012;117:72.
233. Elwood T, et al. *Can J Anaesth*. 2003;50:277.
234. Boushy SF, et al. *Chest*. 1971;59:383.
235. Mittman C. *Am Rev Respir Dis*. 1961;84:197.
236. Reichel J. *Chest*. 1972;62:570.
237. Wong DH, et al. *Anesth Analg*. 1995;80:276.
238. Arozullah AM, et al. *Ann Surg*. 2000;232:242.
239. Arozullah AM, et al. *Ann Intern Med*. 2001;135:847.
240. Matthay RA, et al. *Med Clin North Am*. 1990;74:571.

241. Fedullo PF, et al. *N Engl J Med.* 2001;345:1465.
242. Galie N, et al. *N Engl J Med.* 2005;353:2148.
243. Domino KB, et al. *Anesthesiology.* 1983;59:428.
244. Settipane GA, Dudupakkam RK. *J Allergy Clin Immunol.* 1975;56:215.
245. Centers for Disease Control and Prevention: Cancer statistics for the United States. www.cdc.gov/nchs/products/pubs/pubd/hus/trendtables.htm. 2014 (Accessed 12.06.14.).
246. Aisner J. *J Clin Oncol.* 1996;14:658.
247. Cooper JAD. *Clin Chest Med.* 1990;11:1.
248. Levy JH, et al. *Spine.* 1986;11:282.
249. Kemp SF, Lockey RF. *J Allergy Clin Immunol.* 2002;110:341.
249a. Freundlich RE, et al. *J Clin Anesth.* 2016;35:415.
250. Smith PL, et al. *J Clin Invest.* 1980;66:1072.
251. Delage C, Irey NS. *J Forensic Sci.* 1972;17:525.
252. Bettman MA. *N Engl J Med.* 1987;317:891.
253. Roizen MF, et al. *Anesthesiology.* 1989;71:331.
254. Mertes PM, Laxenaire MC. *Eur J Anaesthesiol.* 2002;19:240.
255. Lieberman P. *J Allergy Clin Immunol.* 2002;110(suppl):S64.
256. Rosow CE, et al. *Anesthesiology.* 1982;56:93.
257. Millbern SM, Bell SD. *Anesthesiology.* 1979;50:56.
258. Halevy S, et al. *Klin Wochenschr.* 1982;60:1021.
258a. Kannan JA, Bernstein JA. *Immunol Allergy Clin North Am.* 2015;35:321.
259. Toogood JH. *J Allergy Clin Immunol.* 1988;81:1.
260. Van Arsdel Jr PP, Larson EB. *Ann Intern Med.* 1989;110:304.
260a. MacBeth LS, et al. *J Clin Anesth.* 2016;34:385.
261. Heyland DK, et al. *JAMA.* 2001;286:944.
261a. Lytvyn L, et al. *J Hosp Infect.* 2016;92:130.
261b. Sawh SC, et al. *PeerJ.* 2016;4:e2429.
261c. Cook DJ, et al. *Trials.* 2016;17:377.
262. *Med Lett Drugs Ther.* 2003;45:57.
262a. Perks A, et al. *Br J Anaesth.* 2012;108:562.
262b. Bhattacharya B, Maung AA. *Anesthesiol Clin.* 2016;34:747.
263. Roberts R. *Curr Opin Neurol.* 1998;11:135.
264. Shaner DM, et al. *Neurology.* 1988;38:202.
265. Schuchat A, et al. *N Engl J Med.* 1997;337:970.
266. Mets B. *Anesth Analg.* 1991;72:557.
267. Muzzi DA, et al. *Anesthesiology.* 1989;71:322.
268. Parkinson Study Group. *Ann Neurol.* 1996;39:37.
269. Goetz CG, et al. *N Engl J Med.* 1989;320:337.
270. Wiklund RA, Ngai SH. *Anesthesiology.* 1971;35:545.
270a. Akbar U, et al. *Expert Rev Neurother.* 2017;17:301.
271. Barry PP, Moskowitz MA. *Arch Intern Med.* 1988;148:1914.
272. Skoog I, et al. *N Engl J Med.* 1993;328:153.
273. Petersen RC, et al. *Arch Neurol.* 1999;56:303.
274. Ross GW, et al. *JAMA.* 1997;277:800.
274a. Alzheimer's A. *Alzheimers Dement.* 2013;9:208.
275. Snowdon DA, et al. *JAMA.* 1997;277:813.
276. *Med Lett Drugs Ther.* 2001;43:53.
277. Jones PM, Soderman RM. *Anaesthesia.* 2007;62:201.
278. Xie Z, Tanzi RE. *Exp Gerontol.* 2006;41:346.
278a. Berger M, et al. *J Cardiothorac Vasc Anesth.* 2014;28:1609.
279. Eckenhoff RG, et al. *Anesthesiology.* 2004;101:703.
280. Wei H, et al. *Anesthesiology.* 2008;108:251.
281. Zhang B, et al. *J Biol Chem.* 2008;283:11866.
282. Hemmelgarn B, et al. *JAMA.* 1997;278:27.
283. Mozkowitz MA. *Neurol Clin.* 1990;8:801.
284. Michel P, et al. *Cephalagia.* 1993;12:54.
285. MacIntyre PD, et al. *Circulation.* 1993;87:401.
286. Shadick NA, et al. *Ann Intern Med.* 1994;121:560.
287. Ferguson RJ, Caplan LR. *Neurol Clin.* 1985;3:373.
288. Ovassapian A, et al. *Anesthesiology.* 1983;58:370.
289. Rudick RA, et al. *N Engl J Med.* 1997;337:1604.
289a. Makris A, et al. *J Anesth.* 2014;28:267.
290. Wipfli M, et al. *J Clin Anesth.* 2013;25:409.
291. Kocabas S, et al. *J Clin Anesth.* 2007;19:299.
292. McKhann GM, et al. *Ann Neurol.* 1988;23:347.
292a. Moran S, et al. *Surg Clin North Am.* 2015;95:417.
293. Toh B-H, et al. *N Engl J Med.* 1997;337:1441.
294. Jensen NF, et al. *Anesth Analg.* 1995;80:591.
295. Kantor G, Rolbin SH. *Can J Anaesth.* 1992;39:282.
296. Meissner PN, et al. *Br J Anaesth.* 1991;66:60.
297. McNeill MJ, Bennet A. *Br J Anaesth.* 1990;64:371.
297a. Bissell DM, et al. *N Engl J Med.* 2017;377:862.
298. Massey JM. *Neurology.* 1997;48:S46.
299. d'Empaire G, et al. *J Thorac Cardiovasc Surg.* 1985;89:592.
300. Eisenkraft JB, et al. *Anesthesiology.* 1988;69:760.
301. Eisenkraft JB, et al. *Anesthesiology.* 1986;65:79.
302. Sungur Ulke Z, et al. *Acta Anaesthesiol Scand.* 2013;57:745.
302a. Chigurupati K, et al. *J Cardiothorac Vasc Anesth.* 2018;32:325.
303. Small S, et al. *Anesthesiology.* 1992;76:142.
303a. Weingarten TN, et al. *J Clin Anesth.* 2014;26:648.
304. Lema G, et al. *Anesthesiology.* 1991;74:373.
305. Ashwood EM, et al. *Anaesthesia.* 1992;47:579.
306. Gutmann DH, Fischbeck KH. *Ann Neurol.* 1989;26:189.
307. Smith CL, Bush GH. *Br J Anaesth.* 1985;57:1113.
307a. Katz JA, Murphy GS. *Curr Opin Anaesthesiol.* 2017;30:435.
307b. Litman RS, et al. *Anesthesiology.* 2018;128:159.
308. Pueschel SM, Scola FH. *Pediatrics.* 1987;80:55.
309. Morray JP, et al. *Anesthesiology.* 1986;65:221.
310. Roizen NJ, Patterson D. *Lancet.* 2003;361:1281.
311. Freeman SB, et al. *Am J Med Genet.* 1998;80:213.
312. Kobel M, et al. *Can J Anaesth.* 1982;29:593.
313. Bedford RF, et al. *Anesth Analg.* 1982;61:430.
314. Treatment guideline. *Med Lett Drugs Ther.* 2003;11:69.
315. Byrick RJ, Rose DK. *Can J Anaesth.* 1990;37:457.
316. Berns AS. *Kidney Int.* 1989;36:730.
317. Myers BD, Moran SM. *N Engl J Med.* 1986;314:97.
318. Thadhani R, et al. *N Engl J Med.* 1996;334:1448.
319. Hebert PC, et al. *N Engl J Med.* 1999;340:409.
320. Koch CG, et al. *Ann Thorac Surg.* 2006;82:13.
321. Coe FL, et al. *N Engl J Med.* 1992;327:1141.
321a. Mazer CD, et al. *N Engl J Med.* 2017;377:2133.
321b. Kanda H, et al. *J Cardiothorac Vasc Anesth.* 2017;31:2251.
322. Kellen M, et al. *Anesth Analg.* 1994;78:134.
323. Novis BK, et al. *Anesth Analg.* 1994;78:143.
324. Lee TH, et al. *Circulation.* 1999;100:1043.
325. Mangano CM, et al. *Ann Intern Med.* 1998;128:194.
325a. McKinlay J, et al. *Anaesthesia.* 2018;73(suppl 1):85.
326. Petroni KC, Cohen NH. *Anesth Analg.* 2002;94:1288.
327. Myers BD, et al. *Kidney Int.* 1988;33:590.
328. Bennett WM, et al. *Am J Kidney Dis.* 1983;3:155.
329. Bennett WM, et al. *Drug Prescribing in Renal Failure: Dosing Guidelines for Adults.* 2nd ed. Philadelphia: American College of Physicians; 1991.
330. Goyal P, et al. *Anaesth Intensive Care.* 2002;30:584.
331. Appel GB, Neu HC. *N Engl J Med.* 1977;296(663):722–784.
332. Rackow EC, Astiz ME. *JAMA.* 1991;266:548.
333. Knaus WA, Wagner DP. *Crit Care Clin.* 1989;5:522.
334. *Med Lett Drugs Ther.* 2004;46:13.
335. Nichol KL, et al. *N Engl J Med.* 2007;357:1373.
335a. Dasta J, et al. *J Crit Care.* 2015;30:1072.
336. Sterns RH. *Ann Intern Med.* 1987;107:656.
337. Surawicz B. *Am Heart J.* 1967;73:814.
338. Rimmer JM, et al. *Arch Intern Med.* 1987;147:867.
339. Busch EH, et al. *South Med J.* 1987;80:1450.
340. Don BR, et al. *N Engl J Med.* 1990;322:1290.
340a. Singla M, et al. *Am J Ther.* 2016;23:e1102.
340b. Saginur M, et al. *Am J Transplant.* 2012;12:3152.
341. Kharasch ED, Bowdle TA. *Anesth Analg.* 1991;72:216.
342. Allon M, et al. *Ann Intern Med.* 1989;110:426.
343. Wong KC, et al. *Can J Anaesth.* 1977;24:203.
344. Lawson DH. *Q J Med.* 1974;43:433.
345. Vitez TS, et al. *Anesthesiology.* 1985;63:130.
346. Hirsch IA, et al. *Anesth Analg.* 1988;67:131.
347. Olson RP, et al. *Can J Anaesth.* 2003;50:553.
348. Schow AJ, et al. *Anesth Analg.* 2002;95:19.
349. Wahr JA, et al. *JAMA.* 1999;281:2203.
350. Cohen JD, et al. *Am J Cardiol.* 1987;60:548.
351. Holland OB, et al. *Am J Med.* 1981;70:762.
352. Kornbluth A, Sachar DB. *Am J Gastroenterol.* 1997;92:204.
353. Kahrilas PJ. *JAMA.* 1996;276:983.
354. Kurz A, et al. *N Engl J Med.* 1996;334:1209.
355. *Med Lett Drugs Ther.* 2001;43:92.
356. Jain NK, et al. *Ann Intern Med.* 1987;107:824.
357. Gorbach SL. *Rev Infect Dis.* 1991;13(suppl 10):S815.
358. Peterson WJ. *West J Med.* 1990;152:167.
358a. Castillo J, et al. *J Cardiothorac Vasc Anesth.* 2018;32:1023.
359. Botero M, et al. *J Clin Anesth.* 2002;14:57.
360. Veall GRQ, et al. *Br J Anaesth.* 1994;72:335.

361. Longnecker M, Roizen MF. *Anesthesiol Clin North Am*. 1987;5:313.
362. Weingarten TN, et al. *Anesth Analg*. 2007;105:1192.
363. Marsh HM, et al. *Anesthesiology*. 1987;66:89.
364. Watson JT, et al. *Can J Anaesth*. 1990;37:798.
365. McCrirrick A, Hickman J. *Can J Anaesth*. 1991;38:339.
366. Quinlivan JK, Roberts WA. *Anesth Analg*. 1994;78:400.
367. Dilger JA, et al. *Anesth Analg*. 2004;98:318.
368. Zimmer C, et al. *Anesthesiology*. 2003;98:1007.
369. Drossman DA, et al. *Gastroenterology*. 1988;95:701.
370. Bunn HF. *N Engl J Med*. 1997;337:762.
371. Adams RJ, et al. *N Engl J Med*. 1998;339:5.
372. Platt OS, et al. *N Engl J Med*. 1991;325:11.
373. Vichinsky EP, et al. *N Engl J Med*. 1995;333:206.
374. Turhan A, et al. *Proc Natl Acad Sci U S A*. 2002;99:3047.
375. Dunn A, et al. *Can J Anaesth*. 1987;34:67.
376. Hemming AE. *J Cardiothorac Vasc Anesth*. 2004;18:663.
377. Messent M. *J Cardiothorac Vasc Anesth*. 2004;18:666.
378. Kark JA, et al. *N Engl J Med*. 1987;317:781.
379. Bischoff RJ, et al. *Ann Surg*. 1988;207:434.
379a. Howard J, et al. *Lancet*. 2013;381:930.
379b. DeBaun MR, et al. *N Engl J Med*. 2014;371:699.
379c. Iughetti L, et al. *World J Clin Pediatr*. 2016;5:25.
380. Tuck SM, et al. *Br J Obstet Gynaecol*. 1987;94:121.
381. Ould Amar K, et al. *Transfus Clin Biol*. 2013;20:30.
382. Beutler E. *JAMA*. 1988;259:2433.
383. Orr D. *Br J Anaesth*. 1967;39:585.
384. Pootrakul P, et al. *N Engl J Med*. 1981;304:1470.
385. Lux SE, Wolfe LC. *Pediatr Clin North Am*. 1980;27:463.
385a. Ngouleun W, et al. *Int J Mycobacteriol*. 2016;5:482.
386. Engelfriet CP, et al. *Semin Hematol*. 1992;29:3.
387. Schilling RF. *JAMA*. 1986;255:1605.
388. Beebe DS, et al. *Anesth Analg*. 1993;76:1144.
389. Goodnough LT, et al. *N Engl J Med*. 1989;321:1163.
389a. Liebman HA, Weitz IC. *Med Clin North Am*. 2017;101:351.
390. Quesenberg PJ, et al. Hematology. In: *American College of Physicians, Editor: Medical Knowledge Self-Assessment*. Philadelphia: American College of Physicians; 1991:374.
391. Tobias JD, Furman WL. *Anesthesiology*. 1991;75:536.
392. Alavi JB, et al. *N Engl J Med*. 1977;296:706.
393. Gabrilove JL, et al. *N Engl J Med*. 1988;318:1414.
394. Quie PG. *Rev Infect Dis*. 1987;9:189.
395. Crawford SW, Fisher L. *Chest*. 1992;101:1257.
396. McCrae KR, et al. *Hematology Am Soc Hematol Educ Program*. 2001;282.
397. Kelton JG. *Ann Intern Med*. 1983;99:796.
398. Douzinas EE, et al. *Crit Care Med*. 1992;20:57.
398a. Sadler JE. *Blood*. 2017;130:1181.
398b. Tanhehco YC, et al. *Curr Opin Hematol*. 2017;24:521.
398c. Krzych LJ, et al. *Anaesthesiol Intensive Ther*. 2015;47:63.
398d. East JM, et al. *Chest*. 2018;154:678–690.
399. Lewis BE, et al. *Circulation*. 2001;103:1838.
400. Bauer KA. *Ann Intern Med*. 2001;135:367.
401. Levine JS, et al. *N Engl J Med*. 2002;346:752.
402. Evans BE. *Mt Sinai J Med*. 1977;44:409.
403. Zauber NP, Levin J. *Medicine (Baltimore)*. 1977;56:213.
404. Brettler DB, Levine PH. *Blood*. 1989;73:2067.
405. Lee KF, et al. *J Thorac Cardiovasc Surg*. 1988;95:216.
406. Dickman CA, et al. *Anesthesiology*. 1990;72:947.
407. Wademan BH, Galvin SD. *Interact Cardiovasc Thorac Surg*. 2014;18:360.
408. Brigden ML, Barnett JB. *West J Med*. 1987;146:580.
409. *Med Lett Drugs Ther*. 1997;39:21.
410. Bishop JM. *Cell*. 1991;64:235.
411. Chung F. *Can J Anaesth*. 1982;29:364.
412. Norwegian Multicenter Study Group. *N Engl J Med*. 1981;304:801.
413. Frishman WH, et al. *N Engl J Med*. 1984;310:830.
414. Bloor BC, Flacke WE. *Anesth Analg*. 1982;61:741.
415. Weinger MB, et al. *Anesthesiology*. 1989;71:242.
416. Maze M, Tranquilli W. *Anesthesiology*. 1991;74:581.
417. Segal IS, et al. *Anesthesiology*. 1991;74:220.
418. Pandharipande PP, et al. *JAMA*. 2007;298:2644.
419. Katz AM. *N Engl J Med*. 1993;328:1244.
420. Merin RG, et al. *Anesthesiology*. 1987;66:140.
421. Kapur PA, et al. *Anesthesiology*. 1987;66:122.
422. *Med Lett Drugs Ther*. 1993;35:65.
423. Huyse FJ, et al. *Psychosomatics*. 2006;47:8.
424. Michaels I, et al. *Anesth Analg*. 1984;63:1014.
425. Evans-Prosser CDG. *Br J Anaesth*. 1968;40:279.
426. Roizen MF. *J Clin Anesth*. 1990;2:293.
427. Noble WH, Baker A. *Can J Anaesth*. 1992;39:1061.
428. Hirshman CA, Linderman KS. *JAMA*. 1989;261:3407.
429. Veith RC, et al. *N Engl J Med*. 1982;306:954.
430. Richelson E, El-Fakahany E. *Mayo Clin Proc*. 1982;57:576.
431. *Med Lett Drugs Ther*. 1996;38:75.
432. Harrah MD, et al. *Anesthesiology*. 1970;33:406.
433. Telivuo L, Katz RL. *Anaesthesia*. 1970;25:30.
434. Miller RD, et al. *Anesthesiology*. 1967;28:1036.
435. Pittinger CB, et al. *Anesth Analg*. 1970;49:487.
436. Singh YN, et al. *Anesthesiology*. 1978;48:418.
437. Pittinger CB, Adamson R. *Annu Rev Pharmacol*. 1972;12:169.
438. Becker LD, Miller RD. *Anesthesiology*. 1976;45:84.
439. Snavely SR, Hodges GR. *Ann Intern Med*. 1984;101:92.
440. McIndewar IC, Marshall RJ. *Br J Anaesth*. 1981;53:785.
441. Navalgund AA, et al. *Anesth Analg*. 1986;65:414.
442. Kannan R, et al. *Clin Pharmacol Ther*. 1982;31:438.
443. *Med Lett Drugs Ther Guidelines*. 2004;20:27.
444. *Med Lett Drugs Ther*. 1982;24:53.
445. *The Medical Letter Handbook of Adverse Drug Interactions*. Medical Letter; 2003.
446. American Diabetes Association. *Diabetes Care*. 2013;36(suppl 1):S11.
447. Handelsman Y, et al. *Endocr Pract*. 2011;17(suppl 2):1.
448. Dellinger RP, et al. *Intensive Care Med*. 2013;39:165.
449. Qaseem A, et al. *Ann Intern Med*. 2011;154:260.
450. Vaquerizo Alonso C, et al. *Nutr Hosp*. 2011;26(suppl 2):46.
451. Societe francaise d'anesthesie et de reanimation, Societe de reanimation de langue francaise. *Ann Fr Anesth Reanim*. 2009;28:410.
452. Lazar HL, et al. *Ann Thorac Surg*. 2009;87:663.

33 Anesthetic Implications of Complementary and Alternative Therapies

SHIQIAN SHEN and LUCY LIN CHEN

KEY POINTS

- Herbal medication use has increased dramatically in the overall population and particularly in preoperative patients.
- Patients might not volunteer information unless they are queried specifically about herbal medication use.
- Although many commonly used herbs have side effects that affect drug metabolism, bleeding, and neuronal function, they are not subject to regulations on purity, safety, and efficacy.
- Knowledge of specific interactions and metabolism of herbs can provide practical guidelines to facilitate perioperative management.
- Other complementary therapies, including acupuncture and music therapy, have become increasingly popular and have shown positive results for certain pain conditions, albeit high-quality data are still lacking.
- Dietary supplements may influence gut microbiota, a consortium of diverse microorganisms residing in the gastrointestinal tract, which represents a new research frontier in perioperative medicine.

Complementary and alternative medicine (CAM) has implications for physicians in general, but has particular importance for the perioperative period because of specific complications associated with certain therapies. Complementary medicine is defined as the addition of nonconventional therapies to accepted treatments; alternative medicine describes the use of nonconventional therapies in lieu of accepted treatments. They have become an important part of contemporary health care. The more popular term of "integrative health or integrative medicine" is used when complementary approaches are incorporated into mainstream health care.

According to a 2012 U.S. National Health Interview Survey (NHIS), 33.2% of adults and 11.6% of children (4-17 years of age) have used CAM.[1,1a] Visits to CAM practitioners exceed those to American primary care physicians,[2] and CAM is even more widely used in Europe, where herbal medicines are prescribed more frequently than conventional drugs are. Furthermore, patients undergoing surgery appear to use CAM more than the general population does.[3] Aside from the widespread use of CAM, perioperative physicians have a special interest in CAM therapies for several reasons. First, several commonly used herbal medications exhibit direct effects on the cardiovascular and coagulation systems. Second, some CAMs can interfere with conventional medications that are commonly given in the postoperative period. Finally, the therapeutic potential of CAM in the perioperative period is increasingly being described in the literature for reducing postoperative nausea, vomiting, and pain.

Despite the public enthusiasm for CAM, scientific knowledge in this area is still incomplete and often confusing for practitioners and patients. One recent study confirmed poor knowledge of this subject among physicians.[4] Recommendations for clinicians are often based on small clinical trials, case reports, animal studies, predictions derived from known pharmacology, and expert opinion. Research is essential because CAM therapies are often widely adopted by the public before adequate data are available to support their safety and efficacy. In 1991, Congress established the Office of Alternative Medicine, which is now known as the National Center for Complementary and Integrative Health. It operates within the National Institutes of Health.

Based on the 2012 NHIS study, the most commonly used CAMs were natural products, deep breathing exercises, meditation, chiropractic or osteopathic manipulation, massage, and yoga. Interestingly, a 2017 NHIS survey noted increases in the use of yoga and meditation by both adults and children (https://nccih.nih.gov/research/statistics/NHIS, Accessed 11/13/2018/tg). CAM practices can be classified into three general categories (Box 33.1).[5] This chapter is not intended as a comprehensive review of CAM. Specific therapies relevant to anesthesia are discussed, with a focus primarily on herbal medicines. Nonherbal dietary supplements, acupuncture, and music are also considered because they are relevant to perioperative care.

BOX 33.1 Three Major Categories of Complementary and Alternative Medicine

1. Natural products: this group includes a variety of products, such as herbs (also known as botanicals),vitamins and minerals, and probiotics. They are widely marketed, readily available to consumers, and often sold as dietary supplements.
2. Mind-body practices: yoga, chiropractic and osteopathic manipulation, meditation, and massage therapy are among the most popular mind and body practices used by adults. Other mind and body practices include acupuncture, relaxation techniques (such as breathing exercises, guided imagery, and progressive muscle relaxation), tai chi, qi gong, and hypnotherapy.
3. Others: traditional healers, Ayurvedic medicine, traditional Chinese medicine, homeopathy, naturopathy, and functional medicine.

Modified from the National Center for Complementary and Integrative Health. https://nccih.nih.gov/health/integrative-health. Accessed April 11, 2018.

Herbal Medicines

Preoperative use of herbal medicines has been associated with adverse perioperative events.[6] Surveys estimate that 22% to 32% of patients undergoing surgery use herbal medications.[7-9] In a recent retrospective review, 23% of surgery patients indicated the use of natural products, and older patients preferred dietary supplements.[10]

Herbal medicines can affect the perioperative period through several classic mechanisms: direct effects (i.e., intrinsic pharmacologic effects), pharmacodynamic interactions (i.e., alteration of the action of conventional drugs at effector sites), and pharmacokinetic interactions (e.g., alteration of the absorption, distribution, metabolism, and elimination of conventional drugs). Because approximately 50% of herbal medicine users take multiple herbs concomitantly[7] and 25% of herbal medicine users take prescription drugs,[11] adverse effects are difficult to predict and attribute.

Herbal medicines are associated with unique problems not usually found with conventional drugs.[12] Many of the issues complicating the understanding of herbal medications derive from the fact that they are classified as dietary supplements under the Dietary Supplement Health and Education Act of 1994. As such, the introduction of herbal medications does not require animal studies, clinical trials, or postmarketing surveillance. Under current law, the burden is shifted to the U.S. Food and Drug Administration (FDA) to prove products unsafe before they can be withdrawn from the market, such as the withdrawal of intranasal Zicam (cold medicine) after more than 130 reports of persistent anosmia.[13] Commercial herbal medicine preparations can have unpredictable pharmacologic effects resulting from inaccurate labeling, misidentified plants, adulterants, variations in natural potency, and unstandardized processing methods.

Two of the major problems confronting herbal medicine research involve quality control and added adulterants. In a recent clinical trial to treat human H1N1 influenza, an herbal formulation containing 12 different Chinese herbal medicines including licorice (genus *Glycyrrhiza*) was used.[14] Some of the other botanicals in the formula were not accurately identified. There are three *Glycyrrhiza* species on the market that may show a twofold difference when the three species are compared.[15]

Labeled active ingredients can vary tenfold in different commercial preparations.[16] In June 2007, the FDA issued regulations for current good manufacturing practices (GMPs) for dietary supplements.[17] This rule requires that proper controls be in place so that dietary supplements are processed in a consistent manner and meet quality standards. Especially emphasized are the identity, purity, strength, and composition of the products. Dietary products adhering to GMPs undoubtedly reduce the potential risk in the use of herbal medicines. Because this rule is somewhat similar to that for prescription drug GMPs, many supplement manufacturers believe that it is not practical for botanicals.[18]

Beyond quality control is the inclusion of biologically active pharmacologic adulterants in herbal medications and supplements. There are clinical consequences when quality control is lacking or herbal preparations are adulterated, as found in a weight-loss remedy study that revealed one manufacturer's incorrect substitution of an herb for another when the carcinogen aristolochic acid led to an outbreak of nephropathy and urothelial carcinoma.[19] In another event, more than 14 million capsules of asexual enhancement supplement were recalled because the compound on the label did not actually exist and the supplement did contain an analogue of sildenafil, which has not been tested in humans.[20] In light of these events, in August 2016, the FDA proposed a new guidance to evaluate the safety of supplements based on their history of use, formulation, proposed daily dose, and recommended duration of use. Although the guidance represents only a fraction of what is necessary for a new drug application, it requires some testing for tolerability in animals, but not in humans,[21] when products are marketed for consumption at doses substantively greater than those historically ingested. Any ingredient formulated or prepared in a novel manner is considered a new ingredient.

In this section, we discuss the preoperative assessment and management of patients who use herbal medicines and examine 11 herbal medicines that have the greatest effect on perioperative patient care: *Echinacea*, ephedra, garlic, ginger, *Ginkgo biloba*, ginseng, green tea, kava, saw palmetto, St. John's wort, and valerian (Table 33.1).

Preoperative Assessment and Management

Preoperative assessment should address the use of herbal medicines (see Table 33.1). One study found that 90% of anesthesia providers do not routinely ask about herbal medicine use.[22] Moreover, more than 70% of patients are not forthcoming about their herbal medicine use during routine preoperative assessment.[7] When a positive history of herbal medicine use is elicited, one in five patients is unable to properly identify the preparation being taken.[23] Asking patients to bring their herbal medicines

TABLE 33.1 Clinically Important Effects, Perioperative Concerns, and Recommendations for Perioperative Discontinuation of 11 Commonly Used Herbal Medicines

Herbs (Common Names)	Pharmacologic Effects	Perioperative Concerns	Discontinue Before Surgery
Echinacea (purple cone-flower root)	Activation of cell-mediated immunity	Allergic reactions Decreases effectiveness of immunosuppressants Potential for immunosuppression with long-term use	No data
Ephedra (ma huang)	Increases heart rate and blood pressure through direct and indirect sympathomimetic effects	Risk of myocardial ischemia and stroke from tachycardia and hypertension Ventricular arrhythmias with halothane Long-term use depletes endogenous catecholamines and may cause intraoperative hemodynamic instability Life-threatening interaction with MAO inhibitors	24 h
Garlic (ajo)	Inhibits platelet aggregation (may be irreversible) Increases fibrinolysis Equivocal antihypertensive activity	May increase risk of bleeding, especially when combined with other medications that inhibit platelet aggregation	7 days
Ginger	Antiemetic Antiplatelet aggregation	May increase risk of bleeding	No data
Ginkgo (duck-foot tree, maidenhair tree, silver apricot)	Inhibits platelet-activating factor	May increase risk of bleeding, especially when combined with other medications that inhibit platelet aggregation	36 h
Ginseng (American ginseng, Asian ginseng, Chinese ginseng, Korean ginseng)	Lowers blood glucose Inhibits platelet aggregation (may be irreversible) Increased PT/PTT in animals	Hypoglycemia May increase risk of bleeding May decrease anticoagulant effect of warfarin	7 days
Green tea	Inhibits platelet aggregation Inhibits thromboxane A2 formation	May increase risk of bleeding May decrease anticoagulant effect of warfarin	7 days
Kava (awa, intoxicating pepper, kawa)	Sedation Anxiolysis	May increase sedative effect of anesthetics Increase in anesthetic requirements with long-term use unstudied	24 h
Saw palmetto (dwarf palm, *Sabal*)	Inhibits 5α-reductase Inhibits cyclooxygenase	May increase risk of bleeding	No data
St. John's wort (amber, goat weed, hardhay, hypericum, Klamath weed)	Inhibits neurotransmitter reuptake MAO inhibition unlikely	Induction of cytochrome P450 enzymes; affects cyclosporine, warfarin, steroids, and protease inhibitors; may affect benzodiazepines, calcium channel blockers, and many other drugs Decreased serum digoxin levels Delayed emergence	5 days
Valerian (all heal, garden heliotrope, vandal root)	Sedation	May increase sedative effect of anesthetics Benzodiazepine-like acute withdrawal May increase anesthetic requirements with long-term use	No data

MAO, Monoamine oxidase; *PT*, prothrombin time; *PTT*, partial thromboplastin time.

and other dietary supplements with them at the time of the preoperative evaluation would be helpful. A positive history of herbal medicine use should alert one to the presence of undiagnosed disorders causing symptoms leading to self-medication. Patients who use herbal medicines may be more likely to avoid conventional diagnosis and therapy.[24]

In general, herbal medicines should be discontinued preoperatively. Patients who require nonelective surgery are not evaluated until the day of surgery or are noncompliant with instructions to discontinue herbal medications preoperatively. In this situation, anesthesia can usually proceed safely at the discretion of the anesthesia provider, who should be familiar with commonly used herbal medicines. For example, recent use of herbal medicines that inhibit platelet function (e.g., garlic, ginseng, *G. biloba*) may warrant specific strategies for procedures with substantial intraoperative blood loss (e.g., platelet transfusion) and those that alter the risk-benefit ratio of using certain anesthetic techniques (e.g., neuraxial blockade).

Preoperative discontinuation of all herbal medicines might not eliminate complications related to their use. Withdrawal of some of the herbal medicines can increase morbidity and mortality after surgery similar to regular medications.[25,26] The danger of abstinence after long-term use may be similar with herbal medicines such as valerian, which can produce acute withdrawal after long-term use.

Although the American Society of Anesthesiologists has no official standard or guideline for the preoperative use of herbal medications, public and professional educational information released by this organization suggests that herbals be discontinued at least 2 weeks before surgery.[25] Our review of the literature favors a more targeted approach. When pharmacokinetic data for the active constituents in an herbal medication are available, the timeframe for preoperative discontinuation can be tailored. Some herbal medications are eliminated quickly and may be discontinued near the time of surgery. For other herbal medicines, 2 weeks is recommended.[27]

Evidence-based estimates of herbal safety in the perioperative period are limited. One study of 601 patients who used traditional Chinese herbal medications suggested an infrequent rate of potential serious complications.[28] Clinicians should be familiar with commonly used herbal medications to recognize and treat any complications that might arise. Table 33.1 summarizes the clinically important effects, perioperative concerns, and recommendations for preoperative discontinuation of the 11 herbal medications that account for 30% of the dietary supplements sold in the United States.[29] The type of surgery and potential perioperative course should be considered in these clinical recommendations.

ECHINACEA

Three species of *Echinacea*, a member of the daisy family, are used for the prophylaxis and treatment of viral (decreasing the incidence and duration of the common cold), bacterial, and fungal infections, particularly those of upper respiratory origin, although its efficacy in fungal infections is doubtful.[30,31] The biological activity of *Echinacea* could be immunostimulatory, immunosuppressive, or antiinflammatory.[32] Although studies have not specifically addressed interactions between *Echinacea* and immunosuppressive drugs, experts generally warn against the concomitant use of *Echinacea* and these drugs because of the probability of diminished effectiveness.[33,34] In contrast to its immunostimulatory effects with short-term use, long-term use of more than 8 weeks is accompanied by the potential for immunosuppression[34] and a theoretically increased risk for postsurgical poor wound healing and opportunistic infections. A recent phytochemical study identified a potential immunosuppressant compound from *Echinacea*—cynarine.[35]

Information about Echinacea's pharmacokinetics is still limited.[36] *Echinacea* significantly reduced plasma concentrations of S-warfarin, but did not significantly affect warfarin pharmacodynamics and platelet aggregation in healthy subjects.[37] However, this herb should be discontinued as far in advance of surgery as possible when compromises in hepatic function or blood flow are anticipated.[38] In the absence of definitive information, patients with preexisting liver dysfunction should be cautious in using *Echinacea*.

EPHEDRA

Ephedra, known as *ma huang* in Chinese medicine, is a shrub native to central Asia. It is used to promote weight loss, increase energy, and treat respiratory conditions such as asthma and bronchitis. Ephedra contains alkaloids, including ephedrine, pseudoephedrine, norephedrine, methylephedrine, and norpseudoephedrine.[25] Commercial preparations can be standardized to a fixed ephedrine content. Publicity about adverse reactions to this herb prompted the FDA to bar its sale in 2004, but ephedra is still widely available via the Internet.

Ephedra causes dose-dependent increases in arterial blood pressure and heart rate. Ephedrine, the predominant active compound, is a noncatecholamine sympathomimetic that exhibits α_1, β_1, and β_2 activity indirectly by releasing endogenous norepinephrine (noradrenaline). These sympathomimetic effects have been associated with more than 1070 reported adverse events, including fatal cardiac and central nervous system complications.[39] Vasoconstriction and, in some cases, vasospasm of coronary and cerebral arteries can cause myocardial infarction and thrombotic stroke.[40] Ephedra can also affect cardiovascular function by causing hypersensitivity myocarditis, characterized by cardiomyopathy with myocardial lymphocyte and eosinophil infiltration.[41] Long-term use results in tachyphylaxis from depletion of endogenous catecholamine stores and can contribute to perioperative hemodynamic instability. In these situations, direct-acting sympathomimetics may be preferred as first-line therapy for intraoperative hypotension and bradycardia. Concomitant use of ephedra and monoamine oxidase inhibitors can result in life-threatening hyperpyrexia, hypertension, and coma. Finally, continuous ephedra is a rare cause of radiolucent kidney stones.[42] Recently, there was a case report describing acute angle-closure glaucoma caused by ephedra.[42a]

The pharmacokinetics of ephedrine have been studied in humans.[43,44] Ephedrine has an elimination half-life of 5.2 hours, with 70% to 80% of the compound excreted unchanged in urine. Based on the pharmacokinetic data and the known cardiovascular risks associated with ephedra, including myocardial infarction, stroke, and cardiovascular collapse from catecholamine depletion, this herb should be discontinued at least 24 hours before surgery.

GARLIC

Garlic is one of the most extensively researched medicinal plants. It has the potential to modify the risk for atherosclerosis by reducing arterial blood pressure, thrombus formation, and serum lipid and cholesterol concentrations.[45] These effects are primarily attributed to its sulfur-containing compounds, particularly allicin and its transformation products. Commercial garlic preparations can be standardized to a fixed alliin and allicin content.

Garlic inhibits platelet aggregation in vivo in a concentration-dependent fashion. The effect of one of its constituents, ajoene, is irreversible and can enhance the effect of other platelet inhibitors such as prostacyclin, forskolin, indomethacin, and dipyridamole.[46] Although the effects are not consistently demonstrated in volunteers, there is one case described in an 80 year old who had a spontaneous epidural hematoma develop that was attributed to continuous garlic use.[47] Garlic has interacted with warfarin, resulting in an increased international normalized ratio (INR).[48]

In addition to bleeding concerns, garlic can decrease systemic and pulmonary vascular resistance in laboratory animals, but this effect is marginal in humans.[49] Although there are insufficient pharmacokinetic data on garlic's constituents, the potential for irreversible inhibition of platelet function may warrant discontinuation of garlic at least 7 days before surgery, especially if postoperative bleeding is a particular concern or other anticoagulants are given. Additionally, garlic's pharmacokinetics should be considered when a risk-benefit analysis is made for neuraxial techniques.

GINGER

Ginger (*Zingiber officinale*) is a popular spice with a long history of use in Chinese, Indian, Arabic, and Greco-Roman herbal medicines. Ginger has a wide range of reported health benefits for those with arthritis, rheumatism, sprains, muscular aches, pains, sore throats, cramps, constipation, indigestion, nausea, vomiting, hypertension, dementia, fever, infectious diseases, and helminthiasis.[50] Ginger contains up to 3% volatile oil, mostly monoterpenoids and sesquiterpenoids.[51] Gingerols are representative compounds in ginger.[52]

Ginger is an antiemetic and has been used to treat motion sickness and to prevent nausea after laparoscopy.[53] The number of postoperative antiemetic medications was significantly reduced after aromatherapy with essential oil of ginger.[54] In another recent trial, ginger supplementation reduced the severity of acute chemotherapy-induced nausea in adult cancer patients and compared favorably to conventional antiemetics.[55]

In an in vitro study, gingerols and related analogues inhibited arachidonic acid–induced human platelet serotonin release and aggregation, with a potency similar to that of aspirin.[52] In another in vitro study, the antiplatelet effects of 20 ginger constituents were evaluated. Five constituents showed antiplatelet activities at relatively low concentrations. One of the ginger compounds (8-paradol) was the most potent cyclooxygenase-1 inhibitor and antiplatelet aggregation drug.[56] In a case report, a ginger-phenprocoumon combination resulted in an increased INR and epistaxis.[57] Although the sample size was relatively small, the platelet inhibition potential of ginger has been suggested in a pilot clinical study.[58] This result may warrant the discontinuation of ginger at least 2 weeks before surgery.

GINKGO

Ginkgo is derived from the leaf of *G. biloba* and has been used for cognitive disorders, peripheral vascular disease, age-related macular degeneration, vertigo, tinnitus, erectile dysfunction, and altitude sickness. Studies have suggested that ginkgo can stabilize or improve cognitive performance in patients with Alzheimer disease and multiinfarct dementia,[59] but not in healthy geriatric patients.[60] The compounds that might be responsible for its pharmacologic effects are the terpenoids and flavonoids. The two ginkgo extracts used in clinical trials are standardized to ginkgo-flavone glycosides and terpenoids.

Ginkgo alters vasoregulation, acts as an antioxidant, modulates neurotransmitter and receptor activity, and inhibits platelet-activating factor. Of these effects, inhibition of platelet-activating factor is of primary concern for the perioperative period. Although bleeding complications have not occurred in clinical trials, four cases of spontaneous intracranial bleeding,[61-63] one case of spontaneous hyphema,[64] and one case of postoperative bleeding after laparoscopic cholecystectomy[65] have been described when ginkgo was being taken.

Terpene trilactones are highly bioavailable when administered orally. The elimination half-lives of the terpene trilactones after oral administration are between 3 and 10 hours. For ginkgolide B, a dosage of 40 mg twice daily resulted in a higher area under the curve, and a longer half-life and residence time, than after a single 80-mg dose. A once daily dose of 80 mg guaranteed a larger maximum concentration peak (T_{max}) that was reached 2 to 3 hours after administration.[66] The pharmacokinetics of terpene trilactones in three different ginkgo preparations in human plasma[67] indicate that ginkgo should be discontinued at least 2 weeks before surgery to avoid bleeding.[38]

GINSENG

Among the several species of ginseng used for their pharmacologic effects, Asian ginseng *(Panax ginseng)* and American ginseng *(Panax quinquefolius)* are the most commonly described.[68] Ginseng has been labeled an "adaptogen" because it reputedly protects the body against stress and restores homeostasis.[69] Because its pharmacologic actions are attributed to the ginsenosides, a group of compounds known as *steroidal saponins*, many commercially available ginseng preparations have been standardized to ginsenoside content.[68,70]

The many heterogeneous and sometimes opposing effects of different ginsenosides[71,72] give ginseng a broad but incompletely understood pharmacologic profile including general health, fatigue, immune function, cancer, cardiovascular disease, diabetes mellitus, cognitive function, viral infections, sexual function, and athletic performance.[69] The underlying mechanism is similar to that classically described for steroid hormones. This herb decreases postprandial blood glucose in both healthy and type 2 diabetes patients,[73] an effect that can create unintended hypoglycemia in patients who have fasted before surgery.

Ginseng can alter coagulation pathways. The antiplatelet activity of panaxynol, a constituent of ginseng, may be irreversible in humans.[74] Ginseng extract and ginsenosides inhibit platelet aggregation in vitro[75,76] and prolong thrombin time and activated partial thromboplastin time in in vivo animal models.[77,78]

The clinical evidence implicating ginseng as a cause of bleeding is weak and based on only a few case reports.[79] Although ginseng may inhibit the coagulation cascade, one case associated its use with a significant decrease in warfarin anticoagulation.[80] Subsequently, a study in volunteers showed that American ginseng interfered with warfarin-induced anticoagulation,[81] reducing its anticoagulant effect. When prescribing warfarin, clinicians should specifically ask about ginseng use. In another clinical trial, warfarin's clearance was moderately increased with Asian ginseng.[82] Because warfarin is often used after orthopedic or vascular procedures, this herbal drug interaction can affect perioperative management in many patients.

In rats, the elimination half-lives are different after an intravenous infusion of ginseng, with ginsenosides Re and Rg1 between 0.7 and 4 hours, and ginsenosides Rb1 and Rd between 19 and 22 hours.[83] After oral administration of ginseng, ginsenoside Rb1 reached the maximum plasma concentration at approximately 4 hours with a prolonged half-life.[84,85] These data suggest that ginseng should be discontinued at least 48 hours before surgery. Because platelet inhibition by ginseng may be irreversible, ginseng use should be stopped at least 2 weeks before surgery.[38]

GREEN TEA

Tea from the *Camellia sinensis* is one of the most ancient and the second most widely consumed beverage in the world.[86,87] Tea can be classified into different types, such as green, oolong, and black. Green tea, which is not fermented and is derived directly from drying and steaming fresh tea leaves, contains polyphenolic compounds. Catechins in green tea account for 16% to 30% of its dry weight. Epigallocatechin-3-gallate (EGCG), the most predominant catechin in green tea, is responsible for much of the biologic activity mediated by green tea.[86]

In an early in vitro and in vivo study, both green tea and EGCG significantly prolonged mouse tail bleeding time in conscious mice. They inhibited adenosine diphosphate- and collagen-induced rat platelet aggregation in a dose-dependent manner.[88] The antiplatelet activity can result from the inhibition of thromboxane A2 formation by preventing arachidonic acid liberation and thromboxane A2 synthase.[89,90] Regarding a possible adverse effect of green tea on platelets, one case reported thrombotic thrombocytopenic purpura developed after a patient consumed a weight-loss product containing green tea.[91] On the other hand, drinking green tea could antagonize the anticoagulant effects of warfarin because green tea contains vitamin K.[92]

The half-life for EGCG in one study was between 1.9 and 4.6 hours[93] and in another study was observed to be between 2.2 and 3.4 hours.[94] Based on pharmacokinetic data and possible antiplatelet activity, green tea should be discontinued at least 7 days before surgery.

KAVA

Kava is derived from the dried root of the pepper plant *Piper methysticum*. Kava has gained widespread popularity as an anxiolytic and sedative. The kavalactones appear to be the source of kava's pharmacologic activity.[95]

Because of its psychomotor effects, kava was one of the first herbal medications expected to interact with anesthetics. The kavalactones can have many effects such as: (1) dose-dependent effects on the central nervous system, including antiepileptic, neuroprotective, and local anesthetic properties; (2) act as a sedative-hypnotic by potentiating inhibitory neurotransmission of γ-aminobutyric acid (GABA); (3) increased barbiturate sleep time in laboratory animals,[96] which might explain the mechanism of a coma attributed to an alprazolam-kava interaction[97]; (4) abuse potential, whether long-term use can result in addiction, tolerance, and acute withdrawal after abstinence is unknown; (5) increased γ-glutamyl transpeptidase levels with potential risk of hepatotoxicity[98]; and (6) produces "kava dermopathy," characterized by reversible scaly cutaneous eruptions.[99]

In an in vitro investigation, a kava compound (+)-kavain suppressed the aggregation of human platelets. Kava inhibits cyclooxygenase with the potential to decrease renal blood flow and to interfere with platelet aggregation. Consumption of kava has potential cardiovascular effects that could manifest in the perioperative period.[100,101] Although kava has been banned in Europe since 2002, it is available in North America and many countries in the Pacific region. A concentration-based response relationship can occur with hepatotoxicity, even leading to numerous cases of liver transplantation.[102-104]

Peak plasma levels occur 1.8 hours after an oral dose, and the elimination half-life of kavalactones is 9 hours.[105] Unchanged kavalactones and their metabolites undergo renal and fecal elimination.[106] Pharmacokinetic data and the possibility for enhancement of the sedative effects from anesthetics suggest that kava should be discontinued at least 24 hours before surgery. Earlier discontinuation probably should be considered when surgical procedures are expected to compromise hepatic function or blood flow.

SAW PALMETTO

Saw palmetto, which is used by more than 2 million men in the United States to treat symptoms associated with benign prostatic hypertrophy, is of questionable efficacy for this purpose.[107] The major constituents of saw palmetto are fatty acids and their glycerides (i.e., triacylglycerides and monoacylglycerides), carbohydrates, steroids, flavonoids, resin, pigment, tannin, and volatile oil. The pharmacologic activity of saw palmetto has not been attributed to a single compound.

Although the mechanism of action of saw palmetto is not known, multiple mechanisms have been proposed.[108] Saw palmetto extract, like finasteride, inhibits 5α-reductase in vitro; however, results of in vivo studies have been inconsistent.[109] Other proposed mechanisms are inhibition of estrogen and androgen receptors, binding of autonomic receptors, blocking of prolactin receptor signal transduction, interference with fibroblast proliferation, induction of apoptosis, inhibition of α_1-adrenergic receptors, and antiinflammatory effects.

In a patient undergoing craniotomy, saw palmetto was associated with excessive intraoperative bleeding that required termination of the procedure.[109] Another case of hematuria and coagulopathy in a patient who used saw palmetto was reported.[110] This complication was attributed to saw palmetto's antiinflammatory effects, specifically the inhibition of cyclooxygenase and subsequent platelet dysfunction. Because there are no pharmacokinetic or clinical data for saw palmetto, specific recommendations for preoperative discontinuation cannot be made.

ST. JOHN'S WORT

St. John's wort is the common name for *Hypericum perforatum*, and has been used for mental health and depression conditions. A multicenter clinical trial concluded that St. John's wort is not effective in the treatment of major depression.[111] The compounds believed to be responsible for its pharmacologic activity are hypericin and hyperforin.[112] Commercial preparations are often standardized to a fixed hypericin content of 0.3%.

St. John's wort exerts its effects by inhibiting reuptake of serotonin, norepinephrine, and dopamine.[113] Concomitant use of this herb with or without serotonin reuptake inhibitors can create a syndrome of central serotonin excess.[114] Although early in vitro data implicated monoamine oxidase inhibition as a possible mechanism of action, a number of later investigations have demonstrated that monoamine oxidase inhibition is insignificant in vivo.[115]

Use of St. John's wort can significantly increase the metabolism of many concomitantly administered drugs, some of which are vital to the perioperative care of certain patients. There is induction of the cytochrome P450 3A4 isoform,[116] and interactions with substrates of the 3A4 isoform, including indinavir sulfate,[117] ethinylestradiol,[118] and cyclosporine,[119] have been documented. There are important clinical consequences of this metabolic effect, particularly in transplant patients. In two case reports of heart transplant patients, after taking St. John's wort the patients' plasma cyclosporine concentrations became subtherapeutic and acute transplant rejection resulted. After stopping St. John's wort, plasma cyclosporine remained within the therapeutic range with no further episodes of rejection (Fig. 33.1).[120] In one series of 45 organ transplant patients, St. John's wort was associated with an average 49% decrease in blood cyclosporine levels.[121] Other P450 3A4 substrates commonly used in the perioperative period include alfentanil, midazolam, lidocaine, calcium channel blockers, and 5-hydroxytryptamine receptor antagonists. In addition, the cytochrome P450 2C9 isoform also may be induced, which results in decreased anticoagulant effect of warfarin, a substrate of the 2C9 isoform, in seven reported cases.[118] Other 2C9 substrates include the nonsteroidal antiinflammatory drugs. Furthermore, the enzyme induction caused by St. John's wort may be more pronounced when other enzyme inducers, which could include other herbal medications, are taken concomitantly. St. John's wort also affects digoxin pharmacokinetics.[115]

The single-dose and steady-state pharmacokinetics of hypericin, pseudohypericin, and hyperforin have been determined in humans.[122,123] After oral administration, peak plasma levels of hypericin and hyperforin are achieved in 6.0 and 3.5 hours, respectively, and their median elimination half-lives are 43.1 and 9.0 hours, respectively. Long half-life and altered metabolism of many drugs make concomitant use of St. John's wort a particular risk in the perioperative setting. Pharmacokinetic data suggest that this herbal medication should be discontinued at least 5 days before surgery. Discontinuation is especially important in patients awaiting organ transplantation or in those who might require oral anticoagulation postoperatively. Moreover, these patients should be advised to avoid taking St. John's wort postoperatively.

VALERIAN

Valerian *(Valeriana officinalis)* is an herb that is native to temperate regions of the Americas, Europe, and Asia. It is used as a sedative, particularly in the treatment of insomnia, and virtually all herbal sleep aids contain valerian.[124] Valerian contains many compounds acting synergistically, but the sesquiterpenes are the primary source of valerian's pharmacologic effects. Commercially available preparations may be standardized to valerenic acid.

Valerian produces dose-dependent sedation and hypnosis.[125] These effects are probably mediated through modulation of GABA neurotransmission and receptor function.[126] Valerian increased barbiturate sleep time in experimental animals.[127] In several randomized, placebo-controlled trials in humans, there was a mild subjective improvement in sleep with valerian, especially when used for 2 weeks or more.[128,129] Objective tests have had less consistent results, with little or no improvement in sleep noted.[130] In one patient, valerian withdrawal appeared to mimic an acute benzodiazepine withdrawal syndrome characterized by

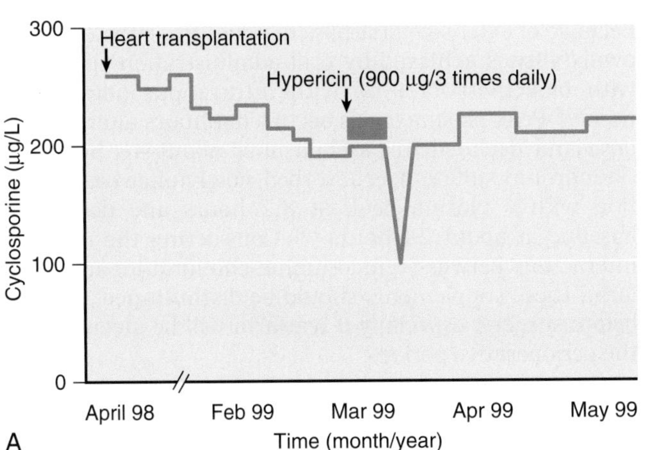

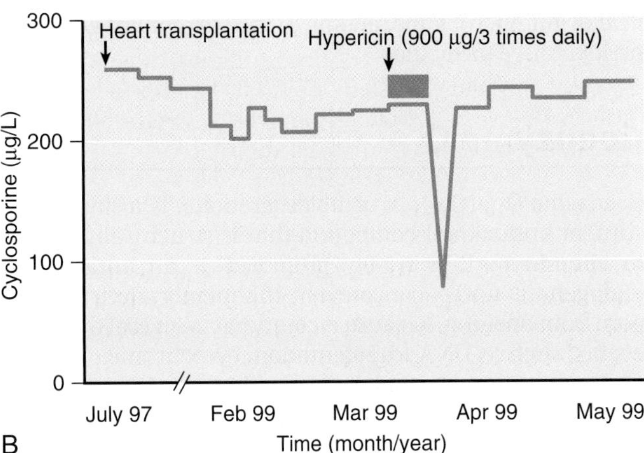

Fig. 33.1 Cyclosporine concentrations in two patients (A and B) after heart transplantation. Treatment with St. John's wort extract containing 900 µg of hypericin was associated with a drop in cyclosporine values below the therapeutic range and acute transplant rejection. (From Breidenbach T, Hoffmann MW, Becker T, et al. Drug interaction of St John's wort with cyclosporine. *Lancet*. 2000;355:1912.)

delirium, cardiac complications after surgery, and attenuation of the symptoms by administration of a benzodiazepine.[131] Based on these findings, valerian should potentiate the sedative effects of anesthetics and adjuvants that act at the GABA receptor, such as midazolam.

The pharmacokinetics of valerian's constituents have not been studied, although their effects may be short-lived. Abrupt discontinuation in patients who may be physically dependent on valerian risks benzodiazepine-like withdrawal. In these individuals, this herbal medication should be gradually decreased with close medical supervision over the course of several weeks before surgery. If such tapering is not feasible, physicians can advise patients to continue taking valerian until the day of surgery. Based on the mechanism of action and a reported case of efficacy,[131] benzodiazepines can treat withdrawal symptoms should they develop in the postoperative period.

OTHER HERBAL MEDICINES

In a survey conducted in 2007,[1] the top 10 herbal medicines also included soy isoflavones, grape seed extract, and milk thistle. There are no reports of adverse effects or perioperative risks from these herbs.

Although boldo *(Peumus boldus)*, Danshen *(Salvia miltiorrhiza)*, Dong quai *(Angelica sinensis)*, and papaya *(Carica papaya)* are encountered less frequently, it may be prudent to discontinue their use 2 weeks before surgery because they have shown antiplatelet aggregation activity and herb-drug interactions.[132]

COMMON DIETARY SUPPLEMENTS

Herbal medicines fall into the broader category of dietary supplements that also includes vitamins, minerals, amino acids, enzymes, animal extracts, prebiotics, and probiotics. Data on the safety of these agents in the perioperative period are scant. High-dose vitamin use, particularly of the fat-soluble vitamins (i.e., A, D, E, and K), can be associated with acute and chronic toxicity. Drug interactions for coenzyme Q_{10}, glucosamine, chondroitin, sulphate, and fish oil have been sufficiently documented to merit inclusion in this chapter. Prebiotics and probiotics have become increasingly popular in research, in the context of the rapidly evolving field of gut microbiome, adding to the current knowledge of perioperative medicine.

Coenzyme Q_{10}

Coenzyme Q_{10} (CoQ_{10}), or ubidecarenone, is a single-constituent antioxidant compound that is structurally related to vitamin K. It is widely promoted as an antioxidant. Endogenous CoQ_{10} can prevent the membrane transition pore from opening, because it counteracts several apoptotic events, such as DNA fragmentation, cytochrome c release, and membrane potential depolarization.[52]

Of importance, this compound interacts with warfarin and was investigated in rats.[133] Following oral administration of 1.5 mg/kg of racemic warfarin to rats during an 8-day oral regimen of CoQ_{10} (10 mg/kg daily), no apparent effect was observed on serum protein binding of warfarin enantiomers. Treatment with CoQ_{10} did not affect the absorption and distribution of the S- and R-enantiomers of warfarin, but it increased total serum clearance of both R- and S-warfarin. The increased clearance values are likely due to acceleration of certain metabolic pathways and renal excretion of the warfarin enantiomers.

An in vitro study showed a predicted 32% and 17% increase in the total clearance of S- and R-warfarin respectively with co-administration of 100 mg CoQ_{10}.[134] CoQ_{10} may decrease the effects of warfarin,[135] but results were inconsistent in another controlled, clinical trial.[136] In 171 patients, co-administration of CoQ_{10} with warfarin appeared to increase the risk of bleeding.[137] Based on the clinical information regarding drug interaction and reported prolonged elimination half-life (38-92 hours) after a single oral dose,[138] CoQ_{10} should be discontinued at least 2 weeks before surgery.

GLUCOSAMINE AND CHONDROITIN SULFATE

Glucosamine and chondroitin sulfate are widely used for joint disorders by many patients undergoing orthopedic procedures. Although their mode of action may be complex, glucosamine and chondroitin sulfate have been widely accepted as supplements in the management of osteoarthritis (OA) because they are the essential components of proteoglycan in normal cartilage.[139] When a large-scale trial evaluated glucosamine and chondroitin sulfate alone or in combination, pain was not reduced in a group of patients with OA of the knee. Exploratory analyses suggested that the two in combination might be effective in a subgroup of patients with moderate-to-severe knee pain.[140]

Long-term clinical data regarding the safety of glucosamine and chondroitin sulfate alone or in combination are limited. Use of chondroitin sulfate alone is well tolerated and without significant adverse drug interaction.[139] One concern regarding the use of glucosamine is its potential to cause or worsen diabetes in animal models[141]; this effect is supported by clinical studies.[142] In a report from the FDA MedWatch database, there were 20 cases of complications involving glucosamine or glucosamine-chondroitin sulfate use with warfarin. Coagulation was altered as manifested by increased INR or increased bleeding or bruising.[143]

When glucosamine is taken orally, 90% is absorbed. Because of extensive first-pass metabolism, only 25% bioavailability is achieved by oral administration compared with bioactivity of 96% with intravenous administration.[144] Peak plasma levels occurred 4 hours after an oral dose and declined to baseline after about 48 hours.[145] Chondroitin sulfate was absorbed slowly after oral ingestion with a plasma peak at 8.7 hours and decline to baseline at about 24 hours.[146] Considering the reported interaction between glucosamine-chondroitin and warfarin, these supplements should be discontinued 2 weeks before surgery, especially if warfarin will be given during the perioperative period.

FISH OIL

Intake of fish oil supplements containing omega-3 fatty acids (eicosapentaenoic acid and docosahexaenoic acid) reduces the incidence of many chronic diseases that involve inflammatory processes, including cardiovascular diseases, inflammatory bowel disease, cancer, rheumatoid arthritis, and neurodegenerative illnesses.[147] However, omega-3 fatty acid did not reduce the rate of death in patients with cardiovascular risk in one study.[148] A metaanalysis of efficacy also concluded that omega-3 polyunsaturated fatty acid supplementation does not decrease the risk of all-cause mortality, cardiac death, sudden death, myocardial infarction, or stroke based on relative and absolute measures of association.[149] This article included many studies of patients with complex risk factors.

Omega-3 fatty acids, however, can inhibit platelet aggregation and increase bleeding risk by the following studies: (1) In vitro experiments have demonstrated an antiplatelet aggregate effect,[150] and inhibition correlated with platelet cyclic adenosine monophosphate levels.[151] (2) In vivo studies have showed decreased platelet aggregation but do not influence bleeding time.[152,153] (3) The inhibition of platelet aggregation was gender specific in a clinical study.[154]

Although evidence for significant bleeding concerns is not found in clinical trials,[155,156] several case reports have illustrated a possible interaction between warfarin and omega-3 fatty acids.[157] Extremely elevated INR associated with warfarin in combination with omega-3 fatty acids was found in two cases.[158,159] These reports suggest that fish oil be discontinued 2 weeks before surgery, especially for patients taking large doses.

PREBIOTICS AND PROBIOTICS

A prebiotic is a nondigestible food ingredient that beneficially affects the host by selectively stimulating the growth and activity of one or a limited number of bacteria in the colon that has the potential to improve host health. A probiotic is a live microbial feed supplement that beneficially affects the host by improving its intestinal microbial balance.[159a] Both prebiotics and probiotics can perturbate the gut microbiota, a consortium of diverse microorganisms residing in the gastrointestinal tract, with significant influence in energy metabolism, immune system development, neurologic function, and behaviors. Research on gut microbiota has made significant progress in recent years owing to the technological advancement of next-generation DNA sequencing and high-throughput data processing.

Targeting gut microbiota using fecal transplantation or fecal capsules to treat recurrent *Clostrisium difficile* infection is under intense investigation, with a few trials indicating promising results.[159b] However, a recent trial comparing oral probiotics with oral antibiotics for elective colorectal surgery showed that conventional oral antibiotics preparation in addition to mechanical bowel preparation is better than oral probiotics with mechanical bowel preparation.[159c] Studies have implicated gut microbiota in visceral hypersensitivity (irritable bowel syndrome), inflammatory pain, and more recently, neuropathic pain.[159d-159f] Moreover, gut microbiota have been shown to modulate the central nervous system function, including anxiety/depression and cognition. Despite the rapidly evolving field of gut microbiome, data on perioperative use of prebiotics and probiotics are scarce. Future research is warranted to investigate potential roles of prebiotics and probiotics in the perioperative setting, particularly in volatile anesthetics sensitivity, postoperative pain control, and postoperative cognitive dysfunction.

Other Dietary Supplements

Other top 10 dietary supplements include flaxseed oil, fiber or psyllium, cranberry, melatonin, methylsulfonylmethane, and lutein.[1] No special concerns have been published associated with bleeding or other perioperative risks from the use of these supplements.

Summary

Commonly used herbal medications can have direct and indirect effects in the perioperative period. Although there is little direct evidence for discontinuation timing, emerging knowledge of the underlying biology of these medications and review of case reports suggest that herbal medications should be considered in the perioperative plan.

Acupuncture

MECHANISM AND GENERAL PRACTICE

Although acupuncture can reduce preoperative anxiolysis, intraoperative anesthetic requirements, and postoperative ileus, and can support cardiovascular function, it has been most widely studied to control postoperative pain and to prevent or treat nausea and vomiting.[160]

Acupuncture has been used in China for more than 3000 years, and in the 1970s, it gained international attention as a treatment for a variety of diseases. In 1974, Dr. Bonica became the first pain physician invited by the Chinese government as a member of an American medical delegation to assess the utility of acupuncture in surgical procedures. He witnessed more than 28 surgeries personally and spoke with a large number of surgeons as well as anesthesia providers. In the report subsequently published in JAMA,[160a] he pointed out, "it (acupuncture) may prove extremely useful in relieving postoperative pain thus obviating the depressant effects of narcotics usually employed for this purpose." Traditional Chinese medicine (TCM) is the basis for acupuncture practice. According to TCM, the human body operates on 12 bilaterally distributed channels (6 yin channels and 6 yang channels) in conjunction with two midline channels in the ventral and dorsal aspects of the body, respectively. Acupuncture is the stimulation of anatomic locations on the skin by a variety of techniques that can be classified as invasive (e.g., needles, injections) or noninvasive (e.g., transcutaneous electrical stimulation, pressure, laser). Needles inserted into the skin can be stimulated by manual manipulation, moxibustion (i.e., burning a substance to produce heat), pressure, laser, and electricity. A scientific basis may exist for acupuncture. Acupuncture stimulates high-threshold, small-diameter nerves that activate the spinal cord, brainstem (i.e., periaqueductal gray area), and hypothalamic (i.e., arcuate) neurons, which trigger endogenous opioid mechanisms.[161] The effect of acupuncture analgesia can be reversed by administration of naloxone.[162] Other mechanisms such as modulation of immune function,[163] inhibition of the inflammatory response,[164] regulation of neuropeptide gene expression,[165] and alteration in hormonal levels[166] have been proposed. The development of neuroimaging tools, such as positron emission tomography[167] and functional magnetic resonance imaging (fMRI),[168,169] make noninvasive studies of acupuncture's effects on human brain activity possible. Studies using positron emission tomography have demonstrated that the thalamic asymmetry present in patients suffering from chronic pain was reduced after acupuncture treatment. Other studies using fMRI have pointed to relationships between particular acupoints and activation of the visual cortex.[170] Using a noninvasive imaging technique called Bi-Digital O-Ring Test, researchers found that each meridian is connected to a representative area in the cerebral cortex, suggesting that the meridian system defined in the theories of Chinese medicine may overlap with distinct supraspinal regions.[170a] Electroacupuncture, particularly at low frequency, is associated with widespread fMRI signal increases in the anterior insula area, limb, and paralimbic structures. These humoral and neuronal changes induced by acupuncture form the basis for its clinical use.

According to the Centers for Disease Control and Prevention, more than 50 million procedures are performed each year in the United States, including more than 1 million hip and knee replacements. Most surgical procedures are associated with postoperative pain, for which opioids are the mainstay of treatment. However, opioid usage is associated with a high incidence of side effects including respiratory depression, reduced gastrointestinal motility, sedation, and itching. Chronic exposure to high-dose opioids can also induce opioid tolerance and dependence. It is therefore highly desirable to develop alternative therapies that provide adequate postoperative pain relief with minimal side effects. In this context, acupuncture for acute postoperative pain control has gained significant interest, including its use for oral-maxillofacial and neck surgeries, sternotomy/thoracotomy, abdominal/pelvic surgeries, and orthopedic and spine surgeries. Studies have shown that acupuncture can lead to improved pain scores or reduced opioid requirements postoperatively. Lao and associates carried out a randomized, double-blinded, and placebo-controlled trial on postoperative dental pain ($N = 39$).[170b] The acupuncture group received acupuncture for about 20 minutes with intermittent manual manipulation to trigger "De Qi" sensation—a sensation of numbness, distension, or electrical tingling at the needling site. The control group underwent placebo acupuncture treatment at the identical acupuncture points to the acupuncture group but without needle insertion into the skin. Mean pain-free postoperative time was significantly longer in the acupuncture group (172.9 minutes) than in the placebo group (93.8 minutes). Pain medication requirements were significantly less in the acupuncture group than in the control group. Of note, this study also ruled out psychological variables as confounders for their observed benefits of acupuncture.

It is important to note that many of the studies on clinical applications of acupuncture have insufficient sample size, high dropout rates, inadequate follow-up, and poorly defined illnesses, enrollment criteria, and outcome measures.[161] Additionally, many of the clinical trials are single center studies, which could potentially demonstrate larger treatment effects than multicenter studies.[170c]

Side effects of acupuncture treatments include bruising or bleeding at the needle insertion site, transient vasovagal response, infection, dermatitis, and retained needle fragments. The occurrence of adverse events during acupuncture treatment is considered extremely low. In a survey that included 34,407 acupuncture treatments, there were no reported events of serious side effects and only 43 cases of significant mild side effects were noted, such as nausea, fainting, and bruising.[170d,e] Recently, the safety of acupuncture was confirmed in a cohort of cancer patients with thrombocytopenia.[170f]

ACUPUNCTURE FOR POSTOPERATIVE NAUSEA AND VOMITING

One of the most promising indications for acupuncture is to prevent postoperative nausea and vomiting (PONV). PONV results in patient dissatisfaction, delayed discharge, unanticipated hospital admission, and the use of resources. Drugs have been the mainstay of management, however these have limited effectiveness, are associated with adverse effects, and can be costly. Acupuncture prevents PONV compared with sham acupuncture or no treatment.[160] In two early controlled trials, acupuncture prevented PONV in the pediatric population[171,172]; however, one literature review of 10 research studies examining the use of acupressure and acupuncture in adults concluded that it is not effective in preventing and managing PONV.[173] Other clinical studies have found that acupuncture prevents PONV and results in a greater degree of adult patient satisfaction.[174,175] For many of the trials in both adults and children, the PONV acupuncture point was P6 or PC6 (i.e., Nei guan or Pericardium 6).[173,176] The P6 acupuncture point is located between the palmaris longus and flexor carpi radialis muscle tendons, 4 cm proximal to the distal wrist crease and 1 cm below the skin (Fig. 33.2). Intraoperative stimulation of the P6 acupuncture point reduced the incidence of PONV, and its efficacy was similar to that of antiemetic drugs.[177] Stimulation of the acupuncture point should be initiated before induction of anesthesia.[178] Postoperative stimulation may be just as or more effective.[179] In children, stimulation immediately before emergence and in the recovery room has been effective. A recent metaanalysis for pediatric tonsillectomy indicated that acupuncture at the P6 acupuncture point is effective in preventing PONV.[179a] Some anesthesiologists anecdotally report tapping a small needle cap or other piece of smooth plastic over the P6 point as an effective means of acupressure stimulation.

Studies often differ in acupuncture method: duration and timing of stimulation, unilateral versus bilateral stimulation, and type of stimulation (i.e., needles with or without additional stimulation, acupressure, transcutaneous electrical stimulation, cutaneous laser stimulation, injection of a 50% dextrose solution, or capsicum plaster). Data to compare the effectiveness, safety, and costs of different methods of stimulation are inadequate.

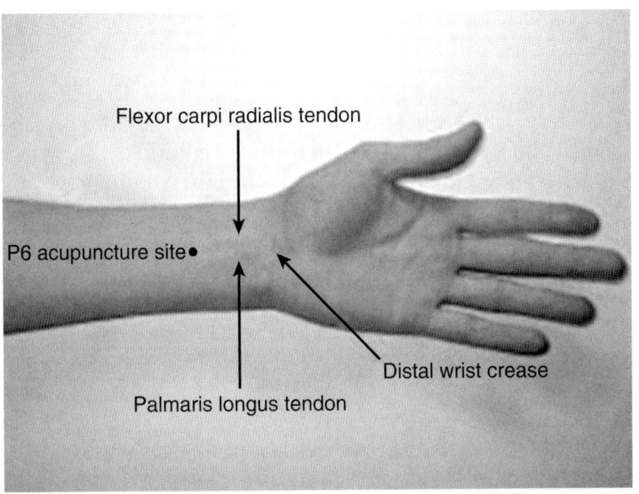

Fig. 33.2 The P6 acupuncture point is located between the palmaris longus and flexor carpi radialis muscle tendons, 4 cm proximal to the distal wrist crease and 1 cm below the skin.

DEEP BREATHING

Deep breathing exercises are performed as part of a relaxation technique. With this method, a subject consciously slows breathing and focuses on taking deep breaths.[180] Deep breathing can help reduce abdominal and surgical pain.[181,182]

Studies of postoperative pain relief with breath control were reported in the 1970s.[183,184] Since then, many studies have reported its efficacy against postoperative pain in adult patients[181,185]; prevented postoperative pulmonary complications[186]; and decreased pain in pediatric patients.[199]

Fast or forced deep breathing can also increase postoperative pain.[187] Thus, those who assist patients in postoperative pain management should encourage deep breathing exercises that are performed slowly, smoothly, and gently. Slow, deep breathing relaxation exercises have been used successfully as an adjunct to opioids for postoperative pain management in patients who had coronary bypass surgery[188]; however, after abdominal surgery, deep breathing was ineffective for pain reduction in older patients because pulmonary complications developed postoperatively.[189] Most patients who receive deep breathing education think it is useful, and the exercise was effective in increasing their feelings of rapport with staff and intention to follow their doctor's directives.[190] Results from a recent trial demonstrated that slow, deep breathing had analgesic effects with increased vagal cardiac activity.[191] Slow, deep breathing relaxation can also decrease the sensation of postoperative nausea.[192,193]

Music Therapy

Music therapy is the clinical, evidence-based use of music interventions to accomplish individualized therapeutic goals. Because music can be used for diverse applications, music therapists practice in a variety of healthcare and education settings.[194] Music for pain relief benefits individuals experiencing a low to moderate amount of pain more than those experiencing a high degree of pain.[195] A patient's preferred music should be considered when it is used for pain relief. The increase of endogenous opioids through music may be the reason for pain relief.[194]

Perioperatively, music can decrease preoperative anxiety, reduce intraoperative sedative and analgesic requirements, and increase patient satisfaction. Patient-selected music can reduce patient-controlled sedative requirements during spinal anesthesia and analgesic requirements during lithotripsy.[196] Music in the preoperative setting can reduce anxiety without affecting physiologic measures of stress.[197,198] Music can also increase patient satisfaction and reduce systolic blood pressure during cataract surgery after retrobulbar block.[199] Perioperative music can reduce arterial pressure, anxiety, and pain among women undergoing mastectomy for breast cancer.[200] As a noninvasive intervention, the low sensory stimulation of music reduced anxiety and increased cooperation in children undergoing induction of anesthesia.[201]

Music therapy interventions that have targeted nausea, both anticipatory or after treatment, have had conflicting results.[194] One study showed that a patient's preferred music for listening during chemotherapy infusion was effective in decreasing the onset and occasion of nausea.[202] In another study, listening to music with a personal message from the physician yielded no difference in chemotherapy-induced side effects compared with not listening to music during chemotherapy.[203] Some studies have found no effect on PONV from music therapy,[204,205] yet PONV was reduced in hospitalized transplant patients postoperatively.[206] Although the exact mechanism is not well understood, music therapy has been an alternative option to mainstream therapies in healthcare settings to reduce patient pain, anxiety, and perioperative stress.[207] Another use of music is in the intensive care unit. A recent clinical trial observed that among patients in the intensive care unit who received acute ventilator support for respiratory failure, patient-directed music intervention resulted in more reduction in anxiety and sedation frequency and intensity compared with usual care.[208] In addition, music can attenuate cardiovascular variability and nociceptive effects.[209,210]

Conclusion

One of the fastest changing aspects of health care is the growing public and scientific interest in CAM. An increasing number of patients and physicians have combined integrative medicine into their treatment plans. Because of the significant increase in demand for CAM therapies, most U.S. medical schools have added coursework on integrative medicine. Anesthesiologists are the physicians to manage these patients perioperatively, and therefore should have updated knowledge for the modalities of complementary and integrative medicine. To manage herbal medications in the perioperative period, their possible direct and indirect effects should be recognized based on an understanding of the underlying pharmacology. Surgery and anesthesia can usually proceed safely if potential complications are anticipated and can be minimized. As CAM therapies

TABLE 33.2 Printed and World Wide Web Sources of Herbal Medicine Information

Source	Comments
Physicians' Desk Reference for Herbal Medicines	
Encyclopedia of Dietary Supplements	
Commission E Monographs	Safety and efficacy information on herbs and phyto-medicinals; published in German, translated to English, 1998
Center for Food Safety and Applied Nutrition, Food and Drug Administration: https://www.fda.gov/AboutFDA/CentersOffices/OfficeofFoods/CFSAN/default.htm	Clinicians should use this site to report adverse events associated with herbal medicines and other dietary supplements. Sections also contain safety, industry, and regulatory information
National Center for Complementary and Alternative Medicine, National Institutes of Health: http://nccam.nih.gov/	This site contains fact sheets about alternative therapies, consensus reports, and databases
Agricultural Research Service, U.S. Department of Agriculture https://www.ars.usda.gov/	The site contains an extensive phytochemical database with search capabilities
Quackwatch: http://www.quackwatch.com	Although this site addresses all aspects of health care, there is a considerable amount of information covering complementary and herbal therapies
National Council Against Health Fraud: http://www.ncahf.org	This site focuses on health fraud with a position paper on over-the-counter herbal remedies
HerbMed: http://www.herbmed.org	This site contains information on numerous herbal medications, with evidence for activity, warnings, preparations, mixtures, and mechanisms of action. There are short summaries of important research publications with Medline links.
ConsumerLab: http://www.consumerlab.com	This site is maintained by a corporation that conducts independent laboratory investigations of dietary supplements and other health products

gain popularity in the United States, patients are likely to accept some alternative modalities during the perioperative period, such as acupuncture, deep breathing, and musical intervention. These modalities are easy to administer, have a rapid onset of action, are cost effective, and produce minimal side effects. Based on preliminary studies, perioperative use of CAM therapies may be an adjunct for management of multiple symptoms including pain, anxiety, and nausea and vomiting, among others. Additional large, well-designed trials are required to verify current observations on the effectiveness of CAM and to answer the concerns of possible side effects. Although medical schools are beginning to incorporate CAM into their curricula, it is important for anesthesiologists to stay informed about CAM therapies (Table 33.2).

Acknowledgment

The editors and publisher would like to thank Drs. Chong-Zhi Wang, Chun-Su Yuan, and Jonathan Moss for contributing a chapter on this topic in the prior edition of this work. It has served as the foundation for the current chapter.

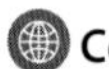 **Complete references available online at expertconsult.com.**

References

1. Clarke TC, et al. National Health Statistics Reports; 2016:1–12.
1a. Nahin RL, et al. National Health Statistics Reports; 2016:1–11.
2. Eisenberg DM, et al. *JAMA*. 1998;280:1569.
3. Wang SM, et al. *Anesth Analg*. 2003;97:1010.
4. Ashar BH, et al. *Arch Intern Med*. 2007;167:966.
5. NIH/NCCAM. *What is complementary and alternative medicine?* 2011. http://nccam.nih.gov/health/whatiscam. Accessed 23.05.12.
6. Ang-Lee MK, et al. *JAMA*. 2001;286:208.
7. Kaye AD, et al. *J Clin Anesth*. 2000;12:468.
8. Tsen LC, et al. *Anesthesiology*. 2000;93:148.
9. Leung JM, et al. *Anesth Analg*. 2001;93:1062.
10. King AR, et al. *BMC Complement Altern Med*. 2009;9:38.
11. Gardiner P, et al. *Arch Intern Med*. 2006;166:1968.
12. De Smet PA. *N Engl J Med*. 2002;347:2046.
13. Food and Drug Administration. *FDA advises consumers not to use certain Zicam cold remedies—intranasal zinc product linked to loss of sense of smell*; 2009. http://www.fda.gov/Newsevents/Newsroom/PressAnnouncements/ucm167065.htm. Accessed 02.06.12.
14. Wang C, et al. *Ann Intern Med*. 2011;155:217.
15. Rauchensteiner F, et al. *J Pharm Biomed Anal*. 2005;38:594.
16. Harkey MR, et al. *Am J Clin Nutr*. 2001;73:1101.
17. Food and Drug Administration. *Dietary supplement current good manufacturing practices (CGMPs) and interim final rule (IFR) facts*; 2007. Accessed 01.05.12. http://www.fda.gov/Food/GuidanceRegulation/CGMP/ucm110858.htm.
18. Shao A. *HerbalGram*. 2010;89(55).
19. Nortier JL, et al. *N Engl J Med*. 2000;342:1686.
20. Cohen PA. *N Engl J Med*. 2012;366:389.
21. Food and Drug Administration. *Draft guidance for industry: dietary supplements: new dietary ingredient notifications and related issues*; 2016. http://www.fda.gov/food/guidanceregulation/guidancedocumentsregulatoryinformation/dietarysupplements/ucm257563.htm. Accessed 09.29.18.
22. McKenzie AG, Simpson KR. *Eur J Anaesthesiol*. 2005;22:597.
23. Kassler WJ, et al. *Arch Intern Med*. 1991;151:2281.
24. Cirigliano M, Sun A. *JAMA*. 1998;280:1565.
25. Kennedy JM, et al. *Br J Clin Pharmacol*. 2000;49:353.
26. Tonnesen H, et al. *BMJ*. 1999;318:1311.
27. Leak JA. *ASA Newsletter*. 2000;64(6).
28. Lee A, et al. *Anesthesiology*. 2006;105:454.
29. Blumenthal M, et al. *HerbalGram*. 2010;90(64).
30. Barrett BP, et al. *Ann Intern Med*. 2002;137:939.
31. Shah SA, et al. *Lancet Infect Dis*. 2007;7:473.
32. Benson JM, et al. *Food Chem Toxicol*. 2010;48:1170.
33. Pepping J. *Am J Health Syst Pharm*. 1999;56:121.
34. Boullata JI. *Nace AM: Pharmacotherapy*. 2000;20:257.
35. Dong GC, et al. *Pharm Res*. 2009;26:375.
36. Toselli F, et al. *Life Sci*. 2009;85(97).
37. Abdul MI, et al. *Br J Clin Pharmacol*. 2010;69:508.
38. Rowe DJ, Baker AC. *Aesthet Surg J*. 2009;29:150.
39. Nightingale SL. *JAMA*. 1997;278(15).
40. Haller CA, Benowitz NL. *N Engl J Med*. 2000;343:1833.
41. Zaacks SM, et al. *J Toxicol Clin Toxicol*. 1999;37:485.
42. Powell T, et al. *Am J Kidney Dis*. 1998;33:153.
42a Ryu SJ, et al. *Medicine*. 2017;96:e9257.
43. White LM, et al. *J Clin Pharmacol*. 1997;37:116.
44. Gurley BJ, et al. *Ther Drug Monit*. 1998;20(439).
45. Stevinson C, et al. *Ann Intern Med*. 2000;133:420.
46. Srivastava KC. *Prostaglandins Leukot Med*. 1986;22:313.
47. Rose KD, et al. *Neurosurgery*. 1990;26:880.
48. Sunter WH. *Pharm J*. 1991;246:722.

49. Silagy CA, Neil HA. *J Hypertens*. 1994;12:463.
50. Coates PM, et al. *Encyclopedia of Dietary Supplements*. 2nd ed. London: Informa Healthcare; 2010.
51. Ali BH, et al. *Food Chem Toxicol*. 2008;46:409.
52. Koo KL, et al. *Thromb Res*. 2001;103(387).
53. Pongrojpaw D, Chiamchanya C. *J Med Assoc Thai*. 2003;86:244.
54. Hunt R, et al. *Anesth Analg*. 2013;117(597).
55. Ryan JL, et al. *Support Care Cancer*. 2012;20:1479.
56. Nurtjahja-Tjendraputra E, et al. *Thromb Res*. 2003;111(259).
57. Kruth P, et al. *Ann Pharmacother*. 2004;38:257.
58. Young HY, et al. *Am J Chin Med*. 2006;34:545.
59. Le Bars PL, et al. *JAMA*. 1997;278:1327.
60. Solomon PR, et al. *JAMA*. 2002;288:835.
61. Rowin J, Lewis SL. *Neurology*. 1996;46:1775.
62. Matthews MK. *Neurology*. 1998;50:1933.
63. Vale S. *Lancet*. 1998;352(36).
64. Rosenblatt M, Mindel J. *N Engl J Med*. 1997;336:1108.
65. Fessenden JM, et al. *Am Surg*. 2001;67:33.
66. Drago F, et al. *J Ocul Pharmacol Ther*. 2002;18:197.
67. Woelkart K, et al. *Phytother Res*. 2010;24:445.
68. Qi LW, et al. *Nat Prod Rep*. 2011;28:467.
69. Attele AS, et al. *Biochem Pharmacol*. 1999;58:1685.
70. Zhang HM, et al. *J Pharm Biomed Anal*. 2012;62:258.
71. Sievenpiper JL, et al. *J Am Coll Nutr*. 2003;22:524.
72. Sengupta S, et al. *Circulation*. 2004;110(1219).
73. Attele AS, et al. *Diabetes*. 2002;51:1851.
74. Teng CM, et al. *Biochim Biophys Acta*. 1989;990:315.
75. Lee WM, et al. *J Pharm Pharmacol*. 2008;60:1531.
76. Lee JG, et al. *Pharmazie*. 2009;64:602.
77. Jin YR, et al. *Basic Clin Pharmacol Toxicol*. 2007;100(170).
78. Endale M, et al. *Br J Pharmacol*. 2012.
79. Beckert BW, et al. *Plast Reconstr Surg*. 2007;120:2044.
80. Janetzky K, Morreale AP. *Am J Health Syst Pharm*. 1997;54:692.
81. Yuan CS, et al. *Ann Intern Med*. 2004;141:23.
82. Jiang X, et al. *J Clin Pharmacol*. 2006;46:1370.
83. Li X, et al. *Biomed Chromatogr*. 2007;21:735.
84. Munekage M, et al. *Drug Metab Dispos*. 2011;39:1784.
85. Wang CZ, et al. *Am J Chin Med*. 2011;39:1161.
86. Wang CZ, et al. *Am J Chin Med*. 2007;35:543.
87. Stote KS, Baer DJ. *J Nutr*. 2008;138:1584S.
88. Kang WS, et al. *Thromb Res*. 1999;96:229.
89. Son DJ, et al. *Prostaglandins Leukot Essent Fatty Acids*. 2004;71(25).
90. Jin YR, et al. *J Cardiovasc Pharmacol*. 2008;51:45.
91. Liatsos GD, et al. *Am J Health Syst Pharm*. 2010;67:531.
92. Taylor JR, Wilt VM. *Ann Pharmacother*. 1999;33:426.
93. Ullmann U, et al. *J Int Med Res*. 2003;31:88.
94. Gawande S, et al. *Phytother Res*. 2008;22:802.
95. Pepping J. *Am J Health Syst Pharm*. 1999;56:957.
96. Jamieson DD, et al. *Arch Int Pharmacodyn Ther*. 1989;301:66.
97. Almeida JC, Grimsley EW. *Ann Intern Med*. 1996;125:940.
98. Brown AC, et al. *Clin Toxicol (Phila)*. 2007;45(549).
99. Norton SA, Ruze P. *J Am Acad Dermatol*. 1994;31:89.
100. Gleitz J, et al. *Planta Med*. 1997;63:27.
101. Raduege KM, et al. *J Clin Anesth*. 2004;16:305.
102. Teschke R, Schulze J. *JAMA*. 2010;304:2174.
103. Escher M, et al. *BMJ*. 2001;322(139).
104. Russmann S, et al. *Ann Intern Med*. 2001;135:68.
105. Chen SE, et al. *Eur J Drug Metab Pharmacokinet*. 1980;5:161.
106. Rasmussen AK, et al. *Xenobiotica*. 1979;9(1).
107. Bent S, et al. *N Engl J Med*. 2006;354:557.
108. Gerber GS. *J Urol*. 2000;163:1408.
109. Cheema P, et al. *J Intern Med*. 2001;250:167.
110. Villanueva S, Gonzalez J. *Bol Asoc Med P R*. 2009;101(48).
111. Shelton RC, et al. *JAMA*. 2001;285:1978.
112. Muller WE, et al. *Pharmacopsychiatry*. 1998;31(suppl 1):16.
113. Neary JT, Bu Y. *Brain Res*. 1999;816(358).
114. Brown TM. *Am J Emerg Med*. 2000;18:231.
115. Johne A, et al. *Clin Pharmacol Ther*. 1999;66:338.
116. Ernst E. *Lancet*. 1999;354:2014.
117. Piscitelli SC, et al. *Lancet*. 2000;355:547.
118. Yue QY, et al. *Lancet*. 2000;355:576.
119. Barone GW, et al. *Ann Pharmacother*. 2000;34:1013.
120. Ruschitzka F, et al. *Lancet*. 2000;355:548.
121. Breidenbach T, et al. *Lancet*. 2000;355:1912.
122. Kerb R, et al. *Antimicrob Agents Chemother*. 1996;40:2087.
123. Biber A, et al. *Pharmacopsychiatry*. 1998;31(suppl 1):36.
124. Houghton PJ. *J Pharm Pharmacol*. 1999;51:505.
125. Hendriks H, et al. *Planta Med*. 1981;42:62.
126. Ortiz JG, et al. *Neurochem Res*. 1999;24:1373.
127. Leuschner J, et al. *Arzneimittelforschung*. 1993;43:638.
128. Gooneratne NS. *Clin Geriatr Med*. 2008;24:121.
129. Taavoni S, et al. *Menopause*. 2011;18:951.
130. Taibi DM, et al. *Sleep Med Rev*. 2007;11:209.
131. Garges HP, et al. *JAMA*. 1998;280:1566.
132. Basila D, Yuan CS. *Thromb Res*. 2005;117:49.
133. Zhou S, Chan E. *Drug Metabol Drug Interact*. 2001;18:99.
134. Zhou Q, et al. *Curr Drug Metab*. 2005;6:67.
135. Spigset O. *Lancet*. 1994;344:1372.
136. Engelsen J, et al. *Ugeskr Laeger*. 2003;165:1868.
137. Shalansky S, et al. *Pharmacotherapy*. 2007;27:1237.
138. Evans M, et al. *J Diet Suppl*. 2010;7:314.
139. Miller KL, Clegg DO. *Rheum Dis Clin North Am*. 2011;37:103.
140. Clegg DO, et al. *N Engl J Med*. 2006;354:795.
141. Tang J, et al. *Diabetes*. 2000;49:1492.
142. Scroggie DA, et al. *Arch Intern Med*. 2003;163:1587.
143. Knudsen JF, Sokol GH. *Pharmacotherapy*. 2008;28:540.
144. Setnikar I, Rovati LC. *Arzneimittelforschung*. 2001;51:699.
145. Persiani S, et al. *Osteoarthritis Cartilage*. 2007;15:764.
146. Volpi N. *Osteoarthritis Cartilage*. 2003;11:433.
147. Wall R, et al. *Nutr Rev*. 2010;68:280.
148. ORIGIN. Trial investigators. *N Engl J Med*. 2012;367:309.
149. Rizos EC, et al. *JAMA*. 2012;308:1024.
150. Dyerberg J. *Philos Trans R Soc Lond B Biol Sci*. 1981;294:373.
151. Lazarus SA, Garg ML. *Asia Pac J Clin Nutr*. 2003;12(suppl):S20.
152. Sarris GE, et al. *Circulation*. 1989;80:I109.
153. Thorwest M, et al. *Thromb Res*. 2000;99:203.
154. Phang M, et al. *Nutr Metab Cardiovasc Dis*. 2012;22:109.
155. Harris WS. *Am J Cardiol*. 2007;99:44C.
156. Salisbury AC, et al. *Am J Cardiol*. 2012;109:13.
157. Stanger MJ, et al. *Nutr Rev*. 2012;70:107.
158. Buckley MS, et al. *Ann Pharmacother*. 2004;38:50.
159. Jalili M, Dehpour AR. *Arch Med Res*. 2007;38:901.
159a. Cerdo T, et al. *Nutrients*. 2017;9.
159b. Kelly CR, et al. *Ann Intern Med*. 2016;165:609.
159c. Sadahiro S, et al. *Surgery*. 2014;155:493.
159d. Luczynski P, et al. *eLife*. 2017;6.
159e. Shen S, et al. *Nat Neurosci*. 2017;20:1213.
159f. Amaral FA, et al. *Proc Natl Acad Sci U S A*. 2008;105:2193.
160. Chernyak GV, Sessler DI. *Anesthesiology*. 2005;102:1031.
160a. Bonica JJ. *JAMA*. 1974;228:1544.
161. Kaptchuk TJ. *Ann Intern Med*. 2002;136:374.
162. Tsunoda Y, et al. *Bull Tokyo Med Dent Univ*. 1980;27:89.
163. Mori H, et al. *Neurosci Lett*. 2002;320:21.
164. Son YS, et al. *Neurosci Lett*. 2002;319:45.
165. Guo HF, et al. *Brain Res Mol Brain Res*. 1996;43:167.
166. Gerhard I, Postneek F. *Gynecol Endocrinol*. 1992;6:171.
167. Hsieh JC, et al. *Neurosci Lett*. 2001;307:105.
168. Wu MT, et al. *Radiology*. 1999;212:133.
169. Hui KK, et al. *Hum Brain Mapp*. 2000;9(13).
170. Shen J. *J Altern Complement Med*. 2001;7(suppl 1):S121.
170a. Omura Y. *Acupunct Electrother Res*. 1989;14:155.
170b. Lao L, et al. *Arch Otolaryngol Head Neck Surg*. 1999;125:567.
170c. Dechartres A, et al. *Ann Intern Med*. 2011;155:39.
170d. White A, et al. *BMJ*. 2001;323:485.
170e. White A, et al. *Acupunct Med*. 2001;19:84.
170f. Cybularz PA, et al. *Med Acupunct*. 2015;27:224–229.
171. Rusy LM, et al. *Anesthesiology*. 2002;96:300.
172. Wang SM, Kain ZN. *Anesthesiology*. 2002;97:359.
173. Abraham J. *J Perioper Pract*. 2008;18:543.
174. El-Deeb AM, Ahmady MS. *J Anesth*. 2011;25:698.
175. Kim YH, et al. *Anesth Analg*. 2011;112:819.
176. Allen TK, Habib AS. *Anesth Analg*. 2008;107:1308.
177. Arnberger M, et al. *Anesthesiology*. 2007;107:903.
178. Dundee JW, et al. *Br J Anaesth*. 1989;63:612.
179. White PF, et al. *Anesth Analg*. 2005;100:367.
179a. Shin HC, et al. *Laryngoscope*. 2016;126:1761.

180. NIH/NCCAM: *Relaxation techniques for health: an introduction*; 2011. http://nccam.nih.gov/sites/nccam.nih.gov/files/D461.pdf. Accessed 16.05.12.
181. Celli BR, et al. *Am Rev Respir Dis*. 1984;130(12).
182. Peretz B, Gluck GM. *J Clin Pediatr Dent*. 1999;24(5).
183. Stewart E. *Am J Nurs*. 1976;76:958.
184. Hudson S. *RN*. 1977;40(37).
185. Heffline MS. *J Post Anesth Nurs*. 1990;5:321.
186. Thomas JA, McIntosh JM. *Phys Ther*. 1994;74(3).
187. Bucciero M, et al. *Anesth Analg*. 2011;113:1266.
188. Friesner SA, et al. *Heart Lung*. 2006;35(269).
189. Shea RA, et al. *Heart Lung*. 2002;31(440).
190. Downey LV, Zun LS. *South Med J*. 2009;102:688.
191. Chalaye P, et al. *Pain Med*. 2009;10:1334.
192. Camu F, et al. *Eur J Anaesthesiol*. 1992;25(suppl 6).
193. Gunta K, et al. *Orthop Nurs*. 2000;19(39).
194. Burns DS, Robb SL. Music therapy. In: Yuan CS, Bieber EJ, Bauer BA, eds. *Textbook of Complementary and Alternative Medicine*. 2nd ed. Abingdon, UK: Informa Healthcare; 2006:271.
195. Engwall M, Duppils GS. *J Perianesth Nurs*. 2009;24:370.
196. Pittman S, Kridli S. *Int Nurs Rev*. 2011;58:157.
197. Wang SM, et al. *Anesth Analg*. 2002;94:1489.
198. Ni CH, et al. *J Clin Nurs*. 2012;21:620.
199. Cruise CJ, et al. *Can J Anaesth*. 1997;44:43.
200. Binns-Turner PG, et al. *AANA J*. 2011;79:S21.
201. Kain ZN, et al. *Anesth Analg*. 2004;98:1260.
202. Ezzone S, et al. *Oncol Nurs Forum*. 1998;25:1551.
203. Sabo CE, Michael SR. *Cancer Nurs*. 1996;19(283).
204. Laurion S, Fetzer SJ. *J Perianesth Nurs*. 2003;18:254.
205. Fetzer SJ, et al. *J Perianesth Nurs*. 2005;20:249.
206. Madson AT, Silverman MJ. *J Music Ther*. 2010;47:220.
207. Nilsson U. *AORN J*. 2008;87:780.
208. Chlan LL, et al. *JAMA*. 2013;309:2335.
209. Bradt J, et al. *Cochrane Database Syst Rev*. 2010:CD006902.
210. Cooke M, et al. *J Nurs Pract*. 2010;16:125.

34

Patient Positioning and Associated Risks

KRISTINE E.W. BREYER and STEVEN ROTH

KEY POINTS

- Patient positioning is a major responsibility that requires the cooperation of the entire surgical team.
- Many patient positions that are used for surgery result in undesirable physiologic consequences including significant cardiovascular and respiratory compromise. Anesthetic agents blunt natural compensatory mechanisms, rendering surgical patients vulnerable to positional changes.
- Peripheral nerve injuries, although rare, represent 22% of cases in the 1990 to 2007 American Society of Anesthesiologists' Closed Claims Project. The mechanisms of injury are stretching, compression, and ischemia. Patient positioning is often a suspected contributory factor, although precautions have usually been taken and no specific cause for the injury is known.
- The American Society of Anesthesiologists first issued a Practice Advisory in 2000 for the prevention of perioperative peripheral neuropathies that was updated in 2019. However, very few of the studies reviewed met the standard for a scientifically proven relationship between intervention and outcome.
- Anesthesia administered outside the operating room presents special challenges with regard to patient positioning because of monitoring and equipment limitations and differences in the work environment and culture.
- Perioperative visual loss (POVL) is a rare but serious injury that appears more frequently after cardiac, spine, and orthopedic joint surgery.
- Causes of POVL include central or branch retinal artery occlusion, anterior and posterior ischemic optic neuropathy, cortical blindness, acute glaucoma, and acute expansion of gas bubbles placed in the eye in retinal surgery.
- Signs and symptoms of visual loss in the postoperative period may be subtle and can be incorrectly attributed to the residual effects of anesthetic drugs. Any patient reporting eye pain, an inability to perceive light or motion, complete or partial loss of visual fields, decreased visual acuity, or loss of pupil reactivity must be evaluated immediately by an ophthalmologist.
- The most common cause of perioperative central and branch retinal artery occlusion is compression of the eye. During cardiac surgery, emboli may occlude the retinal arteries.
- Patients who undergo prolonged operative procedures in the prone position with large blood loss are at increased risk for development of ischemic optic neuropathy. Other factors conferring a risk during spine surgery include male sex, obesity, the use of a Wilson frame, and intravascular fluids administered perioperatively.
- Patients should be informed of the risk for visual loss accompanying lengthy surgical procedures with the patient positioned prone and with anticipated large blood loss. Both anesthesia and surgery personnel, together, should develop a plan by which informed consent for this complication may be facilitated.
- POVL in the presence of focal neurologic signs or the loss of accommodation reflexes or abnormal eye movements suggests a diagnosis of cortical blindness. Neurologic consultation should be obtained.

Introduction

The purpose of patient positioning in the operating room is to facilitate the surgical procedure, however, optimal surgical positioning may put patients at risk of injury or significantly alter intraoperative physiology. Peripheral nerve injuries, pressure injuries, and eye injuries are significant sources of perioperative morbidity.[1-3] Proper patient positioning is imperative and requires the cooperation of the entire surgical team. For this reason the American Society of Anesthesiologists (ASA) requires intraoperative documentation of "patient positioning and actions to reduce the chance of adverse patient effects or complications related to positioning."[4] Preventing positioning complications requires clinical judgement, vigilance, and a cooperative team approach. This chapter will review the most commonly utilized surgical positions, physiologic alterations from positioning, and specific risks and injuries associated with different surgical positions.

Physiologic Considerations of Positioning

Complex physiologic responses have evolved to blunt the hemodynamic effects of positional changes in order to maintain blood pressure within a narrow range. These essential mechanisms maintain perfusion to the brain and vital organs, regardless of posture and position—for example, as a person reclines from an upright to a supine position venous return to the heart increases and initially the increased preload causes an increase in stroke volume and cardiac output. This causes an increase in arterial blood pressure, which activates afferent baroreceptors from the aorta (via the vagus nerve) and within the walls of the carotid sinuses (via the glossopharyngeal nerve). Mechanoreceptors from the atria and ventricles are also activated to decrease sympathetic outflow to muscle and splanchnic vascular beds. Lastly, atrial reflexes are activated to regulate renal sympathetic nerve activity, plasma renin, atrial natriuretic peptide, and arginine vasopressin levels.[5] Ultimately, heart rate and cardiac output are decreased to reach homeostasis in the new position.

Different types of anesthesia and anesthetic agents can blunt these compensatory pathways. Most current inhaled anesthetics, and many intravenous anesthetics, induce vasodilation. The use of spinal or epidural anesthesia causes a significant sympathectomy across all anesthetized dermatomes, independent of the presence of general anesthesia, reducing preload and potentially blunting cardiac response. Therefore, under anesthesia, changes in patient position may cause a more exaggerated hemodynamic response compared with position changes in unanesthetized patients. This can be particularly important for positions that would normally elicit a sympathetic response and vasoconstriction in order to maintain cardiac and cerebral perfusion, such as the sitting position. Interruptions in monitoring to facilitate positioning or turning of the surgical table should be minimized during position changes in order to monitor hemodynamic outcomes. Being aware of the physiologic consequences will help the anesthesiologist anticipate changes in hemodynamics with patient position changes.

Positive-pressure ventilation increases mean intrathoracic pressure, diminishing the venous pressure gradient from peripheral capillaries to the right atrium. This can affect cardiac output as the normal pressure gradients for venous circulation and cardiac preload are relatively low.[6] Positive end-expiratory pressure further increases mean intrathoracic pressure, and possibly further compromises venous return and cardiac output, as do conditions associated with low lung compliance, such as airways disease, obesity, ascites, and light anesthesia.[7] The anesthesia provider needs to anticipate, monitor, and treat these effects, as well as assess the safety of positional changes for each patient.

Normal spontaneous ventilation results from relatively small negative intrathoracic pressure shifts because of diaphragmatic displacement and chest wall movement. Resultant negative intrathoracic pressure also promotes venous return to the heart by reducing the pressure in the great veins and right atrium.[8] With spontaneous ventilation, diaphragmatic movement is greatest adjacent to the most dependent portions of the lung, helping bring new ventilation to the zones of the lung that are preferentially perfused. When a person shifts from standing to a supine position, functional residual capacity decreases in part due to cephalad displacement of the diaphragm. The chest wall contributes less to ventilation in the supine position causing more reliance on diaphragm contribution. Although gravity has some effect on the perfusion and ventilation of the lung, new evidence points to the importance of other factors as well.[9-13]

Under general anesthesia spontaneously breathing patients have reduced tidal volumes, reduced functional residual capacity, and increased closing volumes. This leads to more ventilation perfusion mismatching due to increased atelectasis and a reduced minute ventilation. Using positive-pressure ventilation with muscle relaxation may counter some of the ventilation-perfusion mismatch by ensuring adequate minute ventilation and limiting atelectasis by use of positive end-expiratory pressure.[9] In addition to these effects of anesthesia, patient position has distinct effects on pulmonary function. In particular, any position that limits the movement of the diaphragm, chest wall, or abdomen may increase atelectasis and therefore increase intrapulmonary shunt.

Newer investigations using high-resolution imaging have shown the prone position to provide superior ventilation-perfusion matching in the posterior segments of the lung near the diaphragm when compared with the supine position. Ventilation of these posterior segments is enhanced, while blood flow is maintained, despite their nondependent position.[8,14]

General Positioning Considerations

Coordination of the multidisciplinary surgical team is required in order to achieve proper and safe positioning of patients. Principles include maintaining spine and extremity neutrality as much as possible. The patient should lie on a padded surface, and additional padding should be placed around bony prominences and hard objects, such as intravenous fluid lines, monitoring equipment, and poles.

People who are awake and not sedated change position if they become uncomfortable. Even during normal sleep, some movement is normal in order to prevent pressure or stretch injuries. Anesthetized patients are unable to change position if pressure or stretch causes nociception. Therefore, whenever possible, patients should be placed in a natural position that would be well tolerated if the patient were awake or not sedated. When more extreme positions cannot be avoided, their duration should be limited as much as possible. It is reasonable to ask patients what positions they can tolerate comfortably.

Specific Positions

SUPINE

The most common position for surgery is the supine or dorsal decubitus position (Fig. 34.1). Classically, the head, neck, and spine all retain neutrality. Because the entire body is close to the level of the heart, hemodynamic reserve is well maintained. Tissues overlying all bony prominences,

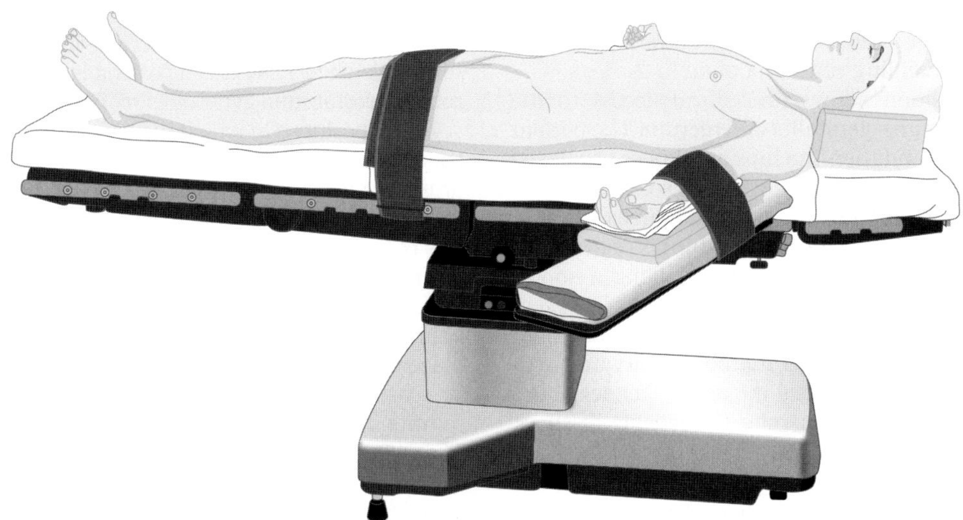

Fig. 34.1 Supine position. The base of the table is asymmetrical. When positioned in the usual direction, the patient's center of gravity is over the base. Weight limits decrease when in reverse orientation to the base.

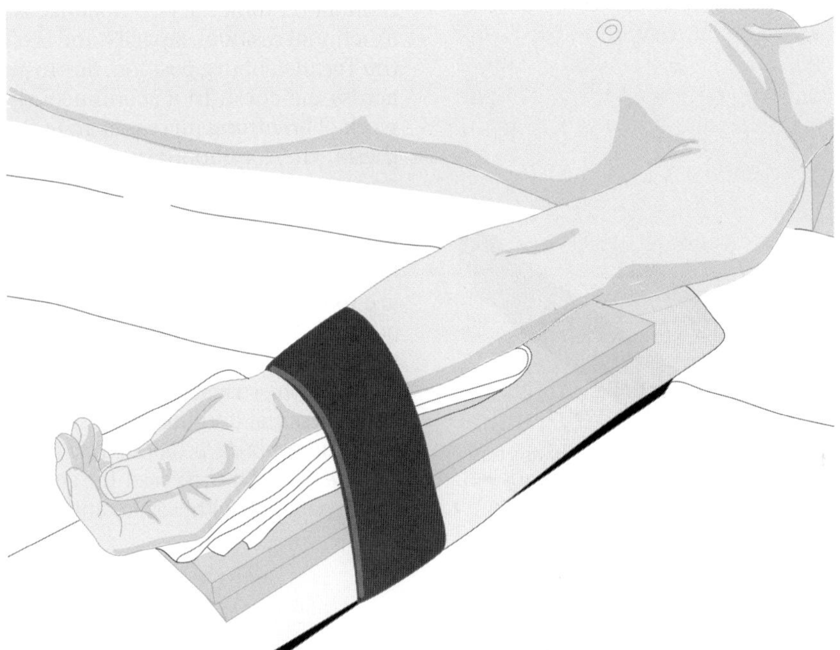

Fig. 34.2 Arm position using the arm board. Abduction of the arm is limited to less than 90 degrees whenever possible. The arm is supinated, and the elbow is padded.

such as the heels and sacrum, must be padded to prevent soft tissue ischemia as a result of pressure, especially during prolonged surgery.[15]

The arms can be abducted, adducted, or one arm abducted and one arm adducted. In any variation, the arms should be placed in as neutral a position as possible, minimizing stretch and over extension.[4] When the arms are adducted, they must remain securely placed next to the body. For abducted arm position, abduction should be limited to less than 90 degrees to minimize the likelihood of brachial plexus injury.[4,16] Hands and forearms can be supinated or kept in a neutral position with the palm toward the body. This also reduces external pressure on the spiral groove of the humerus and the ulnar nerve (Fig. 34.2).[4,17,18] Particular attention should be paid to pad bony prominences, like the elbows, and any protruding objects, such as intravenous fluid lines, monitoring equipment, and poles (Fig. 34.3).

Variations of the Supine Position

Several variations of the supine position are frequently used. These include the lawn (or beach) chair position, frog-leg position, and Trendelenburg and reverse Trendelenburg positions. The lawn chair position (Fig. 34.4) reduces stress on the back, hips, and knees by placing the patient's hips and knees in mild flexion. This position is often better tolerated by patients who are awake or undergoing monitored anesthesia care than the full supine position. The lawn chair position also facilitates lower extremity venous drainage because the legs are placed slightly above the level of the heart. Abdominal wall tension is also reduced because the xiphoid to pubic distance is decreased. Proper positioning involves positioning the patient's hips at the break of the surgical table and avoiding venous pooling in the legs.

The frog-leg position allows procedural access to the perineum, medial thighs, genitalia, and rectum. The patient is positioned supine and then the hips and knees are flexed and the hips are externally rotated with the soles of the feet facing each other. Support of the patient's knees to minimize stress and postoperative pain in the hips is required.

The Trendelenburg position, achieved by tilting a supine patient head down (Fig. 34.5), is linked by name to a 19th-century German surgeon, Friedrich Trendelenburg, who described its use for abdominal surgery. Walter Cannon, a Harvard physiologist, is credited with popularizing the use of Trendelenburg positioning to improve hemodynamics for patients in shock during World War I. Today the Trendelenburg position is frequently utilized to improve exposure during abdominal and laparoscopic surgery, during central line placement to prevent air embolism and distention of the central vein, and to offset hypotension by temporarily increasing venous return. A steep (30-45 degrees) head-down position is now frequently used for robotic prostate and gynecologic surgeries.

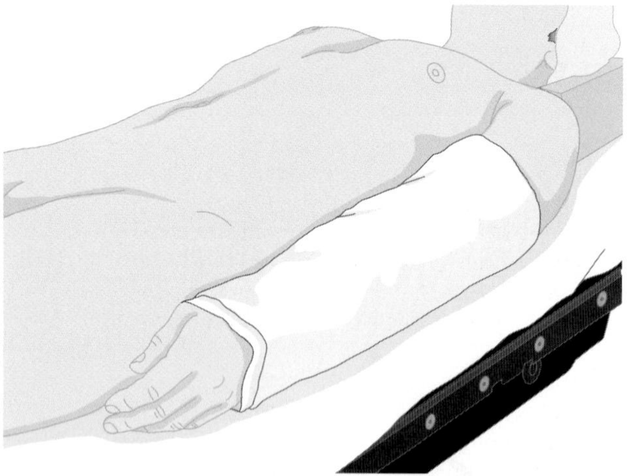

Fig. 34.3 Arm tucked at patient side. The arm is in the neutral position with the palm to the hip. The elbow is padded, and the arm is well supported by the mattress.

For all positions in which the head is at a different level than the heart, the effect of the hydrostatic gradient on cerebral arterial and venous pressures should be considered when estimating cerebral perfusion pressure. Careful documentation of any potential arterial pressure gradient is especially prudent.

The Trendelenburg position does produce hemodynamic and respiratory changes; however, the hemodynamic changes are not as long-lasting as often thought. Initial placement of the patient in head-down supine position will increase cardiac output approximately 9% in less than 1 minute via an autotransfusion from the lower extremities. This effect is not sustained and within approximately 10 minutes the cardiac output begins to return to baseline. Nevertheless, the Trendelenburg position is still considered an essential part of initial resuscitation efforts to treat hypotension and acute hypovolemia.[19] Functional residual capacity is decreased due to gravitational pull of the diaphragm cephalad. Pulmonary compliance is increased by decreased functional residual capacity and is often further decreased in the Trendelenburg position, due to patient-positioning straps across the chest. In a spontaneously breathing patient, the work of breathing increases. In patients under general anesthesia, these pulmonary changes result in higher airway pressures. Changes to the mechanical ventilator settings can compensate for some of the respiratory changes. However, with patient body habitus and variations in positioning, the higher airway pressures, and changes to minute ventilation are too great to safely continue in the steep Trendelenburg position. Testing the position for patient tolerance after anesthetic induction and completed positioning, prior to the initiation of the surgical procedure, is recommended.

Intracranial and intraocular pressures (IOCs) also increase in Trendelenburg position. Trendelenburg is contraindicated in patients with increased intracranial pressures. In fact, for some patients with severe intracranial hypertension, even

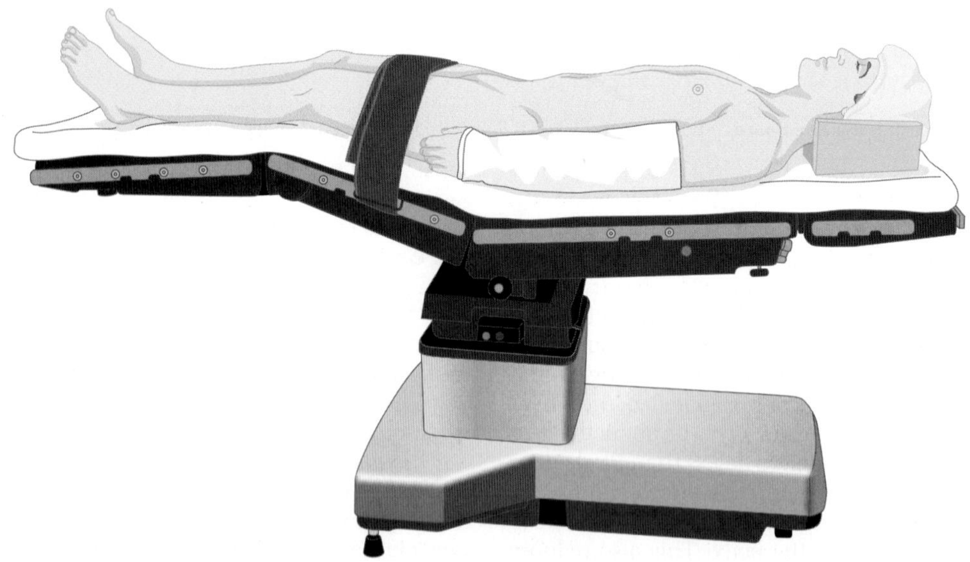

Fig. 34.4 Lawn or beach chair position. Flexion of the hips and knees decreases tension on the back.

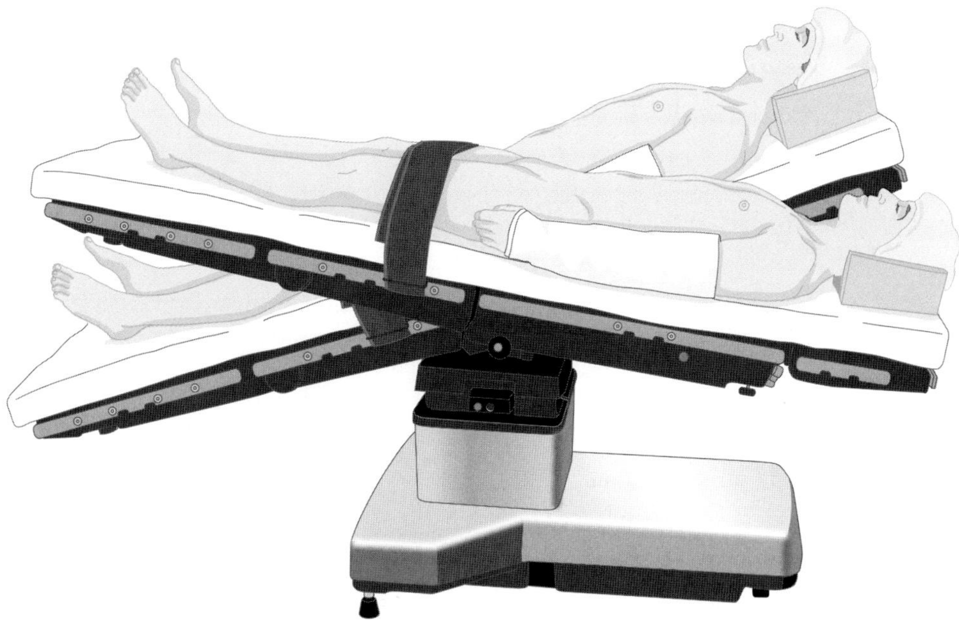

Fig. 34.5 Head-down tilt (Trendelenburg) position and head-up tilt (reverse Trendelenburg) position. Shoulder braces should be avoided to prevent brachial plexus compression injuries.

supine position is not tolerated. Consideration of the impact of positioning on intracranial pressure is important, as it may not only affect intraoperative positioning but also may have consequences on site selection for central line placement. Frequently, femoral vein site selection is preferred in patients with severely elevated intracranial pressure in order to avoid exacerbating intracranial hypertension with patient position changes during line placement.

Prolonged head-down positioning can also lead to swelling of the face, conjunctiva, larynx, and tongue, with an increased potential for postoperative upper airway obstruction. The Trendelenburg position increases intraabdominal pressure and displaces the stomach placing the patient at a higher risk for aspiration. Endotracheal intubation is often preferred in order to prevent aspiration of gastric contents.

Care must be taken to prevent patients in steep head-down positions from slipping cephalad on the surgical instruments.[20,21] Techniques to restrain the patient include antiskid bedding, knee flexion, shoulder braces, beanbag cradling, and padded cross-torso straps.[22] Shoulder braces are specifically not recommended because of the risk of compression injury to the brachial plexus. Beanbag pads become rigid when suction is applied to set the shape, and their use in the Trendelenburg position has been associated with brachial plexus injuries.[23-25] If either shoulder braces or beanbag shoulder immobilization is used to prevent sliding, additional caution is recommended regarding abducting the arm; brachial plexus injuries on the side of the abducted arm have been reported in conjunction with beanbag shoulder immobilization and steep Trendelenburg positioning.[26] These injuries may be due to stretch of the upper and middle trunks of the brachial plexus, as they course around the head of the humerus (Fig. 34.6).

The reverse Trendelenburg position (head-up tilt; see Fig. 34.2) is often used to facilitate upper abdominal surgery by shifting the abdominal contents caudad. This position is increasingly popular because of the growing number of laparoscopic surgeries requiring this position. Again, caution is advised to prevent patients from slipping on the table. As mentioned earlier, any position where the head is above the heart reduces cerebral perfusion pressure and may also cause systemic hypotension. If invasive arterial pressure monitoring is used then the arterial pressure transducer should be zeroed at the level of the Circle of Willis.

Complications of the Supine Position

The base of the surgical table is asymmetric. Classically, the base of the table is directly underneath the patient's torso (see Fig. 34.1). However, sometimes the patient's torso overlies the end of the table without the base underneath it in order to improve surgical access or to facilitate the use of specific equipment such as the C-arm for x-ray. Without the table base under the torso of the patient's body, the table is at risk of tilting or tipping over. This risk is higher with obese patients and when the table is in the Trendelenburg position. The surgical table weight limits are significantly different when the table is reversed and should be strictly observed.

Back pain is common in the supine position because the normal lumbar lordotic curvature is often lost. General anesthesia with muscle relaxation and neuraxial block increases the risk of back pain further due to loss of tone in the paraspinous muscles. Patients with extensive kyphosis, scoliosis, or a history of back pain may require extra padding of the spine or slight flexion at the hip and knee.

Peripheral nerve injury (discussed later in this chapter) is a complex phenomenon with multifactorial causes. The ASA has published several revisions of a practice advisory to help prevent perioperative peripheral neuropathies.[4] Ulnar neuropathy has historically been the most common lesion, although brachial plexus injuries have overtaken ulnar neuropathies in more recent closed claims data associated with general anesthesia.[1,3] Regardless of the position of the upper extremities, maintaining the head in a relatively midline position can help minimize the risk of stretch injury to the brachial plexus.[23] Although no direct evidence suggests

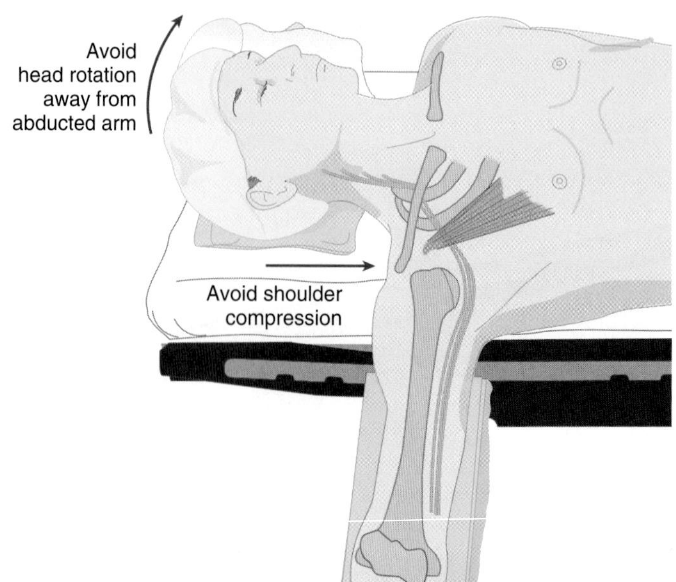

Fig. 34.6 The brachial plexus, shown in *yellow*, is vulnerable to stretch and compression due to its long course. Arm abduction is limited to less than 90 degrees when supine because when the arm is raised the head of the humerus rotates caudad and stretches the plexus. Shoulder braces should be avoided; they may cause direct compression of the plexus medially between the clavicle and first rib or laterally below the head of the humerus. Excessive head rotation should be avoided, especially away from an abducted arm. Abduction of the arm should be avoided when in a steep head-down position if shoulder braces or a beanbag holds the shoulders.

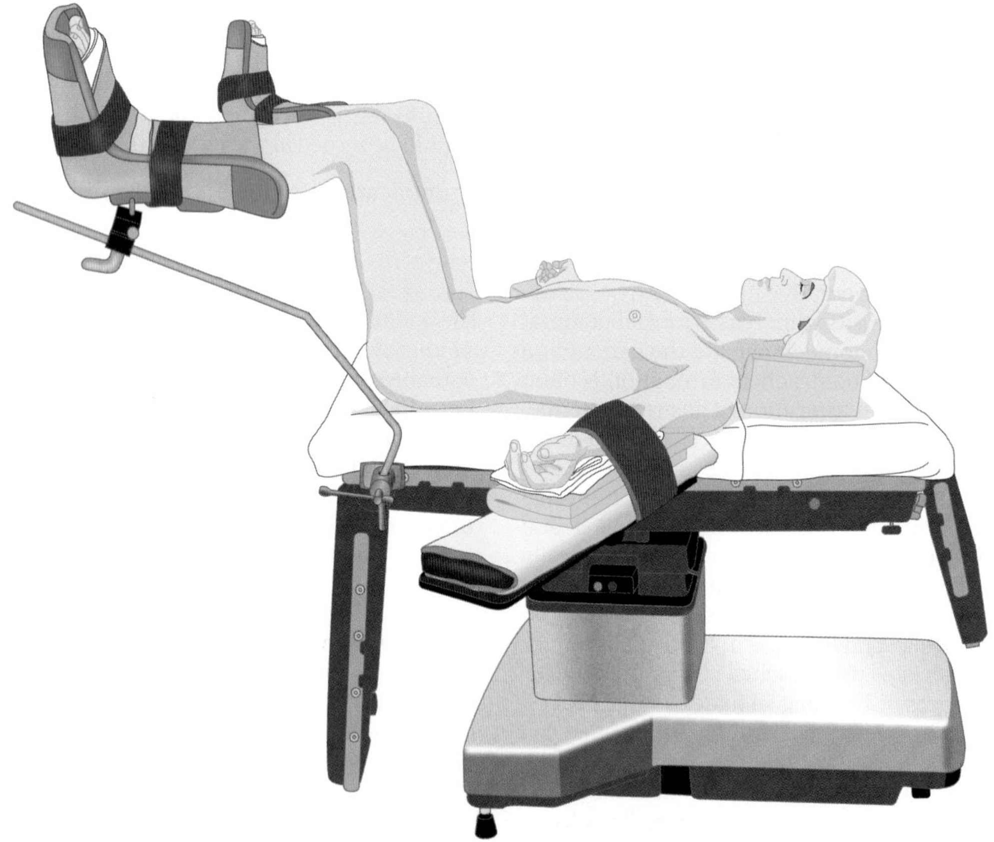

Fig. 34.7 Lithotomy position. Hips are flexed 80 to 100 degrees with the lower leg parallel to the body. Pressure near the fibular head is absent. Arms are on armrests away from the hinge point of the foot section.

that positioning or padding alone can prevent perioperative ulnar neuropathies, the ASA practice advisory recommends limiting arm abduction in the supine patient to less than 90 degrees at the shoulder, with the hand and forearm either supinated or kept in a neutral position.[4]

LITHOTOMY

The classic lithotomy position (Figs. 34.7–34.9) is frequently used during gynecologic, rectal, and urologic surgeries. The patient's hips are flexed 80 to 100 degrees from

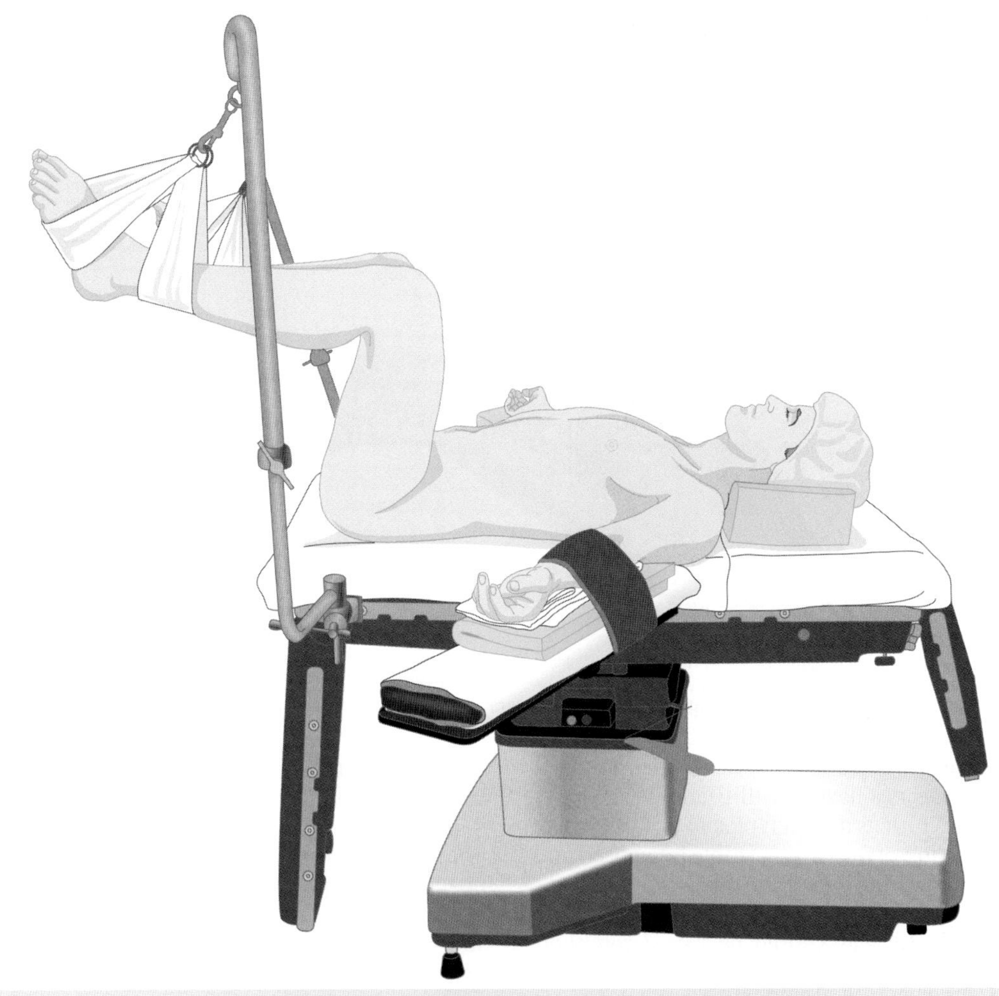

Fig. 34.8 Lithotomy position with "candy cane" stirrup leg holders.

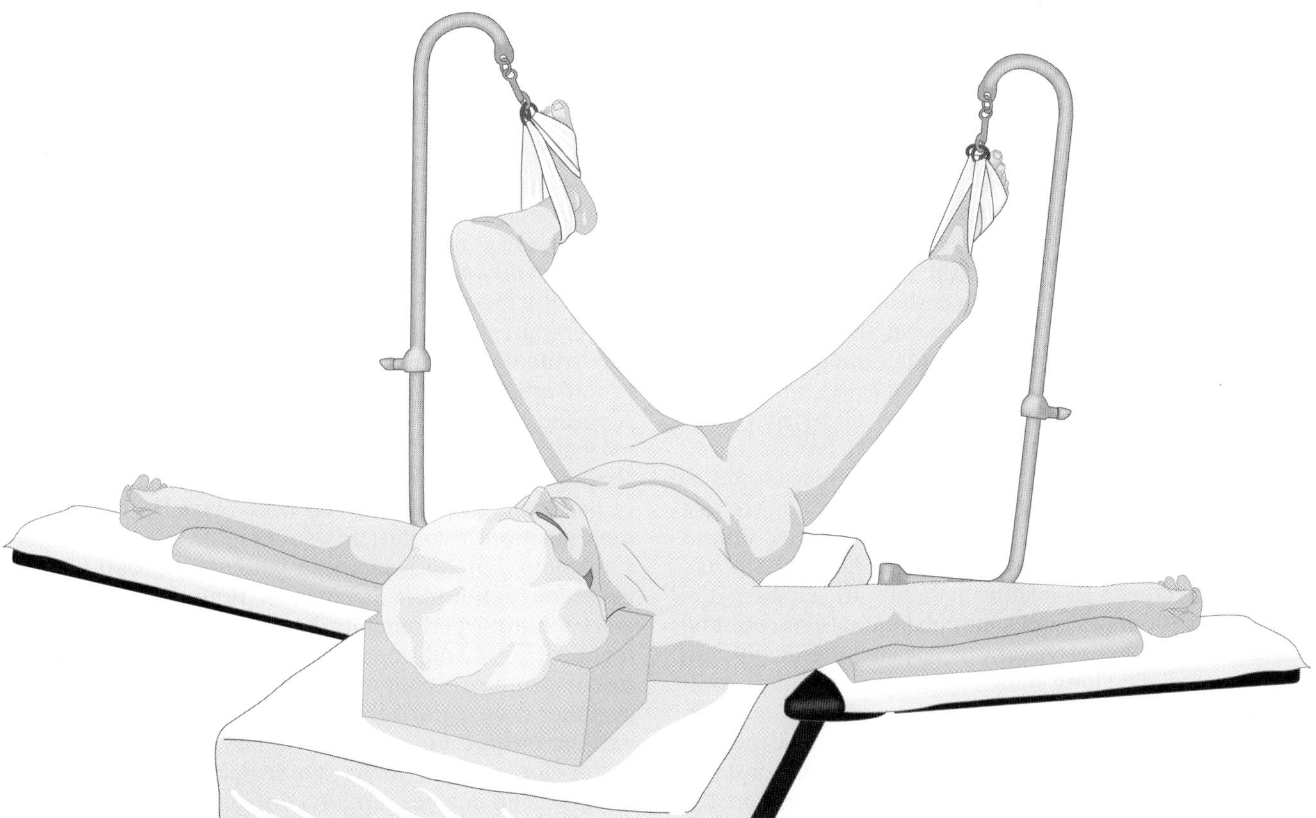

Fig. 34.9 Lithotomy position. The correct position of "candy cane" supports is well away from the lateral fibular head.

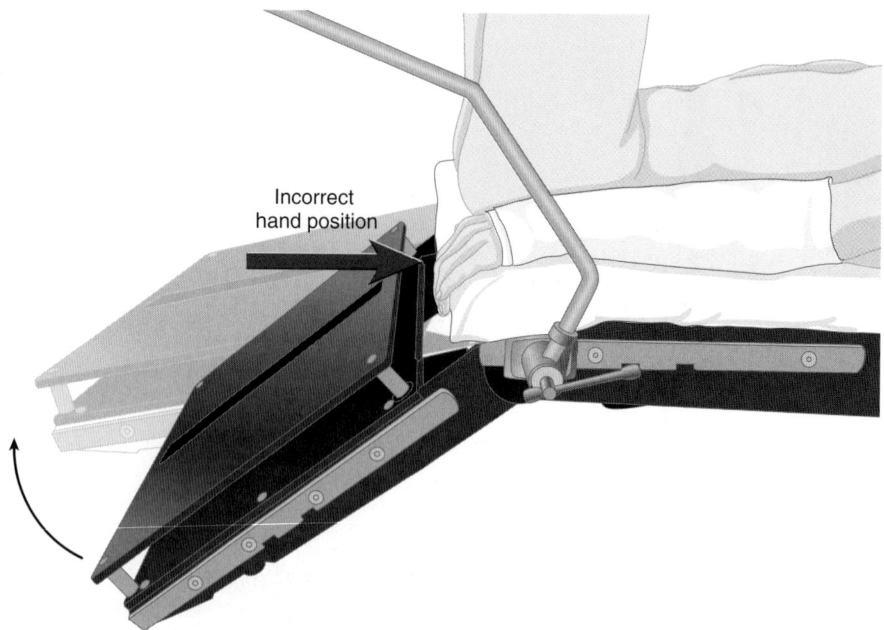

Fig. 34.10 Improper position of arms in lithotomy position. The fingers are at risk for compression when the lower section of the bed is raised.

the trunk, and the legs are abducted 30 to 45 degrees from the midline. The knees are flexed until the lower legs are parallel to the torso. The legs are then placed in supports or stirrups. The foot section of the surgical table is lowered and sometimes removed from the end of the table.

Positioning a patient into and out of lithotomy requires a coordinated team. The legs should be raised together; simultaneously, the knees and hips are flexed. This prevents torsion and injury to the lumbar spine. Padding of the lower extremities is critical, particularly over bony prominences, to prevent compression against the leg supports. The peroneal nerve is particularly prone to injury as it lies between the fibular head and compression from the leg support (see the peripheral nerve injury section of this chapter).

If the arms are tucked or placed alongside the patient, then the patient's hands and fingers are at risk of injury if they lie near the open edge of the lowered section of the table. When the foot of the table is raised at the end of the procedure the fingers near the open edge can get crushed. Strict attention must be paid to the position of the hands to avoid a potentially disastrous crush injury to the fingers (Fig. 34.10). For this reason, the recommended position of the arms is on armrests far from the table hinge point. If the arms must be tucked at the patient's side, then the hands need to be visualized and confirmed to be safe whenever the leg section of the surgical table is manipulated.

The lithotomy position may also cause significant physiologic changes. When the legs are elevated, venous return increases, causing a transient increase in cardiac output and, to a lesser extent, cerebral venous and intracranial pressure in otherwise healthy patients. In addition, the lithotomy position increases intraabdominal pressure and causes the abdominal viscera to displace the diaphragm cephalad, reducing lung compliance and potentially resulting in a decreased tidal volume. In obese patients, or when large abdominal mass is present (e.g., tumor, gravid uterus), abdominal pressure may increase enough to obstruct venous return to the heart. As with the supine position, the curvature of the lumbar spine is lost in lithotomy and can put the patient at risk of back pain.[27]

Lower extremity compartment syndrome is a rare but potentially devastating complication of the lithotomy position. Compartment syndrome is caused by increased tissue pressure within a fascial compartment due to tissue ischemia, edema, and rhabdomyolysis. Inadequate arterial inflow (from lower extremity elevation) and decreased venous outflow (due to direct compression or excessive hip flexion) elevates the risk of compartment syndrome for patients in lithotomy.[28,29] Local arterial pressure decreases 0.78 mm Hg for each centimeter the leg is raised above the right atrium.[30] Reperfusion after ischemic injury further increases edema, exacerbating the problem. In a large retrospective review of 572,498 surgeries, the incidence of compartment syndromes was higher in the lithotomy (1 in 8720) and lateral decubitus (1 in 9711) positions, as compared with the supine (1 in 92,441) position. Long procedure time was the only distinguishing characteristic of the surgeries during which patients developed lower extremity compartment syndromes.[28] A survey of urologists in the United Kingdom suggested that compartment syndrome after surgery in the lithotomy position is underreported and more common than appreciated. Affected patients in this study all had surgical durations greater than 3.5 hours.[31] In a retrospective multicenter review of 185 urologic patients who were placed in high lithotomy position, two patients suffered from compartment syndrome. For both of these patients, operative times exceeded 5 hours.[32] If surgical time extends beyond 2 to 3 hours, periodically lowering the legs is recommended.[32-34] Additional risk includes factors known to compromise tissue oxygenation, such as blood loss, peripheral vascular disease, hypotension, and reduced cardiac output. Elevated body mass index is also a risk factor for compartment syndrome. Intermittent leg compression devices remain controversial.[30,35]

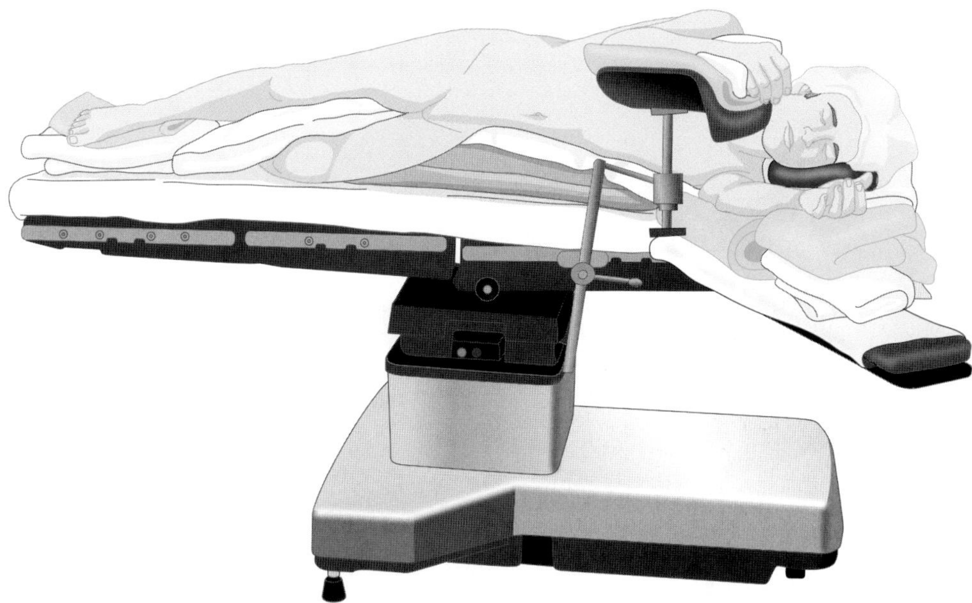

Fig. 34.11 Lateral decubitus position. The lower leg is flexed with padding between the legs, and both arms are supported and padded.

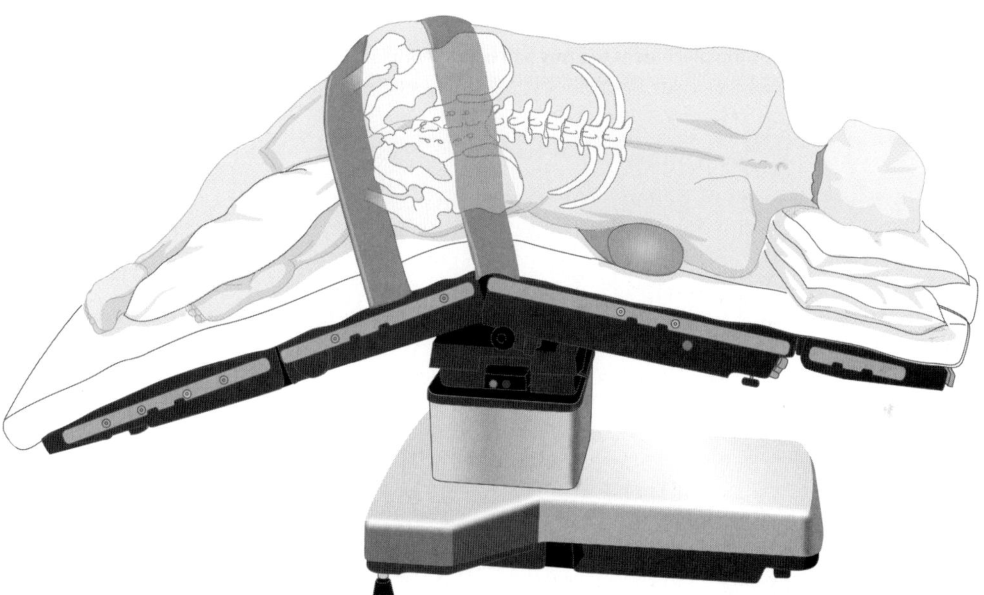

Fig. 34.12 Flexed lateral decubitus position. The point of flexion should lie under the iliac crest, rather than under the flank or lower ribs to optimize ventilation of the dependent lung.

LATERAL DECUBITUS

The lateral decubitus position (Fig. 34.11) is most frequently used for surgery involving the thorax, retroperitoneal structures, and hip. Positioning a patient in the lateral decubitus position requires the cooperation of the entire surgical staff. The nonoperative side is dependent and the dependent leg is flexed to minimize stretch of lower extremity nerves. Padding is placed between the knees to minimize excessive pressure on bony prominences. The torso must be balanced and supported both anteriorly and posteriorly. When a kidney rest is used for this purpose, it must be properly placed under the dependent iliac crest to prevent inadvertent compression of the inferior vena cava.

Patients may be laterally flexed while in the lateral position in order to gain better access to the thoracic cavity or retroperitoneum during renal surgeries. The point of flexion and the kidney rest should lie under the iliac crest rather than the flank or ribcage to minimize compression of the dependent lung (Fig. 34.12). The dependent arm should be placed on a padded arm board perpendicular to the torso. The nondependent arm needs to be carefully supported (Fig. 34.13). Neither arm should be abducted more than 90 degrees. For some high thoracotomies, the nondependent arm may need to be elevated above the shoulder plane for exposure; however, vigilance is warranted to prevent neurovascular compromise. The patient's head must be kept in a neutral position to prevent excessive lateral rotation of the neck and to avoid stretch injuries to the brachial plexus. Often additional head support is required (Fig. 34.14). The dependent ear and eye may be at risk of injury and should be checked regularly.

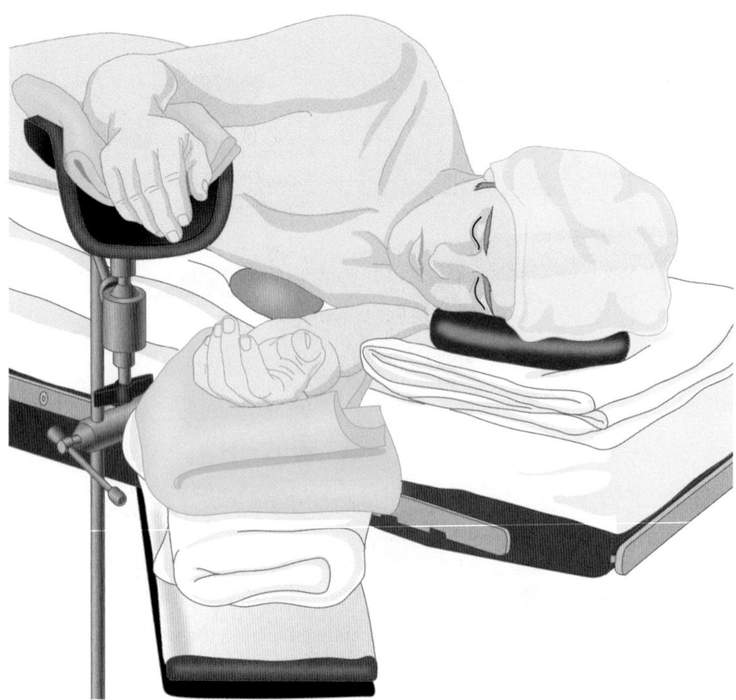

Fig. 34.13 Lateral decubitus position showing placement of arms and head. Additional padding is under the headrest to ensure the alignment of the head with the spine. The headrest is kept away from the dependent eye.

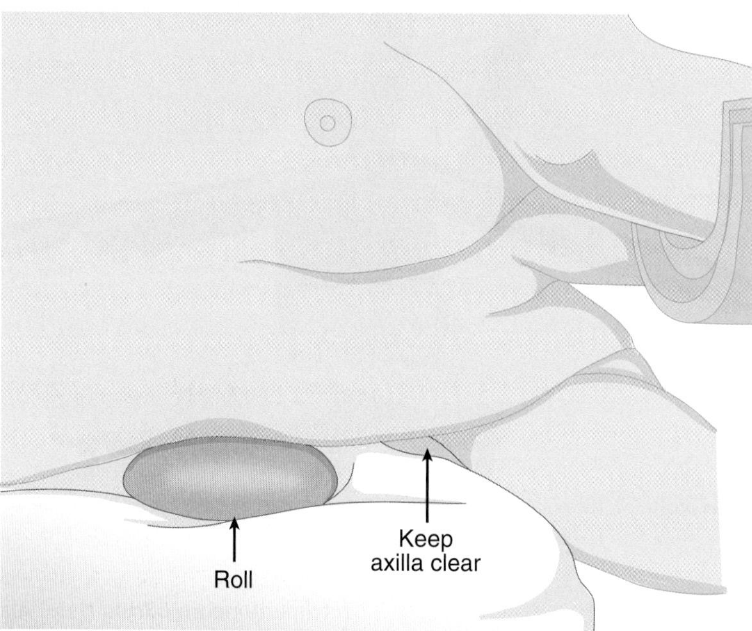

Fig. 34.14 Use of chest roll in the lateral decubitus position. The roll, in this case, is a bag of intravenous fluid and is placed well away from the axilla to prevent compression of the axillary artery and brachial plexus.

The dependent brachial plexus and axillary vascular structures are at particular risk of pressure injury in the lateral decubitus position. In order to avoid compression, an axillary roll is frequently placed between the chest wall and the table just caudal to the dependent axilla (see Fig. 34.13). The purpose of the axillary roll is to protect the dependent shoulder and the axillary contents from the weight of the thorax. The axillary roll should never be placed in the axilla. Sometimes a beanbag is used for positioning without an axillary roll. In this scenario, the axilla should be checked to ensure that it is free from compression. Regardless of the technique, the pulse should be monitored in the dependent arm for early detection of compression to axillary neurovascular structures. Vascular compression and venous outflow obstruction in the dependent arm are risks of the lateral decubitus position. Low pulse oximeter readings can be an early sign of compromised circulation. Similarly, hypotension measured in the dependent arm may be due to axillary arterial compression.

Pulmonary mechanics change in the lateral decubitus position.[36] In a patient who is mechanically ventilated, the

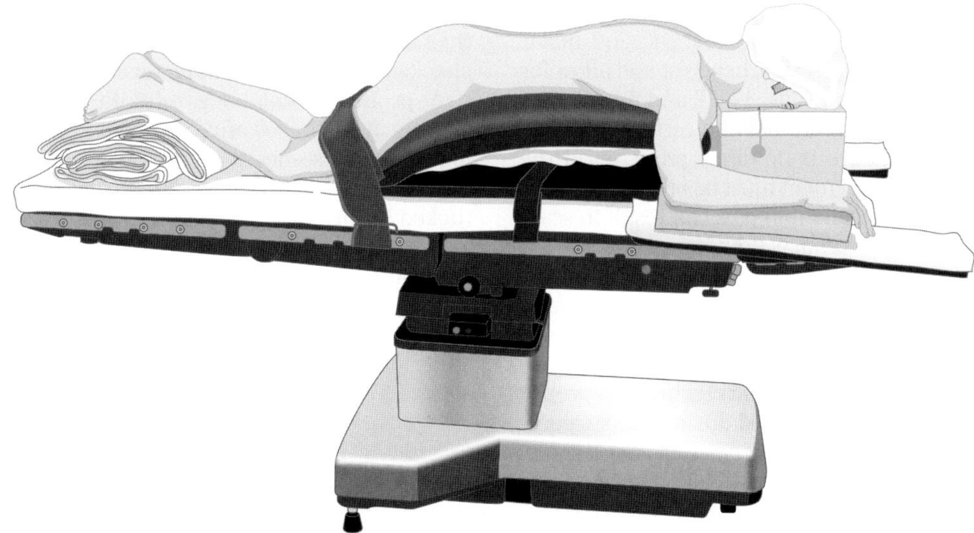

Fig. 34.15 Prone position with Wilson frame. Arms are abducted less than 90 degrees whenever possible, although greater abduction may be better tolerated while prone. Pressure points are padded, and the chest and abdomen are supported away from the bed to minimize abdominal pressure and to preserve pulmonary compliance. Soft head pillow has cutouts for eyes and nose and a slot to permit endotracheal tube exit. Eyes must be checked frequently.

combination of the lateral weight of the mediastinum and the disproportionate cephalad pressure of abdominal contents on the dependent lung favors overventilation of the nondependent lung. At the same time, the effect of gravity causes the pulmonary blood flow to the underventilated, dependent lung to increase. Consequently, ventilation-perfusion matching worsens, potentially affecting gas exchange and ventilation.

The lateral decubitus position is preferred during pulmonary surgery and one-lung ventilation. When the nondependent lung is collapsed, the minute ventilation is allocated to the dependent lung. This, combined with decreased compliance as a result of positioning, may further exacerbate the airway pressure required to achieve adequate ventilation. Head-down tilt in the lateral position worsens pulmonary function yet further, increasing shunt fraction.[37]

PRONE

The prone or ventral decubitus position (Fig. 34.15) is primarily used for surgical access to the posterior fossa of the skull, the posterior spine, the buttocks and perirectal area, and the posterior lower extremities. The patient may receive either monitored anesthesia care or general anesthesia depending on the type of surgery and the patient's body habitus and comorbidities. When general anesthesia is planned, the airway is usually secured via an endotracheal tube while the patient is still supine. Special attention should be paid to securing and taping the endotracheal tube to prevent dislodgement while the patient is prone or during changes in position. Placing an anesthetized patient in the prone position requires the coordination of the entire surgical staff. The anesthesiologist is primarily responsible for coordinating the move while maintaining inline stabilization of the cervical spine and monitoring the endotracheal tube. An exception might be the patient in whom rigid pin fixation is used when the surgeon often holds the pin frame. The endotracheal tube should be disconnected from the circuit during the move from supine to prone in order to prevent dislodgement. Which, and how many, monitors and lines are disconnected during the move is up to the clinical judgement of the anesthesiologist for an individual patient. Lines and monitors connected to the inside arm (the arm moving the least during the move) can often be easily maintained without disconnecting. Ventilation and monitoring should be reestablished as rapidly as possible.

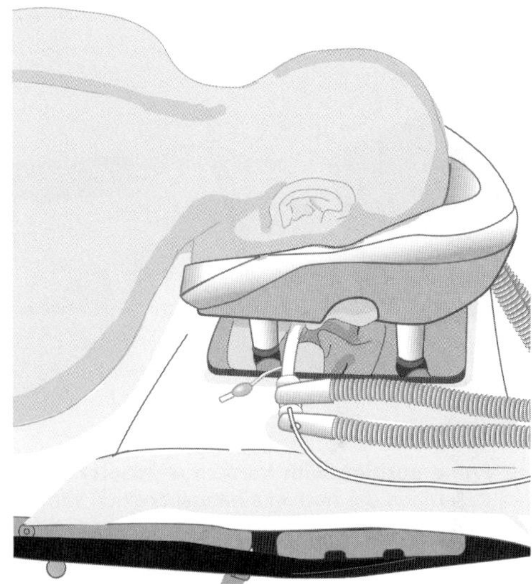

Fig. 34.16 Mirror system for prone position. Bony structures of head and face are supported, and monitoring of the eyes and airway is facilitated with a plastic mirror. Although not illustrated, the eyes should be taped closed.

Prone head position is critical. For patients under sedation, the head may be turned to the side if neck mobility is adequate. During general anesthesia, the head is usually kept neutral using a surgical pillow, horseshoe headrest, or head pins. Weight should be on the bony facial prominences and not soft tissue and especially not on the eyes. The face is not always visible. Mirror systems are available to facilitate intermittent visual confirmation that the eyes are not compressed, although direct visualization or tactile confirmation is prudent (Fig. 34.16). Several commercially available pillows are specially designed for the prone position. Most pillows support the forehead, malar regions, and chin, with a cutout for the eyes, nose, and mouth (see Fig. 34.15). The forehead and malar regions are supported by the horseshoe headrest and allow for reasonable access to the airway (Figs. 34.17 and 34.18). Pin fixation, which is most used in cranial and cervical surgery, is advantageous because there is no direct pressure on the face (Fig. 34.19). Patient movement must be prevented when the head is held in pins; movement in pins can result in scalp lacerations or a cervical spine injury. Both horseshoe and pin headrests attach to the operating room table with adjustable articulating supports. All articulating supports must be fully locked as failure of this bracketing device may lead to complications if the head suddenly drops.

Regardless of the type of head-support technique, proper positioning must be frequently verified during the surgery, checking that there is no pressure on the eyes, that the airway is secure, and that the head weight lies on the bony facial prominences only. The prone position is a risk factor for perioperative visual loss (POVL), which is discussed separately in this chapter. If motor-evoked potentials are used during spine or neurosurgery, then the position of the tongue and placement of bite blocks must be frequently checked; bite injuries can be severe.[38]

A prone patient's legs should be padded and flexed slightly at the knees and hips. The arms may be positioned to the patient's sides or placed outstretched above the head. If the arms are at the patient's sides then they should be tucked in the neutral position. If the arms are outstretched above the head, the arms should be placed on arm boards with slight flexion at the elbows to prevent undue stretch on

Fig. 34.17 Prone position with horseshoe adapter. Head height is adjusted to position the neck in a natural position without undue extension or flexion.

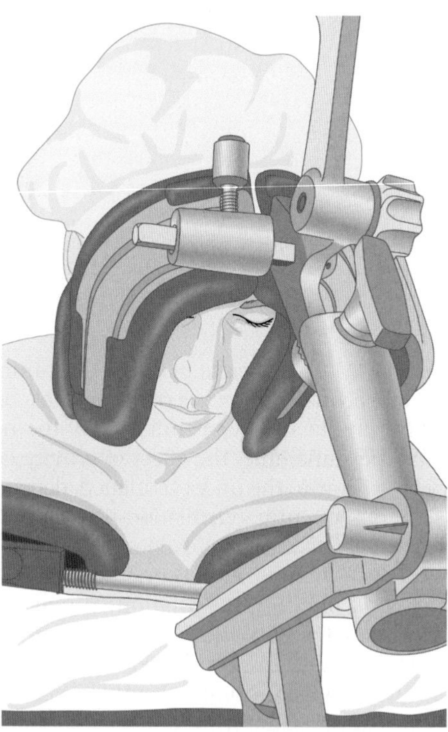

Fig. 34.18 Prone position with horseshoe adapter. The face is seen from below. The horseshoe adapter permits superior access to the airway and visualization of eyes. The width may be adjusted to ensure proper support by facial bones.

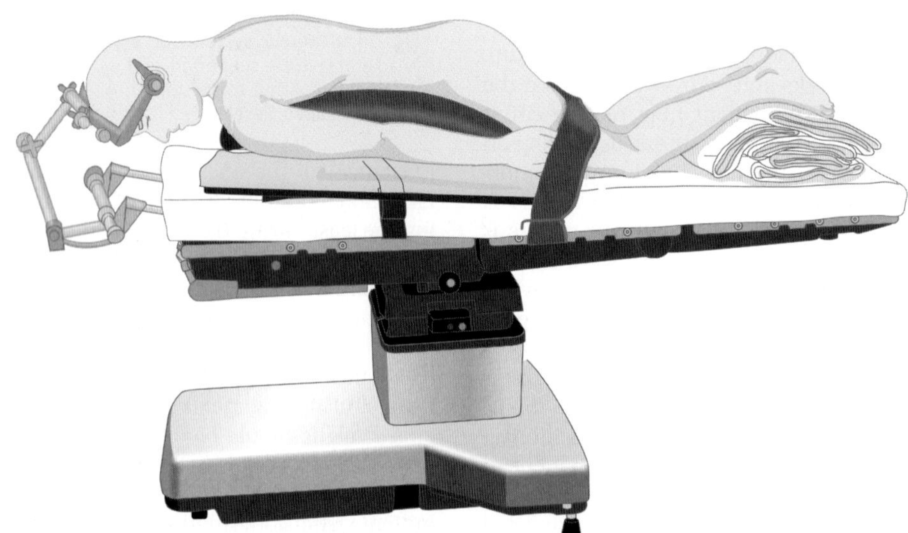

Fig. 34.19 Prone position with Mayfield head pins. Rigid fixation is provided for the cervical spine and posterior intracranial surgeries. The head position may include neck torsion or flexion that affects the depth of the endotracheal tube, and extreme head positions may increase the risk of cervical cord injury.

the peripheral nerves. Extra padding under the elbow may be needed to prevent compression of the ulnar nerve. The arms should not be abducted greater than 90 degrees.

If the legs are in plane with the torso, then hemodynamic reserve is relatively maintained; however, if any significant lowering of the legs or tilting of the entire table occurs, then venous return may increase or decrease accordingly. The prone position does not alter the ability of pulse pressure variation to predict fluid responsiveness. However, the variation has been shown to be augmented at baseline; therefore, fluid responsiveness is observed at a slightly greater level of variation than when supine.[39]

When patients are in the prone position, weight should be distributed to the thoracic cage and bony pelvis, the abdomen should hang freely in order to prevent increases in intraabdominal and intrathoracic pressure. This is accomplished with specific types of prone beds or with gel or foam bolsters. The prone beds and bolsters all place support along each side of the patient from the clavicles to the iliac crests. Placement beyond the iliac crests can cause compression on the femoral vessels and femoral nerve. Some prone beds include the Wilson frame (see Fig. 34.15), Jackson table, Relton frame, and Mouradian/Simmons modification of the Relton frame. Breasts should be placed medially to the prone torso supports (or bolsters), and genitalia should be clear of compression.[40] During posterior spinal surgery, relatively low venous pressure is desirable to minimize bleeding and to facilitate surgical exposure. Elevated abdominal pressure can transmit elevated venous pressures to the abdominal and spine vessels, including the epidural veins, which lack valves. Increased abdominal pressure may also impede venous return through compression of the inferior vena cava, decreasing cardiac output.

Pulmonary function is usually better in the prone position than in the supine position.[41,42] The prone position has been used to improve respiratory function in patients with adult respiratory distress syndrome.[43-45] Under anesthesia, the prone position has advantages over the supine position with regard to lung volumes and oxygenation without adverse effects on lung mechanics,[46,47] including patients who are obese[48] (see also Chapter 58) and pediatric patients (see also Chapter 77).[49] Newer investigations using high-resolution imaging have shown the prone position to provide superior ventilation-perfusion matching in the posterior segments of the lung near the diaphragm when compared with the supine position. The aeration and ventilation of these posterior segments are better, while blood flow is maintained, despite their nondependent position.[8,14]

Other complications of the prone position include airway edema, eye injury, pressure injury, and inadvertent loss of the endotracheal tube, monitoring, and intravenous lines. For long cases, or cases with large intravascular volume shifts, consider checking and documenting an endotracheal cuff leak at the start and end of the case. Lines and tubes need to be placed and should be well secured prior to turning the patient prone.

SITTING

The sitting position offers excellent surgical exposure to the upper posterior cervical spine and posterior fossa. Gravitational venous drainage of blood in the sitting position does decrease blood in the operative field and therefore possibly reduces surgical blood loss.[50] The lawn or beach chair position is a variation of the sitting position and is commonly used for shoulder surgeries (Fig. 34.20). The lawn chair position is really a semi-sitting position, with the head of the patient more reclined than in the traditional sitting position. For the surgeon, its advantages versus the lateral decubitus position are superior access to the shoulder from both the anterior and posterior aspect and the potential for great mobility of the arm at the shoulder joint.[51] Access to the airway is generally excellent in the sitting position, facial swelling is minimized, and pulmonary mechanics are reasonably preserved (Chapter 57).

There are unique risks to the sitting position that require much vigilance. One of the most concerning risks is for venous air embolism (VAE). The veins lie above the level of the heart in this position; therefore, air entrainment through the veins to the heart is a real danger. Furthermore, dural veins are valveless and tented open by the cranium (Fig. 34.21; see also Chapter 57). Other complications from the sitting position include quadriplegia, spinal cord infarction, hemodynamic instability pneumocephalus, macroglossia, and peripheral nerve injuries.[52,53]

Placing an anesthetized patient in the sitting position requires flexion at the torso. Hip flexion should be less than 90 degrees in order to minimize stretch on lower extremity nerves (including the sciatic nerve). Arms are supported so that the shoulders are slightly elevated in order to ensure avoidance of traction on the shoulder muscles and potential stretching of upper extremity neurovascular structures. The knees are also usually slightly flexed for balance and to reduce stretching of the sciatic nerve, and the feet are supported and padded.[54] The patient's head must be specially fixed in the sitting position with either rigid pins or taped into a special headrest.

The head and neck position while in the sitting position has been associated with complications. Surgery in the sitting position was found to be a risk factor for cervical spinal cord injury in a review of the ASA Closed Claims Project database from 1970 to 2007.[55] Although the exact mechanism for cervical spinal cord injury is unknown, cervical hyperextension, cervical hyperflexion, or excessive cervical rotation have been implicated as risk factors. Extreme neck positions can impede both arterial and venous blood flow, causing hypoperfusion or venous congestion of the brain. The patient's cervical range of motion should be examined in the preoperative assessment, and adequate distance should be maintained between the mandible and the sternum when the cervical spine is flexed in order to provide for adequate arterial and venous blood flow.[52,56,57]

VAE is a constant concern in the sitting position due to the position of the surgical field above the level of the heart and the tented open dural venous sinuses. The reported incidence of VAE varies greatly in the literature due to a lack of standardization of measurement and grading scale for VAE. VAE can cause arrhythmias, oxygen (O_2) desaturation, acute pulmonary hypertension, circulatory compromise, and cardiac arrest. If there is a patent foramen ovale (PFO), then the patient is at risk for a paradoxical arterial embolism causing stroke or myocardial infarction. Traditionally, preoperative contrast echocardiography is recommended to evaluate for a PFO. However, failure to detect a PFO on

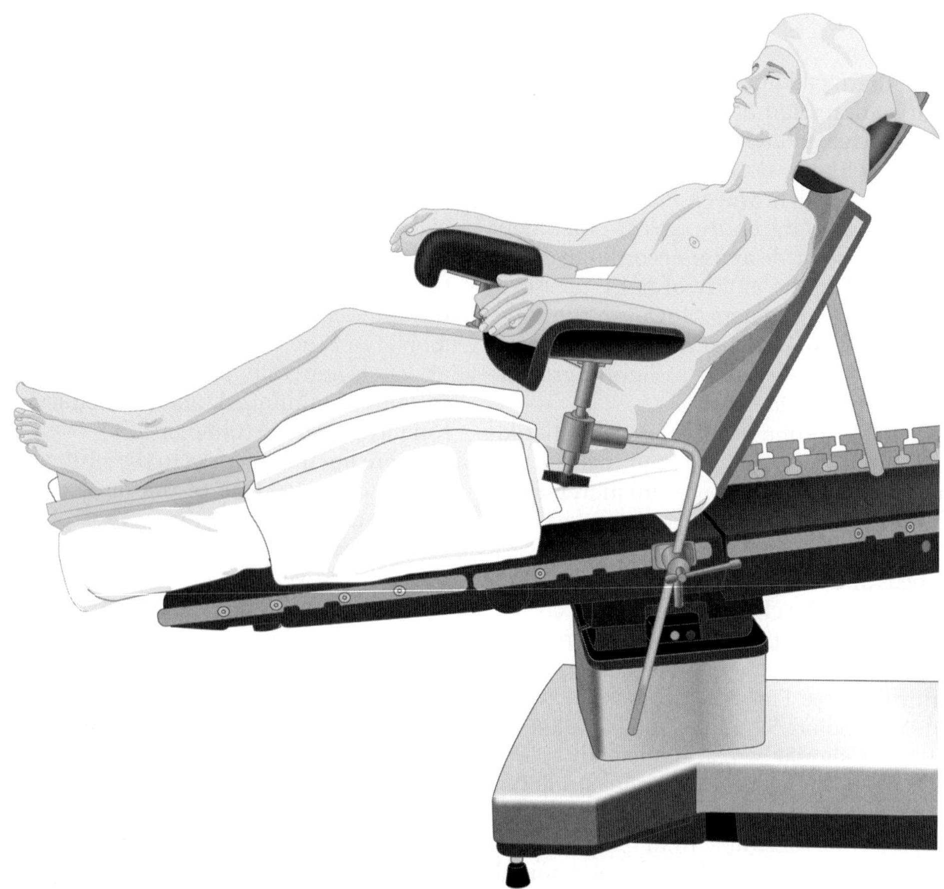

Fig. 34.20 Sitting position adapted for shoulder surgery, often called the lawn or beach chair position. The arms must be supported to prevent stretching of the brachial plexus without pressure on the ulnar area of the elbow. As with all head-up positions, blood pressure should be regulated with the height of the brain in mind.

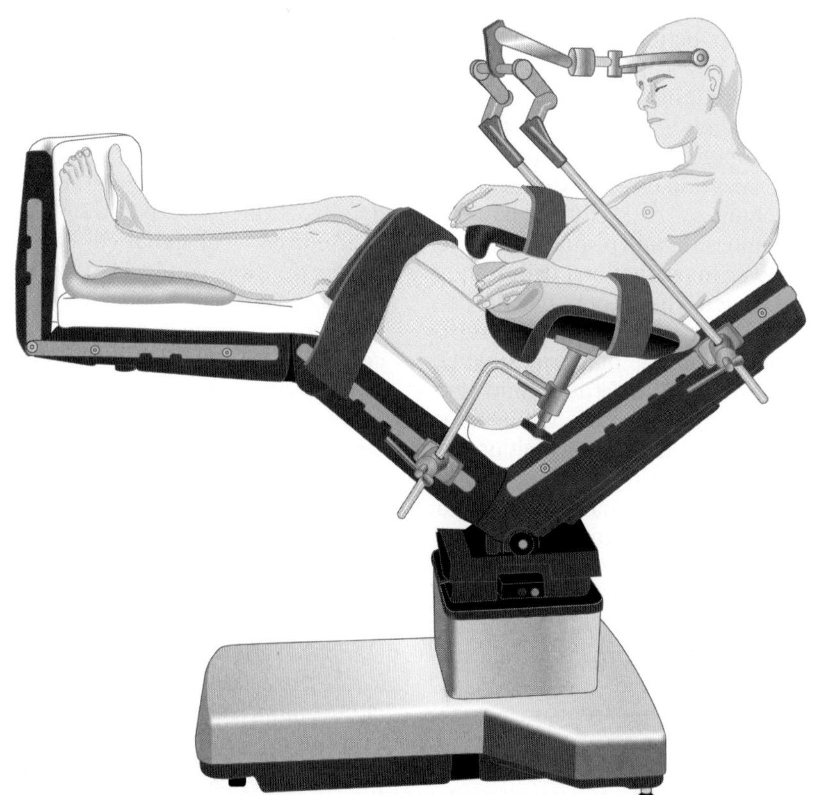

Fig. 34.21 Sitting position with Mayfield head pins. The patient is typically semi-recumbent rather than sitting; the legs are kept as high as possible to promote venous return. Arms must be supported to prevent shoulder traction and stretching of the brachial plexus. In a commonly used variation, the arms are placed on the abdomen and supported. The head support is preferably attached to the back section of the table to allow the back to be adjusted or lowered emergently without first detaching the head holder.

echocardiography does not ensure that the intraatrial septum is intact.[58] The presence of a PFO has generally been considered a contraindication to the sitting position. A recent review suggested that paradoxical VAE is so rare that the presence of a PFO should not necessarily preclude placing the patient in the sitting position. This study found that a VAE was detected in 40% of patients with a known PFO and that no paradoxical embolism was detected.[59] The decision to proceed should be made with patient informed consent and with a discussion between the surgeon and anesthesiologist.

Continuous monitoring for VAE during surgery in the sitting position is essential. There is no standard for type of VAE monitor. Clinical severity of VAE depends on the amount of air and the speed of entrainment. Extrapolation from animal studies suggests that 3 to 5 mL/kg is a lethal amount of air for an adult human, but in reality much less could be required. Transesophageal echocardiography (TEE) is the most sensitive monitor, able to detect as little as 0.02 mL/kg of air. In fact, TEE is so sensitive that some degree of entrained air can be demonstrated in a large majority of patients during neurosurgery in the sitting position.[58,60] Transthoracic Doppler (TTD) is the most sensitive noninvasive monitor with detection rates of approximately 0.05 mL/kg of air. The TTD probe is placed on either the left or right sternal border between the second to fourth intercostal spaces. Transcranial Doppler (TCD) is a monitor of the middle cerebral artery and is nearly as sensitive as TEE. Pulmonary artery catheters, esophageal stethoscopes, and end-tidal carbon dioxide monitors are all much less sensitive monitors. Electrocardiographic and pulse oximeter changes are later findings.[61,62]

Treatment for VAE includes first stopping further air entrainment. The surgeon is asked to stop operating, to flood the field with normal saline, and possibly apply bone wax. The inspired percent of O_2 is changed to 100%. This will aid in treatment during hypoxemia or hypotension and may help reduce the volume of the air embolism via denitrogenation. Hemodynamic compromise is treated with intravenous fluids and vasoactive agents. Consideration is given to placing the patient in left side down and Trendelenburg in order to move an air lock in the right ventricular outflow track (although this can be difficult or impossible in some surgeries).[61] A central venous catheter is often placed preoperatively in order to aspirate entrained air.[58] An ex-vivo study examining different central venous catheter types and positions found that a multiorifice catheter and single orifice catheter both aspirated 50% to 60% of experimentally introduced air.[63]

Pneumocephalus, quadriplegia, spinal cord infarction, cerebral ischemia, and peripheral nerve injuries are all risks of sitting positions. Pneumocephalus is almost universally found on postoperative imaging from cervical or posterior fossa surgery performed in the sitting position. Tension pneumocephalus, which is accumulation of air in the subdural or ventricular space causing pressure on intracranial structures, is very rare but reported after neurosurgery in the sitting position. Prompt diagnosis and surgical evacuation of air is the treatment. Positioning complications causing quadriplegia or spinal cord infarction are thought to be caused by impaired arterial perfusion with hyperextension, hyperflexion, or excessive rotation of the neck. Theories relating the sitting positions to cerebral ischemia include reduced cerebral perfusion caused by reduced cardiac output, deliberate or permissive hypotension, loss of compensatory mechanisms caused by anesthesia, failure to compensate for the height of the head in the regulation of the blood pressure, dynamic vertebral artery narrowing or occlusion with the rotation of the head, and air emboli. Investigators have demonstrated positional effects on cerebral oxygen saturation,[64] as well as transient reductions in cerebral oxygen saturation associated with hypotensive periods during shoulder surgeries in the sitting position that reversed after use of ephedrine and phenylephrine to restore cerebral perfusion pressure.[64-66] One observational study of 124 patients undergoing shoulder arthroscopy demonstrated cerebral desaturation by oximetry in 80% of those who were in the lawn or beach chair position and none in the lateral decubitus position.[67] Cerebral oxygen saturation monitoring may be helpful; however, no gold standard limits exist, and values may change along with alterations in patient position and carbon dioxide concentration. Therefore, if measured, trends in cerebral oxygen saturation are best interpreted during periods of constant ventilation and patient position.[68,69] Reasonable recommendations for patients undergoing surgery in the sitting position are to monitor blood pressure carefully in reference to the level of the brain, avoid and rapidly treat any hypotension or bradycardia, and position the head carefully to avoid extreme positions that may compromise cerebral vessels.[70]

Hypotension is a known and very common problem for anesthetized patients in the sitting position. Pooling of blood in the lower body places anesthetized patients in the sitting position at particular risk to hypotensive episodes. Studies reveal that mean arterial pressure, systolic blood pressure, and cardiac index all decrease in the sitting position.[52] Therefore, placement of the patient into the sitting position should be incremental in order to adjust for hemodynamic changes. Intravenous fluids and vasopressors should be in-line and ready.

ROBOTIC SURGERY

Since its introduction approximately 30 years ago, the use and scope of robotic surgery has expanded greatly. Robotic surgery is now the norm for many types of urologic and gynecologic operations,[71,72] and is extending to other abdominal operations, thoracic surgery, and head and neck operations. Robotic surgery offers technical advantages for surgeons regarding range of motion and accuracy of laparoscopic instrumentation. Once the robot is docked, direct access to the patient is limited. It is therefore imperative that all monitors, lines, and invasive lines are placed prior to docking the robot, and that proper padding and positioning are completed.

Most of the literature about robotic positioning involves urologic and gynecologic operations, which are generally performed with the patient in steep Trendelenburg (30-45 degrees) and lithotomy with arms tucked in neutral position to the sides. The patient must be very well secured in order to avoid slipping in steep Trendelenburg. Non-slip mattresses, chest straps, and shoulder braces may be useful, but shoulder braces are also reported to cause brachial plexus injuries due to stretch between the shoulder and neck. If shoulder braces are employed, monitoring for excessive stretch at the patient's neck is essential. The endotracheal tube should be well secured to avoid migration. Often a tray or table is placed above the patient's face in order to provide protection from laparoscopic equipment.[73-75] It may be prudent to trial the steep Trendelenburg prior to docking the robot to ensure that the patient is properly positioned, does not slip, and can tolerate steep Trendelenburg from a physiologic standpoint.

Physiologic changes during robotic surgery are due to both laparoscopic insufflation as well as positioning. Hemodynamic changes are largely due to laparoscopic insufflation, whereas changes in respiratory mechanics are also affected by positioning. Functional residual capacity is decreased with both laparoscopy and further decreased with the addition of steep Trendelenburg. This is due to a combination of pressure of abdominal contents from laparoscopy and Trendelenburg pushing up on the diaphragm, and can also be worsened by chest fixation that is applied to prevent the patient from slipping off the table. Peak and plateau airway pressures have been shown to rise as much as 50%. Between changes in pulmonary compliance, decreased functional residual capacity, and the need for increased minute ventilation with carbon dioxide insufflation, intraoperative mechanical ventilation can be quite challenging during these cases.[73-76]

The incidence of positioning complications from robotic surgery vary substantially from 0.8% to 6.6%; most studies indicate an incidence of less than 1%.[77-79] One study found longer operative times, higher ASA physical status, and increased intravenous fluid administration to be risk factors for intraoperative positioning complications.[77] A history of prior abdominal surgery was the only associated risk factor found in a study of gynecologic robotic surgeries.[78] Eye injury, peripheral nerve injuries, rhabdomyolysis, and compartment syndrome were the most frequent positioning complications found in patients with robotic assisted radical prostatectomies. Incidence of injury in this study was not different between robotic versus traditional open prostatectomy.[79] In a recent survey of ASA members, 21.7% of responders answered "yes" that they have experienced a "complication related to Trendelenburg positioning (during robotic surgery)." Airway and facial edema, as well as brachial plexus injuries, were the most common recalled complications in this survey.[80] When steep Trendelenburg is used, consideration should be given to documenting the endotracheal tube airway leak at the start and at the end of the surgical procedure prior to extubation.

Peripheral Nerve Injury

Peripheral nerve injury remains a serious perioperative complication and a significant source of professional liability despite its infrequent incidence. The ASA states that "postoperative signs and symptoms related to peripheral nerve injury...may include but are not limited to paresthesias, muscle weakness, tingling, or pain in the extremities."[4] Studies of the ASA Closed Claims Project database (in 1990 and 1999) brought awareness of the incidence of perioperative peripheral nerve injury, which was found to be between 0.03% and 0.11%. However, according to this database, peripheral nerve injuries represented 22% of all claims. In fact, peripheral nerve injury has been second only to death as the leading cause of claims against anesthesiologists.

The overall incidence of peripheral nerve injury claims had increased from 15% in the 1970s.[1,2,81,82] According to a review of 5280 closed claims (from 1990 to 2007), most patients with nerve injuries do recover, however, up to 23% of peripheral nerve injuries remain permanent.[4]

In the closed claims database study, ulnar neuropathy is the most common lesion representing 28% of all peripheral nerve injury claims, followed by the brachial plexus (20%), lumbosacral nerve root (16%), and spinal cord (13%).[2,3] Interestingly, the distribution of nerve injury claims has changed over time. From 1980 through 1984, ulnar neuropathy claims decreased from 37% to 17% in the 1990s, and spinal cord injury claims increased from 8% in 1980 through 1984 to 27% in the 1990s. The incidence of spinal cord injury and lumbosacral nerve root neuropathy increased over this study period and were predominantly associated with regional anesthesia. Epidural hematoma and chemical injuries represented 29% of the known mechanisms of injury among the claims filed.[2,83,84]

In a different retrospective study of 380,680 patients at a single university tertiary care institution, 112 peripheral nerve injuries were observed in the perioperative period, an incidence of 0.3%.[85] Most injuries were sensory (60%) or combined sensory and motor (24%), with only 14% pure motor injuries. This study provides a significantly different numerator and denominator than the ASA Closed Claims Project, and its data contrast with the most recent claims data in which more claims were filed after the administration of regional anesthesia.

Peripheral nerves are made up of bundles of endoneurium wrapped axons bundled into fascicles, which are wrapped in perineurium. Schwann cells provide a myelin sheath to enhance conduction for myelinated nerves. Peripheral nerves are vascular metabolically active structures. The vasa nervorum provides blood flow via a capillary network.[86] Injuries are classified in neurology by the Seddon or Sunderland Classifications. These classifications are based upon neuronal anatomy and can be clinically correlated.[87] There are three main mechanisms for peripheral nerve injury: stretch, compression, and transection. Transection can be partial or complete and can be due to sharp or blunt transection. Compression injuries can be due to compression of vascular structures causing ischemic injury or due to direct nerve or myelin compression.[87] All of these mechanisms can affect sensory and motor nerves.[88]

Perioperative peripheral nerve injury is complex and multifactorial in etiology. Because sensation is blocked by unconsciousness or regional anesthesia, early warning symptoms of pain with normal spontaneous repositioning are absent.[81,89] Patient comorbidities that contribute to peripheral nerve injuries include: hypertension, diabetes, peripheral vascular disease, older age, and heavy alcohol and tobacco use.[4] Extremes of weight, both low body mass index and obesity, are also risk factors. General and epidural anesthesia appeared to be risk factors, compared with monitored anesthesia care, spinal anesthesia, and peripheral nerve blocks. Prolonged surgical times are an additional risk factor.[1,85]

BOX 34.1 Summary of the 2018 American Society of Anesthesiologists Practice Advisory for the Prevention of Perioperative Peripheral Neuropathies

Preoperative Assessment

- Review a patient's preoperative history and perform a physical examination to identify: body habitus, preexisting neurologic symptoms, diabetes mellitus, peripheral vascular disease, alcohol dependency, arthritis, and sex.
- When judged appropriate, ascertain whether patients can comfortably tolerate the anticipated position.

Upper Extremity Positioning

- Positioning Strategies to Reduce Perioperative Brachial Plexus Neuropathy
  - When possible, limit arm abduction in a supine patient to 90 degrees. The prone position may allow patients to comfortably tolerate abduction of their arms to greater than 90 degrees.
- Positioning Strategies to Reduce Perioperative Ulnar Neuropathy
  - Supine Patient with Arm on an Armboard: Position the upper extremity to decrease pressure on the postcondylar groove of the humerus (ulnar groove). Either supination or the neutral forearm positions may be used to facilitate this action.
  - Supine Patient with Arm tucked at Side: Place the forearm in a neutral position.
  - Flexion of the Elbow: When possible, avoid flexion of the elbow to decrease the risk of ulnar neuropathy.
- Positioning Strategies to Reduce Perioperative Radial Neuropathy
  - Avoid prolonged pressure on the radial nerve in the spiral groove of the humerus.
- Positioning Strategies to Reduce Perioperative Median Neuropathy
  - Avoid extension of the elbow beyond the range that is comfortable during the preoperative assessment to prevent stretching of the median nerve.
    - Periodic assessment of upper extremity position during procedures
  - Periodic perioperative assessments may be performed to ensure maintenance of the desired position.

Lower Extremity Positioning

- Positioning Strategies to Reduce Perioperative Sciatic Neuropathy
  - Stretching of the Hamstring Muscle Group: Positions that stretch the hamstring muscle group beyond the range that is comfortable during the preoperative assessment may be avoided to prevent stretching of the sciatic nerve.
  - Limiting Hip Flexion: Since the sciatic nerve or its branches cross both the hip and the knee joints, assess extension and flexion of these joints when determining the degree of hip flexion.
- Positioning Strategies to Reduce Perioperative Femoral Neuropathy
  - When possible, avoid extension or flexion of the hip to decrease the risk of femoral neuropathy.
- Positioning Strategies to Reduce Perioperative Peroneal Neuropathy
  - Avoid prolonged pressure on the peroneal nerve at the fibular head.

Protective Padding

- Padded armboards may be used to decrease the risk of upper extremity neuropathy.
- Chest rolls in the laterally positioned patient may be used to decrease the risk of upper extremity neuropathy.
- Specific padding to prevent pressure of a hard surface against the peroneal nerve at the fibular head may be used to decrease the risk of peroneal neuropathy.
- Avoid the inappropriate use of padding (padding too tight) to decrease the risk of perioperative neuropathy.

Equipment

- When possible, avoid the improper use of automated blood pressure cuffs on the arm to reduce the risk of upper extremity neuropathy.
- When possible, avoid the use of shoulder braces in a steep head-down position to decrease the risk of perioperative neuropathies.

Postoperative Assessment

- Perform a simple postoperative assessment of extremity nerve function for early recognition of peripheral neuropathies.

Documentation

- Document specific perioperative positioning actions that may be useful for continuous improvement processes.

From the Practice Advisory for the prevention of perioperative peripheral neuropathies: an updated report by the American Society of Anesthesiologists Task Force on prevention of perioperative peripheral neuropathies. *Anesthesiology.* 2018;128:11–26.

Ascertaining the presence of preoperative neuropathies and paresthesias is particularly important as injured nerves are more susceptible to injury in a phenomenon described as the double crush syndrome. The theory is that two separate subclinical nerve insults can act synergistically to produce a clinically significant neuropathy.

Usually, the exact mechanism of injury for a particular patient cannot be determined.[2] With the exception of spinal cord injuries, the mechanism of nerve injury remains incompletely explained by scientific studies. Most nerve injuries, particularly those to nerves of the upper extremity such as the ulnar nerve and brachial plexus, occurred in the presence of adequate positioning and padding. Nevertheless, we must prevent nerve injuries to the best of our abilities. The ASA released an updated practice advisory in 2018 to help guide prevention of perioperative nerve injury (Box 34.1).[4] Positions that permit stretching of the nerves and pressure to anatomic locations known to carry nerves prone to injury must be avoided, such as the ulnar cubital tunnel and the peroneal nerve coursing over the fibular head (Table 34.1). Padding and support should distribute weight over as wide an area as possible; however, no padding material has been shown to be superior. Whenever possible, the patient's position should appear natural.

ULNAR NERVE INJURY

The ulnar nerve lies in a superficial position at the elbow. Morbidity associated with ulnar neuropathy can be severe. In a prospective study among 1502 patients undergoing noncardiac surgery, 7 patients developed perioperative ulnar neuropathy, of which 3 patients had residual symptoms after 2 years.[90] In a study on the effect of arm position on the ulnar nerve somatosensory-evoked potentials

TABLE 34.1 Most Common Nerve Injuries in the American Society of Anesthesiologists Closed Claims Database 1990–2010

Nerve Injury	Recommendations for Prevention
Ulnar nerve (14%)	▪ Avoid excessive pressure on the postcondylar groove of the humerus. ▪ Keep the hand and forearm either supinated or in a neutral position.
Brachial plexus (19%)	▪ When utilizing a steep head-down (Trendelenburg) position: ▪ Avoid the use of shoulder braces and beanbags when possible (use nonsliding mattresses). ▪ Avoid abduction of the arm(s) when possible. ▪ Avoid excessive lateral rotation of the head, either in the supine or prone position. ▪ Limit abduction of the arm to <90 degrees in the supine position. ▪ Avoid the placement of high "axillary" roll in the decubitus position—keep the chest roll out of the axilla to avoid neurovascular compression. ▪ Use ultrasound to locate the internal jugular vein for central line placement.
Spinal cord (25%) and lumbosacral nerve root or cord (18%)	▪ Be aware that the fraction of spinal cord injuries is increasing, probably in relation to use of regional anesthesia. ▪ Avoid severe cervical spine flexion or extension when possible. ▪ Follow current guidelines for regional anesthesia in patients on anticoagulant therapy.
Sciatic and peroneal nerves (7%)	▪ Minimize the time in the lithotomy position. ▪ Use two assistants to coordinate simultaneous movement of both legs to and from the lithotomy position. ▪ Avoid excessive flexion of the hips, extension of the knees, or torsion of the lumbar spine. ▪ Avoid excessive pressure on peroneal nerve at the fibular head.

ASA, American Society of Anesthesiologists.
Data from ASA Closed Claims Project 1990 to 2010.
Practice advisory for the prevention of perioperative peripheral neuropathies 2018: An updated report by the American Society of Anesthesiologists Task Force on Prevention of Perioperative Peripheral Neuropathies. *Anesthesiology*. 2018;128:11–26.

(SSEPs) in 15 healthy awake male volunteers, the supinated position was associated with the least pressure on the ulnar nerve, and the neutral position was the next most favorable. When in the neutral position on a surgical armrest, pressure decreased as the arm was abducted between 30 and 90 degrees. Interestingly, not all patients had symptoms of nerve compression when the SSEP was abnormal.[17] Current consensus is that the cause of ulnar nerve palsy is multifactorial and not always preventable.[91,92] In a large retrospective review of perioperative ulnar neuropathy lasting longer than 3 months, the onset of symptoms occurred more than 24 hours postoperatively in 57% of patients; 70% were men and 9% experienced bilateral symptoms. Very thin or obese patients were at increased risk, as were those with prolonged postoperative bed rest. No association with intraoperative patient position or anesthetic technique was confirmed.[93] The ASA Closed Claims Project also demonstrated that perioperative ulnar neuropathy occurred predominately in men, in an older population, and with a delayed onset (median of 3 days).[2] The large predominance of ulnar injury in men may possibly be explained by anatomic differences. Men have a more developed and thickened flexor retinaculum with less protective adipose tissue and a larger tubercle of the coronoid process that can predispose them to nerve compression in the cubital tunnel.[94,95] In the published ASA Closed Claims Project data, only 9% of ulnar injury claims had an explicit mechanism of injury, and in 27% of claims, the padding of the elbows was explicitly documented.[2] Postoperative ulnar nerve palsy can occur without any apparent cause, even when padding and positioning of the patient's arm was carefully managed and documented in the anesthetic record.[18]

BRACHIAL PLEXUS INJURY

The brachial plexus is susceptible to stretching because of its long superficial course from the neck to the arm via the axilla with two points of fixation—the cervical vertebrae and the axillary fascia. The nerves are vulnerable to compression as they pass between the clavicle and the first rib because of the proximity and mobility of both the clavicle and the humerus (see Fig. 34.6). Among patients undergoing noncardiac surgeries, the incidence of brachial plexus injury is reported to be 0.02%.[96] After brachial plexus injury, the patient often complains of sensory deficit in the distribution of the ulnar nerve. This symptom is most commonly associated with intraoperative arm abduction greater than 90 degrees, lateral rotation of the head away from the side of the injury, asymmetric retraction of the sternum for internal mammary artery dissection during cardiac surgery, or direct trauma or compression. To avoid injury, patients should ideally be positioned with the head midline, arms kept at the sides, the elbows mildly flexed, and the forearms supinated, without pressure on the shoulders or the axilla.

Brachial plexus injury is particularly associated with the use of shoulder braces in patients undergoing surgery in the Trendelenburg position. Medial placement of the braces can compress the proximal roots, and lateral placement of the braces can stretch the plexus by displacing the shoulders against the thorax (see Fig. 34.6). The patient with injury often complains of painless motor deficit in the distribution of the radial and median nerves; however, pain may also be present. A report of three cases of upper- and middle-trunk brachial plexopathy after robotic prostatectomy highlights the potential risk of a combination of compression of the shoulder girdle against the thorax in the steep Trendelenburg position with abduction of an arm.[26] Signs of vascular compromise to the upper extremities, such as difficulty obtaining consistent blood pressure or a poor pulse oximetry signal, may be indications of compromise to the neurovascular bundle as reported in a case of bilateral injury related to shoulder braces with abduction of the arms in the Trendelenburg position.[24] Studies of the brachial plexus tension test in human volunteers and nerve strain in cadavers have demonstrated deleterious positional elements including arm abduction, rotation, or flexion of the head away from the affected arm, elbow and wrist extension, and depression of the shoulder girdle.[25] For transaxillary robotic thyroidectomy, a recently developed approach has the arm abducted to 180 degrees. An incidence of brachial plexus injury has been reported to be 0.3%.[97] When an extreme position is used, neurophysiologic monitoring, such as motor-evoked potentials and SSEPs, has been shown to detect an evolving injury and allow for repositioning to prevent permanent damage.[98,99] Nerve function monitoring may therefore become increasingly common with newer surgical techniques that carry increased risk related to patient positioning.

In patients undergoing cardiac surgery requiring median sternotomy, brachial plexus injury has been specifically associated with the C8 to T1 nerve roots. In a prospective study in which the incidence of injury was 4.9%, 73% of the injuries occurred on the same side as the internal jugular vein cannulation; however, this study antedated the widespread use of ultrasound to guide cannulation.[100] Unilateral sternal retraction to harvest the mammary artery is associated with brachial plexus dysfunction, presumably caused by stretching the nerves. SSEP monitoring of the brachial plexus during sternal retraction has been shown to predict injury.[101]

In the 1999 ASA Closed Claims Project report, 10% of brachial plexus injuries were directly attributed to patient positioning. Of those, one half involved the use of shoulder braces in patients in the Trendelenburg position.[2] Consequently, nonsliding mattresses should be used, along with a concerted effort to avoid compression of the shoulders as much as possible.[21,22] Of the 311 brachial plexus injuries in the ASA Closed Claims Project, 59 (19%) occurred after a regional block without general anesthesia, including axillary and interscalene blocks.[2] In those cases, the role of patient positioning cannot be determined.

OTHER UPPER EXTREMITY NERVE INJURY

In a retrospective study of 1000 consecutive spine surgeries that used SSEP monitoring, five arm positions were compared regarding SSEP changes in the upper extremities. A modification of the arm position reversed 92% of upper extremity SSEP changes. The incidence of position-related upper extremity SSEP changes was significantly higher in the prone "superman" (7%) and lateral decubitus (7.5%) positions, compared with the supine arms out, supine arms tucked, and prone arms tucked positions (1.8%-3.2%). Reversible SSEP changes were not associated with postoperative deficits (Chapter 39).[24]

Although quite rare, the radial nerve can be injured from direct pressure as it traverses the spiral groove of the humerus in the lower one third of the arm. The injury often exhibits a wrist drop with an inability to abduct the thumb or extend the metacarpophalangeal joints. An isolated median nerve injury most often occurs during the insertion of an intravenous needle into the antecubital fossa in a patient who has been anesthetized where the nerve is adjacent to the medial cubital and basilic veins. Patients with this injury are unable to oppose the first and fifth digits and have decreased sensation over the palmar surface of the lateral three and a half fingers. Surprisingly, in an evaluation of the ASA Closed Claims Project database from 1970 to 2007, peripheral intravenous and arterial line insertion accounted for 2.1% of all claims filed, particularly among patients who underwent cardiac surgery where the arms were tucked and the lines were not visible for inspection.[102] Nerve injury accounted for 17% of intravenous line complications, second only to skin slough or necrosis (28%) and swelling, inflammation, and infection (17%).

LOWER EXTREMITY NERVE INJURY

Injuries to the sciatic and common peroneal nerves occur most often in the lithotomy position. Because of its fixation between the sciatic notch and the neck of the fibula, the sciatic nerve can be stretched with external rotation of the leg. The sciatic nerve and its branches cross the hip and knee joints and are stretched by hyperflexion of the hips or extension of the knees. The common peroneal nerve, a branch of the sciatic, is most often damaged from the compression between the head of the fibula and an external structure, such as the frame of a leg support. Most often, patients who suffer a peroneal nerve injury will complain of a foot drop and the inability to extend the toes in a dorsal direction or evert the foot. In a prospective study of 991 patients undergoing surgery under general anesthesia in the lithotomy position, the incidence of lower extremity neuropathies was 1.5%, with injuries to the sciatic and peroneal nerves representing 40% of the cases. Interestingly, symptoms were predominantly paresthesia, with onset within 4 hours of surgery and resolution generally within 6 months. No motor deficits were noted, but in a previous retrospective study, the same authors found the incidence of severe motor disability in patients who underwent surgery in the lithotomy position to be 1 in 3608.[103,104]

Injury to the femoral or obturator nerves generally occurs from lower abdominal surgical procedures with excessive retraction. The obturator nerve can also be injured during a difficult forceps delivery or by excessive flexion of the thigh to the groin. A femoral neuropathy will exhibit decreased flexion of the hip, decreased extension of the knee, or a loss of sensation over the superior aspect of the thigh and medial or anteromedial side of the leg. An obturator neuropathy will exhibit an inability to adduct the leg with decreased sensation over the medial side of the thigh.

In a retrospective review of 198,461 patients undergoing surgery in the lithotomy position from 1957 to 1991, injury to the common peroneal nerve was the most common lower extremity motor neuropathy, representing 78% of nerve injuries. A potential cause of the injury was the compression of the nerve between the lateral head of the fibula and the bar holding the legs. When the "candy cane" stirrups are used, special attention must be paid to avoid compression (see Fig. 34.9). The injury was more common with patients who had low body mass index, recent cigarette smoking, or prolonged duration of surgery.[103] Perhaps as a result of an increased awareness of potential injuries, no lower extremity motor neuropathies were reported in a prospective review of 991 patients undergoing surgery in the lithotomy position from 1997 to 1998. Paresthesias in the distribution of the obturator, lateral femoral cutaneous, sciatic, and peroneal nerves were reported in 1.5% of patients, and nearly all recovered. Surgical times longer than 2 hours were significantly associated with this complication.[104]

EVALUATION AND TREATMENT OF PERIOPERATIVE NEUROPATHIES

When a nerve injury becomes apparent postoperatively, it is essential to perform and document a directed physical examination to correlate the extent of sensory or motor deficits with the preoperative examination as well as any intraoperative events. It is prudent to seek neurologic consultation to help define the neurogenic basis, localize the site of the lesion, and determine the severity of injury for guiding prognostication. With proper diagnosis and management, most injuries resolve, but months to years may be required.[88,105,106] In addition, perioperative neuropathies associated with pain must be differentiated from surgically induced neuropathic pain, which is receiving increasing attention by surgeons because it affects an estimated 10% to 40% of surgical patients postoperatively.[107]

If a new sensory or motor deficit is found postoperatively, then electrophysiologic evaluation by a neurologist within the first week may provide useful information concerning the characteristic and temporal pattern of the injury. Another examination after 4 weeks, when enough time has elapsed for the electrophysiologic changes to evolve, will provide more definitive information about the site and severity of the nerve injury. Regardless, electrophysiologic testing must be interpreted within the clinical context. No single test can define the cause of injury. Nerve conduction studies may be useful to evaluate potential peripheral nerve injuries, as they permit the assessment of both motor and sensory nerves. To evaluate motor integrity, the nerve is supramaximally stimulated at two points along its course, and a recording is made of the electrical response of one of the muscles that it innervates. The size of the muscle action potential provides an estimate of the number of motor axons and muscle fibers that are activated by the stimulus. For sensory conduction studies, the nerve fiber is supramaximally stimulated at one point and the sensory nerve action potential is recorded from another point. The latency of the response can be interpreted as a reflection of the number of functioning sensory axons. Nerve conduction studies are useful for several reasons; they may reveal the presence of a subclinical polyneuropathy that made the individual nerves more susceptible to injury and help distinguish between axon loss and demyelination, which has significant implications regarding course and overall prognosis.

For motor neuropathy, an electromyogram can be performed to characterize the injury. An electromyographic examination involves recording the electrical activity of a muscle from a needle electrode inserted within it. If present, abnormalities may point to the affected component in the motor unit, which consists of the anterior horn cell, its axon and neuromuscular junctions, and the muscle fibers that it innervates. Certain findings are suggestive of denervation, including the presence of abnormal spontaneous activity in the resting muscle (fibrillation potentials and positive sharp waves, which results from muscle irritability) and increased insertion activity. Insertion activity increases within a few days of muscle denervation, whereas abnormal spontaneous activity takes 1 to 4 weeks to develop, depending on the distance from the nerve lesion to the muscle. Depending on the pattern of abnormalities, an electromyographic study may distinguish between radiculopathies, plexopathies, and neuropathies.

Most sensory neuropathies are generally transient and require only reassurance to the patient with follow-up visits, whereas most motor neuropathies include demyelination of peripheral fibers of a nerve trunk (neurapraxia) and generally take 4 to 6 weeks for recovery. Injury to the axon within an intact nerve sheath (axonotmesis) or complete nerve disruption (neurotmesis) can cause severe pain and disability. When reversible, recovery often takes 3 to 12 months. Interim physical therapy is recommended to prevent contractures and muscle atrophy.[105,106]

Pressure Injuries

Pressure injuries are a significant source of patient morbidity and healthcare expenditures in the United States and internationally. Approximately 23% of all pressure ulcers occur while patients are in operating rooms.[108] General anesthesia and length of surgical procedure are both risk factors for pressure injury development. The National Pressure Ulcer Advisory Panel recently revised their definitions and classification scales for pressure injuries, formerly referred to as pressure ulcers.[109] Pressure injury is injury to the skin, and/or underlying tissue, due to pressure or shearing forces. Currently, there are no universal guidelines for pressure injury prevention. The Association of Perioperative Registered Nurses and the Joint Commission have statements issued stating that the prevention of pressure injuries is a joint responsibility shared by all members of the healthcare team. Understanding the risks of pressure injury is essential to preventing their occurrence.

Often early signs of pressure injury start with nonblanching skin erythema. The skin is more resistant to pressure injury than muscle and can actually mask a more extensive injury underneath.[110] This is likely due to increased O_2 requirements of muscle. Pressure injuries associated with operations are often not seen at the time of operation but could be diagnosed days after.[111,112] In the supine position, areas most at risk include the sacrum, heels, and occiput. In the prone position, the chest and knees are at highest risk for pressure injury, and in the sitting position, the ischial tuberosities are at greatest risk.[74]

Factors contributing to the development of pressure injuries include pressure over bony prominences, shear force, skin breakdown, compromised blood flow, immobility, and decreased sensation. Infection, inflammation, edema, and steroids are all also contributing factors.[113] Patient comorbidities such as diabetes, peripheral vascular disease, obesity, low body mass index, and poor nutrition are also known risks.[108]

There are case reports, and very few larger studies, assessing specific medical device-related pressure injuries. One retrospective study found that approximately 0.65% of all pressure injuries were due to medical devices. Nasal cannulas, endotracheal tubes, nasogastric tubes, and cervical collars were all associated with pressure injuries.[114]

Hypothermia and hypotension during surgery, such as during cardiopulmonary bypass (CPB) surgery, may increase the incidence of these complications. Pressure alopecia, caused by ischemic hair follicles, is related to prolonged immobilization of the head with its full weight falling on a limited area, usually the occiput. Hard objects should not be placed under the head as they may create focal areas of pressure. Consequently, ample cushioning of the head and, if possible during prolonged surgery, periodic rotation of the head, are prudent to redistribute the weight.

Bite Injuries

Transcranial motor-evoked potentials (Tc-MEPs) are increasingly used for both spine surgical procedures and also neurosurgical procedures. Tc-MEPs involve contraction of the temporalis and masseter muscle, which has been implicated in tongue, lip, and even tooth injuries due to biting motion. Two large retrospective reviews, each with more than 170,000 cases employing Tc-MEPs, found an overall incidence of 0.14% to 0.63%, and the tongue was most frequently injured (~80% of all associated injuries).[38,115] Injury severity ranged from minor bruising to necessity of laceration repair by suture in 15% to 23% of patients.

Macroglossia following surgery in the sitting position has been reported, presumably due to pressure, ischemia, and decreased venous outflow. A recent review of case reports for macroglossia after neurosurgical procedures found macroglossia was associated with prolonged operative times (50% of cases were over 8 hours) and suboccipital and posterior fossa surgeries (40%).[116] Excessive neck flexion can also obstruct the endotracheal tube and place significant pressure on the tongue, leading to edema. Classically, two finger breadth distance between the chin and chest is recommended. Extra caution is advised in cases with neck flexion if TEE is used for air embolism monitoring, because the esophageal probe lies between the flexed spine and the airway and endotracheal tube, adding to the potential for compression of laryngeal structures and the tongue.

At this time there are no specific recommendations for prevention of bite injuries or macroglossia. Double-sided bite blocks may help in surgical procedures using Tc-MEP, although studies of macroglossia document bite blocks in 50% of patients. The most important prevention measures are ensuring proper placement of bite blocks and rechecking placement throughout the case.

Anesthesia Outside the Operating Room

Anesthesia providers are increasingly involved with gastrointestinal endoscopy, cardiac catheterization, interventional radiology, neuroradiology, magnetic resonance imaging, and computed tomography in hospital locations outside the operating room, as well as for office-based procedures (Chapter 73).[117] Anesthesia care may be specifically requested if an individual is not expected to tolerate the position required for the procedure because of comorbidities such as congestive heart failure, pulmonary disease, or morbid obesity. In addition, although positions customarily used for procedures without anesthesia may be generally safe for patients who are awake, they may pose serious risks to those under anesthesia.

Because of the less familiar environment, relative lack of positioning equipment, and a variability in staff and nursing training with regard to patient positioning, planning, and continued vigilance are particularly important in settings outside the operating room. Diagnostic tables may not lend themselves to established intraoperative solutions to patient positioning challenges. The ability to initiate the Trendelenburg position to augment venous return and cardiac output rapidly is often lacking. In such an environment, where practice patterns often evolve in the context of nonanesthetized patients, the anesthesiologist must verify the safety of each patient's position.

Perioperative Visual Loss

POVL is a rare but serious complication. Ischemic optic neuropathy (ION), and retinal arterial occlusion (RAO) are the main causes.[118,119] Other causes include cortical blindness,[120] acute glaucoma,[121] choroidal and vitreous hemorrhage,[122] and gas bubble expansion after retinal surgery.[123] The discussion here is confined to visual loss that follows nonocular surgery because eye damage after ocular surgery is well described in the ophthalmology literature. Most of our attention is focused on retinal artery occlusion and ION.

Retrospective studies, surveys, and case reports provide much of the current knowledge on POVL. Two large studies showed that perioperative ION is rare, occurring in approximately 1 in 60,000 to 125,000 anesthetic procedures in the overall surgical population.[124,125] Spine fusion and cardiac surgery are associated with higher incidence of POVL than other operative procedures. Shen examined the POVL prevalence in the US Nationwide Inpatient Sample, for the eight most commonly performed surgical procedures, excluding obstetric and gynecologic surgery. ION occurred most frequently in spine (3.09/10,000, 0.03%) and cardiac surgery (8.64/10,000, 0.086%).[126] The yearly rates of POVL have been decreasing in the 10-year period from 1996 to 2005, and for spine surgery have continued to decline as well.[126,127] Patil found an overall rate of 0.094% in spine surgery.[128] In previous, smaller case series, Stevens found ION in 4 of 3450 spine surgeries (0.1%).[129] Chang and Miller reviewed 14,102 spine surgery procedures in one hospital, identifying 4 with ION (0.028%).[130] After cardiac surgery, the incidence may be as high as 1.3%,[131] but is between 0.06% to 0.113% in more recent, larger retrospective studies.[132-134]

Myers conducted a retrospective case-control study of 28 patients with visual loss after spine surgery.[135] The ASA Postoperative Visual Loss Registry reported 93 cases of visual loss after spine surgery.[136] Nuttall performed a retrospective case-control study of cardiac surgery patients at the Mayo Clinic.[132] A retrospective, case-controlled study of risk factors in perioperative ION in spine surgery, a collaborative effort of 17 American and Canadian medical centers, has been reported.[137] These studies are described in detail in subsequent sections of this chapter.

RETINAL ISCHEMIA: BRANCH AND CENTRAL RETINAL ARTERY OCCLUSION

Central retinal artery occlusion (CRAO) decreases blood supply to the entire retina, whereas branch retinal artery occlusion

TABLE 34.2 Differential Diagnosis: Eye Examination in Retinal, Optic Nerve, or Visual Cortex Injury*

	AION	PION	Cortical Blindness	CRAO	BRAO
Optic disk	Pale swelling, peripapillary flame-shaped hemorrhages, edema of optic nerve head Late: Optic atrophy	Initially normal Late: Optic atrophy	Normal	Normal Late: Optic atrophy	Normal Late: Optic atrophy
Retina	Normal; may have attenuated arterioles	Normal; may have attenuated arterioles	Normal	Cherry-red macula†; pallor and edema, narrowed retinal arteries	Emboli may be present‡; partial retinal whitening and edema
Light reflex	Absent or RAPD	Absent or RAPD	Normal	Absent or RAPD	Normal or RAPD
Fixation and accommodation	Normal	Normal	Impaired	May be impaired with external compression	May be impaired with external compression
Opticokinetic nystagmus	Normal	Normal	Absent	Normal	Normal
Response to visual threat	Yes, if some vision remains	Yes, if some vision remains	No	Yes	Yes
Object tracking	Normal, if some vision remains	Normal, if some vision remains	Absent	Normal	Normal
Ocular muscle function	Normal	Normal	Normal	May be impaired if results from external compression	May be impaired if results from external compression
Perimetry	Altitudinal defect; scotoma	Altitudinal defect; blind; scotoma; Often no light perception	Hemianopia (depending on lesion location); periphery affected usually	Usually blind	Scotoma; usually normal periphery

*Typical symptoms and signs are listed. Some patients may have varying findings as a result, among other factors, of timing of examination relative to symptom onset.
†Because of a lack of overlying inner retinal cells in the fovea, the intact choroidal circulation is visible as a cherry-red spot.
‡Cholesterol, platelet-fibrin emboli, calcified atheromatous material.
AION, Anterior ischemic optic neuropathy; *BRAO,* occlusion of a retinal arterial branch; *CRAO,* central retinal arterial occlusion; *PION,* posterior ischemic optic neuropathy; *RAPD,* relative afferent pupillary defect.

(BRAO) is a localized injury; these are generally unilateral. There are four mechanisms: (1) external compression of the eye, (2) decreased arterial supply (embolism to retinal arterial circulation or decreased systemic blood flow), (3) impaired venous drainage, and (4) thrombosis from a coagulation disorder.[138] The most common in the perioperative period is improper positioning with external compression producing sufficiently high IOP to stop blood flow in the central retinal artery. It most often occurs during spine surgery performed with the patient in the prone position. Pressure within the orbit also can be increased after retrobulbar hemorrhage, associated usually with vascular injury from sinus or nasal surgery.[139]

Although rare in most surgical procedures, emboli can directly impair blood flow in the central retinal artery or produce BRAO. Paradoxical embolism from the operative site reaching the arterial circulation through a patent foramen ovale has been reported in perioperative retinal vascular occlusion.[140] Venous drainage can be impaired after radical neck surgery by jugular vein ligation.[141] Retinal microemboli, however, are common during open heart surgery.[142]

Clinical Findings

There is painless visual loss, abnormal pupil reactivity, opacification or whitening of the ischemic retina, and narrowing of retinal arterioles.[143] BRAO is characterized by cholesterol, and calcific or pale platelet fibrin emboli. A cherry-red macula with a white ground-glass appearance of the retina and attenuated arterioles is a "classic" sign.[144] Pallor in the ischemic, overlying retina makes visible the red color of the intact, underlying choroidal circulation, but its absence does not rule out RAO. Differential diagnosis from other causes of visual loss is presented in Table 34.2.

Mechanisms of Retinal Ischemia

The retinal blood supply is derived from the retinal and choroidal vessels.[145] After RAO, some O_2 may still be supplied by diffusion from outer retinal layers via the choroid. In monkeys, eyes with CRAO showed little damage in the macular retina after 97 minutes of ischemia. After 240 minutes, damage was profound and irreversible.[146] But proximal occlusion of the central retinal artery may not necessarily extrapolate to external compression of the eye.[147] Increased IOP from external compression is a more severe insult because of the profound simultaneous decreases in both retinal and choroidal blood flows,[148,149] and the greater susceptibility of the inner retinal cells to damage from pressure.[150] Ischemic tolerance time is probably shorter with external compression.[151,152]

Central Retinal Artery Occlusion

The cause of perioperative CRAO is usually external compression of the eye, although it may also occur in cardiac surgery, suspected from emboli.[153,154] Altered facial anatomy may predispose to damage by pressure from anesthesia masks or headrests. In osteogenesis imperfecta, for example, fibrous coats of the eye are thin and immature because of deficiency of collagen fibers, persistent reticulin fibers, and increased mucopolysaccharide ground substance.[155] Sclerae and corneas are thin and exophthalmos common, rendering the eye more vulnerable to damage from external pressure.[156] The horseshoe headrest leaves limited space for eyes, and the eye may inadvertently contact the headrest. Rectangular and horseshoe headrests were implicated in most reports of external compression.[157,158] Kumar reviewed CRAO cases after spine surgery, noting that signs and symptoms included unilateral vision loss, no light perception, afferent pupil defect, periorbital or eyelid edema, chemosis, proptosis, ptosis, supraorbital paresthesia, hazy or cloudy cornea, corneal abrasion, loss of eye movements, ecchymosis, or other trauma near the eye.[159] Macular or retinal edema, a cherry-red spot, or attenuated retinal vessels were often present. Four patients with external compression had retinal pigmentary alterations, suggesting simultaneous choroidal circulatory ischemia.[160,161] Early orbital computed tomography or magnetic resonance imaging showed proptosis and extraocular muscle swelling.[159] Findings were similar to "Saturday night retinopathy" in intoxicated individuals with ocular compression.[162]

Hollenhorst described unilateral blindness in patients positioned prone for neurosurgery and replicated the findings in monkeys with 60 minutes of elevated IOP together with hypotension (six of the eight human subjects did not have hypotension). In the monkey, histologic findings were retinal edema and dilated vascular channels, followed by retinal structural damage, and axonal loss in the optic nerve 4 months later, due to retrograde axonal degeneration after the death of retinal ganglion cells.[163]

Bui documented that during acute IOP increases in rats, changes in visual function assessed by electroretinography progressed from inner to outer retina, that is, retinal ganglion cells were the most sensitive, abnormal at IOPs 30 to 50 mm Hg; photoreceptors were not affected until IOP was higher.[164] The duration of increased IOP that injures the retina varies, with ischemic times as short as 20 or more than 30 or 45 minutes (Table 34.3).[165,166]

Modern head-positioning devices such as square or circular foam headrests with cutouts for the eyes and a mirror to view the eyes should prevent ocular compression.[167] However, unilateral RAO in a prone-positioned patient whose head was in a square foam headrest with goggles covering the eyes has been reported. There is limited space between the headrest and goggles. The patient exhibited signs of direct compression of the eye by the goggles, which, ironically, were designed as eye protectors.[168]

Orbital compartment syndrome, an acute ophthalmologic injury, requiring prompt decompression to relieve the increased IOP, can occur from perioperative intraorbital hemorrhage, orbital emphysema, or intraorbital bacitracin ointment and has been described during endoscopic sinus surgery.[169] There have also been several case reports[170-172] where its occurrence may have been related to positioning, such as in a patient undergoing spine surgery and positioned prone.

Cardiac Surgery and Retinal Arterial Occlusion

The largest case series of perioperative RAO is in cardiac surgery.[153] This recent study retrospectively examined RAO (CRAO and BRAO) in cardiac surgery using the Nationwide Inpatient Sample. More than 5.8 million cardiac operative procedures were estimated from 1998 to 2013, with 4564 RAO cases, an incidence of 7.8/10,000. Associated with increased RAO were giant cell arteritis, transient cerebral ischemia, carotid artery stenosis, embolic stroke, hypercoagulability, myxoma, diabetes mellitus with ophthalmic complications, and aortic insufficiency. Perioperative factors were bleeding, aortic and mitral valve surgery, and septal surgery. These results indicate that conditions that predispose to embolic phenomena, such as carotid disease, opening of the heart during surgery, and preexisting abnormal retinal vasculature (diabetic retinopathy) are potential predictors for RAO in cardiac surgery. Embolization during CPB remains a cause of retinal vascular occlusion. Better means for detecting and preventing this complication are needed.

Branch Retinal Artery Occlusion

BRAO usually leads to permanent ischemic retinal damage with partial visual field loss. Symptoms may not be immediately apparent if the visual field loss is peripheral or when only a small scotoma is present. BRAO is primarily from emboli and, less often, vasospasm. Most case reports describe embolization from intravascular injections, the surgical field, or CPB in cardiac surgery. Microemboli during CPB have been shown by retinal fluorescein angiography.[173] With a bubble oxygenator, all patients had perfusion defects versus 50% with a membrane oxygenator.[174] In coronary artery bypass graft surgery, multiple calcific emboli in branches of the central retinal artery are not unusual, resulting in visual field deficits of varying size and location.[175] In pigs, mechanisms of air embolism during CPB included nonperfusion, vascular leakage and spasm, red blood cell sludging, and hemorrhage. Priming with perfluorocarbons blocked many of these mechanisms.[176]

BRAO was described in a patient in the prone position for spine surgery. After surgery a patent foramen ovale was

TABLE 34.3 Animal Studies of Retinal Ischemia and Time Required to Produce Injury

Author	Animal	Ischemia Method	Ischemia Time
Hayreh et al. (1980, 2004)[146,147]	Monkey	Central retinal artery ligation	>100-240 min
Ettaiche et al. (2001)[151]	Rat (brown Norway)	Increased intraocular pressure	20 and 40 min
Roth et al., Zhang et al. (1998, 2002)[152,165]	Rat (S-D)	Central retinal artery ligation, increased intraocular pressure	45 and 60 min
Zhu et al. (2002)[166]	Mouse (ND4)	Increased intraocular pressure	30, 45, 60 min

discovered. The patient likely sustained a paradoxical air, fat, or bone marrow embolization from the operative site in the lumbar spine.[140] A large retrospective series on RAO in spine surgery has also recently been published.[154]

Considerations in Head and Neck Surgery

The incidence of orbital complications after endoscopic sinus surgery is estimated at 0.12%.[177] Vascular injury during the procedure can cause orbital compartment syndrome with compression of the arterial and venous circulations and in CRAO and optic nerve injury.[178] Indirect damage to the central retinal artery from intraarterial injections of 1% lidocaine with epinephrine has also been described; the mechanism is thought to be arterial spasm or embolism.[179] Orbital surgery is associated with an estimated 0.84% incidence of vision loss.[180] Risk is higher in patients undergoing facial polytrauma repair, optic canal decompression, or orbital apex surgery from an intracranial approach.[181]

Case reports have described sudden irreversible blindness due to BRAO following injection of various drugs into the head and neck region.[182] Super-selective carmustine injection into the internal carotid artery to treat gliomas, or fat injected into the orbit for cosmetic surgery, also have been complicated by visual loss from RAO. This complication can also occur from a neuroradiologic or angiographic or embolism procedure in the head and neck.[183,184]

Prognosis, Treatment, and Prevention

Perioperative RAO results in permanent loss of vision in most cases. Currently available treatment is unsatisfactory. Ocular massage to more peripheral arterial branches could be instituted to decrease IOP and dislodge emboli, if present.[143] Intravenous acetazolamide may increase retinal blood flow. Five percent carbon dioxide in 95% O_2 can enhance dilation and increase O_2 delivery from retinal and choroidal vessels.[185] Further treatment may include thrombolysis, contraindicated after certain surgical procedures. Fibrinolysis through a catheter in the ophthalmic artery within 6 to 8 hours after spontaneous CRAO was associated with improved visual outcome; pooled analysis of trials showed promising results particularly in incomplete CRAO.[186-189] Localized hypothermia to the eye is a simple technique that has decreased injury in animal studies after ischemia, and probably should be instituted because of its minimal risk.[190-192]

In patients positioned prone for surgery, a foam headrest should be used with the eyes properly placed in the opening; the position of the head and the eyes should be checked intermittently about every 20 minutes by palpation or visualization. A headrest that combines a foam headrest with a mirror immediately below, which enables the eyes to be seen easily during surgery, is useful. The use of goggles to cover the eyes is not advised when the head is positioned prone in a conventional square foam headrest. The horseshoe headrest must be used with great caution, and safer choices are available. For the patient positioned prone for cervical spine surgery, this headrest should not be used because of the likelihood of head movement and compression of the eye. Rather, the most effective method for preventing head movement is to place the head in pins. For most procedures in which the patient is prone, any of the commercially available square foam headrests are recommended, where the head is positioned straight down in the neutral position.

In nasal and sinus surgery and in neuroradiologic procedures, the most important principles are avoidance of inadvertent injections into, or compromise of, the ocular circulation. After endoscopic sinus surgery, patients should be checked for signs of acutely elevated IOP (such as blurred vision, eye pain, and nausea) suggestive of orbital hemorrhage. If present, immediate ophthalmologic consultation should be obtained.

ISCHEMIC OPTIC NEUROPATHY

ION, primarily manifesting spontaneously without warning signs, is the leading cause of sudden visual loss in patients older than 50 years of age, with an estimated annual incidence of nonarteritic ION in the United States of 2.3/100,000.[193] Two types of ION—anterior (AION) and posterior (PION)—have been described and can be arteritic or nonarteritic by mechanism. Arteritic AION, caused by temporal arteritis, is a systemic disease, which generally occurs in patients older than 60 years of age, and has a female preponderance. Spontaneously occurring ION, unrelated to surgical procedures, is usually caused by AION.[194]

Nonarteritic ION is overwhelmingly the type found perioperatively. It has been reported after a wide variety of surgical procedures, most after cardiac surgery,[195] spinal fusion,[137] head and neck surgery,[196,197] orthopedic joint procedures,[198] and surgery on the nose or sinuses.[199] Cases also have been described after vascular surgery, general surgical and urologic procedures (radical prostatectomy), cesarean section and gynecologic surgery, and liposuction.[200] The lack of controlled studies, and poorly defined pathologic and risk factors, still limit understanding of perioperative ION, although a number of recent retrospective case-control studies in spine and in cardiac surgery are yielding increasing knowledge of risk factors.[127,134] An animal model of perioperative ION has recently been described as well.[201]

Mechanisms

Disruption of the blood-brain barrier occurs early in AION. There are sparse studies of PION; thus most of this discussion concerns AION. Fluorescein angiography showed dye leakage in the optic nerve head,[202] correlating with early onset of optic disk edema, even before symptoms. [203] The relationship between disruption of the blood-brain barrier and ischemic injury is not known. Earlier studies showed classic blood-brain barrier properties in the optic nerve head[204]; however, more recent immunohistochemical studies of microvessels in the monkey and human optic nerve head suggest a lack of classic blood-brain barrier characteristics in the prelaminar region,[204] which could explain the early edema.

Guy showed that carotid artery occlusion in rats produced a swollen optic nerve within 24 hours.[205] Positive nitrotyrosine immunostaining in the ischemic optic nerve suggests a possible role for nitric oxide (NO) and O_2 free radicals, expected to increase disruption of the blood-brain barrier. Bernstein produced rodent AION by photothrombotic vessel occlusion, and circulation to the optic nerve was lost within 30 minutes; edema peaked 1 to 2 days later and resolved by 5 days.[206] A pale, shrunken optic nerve resembled the limited pathologic studies of human AION.[207] After 6 days, the optic nerve showed axonal swelling and collapse. By 37 days, the retinal ganglion cells were reduced by approximately 40%. Permanent changes included septal thickening and axonal loss, most evident in the center, also similar to that in the human optic nerve. Presently, the number of cases of ION with documented histopathological study is limited.[208]

Clinical studies of AION with fluorescein angiography showed delayed filling of the prelaminar optic disk in 76% of subjects and was not found in normal eyes. This suggests that delayed filling is the primary process, not disk edema,[194] while Hayreh attributed AION to individual variations in blood supply to the optic nerve.[209] This theory is supported by anatomic studies and the variability of visual loss in AION. But the watershed concept—that impaired perfusion and distribution within a posterior ciliary artery predisposes the optic disk to infarction—is disputed. Arnold and Hepler demonstrated that delayed filling of watershed zones was more common in normal eyes than in patients with AION.[202] Thus reduced perfusion pressure in the region of the paraoptic branches of the short posterior ciliary arteries results in optic disk hypoperfusion, rather than a watershed event.[210] Histopathologic examination in AION showed that the infarction was mainly in the retrolaminar region.[211] This implicates as the source of decreased blood flow the short posterior ciliary arteries as directly supplying the optic disk.

A small optic disk (small cup-to-disk ratio) may increase susceptibility to AION because axons of the optic nerve pass through a narrower opening as they exit the eye. Mechanisms of injury resulting from a crowded disk include mechanical axoplasmic flow obstruction, stiff cribriform plate, and decreased availability of neurotrophic factors to retinal ganglion cells.[212-214]

Blood Supply to the Optic Nerve

ION affects the anterior portion of the optic nerve in AION or beyond the retrolaminar region, and behind the eye in PION. Anatomy of and blood supply to the anterior and posterior optic nerves differ.[209] The anterior portion is proximal to the lamina cribrosa, an elastic, collagenous tissue through which the optic nerve, central retinal artery, and central retinal vein pass as they enter the optic disk. The anterior portion includes the superficial nerve fiber layer and the prelaminar region, a thick tissue that constitutes most of the optic disk volume.[215] The superficial nerve fiber layer, composed of axons extending from the retinal ganglion cells, is anterior to the plane extending across the optic nerve from the peripapillary Bruch membrane. Immediately posterior is the prelaminar region, adjacent to the peripapillary choroid. The laminar region is a transition zone between columns of glial cells and dense connective tissue plates. Astrocytes are predominant in the anterior optic nerve, and oligodendrocytes and microglial cells are more common in the posterior or retrobulbar optic nerve. Neural fibers transit the laminar region through fenestrations. The retrolaminar region is the posterior portion of the optic nerve and consists of meningeal sheaths and myelinated axons. The diameter of the optic nerve is enlarged in this area to approximately 3 mm.

The superficial nerve fiber layer derives its blood supply mainly from arterioles in the retina, although in the temporal regions it may receive blood from the posterior ciliary arteries. The prelaminar region is perfused by centripetal branches of the peripapillary choroid and vessels from the circle of Zinn-Haller (Fig. 34.22), which are not found in every eye.[209] Whether the region has a choroid-derived source of blood is controversial. The laminar region is supplied by centripetal branches from the short posterior ciliary arteries or by the circle of Zinn-Haller, but the short posterior ciliary arteries are the primary inputs. Longitudinal anastomoses of capillaries can be seen in the prelaminar and laminar regions and may provide some circulation, although their functional importance is not clearly known.

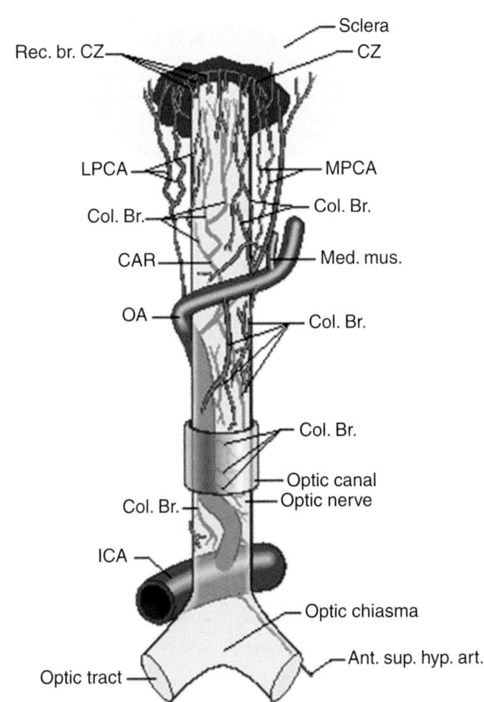

Fig. 34.22 The origin, course, and branches of the ophthalmic artery, including the posterior ciliary arteries, as seen from above. *Ant. sup. hyp. art.*, Anterior superior hypophyseal artery; *CAR*, central retinal artery; *Col. Br.*, collateral branches; *CZ*, circle of Zinn and Haller; *ICA*, internal carotid artery; *LPCA*, lateral posterior ciliary artery; *Med. mus.*, medial muscular artery; *MPCA*, medial posterior ciliary artery; *OA*, ophthalmic artery; *Rec. br.*, recurring branches. (From Pillanut LE, Harris A, Anderson DR, et al, eds. *Current Concepts on Ocular Blood Flow in Glaucoma*. The Hague, Netherlands: Kugler; 1999.)

The retrolaminar, posterior portion of the optic nerve, which is affected in PION (Fig. 34.23), is perfused by two main vascular supplies. The peripheral centripetal vascular system is the major supply and is found in all optic nerves; it is formed by recurrent branches of the peripapillary choroid and the circle of Zinn-Haller. Pial branches of the central retinal artery and other orbital arteries, the ophthalmic artery, and the posterior ciliary arteries also contribute. Branches of the pial vasculature run in the septa of the nerve. The axial centrifugal vascular system is formed by small branches from the intraneural part of the central retinal artery and is not present in every eye; thus differences in blood supply in the posterior optic nerve may render some individuals more susceptible to PION.[216]

Control of Blood Flow

Studies of autoregulation of blood flow in the optic nerve head have yielded conflicting results because of limited

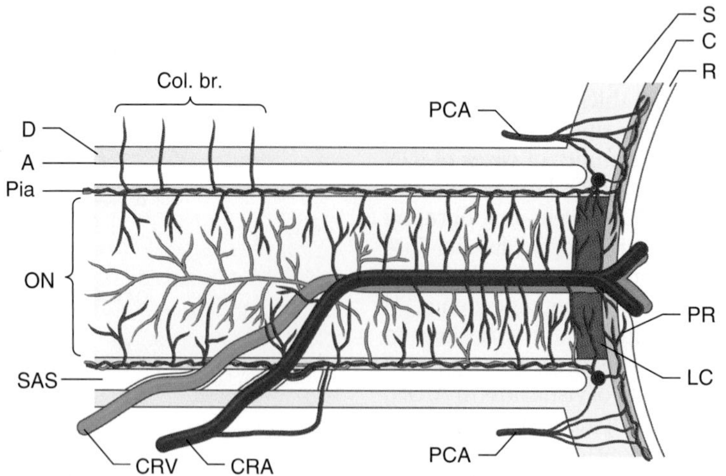

Fig. 34.23 The blood supply to the optic nerve. The anterior portion of the optic nerve is located to the left, whereas the posterior portion (closer to the brain) is on the right. The anterior portion of the nerve derives its blood supply from the posterior ciliary arteries *(PCA)* and the choroid *(C)*, whereas the posterior optic nerve derives its blood supply from penetrating pial arteries (collateral branches *[Col. br.]*) and branches of the central retinal artery *(CRA)*. *A*, Arachnoid; *CRV*, central retinal vein; *D*, dura; *LC*, long ciliary artery; *ON*, optic nerve; *PR*, short posterior ciliary artery; *R*, retina; *S*, sclera; *SAS*, subarachnoid space. (From Hayreh SS. Ischemic optic neuropathy. Department of Ophthalmology, University of Iowa. http://www.medicine.uiowa.edu/eye/AION-part2. Accessed August 8, 2014)

measurement techniques. Blood flow in the optic nerve head is autoregulated within a range of perfusion pressures similar to those in the brain of monkeys and sheep. In a small sample of atherosclerotic monkeys, however, autoregulation was defective.[217] This study did not directly measure blood flow; rather, it measured glucose consumption, and the sample size was small. Other evidence of autoregulation is seen in the posterior portion of the optic nerve. In cats, blood flow in the optic nerve measured directly by autoradiography remained constant in the prelaminar, laminar, and postlaminar nerve across a range of systemic mean arterial blood pressure values from 40 to more than 200 mm Hg.[218]

In 13 healthy volunteers, blood flow in the optic nerve head measured by laser Doppler flowmetry was constant between ocular perfusion pressures of 56 to 80 mm Hg.[219]; in another study, flow was preserved at extremely high IOP that resulted in a minimal perfusion pressure of 22 mm Hg.[220] Other investigators found that flow was preserved in the optic nerve head until ocular pressure reached levels of 40 mm Hg. However, 2 of 10 young healthy volunteers in the study failed to demonstrate autoregulation.[221] Using color Doppler imaging in humans, another group showed that flow velocity in the posterior ciliary arteries decreased at extremely high IOP. These findings seem to support the theory that "watershed" areas in the distribution of the posterior ciliary arteries predispose some patients, including otherwise healthy ones with no known vascular disease, to damage to the anterior portion of the optic nerve when perfusion pressure is decreased, either after systemic blood pressure decreases or IOP is elevated. At present, however, no clinical technique can reliably detect such patients.

Histopathologic Findings

There are few reports on the histopathologic examination of the optic nerve in ION. Of three PION cases evaluated after surgical procedures, all showed infarcts in the intraorbital portion of the optic nerve, but results were not consistent. Two patients had lesions in the central axial portion with peripheral axonal sparing; the other had the opposite pattern in one eye and complete axonal loss in the other.[200] Despite a larger autopsy series in AION, the location of the infarct has also not been documented. Tesser and colleagues[207] showed that in a patient with spontaneous AION, axonal loss was in the superior optic nerve, encircling the central retinal artery. The infarct was in the intrascleral portion of the nerve, extending 1.5 mm posteriorly.

Patient Characteristics in Perioperative Ischemic Optic Neuropathy

Most of the cases occurring after spine surgery have been PION.[200] AION occurs more frequently after cardiac surgery. ION's onset is typically within the first 24 to 48 hours after surgery and is frequently noted on awakening, although later onset has been described, particularly in sedated patients.[137] Patients present typically with painless visual loss, afferent pupil defect or nonreactive pupils, complete visual loss, no light perception, or visual field deficits. Color vision is decreased or absent. In AION, altitudinal visual field deficits may be present. Optic disk edema and hemorrhages are seen on symptom onset in AION; in PION, the optic disk appears normal even though the patient reports visual loss. Over a span of weeks to months, optic atrophy develops. The lesion may be unilateral or bilateral, but most post–spine surgery ION cases are bilateral. Orbital magnetic resonance imaging is frequently nondiagnostic, although some have described changes including enlargement of the nerve from edema or perineural enhancement.[222,223] Visual evoked potential and pattern evoked electroretinogram are abnormal.[224]

Retrospective Case Series

Buono and Foroozan reviewed 83 reported cases of PION, some of which were perioperative.[200] Approximately 54% followed spine surgery, 13% radical neck dissection, and 33% other surgery. Mean age was 52 years; patients who had spine surgery were younger (mean age, 44 years) than those in the other groups. Approximately two thirds were men. In 75%, visual loss was apparent within 24 hours. For 54% of affected eyes, initial visual acuity was light perception, with greater than 60% bilateral. In 38%, vision improved, but of 14 patients with no light perception initially, 12 (85%) had no improvement. Mean lowest hemoglobin was 9.5 g/dL (range: 5.8-14.2 g/dL), mean lowest systolic blood pressure was 77 (48-120 mm Hg), mean intraoperative blood loss was 3.7 L (0.8-16 L), and mean operative duration was 8.7 hours (3.5-23 hours). The drawback of this study is the limited amount of information on perioperative ION and its reliance on previously reported cases.

Spine Surgery

Ho reviewed cases of AION and PION after spine surgery. In the 5 AION and 17 PION cases, median ages were 53 and 43 years, respectively.[225] Most followed lumbar spine fusion. Mean operative time for AION was 522 minutes and for PION was 456 minutes. For AION, the range of the lowest mean arterial pressure was 62 to 78 mm Hg; for PION, it was 52 to 85 mm Hg. Mean lowest intraoperative hematocrit was 27% in PION. Mean blood loss was 1.7 and 5 L for AION and PION, respectively. Crystalloid/colloid volumes averaged 6.0/0.8 and 8.0/2.2 L for AION and PION, respectively. Sixty percent with AION and 27% with PION had diabetes mellitus; coronary artery disease was noted in 20% of patients with AION and in none with PION. Prevalence of hypertension was similar (40% or 53%). Symptoms were reported within 24 hours of surgery in 40% of patients with AION; 59% of patients with PION reported symptoms immediately on awakening and 88% within 24 hours. Visual acuity improved somewhat in 60% of AION and 65% of PION cases. This study is limited by its reliance upon literature reports.

In a retrospective case-control study of 28 patients with visual loss after spine surgery, Myers and colleagues found no difference in lowest systolic blood pressure or hematocrit in the affected versus unaffected patients.[135] Approximately 40% of these patients had no risk factors for vascular disease preoperatively; a similar percentage in the two groups had hypertension or were smokers. This study's limitations were that controls were not randomly chosen and matching of controls to cases was not adequately explained.

Spine surgery patients with ION in the ASA Postoperative Visual Loss Registry had an average blood loss of 2.0 L, and the lowest hematocrit was 26%.[136] Decreases in blood pressure varied widely from preoperative baseline: in 33%, the lowest systolic blood pressures were greater than 90 mm Hg; in 20%, the lowest was 80 mm Hg or less. Approximately 57% of patients had systolic or mean arterial blood pressure 20% to 39% below preoperative baseline, and 25% of patients were at 40% to 49% below preoperative baseline. Deliberate hypotension was used in approximately 25% of patients. Nearly all cases involved surgery exceeding 6 hours. In the majority of patients, estimated blood loss was greater than 1 L, the median estimated blood loss was 2 L, and the median lowest hematocrit was 26%. Large-volume fluid resuscitation was typical, with median crystalloid administration of approximately 10 L. Most of the patients underwent thoracic, lumbar, or lumbar-sacral fusion procedures that were often repeat operations that involved multilevel surgery. Surgical positioning devices included the

TABLE 34.4 Factors Increasing the Odds Ratio of Developing Perioperative ION in Lumbar Spine Fusion Surgery

	Odds Ratio	*P* Value
Male	2.53 (1.35-4.91)	.005
Obesity	2.83 (1.52-5.39)	.001
Wilson frame	4.30 (2.13-8.75)	<.001
Anesthesia duration, per hour	1.39 (1.22-1.58)	<.001
Estimated blood loss, per 1 L	1.34 (1.13-1.61)	.001
Colloid as percent of nonblood replacement, per 5%	0.67 (0.52-0.82)	<.001

Wilson frame (30%), Jackson spinal table (27%), and soft chest rolls (20%). A foam pad was used for head positioning for 57%; 19% had the head in a Mayfield head holder. PION accounted for the majority of cases, compared with AION. Patients in ASA physical status 1 or 2 accounted for 64% of cases. The mean age was 50 years. Approximately, 41% had hypertension, 16% diabetes mellitus, and 10% coronary artery disease. Limitations of this study are related to data collection and lack of control nonaffected cases for comparison.

This limitation was addressed by a follow-up comparison of the ION spine dataset with randomly selected, matched controls from 17 academic medical centers in North America. Results are summarized in Table 34.4. After multivariable analysis, six factors conferred higher risk for ION in lumbar spine fusion: male gender, obesity, Wilson frame positioning, anesthesia duration, large blood loss, and a relatively low ratio of colloid to crystalloid fluid resuscitation.[137] This study was the first large and well-matched case control study of perioperative ION. The limitations are the relatively limited amount of preoperative data, no distinction between AION and PION, and the possibility that controls did not represent a population-matched sample.

The Nationwide Inpatient Sample is a random sample of discharge data from 20% of US hospitals. Rubin and colleagues analyzed trends in ION incidence in spine fusion from 1998 to 2012 (more than 2.5 million discharges). ION prevalence was 1.02/10,000, with an encouraging, still unexplained, significant decrease over time.[127] Significantly associated with ION were age, blood transfusion, and obesity; female sex was inversely associated. These results are important because they were obtained from a very large, randomly collected sample, and suggested the importance of specific preoperative factors. But there are limitations. The Nationwide Inpatient Sample relies on the accuracy of diagnosis and coding. Verification of medical diagnoses are not possible. Both over- and under-coding are possible. The coding depends on entry of the data by professional coders; however, the accuracy depends upon the diagnoses recorded by physicians and the procedure description provided by the surgeon.[226]

Cardiac Surgery

Shapira and colleagues studied 602 patients undergoing CPB at a single institution under moderate systemic hypothermia (25°C) with pulsatile flow and a membrane oxygenator.[131] Phenylephrine maintained perfusion pressure above 50 mm Hg. Eight patients (1.2%) had AION. There were no differences in preoperative vascular risk factors in those with or without visual loss. CPB time was longer in patients with AION (252 vs. 164 minutes), and minimum hematocrit was lower (18% vs. 21%) compared with unaffected patients. There were no differences in flow indices, perfusion pressures, and carbon dioxide tension. Patients with AION had a greater 24-hour postoperative weight gain (18% vs. 11%) and required more vasoactive drugs to maintain hemodynamics than did patients with unaffected vision. Visual symptoms were usually reported between days 1 and 3 postoperatively, soon after removal of mechanical ventilatory support. This study is limited due to the small sample size and single institution design.

Nuttall and colleagues performed a larger retrospective case-control study of approximately 28,000 patients who had cardiac surgery at the Mayo Clinic from 1976 to 1994, with 17 patients with ION (0.06%).[132] By univariate analysis, significant risk factors included lower minimum postoperative hemoglobin, clinically severe vascular disease, preoperative angiogram within 48 hours of CPB, longer CPB duration, red blood cell transfusions, and the use of non–red blood cell blood components. Patients with ION underwent longer CPB runs; no differences were found in pre-CPB or post-CPB systemic blood pressures. Nine cases of bilateral ION were reported; disk edema was not found in 5 patients (29%), who may have had PION. Small cup-to-disk ratio (<0.3) was identified in 5 patients (29%) with ION. This study was limited by a large number of comparisons, small sample, single institution design, and no distinction between AION and PION. A more recent series by Holy and colleagues showed similar results, but it included other surgical procedures, complicating interpretation of the results with cardiac surgery.[227] Kalyani and colleagues reviewed cases of ION after 9701 cardiac surgeries over 9-year period at a single institution. Specific risk factors could not be determined from the 11 patients (0.11%) with ION.[133]

Rubin examined ION in the largest series of cardiac surgery cases to date, using the Nationwide Inpatient Sample (1998-2012), as described earlier.[134] There were more than 5 million discharges meeting inclusion criteria with 794 (0.014%) ION cases. Average yearly incidence was 1.43 of 10,000 cardiac procedures. Increasing risk were carotid artery stenosis, stroke, diabetic or hypertensive retinopathy, macular degeneration, glaucoma, and cataract. Female sex and uncomplicated diabetes mellitus type 2 decreased risk. This study was large but has the same limitations as other studies using the National Inpatient Sample. Intriguingly, it does suggest that preoperative degenerative eye diseases may predict patients that will develop ION.

Controversies and Anesthesia Management Recommendations

This discussion will primarily concern spinal fusion procedures, where the largest number of cases have been described. For more detail, the reader is referred to the practice advisories of the ASA.[228-230]

Length of Surgery. Both Myers[135] and the Postoperative Visual Loss (POVL) Study Group[137] reported increased risk with long duration of spine fusion surgery. Therefore, staging of spinal fusion procedures, particularly those for anterior and posterior surgery, may be advisable (but see later). A discussion between the surgeon and anesthesia provider should occur in selected cases. Revision spinal fusion procedures are common, and these operations may be longer in duration and involve larger blood loss.[231]

Hypotension. Intraoperative hypotension has been cited as a risk factor by a number of authors of case reports,[232,233] but this risk has not been confirmed by case control studies, with one exception.[135,137,227] Patil and colleagues reported a higher odds ratio for ION in patients who sustained hypotension.[128] However, the diagnostic coding of hypotension in this study from the Nationwide Inpatient Sample is not defined, cannot be confirmed, and the timing (during the perioperative period or not) and the degree of hypotension are not specified.[234]

Hypotension can potentially lead to a decrease in perfusion pressure in the optic nerve and to ischemic injury because of either anatomic variation in the circulation or abnormal autoregulation and an inability to adequately compensate for decreased perfusion pressure. The degree of hypotension that is potentially dangerous is difficult to determine because of the lack of data.[230] Judgment and discussion are thus advisable when surgeons request a decrease in blood pressure to decrease blood loss in spine surgery. In cardiac surgery, special considerations exist regarding the optimal systemic perfusion pressures to be maintained during CPB.[235]

Hemodilution and Blood Loss. Clinical blood transfusion practice in surgical patients, based on ASA practice guidelines,[236] suggests that transfusion is not generally required for hemoglobin values higher than 8.0 g/dL, and thus isovolumic hemodilution is common in patients undergoing spine fusion. The Society of Thoracic Surgeons and the Society of Cardiovascular Anesthesiologists reviewed the available evidence with respect to cardiac surgery, and has issued a similar clinical practice guideline.[237] Some authors suggested that allowing hemoglobin to decrease, as is common in anesthesia practice, may increase the risk for ION[238]; however, whether this practice should be changed in surgical procedures such as spine or heart surgery—or in any operative procedure—remains controversial.

In uncontrolled hemorrhage in which blood volume is not maintained, decreased O_2 delivery to the optic nerve could result in either AION or PION.[239] But how low or for how long the hemoglobin concentration must decrease to lead to this complication is not known. However, the presence of recurrent and profound hemorrhage has been described in many reports. The argument that blood loss in the presence of maintained intravascular volume (hemodilution) is harmful seems less scientifically grounded. It has been shown experimentally in miniature pigs that blood flow in the optic nerve head, as measured by laser Doppler imaging, was maintained during isovolumic hemodilution with a 30% decrease in hematocrit. Moreover, O_2 tension at the vitreal surface increased 15%.[240] Also, Lee and colleagues demonstrated that extreme decreases in hematocrit (15%) and mean arterial pressure (50 mm Hg) in adult pigs resulted in significant reductions in blood flow to the optic nerve. But no histologic or optic nerve function was studied, and the pig brain and eye circulation significantly differ from that of humans.[241] Roth and associates showed that hemodilution and extreme head-down tilt in rats resulted in significant changes in visual evoked potentials, electrical activity originating in retinal ganglion cells, and increased glial reactivity in the optic nerve; thus, if extrapolated to humans, caution is in order during extreme hemodilution with the head-down tilt.[201]

Head Positioning. Many reports of ION include patients who were in the prone position, raising the possibility that positioning itself contributes to altered venous hemodynamics within the optic nerve. The patient's head should be level with or above the heart, when possible, and in a neutral position during spine surgery performed with the patient in the prone position. When the patient is positioned for spine surgery in the Wilson frame, the head may be below the level of the back; the head can be elevated using pillows or the bed placed in reverse Trendelenberg.[242] With the Jackson table, the head is maintained at the level with the back.[229]

Several studies found that IOP increased in the prone position and was influenced by the position of the operating room table. However, there has been no correlation between IOP changes and visual outcome or visual function.[242] Cheng and colleagues found that in anesthetized patients, mean (± standard deviations) IOP increased significantly on initial prone positioning relative to supine (27 ± 2 vs. 13 ± 1 mm Hg). After 5 hours in the prone position, IOP remained increased at 40 ± 2 mm Hg. None of the 20 patients in the study experienced visual loss. The largest increases in IOP were evident near the time patients were awakening.[243] Although these data suggest that ocular perfusion pressure may decline even during maintenance of normotension, some experimental design issues must be considered in interpreting these results. The main issue is that the largest increases in IOP were evident near the time of awakening from anesthesia. Accordingly, IOP could have increased because of light anesthesia. Moreover, the study did not include a supine group to control for the effects of fluid administration on IOP. Such control is important because prone positioning itself may not explain the large increases in IOP. These results are valuable as well as of concern, but further studies are needed to fully evaluate their significance.

External pressure on the eye is a potential concern when a patient is positioned prone for surgery. Many cases of ION have occurred when pressure could not have been placed on the eye. Such cases include patients in pin head holders[244] and those in whom the head was turned with the affected eye placed upward.[245] But ION would not occur without retinal damage in a situation in which external compression was applied (see earlier discussion). Although we demonstrated that high IOP decreased retinal and choroidal blood flows in cats,[148] Geijer and Bill specifically measured the impact of graded increases in IOP on blood flow in the retina and optic nerve in monkeys.[246] When IOP was elevated such that perfusion pressure was decreased to levels above 40 cm H_2O, small effects on retinal blood flow and in the prelaminar portion of the optic nerve were noted. When perfusion pressure was less than 40 cm H_2O, retinal and prelaminar flows were proportional to the perfusion pressure. At very high IOP, blood flow stopped in the retina and the prelaminar area, but flow in the retrolaminar region increased. High IOP results in a redistribution of blood flow that favors the retrolaminar portion of the optic nerve. Therefore, an increase in IOP would not produce an isolated ION without also causing retinal damage. Further support is that sustained increases in IOP significantly decreased both retinal and choroidal blood flow, and even small increases in IOP damaged the retinal ganglion cells, which are sensitive to pressure alterations.[247,248]

Fluid Administration. The theory that massive intravascular fluid resuscitation could be a pathogenic factor in perioperative ION remains speculative, but it does have some merit. Conceivably, fluid administration could result in increased IOP, accumulation of fluid in the optic nerve, or both. Because the central retinal vein exits out of the optic nerve, an internal compartment syndrome may occur in the optic nerve. Alternatively, fluid accumulation in the vicinity of the lamina cribrosa may compress axons as they transit this region. In the report by Cullinane and colleagues,[249] trauma patients who were acidotic received massive blood replacement and most had abdominal compartment syndrome. Analysis of these patients is complicated because of the presence of numerous systemic alterations. Sullivan and colleagues described a retrospective series of 13 burn patients with 25% or greater body surface area burns and massive fluid resuscitation. IOP was elevated more than 30 mm Hg in four patients at 48 hours after admission, all of whom received more than 27 L of intravenous fluid. Eye findings and vision diagnoses were not described.[250] Large-volume fluid replacement is generally seen in spinal fusion surgery.[251] Patients in the ASA Postoperative Visual Loss Registry received on average 9.7 L of crystalloid intraoperatively,[137] and increased postoperative weight gain was identified in a case-control study of visual loss after heart surgery,[131] suggesting, although not proving, that fluid replacement may play a role. The finding of the POVL Study Group was that the odds ratio for developing ION was increased as the percent colloid of nonblood replacement decreased.[137] It is possible that the use of colloids may decrease edema in the optic nerve during surgery, particularly when the patient is placed prone for surgery. However, at present, such edema has not yet been demonstrated. In healthy volunteer subjects, placement in the prone position led to an increase in diameter of the optic nerve.[242] This could be due to venous hypertension. New magnetic resonance imaging methods may enable the study of edema and venous hemodynamics in the optic nerve in the near future. Animal models also may provide a means to study these perioperative factors. No study has shown any relationship among periorbital edema, IOP, and ION. Fluid administration could be a pathogenic factor in ION, especially in patients positioned prone or undergoing cardiac surgery, but the mechanisms involved, in addition to the amounts and nature of fluid required, remain undefined.

Anatomic Variation. Anatomic variation in the circulation of the optic nerve may potentially predispose patients to the development of ION. The location of potential watershed zones in the anterior and posterior circulation and the presence of disturbed autoregulation, even in normal patients,[108] are of concern but at present cannot be predicted clinically. Few human studies have been conducted on the relationship between perfusion pressure and changes in blood flow in the optic nerve. Human studies generally show preserved blood flow at clinically used or even lower ranges of perfusion pressure, but these studies have focused primarily on the anterior portion of the optic nerve.[219] In the studies that used laser Doppler flowmetry, depth of penetration of the measuring device is critical. Measurements might have been closer to the retinal blood vessels than the optic nerve head, and these do not measure optic nerve circulation. It is not currently feasible to measure blood flow in the human retrolaminar optic nerve. In animal studies, blood flow is preserved in various layers of the optic nerve, including the retrolaminar area, at a mean arterial blood pressure as low as 40 mm Hg.[218]

Vasoconstrictors. Hayreh and colleagues theorized that AION is related to excessive secretion of vasoconstrictors, which in turn could lower optic nerve perfusion to dangerously low levels.[252] However, the theory was based on the development of AION in patients who sustained massive hemorrhage. Vasopressors are used to maintain blood pressure in circumstances, such as after cardiac surgery and in cases in which vasomotor tone is decreased. Shapira and colleagues showed an association between prolonged use of epinephrine or long bypass time and ION in patients undergoing open heart surgery.[131] Lee and Lam reported a case of ION in a patient after lumbar spine fusion during which phenylephrine infusion was used to maintain blood pressure.[253] They later presented a series of four case reports of ION in critically ill patients with significant systemic illness who required prolonged use of vasopressors and inotropic agents to maintain blood pressure and cardiac output. However, α-adrenergic receptors are not located in the optic nerve and the blood-brain barrier prevents entry of systemically administered agents, except possibly in the prelaminar zone of the nerve. Therefore, the role of vasopressor use in ION remains unclear, and no clear guidance with respect to risk for ION can be provided at this time.

Informed Consent. A single institution survey reported that patients prefer to be informed of the risk of visual loss in spine surgery.[254] It seems advisable to have the discussion with patients that are at higher risk of developing ION. Often it is difficult to do when, as is common, the patient is first seen soon before surgery. It may be preferable for anesthesiologists and surgeons to develop a means to inform patients earlier of the risk of ION.

Staging and Minimally Invasive Spine Fusion. Increasingly, neurosurgeons have been using minimally invasive surgical techniques for lumbar spine surgery and fusion.[255] These methods reduce the amount of blood loss and fluid requirements, but cases of ION have arisen under these circumstances as well.[256] Another strategy not under the direct control of the anesthesia provider is to consider staging of complex spine procedures. However, in some instances the anesthesiologist may be able to persuade a surgeon to follow a less ambitious surgical plan. This decision requires an assessment of the associated increased risks for multiple surgeries (infection, spinal instability) but may significantly shorten the duration of each procedure. However, perioperative complications such as infection and deep vein thrombosis may be increased.[257-261] Another strategy is to advocate for patients by regular preoperative conferencing with surgeons. Anticipating high blood loss and other risks may enhance perioperative planning and care in spine surgery patients.

Prognosis, Treatment, and Prevention

No effective treatment exists for ION. A few cases of treating perioperative ION have been reported. Acetazolamide decreases IOP and may improve flow to the optic nerve head and retina. Diuretics such as mannitol or furosemide reduce edema.[262] In the acute phase, corticosteroids may reduce axonal swelling, but in the postoperative period they may increase wound infection. Because steroids are of unproven benefit, their use must be carefully weighed.[263] Increasing ocular perfusion pressure or hemoglobin concentration may be appropriate when ION is found in conjunction with significant decreases in blood pressure and hemoglobin concentration. Maintaining the patient in a head-up position if increased ocular venous pressure is suspected may be advantageous, but its use must be balanced against decreased arterial supply with the head-up position. Clearly, if a patient has visual loss from ocular compartment syndrome, immediate decompression (lateral canthotomy) is indicated.

In their review of perioperative PION reports in the literature, Buono and Foroozan summarized the lack of proof that treatment altered the course of PION. In a few anecdotal case reports, increasing blood pressure or hemoglobin, or applying hyperbaric O_2, improved visual outcome.[200] The use of neuroprotective agents or drugs that lower IOP, valuable in theory, has never been shown to result in improvement.[248] Stevens and colleagues, who compiled a report of ION in patients after spine surgery, had apparent improvement of vision in two patients when anemia and hypotension were corrected.[129] One patient demonstrated partial improvement that subsequently regressed, and one patient showed more clear signs of improvement. However, as Buono and Foroozan mentioned, it is difficult to ascertain if improvement came from treatment, because some patients recover vision spontaneously after PION.[200]

American Society of Anesthesiologists Advisories (Updated With 2019 Advisory)

The 2006 ASA Task Force on Perioperative Blindness concluded that high-risk patients who have surgery that is prolonged in duration and/or have large blood loss have an increased risk of POVL.[228] Yet POVL was not related to blood loss per se, hemoglobin levels, or the use of crystalloids. In 2012, another ASA Task Force published an update regarding POVL primarily associated with spine surgery.[229] While major changes were not made, analysis of the literature was updated and the recommendations were more detailed. For example, the 2006 Summary had 7 bullet points. In contrast, the 2012 Summary of Advisory Statements has 22 bullet points subdivided into Preoperative, Intraoperative, Staging of Surgical Procedures, and Postoperative Management (Box 34.2). The 2012 ASA Task Force on POVL reviewed the additional literature and concluded that newer findings and the literature do not justify major

BOX 34.2 American Society of Anesthesiologists 2012 Task Force Summary of Advisory Statements

I. Preoperative Considerations

- At this time, there were no identifiable preoperative patient characteristics that predispose patients to perioperative posterior ischemic optic neuropathy (ION).
- There is no evidence that an ophthalmic or neuro-ophthalmic evaluation would be useful in identifying patients at risk for perioperative visual loss.
- The risk of perioperative ION may be increased in patients who undergo prolonged procedures, have substantial blood loss, or both.
- Prolonged procedures, substantial blood loss, or both are associated with a small, unpredictable risk of perioperative visual loss.
- Because the frequency of visual loss after spine surgery of short duration is infrequent, the decision to inform patients who are *not* anticipated to be "high risk" for visual loss should be determined on a case-by-case basis.

Intraoperative Management

Blood Pressure Management

- Arterial blood pressure should be monitored continually in high-risk patients.
- The use of deliberate hypotensive techniques during spine surgery can be associated with the development of perioperative visual loss. Therefore the use of deliberate hypotension for these patients should be determined on a case-by-case basis.
- Central venous pressure monitoring should be considered in high-risk patients. Colloids should be used along with crystalloids to maintain intravascular volume in patients who have substantial blood loss.

Management of Anemia

- Hemoglobin or hematocrit values should be monitored periodically during surgery in high-risk patients who experience substantial blood loss. A transfusion threshold that would eliminate the risk of perioperative visual loss related to anemia cannot be established at this time.

Use of Vasopressors

- There is insufficient evidence to provide guidance for the use of α-adrenergic agonists in high-risk patients during spine surgery.

Patient Positioning

- The Task Force believes that there is no pathophysiologic mechanism by which facial edema can cause perioperative ION. There is no evidence that ocular compression causes isolated perioperative anterior ION or posterior ION. However, direct pressure on the eye should be avoided to prevent central retinal artery occlusion (CRAO).
- The high-risk patient should be positioned so that the head is level with or higher than the heart when possible.

Staging of Surgical Procedures

- Although the use of staged spine surgery procedures in high-risk patients may entail additional costs and patient risks (e.g., infection, thromboembolism, or neurologic injury), it also may decrease these risks and the risk of perioperative visual loss in some patients.

Postoperative Management

- The consensus of the Task Force is that a high-risk patient's vision should be assessed when the patient becomes alert.
- If there is concern regarding potential visual loss, an urgent ophthalmologic consultation should be obtained to determine its cause.
- There is no role for antiplatelet drugs, steroids, or intraocular pressure-decreasing drugs in the treatment of perioperative ION.

From Practice advisory for perioperative visual loss associated with spine surgery: an updated report by the American Society of Anesthesiologists Task Force on Perioperative Visual Loss. *Anesthesiology*. 2012; 116: 274–285.

changes in the 2006 recommendations. A further update was published in 2019.[230]

VISUAL LOSS AFTER VITRECTOMY AND VITREAL GAS BUBBLE TAMPONADE

Patients who have undergone vitrectomy with perfluorocarbon gas tamponade (C_3F_8) are at risk for gas bubble expansion and loss of vision from acutely increased IOP. Patients anesthetized for a subsequent surgical procedure with gas mixtures containing nitrous oxide (N_2O) after vitrectomy sustained retinal vascular occlusion from acute gas bubble expansion. N_2O anesthesia affects the size of the intraocular gas bubble. Wolf and colleagues demonstrated that N_2O and O_2 resulted in a more than threefold increase in SF_6 gas bubble volume, in contrast to a 50% increase with air ventilation and 35% increase with O_2 ventilation alone.[264] Perfluorocarbon gas remains in the eye for at least 28 days. Visual loss has been reported with N_2O anesthesia administered as long as 41 days after vitrectomy and gas bubble tamponade. Therefore, patients should wear a warning tag to alert the anesthesiologist to the presence of the gas bubble in the vitreous, and N_2O should not be used in patients who have had recent vitrectomy and gas bubble tamponade.[265,266]

Conclusion

The positioning of patients under anesthesia care is a major responsibility requiring great attention to detail and constant vigilance. Positioning for optimal surgical exposure but the potential for lasting harm to patients from improper positioning must guide our actions. Each position has significant physiologic effects on ventilation and circulation. In addition, despite increased awareness, position-related complications, including peripheral nerve injuries, continue to remain a significant source of patient morbidity. As surgical techniques evolve, extreme positions sometimes permit advantages, such as smaller incisions and more effective displacement of internal organs to facilitate surgical exposure. Unfortunately, associated risks may increase with positions that would not be tolerated when patients are awake. Anesthesiologists and surgeons must work together with all operating room staff when each patient is positioned to promote comfort and safety in addition to securing the desired surgical exposure. Ideally, the final position should appear natural; that is, a position that the patient would comfortably tolerate if awake and unsedated for the anticipated duration of the procedure.

Disclosure

Dr. Roth's research on vision loss is supported by National Institutes of Health Grants EY10343, EY027447, the Michael Reese Foundation Pioneers Award, and by the North American Neuro-ophthalmological Society. Dr. Roth discloses that he has provided expert witness evaluation and testimony in cases of perioperative visual loss on behalf of patients, hospitals, and healthcare providers.

Acknowledgment

This chapter is a consolidation of two chapters in the 8th edition, Chapter 41, "Patient Positioning and Associated Risks," and Chapter 100, "Postoperative Visual Loss." The editors and publisher would like to thank authors Lydia Cassorla and Jae-Woo Lee, as well as returning author Dr. Steven Roth for their contributions to the prior edition of this work. It has served as the foundation for the current chapter.

 **Complete references available online at expertconsult.com.**

References

1. Metzner J, et al. *Best Pract Res Clin Anaesthesiol.* 2011;25:263.
2. Cheney FW, et al. *Anesthesiology.* 1999;90:1062.
3. Warner MA. *Mayo Clin Proc.* 1998;73:567.
4. Practice advisory for the prevention of perioperative peripheral neuropathies 2018. *Anesthesiology.* 2018;128:11–26.
5. O'Brien TJ, Ebert TJ. In: Martin JT, Warner MA, eds. *Positioning in Anesthesia and Surgery.* 3rd ed. Philadelphia: Saunders; 1997.
6. Gelman S. *Anesthesiology.* 2008;108:735.
7. Luecke T, Pelosi P. *Crit Care.* 2005;9:607.
8. Froese AB. *Anesthesiology.* 2006;104:193.
9. Glenny RW. *Intensive Care Med.* 2009;35:1833.
10. Hakim TS, et al. *J Appl Physiol.* 1987;63:1114.
11. Burrowes KS, Tawhai MH. *Respir Physiol Neurobiol.* 2006;154:515.
12. Galvin I, et al. *Br J Anaesth.* 2007;98:420.
13. Petersson J, et al. *Respir Physiol Neurobiol.* 2009;166:54–60.
14. Nyren S, et al. *Anesthesiology.* 2010;112:682–687.
15. Warner MA. *Supine Positions.* 3rd ed. Philadelphia: Saunders; 1997.
16. Britt BA, Gordon RA. *Can Anaesth Soc J.* 1964;11:514.
17. Prielipp RC, et al. *Anesthesiology.* 1999;91:345.
18. Stewart JD, Shantz SH. *Can J Neurol Sci.* 2003;30:15.
19. Geerts BF, et al. *J Clin Anesth.* 2012;24:668–674.
20. Cestari A, et al. *Eur Urol.* 2010;57:530.
21. Klauschie J, et al. *J Minim Invasive Gynecol.* 2010;17:504.
22. Phong LK, Koh LK. *Anaesth Intensive Care.* 2007;35:281.
23. Coppieters MW, et al. *Anesthesiology.* 2002;97:75.
24. Kent CD, Cheney FW. *J Clin Anesth.* 2007;19:482.
25. Coppieters MW. *Anesthesiology.* 2006;104:1351.
26. Devarajan J, et al. *Anesth Analg.* 2012;115:867.
27. Martin JT. In: Martin JT, Warner MA, eds. *Positioning in Anesthesia and Surgery.* 3rd ed. Philadelphia: Saunders; 1997.
28. Warner ME, et al. *Anesthesiology.* 2001;94:705.
29. Wassenaar EB, et al. *Dis Colon Rectum.* 2006;49:1449.
30. Mumtaz FH, et al. *BJU Int.* 2002;90:792.
31. Simms MS, Terry TR. *Postgrad Med J.* 2005;81:534.
32. Anema JG, et al. *J Urol.* 2000;164:360–363.
33. Chase J, et al. *Dis Colon Rectum.* 2000;43:678.
34. Turnbull D, et al. *Anaesthesia.* 2002;57:905.
35. Akhavan A, et al. *Urology.* 2010;76:1309.
36. Dunn PF. *Int Anesthesiol Clin.* 2000;38:25.
37. Choi YS, et al. *J Thorac Cardiovasc Surg.* 2007;134:613.
38. Tamkus A, Rice K. *Anesth Analg.* 2012;115:663.
39. Biais M, et al. *Br J Anaesth.* 2010;104:407.
40. Martin JT. In: Martin JT, Warner MA, eds. *Positioning in Anesthesia and Surgery.* 3rd ed. Philadelphia: Saunders; 1997.
41. Douglas, et al. *Am Rev Respir Dis.* 1977;115:559.
42. Lumb AB, Nunn JF. *Anesth Analg.* 1991;73:422.
43. Girard TD, Bernard GR. *Chest.* 2007;131:921–929.
44. Alsaghir AH, Martin CM. *Crit Care Med.* 2008;36:603–609.
45. Guerin C, et al. *N Engl J Med.* 2013;368:2159–2168.
46. Pelosi P, et al. *Anesth Analg.* 1995;80:955–960.
47. Soro M, et al. *Eur J Anaesthesiol.* 2007;24:431–437.
48. Pelosi P, et al. *Anesth Analg.* 1996;83:578–583.
49. von Ungern-Sternberg BS, et al. *Intensive Care Med.* 2007;33:1771–1777.
50. Black S, et al. *Anesthesiology.* 1988;69:49–56.
51. Peruto CM, et al. *Arthroscopy.* 2009;25:891.
52. Porter JM, et al. *Br J Anaesth.* 1999;82:117–128.
53. Himes BT, et al. *J Neurosurg.* 2017;127:182–188.
54. Newberg Milde L: In: *Positioning in Anesthesia and Surgery.* 3rd ed. Edited by Martin JT, Warner MA. Philadelphia: Saunders; 1997: 1009
55. Hindman BJ, et al. *Anesthesiology.* 2011;114:782–795.
56. Warner MA. In: Martin JT, Warner MA, eds. *Positioning in Anesthesia and Surgery.* 3rd ed. Philadelphia: Saunders; 1997.
57. Rozet I, Vavilala MS. *Anesthesiol Clin.* 2007;25. 631-53, x.
58. Mammoto T, et al. *Acta Anaesthesiol Scand.* 1998;42:643–647.
59. Klein J, et al. *World Neurosurg.* 2018;115:196–200.
60. Papadopoulos G, et al. *Acta Neurochir (Wien).* 1994;126:140–143.
61. Mirski MA, et al. *Anesthesiology.* 2007;106:164–177.
62. Gunther F, et al. *Acta Neurochir (Wien).* 2017;159:339–346.
63. Hanna PG, et al. *J Clin Anesth.* 1991;3:290–294.
64. Pohl A, Cullen DJ. *J Clin Anesth.* 2005;17:463.
65. Pollard V, et al. *Anesth Analg.* 1996;82:278.
66. Fischer GW. *Pain Pract.* 2009;9:304.
65. Dippman C, et al. *Arthroscopy.* 2010;26(suppl 9):S148.
66. Drummond JC, et al. *Anesth Analg.* 2012;114:1301.
67. Lam AM, Baldwin G. *Anesth Analg.* 2012;114:1156.
68. Murphy GS, et al. *Anesth Analg.* 2010;111:496.
69. Ghosh A, et al. *Anesth Analg.* 2012;115:1373.
70. Rains DD, et al. *Arthroscopy.* 2011;27:532–541.
71. Hu JC, et al. *JAMA.* 2009;302:1557–1564.
72. Wright JD, et al. *JAMA.* 2013;309:689–698.
73. Gainsburg DM. *Minerva Anestesiol.* 2012;78:596–604.
74. Hsu RL, et al. *Rev Urol.* 2013;15:178–184.
75. Kalmar AF, De Wolf A, Hendrickx JF. *Adv Anesth.* 2012;20:75–96.
76. Lestar M, et al. *Anesth Analg.* 2011;113:1069–1075.
77. Mills JT, et al. *J Urol.* 2013;190:580–584.
78. Ulm MA, et al. *Gynecol Oncol.* 2014;135:534–538.
79. Wen T, et al. *J Endourol.* 2014;28:660–667.
80. Souki FG, et al. *BMC Anesthesiol.* 2018;18:117.
81. Cheney FW. *Anesthesiology.* 1999;91:552–556.
82. Kroll DA, et al. *Anesthesiology.* 1990;73:202–207.
83. Lee LA, et al. *Anesthesiology.* 2004;101:143–152.
84. Fitzgibbon DR, et al. *Anesthesiology.* 2004;100:98–105.
85. Kamel IR, et al. *Anesth Analg.* 2006;102:1538–1542.
86. Chui J, et al. *Anesth Analg.* 2018;127:134–143.
87. Goubier J, Teboul F. Nerves and Nerve Injuries. In: Tubbs R, Shoja M, Barbaro N, Rizk E, Loukas M, Spinner R, eds. *Amsterdam.* Elsevier; 2015.
88. Winfree CJ, Kline DG. *Surg Neurol.* 2005;63:5.
89. Welch MB, et al. *Anesthesiology.* 2009;111:490.
90. Warner MA, et al. *Anesthesiology.* 1999;90:54.
91. Prielipp RC, et al. *Anesthesiology Clin N Am.* 2002;20:589.
92. Cheney FW. *ASA Newsletter.* 1998;62(6):10.
93. Warner MA, et al. *Anesthesiology.* 1994;81:1332.
94. Contreras MG, et al. *Clin Anat.* 1998;11:372.
95. Morell RC, et al. *Anesth Analg.* 2003;97:1183.
96. Cooper DE, et al. *Clin Orthop Relat Res.* 1988;228:33.
97. Kang SW, et al. *Surgery.* 2009;146:1048–1055.
98. Luginbuhl A, et al. *Laryngoscope.* 2012;122:110.
99. Davis SF, et al. *Am J Electroneurodiagnostic Technol.* 2011;51:274.
100. Hanson MR, et al. *Ann Thorac Surg.* 1983;36:675.
101. Jellish WS, et al. *J Cardiothorac Vasc Anesth.* 1994;8:398.
102. Liau DW. *ASA Newsletter.* 2006;70:11–13, 16.
103. Warner MA, et al. *Anesthesiology.* 1994;81:6–12.
104. Warner MA, et al. *Anesthesiology.* 2000;92:614.
105. Aminoff MJ. *Anesthesiology.* 2004;100:1298.
106. Dylewsky W, McAlpine FS. In: Martin JT, Warner MA, eds. *Positioning in Anesthesia and Surgery.* 3rd ed. Philadelphia: Saunders; 1997.

107. Borsook D, et al. *Ann Surg*. 2013;257:403.
108. Primiano M, et al. *AORN J*. 2011;94:555–566.
109. Edsberg LE, et al. *J Wound Ostomy Continence Nurs*. 2016;43:585–597.
110. Cushing CA, Phillips LG. *Plast Reconstr Surg*. 2013;132:1720–1732.
111. Aronovitch SA. *J Wound Ostomy Continence Nurs*. 1999;26:130–136.
112. Hayes RM, et al. *Am J Med Qual*. 2015;30:591–597.
113. Campbell C, Parish LC. *Clin Dermatol*. 2010;28:527–532.
114. Kayser SA, et al. *Adv Skin Wound Care*. 2018;31:276–285.
115. Schwartz DM, et al. *Spine (Phila Pa 1976)*. 2011;36:1046–1049.
116. Brockerville M, et al. *J Neuroanesth Crit Care*. 2017;4:78–84.
117. Lalwani K. *Curr Opin Anaesthesiol*. 2006;19:430.
118. Biousse V, et al. *Ophthalmology*. 2018;125:1597–1607.
119. Biousse V, Newman NJ. *N Engl J Med*. 2015;373:1677.
120. De la Garza-Ramos R, et al. *Spine J*. 2016;16:516–522.
121. Gayat E, et al. *Anesth Analg*. 2011;112:126–128.
122. Frenkel RE, Shin DH. *Arch Ophthalmol*. 1986;104:1459–1463.
123. Hart RH, et al. *Am J Ophthalmol*. 2002;134:761–763.
124. Roth S, et al. *Anesthesiology*. 1996;85:1020–1027.
125. Warner ME, et al. *Anesth Analg*. 2001;93:1417.
126. Roth S, et al. *Anesthesiology*. 1996;85:1020.
127. Shen Y, et al. *Anesth Analg*. 2009;109:1534.
128. Patil CG, et al. *Spine*. 2008;33:1491.
129. Stevens WR, et al. *Spine*. 1997;22:1319.
130. Chang SH, et al. *Spine*. 2005;30:1299.
131. Shapira OM, et al. *Ann Thorac Surg*. 1996;61:660.
132. Nuttall GA, et al. *Anesth Analg*. 2001;93:1410.
133. Kalyani SD, et al. *Ann Thorac Surg*. 2004;78:34.
134. Rubin DS, et al. *Anesthesiology*. 2017;126:810–821.
135. Myers MA, et al. *Spine*. 1997;22:1325.
136. Lee LA, et al. *Anesthesiology*. 2006;105:652.
137. Postoperative visual loss study group. *Anesthesiology*. 2012;116:15.
138. Dattilo M, et al. *Neurol Clin*. 2017;35:83–100.
139. Goldsmith MO. *Ophthalmologica*. 1967;153:191–196.
140. Katz DA, et al. *Spine*. 2005;30:E83.
141. Marks SC, et al. *Head Neck*. 1990;12:342–345.
142. Blauth CI, et al. *J Thoracic Cardiovasc Surg*. 1988;95:668.
143. Wray SH. *J Neurol Neurosurg Psychiatry*. 1993;56:234–240.
144. Tobalem S, et al. *BMC Ophthalmol*. 2018;18:101.
145. Alm A, et al. In: Moses A, Hart C, eds. *Adler's Physiology of the Eye*. 8th ed. St. Louis: CV Mosby; 1987:183.
146. Hayreh SS, et al. *Exp Eye Res*. 2004;78:723.
147. Hayreh SS, et al. *Br J Ophthalmol*. 1980;64:818.
148. Roth S, et al. *Invest Ophthalmol Vis Sci*. 1994;35:3209.
149. Lin J, et al. *Invest Ophthalmol Vis Sci*. 1999;40:2925.
150. Chen X, et al. *Invest Ophthalmol Vis Sci*. 2005;46:2611.
151. Ettaiche M, et al. *Brain Res*. 2001;890:118.
152. Roth S, et al. *Invest Ophthalmol Vis Sci*. 1998;39:775.
153. Calway T, et al. *Ophthalmology*. 2017;124:189–196.
154. Calway T, et al. *J Neuroophthalmol*. 2018;38:36–41.
155. Van Dijk FS, Sillence DO. *Am J Med Genet A*. 2014;164a:1470–1481.
156. Cole DE, Carpenter TO. *J Pediatr*. 1987;110:76–80.
157. Sys J, et al. *Eur Spine J*. 1996;5:74.
158. Grossman W, et al. *Spine*. 1993;18:1226.
159. Kumar N, et al. *Am J Ophthalmol*. 2004;138:889.
160. Carr RE, et al. *Arch Ophthalmol*. 1973;90:21.
161. Jampol LM, et al. *Arch Ophthalmol*. 1975;93:1311.
162. Jayam AV, et al. *J Neurol Sci*. 1974;22:413.
163. Hollenhorst RW, et al. *Arch Ophthalmol*. 1954;52:819.
164. Bui BV, et al. *Invest Ophthalmol Vis Sci*. 2005;46:202.
165. Zhang C, et al. *Invest Ophthalmol Vis Sci*. 2002;43:3059–3066.
166. Zhu Y, et al. *Invest Ophthalmol Vis Sci*. 2002;43:1903–1911.
167. Grant GP, et al. *Anesth Analg*. 2006;103:499–500.
168. Roth S, et al. *Anesth Analg*. 2007;104:1185.
169. Rubinstein A, et al. *Arch Ophthalmol*. 2005;123:1452.
170. Amorim Correa JL, Acioly MA. *World Neurosurg*. 2018;110:309–314.
171. Habets JGV, et al. *World Neurosurg*. 2018;114:72–75.
172. Pahl FH, et al. *World Neurosurg*. 2018;109:218–221.
173. Rimpilainen R, et al. *Perfusion*. 2011;26:479–486.
174. Blauth CI, et al. *J Thorac Cardiovasc Surg*. 1990;99:61.
175. Slaughter MS, et al. *Artif Organs*. 2008;32:880–884.
176. Herren JI, et al. *Stroke*. 1998;29:2396.
177. Bhatti MT, et al. *Surv Ophthalmol*. 2003;48:389.
178. Haller D, et al. *Rhinology*. 2006;44:216.
179. Savino PJ, et al. *J Clin Neuroophthalmol*. 1990;10:140–144.
180. Jacobs SM, et al. *Ophthalmology*. 2018;125:1100–1108.
181. Christie B, et al. *J Plast Reconstr Aesthet Surg*. 2018;71:155–161.
182. Moss WJ, et al. *Laryngoscope*. 2015;125:796–800.
183. Byers B. *Arch Ophthalmol*. 1979;97:79.
184. Watanabe W, et al. *Graefs Arch Clin Exp Ophthalmol*. 2002;240:1033.
185. Anderson Jr B. *Trans Am Ophthalmol Soc*. 1968;66:423–474.
186. Ahn SJ, et al. *Invest Ophthalmol Vis Sci*. 2013;54:7746–7755.
187. Nedelmann M, et al. *Stroke*. 2015;46:2322–2324.
188. Schrag M, et al. *JAMA Neurol*. 2015;72:1148–1154.
189. Page PS, et al. *Front Neurol*. 2018;9:76.
190. Tamai K, et al. *Br J Ophthalmol*. 1997;81:789–794.
191. Schultheiss M, et al. *PLoS One*. 2016;11:e0148616.
192. Reinhard K, et al. *Invest Ophthalmol Vis Sci*. 2016;57:658–663.
193. Johnson LJ, et al. *J Clin Neuroophthalmol*. 1994;14:38.
194. Arnold AC. *J Neuroophthalmol*. 2003;23:157.
195. Tice DA. *Ann Thorac Surg*. 1987;44:677.
196. Schobel GA, et al. *Int J Oral Maxillofac Surg*. 1995;24:283.
197. Fenton S, et al. *J Laryngol Otol*. 2001;115:158–160.
198. Kaeser PF, Borruat FX. *J Arthroplasty*. 2011;26. 338.e17-9.
199. Huang TW, et al. *Otolaryngol Head Neck Surg*. 2003;129:448–450.
200. Buono LM, Foroozan R, et al. *Surv Ophthalmol*. 2005;50:15–26.
201. Roth S, et al. *Eur J Anaesthesiol*. 2018;35:840–847.
202. Arnold AC, et al. *Am J Ophthalmol*. 1994;117:222.
203. Subramanian PS, et al. *Br J Ophthalmol*. 2017;101:671–675.
204. Grieshaber MC, et al. *Surv Ophthalmol*. 2007;52:S115.
205. Guy J. *Curr Opin Ophthalmol*. 2000;11:421.
206. Bernstein SL, et al. *Invest Ophthalmol Vis Sci*. 2003;44:4153–4162.
207. Tesser RA, et al. *Ophthalmology*. 2003;110:2031.
208. Patel HR, Margo CE. *Arch Pathol Lab Med*. 2017;141:162–166.
209. Hayreh SS. In: Pillunat LE, Harris A, Anderson DR, et al., eds. *Current Concepts in Ocular Blood Flow in Glaucoma*. The Hague, Netherlands: Kugler; 1999:3.
210. Olver JM, et al. *Eye*. 1990;4:7.
211. Knox DL, et al. *Trans Am Ophthalmol Soc*. 2000;98:203.
212. Hayreh SS, Zimmerman MB. *Ophthalmology*. 2008;115:2275–2281.
213. Saito H, et al. *Ophthalmology*. 2008;115:1585–1590.
214. Beck RW, et al. *Ophthalmology*. 1987;94:1503.
215. Hayreh SS, Jonas JB. *Ophthalmology*. 2001;108:1586–1594.
216. Isayama Y, et al. *Ophthalmologica*. 1983;186:197–203.
217. Hayreh SS, et al. *Graefes Arch Clin Exp Ophthalmol*. 1994;232:745–752.
218. Weinstein JM, et al. *Invest Ophthalmol Vis Sci*. 1983;24:1559–1565.
219. Movaffaghy A, et al. *Exp Eye Res*. 1998;67:561–568.
220. Riva CE, et al. *Graefes Arch Clin Exp Ophthalmol*. 1997;235:618–626.
221. Pillunat LE, et al. *Exp Eye Res*. 1997;64:737–744.
222. Vaphiades MS. *J Neuroophthalmol*. 2004;24:235.
223. Bolacchi F, et al. *Invest Ophthalmol Vis Sci*. 2012;53:4191.
224. Parisi V, et al. *Eur J Neurol*. 2008;15:839–845.
225. Ho VTG, et al. *J Neurosurg Anesthesiol*. 2005;17:38.
226. Golinvaux NS, et al. *Spine (Phila Pa 1976)*. 2014;39:2019–2023.
227. Holy SE, et al. *Anesthesiology*. 2009;110:246.
228. Practice advisory for perioperative visual loss associated with spine surgery. *Anesthesiology*. 2006;104:1319–1328.
229. Practice advisory for perioperative visual loss associated with spine surgery. *Anesthesiology*. 2012;116:274–285.
230. Practice advisory for perioperative visual loss associated with spine surgery 2019. *Anesthesiology*. 2019;130:12–30.
231. Farshad M, et al. *Spine J*. 2018;18:1625–1631.
232. Brown RH, et al. *Anesthesiology*. 1994;80:222.
233. Katz DM, et al. *Arch Ophthalmol*. 1994;112:925.
234. Shen Y, et al. *J Neurosurg Anesthesiol*. 2009;21:21–30.
235. Murphy GS, et al. *Anesth Analg*. 2009;108:1394–1417.
236. Practice guidelines for perioperative blood management. *Anesthesiology*. 2015;122:241–275.
237. Ferraris VA, et al. *Ann Thorac Surg*. 2007;83:S27–86.
238. Williams EL, et al. *Anesth Analg*. 1995;80:1018–1029.
239. Hayreh SS. *Ophthalmology*. 1987;94:1488–1502.
240. Chamot SR. *Klin Monbl Augenheilkd*. 2002;219:292–295.
241. Lee LA, et al. *Anesthesiology*. 2008;108:864–872.
242. Grant GP, et al. *Anesthesiology*. 2010;112:57–65.
243. Cheng MA, et al. *Anesthesiology*. 2001;95:1351–1355.
244. Murphy MA. *Ophthalmology*. 2003;110:1454–1457.
245. Roth S, et al. *J Neurosurg Anesthesiol*. 1997;9:346–348.
246. Geijer C, Bill A. *Invest Ophthalmol Vis Sci*. 1979;18:1030–1042.
247. He Z, et al. *Invest Ophthalmol Vis Sci*. 2006;47:4872–4880.

248. Bui BV, Fortune B. *J Physiol*. 2004;555:153–173.
249. Cullinane DC, et al. *J Trauma*. 2000;48:381.
250. Sullivan SR, et al. *J Trauma*. 2006;60:72–76.
251. Alian AA, et al. *Anesth Analg*. 2016;123:346–356.
252. Hayreh SS, et al. *Am J Ophthalmol*. 1994;118:766–780.
253. Lee LA, et al. *Anesthesiology*. 2001;95:793.
254. Corda DM, et al. *Mayo Clin Proc*. 2011;86:865–868.
255. Bae J, Lee SH. *Neurospine*. 2018;15:18–24.
256. Hussain NS, Perez-Cruet MJ. *Neurosurg Focus*. 2011;31:E2.
257. Edwards 2nd CC, et al. *Spine Deform*. 2018;6:141–147.
258. Hassanzadeh H, et al. *Spine J*. 2013;13:1717–1722.
259. Maddox JJ, et al. *Spine J*. 2014;14:1159–1165.
260. Passias PG, et al. *Spine J*. 2017;17:1091–1099.
261. Siemionow K, et al. *Neurol Neurochir Pol*. 2014;48:403–409.
262. Hayreh SS. *Br J Ophthalmol*. 1974;58:981.
264. Wolf GL, et al. *Anesthesiology*. 1983;59:547.
265. Vote BJ, et al. *Anesthesiology*. 2002;97:1305.
266. Seaberg RR, et al. *Anesthesiology*. 2002;97:1309.

35 Neuromuscular Disorders Including Malignant Hyperthermia and Other Genetic Disorders

JIE ZHOU, ALA NOZARI, BRIAN BATEMAN, PAUL DENNEY ALLEN, and ISAAC NESS PESSAH

KEY POINTS

- Malignant hyperthermia (MH) is a pharmacogenetic disorder inherited primarily in an autosomal dominant pattern.
- MH susceptibility is linked to 230 mutations in the skeletal muscle ryanodine receptor (RyR1) and four mutations in the calcium voltage-gated channel subunit alpha1 S (CACNA1S) genes that encode two Ca^{2+} channels necessary for skeletal muscle excitation-contraction coupling.
- Physical interactions between L-type Ca^{2+} channel ($Ca_V1.1$) and RyR1 tightly regulate initiation and termination of skeletal muscle excitation-contraction coupling.
- Skeletal muscle accounts for approximately 40% of body weight and inherent changes in its metabolism have profound impacts on whole-body metabolism and physiology.
- Carriers of MH mutations can exhibit mild to moderate muscle impairments in the absence of triggering agents but are rarely diagnosed.
- Carriers of MH mutations are susceptible to anesthetic-triggered runaway skeletal muscle metabolism, which if not promptly treated is lethal.
- Signs of MH, including increased end-tidal CO_2, increased core temperature, muscle rigidity, tachycardia, and more, are consequences of the fulminant hypermetabolic crisis.
- Exposure to triggering agents or heat stress leads to acute loss of RyR1/$Ca_V1.1$ channel regulation, rapid accumulation of Ca^{2+} within the sarcoplasm, and a hypermetabolic crisis that stimulates adenosine triphosphate (ATP) utilization by pumps attempting to restore resting Ca^{2+} balance among sarcoplasmic reticulum, mitochondrial, and extracellular compartments.
- Dantrolene markedly attenuates myoplasmic calcium (Ca^{2+}) concentrations and thereby restores resting Ca^{2+} balance and metabolism, with reversal of clinical signs.
- Evaluation of persons susceptible to MH includes an in vitro contracture test (IVCT) and caffeine/halothane contracture test (CHCT), and evaluation of DNA to identify mutations.
- Currently DNA testing alone can be used to evaluate 42 human mutations and all swine, equine, and canine MH.
- Future MH goals include advancement of genetic evaluations in North American and European medical programs and stronger finances to support genetic studies, the identification of the mode of action of dantrolene, a determination of the immediate cause of triggering MH, and the development of effective, noninvasive tests for MH susceptibility.
- The absence of mutations in dystrophin, along with dystrophin-associated glycoproteins, is involved in sarcolemmal stability. Its defects are responsible for Duchenne muscular dystrophy (DMD) and Becker muscular dystrophy (BMD).
- Whereas the risk for an MH mutation in DMD and BMD patients is similar to that in the general population, the incidence of MH-like anesthetic events has been reported to be 0.002 with DMD and 0.00036 with BMD.
- Succinylcholine is contraindicated in DMD and BMD patients because of the risk of rhabdomyolysis and hyperkalemia as a result of their unstable sarcolemmal membrane.
- Reversal of neuromuscular blockade with sugammadex is a practical alternative to the management of many of these disorders, if rocuronium or vecuronium is used. The combination of rocuronium and sugammadex has improved the anesthetic management for some of these challenging disorders.

Malignant Hyperthermia

Malignant hyperthermia (MH) is one of the most devastating anesthesia-related complications. The fulminant MH syndrome is elicited by the administration of triggering anesthetic agents, such as volatile halogenated anesthetics or depolarizing neuromuscular blocking agents (NMBAs). MH has been and continues to be a life-threatening complication of anesthesia if the diagnosis is not made promptly and treatment is not begun in a timely fashion. Unlike other disorders described in this chapter, MH has virtually no characteristic phenotype before exposure to the triggering agent and is truly an example of the interaction of genes and the environment. Also covered in this chapter are some of the neuromuscular disorders, although rarely encountered in a routine anesthetic practice. This group of disorders challenges both perioperative management and intensive care. They affect the normal function of peripheral nerves, the neuromuscular junction, and/or muscles. Although such diseases are thought to be rare, the number of patients that a clinician may encounter is increasing because of better medical care, increasing longevity, and other possible unidentified factors. Neuromuscular disorders have significant potential to interact with an improper anesthetic plan, and all affected patients require special perioperative attention for anesthetic management. In this area, the armamentarium of invasive and noninvasive diagnostic tools is being developed, especially in genetics.

MH is a pharmacogenetic clinical syndrome that, in its classic form, occurs during anesthesia with volatile halogenated alkanes such as halothane, isoflurane/sevoflurane, /desflurane, and/or administration of the depolarizing muscle relaxant succinylcholine. The fulminant MH episode observed clinically produces muscle hypermetabolism with rapidly increasing body temperature, by as much as 1°C in 5 minutes, and extreme acidosis as a result of acute loss of control of intracellular ionized calcium (Ca^{2+}). It is the sustained high levels of sarcoplasmic Ca^{2+} that rapidly drives skeletal muscle into a hypermetabolic state that may proceed to severe rhabdomyolysis. Although MH was initially associated with a mortality rate of 60%, earlier diagnosis and the use of dantrolene have reduced the mortality to less than 1.4%.[1] Current cases of MH are restricted in severity because of diagnostic awareness, early detection through end-expired carbon dioxide (CO_2), the use of less potent anesthetic triggers, and prior administration of drugs that attenuate the progression of the fulminant episode. Estimates of the incidence of fulminant MH vary widely from one case per 10,000 to 1:250,000 anesthetics administered.[2] The prevalence of MH events in Japan was calculated to be between 1:60,000 and 1:73,000.[3,4] However, the prevalence of MH mutations within kindred known to transmit MH-susceptibility (MHS) mutations may be as high as 1:2000.[5] Males appear to be more susceptible to developing a clinical MH episode than females.[3,6] A gender difference in MHS has also been demonstrated in knock-in mice expressing human MH mutation RyR1-T4825I.[7] The pediatric population accounts for 52.1% of all MH reactions.[8,9]

Between 50% and 80% of genotyped patients who have had a clinical MH syndrome and a positive muscle biopsy have had their disease linked to one of more than 230 mutations in the type 1 ryanodine receptor (RyR1; sarcoplasmic reticulum [SR] Ca^{2+} release channel) gene and four mutations in L-type Ca^{2+} channel ($Ca_V1.1$), the pore subunit of the slowly inactivating L-type Ca^{2+} channel encoded by Calcium Voltage-Gated Channel Subunit Alpha1 S (CACNA1S) (also referred to as the dihydropyridine receptor [DHPR]).[10] The genetics of MHS and the related abnormal function of RyR1, the DHPR, and associated proteins are being investigated at the molecular biologic level, with a porcine model and several new mouse models providing intricate details about the etiology of the disorder. Parallel studies in humans are limited by scarce material for scientific study and are complicated by the fact that phenotypes within a single genotype vary as a result of sex, age, genetic, epigenetic, and environmental modifiers.

Public education and communication in the United States are provided by Malignant Hyperthermia Association of the United States (MHAUS, 11 E. State Street, P.O. Box 1069, Sherburne, NY 13460, U.S.A.; telephone: (+1) 607-674-7901; fax: (+1) 607-674-7910; e-mail: info@mhaus.org; website: http://www.mhaus.org), and by emergency consultation with the MH Hotline (1-800-MHHYPER, or 1-800-644-9737). The North American Malignant Hyperthermia Registry (NAMHR), a professional subsidiary of MHAUS, collates findings from muscle biopsy centers in Canada and the United States (NAMHR, 1345 SW Center Drive, P.O. Box 100254, Gainesville, FL 32610, U.S.A.); telephone: (+1) 888-274-7899; fax: (+1) 352-392-7029.; website http://anest.ufl.edu/namhr/).

HISTORY

Between 1915 and 1925, one family experienced three anesthetic-induced MH deaths with rigidity and hyperthermia and was puzzled for decades regarding the cause of these deaths.[11,12] MHS was eventually confirmed in three descendants by in vitro muscle biopsy tests.[11] In 1929, Ombrédanne described anesthesia-induced postoperative hyperthermia and pallor in children accompanied by significant mortality but did not detect any familial relationships.[13] Critical worldwide attention to MH began in 1960 when Denborough and associates reported a 21-year-old Australian with an open leg fracture who was more anxious about anesthesia than about surgery because 10 of his relatives died during or after anesthesia.[14] Denborough and colleagues initially anesthetized him with the then-new agent halothane, halted it when signs of MH appeared, successfully treated the symptoms, aborted the syndrome, and subsequently used spinal anesthesia. Further evaluations by George Locher in Wausau, Wisconsin, and Beverly Britt in Toronto, Canada, led to the discovery that MH risk was indeed familial.[15] It was also found that the cause of the syndrome was the result of skeletal muscle involvement rather than central loss of temperature control by the recognition of increased muscle metabolism or muscle rigidity early in the syndrome, low-threshold contracture responses, and elevated creatine kinase (CK) values.[16]

Interestingly, a similar syndrome was discovered in swine inbred with breeding patterns designed to produce a rapid growth rate and superior muscle development (e.g., Landrace, Piétrain, Duroc, and Poland China). *Porcine stress syndrome*,[17] which is associated with increased metabolism, acidosis, rigidity, fever, and death from rapid deterioration of muscle and results in pale, soft, exudative pork,[18] can be triggered by any stress, such as separation, shipping conditions, weaning, fighting, coitus, or preparation for slaughter, and had become a significant problem for meat production. In 1966, Hall and coworkers reported that a syndrome that appeared to be identical to MH could be induced in stress-susceptible swine by the administration of halothane and succinylcholine.[19] The cause of this syndrome in pigs was discovered to be a single missense mutation in RyR1, and all susceptible swine have the same Arg615Cys mutation in the SR calcium release channel RyR1.[20]

In 1975, Harrison described the efficacy of dantrolene in preventing and treating porcine MH,[21] which was rapidly confirmed in humans by a multihospital evaluation of dantrolene used to treat anesthetic-induced MH episodes.[22] Today, dantrolene still remains the primary pharmacologic approach for successful MH therapy.

PHYSIOLOGY AND PATHOPHYSIOLOGY OF EXCITATION-CONTRACTION COUPLING AND MALIGNANT HYPERTHERMIA

MH is a syndrome caused by dysregulation of excitation-contraction (EC) coupling in skeletal muscle. Normal muscle contraction is initiated by nerve impulses arriving at the neuromuscular junction (i.e., the motor end plate) that trigger the release of acetylcholine from the nerve terminal. Acetylcholine activates nicotinic cholinergic receptors (nAChR), nonselective cation channels located at the postsynaptic neuromuscular junction, that are essential for local depolarization of the surface muscle membrane (sarcolemma) and initiating action potentials that propagate rapidly along the sarcolemma of muscle cells. Invaginations of the sarcolemma (termed transverse or T tubules) act as conduits to rapidly and uniformly direct-action potentials deep within the myofibrils where they transduce a conformational change in the "voltage sensor" protein $Ca_V1.1$. A central T-tubule is flanked on both sides by a terminal cisternae element from the SR that contains the Ca^{2+} release channels (RyR1). Conformational changes in $Ca_V1.1$ residing within the T-tubule are mechanically transmitted to RyR1 residing in the junctional face of the SR. More specifically, physical coupling of four $Ca_V1.1$ (dihydropyridine receptor) units to every second RyR1 channel form linear arrays at specialized junctions (*triadic junctions*) that are essential for linking electrical signals at the T tubules with the release of Ca^{2+} stored within the SR. Release of SR Ca^{2+} causes the free, cytoplasmic (sarcoplasmic) Ca^{2+} concentration to increase from 10^{-7} M to about 10^{-5} M. This released Ca^{2+} binds to contractile proteins (troponin C and tropomyosin) in the thin filament to expose myosin's actin binding sites which allow shortening and force development by the muscle fibers (i.e., muscle contraction). The entire process is termed excitation-contraction coupling (EC coupling) Intracellular Ca^{2+} pumps (i.e., sarcoplasmic/endoplasmic reticulum Ca^{2+}-adenosine triphosphatase [ATPase], or SERCA) rapidly sequester Ca^{2+} back into the SR lumen, and muscle relaxation begins when the Ca^{2+} concentration falls below 10^{-6} M and ends when the resting sarcoplasmic Ca^{2+} concentration is restored to 10^{-7} M. Because both contraction and relaxation are energy-related processes that consume adenosine triphosphate (ATP), knowing the molecular events contributing to EC coupling and the subsequent relaxation phase is essential to understanding the cause of MH (Fig. 35.1). Clinical and laboratory data from humans, swine, and mice with knock-in mutations indicate that the fulminant MH syndrome is associated with a persistent increase in the concentration of sarcoplasmic Ca^{2+}.[23-26] The increased activity of pumps and exchangers trying to

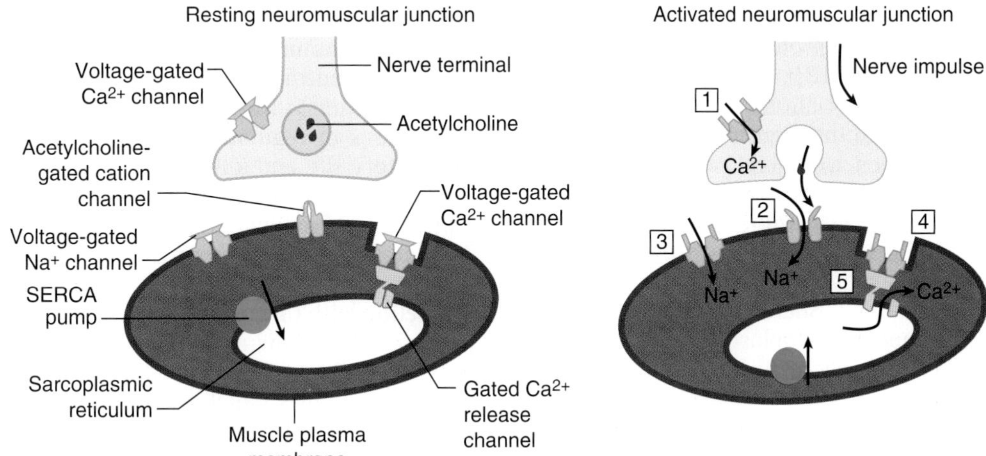

Fig. 35.1 Key ion channels involved in neuromuscular transmission and excitation-contraction coupling. Nerve impulses arriving at the nerve terminal activate voltage-gated Ca^{2+} channels (1). The resulting increase in cytoplasmic Ca^{2+} concentration is essential for the exocytosis of acetylcholine. Binding of acetylcholine to postsynaptic nicotinic cholinergic receptors (nAChR) activates an integral nonselective cation channel that depolarizes the sarcolemma (2). Depolarizing the sarcolemma to threshold activates voltage-gated Na^+ channels (3), which initiates action potential impulses that propagate deep into the muscle through the transverse tubule system. Within the transverse tubule system, L-type voltage-gated Ca^{2+} channels sense membrane depolarization and undergo a conformational change (4). A physical link between these voltage sensors and the ryanodine receptor (RyR1) sarcoplasmic reticulum Ca^{2+} channel is the means by which the electrical signal is transferred from the T tubule to Ca^{2+} release from the sarcoplasmic reticulum (5). (Modified from Alberts B, Bray D, Lewis J, et al. *Molecular Biology of the Cell*. 3rd ed. New York: Garland Press; 1994.)

correct the increase in sarcoplasmic Ca^{2+} associated with triggered MH increases the need for ATP, which in turn produces heat. Thus the common etiological feature of the disorder is hyperthermia. The rigidity that is frequently seen during a fulminant MH episode is the result of the inability of the Ca^{2+} pumps and transporters to reduce the unbound sarcoplasmic Ca^{2+} below the contractile threshold (10^{-6} M). Dantrolene is an effective therapeutic for treatment of fulminant MH because it reduces the concentration of sarcoplasmic Ca^{2+} to below contractile threshold. However, the pathway by which dantrolene lowers sarcoplasmic Ca^{2+} is complex and still not fully understood. Dantrolene's ability to suppress Ca^{2+} release from SR appears to depend on elevated sarcoplasmic Mg^{2+} concentration[27]; however the drug also attenuates depolarized-triggered Ca^{2+} entry mediated by $Ca_V1.1$, which is exacerbated in MHS muscle cells and MH normal muscle cells exposed to ryanodine.[28] Thus whether dantrolene directly inhibits RyR1 or requires additional intermediates within the triad junctions remains to be clarified.

Malignant Hyperthermia Is the Result of Abnormal Function of Muscle Calcium Release Units

RYANODINE RECEPTORS

Ryanodine receptors (RyRs) within the muscle are synonymous with the junctional foot protein/SR calcium release channel, and are so named because they specifically bind the toxic plant alkaloid ryanodine, which can activate or inhibit the channel depending on its concentration.[29,30] In all mammals there are three RyR isoforms. In humans, they are encoded by three genes located on chromosomes 19q13.1,[31] 1q42.1-q43,[32] and 15q14-q15,[33] for the "skeletal" (RyR1), "cardiac" (RyR2), and "brain" (RyR3) isoforms, respectively. Each functional RyR is a homotetramer consisting of four identical subunits (~5000 amino acids each), and an accessory protein, calstabin 1 (FK506 12-kd binding protein [FKBP12]).[34-37]. The total mass of the tetramer exceeds 2 mega-Daltons. Thus it is one of the largest known proteins and the largest known channel in mammalian species. Evidence of direct coupling of $Ca_V1.1$ and RyR1 has been demonstrated both by expressing chimeric $Ca_V1.1/Ca_V1.2$ cDNA in dysgenic myotubes that lack constitutive expression of $Ca_V1.1$[38,39] and chimeric RyR1/RyR2/3 cDNA in dyspedic myotubes that lack constitutive expression of RyR1, 2, and 3. Such studies have provided compelling evidence that the cytoplasmic region between repeats II and III (i.e., cytosolic II-III loop) of $Ca_V1.1$ contains a stretch of 46 amino acids (L720 to Q765) and multiple regions of RyR1 that are essential for engaging bidirectional signaling between $Ca_V1.1$ and RyR1.[40-42]

In the last two decades, our understanding of EC coupling has increased significantly by identifying protein-protein interactions that regulate both the release and sequestration of Ca^{2+} within skeletal muscle. The elemental unit of function has been named the Ca^{2+} release unit (CRU), and it is localized within junctional regions of T-tubule and SR membranes.[43] The CRU is a macromolecular assembly of interacting proteins that participate in regulating EC coupling. RyR1 is a high-conductance channel that regulates release of SR Ca^{2+} and is the central component of the CRU. The functional RyR1 tetramer anchored within the SR membrane physically spans the junctional space to interact with tetrads composed of four voltage-activated $Ca_V1.1$ subunits within the T-tubule membrane. This physical interaction engages a form of bidirectional signaling that tightly regulates the function of both proteins. Moreover, interaction of $Ca_V1.1$ and RyR1 does not occur in isolation, but are further subject to regulation by a number of proteins localized within the triad junction, including Homer 1, which physically binds and functionally couples target proteins, calstabin 1, triadin, junctin, Mg29, junctophilin 1 and 2, calsequestrin, calmodulin, STAC 3, the catalytic and regulatory subunits of protein kinase A, and protein phosphatase 1.[44-50]. It is likely that this list is not complete and that there are other critical components which make up this tightly regulated macromolecular complex. More importantly, there is increasing experimental evidence that mutations found in RyR1 ($_{MH}$RyR) or $Ca_V1.1$ ($_{MH}Ca_V1.1$) can alter protein-protein interactions in the CRU,[51-53] as well as alter the functional fidelity of bidirectional signals.[54-58]

In the presence of certain chemical substances, MH mutations in RyR1 or DHPR cause severe dysregulation of RyR1 channel function. This can be seen in vitro as a heightened sensitivity to volatile anesthetics, 4-chloro-*m*-cresol, caffeine, ryanodine, and potassium depolarization.[59-61] Chemically induced dysfunction of the RyR1 complex appears to be the principal cause of triggering uncontrolled skeletal muscle metabolic acidosis (aerobic and glycolytic), rigidity, and hyperkalemia, but the mechanisms governing the syndrome are unclear. Also unclear is the relationship among exertional heat illness, exertional rhabdomyolysis, and MHS, an area that requires more investigation and, if possible, controlled clinical studies.[62]

Two essential cations greatly shape the kinetics and magnitude of Ca^{2+} release in response to depolarizing triggers: Ca^{2+} itself and Mg^{2+}. The normal RyR1 complex responds to Ca^{2+} in a biphasic manner. First, Ca^{2+} activates the channel in a graded manner between 100 nM and 100 μM, whereas higher concentrations inhibit channel activity.[63,64] This biphasic action is thought to occur via binding of Ca^{2+} to two classes of regulatory sites on RyR1, a high-affinity stimulatory site and a low-affinity inhibitory site.[46] Mg^{2+}-induced inhibition is the second important physiologic regulator of RyR1 activity in skeletal muscle.[65,66] Mg^{2+} inhibits RyR1 in a cooperative manner ($n_H \approx 2$; 50% inhibitory concentration [IC_{50}] ≈ 650 μM). It is likely that Mg^{2+} acts by competing with Ca^{2+} at its activator sites and by binding to yet unidentified low-affinity inhibitory sites.[67,68] It is possible that MH mutations introduce allosteric instability into the RyR1 complex which leads to a reduction of inhibition rather than directly altering the binding properties of Ca^{2+} or Mg^{2+}, or both, at the activator or inhibitor sites. Therefore hypersensitivity to pharmacologic agents is likely to be closely tied to altered responses to physiologic ligands. However, whether MHS channels are primarily hyposensitive to inhibition by Mg^{2+} or Ca^{2+} (or both),[69,70] are hypersensitive to activation by Ca^{2+}, or exhibit altered sensitivities in both directions to both ions seems to be highly dependent on the location of the MH mutation.[71,72] Studies have also pursued the "leaky channel" hypothesis by examining

SR preparations from homozygous R615C MHS pigs and heterozygous R163C and C512S mice. They observed a significantly lower Ca^{2+} loading capacity (38%, 23%, and 22% lower than matched wild type mice, respectively) primarily mediated by the presence of leaky channels that remain active even with 100 nM extravesicular Ca^{2+}.[73,74] Recent studies indicated that expression of $Ca_V1.1$ represses the basal activity of the ryanodine-insensitive RyR1 leaky state.[56] It is important that MHS mutations appear to not only alter bidirectional signaling during EC coupling [57,58] and inherent regulation of RyR1 channel functions,[71,72] but also weaken negative regulation conferred by $Ca_V1.1$ on RyR1 Ca^{2+} leak under nontriggering conditions.[54] These findings at the molecular and cellular level using knock-in MHS mice confirm earlier measurements made in porcine and human MHS muscles, myotubes, and myoball preparations and in dyspedic myotubes expressing $_{MH}$RyR1 cDNAs, all of which have been shown to have chronically elevated resting cytoplasmic $[Ca^{2+}]_i$.[53,60,75]

Results from both functional and structural evidence suggests that long-range interdomain interactions between regions of RyR1 are involved in channel regulation by stabilizing protein conformations critical for normal channel transitions.[76] A three-dimensional reconstruction of RyR1 by Samso and coworkers shows that the RyR1 architecture is designed to support long-range allosteric pathways such as coupling with $Ca_V1.1$ and binding to ligands such as calmodulin and FKBP12.[77] This structural model for gating has been recently confirmed at molecular scale resolution by several laboratories.[78]

VOLTAGE-GATED CALCIUM CHANNELS: ROLE OF $CA_V1.1$

Although the majority of mutations that confer MHS reside in the RyR1 gene, three mutations in the *CACNA1S* gene encoding for the $Ca_V1.1$ subunit of skeletal muscle have been linked to human MHS.[5,79-81] The Arg1086His mutation in the intracellular loop connecting homologous repeats III and IV of $Ca_V1.1$ represented the first MH-causing mutation so far identified in a protein other than RyR1. Physiological characterization of the R1086H mutation further demonstrated that sensitivity of RyR1 activity was significantly enhanced by membrane depolarization or by pharmacologic activators of RyR1 (e.g., caffeine).[82] In addition, Pirone and associates have identified an MHS-causing Thr1354Ser mutation in the S5-S6 extracellular pore-loop region of the homologous repeat IV of $Ca_V1.1$ Expression of the T1354S mutation also accelerated L-type Ca^{2+} current kinetics and also contributed to an increase in RyR1-mediated Ca^{2+} release.[81] The Arg174Trp $Ca_V1.1$ MH mutation occurs at the innermost basic residue of the IS4 voltage-sensing helix, a residue conserved among all Ca_V channels. Unlike the other $Ca_V1.1$ MHS mutations, homozygous expression of R174W completely ablates the L-type current, but despite this, has no influence on normal EC coupling. In murine studies, muscle fibers from Het R174W animals verify the increased sensitivity of Ca^{2+} release to caffeine and halothane compared with myotubes expressing wild type $Ca_V1.1$,[54,83] but whether this mutation is sufficient to confer anesthetic- or heat-triggered fulminant MH remains to be tested.

FACTORS OTHER THAN RYANODINE RECEPTOR ABNORMALITIES

Other cellular processes can affect MH episodes. It has been demonstrated that concurrent administration of nondepolarizing neuromuscular blocking drugs at the same time as triggering agents can delay or prevent the onset of clinical MH syndrome. Pretreatment of MHS pigs with sufficient nondepolarizing neuromuscular blocking agent, which is used to completely abolish muscle twitch elicited by electrical stimulation of the nerve, prevented halothane from triggering the clinical syndrome for 90 minutes, the longest time point tested.[84] However, in the continued presence of halothane, when function of the neuromuscular junction was restored by administration of the cholinesterase inhibitor neostigmine, clinical MH was triggered immediately. This suggested a close relationship between functional neuromuscular junctions or depolarization of the sarcolemma (or both) and the clinical syndrome.

In myotubes, sarcolemmal excitation-coupled Ca^{2+} entry (ECCE) is sensitive to the conformation of the RyR1 and is enhanced by several mutations in RyR1, including MH mutations.[44,52,85] ECCE appears to be an inherent property of $Ca_V1.1$ during long or repetitive depolarization of myotubes,[86] possibly mediated by shifting $Ca_V1.1$ to the mode 2 gating conformation. Nevertheless, enhanced ECCE in MHS muscle may contribute to an increased sensitivity to depolarization and appears to be one target for dantrolene's abrogation of responses to both electrical and potassium chloride depolarization.[51] Although CACNA1S expression undergoes developmental switching to a splice variant that downregulates Ca^{2+} current density of $Ca_V1.1$ channels in adult fibers, mutations that maintain Ca^{2+} current density more similar to those measured with embryonic myotubes has recently been shown to promote muscle pathology.[87]

In addition to ECCE, classic store-operated capacitive Ca^{2+} entry pathways similar to the store-operated Ca^{2+} entry (SOCE) seen in nonexcitable cells[88] have been shown to be present in skeletal muscle[89-91] and appear to be more active in MHS muscles both at rest as a response to chronic store depletion and during an MH crisis. These SOCE channels have also been suggested to be a target for dantrolene, but this has not been validated by other studies.[92] Together, these data suggest that $_{MH}$RyRs or $_{MH}Ca_V1.1$ assume a conformation that enhances Ca^{2+} entry via ECCE or SOCE (or both). This enhanced entry, when combined with decreased sensitivity of $_{MH}$RyRs to Ca^{2+} and Mg^{2+} inhibition, could provide cellular conditions that heighten sensitivity to triggering agents and perpetuate the fulminant clinical MH syndrome.

DANTROLENE

Dantrolene is the only medication that has been shown to be effective in reversing the symptoms of MH. Preadministration of dantrolene will also prevent the development of fulminant MH in homozygous pigs or MH mice when exposed to a triggering stimulus. Dantrolene sodium is a hydantoin derivative (1-[5-(4-nitrophenyl)-2-furanyl]methylene] imino]-2,4-imidazolidinedione) that does not block neuromuscular transmission, but causes muscle weakness by direct muscular action. The properties of dantrolene have been closely correlated with its ability to reduce efflux of Ca^{2+} from the SR in vitro.[93] Dantrolene (20 μM) counteracts the effect of reduced Mg^{2+} inhibition in MH-affected muscle.[94] Dantrolene (20 μM) can inhibit the enhanced sensitivity to caffeine seen in MH muscles, and both dantrolene and its more water-soluble analog azumolene (150 μM) have been shown to reduce depolarization-induced release of Ca^{2+}, both in muscle and in triadic vesicles.[95] The idea that dantrolene suppresses SR Ca^{2+} release as a result of direct interactions with RyR1 is somewhat controversial. Paul-Pletzer and associates demonstrated that [^{3}H]azidodantrolene specifically labels the amino terminus of RyR1 defined by the 1400-amino acid residue N-terminal calpain digestion fragment of RyR1.[96] More detailed analysis further localized the [^{3}H]azidodantrolene binding site to a single domain containing the core sequence corresponding to amino acid residues 590 through 609 of RyR1.[96] However, to date, we lack evidence of a direct action of dantrolene on single RyR1 channels studied in lipid bilayers, even though they are reconstituted with calstabin 1, ATP, and activating concentrations of Ca^{2+}, which suggests that dantrolene's main action is to alter key protein-protein interactions. The recent discovery that inhibition of SR Ca^{2+} release by dantrolene requires Mg^{2+} may help resolve the controversy of the conflicting observations on dantrolene inhibition of RyR1 channel activity in Mg^{2+}-free bilayer experiments.[27]

Genetics

RyR1 mutations have been found in 50% to 80% of patients and relatives who are labeled MHS by positive contracture tests and in almost all families with central core disease (CCD) and King-Denborough syndrome (KDS). More than 210 missense mutations and 8 deletions associated with MH have thus far been detected. Another 29 missense mutations are associated with CCD and multiminicore disease (MMD) in patients with unknown MH testing status.[10] Interestingly, 40% of missense *RyR1* mutations occur at CpG dinucleotide sequences. Five other loci (17q21-24, 1q32, 3q13, 7q21-24, and 5p) have been linked to families with both positive contracture tests and an unusual response to anesthesia, and have been designated MHS loci 2 through 6, respectively. However, of these five, the only gene that has been shown to be associated with MH is *CACNA1S*,[97] which codes for $Ca_V1.1$ (the α_{1S}-subunit of DHPR) in the MHS3 locus. Two causative mutations in this gene are linked to less than 1% of MHS families worldwide. In some of the other loci, all genes within the locus have been ruled out as causing susceptibility to MH. Hence for practical reasons, the *RyR1* gene remains the primary target for current clinical genetic analysis.

DISTRIBUTION OF *RyR1* MUTATIONS

The missense mutations associated with MHS, CCD, or, in some cases, both, are dispersed throughout the coding region of the *RyR1* gene, and all allow transcription of a protein that is putatively functional.[10,98] Until recently, it was thought that most *RyR1* mutations were clustered in three "hot spots:" between amino acid residues 35 and 614 (MH/CCD region 1), between amino acid residues 2163 and 2458 (MH/CCD region 2) in the sarcoplasmic foot region of the protein, and between amino acids 4643 and 4898 in the carboxyl-terminal transmembrane loop or pore region (MHS/CCD region 3) (Fig. 35.2).[99] It appears that the supposition that there were "hot spots" was simply due to bias in sample analysis inasmuch as the missense mutations associated with MH or CCD (or both) are scattered over 54 of the 107 exons of *RyR1*. Approximately 41% of reported MH

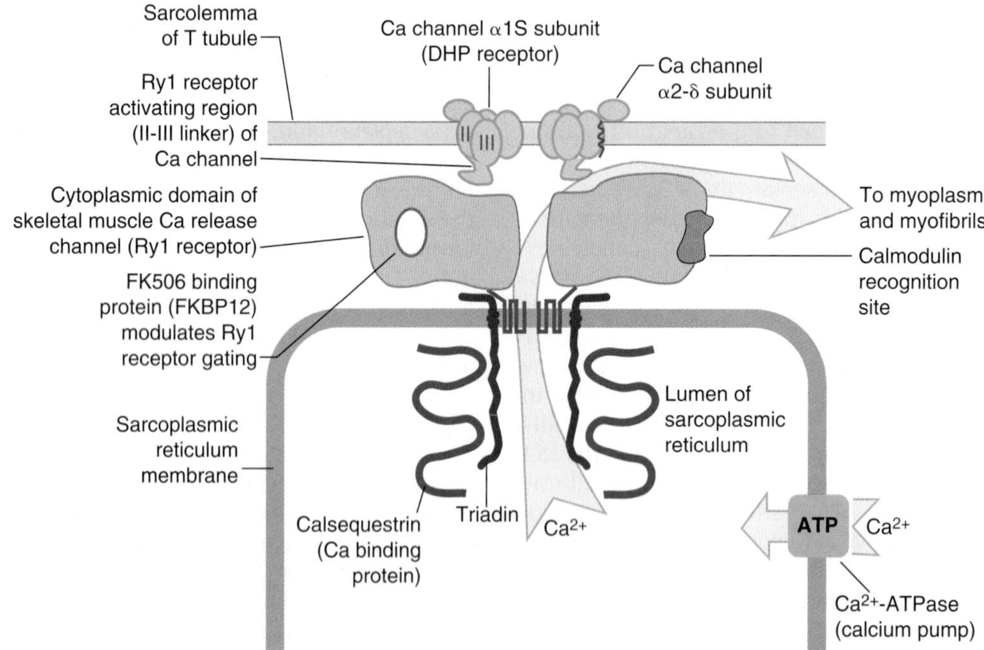

Fig. 35.2 Schematic representation of the triad junction of skeletal muscle shows the junctional foot protein (ryanodine [RyR1] receptor) and its associated proteins. In skeletal muscle, the α_{1S}-subunit of the dihydropyridine receptor *(DHPR)* participates in excitation-contraction coupling. These physical links transmit essential signals across the narrow gap of the triadic junction that activate the RyR1 and release Ca^{2+} from the sarcoplasmic reticulum. (Modified from Pessah IN, Lynch C III, Gronert GA: Complex pharmacology of malignant hyperthermia. *Anesthesiology* 1996;84:1275.)

mutations are found in multiple families. CCD mutations are predominantly found in the C-terminal region of the gene (exons 85-103), and only 10 mutations (17%) have been described in more than one family: R4861H (n = 14), V4849I (n = 9), I4898T (n = 7), L4824P (n = 4), A4940T (n = 4), G4638D (n = 3), R4893W (n = 3), R4861C (n = 2), R4893Q (n = 2), and G4899E (n = 2).

The true ethnic distribution of MH and CCD is difficult to ascertain. MH and CCD have been reported in Western populations predominantly, but this is likely the result of the manner and frequency in which cases are reported. It does appear that some mutations are clustered in a given region of the world, but the distribution and frequency appear to be somewhat population specific. In the United Kingdom, 69 *RyR1* mutations have been discovered, 25 of which are found only in a single family. G2434R is found in approximately 40% of the 434 mutation-positive MH families investigated in the United Kingdom, with the next most common mutations being T2206M (10%) and G341R (8%). In Switzerland, V2168M and I2336H are the predominant mutations,[100] and in Germany, R163C (MH and CCD), R614C (MH), T2206M (MH), G2434R (MH), and R2454H (MH) have each been detected in five or more independent cases.[101,102] G341R and R614C are common in France,[103] and R614C has also been found in several MH families from Italy[103] and Canada.[104] G341R has been found frequently in Belgium.[103] The mutation common to Europe and North America is G2434R, which occurs in 4% to 7% of European and 5.5% of North American families.[105] Single-family mutations are the most common mutations reported in Japanese, Chinese, Taiwanese, Australian, and New Zealand MH families with the exception of the R163C mutation reported in a large population in rural New South Wales in Australia and the T4826I mutation which is found in numerous families in the Maori population of New Zealand.[106-108] However, despite these two exceptions, it is likely that the reason for unique family mutations in Asia and Australasia may reflect the small number of cases investigated there. Because genetic screening in European and North American studies has predominantly targeted only regions 1 and 2 of the original hot spots in the gene, the absence of *RyR1* mutations in some of the screened population could be explained by *RyR1* mutations located outside these two regions or by involvement of other genes.

INHERITANCE AND PENETRANCE OF MALIGNANT HYPERTHERMIA

Inheritance of human MH can no longer be considered to be solely autosomal dominant with variable penetrance because more than one MH-linked mutation has been identified in some probands and families. Six non-consanguineous families harbor at least two *RyR1* mutations that have both been linked to MHS, and in two of those families, one is an *RyR1* mutation and the second is a $Ca_V1.1$ mutation.[5] Although MHS homozygotes are common in affected pigs, they are rare in humans and only found in 50% of currently available transgenic mouse populations. The known MHS homozygous humans also appear clinically normal, but exhibit stronger responses to in vitro contracture test (IVCT) and caffeine/halothane contracture tests (CHCTs) than heterozygous individuals do.[109-112] Homozygosity of two MH mutations in "hot spot" 1 leads to perinatal lethality in mice.[73,74] Double heterozygous individuals do not appear to show any additive effect of the second mutation on IVCT.[5]

IN VITRO CONTRACTURE TEST AND CAFFEINE HALOTHANE CONTRACTURE TEST

The gold standard for diagnosis of MH is the halothane and caffeine muscle contracture test, also known as the IVCT or the CHCT. There are two protocols developed by the European Malignant Hyperthermia Group (EMHG) and the North American Malignant Hyperthermia Group (NAMHG), respectively.[9] The two protocols are similar, but not identical. For the purpose of differentiation, we designate IVCT to the EMHG protocol and CHCT to the NAMHG protocol.

For IVCT, the muscle biopsy will be performed on the quadriceps (either vastus medialis or vastus lateralis)[113,114] and consists of three parts: a static caffeine test, a static halothane test, and a dynamic halothane test.[114] For the static caffeine test, a stepwise increased concentration (0.5, 1, 1.5, 2, 3, 4, and 32 mmol/L) is applied. The lowest concentration of caffeine which produces a sustained increase of at least 0.2 g in baseline tension is reported as the caffeine threshold. Then, the halothane threshold is obtained using the same method by exposing the muscle to halothane concentrations of 0.5%, 1%, 2%, and 3% v/v. The dynamic halothane test is performed with the muscle stretched at a constant rate of 4 mm/min to achieve a force of approximately 3 g and held at the new length for 1 min for a 3 min exposure to halothane. For each cycle, halothane concentration will be increased from 0.5%, 1%, 2%, to 3% v/v: volume (solute) per volume (solvent). The concentration of halothane which produces a sustained increase of at least 0.2 g in the muscle tension compared to the pre-halothane control is defined as the dynamic halothane threshold.[114] The IVCT protocol classifies the patients into three groups: MH Susceptible (MHS_{HC}) group with a caffeine threshold at the caffeine concentration of 2 mmol or less and a halothane threshold of 2% v/v halothane or less; MH Normal (MHN) group with a caffeine threshold at the caffeine concentration of 3 mmol or more without a halothane response at 2% v/v; MHS_H and MHS_C groups which describe individuals that used to be classified as MHE (equivocal) who are only responsive to either halothane or caffeine alone.[113,114] The MHE descriptor was dropped because use of the 'equivocal' label outside of its laboratory context has the potential to confuse patients and clinicians unfamiliar with its derivation.[115]

For CHCT, a muscle biopsy can be taken from the following sites in the order of preference: (1) the vastus group, (2) the rectus abdominis, and (3) other muscle groups under special circumstances.[116] Required tests include exposure of muscle to 3% v/v halothane alone and to incremental caffeine concentrations (0.5, 1, 2, 4 mmol, and 8.0 mmol if the response at 4 mmol is <1 g, and 32 mmol) alone. Optional tests include exposure of muscle to a combination of both 1% halothane and incremental caffeine concentrations, and to 2% v/v halothane alone.[116] According to CHCT protocol, an individual is MHS when either of the halothane or the caffeine test is positive, and MHN when both tests are negative.[116]

The sensitivity of IVCT was reported to be 99.0% (95% confidence interval [CI] 94.8%-100%) if the MHE group is considered susceptible and the specificity of IVCT was 93.6% (95% CI 89.2%-96.5%),[114] while the sensitivity and specificity of CHCT was 97% (95% CI 84%-100%) and 78% (95% CI 69%-85%), respectively.[117] Recently, fluoroquinolones and statins, 3-hydroxy-3-methylglutaryl-coenzyme A (HMG-CoA) reductase inhibitors, were found to induce significant contractures in MHS muscle bundles, but not in MHN.[118,119] Ondansetron and 3,4-methylenedioxymethamphetamine (MDMA) may also dose-dependently induce contracture or increase the sensitivity of the contractile apparatus to calcium in both MHS and MHN fibers.[120,121] Modifications to the IVCT protocol by adding ryanodine[122] or 4-chloro-*m*-cresol,[114,123] a RyR-specific agonist, has been reported, but has not been included in the standard protocol. Furthermore, Metterlein and associates studied the possibility of replacing halothane with newer volatile agents in IVCT. At increasing concentration, except for sevoflurane, all newer volatile agents, including enflurane, isoflurane, and desflurane, induced significantly greater contractures in MHS muscle compared to MHN bundles. However, within the MHS muscle bundles, halothane produced significantly higher contractures, and was considered the strongest discriminator for MH using the IVCT protocol.[124] A direct application of high sevoflurane concentration of 8%, instead of the stepwise application, has been shown to induce significantly stronger contractures in MHS subjects.[125] Nevertheless, from the retrospective analysis of the Japanese MH database, there was no evidence between the severity of MH triggered by sevoflurane and isoflurane, or other agents, suggesting sevoflurane is a weak or weaker MH triggering agent.[126]

DISCORDANCE BETWEEN GENETIC AND IN VITRO CONTRACTURE TEST/CAFFEINE/HALOTHANE CONTRACTURE TESTS MALIGNANT HYPERTHERMIA TESTING

Discordance has confounded linkage analysis worldwide. Examples include MHN patients carrying an *RyR1* mutation associated with MH and MHS patients who do not carry the familial *RyR1* mutation. Several explanations are possible, the most likely being that IVCT/CHCT is not clinically precise and that the thresholds for IVCT or CHCT are inexact. This would lead to errors in determining whether a patient was MHN or MHS. A second possibility is variable penetrance with possible allelic silencing,[127] and a third is that individuals with discordance have mutations in other unknown genes or modifier genes that affect the function of *RyR1* and its phenotypic penetrance. The discrepancy between the incidence estimates of MH events and the prevalence estimates also points to possible epigenetic factors at work. Carpenter and associates have suggested that the severity of MHS may be related to the *RyR1* variant and mutation found within the highly conserved regions of *RyR1* gene.[79] The rarity of large kindreds with MH makes linkage analysis and understanding variability in clinical manifestations difficult. Robinson and associates demonstrated by the transmission disequilibrium test that loci on chromosomes 5 and 7 and, to a lesser extent, loci on chromosomes 1 and 7 influence susceptibility to MH.[103]

GUIDELINES FOR GENETIC SCREENING

In 2000, the European MH group (EMHG) formulated guidelines for *RyR1* mutation screening with linkage data to other loci for some MH families, but all MH investigators emphasized the vital role of IVCT in the diagnosis of MH.[128] These guidelines for screening have reduced the number of relatives requiring contracture testing without increasing the risk of misdiagnosis.[129,130] In 2015, the EMHG published a revision of the guidelines for the investigation of MHS. This updated guideline provided a detailed patient referral criteria and clinical interpretation of IVCT results (https://www.emhg.org/testing-for-mh-1).

Only a small number of MHS families have been investigated extensively in North America by phenotyping, linkage analysis, and screening of specific genes. Collaborative protocols over the past several years between MH biopsy centers and molecular biologists have screened 209 unrelated MHS subjects for mutations in the *RyR1* gene (see Distribution of *RyR1* Mutations).

Larach and coworkers reported a 34.8% morbidity rate in 181 MH cases reported to the NAMHR between January 1987 and December 2006. They also reported that the occurrence was more frequent in young males (75%) (median age of 22.0) and 75% of these patients had undergone at least one general anesthetic with no observed signs of MHS.[131] This underscores the complication of determining the prevalence of MHS in the absence of an inexpensive MH diagnostic test.

Fulminant Malignant Hyperthermia

Fulminant MH is rare. Acute episodes of MH depend on four variables: a genetic (perhaps rarely acquired) predisposition, the absence of inhibiting factors, the presence of an anesthetic or nonanesthetic trigger, and the presence of environmental factors that could potentiate the action of one or more of the other three variables.

ANESTHETIC TRIGGERING

Anesthetic drugs that trigger MH include ether, halothane, enflurane, isoflurane, desflurane, sevoflurane, and depolarizing muscle relaxants, the only currently used of which is succinylcholine. Desflurane and sevoflurane appear to be less potent triggers than halothane and produce a more gradual onset of MH.[132,133] The onset may be explosive if succinylcholine is used. MHS swine were traditionally screened by induction with a volatile anesthetic, which led to pronounced hind limb rigidity within 5 minutes, frequently sooner.[134] Prior exercise even an hour before induction of anesthesia increased the severity and hastened the onset of rigidity in swine.[134] Similarly, in the new knock-in mouse models, the onset of limb rigidity after commencing exposure to volatile anesthetics is very rapid. There are also several modifying factors that are more likely to be present in humans than in pigs or mice and can alter (or even prevent) the onset of clinical MH. Mild hypothermia and preadministration of barbiturates, tranquilizers, propofol, or nondepolarizing neuromuscular blockers delay or prevent the onset of MH[25,134-136] in MHS humans, thus making them respond less predictably than swine or MH knock-in mice. There have been many instances in which fulminant MH has been reported in patients who have previously tolerated potent triggers without difficulty.[137] The reason behind why this occurs is unknown, but it is likely to be related to prior or concurrent administration of drugs that prevent or delay onset of the syndrome, as described earlier, or unknown environmental influences that help provoke the positive incident. Thus onset of the syndrome in humans is extremely variable both in initial symptoms and in the time of onset of the syndrome. Its onset is so variable that making the diagnosis in the setting of a clinical anesthetic can be quite difficult. Although not perfect, the clinical grading scale developed by Larach and colleagues[138] is a useful way for clinicians to retrospectively determine whether a patient who responded abnormally to anesthesia is in any way likely to actually have had a clinical MH episode. However, MH is most easily diagnosed prospectively by vigilance, recognizing its signs and symptoms, and knowing how to treat the syndrome.

The two classic clinical manifestations of fulminant MH syndrome may start in one of the following two scenarios.

1. Rigidity after induction with thiopental and succinylcholine, but successful intubation, followed rapidly by the symptoms listed after scenario 2.
2. Normal response to induction of anesthesia and uneventful anesthetic course until onset of the following symptoms:

- Unexplained sinus tachycardia or ventricular arrhythmias, or both
- Tachypnea if spontaneous ventilation is present
- Unexplained decrease in O_2 saturation (because of a decrease in venous O_2 saturation)
- Increased end-tidal PCO_2 with adequate ventilation (and in most cases unchanged ventilation)
- Unexpected metabolic and respiratory acidosis
- Central venous desaturation
- Increase in body temperature above 38.8°C with no obvious cause

The usually muted onset of MH (scenario 2) is in most cases detected quickly by the development of tachycardia, increased levels of expired CO_2, and muscle rigidity. It can be delayed for several reasons and may not be overt until the patient is in the recovery room. Once initiated, the course of MH can be rapid. When clinical signs such as increased expired CO_2, muscle rigidity, tachycardia, and fever suggest MH, more than one abnormal sign must be observed before making the diagnosis because according to a metaanalysis of many reported cases, a single adverse sign does not usually indicate MH.[138] The mechanism by which anesthetics and depolarizing muscle relaxants trigger MH is unsolved, *but* it cannot be ignored that they are etiologic agents and that early diagnosis is critical for successful treatment.

NONANESTHETIC MALIGNANT HYPERTHERMIA

MH can be triggered by stress such as exercise and overheating, known as "awake" MH. Numerous anecdotal reports of MH-like episodes in humans after stressful situations were reported.[139-144] Measurement of plasma catecholamine levels during exercise showed no differences between MHS and normal individuals.[145,146] Therefore it is unlikely that these responses were provoked by sympathetic overdrive or catecholamine surge.[147]

Wappler and associates reported *RyR1* mutations in three of twelve unrelated patients with exercise-induced rhabdomyolysis (ER); and 10 of those same 12 patients produced abnormal contracture response with IVCT.[148] One had an equivocal response. In susceptible swine, environmental stress such as exercise, heat, anoxia, apprehension, and excitement triggers fulminant MH (see History).[9,134] These responses are related to muscle movement or to increased temperature. Increased ambient temperature triggers fulminant MH in four strains of heterozygous MH mice and in two homozygous strains.[74,75] Epidemiologic studies have shown that exercise-induced symptoms, including rhabdomyolysis, may occur more frequently in MHS patients[148]; and an Arg401Cys *RyR1* mutation was present in three cases of exercise-induced rhabdomyolysis.[106] Other reports are largely anecdotal and relate heat stroke, sudden and unexpected death, unusual stress and fatigue, or myalgias to possible "awake" MH episodes. Stresses associated with these episodes include exercise and environmental exposure to volatile nonanesthetic vapors.[141,149,150] In the United States, MHAUS provided recommendations of adverse effects of heat and exercise in relation to MHS.[151]

Malignant Hyperthermia–Associated Syndromes

MASSETER SPASM ("THIOPENTAL-SUCCINYLCHOLINE OR HALOTHANE-SUCCINYLCHOLINE RIGIDITY")

A masseter spasm or trismus is defined as jaw muscle rigidity in association with limb muscle flaccidity after the administration of succinylcholine. The masseter and lateral pterygoid muscles contain slow tonic fibers that can respond to depolarizing neuromuscular blockers with a contracture.[152,153] This is manifested clinically on exposure to succinylcholine as an increase in jaw muscle tone, and was well defined by van der Spek and associates.[154] There is a spectrum of responses, for example, a tight jaw that becomes a rigid jaw and then a very rigid jaw (Fig. 35.3). This jaw rigidity may occur even after pretreatment with a "defasciculating" dose of a nondepolarizing relaxant. If there is rigidity of other muscles in addition to trismus, the association with MH is absolute; anesthesia should be halted as soon as possible and treatment of MH begun.

However, in more than 80% of patients with trismus but no rigidity of other muscles, it is a variant found in normal patients. If trismus occurs, proper monitoring should include end-expired CO_2, examination for pigmenturia, and arterial or venous blood sampling for CK, acid-base status, and electrolyte levels, particularly potassium. Although scientifically unproven, it is thought that the initial tightness of the jaw and its duration may predict the gravity of the response. MHAUS recommends following CK and urine myoglobin for 36 hours with 6-hour intervals. Patients with masseter spasm should be observed closely for at least 12 hours.

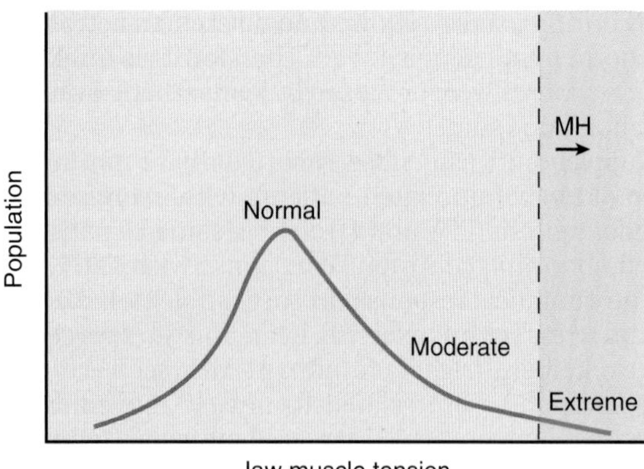

Fig. 35.3 Succinylcholine usually increases jaw muscle tone slightly. In some patients this increase is moderate, and in very few, the effect is extreme (i.e., "jaws of steel"). As many as 50% of this latter group may be susceptible to malignant hyperthermia *(MH)*. Somewhere in the area of the declining curve is the boundary for the MH population.

CORE MYOPATHIES

CCD is a rare hereditary disease. It was first reported in 1956 by Magee and Shy.[155] A recent population study in northern England revealed a prevalence of 1:250,000.[156] In 1971, Engel and colleagues reported a related congenital myopathy, multicore disease.[157,158] Subsequently, various designations of the terms were reported for the variations of the disease, including minicore myopathy and multiminicore myopathy.[157] MmD is now the most official term for these variations sponsored by the European Neuromuscular Centre.[157]

As mentioned, most CCD cases are due to dominant missense mutations in the RyR1 gene. Clinically, CCD patients present with muscle weakness of variable degree and histologically with central cores in the skeleton muscle type I fibers.[159] MmD is considered a recessively inherited myopathy with severe axial weakness, while respirator, bulbar, and extraocular muscles are commonly affected.[159] MmD has a heterogenous genetic association with a recessive mutation in the SEPN1 gene on chromosome 1p36 and in the RyR1 gene.[159] Both type 1 and type 2 fibers may be affected.[157]

Serum CK levels in CCD patients are often normal but may be elevated up to 6 to 14 times in rare cases. Muscle ultrasound often demonstrates increased echogenicity in the quadriceps muscle with relative sparing of the rectus muscle. This characteristic pattern of selective involvement can also be seen on the muscle MRI and has been reported in the patients with typical CCD,[157] which seems to be distinctive to conditions linked to *RyR1* locus.

The relationship between CCD and MHS is complex. A positive IVCT test has been confirmed in many patients with CCD, whereas MHS has been excluded in some. In consideration of the strong link and potential risk, it is advisable to consider all patients with CCD at risk for MH unless the patient has a negative IVCT. Although MHS has not been reported in *SEPN1*-related myopathies, it is prudent to apply a nontriggering approach to MmD patients, given the potential risk in *RyR1*-related MmD. Clinical MH reactions have been reported in MmD patients.[160,161]

KING-DENBOROUGH SYNDROME

To address the KDS, we first introduce Noonan syndrome, an autosomal dominant condition involving the face, cardiovascular, hematological, and skeletal systems. Named after Dr. Jacquline Anne Noonan, a pediatric cardiologist, typical Noonan syndrome features delayed puberty, down-slanting or wide-set eyes, hearing loss, low-set or abnormal shaped ears, mild mental retardation (in about 25% of the cases), ptosis, short statue, small penis and undescended testicles in males, pectus excavatum, and a webbed and short neck. The incidence is 1:1000-1:2500 live births.[162] Fifty percent of the patients have protein-tyrosine phosphatase, nonreceptor-type II (*PTPN2*) mutations.[163] Other genes involved are *SOS1*, *KRAS*, *RAF1*, *BRAF*, *MEK1*, and *NRAS*, and they encode proteins that are part of the Ras (a GTPase)-mitogen activated protein kinase (RAS-MAPK) signaling pathway.[164] Noonan syndrome was recently defined as part of the neuro-cardio-facial-cutaneous syndrome family.[165] An earlier study with a series of 27 patients demonstrated one case of mildly elevated CK despite multiple uneventful cases of general anesthesia with halothane and succinylcholine.[166] Although there is weak evidence for MHS for patients with Noonan syndrome, its resemblances to KDS should raise the concern for the confirmation of the diagnosis. Prevalence of bleeding disorders in Noonan syndrome was reported to be from 20% to 89%,[164] ranging from thrombocytopenia to platelet dysfunction to von Willebrand disease to factor deficiencies. Routine screening including, but not limited to, bleeding history, platelet count, coagulation panel, and factor XI level, was recommended.[165,167] Hematological consultation becomes appropriate if any of these tests are abnormal. The high palatal arch, dental malocclusion, and the webbed neck of Noonan syndrome make tracheal intubation potentially risky.[168] Nevertheless, odontoid hypoplasia and atlantoaxial instability may result in cervical cord compression. Preoperative cervical spine evaluation is advisable.[169] Right ventricular function needs to be monitored closely because 30% to 50% of the patients with Noonan syndrome have pulmonary stenosis.[170] Regional anesthesia in Noonan patients may be technically challenging due to the prevalence of scoliosis. The spread of local anesthetic can be unpredictable.[169,171]

KDS features the dysmorphic facial and skeletal abnormalities similar to Noonan syndrome and congenital myopathy with proximal muscle weakness.[163] Sporadic cases have been reported in the literature.[172-181] The inheritance pattern of the disease is not clear. Elevated baseline CK appears in approximately one half of the KDS patients. A heterozygous A97G point mutation in exon 2 of the *RyR1*, causing a substitution of lysine for glutamine at amino acid residue 33 (Lys33Glu), was reported.[182] This substitution creates a major polarity change, from positive to negative, in a known hot spot for an MH causative mutation. Dowling and associates recently identified *RyR1* mutation in three out of the four patients with KDS, which supports the hypothesis of its genetic heterogeneity.[183] Given the strong evidence for MHS in KDS patients, MH triggering agents should be avoided for anesthesia on KDS patients.

BOX 35.1 Clinical Signs of Malignant Hyperthermia

Early Signs

Elevated end-tidal CO_2
Tachypnea and/or tachycardia
Masseter spasm if succinylcholine has been used
Generalized muscle rigidity
Mixed metabolic and respiratory acidosis
Profuse sweating
Mottling of skin
Cardiac arrhythmias
Unstable blood pressure

Late Signs

Hyperkalemia
Rapid increase of core body temperature
Elevated creatine phosphokinase levels
Gross myoglobinemia and myoglobinuria
Cardiac arrest
Disseminated intravascular coagulation

BOX 35.2 Conditions and Disorders that May Mimic Malignant Hyperthermia

Anaphylactic reaction
Alcohol therapy for limb arteriovenous malformation
Contrast dye injection
Cystinosis
Diabetic coma
Drug toxicity or abuse
Elevated end-tidal CO_2 due to laparoscopic operation
Environmental heat gain more than loss
Equipment malfunction with increased carbon dioxide
Exercise hyperthermia
Freeman-Sheldon syndrome
Generalized muscle rigidity
Heat stroke
Hyperthyroidism
Hyperkalemia
Hypokalemic periodic paralysis
Hypoventilation or low fresh gas flow
Increased $ETCO_2$ from laparoscopic surgery
Insufficient anesthesia and/or analgesia
Malignant neuroleptic syndrome
Muscular dystrophies (Duchenne and Becker)
Myoglobinuria
Myotonias
Osteogenesis imperfecta
Pheochromocytoma
Prader-Willi syndrome
Recreational drugs
Rhabdomyolysis
Sepsis
Serotonin syndrome
Stroke
Thyroid crisis
Ventilation problems
Wolf-Hirschhorn syndrome

Diagnosis in the Operating Room and Postanesthesia Care Unit

As stated earlier, fulminant MH is rare, and early signs of clinical MH may be subtle (Box 35.1). These signs must be distinguished from other disorders with similar signs (Box 35.2).

When the diagnosis is obvious (i.e., fulminant MH or succinylcholine-induced rigidity with rapid metabolic changes), marked hypermetabolism and heat production occur, and there may be little time left for specific therapy to prevent death or irreversible morbidity. If the syndrome begins with slowly increasing end-tidal CO_2 (defined earlier), specific therapy can await a complete clinical workup before treatment. In general, MH is not expected to occur when no triggers are administered (see "Anesthesia for Susceptible Patients"). However, several confirmed fulminant nonanesthetic cases of MH that resulted in death have been reported (see "Nonanesthetic Malignant Hyperthermia").[148]

When volatile anesthetics or succinylcholine are used, MH should be suspected whenever there is an unexpected increase in end-tidal CO_2 ($ETCO_2$), undue tachycardia, tachypnea, arrhythmias, mottling of the skin, cyanosis, muscle rigidity, sweating, increased body temperature, or unstable blood pressure. If any of these occur, signs of increased metabolism, acidosis, or hyperkalemia must be sought. The most common cause for sudden $ETCO_2$ during general anesthesia and sedation is hypoventilation. Increased minute ventilation should be able to correct such a problem.

The diagnosis of MH can be supported by the analysis of arterial or venous blood gases which demonstrates a mixed respiratory and metabolic acidosis;[184] however, the respiratory component of acidosis may be predominate in the very early stage of the onset of fulminant MH. O_2 and CO_2 change more markedly in the central venous compartment than in arterial blood; therefore end-expired or venous CO_2 levels more accurately reflect whole-body stores. Venous CO_2, unless the blood drains an area of increased metabolic activity, should have PCO_2 levels of only about 5 mm Hg greater than that of expected or measured $PaCO_2$. In small children, particularly those without oral food or fluid for a prolonged period, the base deficit may be 5 mEq/L because of their smaller energy stores.

Any patient suspected of having an MH episode should be reported to the North American MH Registry via the adverse metabolic/muscular reaction to anesthesia (AMRA) report available from the website at http://anest.ufl.edu/namhr/namhr-report-forms/.

TREATMENT

Acute management for MH can be summarized as follows:

1. Discontinue all triggering anesthetics, maintain intravenous agents, such as sedatives, opioids, and nondepolarizing muscular blockers as needed, and hyperventilate with 100% oxygen with a fresh flow to at least 10 L/min. With increased aerobic metabolism, normal ventilation must increase. However, CO_2 production is also increased because of neutralization of fixed acid by bicarbonate; hyperventilation removes this additional CO_2.
2. Administer dantrolene rapidly (2.5 mg/kg intravenously [IV] to a total dose of 10 mg/kg IV) every 5 to 10 minutes until the initial symptoms subside.

3. Administer bicarbonate (1-4 mEq/kg IV) to correct the metabolic acidosis with frequent monitoring of blood gases and pH.
4. Control fever by administering iced fluids, cooling the body surface, cooling body cavities with sterile iced fluids, and if necessary, using a heat exchanger with a pump oxygenator. Cooling should be halted at 38°C to prevent inadvertent hypothermia.
5. Monitor and treat arrhythmia. Advanced cardiac life support protocol may be applied.
6. Monitor and maintain urinary output to greater than 1 to 2 mL/kg/h and establish diuresis if urine output is inadequate. Administer bicarbonate to alkalinize urine to protect the kidney from myoglobinuria-induced renal failure.
7. Further therapy is guided by blood gases, electrolytes, CK, temperature, muscle tone, and urinary output. Hyperkalemia should be treated with bicarbonate, glucose, and insulin, typically 10 units of regular insulin and 50 mL of 50% dextrose for adult patients. The most effective way to lower serum potassium is reversal of MH by effective doses (ED) of dantrolene. In severe cases, calcium chloride or calcium gluconate may be used.
8. Recent data demonstrated that magnesium level could be a prerequisite for dantrolene efficacy in managing MH crisis.
9. Analyze coagulation studies (e.g., international normalized ratio [INR], platelet count, prothrombin time, fibrinogen, fibrin split, or degradation products).
10. Once the initial reaction is controlled, continued monitoring in the intensive care unit for 24 to 48 hours is usually recommended.

Adequate personnel support is critical to the successful management of such a crisis. Discontinuation of the trigger may be adequate therapy for acute MH if the onset is slow or if exposure was brief. Changing the breathing circuit and CO_2 absorbent can be time-consuming. However, application of activated charcoal filters may rapidly reduce the volatile anesthetic concentration to an acceptable level in less than2 minutes, if they are readily available.[185]

Dantrolene used to be packaged in 20-mg bottles with sodium hydroxide for a pH of 9.5 (otherwise it will not dissolve) and with 3 g of mannitol (converts the hypotonic solution to isotonic). The initial dose should be 2.5 mg/kg dantrolene reconstituted in sterile water and administered intravenously. Dantrolene *must* be reconstituted in sterile water rather than salt solutions or it will precipitate. It has been shown that prewarming of sterile water may expedite the solubilization of dantrolene compared to water in ambient temperature.[186] In 2009, a newer, rapid soluble lyophilized powder form of dantrolene became available for intravenous use. It reconstitutes in less than a minute which is much faster than the older version.[187] The higher dosing capacity, 250 mg per vial, of the newer version of dantrolene also reduces the storage space with a similar recommended shelf life as the older versions.

In awake, healthy volunteers, the maximum twitch depression occurs at a dantrolene dose of 2.4 mg/kg.[188] Therefore it is not surprising that at therapeutic concentrations, dantrolene may prolong the need for intubation and assisted ventilation. Brandom and associates reviewed the complications associated with the administration of dantrolene from 1987 to 2006 using the dataset in the NAMHR via the AMRA reports and found that the most frequent complications of dantrolene were muscle weakness (21.7%), phlebitis (9%), gastrointestinal upset (4.1%), respiratory failure (3.8%), hyperkalemia (3.3%), and excessive secretions (8.2%).[189] Given its high pH, it is advisable to administer dantrolene through a large bore IV line. It has been demonstrated that dantrolene interferes with EC coupling of murine intestinal smooth muscle cells,[190] rat gastric fundus, and colon,[191] which in part explains its gastrointestinal side effect. Caution should be used when ondansetron is to be used in this setting. As a serotonin antagonist, ondansetron may increase serotonin at the 5-HT_{2A} receptor in the presynaptic space. In MHS individuals, agonism of 5-HT_{2A} receptor may produce a deranged response, precipitating MH.[192]

The clinical course will determine further therapy and studies. Dantrolene should probably be repeated at least every 10 to 15 hours, since it has a half-life of at least 10 hours in children and adults.[188,193] The total dose of dantrolene that can be used is up to 30 mg/kg in some cases. Recrudescence of MH can approach 50%, usually within 6.5 hours.[194,195] When indicated, calcium and cardiac glycosides may be used safely. They can be lifesaving during persistent hyperkalemia. Slow voltage-gated calcium channel blockers do not increase porcine survival.[196,197] Instead, a recent study by Migita demonstrated that calcium channel blockers, including dihydropyridine (i.e., nifedipine), phenylalkylamine (i.e., verapamil), and benzothiazepine (i.e., diltiazem), led to increased $[Ca^{2+}]_i$ in human skeletal muscle cells. Interestingly, the potency of such calcium release is correlated with the number of binding sites on DHPR (i.e., nifedipine > verapamil > diltiazem).[198] Clinical doses of dantrolene were only able to attenuate 20% of the nifedipine-induced $[Ca^{2+}]_i$ surge. [198] Current recommendations of MHAUS discourage the use of calcium channel blockers in the presence of dantrolene because they can worsen the hyperkalemia resulting in cardiac arrest. Although administration of magnesium sulfate could not prevent the development of MH and did not influence the clinical course in succinylcholine-induced MH,[199] recent data suggested that dantrolene might require magnesium to arrest the course of MH triggered by halothane.[200] Permanent neurologic sequelae, such as coma or paralysis, may occur in advanced cases, probably because of inadequate cerebral oxygenation and perfusion for the increased metabolism and because of the fever, acidosis, hypo-osmolality with fluid shifts, and potassium release.

For MH cases diagnosed in the ambulatory surgical centers, guidelines have been recently proposed for the transferring of care to receiving hospital facilities.[201] Although it is preferable that immediate treatment and stabilization of the patient be achieved onsite, several factors need to be considered before implementation of a transfer plan, which include capabilities of the available professionals at the initial treatment and receiving facilities, clinical best interests of patients, and capabilities of the transfer team.[202] The validity of stocking dantrolene in ambulatory surgery centers was confirmed with a cost-effectiveness analysis.[203]

Anesthesia for Susceptible Patients

Safe anesthetics consist of nitrous oxide, barbiturates, etomidate, propofol, opiates, tranquilizers, and nondepolarizing muscle relaxants. Potent volatile anesthetics and succinylcholine must be avoided, even in the presence of dantrolene. There are anecdotal reports that some human patients have experienced a hypermetabolic state despite these precautions, but they have always responded favorably to the administration of intravenous dantrolene. Preoperative dantrolene is never needed because the use of nontriggering agents is almost always associated with uneventful anesthesia. Regional anesthesia is safe and may be preferred. Amide anesthetics such as lidocaine were once considered dangerous in susceptible patients because they were thought to induce or worsen muscle contractures in vitro as a result of their effect of increasing calcium efflux from the SR. Porcine and human studies have consistently demonstrated the lack of danger of amide anesthetics.

Before being used for MHS patients, anesthetic machines may be "cleansed" of potent volatile agents by disconnecting or removing the vaporizers from the anesthesia workstation, renewing the CO_2 absorbent, using a new, disposable breathing circuit, and, if possible, a fresh gas hose. If there is no dedicated machine for MHS patients, flushing the anesthesia workstation to less than5 parts per million (ppm) of the volatile anesthetic agents concentration is generally accepted.[204] It may take 10 to 104 min with different machines.[185,205-214] This preparation process also should be directed based on the halogenated volatile agents that have been used. Jones and colleagues demonstrated that desflurane required longer purge time than sevoflurane on both the Datex-Ohmeda Aestiva and Aisys machines.[213] Application of activated charcoal filters have been shown to successfully accelerate the process of cleansing.[185,215-217] Such filters should be placed on both the inspiratory and expiratory limbs of the anesthesia machine with replacement of a new set every 60 minutes on patients who are exhaling volatile anesthetics.[185] MHAUS recommends flushing and preparing the anesthesia workstation according to the manufacturer's recommendations or published studies.[218] During the case, lowering the fresh gas rate after the washout period may allow the concentration of volatile anesthetic agents to reaccumulate.[209] Fresh gas flow should be kept to at least 10 L/min to avoid this rebound.

It is important to be aware that the National Institute for Occupational Safety and Health issued "Criteria for a Recommended Standard- Occupational Exposure to Waste Anesthetic Gases (WAGs) and Vapors."[219] No worker is exposed to halogenated anesthetic agents at concentrations greater than 2 ppm when used alone or greater than 0.5 ppm when used in combination with nitrous oxide over a sampling period not to exceed 1 hour. Anesthetic gas machines, non-rebreathing systems, and T-tube devices shall have an effective scavenging device that collects all WAGs. Occupational Safety and Health Administration also has guidelines for workplace exposures.[220]

The anesthesiologist should confidently discuss anesthetic care with MHS patients and assure them that all will be done to avoid difficulties with MH and that the appropriate drugs, knowledge, and skills are immediately at hand if any problems occur. Many of these patients have undergone procedures uneventfully, such as dental analgesia and obstetric anesthesia, before the diagnosis of susceptibility was made. The patient can enter the therapeutic environment in a reassured, relaxed, and comfortable state. Outpatient procedures are feasible in most environments; the time of discharge depends on the usual outpatient criteria.

Any facility using MH triggers on an inpatient or outpatient basis should have dantrolene available immediately. The current recommendation by MHAUS to stock 36 vials of 20 mg dantrolene Dantrium/Revonto is based on dantrolene needed to treat an MH crisis on a 70-kg patient.[187] FDA approved the Ryanodex in 2014. Administration of three vials of 250 mg Ryanodex injectable suspension is the alternative preparation plan.

EVALUATION OF SUSCEPTIBILITY

Evaluation of susceptibility includes a history and physical examination to detect any subclinical abnormality. A genealogy with specific information about anesthetic exposure and agents can estimate the likelihood of exposure to triggering agents. Blood CK values, when determined in a resting, fasting state without recent trauma, reflect muscle membrane stability. When the CK level is elevated in a close relative of a person with known MHS, the relative may be considered to have MHS without contracture testing. If the CK level is normal on several occasions, there is no predictive value, and contracture studies are necessary. The patient must travel to the test center for a surgical biopsy to ensure viability and accurate results. Muscle biopsy contracture studies, performed at about 30 centers around the world, involve exposure of the muscle biopsy sample to halothane, caffeine, and, in the North American test, to halothane plus caffeine.[128] Sensitivity to 4-chloro-*m*-cresol or ryanodine have also been used by some centers.[52] It is also important to note that contracture responses are sometimes positive in patients with myopathies that bear no direct relationship to MH and therefore may not indicate susceptibility. Dantrolene must be avoided before biopsy because it masks the response to contracture-producing drugs. After a patient is diagnosed as being MHS, DNA testing for mutations should follow. When a mutation is detected, other relatives with that mutation should be considered to be MHS without the need for an invasive contracture test, and they need not travel to a testing center (see Genetics).

MHS patients and all patients who are not biopsy tested, but who present with a clinical picture that suggests a high probability for MHS, should be given advice. Precautions are necessary in regard to general anesthesia, and triggers include all potent volatile agents and succinylcholine. Awake episodes are uncommon, and if not experienced before diagnosis, they are an unlikely problem. The true predictive value (i.e., percentage of positive results that are true positives) or efficiency (i.e., percentage of all results that are true, whether positive or negative) of contracture testing in determining susceptibility in the general population cannot be estimated because of the selection process that has been used to date for testing (i.e., limited to those with anesthesia reactions who do not have any other muscle disease pathology). False-positive results from cautious interpretation or decreased specificity are masked because the patient will never be exposed to triggering agents. A promising innovative in vivo human application involves physiologically based microdialysis infusion of caffeine or halothane into muscle of MHS patients to trigger exaggerated localized changes in acid-base balance.[221-225] White blood cells express RyR1-MHS and provide a substrate for a less invasive analysis for susceptibility but have the limitation that not all causative mutations are expressed in the white blood cells.[226-230] Nuclear magnetic resonance has promise,[231,232] but to date it has been difficult to standardize a stress, such as forearm ischemia, that can differentiate susceptibles from normals.

For anesthesia assessment of the non-MHS pregnant patient carrying a potential MHS fetus, the parturient should be treated as MHS until the fetus is delivered.[233-235] For emergencies in such patients, the use of succinylcholine, although little of the drug crosses the placenta, is controversial.[236]

Multiple Sclerosis

Multiple sclerosis (MS) is an autoimmune disorder characterized by T-cell–mediated autoantibodies against myelin and a subsequent inflammatory response within the central nervous system (CNS: brain and spinal cord), where it primarily affects the optic nerve, the corticospinal tract, or posterior columns. Thus MS is a disorder of the myelinated part of the axon that leads to secondary nerve conduction failure. It is characterized by sensitization of the peripheral leukocytes to the myelin antigen and a subsequent inflammatory response, monocytic and lymphocytic perivascular cuffing, and glial scars with plaque formation within the central nervous system, especially in the periventricular white matter. The disease affects mainly women, primarily between 20 and 40 or 45 and 60 years of age. Although the etiology is unknown, it has been speculated that MS is caused by environmental factors combined with a genetic predisposition. Naturally, researchers have focused on identifying key events and the genetic origin of the disorder to provide diagnostic and possibly also therapeutic tools for the management of MS patients.

Its clinical course is characterized by exacerbations and remissions in most patients, but continuous neurological deterioration has been reported in up to 10% of cases (primary progressive MS). Patients with MS frequently report paresthesias, muscle weakness, and sensory disturbances. Acute symptoms, which are related to the site and extent of sclerosing CNS plaques, commonly include visual disturbances (diplopia, blurring, and field cuts), sensory abnormalities with numbness and paresthesia, pain, and electric shock sensation that radiates down the spine and into the limbs upon flexion of the neck (Lhermitte sign). Cranial nerve dysfunction, ataxia, and bladder and bowel disturbances are also common. Typically, there is a localized or, late in the course of disease, generalized muscle weakness with the legs affected more than the arms. Chronic symptoms can also include spastic paraparesis, appendicular tremor, psychiatric disturbances such as depression or euphoria (la belle indifference), and dementia. In severe cases, respiration may be involved with the development of hypoxemia. As a rule, symptoms are closely related to the site affected within the CNS, and the number of symptoms is related to the extent of sclerosing CNS plaques. Notably, MS can be associated with impaired autonomic function, and hence an increased risk for exaggerated hemodynamic response to anesthetic induction agents, vasodilators, and sympathomimetic drugs.[237]

Diagnosing MS after a single, acute remitting clinically isolated syndrome is discouraged, whereas repeated attacks with increased CSF IgG and multifocal MRI abnormalities are strongly supportive of the diagnosis.[238] Acute attacks are treated with various combinations of immunosuppression modalities including glucocorticoids or plasma exchange therapy, which have been shown to increase the rate of recovery but not the overall level of recovered function. Disease progression can, nevertheless, be modified with a novel humanized CD20 monoclonal antibody (ocrelizumab) in patients with primary-progressive or relapsing-remitting forms of MS. Other immunomodulatory treatment options include interferon β1a or glatiramer acetate (a mixture of polypeptides synthesized to mimic myelin basic protein) in individuals with the relapsing-remitting MS, fingolimod, teriflunomide, or natalizumab, and the antineoplastic agent mitoxantrone. Teriflunomide is associated with hepatic injury, while mitoxantrone can be associated with cardiomyopathy. These patients may also receive treatments aimed at reducing spasticity (baclofen and benzodiazepines), as well as anticonvulsants or propranolol for tremor, oxybutynin and propantheline for bladder spasticity, and SSRIs or other antidepressive agents for mood disorders.

ANESTHETIC CONSIDERATIONS

It has been speculated that general anesthesia and surgery may increase the risk for aggravation of MS.[239] Presently, there is no general consensus on this matter, and patients should therefore be informed of the potential for aggravated symptoms in the postoperative period. In general, preoperative chronic immunosuppressive medication should be continued during the perioperative period. Patients with MS are sensitive to physical (pain, fever, infection) and emotional stress, which makes it more likely that symptoms will be intensified in the perioperative period. Increased body temperature is often cited as an offending mechanism, possibly by causing a complete block of conduction in demyelinated nerves. Body temperature should therefore be closely monitored and controlled during the perioperative period. Great care must be exercised to minimize changes in fluid homeostasis, and central hemodynamics (preload, afterload) and to maintain respiration. Although intravenous induction agents and volatile anesthetics have been used safely, it is wise to avoid administering depolarizing neuromuscular blocking drugs to MS patients. MS-induced denervation, or misuse myopathy, may lead to a risk for succinylcholine-induced hyperkalemia, which can result in fatal cardiac arrhythmias. Nondepolarizing neuromuscular blockers are safe to use but should be dosed cautiously as both prolonged responses (increased sensitivity in patients with preexisting muscle weakness) and resistance to these NMBAs have

BOX 35.3 Perioperative Considerations for Patients with Multiple Sclerosis

1. Thoroughly inform the patient and family of the natural course of MS, and the risk for perioperative worsening of symptoms
2. Continue preoperative immunosuppressive therapy
3. Type of general anesthetics is unlikely to affect the course of disease
4. Minimize perioperative changes in fluid homeostasis and hemodynamics
5. Monitor body temperature closely, avoid hyperthermia
6. It is reasonable to avoid depolarizing neuromuscular blocking agents (NMBAs)
7. Nondepolarizing NMBAs can be used, but should be dosed cautiously with monitoring of the neuromuscular transmission
8. Epidural anesthesia has been used successfully, but spinal anesthesia is usually not recommended
9. Consider extended postoperative care in a monitored setting if patient has severe preoperative weakness or respiratory compromise

been reported. The use of rocuronium with sugammadex to ensure full reversal has been suggested as a safe alternative.[240] It is speculated that the demyelination associated with MS renders the spinal cord susceptible to the neurotoxic effects of the local anesthetics. Epidural application of low concentrations of local anesthetics has, nevertheless, been successfully used in MS patients.[239] Spinal anesthesia, on the other hand, has been implicated in postoperative exacerbations of symptoms in MS. As the blood–brain barrier may also be damaged by demyelination, spinal anesthesia is usually not recommended for these patients. A recent metaanalysis of 37 reports found that the MS symptoms were worsened in 10 of 231 patients, but despite the association no clear cause-effect relationship could be identified.[241] Notably, postpartum worsening of MS symptoms is noted in 20% of females. The need for postoperative care is dependent on the preoperative symptoms, type of surgery, and status of the patient at the end of the surgical procedure. In this context, MS patients with severe weakness and respiratory distress, including pharyngeal dysfunction, may need extended postoperative care, such as noninvasive respiratory support and intense physiotherapy, to avoid further impairment of their pulmonary function (Box 35.3).

Motor Neuron Disorders

Motor neuron disorders involve either the upper or the lower motor neurons of the cerebral cortex, brainstem, and spinal cord. Some forms are mixed, whereas others have predominately upper or lower motor neuron involvement. Amyotrophic lateral sclerosis (ALS, also known as Lou Gehrig's disease) is the most common disease within this group and involves both upper and lower motor neurons. Other examples of motor neuron disease are Kennedy disease (spinobulbar muscular atrophy), Friedreich ataxia (mixed upper and lower motor neurons), and spinal muscular atrophy (lower motor neurons).

ALS is characterized by degeneration of the anterior horn α-motoneurons in the spinal cord and brainstem motor nuclei, as well as the primary descending upper motor neurons of the corticospinal tract. Degenerative loss of these neurons leads to progressive muscle weakness, muscle atrophy, and loss of neuronal mass in these locations. Patients present with gradually spreading focal weakness and muscle atrophy (typically of the hands), spasticity, and hyperreflexia of lower extremities. Dysarthria and dysphagia, tongue atrophy, and fasciculations may also occur. Progressive weakness can lead to respiratory failure and death. Sensory functions, including intellectual capacity and cognition, as well as bowel and bladder function, are not usually affected in ALS.

ALS has an incidence of about 2 in 100,000, and onset of the disease usually takes place around 40 to 50 years of age, with males more often affected than females. Most cases are sporadic, but rare familial forms (autosomal dominant and recessive forms) do exist. The underlying mechanism or mechanisms for this selective and progressive motor neuronal death are thus far unclear, but it has recently been suggested that superoxide dismutase (SOD) mutations may have a key role in the increased formation of free radicals seen in subsets of patients. SOD is an important antioxidant and its mutation can lead to decreased clearance of free radicals, increased oxidative stress, and mitochondrial dysfunction. Most familial forms are associated with the mutation of C9ORF72 on 9p21, TDP43, FUS, and VCP genes. The diagnosis is made by electrophysiology (electromyography [EMG] and electroneurography), neurologic examination, MRI imaging, and CSF analysis, which demonstrates early spastic weakness of the upper and lower extremities, typical subcutaneous muscle fasciculations, and bulbar involvement affecting pharyngeal function, speech, and the facial muscles. No curative treatment is currently available, and patients are therefore treated symptomatically. Riluzole, a glutamate release inhibitor, may provide neuroprotection and extend survival in these patients.[242] More recently, the antioxidant edaravone was shown to reduce the decline in daily functioning associated with ALS.[243] Patients may also receive spasmolytic and analgesic agents. Those with advanced disease will ultimately require tracheostomy and gastrostomy surgeries and other supportive treatments including mechanical ventilation.

ANESTHETIC CONSIDERATIONS

Bulbar involvement in combination with respiratory muscle weakness leads to a risk for aspiration and pulmonary complications. Notably, these patients may have increased sensitivity to the respiratory depressant effects of sedatives and hypnotics. There are reports of sympathetic hyperreactivity and autonomic failure.[244] Sympathetic hyperreactivity and autonomic dysfunction, often manifested as orthostatic hypotension and resting tachycardia but also significant hypotension or even pulseless electrical activity upon anesthesia induction, have been reported,[245] and should be considered during the perioperative management of these patients.[244] Succinylcholine should be avoided because of the risk for hyperkalemia as a result of denervation and immobilization. Nondepolarizing NMBA may cause prolonged and pronounced neuromuscular blockade and hence should be used with great caution.[246] General anesthesia may be associated with exaggerated ventilatory depression. Regional anesthesia is also often avoided

BOX 35.4 Perioperative Considerations for Patients with Amyotrophic Lateral Sclerosis

1. Exaggerated respiratory depression and sensitivity to sedatives and hypnotics
2. Higher risk for aspiration and pulmonary complications
3. Autonomic dysfunction with risk for hemodynamic instability
4. Avoid depolarizing neuromuscular blocking agents (NMBAs) (risk for hyperkalemia); nondepolarizing NMBAs may cause prolonged and profound neuromuscular blockade
5. General and epidural anesthesia have been successfully administered; spinal anesthesia is often avoided

for fear of exacerbating disease symptoms. Both general and epidural anesthesia have, however, been successfully administered to these patients without reported complications (Box 35.4).

Guillain-Barré Syndrome

Guillain-Barré syndrome or acute inflammatory demyelinating polyradiculopathy is an acute inflammatory polyneuritis that is triggered by humoral and cell-mediated autoimmune response to a sensitizing event. Although the etiology is unknown, in many cases a timely association with a viral (influenza-like) or bacterial infection or even lymphomatous disease can be demonstrated.[247] It typically presents as an ascending paralysis characterized by symmetric weakness that can vary from mild difficulty with walking to nearly complete paralysis of all extremities, facial, respiratory, and bulbar muscles. Mild variants can present with ataxia, ophthalmoplegia, or hyporeflexia without significant appendicular weakness. Fulminant cases can present with severe ascending weakness leading to complete tetraplegia, and paralysis of cranial nerves and phrenic and intercostal nerves with facial and respiratory muscle weakness necessitating tracheostomy and ventilatory support.[248] Importantly, patients may also have autonomic involvement that could lead to hemodynamic instability and arrhythmias with risk for sudden circulatory collapse and fatal cardiac.

The diagnosis is made after careful neurologic examination such as areflexia and progressive motor weakness, clinical and electrophysiological studies,[249] and CSF analysis. CSF analysis may show a typical increase in CSF protein in combination with a normal cell count, which is a classic sign of the disease. Electromyogram (EMG) and nerve conduction studies may be normal in the early acute period, but characteristic segmental demyelination and reduction of conduction velocity and dispersion or absence of F-waves are usually seen within 1 to 2 weeks.

Management is primarily supportive and includes nutritional support, respiratory support, and measures to prevent aspiration. Early plasma exchange, typically five exchanges with 5% albumin repletion, may mitigate the course but is contraindicated in setting of hemodynamic instability, marked dysautonomia, and active bleeding.[250] Intravenous immunoglobulin (IVIG) is typically administered in the setting of dysautonomia, or if plasmapheresis and exchange transfusion are contraindicated.

BOX 35.5 Perioperative Considerations for Patients with Acute Inflammatory Demyelinating Polyradiculopathy

1. Autonomic dysfunction may be associated with hemodynamic instability and an exaggerated response to anesthesia induction agents, or to stimulating interventions such as laryngoscopy
2. Depolarizing neuromuscular blocking agents (NMBAs) should be avoided due to an upregulation of the acetylcholine receptors and risk for hyperkalemic response
3. Nondepolarizing NMBAs can be used but are commonly also avoided because of the risk for prolonged weakness
4. The use of regional anesthesia is controversial and may be associated with worsening symptoms

ANESTHETIC CONSIDERATIONS

Cranial nerve paralysis and autonomic dysfunction predispose these patients to an increased risk for aspiration. Aspiration precautions, including decompression of the stomach, should therefore be considered before the induction of anesthesia. Absence of compensatory cardiovascular responses may be associated with exaggerated hypotension at anesthesia induction or in response to hypovolemia. Conversely, laryngoscopy or noxious stimuli can be associated with an exaggerated increase in blood pressure. The hemodynamic instability is typically short-lived and self-limited, but small doses of short-acting and titratable vasoactive medications may be required.[251] Careful hemodynamic monitoring is essential and continuous monitoring of the blood pressure with an arterial catheter is often considered. These patients may also exhibit abnormal responses to NMBA; succinylcholine should not be used because of the risk of hyperkalemia. Nondepolarizing muscle relaxants are not contraindicated but should be avoided as a result of the increased sensitivity and risk for prolonged muscle weakness in the postoperative period. The risk for autonomic dysfunction, respiratory failure, and aspiration may require assisted or mechanical ventilation, even in the postoperative period. If these agents are used, the neuromuscular transmission should be closely monitored with a nerve stimulator as both resistance and sensitivity to these agents have been reported. Great care should be taken to maintain circulatory stability, including adequate cardiac preload and afterload. Careful hemodynamic monitoring is therefore essential in these patients.

Regional anesthesia is employed by some practitioners[252] but its use remains controversial as it has been reported to cause worsening of neurological symptoms.[253] General anesthesia can be used; however, the combination of general anesthesia and epidural anesthesia is more controversial (Box 35.5).[254]

CRITICAL ILLNESS POLYNEUROPATHY AND CRITICAL ILLNESS MYOPATHY

Despite earlier reports of a rapid development of weakness, muscle atrophy, and polyneuropathy in critically ill patients, it was not until the 1987 report by Bolton and associates that the characteristic widespread axonal degeneration of motor and sensory fibers and the extensive denervation atrophy of limb and respiratory muscle associated with this polyneuropathy were clearly identified.[255] Although the

BOX 35.6 Perioperative Considerations for Patients with Critical Illness Polyneuropathy

1. Particular attention should be made to protect peripheral nerves, in particular the ulnar and peroneal nerves, during positioning of these patients
2. Monitor and correct electrolyte and glucose abnormalities
3. Steroids have been implicated in the pathophysiology of the disease and should therefore be avoided
4. Neuromuscular blocking agents are best avoided altogether, but if needed only nondepolarizing agents should be considered

true incidence of critical illness polyneuropathy (CIP) is difficult to determine, critical illness neuropathy and myopathy are believed to affect up to 50% of all patients remaining in the intensive care unit for more than 2 weeks.[256] It is typically manifested as profound symmetric limb weakness, with reduced or absent tendon reflexes and diaphragmatic and intercostal weakness. It affects the lower extremities to a greater extent than upper extremities, and distal muscle groups more severely than the proximal. The autonomic function is not affected and the extraocular eye movements remain intact. In CIP, there is no evidence of neuromuscular junction disorder and the electromyography and nerve conduction study findings are consistent with axonal motor and sensory polyneuropathy, with amplitude reduction of motor and sensory action potentials, and slowed conduction velocities. Serum CK levels are usually normal. Conversely, a sensory nerve action potential is often normal in critical illness myopathy but compound muscle action potentials are diminished and electromyography is consistent with myopathy. Serum CK levels may be elevated. No specific treatments are currently available, and management is supportive with aggressive and early rehabilitation. Use of sedation, paralytics, and corticosteroids should be limited,[257] and aggressive control of hyperglycemia has been suggested to reduce the incidence of CIP by 44%.[258]

ANESTHETIC CONSIDERATIONS

Anesthetic considerations in CIP patients are similar to those with other acquired neuropathies (see above), and include protection of nerve compression sites, particularly the ulnar and peroneal nerves. Prolonged immobility in critically ill patients is associated with a relative increase in immature acetylcholine receptors that can lead to an insensitivity to nondepolarizing NMBA.[259] Conversely, the sensitivity to depolarizing neuromuscular blockers is increased, with a risk for increased potassium efflux after succinylcholine administration (Box 35.6).[260]

Hereditary Motor-Sensory Neuropathies, including Charcot-Marie-Tooth Disease

Hereditary motor-sensory neuropathies include a spectrum of peripheral neurologic disorders, among which Charcot-Marie-Tooth (CMT) disease is often listed. They are caused by a specific mutation in one of several myelin genes that result in defects in myelin structure, maintenance, and formation. Hereditary motor-sensory neuropathies have been classified into seven types and multiple subtypes according to the age at onset, mode of inheritance, predominately involved muscle groups, and genotypes.[261,262] CMT types 1 and 2 are the most common hereditary peripheral neuropathies, with an estimated prevalence of 40 per 100,000.[262] Patients with CMT disease typically experience slow and progressive distal muscle weakness and wasting. Damage to sensory axons may also lead to sensory loss resulting in frequent tripping and falls. Neuropathic pain may develop in some patients. CMT patients usually have normal life expectancy. CMT type 3, also known as Dejerine-Sottas disease, is a very severe condition with an early onset of hypotonia during infancy. Nerve conduction velocity is typically significantly reduced to less than 10 ms.[262] The genetic inheritance pattern for CMT disease is heterogeneous.

ANESTHETIC CONSIDERATIONS

The anesthesia experience in patients with CMT disease is limited because of the small number of cases. Major considerations include the use of hypnotic agents, muscle relaxants, volatile agents, and neuraxial techniques. CMT type 1 patients have been reported to have significantly increased sensitivity to thiopental at induction that correlates with the severity of both motor and sensory defects. However, total intravenous anesthesia (TIVA) has been performed successfully in a number of cases without any reported problems.[263-265]

Because of the reduced number of acetylcholine receptors, sensitivity to nondepolarizing muscle relaxants is elevated and the response to succinylcholine is also reduced.[266] Although succinylcholine has been used without adverse effect,[267,268] the risk of an exaggerated hyperkalemic response may be sufficient to preclude it from being used in patients with suspected muscular denervation.[268] Prolonged neuromuscular blockade with vecuronium has been reported.[269] As a result of the large variety of disabilities in this patient group, careful baseline assessment of neuromuscular status should be conducted before the use of nondepolarizing neuromuscular relaxants. Normal response to atracurium and mivacurium has been demonstrated.[270,271] Both TIVA and volatile anesthetics have been used safely in CMT patients in a series of cases.[267] Neuraxial techniques for obstetric procedures have been reported to generally be successful in CMT patients.[272-275] However, the use of regional anesthesia can be controversial given that the possible complications may exacerbate the neurologic symptoms.[276] Similar medicolegal concerns may apply to the surgical and anesthesia positioning of CMT patients because of the sensory deficits and limb deformities.

Duchenne Muscular Dystrophy and Becker Muscular Dystrophy

Duchenne muscular dystrophy (DMD) is the most common and severe type of muscular dystrophy, with an incidence of 1 per 3500 live male births[277] and a total male prevalence of about 50 to 60 × 10^{-6}.[278] Becker muscular dystrophy (BMD) is relatively rare and has an incidence of about 1 in

18,000 live male births and a prevalence of 23.8×10^{-6}.[278] Both DMD and BMD are X-linked recessive diseases. The defect is located on the short arm of the X chromosome at the Xp21 region, which contains the gene for the large protein Dp427, also known as dystrophin. The dystrophin gene is 2500 kilobases long with more than 70 exons.[278] Dystrophin is distributed not only in skeletal, cardiac, and smooth muscle but also in the brain.[279] Because of the large size of the dystrophin gene, spontaneous new mutations are common and account for a third of new cases.[280]

The most common form of mutation is a deletion within the gene (65%-70% of cases of DMD and >80% of BMD). Duplication and point mutations are responsible for the rest. It also appears that there are "hot spots" within the first 20 exons and in the central region of the gene (exons 45-55) where deletion and duplication are likely to occur.[278] Female cases of DMD have been reported with the 45,X and 46,XX karyotypes. The disease mechanism for the female 46,XX karyotype was thought to be preferential loss of the paternal X chromosome by postzygotic nondisjunction and manifestation of the DMD gene from the maternal X chromosome in muscle cells.[281] BMD is usually milder in severity than DMD because disruption of the translation process occurs in the relatively distal part of the gene, which leads to a reduced amount of truncated dystrophin protein.[278,282]

Dystrophin, along with dystrophin-associated glycoproteins (DAGs), is involved in sarcolemmal stability. Dystrophin is responsible for maintenance of muscle membrane integrity despite the fact that it accounts for only approximately 0.002% of the protein in striated muscle.[283] Dystrophin aggregates and links to actin (at its N terminus) and the DAG complex (at its C terminus) to form a stable structure that interacts with laminin in the extracellular matrix (Fig. 35.4). Lack or dysfunction of dystrophin leads to cellular and membrane instability, with progressive leakage of intracellular components and elevation of creatine phosphokinase (CPK) levels. Eventually, damaged muscle cell units are invaded by macrophages and destroyed. Current study suggests that cytotoxic T cells are probably the culprit. Consequently, clinical pseudohypertrophy of the muscle occurs when the dead muscle shells are replaced by fibrofatty infiltrates. Loss of muscle units accounts for the weakness and contracture.[279]

Both DMD and BMD are characterized by progressive weakness and wasting of predominantly the proximal musculature. Pseudohypertrophy of the calves and other muscle groups is common. As the more severe of the two diseases, DMD tends to be symptomatic early in life. Seventy-four percent of children with DMD were found to manifest the disease by 4 years of age.[277] DMD patients do not usually begin to walk until they are about 18 months of age or later.

The initial clinical findings include a waddling gait, frequent falling, and difficulty climbing stairs because of proximal muscle weakness in the pelvic girdle. The classic Gower maneuver describes rising from a sitting to a standing position with the help of both arms. Patients may also show weakness in the shoulder girdle and trunk erectors that leads to thoracolumbar scoliosis. The earlier the onset of disease, the more rapid the disease will take its course. In most cases, children with DMD are unable to walk by the age of 9 to 11. Proximal deep tendon reflexes in the upper extremities and patella may also disappear despite the lack of denervation.[282] Nevertheless, the Achilles tendon reflex remains intact even in later stages of the disease. Sixty percent of patients will have pseudohypertrophy of the calves, and thirty percent will have macroglossia. Some may also suffer from pain in the calves with activity.

The intellectual impairment that can be associated with the disease was thought to be related to limitation of educational opportunities. However, with equalization of educational opportunities, psychometric studies have revealed a significantly lower average intelligence quotient in DMD

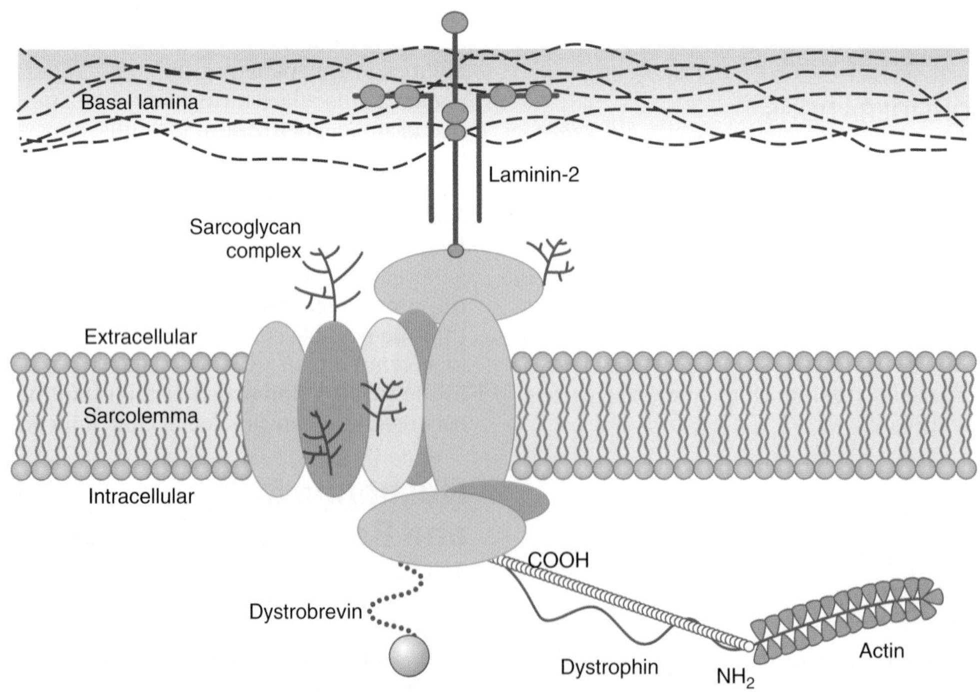

Fig. 35.4 Diagram of the cell–surface and cytoskeleton protein complex.

patients than in healthy groups.[284] This implies a possible effect of dysfunctional dystrophin in the brain on learning.

Death in patients with DMD is commonly due to cardiopulmonary compromise in their 30s.[277] BMD is a mild form of DMD. The mutation that causes BMD produces dystrophin that retains partial function. The onset of symptoms occurs in the second or third decade of life. As a result, the life span of BMD patients can reach the early 40s. Pneumonia is the most common cause of death (Fig. 35.5).[282]

The heart is also affected to various degrees, depending on the stage of the disease and the type of mutation. Cardiac degeneration is due to replacement of myocardium by connective tissue or fat, which leads to dilated cardiomyopathy.[285] Cardiac involvement starts early in the course of the disease, although clinical signs are not usually obvious in the early stage. No correlation has been established between the severity of cardiac disease and the severity of skeletal disease. Studies of necropsy have shown that the cardiomyopathy in DMD involves the posterobasal and contiguous lateral left ventricular walls as initial and primary sites of myocardial dystrophy in the absence of small vessel coronary artery disease in these areas.[286] Typical initial manifestations on the electrocardiogram (ECG) in DMD and BMD are sinus tachycardia, tall R waves in the right precordial leads, prominent left precordial Q waves, increased QT dispersion, and inverted T waves from scarring of the posterobasal portion of the left ventricle. Initially, the echocardiography is normal or shows regional wall motion abnormalities in areas of fibrosis. With the spreading of fibrosis, left ventricular dysfunction can be seen and ventricular arrhythmias frequently occur as well. In the final stages of the disease, systolic dysfunction may lead to heart failure and sudden death. Subclinical or clinical cardiac involvement is present in about 90% of DMD/BMD patients, but it is the cause of death in only 20% of DMD and 50% of BMD patients. Angiotensin-converting enzyme inhibitors are recommended in early stages of the disease, and β-blockers may be an additional option if indicated.[285]

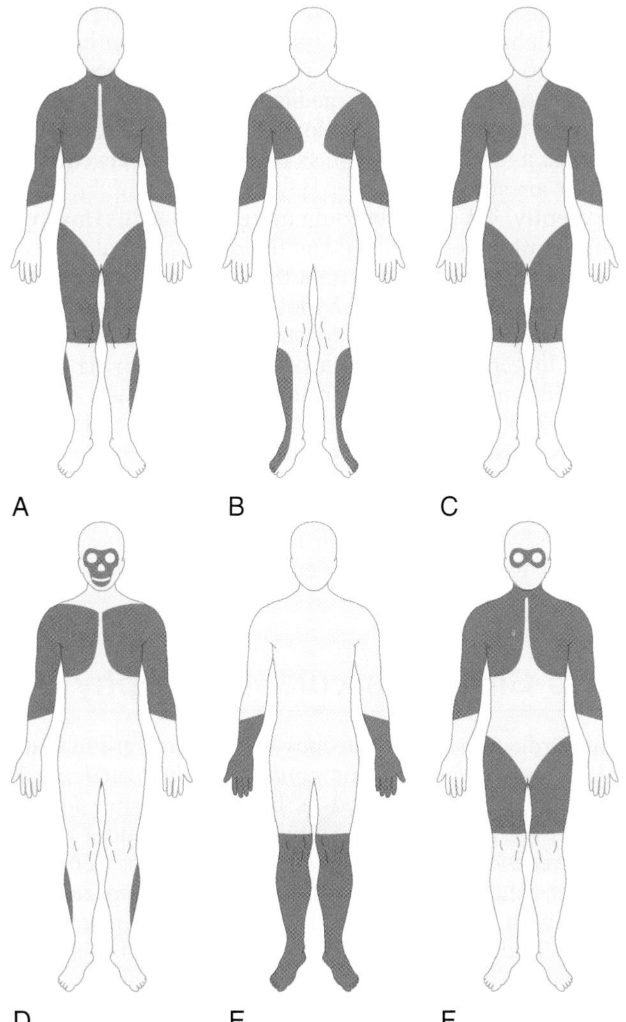

Fig. 35.5 Distribution of predominant muscle weakness in different types of dystrophy: (A) Duchenne type and Becker type; (B) Emery-Dreifuss; (C) limb girdle; (D) facioscapulohumeral; (E) distal; and (F) oculopharyngeal. (Redrawn from Emery AE. The muscular dystrophies. *BMJ* 1998;317:991–995.)

Pulmonary insufficiency is a leading cause of morbidity and mortality in DMD.[287] Usually, expiratory muscle function is affected first, because of the early onset of abdominal muscle weakness. By contrast, inspiratory muscle function is relatively preserved in the first decade, implying sparing of the diaphragm.[288] Vital capacity (VC) increases in the first decade because of overall body growth, plateaus in early adolescence, and then declines dramatically as the diaphragmatic weakness progresses.[288] Other measured lung volumes such as inspiratory reserve volume and total lung capacity (TLC) follow the same pattern. A disproportionate loss of VC and TLC relative to the respiratory muscle dysfunction results in part from additional factors, such as altered chest wall and lung mechanics, modifications in the distribution of surfactant, micro-atelectasis, and local fibrosis secondary to recurrent pneumonia.[288] Scoliosis further impairs pulmonary function. On average, for each 10 degrees of thoracic scoliosis curvature, forced vital capacity (FVC) decreases by 4%.[283] In 90% of patients, a curvature of greater than 20 degrees develops 3 to 4 years after they are wheelchair bound. Respiratory failure inevitably occurs in the second decade of life and is the most common cause of death.[289]

DIAGNOSIS AND DIFFERENTIAL DIAGNOSIS

Chronic elevation of the serum CPK level is a general indication of muscle disease. Three serum tests showing elevated CPK levels obtained one month apart is diagnostic of muscular dystrophy. CPK represents leakage of enzyme from muscle cells and does not correlate with severity of the disease. CPK could reach 50 to 300 times the normal value in early stages of the disease. The level tends to decrease with the loss of muscle mass. Elevation of the MB fraction of CK precludes its use as a marker for cardiac injury.[282] EMG can be supportive of the diagnosis; however, it can be very difficult to perform on children. Muscle biopsy, followed by immunostaining or Western blot analysis for dystrophin, is recommended for diagnostic testing. Multiple polymerase chain reactions are also useful in detecting more than 98% of the existing deletions.[279] The result is usually available within 24 hours, which may render muscle biopsy, the old "gold standard," obsolete.

ANESTHETIC CONSIDERATIONS

Patients with DMD and BMD may require anesthesia for muscle biopsy, correction of scoliosis, release of contractures, and exploratory laparotomy for ileus,[282] as well as for dental[290] and obstetric[291] procedures. As the natural course of the disease progresses, the risk of surgery increases concomitant with the increased comorbid conditions associated with the later phase of the disease. However, perioperative complications are not proportional to the severity of the disease. They occur even in mildly affected patients. Consequently, patients should undergo careful preoperative consultation and evaluation.

Fifty to seventy percent of patients with muscular dystrophy demonstrate some cardiac abnormality, although it is clinically significant in only ten percent.[282] Preoperative cardiology assessment with an ECG and echocardiography is essential. Continuous cardiac Holter monitoring is necessary if an arrhythmia is captured on the ECG or if the patient describes symptoms that can be related to cardiac arrhythmias. An echocardiography will demonstrate mitral valve prolapse in 10% to 25% of patients. It may also show posterobasilar hypokinesis in a thin-walled ventricle and a slow relaxation phase with normal contraction characterizing the cardiomyopathy seen in DMD.[282] However, echocardiography may not always reflect the ability of the diseased myocardium to respond to perioperative stress. A stress echocardiography using angiotensin to detect latent heart failure and identify inducible contraction abnormalities has been advocated.[292]

An estimated 30% of deaths in individuals with DMD are due to respiratory causes.[293] Therefore careful preoperative pulmonary assessment is important. Webster demonstrated that the manual muscle strength test has a strong statistical correlation with all of the timed functional tests. Peak expiratory flow was not only easy to perform, but also correlated statistically with all timed functional tests.[294] The correlation was not significant for VC or forced expiratory volume in 1 second (FEV_1).

Intraoperatively, in terms of airway management, patients with DMD and BMD may have decreased laryngeal reflexes and prolonged gastric emptying time, which increases the risk for aspiration.[295] Decreased ability to cough up the accumulation of oral secretions predisposes muscular dystrophy patients to postoperative respiratory tract infections.[282] Masseter spasm is also a possible complication during induction of anesthesia in these patients.[296] Preparedness for a difficult airway is necessary, especially in patients with potential airway problems.

Postoperatively, DMD patients are at an increased risk for respiratory compromise.[297] Retrospective reviews have indicated that the incidence of prolonged postoperative ventilation (>36 hours) was greatest in DMD patients who had a preoperative FVC of less than 40% of the predicted value.[298,299] Preoperative pulmonary function studies are valuable in determining the postoperative course. Patients with a VC of greater than 30% of the predicted value can usually be extubated immediately after surgery.[282] Sleep apnea may also compound the condition and contribute to the development of pulmonary hypertension. Continuous positive airway pressure and bilevel positive airway pressure have been demonstrated to be effective in the management of postoperative respiratory depression. Delayed pulmonary insufficiency may occur up to 36 hours postoperatively despite the apparent recovery of skeletal muscle strength.[300]

Reports have suggested a relationship between DMD/BMD and MH, but this association is not based on good rational grounds.[301] Whereas the risk for an MH mutation in DMD/BMD patients is similar to that of the general population, the incidence of MH-like anesthetic events has been reported to be 0.002 with DMD and 0.00036 with BMD. Unexplained cardiac arrest[296,302] and acute heart failure[303] have been reported in DMD/BMD patients. Succinylcholine is contraindicated in these patients because of the potential for rhabdomyolysis and hyperkalemia as a result of their unstable sarcolemmal membranes. Succinylcholine-induced hyperkalemia during acute rhabdomyolysis is more likely to result in cardiac arrest and unsuccessful resuscitation than is the potassium efflux resulting from upregulation of acetylcholine receptors in burn patients.[300] Although the use of nondepolarizing muscle relaxants is usually accompanied by an increase in both maximal effect and duration of action,[304] proper and rapid reversal with sugammadex may put some of these concerns to rest. Current off-label experience in infants and children has been favorable. Narcotics can be used, but small incremental dosing and short-acting medications are recommended given the respiratory depression associated with these medications, as well as the reports of inadvertent reactions to volatile anesthetics.[282]

Recently, TIVA has become more popular.[305] However, consideration needs to be given to the myocardial status of the patient when propofol or barbiturates are used because they may lead to profound hypotension and reduced organ perfusion.[282,306] Regional anesthesia may be a good alternative to general anesthesia because it avoids the risk of triggering agents and respiratory depression and enables the use of local anesthetics for postoperative analgesia. It may also facilitate chest physiotherapy.[307]

Recent breakthroughs in gene therapy are shining new lights into the management of these relatively common disorders. We have not seen reports on anesthesia management for DMD/BMD patients who had received gene therapy.

Limb-Girdle Muscular Dystrophy

Limb-girdle muscular dystrophy (LGMD) is a group of disorders with heterogeneous causes. To date, at least 18 genes have been identified as being responsible for this disease, with 7 being autosomal dominant and 11 autosomal recessive.[308] Mutations within the same gene may result in different phenotypes that sometimes are not consistent with LGMD. Proximal muscle (shoulder or pelvic) girdle weakness is the characteristic feature of this group of diseases. Given the marked genetic heterogeneity, clinical manifestations of the disease vary. Autosomal recessive forms are about 10 times more common than autosomal dominant forms. Fukutin-related protein (*FKRP*) and calpain 3 (*CAPN3*) gene mutations have been associated with LGMD. In addition, a number of other disorders, not strictly included under LGMD in this classification, may have

LGMD-like phenotypes.[308] Sporadic cases of LGMD have been reported in the anesthesia literature.[309-311] General approaches to these patients are the same as those for DMD/BMD.

Myotonic Dystrophy

Myotonic dystrophy (MD) is an inherited muscular disorder characterized by progressive muscle weakness and wasting. Two types of MD result from a mutation in either the dystrophia myotonica–protein kinase (*DMPK*) gene, located on chromosome 19q13.3 (MD1, also known as Steinert disease), or the CysCysHisCys (CCHC)-type zinc finger, nucleic acid binding protein (*CNBP*) gene, located on chromosome 3q21 (MD2).[312]

The incidence of MD is 1 in 8000. MD1 is by far the most common of the two types and accounts for about 98% of all cases. MD1 is caused by expansion of a CTG trinucleotide repeat in the *DMPK* gene and is inherited in an autosomal dominant manner.[312] Typical signs and symptoms include muscle weakness and wasting (most prominent in the cranial and distal limb musculature), periodic myotonia, progressive myopathy, insulin resistance, defects in cardiac conduction, neuropsychiatric impairment, cataracts, testicular atrophy, and frontal balding in males. The typical cranial muscle weakness and wasting are manifested not only in the facial, temporalis, masseter, and sternocleidomastoid muscles but also in the vocal cord apparatus. Mitral valve prolapse is found in 20% of patients.[300] The severity of the disease is related to the number of extra trinucleotide repeats.[94] MD1 patients may also have mildly elevated CK levels. Myotonic discharges can be identified on EMG, as well as an inability to relax from a handgrip. During pregnancy, the symptoms may be exacerbated. Uterine atony and a retained placenta may also complicate vaginal delivery. First-degree atrioventricular heart block is a common finding on the ECG before the onset of symptoms.[300]

MD2 is also called proximal myotonic myopathy. Intron 1 of the *CNBP* gene contains a complex repeat motif, (TG)n(TCTG)n(CCTG)n, and expansion of the CCTG repeat was determined as the cause of MD2. Patients with MD2 suffer from myotonia (90% of those affected), muscle dysfunction (82% weakness, pain, and stiffness), and less commonly, cardiac conduction defects, iridescent posterior subcapsular cataracts, insulin-insensitive type 2 diabetes mellitus, and testicular failure.

There is no case report in the literature linking MD to MH.[313] Lehmann-Horn and associates performed IVCT in 44 patients with myotonias and periodic paralyses, which revealed 4 positive, 10 equivocal, and 30 negative results.[314]

ANESTHETIC CONSIDERATIONS

General considerations for MD are similar to those for other muscular dystrophies. Mathieu and coworkers conducted a retrospective study on the anesthetic and surgical complications of MD. The majority of complications were found to be pulmonary related and significantly more frequent in patients undergoing upper abdominal operations and those with severe disability, as assessed by the presence of proximal limb weakness.[315] The pulmonary complications of MD are the result of hypotonia, chronic aspiration, and central and peripheral hypoventilation.[282] Smooth muscle atrophy, which leads to poor gastric motility, when coupled with a diminished cough reflex, promotes aspiration.

Succinylcholine will produce contractions lasting for several minutes, thus making intubation and ventilation a challenge. These contractions are not antagonized by nondepolarizing muscle relaxants. Other agents, including methohexital, etomidate, propofol, and even neostigmine, may also induce myotonic reactions. Short-acting nondepolarizing muscle relaxants or avoidance of relaxation is therefore advised.[282] Case reports have demonstrated normal responses to sugammadex when rocuronium was used as the neuromuscular blockade.[316-318]

Triggering factors, such as hypothermia, shivering, and mechanical or electrical stimulation, may cause a myotonic reaction.[319] The reaction can be treated with phenytoin (4-6 mg/kg/day) or quinine (0.3-1.5 g/day).[282] Furthermore, MD patients can be very sensitive to anesthetic agents, with hypersomnolence and CO_2 retention sometimes being observed. Careful titration with relatively short-acting anesthetic agents may be beneficial. Close cardiac monitoring is required for MD patients. Pacing equipment should be readily available because a third of first-degree atrioventricular blocks may not respond to atropine.[282] All patients should be treated as though they have both cardiomyopathy and conduction defects.

Myotonia Congenita

Myotonia congenita (MC) is a congenital form of muscular dystrophy characterized by uncontrolled temporary skeleton muscle excitability as a result of mutations in the muscle chloride channel gene (*CLCN1*). There are two forms of MC, one with autosomal dominant and the other with recessive inheritance. The former is also known as Thomsen disease and the later as Becker myotonia. The myotonia in MC patients is usually initiated by a forceful muscle contraction, particularly after being at rest for at least 10 minutes. The myotonic muscle stiffness then becomes increasingly obvious after a second and third short, but forceful contraction. Further contractions usually dampen the myotonia.[320]

Thomsen disease was the first myotonic disease to be described. Patients may have a hypertrophic and athletic appearance. The sign of percussion myotonia is described as an indenting-appearing myotonia triggered by tapping the muscle. Lid lag is common and muscle stretch reflexes are normal.[320] Myotonia symptoms in Becker myotonia usually start at 10 to 14 years of age or even later and are more severe than those of Thomsen disease. Becker myotonia may be associated with severe generalized stiffness resulting in falling. It can frequently be misdiagnosed as epilepsy. Antiepileptic medications do improve the symptoms, however.[320]

ANESTHETIC CONSIDERATIONS

As with many muscle diseases, there have been reports that MC patients are predisposed to MH, but as is the case for almost all of them, there are no data to support this hypothesis.[321-323] However, depolarizing muscle relaxants can lead to severe masseter spasms in MC patients. Generalized spasms involving the respiratory and skeletal muscles have been reported.[321] The findings resemble those of MH, so dantrolene is sometimes administered.[320] Because dantrolene is an inhibitor of calcium release from the SR, it can usually abolish the myotonia effectively.[321,322] Some believe that local anesthetics and class Ib antiarrhythmic drugs such as lidocaine should be used for myotonic reactions rather than dantrolene.[324] Because shivering in the operating room can trigger the myotonic reaction, MC patients should be kept normothermic during surgery.[320]

Myotubular Myopathy

Myotubular myopathy (MTM) is pathologically defined by the presence of centrally placed nuclei in the majority of extrafusal muscle fibers, an appearance resembling fetal myotubes during normal muscle development. Consequently, MTM is also called centronuclear myopathy (CNM).[325] However, MTM now mostly refers to the X-linked form of the disease, whereas CNM is used for the autosomal form.[325]

MTM and CNM are rare. The estimated incidence of MTM is 1 in 50,000 newborn males.[325] MTM has been linked to the myotubularin (*MTM1*) gene on Xq28. Pregnancy is often complicated by polyhydramnios and reduced fetal movements. Affected males typically have severe floppiness and weakness and respiratory distress at birth. Cardiac muscles are not generally involved. The patient usually has a normal response to pain, but tendon reflexes are absent. The long-term prognosis for MTM is extremely poor.[325] In patients who survive the first year of life, most are either completely or partially ventilator dependent.[326] These patients often have abnormal liver function.[326] Both autosomal recessive and autosomal dominant forms have been observed in CNM patients. Its clinical features include respiratory distress, hypotonia, bulbar weakness, ophthalmoplegia, ptosis, and facial diplegia. Although the exact genetic mechanism is not fully understood, the *MTM1*, myotubularin-related protein (*MTMR2*), and myotubularin-related phosphatase (*MTMR3*) genes have been implicated.[325] Pathologically, MTM and CNM share a similar, characteristic histologic feature: predominantly type 1 fiber with centrally placed nuclei seen on hematoxylin-eosin staining of formalin-fixed, paraffin-embedded tissue.[325]

ANESTHETIC CONSIDERATIONS

Reports of anesthesia for patients with MTM are sparse.[327-332] Nontriggering general anesthesia has been used because of the unfounded concern of possible susceptibility to MH. Agents such as propofol, fentanyl, remifentanil, and nitrous oxide have been used successfully without adverse effects.[327-332] The possibility of a prolonged effect of nondepolarizing muscle relaxants has been suggested with mechanomyography.[327-332] However, in reality, intubation of such patients may not require any muscle relaxant because of their hypotonic state. Costi and van der Walt suspected that the defect in MTM is distal to the neuromuscular junction,[328] whereas Dorchies and coworkers suggested that muscles in MTM might be intrinsically normal, with myotubularin-deficient motor neurons involved in development of the disease.[333]

Metabolic Myopathies

Two major energy sources for muscle exist: glycogen and fatty acid. Glycogen serves as a dynamic, but limited reservoir of glucose, mainly stored in skeletal muscle and liver. Glycogen storage disorders (GSDs) are a group of metabolism disorders caused by enzyme deficiency or dysfunction. They reduce effective glucose storage by interfering with normal glycogen synthesis and degradation. Synthetic errors cause decreased normal glycogen, whereas degradation errors tend to block the breakdown of glycogen. Subsequently, hypoglycemia and accumulation of glycogen in tissues could occur as a result of substrate use. There are more than 12 types of GSD that are assigned roman numerals based on the enzyme deficiencies. Types I and II are discussed here.

Glycogen Storage Disease Type I

The incidence of GSD I is approximately 1 in 100,000 live newborns.[334] The incidence in non-Ashkenazi Jews from North Africa may be as high as 1 in 5420 people.[334] The defective enzyme causing the disease is glucose-6-phosphatase, which is the enzyme that converts glucose 6-phosphate (G6P) to glucose in the liver. Type Ia (von Gierke disease) is due to a deficiency in G6P hydrolase (catalytic subunit) activity and accounts for more than 80% of cases. Types Ib (G6P transporter deficiency), Ic, and Id represent allelic defects in the translocase associated with G6P. Their inheritance is autosomal recessive. The G6P gene (*G6PC*) encoding the hydrolase resides at 17q21, with the gene encoding G6P translocase (*G6PT*) located at 11q23. Mutations responsible for GSD I have been described in both type Ia and Ib patients.[334]

Impaired glycogenolysis results in accumulation of glycogen and G6P in the liver, kidney, intestine, skeletal muscle, and heart and is manifested as hepatomegaly, renomegaly, proximal tubular dysfunction, and diarrhea.[335] Fasting hypoglycemia is the initial manifestation of the disease. As a result, upregulation of the synthesis and transport of counter-regulatory hormones, such as glucagon, cortisol, catecholamines, and growth hormone, becomes obvious and leads to the release of pyruvate, lactate, and free fatty acid. Lipid deposition in lean tissues such as the liver, skeletal muscle, cardiac muscle, and pancreas results in lipotoxicity and organ failure, including pulmonary hypertension, steatohepatitis, end-stage renal disease, insulin resistance, cardiac contractile dysfunction, and pancreatic β cell failure.[334] For type Ib disease, specific problems such as neutropenia and neutrophil dysfunction are prominent. Patients may have recurrent infections and inflammatory bowel disease.[336]

ANESTHESIA CONSIDERATIONS

Anesthesia case reports for GSD I patients are rare.[337,338] Patients with GSD I diseases should be given intravenous glucose-containing fluid preoperatively when they have fasted. Lactate-containing solutions should be avoided because these patients are not able to convert the lactic acid to glycogen.[282] Patients need to be monitored frequently to avoid hypoglycemia.

Glycogen Storage Disease Type II (Acid Maltase Deficiency)

The incidence of acid maltase deficiency (AMD) is estimated to be 1 in every 14,000 to 40,000 births. Its inheritance is autosomal recessive with a few exceptions.[339,340] Mutations of the acid maltase gene on chromosome 17q25 cause deficiency of lysosomal acid maltase (acid α-1,4-glucosidase).[340] Cases of AMD have been arbitrarily classified into three groups—infantile, childhood, and adult—according to the age at onset or death, rate of progression, and tissue-organ involvement.[340]

Acid maltase is a lysosomal enzyme that catalyzes the one-way hydrogenation of glycogen to G6P and is found in all tissues, including skeletal and cardiac muscle.[341] Consequently, glycogen accumulates within the muscle tissues of maltase-deficient patients. Infantile AMD, also known as Pompe disease, is usually manifested within the first few months of life as rapidly progressive weakness and hypotonia and enlargement of the tongue, heart, and liver. Massive amounts of glycogen (8%-15% of the wet weight of the tissue) accumulate in the heart, liver, and skeletal muscle, with relatively smaller deposits in smooth muscle, eyes, kidneys, endothelial cells, lymphocytes, brain, and spinal cord. Accumulation of glycogen in cardiac muscle leads to cardiac failure in the infantile form.[340] Echocardiography demonstrates marked thickening of the interventricular septum and posterior left ventricular wall, left ventricular outflow obstruction, and trabecular hypertrophy.[340] Ventricular wall thickness may be increased to up to 25 mm.[342] Wolff-Parkinson-White syndrome has been reported.[343] The signs and symptoms of infantile AMD may resemble those of DMD. Death usually results from cardiorespiratory decompensation within several years of disease progression.[344]

Childhood AMD occurs in infancy to early childhood and is manifested by clinical signs of myopathy. Respiratory muscles tend to be selectively affected. Calf enlargement can also occur. The disease progresses relatively slowly in this form, with a few patients surviving beyond the second decade of life.[340] Tongue, heart, and liver enlargement occur infrequently.[345] However, involvement of vascular smooth muscle is more severe than in the infantile form. There has been a report of extensive glycogen deposition in the arterial wall causing basilar aneurysms.[345]

Adult AMD usually occurs after age 20 and is characterized by slow progressive myopathy or symptoms of respiratory failure.[340] The weakness in proximal muscles is more prominent than the weakness in distal muscles. A third of adult AMD patients suffer from respiratory failure with a restrictive pattern. Weakness in the diaphragm causes extensive atelectasis. VC may be significantly reduced.[340]

ANESTHETIC CONSIDERATIONS

Anesthesia reports in AMD patients are rare.[346-349] Isolated intraoperative cardiac arrest during halothane anesthesia in infantile AMD has been documented.[349] Despite the problem noted with halothane, enflurane[347] and sevoflurane[348] have been used without complications. Theoretically, total intravenous general anesthesia with propofol may cause a reduction in afterload leading to an increased risk for myocardial ischemia. This may become significant when the patient is tachycardic.[348]

Subendocardial ischemia may occur in patients with a thickened ventricular wall and results in higher left ventricular end-diastolic pressure at lower ventricular volume.[348,350] Close cardiac monitoring is therefore necessary. A central venous or pulmonary artery catheter is not essential in patients who are normovolemic without preexisting heart failure.[348] Adequate filling pressure and normal to high systemic vascular resistance (SVR) are required to ensure effective coronary perfusion.[348] Ketamine has been used successfully in a number of cases because of its ability to maintain SVR and contractility. Respiratory failure and muscle weakness are the other concerns for anesthesiologists. A spectrum of uses of muscle relaxants from none[347] to atracurium[346] to rocuronium[348] have been attempted. Low-dose rocuronium, 0.5 mg/kg, with close monitoring of neuromuscular function and adequate use of reversal agents, has been sufficient to prevent prolonged postoperative weakness.[348] Depolarizing agents should be avoided because of the potential risk of hyperkalemia and rhabdomyolysis.[348,349]

Mitochondrial Myopathies

Mitochondrial diseases refer to defects in the five main steps of mitochondrial metabolism: substrate transport, substrate utilization, the Krebs cycle, the electron transport chain, and oxidation-phosphorylation coupling.[351] However, the term *mitochondrial myopathy* has been reserved for disorders caused by defects in the respiratory chain.[351] The respiratory chain is composed of five multimeric complexes (I-V) embedded in the inner mitochondrial membrane, plus two small mobile electron carriers, coenzyme Q_{10} (CoQ_{10}) and cytochrome *c*, for a total of more than 80 proteins,[351] among which 13 are encoded by mitochondrial DNA (mtDNA) and all others by nuclear DNA (nDNA). mtDNA is different from nDNA in several aspects: (1) mtDNA is circular and contains no intron, (2) it has larger numbers of copies than nDNA does and a much higher spontaneous mutation rate, and (3) its inheritance is maternal. Diagnosis of mitochondrial diseases is difficult because of their clinical heterogeneity.

Primary mtDNA mutations may include point mutations in polypeptide, tRNA, or rRNA encoding regions and large-scale rearrangements, duplications, or deletions.[352] Some of the common conditions caused by point mutations include myoclonic epilepsy with ragged-red fibers (MERRF); mitochondrial encephalopathy, lactic acidosis, and stroke-like episodes (MELAS); neuropathy, ataxia, and retinitis pigmentosa (NARP); maternally inherited Leigh syndrome; and Leber hereditary optic neuropathy.[351] Sporadic large-scale mutations may lead to Kearns-Sayre syndrome, progressive external ophthalmoplegia, and Pearson syndrome.[351] nDNA mutations can cause deficiencies in complexes I to IV and CoQ_{10} of the electron transport chain.[351]

Mitochondrial diseases present a diagnostic challenge due to their clinical heterogeneity. Since mitochondria are ubiquitous; every tissue in the body can be affected by mtDNA mutations. Disorders due to nDNA mutations follow a Mendelian pattern and are thus phenotypically "all or none," while inheritance of mtDNA is stochastic, leading to greater variability. Mitochondrial myopathy is estimated to have an incidence of 1 in 4000.[353] Among all the mitochondrial functions, abnormalities in electron transport and oxidative phosphorylation are the most common causes of mitochondrial myopathies.[354] Mitochondrial myopathies are characterized by proximal muscle weakness. Common laboratory findings include a very high lactate to pyruvate ratio (50-250:1 instead of a normal ratio of <25:1), increased blood levels of free carnitine, and occasionally low levels of folate (for instance in Kearns-Sayre syndrome). The hallmark of mitochondrial myopathies is the "ragged red fiber" when muscle biopsy specimens are stained with modified Gomori trichrome stain,[355] and specific defects in the activity of these enzymes have been demonstrated in patients with mitochondrial disease.[356] Fatigue and poor stamina are prominent clinical features. Movement disorders such as ataxia, dystonia, myoclonus, chorea, athetosis, and tremors have also been described as being due to mitochondrial abnormalities.[356] CT and MRI scans of the brain may be very helpful—for example, patients with MELAS demonstrate basal ganglia calcifications and stroke-like patterns not confined to vascular territories.[357] Clinical features of two relatively common encephalomyopathies, MELAS and MERRF, are briefly discussed below.

MITOCHONDRIAL MYOPATHY, ENCEPHALOPATHY, LACTIC ACIDOSIS, AND STROKE-LIKE EPISODES

MELAS is the most common mitochondrial encephalomyopathy. Onset is most commonly before age 20. Seizures are common and stroke-like episodes ("stroke-like" because they do not conform to vascular distributions) may produce hemiparesis, hemianopia, and cortical blindness. Any patient with a stroke below the age of 40 should be worked up for MELAS. Associated findings include diabetes mellitus, hearing loss, pituitary and thyroid hypofunction, and lack of secondary sexual characteristics. In its full expression, MELAS leads to dementia, a bedridden state, and death. There is no specific treatment.[358]

MYOCLONIC EPILEPSY WITH RAGGED RED FIBERS

MERRF is a multisystem disorder characterized by myoclonus, generalized epilepsy, ataxia, and ragged red fibers on muscle biopsy. Other clinical features may include hearing loss, peripheral neuropathy, optic atrophy, dementia, short stature, and exercise intolerance.[359] Cardiomyopathy is occasionally present. Laboratory features include an increased lactate at rest and exercise, and a myopathic picture on EMG and electroencephalogram showing generalized spike and wave discharges with background slowing. Only supportive treatment is available.

ANESTHETIC CONSIDERATIONS

The anesthesiologist may be involved in the care of patients with mitochondrial disease in multiple situations—often in the setting of obtaining a muscle biopsy in a child with an undiagnosed myopathy.[360] These patients may also present for surgery for procedures related to the disease (such as implantation of a permanent pacemaker in a patient with KSS[361]), for incidental medical problems, as well as in the labor and delivery suite for labor analgesia.[362] The diversity of clinical presentations encountered in the mitochondrial myopathies discourages a "one size fits all" approach to anesthesia. Rather, each patient should be thoroughly evaluated and the anesthetic plan tailored to the patient's specific needs.

PREOPERATIVE EVALUATION

Given the heterogeneous types of mitochondrial disease, patients with mitochondrial disease will need a comprehensive preoperative evaluation with a particular focus on neurologic, cardiac, respiratory, musculoskeletal, endocrinopathic, and metabolic compromise. An ECG and echocardiogram should be considered in patients with signs and symptoms of cardiomyopathy or conduction defects (or both). Although normal lactate and glucose levels cannot rule out mitochondrial diseases, laboratory studies consisting of glucose, electrolytes with anion gap, complete blood count, blood urea nitrogen, lactate, pyruvate, ammonia, CK, biotinidase, acyl carnitines, and blood and urine amino and organic acids could be used as initial investigation for suspected mitochondrial disorders.[363] Further workup should include an erythrocyte sedimentation rate, glycosylated hemoglobin (HbA_{1C}), liver and renal profiles, thyroid function tests, arterial blood gas, and urinalysis.[353,356] Multidisciplinary consultation with special laboratory and imaging studies may be required.[356]

INDUCTION AND MAINTENANCE OF ANESTHESIA

Anesthesia has a significant impact on mitochondrial function. Both barbiturates and propofol inhibit complex I of the electron transport chain.[363] Local anesthetics have been demonstrated to disrupt oxidative phosphorylation and decrease the bioenergetic capacity of mitochondria.[363] Sensitivity to intravenous barbiturates and etomidate has been reported.[364,365] Fortunately, notwithstanding the potential pitfalls mentioned above, almost every anesthetic technique has been safely used in patients with mitochondrial disease.[366,367] Midazolam,[368] thiopental,[369] propofol,[370,371] remifentanil,[372] and ketamine[371] have all been used safely. Notably, propofol and midazolam are known to inhibit the mitochondrial respiratory chain in a dose-dependent manner.[373] Indeed, mitochondrial dysfunction has been postulated as a mechanism for the propofol infusion syndrome.[374] It is safe to use propofol as an anesthetic induction agent, but the use of a propofol infusion for long periods should probably be avoided.

Premedication should avoid respiratory depression caused by impaired respiratory responses to hypoxemia. Volatile agents such as halothane, isoflurane, and sevoflurane have been shown to inhibit complex I.[363] This direct inhibition of mitochondrial electron transport system enzymes and altered mitochondrial bioenergetics in the heart were thought to be the mechanism of cardiac preconditioning by volatile anesthetics.[375,376] Inhaled sevoflurane has been widely used for induction because of its low pungency.[377] In some cases, halothane[368] and isoflurane[368,378] have also been used. Isoflurane has been recommended as the agent of choice in patients with Kearns-Sayre syndrome because rhythm disturbances have been reported with halothane in such patients.[368,378] In addition, artificial pacing capability is recommended when dealing with this specific subset of patients.[377] With use of the bispectral index, higher sensitivity to volatile agents has been suggested in children with mitochondrial diseases, especially with dysfunction of complex I.[379] However, its methodology has been criticized.[380] A decreased minimum alveolar concentration of halothane in patients with mental retardation has also been reported.[381]

Despite no real evidence and the fact that volatile anesthetics are frequently the anesthetic of choice when muscle relaxants are considered, several papers have expressed concern that these myopathies are associated with increased sensitivity to MH. This conclusion is not supported by any data. Increased sensitivity to nondepolarizing muscle relaxants has been documented for mivacurium,[382] atracurium,[383] and rocuronium.[383,384] In contrast, normal responses to depolarizing and nondepolarizing neuromuscular blockers such as pancuronium,[385] vecuronium,[386] and atracurium[370,387] are also reported. Although muscle relaxants are not absolutely contraindicated based on current literature and research, it is necessary for anesthesia practitioners to cautiously administer depolarizing or nondepolarizing neuromuscular blockers to those patients with mitochondrial diseases and to use neuromuscular monitoring.[353] Presently, there is no evidence to support an association between MH and mitochondrial disease. However, it may be prudent to avoid succinylcholine in patients with extensive myopathy to minimize the risk of hyperkalemia, although the safe use of succinylcholine has been documented in at least one patient with KSS.[385]

Nonsteroidal antiinflammatory drugs[377] and regional techniques consisting of local,[377,388] spinal,[389] and epidural administration have been reported. However, it is suggested that regional anesthesia be performed when neurologic abnormalities of the spinal cord and peripheral nerves have definitely been ruled out.[389] Importantly, coagulation function should be assessed because of the possibility of hepatic dysfunction.[377]

Opioids should be used with caution because of the increased risk for respiratory depression and their potential to induce respiratory acidosis in addition to the underlying metabolic acidosis.[377] Because patients with mitochondrial diseases have dysfunctional aerobic metabolism, any increase in the basic metabolic rate should be prevented.[356] Shivering, hypoxia, fasting, and hypotension in such patients may exacerbate the lactic acidosis and should therefore be avoided.[390] Finally, the increased postoperative infection rate in patients with mitochondrial diseases may be due to low hepatic mitochondrial activity, phagocytosis by Kupffer cells, and decreased activity of the reticuloendothelial system.[391]

Perhaps more important than the specific choice of anesthetic agents are the implications of patients' comorbidities and metabolic status. Normothermia should be maintained during surgeries, and intravenous fluids should be warmed to body temperature. Lactated Ringer (LR) should probably be avoided given the risk of preexisting lactic acidosis (although there is no evidence that LR has worsened acidosis when it has been used[366]). There have been multiple reports of hyponatremia (and occasional hyperkalemia) in these patients.[366,392,393] Adrenal insufficiency should be considered in such a picture, particularly when accompanied by hypotension.[366] Finally, these patients are at increased risk of cardiac conduction abnormalities and cardiomyopathy that should be taken into consideration while formulating an anesthetic plan (Box 35.7).

BOX 35.7 Perioperative Considerations for Patients with Mitochondrial Disease

1. Carefully assess and document the extent of organ system involvement preoperatively (including cardiac abnormalities in the KSS patients).
2. Minimize fasting period, avoid hypovolemia and glucose store depletion.
3. Minimize perioperative stress that may provoke increased energy requirement.
4. Pay particular attention to perioperative temperature control given that the mitochondrial respiratory chain is responsible for thermogenesis.
5. It is reasonable to administer glucose-containing solutions perioperatively, and to avoid lactate-containing fluids (e.g., lactated Ringer solution), particularly in children who are prone to lactic acidosis.
6. Every class of anesthetic agents is associated with theoretical risk of complications, but both volatile anesthetics and propofol have been successfully used in these patients.
7. Although there is no clear evidence of an association between malignant hyperthermia and mitochondrial disease, it is important to avoid succinylcholine.
8. Neuraxial anesthesia can be considered, but requires careful attention to preoperative neurologic dysfunction.

Myasthenia Gravis

Myasthenia gravis (MG) is an autoimmune disorder of the neuromuscular junction. Autoantibodies against the α-subunit of the muscle-type nicotinic acetylcholine receptor destroy acetylcholine receptors of the neuromuscular junction and cause classic transmission failure with muscle weakness and fatigue. Sparing of other α-subunits of neuronal-type nicotinic acetylcholine receptors provides an explanation for the lack of autonomic or CNS involvement of the disease. The incidence of MG varies between geographic regions, being 1.2 per million in Japan and about 14 per 100,000 in some areas of the United States.[394,395] In younger age groups, females are affected more often than males, whereas in elderly age groups (>60 years), males are more frequently affected.

There is a striking association between MG and hyperplasia of the thymus, with more than 70% of MG patients having thymus hyperplasia and 10% having thymomas.[395] MG may also be seen as a part of a paraneoplastic syndrome.[395]

Typically, patients first report bulbar symptoms consisting of diplopia and ptosis. The bulbar symptoms are often followed by unevenly distributed muscle weakness and fatigue of the extremities and face. Speech and chewing may be affected, as well as pharyngeal function and coordination of swallowing, with a subsequent increased frequency of aspiration of oral contents. The muscle weakness is often

BOX 35.8 Risk Factors of Postoperative Ventilation for Patients with Myasthenia Gravis[396]

Vital capacity <2-2.9 L
Duration of MG >6 years
Pyridostigmine dosage >750 mg/day
History of chronic pulmonary disease
Preoperative bulbar symptoms
History of myasthenic crisis
Intraoperative blood loss >1000 mL
Serum antiacetylcholine receptor antibody >100 nmol/mL
Pronounced decremental response on low frequency repetitive nerve stimulation

MG, Myasthenia gravis.
Modified from Anesthesia for the patient with myasthenia gravis. https://www.uptodate.com/contents/anesthesia-for-the-patient-with-myasthenia-gravis; 2018. Accessed April 8, 2019.

exacerbated during exercise and throughout the course of the day. Apart from the patchy distribution of muscle weakness, symptoms may also vary from day to day, and there may be periods of remission of varying duration.

The diagnosis of MG is made by neurologic examination and testing of the tendency to fatigue and exhibit increased weakness during exercise or repeated contractions. The diagnosis can be confirmed by the Tensilon test (administration of an anticholinesterase, e.g., edrophonium). Improvement is usually seen within 5 minutes after administration of the drug and lasts for about 10 minutes. In addition, electrophysiologic evaluation is often performed and shows a classic decrement in the compound muscle action potential after repetitive nerve stimulation (Box 35.8).[396]

ANESTHETIC CONSIDERATIONS

Ideally, careful neurologic consultation in addition to preoperative evaluation should be performed on MG patients with the aim of optimizing drug therapy and preparing for postoperative care. Pulmonary function tests may be indicated to determine the need for mechanical ventilation postoperatively.[382] In addition, a number of risk factors have been associated with the necessity for postoperative ventilation.

As a general rule, patients should keep taking their anticholinesterase medication and be informed about the possibility of postoperative ventilator support. Succinylcholine can be used if needed for rapid tracheal intubation. However, patients with MG might need larger than normal doses (1.5-2.0 mg/kg body weight) because of the decreased number of functional acetylcholine receptors.[397] On the other hand, as a result of the decrease in cholinesterase activity achieved by anticholinesterase treatment, neuromuscular blocks with succinylcholine or mivacurium are frequently prolonged.[398,399] Traditionally, nondepolarizing neuromuscular blockers can be used in patients with MG but should be given with caution because their effects are highly unpredictable and the distribution of muscle weakness is often uneven. Most anesthesiologists used to dose nondepolarizing muscle relaxants in small increments corresponding to 0.1 to 0.2 times the 95% effective dose (ED_{95}) until the desired neuromuscular blocking effect is achieved. Perioperative anticholinesterase treatment will modify the response to traditional reversal agents, because of the already existing acetylcholinesterase block, and in some cases, will reportedly prolong the recovery of neuromuscular function after the administration of a reversal agent.[400] With the adoption of a newly modified γ-cyclodextrin neuromuscular reversal agent, sugammadex, the management of airway and steroidal neuromuscular blockade agents, such as rocuronium or vecuronium, becomes simplified in patients with MG.[401,402]

Sugammadex has a lower affinity to vecuronium than rocuronium; however, the reversal with sugammadex for vecuronium is still very satisfactory because fewer vecuronium molecules are present for equivalent blockade due to its higher potency to rocuronium. Although FDA has not approved its use in pediatric populations, current reported cases were favorable. On a separate note, sugammadex does have conflicting effects on progesterone, cortisol, aldosterone, and testosterone levels and may alter some coagulation parameters such as activated thromboplastin time and prothrombin time, or INR.[403]

Potent volatile anesthetics have been used successfully in MG patients. Because of the impaired margin of safety at the neuromuscular junction, a volatile anesthetic usually provides adequate muscular paralysis to allow most surgical procedures to be performed without the need for a neuromuscular blocking agent. Epidural and spinal anesthesia can be used in MG patients in addition to general anesthesia, provided that muscle function and ventilation are carefully monitored perioperatively. For a more detailed review, see Baraka[404] and Abel and Eisenkraft.[405]

EATON-LAMBERT MYASTHENIC SYNDROME

Eaton-Lambert myasthenic syndrome (ELMS) is an immune-mediated channelopathy caused by decreased release of acetylcholine as a result of autoantibodies against presynaptic voltage-gated calcium channels and other presynaptic elements.[406] Patients with ELMS have muscle weakness and fatigability, generally of the proximal limb muscles, with the lower extremities affected more often than the extraocular and bulbar muscle groups. The syndrome is frequently part of a paraneoplastic phenomenon, usually combined with small cell lung carcinoma. Unlike MG, patients with ELMS are usually worse in the morning with gradual improvement throughout the day. Improvement of muscle function with exercise is due to the accumulation of presynaptic calcium and subsequent improved release of acetylcholine.[407] A minority of patients exhibit autonomic dysfunction. The diagnosis of ELMS is made by careful physical examination combined with clinical electrophysiology showing the typical facilitation of motor action potential with high-frequency nerve stimulation (30-50 Hz). Anticholinesterase treatment has little effect on patients with ELMS. Plasmapheresis, immunoglobulin therapy, and 3,4-diaminopyridine (DAP) result in transient improvement.

ANESTHETIC CONSIDERATIONS

As in patients with MG, those with ELMS should be carefully evaluated for the risk of postoperative respiratory failure and the need for prolonged respiratory monitoring in the postoperative period. Sensitivity to depolarizing and nondepolarizing NMBA is usually increased. In patients treated with DAP or an anticholinesterase agent, reversal of a neuromuscular blockade may be ineffective.

Periodic Paralysis (Hyperkalemic, Hypokalemic, and Normokalemic)

The periodic paralyses are a group of disorders that are characterized by alterations of function in voltage-gated ion channels; hence these diseases are sometimes termed "skeletal muscle channelopathies."[408] The symptomatology of the particular channelopathy depends on the specific ion channel involved and can be divided into three broad categories: (1) chloride channelopathies (myotonia without paralysis e.g., MC, see earlier), (2) sodium channelopathies (myotonia with paralysis, such as hyperkalemic periodic paralysis [HyperPP]), and (3) other cation channelopathies (paralysis without myotonia, such as hypokalemic periodic paralysis [HypoPP]).[409]

HyperPP is an autosomal dominant disorder first described by Tyler and associates in 1951.[320] It is characterized by attacks of flaccid weakness associated with increased serum potassium.[410] Precipitating factors include potassium rich foods, and rest after exercise. In addition, a cold environment, emotional stress, fasting, glucocorticoids, and pregnancy can provoke or worsen the attacks. The paralysis may last for 15 minutes to an hour, with decreased tendon reflexes. In the interictal state, HyperPP is usually associated with mild myotonia that does not impede voluntary movements.[320]

The pathogenesis of HyperPP involves mutations in *SCN4A*, encoding the voltage-gated sodium channel $Na_V1.4$ of mature muscle fibers; and such mutations lead to pathologically increased sodium current and an increased tendency of the muscle fiber to become depolarized.[320,410] Influx of sodium into the muscle is accompanied by simultaneous efflux of potassium and hyperkalemia. Mutant channels exhibit sustained sodium currents that lead to prolonged membrane depolarization, which will then cause myotonia followed by membrane desensitization (or inactivation) and will eventually result in paralysis. In HyperPP patients, serum CK can be elevated, sometimes 5 to 10 times above the normal limit, whereas serum sodium and potassium levels are normal in the interictal state.[320] EMG recordings will often show myotonic discharges during and between attacks. Muscle biopsies may show small peripheral vacuoles in the sarcoplasm. Recent studies supported that normokalemic periodic paralysis is a variant of the HyperPP, not a distinct disease, because all the subjects exhibited clinical and laboratory features of the HyperPP.[411-413] Treatment includes medication with acetazolamide (a carbonic anhydrase inhibitor) and mexiletine (an antiarrhythmic with a mechanism of action similar to lidocaine). Behavioral modification, such as avoiding potassium containing foods, strenuous exercise, fasting, and exposure to cold are also important.[409]

HypoPP is characterized by a decrease in potassium levels in blood. Attacks of HypoPP can be triggered by rigorous exercise, stress, high-carbohydrate or high-salt meals, pregnancy, menstruation, hypothermia, or drugs such as insulin.[414,415] EMG does not usually show myotonia.[410] The severity of attacks is usually greater than those occurring in patients with HyperPP. HypoPP is an autosomal dominant disease with higher penetration in males. The disease is due to loss of function of one of the two different ion channel types: $Ca_V1.1$ and $Na_V1.4$.[410] The most common muscle groups affected are those in the arms and legs; however, the disorder can also affect swallowing and respiratory muscles, which can be fatal in severe cases. The diagnosis of HypoPP is made by laboratory tests demonstrating hypokalemia during attacks and normokalemia between attacks. Mutations in the skeletal muscle voltage-gated calcium channel encoded by *CACNA1S* (HypoPP type 1) and *SCN4A* (HypoPP type 2) have been identified.[313] Theoretical association of HypoPP to MH was made because a few MH patients were known to have mutations in the *CACNA1S*.[313] It is generally accepted that the risk of susceptibility of HypoPP patients to MH is similar to that of the general population. It is still unclear the exact mechanisms that lead to hypokalemic paralysis. It is important to remain aware of the differences in the clinical features between HyperPP and HypoPP. HypoPP is not associated with myotonia, a spontaneous attack is associated with hypokalemia (a diagnostic criterion), potassium is a remedy, and glucose triggers an attack.[409] Treatment is centered on the identification and avoidance of triggers. Potassium administration can be useful in the treatment of an acute attack. The prophylactic medication of choice in HypoPP type 1 is acetazolamide[416]—however, acetazolamide can worsen symptoms in type 2 HypoPP.[417] Such patients may respond to potassium-sparing diuretics such as spironolactone.[418]

Clinically resembling HypoPP, thyrotoxic periodic paralysis (TPP) occurs later in life than HypoPP. It has a strong male predominance, and is much more common in patients of oriental descent. Loss of function mutations in the inward rectifying potassium channel ($K_{ir}2.6$) may be involved in some cases of TPP.[419] The condition responds to antithyroid medications such as methimazole.[409]

ANESTHETIC CONSIDERATIONS

Potassium, cholinesterase inhibitors, and depolarizing muscle relaxants will aggravate the myotonia in HyperPP patients.[320] Prolonged muscle weakness has been reported when succinylcholine is used.[420] Although one third of patients had no signs of myotonia,[421] masseter spasm and respiratory and skeletal muscles stiffness could still occur during intubation and ventilation.[320] Therefore neostigmine and succinylcholine should be contraindicated in HyperPP patients. Nondepolarizing muscle relaxants may be safely used.[422,423] The safe use of both volatile agents and propofol has been documented.[422-424] Ideally, all patients with HyperPP need to be admitted preoperatively so that proper preoperative fasting can be accompanied by the administration of dextrose-containing potassium-free maintenance fluid.[423] Postoperatively, HyperPP patients may remain paralyzed for up to several hours. Preventive measures such as maintaining normal body temperature and low serum potassium levels and avoiding hypoglycemia are helpful in limiting such paralysis.[422] Although patients with sodium channel pathology have often been considered to be susceptible to MH, there is no increased risk for MH in these patients.[314] General anesthesia with and without nondepolarizing muscle relaxants has been shown to have satisfactory outcomes.[420,422,423,425,426] Regional techniques may also be appropriate for this patient group.[421,425,426] Abortion of the hyperkalemic attack may be accomplished by administering glucose, insulin, epinephrine, and calcium supplements, or, alternatively, glucagon may be used. β-Adrenergic treatment with metaproterenol has also been shown to prevent attacks and facilitate recovery.[423]

Management of HypoPP patients should focus on avoiding triggers and medications causing a shift of potassium. General anesthesia, postoperative stress, glucose-containing intravenous solutions, and long-acting neuromuscular blockers are associated with postoperative paralytic events.[414] Patients with HypoPP undergoing general anesthesia have been reported to exhibit weakness and respiratory distress in the postoperative period.[427,428] While safe use of intermediate and short-acting nondepolarizing muscle relaxants, such as atracurium and mivacurium, have been documented,[429-431] and it is probably prudent to avoid long-acting muscle relaxants.[432] Epidural analgesia has been shown to reduce both pain-related hyperventilation and serum catecholamines, thereby minimizing changes in serum potassium levels.[414] The sympathomimetic effect of epinephrine-containing local anesthetics may also precipitate hypokalemia.[414] Unlike HyperPP, an association between HypoPP and MH cannot be categorically ruled out,[433] although the use of isoflurane in HypoPP has been reported.[431] There are a number of reports of MH-like metabolic crises in patients with HypoPP.[434-436] Contracture-like responses to succinylcholine have also been described.[437] In one of the above descriptions, it seemed likely that there were two unrelated mutations conferring both HypoPP and sensitivity to MH in the same patient.[436] Therefore while the probability of MH in a given patient with HypoPP is likely to be remote, it cannot be ruled out, and the safest course might be the use of a nontriggering anesthetic. If volatile agents are used, they should be used with extra vigilance.[433]

Summary

MH is a subclinical myopathy featuring an eerie and erratic metabolic mayhem that is unmasked on exposure to potent volatile anesthetics or succinylcholine. Skeletal muscle acutely and unexpectedly increases its sarcoplasmic Ca^{2+} concentration, thereby leading to increased oxygen consumption and lactate production, and resulting in greater heat production, respiratory and metabolic acidosis, muscle rigidity, sympathetic stimulation, and increased cellular permeability. MHS skeletal muscle differs from normal muscle in that it is always closer to loss of control of Ca^{2+} concentration within the muscle fiber, and it can involve a generalized alteration in cellular or subcellular membrane permeability. This is an EC coupling defect resulting from an alteration in protein-protein interaction in the CRU. It is a homozygous, single point mutation of *RyR1* in swine and a heterozygous disorder in humans, in whom there may also be a modification of RyR1 protein function by interacting structures, membranes, or enzymes. Diagnosis rests on acute awareness of the signs and symptoms of this syndrome, of which hyperthermia is a late sign. Specific treatment includes administration of dantrolene to lower muscle Ca^{2+} levels, and symptomatic treatment consists of reversal of the acid-base and temperature changes. Evaluation of affected families is guided by analysis of drug-induced muscle contractures (by European IVCT and North American CHCT protocols) and genetic testing of DNA samples. General or regional anesthesia is safe for patients susceptible to MH, provided that care is taken to specially prepare the anesthesia machine and avoid all potent volatile anesthetics and succinylcholine. Research on MH has yielded insight into the physiology of metabolism and into the molecular biology of genetic muscle disorders. Challenges that remain include identification of all genetic mutations responsible for human MH, elucidation of the mechanism that links exposure to subsequent loss of control of Ca^{2+}, development of noninvasive and nondestructive testing for susceptibility, and determination of the mode of action of dantrolene.

Acknowledgment

This chapter is a consolidation of two chapters in the 8th edition, Chapter 42, Neuromuscular Disorders and other Genetic Disorders and Chapter 43, Malignant Hyperthermia and Muscle-Related Disorders. The editors, publisher, and the returning authors, would like to thank the following authors: Aranya Bagchi, Richa Saxena, and Diptiman Bose for their contributions to the prior edition of this work. It has served as the foundation for the current.

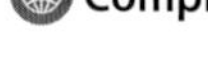

Complete references available online at expertconsult.com.

References

1. Lerman J. *Br J Anaesth*. 2011;107(suppl 1):i79.
2. Rosenberg H, Pollock N, Schiemann A, Bulger T, Stowell K. Malignant hyperthermia: a review. *Orphanet J Rare Dis*. 2015;10:93.
3. Sumitani M, et al. *Anesthesiology*. 2011;114:84.
4. Suyama H, et al. *J Anesth*. 2002;16:207.
5. Monnier N, et al. *Anesthesiology*. 2002;97:1067.
6. Brady JE, et al. *Anesth Analg*. 2009;109:1162.
7. Yuen B, et al. *FASEB J*. 2012;26:1311.
8. Rosenberg H, Shutack JG. *Paediatr Anaesth*. 1996;6:87.
9. Rosenberg H, et al. *Orphanet J Rare Dis*. 2007;2:21.
10. Robinson R, et al. *Hum Mutat*. 2006;27:977.
11. Harrison GG, Isaacs H. *Anaesthesia*. 1992;47:54.
12. Gronert BJ, Antognini JF. Malignant hyperthermia. In: Miller RD, ed. *Anesthesia*. New York: Churchill Livingstone; 1994:1075.
13. Ombrédanne L. *Rev Med Française*. 1929;10:617.
14. Denborough MA, et al. *Br J Anaesth*. 1962;34:395.
15. Kalow W, et al. *Lancet*. 1970;296:895.
16. Britt BA, et al. *Can Anaesth Soc J*. 1969;16:89.
17. Ball RA, et al. *Vet Med Small Anim Clin*. 1973;68:1156.
18. Briskey EJ. *Adv Food Res*. 1964;13:89.
19. Hall LW, et al. *Br Med J*. 1966;2:1305.
20. Fujii J, et al. *Science*. 1991;253:448.
21. Harrison GG. *Br J Anaesth*. 1975;47:62.
22. Kolb ME, et al. *Anesthesiology*. 1982;56:254.
23. Lopez JR, et al. *Acta Cient Venez*. 1985;36:102.
24. Lopez JR, et al. *Muscle Nerve*. 1986;9:85.
25. Lopez JR, et al. *Muscle Nerve*. 1988;11:82.
26. Lopez JR, et al. *Anesthesiology*. 1992;76:711.
27. Choi RH, et al. *Proc Natl Acad Sci U S A*. 2017;114:4811.
28. Cherednichenko G, et al. *Molecular Pharmacology*. 2008;73:1203.
29. Pessah IN, et al. *Biochem Biophys Res Commun*. 1985;128:449.

30. Pessah IN, et al. *Biochem Biophys Res Commun.* 1986;139:235.
31. MacKenzie AE, et al. *Am J Hum Genet.* 1990;46:1082.
32. Otsu K, et al. *Genomics.* 1993;17:507.
33. Sorrentino V, et al. *Genomics.* 1993;18:163.
34. Collins JH. *Biochem Biophys Res Commun.* 1991;178:1288.
35. Jayaraman T, et al. *J Biol Chem.* 1992;267:9474.
36. Lam E, et al. *J Biol Chem.* 1995;270:26511.
37. Timerman AP, et al. *J Biol Chem.* 1996;271:20385.
38. Beam KG, et al. *Ann N Y Acad Sci.* 1989;560:127.
39. Tanabe T, et al. *Nature.* 1990;346:567.
40. Nakai J, et al. *J Biol Chem.* 1998;273:24983.
41. Nakai J, et al. *Two Regions of the Ryanodine Receptor Involved in Coupling with L-Type Ca2+ Channels.* 1998.
42. Sheridan DC, et al. *Proc Natl Acad Sci U S A.* 2006;103:19760.
43. Flucher BE, Franzini-Armstrong C. *Proc Natl Acad Sci U S A.* 1996;93:8101.
44. Cherednichenko G, et al. *Proc Natl Acad Sci U S A.* 2004;101:15793.
45. Gaburjakova M, et al. *J Biol Chem.* 2001;276:16931.
46. Meissner G. *Front Biosci.* 2002;7:d2072.
47. Ward CW, et al. *J Biol Chem.* 2004;279:5781.
48. Pessah IN, et al. *Pharmacol Ther.* 2010;125:260.
49. Perni S, et al. *De Novo Reconstitution Reveals the Proteins Required for Skeletal Muscle Voltage-Induced Ca(2+) Release.* 2017.
50. Polster A, et al. *Proc Natl Acad Sci U S A.* 2016;113:10986.
51. Cherednichenko G, et al. *Mol Pharmacol.* 2008;73:1203–1212.
52. Yang T, et al. *J Biol Chem.* 2007;282:37471.
53. Yang T, et al. *Am J Physiol Cell Physiol.* 2007;292:C1591.
54. Eltit JM, et al. *Proc Natl Acad Sci U S A.* 2012;109:7923.
55. Eltit JM, et al. *J Biol Chem.* 2010;285:38453.
56. Eltit JM, et al. *Proc Natl Acad Sci U S A.* 2011;108:7046.
57. Bannister RA, et al. *J Gen Physiol.* 2010;135:629.
58. Esteve E, et al. *J Gen Physiol.* 2010;135:619.
59. Wappler F, et al. *Eur J Anaesthesiol.* 2003;20:528.
60. Yang T, et al. *J Biol Chem.* 2003;278:25722.
61. Reuter DA, et al. *Can J Anaesth.* 2003;50:643.
62. Capacchione JF, Muldoon SM. *Anesth Analg.* 2009;109:1065.
63. Pessah IN, et al. *Mol Pharmacol.* 1987;31:232.
64. Zimanyi I, Pessah IN. *Brain Res.* 1991;561:181.
65. Jona I, et al. *Pflugers Arch.* 2001;441:729.
66. Laver D. *Clin Exp Pharmacol Physiol.* 2001;28:675.
67. Laver DR, et al. *J Membr Biol.* 1997;156:213.
68. Voss AA, et al. *Biochem Biophys Res Commun.* 2008;366:988.
69. Lamb GD. *J Muscle Res Cell Motil.* 1993;14:554.
70. Laver DR, et al. *Biophys J.* 1997;73:1913.
71. Barrientos GC, et al. *J Biol Chem.* 2012;287:2863.
72. Feng W, et al. *Mol Pharmacol.* 2011;79:420.
73. Chelu MG, et al. *FASEB J.* 2006;20:329.
74. Yang T, et al. *Anesthesiology.* 2006;105:1164.
75. Lopez JR, et al. *Am J Physiol Cell Physiol.* 2005;288:C606.
76. Ikemoto N, Yamamoto T. *Front Biosci.* 2002;7:d671.
77. Samso M, et al. *PLoS Biol.* 2009;7:e85.
78. Zalk R, Marks AR. *Ca(2+) Release Channels Join the 'Resolution Revolution'.* 2017.
79. Carpenter D, et al. *BMC Med Genet.* 2009;10:104.
80. Toppin PJ, et al. *Can J Anaesth.* 2010;57:689.
81. Pirone A, et al. *Am J Physiol Cell Physiol.* 2010;299:C1345.
82. Weiss RG, et al. *Am J Physiol Cell Physiol.* 2004;287:C1094.
83. Bannister RA, Beam KG. *J Muscle Res Cell Motil.* 2009;30:217.
84. Jones DE, et al. *Anesthesiology.* 1988;83:A344.
85. Hurne AM, et al. *J Biol Chem.* 2005;280:36994.
86. Bannister RA, et al. *J Gen Physiol.* 2009;133:79.
87. Sultana N, et al. *Development.* 2016;143:1547.
88. Putney JW, et al. *J Cell Sci.* 2001;114:2223.
89. Kurebayashi N, Ogawa Y. *J Physiol.* 2001;533:185.
90. Ma J, Pan Z. *Front Biosci.* 2003;8:d242.
91. Pan Z, et al. *Nat Cell Biol.* 2002;4:379.
92. Zhao X, et al. *J Biol Chem.* 2006;281:33477.
93. Desmedt JE, Hainaut K. *J Physiol.* 1977;265:565.
94. Krivickas LS, et al. *Muscle Nerve.* 2000;23:529.
95. Yamaguchi N, et al. *J Biochem. (Tokyo).* 1997;121:432.
96. Paul-Pletzer K, et al. *J Biol Chem.* 2002;277:34918.
97. Monnier N, et al. *Am J Hum Genet.* 1997;60:1316.
98. Sambuughin N, et al. *Anesthesiology.* 2001;95:594.
99. Brown RL, et al. *Hum Mol Genet.* 2000;9:1515.
100. Girard T, et al. *Hum Mutat.* 2001;18:357.
101. Brandt A, et al. *Hum Mol Genet.* 1999;8:2055.
102. Rueffert H, et al. *Am J Med Genet A.* 2004;124:248.
103. Robinson R, et al. *Hum Genet.* 2003;112:217.
104. Gillard EF, et al. *Genomics.* 1991;11:751.
105. Sei Y, et al. *Anesthesiology.* 2004;101:824.
106. Davis M, et al. *Br J Anaesth.* 2002;88:508.
107. Oyamada H, et al. *Jpn J Pharmacol.* 2002;88:159.
108. Yeh HM, et al. *Anesth Analg.* 2005;101:1401.
109. Fletcher JE, et al. *Br J Anaesth.* 1995;75:307.
110. Lynch PJ, et al. *Anesthesiology.* 1997;86:620.
111. Monnier N, et al. *Hum Mol Genet.* 2003;12:1171.
112. Rueffert H, et al. *Br J Anaesth.* 2001;87:240.
113. No authors listed. A protocol for the investigation of malignant hyperpyrexia (MH) susceptibility. *Br J Anaesth.* 1984;56:1267.
114. Ording H, et al. *Acta Anaesthesiol Scand.* 1997;41:955.
115. Hopkins PM, et al. *Br J Anaesth.* 2015;115:531.
116. Larach MG. *Anesth Analg.* 1989;69:511.
117. Allen GC, et al. *Anesthesiology.* 1998;88:579.
118. Metterlein T, et al. *Cardiovasc Ther.* 2010;28:356.
119. Metterlein T, et al. *Muscle Nerve.* 2011;44:208.
120. Gerbershagen MU, et al. *Eur J Anaesthesiol.* 2011;29:42.
121. Johannsen S, et al. *Anesth Analg.* 2012;115:925.
122. Bendahan D, et al. *Acta Anaesthesiol Scand.* 2004;48:1019.
123. Baur CP, et al. *Anesth Analg.* 2000;90:200.
124. Metterlein T, et al. *Eur J Anaesthesiol.* 2011;28:251.
125. Metterlein T, et al. *Minerva Anestesiol.* 2011;77:768.
126. Migita T, et al. *Acta Anaesthesiol Scand.* 2011;56:351.
127. Zhou H, et al. *Am J Hum Genet.* 2006;79:859.
128. Urwyler A, et al. *Br J Anaesth.* 2001;86:283.
129. Robinson RL, et al. *Hum Mutat.* 2002;20:88.
130. Rueffert H, et al. *Acta Anaesthesiol Scand.* 2002;46:692.
131. Larach MG, et al. *Anesth Analg.* 2010;110:498.
132. Allen GC, Brubaker CL. *Anesth Analg.* 1998;86:1328.
133. Shulman M, et al. *Anesthesiology.* 1981;54:259.
134. Gronert GA. *Anesthesiology.* 1980;53:395.
135. Hall GM, et al. *Br J Anaesth.* 1976;48:270.
136. Denborough M, Hopkinson KC. *Lancet.* 1988;1:191.
137. Bendixen D, et al. *Acta Anaesthesiol Scand.* 1997;41:480.
138. Larach MG, et al. *Anesthesiology.* 1994;80:771.
139. Gronert GA, et al. *Anesth Analg.* 1980;59:377.
140. Haverkort-Poels PJ, et al. *Muscle Nerve.* 1987;10:45.
141. Denborough MA, et al. *Br Med J (Clin Res Ed).* 1988;296:1442.
142. Hackl W, et al. *Br J Anaesth.* 1991;66:138.
143. Hopkins PM, et al. *Lancet.* 1991;338:1491.
144. Kochling A, et al. *Anaesth Intensive Care.* 1998;26:315.
145. Reynolds AC, et al. *Lancet.* 1981;2:303.
146. Gronert GA, et al. *Anesthesiology.* 1977;47:411.
147. Gronert GA, White DA. *Pflugers Arch.* 1988;411:226.
148. Wappler F, et al. *Anesthesiology.* 2001;94:95.
149. Anetseder M, et al. *Neurology.* 1994;44:2393.
150. Ryan JF, Tedeschi LG. *J Clin Anesth.* 1997;9:66.
151. *Adverse Effects of Heat and Exercise in Relation to MH Susceptibility.* 2018. https://www.mhaus.org/healthcare-professionals/mhaus-recommendations/adverse-effects-of-heat-and-exercise-in-relation-to-mh-susceptibility/.
152. Butler-Browne GS, et al. *Muscle Nerve.* 1988;11:610.
153. Morgan DL, Proske U. *Physiol Rev.* 1984;64:103.
154. van der Spek AF, et al. *Br J Anaesth.* 1990;64:21.
155. Magee KR, Shy GM. *Brain.* 1956;79:610.
156. Norwood FL, et al. *Brain.* 2009;132:3175.
157. Jungbluth H, et al. *Semin Pediatr Neurol.* 2011;18:239.
158. Engel AG, et al. *Mayo Clin Proc.* 1971;46:666.
159. Klingler W, et al. *Anesth Analg.* 2009;109:1167.
160. Koch BM, et al. *Arch Neurol.* 1985;42:1204.
161. Osada H, et al. *Gynecol Obstet Invest.* 2004;58:32.
162. Allanson JE. Noonan syndrome. *J Med Genet.* 1987;24:9–13.
163. Benca J, Hogan K. *Anesth Analg.* 2009;109:1049.
164. Briggs BJ, Dickerman JD. *Pediatr Blood Cancer.* 2012;58:167.
165. Tartaglia M, et al. *Mol Syndromol.* 2010;1:2.
166. Hunter A, Pinsky L. *J Pediatr.* 1975;86:412.
167. Sharathkumar AA. *Pediatr Blood Cancer.* 2012;59:592.
168. Bajwa SJ, et al. *Saudi J Anaesth.* 2011;5:345.
169. Dadabhoy ZP, Winnie AP. *Anesthesiology.* 1988;68:636.
170. Campbell AM, Bousfield JD. *Anaesthesia.* 1992;47:131.
171. McBain J, et al. *Can J Anaesth.* 2006;53:274.

172. Isaacs H, Badenhorst ME. *Muscle Nerve*. 1992;15:740.
173. Heiman-Patterson TD, et al. *Pediatr Neurol*. 1986;2:175.
174. King JO, Denborough MA. *J Pediatr*. 1973;83:37.
175. McPherson EW, Taylor CA. *Am J Med Genet*. 1981;8:159.
176. Kaplan AM, et al. *J Pediatr*. 1977;91:431.
177. Isaacs H, Barlow MB. *Br J Anaesth*. 1973;45:901.
178. Isaacs H, et al. *Br J Anaesth*. 1973;45:860.
179. Isaacs H, Barlow MB. *J Neurol Neurosurg Psychiatry*. 1973;36:228.
180. Reed W, et al. *Blood*. 2003;101:351.
181. Habib AS, et al. *Can J Anaesth*. 2003;50:589.
182. D'Arcy CE, et al. *Neurology*. 2008;71:776.
183. Dowling JJ, et al. *Neuromuscul Disord*. 2011;21:420.
184. Glahn KP, et al. *Br J Anaesth*. 2010;105:417.
185. Birgenheier N, et al. *Anesth Analg* 112:1363.
186. Kugler Y, Russell WJ. *Anaesth Intensive Care*. 2011;39:84.
187. Rosenberg H. *Anesthesiol*. 2010;20. News.
188. Flewellen EH, et al. *Anesthesiology*. 1983;59:275.
189. Brandom BW, et al. *Anesth Analg*. 2011;112:1115.
190. Oh ST, et al. *J Surg Res*. 1997;71:79.
191. Korolkiewicz RP, et al. *J Physiol Pharmacol*. 2000;51:821.
192. Gener B, et al. *Pediatrics*. 2010;125:e1514.
193. Lerman J, et al. *Anesthesiology*. 1989;70:625.
194. Burkman JM, et al. *Anesthesiology*. 2007;106:901; quiz 1077.
195. Hopkins PM. *Anesthesiology*. 2007;106:893.
196. Gallant EM, et al. *Anesth Analg*. 1985;64:601.
197. Harrison GG, et al. *Anaesth Intensive Care*. 1988;16:197.
198. Migita T, et al. *J Anesth*. 2012;26:579.
199. Metterlein T, et al. *Anesth Analg*. 2011;112:1174.
200. Choi RH, et al. *Proceedings of the National Academy of Sciences*; 2017:4811.
201. Larach MG, et al. *Anesth Analg*. 2012;114:94.
202. Wong CA, Denholm B. *Anesthsiol News*. 2011;17.
203. Aderibigbe T, et al. *Anesthesiology*. 2014;120:1333.
204. Maccani RM, et al. *Anesth Analg*. 1996;82:790.
205. McGraw TT, Keon TP. *Can J Anaesth*. 1989;36:530.
206. Whitty RJ, et al. *Can J Anaesth*. 2009;56:497.
207. Crawford MW, et al. *Anesthesiology*. 2007;106:289.
208. Prinzhausen H, et al. *Can J Anaesth*. 2006;53:885.
209. Petroz GC, Lerman J. *Anesthesiology*. 2002;96:941.
210. Brunner HW, et al. *Acta Anaesthesiol Scand*. 2011;55:1118.
211. Shanahan H, et al. *Eur J Anaesthesiol*. 2012;29:229.
212. Gunter JB, et al. *Anesth Analg*. 2008;107:1936.
213. Jones C, et al. *Anaesth Intensive Care*. 2012;40:490.
214. Schonell LH, et al. *Anaesth Intensive Care*. 2003;31:58.
215. Feldman JM. *Anesthesiology*. 2011;115:434; author reply 6.
216. Block FE. *Anesth Analg*. 2011;112:1270.
217. Jantzen JP, et al. *Anaesthesist*. 1989;38:639.
218. Preparation of Anesthesia Workstations to Anesthetize MH Susceptible Patients. https://www.mhaus.org/healthcare-professionals/mhaus-recommendations/preparation-of-anesthesia-workstations-to-anesthetize-mh-susceptible-patients/. Accessed 30.05.18.
219. Criteria for a recommended standard. *Occupational Exposure to Waste Anesthetic Gases and Vapors*; 1977. http://www.cdc.gov/niosh/pdfs/77-140a.pdf
220. Anesthetic Gases. *Guidelines for Workplace Exposures*; 2000. https://www.osha.gov/dts/osta/anestheticgases/index.html
221. Anetseder M, et al. *Lancet*. 2003;362:494.
222. Bina S, et al. *Anesthesiology*. 2006;104:90.
223. Schuster F, et al. *Anesthesiology*. 2007;107:616.
224. Schuster F, et al. *Anesth Analg*. 2006;102:468.
225. Bina S, et al. *Eur J Anaesthesiol*. 2007;25:48.
226. Girard T, et al. *J Biol Chem*. 2001;276:48077.
227. Litman RS, Rosenberg H. *JAMA*. 2005;293:2918.
228. McKinney LC, et al. *Anesthesiology*. 2006;104:1191.
229. Ording H, et al. *Br J Anaesth*. 1990;64:341.
230. Sei Y, et al. *Anesthesiology*. 2002;97:1052.
231. Gareau PJ, et al. *Free Radic Res Commun*. 1993;19:43.
232. Payen JF, et al. *Anesthesiology*. 1993;78:848.
233. Nanson JK, Sheikh A. *Int J Obstet Anesth*. 2000;9:276.
234. Stowell K, et al. *Anaesth Intensive Care*. 2007;35:454.
235. Girard T, et al. *Anesthesiology*. 2006;104:1353.
236. Suggested guidelines for management of the pregnant-patient not believed to be at risk for MH, but whose partners is susceptible to malignant hyperthermia. 2009. https://www.mhaus.org/healthcare-professionals/mhaus-recommendations/parturient-with-mhs-partner/.
237. Tombul T, et al. *Acta neurologica Belgica*. 2011;111:116.
238. Freedman MS, et al. *Arch Neurol*. 2005;62:865.
239. Bader AM, et al. *J Clin Anesth*. 1988;1:21.
240. Staikou C, Rekatsina M. *Saudi J Anaesth*. 2017;11:472.
241. Bornemann-Cimenti H, et al. *Rev Bras Anestesiol*. 2016;67:404.
242. Ludolph AC, et al. *Curr Opin Neurol*. 2012;25:530.
243. Rothstein JD. *Cell*. 2017;171:725.
244. Shimizu T, et al. *Neurology*. 2000;54:1534.
245. You TM, Kim S. *J Dent Anesth Pain Med*. 2017;17:235.
246. Rosenbaum KJ, et al. *Anesthesiology*. 1971;35:638.
247. Jacobs BC, et al. *Neurology*. 1998;51:1110.
248. Lawn ND, et al. *Arch Neurol*. 2001;58:893.
249. Asbury AK. *Arch Neurol*. 1981;(suppl 9):1.
250. Hughes RA, et al. *Cochrane Database Syst Rev*. 2012;7:CD002063.
251. Asahina M, et al. *Acta Neurol Scand*. 2002;105:44.
252. McGrady EM. *Anaesthesia*. 1987;42:899.
253. Steiner I, et al. *Neurology*. 1985;35:1473.
254. Brooks H, et al. *Anaesthesia*. 2000;55:894.
255. Zochodne DW, et al. *Brain*. 1987;110(Pt 4):819.
256. Bolton CF. *Muscle Nerve*. 2005;32:140.
257. Dodson BA, et al. *Crit Care Med*. 1995;23:815.
258. Hermans G, et al. *Am J Respir Crit Care Med*. 2007;175:480.
259. Gronert GA. *Anesthesiology*. 1981;55:547.
260. O'Neill GN. *Int Anesthesiol Clin*. 2006;44:107.
261. Rudnik-Schneborn S, et al. Spinal muscular atrophies. In Engel A, Franzini-Armstrong C, eds: *Myology*, 3rd ed, New York: McGraw-Hill; 20041845.
262. Charcot-Marie-Tooth disease. Genetics, clinical features, and diagnosis. *UpToDate*. 2018. https://www.uptodate.com/contents/charcot-marie-tooth-disease-genetics-clinical-features-and-diagnosis.
263. Ginz HF, et al. *Anaesthesist*. 2001;50:767.
264. Gratarola A, et al. *Minerva Anestesiol*. 1998;64:357.
265. Sugino S, et al. *Masui*. 2002;51:1016.
266. Baur CP, et al. *Anasthesiol Intensivmed Notfallmed Schmerzther*. 2002;37:125.
267. Antognini JF. *Can J Anaesth*. 1992;39:398.
268. Baranov D, et al. Neurological diseases. In: Fleisher L, ed. *Anesthesia and Uncommon Diseases*. 5th ed. Philadelphia: Saunders; 2006.
269. Pogson D, et al. *Br J Anaesth*. 2000;85:914.
270. Naguib M, Samarkandi AH. *Can J Anaesth*. 1998;45:56.
271. Schmitt HJ, Munster T. *Can J Anaesth*. 2006;53:984.
272. Reah G, et al. *Anaesthesia*. 1998;53:586.
273. Scull T, Weeks S. *Can J Anaesth*. 1996;43:1150.
274. Sugai K, Sugai Y. *Masui*. 1989;38:688.
275. Tanaka S, et al. *Masui*. 1994;43:931.
276. Schmitt HJ, et al. *Can J Anaesth*. 2004;51:1049.
277. Dubowitz V. *Muscle Disorders in Childhood*. 2nd ed. Philadelphia: Saunders; 1995.
278. Dalakas M, et al. The muscular dystrophies. In: Barnes P, Hilton-Jones D, eds. *Myopathies in Clinical Practice*. 1st ed. London: Martin Dunitz; 2003.
279. *Muscular Dystrophy*. 2017. https://emedicine.medscape.com/article/1259041-overview.
280. Emery A. *Neuromuscul Disord*. 1991;1:19.
281. Sano M, et al. *Jinrui Idengaku Zasshi*. 1987;32:257.
282. Urban M, Lahlou S. Muscle diseases. In Fleisher L, ed. *Anesthesia and Uncommon Diseases*. Philadelphia: Saunders; 2006:303.
283. Hoffman E. *Cell*. 1987;51:919.
284. Leibowitz D, Dubowitz V. *Dev Med Child Neurol*. 1981;23:577.
285. Finsterer J, Stollberger C. *Cardiology*. 2003;99:1.
286. Perloff JK, et al. *Circulation*. 1984;(69):33.
287. Morris P. *Paediatr Anaesth*. 1997;7:1.
288. Hahn A, et al. *Arch Phys Med Rehabil*. 1997;78:1.
289. Ames WA, et al. *Paediatr Anaesth*. 2005;15:3.
290. Kawaai H, et al. *Anesth Prog*. 2005;52:12.
291. Molyneux MK. *Int J Obstet Anesth*. 2005;14:58.
292. Angermann C, et al. *Z Kardiol*. 1986;75:542.
293. Smith CL, Bush GH. *Br J Anaesth*. 1985;57:1113.
294. Webster R. *Respiratory Function as a Measure of Muscle Strength in Young Boys with Duchenne Muscular Dystrophy*. School of Women and Children's Health, University of N.S.W; 2003.
295. Stevens RD. *Curr Opin Anaesthesiol*. 2001;14:693.
296. Breucking E, et al. *Anaesthesist*. 2000;49:187.

297. Benson ER, et al. *Spine*. 1998;23:2308.
298. Miller F, et al. *Dev Med Child Neurol*. 1992;34:775.
299. Jenkins JG, et al. *Crit Care Med*. 1982;10:645.
300. Stoelting R, Dierdorf S. In: *Anesthesia and Co-Existing Disease*. Philadelphia: Churchill Livingstone; 2002:505.
301. Gurnaney H, et al. *Anesth Analg*. 2009;109:1043.
302. Farell PT. *Anaesth Intensive Care*. 1994;22:597.
303. Schummer W, Schummer C. *Br J Anaesth*. 2004;92:149.
304. Ririe DG, et al. *Anesthesiology*. 1998;88:351.
305. Yemen TA, McClain C. *Paediatr Anaesth*. 2006;16:105.
306. Fairfield MC. *Anaesthesia*. 1993;48:1013.
307. Murat I, et al. *Anesthesiology*. 1987;67:249.
308. Kirschner J, Bonnemann CG. *Arch Neurol*. 2004;61:189.
309. Moro C, et al. *Ann Fr Anesth Reanim*. 2007;26:359.
310. Egi M, et al. *Masui*. 2002;51:196.
311. Pash MP, et al. *Can J Anaesth*. 1996;43:959.
312. Myotonic dystrophy. *Etiology, Clinical Features, and Diagnosis*. 2018. https://www.uptodate.com/contents/myotonic-dystrophy-etiology-clinical-features-and-diagnosis.
313. Parness J, et al. *Anesth Analg*. 2009;109:1054.
314. Lehmann-Horn F, Iaizzo PA. *Br J Anaesth*. 1990;65:692.
315. Mathieu J, et al. *Neurology*. 1997;49:1646.
316. Matsuki Y, et al. *Eur J Anaesthesiol*. 2011;28:145.
317. Stourac P, et al. *Br J Anaesth*. 2013;110:657.
318. Ahmed S, et al. *Cardiol Res*. 2018;9:50.
319. Catena V, et al. *Minerva Anestesiol*. 2007;73:475.
320. Lehmann-Horn F, et al. Nondystrophic myotonias and periodic paralyses. In: Engel A, Franzini-Armstrong C, eds. *Myology*. 3rd ed. New York: McGraw-Hill; 2004:1257–1300.
321. Farbu E, et al. *Acta Anaesthesiol Scand*. 2003;47:630.
322. Newberg LA, et al. *Br J Anaesth*. 1983;55:57.
323. Beck CL, et al. *Proc Natl Acad Sci U S A*. 1996;93:11248.
324. Rosenbaum HK. *Anesthesiol Clin North America*. 2002;20:623.
325. North K. Congenital myopathies. In: Engel A, Franzini-Armstrong C, eds. *Myology*. New York: McGraw-Hill; 2004:1473.
326. Herman GE, et al. *J Pediatr*. 1999;134:206.
327. Breslin D, et al. *Anaesthesia*. 2000;55:471.
328. Costi D, van der Walt JH. *Paediatr Anaesth*. 2004;14:964.
329. Garcia-Aguado R, et al. *Rev Esp Anestesiol Reanim*. 1994;41:302.
330. Gottschalk A, et al. *Anesthesiology*. 1998;89:1018.
331. Schmid E. *Paediatr Anaesth*. 2006;16:218.
332. Tokarz A, et al. *Eur J Anaesthesiol*. 2002;19:842.
333. Dorchies OM, et al. *Neuromuscul Disord*. 2001;11:736.
334. Glucose-6-phosphatase deficiency (glycogen storage disease I, von Gierke disease). 2018. https://www.uptodate.com/contents/glucose-6-phosphatase-deficiency-glycogen-storage-disease-i-von-gierke-disease. Accessed 30.05.18.
335. Rake JP, et al. *Eur J Pediatr*. 2002;161(suppl 1):S112.
336. Visser G, et al. *Eur J Pediatr*. 2002;161(suppl 1):S120.
337. Kakinohana M, et al. *Masui*. 1998;47:1104.
338. Kawai T. *Masui*. 2005;54:924.
339. Loonen MC, et al. *Neurology*. 1981;31:1209.
340. Engel A, et al. Acid maltase deficiency. In: Engel A, Franzini-Armstrong C, eds. *Myology*. New York: McGraw-Hill; 2004:1559.
341. Type II glycogen storage disease (pompe disease). https://emedicine.medscape.com/article/119506-overview. 2017.
342. Ehlers KH, et al. *Circulation*. 1962;25:96.
343. Bulkley BH, Hutchins GM. *Am Heart J*. 1978;96:246.
344. Weinik M, King F. Acid maltase deficiency myopathy. *eMedicine*. 2012.
345. Makos MM, et al. *Ann Neurol*. 1987;22:629.
346. Gitlin MC, et al. *Anesth Analg*. 1993;77:392.
347. Kotani N, et al. *Anesth Analg*. 1996;82:182.
348. Ing RJ, et al. *Paediatr Anaesth*. 2004;14:514.
349. McFarlane HJ, Soni N. *Anaesthesia*. 1986;41:1219.
350. Mohiddin SA, Fananapazir L. *Tex Heart Inst J*. 2002;29:290.
351. DiMauro S, Bonilla E. Mitochondrial encephalomyopathies. In: Engel A, Franzini-Armstrong C, eds. *Myology*. 3rd ed. New York: McGraw-Hill; 2004:1623.
352. Siciliano G, et al. *Biosci Rep*. 2007;27:53.
353. Wisely NA, Cook PR. *Eur J Anaesthesiol*. 2001;18:333.
354. Mehndiratta MM, et al. *Neurol India*. 2002;50:162.
355. Swash M, et al. *J Neurol Sci*. 1978;38:347.
356. Shipton EA, Prosser DO. *Eur J Anaesthesiol*. 2004;21:173.
357. Swash M, et al. *J Neurol Sci*. 1978;38:347.
358. Amato AA, Brown RH. Muscle dystrophies and other muscle diseases. In: Longo DL, Fauci AS, Kasper DL, Hauser SL, Jameson JL, eds. *Harrison's Priciples of Internal Medicine*. 18th ed. McGraw-Hill; 2012.
359. DiMauro S, Bonilla E. Mitochondrial encephalomyopathies. In: Engel AG, Franzini-Armstrong C, eds. *Myology*. 3rd ed. McGraw-Hill; 2004:1623–1662.
360. Allison KR. Muscular dystrophy versus mitochondrial myopathy: the dilemma of the undiagnosed hypotonic child. In: *Paediatric Anaesthesia*. 2007; 17:1–6.
361. Hara K, et al. *J Clin Anesth*. 2004;16:539.
362. Maurtua M, et al. *Int J Obstet Anesth*. 2008;17:370.
363. Levy E, Muravchick S. Mitochondrial diseases. In: Fleisher L, ed. *Anesthesia and Uncommon Diseases*. Philadelphia: Saunders; 2006:455.
364. James RH. *Anaesthesia*. 1985;40:88.
365. James RH. *Anaesthesia*. 1986;41:216.
366. Gurrieri C, et al. *Can J Anaesth*. 2011;58:751.
367. Footitt EJ, et al. *Br J Anaesth*. 2008;100:436.
368. Driessen J, et al. *Paediatr Anaesth*. 2007;17:16.
369. Burns AM, Shelly MP. *Anaesthesia*. 1989;44:975.
370. Kelly A, O'Connor M. *Anaesthesia*. 1990;45:596.
371. Ramchandra DS, et al. *Can J Anaesth*. 1990;37:474.
372. Guasch E, et al. *Anaesthesia*. 2003;58:607.
373. Sharma AD, et al. *Paediatr Anaesth*. 2001;11:488.
374. Vanlander AV, et al. *Acta Anaesthesiol Scand*. 2012;56:520.
375. Stowe DF, Kevin LG. *Antioxid Redox Signal*. 2004;6:439.
376. Stadnicka A, et al. *J Anesth*. 2007;21:212.
377. Wallace JJ, et al. *Paediatr Anaesth*. 1998;8:249–254.
378. Lauwers MH, et al. *Anaesthesia*. 1994;49:876.
379. Morgan PG, et al. *Anesthesiology*. 2002;96:1268.
380. Allen GC. *Anesthesiology*. 2003;98:282.
381. Frei FJ, et al. *Anaesthesia*. 1997;52:1056.
382. Naguib M, et al. *Anesthesiology*. 1996;84:1506.
383. Finsterer J, et al. *Can J Anaesth*. 1998;45:781.
384. Sharma AD, et al. *Paediatr Anaesth*. 2001;11:488.
385. D'Ambra MN, et al. *Anesthesiology*. 1979;51:343.
386. Wiesel S, et al. *Anesth Analg*. 1991;72:696.
387. Rowe RW, Helander E. *Anesth Analg*. 1990;71:295.
388. Rosaeg OP, et al. *Can J Anaesth*. 1994;43:403.
389. Hsiao PN, et al. *Acta Anaesthesiol Sin*. 2000;38:107.
390. Sasano N, et al. *J Anesth*. 2007;21:72.
391. Farag E, et al. *Can J Anaesth*. 2002;49:958.
392. Sasano N, et al. *J Anesth*. 2009;23:587.
393. Kubota H, et al. *J Child Neurol*. 2005;20:116.
394. Vincent A, et al. *Lancet*. 2001;357:2122.
395. Lindstrom JM. *Muscle Nerve*. 2000;23:453.
396. Anesthesia for the patient with myasthenia gravis. 2018. https://www.uptodate.com/contents/anesthesia-for-the-patient-with-myasthenia-gravis. Accessed April 8, 2019.
397. Eisenkraft JB, et al. *Anesthesiology*. 1988;69:760.
398. Baraka A. *Anaesthesia*. 1992;47:217.
399. Seigne RD, Scott RP. *Br J Anaesth*. 1994;72:468.
400. Kim JM, Mangold J. *Br J Anaesth*. 1989;63:497.
401. Sungur Ulke Z, et al. *Acta Anaesthesiol Scand*. 2013;57:745.
402. de Boer HD, et al. *Rev Esp Anestesiol Reanim*. 2010;57:181.
403. *BRIDION(R) (sugammadex) Injection - First and Only Selective Relaxant Binding Agent - Approved in European Union*. 2008. http://www.evaluategroup.com/Universal/View.aspx?type=Story&id=160887.
404. Baraka A. *Br J Anaesth*. 1992;69:227
405. Abel M, Eisenkraft JB. *Mt Sinai J Med*. 2002;69:31.
406. Takamori M, et al. *Neurosci Res*. 2000;36:183.
407. Hewett SJ, Atchison WD. *Brain Res*. 1991;566:320.
408. Burge JA, Hanna MG. *Curr Neurol Neurosci Rep*. 2012;12:62.
409. Lehmann-Horn F, Rudel R, Jurkat-Rott K. Nondystrophic myotonias and periodic paralyses. In: Engel AG, Franzini-Armstrong C, eds. *Myology*. McGraw-Hill; 2004:1257–1300.
410. Jurkat-Rott K, Lehmann-Horn F. *J Neurol*. 2006;253:1391.
411. Chinnery PF, et al. *Ann Neurol*. 2002;52:251.
412. Song YW, et al. *Muscle Nerve*. 2012;46:914.
413. Vicart S, et al. *Neurology*. 2004;63:2120.
414. Viscomi CM, et al. *Anesth Analg*. 1999;88:1081.
415. Robinson JE, et al. *Can J Anaesth*. 2000;47:160.
416. Griggs RC, et al. *Ann Intern Med*. 1970;73:39.
417. Bendahhou S, et al. *Ann Neurol*. 2001;50:417.
418. LoVecchio F, Jacobson S. *Emerg Med Clin North Am*. 1997;15:605.

419. Lin SH, Huang CL. *J Am Soc Nephrol*. 2012;23:985.
420. Depoix JP, et al. *Anesth Analg*. 2004;99:302.
421. Aouad R, Atanassoff PG. *Can J Anaesth*. 2004;51:92.
422. Ashwood EM, et al. *Anaesthesia*. 1992;47:579.
423. Aarons JJ, et al. *Anesthesiology*. 1989;71:303.
424. Cone AM, Sansome AJ. *Anaesthesia*. 1992;47:1097.
425. Weller JF, et al. *Anesthesiology*. 2002;97:259.
426. Barker MC. *AANA J*. 2012;78:191.
427. Siler JN, Discavage WJ. *Anesthesiology*. 1975;43:489.
428. Melnick B, et al. *Anesthesiology*. 1983;58:263.
429. Rooney RT, et al. *Anesth Analg*. 1988;67:782.
430. Hofer C, et al. *Anaesthesia*. 2001;56:1082.
431. Chitra S, Korula G. *Indian J Anaesth*. 2009;53:226.
432. Viscomi CM, et al. *Anesth Analg*. 1999;88:1081.
433. Parness J, et al. *Anesth Analg*. 2009;109:1054.
434. Lambert C, et al. *Anesth Analg*. 1994;79:1012.
435. Rajabally YA, El Lahawi M. *Muscle Nerve*. 2002;25:453.
436. Marchant CL, et al. *Muscle Nerve*. 2004;30:114.
437. Neuman GG, Kopman AF. *Anesth Analg*. 1993;76:426.

36 Cardiovascular Monitoring

BECKY SCHROEDER, JONATHAN MARK, and ATILIO BARBEITO

KEY POINTS

- Monitoring of the electrocardiogram (ECG) provides continuous monitoring of heart rate, identification of arrhythmias and conduction abnormalities, and detection of myocardial ischemia.
- Accurate and reliable ECG monitoring requires attention to lead placement and selection, choice of filter, and gain that will influence the displayed ECG tracing.
- An anterolateral precordial lead (V_3, V_4, or V_5) should be selected for the most sensitive detection of myocardial ischemia.
- Demand-mediated subendocardial ischemia resulting in ST-segment depression is the most commonly observed form of perioperative ischemia. ST-segment depression is most commonly observed in an anterolateral precordial lead regardless of the coronary territory responsible.
- Supply-mediated transmural ischemia resulting in ST-segment elevation is uncommonly observed intraoperatively except during cardiac operations. In contrast to ST-segment depression, ST-segment elevation is indicative of the myocardial territory and coronary artery involved.
- Most automated noninvasive arterial blood pressure measuring devices use an oscillometric measurement technique and rarely cause complications. Caution should be exercised in patients who cannot complain of arm pain, those with irregular rhythms that force repeated cuff inflation, and those receiving anticoagulant therapy.
- The Allen test for palmar arch collateral arterial flow is not a reliable method to predict complications from radial artery cannulation. Despite the absence of anatomic collateral flow at the elbow, brachial artery catheterization for perioperative blood pressure monitoring is a safe alternative to radial or femoral arterial catheterization.
- The accuracy of a directly recorded arterial pressure waveform is determined by the natural frequency and damping coefficient of the pressure monitoring system. Optimal dynamic response of the system will be achieved when the natural frequency is high, thereby allowing accurate pressure recording across a wide range of damping coefficients.
- The preferred position for alignment (or "leveling") of external pressure transducers for measuring arterial or central venous pressure (CVP), which eliminates confounding hydrostatic pressure artifacts, lies approximately 5 cm posterior to the sternomanubrial junction. The more conventional location for the reference level used for hemodynamic monitoring including central venous and pulmonary artery pressures, is the mid-thoracic level, which corresponds most closely to the mid-left atrial position and is located halfway between the anterior sternum and the bed surface in the supine patient.
- Because of wave reflection and other physical phenomena, the arterial blood pressure recorded from peripheral sites has a wider pulse pressure than when measured more centrally.
- Dynamic measures of cardiac preload, such as stroke volume and pulse pressure variation, are better predictors of intravascular volume responsiveness than static indicators, such as CVP and pulmonary capillary wedge pressure.
- Selecting the best site, catheter, and method for safe and effective central venous cannulation requires that the physician consider the purpose of catheterization, the patient's underlying medical condition, the intended operation, and the skill and experience of the physician performing the procedure. Right internal jugular vein cannulation is preferred due to its consistent, predictable anatomic location and its relative ease of access intraoperatively.
- Mechanical complications from central venous catheters can be decreased by the use of ultrasound vessel localization, venous pressure measurement before large catheter insertion, and radiographic confirmation that the catheter tip lies outside the pericardium and parallel to the walls of the superior vena cava.
- CVP is the result of a complex and diverse interplay among many different physiologic variables, the main ones being venous return and cardiac function. No simple relationship exists between CVP and circulating blood volume. Despite this, important pathophysiologic information can be obtained by careful assessment of the CVP waveform morphology.
- Catheter misuse and data misinterpretation are among the most common complications of central venous and pulmonary artery catheters.
- Pulmonary artery wedge pressure is a delayed and damped reflection of left atrial pressure. The wedge pressure provides a close estimate for pulmonary capillary pressure in many cases, but it may underestimate capillary pressure when postcapillary pulmonary vascular resistance is increased, as in patients with sepsis.

- Use of central venous, pulmonary artery diastolic, or pulmonary artery wedge pressures as estimates of left ventricular preload is subject to many confounding factors, including changes in diastolic ventricular compliance and juxtacardiac pressure.
- Pulmonary artery catheter monitoring has not been shown to improve patient outcomes. Reasons cited for these results include misinterpretation of catheter-derived data and failure of hemodynamic therapies that are guided by specific hemodynamic indices.
- Thermodilution cardiac output monitoring, the most widely used clinical technique, is subject to measurement errors introduced by rapid intravenous fluid administration, intracardiac shunts, and tricuspid valve regurgitation.
- Mixed venous hemoglobin oxygen saturation is a measure of the adequacy of cardiac output relative to body oxygen requirements. This measurement is also dependent on the arterial hemoglobin oxygen saturation and hemoglobin concentration.

Introduction to Cardiovascular Monitoring: Focused Physical Examination

Electronic devices currently provide the vast majority of information used in monitoring a patient's cardiovascular status. However, the physician's senses, augmented by clinical context, continue to provide global insight into the patient's condition and remain critical in evaluating, and interpreting data derived from other sources.[1] Manual palpation of an arterial pulse will differentiate true asystole from monitoring artifact more efficiently than troubleshooting any monitor. Regardless of the manner used, though, it is important to understand the strengths and limitations of monitoring techniques.

Heart Rate and Pulse Rate Monitoring

The ability to estimate the heart rate quickly with a "finger on the pulse" is as important as this expression is common despite near-universal use of electronic devices for continuous monitoring. The electrocardiogram (ECG) is the most common heart rate monitoring method used in the operating room, even though any device measuring the period of the cardiac cycle will suffice. Accurate detection of the R wave and measurement of the interval from the peak of one QRS complex to the peak of the next on an ECG (R-R interval) serve as the basis from which digitally displayed values are derived and periodically updated (e.g., at 5- to 15-second intervals) (Fig. 36.1).[2]

The distinction between heart rate and pulse rate lies in the difference between electrical depolarization with systolic contraction of the heart (heart rate) and a detectable peripheral arterial pulsation (pulse rate). Pulse deficit describes the extent to which the pulse rate is less than the heart rate and may arise in conditions such as atrial fibrillation in which stroke volume is periodically compromised by a very short R-R interval to such an extent that no arterial pulse is detectable for that systolic ejection. Electrical-mechanical dissociation and pulseless electrical activity are extreme examples of pulse deficit in which cardiac contraction is completely unable to generate a palpable peripheral pulse. The heart rate is reported from the ECG trace and the pulse rate from the pulse oximeter plethysmograph or arterial blood pressure monitor. Considering both in monitoring and clinical evaluation improves accuracy and reduces measurement errors and false alarms.[3]

Electrocardiography Monitoring

The value and importance of intraoperative monitoring of the ECG is evidenced by its requirement as a basic circulatory monitoring standard by the American Society of Anesthesiologists (ASA)[4]: "Every patient receiving anesthesia shall have the ECG continuously displayed from the beginning of anesthesia until preparing to leave the anesthetizing location." Similar recommendations have been recently updated by the American Heart Association (AHA) to guide indications, duration, and implementation of ECG monitoring in hospitalized patients outside of the operating room.[5]

The three primary reasons for ECG monitoring are continuous monitoring of heart rate, identification of arrhythmias and conduction abnormalities, and detection of myocardial ischemia. Furthermore, with many patients coming to surgery with pacemakers or implantable cardiac defibrillators in place, the ECG monitor enables the anesthesiologist to follow the proper function of these devices during the perioperative period. (Perioperative management of these devices is described in Chapter 38.) In order for bedside ECG monitoring to be accurate and effective, the clinician must attend to proper lead placement and selection, filter mode, and gain adjustment.

ELECTROCARDIOGRAM LEAD PLACEMENT AND SELECTION

Standard Lead Systems

Current operating room and intensive care monitoring systems have five leads that allow monitoring of the standard limb leads (I, II, III), the augmented limb leads (aVR, aVL, aVF), and a single precordial lead (V_1, V_2, V_3, V_4, V_5, or V_6). Typically, two of these 12 standard leads are simultaneously displayed on the bedside monitor. Historically, the augmented limb leads and precordial leads were described as *unipolar*, whereas the standard limb leads were described as *bipolar*. A recent scientific statement from the AHA and others[6] discourages this distinction because in effect, all the lead configurations are effectively bipolar in their recording of surface electrical potentials.

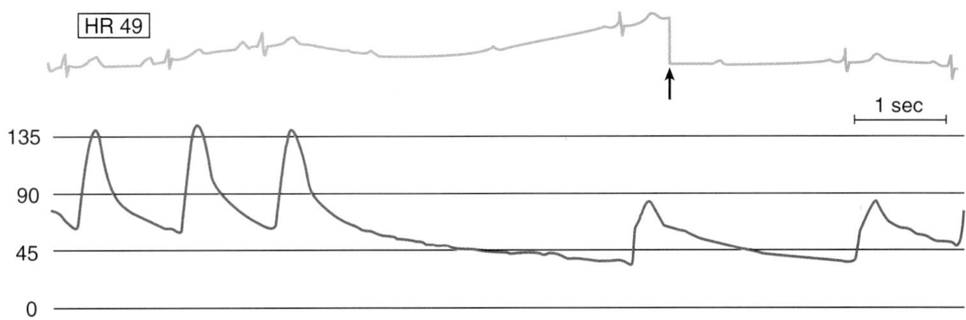

Fig. 36.1 Digital heart rate *(HR)* displays may fail to warn of dangerous bradyarrhythmias. Direct observation of the electrocardiogram (ECG) and the arterial blood pressure traces reveals complete heart block and a 4-second period of asystole, whereas the digital display reports an HR of 49 beats/min. Note that the ECG filter *(arrow)* corrects the baseline drift so that the trace remains on the recording screen. (From Mark JB. *Atlas of Cardiovascular Monitoring*. New York: Churchill Livingstone; 1998.)

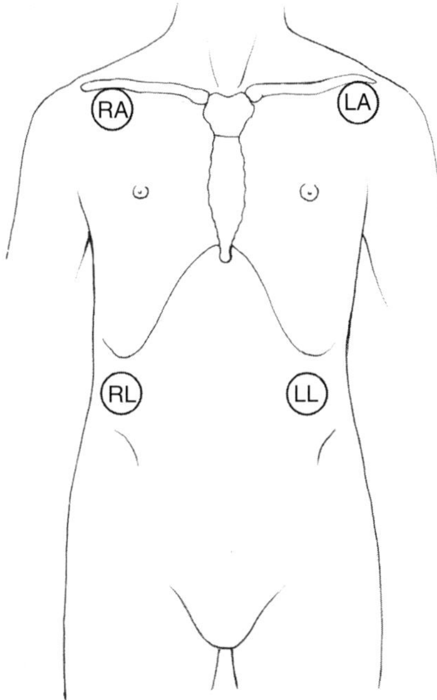

Fig. 36.2 Standard ECG limb lead placement for patient monitoring. *LA*, Left arm; *LL*, left leg; *RA*, right arm; *RL*, right leg. (From Mark JB. *Atlas of Cardiovascular Monitoring*. New York: Churchill Livingstone;1998.)

Based on AHA guidelines, ECG monitoring leads have a standard color-coding system: right arm (white), left arm (black), right leg (green), left leg (red), and precordial lead (brown). Of note, this color scheme is not the same used internationally or the one recommended by the International Electrotechnical Commission. Unlike recording a standard 12-lead ECG, where the limb leads are attached to electrodes placed on the wrists and ankles or arms and legs, when monitoring patients in the operating room or intensive care unit (ICU), the limb leads are typically placed on the torso, with the right and left arm leads placed just below the clavicles and the leg leads placed above the hips (Fig. 36.2). Of note, placement of the right leg lead (green lead) can be anywhere on the body because it is a ground electrode, and its location will not alter the display of any of the selected standard leads.[7]

Placement of the limb electrodes on the torso has been utilized since 1966, when Mason and Likar introduced a variation on positioning the standard limb electrodes of the 12-lead ECG during exercise stress testing to minimize artifacts in the limb leads caused by movement.[8] Although the limb lead QRS complexes are slightly different in amplitude and axis, and the precordial leads may vary slightly from the standard 12-lead ECG recording, studies have shown that the ST-segment measurements during exercise stress testing were generally similar when the Mason-Likar 12-lead ECG system is used, as compared with the standard 12-lead ECG.[8-11] Consequently, torso-positioned limb leads have become standard for monitoring in the operating room and ICU because of convenience and the potential to obviate motion artifact.

In some cases, surgical incisions, patient positioning, or other procedural aspects may mandate adjusting these limb lead electrode locations. However, for reliable recording of standard limb leads, the electrodes must be outside the cardiac borders, in the transverse plane above and below the heart, and in the sagittal plane to the left and right of the heart (Fig. 36.3). In practice, limb lead placement closer to the heart may lead to unintended distortion of the ECG tracings.[10]

Placement of the precordial lead (brown) electrode requires more attention than the limb leads, since this lead is often misplaced and its position is critical for the reliable and sensitive detection of myocardial ischemia. The V_5 precordial lead is the one most commonly chosen for monitoring patients at risk for myocardial ischemia, since historically it has been shown to be the most sensitive single lead for detecting ischemia during exercise stress testing[12,13] and during anesthesia.[14,15] Importantly, the V_5 precordial lead can be monitored during cardiac operations without interfering with the surgical prep and median sternotomy incision. For patients undergoing other operations, particularly high-risk patients undergoing vascular procedures, leads V_4 or V_3 may be chosen because there is good evidence that these leads are even more sensitive for detecting prolonged postoperative myocardial ischemia.[16]

Standard locations for the six precordial lead electrodes are shown in Fig. 36.4. Given that there is considerable evidence that precordial lead placement is inaccurate even during diagnostic 12-lead ECG recordings,[6] it is likely that this is also commonplace during ECG monitoring in the operating room and ICU. Accurate lead placement is facilitated by locating the manubrial-sternal junction, its immediately inferior rib interspace (the second), and then palpating down to identify the fourth and fifth interspaces for accurate precordial lead location. Note that lead V_4 lies

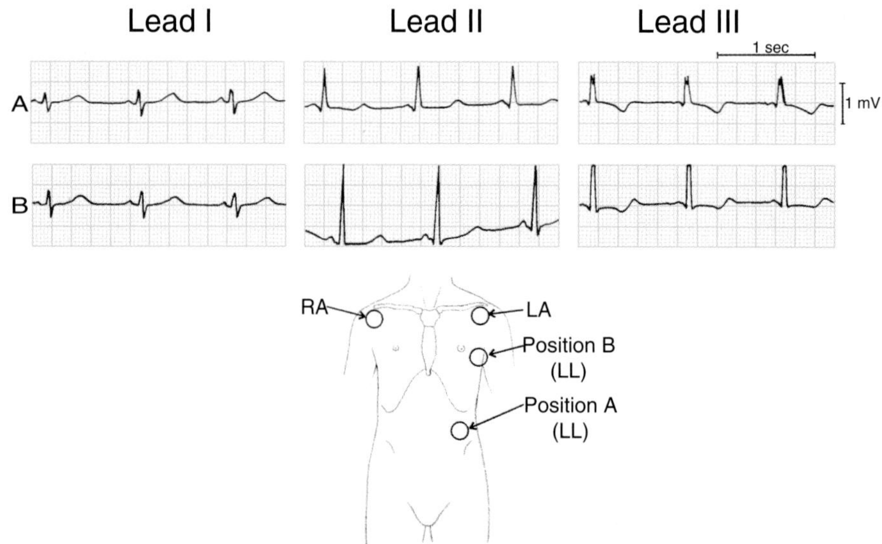

Fig. 36.3 Importance of ECG limb lead placement. ECG recording of leads I, II, and III from position A, with the left leg *(LL)* lead in the standard location below the heart near the left iliac crest compared with position B, with the LL lead placed over the precordium (near the V_5 position). Standard ECG limb lead positioning should be outside the cardiac borders, as shown here in position A. If the LL lead electrode is placed inappropriately in position B, the recording of leads II and III will be modified. Note, however, that the recording of lead I is not affected by the misplaced LL lead, since lead I measures the difference between left arm *(LA)* and right arm *(RA)* electrodes. (From Mark JB. *Atlas of Cardiovascular Monitoring.* New York: Churchill Livingstone;1998.)

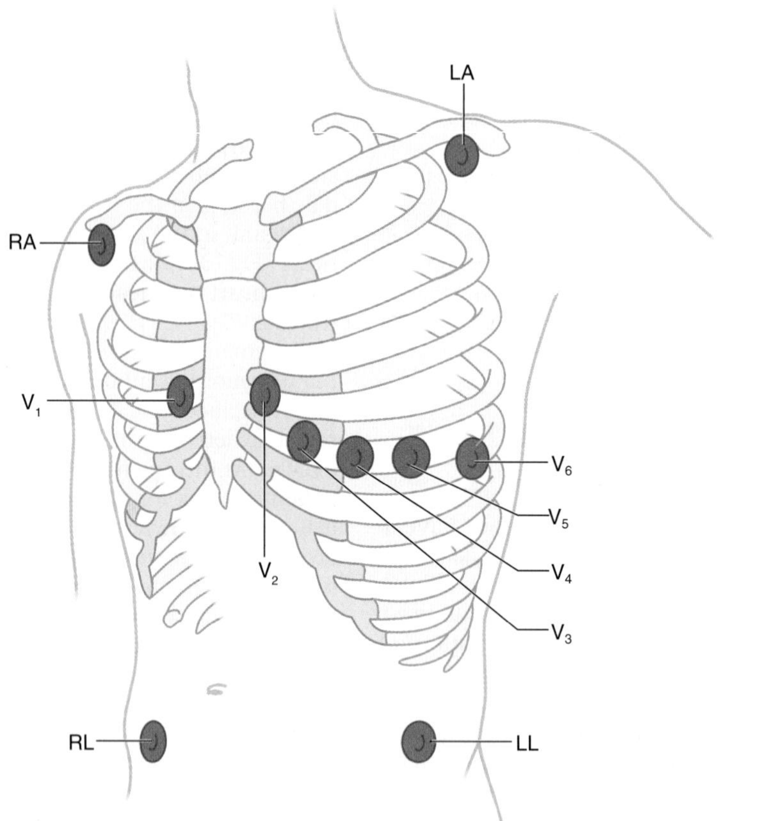

Fig. 36.4 Proper anatomic location of the six standard precordial ECG leads. Precise positioning of the lateral precordial leads is ensured by identifying the fifth intercostal space in the mid-clavicular line for lead V_4, moving laterally to the anterior axillary line for V_5, and further laterally to the mid-axillary line for V_6. *LA*, Left arm; *LL*, left leg; *RA*, right arm; *RL*, right leg.

in the fifth interspace at the mid-clavicular line, and leads V_5 and V_6 are located directly lateral to V_4 in the anterior and mid-axillary lines, respectively.

Given anatomic considerations and the strong evidence that the mid-precordial leads (V_3, V_4, V_5) are best for detection of ischemia, it is important that the precordial lead not be placed haphazardly or too laterally. In some cases (e.g., patients undergoing left thoracotomy), none of these precordial lead placement sites are possible. In this instance, it is reasonable to choose another standard lead position, such as V_1, but it is important that the clinician recognize that ECG monitoring for ischemia will not be as sensitive.

Alternative Lead Systems

Electrocardiographic evidence for right ventricular (RV) ischemia and infarction is best identified by right-sided precordial leads, particularly lead V_{4R}, a mirror image of the V_4 lead, positioned in the fourth intercostal space at the midclavicular line. Although never chosen for routine ischemia monitoring, this lead has proven valuable for detecting RV ischemia and infarction, and might be chosen to monitor patients at risk for inferior left ventricular (LV) ischemia, which is commonly accompanied by RV involvement.[6,17]

Three-lead ECG monitoring systems, while less common today than five-lead systems, remain available particularly in non-operating room procedural settings and for patient transport. A three-lead system is also the standard ECG monitoring system incorporated in external defibrillator devices. The three leads (right arm, left arm, left leg) can be placed in similar locations to their five-lead system counterparts, and this allows reliable monitoring of heart rate, detection of R waves for synchronized direct current cardioversion, and monitoring for potentially life-threatening arrhythmias such as ventricular fibrillation. These systems are more limited than five-lead systems (or standard 12-lead ECG recordings) for diagnosing more complex arrhythmias and detection of myocardial ischemia. Modifications of these standard limb leads allow better sensitivity for ischemia monitoring by placing the positive (left arm) electrode in the standard precordial V_5 position and selecting an appropriate limb lead (usually lead I) to create this modified lead recording. These three-lead variations useful for ischemia monitoring are created by placing the right arm lead in the following locations: CS_5 (central subclavicular), CM_5 (central manubrial), CB_5 (central back), and CC_5 (central chest) (Fig. 36.5). Each of these lead recordings will be a modification of the standard precordial V_5 lead, and owing to differences in R-wave amplitude and ST-segment morphology, may lead to over- or underestimation of ST-segment changes.[18]

Another modified three-lead system is a surrogate for precordial lead V_1. This lead (MCL_1) is recorded by placing the left arm lead in standard position, the left leg lead at the V_1 position, and selecting lead III (see Fig. 36.5). This modified lead system is useful for monitoring in the ICU or other circumstances where detection of P-wave morphology and arrhythmias is of paramount importance.

Following cardiac surgical procedures, recording the ECG signal from an epicardial atrial pacing wire may also be useful for detecting P waves that may not be as evident from skin surface ECG recordings (Fig. 36.6). This alternative lead recording is usually performed in the ICU using a 12-lead ECG system and attaching one of the atrial pacing wires to a precordial lead wire.

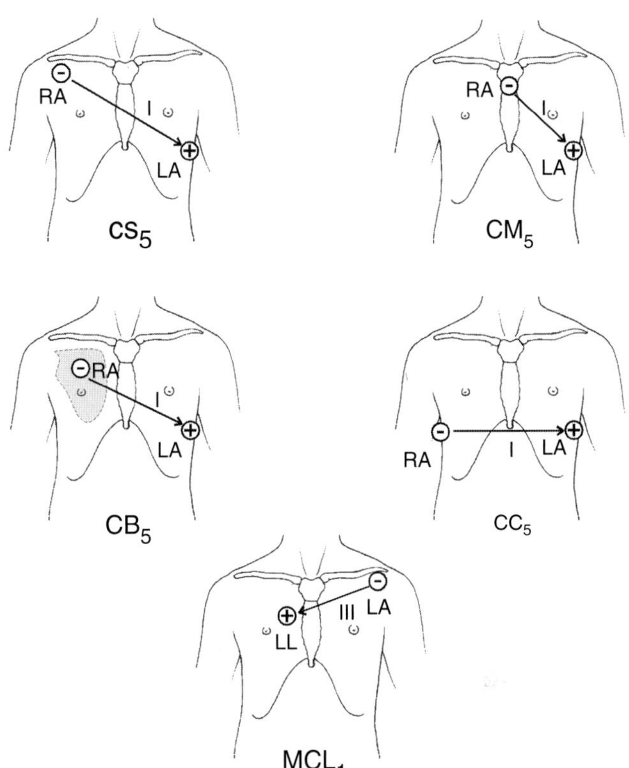

Fig. 36.5 When only a three-electrode lead set is available, modified bipolar limb leads may be recorded as surrogates for standard precordial leads. Alternatives to precordial lead V_5 are recorded by selecting lead I on the bedside monitor and placing the positive exploring left arm *(LA)* electrode in the V_5 position. The nomenclature describing these leads derives from the location of the positive exploring electrode located in the V_5 position and the negative right arm *(RA)* electrode position being located as follows: *(CS_5)* central subclavicular, *(CM_5)* central manubrial, *(CB_5)* central back (shown overlying the right scapula), and *(CC_5)* central chest. In contrast, note that the *(MCL_1)* lead (modified central lead 1) is recorded by selecting lead III on the bedside monitor and placing the positive exploring left leg *(LL)* electrode in the V_1 position with the negative LA lead in a modified position beneath the left clavicle. (From Mark JB. *Atlas of Cardiovascular Monitoring*. New York: Churchill Livingstone;1998.)

ELECTROCARDIOGRAM FILTER SELECTION

The ECG signal is subject to artifacts (noise) both in the low-frequency and high-frequency ranges. Consequently, all ECG monitors use bandpass filters to narrow the signal bandwidth, preserving the signal of interest while reducing artifacts and improving signal quality. As the name suggests, a bandpass filter allows signal frequencies within a certain range to pass or be displayed, while attenuating or functionally eliminating signal frequencies both at a low range and a high range.

Low-frequency artifact is typically caused by respiration or patient movement that causes the ECG tracing to wander above and below the baseline (Fig. 36.7). Often this will appear as the ECG tracing being cut off or only partially displayed on the bedside monitor channel. Therefore, low-frequency filters (also called high-pass filters) are used in ECG monitoring. The heart rate forms a rough lower bound for the frequency content of the ECG signal and is measured in Hertz (Hz, cycles per second). Since heart rates slower than 40 beats per minute (bpm) (0.67 Hz) are uncommon, traditional low-frequency analog filters are used to cut off signals at frequencies below 0.5 Hz. However, such filters may introduce considerable distortion into the ECG, particularly with respect to the level of the ST segment, resulting from phase nonlinearities that occur in areas of the ECG signal where frequency content and wave amplitude abruptly change, as occurs where the end of the QRS complex meets the ST segment. The 1975 AHA recommendations included

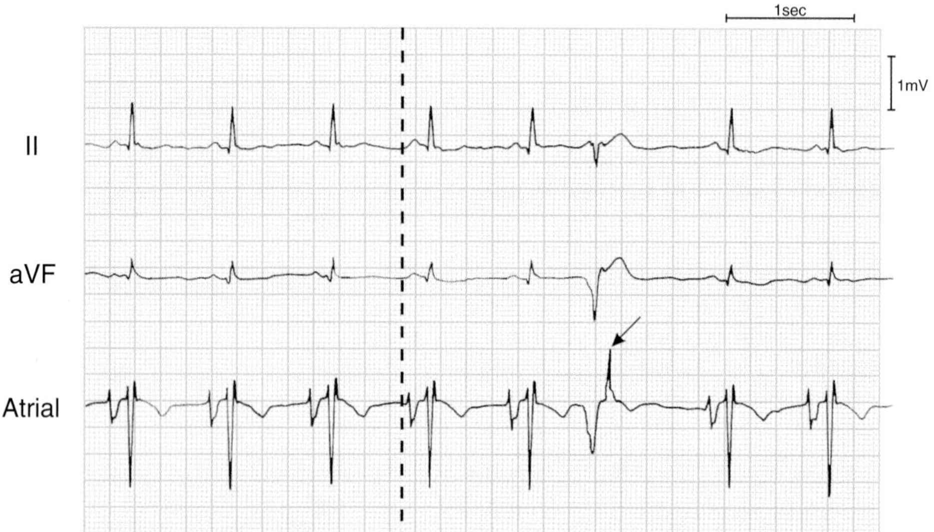

Fig. 36.6 Simultaneous recording of surface ECG leads II and aVF and an atrial epicardial lead *(atrial)* recorded from a pacing wire attached to the surface of the right atrium. Onset of atrial electrical activity is denoted by the P wave in the surface leads and marked by the dashed vertical line. Note that the amplitude of the atrial electrical signal is greatest in the atrial lead recording. In addition, the sixth beat is a ventricular premature beat, and the resulting retrograde atrial depolarization is clearly evident in the atrial lead *(arrow)* but not seen as easily in standard surface ECG leads II or aVF. (From Mark JB. *Atlas of Cardiovascular Monitoring*. New York: Churchill Livingstone;1998.)

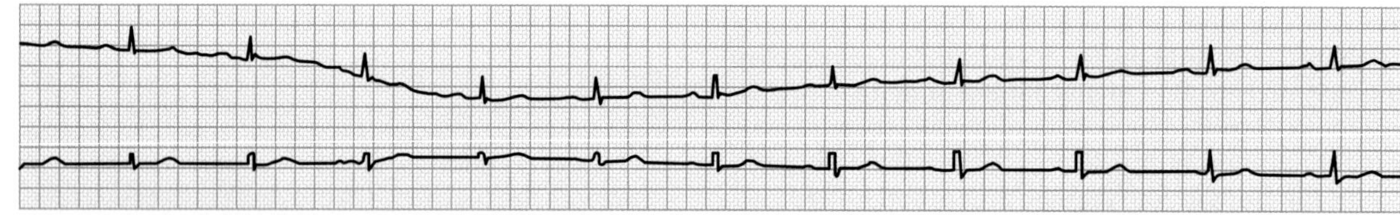

Fig. 36.7 ECG recording of lead II *(top)* and lead V_5 *(bottom)* at standard speed (25 mm/s) and gain (10 mm/mV) with a diagnostic bandpass filter. The respiratory artifact is evident from the varying or wandering baseline most noticeable in lead II. This artifact will be eliminated by using the monitor bandpass filter.

a 0.05-Hz low-frequency cutoff for diagnostic ECGs. This recommendation preserves the fidelity of repolarization, but baseline drift can still be a problem. Current modern digital filtering provides more sophisticated methods for a higher cutoff for low-frequency filtration without those phase distortions observed with analog filtering. Thus, to reduce artifactual distortion of the ST segment, current AHA recommendations suggest the low-frequency cutoff should be either 0.05 Hz for monitors with analog filters or 0.67 Hz or below for monitors and ECG recording devices with linear digital filters with zero phase distortion.[6]

High-frequency ECG artifacts are typically caused by muscle fasciculations, tremors, and most importantly, the ever present 60 cycle (Hz) electromagnetic interference from other electrical equipment in the monitoring environment. These artifacts can be eliminated with high-frequency filters (also termed low-pass filters), but like low-frequency filters, the high-frequency filters may distort the ECG signal in undesirable ways. The higher frequencies in the ECG signal include features such as rapid upstroke velocity (QRS complex), peak amplitude (R wave), and waves of short duration. Most importantly, pacing spikes, which by definition are high frequency and low amplitude, are often eliminated by high-frequency filters and make bedside identification of pacemaker function impossible. A high-frequency cutoff of 100 Hz was considered adequate by the AHA in 1975 to maintain diagnostic accuracy during visual inspection of an ECG, although it has long been recognized that higher-frequency components of the QRS complex may have clinical significance in patients with various forms of heart disease. According to current AHA recommendations, to measure routine duration and amplitudes accurately in adults, adolescents, and children, an upper frequency cutoff of at least 150 Hz is required, and an upper frequency cutoff of 250 Hz is more appropriate for infants.[6]

Current ECG monitors allow the clinician a choice among several filtering modes or bandwidths. The actual filter frequencies tend to vary among manufacturers, but in general there are three different filters that may be selected, termed diagnostic mode, monitoring mode, and filter mode. The ***diagnostic mode*** typically has a bandpass of 0.05 to 150 Hz, and this filter should always be selected for the most undistorted and accurate display of the ST segment and the identification of pacing spikes. The ***monitor mode*** typically has a bandpass of 0.5 to 40 Hz, and while both low-frequency (respiratory drift) and high-frequency (60 Hz) noise is reduced or attenuated, the ST segments are often distorted and typically show an exaggerated deviation that is artifactually introduced by the filter (Figs. 36.8A and B).[19] The ***filter mode*** bandpass is 0.5 to 20 Hz and may incorporate a notch filter aimed at further attenuating and eliminating 60 Hz interference from nearby electrical equipment.

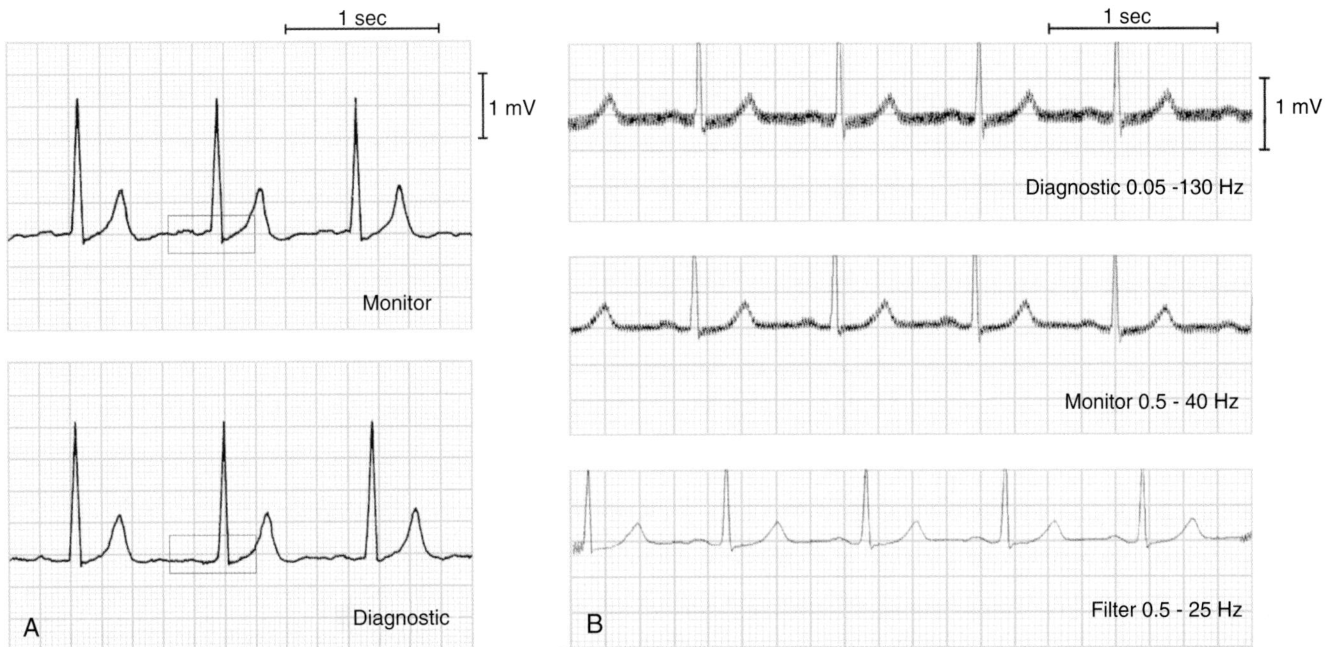

Fig. 36.8 Effects of filter selection on the ST segment. Application of the monitor mode filter (8A, *top panel*) produces artifactual J-point depression and upsloping ST-segment depression *(box)*. These abnormalities are not seen when the diagnostic mode filter (8A, *bottom panel*) is used to record the ECG. Filter selection also effects ECG electrical interference originating from the wall power source (8B). Compared to the diagnostic mode filter (bandpass 0.05-130 Hz), the narrower bandpass of the monitor mode (0.5-40 Hz) reduces this high-frequency artifact, and the filter mode (0.5-25 Hz) that incorporates an additional notch filter at 60 Hz eliminates this electrical artifact entirely. (From Mark JB. *Atlas of Cardiovascular Monitoring*. New York: Churchill Livingstone;1998.)

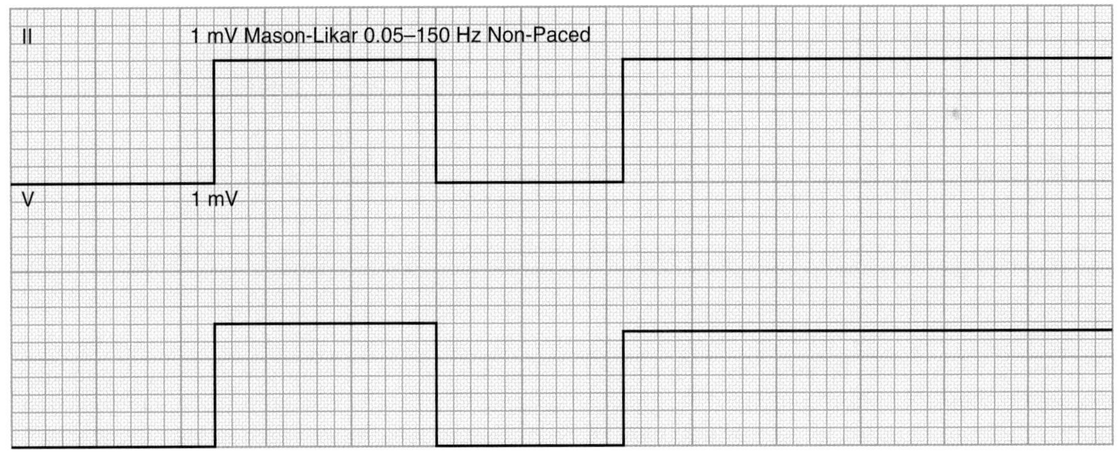

Fig. 36.9 ECG gain is indicated by a 1 mV rectangular calibration signal on a paper recording or by a 1 mV vertical marker at the edge of the bedside monitor ECG waveform. In this example, the ECG is shown at standard gain, 10 mm/mV.

ELECTROCARDIOGRAM GAIN SELECTION

In addition to lead and filter selection, bedside monitors also allow adjustment and selection of the ECG signal gain. A standard ECG is recorded at a gain of 10 mm/mV and is indicated by a 1 mV rectangular calibration signal on a paper recording (Fig. 36.9) or by a 1 mV vertical marker at the edge of the bedside monitor ECG waveform. Bedside monitors may be set to an autogain mode, where the available display space is filled by the ECG tracing and the corresponding increase or decrease from standard gain is indicated by the vertical marker. Alternatively, the clinician may adjust the ECG signal gain manually. This is done when the monitor detection of heart rate is inaccurate. For example, one might reduce the ECG signal gain when the monitor is inappropriately counting a tall T wave as an R wave and displaying an artifactual heart rate that is twice the true rate. Conversely, one would increase the ECG gain when there are very small R waves and the monitor cannot record and display the heart rate.

Gain adjustment is important because all features of the ECG are equally amplified or reduced when the gain is changed from the 10 mm/mV standard. As a consequence, ST-segment deviations can be obscured when gain is reduced and thereby impair clinical observation of important ST-segment changes. Alternatively, if the gain is

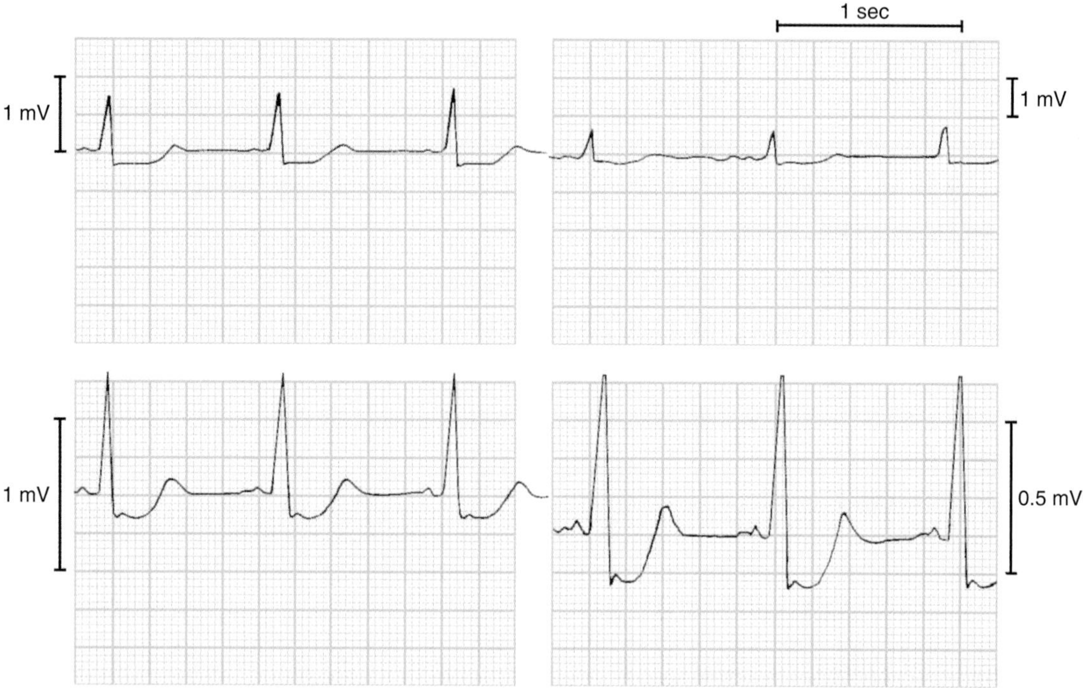

Fig. 36.10 Effect of gain adjustment on the magnitude of ST-segment shift. The magnitude of ST-segment depression and R-wave amplitude vary in direct proportion to overall signal gain denoted by the vertical calibration signals adjacent to the traces (10 mm/mV, *upper left panel*; 5 mm/mV, *upper right panel*; 20 mm/mV, *lower left panel*; 20 mm/0.5 mV or 40 mm/mV, *lower right panel*). Note that at four times standard gain *(lower right panel)*, the ST depression increases to 6 mm but R-wave amplitude only increases to 21 mm because the R-wave peak is "cut off" at the upper limits of the recording display. (From Mark JB. *Atlas of Cardiovascular Monitoring*. New York: Churchill Livingstone;1998.)

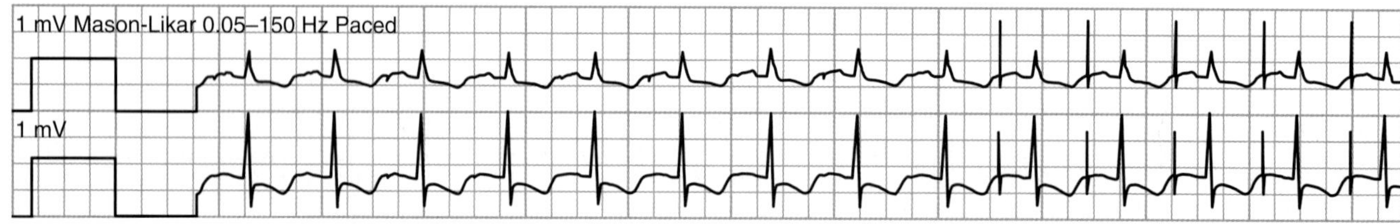

Fig. 36.11 Leads II *(top)* and V_5 *(bottom)* are recorded during atrial pacing (86 beats/min) at standard speed (25 mm/ms) and gain (10 mm/mV). Atrial pacing spikes are small and difficult to discern, particularly in lead V_5. Prior to the 10th beat, the *Pacing Mode* is selected and the monitor marks the atrial pacing spikes clearly on the remaining five beats.

increased, ST deviations will also be amplified proportionally. While common clinical communication of ST-segment shifts is always described in terms of millimeters (mm) of depression or elevation, interpretation of bedside monitor ECG tracings must always be tempered by consideration of the display gain (Fig. 36.10).

ELECTROCARDIOGRAM PACING MODE

While older ECG monitors recorded analog (continuous) signals, current devices convert the analog ECG signal to digital form by sampling the signal at very high rates up to 15,000 times per second.[6] This oversampling of the ECG signal was originally introduced to allow identification and recording of pacemaker stimulus outputs (pacing spikes), which are generally shorter than 0.5 ms, but current systems do not always detect these small-amplitude high-frequency signals reliably. As a result, most bedside ECG monitors now include a ***pacing mode*** selection, which when activated, employs an algorithm to detect and highlight these pacing spikes, making detection of pacemaker function easier. When this monitoring mode is selected, clinicians should recognize that the displayed ECG tracing shows regular markers, often in a different color than the ECG tracing, that indicate and highlight presence of a pacemaker stimulus output. These are not amplified pacemaker signals, but rather monitor-generated markers of their detection. While very helpful to the clinician at the bedside, pacemaker mode monitoring may not reliably detect pacemaker spikes in all patients. In other instances, the intrinsic features of the pacemaker stimulus in different leads might allow their detection in some leads but not others (Fig. 36.11).

ELECTROCARDIOGRAM DISPLAYS AND RECORDINGS

Monitoring the ECG during anesthesia and in the ICU includes both observation of the bedside monitor display and periodic recording of the ECG "rhythm strip" for documentation or more careful analysis. The most common bedside recording system provides a 2-inch strip that records two

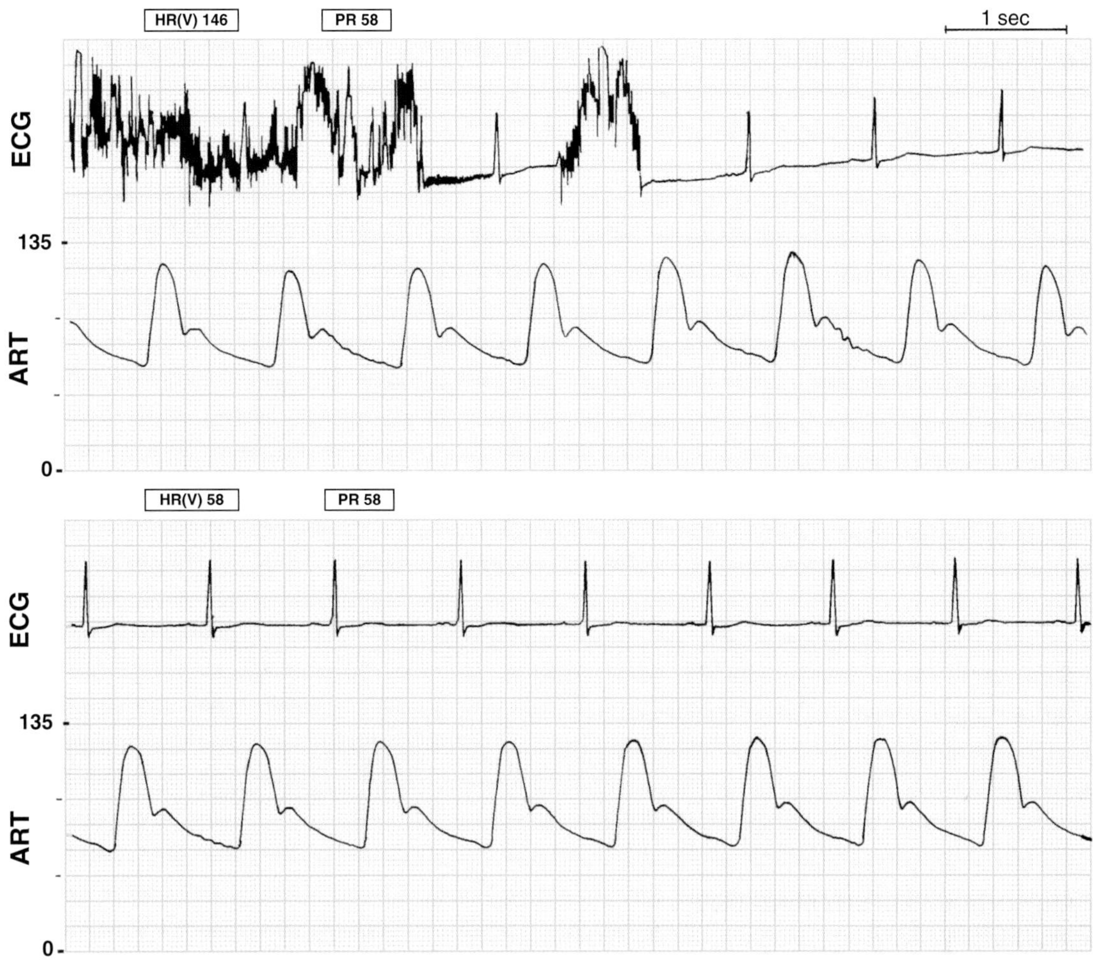

Fig. 36.12 Electrosurgical unit interference with heart rate measurement from the ECG. *(Top panel)* The ECG signal from lead V is distorted by the electrosurgical unit. As a result, the digital value for heart rate *(HR)* is erroneous (146 beats/min), although the pulse rate *(PR)* is measured accurately by the monitor from the arterial blood pressure waveform (58 beats/min). *(Lower panel)* Correct (and identical) digital values for both HR and PR are displayed by the monitor. *ART*, Arterial blood pressure. (From Mark JB. *Atlas of Cardiovascular Monitoring.* New York: Churchill Livingstone;1998.)

ECG leads (see Fig. 36.11), but other recording systems may provide larger formats for multi-lead or multi-waveform recording. Monitoring systems may also have "full disclosure" capability whereby monitored ECG (and other) waveforms are stored for up to 24 hours and can be retrieved and printed for review. This last system is particularly useful for the retrospective identification, interpretation, and documentation of arrhythmias or other cardiovascular changes that may have escaped detection in real time by clinicians at the bedside.

The ECG tracing on the bedside monitor can be displayed at varying sweep speeds, but most typically is displayed at 25 mm/s, the same speed as a standard 12-lead ECG tracing. As described previously, the ECG gain can be adjusted and the displayed gain should be indicated by a vertical marker overlying the ECG tracing, the standard being 10 mm/mV.

Paper recordings of the ECG should have standard millimeter grids, such that with a standard sweep speed of 25 mm/s, each 1 mm is a 40 ms interval, and a darker line appearing every 5 mm indicates a 200 ms interval (see Fig. 36.11). As noted, the recorded gain is indicated by a 1 mV rectangular calibration signal, the standard being 10 mm/mV.

ELECTROCARDIOGRAM ARTIFACTS

As is the case for all bedside monitoring,[20] artifacts commonly distort the monitored ECG tracing and must be identified to prevent misinterpretation or inappropriate treatment. In the operating room, the most common cause of ECG artifact is the electrosurgical unit (ESU). Since some of the frequencies generated by the ESU fall within the QRS frequency range, and the amplitude of these signals can be very high (1 kV or 1 million times the typical QRS amplitude of 1 mV),[21] even the best current advanced filtering techniques cannot eliminate this artifact that often totally masks the ECG signal (Fig. 36.12). This not only precludes identification of any ECG waveform features, but it can also prevent ECG monitoring of heart rate. The almost universal availability of additional simultaneously displayed waveforms, such as the pulse oximetry plethysmogram or an arterial blood pressure waveform, allow safe patient monitoring during these brief periods of ESU deployment (Fig. 36.12).

Other common ECG artifacts have been identified, and include common sources such as the 60 Hz interference from other medical devices near the patient (see Fig. 36.8B) and less common sources such as the cardiopulmonary

BOX 36.1 Equipment or Component-Related Electrocardiographic Artifacts

- Monitor/components
  - Manufacturing problems (50/60-Hz filter)
  - Defective monitor insulation
- Orthopedic shaver
- Intraoperative MRI
- Sinus endoscope
- Pressure-controlled irrigation pumps
- Flexible bronchoscopes
- ESWL
- Digital urine output-core temperature monitors
- Intravenous fluid warmer/warming sets
- Cardiopulmonary bypass machine
- Ventilator—HFOV
- Electrostimulators
  - Spinal cord, peripheral nerve, thalamic, vagal nerve, transcutaneous nerve, other
- Evoked potential monitoring units
- Hemodialysis machines
- Cellular telephones

ESWL, Extracorporeal shock-wave lithotripsy; *HFOV*, high-frequency oscillatory ventilation; *MRI*, magnetic resonance imaging.

Adapted from Patel SI, Souter MJ. Equipment-related electrocardiographic artifacts: causes, characteristics, consequences, and correction. *Anesthesiology*. 2008;108(1):138–148.

bypass machine.[22] Patel and Souter provide a comprehensive list of reported sources of ECG artifact (Box 36.1).[23]

ELECTROCARDIOGRAM MONITORING FOR MYOCARDIAL ISCHEMIA

The ST segment, representing myocardial repolarization, is the ECG component most sensitive to acute myocardial ischemia. ST elevation, with or without tall positive (hyperacute) T waves, indicates transmural ischemia and is most often the result of acute coronary artery occlusion either by coronary thrombosis or vasospasm (Prinzmetal-variant angina). Reciprocal ST-segment depression may appear in the contralateral leads. Ischemia confined to the subendocardial area is usually denoted by ST-segment depression. Subendocardial, ST-depression–type ischemia typically occurs during episodes of symptomatic or asymptomatic (*silent*) stable angina pectoris, and is characteristic of ischemia occurring during exercise, tachycardia, or pharmacologic stress testing in patients with significant but stable coronary artery disease.

Automated Real-Time ST-Segment Monitoring

Real-time ST-segment analysis first appeared in cardiac monitoring in the mid-1980s and is currently standard in most ECG monitors. On some monitors, the ST-segment analysis is set up to turn on automatically, but while ST-segment analysis is commonplace in the operating room, it is underutilized in other monitoring settings. A recent study has shown that even among coronary care units, less than 50% routinely use ST-segment monitoring for the detection of myocardial ischemia in patients admitted with acute coronary syndromes.[24] Chief among the reasons for the underuse of ST-segment analysis are the frequent number of false alarms and the lack of education on how to use the technology. In addition, no evidence exists as to whether the addition of computerized ST-segment ischemia monitoring improves patient outcomes after surgery.

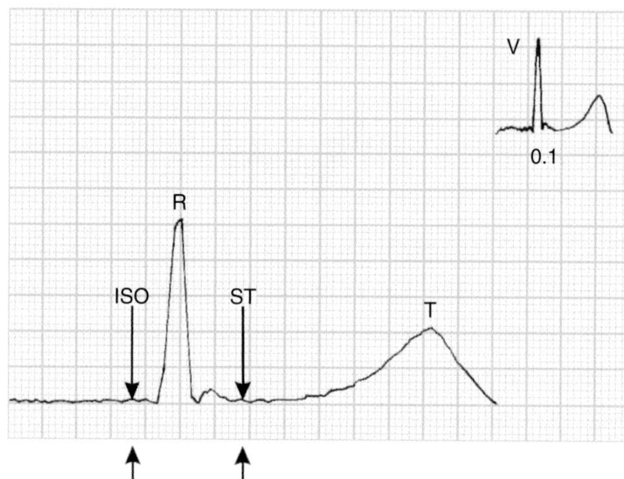

Fig. 36.13 Enlarged display of ECG lead V, showing the isoelectric *(ISO)* and ST-segment *(ST)* measurement points during continuous computer-aided ST-segment monitoring. The ECG R and T waves are also identified. This V lead ECG complex is shown at standard gain (10 mm/mV) in the upper right corner of the panel. The computer measures and displays 0.1 mm (0.01 mV) of ST-segment elevation in this lead. (From Mark JB. *Atlas of Cardiovascular Monitoring*. New York: Churchill Livingstone;1998.)

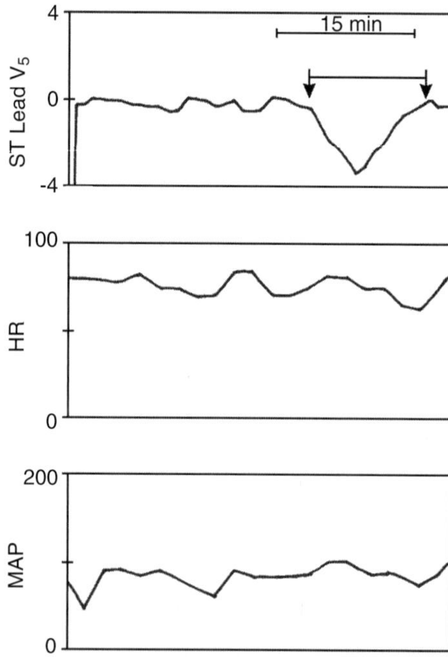

Fig. 36.14 One-hour trend displays for computer-aided continuous ST-segment monitoring in lead V_5, heart rate (*HR*, beats/min), and mean arterial pressure (*MAP*, mm Hg). A 15-minute episode of ST-segment depression *(arrows)* occurs without significant accompanying changes in HR or MAP. (From Mark JB. *Atlas of Cardiovascular Monitoring*. New York: Churchill Livingstone;1998.)

Computerized ST-segment analysis is achieved by the monitor measuring the ST segment at 60 or 80 ms after the J point (termed as J+60 or J+80 ms) and comparing it with the isoelectric point measured during the PR interval (Fig. 36.13). One millimeter of ST-segment deviation is equivalent to a 0.1 mV difference. The changes in ST-segment level over time in each lead can be displayed as ST-segment trends, just like trend displays of other hemodynamic variables (Fig. 36.14).

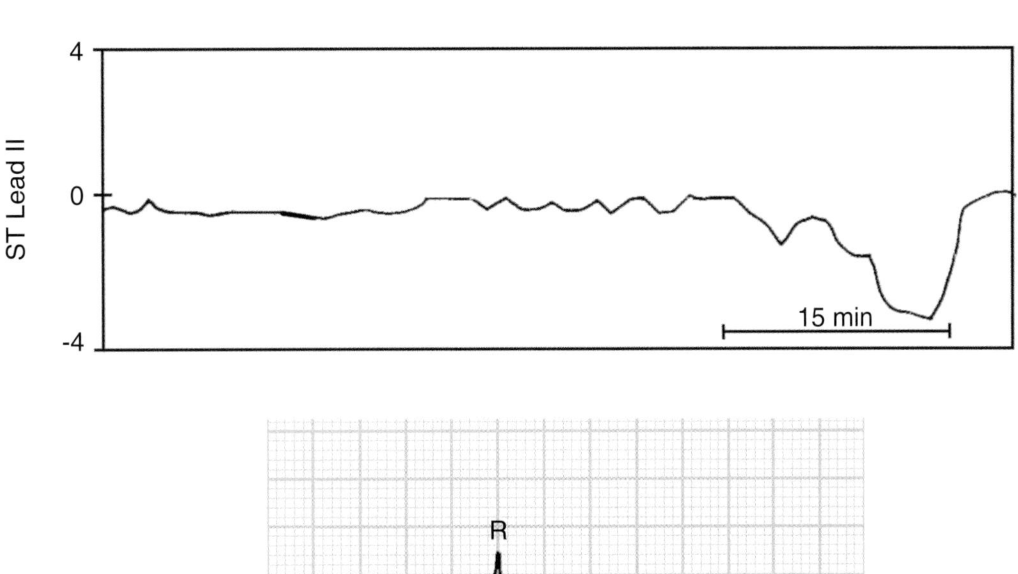

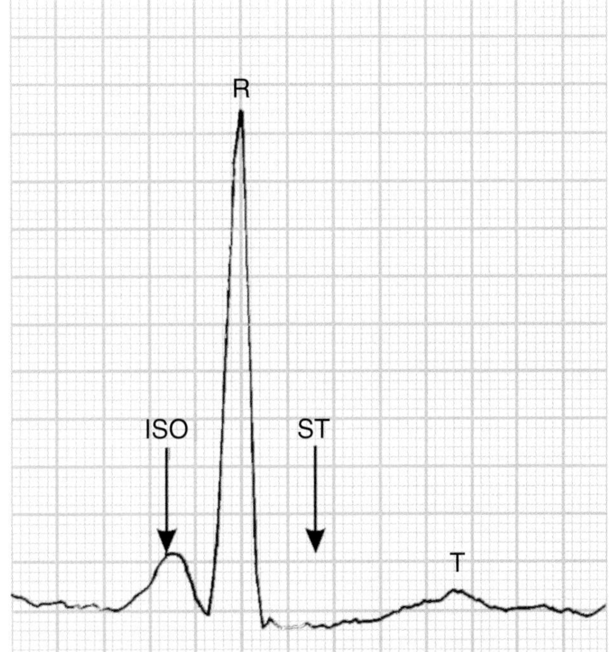

Fig. 36.15 Erroneous identification of the isoelectric *(ISO)* point measurement during computer-aided continuous ST-segment monitoring. A 1-hour trend recording of ST-segment deviations in lead II, displayed as millimeters of ST displacement, shows approximately 15 minutes of ST-segment depression, which reaches 3 mm in magnitude during this episode *(top panel)*. The enlarged display of ECG lead II showing the ISO and ST-segment *(ST)* measurement points during the episode of ST-segment depression reveals that the ISO point is identified inappropriately at the peak of the P wave, thereby producing artifactual ST-segment depression *(bottom panel)*. (From Mark JB. *Atlas of Cardiovascular Monitoring*. New York: Churchill Livingstone;1998.)

When the computer misidentifies the appropriate isoelectric or ST monitoring point, the clinician can manually adjust the J-point or the ST-segment measurement point (Fig. 36.15).

One major advantage of continuous ST-segment monitoring is that the electrodes stay in place and do not vary as they may with serial 12-lead ECG recordings. However, for improved diagnostic accuracy of ST-segment monitoring, the following points should be recognized:

1. Changes in body position may cause ST-segment changes and lead to false ST-segment alarms. However, changes in the QRS complex almost always accompany these positional ST-segment changes and therefore can be easily distinguished from true ST-segment deviations (Fig. 36.16). Changes in position of the heart in the mediastinum have also shown to affect the ST segment. Mark and associates observed that placement of a sternal retractor during cardiac surgery was associated with a reduction in V_5 R-wave amplitude (Fig. 36.17).[25] Simultaneously, V_5 S-wave amplitude and absolute ST-segment deviation were reduced. These investigators concluded that inclusion of an R-wave gain factor might improve perioperative ECG ischemia monitoring.
2. Many patients have preexisting ECG abnormalities that confound interpretation of ST-segment changes. Early repolarization (a normal variant), intraventricular conduction delays, LV hypertrophy, digitalis, pericarditis, and other conditions may cause baseline ST-segment abnormalities. In these conditions, standard ECG criteria for diagnosing myocardial ischemia are less specific.
3. Most cardiac monitors with ST-segment monitoring software provide displays of ST-segment trends in a single lead or the sum of absolute ST-segment deviations from multiple leads (Fig. 36.18). Although such graphic trends are convenient for the quick identification of potential ischemic events, analysis of the ECG waveform on the monitor screen or by recording the ECG tracing is of paramount importance for verification.

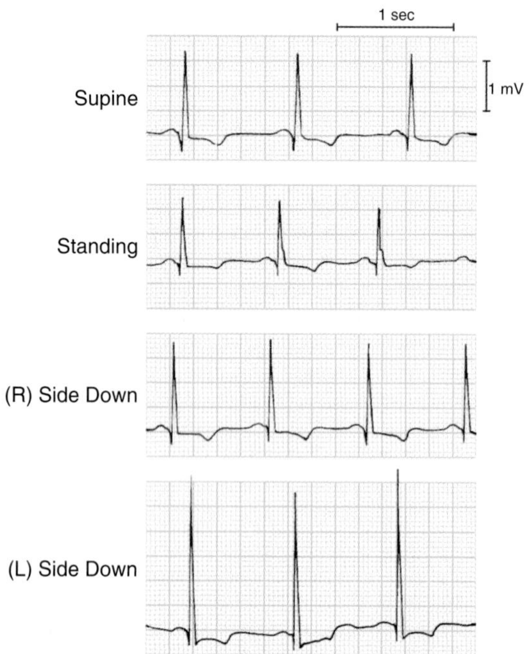

Fig. 36.16 Effect of changing body position on the ECG in a patient with preexisting ST-segment depression. Lead CC_5, a surrogate for lead V_5, is recorded with the patient in four different positions: supine, standing, right *(R)* side down, and left *(L)* side down. The magnitude of ST-segment depression changes in direct proportion to the R-wave amplitude. (From Mark JB. *Atlas of Cardiovascular Monitoring*. New York: Churchill Livingstone;1998.)

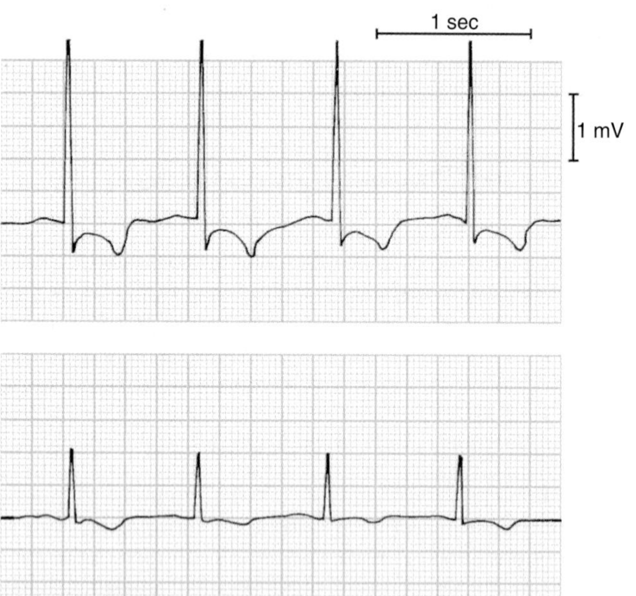

Fig. 36.17 Effect of surgical retraction on the ECG. Baseline lead V_5 recording shows 2 mm ST-segment depression and 27 mm R-wave amplitude *(top panel)*. Placement of a sternal retractor during cardiac surgery displaces the precordial lead electrode relative to the heart, resulting in a marked reduction in R-wave amplitude to 10 mm and a proportional reduction in the magnitude of ST-segment displacement *(bottom panel)*. (From Mark JB. *Atlas of Cardiovascular Monitoring*. New York: Churchill Livingstone;1998.)

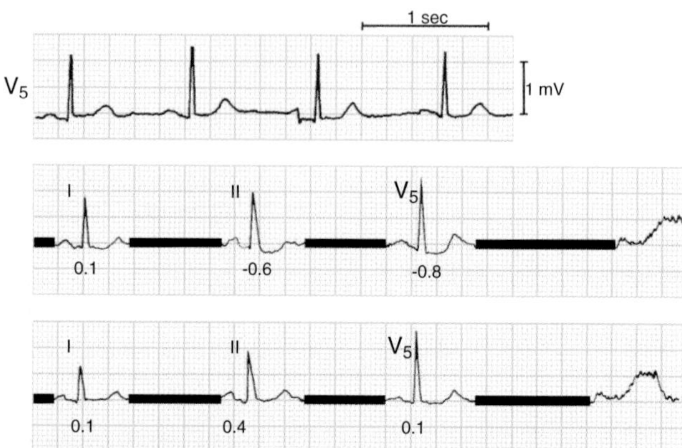

Fig. 36.18 Computer-aided continuous ST-segment monitoring. A baseline recording of lead V_5 shows isoelectric ST segments *(top panel)*. Shortly after induction of anesthesia, the ST-segment monitoring display shows the three monitored leads I, II, and V_5 and the absolute amount of ST-segment elevation (0.1 mm in lead I) or depression (−0.6 mm in lead II, −0.8 mm in lead V_5) in each lead *(middle panel)*. A trend line is displayed on the right side of the panel and demonstrates that the sum of ST-segment deviations in these three monitored leads has increased and reached a plateau over the previous few minutes. Another ST-segment display recorded 5 minutes later shows resolution of these subtle ST changes *(bottom panel)*. Note that the appearance of lead V_5 in this last display closely resembles the baseline recording and that the trend line has returned to pre-induction baseline level. (From Mark JB. *Atlas of Cardiovascular Monitoring*. New York: Churchill Livingstone;1998.)

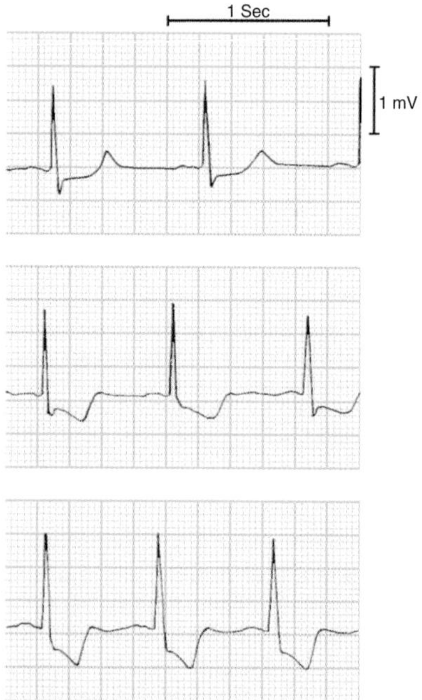

Fig. 36.19 Subendocardial ischemia produces ST-segment depression. As heart rate increases progressively from 63 beats/min *(top panel)* to 75 beats/min *(middle panel)* and finally to 86 beats/min *(bottom, panel)* in this patient with left main coronary artery disease, the ST segment becomes more depressed and more downsloping, owing to an increase in myocardial oxygen demand. (From Mark JB. *Atlas of Cardiovascular Monitoring*. New York: Churchill Livingstone;1998.)

Electrocardiogram Criteria for Acute Myocardial Ischemia

The ECG criteria most accepted for detecting myocardial ischemia during continuous ECG monitoring are those established and validated during exercise stress testing.[26] During stress testing and with acute subendocardial ischemia, the electrical forces responsible for the ST segment are deviated toward the inner layer of the heart, causing ST-segment depression or demand-mediated ischemia (Fig. 36.19). With acute transmural epicardial ischemia, the electrical forces in the ischemic area are deviated toward the outer layer of the heart, causing ST-segment elevation or supply-mediated ischemia in

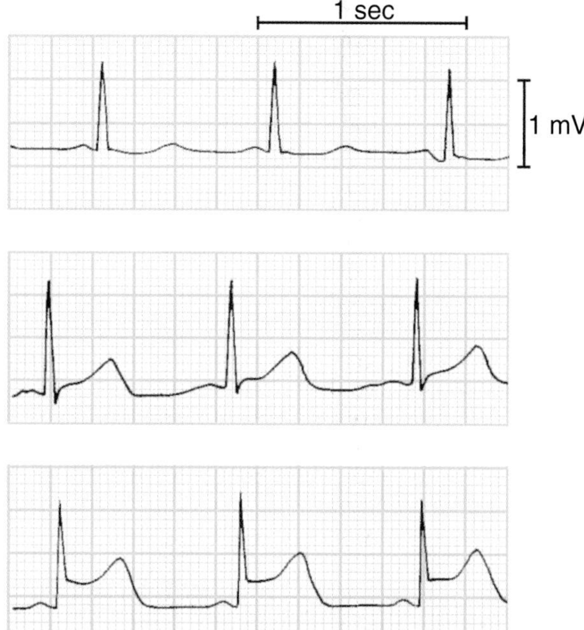

Fig. 36.20 Transmural ischemia produces ST-segment elevation. Occlusion of a patent saphenous vein graft during repeat coronary artery bypass surgery causes an abrupt reduction of coronary blood supply and results in progressive ST-segment elevation *(middle and bottom panels)*. (From Mark JB. *Atlas of Cardiovascular Monitoring*. New York: Churchill Livingstone;1998.)

the overlying leads (Fig. 36.20). Note that most commonly, intraoperative or perioperative ischemia is demand-mediated subendocardial ischemia, which is manifest as ST-segment depression.[27] Although the anterolateral precordial leads are most sensitive for detecting these changes, they are **nonlocalizing** as to the coronary distribution responsible. In contrast, supply-mediated transmural ischemia, while much less common perioperatively, causes ST-segment elevation in leads overlying the involved coronary bed and thus are able to **localize** the responsible coronary territory (e.g., ST elevations in inferior leads II, III, aVF suggest occlusion of the right or posterior descending coronary artery).

With demand-mediated ischemia, as heart rate increases, J-point depression and upsloping ST-segment depression occurs. As the severity of ischemia progresses, the ST segment typically becomes horizontal (flattens) and the extent of ST-segment depression may increase and the ST segment may become downsloping (see Fig. 36.19). Standard criteria for stress-induced ischemia are 1 mm (0.1 mV) or more of horizontal or downsloping ST-segment depression measured 60 to 80 ms after the J point. As noted earlier, patients with preexisting ST-segment abnormalities make ST-segment interpretation more difficult.

During the perioperative period, ECG monitoring most commonly identifies stress-induced, ST-depression, demand-mediated ischemia, or other causes of supply-demand imbalance such as prolonged or severe hypotension. Such ECG changes do not provide information about the location of the ischemic myocardial area. In contrast, ST-segment elevation indicating transmural or supply-mediated ischemia, observed particularly during cardiac surgery, provides useful information about the myocardial segment and coronary perfusion territory responsible for the ischemic episode. Because the majority of modern patient-monitoring systems do not simultaneously monitor all 12 ECG leads, selecting which chest leads to monitor is of great importance, particularly in noncardiac surgery. During exercise stress testing, investigators have identified leads V_4 and V_5 as the most sensitive leads to detect exercise-induced ischemia (90%-100% sensitivity).[28] London and colleagues studied high-risk patients undergoing noncardiac surgery and showed that the greatest sensitivity for ischemia was obtained with lead V_5 (75%), followed by lead V_4 (61%).[15] Combining leads V_4 and V_5 increased the sensitivity to 90%, whereas with the standard lead II and V_5 combination, the sensitivity was only 80%. They also suggested that if three leads (II, V_4, and V_5) could be simultaneously examined, the sensitivity would increase to 98%. More recently, Landesberg and associates monitored continuous 12-lead ST-segment changes greater than 0.2 mV from baseline in a single lead or more than 0.1 mV in two contiguous leads at J+60 ms, lasting longer than 10 minutes in patients undergoing major vascular surgery.[16] They showed that leads V_3 and V_4 were more sensitive than V_5 in detecting perioperative ischemia (87%, 79%, and 66%, respectively). As a result of these and other investigations, it appears most appropriate to monitor lead V_3, V_4, or V_5 for optimal detection of perioperative ST-segment depression, choosing the specific lead location based on whether the lead placement might interfere with the surgical prep and procedure.

Blood Pressure Monitoring

Like heart rate, blood pressure has long been a fundamental cardiovascular vital sign included in the mandated standards for basic anesthetic monitoring.[29] Measuring blood pressure is primarily performed with either indirect cuff devices or direct arterial cannulation with pressure transduction. These techniques measure different physical signals and differ in their degree of invasiveness, but both are subject to numerous confounding factors that often result in significant discrepancies among simultaneous measurements.[30]

INDIRECT MEASUREMENT OF ARTERIAL BLOOD PRESSURE

Manual Intermittent Techniques

Most indirect methods of blood pressure measurement utilize a sphygmomanometer, first described by Riva-Rocci in 1896.[31] The systolic pressure was identified using an inflatable elastic cuff around the arm and a mercury manometer to measure cuff pressure, while the radial arterial pulse was palpated as the cuff pressure was increased or rapidly decreased. The technique was later modified to detect both systolic and diastolic pressure with description of auscultatory method of blood pressure measurement by Korotkoff in 1905.[32] Korotkoff sounds are a complex series of audible frequencies produced by turbulent flow beyond the partially occluding cuff. Put simply, the systolic pressure is associated with first sound heard (beginning of turbulent flow through the vessel) and diastolic pressure at the point when the sounds disappear (when vessel flow becomes laminar).[33] Mean blood pressure cannot be measured using this technique.

A fundamental principle of the auscultatory method is its reliance on blood flow to generate Korotkoff sounds. Physiologic conditions that interfere with sound detection (e.g., severe edema, obesity, abnormal compliance of overlying tissue) or blood flow (shock, intense vasoconstriction) will frustrate manual blood pressure measurement.[33-37] Furthermore, the cuff must also be snugly fitted, with a bladder that measures 40% of arm circumference and 80% of length of the upper arm, and centered over the artery. A cuff that is too large will often yield acceptable results when used for *manual* measurements, but a small cuff will usually yield falsely high readings.[36]

Automated Intermittent Techniques

Automated noninvasive blood pressure (NIBP) devices are the most commonly used means of measuring blood pressure in the operating room. Small oscillations in pressure amplitude are measured in an air-filled cuff that slowly deflates from a pressure well in excess of that needed to collapse the underlying artery. The point of maximal oscillation marks the mean arterial blood pressure (MAP), with systolic and diastolic being calculated by various proprietary algorithms specific to individual device manufacturers.[33,35,36] In general, a cuff that is too large will underestimate the blood pressure while a small cuff will overestimate.[36,38] Of the three possible measurements, systolic has the poorest agreement with invasive blood pressure values.[38,39]

Although automated NIBP measurements have generally been shown to approximate directly measured arterial pressures, there are also important shortcomings to keep in mind.[36,38] For reasons involving the ethics of validation against invasive measurements, standards for device performance established by the Association for the Advancement of Medical Instrumentation (AAMI) and the British Hypertension Society are defined by auscultation.[40] New devices must demonstrate average differences ≤ ± 5 mm Hg and standard deviations ≤ 8 mm Hg, which means that deviations of up to 20 mm Hg are still considered "acceptable performance."[41]

Clinical studies comparing NIBP with direct arterial pressure measurements reflect the problematic nature of NIBP monitoring. Direct comparisons of oscillometric devices to invasive monitoring have shown that mean blood pressure measurements generally show the greatest degree of agreement with invasive blood pressure readings while systolic measurements are the most divergent.[39,42-44] Agreement is especially problematic in critically ill or older patients.[38,42-44]

Oscillometric NIBP values tend to underestimate MAP values during periods of hypertension and overestimate during hypotension, potentially biasing clinical decisions in unstable patients.[45] And they often underestimate the systolic while overestimating the diastolic measurements.[46] A well-fitted arm cuff does appear to be helpful in identifying hypotension in unstable patients and differentiating responses to therapy in such situations, but below a MAP of 65 mm Hg, it is not useful for titration of therapy, and a more frequent interval of measurement is probably required to be considered reliable.[38,42,47,48] Dysrhythmia may also result in significant error in blood pressure measurement, especially in systolic and diastolic estimation, although averaging three measurements seems to minimize the clinical impact.[49,50]

While the upper arm is the most common cuff location, various factors may force choice of an alternative site. In obese patients, there is little agreement between any alternate location and invasively measured pressures while ankle, calf, and thigh cuffs have never been validated at all.[51] Interestingly, the forearm may be a preferable site to upper arm in obese patients, although such cuffs display a reversed pattern of bias; overestimation of the systolic and underestimation of the diastolic pressure.[48]

It is important to remember the auscultatory method measures the systolic and diastolic pressures while oscillometric devices measure the mean and calculate the systolic and diastolic, albeit in different and non-interchangeable ways. Furthermore, directly-measured arterial pressure measurements utilize another technique altogether. In some authors' opinions, "current protocols for validating blood pressure monitors give no guarantee of accuracy in clinical practice."[40,52] Expecting them to yield identical values is unrealistic, especially in complex and unstable clinical situations. The sources of error vary significantly for each of these measurement techniques and should closely guide evaluation and therapeutic intervention, especially when there is discrepancy between the measured values or between measurements and clinical conditions.

BOX 36.2 Complications of Noninvasive Blood Pressure (NIBP) Measurement

Pain
Petechiae and ecchymoses
Limb edema
Venous stasis and thrombophlebitis
Peripheral neuropathy
Compartment syndrome

Complications of Noninvasive Blood Pressure Measurement

Although automated NIBP measurement is generally safe, there have been reports of rare but severe complications (Box 36.2).[53] Compartment syndrome is possible after prolonged periods of frequent cycling and is most likely related to trauma or impaired distal limb perfusion. Caution should be exercised in cases of peripheral neuropathy, arterial or venous insufficiency, severe coagulopathies, or recent use of thrombolytic therapy.

Automated Continuous Techniques

Continuous methods for NIBP monitoring are being developed with various degrees of success. The most current version is based on the volume clamp technique and involves photoplethysmography and closed loop continuous control of a pressure cuff around a finger. This creates a stable arterial pressure waveform via quantification of an infrared beam applied distal to the finger cuff. Many of these require initial calibration with a standard NIBP

BOX 36.3 Indications for Arterial Cannulation

Continuous, real-time blood pressure monitoring
Anticipated pharmacologic or mechanical cardiovascular manipulation
Repeated blood sampling
Failure of indirect arterial blood pressure measurement
Supplementary diagnostic information from the arterial waveform

cuff, and all are significantly affected by changes in vascular tone and perfusion in the finger, as well as movement, vascular disease, and a host of other factors.[54] While none of these devices technically meet AAMI standards when compared with invasive pressures, clinical studies have shown their correlation to be reasonable in a variety of operative cases.[35,55-58]

Other devices use technologies related to pulse transit time or arterial tonometry.[59,60] All of these techniques, however, have limitations, including need for calibration, sensitivity to motion artifact, and limited applicability in critically ill patients.[36,61,62] It remains unclear whether any noninvasive technique will reduce the need for direct arterial pressure monitoring during anesthesia or critical care, but with continued development and technical refinement, they remain promising.

DIRECT MEASUREMENT OF ARTERIAL BLOOD PRESSURE

Arterial cannulation with continuous pressure transduction remains the accepted reference standard for blood pressure monitoring despite its risk, cost, and need for technical expertise for placement and management (Box 36.3). Its superiority over noninvasive techniques for early detection of interoperative hypotension was confirmed by The Australian Incident Monitoring Study of 1993.[42,63] More recently, though, the use of waveform analysis in physiologic monitoring has become more popular. This was initially proposed more than a half century ago by Eather and associates, who advocated monitoring of "arterial pressure and pressure pulse contours" in anesthetized patients.[64] Arterial pressure waveform characteristics used in current clinical practice include the dicrotic notch as a trigger for intra-aortic balloon counterpulsation as well as respiratory-induced variation in an array of directly-measured and derived pressure measurements to indicate preload reserve and volume responsiveness.[65-68] Rates of intraoperative direct arterial blood pressure measurement vary significantly across clinical environments even for similar procedures.[69]

Percutaneous Radial Artery Cannulation

The radial artery is the most common site for invasive blood pressure monitoring because it is technically easy to cannulate and complications are rare.[70,71] Slogoff et al. described 1700 cardiovascular surgical patients who underwent radial artery cannulation without ischemic complications despite evidence of arterial occlusion after decannulation in more than 25% of patients.[72] Furthermore, most investigations of hand perfusion following radial artery harvest have reported no significant decrease relative to the contralateral hand in either the early or late postoperative periods.[73-78]

Before radial artery cannulation, some clinicians assess collateral blood flow to the hand by performing a modified Allen test, originally described in 1929 to assess arterial stenosis in patients suffering from thromboangiitis obliterans.[79] The radial and ulnar arteries are both compressed while the patient makes a tight fist to exsanguinate the palm and then slowly reopens it. As occlusion of the ulnar artery is released, the color of the open palm is observed. Normally, the color will return to the palm within several seconds; severely reduced collateral flow is present when the palm remains pale for more than 6 to 10 seconds. Unfortunately, the predictive value of this test is poor. There are numerous reports of ischemic sequelae in the face of a normal Allen test, and conversely, reports of uncomplicated radial catheter use and even harvest for bypass grafting in the presence of an abnormal result.[72,73,80,81] In recent years, the radial artery has become more popular for coronary catheterization and stenting access, even in individuals with abnormal Allen tests.[82] Overall, the diagnostic accuracy of the modified Allen test with a 5-second threshold is only 80% with 76% sensitivity and 82% specificity. It appears that the test is unable to provide a cutoff point below which perfusion can be deemed vulnerable.[83] Use of pulse oximetry, plethysmography, or Doppler ultrasound as adjuncts does not seem to improve its accuracy. Oximetry detects blood flows at extremely low flows, leading to poor specificity, while there are no established ultrasound criteria by which to evaluate radial or ulnar blood flow.[73,84,85] In general, it seems that while a normal modified Allen test may be useful in identifying patients unacceptable for radial artery use for bypass graft or coronary angiography, there is no evidence that it predicts clinical outcomes following cannulation for blood pressure monitoring.[73]

Techniques for radial artery cannulation have been unchanged for decades with the notable exception of the use of ultrasound in guiding catheter placement. Evidence supports its use, especially as a rescue method following a failed attempt.[86] Although evidence in the critical care setting suggests that ultrasound techniques improve first-pass cannulation success rates, it is not clear that this translates to improved clinical outcomes, nor that the impact on time required to perform the procedure or other factors warrants routine intraoperative use.[87-90] Ultrasound guidance in catheterization of other vessels other than the radial artery or in special populations, such as those on mechanical support without pulsatile flow, is more likely to be of substantial benefit.[91]

Alternative Arterial Pressure Monitoring Sites

If the radial arteries are unsuitable or unavailable, there are multiple alternatives. The *ulnar artery* has been used safely even following failed attempts to access the ipsilateral radial artery.[72,92] Similarly, the *brachial artery*, while lacking collateral branches to protect the hand, has a long track record of safe use. Several investigators have reported large series of brachial artery catheters in patients undergoing cardiac surgery with very few vascular, neurologic, or thrombotic sequelae.[93,94] The *axillary artery* has the advantages of patient comfort and mobility, and complications appear to be similar in incidence to those for radial and femoral

BOX 36.4 Complications of Direct Arterial Pressure Monitoring

Distal ischemia, pseudoaneurysm, arteriovenous fistula
Hemorrhage
Arterial embolization
Infection
Peripheral neuropathy
Misinterpretation of data
Misuse of equipment

arteries.[71] A slightly longer catheter is preferred for the brachial or axillary sites due to their relatively deeper and more mobile anatomic locations. Clinicians should be aware, however, that the risk of cerebral embolization is significantly increased when more central vessels are utilized.

The *femoral artery* is the largest vessel in common use for blood pressure monitoring but its safety profile seems comparable to other sites.[71] Catheterization of the femoral artery is best achieved with a guidewire technique and the point of vessel entry must be distal to the inguinal ligament to minimize the risk of arterial injury, hidden hematoma formation, or even uncontrolled hemorrhage into the pelvis or retroperitoneum.[95]

Less commonly used alternatives include the *dorsalis pedis, posterior tibial*, and *superficial temporal arteries*, with the pedal vessels being more popular in pediatric patients. Lower extremity vessels tend to demonstrate greater with disagreement noninvasively acquired data, with diastolic and mean measurements being the most affected.[96]

Complications of Direct Arterial Pressure Monitoring

Although large clinical investigations confirm the low incidence of long-term complications after radial arterial pressure monitoring, factors that may increase such risks include vasospastic arterial disease, previous arterial injury, thrombocytosis, protracted shock, high-dose vasopressor administration, prolonged cannulation, and infection.[70-73,97,98]

Rare but serious complications have been reported after arterial cannulation at all locations (Box 36.4). In most cases, catheter placement was technically difficult or there were contributory factors such as shock or coagulopathy. In a large observational study of 2000 untoward clinical events resulting from any kind of vascular access, only 13 were related to peripheral arterial cannulation, fewer than those associated with central venous (18) or even peripheral venous cannulation (33). The events involved equipment problems, inadvertent drug administration, or disruption/kinking of the catheter itself. In only 1 case did transient vasospasm follow radial artery cannulation. An additional 10 cases were noted to involve problems with incorrect device calibration or erroneous data interpretation.[63,99] Data from the anesthesia closed claims reports have shown that claims related to arterial pressure monitoring constitute only 8% of all claims related to any vascular access (2% of total claims). Of this small number, almost 54% were related to radial artery use (ischemic injury, median or radial nerve injury, or retained wire fragment), less than 8% were associated with use of the brachial artery, and the remainder involved severe thrombotic or hemorrhagic complications following femoral artery monitoring.[100] While patient physiology is important, equipment misuse, poor placement technique or catheter care, as well as improper data interpretation play important roles in most complications related to arterial pressure monitoring.

Technical Aspects of Direct Blood Pressure Measurement

There are a variety of factors, including extension tubing, stopcocks, flush devices, recorders, amplifiers, and transducers that may confound the process by which pressure waveforms are reproduced for measurement and display.[101]

Most invasive blood pressure monitoring systems are underdamped second-order dynamic systems that demonstrate simple harmonic motion dependent on *elasticity, mass*, and *friction*.[101-103] These three properties determine the system operating characteristics (i.e., *frequency response* or *dynamic response*) which in turn are characterized by *natural frequency* and *damping coefficient*. The natural frequency of a system determines how rapidly the system oscillates after a perturbation, while the damping coefficient reflects how rapidly it returns to its prior resting state. Both parameters may be estimated or measured at the bedside and dramatically influence the appearance of the displayed pressure waveform.

Natural Frequency, Damping Coefficient, and Dynamic Response of Pressure Monitoring Systems

The displayed pressure waveform is a periodic complex wave produced via Fourier analysis of a summation of multiple propagated and reflected pressure waves. As such, it is a mathematical re-creation of the original complex pressure wave created and propagated by stroke volume ejection.[104,105] The original pressure wave is characterized by its fundamental frequency, a characteristic manifested clinically as the pulse rate and expressed as cycles/second (Hertz).

The sine waves that sum to produce the final complex wave have frequencies that are multiples or harmonics of the fundamental frequency (i.e., pulse rate). A very crude arterial waveform depicting a systolic upstroke and peak, dicrotic notch, and so forth can be reconstructed with reasonable accuracy from only two sine waves, the fundamental frequency and the second harmonic (Fig. 36.21). As a general rule, though, 6 to 10 harmonics are required to provide distortion-free reproductions of most arterial pressure waveforms.[104,106] Consequently, accurate blood pressure measurement in a patient with a pulse rate of 120 beats/min (2 cycles/s or 2 Hz) requires a monitoring system dynamic response of 12 to 20 Hz (i.e., 6 to 10 waveforms X 2 Hz). The faster the heart rate and the steeper the systolic pressure upstroke, the greater the demands on the monitoring system.

Natural frequency and damping coefficient are intrinsic characteristics of all monitoring systems. If the system's natural frequency is too low, the system will resonate, and pressure waveforms recorded on the monitor will be exaggerated or amplified versions of true intraarterial pressure. An underdamped system may combine elements of the measurement system itself with the measured sine waves

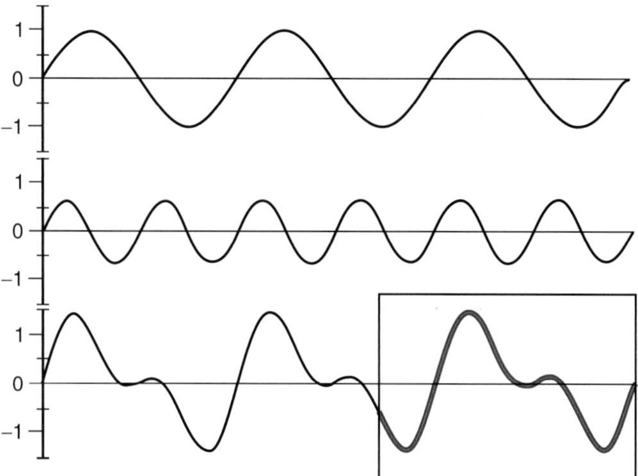

Fig. 36.21 **Arterial blood pressure waveform produced by summation of sine waves.** The fundamental wave *(top)* added to 63% of the second harmonic wave *(middle)* results in a pressure wave *(bottom)* resembling a typical arterial blood pressure waveform *(box)*. (From Mark JB. *Atlas of Cardiovascular Monitoring*. New York: Churchill Livingstone; 1998.)

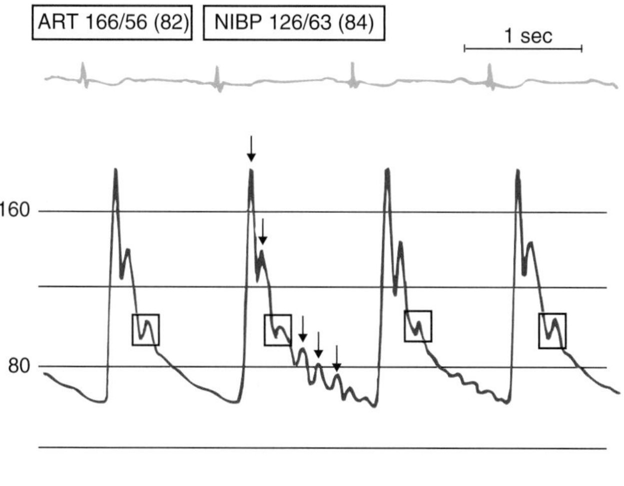

Fig. 36.22 **Underdamped arterial pressure waveform.** Systolic pressure overshoot and additional small, nonphysiologic pressure waves *(arrows)* distort the waveform and make it hard to discern the dicrotic notch *(boxes)*. Digital values displayed for direct arterial blood pressure (*ART* 166/56, mean 82 mm Hg) and noninvasive blood pressure (*NIBP* 126/63, mean 84 mm Hg) show the characteristic relationship between the two measurement techniques in the presence of an underdamped system. (From Mark JB. *Atlas of Cardiovascular Monitoring*. New York: Churchill Livingstone; 1998.)

and display systolic pressure overshoot (Fig. 36.22). In contrast, an overdamped waveform exhibits a slurred upstroke, absent dicrotic notch, and loss of fine detail. In such cases, the pulse pressure will be falsely narrow but MAP may remain reasonably accurate (Fig. 36.23).

The interplay between natural frequency and damping coefficients is complex, but in general, the lower the natural frequency of the system, the narrower the range of acceptable damping coefficients. It follows logically that for any specific system, the highest possible natural frequency yields the optimal result.[105] In theory, this is best achieved by using short lengths of stiff pressure tubing and limiting

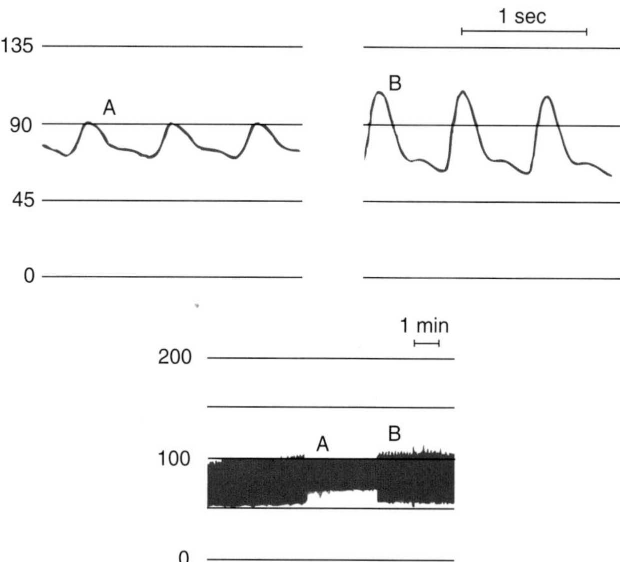

Fig. 36.23 **Overdamped arterial pressure waveform.** The overdamped pressure waveform (A) shows a diminished pulse pressure compared with the normal waveform (B). The slow-speed recording *(bottom)* demonstrates a 3-minute period of damped arterial pressure. Note that despite the damped system, mean arterial pressure remains unchanged. (From Mark JB. *Atlas of Cardiovascular Monitoring*. New York: Churchill Livingstone; 1998.)

additions or connections to the system such as stopcocks. While adding an air bubble to the monitoring system will increase damping, it simultaneously lowers natural frequency and may actually increase the intrinsic system resonance and worsen systolic pressure overshoot (Fig. 36.24).

The fast-flush test provides a convenient bedside method for determining system dynamic response and assessing signal distortion.[101,103,105] The nature and duration of the flush artifact following a brief opening of the fast-flush valve are noted visually with shorter oscillation cycles indicating a higher natural frequency and the damping coefficient being related to the resulting pattern of peak amplitudes (Fig. 36.25).[101,105] Thus, an adequate fast-flush test pattern has short oscillation cycles (<30 ms) and a pattern of amplitudes that rapidly return to rest. The clinical impact of resonance and under- or over-damping is common, occurring in up to 30% of surgical patients and 44.5% of patients admitted to the ICU. Interestingly, it appears to be more significant for systolic blood pressure measurement than mean or diastolic, and is associated with preexisting arteriopathy, lung disease, hypertension, and smaller-gauge arterial catheters.[107] Distortion of the arterial waveform is common in clinical practice, particularly systolic pressure overshoot secondary to underdamped systems.[101,108]

Pressure Monitoring System Components

Arterial pressure monitoring systems have a number of components, including the intraarterial catheter itself, stopcocks for blood sampling and transducer zeroing, in-line blood sampling ports, a pressure transducer, continuous-flush device, and electronic cable. Innovation to the basic system such as needleless ports and closed aspiration systems, while intended to improve safety, may also degrade the dynamic response of the monitoring system and further exacerbate systolic arterial pressure overshoot.

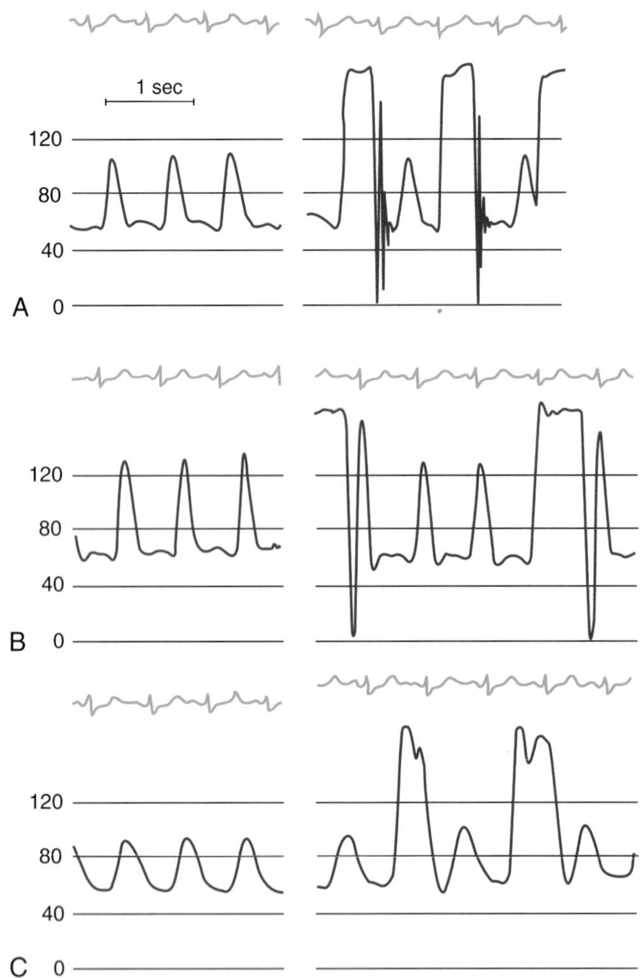

Fig. 36.24 **Effect of small air bubbles within arterial pressure monitoring systems.** Arterial pressure waveforms are displayed, along with superimposed fast-flush square-wave artifacts. (A) Original monitoring system has an adequate dynamic response (natural frequency 17 Hz, damping coefficient 0.2). (B) A small 0.1-mL air bubble added to the monitoring system produces a paradoxical increase in arterial blood pressure. Note decreased natural frequency of the system. (C) A larger 0.5-mL air bubble further degrades dynamic response and produces spurious arterial hypotension. (From Mark JB. *Atlas of Cardiovascular Monitoring*. New York: Churchill Livingstone; 1998.)

The flush device provides a continuous, slow (1-3 mL/h) infusion of saline to purge the monitoring system and prevent thrombus formation within the system. Dextrose solutions should not be used, since flush contamination of sampled blood may cause serious errors in blood glucose measurement.[109] The flush device not only ensures continuous slow flushing of the system but also includes a spring-loaded valve for periodic, high-pressure flushing following sample collection or to restore the system's dynamic response to baseline.[110]

Transducer Setup: Zeroing and Leveling

Prior to use, pressure transducers must be zeroed, calibrated, and leveled to the appropriate position, a maneuver accomplished by exposing the transducer to atmospheric pressure and performing the zero procedure as defined by each device manufacturer. It is important to recognize that the *zero pressure locus* should be positioned appropriately given the specific clinical context, that it is positioned relative to the patient, that the zero reference point is local atmospheric pressure, and that the zero should be checked and re-zeroed periodically.[105] Occasionally, a faulty transducer, cable, or monitor will cause the zero baseline to drift, introducing significant error until the zero reference is reestablished.[111,112] Because current disposable pressure transducers meet accuracy standards established by the AAMI and the American National Standards Institute, formal bedside transducer calibration is no longer routinely performed. However, it remains good practice to routinely compare pressures obtained via a newly placed arterial catheter with a blood pressure obtained via other means.[111,112]

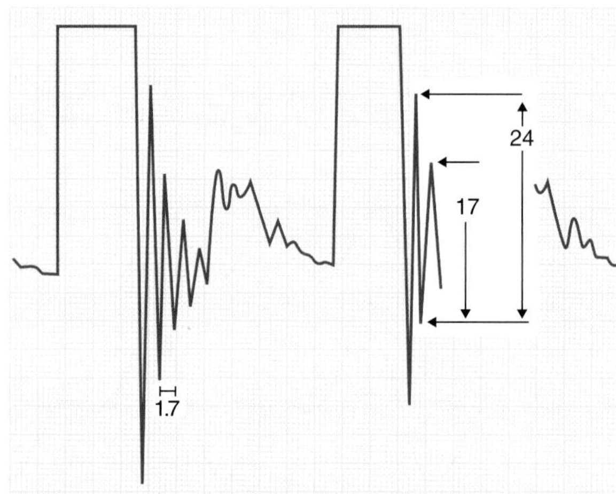

Fig. 36.25 **Clinical measurement of natural frequency and damping coefficient.** Two square-wave fast-flush artifacts interrupt an arterial pressure waveform recorded on standard 1-mm grid paper at a speed of 25 mm/s. Natural frequency is determined by measuring the period of one cycle of adjacent oscillation peaks (1.7 mm). Damping coefficient is determined by measuring the heights of adjacent oscillation peaks (17 and 24 mm). From these measurements, a natural frequency of 14.7 Hz and an amplitude ratio of 0.71 may be calculated. (From Mark JB. *Atlas of Cardiovascular Monitoring*. New York: Churchill Livingstone; 1998.)

Choosing the appropriate level at which to establish the zero point must be done with respect to the patient and the clinical context. Note that transducer zeroing and leveling are distinct and separate. Zeroing establishes the zero reference point as ambient atmospheric pressure, while leveling aligns this reference point relative to the patient's body, determining where the value "0" will be. This is even more important when monitoring values for which the physiologic range is small, such as central venous or intracranial pressure. In such cases, small zeroing or leveling errors may translate to large relative errors in measurement.

In most cases, arterial pressure transducers should be placed to best estimate aortic root pressure. In general, the best position for this is approximately 5 cm posterior to the sternal border.[113,114] However, a more conventional location for the reference level used for all hemodynamic monitoring, including central venous and pulmonary artery pressures (PAPs), is the mid-thoracic level, which corresponds most closely to the mid-left atrial position and is located halfway between the anterior sternum and the bed surface in the supine patient.[115,116] The most critical point, regardless of where the clinician chooses to assign the reference level, is that it is consistently maintained throughout the monitoring period.

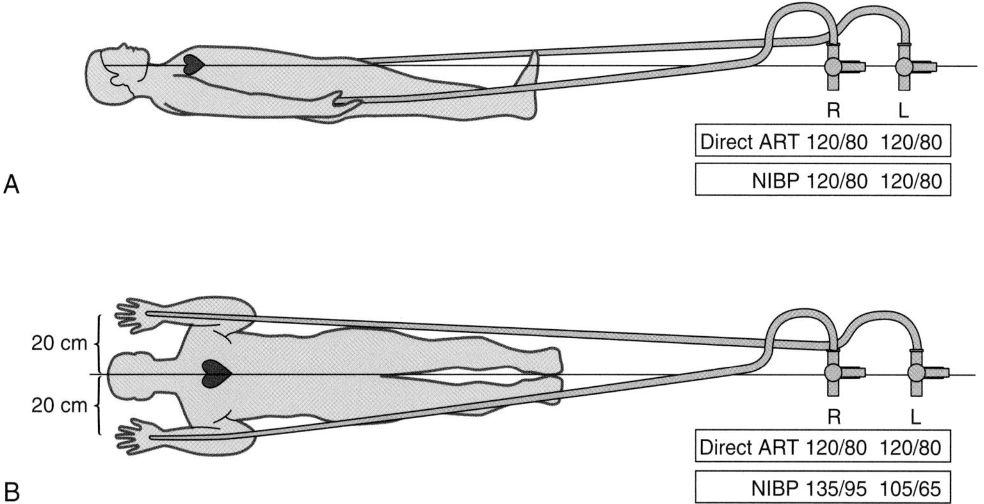

Fig. 36.26 Effect of patient position on the relation between direct arterial blood pressure *(ART)* and indirect noninvasive blood pressure *(NIBP)* measurements. (A) In the supine patient, pressures measured from the right *(R)* or left *(L)* arms by either technique will be the same. (B) In the right lateral decubitus position, ART pressures recorded directly from the right and left radial arteries will remain unchanged so long as the respective pressure transducers remain at heart level. However, NIBP will be higher in the dependent right arm and lower in the nondependent left arm. Differences in NIBP are determined by the positions of the arms above and below the level of the heart and are equal to the hydrostatic pressure differences between the level of the heart and the respective arm. A 20-cm difference in height produces a 15-mm Hg difference in pressure. (From Mark JB. *Atlas of Cardiovascular Monitoring.* New York; Churchill Livingstone; 1998.)

In specific circumstances, though, clinicians may choose to place the transducer at a level different from the standard. For example, during a sitting neurosurgical procedure, it may be more informative to place it at the level of the patient's ear to approximate the level of the Circle of Willis. In such cases, the blood pressure at the level of the brain is being measured and displayed rather than that of the aortic root, which will be significantly higher. Fixing the transducer to a pole rather than the bed risks introducing error when the bed height or position is changed.

For proper interpretation of blood pressure measurements from a patient in the lateral decubitus position, differentiating zeroing and leveling pressure transducers and appreciating the differences between noninvasive and invasive blood pressure measurement is an informative exercise. In this position, while the aortic root remains stationary, one arm is necessarily higher than the other. However, as long as the pressure transducer remains *fixed at the level of the heart,* the measured pressure remains completely unaffected by the position of the arms, or location of the arterial catheter. Conversely, non-invasive cuff blood pressure measurements will differ in the two arms, being higher in the dependent (down) arm and lower in the non-dependent (up) arm (Fig. 36.26). This relationship must be taken into account when using the cuff to calibrate an invasively measured pressure.

Normal Arterial Pressure Waveforms

The systemic arterial pressure waveform results from ejection of blood from the left ventricle during systole followed by peripheral runoff during diastole. The systolic waveform immediately follows the ECG R wave and consists of a steep pressure upstroke, peak, and ensuing decline. The downslope of the arterial pressure waveform is interrupted by the dicrotic notch, continues its decline during diastole after the ECG T wave, and reaches its nadir at end-diastole

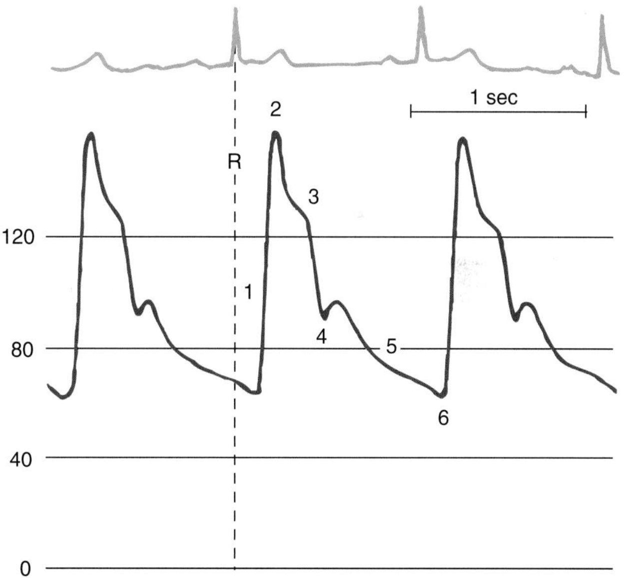

Fig. 36.27 Normal arterial blood pressure waveform and its relation to the electrocardiographic R wave. *(1)* Systolic upstroke, *(2)* systolic peak pressure, *(3)* systolic decline, *(4)* dicrotic notch, *(5)* diastolic runoff, and *(6)* end-diastolic pressure. (From Mark JB. *Atlas of Cardiovascular Monitoring.* New York: Churchill Livingstone; 1998.)

(Fig. 36.27). The dicrotic notch of a central aortic pressure waveform is sharply defined and thought to result from aortic valve closure.[117] In contrast, more peripheral arterial waveforms generally display a slightly delayed and mildly blunted dicrotic notch that is more dependent on properties of the arterial wall. Note that the systolic upstroke starts 120 to 180 ms after beginning of the R wave, reflecting the time required for LV depolarization, isovolumic contraction, opening of the aortic valve, LV ejection, and propagation of the pressure wave through the aorta to the pressure transducer (see Fig. 36.27).

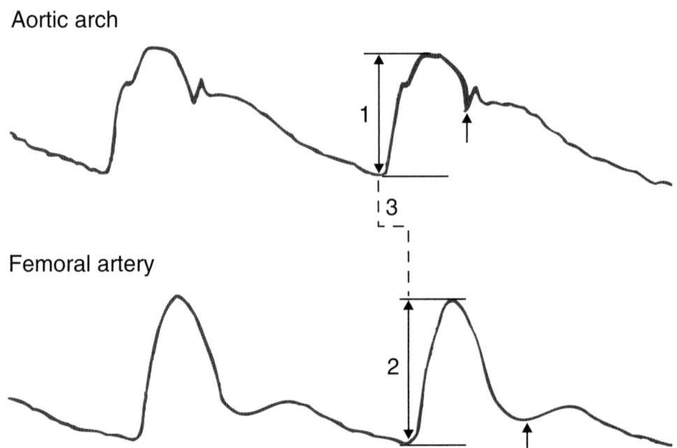

Fig. 36.28 Distal pulse wave amplification of the arterial pressure waveform. Compared with pressure in the aortic arch, the more peripherally recorded femoral artery pressure waveform demonstrates a wider pulse pressure (compare *1* and *2*), a delayed start to the systolic upstroke *(3)*, a delayed, slurred dicrotic notch (compare *arrows*), and a more prominent diastolic wave. (From Mark JB. *Atlas of Cardiovascular Monitoring*. New York: Churchill Livingstone; 1998.)

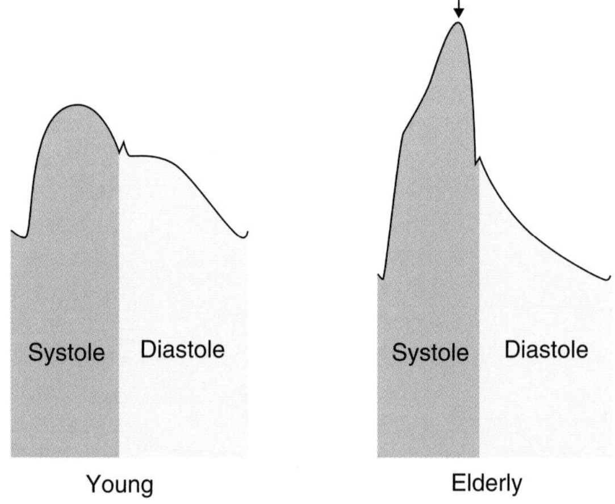

Fig. 36.29 Impact of pressure wave reflection on arterial pressure waveforms. In older individuals with reduced arterial compliance, early return of peripherally reflected waves increases pulse pressure, produces a late systolic pressure peak *(arrow)*, attenuates the diastolic pressure wave, and at times, distorts the smooth upstroke with an early systolic hump.

The bedside monitor displays values for the systolic peak and end-diastolic nadir pressures. In simplest terms, MAP reflects the area beneath the arterial pressure curve divided by the beat period, averaged over multiple cardiac cycles, but is dependent on device-specific algorithms. MAP is sometimes estimated as diastolic pressure plus one third of the pulse pressure but this shortcut is only valid at slower heart rates, because the duration of diastole decreases as the heart rate increases.[118]

The morphology of the arterial waveform and the precise values of systolic and diastolic blood pressure vary throughout the arterial system even under normal conditions in healthy individuals in a variety of ways. Distal pulse amplification is one such example. Pressure waveforms recorded simultaneously from different sites have different morphologies due to the physical characteristics of the vascular tree, namely, impedance and harmonic resonance (Fig. 36.28).[62,119] As the pressure wave travels from the central aorta to the periphery, the arterial upstroke becomes steeper, the systolic peak rises, the dicrotic notch appears later, the diastolic wave becomes more prominent, and end-diastolic pressure falls. As a result, peripheral arterial waveforms have higher systolic, lower diastolic, and wider pulse pressures compared with central aortic waveforms. Interestingly, the displayed MAP is only slight increased.

Reflection of pressure waves within the arterial tree significantly affects the arterial pressure waveform as it travels peripherally.[119] As blood flows from the aorta to the radial artery, MAP decreases only slightly because there is little resistance to flow in the major conducting arteries. At the arteriolar level, though, resistance to flow shrinks pressure pulsations in smaller downstream vessels but augments upstream arterial pressure pulses due to reflected pressure waves.[120] It is the summation of these antegrade and reflected waves that determines the shape of the displayed waveform. For example, reduced arterial compliance causes extremely rapid return of reflected pressure waves, resulting in arterial pressure waveforms with increased pulse pressure, a late systolic pressure peak, attenuated diastolic pressure waves, and at times, an early systolic hump distorting the smooth upstroke (Fig. 36.29).

Arterial Blood Pressure Gradients

Numerous pathophysiologic conditions cause exaggerated arterial pressure gradients between monitoring sites, be they real, iatrogenic, or artifactual. Frank and coworkers found that 21% of patients undergoing peripheral vascular surgery had a blood pressure difference between the two arms that exceeded 20 mm Hg.[121] Atherosclerosis, arterial dissection, stenosis, or embolism may exclude certain locations as reliable sites for invasive monitoring. In addition, certain patient positions, surgical retraction, or clamp placement may compromise perfusion in regional or local areas, precluding specific sites from use for invasive monitoring.[122,123]

Pathologic changes in peripheral vascular resistance may also produce generalized arterial pressure gradients that can affect the choice of site for arterial pressure monitoring. In patients receiving vasopressor infusions for septic shock, the femoral arterial pressure may exceed the radial pressure by greater than 50 mm Hg.[124] Less severe gradients have been noted with general anesthesia, neuraxial blocks, and changes in patient temperature.[62] During hypothermia, vasoconstriction causes systolic pressure in the radial artery to exceed that in the femoral artery, whereas during rewarming, vasodilation reverses the gradient.[125]

Characteristic gradients between central and peripheral sites have also been described during cardiopulmonary bypass (Fig. 36.30). The mean radial artery pressure falls on initiation of bypass and remains lower than mean femoral artery pressure throughout the bypass period and into the initial postbypass period, often by more than 20 mm Hg.[126,127] In most patients, this gradient resolves within the first hour, but occasionally remains well into the postoperative period.

Abnormal Arterial Pressure Waveforms

The morphologic features of individual arterial pressure waveforms can provide important diagnostic information (Table 36.1) (Fig. 36.31A–D). Aortic stenosis produces a

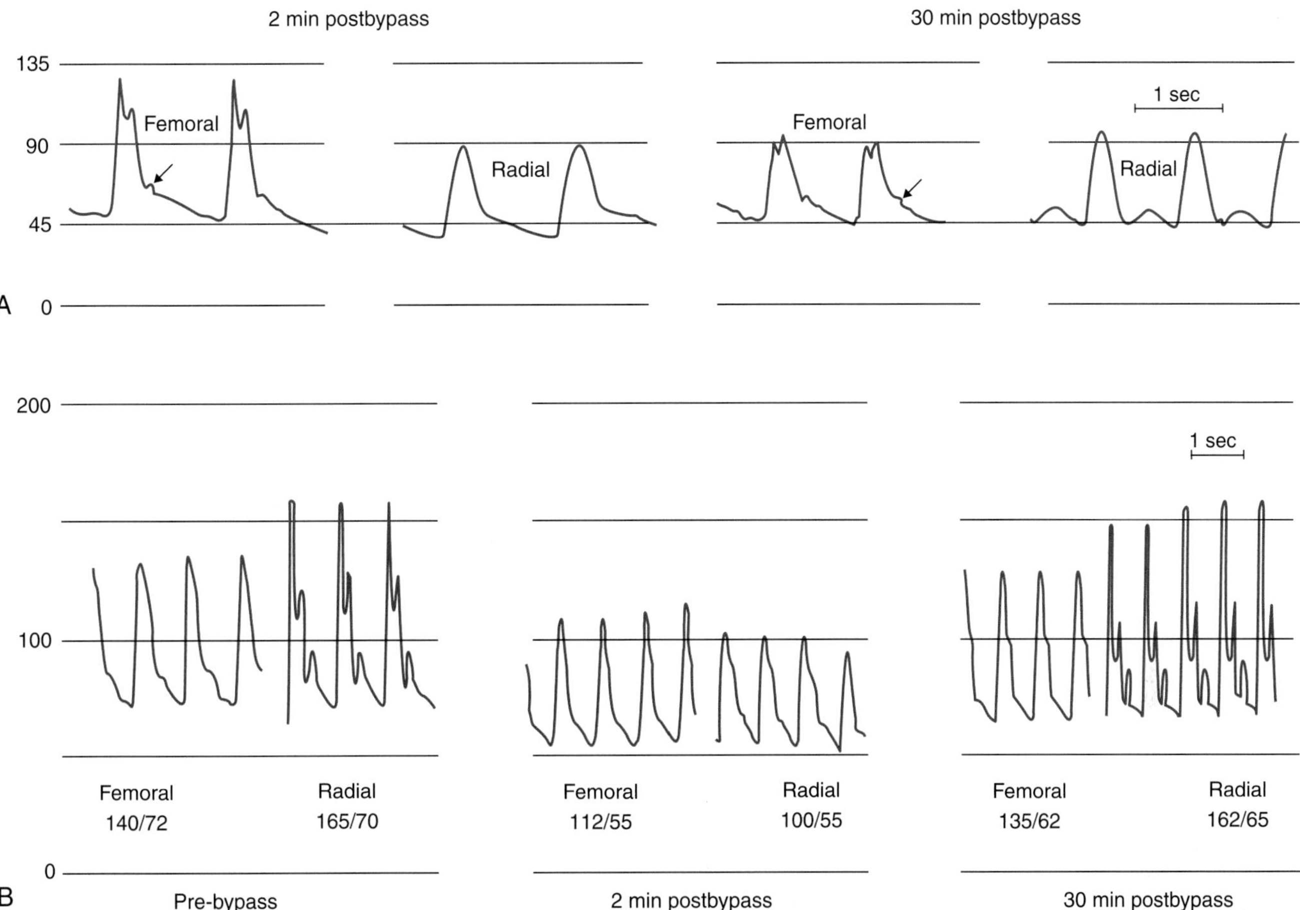

Fig. 36.30 Arterial pressure gradients following cardiopulmonary bypass. (A) Femoral and radial artery pressure traces recorded 2 minutes after bypass (2 min postbypass), when radial artery pressure underestimates the more centrally measured femoral artery pressure and 30 minutes later (30 min postbypass), when radial and femoral arterial pressures have equalized and radial pressure has resumed a more typical morphology. Note that dicrotic notch *(arrows)* is visible in the femoral pressure trace immediately after bypass, but is delayed in the radial pressure trace. (B) Femoral and radial artery pressure traces recorded before cardiopulmonary bypass (pre-bypass), 2 minutes following bypass (2 min postbypass), and 30 minutes following bypass (30 min postbypass). Note changing relationship between femoral and radial artery pressure measurements at these different times.

TABLE 36.1 Arterial Blood Pressure Waveform Abnormalities

Condition	Characteristics
Aortic stenosis	Pulsus parvus (narrow pulse pressure) Pulsus tardus (delayed upstroke)
Aortic regurgitation	Bisferiens pulse (double peak) Wide pulse pressure
Hypertrophic cardiomyopathy	Spike and dome (mid-systolic obstruction)
Systolic left ventricular failure	Pulsus alternans (alternating pulse pressure amplitude)
Cardiac tamponade	Pulsus paradoxus (exaggerated decrease in systolic blood pressure during spontaneous inspiration)

fixed obstruction to ejection resulting in reduced stroke volume and a slowed rate of ejection. As a result, the waveform is small in amplitude *(pulsus parvus)*, has a slowly rising systolic upstroke *(pulsus tardus)*, and a delayed peak in systole (see Fig. 36.31B). A distinct shoulder, termed the anacrotic notch, often distorts the pressure upstroke and the dicrotic notch may not be discernible. These features may make the arterial pressure waveform appear overdamped.

In aortic regurgitation, the arterial pressure wave displays a sharp rise, wide pulse pressure, and low diastolic pressure owing to the diastolic runoff of blood both antegrade into the aortic root and retrograde into the left ventricle. The arterial pressure pulse may have two systolic peaks *(bisferiens pulse)*, with the first peak resulting from antegrade ejection and the second from a wave reflected from the periphery (see Fig. 36.31C). In hypertrophic cardiomyopathy, the waveform assumes a peculiar bifid shape termed a "spike-and-dome" configuration. After an initial sharp blood pressure increase resulting from rapid, early systolic ejection, arterial pressure abruptly falls as mid-systolic LV outflow obstruction interrupts stroke volume ejection. This is finally followed by a second, late-systolic increase associated with arrival of reflected waves from the periphery (see Fig. 36.31D).

Changes in arterial waveform patterns over time are also valuable. *Pulsus alternans* is a pattern of alternating larger and smaller pressure waves that appear to vary with the respiratory cycle and is generally associated with severe LV systolic dysfunction or aortic stenosis (Fig. 36.32A).

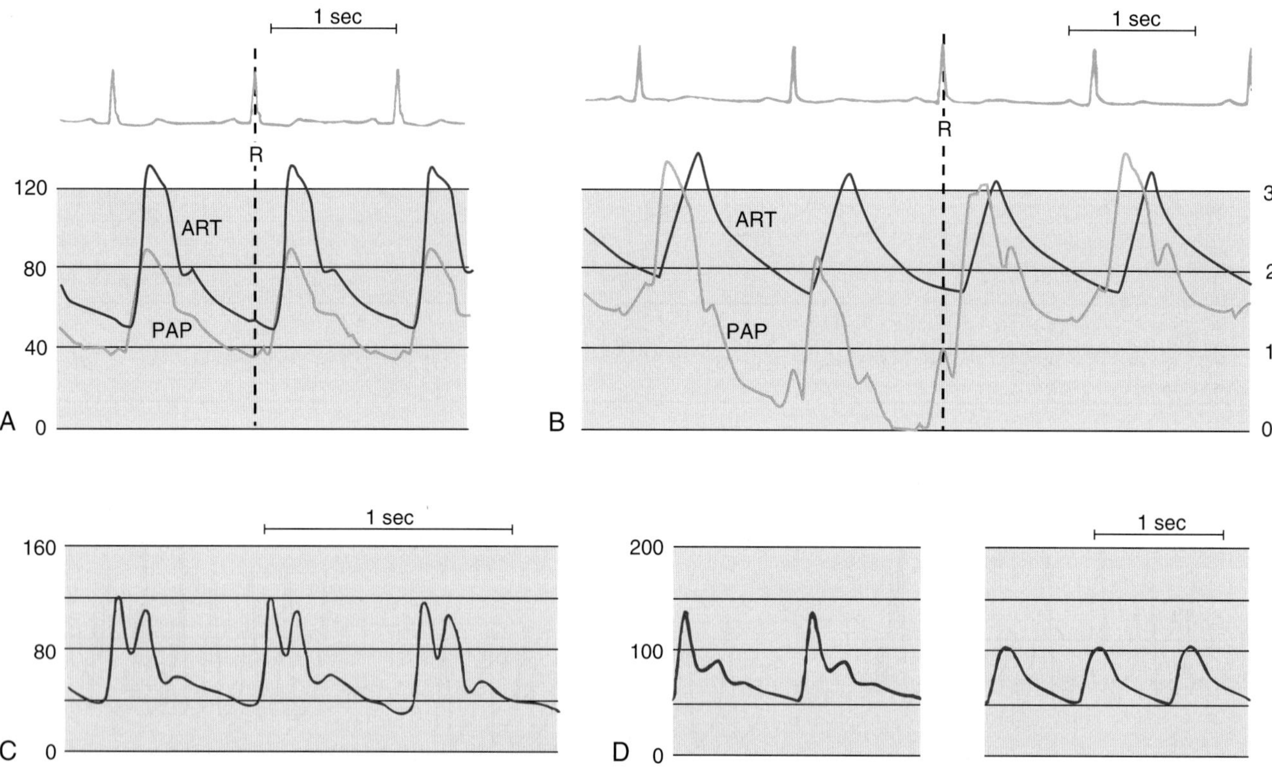

Fig. 36.31 Influence of pathologic conditions on arterial pressure *(ART)* waveform morphology. (A) Normal ART and pulmonary artery pressure *(PAP)* waveform morphologies demonstrating the similar timing of these waveforms relative to the electrocardiographic R wave. (B) In aortic stenosis, the ART waveform is distorted with a slurred upstroke and delayed systolic peak. These changes are particularly striking in comparison with the normal PAP waveform. Note the beat-to-beat respiratory variation in the PAP waveform. For A and B, the ART scale is on the left and the PAP scale is on the right. (C) Aortic regurgitation produces a bisferiens pulse and a wide pulse pressure. (D) Arterial pressure waveform in hypertrophic cardiomyopathy shows a peculiar spike-and-dome configuration. The waveform assumes a more normal morphology following surgical correction of this condition. (From Mark JB. *Atlas of Cardiovascular Monitoring*. New York: Churchill Livingstone; 1998.)

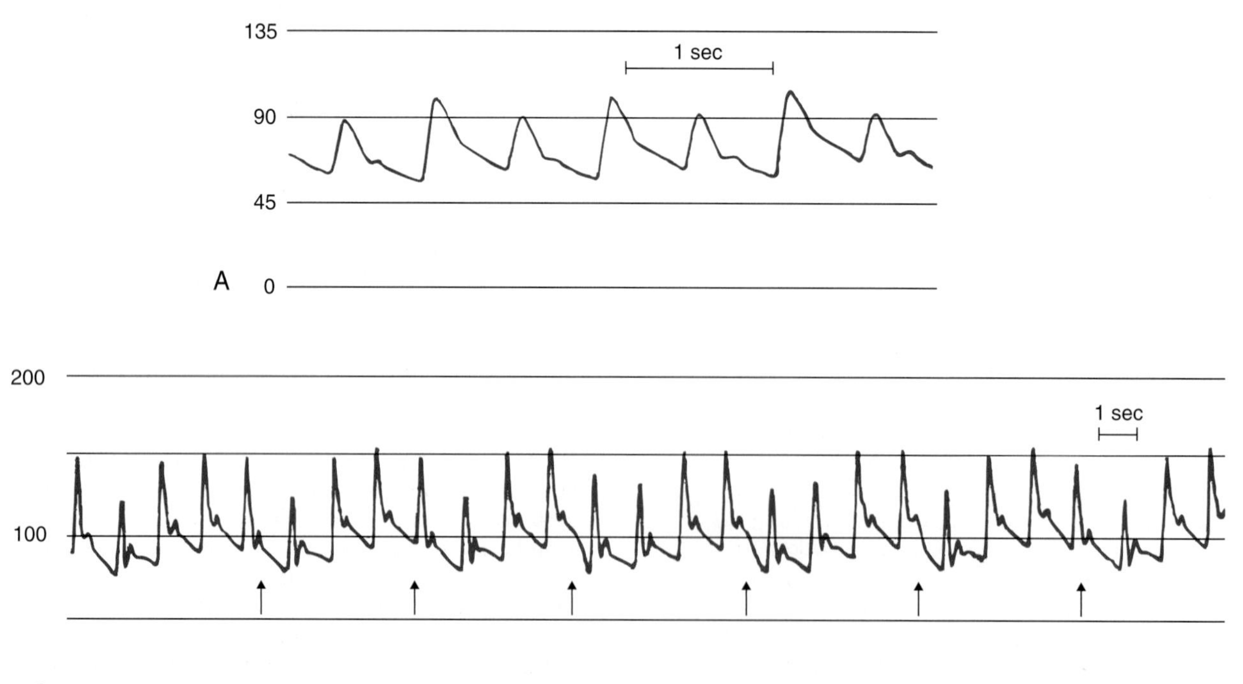

Fig. 36.32 Beat-to-beat variability in arterial pressure waveform morphologies. (A) Pulsus alternans. (B) Pulsus paradoxus. The marked decline in both systolic blood pressure and pulse pressure during spontaneous inspiration *(arrows)* is characteristic of cardiac tamponade. (From Mark JB. *Atlas of Cardiovascular Monitoring*. New York: Churchill Livingstone; 1998.)

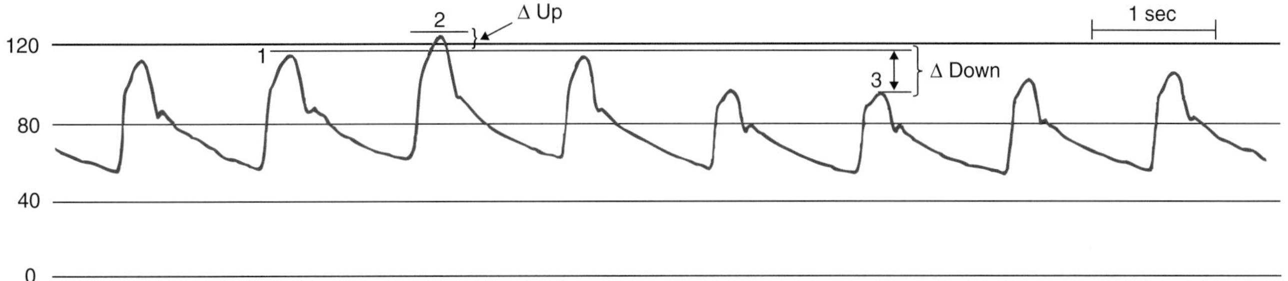

Fig. 36.33 Systolic pressure variation. Compared with systolic blood pressure recorded at end expiration *(1)* a small increase occurs during positive-pressure inspiration (*2*, Δ Up) followed by a decrease (*3*, Δ Down). Normally, systolic pressure variation does not exceed 10 mm Hg. In this instance, the large Δ Down indicates hypovolemia even though systolic arterial pressure and heart rate are relatively normal. (From Mark JB. *Atlas of Cardiovascular Monitoring*. New York: Churchill Livingstone; 1998.)

Pulsus paradoxus is an exaggerated variation in arterial pressure (>10-12 mm Hg) during quiet breathing (see Fig. 36.32B).[128,129] *Pulsus paradoxus* is not truly paradoxical, but rather an exaggeration of a normal variation in blood pressure that accompanies spontaneous ventilation. *Pulsus paradoxus* is a common and important sign in cardiac tamponade but may also be seen with pericardial constriction, severe airway obstruction, bronchospasm, dyspnea, or any condition that involves large swings in intrathoracic pressure. Importantly, though, in cases of cardiac tamponade, the *pulse pressure* and *left ventricular stroke volume* decrease during inspiration, in contrast to the pattern observed associated with large variations in intrathoracic pressure in which *pulse pressure* remains constant.[130]

Arterial Pressure Monitoring and Waveform Analysis for Prediction of Volume Responsiveness

The starting point for volume resuscitation begins with optimizing cardiac preload, or more precisely, identifying the presence of residual preload reserve. The limitations and potential confounders of static indicators of preload such as central venous pressure (CVP) are well documented.[131] A wide array of dynamic markers of preload reserve and volume responsiveness have been described and evaluated for their ability to discriminate patients for whom volume expansion would be beneficial from those for whom it would not. These are largely based on cyclic variations in arterial blood pressure resulting from respiratory-induced changes in intrathoracic pressure.

During the inspiratory phase of a positive pressure breath, the increase in intrathoracic pressure simultaneously decreases LV afterload while increasing total lung volume which displaces blood from the pulmonary venous reservoir forward into the left side of the heart and increases LV preload. The increase in LV preload and decrease in afterload produce an increase in LV stroke volume, an increase in cardiac output, and in the absence of changes in system resistance, an increase in systemic arterial pressure. In most patients the preload effects predominate, but in patients with severe LV systolic failure, the reduction in afterload facilitates ventricular ejection. At the same time, rising intrathoracic pressure impairs systemic venous return and RV preload, possibly increasing RV afterload by slightly increasing pulmonary vascular resistance. These effects combine to reduce RV ejection during the early phase of inspiration. During the expiratory phase, however, the situation is reversed. The smaller stroke volume ejected from the RV during inspiration traverses the pulmonary vascular bed and enters the left heart, resulting in reduced LV filling, reduced LV stroke volume, and a fall in systemic arterial blood pressure. This cycle of increasing and decreasing stroke volume and systemic arterial blood pressure in response to inspiration and expiration is known as the *systolic pressure variation* (SPV).

SPV is often subdivided into inspiratory and expiratory components by measuring the increase (Δ Up) and decrease (Δ Down) in systolic pressure relative to the end-expiratory, apneic baseline pressure (Fig. 36.33). In a mechanically ventilated patient, normal SPV is 7 to 10 mm Hg, with Δ Up being 2 to 4 mm Hg and Δ Down being 5 to 6 mm Hg. Values greater than this are felt to indicate hypovolemia.[66,67] Both in experimental animals and critically ill patients, hypovolemia causes a dramatic increase in SPV, particularly the Δ Down component. Patients who manifest increased SPV during positive pressure mechanical ventilation may be described clinically as having residual preload reserve or being "volume responsive." While not synonymous with hypovolemia, preload reserve describes a physiologic state in which volume expansion or fluid challenge shifts the patient upward on the Frank-Starling curve resulting in increased stroke volume and increased cardiac output as long as systemic vascular resistance remains unchanged. Indeed, in a heterogeneous group of intensive care patients, Marik demonstrated that a large SPV (>15 mm Hg) was highly predictive of a low pulmonary artery wedge pressure (PAWP; <10 mm Hg), a surrogate for LV preload reserve.[132]

Pulse pressure variation (PPV), another dynamic indicator of preload reserve, is now available as part of standard monitoring software packages whenever an invasive arterial catheter is in use. In general, normal PPV is less than 13% to 17% (Fig. 36.34).[133-137] More sophisticated methods of pulse contour analysis allow real-time measurement of *stroke volume variation* (SVV), as well as calculation of a *stroke volume variation index*. When these measures exceed 10% to 13%, the patient is likely to have a positive response to volume expansion.[136,138] Although all of these dynamic measures are thought to indicate preload reserve, they are not interchangeable. PPV has been shown to diverge from SVV in the setting of vasopressor use or when the autonomic nervous system intervenes to preserve perfusion pressure in the face of falling stroke volume. In such cases, PPV will remain low while SVV increases.[139,140]

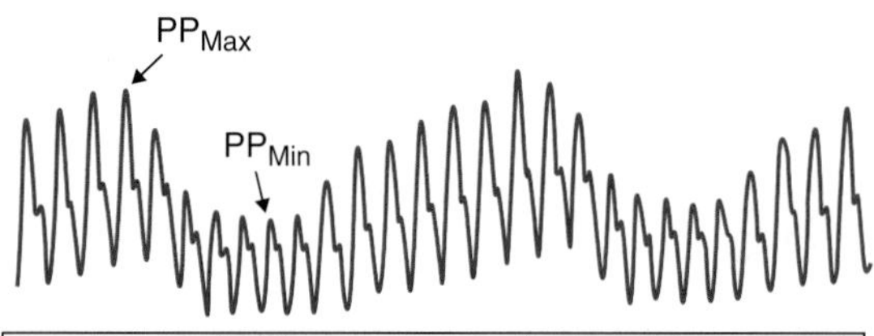

$PP_{Max} = 150–70 = 80$

$PP_{Min} = 120–60 = 60$

$PPV = (PP_{Max} – PP_{Min})/([PP_{Max} + PP_{Min}]/2)$

$PPV = 80–60/([80+60]/2) = 29\%$

Fig. 36.34 Pulse pressure variation. Pulse pressure variation *(PPV)* is calculated as the difference between maximal *(PP_{Max})* and minimal *(PP_{Min})* pulse pressure values during a single mechanical respiratory cycle, divided by the average of these two values. (Note that the arterial blood pressure trace is drawn for illustrative purposes and not to scale.)

Devices based on respiratory cycle-induced variation in the pulse plethysmogram have been developed as a similar but less invasive alternative for assessing preload reserve or volume responsiveness. Measures such as *photoplethysmography variation* (ΔPOP) or the *plethysmography variability index* appear to be useful when clinical and environmental conditions are optimal, but the transcutaneous oximetry signal is even more subject to confounding influences than the arterial blood pressure waveform.[135,141,142] Tidal volume, core and peripheral temperature, ambient light, and cardiac dysrhythmias pose significant impediments to valid and reproducible data collection and interpretation. There is no consensus regarding meaningful threshold values, and validity seems especially poor in children, in settings where patients are ventilated and sedated but not paralyzed, or in the setting of an open abdomen.[142] Furthermore, there are sophisticated auto-gaining features incorporated in most commercially available monitoring systems to optimize signal display. As such, the degree of variation visible to the naked eye may not correlate with true signal variation, resulting in erroneous clinical decisions and incorrect therapy.

Evidence is accumulating that dynamic measures are significantly superior to static indices of intravascular volume, especially in critically ill patients. Both PVV and SVV have been shown to be accurate following cardiac surgery in patients with normal and reduced ventricular function, while PPV was validated in assessing fluid responsiveness in patients with septic shock.[143,144] Intraoperative use has also been examined with similar results.[145,146] Indeed, the ability of clinicians to "eyeball" respiratory variation in the arterial blood pressure waveform as displayed on the monitor seems reasonably accurate. Subjective estimates of such pressure variation were incorrect only 4.4% of the time, a rate that would have resulted in only 1% of treatments being erroneous.[137]

There is disagreement on precise threshold values that differentiate fluid responders from non-responders, and the variety of techniques, devices, and approaches have not been standardized.[135] In a recent systematic review, mean discriminatory thresholds defining volume responsiveness for PVV and SVV were found to be 12.5% ± 1.6% and 11.6% ± 1.9%, respectively, with acceptable sensitivities and specificities (89%, 88% and 82%, 86%, respectively).[147] However, simply differentiating patients who will respond from those who will not fails to take into account the nature of the clinical intervention at issue. Volume expansion does not result in a dichotomous outcome, and the asymmetric nature of the Frank-Starling curve dictates that the cost-benefit ratio of acting in one direction will be different from acting in the other. For any given change in preload, the change in stroke volume will be different depending on the direction of the preload change, with that differential being dependent on how close to the peak of the curve the patient begins. Consequently, the concept of the "gray zone" has been proposed that defines a range of values between which evidence-based decision making is not possible.[148] For PPV, this zone has been described as 9% to 13% such that those above 13% should receive volume expansion while those below 9% should not. Between those two values, the measurement is not able to provide meaningful guidance and the decision should be based on other criteria.[136,149]

Continuous display of PPV is now routine on bedside monitors, a feature that has facilitated rapid adoption of dynamic preload reserve assessment.[150,151] As such, while its use is clinically relevant, it is even more important to understand the shortcomings of all respiratory-induced dynamic indicators and the clinical conditions under which they were originally studied and validated. While PPV appears to be valid in the setting of liver failure, it is significantly affected by increased abdominal pressure; patient position, including steep Trendelenburg, prone, or lateral positions; and use of vasopressors.[136,140,152-154] Variability in diastolic filling causing variable stroke volumes makes irregular heart rhythms highly problematic in the use of all dynamic preload reserve indicators.[155,156] In addition, there is evidence that patients with pulmonary hypertension or reduced RV ejection fraction may not have reliable responses to changes in intrathoracic pressure, increasing the risk of over-hydration and worsening right heart failure.[157] Dynamic indices are of marginal value in the setting of either minimally invasive or open thoracic surgery, and their use in children is considered unreliable due to the increased compliance of the myocardium and the chest wall in younger patients.[158,159] It has even been suggested that tachypnea, (especially in the setting of respiratory failure), or significant bradycardia may disrupt the relationship between respiratory-cycle–induced changes in intrathoracic pressure and cardiac chamber volumes, thus invalidating the theoretical basis for blood pressure variation analysis.[136]

Most importantly, though, is the profound effect of protective lung ventilation on the predictive power of respiratory-induced SPV, PPV, or SVV to identify a patient with residual preload reserve.[160-162] Mechanical ventilation with tidal volume of 8 to 10 mL/kg, positive end-expiratory pressure ≥ 5 mm Hg, regular cardiac rhythm, normal intra-abdominal pressure, and a closed chest are necessary to duplicate the experimental conditions under which most of these indices have been investigated, and these conditions are largely inconsistent with ventilatory parameters chosen for lung protective ventilation. Clinical trials have found waveform analysis to be of limited utility in this setting.[160-162] However, measuring PPV or SVV during or immediately following a recruitment maneuver increased its sensitivity and specificity in predicting fluid responsiveness, although a broader gray zone of up to 26% should be considered.[163,164]

As noted above, respiratory-cycle–induced arterial pressure variations are dependent on changes in LV preload and, to a lesser degree, afterload. Indeed, decreased arterial compliance and the resultant increased pulse pressure that accompanies both normal and pathologic vascular aging results in an exaggerated PPV response to any change in stroke volume. As such, it is possible that PPV thresholds should be higher in such patients than in those with greater elastance in their vascular trees.[165,166]

Central Venous Pressure Monitoring

Cannulation of a central vein and direct measurement of CVP are frequently performed in hemodynamically unstable patients and those undergoing major operations. A central venous catheter may be inserted to provide secure vascular access for administration of vasoactive drugs or fluids, CVP monitoring, transvenous cardiac pacing, temporary hemodialysis, pulmonary artery catheterization (PAC) for more comprehensive cardiac monitoring, or aspiration of entrained air in patients at risk for venous air emboli. A central venous catheter may also be inserted when no peripheral access can be obtained, or when repeated venous blood sampling is required (Box 36.5).

BOX 36.5 Indications for Central Venous Cannulation

- Central venous pressure monitoring
- Pulmonary artery catheterization and monitoring
- Transvenous cardiac pacing
- Temporary hemodialysis
- Drug administration
  - Concentrated vasoactive drugs
  - Hyperalimentation
  - Chemotherapy
  - Agents irritating to peripheral veins
  - Prolonged antibiotic therapy (e.g., endocarditis)
- Rapid infusion of fluids (via large cannulas)
  - Trauma
  - Major surgery
- Aspiration of air emboli
- Inadequate peripheral intravenous access
- Sampling site for repeated blood testing

CENTRAL VENOUS CANNULATION

When required in the intraoperative period, the decision to perform central venous cannulation before or after induction of anesthesia is guided most often by individual patient and physician preferences or institutional practice.

CHOOSING THE CATHETER, SITE, AND METHOD FOR CENTRAL VENOUS CANNULATION

Central venous catheters come in a variety of lengths, gauges, compositions, and lumen numbers.[167,168] This makes it critical for the physician to choose the best catheter for any given application. Multiport catheters, which allow monitoring of CVP and infusion of drugs and fluids simultaneously, are the most common,[169] but introducer sheaths with one or two integrated ports for multiple drug infusions are an alternative. Introducer sheaths allow insertion of a single-lumen catheter through the hemostasis valve for continuous CVP monitoring and rapid placement of a pacing wire or PAC for more intensive monitoring should the need arise.

Selecting the best site for safe and effective central venous cannulation ultimately requires consideration of the indication for catheterization (pressure monitoring versus drug or fluid administration), the patient's underlying medical condition, the clinical setting, and the skill and experience of the physician performing the procedure. In patients with severe bleeding diatheses, it is best to choose a puncture site where bleeding from the vein or adjacent artery is easily detected and controlled with local compression. In such a patient, an internal or external jugular approach would be preferable to a subclavian site. Likewise, patients with severe emphysema or others who would be severely compromised by a pneumothorax would be better candidates for internal jugular than subclavian cannulation, owing to the higher risk with the latter approach. If transvenous cardiac pacing is required in an emergency situation, catheterization of the right internal jugular vein is recommended, as it provides the most direct route to the right ventricle. Trauma patients, with their necks immobilized in a hard cervical collar, are best resuscitated using a femoral or subclavian approach; the latter may be placed even more safely if the risk of pneumothorax is obviated by prior placement of a thoracostomy tube. The physician must recognize that the length of catheter inserted to position the catheter tip properly in the superior vena cava will vary according to puncture site, being slightly (3-5 cm) greater when the left internal or external jugular veins are chosen, compared with the right internal jugular vein.[170] Finally, a physician's personal experience undoubtedly plays a significant role in determining the safest site for central venous cannulation, particularly when the procedure is performed under urgent or emergent circumstances.

A central vein may be cannulated using either a landmark technique or ultrasound guidance. Ultrasound technology is now widely available and is strongly recommended for central line placement.[171-173] The reader is referred to other sources for detailed descriptions and tutorials on the various insertion techniques for different access sites.[169,174-176] Regardless of the insertion technique used or the cannulation site chosen, certain general principles should be emphasized. Ideally, a protocol or checklist describing the basic procedural steps for central line insertion should be in place at every institution, and all staff members should feel empowered to speak up when they witness a protocol violation. Standardized equipment, routine use of an assistant, hand washing, and maximal barrier precautions all contribute to the sterility of the procedure.[172] The use of real-time ultrasound guidance for vessel localization and venipuncture should be routine or at least strongly considered, especially when the internal jugular vein site is selected. Waveform manometry or pressure measurement

BOX 36.6 Complications of Central Venous Pressure Monitoring

- Mechanical
  - Vascular injury
    - Arterial
    - Venous
    - Cardiac tamponade
  - Respiratory compromise
    - Airway compression from hematoma
    - Pneumothorax
  - Nerve injury
  - Arrhythmias
- Thromboembolic
  - Venous thrombosis
  - Pulmonary embolism
  - Arterial thrombosis and embolism
  - Catheter or guidewire embolism
- Infectious
  - Insertion site infection
  - Catheter infection
  - Bloodstream infection
  - Endocarditis
- Misinterpretation of data
- Misuse of equipment

should be used to confirm venous placement of the catheter before use. Finally, the position of the catheter tip should be verified as soon as clinically appropriate to avoid delayed complications.

COMPLICATIONS OF CENTRAL VENOUS PRESSURE MONITORING

Complications of central venous cannulation are becoming increasingly recognized as major sources of morbidity with more than 15% of patients experiencing some sort of related adverse event.[177,178] Although serious immediate complications are infrequent when these procedures are performed by well-trained, experienced clinicians, use of CVP catheters continues to result in significant morbidity and mortality. Complications are often divided into mechanical, thromboembolic, and infectious etiologies (Box 36.6).

Mechanical Complications of Central Venous Catheterization

The incidence of complications depends on a number of factors including the catheter insertion site and the patient's medical condition. Large retrospective and observational studies provide the best estimates of incidence and frequency.

Vascular injuries from central venous catheterization have a range of clinical consequences. The most common minor complications are localized hematoma or injury to the venous valves.[179] More serious complications include perforation into the pleural space or mediastinum, resulting in hydrothorax, hemothorax, hydromediastinum, hemomediastinum, and or chylothorax.[180-186]

In general, *unintended arterial puncture* is the most common acute mechanical complication, ranging from 1.9 to 15%.[187] Many of these injuries result in localized hematoma formation, but in rare occasions even small-gauge-needle punctures may lead to serious complications such as arterial thromboembolism.[188] Delayed vascular complications following central venous catheterization are uncommon but should be considered as consequences of this procedure. A number of these have been described in the literature, including aorto-atrial fistula, venobronchial fistula, carotid artery–internal jugular vein fistula, and pseudoaneurysm formation.[189-192]

The most important life-threatening vascular complication of central venous catheterization is **cardiac tamponade** resulting from perforation of the intrapericardial superior vena cava, right atrium, or right ventricle, and resulting hemopericardium or unintentional pericardial instillation of intravenous fluid.[193] Most reports document the avoidable nature of this catastrophic event and highlight that patients are predisposed to this complication when central venous catheter tips are malpositioned within the heart chambers or abutting the wall of the superior vena cava at a steep angle. This latter position can be recognized radiographically as a gentle curvature of the catheter tip within the superior vena cava.[194] These observations emphasize that objective confirmation of proper catheter tip location is mandatory, regardless of whether the catheter is inserted from a central or peripheral site.

Pneumothorax is often cited as the most common complication of subclavian vein cannulation, although it appears that unintended arterial puncture is actually more frequent.[99,195] Mansfield et al. reported 821 patients who underwent attempted subclavian venous cannulation, with a 1.5% incidence of pneumothorax and a 3.7% incidence of arterial puncture when using the landmark technique.[195] Pneumothorax is even less frequent with the internal jugular approach. Shah et al. reported an incidence of pneumothorax of 0.5% in their series of nearly 6000 internal jugular catheterizations.[187] This is most likely a high estimate, as these patients had undergone sternotomy for cardiac surgery, a procedure that may have been responsible for the pneumothorax in many cases.

Nerve injury is another potential complication of central venous cannulation. Damage may occur to the brachial plexus, stellate ganglion, phrenic nerve, or vocal cords.[196-198] In addition, chronic pain syndromes have been attributed to this procedure.[199]

Thromboembolic Complications of Central Venous Catheterization

Catheter-related thrombosis varies according to the site of central venous catheterization, occurring in as many as 21.5% of patients with femoral venous catheters and 1.9% of those with subclavian venous catheters.[200] Catheters that are positioned low in the right atrium may be more prone to thrombus formation, possibly due to mechanical irritation of the right atrial endocardium by the catheter.[201] Thrombi that form at the catheter tip or adhere to the endocardium have the potential to become a nidus for infection, cause superior vena cava syndrome, or embolize into the pulmonary circulation.[202-204] Occasionally, surgical removal is required.[205]

In addition to thromboembolism, other reported embolic complications of central venous catheterization include embolism of portions of the catheter or guidewire, and air embolism.[206,207] Almost invariably, these are the result of misuse of equipment, highlighting the need for proper education and training of nurses and physicians responsible for the use of these devices.

Infectious Complications of Central Venous Catheterization

By far, the most common major late complication of central venous cannulation is *infection*. Major progress has been made in the control of central line-associated blood stream infections (CLABSI), likely due to a focus on evidence-based best practices for catheter insertion and maintenance.[208] In fact, CLABSI rates have declined by about 50% between 2008 and 2016.[209] The majority of CLABSIs are occurring in inpatient wards and outpatients receiving hemodialysis, but approximately one third of these cases still occur in the ICU, a cohort that likely includes most of the catheters placed intraoperatively.[209-211]

As previously noted, the starting point for prevention of infection is meticulous attention to aseptic technique.[212] Multilumen catheters may carry a higher risk of infection than single-lumen catheters although the added clinical functionality of such catheters often mandates their use.[178,213] Catheters are made from materials such as silicone, polyvinyl chloride, Teflon, and polyurethane. Furthermore, catheters of the same material may be manufactured differently, which influences their surfaces and the frequency of bacterial adherence to the surface.[214] Heparin-bonded central venous catheters have been shown to reduce the incidence of catheter-related thrombosis and infection in children and adults.[215,216] The incorporation of antimicrobial treatments such as silver (this metal has broad antimicrobial activity and is nontoxic), combinations of the antiseptics chlorhexidine and silver sulfadiazine, or the antibiotics minocycline and rifampin onto the catheter surfaces have been shown to reduce rates of catheter colonization and in some cases blood stream infection.[216-218] The added expense has prevented more widespread adoption of these catheters, although an analysis has suggested their cost-effectiveness in settings in which the rate of catheter-related infections remains high (more than 3.3 per 1000 catheter days).[219]

A chlorhexidine gluconate-impregnated sponge dressing has been shown to reduce catheter colonization in infants and children, but does not reduce the rate of catheter-associated bloodstream infections.[220,221] Current guidelines from the Centers for Disease Control and Prevention do not support routine catheter site changes or scheduled changes over a guidewire and provide other detailed recommendations for catheter management to reduce the risk of infectious complications.[213,222]

Overall, there does not appear to be an ideal site for central venous cannulation with respect to prevention of complications given that, taken together, the risk of mechanical, thrombotic, and infectious complications is similar among the three insertion sites. This was illustrated by a recent prospective, randomized, multicenter trial in adult ICU patients, where catheterization of the subclavian vein is associated with the lowest risk of infectious complications and deep vein thrombosis, but the highest risk of mechanical complications.[223]

TABLE 36.2 Normal Cardiovascular Pressures

Pressures	Average (mm Hg)	Range (mm Hg)
RIGHT ATRIUM		
a wave	6	2-7
v wave	5	2-7
Mean	3	1-5
RIGHT VENTRICLE		
Peak systolic	25	15-30
End-diastolic	6	1-7
PULMONARY ARTERY		
Peak systolic	25	15-30
End-diastolic	9	4-12
Mean	15	9-19
PULMONARY ARTERY WEDGE		
Mean	9	4-12
LEFT ATRIUM		
a wave	10	4-16
v wave	12	6-21
Mean	8	2-12
LEFT VENTRICLE		
Peak systolic	130	90-140
End-diastolic	8	5-12
Central aorta		
Peak systolic	130	90-140
End-diastolic	70	60-90
Mean	90	70-105

Other Complications of Central Venous Catheterization

Although many complications of CVP monitoring relate to equipment misuse, the frequency of complications caused by data misinterpretation remains unknown. It is extremely likely, however, that clinicians misinterpret CVP measurements and have suboptimal understanding of CVP monitoring, just as has been demonstrated repeatedly for PAC monitoring (see discussion later). Safe and effective use of CVP monitoring requires a detailed understanding of cardiovascular physiology, normal CVP waveforms, and common pathologic abnormalities in these measurements.

PHYSIOLOGIC CONSIDERATIONS FOR CENTRAL VENOUS PRESSURE MONITORING

Cardiac filling pressures are measured directly from a number of sites in the vascular system. CVP monitoring is the least invasive method, followed by pulmonary artery and left atrial pressure monitoring. Proper interpretation of all cardiac filling pressures requires knowledge of normal values for these pressures, as well as pressures in the cardiac chambers, the great vessels, and other measured and derived hemodynamic variables (Table 36.2).

Two prerequisites must be met in order to correctly interpret the information provided by the CVP monitor: (a) the clinician must possess a thorough understanding of all the variables that affect right atrial pressure; and (b) measurements need to be made with extreme attention to detail.

CVP is determined by the interaction of the venous return function of the circulatory system and the cardiac function.[224] An increase in cardiac function with an increase in venous return will result in an increase in cardiac output and *rise* in CVP. An increase in cardiac function *without* an increase in venous return will result in an increase in cardiac output and a *fall* in CVP. In other words, an isolated CVP measurement has very little meaning unless the information is interpreted in the context of some estimation of cardiac function.

Central Venous Pressure and Venous Return

What determines venous return to the heart? The relationship among the multiple variables that affect blood return to the right atrium is complex. In short, venous return is mostly determined by the gradient between the *mean circulatory filling pressure* (MCFP) and CVP.[131] MCFP results from the elastic recoil pressure from distended small veins and venules and is the force that drives blood back to the right atrium.[224] This pressure has been estimated to be between 8 and 10 mm Hg in healthy individuals at rest, but it cannot be measured in the clinical setting.[225] MCFP rises when volume is administered intravenously, but also in many other circumstances such as when venous tone changes in response to venoconstrictors or endogenous catecholamines, or when there is a shift of blood volume from the splanchnic system into the systemic circulation.[131] The CVP, typically 2 to 3 mm Hg in healthy individuals, is the downstream pressure. Two important corollaries emerge: right atrial pressure is key for maintaining cardiac output, and the body will compensate through the mechanisms described above and others to preserve venous return. This explains why a patient may lose 10% to 12% of his circulating blood volume without exhibiting changes in blood pressure or CVP. Secondly, the difference between MCFP and CVP is only 6 to 8 mm Hg, and hence small changes in CVP may have profound hemodynamic consequences.

Central Venous Pressure and Cardiac Function

The exact same amount of blood returning to the heart can result in very different CVP values at different cardiac function states. This may be explained by the classic diastolic pressure-volume relationship. This curve is one limb of a pressure-volume loop that describes the relation between pressure and volume for the left or right ventricle during an entire cardiac cycle. When a ventricle is operating along the flat portion of its diastolic filling curve it will exhibit only a small increase in filling pressure (CVP in the case of the right ventricle) after significant increases in filling volume or preload. The same increase in filling volume causes a significant increase in filling pressure when the ventricle is operating on the steep portion of its curve.[226] An even more confusing situation arises when the diastolic pressure-volume relation of the ventricle changes, for example with the onset of myocardial ischemia. Rather than moving along the same diastolic pressure-volume curve, the ventricle now shifts to a different, steeper curve where, somewhat paradoxically, an increase in filling pressure may accompany a decrease in filling volume.[227] As in this example, not only can one not assume that a given measured change in cardiac filling pressure reflects a proportional change in ventricular preload, it cannot even be assumed that pressure and volume change in the same direction.[227] In summary, changes in CVP may be the sole result of changes in inotropic state or compliance of the ventricle, independent of the total circulating volume or venous return to the heart.

To summarize, CVP is the result of a complex and diverse interplay among many different physiologic variables, many of which are impossible to measure in the operating room or ICU. It is therefore not surprising that studies assessing the value of CVP as a predictor of volume status or fluid responsiveness have failed to demonstrate a relationship. There is, in fact, no simple relationship between CVP and circulating blood volume.[131]

Further complicating the analysis are the effects of intrathoracic and intrapericardial pressures on filling pressures such as CVP.[226,228] In general, all intravascular pressures measured in clinical practice are referenced to ambient atmospheric pressure. Thus, a cardiac filling pressure of 10 mm Hg is 10 mm Hg higher than ambient atmospheric pressure. Does this pressure value accurately represent the distending force across the cardiac chamber wall at end-diastole?

To answer this question, one needs to consider transmural pressure. The cardiac chambers are all contained within the pericardium and thorax. Changes in pressure in the structures surrounding the heart will influence pressures recorded within the heart. Transmural pressure is the difference between chamber pressure and juxtacardiac or pericardial pressure. This transmural pressure determines ventricular preload, end-diastolic volume, or fiber length. The same measured filling pressure, referenced to atmospheric pressure, can be associated with markedly different transmural pressures and chamber volumes, depending on whether juxtacardiac pressure is high or low. Although juxtacardiac pressure can be ignored under some circumstances, marked alterations in pleural and pericardial pressures occur commonly and must be considered when any cardiac filling pressure is interpreted. Transmural pressure is always the pressure of physiologic interest. Because juxtacardiac pressure is not measured routinely, one must always consider that the measured central vascular pressure, referenced to the ambient atmosphere, may be a poor estimate of transmural pressure.[226,228]

During spontaneous breathing, inspiration causes a decrease in pleural and juxtacardiac pressures which is transmitted, in part, to the right atrium, and lowers CVP. This same decrease in pleural pressure will influence other measured central vascular pressures in a similar fashion. Note a subtle but critically important observation about the measurement of central vascular pressures. Although CVP measured relative to atmospheric pressure decreases during the inspiratory phase of spontaneous ventilation, transmural CVP, the difference between right atrial pressure and juxtacardiac pressure may actually increase slightly as more blood is drawn into the right atrium. The opposite pattern is observed during positive-pressure ventilation, in which inspiration increases intrathoracic pressure while raising the measured CVP, but decreases transmural CVP,

TABLE 36.3 Central Venous Pressure Waveform Components

Waveform Component	Phase of Cardiac Cycle	Mechanical Event
a wave	End-diastole	Atrial contraction
c wave	Early systole	Isovolumic ventricular contraction, tricuspid motion toward right atrium
v wave	Late systole	Systolic filling of atrium
h wave	Mid- to late diastole	Diastolic plateau
x descent	Mid-systole	Atrial relaxation, descent of the base, systolic collapse
y descent	Early diastole	Early ventricular filling, diastolic collapse

because the elevated intrathoracic pressure reduces venous return. As mentioned before, transmural pressures are rarely measured in clinical practice owing to difficulties in assessing juxtacardiac or intrathoracic pressure. Instead, end-expiratory values for cardiac filling pressures should be recorded in all patients, to provide the best estimate of transmural pressure. At the end of expiration, intrathoracic and juxtacardiac pressures approach atmospheric pressure regardless of ventilatory status and the CVP values will coincide. Proper pressure values can also be determined by visual inspection of the CVP waveform on a calibrated monitor screen or paper recording. This facilitates comparison of CVP values (and other cardiac filling pressures) obtained from the same patient under varying patterns of ventilation, a common situation in anesthesia and critical care.

The second prerequisite for interpretation of CVP values is correct measurement. Details about the correct zeroing and leveling of the transducer are discussed elsewhere in this text. (See Technical Aspects of Direct Blood Pressure Measurement.). Leveling of the transducer for accurate CVP measurements is best achieved by aligning the stopcock (not the transducer) to a point 5 cm below the sternal angle, as opposed to the more commonly used mid-axillary line at the fourth intercostal space. When this reference point is used, measurements can be done in both the supine position or with the patient sitting up (up to an angle of 60 degrees),[116,229,230] and better represent the upper fluid level of the right atrium. Regardless of the position chosen, it is most important to be consistent throughout the monitoring period to maintain the same reference point.

Despite these limitations, there is still a great deal of information that may be gathered from careful interpretation of the CVP waveform. For this, it is essential to understand the components of the normal CVP waveform.

NORMAL CENTRAL VENOUS PRESSURE WAVEFORMS

Mechanical events during the cardiac cycle are responsible for the sequence of waves seen in a typical CVP trace. The CVP waveform consists of five phasic events, three peaks (a, c, v) and two descents (x, y) (Table 36.3, Fig. 36.35).[231,232] The most prominent wave is the **a wave** of atrial contraction, which occurs at end-diastole following the ECG P wave. Atrial contraction increases atrial pressure and provides the "atrial kick" to fill the right ventricle through the open tricuspid valve. Atrial pressure decreases following the a wave, as the atrium relaxes. This smooth decline in pressure is interrupted by the **c wave**. This wave is a transient increase in atrial pressure produced by isovolumic ventricular contraction, which closes the tricuspid valve and displaces it toward the atrium. The c wave always follows the ECG R wave because it is generated during onset of ventricular systole. (Note that the c wave observed in a jugular venous pressure trace might have a slightly more complex origin. This wave has been attributed to early systolic pressure transmission from the adjacent carotid artery and may be termed a carotid impact wave.[233] Because the jugular venous pressure also reflects right atrial pressure, however, this c wave likely represents both arterial [carotid impact] and venous [tricuspid motion] origins.) Atrial pressure continues its decline during ventricular systole, owing to continued atrial relaxation and changes in atrial geometry produced by ventricular contraction and ejection that draw the tricuspid annulus toward the cardiac apex. This is the **x descent** or systolic collapse in atrial pressure. The x descent can be divided into two portions, x and x′, corresponding to the segments before and after the c wave. The last atrial pressure peak is the **v wave**, and is caused by venous filling of the atrium during late

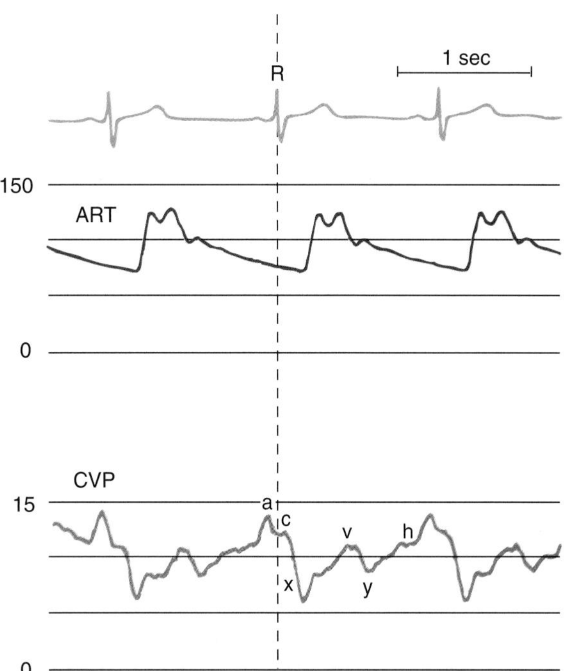

Fig. 36.35 Normal central venous pressure *(CVP)* waveform. The diastolic components (y descent, end-diastolic a wave) and the systolic components (c wave, x descent, end-systolic v wave) are all clearly delineated. A mid-diastolic plateau wave, the h wave, is also seen because heart rate is slow. Waveform identification is aided by timing the relation between individual waveform components and the electrocardiographic R wave. Waveform timing using the arterial *(ART)* pressure trace is more confusing, owing to the relative delay in the systolic arterial pressure upstroke. (From Mark JB. *Atlas of Cardiovascular Monitoring*. New York: Churchill Livingstone; 1998.)

systole while the tricuspid valve remains closed. The v wave usually peaks just after the ECG T wave. Atrial pressure then decreases, inscribing the **y descent** or diastolic collapse, as the tricuspid valve opens and blood flows from atrium to ventricle. (A final component of the CVP waveform, the **h wave**, occasionally appears as a pressure plateau in mid- to late diastole. The h wave is not normally seen unless the heart rate is slow and venous pressure is elevated.)[233,234] In summary, the normal venous waveform components may be remembered as follows: the a wave results from atrial contraction; the c wave from tricuspid valve closure and isovolumic RV contraction; the x descent is the systolic decrease in atrial pressure due to atrial relaxation and ventricular contraction; the v wave from ventricular ejection, which drives venous filling of the atrium; and the y descent is the diastolic decrease in atrial pressure due to flow across the open tricuspid valve.

In relation to the cardiac cycle and ventricular mechanical actions, the CVP waveform can be considered to have three systolic components (c wave, x descent, v wave) and two diastolic components (y descent, a wave). By recalling the mechanical actions that generate the pressure peaks and troughs, it is easy to identify these waveform components properly by aligning the CVP waveform and the ECG trace and using the ECG R wave to mark end-diastole and onset of systole. When the radial artery pressure trace is used for CVP waveform timing instead of the ECG, confusion may arise because the arterial pressure upstroke occurs nearly 200 ms after the ECG R wave (see Fig. 36.35). This normal physiologic delay reflects the times required for the spread of the electrical depolarization through the ventricle (≈60 ms), isovolumic LV contraction (≈60 ms), transmission of aortic pressure rise to the radial artery (≈50 ms), and transmission of the radial artery pressure rise through fluid-filled tubing to the transducer (≈10 ms).[117,235]

The normal CVP peaks are designated systolic (c, v) or diastolic (a) according to the phase of the cardiac cycle in which the wave begins. However, one generally identifies these waves not by their onset or upstroke, but rather by the location of their peaks. For instance, the a wave generally begins and peaks in end-diastole, but the peak may appear delayed to coincide with the ECG R wave, especially in a patient with a short PR interval. In this instance, a and c waves merge, and this composite wave is termed an a-c-wave. Designation of the CVP v wave as a systolic event may be even more confusing. Although the ascent of the v wave begins during late systole, the peak of the v wave occurs during isovolumic ventricular relaxation, immediately prior to atrioventricular valve opening and the y descent. Consequently, the most precise description would be that the v wave begins in late systole, but peaks during isovolumic ventricular relaxation, the earliest portion of diastole. For clinical purposes, it is simplest to consider the v wave to be a systolic wave.

Although three distinct CVP peaks (a, c, v) and two troughs (x, y) are discernible in the normal venous pressure trace, heart rate changes and conduction abnormalities alter this pattern. A short ECG PR interval causes fusion of a and c waves, and tachycardia reduces the length of diastole and the duration of the y descent, causing v and a waves to merge. In contrast, bradycardia causes each wave to become more distinct with separate x and x' descents visible and a more prominent h wave. Although there are circumstances in which other pathologic waves may be evident in the CVP trace, one should resist the temptation to assign physiologic significance to each small pressure peak, as many will arise as artifacts of fluid-filled tubing-transducer monitoring systems. It is more useful to search for the expected waveform components, including those waveforms that are characteristic of the pathologic conditions suspected.

TABLE 36.4 Central Venous Pressure Waveform Abnormalities

Condition	Characteristics
Atrial fibrillation	Loss of a wave Prominent c wave
Atrioventricular dissociation	Cannon a wave
Tricuspid regurgitation	Tall systolic c-v-wave Loss of x descent
Tricuspid stenosis	Tall a wave Attenuation of y descent
Right ventricular ischemia	Tall a and v waves Steep x and y descents M or W configuration
Pericardial constriction	Tall a and v waves Steep x and y descents M or W configuration
Cardiac tamponade	Dominant x descent Attenuated y descent
Respiratory variation during spontaneous or positive-pressure ventilation	Measure pressures at end-expiration

ABNORMAL CENTRAL VENOUS PRESSURE WAVEFORMS

Various pathophysiologic conditions may be diagnosed or confirmed by examination of the CVP waveform (Table 36.4). One of the most common applications is the rapid diagnosis of cardiac arrhythmias.[236] In **atrial fibrillation** (Fig. 36.36A), the a wave disappears and the c wave becomes more prominent because atrial volume is greater at end-diastole and onset of systole, owing to the absence of effective atrial contraction. Occasionally, atrial fibrillation or flutter waves may be seen in the CVP trace when the ventricular rate is slow. Isorhythmic **atrioventricular dissociation or accelerated junctional (nodal) rhythm** (see Fig. 36.36B) alters the normal sequence of atrial contraction prior to ventricular contraction. Instead, atrial contraction now occurs during ventricular systole when the tricuspid valve is closed, thereby inscribing a tall "cannon" a wave in the CVP waveform. Absence of normal atrioventricular synchrony during ventricular pacing (see Fig. 36.36C) can be identified in a similar fashion by searching for cannon waves in the venous pressure trace. In these instances, the CVP helps diagnose the cause of arterial hypotension; loss of the normal end-diastolic atrial kick may not be as evident in the ECG trace as it is in the CVP waveform.

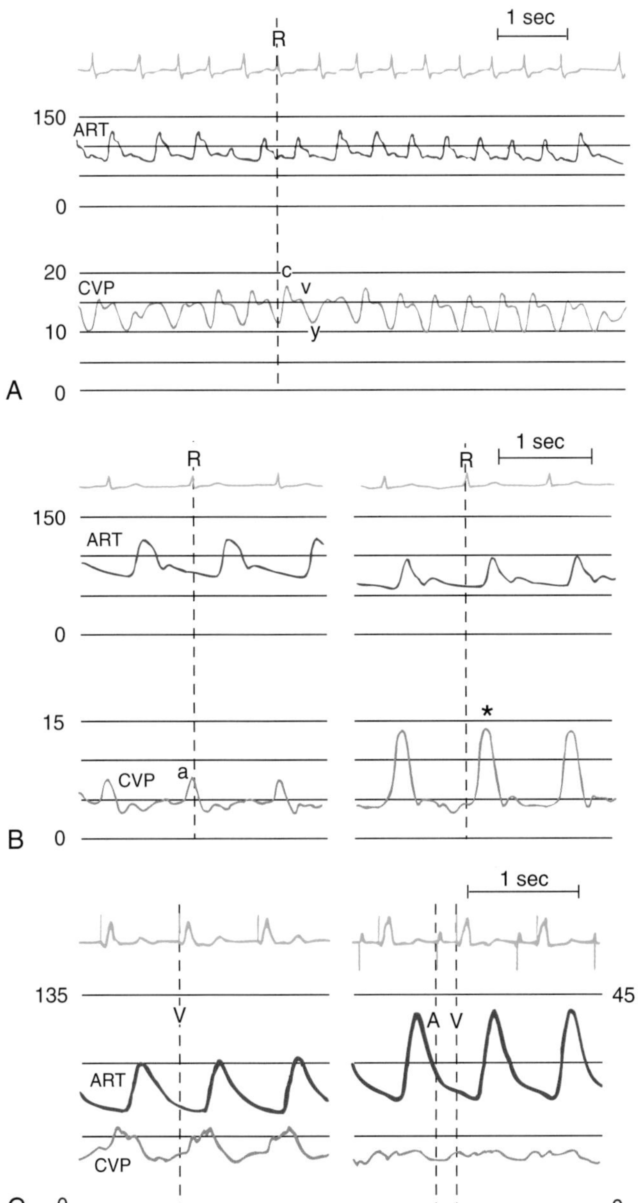

Fig. 36.36 Central venous pressure *(CVP)* changes caused by cardiac arrhythmias. (A) Atrial fibrillation. Note absence of the a wave, a prominent c wave, and a preserved v wave and y descent. This arrhythmia also causes variation in the electrocardiographic (ECG) R-R interval and left ventricular stroke volume, which can be seen in the ECG and arterial *(ART)* pressure traces. (B) Isorhythmic atrioventricular dissociation. In contrast to the normal end-diastolic a wave in the CVP trace *(left panel)*, an early systolic cannon wave is inscribed (*, *right panel*). Reduced ventricular filling accompanying this arrhythmia causes a decreased arterial blood pressure. (C) Ventricular pacing. Systolic cannon waves are evident in the CVP trace during ventricular pacing *(left panel)*. Atrioventricular sequential pacing restores the normal venous waveform and increases arterial blood pressure *(right panel)*. ART scale left, CVP scale right. (From Mark JB. *Atlas of Cardiovascular Monitoring*. New York: Churchill Livingstone; 1998.)

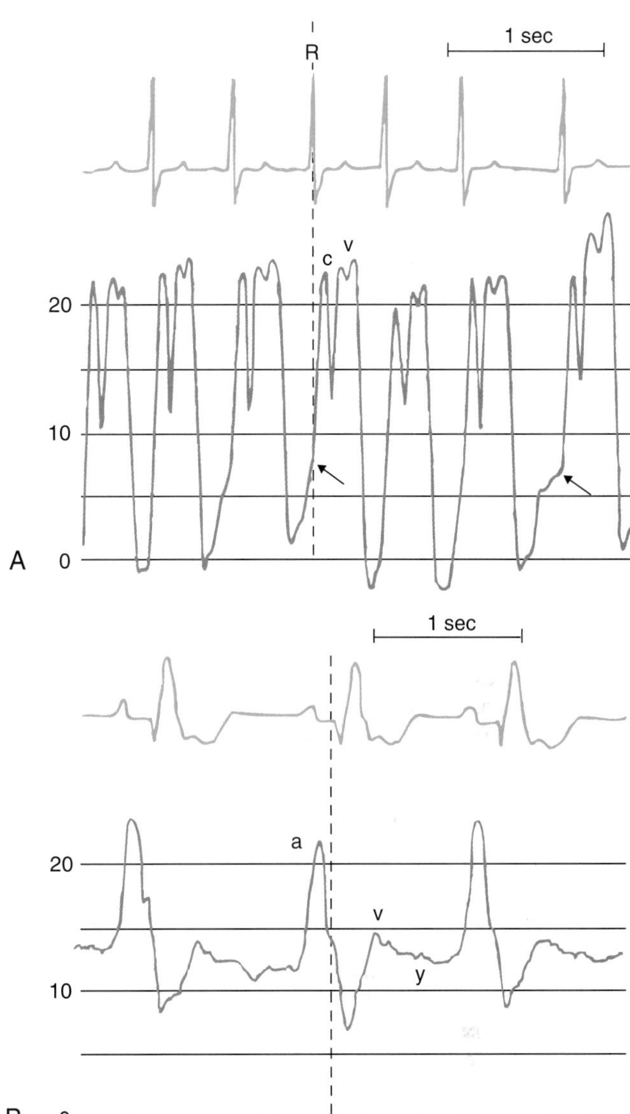

Fig. 36.37 Central venous pressure (CVP) changes in tricuspid valve disease. (A) Tricuspid regurgitation increases mean CVP, and the waveform displays a tall systolic c-v-wave that obliterates the x descent. In this example, the a wave is not seen because of atrial fibrillation. Right ventricular end-diastolic pressure is estimated best at the time of the electrocardiographic R wave *(arrows)* and is lower than mean CVP. (B) Tricuspid stenosis increases mean CVP, the diastolic y descent is attenuated, and the end-diastolic a wave is prominent. (From Mark JB. *Atlas of Cardiovascular Monitoring*. New York: Churchill Livingstone; 1998.)

Right-sided valvular heart diseases alter the CVP waveform in different ways.[237] **Tricuspid regurgitation** (Fig. 36.37A) produces abnormal systolic filling of the right atrium through the incompetent valve. A broad, tall systolic c-v-wave results, beginning in early systole and obliterating the systolic x descent in atrial pressure. The CVP trace is said to be ventricularized, resembling RV pressure. Note that this regurgitant wave differs in onset, duration, and magnitude from a normal v wave caused by end-systolic atrial filling from the venae cavae. In patients with tricuspid regurgitation, RV end-diastolic pressure is overestimated by the numeric display on the bedside monitor, which reports a single mean value for CVP. Instead, RV end-diastolic pressure is estimated best by measuring the CVP value at the time of the ECG R wave, prior to the regurgitant systolic wave (see Fig. 36.37A). Unlike tricuspid regurgitation, **tricuspid stenosis** produces a diastolic defect in atrial emptying and ventricular filling (see Fig. 36.37B). Mean CVP is elevated, and a pressure gradient exists throughout diastole between right atrium and ventricle. The a wave is unusually prominent and the

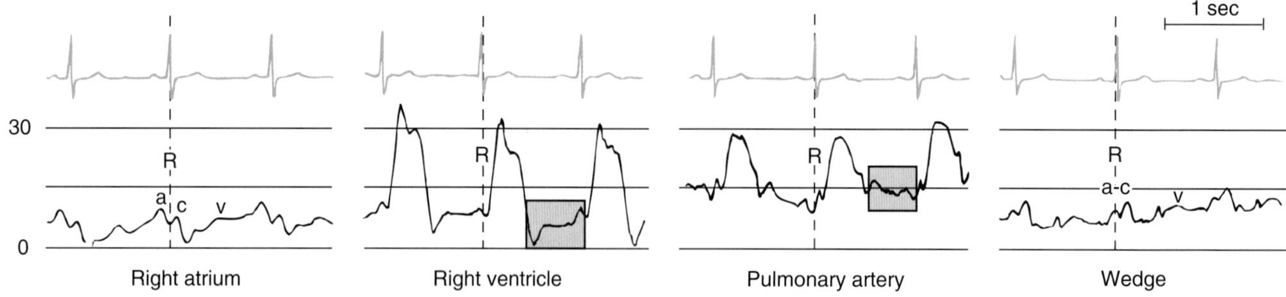

Fig. 36.38 Characteristic waveforms recorded during passage of the pulmonary artery catheter. The right atrial pressure resembles a central venous pressure waveform and displays a, c, and v waves. Right ventricular pressure shows a higher systolic pressure than seen in the right atrium, although the end-diastolic pressures are equal in these two chambers. Pulmonary artery pressure shows a diastolic step-up compared with ventricular pressure. Note also that right ventricular pressure increases during diastole, whereas pulmonary artery pressure decreases during diastole *(shaded boxes)*. Pulmonary artery wedge pressure has a similar morphology to right atrial pressure, although the a-c and v waves appear later in the cardiac cycle relative to the electrocardiogram. (From Mark JB. *Atlas of Cardiovascular Monitoring*. New York: Churchill Livingstone; 1998.)

y descent is attenuated, owing to the impaired diastolic egress of blood from the atrium. Other conditions that reduce RV compliance, such as RV ischemia, pulmonary hypertension, or pulmonic valve stenosis, may produce a prominent end-diastolic a wave in the CVP trace but do not attenuate the early diastolic y descent. CVP waveform morphology changes in other characteristic ways in the presence of pericardial diseases and RV infarction. These patterns are interpreted best in conjunction with PAP monitoring, which is discussed below.

Perhaps the most important traditional application of CVP monitoring is to provide an estimate of the adequacy of the circulating blood volume. Several randomized trials and systematic reviews have demonstrated a very poor relationship between CVP and circulating blood volume, as well as the inability of a static CVP value to predict the hemodynamic response to a fluid challenge.[238-240] This is not surprising in light of the factors described above. Some have argued that the important clinical question with regard to volume responsiveness should be phrased in the negative, that is, whether a patient is *unlikely* to respond to fluids. The subset of patients that will derive all the deleterious effects of fluid administration (capillary leak and tissue edema) and no benefit (increased cardiac output) is in most instances the group of clinical interest. In this regard, the lack of an inspiratory fall in CVP in patients who have spontaneous inspiratory efforts (provided the inspiratory effort is adequate, i.e., >2 mm Hg fall in PAOP with inspiration) was able to predict no improvement in cardiac output following fluid administration.[241]

Pulmonary Artery Catheter Monitoring

In 1970, Swan, Ganz, and colleagues introduced PAC into clinical practice for the hemodynamic assessment of patients with acute myocardial infarction.[242] This device allowed accurate bedside measurement of important cardiovascular physiologic variables, and its popularity soared. While the PAC provides measurements of several hemodynamic variables that clinicians find it hard to predict accurately from standard clinical signs and symptoms,[243] it remains uncertain whether PAC monitoring leads to improved patient outcome.[244]

PULMONARY ARTERY CATHETER INSERTION

The standard PAC has a 7.0 to 9.0 Fr circumference, is 110 cm in length marked at 10-cm intervals, and contains four internal lumens. The distal port at the catheter tip is used for PAP monitoring, while the second is 30 cm more proximal and is used for CVP monitoring. The third lumen leads to a balloon near the tip which is used to float the catheter through the cardiac chambers, and the fourth houses wires for a temperature thermistor, the end of which lies just proximal to the balloon.[245]

PACs can be placed from any of the central venous cannulation sites described earlier, but the right internal jugular vein provides the most direct route to the right heart chambers. The balloon at the tip of the catheter is inflated with air, and the catheter is advanced into the right atrium, through the tricuspid valve, the right ventricle, the pulmonic valve, into the pulmonary artery, and finally into the wedge position. Characteristic waveforms from each of these locations confirm proper catheter passage and placement (Fig. 36.38).

After the PAWP is measured, the balloon is deflated, and the PAP waveform should reappear. Catheter position is confirmed with a chest radiograph. The tip of the PAC should be within 2 cm of the cardiac silhouette on a standard anteroposterior chest film.[246]

If an RV waveform is not observed after inserting the catheter 40 cm, coiling in the right atrium is likely. Similarly, if a pulmonary artery waveform is not observed after inserting the catheter to 50 cm, coiling in the right ventricle has probably occurred. The balloon should be deflated, the catheter withdrawn to 20 cm, and the PAC floating sequence repeated.

A few additional points might aid successful positioning of the PAC. The air-filled balloon tends to float to nondependent regions as it passes through the heart into the pulmonary vasculature. Consequently, positioning a patient head down will aid flotation across the tricuspid valve, and tilting the patient onto the right side and placing the head up will encourage flotation out of the right ventricle, as well as reduce the incidence of arrhythmias during insertion.[247,248] Deep inspiration during spontaneous ventilation will increase venous return and RV output transiently, and may facilitate catheter flotation in a patient with low cardiac output. On occasion, a catheter may be floated to

BOX 36.7 Complications of Pulmonary Artery Catheter Monitoring

Catheterization
- Arrhythmias, ventricular fibrillation
- Right bundle branch block, complete heart block (if preexisting left bundle branch block)

Catheter residence
- Mechanical: catheter knots, entangling with or dislodgement of pacing wires
- Thromboembolism
- Pulmonary infarction
- Infection, endocarditis
- Endocardial damage, cardiac valve injury
- Pulmonary artery rupture
- Pulmonary artery pseudoaneurysm

Misinterpretation of data
- Misuse of equipment

proper position when stiffened by injecting 10 to 20 mL of ice cold solution through the distal lumen. Finally, maneuvering of the PAC can also be guided by transesophageal or transthoracic echocardiography, demonstrating the catheter passage through the right heart.[249,250]

COMPLICATIONS OF PULMONARY ARTERY CATHETER MONITORING

Complications of PAC use may be divided into those resulting from catheter placement, those associated with the *in-vivo* presence of the catheter, and those resulting from catheter use and misuse. For the most part, problems encountered during catheter placement are the same for both PAC and CVP monitoring (see Box 36.6). However, catheterization of the right ventricle and pulmonary artery causes complications uniquely associated with PACs (Box 36.7).[251]

When all adverse effects from PAC use are considered, including self-limited arrhythmias observed during catheter insertion, it appears that minor complications occur in more than 50% of catheterized patients.[252] However, major morbidity specifically attributable to PAC use is uncommon.[253] In both an initial exhaustive review of the literature and in its 2003 update, the ASA Task Force on Pulmonary Artery Catheterization emphasized that the reported incidence of complications from PAC monitoring varies widely, although it seems that serious complications occur in 0.1% to 0.5 % of PAC-monitored surgical patients.[252] In 1984, Shah et al. reported use of PACs in 6245 patients undergoing cardiac and noncardiac operations.[187] Quite remarkably, only 10 patients (0.16%) had serious complications resulting in morbidity and only 1 patient (0.016%) died as a result of PAC. Furthermore, a 1998 European report of PAC use in 5306 patients undergoing cardiac surgery confirms this low incidence of major morbidity, with injury of the right ventricle or PA occurring in only 4 patients (0.07%).[254] Finally, only 1 of 2000 adverse events reported in the Australian Incident Monitoring Study of 1993 involved use of a PAC, in contrast to 64 adverse events involving access to the arterial or venous systems.[99] However, it is important to acknowledge that although these large studies indicate a low incidence of serious complications attributable to the use of PACs, the frequency of complications in a particular clinical setting or patient group remains unknown.

A more insidious but possibly more common complication of PAC use is **misinterpretation of data.**[255,256] Although the magnitude of the problem is not clear, studies show widespread knowledge deficits among practitioners who use PACs. In 1990, Iberti and associates reported the results of a 31-question multiple-choice examination given to 496 physicians. They found a poor overall level of knowledge of PACs, as evidenced by a mean score of only 67% correct answers. Although higher scores were demonstrated by individuals with more training and more experience inserting and using PACs, none of these factors ensured a high level of knowledge.[257] These results have been duplicated in a variety of other specialty care groups.[258] It is especially concerning that PAWP measurement was performed incorrectly by 30% to 50% of the clinicians in these studies and that educational programs failed to improve performance.[259,260] Taken together, these observations highlight the fact that effective use of PACs requires a great deal of expertise and clinical experience, and even measuring the most fundamental PAC-derived variable, namely wedge pressure, is a complicated endeavor.[261]

NORMAL PULMONARY ARTERY PRESSURES AND WAVEFORMS

As the balloon-tipped PAC is floated to its proper position in the pulmonary artery, characteristic pressure waveforms are recorded (see Fig. 36.38). In the superior vena cava or right atrium, a CVP waveform with characteristic a-, c-, and v waves and low mean pressure should be observed. RV pressure is characterized by a rapid systolic upstroke, a wide pulse pressure, and low diastolic pressure. Entry of the PAC into the pulmonary artery is heralded by a step-up in diastolic pressure and a change in waveform morphology.

On occasion, it may be difficult to distinguish RV pressure from PAP, particularly if only the numeric values for these pressures are examined. However, careful observation of the pressure waveforms, focusing on the diastolic pressure contours, allows differentiation. During diastole, the PAP will fall owing to continuous runoff flow to the lung, while the pressure in the right ventricle will increase due to filling from the right atrium (see Fig. 36.38).[262]

As noted above, the wedge pressure is an indirect measurement of pulmonary venous pressure and left atrial pressure and should therefore resemble these venous waveforms with characteristic a and v waves and x and y descents. However, owing to the pulmonary vascular bed interposed between the PAC tip and left atrium, wedge pressure is a delayed and damped representation of left atrial pressure.[263]

The terms PAWP and pulmonary artery occlusion pressure are used interchangeably and refer to the same measurement obtained from the tip of a PAC following balloon inflation and flotation to the wedged position. However, pulmonary capillary pressure must not be confused with wedge pressure or left atrial pressure, nor should the term *pulmonary capillary wedge pressure* be used at all. The hydrostatic pressure in the pulmonary capillaries that causes edema formation according to the Starling equation is different from left arterial pressure (LAP). This is the pressure that must exceed

LAP in order to maintain antegrade blood flow through the lungs. Although the magnitude of the difference between pulmonary capillary pressure and wedge pressure is generally small, it can increase markedly when resistance to flow in the pulmonary veins is elevated.[264] In most situations, the major component of pulmonary vascular resistance occurs at the precapillary, pulmonary arteriolar level. However, rare conditions like pulmonary venoocclusive disease may cause a marked increase in postcapillary resistance to flow. Similar situations arise in conditions that disproportionately increase pulmonary venous resistance, such as central nervous system injury, acute lung injury, hypovolemic shock, endotoxemia, and norepinephrine infusion.[265,266] Under these conditions, measurement of wedge pressure will underestimate pulmonary capillary pressure substantially and thereby underestimate the risk of hydrostatic pulmonary edema.

ABNORMAL PULMONARY ARTERY AND WEDGE PRESSURE WAVEFORMS

PAC monitoring is subject to the same technical artifacts inherent in all invasive pressure monitoring techniques as well as some additional problems unique to this method.[267-269] Because the PAC is longer and passes through the cardiac chambers, it is more prone to distortions from clot or air bubbles, and motion-related artifacts are more problematic. Artifactual pressure spikes may be distinguished from the underlying physiologic pressure waveform by their unique morphology and timing.

At the onset of systole, tricuspid valve closure accompanied by RV contraction and ejection result in excessive **catheter motion** causing the most common PAC trace artifact.[268,270] This pressure artifact may produce an artificially low pressure, erroneously designated as the pulmonary artery diastolic (PAD) pressure (Fig. 36.39). Repositioning the PAC often solves the problem.

Another common artifact in PAC pressure measurement occurs when the balloon is overinflated and occludes the distal lumen orifice. This phenomenon is termed **overwedging** and usually is caused by distal catheter migration and eccentric balloon inflation that forces the catheter tip against the vessel wall. The catheter now records a gradually rising, non-pulsatile pressure as the continuous flush system builds up pressure against the obstructed distal opening (Fig. 36.40). When observed, this should be corrected immediately by gentle catheter withdrawal to a more proximal location in the pulmonary artery.

As emphasized earlier, with each PAC balloon inflation and wedge measurement, the catheter tip migrates distally. When a wedge pressure tracing appears during partial balloon inflation, it suggests that the PAC is inappropriately located in a smaller, distal branch of the pulmonary artery. The catheter should be withdrawn slightly before overwedging can occur and result in vascular injury or pulmonary infarction.

Pathophysiologic conditions involving the left-sided cardiac chambers or valves produce characteristic changes in the pulmonary artery and wedge pressure waveforms. One of the most easily recognized patterns is the tall v wave of **mitral regurgitation**. Unlike a normal wedge pressure v wave produced by late systolic pulmonary venous inflow, the prominent v wave of mitral regurgitation begins in early systole. Mitral regurgitation causes fusion of c and v waves and obliteration of the systolic x descent, as the isovolumic phase of LV systole is eliminated owing to the retrograde ejection of blood into the left atrium.[237] Because the prominent v wave of mitral regurgitation is generated during

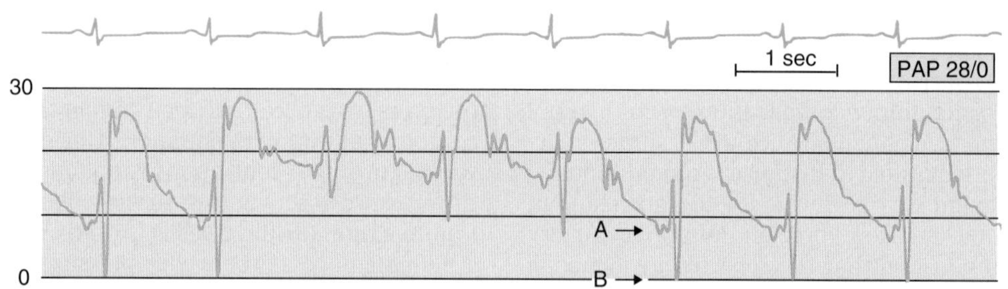

Fig. 36.39 Artifactual pressure peaks and troughs in the pulmonary artery pressure *(PAP)* waveform caused by catheter motion. The correct value for pulmonary artery end-diastolic pressure is 8 mm Hg (A), although the monitor digital display erroneously reports the PAP as 28/0 mm Hg (B). (From Mark JB. *Atlas of Cardiovascular Monitoring*. New York: Churchill Livingstone; 1998.)

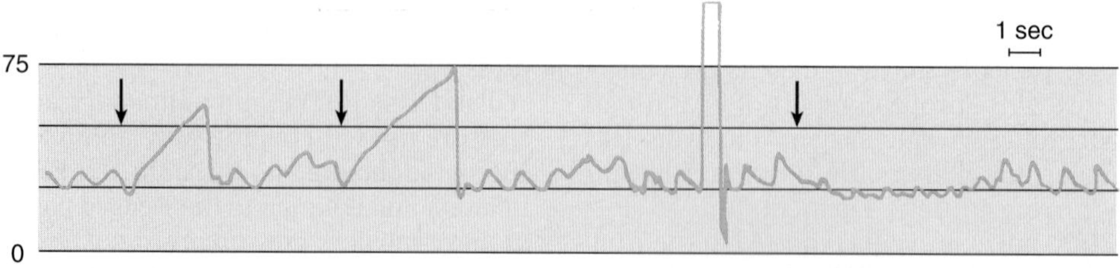

Fig. 36.40 Overwedging of the pulmonary artery (PA) catheter causes artifactual waveform recordings. The first two attempts to inflate the PA catheter balloon *(first two arrows)* produce a nonpulsatile increasing pressure caused by an occluded catheter tip. After the catheter is withdrawn slightly, balloon inflation allows proper wedge pressure measurement *(third arrow)*. Before the third attempt at balloon inflation, the PA pressure lumen is flushed. This restores the appropriate pulsatile nature to the PA and wedge pressure waveforms on the right side of the trace. (From Mark JB. *Atlas of Cardiovascular Monitoring*. New York: Churchill Livingstone; 1998.)

ventricular systole, the mean wedge pressure overestimates LV end-diastolic filling pressure, which is better estimated by the pressure value prior to onset of the regurgitant v wave (Fig. 36.41). However, it remains a good approximation for mean left atrial pressure and the subsequent risk of hydrostatic pulmonary edema.

It should be noted that although the height of the v wave in the wedge pressure trace will be affected by the volume of regurgitant blood entering the left atrium, it also depends on the left atrial volume and compliance (Fig. 36.42). This may explain why patients with acute mitral regurgitation tend to have tall wedge pressure v waves—they have smaller, stiffer left atria with poorer compliance compared to patients with longstanding disease. Therefore, the height of the wedge pressure v wave is neither a sensitive nor a specific indicator of mitral regurgitation severity.[271]

In contrast to mitral regurgitation, which distorts the systolic portion of the wedge pressure waveform, **mitral stenosis** alters its diastolic aspect. In this condition, the holo-diastolic pressure gradient across the mitral valve results in an increased mean wedge pressure, a slurred early diastolic y descent, and a tall end-diastolic a wave. Similar hemodynamic abnormalities are seen in patients with left atrial myxoma or whenever there is obstruction to mitral flow. Diseases that increase LV stiffness (e.g., LV infarction, pericardial constriction, aortic stenosis, and systemic hypertension) produce changes in the wedge pressure that resemble in part those seen in mitral stenosis. In these conditions, mean wedge pressure is increased and the trace displays a prominent a wave, but the y descent remains steep because there is no obstruction to flow across the mitral valve during diastole. Because patients with advanced mitral stenosis often have coexisting atrial fibrillation, the a wave will not be present in many of these cases (Fig. 36.43).[237]

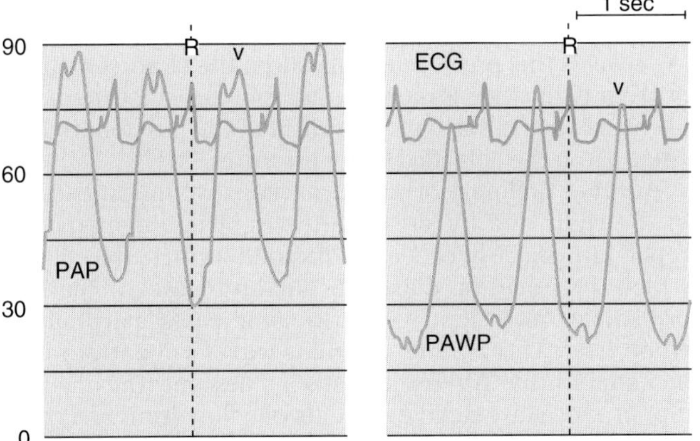

Fig. 36.41 Severe mitral regurgitation. A tall systolic v wave *(v)* is inscribed in the pulmonary artery wedge pressure *(PAWP)* trace and also distorts the pulmonary artery pressure *(PAP)* trace, giving it a bifid appearance. The electrocardiogram *(ECG)* is abnormal owing to ventricular pacing. Left ventricular end-diastolic pressure is estimated best by measuring PAWP at the time of the electrocardiographic R wave, before onset of the regurgitant v wave. Note that mean PAWP exceeds left ventricular end-diastolic pressure in this condition. (From Mark JB. *Atlas of Cardiovascular Monitoring.* New York: Churchill Livingstone; 1998.)

Myocardial ischemia may be detected by PAC in several ways. Ischemia itself impairs LV relaxation resulting in diastolic dysfunction, a pattern particularly characteristic of demand ischemia associated with tachycardia or induced by rapid atrial pacing.[227,272,273] Impaired ventricular relaxation results in a stiffer, less compliant left ventricle, resulting in an increased LV end-diastolic pressure. This will result in a tall a wave on the wedge trace, as the left atrium contracts into a stiff, incompletely relaxed left ventricle (Fig. 36.44).[274]

Myocardial ischemia can also produce LV systolic dysfunction, typically as a result of supply ischemia, caused by a sudden reduction or cessation of coronary blood flow to a region of the myocardium.[273,275] As ejection fraction falls significantly, LV end-diastolic volume and pressure rise, and elevated pulmonary diastolic and wedge pressures develop.[276] Distortion of LV geometry or ischemia of the myocardium underlying the papillary muscles can lead to acute mitral regurgitation with its characteristic PAP trace changes described above (see Fig. 36.41).[277]

Whether the PAC should be used in high-risk patients as a supplemental monitor for detection of myocardial ischemia remains controversial. Although patients with LV ischemia are likely to have higher mean wedge pressures than those without ischemia, these differences are small, may be difficult to detect clinically, and no clear quantitative threshold values for diagnosis of ischemia have been identified.[278]

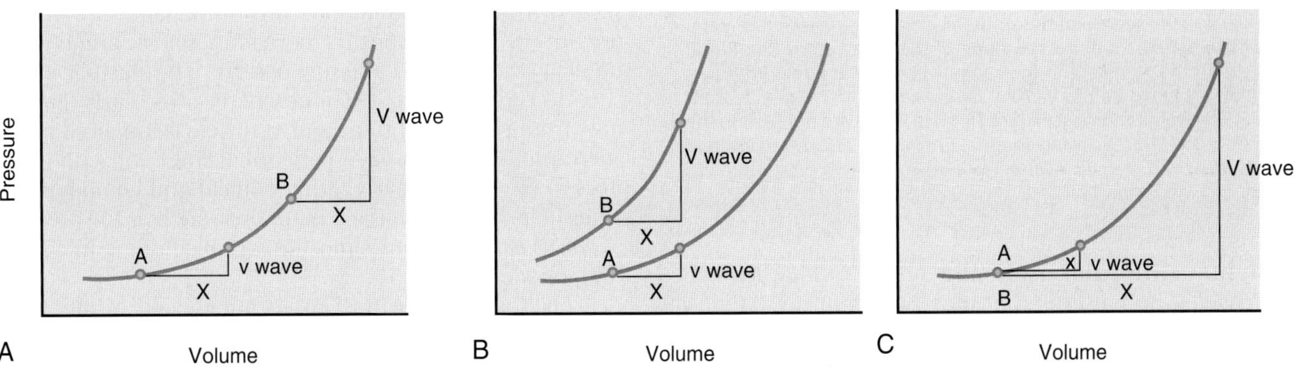

Fig. 36.42 V-wave height as an indicator of mitral regurgitation severity. Left atrial pressure-volume curves describe the three factors that determine v-wave height. (A) Influence of left atrial volume. For the same regurgitant volume (X), the left atrial v wave will be taller if baseline atrial volume is greater (point B versus point A). (B) Influence of left atrial compliance. For the same regurgitant volume (X), the left atrial v wave will be taller if baseline atrial compliance is reduced (point B versus point A). (C) Influence of regurgitant volume. Beginning at the same baseline left atrial volume (points A and B), if regurgitant volume increases (X versus x), the left atrial pressure v wave will increase (V versus v). (From Mark JB. *Atlas of Cardiovascular Monitoring.* New York: Churchill Livingstone; 1998.)

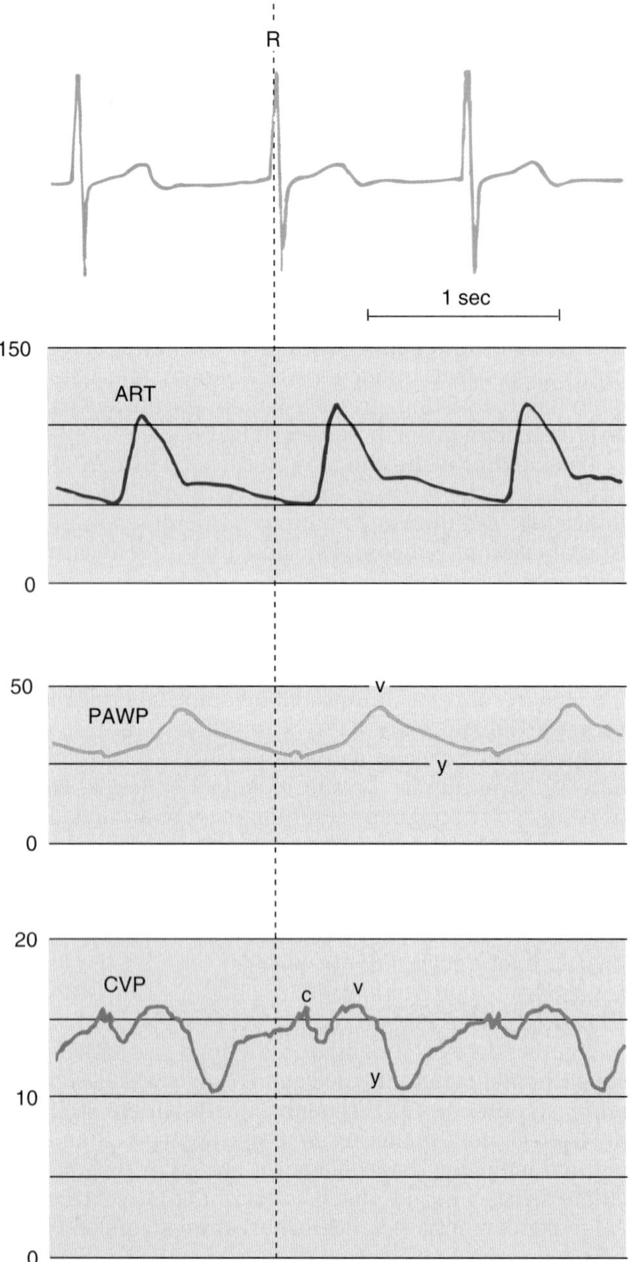

Fig. 36.43 Mitral stenosis. Mean pulmonary artery wedge pressure *(PAWP)* is increased (35 mm Hg), and the diastolic y descent is markedly attenuated. Compare the slope of the y descent in the PAWP trace with the y descent in the central venous pressure *(CVP)* trace. In addition, compare this PAWP y descent with the PAWP y descent in mitral regurgitation (see Figure 36.41); a waves are not seen in the PAWP or CVP traces, owing to atrial fibrillation. *ART,* Arterial blood pressure. (From Mark JB. *Atlas of Cardiovascular Monitoring.* New York: Churchill Livingstone; 1998.)

Right ventricular ischemia produces characteristic PAC waveform patterns that may be helpful in diagnosis and management. Just as LV ischemia increases PAWP, RV ischemia increases CVP. In fact, this is one of the few situations in which CVP may be higher than wedge pressure. In addition, CVP waveforms may display a prominent a wave resulting from RV diastolic dysfunction, and a prominent v wave resulting from ischemia-induced tricuspid regurgitation.[279,280] This particular CVP waveform is described as having an M or W configuration, referring to the tall a and v waves and interposed steep x and y descents. Severe pulmonary artery hypertension may also result in RV ischemia and dysfunction as well as increased CVP, but this is distinguished from primary RV dysfunction in that the PAP and calculated pulmonary vascular resistance are normal in primary RV failure.

The CVP waveform in RV infarction is similar to that from a patient with restrictive cardiomyopathy or **pericardial constriction**, including elevated mean pressure, prominent a and v waves, and steep x and y descents.[281] The cardinal feature common to these conditions is impaired RV diastolic compliance, often termed "restrictive physiology." In restrictive cardiomyopathy and RV infarction, diastolic dysfunction impairs ventricular relaxation and decreases chamber compliance, whereas in constrictive pericarditis cardiac filling is limited by the rigid, often calcified pericardial shell. Impaired venous return decreases end-diastolic volume, stroke volume, and cardiac output. Despite reduced cardiac volumes, cardiac filling pressures are markedly elevated and equal in all four chambers of the heart at end-diastole (Fig. 36.45). Although PAC monitoring reveals this pressure equalization, the characteristic M or W configuration is more apparent in the CVP trace, most likely because of the damping effect of the pulmonary vasculature on the left-sided filling pressures.[282-284]

Another hallmark of pericardial constriction is observed in the right and LV pressure traces. These demonstrate rapid but short-lived early diastolic ventricular filling, which produces a diastolic "dip-and-plateau" pattern or "square root sign."[129,285] In some cases, particularly when heart rate is slow, a similar waveform pattern may be noted in the CVP trace: a steep y descent (the diastolic dip) produced by rapid early diastolic flow from atrium to ventricle, followed by a mid-diastolic h wave (the plateau) from the interruption in flow imposed by the restrictive pericardial shell (see Fig. 36.45).

Like pericardial constriction, **cardiac tamponade** impairs cardiac filling, but in the case of tamponade, a compressive pericardial fluid collection produces this effect. This results in a marked increase in CVP and a reduced diastolic volume, stroke volume, and cardiac output. Despite many similar hemodynamic features, tamponade and constriction may be distinguished by the different CVP waveforms seen in these two conditions. In tamponade, the venous pressure waveform appears more monophasic and is dominated by the systolic x pressure descent. The diastolic y pressure descent is attenuated or absent, because early diastolic flow from right atrium to right ventricle is impaired by the surrounding compressive pericardial fluid collection (Fig. 36.46).[282,286,287] Clearly, other clinical and hemodynamic clues help distinguish these diagnoses, such as the presence of *pulsus paradoxus*, an almost invariable finding in cardiac tamponade (see Fig. 36.32).[288]

Probably the single most important waveform abnormality or interpretive problem in PAC monitoring is discerning the correct pressure measurement in patients with large intrathoracic pressure swings like those receiving **positive pressure ventilation** or those with labored spontaneous breathing. During positive pressure ventilation, inspiration increases pulmonary artery and wedge pressures. By measuring these pressures at end-expiration, the confounding

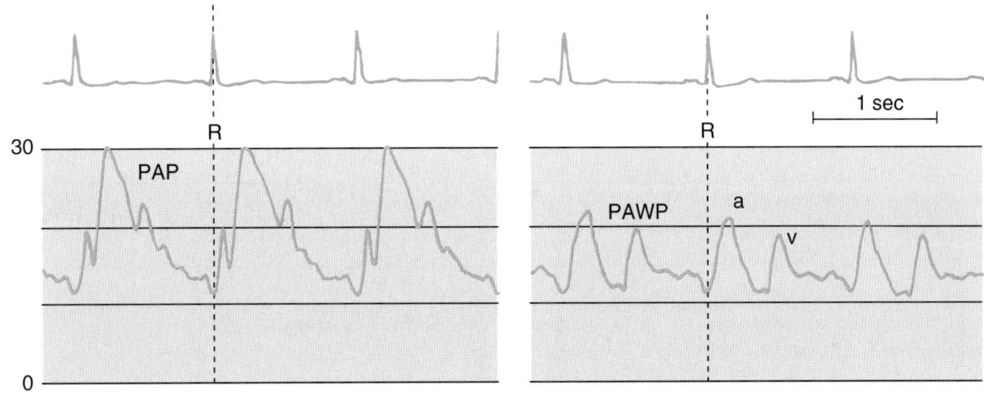

Fig. 36.44 Myocardial ischemia. Pulmonary artery pressure *(PAP)* is relatively normal and mean pulmonary artery wedge pressure *(PAWP)* is only slightly elevated (15 mm Hg). However, PAWP morphology is markedly abnormal with tall a waves (21 mm Hg) resulting from the diastolic dysfunction seen in this condition. (From Mark JB. *Atlas of Cardiovascular Monitoring*. New York: Churchill Livingstone; 1998.)

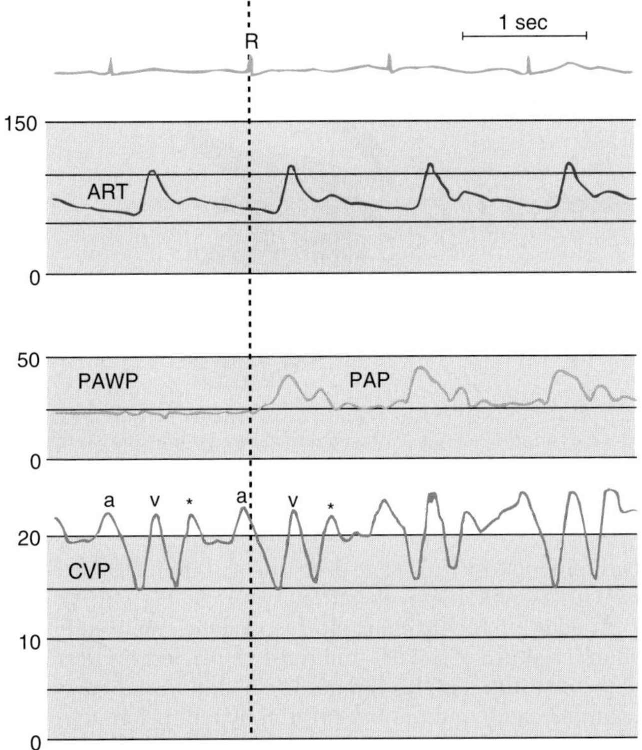

Fig. 36.45 Pericardial constriction. This condition causes elevation and equalization of diastolic filling pressures in the pulmonary artery pressure *(PAP)*, pulmonary artery wedge pressure *(PAWP)*, and central venous pressure *(CVP)* traces. The CVP waveform reveals tall a and v waves with steep x and y descents and a mid-diastolic plateau wave (*) or h wave. *ART*, Arterial blood pressure. (From Mark JB. *Atlas of Cardiovascular Monitoring*. New York: Churchill Livingstone; 1998.)

effect of this inspiratory increase in intrathoracic pressure is minimized (Fig. 36.47).[228] Forceful inspiration during spontaneous ventilation has the opposite effect, but again, measurement of these pressures at end-expiration eliminates this confounding factor. Bedside monitors are designed with algorithms that aim to identify and report the numeric values for end-expiratory pressures but are often inaccurate.[289,290] The most reliable method for measuring central vascular pressures at end-expiration is examination of the waveforms on a calibrated monitor screen or paper recording.[290,291]

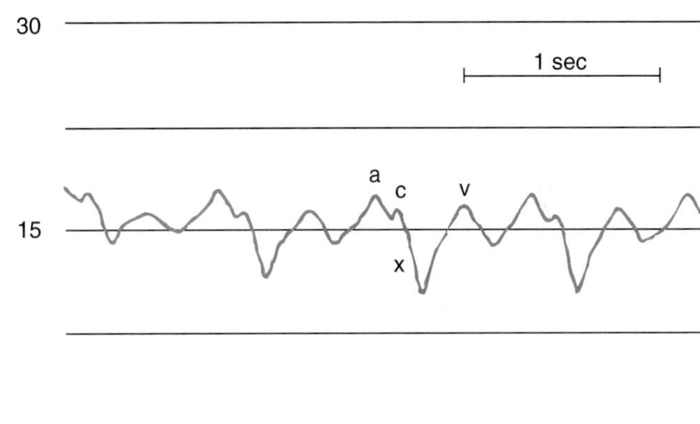

Fig. 36.46 Cardiac tamponade. The central venous pressure waveform shows an increased mean pressure (16 mm Hg) and attenuation of the y descent. Compare with Figure 36.45. (From Mark JB. *Atlas of Cardiovascular Monitoring*. New York: Churchill Livingstone; 1998.)

PHYSIOLOGIC CONSIDERATIONS FOR PULMONARY ARTERY CATHETER MONITORING: PREDICTION OF LEFT VENTRICULAR PRELOAD

One reason to measure PAD and wedge pressures is to be able to estimate LV end-diastolic pressure, the closest surrogate to LV end-diastolic volume, which is the true LV preload. When a PAC floats to the wedge position, the inflated balloon isolates the distal pressure-monitoring orifice from upstream PAP. A continuous static column of blood now connects the wedged PAC tip to the junction of the pulmonary veins and left atrium. Thus, wedging the PAC, in effect, extends the catheter tip to measure the pressure at the point at which blood flow resumes on the venous side of the pulmonary circuit. Because resistance in the large pulmonary veins is negligible, PAWP provides an indirect measurement of both pulmonary venous pressure and left atrial pressure.[292,293] For the column of blood connecting the tip of the wedged catheter and the draining pulmonary vein to be continuous, however, external compression by surrounding alveoli should be negligible (i.e., the catheter needs to reside in the so-called West zone 3 of the lung) (Fig. 36.48).[293]

PAD pressure is often used as an alternative to PAWP to estimate LV filling pressure. This is acceptable under normal circumstances because when pulmonary venous

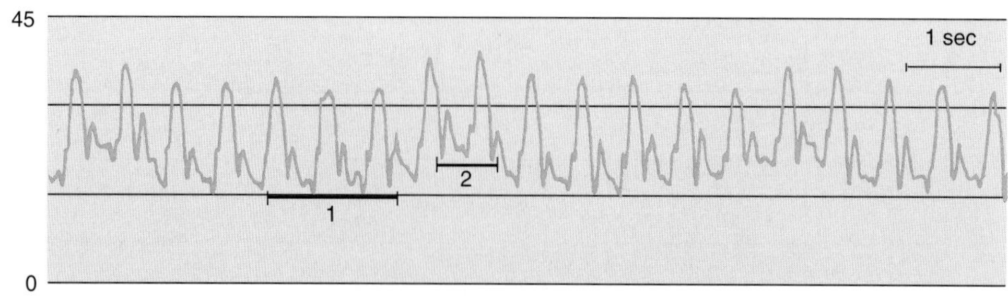

Fig. 36.47 Influence of positive-pressure mechanical ventilation on pulmonary artery pressure. Pulmonary artery pressure should be measured at end expiration (*1*, 15 mm Hg) in order to obviate the artifact caused by positive-pressure inspiration (*2*, 22 mm Hg). (From Mark JB. *Atlas of Cardiovascular Monitoring*. New York: Churchill Livingstone; 1998.)

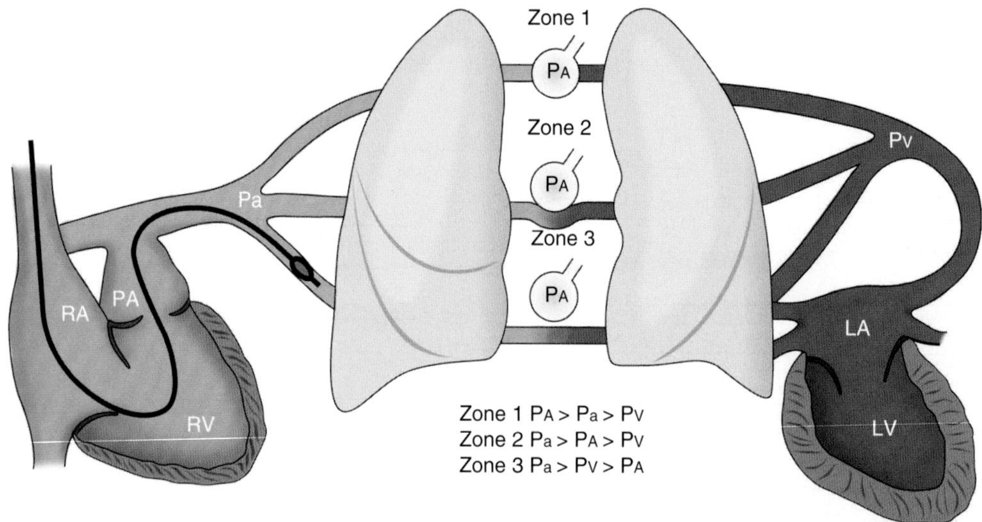

Fig. 36.48 The pulmonary artery catheter tip must be wedged in lung zone 3 to provide an accurate measure of pulmonary venous *(Pv)* or left atrial *(LA)* pressure. When alveolar pressure *(P_A)* rises above Pv in lung zone 2, or above pulmonary arterial pressure *(Pa)* in lung zone 1, wedge pressure will reflect alveolar pressure rather than intravascular pressure. *RA*, Right atrium; *RV*, right ventricle; *PA*, pulmonary artery; *LV*, left ventricle. (From Mark JB. *Atlas of Cardiovascular Monitoring*. New York: Churchill Livingstone; 1998, Fig. 6–10.)

resistance is low, the pressure in the pulmonary artery at end of diastole will equilibrate with downstream pressure in the pulmonary veins and left atrium.[294,295] From a monitoring standpoint, PAD has the added advantage of being available for continuous monitoring whereas PAWP is only measured intermittently.

In many situations, LV end-diastolic pressure can be either underestimated or overestimated by the PAWP and/or PAD. These situations are summarized in Figure 36.49 and Tables 36.5 and 36.6. The interested reader is referred to several excellent references for further discussion of this topic.[292,293,296]

However, even when PAD and wedge pressure accurately estimate LV end-diastolic pressure, many factors can influence the relationship between end-diastolic pressure and end-diastolic chamber volume, which is the true preload. Proper interpretation of filling pressures requires assessment of juxtacardiac pressure as well as ventricular compliance. When both are normal, a wedge pressure of 20 mm Hg is interpreted as hypervolemia, with an increased LV end-diastolic volume causing the increased PAWP. However, if juxtacardiac pressure is increased (e.g., due to cardiac tamponade, pericardial constriction, or positive pressure ventilation), or ventricular compliance is decreased (e.g., with myocardial ischemia, hypertrophy, or cardiomyopathy), a wedge pressure of 20 mm Hg can coexist with a small, hypovolemic left ventricle (Fig. 36.50).

In addition, ventricular interdependence (caused by the shared septum of the left and right ventricles) and pericardial constraint couple changes in RV and LV function. For example, acute pulmonary arterial hypertension increases RV end-diastolic volume and pressure, and shifts the ventricular septum leftward, thus increasing LV end-diastolic pressure while simultaneously decreasing LV end-diastolic volume. Conversely, primary changes on the left side can adversely affect the right heart structures in similar ways. With all these considerations in mind, it should be of no surprise that various studies have repeatedly shown that both CVP and PAWP may not always correlate with cardiac preload and do not necessarily predict the cardiac output response to a fluid challenge.[238,297] In contrast, in patients with systolic ventricular dysfunction, filling pressures were found more accurate than cardiac volume indices in predicting fluid responsiveness.[298]

PULMONARY ARTERY CATHETER-DERIVED HEMODYNAMIC VARIABLES

The cardiovascular system is often modeled as an electrical circuit, with the relationship between cardiac output, blood

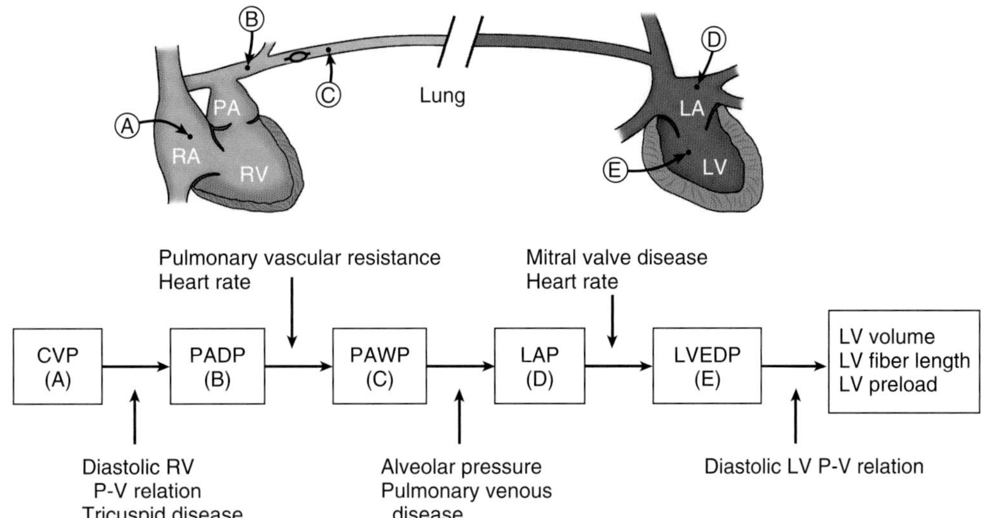

Fig. 36.49 Anatomic and physiologic factors that influence the relations between various measures of left ventricular *(LV)* filling and true LV preload. The further upstream the filling pressure is measured, the more confounding factors may influence the relation between this measurement and LV preload. *CVP*, Central venous pressure; *LA*, left atrium; *LAP*, left atrial pressure; *LVEDP*, left ventricular end-diastolic pressure; *PA*, pulmonary artery; *PADP*, pulmonary artery diastolic pressure; *PAWP*, pulmonary artery wedge pressure; *P-V*, pressure-volume; *RA*, right atrium; *RV*, right ventricle. (From Mark JB. *Atlas of Cardiovascular Monitoring*. New York: Churchill Livingstone; 1998.)

TABLE 36.5 Underestimation of Left Ventricular End-Diastolic Pressure

Condition	Site of Discrepancy	Cause of Discrepancy
Diastolic dysfunction	Mean LAP <LVEDP	Increased end-diastolic a wave
Aortic regurgitation	LAP a wave <LVEDP	Mitral valve closure before end-diastole
Pulmonic regurgitation	PADP <LVEDP	Bidirectional runoff for pulmonary artery flow
Right bundle branch block	PADP <LVEDP	Delayed pulmonic valve opening
Post-pneumonectomy	PAWP <LAP or LVEDP	Obstruction of pulmonary blood flow

LAP, Left atrial pressure; *LVEDP*, left ventricular end-diastolic pressure; *PADP*, pulmonary artery diastolic pressure; *PAWP*, pulmonary artery wedge pressure.

Modified from Mark JB. Predicting left ventricular end-diastolic pressure. In: Mark JB, ed. *Atlas of Cardiovascular Monitoring*. New York: Churchill Livingstone; 1998:59.

pressure, and resistance to flow related in a manner similar to Ohm's law:

$$PVR = \frac{MPAP - PAWP}{CO} \bullet (80)$$
$$SVR = \frac{MAP - CVP}{CO} \bullet (80) \quad (36.1)$$

Where,
SVR = systemic vascular resistance (dyne•s/cm^5)
PVR= pulmonary vascular resistance (dyne•s/cm^5)
MAP = mean arterial pressure (mm Hg)
CVP = central venous pressure (mm Hg)
MPAP = mean pulmonary artery pressure (mm Hg)
PAWP = pulmonary artery wedge pressure (mm Hg)
CO = cardiac output (L/min)

Normal values for SVR and PVR are given in Table 36.7. Note that these calculations of systemic and pulmonary vascular resistance are based on a hydraulic fluid model that assumes continuous, laminar flow through a series of rigid pipes.[299] This is an oversimplification. A more physiologic model of the systemic circulation considers the vasculature to be a series of collapsible vessels with intrinsic tone. This model, also called the vascular waterfall, describes a critical closing pressure in the downstream end of the circuit that exceeds right atrial pressure and serves to limit flow—an effective downstream pressure that is higher than the right

TABLE 36.6 Overestimation of Left Ventricular End-Diastolic Pressure

Condition	Site of Discrepancy	Cause of Discrepancy
Positive end-expiratory pressure	Mean PAWP >Mean LAP	Creation of lung zone 1 or 2, or pericardial pressure changes
Pulmonary arterial hypertension	PADP >Mean PAWP	Increased pulmonary vascular resistance
Pulmonary venoocclusive disease	Mean PAWP >Mean LAP	Obstruction to flow in large pulmonary veins
Mitral stenosis	Mean LAP >LVEDP	Obstruction to flow across mitral valve
Mitral regurgitation	Mean LAP >LVEDP	Retrograde systolic v wave raises mean atrial pressure
Ventricular septal defect	Mean LAP >LVEDP	Antegrade systolic v wave raises mean atrial pressure
Tachycardia	PADP >Mean LAP >LVEDP	Short diastole creates pulmonary vascular and mitral valve gradients

LAP, Left atrial pressure; *LVEDP*, left ventricular end-diastolic pressure; *PADP*, pulmonary artery diastolic pressure; *PAWP*, pulmonary artery wedge pressure.

Modified from Mark JB. Predicting left ventricular end-diastolic pressure. In: Mark JB, ed. *Atlas of Cardiovascular Monitoring*. New York: Churchill Livingstone; 1998:59.

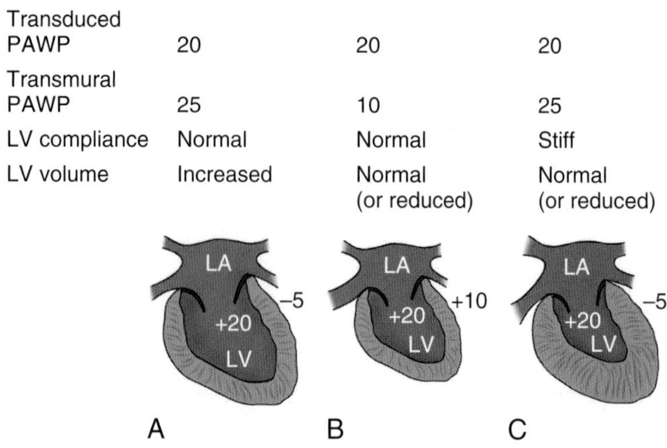

Fig. 36.50 Influence of juxtacardiac pressure and ventricular compliance on left ventricular *(LV)* preload. Three interpretations of an increased transduced pulmonary artery wedge pressure (*PAWP*, 20 mm Hg) are possible. (A) Juxtacardiac pressure (−5 mm Hg) and LV compliance are normal, transmural PAWP is increased (25 mm Hg), and LV volume is increased. (B) Juxtacardiac pressure is increased (+10 mm Hg), LV compliance is normal, transmural PAWP is decreased (10 mm Hg), and LV volume is normal or decreased. (C) Juxtacardiac pressure is normal, LV compliance is decreased, transmural PAWP is increased (25 mm Hg), and LV volume is normal or decreased. *LA*, Left atrial. (From Mark JB. *Atlas of Cardiovascular Monitoring*. New York: Churchill Livingstone; 1998.)

atrial pressure used in the SVR formula. A detailed consideration of these issues is beyond the scope of this discussion and is available in other sources.[300,301] The important point for clinicians, though, is that therapy focused on the fine adjustment of SVR may be very misleading and should be avoided.

Additional problems arise in considering the pulmonary vasculature and using the above formulae as a measure of resistance to flow through the lung.[302] The pulmonary vasculature is more compliant than the systemic vasculature, and marked increases in pulmonary blood flow may not produce any significant increase in PAP. In addition, flow usually ceases at end-diastole in the low resistance pulmonary circuit. Thus, changes in pulmonary vascular resistance may result from intrinsic alterations in pulmonary vascular tone (constriction or dilation), vascular recruitment, or rheologic changes. For the pulmonary circuit, a better approach to evaluating the changes in pulmonary vascular resistance may be to examine the pressure gradient between the PAD and wedge pressures, or the gradient between the mean pulmonary artery and wedge pressures (also termed the trans-pulmonary gradient).

Another set of common calculations derived from standard hemodynamic variables adjusts these measurements for the patient's body surface area (BSA) in an attempt to normalize these measurements for patients of different sizes. The BSA is generally determined from a standard nomogram based on height and weight. The most commonly indexed variables are the cardiac index (cardiac index = cardiac output/body surface area) and stroke volume index (stroke volume index = stroke volume/body surface area). On occasion, the systemic and pulmonary vascular resistances are indexed as well by multiplying by BSA. In theory, normalizing hemodynamic values through "indexing" should help clinicians determine appropriate normal physiologic ranges

TABLE 36.7 Normal Hemodynamic Values

	Average	Range
Cardiac output (L/min)	5.0	4.0-6.5
Stroke volume (mL)	75	60-90
Systemic vascular resistance (Wood units) (Dynes-sec-cm^{-5})	1200	800-1600
Pulmonary vascular resistance (Wood units) (Dynes-sec-cm^{-5})	80	40-180
Arterial oxygen content (mL/dL)	18	16-20
Mixed venous oxygen content (mL/dL)	14	13-15
Mixed venous oxygen saturation (%)	75	70-80
Arteriovenous oxygen difference (mL/dL)	4	3-5
Oxygen consumption (mL/min)	225	200-250

to help guide therapy. Unfortunately, there is little evidence that these additional calculations provide valid normalizing adjustments. BSA is a biometric measurement with an obscure relationship to blood flow and cardiac output, and it does not adjust for variations between individuals based on age, sex, body habitus, or metabolic rate.[303] Although it is important to be aware of a patient's size and medical history in interpreting and treating changes in any of the measured or calculated hemodynamic variables, it is not appropriate to target therapy solely at achieving normal indexed values.

PULMONARY ARTERY CATHETERIZATION: INDICATIONS AND OUTCOME CONTROVERSY

The PAC allows continuous tracking of hemodynamic variables, which seems particularly valuable in critically ill high-risk patients with circulatory dysfunction. Measurement of cardiac output (see below section on Thermodilution cardiac output) can separate shock states into hypovolemic etiology (low cardiac output with low filling pressures), cardiogenic etiology (low cardiac output and high filling pressures), and distributive etiology (high cardiac output and low SVR). Through measurement of cardiac output and left and right filling pressures (PAWP and CVP, respectively), it can separate out predominantly LV or RV dysfunction or global dysfunction. For RV dysfunction, the PAC allows distinction of RV dysfunction predominantly related to increased afterload (high PAP) versus dysfunction related mostly to pump failure (high CVP and low PAP).[304,305]

Despite these advantages, the PAC has stimulated a great deal of vigorous controversy.[306,307] It is an expensive, invasive technique that is widely used but still not proven to improve patient outcomes. This controversy was much fueled by a study published by Connors and associates in 1996, showing that PAC-monitored patients in the ICU had 20% increased mortality, increased length of hospital stay, and incurred increased costs.[308] The publication of this study was accompanied by a strongly worded editorial calling for a moratorium on PAC use or a randomized controlled trial to define its efficacy.[309]

Surrounding that time and in subsequent years, several large, randomized, adequately powered studies have been published regarding the use of the PAC in various settings: general non-cardiac surgery,[244] vascular surgery,[310] CABG surgery,[311,312] non-surgical patients with congestive heart failure,[313] patients with acute lung injury,[314] and critically ill patients in the ICU.[315] Generally, these studies have shown no benefit to PAC use, but also no increase in mortality or in hospital or ICU length of stay.

One common drawback to most of these large randomized studies is that they have necessarily examined the routine use of PAC and enrolled a sequential cohort of patients, most of them with a relatively moderate risk of death or complications. Also, not all of them have employed a specific therapeutic intervention protocol.[316] Indeed, in especially high-risk patients, marked either by old age, severe comorbidity, or increased disease acuity, several recent nonrandomized studies were indeed able to demonstrate a clinical benefit from PAC use.[317-320]

The most recent recommendations pertaining to the perioperative use of PACs are the ASA practice guidelines published in 2003.[252] The task force considered PAC monitoring to be appropriate in high-risk surgical patients undergoing high-risk procedures. Furthermore, the specific practice setting as well as the proficiency and experience of clinicians should be considered.

PAC use must be tailored to the degree of risk for the patient and the risk posed by the procedure itself. For example, a patient with advanced ischemic cardiomyopathy who needs lower extremity amputation under regional anesthesia would not warrant PAC monitoring while a patient with stable ischemic heart disease scheduled for extensive abdominal cancer resection may benefit from perioperative use. Furthermore, practice setting must be considered such as the operators' technical skill, knowledge, and experience in PAC use.[252]

A reasonable conclusion from the bulk of published research would be that PAC use should be limited, although a moratorium on use is ill-advised. Indeed, data demonstrate a significant and continuing decrease in PAC usage.[321] Use should be reserved to centers with significant experience and expertise. The PAC generally should be used to monitor and guide therapy in patients at high risk for hemodynamic instability, those who are judged more critically ill by a variety of clinical means, and those who are in shock, especially if elderly and suffering from other systemic diseases.

Obviously, the PAC itself has no potential for benefit unless it guides therapies that improve patient outcomes. Future research should focus on defining subgroups of patients who might benefit from use of the PAC, as well as defining effective therapeutic interventions based on the hemodynamic information gained from the PAC.[316,322,323] Heart failure patients in shock are one such population for which data from clinical registries suggest benefit despite lack of confirmatory evidence from randomized trials.[323,324]

SPECIAL TYPES OF PULMONARY ARTERY CATHETERS

Specific PAC modifications were designed to allow for continuous cardiac output (CCO) measurement (described in the Cardiac Output section), mixed venous oxygen saturation monitoring, or right heart function evaluation, vastly expanding the types of physiologic information available to those caring for critically ill patients.

Mixed Venous Oximetry Pulmonary Artery Catheter

Although the formal Fick cardiac output method is not widely applied in clinical practice outside the cardiac catheterization laboratory, the physiologic relations described by the Fick equation form the basis for another PAC-based monitoring technique termed continuous mixed venous oximetry.[325] Rearrangement of the Fick equation reveals the four determinants of mixed venous hemoglobin saturation ($S_{\bar{v}}O_2$):

$$S_{\bar{v}}O_2 = S_aO_2 - \frac{\dot{V}O_2}{\dot{Q} \bullet 1.36 \bullet Hgb} \qquad (36.2)$$

Where,

$S_{\bar{v}}O_2$ = mixed venous hemoglobin saturation (%)
S_aO_2 = arterial hemoglobin saturation (%)
$\dot{V}O_2$ = oxygen consumption (mL•O_2/min)
$\dot{Q}$ = cardiac output (L/min)
Hgb = hemoglobin concentration (g/dL)

To the extent that arterial hemoglobin saturation, oxygen consumption, and hemoglobin concentration remain stable, mixed venous hemoglobin saturation may be used as an indirect indicator of cardiac output. Thus, when cardiac output falls, tissue oxygen extraction increases and the mixed venous blood will have a lower hemoglobin oxygen saturation. Monitoring this variable provides more comprehensive information about the balance of oxygen delivery and consumption by the body—not just the cardiac output value, but also the adequacy of that cardiac output compared to tissue oxygen requirements.[325] It is important to remember that mixed venous hemoglobin saturation values reflect global, whole-body measurement. Therefore, regionally inadequate blood flow and tissue oxygen delivery (like limb or intestinal ischemia) can coexist with a normal or high mixed venous hemoglobin saturation.

Although mixed venous hemoglobin saturation may be determined by intermittent blood sampling from the distal port of the PAC, a specially designed PAC can provide this information reliably and continuously. Fiberoptic bundles incorporated into the PAC determine the hemoglobin oxygen saturation in pulmonary artery blood based on the principles of reflectance oximetry using either a two or three wavelength system. A special computer connected to this PAC displays the mixed venous hemoglobin saturation continuously. The technology is typically incorporated into the standard PAC or the CCO PAC (see later), in the latter case providing both CCO and venous oximetry data. These catheters are calibrated at the bedside prior to use but may also be calibrated in vivo from a pulmonary artery blood gas sample. Recalibration every 24 hours is usually recommended due to a drift artifact.

Recently, the technology to continuously measure oxygen saturation has been incorporated into central venous catheters as well. These catheters measure central venous saturation, measured in the superior vena cava. Normally, this saturation is around 70% versus 75% in the pulmonary artery.[325] Low central venous saturation has been associated with increased complications both in trauma patients and in major surgery patients.[326,327]

The real value of measuring venous oxygen saturation lies in its ability to guide therapeutic interventions. Because one of the body's physiologic compensations for anemia is increased oxygen extraction, low venous hemoglobin saturation has been used to guide the need for blood transfusion.[328] Several studies have used venous hemoglobin saturation to guide interventions aimed at increasing cardiac output—a goal-directed approach. A study in patients undergoing cardiac surgery has shown better outcomes in patients randomized to protocol-driven interventions aimed at achieving mixed venous hemoglobin saturation above 70% (and blood lactate <2mg/dL).[329] Similarly, optimizing the central venous oxygen saturation has been shown to improve outcome in high-risk non-cardiac and off-pump cardiac surgical patients.[330,331] Although an early study showed similar benefit in patients with early sepsis,[332] a more recent study could not confirm these results.[333]

It is important to note that these studies have employed strict protocol-driven therapeutic interventions. In contrast, a large Veterans Affairs observational trial of 3265 cardiac surgical patients noted that 49% of patients received continuous mixed venous oximetry PACs, and use of this catheter was associated with increased cost but no better outcome than the standard PAC group.[334] In this study, however, no protocol was used to guide therapeutic interventions based on monitoring results.

Right Ventricular Ejection Fraction Pulmonary Artery Catheter

Although cardiovascular monitoring has focused predominantly on LV performance, in some instances RV dysfunction may be the more important factor limiting circulation. Patient populations at increased risk for RV dysfunction include those with chronic obstructive pulmonary disease, adult respiratory distress syndrome, pulmonary hypertension, and RV ischemia and infarction.[335]

Measurement of right ventricular ejection fraction (RVEF) with a specially designed PAC offers another method for evaluating RV function. This method uses a standard PAC equipped with a rapid response thermistor that detects and quantifies the small changes in pulmonary artery blood temperature that occur with each heartbeat, in a manner somewhat analogous to a standard CCO PAC. The cardiac output computer measures the residual fraction of thermal signal following each heart beat and derives the RVEF.[336] RV end-diastolic volume can be calculated from RVEF and stroke volume, and can be used as an index of RV preload. Clearly, all factors that confound standard thermodilution cardiac output measurement (described later) will also interfere with accurate determination of RVEF. In addition, because the temperature changes measured by the RVEF PAC are small beat-to-beat changes, the method will not work if the ECG R waves cannot be detected accurately, the R-R interval is short owing to tachycardia, or the cardiac rhythm is irregular.[337]

Clinical use of the RVEF PAC has been described in critically ill patients, especially in those with respiratory failure,[338,339] as well as intraoperatively during cardiac surgery, where a reduced RVEF has been noted following cardiopulmonary bypass, particularly in patients with preexisting right coronary artery obstruction.[340] However, as in the case of standard PAC monitoring, the benefit of RVEF PAC monitoring in terms of patient outcomes remains unproven.[252]

Cardiac Output Monitoring

Cardiac output is the total blood flow generated by the heart, and in a normal adult at rest ranges from 4.0 to 6.5 L/min. Measurement of cardiac output provides a global assessment of the circulation, and in combination with other hemodynamic measurements (heart rate, arterial blood pressure, CVP, PAP, and wedge pressure), it allows calculation of additional important circulatory variables, such as systemic and pulmonary vascular resistance and ventricular stroke work (see Table 36.7).

Three factors have driven efforts to measure cardiac output in clinical practice. The first is the recognition that in many critically ill patients, low cardiac output leads to significant morbidity and mortality.[341] Secondly, clinical assessment of cardiac output is often inaccurate; for example, seriously ill patients with decreased cardiac output might have normal systemic arterial blood pressures.[342] Finally, newer techniques for cardiac output measurement are becoming less invasive and thus might provide benefit to many patients without the attendant risks of invasive monitoring.[342,343] The advantages and disadvantages of each technique must be appreciated for proper clinical application.

THERMODILUTION CARDIAC OUTPUT MONITORING

The thermodilution technique is considered the gold standard for measuring cardiac output because of its ease of implementation and the long clinical experience with its use in various settings. It is a variant of the **indicator dilution** method, in which a known amount of a tracer substance is injected into the blood stream and its concentration change is measured over time at a downstream site.[344] For thermodilution, a known volume of room temperature fluid is injected as a bolus into the proximal (right atrium) lumen of the PAC, and the resulting change in the pulmonary artery blood temperature is recorded by the thermistor at the catheter tip. In adults, an injectate volume of 10 mL should be used, while in children, an injectate volume of 0.15 mL/kg is recommended.[345] As in all other forms of cardiovascular monitoring, it is important to have a real-time display of the thermodilution curve resulting from each cardiac output measurement.[345] This allows the clinician to discern artifacts that would invalidate the cardiac output measurement, such as unstable blood temperature, recirculation, or incomplete indicator injection.

Usually three cardiac output measurements performed in rapid succession are averaged to provide a more reliable result. If only a single injection is used to determine cardiac output, a difference between sequential cardiac output measurements of 22% is required to suggest a clinically significant change. In contrast, when three injections are

BOX 36.8 Factors Influencing Accuracy of Thermodilution Cardiac Output Measurement

Intracardiac shunts
Tricuspid or pulmonic valve regurgitation
Inadequate delivery of thermal indicator
  Central venous injection site within catheter introducer sheath
  Warming of iced injectate
Thermistor malfunction from fibrin or clot
Pulmonary artery blood temperature fluctuations
  Following cardiopulmonary bypass
  Rapid intravenous fluid administration
Respiratory cycle influences

averaged to determine the thermodilution measurement, a change greater than 13% indicates a clinically significant change in cardiac output.[346]

Even when carefully performed, some studies have found that thermodilution cardiac output measurements may not agree with other reference methods.[347,348] However, few complications are directly attributable to the technique itself, and following the trend in cardiac output is probably more clinically useful than emphasizing any absolute value.

Sources of Error in Thermodilution Cardiac Output Monitoring

Several important technical issues and potential sources of error must be considered to interpret thermodilution cardiac output measurements properly (Box 36.8).[344,345] The thermodilution technique measures RV output. With **intracardiac shunt**, RV and LV outputs will not be equal.

Patients with **tricuspid or pulmonic valve regurgitation** pose additional problems for thermodilution cardiac output measurement owing to recirculation of the indicator across the incompetent valve. Although minor degrees of valvular regurgitation have little effect on thermodilution cardiac output monitoring, these values are unreliable with more severe valvular regurgitation, either underestimated or overestimated, depending on the severity of valvular regurgitation and the magnitude of the cardiac output.[345,349]

Unrecognized **fluctuation in blood temperature** may also influence cardiac output measurement. In most patients, pulmonary artery blood temperature falls somewhat in the initial minutes **following cardiopulmonary bypass,** when the rewarmed vascular and vessel rich tissues redistribute the heat gained to the less well perfused body core. Therefore, the thermal baseline is unstable and measurements made in the minutes following bypass are notoriously unreliable, most often leading to marked underestimation of the true cardiac output.[350] Pulmonary artery blood temperature can also change due to **rapid fluid infusion.**[351]

One controversy surrounding bolus thermodilution cardiac output monitoring is the proper timing of measurement in relation to the **respiratory cycle**, particularly in patients receiving positive pressure mechanical ventilation, because RV stroke output varies as much as 50% during the respiratory cycle. Although reproducibility of consecutive measurements improves markedly when the bolus injections are synchronized to the same phase of the respiratory cycle, an accurate measurement of average cardiac output is achieved more reliably by making multiple injections during the different phases of the respiratory cycle and then averaging the results.[345,352]

Last, the measured thermodilution cardiac output can overestimate true cardiac output during low flow states because of significant heat loss from slow injectate transit.[353]

Continuous Thermodilution Cardiac Output Monitoring

Newer technologies applied to PAC monitoring allow nearly continuous cardiac output monitoring using warm thermal indicator.[344,354] In brief, small quantities of heat are released from a 10-cm thermal filament incorporated into the RV portion of a PAC, approximately 15 to 25 cm from the catheter tip, and the resulting thermal signal is measured by the thermistor at the tip of the catheter in the pulmonary artery. The heating filament is cycled on and off in a pseudorandom binary sequence, and the cardiac output is derived from cross correlation of the measured pulmonary artery temperature with the known sequence of heating filament activation.[354] Typically, the displayed value for cardiac output is updated every 30 to 60 seconds and represents the average value for the cardiac output measured over the previous 3 to 6 minutes. On the one hand, this will lead to a delayed response during unstable hemodynamic conditions.[355] On the other hand, reproducibility and precision appear to be better compared with the single instantaneous bolus thermodilution technique, especially during positive pressure ventilation.[356,357]

The CCO PAC has been widely accepted into clinical use for a number of practical reasons. Although these catheters are more expensive than standard PACs, obviating the need for bolus injections reduces nursing workload and the potential risk of fluid overload or infection. However, like cold bolus thermodilution techniques, warm thermal CCO has certain methodological pitfalls that must be recognized and avoided. The CCO computer and catheter require a significant amount of time to warm up and may work poorly in an environment where there is a great deal of thermal noise, such as the cardiac operating room. Recent observations also suggest that the use of pneumatic compression devices may introduce artifacts that appear as large variations (oscillations) in CCO values in otherwise stable patients.[358] As already emphasized, CCO monitors have an inherent 5- to 15-minute delay in responding to abrupt changes in cardiac output, and the magnitude of this delay depends on the type of physiologic perturbation, as well as the CCO computer monitor algorithm.[355] Although modifications of CCO algorithms provide a "STAT Mode" rapid response time, acute changes in cardiac output are still detected more slowly by CCO monitoring than by other methods, such as direct arterial pressure or mixed venous oximetry. In effect, the CCO technique involves a fundamental tradeoff between rapid response time and overall accuracy and stability of the displayed value.[356] While it might be useful for clinical decision making, no studies exist that demonstrate improved patient outcomes from use of the CCO PAC.

Transpulmonary Thermodilution Cardiac Output

For transpulmonary thermodilution measurement, ice-cold saline is injected into a central venous line while the change in temperature is measured in a large peripheral artery (femoral, axillary, or brachial artery) via a special arterial catheter equipped with a thermistor.[359] Several studies have shown adequate agreement with standard thermodilution cardiac output.[360,361] In contrast to the standard thermodilution method, the transpulmonary thermodilution measurement lasts over several respiratory cycles and thereby obviates the respiratory effects on stroke volume and measured cardiac output.[362]

Mathematical derivation from the transpulmonary thermodilution curve can produce several additional useful indices. Extravascular lung water is a measure of pulmonary edema and can be used to guide fluid therapy in patients with acute lung injury or sepsis.[363-365] Other derived indices are the global end-diastolic volume and intrathoracic blood volume. Several studies have found these indices to be a better measure of cardiac preload than traditional measurements such as CVP or PAWP.[366,367] However, it appears that these indices still cannot predict cardiac output response to fluid loading.[368] Another parameter derived from the transpulmonary thermodilution curve is the cardiac function index, calculated using cardiac output and the intrathoracic blood volume. In patients without RV failure, it has been shown to correlate with LV ejection fraction and its response to inotropic therapy.[369]

LITHIUM DILUTION CARDIAC OUTPUT MONITORING

The lithium dilution technique is another cardiac output monitoring method that derives its fundamental basis from indicator dilution principles.[370] In brief, following an intravenous bolus injection of a small dose of lithium chloride, an ion-selective electrode attached to a peripheral arterial catheter measures the lithium dilution curve, from which the cardiac output is derived. Several studies have shown that this is an accurate technique compared with standard thermodilution or electromagnetic flowmetry.[371,372] The lithium indicator can be injected through a peripheral intravenous catheter with similar measurement accuracy, thus eliminating the need for a central venous line.[373] This technique can also be used in children.[374] Lithium dilution cannot be used in patients who are taking lithium or those who have just received nondepolarizing neuromuscular blockers, since the latter also alter the lithium sensor electrode measurement.

OTHER METHODS FOR MONITORING CARDIAC OUTPUT AND PERFUSION

In recent years, much work has been dedicated to developing minimal or non-invasive methods to measure cardiac output. While it seems that these methods' overall agreement with the traditional thermodilution method is not very high,[375] they do offer other advantages. Some of these newer methods are discussed herein.

Esophageal Doppler Cardiac Output Monitoring

All of the ultrasound-based methods for cardiac output monitoring employ the Doppler principle as described in detail in Chapter 37. While cardiac output can be intermittently measured by the Doppler technique during transthoracic or transesophageal echocardiography examinations, for monitoring purposes, a special esophageal Doppler probe has been developed that allows continuous monitoring of cardiac output by measuring the Doppler shift of the interrogated blood flow in the descending thoracic aorta. The Doppler probe is inserted into the esophagus to a depth of approximately 35 cm from the incisor teeth and is adjusted to optimize the audible Doppler flow sound from the descending aorta, which lies in close proximity and runs essentially parallel to the esophagus at this location.[376]

Several limitations of the esophageal Doppler technique must be appreciated by the physician to avoid pitfalls in data interpretation. This monitoring method interrogates blood flow in the descending thoracic aorta and therefore only measures a fraction of total cardiac output. To report total cardiac output, either the esophageal Doppler measurement must be "calibrated" by some alternative method, or an empirically determined correction constant of 1.4 is used.[376] This constant is accurate for most patients but does not apply universally, especially in the presence of conditions that redistribute blood flow, such as pregnancy, aortic cross-clamping, and following cardiopulmonary bypass.[377,378] In addition, the descending thoracic aorta diameter is either measured using A-mode ultrasound or calculated from a nomogram based on the patient's age, sex, height, and weight.[376] When calculated, it is assumed that the aortic diameter does not change throughout the cardiac cycle. In addition to these considerations, the technique is likely to be inaccurate in the presence of aortic valve stenosis or regurgitation, or in patients with thoracic aortic disease. It is not easily applied in nontracheally intubated non-sedated patients, and it cannot be used in individuals with esophageal pathology. Finally, like all ultrasound techniques, the acoustic window needed to acquire the Doppler signal may not be adequate in some individuals, thereby precluding use of this method.

Advantages of the esophageal Doppler monitoring technique include its ease of use, minimal invasiveness, and inherent safety. It appears that limited experience is needed for clinical success—as few as 10 to 12 cases for accurate application of the technique.[377] A review of 25 clinical trials comparing esophageal Doppler cardiac output measurement with PAC thermodilution measurements noted that the Doppler cardiac output values correlated well with thermodilution measurements and showed minimal overall bias and good tracking of directional changes in thermodilution cardiac output with low intra- and inter-observer measurement variability.[377]

Recently, the esophageal Doppler method has seen renewed popularity.[379,380] Current devices provide a clear visual display of the spectral Doppler waveform and also calculate and display additional hemodynamic variables including the peak blood flow velocity, flow acceleration, and heart rate-corrected flow time (Fig. 36.51). Some studies have shown that these additional measures provide useful information about LV preload, fluid responsiveness, contractility, and systemic vascular resistance.[381-383] Additionally, respiratory variability of the aortic blood flow velocity can be used to predict cardiac output response to a fluid bolus.[384] One of the more important benefits of this monitor may be focusing clinical attention on optimizing

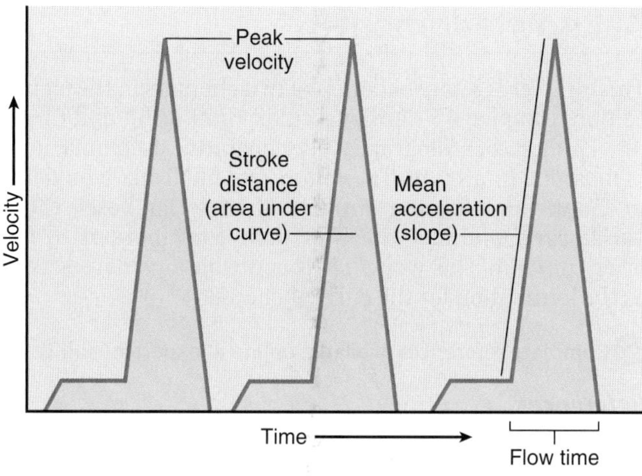

Predominant change in waveform

Physiologic change from baseline state	FTc	SD	PV
↑ Preload	↑	↑	↔
↓ Preload	↓	↓	↔
↑ Afterload	↓	↓	↓
↓ Afterload	↑	↑	↑
↑ Contractility	↔	↑	↑
↓ Contractility	↔	↔ *	↓

* Rounding of waveform

Fig. 36.51 The velocity-time waveform displayed by esophageal Doppler cardiac output monitoring devices reflects alterations in contractility, preload, and afterload. Stroke distance *(SD)* is directly related to calculated stroke volume and provides a useful surrogate measure of cardiac output. *FTc,* Systolic flow time corrected for heart rate; *PV,* peak velocity.

stroke volume rather than total cardiac output. Indeed, in critically ill patients, complications may be better predicted by low stroke volume than by low cardiac output.[385] Several studies have shown that hemodynamic optimization, guided by maximizing esophageal Doppler-measured stroke volume in moderate-risk surgical patients, reduces perioperative morbidity and shortens hospital stay.[379,380,386]

Bioimpedance and Bioreactance Cardiac Output Monitoring

The technique of bioimpedance cardiac output monitoring was first described by Kubicek and associates and is based on changes in electrical impedance of the thoracic cavity or the whole body occurring with ejection of blood during cardiac systole.[387] As blood has a significantly lower electrical resistance compared with tissues, changes in impedance to electrical flow reflect a change in blood volume, and this can be used to calculate stroke volume.[388]

For bioimpedance measurement, disposable electrodes are applied to the skin surface along the sides of the neck and lateral aspect of the costal margin (thoracic bioimpedance) or to the four limbs (whole body bioimpedance); a high-frequency, low-amplitude electrical current is applied; and the voltage change is measured. Patient height, weight, and gender are used to calculate the volume of the thoracic cavity. Bioimpedance cardiac output is computed for each cardiac cycle and continuously displayed as an average value over several heart beats.

Although many studies suggest that the bioimpedance method is accurate in healthy volunteers, its reliability deteriorates in surgical and critically ill patients.[389] This led to attempts at improving the technology used. A newer technique, termed bioreactance cardiac output monitoring, measures not only the amplitude change of the received signal, but also its phase shift compared to the applied electrical signal. It utilizes four dual-electrode patches, placed two on each side of the body.[388] Compared to the standard bioimpedance method, the bioreactance method shows somewhat better agreement with traditional cardiac output calculations. Several clinical scenarios where this new method has been validated include the prediction of fluid responsiveness when using the passive leg raising test in patients after cardiac surgery and evaluating cardiac output change during exercise stress testing.[388]

Partial CO_2 Rebreathing Cardiac Output Monitoring

Another method for cardiac output monitoring that does not require a PAC is the partial CO_2 rebreathing technique.[390,391] Owing to the difficulty encountered in the standard Fick method involving measuring oxygen consumption and mixed venous hemoglobin saturation, this alternative technique is based upon a restatement of the Fick Equation for carbon dioxide elimination rather than oxygen uptake.

$$\dot{Q} = \frac{\dot{V}CO_2}{(C_{\bar{v}}CO_2 - C_aCO_2)} \qquad (36.3)$$

Where,

$\dot{Q}$ = cardiac output
$\dot{V}CO_2$ = rate of carbon dioxide elimination
$C_{\bar{v}}CO_2$ = carbon dioxide content of mixed venous blood
C_aCO_2 = carbon dioxide content of arterial blood

This method uses the change in CO_2 production and end-tidal CO_2 concentration in response to a brief, sudden change in minute ventilation. With a specifically designed breathing system and monitoring computer, this measurement is easily performed in any tracheally intubated patient. Changes in end-tidal CO_2 in response to the rebreathing maneuver are used to calculate cardiac output by a differential version of the Fick equation for carbon dioxide. The attractive features of this method are that it is entirely noninvasive, it can be performed every few minutes, and the brief episodes of rebreathing pose no substantial risk to most patients, with end-tidal CO_2 measurements increasing by less than 3 mm Hg. However, as currently designed, accurate measurements with this technique require tracheal intubation for precise measurement of exhaled gasses. Furthermore, changing patterns of ventilation may have an unpredictable influence on the measurement. As with all Fick-based techniques, the partial CO_2 rebreathing method measures pulmonary capillary blood flow as an indicator of total cardiac output and thus requires correction for pulmonary shunt.

Initial clinical trials suggested reasonably good agreement between the partial rebreathing CO_2 cardiac output method and other techniques, such as thermodilution. However, as with most of these alternative monitoring methods, the clinical trials are small and mainly focused on specific patient groups, particularly coronary artery bypass surgery patients.[392] At present, the clinical role for this technique is mainly focused on short-term intraoperative applications or mechanically ventilated postoperative patients. Due to the mandatory increase in arterial pCO_2, the technique is relatively contraindicated in patients with increased intracranial pressure.

Pulse Contour Cardiac Output Monitoring

Much of recent development in the area of cardiac output monitoring has been focused on continuous measurement of cardiac output derived from the analysis of the arterial pulse pressure waveform. These methods, generally termed pulse contour cardiac output, determine stroke volume from computerized analysis of the area under the arterial pressure waveform recorded from an arterial catheter or even a noninvasive finger blood pressure waveform.[393-396] Pulse contour methods offer the potential for non-invasive, continuous, beat-to-beat cardiac output monitoring. Also, the change in stroke volume from beat to beat (termed SVV) in response to tidal ventilation can be used to evaluate volume status in ventilated patients.[147,397]

However, several shortcomings need to be considered.[398,399] First, a baseline calibration with a known cardiac output is required to account for individual differences in vascular resistance, impedance, and wave reflectance. Additionally, recalibration is required every 8 to 12 hours to account for changes in vascular characteristics over time. Also, the use of vasopressors might affect the accuracy of pulse contour methods.[400] This need for external calibration might require the use of a more invasive technique, negating the non-invasiveness advantage of pulse contour methods. Recently, several systems were developed with the capability for an auto-calibration based on a patient's demographic variables. However, the accuracy of this auto-calibration in various clinical situations is questionable.[401] A reasonably well-defined arterial pressure waveform with a discernible dicrotic notch is required for accurate identification of systole and diastole, a condition that might not exist under severe tachycardia or dysrhythmia, or other very low-output states. Last, for a meaningful use of beat-to-beat variation in stroke volume (as well as systolic pressure or PPV), the patient needs to be on controlled mechanical ventilation with a tidal volume of at least 8 mL/kg body weight and to be in a regular cardiac rhythm.[402]

Notwithstanding these shortcomings, clinical trials in surgical patients have shown that the pulse contour cardiac output methods provide an acceptable level of accuracy with a bias of less than 0.5 L/min compared to thermodilution cardiac output.[395,403,404] SVV above 10% has been shown to be a useful predictor of fluid responsiveness.[138] Last, several recent studies have shown that goal-directed therapy based on either maximizing pulse contour derived cardiac output or minimizing SVV results in improved perioperative outcomes.[405-407]

Acknowledgment

This chapter is a consolidation of two chapters in the eighth edition, Chapter 45 Cardiovascular Monitoring and Chapter 47 Electrocardiography, Perioperative Ischemia, and Myocardial Infarction. The editors and publisher would like to thank the following authors: Shahar Bar-Yosef, Giora Landesberg, and Zak Hillel for their contributions to the prior edition of this work. Their contributions have served as the foundation for the current chapter.

Complete references available online at expertconsult.com.

References

1. Gravenstein JS. *J Clin Monit Comput*. 1998;14:451.
2. Block FE. *J Clin Monit*. 1994;10:366.
3. Zong W, et al. *Med Biol Eng Comput*. 2004;42(5):698.
4. American Society of Anesthesiologists. *Standards for basic anesthetic monitoring. ASA standards, guidelines and statements*. Park Ridge, Illinois: American Society of Anesthesiologists; 1993:5.
5. Sandau KE, et al. *Circ*. 2017;136:e273–e344.
6. Kligfield P, et al. *Journal of the American College of Cardiology*. 2007;49:1109–1127.
7. Ortega R, et al. *N Engl J Med*. 2015;372:e11.
8. Mason RE, Likar I. *Am Heart Jnl*. 1966;71:196–205.
9. Krucoff MW, et al. *Am J Card*. 1994;74:997–1001.
10. Drew BJ. *Cardiol Clin*. 2006;24:309–315. vii.
11. Chaitman BR, Hanson JS. *Am J Card*. 1981;47:1335–1349.
12. Blackburn H, Katigbak R. *Am Heart Jnl*. 1964;67:184–185.
13. Kubota I, et al. *Am Heart Jnl*. 1985;110:949–955.
14. Kaplan JA, et al. *Anesth Analg*. 1978;57:364–367.
15. London MJ, et al. *Anesthesiology*. 1988;69:232–241.
16. Landesberg G, et al. *Anesthesiology*. 2002;96:264–270.
17. Klein HO, et al. *Circ*. 1983;67:558–565.
18. Griffin RM, Kaplan JA. *Anaesthesia*. 1987;42:155–159.
19. Slogoff S, et al. *Anesthesiology*. 1990;73:1074–1081.
20. Takla G, et al. *Anesth Analg*. 2006;103:1196–1204.
21. Weinfurt PT. *J Clin Monitor*. 1990;6:132–138.
22. Khambatta HJ, et al. *Anesth Analg*. 1990;71:88–91.
23. Patel SI, Souter MJ. *Anesthesiology*. 2008;108:138–148.
24. Patton JA, et al. *Am J Crit Care: an official publication, American Association of Critical-Care Nurses*. 2001;10:23–32. quiz 3-4.
25. Mark JB, et al. *Anesth Analg*. 1992;74:26–31.
26. Stern S. *Card Electro Rev*. 2002;6:204–208.
27. Helwani MA, et al. *Anesthesiology*. 2018;128:1084–1091.
28. Miller TD, et al. *J Electrocard*. 1987;20:131–137.
29. ASA, Standards for Basic Anesthetic Monitoring. 2005. (Accessed May 5, 2008, 2008, at http://www.asahq.org/publicationsAndServices/standards/02.pdf.)
30. Bruner JMR, et al. *Med Instrum*. 1981;15:11.
31. Riva-Rocci S. *Gaz Med Torino*. 1896;47:981.
32. Korotkoff NS. *Bull Imp Med Acad St Petersburg*. 1905;11:365.
33. Kuck K, Baker PD. *Anesth Analg*. 2018 Aug;127(2):408–411.
34. Alpert BS, et al. *J Am Soc Hyper: JASH*. 2014;8:930–938.
35. Lakhal K, et al. *Chest*. 2017.
36. Pickering TG, et al. *Hypertension*. 2005;45(1):142.
37. Cohn JN. *JAMA*. 1967;199:972.
38. Lakhal K, et al. *Crit Care Med*. 2012;40(4):1207.
39. Ribezzo S, et al. *Sci World Jnl*. 2014;2014:353628.
40. Wan Y, et al. *J Hum Hypertens*. 2010;24(7):431.
41. AAMI. American national standard for non-invasive sphygmomanometers—part 2: clinical validation of automated measurement type. *AAMI*. 2009;25.
42. Lakhal K, et al. *Anesth Analg*. 2009;109(2):494.
43. Liu B, et al. *Blood pressure*. 2016;25:155–161.
44. Riley LE, et al. *Blood pressure monitoring*. 2017;22:202–207.
45. Wax DB, et al. *Anesthesiology*. 2011;115(5):973.
46. Jankowski P, et al. *Hypertension*. 2008;51:848–855.
47. Min JY, et al. *BMC anesthesiology*. 2017;17:110.
48. Leblanc ME, et al. *Obesity (Silver Spring, Md)*. 2013;21:E533–E541.
49. Celler BG, et al. *Annual Conference*. 2015;2015:5964–5967.
50. Lakhal K, et al. *J Clin Monit Comput*. 2017.

51. Anast N, et al. *Can J Anesth* 2016;63:298-306.
52. Benmira A, et al. *Expert review of medical devices*. 2016;13:179–189.
53. Alford JW, et al. *J Clin Monit Comput*. 2002;17:163.
54. Kuck K, et al. *J Clin Monit*. 1997;13:424.
55. Tobias JD, et al. *Anesthesia*. 2014;28:861–865.
56. Kim SH, et al. *Anesthesiology*. 2014;120:1080–1097.
57. Balzer F, et al. *J Int Med Res*. 2016;44:832–843.
58. Benes J, et al. *J Clin Monit Comput*. 2015;29:11–17.
59. Bilo G, et al. *Blood Pressure Monitoring*. 2015;20:291–294.
60. Dueck R, et al. *J Clin Monit Comput*. 2012;26:75–83.
61. Belani K, et al. *Anesthesiology*. 1999;91(3):686.
62. Weiss BM, Pasch T. *Curr Opin Anaesthesiol*. 1997;10:459.
63. Cockings JGL, et al. *Anaesth Intensive Care*. 1993;21:565.
64. Eather KF, et al. *Anesthesiology*. 1949;10:125.
65. Mark JB. *Atlas of cardiovascular monitoring*. New York: Churchill Livingstone; 1998.
66. Perel A. *Anesthesiology*. 1998;89:1309–1310.
67. Rooke GA. *Curr Opin Anesth*. 1995;8:511–515.
68. Thiele RH, et al. *Can J Anesth*. 2015;62:169–181.
69. Gabriel RA, et al. *J Clin Monit Comput*. 2017;31:877–884.
70. Mandel MA, Dauchot PJ. *J Hand Surg*. 1977;2(6):482.
71. Scheer B, et al. *Crit Care*. 2002;6(3):199.
72. Slogoff S, et al. *Anesthesiology*. 1983;59:42.
73. Brzezinski M, et al. *Anesth Analg*. 2009;109(6):1763.
74. Knobloch K, et al. *Ann Thorac Surg*. 2005;80(3):918.
75. Knobloch K, et al. *Ann Thorac Surg*. 2005;79(3):1026. discussion 30.
76. Ciria-Llorens G, et al. *Surg Radiol Anat*. 1998;20(5):377.
77. Ciria-Llorens G, et al. *Br J Plast Surg*. 1999;52(6):440.
78. Richardson D, et al. *Plast Reconstr Surg*. 1997;99(1):109.
79. Allen EV. *Am J Med Sci*. 1929;178:237.
80. Wilkins RG. *Anaesthesia*. 1985;40(9):896.
81. Abu-Omar Y, et al. *Ann Thorac Surg*. 2004;77(1):116.
82. Barbeau GR, et al. *Am Heart J*. 2004;147(3):489.
83. Jarvis MA, et al. *Ann Thorac Surg*. 2000;70(4):1362.
84. Rozenberg B, et al. *Anaesthesia*. 1988;43(6):515.
85. Williams JS, et al. *N Engl J Med*. 2009;360(5):e6.
86. Levin PD, et al. *Crit Care Med*. 2003;31(2):481.
87. Ganesh A, et al. *Pediatr Crit Care Med*. 2009;10(1):45.
88. Shiver S, et al. *Acad Emerg Med*. 2006;13(12):1275.
89. Ueda K, et al. *Anaesthesia*. 2015;70:1039–1044.
90. Gu WJ, et al. *Chest*. 2016;149:166–179.
91. Htet N, et al. *J Crit Care*. 2017;41:194–197.
92. Karacalar S, et al. *J Clin Anesth*. 2007;19(3):209.
93. Bazaral MG, et al. *Anesthesiology*. 1990;73:38.
94. Singh A, et al. *Anesthesiology*. 2017;126:1065–1076.
95. Muralidhar K. *J Cardiothorac Vasc Anesth*. 1998;12(1):128.
96. Chen Y, et al. *Blood pressure monitoring*. 2016;21:27–32.
97. Rehfeldt KH, Sanders MS. *Anesth Analg*. 2000;90:45.
98. Rose SH. *Anesthesiology*. 1993;78:587.
99. Singleton RJ, et al. *Anaesth Intensive Care*. 1993;21:664.
100. Bhananker SM, et al. *Anesth Analg*. 2009;109(1):124.
101. Gardner RM. *Anesthesiology*. 1981;54:227.
102. Kleinman B. *J Clin Monit*. 1989;5:137.
103. Kleinman B, et al. *Anesthesiology*. 1992;77:1215.
104. O'Quin R, Marini JJ. *Am Rev Respir Dis*. 1983;128:319.
105. Mark JB. Technical requirements for direct blood pressure measurement. In: Mark JB, ed. *Atlas of cardiovascular monitoring*. New York: Churchill Livingstone; 1998:99.
106. Geddes LA. *Handbook of blood pressure measurement*. Clifton, NJ: Humana Press; 1991.
107. Romagnoli S, et al. *Crit Care (London, England)*. 2014;18:644.
108. Schwid HA. *J Clin Monit*. 1988;4:181.
109. Sinha S, et al. *Anaesthesia*. 2007;62(6):615.
110. Promonet C, et al. *Anesthesiology*. 2000;92(1):208.
111. Gardner RM. *Crit Care Med*. 1996;24(5):879.
112. Skidmore K, et al. *Anesth Analg*. 2002;95:1192.
113. Courtois M, et al. *Circulation*. 1995;92:1994.
114. Seo JH, et al. *Anesthesiology*. 2007;107(2):260.
115. Ortega R, et al. *N Engl J Med*. 2017;376:e26.
116. Kovacs G, et al. *Euro Resp J*. 2013;42:1586–1594.
117. Braunwald E, et al. *Circ Res*. 1956;4:100.
118. Stouffer G. Arterial Pressure. In: Stouffer G, ed. *Cardiovascular hemodynamics for the clinician*. Malden, Mass: Blackwell Futura; 2008:57.
119. O'Rourke MF, Gallagher DE. *J Hyper*. 1996;14:S147–S157.
120. Franklin SS, Weber MA. *Am Heart J*. 1994;128:793.
121. Frank SM, et al. *Anesthesiology*. 1991;75:457.
122. Kinzer JB, et al. *Anesth Analg*. 1985;64:1134.
123. Mark JB. Arterial blood pressure. Direct vs. indirect measurement. In: Mark JB, ed. *Atlas of cardiovascular monitoring*. New York: Churchill Livingstone; 1998:81.
124. Dorman T, et al. *Crit Care Med*. 1998;26:1646.
125. Urzua J, et al. *J Clin Monit*. 1994;10:229.
126. Chauhan S, et al. *J Cardiothorac Vasc Anesth*. 2000;14(3):274.
127. Hynson JM, et al. *Crit Care Med*. 1998;26:1623.
128. McGregor M. *N Engl J Med*. 1979;301(480).
129. Shabetai R, et al. *Am J Cardiol*. 1970;26:480.
130. Mark JB. Pericardial constriction and cardiac tamponade. In: Mark JB, ed. *Atlas of cardiovascular monitoring*. New York: Churchill Livingstone; 1998:313.
131. Gelman S. *Anesthesiology*. 2008;108(4):735.
132. Marik PE. *Anaesth Intensive Care*. 1993;21:405.
133. Gunn SR, Pinsky MR. *Curr Opin Crit Care*. 2001;7:212.
134. Preisman S, et al. *Br J Anaesth*. 2005;95(6):746.
135. Perel A. *Anesth Analg*. 2008;106(4):1031.
136. Hofer CK, Cannesson M. *Acta Anaesthesiol Taiwan*. 2011;49(2):59.
137. Thiele RH, et al. *Anesth Analg*. 2012;115(1):176.
138. Berkenstadt H, et al. *Anesth Analg*. 2001;92(4):984.
139. Phillips R, Brierley J. *J Clin Monit Comput*. 2015;29:197–200.
140. Kong R, et al. *J Clin Monit Comput*. 2016;30:81–86.
141. Cannesson M, et al. *Anesth Analg*. 2008;106(4):1189.
142. Antonsen LP, Kirkeboen KA. *Anesthesiol Res Pract*. 2012;617380:2012.
143. Cannesson M, et al. *J Clin Monit Comput*. 2011;25(1):45.
144. Michard F, et al. *Am J Respir Crit Care Med*. 2000;162(1):134.
145. Biais M, et al. *Br J Anaesth*. 2010;104(4):407.
146. Mahjoub Y, et al. *Intensive Care Med*. 2011;37(2):360.
147. Marik PE, et al. *Crit Care Med*. 2009;37:2642–2647.
148. De Hert SG. *Anesthesiology*. 2011;115:229–230.
149. Cannesson M. *J Card Vasc Anesth*. 2010;24:487–497.
150. Cannesson M, et al. *Anesth Analg*. 2008;106(4):1195.
151. Auler Jr JO, et al. *Anesth Analg*. 2008;106(4):1201.
152. Min JJ, et al. *J Clin Monit Comput*. 2017;31:397–405.
153. Audimoolam VK, et al. *Anesth Analg*. 2017;124:480–486.
154. Royer P, et al. *J Trauma Acute Care Surg*. 2015;78:994–999.
155. Wyffels PA, et al. *Am J Phys Hrt Circ Phys*. 2016;310:H1194–H1200.
156. Ho KM. *Anesth Int Care*. 2016;44:14–19.
157. Wyler von Ballmoos M, et al. *Crit Care*. 2010;14(3):R111.
158. Yi L, et al. *PLoS One*. 2017;12:e0177590.
159. Jeong DM, et al. *Anesthesia and analgesia*. 2017;125:1158–1165.
160. Hennings LI, et al. *Danish medical journal*. 2015;62.
161. Ikeda K, et al. *Sem Card Vasc Anesth*. 2016;20:188–196.
162. Myatra SN, et al. *Crit Care Med*. 2017;45:415–421.
163. Biais M, et al. *Anesthesiology*. 2017;126:260–267.
164. De Broca B, et al. *Medicine*. 2016;95:e4259.
165. Augusto JF, et al. *Intensive Care Med*. 2011;37(3):411.
166. Barodka VM, et al. *Anesth Analg*. 2011;112(5):1048.
167. Gravenstein N, Blackshear RH. *J Clin Monit*. 1991;7(1).
168. Fisher KL, Leung AN. *AJR Am J Roentgenol*. 1996;166(2):329.
169. Graham AS, et al. *N Engl J Med*. 2007;356(21):e21.
170. Peres PW. *Anaesth Intensive Care*. 1990;18(4):536.
171. Rupp SM, et al. *Anesthesiology*. 2012;116(3):539.
172. Troianos CA, et al. *Anesth Analg*. 2012;114(1):46.
173. Rothschild JM. *Ultrasound guidance of central vein catheterization. Evidence report/technology assessment, No. 43. Making health care safer. A critical analysis of patient safety practices*. Rockville, MD: Agency for Healthcare Research and Quality; 2001:245.
174. Schulman PM, et al. *N Engl J Med*. 2018;379:e1.
175. Tsui JY, et al. *N Engl J Med*. 2008;358:e30.
176. Ortega R, et al. *N Engl J Med*. 2010;362:e57.
177. Taylor RW, Palagiri AV. *Crit Care Med*. 2007;35:1390–1396.
178. McGee DC, Gould MK. *N Engl J Med*. 2003;348:1123–1133.
179. Imai M, et al. *Anesth Analg*. 1994;78:1041.
180. Wetzel LR, et al. *A & A case reports*. 2017;9:16–19.
181. Kainuma A, et al. *A & A case reports*. 2017;9:258–261.
182. Beilin Y, et al. *Anesthesiology*. 1998;88(5):1399.
183. Bernard RW, Stahl WM. *NY State J Med*. 1974;74:83–86.
184. Khalil KG, et al. *JAMA*. 1972;221:908–909.
185. Naguib M, et al. *Can Anaesth Soc J*. 1985;32(4):412.
186. Rudge CJ, et al. *Br Med J*. 1973;3:23.

187. Shah KB, et al. *Anesthesiology*. 1984;61(3):271.
188. Heath KJ, et al. *Anesthesiology*. 1998;89(5):1273.
189. Ezri T, et al. *J Cardiothorac Vasc Anesth*. 2001;15(2):231.
190. Brennan MF, et al. *Arch Surg*. 1973;106:871.
191. Caron NR, et al. *Chest*. 1994;106:1917.
192. Danenberg HD, et al. *Euro Heart J*. 1995;16(2):279.
193. Collier PE, et al. *Angiology*. 1984;35:595.
194. Tocino IM, Watanabe A. *AJR Am J Roentgenol*. 1986;146(3):487.
195. Mansfield PF, et al. *N Engl J Med*. 1994;331(26):1735.
196. Gozubuyuk E, et al. *A & A case reports*. 2017;9:207–211.
197. Butsch JL, et al. *Arch Surg*. 1976;111:828.
198. Drachler DH, et al. *JAMA*. 1976;236(25):2880.
199. Burton AW, et al. *Anesthesiology*. 1998;89(3):804.
200. Merrer J, et al. *JAMA*. 2001;286:700–707.
201. Gilon D, et al. *Am Heart J*. 1998;135(3):457.
202. Ghani MK, et al. *Intensive Care Med*. 2003;29(10):1829.
203. Roguin A, Reisner SA. *Eur J Echocardiogr*. 2000;1:222.
204. Barbeito A, et al. *Can J Anaesth*. 2008;55(11):774.
205. Horner SM, et al. *Eur Heart J*. 1993;14(1):138.
206. Reynen K. *New Engl J Med*. 1993;329(13):970.
207. Grace DM. *Can J Surg*. 1977;20:51.
208. Miller SE, Maragakis LL. *Curr Opin Inf Dis*. 2012;25:412–422.
209. Healthcare-associated infections in the United States, 2006-2016: a story of progress. In: *Promotion DoHQa*. Atlanta, GA: National Center for Emerging and Zoonotic infectious Diseases (NCEZID); 2018.
210. Marschall J. *Am J Infect Control*. 2008;36(10):S172 e5.
211. Zingg W, Pittet D. *Int J Antimicrob Agents*. 2009;34(suppl 4):S38.
212. Corona ML, et al. *Mayo Clin Proc*. 1990;65(July):979.
213. O'Grady NP, et al. *MMWR*. 2002;51:1–29.
214. Tebbs SE, et al. *Br J Anaesth*. 1994;72(5):587.
215. Long DA, Coulthard MG. *Anaesth Intensive Care*. 2006;34(4):481.
216. Gilbert RE, Harden M. *Curr Opin Infect Dis*. 2008;21(3):235.
217. Darouiche RO, et al. *N Engl J Med*. 1999;340(1):1.
218. Maki DG, et al. *Ann Intern Med*. 1997;127(4):257.
219. Veenstra DL, et al. *JAMA*. 1999;282(6):554.
220. Levy I, et al. *Pediatr Infect Dis J*. 2005;24(8):676.
221. Garland JS, et al. *Pediatrics*. 2001;107(6):1431.
222. O'Grady NP, et al. *Am J Infec Cont*. 2011;39:S1–34.
223. Parienti JJ, et al. *N Engl J Med*. 2015;373:1220–1229.
224. Magder S. *Crit Care Med*. 2006;34(8):2224.
225. Magder S, et al. *Crit Care Med*. 1998;26:1061–1064.
226. Mark JB. Pressure-volume relations, transmural pressure, and preload. In: Mark JB, ed. *Atlas of cardiovascular monitoring*. New York: Churchill Livingstone; 1998:247–259.
227. Dwyer EM. *Circ*. 1970;42:1111–1122.
228. Mark JB. Respiratory-circulatory interactions. In: Mark JB, ed. *Atlas of cardiovascular monitoring*. New York: Churchill Livingstone; 1998:261–285.
229. Magder S. *Curr Opin Crit Care*. 2006;12(3):219.
230. Kovacs G, et al. *Am J Resp Crit Care Med*. 2014;190:252–257.
231. Mark JB. Getting the most from your central venous pressure catheter. In: Barash PG, ed. *ASA refresher courses in anesthesiology*. Philadelphia: Lippincott-Raven; 1995:157–175.
232. Mark JB. *J Cardiothorac Vasc Anesth*. 1991;5:163.
233. O'Rourke RA, et al. General examination of the patient. In: Schlant RC, Alexander RW, eds. *The heart, arteries, and veins*. New York: McGraw-Hill; 1994:238.
234. Mackay IFS, Walker RL. *Am Heart J*. 1966;71(2):228.
235. Shinozaki T, et al. *Anesthesiology*. 1980;53:498.
236. Mark JB. Arrhythmias. An integrated ECG and hemodynamic approach. In: Mark JB, ed. *Atlas of cardiovascular monitoring*. New York: Churchill Livingstone; 1998:219.
237. Mark JB. Patterns of valvular heart disease. In: Mark JB, ed. *Atlas of cardiovascular monitoring*. New York: Churchill Livingstone; 1998:287.
238. Marik PE, et al. *Chest*. 2008;134(1):172.
239. Kuntscher MV, et al. *Resuscitation*. 2006;70:37–43.
240. Wiesenack C, et al. *Eur J Anaesthesiol*. 2005;22(9):658.
241. Coudray A, et al. *Crit Care Med*. 2005;33:2757–2762.
242. Swan HJC, et al. *N Engl J Med*. 1970;283(9):447.
243. Connors AF, et al. *N Engl J Med*. 1983;308(5):263.
244. Sandham JD, et al. *N Engl J Med*. 2003;348(1):5.
245. Kelly CR, Rabbani LE. *N Engl J Med*. 2013;369:e35.
246. Bennett D, et al. *Intensive Care Med*. 1991;17(1):I.
247. Szabo Z. *Br J Anaesth*. 2003;90(6):794.
248. Pipanmekaporn T. *J Cardiothorac Vasc Anesth*. 2012;26(3):391.
249. Tan CO. *World Anesthesiology*. 2015;4:30.
250. Cronin B, et al. *J Card Vasc Anesth*. 2017;31:178–183.
251. Evans DC, et al. *Scand J Surg*. 2009;98(4):199.
252. Roizen MF, et al. *Anesthesiology*. 2003;99(4):988.
253. Damen J, Bolton D. *Acta Anaesthesiol Scand*. 1986;30:386.
254. Procaccini B, et al. *Br J Anaesth*. 1998;80(suppl 2):A26.
255. Jain M, et al. *Intensive Care Med*. 2003;29:2059.
256. Squara P, et al. *Chest*. 2002;121(6):2009.
257. Iberti TJ, et al. *JAMA*. 1990;264(22):2928.
258. Gnaegi A, et al. *Crit Care Med*. 1997;25(2):213.
259. Jacka MJ, et al. *Crit Care Med*. 2002;30(6):1197.
260. Zarich S, et al. *Intensive Care Med*. 2000;26:698.
261. Marik P, et al. *Crit Care Med*. 1998;26(10):1761.
262. Mark JB. Pulmonary artery pressure. In: Mark JB, ed. *Atlas of Cardiovascular Monitoring*. New York: Churchill Livingstone; 1998:27–37.
263. Mark JB. Pulmonary artery wedge pressure. In: Mark JB, ed. *Atlas of cardiovascular monitoring*. New York: Churchill Livingstone; 1998:39.
264. Levy MM. *Crit Care Clin*. 1996;12(4):819.
265. Mark JB, Chetham PM. *Anesthesiology*. 1991;74:375.
266. Zahorec R, Holoman M. *Eur J Cardiothorac Surg*. 1997;11(2):379.
267. Shin B, et al. *Crit Care Med*. 1977;5(3):125.
268. Mark JB. Pulmonary artery and wedge pressure artifacts. In: Mark JB, ed. *Atlas of cardiovascular monitoring*. New York: Churchill Livingstone; 1998:49.
269. Morris AH, et al. *Crit Care Med*. 1984;12:164.
270. Bashein G. *Anesthesiology*. 1988;68:310.
271. Fuchs RM, et al. *Am J Cardiol*. 1982;49:849.
272. Braunwald E, Awe WC. *Circ*. 1963;27:29.
273. Grossman W. *N Engl J Med*. 1991;325:1557.
274. Stott DK, et al. *Circ*. 1970;41:1031.
275. Wohlgelernter D, et al. *J Am Coll Cardiol*. 1978;10:491.
276. Leung JM, et al. *Anesthesiology*. 1990;73:802.
277. Sabbah HN, et al. *Am J Cardiol*. 1993;72:1074.
278. van Daele MERM, et al. *Circ*. 1990;81:865.
279. Goldstein JA, et al. *Circ*. 1990;82:359.
280. Trager MA, et al. *J Cardiothorac Anesth*. 1987;1:123.
281. Kushwaha SS, et al. *N Engl J Med*. 1997;336:267.
282. Kern MJ, Aguirre F. *Cathet Cardiovasc Diagn*. 1992;25:336.
283. Kern MJ, Aguirre F. *Cathet Cardiovasc Diagn*. 1992;26:34.
284. Kern MJ, Aguirre F. *Cathet Cardiovasc Diagn*. 1992;26:152.
285. Hirschmann JV. *Am Heart J*. 1978;96:110.
286. Beloucif S, et al. *Am J Physiol*. 1992;263:H125.
287. Lorell BH, Braunwald E. Pericardial disease. In: Braunwald E, ed. *Heart disease. A textbook of cardiovascular medicine*. Philadelphia: Saunders; 1992:1465.
288. Fowler NO. *Circ*. 1993;87:1738.
289. Mitchell MM, et al. *Anesthesiology*. 1987;67:294.
290. Teplick RS. *Anesthesiology*. 1987;67:289.
291. Cengiz M, et al. *Crit Care Med*. 1983;11:502.
292. Pinsky MR. *Intensive Care Med*. 2003;29(1):19.
293. Gidwani UK, et al. *Card Clin*. 2013;31:545–565.
294. Falicov RE, Resnekov L. *Circ*. 1970;42:65.
295. Scheinman M, et al. *Circ*. 1973;47:317.
296. Mark JB. Predicting left ventricular end-diastolic pressure. In: Mark JB, ed. *Atlas of cardiovascular monitoring*. New York: Churchill Livingstone; 1998:59.
297. Osman D, et al. *Crit Care Med*. 2007;35(1):64.
298. Trof RJ, et al. *Crit Care*. 2011;15. R73-R.
299. McGregor M, Sniderman A. *Am J Cardiol*. 1985;55:217.
300. Permutt S, Riley RL. *J Appl Phys*. 1963;34:924.
301. Brengelmann GL. *J Appl Physiol*. 2006;101(5):1525. discussion 1526.
302. Naeije R. *Intensive Care Med*. 2003;29(4):526.
303. Reeves JT, et al. *J Appl Physiol*. 1961;16:276.
304. De Backer D, et al. *Int Care Med*. 2018;44:960–962.
305. De Backer D, Vincent JL. *Curr Opin Crit Care*. 2018;24:204–208.
306. Youssef N, Whitlock RP. *Can J Card*. 2017;33:135–141.
307. Lee M, et al. *Can J Card*. 2017;33:142–147.
308. Connors AF, et al. *JAMA*. 1996;276:889–897.
309. Dalen JE, Bone RC. *JAMA*. 1996;276:916.
310. Valentine RJ, et al. *J Vasc Surg*. 1998;27(2):203. discussion 211.
311. Tuman KJ, et al. *J Cardiothorac Anesth*. 1989;3:625–641.
312. Connors AF, et al. *JAMA*. 1997;277:113–114.

313. Binanay C, et al. *JAMA*. 2005;294(13):1625.
314. Wheeler AP, et al. *N Engl J Med*. 2006;354(21):2213.
315. Harvey S, et al. *Lancet*. 2005;366(9484):472.
316. De Backer D. *Intensive Care Med*. 2003;29(11):1865.
317. Friese RS, et al. *Crit Care Med*. 2006;34(6):1597.
318. Chittock DR, et al. *Crit Care Med*. 2004;32(4):911.
319. Kavarana MN, et al. *Am Surg*. 2003;69(5):411.
320. Sotomi Y, et al. *Int J Card*. 2014;172:165–172.
321. Ikuta K, et al. *JAMA Cardiology*. 2017;2.
322. Pinsky MR, Vincent JL. *Crit Care Med*. 2005;33(5):1119.
323. Sotomi Y, et al. *Int J Card*. 2014;172:165–172.
324. Allen LA, et al. *J Card Fail*. 2008;14:661–669.
325. Hartog C, Bloos F. *Anaesthesiology*. 2014;28:419–428.
326. Scalea TM, et al. *J Trauma*. 1990;30(12):1539.
327. Pearse R, et al. *Crit Care*. 2005;9(6):R694.
328. Vallet B, et al. *Crit Care*. 2010;14(2):213.
329. Pölönen P, et al. *Anesth Analg*. 2000;90:1052.
330. Donati A, et al. *Chest*. 2007;132(6):1817.
331. Smetkin AA, et al. *Acta Anaesthesiol Scand*. 2009;53(4):505.
332. Rivers E, et al. *N Engl J Med*. 2001;345(19):1368.
333. Pro CI, et al. *N Engl J Med*. 2014;370:1683–1693.
334. London MJ, et al. *Anesthesiology*. 2002;96(4):860.
335. Haddad F, et al. *Circ*. 2008;117(13):1717.
336. Dhainaut J-F, et al. *Crit Care Med*. 1987;15(2):148.
337. Nelson LD. *New Horizons*. 1997;5:251–258.
338. Chang MC, et al. *Arch Surg*. 1996;131(7):728.
339. Her C, Lees DE. *Crit Care Med*. 1993;21(11):1665.
340. Boldt J, et al. *Crit Care Med*. 1989;17:518–522.
341. Dupont H, Squara P. *Curr Opin Anaesthesiol*. 1996;9:490.
342. Linton RAF, et al. *J Cardiothorac Vasc Anesth*. 2002;16(1):4.
343. Funk DJ, et al. *Anesth Analg*. 2009;108(3):887.
344. Reuter DA, et al. *Anesth Analg*. 2010;110(3):799.
345. Nishikawa T, Dohi S. *Can J Anaesth*. 1993;40(2):142.
336. Stetz CW, et al. *Am Rev Respir Dis*. 1982;126(6):1001.
347. Dhingra VK, et al. *Chest*. 2002;122(3):990.
348. Ganz W, et al. *Am J Cardiol*. 1971;27:392.
349. Heerdt PM, et al. *J Cardiothorac Vasc Anesth*. 2001;15(2):183.
350. Bazaral MG, et al. *Anesthesiology*. 1992;77(1):31.
351. Wetzel RC, Latson TW. *Anesthesiology*. 1985;62(5):684.
352. Groeneveld ABJ, et al. *J Appl Physiol*. 2000;89:89.
353. van Grondelle A, et al. *Am J Physiol*. 1983;245(4):H690.
354. Yelderman M. *J Clin Monit*. 1990;6(4):322.
355. Siegel LC, et al. *Anesth Analg*. 1996;83:1173.
356. Gardner RM. *Crit Care Med*. 1998;26(8):1302.
357. Le Tulzo Y, et al. *J Clin Monit*. 1996;12(5):379.
358. Hatton KW, et al. *J Cardiothorac Vasc Anesth*. 2017;31:e61–e62.
359. Monnet X, Teboul J-L. *Crit Care*. 2017;21.
360. Mielck F, et al. *J Cardiothorac Vasc Anesth*. 2003;17(2):211.
361. Segal E, et al. *J Clin Anesth*. 2002;14(3):210.
362. von Spiegel T, et al. *Anaesthesist*. 1996;45(11):1045.
363. Michard F. *Crit Care Med*. 2007;35(4):1186.
354. Matejovic M, et al. *Acta Anaesthesiol Scand*. 2004;48(1):69.
365. Mitchell JP, et al. *Am Rev Respir Dis*. 1992;145(5):990.
366. Hoeft A, et al. *Anesthesiology*. 1994;81(1):76.
367. Wiesenack C, et al. *J Cardiothorac Vasc Anesth*. 2001;15(5):584.
368. Briegel J, et al. *Anaesthesist*. 2009;58(2):122.
369. Perny J, et al. *BioMed Res Intl*. 2014;2014:1–7.
370. Linton RAF, et al. *Br J Anaesth*. 1993;71:262.
371. Kurita T, et al. *Br J Anaesth*. 1997;79:770.
372. Linton R, et al. *Crit Care Med*. 1997;25(11):1796.
373. Garcia-Rodriguez C, et al. *Crit Care Med*. 2002;30(10):2199.
374. Linton RA, et al. *Intensive Care Med*. 2000;26(10):1507.
375. Joosten A, et al. *Br J Anaesth*. 2017;118:298–310.
376. Colquhoun DA, Roche AM. *Anaesthesiology*. 2014;28:353–362.
377. Laupland KB, Bands CJ. *Can J Anaesth*. 2002;49(4):393.
378. Mark JB, et al. *Anesth Analg*. 1986;65:1013.
379. Roche AM, et al. *Best Pract Res Clin Anaesthesiol*. 2009;23(3):327.
380. Abbas SM, Hill AG. *Anaesthesia*. 2008;63(1):44.
381. Singer M. *Int Anesthesiol Clin*. 1993;31:99–125.
382. Thys DM, Hillel Z. *Anesthesiology*. 1988;69:728.
383. Lee JH, et al. *Br J Anaesth*. 2007;99(3):343.
384. Guinot P-G, et al. *Br J Anaesth*. 2013;110:28–33.
385. Poeze M, et al. *Crit Care Med*. 1999;27(7):1288.
386. Calvo-Vecino JM, et al. *Br J Anaesth*. 2018;120:734–744.
387. Kubicek WG, et al. *Aviat Space Environ Med*. 1966;37(12):1208.
388. Jakovljevic DG, et al. *Anaesthesiology*. 2014;28:381–394.
389. Peyton PJ, Chong SW. *Anesthesiology*. 2010;113:1220–1235.
390. Jaffe MB. *J Clin Monit*. 1999;15:387.
391. Orr J, et al. *J Clin Monit*. 1996;12:464.
392. Osterlund B, et al. *Acta Anaesthesiol Scand*. 1995;39(6):727.
393. Thiele RH, Durieux ME. *Anesth Analg*. 2011;113(4):766.
394. Wesseling KH, et al. *J Appl Physiol*. 1993;74(5):2566.
395. Linton NWF, Linton RAF. *Br J Anaesth*. 2001;86(4):486.
396. Bogert LW, et al. *Anaesthesia*. 2010;65(11):1119.
397. Michard F. *Anesthesiology*. 2005;103(2):419. quiz 449.
398. Lieshout JJ, Wesseling KH. *Br J Anaesth*. 2001;86(4):467.
399. Cecconi M, et al. *Int Care Med*. 2013;39:787–789.
400. Monnet X, et al. *Br J Anaesth*. 2012;108:615–622.
401. Camporota L, Beale R. *Crit Care*. 2010;14(2):124.
402. De Backer D, et al. *Intensive Care Med*. 2005;31(4):517.
403. Goedje O, et al. *Crit Care Med*. 1999;27(11):2407.
404. Pittman J, et al. *Crit Care Med*. 2005;33(9):2015.
405. Benes J, et al. *Crit Care*. 2010;14(3):R118.
406. Mayer J, et al. *Crit Care*. 2010;14(1):R18.
407. Salzwedel C, et al. *Crit Care*. 2013;17:1.

37 Perioperative Echocardiography

MEGAN L. KRAJEWSKI and FEROZE MAHMOOD

KEY POINTS

- Perioperative applications of transesophageal echocardiography (TEE) include monitoring, diagnosis, and procedural guidance. The role of TEE in cardiac surgery, noncardiac surgery, interventional procedures, and critical care continues to evolve.
- In noncardiac surgery, intraoperative TEE serves as a routine monitor or as a rescue tool in life-threatening emergencies.
- TEE aids in decision making during cardiac surgery, and three-dimensional (3-D) TEE adds incremental value in intraoperative assessments.
- TEE is integral to structural heart interventions and is a key component of multimodality imaging.
- Echocardiography plays a vital role in the diagnosis and management of shock.
- Applications of transthoracic echocardiography (TTE) in the perioperative setting are expanding.
- Focused cardiac ultrasound is performed and interpreted at the point of care, and addresses specific questions relevant to the clinical context.
- Critical care societies have proposed distinct competencies and guidelines for critical care echocardiography beyond those included in perioperative TEE guidelines. The skill set of the intensivist performing echocardiography overlaps with that of the intraoperative echocardiographer and includes other unique components.
- Basic knowledge of echocardiography is an expectation of anesthesiology training.
- Simulation is an effective training tool when integrated within a multimodal, curriculum-based approach to echocardiography education.

Introduction

Echocardiography is an invaluable tool used throughout the perioperative period. Image acquisition and interpretation occur at the point of care, enabling real-time integration of the findings in the context of the patient's clinical condition. Transesophageal echocardiography (TEE) has broad functionality in the perioperative environment. TEE serves as an intraoperative monitor, provides detailed structural and functional information, facilitates diagnosis of pathology, and guides percutaneous interventions. Applications of TEE have expanded within cardiac surgery, and into the realms of noncardiac surgery, catheter-based procedures, and critical care. As the use of clinical ultrasound grows in modern anesthetic practice, perioperative clinicians are also beginning to embrace transthoracic echocardiography (TTE). Critical care echocardiography shares many similarities with intraoperative echocardiography, but is simultaneously evolving under the larger umbrella of critical care ultrasonography. This chapter provides a historical synopsis and summary of imaging techniques and echocardiographic views and discusses applications of TEE and TTE in perioperative care.

History of Perioperative Echocardiography

INTRAOPERATIVE TRANSESOPHAGEAL ECHOCARDIOGRAPHY

Decades of evolution and advancement have led to the current state of perioperative TEE (Fig. 37.1).[1] Clinical echocardiography first emerged in the 1950s with the use of motion mode (M-mode) ultrasound to record signals from cardiac structures.[2] Nearly two decades later, the first intraoperative echocardiography was performed with epicardial imaging.[3] The first practical clinical application of TEE was reported in 1976.[4] Soon after, a group reported the first use of intraoperative TEE[5] and described its utility in monitoring left ventricular (LV) function during cardiac surgery.[6] In the 1980s, the mounting of two-dimensional (2-D) transducers onto modified flexible gastroscopes[7,8] created more versatile probes, and pioneering anesthesiologists and cardiologists began to demonstrate the usefulness of TEE as an intraoperative monitor.[9-11] Further advancements such as transducers with combined 2-D and Doppler capabilities,[12,13] biplane imaging,[14] multiplane imaging,[15] and pediatric probes[16] unlocked the diagnostic potential of intraoperative TEE. Real-time three-dimensional imaging (RT-3D) entered the scene in the mid-2000s,[17] and since then its intraoperative use has grown exponentially. Advances in probe technology and improved computing power continue to further the practicality of three-dimensional (3-D) image acquisition.

CRITICAL CARE ECHOCARDIOGRAPHY

Prior to the introduction of TEE in 1976, significant advances in 2-D transthoracic imaging occurred, leading to better visualization of cardiac structures.[18-22] Production of commercially available instruments soon followed. In the intensive care units (ICUs), some clinicians incorporated echocardiography in the evaluation of cardiac function in acute respiratory distress syndrome and sepsis.[23,24]

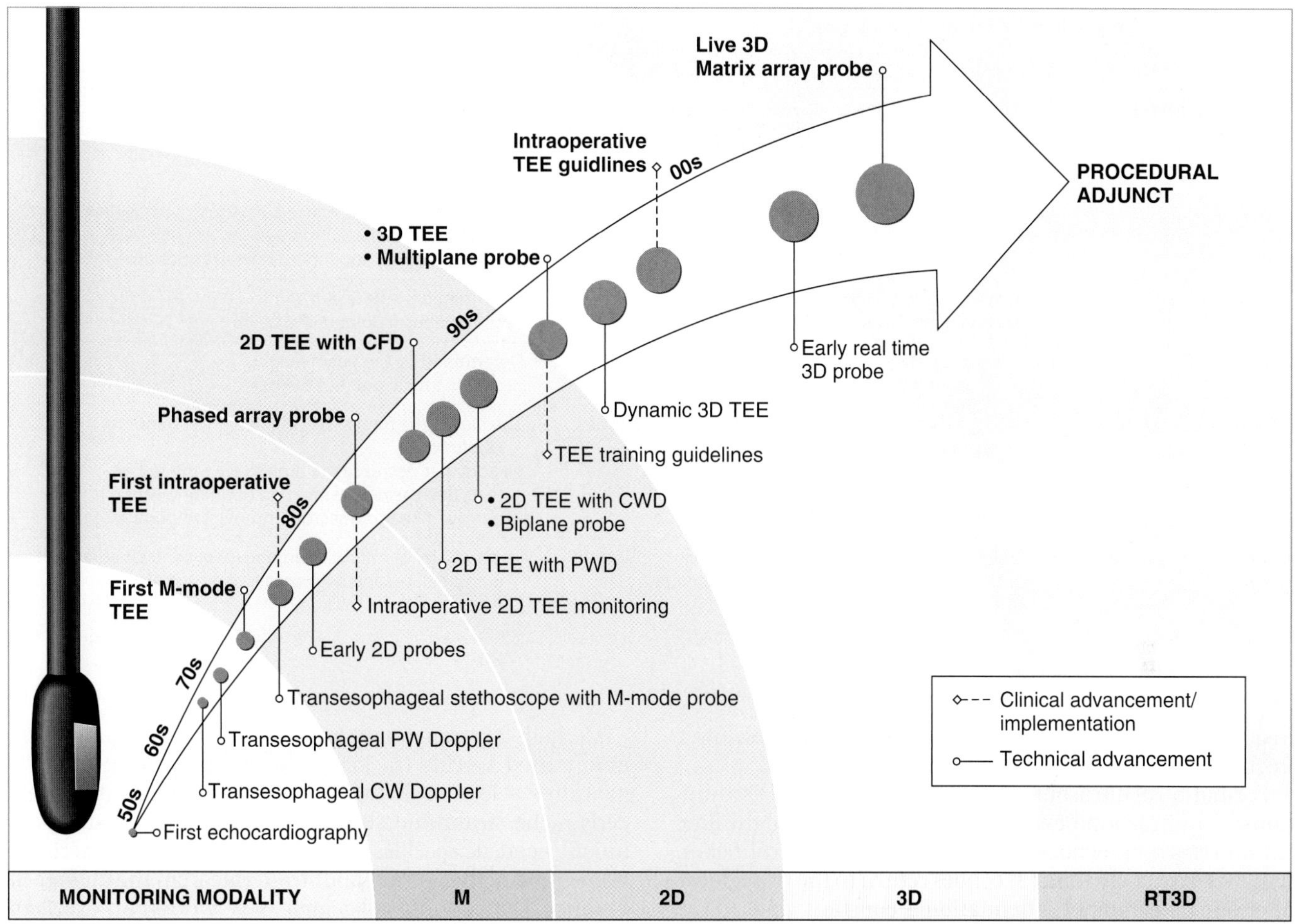

Fig. 37.1 Evolution of transesophageal echocardiography *(TEE)* over the years from a monitoring modality to procedural adjunct. *2D,* two-dimensional; *3D,* three-dimensional; *CFD,* color flow Doppler; *CWD,* continuous wave Doppler; *RT3D,* real-time 3D. (Modified with permission from, Mahmood F, Shernan SK. Perioperative transoesophageal echocardiography: current status and future directions. *Heart.* 2016;102(15):1159–1167.)

TTE was not widely disseminated in ICUs, however, as the intensivist's tool of choice at the time was the pulmonary artery catheter.[25-27] During the late 1990s to 2000s, the use of pulmonary artery catheters declined,[28-32] and TTE simultaneously gained more traction in the ICUs. With the miniaturization of equipment and emphasis on point-of-care ultrasound, use of echocardiography as a hemodynamic monitor and diagnostic tool in the ICU continues to increase.

Principles of Ultrasound

While a thorough discussion of ultrasound physics is beyond the scope of this chapter, a basic understanding of fundamental concepts is requisite for any echocardiographer. Sound is a mechanical, longitudinal wave of vibrations propagated through a medium. Several parameters describe sound waves including frequency, wavelength, amplitude, and propagation speed. Ultrasound waves are sound waves with frequencies above the audible human range (20-20,000 hertz [Hz]). Echocardiography typically uses frequencies between 2 and 12 megahertz (MHz). Ultrasound transducers use piezoelectric elements to convert ultrasound energy into electrical energy and vice versa. Transducers function both as transmitters and receivers of ultrasound signals. 2-D echocardiography uses a phased-array transducer, which has a row of electrically interconnected piezoelectric elements.

As ultrasound energy propagates through tissue, interactions between the wave and tissue result in absorption, divergence, reflection, and scattering of the energy. Reflection of ultrasound energy at tissue interfaces forms the basis of image generation. These sound-tissue interactions reduce the intensity of the ultrasound signal, and this attenuation limits the depth of imaging. Transmitted energy at tissue interfaces often undergoes refraction and changes directions, contributing to imaging artifacts.

The accurate display of an image depends on imaging resolution, components of which include spatial resolution, temporal resolution, and contrast resolution (Table 37.1). Spatial resolution can be described according to the three beam dimensions: axial, lateral, and elevational. Image formation involves a tradeoff between spatial resolution and depth of penetration. Higher frequency (shorter wavelength) transducers provide superior axial resolution, but limited penetration depth due to attenuation. Lower frequencies (longer wavelengths) penetrate more deeply at the expense of axial resolution. Higher

TABLE 37.1 Components of Imaging Resolution

	Description	Practical points
Spatial resolution	The ability to discriminate between two closely-spaced objects The minimum distance necessary between two structures so that they are displayed as separate objects	Determines image details Factors that improve spatial resolution often come at the expense of decreased temporal resolution and vice versa
Axial	Differentiates between objects along the length of the ultrasound beam	Higher frequency transducers have shorter wavelengths and better axial resolution Axial resolution is superior to lateral resolution
Lateral	Discriminates side-to-side (or horizontal) relative to the direction of the beam	Determined by the beam width Best at the focal point of the beam
Elevational	Discriminates between objects vertical to the plane of the ultrasound beam	Determined by the beam height Best at the focal point of the beam
Temporal resolution	The ability to accurately display a structure's motion with respect to time	The higher the frame rate, the better the temporal resolution Factors that decrease the time to scan the sector (e.g., decreasing the imaging depth or creating a narrower imaging sector) improve temporal resolution
Contrast resolution	The ability to resolve subtle differences in echogenicity, which are displayed as different shades of gray	Improved by harmonic imaging, use of contrast agents, B-color maps, and post-processing controls

frequencies are better for imaging superficial structures; lower frequencies are better for deeper structures.

Formation of ultrasound images relies on several assumptions: (1) ultrasound energy propagates in a straight line; (2) all returning echoes originate from the central beam, which is extremely thin; (3) echoes return to the transducer after one reflection; (4) attenuation is constant; and (5) the speed of sound is constant, therefore the depth of a reflector is proportional to the round-trip transit time.[33] Violations of these assumptions result in imaging artifacts. Spectral and color flow Doppler (CFD) and 3-D images are also susceptible to imaging artifacts.

Ultrasound Modalities

Key ultrasound modalities used in echocardiography include motion mode (M-mode), 2-D imaging, Doppler (spectral and color flow), and Doppler tissue imaging (DTI). Table 37.2 highlights important aspects of these techniques. Additional techniques may be applied in specific contexts and are introduced in the next section.

STRAIN AND STRAIN-RATE IMAGING

Strain and strain-rate imaging techniques (also called cardiac mechanics or myocardial deformation) are used to quantify global and regional ventricular function. Strain is the relative change in shape or size of an object as a result of an applied force. In the context of the myocardium, it is the fractional change in the length of a segment relative to its baseline and expressed as a percentage. Positive strain indicates lengthening or thickening and negative strain represents shortening or thinning. Three axes are relevant to myocardial deformation: longitudinal, circumferential, and radial. Normal deformation patterns during systole are longitudinal shortening (negative strain), circumferential shortening (negative strain), and radial thickening (positive strain).

Methods for strain analysis include DTI and the more commonly used speckle tracking echocardiography (STE). DTI measures velocities at two points in the myocardium and derives the strain and strain rate. STE, in contrast, tracks unique acoustic speckles in the myocardium over a series of frames and derives strain and strain rate from the change in distance. Duncan and colleagues have written an excellent review on perioperative strain and strain-rate imaging.[34]

HARMONIC IMAGING

Harmonic imaging is a processing technique used to improve the quality of 2-D images.[35] A sound wave propagates nonlinearly through tissue, distorting the wave's shape. This produces harmonic frequencies, which are integer multiples of the fundamental frequency originally transmitted by transducer. Signals return to the transducer at both the fundamental frequency and harmonic frequencies. Harmonic imaging typically creates images from the second harmonic frequency and filters the fundamental frequency signals. Harmonic imaging increases contrast resolution, improves signal-to-noise ratio, and decreases some artifacts. Disadvantages include slightly decreased spatial resolution and thickened appearance of some cardiac structures.[36,37]

CONTRAST ECHOCARDIOGRAPHY

Contrast echocardiography can be used to improve diagnostic evaluation and enhance suboptimal images.[38,39] Two methods of contrast echocardiography include injection of agitated saline or injection of commercially available contrast agents. Agitated saline can be used to identify the presence of intracardiac right-to-left shunt, because microbubbles created by agitation do not cross the pulmonary circulation.[40] Commercially available contrast agents use encapsulated microbubbles of high-density gas and are able to traverse the pulmonary circulation, allowing for opacification of the left side of the heart. Perioperative applications

TABLE 37.2 Ultrasound Modalities

Modality	Description/Features
Brightness Mode (B-mode)	▪ Depicts the strength of returning sound signals using corresponding degrees of brightness ▪ M-mode and 2D imaging are modifications of original B-mode imaging
Motion Mode (M-mode)	▪ Displays a one-dimensional image of the motion of cardiac structures relative to time ▪ Very high temporal resolution ▪ Provides limited spatial information ▪ Greatest utility in providing information about rapidly moving structures (e.g., valves, walls) in relation to the timing of the cardiac cycle
Two-Dimensional (2D)	▪ The mainstay of the echocardiographic examination ▪ Scanning of repeated pulses generates an image representative of the cardiac structures with real-time motion ▪ Images are produced in a sector format ▪ Temporal resolution is less than that of M-mode
Doppler	▪ Ultrasound energy scattered from moving red blood cells shifts to a higher frequency when moving toward the transducer and a lower frequency when moving away ▪ Doppler modes analyze this frequency shift and use the Doppler equation to estimate velocities of blood flow ▪ Velocity (*v*) can be calculated as follows: $v = \frac{c * \Delta f}{2 f_t * cos\theta}$ Where *c* = the propagation speed of sound in blood (1540 m/s), Δf is the difference between the transmitted frequency (f_t) and the received frequency, and cosθ is the angle of incidence between the ultrasound beam and blood flow ▪ Angle-dependent ▪ Maximum Doppler shift occurs when blood flow is directly parallel to the beam. When the incident angle is ≤ 20 degrees, the percentage error in estimating the velocity is ≤ 6%. At greater incident angles the error significantly increases. ▪ Includes spectral (pulsed-wave, continuous wave) and color flow Doppler
Pulsed-Wave Doppler (PWD)	▪ Samples blood flow velocities at a specific location ▪ The frequency of sampling determines the maximum velocity that can be detected and depends on imaging depth ▪ This maximum velocity is half of the pulse repetition frequency and referred to as the Nyquist limit ▪ Above the Nyquist limit, *aliasing* occurs. The Doppler information is displayed ambiguously, displaying both positive and negative velocities
Continuous Wave Doppler (CWD)	▪ Transducer continuously transmits and receives ultrasound energy along the length of the ultrasound beam ▪ Allows measurement of higher velocity flows, such as those that are encountered with stenotic or regurgitant lesions ▪ The location of the high velocity flow may occur anywhere along the length of the beam, a limitation referred to as *range ambiguity*
Color Flow Doppler (CFD)	▪ A form of pulsed-wave Doppler ▪ The direction and velocity of flow are measured in multiple sample volumes within an imaging sector. The direction and velocity information are displayed according to a color scale ▪ Flow data are superimposed on the corresponding 2D image ▪ Limited by aliasing ▪ Lower temporal resolution than 2D imaging
Doppler Tissue Imaging (DTI)	▪ Used to assess myocardial motion ▪ Eliminates the high-velocity, low-amplitude signals from red blood cells and displays the low-velocity, high-amplitude signals from tissue ▪ Angle-dependent ▪ Does not distinguish between translational motion and contraction

of contrast echocardiography include improved endocardial border delineation for assessment of function, assessment of regional wall motion, and exclusion of intracardiac thrombus or mass.

Three-Dimensional Image Acquisition

3-D imaging provides information that complements the findings from the 2-D examination. Transducers with 3-D capabilities contain thousands of piezoelectric elements in a rectangular (or matrix) array configuration and create pyramidal-shaped images. The optimal 3-D image involves tradeoffs between temporal resolution, spatial resolution, and sector size. 3-D imaging is susceptible to the same artifacts as 2-D imaging and additional artifacts unique to 3-D image construction. We encourage the interested reader to refer to published 3-D echocardiography guidelines[41] as well as a practical overview focused on intraoperative 3-D image acquisition.[42]

IMAGING MODES

Two-Dimensional Multiplane Acquisition

Matrix array (3-D) transducers have multiplane imaging capabilities and can simultaneously display two or

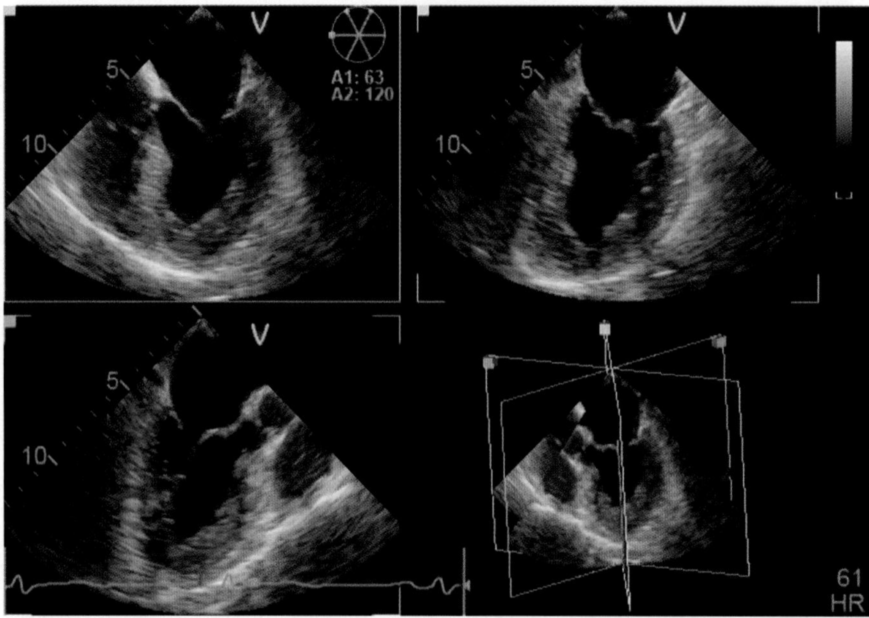

Fig. 37.2 Simultaneous display of multiple two-dimensional scan planes by multiplane imaging. The upper left panel *(yellow panel)* displays the primary reference imaging plane. The circular icon in this panel indicates the positions of the secondary imaging planes. Images from the secondary planes are displayed at the top right *(white panel)* and bottom left *(green panel)*. A three-dimensional representation of the imaging planes and their angulation is displayed at the bottom right.

BOX 37.1 Perioperative Applications of Multiplane Imaging

- Simultaneous visualization of segmental wall motion
- Characterization of the mechanism and origin of valvular regurgitation
- Procedural guidance during percutaneous closure of atrial septal defect
- Guidance of transseptal puncture for transcatheter left atrial appendage and mitral valve procedures
- Evaluation of the left atrial appendage morphology and exclusion of thrombus

more live 2-D imaging planes. In biplane imaging, the first image serves as the reference view, and the second image is obtained by rotating the scanning plane around the longitudinal axis of the reference view. The secondary image can also be adjusted by tilting the imaging plane in the elevational or lateral axis. Multiplane imaging allows simultaneous display of multiple rotatable imaging planes (Fig. 37.2). Box 37.1 lists common perioperative applications of multiplane imaging.

Real-Time Three-Dimensional Imaging

3-D images can be displayed live or in "real time." RT-3D imaging acquires data over a single heartbeat; some authors refer to this as 4-D imaging. The proprietary nomenclature varies, but there are three main RT-3D modes of differing sector size:

- Narrow sector: this mode displays a pyramidal volume with the best temporal and spatial resolution of the live modes. The major limitation is that it often does not capture an entire structure of interest (Fig. 37.3).
- Wide sector: this mode "zooms in" on a selected region of interest. There is a decrease in temporal and spatial resolution compared to narrow sector imaging. Images are easy to acquire. This mode is ideal for real-time image manipulation (see Fig. 37.3).
- Full-volume: full-volume mode has the largest imaging sector. Live full-volume images have reduced temporal and spatial resolution. Ideally, acquisition of full-volume images occurs over multiple beats. Live full-volume mode has utility when multiple-beat acquisition is not feasible.

Gated Acquisition

Gated acquisition divides the imaging volume into multiple narrow subvolumes that are acquired over a specified number of heartbeats. "Stitching" the subvolumes together creates the final image. In order to obtain the subvolumes at the same time in the cardiac cycle, image acquisition is gated to the R-wave of the electrocardiogram (ECG). Gated acquisition requires normal cardiac rhythm and the absence of electrical interference and respiratory variation.

- Wide sector: multiple-beat gated acquisition using wide sector mode significantly improves the temporal resolution of the "zoomed in" view. Spatial resolution marginally improves.
- Full-volume: this mode has the largest sector size with optimal spatial resolution and high temporal resolution (Fig. 37.4; Video 37.1).

Color Flow Doppler

CFD may be incorporated with any of the modalities, but leads to a reduction in temporal resolution. Optimal CFD images are obtained using R-wave gated multiple beat acquisitions.

QUANTITATIVE ANALYSIS

Multiplanar Reformatting

Multiplanar reformatting enables alignment of orthogonal planes to accurately measure linear dimensions and areas (e.g., planimetry of stenotic orifice, annular area).

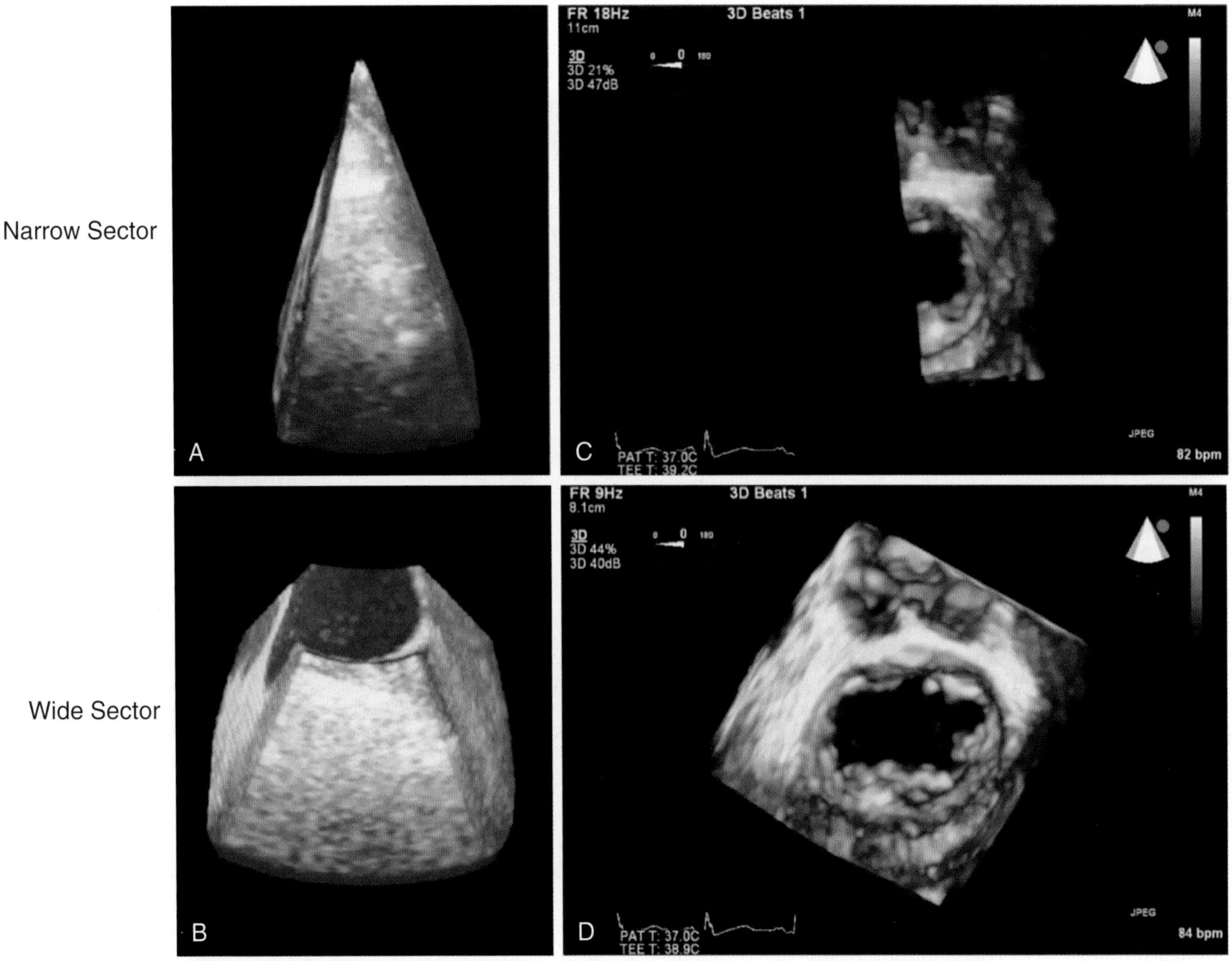

Fig. 37.3 Real-time three-dimensional imaging using narrow sector *(top)* and wide sector *(bottom)* modes. (A) Narrow sector imaging displays a narrow, pyramidal volume. (B) Wide sector imaging displays a defined region of interest selected from a larger pyramidal volume. (C) Narrow sector image of the mitral valve after cropping and rotating. Only a portion of the mitral valve structure is visualized. (D) Wide sector image of the mitral valve after cropping and rotating. The entire mitral valve structure is visualized, but at the expense of decreased spatial and temporal resolution.

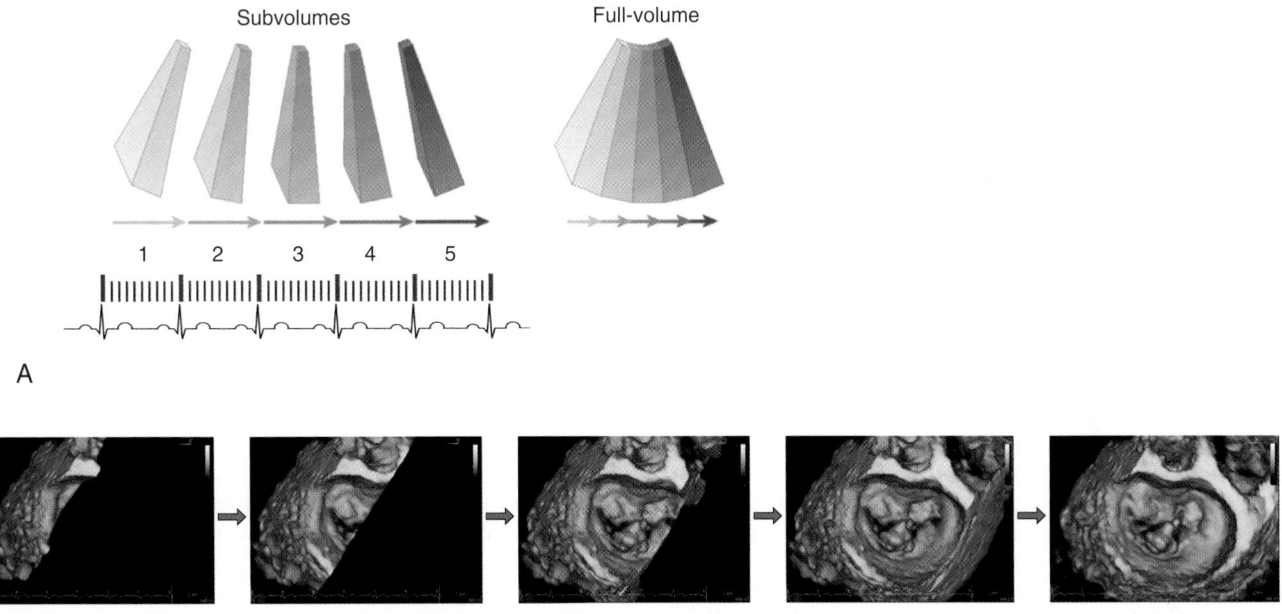

Fig. 37.4 (A) Schematic of multibeat gated full-volume image acquisition. Subvolume acquisition is gated to the R-wave of the electrocardiogram. In this example, subvolume acquisition occurs over five consecutive heartbeats. The individual subvolumes are then synchronized and "stitched" together to create a larger full-volume three-dimensional image. (B) Creation of the three-dimensional (3D) full-volume image from narrow subvolumes. (Modified from Desjardins G. Perioperative echocardiography. In: Miller R, ed. *Miller's Anesthesia*. 8th ed. Philadelphia, PA: Elsevier/Saunders; 2015:1396–1428.)

Advanced Applications

Quantitative applications exist for 3-D imaging and eliminate some of the geometric assumptions required in 2-D imaging calculations. Example analyses include calculation of ventricular ejection fraction (EF), analysis of mitral valve structure, and dynamic annular measurements. The degree of automation and need for post-processing manipulation vary. Some analyses are performed exclusively offline, making them useful in research, but less applicable to intraoperative decision making.

Indications and Practice Guidelines

PERIOPERATIVE TRANSESOPHAGEAL ECHOCARDIOGRAPHY

The American Society of Anesthesiology (ASA) and Society of Cardiovascular Anesthesiologists (SCA) issued perioperative TEE practice guidelines in 1996, categorizing indications for TEE in various clinical settings.[43] An updated version in 2010 recommended the indications for perioperative TEE based on literature review and expert opinion.[44] In the absence of contraindications, TEE should be used in all adult open heart and thoracic aortic surgical procedures. It should be considered in coronary artery bypass graft surgeries to confirm diagnostic information, detect pathology, influence the anesthetic or surgical plan, and assess surgical results. It is recommended that TEE be considered on a case-by-case basis in small children undergoing cardiac surgery due to unique risks in this population. For catheter-based intracardiac procedures, the 2010 guidelines state TEE may be used. Separate guidelines focus specifically on the role of echocardiography in interventional and catheter-based procedures.[45,46] In noncardiac surgery, TEE is indicated in the setting of persistent unexplained life-threatening circulatory instability. If the surgical procedure or the patient's known or suspected pathology could result in severe hemodynamic, pulmonary, or neurologic compromise, TEE may be used. TEE is recommended in critical care if the diagnostic information is expected to alter management and cannot be obtained by other modalities expediently. European guidelines offer similar recommendations for the use of perioperative TEE,[47-49] while the American Heart Association (AHA) and American College of Cardiology (ACC) make more limited recommendations regarding specific indications for intraoperative TEE.[50,51]

In addition to describing indications for perioperative TEE, the 1996 ASA/SCA guidelines also distinguish between basic and advanced levels of training.[43] In 2002, an American Society of Echocardiography (ASE)/SCA Joint Task Force authored guidelines for training in perioperative echocardiography, defined as TEE, epicardial echocardiography, or epiaortic ultrasonography performed in surgical patients immediately before, during, or after surgery.[52] These guidelines do not include TTE. Expectations for cognitive and technical skills of both basic and advanced training are outlined with recommendations for the minimum numbers of echocardiographic examinations performed. Further discussion of training and certification occurs at the end of the chapter.

TABLE 37.3 List of Contraindications to Transesophageal Echocardiography

Absolute Contraindications	Relative Contraindications
Esophageal pathology ▪ Diverticulum ▪ Laceration ▪ Stricture ▪ Tumor	History of: ▪ Dysphagia ▪ Radiation to neck and chest ▪ Upper gastrointestinal surgery
Active upper gastrointestinal bleeding	Recent upper gastrointestinal bleeding
History of esophagectomy	Active peptic ulcer disease, esophagitis
Perforated viscus	Esophageal varices Barrett's esophagus Symptomatic hiatal hernia Restricted cervical spine mobility ▪ Atlantoaxial instability ▪ Severe cervical arthritis Coagulopathy or thrombocytopenia

Adapted from Hahn RT, Abraham T, Adams MS, et al. Guidelines for performing a comprehensive transesophageal echocardiographic examination: recommendations from the American Society of Echocardiography and the Society of Cardiovascular Anesthesiologists. *J Am Soc Echocardiogr.* 2013;26(9):921–964.

CRITICAL CARE

Critical care societies have further defined competencies and applications of echocardiography in critical care beyond that established by the ASA/SCA guidelines. Several internationally based expert panels have proposed training objectives and competency-based training standards in consensus statements. Similar to the distinction between basic and advanced training in perioperative echocardiography, these statements distinguish between basic and advanced critical care echocardiography,[53-56] or a basic and expert skill set.[57] The Society of Critical Care Medicine has provided evidence-based recommendations for the use of bedside echocardiography (TEE and TTE) in the evaluation of the critically ill patient.[57]

Transesophageal Echocardiography Examination

CONTRAINDICATIONS AND COMPLICATIONS

TEE is a safe and relatively minimally invasive procedure, although echocardiographers should be aware of potential complications resulting from probe insertion and manipulation. Table 37.3 lists absolute and relative contraindications to TEE. The risks and benefits must be carefully considered in patients with oral, esophageal, or gastric disease. Hilberath and associates provide an excellent summary on the safety of TEE, with reviewed studies reporting an overall complication rate in adults of 0.18% to 2.8% and major complication rate of 0.2% to 1.2%.[58] A 2017 retrospective study reviewed recent data regarding complications in a contemporary cardiac surgery cohort.[59] Of the 7948 patients that underwent

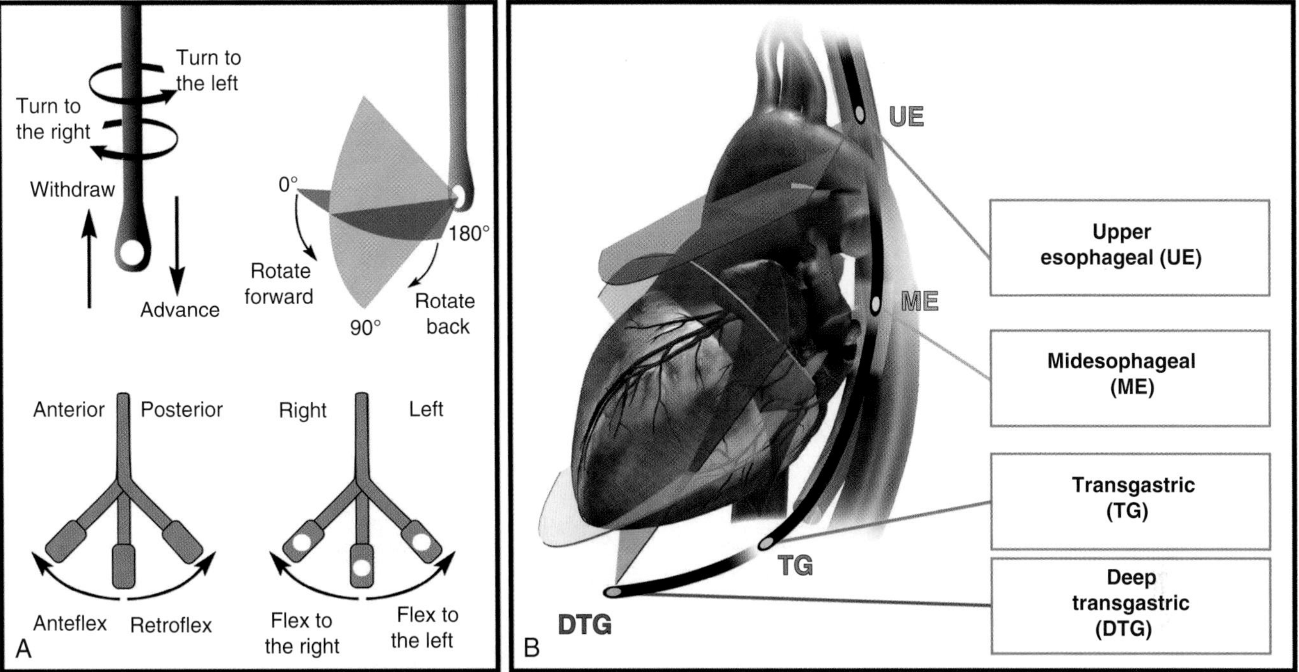

Fig. 37.5 Terminology used to describe manipulation of the transesophageal echocardiographic probe during image acquisition. (A) Terminology used for the manipulation of the transesophageal echocardiographic probe. (B) Four standard transducer positions within the esophagus and stomach and the associated imaging planes. (From Hahn RT, Abraham T, Adams MS, et al. Guidelines for performing a comprehensive transesophageal echocardiographic examination: recommendations from the American Society of Echocardiography and the Society of Cardiovascular Anesthesiologists. *J Am Soc Echocardiogr.* 2013;26(9):921–964.)

TEE, 111 (1.4%) were identified as having complications likely attributable to TEE (no other cause identified). Incidence of significant dysphagia was 0.3% and esophageal or gastric complications 0.9%. Independent risk factors associated with complications were age, body mass index, previous stroke, procedure other than isolated coronary artery bypass grafting (CABG), cardiopulmonary bypass time, and return to the operating room for any reason.

TRANSESOPHAGEAL ECHOCARDIOGRAPHY IMAGE ACQUISITION

Probe Manipulation and Imaging Planes

TEE probe manipulation includes withdrawal/advancement, turning left/right, and angle adjustment. The large knob on the handle controls anteflexion/retroflexion and the smaller knob allows flexion to the left and right. TEE image acquisition occurs at four different levels: upper esophageal (UE), midesophageal (ME), transgastric (TG), and deep transgastric (DTG) (Fig. 37.5).

Basic Examination

The basic perioperative TEE examination serves as an intraoperative monitoring tool used to identify cardiac causes of hemodynamic or respiratory instability.[60] The basic perioperative examination includes 11 views suited to evaluating hemodynamic instability. A suggested examination sequence progresses through the 11 views as follows: ME four-chamber (ME 4C), ME two-chamber (ME 2C), ME long axis (ME LAX), ME ascending aorta long-axis, ME ascending aorta short-axis, ME aortic valve short-axis (ME AV SAX), ME right ventricular inflow-outflow (ME RV Inflow-Outflow), ME bicaval, TG midpapillary short-axis (TG SAX), descending aorta short-axis, and descending aorta long-axis.

Comprehensive Examination

A comprehensive TEE examination enables practitioners with appropriate training to fully utilize the diagnostic capabilities of TEE. Twenty-eight views (including the 11 basic views) are recommended for comprehensive assessment (Fig. 37.6). Technical aspects of image acquisition have been extensively reviewed elsewhere.[61] Echocardiographers should complete their examinations systematically to avoid missing key findings. As a result of individual patient anatomy and the time constraints of the intraoperative environment, not all views are obtained in every examination.

Epicardial and Epiaortic Imaging

While epicardial echocardiography ushered in the era of intraoperative echocardiography, its use was supplanted by TEE. In the setting of contraindications to TEE or the need for better visualization of anterior structures, epicardial echocardiography remains an alternative modality.[62]

Epiaortic ultrasound (EAU) serves as an imaging adjunct, allowing visualization of the ascending aorta and aortic arch, regions that are unable to be visualized on TEE. Detection of ascending aorta atheroma is superior with

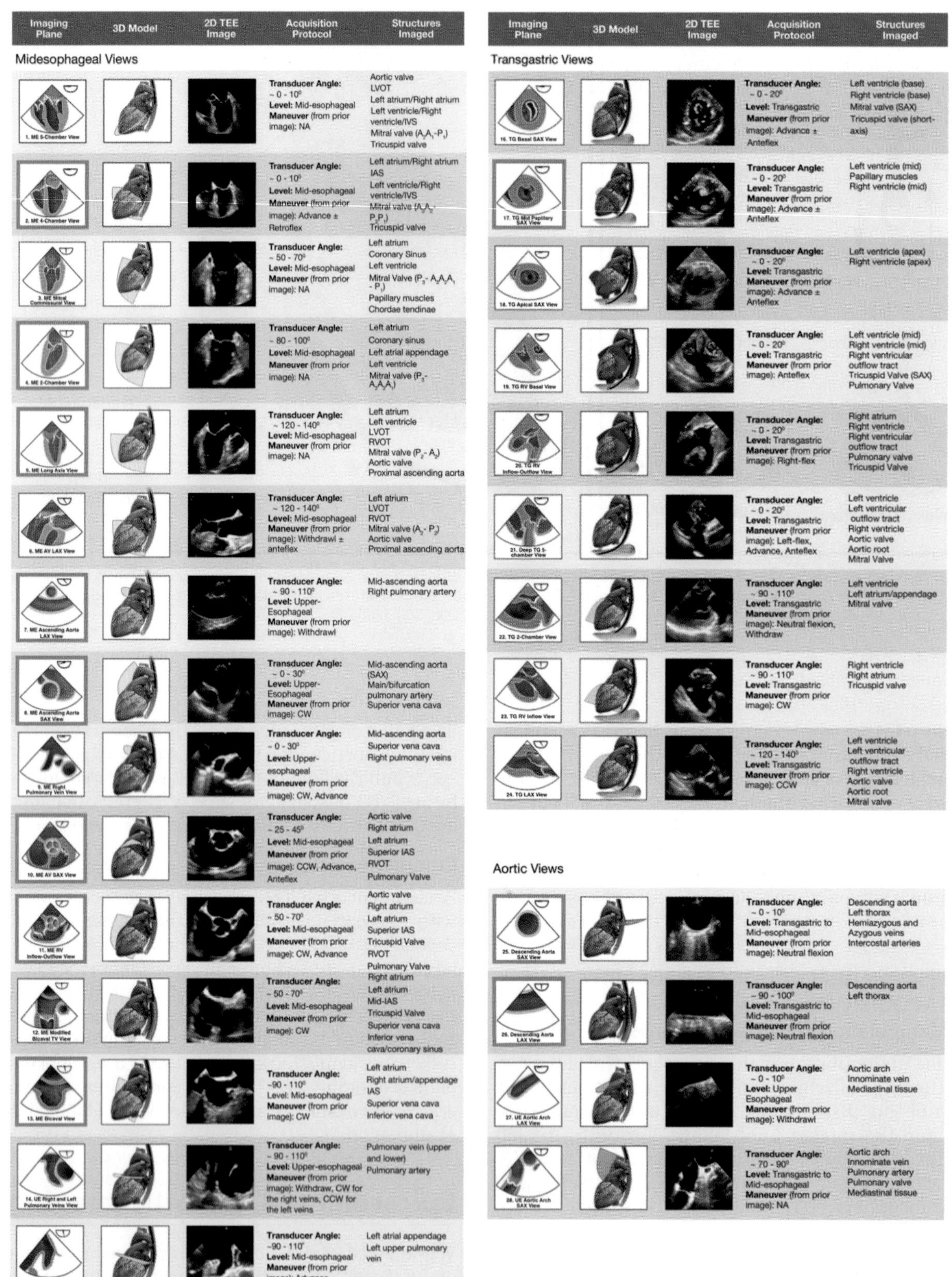

Imaging Plane	3D Model	2D TEE Image	Acquisition Protocol	Structures Imaged
Midesophageal Views				
1. ME 5-Chamber View			**Transducer Angle:** ~0 - 10º **Level:** Mid-esophageal **Maneuver** (from prior image): NA	Aortic valve, LVOT, Left atrium/Right atrium, Left ventricle/Right ventricle/IVS, Mitral valve (A_2A_1-P_1), Tricuspid valve
2. ME 4-Chamber View			**Transducer Angle:** ~0 - 10º **Level:** Mid-esophageal **Maneuver** (from prior image): Advance ± Retroflex	Left atrium/Right atrium, IAS, Left ventricle/Right ventricle/IVS, Mitral valve (A_2A_1-P_2P_1), Tricuspid valve
3. ME Mitral Commissural View			**Transducer Angle:** ~50 - 70º **Level:** Mid-esophageal **Maneuver** (from prior image): NA	Left atrium, Coronary Sinus, Left ventricle, Mitral Valve (P_3-$A_3A_2A_1$-P_1), Papillary muscles, Chordae tendinae
4. ME 2-Chamber View			**Transducer Angle:** ~80 - 100º **Level:** Mid-esophageal **Maneuver** (from prior image): NA	Left atrium, Coronary sinus, Left atrial appendage, Left ventricle, Mitral valve (P_3-$A_3A_2A_1$)
5. ME Long Axis View			**Transducer Angle:** ~120 - 140º **Level:** Mid-esophageal **Maneuver** (from prior image): NA	Left atrium, Left ventricle, LVOT, RVOT, Mitral valve (P_2-A_2), Aortic valve, Proximal ascending aorta
6. ME AV LAX View			**Transducer Angle:** ~120 - 140º **Level:** Mid-esophageal **Maneuver** (from prior image): Withdrawl ± anteflex	Left atrium, LVOT, RVOT, Mitral valve (A_2-P_2), Aortic valve, Proximal ascending aorta
7. ME Ascending Aorta LAX View			**Transducer Angle:** ~90 - 110º **Level:** Upper-Esophageal **Maneuver** (from prior image): Withdrawl	Mid-ascending aorta, Right pulmonary artery
8. ME Ascending Aorta SAX View			**Transducer Angle:** ~0 - 30º **Level:** Upper-Esophageal **Maneuver** (from prior image): CW	Mid-ascending aorta (SAX), Main/bifurcation pulmonary artery, Superior vena cava
9. ME Right Pulmonary Vein View			**Transducer Angle:** ~0 - 30º **Level:** Upper-esophageal **Maneuver** (from prior image): CW, Advance	Mid-ascending aorta, Superior vena cava, Right pulmonary veins
10. ME AV SAX View			**Transducer Angle:** ~25 - 45º **Level:** Mid-esophageal **Maneuver** (from prior image): CCW, Advance, Anteflex	Aortic valve, Right atrium, Left atrium, Superior IAS, RVOT, Pulmonary Valve
11. ME RV Inflow-Outflow View			**Transducer Angle:** ~50 - 70º **Level:** Mid-esophageal **Maneuver** (from prior image): CW, Advance	Aortic valve, Right atrium, Left atrium, Superior IAS, Tricuspid Valve, RVOT, Pulmonary Valve
12. ME Modified Bicaval TV View			**Transducer Angle:** ~50 - 70º **Level:** Mid-esophageal **Maneuver** (from prior image): CW	Right atrium, Left atrium, Mid-IAS, Tricuspid Valve, Superior vena cava, Inferior vena cava/coronary sinus
13. ME Bicaval View			**Transducer Angle:** ~90 - 110º Level: Mid-esophageal **Maneuver** (from prior image): CW	Left atrium, Right atrium/appendage, IAS, Superior vena cava, Inferior vena cava
14. UE Right and Left Pulmonary Veins View			**Transducer Angle:** ~90 - 110º **Level:** Upper-esophageal **Maneuver** (from prior image): Withdraw, CW for the right veins, CCW for the left veins	Pulmonary vein (upper and lower), Pulmonary artery
15. ME Left Atrial Appendage View			**Transducer Angle:** ~90 - 110º **Level:** Mid-esophageal **Maneuver** (from prior image): Advance	Left atrial appendage, Left upper pulmonary vein
Transgastric Views				
16. TG Basal SAX View			**Transducer Angle:** ~0 - 20º **Level:** Transgastric **Maneuver** (from prior image): Advance ± Anteflex	Left ventricle (base), Right ventricle (base), Mitral valve (SAX), Tricuspid valve (short-axis)
17. TG Mid Papillary SAX View			**Transducer Angle:** ~0 - 20º **Level:** Transgastric **Maneuver** (from prior image): Advance ± Anteflex	Left ventricle (mid), Papillary muscles, Right ventricle (mid)
18. TG Apical SAX View			**Transducer Angle:** ~0 - 20º **Level:** Transgastric **Maneuver** (from prior image): Advance ± Anteflex	Left ventricle (apex), Right ventricle (apex)
19. TG RV Basal View			**Transducer Angle:** ~0 - 20º **Level:** Transgastric **Maneuver** (from prior image): Anteflex	Left ventricle (mid), Right ventricle (mid), Right ventricular outflow tract, Tricuspid Valve (SAX), Pulmonary Valve
20. TG RV Inflow-Outflow View			**Transducer Angle:** ~0 - 20º **Level:** Transgastric **Maneuver** (from prior image): Right-flex	Right atrium, Right ventricle, Right ventricular outflow tract, Pulmonary valve, Tricuspid Valve
21. Deep TG 5-chamber View			**Transducer Angle:** ~0 - 20º **Level:** Transgastric **Maneuver** (from prior image): Left-flex, Advance, Anteflex	Left ventricle, Left ventricular outflow tract, Right ventricle, Aortic valve, Aortic root, Mitral Valve
22. TG 2-Chamber View			**Transducer Angle:** ~90 - 110º **Level:** Transgastric **Maneuver** (from prior image): Neutral flexion, Withdraw	Left ventricle, Left atrium/appendage, Mitral valve
23. TG RV Inflow View			**Transducer Angle:** ~90 - 110º **Level:** Transgastric **Maneuver** (from prior image): CW	Right ventricle, Right atrium, Tricuspid valve
24. TG LAX View			**Transducer Angle:** ~120 - 140º **Level:** Transgastric **Maneuver** (from prior image): CCW	Left ventricle, Left ventricular outflow tract, Right ventricle, Aortic valve, Aortic root, Mitral valve
Aortic Views				
25. Descending Aorta SAX View			**Transducer Angle:** ~0 - 10º **Level:** Transgastric to Mid-esophageal **Maneuver** (from prior image): Neutral flexion	Descending aorta, Left thorax, Hemiazygous and Azygous veins, Intercostal arteries
26. Descending Aorta LAX View			**Transducer Angle:** ~90 - 100º **Level:** Transgastric to Mid-esophageal **Maneuver** (from prior image): Neutral flexion	Descending aorta, Left thorax
27. UE Aortic Arch LAX View			**Transducer Angle:** ~0 - 10º **Level:** Upper Esophageal **Maneuver** (from prior image): Withdrawl	Aortic arch, Innominate vein, Mediastinal tissue
28. UE Aortic Arch SAX View			**Transducer Angle:** ~70 - 90º **Level:** Transgastric to Mid-esophageal **Maneuver** (from prior image): NA	Aortic arch, Innominate vein, Pulmonary artery, Pulmonary valve, Mediastinal tissue

Fig. 37.6 The 28 suggested views of the comprehensive transesophageal echocardiographic *(TEE)* examination. Each view is shown as a 3D image, the corresponding imaging plane, and a 2D image. The acquisition protocol and the structures imaged in each view are listed in the subsequent columns. The green boxes indicate the 11 views of the basic TEE examination. (Modified from Hahn RT, Abraham T, Adams MS, et al. Guidelines for performing a comprehensive transesophageal echocardiographic examination: recommendations from the American Society of Echocardiography and the Society of Cardiovascular Anesthesiologists. *J Am Soc Echocardiogr*. 2013;26(9):921–964.)

EAU compared to that of TEE or manual palpation.[63-65] EAU impacts surgical strategy, but data as to whether this translates into improved clinical outcomes are limited and heterogeneous.[63-65] Examination guidelines and example imaging views are available.[66]

Transthoracic Echocardiography Examination

TRANSTHORACIC ECHOCARDIOGRAPHY IMAGE ACQUISITION

Three elements describe transthoracic sonographic views: (1) transducer position or window, (2) imaging plane, and (3) structures imaged. When feasible, patients should turn to their left side with the left hand resting behind the head. The main windows are parasternal, apical, subcostal, and suprasternal. Imaging motions include translation (sliding), tilting, angulation, and rotation.

Focused Cardiac Ultrasound Versus Limited Examination

With increasing use of ultrasonography at the point of care, it is important for the clinician to recognize the distinction between focused cardiac ultrasound (FoCUS, FCU) and limited TTE examination. Guidelines endorsed by several societies describe the key differences between the two examinations.[67,68] FoCUS is a simplified, point-of-care ultrasound examination that complements the physical examination (Box 37.2). FoCUS addresses specific questions within a given clinical context. Relevant abnormalities are characterized as present or absent, and questions are answered in a yes/no format. In contrast, limited TTE is broad in scope. Interpretation includes normal, pathological, and incidental findings, and quantitative techniques may be employed. Fewer images are acquired in a limited examination compared to a comprehensive examination.[67] Limited TTE requires a practitioner with advanced training and expertise.

Abnormalities identified by FoCUS require follow-up with formal comprehensive echocardiography. If FoCUS does not reveal pathology but there is clinical suggestion of cardiac disease, formal comprehensive echocardiography should also be pursued. Many FoCUS protocols exist, most including five key views: parasternal long-axis (PLAX), parasternal short-axis (PSAX), apical four-chamber (A4C), subcostal four-chamber (SC4), and subcostal inferior vena cava (SIVC) (Fig. 37.7 through 37.10; Video 37.2). Protocols often incorporate lung ultrasound. For those interested in details of image acquisition, we refer the reader to a practical introductory primer.[69]

Comprehensive Examination

A minority of anesthesiologists have the necessary training required to perform and/or formally interpret comprehensive TTE examinations. Standard imaging views occur at the parasternal, apical, and subcostal windows, plus the suprasternal notch. In addition to the views included in FoCUS, a comprehensive TTE examination includes the

BOX 37.2 Features of Focused Cardiac Ultrasound

- Goal-directed
- Problem-oriented
- Limited in scope
- Simplified
- Time sensitive and repeatable
- Qualitative or semiquantitative
- Performed at the point of care
- Usually performed by clinicians

FoCUS, Focused Cardiac Ultrasound.

Adapted from Via G, Hussain A, Wells M, et al. International evidence-based recommendations for focused cardiac ultrasound. *J Am Soc Echocardiogr*. 2014;27(7):683 e681–683 e633.

PLAX right ventricular outflow, PLAX right ventricular inflow, PSAX apical, PSAX mitral (basal), PSAX aortic, apical right ventricle-focused, apical five-chamber (A5C), apical two-chamber (A2C), apical three-chamber (A3C), and suprasternal notch long axis views.[70]

Qualitative Assessment

VENTRICULAR SIZE AND FUNCTION

Left Ventricle

Qualitative visual assessment of LV systolic function is the mainstay of perioperative echocardiography. Visual estimation of EF by TTE correlates well with quantitative methods[71,72] and real-time intraoperative TEE interpretation can reasonably estimate function compared to formal offline methods.[73] Wall thickening is symmetric and vigorous when LV systolic function is normal (Video 37.3). The key TEE views for global assessment of LV function include the TG SAX (Fig. 37.11), ME 4C, ME 2C, and ME LAX views (Fig. 37.12). Analogous TTE views are PSAX, A4C, A2C, and PLAX views. The TG SAX and PSAX views display distributions of all three coronary arteries.

Assessment of regional function focuses on the thickening and shortening of individual segments. Translational motion, tethering, or dyssynchrony due to conduction delay or pacing can make interpretation challenging. A 17-segment model divides the heart into six basal segments (from the mitral valve annulus to the tips of the papillary muscles), six midpapillary level segments (from the tips to the base of the papillary muscles), four apical (or distal) segments (from the base of the papillary muscles to the LV apex), and the apical cap.[74] The apical cap is difficult to visualize with TEE due to foreshortening. Segmental thickening should be assessed in the context of coronary distribution, recognizing variability among individuals. The left anterior descending artery (LAD) consistently supplies the anterior and anteroseptal segments and apical cap (Fig. 37.13). The right coronary artery (RCA) supplies the right ventricle (RV) and the basal inferior, basal inferoseptal, and mid-inferior and possibly the mid-inferoseptal segments, the latter of which may be supplied by the LAD. The left circumflex typically supplies the lateral segments, although

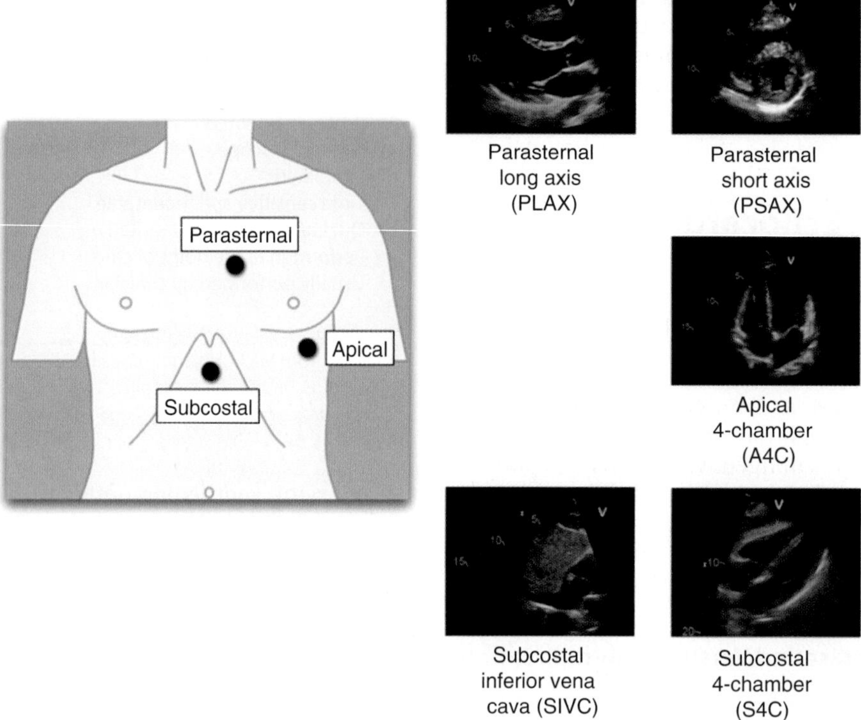

Fig. 37.7 Views included in the focused cardiac ultrasound *(FoCUS)* examination: parasternal long axis *(PLAX)*, parasternal short axis *(PSAX)*, apical 4-chamber *(A4C)*, subcostal 4-chamber *(S4C)*, and subcostal inferior vena cava *(SIVC)*. The parasternal window is between the third through fifth intercostal space to the left of the sternum. The apical window is near the point of maximal impulse along the mid-axillary line, often near the fifth intercostal space. The subcostal window is just below the xiphoid, along the midline or slightly to the patient's right. (Adapted from Via G, Hussain A, Wells M, et al. International evidence-based recommendations for focused cardiac ultrasound. *J Am Soc Echocardiogr*. 2014;27(7):683 e681–683 e633.)

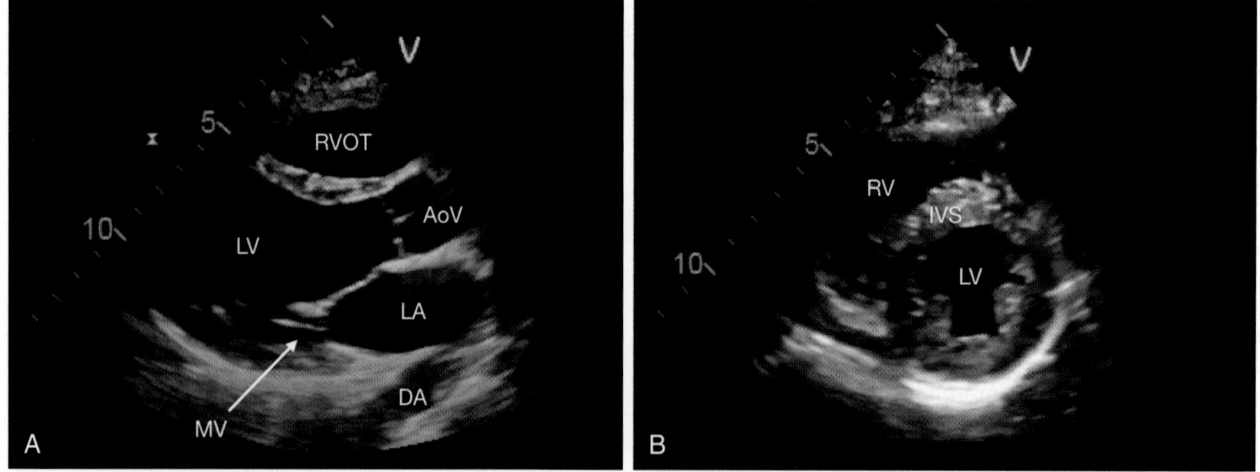

Fig. 37.8 Transthoracic parasternal views included in focused cardiac ultrasound. (A) The parasternal long axis view is shown. This view is analogous to the transesophageal midesophageal long axis view. In transthoracic imaging, anterior structures are closest to the transducer (and therefore displayed at the top of the image), while in transesophageal imaging, posterior structures are in closest proximity to the transducer (and displayed at the top of the image). (B) The parasternal short axis view is shown. This view is analogous to the transesophageal transgastric mid-papillary short axis view. *AoV,* Aortic valve; *DA,* descending aorta; *IVS,* interventricular septum; *LA,* left atrium; *LV,* left ventricle; *MV,* mitral valve; *RV,* right ventricle; *RVOT,* right ventricular outflow tract.

contributions from the LAD to the anterolateral segments or RCA to the inferolateral segments are not uncommon.[75] Each segment should be evaluated as normal/hyperkinetic, hypokinetic (reduced thickening), akinetic (minimal or absent thickening), or dyskinetic (thinning, stretching, or aneurysmal). Echocardiography is more sensitive than the ECG in detecting ischemic changes.[76]

Right Ventricle

The complex geometry of the RV makes assessment more challenging. Qualitatively, the RV should appear approximately two-thirds the size of the left ventricle, assessed in ME 4C and A4C views. Typically the right ventricle does not extend to the LV apex. RV hypertrophy suggests chronic pulmonary hypertension or the presence of cardiomyopathies.

The interventricular septum provides additional information about RV pathology. Normally, the septum curves toward the RV, and the LV cavity appears circular in short axis. In states of RV *volume* overload, the septum shifts away from the RV and flattens resulting in a D-shaped LV cavity mainly in *mid-to-late diastole* (Video 37.4). RV *pressure* overload leads to leftward septal shift and septal flattening throughout the cardiac cycle, with the changes most pronounced at *end-systole* (Video 37.5).[77]

VALVULAR FUNCTION

Qualitative assessment of valvular function begins with sequential assessment of the valve in multiple imaging planes, noting the motion of the leaflets, presence of leaflet thickening or calcification, vegetations or masses, and additional structural abnormalities (Fig. 37.14). Malcoaptation and annular dilation help define the etiology of dysfunction in regurgitant lesions. 3-D imaging modalities clarify the location of structure abnormalities.

CFD provides visual information about flow through valves. Aliasing or turbulence of forward flow through a valve should prompt evaluation for additional signs of stenosis. Further characterization of stenotic lesions is primarily quantitative in nature. Color Doppler imaging also detects

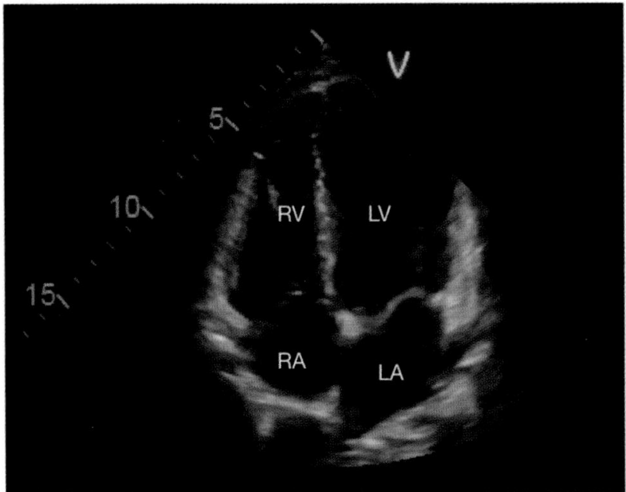

Fig. 37.9 Transthoracic apical four-chamber view. This view is analogous to the midesophageal four-chamber view in transesophageal echocardiography. *LA*, Left atrium; *LV*, left ventricle; *RA*, right atrium; *RV*, right ventricle.

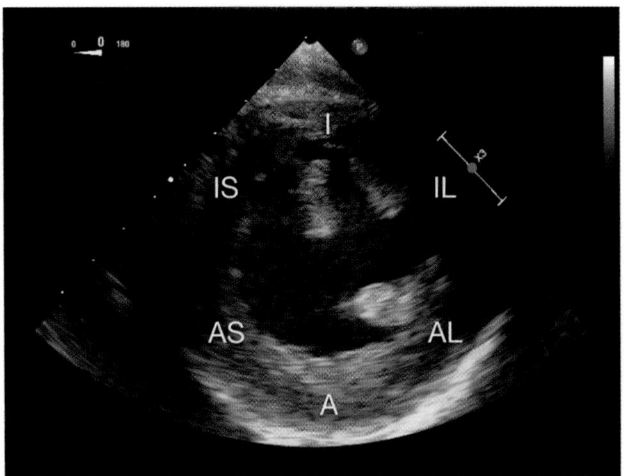

Fig. 37.11 The transesophageal transgastric mid-papillary short axis view (TG SAX) is a common view for qualitative evaluation of global left ventricular systolic function. Basal and apical segments are not visualized in this view, so midesophageal or TG LAX views should also be obtained to provide a more complete picture of the overall function. The TG SAX view includes myocardial segments supplied by each of the coronary arteries, making it useful for detection of new ischemia. The TG SAX view displays the mid inferior *(I)*, mid inferolateral *(IL)*, mid anterolateral *(AL)*, mid anterior *(A)*, mid anteroseptal *(AS)*, and mid inferoseptal *(IS)* segments.

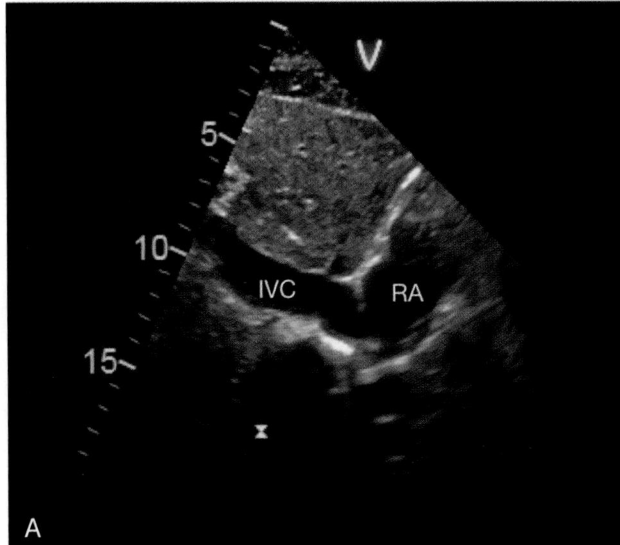

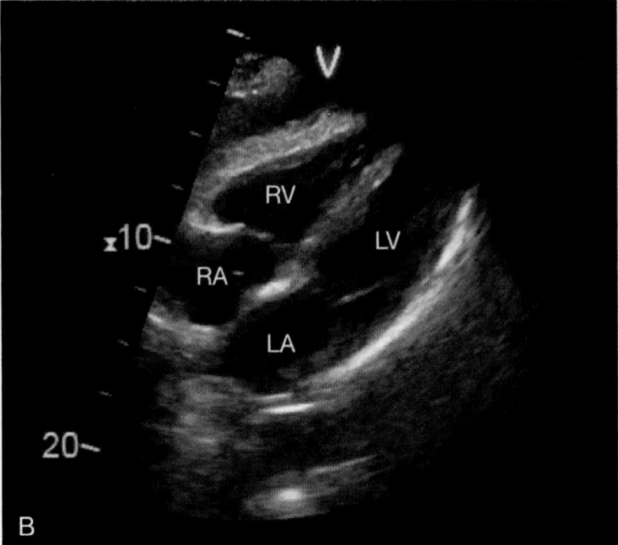

Fig. 37.10 Transthoracic subcostal views included in focused cardiac ultrasound. (A) The subcostal inferior vena cava *(IVC)* view is shown. The IVC diameter and collapsibility index are measured in this view to estimate right atrial pressure in spontaneously breathing individuals (see text). (B) The subcostal four-chamber view is shown. This view is useful for ultrasonographic examination during cardiac arrest, because it can be performed without interrupting chest compressions. *LA*, Left atrium; *LV*, left ventricle; *RA*, right atrium; *RV*, right ventricle.

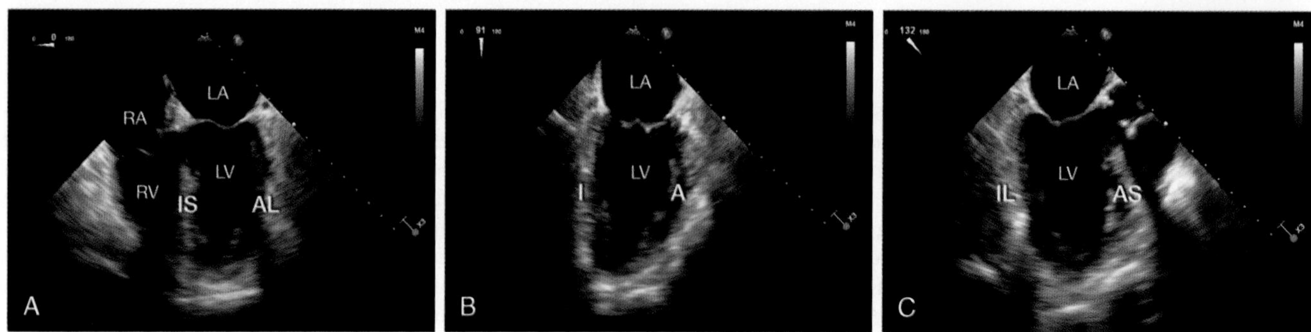

Fig. 37.12 Midesophageal views for assessing left ventricular function using transesophageal echocardiography. (A) The midesophageal four-chamber (ME 4C) view displays the inferoseptal *(IS)* and anterolateral *(AL)* walls. (B) The midesophageal two-chamber (ME 2C) view displays the inferior *(I)* and anterior *(A)* walls. (C) The midesophageal long axis view (ME LAX) displays the inferolateral *(IL)* and anteroseptal *(AS)* walls. *LA,* Left atrium; *LV,* left ventricle; *RA,* right atrium; *RV,* right ventricle.

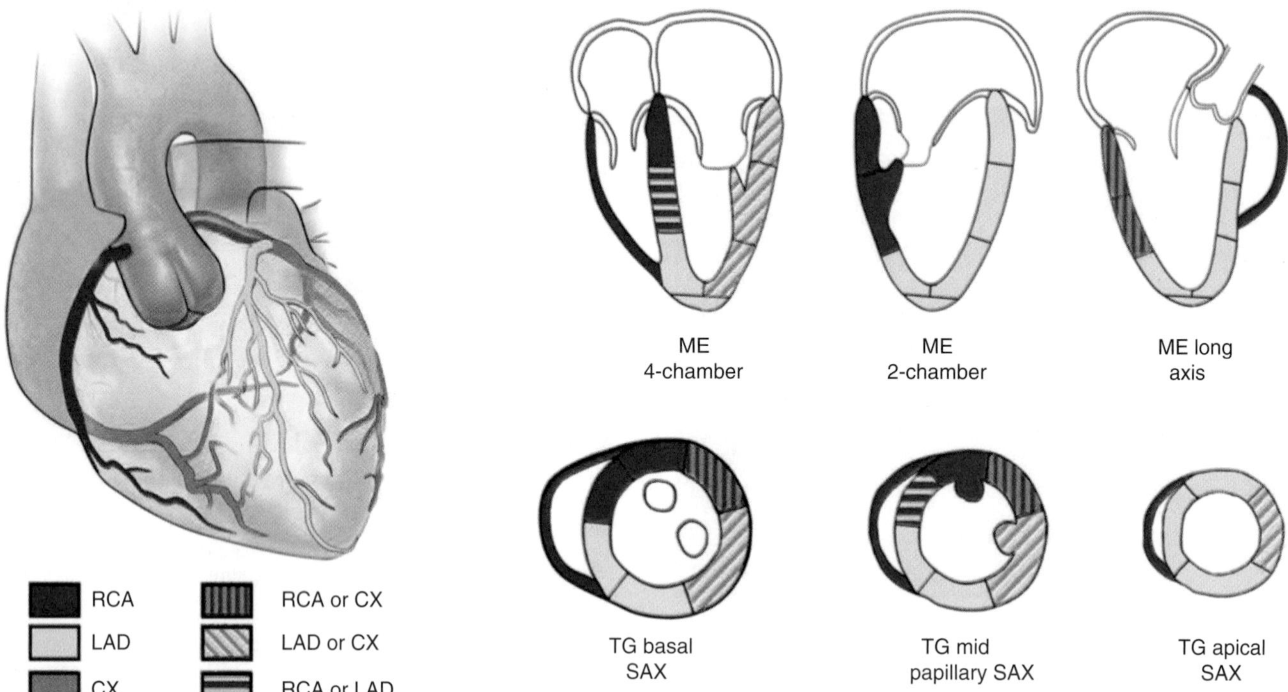

Fig. 37.13 Typical distributions of the right coronary artery *(RCA)*, the left anterior descending coronary artery *(LAD)*, and the circumflex coronary artery *(CX)* from transesophageal views of heart. The arterial distribution varies among patients. Some segments have variable coronary perfusion. *ME,* Mid-esophageal; *TG,* transgastric; *SAX,* short axis. (Modified from Lang RM, Badano LP, Mor-Avi V, et al. Recommendations for cardiac chamber quantification by echocardiography in adults: an update from the American Society of Echocardiography and the European Association of Cardiovascular Imaging. *J Am Soc Echocardiogr.* 2015;28(1):1–39 e14.)

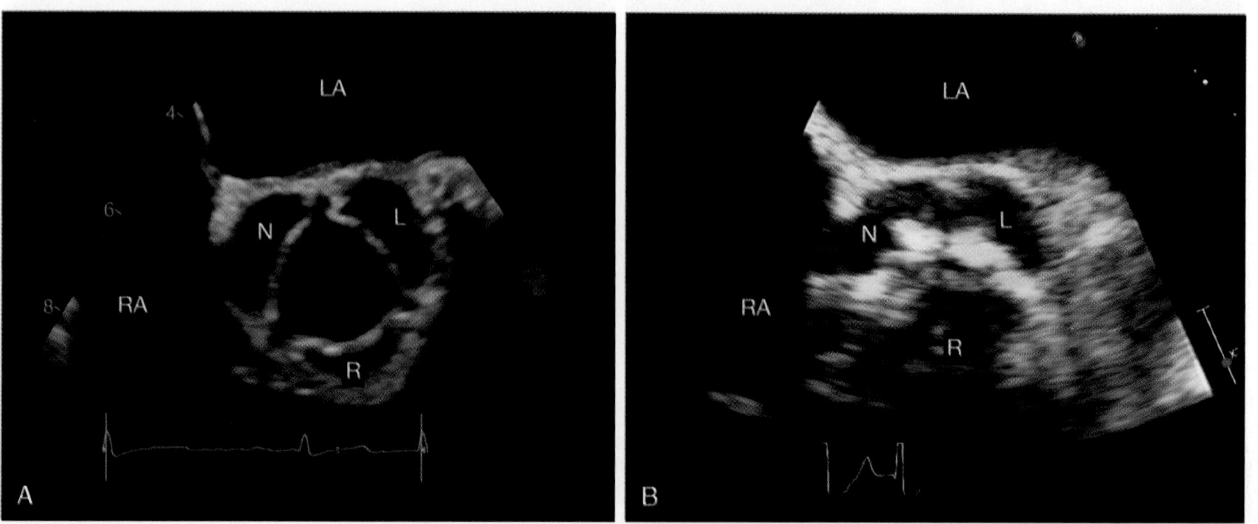

Fig. 37.14 Qualitative assessment of the aortic valve (zoomed-in transesophageal aortic valve short axis view) (A) There are three valve leaflets of normal thickness. Leaflet excursion appears normal. (B) There are three aortic valve leaflets which are severely thickened. Leaflet excursion is reduced. These qualitative findings should prompt additional quantitative assessment of valvular stenosis. *L,* Left coronary cusp; *LA,* left atrium; *N,* non-coronary cusp; *R,* right coronary cusp; *RA,* right atrium

the presence of valvular regurgitation. The three color Doppler components of a regurgitant jet are proximal flow convergence, vena contracta, and jet area (Figure. 37.15). As blood approaches the regurgitant orifice, it accelerates, forming a series of hemispheric shells of increasing velocity and decreasing area. This flow convergence region provides qualitative information about regurgitation severity and is also utilized in quantitative assessments. The vena contracta is the narrowest portion of a regurgitant jet at or immediately downstream of the regurgitant orifice.[78,79] The jet area provides information about the mechanism of regurgitation. For example eccentric regurgitation often arises from structural abnormalities while centrally originating regurgitation may be secondary in nature. The size of the jet area is subject to both technical and hemodynamic limitations, so visual estimation of jet area alone is not a reliable means of assessing regurgitation severity.

Atrial and ventricular dilation suggest chronicity of severe regurgitation; normal chamber size would be unusual in the presence of chronic severe regurgitation. Density and shape of the continuous-wave Doppler (CWD) recording of the regurgitant jet provide additional qualitative information.[79]

An important limitation of intraoperative assessment of valvular regurgitation is the hemodynamic consequences of general anesthesia, resulting in reduced preload, afterload, and contractility. General anesthesia commonly reduces the severity of MR. Pharmacologic increase of afterload may provide more representative measurements, but may also lead to significant overestimation of regurgitation severity.[80]

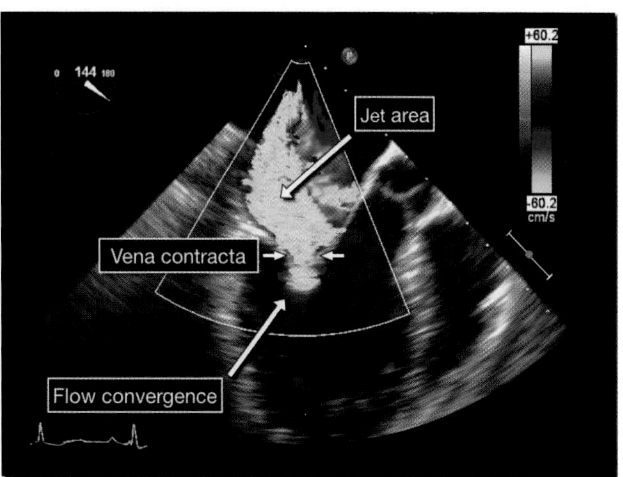

Fig. 37.15 Mitral regurgitation displaying the three components of a regurgitant jet: (1) flow convergence, (2) the vena contracta, and (3) the regurgitant jet area.

TABLE 37.4 Classification of Left Ventricular Systolic Function According to Ejection Fraction

Systolic Function	Male	Female
Normal	52%–72%	54%–74%
Mild dysfunction	41%–51%	41%–53%
Moderate dysfunction	30%–40%	30%–40%
Severe dysfunction	<30%	<30%

From Lang RM, Badano LP, Mor-Avi V, et al. Recommendations for cardiac chamber quantification by echocardiography in adults: an update from the American Society of Echocardiography and the European Association of Cardiovascular Imaging. *J Am Soc Echocardiogr*. 2015;28(1):1–39 e14.

Quantitative Assessment

VENTRICULAR SIZE AND FUNCTION

Left Ventricle

Most indices of systolic function used in routine evaluation are load-dependent, necessitating interpretation in context and serial assessments due to changing intraoperative conditions. Global systolic function is assessed by measuring the difference between an end-diastolic and end-systolic value of a parameter and dividing by the end-diastolic value. Fractional shortening uses length measurements and fractional area change (FAC) uses area measurements. Both approaches have limitations in the setting of regional wall motion abnormalities (RWMAs). Ejection fraction (EF) is the difference between the end-diastolic volume (EDV) and end-systolic volume (ESV), divided by EDV:

$$EF = \frac{(EDV - ESV)}{EDV}$$

The recommended method for 2-D calculation of EF is the biplane method of disks (modified Simpson rule).[81] This requires tracing the endocardial border in two perpendicular views and assumes the LV volume consists of a stack of elliptical disks. The upper limit of normal for EDV is 74 mL/m^2 for males and 61 mL/m^2 for females; ESV is 31 mL/m^2 for males and 24 mL/m^2 for females.[81] Table 37.4 presents updated reference ranges for LVEF.[81] Assessment of EF using 3-D echocardiography (Fig. 37.16) is more accurate than 2-D echocardiography.[41] In the presence of significant valvular regurgitation, myocardial contractility may be depressed and forward cardiac output low despite a normal EF.

Additional indices of LV systolic function include DTI of the mitral annular systolic velocity (s′), myocardial performance index (MPI), and the change in LV pressure over time (dP/dt). Pulsed-wave DTI of the myocardium at the level of the mitral annulus yields a myocardial velocity profile (Fig. 37.17). The systolic velocity wave (s′) reflects the apically-directed motion of the myocardium and correlates with EF. Normal s′ reference ranges vary based on sex, age, and mitral annulus measurement size.[82] MPI assesses both systolic and diastolic performance and is calculated by the sum of isovolumetric contraction and relaxation times divided by ejection time. MPI identifies impaired global function and has prognostic value, however it is not routinely part of the perioperative examination. The change in LV pressure over time (dP/dt) derived from the CWD signal of MR provides information about LV contractility. Normal LV dP/dt is greater than 1200 mm mmHg/s; dP/dt less than 800 mmHg/s is consistent with severe dysfunction.[83] Global longitudinal strain is emerging as a technique with utility in identifying systolic dysfunction prior to decrement in EF. Normal values vary across vendor platforms, but in general, a value of −20% (or more negative) would be expected in normal systolic function (Fig. 37.18).

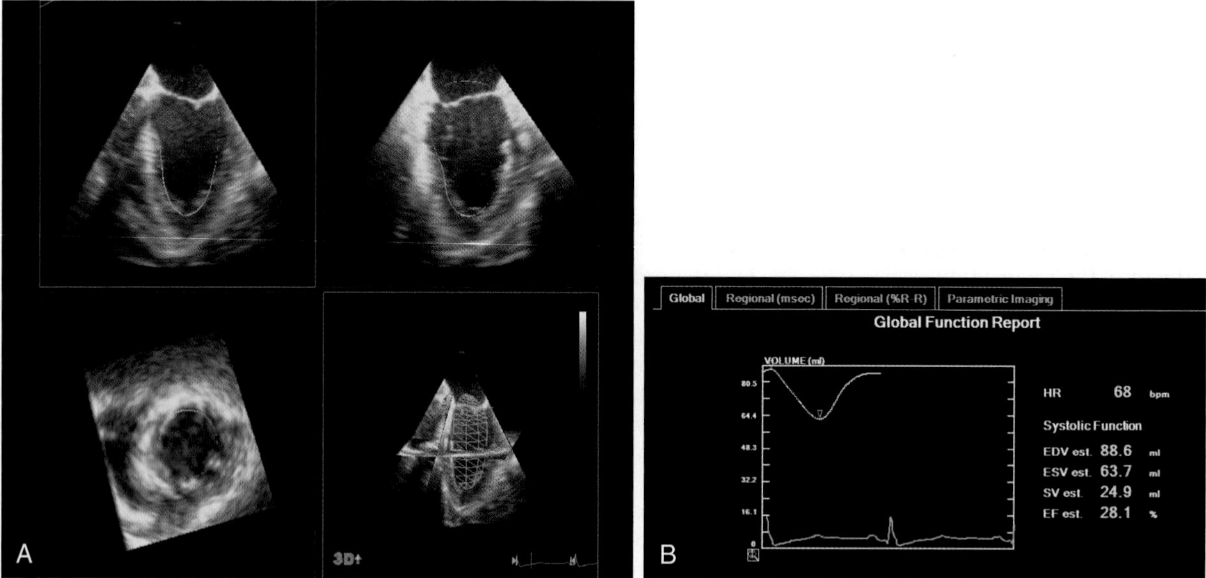

Fig. 37.16 Three-dimensional (3D) transesophageal echocardiographic measurement of left ventricular ejection fraction. (A) A full-volume data set of the left ventricle is displayed using multiplanar reconstruction. After manual tracing of the endocardial borders at end-diastole and end-systole in the planes displayed in the top two panels, a semi-automated endocardial border detection algorithm tracks the borders in the remaining frames. (B) The *yellow line* displays the left ventricular volume over the duration of the cardiac cycle. Measurements reported include end-diastolic volume, end-systolic volume, stroke volume, and ejection fraction. Segmental changes in volume over the course of the cardiac cycle can also be displayed.

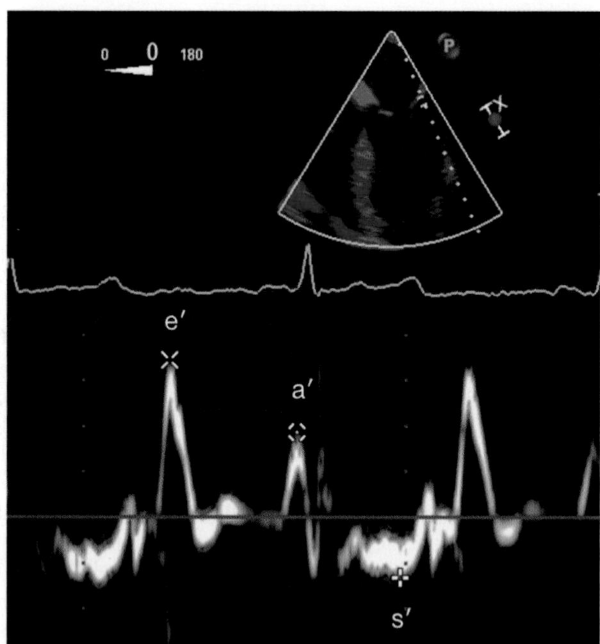

Fig. 37.17 Spectral Doppler tissue imaging obtained at the lateral mitral annulus in the midesophageal four-chamber view. The systolic waveform (s′) corresponds to the systolic tissue velocity. The two diastolic waveforms correspond to the early diastolic tissue velocity (e′) and the late (atrial) diastolic tissue velocity (a′). When obtained using TEE, s′ is a negative waveform (directed away from the transducer), while e′ and a′ are positive waveforms. Transthoracic acquisition of mitral annular velocity is performed in the apical four-chamber view. In TTE acquisition, the s′ waveform is positive, while e′ and a′ are negative.

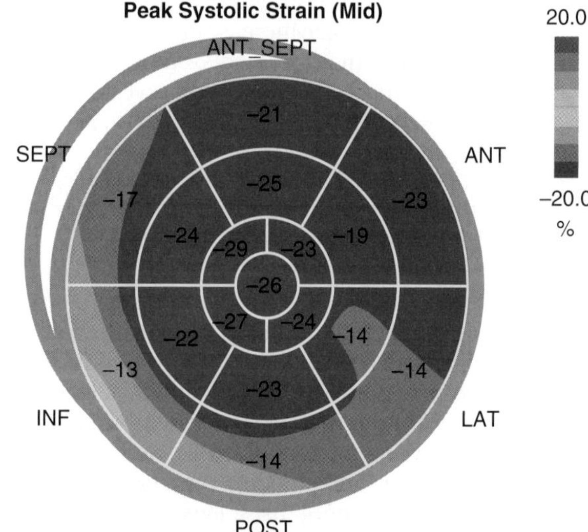

Fig. 37.18 A transthoracic "bulls-eye" plot of speckle tracking-derived global longitudinal strain obtained with transthoracic echocardiography. The image depicts the 17 segments of the left ventricle and the peak segmental systolic strain for each segment. The dark red areas represent normal strain, while the light red and pink areas represent abnormal strain. The average global longitudinal strain in this example is normal (−20.8%, not displayed in the image).

Right Ventricle

Parameters for assessment of RV function include FAC, volumetric assessments (EF), tricuspid annular plane systolic excursion (TAPSE), DTI of the tricuspid annular systolic velocity (s′), and MPI. RV FAC is obtained by tracing the endocardial border in diastole and systole, from the annulus along the free wall (excluding trabeculations) to the apex, from the apex to the annulus along the interventricular septum, and then returning to the annular starting point. RV FAC is calculated as:

$$\text{RV FAC} = \frac{\text{RV EDA} - \text{RV ESA}}{\text{RV EDA}} * 100$$

RV FAC is expressed as a percentage and has a lower limit of normal of 35%.[77] Estimation of RV EF using 2-D echocardiography requires geometric assumptions, and guidelines do not recommend its use.[77] When expertise is available 3-D RV EF is recommended, with less than 45% usually representing abnormal function.[81]

TAPSE is commonly used in TTE for evaluating RV longitudinal function, measured by aligning the M-mode cursor parallel to the tricuspid annular motion in the A4C view.[81] TAPSE less than 17 mm is consistent with RV systolic dysfunction. Parallel alignment of the tricuspid annulus with the M-mode cursor is difficult in TEE, and ME 4C measurements of TAPSE correlate poorly with TTE measurements. Alternative methods for measuring tricuspid annular motion with TEE have been explored. Anatomical M-mode measurements in ME 4C and DTG 4-chamber 0-degree views demonstrate agreement with TTE TAPSE.[84] TEE speckle tracking of tricuspid annular motion has also been demonstrated to correlate well with TTE TAPSE[85,86]; whether this will have practical perioperative applications requires further investigation. Reduction in TAPSE following cardiac surgery is well described. Whether reduced TAPSE reflects a true decrement in RV systolic function or rather geometric alteration from pericardiotomy remains controversial.[87,88]

An s′ of less than 9.5 cm/s is consistent with RV dysfunction, but like TAPSE is an index of longitudinal excursion and may be reduced after cardiac surgery. A right ventricular myocardial performance index (MPI) of greater than 0.43 by pulsed-wave Doppler (PWD) or greater than 0.54 by DTI reflects abnormal RV function.[81] RV strain and strain rate are emerging as prognostic parameters in the cardiology literature, but reference values are vendor specific and measurements are not yet routinely part of the perioperative examination.

Diastolic Function

Many complex interactions contribute to ventricular filling during diastole, but the echocardiographer should have a basic understanding of diastolic physiology and the progression of LV filling abnormalities along a continuum of impaired relaxation and decreased compliance. Myocardial relaxation primarily affects LV filling during early diastole (isovolumetric relaxation and early rapid filling), whereas the effects of ventricular compliance predominate in late diastole (diastasis and atrial contraction).

Transmitral PWD flow patterns reflect changes in LV filling and are used to characterize the stages of diastolic dysfunction. Two waveforms correspond to early rapid filling (E wave) and atrial contraction (A wave), respectively. (Fig. 37.19). The E:A ratio changes with progressive diastolic dysfunction (Fig. 37.20), and traditionally, other parameters such as isovolumetric relaxation time, deceleration time, pulmonary venous flow profiles, and propagation velocities have provided supportive information when grading diastolic dysfunction. Under normal conditions, most ventricular filling occurs during early diastole (resulting from relaxation and suction forces), and the E:A is ratio greater than 1. Grade 1 diastolic dysfunction manifests as *impaired relaxation* with decreased early diastolic filling and a compensatory increase in late diastolic filling (E < A). Relaxation remains impaired in more advanced degrees of diastolic dysfunction. In grade 2 diastolic dysfunction *(pseudonormal pattern)*, decreasing LV compliance leads to a rise in LV end-diastolic pressure (LVEDP). Ultimately an increase in left atrial pressure (LAP) increases driving pressures across the mitral valve, increasing early filling, and "normalizing" the E:A ratio. With progression to a *restrictive* pattern (grade 3 dysfunction), markedly decreased LV compliance and significantly elevated LVEDP and LAP result in very elevated peak E-wave velocity (E:A > 2) and rapid equilibration of LV and LAPs.

DTI is an important technique for evaluating diastolic function. DTI of mitral annular myocardial velocities produces two diastolic waveforms: e′ (early diastolic tissue velocity) and a′ (late diastolic tissue velocity), as shown in Fig. 37.17. Preload conditions have less effect on e′ than on the transmitral E wave. DTI e′ is reduced when impaired relaxation is present, making

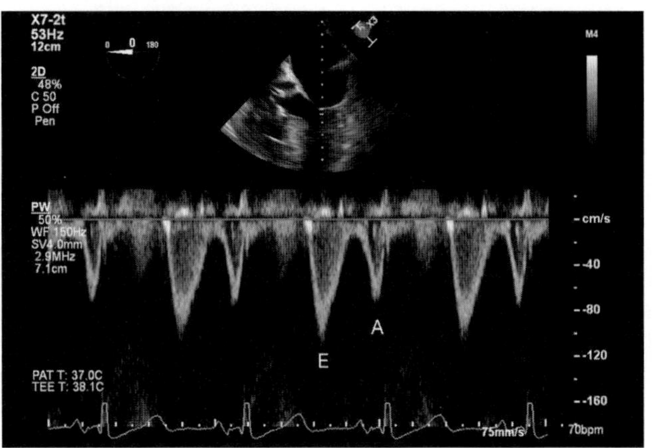

Fig. 37.19 Transmitral pulsed-wave Doppler profile demonstrating the peak early filling (E-wave) and flow due to atrial contraction (A-wave).

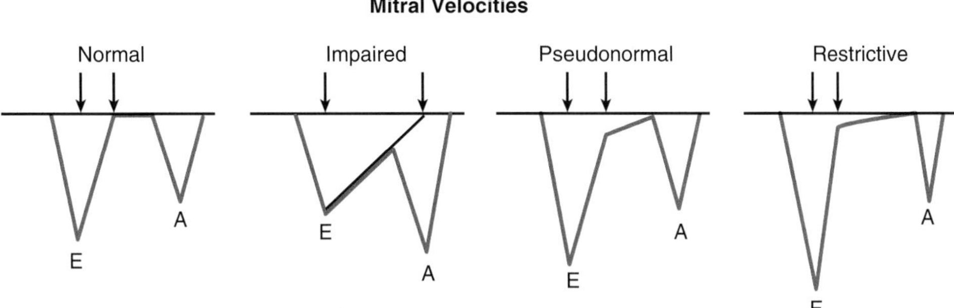

Fig. 37.20 Line drawings representing simultaneous transesophageal pulsed-wave Doppler recordings from the mitral annulus are shown for normal, impaired, pseudonormal, and restrictive left ventricular diastolic function. The black arrows mark the deceleration time of early filling, which is the interval between the peak E velocity and the point where the deceleration slope intersects the baseline. (Modified from Fig. 46.32, Desjardins G. Perioperative echocardiography. In: Miller R, ed. *Miller's Anesthesia*. 8th ed. Philadelphia, PA: Elsevier/Saunders; 2015:1396–1428.

this a useful parameter for assessing whether diastolic dysfunction is present or absent. Much has been published about site of measurement (septal vs. lateral vs. averaged) and corresponding normal thresholds. A lateral e′ velocity of 10 cm/s or greater virtually excludes diastolic dysfunction (pericardial constriction being an exception). The E:e′ ratio provides information about LV filling pressures: usually filling pressures are normal when the average E:e′ is less than 8, whereas average E:e′ greater than 14 usually reflects elevated filling pressures. However, many factors limit the interpretation of e′, including mitral stenosis, significant mitral annular calcification, mitral valve prosthesis or ring, left bundle branch block, ventricular pacing, and significant MR.[89]

Updated ASE guidelines address the perceived complexities of diastolic function assessment and propose a simplified approach to evaluation. In patients with preserved EF, four parameters should be assessed initially: e′, E:A ratio, left atrial volume index, and peak tricuspid jet annular velocity.[90] These updates reflect an appreciation that increased LA size serves as a marker of chronically elevated LVEDP. In patients with reduced EF, characterization of diastolic dysfunction begins with transmitral E:A ratio. These updated guidelines may not be generalizable to the perioperative period, and moreover, TEE cannot reliably assess LA size. There are several algorithms relevant to the perioperative period that can be referenced for a more in-depth review of diastolic dysfunction.[91-93]

VALVULAR FUNCTION

Stenosis

Aortic and mitral stenosis are the most common stenotic lesions in the perioperative setting. Fundamental to the quantitative evaluation of valvular stenosis is Doppler echocardiography. Two key concepts underlying Doppler hemodynamic measurements are the continuity principle and the pressure-velocity relationship (see *Hemodynamic measurements* section). Recommended parameters for the assessment of aortic stenosis include peak aortic velocity, mean transvalvular gradient, and valve area calculation by continuity equation (Table 37.5).[94] The peak gradient derived using echocardiography estimates the instantaneous peak pressure difference across the valve, whereas conventional catheterization data report the difference between peak LV and peak aortic pressures (peak-to-peak gradient). Dimensionless index and 3-D planimetry corroborate findings obtained by recommended methods. Discordant grading of aortic stenosis by valve area and mean gradient requires additional evaluation of LV function, stroke volume (SV), and assessment of flow reserve. Recommended parameters for assessing mitral stenosis include gradient measurements, planimetry, and pressure half-time.[95] The continuity equation and the proximal isovelocity surface area (PISA) method may be used for additional information.

Limitations exist with quantitative methods. Geometric assumptions made when using the continuity equation may lead to an underestimation of calculated valve area. Loading conditions impact flow, and as a result, impact peak velocities and calculated pressure gradients. Under general anesthesia, gradients may underestimate the severity of stenosis. In high-flow states, elevated gradients may reflect high cardiac output.

TABLE 37.5 Parameters for Evaluating Severity of Aortic Stenosis

	SEVERITY OF STENOSIS		
Parameter	**Mild**	**Moderate**	**Severe**
Peak velocity (m/s)	2.6–2.9	3.0–4.0	≥4.0
Mean gradient (mm Hg)	<20	20–40	≥40
AVA (cm^2)	>1.5	1.0–1.5	<1.0
Indexed AVA (cm^2/m^2)*	>0.85	0.6–0.85	<0.6

*In patients with small body size, aortic valve area (AVA) should be indexed to body surface area. A small valve area in a small patient may only represent moderate stenosis. Indexing to very large body surface area is controversial.

Adapted from: Baumgartner H, Hung J, Bermejo J, et al. Recommendations on the echocardiographic assessment of aortic valve stenosis: a focused update from the European Association of Cardiovascular Imaging and the American Society of Echocardiography. *J Am Soc Echocardiogr*. 2017;30(4):372–392.

Regurgitation

Recall that the vena contracta is the narrowest portion of a regurgitant jet at or downstream of the regurgitant orifice. The vena contracta width is a semiquantitative parameter for grading regurgitation severity, with cutoff values differing between valves. Pulsed-wave interrogation of flow patterns provides additional semiquantitative information. Pulmonary vein systolic flow reversal is specific for severe mitral regurgitation (MR) and hepatic vein systolic flow reversal is specific for severe tricuspid regurgitation[78].* Holodiastolic flow reversal in the descending aorta with velocities sustained above 20 cm/s is specific for severe aortic insufficiency.

Quantitative methods for grading regurgitation include calculation of regurgitant volume, regurgitant fraction, and effective regurgitant orifice area (EROA). Approaches include the stroke volume method, ventricular volumetric method, and the proximal isovelocity surface area (PISA) method. The radius of the previously mentioned flow convergence region is included in the PISA calculation. The details of these approaches are beyond the scope of this chapter. 3-D echocardiography allows for measurement of vena contracta area, which may be advantageous in the case of multiple jets or noncircular regurgitant orifices.

HEMODYNAMIC MEASUREMENTS

Cardiac Output

Doppler-based methods can be used to estimate SV and cardiac output (Fig. 37.21). Volumetric flow or SV can be calculated as a cylindrical volume as follows:

$$\mathrm{SV}\ \left(\mathrm{cm}^3\right) = \mathrm{CSA}\ \left(\mathrm{cm}^2\right) * \mathrm{VTI}\ (\mathrm{cm}),$$

where CSA is the cross-sectional area through which the blood flows and VTI is the velocity time integral of blood flow at that location. The VTI represents the distance the average blood cell travels during one cardiac cycle, and is

* in the absence of conditions such as atrial fibrillation, atrioventricular dissociation, or pacing with ventriculoatrial conduction.

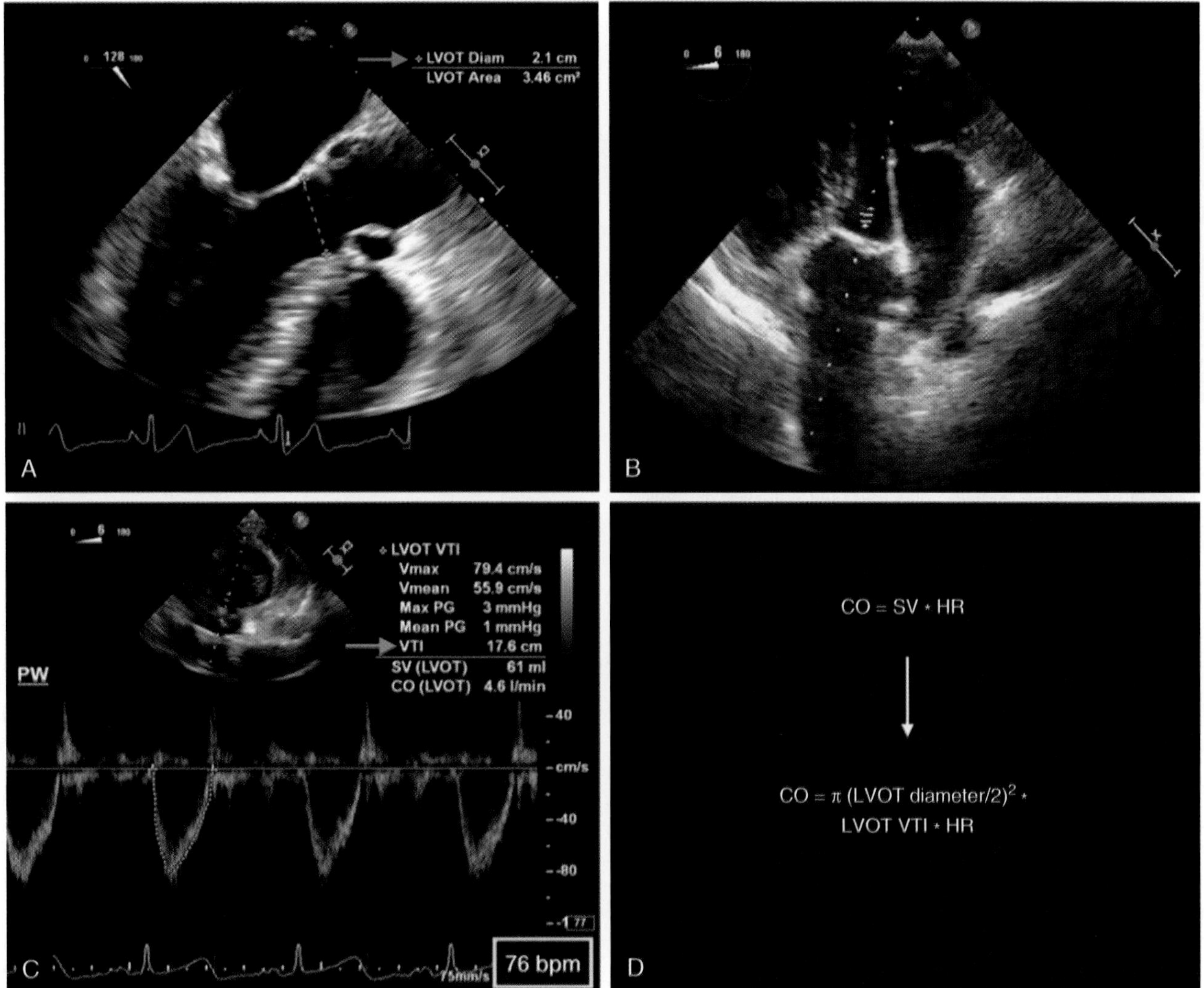

Fig. 37.21 Calculation of cardiac output (CO) using transesophageal echocardiography. (A) The left ventricular outflow tract (LVOT) diameter is measured in the midesophageal aortic valve long axis view. The cross-sectional area (CSA) of the LVOT is assumed to be circular, and is calculated as: $CSA_{LVOT} = \pi \left(\frac{\text{LVOT Diameter}}{2}\right)^2$. In this example, $CSA_{LVOT} = 3.14 * \left(\frac{2.1\text{ cm}}{1}\right)^2 = 3.46\text{ cm}^2$. (B) Velocity of blood flow through the LVOT is measured using pulsed-wave Doppler in the deep transgastric view. The velocity and diameter measurements should be performed at the same anatomic location. (C) The spectral envelope is traced to determine the area under the curve, which is equal to the velocity time integral (VTI). This represents the distance the column of blood travels with each beat and is sometimes referred to as "stroke distance." Stroke volume (SV) is the product of the cross-sectional area of the LVOT and the LVOT VTI, or $SV = CSA_{LVOT} * \text{LVOT VTI}$. (D) CO is derived by multiplying the stroke volume *(SV)* by heart rate *(HR)*, or $CO = 3.46\ cm^2 * 17.6\ cm * 76\ bpm = 4{,}628\frac{ml}{min}$. In the example provided, the machine is configured to automatically calculate stroke volume and cardiac output as displayed in panel C.

the area under the spectral Doppler envelope. Cardiac output is the product of SV and heart rate.

Cardiac output calculation is typically performed at the LV outflow tract (LVOT). The diameter is measured in the ME AV LAX view using TEE and the parasternal LAX view using TTE. The LVOT VTI is obtained in the Deep TG LAX using TEE and the A5C using TTE. Potential sources of error include inaccurate measurement of the LVOT diameter (with a squaring of any error when calculating the cross-sectional area), poor Doppler alignment with the blood flow, and measurement of the area and velocity measurements at different anatomic locations.

Many studies in surgical and ICU patients have compared Doppler-derived cardiac output (CO) to CO by thermodilution. Some authors interpret the literature to indicate Doppler-derived measurements have good agreement with CO by thermodilution.[96] Other authors, however, highlight the methodological limitations and heterogeneity of studies, and argue echocardiographic and thermodilution-derived CO cannot be used interchangeably.[97] Stronger evidence supports the use of echocardiographic-derived CO for assessing trends over time.[97]

Continuity Principle

The continuity principle states that flow rate proximal to a restricted orifice equals the flow rate through the orifice. Applying this principle to pulsatile intracardiac flow, the stroke volumes proximal to (SV_1) and at a restricted orifice (SV_2) are the same.

$$SV_1 = SV_2$$

and therefore

$$CSA_1 * VTI_1 = CSA_2 * VTI_2$$

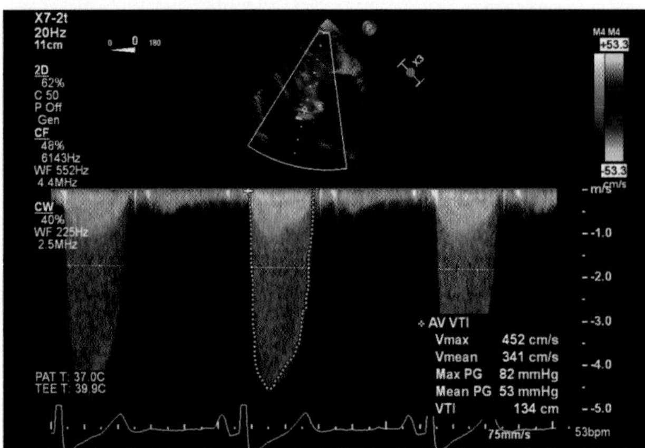

Fig. 37.22 The transvalvular pressure gradient across a stenotic aortic valve is estimated using continuous wave Doppler in the transesophageal deep transgastric view. The peak gradient is derived from the peak velocity of the spectral Doppler signal using the simplified Bernoulli equation. The mean gradient is the average of the instantaneous peak gradients throughout systole and is obtained by tracing the Doppler envelope. The ultrasound system will automatically calculate the mean pressure gradient from the tracing. The measurements in this example are consistent with severe aortic stenosis.

Common clinical applications of this equation include calculation of stenotic valve areas, prosthetic valve areas, and regurgitant orifice areas.

Bernoulli Equation

Pressure cannot be measured directly using echocardiography, however applications of the Bernoulli principle allow for estimation of gradients from velocity information (Fig. 37.22). This technique is commonly applied to quantify the severity of stenosis. The modified Bernoulli equation estimates the transvalvular pressure gradient (ΔP) as follows:

$$\Delta P = 4\left(V_2^2 - V_1^2\right)$$

where V_2 represents the peak velocity at the valve and V_1 represents the peak velocity proximal to the valve. V_1 is usually much lower than V_2 and can be ignored, simplifying the equation to:

$$\Delta P = 4V^2$$

If V_1 exceeds 1.5 m/s it should be included in the calculation.[94]

Intracardiac Pressure Estimates

Right Atrial Pressure. In *spontaneously* breathing individuals, right atrial pressure (RAP) can be estimated from the inferior vena cava (IVC) diameter and collapsibility of the IVC during inspiration ("sniff" maneuver). The IVC collapsibility index (cIVC) is defined as:

$$\text{cIVC} = \frac{(D_{max} - D_{min})}{D_{max}} * 100\,\%$$

where D_{max} is the maximum diameter on expiration and D_{min} is the minimum diameter on inspiration. Table 37.6 presents a simplified approach to estimating RAP using IVC diameter and cIVC recommended by Rudski and associates.[77] In cases of intermediate RAP estimates, it is recommended to use secondary indices of elevated RAP to downgrade or upgrade the estimate.[77]

TABLE 37.6 Echocardiographic Estimation of Right Atrial Pressures*

RAP	Estimated RAP (Range) (mm Hg)	IVC Diameter (cm)	cIVC
Normal	3 (0–5)	≤2.1	>50%
Intermediate	8 (5–10)	≤2.1	<50%
Intermediate	8 (5–10)	>2.1	>50%
Elevated	15 (10–20)	>2.1	<50%

*In spontaneously breathing individuals.

In the case of intermediate estimates, the presence or absence of secondary indices of elevated RAP can be used to better characterize the pressure estimate. *cIVC*, IVC collapsibility index (see text for definition); *IVC*, inferior vena cava; *RAP*, right atrial pressures.

As proposed by/adapted from Table 3 in Rudski LG, Lai WW, Afilalo J, et al. Guidelines for the echocardiographic assessment of the right heart in adults: a report from the American Society of Echocardiography endorsed by the European Association of Echocardiography, a registered branch of the European Society of Cardiology, and the Canadian Society of Echocardiography. *J Am Soc Echocardiogr*. 2010;23(7):685–713; quiz 786–688.

Chamber Pressures. Velocity measurements of valvular regurgitation or shunt can be used to estimate chamber pressures using the simplified Bernoulli equation. The pressure gradient (ΔP) reflects the pressure difference between the chamber where blood flow originates and blood flow is received. This is expressed as:

$$P_{OC} - P_{RC} = 4V^2$$

where P_{OC} is the pressure in the originating chamber and P_{RC} is the pressure in the receiving chamber. The equation can then be rearranged to:

$$P_{OC} = 4V^2 + P_{RC}$$

A common application is estimation of pulmonary artery systolic pressure (PASP) from the maximal tricuspid regurgitant jet velocity (Fig. 37.23). Pulmonary hypertension is defined as a mean pulmonary arterial pressure (mPAP) of 25 mm Hg or greater, which corresponds to a PASP of 38 mm Hg. mPAP can be estimated from PASP as follows: mPAP = (0.61 × PASP) + 2 mm Hg.[98] Alternatively, mPAP can be estimated using the simplified Bernoulli equation and the peak velocity of pulmonary regurgitation.

Hemodynamic Failure and Shock

Hemodynamic instability and circulatory failure may occur at any phase in a patient's perioperative care, and echocardiography provides valuable information to the operating room anesthesiologist and intensivist alike. Echocardiography enables characterization of the mechanism of shock (cardiogenic, hypovolemic, distributive, and/or obstructive)[99] and can be used for serial assessment of response to therapies.[100] Most clinicians will apply qualitative techniques during echocardiographic assessment; quantitative approaches also add valuable information when used by appropriately trained individuals.

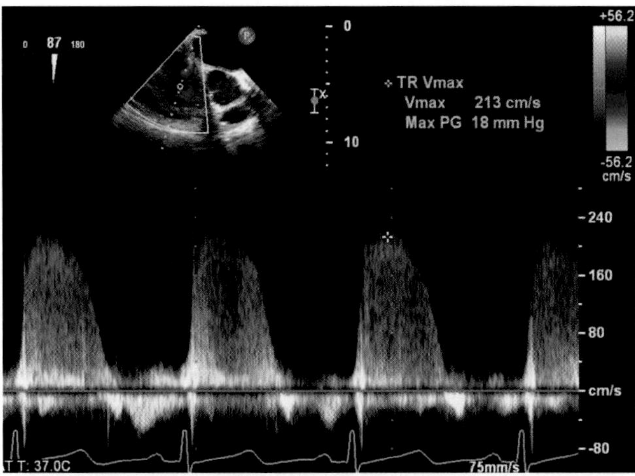

Fig. 37.23 A midesophageal modified bicaval view aligns the Doppler cursor with the tricuspid regurgitant jet. Continuous wave Doppler measures the peak systolic velocity of the tricuspid regurgitation (V_{TR}). V_{TR} reflects difference between the right ventricular systolic pressure (RVSP) and right atrial pressure (RAP), so RVSP = 4 V_{TR}^2 + RAP. In the absence of right ventricular outflow tract obstruction or pulmonary stenosis, RVSP and pulmonary artery systolic pressure (PASP) are essentially equal. In this example, the estimated PASP = 18 mm Hg + RAP.

VENTRICULAR DYSFUNCTION

Qualitative evaluation of biventricular systolic function is central to identifying the etiology of shock or hemodynamic instability. As previously mentioned, visual estimation of LVEF by experienced individuals correlates well with quantitative methods,[71,72] and can be learned easily with proper feedback.[101] A focused examination should identify whether significant myocardial dysfunction is present. Further assessment may suggest myocardial stunning or ischemia, especially if in a segmental distribution or acute in onset. This is not without limitations however, as acute decreases in preload can cause new RWMAs in the absence of ischemia.[102]

Takotsubo cardiomyopathy, a form of stress cardiomyopathy thought to result from excess catecholamine stimulation, may occur with a perioperative incidence of 1 in 6700.[103] Classically described as apical ballooning and basal hyperkinesis in the absence of obstructive coronary disease (Video 37.6), it derives its name from the similarly appearing Japanese takotsubo octopus pot trap. Additional patterns of regional involvement in stress cardiomyopathy include midventricular, basal, localized, or global.[104] Echocardiography allows evaluation of LV morphology and segmental wall motion, right ventricular involvement, and complications such as MR, LVOT obstruction, intracardiac thrombus, and cardiac rupture.[104]

SEVERE HYPOVOLEMIA

Hypovolemia leads to a decrease in LV end-diastolic area (EDA) and end-systolic area (ESA), but at baseline there is wide variability in the normal ranges.[105] For practical purposes, qualitative assessment of chamber size provides the most useful information if monitored serially in the operating room or in the setting of significant hypovolemia, where EDA will be markedly reduced. It is important to distinguish hypovolemia from distributive shock, where ESA is also decreased but the EDA area will be normal.[106] End-systolic cavity obliteration (sometimes described as "kissing walls") is frequently associated with decreased EDA and hypovolemia, but may also occur in high inotropic or vasodilatory states.[105]

As previously described, IVC diameter and cIVC can be used to estimate the RAP in spontaneously breathing individuals.[77] Central venous pressure, however, is a poor predictor of fluid responsiveness.[107] Whether cIVC predicts fluid responsiveness during spontaneous ventilation is an area of active debate,[108–111] and has been examined in several studies.[112–117] In many instances, spontaneously breathing patients with cIVC of more than 40% to 50% will respond to fluid administration,[112,115,117] but this is not found consistently,[113,114] and does not necessarily identify nonresponders.[112,115] We would encourage the reader to read the primary literature to gain a more in-depth understanding of the topic prior to attempting to use cIVC in the assessment of hypovolemia.

Predictors of fluid responsiveness applicable in patients who undergo passive mechanical ventilation, typically in the setting of critical illness, are covered in the *Critical Care* section of the chapter.

LEFT VENTRICULAR OUTFLOW TRACT OBSTRUCTION

LVOT obstruction may precipitate significant hemodynamic compromise, creating a perplexing scenario of worsening instability despite aggressive inotropic resuscitation. LVOT obstruction and systolic anterior motion (SAM) of the mitral valve are classically associated with hypertrophic cardiomyopathy. In the perioperative setting, LVOT obstruction and SAM often occur following mitral valve repair. The presence of LVOT obstruction in other susceptible populations is likely underappreciated, and probably results from a combination of anatomic predisposition and precipitating hemodynamic factors associated with enhanced LV contractility (hypovolemia, hyperkinesis, inotropes). Anatomic factors include small LV cavity, basal septal hypertrophy, and an anteriorly-displaced mitral valve coaptation zone with redundant leaflet tissue.[118] One series observed LVOT obstruction in over 20% of patients admitted in septic shock, and the presence of LVOT obstruction was associated with higher mortality.[119] SAM was present in only two-thirds of the cases of LVOT obstruction, underscoring the complex mechanisms leading to clinically relevant obstruction. In a series of perioperative rescue echocardiograms, LVOT obstruction was present in 3.6% of cases.[120]

LVOT obstruction produces high-velocity flow in the LVOT. Interrogation of the LVOT with CFD reveals flow acceleration and turbulence. Blood flow velocity exceeds the Nyquist limit of PWD, so CWD is required for quantification. Visual assessment of CFD and gradual movement of the PW sampling volume through the LV cavity and LVOT can be used to estimate the location of the obstruction. In the presence of LVOT obstruction, the spectral Doppler profile of systolic blood flow across the LVOT is dagger-shaped and mid-to-late peaking (Fig. 37.24). The

M-mode of the aortic valve will demonstrate premature leaflet closure during mid-systole (Fig. 37.25*B*). Findings consistent with SAM include anterior displacement of the mitral leaflet during systole with entrainment in the LVOT (Fig. 37.26; Video 37.7). Variable degrees of MR may be present.

CARDIAC TAMPONADE

Echocardiography readily detects pericardial fluid, which appears as an echolucent space adjacent to the heart. The physiologic significance of a pericardial effusion depends on both the volume and rate of accumulation. A large effusion may develop slowly with minimal consequence, whereas a rapidly accumulating effusion of small volume can have profound hemodynamic impact. Cardiac tamponade develops when intrapericardial pressure exceeds cardiac chamber pressures, thereby compressing the cardiac chambers. This impairs chamber filling ultimately compromising cardiac output. Hemodynamic effects of tamponade occur along a continuum.[121]

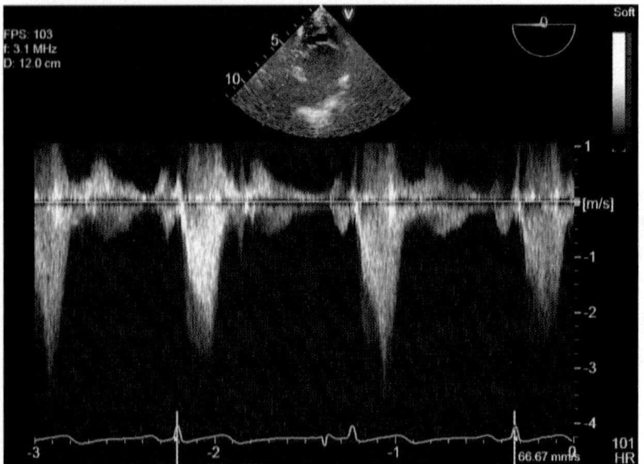

Fig. 37.24 A continuous wave Doppler signal characteristic of left ventricular outflow tract obstruction. The signal appears "dagger-shaped," with the peak velocity occurring in mid-to-late systole. In the perioperative setting, obstruction may be dynamic and unmasked by precipitating factors in susceptible individuals.

Echocardiographic findings can support the diagnosis of cardiac tamponade in the context of relevant clinical findings. When intrapericardial pressure exceeds cardiac chamber pressures, chamber collapse may occur during the respective relaxation phases. The thin right atrium typically has the lowest pressure and usually is the first chamber to show collapse or inversion, which is observed in ventricular systole (Fig. 37.27*A*; Video 37.8).[122,123] Importantly, transient right atrial collapse may be present in the absence of tamponade, and therefore is a nonspecific finding. A longer duration of atrial collapse improves the specificity of this finding.[122] RV diastolic collapse (Video 37.9; see Fig. 37.27*B*) occurs later than right atrial collapse in the progression of tamponade, and is a more specific finding. In a series of patients with moderate or large pericardial effusions, the absence of any right-sided chamber collapse had a high negative predictive value for clinical tamponade.[124] Collapse of right heart chambers may not occur in settings where baseline right-sided pressures are elevated, such as in patients with pulmonary hypertension. Following cardiac surgery, echocardiographic findings in the setting of tamponade may be atypical, including localized compression of cardiac chambers and accumulation of clot.

In spontaneously breathing patients, a dilated IVC with less than a 50% decrease in diameter with deep inspiration is a sensitive sign for tamponade. This combination of findings has poor specificity, however, because it reflects elevated central venous pressure.[125] During spontaneous ventilation in the absence of pathology, there is a normal

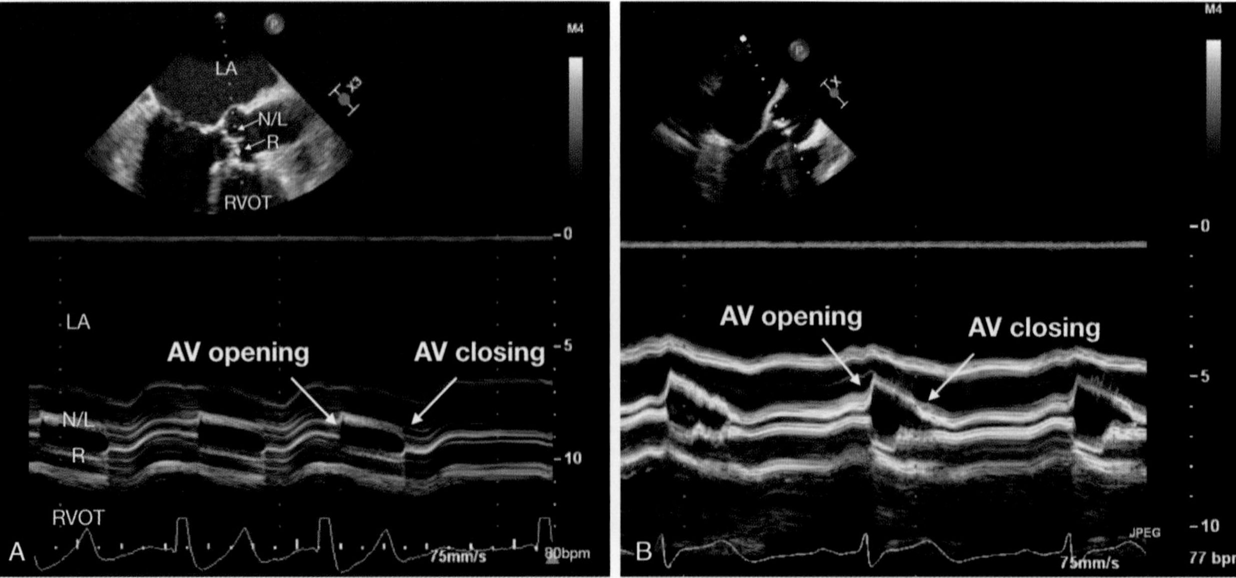

Fig. 37.25 M-mode interrogation of the aortic valve in the midesophageal aortic valve long axis view. The cursor passes through the left atrium *(LA)*, posterior aortic root, the non or left coronary cusp *(N/L)*, the right coronary cusp *(R)*, the anterior aortic root, and the right ventricular outflow tract *(RVOT)*. (A) In the absence of obstruction to flow (or other aortic valve pathology), the motion of the aortic valve leaflets during systole creates a rectangular shape. (B) In the presence of left ventricular outflow tract obstruction, the aortic valve opens normally, but closes prematurely.

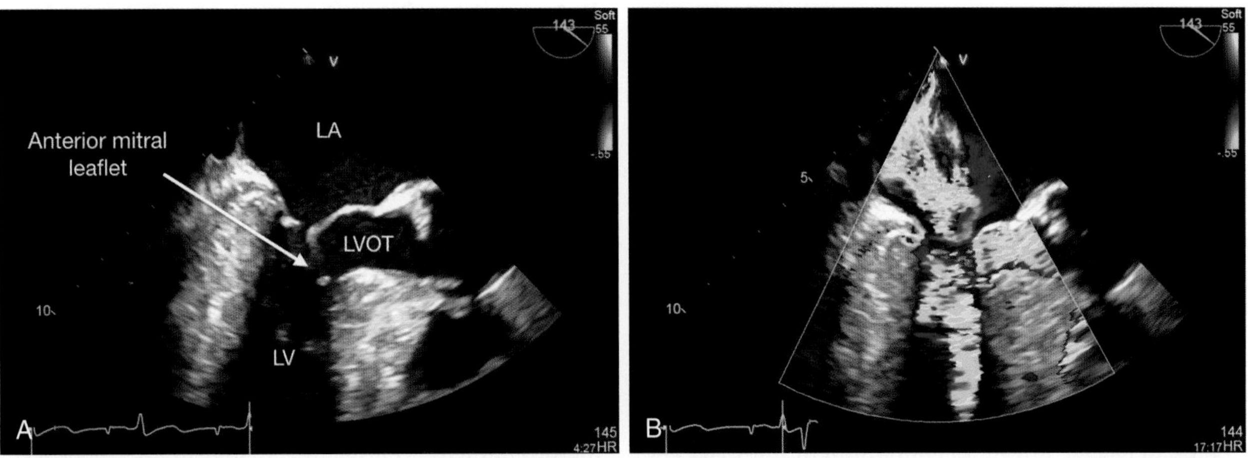

Fig. 37.26 Midesophageal long axis views without (A) and with color (B) demonstrating systolic anterior motion of the mitral valve (SAM). (A) Instead of coapting normally, the anterior mitral leaflet *(arrow)* moves into the left ventricular outflow tract *(LVOT)* during systole. This narrows the effective outflow tract and can lead to dynamic obstruction to flow. (B) Turbulent flow is visualized by color Doppler in the LVOT. In this example, there is significant mitral regurgitation associated with SAM. *LA*, Left atrium; *LV*, left ventricle.

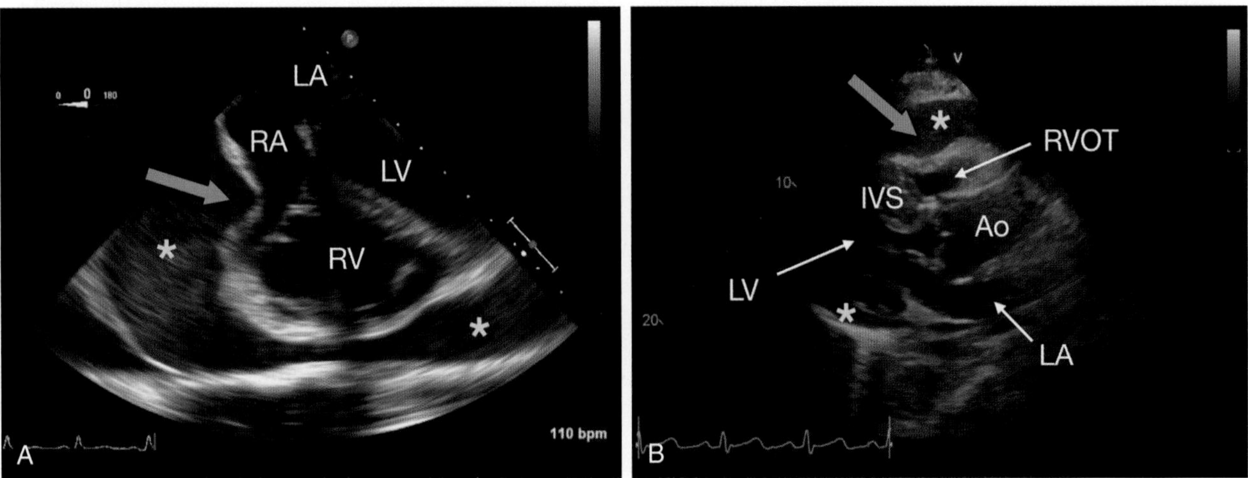

Fig. 37.27 Echocardiographic features supporting the clinical diagnosis of tamponade. (A) Transesophageal midesophageal four-chamber view demonstrating a large echolucent pericardial effusion (*). Right atrial collapse *(blue arrow)* is present during ventricular systole (note the red marker on the ECG tracing after the R-wave). (B) Transthoracic parasternal long axis view also demonstrating a large pericardial effusion (*). Right ventricular collapse *(green arrow)* during diastole is present (note the red marker on the p-wave of the ECG tracing). Right ventricular collapse is more specific for tamponade than right atrial collapse. *Ao*, Ascending aorta; *IVS*, interventricular septum; *LA*, left atrium; *LV*, left ventricle; *RA*, right atrium; *RV*, right ventricle.

variation in the peak transvalvular flow velocities, with transtricuspid velocities increasing during inspiration and transmitral velocities decreasing. Exaggerated respiratory variation in transvalvular flow velocities occurs in tamponade, calculated as a percentage change from expiration velocity.[121] In tamponade, there is usually a greater than 30% variation in mitral inflow velocities, and greater than 60% (absolute) variation in tricuspid inflow velocities. Exaggerated respirophasic changes in transvalvular velocities alone are insufficient to support a diagnosis of tamponade. Additionally, these findings have not been validated in patients receiving positive pressure ventilation. In fact, in an experimental animal model of tamponade, the greatest variation in mitral inflow velocities was observed during the control phase, with attenuation of the variation during tamponade.[126] Abnormal venous flow patterns in the superior vena cava (SVC) and hepatic veins can also provide supportive evidence of tamponade; however, analysis may not be feasible in at least one-third of patients due to the presence of TR, atrial fibrillation, paced rhythm, or technical inadequacy.[124] Echocardiography frequently guides pericardiocentesis procedures.

PULMONARY EMBOLISM

Acute pulmonary embolism (PE) is classified into three subgroups: high-risk (massive), intermediate-risk (submassive), and low-risk.[127,128] The presence of sustained hypotension or shock (not explained by other causes) defines massive PE. Patients with intermediate- and low-risk PE by definition are normotensive. The groups are further delineated according to RV dysfunction, myocardial injury, and other clinical features. When PE is suspected, the recommended first-line imaging modality is computed tomography angiography (CTA).[128] Echocardiography, in contrast, is not recommended in the initial diagnostic evaluation of PE.[129] When the diagnosis of PE is established, echocardiography has utility in risk stratification, prognostication, and response to therapy.[128,130]

In cases of suspected PE with hemodynamic instability or shock, obtaining a CTA may not be feasible. In this context, echocardiography has a role in refining the diagnostic assessment and management decisions.[128,131] Freely mobile intracardiac thrombus, or "clot in transit," is visualized rarely on echocardiography (<4% of cases), but more commonly in high-risk PE (22%) and is associated with worse prognosis.[132] Indirect signs of PE include RV dilation, RV dysfunction, and the 60/60 sign, which is a pulmonary ejection acceleration time of less than 60 ms with a mid-systolic notch and a TR peak gradient between 30 and 60 mm Hg.[130] Several parameters may be used to assess RV dysfunction, including "McConnell's sign," TAPSE, increased end-diastolic RV-to-LV diameter ratio (≥0.9 or 1.0), and interventricular septal flattening during systole, indicative of pressure overload.[128,130] Myocardial deformation as a marker of RV dysfunction is not widely used but is an area of investigation.[130,133]

"McConnell's sign" is an echocardiographic finding of RV hypokinesis or akinesis with apical sparing (Video 37.10). It was originally reported as having a high sensitivity and specificity for acute PE,[134] however several subsequent studies have demonstrated this finding to lack sensitivity.[135] The absence of McConnell's sign does not exclude acute PE. In many populations, McConnell's sign is highly specific. Important exceptions include patients with RV infarction[136] or pulmonary hypertension,[133] where McConnell's sign may be observed in the absence of acute PE (i.e., a nonspecific finding).

Few studies focus specifically on echocardiographic findings in the high-risk subgroup. However, in a series of 511 patients with confirmed PE, 16 of the patients met high-risk criteria.[137] Interestingly, all 16 patients had RV enlargement and hypokinesis, and at least one of the following: McConnell's sign, 60/60 sign, or right heart thrombus. Flattened interventricular system, RV free wall hypokinesis plus a RV-to-LV diameter ratio greater than 0.9, McConnell's sign, and right heart thrombus were observed significantly more frequently in patients with high-risk PE than those without.

Recent work has sought to better define the diagnostic utility of echocardiography in PE (including all risk categories), especially in light of the increasing use of point-of-care ultrasound. Meta-analysis of both formal and point-of-care TTE examinations in patients with clinical concern for PE found that echocardiographic signs of right heart strain (variably defined) had a sensitivity of 53% and a specificity of 83%.[135] In the previously mentioned series of 511 patients, over one-third of the non-high-risk patients demonstrated completely normal RV morphology and function.[137]

Intraoperative Transesophageal Echocardiography - Noncardiac Surgery

In noncardiac surgery, TEE serves two main roles: an intraoperative monitor and a rescue tool. TEE has been used in diverse operative settings including vascular, orthopedic, and transplant surgery. A comprehensive review on the topic has been published by Mahmood and colleagues.[138] The impact of TEE tends to be greater when it is used as a rescue tool versus as a monitor.[139] The extent of the therapeutic impact is difficult to quantify, however, in part because interpretation of "impact" is not uniform. Supportive or confirmatory information adds substantial value in many contexts. Therapeutic modifications reported as a result of TEE findings include initiation of pharmacologic therapy, fluid administration, and alteration in anesthetic plan or surgical procedure.[138,140,141] Continuation of patient management without changes may also be considered a relevant impact.

MONITORING ROLE

Myocardial Ischemia

Echocardiographic changes of myocardial ischemia manifest earlier than ECG changes, suggesting a potential role for TEE in the early detection of intraoperative ischemia. Current practice is to perform TEE monitoring selectively in patients with known risk factors or undergoing high-risk procedures. Early research demonstrated a 20% incidence of new or worsening RWMAs in high-risk patients.[142] Intraoperative RWMAs were infrequently associated with postoperative myocardial infarction (MI) and overall complication rate was low. Another study in the 1990s concluded that changes detected by intraoperative TEE added little incremental value in predicting risk of postoperative ischemic outcomes (death, nonfatal MI, unstable angina) compared with preoperative data and two-lead ECG monitoring.[143] The imaging capabilities of current transducers are vastly enhanced compared to those used in earlier decades, and may not reflect TEE's utility as a monitor of ischemia in the current era. A study of 54 high-risk patients undergoing vascular surgery demonstrated new RWMAs on intraoperative TEE in 43% of cases.[144] Overall incidence of postoperative MI was 11%, and all patients with MI demonstrated intraoperative RMWAs. Intraoperative TEE was a sensitive indicator of risk for postoperative MI, although there still were a substantial number of patients with "false positive" echocardiographic changes. Many questions surrounding the optimal use and potential impact of TEE as a monitor for ischemia in high-risk settings remain unanswered. In the absence of patient-specific or procedural risk factors, the routine use of TEE during noncardiac surgery to monitor for myocardial ischemia is not recommended.[51]

Liver Transplantation

Hemodynamic management during orthotopic liver transplantation is complex, with frequent periods of instability from potentially numerous causes.[145,146] At baseline, patients often have high cardiac output and low systemic vascular resistance with significant comorbidities. In the preanhepatic phase (from incision to occlusion of vascular inflow to the liver), hemodynamic alterations may result from an abrupt change in preload due to drainage of large volume ascites, hemorrhage, or surgical caval compression. TEE examination during this phase allows for characterization of dynamic changes, as well as baseline evaluation of biventricular and valvular function. During the anhepatic phase (occlusion of inflow to the liver to unclamping of the portal vein), preload to the heart is decreased. If an end-to-end interposition of the IVC is performed, complete caval occlusion is required and venovenous bypass may be used to improve preload and decrease venous congestion. A piggyback technique only requires partial caval occlusion and venous return to the heart is usually adequate without bypass. TEE findings of ventricular dysfunction, diminished cardiac output, hypovolemia, and intracardiac thrombi may be present regardless of the surgical technique. The reperfusion phase begins with release of the cross clamp from the portal vein, resulting in infusion of cold, hyperkalemic, acidotic blood. Profound instability may result and even progress to cardiac arrest. TEE provides real-time visualization of cardiac function and filling. Over 40% of liver transplant patients demonstrate evidence of inducible LVOT obstruction on preoperative dobutamine stress echocardiography,[147] making this an important diagnosis to exclude in the setting of refractory hypotension. Inspection of the IVC for high-velocity or turbulent flow is also possible with TEE.

Esophageal varices are a relative contraindication to TEE and are a relevant concern in the liver transplant population. However, the reported rate of TEE complications in liver transplantation is low, even in patients with known esophageal varices or history of upper gastrointestinal bleeding. A recent review suggests TEE to be safe in patients without grade 3 varices or active gastrointestinal bleeding.[146] Approaches to minimize risk include limited probe manipulation during the anhepatic phase and avoidance of TG and DTG views.

Lung Transplantation

Intraoperative TEE provides key information in each phase of lung transplantation in a patient population with impaired cardiopulmonary reserve.[148] Initial assessment includes evaluation for RV dilation, hypertrophy, and dysfunction, which result from long-standing pulmonary hypertension. Identification of a patent foramen ovale (PFO) may have clinical consequence if right-sided pressures exceed left-sided pressures, impacting the surgical plan. Common problems during one-lung ventilation and graft implantation include hypoxemia, hypercapnia, and elevated pulmonary vascular resistance, which may precipitate acute RV failure. Recognition of deteriorating RV function by TEE prompts initiation of inotropes or pulmonary vasodilators. Should profound instability result, TEE may provide information leading to initiation of cardiopulmonary bypass or help guide cannula placement for extracorporeal membrane oxygenation (ECMO). After reperfusion, in addition to continued assessment of biventricular function, attention turns to the pulmonary artery anastomosis and the pulmonary veins[149] for findings suggestive of kinking, thrombus, or stenosis.

Vascular Surgery/Endovascular Procedures

Patients undergoing vascular procedures are at increased risk of perioperative cardiovascular morbidity and mortality. Applications of TEE in this setting include monitoring for ischemia, assessment of systolic and diastolic function, and guidance for fluid resuscitation. In open abdominal aortic aneurysm repair, significant increases in afterload and wall tension occur with application of the cross clamp. After aortic occlusion, LVEF significantly decreases and EDV and ESV increase.[150] New or worsening RWMAs have been reported in up to one-third of patients, and occur more frequently with suprarenal versus infrarenal clamping.[151] Persistent RWMAs after several hours have been associated with postoperative MI.[151] With unclamping of vessels and ensuing instability, TEE serves as an adjunctive monitor as resuscitation proceeds. Over the past two decades, there has been a dramatic increase in endovascular repairs and a decline in open vascular procedures, consequently impacting the anticipated anesthetic concerns. Potential profound instability may be dramatically reduced, diminishing the value of intraoperative TEE in that context. However, TEE may be used to identify aortic pathology, identify landing zones, and evaluate for endoleaks.[138]

RESCUE ROLE

TEE used in the setting of unanticipated hemodynamic instability or cardiopulmonary arrest, also called "rescue" TEE, rapidly provides valuable information. Rescue TEE identifies causes of shock described earlier in the chapter (e.g., ventricular dysfunction, severe hypovolemia, LVOT obstruction, tamponade, and PE). Embolic phenomena relatively unique to the operative setting include air emboli during upright neurosurgical procedures and fat or cement emboli in orthopedic and spine surgeries.

Several series report the value of rescue echocardiography, describing its ability to identify a cause for instability or confirm expected diagnoses.[152-154] TEE aided or impacted clinical management in the majority of the cases. Rescue TEE commonly implicates LV dysfunction and hypovolemia in instability, although no diagnosis occurs with enough frequency to be predictive without performing an echocardiographic examination. In fact, in one series the most frequent finding was a normal examination or demonstration of known pathology (48%).[155] Despite a "negative" result, the TEE findings influenced management in more than half of these cases, suggesting the impact of TEE is not confined to cases demonstrating pathology. The largest reported study includes 364 rescue studies (96% TEE) performed throughout the perioperative period (55% intraoperatively).[120] The most common findings intraoperatively were hypovolemia (32%) and LV dysfunction (11%), whereas postoperatively RV (24%) and LV (22%) systolic dysfunction predominated. The findings influenced management in 59% of cases. Information can be obtained quickly (<5 minutes)[154] and may make an immediate impact. The sequence of examination and included views may vary among providers, but these should provide information swiftly. One proposed rescue protocol includes a sequence of five views: ME 4C, ME AV LAX, ME bicaval, TG SAX, and descending aorta SAX.[155]

Intraoperative Transesophageal Echocardiography - Cardiac Surgery

Numerous observational studies demonstrate the impact of intraoperative TEE on decision making in cardiac surgery. In a retrospective study of 12,566 patients, new echocardiographic findings on TEE prior to cardiopulmonary bypass (CPB) led to changes in surgical management in 7% of cases.[156] After CPB, TEE findings prompted return to CPB in 2.2% of cases. When analyzed according to surgical procedure, influential new findings were demonstrated in 5.4% of 3853 isolated CABG cases pre-CPB, and in 1.5% of CABG cases post-CPB with 0.8% requiring graft revision. A study of 521 patients undergoing CABG demonstrated new pre-CPB findings influencing the surgical plan in 11.9% of cases, and in 0.7% of cases post-CPB.[157] In valvular surgery, an analysis of 8 studies including 15,540 patients demonstrated the influence of TEE findings on surgical decision making in 11% of cases pre-CPB and 4% of cases post-CPB.[64]

When considering the impact of TEE findings on surgical interventions, limitations should be recognized. Selection bias for the use of TEE may be present in cases where it is anticipated to alter decision making, especially in CABG. Also, many studies included PFO as a diagnosis influencing the surgical plan. In the absence of high risk for hypoxemia and right-to-left shunting, optimal management of PFO when the surgical procedure does not involve atriotomy is unclear.[158] In an observational study of patients undergoing cardiac surgery, newly diagnosed PFO was not associated with increased perioperative morbidity or mortality.[159] PFO closure did not influence long-term survival, but was associated with higher risk of intraoperative stroke.

Intraoperative TEE findings provide prognostic value. Detection of RWMAs by TEE at any time during CABG is an independent predictor of postoperative MI.[160] Deterioration of regional wall motion on intraoperative TEE following revascularization is associated with higher risk of both short-term[161] and long-term[162] adverse cardiovascular events.

A general framework is useful when conducting pre-CPB and post-CPB examinations. Prior to initiation of CPB, evaluation includes assessment of overall biventricular function, aortic pathology that may affect cannulation strategy, presence of aortic regurgitation, and identification of unanticipated findings (e.g., severe valvular lesions, intracardiac thrombus). In the case of valvular surgery, diagnosis is confirmed and additional information regarding the mechanism of dysfunction is communicated to the surgeon. In minimally invasive cardiac surgery, TEE enables visualization of wires for cannulae placement and can guide percutaneous coronary sinus catheter placement. Post-CPB examination includes assessment of global and regional ventricular function, appropriate seating and function of newly implanted prosthetic valves,[163] identification of any new valvular abnormalities requiring intervention, and exclusion of iatrogenic aortic injury. Applications of TEE in the context of specific pathology and surgical procedures are outlined in the sections that follow.

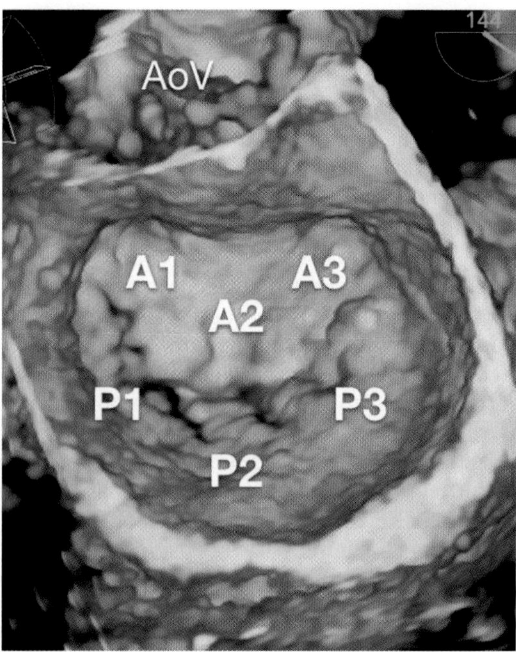

Fig. 37.28 En face display of a three-dimensional image of the mitral valve. This orientation is analogous to the viewpoint of the surgeon, and facilitates communication regarding the location of structural pathology. The scallops of the anterior *(A1, A2, A3)* and posterior *(P1, P2, P3)* mitral leaflets are labeled. *AoV*, Aortic valve.

MITRAL VALVE REPAIR

TEE imaging of the mitral valve has transformed surgical planning, particularly when assessing the suitability of attempted repair versus valve replacement for MR. Assessment of the regurgitant valve begins with examination of the structure of the valve leaflets and valvular apparatus. Primary (degenerative) MR involves abnormality of the leaflets or valvular apparatus, whereas in secondary (functional) regurgitation, the valve is structurally normal with insufficient coaptation resulting from ventricular remodeling. The mechanism of MR is classified according to Carpentier's classification of leaflet motion: type I-normal leaflet motion, type II-excessive leaflet motion, and type III-restricted leaflet motion (IIIa-restricted in systole and diastole, while IIIb is restricted in systole).[164] Quantitative assessment is performed, recognizing that intraoperative conditions often lead to underestimation of the severity of regurgitation.[80] 3-D TEE offers enhanced spatial resolution and superior accuracy in localizing leaflet pathology compared to 2-D TEE.[165-167] "En face" display of 3-D images analogous to the surgeon's intraoperative view facilitates communication regarding structural details (Fig. 37.28). The origin of the regurgitation can be precisely identified using multiplanar reformatting 3-D technology. Vena contracta area, regurgitant volume, and EROA can be quantified using 3-D techniques with potentially improved accuracy. At present, 3-D quantitative analyses are labor-intensive and time consuming, making them largely impractical for routine intraoperative assessments.

Valve repair is often feasible in degenerative disease with isolated prolapse or flail, and moderate or less annular dilation.[79] Bileaflet disease (Barlow disease), severe annular dilation, rheumatic deformities, and severe mitral annular calcification are predictors of unsuccessful repair.[168] Regurgitation recurs in a substantial proportion of patients with ischemic MR following repair. LV remodeling and leaflet tethering with apical displacement of the coaptation point impact the feasibility of repair of ischemic MR. Quantitative measurements include assessment of the tenting height (the perpendicular distance from the plane of the mitral annulus to the point of leaflet coaptation) and systolic tenting area (area enclosed by the mitral annular plane and closed leaflets). Tenting height of 11 mm or greater is associated with recurrent MR. On intraoperative TEE, mitral diastolic annular diameter of 37 mm or greater, tenting area of 1.6 cm^2 or greater, and severe MR are associated with high probability of repair failure.[168]

Additional considerations in the pre-bypass echocardiographic evaluation include predictors of post-repair SAM of the anterior mitral leaflet, which commonly reflect anterior displacement of the coaptation point. This may take the form of reduction in distance between the coaptation point and the septum (C-sept distance < 2.5 cm) or a relatively elongated posterior leaflet (anterior to posterior leaflet ratio of ≤ 1.3 or posterior leaflet height > 1.5 cm), and narrow aorto-mitral angle.[169,170] Other SAM predictors include basal septal hypertrophy (>15 mm), small LV cavity, and anterior displacement of the papillary muscles.

Immediately following separation from CPB, echocardiography assesses for significant regurgitation, stenosis, or dynamic LVOT obstruction due to SAM. Stability of the ring and normal leaflet motion should be demonstrated. Any residual regurgitation should be no more than mild and transvalvular. Should SAM occur, management steps include administration of fluid and discontinuation of any inotropes. If SAM persists, the next therapeutic maneuvers are administration of beta blockers and increase in afterload. The effect of these interventions can be readily observed on TEE. SAM will improve or resolve in most patients, and long-term follow-up demonstrates low incidence of SAM, favoring conservative management.[171] Persistence of significant SAM requires revision. Assessment of mitral inflow typically involves measurement of transvalvular gradient, recognizing this is dependent on cardiac output.

TRICUSPID VALVE REPAIR

Increased recognition of the adverse prognostic effects of TR has stimulated interest in tricuspid valve pathology. After surgical correction of left-sided valvular heart disease, severe secondary TR often fails to improve. Even mild or moderate secondary TR may progress if uncorrected. Current AHA/ACC guidelines recommend tricuspid valve repair for severe TR at the time of left-sided valve surgery.[50]

The decision to intervene upon less than severe TR at the time of left-sided valve surgery is more complex. When not intervened upon at the time of left-sided valve surgery, mild or moderate TR progresses in approximately 25% of individuals.[50] Annular dilation strongly factors in the decision to intervene early. Individuals with mild or greater TR and either annular dilation (diastolic diameter of > 40 mm or > 21 mm/m^2) or evidence of prior right-sided heart failure can benefit from concomitant tricuspid valve repair (type IIa recommendation). In the absence of tricuspid annular dilation, tricuspid valve repair may be considered during left-sided surgery when moderate TR and pulmonary hypertension are present (type IIb recommendation).

The structure of the tricuspid valve is complex. Because the annulus is nonplanar and the valve leaflets unequal in size, it can be difficult to visualize all three leaflets in the same 2-D imaging plane. The anterior location of the valve (far field in the scanning plane) and the thin leaflets also limit 2-D TEE imaging. Measurement of annular diameter by 2-D TTE typically occurs in the A4C view,[172] however this one measurement may not accurately reflect the degree of dilation and has underestimated maximal diameter compared to 3-D TEE.[173] Studies of 3-D TEE have enhanced our understanding of annular dilation in the septal-to-lateral dimension, the progression from an oval to more circular shape, and the accompanying changes in annular dynamism.[174,175] Use of 3-D color may improve quantitative assessment of regurgitation severity,[172] however in the intraoperative environment, underestimation of TR is not unexpected. Technologies using 3-D TEE will continue to fill a larger role in the evaluation of TR.

AORTIC DISSECTION

Acute type A aortic dissection has high morbidity and mortality. Accurate diagnosis is paramount to rapid treatment. The preferred diagnostic approach under most circumstances is CTA, which identifies dissection with a sensitivity of 100% and specificity of 98%.[176] In some cases, TEE may be performed more readily than CTA. TEE performs with slightly lower sensitivity (86%-100%) and specificity (90%-100%), although in many studies TEE performs with comparable specificity to CTA.[176,177] TEE imaging challenges include a blind spot in visualization of the distal ascending aorta and proximal arch due to interposition of the left mainstem bronchus between the aorta and esophagus. Imaging artifacts in the near field are common because of reverberation and refraction (especially in the presence of a pulmonary artery catheter) and may be erroneously interpreted as an intimal flap.

Intraoperative TEE during surgical intervention further defines features of the dissection. Measurements of the aortic annulus and root are performed, effacement of the sinotubular junction excluded, and structure and function of the aortic valve assessed. Mechanisms of aortic insufficiency include regurgitation due to a bicuspid valve, extension of the intimal flap to the annulus causing asymmetric leaflet prolapse, malcoaptation due to root dilation, and prolapse of the intimal flap preventing complete leaflet closure.[178] This mechanistic information influences whether valve repair is feasible and may lead to modification of the planned surgical procedure.[179] Further assessment includes examination of the true and false lumens. Blood flow may be visualized across the intimal flap. Usually the true lumen will expand during systole, which can be appreciated using M-mode echocardiography. The false lumen often demonstrates diastolic expansion and spontaneous echo contrast. Due to the complex nature of some dissections, it may be difficult to determine the true and false lumens accurately.

MECHANICAL CIRCULATORY SUPPORT (MCS)

Durable Mechanical Circulatory Support

Approximately 2500 durable left ventricular assist devices (LVADs) are implanted annually in North America, nearly half of which are destination therapy.[180] Intraoperative TEE confirms known pathology and is integral for identifying abnormalities that may require additional intervention.[181-183] Prior to implantation, echocardiographic assessment includes examination of biventricular size and function, and evaluation for intracardiac shunt (including PFO) and intracardiac thrombus. Preexisting valvular dysfunction is characterized. Greater than mild aortic insufficiency, moderate or greater mitral stenosis, and moderate or greater tricuspid insufficiency may require additional valvular procedures. An existing mechanical aortic valve may require replacement due to the risk for thrombus formation secondary to decreased transvalvular flow after LVAD implantation. Echocardiographic predictors of RV failure following LVAD implantation have been an area of considerable investigation, including the newer myocardial deformation techniques. At this time no measures reliably predict the need for biventricular mechanical support.[183]

During device implantation, TEE guidance facilitates appropriate apical positioning of the inflow cannula. Postimplantation assessment includes LV size, degree of LV decompression, RV function, reassessment for PFO, and frequency and extent of aortic valve opening. Assessment of LV unloading includes determination of overall chamber size and the position of the interventricular septum, which should be midline rather than bowing toward either chamber. As LVAD speeds are increased, parameters are frequently reassessed, especially if there is concern for marginal RV function. An appropriately positioned inflow cannula should be in the apex, directed toward the mitral valve, and should not interfere with the subvalvular apparatus. Acute angulation of the inflow cannula toward the septum may lead to cannula obstruction. Typical inflow velocity is 1.5 m/s or less. Imaging artifacts with newer-generation LVADs may preclude spectral Doppler and color flow assessment of the cannula. The outflow graft–ascending aorta anastomosis may be visualized in ME or UE views. An outflow velocity of 2 m/s or greater raises concern for obstruction, although normal values for newer generation devices may be higher.[183,184] The mid-portion of the outflow graft can also be visualized along the right side of the heart, but should not cause compression.

Temporary Mechanical Circulatory Support

Common percutaneous devices for temporary MCS include intraaortic balloon pumps, ECMO, Impella percutaneous ventricular assist devices (Abiomed, Danvers, MA), and TandemHeart percutaneous ventricular assist devices (CardiacAssist, Pittsburgh, PA). Surgically implanted devices are options when longer duration of temporary support is anticipated. Appropriate device position depends on the specific technology and may be facilitated by TEE guidance.[183,185] When assessing for myocardial recovery, TEE may add to the information provided by hemodynamics and has been incorporated into some venoarterial extracorporeal membrane oxygenation weaning protocols.[186]

CONGENITAL HEART SURGERY

In congenital heart surgery, TEE provides diagnostic information, contributes to surgical planning, identifies residual defects after repair, and influences postoperative medical management.[187] As TEE has been more widely applied in congenital heart surgery, contemporary studies report pre-CPB findings altering the surgical procedure in approximately 1% to 9% of cases and residual lesions requiring surgical revision in approximately 4% to 6% of cases, with greater impact in more complex cases.[188-191] When including return to CPB for brief ventricular support or an assist device, TEE has impacted surgical interventions in close to 13% of cases.[189] TEE further influences pharmacologic management and provides new diagnostic information. Epicardial imaging may provide complementary information to TEE when assessing pulmonary arteries and coronary arteries during pediatric congenital heart surgery.[192] There is a limited body of literature suggesting that intraoperative TEE in pediatric cardiac surgery has cost-saving benefits.[193]

OTHER SURGICAL PROCEDURES

The intraoperative echocardiographer encounters many scenarios where valvular disease requires surgical intervention, including native and prosthetic valve dysfunction. TEE confirms the preprocedure diagnosis and may refine the location of structural abnormalities. Surgical intervention for endocarditis prompts TEE evaluation for vegetations on other valves and the presence of abscess cavities. Other cardiac surgical procedures that commonly rely on intraoperative TEE include minimally invasive approaches (valve repair/replacement and CABG), cardiac mass removal, heart transplantation, and pulmonary thromboendarterectomy.

Intraprocedural Transesophageal Echocardiography- Structural Heart Interventions

Innovations in percutaneous technologies have led to exciting growth in the management of structural heart disease, extending treatment to patients with previously limited therapeutic options. The section that follows elaborates on the role of echocardiography in a few of these percutaneous procedures.

TRANSCATHETER AORTIC VALVE REPLACEMENT

First approved for commercial use in Europe in 2007 and the United States in 2011,[194] transcatheter aortic valve replacement (TAVR) has revolutionized the treatment paradigm for aortic stenosis. TAVR is indicated for the treatment of extreme- and high-risk populations with severe symptomatic aortic stenosis and it is a reasonable alternative in patients with intermediate surgical risk.[195] The number of procedures performed annually continues to grow.[196] Comprehensive resources are available detailing the periprocedural echocardiographic imaging for TAVR.[197,198]

Valve Sizing

Annular dimensions guide appropriate sizing of the transcatheter valve. The preferred imaging modality for annular size measurements is multidetector computed tomography (MDCT).[199] As compared to MDCT, 2-D TTE and TEE routinely underestimate annular size because of the elliptical shape of the aortic valvular complex.[200,201] 3-D TEE yields larger annular size measurements than 2-D TEE.[202,203] Measurements obtained by 3-D TEE may underestimate[204-206] or be comparable to[200,203,207] MDCT measurements. Both MDCT[208,209] and 3-D TEE[205,210] have been used to predict postimplantation paravalvular regurgitation. Automated 3-D TEE software is under investigation, demonstrating reproducibility and good agreement with MDCT-based prosthesis sizing.[211,212]

Intraprocedural Examination

At the beginning of the procedure, echocardiographic assessment includes not only evaluation of the aortic valve, but also determination of biventricular function, assessment of other valvular abnormalities, characterization of any preexisting pericardial effusion, and identification of other features of procedural significance, including small LV cavity and basal septal hypertrophy. When the procedure is underway, wire and device position can be guided with echocardiography, although often fluoroscopy is the primary tool. Ideal valve position prior to deployment depends on valve design (e.g. self-expanding or balloon-expandable).

Following implantation of the valve, an integrated assessment using fluoroscopy, invasive hemodynamics, and echocardiography provides information about valve position, severity of paravalvular regurgitation, and transvalvular gradients. Early recognition of unfavorable results allows for further interventions such as balloon dilation or implantation of a second device. Echocardiography excludes other complications, including functional mitral stenosis, new pericardial effusion, new RWMAs (potentially due to coronary obstruction), and aortic injury.

Transesophageal Echocardiography Versus Transthoracic Echocardiography

Active debate surrounds the optimal anesthetic approach[213] and intraprocedural imaging strategy[214] for transfemoral TAVR. Original TAVR clinical trials were performed under general anesthesia with intraprocedural TEE.[215,216] However technology has improved and procedures are of shorter duration, making procedures under monitored anesthesia care or with nursing-administered sedation feasible. High-volume centers employ these techniques along a spectrum, ranging from 100% general anesthesia, to using both sedation and general anesthesia, to nearly 100% of cases with sedation.[217] In the United States from 2012 to 2015, use of general anesthesia decreased from 97.6% to 82.6%, while use of moderate sedation increased from 2.2% to 16.6%.[196] In a 2015 survey of 250 centers representing 38 countries, general anesthesia was the most common technique in 60.1% of centers, with 39.5% of the total centers reporting exclusive use of general anesthesia.[218] Forty-six percent of centers reported systematic use of intraprocedural TEE; 62% and 31% of centers reported use of TEE and TTE, respectively, for assessment of aortic regurgitation following device implantation.[218] Despite the increasing shift away from general anesthesia and consequently TEE, use of intraprocedural TEE may be preferable for monitoring patients at high risk for coronary occlusion or annular rupture, reducing intravenous contrast exposure in high-risk patients, and providing secondary measurements for valve sizing.[219]

Because intraprocedural TEE is often performed in the setting of general anesthesia, it is difficult to assess the independent effects of general anesthesia or echocardiographic modality on outcomes. In a study comparing general anesthesia to nongeneral anesthesia in transfemoral TAVR, the majority of patients receiving general anesthesia had intraprocedural TEE, while TEE was performed in a minority of cases without general anesthesia. Propensity-matched analysis adjusted for type of anesthetic did not demonstrate significant differences in rates of successful valve deployment, more-than-mild aortic regurgitation, or other complications in patients that had an intraprocedural TEE versus those that did not.[220] A retrospective study of 454 consecutive patients undergoing transfemoral TAVR with either TTE under moderate sedation (n = 234) or TEE under general anesthesia (n = 220) showed no difference in the incidence of at least mild paravalvular regurgitation at hospital discharge (33% in TTE group vs. 38% TEE group, respectively P = .326).[221] The TTE group did however have a significantly higher incidence of second valve implantation (7% vs. 2%, P = .026) and postdilation (38% vs. 17%, P < .001).[221] Many retrospective studies are confounded by chronology bias—use of primarily TEE early on with a transition to TTE occurring after the development of procedural expertise. Additionally, findings with earlier generations of valves may not be applicable to the current generation used in clinical practice. While current studies do not allow definitive conclusions to be drawn about TEE versus TTE in TAVR, they represent initial steps in tackling these questions.

TRANSCATHETER MITRAL VALVE REPAIR

Percutaneous treatment of MR with the MitraClip procedure (Abbott Vascular-Structural Heart, Menlo Park, CA) uses a clip to grasp and appose the free edges of the anterior and posterior mitral leaflets at the site of regurgitation, creating a double orifice similar to that of the surgical Alfieri technique. In the United States, MitraClip was initially approved for the treatment of severe primary (degenerative) MR in patients with prohibitive surgical risk. In Europe, percutaneous valve repair has also been used for the treatment of secondary (functional) MR. In both patient populations, impact of treatment and long term outcomes are areas of active investigation.[222] Several randomized trials now include patients with secondary MR[223–225], and the body of literature is rapidly growing. As of 2019, indications for MitraClip therapy in the United States have expanded to include patients with significant secondary MR despite optimal medical therapy.

Echocardiographic imaging is essential in determining the suitability for the procedure, providing intraprocedural guidance, and evaluating procedural success.[226] Preoperative echocardiography characterizes the anatomic features of the valve, examines the subvalvular apparatus, and provides qualitative and quantitative assessments of the severity of the regurgitation. Optimal morphologic features

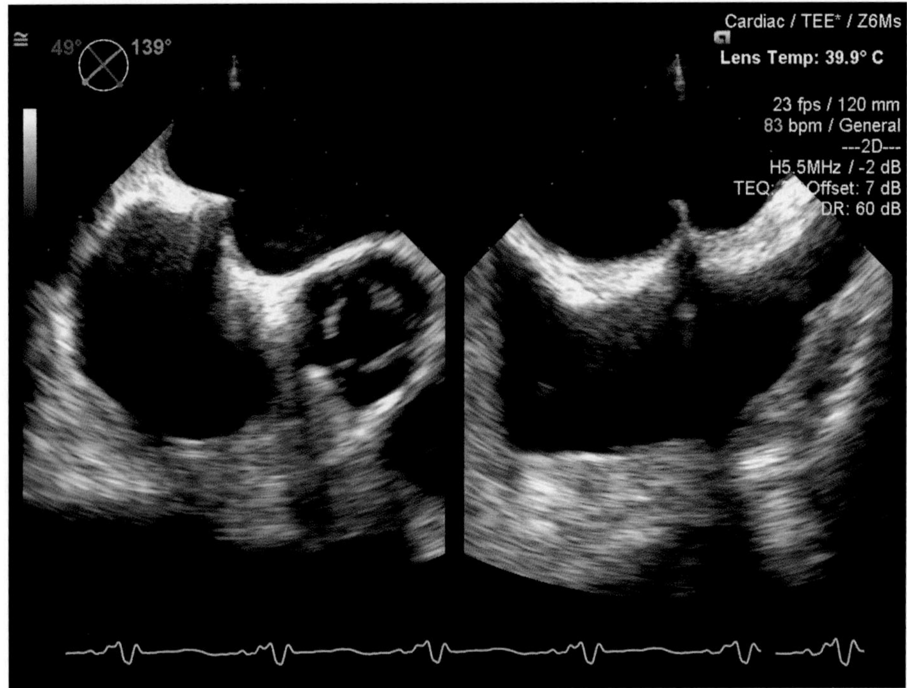

Fig. 37.29 Biplane imaging of modified midesophageal aortic valve short axis *(left)* and bicaval *(right)* views. Live biplane imaging is an essential tool in guiding puncture of the interatrial septum in catheter-based procedures entering the left side of the heart.

are based on the EVEREST study inclusion and exclusion criteria, and include regurgitation central in origin (A2/P2), lack of calcification in grasping area, mitral valve area greater than 4 cm^2, small flail gap (<10 mm), and narrow flail width (<15 mm).[227] Intraprocedural TEE, in combination with fluoroscopy, guides interatrial septal puncture and advancement of the catheter into the LA (Fig. 37.29). Under TEE guidance, the clip is aligned above the leaflets with the arms perpendicular to the line of coaptation. Once satisfactory position is obtained, the device system is advanced into the left ventricle (Fig. 37.30). Live echocardiographic imaging is often utilized as the system is slightly withdrawn so the clip grasps the leaflets; confirmation of bileaflet capture and assessment of the regurgitation severity is performed prior to clip deployment. Presence of significant residual or worsened MR, or evidence of mitral stenosis by echocardiography may prompt repositioning of the clip. Regurgitation and stenosis are quantified after deployment; placement of a second clip may be indicated if significant MR remains.

OTHER PERCUTANEOUS STRUCTURAL HEART PROCEDURES

TEE serves as a standard imaging modality in numerous other catheter-based procedures, including atrial septal defect closures, ventricular septal defect closures, LA appendage occlusion, valve-in-valve therapies for failed prostheses, and paravalvular leak closures. Echocardiography during these procedures assesses the suitability of the intervention, provides real-time guidance, and assesses the effectiveness of the intervention. Transcatheter techniques under investigation include mitral valve replacement[228] and therapies directed at TR, including valve annuloplasty, techniques targeting leaflet coaptation, and caval valve implantation.[229,230]

Emerging Technologies

FUSION IMAGING

Multimodality imaging is essential for planning and execution of percutaneous structural heart procedures. Interventional cardiologists use echocardiographic and fluoroscopic data simultaneously to guide catheter manipulation and device deployment. Often these images are displayed on separate screens, which can provide challenges as the proceduralist must combine the information to reconstruct a mental 3-D representation of the structures. Fusion of echocardiographic and fluoroscopic images provides simultaneous visualization of catheter movements with cardiac structures. Currently a technology in development, the optimal applications will be better characterized in the coming years.[231,232]

THREE-DIMENSIONAL PRINTING

3-D models of valvular structures and complex congenital heart defects can be printed from echocardiographic and other imaging data sets. Visual and tactile interactions with the models allow for improved understanding of structural interactions and abnormalities. At present, 3-D printing in this context is most relevant as a training and simulation tool, but patient-specific models can be used to optimize preprocedural planning.[233] Model quality depends on the quality of the imaging data. High cost, long printing times, and lack of materials capable of replicating tissue structural properties limit perioperative applications of 3-D printing.[234]

ARTIFICIAL INTELLIGENCE/MACHINE LEARNING

Artificial intelligence and its subfield, machine learning, permeate everyday life. The quest to apply these

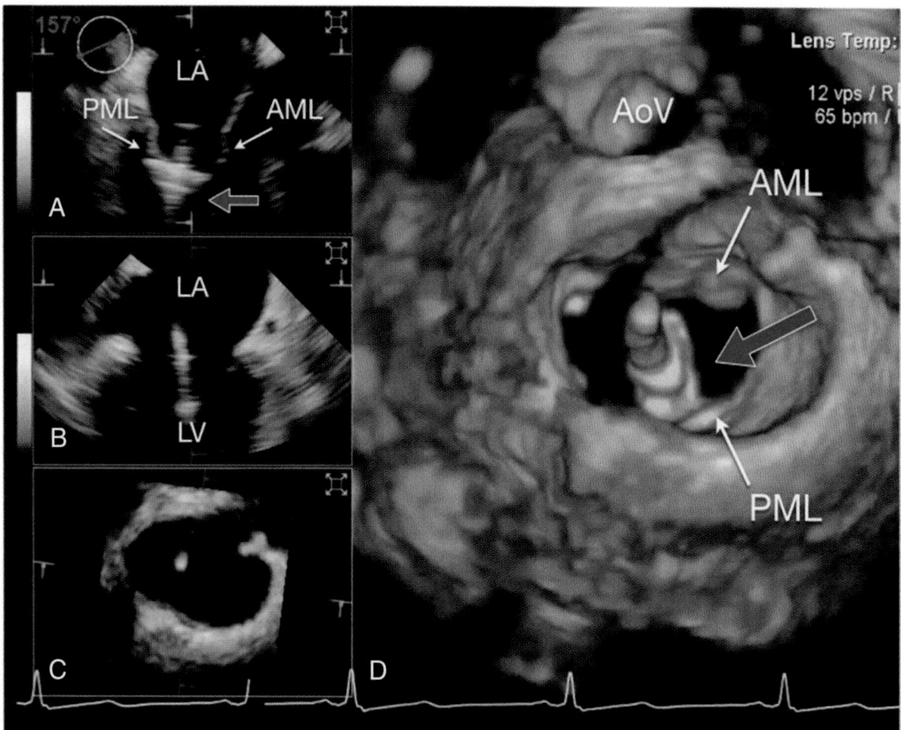

Fig. 37.30 Simultaneous live display of two-dimensional reference planes (Panels A-C) and the three-dimensional volume (Panel D) during a MitraClip procedure. The clip *(blue arrow)* should be aligned orthogonally to the line of coaptation of the mitral valve. Real-time imaging facilitates optimal device positioning by providing visual feedback following changes in catheter and device position. *AML*, Anterior mitral leaflet; *AoV*, aortic valve; *LA*, left atrium; *LV*, left ventricle; *PML*, posterior mitral leaflet.

technologies to questions in medicine is no exception. Artificial intelligence is a branch of computer science focused on development of computer systems capable of emulating human intelligence, including aspects such as learning, knowledge retention, problem solving, and reasoning.[235] Machine learning focuses on the development of predictive models where rules are learned from data rather than explicitly programmed.[236] Currently, many 3-D echocardiography platforms require manual, time-consuming user input for quantitative analysis, making their routine use in the operating room impractical. While not yet mainstream, automated analysis platforms using artificial intelligence in echocardiography exist, including mitral and aortic valve analysis in 3-D TEE[237] (Fig. 37.31) and automated chamber quantification in 3-D TTE.[238-240] Outside of the perioperative arena, machine learning has been applied to 2-D TTE assessment of LV hypertrophy phenotypes.[241] Refinement and continued development of such technologies conceivably could provide complex, quantitative valvular and ventricular analyses under dynamic conditions, improving accuracy and reducing inconsistencies in interpretation.

Perioperative Transthoracic Echocardiography and Focused Cardiac Ultrasound

While TEE has historically been the principal modality of perioperative echocardiography, TTE is emerging as a relevant and feasible counterpart. Anesthesiologists with substantial echocardiography experience have initiated preoperative TTE consult services, providing echocardiographic examination and interpretation when indicated during preoperative evaluation.[242-245] Echocardiographic findings have led to management changes in 54% to 84% of cases, including modification of the planned anesthetic approach and influencing decision making regarding the need for additional preoperative consultation or intraoperative monitoring.[242-244] Interpretation of the images by cardiologists[244] and formal TTE imaging in a subset of patients confirmed the major findings of the focused TTE examination in the majority of cases.[242,243] Standard preoperative echocardiography in patients undergoing major surgery has failed to demonstrate an association with improved outcomes,[246] so the value of preoperative anesthesiologist-performed TTE in guiding interventions or prognostication needs further characterization. As these consult services develop, important considerations include the intended scope of the examination and the experience of the individuals performing and interpreting the studies.

Several small investigations demonstrate the feasibility of FoCUS* prior to urgent or emergent surgical procedures, resulting in changes to the anesthetic technique or management plan.[247-249] Specific patient populations, such as patients sustaining hip fractures, may be optimally suited for FoCUS. Delay in surgery for hip fractures is associated with increased risk of mortality,[250,251] and preoperative echocardiographic examination through standard channels has been associated with delayed surgery.[252] A multi-center,

*These studies described the use of "focused transthoracic echocardiography." To maintain consistency with terminology proposed in published guidelines, we described these studies as FoCUS.

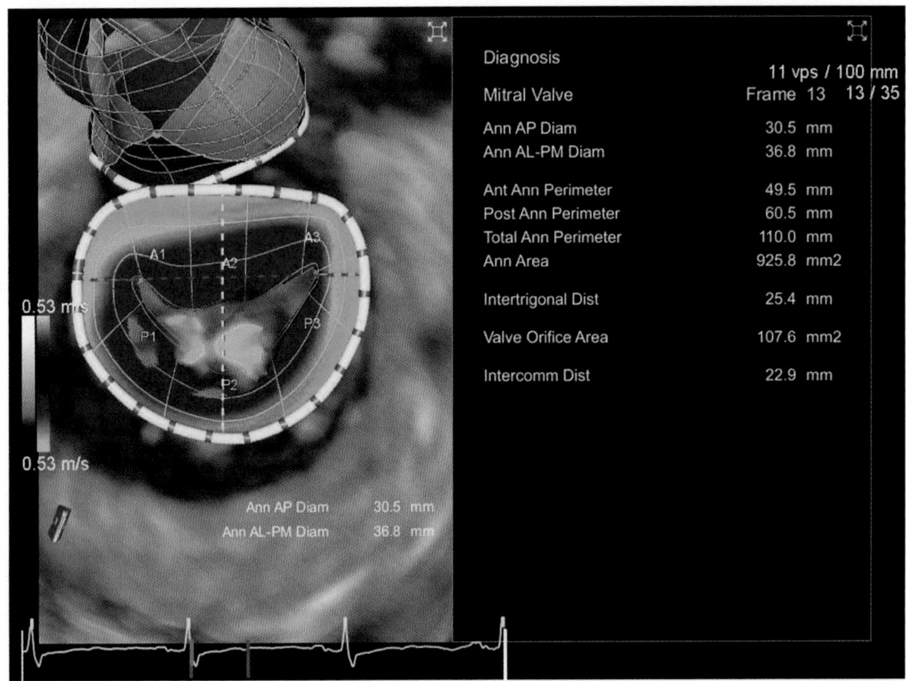

Fig. 37.31 Example of valve analysis program using artificial intelligence. Dynamic measurements of mitral annular geometry are provided throughout the cardiac cycle.

randomized pilot study of preoperative FoCUS in hip surgery has been completed, providing the groundwork for a larger, definitive randomized controlled trial.[253]

The operating theater, with the sterile surgical field and limited patient accessibility, is not necessarily conducive to transthoracic imaging. Despite the perceived challenges, small studies have prospectively demonstrated the feasibility of FoCUS during surgery. In a series that included stable and unstable patients undergoing a range of surgeries (orthopedics/trauma, abdominal/vascular, urology/gynecology, and head or ear, nose, and throat), focused examination was feasible in more than 90% of cases.[254] Patients with chronic obstructive pulmonary disease and those undergoing abdominal surgery had significantly worse image quality. Subsequent studies have demonstrated feasibility in thoracic surgery,[255] and an impact on intraoperative management in 22% to 66% of patients.[255,256]

There is increasing interest in FoCUS and TTE for hemodynamic monitoring and diagnostic assessments in the peripartum anesthetic management of pregnant women.[257] The leftward displacement of the heart and left tilt to avoid aortocaval compression are favorable for parasternal and apical imaging windows.[257] Postpartum hemorrhage, preeclampsia, and cardiomyopathy can all result in hemodynamic derangements detectable by cardiac ultrasound.[258]

Despite the recognized value of FoCUS,[259] it is not yet a routine aspect of anesthesiology practice. A survey of cardiothoracic anesthesiologists revealed a familiarity with FoCUS (81%), but only 47% of respondents use it in their clinical practice.[260] While the study has limitations, including low response rate, it provides insight into current practice patterns. The most frequently cited obstacle to use of FoCUS was lack of training, followed by concerns about missed diagnosis, lack of equipment, and lack of a certification process. As the majority of these anesthesiologists had prior formal echocardiography training (TEE, TTE, or FoCUS), it is likely the obstacles would be further amplified for anesthesiologists without this exposure.

Critical Care

Echocardiography performed and interpreted at the point of care is feasible and influential in the care of critically ill surgical and nonsurgical patients. Both TTE and TEE findings impact the management of patients in shock, influence diagnostic and therapeutic management,[261-263] and provide prognostic information.[264,265] In a study of 110 patients in undifferentiated shock, early resuscitation guided by echocardiography was associated with improved survival, less fluid administration, and greater inotrope use compared to 110 control patients examined retrospectively.[266] Although this does not indicate causality, it highlights the potential value of echocardiography in resuscitation, especially in light of the association between positive fluid balance and mortality.[267-269] TTE use is more prevalent than TEE in the ICU,[270] and European and Australian intensivists use TEE more commonly than their North American counterparts.[271] TEE offers improved diagnostic accuracy in the setting of mechanical ventilation,[261] however several groups have obtained adequate transthoracic images for focused studies in the majority of mechanically ventilated patients.[262,272,273] TEE provides superior imaging for the evaluation of suspected endocarditis or intracardiac mass, evaluation of great vessel pathology, and assessment of valvular dysfunction.[56]

Similar to perioperative TEE, there are proposed basic and advanced applications of critical care echocardiography.[54,57] Basic applications include assessment of global biventricular size and function, identification of pericardial fluid or tamponade, identification of severe valvular regurgitation, and as guidance for resuscitative efforts during and after cardiac arrest. Advanced applications include quantitative assessments of function and filling pressures, evaluation of fluid responsiveness, and detection of abnormalities including cardiac source of embolism, endocarditis, acute aortic pathology or injury, intracardiac shunt, and complications of MI. Evaluation of suspected endocarditis, great vessel pathology or injury, and PE may be considered basic or advanced applications.

FLUID RESPONSIVENESS

When assessing a patient in shock, the decision to administer, withhold, or stop fluids is often challenging. Patients who are fluid responsive will demonstrate an increase in SV or cardiac output in response to a fluid challenge,[107] and dynamic indices (such as heart-lung interactions or the passive leg raise maneuver) temporarily induce changes in preload to assess for this response. In patients receiving passive mechanical ventilation, several echocardiographic dynamic parameters have been used to predict fluid responsiveness and aid in clinical decision making:

- *Inferior vena cava distensibility index:* During positive pressure ventilation, inspiration causes a rise in intrathoracic pressure, which decreases the venous return to the heart and leads to IVC distension. During expiration, IVC diameter is at a minimum. Two IVC distensibility indices (dIVC or ΔIVC) relating the maximum (D_{max}) and minimum (D_{min}) diameters during the respiratory cycle have been described:

$$\Delta IVC = \frac{D_{max} - D_{min}}{D_{min}} * 100\,\%$$

  where a threshold of 18% or greater discriminated between responders and nonresponders,[274]

  and

$$\Delta IVC = \frac{D_{max} - D_{min}}{(D_{max} + D_{min})\,/2} * 100\,\%$$

  where a threshold of 12% or greater discriminated between responders and nonresponders.[275]

  Use of the first equation is most common.[276] In more heterogeneous populations, ΔIVC performs less accurately (two subsequent studies report an area under the receiver operating characteristic curve of 0.43 and 0.635, respectively).[277,278] The reported optimal thresholds for discriminating responders from nonresponders also vary. In general, ΔIVC has greater specificity than sensitivity.

  Several preconditions must be met for ΔIVC to be a useful tool, including absence of spontaneous respiratory effort, 8 to 12 mL/kg tidal volumes (necessary to increase the pleural pressure to affect the IVC diameter), absence of cor pulmonale, and absence of intraabdominal hypertension.[108] Highlighting the importance of these conditions, ΔIVC accurately predicts fluid responsiveness in patients ventilated with tidal volumes of 8 to 10 mL/kg and PEEP of 5 cm H_2O or less but poorly predicts fluid responsiveness in patients receiving tidal volumes less than 8 mL/kg or PEEP greater than 5 cm H_2O.[276]

- *Superior vena cava collapsibility index:* During positive pressure ventilation, the SVC collapses during inspiration due to increased intrathoracic pressure (a pattern opposite that of the IVC). An initial study of patients with septic shock evaluated the SVC collapsibility index (ΔSVC), defined as:

$$\Delta SVC = \frac{D_{max} - D_{min}}{D_{max}} * 100\,\%$$

  where D_{max} is the maximum diameter on expiration and D_{min} is the minimum diameter on inspiration.[279] A threshold of more than 36% distinguished fluid responders from nonresponders with 90% sensitivity and 100% specificity. In a larger cohort including mechanically ventilated patients with any type of shock, ΔSVC of 21% or greater predicted fluid responsiveness with 61% sensitivity and 84% specificity.[278] When compared in the same patients, ΔSVC has greater diagnostic accuracy than ΔIVC_1.[277,278] TEE imaging is required to determine ΔSVC.
- *Variation in peak aortic/LVOT velocity:* Positive pressure ventilation results in cyclical changes in the maximum velocity of flow in the LVOT and across the aortic valve. Application of PWD at the level of the aortic valve[280] or in the LVOT[278] allows for measurement of the highest (V_{max}) and lowest (V_{min}) peak velocities over the course of the respiratory cycle. The difference between the two is divided by their mean and expressed as a percentage as follows:

$$\Delta V_{max}Ao = \frac{V_{max} - V_{min}}{(V_{max} + V_{min})\,/2} * 100\,\%$$

  A threshold of 12% or more discriminated between responders and nonresponders in initial investigations.[280] Similar to other dynamic indices, in larger, diverse populations, this parameter does not perform as accurately as originally reported. When compared in the same cohort, $\Delta V_{max}Ao$ had the highest sensitivity, whereas ΔSVC had the highest specificity for predicting fluid responsiveness.[278]

Additional echocardiographic assessments utilizing heart-lung interactions and dynamic parameters are an area of active research. End-expiratory occlusion maneuvers alone or in combination with end-inspiratory occlusions have been used to predict fluid responsiveness as assessed by changes in LVOT velocity time integral and/or maximum aortic velocity.[281,282] These approaches are not currently widely applied and require further validation in varying patient populations. With any of these indices, the clinician should interpret these findings within the overall context of the patient's status and with an awareness of the limitations.

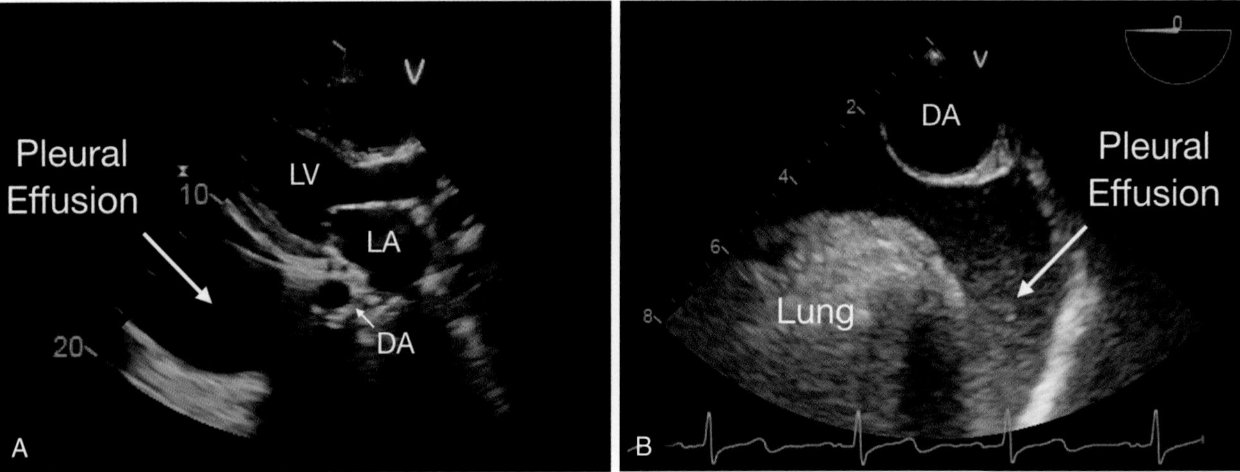

Fig. 37.32 Pleural effusions demonstrated by echocardiography. (A) This transthoracic parasternal long axis view demonstrates an echolucent space posterior to the DA, consistent with a large left pleural effusion. A pericardial effusion (not present in this image) would be seen as an echolucent space anterior to the descending aorta. (B) A transesophageal descending aorta short axis view demonstrating an echolucent space consistent with a left pleural effusion. Note the atelectatic lung at the left of the image. *DA*, Descending aorta; *LA*, left atrium; *LV*, left ventricle.

POST-CARDIAC SURGERY

A 2016 systematic review of 15 studies examining TTE and TEE after cardiac surgery demonstrated that echocardiography (performed by a mix of novice and expert sonographers) was feasible and that findings frequently led to management changes.[283] In hemodynamically unstable postoperative cardiac surgical patients, significant discordance has been demonstrated between diagnoses obtained from continuous TEE and diagnoses obtained from hemodynamic measurements.[284] TEE-based diagnoses have greater interobserver agreement, suggesting that echocardiography may add valuable diagnostic information even in the presence of invasive hemodynamic monitors.

TRAUMA AND RESUSCITATION

For decades, cardiac ultrasound via the subcostal window has been part of the evaluation of the trauma patient within the Focused Assessment with Sonography for Trauma (FAST) examination.[285] FoCUS extends this cardiac examination and has been adopted as a tool to guide resuscitation of trauma patients. A trial randomizing trauma patients to FoCUS or no FoCUS as part of the initial evaluation demonstrated significantly less fluid administration, shorter time from the trauma bay to the operating room, and higher rate of ICU admissions in the FoCUS group.[286] In blunt or penetrating chest trauma, echocardiography reveals complications such as cardiac rupture, dysfunction (due to contusion), valvular injury, hemopericardium, and aortic disruption.[287]

OTHER CLINICAL APPLICATIONS

Echocardiography may identify causes of hypoxia, such as right-to-left intracardiac shunt or pleural effusion (Fig. 37.32). Clinicians often incorporate lung ultrasound with echocardiography when evaluating cardiopulmonary failure (also see Chapter 83).[288]

Novel applications of echocardiography in critical care are emerging. Areas of active research include strain imaging in sepsis[289] and the use of echocardiography in evaluating patients that fail to liberate from mechanical ventilation.[290]

HANDHELD CARDIAC ULTRASOUND

With their compact size and portability, handheld echocardiography devices are ideal for point-of-care assessments.[291] Intensivists with limited echocardiography training have performed and interpreted focused handheld examinations, estimating LV systolic function with reasonable accuracy compared to formal TTE performed by a sonographer and interpreted by an echocardiographer.[292] When performed by intensivists experienced in echocardiography, handheld echocardiographic examinations offer similar 2-D diagnostic capabilities to full-platform TTE in mechanically ventilated, critically ill patients, with limitations due to lack of spectral Doppler.[293]

MINIATURE TEE PROBES

Miniature TEE probes have promise as tools for hemodynamic monitoring or characterization of cardiopulmonary failure in the critical care setting.[294,295] Examination with miniaturized multiplane TEE probes is feasible and well tolerated in ventilated, critically ill patients.[295] When compared to standard TEE, miniature probes enable concordant diagnostic assessments of causes of cardiorespiratory failure, albeit with lesser image quality. Consequent to the diminished image quality, common hemodynamic measurements can be performed less frequently, but when possible, the results agree with those obtained by standard TEE. Larger studies and evaluation of resulting clinical impact are necessary prior to widespread adoption of miniature TEE.

Training and Certification

KNOWLEDGE EXPECTATIONS AND TRAINING

Across the field of anesthesiology, there is a growing impetus for formalized training in perioperative ultrasound including echocardiography. The American Council for Graduate Medical Education requires anesthesiology residents to demonstrate competency in the acquisition of standard transesophageal and transthoracic echocardiographic views.[296] Certification by the American Board of Anesthesiology requires basic knowledge of TEE, assessed both in the written examination[297] and the Objective Structured Clinical Exam.[298] Accredited Anesthesiology Critical Care Medicine programs require fellows to demonstrate knowledge of ultrasound principles and proficiency in TEE and TTE.[299]

Formalized echocardiography training requires curriculum development and educational initiatives. For some trainees, exposure to ultrasound now begins in medical school. Several institutions include cardiac ultrasound in their educational programs, initially using it to teach anatomy and function, and later as an adjunct to the physical examination.[300] Many residency programs are developing multimodal longitudinal curricula including didactic lectures, hands-on workshops, online modules, simulation, and formal echocardiography rotations.[301-304] Online virtual simulation provides users an interactive format to learn standard views and spatial relationships.[305,306] Mannequin-based simulation is an effective method for improving the acquisition of cognitive and technical skills both in TEE[307-312] and TTE,[308,313,314] and may be a useful educational tool for learners early in training. In addition to these multimodal didactic approaches, practical clinical experience under supervision remains a key part of the training process. In North America, advanced training in TEE usually occurs in the context of the cardiothoracic anesthesiology fellowship.

The coming years will likely include increasing emphasis on FoCUS training in anesthesiology. In a survey of US anesthesiology residency program directors and trainees, the majority of respondents indicated FoCUS should be a standard component of training, while only a minority of the programs incorporated such training.[315] A different survey of Canadian residency program directors indicated FoCUS training should be compulsory, and while most of the programs had training opportunities, only a minority included mandatory rotations.[316] The challenge to the specialty is how to best incorporate FoCUS, to define minimum training standards and competencies, and to provide education for trainees as well as anesthesiologists already in practice. The European Association of Cardiovascular Imaging has published a reference curriculum and syllabus for FoCUS education and training.[317] Clinicians must clearly understand the narrow scope of FoCUS, recognizing the limitations and indications for expert consultation. Many examples of the applicability of perioperative FoCUS are in the hands of experienced echocardiographers—whether this translates to operators with less experience and less formal training will need to be examined. After the initial acquisition of cognitive and technical skills in ultrasound, continued use is important to ensure proficiency; when these skills are not used for over a year, significant attrition occurs.[318]

CERTIFICATION

The National Board of Echocardiography offers examination and certification in basic (Basic PTEeXAM) and advanced (Advanced PTEeXAM) perioperative TEE.[319] Individuals that pass the examination achieve testamur status. Testamurs can achieve basic certification via supervised training, practice experience, or extended continuing medical education. Advanced PTEeXAM testamurs can receive certification by completing an accredited cardiothoracic anesthesiology pathway; a practice experience pathway is only available to individuals that completed training prior to 2009. There is no certification for perioperative TTE, however, qualified individuals can take the Examination of Special Competence in Adult Comprehensive Echocardiography (ASCeXAM) and achieve testamur status. In Europe, the European Association of Cardiovascular Imaging and European Association of Cardiothoracic Anaesthesiology jointly offer certification in adult TEE.[320] General critical care ultrasound and basic critical care echocardiography are now considered to be within the scope of practice of intensivists, while certification has been proposed for those obtaining advanced training.[55,56] As of 2019, the National Board of Echocardiography now offers an Examination of Special Competence in Critical Care Echocardiography (CCEeXAM).[321]

Future Directions

The evolution of perioperative echocardiography is at a transformative juncture. The landscape is one of growth, innovation, and accessibility. From its perioperative origin as a monitor in cardiac surgery decades ago, TEE has become integral to the practice of cardiac anesthesia and surgical decision making. More sophisticated and automated platforms will pave the way for increasingly complex, quantitative analyses to be performed in real time. Catheter-based procedures push the boundaries of treatable pathologies, and echocardiography is central to the multimodal imaging techniques employed by structural heart teams. Many cardiac anesthesiologists have an interest in TTE, which complements and builds upon their already established cognitive and technical skills.

Outside of the cardiac arena, anesthesiologists use TEE as an intraoperative monitor in high-risk procedures or populations. Basic knowledge of TEE is now expected of anesthesiology trainees. In the future, knowledge of transthoracic imaging in the form of FoCUS may too become a requirement. Increased portability of ultrasound machines and newer technologies like capacitive micromachined ultrasound transducers make the potential for widespread point-of-care imaging an imminent reality. With the growing interest and investment in ultrasonography, a basic skill set may soon be within the purview of all anesthesiologists. Opportunities for research into education and the impact of anesthesiologist-performed examinations abound. Critical care training objectives now include basic proficiency in echocardiography in the larger context of critical care ultrasound. Similar to advanced perioperative TEE, proficiency in advanced critical care echocardiography requires additional dedicated training and allows comprehensive evaluation of cardiac structure and function, and hemodynamic assessments in the context of the critically ill patient. Whether applied as a routine monitor, a more advanced diagnostic tool, or used in procedural guidance, echocardiography is an essential component of the modern perioperative physician's armamentarium.

Acknowledgment

The editors and publisher would like to thank Drs. Georges Desjardins, Daniel P. Vezina, Ken B. Johnson and Michael K. Cahalan for contributing a chapter on this topic in the prior edition of this work. It has served as the foundation for the current chapter.

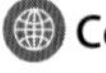 **Complete references available online at expertconsult.com.**

References

1. Mahmood F, Shernan SK. *Heart.* 2016;102(15):1159–1167.
2. Edler I, Hertz CH. *Clin Physiol Funct Imaging.* 2004;24(3):118–136.
3. Johnson ML, et al. *J Thorac Cardiovasc Surg.* 1972;64(6):922–934.
4. Frazin L, et al. *Circulation.* 1976;54(1):102–108.
5. Matsumoto M, et al. *N Y State J Med.* 1979;79(1):19–21.
6. Matsumoto M, et al. *Am J Cardiol.* 1980;46(1):95–105.
7. Souquet J, et al. *IEEE Trans Biomed Eng.* 1982;29(10):707–712.
8. Schluter M, et al. *Br Heart J.* 1982;48(1):67–72.
9. Roizen MF, et al. *J Vasc Surg.* 1984;1(2):300–305.
10. Beaupre PN, et al. *Am Heart J.* 1984;107(5 Pt 1):1021–1023.
11. Cucchiara RF, et al. *Anesthesiology.* 1984;60(4):353–355.
12. de Bruijn NP, et al. *Anesth Analg.* 1987;66(5):386–390.
13. Roewer N, et al. *J Cardiothorac Anesth.* 1987;1(5):418–428.
14. Omoto R, et al. *Int J Card Imaging.* 1989;4(1):57–58.
15. Flachskampf FA, et al. *Eur Heart J.* 1992;13(9):1201–1206.
16. Kyo S, et al. *Int J Card Imaging.* 1989;4(1):41–42.
17. Pothineni KR, et al. *Echocardiography.* 2007;24(10):1099–1104.
18. Kloster FE, et al. *Circulation.* 1973;48(5):1075–1084.
19. Griffith JM, Henry WL. *Circulation.* 1974;49(6):1147–1152.
20. vonRamm OT, Thurstone FL. *Circulation.* 1976;53(2):258–262.
21. Kisslo J, et al. *Circulation.* 1976;53(2):262–267.
22. Feigenbaum H. *Circulation.* 1996;93(7):1321–1327.
23. Jardin F, et al. *Crit Care Med.* 1985;13(11):952–956.
24. Jardin F, et al. *Crit Care Med.* 1990;18(10):1055–1060.
25. Swan HJ, et al. *N Engl J Med.* 1970;283(9):447–451.
26. Connors Jr AF, et al. *N Engl J Med.* 1983;308(5):263–267.
27. Eisenberg PR, et al. *Crit Care Med.* 1984;12(7):549–553.
28. Connors Jr AF, et al. *JAMA.* 1996;276(11):889–897.
29. Dalen JE, Bone RC. *JAMA.* 1996;276(11):916–918.
30. Richard C, et al. *JAMA.* 2003;290(20):2713–2720.
31. Sandham JD, et al. *N Engl J Med.* 2003;348(1):5–14.
32. Wiener RS, Welch HG. *JAMA.* 2007;298(4):423–429.
33. Le HT, et al. *Anesth Analg.* 2016;122(3):633–646.
34. Duncan AE,A, et al. *Anesth Analg.* 2014;118(3):525–544.
35. Thomas JD, Rubin DN. *J Am Soc Echocardiogr.* 1998;11(8):803–808.
36. Turner SP, Monaghan MJ. *Eur J Echocardiogr.* 2006;7(1):9–15.
37. Hawkins K, et al. *Echocardiography.* 2008;25(2):119–123.
38. Porter TR, et al. *J Am Soc Echocardiogr.* 2018;31(3):241–274.
39. Bhatia VK, Senior R. *J Am Soc Echocardiogr.* 2008;21(5):409–416.
40. Porter TR, et al. *J Am Soc Echocardiogr.* 2014;27(8):797–810.
41. Lang RM, et al. *J Am Soc Echocardiogr.* 2012;25(1):3–46.
42. Mahmood F, et al. *J Cardiothorac Vasc Anesth.* 2016;30(2):470–490.
43. Practice guidelines for perioperative transesophageal echocardiography. A report by the American Society of Anesthesiologists and the Society of Cardiovascular Anesthesiologists Task Force on Transesophageal Echocardiography. *Anesthesiology.* 1996;84(4):986–1006.
44. American Society of Anesthesiologists and Society of Cardiovascular Anesthesiologists Task Force on Transesophageal Echocardiography. Practice guidelines for perioperative transesophageal echocardiography. An updated report by the American Society of Anesthesiologists and the Society of Cardiovascular Anesthesiologists Task Force on Transesophageal Echocardiography. *Anesthesiology.* 2010;112(5):1084–1096.
45. Silvestry FE, et al. *J Am Soc Echocardiogr.* 2009;22(3):213–231; quiz 316-217.
46. Zamorano JL, et al. *J Am Soc Echocardiogr.* 2011;24(9):937–965.
47. Flachskampf FA, et al. *Eur J Echocardiogr.* 2001;2(1):8–21.
48. Flachskampf FA, et al. *Eur J Echocardiogr.* 2010;11(7):557–576.
49. Kristensen SD, et al. *Eur Heart J.* 2014;35(35):2383–2431.
50. Nishimura RA, et al. *Circulation.* 2014;129(23):e521–643.
51. Fleisher LA, et al. *Circulation.* 2014;130(24):2215–2245.
52. Cahalan MK, et al. *J Am Soc Echocardiogr.* 2002;15(6):647–652.
53. Price S, et al. *Cardiovasc Ultrasound.* 2008;6:49.
54. Mayo PH, et al. *Chest.* 2009;135(4):1050–1060.
55. Expert Round Table on Ultrasound in ICU. *Intensive Care Med.* 2011;37(7):1077–1083.
56. Expert Round Table on Echocardiography in ICU. *Intensive Care Med.* 2014;40(5):654–666.
57. Levitov A, et al. *Crit Care Med.* 2016;44(6):1206–1227.
58. Hilberath JN, et al. *J Am Soc Echocardiogr.* 2010;23(11):1115–1127.
59. Purza R, et al. *Ann Thorac Surg.* 2017;103(3):795–802.
60. Reeves ST, et al. *Anesth Analg.* 2013;117(3):543–558.
61. Hahn RT, et al. *J Am Soc Echocardiogr.* 2013;26(9):921–964.
62. Reeves ST, et al. *J Am Soc Echocardiogr.* 2007;20(4):427–437.
63. Royse AG, Royse CF. *Best Pract Res Clin Anaesthesiol.* 2009;23(3): 335–341.
64. Michelena HI, et al. *Mayo Clin Proc.* 2010;85(7):646–655.
65. Ikram A, et al. *J Clin Neurosci.* 2018;50:30–34.
66. Glas KE, et al. *J Am Soc Echocardiogr.* 2007;20(11):1227–1235.
67. Spencer KT, et al. *J Am Soc Echocardiogr.* 2013;26(6):567–581.
68. Via G, et al. *J Am Soc Echocardiogr.* 2014;27(7): 683.e681-683.e633.
69. Zimmerman JM, Coker BJ. *Anesth Analg.* 2017;124(3):753–760.
70. Mitchell C, et al. *J Am Soc Echocardiogr.* 2018.
71. Gudmundsson P, et al. *Int J Cardiol.* 2005;101(2):209–212.
72. Shahgaldi K, et al. *Cardiovasc Ultrasound.* 2009;7:41.
73. Mathew JP, et al. *Anesth Analg.* 2002;94(2):302–309.
74. Cerqueira MD, et al. *J Nucl Cardiol.* 2002;9(2):240–245.
75. Ortiz-Perez JT, et al. *JACC Cardiovasc Imaging.* 2008;1(3):282–293.
76. Hauser AM, et al. *J Am Coll Cardiol.* 1985;5(2 Pt 1):193–197.
77. Rudski LG, et al. *J Am Soc Echocardiogr.* 2010;23(7):685–713; quiz 786-688.
78. Zoghbi WA, et al. *J Am Soc Echocardiogr.* 2017;30(4):303–371.
79. Lancellotti P, et al. *Eur Heart J Cardiovasc Imaging.* 2013;14(7):611–644.
80. Sanfilippo F, et al. *J Cardiothorac Vasc Anesth.* 2017;31(5):1681–1691.
81. Lang RM, et al. *J Am Soc Echocardiogr.* 2015;28(1):1–39.e14.
82. Caballero L, et al. *Eur Heart J Cardiovasc Imaging.* 2015;16(9):1031–1041.
83. Nishimura RA, Tajik AJ. *Prog Cardiovasc Dis.* 1994;36(4):309–342.
84. Forner AF, et al. *Int J Cardiovasc Imaging.* 2017;33(9):1385–1394.
85. Shen T, et al. *Anesth Analg.* 2018;126(1):62–67.
86. Markin NW, et al. *J Am Soc Echocardiogr.* 2017;30(2):180–188.
87. Tamborini G, et al. *Eur J Echocardiogr.* 2009;10(5):630–634.
88. Unsworth B, et al. *Int J Cardiol.* 2013;165(1):151–160.
89. Nagueh SF. *Curr Heart Fail Rep.* 2009;6(3):154–159.
90. Nagueh SF, et al. *J Am Soc Echocardiogr.* 2016;29(4):277–314.
91. Swaminathan M, et al. *Ann Thorac Surg.* 2011;91(6):1844–1850.
92. Matyal R, et al. *Anesth Analg.* 2011;113(3):449–472.
93. McIlroy DR, et al. *J Cardiothorac Vasc Anesth.* 2015;29(4):1033–1043.
94. Baumgartner H, et al. *J Am Soc Echocardiogr.* 2017;30(4):372–392.
95. Baumgartner H, et al. *J Am Soc Echocardiogr.* 2009;22(1):1–23; quiz 101-102.
96. Brown JM. *Crit Care Med.* 2002;30(6):1361–1364.
97. Wetterslev M, et al. *Intensive Care Med.* 2016;42(8):1223–1233.
98. Amsallem M, et al. *J Am Soc Echocardiogr.* 2016;29(2):93–102.
99. Vincent JL, De Backer D. *N Engl J Med.* 2014;370(6):583.
100. Cecconi M, et al. 2014;40(12):1795–1815.
101. Akinboboye O, et al. *Clin Cardiol.* 1995;18(12):726–729.
102. Seeberger MD, et al. *Anesth Analg.* 1997;85(6):1252–1257.
103. Hessel 2nd EA. *Can J Anaesth.* 2016;63(9):1059–1074.
104. Citro R, et al. *J Am Soc Echocardiogr.* 2015;28(1):57–74.
105. Leung JM, Levine EH. *Anesthesiology.* 1994;81(5):1102–1109.
106. Porter TR, et al. *J Am Soc Echocardiogr.* 2015;28(1):40–56.
107. Marik PE, Cavallazzi R. *Crit Care Med.* 2013;41(7):1774–1781.
108. Schmidt GA. *Chest.* 2017;151(3):531–532.
109. Kory P. *Chest.* 2017;151(3):533–536.
110. Schmidt GA. *Chest.* 2017;151(3):536–537.
111. Kory P. *Chest.* 2017;151(3):537–538.
112. Muller L, et al. *Crit Care.* 2012;16(5):R188.
113. Corl K, et al. *Emerg Med Australas.* 2012;24(5):534–539.
114. de Valk S, et al. *BMC Anesthesiol.* 2014;14:114.
115. Airapetian N, et al. *Crit Care.* 2015;19:400.
116. Corl KA, et al. *J Crit Care.* 2017;41:130–137.
117. Preau S, et al. *Crit Care Med.* 2017;45(3):e290–e297.

118. Evans JS, et al. *Anaesth Intensive Care.* 2017;45(1):12–20.
119. Chauvet JL, et al. *Crit Care.* 2015;19:262.
120. Markin NW, et al. *J Cardiothorac Vasc Anesth.* 2015;29(1):82–88.
121. Klein AL, et al. *J Am Soc Echocardiogr.* 2013;26(9):965–1012.e1015.
122. Gillam LD, et al. *Circulation.* 1983;68(2):294–301.
123. Kronzon I, et al. *J Am Coll Cardiol.* 1983;2(4):770–775.
124. Merce J, et al. *J. Am Heart J.* 1999;138(4 Pt 1):759–764.
125. Himelman RB, et al. *J Am Coll Cardiol.* 1988;12(6):1470–1477.
126. Faehnrich JA, et al. *J Cardiothorac Vasc Anesth.* 2003;17(1):45–50.
127. Jaff MR, et al. *Circulation.* 2011;123(16):1788–1830.
128. Konstantinides SV, et al. *Eur Heart J.* 2014;35(43):3033–3069.
129. American College of Cardiology Foundation Appropriate Use Criteria Task F, et al. *J Am Soc Echocardiogr.* 2011;24(3):229–267.
130. Shafiq Q, et al. *J Echocardiogr.* 2016;14(4):146–155.
131. Labovitz AJ, et al. *J Am Soc Echocardiogr.* 2010;23(12):1225–1230.
132. Mansencal N, et al. *Eur Radiol.* 2011;21(2):240–245.
133. Mediratta A, et al. 2016;33(5):696–702.
134. McConnell MV, et al. *Am J Cardiol.* 1996;78(4):469–473.
135. Fields JM, et al. *J Am Soc Echocardiogr.* 2017;30(7):714–723.e714.
136. Casazza F, et al. *Eur J Echocardiogr.* 2005;6(1):11–14.
137. Kurnicka K, et al. *J Am Soc Echocardiogr.* 2016;29(9):907–913.
138. Mahmood F, et al. *Semin Cardiothorac Vasc Anesth.* 2008;12(4):265–289.
139. Denault AY, et al. *Can J Anaesth.* 2002;49(3):287–293.
140. Suriani RJ, et al. *J Cardiothorac Vasc Anesth.* 1998;12(3):274–280.
141. Hofer CK, et al. *Anaesthesia.* 2004;59(1):3–9.
142. London MJ, et al. *Anesthesiology.* 1990;73(4):644–655.
143. Eisenberg MJ, et al. *JAMA.* 1992;268(2):210–216.
144. Galal W, et al. *Anesthesiology.* 2010;112(3):557–566.
145. Robertson AC, Eagle SS. *J Cardiothorac Vasc Anesth.* 2014;28(1):141–154.
146. Dalia AA, et al. *J Cardiothorac Vasc Anesth.* 2018.
147. Maraj S, et al. *Echocardiography.* 2004;21(8):681–685.
148. Nicoara A, Anderson-Dam J. *Anesthesiol Clin.* 2017;35(3):473–489.
149. Cartwright BL, et al. *J Cardiothorac Vasc Anesth.* 2013;27(1):111–120.
150. Harpole DH, et al. *Ann Surg.* 1989;209(3):356–362.
151. Koolen JJ, et al. *Eur Heart J.* 1992;13(8):1028–1033.
152. Memtsoudis SG, et al. *Anesth Analg.* 2006;102(6):1653–1657.
153. Shillcutt SK, et al. *J Cardiothorac Vasc Anesth.* 2012;26(3):362–370.
154. Schulmeyer C, et al. *Rev Bras Anestesiol.* 2010;60(5):513–521.
155. Staudt GE, Shelton K. *Anesth Analg.* 2018.
156. Eltzschig HK, et al. *Ann Thorac Surg.* 2008;85(3):845–852.
157. Guarracino F, et al. *HSR Proc Intensive Care Cardiovasc Anesth.* 2010;2(1):43–49.
158. Ramakrishna H, et al. *J Cardiothorac Vasc Anesth.* 2014;28(6):1691–1695.
159. Krasuski RA, Hart SA, Allen D, et al. *JAMA.* 2009;302(3):290–297.
160. Comunale ME, Body SC, Ley C, et al. *Anesthesiology.* 1998;88(4):945–954.
161. Leung JM, et al. *Anesthesiology.* 1989;71(1):16–25.
162. Swaminathan M, et al. *Anesthesiology.* 2007;107(5):739–745.
163. Mahmood F, et al. *J Cardiothorac Vasc Anesth.* 2018;32(2):823–837.
164. Carpentier A. *J Thorac Cardiovasc Surg.* 1983;86(3):323–337.
165. Grewal J, et al. *J Am Soc Echocardiogr.* 2009;22(1):34–41.
166. Ben Zekry S, et al. *J Am Soc Echocardiogr.* 2011;24(10):1079–1085.
167. Hien MD, et al. *Anesth Analg.* 2013;116(2):287–295.
168. Mahmood F, Matyal R. *Anesth Analg.* 2015;121(1):34–58.
169. Maslow AD, et al. *J Am Coll Cardiol.* 1999;34(7):2096–2104.
170. Varghese R, et al. *Eur J Cardiothorac Surg.* 2014;45(1):132–137; discussion 137-138.
171. Kuperstein R, et al. *J Thorac Cardiovasc Surg.* 2015;149(2):471–476.
172. Hahn RT. *Circ Cardiovasc Imaging.* 2016;9(12).
173. Dreyfus J, et al. *Circ Cardiovasc Imaging.* 2015;8(7):e003241.
174. Ring L, et al. *Eur Heart J Cardiovasc Imaging.* 2012;13(9):756–762.
175. Hai T, et al. *J Cardiothorac Vasc Anesth.* 2017;31(6):2106–2114.
176. Bhave NM, et al. *JACC Cardiovasc Imaging.* 2018;11(6):902–919.
177. Mussa FF, et al. *JAMA.* 2016;316(7):754–763.
178. Tan CN, Fraser AG. *Can J Anaesth.* 2014;61(4):362–378.
179. Thorsgard ME, et al. *J Cardiothorac Vasc Anesth.* 2014;28(5):1203–1207.
180. Kirklin JK, et al. *J Heart Lung Transplant.* 2017;36(10):1080–1086.
181. Estep JD, et al. *JACC Cardiovasc Imaging.* 2010;3(10):1049–1064.
182. Flores AS, et al. *J Thorac Dis.* 2015;7(12):2139–2150.
183. Stainback RF, et al. *J Am Soc Echocardiogr.* 2015;28(8):853–909.
184. Grinstein J, et al. *J Card Fail.* 2016;22(10):808–814.
185. Platts DG, et al. *J Am Soc Echocardiogr.* 2012;25(2):131–141.
186. Cavarocchi NC, et al. *J Thorac Cardiovasc Surg.* 2013;146(6):1474–1479.
187. Kamra K, et al. *Paediatr Anaesth.* 2011;21(5):479–493.
188. Randolph GR, et al. *J Thorac Cardiovasc Surg.* 2002;124(6):1176–1182.
189. Bettex DA, et al. *Anesth Analg.* 2003;97(5):1275–1282.
190. Guzeltas A, et al. *Congenit Heart Dis.* 2014;9(4):300–306.
191. Jijeh AM, et al. *J Saudi Heart Assoc.* 2016;28(2):89–94.
192. Dragulescu A, et al. *J Thorac Cardiovasc Surg.* 2012;143(2):361–367.
193. Levin DN, Taras J, Taylor K. *Paediatr Anaesth.* 2016;26(7):682–693.
194. Dvir D, et al. *Arch Cardiovasc Dis.* 2012;105(3):160–164.
195. Nishimura RA, et al. *J Am Coll Cardiol.* 2017;70(2):252–289.
196. Grover FL, et al. *J Am Coll Cardiol.* 2017;69(10):1215–1230.
197. Hahn RT, et al. *JACC Cardiovasc Imaging.* 2015;8(3):261–287.
198. Hahn RT, et al. *J Am Soc Echocardiogr.* 2018;31(4):405–433.
199. Otto CM, et al. *J Am Coll Cardiol.* 2017;69(10):1313–1346.
200. Altiok E, et al. *Heart.* 2011;97(19):1578–1584.
201. Gurvitch R, et al. *JACC Cardiovasc Interv.* 2011;4(11):1235–1245.
202. Husser O, et al. *Catheter Cardiovasc Interv.* 2012;80(6):956–963.
203. Smith LA, et al. *J Am Soc Echocardiogr.* 2013;26(4):359–369.
204. Ng AC, et al. *Circ Cardiovasc Imaging.* 2010;3(1):94–102.
205. Jilaihawi H, et al. *J Am Coll Cardiol.* 2013;61(9):908–916.
206. Vaquerizo B, et al. *Eur Heart J Cardiovasc Imaging.* 2016;17(1):15–23.
207. Khalique OK, et al. *Circ Cardiovasc Imaging.* 2014;7(1):155–163.
208. Jilaihawi H, et al. *J Am Coll Cardiol.* 2012;59(14):1275–1286.
209. Willson AB, et al. *J Am Coll Cardiol.* 2012;59(14):1287–1294.
210. Gripari P, et al. *Heart.* 2012;98(16):1229–1236.
211. Queiros S, et al. *J Am Soc Echocardiogr.* 2018;31(4):515–525.e515.
212. Prihadi EA, et al. *J Am Soc Echocardiogr.* 2018;31(4):505–514.e503.
213. Neuburger PJ, Patel PA. *J Cardiothorac Vasc Anesth.* 2017;31(6):2175–2182.
214. Kronzon I, et al. *JACC Cardiovasc Imaging.* 2015;8(3):361–370.
215. Leon MB, et al. *N Engl J Med.* 2010;363(17):1597–1607.
216. Smith CR, et al. *N Engl J Med.* 2011;364(23):2187–2198.
217. Patel PA, et al. *J Cardiothorac Vasc Anesth.* 2017;31(3):777–790.
218. Cerrato E, et al. *Int J Cardiol.* 2017;228:640–647.
219. Vahl TP, et al. *J Am Coll Cardiol.* 2016;67(12):1472–1487.
220. Eskandari M, et al. *Heart.* 2018.
221. Hayek SS, et al. *J Am Soc Echocardiogr.* 2017;30(6):533–540.
222. Chiarito M, et al. *Heart.* 2018;104(4):306–312.
223. Obadia JF, et al. *EuroIntervention.* 2015;10(11):1354–1360.
224. Cardiovascular Outcomes Assessment of the MitraClip Percutaneous Therapy for Heart Failure Patients With Functional Mitral Regurgitation (The COAPT Trial). https://ClinicalTrials.gov/show/NCT01626079. Accessed June 6, 2018.
225. A Multicenter, Randomized, Controlled Study to Assess Mitral vAlve reconsTrucTion for advancEd Insufficiency of Functional or iscHemic ORigiN. https://ClinicalTrials.gov/show/NCT02371512. Accessed June 6, 2018.
226. Nyman CB, et al. *J Am Soc Echocardiogr.* 2018;31(4):434–453.
227. Mauri L, et al. *Am Heart J.* 2010;160(1):23–29.
228. Bapat V, et al. *J Am Coll Cardiol.* 2018;71(1):12–21.
229. Rodes-Cabau J, et al. *J Am Coll Cardiol.* 2016;67(15):1829–1845.
230. Prihadi EA, et al. *JACC Cardiovasc Imaging.* 2018;11(5):736–754.
231. Thaden JJ, et al. *J Am Soc Echocardiogr.* 2016;29(6):503–512.
232. Faletra FF, et al. *J Am Soc Echocardiogr.* 2017;30(9):886–895.
233. Giannopoulos AA, et al. *Nat Rev Cardiol.* 2016;13(12):701–718.
234. Ginty O, et al. *J Cardiothorac Vasc Anesth.* 2018;32(3):1368–1373.
235. Krittanawong C, et al. *J Am Coll Cardiol.* 2017;69(21):2657–2664.
236. Henglin M, et al. *Circ Cardiovasc Imaging.* 2017;10(10).
237. Jeganathan J, et al. *Ann Card Anaesth.* 2017;20(2):129–134.
238. Medvedofsky D, et al. *Eur Heart J Cardiovasc Imaging.* 2018;19(1):47–58.
239. Tsang W, et al. *JACC Cardiovasc Imaging.* 2016;9(7):769–782.
240. Otani K, et al. *J Am Soc Echocardiogr.* 2016;29(10):955–965.
241. Narula S, et al. *J Am Coll Cardiol.* 2016;68(21):2287–2295.
242. Cowie B. *J Cardiothorac Vasc Anesth.* 2009;23(4):450–456.
243. Cowie B. *Anaesthesia.* 2011;66(4):268–273.
244. Canty DJ, et al. *Anaesthesia.* 2012;67(6):618–625.
245. Shillcutt SK, et al. *Anesth Analg.* 2017;125(5):1479–1481.
246. Wijeysundera DN, et al. *BMJ.* 2011;342:d3695.
247. Canty DJ, et al. *Anaesthesia.* 2012;67(7):714–720.

248. Canty DJ, et al. *Anaesthesia.* 2012;67(11):1202–1209.
249. Botker MT, et al. *Acta Anaesthesiol Scand.* 2014;58(7):807–814.
250. Moja L, et al. *PLoS One.* 2012;7(10):e46175.
251. Pincus D, et al. *JAMA.* 2017;318(20):1994–2003.
252. O'HEireamhoin S, et al. *J Trauma.* 2011;71(5):1345–1347.
253. Canty DJ, et al. *Anaesthesia.* 2018;73(4):428–437.
254. Kratz T, et al. *Minerva Anestesiol.* 2015;81(5):490–496.
255. Kratz T, et al. *J Cardiothorac Vasc Anesth.* 2018;32(2):848–852.
256. Kratz T, et al. *J Cardiothorac Vasc Anesth.* 2017;31(2):602–609.
257. Dennis AT. *Int J Obstet Anesth.* 2011;20(2):160–168.
258. Dennis AT. *Curr Opin Anaesthesiol.* 2015;28(3):254–260.
259. Coker BJ, Zimmerman JM. *Anesth Analg.* 2017;124(3):761–765.
260. Conlin F, et al. *Anesth Analg.* 2017;125(6):1878–1882.
261. Vignon P, et al. *Chest.* 1994;106(6):1829–1834.
262. Orme RM, et al. *Br J Anaesth.* 2009;102(3):340–344.
263. Huttemann E. *Minerva Anestesiol.* 2006;72(11):891–913.
264. Heidenreich PA, et al. *J Am Coll Cardiol.* 1995;26(1):152–158.
265. Reichert CL, et al. *J Cardiothorac Vasc Anesth.* 1992;6(4):429–432.
266. Kanji HD, et al. *J Crit Care.* 2014;29(5):700–705.
267. Vincent JL, et al. *Crit Care Med.* 2006;34(2):344–353.
268. Boyd JH, et al. *Crit Care Med.* 2011;39(2):259–265.
269. Benes J, et al. *Biomed Res Int.* 2015;2015:729075.
270. Zieleskiewicz L, et al. *Intensive Care Med.* 2015;41(9):1638–1647.
271. Mayo PH, et al. *Chest.* 2015;148(5):1323–1332.
272. Jensen MB, et al. *Eur J Anaesthesiol.* 2004;21(9):700–707.
273. Joseph MX, et al. *Chest.* 2004;126(5):1592–1597.
274. Barbier C, et al. *Intensive Care Med.* 2004;30(9):1740–1746.
275. Feissel M, et al. *Intensive Care Med.* 2004;30(9):1834–1837.
276. Si X, et al. *Anesth Analg.* 2018;127(5):1147–1164.
277. Charbonneau H, et al. *Crit Care.* 2014;18(5):473.
278. Vignon P, et al. *Am J Respir Crit Care Med.* 2017;195(8):1022–1032.
279. Vieillard-Baron A, et al. *Intensive Care Med.* 2004;30(9):1734–1739.
280. Feissel M, et al. *Chest.* 2001;119(3):867–873.
281. Jozwiak M, Depret F, Teboul JL, et al. *Crit Care Med.* 2017;45(11): e1131–e1138.
282. Georges D, et al. *Crit Care.* 2018;22(1):32.
283. Heiberg J, et al. *Anaesthesia.* 2016;71(10):1210–1221.
284. Costachescu T, et al. *Crit Care Med.* 2002;30(6):1214–1223.
285. Scalea TM, et al. *J Trauma.* 1999;46(3):466–472.
286. Ferrada P, et al. *J Ultrasound Med.* 2014;33(10):1829–1832.
287. Saranteas T, et al. *J Crit Care.* 2017;38:144–151.
288. Lichtenstein DA. *Chest.* 2015;147(6):1659–1670.
289. Ehrman RR, et al. *Crit Care.* 2018;22(1):112.
290. Vignon P, et al. *Crit Care.* 2016;20(1):228.
291. Chamsi-Pasha MA, et al. *Circulation.* 2017;136(22):2178–2188.
292. Melamed R, et al. *Chest.* 2009;135(6):1416–1420.
293. Vignon P, et al. *Crit Care.* 2003;7(5):R84–91.
294. Vieillard-Baron A, et al. *Intensive Care Med.* 2013;39(4):629–635.
295. Begot E, al Det. *Intensive Care Med.* 2015;41(11):1886–1894.
296. ACGME Program Requirements for Graduate Medical Education in Anesthesiology. Available at: https://www.acgme.org/Portals/0/PFAssets/ProgramRequirements/040Anesthesiology2018.pdf?ver=2018-06-14-142529-527. Approved focused revision June 10, 2018. Effective July 1, 2018. Accessed July 15, 2018.
297. ABA Primary Certification in Anesthesiology -Content Outline. Available at: http://www.theaba.org/PDFs/ADVANCED-Exam/Basic-and-Advanced-ContentOutline. Revised April 2018. Accessed July 01, 2018.
298. ABA APPLIED Examination - OSCE Content Outline. Available at: http://www.theaba.org/PDFs/APPLIED-Exam/APPLIED-OSCE-ContentOutline. Accessed February 07, 2018.
299. ACGME Program Requirements for Graduate Medical Education in Anesthesiology Critical Care Medicine. Available at: https://www.acgme.org/Portals/0/PFAssets/ProgramRequirements/045_critical_care_anes_2017-07-01.pdf?ver=2017-05-17-155711-140. Approved September 29, 2013. Revised July 1, 2017. Accessed March 1, 2018.
300. Johri AM, et al. *J Am Soc Echocardiogr.* 2018.
301. Zimmerman J. *J Cardiothorac Vasc Anesth.* 2017.
302. Mitchell JD, et al. *J Cardiothorac Vasc Anesth.* 2014;28(3):800–809.
303. Tanzola RC, et al. *Can J Anaesth.* 2013;60(1):32–37.
304. Mitchell JD, et al. *J Cardiothorac Vasc Anesth.* 2015;29(2):402–409.
305. Jerath A, et al. *Can J Anaesth.* 2011;58(1):14–21.
306. Vegas A, et al. *J Cardiothorac Vasc Anesth.* 2013;27(3):531–535.
307. Bose RR, et al. *J Cardiothorac Vasc Anesth.* 2011;25(2):212–215.
308. Platts DG, et al. *Heart Lung Circ.* 2012;21(5):267–274.
309. Sharma V, et al. *Anaesthesia.* 2013;68(6):621–627.
310. Jelacic S, et al. *J Cardiothorac Vasc Anesth.* 2013;27(4):670–675.
311. Ferrero NA, et al. *Anesthesiology.* 2014;120(1):149–159.
312. Matyal R, et al. *Anesthesiology.* 2014;121(2):389–399.
313. Neelankavil J, et al. *Anesth Analg.* 2012;115(5):1042–1051.
314. Edrich T, et al. *J Cardiothorac Vasc Anesth.* 2014;28(1):49–53.
315. Conlin F, et al. *J Cardiothorac Vasc Anesth.* 2016;30(1):102–106.
316. Mizubuti G, et al. *Can J Anaesth.* 2017;64(4):441–442.
317. Neskovic AN, et al. *Eur Heart J Cardiovasc Imaging.* 2018.
318. Kimura BJ, et al. *J Am Soc Echocardiogr.* 2016;29(10):992–997.
319. National Board of Echocardiography, Inc. NBE Certification General Instructions. http://echoboards.org/Echoboards/Certifications/General_Instructions.aspx. Accessed May 1, 2018.
320. https://www.escardio.org/Education/Career-Development/Certification/Adult-Transoesophageal-Echo. Accessed May 1, 2018.
321. Diaz-Gomez JL, et al. *Crit Care Med.* 2017;45(11):1801–1804.

38 Implantable Cardiac Pulse Generators: Pacemakers and Cardioverter-Defibrillators

AMAN MAHAJAN and JACQUES PRINCE NEELANKAVIL

KEY POINTS[a]

- Identify the type of cardiovascular implantable electronic device (CIED) (pacemaker, transvenous defibrillator, subcutaneous defibrillator), as well as the generator manufacturer and model of the CIED.
- Contact the physician or clinic managing the patient's CIED in the preoperative period to obtain appropriate records and a perioperative recommendation (Heart Rhythm Society [HRS]).
- Obtain a copy of this interrogation and the perioperative recommendation from the CIED physician (HRS). Ensure that the implantable cardioverter-defibrillator (ICD) treatment settings are appropriate and that the CIED will pace the heart.
- Consider replacing any CIED near its elective replacement period in a patient scheduled to undergo either a major surgical procedure or a surgical procedure where monopolar electrosurgery will be used within 15 cm of the generator.
- Determine the patient's underlying rate and rhythm to determine the need for backup (external) pacing support.
- Ensure that all magnet behavior (pacing, suspension of shock therapy) is appropriate if magnet use is planned.
- Program minute ventilation rate responsiveness "off," if present.
- Consider disabling all rate enhancements to prevent misinterpretation of cardiac rhythm.
- Consider increasing the lower rate limit to provide optimal oxygen delivery for major procedures.
- If electromagnetic interference is likely, (1) disable antitachycardia therapy if a defibrillator is present and (2) consider asynchronous pacing for some pacing-dependent patients. Magnet application may be acceptable for some ICDs (disable antitachycardia therapy) or pacemakers (provide asynchronous pacing). Asynchronous pacing from an ICD always requires reprogramming.
- Monitor cardiac rhythm with the pulse oximeter (plethysmography) or arterial waveform analysis.
- Use a bipolar electrosurgical unit (ESU), if possible; if not possible, then pure "cut" electrosurgery is better than "blend" or "coag," and ESU should be applied in short bursts (<4 seconds) separated by at least 2 seconds.
- Place the ESU dispersive electrode in such a way to prevent electricity from crossing the generator-heart circuit.
- If the ESU causes ventricular oversensing with pacing quiescence or atrial oversensing with inappropriate ventricular pacing, limit the effect by using short ESU bursts, relocating the dispersive electrode, or placing a magnet over the pacemaker (not indicated for ICDs).
- Some patients require postoperative interrogation, especially if preoperative reprogramming took place. For "low-risk cases," HRS (but not ASA) states that this interrogation can take place in an ambulatory setting up to 1 month postoperatively. Some rate enhancements can be reinitiated, and a determination of optimum heart rate and pacing parameters should be made. Any patient with disabled antitachycardia therapy must be monitored until the antitachycardia therapy is restored.

[a]Adapted from the American Society of Anesthesiologists (ASA) *Practice Advisory* (2005, revised 2011) and the Heart Rhythm Society (HRS), formerly the North American Society of Pacing and Electrophysiology (NASPE) and ASA *Consensus Statement* (2011) *for Perioperative Management of Patients With a Pacemaker or Defibrillator.*

Introduction

Cardiac implantable electronic devices (CIEDs) refer to a permanently implanted cardiac pacemaker, an implantable cardioverter-defibrillator (ICD), or a cardiac resynchronization therapy (CRT) device. Evolving technology for CIEDs and their widespread use for bradyarrhythmias, tachyarrhythmias, and congestive heart failure management have made the perioperative management of these devices critical for anesthesiologists. It is estimated that more than 3 million people in the United States have a pacemaker and more than 300,000 people have an ICD.[1,2] With approximately 1 million patients worldwide receiving a pacemaker or ICD every year, patients with CIEDs are a growing population in the perioperative arena. The prevalence of cardiovascular disease in an aging population is an important driver for the increased utilization of CIEDs.

Historically, there was little guidance for anesthesiologists caring for patients with CIEDs because of the conflicting consensus statements regarding the perioperative management of CIEDs. In 2011, the Heart Rhythm Society (HRS)/American Society of Anesthesiologists (ASA) published an Expert Consensus Statement on the perioperative management of patients with CIEDs. This statement was in collaboration with the American Heart Association (AHA) and the Society of Thoracic Surgeons (STS).[3] This article provides information and a guided team approach to best manage this patient population, and it has become an important piece of literature for anesthesiologists. In this chapter, we will review basic CIED function, the perioperative management of these devices, and emerging technology of CIEDs.

Basic Cardiac Implantable Electronic Device Function

PACEMAKERS

Pacemakers are devices placed for bradyarrhythmias, and they remain the only effective treatment for ameliorating symptomatic bradycardia due to sinus node dysfunction (e.g., sick sinus syndrome) or a failure of impulse propagation (e.g., complete heart block). Advances in technology and understanding of cardiac conduction physiology have led to the development of more physiologic pacing. Pacemakers have become sophisticated at maintaining the normal atrial-ventricular activation over various heart rate ranges, varying the heart rate in response to metabolic demands, and preserving natural ventricular activation. Pacemakers have many additional features that correspond to the changing needs of patients throughout the day, including rate responsiveness to increase pacing during times of increased physical exertion and sleep functions to decrease pacing rate during times of rest. Standard pacemakers have either one or two (atrial and ventricular) leads. A patient is considered to be pacemaker dependent if they suffer significant symptoms or even cardiac arrest upon the cessation of pacing.[4,5]

The dual chamber pacemakers are capable of pacing and sensing in both the ventricle and the atrium. Such capability permits the pacemaker to ensure not only an adequate ventricular rate, but to preserve the atrial contraction before each ventricular contraction. These pacemakers guarantee a minimum atrial rate and also ensure that a ventricular contraction occurs within a specified amount of time after each atrial contraction. Limitations on ventricular rate are usually built in the circuitry and are programmable. Most pacemakers have the capability of varying the pacing rate. In the rate adaptive mode, the pacemakers sense the patient's level of activity and accordingly adjust the pacing rate using sensors that are typically piezoelectric and detect body motion transmitted from underlying muscles. Another method of determining the presence of physical activity utilizes detection of the respiratory rate and/or volume using bioimpedance sensors.

All pacemakers generate a pulse of current to depolarize a small region of the myocardium; the wave then spontaneously spreads to the rest of the myocardium. The pacing capture threshold is the minimum electrical energy needed to consistently capture the heart outside of the refractory period and is determined by (1) the intrinsic excitability of the myocardium, (2) the current density at the electrode-tissue interface, and (3) the duration of the electric pulse.

The North American Society of Pacing and Electrophysiology (NASPE) and the British Pacing and Electrophysiology Group (BPEG) initially published a generic pacemaker code (NBG code) in 1987. In 2002 the NBG code was subsequently revised (Table 38.1).[6] Common perioperative pacing modes include dual chamber, adaptive-rate pacing (DDDR), dual chamber pacing without atrium synchronous ventricular pacing (DDIR), and dual chamber asynchronous pacing with no rate modulation or multisite pacing (DOO).

1. DDDR pacing defines a pacemaker programmed to pace the atrium and/or ventricle, sense the atrium and/or ventricle, inhibit or trigger pacing output in response to a sensed event, and have a rate responsive sensor that is able to alter paced rates due to changes in perceived metabolic demand. DDDR is a very common program configuration for patients with sick sinus syndrome and/or heart block.

TABLE 38.1 2002 NASPE/BPEG Generic Code for Antibradycardic Pacing

Position	I	II	III	IV	V
Description	Chamber Paced	Chamber Sensed	Response to Sensing	Rate Modulation	Multisite Pacing
Possible designations	D = Dual (A+V) A = Atrium V = Ventricle O = None	D = Dual (A+V) A = Atrium V = Ventricle O = None	D = Dual (T+I) T = Triggered I = Inhibited O = None	R = rate modulation O = None	D = Dual (A+V) A = Atrium V = Ventricle O = None

2. DDIR is a common pacing mode for patients with supraventricular tachyarrhythmias (SVTs). If a patient is set to DDD, the ventricle response depends on the atrial rate. During SVT in DDD mode, rapid ventricular pacing may occur. In DDI, the pacemaker paces and senses both the atrium and ventricle; however, the device will not pace the ventricle at an identical rate if the patient has SVT. The response to a fast rate in the atrium will lead to inhibition of pacing in the ventricle—hence the *I* in the third designation. Most modern pacemakers have built-in automatic mode switching during episodes of SVT. They will switch from DDD to DDI to avoid SVT with a rapid ventricular response.
3. For some perioperative care, devices will be placed in an asynchronous mode like DOO. An asynchronous mode or nontracking mode will pace the atrium and ventricle at a set rate, regardless of the underlying rate and rhythm. This is advantageous in the perioperative environment in order to avoid the pacemaker from oversensing the monopolar electrocautery as intrinsic cardiac conduction. Asynchronous modes avoid oversensing (and under pacing) hearts that are pacemaker dependent and inhibited from pacing due to monopolar electrocautery (Table 38.2).

IMPLANTABLE CARDIOVERTER-DEFIBRILLATORS

ICDs are implanted in patients for primary or secondary prevention of cardiac arrest. Primary prevention refers to ICD placement for patients who have not had any episodes of ventricular arrhythmias but who are at risk for future events. Secondary prevention refers to ICD placement for patients who have had prior ventricular arrhythmias. There is strong evidence that ICDs implanted for primary prevention improve mortality in high-risk patients, including patients with a left ventricular ejection fraction less than 40% who are on optimal medical therapy.[7-11] For patients with ischemic and nonischemic cardiomyopathy, ICDs reduce mortality approximately 23% to 55%.[12,13] Certain groups of patients do not benefit from ICD implantation, including patients with recent myocardial infarction and patients who have received coronary artery bypass grafting.[14] In addition, many of the patients in the decisive trials for ICD placement were younger (mean or median age between 58 and 67 years for the MADIT-II, CABG-PATCH, DINAMIT), whereas many patients currently receiving ICDs are over the age of 70.[15]

ICDs have four main functions. They sense atrial or ventricular electrical activity, classify these signals to various programmed "heart rate zones," deliver tiered therapies to terminate ventricular tachycardia (VT) or fibrillation, and pace for bradycardia. All modern ICDs are pacemakers, and this has important perioperative applications. Although ICDs improve survival in many patients, unnecessary shocks are very detrimental. They are proarrhythmic, can lead to anxiety and depression, and decrease patient quality of life. Inappropriate shocks are common (30% to 50% of all shocks) as a result of inappropriate treatment of SVT, oversensing physiologic T waves, or lead fracture.[16] The discrimination between VT and SVT is critical for ICDs to avoid inappropriate therapy. There are several methods by which ICDs discriminate between SVT and VT. Single chamber ventricular ICDs utilize ventricular–ventricular timing intervals and QRS morphology. Dual chamber ICDs use atrial–atrial timing intervals and the chamber of onset. Subcutaneous ICDs assess surface electrocardiogram (ECG). The sensitivity and specificity for VT detection by QRS morphology is more than 90%.[16]

ICDs terminate ventricular arrhythmias by either antitachycardiac pacing (ATP) or defibrillation. ATP terminates reentrant VT by blocking reentry and it terminates slow VT (<188 to 200) approximately 90% of the time. ATP is desirable because it reduces inappropriate shocks and prolongs battery life. For VT that is not terminated by ATP or for ventricular fibrillation (VF), defibrillation is the treatment of choice. The energy for defibrillation may be incrementally increased or set to maximum energy for each shock.[17]

TABLE 38.2 Common Pacemaker Settings

Examples	Chamber Paced	Chamber Sensed	Response to Sensing	Rate Modulation	Multisite Pacing	Common Clinical Utilization
AAI	Atrium	Atrium	Intrinsic atrial beat inhibits atrial pacing	None	None	Sick sinus syndrome with intact atrioventricular conduction
DDDR	Both	Both	Intrinsic beat will inhibit output; atrial beat will trigger ventricular pacing if lack of intrinsic ventricular beat	Present	None	Atrioventricular block
VVIRV	Ventricle	Ventricle	Intrinsic ventricular beat will inhibit ventricular pacing	Present	Multisite ventricular pacing	Heart failure with prolonged QRS
DOO	Both	None	None	None	None	Perioperative asynchronous setting to avoid electromagnetic interference

CARDIAC RESYNCHRONIZATION THERAPY DEVICES

CRT plays an important role in the management of heart failure and is becoming a device commonly encountered by anesthesiologists because of the large prevalence of heart failure in this country. These devices are indicated in select patients with heart failure, systolic dysfunction, and a prolonged QRS. Conduction abnormalities are frequently seen in systolic heart failure, with approximately 25% to 40% of these patients having a prolonged QRS complex (>120 ms).[18] In these patients, cardiac depolarization spreads slowly through the myocardium without a healthy Purkinje conduction system, leading to intraventricular dyssynchrony. During intraventricular dyssynchrony, the left ventricular (LV) septal wall contracts earlier than the lateral wall, which leads to less efficient ejection from the left ventricle in addition to decreased diastolic filling. The goal of CRT is to restore synchronous contraction of the left ventricle and to optimize timing of LV and right ventricular (RV) ejection. This is accomplished through biventricular pacing using a standard RV lead and an LV lead placed adjacent to the lateral wall via the coronary sinus. Biventricular pacing in the right ventricle and the left ventricle leads to improved hemodynamic variables, including systolic blood pressure, stroke volume, cardiac output, and rate of rise of LV pressure (dP/dt). In contrast to pharmacologic means of improving systolic function, CRT improves cardiac performance with reductions rather than with increases in myocardial metabolic demand. In addition, CRT has been shown to improve mitral regurgitation (MR) and New York Heart Association (NYHA) function class because of reverse ventricular remodeling over time.[19] Standard indications for CRT are LV ejection fraction (LVEF) less than 35% with QRS greater than 120 ms, sinus rhythm, and NYHA class III or IV after optimal medical therapy. Left bundle branch block is the most common conduction abnormality in patients undergoing CRT. Approximately 30% of patients meeting selection criteria for CRT do not respond to biventricular pacing. Risk factors for failure to respond to CRT include ischemic cardiomyopathy, sustained VT, severe MR, and dilated LV cavity.[20] CRT has been shown to reduce mortality, heart failure symptoms, and also heart failure hospitalizations. Patients with CRT should be considered pacemaker-dependent because of the constant pacing they undergo to synchronize the ventricle.

Perioperative Considerations

PREOPERATIVE ASSESSMENT

As perioperative physicians, the preoperative assessment of patients with CIEDs is critical to safe and time-efficient care. The key to the preoperative assessment is timely communication between the anesthesia provider and the CIED team that usually manages the device programming and function. The CIED team may include a cardiologist, an electrophysiologist, and/or a physician extender such as a nurse or nurse practitioner. The CIED team needs to know various information about the surgical case and postoperative disposition in order to create an individualized care plan for the patient. The anesthesiology provider must communicate the specifics of perioperative care to the CIED team in order to ensure a proper plan specific to that patient and the surgical case. Unfortunately, there is no single prescription for CIED management that can be applied to all patients coming for surgery. In addition, it is not recommended that an industry-employed allied profession determine the perioperative plan for a particular CIED.[21]

The perioperative team must convey to the CIED team important information regarding the presence of electromagnetic interference (EMI), the likelihood of cardioversion or defibrillation, patient position, location of surgery that may damage or encroach upon the CIED leads, and postoperative disposition. The CIED team must communicate with the anesthesiology team the date of last interrogation, the type of CIED device, the indication for CIED placement, the battery life, pacemaker dependence, and magnet response. Each of these vital perioperative parameters are discussed in detail in this chapter.

The goal of a thorough preoperative evaluation between the CIED and anesthesia teams is to avoid CIED complications in the perioperative period, such as damage to the device, inability of the device to deliver pacing or shocks, lead-tissue interface damage, changes in pacing behavior, electrical reset to the backup pacing mode, or inappropriate ICD therapies. Any of the these complications can lead to poor patient outcomes, including hypotension, arrhythmias, and myocardial ischemia.

PREOPERATIVE INFORMATION TRANSFER

The ACCF/AHA/HRS 2011 guidelines emphasize that a team approach should be utilized when caring for patients with CIEDs. Patients coming for surgery with CIEDs do not need routine interrogations prior to surgery unless there has been a change in clinical presentation. For patients with a pacemaker, they should have an interrogation report within the last 12 months; patients with an ICD or CRT should have a report within the previous 6 months. The different time courses for interrogations between pacemakers and ICDs and CRT devices reflect the overall cardiovascular comorbidities of these respective patient populations. By definition, patients with ICDs and CRT devices have decreased systolic function and heart failure, and they are more likely to have clinical decompensation compared to patients with isolated pacemakers. Worsening cardiovascular function might negatively impact CIED performance. The preoperative evaluation begins with general considerations, such as establishing whether a patient has a CIED and defining the type of device. A focused history and physical, including rhythm strips and ECGs, can usually answer important basic questions about the patient's CIED. After these are completed, it is important to define the type of the device to be used. If the patient has been seen by the CIED team, they will leave a detailed note.

Within the interrogation report, it is important to note the type of device. Patients with pacemakers have different clinical risk profiles compared with those with ICDs and CRTs. In addition, the goals of perioperative management for these devices are different. Most pacemakers encourage intrinsic cardiac conduction because this maintains atrial–ventricular synchrony, LV-RV synchrony, and septal

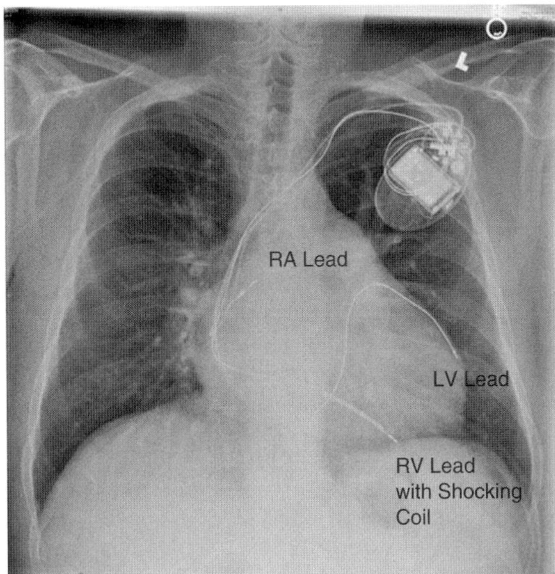

Fig. 38.1 Chest radiograph: the pulse generator is located in the left deltopectoral groove. There are three leads visualized: a lead in the right atrium *(RA)*, a lead in the left ventricle *(LV)* via the coronary sinus, and a lead in the right ventricle *(RV)*. The RV lead has a thicker diameter toward the tip, indicating it is an implantable cardioverter-defibrillator lead.

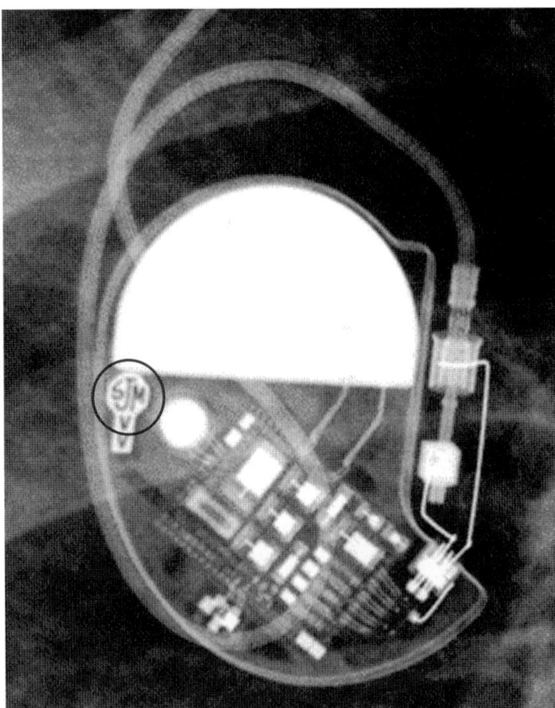

Fig. 38.2 Chest radiograph of the cardiovascular implantable electronic device generator. The letter designation on the generator allows the physician to identify this manufacturer as St. Jude Medical.

LV–lateral LV synchrony. Although DDD pacing of both atrium and ventricle in a dual-chamber pacemaker maintains atrioventricular (AV) synchrony, it creates RV-LV dyssynchrony and LV-LV dyssynchrony because pacing begins in the right ventricle and crosses the septum before activating the LV lateral wall. Preserved synchrony optimizes stroke volume, which is desirable during the perioperative environment. Therefore, in the perioperative environment, it is advantageous to maintain intrinsic cardiac conduction as much as possible if the surgical procedure and use of EMI permits. In contrast, CRT devices attempt to ensure pacing 100% of the time in order to optimize stroke volume.

The manufacturer and model should be noted, along with the indication for placement of the CIED, in order to troubleshoot problems. Theoretically all patients with CIEDs should carry identification cards that identify the type of CIED, the manufacturer, the model, and date of implantation. In practice, many patients do not carry their CIED cards, and it is left to the anesthesia provider to identify these parameters. There are several methods for obtaining this information. Frequently an interrogation note from the CIED team will identify all these parameters. Occasionally, patients present for elective surgery without CIED team communication. In this subset of patients, there are several options. One option for identifying the type of device and manufacturer is the use of chest radiographs (Fig. 38.1). Chest radiographs can identify pacemakers versus ICDs, due to the increased thickness of the shocking coil in ICDs. Chest radiographs can also identify CRT devices due to the lead in the coronary sinus. With some training, the manufacturer can also be identified via chest radiograph (Fig. 38.2). In situations where the patient does not have his or her card, or there is no CIED note and there is no chest radiograph available or it cannot be interpreted, then contact with the CIED manufacturers can be initiated, since they all keep clinical records of their patients. Communicating directly with the manufacturer can disclose information about the type of CIED, date of implantation, and original settings. Unfortunately, current information about pacemaker dependence and battery life is not usually available by phone.

Battery longevity is important to consider as an anesthesia provider. Three months of battery duration is reasonable in the perioperative period. This time point is chosen because battery life depends on the amount of pacing and the number of shocks delivered for pacemakers and ICDs, respectively. The burden of pacing in the perioperative period may be very different than the patient's normal requirements. Sinoatrial (SA) and AV nodal suppressing agents such as opioids, beta-blockers, and calcium channel blockers administered in the hospital may increase pacing requirements; therefore it is prudent to have several months of battery life remaining. In addition, there may be unexpected postoperative complications leading to the increased duration of hospitalization. If a patient is presenting for elective surgery with a diminished battery life, the generator should be replaced prior to the surgery.

It is important to establish if the patient is pacemaker-dependent, which is defined as the absence of a perfusing rhythm without pacing. In order to establish pacemaker dependence, a history and chart review may identify an episode of bradyarrhythmia leading to syncope. In addition, for patients with refractory SVT, they will occasionally have an AV nodal ablation. This is a therapeutic procedure that establishes complete heart block to eliminate rapid ventricular response to SVT. This patient population is pacemaker-dependent. Patients with CRT devices can be considered pacemaker-dependent even if they have a normal sinus rate and intact AV conduction due to

TABLE 38.3 Summary of Information Anesthesiology Team Should Identify Prior to Surgery

Perioperative Considerations	Comments
Last CIED interrogation	12 months for pacemakers 6 months for ICD/CRT
Type of device	Pacemaker ICD CRT Loop recorder
Manufacturer	Obtained via patient card, history, CIED note, chest radiograph, or telephone call to manufacturer
Battery life	Suggested >3 months
Pacemaker dependence	Underlying rhythm CRT devices should be paced 100%
Magnet response	Differs by manufacturer and battery life
Pacing threshold	Should be set several times higher for safety

CIED, Cardiac implantable electronic devices; *CRT*, cardiac resynchronization therapy; *ICD*, implantable cardioverter-defibrillator.

the hemodynamic deterioration they suffer with dyssynchrony of the RV-LV and LV-LV. Pacemaker dependence can be established by the CIED team preoperatively. They can decrease the pacing rate in a stepwise fashion to search for intrinsic electrical activity. If no intrinsic rate is present around 40 to 45 beats/min or the patient develops symptoms, the patient may be considered pacemaker-dependent. Some patients who are not pacemaker-dependent may become pacemaker-dependent in the perioperative period due to SA and AV nodal blocking agents; therefore, it is important to be prepared to address this clinical scenario. If the patient is deemed to be pacemaker-dependent, a secondary method for pacing the patient should be considered in the event of a pacemaker failure. Alternative methods of pacing patients intraoperatively include transesophageal pacing, transcutaneous pacing, or transvenous pacing through a pacing pulmonary artery catheter or through a temporary transvenous pacing wire. Transesophageal pacing activates the left atrium, which is in close proximity to the esophagus, so this type of pacing depends on intact AV node conduction. It will not work for heart block. Transcutaneous pacing depends on correct pad position and high pacing outputs, which can be very uncomfortable in a nonsedated patient. Transvenous pacing and pacing pulmonary artery catheters can be time consuming, and they are not ideal choices for emergent pacing. Whatever method is chosen, it is important to have the necessary equipment and support organized and available prior to beginning the procedure. A summary of important information for the anesthesia team to identify is summarized in Table 38.3.

ELECTROMAGNETIC INTERFERENCE

EMI in the preoperative setting can interfere with the functioning of both pacemakers and ICDs.[22,23] EMI may inhibit pacing, damage the lead-tissue interface, damage the pulse generator, and/or trigger an electric reset mode, particularly if the source of EMI is within 6 inches (15 cm) of the CIED generator.[24] Although there are several potential sources of EMI, the most commonly encountered source is monopolar electrocautery. Monopolar electrocautery is the most frequently used type of electrocautery because it has both cutting as well as coagulation capabilities. Monopolar electrocautery creates a current that passes from the probe to the tissue and returns through the patient to the return pad to create an electrical circuit. Bipolar electrocautery is usually not a concern[25]; the electrical current field is small and limited to the two poles at the end of the electrode. Unfortunately, bipolar is less frequently used compared with monopolar electrocautery and is usually reserved for neurosurgery, ophthalmology, and head and neck procedures. Bipolar electrocautery does not cause EMI of CIEDs unless it is applied directly to a CIED, and there are minimal clinical circumstances where that would be indicated. The vast majority of electrocautery encountered in the operating suite is monopolar due to its versatility.

Modern CIEDs have evolved to produce better shielding from EMI, and adverse events from EMI are much less common with improvements in CIED technology.[24-27] Shielding reduces the potential to induce oversensing in the CIED. Oversensing in a pacemaker means the pacemaker "sees" the EMI-generated artifacts as intrinsic cardiac electrical activity and therefore does not initiate a paced rhythm. Such failure to initiate a paced rhythm (inhibition of the pacemaker) can compromise hemodynamics in a pacemaker-dependent patient. If oversensing occurs in an ICD, EMI may be misinterpreted by the ICD as a malignant tachyarrhythmia, which may cause the patient to receive an inappropriate shock. It is important to note that it is not only the location of monopolar electrocautery that is critical to proper CIED function, but it is also the location of the grounding pad that is critical to avoid CIED malfunction. The HRS/ASA Expert Consensus Statement suggests that due to the decreased likelihood of EMI-related interference seen when surgery is below the umbilicus, the patient should proceed to surgery with no magnet application to the device or reprogramming. This assumes that the monopolar electrocautery grounding pad or return pad is also placed below the level of the umbilicus. If current is traveling above the level of the umbilicus, there is significant risk of EMI of the CIED. For procedures above the umbilicus with no EMI from the surgical procedure, the patient may also proceed for surgery without routine magnet use or device reprogramming. For all patients presenting for surgery with CIEDs, there should be a magnet available with the magnet function of the device known in case of a change in the surgical plan or unexpected EMI. Magnet function is discussed in the next section.

MAGNETS

Magnet applications for CIEDs were originally intended to investigate battery life of the device, and they were not created for perioperative management of CIEDs, although that is probably their most common utilization at this time. When magnets are applied to the pacemaker, the effect on the device depends on the manufacturer, in addition to the battery life. For example, when a magnet is applied to a Medtronic pacemaker, the device will pace asynchronously. If the Medtronic device is a single-chamber pacemaker, it will pace that single chamber asynchronously. If the Medtronic device is a dual-chamber pacemaker, it will pace both chambers asynchronously. However, the rate at which the pacemaker will pace depends on battery life. If the Medtronic pacemaker has adequate battery life, the device will pace at 85 beats/min. However, if the battery life is at the elective replacement interval, the device will pace at 65 beats/min. The change in rate is binary, meaning that the rate goes from 85 to 65 beats/min when the battery enters its elective replacement interval. Different manufacturers have difference responses to magnet application. St. Jude pacemakers will pace asynchronously during magnet application if the magnet response is turned on. It is important to note that magnet application is programmable—that is, with some devices, magnet application will have no effect. The effect of magnet response is an important piece of information to obtain from the CIED team. For a St. Jude pacemaker with magnet response programmed on, magnet application will program the device to pace asynchronously at a rate of 100 beats/min if the battery life is normal or a rate of 85 beats/min if the device is at its battery elective replacement interval. Unlike Medtronic devices, the rate change from 100 to 85 beats/min is not binary; it is a gradual reduction from 100 to 85 beats/min.[3]

Magnets continue to be very popular in everyday practice for the management of CIEDs. This is a relatively easy way to render the pacemaker asynchronous, with the added benefit of the device reverting back to its programmed settings once the magnet is removed. Importantly, the asynchronous rate provided by magnet placement may not be appropriate for the patient for a particular procedure. At times, patients require a higher heart rate in order to increase tissue oxygen delivery. To the contrary, most magnet rates are typically around 90 beats/min, which may not be appropriate for a large subset of patients—that is, those with aortic stenosis or coronary artery disease. These variables make it important to confirm the magnet effect on each individual patient's device before the procedure, and to have an individualized plan for each patient.

The choice of reprogramming versus magnet application largely depends on the type of surgery, patient position, accessibility of a programmer, and knowledge of magnet function of a particular patient's device. It should be emphasized that a magnet has different effects when applied to a pacemaker or to an ICD. In a majority of pacemakers, magnet application induces an asynchronous mode. Magnet application to an ICD inhibits tachyarrhythmia detection, thus preventing therapy (i.e., delivery of shocks). However, it does *not* change the mode of the underlying pacemaker. Therefore, a magnet placed over an ICD will not induce asynchronous mode in the underlying pacemaker. For patients with an ICD who are pacemaker dependent, reprogramming is the preferred option if EMI is a significant concern. One advantage of reprogramming are that if the patient is not in the supine position, it may be difficult to maintain the magnet in a location over the device to render it asynchronous. This is particularly true in the prone position. If the patient has a normal sinus rate, adequate chronotropy, and intact AV node conduction, magnet application may compete with the patient's own heart rate if surgical stimulation increases the sinus rate. This can lead to significant arrhythmias caused by depolarization of the ventricle by the pacemaker during a refractory period, due to intrinsic electrical activity. The principal disadvantage of reprogramming versus magnet application is that the changes made with the programmer are not as easily reversed. If the patient develops an arrhythmia or has an increased sinus rate, it may be difficult to reprogram the device intraoperatively, depending on programmer availability and CIED team presence. The other disadvantage of reprogramming a CIED compared with magnet application involves the human factor. Failure to re-enable tachyarrhythmia therapy following surgery can lead to catastrophic consequences for patients with CIEDs. It is important to understand the risks and benefits of magnet application versus reprogramming, and create a perioperative plan that suits the patient.

ELECTROMAGNETIC INTERFERENCE DAMAGE TO THE CARDIAC IMPLANTABLE ELECTRONIC DEVICE

EMI is an important consideration for anesthesiology providers because of oversensing. It is uncommon for modern CIEDs to be damaged by EMI from the operative environment; however, some particular complications will be discussed. Monopolar electrocautery that is done in very close proximity to the pulse generator may directly damage the myocardium at the interface with the CIED lead. This can trigger arrhythmias or loss of pacing capture due to increases in pacing thresholds.[28] Therefore, it is recommended that bipolar electrocautery should be used when electrocautery is performed in close proximity to the pulse generator. Another complication that may happen due to ionizing radiation is device reset.[29,30] It is uncommon for even monopolar electrocautery to cause reset. In the perioperative setting, this very rarely occurs when an energy surge directly contacts the pulse generator, resulting in a major hardware/software failure. The reset mode is unique to each manufacturer and serves as a safety backup in the case of catastrophic failure. Unfortunately, magnet application and device reprogramming will not prevent electrical reset. The best way to prevent reset is to ensure that EMI is as far as possible from the pulse generator (ideally >15 cm). If a patient's CIED does go into reset mode, the pacemaker will commonly revert to a ventricular demand pacing (VVI) mode between 65 and 70 beats/min. Magnet response in reset mode will also vary among manufacturers. ICDs will have a wide range of rate cutoffs for VT detection in the reset mode. ICD pacing will be typically in a VVI mode again around 65 to 70 beats/min. Electrical reset should prompt consultation with a CIED team to ensure proper device functionality.

INTRAOPERATIVE MANAGEMENT

The intraoperative management of CIEDs naturally evolves from a thoughtful preoperative plan. A pathway for management of CIEDs during nonemergent surgery is outlined in Fig. 38.3. Pacemaker patients who are pacemaker-dependent and who are having surgery with monopolar electrocautery within 15 cm of the generator should have their

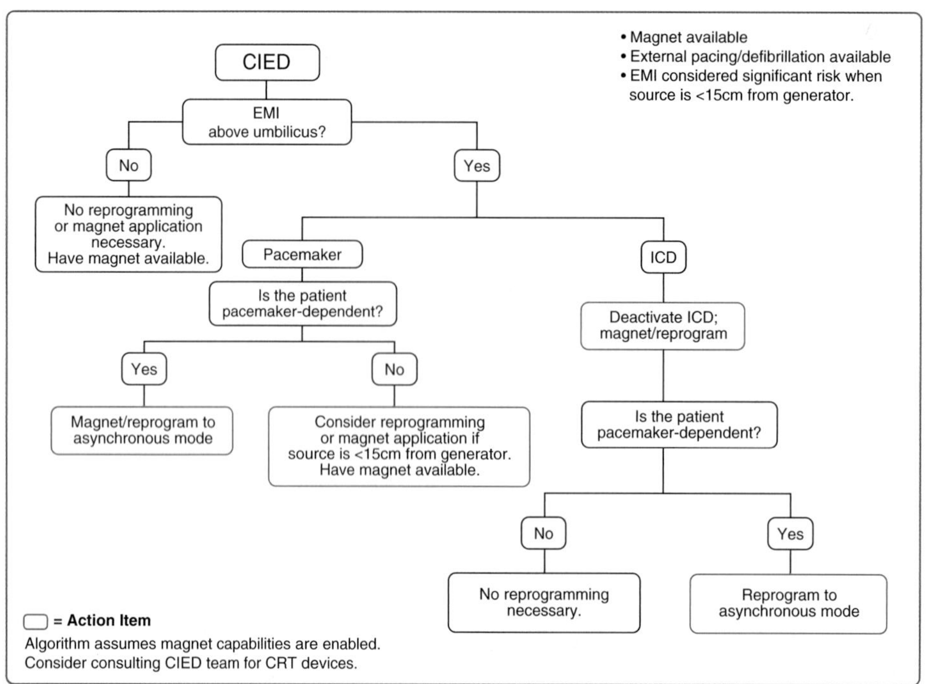

Fig. 38.3 Cardiovascular Implantable Electronic Device pathway for nonemergent surgery. *CIED*, Cardiac implantable electronic devices; *CRT*, cardiac resynchronization therapy; *ICD*, implantable cardioverter-defibrillator; *EMI*, electromagnetic interference. Thompson A, Neelankavil JP, Mahajan A. Current Anesthesiology Reports, 2013, Vol 3, Issue 3, 139–143. (Courtesy Dr. Annemarie Thompson.)

device reprogrammed to avoid pacemaker oversensing of electrocautery as intrinsic cardiac function. This could lead to underpacing and hemodynamic collapse in pacemaker-dependent patients. For patients in the supine position with known magnet function who have magnet rates appropriate for their concurrent comorbidities, placement of a magnet over a pacemaker is a reasonable approach for patients at risk for monopolar electrocautery oversensing. Whether the prescription plan is reprogramming or magnet application, the rate responsive features of the device should be disabled. The rate response is the fourth letter in the 2002 NAPSE guidelines and refers to increasing the heart rate above the lower rate limit when the patient has increased metabolic demand (e.g., exercise). Rate response sensors commonly use minute ventilation or thoracic impedance to increase rate, and both may be affected intraoperatively. Patients on mechanical ventilation will see increases in heart rate if the minute ventilation is increased with these sensors. For patients with thoracic impedance sensors, electrocautery may lead to increases in heart rate. Although these increases in heart rate may be transient, they may be detrimental for patients in whom strict heart rate control is optimal. In addition, these changes in heart rate may be distracting for the anesthesia provider, who may perceive the heart rate fluctuations as CIED malfunction. Patients with ICDs should have their tachyarrhythmia therapies disabled to avoid inappropriate shocks from monopolar cautery oversensing by either reprogramming or magnet application if EMI (or the return pad) is used above the umbilicus. Patients with ICDs who are pacemaker dependent with close EMI to the generator are a special group that must have their devices reprogrammed. Magnet application is not a reasonable strategy in these patients, since the magnet will not make the pacemaker asynchronous. Patients who have CRT devices are another special classification of patients presenting for surgery. Again, most dual-chamber pacemakers are programmed to minimize RV pacing. CRT devices are programmed to achieve ventricular pacing 100% of the time to improve cardiac output, systolic, and diastolic function. Even though CRT devices are pacing the ventricle 100% of the time, they will not have the characteristic wide complex QRS found in RV pacing alone. Programming the CRT device to an asynchronous mode above the intrinsic rate is a reasonable intraoperative management strategy. Since almost all CRT devices are ICDs, magnet application to the device will deactivate tachyarrhythmia therapy but will not make the CRT device asynchronous. It is critical to reprogram CRT devices to an asynchronous mode if EMI is used above the umbilicus. Brief periods of monopolar electrocautery may be tolerated in patients with CRT devices who have a reasonable sinus rate and normal conduction if the device is not reprogrammed. However, prolonged use of monopolar electrocautery will lead to hemodynamic deterioration due to a loss of synchrony between the RV and LV and the LV septal and lateral walls.

Intraoperative monitoring mirrors standard American Society of Anesthesiology (ASA) guidelines. Plethysmographic pulse oximetry is invaluable for patients with CIEDs undergoing surgery because it is the best clinical indicator that the pacemaker is capturing and creating cardiac output. With monopolar electrocautery, monitoring for pacemaker capture with ECG can be challenging. Due to ECG technology, the ECG rate will sometimes double count the heart rate due to counting of a pacemaker spike and the resulting QRS complex. Double counting of the heart rate may lead to erroneous patient management. In addition, pacemaker spikes may be difficult to see due to their low voltage. Pacemaker spikes may be accentuated with various patient monitors; however, they may inaccurately identify a pacemaker spike. It is important to ensure that each pacemaker spike is capturing the myocardium. Ensuring the paced rate of the device is the same as the pulse oximetry rate ensures proper capture of the myocardium and appropriate cardiac output. While arterial lines accurately display pacemaker capture and cardiac output, patients with CIEDs do not need routine arterial line placement unless patient acuity or surgical complexity deems it necessary.

If a patient requires central venous access or a pulmonary artery catheter, it is important to be mindful of CIED leads placed within 1 to 2 months prior to the planned surgical procedure. The risk for dislodging new leads in the right atrium and right ventricle is higher until the leads become fixed within the myocardium. Patients with CRT devices have a coronary sinus lead that can be more easily dislodged when compared with a chamber lead, since there is no mechanism of lead fixation in the coronary sinus.

POSTOPERATIVE MANAGEMENT

Patients with CIEDs should be appropriately monitored in a clinical environment that is tailored to their postoperative risk. There does not need to be escalation of postoperative disposition based on the presence of a CIED alone. The patient acuity and operative course should be the major drivers for postoperative disposition. For example, patients presenting for outpatient surgery require routine postoperative continuous monitoring until they meet discharge criteria. Most patients with CIEDs do not require routine interrogation following surgery; however, there are notable exceptions. It is reasonable to evaluate patients with CIEDs within 1 month of their surgery on an outpatient basis.[3] For some patients, they must have their device interrogated prior to leaving a monitored setting, whether that is the postanesthesia care unit or a monitored bed. Patients who have had their tachyarrhythmia therapy disabled for surgery must have their device reprogrammed and their tachyarrhythmia therapy re-enabled prior to leaving a monitored setting. In addition, patients who have undergone hemodynamically significant procedures with large volume shifts should have their device interrogated to ensure proper sensing and capture. Patients receiving cardioversion, defibrillation, and therapeutic radiation are at risk for device reset, and should have interrogations as well in the immediate postoperative period.[3] Patients who fall into high-risk categories are more likely to have a change in CIED functionality. Part of the preoperative communication between the CIED team and the anesthesia team should address the need for CIED interrogation postoperatively. Identifying patients who need CIED interrogation prior to discharge avoids lapses in communication in the postoperative period.

EMERGENCY PROTOCOL

Patients with CIEDs may present for urgent or emergent surgery. In these instances, the bidirectional communication between the CIED and anesthesiology teams may not be feasible. When these clinical scenarios present themselves, it is important for the anesthesiology team to identify several components of the CIED in a time efficient manner (Table 38.4). As described previously, the anesthesiology team can get this information from the patient's CIED wallet card, medical records, or CIED team note, or from the chest radiograph. If these methods do not provide pertinent information, the anesthesiology team should call the device manufacturer to obtain basic information regarding the type of device and date of implantation (Table 38.5).

During an emergency procedure, it is important to establish whether the patient is pacemaker dependent. In the absence of a CIED note, a 12-lead ECG or rhythm strip can be examined to look for pacemaker spikes. If the majority of QRS complexes are preceded by a pacing spike, the patient should be treated as pacemaker dependent. The risk of EMI to the CIED should be established using the criteria previously presented, including the use of monopolar versus bipolar electrocautery, in addition to the location of EMI and the return pad. For pacemaker patients who are pacemaker dependent, it is reasonable to use a magnet for surgeries requiring EMI above the umbilicus. However, it is important to remember that a minority of pacemakers will have the magnet function turned off. Therefore, the anesthesiologist should monitor the pulse oximeter to ensure that there is no oversensing of the EMI leading to a lack of pacing in pacemaker-dependent patients, even when the magnet is applied to the device. For patients who are not pacemaker dependent, it is reasonable to have a magnet available in case the patient requires asynchronous pacing. For patients with ICDs, defibrillator pads should be placed on the patient during emergency procedures. Magnet application should be applied for cases with EMI above the level of the umbilicus. Since this will not render the pacemaker asynchronous, if monopolar EMI is used above the umbilicus, it is critical for the surgeon to use short bursts (<5 seconds) of monopolar electrocautery to avoid pacemaker

TABLE 38.4 Cardiovascular Implantable Electronic Device Information for Emergency Surgery

Important Information to Obtain for Emergency Surgery	How to Obtain Information
Type of device	Wallet card Medical record Chest radiograph Manufacturer 1-800 number Device programmer
Pacemaker dependence	Medical record Electrocardiogram Rhythm strip Device programmer
Risk of electromagnetic interference	Discussion with surgeon
Magnet function	Medical record Device programmer

TABLE 38.5 Manufacturer Contact Information

Manufacturer	Phone Number
Medtronic	1-800-633-8766
St. Jude	1-800-722-3423
Boston Scientific	1-800-227-3422
Biotronik	1-800-547-0394

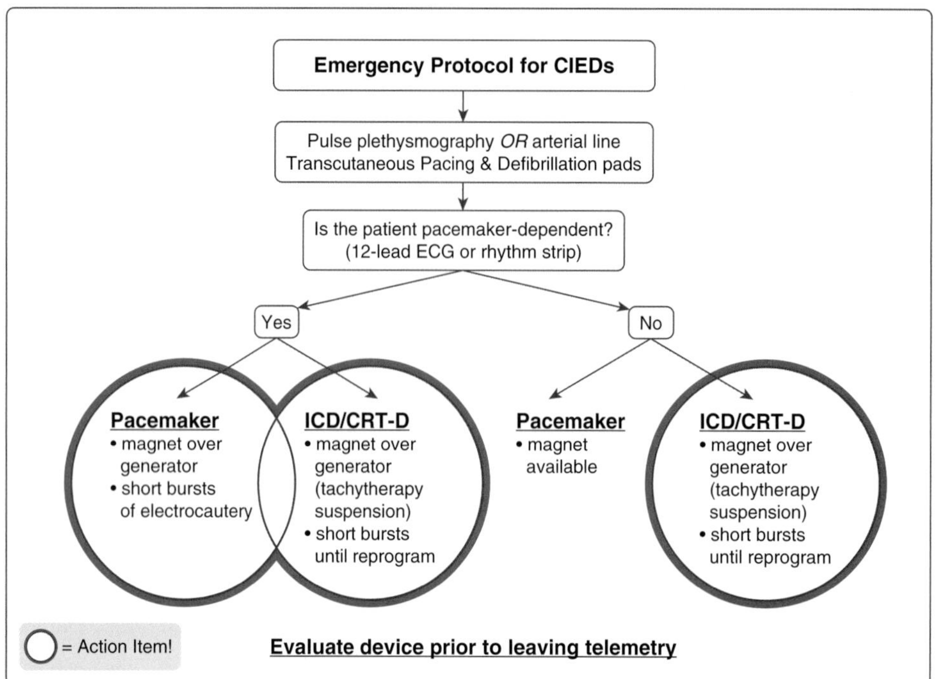

Fig. 38.4 Cardiac implantable electronic device *(CIED)* pathway for emergency surgery. *CRT*, Cardiac resynchronization therapy; *ECG*, electrocardiogram; *ICD*, implantable cardioverter-defibrillator. (Courtesy Dr. Annemarie Thompson.)

oversensing. Interrogation of the CIED under the direction of a physician knowledgeable in the function of these devices should be done as soon as possible. The emergency protocol is described in the HRS/ASA Expert Consensus Statement. A suggested emergency algorithm is shown in Fig. 38.4.

It may be challenging for anesthesiology providers to feel comfortable reprogramming CIEDs in the perioperative environment. Having a structured CIED team that is willing to work with anesthesiologists is a great way to learn how to reprogram devices. Even if one does not feel comfortable reprogramming CIEDs in the perioperative environment, it may be very important for the anesthesiologist to know how to turn on a programmer to obtain important information about a device during an emergency procedure. Interrogating a device and simply reading the home screen can provide critical information regarding the type of device (pacemaker, ICD, CRT), the pacemaker mode, histograms of percentage of time the patient is being paced, battery life, and lead impedance. This is relatively easy to do if one has access to a device programmer in one's institution. Sample images of home screens are shown in Fig. 38.5.

SPECIFIC SURGICAL PROCEDURES

The general perioperative recommendations as outlined before cover the majority of clinical scenarios encountered by anesthesia providers caring for patients with CIEDs. However, there are specific surgical procedures that convey increased risk for CIED malfunction or damage due to high therapeutic energy transfer to the CIED.

Cardioversion

External cardioversion may occur as a planned procedure or as part of advanced cardiovascular life support (ACLS) to treat unstable arrhythmias. Historically, there was increased concern for CIED function because of the use of unipolar leads. With these older leads, the current traveled from the generator (one pole) to the tip of the lead (second pole). There were reports of loss of capture and electrical reset when the cardioversion pads were placed in an anterior and lateral orientation.[31,32] With newer leads, which have a bipolar configuration (both poles located in the tip of the lead), it is uncommon for cardioversion to affect CIED function. In a study with 44 patients, no CIED malfunction was observed during cardioversion with an anterior–posterior pad orientation with the anterior pad more than 8 cm from the CIED generator.[33]

Radiofrequency Ablation

Many patients with CIEDs present to the electrophysiology laboratory for electrophysiology studies and catheter ablation. It is uncommon to have CIED malfunction with radiofrequency ablation (RFA); however, if complications occur, they involve electrical reset, oversensing, and undersensing due to energy delivery near CIEDs. Recommendations include avoiding direct contact between the ablation catheter and the pulse generator and leads, and keeping the path of radiofrequency current (electrode tip to current return pad) as far away from the pulse generator and leads as possible.[34,35]

Lithotripsy

Extracorporeal shockwave lithotripsy is used for disintegrating renal calculi. From the initial use of lithotripsy, there was theoretical concern that the shockwaves and EMI would damage CIEDs; therefore, CIED presence was originally a contraindication to lithotripsy. As technology has evolved, current lithotripsy requires less energy transfer to the patient with improved focus of energy, as well to the renal calculi. Guidelines from Canada recommend a

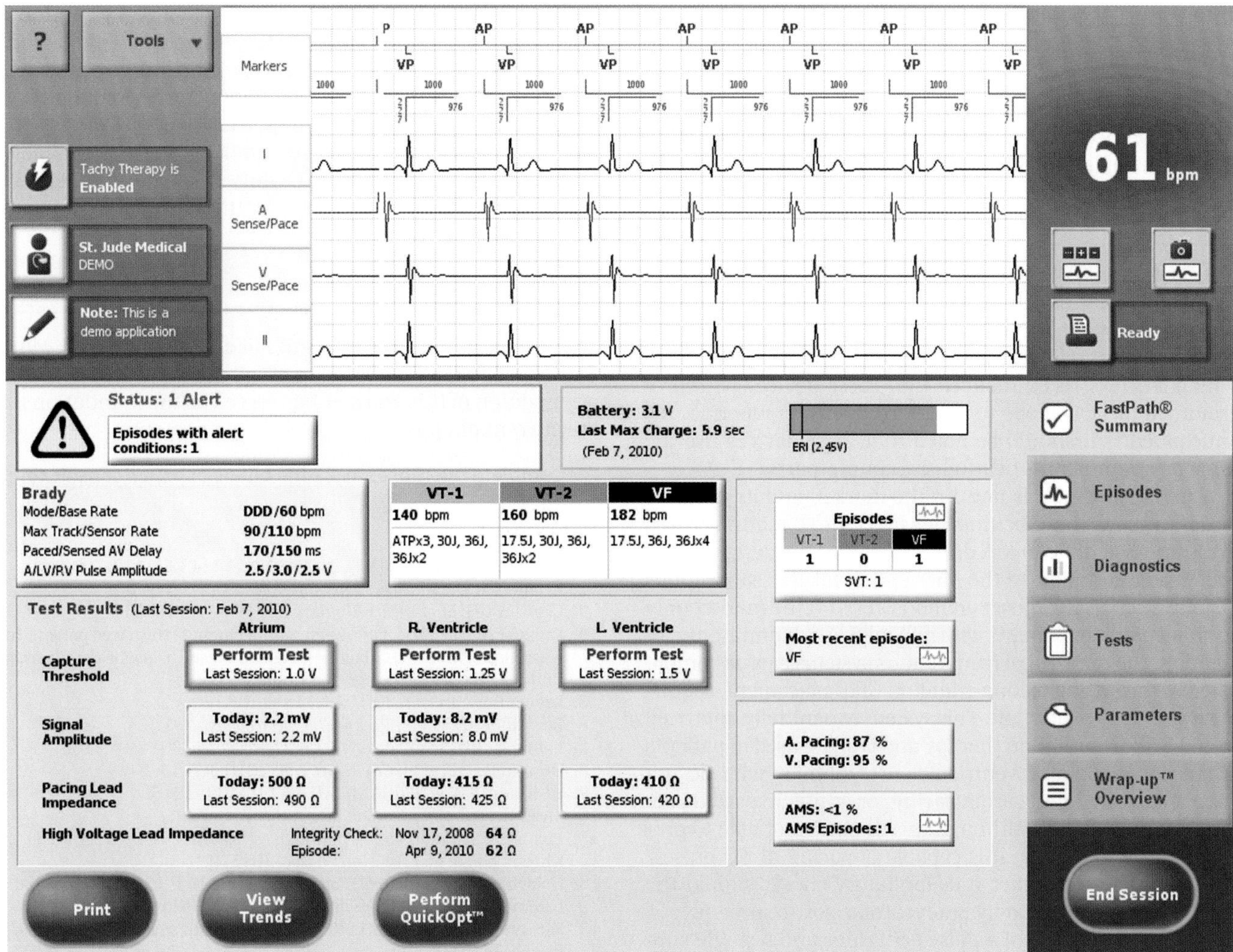

Fig. 38.5 Representative image of pacemaker programmer. Battery life, pacemaker settings, implantable cardioverter-defibrillator therapy, and percentage of atrial and ventricular pacing are readily found on the home screen.

distance of 15 cm from the device to treatment area and that abdominal CIEDs are contraindicated.[36] Another study suggests that with improved technology for lithotripsy, most CIEDs do not have complications; however, if complications arise, the device should be reprogrammed immediately by a member of the CIED team.[37]

Radiation

Diagnostic radiation usually does not significantly affect CIEDs. On the other hand, therapeutic radiation can significantly affect CIED function if directed onto the pulse generator.[38-40] If radiation therapy is performed, position the device outside the field of radiation. The concern with therapeutic radiation and CIEDs is that the circuit of the CIED may be damaged directly by the radiation. Direct radiation of CIEDs should be avoided, and accumulated doses should be kept under 5 Gy.[3] In some instances, the pulse generator will require surgical relocation prior to commencing radiation.

Electroconvulsive Therapy

Electroconvulsive therapy (ECT) involves direct electric current to the brain for the treatment of depression. There are no reports of direct damage to the CIED; however, the concern is pacemaker oversensing of the electric current leading to underpacing in pacemaker-dependent patients. The medical decision to use ECT should consider the duration of its application. If the therapy is going to be short (<5 seconds), it is unlikely that hemodynamically significant oversensing will occur. It is also unlikely that the patient will receive an inappropriate shock. If prolonged ECT exposure is required, the device should be placed in asynchronous pacing mode and antitachyarrhythmia function should be disabled. A discussion between the CIED team and the psychiatrist may facilitate treatment plans, since these patients usually undergo multiple treatments of ECT. ECT may lead to significant hemodynamic effects unrelated to the CIED, including sinus tachycardia from the seizure and ventricular arrhythmias. A magnet should be available for all patients undergoing ECT in the event that oversensing of myopotentials or inappropriate therapy for sinus tachycardia occurs.[3]

Endoscopy

Most upper and lower endoscopies do not use electrocautery, and for those cases, CIED management is straightforward. However, occasionally, electrocautery is used for some patients. There are case reports of inappropriate ICD therapy in these patients. When electrocautery is planned for endoscopy, the same guidelines as previously presented apply with regard to CIED team communication and the assessment of EMI risk to the CIED.

Emerging Technologies

The past couple of years have seen the advent of a new, leadless pacemaker. The impetus for the development of a leadless pacemaker stems from the fact that many pacemaker complications are related to the leads themselves, including lead fracture and infection. Currently, the Medtronic Micra is the only leadless pacemaker approved for use in the United States. The Micra is a single-chamber device placed in the right ventricle via the femoral vein. Its modes include VVIR, VVI, VOO, and OVO. Because these devices are so new, there is very little data on how to manage these patients in the perioperative period. Because of their small size, these devices do not have a magnet sensor and thus will not respond to a magnet. It is recommended that these devices be reprogrammed to VOO mode to reduce oversensing when EMI is anticipated.[41] It should be noted that these devices use the same programmer as their full-size counterparts.

A new type of ICD is now on the market, and its use continues to grow: the subcutaneous ICD (S-ICD) manufactured by Boston Scientific Inc. A driving force for the design of this pacemaker is similar to the Micra pacemaker. Transvenous systems such as the most common CIEDs on the market may be challenging in patients with difficult vascular anatomy. In addition, the removal of transvenous systems can be complicated in the setting of long-standing CIED placement, requiring a laser lead extraction. This system was initially approved in 2012 as defibrillation therapy and is being used in patients at risk for malignant ventricular arrhythmias who do not have a need for bradycardia pacing, or antitachycardia pacing to manage VT.[42] Although this device is not able to provide long-term pacing, it is capable of pacing at 50 pulses/min for 30 seconds after a defibrillatory shock, should the patient become profoundly bradycardiac posttreatment.[43]

The S-ICD consists of a pulse generator and a single subcutaneous lead. Both the pulse generator and the lead are implanted in the subcutaneous tissue and are extrathoracic.[44] Currently, the S-ICD can only be implanted in the left chest. The pulse generator is usually implanted between the anterior and midaxillary lines at the level of the sixth intercostal space. The lead is then tunneled medially from the pulse generator pocket to the xiphoid process and then superiorly along the left parasternal border.

Although different in its makeup, the S-ICD has the same response to a magnet as a traditional ICD. That is, magnet application over the pulse generator will turn off the antiarrhythmic features of the device, and removing the magnet will revert the device to its prior programmed state. A feature the S-ICD has that ensures the magnet is properly positioned is a beeping sound that indicates that arrhythmia detection and shock therapy have been suspended. If the beep is not heard with magnet application, the magnet should be repositioned over the device until a beep is elicited. Due to the location of the ICD at the midaxillary line, it is best to reprogram this device in the perioperative setting to turn off the antitachycardic function. When the device is reprogrammed, defibrillator pads should be placed on the patient.

Conclusions

Anesthesiologists should have a basic understanding of CIEDs and also the nuances of managing this subset of patients in the perioperative period. As technology continues to evolve, and as the population lives longer and indications for CIED therapy continue to grow, perioperative physicians will encounter this patient population more frequently. It should also be noted that at times, trained CIED experts (cardiologists, manufacturer representatives) are not available, making it the anesthesiologist's duty as a true perioperative physician to be able to fully care for these patients.

Acknowledgment

The editors and publisher would like to recognize Dr. Marc A. Rozner for contributing a chapter on this topic in the prior edition of this work. It has served as the foundation for the current chapter.

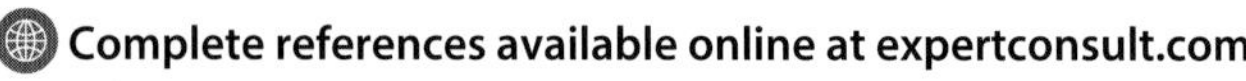

Complete references available online at expertconsult.com.

References

1. Porkorney SD, et al. *JAMA*. 2015;313(24):2433–2440.
2. Kremers MS, et al. *Heart Rhythm*. 2013;10(4):e59–e65.
3. Crossley GH, et al. *Heart Rhythm*. 2011;8(7):1114–1154.
4. Levine PA, Isaeff DM. Follow-up management of the paced patient. In: Kusumoto FM, Goldschlager NF, eds. *Cardiac Pacing for the Clinician*. 2nd ed. New York: Springer; 2008:p647–p694.
5. Levine PA. *Cardiol J*. 2007;14:318–320.
6. Bernstein AD, et al. *J Pacing Clin Electrophys*. 2002;25.
7. Lambiase PD, Srinivasan NT. *Curr Cardiol Rep*. 2014;16:516.
8. Hernandez AF, et al. *Circ Heart Fail*. 2010;3:7–13. 21.
9. Al-Khatib SM, et al. *JAMA*. 2014;311:2209–2215.
10. Mezu U, et al. *Am J Cardiol*. 2011;108:718–722.
11. Pokorney SD, et al. *Circ Arrhythm Electrophysiol*. 2015;8:145–151.
12. Khazanie P, et al. *J Am Heart Assoc*. 2015;4(8):e002061.
13. Goldenberg I, et al. *Circulation*. 2010;122:1265–1271.
14. Hiremath S, et al. *Am J Nephrol*. 2010;32:305–310.
15. Kusumoto FM, et al. *J Am Coll Cardiol*. 2017. https://doi.org/10.1016/j.jacc.2017.10.052.
16. Kramer DB, et al. *Circ Cardiovasc Qual Outcomes*. 2013;6:488–497.
17. Madhavan M, et al. *Circulation*. 2013;128:659–672.
18. Ho J, Mahajan A. *Cardiac Resynchronization Therapy*. A&A; 2010.
19. Ypenburg C, et al. *Eur Heart J*. 2008;29:757–765.
20. Kanzaki H, et al. *J Am Coll Cardiol*. 2004;44:1619–1625.
21. Lindsay BD, et al. *Heart Rhythm*. 2005.
22. Niehous M, Tebbenjohanns J. *Heart*. 2001;86:246–248.
23. Lee D, et al. *Urology*. 2005;66:194.
24. Wilson JH, et al. *Ann Thorac Surg*. 1991;51:225–226.
25. Bayes J. *Anesth Analg*. 2010;103:1615–1616.
26. Lamas GA, et al. *Ann Thorac Surg*. 1986;41:155–157.
27. Mangar D, et al. *Br J Anaesth*. 1991;38:616–618.
28. Snow JS, et al. *J Invasive Cardiol*. 1995;7:25–32.
29. Furman S, Fisher JD. *Pacing Clin Electrophysiol*. 1982;5:486–489.
30. Katzenberg CA, et al. *Pacing Clin Electrophysiol*. 1982;5:156–159.
31. Levine PA, et al. *JACC*. 1983;1:1413–1422.
32. Altamura G, et al. *Pacing Clin Electrophysiol*. 1995;18:1–8.
33. Manegold JC, et al. *Eur Heart J*. 2007;28:1731–1738.
34. Lakkireddy D, et al. *Heart Rhythm*. 2005;2:1309–1316.
35. Ellenbogen KA, et al. *Pacing Clin Electrophysiol*. 1996;19:1287–1295.
36. Health Canada Health Products and Food Branch. http://www.healthycanadians.gc.ca/recall-alert-rappel-avis/hc-sc/2005/14340a-eng.php.
37. Platonov M, et al. *J Endourol*. 2008;22.
38. Hayes DL, et al. *JACC*. 1987;10:782–786.
39. Brook C, Mutter M. *Am J Emerg Med*. 1988;6:591–593.
40. Adamec R, et al. *Pacing Clin Electrophysiol*. 1982;5:145–150.
41. Medtronic Micra Model MC1VR01 Manual. Available at: http://manuals.medtronic.com/wcm/groups/mdtcom_sg/@emanuals/@era/@crdm/documents/documents/contrib_231758.pdf.
42. Burke MC, et al. *J Am Coll Cariol*. 2015;65:1605–1615.
43. Weiss R, et al. *Circulation*. 2013;128:944–953.
44. Lambiase PD, Srinivasan NT. *Curr Cardiol Rep*. 2014;16:516.

39 *Neurologic Monitoring*

CHRISTOPH N. SEUBERT, JOHN J. MCAULIFFE III, and
MICHAEL MAHLA

KEY POINTS

- There are four key principles of intraoperative neurologic monitoring.
  - The pathway at risk during the surgical procedure must be amenable to monitoring.
  - The monitor must provide reliable and reproducible data.
  - If evidence of injury to the pathway is detected, there must be some intervention possible.
  - If changes in the neurologic monitor are detected, and no intervention is possible, although the monitor may be of prognostic value, it does not have the potential to provide direct benefit to the patient from early detection of impending neurologic injury.
- There are few randomized prospective studies evaluating the efficacy of neurologic monitoring modalities.
- Anesthesiologists can improve the efficacy of monitoring by maintaining good physiologic homeostasis and stable levels of anesthesia during parts of the surgical procedure that place the nervous system at greatest risk.
- Based on clinical experience and nonrandomized studies, four practice patterns for use of neurologic monitoring have emerged:
  - There are procedures for which monitoring is recommended and used by most centers.
  - There are procedures for which monitoring is used frequently in some centers, but not in others.
  - There are procedures for which there is no clear clinical experience or evidence indicating that monitoring is useful at all (experimental use).
  - There are procedures in which monitoring is used selectively for patients believed to be at higher-than-usual risk for intraoperative neurologic injury.
- Good communication between surgeon, anesthesiologist, and neurophysiologist is essential to optimizing the utility of monitoring.

Neurologic monitoring during anesthesia care for a patient spans a wide spectrum of techniques, diverse procedures, and various intraoperative or even postoperative settings. Techniques for monitoring fall into two broad categories: techniques to assess metabolic integrity of the nervous system, which typically entail either global or regional determinations of blood flow or oxygenation; or techniques to assess functional integrity, which likewise may be global or focused on specific anatomic pathways or structures of the nervous system. Neurologic monitoring implies that the data for the assessment of the integrity of the nervous system are acquired on a continuous or frequent intermittent basis rather than just at the beginning and end of a procedure.

The procedures and settings in which neurologic monitoring is typically applied all share the characteristic that changes in the monitored parameters can be corrected or minimized by either modifying the surgical approach or manipulating parameters under the control of the anesthesiologist. Monitored procedures range from procedures where monitoring dictates the surgical approach, such as localization of the motor strip during tumor surgery or the neurologic examination during an "awake" craniotomy, to procedures that by their nature put parts of the nervous system at increased risk.

In many procedures that require neurologic monitoring, the anatomical target is also susceptible to drugs administered in the course of an anesthetic. The anesthesiologist and the surgeon need to be aware not only of limitations inherent in individual monitoring techniques, but also of nonsurgical factors that influence the monitoring results. The monitoring approach ideally should anticipate nonsurgical factors by providing a degree of redundancy that helps distinguish a localized surgical trespass from a systemic event.

The application of neurologic monitoring to a surgical procedure may be organized in different ways. It may simply consist in setting up a piece of monitoring equipment, such as a facial nerve monitor that provides acoustic feedback to the surgeon. At the other end of the spectrum, it may require the dedicated services of a technologist and a neurophysiologist in addition to the surgical and anesthesia teams as would be the case during the mapping phase of the resection of a brain tumor. Between those extremes are a variety of delivery models for intraoperative neurophysiologic monitoring that may entail components of telemedicine. Regardless of the organizational structure, the utility of intraoperative neuromonitoring will depend on a shared understanding of surgical objectives, anesthetic constraints, and limitations of monitoring. This shared understanding will then need to be supported by open lines of communications by all involved, particularly during critical phases of an operation.[1]

For some procedures, neurologic monitoring is a marker of the quality of care and is routinely employed because outcome data support its use. Examples include correction of scoliosis and resection of vestibular schwannomas. More frequently, the approach to monitoring is based on local conventions and surgical expectations. In this latter case, monitoring utility depends even more on a good understanding of the technique's capabilities and limitations by anesthesiologists, surgeons, and the intraoperative monitoring team; on good communication; and on their mutual collaboration to allow corrective action in the face of changing signals or to prevent false alarms that disrupt surgery.

This chapter first discusses individual monitoring modalities in isolation so that the clinician can appreciate the inherent strengths and weaknesses of each. Subsequent sections apply this information by describing suitable approaches to various clinical settings that combine and integrate individual techniques to optimize neurologic outcome for patients. The chapter ends with a brief discussion of how neurologic monitoring is believed to be useful today, and where more work is needed to determine whether monitoring has a role in surgical patients in the future.

Monitoring Modalities

MONITORS OF ADEQUACY OF NERVOUS SYSTEM BLOOD FLOW

Adequacy of cerebral blood flow (CBF) can be monitored by two principal methods. The first method assesses blood flow itself with the implicit assumption that "normal" flow provides adequately for the metabolic needs of the brain. The second approach assesses oxygen delivery either locally or globally with the implicit assumption that normal oxygen delivery at the site of measurement reflects adequate blood supply throughout the central nervous system (CNS). To illustrate the limitations imposed by such implicit assumptions, let us examine global or hemispheric CBF in the context of a patient's disease process.

In normal brain, values of hemispheric CBF of approximately 50 mL/100 g/min reflect adequate oxygen delivery for maintaining structural integrity and function. Values of less than 20 to 25 mL/100 g/min are associated first with failure of function and on further decrease with structural damage.[2] In neurosurgical patients, structural integrity and function may be altered by disease processes and anesthetics, which have an impact on the interpretation of measured CBF. A CBF of 40 mL/100 g/min in a patient in barbiturate coma after resection of an arteriovenous malformation may represent hyperemia (because metabolic demand is very low), whereas the same CBF in a patient with a mass lesion may reflect a modest decrease in cerebral perfusion pressure secondary to increasing intracranial pressure. Thus the clinical response to an abnormal value requires context and clinical judgement.

Global Blood Flow Monitoring Techniques (Noninvasive)

Intravascular Tracer Compounds. Direct measurement of CBF is possible by determining kinetics of wash-in and/or wash-out of an inert tracer compound, a method originally described by Kety and Schmidt.[3] A widely used modern variation of the same concept is the imaging of the first passage of intravascular contrast agents during computer tomographic or magnetic resonance imaging for determining loco-regional blood flow (Fig. 39.1). These techniques share the limitation of providing a snapshot of CBF in time instead of continuous assessment of flow over time.

Transcranial Doppler Ultrasound. Transcranial Doppler (TCD) ultrasound is a technique that infers CBF from measurements of the blood flow velocity in the large conducting arteries of the brain. The TCD probe transmits pulses of sound waves through the thin temporal bone in a variation of the pulsed wave Doppler technique with which anesthesiologists may be familiar from echocardiography. When these sound waves are reflected off the red blood cells back toward the TCD probe, the velocity of the reflected sound waves is changed because the blood cells themselves are in motion toward or away from the probe. This phenomenon is known as the "Doppler shift," and is directly related to flow velocity and flow direction of the blood cells. Blood flow is faster during systole and in the center of a vessel whereas it is slower in diastole and near the vessel wall. TCD records a spectrum of flow velocities whose outline resembles an arterial waveform tracing. These concepts are illustrated in Fig. 39.2.

Intraoperatively, TCD measurements are most commonly and easily made by continuous monitoring of the middle cerebral artery for the purpose of detecting either significant changes in flow velocity or the presence of particulate emboli.[4] As a diagnostic study, segments of all proximal intracranial arteries and the internal carotid artery of the neck can be insonated. An important limitation of TCD results from the fact that most of the examination is done through the temporal bone, which may be thick enough to preclude an adequate examination in 10% to 20% of patients.[5,6]

Two assumptions that are intuitive and plausible, but ultimately unproven, must be made for TCD-measured blood flow velocity to have a direct relationship to CBF. First, blood flow velocity is directly related to blood flow only if the diameter of the artery where the flow velocity is measured and the measurement angle of the Doppler probe remain constant. In practical terms, the difficulty with this assumption lies in finding a means to affix the TCD probe in a way that prevents dislodgment or movement during monitoring. The second assumption requires that CBF in the basal arteries of the brain is directly related to cortical CBF. Because TCD monitoring is typically done using the middle cerebral artery, this assumption may be invalid if collateral blood flow by leptomeningeal collaterals from anterior and posterior cerebral artery territories is adequate. Although these two assumptions constrain the utility of TCD as a stand-alone monitor of CBF, the changes in flow velocity seen in typical applications (discussed subsequently) are large enough to provide useful clinical information.

More importantly, TCD is the only continuous neurologic monitoring technique that provides early warning for hyperperfusion and for the number of emboli delivered to the brain during various phases of an operation. Because of their high echogenicity, emboli show up in the TCD spectrum as high-intensity transient signals (see Fig. 39.2) and are easily identified as brief beeps or chirps within the background of the Doppler sounds.

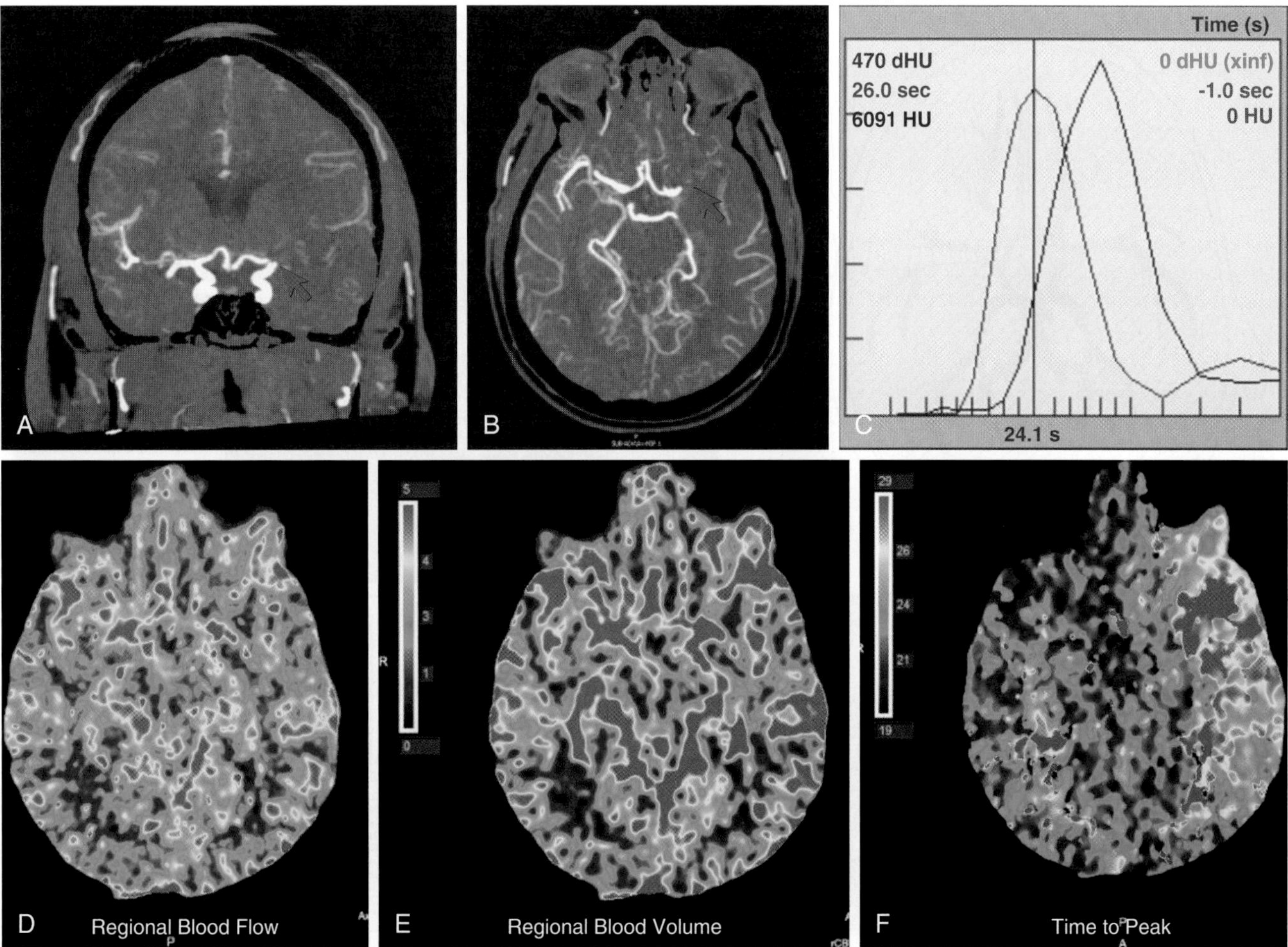

Fig. 39.1 Determination of cerebral blood flow by means of an intravascular tracer. Shown are computer tomographic images of a patient 90 minutes after onset of a left middle cerebral artery stroke. The site of the occlusion in coronal (A) and axial (B) planes is indicated by a red arrow. Panel C shows the arterial inflow function and venous outflow function derived by repeated imaging of the passage of radiopaque contrast through a volume element (voxel) representative of arterial and venous territory, respectively. The A2 segment of the anterior cerebral artery is typically chosen as a voxel for the arterial inflow function and the superior sagittal sinus for the venous outflow function. Based on these functions, blood flow, volume, and flow kinetics can be calculated for other areas of the image. The cerebral blood flow map (D) shows symmetrical flow in both hemispheres, with warmer colors indicating areas of higher flow consistent with grey matter. Blood volume (E) is symmetrical as well, but the time to the peak concentration of contrast (F) is significantly delayed for brain affected by the stroke.

Jugular Bulb Venous Oxygen Saturation. The degree of oxygen extraction by an organ can be monitored by following the oxygen saturation of the mixed venous blood that drains that organ. In the case of the brain, jugular bulb venous oxygen saturation ($Sjvo_2$) is believed to measure the degree of oxygen extraction by the brain and to represent the balance between cerebral oxygen supply and demand. To monitor $Sjvo_2$, a fiberoptic catheter is placed in a retrograde fashion into the jugular bulb through the internal jugular vein under fluoroscopic guidance. Correct tip placement is crucial to minimize admixture of extracranial venous blood. To decrease the risk of complications, usually only one side is monitored.

Several theoretical limitations of the technique must be borne in mind to interpret $Sjvo_2$ values and trends properly. Although nearly all blood from the brain drains via the jugular veins, intracranial mixing of venous blood is incomplete and may result in differences between right-sided and left-sided measurements. The dominant jugular vein (i.e., the right for most patients) drains predominantly cortical venous blood, whereas the contralateral jugular vein drains more of the subcortical regions.[7] Despite such regional differences, $Sjvo_2$ must be considered a monitor of global cerebral oxygenation because inadequate perfusion to a focal brain region may not decrease $Sjvo_2$ values below the normal range of 55% to 75%. Because $Sjvo_2$ represents the balance between supply and demand, interpretation of the absolute value of $Sjvo_2$ must take the clinical circumstances into account.

Cerebral Oximetry. Cerebral oximetry is a noninvasive technique that, similar to $Sjvo_2$, uses reflectance oximetry to measure the oxygen saturation of the tissues underneath the sensor. Typically, two sensors are applied to both sides of the forehead. The light passes not only through parts of the frontal brain, but also through the overlying skull and scalp. Contamination of the oximetry signal by extracranial blood sources is a serious concern, although the use of two sensing diodes with different distances from the light source within one sensor patch and adjustments of the algorithm of the oximeter may minimize this problem.[8,9]

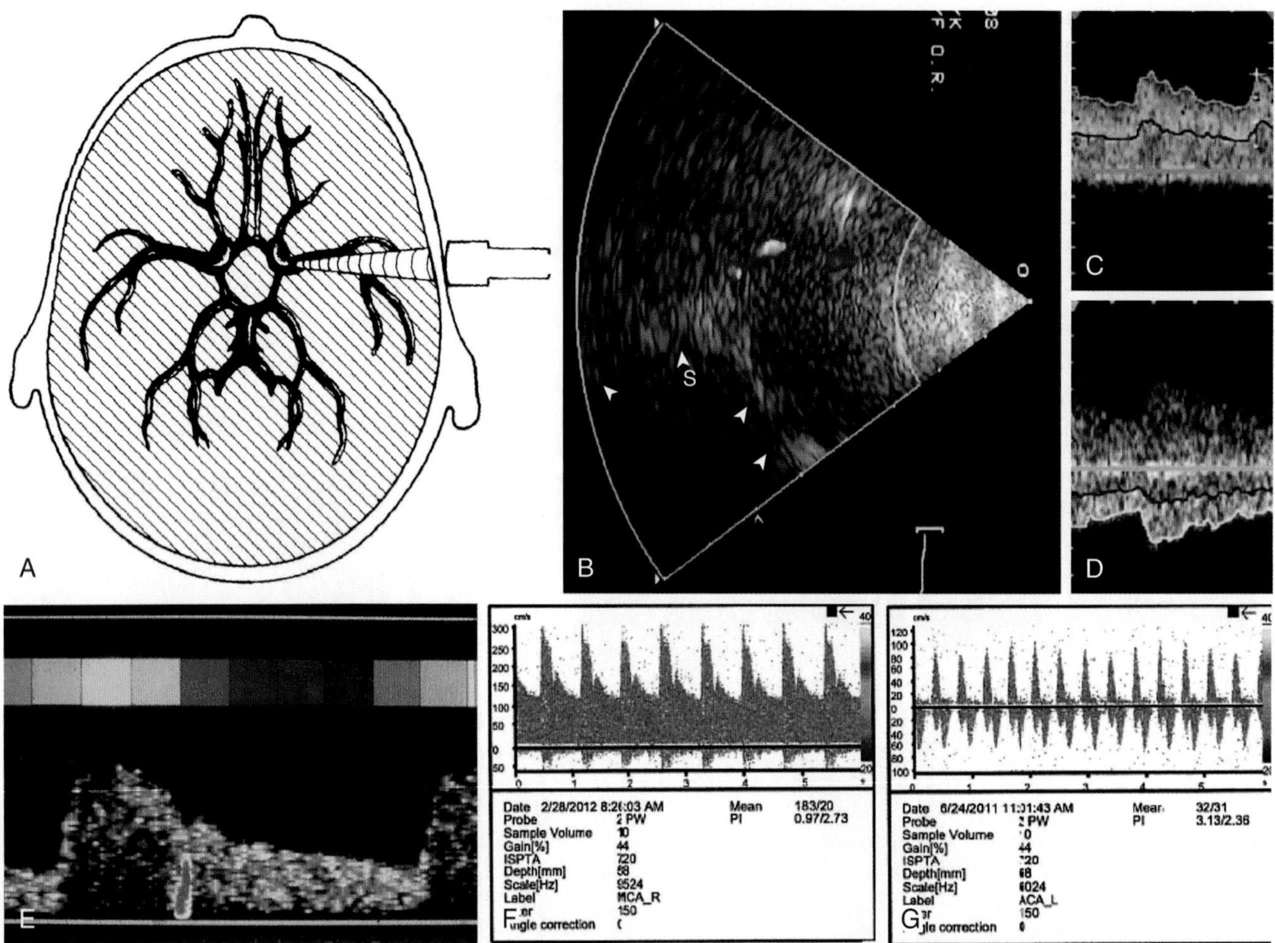

Fig. 39.2 (A) Transcranial Doppler monitoring is done by insonating the arteries at the base of the brain through a thin part of the temporal bone. (B) If this procedure is performed with an imaging probe, some intracranial structures, such as the cerebral peduncles (white triangles) or the sella complex (white triangle labeled "S"), can be visualized. The captured Doppler signals originate from the right middle, right anterior, and left anterior cerebral arteries. (C) Normal Doppler spectrum obtained from the middle cerebral artery. By convention, flow toward the probe is displayed as a waveform above the baseline. (D) Doppler profile of the bifurcation of the terminal internal carotid artery as it branches into the middle cerebral artery (flowing toward the transducer) and the anterior cerebral artery (flowing away). This flow signal can be obtained if the transducer is focused as shown in A. (E–G) Examples of three clinical applications of transcranial Doppler. (E) Emboli are highly echogenic and appear as high-energy transient signals. On the audible output, these emboli are easily noticed as brief beeps or chirps. (F) Doppler profile of a middle cerebral artery in a patient with severe vasospasm after an aneurysmal subarachnoid hemorrhage (compare with C). (G) Transcranial Doppler examination consistent with intracranial circulatory arrest. There is a brief systolic inflow followed by retrograde flow during diastole.

Because 66% to 80% of the cerebral blood volume is venous blood, cerebral oximetry determines predominantly "local venous oxygen saturation." The simplicity of its use, and the familiarity with the principles of treating decreases in systemic mixed venous oxygen saturation, have made cerebral oximetry a popular trend monitor in operations that potentially cause decreases in blood flow to the vessels of the head.[10] There are some significant limitations, however, of the use of cerebral oximetry during such procedures. First, adequacy of global cerebral perfusion is inferred from measurements over the frontopolar brain. Second, normative data on normal values or expected changes for cerebral oximetry are largely absent, but preoperative application of the sensors allows the start of a trend in conjunction with a neurologic baseline examination.[11]

An example of how these limitations play out is provided by a study of the use of cerebral oximetry during 100 carotid endarterectomies in awake patients.[12] Cerebral oximetry was able to identify 97.4% of patients with adequate CBF as indicated by the absence of clinical symptoms. The monitor frequently indicated inadequate CBF, defined as a 20% decrease in cerebral oxygen saturation from the pre-clamp baseline, although the patient had no clinical symptoms of inadequate CBF. The false-positive rate of 66.7% may simply illustrate the fact that oxygen extraction increases before function fails. The real problem is that the lower limit for acceptable regional oxygen saturation is unknown in a large population of patients.[13] Acceptable values may be different from patient to patient, and addition of anesthetic drugs that influence cerebral metabolism may confuse the picture further.

Tissue-Level Blood Flow Monitoring Techniques (Invasive)

Tissue-level monitoring for the brain is by definition invasive. All monitors in current clinical or research use are implanted through a burr hole, extend either into the white matter or ventricular system, and typically use a bolt for stabilization. They all share a 1% to 2% risk of bleeding, infection, or ischemia owing to the implantation procedure.[14]

A second shared feature is their limited spatial resolution (i.e., each monitoring probe monitors only a limited area of brain surrounding the probe). When these monitors were first developed, there was considerable debate regarding the optimal placement of the device given such limited spatial resolution. Based on today's appreciation for the impact of secondary neurologic insults on the ultimate outcome, there is growing agreement that tissue-level monitoring is best performed in morphologically and functionally normal tissue that is part of the penumbra or vulnerable zone of interest.[15-17]

Of the tissue-level monitors, tissue partial pressure of oxygen (Po_2) monitoring has undergone sufficient refinement to be in wider clinical use. Thermal diffusion blood flow measurement and laser Doppler flow measurement are experimental and not in widespread clinical use.

Tissue Partial Pressure of Oxygen Monitoring

Localized monitoring of tissue Po_2 is based on an oxygen-sensitive electrode originally described by Clark.[18] The diffusion of oxygen molecules through an oxygen-permeable membrane into an electrolyte solution causes an electric current that is proportional to Po_2. Currently available catheter-based electrodes placed into the subcortical white matter provide stable recording conditions over long periods.

Most of the data on brain tissue oxygen levels ($P_{Br}o_2$) come from studies in patients with head trauma.[19] Comparison with stable xenon CT for assessment of CBF and studies during temporal clipping in aneurysm surgery show good correlation between $P_{Br}o_2$ and CBF.[20,21] Similarly, the time course of changes in $P_{Br}o_2$ after traumatic brain injury resembles that of CBF.[22,23] Critics of the technique argue that $P_{Br}o_2$ values are highly influenced by the partial pressure of arterial oxygen (Pao_2) and are merely an elaborate indicator of the quality of patient ventilation. This view is supported by the observation that increasing the fraction of inspired oxygen (Fio_2) increases $P_{Br}o_2$, but likely represents an oversimplification.[24] Concurrent microdialysis studies have shown that increasing Fio_2 not only increases $P_{Br}o_2$, but also decreases tissue lactate levels, suggesting a true improvement in the metabolic milieu of the brain tissue itself.[25,26] While decreases in $P_{Br}o_2$ are associated with worse outcomes in traumatic brain injury patients, the role of $P_{Br}o_2$-directed therapy is still investigational.[27]

MONITORS OF NERVOUS SYSTEM FUNCTION

The most commonly used monitors of function are the electroencephalogram (EEG), sensory-evoked responses (SERs), motor evoked responses, and the electromyogram (EMG). The EEG is a surface recording of the summation of excitatory and inhibitory postsynaptic potentials spontaneously generated by the pyramidal cells in the cerebral cortex. The signals are very small, and each recording electrode records information both directly beneath the electrode and information volume conducted from deeper tissue.[28] Monitoring the EEG is usually directed toward one or more of four perioperative uses. First, the EEG is used to help identify inadequate blood flow to the cerebral cortex caused by either a surgically induced or anesthetic-induced reduction in blood flow or retraction on cerebral tissue. Second, the EEG may be used to guide an anesthetic-induced reduction of cerebral metabolism either in anticipation of a loss of CBF or in the treatment of high intracranial pressure, when a reduction in CBF and blood volume is desired. Third, the EEG may be used to predict neurologic outcome after a brain insult. Finally, the EEG may be used to gauge the depth of the hypnotic state of the patient under general anesthesia (see Chapter 40).

More than 50 years of experience monitoring the EEG has led to many known correlations of EEG patterns with clinical states of the normal and diseased cerebral cortex. The electroencephalographer can accurately identify consciousness, unconsciousness, seizure activity, stages of sleep, and coma. In the absence of significant changes in anesthetic technique, the electroencephalographer also can accurately identify inadequate oxygen delivery to the brain (from either hypoxemia or ischemia). By using high-speed computerized EEG analysis and statistical methods, EEG patterns in the continuum from awake to deeply anesthetized are becoming, with few exceptions, much better understood. In addition, computer advances have made possible high-speed mathematic manipulation of the EEG signal to present the data in a manner more suitable to continuous trends for use during surgical or anesthetic monitoring.

Evoked potentials are electrical activity generated in response to either a sensory or a motor stimulus. Measurements of evoked responses may be made at multiple points along an involved nervous system pathway. The evoked responses are generally smaller than other electric activity generated in nearby tissue (muscle or brain) and are readily obscured by these other biologic signals. In the case of SERs, repeated sampling and sophisticated electronic summation and averaging techniques are needed to extract the desired evoked potential signal from background biologic signals. Motor-evoked responses are generally larger and commonly do not require averaging.

SERs are the most common type of evoked potentials monitored intraoperatively. During the last three decades, much research has been done on the use of intraoperative motor-evoked potentials (MEPs), and use of MEPs during both intracranial and spinal surgery is now no longer considered experimental. There are three basic types of SERs: somatosensory-evoked potentials (SSEPs), brainstem auditory-evoked potentials (BAEPs), and visual-evoked potentials (VEPs).

Electroencephalogram

Basic Unprocessed Electroencephalogram Concepts. The EEG is produced by a summation of excitatory and inhibitory postsynaptic potentials produced in cortical gray matter. Because the EEG signal is generated only by postsynaptic potentials and is much smaller than action potentials recorded over nerves or from heart muscle, extreme care must be taken when placing electrodes to ensure proper placement and excellent contact with the skin to avoid significant signal loss. Alternatively, subdermal needle electrodes may be used, particularly when sterile application of an electrode close to a surgical field is necessary. When electrodes are applied directly to the surface of the brain, impedance is minimized by close electrode contact and saturation of the area with an electrolyte solution.

EEG electrodes generally are placed according to a mapping system that relates surface head anatomy to underlying brain cortical regions. The placement pattern of recording electrodes is called a montage. Use of a standard recording montage permits anatomic localization of signals produced by the brain and allows development of normative EEG patterns and comparison of EEG recordings made at different times. The standard EEG "map" is called the 10 to 20 system for EEG electrode placement (Fig. 39.3). This system is a symmetric array of scalp electrodes placed systematically based on the distance from the nasion to the inion and from the pretragal bony indentations associated with both temporomandibular joints. Based on 10% or 20% of these distances, recording electrodes are placed systematically over the frontal (F), parietal (P), temporal (T), and occipital (O) regions at increasing distances from the midline. Left-sided electrodes are given odd number subscripts, and right-sided electrodes are given even number subscripts. Increasing numbers indicate a greater distance from the midline. Midline electrodes are designated with a "z" subscript. The standard diagnostic EEG uses at least 16 channels of information,[29] but intraoperative recordings have been reported using 1 to 32 discreet channels.

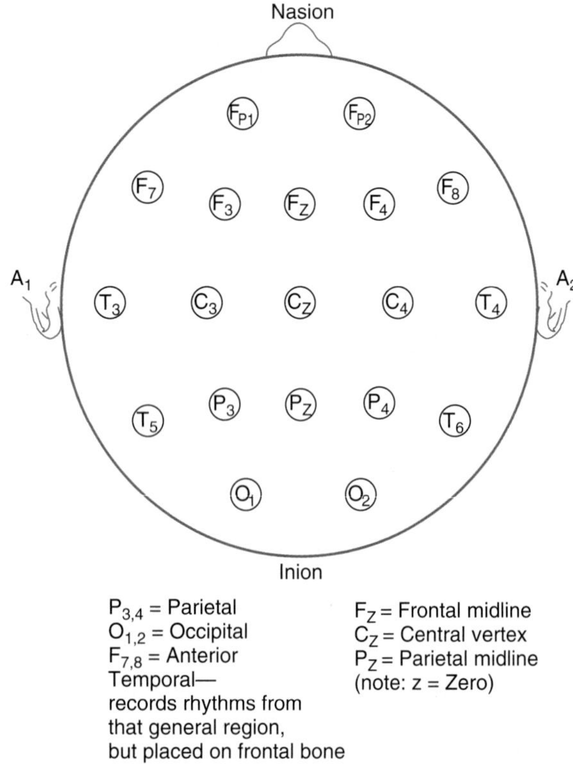

Fig. 39.3 International 10 to 20 system of electrode placement for recording electroencephalogram and sensory-evoked responses. (From Hughes JR. *EEG in Clinical Practice.* 2nd ed. Newton, MA: Butterworth-Heinemann; 1994.)

The intraoperative EEG is most commonly recorded from electrodes placed on the scalp. Recordings also may be made from electrodes placed on the surface of the brain (electrocorticography), or from microelectrodes placed transcortically to record from individual neurons (e.g., during surgery for Parkinson disease).[30,31] The EEG signal is described using three basic parameters: amplitude, frequency, and time. Amplitude is the size, or voltage, of the recorded signal and ranges commonly from 5 to 500 μV (vs. 1-2 mV for the electrocardiogram signal). Because neurons are irreversibly lost during the normal aging process, EEG amplitude decreases with age. Frequency can be thought of simply as the number of times per second the signal oscillates or crosses the zero voltage line. Time is the duration of the sampling of the signal; this is continuous and real time in the standard paper or digital EEG, but is a sampling epoch in the processed EEG (see later).

Normal Electroencephalogram. Normal patterns seen on the EEG vary among normal individuals, but are consistent enough to allow for accurate recognition of normal and pathologic patterns. The usual base frequency in an awake patient is the beta range (>13 Hz). This high-frequency and usually low-amplitude signal is common from an alert attentive brain and may be recorded from all regions. With eye closure, higher amplitude signals in the alpha frequency range (8-13 Hz), seen best in the occipital region, appear (Fig. 39.4). This "eyes closed" resting pattern is the

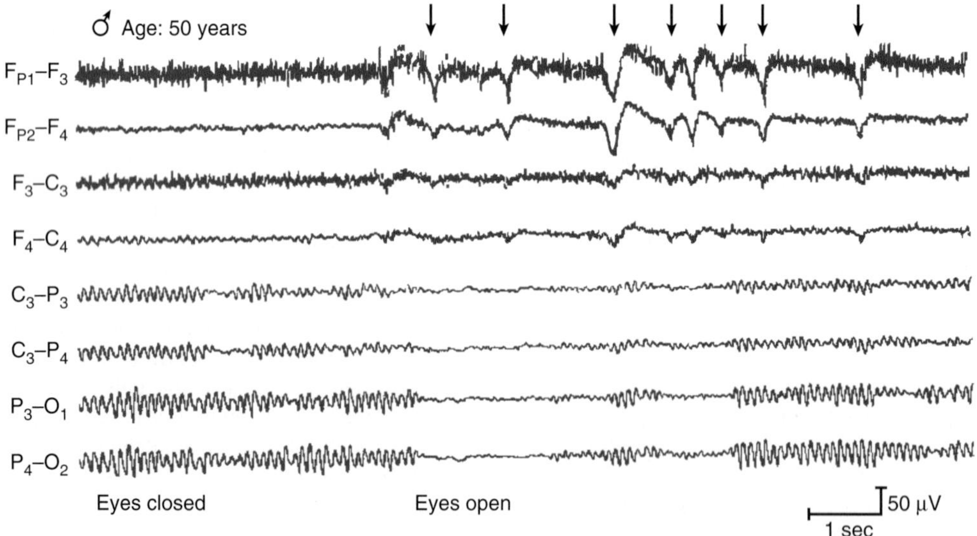

Fig. 39.4 The loss and return of alpha activity as the eyes open and close can be seen. The large spikes (↓) are muscle artifact from eye blinks and hence are best visible in channels that incorporate frontal electrodes (designated F).

baseline awake pattern used when anesthetic effects on the EEG are described. When events that lead the brain to produce higher frequencies and larger amplitudes occur, the EEG is described as "activated," and when slower frequencies are produced (theta = 4-7 Hz, and delta = <4 Hz), the EEG is said to be "depressed." The EEG during natural sleep may contain all of these frequencies at various times. The slower frequencies occur during deep natural sleep with "sleep spindles" (Fig. 39.5), but during light sleep or rapid eye movement sleep, the EEG becomes activated, and the eye muscle EMG appears on the EEG.

In the normal EEG in awake and asleep patients, patterns recorded from corresponding electrodes on each hemisphere are symmetric in terms of frequency and amplitude, the patterns are predictable if clinical states are known, and spike (epileptic) waveforms are absent. In most cases, normal EEG patterns are associated with normal underlying brain function in awake and asleep patients.

Abnormal Electroencephalogram. General characteristics of the "abnormal" EEG include asymmetry with respect to frequency, amplitude, or both, recorded from corresponding electrodes on each hemisphere, and patterns of amplitude and frequency that are unpredictable or unexpected in the normal recording. These abnormal patterns reflect either anatomic or metabolic alterations in the underlying brain. Regional asymmetry can be seen with tumors, epilepsy, and cerebral ischemia or infarction. Epilepsy may be recognized by high-voltage spike and slow waves, whereas cerebral ischemia manifests first with EEG slowing with preservation of voltage. Further slowing and loss of voltage occurs as ischemia becomes more severe. Factors affecting the entire brain may produce symmetric abnormalities of the signal. Identifying pathologic abnormal patterns in the global EEG signal is very important, although sometimes quite difficult, in the clinical situation. Many of the normal global pattern changes produced by anesthetic drugs are similar to pathologic patterns produced by ischemia or

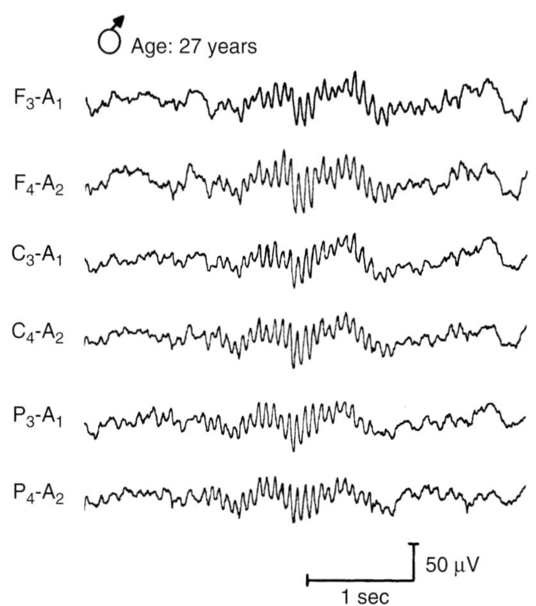

Fig. 39.5 Characteristic sleep spindles in normal sleep are shown in the center.

hypoxemia. Control of anesthetic technique is very important when the EEG is being used for clinical monitoring of the nervous system.

Processed Electroencephalogram Concepts. Numerous limitations are introduced when moving from the raw EEG domain to the processed EEG domain. First, artifact is processed in many cases along with desired signal leading to a perfectly believable processed EEG display that is materially incorrect. Second, the standard 16-channel EEG montage provides more information than can be practically analyzed or displayed by most processed EEG monitors and perhaps more than is needed for routine intraoperative use. Most available processed EEG devices used by anesthesiologists use four or fewer channels of information—translating to at most two channels per hemisphere. Processed EEG devices generally monitor less cerebral territory than a standard 16-channel EEG. Third, some intraoperative changes are unilateral (e.g., regional ischemia owing to carotid clamping), and some are bilateral (e.g., EEG depression by bolus administration of an anesthetic). Display of the activity of both hemispheres is necessary to delineate unilateral from bilateral changes. An appropriate number of leads over both hemispheres is needed. Most early studies validating intraoperative EEG monitoring used continuous visual inspection of a 16- to 32-channel analog EEG by an experienced electroencephalographer—such monitoring was considered the gold standard.[32,33] Adequate studies comparing the processed EEG with fewer channels with this gold standard across multiple uses and operations have not been done, although limited data using processed EEG monitoring during carotid surgery suggest that two- or four-channel instruments would detect most significant changes,[34,35] provided that the electrodes are appropriately placed over watershed areas of blood supply.

Devices. EEG processing for intraoperative monitoring is typically based on power analysis of a segment of raw EEG, referred to as an epoch. Power analysis uses Fourier transformation to convert the digitized raw EEG signal into component sine waves of identifiable frequency and amplitude. The raw EEG data, which is a plot of voltage versus time, is converted to a plot of frequency and amplitude versus time. Many commercially available processed EEG machines display power (voltage or amplitude squared) as a function of frequency and time. These monitors display the data in two general forms, either compressed spectral array or density spectral array. In compressed spectral array, frequency is displayed along the x axis, and power is displayed along the y axis with height of the waveform equal to the power at that frequency. Time is displayed along the z axis. Tracings overlap each other, with the most recent information in front (Fig. 39.6). Density spectral array also displays frequency along the x axis, time is displayed along the y axis, and power is reflected either by the density of the dots at each frequency or by a spectrum of colors. Each display format provides the same data, and choice depends on the preference of the user.

Many changes that occur during anesthesia and surgery are reflected as changes in amplitude, frequency, or both. These changes can be clearly seen in these displays if adequate and appropriate channels are monitored. Power

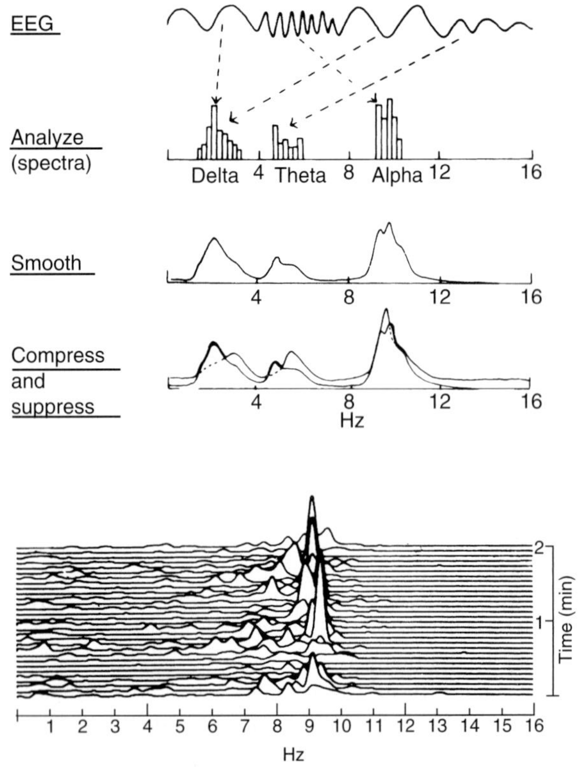

Fig. 39.6 Diagram of a technique used to generate compressed spectral array. Example at the bottom of the figure shows compressed spectra of the alpha rhythm from a normal subject. *EEG*, Electroencephalogram. (From Stockard JJ, Bickford RG. The neurophysiology of anaesthesia. In: Gordon E, ed. *A Basis and Practice of Neuroanesthesia*. New York: Elsevier; 1981:3.)

analysis has been used clinically for many years as a diagnostic tool during procedures with risk for intraoperative cerebral ischemia, such as carotid endarterectomy and cardiopulmonary bypass (CPB). Power analysis has proven to be a sensitive and reliable monitor in the hands of experienced operators using an adequate number of channels. In addition, parameters obtained from power analysis have been investigated as monitors for depth of anesthesia.[36-39]

Data Acquisition Period. An important consideration in the processed EEG is time. Raw EEG is continuous in real time. The processed EEG samples data over a given time period (epoch), processes the data, and then displays information in various formats. There is a relationship between epoch length and spectral resolution. If a long epoch length is chosen, the waveform can be described precisely, but the time required for data processing is long and not real time. If a short length of data is sampled, analysis may be done in near real time, but the epoch chosen for analysis may not be representative of the overall waveform (i.e., the condition of the patient). There also may be insufficient data points for meaningful Fourier transformation. This issue, as related to the use of intraoperative EEG for analysis of anesthetic depth, has been studied by Levy.[40] A longer epoch may produce less epoch-to-epoch variability and allow more precise description of frequency and power; however, the longer epoch increases the delay before new information is processed and displayed, reducing the amount and timeliness of information available for clinical decision making. In studying EEG epochs of 2 to 32 seconds, Levy[40] concluded that 2-second epochs are appropriate during general anesthesia. Many commercially available devices have used 2-second epoch lengths, updated at varying user-selected intervals. With better and faster computers, continuous monitoring of 2-second epochs and now even longer epochs is possible.

Evoked Potentials

Basic Concepts Common to All Modalities. EEG signals provide information about cortical function, but little to no information about subcortical neural pathways crucial to normal neurologic function. Intraoperative monitoring of SERs has gained increasing popularity over the last 35 years because it provides the ability to monitor the functional integrity of sensory pathways in an anesthetized patient undergoing surgical procedures placing these pathways at risk. Because motor pathways are often adjacent anatomically to these sensory pathways or supplied by the same blood vessels, or both, function of motor pathways may be inferred, albeit imperfectly, from the function of these sensory pathways. Today, MEPs are monitored together with SERs to provide direct information about function of motor pathways. SERs are typically 100-fold smaller in amplitude than the EEG. Recording SERs in an environment such as an operating room with its myriad electrical devices is challenging and requires substantial technical expertise.

Sensory-Evoked Responses. SERs are electric CNS responses to electric, auditory, or visual stimuli. SERs are produced by stimulating a sensory system and recording the resulting electric responses at various sites along the sensory pathway up to and including the cerebral cortex. Because of the very low amplitude of SERs (0.1-10 μV), it is often impossible to distinguish SERs from other background biologic signals, such as the EEG or EMG, which may be considered in this case undesirable "noise." To extract the SER from the background noise, the recorded signal is digitized, and signal averaging is applied. With this technique, signal recording is time-locked to the application of the sensory stimulus. For example, during intraoperative posterior tibial nerve SER monitoring, after nerve stimulation at the ankle, only signal information occurring less than 90 ms after the stimulus is recorded (Fig. 39.7). The SER occurs at a constant time after the stimulus application; other electric activity, such as spontaneous EEG, occurs at random intervals after the sensory stimulus. The averaging technique improves the SER signal-to-noise ratio by eliminating random elements and enhancing the SER. This enhancing effect increases directly with the square root of the number of responses added into the averaged response.

SER recordings are of two general types determined by the distance of the recording electrode from the neural generator of the evoked response. SERs recorded from electrodes close to the neural generators (within approximately 3-4 cm in the average adult) are termed "near-field potentials."[41] Near-field potentials are recorded from electrodes placed very close to the actual signal generator site,[42] and the morphology is directly affected by electrode location.[41] Far-field potentials are recorded from electrodes located a greater distance from the neural generator and are conducted to the recording electrode through a volume

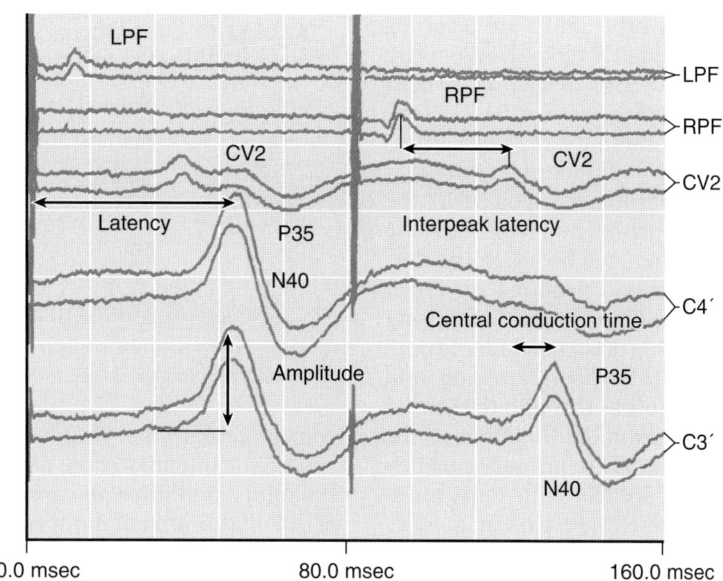

Fig. 39.7 Sensory-evoked responses are described in terms of latency and amplitude. Interpeak latency is the measured time between two peaks. Interpeak latency may be measured between two peaks in the same channel or between peaks in different channels (shown in figure). Note that the polarity of peaks is displayed contrary to standard convention (see text). The example shows a recording of posterior tibial somatosensory-evoked potentials. Each tracing is reproduced twice because reproducibility of a waveform helps distinguish signal from artefact. Left and right posterior tibial nerves are stimulated at 0 and 90 ms, respectively. The first evoked response is recorded from left and right popliteal fossa (*LPF* and *RPF*, respectively). The peak labeled CV2 represents the brainstem response recorded at the craniocervical junction. As a far-field potential, the potential looks similar for right- and left-sided stimulation. The primary cortical responses are recorded from the contralateral hemisphere (labeled P35 and N40).

conductor (brain, cerebrospinal fluid, and membranes). Because the current spreads diffusely throughout the conducting medium, it is more difficult to locate the source of the recorded signal and the electrode position has little effect on the morphology of the recorded evoked potential (see Fig. 39.7).[41,42] As the distance between the recording electrode and the neural generator increases, the recorded SER becomes smaller. More responses have to be averaged to record far-field potentials (several thousand) than near-field potentials (50–100).[41,42]

SERs also may be described as cortical or subcortical in origin. Cortical SERs are generated by the arrival at the cortex of the volley of action potentials generated by stimulating the sensory system. Because they are recorded as a near-field potential, they are typically easy to identify by elapsed time, waveform morphology, and amplitude. Subcortical responses may arise from many different structures depending on the type of response, including peripheral nerves, spinal cord, brainstem, thalamus, cranial nerves, and others. Cortical SERs are usually recorded from scalp electrodes placed according to the standard 10 to 20 system for EEG recordings (see Fig. 39.3). Subcortical evoked responses also may be recorded as far-field potentials from scalp electrodes or, as appropriate, from electrodes placed over the spinal column or peripheral nerve.

Evoked potentials of all types (sensory or motor) are described in terms of latency and amplitude (see Fig. 39.7). Latency is defined as the time measured from the application of the stimulus to the onset or peak (depending on convention used) of the response. The amplitude is simply the voltage of the recorded response. According to convention, deflections below the baseline are labeled "positive (P)," and deflections above the baseline are labeled "negative (N)." Because amplitude and latency change with recording circumstances, normal values must be established for each neurologic monitoring laboratory, and may differ from values recorded in other laboratories.

SERs used for intraoperative monitoring include SSEPs, BAEPs, and rarely VEPs. For all these techniques, cortical recording electrodes are placed on the scalp, using the same standard 10 to 20 system as for recording the EEG, whereas recordings for subcortical and peripheral signals are placed in various standardized anatomic locations. The surgical incision and the need for sterility may necessitate nonstandard electrode placements. Such deviations must be considered when interpreting baseline and subsequent SERs. In the case of MEPs, stimulating electrodes also are placed according to the 10 to 20 system of electrode placement, but over the motor cortex instead. Recording electrodes may be placed over the spinal column, peripheral nerve, and (most commonly) innervated muscle.

One of the most important principles of recording SERs intraoperatively is that reproducible, reliable tracings must be obtained at baseline before any intervention likely to cause changes in the evoked response. If good-quality tracings with identifiable waveforms cannot be recorded and reproduced at baseline, evoked-response monitoring would be of little use in monitoring the integrity of the CNS intraoperatively. If significant variability exists, or waveforms are difficult to identify, it will be impossible intraoperatively to distinguish SER changes that are clinically significant from a preexisting baseline variability of waveforms. When good, reproducible responses cannot be recorded at baseline, monitoring should not be used for clinical decision making. It is helpful to comment on the quality of the baseline SERs during the preincision time out so that the whole team is better positioned to put changes in SERs into context.

Somatosensory-Evoked Potentials. SSEPs are recorded after electric stimulation of a peripheral mixed nerve using needles or surface gel electrodes. SSEP responses consist of short-latency and long-latency waveforms. Cortical short-latency SSEPs are most commonly recorded intraoperatively because they are less influenced by changes in anesthetic drug levels. The pathways involved in the generation of upper extremity short-latency SSEPs include large-fiber sensory nerves with their cell bodies in the dorsal root ganglia and central processes traveling rostrally in the ipsilateral posterior column of the spinal cord synapsing in the dorsal column nuclei at the cervicomedullary junction (first-order fibers), second-order fibers crossing and traveling to the contralateral thalamus through the medial lemniscus, and third-order fibers from the thalamus to the frontoparietal sensorimotor cortex. These primary cortical-evoked responses, which are recordable with most anesthetic techniques, result from the earliest electric activity generated by the cortical neurons and are thought to arise from the postcentral sulcus parietal neurons. The longer-latency secondary cortical waves are thought to arise in the association cortex. These responses have much greater variability in an awake patient,[42] habituate rapidly on repetitive stimulation,[41] and are only poorly reproducible during general anesthesia. Cortical SSEPs other than the primary cortical response are not monitored or interpreted intraoperatively because they are severely altered by general anesthesia.[41]

Although most evidence indicates that upper extremity evoked potentials are conducted rostrally in the spinal cord through dorsal column pathways, some data suggest that lower extremity SSEPs are conducted at least partially by the lateral funiculus.[43] Stimulation of the posterior tibial nerve or common peroneal nerve at or above motor threshold activates group I fibers that synapse and travel rostrally through the dorsal spinocerebellar tract. After synapsing in nucleus Z at the spinomedullary junction, the pathway crosses and projects onto the ventral posterolateral thalamic nucleus.[44] This pathway difference is important because the dorsal lateral funiculus is supplied primarily by the anterior spinal artery, the artery that also supplies the descending motor pathway and neurons in the spinal cord. Manipulations, such as distraction of the spinal column to correct scoliosis, which may secondarily compress or distort radicular blood supply to the anterior spinal cord, should cause changes in the SSEP in the event blood supply is reduced to critical levels. This hypothesis is verified by the very low, but not zero, incidence of postoperative paraplegia on awakening without any intraoperative changes in SSEPs.

For SSEP recordings with median nerve stimulation, recording electrodes are first placed at Erb point, just above the midpoint of the clavicle. This point overlies the brachial plexus, and signals recorded here assure the clinician that the stimulus is actually being delivered properly to the patient. The next electrode is placed midline posteriorly over the neck at level of the second cervical vertebra, relatively near the dorsal column nuclei. Signals recorded here ensure proper transmission of the response from the peripheral nervous system into the spinal cord and rostral along the spinal cord to the lower medulla. The final electrodes are placed on the scalp overlying the sensory (parietal) cortex contralateral to the stimulated limb. Signals recorded here ensure the integrity of the pathway through the brainstem, thalamus, and internal capsule, and may assess adequacy of CBF in this area of the cortex.[45-49]

TABLE 39.1 Generators of Somatosensory-Evoked Potentials After Median Nerve Stimulation

Peak	Generators
N9 (EP)	Brachial plexus*
N11	Posterior columns or spinal roots
N13/P13	Dorsal column nuclei*
N14, 15	Brainstem or thalamus
N19/P22	Parietal sensory cortex*

*Indicates sites commonly recorded during surgical procedures. All other waveforms indicated are not commonly monitored.

To record SSEPs after posterior tibial nerve stimulation, electrodes are placed first over the popliteal fossa to ensure proper stimulus delivery to the nervous system. Electrodes also may be placed over the lower lumbar spine to ensure proper transmission of the signal into the spinal cord itself, but this site is not commonly used because of the proximity of sterile surgical incisions. Cervical spine and scalp recording electrodes are placed in a similar fashion as described previously, although different locations may be used as required by the surgical incision. More invasive recording methods, such as epidural electrodes, also may be used intraoperatively.

Purported generators for short-latency SSEPs are listed in Table 39.1 and shown in Fig. 39.8.[41,50] Induction of anesthesia, a patient's neurological disease or age, and use of different recording electrode locations (montage), necessitated by the surgical incision, may significantly alter the appearance of the SSEP. In these cases, attribution of a particular generator to a given wave on the tracing may be quite difficult. During neurologic monitoring, such precision is not needed, and recorded waveforms are compared with tracings obtained at baseline and during earlier portions of the surgical procedure. After lower limb stimulation, absolute latencies are increased because of the greater distance the response to stimulation must travel along the peripheral sensory nerve and spinal cord. Interpeak latencies (see Fig. 39.7) also are evaluated to assess specific conduction times, such as N9 to N14 conduction time, reflecting transmission time from the brachial plexus to brainstem, or N14 to N20 conduction time, reflecting transmission time between the dorsal column nuclei and the primary sensory cortex.[51] Latencies are also significantly affected by age at both extremes of life and many neurologic disorders.

Brainstem Auditory-Evoked Potentials. BAEPs are produced in the diagnostic laboratory by delivering repetitive clicks or tones via headphones. Headphones are not practical for surgical monitoring of neurosurgical procedures, and click stimuli are delivered using foam ear inserts attached to stimulus transducers (Fig. 39.9). Stimulus intensity is usually set at 60 to 70 dB above the patient's click-hearing threshold, although, practically speaking, many intraoperative laboratories establish monitoring after induction of anesthesia and instead begin with a stimulus

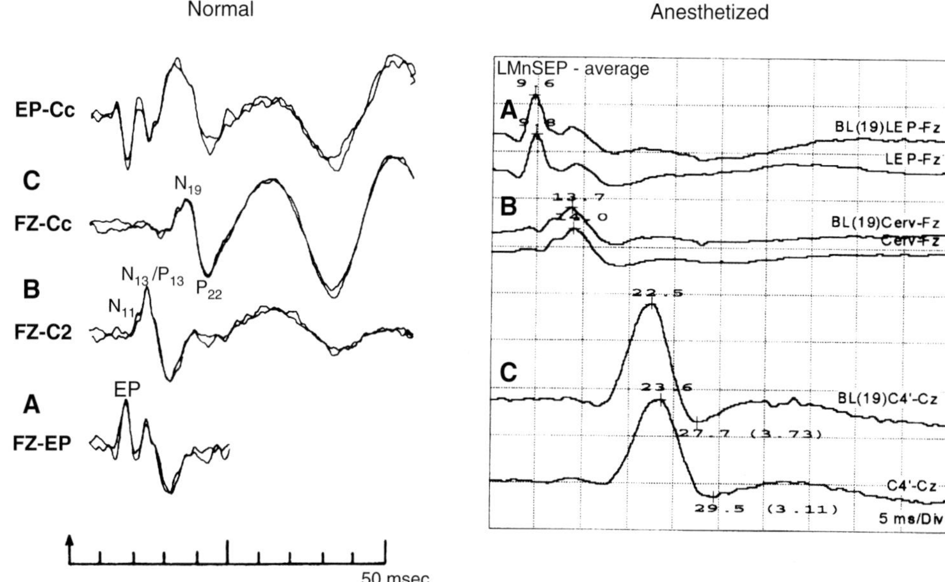

Fig. 39.8 Short-latency somatosensory-evoked potentials *(SEP)* produced by stimulation of the left median nerve *(LMn)* at the wrist. The ability to identify each of the labeled peaks shown in the tracing from the awake patient is compromised by the anesthetic state and use of different recording electrode locations (A–C). Corresponding tracings are labeled with the same letter. (From Chiappa KH, Ropper AH. Evoked potentials in clinical medicine. *N Engl J Med*. 1982;306:1205.)

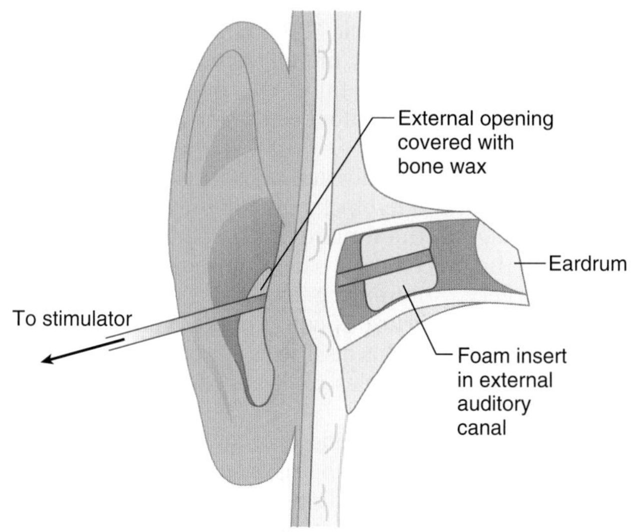

Fig. 39.9 Schematic of brainstem auditory-evoked potential-stimulating apparatus. Loud click stimuli are delivered directly to the eardrum through the ear insert.

intensity of 90 dB nHL (normal hearing level). The duration of the click is approximately 100 μs, and the stimulus is given usually 10 to 15 times per second. Clicks are delivered using different "polarities"—that is, the click may cause initial movement of the tympanic membrane away from the transducer (rarefaction) or toward the transducer (condensation). Use of these two different methods commonly produces very different waveforms, amplitudes, and latencies in individual patients, and the method that produces the largest reproducible response is chosen. If stimulus artifact is a serious problem, clicks of alternating polarity may be used to decrease the artifact, but the waveforms produced are an average of those produced by either stimulating technique alone and may be more difficult to monitor.

Rate and intensity of stimulus delivery affect BAEPs.[41,52] Unilateral stimulation is used because responses from the other ear, which may remain normal during surgery, may obscure any abnormal responses from the monitored ear. Recording electrodes are placed on the lobe of the stimulated ear and on the top of the head (vertex).[52] White noise may be delivered to the contralateral ear to prevent bone conduction from stimulation of the monitored ear from producing an evoked response from the contralateral ear. On average, 500 to 2000 repetitions are required because BAEPs recorded from the scalp are far-field potentials and extremely small (often <0.3 μV).[41,52]

Peaks in recordings of BAEPs are labeled I through VII; the purported neural generators for these peaks and the auditory pathway are shown in Fig. 39.10. The anatomic auditory pathway would predict that BAEP monitoring would be most useful for surgical procedures in the posterior fossa that risk hearing or structures in the upper medulla, pons, and midbrain. As with other SERs, amplitude, absolute latencies, and interpeak latencies are evaluated to assess integrity of the auditory system, localize the functional defect when it occurs, and assess peripheral and central conduction times. Because waves VI and VII are inconsistent and variable, they are not routinely monitored,[52] and most articles reporting use of BAEP for surgical monitoring in the operating room monitor waves only up to wave V.[53-55]

Visual-Evoked Potentials. VEPs are recorded after monocular stimulation with recording electrodes over the occipital, parietal, and central scalp.[56] Flash stimulation of the retina using light-emitting diodes embedded in soft plastic goggles through closed eyelids or as needed via contact lenses with built-in light-emitting diodes is provided. VEPs are cortical SERs, which vary with the type of stimulus, part of the retina stimulated, degree of pupil

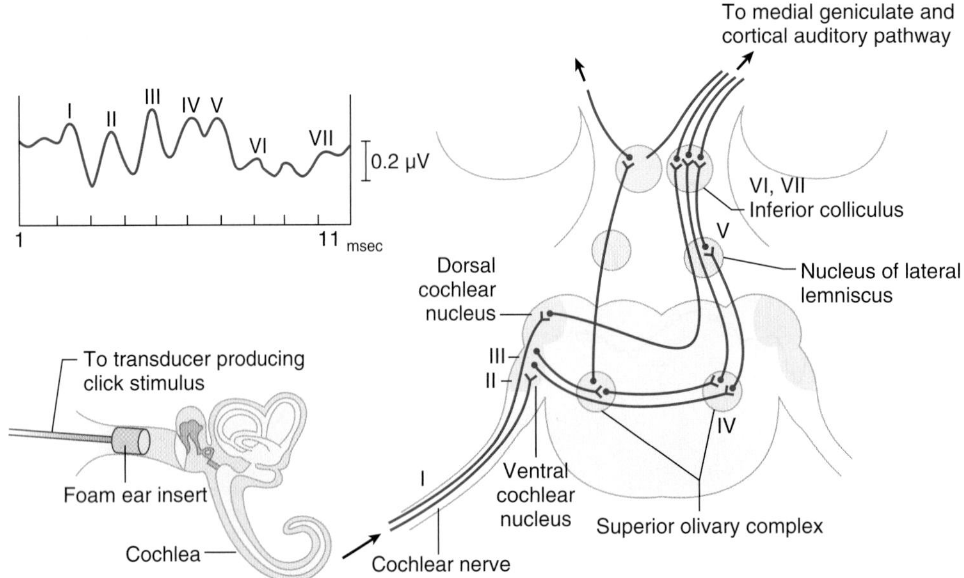

Fig. 39.10 Schematic of auditory neural pathway. The brainstem auditory-evoked potential is initiated by stimulation of the cochlea with a broadband click stimulus given through an ear insert in the external auditory canal. Neural generators of the brainstem auditory-evoked potential peaks are shown.

dilation, and patient's attention level.[41] Because some of these factors change commonly and even constantly during the course of every anesthetic, VEPs would be expected to be highly variable during surgery even when no surgical trespass on the visual system occurs. VEPs are the least commonly used evoked-response monitoring technique intraoperatively. However, some investigators have recently been able to generate reproducible intraoperative VEPs using multiple red light-emitting diodes embedded in a soft silicone disk placed directly on the cornea for stimulating the retina.[56] This technique may allow for further studies which will determine the clinical utility of this modality. However, flash stimuli generate potentials in all areas of the primary visual cortex at once making it difficult detect an injury to a small area of cortex.

Motor-Evoked Potentials. MEPs are generated most commonly by the application of a transcranial train of electric stimuli, and responses are recorded at various points along the spinal column, peripheral nerve, and innervated muscle.

Transcranial Motor-Evoked Potentials. Monitoring of the integrity of the motor tracts within the spinal cord is a technique with great potential benefit, and even during the relative short history of MEP monitoring, there are reported cases of loss of MEPs with preservation of the SSEP.[57-62] This technique is used extensively in spinal surgery, in which transmission across the operative field can be assessed, and in aortic surgery, with the potential for impairment of the blood supply to the vulnerable anterior spinal cord. Relative to SER monitoring, MEP monitoring is quite invasive and, in the case of transcranial stimulation, uses much higher stimulus intensity (≥400 V). Special stimulation techniques may be used to obtain transcranial MEPs (tcMEPs) from young children or adults with some degree of neurologic compromise at baseline.

Several variants of MEP monitoring exist. The most common method involves transcranial electrical stimulation. During transcranial electric MEP monitoring, stimulating electrodes (usually small, metallic screw-type electrodes similar to those used in fetal monitoring) are placed into the scalp overlying the motor cortex, and a train of electric stimuli (usually around 400–500 V) is applied to the scalp. This stimulation definitely activates muscles of mastication, and bilateral bite-blocks must be placed to prevent serious damage to the tongue during stimulation. Alternatively, if the precentral gyrus or motor strip is exposed during surgery, stimulating electrodes may be placed directly onto the cortex. Because approximately 90% of the transcranial stimulus dissipates across scalp and skull, typical stimulus intensities of direct cortical stimulation are 40 to 50 V.

Both stimulating methods also activate surrounding cortical structures and subcortical white matter pathways (sensory and motor). In fact, tcMEPs can frequently be recorded from patients with cerebral palsy, despite the disruption of their cortical neuronal architecture. Distal antidromic propagation of the transcranially applied stimulus is blocked by synapses in all of the ascending sensory pathways. The stimulus is propagated easily orthodromically through descending motor pathways. It is important to note that only the largest diameter fibers, 2% to 3% of all fibers in the corticospinal tract, propagate the impulses associated with tcMEPs. The evoked responses may be recorded over the spinal cord, the peripheral nerve, and, most commonly, the muscle itself. To enhance the MEP, these responses may be averaged in the same manner as SERs, but averaging is almost always unnecessary. Activation of the corticospinal tract well below the motor cortex may limit the utility of tcMEP to assess the adequacy of CBF to the motor cortex, because activation may be distal to the site of ischemia and part of a different vascular bed.

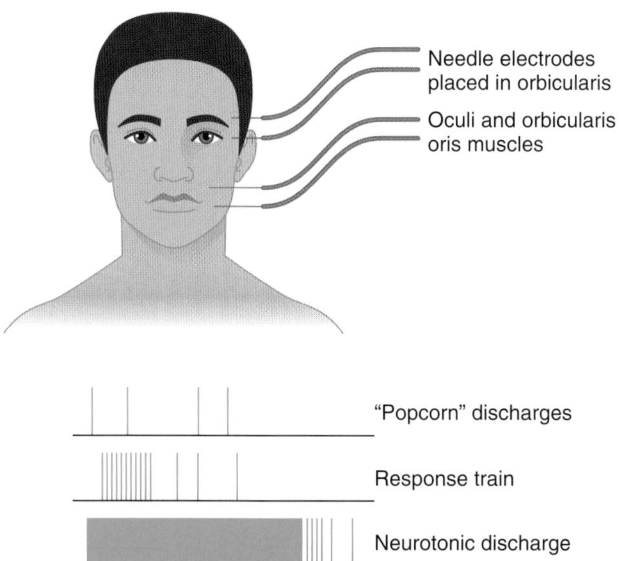

Fig. 39.11 Schematic of facial nerve monitoring and typical responses seen during surgery.

Electromyography. Intraoperative monitoring of EMG responses generated by cranial and peripheral motor nerves allows early detection of surgically induced nerve damage and assessment of level of nerve function intraoperatively. In these cases, the ability of a nerve to produce a response in the innervated muscle is used to assess the health of a cranial or peripheral nerve at risk during surgery. Recordings are made from either surface (electrocardiogram or gold cup) electrodes or needle electrodes placed directly in the innervated muscle of interest. Sensitivity of EMG recordings is best if recordings are made from needles within the muscle itself. Surface electrodes and, to a lesser extent, subdermal needle electrodes may completely miss neurotonic discharges that indicate damage to a nerve.[63] The most experience with this monitoring modality has been obtained during facial nerve monitoring.

EMG monitoring may be either active or passive. During active monitoring, a cranial or peripheral nerve is stimulated electrically, and the evoked EMG (compound muscle action potential) response from the muscle is recorded. Stimulation of the nerve proximal to the operative area or tumor can be used to assess functional integrity of the nerve.[64] Nerve function also may be assessed by noting the intensity of nerve stimulus needed to evoke a muscle response and by the morphology of the compound muscle action potential. Nerve function may be monitored passively during surgery with continuous recording of all generated responses from innervated muscle groups. "Popcorn" EMG discharges are produced by simple, benign contact with the monitored nerve. Response trains are produced with more significant nerve irritation. Neurotonic discharges are produced by significant nerve irritation or damage or both (Fig. 39.11).[65] When these EMG responses reach a certain voltage threshold, they are usually converted into audible signals that provide immediate feedback to the surgeon and warn of impending nerve damage in real time. Real-time feedback is key because density and frequency of neurotonic discharges may correlate with degree of postoperative nerve dysfunction, as shown by data obtained from patients undergoing resection of acoustic tumors.[64] One caveat of EMG monitoring is that sharp section of a nerve may produce no EMG discharge at all.

Intraoperative monitoring of the motor component of other cranial nerves also has been successfully performed. EMG monitoring of the trigeminal nerve can be accomplished with electrodes placed over or in the temporalis or masseter muscles. Trigeminal nerve motor monitoring has been used during nerve section for tic douloureux to ensure preservation of the motor branch of the trigeminal nerve and in combination with facial nerve monitoring during resection of large posterior fossa lesions.[65] Using recording electrodes placed in or over the trapezius or sternocleidomastoid muscles, the spinal accessory nerve has been successfully monitored during resection of large meningiomas, glomus jugulare tumors, and neck carcinomas.[65] EMG monitoring of the hypoglossal nerve with needle electrodes placed in the tongue has been infrequently used for large posterior fossa lesions and clivus tumors.[65] EMG monitoring of the eye muscles can be performed using tiny hook wires for recording; however it is rarely used in practice.

Monitoring of peripheral motor nerves has been performed by placing needle electrodes in or over the muscles innervated by nerves that traverse the operative area and are at risk from the planned surgical procedure. Auditory feedback from EMG monitoring can warn the surgeon of unexpected surgical trespass of the nerve, help locate a nerve within the field (e.g., during untethering of the spinal cord), and localize the level of any conduction block or delay. Because radiculopathies have been reported to occur after spine surgery, particularly because of incorrect pedicle screw placement, EMG monitoring of peripheral nerves has been used in patients undergoing spine surgery to decrease the risk of nerve root injury during the procedure.[65] During pedicle screw placement, the surgeon can stimulate the screw directly with a small amount of current. If EMG responses are produced with only a small amount of current, the screw has likely been placed outside the bony pedicle.

Reactions to Intraoperative Changes in Monitored Responses

Intraoperative changes in evoked responses, such as decreased amplitude, increased latency, or complete loss of the waveform, may result from surgical trespass, such as retractor placement or ischemia, or they may reflect systemic changes, such as changes in anesthetic drug administration, temperature changes, or hypoperfusion. When these changes are detected and considered to be significant, the surgeon or anesthesiologist can make changes to relieve or lessen the insult to the monitored pathway (and presumably surrounding neural structures). Interventions by the anesthesiologist are directed at improving perfusion to the nervous tissue at risk and include increasing arterial blood pressure, especially if induced hypotension is used, or if the patient's blood pressure has decreased significantly from preoperative values; transfusion, if significant anemia is present; volume expansion; augmentation of cardiac output; and normalization of abnormal arterial blood gas tensions. Changes in evoked potentials after retractor

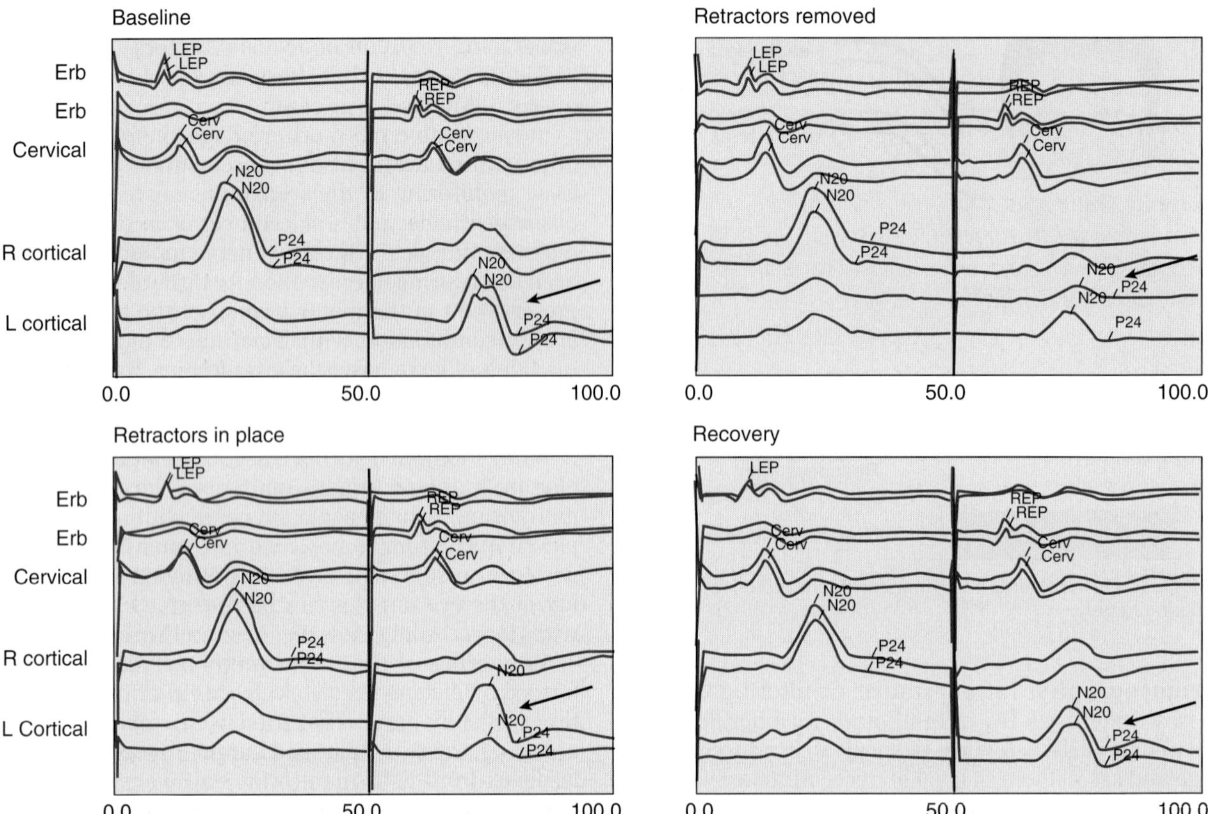

Fig. 39.12 Somatosensory-evoked potentials during aneurysm clipping. Responses generated by the cortex at risk are indicated by arrows. Baseline, after retractor placement, after retractor removal, and recovery traces are shown. The initial evoked response change occurred 4 minutes after retractor placement. Note loss of voltage of cortical-evoked response caused by inadvertent compression of the middle cerebral artery. *Cerv*, Cervical; *LEP*, left Erb point; *REP*, right Erb point.

placement during a craniotomy or after compression of the blood supply to the spinal cord from spinal column distraction promptly allow the surgeon and the anesthesiologist to make appropriate changes to the operative procedure and anesthetic management that may prevent or minimize any postoperative neurologic deficit (Fig. 39.12). It is imperative that clear communication occur between all parties in the operating room when significant intraoperative changes in evoked potentials occur. If expected results of an intervention are not observed the underlying hypothesis as to the cause of the changes must be reevaluated. This can only happen when lines of communication are open between all participants.[66]

Tolerance limits for degree of change in evoked response signals or duration of complete loss of waveform before permanent neurologic dysfunction are becoming better defined, and position statements have been issued by the American Society of Neurophysiologic Monitoring (http://www.asnm.org/page/PositionStatements). Tolerance limits for degree of change are especially unclear for tcMEPs. Such ambiguity is common among intraoperative monitors. Although we do know that increased frequency and duration of ST segment depression during coronary bypass surgery is associated with an increased risk of perioperative infarction, exact limits for degree and duration of ST segment depression for surgery do not exist, and likely vary significantly from patient to patient. The same problem may be exhibited with neurologic monitors.

Many centers using intraoperative SER monitoring define decreases in amplitude of 50% or more from baseline associated with a less than 10% prolongation in latency as clinically significant SER changes. Uncorrected, such changes are associated in clinical series and in case reports with onset of new postoperative neurologic deficits. As a result, such changes are immediately investigated. In practice, any SER changes directly associated with a surgical event are considered clinically significant, however, even if the magnitude of change is less than just described. Changes in SER that do not progress to complete loss of the waveform are less likely to be associated with a major new postoperative neurologic deficit. Complete loss of the SER waveform intraoperatively without recovery is highly likely to be associated with a major new deficit. If the SER recovers either spontaneously or after intraoperative interventions, the likelihood of neurologic injury depends on the procedure, the duration of the SER loss, and on whether the SER is mainly used to judge integrity of adjacent unmonitored structures. These problems are illustrated in one study of intracranial aneurysm surgery in which SSEPs were monitored to predict/prevent postoperative motor deficits. Loss of the SSEP waveform for less than 15 minutes was not associated with a new permanent neurologic deficit, whereas complete loss of the SSEP for longer periods was increasingly likely to reflect permanent neurologic injury, even if the response recovered completely to its intraoperative baseline during surgery.[67]

Clinical Applications of Neurologic Monitoring

NEUROVASCULAR SURGERY (ALSO SEE CHAPTERS 56 AND 57)

Extracranial Neurovascular Surgery: Carotid Vascular Surgery (Monitors: Electroencephalogram, Somatosensory-Evoked Potentials, Transcranial Doppler, Cerebral Oximetry)

Carotid vascular surgery typically requires transient interruption of blood flow to the brain through the affected carotid artery. Although the risk of stroke associated with carotid vascular surgery has been declining,[68] the residual risk varies greatly based on the indication for the procedure. It is lowest for asymptomatic patients and highest after a recent revascularization for ischemic stroke.[69]

Electroencephalogram. The use of the EEG as a monitor of the adequacy of hemispheric blood flow during carotid endarterectomy has been established for many years. In a large series of patients undergoing carotid endarterectomy at the Mayo Clinic,[33] the EEG was compared with regional CBF using the Xe washout method. This study validated the EEG as an indicator of the adequacy of regional CBF.

Normal CBF in gray and white matter averages 50 mL/100 g/min. With most anesthetic techniques, the EEG begins to become abnormal when CBF decreases to 20 mL/100 g/min. Cellular survival is not threatened until CBF decreases to 12 mL/100 g/min. The difference in blood flow between when the EEG becomes abnormal and the blood flow at which cellular damage begins to occur provides a rational basis for monitoring the EEG during carotid surgery. In many cases, prompt detection of EEG changes may allow intervention (e.g., shunting, increasing cerebral perfusion pressure) to restore CBF before onset of permanent neurologic damage.

Serious intraoperative reduction in cerebral oxygen supply may result from surgical factors (e.g., carotid cross-clamping) that are usually beyond the anesthesiologist's control, and from factors that the anesthesiologist can correct. Reduction in CBF produced by hyperventilation, hypotension, or temporary occlusion of major blood vessels may be corrected by reducing ventilation, by restoring normal blood pressure, or, in the case of temporary vessel occlusion, by increasing blood pressure above normal. Because the EEG may readily detect cerebral ischemia, continuous EEG monitoring may be used to evaluate the effectiveness of therapy instituted to correct ischemia.

Should the patient undergoing carotid endarterectomy have EEG monitoring? That question cannot be answered based on available data. EEG monitoring provides information about CBF that would not otherwise be available. The clinician has an opportunity to intervene to increase inadequate blood flow when it occurs. Anecdotally, many clinicians have found such monitoring useful and use it routinely. Population studies do not support routine use, reflecting the fact that strokes in carotid vascular surgery are infrequent and the majority are caused by embolism, which may not be adequately treated by simply increasing CBF.

In a large series of patients undergoing carotid endarterectomy with selective shunting who were monitored with 16-channel unprocessed EEG, no patient awakened with a new neurologic deficit that was not predicted by EEG.[70] Transient, correctable EEG changes were not associated with stroke. Persistent changes were associated with stroke. This study had no comparison group, however, analyzing stroke rate when EEG monitoring was not used during surgery. Conversely, in the North American Symptomatic Carotid Endarterectomy Trial and the European Carotid Surgery Trial, retrospective comparisons of patients receiving EEG monitoring and patients not receiving EEG monitoring failed to show a significant difference in outcome.[71,72]

Even more difficult to prove is that EEG monitoring is useful when all patients are shunted during carotid clamping. Such monitoring has detected correctable shunt malfunction, and investigators have described hypotension-related EEG changes in patients with critical stenoses and poor collateral circulation.[73] Advocates of selective shunting based on EEG (or other monitoring) criteria claim that inserting a shunt unnecessarily through a region of diseased vessel would surely increase embolization. A multicenter study of 1495 carotid endarterectomies provides some evidence that shunting of patients without evidence of decreased cerebral perfusion increases the incidence of stroke more than sixfold.[74] Although this study and other more recent studies[75-77] advocate that selective shunting using some form of monitoring of the adequacy of CBF should improve perioperative stroke rate, an analysis by the Cochrane Stroke Group[78] failed to show sufficient evidence to advocate for routine shunting, selective shunting, or even no shunting at all. In addition, this review failed to demonstrate that any type of monitoring for cerebral ischemia was superior to another.

Processed EEG also has been used during carotid vascular surgery. Two issues affect the efficacy and reliability of processed EEG as a monitor for cerebral ischemia. First, what is the minimum number of channels (or areas of the brain) to be monitored? Clinical experience and clinical investigations suggest that four channels (two per side) are the minimum number of channels for adequate sensitivity and specificity.[34] When a limited number of channels were compared with 16-channel EEG monitoring, 100% sensitivity and specificity were obtained using 2 channels per hemisphere, provided that those channels monitored the middle cerebral artery territory. These results were obtained with a frontoparietal channel combined with a frontotemporal channel.[34]

The second issue is the experience level of the observer monitoring the processed EEG. Is a dedicated, experienced technician or electroencephalographer needed? In a study addressing this question, the 16-channel unprocessed EEG monitored by a dedicated technician was compared with a processed EEG reviewed by three anesthesiologists of differing levels of experience with processed EEG.[35] The three anesthesiologists interpreted the tracings without knowledge of the case. They were presented only with the written trace with an indication of the point at which the carotid artery was clamped. In these cases, the most important interpretation pitfall to avoid is the "false-negative" pattern. If the clinician interprets the EEG as showing adequate CBF when in fact it does not, the surgeon may fail to shunt

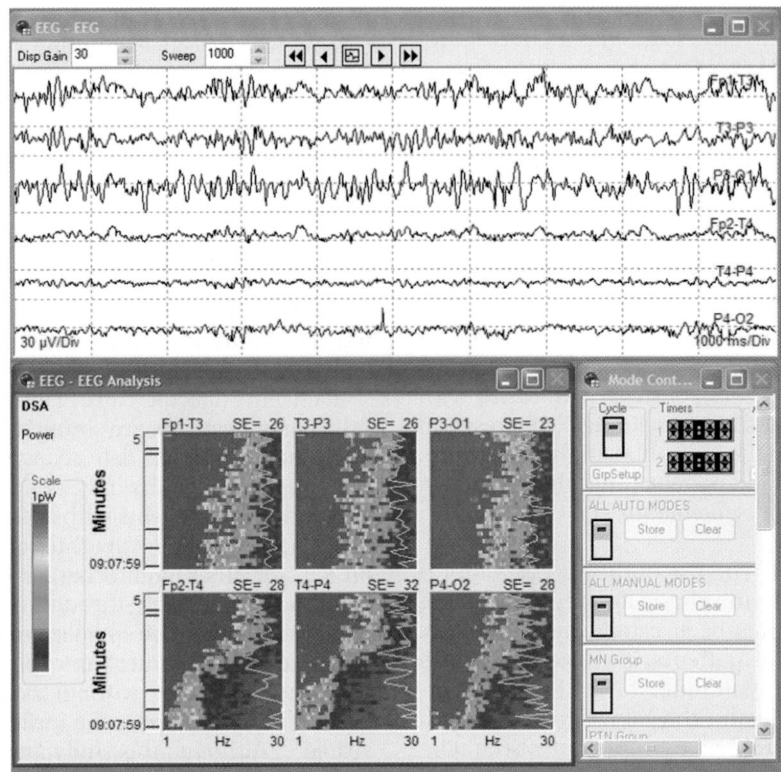

Fig. 39.13 Hemispheric ischemia after clamping of the internal carotid artery. The top panel shows three channels of electroencephalogram *(EEG)* for each hemisphere. The right-sided channels (bottom three tracings) show nearly suppressed *EEG* activity due to ischemia. The bottom panel shows the corresponding density spectral array, where *EEG* power in each frequency is coded in color, with red indicating greater power. The oldest data is at the top of each field and the most recent at the bottom. The lower row of three density spectral array *(DSA)* panels corresponds to the right-sided *EEG* leads. Halfway through the panel there is a dramatic reduction in *EEG* power after clamp placement. The bottom spectrum corresponds to the raw *EEG* shown tracings shown in the top panel. (Image courtesy of Reza Gorji, MD.)

an ischemic patient. A false-positive result may be less of a problem because that patient is not ischemic but is given a shunt anyway. In this case, only the risk of emboli from the "unnecessary" shunt is incurred. The positive predictive value of the anesthesiologist correctly interpreting the trace as unchanged after clamping was 91% to 98%, which indicates that the device can be used by novice interpreters with fair accuracy to determine the presence of cerebral ischemia at the time of carotid occlusion (Fig. 39.13).

Somatosensory-Evoked Potentials. SSEP monitoring also has been used to gauge adequacy of CBF to the cerebral cortex and subcortical pathways during carotid vascular surgery.[49,79,80] SSEPs have been found in the laboratory to have a similar but slightly lower threshold for electrical failure compared with the EEG when CBF is reduced. SSEPs are generally intact until the cortical blood flow decreases to less than 15 mL/100 g/min.[47] A recent review (meta-analysis) of shunting during carotid vascular surgery suggests that selective shunting based on SSEP monitoring results in a perioperative stroke rate similar to when EEG monitoring is used as the basis for shunting.[81] However, logic would also suggest that changes in SSEP are unlikely, for example, with ischemia involving the anterior portions of either the frontal or temporal lobe, which could readily be detected by an appropriately placed EEG electrode. There is even less outcome evidence to support the use of SSEPs during carotid surgery than there is for the EEG, but the authors and others have found SSEPs to be useful as a simultaneous monitor with EEG to detect subcortical ischemia.[82]

Transcranial Doppler. TCD monitoring during carotid vascular surgery is based on measurement of two primary parameters—blood flow velocity in the middle cerebral artery and the number of emboli detected in the same artery. The hypothesis justifying the use of this monitoring during carotid vascular surgery has two components: blood flow velocity correlates with CBF, and increasing numbers of emboli increase the likelihood of embolic stroke. Intraoperative use of TCD has not been widely adopted for many reasons. As previously noted, good TCD signals cannot be obtained in up to 20% of individuals who could benefit from monitoring. Also, TCD probe motion during surgery causes major problems with loss of signal or with angle of insonation–induced changes in the relationship between blood flow velocity and blood flow. Nonetheless, multiple series of carotid endarterectomies with TCD monitoring have been reported with good success, quoting a critical blood flow velocity reduction around 50% as indicative of inadequate CBF requiring intervention (shunt or increased blood pressure or both).[83-89] The relationship between emboli count and stroke is better established. Multiple studies conducted in the preoperative, intraoperative, and postoperative periods indicate that higher emboli counts are associated with higher stroke risk and warrant intervention.[83-89] TCD is the only monitor able to detect dangerous hyperemia, also known as normal perfusion pressure breakthrough, after removal of a severe, flow-limiting carotid stenosis. Typically, a sustained doubling of flow velocity after unclamping should prompt the anesthesiologist to consider lowering the blood pressure. There are no good outcome data supporting TCD use intraoperatively, but data regarding emboli count and risk of stroke suggest that if technical issues with probe attachment to the patient can be overcome, TCD may be useful as a predictor of impending stroke in the preoperative, postoperative, and perhaps intraoperative periods.

Cerebral Oximetry (Near-Infrared Spectroscopy). Near-infrared spectroscopy (NIRS) is an attractive monitor during carotid endarterectomy because of its ease of application and lack of training required for interpretation. The hypothesis governing its use is very simple: as oxygen delivery to the brain decreases, oxygen extraction from arterial blood increases, and the oxygen saturation in cerebral venous blood decreases. Multiple case reports and series document the use of cerebral oximetry during neurovascular surgery, but several major questions surrounding use of NIRS during carotid surgery remain unanswered.

The first and most important question is what degree of decrease in oxygen saturation can be tolerated before intervention is necessary. Because most interventions involve some risk (e.g., shunt → emboli, increased BP → myocardial ischemia), the answer to this question is important. The answer does not yet exist, however, and may vary from patient to patient. Two studies in awake patients showed that the saturation value at which any patient would develop symptoms varied from patient to patient,[12,13] and an absolute value that required shunting could not be determined. Another study showed that cerebral oxygen saturation decreased before the EEG developed changes, and the authors used this observation to claim superiority for NIRS monitoring of the brain during carotid surgery.[90] This finding should not be surprising, however, because function of the brain (in this case, electric function) does not fail until increased extraction of oxygen no longer meets metabolic demands for the tissue. If metabolic demands are being met by increased extraction, it is unclear that intervention is needed.

Finally, a study by Friedell and colleagues[91] compared NIRS with EEG and SSEP monitoring during carotid surgery. In 24 of 323 patients, significant differences were observed between NIRS and monitors of electric function. Seventeen patients showed no changes in electric function with significant decreases in cerebral oxygen saturation. In seven patients, no change in cerebral oxygen saturation occurred despite significant change in the EEG and SSEP. The latter finding may be due to the fact that NIRS and EEG/SSEP monitor different vascular territories. These data in combination with the data from studies in awake patients suggest that use of NIRS alone during carotid vascular surgery may be inappropriate. In addition, an aggregate of studies and case reports available in the literature suggests that there is no clear cutoff value of regional oxygen saturation which would mandate shunt placement or increasing the cerebral perfusion pressure.

Intracranial Neurovascular Surgery (Monitors: Somatosensory-Evoked Potentials, Motor-Evoked Potentials)

Somatosensory-Evoked Potentials. SSEPs have been extensively studied during cerebral aneurysm surgery. During these procedures, the surgical incision and brain retraction diminishes the utility of placing EEG scalp or brain surface electrodes that could detect cerebral ischemia in at-risk cortex. Recording electrodes placed on the surface of the brain have been used successfully, but they are commonly considered “in the way” by neurosurgeons. Thus EEG is typically used only to confirm metabolic suppression during temporary clip placement. Scalp electrodes for SSEP monitoring may be placed more easily, although the recording montage is frequently not the same as that used in an awake patient.

For aneurysms involving the anterior cerebral circulation, SSEP monitoring has an excellent, but not perfect, record for predicting postoperative neurologic function. Most patients without surgically induced SSEP changes during the procedure awaken with an unchanged neurologic examination. Patients with significant SSEP changes that do not revert to normal awaken with a new neurologic deficit. Patients with significant intraoperative SSEP changes that return to normal may show at least a transient postoperative deficit, with the severity and duration of that deficit increasing as the severity of the SSEP change increases. Many authors have reported significant utility of SSEP monitoring in detecting improper aneurysm clip placement (see Fig. 39.12) and in guiding intraoperative blood pressure management, particularly in patients already showing, or at significant risk for, vasospasm after subarachnoid hemorrhage.[48,92-97] The same success cannot be reported, however, for posterior circulation aneurysms. In these cases, many areas of the cortex and subcortical structures are at risk for damage that cannot be monitored at all by somatosensory pathway function. A significant false-negative monitoring pattern exists for these patients, but changes can still be detected when a surgical insult is sufficiently severe to involve large portions of the brain.[98-101]

An important concern during aneurysm surgery is injury to perforating vessels near the aneurysm, which risks damage to subcortical pathways in the internal capsule and may account for half the new neurologic deficits immediately postoperatively.[102] Anatomically, the motor pathway runs anterior to the sensory pathway in the internal capsule and is at greater risk if the anterior choroidal artery, lenticulostriate perforator vessels, or even perforating branches of the anterior cerebral artery are injured during dissection and clip placement. Two concerns need to be addressed if tcMEP is to be incorporated successfully in these cases. First, motion caused by stimulation needs to be minimized to not interfere with the surgery. Second and more importantly, stimulus parameters need to be set to limit deep current spread that would activate the corticospinal tract distal to the internal capsule and obscure ischemia of the proximal pathway. The use of longer stimulus trains at intensities close to the motor threshold addresses both concerns[103] and have made tcMEP monitoring a useful adjunct during aneurysm surgery in many centers.[104]

SUPRATENTORIAL INTRACRANIAL NONVASCULAR SURGERY (MONITORS: AWAKE PATIENT, ELECTROENCEPHALOGRAM, SOMATOSENSORY-EVOKED POTENTIALS)

The most comprehensive approach to the problem of functional localization of brain structures that need to be preserved to achieve a good outcome is to perform entire segments of a supratentorial craniotomy in an awake patient, who is undergoing repeated neurologic examinations targeted to assess the eloquent area at risk. Such procedures are typically divided into exposure, mapping, and resection phases, and can be done with the patient entirely awake or awake only during periods when the neurologic examination needs to be assessed.[105] Common to all these approaches is the need for meticulous locoregional anesthesia of the scalp at the craniotomy site and the pin sites of the head holder. A second requirement is a patient who is well informed about the awake parts of the procedure and willing and able to cooperate. Dexmedetomidine, propofol, and remifentanil are the agents most frequently incorporated into the anesthetic regimens for awake craniotomy.[106] Complications of awake craniotomy include nausea and vomiting, respiratory problems, and "tight" brain, but are typically mild and occur in less than 10% of cases in experienced centers. Seizures triggered by cortical stimulation can be stopped by the application of iced saline to the exposed cortex or a small amount of barbiturate or propofol.

Seizure Focus Localization Surgery

Patients with epilepsy who have seizures that generalize from an anatomically distinct focus may benefit greatly from the surgical resection of that seizure focus.[107] Precise localization of a seizure focus is important for achieving the therapeutic objective of seizure control and for minimizing complications from the resection. With sensitive magnetic resonance tomography techniques, neuronavigation, and recordings of typical seizure activity in the awake patient after placement of subdural and depth electrodes, the anatomic location and the appropriate extent of the resection frequently can be determined preoperatively.[108] These developments have diminished the role of intraoperative recordings from the epileptogenic zone using electrocorticography.

Electrocorticography is done by placing a grid of subdural electrodes onto the exposed brain surface and recording spontaneous electric activity. Electrocorticography is constrained by several limitations. The time for such recordings is limited to a few minutes; recordings are limited to interictal discharges, which may not correlate with the epileptogenic focus; and recordings need to be obtained from a brain that is under the effects of general anesthetic agents, which alter the EEG.

To provide good conditions during the recording, the level of anesthesia is lightened (e.g., by use of a strict nitrous oxide–narcotic technique or low concentrations of volatile anesthetic drugs). Provocative techniques, such as hyperventilation or administration of a small dose of methohexital, may be useful to activate the seizure focus. Intraoperative seizure mapping requires the involvement of an expert electroencephalographer familiar with this technique.

Motor Strip Localization

Electrophysiologic monitoring of the somatosensory system in anesthetized patients can provide a simple anatomic guide to the location of the rolandic fissure, which separates the parietal primary sensory and frontal primary motor cortex. The fissure is located by recording cortical SSEPs from a subdural strip electrode that is placed perpendicular to the presumed location of the fissure. The exact location of the fissure is characterized by a reversal in the polarity of the primary cortical response between the electrodes straddling the fissure, as illustrated in the clinical example in Fig. 39.14. Subsequent placement of the electrode strip onto the primary motor area of the precentral gyrus allows subsequent monitoring of the corticospinal tract through direct cortical stimulation.

POSTERIOR FOSSA SURGERY (MONITORS: BRAINSTEM AUDITORY-EVOKED POTENTIALS, CRANIAL NERVE MONITORING, SOMATOSENORY-EVOKED POTENTIALS, MOTOR-EVOKED POTENTIALS)

Besides the cerebellum, the posterior fossa contains within the narrow space of the brainstem many crucial neural structures, including the following: the ascending and descending sensorimotor pathways; cranial nerve nuclei; cardiorespiratory centers; the reticular activating system; and the neural networks that underlie crucial protective reflexes, such as eye blink, swallowing, gag, and cough. Posterior fossa surgery is not undertaken lightly, and even small injuries can leave significant neurologic deficits. Although some of these neural structures, such as the sensory, voluntary motor, or auditory pathway, can be monitored consistently, intraoperative integrity of other neural structures is frequently only inferred from the well-being of neighboring structures amenable to monitoring.

Microvascular Decompression of Cranial Nerves V, VII, and IX

Microvascular decompression is done most frequently for trigeminal neuralgia (cranial nerve V) in patients who present acceptable medical risks for a posterior fossa craniotomy. More rarely, the same approach is used to treat hemifacial spasm or neurovascular compromise of lower cranial nerves. The surgery entails dissecting along the intracranial portion of the nerve, identifying offending blood vessels that encroach on the nerve, and placing an insulating Teflon pad between vessel and nerve. The surgery risks ischemic damage to perforating vessels arising from the offending arteries and cerebellar retraction–related damage to cranial nerves. The facial and vestibulocochlear nerves are at particular risk for stretch-induced injury caused by medial retraction of the cerebellum. Retraction-induced stretch produces a prolongation of the interpeak latency between peaks I and V of the BAEP waveform, ultimately leading to a complete loss of all waves beyond wave I (Fig. 39.15). Failure to release retraction in a timely manner results in postoperative hearing loss. Such monitoring increases the chances for preserved hearing after microvascular decompression.[109-113] During microvascular decompression of the facial nerve for hemifacial spasm, recent developments using EMG monitoring

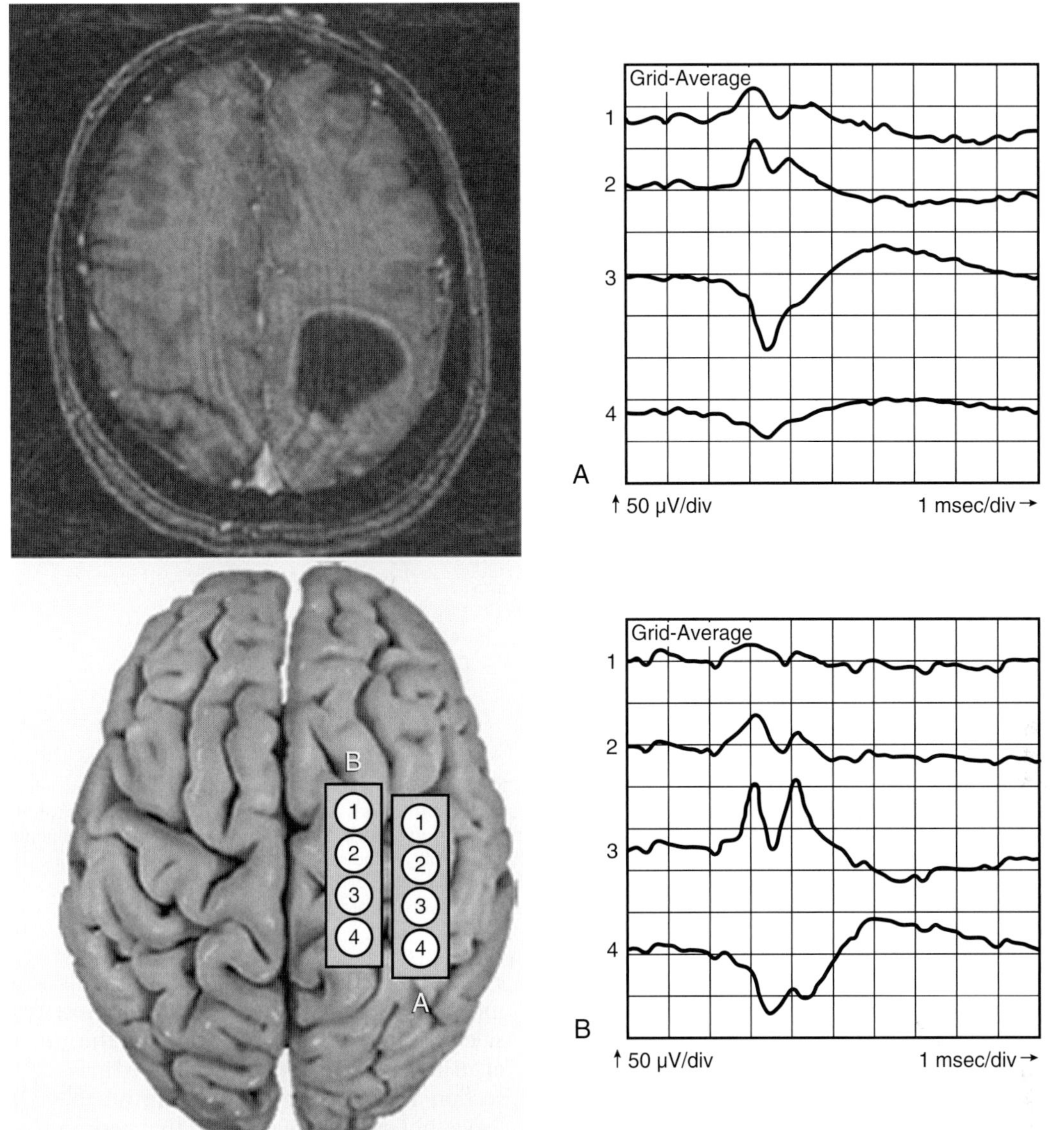

Fig. 39.14 Intraoperative localization of the rolandic fissure separating the primary sensory and motor cortex. The clinical example is from a patient with a large parietal tumor shown in the scan. Two of the recordings made from a four-contact subdural electrode strip are shown. The relative positions of the strip electrode are labeled B and A. In recording A, the primary cortical response from the electrodes anterior to the rolandic fissure shows an upward deflection, whereas the response from electrodes posterior to the fissure shows a downward deflection. Moving the strip electrode anteriorly (recording B) moves this "phase reversal" between electrodes 3 and 4.

have enabled better documentation of the adequacy of nerve decompression and lessen the likelihood of persistence or recurrence of hemifacial spasm postoperatively. This new technique monitors the so-called lateral spread response (LSR) of the facial nerve. A peripheral branch of the facial nerve is stimulated. In the normal patient, this stimulation would not result in a recordable EMG response in a muscle innervated by a different branch of the facial nerve. In patients with hemifacial spasm, EMG responses can be recorded in muscles innervated by a different branch of the facial nerve (an LSR) indicating abnormal crossover of electrical activity. Decompression of the facial nerve has been shown in multiple studies to result in a great decrease or elimination of this LSR, and studies have indicated that elimination of the LSR is highly predictive of immediate postoperative relief of hemifacial spasm.[114]

Vestibular Nerve Schwannoma

Vestibular nerve schwannomas are the most common tumors located in the cerebellopontine angle. Because of the common origin of the cochlear component of cranial nerve VIII and the essentially identical intracranial trajectory of the facial nerve, hearing loss and facial nerve palsy are concerns during surgical resection of these tumors. Size and preoperative auditory function are the best predictors of postoperative hearing.[115] For tumors up to about 1.5 cm in diameter, monitoring of BAEPs can increase the chances of preserving hearing.[116] In addition to BAEPs, the facial nerve is monitored through spontaneous and stimulated EMG. Prospective trials have shown a higher percentage of patients with a functional facial nerve 1 year after surgery if facial nerve monitoring was used. Tonic discharges warn of impending damage caused by stretch or heat

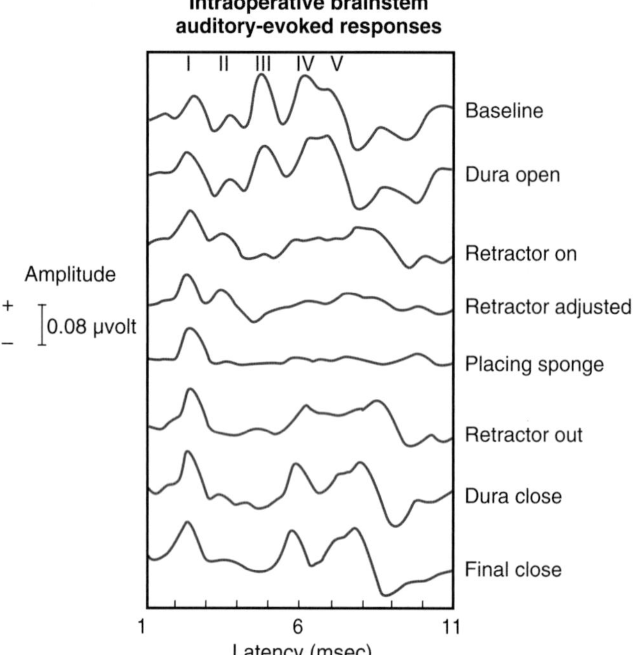

Fig. 39.15 Intraoperative monitoring of brainstem auditory-evoked responses during microvascular decompression. The baseline recording shows the typical five waves of the brainstem auditory-evoked potential response. Intraoperative events are designated to the right of each trace. Placement of the retractor causes a severe increase in latency of wave V even after adjustment of retraction. During placement of the sponge, all waves subsequent to wave I, which originates in the inner ear, are nearly completely lost. Removal of the retractor causes brainstem auditory-evoked potentials to revert toward baseline.

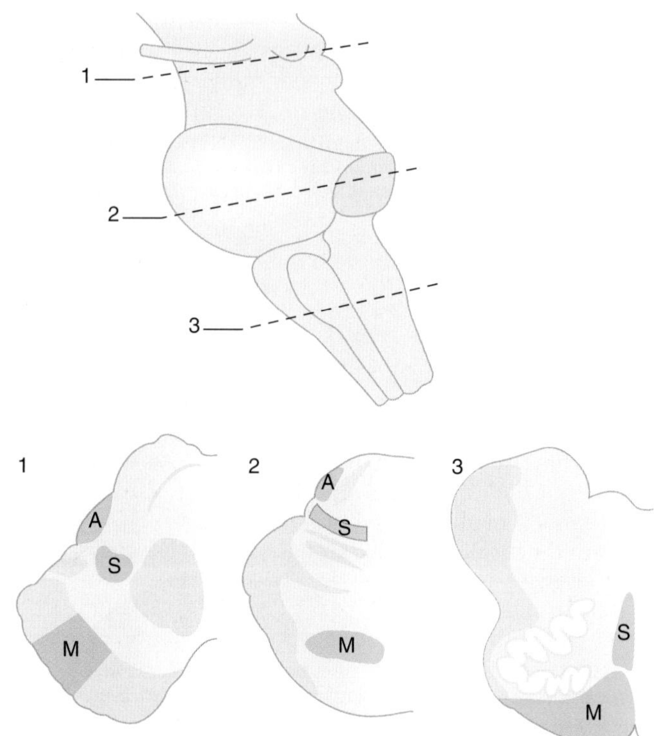

Fig. 39.16 Monitoring of the brainstem with evoked potentials. Evoked potentials monitor specific tracts that encompass defined areas in the brainstem. This is shown in three transverse sections approximately at the levels indicated in the drawings. The areas directly monitored by a given modality are indicated in blue and labeled *M* (motor), *S* (somatosensory), and *A* (auditory). Conclusions about the well-being of the remainder of the brainstem are made by inference from the monitored areas.

(e.g., electrocautery). Sharp section of the nerve may elicit no discharge, and neuromuscular blockade may eliminate the ability to monitor. If the course of the nerve is displaced by the tumor, the surgeon can map its course with a handheld stimulator and real-time auditory feedback.

Other Posterior Fossa Neoplasms

Monitoring for operations on other neoplasms located in the brainstem typically is individualized to each particular case or to the particular surgical approach. EMG and compound muscle action potentials may be recorded not only from the territory of the facial nerve, but also from the tongue to monitor the hypoglossal nerve, and from the glottis through electrodes embedded into a specialized endotracheal tube to monitor the vagus nerve. Such a setup can be used to map the floor of the fourth ventricle functionally, if it is distorted by a tumor.[117] Such monitoring may be insufficient to preserve vital reflexes because only the efferent limb of these reflexes is monitored by recording EMG from innervated muscle. MEPs can be recorded from orbicular oris, or mentalis, to assess the integrity of the facial nerve motor nucleus as well as the proximal facial nerve when tumors prevent visualization of the proximal portion of cranial nerve VII. MEPs can also be recorded from tongue as well. Obtaining these responses relies on placement of additional stimulating electrodes and optimization of stimulating conditions.

Use of neurologic monitoring for brainstem ischemia, although done in some centers, is not well documented or supported by clinical studies. Global well-being of the brainstem may be monitored by combining multiple modalities of evoked potentials, such as BAEPs, SSEPs, and MEPs. Each modality monitors a function whose integrity would be considered important in its own right for the functional outcome of an individual patient. As illustrated in Fig. 39.16, the cross-section monitored by combining all these modalities still leaves out crucial areas. Given that perfusion occurs through perforating vessels, it is easy to see that monitoring may indicate that all is well or, more likely, that a therapeutic intervention was helpful in restoring function, when clinically the patient is still left with a significant deficit. This occurrence invalidates neither monitoring nor the therapeutic intervention, but indicates only that the monitored pathway was not located in an area at risk from the surgical procedure. Because of such obligatory "false-negative" results, few studies address the utility of such monitoring. Given that each individual monitoring modality comes with its own constraints, such an approach typically requires a dedicated neurophysiologist for interpretation and troubleshooting.

SPINAL COLUMN AND SPINAL CORD SURGERY (MONITORS: SOMATOSENSORY-EVOKED POTENTIALS, MOTOR-EVOKED POTENTIALS, ELECTROMYOGRAM, AND BULBOCAVERNOSUS REFLEX)

Intraoperative monitoring of SSEPs has been used most extensively in patients undergoing surgical procedures involving the spinal column or spinal cord, or both. Extensive experience has been gained in patients who have decompressive laminectomies or who have undergone corrective procedures for scoliosis. Intraoperative changes in SSEPs have been noted in 2.5% to 65% of patients undergoing surgical procedures on the spine or spinal cord.[118-121] When these changes are promptly reversed either spontaneously or with interventions by the surgeon or anesthesiologist (e.g., lessening the degree of spine straightening in scoliosis surgery or increasing arterial blood pressure), the patients most often have preserved neurologic function postoperatively. When these changes persisted, however, the patients most often awakened with worsened neurologic function.

False-negative (rare) and false-positive (common) results have been reported with SSEP monitoring during spine surgery. Patients with intact SSEPs throughout the procedure have awakened with a new significant neurologic deficit, but the total reported incidence of this finding is far less than 1% of all cases monitored. Patients with no postoperative neurologic deficit commonly experience significant changes in intraoperative SSEPs.[70] This monitoring pattern is most commonly caused by failure to control for other, nonpathologic factors that may alter the SSEP. Overall, the reliability of properly performed SSEP monitoring to predict the postoperative sensory and motor function has been reported to be excellent.[41,121,122] Motor tracts are not directly monitored by SSEPs, however. In addition, the blood supply to the dorsal columns of the spinal cord, which carries all of the upper extremity SSEPs and at least a portion of the lower extremity SSEPs, is derived primarily from the posterior spinal arteries. The blood supply to motor tracts and neurons is derived primarily from the anterior spinal artery. It is possible for a significant motor deficit to develop postoperatively in patients with intact SSEPs throughout the operative course. Such events have been reported.[123,124]

In operations on the spinal column and after acute spinal cord injury, the sensory and motor changes generally correlate well;[41] however, in patients with neurologic dysfunction after thoracic aortic vascular surgery, frequently posterior spinal cord function (proprioception, vibration, light touch) is left intact when motor and other sensory functions (pain, temperature) are impaired. This result occurred in 32% of patients with neurologic injury after aortic aneurysm repair in one series,[125] with similar results in many other series. Intraoperative SSEP monitoring in these patients carries a significant risk for false-negative results, and as a result, such monitoring is not widely used.

Multiple anecdotal reports and an increasing number of case series suggest that MEP monitoring during surgery on the spine or its blood supply is useful. Several series have reported significant changes in MEPs without changes in SSEPs. These series suggest that combined use of SSEP monitoring and MEP monitoring may eliminate false-negative monitoring patterns during spine surgery.[126-131] In a consensus statement, the American Society of Neurophysiologic Monitoring concluded that use of MEP monitoring in combination with SSEP monitoring is well established to prevent injury to sensory and motor tracts during spinal column surgery.[132] In the case of monitoring paraplegia risk during thoracoabdominal aneurysm surgery, the literature shows mixed but improving support for the use of MEP monitoring. Two earlier studies suggested that MEPs may not be as effective as hoped. The first study recorded MEPs from the lumbar spinal cord in dogs produced by transcranial electric stimulation.[133] Elmore and associates found that these spinally recorded potentials did not accurately predict postoperative motor function. In a second study, Reuter and colleagues[134] recorded MEPs at the spinal cord and the peripheral nerve level in dogs produced by transcranial electric stimulation. They also found that the spinally recorded responses were inaccurate in predicting motor function postoperatively. The peripheral nerve responses disappeared in all animals and were not present 24 hours later regardless of whether the animal could move its lower extremities.

These studies suggest that the spinally recorded MEP likely represents a response generated by the descending corticospinal tract. This white matter pathway is resistant to ischemia compared with the more metabolically active anterior horn cells (gray matter). Recovery of this white matter–generated MEP response could occur after reperfusion of the cord, whereas the gray matter might not recover. Responses recorded from the peripheral nerve would reflect postsynaptic anterior horn cell function, but lower extremity ischemia occurring after aortic cross-clamping may preclude recording this or the response from muscles during surgery.

More recent clinical series have shown much greater success with MEP monitoring during aortic vascular surgery in correctly detecting inadequate spinal cord blood flow and in improving operative outcome. The technique has proven useful, particularly when operative strategies such as reimplantation of crucial intercostal vessels based on results of MEP monitoring, alteration of spinal cord perfusion pressure (blood pressure increase or cerebrospinal fluid drainage or both), spinal cord cooling, and other methods are used.[135] Additional studies, particularly with the use of endovascular stent repair of thoracoabdominal aneurysms, have found MEPs very useful in guiding therapy and improving outcome.[136,137]

For surgeries involving the conus medullaris and sacral nerve roots such as untethering of the spinal cord or resection of a lipoma of the filum terminale, tcMEPs can be recorded from the anal sphincter. In addition, the reflex arc of the bulbocavernosus reflex can be recorded, by stimulating the pudendal nerve and recording a motor response from the anal sphincter.[138]

PERIPHERAL NERVE SURGERY (MONITORS: ELECTROMYOGRAM, NERVE ACTION POTENTIAL)

Neurologic monitoring for surgeries involving peripheral nerves can be done in two different settings. In the first setting, the peripheral nerve is intact, but threatened by the surgery. Examples would be an intrinsic nerve tumor, such as a schwannoma or an extensive soft tissue tumor, particularly if it displaces the normal anatomic course of a nerve. Monitoring of spontaneous and stimulated muscle responses from muscle groups innervated by the nerve in question can be used to guide the resection. Spontaneous EMG discharges can be generated by stretch or compression of the nerve, by local heating from electrocautery, or from ischemia. Two caveats apply to the monitoring

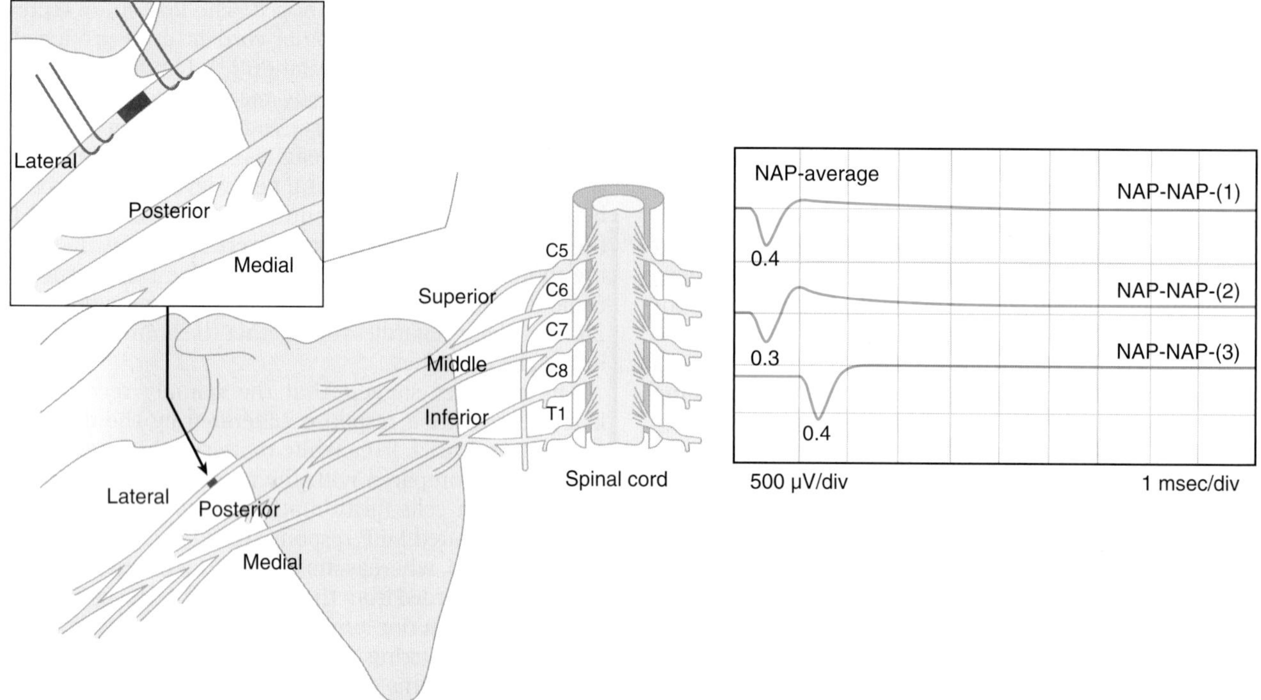

Fig. 39.17 Recording a nerve action potential *(NAP)* during a brachial plexus exploration. The site of the injury on the lateral fascicle is indicated in red. As shown in the inset, the surgeon places hook electrodes on either side of the exposed part of the nerve. If the injury is limited to an axonotmesis, proximal stimulation will result in a distal NAP similar to the ones shown in the recording to the right. The delay in the response in the third tracing is simply the result of a change in technical settings.

of spontaneous EMG. First, the neuromuscular junction is part of the monitored pathway, and muscle relaxation decreases/abolishes the sensitivity of monitoring in a dose-dependent manner. Second, sharp section of the nerve may not result in a noticeable discharge. To search out the course of the nerve intraoperatively, the surgeon may stimulate the wound area with a hand-held probe and listen for stimulated EMG or palpate for muscle contraction. The underlying concept should be familiar to anesthesiologists from the use of nerve stimulators in regional anesthesia.

A variation of this technique of monitoring that is in widespread use, because it is conceptually simple, is monitoring of pedicle screw placement during spinal instrumentation with the aim of avoiding nerve root injuries owing to malpositioned pedicle screws.[139,140] The aim is to avoid malpositioned screws that weaken the construct or cause postoperative radicular pain. Typically, the pilot hole or, less desirable, the shank of an implanted pedicle screw is stimulated repetitively with increasing current to determine the threshold for eliciting a dermatomal compound muscle potential. The interpretation of responses is complicated by the fact that the anatomical relationship between pedicles and nerve roots depends on the level of the spinal cord because the spinal cord is shorter than the bony spinal column. Thus a medially misplaced screw in the lumbar region will come to lie next to a nerve root, whereas in the thoracic spine, a medial misplacement puts the screw next to the corticospinal tract, which cannot be activated by single stimuli. Because thresholds vary among cervical, thoracic, and lumbar spine, as well as between healthy and diseased nerve roots, this technique has limitations but is widely thought to be useful.[141]

A second setting where monitoring of peripheral nerves is used is in patients with prolonged weakness and sensory loss after nerve injury undergoing nerve exploration.[142] The aim is to determine whether nerve reconstruction may improve outcome. The area of the lesion is determined by preoperative nerve conduction studies. Intraoperatively, the nerve is first stimulated proximal to the lesion, and a recording of the nerve action potential is made directly from the nerve distal to the lesion, as illustrated in Fig. 39.17. If there is nerve conduction across the lesion, lysis of scar is performed, and the incision is closed. Natural recovery by means of axonal regrowth produces the best outcome. If conduction does not occur across the lesion, resection of the damaged nerve and nerve cable grafting is performed.[65,143,144]

APPLICATIONS OF INTRAOPERATIVE MONITORING TO PEDIATRIC PATIENTS

In recent years many of the techniques described above have been used during surgery on children as young as 6 weeks of age. Very young children present special challenges due to the immaturity of the CNS. Incomplete myelination of specific tracts that carry sensory or motor signals is the primary source of the challenges. While light anesthesia (0.5 minimum alveolar concentration [MAC] volatile anesthetic) allows MEPs to be elicited from healthy adolescents, infants and young children are exquisitely sensitive to the effects of volatile anesthetic drugs. Therefore total intravenous anesthesia (TIVA) techniques are the anesthetics of choice when recording evoked potentials from these patients. In addition, adaptive strategies need to be applied by the monitoring team to overcome the effects of myelination delays and other developmental factors (Table 39.2).

TABLE 39.2 Additional Considerations When Monitoring Infants and Young Children

Modality	Observation	Developmental Neurophysiology	Compensation Strategy
SSEPs—MN & UN	Prolonged Erb's to cortical or cervical to cortical inter-peak latency	Incomplete myelination of medial lemniscus and thalamocortical pathways	Avoid volatile anesthetic drugs, avoid burst suppression, reduce stimulation rate
SSEP—PTN	Difficult to obtain; low amplitude	Incomplete myelination of dorsal columns; asynchronous volleys	As above, increase pulse length; optimize signal:noise ratio
tcMEP		Cortical and spinal cord motor neurons very susceptible to effects of volatile agents. Variance in conduction velocity of large CST fibers exceeds mean conduction velocity	TIVA, may need low-dose ketamine to help support BP. Double-train stimulation with unequal train lengths; optimizing inter-train interval
D-wave	Difficult to obtain in children under 24 months of age	Signal dispersion due to large variance in conduction velocities	Electrodes with larger surface area may be helpful
ABR	Low quality signals with volatile agents	uncertain	TIVA for ABR for less than 24 months
Bulbocavernosus Reflex	Very susceptible to effects of volatile agents	Oligosynaptic reflex; sensitivity to volatile agents persists	Double pulse train with large inter-train interval

ABR, Auditory brainstem response; *D-wave,* positive or negative deflection recorded from electrodes placed directly over the spinal cord; *SSEPs,* somatosensory-evoked potentials; *tcMEP,* transcranial motor-evoked potential; *TIVA,* total intravenous anesthesia.
Modified from Francis L, Busso V, McAuliffe JJ. Intraoperative neuromonitoring in pediatric surgery. In: Koth A, Sloan TB, Toleikis JR, eds. *Monitoring the Nervous System for Anesthesiologists and Other Health Care Professionals.* Cham: Springer Int; 2017.

Some monitored surgical procedures are performed almost exclusively in children. One example is selective dorsal rhizotomies for relief of spasticity associated with cerebral palsy. This procedure involves interrogation of lower extremity dorsal root subdivisions (rootlets) and evaluating the compound action potentials generated in response. This technique is best performed with a TIVA technique. Infant/toddler hearing evaluations may require the use of auditory brainstem response tests under anesthesia. Experience at the Cincinnati Children's Hospital Medical Center (CCHMC) suggests that a propofol infusion anesthetic yields a more reliable assessment of wave V than a sevoflurane-based anesthetic.

It is important to recognize that the EEG patterns associated with an anesthetic state in adults do not apply to infants under anesthesia. Infants less than 3 months have almost no change in their EEGs when transitioning from a quiet resting state to an anesthetized state as slow wave patterns dominate both states. Alpha and theta patterns emerge under anesthesia at 4 months of age but differ from those of older children and adults.[145]

In summary, infants and young children can benefit from intraoperative neurophysiological monitoring if both monitoring and anesthetic techniques are appropriately modified.

NONNEUROLOGIC SURGERY THAT RISKS DAMAGE TO THE CENTRAL NERVOUS SYSTEM (MONITORS: ELECTROENCEPHALOGRAM, TRANSCRANIAL DOPPLER, CEREBRAL OXIMETRY, JUGULAR VENOUS OXYGEN SATURATION)

Cardiopulmonary Bypass

Electroencephalogram. In humans, changes that occur with the institution of CPB may alter the EEG by multiple different mechanisms. Plasma and brain concentrations of anesthetic drugs may be altered by CPB or by anesthetic drugs commonly given during CPB, alterations in arterial carbon dioxide tension and arterial blood pressure may occur, and hemodilution with hypothermic perfusate nearly always occurs. These effects, all of which may produce EEG changes similar to pathologic changes seen with ischemia, make it difficult to interpret EEG changes occurring during CPB.

Levy and others[146,147] tried to distinguish the normal effects of hypothermia from other events occurring at the institution and conclusion of CPB. Initially, Levy concluded that only a qualitative relationship could be determined, but later, with the use of a much more sophisticated EEG analysis technique (approximate entropy), EEG changes associated with changes in temperature could be quantified.

Chabot and colleagues[148] and Edmonds and colleagues[149] have attempted to use quantitative (processed, multiple-channel) EEG during CPB to detect cerebral hypoperfusion and relate these changes to postoperative neurologic function. In addition, some minimal work has been done with intervention after detection of cerebral hypoperfusion using quantitative EEG. Although the data seem promising, only a few patients have been studied, with very few corroborating studies. In addition, this type of monitoring is extremely costly in time, personnel, and equipment. Given the lack of convincing outcome data, the cost-to-benefit ratio is unclear at best. Some other investigators failed to show any convincing relationship between intraoperative EEG parameters and postoperative neurologic function, especially in small infants and children.[150,151] Whether the processed, quantitative EEG provides useful information for clinical management of patients during CPB is not clear. None of the currently available studies and recommendations would support an evidence-based justification for their routine application. However, use of EEG to document electrocortical silence and maximum reduction of cerebral metabolism prior to institution of circulatory arrest seems logical.

Transcranial Doppler. TCD ultrasound can monitor the cerebral circulation during CPB. Anecdotal reports and case series document the use of TCD for determining adequacy of CBF, detection of emboli, and detection of improper cannula placement.[152] Only very limited outcome data exist, and use of TCD ultrasound during CPB does not stand up to evidence-based examination, primarily because of lack of information. Probe placement instability and inability to obtain signals in some patients also have limited the use of this monitor intraoperatively. Finally, although the hypothesis that cerebral microemboli are at least part of the pathogenesis of postoperative cognitive decline following CPB is attractive, a recent study failed to demonstrate any relationship between CPB counts of presumed emboli and postoperative cognitive dysfunction.[153]

Cerebral Oximetry and Jugular Venous Oxygen Saturation. As is the case with EEG monitoring during CPB, there are multiple case reports and several series that advocate the use of NIRS or jugular venous oxygen saturation ($Sjvo_2$) as indicators of adequate perfusion of the brain during CPB.[154,155] Incorrect placement of CPB cannulae has been detected clinically and in laboratory studies. One more recent series of patients undergoing CPB for coronary bypass surgery showed a higher incidence of major organ system dysfunction and longer hospital stays in patients with lower baseline and intraoperative cerebral oxygen saturation values.[156] The same questions exist for this application of NIRS, however, as do for the use of NIRS during carotid vascular surgical procedures. Although a recent systematic review of the use of NIRS during CPB showed that data are insufficient to conclude that interventions based on low cerebral oxygen saturation values prevent either stroke or postoperative cognitive dysfunction,[157] several more recent studies suggest significant promise for this modality when used in combination with TCD ultrasound. Use of NIRS and TCD ultrasound together identified a significant percentage of patients undergoing CPB with impaired autoregulation who were at higher risk for postoperative cognitive dysfunction and/or stroke.[158-160] This patient population may benefit from higher mean arterial pressure (MAP) during CPB. Use of NIRS during CPB clearly provides information that would not otherwise be available, but more work is needed before we fully understand the role of this monitor during CPB.

$Sjvo_2$ is very invasive. Although data from case reports and studies suggest that $Sjvo_2$ may have utility in detecting inadequate CBF, lack of outcome data, lack of clearly defined critical values at different temperatures during CPB, and availability of less invasive modalities (EEG, cerebral oximetry) have resulted in only limited use of this monitoring method during CPB. Based on current information, no neurologic monitoring techniques, either alone or in combination, are clearly useful in improving outcome during surgical procedures requiring CPB. Further research is needed before the cost in personnel and equipment of neurologic monitoring during CPB can be justified.

INTENSIVE CARE APPLICATIONS OF NEUROLOGIC MONITORING (MONITORS: ELECTROENCEPHALOGRAM, EVOKED POTENTIALS, TRANSCRANIAL DOPPLER, JUGULAR VENOUS OXYGEN SATURATION)

Secondary injury to the CNS has been recognized in past decades as a major modifiable risk factor in patients with CNS disease. Aneurysmal subarachnoid hemorrhage, stroke, and traumatic brain injury are examples of CNS insults in which secondary injury has important implications for the ultimate functional outcome.[161-163] These same diseases frequently result in a primary insult to the CNS that severely constrains the utility of the clinical neurologic examination because of the need for mechanical ventilation and sedation. Many techniques of neurologic monitoring discussed earlier are used in the intensive care unit. Generally, however, techniques that require the continued presence of skilled technologists, such as monitoring of evoked potentials, are prohibitively expensive and of less practical value than techniques that provide data that easily integrates into the physiologic support provided through intensive care or techniques that can be performed as daily assessments. Some of this neurophysiologic data can provide important prognostic information in comatose patients and guide decision making.

Continuous Electroencephalogram Monitoring

Continuous EEG monitoring may be of benefit in comatose patients. It facilitates timely intervention for specific diagnoses, such as nonconvulsive seizures, as the underlying cause of a fluctuating neurologic status, or point to focal problems such as regional ischemia due to vasospasm after subarachnoid hemorrhage.[164] The perceived utility of continuous EEG monitoring has led to a degree of standardization in indications and the logistics of the application of this technique in the intensive care unit.[165,166]

Cerebral Ischemia

Cerebral ischemia is an important cause of secondary injury to the CNS. It can be difficult to detect in patients who are either comatose or sedated, but can occur even in patients with adequate cerebral perfusion pressure.[167,168] Three techniques may provide intensivists with additional information about cerebral perfusion. None of the monitors is considered "standard of care." As with all monitors, the impact of the monitor on outcome depends on the quality of the therapeutic interventions that result from integration of the additional data into the clinical management of a given patient.

$Sjvo_2$ monitoring is used most extensively in the intensive care unit to monitor patients with traumatic brain injury. The data have been used to guide blood pressure and ventilatory management to optimize blood flow. $Sjvo_2$ monitoring has had a major effect on ventilatory management of head-injured patients and has significantly reduced the routine use of hyperventilation in neurosurgical patients.[169-172] $Sjvo_2$ values of less than 50% generally indicate cerebral ischemia. Increases in $Sjvo_2$ may occur in response to therapy, or they may be an ominous sign if the increase is caused by falling demand because of neuronal death.

Similar to $Sjvo_2$ monitoring, monitoring of $P_{Br}o_2$ and blood flow is used most frequently in patients with traumatic brain injury. $P_{Br}o_2$ performs well in clinical practice. Decreases to less than 10 to 15 mm Hg are associated with worsening outcome,[22,173] whereas $P_{Br}o_2$-targeted treatment strategies may improve outcome.[174]

TCD ultrasound is widely used in the intensive care unit to document the presence and severity of cerebral vasospasm after subarachnoid hemorrhage. As the major cerebral arteries narrow, flow velocity within the lumen must increase if blood flow is to be maintained. Such narrowing occurs 12 to 24 hours before the onset of clinical symptoms, thus allowing therapy to be initiated before the onset of clinical symptoms.[175-179] Mean flow velocities of more than 120 cm/s seem to correlate well with angiographic vasospasm,[180,181] although intracranial pressure and concurrent therapy to raise cerebral perfusion pressure modify the flow velocity. The latter two factors result in characteristic changes of the TCD waveform, however, and preserve the utility of the examination.

Prognosis in Coma and Determination of Brain Death

EEG monitoring may help to assess the clinical course and the prognosis of comatose patients. Assessment of prognosis must be separated from the insult that precipitated the coma by more than 24 hours. If not, the EEG may reflect predominantly the effect of the insult and may not predict prognosis. More than 24 hours after the insult, spontaneous sustained burst suppression correlates strongly with severe irreversible brain injury.[182] Absence of EEG variability portends a high likelihood of persistent vegetative state or death,[182,183] whereas spontaneous variability, reactivity to external stimuli, and typical sleep patterns are associated with more favorable outcomes.[184-186]

A specific indication for EEG monitoring is the therapeutic induction of a coma by barbiturate administration. Because neither blood nor cerebrospinal fluid concentrations of barbiturates reliably predict burst suppression and near-maximal reduction in cerebral metabolic rate of oxygen consumption,[187] and because barbiturate administration usually requires an increase in cardiovascular support, documentation of a burst suppression pattern on EEG allows the use of the minimal effective dose of barbiturate.

Similar to EEG, evoked potential studies have a place in predicting prognosis in comatose patients.[188] The presence of normal SSEPs bilaterally is an excellent prognostic sign, whereas the absence of any SSEP cortical response is a poor prognostic indicator. The degree of bad outcome can be predicted by BAEPs. Intact and normal BAEPs with absent cortical SSEPs predict a best outcome of a chronic vegetative state. Outcome may be worse, however, because BAEPs commonly deteriorate later with rostral-to-caudal deterioration. Absent BAEP responses beyond wave I predict a high likelihood of brain death. Present but abnormal SSEPs are associated with outcomes intermediate between good to high function and a chronic vegetative state.[189-198]

TCD ultrasound also has been used in the intensive care unit as an aid to the diagnosis of brain death. As intracranial pressure increases, the pulsatility of the TCD waveform increases, accentuating the systolic peak and diminishing flow during diastole. With further increases in intracranial pressure, a characteristic to-and-fro pattern of flow is established, which is consistent with clinical brain death.[199] TCD studies are easily performed at the bedside and can minimize the need for unnecessary transports of the patient for definitive radiologic studies.

Nonsurgical Factors Influencing Monitoring Results

ANESTHESIA AND THE ELECTROENCEPHALOGRAM

Anesthetic drugs affect the frequency and amplitude of EEG waveforms. Although each drug class and each specific drug has some specific, dose-related EEG effects (Table 39.3), some basic anesthesia-related EEG patterns may be described. Subanesthetic doses of intravenous and inhaled anesthetics usually produce an increase in frontal beta activity and abolish the alpha activity normally seen in the occipital leads in an awake, relaxed patient with the eyes closed. As the patient loses consciousness with general anesthesia, the brain waves become larger in amplitude and slower in frequency. In the frontal areas, small beta activity seen in an awake patient slows to the alpha range and increases in size. In combination with the loss of the occipital alpha activity, this phenomenon produces the appearance of a "shift" of the alpha activity from the posterior cortex to the anterior cortex. Further increases in the dose of inhaled or intravenous anesthetic drugs produce further slowing of the EEG. Some anesthetic drugs suppress EEG activity totally (see Table 39.3). Other anesthetic drugs never produce burst suppression or an isoelectric EEG, despite increasing dose, either because they are incapable of completely suppressing the EEG (e.g., opioids, benzodiazepines) or because cardiovascular toxicity of the drug (e.g., halothane) prevents administration of a large enough dose.

Intravenous Anesthetic Drugs

Barbiturates, Propofol, and Etomidate. Despite widely varying potencies and durations of action, barbiturates, propofol, and etomidate produce similar EEG patterns (Fig. 39.18 shows EEG effects of thiopental). These drugs all follow the basic anesthesia-related EEG pattern described previously with initial EEG activation (see Fig. 39.18A), followed by dose-related depression. As the patient loses consciousness, characteristic frontal spindles are seen (see Fig. 39.18B), which are replaced by polymorphic 1- to 3-Hz activity (see Fig. 39.18C) as the drug dose is increased. Further increases in dose result in lengthening periods of suppression interspersed with periods of activity (burst suppression). With a very high dose, EEG silence results. All of these drugs have been reported to cause epileptiform activity in humans, but epileptiform activity is clinically significant only after methohexital and etomidate when given in subhypnotic doses.

Ketamine. Ketamine does not follow the basic anesthesia-related EEG pattern. Anesthesia with ketamine is characterized by frontally dominant rhythmic, high-amplitude theta activity. Increasing doses produce intermittent polymorphic delta activity of very large amplitude interspersed with low-amplitude beta activity.[200] Electrocortical silence cannot be produced with ketamine. EEG activity may be very disorganized and variable at all doses. This disorganization of the EEG with ketamine is responsible for the failure of the bispectral index (BIS) to be useful in looking at the effect of ketamine on consciousness.[201] Recovery of normal EEG

TABLE 39.3 Anesthetic Drugs and Electroencephalogram

Drug	Effect on EEG Frequency	Effect on EEG Amplitude	Burst Suppression?
Isoflurane, Sevoflurane, Desflurane			Yes, >1.5 MAC
Subanesthetic	Loss of alpha, ↑frontal beta		
Anesthetic	Frontal 4-13 Hz activity		
Increasing dose >1.5 MAC	Diffuse theta and delta → burst suppression → silence	↓0	
Nitrous oxide (alone)	Frontal fast oscillatory activity (>30 Hz)	↓, especially with inspired concentration >50%	No
Barbiturates			Yes, with high doses
Low dose	Fast frontal ↑ beta activity	Slight	
Moderate dose	↑Frontal alpha frequency spindles		
Increasing high dose	Diffuse delta → burst suppression → silence	↓0	
Etomidate			Yes, with high doses
Low dose	Fast frontal beta activity		
Moderate dose	Frontal alpha frequency spindles		
Increasing high dose	Diffuse delta → burst suppression → silence	↓0	
Propofol			Yes, with high doses
Low dose	Loss of alpha; frontal beta		
Moderate dose	Frontal delta; waxing/waning alpha		
Increasing high dose	Diffuse delta → burst suppression → silence	↓0	
Ketamine			No
Low dose	Loss of alpha, variability	↓	
Moderate dose	Frontal rhythmic delta		
High dose	Polymorphic delta; some beta	Beta is low amplitude	
Benzodiazepines			No
Low dose	Loss of alpha; increased frontal beta activity		
High dose	Frontally dominant delta and theta		
Opioids			No
Low dose	Loss of beta; alpha slows	None	
Moderate dose	Diffuse theta, some delta		
High dose	Delta, often synchronized		
Dexmedetomidine	Moderate slowing, prominent spindles		No

Alpha =8-13 Hz frequency; beta =>13 Hz frequency; delta =<4 Hz frequency; theta = 4-7 Hz frequency. *EEG*, Electroencephalogram; *MAC*, minimum alveolar concentration.

activity even after a single bolus dose of ketamine is slow compared with barbiturates. There is no information available about the relationship between emergence reactions after ketamine and the EEG. Ketamine also has been associated with increased epileptiform activity.[200]

Benzodiazepines. Despite varying potencies and durations of action, benzodiazepines also follow the basic anesthesia-related EEG pattern. As a class, however, these drugs are incapable of producing burst suppression or an isoelectric EEG.

Opioids. As a class, opioids do not follow the basic anesthesia-related EEG pattern. Opioids generally produce a dose-related decrease in frequency and increase in amplitude of the EEG. If no further doses of opiates are given, alpha and beta activity return as drug redistribution occurs. The rapidity of return depends on the initial dose and on the drug. In rats, remifentanil is associated with the most rapid return to normal.[202] Complete suppression of the EEG cannot be obtained with opioids. Epileptiform activity occurs in humans and in animals receiving large to supraclinical doses of opioids. Sharp wave activity is common after induction of anesthesia with fentanyl, with 20% of patients showing this phenomenon after 30 μg/kg; 60%, after 50 μg/kg; 58%, after 60 μg/kg; and 80%, after 70 μg/kg.[203] Alfentanil bolus has been used clinically to activate seizure foci during epilepsy surgery.[204] This epileptiform activity is mainly noted in the frontotemporal region.

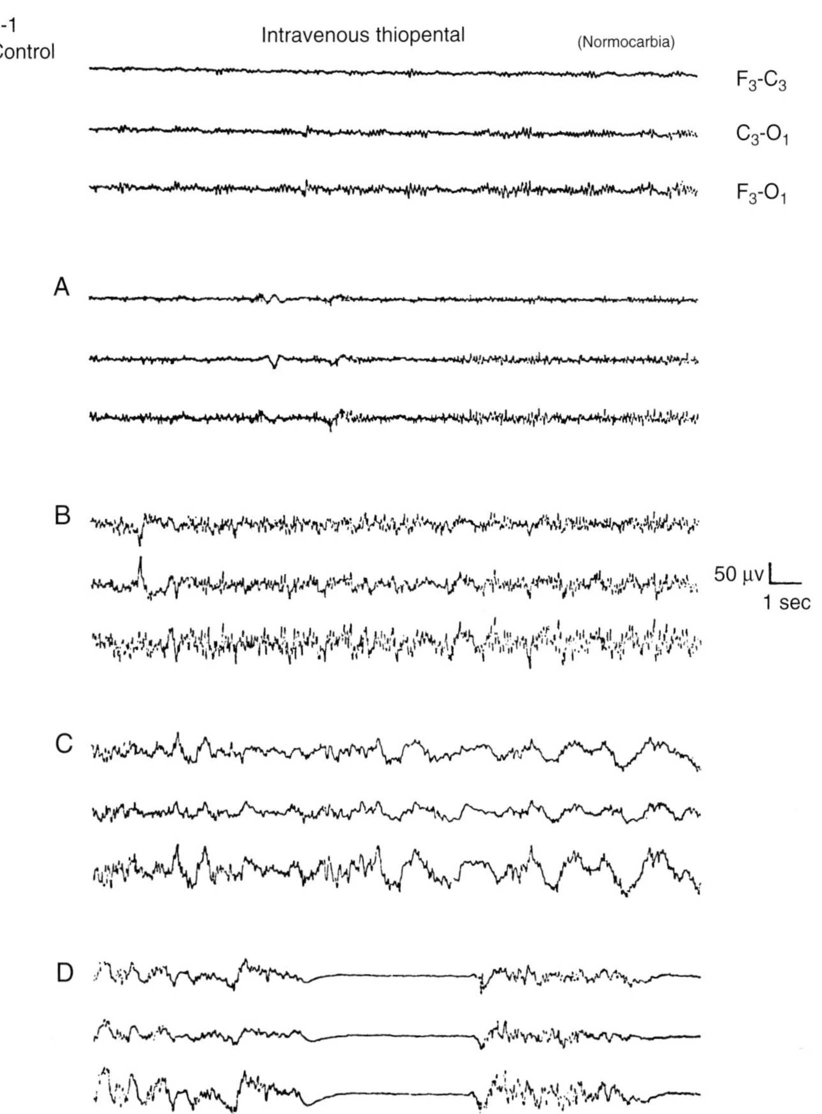

Fig. 39.18 Electroencephalogram effects of intravenous administration of thiopental in humans. (A) Rapid activity. (B) Barbiturate spindles. (C) Slow waves. and (D) Burst suppression. (From Clark DL, Rosner BS. Neurophysiologic effects of general anesthetics. *Anesthesiology*. 1973;38:564.)

Dexmedetomidine. Dexmedetomidine is being increasingly used for sedation in the operating room and in the intensive care unit, and is also used for sedation during diagnostic EEG studies in children. EEG studies of patients undergoing sedation with dexmedetomidine alone show patterns similar to those seen in normal human sleep with increased slow-wave activity and sleep spindles prominent.[205] Burst suppression or an isoelectric EEG pattern cannot be produced even with high doses of the drug. Level of sedation with dexmedetomidine can be effectively monitored using processed EEG parameters and has been reported using BIS and entropy techniques.[206] Interestingly, BIS values at comparable levels of sedation appear to be lower with dexmedetomidine than propofol.[207]

Inhaled Anesthetics

Nitrous Oxide. Used alone, nitrous oxide causes a decrease in amplitude and frequency of the dominant occipital alpha rhythm. With the onset of analgesia and depressed consciousness, frontally dominant fast oscillatory activity (>30 Hz) is frequently seen.[208] This activity may persist to some extent for 50 minutes after discontinuation of nitrous oxide. When nitrous oxide is used in combination with other agents, it increases the effects that would be associated with the agent alone clinically and with respect to the EEG pattern seen.

Isoflurane, Sevoflurane, and Desflurane. Potent inhaled anesthetic drugs, including halothane and enflurane, which are no longer available, follow the basic anesthesia-related EEG pattern. Isoflurane initially causes an activation of the EEG followed by a slowing of the EEG activity that is more marked with increasing dose. Isoflurane begins to produce periods of EEG suppression at 1.5 MAC, which become longer with increasing dose until electric silence is produced at 2 to 2.5 MAC. Isolated epileptiform patterns sometimes can be seen during intersuppression activity at 1.5 to 2 MAC isoflurane.[209] Sevoflurane causes similar dose-dependent EEG effects. Equi-MAC concentrations of sevoflurane and isoflurane

TABLE 39.4 Ability of an Individual Anesthetic Drug to Produce a Change in Sensory- and Motor-Evoked Potentials That Could Be Mistaken for a Surgically Induced Change

	SSEPS		BAEPS		VEPS		TRANSCRANIAL MEPS	
Drug	**LAT**	**AMP**	**LAT**	**AMP**	**LAT**	**AMP**	**LAT**	**AMP**
Isoflurane	Yes	Yes	No	No	Yes	Yes	Yes	Yes
Nitrous oxide*	Yes	Yes	No	No	Yes	Yes	Yes	Yes
Barbiturates	Yes	Yes	No	No	Yes	Yes	Yes	Yes
Etomidate	No	No	No	No	Yes	Yes	No	No
Propofol	Yes	Yes	No	No	Yes	Yes	Yes	Yes
Diazepam	Yes	Yes	No	No	Yes	Yes	Yes	Yes
Midazolam	Yes	Yes	No	No	Yes	Yes	Yes	Yes
Ketamine	No	No	No	No	Yes	Yes	No	No
Opioids	No	No	No	No	No	No	No	No
Dexmedetomidine	No	No	No	No	No	ND	ND	No

*Increases the anesthetic effect of the drug or drugs with which it is used.

Note. This table is not quantitative in any way. "Yes" or "No" designations indicate whether an individual drug is capable of producing an effect on any portion of the evoked response that could be mistaken for a surgically induced change.

AMP, Amplitude; *BAEPs,* brainstem auditory-evoked potentials; *LAT,* latency; *MEPs,* motor-evoked potentials; *ND,* no data available from the literature; *SSEPs,* somatosensory-evoked potentials; *VEPs,* visual-evoked potentials.

cause similar EEG changes.[210] Epileptiform activity has been induced by administration of sevoflurane in patients without epilepsy, and seizure activity on EEG, but not clinical seizure activity, has been reported in pediatric patients with a history of epilepsy during induction of anesthesia with sevoflurane.[211,212] Despite these observations, sevoflurane, similar to other inhalation drugs, is not suitable for use during electrocorticography for localization of seizure foci.[213] EEG patterns seen with enflurane are similar to the patterns seen with isoflurane except that epileptiform activity is considerably more prominent. At 2 to 3 MAC, burst suppression is seen, but virtually all intersuppression activity consists of large spike/wave pattern discharges. Hyperventilation with high concentrations of enflurane increases the length of suppression, decreases the duration of bursts, but increases the amplitude and main frequency component of the intersuppression epileptiform activity. Frank EEG seizures also may occur with enflurane that produce the same cerebral metabolic effects as pentylenetetrazol, a known convulsant.

Halothane also produces EEG patterns similar to those of isoflurane, but dosages of halothane that would produce burst suppression in the EEG (3-4 MAC) are associated with profound cardiovascular toxicity. Desflurane produces EEG changes similar in nature to equi-MAC concentrations of isoflurane. In limited clinical studies, there has been no evidence of epileptiform activity with desflurane, despite hyperventilation and 1.6 MAC dosage,[214] and desflurane has been used as a treatment of refractory status epilepticus.[215]

Clinical studies have shown that the EEG effects of inhaled anesthetic drugs are influenced by age and baseline EEG characteristics. Older patients and patients with EEG slowing at baseline were more sensitive to the EEG effects of isoflurane and desflurane. As anesthesia was deepened, similar EEG pattern changes were noted, but these changes occurred at lower end-tidal anesthetic concentrations.[216]

BOX 39.1 Guidelines for Choosing Anesthetic Techniques During Procedures in Which Sensory-Evoked Responses Are Monitored

1. Intravenous drugs have significantly less effect than "equipotent" doses of inhaled anesthetics
2. Combinations of drugs generally produce "additive" effects
3. Subcortical (spinal or brainstem) sensory-evoked responses are very resistant to the effects of anesthetic drugs. If subcortical responses provide sufficient information for the surgical procedure, anesthetic technique is not important, and effects on cortically recorded responses may be ignored

ANESTHESIA AND SENSORY-EVOKED RESPONSES

Volatile Anesthetics

Multiple drugs used in the perioperative period can influence the ability to monitor SERs accurately (Table 39.4). An extensive review from 2003 provides the interested clinician with a detailed analysis of all drug effects on SERs,[217] which is beyond the scope of this chapter. Table 39.4 does not quantify drug effects, but rather lists whether an individual drug is capable of producing a change in any part of an evoked response that could be mistaken for a surgically induced change. A "no" designation in this table does not mean that there are no effects of a given drug on SERs. The "no" designation indicates that any effects that do occur would not be called clinically significant by *clinicians experienced in intraoperative monitoring*. Several general concepts (Box 39.1) help the clinician who is trying to determine the best choice of drugs for use during monitored cases.

The volatile anesthetics isoflurane, sevoflurane, desflurane, enflurane, and halothane have similar effects in differing degrees on all types of SERs. VEPs are the most sensitive

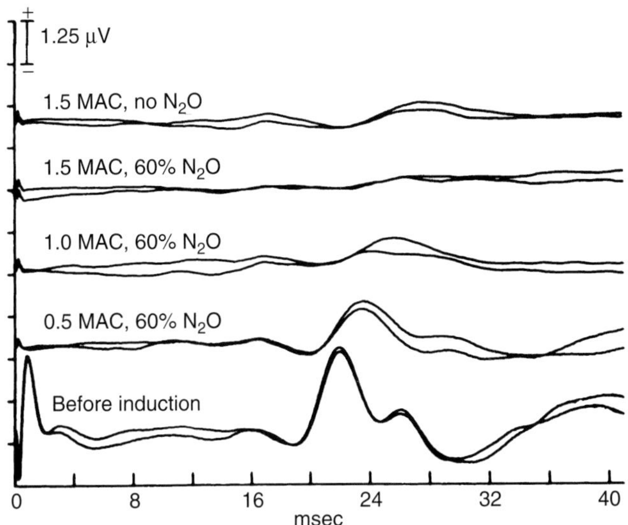

Fig. 39.19 Representative somatosensory-evoked potential cortical responses (C-3, C-4-FPz) at various minimum alveolar concentration *(MAC)* levels of isoflurane. (From Peterson DO, Drummond JC, Todd MM. Effects of halothane, enflurane, isoflurane, and nitrous oxide on somatosensory-evoked potentials in humans. *Anesthesiology*. 1986;65:35.)

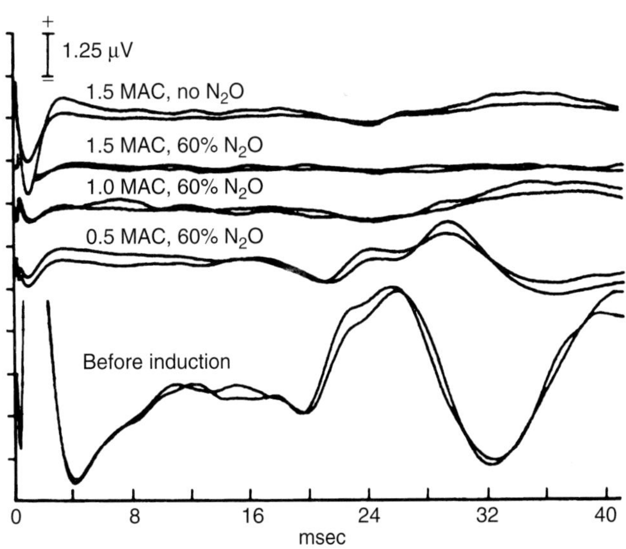

Fig. 39.20 Representative somatosensory-evoked potential cortical responses (C-3, or C-4-FPz) at various minimum alveolar concentration *(MAC)* levels of enflurane. (From Peterson DO, Drummond JC, Todd MM. Effects of halothane, enflurane, isoflurane, and nitrous oxide on somatosensory-evoked potentials in humans. *Anesthesiology*. 1986;65:35.)

to the effects of volatile anesthetics, and BAEPs are the most resistant to anesthetic-induced changes. Spinal and subcortical SSEP responses are significantly less affected than cortical potentials.[218-220]

SSEPs, because they are the most widely used intraoperative SER technique, are the most completely studied with respect to the effects of anesthetic drugs. The effects of the currently used volatile anesthetics on cortical SSEPs are dose-dependent increases in latency and conduction times and a decrease in amplitude of cortically, but not subcortically recorded signals.[221] When comparing the different volatile agents, studies have reported conflicting results.[218,220] None of these differences are clinically important and may be ignored by the practicing clinician. With respect to the newer agents, desflurane and sevoflurane seem to have qualitatively and quantitatively similar effects on SERs as isoflurane.[222-225] In neurologically normal patients, 0.5 to 1 MAC of any of the potent inhaled agents in the presence of nitrous oxide is compatible with monitoring of cortical SSEPs (Figs. 39.19–39.21).[217] Neurologically impaired patients may show a significantly greater sensitivity to inhaled agents, even to the point of not tolerating any recordable level of inhaled agent. Generally, better monitoring conditions are obtained, however, with narcotic-based anesthetics with less than 1 MAC total (nitrous oxide plus potent agent) end-tidal inhaled anesthetic concentration.

The volatile anesthetics result in increases in latency of BAEPs without significantly affecting the amplitude.[226-228] Volatile anesthetics cause increases in latency and decreases in amplitude in the early (middle latency) cortical responses after auditory stimulation,[227] however, and these middle latency responses are now being used to monitor the hypnotic component of general anesthetics.[228] Adequate monitoring of BAEPs is possible with any clinically useful concentrations of inhaled agents (with or without nitrous oxide) (Figs. 39.22 and 39.23).

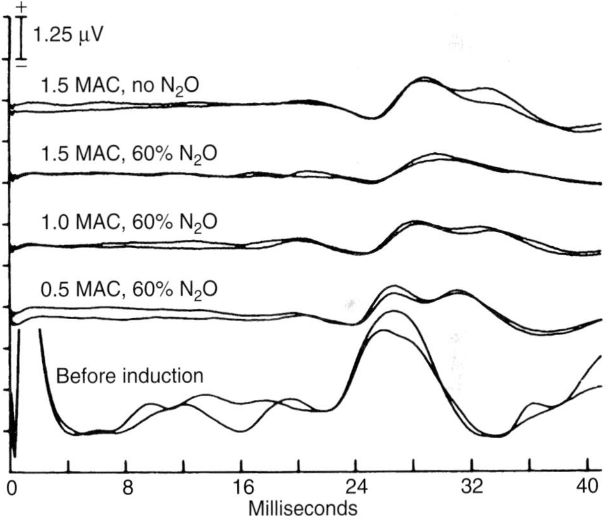

Fig. 39.21 Representative somatosensory-evoked potential cortical responses (C-3, C-4-FPz) at various minimum alveolar concentration *(MAC)* levels of halothane. (From Peterson DO, Drummond JC, Todd MM. Effects of halothane, enflurane, isoflurane, and nitrous oxide on somatosensory-evoked potentials in humans. *Anesthesiology*. 1986;65:35.)

Use of the volatile anesthetic drugs during monitoring of VEPs results in dose-dependent increases in latency with or without changes in amplitude.[229] Isoflurane results in dose-dependent increases in latency and decreases in amplitude up to 1.8% in 100% oxygen, at which time the waveform is lost.[221] More recent studies report some success in recording intraoperative VEPs from patients with normal eyesight, but waveform variability and potent depression of waveforms by volatile agents remain concerns.[230,231] In the opinion of many experts, the variability of VEPs in anesthetized patients is so great that satisfactory monitoring is impossible using any anesthetic technique.

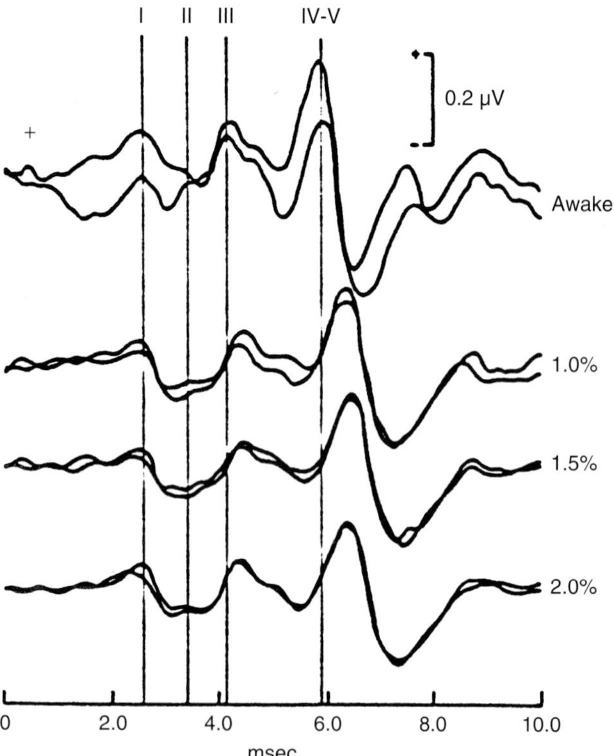

Fig. 39.22 Influence of isoflurane alone on brainstem auditory-evoked potential in a typical subject. Latency of peaks III and IV to V increased at 1.0% but stabilized with increasing anesthetic depth. (From Manninen PH, Lam AM, Nicholas JF. The effects of isoflurane–nitrous oxide anesthesia on brainstem auditory evoked potentials in humans. *Anesth Analg.* 1985;64:43.)

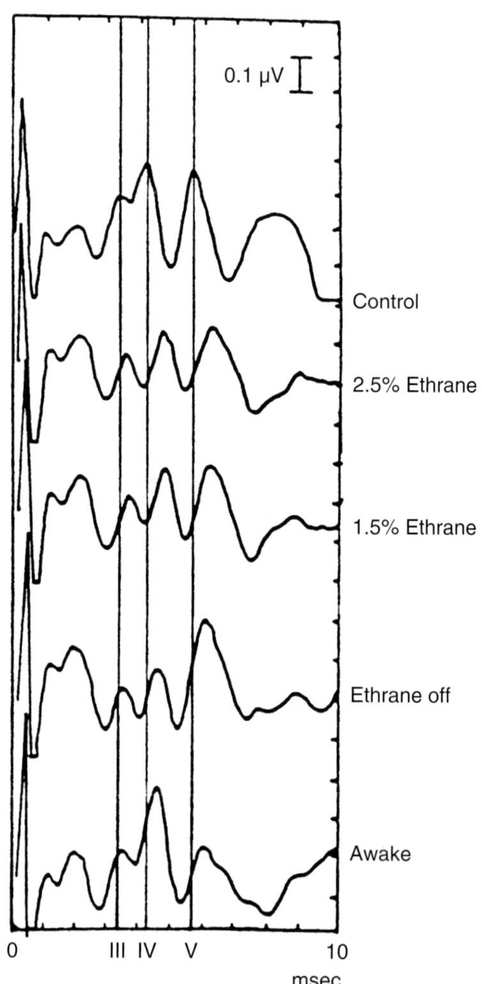

Fig. 39.23 Brainstem auditory-evoked potential recording obtained in one patient at different enflurane (Ethrane)-inspired concentrations. (From Dubois MY, Sato S, Chassy J, et al. Effects of enflurane on brainstem auditory evoked responses in humans. *Anesth Analg.* 1982;61:898.)

Although volatile anesthetics cause significant changes in the SER waveforms, it is possible to provide adequate monitoring intraoperatively in the presence of anesthetic doses of volatile anesthetics. Doses of anesthetic drugs causing significant depression of the response to be monitored must be prevented. In our experience, end-tidal concentrations of inhaled anesthetic drugs totaling greater than 1.3 MAC have a dose-related, increasing probability of obliterating cortical SSEPs even in neurologically normal patients. Equally important, anesthetic concentration should not be changed during the critical periods of intraoperative monitoring. Critical periods are defined as periods in which surgical interventions are most likely to result in damage to neurologic tissue and changes in the SERs. Because the volatile anesthetic-induced changes in SERs are dose dependent, increasing anesthetic dosage at a crucial point in the operative procedure can result in confusing changes in the SERs that potentially may be caused by the anesthetic, the surgical procedure, or both. The appropriate intervention is difficult to determine.

As with the volatile anesthetics, nitrous oxide causes differing effects on the SERs depending on the sensory system monitored. It causes decreases in amplitude without significant changes in latency in SSEPs when used alone or when added to a narcotic-based or volatile anesthetic.[217,218,232] The addition of nitrous oxide to a maintenance volatile anesthetic during the monitoring of BAEPs causes no further change.[226] Likewise, use of nitrous oxide alone causes no change in BAEPs, unless gas accumulates in the middle ear.[232] Use of nitrous oxide alone results in an increase in latency and a decrease in amplitude in VEPs, but when it is added to a volatile anesthetic technique, it causes no further changes in VEPs.[229,232]

Intravenous Anesthetics

The effects of propofol on SERs have been studied in many different settings. At typical clinical doses required for general anesthesia, propofol has minimal effects on somatosensory-evoked responses recorded along the somatosensory pathway up to the early cortical potentials.[233,234] Thus propofol-based TIVA is frequently used as the preferred technique to optimize signal-to-noise ratio for SSEPs and provide rapid feedback to the surgeon.[235] BAEPs under propofol anesthesia show minor increases in interpeak latencies and decreases in amplitude that are insufficient to interfere with clinical monitoring of auditory function.[236,237]

The effects of barbiturates on SERs have been studied in animals and humans. Increasing doses of thiopental in patients result in progressive dose-dependent increases in latency, decreases in amplitude of SSEPs, and progressive increases in latency of wave V in BAEPs. The changes in SSEPs are more pronounced than the changes in BAEPs, and waveforms beyond the initial primary cortical response are quickly obliterated. This finding is consistent with the theories that barbiturates affect synaptic transmission more than axonal conduction. Early waveforms in SERs result primarily from axonal transmission, and later waves depend on multisynaptic pathways in addition to axonal transmission. At doses of thiopental far greater than doses producing an isoelectric EEG, adequate monitoring of early cortical and subcortical SSEPs and BAEPs was preserved.[238] Other barbiturate compounds show similar effects.[239] This observation is important, especially when attempting to monitor the adequacy of CBF during cerebrovascular surgery when the patient has been given large, "protective" doses of barbiturates. The EEG is isoelectric and not helpful for monitoring. The early cortical SSEP waveforms are still preserved, however, and may be very helpful in determining adequacy of CBF. Preserved ability to monitor SSEPs in head-injured patients receiving therapeutic thiopental infusions has been demonstrated.[240] VEPs are much more sensitive to barbiturates. Low barbiturate doses obliterate all except the earliest waveforms. In cats, the early potentials persisted with increases in latency even to very high pentobarbital doses.[241] Except for VEPs, adequate perioperative monitoring of SERs is possible even in the presence of high-dose barbiturate therapy as long as the effects of the drug (increased latency with moderately decreased amplitude) are considered.

After bolus administration and intravenous infusions, etomidate causes increases in latency of all waves and prolongation of central conduction time in SSEPs. In contrast to virtually all other commonly used anesthetics, etomidate causes increases in amplitude of the cortical SSEP.[242,243] This effect may be due to an alteration in the balance of inhibitory and excitatory influences or an increase in the irritability of the CNS. This effect seems to be present in the cortex, but not in the spinal cord. Etomidate infusions have been used to enhance SSEP recording in patients when it was impossible to obtain reproducible responses at the beginning of intraoperative monitoring because of the pathology (Fig. 39.24). Following baseline responses that could not be monitored, the etomidate augmentation of the SSEP allowed adequate monitoring and detection of intraoperative events leading to compromise of the spinal cord.[243] The effects of etomidate on BAEPs are dose-dependent increases in latency and decreases in amplitude that are not clinically significant.[244]

Benzodiazepines also can cause changes in SERs.[245,246] Diazepam causes increases in latency and decreases in amplitude of SSEPs, increases in latency in the cortical response after auditory stimulation, and no change in BAEPs. Midazolam causes decreases in amplitude without changes in latency of SSEPs.[242]

Generally, opioids cause small dose-dependent increases in latency and decreases in amplitude of SSEPs. These changes are not clinically significant. Effects on amplitude are more variable than the latency increases.[247,248] Even at large doses of fentanyl (60 μg/kg), reproducible SSEPs can be recorded. Other opioids cause similar dose-dependent changes in SSEPs.[249] Opioids can be used even in high doses in patients requiring intraoperative SSEP monitoring without impairment of ability to monitor neurologic function adequately. Opioid-induced changes must be taken into account, however, when evaluating the recordings. Large intravenous bolus administration of opioids should be avoided at times of potential surgical compromise to neurologic function to prevent confusing the interpretation of SEP changes if they develop. BAEPs were resistant to doses

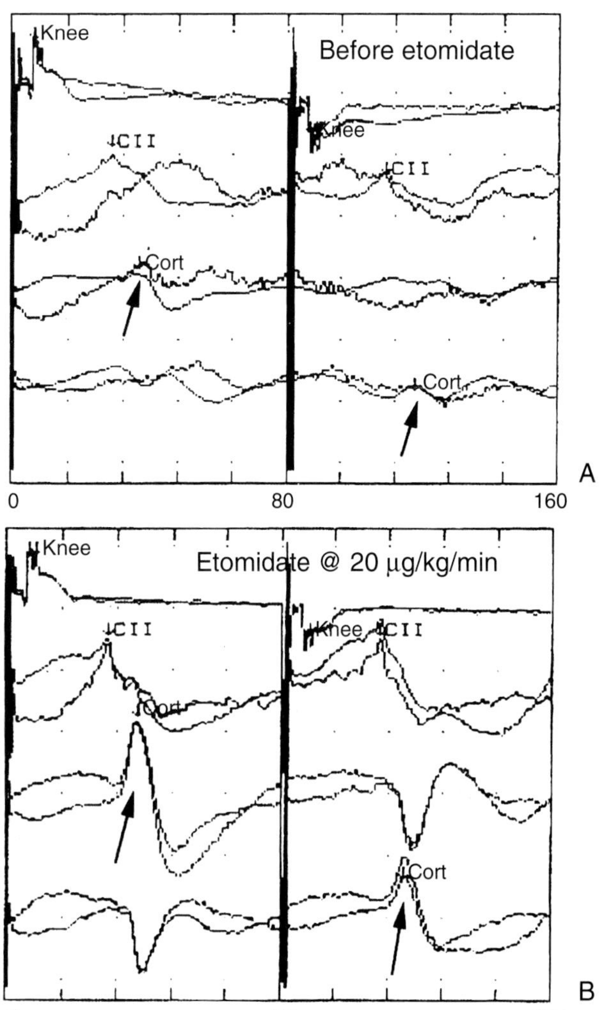

Fig. 39.24 Effects of etomidate on somatosensory-evoked potential. (A) These tracings were obtained from a mildly mentally impaired patient with severe kyphoscoliosis during the early maintenance phase of anesthesia using isoflurane and fentanyl. (B) These tracings were obtained after discontinuing isoflurane and instituting an etomidate infusion at 20 μg/kg/minute. Note dramatically increased amplitude and clarity of the signal in the cortical *(Cort)* channels (marked by *arrows*), which both are recorded with the same amplification scale.

of fentanyl of 50 μg/kg with no changes observed in absolute latency, interpeak latency, or amplitude.[250]

Based on several case reports and small series, dexmedetomidine is compatible with all types of evoked potential monitoring,[251] although data regarding MEPs are not entirely consistent. One recent study demonstrated significant attenuation of MEPs during scoliosis surgery when dexmedetomidine was used as an adjunct to propofol and remifentanil.[252] Data are limited, and large studies are lacking entirely. As the use of this drug increases, more data should become available, but at this time, use of dexmedetomidine does not seem to be clearly problematic.

ANESTHESIA AND MOTOR-EVOKED POTENTIALS

Effects of anesthetics on tcMEPs recorded from muscle are surprisingly profound (see Table 39.4).[253-257] Anesthetic techniques typically used by most anesthesiologists for spine surgery would produce prohibitive depression of the MEP.[258,259] Investigators showed in several studies that intravenous anesthetic drugs produce significantly less depression, and techniques using any of a combination of ketamine, opiates, etomidate, and propofol have been described.[255,256,260-263] The authors have had excellent experience with a combination of propofol and remifentanil, which also is supported in the literature.

Anesthetic effects on MEP responses recorded at spinal levels seem to be less serious. When responses are recorded from muscle, neuromuscular blocking drugs should be monitored quantitatively, maintaining T1 twitch height at around 30% of control values to prevent excessive movement during the operation.[126,254] When responses are not recorded from muscle, profound relaxation is desirable because gross muscle movement produced by MEP stimulation is eliminated, facilitating the surgical procedure. More recent studies using rapid trains of stimuli with transcranial electric and magnetic stimulus techniques have produced responses that are more resistant to the effects of anesthetic drugs, and more "traditional" techniques using inhaled anesthetics and narcotics may be used.[263-265] Most studies support the use of TIVA as preferable to techniques using nitrous oxide or potent inhaled anesthetic drugs, however. Precise control of the anesthetic and avoidance of boluses during critical monitoring periods seem to be even more important than for SSEPs, and active cooperation of the anesthesia care team is essential for good, reproducible results. Fig. 39.25 shows the dramatic effect of introduction of 0.3 MAC isoflurane to a total intravenous technique using propofol and remifentanil. Given ability to monitor the hypnotic component of a TIVA technique with several different available monitors, the authors recommend a total intravenous technique without relaxant whenever possible.

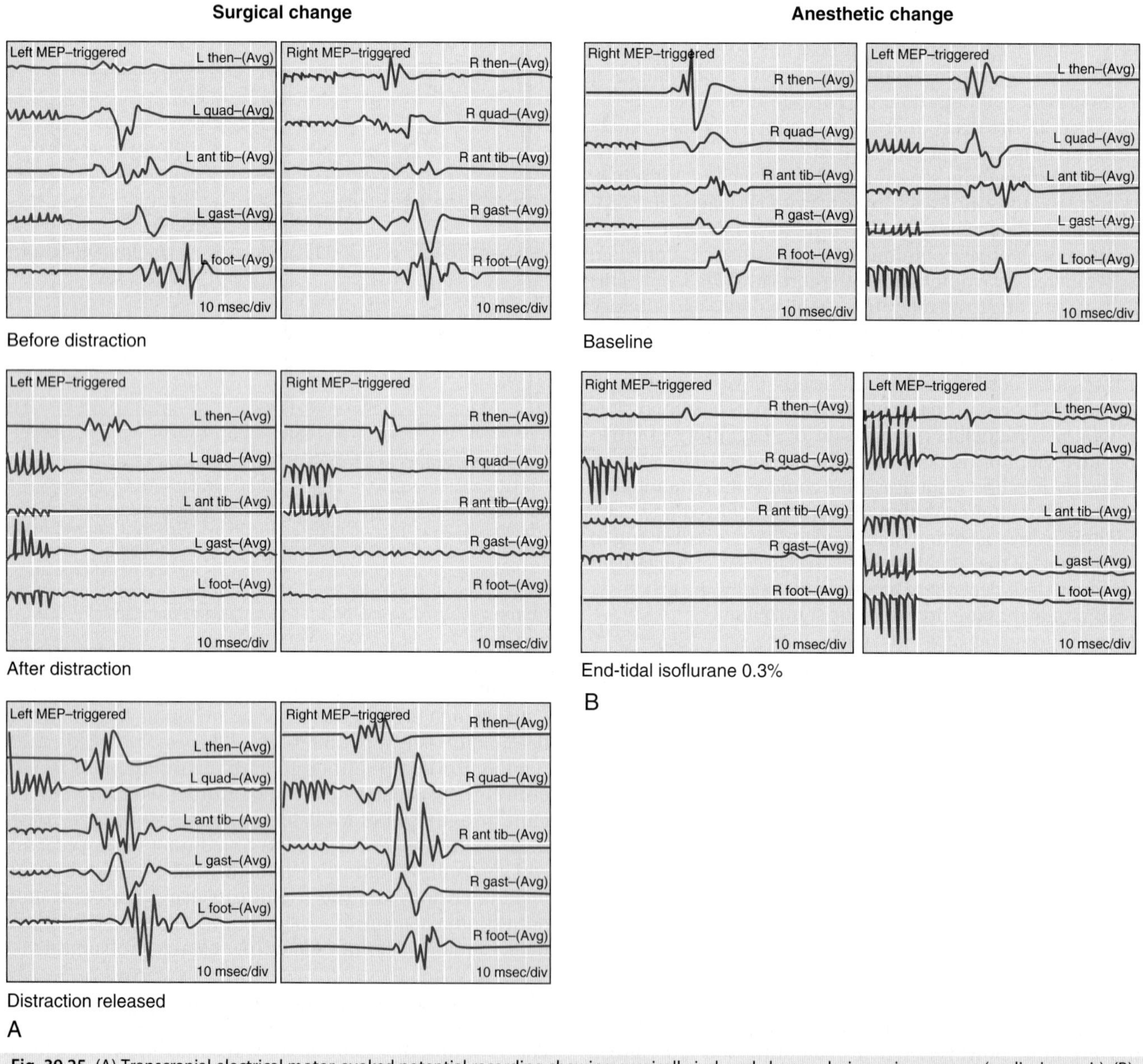

Surgical change

Before distraction

After distraction

Distraction released

A

Anesthetic change

Baseline

End-tidal isoflurane 0.3%

B

Fig. 39.25 (A) Transcranial electrical motor-evoked potential recording showing surgically induced change during spine surgery (scoliosis repair). (B) Motor-evoked potential with an anesthetic-induced change. Note similarity of the change pattern, except that in the anesthetic-induced change, the responses in the upper extremity also changed. Left-sided and right-sided responses are shown on the corresponding panel. A single upper extremity response is shown (top tracing) in each panel. Responses from four muscle groups in each lower extremity are shown directly below. *Ant tib,* M tibialis anterior; *gast,* m gastrocnemius; *L,* left; *quad,* m quadriceps femoris; *R,* right; *then,* thenar.

PATHOPHYSIOLOGIC EFFECTS ON THE ELECTROENCEPHALOGRAM

Hypoxia

Hypoxia may produce inadequate delivery of oxygen to the cerebral cortex generating EEG, and changes similar to those occurring with ischemia result. Initially, hypoxemia may not result in any EEG changes because the brain can increase blood flow to compensate. When the hypoxemia becomes severe enough, further increases in flow are impossible, and EEG changes occur. "Slowing" of the EEG during hypoxia is a nonspecific global effect. Fast frequencies are lost, and low frequencies dominate. Eventually, the EEG is abolished as the brain shuts down electric activity and diverts all oxygen delivered to maintenance of cellular integrity.

Hypotension

In a normal, awake patient, significant levels of hypotension are needed to cause the earliest of CNS signs, as measured by discrimination tests such as the flicker-fusion test. This test examines the flicker rate at which the observer perceives the light to be continuous. In the early days of deliberate hypotension, this test was part of the preoperative evaluation to judge how far the pressure could be reduced during the operation. Clear signs of confusion and inability to concentrate or respond properly to simple commands generally represent very low levels of cerebral perfusion when caused by hypotension because the normal cerebral circulation has a large capacity to vasodilate and maintain normal flow in the face of significant hypotension.

The EEG changes associated with even this level of hypotension are not dramatic, although they are clear by comparison with a previously active recording. Herein lies the problem with using intraoperative EEG to determine whether a given level of hypotension has resulted in brain ischemia. EEG changes are not very pronounced and are bilateral. These changes also are nearly identical to the changes caused by increasing doses of many anesthetic drugs. EEG changes associated with hypotension can be detected, but when the hypotension is induced slowly and associated with changes in anesthetic drugs (e.g., use of isoflurane to reduce blood pressure), the changes are very difficult to interpret. EEG changes associated with acute, severe hypotension such as may be caused by sudden arrhythmias are easier to read. Many patients undergoing surgery do not have a normal cerebral circulation, however. In these individuals, even mild hypotension may result in significant cerebral ischemia. In these individuals, monitoring the EEG during planned hypotension may be helpful, provided that other causes of similar EEG changes may be carefully controlled. There remains little literature to support the use of EEG monitoring during hypotension, but in our opinion, when the EEG is being monitored (e.g., during carotid surgery), EEG changes secondary to hypotension really do represent cerebral ischemia of a significant degree and should be considered an important finding.

Hypothermia

During cooling on CPB, the total power and peak power frequency of the high-frequency band were highly correlated with temperature using Fourier analysis and spectral edge data; however, significant variability was noted among subjects, especially during cooling.[266] Complete EEG suppression usually develops at 15°C to 18°C. Levy and colleagues[147] showed an improved ability to quantify the effects of hypothermia on the EEG using an EEG processing technique known as "approximate entropy."

Hypercarbia and Hypocarbia

Hypocapnia is known to activate excitable seizure foci, and in rare cases may produce EEG evidence of cerebral ischemia even in awake subjects.[267] Hypercapnia, unless severe and associated with hypoxemia, has only indirect effects secondary to increased CBF. In an anesthetized patient, hypercarbia-associated increases in CBF may have similar effects to the effects seen with increasing end-tidal tension of volatile anesthetics.[268]

Untoward Events

One of the suggested reasons for monitoring the brain of an anesthetized patient is to enable detection of injuries to the nervous system that would not be otherwise apparent. Although hundreds of such case reports are in the literature, as well as many in our experience, cost-effectiveness of such monitoring is unclear. In a more recent case at our institution, severe EEG changes occurred at the beginning of a carotid endarterectomy, before surgical incision, and were unassociated with any other vital sign changes or hypotension. Immediate angiography revealed acute carotid occlusion and completely changed the operation performed with this patient, and the patient recovered completely. There are intraoperative events that could lead to CNS insult, which, if detected early, could be rapidly reversed or treated to prevent permanent injury. Given the rarity of such events, however, it is extremely unlikely that such monitoring would be shown to be beneficial in any foreseeable randomized trial. If the "at-risk" patient could be identified preoperatively, perhaps the EEG or other types of neuromonitoring could be useful in detecting untoward CNS events during anesthesia, such as a new stroke after elective general surgery.

PHYSIOLOGIC FACTORS INFLUENCING SENSORY-EVOKED RESPONSES

Numerous physiologic variables, including systemic arterial blood pressure, temperature (local and systemic), and blood gas tensions, can influence SEP recordings. With decreases in mean arterial blood pressure to below levels of cerebral autoregulation owing to either blood loss or vasoactive drugs, progressive changes in SERs have been noted. SSEP changes observed are progressive decreases in amplitude until loss of the waveform with no changes in latency.[269,270] BAEPs are resistant to even profound levels of hypotension (MAP of 20 mm Hg in dogs).[269] Cortical (synaptic) function necessary to produce cortical SERs seems to be more sensitive to hypoperfusion than spinal cord or brainstem, nonsynaptic transmission.[270] Rapid decreases in arterial blood pressure to levels above the lower limit of autoregulation also have been associated with transient SSEP changes of decreased amplitude that resolve after several minutes of continued hypotension at the same level.[271] Reversible SSEP changes at systemic pressures within the normal range have been observed in patients undergoing spinal distraction during scoliosis surgery. These changes resolved with increases of systemic arterial blood pressure to slightly higher than the patient's normal pressure, suggesting that the combination of surgical manipulation with levels of hypotension generally considered "safe" could result in spinal cord ischemia.[272]

Changes in temperature also affect SERs. Hypothermia causes increases in latency and decreases in amplitude of cortical and subcortical SERs after all types of stimulation.[273-275] Hyperthermia also alters SERs, with increases in temperature leading to decreases in amplitude in SSEPs and loss of SSEPs at 42°C during induced hyperthermia.[276]

Changes in arterial blood gas tensions can alter SERs, probably in relation to changes in blood flow or oxygen delivery to neural structures.[277,278] Hypoxia produces SSEP changes (decreased amplitude) similar to the changes seen with ischemia.[278] Decreased oxygen delivery associated with anemia during isovolemic hemodilution results in progressive increases in latency of SSEPs and VEPs that become significant at hematocrit values lower than 15%. Changes in amplitude were variable until very low hematocrit values (approximately 7%) were reached, at which point the amplitude of all waveforms decreased.[279]

Summary

Regardless of the type of intraoperative neurologic monitor, several principles must be observed for neurologic monitoring to provide potential benefit to the patient. First, the pathway at risk during the surgical procedure must be amenable to monitoring. Second, if evidence of injury to the pathway is detected, some intervention must be possible. If changes in the neurologic monitor are detected, and no intervention is possible, although the monitor may be of prognostic value, it does not have the potential to provide direct benefit to the patient from early detection of impending neurologic injury. Third, the monitor must provide reliable and reproducible data. If the data have a high degree of variability in the absence of clinical interventions, their utility for detecting clinically significant events is limited.

This chapter reviews the most common clinically used intraoperative neurologic monitors. Ideally, clinical studies would provide outcome data on the efficacy of a neurologic monitor in a given procedure to improve neurologic outcome. Although there is a wealth of clinical experience with many of these monitoring modalities, there is little in the way of randomized prospective studies evaluating the efficacy of neurologic monitoring. Based on clinical experience with neurologic monitoring and nonrandomized clinical studies in which neurologic monitoring is used and generally compared with historical controls, practice patterns for use of neurologic monitoring have developed. In certain procedures, neurologic monitoring is recommended and used by most centers; in other procedures, monitoring is used almost routinely in some centers, but not in others; and in some procedures, no clear clinical experience or evidence indicates that monitoring is useful at all (experimental use). Finally, there are procedures in which monitoring is used selectively for patients believed to be at higher-than-usual risk for intraoperative neurologic injury. Table 39.5 provides a summary of current clinical practice.

Complete references available online at expertconsult.com.

TABLE 39.5 Current Practices in Neurologic Monitoring

Procedure	Monitors	Current Practice
Carotid endarterectomy	Awake patient neurologic examination, EEG, SSEP, TCD	NIH recommends use of one of these four available monitors
	CO	Threshold value not determined, inadequate normative population data
Scoliosis surgical treatment	SSEP	Monitoring recommended and may substitute for wake-up testing
	Wake-up test	Largely abandoned in centers using electrophysiologic monitoring; monitoring is not continuous, and false-negative monitoring patterns reported
	MEP	Increased clinical use now that transcranial electrical stimulation is FDA approved; useful in combination with SSEP
Acoustic neuroma	Facial nerve monitor	Facial nerve monitoring recommended
	BAEP	BAEP showing some clinical evidence of improved outcome in some procedures
Intracranial aneurysm clipping	SSEP, EEG, tcMEP	Used routinely in some centers; limited clinical data on outcome, but appears clinically useful during anterior circulation procedures
Cranial nerve V decompression	BAEP	Used in some centers; reduces hearing loss
Cranial nerve VII decompression	BAEP, facial nerve monitor	Data from small series showing improved hearing preservation
Supratentorial mass lesions	SSEP, tcMEP	Used in some centers in selected high-risk procedures
Infratentorial mass lesions	BAEP, SSEP, tcMEP	BAEP to detect retractor-related cranial nerve VIII injury; SSEP and tcMEP in rare, high-risk lesions adjacent to ascending sensory or descending motor pathways
Decompression of spinal stenosis	SSEP, tcMEP	Used in some centers in high-risk procedures (more often cervical)
Spinal cord trauma	SSEP, MEP	Used in some centers in high-risk procedures
Cardiopulmonary bypass	EEG, TCD, $Sjvo_2$, CO	Used routinely in some centers; actively studied, but no outcome data yet
Aortic coarctation	SSEP	Used routinely in a few centers; no widespread acceptance
Aortic aneurysm repair	SSEP, MEP	Used routinely in a few centers; no widespread acceptance

BAEP, Brainstem auditory-evoked potential; *CO*, cerebral oximetry; *EEG*, electroencephalogram; *FDA*, U.S. Food and Drug Administration; *MEP*, motor-evoked potential; *NIH*, National Institutes of Health; $Sjvo_2$, jugular bulb venous oxygen saturation; *SSEP*, somatosensory-evoked potential; *TCD*, transcranial Doppler; *tcMEP*, transcranial motor-evoked potential.

References

1. Skinner SA, et al. *J Clin Monit Comput*. 2014;28:103. 2014.
2. Martin NA, Doberstein C. *Neurosurg Clin North Am*. 1994;5:607. 1994.
3. Kety SS, Schmidt CF. *Am J Physiol*. 1945;143:53. 1945.
4. Udesh R, et al. *J Ultrasound Med*. 2017;36:621. 2017.
5. Bass A, et al. *J Vasc Surg*. 1989;10:549. 1989.
6. Manno EM. *Crit Care Clin*. 1997;79. 199713.
7. White H, Baker A. *Can J Anaesth*. 2002;49:623. 2002.
8. Hongo K, et al. *Neurol Res*. 1995;17:89. 1995.
9. Davie SN, Grocott HP. *Anesthesiology*. 2012;116:834. 2012.
10. Zheng F, et al. *Anesth Analg*. 2013;116:663. 2013.
11. Bickler P, et al. *Anesth Analg*. 2017;124:72–82. 2017.
12. Samra SK, et al. *Anesthesiology*. 2000;93:964. 2000.
13. Rigamonti A, et al. *J Clin Anesth*. 2005;17:426. 2005.
14. Dings J, et al. *Neurosurgery*. 1998;43:1082. 1998, PMID.
15. Vajkoczy P, et al. *J Neurosurg*. 2003;98:1227. 2003.
16. Lang EW, et al. *Neurosurg Rev*. 2007;30:99. 2007.
17. Vajkoczy P, et al. *J Neurosurg*. 2000;93:265. 2000.
18. Clark LC. *Trans Am Soc Artif Int Org*. 1956;2:41. 1956.
19. Ngwenya LB, et al. *Respir Care*. 2016;61:1232. 2016.
20. Menzel M, et al. *J Neurosurg Anesthesiol*. 1999;11:240. 1999.
21. Gopinath SP, et al. *Crit Care Med*. 1999;27:2337. 1999.
22. Valadka AB, et al. *Crit Care Med*. 1998;26:1576. 1998.
23. Sarrafzadeh AS, et al. *Acta Neurochir Suppl (Wien)*. 1998;71:186. 1998.
24. Rosenthal G, et al. *Crit Care Med*. 2008;36:1917. 2008.
25. Menzel M, et al. *J Neurosurg*. 1999;91(1). 1999.
26. Menzel M, et al. *J Neurosurg Anesthesiol*. 1999;11:240. 1999.
27. Carney N, et al. *Neurosurgery*. 2017;80(6). 2017.
28. Gloor P. In: Wieser HG, Elger CE, eds. *Presurgical Evaluation of Epileptics*. Berlin: Springer; 1987.
29. Hughes JR. *EEG in clinical practice*. Newton, Mass: Butterworth-Heinemann; 1994. 1994.
30. Vitek JL, et al. *J Neurosurg*. 1998;88:1027.
31. Garonzik IM, et al. *Mov Disord*. 2002;17(suppl 3):S135. 2002.
32. Martin JT, et al. *Anesthesiology*. 1959;20:359. 1959.
33. Sharbrough FW, et al. *Stroke*. 1973;4:674. 1973.
34. Craft RM, et al. *J Neurosurg Anesthesiol*. 1994;6:301. 1994.
35. Spackman TN, et al. *Anesthesiology*. 1987;66:229. 1987.
36. Billard V, et al. *Clin Pharmacol Ther*. 1997;61:45. 1997.
37. Schmidt GN, et al. *Anesthesiology*. 2003;99:1072. 2003.
38. Willmann K, et al. *J Clin Monit Comput*. 2002;17:345. 2002.
39. Drover DR, et al. *Anesthesiology*. 2002;97:82. 2002.
40. Levy WJ. *Anesthesiology*. 1987;66:489. 1987.
41. Grundy BL. *Neurosurgery*. 1982;11:556. 1982.
42. Greenberg RP, Ducker TB. *J Neurosurg*. 1982;56(1). 1982.
43. Cohen AR, et al. *Neurosurgery*. 1981;9:157. 1981.
44. York DH. *Progr Neurobiol*. 1985;25(1). 1985.
45. Bundo M, et al. *Stroke*. 2002;33:61. 2002.
46. Symon L. *Br J Anaesth*. 1985;57:34. 1985.
47. Brainston NM, et al. *J Cereb Blood Flow Metab*. 1984;4:68. 1984.
48. Lopez JR, et al. *J Neurol Neurosurg Psychiatry*. 1999;66:189. 1999.
49. Guerit JM, et al. *Electroencephalogr Clin Neurophysiol*. 1997;104:459. 1997.
50. Chiappa KH, Ropper AH. *N Engl J Med*. 1982;306:1140. 1982.
51. Ganes T. *Electroencephalogr Clin Neurophysiol*. 1980;49:446. 1980.
52. Chiappa KH, Ropper AH. *N Engl J Med*. 1982;306:1140. 1982.
53. Grundy BL, et al. *J Neurosurg*. 1982;57:674. 1982.
54. Raudzens PA, Shetter AG. *J Neurosurg*. 1982;57:341. 1982.
55. Duncan PG, et al. *Can Anaesth Soc J*. 1979;26:492. 1979.
56. Sasaki T, et al. *J Neurosurg*. 2010;112:273. 2010.
57. Levy WJ, et al. *Neurosurgery*. 1984;15:287. 1984.
58. Legatt AD. *J Clin Neurophysiol*. 2002;19:454. 2002.
59. MacDonald DB, et al. *Spine*. 2003;28:194. 2003.
60. Szelenyi A, et al. *J Neurosurg*. 2003;99:575. 2003.
61. Meylaerts S, et al. *Ann Surg*. 1999;230:742. 1999.
62. Pelosi L, et al. *Clin Neurophysiol*. 2002;113:1082. 2002.
63. Skinner SA, et al. *J Clin Monit Comp*. 2008;22:131. 2008 .
64. Harner SG, et al. *Mayo Clin Proc*. 1987;62:92. 1987.
65. Harper CM, Daube RJ. In: Desmedt JE, ed. *Neuromonitoring in Surgery*. New York: Elsevier Science; 1989:275–297. 1989.
66. Skinner S, et al. *J Clin Neurophysiol*. 2017;34:477. 2017.
67. Freedman WA, et al. *Neurosurgery*. 1991;29:98. 1991.
68. Lokuge K, et al. *Br J Surg*. 2018;105:26. 2018.
69. De Rango P, et al. *Stroke*. 2015;46:3423. 2015.
70. Sundt TW Jr, et al. *Mayo Clin Proc*. 1981;56:533. 1981.
71. Bond R, et al. *Eur J Vasc Endovasc Surg*. 2002;23:117. 2002.
72. Kalkman CJ. *J Cardiothorac Vasc Anesth*. 2004;18:381. 2004.
73. Plestis KA, et al. *J Vasc Surg*. 1997;25:620. 1997.
74. Halsey JH Jr. *Stroke*. 1992;23:1583. 1992.
75. Roseborough GS. *J Cardiothorac Vasc Anesth*. 2004;18:375. 2004.
76. Schneider JR, et al. *J Vasc Surg*. 2002;35:1114. 2002.
77. Woodworth GF, et al. *Neurosurgery*. 2007;61:1170. 2007.
78. Chongruksut W, et al. *Cochrane Database Syst Rev*. 2014;6:CD000190. 2014.
79. Lam AM, et al. *Anesthesiology*. 1991;75(15). 1991.
80. Ackerstaff RG, van de Vlasakker CJ. *J Cardiothorac Vasc Anesth*. 1998;12:341. 1998.
81. AbuRahma AF, et al. *J Vasc Surg*. 2011;54:1502. 2011.
82. Thirumala PD, et al. *Neurol Res*. 2016;38:698. 2016.
83. Ackerstaff RG, et al. *Stroke*. 2000;31:1817. 2000.
84. Ogasawara K, et al. *Stroke*. 2008;39:3088. 2008.
85. Mueller M, et al. *Acta Neurol Scand*. 1998;97:110. 1998.
86. Abbott AL, et al. *Cerebrovasc Dis*. 2007;23:362. 2007.
87. Dunne VG, et al. *J Clin Neurosci*. 2001;8:140. 2001.
88. Spencer MP. *Stroke*. 1997;28:685. 1997.
89. Gaunte ME. *Ann R Coll Surg Engl*. 1998;80:377. 1998.
90. Calderon-Arnulphi M, et al. *J Neurosurg*. 2007;106:283. 2007.
91. Friedell ML, et al. *J Vasc Surg*. 2008;48:601. 2008.
92. Friedman WA, et al. *Neurosurgery*. 1991;29:83. 1991.
93. Mizoi K, Yoshimoto T. *Neurol Med Chir (Tokyo)*. 1991;31:318. 1991.
94. Misoi K, Yoshimoto T. *Neurosurgery*. 1993;33:434. 1993.
95. Holland NR. *J Clin Neurophysiol*. 1998;15:439. 1998.
96. Schramm J, et al. *Neurol Res*. 1994;16:20. 1994.
97. Wiedemayer H, et al. *J Neurosurg*. 2002;96:255. 2002.
98. Manninen PH, et al. *Can J Anaesth*. 1994;41:92. 1994.
99. Manninen PH, et al. *Can J Anaesth*. 1990;37:S23. 1990.
100. Friedman WA, et al. *Neurosurgery*. 1987;20:678.
101. Little JR, et al. *Neurosurgery*. 1987;20:421. 1987.
102. Sasaki T, et al. *J Neurosurg*. 2007;107:60. 2007.
103. Hemmer LB, et al. *World Neurosurg*. 2014;81:99. 2014.
104. Thomas B, Guo D. *World Neurosurg*. 2017;103:829. 2017.
105. Meng L, et al. *Can J Anaesth*. 2017;64:517. 2017.
106. Stevanovic A, et al. *PLoS One*. 2016;11:e0156448. 2016.
107. West S, et al. *Epileptic Disord*. 2016;18:113. 2016.
108. Ryvlin P, et al. *Lancet Neurol*. 2014;13:1114.
109. Ramnarayan R, Mackenzie I. *Neurol India*. 2006;54:250. 2006.
110. Sindou MP. *Acta Neurochir (Wien)*. 2005;147:1019. 2005.
111. Brock S, et al. *Stereotact Funct Neurosurg*. 2004;82:199. 2004.
112. Sindou M, et al. *Laryngoscope*. 1992;102:678. 1992.
113. Friedman WA, et al. *J Neurosurg*. 1985;62:552. 1985.
114. Thirumala PD, et al. *J Clin Neurophys*. 2011;28:56. 2011.
115. Khrais T, Sanna M. *J Laryngol Otol*. 2006;120:366. 2006.
116. Vivas EX, et al. *Neurosurgery*. 2018;82:E44. 2018.
117. Sala F, et al. *Childs Nerv Syst*. 2015;31:1791. 2015.
118. McCallum JE, Bennett MH. *Surg Forum*. 1975;26:469. 1975.
119. Maccabee PJ, et al. *Electroencephalogr Clin Neurophysiol*. 1982;53: P32. 1982.
120. Luederes H, et al. *Spine*. 1982;7:110. 1982.
121. Raudzens PA. *Ann N Y Acad Sci*. 1982;388:308. 1982.
122. Grundy BL. In: Nodar RH, Barber C, eds. *Evoked potentials II*. Boston: Butterworth; 1984:624. 1984.
123. Deutsch H, et al. *J Neurosurg*. 2000;92(suppl 2):155. 2000.
124. Ben-David B, et al. *Spine*. 1987;12:536. 1987.
125. Szilagyi DE, et al. *Surgery*. 1978;83:38. 1978.
126. Edmonds HL, et al. *Spine*. 1989;14:683. 1989.
127. Boyd SG, et al. *J Neurol Neurosurg Psychiatry*. 1986;49:251. 1986.
128. Sloan TB, et al. *Curr Opin Anesthesiol*. 2008;21:560. 2008.
129. Padberg AM, et al. *Spine*. 1998;23:1392. 1998.
130. Schwartz DM, et al. *J Bone Joint Surg Am*. 2007;89:2440. 2007.
131. MacDonald DB, et al. *Spine*. 2003;28:194. 2003.
132. MacDonald DB, et al. *Clin Neurophysiol*. 2013;124:2291. 2013.
133. Elmore JR, et al. *J Vasc Surg*. 1991;14:131. 1991.
134. Reuter DG, et al. *J Thorac Cardiovasc Surg*. 1992;104:262. 1992.
135. Conrad MF, et al. *J Vasc Surg*. 2011;53:1195. 2011.
136. Weigang E, et al. *Ann Thorac Surg*. 2006;82:1679. 2006.
137. Etz CD, et al. *Ann Thorac Surg*. 2006;82:1670. 2006.
138. Skinner SA, Vodušek DB. *J Clin Neurophysiol*. 2014;31:313. 2014.
139. Raynor BL, et al. *Spine*. 2007;32:2673. 2007.
140. Shi YB, et al. *Spine*. 2003;28:595. 2003.
141. Isley MR, et al. *Neurodiagn J*. 2012;52:100. 2012.
142. Shin AY, et al. *J Am Acad Orthop Surg*. 2005;13:382. 2005.

143. Kline DG, et al. *J Neurosurg*. 1998;89(13). 1998.
144. Kim DH, et al. *J Neurosurg*. 2003;98:1005. 2003.
145. Cornelissen L, et al. *Elife*. 2015;23(4):e06513. 2015.
146. Levy WJ. *Anesthesiology*. 1984;60:291. 1984.
147. Levy WJ, et al. *Anesthesiology*. 2003;98:53. 2003.
148. Chabot RJ, et al. *Clin Electroencephalogr*. 1997;28:98. 1997.
149. Edmonds HL Jr, et al. *J Thorac Cardiovasc Surg*. 1992;103:555. 1992.
150. Miller G, et al. *Pediatr Neurol*. 1994;10:124. 1994.
151. Hirsch JC, et al. *Ann Thorac Surg*. 2012;94:1365. 2012.
152. Doblar DD. *Semin Cardiothorac Vasc Anesth*. 2004;8:127. 2004.
153. Rodriguez PA, et al. *Stroke*. 2010;41:2229. 2010.
154. Sakamoto T, et al. *J Cardiothorac Vasc Anesth*. 2004;18:293. 2004.
155. Kussman BD, et al. *Anesth Analg*. 2005;101:1294. 2005.
156. Murkin JM, et al. *Anesth Analg*. 2007;104:51. 2007.
157. Zheng F, et al. *Anesth Analg*. 2013;163:663. 2013.
158. Ono M, et al. *Br J Anesth*. 2012;109:391. 2012.
159. Colak Z, et al. *Eur J Cardiothorac Surg*. 2015;47:447. 2015.
160. Brady K, et al. *Stroke*. 2010;41:1951. 2010.
161. Gopinath SP, et al. *J Neurol Neurosurg Psychiatry*. 1994;57:717. 1994.
162. Fandino J, et al. *J Clin Neurosci*. 2000;7:226. 2000.
163. Cormio M, et al. *J Neurosurg*. 1999;90(9). 1999.
164. Hilkman DM, et al. *Curr Opin Anaesthesiol*. 2017;30:192. 2017.
165. Herman ST, et al. *J Clin Neurophysiol*. 2015;32:87. 2015.
166. Herman ST, et al. *J Clin Neurophysiol*. 2015;32:96. 2015.
167. Cremer OL, et al. *Crit Care Med*. 2005;33:2207. 2005.
168. Stiefel MF, et al. *J Neurosurg*. 2006;105:568.
169. Fortune JB, et al. *J Trauma*. 1995;39:1091. 1995.
170. Skippen P, et al. *Crit Care Med*. 1997;25:1402. 1997.
171. Imberti R, et al. *J Neurosurg*. 2002;96:97. 2002.
172. Coles JP, et al. *Crit Care Med*. 2002;30:1950. 2002.
173. van den Brink WA, et al. *Neurosurgery*. 2000;46:868. 2000.
174. Stiefel MF, et al. *J Neurosurg*. 2005;103:805. 2005.
175. Suarez JI, et al. *Crit Care Med*. 2002;30:1348. 2002.
176. Topcuoglu MA, et al. *Curr Treat Options Cardiovasc Med*. 2002;4:3731. 2002.
177. Jarus-Dziedzic K, et al. *Neurol Res*. 2002;24:5822. 2002.
178. Aaslid R. *Eur J Ultrasound*. 2002;16(3). 2002.
179. Mascia L, et al. *Intensive Care Med*. 2003;29:1088. 2003.
180. Sloan MA, et al. *Neurology*. 1989;39:1514. 1989.
181. Sekhar LN, et al. *Neurosurgery*. 1988;22:813. 1988.
182. Vespa PM, et al. *J Clin Neurophysiol*. 1999;16(1). 1999.
183. Bricolo A, et al. *Electroencephalogr Clin Neurophysiol*. 1978;45:211. 1978.
184. Gutling E, et al. *Neurology*. 1995;45:915. 1995.
185. Alexandre A, et al. *Acta Neurochir Suppl (Wien)*. 1979;28:188. 1979.
186. Bergamasco B, et al. *Electroencephalogr Clin Neurophysiol*. 1968;24:374. 1968.
187. Winer JW, et al. *Neurosurgery*. 1991;29:739. 1991.
188. Koenig MA, Kaplan PW. *J Clin Neurophysiol*. 2015;32:472. 2015.
189. Facco E, et al. *Neurophysiol Clin*. 1993;23:237. 1993.
190. Pohlmann-Eden B, et al. *Intensive Care Med*. 1997;23:301. 1997.
191. Ruiz-Lopez MJ, et al. *Crit Care Med*. 1999;27:412. 1999.
192. Goodwin SR, et al. *Crit Care Med*. 1991;19:518. 1991.
193. Morgalla MH, et al. *Anaesthesist*. 2006;55:760. 2006.
194. Nuwer MR. *Neurosurg Clin North Am*. 1994;5:647. 1994.
195. Lew HL, et al. *J Head Trauma Rehabil*. 2006;21:350. 2006.
196. Carter BG, Butt W. *Crit Care Med*. 2001;29:178. 2001.
197. Carter BG, Butt W. *Intensive Care Med*. 2005;31:765. 2005.
198. Fischer C, Luaute J. *Neuropsychol Rehabil*. 2005;15:372. 2005.
199. Petty GW, et al. *Neurology*. 1990;40:300. 1990.
200. Rosen I, Hagerdal M. *Acta Anaesthesiol Scand*. 1976;20:32. 1976.
201. Akeju Oluwaseun, et al. *Clin Neurophysiol*. 2016;127:2414. 2016.
202. McGuire G, et al. *Br J Anaesth*. 2003;91:651. 2003.
203. La Marca S, et al. *Psychopharmacology (Berl)*. 1995;120:426. 1995.
204. Sebel PS, et al. *Anesthesiology*. 1981;55:203. 1981.
205. Hyypponen E, et al. *Acta Anaesthesiol Scand*. 2008;52:289. 2008.
206. Maksimow A, et al. *Acta Anaesthesiol Scand*. 2007;51:22. 2007.
207. Kasuya Y, et al. *Anesth Analg*. 2009;109:2009. 1811.
208. Yamamura T, et al. *Anesth Analg*. 1981;60:283. 1981.
209. Clark DL, et al. *Anesthesiology*. 1973;39:261. 1973.
210. Artru AA, et al. *Anesth Analg*. 1997;85:587. 1997.
211. Komatsu H, et al. *Anesthesiology*. 1994;81:1535. 1994.
212. Jaaskelainen SK, et al. *Neurology*. 2003;61:1073. 2003.
213. Endo T, et al. *J Neurosurg Anesthesiol*. 2002;14:59. 2002.
214. Rampil IJ, et al. *Anesthesiology*. 1991;74:434. 1991.
215. Sharpe MD, et al. *Anesthesiology*. 2002;97:261. 2002.
216. Hoffman WE, Edelman G. *Anesth Analg*. 1995;81:811. 1995.
217. Banoub M, et al. *Anesthesiology*. 2003;99:716. 2003.
218. Peterson DO, et al. *Anesthesiology*. 1986;65:35. 1986.
219. McPherson RW, et al. *Anesthesiology*. 1985;62:626. 1985.
220. Pathak KS, et al. *Anesthesiology*. 1989;70:207. 1989.
221. Samra SK, et al. *Anesthesiology*. 1987;66:29. 1987.
222. Haghighi SS, et al. *J Neurosurg Anesthesiol*. 1996;8:148. 1996.
223. Bernard JM, et al. *Anesthesiology*. 1996;85:1013. 1996.
224. Boisseau N, et al. *Br J Anaesth*. 2002;88:785. 2002.
225. Vaugha DJ, et al. *Br J Anaesth*. 2001;86:59. 2001.
226. Manninen PH, et al. *Anesth Analg*. 1985;64:43. 1985.
227. Thornton C, et al. *Br J Anaesth*. 1983;55:479. 1983.
228. Matsushita S, et al. *J Clin Monit Comput*. 2015;29:621. 2015.
229. Chi OZ, Field C. *Anesthesiology*. 1986;65:328. 1986.
230. Soffin EM, et al. *J Clin Monit Comput*. 2017.
231. Uribe AA, et al. *Clin Neurophysiol*. 2017;128:2006. 2017.
232. Sebel PS, et al. *Br J Anaesth*. 1984;56:1403. 1984.
233. Liu EH, et al. *Br J Anaesth*. 2005;94:193. 2005.
234. Boisseau N, et al. *Br J Anaesth*. 2002;88:785. 2002.
235. Taniguchi M, et al. *Neurosurgery*. 1992;31:891. 1992.
236. Chassard D, et al. *Br J Anaesth*. 1989;62:522.
237. Purdie JA, Cullen PM. *Anaesthesia*. 1993;48:192. 1993.
238. Drummond JC, et al. *Anesthesiology*. 1985;63:249. 1985.
239. Shimoji K, et al. *Anesthesiology*. 1974;40:234. 1974.
240. Ganes T, Lundar T. *J Neurol Neurosurg Psychiatry*. 1983;46:509. 1983.
241. Sutton LN, et al. *J Neurosurg*. 1982;57:178. 1982.
242. Koht A, et al. *Anesth Analg*. 1988;67:435. 1988.
243. Sloan TB, et al. *Anesth Analg*. 1988;67:582. 1988.
244. Heneghan CPH, et al. *Br J Anaesth*. 1985;57:554. 1985.
245. Doring WH, Daub D. *Arch Otorhinolaryngol*. 1980;227:522. 1980.
246. Grundy BL, et al. *Anesthesiology*. 1979;538. 197951.
247. Pathak KS, et al. *Anesth Analg*. 1984;63:833. 1984.
248. Schubert A, et al. *Anesth Analg*. 1986;65:S136. 1986.
249. Grundy BL, Brown RH. *Electroencephalogr Clin Neurophysiol*. 1980;50:177. 1980.
250. Samra SK, et al. *Anesthesiology*. 1984;61:261. 1984.
251. Bala E, et al. *Anesthesiology*. 2008;109:417. 2008.
252. Mahmoud M, et al. *Anesthesiology*. 2010;112:1364. 2010.
253. Zentner J, et al. *Neurosurgery*. 1989;24:253. 1989.
254. Jellinek D, et al. *Neurosurgery*. 1991;29:551. 1991.
255. Taniguchi M, et al. *Neurosurgery*. 1993;33:407. 1993.
256. Ubags LH, et al. *J Neurosurg Anesthesiol*. 1997;9:228. 1997.
257. Kalkman CJ, et al. *Neurosurgery*. 1994;35:1066. 1994.
258. Sloan TB, Heyer EJ. *J Clin Neurophysiol*. 2002;19:430. 2002.
259. Zentner J, et al. *Spine*. 1997;22:1002. 1997.
260. Nathan N, et al. *Br J Anaesth*. 2003;91:493. 2003.
261. Ghaly RF, et al. *Neurol Res*. 2001;23:881. 2001.
262. Scheufler KM, Zentner J. *J Neurosurg*. 2002;96:571.
263. Pechstein U, et al. *Electroencephalogr Clin Neurophysiol*. 1998;108:175. 1998.
264. Pelosi L, et al. *Clin Neurophysiol*. 2001;112:1076. 2001.
265. Ubaga LH, et al. *Neurosurgery*. 1998;43:90. 1998.
266. Stockard JJ, Bickford RG. In: Gordon E, ed. *A Basis and Practice of Neuroanesthesia*. New York: Elsevier; 1981:3. 1981.
267. Kraaier V, et al. *Electroencephalogr Clin Neurophysiol*. 1988;70:377. 1988.
268. Clowes GHA, et al. *Ann Surg*. 1953;138:558. 1953.
269. Eng DY, et al. *Anesthesiology*. 1980;53:S92. 1980.
270. Kobrine AI, et al. *J Neurol Sci*. 1980;45:65. 1980.
271. Bunegin L, et al. *Anesthesiology*. 1981;55:A232. 1981.
272. Grundy BL, et al. *Anesthesiology*. 1981;54:249. 1981.
273. Russ W, et al. *Anesthesiology*. 1984;61:207. 1984.
274. Stockard JJ, et al. *Ann Neurol*. 1978;3:368. 1978.
275. Spetzler RF, et al. *J Neurosurg*. 1988;68:868. 1988.
276. Dubois M, et al. *Electroencephalogr Clin Neurophysiol*. 1981;52:157. 1981.
277. Nakagawa Y, et al. *Stroke*. 1984;25:275. 1984.
278. Grundy BL, et al. *Anesth Analg*. 1981;60:437. 1981.
279. Nagao S, et al. *J Surg Res*. 1978;25:530. 1978.

40 Monitoring the State of the Brain and Central Nervous System During General Anesthesia and Sedation

EMERY N. BROWN, PATRICK L. PURDON, OLUWASEUN AKEJU, and KEN SOLT

KEY POINTS

- Anesthesiologists rely extensively on physiologic signals and anesthetic dosing strategies to infer and to track states of the brain and central nervous system under general anesthesia.
- Heart rate and systemic arterial blood pressure changes are the principal physiologic signals used to monitor the anesthetic state of patients receiving general anesthesia.
- Use of the neurologic examination during induction of and emergence from general anesthesia can provide information regarding loss and recovery of consciousness.
- Electroencephalogram (EEG)–based indices are used to track the level of unconsciousness of patients receiving general anesthesia. The most commonly used EEG-based indices are the bispectral index (BIS), the Patient Safety Index (PSI), Narcotrend, and Entropy.
- Real-time analysis of the unprocessed EEG and the spectrogram (density spectral array) is a highly informative way to monitor the level of unconsciousness of patients receiving general anesthesia.
- Use of the unprocessed EEG and spectrogram for real-time monitoring of the level of unconsciousness is made possible by the fact that the EEG oscillations of anesthetized patients change systematically with anesthetic dose, with anesthetic class (mechanism of action), and patient age.
- Anesthetic-induced oscillations are one of the primary mechanisms through which these agents induce altered arousal states such as sedation and unconsciousness. Therefore, real-time monitoring of the unprocessed EEG and the spectrogram provide a scientifically based, practical, and patient-specific way to track sedation and unconsciousness in the operating room.
- Normalized symbolic transfer entropy (NSTE) is an approach for quantifying how changes in frontoparietal functional connectivity relate to anesthesia-induced changes in consciousness.
- In the future, closed-loop anesthetic delivery (CLAD) systems may provide highly accurate ways to control states of general anesthesia, medical coma, and sedation.
- Obtaining reliable quantitative markers of nociception is an active area of investigation.

General anesthesia is a drug-induced reversible condition composed of four behavioral and physiologic states: antinociception, unconsciousness, amnesia, immobility; and stability of the physiologic systems, including the autonomic, cardiovascular, respiratory, and thermoregulatory systems.[1-3] Continuously monitoring the status of the patient during general anesthesia is crucial for safe and proper delivery of anesthesia care. The physiologic state of the patient under general anesthesia is commonly monitored using the electrocardiogram and an arterial blood pressure cuff, or an arterial catheter, to monitor the cardiovascular system. In more complex cases, a central venous catheter can be used to monitor central venous pressures, and a pulmonary artery catheter can be placed to monitor cardiac output and pressures in the heart and pulmonary circulation. Transesophageal echocardiography can be used intermittently to gain direct visual information about the anatomy and function of the heart. The capnogram provides a continuous readout of the level of expired carbon dioxide and respiration. In intubated patients, more detailed information about the state of the lungs can be acquired from the pressure and volume tracings on the ventilator. The pulse oximeter estimates the level of hemoglobin saturation in the arterial blood, and the thermometer tracks body temperature. Muscle relaxation, or immobility, is monitored primarily using a train-of-four stimulation device, and more grossly by observing changes in muscle tone or movement.

Monitoring the behavioral states is more challenging. During general anesthesia, amnesia is not monitored directly but implicitly by the extent to which unconsciousness is achieved. If the patient is unconscious and not simply conscious but unresponsive, the patient will likely have amnesia. In this chapter, we discuss approaches for monitoring unconsciousness and analgesia, or more accurately stated antinociception, and each of the three phases of general anesthesia: induction, maintenance, and emergence. This chapter's focus is on physiologic signs and neurologic examination findings, and the electroencephalogram (EEG)–based measures, used to track these states of general anesthesia.

Induction of General Anesthesia

Monitoring of a patient's level of consciousness begins at induction of general anesthesia. Induction is usually achieved by an intravenous bolus dose of a hypnotic drug such as propofol, a barbiturate, ketamine, or etomidate. Unconsciousness usually occurs in 10 to 30 seconds. The brain state of the patient, which in this case is the transition into unconsciousness, is tracked by monitoring the patient's physiologic signs and the EEG-based index.

PHYSIOLOGIC SIGNS OF LOSS OF CONSCIOUSNESS

When a hypnotic drug is administered to induce general anesthesia—usually as an intravenous bolus over a 5- to 10-second period—several physiologic signs are observed. If asked to count backwards from 100, the patient typically does not get beyond 85 to 90. This transition into unconsciousness can be followed easily by asking the patient to perform smooth pursuit of the anesthesiologist's finger.[1] In smooth pursuit, the patient is instructed to move his or her eyes to track the position of the anesthesiologist's finger. As loss of consciousness ensues, the lateral excursions of the eyes during smooth pursuit decrease, nystagmus may appear, blinking increases, and the eyes fix abruptly in the midline. The oculocephalic reflex and the corneal reflex are lost, but the pupillary response to light can remain intact. The patient typically becomes apneic, atonic, and unresponsive at the point when the oculocephalic reflex is lost.

The oculocephalic reflex is assessed by turning the patient's head from side to side, while lifting the eyelids. Before administration of the induction anesthetic, when the reflex is intact in a patient with no neurologic deficits, the eyes move in the direction opposite the motion of the head. When the reflex is lost, the eyes stay fixed in the midline.[4] The oculocephalic reflex requires the circuits of cranial nerves III, IV, VI, and VIII to be intact. The motor nuclei associated with cranial nerves III and IV are located in the midbrain, whereas the nucleus of cranial nerve VI is located in the pons. The corneal reflex has traditionally been assessed using a wisp of cotton at the corner of the eye to stroke the cornea. An easier way to assess the reflex is to allow a drop of sterile water to fall on the cornea. Using a drop of sterile water may be safer than using the wisp of cotton, because the former is less likely to cause a corneal abrasion. With either approach, the reflex is intact if the eyes blink consensually, is impaired if there is a blink in one eye and not the other, and is absent if there is no blink. The afferent component of the corneal reflex travels to the sensory nucleus of the cranial nerve V through the ophthalmic branch, whereas the efferent component arises from the motor nucleus of the cranial nerve VII. The nuclei for these nerves associated with the oculocephalic reflex and the corneal reflex lie in close proximity to the arousal centers in the midbrain, pons, hypothalamus, and basal forebrain.[4]

Loss of the oculocephalic reflex suggests that the motor nuclei required for eye movements have been affected by the anesthetic. Similarly, loss of the corneal reflex suggests that the nuclei that control sensation and motor responses to sensation on the eyes and the face have also been affected. Because the loss of the oculocephalic and corneal reflexes occur concomitantly with the loss of responsiveness, the anesthesiologists can also infer that the loss of consciousness is due at least in part to the effects of the anesthetics on the nearby arousal centers.[1,4,5] Apnea, which commonly occurs on induction of general anesthesia with bolus administration of a hypnotic agent, is most likely due to the inhibitory effects of the anesthetic on the dorsal and ventral respiratory groups in the medulla and pons, respectively.[6] Atonia can be due to anesthetic action at any one of multiple sites in the motor pathways between the primary motor areas and the spinal cord. The most likely brainstem sites are the pontine and medullary reticular nuclei.[2]

Loss of the oculocephalic reflex, the corneal reflex, apnea, and atonia occur concomitantly with loss of consciousness on induction of general anesthesia because of the actions of the hypnotic drug in the brainstem after an intravenous bolus. Blood containing the anesthetic reaches the brainstem through the basilar artery, which supplies the posterior cerebral arteries that provide the posterior input to the circle of Willis.[5] Before terminating in the posterior cerebral arteries, the basilar artery runs on the dorsal surface of the brainstem and gives off multiple penetrating arteries that perfuse the brainstem nuclei with the anesthetic leading to the observed physiological effects.

ELECTROENCEPHALOGRAM-MARKERS OF LOSS OF CONSCIOUSNESS

EEG-based indices are among the most commonly used methods for tracking loss of consciousness induced by general anesthesia.[7] With induction of general anesthesia, these indices usually change from high values that indicate the awake state to lower values that indicate states of sedation and unconsciousness.

Maintenance of General Anesthesia: Physiologic Signs and the Nociceptive-Medullary-Autonomic Pathway

Despite the many advances in anesthesia care, the physiologic signs of changes in heart rate, arterial blood pressure, and movement are the measurements most commonly used to track the anesthetic state during maintenance of general anesthesia.[8] When the state of general anesthesia is not adequate for the level of surgical (nociceptive) stimulation, heart rate and arterial blood pressure can increase dramatically. The changes in heart rate and arterial blood pressure that anesthetized patients show in response to a nociceptive stimulus can be explained in terms of the nociceptive-medullary-autonomic (NMA) circuit composed of the spinoreticular tract, the brainstem arousal circuits, and the sympathetic and parasympathetic efferent pathways (Fig. 40.1).[1,9] It is important to understand how the NMA circuit works because it is the pathway most used by anesthesiologists for monitoring the patient's level of unconsciousness and antinociception. One example is a description of the NMA pathway in a clinical context that is commonly observed in the operating room.

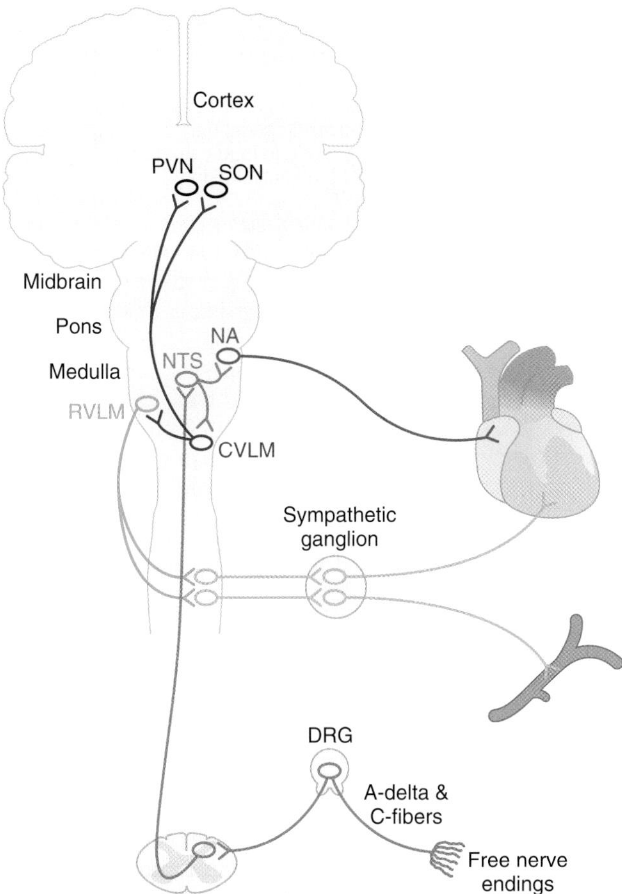

Fig. 40.1 Nociceptive medullary autonomic circuit. The ascending nociceptive (pain) pathway starts with C fibers and A-delta peripheral afferent fibers that synapse on projection neurons (PNs) in the dorsal horn. The PNs cross the midline, course to the brain where they synapse at several targets, including the nucleus of the tractus solitarius *(NTS)* in the medulla. The NTS mediates the autonomic response to a nociceptive stimulus by increasing sympathetic output through the rostral ventral lateral medulla *(RVLM)* and the caudal ventral lateral medulla *(CVLM)*, which projects to the thoracolumbar sympathetic ganglia. The ganglia project to peripheral blood vessels and the heart. The nucleus ambiguous *(NA)* mediates the parasympathetic output to the sinoatrial node of the heart through the vagus nerve. The NTS projects also to the supraoptic nucleus *(SON)* and periventricular nucleus *(PVN)* in the hypothalamus. The NMA circuit is the reason why anesthesiologists use increases in blood pressure and heart rate as markers of increases in nociceptive stimulation and, possibly, a level of general anesthesia that is inadequate. *DRG,* Dorsal root ganglion. (Redrawn from Brown EN, Lydic R, Schiff ND. General anesthesia, sleep, and coma. *N Engl J Med.* 2010;363:2638–2650.)

Suppose that a patient is in a stable state of general anesthesia when, to gain better exposure, the surgeon moves the retractor. Suppose also that this maneuver induces an immediate increase in heart rate and arterial blood pressure. Assuming, that there are no occult hemodynamic or respiratory problems or other common issues that increase heart rate and arterial blood pressure, then these increases likely occurred because the level of general anesthesia did not maintain an adequate level of antinociception. By simultaneously monitoring, in addition, the level of muscle relaxation and oxygen saturation, and oxygen delivery, along with EEG-based indices to track level of unconsciousness, the anesthesia provider can determine that these increases are due to inadequate antinociception and decide to administer more analgesic.

The ascending nociceptive (pain) pathway begins with A-delta and C-fibers whose free nerve endings bring nociceptive information from the periphery to the spinal cord (see Fig. 40.1).[10] In the spinal cord, these fibers synapse in the dorsal horn on projection neurons that travel through the anterolateral fasciculus and synapse at multiple sites in the brainstem, including the nucleus of the tractus solitarius in the medulla.[1,9] The autonomic response to a nociceptive stimulus is initiated from the nucleus of the tractus solitarius, which mediates sympathetic output through the rostral ventral lateral medulla and the caudal ventral lateral medulla to the heart and peripheral blood vessels through projections to the thoracolumbar sympathetic ganglia.[1] The parasympathetic output from the nucleus of the tractus solitarius is mediated through the nucleus ambiguous, which projects through the vagus nerve to the sinoatrial node of the heart.[1] The nucleus of the tractus solitarius also projects to the periventricular nucleus and supraoptic nucleus in the hypothalamus. Thus the nociceptive stimulus of moving the retractor initiates an increase in sympathetic output and a decrease in parasympathetic output through the NMA circuit that rapidly results in the observed increases in heart rate and arterial blood pressure.

The NMA circuit explains why increases in heart rate and arterial blood pressure are used as a rapid indicator of an inadequate level of antinociception. If unconsciousness is sufficiently well maintained, then no EEG changes will likely be observed. If no acute changes in physiology occur for other reasons, such as bleeding, hypoxemia, disconnection of the breathing circuit, or inadequate dosing of the muscle relaxant, the appropriate treatment is administration of more analgesic medication.

Activity in the NMA circuit can be observed rapidly when a patient is under general anesthesia,[11] because this pathway is a fundamental component of the fight-or-flight response.[12] This circuit is used as a sentinel for detecting nociceptive stimuli that can lead to autonomic, stress, and arousal responses. Heart rate and arterial blood pressure changes are the principal markers of activity under general anesthesia because motor responses are often blocked by muscle relaxation. Neurologists frequently test the NMA circuit with nociceptive stimuli, such as total body pinches, nail bed pinches, and sternal rubs, to evaluate the level of arousal of patients with brain injuries that affect the level of consciousness.[4,13,14]

Other signs of inadequate antinociception are perspiration, tearing, pupil dilation, and return of muscle tone and movement.[8] Changes in muscle tone and movement are not observed if the patient is receiving a muscle relaxant. The galvanic skin response has also been studied as a potentially more objective measure of antinociception. However, it is not used in clinical practice.[15]

Maintenance of General Anesthesia: Electroencephalogram-Based Indices of Level of Consciousness

It is widely recognized that the EEG changes systematically in relation to the dose of anesthetic drug administered (Fig. 40.2).[1,7,16-18] As a consequence, the unprocessed EEG and

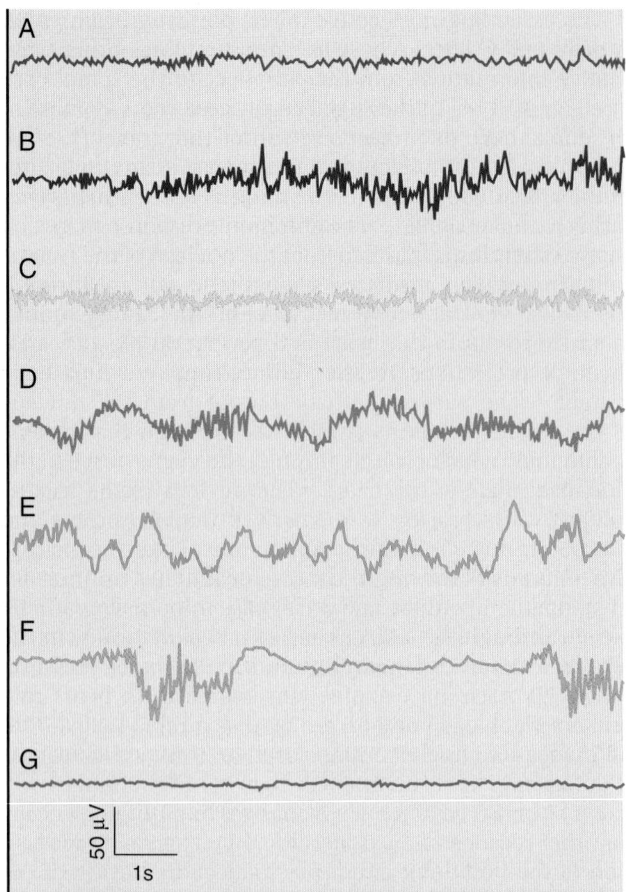

Fig. 40.2 Anesthetic states and electroencephalogram signatures of propofol. (A) Awake electroencephalogram pattern with eyes open. (B) State of paradoxical excitation. (C) Beta (13-25 Hz) oscillations frequently associated with an arousable state of sedation. (D) Slow (0.1-1 Hz), delta (1-4 Hz), and alpha (8-12 Hz) oscillations commonly seen during unconsciousness at surgical planes. (E) Slow oscillations typically recorded during propofol induction and during deep dexmedetomidine sedation (see Fig. 40.8, *D*). (F) Burst suppression, a state of profound anesthetic-induced brain inactivation, seen commonly in the elderly during normal maintenance, anesthetic-induced coma, and hypothermia. (G) Isoelectric electroencephalogram pattern commonly observed in brief periods during normal maintenance, in anesthetic-induced coma, and profound hypothermia.

various forms of processed EEG have been used to track the level of unconsciousness of patients receiving general anesthesia and sedation. Several EEG-based index systems have been studied and used in clinical practice. These systems process the EEG and provide an index value or set of values in real time or near real time that can be used to track the level consciousness. In general, the indices are designed to decrease with decreasing level of consciousness and increase as consciousness returns. In this way, the anesthesia provider can use these indices along with the physiological signs to track the patient's state of unconsciousness and, to some degree, antinociception. A summary of the EEG-based indices that have received the most use in clinical practice and clinical studies follows.

BISPECTRAL INDEX

The bispectral index (BIS) is an empirically derived scale that was proposed in 1994 by Aspect Medical Systems

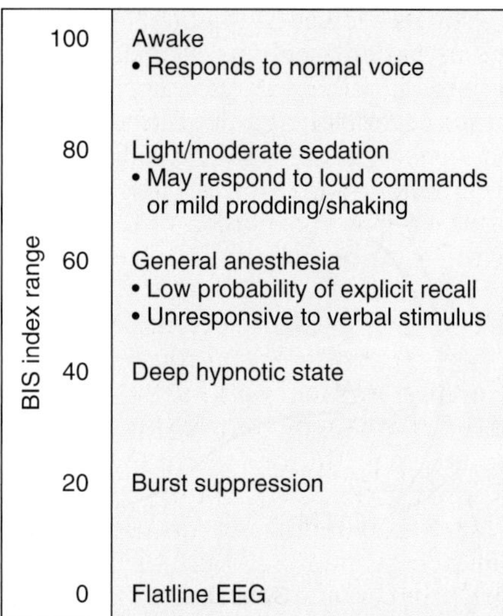

Fig. 40.3 Anesthetic states and the bispectral index (*BIS*). The chart provides a behavioral interpretation of the values of the BIS. *EEG*, Electroencephalogram. (Redrawn from Kelley SD. *Monitoring Consciousness: Using the Bispectral Index*. 2nd ed. Boulder, CO: Covidien; 2010.)

(later acquired by Covidien [Boulder, Colorado] and lastly by Medtronic [Minneapolis, Minnesota]) as a novel way to monitor anesthetic state in patients receiving general anesthesia and sedation.[19,20] The algorithm processes the EEG in near real time and computes an index value between 0 and 100 that indicates the patient's anesthetic state (Fig. 40.3).[21,22] A value of 100 corresponds to being completely awake, whereas 0 corresponds to a profound state of coma or unconsciousness that is reflected by an isoelectric or flat EEG. The BIS algorithm is proprietary, and the actual computation through which the index is derived is not public knowledge. However, it is known that BIS combines information from three EEG analyses: the spectrogram, the bispectrum, and a time domain assessment of burst suppression.[21-23] The spectrogram is a decomposition of the EEG into its power content by frequency as a function of time.[21] The bispectrum measures the degree of nonlinear coupling between pairs of frequencies in the spectrogram.[21] The BIS algorithm works by measuring specific features of the spectrogram, the bispectrum, and the level of burst suppression, and uses a predetermined weighting scheme to convert these features into the index value. The EEG also undergoes various artifact corrections. Along with the index value, the unprocessed EEG, the spectrogram, and the level of electromyographic activity are displayed on the monitor. Production of the index is computationally intensive, so that there is a 20- to 30-second lag between the time the EEG is observed and the computation of the corresponding BIS value.[24] A patient is considered to be appropriately anesthetized (i.e., unconscious) when the value of the BIS is between 40 and 60 (see Fig. 40.3).[22,25] The EEG is recorded from a four-lead frontal montage.

Since its approval by the US Food and Drug Administration (FDA) in 1996, the BIS monitor has been studied extensively in clinical trials and used widely in anesthesiology practice. The changes in the index are correlated with the level of sedation and unconsciousness (see Fig. 40.3), primarily because for many anesthetics, the EEG shows lower-frequency, higher-amplitude oscillations as patients achieve deeper states of unconsciousness (see Fig. 40.2). Three exceptions are the anesthetics ketamine, nitrous oxide, and dexmedetomidine. The dissociative anesthetic state produced by ketamine is associated with prominent high-frequency oscillations rather than slow wave oscillations.[26] As a consequence, patients can be unconscious with ketamine but have high index values.[27]

The effect of nitrous oxide on the BIS index is ambiguous. Most recent studies state that nitrous oxide increases the amplitude of high-frequency EEG activity[28] and decreases the amplitude of low-frequency EEG activity,[29] yet it has little to no effect on the BIS index.[22,30] However, these studies have not taken into account the state of profound transient large-amplitude slow oscillations, followed by lower amplitude gamma oscillations that have now been documented to be common features observed when nitrous oxide is administered in high-dose (>50%).[31] In the case of dexmedetomidine, slow oscillations and an appreciable decrease in beta oscillation power[32,33] are prominent during sedation.[34-36] These dynamics most likely lead to BIS values that are typically in the unconscious range, even though the patient can be aroused by verbal commands or light shaking.

As we discuss in the "Changes in EEG Signatures with Aging" section, anesthetic-induced EEG oscillations change systematically with age.[26,37] BIS appears to work poorly in older adults (>60), as patients in this age cohort tend to have lower amplitude oscillations, which the BIS algorithm can interpret as an awake state or state of unconsciousness. Similarly, the BIS algorithm is known to inaccurately reflect the anesthetic state of children because they generally have much more power across a broader range of frequency bands when appropriately anesthetized compared with adults in the 18 to 59 year age range.[37,38] Hence, even though the children may be well anesthetized, the BIS algorithm provides numbers suggesting a state of sedation rather than unconsciousness.

Use of the BIS monitor has been proposed as a way to prevent intraoperative awareness, which is defined as the patient having explicit recall of events that transpired during the time that he or she was under general anesthesia. Use of the BIS monitor as a way to prevent intraoperative awareness was studied in the B-Aware Trial.[39] This study compared patients at high risk for awareness who were randomly assigned to monitoring with BIS using a target range of 40 to 60 and patients monitored with the standard of care at that particular institution. The patients in the BIS group had a significantly lower incidence of awareness.

The findings from this study were called into question because of several design concerns, and for this reason the B-Unaware Trial was conducted.[40] The B-Unaware Trial was a multicenter investigation that randomly assigned patients to either BIS monitoring or monitoring of the end-tidal anesthetic gas concentration to compare the two approaches for preventing awareness. The end-tidal gas concentration was maintained between 0.7 and 1.3 of the age-adjusted minimum alveolar concentration (MAC) of the anesthetic administered to the patient (discussed under End-Tidal Anesthetic Concentration). As in the B-Aware Trial, the objective in the BIS-monitored group was maintenance of the BIS value between 40 and 60. This study found no significant difference in the incidence of awareness among the patients monitored with BIS compared with those monitored with the end-tidal gas concentration. The authors interpreted these findings to mean that BIS monitoring was not more effective than the end-tidal anesthetic criterion in preventing awareness in patients receiving general anesthesia using volatile anesthetics. Several concerns were expressed about the findings of this study as well. The most notable were subject selection and whether the study had sufficient power to detect actual differences, had they been present.[41,42]

As a follow-up to this study, the investigators in the B-Unaware Trail conducted the BIS or Anesthetic Gas to Reduce Explicit Recall (BAG-RECALL) trial, a second trial investigating whether BIS was superior to the end-tidal anesthetic gas concentration in preventing intraoperative awareness in a larger group of patients at high risk for awareness.[41] In this trial, the investigators found that the BIS-guided protocol was not superior to the end-tidal anesthetic concentration-guided protocol in preventing awareness. Because the B-Unaware trial and the BAG-RECALL trial used inhaled anesthetics as the primary agents, their conclusions do not apply to patients receiving total intravenous anesthesia.

Preventing awareness under general anesthesia is a solvable problem if strategies used to monitor the brain states of patients use markers that relate directly rather than indirectly to the mechanisms through which the anesthetics act at specific receptors and neural circuits to alter level of arousal.[1,43,44] Unlike the current EEG-based indices, these markers will differ with patient age and different anesthetics, (See the Unprocessed EEG and the Spectrogram section).

PATIENT SAFETY INDEX

The Patient Safety Index (PSI) is like the BIS index—a proprietary algorithm that assesses anesthetic state based on the EEG for patients receiving general anesthesia or sedation. The PSI was approved by the FDA in 2000 and was originally developed by Physiometrix (North Billerica, Massachusetts), and was ultimately acquired by Masimo (Irvine, California). The development of the PSI was the outgrowth of several years of research conducted by E. Roy John at the Brain Research Laboratory at the New York University School of Medicine.[45] Like the BIS index, the PSI is also scaled between 0 and 100 (Fig. 40.4). However, the PSI range to ensure that the patient is unconscious is between 25 and 50.[46]

The original formulation of the PSI used an electrode montage that included occipital and frontal EEG leads to monitor the phenomenon of anteriorization as a marker of change in anesthetic state. Anteriorization is the forward shift of spectral power from the occipital area to the frontal area during loss of consciousness and the posterior shift of this power from the frontal areas to the occipital areas during the return of consciousness.[44,47-49] The current formulation of the PSI uses a four-lead frontal EEG montage. In addition to displaying the PSI, this monitor also shows

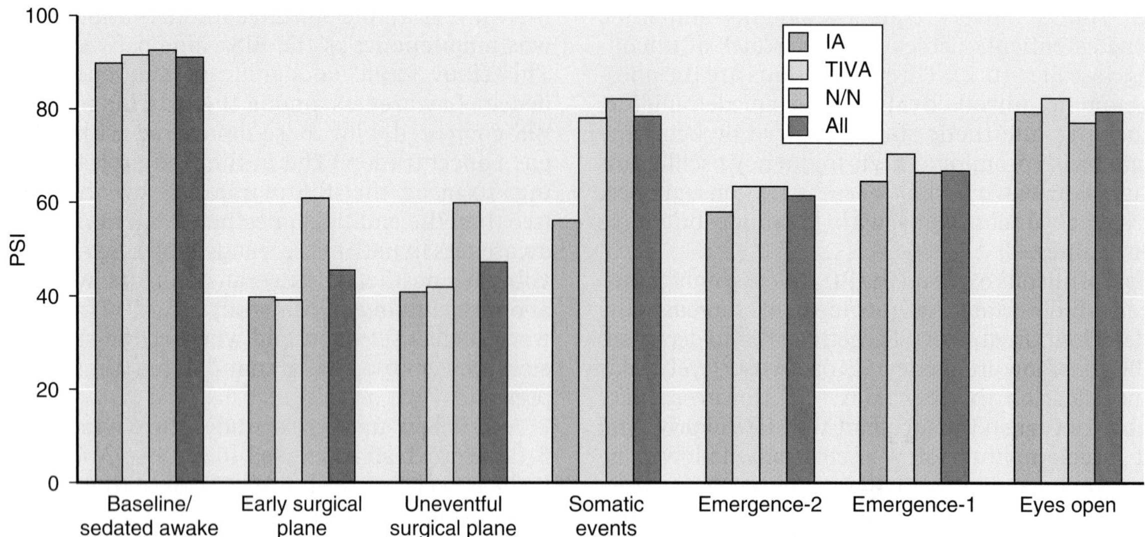

Fig. 40.4 Anesthetic states and the patient safety index *(PSI)*. The histogram provides the anesthetic state interpretation of the values of the PSI. *IA*, Inhaled anesthetics; *N/N*, nitrous narcotic; *TIVA*, total intravenous anesthesia. (Redrawn from Drover D, Ortega HR. Patient state index. *Best Pract Res Clin Anaesthesiol.* 2006;20:121–128.)

in real time the unprocessed EEG and its spectrogram from both the left and right sides of the head, the level of electromyographic activity, an artifact index, and the suppression ratio. The suppression ratio is a number between 0 and 100 that measures the fraction of time the EEG is in burst suppression. The monitor also allows the user to change the viewing screen among various combinations of the unprocessed EEG traces, the spectrogram, and the time series of the PSI values.

In head-to-head comparisons, the PSI correlates strongly with the BIS readings in terms of tracking a patient's anesthetic state.[50-52] This monitor has been less frequently studied in clinical investigations and has not received the same level of clinical use as the BIS monitor. In our experience, the PSI can also give ambiguous information for ketamine, nitrous oxide, dexmedetomidine, and pediatric patients.

NARCOTREND

The Narcotrend, produced by MonitorTechnik (Bad Bramstedt, Germany), is an EEG-based device designed to monitor the anesthetic state in patients receiving general anesthesia or sedation.[53] This monitor was developed at the University Medical School of Hanover, Germany, and has been approved by the FDA for use in the United States for patient care. Like the BIS and PSI, the Narcotrend uses a proprietary algorithm that converts the EEG into different states, denoted as *A* to *F* (Table 40.1).[54] Stage A corresponds to the patient being wide-awake, whereas stage F corresponds to increasing burst suppression down to an isoelectric state. The newer version of the Narcotrend monitor includes a Narcotrend Index, which is scaled between 0 and 100.[51] In addition, the Narcotrend monitor displays the unprocessed EEG signal and its spectrogram. This monitor has also been validated with respect to the BIS index and separately. Its performance has been variable.[24,55,56] Narcotrend has received less clinical use than BIS and PSI.

TABLE 40.1 Anesthetic States, the Narcotrend Stages, and Narcotrend Index Ranges

	Narcotrend Stage	Narcotrend Index
Awake	A	95-100
	B_0	90-94
Sedated	B_1	85-89
	B_2	80-84
Light anesthesia	C_0	75-79
	C_1	70-74
	C_2	65-69
General anesthesia	D_0	57-64
	D_1	47-56
	D_2	37-46
General anesthesia with deep hypnosis	E_0	27-36
	E_1	20-26
	E_2	13-19
General anesthesia with increasing burst suppression	F_0	5-12
	F_1	1-4

The table provides the anesthetic state interpretation of the Narcotrend Stages and the Narcotrend Index values.

From Kreuer S, Wilhelm W. The Narcotrend monitor. *Best Pract Res Clin Anaesthesiol.* 2006;20:111–119.

ENTROPY

The use of entropy to track the anesthetic state of patients is a relatively new monitoring approach. Entropy is a well-known concept in the physical sciences, mathematics, and information theory. Entropy measures the degree of disorder or the lack of synchrony or consistency in a system.[57] Entropy-based analyses have been applied to the EEG and have been used to construct EEG-based indices meant to indicate the depth of anesthesia. The Entropy monitor was developed by Datex-Ohmeda, which is now part of GE Healthcare (Little Chalfont, United Kingdom). The algorithm in the GE device uses frequency domain analysis,

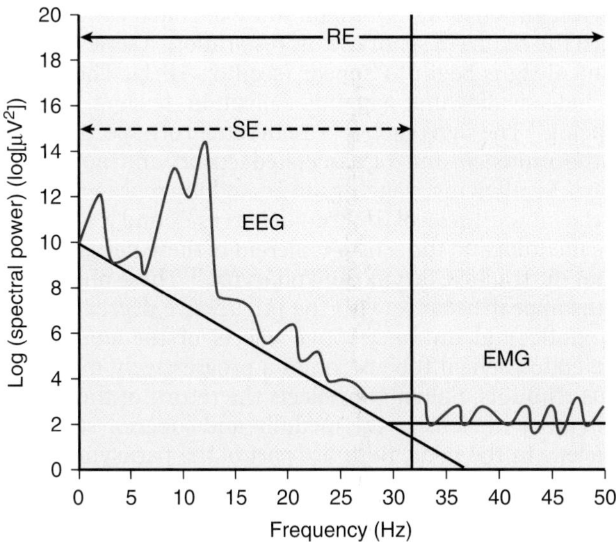

Fig. 40.5 Schematic representation of the spectral entropy. The response entropy *(RE)* is computed from the power in the frequencies between 0 and 47 Hz. The state entropy *(SE)* is computed from the power in the frequencies between 0 and 32 Hz. The power between 32 and 47 Hz is assumed to represent artifacts coming from the electromyogram *(EMG)*. The difference between the RE and SE allows the anesthesiologist to distinguish between electroencephalogram *(EEG)* changes related to changes in the anesthetic state and changes that are due to artifact or movement. (Redrawn from Bein B. Entropy. *Best Pract Res Clin Anaesthesiol.* 2006;20:101–109.)

combined with burst suppression to measure the entropy of the EEG in patients receiving anesthetic drugs. Unlike several of the other algorithms we have discussed, the entropy algorithm used in the GE entropy device is publicly available.[58,59]

A readily apparent feature of the EEG, as patients proceed through deeper anesthetic states, is that the patterns become more regular and ordered (see Fig. 40.2). That is, we observe an apparent decrease in the entropy of the EEG signal. The Entropy monitor reports two entropy numbers to aid in interpreting this monitor's EEG analysis (Fig. 40.5).[60] The first is the response entropy (RE) and the second is the state entropy (SE). The RE tracks the changes in the EEG power in the higher frequency range 0.8 to 47 Hz, whereas the SE tracks the changes in the EEG power in the lower frequency range of 0.8 to 32 Hz.[58] The relative changes in the RE and the SE have been proposed as a way to distinguish between real brain state changes versus those that are due to muscle activity on the electromyogram.[58] In general, electromyographic activity shows up in the higher frequency range tracked by the RE. As a patient becomes more profoundly unconscious, the RE declines faster than the SE, thereby making it possible to distinguish unconsciousness from movement artifacts. Monitoring entropy is consistent with changes with the BIS.[61]

Like the BIS, PSI, and Narcotrend, the Entropy scores correlate with anesthetic state. The Entropy monitor, like BIS and the PSI, can show paradoxically high readings for ketamine and nitrous oxide. The Entropy scores can be misleading when the patient is receiving dexmedetomidine, because the highly ordered slow waves that are present commonly during deep sedation with dexmedetomidine do not necessarily indicate a profound state of unconsciousness.

END-TIDAL ANESTHETIC CONCENTRATION

In 1965, Eger and colleagues first introduced the concept of the MAC of an inhaled anesthetic required for immobility (defined as lack of movement in response to noxious stimulation).[62] Five years later, Eger's group also introduced the concept of MAC-awake, or the MAC of inhaled anesthetic necessary to ablate response to a verbal command.[63] The median MAC value (i.e., the MAC of inhaled anesthetic required for immobility in 50% of patients) remains the gold standard for dosing inhaled anesthetics, and some modern anesthesia machines calculate age-adjusted MAC values based on the patient's end-tidal anesthetic gas concentration. However, the ratio of MAC to MAC-awake varies widely among general anesthetics,[64] suggesting that MAC cannot be used to define or predict brain states in anesthetized patients. This has been confirmed by animal experiments demonstrating that there is no clear association between anesthetic-induced EEG patterns and immobility,[65] and that inhaled anesthetics produce immobility primarily through their actions in the spinal cord, rather than the brain.[66,67] Nevertheless, the widely accepted concept of MAC has led to the use of end-tidal anesthetic concentration as a way to monitor anesthetic state induced by inhaled anesthetics.

As mentioned previously, this use of MAC has been supported by the B-Unaware Trial, which reported no difference in the incidence of intraoperative awareness with an anesthetic protocol that maintained the BIS value between 40 and 60, and a protocol that maintained an end-tidal anesthetic concentration between 0.7 and 1.3 MAC.[40] Similarly, the BAG-RECALL Trial limited enrollment to patients at high risk for intraoperative awareness. Patients with BIS-guided general anesthesia experienced a small but statistically significant higher incidence of intraoperative awareness than patients receiving general anesthesia guided by an end-tidal anesthetic criterion.[41]

Unlike the BIS, PI, Entropy, and Narcotrend, which provide EEG-based measures of brain activity, the end-tidal anesthetic concentration is related to brain activity through the concentration of inhaled anesthetic expired in the lungs. This assumes that the lung anesthetic concentration is in equilibrium with the brain concentration. Moreover, this assumes that, except for age adjustment, the same brain concentration in every patient, regardless of brain health or physiological state, defines the same anesthetic state. The end-tidal anesthetic concentration is thus an indirect and less nuanced measure of anesthetic state, given that the relevant effects of the anesthetics for inducing unconsciousness are in the brain and not in the lungs. That an EEG-based criterion and a lung-gas criterion are comparable for monitoring the level of consciousness under general anesthesia suggests more of a flaw in the design of the EEG-based marker, rather than the accuracy of the end-tidal anesthetic concentration. Because it is a more indirect measure of anesthetic state, the success of the end-tidal anesthetic concentration in preventing awareness comes likely at the expense of overdosing some patients. A key drawback of the end-tidal anesthetic concentration is that it cannot be used with total intravenous anesthesia.

OTHER STRATEGIES FOR MONITORING LEVEL OF CONSCIOUSNESS

Other strategies for monitoring level of consciousness during general anesthesia and sedation have been studied. For example, the Cerebral State Monitor,[68] the SNAP Index,[69] and the AEP Index[70] are other EEG-based approaches that have been studied and applied in clinical practice.

Emergence From General Anesthesia

ELECTROENCEPHALOGRAM-BASED INDICES AND RETURN OF CONSCIOUSNESS

As stated earlier, the EEG-based indices typically specify a range for maintenance of anesthetic state (see Figs. 40.3 to 40.5, and Table 40.1). When delivery of the anesthetic drugs is decreased or terminated, the indices increase toward values that are consistent with the awake state. As the values of the indices increase, the patient is more likely to become conscious. In this way, the EEG-based indices can be used to monitor changes in anesthetic state during emergence from general anesthesia. Although the values of the indices increase during emergence, none of the indices has a value at which the patient is certain to regain consciousness. The lack of any mechanistic relationship between the values of the EEG-based index and level of consciousness is due to imprecision in the definition of the indices, in that many different anesthetic states are presumed to map to the same index value. Friedman and colleagues and Joiner and colleagues found that neural inertia can play a role with inhaled anesthetics.[71,72] Neural inertia is the extent to which equal brain concentrations of anesthetic on induction and emergence often yield different behavioral states. In other words, the history of the brain states helps determine arousability.

PHYSIOLOGIC SIGNS AND RETURN OF CONSCIOUSNESS

The state of the patient during emergence from general anesthesia can be tracked reliably by monitoring the patient's physiologic signs and performing neurologic examinations.[1] Many of these physiologic changes relate to the return of brainstem function (Box 40.1). Therefore, by relating the physiologic signs and the findings from the neurologic examinations to the brainstem centers responsible for them, anesthesia providers can track the return of function to specific brainstem sites during emergence from general anesthesia. Once neuromuscular blockade has been reversed, the patient may breathe unassisted. As the level of carbon dioxide in the cerebral circulation increases, most patients begin to breathe spontaneously. As the patient emerges from general anesthesia, the respiratory pattern can transition from one that is irregular with small tidal volumes to one that is regular with full normal tidal volumes.[1] Return of spontaneous breathing is a distinct indicator of return of function in the medulla and lower pons, as these are the locations of the dorsal and ventral respiratory groups, respectively.[6]

Over the ensuing several minutes and often concomitant with the return of spontaneous respiration, a series of other clinical signs begin to appear (see Box 40.1). These signs include swallowing, gagging, salivation, tearing, and grimacing.[1] The signs each represent return of a specific center in the brainstem and the associated sensory and motor pathways. Swallowing, gagging, and coughing represent return of the motor nuclei of the cranial nerves IX and X located in the medulla and the sensory afferent of these nerves arising from the trachea, larynx, and pharynx.[10] These physiologic signs appear because with the progressive decrease in the hypnotic and antinociceptive effects of the anesthetics, the endotracheal tube becomes a progressively more noxious stimulus. Salivation reflects the return of the inferior salivatory nucleus in the medulla and superior salivatory nucleus in the pons. Both are part of the parasympathetic nervous system. The efferent pathways from these nuclei travel in cranial nerves VII and IX, respectively.[9] Tearing also reflects the return of function in the superior salivatory nucleus. Grimacing, the use of muscles of facial expression, represents the return of function to the motor nucleus of cranial nerve VII, located in the pons.[10] Return of muscle tone to the upper and lower extremities is another important clinical sign that clearly reflects return of function in a number of circuits including the spinal cord, the reticulospinal tract, the basal ganglia, and the primary motor tracts.[1] In addition, as the endotracheal tube is perceived as more noxious and motor tone has returned, the patient may commonly exhibit defensive posturing indicated by reaching for the endotracheal tube.

These physiologic signs are often present in advance of the patient responding to any verbal commands. The patient need not respond to commands to be extubated. Tracheal extubation only requires that the patient have sufficient return of airway reflexes and motor function to ventilate and oxygenate adequately with spontaneous breathing. To meet the criteria for extubation of the trachea, a patient can be in a vegetative state as defined by the criteria used by neurologists and rehabilitation specialists to assess the brain states of patients recovering from coma (see Box 40.1).[13,14,73]

The corneal reflex typically returns before the oculocephalic reflex.[1] Return of the corneal reflex indicates return of function in the sensory nucleus of cranial nerve V and the motor nucleus of cranial nerve VII.[4] The afferent pathway in the corneal reflex is the ophthalmic branch of cranial nerve V that projects to the trigeminal (cranial nerve V) nucleus, whereas the efferent pathway arises from the facial nerve (cranial nerve VII) nucleus. The consensual response in the corneal reflex indicates bilateral return of the sensory and motor components of this pathway. The trigeminal nucleus and the motor nucleus of cranial nerve VII lie in the pons. Return of the oculocephalic reflex indicates return of activity in the oculomotor (III), trochlear (IV), and abducens (VI) cranial nerves, which control movement of the eyes.[4] The cranial nerves III and IV nerve nuclei are located in the midbrain, whereas the cranial nerve VI nerve nucleus is in the pons. Return of the oculocephalic and corneal reflexes provides indirect evidence that the nearby arousal centers in the pons, midbrain, hypothalamus, and basal forebrain, may have also recovered function.[1] The oculocephalic reflex may not return even though the patient is extubated.

BOX 40.1 Phases of Emergence From General Anesthesia and States of Coma Recovery

General Anesthesia
Stable administration of anesthetic drugs
Arousal not possible, unresponsive; eyes closed, with reactive pupils
Analgesia, akinesia
Drug-controlled blood pressure and heart rate
Mechanically controlled ventilation
EEG patterns ranging from delta and alpha activity to burst suppression

Brain-Stem Death
No respiratory response to apneic oxygenation test
Total loss of brain-stem reflexes
Isoelectric EEG pattern

Coma
Structural brain damage to both cerebral hemispheres, with or without injuries to tegmental midbrain, rostral pons, or both
Isolated bilateral injuries to midline tegmental midbrain, rostral pons, or both
Arousal not possible, unresponsive
Functionally intact brain stem, normal arterial blood gases
EEG pattern of low-amplitude delta activity and intermittent bursts of theta and alpha activity or possibly burst suppression

Emergence, Phase 1
Cessation of anesthetic drugs
Reversal of peripheral-muscle relaxation (akinesis)
Transition from apnea to irregular breathing to regular breathing
Increased alpha and beta activity on EEG

Vegetative State
Spontaneous cycling of eye opening and closing
Grimacing and nonpurposeful movements
EEG pattern of high-amplitude delta and theta activity
Absence of EEG features of sleep
Usually able to ventilate without mechanical support

Emergence, Phase 2
Increased heart rate and blood pressure
Return of autonomic responsiveness
Responsiveness to painful stimulation
Salivation (CN VII and IX nuclei)
Tearing (CN VII nuclei)
Grimacing (CN V and VII nuclei)
Swallowing, gagging, coughing (CN IX and X nuclei)
Return of muscle tone (spinal cord, reticulospinal tract, basal ganglia, and primary motor tracts)
Defensive posturing
Further increase in alpha and beta activity on EEG
Extubation possible

Emergence, Phase 3
Eye opening
Responses to some oral commands
Awake patterns on EEG
Extubation possible

Minimally Conscious State
Purposeful guarding movements, eye tracking
Inconsistent communication, verbalizations
Following oral commands
Return of sleep–wake cycles
Recovery of some EEG features of normal sleep–wake architecture

General anesthesia is a drug-induced, reversible coma. The physiological signs observed in the phases of emergence from general anesthesia can be related to changes in activity in specific brainstem nuclei. Emergence from general anesthesia has similarities and differences with recovery from coma due to a brain injury.
CN, Cranial nerve; ***EEG***, electroencephalogram.
From Brown EN, Lydic R, Schiff ND. General anesthesia, sleep, and coma. N Engl J Med. 2010;363:2638–2650.

Patients commonly leave the operating room without return of this reflex, suggesting persistent sedation of the brainstem arousal centers. The pupils can remain pinpoint if the patient has received a substantial dose of an opioid. The pupillary light reflex can remain intact even when the patient is profoundly unconscious under general anesthesia[4]; therefore, the presence of the pupillary light reflex might not indicate a change in the level of consciousness while under general anesthesia.

Responding correctly to verbal commands, a criterion that is commonly used to assess the extent to which a patient has recovered from general anesthesia, and hence the patient's readiness for extubation, suggests a return of integrated function between the brainstem, the thalamus and cortex, and among cortical regions.[1,74,75] Responding correctly to verbal commands means that the patient is correctly interpreting auditory information and that the cranial nerve VIII nuclei located in the pons and the auditory pathways from the pons to the cortex and the relevant effector pathways have regained substantial function. If the patient inconsistently follows motor commands, then he or she is classified as being in a minimally conscious state by the criteria neurologists use in examining patients recovering from coma (see Box 40.1).[13,14,73] With emergence, the physiologic signs and neurologic findings can be related to changes in activity in specific brainstem centers. Although the EEG shows the resumption of high-frequency activity consistent with the return of cognitive processing, normal brainstem-cortical, brainstem-thalamic, thalamocortical, and intracortical communication must clearly return for full return of consciousness.[44,75-78] Current clinical monitoring approaches do not allow us to monitor these changes adequately.

Opening of the eyes is typically one of the last physiologic signs observed in patients emerging from general anesthesia. In particular, patients may respond reliably to verbal commands, have substantial return of motor functions, yet not necessarily open their eyes.[1] In general, patients tend to keep their eyes closed even when consciousness has returned. In contrast, during coma recovery, patients can have their eyes open in a vegetative state (see Box 40.1).

Emerging Strategies for Monitoring the Brain States of General Anesthesia and Sedation

In the last several years, there has been strong growth in research on the neuroscience of general anesthesia. As a result, there are several reports of new approaches to monitoring the brain states under general anesthesia.

UNPROCESSED ELECTROENCEPHALOGRAM AND THE SPECTROGRAM

Different anesthetics have different receptor targets[79] and neural circuit mechanisms of action.[1,43] These differences in targets and neural circuits translate into different patterns of activity in the brain that are readily visible in the unprocessed EEG or its spectrogram.[26] The spectrum of a segment of EEG is the decomposition of the EEG signal into its power content by frequency.[26] Power is typically expressed in decibels which is 10 times the base 10 logarithm of the square of the amplitude of a given frequency component.[26] When the spectrum is computed on successive nonoverlapping or overlapping segments of EEG data, it is termed the *spectrogram*[26]; it is called the *compressed spectral array* when the spectrogram is plotted in three dimensions[80] and the *density spectral array* when it is plotted in two dimensions.[81]

The EEG patterns of propofol have been related to its neural circuit mechanisms. The brain states under propofol are readily visible in the unprocessed EEG and the spectrogram (see Figs. 40.2, 40.6 and 40.7, *A*). Propofol acts primarily at $GABA_A$ receptors throughout the brain and spinal cord to enhance inhibition in neural circuits.[79,82] When patients are unconscious from propofol, the EEG shows a characteristic alpha (8-12 Hz) oscillation pattern along with slow (0.1-1 Hz) and delta (1-4 Hz) oscillation patterns (see Fig. 40.7 *A*).[44,49,83,84] Another phenomenon that is observed in patients who are unconscious from propofol and several other anesthetics is anteriorization—the increase in power in the alpha and beta frequency ranges during unconsciousness across the front of the scalp relative to other areas of the scalp (see Fig. 40.6, *C* and *D*).[44,47,49]

During unconsciousness, the alpha oscillations are highly coherent across the front of the scalp, whereas the slow and gamma oscillations are not coherent.[44,49,84] Highly coherent alpha oscillations have also been identified in animal studies of inhaled anesthetics during unconsciousness.[85] The coherent structure in the alpha oscillations is most likely due to strong alpha oscillations between the thalamus and frontal cortex.[86] The slow oscillations are a marker of fragmented intracortical communication because in the presence of the slow oscillations, cortical neurons spike only in a limited phase dictated by their local slow oscillations.[84] As the slow oscillations are spatially incoherent and spiking is phase limited, neuronal communication among brain regions that are separated by more than 1 cm is greatly impeded. There is a strong modulation of the alpha oscillation amplitude by the phase of the slow-delta oscillation[44]. Patients are profoundly unconscious when the maximum amplitude of the alpha oscillations occurs at the peak of the slow oscillation waveform.[44] In contrast, patients are likely to be arousable when the maximum amplitude of the alpha oscillations occurs at the trough of the slow oscillation waveform.[44] With return of consciousness, the alpha and slow oscillations dissipate (see Fig. 40.6.*B*). A mechanism by which propofol produces unconsciousness is through hypersynchronous alpha oscillations impeding communication between the thalamus and prefrontal cortex and through highly desynchronous slow oscillations impeding intracortical communication.[44,84,86,87]

Similarly, the EEG patterns of ketamine (see Fig. 40.7, *B*)[27] and dexmedetomidine (Fig. 40.8, *A* and*B*)[34] are distinctive and can be related to the mechanisms of actions of these drugs in the brain and central nervous system.[1,3,43] Ketamine acts principally by binding to *N*-methyl-D-aspartate (NMDA) receptors.[43,88] Thus, with small to moderate doses, ketamine has its primary effect by blocking excitatory glutamatergic inputs to inhibitory interneurons.[89,90] Impaired control over pyramidal neurons is why increases in cerebral metabolism, and the appearance of altered behavioral states including hallucinations, dissociative states, euphoria, and dysphoria, are common with low-dose ketamine. Brain regions, such as the limbic system, cortex, and thalamus, continue to communicate but with much less regulatory control from the inhibitory interneurons—that is, information processing proceeds in the absence of proper coordination in time and space.[1,43] Increasing the dose of ketamine blocks the NMDA receptors on the excitatory glutamatergic neurons, and eventual loss of consciousness, as when ketamine is used to induce anesthesia.[91] The increased activity of pyramidal neurons throughout the brain is consistent with the high frequency (20-30 Hz) oscillations that are commonly observed in the EEG of patients receiving ketamine (see Fig. 40.7 *B*).[27,92] This high-frequency EEG activity helps explain why EEG-based indices often give high values in patients receiving ketamine.

Dexmedetomidine induces its sedative effects primarily by actions on presynaptic α2-adrenergic receptors on neurons that project from the locus ceruleus.[93-95] Binding of dexmedetomidine results in a decrease in the release of norepinephrine from these neurons.[96-98] Loss of the norepinephrine-mediated inhibition to the preoptic area of the hypothalamus leads to activation of the preoptic area's GABAergic and galanergic inhibitory inputs to most of the principal arousal centers in the midbrain, pons, basal forebrain, and hypothalamus.[99] Activation of inhibitory inputs from the preoptic area is postulated to be a component of how nonrapid eye movement (NREM) sleep is initiated.[100,101] This suggests why light sedation with dexmedetomidine shows spindles, intermittent bursts of 9 to 15 Hz oscillations, and slow-wave patterns in the EEG that closely resemble NREM sleep stage 2 (see Fig. 40.8, *A*). Recent studies have demonstrated that deep sedation with dexmedetomidine also shows the combined spindle and slow-delta oscillation patterns seen with light dexmedetomidine sedation (see Fig. 40.8, *A*), along with an appreciable decrease in beta oscillation power.[32,33,102] Deep

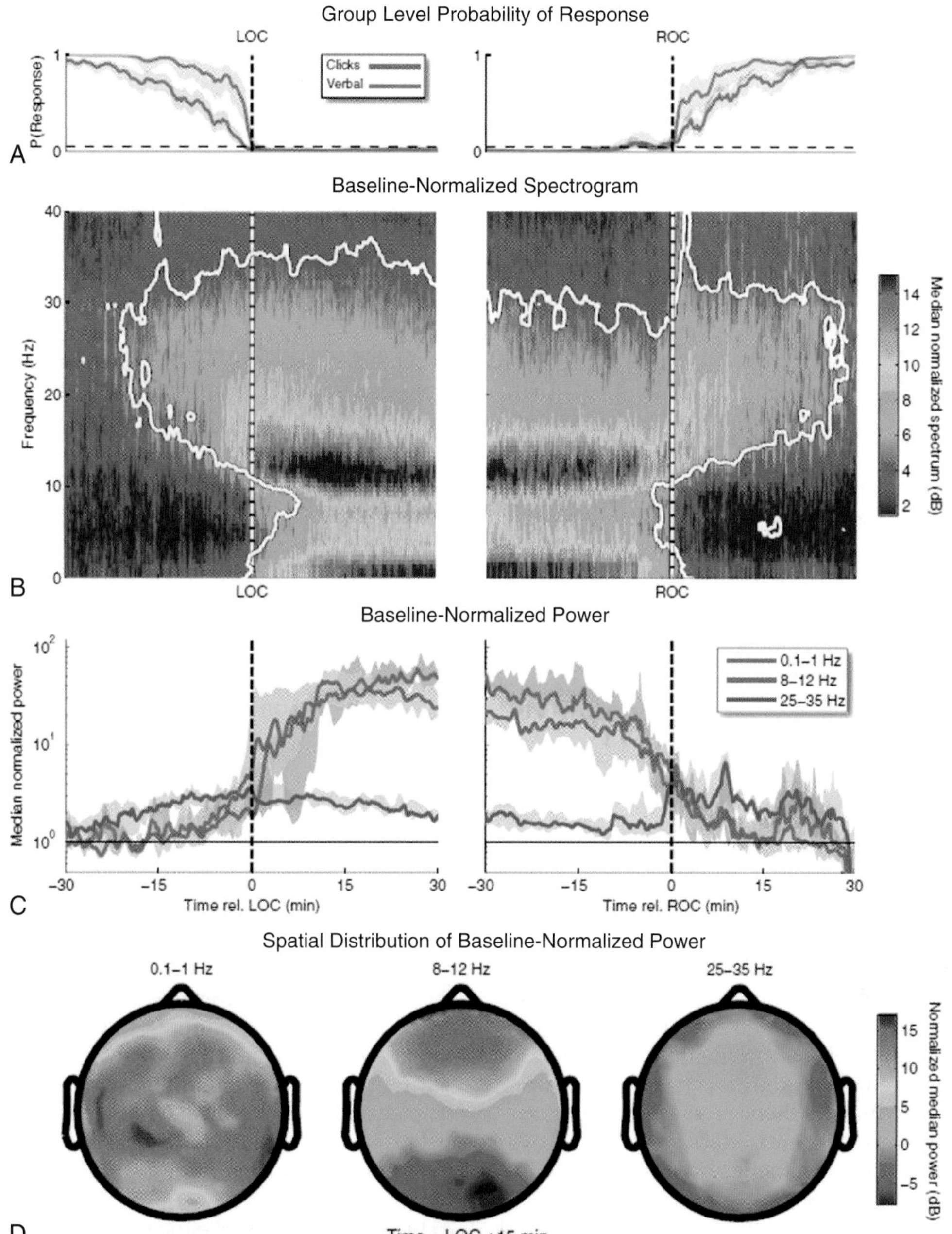

Fig. 40.6 Behavioral and electroencephalogram dynamics of loss and recovery of consciousness from propofol. (A) Group-level (10 subjects) click or nonsalient stimulus *(blue, P_{clicks})* and verbal or salient stimulus *(red, P_{verbal})* response-probability curves. (B) Group-level spectrograms computed by baseline-normalization from a frontal channel (approximately *Fz*, using nearest-neighbor Laplacian reference) aligned across subject with respect to loss of consciousness *(LOC)*. Area enclosed within the white borders show where power is significantly different from baseline ($P < .05$, sign test) and shows significant power increases spanning slow (0.1-1 Hz) through gamma (25-35 Hz) bands. (C) Time course of group-level power in slow, alpha (8-12 Hz), and gamma bands aligned with respect to LOC and recovery of consciousness *(ROC)*. (D) Group-level spatial distribution of slow, alpha, and gamma power during unconsciousness (LOC + 15 min). The frontal increase in alpha power is termed *anteriorization*. These analyses illustrate that changes in broad-band gamma/beta power occur with the behavioral changes before LOC and after ROC, whereas changes in slow and alpha power occur with LOC and ROC. (From Purdon PL, Pierce ET, Mukamel EA, et al. Electroencephalogram signatures of loss and recovery of consciousness from propofol. *Proc Natl Acad Sci U S A.* 2013;110:E1142–E1151.)

sedation with dexmedetomidine can also show a slow-delta oscillation EEG pattern that closely resembles the patterns observed in NREM sleep stage 3 or slow-wave sleep (see Fig. 40.8 *B*).[26]

Sevoflurane, like the other inhaled ether anesthetics, produces its physiologic and behavioral effects by binding at multiple targets in the brain and spinal cord. These include binding to $GABA_A$ receptors and enhancing GABAergic inhibition, and blocking glutamate release by binding to NMDA receptors, along with activating two-pore potassium channels and hyperpolarization-activated cyclic nucleotide-gated channels.[79] Although debates still exist over the relative importance of these targets, sevoflurane and the other ether anesthetics have distinct EEG signatures.

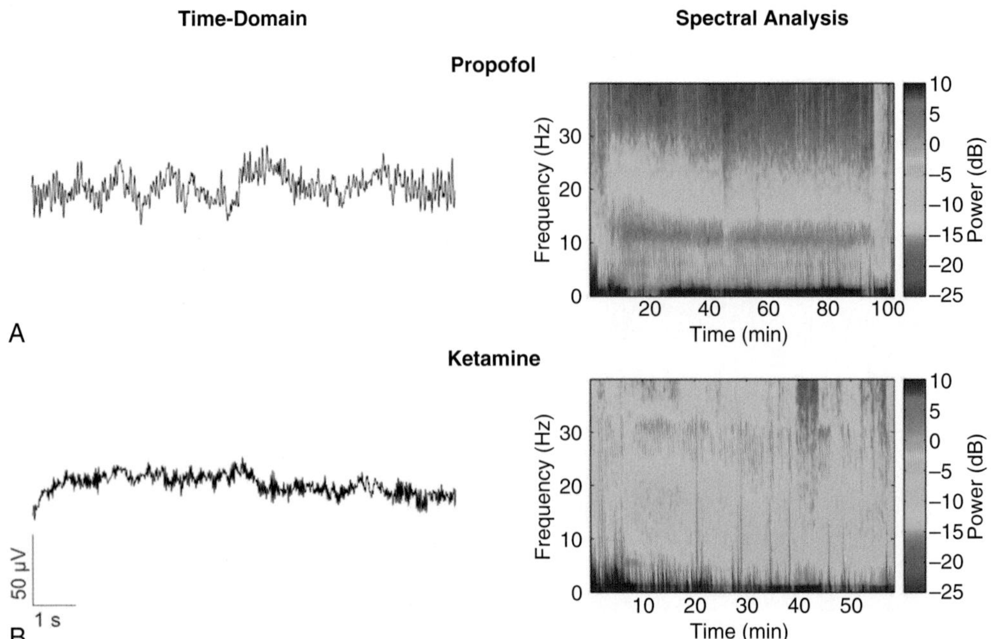

Fig. 40.7 Time-domain and spectral electroencephalogram (EEG) signatures of common anesthetics. The left column shows a 10-s time-domain (unprocessed) segment of the EEG for each anesthetic. The right column shows several minutes of the spectrogram (density spectral array) computed from the EEG for each anesthetic. (A) The EEG and spectrogram of propofol show its characteristic alpha (8-12 Hz) and slow-delta (0.1-4 Hz) oscillation pattern. (B) The ketamine EEG and spectrogram show high frequency oscillations in the high beta (20-24 Hz) and low gamma (25-35 Hz) range.

At doses of sevoflurane appropriate for general anesthesia, the EEG shows strong alpha and slow oscillations like propofol, in addition to a strong theta (4-8 Hz) oscillation (see Fig. 40.8 *C*). The presence of the theta oscillations creates a distinctive pattern of evenly distributed EEG power from the slow oscillation through the alpha oscillation range. The predominance of the alpha and slow oscillations in the sevoflurane spectrogram and those of the other inhaled ethers suggest that $GABA_A$-mediated inhibition is a primary mechanism of action of these anesthetics. This spectrogram pattern further suggests that a primary mechanism through which the inhaled ethers produce unconsciousness is largely similar to that of propofol.[44,84,86,87]

Nitrous oxide has a highly distinctive EEG dynamic. A common practice in our institution, at the end of surgery, is to switch from the inhaled ether, isoflurane, to nitrous oxide to facilitate emergence from general anesthesia (Fig. 40.9 *A*). When nitrous oxide is administered at high doses (greater than 50%), it produces large slow-delta oscillations that last from 3 to 12 minutes before converting to high-frequency gamma oscillations (see Fig. 40.9 *B*).[26,31,103,104] Why the slow-delta oscillations are transient is unknown. Nitrous oxide is known to act by blocking NMDA glutamate receptors.[31,79,105,106] It is likely that the slow-delta oscillations reflect a transient profound state of unconsciousness most likely mediated through inactivation of key NMDA glutamate projections from the parabrachial nucleus and from the median pontine reticular formation into the central thalamus and basal forebrain.[31,107]

Although the unprocessed EEG recordings of the anesthetics can look similar, the spectrograms make clear that each anesthetic has a distinct EEG signature. These signatures can be related to the mechanisms through which the drugs act at specific receptors in specific neural circuits to alter arousal. Using the spectrogram to monitor brain function under general anesthesia and sedation is fundamentally different from using EEG-based indices that are predicated on the assumption that different anesthetics can create the same anesthetic state irrespective of mechanism. The differences in the spectral signatures between propofol (see Fig. 40.7 *A*) and ketamine (see Fig. 40.7 *B*) illustrate why the latter often gives a high index reading when clinically the patient is clearly sedated. Similarly, the predominance of the slow-wave oscillations observed during deep dexmedetomidine (see Fig. 40.8, *B*) sedation helps explain why this drug gives low index values consistent with profound unconsciousness yet the patient remains arousable.

CHANGES IN ELECTROENCEPHALOGRAM SIGNATURES WITH AGING

In addition to changing systematically with anesthetic class, the EEG signatures of patients under general anesthesia change systematically with age. Fig. 40.10 shows the spectrogram of patients of different ages anesthetized with propofol. There are three principal changes in the EEG signatures of propofol with age. First, the EEG of children between 0 to 3 months of age, anesthetized with propofol or another GABAergic drug such as sevoflurane as the primary hypnotic, show only slow-delta oscillations (see Fig. 40.10, *A* and *B*).[108] Slow-delta and alpha oscillations do not appear together until children are at least 4 months of age or older (see Fig. 40.10 *C*).[108] The alpha oscillations become coherent and show anteriorization specifically at the alpha frequency, at approximately 1 year of age.[37,38,108,109] Coherence means the oscillations are highly synchronized, whereas anteriorization means that the oscillations are predominant in the

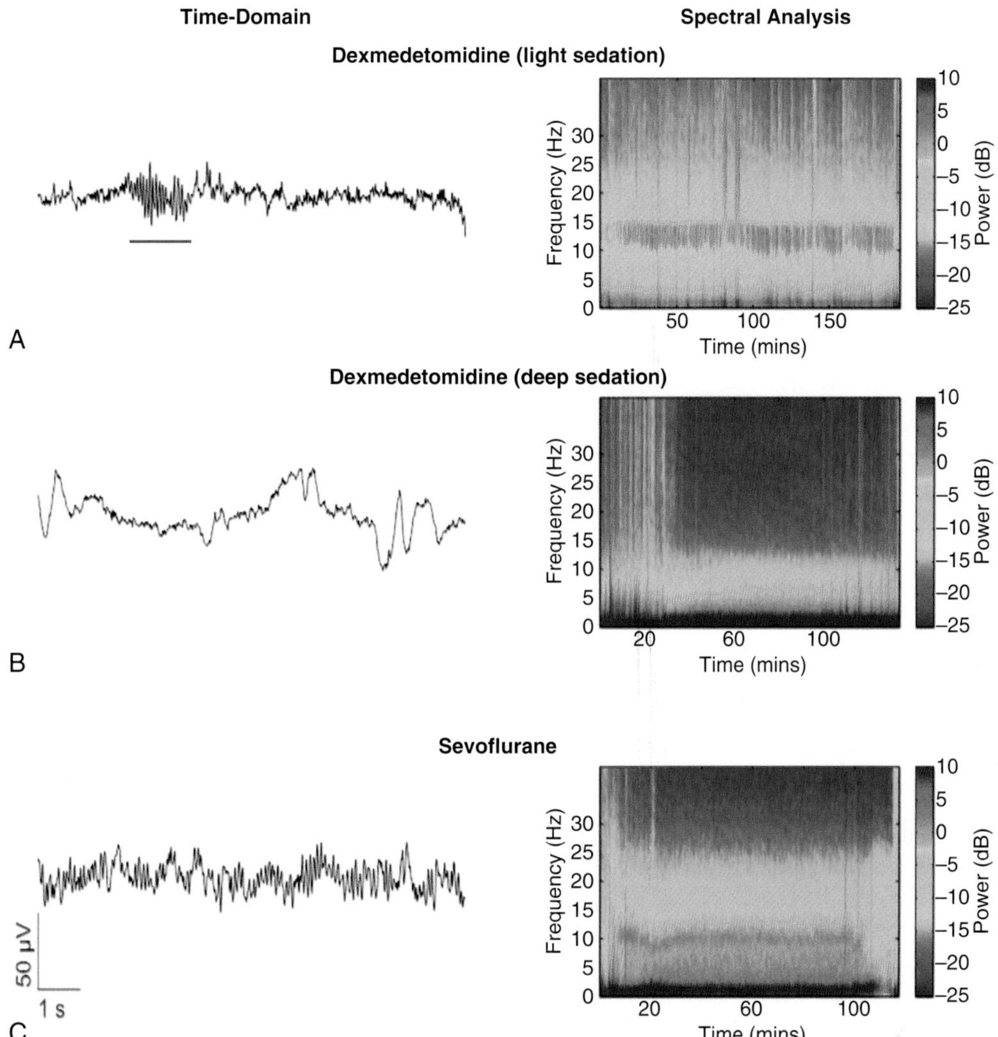

Fig. 40.8 Time-domain and spectral electroencephalogram (EEG) signatures of common anesthetics. The *left column* shows a 10-second time domain (unprocessed) segment of the EEG for each anesthetic. The *right column* shows several minutes of the spectrogram (density spectral array) computed from the EEG for each anesthetic. (A) The dexmedetomidine EEG and spectrogram for light sedation shows spindle (9-15 Hz) oscillations, and the slow (0.1-1 Hz) oscillations, and delta (1-4 Hz) oscillations similar to the EEG patterns observed in nonrapid eye movement (NREM) sleep stage 2. The spindle is apparent in the unprocessed EEG trace (red underscore). The spindles are intermittent and have less intensity than the alpha oscillations observed with propofol. (B) The EEG and spectrogram for deep dexmedetomidine sedation can be associated with an absence of spindles and a predominance of slow and delta waves similar to the slow waves seen in NREM sleep stage 3, termed *slow-wave sleep.* (C) The sevoflurane spectrogram is similar to propofol with the addition of oscillatory activity in the theta band from 4 to 8 Hz.

frontal EEG leads and completely absent in the occipital leads. The mechanisms underlying these age-dependent changes are unclear, but they almost certainly reflect development of underlying brain circuits in children.[37,38,110] According to computational modeling studies propofol can generate alpha oscillations as a result of increasing inhibition in cortical networks.[111] When thalamocortical components are added to this model, the alpha oscillations become highly coherent.[86] Hence, the development of propofol- and sevoflurane-induced alpha oscillations in the first 6 months of life could reflect developing inhibition, particularly within cortical circuits.[110] The later development of coherent alpha oscillations could reflect developing thalamocortical connections that facilitate coherent alpha oscillations.[86,112] Although not shown in the figures presented here, the total power in the spectrogram increases with age from 0 months to a maximum at approximately 6 to 8 years and then declines from there with each year of age.[37,38]

Second, the alpha band is characteristic of young adults (approximately 18-35 years of age) and ranges from 8 to 15 Hz for this group (see Fig. 40.10 *F*). The corresponding band for ages below 18 years falls generally over a broader frequency range, 10 to 20 Hz (see Fig. 40.10, *D* and*E*), and has higher power relative to the alpha band of the young adults (see Fig. 40.10 *F*). The corresponding band for ages greater than 35 years falls generally over a narrower frequency range, 6 to 10 Hz (see Fig. 40.10 G), and has less power relative to the alpha band of the young adults (see Fig. 40.10 *F*). Third, the alpha oscillations in adults 55 years or older may be diminished and in the lower frequency range from 6 to 10 Hz or nearly absent (see Fig. 40.10, *G-I*).

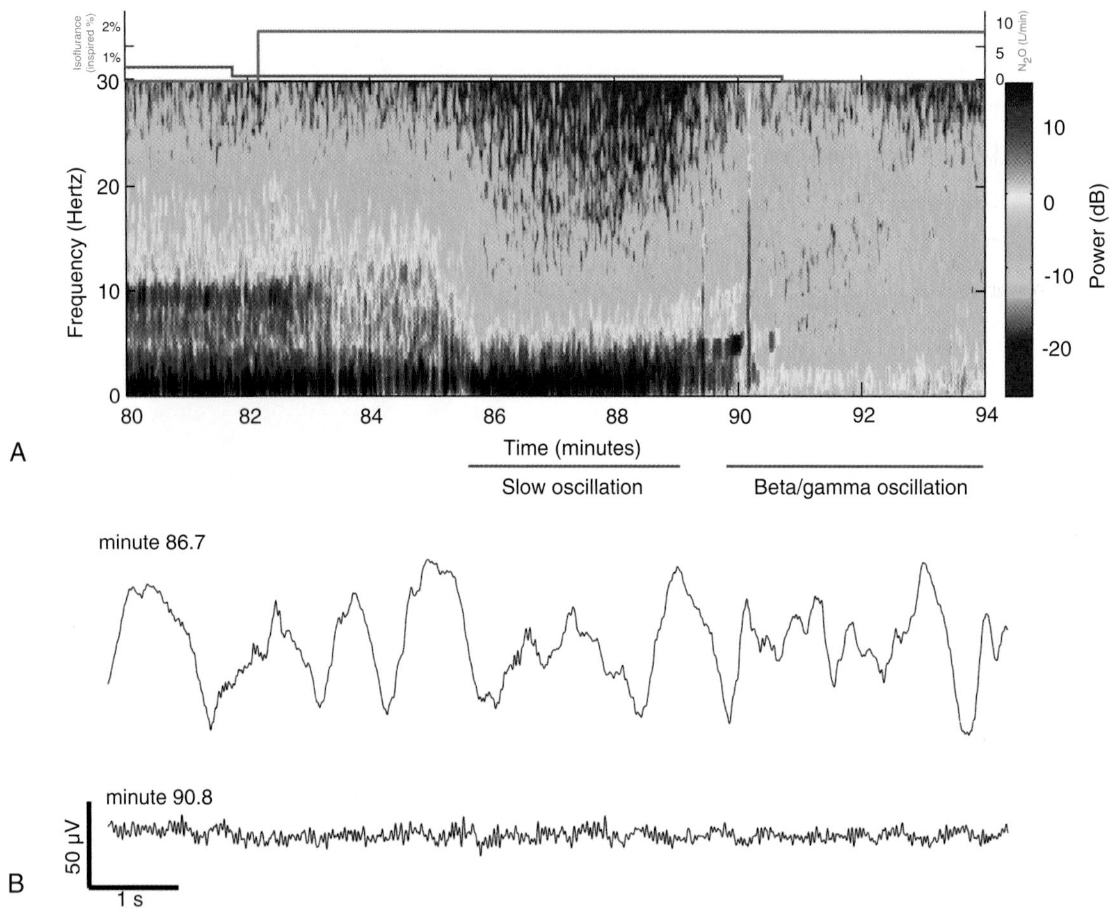

Fig. 40.9 Spectrogram displays of nitrous oxide-induced slow-delta and beta-gamma oscillations. (A) To facilitate emergence, a patient maintained on a mixture of 0.5% isoflurane and 58% oxygen at 3 L/min was changed to 75% nitrous oxide and 24% oxygen at 7 L/min. Between minutes 83 and 85 the slow-delta, theta, and alpha oscillation power decreased. The beta and theta band power appreciably decreased whereas the slow-delta oscillation power substantially increased beginning at minute 86. By minute 90 the slow-delta oscillation power has noticeably decreased, and beta-gamma oscillations begin to appear. (B) Electroencephalogram traces of the slow-delta oscillations recorded at minute 86.7 and the beta-gamma oscillations recorded at minute 90.8. Each trace is 10 s.

The changes in the slow-delta oscillations follow similar changes to the alpha oscillations band in that the band is broad with high power at younger ages (see Fig. 40.10, *C-E*) and becomes narrower with lower power with aging (see Fig. 40.10, *F-I*). Indeed, the alpha and slow-delta oscillations of the 56-year old patient and of the 81-year old patient are barely perceptible (see Fig. 40.10).

Fig. 40.10, *F-G* show that there can be significant between-person variation in power for patients of approximately the same age. The 57-year-old patient (see Fig. 40.10 *G*) has alpha and slow-delta oscillations that resemble the pattern seen in the 30-year-old patient (see Fig. 40.10 *F*), whereas the alpha and slow-delta oscillations of the 56-year-old patient (see Fig. 40.10 *H*) resemble those of the 81-year-old patient (see Fig. 40.10 *I*). We conjecture that these differences in oscillatory dynamics induced by propofol reflect between - individual variation in normal brain aging.[113] The age-related EEG changes of sevoflurane, and presumably those associated with isoflurane and desflurane, are similar to those of propofol, given that all of these agents have primary GABAergic mechanisms of action.

IMPLICATIONS FOR MONITORING ANESTHETIC STATE

These observations suggest that the unprocessed EEG and the spectrogram can be used to monitor the brain states of patients receiving anesthesia care (see Figs. 40.6 to 40.10). The unprocessed EEG waveform has been advocated as a tool for monitoring "depth of anesthesia" since 1937.[16,17,26,114,115] Although the spectrogram is easy to compute in real time and has been reported in studies of anesthetics,[80,81,116] a strategy to use it in conjunction with the unprocessed EEG and the EEG-based indices for management of patients receiving anesthesia care is now being developed. Many of the current EEG brain function monitors display both the unprocessed EEG and the spectrogram.[22,54,117] Training anesthesia providers to track brain states under general anesthesia and sedation by reading the unprocessed EEG and the spectrogram is a program being pursued currently in the Department of Anesthesia, Critical Care and Pain Medicine, of Massachusetts General Hospital in collaboration with the International Anesthesia Research Society (www.eegforanesthesia.iars.org).

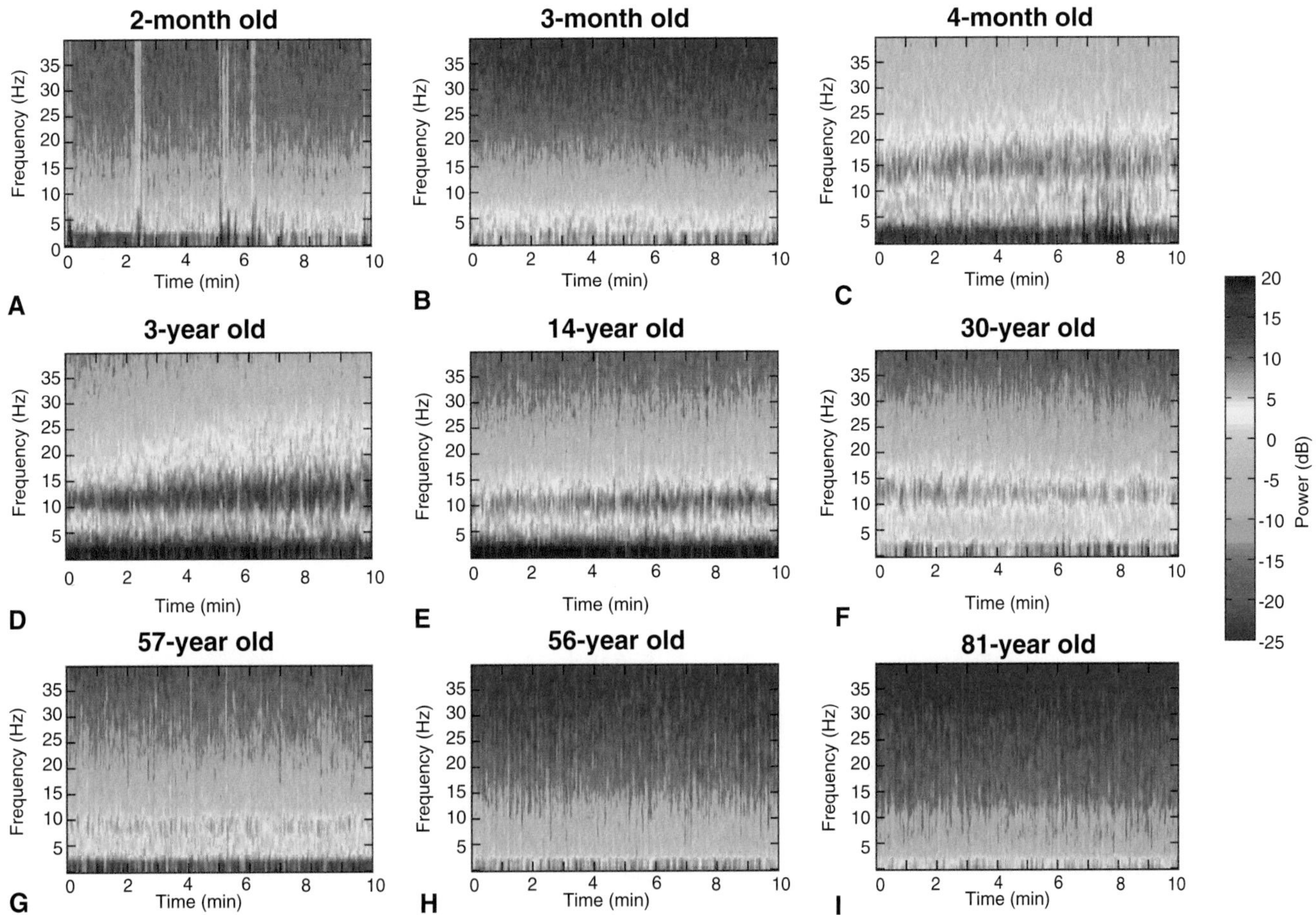

Fig. 40.10 Spectral electroencephalogram signatures of propofol as a function of age. Each panel is a 10-minute segment recorded from a patient receiving a propofol infusion as the primary anesthetic to maintain unconsciousness. The spectral power in all of the panels are plotted on the same decibel scale. (A) A 2-month-old patient. (B) A 3-month-old patient. (C) A 4-month-old patient. (D) A 3-year-old patient. (E) A 14-year-old patient. (F) A 30-year-old patient. (G) A 57-year-old patient. (H) A 56-year-old patient. (I) An 81-year-old patient. Children less than 4 months of age show only slow-delta oscillations. Alpha oscillations appear at 4 months of age. Although children greater than 4 months of age and adults from 18 to 55 years of age show both slow-delta and alpha oscillation patterns under propofol, the frequency range of the alpha oscillations and the power content changes with age. Elderly patients often have a noticeable decrease in or absence of alpha oscillations.

Another EEG education resource has been developed at Washington University (icetap.org). Highly structured oscillations are the sine qua non of anesthetic states. Therefore, use of the spectrogram to track level of consciousness under general anesthesia and sedation facilitates direct integration of clinical and research observations from EEG recordings with experimental studies and biophysically-based modeling studies that help define the neural circuit mechanisms of anesthetic actions.[86,111,118,119]

NORMALIZED SYMBOLIC TRANSFER ENTROPY

A growing body of information suggests that a key marker or mechanism of unconsciousness under general anesthesia is loss of intracortical connectivity.[74,75,84,91,120,121] The loss of functional connectivity between the frontal and parietal areas is associated with unconsciousness.[91,120] By using the EEG recorded from a montage that includes both frontal and parietal electrodes, a mutual information technique termed normalized symbolic transfer entropy (NSTE) can be used to measure this loss of functional connectivity (Fig. 40.11). When NSTE is used to assess functional connectivity from the parietal area to the frontal cortical area, it is termed *feedforward functional connectivity*, whereas when it is used to assess functional connectivity from the frontal area to the parietal area, it is termed *feedback functional connectivity*.

Unconsciousness induced by propofol, sevoflurane, or ketamine has been associated with loss of feedback functional connectivity (see Fig. 40.11).[91,120] As a consequence, measuring NSTE to assess functional connectivity could provide a means of monitoring the level of consciousness in patients receiving general anesthesia. The loss of feedback functional connectivity is present for unconsciousness induced by all three anesthetics, suggesting that NSTE does not distinguish among the mechanisms of actions of these anesthetics.[120] Nevertheless, NSTE could still offer a way to track levels of unconsciousness.

A partial answer regarding the mechanism of loss of the feedback functional connectivity for unconsciousness induced by propofol and the inhaled ether anesthetics may be related to anteriorization (see Fig. 40.6, *D*). The model by Vijayan and colleagues[119] shows that anteriorization can be explained by the differences in the electrophysiologic

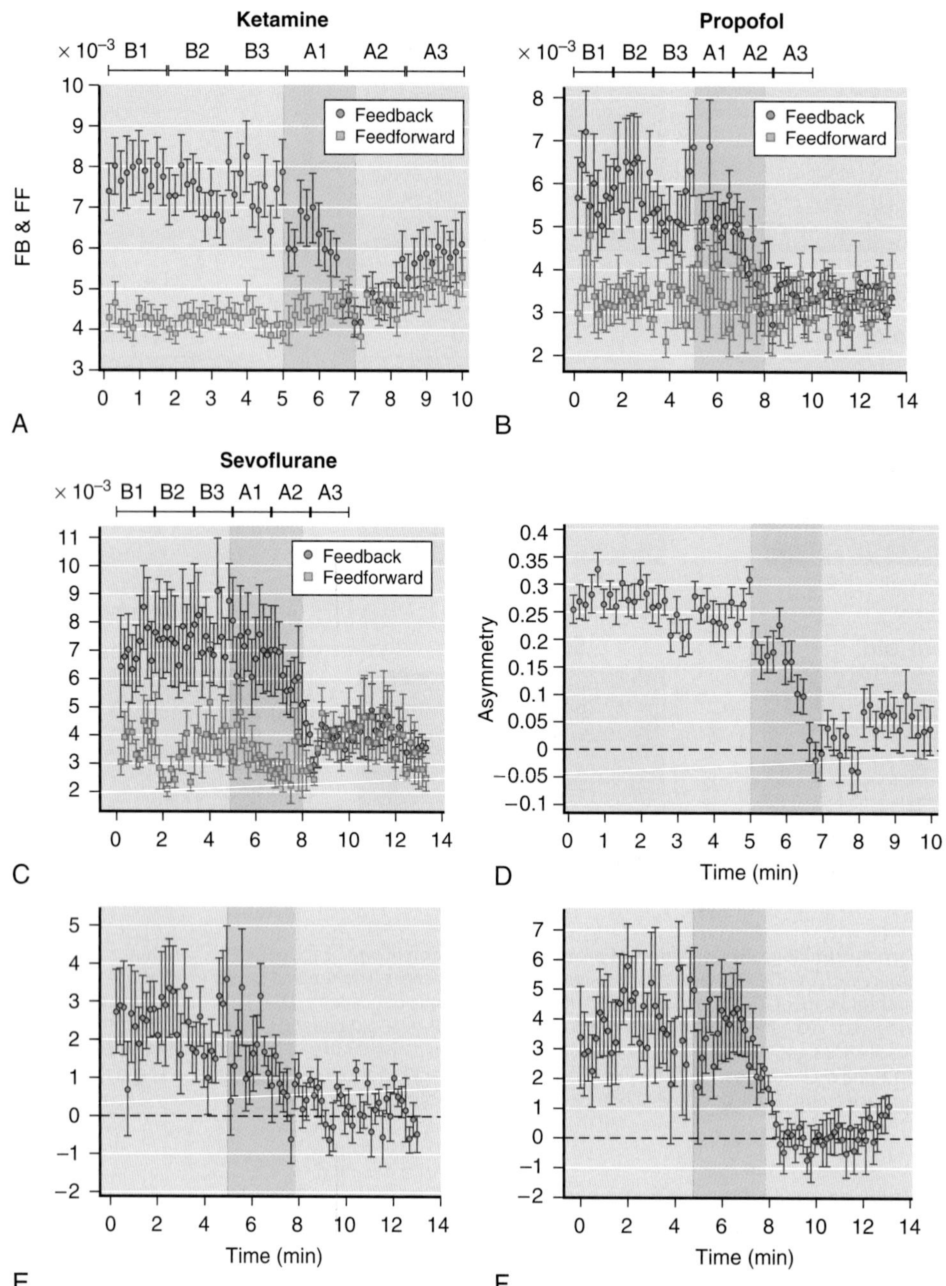

Fig. 40.11 Normalized symbolic transfer entropy. An analysis of loss of consciousness induced by ketamine, propofol, and sevoflurane using normalized symbolic transfer entropy. Asymmetry in the change of feedforward *(FF)* and feedback *(FB)* connectivity is common to all three anesthetics. The FF *(blue)*/FB *(red)* connections (A–C) and their associated asymmetry (D–F) in the frontal–parietal network displayed for (A and D) ketamine, (B and E) propofol, and (C and F) sevoflurane. Green shading highlights induction of general anesthesia. *B1 to B3* define baseline substates. *A1 to A3* define anesthetized substates. There were 30, 9, and 9 subjects in the ketamine, propofol, and sevoflurane groups, respectively. All three anesthetics show a greater loss in FB frontal-parietal connectivity than FF connectivity at loss of consciousness. (Redrawn from Lee U, Ku S, Noh G, et al. Disruption of frontal-parietal communication by ketamine, propofol, and sevoflurane. *Anesthesiology* 2013;118:1264–1275.)

properties, such as the resting membrane potentials and ionic currents, in the frontal thalamocortical connections compared with the posterior thalamocortical connections. If the parietal circuits resemble their nearby occipital counterparts neurophysiologically, then the neurophysiologic dynamics that lead to anteriorization could also contribute to loss of feedback functional connectivity. Studies of functional connectivity changes during loss of consciousness due to general anesthesia using the Vijayan model may shed mechanistic light on the differences between changes in feedback connectivity and feedforward connectivity.

At present, the use of NSTE in the operating room is not tractable because it is not possible to compute these mutual information measures in real time.[91] Moreover, the use of NSTE in its current form requires an EEG montage with both frontal and parietal electrodes, unlike the montages used with most current brain function monitors, which require only frontal electrodes.

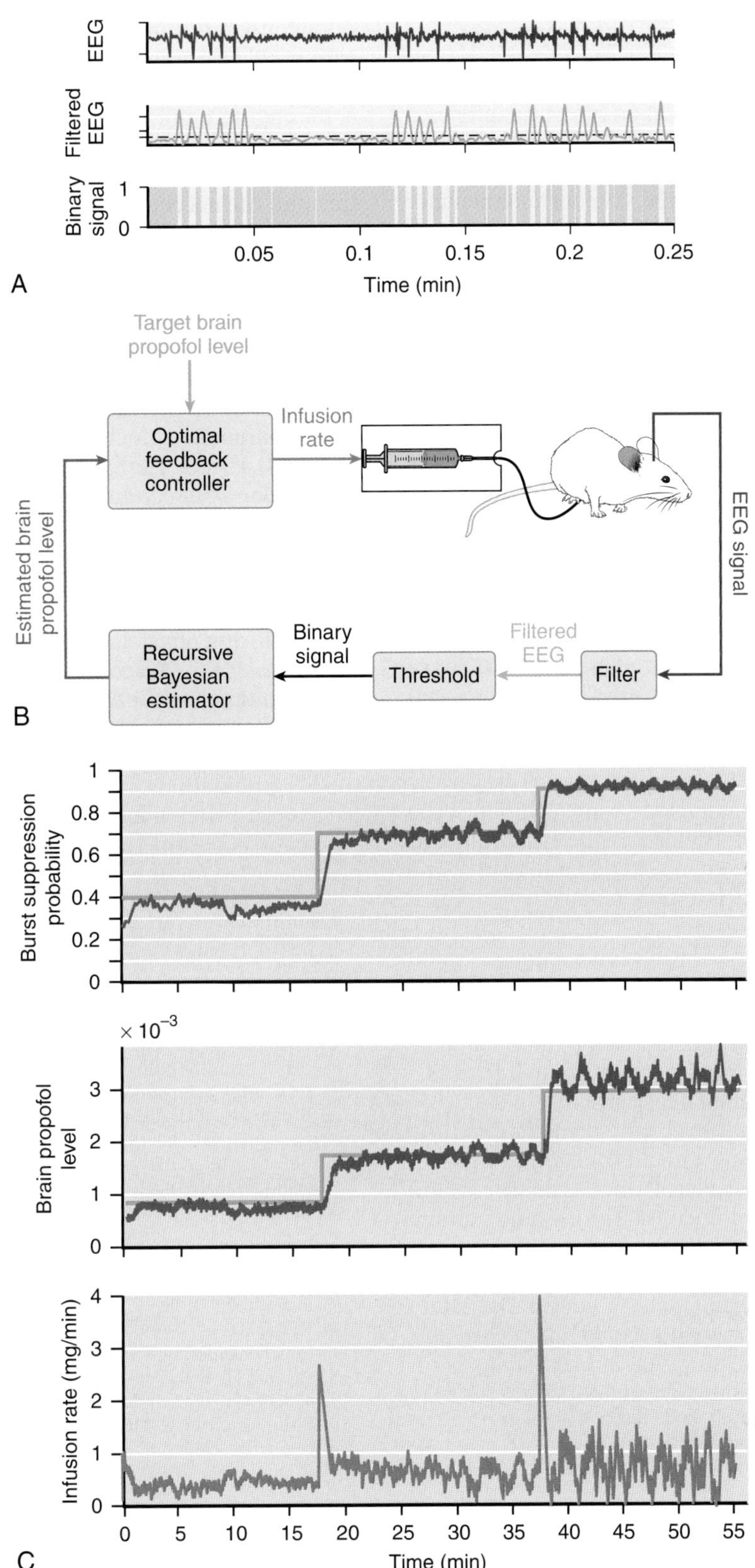

Fig. 40.12 An experimental closed loop anesthetic delivery system for control of medical coma by controlling burst suppression. (A) The electroencephalogram *(EEG)* of the rat in burst suppression is filtered, thresholded, and converted into binary observations (i.e., 0 for a burst and 1 for a suppression). (B) A target brain level of propofol is set by specifying a burst suppression probability. The Bayesian algorithm estimates the brain level of propofol from the EEG. The controller compares the estimated propofol level with the target level and adjusts the infusion rate every second to maintain the specified target burst suppression probability or, equivalently, the target brain propofol level. (C) The *top panel* shows that the target burst suppression probability *(green line)* was maintained at 0.4 for 20 minutes, changed to 0.7 for 20 minutes, and then changed to 0.9 for 15 minutes. The estimated burst suppression probability *(purple curve)* tracks exactly the targeted level. The *middle panel* shows the equivalent close tracking of the target brain propofol level *(green line)* by the estimated propofol level *(purple curve)*. The *bottom panel* shows how the controller instantaneously changed the infusion rate to maintain the targeted level of burst suppression. This experimental study establishes the feasibility of real-time control of burst suppression and most likely other states of general anesthesia. (Redrawn from Shanechi M, Chemali JJ, Liberman M, et al. A brain-machine interface for control of medically-induced coma. *PLoS Comput Biol.* 2013;9:e1003284.)

CLOSED-LOOP ANESTHETIC DELIVERY SYSTEMS

Closed-loop anesthetic delivery (CLAD) systems for maintenance of general anesthesia and sedation have been proposed since the early 1950s. These studies have been summarized.[122,123] The CLAD systems work by using an EEG marker of anesthetic state to define a desired state for maintenance during surgery. The EEG is monitored, the marker is computed from the EEG, and a computer-controlled infusion delivering the anesthetic drug is automatically changed based on the difference between the targeted level of the EEG marker and the actual level of the marker computed from the EEG analysis. Although numerous EEG markers have been used to guide delivery of anesthetics in CLAD systems, the most widely used marker is the BIS index.[25,124] Use of the BIS requires a 20- to 30-second delay in computing updates.[24] Use of a CLAD system leads to maintenance of the desired anesthetic state while delivering significantly less anesthetic drug.[25,125-127] Although most CLAD systems have focused on maintenance of unconsciousness, a recently developed control system has studied maintenance of unconsciousness and antinociception.[128,129]

Recent simulation studies using rodent and human models, as well as recent experimental studies in rodents, have shown that highly reliable and accurate CLAD systems can be devised to maintain medical coma by using burst suppression (see Fig. 40.2 *F*) as the control variable.[122,123] A CLAD system developed by Shanechi and colleagues[130] uses a stochastic control framework and, as the control variable, the burst suppression probability, which is the instantaneous probability that the brain is suppressed (Fig. 40.12).[110] The burst suppression probability is a more reliable way to track burst suppression than the suppression ratio. The CLAD system precisely tracked the target level of burst suppression. If these results are successfully reproduced in human studies, the CLAD system could offer an automatic and highly efficient way to maintain medical coma in the many patients who require this therapy for multiple days to treat intractable status epilepticus or intracranial hypertension.

Several clinical studies have recently demonstrated the feasibility of CLAD systems as a means of controlling level of unconsciousness alone, level of unconsciousness and antinociception, and level of unconsciousness and volume status.[131-133] All of these studies have been conducted outside of the United States, as the FDA has not approved any CLAD system for administering general anesthesia. Many new findings and approaches will probably be reported in the near future because the study of CLAD systems is an active area of research by many investigators.

MONITORING ANTINOCICEPTION

The discussion of monitoring brain states under general anesthesia and sedation has focused largely on monitoring level of unconsciousness. Monitoring antinociception is an important, growing area of investigation. In the introduction, we modified the definition of general anesthesia given previously by Brown and colleagues[1] by substituting antinociception for analgesia.[3] We did so to make a precise distinction between the concept of nociception, which is transmission of potentially harmful and noxious stimuli through the sensory system, and pain, which is conscious processing of nociceptive information. When a patient is unconscious under general anesthesia, the anesthesia care provider is managing nociception, whereas when the patient is awake at the end of surgery, the care provider is managing pain. Antinociception is therefore the extent to which anesthetic and analgesic agents impede the flow of information regarding harmful and noxious stimuli through the nervous system.

At present, movement and the physiological responses of changes in heart rate, blood pressure, and perhaps respiratory rate, are the most commonly used markers of nociception. The changes in these physiological markers are a consequence of the NMA circuit responses to nociceptive information transmission in the central nervous system (see Fig. 40.1). Investigations are using multiple physiologic parameters including heart rate, heart rate variability (0.15-0.4 Hz band power), plethysmograph wave amplitude, skin conductance, skin conductance fluctuations, and the derivatives of these signals to track antinociception.[134,135] In addition, nociception can be tracked by using infrared pupillometry to record pupillary activity.[136] Commercial monitors that track level of antinociception by monitoring physiologic variables are now commercially available.[137-140] A recent report suggests that monitoring simultaneously unconsciousness and antinociception together allows the implementation of more principled multimodal strategies for choosing and administering anesthetic combinations.[3] This new strategy offers the potential to achieve better nociceptive control intraoperatively and pain control postoperatively, and to reduce the likelihood of postoperative cognitive dysfunction and opioid overuse.

Complete references available online at expertconsult.com.

References

1. Brown EN, et al. *N Engl J Med.* 2010;363:2638–2650.
2. Cellular and molecular mechanisms of anesthesia. In: Evers AS, PG Barash, BF Cullen, RK Stoelting ed. *Clinical Anesthesia.* 3rd ed. Philadelphia: Lipponcott-Raven; 1997.
3. Brown EN, et al. *Anesth Analg.*2018; 127: 1246-1258.
4. Posner J, et al. Oxford University Press; 2007.
5. Cote CJ, et al. *Anesthesiology.* 1981;55:703–705.
6. Feldman JL, Del Negro CA. *Nat Rev Neurosci.* 2006;7:232–242.
7. Palanca BJ, et al. *Curr Opin Anaesthesiol.* 2009;22:553–559.
8. Prys-Roberts C. *Br J Anaesth.* 1987;59:1341–1345.
9. Price DD. *Science.* 2000;288:1769–1772.
10. Purves D, et al. *Neuroscience.* 4th ed. Sunderland, MA: Sinauer Associates, Inc.; 2008.
11. Kertai MD, et al. *Anesth Analg.* 2012;114:533–546.
12. Pfaff D. Cambridge: Harvard University Press; 2005.
13. Giacino JT, et al. *Neurology.* 2002;58:349–353.
14. Giacino JT, et al. *Arch Phys Med Rehabil.* 2004;85:2020–2029.
15. Storm H. *Curr Opin Anaesthesiol.* 2008;21:796–804.
16. Bennett C, et al. *Anesth Analg.* 2009;109:539–550.
17. Gibbs FA, et al. *Arch Intern Med.* 1937;60:154–166.
18. Kiersey DK, et al. *Br J Anaesth.* 1951;23:141–152.
19. Kearse Jr LA, et al. *Anesthesiology.* 1994;81:1365–1370.
20. Glass PS, et al. *Anesthesiology.* 1997;86:836–847.
21. Rampil IJ. *Anesthesiology.* 1998;89:980–1002.
22. Kelley SD. *Monitoring Consciousness: Using the Bispectral Index.* 2nd ed. Boulder, CO: Covidien; 2010.
23. Bruhn J, et al. *J Clin Mon Comp.* 2000;16:593–596.
24. Pilge S, et al. *Anesthesiology.* 2006;104:488–494.
25. Struys MM, et al. *Anesthesiology.* 2001;95:6–17.
26. Purdon PL, et al. *Anesthesiology.* 2015;123:937–960.
27. Hayashi K, et al. *Br J Anaesth.* 2007;99:389–395.
28. Yamamura T, et al. *Anesth Analg.* 1981;60:283–288.
29. Foster BL, Liley DT. *Anesth Analg.* 2011;113:758–765.
30. Ozcan MS, et al. *J Neurosurg Anesthesiol.* 2010;22:309–315.

31. Pavone KJ, et al. *Clin Neurophysiol.* 2016;127:556–564.
32. Sleigh JW, et al. *Anesth Analg.* 2018;127:951–959.
33. Xi C, et al. *PLoS One.* 2018;13:e0199120.
34. Huupponen E, et al. *Acta Anaesthesiol Scand.* 2008;52:289–294.
35. Aksu R, et al. *Paediatr Anaesth.* 2011;21:373–378.
36. Mason KP, et al. *Paediatr Anaesth.* 2009;19:1175–1183.
37. Akeju O, et al. *Br J Anaesth.* 2015;115(suppl 1):i66–i76.
38. Lee JM, et al. *Anesthesiology.* 2017;127:293–306.
39. Myles PS, et al. *Lancet.* 2004;363:1757–1763.
40. Avidan MS, et al. *N Engl J Med.* 2008;358:1097–1108.
41. Avidan MS, et al. *N Engl J Med.* 2011;365:591–600.
42. Myles PS, et al. *N Engl J Med.* 2008;359:428–429; author reply 30-1.
43. Brown EN, et al. *Annu Rev Neurosci.* 2011;34:601–628.
44. Purdon PL, et al. *Proc Natl Acad Sci U S A.* 2013;110:E1142–E1151.
45. Prichep LS, et al. *Br J Anaesth.* 2004;92:393–399.
46. Drover D, Ortega HR. *Best Pract Res Clin Anaesthesiol.* 2006;20: 121–128.
47. Tinker JH, et al. *Anesthesiology.* 1977;46:252–259.
48. Kochs E, et al. *Anesthesiology.* 1994;80:1026–1034.
49. Cimenser A, et al. *Proc Natl Acad Sci U S A.* 2011;108:8832–8837.
50. Chen X, et al. *Anesth Analg.* 2002;95:1669–1674, table of contents.
51. Soehle M, et al. *Br J Anaesth.* 2010;105:172–178.
52. Adesanya AO, et al. *J Crit Care.* 2009;24:322–328.
53. Schultz B, et al. *Anaesthesist.* 2003;52:1143–1148.
54. Kreuer S, Wilhelm W. *Best Pract Res Clin Anaesthesiol.* 2006;20: 111–119.
55. Schneider G, et al. *Br J Anaesth.* 2003;91:329–335.
56. Schneider G, et al. *Anesthesiology.* 2004;101:1105–1111.
57. Bruhn J, et al. *Anesthesiology.* 2001;95:30–35.
58. Viertio-Oja H, et al. *Acta Anaesthesiol Scand.* 2004;48:154–161.
59. Jantti V, Alahuhta S. *Br J Anaesth.* 2004;93:150–151; author reply 1-2.
60. Bein B. *Best Pract Res Clin Anaesthesiol.* 2006;20:101–109.
61. Gruenewald M, et al. *Anaesthesia.* 2007;62:1224–1229.
62. Eger 2nd EI, et al. *Anesthesiology.* 1965;26:756–763.
63. Stoelting RK, et al. *Anesthesiology.* 1970;33:5–9.
64. Solt K, Forman SA. *Curr Opin Anaesthesiol.* 2007;20:300–306.
65. Rampil IJ, Laster MJ. *Anesthesiology.* 1992;77:920–925.
66. Antognini JF, Schwartz K. *Anesthesiology.* 1993;79:1244–1249.
67. Rampil IJ. *Anesthesiology.* 1994;80:606–610.
68. Anderson RE, Jakobsson JG. *Eur J Anaesthesiol.* 2006;23:208–212.
69. Schmidt GN, et al. *Anaesthesia.* 2005;60:228–234.
70. Kreuer S, et al. *Br J Anaesth.* 2003;91:336–340.
71. Friedman EB, et al. *PLoS One.* 2010;5:e11903.
72. Joiner WJ, et al. *PLoS Genet.* 2013;9:e1003605.
73. Hirschberg R, Giacino JT. *Neurol Clin.* 2011;29:773–786.
74. Alkire MT, et al. *Science.* 2008;322:876–880.
75. Hudetz AG. *Brain Connect.* 2012;2:291–302.
76. Langsjo JW, et al. *J Neurosci.* 2012;32:4935–4943.
77. Mhuircheartaigh RN, et al. *J Neurosci.* 2010;30:9095–9102.
78. Breshears JD, et al. *Proc Natl Acad Sci U S A.* 2010;107: 21170–21175.
79. Hemmings Jr HC, et al. *Trends Pharmacol Sci.* 2005;26:503–510.
80. Bickford RG, et al. *Trans Am Neurol Assoc.* 1971;96:118–122.
81. Fleming RA, Smith NT. *Anesthesiology.* 1979;50:456–460.
82. Bai D, et al. *J Neurosci.* 1999;19:10635–10646.
83. Feshchenko VA, et al. *Neuropsychobiology.* 2004;50:257–266.
84. Lewis LD, et al. *Proc Natl Acad Sci U S A.* 2012;109:E3377–E3386.
85. Li D, et al. *Anesthesiology.* 2013;119:81–88.
86. Ching S, et al. *Proc Natl Acad Sci U S A.* 2010;107:22665–22670.
87. Soplata AE, et al. *PLoS Comput Biol.* 2017;13:e1005879.
88. Sinner B, Graf BM. *Handb Exp Pharmacol.* 2008:313–333.
89. Olney JW, Farber NB. *Arch Gen Psychiatry.* 1995;52:998–1007.
90. Seamans J. *Nat Chem Biol.* 2008;4:91–93.
91. Lee U, et al. *Anesthesiology.* 2013;118:1264–1275.
92. Tsuda N, et al. *Acta Anaesthesiol Scand.* 2007;51:472–481.
93. Correa-Sales C, et al. *Anesthesiology.* 1992;76:948–952.
94. Chiu TH, et al. *Eur J Pharmacol.* 1995;285:261–268.
95. Mizobe T, et al. *J Clin Invest.* 1996;98:1076–1080.
96. Jorm CM, Stamford JA. *Br J Anaesth.* 1993;71:447–449.
97. Nacif-Coelho C, et al. *Anesthesiology.* 1994;81:1527–1534.
98. Nelson LE, et al. *Anesthesiology.* 2003;98:428–436.
99. Saper CB, et al. *Nature.* 2005;437:1257–1263.
100. Sherin JE, et al. *J Neurosci.* 1998;18:4705–4721.
101. Morairty S, et al. *Neuroscience.* 2004;123:451–457.
102. Scheinin A, et al. *Anesthesiology.* 2018;129:22–36.
103. Avramov MN, et al. *Anesth Analg.* 1990;70:369–374.
104. Hagihira S, et al. *Anesth Analg.* 2012;115:572–577.
105. Mennerick S, et al. *J Neurosci.* 1998;18:9716–9726.
106. Jevtovic-Todorovic V, et al. *Nat Med.* 1998;4:460–463.
107. Boon JA, Milsom WK. *Resp Phys Neurobiol.* 2008;162:63–72.
108. Cornelissen L, et al. *Elife.* 2015;4:e06513.
109. Cornelissen L, et al. *Br J Anaesth.* 2018;120:1274–1286.
110. Purdon PL. In: Benasich AA, Ribary U, eds. *Emergent Brain Dynamics: Prebirth to Adolescence.* Cambridge, MA: MIT Press; 2018.
111. McCarthy MM, et al. *J Neurosci.* 2008;28:13488–13504.
112. Flores FJ, et al. *Proc Natl Acad Sci U S A.* 2017;114:E6660–E6668.
113. Brown EN, Purdon PL. *Curr Opin Anaesthesiol.* 2013;26:414–419.
114. Martin JT, et al. *Anesthesiology.* 1959;20:359–376.
115. Wildes TS, et al. *BMJ Open.* 2016;6:e011505.
116. Levy WJ. *Anesthesiology.* 1984;60:430–434.
117. Drover DR, et al. *J Clin Mon Comp.* 2011;25:175–181.
118. Ching S, et al. *Proc Natl Acad Sci U S A.* 2012;109:3095–3100.
119. Vijayan S, et al. *J Neurosci.* 2013;33:11070–11075.
120. Ku SW, et al. *PLoS One.* 2011;6:e25155.
121. Casali AG, et al. *Sci Transl Med.* 2013;5:198ra05.
122. Ching S, et al. *Anesthesiology.* 2013.
123. Liberman MY, et al. *J Neural Eng.* 2013;10:046004.
124. Mortier E, et al. *Anaesthesia.* 1998;53:749–754.
125. Agarwal J, et al. *Acta Anaesthesiol Scand.* 2009;53:390–397.
126. Puri GD, et al. *Anaesth Intensive Care.* 2007;35:357–362.
127. Hemmerling TM, et al. *Can J Anaesth.* 2010;57:725–735.
128. Liu N, et al. *Anesth Analg.* 2011;112:546–557.
129. Liu N, et al. *Anesthesiology.* 2012;116:286–295.
130. Shanechi M, et al. *PLoS Comp Bio.* 2013.
131. Dutta A, et al. *Anesth Analg.* 2018.
132. Joosten A, et al. *Anesth Analg.* 2018.
133. West N, et al. *Anesth Analg.* 2018;127:883–894.
134. Ben-Israel N, et al. *J Clin Mon CompJ.* 2013.
135. Ledowski T, et al. *Anaesthesia.* 2010;65:1001–1006.
136. Neice AE, et al. *Anesth Analg.* 2017;124:915–921.
137. The Dolosys Paintracker. (Accessed June 29, 2017, at http://www.dolosys.de/Products-EN.htm.)
138. ANI (Analgesia Nociception Index). (Accessed June 29, 2017, at https://www.mdoloris.com/en/technologies/ani-analgesia-nociception-index/.)
139. Storm H. Med-Storm, PainMonitorTM. 2016.
140. Huiku M, et al. *Surgical Plethysmographic Index (SPI) in Anesthesia Practice*; 2014.

41 Respiratory Monitoring

DAVID W. KACZKA, HOVIG V. CHITILIAN, and MARCOS F. VIDAL MELO

KEY POINTS

- Intraoperative respiratory monitoring is a fundamental component of the American Society of Anesthesiologists' standards for basic anesthetic monitoring. Monitoring of oxygenation and ventilation is essential for the safe conduct of an anesthetic.
- A thorough understanding of the physiological and technological principles underlying respiratory monitoring is essential for its appropriate clinical application.
- The majority of respiratory monitors in clinical use provide information at the systemic and whole-lung level from which inferences are made regarding the regional lung and tissue-level conditions.
- The degree of invasiveness of utilized monitors should be determined by clinical requirements.
- Pulse oximetry is a noninvasive, reliable, and simple method for continuously monitoring the fractional arterial oxygen saturation.
- Ventilation-perfusion mismatch, shunt, and hypoventilation are the most common causes of hypoxemia in the perioperative period. Monitoring of gas exchange, and its response to various interventions, may differentiate etiologies for hypoxemia.
- Mixed venous oxygen saturation ($S\bar{v}O_2$) allows for monitoring of the global balance between oxygen delivery and consumption. Its measurement provides information on gas exchange, cardiac output, and global oxygen consumption.
- Systems utilizing near infrared spectroscopy are used clinically to monitor regional tissue oxygenation, particularly in the brain. The value of regional tissue oxygenation monitoring for clinical management is currently being established.
- Capnography is the primary quantitative method to assess ventilation in the perioperative period. Besides providing physiologic information on ventilation, pulmonary blood flow, and aerobic metabolism, capnography is important for verifying the endotracheal tube positioning, and determining the integrity of the breathing circuit.
- End-tidal carbon dioxide (CO_2) is not always a reliable approximation of arterial CO_2 tension, especially in the presence of significant heterogeneity in the distribution of ventilation and perfusion.
- Measurement of the pressures, flows, and volumes associated with ventilation is necessary to optimize mechanical ventilation, as well as to detect pathophysiologic mechanical derangements of the respiratory system (i.e., increased airway resistance or reduced lung compliance).
- Imaging techniques have emerged as important tools for respiratory monitoring. Lung ultrasonography is increasingly utilized in emergency and perioperative settings, allowing for prompt bedside assessments of pulmonary abnormalities such as pneumothorax, lung edema, consolidation, and pleural effusions. Electrical impedance tomography is another noninvasive imaging technique that provides information on lung aeration and recruitment.
- Current approaches to respiratory monitoring primarily assess pulmonary mechanical and global gas exchange processes. The monitoring of tissue and subcellular respiration remains a desirable goal for future innovation.

Overview of Respiratory Monitoring

Respiratory monitoring is essential to every anesthetic. Its major relevance for maintenance of homeostasis and patient safety is acknowledged by its mandatory position in national and international standards for anesthetic monitoring.[1,2] Through the decades, advances in respiratory monitoring have resulted in substantial reduction in anesthetic morbidity and mortality, and opened a new era of safe anesthetic practice.[3]

Respiration is the transport of oxygen (O_2) from the environment to the body cells and the transport of carbon dioxide (CO_2) from those cells to the environment. The concept includes a component of cellular respiration, the process by which cells obtain energy in the form of adenosine triphosphate from the controlled reaction of hydrogen with O_2 to form water.[4] Thus, in its broadest sense, respiratory monitoring refers to the continuous or periodic assessment of processes involved with the exchange of respiratory gases between the environment and the subcellular pathways where those gases are utilized and produced (Fig. 41.1).[4]

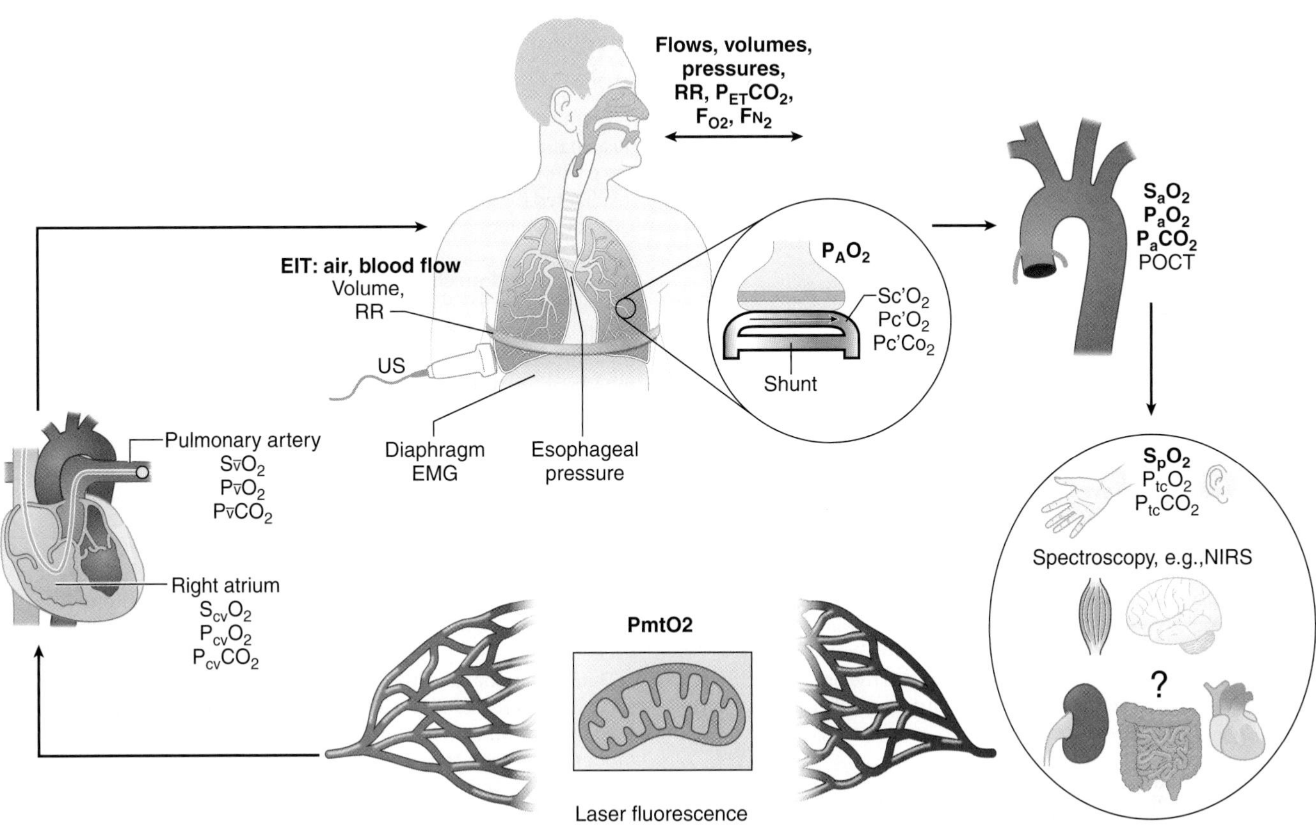

Fig. 41.1 Respiratory Processes and Measurement Sites for Current Respiratory Monitoring Techniques. Most monitored variables are derived from sites at the entrance of the airway and systemic blood (bold) and assess the elements of respiration related to global pulmonary mechanics and gas exchange. Pulse oximetry represents a transition between systemic and local tissue oxygenation assessment. Methods for routine and reliable clinical monitoring of respiratory processes at the tissue, cellular, and subcellular levels are limited. *EMG,* Electromyography; *EIT,* electrical impedance tomography; *FN_2,* nitrogen fraction; *F_{O2},* oxygen fraction; *NIRS,* near-infrared spectroscopy; *P_aCO_2,* arterial partial pressure of carbon dioxide; *P_aO_2,* arterial partial pressure of oxygen; *P_AO_2,* alveolar partial pressure of oxygen; *$Pc'Co_2$,* end-capillary partial pressure of carbon dioxide; *$Pc'O_2$,* end-capillary partial pressure of oxygen; *$P_{cv}CO_2$,* central venous partial pressure of carbon dioxide; *$P_{cv}O_2$,* central venous partial pressure of oxygen; *$P_{ET}CO_2$,* end-tidal partial pressure of carbon dioxide; , mixed venous partial pressure of carbon dioxide;, mixed venous partial pressure of oxygen; *POCT,* point of care testing; *$P_{tc}Co_2$,* transcutaneous partial pressure of carbon dioxide; *$P_{tc}O_2$,* transcutaneous partial pressure of oxygen; *RR,* respiratory rate; *S_aO_2,* arterial oxygen saturation; *$S_c'O_2$,* end-capillary oxygen saturation; *$S_{cv}O_2$,* central venous oxygen saturation; *$S\bar{v}O_2$,* mixed venous oxygen saturation; *S_pO_2,* peripheral oxygen saturation; *US,* ultrasound.

Respiratory monitoring includes assessment of (1) convective and diffusive gas transport through the branching airway tree and alveoli, (2) equilibration of gases between alveoli and pulmonary capillary blood, (3) mass balance of the distinct regional ventilation and perfusion contributions to produce expired gases and arterial and mixed venous blood, (4) gas transport between the blood and body tissues through the microcirculation, (5) gas diffusion between tissues and mitochondria, and (6) cellular respiration with O_2 use and CO_2 production.

Advances in physiologic measurements have enhanced our understanding of these stages of respiratory function during anesthesia. This chapter provides an overview of current and emerging techniques of respiratory monitoring. Despite these technical advancements, current instrumentation is limited in providing accurate and comprehensive information on respiratory function in anesthetized and critically ill patients. The area is therefore rich for research to advance the monitoring of all components of respiration.[5,6]

AMERICAN SOCIETY OF ANESTHESIOLOGISTS STANDARDS

The word *monitoring* is often associated with electronic instrumentation, and it is noteworthy that the current American Society of Anesthesiologists' (ASA) Standards for Basic Anesthetic Monitoring states in Standard I that "Qualified anesthesia personnel shall be present in the room throughout the conduct of all general anesthetics, regional anesthetics, and monitored anesthesia care" (Box 41.1). This precedes reliance on any instrumentation (as implied in Standard II), and clearly indicates that the anesthesia provider brings essential expertise and interpretation to monitoring beyond information provided by equipment. Increased safety in our specialty lies primarily in high-quality training and environments that encourage continuing education, and not exclusively on new technology.[7] The ASA Standards for Basic Anesthetic Monitoring reflect monitoring principles during anesthesia established in the 1980s[3] and should be systematically followed. The

BOX 41.1 American Society of Anesthesiologists Standards for Basic Anesthetic Monitoring Related to Respiratory Monitoring

Standard I

Qualified anesthesia personnel shall be present in the room throughout the conduct of all general anesthetics, regional anesthetics, and monitored anesthesia care.

Standard II

During all anesthetics, the patient's oxygenation, ventilation, circulation, and temperature shall be continually† evaluated.

Oxygenation

Objective: To ensure adequate oxygen concentration in the inspired gas and the blood during all anesthetics.

Methods

Inspired gas: During every administration of general anesthesia using an anesthesia machine, the concentration of oxygen in the patient breathing system shall be measured by an oxygen analyzer with a low oxygen concentration limit alarm in use.*

Blood oxygenation: During all anesthetics, a quantitative method of assessing oxygenation such as pulse oximetry will be employed.* When the pulse oximeter is utilized, the variable pitch pulse tone and the low threshold alarm will be audible to the anesthesiologist or the anesthesia care team personnel.* Adequate illumination and exposure of the patient are necessary to assess color.*

Ventilation

Objective: To ensure adequate ventilation of the patient during all anesthetics.

Methods

Every patient receiving general anesthesia will have the adequacy of ventilation continually evaluated. Qualitative clinical signs such as chest excursion, observation of the reservoir breathing bag and auscultation of breath sounds are useful. Continual monitoring for the presence of expired carbon dioxide will be performed unless invalidated by the nature of the patient, procedure, or equipment. Quantitative monitoring of the volume of expired gas is strongly encouraged.*

When an endotracheal tube or laryngeal mask is inserted, its correct positioning must be verified by clinical assessment and by identification of carbon dioxide in the expired gas. Continual end-tidal carbon dioxide analysis, in use from the time of endotracheal tube/laryngeal mask placement, until extubation/removal or initiating transfer to a postoperative care location, will be performed using a quantitative method such as capnography, capnometry, or mass spectroscopy.* When capnography or capnometry is utilized, the end tidal CO_2 alarm will be audible to the anesthesiologist or the anesthesia care team personnel.†

When ventilation is controlled by a mechanical ventilator, there will be in continuous use a device that is capable of detecting disconnection of components of the breathing system. The device must give an audible signal when its alarm threshold is exceeded.

During regional anesthesia (with no sedation) or local anesthesia (with no sedation), the adequacy of ventilation will be evaluated by continual observation of qualitative clinical signs. During moderate or deep sedation the adequacy of ventilation will be evaluated by continual observation of qualitative clinical signs and monitoring for the presence of exhaled carbon dioxide unless precluded or invalidated by the nature of the patient, procedure, or equipment.

† Note that "continual" is defined as "repeated regularly and frequently in steady rapid succession" whereas "continuous" means "prolonged without any interruption at any time."

*Under extenuating circumstances, the responsible anesthesiologist may waive the requirements marked with an asterisk (*); it is recommended that when this is done, it should be so stated (including the reasons) in a note in the patient's medical record.

standards represent a foundation to additional monitoring according to clinical requirements.

The Physical Examination

Physical examination remains an essential component of perioperative respiratory monitoring. It provides essential information for diagnosis and treatment, and may be the first indication of changes in patient status requiring intervention. Physical examination has limitations, but it routinely allows for detection of information relevant for the management of the patient.

Respiratory monitoring starts with inspection of the patient, either awake or during anesthesia. In elective cases, the anesthesiologist will have time to investigate causes for abnormal presentations. In emergent situations, careful inspection may be the only source of information for timely and accurate anesthetic management. The observation of respiratory distress should prompt immediate search for specific causes. Assessment of the respiratory rate provides a measure of the breathing pattern. For example, during sepsis, respiratory rate is significantly correlated with disease severity.[8] Anatomic signs relevant to respiration include (but are not limited to) deformities of the chest wall and spine, goiter, tracheostomy scar, and tracheal deviation. Functional elements to be noticed include the components of inspiration and expiration (diaphragmatic versus thoracic), duration and difficulty of inspiration and expiration, paradoxical chest wall motion, use of accessory muscles, central and peripheral cyanosis, pallor, wheezing, stridor, cough and sputum, aphonia, splinting, and clubbed fingers. Neck vein distension should be examined for a potential cardiovascular contribution to respiratory distress, noting that it is a less reliable indicator of central venous pressure during significant dyspnea. Attention should be paid to painful respiration in trauma patients, as well as the possibility of flail chest, pericardial tamponade, hemothorax, pneumothorax, pulmonary contusion, and tension pneumothorax.

Auscultation of the lung during anesthesia is another essential skill in physical diagnosis. Ambient noise, individual hearing limitations, and the acoustic properties of the stethoscope all influence the anesthesiologist's clinical judgment. A stethoscope of sufficient quality will allow for identification of distinctive normal and abnormal breath sounds: vesicular sounds, ronchi, wheezes, fine and coarse crackles, inspiratory stridor, and pleural friction. A clear understanding of the acoustic mechanisms for each of these sounds is essential for adequate clinical assessment.[9,10]

Pulse Oximetry

PHYSIOLOGIC FUNDAMENTALS

The primary role of the cardiorespiratory system is the transport of O_2 and CO_2 throughout the body. O_2 delivery is quantified as the product of arterial O_2 content and cardiac output (see Chapter 13, "Respiratory Physiology and Pathophysiology"). Arterial O_2 content (C_aO_2, in mL of O_2 per 100 mL of blood [hemoglobin—Hb], mL/100 mL) is calculated as

$$C_aO_2 = (1.34 \times S_aO_2 \times Hb) + 0.0031 \times P_aO_2 \quad (41.1)$$

where 1.34 mL/g is the O_2 binding capacity of Hb (i.e., Hüfner constant, theoretically equal to 1.39 mL/g but experimental range between 1.31 and 1.37 mL/g because of the presence of small amounts of other Hb species[11]); S_aO_2 is the O_2 saturation of Hb in the arterial blood (percent saturation/100); Hb is the concentration of Hb in the arterial blood (g/dL); 0.0031 is the solubility of O_2 in blood (mL/100 mL/mm Hg); and P_aO_2 is the arterial partial pressure of O_2 (mm Hg). As can be inferred from Eq. (41.1), S_aO_2 and Hb are the major determinants of O_2 content in the blood and consequently O_2 delivery to the tissues.

Five species of Hb are found in adult blood: oxygenated Hb (O_2Hb), deoxygenated Hb (deO_2Hb); carboxyhemoglobin (COHb); methemoglobin (MetHb); and sulfhemoglobin (SHb). Under normal circumstances, the concentrations of COHb, MetHb, and SHb are small (1%-3% for COHb and less than 1% for MetHb and SHb). *Functional* O_2 saturation (S_aO_2) refers to the amount of O_2Hb as a fraction of the total amount of O_2Hb and deO_2Hb and is expressed as

$$\text{Functional } S_aO_2 = \frac{[O_2Hb]}{[O_2Hb] + [deO_2Hb]} \times 100\% \quad (41.2)$$

The O_2Hb fraction or *fractional* saturation is defined as the amount of O_2Hb as a fraction of the total amount of Hb[12]:

$$\text{Fractional } S_aO_2 = \frac{[O_2Hb]}{[O_2Hb] + [deO_2Hb] + [COHb] + [MetHb] + [SHb]} \times 100\% \quad (41.3)$$

S_aO_2 is a function of the P_aO_2. The relationship between the two is described by the O_2Hb dissociation curve (Fig. 41.2). As can be appreciated by inspection of the curve, the relationship is not linear. This has important consequences. First, a high S_aO_2 cannot discriminate between normoxic and hyperoxic conditions; this can be relevant when attempting to limit O_2 exposure in neonates or patients at risk for O_2 toxicity. Second, a large numeric change in P_aO_2 at the flat portion of the curve (P_aO_2 approximately above 70 mm Hg) has relatively small consequences in terms of blood O_2 content. Furthermore, changes in temperature, pH, P_aCO_2, and erythrocyte 2,3-diphosphoglycerate concentration can shift the curve such that the same S_aO_2 can be present under a range of different oxygen partial pressures (PO_2). This may be relevant, given that diffusion from the microcirculation to tissue depends on PO_2 gradients.

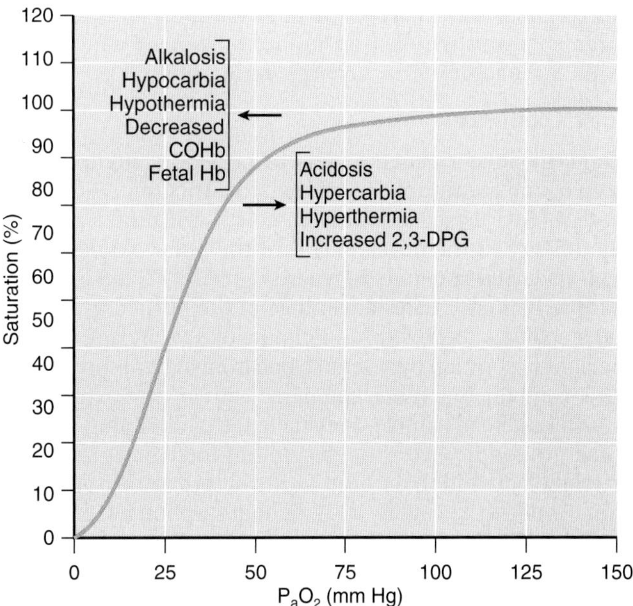

Fig. 41.2 Oxyhemoglobin Dissociation Curve. The relationship between oxyhemoglobin saturation and arterial partial pressure of oxygen is nonlinear and affected by a number of different factors such as pH, PCO_2, and temperature. Given the nonlinear nature of the curve, it is difficult to determine the partial pressure of oxygen at the higher range of oxygen saturations. *2,3-DPG,* 2,3-diphospoglycerate; *COHb,* carboxyhemoglobin. (Redrawn from Longnecker DE, Brown DL, Newman MF, Zapol WM, eds. *Anesthesiology.* 2nd ed. New York, NY: McGraw-Hill; 2012.)

MEASUREMENT PRINCIPLES

Oximetry

Oximetry is the measurement of the O_2 saturation of Hb. It is an application of the Beer-Lambert law (Eq. 41.4), which relates the transmission of light through a solution to the concentration of the solute in the solution.[13] For each solute in a solution,

$$I_{trans} = I_{in} e^{-DC\varepsilon} \quad (41.4)$$

where I_{trans} is the intensity of transmitted light, I_{in} is the intensity of the incident light, e is the base of the natural logarithm, D is the distance the light is transmitted through the solution, C is the concentration of the solute, and ε is the extinction coefficient of the solute.

The concentration of a single solute in solution can be calculated by measuring the amount of light transmitted through the solution as long as the other variables are known. For a solution containing multiple solutes, the calculation of the concentrations of the different solutes requires that light absorption be measured at a number of different wavelengths at least equal to the number of solutes. In a sample of blood in a cuvette, the absorption of a given wavelength of light passing through the blood will depend on the concentrations of the different species of Hb. Fig. 41.3*A* illustrates the absorption spectra of the five species of Hb for wavelengths of light along the visible spectrum. To measure the concentrations of all five species of Hb in a sample of blood, light absorption of at least five different wavelengths must be measured. This measurement is typically conducted using a co-oximeter. A co-oximeter uses the principle of oximetry to measure the S_aO_2 as well as the concentrations of other Hb species in a blood sample.

Co-oximetry is considered the gold standard for S_aO_2 measurements and is relied on in circumstances when pulse oximetry readings are inaccurate or unobtainable.

Pulse Oximetry

Standard pulse oximetry aims to provide a noninvasive, in vivo, and continuous assessment of functional S_aO_2. Estimates of S_aO_2 based on pulse oximetry are denoted as S_pO_2. The history of the development of the pulse oximetry has been reviewed in detail elsewhere.[14]

Pulse oximetry takes advantage of the pulsatility of arterial blood flow to provide an estimate of S_aO_2 by differentiating light absorption by arterial blood from light absorption by other components. When compared with in vitro oximetry of an arterial blood sample, the challenge of obtaining arterial O_2 saturation in vivo is to ensure that the light is sampling arterial blood and to account for its absorption by other tissues. As illustrated in Fig. 41.4, light absorption by tissue can be divided into a time-varying (pulsatile) component, historically referred to as "AC" (from "alternating current"), and a steady (nonpulsatile) component, referred to as "DC" ("direct current"). In conventional pulse oximetry, the ratio (R) of AC and DC light absorption at two different wavelengths is calculated. The wavelengths of light are selected to maximize the difference between the ratios of the absorbances of O_2Hb and deO_2Hb (see Fig. 41.3*B*). The most commonly used wavelengths of light are 660 nm and 940 nm. At 660 nm, there is greater light absorption by deO_2Hb than by O_2Hb. At 940 nm, there is greater light absorption by O_2Hb than by deO_2Hb,

$$R = \frac{AC_{660}/DC_{660}}{AC_{940}/DC_{940}} \tag{41.5}$$

where AC_{660}, AC_{940}, DC_{660}, and DC_{940} denote the corresponding AC and DC components of the 640-nm and 940-nm wavelengths.

The ratio R is then empirically related to O_2 saturation based on a calibration curve internal to each pulse oximeter (Fig. 41.5).[13] Each manufacturer develops its own calibration curve by having volunteers breathe hypoxic gas mixtures to create a range of S_aO_2 values between 70% and 100%. The FDA

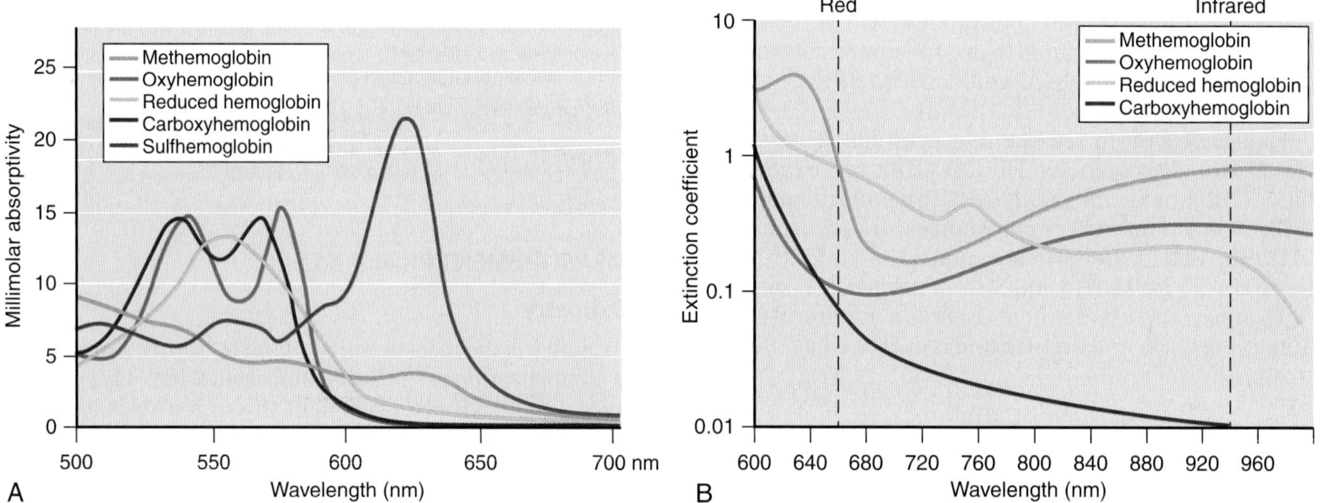

Fig. 41.3 (A) Absorption spectra of five species of hemoglobin for wavelengths of light across the visible spectrum. (B) Extinction coefficients of the most frequently measured hemoglobin species extending to infrared wavelengths used for pulse oximetry. The vertical lines indicate specific wavelengths for red and infrared light applied in pulse oximeters. The differences in the extinction coefficients of oxyhemoglobin and reduced hemoglobin (deoxygenated hemoglobin) are pronounced at these wavelengths. Note that the extinction coefficients of carboxyhemoglobin and methemoglobin are similar to those of oxyhemoglobin and reduced hemoglobin, respectively, at 660 nm. ([A] Redrawn from Zwart A, van Kampen EJ, Zijlstram WG. Results of routine determination of clinically significant hemoglobin derivatives by multicompartment analysis. *Clin Chem.* 1986;32:972–978. [B] Modified from Tremper KK, Barker SJ. Pulse oximetry. *Anesthesiology.* 1989;70:98–108.)

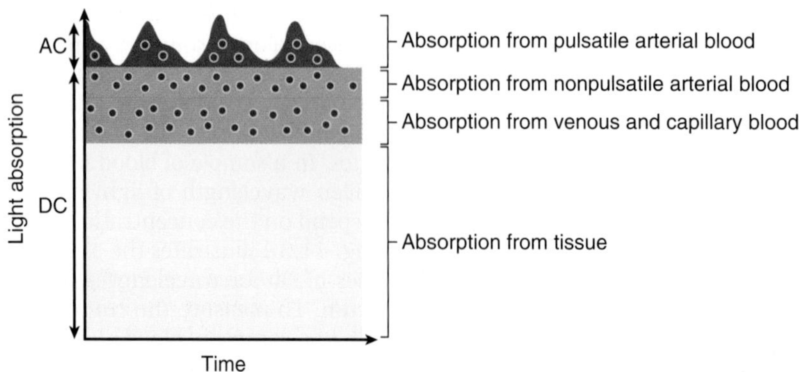

Fig. 41.4 Schematic of the Pulse Principle. Absorption of light passing through tissue is characterized by a pulsatile component (AC) and a nonpulsatile component (DC). The pulsatile component of absorption is due to arterial blood. The nonpulsatile component is due to venous blood and the remainder of the tissues. (Redrawn from Severinghaus JW. Nomenclature of oxygen saturation. *Adv Exp Med Biol.* 1994;345:921–923)

recommends root mean square differences between measured values (S_pO_2) and reference values (S_aO_2) under normal conditions ranging from 70% to 100% S_pO_2 of ≤3.0% for transmittance, wrap and clip pulse oximeter sensors and of ≤3.5% for ear clip and reflectance sensors.[14a] Most manufacturing literature reports an accuracy of ± 2% to 3% S_pO_2 over this range.[15] The dependence of S_pO_2 on pulsatility may result in inaccurate estimates of S_aO_2 when pulsatility is reduced or absent.

A pulse oximeter probe is composed of a light emitter and a photodetector. Transmission pulse oximetry involves the placement of the emitter and detector on opposite sides of the tissue being measured, usually of a finger. Reflectance pulse oximetry probes have the emitters and detector arranged on the same side. They are typically placed on the forehead. In a typical pulse oximeter, two light-emitting diodes (LEDs) are used to emit light at the two wavelengths. During operation, each LED is turned on and off in sequence. The photodetector measures transmission of light from each LED. When both LEDs are turned off, the photodetector measures ambient light and subtracts it from the signals obtained throughout the remainder of the cycle.[16]

Pulse oximetry has been an integral component of intraoperative anesthetic management since the first anesthetic monitoring standards were introduced in 1986.[3] It was adopted as a minimum monitoring standard by the ASA the same year and has subsequently been defined as a minimum standard for intraoperative monitoring by the World Federation of Societies of Anaesthesiologists and the World Health Organization (WHO).[17] The use of pulse oximetry is a part of the WHO safe surgery checklist.[18]

Multiwavelength pulse oximeters—that is, pulse oximeters with additional wavelengths of light to allow for the continuous noninvasive measurement of total hemoglobin concentration (S_pHb)[19]—as well as concentrations of MetHb and COHb utilizing up to 12 wavelengths have been developed.[20,21] S_pHb in the surgical and intensive care unit (ICU) settings has shown reasonable bias and precision when compared with laboratory measurements.[22-24] However, few of the measurements were obtained in patients with Hb concentrations within the clinically relevant range of 6 to 10 mg/dL.[25] Another limitation of S_pHb may be its absent or unreliable signal under conditions of low peripheral perfusion.[26] To date, noninvasive COHb measurements have not shown enough precision to replace laboratory measurements.[26,27] Accuracy has improved at hypoxic O_2 levels, but detecting COHb for S_aO_2 less than 87% is still unreliable.[28,29] Pulse oximetry-based MetHb measurements with a newer device are accurate, even under conditions of hypoxia.[30]

Universal pulse oximetry has been recommended by the US Secretary of Health and Human Services to screen newborns for critical congenital heart disease.[31,32] Use of a clinical algorithm based on detection of S_pO_2 lower than 95% in either right upper or lower limbs, or more than a 2% difference led to a sensitivity of 75% in suspected cases and 58% in cases that were not suspected. When this modality is combined with a routine anomaly scan and newborn physical examination screening, 92% of critical congenital heart disease lesions can be identified.[33,34]

Photoplethysmography. Along with measuring O_2 saturation, the pulse oximeter can also be used as a photoplethysmograph. Because the absorption of light is proportional to the amount of blood between the transmitter and photodetector, changes in the blood volume are reflected in the pulse oximeter trace (Fig. 41.6).[35] During anesthesia, the plethysmographic trace is affected by changes in blood volume pulsations, which depends on the distensibility of the vessel wall, as well as on the intravascular pulse pressure.[35] Variations in the amplitude of the pulse oximetry plethysmographic waveform (ΔPOP) have been shown to predict fluid responsiveness in mechanically ventilated patients.[36] An index derived from the percent difference between the maximum and minimum amplitudes of the plethysmographic waveform during a respiratory cycle (PVI, Pleth Variability Index) has been incorporated into a commercially available pulse oximeter and used to quantify ΔPOP and predict fluid responsiveness.[37,38] A number of studies have shown it to be a reasonably reliable indicator of fluid responsiveness perioperatively and in critically ill patients.[39,40] The technique does have greater reliability in mechanically ventilated patients compared with spontaneously breathing patients, but its accuracy may be compromised by the presence of cardiac arrhythmias.[39] Its accuracy has also been shown to be better for 500 mL fluid challenges compared with 250 mL.[41] Goal-directed fluid management based on PVI has been shown to improve outcomes in major abdominal surgery.[42]

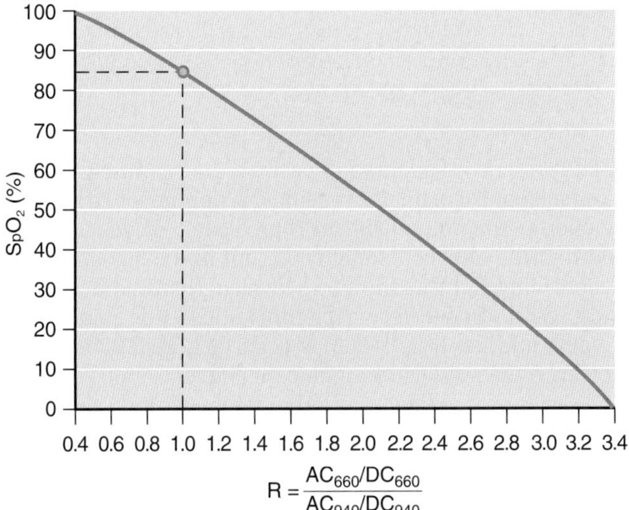

Fig. 41.5 Typical Pulse Oximeter Calibration Curve Relating Oxygen Saturation to the R Value. These curves are developed using healthy volunteers and incorporated into the pulse oximeter. *R*, Ratio of AC and DC light absorption; S_pO_2, peripheral oxygen saturation. [Tremper KK and Barker SJ. Pulse Oximetry. *Anesthesiology.* 1989;70:90-108.]

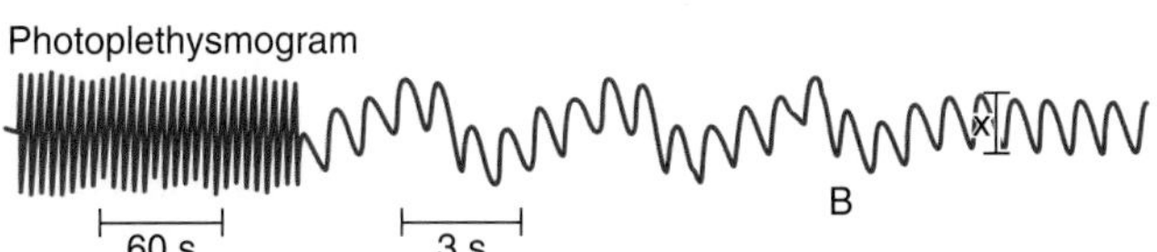

Fig. 41.6 Photoplethysmograph Recorded at Two Speeds Demonstrating Respiratory Variation. At time point (B) ventilation has been stopped, and no variation is observed. The plot illustrates the effect of intrathoracic blood volume in the pulse oximeter trace. The variation in the trace with respiration is associated with the fluid responsiveness of the patient. (Redrawn from Dorlas JC, Nijboer JA. Photo-electric plethysmography as a monitoring device in anaesthesia. Application and interpretation. *Br J Anaesth.* 1985;57:524–530.)

LIMITATIONS AND SOURCES OF ERROR

S_pO_2 is an estimate of S_aO_2 of circulating hemoglobin. As a consequence, it does not provide information about *tissue* oxygenation. Because S_pO_2 is a measurement of functional and not fractional S_aO_2, the presence of other Hb variants can significantly affect its accuracy. The nonlinearity of the Hb dissociation curve prevents the detection of hyperoxia with S_pO_2 for high S_aO_2, whereas for low saturations such as at altitude, small changes in P_aO_2 can produce large changes in S_pO_2. There is significant variability in the actual in vivo Hb dissociation curve.[43] Thus changes in S_pO_2 are not necessarily well correlated with changes in S_aO_2.[44,45] These measurements illustrate that knowledge of the individual Hb dissociation curve is important for correct interpretation of S_aO_2 and P_aO_2. More importantly, pulse oximetry does not provide information about ventilation or acid-base status.

A number of conditions can lead to inaccuracies in pulse oximeter readings (Table 41.1). These conditions include decreased perfusion, motion artifact, venous pulsation, low S_aO_2, variant Hb species, the presence of intravascular dyes, and the presence of nail polish.

Despite the recommendations of numerous boards and guidelines, there is no evidence that the use of pulse oximetry improves patient outcomes, not during transfers to ICUs nor in terms of improving patient mortality.[45a,b] There is evidence that pulse oximetry reduces the incidence of hypoxemia,[45a] and the duration and cost of ICU stay, suggesting it allows for early intervention.[45c]

The calibration of pulse oximeters is based on curves obtained in normal individuals under experimental conditions with S_aO_2 as low as 70%. As such, pulse oximeters have limited accuracy for S_aO_2 values less than 70%. Moreover, systematic errors in S_pO_2 tend to increase as S_aO_2 falls below 90%.[46] At S_aO_2 levels under 70%, a positive or negative bias of the S_pO_2 value can be observed, depending on the manufacturer of the pulse oximeter.[47] Manufacturers have developed pulse oximeters with increased accuracy at saturations as low as 60%. Preliminary data suggest that these probes may be useful in neonates with cyanotic congenital heart disease.[48]

Hypoperfusion leads to a reduction in the amplitude of the pulsatile component of the light absorbance waveform, the essential signal for pulse oximetry, consequently giving rise to absent or inaccurate readings. Significantly erroneous reductions in S_pO_2 may be observed for systolic blood pressures lower than 80 mm Hg.[49] Motion artifact can produce considerable error in the pulse oximeter reading. Manufacturers have developed advanced proprietary signal processing algorithms that effectively filter out noise caused by motion.[50,51]

With continued clinical use, the performance of the LEDs in the probe may be degraded, leading to inaccuracy in the S_pO_2 value outside of the range specified by the manufacturer. These inaccuracies are expected to be more pronounced at lower saturations (i.e., <90%).[15]

Venous pulsations may result in the detection of venous O_2Hb saturation by the pulse oximeter, resulting in artifactual reduction of the presumed arterial S_pO_2 being measured. Venous pulsations can be due to excessively tight placement of adhesive finger probes, severe tricuspid regurgitation, probe placement in dependent positions (e.g., forehead during Trendelenburg position), and possibly in distributive shock when vasodilation may result in physiologic arteriovenous shunting.[18,19,52]

TABLE 41.1 Potential Sources of Artifacts in Pulse Oximetry and Their Effects on Measurements

Source of Error	Effect on S_pO_2 Relative to S_aO_2
Hypotension	↓
Anemia	↓
Polycythemia	No significant effect
Motion	↓
Low S_aO_2	variable
Methemoglobinemia	↓/↑ (S_pO_2 approaches 85%)
Carboxyhemoglobinemia	↑
Cyanmethemoglobin	No significant effect
Sulfhemoglobin	No significant effect
Hemoglobin F	No significant effect
Hemoglobin H	No significant effect
Hemoglobin K	↓
Hemoglobin S	No significant effect
Methylene blue	↓
Indigo carmine	↓
Indocyanine green	↓
Isosulfan blue	No significant effect/↓
Fluorescein	No significant effect
Nail polish	Black, dark blue, purple ↓
Acrylic fingernails	No significant effect
Henna	Red—No significant effect ↓
Skin pigmentation	At S_aO_2 >80%, no significant effect At S_aO_2 <80%, ↑
Jaundice	No significant effect
Ambient light	No significant effect
Sensor contact	↓
IABP	↑

IABP, Intraaortic balloon pump; *S_aO_2*, arterial oxygen saturation; *S_pO_2*, peripheral oxygen saturation.

The presence of additional species of Hb can also generate erroneous pulse oximeter readings. As outlined earlier, the function of the pulse oximeter is predicated on the assumption that the only components present in the blood capable of absorbing light at the two wavelengths used are O_2Hb and deO_2Hb. Under normal circumstances, this assumption is valid, and the S_pO_2 readings accurately reflect the S_aO_2. However, the presence of significant concentrations of other Hb species or substances absorbing light at the used wavelengths will lead to erroneous S_pO_2 readings. As illustrated in Fig. 41.3, both COHb and MetHb absorb light at one or both of the wavelengths used by the pulse oximeter. Accordingly, the presence of these Hb species will produce errors in S_pO_2. The absorption of light at 660 nm by COHb is similar to that of O_2Hb. At 940 nm, COHb absorbs virtually no light. Thus, in a patient with carbon monoxide poisoning, the S_pO_2 will be falsely elevated.[53] MetHb absorbs a significant amount of light at both 660 nm and 940 nm. As a result, in its presence, the ratio of light absorption R (Eq. 41.5) approaches unity. An R-value of 1 represents the presence of equal concentrations of O_2Hb and deO_2Hb and corresponds to an S_pO_2 of 85%. Thus, in a patient with methemoglobinemia, the S_pO_2 will be 80% to 85%, irrespective of the S_aO_2.[54] SHb absorbs red light (660 nm) more than deoxyhemoglobin (HHb) or MetHb, and likely as much near the infrared spectrum.[52] This results in S_pO_2 values close to 85% in severe cases of sulfhemoglobinemia. Although newer generations of co-oximeters can detect SHb, most existing co-oximeters cannot; consequently, additional clinical laboratory testing may be required if sulfhemoglobinemia is suspected.[52]

With normal S_aO_2, anemia has little effect on S_pO_2.[55] However, in the presence of hypoxia, S_pO_2 readings underestimate S_aO_2 in anemic patients with true hypoxemia.[56] Pulse oximeters are sufficiently accurate in adult patients with sickle cell disease,[57] as well as in the presence of fetal Hb.[58] However caution is warranted when using pulse oximetry in patients with sickle cell disease, because heme metabolism may result in elevated COHb.[52] Some studies also suggest that S_pO_2 may overestimate S_aO_2 during vaso-occlusive crises.[59,60] Another relevant point is that in patients with sickle cell disease, the affinity of O_2 for Hb is normal under normoxic conditions but becomes low during hypoxia.

A relatively uncommon cause for reduced S_pO_2 readings is the presence of congenital variants of Hb. Some variants, such as Hb Bassett, Hb Rothschild, and Hb Canabiere, have a reduced affinity for O_2, and changes in S_pO_2 appropriately reflect changes in S_aO_2.[61] Other variants, such as Hb Lansing, Hb Bonn, Hb Koln, Hb Cheverly, and Hb Hammersmith, have altered absorption spectra (closer to HHb) that result in low S_pO_2 readings in the setting of normal S_aO_2.[61]

The administration of intravenous dyes can result in inaccurate S_pO_2 readings. Methylene blue leads to a transient, marked decrease in S_pO_2 down to 65% due to its peak light absorption at 668 nm, which is very close to that of HHb. Indigo carmine and indocyanine green also artificially decrease S_pO_2 measurements, although to a lesser extent than methylene blue, because they do not substantially absorb red light.[62] Isosulfan blue can produce a prolonged reduction at higher doses.[62]

Although all colors of nail polish can reduce the calculated value of S_pO_2, black, purple, and dark blue colors have the greatest effect. Nonetheless, the error generally remains within 2%.[63] Depending on the brand of pulse oximeter, artificial acrylic nails may impair S_pO_2 readings, although generally not to a clinically significant extent.[64] Under conditions of normal S_aO_2, skin pigmentation has no effect on S_pO_2 estimates.[65] However, increased skin pigmentation is associated with S_pO_2 values that overestimate S_aO_2 by as much as 8% for S_aO_2 less than 80%.[47,66]

In the presence of severe hyperbilirubinemia (30 mg/dL or greater) caused by increased hemolysis or liver disease, the fraction of oxygenated hemoglobin (FO_2Hb) may be falsely low by artifactual increase in MetHb and COHb, resulting in more accurate S_pO_2 than FO_2Hb measurements.[52] Although earlier case reports and small studies have suggested that ambient light may interfere with the accuracy of S_pO_2 readings,[67,68] a large prospective study found no significant effect on S_pO_2 accuracy with exposure to five types of light sources: quartz-halogen, incandescent, fluorescent, infant bilirubin lamp, and infrared.[69] Infrared light pulses from image guidance systems used for navigational neurosurgery can interfere with pulse oximetry readings by causing decreased readings or disruptions in S_pO_2 waveform detection.[70] Different pulse oximeters show variable susceptibility to such interference.[71] Shielding the probe with a single layer of aluminum foil can protect from this effect.[70,71] Misplacement of the probe can allow for direct detection of LED light by the photodetector. This optical shunt gives rise to an S_pO_2 reading of 85%.[72]

In patients with intraaortic balloon pump support, S_pO_2 accuracy depends on the brand of pulse oximeter used as well as the support ratio. Accuracy is generally reduced in the setting of higher support ratios.[73] In patients with continuous flow ventricular assist devices, pulse oximetry may not be possible because of the absence of pulsatile flow. In these cases, the use of cerebral oximetry as an adjunct is advocated.[74]

Pulse Oximeter Probes

Probes are usually applied to accessible body areas with high vascularity, such as the finger, nose, ear lobe, or forehead. The probes may be reusable or disposable. The advantages of reusable clip probes are that they are more cost-effective compared with disposable adhesive probes, can be rapidly applied, and are amenable to multiple applications in cases of low signal-to-noise ratio at the specified wavelengths. However, disposable probes allow for more secure placement (in case of patient movement) and provide the capability of monitor sites other than acral areas. Although reduced infectious transmission is a purported benefit of disposable probes, evidence is limited, and one must consider that pulse oximetry probes represent a small fraction of anesthetic equipment requiring decontamination.[75] Accordingly, different probe models may be advantageous in specific conditions. For instance, ear and forehead probes may be more reliable during vasoconstriction compared with finger probes, given that the arterial vessels of such regions are less responsive to circulating catecholamines. As an example, in hypotensive patients that require vasopressors, ear and forehead probes may provide more accurate value of S_pO_2, because these areas are less likely to vasoconstrict with endogenous and exogenous catecholamines compared to fingers or toes.[76,77] During hypothermia with secondary vasoconstriction, the forehead probe is more reliable compared with the finger probe.[78,79]

Emerging Techniques: Pulse spectroscopy is a new technique that utilizes hundreds of wavelengths to assess normal and dysfunctional hemoglobins. Initial results are promising with accurate S_pO_2 determinations, as well as COHb and MetHb assessment during normoxia and hypoxia.[80]

Mixed Venous Oxygen Saturation

PHYSIOLOGIC FUNDAMENTALS

Mixed venous oxygen saturation ($S\bar{v}O_2$) is the O_2 saturation of blood at the proximal pulmonary artery. It has been a frequently monitored variable in critically ill patients, since it reflects the average O_2 saturation of the blood returning from the body to the right heart, weighted by the respective regional blood flows. As such, it is a measure of the balance between global oxygen delivery (DO_2) and global oxygen uptake ($\dot{V}_{O_2}$), and a useful resuscitation target.[81] Factors that influence the $S\bar{v}O_2$ can be illustrated through a derivation of the mixed venous O_2 content equation.

$\dot{V}_{O_2}$ (mL/min) is defined as

$$\dot{V}_{O_2} = 10 \times \dot{Q}_T \times (C_aO_2 - C\bar{v}O_2) \quad (41.6)$$

where $\dot{Q}_T$ is the cardiac output (L/min), and $C\bar{v}O_2$ is the O_2 content of the mixed venous blood (mL/100 mL).

Rearranging Eq. (41.6) to solve for $C\bar{v}O_2$ yields

$$C\bar{v}O_2 = C_aO_2 - \dot{V}_{O_2}/\dot{Q}_T \quad (41.7)$$

The contribution of dissolved O_2 to the blood O_2 content is small. By expanding the definition of O_2 content (Eq. 41.1) and ignoring the term for dissolved O_2, Eq. (41.7) can be rewritten as

$$S\bar{v}O_2 = S_aO_2 - \dot{V}_{O_2}/(1.34 \cdot Hb \cdot Q_T) \quad (41.8)$$

Normal values of $S\bar{v}O_2$ range between 65% and 80%.[82,83] Values close to 40% are associated with tissue hypoxia, anaerobic metabolism, and lactate production. $P\bar{v}O_2$ can be derived from $S\bar{v}O_2$ values by utilizing the O_2Hb dissociation curve adjusted to mixed-venous pH, PCO_2, and temperature (see Fig. 41.2). The normal value of $P\bar{v}O_2$ is 40 mm Hg.

DO_2 is defined as

$$DO_2 = Q_T \times C_aO_2 \quad (41.9)$$

As is evident from Eq. (41.8), a low $S\bar{v}O_2$ indicates either a reduction in DO_2 secondary to low S_aO_2, low Hb, or low $\dot{Q}_T$, or an increase in $\dot{V}_{O_2}$. The association among $S\bar{v}O_2$, DO_2, and $\dot{V}_{O_2}$ can be illustrated by expressing $S\bar{v}O_2$ as a function of the O_2 extraction ratio, ERO_2.

$$ERO_2 = \dot{V}_{O_2}/DO_2 \quad (41.10)$$

Expanding the terms yields

$$ERO_2 = 1 - C\bar{v}O_2/C_aO_2 \quad (41.11)$$

Assuming that the O_2 dissolved in plasma is a negligible component to total O_2 content dissolved in the arterial or mixed venous blood, Eq. (41.11) can be rewritten as

$$ERO_2 = 1 - S\bar{v}O_2/S_aO_2 \quad (41.12)$$

For conditions in which the arterial blood is fully saturated, Eq. (41.12) may be further simplified:

$$ERO_2 = 1 - S\bar{v}O_2 \quad (41.13)$$

Solving for $S\bar{v}O_2$ yields

$$S\bar{v}O_2 = 1 - ERO_2 \quad (41.14)$$

Thus a reduction in $S\bar{v}O_2$ results from an increase in ERO_2, from either an increased $\dot{V}_{O_2}$ or a decreased DO_2 (Fig. 41.7). A decrease in DO_2 occurs in conditions such as hemorrhagic or hypovolemic shock. An increase in $\dot{V}_{O_2}$ may occur in conditions such as stress, pain, shivering, sepsis, and thyrotoxicosis. Conversely, an increase in $S\bar{v}O_2$ indicates either an increase in O_2 supply (elevated S_aO_2, Hb, or $\dot{Q}_T$) or a reduction in $\dot{V}_{O_2}$, as occurs during hypothermia.

There are some subtle considerations in the interpretation of changes in $S\bar{v}O_2$. At PO_2 values typical of venous blood, small increases in the fraction of inspired oxygen (F_IO_2) can cause significant increases in $S\bar{v}O_2$ because of the shape of the O_2Hb dissociation curve (Fig. 41.2). Therefore, when $S\bar{v}O_2$ is tracked as a measure of cardiac function, changes in F_IO_2 must be taken into account during its interpretation.[84] In the setting of septic shock, impairment in O_2 extraction may yield normal $S\bar{v}O_2$ values, despite the presence of tissue hypoxia.

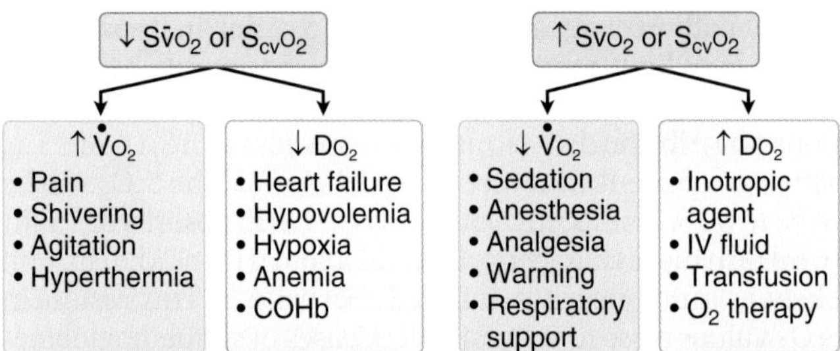

Fig. 41.7 Mixed venous saturation is a measure of the balance between global oxygen delivery and uptake. Conditions which increase $\dot{V}_{O_2}$ or decrease DO_2 will lead to a reduction in $S\bar{v}O_2$. Conversely, conditions which decrease $\dot{V}_{O_2}$ or improve DO_2 will lead to an increase in the $S\bar{v}O_2$. (Modified from Shepherd SJ, Pearse RM. Role of central and mixed venous oxygen saturation measurement in perioperative care. *Anesthesiology*. 2009;111:649–656.)

Direct measurement of $S\bar{v}O_2$ requires the insertion of a pulmonary artery catheter, a procedure associated with some morbidity. However, in most clinical situations, the O_2 saturation of a blood sample drawn from a central venous catheter will suffice. Thus the use of central venous saturation can be a surrogate for $S\bar{v}O_2$. The saturation of blood at the level of a central venous catheter placed in the superior vena cava ($S_{cv}O_2$) reflects the balance between O_2 supply and demand in the brain and upper extremities. Under normal physiologic conditions, $S_{CV}O_2$ is typically 2% to 5% less than $S\bar{v}O_2$, primarily because of the higher O_2 content of splanchnic and renal venous blood.[85] However, during hemodynamic instability, as circulation is redistributed to the upper body, the relationship between $S\bar{v}O_2$ and $S_{CV}O_2$ may reverse, and the difference between the two may increase significantly.[86-88] Although trends in $S_{CV}O_2$ may reflect those in $S\bar{v}O_2$, the two measures cannot be used interchangeably.[88-96]

Mixed venous CO_2 has been used to compute the arteriovenous CO_2 difference ($\Delta PCO_2 = P\bar{v}CO_2 - P_aCO_2$). In conditions of steady-state CO_2 production, ΔPCO_2 changes inversely and nonlinearly with cardiac output as a result of the Fick equation.[97] Accordingly, ΔPCO_2 is an indicator of the adequacy of cardiac output to provide adequate clearance of tissue CO_2. However, because of several limitations, the parameter has not yet found widespread clinical use.[97]

MEASUREMENT PRINCIPLES

The measurement of venous O2 saturation can be performed intermittently by co-oximetry of blood sampled from the distal tip of a pulmonary artery catheter ($S\bar{v}O_2$) or a central venous catheter ($S_{CV}O_2$). Falsely increased values can occur in the presence of a wedged pulmonary artery tip, mitral regurgitation, or left-to-right shunts.[98] Venous saturations can also be measured continuously by spectrophotometry using specialized fiberoptic catheters, which transmit infrared light and detect the amount of light reflected from red blood cells.[99,100] Specialized venous oximetry catheters are available for both pulmonary artery and central venous monitoring and have the advantage of providing continuous measurements of O_2 saturation. Their disadvantage is the cost. Although continuous venous oximetry catheters trend changes, their reported absolute values are not equivalent to concurrently obtained co-oximetry measurements.[101-103]

APPLICATIONS AND INTERPRETATION

In patients undergoing major abdominal or cardiac surgery, intraoperative reductions in $S\bar{v}O_2$ and $S_{CV}O_2$ have been associated with postoperative complications.[104-108] Protocol-based interventions that target specific values of $S\bar{v}O_2$ or $S_{CV}O_2$ have been shown to reduce the length of stay, organ dysfunction, and mortality in patients undergoing major surgery and patients presenting with sepsis.[109-111] Goal-directed therapy based on $S_{cv}O_2$ has been advocated for the management of sepsis, and the implementation of such protocols is associated with improvements in mortality.[112,113] The use of $S_{CV}O_2$ as a therapeutic endpoint remains controversial for several reasons: $S_{CV}O_2$ may be increased in sepsis because of impaired tissue O_2 extraction[114]; the increased cost associated with the use of $S_{CV}O_2$-measuring catheters[115]; and other measures, such as lactate clearance, are less costly while leading to similar outcomes.[116] Furthermore, the management of sepsis without an $S_{CV}O_2$ endpoint can yield equally favorable results.[115] The difference between $S\bar{v}O_2$ and $S_{CV}O_2$ has been proposed as a marker of complications after cardiac surgery.[117]

Tissue Oxygenation

Arterial and venous O_2 saturations are measures of DO_2 and uptake by the whole body. Although useful, these global measures do not provide information regarding organ or tissue oxygenation, which reflects the important local balance between O_2 supply and demand. Regional O_2 balance can differ both among organs as well as within regions of the same organ.[118] Current noninvasive methods for the assessment of microcirculatory oxygenation make use of reflectance spectroscopy using light either in the visible spectrum (VLS) or in the near-infrared spectrum (NIRS). A recent technique based on the protoporphyrin IX triplet state lifetime aims at the assessment of mitochondrial O_2 tension in vivo, and opens the prospect of future clinical monitoring (see Fig. 41.1).[119]

Reflectance spectroscopy probes have light emitters and receivers positioned in line (Fig. 41.8). When they are placed on a tissue surface, light transmission through the tissue is affected by reflection, absorption, and scatter. Reflection depends on the angle of incidence of the light beam and the wavelength of light, whereas scatter depends on the number and type of tissue interfaces. As previously outlined, the Beer-Lambert law relates the absorption of light by the tissue to the concentration of tissue chromophores, the extinction coefficient of each, and the pathlength of the light through the tissue.[120] The predominant tissue chromophore is hemoglobin. The pathlength of the

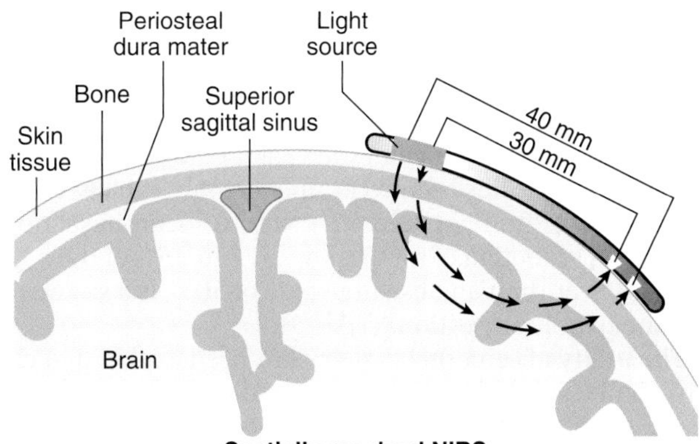

Fig. 41.8 Near Infrared Spectroscopy Applied to Cerebral Oximetry. In this case, a reflectance oximeter is placed on the forehead. Near infrared wavelength light is emitted from the light source and enters the underlying tissue. Light is scattered, reflected, and absorbed. Light that reaches the photodetector travels an arc-shaped path. The depth of the path is a function of the distance between the emitter and the detector. The measured value is the oxygen saturation of the tissue through which the light travels on its way to the detector. It is a primarily venous-weighted value. *NIRS*, Near infrared spectroscopy. (Redrawn from Casati A, Spreafico E, Putzu M, et al. New technology for noninvasive brain monitoring: continuous cerebral oximetry. *Minerva Anestesiol.* 2006;72:605–625.)

light is affected by both reflection and scatter, so it cannot be measured directly, but rather must be estimated. Most of the detected photons travel in an arc between the two detectors (see Fig. 41.8). The depth of penetration of the arc into the tissue is proportional to the wavelength of light and the distance between the transmitter and detector.[120,121]

VLS makes use of white light with wavelengths of 500 to 800 nm, whereas NIRS employs light in the 700 to 1100 nm range.[122] In general, the depth of penetration of VLS is less than that of NIRS, thus allowing superficial measurements of up to 16 mm and making it suitable for measurements of small subsurface volumes. NIRS can penetrate tissue to a depth of several centimeters and allows sampling of a larger volume of tissue.[123] The O_2 saturation displayed is that of a volume of tissue. This volume includes arteries, capillaries, and veins, and has a predominantly venous weighting.[124]

CLINICAL APPLICATIONS

A number of applications have been described for VLS. Buccal microvascular Hb saturation has been associated with survival in patients with sepsis.[125] VLS has also been used for monitoring flap viability following reconstructive surgery.[126] During gastrointestinal and esophageal surgery, reductions in gastrointestinal tissue saturation, measured by VLS, have been associated with postoperative anastomotic complications.[127,128] Endoscopic VLS differentiates between normal and ischemic areas of colon,[129] and it may be useful for the diagnosis of mesenteric ischemia.[130] In addition, mucosal O_2 saturation of the gastric conduit following esophagectomy is useful and explores the benefits of ischemic preconditioning.[131]

The most widespread application of NIRS has been in cerebral oximetry,[118] with probes placed on the forehead to measure frontal cortical oxygenation (rSO_2). Several NIRS systems are commercially available, with each manufacturer offering a different specific technology. As there is no gold standard for cerebral oximetry, it is difficult to compare the accuracy of the devices. Furthermore, each device has its own set of "normal" values. For this reason, acquisition of baseline values for each patient at the start of the procedure has been recommended.[132] Typical values of rSO_2 range from 51% to 82% with a mean baseline of 66%.[133] A reduction of rSO_2 below 20% to 25% of the baseline, or lower than an absolute value of 50%, is a suggested threshold for intervention.[134,135]

The utility of cerebral oximetry has been explored in cardiovascular, abdominal, thoracic, and orthopedic surgery. In the cardiac surgical setting, intraoperative reductions in rSO_2 have been associated with early postoperative cognitive dysfunction and prolonged ICU and hospital lengths of stay.[135-138] Baseline rSO_2 measurements have been associated with 30-day mortality after left ventricular assist device surgery.[139] As a guide to therapy, interventions for rSO_2 reductions less than 75% of baseline in patients undergoing coronary artery bypass graft surgery have been shown to significantly reduce the incidence of major organ morbidity and mortality, as well as ICU length of stay.[134]

During carotid endarterectomy, intraoperative reductions in rSO_2 correlate well with changes in transcranial Doppler measurements,[140-144] electroencephalographic waveforms,[145-147] and stump pressure[144,148,149], which are consistent with ischemia. Although some studies indicate that reductions in rSO_2 that are less than 20% of baseline are well tolerated, data are lacking for a clear rSO_2 threshold for carotid shunt placement.[150,151] NIRS has also been preliminarily used during and following ICU open thoracoabdominal aortic aneurysm repair for continuous monitoring of spinal cord oxygenation[152].

In elderly patients undergoing major abdominal surgery, protocol-based intraoperative treatment of reductions in rSO_2 results in decreases in postoperative cognitive decline and hospital length of stay.[153] In patients undergoing thoracic surgical procedures with single-lung ventilation, early postoperative cognitive dysfunction is directly related to intraoperative exposure time to rSO_2 less than 65%.[154] Patients undergoing shoulder surgery in the beach chair position have a lower baseline rSO_2 and a larger number of episodes of cerebral desaturation, although the clinical implications of these findings are unclear.[155-157]

Shock is a condition in which patients may have inadequate *regional* perfusion in the setting of normal *global* perfusion parameters. In such circumstances, the use of NIRS to monitor tissue perfusion holds some promise. Values obtained by the application of an NIRS probe to the thenar eminence (S_tO_2) discriminate between healthy volunteers and patients with shock.[158] Furthermore, in patients with major trauma who present with shock, S_tO_2 values can identify patients who proceed to develop multiorgan dysfunction or actually die.[159,160]

Overall, available information is still limited to warrant clinical decision making exclusively based on NIRS measurements. Currently there is insufficient evidence to support the use of perioperative NIRS monitoring in adults to reduce short-term or mild postoperative cognitive dysfunction, postoperative stroke, delirium, or death.[161] Of note, in a 2015 retrospective study, patients who self-identified as African American had lower rSO_2 compared with those who self-identified as Caucasian, a finding attributed to light attenuation by skin pigmentation.[162] Further investigations are necessary to improve our understanding of NIRS and its relevance for clinical management.

Capnometry and Capnography

GENERAL CONCEPTS

The presence CO_2 in exhaled breath reflects the fundamental physiologic processes of ventilation, pulmonary blood flow, and aerobic metabolism. Its continued monitoring ensures the anesthesiologist of correct placement of an endotracheal tube (ETT) or laryngeal mask airway (LMA), as well as the integrity of a breathing circuit. Exhaled CO_2 provides information primarily on ventilation. It is also used to estimate the adequacy of cardiac output. In combination with P_aCO_2, exhaled CO_2 can be used to estimate the ratio of physiologic dead space (V_D) to tidal volume (V_T) by using the Bohr equation[163]:

$$\frac{V_D}{V_T} = \left(\frac{P_aCO_2 - P_{\bar{E}}CO_2}{P_aCO_2}\right) \qquad (41.15)$$

where $P_{\bar{E}}CO_2$ is the mixed expired CO_2 partial pressure, such as measured in exhaled air collected in a mixing bag chamber, or computed from a volumetric capnogram. The ability to detect and quantify CO_2 is a crucial component of respiratory monitoring in anesthesia and critical care medicine.

Considerable confusion arises from inconsistent and interchangeable terminology as applied to medical CO_2 gas analysis.[163-165] In a very general sense, *capnometry* refers to the measurement and quantification of inhaled or exhaled CO_2 concentrations at the airway opening. *Capnography*, however, refers not only to the method of CO_2 measurement, but also to its graphic display as a function of time or volume. A *capnometer* is simply a device that measures CO_2 concentrations. A capnometer may display a numeric value for inspired or exhaled CO_2. A *capnograph*, however, is a device that records and displays CO_2 concentrations, usually as a function of time. A *capnogram* refers to the graphic display that the capnograph generates. Fig. 41.9 illustrates a typical CO_2 concentration profile for three breaths as a function of time.

MEASUREMENT PRINCIPLES

Various methods exist for detecting and quantifying CO_2 concentrations in respiratory gases, such as mass spectrometry, Raman spectrometry, or gas chromatography.[166,167] The most commonly used method in clinical environments relies on nondispersive infrared absorption.[168] With this technique, a beam of infrared light is passed through a gas sample, and the resulting intensity of the transmitted light is measured by a photodetector.[164] Gaseous CO_2 absorbs light over a very narrow bandwidth centered around 4.26 μm. Its presence in the sample cell decreases the amount of infrared light at this wavelength that reaches the detector in proportion to its concentration. Because the absorption spectrum for CO_2 partially overlaps with the spectra of other gaseous species commonly encountered in anesthesia (i.e., water and nitrous oxide[169]), infrared filters and

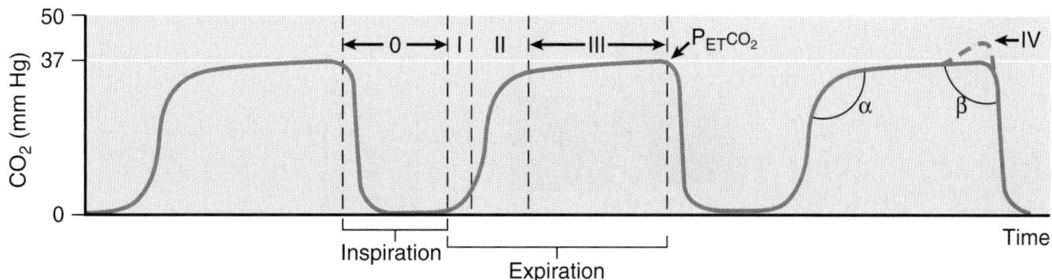

Fig. 41.9 Representative Time Capnogram for Three Breaths. The expiratory segment is divided into phases I, II, III, and IV. The inspiratory segment is referred to as phase 0 in this figure. α denotes the angle between phases II and III, whereas β denotes the angle between phase III and the descending limb of phase 0. Phase IV (*dashed line* in third breath) denotes the upstroke observed at the end of phase III in some patients. $P_{ET}CO_2$, Partial pressure of end-tidal carbon dioxide. (Courtesy Respironics, Inc., Murraysville, PA, with permission.)

compensation algorithms are used to minimize this interference and improve accuracy.[170]

Most capnometers rely on infrared-light source that is focused on a chopper disk that rotates at approximately 60 revolutions per second. The chopper allows the beam to be alternately directed through (1) the sample cell with the gas to be analyzed and (2) a reference cell with no detectable CO_2. In addition, the light source is completely blocked at various points during the revolution of the chopper disk. The photodetector and associated circuitry process these three signals to estimate the changes in CO_2 concentration continuously in the sample cell. Alternatively, CO_2 concentration may be estimated with solid-state technology, using a beam splitter instead of a chopper wheel. The splitter allows for the measurement of infrared energy at wavelengths within and outside the absorption spectrum of CO_2.

Capnometers fall into two general categories: sidestream (diverting) and mainstream (nondiverting). Sidestream analyzers are more frequently used in clinical environments. Their CO_2 sensors are physically located away from the airway gases to be measured. Sidestream analyzers incorporate a pump or compressor that aspirates gases into a sample cell located at the unit's console (Fig. 41.10*A*). Typical tubing length for this aspiration may be 6 feet, and gas withdrawal rates may vary from 30 to 500 mL/min. This lost gas volume may need to be considered during closed-circuit anesthesia or during ventilation of neonates and infants. The volume can be returned to the circuit, or it can be routed to a scavenger to prevent contamination of the environment with anesthetic or waste gases. Gases must also pass through various filters and water traps before they are presented to the sample cell.[164] Sidestream capnometers have a transport delay time corresponding to the rate at which gas is sampled and the washout of the analyzing chamber (see Fig. 41.10*B*). The capnograms generated by sidestream analyzers also have an associated rise time, defined as the time required for the analyzer to respond to a sudden change in CO_2 concentration.[171] By convention, this is usually the time interval required for the for the analyzer output to change from 10% to 70% of its final value.[*,171] Typical rise times for commercially available capnometers range from 10 to 400 ms, and they can depend on the rotation of the chopper wheel, the rate of gas aspiration, the volume of aspiration tubing and water traps, and the dynamic response of the infrared filters and other electronics.

With mainstream analyzers, the sample cell is placed directly into the patient's breathing circuit. Thus the inspiratory or expiratory gases pass directly through the infrared light path (see Fig. 41.10*C*). An advantage of mainstream analyzers is that they have no delay time (see Fig. 41.10*D*). Moreover, their rise time is generally faster than that of sidestream analyzers.[171] A disadvantage is the potential increase in dead space, although recent developments in solid-state electronics have made this much less of an issue.[172] In addition, the sample cell is usually heated to 40°C to minimize the condensation of water vapor, which can bias the measurement. This increase in temperature, combined with the proximity of the sensor to the patient's airway, can potentially increase the risk of facial burns.

TIME CAPNOGRAM

The simplest and most widely used form of display for exhaled CO_2 is the *time capnogram*. The time capnogram displays both inspiratory and expiratory phases. Fig. 41.9 shows a typical time capnogram for three breaths. The expiratory phase is divided into three distinct components. Phase I corresponds to the exhalation of dead space gas from the central conducting airways or any equipment distal to the sampling site, which ideally should have no detectable CO_2 (i.e., partial pressure of CO_2, $PCO_2 \sim 0$). During phase II, a sharp rise in PCO_2 to a plateau indicates the sampling of transitional gas between the airways and alveoli. The plateau region of the capnogram, phase III, corresponds to the PCO_2 in the alveolar compartment. For a lung with relatively homogeneous ventilation, phase III is approximately flat throughout expiration. In fact, various mechanisms contribute to the slight upsloping of CO_2 concentration versus time during phase III. Most of these mechanisms reflect a heterogeneous distribution of ventilation-perfusion ($\dot{V}/\dot{Q}$) or alveolar CO_2 partial pressure (P_ACO_2) throughout the lung. Well-ventilated and well-matched $\dot{V}/\dot{Q}$ regions tend to have lower PCO_2 and shorter time constants, and they empty earlier during the expiratory phase. Less well-ventilated and poorly matched $\dot{V}/\dot{Q}$ regions have higher CO_2 levels, and they empty later in the expiratory cycle. Respiratory pathologies associated with an increase in ventilation heterogeneity, such as asthma, chronic obstructive pulmonary disease (COPD), or acute lung injury,[173] yield a steeper upslope of phase III. Interventions that improve ventilation

*Rise time may also be defined as the time required for the analyzer output to change from 10% to 90% of its final value.

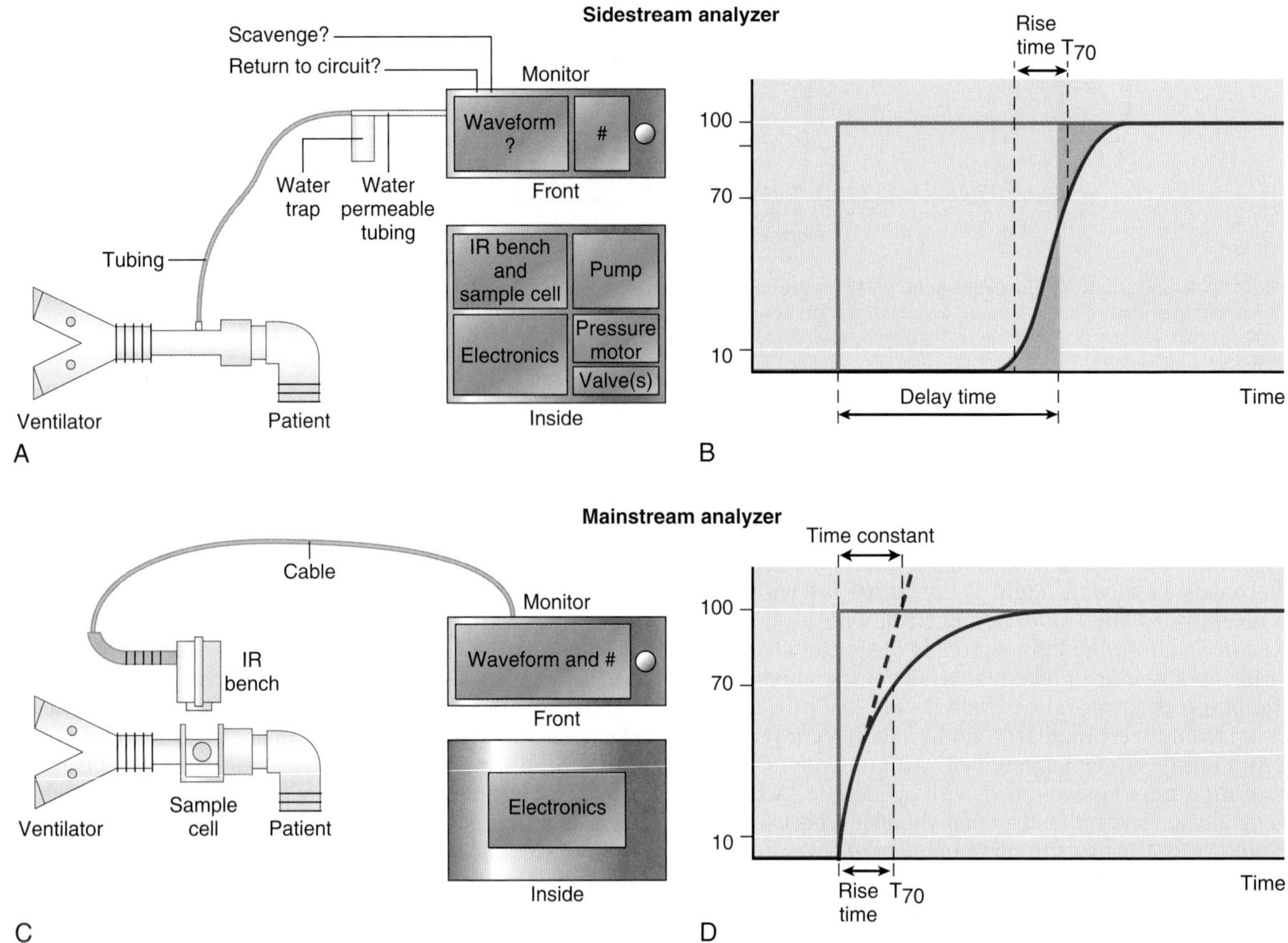

Fig. 41.10 Schematics of sidestream (A) and mainstream (C) capnometry sampling methods, along with corresponding representative time capnograms (*curves* in B and D) following a step increase in CO_2 concentration *(blue lines)*. Rise time *(T_{70})* corresponds to the time required for either sensor to change from 10% to 70% of its final value. A delay time is observed for the sidestream analyzer, corresponding to the aspiration rate of the sampled gas and the washout of the analyzing chamber. *IR*, Infrared. (Modified from Jaffe MB. Mainstream or sidestream capnography? Technical considerations. Wallingford, CT: Respironics Novametric, Inc; 2002;; and Brunner JX, Westenskow DR. How the rise time of carbon dioxide analysers influences the accuracy of carbon dioxide measurements. *Br J Anaesth.* 1988;61:628–638.)

homogeneity, such as positive end-expiratory pressure (PEEP) or bronchodilators, flatten phase III. Mechanical disturbances may also be present during phase III, reflecting processes such as spontaneous breathing efforts, cardiogenic oscillations, or surgical manipulation (Fig. 41.11). Following phase III, a sharp downstroke of PCO_2 occurs as fresh inspired gas moves past the sampling site and washes out the remaining CO_2. This is referred to as the beginning of phase 0 by some authors,[165,174] or phase IV by others.[166] Occasionally, a sharp upstroke in PCO_2 is observed at the very end of phase III, which is termed phase IV or IV′, depending on the author.[175] This upstroke probably results from the closure of lung units with relatively low PCO_2 and allows for regions of higher CO_2 to contribute a greater proportion of the exhaled gas to be sampled.[165] Additional insights into various abnormalities in ventilation or perfusion are also obtained by trending time capnograms over many breaths for long periods (Fig. 41.12).

The term "end-tidal" CO_2 ($P_{ET}CO_2$) generally refers to the final value of the exhaled PCO_2 curve, at the very end of the expiratory phase. The method used to determine this number is not universal, and varies according to the manufacturer of the particular capnograph in use. For example, $P_{ET}CO_2$ may simply be (1) the PCO_2 value just before inspiration, (2) the largest PCO_2 value during a single exhalation cycle, or (3) the PCO_2 value at a specified time in the capnogram averaged across several breaths. If $P_{ET}CO_2$ is measured during a reasonably flat and undistorted phase III, it may be well correlated with P_aCO_2.[170] This may not be the case if the duration of phase III is truncated, or if CO_2 is measured from gas that is contaminated with room or O_2-enriched air (i.e., during spontaneous breathing with a nasal cannula or facemask). Potential causes of increased or decreased $P_{ET}CO_2$ are listed in Table 41.2. In healthy individuals with homogeneous ventilation, the difference between P_aCO_2 and $P_{ET}CO_2$ is usually less than 5 mm Hg, thereby expressing the equilibration between alveolar and pulmonary capillary blood. Several disease states compromise this equilibration and produce increased $P_aCO_2 - P_{ET}CO_2$ difference (Box 41.2). There are situations in which $P_{ET}CO_2$ can be greater than P_aCO_2, especially in the presence of severe ventilation heterogeneity and lung units with very low $\dot{V}/\dot{Q}$. For steady-state conditions, the $P_{ET}CO_2$ usually reflects the relative balance between CO_2 production and alveolar ventilation.

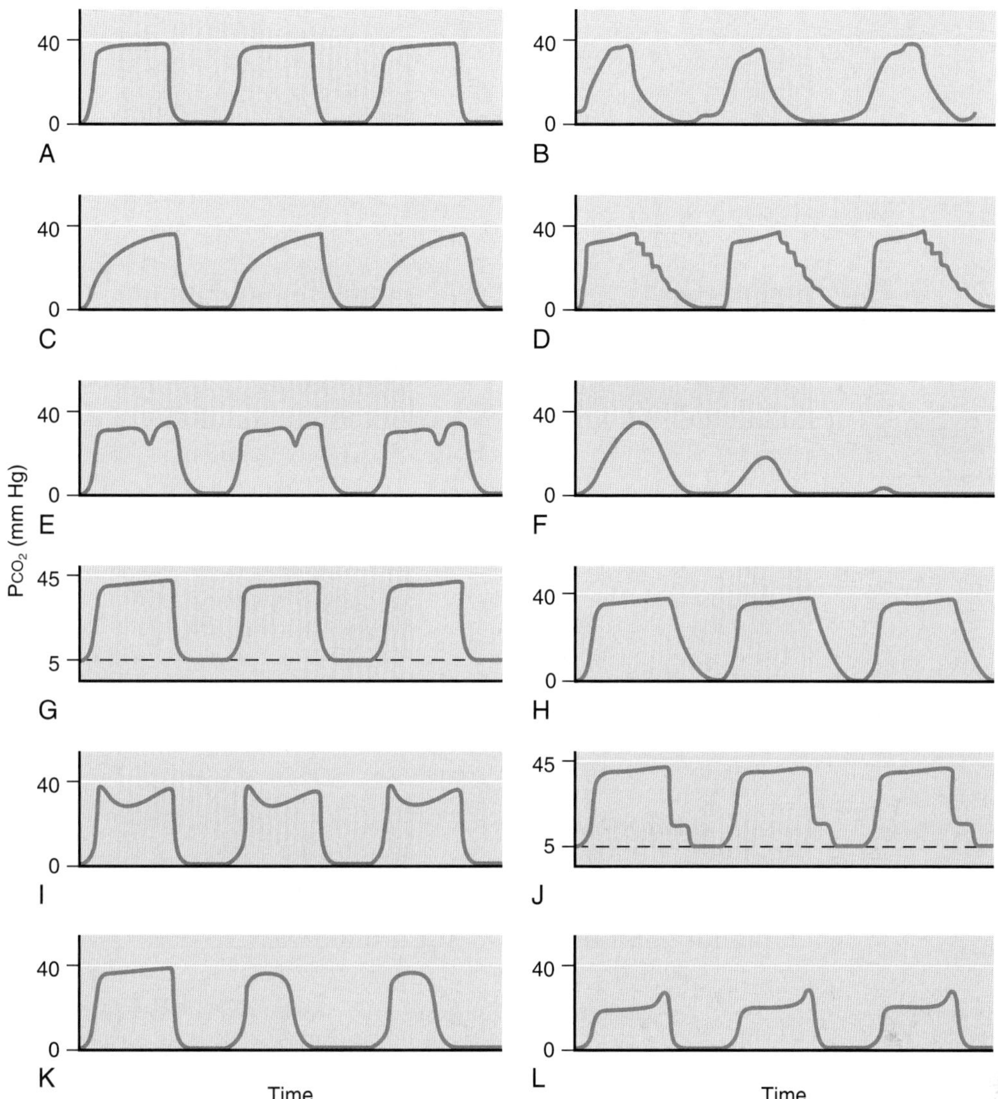

Fig. 41.11 Representative Time Capnograms under Normal and Abnormal Conditions. (A) Normal capnogram during controlled mechanical ventilation; (B) normal capnogram during spontaneous breathing; (C) increased upslope of phase III, as may occur during bronchospasm (asthma, chronic obstructive pulmonary disease), or partially obstructed endotracheal tube/breathing circuit; (D) cardiogenic oscillations at the end of exhalation as flow decreases to zero and the beating heart causes emptying of different lung regions and back-and-forth motion between exhaled and fresh gas; (E) clefts during phase III indicating spontaneous breathing efforts during controlled mechanical ventilation; (F) esophageal intubation; (G) rebreathing of CO_2, as may occur with faulty expiratory valve or exhausted absorber system. Inspiratory CO_2 is consistently above 0; (H) faulty inspiratory valve, resulting in a slower downslope, which extends into the inhalation phase (phase 0) as CO_2 in the inspiratory limb is rebreathed; (I) two peaks in phase III suggestive of sequential emptying of two heterogeneous compartments, as may be seen in a patient with a single lung transplant; (J) faulty inspiratory valve; (K) sudden shortening of the duration of phase III during controlled mechanical ventilation, suggesting the abrupt onset of a ruptured or leaking endotracheal tube cuff; (L) dual plateau in phase III, suggesting the presence of a leak in a sidestream sample line. Early portion of phase III abnormally low due to dilution of exhaled gas with ambient air. The sharp increase in CO_2 at the end of phase III reflects a diminished leak resulting from the increased circuit pressure at the onset of inspiration. *PCO_2*, Partial pressure of carbon dioxide. (Modified from Hess D. Capnometry and capnography: technical aspects, physiologic aspects, and clinical applications. *Respir Care.* 1990;35:557–576; Roberts WA, Maniscalco WM, Cohen AR, et al. The use of capnography for recognition of esophageal intubation in the neonatal intensive care unit. *Pediatr Pulmonol.* 1995;19:262–268; and Eskaros SM, Papadakos PJ, Lachmann B. Respiratory monitoring. In: Miller RD, Eriksson LI, Fleisher LA, eds. *Miller's Anesthesia.* 7th ed. New York, NY: Churchill Livingstone; 2010:1427.)

VOLUME CAPNOGRAM

Although time capnography is relatively straightforward to monitor in clinical environments, a major limitation of the technique is its lack of information regarding respiratory flows or volumes.[174] The *volume capnogram* is a graphic display of CO_2 concentration or partial pressure versus exhaled volume.[166] The inspiratory phase is not defined in a volume capnogram. Similar to its temporal counterpart, it is also partitioned into three distinct phases (I, II, and III) corresponding to anatomic dead space, transitional, and alveolar gas samples (Fig. 41.13). However, it possesses several advantages over the time capnogram. First, it allows for estimation of the relative contributions of anatomic and alveolar components of physiologic dead space.[175a,176] Second, it is more sensitive than the time capnogram in detecting subtle changes in dead space that are caused by alterations in PEEP, pulmonary blood flow, or ventilation heterogeneity (Fig. 41.14). Finally, the numeric integral of PCO_2 as a function of volume allows for determination of

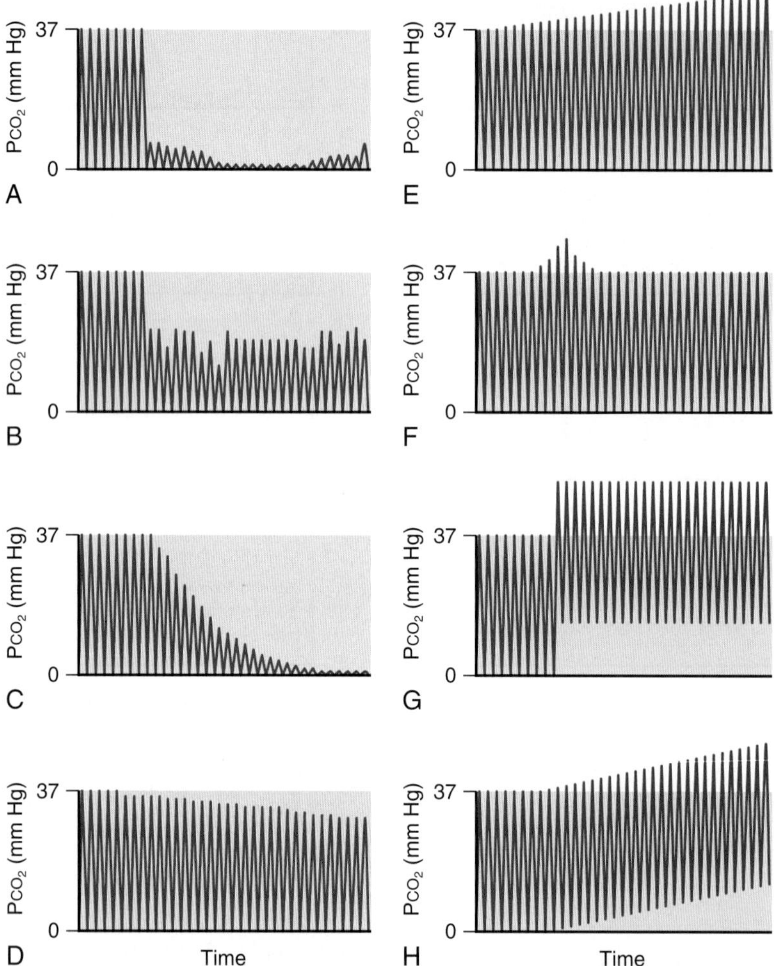

Fig. 41.12 Representative time capnograms trended over many breaths, illustrating various abnormalities in ventilation and/or perfusion. (A) sudden drop in CO_2 due to catastrophic loss of ventilation; (B) leak or partial obstruction in breathing circuit; (C) sudden interruption in pulmonary perfusion, as may occur during cardiac arrest; (D) gradual decrease in CO_2 due to hyperventilation, decreased metabolism, or decreased pulmonary perfusion; (E) gradual increase in CO_2 as may occur during hypoventilation, laparoscopic insufflation, increased metabolism, or increased pulmonary perfusion; (F) transient rise in CO_2 indicated acute increase in CO_2 delivery to the lungs, as may occur during release of a tourniquet or administration of a bicarbonate bolus; (G) rise in both the baseline and end-tidal CO_2, consistent with a contaminated sample cell; (H) gradual rise in baseline and end-tidal CO_2, consistent with rebreathing. *PCO_2*, Partial pressure of CO_2. (Modified from Swedlow DB. Capnometry and capnography: the anesthesia disaster early warning system. *Semin Anesth.* 1986;5:194–205.)

the total mass of CO_2 exhaled during a breath and provides for the estimation of $\dot{V}_{CO_2}$.

Blood Gas Analysis

PHYSIOLOGIC FUNDAMENTALS

Arterial blood gas analysis is used to assess oxygenation, ventilation, and acid-base status. This section focuses on the use of arterial blood gases to assess oxygenation and ventilation. For a discussion of acid-base status, see Chapter 48, "Perioperative Acid-Base Balance."

Oxygenation is reflected in the P_aO_2, which is a function of the alveolar partial pressure of O_2 (P_AO_2) and the efficiency of O_2 transfer from alveoli to the pulmonary capillary blood. In healthy adults breathing room air at sea level, P_aO_2 ranges between 80 and 100 mm Hg. The normal value of P_aO_2 decreases with increasing age and increasing altitude. Hypoxemia is defined as a P_aO_2 less than 80 mm Hg. There are five physiologic causes of hypoxemia: (1) hypoventilation, (2) $\dot{V}/\dot{Q}$ mismatching, (3) right-to-left shunt, (4) diffusion limitation, and (5) diffusion-perfusion mismatch. The first three causes explain the majority of hypoxemia in the perioperative setting. Reduced inspired PO_2 (e.g., in faulty closed or partially closed anesthesia breathing circuits or at high altitude) is an additional cause of hypoxemia.

These factors produce hypoxemia by affecting different steps of O_2 transport from the environment to the arterial blood. A low inspired PO_2, as well as hypoventilation, reduces the P_AO_2. $\dot{V}/\dot{Q}$ mismatch, right-to-left shunt, and alveolar diffusion limitation affect the efficiency of O_2 exchange. Diffusion limitation plays a role in conditions that thicken the alveolar-capillary barrier, such as interstitial lung diseases, and in hypoxemia induced by exercise or altitude.[177,178] In the clinical setting, impairment of diffusion of O_2 or CO_2 rarely occurs to a significant extent. The remainder of this section focuses on $\dot{V}/\dot{Q}$ mismatch and right-to-left shunt.

TABLE 41.2 Causes of Changes in Partial Pressure of End-Tidal Carbon Dioxide

↑$P_{ET}CO_2$	↓$P_{ET}CO_2$
↑CO_2 Production and Delivery to the Lungs	**↓CO_2 Production and Delivery to the Lungs**
Increased metabolic rate	Hypothermia
Fever	Pulmonary hypoperfusion
Sepsis	Cardiac arrest
Seizures	Pulmonary embolism
Malignant hyperthermia	Hemorrhage
Thyrotoxicosis	Hypotension
Increased cardiac output (e.g., during CPR)	
Bicarbonate administration	
↓Alveolar Ventilation	**↑Alveolar Ventilation**
Hypoventilation	Hyperventilation
Respiratory center depression	
Partial muscular paralysis	
Neuromuscular disease	
High spinal anesthesia	
COPD	
Equipment Malfunction	**Equipment Malfunction**
Rebreathing	Ventilator disconnect
Exhausted CO_2 absorber	Esophageal intubation
Leak in ventilator circuit	Complete airway obstruction
Faulty inspiratory/expiratory valve	Poor sampling
	Leak around endotracheal tube cuff

CO_2, Carbon dioxide; *COPD*, chronic obstructive pulmonary disease; *CPR*, cardiopulmonary resuscitation; *$P_{ET}CO_2$*, partial pressure of end-tidal carbon dioxide. Modified from Hess D. Capnometry and capnography: technical aspects, physiologic aspects, and clinical applications. *Respir Care*. 1990;35:557–576.

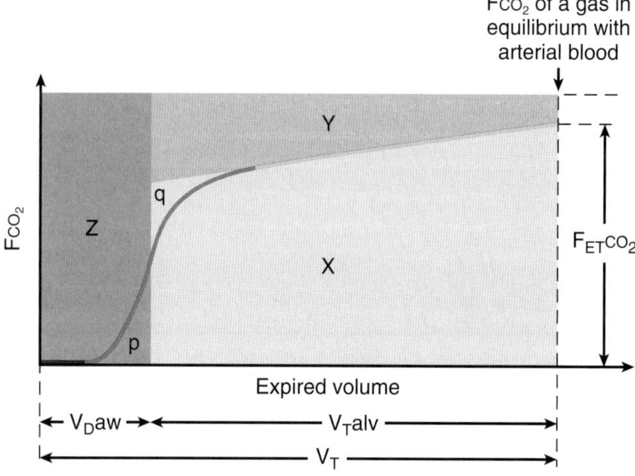

Fig. 41.13 The volume capnogram is a plot of the fraction of CO_2 *(FCO_2)* in exhaled gas versus exhaled volume. It is divided into three phases, which reflect the same sources of expired gas as present in the time capnograph: anatomic dead space (phase I, *red*), transitional (phase II, *blue*), and alveolar gas (phase III, *green*). The volume capnogram allows for the partition of total tidal volume *(V_T)* into airway dead space volume *(V_Daw)* and an effective alveolar tidal volume *(V_Talv)* by a vertical line through Phase II, positioned such that the approximately triangular areas p and q are equal. It also provides the slope of phase III as a quantitative measure of the heterogeneity of alveolar ventilation. The total area below the horizontal line (denoting the FCO_2 of a gas in equilibrium with arterial blood) can be divided into three distinct areas: *X*, *Y*, and *Z*. Area X corresponds to the total volume of CO_2 exhaled over a tidal breath. This value can be used to compute the CO_2 production ($\dot{V}_{CO_2}$), and the mixed expired CO_2 fraction or partial pressure to be used in the Bohr equation (Eq. [41.15]) based on the division of the exhaled CO_2 volume by the exhaled tidal volume. Area Y represents wasted ventilation due to alveolar dead space, while area Z corresponds to wasted ventilation due to anatomic deadspace (V_Daw). Thus areas Y + Z represent the total physiologic dead space. The volume capnogram can also be plotted as a PCO_2 versus exhaled volume curve. *$F_{ET}CO_2$*, Fraction of end-tidal carbon dioxide. (Modified from Fletcher R, Jonson B, Cumming G, et al. The concept of deadspace with special reference to the single breath test for carbon dioxide. *Br J Anaesth*. 1981;53:77–88.)

BOX 41.2 Causes of Increased Arterial-to-End-Tidal Carbon Dioxide Pressure Difference $P_{(a\text{-}ET)CO2}$

- Increased ventilation-perfusion heterogeneity, particularly with high V/Q regions
- Pulmonary hypoperfusion
- Pulmonary embolism
- Cardiac arrest
- Positive pressure ventilation (especially with PEEP)
- High-rate low-tidal-volume ventilation

PEEP, Positive end-expiratory pressure. Modified from Hess D. Capnometry and capnography: technical aspects, physiologic aspects, and clinical applications. *Respir Care*. 1990;35:557–576.

$\dot{V}/\dot{Q}$ mismatch is the most common cause of hypoxemia in the clinical setting. Ventilation and perfusion are nonuniformly distributed throughout the normal lung, with worsening mismatch in the setting of lung disease, general anesthesia, and mechanical ventilation. Areas with low or zero $\dot{V}/\dot{Q}$ yield low end-capillary PO_2, whereas areas with normal or high $\dot{V}/\dot{Q}$ produce higher end-capillary PO_2. However, because of the plateau of the O_2Hb dissociation curve (see Fig. 41.2), the normal and high $\dot{V}/\dot{Q}$ regions are limited in the extent to which they increase the O_2 content and compensate for the low $\dot{V}/\dot{Q}$ regions (Fig. 41.15). Consequently, $\dot{V}/\dot{Q}$ mismatch results in hypoxemia.

Right-to left shunt is the amount of blood that flows from the pulmonary artery to the systemic arterial circulation without undergoing pulmonary gas exchange. It represents an extreme case of $\dot{V}/\dot{Q}$ mismatch in which the ratio equals zero and the end-capillary gas partial pressures are equal to the values found in mixed venous blood. In healthy awake spontaneously breathing subjects, intrapulmonary shunt is negligible,[179] and a small (<1% of cardiac output) extrapulmonary shunt results from drainage of the bronchial and Thebesian veins into the arterial side of the circulation.[180] During general anesthesia, a right-to-left shunt can develop as a result of atelectasis.[181,182] Right-to-left shunt can also be seen in pathologic conditions such as pneumonia and acute lung injury. The effect of the shunt on P_aO_2 is a function of the magnitude of the shunt, F_IO_2, and the cardiac output (Fig. 41.16). Importantly, increases in F_IO_2 have a small effect on P_aO_2 in the presence of large true right-to-left shunt (see Fig. 41.16).

The traditional method to estimate flow through shunting regions ($\dot{Q}_S$) as a fraction of the total cardiac output ($\dot{Q}_T$) is based on the modeling of the lung as a three-compartment system (Fig. 41.17).[183] The three compartments represent (1) lung regions receiving both ventilation and perfusion,

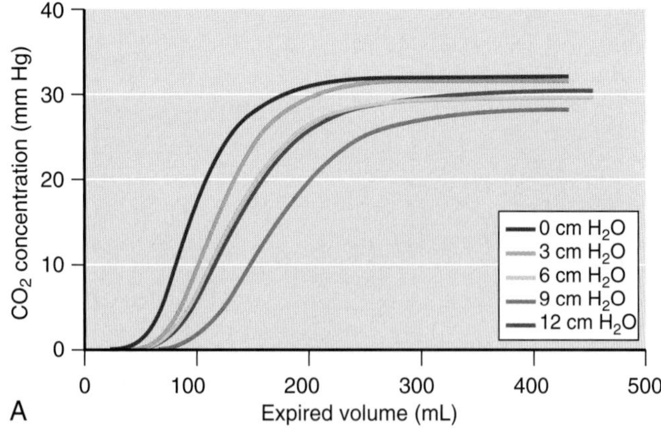

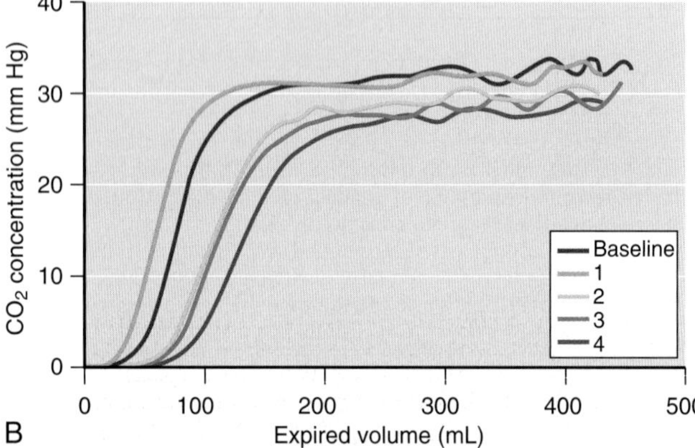

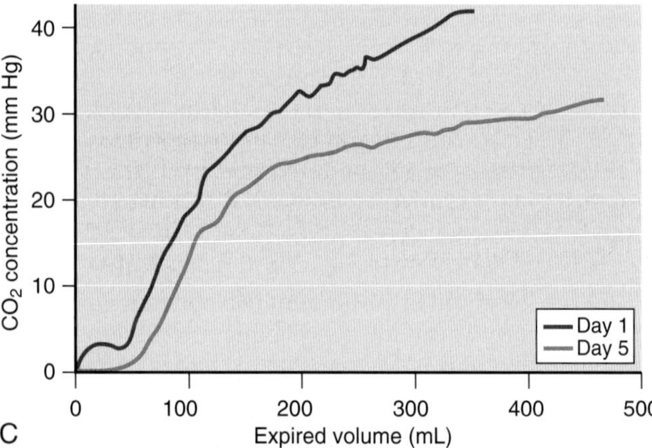

Fig. 41.14 Representative Single-breath Volume Capnograms, Illustrating Various Abnormalities in Ventilation or Perfusion. (A) alterations in phases II and III with corresponding changes in positive end-expiratory pressure (0, 3, 6, 9, and 12 cm H_2O) during positive pressure ventilation; (B) alterations in phases II and III with corresponding changes in pulmonary perfusion (increasing numbers correspond to decreasing pulmonary blood flow); (C) pronounced positive slope of phase III during acute bronchospasm (Day 1). Following resolution (Day 5), there is a noticeable reduction in the slope phase III. *CO_2,* Carbon dioxide. (Modified from Thompson JE, Jaffe MB. Capnographic waveforms in the mechanically ventilated patient. *Respir Care.* 2005;50:100–108.)

(2) a shunt compartment ($\dot{V}/\dot{Q} = 0$), and (3) a dead space compartment with ventilation but no perfusion ($\dot{V}/\dot{Q}$ = infinity). The application of the concept of mass balance to this model yields the shunt fraction ($\dot{Q}_s/\dot{Q}_T$) expression

$$\dot{Q}_S/\dot{Q}_T = \frac{(Cc'O_2 - Ca\,O_2)}{(Cc'O_2 - C\bar{v}O_2)} \qquad (41.16)$$

where $\dot{Q}_s$ is the shunted blood flow, and $Cc'O_2$ is the end-capillary O_2 content. $Cc'O_2$ is calculated using Eq. (41.1), assuming equilibration between the end-capillary blood and alveolar gas. The P_AO_2 is calculated using the ideal alveolar gas equation:

$$P_AO_2 = F_IO_2 \cdot (P_{atm} - P_{H_2O}) - P_aCO_2/R \qquad (41.17)$$

where F_IO_2 is the inspired O_2 fraction, P_{atm} is barometric pressure (typically assumed to be the pressure of one standard atmosphere at sea level, 760 mm Hg), and P_{H_2O} is partial pressure of water vapor (47 mm Hg at 37°C). R, the respiratory quotient, is the ratio of pulmonary CO_2 elimination to O_2 uptake ($R = \dot{V}_{CO_2}/\dot{V}_{O_2}$), which equals the value of 0.8 under normal diet and metabolic conditions.

The three-compartment model is a simplification of the real lung. As a result, under conditions of F_IO_2 less than 100%, $\dot{Q}_S/\dot{Q}_T$ computed with Eq. (41.16) represents a combination of all factors producing hypoxemia, predominantly true right-to-left shunt and $\dot{V}/\dot{Q}$ mismatch. Under such conditions, $\dot{Q}_S/\dot{Q}_T$ is referred to as venous admixture. When F_IO_2 is 100%, the effects of $\dot{V}/\dot{Q}$ heterogeneity on O_2 exchange are eliminated and the equation exclusively yields the right-to-left shunt fraction.[184] The administration of 100% O_2 (i.e., F_IO_2 of 1.0) can lead to the development of absorption atelectasis in compartments with very low $\dot{V}/\dot{Q}$, thus leading to an increase in true right-to-left shunt.[184]

If the assumptions are made that end-capillary blood has an O_2 saturation of 100% and the O_2 content of blood is predominantly determined by Hb saturation, the shunt fraction equation can be simplified to

$$\dot{Q}_S/\dot{Q}_T = \frac{(1 - S_aO_2)}{(1 - S\bar{v}O_2)} \qquad (41.18)$$

where S_aO_2 is arterial saturation, and $S\bar{v}O2$ is mixed venous saturation.

Other indices of oxygenation: The calculation of the shunt fraction is a fundamental measure of O_2 exchange impairment. However, a pulmonary artery catheter is required for the measurement of $S\bar{v}O2$. For this reason, indices of oxygenation that rely on less invasive measures have been developed. An ideal index should reflect the efficiency of oxygenation, change with changes in lung function, remain constant with changes in extrapulmonary conditions (such as F_IO_2), and provide clinically useful diagnostic and prognostic information.[185] Although P_aO_2 certainly reflects arterial blood oxygenation, it is limited in providing a measure of the magnitude of the O_2 exchange deficiency because of its dependence on the F_IO_2 and to the nonlinear relationship between P_aO_2 and blood O_2 content.[185] As a consequence, several indices based on the P_aO_2 that account for the F_IO_2 or the P_AO_2 have been developed: the alveolar-arterial partial pressure gradient of O_2 ($[A-a]PO_2$), the respiratory index ($[A-a]PO_2/P_aO_2$), the arterial-alveolar ratio of O_2 partial pressures (P_aO_2/P_AO_2), and the ratio between P_aO_2 and F_IO_2 (P_aO_2/F_IO_2).[185]

The advantages of indices based on P_aO_2 are that their calculations are fairly simple and require only arterial blood sampling. However, an important limitation is that these indices vary with the F_IO_2, P_aCO_2, Hb, and O_2 consumption ($\dot{V}_{O_2}$).[186,187] Consequently, changes in those variables can lead to changes in the values of the indices in the absence of

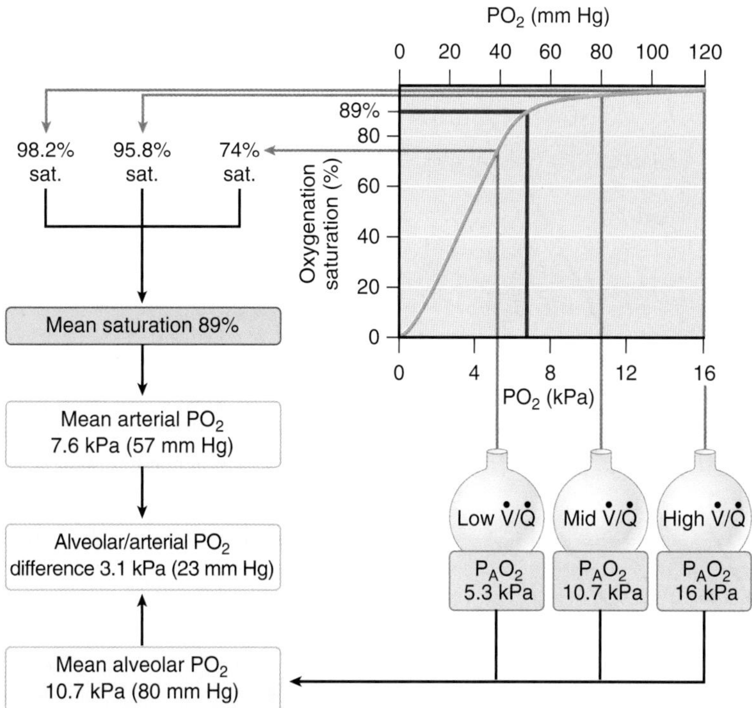

Fig. 41.15 Effect of Different Ventilation-Perfusion ($\dot{V}/\dot{Q}$) Regions on Partial Pressure of Arterial Oxygen (P_aO_2). Because of the shape of the oxyhemoglobin dissociation curve, regions of lung with low $\dot{V}/\dot{Q}$ have a disproportionately greater effect on lowering the arterial saturation than do regions of lung with normal or higher $\dot{V}/\dot{Q}$ to increase P_aO_2. Assuming equal blood flow, the average partial pressure of alveolar oxygen (P_AO_2) of the V/Q regions represented in the illustration is 10.7 kPa (80 mm Hg). Based on the oxyhemoglobin dissociation curve, however, the average saturation of the arterial blood is 89%, producing an average P_aO_2 equal to 7.6 kPa (57 mm Hg). *PO_2,* Partial pressure of oxygen. (Modified from Lumb AB. *Nunn's Applied Respiratory Physiology.* 6th ed. Philadelphia: Elsevier/Butterworth Heinemann; 2005.)

any change in lung gas exchange function. Another limitation is the failure of these indices to account for changes in $\dot{V}/\dot{Q}$ matching resulting from changes in the F_IO_2. In addition, indices that use P_AO_2 rely on the assumptions of the alveolar gas equation, including $P_ACO_2 = P_aCO_2$, which may not hold true in pathologic conditions.

An early index developed to assess oxygenation that used only peripheral blood sampling was the (A-a)PO_2.[188] The (A-a)PO_2 can help to differentiate $\dot{V}/\dot{Q}$ mismatch, shunt, and diffusion limitation from hypoventilation and low F_IO_2 as causes of hypoxemia. This is because the (A-a) PO_2 is unchanged under conditions of decreased F_IO_2 and hypoventilation but increased with $\dot{V}/\dot{Q}$ mismatch, shunt, and diffusion limitation.

The A-a gradient of O_2 is calculated as

$$\text{(A-a) } PO_2 = P_AO_2 - P_aO_2 \tag{41.19}$$

The normal value of the (A-a)PO_2 is less than 10 mm Hg in young adults breathing room air, and it increases with age and the administration of supplemental O_2. The change in (A-a)PO_2 with age can be estimated by[189]

$$\text{(A-a) } PO_2 = 0.21 \cdot (\text{age} + 2.5) \tag{41.20}$$

The (A-a)PO_2 varies significantly with the F_IO_2 such that the application of supplemental O_2 can lead to an increase in the (A-a)PO_2 independent of pulmonary disease.[186] Like the (A-a)PO_2, the respiratory index (A-a)PO_2/P_aO_2 and the P_aO_2/P_AO_2 are sensitive to F_IO_2, especially in the presence of a high degree of $\dot{V}/\dot{Q}$ mismatch, such as during acute respiratory distress syndrome (ARDS), and less so in the absence of true shunt or when low $\dot{V}/\dot{Q}$ regions are minimal (e.g., in healthy lung or pulmonary embolus).[190]

Unlike the other indices based on partial pressures, the P_aO_2/F_IO_2 ratio does not use the P_AO_2 and its associated assumptions. This index is more stable, particularly under conditions relevant to ARDS such as P_aO_2 lower than 100 mm Hg in the setting of an F_IO_2 greater than 0.5.[186,187] P_aO_2/F_IO_2 values are part of the diagnostic criteria for ARDS and have been correlated with outcomes in these patients.[191] When repeated arterial blood sampling is not possible, the S_pO_2/F_IO_2 (also referred to as SF) ratio may be useful. SF ratio values have shown good correlation with P_aO_2/F_IO_2 values in both adults and children with respiratory failure who have S_pO_2 values in the range of 80% to 97%.[192,193]

The P_aO_2/F_IO_2 ratio does not characterize factors associated with the severity of respiratory failure such as ventilator settings or respiratory system mechanics.[194-196] Another drawback of the P_aO_2/F_IO_2 ratio is its dependence on PEEP or mean airway pressure, because increases in these variables result in lung recruitment and improved oxygenation. As a consequence, the oxygenation index (OI) was proposed as a more robust alternative to the P_aO_2/F_IO_2 ratio[197]:

$$OI = 100\,\% \times \frac{F_IO_2\bar{P}_{ao}}{P_aO_2} \tag{41.21}$$

where $\bar{P}_{ao}$ denotes the mean airway pressure. The OI has been used as a prognostic indicator in pediatric patients

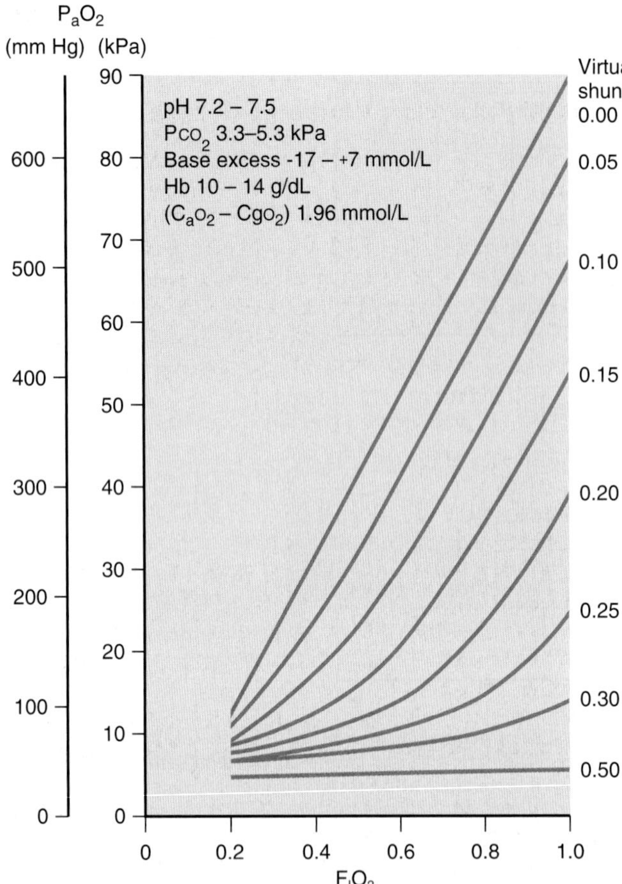

Fig. 41.16 Relationship between partial pressure of arterial oxygen *(P_aO_2)* and fraction of inspired oxygen *(F_IO_2)* for different values of shunt fraction computed for normal values of barometric pressure, pH, partial pressure of carbon dioxide *(PCO_2)*, base excess, hemoglobin *(Hb)* concentration, and arterial-mixed venous oxygen content difference (C_aO_2 – CgO_2). Note the small increase in P_aO_2 with F_IO_2 in the presence of large shunt. This graph corresponds to the so-called isoshunt diagram presented by Lawler and Nunn. (From Welsby PD, Earis JE. Some high pitched thoughts on chest examination. *Postgrad Med J.* 2001;77:617–620.)

with acute hypoxemic respiratory failure,[198] as a predictor of mortality in adult ARDS,[196,199] and as an index of enhanced lung recruitment during oscillatory ventilation.[200] An alternative "oxygenation saturation index" (OSI) has also been recently proposed:

$$OSI = 100\,\% \times \frac{F_IO_2\bar{P}_{ao}}{S_pO_2} \tag{41.22}$$

Similar to the pulse oximetric saturation S_pO_2/F_IO_2 (SF) ratio, the OSI eliminates the need for invasive arterial blood gas sampling by using pulse oximetry. When computed on the day of ARDS diagnosis, it correlates well with the OI and is associated with increased mortality and fewer ventilator free days.[194]

Unlike P_aO_2, P_aCO_2 can be maintained in the normal range in the presence of significant $\dot{V}/\dot{Q}$ mismatching. The reason is that the CO_2 content curve has no plateau. In this way, compensatory hyperventilation can be used to reduce elevations in P_aCO_2.[201] The dependence of P_aCO_2 on CO_2 elimination ($\dot{V}_{CO_2}$) and alveolar ventilation ($\dot{V}_A$), with

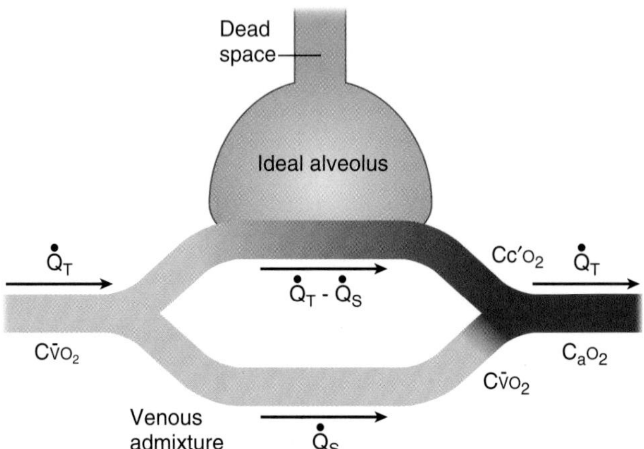

Fig. 41.17 Three-Compartment Model of Gas Exchange. The lung is represented as three functional units: alveolar dead space, "ideal" alveoli, and venous admixture (shunt). Note that the model doesn't differentiate between true shunt or true dead space and components of shunt and dead space that are caused by ventilation-perfusion ($\dot{V}/\dot{Q}$) mismatch. *CaO_2*, Arterial oxygen content; *$Cc'O_2$*, oxygen content of end pulmonary capillary blood; $C\bar{v}O_2$, mixed venous oxygen content; $\dot{Q}_S$, shunted blood flow; $\dot{Q}_T$, total blood flow. (From Lumb AB. *Nunn's Applied Respiratory Physiology.* 6th ed. Philadelphia: Elsevier/Butterworth Heinemann; 2005.)

k in the equation as a conversion factor equal to 0.863, is expressed by

$$P_aCO_2 = k \times \left(\dot{V}_{CO_2}/\dot{V}_A\right) \tag{41.23}$$

In steady-state conditions (constant $\dot{V}_{CO_2}$), P_aCO_2 changes inversely with the alveolar ventilation. The traditional measure of ventilation inefficiency has been the fraction of dead space to tidal volume (V_D/V_T) as calculated using the Bohr equation (Eq. 41.15) and the assumption that the arterial and alveolar partial pressures of CO_2 are equivalent (i.e., $P_ACO_2 = P_aCO_2$). The dead space fraction determined in this manner includes alveolar (i.e., nonperfused alveoli) and anatomic dead space, as well as regions of high $\dot{V}/\dot{Q}$ ratio. As with the discussion on shunt, the dead space fraction characterizes not only real anatomic dead space, but also areas of inefficient ventilation (see Fig. 41.17).

MEASUREMENT PRINCIPLES

P_aO_2 is measured using a Clark electrode. The electrode consists of a cathode (either platinum or gold) and an anode in an electrolytic bath, surrounded by a thin O_2 permeable membrane. The electrode is inserted into the sample, and O_2 diffuses through the membrane and is reduced by the cathode, generating a current. The current is proportional to the PO_2 in the sample.[202] The PCO_2 electrode measures the change in pH brought about by the equilibration of blood with a bicarbonate solution.[203]

Effect of Temperature

The solubility of CO_2 and O_2 in blood is affected by temperature. At lower temperatures, solubility is increased, leading to a reduction in partial pressure. Blood gas analyzers measure gas partial pressures at 37°C. As blood from a hypothermic patient is warmed to 37°C by the analyzer, CO_2 and O_2 will come out of solution, leading to P_aCO_2 and P_aO_2

higher than those present in the patient. Blood gas analyzers make use of algorithms to correct the reported values to the patient's actual temperature.[204] The temperature effects on blood gas analysis are most relevant during management of hypothermic patients, such as during hypothermic cardiopulmonary bypass (HCPB) or deep hypothermic circulatory arrest (DHCA).

Two strategies have been developed for the management of arterial gas partial pressures under these conditions: alpha-stat and pH-stat. During alpha-stat management, blood gas measurements obtained after the analyzer warms the sample to 37°C are used for acid-base and gas exchange management. Potential benefits of alpha-stat management include the preservation of cerebral autoregulation and the maintenance of protein function.[205] During pH-stat management, measurements are corrected to the patient's temperature before they are used for acid-base and gas exchange management. Because patients are hypothermic, the P_aO_2 and P_aCO_2 at the patient's temperature are lower and the pH higher than those measured in the analyzer at 37°C. CO_2 is usually added to the oxygenator to maintain the temperature-corrected P_aCO_2 and pH at normothermic values. The theoretical benefits of pH-stat management are increased cerebral vasodilation leading to more homogenous cerebral cooling.[206]

Studies have compared the two strategies with respect to outcomes with varying results.[207-214] In general, clinical studies support the use of pH-stat management in pediatric cardiac surgical procedures during HCPB or DHCA.[209,213,215] In adult patients, the use of alpha-stat management is supported for HCPB.[216] For procedures involving DHCA in adults, the use of pH-stat management has been suggested to increase the rate and uniformity of cooling and alpha-stat management during rewarming.[217]

LIMITATIONS AND SOURCES OF ERRORS

Proper handling of arterial blood gas samples is important to prevent errors. Two common sources of error are delays in sample analysis and the presence of air in the sampling syringe.[218] A delay in sample analysis by 20 minutes at room temperature or at 4°C can lead to a decline in P_aO_2.[218] The decline is attributed to the metabolic activity of leukocytes and is not observed in samples placed on ice. The presence of an air bubble in the syringe can lead to a change in the measured P_aO_2 toward the PO_2 of the bubble and decline in P_aCO_2.[218]

Monitoring Lung Flows, Volumes, and Pressures:

As an organ of gas exchange, the human respiratory system relies on convective and diffusive gas transport processes for VO_2 and elimination of CO_2. The transport of air to the alveoli and alveolar gas to the environment requires the creation of a pressure gradient, which results in volume changes in the elastic components of the respiratory system, flow in the airways, velocity of moving tissues, and acceleration of air and tissues. The lung consists of a complex branching network of airway segments and viscoelastic tissues that, during the processes of spontaneous breathing or mechanical ventilation, gives rise to tremendous variations in gas velocities and flow regimens. The movement of gas flow ($\dot{V}$) into and out of the lungs requires pressure (P) to overcome the resistive (P_R), elastic (P_E), and at times inertial (P_I) forces offered by the airway tree, parenchymal tissues, and chest wall:

$$P = P_R + P_E + P_I \tag{41.24}$$

Eq. (41.24) can be used to describe the mechanical behavior of the total respiratory system, the lungs alone, or the chest wall, depending on whether P refers to airway pressure relative to atmosphere (transrespiratory pressure), airway pressure relative to pleural pressure (transpulmonary pressure), or pleural pressure alone.[219-221]

DYNAMIC RESPIRATORY MECHANICS

As a first approximation to Eq. (41.24), the mechanical behavior of the respiratory system during breathing or ventilation can be described according to the simple equation of motion that encompasses its resistive (R), elastic (E), and inertial (I) properties[219,222]:

$$P = R\dot{V} + EV + I\ddot{V} + P_o \tag{41.25}$$

where V is volume, $\ddot{V}$ denotes volume acceleration (i.e., the first time-derivative of flow or the second time-derivative of volume), and P_o is the distending pressure at end expiration. The coefficients R, E, and I in Eq. (41.25) may refer to the mechanical properties of the total respiratory system (rs), the lungs alone (L), or the chest wall (cw), depending on whether P refers to transrespiratory pressure, transpulmonary pressure, or intrapleural pressure, respectively.[221] The resistive properties of the respiratory system (R_{rs}) are generally assumed to arise from viscous and turbulent losses associated with gas flowing through the airway tree and the deformation of parenchymal and chest wall tissues. Hence, airway resistance may reflect airway caliber.[223] Provided that variations in flow are small, resistive pressure losses are assumed to be linearly related to flow according to the first term of Eq. (41.25). With more rapid flow rates, as may be seen during exercise or forced vital capacity maneuvers, resistive losses vary nonlinearly with flow, which may more accurately be described according to[224]

$$P_R = K_1\dot{V} + K_2\dot{V}^2 \tag{41.26}$$

where K_1 and K_2 are empirically determined constants. Additional energy losses arise from the tension within the alveolar surface film,[225] friction within the pleural space, and various tissue components of the parenchyma and chest wall,[220] as well as cross-bridge cycling of contractile elements within the airway walls and lung tissues.[226,227] Such losses are collectively termed "tissue resistance."[228,229] If these tissue resistive losses are assumed to be proportional to flow according to Eq. (41.25), one will observe that they vary inversely with breathing frequency,[226,230] a phenomenon commonly associated with viscoelastic materials.[220] In adult patients, lung tissue resistance comprises about 60% of subglottal total lung resistance at typical breathing rates.[231] During volume-cycled ventilation with an end-inspiratory pause, resistance can quickly be estimated from the difference between the peak (P_{peak}) and plateau (P_{plat}) airway pressures (i.e., the resistive pressure loss P_R) divided

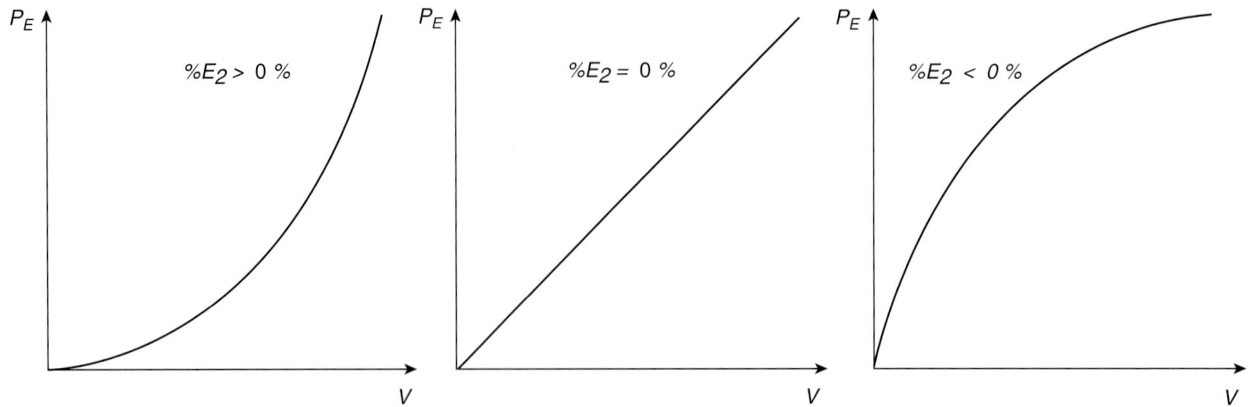

Fig. 41.18 Example elastic pressure *(P_E)* versus volume *(V)* curves and corresponding percentage of volume-dependent respiratory system elastance *($\%E_2$)* values. (Modified from D'Antini D, Huhle R, Herrmann J, et al. Respiratory system mechanics during low versus high positive end-expiratory pressure in open abdominal surgery: a substudy of PROVHILO randomized controlled trial. *Anesth Analg.* 2018;126:143–149.)

by the inspiratory flow ($\dot{V}_I$) immediately before the end-inspiratory pause:

$$R = \frac{P_{peak} - P_{plat}}{\dot{V}_I} = \frac{P_R}{\dot{V}_I} \tag{41.27}$$

Thus, for a specified flow rate, alterations in P_R may reflect changes in airway caliber, as may occur during an intraoperative asthma exacerbation (Fig. 41.18, center panel), or obstruction within the ETT or breathing circuit.

Elastic pressures arise from the recoil of the lungs and chest wall when their normal anatomic configurations are deformed, either by contraction of the diaphragm and intercostal muscles, or by some external force such as a ventilator.[232] Elastance is defined as the change in distending pressure (transrespiratory, transpulmonary, or intrapleural) for a given change in volume. *Dynamic elastance* refers to the change in elastic (i.e., nonresistive) distending pressure per unit volume during the process of breathing or ventilation.†Elastance of the total respiratory system (E_{rs}) comprises both lung (E_L) and chest wall (E_{cw}) elastances:

$$E_{rs} = E_L + E_{cw} \tag{41.28}$$

In clinical settings, elastance is usually expressed as its reciprocal, compliance (i.e., change in volume per unit change in pressure). This leads to an alternate form of Eq. (41.28), expressing the relationships of the compliant components of the total respiratory system (C_{rs}), lungs (C_L), and chest wall (C_{cw}):

$$\frac{1}{C_{rs}} = \frac{1}{C_L} + \frac{1}{C_{cw}} \tag{41.29}$$

Factors that increase total respiratory or lung elastance (or likewise reduce the corresponding total respiratory or lung compliance) include consolidation, pulmonary edema, pneumothorax, atelectasis, interstitial disease, pneumonectomy or surgical resection, lung overdistension, and mainstem intubation. Lung compliance generally increases in emphysema. Factors that reduce chest wall compliance are abdominal distension, abdominal compartment syndrome, chest wall edema, thoracic deformity, muscle tone, and extensive thoracic or abdominal scar (e.g., from burns); C_{cw} is reduced with muscle relaxation and flail chest.

In some situations, the magnitude of V_T, relative to the functional lung size, may be such that the linear dependence of P_E on V (Eq. [41.24] and [41.25]) is no longer an accurate description of the pressure-volume (PV) relationship of the lungs and/or chest wall. In these cases, elastic pressure may be more accurately described by a quadratic relationship with volume[232a,232b]:

$$P_E = E_1 V + E_2 V^2 \tag{41.30}$$

in which E_1 and E_2 denote the so-called volume-independent and volume-dependent components of elastance, respectively, since P_E will be reduced to $E_1 V$ when E_2 is negligible (Eq. [41.23]). An advantage of using Equation 41.30 is that it readily allows for the determination of the percentage of volume-dependent elastance contributing to P_E[232c]:

$$\% E_2 = \frac{E_2 V_T}{E_1 + E_2 V_T} \times 100\,\% \tag{41.31}$$

Since the $\%E_2$ index quantifies the deviation of linearity between P_E and V, it may provide quantitative information on the degree of intratidal recruitment or overdistention occurring during a mechanical breath.[232d] For example, positive values of $\%E_2$ (see Fig. 41.18*A*) indicate a convex P_E-V relationship, with probable overdistention occurring for $\%E_2$ greater than 30%.[232c] By contrast, negative values of $\%E_2$ (see Fig. 41.18*C*) indicate concave P_E-V relationship, with likely intratidal recruitment occurring during the breath.[232e]

For the special case of constant inspiratory flow during volume-cycled ventilation, the curvature of the inspiratory pressure-time profile can also be used to infer the processes of intratidal recruitment and overdistention. Raneiri and associates[232f] described this relationship using a simple power law expression:

$$P = at^b + c \tag{41.32}$$

where, similar to Eq. (41.24), P may refer to either transrespiratory or transpulmonary pressure, and t is time. The constants a, b, and c can be estimated from the inspiratory pressure profile using various nonlinear regression techniques.[232g] The exponent b is referred to as the "stress

†Certain conventions of nomenclature incorrectly define dynamic elastance as the *peak* airway pressure divided by tidal volume. However, such a definition of dynamic elastance includes both resistive *and* elastic pressures, and thus is not an index of purely elastic processes.

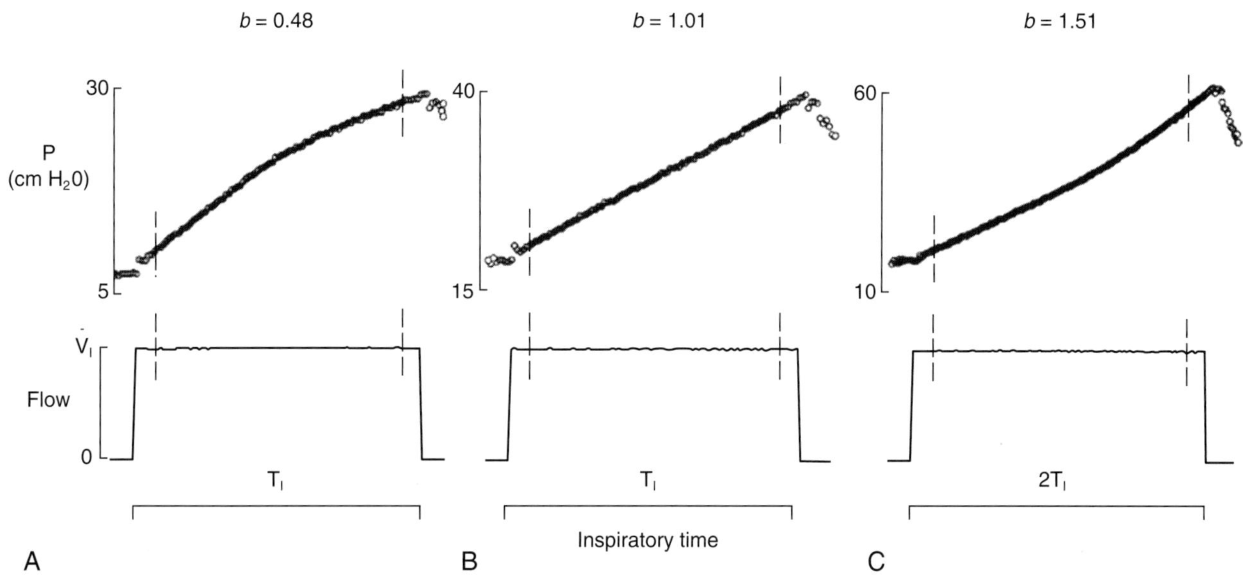

Fig. 41.19 Conceptual example of the stress index during constant inspiratory flow levels of $\dot{V}_I$ over durations of T_I and $2T_I$, assuming that the power law $P = at^b + c$ can describe the pressure-time (P-t) curve. (A) b <1.0, yielding a convex P-t curve, suggesting the dominance of intratidal recruitment; (B) b ~ 1.0, yielding a straight P-t line, suggesting minimal recruitment or overdistension; and (C) b >1.0, yielding a concave P-t curve, suggesting the dominance of parenchymal overdistension. (Modified from Ranieri VM, Zhang H, Mascia L, et al. Pressure-time curve predicts minimally injurious ventilatory strategy in an isolated rat lung model. *Anesthesiology*. 2000:93:1320–1328.)

index," and its estimated value characterizes the convexity (b <1.0), concavity (b >1.0), or linearity (b = 1.0) of the inspiratory pressure with time (Fig. 41.19). Similar to %E_2, b may also provide some insight into the relative contributions of intratidal recruitment (b <1.0) and parenchymal overdistention (b >1.0) to inspiratory pressure, or when these processes may be appropriately balanced (b ~ 1). However, as noted, the stress index is only interpretable during volume-cycled with constant inspiratory flows, in contrast to the %E_2 index, which can be used during other ventilatory modalities.[232h] Moreover, the interpretation of the stress index may be obscured during certain clinical situations, such as abdominal insufflation, abdominal compartment syndrome, or pleural effusion.[232i,j,k]

Similar to Eq. (41.27) to estimate R_{rs}, linear approximations to respiratory system elastance (E_{rs}) can be easily determined during volume-cycled ventilation for periods of zero-flow (i.e., during an end-inspiratory pause, when resistive pressures are zero) as the difference between P_{plat} and PEEP (i.e., the elastic pressure P_E) divided by the V_T:

$$E_{rs} = \frac{P_{plat} - PEEP}{V_T} = \frac{P_E}{V_T} \qquad (41.33)$$

Since the value of E_{rs} in Eq. (41.33) is obtained during zero-flow, it is often referred to as "static elastance." The corresponding static C_{rs} is usually between 50 and 100 mL/cm H_2O in normal mechanically ventilated lungs. Alterations in P_E for a specified V_T may be observed during processes that alter lung or chest wall elastance, such as a pneumothorax during thoracotomy or abdominal insufflation during laparoscopic surgical procedures (Fig. 41.20, *right panel*). In contrast to static E_{rs}, dynamic E_{rs} is estimated during periods of nonzero-flow by using multiple linear regression techniques (see later), and is higher than static elastance because of viscoelasticity[222] and gas redistribution.[233] Both the apparent static or dynamic E_{rs} will decrease following a recruitment maneuver because of an increase in aerated or functional lung volume. However, E_{rs} may also be increased due to *strain stiffening* of the lung tissues,[233a] in which collagen fibers within the extracellular matrix of the parenchyma become progressively recruited with increasing strain. Recruitment of stiff collagen fibers results in their dominance of load-bearing within the lung, in contrast to the more stretchable elastin fibers that are the main load-bearing elements during low levels of tissue strain.[233b] Such behavior may allow for titration of PEEP to achieve an optimal balance between intratidal recruitment and parenchymal overdistention—that is, the PEEP for which E_{rs} is minimized or, equivalently, C_{rs} is maximized.[232b,c,233c-f] The clinical utility of such PEEP titration in patients with ARDS is still not entirely established.[233e,233g]

Finally, inertial pressures are associated with the kinetic energy of accelerating the gas column in the central airways, as well as the motion of the respiratory tissues.[234] Inertial pressures are typically expressed as the product of a lumped "inertia" parameter and volume acceleration (Eq. [41.25]). Inertia is usually not a significant contributor to the apparent airway pressure or the work of breathing, except during sudden changes in air flow, as may occur during inspiratory step profiles or various modalities of high-frequency ventilation (HFV).[235,235a,b]

Eqs. (41.27) and (41.33) cannot be used to estimate R_{rs} and E_{rs} if an end-inspiratory pause is not present in the ventilator waveform. This is because one cannot easily separate the resistive and elastic pressures by visual inspection alone. For example, during pressure-controlled ventilation (PCV), the airway opening is exposed to a constant inflation pressure during inspiration (Fig. 41.21). Airway flow and V_T during PCV are determined not by the ventilator, but rather by the gradient between airway and alveolar pressures. Thus a more robust method of estimating respiratory

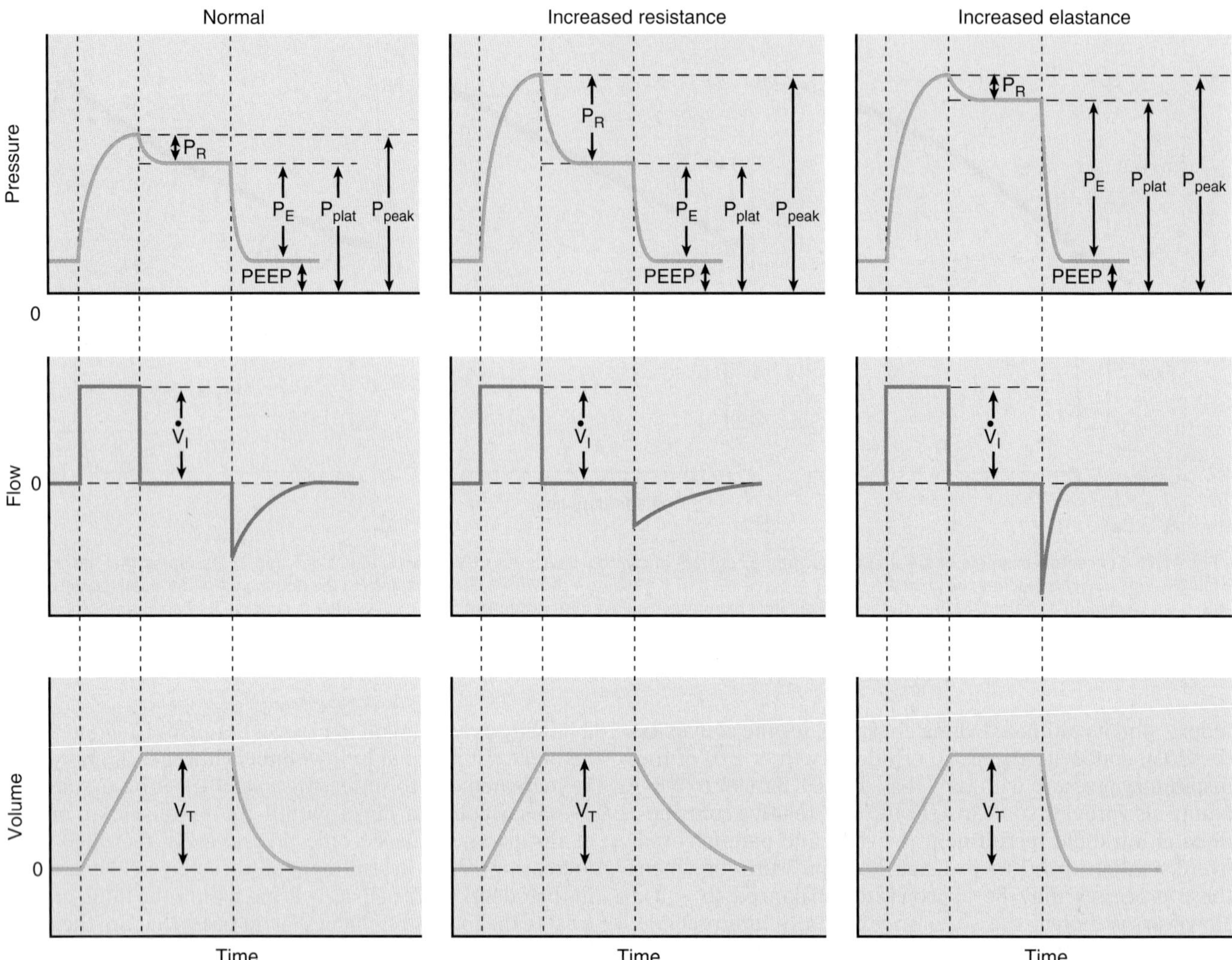

Fig. 41.20 Airway pressure, flow, and volume waveforms during constant-flow volume-cycled ventilation with an end-inspiratory pause. The components of the peak inspiratory pressure *(P_{peak})* and the plateau pressure *(P_{plat})* are presented: P_R, resistive pressure; P_E, elastic pressure; and *PEEP*, positive end-expiratory pressure. The same peak flow ($\dot{V}_I$) and tidal volume *(V_T)* are delivered by the mechanical ventilator in each case. Leftmost panels represent waveforms in a healthy patient. There is a small resistive pressure component, with most of the peak pressure comprised of elastic pressure. Expiratory flow decreases to zero before the start of the next inspiration, indicating appropriate I:E ratio and the absence of slowly emptying lung regions. Volume, as the integral of flow, also returns to zero before the initiation of the next breath. Middle panels represent waveforms in a patient with an increase in airways resistance. There is a significant increase in the resistive component P_R, and consequently P_{peak}. The elastic component is unchanged, as reflected in identical P_{plat} as compared with the healthy condition. Because increased resistance slows the process of lung emptying, the expiratory phase of the flow and volume curves now take longer to reach the zero. In several cases, the zero will not be reached, and a change in the I:E ratio will be necessary to avoid volume trapping and auto-PEEP. Rightmost panels represent a subject with increased P_E, as may occur during laparoscopic insufflation or pneumothorax. There is an increase in P_{plat} consistent with the increased elastance of the respiratory system, and a fast emptying of the lungs during exhalation.

R_{rs} and E_{rs} involves multiple linear regression of the coefficients in Eq. (41.25) on sampled flow and pressure data.[236-238] Such numerical approaches are present in commercially available respiratory mechanics monitors, and they can be used on almost all ventilator waveforms. Moreover, estimates of mechanical properties based on linear regression are not restricted to volume- or time-cycled waveforms with an end-inspiratory pause. One can separately estimate R_{rs} and E_{rs} during the inspiratory and expiratory phases, which may be different in some patients because of dynamic airway compression or derecruitment.[239,240]

Dynamic estimates of total respiratory R_{rs} and E_{rs} based on positive airway opening pressures are valid only during controlled modes of ventilation when the chest wall is relaxed. Although this is certainly the case during general anesthesia with neuromuscular blockade, the situation is more complicated during spontaneous breathing or assisted modes of ventilation. In such situations, the mechanics of the chest wall can be accounted for, if transpulmonary pressure is estimated using esophageal manometry, as described later.

STATIC RESPIRATORY MECHANICS

As previously illustrated, elastance (or compliance) is most easily measured during periods of zero flow because during these conditions the measured distending pressure is exclusively associated with elastic processes. However, a

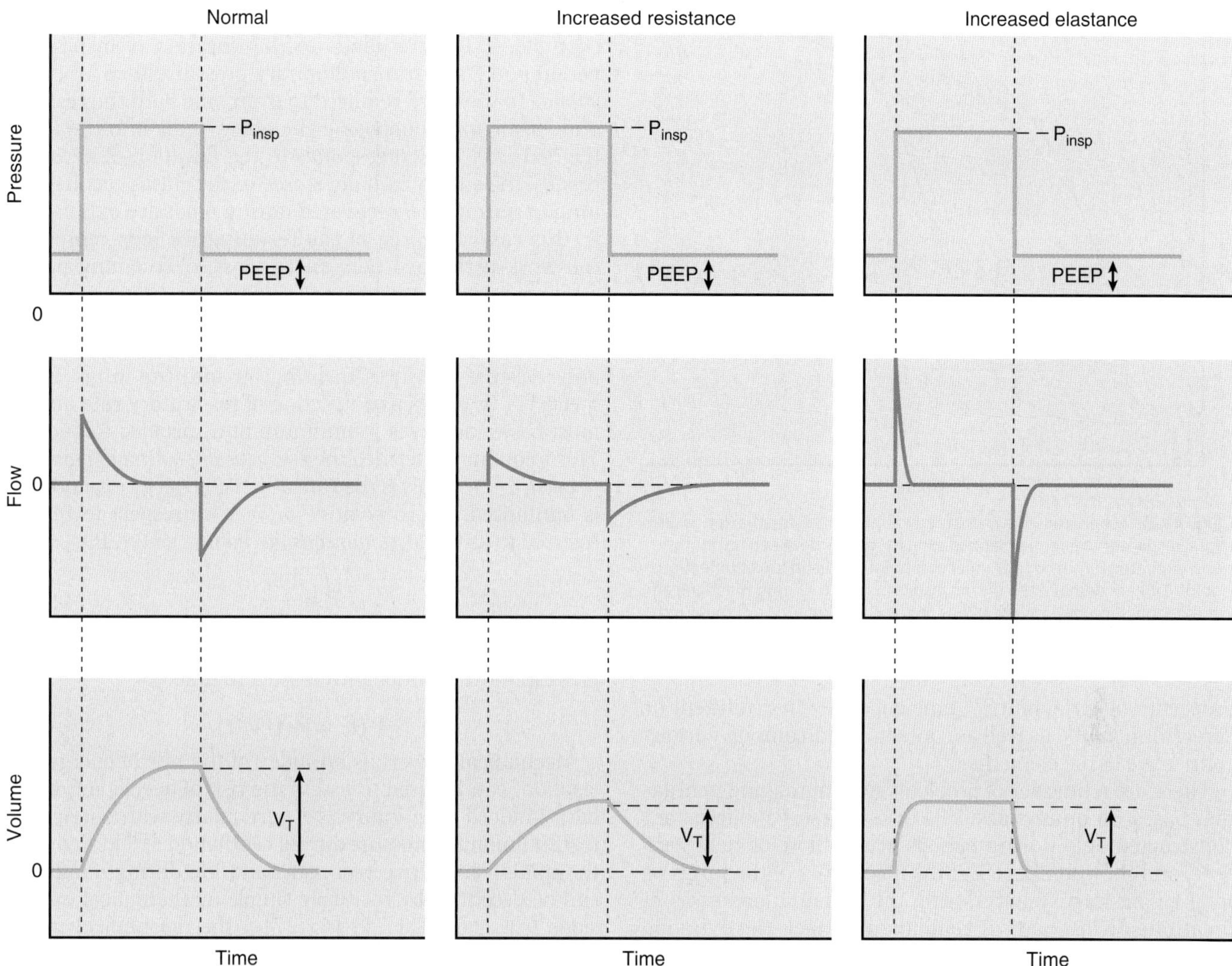

Fig. 41.21 Airway pressure, flow, and volume waveforms during pressure-controlled ventilation for the same patients depicted in Fig. 41.18. In this ventilatory mode, the ventilator delivers a fixed pressure during the inspiratory phase, irrespective of the resistance and compliance. Airflow and tidal volume will consequently change with changes in those parameters. Leftmost panels represent waveforms in a patient with normal lungs. Middle panels represent waveforms in a patient with airway obstruction. Note the absence of a peak-plateau difference as compared with the volume-controlled mode, a lower V_T, and a prolonged time for airflow to reach zero during exhalation as compared to the normal patient. Rightmost panels represent a subject with increased elastance, as may occur during laparoscopic insufflation or pneumothorax. Note a reduction in V_T and a shorter time to reach zero flow consistent with a more rigid lung. *PEEP,* positive end-expiratory pressure; P_{insp}, inspiratory pressure; V_T, tidal volume.

more comprehensive characterization of elastance can be obtained by plotting cumulative inspired or expired lung volume against the distending pressure across the lungs or total respiratory system. This quasi-static PV curve can be constructed during very slow inflations or deflations[241] (when resistive pressures are negligible), or during periodic flow occlusions.[242] For example, the expiratory limb of the PV curve can be constructed by inflating the lungs to a specified volume (usually total lung capacity) and then allowing a passive deflation with flow interruptions of 1 to 2 seconds.

The quasi-static PV curves of the lungs or total respiratory system are inherently nonlinear (Fig. 41.22); that is, compliance, defined as the local slope (dP/dV) of the PV curve, varies with lung volume. Empirically, PV curves are described using single exponential[243] or sigmoidal[244] functions. When they are described using sigmoidal functions, two points are usually demarcated on such curves, which have traditionally been termed the upper inflection point (UIP) and lower inflection point (LIP)[‡] The UIP is thought to represent the point at which lung overdistention occurs, as during parenchymal strain-stiffening,[220] The LIP is thought to reflect the process of maximum alveolar recruitment. During protective ventilation, one seeks to ventilate a patient in the most linear region of the PV curve.

Enough PEEP needs to be applied to avoid the LIP, where cyclic recruitment and derecruitment occur, along with lower V_Ts to avoid the UIP and overdistention.[242] Also, PV curves exhibit hysteresis, a phenomenon in which the lung volume at a specified pressure depends on the direction from which the distending pressure is approached (i.e., either inspiration or expiration). The reasons that the PV curve of the lungs or total respiratory system exhibits hysteresis are numerous and complex, and include the biophysical

‡The formal mathematical definition of an inflection point is a point on a curve at which its concavity (i.e., its second derivative) changes sign from positive to negative or vice versa.

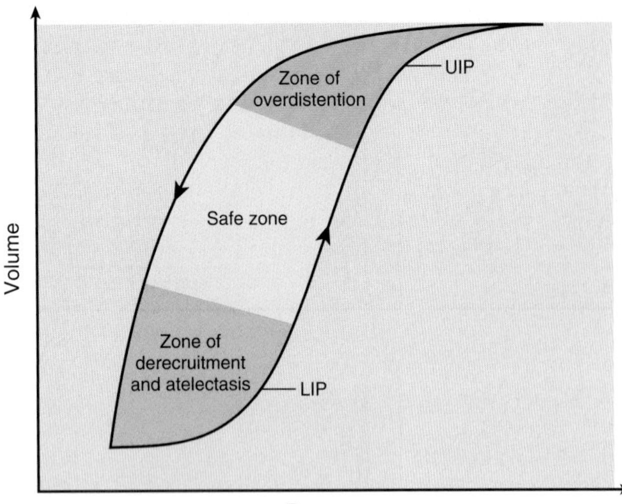

Fig. 41.22 Schematic of a pressure–volume curve for the lungs or total respiratory system, demonstrating hysteresis between inspiratory and expiratory limbs. Upper inflection point *(UIP)* and lower inflection point *(LIP)* are demarcated on the inspiratory limb. During mechanical ventilation, lung regions should be in the Safe Zone for optimal lung protection.

properties of surfactant,[245] time-dependent recruitment or derecruitment,[246] as well as contact friction among various connective tissue elements.[247]

There are a number of problems with managing ventilation based on quasi-static PV curves. First, PV curves are constructed only during periods of zero flow or near zero flow, and they do not reflect the mechanics of the lungs or total respiratory system during the dynamic processes of breathing or mechanical ventilation. In fact, the dynamic PV relationships for the same patient may be very different. Second, the UIP and LIP are not always visually apparent. Finally, a PV curve for the lungs or total respiratory system represents the averaged static behavior of a population of many lung units, with each operating on different portions of their own individual PV curves.

WORK OF BREATHING AND MECHANICAL POWER

The work of breathing (W) represents the energy required to inflate or deflate the lungs, or chest wall, or both, by a specified volume. In its simplest form, it can be represented as the product of the applied distending pressure and resulting volume change:

$$W = PV \tag{41.34}$$

However, when pressure and volume vary as functions of time (as during the course of a spontaneous or controlled breath), work may be expressed as the cumulative product[248]

$$W = \int PdV \tag{41.35}$$

or equivalently as the integral of the pressure-flow product with respect to time[249]

$$W = \int_{t=0}^{T} P(t)\,\dot{V}(t)dt \tag{41.36}$$

where T is the duration over which W is determined. For example, if T corresponds to the duration of inspiratory period and P the transpulmonary pressure, then W corresponds to the work required to overcome both the resistive and elastic forces opposing the entry of air into the lungs (Fig. 41.23). If T corresponds to the duration of an entire breath, the energy initially stored in the elastic recoil of the lung tissues will be recovered during a passive exhalation. In this case, the area of the resulting PV loop represents the work performed (i.e., energy lost) overcoming purely resistive losses in the airways and tissues. In general, W is assessed during inspiration only because the respiratory musculature (or a ventilator) must overcome both elastic and resistive pressures to bring air into the lungs. For a given V_T, W varies as a function of respiratory rate and, in most cases, achieves a minimum at a specified frequency. This frequency is termed the *energetically optimum breathing frequency*,[249] as this is the rate at which energy expenditure is minimized. The derivative of W with respect to time is referred to as the *instantaneous mechanical power*, P,

$$P = \frac{dW}{dt} \tag{41.37}$$

which, based on Eq. (41.31), can simply be expressed as the pressure-flow product with respect to time:

$$P(t) = P(t)\,\dot{V}(t) \tag{41.38}$$

Mechanical power, as an index of the *rate* of energy dissipation, can be used to assess the risk of developing ventilator-induced lung injury,[249a] particularly with changes in transpulmonary pressure during ventilation.[249b] Moreover, if the relationship between pressure and flow during ventilation can be described by relatively simple mathematical expressions (e.g., Eqs. [41.25]–[41.27]), the mechanical power likewise can be embodied by simple analytic formulæ.[249c,d]

MONITORING OF RESPIRATORY PRESSURES

Fundamental to any quantitative assessment of respiratory mechanics is the measurement of pressure. Such pressures may include those measured in the inspiratory or expiratory limb of the anesthesia machine, at the proximal end of an ETT, or within the trachea or esophagus. Pressure allows for the inference of the forces associated with the movement of gases through the airway tree, as well as the distension of the parenchymal tissues and chest wall, according to the elements described in Eq. (41.24). The most accessible and familiar pressure to the anesthesiologist or intensivist is the airway pressure during controlled mechanical ventilation. Ideally, this should be the pressure measured in the trachea or at the airway opening, exclusive of any distortions from airway devices or breathing circuits. However, for practical reasons, this "airway" pressure is not the actual pressure at the airway opening or within the trachea, but is the pressure transduced at the anesthesia machine or ventilator and reflects the resistive and compliant properties of the breathing circuit and face mask or ETT, as well as the mechanical properties of the respiratory system. Although many ventilators now use computer algorithms to provide some compensation for flow and pressure losses in the breathing circuit,[250] such approaches often rely on idealized, linear models that do not truly reflect the complex

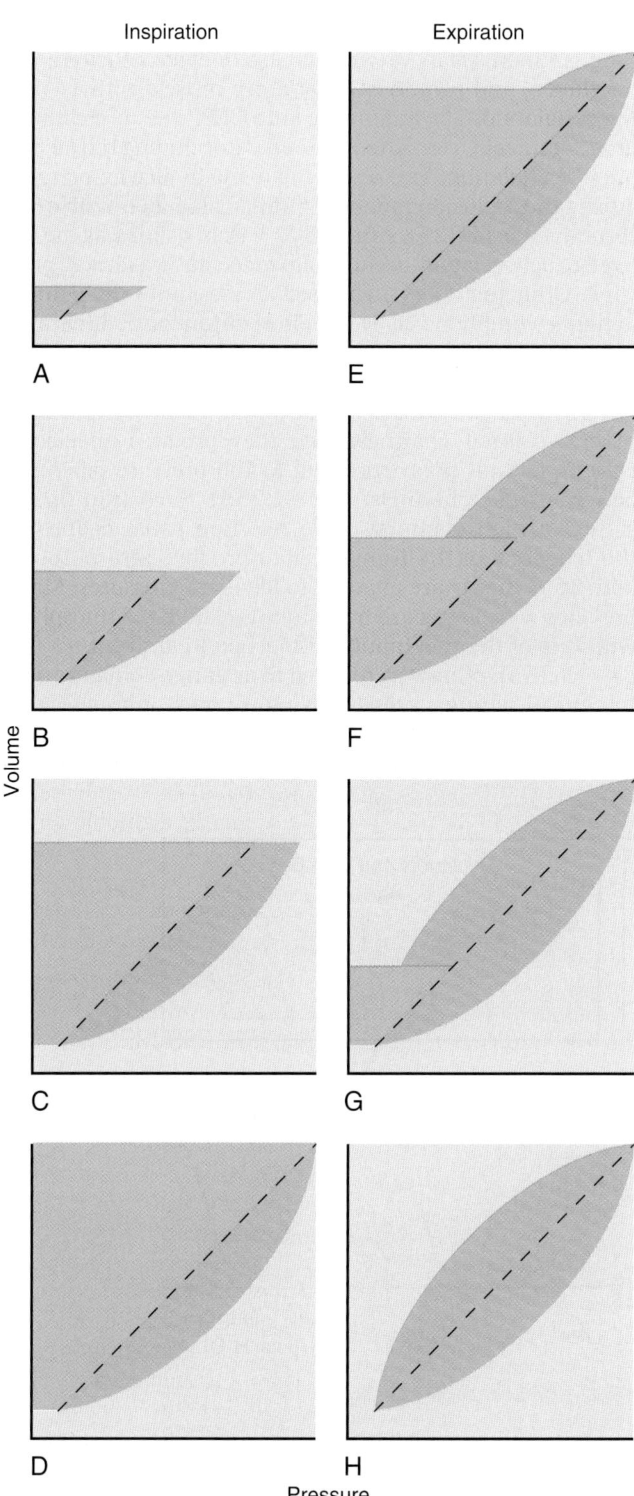

Fig. 41.23 Volume plotted against transpulmonary or (transrespiratory) pressure during the course of a single breath. Plots are shown during inspiration (panels A through D) and expiration (panels E through H). *Gray area* denotes the work of breathing due to tissue elasticity, while the *hatched area* denotes the work of breathing due to airways and tissue resistance. Energy stored in elastic recoil at the end of inspiration will be entirely recovered during expiration. However, resistive energy will always be lost during both inspiration and expiration.

processes of turbulent air flow, polytropic gas compression, or viscoelastic tubing walls.[251,252] Therefore, one must use caution when making physiologic inferences based on airway pressures and volumes reported by a ventilator.

Often airway pressure is improperly used as a surrogate for lung distention. *Transrespiratory pressure* refers to the pressure drop across the lungs and chest wall, which during positive-pressure ventilation is usually determined by the difference between airway pressure and atmospheric pressure. Several processes that may contribute to increased transrespiratory pressure do not correspond to excessive lung inflation. For example, obesity, abdominal insufflation, or steep Trendelenburg position all may contribute to high airway opening pressures, but they do not necessarily indicate parenchymal overdistention.

By contrast, *transpulmonary pressure* refers to the distending pressure across the lungs alone. Its determination requires not only measurement of airway opening pressure, but also estimates of the pressure within the pleural space. This can be obtained relatively noninvasively using an esophageal balloon catheter, because the pressure measured within the esophagus is relatively close to intrapleural pressure.[253,253a] Such catheters are typically 100 cm long, with side holes in the distal tip covered by a thin-walled balloon (Fig. 41.24). The catheter can be placed through the mouth or nares and positioned in the middle-to-distal third of the esophagus. The catheter is connected to a transducer by a three-way stopcock, and a small amount of air is injected into the balloon such that its walls remain flaccid and do not contribute an additional recoil pressure to the measurement. Because the local values of pleural pressure vary depending on gravity, the balloon should be several centimeters in length to provide an average estimate of the pressure field surrounding the lungs. Estimating pleural pressure based on esophageal manometry has several limitations, including mediastinal compression of the balloon in supine patients, catheter migration, and cardiac artifact on the tracing.[254,255] Nonetheless, its use in critically ill patients and under certain special conditions such as obesity, abdominal hypertension (primary or during laparoscopic insufflation), and extreme Trendelenburg position may be valuable in the adjustment of appropriate levels of PEEP.[256,256a] Peak and plateau pressures, which are typical in clinical practice, are obtained from the *transrespiratory* pressure. Accordingly, they do not characterize the pressures acting exclusively on the lungs, but on the whole respiratory system. Current recommendations suggest limiting transrespiratory plateau pressures to 26 to 30 cm H_2O, to minimize alveolar overdistension.[257] However, such recommendations should be applied in appropriate clinical context, given that the same plateau pressure could correspond to very different transpulmonary pressures, and consequently to very different degrees of risk for lung injury, depending on the partitioning between lung and chest wall pressure components.[257a,b]

More recent studies suggest that the "driving pressure"—that is, the V_T normalized by the respiratory system compliance ($\Delta P = V_T/C_{rs}$)—may be one of the most important ventilatory variables to consider when stratifying mortality risk during ARDS.[257c,d] Its relationship to postoperative pulmonary complications in surgical patients has also been demonstrated.[258,259] In practice, driving pressure may be computed as the difference between P_{plat} and PEEP.[257c]

Auto-PEEP or *intrinsic-PEEP* is the positive pressure present within the alveoli at end-exhalation and is typically observed in ventilated patients with COPD, who demonstrate dynamic airway compression and expiratory flow limitation, as well as a significant portion of patients with ARDS, sepsis, and respiratory muscle weakness.[260] Auto-PEEP can promote significant respiratory and hemodynamic compromise. It is usually caused by a combination of increased airway resistance and reduced lung elastic recoil (i.e., an increase in the expiratory time constant of the respiratory system). Other factors are a decrease in expiratory time, an increase in V_T, an increase in external expiratory resistance, and persistent inspiratory muscle activity during exhalation. The amount of auto-PEEP can be estimated in mechanically ventilated patients by occluding the airway at end exhalation, and observing a rise in airway pressure during the occlusion maneuver until a plateau is visible (<4 seconds) (Fig. 41.25). Auto-PEEP is then defined as the difference between end-occlusion to preocclusion airway pressures. Other methods can be used to assess auto-PEEP under dynamic conditions, as well as in spontaneously breathing patients with the use of an esophageal balloon.[260,261]

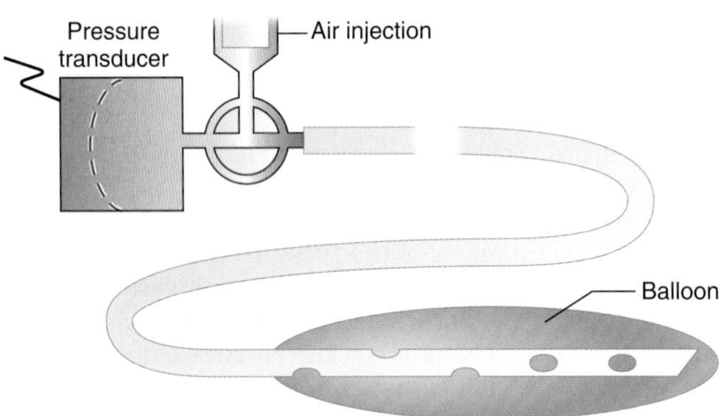

Fig. 41.24 Example of an Esophageal Balloon Catheter. The proximal end of the catheter is connected to a pressure transducer, and air is injected into the balloon via a three-way stopcock. (Modified from Bates JHT. *Lung Mechanics: an Inverse Modeling Approach*. Cambridge: Cambridge University Press; 2009:220.)

Any measurement of pressure requires pressure transducers. Most pressure transducers are differential sensors with two input channels, and they produce an electrical output that is proportional to the pressure difference between these channels (Fig. 41.26*A*). Such transducers exhibit a high common-mode rejection ratio, defined as the tendency of the transducer to produce zero output if both of its inputs are exposed to identical pressures. Many pressure waveforms are transduced relative to atmosphere with one of the two inputs left opened to ambient air (see Fig. 41.26*B*), otherwise referred to as gauge configuration. In clinical settings, pressure is most commonly measured using relatively inexpensive, piezoresistive transducers.[222] These devices rely on a pressure-sensing diaphragm

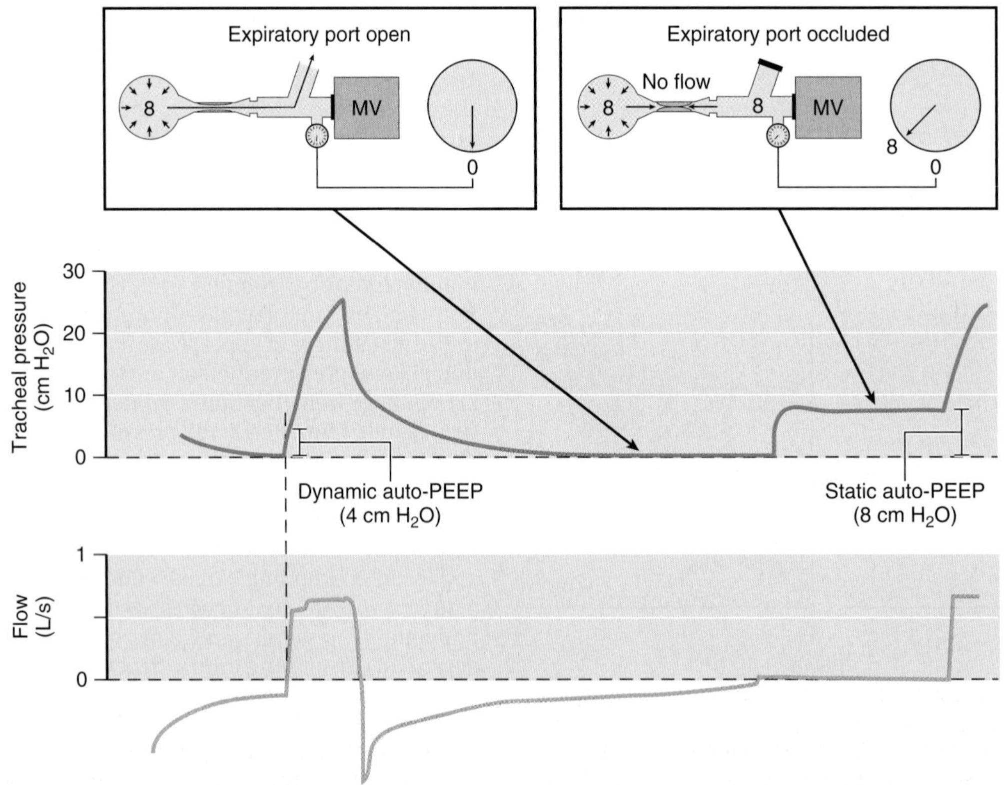

Fig. 41.25 Concept of Intrinsic Positive End-Expiratory Pressure (auto-PEEP). Shown are tracheal pressure and flow waveforms during controlled mechanical ventilation. Dynamic auto-PEEP can be estimated at the beginning of inspiration as the tracheal pressure when the flow trace equals zero. Static auto-PEEP can be estimated as the tracheal pressure following a prolonged expiratory occlusion. (Modified from Blanch L, Bernabé F, Lucangelo U. Measurement of air trapping, intrinsic positive end-expiratory pressure, and dynamic hyperinflation in mechanically ventilated patients. *Respir Care.* 2005;50:110–123; and Moon RE, Camporesi EM. Respiratory monitoring. In: Miller RD, Fleisher LA, Johns RA, eds. *Miller's Anesthesia.* 6th ed. New York, NY: Churchill Livingstone; 2005:1255, 1295.)

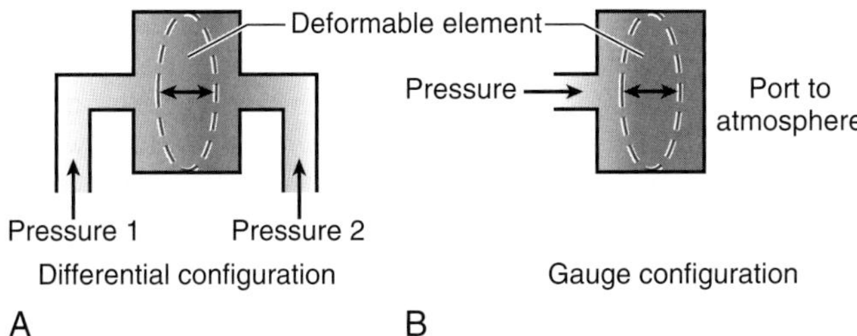

Fig. 41.26 **Pressure transducers arranged in differential (A) or gauge (B) configurations.** (Modified from Bates JHT. *Lung Mechanics: An Inverse Modeling Approach*. Cambridge: Cambridge University Press; 2009:220.)

whose electrical resistance changes when it is deformed in response to a differential pressure. This change in electrical resistance can be sensed with a standard Wheatstone bridge circuit, which produces an output-voltage signal appropriate for amplification and filtering. In general, piezoresistive transducers have adequate frequency responses sufficient for most respiratory applications.[262,263] However, this frequency response can be easily degraded if the transducer is connected to the pressure-sensing location with long, compliant tubing.[264]

MONITORING OF RESPIRATORY FLOWS

Ideally, any measurement of flow should indicate the exact rate at which gas is entering and leaving the patient's lungs. This can be most easily accomplished by placing the flow-measuring device as close to the patient as possible, such as between the circuit Y-connector and the proximal end of the ETT or LMA. However, for practical reasons, most ventilators and anesthesia machines measure flow close to the machine console. This flow can be considerably different from that close to the patient because of the effects of gas compression, wall distention of the breathing circuit, and changes in gas humidity.

An important clinical use of flow monitoring is the detection of nonzero end-expiratory flows. This indicates that a gradient of pressure exists between alveolar regions and the upper airway with incomplete lung emptying at end-expiration, characteristic of auto-PEEP (PVolFl-7). As a consequence, end-expiratory lung volumes would be larger than those in the absence of auto-PEEP, with risk of dynamic lung hyperinflation and reduction of venous return. Increase in expiratory time and reduction of V_T or respiratory rate should be considered to eliminate the issue.

During ventilation, airway flow can often be inferred according to time-dependent changes in delivered or inspired V_T or from the displacement waveform of a piston or cylinder arrangement or bellows.[265-267] Preferably, flow is measured using transducers designed specifically for this task. The most common method involves the measurement of a differential pressure decrease (ΔP) across a fluid resistive element. Ideally, this ΔP is linearly related to the corresponding flow through the device. Such a principle forms the basis for one of the oldest and most widely used flowmeters, the pneumotachograph. Although the instruments provide accurate measurement of flow, pneumotachographs are very sensitive to changes in temperature, humidity, and gas composition,[268] and require frequent calibration using various electronic or software-based techniques to ensure accurate measurements.[269,270] This sensitivity, combined with difficulties in cleaning and sterilization, limits the routine use of these instruments in clinical environments. Orifice flowmeters also have the advantage of having relatively large internal diameters that limit the formation of condensation and minimize obstruction with secretions. Given that these devices can be manufactured using inexpensive plastic injection molding techniques, many orifice flowmeters are designed to be disposable, thus making their use increasingly popular for respiratory applications in clinical environments.[271]

Most anesthesia machines use hot wire anemometers for flow measurement,[272] which rely on temperature-dependent changes in the electrical resistance of a current carrying wire. When gas flows past the wire, the corresponding temperature drop changes the conductivity of the filament, which can be sensed with appropriate electronic circuits.[273] Because a single wire filament cannot sense the direction of flow, two different anemometers can be used in the ventilator circuit: one for the inspiratory limb, and the other for the expiratory limb. Alternatively, two wires in series must be used for sensing bidirectional flow through a single conduit,[274] with the flow direction determined according to which wire is cooled first. In general, hot wire anemometers have a better dynamic response compared with pneumotachographs or orifice flowmeters,[275] making them ideal for flow measurement during HFV.[235a,276] However, these devices must also be calibrated to account for variations in gas density or humidity as well.[276a]

MONITORING OF RESPIRATORY VOLUME

Similar to flow measurement, the ideal measurement of volume should be an accurate accounting of the gas quantity moving into and out of the patient. However, delivered or exhaled V_T measurement is subjected to the same limitations of flow measurement because most anesthesia machines and ventilators determine volume by electrically or numerically integrating the corresponding flow signal.[222] Care must be taken to ensure any drifts or offsets from the flow transducer are minimized, given that their integration will result in errors in estimated volume. This may be accomplished by appropriately zeroing the transducer periodically, such as at the end of a breath. Although electronic or digital high-pass filters may be used to remove drifts and offsets in real-time, these tend to have long transient responses.[276b,c]

Finally, besides the pathophysiologic and monitoring applications described in this section, monitoring of pressures, volumes, and flows has been applied to monitoring, training, and education for neonatal resuscitation.[277]

Plethysmographic Monitoring

Respiratory inductance plethysmography (RIP) is a noninvasive respiratory monitoring technique that quantifies changes in the cross-sectional area of the chest wall and the abdominal compartments. The method is used to assess V_T, respiratory rate, adequacy of high-frequency oscillatory ventilation (HFOV), lung volume changes during tracheobronchial suctioning, and thoracoabdominal synchrony.[278] RIP relies on the principle that a current applied through a loop of wire generates a magnetic field normal to the orientation of the loop (Faraday's law) and that a change in the area enclosed by the loop creates an opposing current within the loop directly proportional to the change in the area (Lenz's law). Two elastic bands containing a conductor are used: one typically placed around the patient's chest, 3 cm above the xiphoid process; and the other around the abdomen. Each of these bands produces an independent signal representative of the thoracic and abdominal cross-sectional area, and the sum of these two signals calibrated against a known gas volume yields lung volume change.

There have been several pediatric applications of RIP to monitor V_T and respiratory rate, building on the advantage that a facemask, LMA, or ETT is not required for measurements.[279-281] The technique could also guide lung-protective ventilation strategies by facilitating the construction of PV curves for individual patients. These can be used to optimize lung recruitment, maintain an open lung, and limit overdistension (see the section on "Static Respiratory Mechanics"). RIP has found several applications in sleep studies.

Intraoperatively, RIP may be useful in areas for which accurate monitoring of V_T is required but not possible with the usual anesthesia machine monitors. This could occur with a shared airway (e.g., laryngotracheal surgery,[282] flexible and rigid bronchoscopy[283]), or a patient whose trachea is not intubated (e.g., monitored anesthesia care and noninvasive pressure support ventilation).

Limitations of intraoperative RIP include the fact that it cannot be used during thoracic and abdominal surgery, because of the need for the measurement bands. Also, the calibration characteristics of the device are affected by changes in the pattern of breathing.[284]

Respiratory Rate Monitoring: Apnea Monitoring

Apnea and bradypnea are life-threatening events frequently observed in the intraoperative and postoperative periods of anesthesia. Prematurity, morbid obesity, age, obstructive sleep apnea, and central nervous system depressant medications have been associated with risk of apnea or bradypnea.[285,286] Accordingly, many different approaches have been developed for detecting those events.[287,288] Two main types of apnea are observed: central and obstructive. Central apnea is defined as apnea resulting from a failure of the central nervous system to drive respiration. Obstructive apnea is that resulting from upper airway obstruction. Current monitors assess at least one of three processes occurring during breathing to detect apnea[288]: chest wall expansion, gas flow, and gas exchange.

Chest wall expansion is usually measured as follows:

1. Changes in thoracic electrical impedance (impedance pneumography) of the chest wall. The method is based on the changes in electrical conductivity of the chest to an electrical current as air moves in and out of the lungs during breathing and blood volume changes in the same period. This is because air is a poor electrical conductor and blood is a good electrical conductor. A low electrical current at high frequency is applied in two chest electrodes, corresponding changes in voltage of the chest are measured, and the impedance is continuously calculated from these. The technique is implemented in several commercial systems using routine electrocardiographic leads and is also used in home monitoring of neonatal apnea.
2. Inductive plethysmography (as described earlier).
3. Abdominal and chest fiberoptic and resistive strain gauges (a pressure pad placed alongside the infant's rib cage, pneumatic abdominal sensors) are used.
4. Electromyographic signal of respiratory muscles is not frequently used because of the low signal-to-noise ratio.

An important drawback of techniques based on chest expansion is their inaccuracy in the presence of movement. Thus obstructive apnea may be falsely assessed as normal respirations.[289]

Gas flow methods are based on measurements of different variables directly related to the presence of air flow in the airway:

1. Pressure gradients along the breathing circuit. This approach uses the Poiseuille principle ($\Delta P = k \times V$) and differential pressure transducers to detect flow.
2. Temperature of the breathed air in the nose or mouth is used.
3. Rapid response hygrometer is based on assessment of humidity in the exhaled air.

Techniques based on gas exchange focus essentially on exhaled CO_2, as routinely used in intubated patients in the operating room. In nonintubated patients, the use of specifically designed cannulae combining DO_2 and breathed gas sampling facilitates the monitoring of exhaled CO_2. Capnography allows for early detection of respiratory depression before O_2 desaturation, particularly when supplemental O_2 is administered.[290,290a] Off-line or in-line infrared sensors are the most common technique. Respiratory rate measurements using these techniques were more accurate than those obtained with thoracic impedance tomography in extubated patients in postanesthesia care units, even with supplemental O_2 at high flows.[291] Accurate end-tidal CO_2 measurements through a nasal cannula may be difficult in mouth breathers, including obese patients and those with obstructive sleep apnea. In such cases, a nasal cannula with an oral guide may improve measurement accuracy.[292] Simulation studies indicated that respiratory rate can be accurately monitored during esophagogastroduodenoscopies using a CO_2 sampling bite block or a nasal cannula with oral cup. The accuracy of $P_{ET}CO_2$ measurements depends on the device used, O_2 flow, the intensity of oral breathing, and minute ventilation.[293]

Pulse oximetry cannot be used as the primary monitor of apnea or bradypnea because O_2 desaturation occurs only late in a well-oxygenated apneic patient. However, pulse oximetry adds an additional level of safety combined with primary monitors of ventilation. For example, in a study using pulse oximetry and noninvasive capnography for continuous monitoring of 178 patients receiving patient-controlled analgesia, respiratory depression measured by O_2 desaturation occurred in 12% of the patients, in line with previous studies.[285] In contrast to previous estimates, episodes of bradypnea (respiratory rate < 10 breaths/min) were present in 41% of patients, far more frequently than the previously reported 1% to 2%.[294-296]

Respiratory rate monitoring is also critical to infant apnea monitoring. Combinations of transthoracic impedance and pulse oximetry may maximize the detection of true episodes of apnea in home monitors for neonatal apnea.[297] This is because pulse oximetry provides an additional level of monitoring in cases of poor performance of transthoracic impedance secondary to motion artifacts. The value of combining monitors of ventilation such as capnography with pulse oximetry to maximize the detection of alveolar hypoventilation has been confirmed.[298] Capnography allowed for early detection of arterial O_2 desaturation in cases of alveolar hypoventilation in the presence of supplemental O_2.

False-positive and false-negative alarms occur during apnea monitoring. The most dangerous conditions occur when artifacts are detected as breathing and alarms are not activated. Such artifacts include vibrations, cardiac motion, patient movement, and electromagnetic interference from other instrumentation. Impedance pneumographs are subject to cardiovascular artifacts, whereas pressure pads are subject to patient motion artifacts. A more common (yet less dangerous) problem is when an alarm sounds in a patient without apnea. Frequent causes include inadequate sensitivity settings, malfunctioning electrodes, and movement of the patient. Motion transducers based on sensing of acceleration were used in neonates undergoing HFOV, and results showed that monitoring of regional tidal displacement may enable the early recognition of deteriorating ventilation during HFOV that eventually leads to hypoxemia.[299] This study found that in approximately half of the cases, hypoxemia had causes other than slowly deteriorating ventilation.[299]

Current recommendations of the Anesthesia Patient Safety Foundation for Essential Monitoring Strategies to Detect Clinically Significant Drug-Induced Respiratory Depression in the Postoperative Period (http://www.apsf.org/initiatives.php), including opioid-induced ventilatory impairment, state that continuous electronic monitoring of oxygenation and ventilation should be available and considered for all patients, not only those at risk for postoperative respiratory insufficiency. This is because selective monitoring is likely to miss respiratory depression in patients without risk factors. These recommendations stress that maintaining status quo while awaiting newer technology is not acceptable, and that intermittent "spot checks" of oxygenation (pulse oximetry) and ventilation (nursing assessment) are not adequate for reliably recognizing clinically significant evolving drug-induced respiratory depression. Continuous electronic monitoring should not replace traditional intermittent nursing assessment and vigilance. All patients should have oxygenation continuously monitored by pulse oximetry. Capnography or other monitoring modalities that measure ventilation and airflow are indicated when supplemental O_2 is needed to maintain acceptable O_2 saturations. The recommendations also call attention to threshold-based alarm limits on individual physiologic variables, which may result in failure to recognize early signs of progressive hypoventilation by either being insufficiently, or too, sensitive (excess false alarms).

Unexpected death has been associated with three patterns of respiratory depression.[300-302] (1) Hyperventilation compensated respiratory distress (e.g., from sepsis, pulmonary embolus, or congestive heart failure): patients present initially with stable S_pO_2 and decreasing P_aCO_2 as metabolic acidosis develops with associated compensatory hyperventilation. High respiratory rate is typical of this pattern. Ultimately, a slow desaturation is followed by an abrupt fall in oxygenation as the ventilatory response to worsening acidosis fails. (2) Progressive unidirectional hypoventilation or CO_2 narcosis: frequently due to opioid or other sedative overdose, it is characterized by a rise in P_aCO_2 (and $P_{ET}CO_2$) initially because of decreased minute ventilation, often while S_pO_2 remains above 90%. (3) Sentinel rapid airflow/O_2 saturation reduction with precipitous S_pO_2 fall: observed in patients with obstructive sleep apnea, who are dependent on the arousal state to maintain oxygenation. Sleep results in precipitous hypoxemia during apnea with potential sudden arrest.

Imaging for Respiratory Monitoring

Imaging as a monitoring technique provides tremendous insight into pulmonary structure, function, and inflammation in both health and disease.[303-305] However, exposure to radiation and bulky devices has prevented its use at the bedside. Technologic advances have led to the introduction of new modalities with more compact equipment for clinical use. This may herald an important shift in respiratory monitoring toward the increased use of bedside imaging. Such improvements come with the advantages of less radiation exposure, noninvasiveness, and more detailed physiologic information.

CHEST RADIOGRAPHY

Chest radiography has been the traditional imaging method to assess intrathoracic conditions in the operating room, postoperative anesthesia care unit, and ICUs. Anesthesiologists should be familiar with basic radiologic findings representative of important pulmonary conditions such as interstitial infiltrates, hyperinflation, pneumothorax, pleural effusion, and consolidation. The image during chest radiography, as well as computed tomography, is based on the physical principle that x-rays reaching a detector (e.g., film) depend on tissue absorption, which varies linearly with tissue density. However, radiation exposure restricts frequency of use. Furthermore, technical difficulties limit image quality. These difficulties include reduced resolution caused by patient movement during acquisition, and image distortion related to proximity of the x-ray beam source to the film/detector and posterior position of the film cassette.

ULTRASONOGRAPHY

Lung ultrasonography is a technique increasingly used in the perioperative, critical care, and emergency settings in adults and children.[306-309] Critical and systematic approaches have proven that important clinical information can be obtained with lung ultrasonography at levels

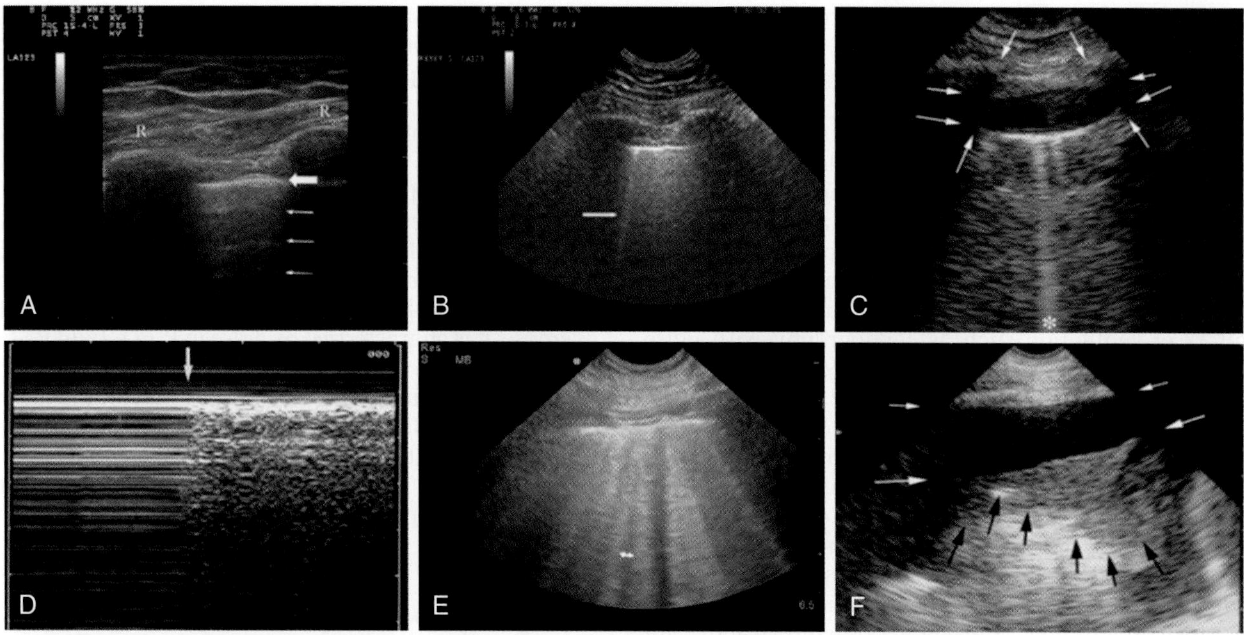

Fig. 41.27 (A) Typical thoracic view depicting adjacent ribs (R) producing acoustic shadowing. The white echogenic pleural line *(block arrow)*, is approximately 0.5 cm below the ribs. A-line artifacts *(line arrows)* are seen at equidistant spaces below the pleural line; (B) B-line, or comet-tail artifact *(line arrow)*, is the hyperechoic artifact extending from the pleural line to the edge of the screen, erasing the A-line. A solitary B-line is a usual finding in normal lungs; (C) pleural effusion: image obtained at the posterolateral region showing the parietal pleural *(upper horizontal arrows)*, the rib shadows *(vertical arrows)*, and the visceral pleura (line indicated by the *lower horizontal arrows*) with the underlying lung. The dark anechoic region between the parietal and visceral pleura represents the pleural effusion. A B-line artifact *(asterisk)* originates from the lung and not from the pleural line, implying the presence of aeration; (D) M-mode of lung of lung ultrasound illustrative of the "lung point" for diagnosis of pneumothorax. The sudden inspiratory transition from a parallel line pattern indicative of absence of lung motion (pneumothorax) to a granular pattern indicative of lung tissue can be observed *(arrow)*; (E) Interstitial syndrome case showing B-lines 7 mm or less apart. Notice the increased number of B-lines as compared to panel (B). The pleural line *(arrow)* and ribs are also appreciated; (F) Lung consolidation with pleural effusion. As in (C), the image was obtained at the posterolateral region showing the parietal pleura *(upper horizontal arrows)* and the visceral pleura and lung *(lower horizontal arrows)* with an anechoic pleural effusion between them. Lung tissue denser than that presented in (C) with gas barriers *(vertical arrows)*. This indicates pleural fluid with alveolar fluid often seen in critically ill patients. ([A, B, D, E] From Turner JP, Dankoff J. Thoracic ultrasound. *Emerg Med Clin North Am*. 2012;30:451–473, ix. [C, F] From Lichtenstein DA. BLUE-protocol and FALLS-protocol: two applications of lung ultrasound in the critically ill. *Chest*. 2015;147[6]:1659–1670. doi: 10.1378/chest.14-1313.)

comparable to computed tomography.[309] Such features add to the advantages of practicality, low cost, and absence of radiation or other significant biologic side effects. Excellent reviews have been published, and the reader should refer to those for additional learning.[308,309]

Lung ultrasonography has been applied successfully in the assessment of pneumothorax, interstitial syndrome (i.e., cardiogenic and permeability pulmonary edema), lung consolidation, and pleural effusion. Currently available multipurpose ultrasonography probes can be used for specific portions of the pulmonary exam according to their characteristics. For instance, the high-frequency (10-12 MHz) linear array probe allows for detailed examination of the pleura and superficial changes, such as pneumothorax. This probe's limitations include its size, which impedes access to larger areas of lung tissue because of the interference of the ribs, and high frequency, which limits assessment of deeper structures. A lower frequency (1-5 MHz) probe provides improved depth penetration and is used to assess supradiaphragmatic structures (pleural space, lung). To optimize lung visualization with a single probe, frequently probes with emission frequencies of 5 to 7 MHz are used and are usually small with a tip shaped so that an acoustic window on the lung parenchyma can be obtained on intercostal spaces. The 5 MHz microconvex probe is frequently favored,[306,307] although curvilinear and phased-array probes are also appropriate.[308]

When examining the patient, a methodical approach should be used to ensure comprehensive assessment of lung structure and function. The I-AIM (Indication, Acquisition, Interpretation, Medical Decision-Making) framework has been recently proposed for point of care lung ultrasound.[308] A complete exam involves the bilateral assessment of the anterior, lateral, and posterior lung. Although protocols vary, in the supine patient, each hemithorax should be assessed in at least six zones during emergencies: two anterior (separated by the third intercostal space), two lateral, and two posterior. In routine assessments, 8-zone and 12-zone protocols are most commonly used.[308,310,311] Because of the significant acoustic impedance differences between air, tissue, and bone (ribs), thoracic ultrasound is based primarily on characteristic artifacts and not only on the visualization of anatomic structures.[312] Videos of 1 to 2 breaths should be acquired to take advantage of the lung dynamics in the findings. Machine settings should be optimized at the start of the examination.[308] Usually, studies are initiated with the identification of the ribs as hyperechoic lines producing significant ultrasonography shadow (Fig. 41.27*A*), followed by visualization of the pleural line approximately 0.5 to 1.0 cm deeper and between the ribs. This is typically a bright, slightly curved line. These are major structures to be identified, because many pathologies of relevance to the anesthesiologist affect their observed pattern. In the normal lung, lung sliding represents the

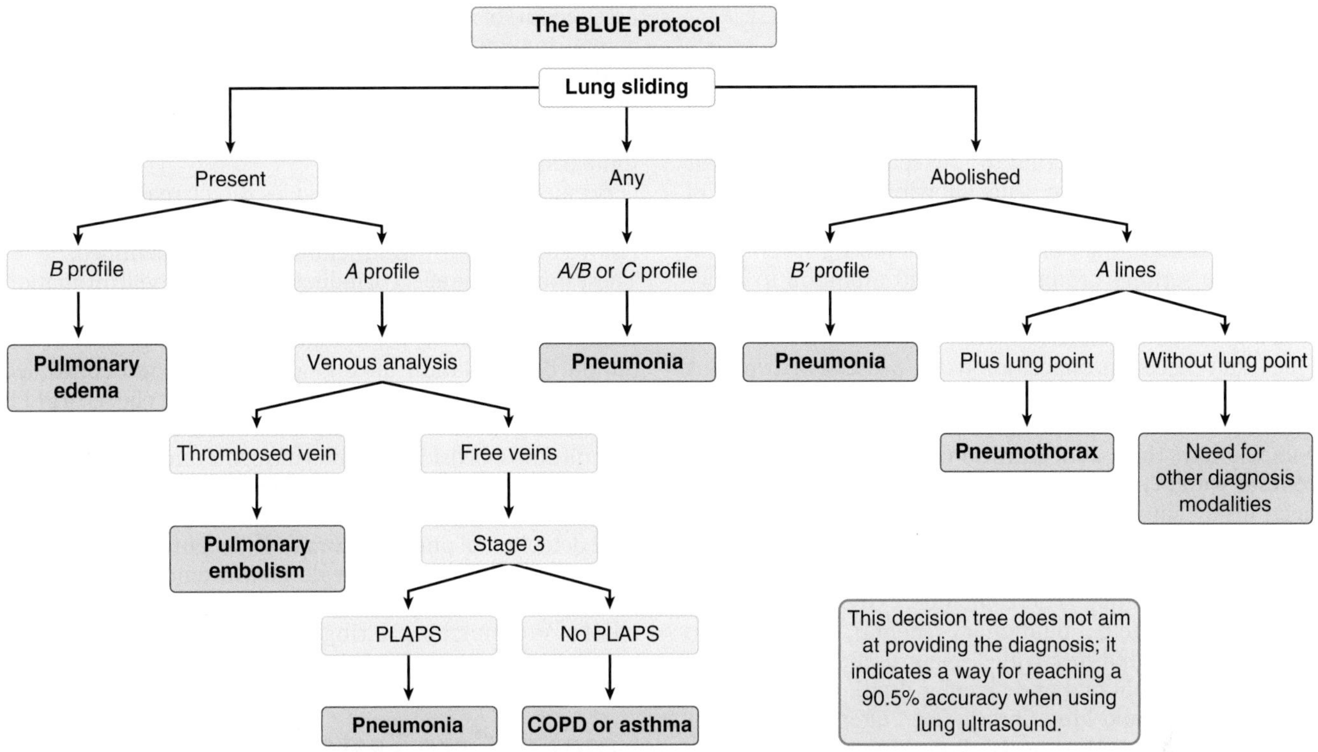

Fig. 41.28 **The BLUE protocol algorithm based on the particular ultrasound profile of the different kinds of respiratory failure. It uses three lung ultrasound signs with binary answers: anterior lung sliding, multiple B-lines visible between two ribs in the anterior lung, and posterior and/or lateral alveolar and/or pleural syndrome. These are combined with venous analysis to yield 90.5% accuracy in the diagnosis of respiratory failure.** ***COPD*, Chronic obstructive pulmonary disease; *PLAPS*, posterolateral alveolar and/or pleural syndrome.** (Redrawn from Lichtenstein DA, Mezière GA. Relevance of lung ultrasound in the diagnosis of acute respiratory failure: the BLUE protocol. *Chest.* 2008;134:117–125; Milner QJ, Mathews GR. An assessment of the accuracy of pulse oximeters. *Anaesthesia.* 2012;67:396–401; and Pologe JA. Pulse oximetry: technical aspects of machine design. *Int Anesthesiol Clin.* 1987;25:137–153.)

movement of the visceral on the parietal pleura during respiration and is another key sonographic finding to be appreciated. The magnitude of the movement is larger in regions closer to the diaphragm than those near the lung apex.

Below the pleura, hyperechoic horizontal reverberation artifacts at regular distances are referred to as A lines (see Fig. 41.27*A*). Another artifact is the B line, a discrete laser-like vertical hyperechoic reverberation artifact that arises from the pleural line (previously described as "comet tails"), extends to the bottom of the screen without fading, moves synchronously with lung sliding, and erases A lines (see Fig. 41.27*B* and *C*). Solitary B lines are a normal finding in the normal lung, and increased numbers are observed in disease. Based on the recognition of such artifacts, pathologic conditions are identified.[306-308,313] Most acute disorders involve the lung surface, and this explains the utility of thoracic ultrasound in visualizing them. Ultrasonography findings for pneumothorax are the absence of lung sliding, B lines, and lung pulse, and the presence of lung points.

Pleural effusions are characterized by a usually anechoic space between the parietal and visceral pleurae (see Fig. 41.27*C* and *F*) and by respiratory movement of the lung within the effusion ("sinusoid sign"). The presence of echogenic material within the effusion suggests an exudate or hemorrhage, although some exudates are anechoic. Most transudates are anechoic. The M-mode ultrasound scan shows parallel lines indicative of no moving structure underlying the probe. The ultrasonographic finding designated as a lung point is found in the presence of pneumothorax and represents the imaging of the cyclic transition during breathing from the absence of any sliding or moving B lines at a physical location (i.e., air with no lung parenchyma) to the visualization of lung sliding, B lines, or altered A lines indicative of lung tissue (see Fig. 41.27*D*).[307,314] Bedside ultrasound scans can detect pneumothorax with sensitivity similar to a CT scan.[306,307]

An interstitial syndrome is characterized by the presence of multiple B lines. A positive region is defined by three or more B lines in a longitudinal plane between two ribs (see Fig. 41.27*E*).[307] Lung consolidation is characterized sonographically by a subpleural echo-poor region or one with tissue-like echo-texture (see Fig. 41.27*F*). Lung consolidations may be caused by infection, pulmonary embolism, lung cancer and metastasis, compression atelectasis, obstructive atelectasis, and lung contusion. Additional sonographic signs that may help determine the cause of lung consolidation include the quality of the deep margins of the consolidation, the presence of comet-tail reverberation artifacts at the far-field margin, the presence of air or fluid bronchograms, and the vascular pattern within the consolidation. Advances in clinical research and experience in lung ultrasonography allowed for the proposal of an algorithm to assess severe dyspnea in the acute setting (Fig. 41.28). The denominated BLUE protocol is a stepwise ultrasonographic approach to the patient with acute respiratory failure that aims at expeditious diagnosis with 90.5% accuracy.[309,313,315]

ELECTRICAL IMPEDANCE TOMOGRAPHY

Electrical impedance tomography (EIT) is a noninvasive and radiation-free imaging modality used to assess regional lung function at the bedside. The method is clinically available and has moderate to low spatial resolution but high temporal resolution, thus allowing for assessment of regional ventilation in real-time.[235a,305,316] Its use in estimating regional lung volume and optimizing mechanical ventilation settings brought significant attention to applications in ICUs and operating rooms.[305]

EIT is based on electrical impedance, a physical variable that reflects the opposition to the passage of a current through an object when a voltage is applied across it.[317] The impedance of biological tissues depends on the tissue composition. High concentrations of electrolytes, extracellular water content, large cells, and number of cell connections by gap junctions as present in blood and muscles reduce impedance. Air, fat, and bone have high electrical impedance. Pathologic changes of tissue composition influence impedance. These include extravascular lung water (EVLW) (e.g., pulmonary edema), intrathoracic blood volume, fluid in cavities (pleural effusion, pericardial effusion, bronchial and alveolar fluid), foreign bodies (pleural drain), and lung fibrosis (e.g., after ARDs or as a primary disorder). During the breathing cycle, thoracic bioimpedance is influenced fundamentally by both ventilation and perfusion.

EIT relies on an array of electrodes (typically 16-32) around the chest region of interest. The location is chosen based on the clinical information desired, usually at the fifth intercostal space for standard lung assessment. The impedance information is provided in the form of a functional EIT image, or EIT waveforms that quantify changes in lung volume or perfusion in the studied thoracic cross section. Usually, images are presented with pixels representing relative impedance change, so-called functional EIT, because air corresponds to high impedances and fluid and tissue to low impedances, and the image represents regional lung ventilation. Absolute EIT (a-EIT) is the modality in which the image represents the actual impedance values. Direct assessment of lung conditions can be accomplished by comparing low impedance (e.g., hemothorax, pleural effusion, atelectasis and lung edema) with high impedance (e.g., pneumothorax, emphysema).[318] EIT has compared successfully with standard methods, including computed tomography.[319]

Because the technique provides direct real-time assessment of changes in regional aeration, several applications related to regional lung function have been identified.[316,319] These include the effect of induction and tracheal intubation on the expiratory lung level and regional ventilation in children (Fig. 41.29)[320]; perioperative monitoring of the distribution of ventilation during spontaneous and controlled breathing,[321,322] including HFOV[235a,278,323]; effects of PEEP on regional ventilation during laparoscopic surgery[324]; the magnitude of bedside lung recruitment; and PEEP titration with assessment of alveolar collapse and hyperdistention in ARDS[325] and obese patients.[326] EIT may also allow for real-time detection of pneumothorax.[327] Recent advances show the potential of EIT to provide measurements of regional perfusion,[319,328] which could be valuable for bedside assessment of $\dot{V}/\dot{Q}$ matching during spontaneous and mechanical ventilation.

Point of Care Tests

Point-of-care testing (POCT) is the performance of laboratory measurements near the site of patient care. POCT technology includes portable analyzers and use of small blood samples. For the anesthesiologist, it implies the availability of rapid, precise, and accurate measurements in operating rooms and ICUs. POCT yields improvements in patient outcome through expeditious detection of physiologic deterioration and prompt treatment. Respiratory monitoring is a major element of POCT and includes analysis of arterial blood gases (P_aO_2, P_aCO_2, pH), Hb, and lactate.

Blood gas measurements can be obtained with acceptable levels of accuracy and precision with POCT.[329-331] For instance, different platforms for arterial blood gases and Hb were found to show coefficients of variation of

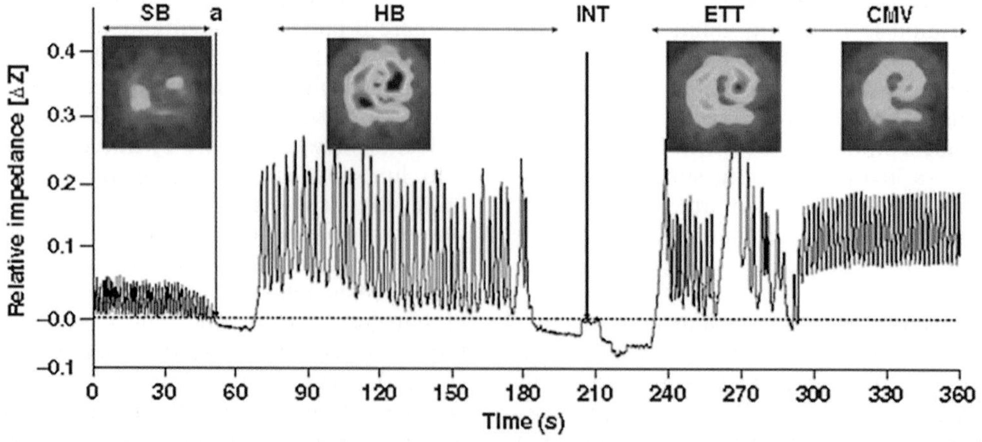

Fig. 41.29 Relative impedance signal at five key stages during induction of anesthesia in children. (a) There is a small impedance signal during spontaneous breathing *(SB)* as muscle paralysis develops. Effective hand bagging *(HB)* produces a high intensity signal, which is zeroed during tracheal intubation *(INT)*. Distribution of regional impedances during hand bagging with the endotracheal tube *(ETT)* and conventional mechanical ventilation *(CMV)* are also visualized. (From Humphreys S, Pham TM, Stocker C, Schibler A. The effect of induction of anesthesia and intubation on end-expiratory lung level and regional ventilation distribution in cardiac children. *Paediatr Anaesth*. 2011;21:887–893.)

approximately 3% to 6%.[330,331] Accuracy is present in wide ranges of P_aO_2 and pH[329-331], and shows bias of some devices for P_aCO_2.[331]

Hb is measured using either conductivity-based methods where hematocrit is assessed and the Hb concentration calculated (Hb [g/dL] = hematocrit × 0.34) or with optical methods, such as using the azide-metHb reaction and photometry absorbance.[332] Conductivity-based Hb measurements can be less than those reported by standard systems, with a clinically significant bias of at least −1.2 g/dL in the Hb range of 8.5 to 14.2 g/dL and a trend to underestimate the Hb value at low ranges.[330,331] Variable measurement agreement across devices, and bias resulting from inspired O_2 fraction are issues that still limit noninvasive Hb assessment.[331,333,334]

The site of blood sampling can influence POCT results. For capillary blood samples obtained from finger and ear punctures, a significant correlation exists between optical-based and automated laboratory Hb analysis, with a nonsignificant bias. Fingerstick samples may approximate standard laboratory Hb measurements better than earlobe samples.[22] Capillary blood samples (lancet puncture to middle or ring finger and fourth drop used) in patients with gastrointestinal bleeding resulted in high deviations (>1 g/dL) in 21% of cases and very high deviations (>2 g/dL) in 4% of cases.[335] In critically ill patients, poor agreement with reference measurements is reported,[336] especially with capillary blood samples and in patients with extremity pitting edema. POCT proved relevant in the assessment of arterial blood gases during pseudohypoxemia (also called "spurious hypoxemia" and "leukocyte larceny"). This is a known cause of inaccurate blood gas measurements and occurs when P_aO_2 is reduced by increased O_2 consumption as a result of markedly elevated white blood cell counts in the arterial blood sample. Measurement error is further aggravated by delayed laboratory analysis or incorrect sampling. Pseudohypoxemia occurs not only in hyperleukocytosis but also in thrombocytosis associated with polycythemia vera.

As POCT progresses, relevant limitations will need to be addressed, including cost, accuracy, data management, and evidence for improved outcomes. Contrary to some expectations, availability of POCT in academic centers does not increase the number of tests performed.[337] Characteristics of individual institutions should be considered before POCT is implemented. For instance, POCT blood-gas analysis may offer minimal time savings and cost benefits compared with central laboratory analysis in an institution with short turnaround time.

Respiratory Monitoring in Special Conditions

As methods for life support are advanced, the physiologic patterns that serve as the basis for assessment of gas exchange and respiratory mechanics can be dramatically changed. This occurs, for instance, during HFV when significant reductions in V_T are combined with large increases in respiratory rate. During rigid bronchoscopy or laryngeal interventions, the anesthesiologist is required to share management of the airway with the surgeon. This may result in intermittent loss of information regarding airway flow, volume, and pressure, as well as end-tidal gas concentration. In these situations, clinical assessment based on physical examination (i.e., inspection, auscultation) becomes paramount. Specific considerations for respiratory monitoring in special conditions are detailed in the next section.

HIGH-FREQUENCY VENTILATION

HFV is a ventilatory mode using V_T smaller than the anatomic dead space, 10-fold to 50-fold higher respiratory frequencies, and high instantaneous flow rates. The HFV is a broad term encompassing various modalities. These include high-frequency jet ventilation (HFJV) and high-frequency percussive ventilation (HFPV), both of which allow for passive exhalation, as well as HFOV, in which exhalation is actively driven by the device. The mechanisms for gas exchange during HFV are complex and include convective transport, turbulence, pendelluft, velocity profile distortion and asymmetry, Taylor dispersion, molecular diffusion, collateral ventilation, and cardiogenic mixing.[338-340] This method results in a fundamentally different relationship for CO_2 elimination ($\dot{V}_{CO_2}$) compared with conventional ventilation.[341] For example, during conventional ventilation,

$$\dot{V}_{CO_2} \propto f\,(V_T - V_D) \tag{41.39}$$

where f is the breathing frequency and V_D is dead space volume. However, during HFOV[342,342a],

$$\dot{V}_{CO_2} \propto f\frac{V_T^2}{V_D} \tag{41.40}$$

The use of HFOV for neonates in respiratory distress failing conventional ventilation is common.[343-345] However, its use in adult patients with ARDS has been limited in light of recent clinical trials,[345a,b] despite the sound physiologic rationale of using high mean airway pressures and low V_T to achieve alveolar recruitment without overdistention.[346-350]

Most high-frequency oscillators use pistons to actively drive flow into and out of the airway at respiratory rates between 3 to 20 Hz.[351,352] However, some oscillators, and most jet ventilators, rely on solenoid valves.[353-355] With HFOV, fresh gas and CO_2 may be removed by a continuous bias flow of warmed, humidified gas past the proximal end of the ETT, and mean airway pressure is regulated by an adjustable valve venting the bias flow and exhaled gas from the circuit. These devices may be either pressure or time cycled, and both the mean airway pressure and oscillatory pressure amplitude are displayed on the console to the clinician. However, for the frequencies used during HFV, a significant portion of the oscillatory pressure amplitude results from the inertia of the gas column contained in the breathing circuit and the patient's airways, and thus it should not be used as a surrogate for lung distention.

Clinically useful physiologic information inferred from airway flow and pressure measurements is somewhat limited during HFV. During conventional mechanical ventilation, airway pressure and flow are related according to basic mechanical properties of the respiratory system, such as airway resistance and tissue compliance. However, during HFV, airway pressure and flow reflect complex resistive and inertial gas properties in the central airways. Many investigators have assessed respiratory mechanics during HFV by transiently switching patients to conventional mechanical ventilation to obtain basic estimates of resistance and compliance,[356] or even making intermittent low-frequency oscillatory measurements to measure airway and tissue properties.[357] The pressure transmission index, defined as the ratio of the pressure measured directly in the trachea to the pressure at the proximal end of the breathing circuit (i.e., the pressure amplitude measured at the oscillator), is strongly correlated with tissue elastance.[357,358]

An important component of monitoring during any form of HFV is the assessment of mechanical function. Many important physiologic parameters, such as mean airway pressure and V_T, are not explicitly controlled by most high-frequency ventilators.[358a,b] Thus the relationship between pressure transduced at the proximal end of the breathing circuit and the V_T delivered to the patient is difficult to assess. Indeed, this relationship is highly nonlinear,[343] and it depends on frequency, gas composition and inertia, and the overall mechanics of the patient's respiratory system.[235,276] Given the important role that V_T plays in CO_2 elimination during HFV (Eq. [41.40]), accurate measurement of airway flow is important for the development and standardization of clinical trials.[359] Hot wire anemometry yields the most accurate estimates of airway flow and delivered V_T during HFOV compared with other measuring devices.[235,276]

Adequacy of gas exchange is essential during HFV. Analysis of arterial blood gas measurements should be performed within 30 minutes of any change in ventilator settings, and at least twice per day on stable settings.[346] Whereas oxygenation is usually assessed with continuous pulse oximetry, CO_2 elimination is more technically challenging to monitor. Attempts have been made to incorporate various forms of capnography into HFV circuits,[360-363] with varying degrees of success. Depending on where exhaled gases are sampled, there may be adequate correlation between $P_{ET}CO_2$ and P_aCO_2 during HFV.[362,363] This is often a reflection of the slower response time of many sidestream CO_2 analyzers.[171]. The PCO_2 sampled at the airway opening may thus underestimate the true alveolar CO_2 levels.[361] The most accurate measurement of alveolar PCO_2 is obtained when it is measured at the very distal tip of the ETT,[364] although this is not always clinically feasible. Transcutaneous measurements of PCO_2 may hold considerable promise for assessment of CO_2 clearance during HFV.[365]

Although HFOV has not been shown to improve outcomes in adult patients with ARDS,[345a,b] this finding may reflect the variable effects of frequency, amplitude, and mean airway pressure with oscillating of a heterogeneously injured lung,[342a,348] as well as the poorly understood phenomena of gas distribution, volume recruitment, and $\dot{V}/\dot{Q}$ matching in individual patients. Recent studies suggest that oscillation using multiple simultaneous frequencies may improve the efficiency of gas exchange, reduce the heterogeneity of parenchymal strain, and maintain lung recruitment at lower mean airway pressures.[235a,365a] Despite significant gaps in our understanding of the use of HFOV in acute respiratory failure, this modality may still have some clinical application as part of a lung-protective ventilatory strategy, particularly in patients with severe hypoxemia.[290a] Future clinical trials will guide both therapy and technologic development of HFOV,[347] thus providing a scientific basis for the rational use of this technology in critically ill patients.

JET VENTILATION

Jet ventilation is commonly used for procedures in which the surgeon requires unobstructed access to the airway.[366] During inspiration, O_2 or an O_2-air mixture is applied under high pressure to the airway through either a specialized catheter or a rigid bronchoscope. This jet of gas, along with entrained air from the surrounding environment, leads to insufflation of the lungs. Expiration takes place through passive recoil. The entire system is open to the environment, thus leading to significant escape of respiratory gases.[354]

Oxygenation during jet ventilation can be adequately monitored using pulse oximetry. Ascertaining the presence and adequacy of ventilation, especially during HFJV, is more challenging because the composition and volume of the exhaled gases cannot be directly measured. Arterial sampling of P_aCO_2 is accurate but intermittent and invasive. Gas can be sampled at the distal end of the catheter or rigid bronchoscope through a dedicated channel. Quantitative capnography during HFJV does not accurately reflect P_aCO_2 because V_T is smaller than dead space.[367] This problem can be overcome by the intermittent suspension of HFJV or reduction in frequency to 10 breaths/min or less. $P_{ET}CO_2$ measurements obtained in this manner accurately reflect the P_aCO_2 and allow the intermittent monitoring of ventilation.[363,368-370] The measurement of transcutaneous PCO_2 ($P_{tc}CO_2$) is noninvasive and continuous. Although $P_{tc}CO_2$ is not as accurate as capnometry and has a slower response time to changes in P_aCO_2, its use may allow for tracking of changes in P_aCO_2.[370] The absence of V_T and continuous $P_{ET}CO_2$ monitoring precludes standard ventilator disconnect monitoring during intraoperative HFJV. RIP, which uses changes in the inductance of bands placed around the chest to monitor respirations, has been demonstrated to discriminate reliably between the presence and absence of HFJV and may be developed as a monitor to detect disconnect or the absence of adequate thoracic excursion during HFJV.[282]

PATIENT TRANSPORT

Intrahospital transport of critically ill patients is a frequent occurrence. Transport of adult and pediatric patients from locations with advanced monitoring to more remote locations is fraught with difficulty, ranging from simple equipment malfunction to major disasters.[371-373] Complex monitoring and numerous pieces of equipment are often required for safe transfer, especially when additional devices such as extracorporeal membrane oxygenators and ventricular assist devices are present. The lack of standardized monitoring techniques and terminology explains the widely reported discrepancies in the incidence of adverse events. Overall, a high incidence of respiratory complications following transport has been reported.[372-374]

Respiratory monitoring during transport should ideally be the same as that in the operating room or ICU before relocation. In practice, at least clinical signs (e.g., skin color, chest expansion, auscultation, endotracheal secretions), pulse oximetry, and respiratory rate, together with EKGp and blood pressure, should be monitored throughout intrahospital transport. If a transport ventilator is used, airway pressures should be readily available in numeric or graphic formats. Human factors are essential during transport, and a specialized transport team using standardized management procedures with preparatory, transfer, and post-transport stabilization phases likely limits the frequency of adverse events.[375-377] This is particularly important when high-risk patients are involved.[376] Equipment and medications needed to establish and maintain a secure airway and hemodynamics should be available during any transfer. Adequate O_2 supply with functioning low-pressure alarms should be verified during pretransport preparation. A transport ventilator can provide better oxygenation and reduce variability in pH and PCO_2 compared with manual ventilation.[374,378] The transfer phase may require several professionals under the coordination and supervision of an attending anesthesiologist.

Automated Data Systems

Electronic anesthesia records are part of routine clinical practice in many institutions. Such systems provide data from medical devices, clinical information management systems, and laboratory data. The availability of large amounts of real-time data in digital form allows for introduction of new approaches to monitoring that may have been conceptualized, but not yet clinically implemented. In fact, although decision-support research has been done for years, little progress has been made in clinical decision support for the acute management of unstable patients, a major challenge in the operating room and ICU.[379-381] Computerized monitoring has significant potential to improve clinical monitoring.[379,382] However, it has limitations resulting from typical requirements not well-suited for human performance, such as monitoring graphic displays over extended periods, or the execution of overt responses to low-probability events. Humans are limited in their ability to analyze large quantities of data accurately and continuously. Accordingly, computer algorithms that identify subtle but meaningful trends in physiologic data are desirable. Such tools require relevant contextualization of measurement to improve accuracy, as well as minimization of false-negative and false-positive alarms. This automated monitoring should depend not only on timely measurements, but also on prior information. Alarms should not be fixed to specified thresholds, but rather dynamically adapted to information as it becomes available. Algorithms with established clinical rules provide the opportunity to detect subtle changes in time-series data,[383] which exceed human discrimination.[384] Such automated systems minimize monitoring failures and promote timely responses, thus enhancing the performance of anesthesia delivery during long periods. Some tools of respiratory monitoring have been assessed in adult and pediatric populations.[379,385-387] Data banks have been developed for research.[381] Another potential interest in these systems is that of creating closed-loop systems, such as those currently implemented to adjust settings in commercial mechanical ventilators.[386,388]

Although these methods are not currently established for clinical use, they are expected to find increasing application as reliable monitoring algorithms are implemented and validated. Such automated systems allow for the implementation of additional levels of safety. The detection of potentially dangerous events, such as continuously low S_aO_2 or the absence of $P_{ET}CO_2$ measurements for several breaths, can generate an automated alarm, a screen alert, or an automated page to the supervising anesthesiologist.[389] In a different condition, for example when changes in oxygenation occur over a period of minutes, improved processes should be directed to the anesthesia provider in direct contact with the patient, to initiate prompt treatment, assess artifacts, and/or call for assistance.[389]

Additional Monitored Variables

NITROGEN WASHOUT AND END-EXPIRATORY LUNG VOLUME

There has been a resurgence of interest in the use of nitrogen washout methods for adult[390,391] and pediatric[392] patients. Nitrogen washout techniques are found in commercial mechanical ventilators for intensive care use. The main parameter of interest has been the end-expiratory lung volume, a potentially valuable measurement to optimize lung expansion during mechanical ventilation, and for the assessment of ventilatory interventions such as PEEP adjustment.[391] The measurements are performed by introducing a step change in the inspired air (traditionally from room air to 100% O_2, in current systems a nitrogen washout/wash-in method with 10% to 20% change in F_IO_2) and solving mass balance equations for the lung volume. In patients with ARDS, measurements of end-expiratory lung volume demonstrated good accuracy and reproducibility, with a coefficient of variation of less than 4%.[391] In 30 intensive care patients undergoing computed tomography for clinical reasons, the end-expiratory lung volume measured with the modified nitrogen washout/wash-in technique was well correlated ($r^2 = 0.89$) with computed tomography measurements with a bias of 94 ± 143 mL (15 ± 18%, $P = .001$), within the limits of accuracy provided by the manufacturer.[390] Nitrogen washouts can also provide measures of ventilation heterogeneity.[392]

TRANSCUTANEOUS MEASUREMENTS OF PARTIAL PRESSURES OF OXYGEN AND CARBON DIOXIDE

Gas exchange is a dynamic and at times rapidly changing process. Conventional direct measurements of arterial blood gases, although still the gold standard for P_aO_2, P_aCO_2, and pH monitoring, provide only an isolated picture of that process. Expeditious assessment of circulating blood gases could facilitate faster initiation of required therapy and adjustment of implemented ventilation. A method for noninvasive continuous monitoring of P_aO_2 and P_aCO_2 is a current clinical need.

Transcutaneous measurements of PCO_2 ($P_{tc}CO_2$), in addition to transcutaneous PO_2 ($P_{tc}O_2$), aim to provide noninvasive estimates of arterial CO_2 and O_2, or at least trends associated with them. These measurements have been useful in intensive care management of neonates and infants,[393] and in the fields of wound healing and hyperbaric O_2 therapy. An advantage is that transcutaneous monitoring can be applied when expired gas sampling is limited such as during HFOV, apnea testing, and noninvasive ventilation. The measurements are based on the diffusion of O_2 and CO_2 through the skin. Because the skin is not entirely permeable to gases, warming is used to facilitate gas diffusion. Such an increase in temperature (usually 42°C-45°C) promotes increased O_2 and CO_2 partial pressure at the skin surface resulting from changes in structure of the stratum corneum that increase diffusion and dermal hyperemia and shift the Hb dissociation curve. This process ultimately results in arterialization of the regional blood. $P_{tc}O_2$ and $P_{tc}CO_2$ are influenced not only by the arterial gas partial pressures but also by skin O_2 consumption, CO_2 production, and regional blood flow. Accordingly, $P_{tc}O_2$ is usually lower than P_aO_2, and $P_{tc}CO_2$ is usually higher than P_aCO_2.

O_2 transducers are electrochemical polarographic Clark-type electrodes in which the rate of chemical reaction is related to an electrical signal proportional to the O_2 concentration. For CO_2, a transducer using a pH electrode to measure PCO_2 (Stow-Severinghaus electrode) is used, where a change in pH is proportional to the logarithm of the PCO_2 change. For CO_2 monitors, a temperature correction factor is used to estimate P_aCO_2 from $P_{tc}CO_2$. In vivo correction is available in some devices based on arterial blood gases. The thin epidermal layer of infants facilitates the measurements, in contrast to the diffusion barrier introduced by the thicker adult skin. A lower electrode temperature in $P_{tc}CO_2$ monitoring produces systematic bias of the transcutaneous electrode. However, in very preterm babies, monitoring at 40°C or 41°C to reduce the risk of burns is possible, provided a bias correction of 12% to 15% is applied.[394]

The main application of $P_{tc}CO_2$ is in the neonatal ICU population.[393] Even in very low-birth-weight infants, the mean difference between $P_{tc}CO_2$ and P_aCO_2 is 3.0 mm Hg (95% confidence interval, 0.2 to 6.0 mm Hg; $P < .05$).[395] In addition, $P_{tc}CO_2$ may be used to assess the efficacy of mechanical ventilation continuously during respiratory failure. In this setting, in children 1 to 16 years, $P_{tc}CO_2$ was more accurate and precise than $P_{ET}CO_2$ in relation to P_aCO_2. $P_{tc}CO_2$-P_aCO_2 differences were 2.3 ± 1.3 mm Hg in children 1 to 3.4 years old and 2.6 ± 2.0 mm Hg in children 4 to 16 years old.[393] $P_{ET}CO_2$−P_aCO_2 differences were larger (6.8 ± 5.1 and 6.4 ± 6.3 mm Hg) for the same age ranges. When compared with $P_{ET}CO_2$, $P_{tc}CO_2$ monitoring is equally accurate in patients with normal respiratory function. Accuracy and precision in the perioperative period of cardiac surgery for congenital heart disease in infants and children were better for $P_{tc}CO_2$ than $P_{ET}CO_2$ in relation to P_aCO_2, with the exception of patients receiving significant amounts of vasoactive medications and in low cardiac output states.

In adults, $P_{tc}CO_2$ has proven to be a less accurate and precise surrogate for P_aCO_2. Nonetheless, $P_{tc}CO_2$ could be suitable for specific conditions. Laparoscopic surgery with prolonged pneumoperitoneum is one condition in which $P_{tc}CO_2$ may be a more accurate estimate of P_aCO_2 compared with $P_{ET}CO_2$,[396] even for trending P_aCO_2.[397] During deep sedation for ambulatory hysteroscopy in healthy patients, earlobe $P_{tc}CO_2$ agreed better with P_aCO_2 than did nasal sidestream $P_{ET}CO_2$, with lower bias (1.7 vs. −7.0 mm Hg) and smaller mean differences to $PaCO_2$ (3.2 ± 2.6 vs. 8.0 ± 6.0 mm Hg).[398] The sensitivity of the $P_{tc}CO_2$ monitor for detecting P_aCO_2 values higher than 50 mm Hg was also greater than for $P_{ET}CO_2$ (66.7% vs. 33.3%; $P < .01$).[398] $P_{tc}CO_2$ is also helpful during weaning from mechanical ventilation after off-pump coronary artery bypass graft.[399] In adults admitted to an emergency department for acute respiratory failure, agreement between P_aCO_2 and $P_{tc}CO_2$ was 0.1 mm Hg, and the limits of agreement were from −6.0 to 6.2 mm Hg). In patients undergoing noninvasive ventilation, unacceptably wide variability may be observed.[400] In mechanically ventilated ICU patients, $P_{tc}CO_2$ correlated better and with less bias to P_aCO_2 than $P_{ET}CO_2$ even if still with sizeable variability (mean $P_{tc}CO_2 - P_aCO_2 = 2.2 \pm 5.7$ mm Hg).[401] $P_{tc}CO_2$ does not replace $P_{ET}CO_2$ monitoring, which remains the standard of care to confirm intratracheal placement of the ETT following intubation, or to actuate a disconnect alarm in the operating room.

$P_{tc}O_2$ from normal to extremely low-birth-weight infants agreed well with P_aO_2 measurements, with mean $P_{tc}O_2$−P_aO_2 difference 2.3 (−1.5 to 6.8) mm Hg, clinically acceptable in current neonational ICUs. $P_{tc}O_2$ in neonates is additionally important to detect hyperoxia, which is not feasible with pulse oximetry. The use of $P_{tc}O_2$ in adults has been focused on wound management, peripheral vascular disease, and hyperbaric medicine. Although attempts for applications in adults were promising, such as the use of $P_{tc}O_2$ to support resuscitative efforts,[402] measurements following off-pump coronary artery surgical procedures still present very high variability.[403] The dependence of $P_{tc}O_2$ on low-flow states has been used in conjunction with analysis of arterial blood gases to estimate adequacy of cutaneous blood flow and, by inference hemodynamic, stability.[404,405]

In summary, transcutaneous measurements are favorably positioned for continuous gas exchange monitoring in neonates and infants. In contrast, widespread applications of transcutaneous techniques in the perioperative settings are still hindered by limitations, such as poor cutaneous blood flow, need for frequent calibration, slow response time, and risk for skin burns with prolonged application.

LUNG WATER

Pulmonary edema is a hallmark of lung injury. It can result from increased hydrostatic pressure in the pulmonary capillaries (cardiogenic), increased permeability of the alveolar capillary membrane (noncardiogenic), and reduced lymphatic drainage from the lungs. Such mechanisms can be caused by pulmonary or extrapulmonary factors. For these reasons, interest in the development of methods to quantify EVLW has been considered, because this may assist in the diagnosis and management of those conditions, including early detection, differential diagnosis, fluid therapy, diuretics, and mechanical ventilation.[406] In patients, assessment of pulmonary edema is made with imaging techniques (e.g., chest radiography, ultrasonography, and computed tomography), thermodilution, bioimpedance, bioreactance, and remote dielectric sensing.

Imaging Techniques

The method used primarily in clinical practice remains bedside chest radiograph. It allows for semiquantitative assessment of EVLW, its distribution, and its possible etiology. The chest radiograph has limited diagnostic accuracy. This is because (1) edema may not be visible until the amount of lung water increases by 30%[407]; (2) any radiolucent material that fills the air spaces (e.g., alveolar hemorrhage, pus, and bronchoalveolar carcinoma) will produce a radiographic image similar to that of pulmonary edema; (3) technical issues including rotation, inspiration, positive-pressure ventilation, patient position, and underpenetration or overpenetration can reduce sensitivity and specificity; and (4) substantial interobserver variability exists in interpretation of chest radiographs.[408,409] Computed tomography is another radiographic technique to quantify EVLW. In animal experiments, computed tomography densitometry could detect an increase in EVLW by as little as 50%.[162] Computed tomography-based studies indicated that significant hypoxemia secondary to pulmonary edema may not develop until the increase in EVLW approaches 200% to 300%.[163] Lack of portability and high radiation exposure limit the use of computed tomography as a continuous intraoperative monitor. Positron emission tomography[165] and nuclear magnetic resonance[166] are imaging techniques that can assess lung water. However, they are not amenable for routine clinical use in the perioperative setting. Lung ultrasonography is garnering greater acceptance as another method for assessing lung edema.

Indicator Dilution Methods

Such measurements of EVLW have been expected to be superior to blood oxygenation and chest radiography. They are based on the kinetics of one or two tracers injected centrally and measured in an artery. Initial techniques were based on a double-indicator dilution method. These techniques gained renewed attention with the introduction of a clinical device to assess EVLW using the transpulmonary thermodilution technology, which facilitated bedside measurements.[410] The device uses cold saline as the single indicator injected in a central venous line. EVLW and additional hemodynamic parameters (i.e., cardiac output) are computed from the curve of temperature in the peripheral artery.[411] Good reproducibility and correlation can occur with gravimetric methods and can be a useful clinical and research tool. EVLW may be a predictor of mortality in patients with severe sepsis[412] and ARDS.[413,414] It is a diagnostic tool in detecting early pulmonary edema,[415,416] including reperfusion edema after pulmonary endarterectomy,[417] after lung transplantation,[418] and in evaluating the effect of ventilatory modes during esophagectomy.[419] The measurement has also been proposed to guide fluid therapy in ARDS[420] and subarachnoid hemorrhage,[421] as well as assess the effect of steroids during cardiac surgery.[422] EVLW was the primary outcome variable in clinical trials to study the efficacy of salbutamol to resolve pulmonary edema in patients with ARDS (the Beta-Agonist Lung Injury Trial)[423] and lung resection.[424]

The limitations on this technique derive from the considerable and at times conflicting assumptions.[411,425] Measurement premises include that the thermal indicator reaches all lung regions and equilibrates in all of them and that the central circulation volumes between the injection and temperature measurement sites can be described as a small number of individual well-mixed compartments, each showing a monoexponential decay of temperature with time. Experimental evidence indicated that assumptions for the method do not apply to all conditions; an important factor is the changes in the regional distribution of perfusion during lung injury.[411,426,427] These changes may compromise the measurement.[425] Indeed, redistribution of lung perfusion can produce measurement changes larger than those seen in the Beta-Agonist Lung Injury Trial between treatment and control groups.[423,426] Such results are also consistent with the influence of the type of lung injury on the accuracy of EVLW measurements,[428-430] as well as with the poor correlation between transpulmonary thermodilution EVLW and computed tomographic estimates of EVLW.[431,432] Thus the expected reliability of transpulmonary thermodilution EVLW to follow trends[433] cannot be taken for granted, and it requires interpretation in light of potential simultaneous changes in regional perfusion. Finally, the technique requires placement of arterial and central venous catheters, thereby increasing invasiveness.

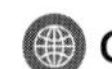 **Complete references available online at expertconsult.com.**

References

1. American Society of Anesthesiologists. *Standards for Basic Anesthetic Monitoring*; 2011.
2. International Task Force on Anaesthesia Safety. *World Federation of Societies of Anaesthesiologists: International Standards for a Safe Practice of Anaesthesia*; 2010.
3. Eichhorn JH, et al. *JAMA*. 1986;256:1017.
4. Botham KM, Mayes PA. Biologic oxidation, Harper's illustrated biochemistry. In: Murray RK, Rodwell VW, Bender D, Botham KM, Weil PA, Kennelly PJ, eds. *eBook Collection (EBSCOhost)*. 28th ed. McGraw-Hill Medical; 2009:98.
5. Severinghaus JW. *J Clin Monit Comput*. 2011;25:155.
6. Severinghaus JW. *Anesthesiology*. 2009;110:721.
7. Campbell S, et al. *Paediatr Anaesth*. 2011;21:815.
8. Kenzaka T, et al. *Intern Med*. 2012;51:871.
9. Welsby PD, Earis JE. *Postgrad Med J*. 2001;77:617.
10. Epstein O, et al. The respiratory system, Clinical examination. In: *Anonymous*. 4th ed. Elsevier Health Sciences; 2008.
11. Thomas C, Lumb AB. *Contin Educ Anaesth Crit Care Pain*. 2012;12:251.
12. Severinghaus JW. *Adv Exp Med Biol*. 1994;345:921.
13. Tremper KK, Barker SJ. *Anesthesiology*. 1989;70:98.
14. Severinghaus JW, Honda Y. *Int Anesthesiol Clin*. 1987;25:205.

14a. Pulse Oximeters https://www.fda.gov/RegulatoryInformation/Guidances/ucm341718.htm.

15. Milner QJ, Mathews GR. *Anaesthesia*. 2012;67:396.
16. Pologe JA. *Int Anesthesiol Clin*. 1987;25:137.
17. Merry AF, et al. *Can J Anaesth*. 2010;57:1027.
18. Haynes AB, et al. *N Engl J Med*. 2009;360:491.
19. Macknet MR, et al. *Anesth Analg*. 2010;111:1424.
20. Barker SJ, et al. *Anesthesiology*. 2006;105:892.
21. Roth D, et al. *Ann Emerg Med*. 2011;58:74.
22. Lamhaut L, et al. *Anesthesiology*. 2011;115:548.
23. Frasca D, et al. *Crit Care Med*. 2011;39:2277.
24. Berkow L, et al. *Anesth Analg*. 2011;113:1396.
25. Morey TE, et al. *Anesth Analg*. 2011;113:1289.
26. Shamir MY, et al. *Anesth Analg*. 2012;114:972.
27. Maisel WH, Lewis RJ. *Ann Emerg Med*. 2010;56:389.
28. Caboot JB, et al. *Pediatr Pulmonol*. 2012;47:808.
29. Feiner JR, et al. *Anesth Analg*. 2013;117:847.
30. Feiner JR, Bickler PE. *Anesth Analg*. 2010;111:1160.
31. Mahle WT, et al. *Circulation*. 2009;120:447.
32. Mahle WT, et al. *Pediatrics*. 2012;129:190.
33. Ewer AK, et al. *Lancet*. 2011;378:785.
34. Thangaratinam S, et al. *Lancet*. 2012;379:2459.
35. Dorlas JC, Nijboer JA. *Br J Anaesth*. 1985;57:524.
36. Cannesson M, et al. *Anesthesiology*. 2007;106:1105.
37. Cannesson M, et al. *Anesth Analg*. 2008;106:1189.
38. Cannesson M, et al. *Anesth Analg*. 2008;106:1195.
39. Yin JY, Ho KM. *Anaesthesia*. 2012;67:777.

40. Wu CY, et al. *Eur J Anaesthesiol.* 2016;33:645.
41. Sandroni C, et al. *Intensive Care Med.* 2012;38:1429.
42. Forget P, et al. *Anesth Analg.* 2010;111:910.
43. Gothgen IH, et al. *Scand J Clin Lab Invest Suppl.* 1990;203:87.
44. Perkins GD, et al. *Crit Care.* 2003;7:R67.
45. Van de Louw A, et al. *Intensive Care Med.* 2001;27:1606.
45a. Pedersen T, et al. *Cochrane Database Syst Rev.* 2014;(3):CD002013.
45b. Moller JT, et al. *Anesthesiology.* 1993;78(3):445.
45c. Ochroch EA, et al. *Anesth Analg.* 2006;102(3):868.
46. Mannheimer PD. *Anesth Analg.* 2007;105:S10.
47. Feiner JR, et al. *Anesth Analg.* 2007;105:S18.
48. Cox P. *Anesthesiology.* 2007;107:A1540.
49. Hinkelbein J, et al. *Resuscitation.* 2005;64:315.
50. Barker SJ. *Anesth Analg.* 2002;95:967.
51. Shah N, et al. *J Clin Anesth.* 2012;24:385.
52. Chan ED, et al. *Respir Med.* 2013;107:789.
53. Hampson NB. *Chest.* 1998;114:1036.
54. Eisenkraft JB. *Anesthesiology.* 1988;68:279.
55. Jay GD, et al. *Ann Emerg Med.* 1994;24:32.
56. Severinghaus JW, Koh SO. *J Clin Monit.* 1990;6:85.
57. Ortiz FO, et al. *Am J Respir Crit Care Med.* 1999;159:447.
58. Rajadurai VS, et al. *J Paediatr Child Health.* 1992;28:43.
59. Ahmed S, et al. *Eur J Haematol.* 2005;309:74.
60. Comber JT, Lopez BL. *Am J Emerg Med.* 1996;14:16.
61. Verhovsek M, et al. *Am J Hematol.* 2010;85:882.
62. Scheller MS, et al. *Anesthesiology.* 1986;65:550.
63. Hinkelbein J, et al. *Resuscitation.* 2007;72:82.
64. Hinkelbein J, et al. *Resuscitation.* 2007;74:75.
65. Adler JN, et al. *Acad Emerg Med.* 1998;5:965.
66. Bickler PE, et al. *Anesthesiology.* 2005;102:715.
67. Amar D, et al. *J Clin Monit.* 1989;5:135.
68. Trivedi NS, et al. *J Clin Anesth.* 1997;9:179.
69. Fluck RR Jr, et al. *Respir Care.* 2003;48:677.
70. van Oostrom JH, et al. *Can J Anaesth.* 2005;52:379.
71. Mathes AM, et al. *Anesth Analg.* 2008;107:541.
72. Kelleher JF, Ruff RH. *Anesthesiology.* 1989;71:787.
73. Zoremba N, et al. *Acta Anaesthesiol Scand.* 2011;55:322.
74. Oleyar M, et al. *J Cardiothorac Vasc Anesth.* 2010;24:820.
75. Mabadeje O, et al. *J Hosp Infect.* 2010;76:93.
76. Evans ML, Geddes LA. *Med Instrum.* 1988;22:29.
77. Sinex JE. *Am J Emerg Med.* 1999;17:59.
78. Berkenbosch JW, Tobias JD. *Respir Care.* 2006;51:726.
79. MacLeod DB, et al. *Anaesthesia.* 2005;60:65.
80. Kulcke A, et al. *Anesth Analg.* 2016;122:1856.
81. Smit M, al ety. *J Cardiothorac Vasc Anesth.* 2016;30:379.
82. Jenstrup M, et al. *Acta Anaesthesiol Scand Suppl.* 1995;107:29.
83. Harms MP, et al. *Exp Physiol.* 2003;88:611.
84. Ho KM, et al. *Shock.* 2008;29:3.
85. Dahn MS, et al. *Intensive Care Med.* 1988;14:373.
86. Martin C, et al. *Intensive Care Med.* 1992;18:101.
87. Varpula M, et al. *Intensive Care Med.* 2006;32:1336.
88. Ho KM, et al. *J Cardiothorac Vasc Anesth.* 2010;24:434.
89. Reinhart K, et al. *Chest.* 1989;95:1216.
90. Chawla LS, et al. *Chest.* 2004;126:1891.
91. Dueck MH, et al. *Anesthesiology.* 2005;103:249.
92. Lorentzen AG, et al. *J Cardiothorac Vasc Anesth.* 2008;22:853.
93. Grissom CK, et al. *Crit Care Med.* 2009;37:2720.
94. Kopterides P, et al. *Shock.* 2009;31:561.
95. Dahmani S, et al. *Eur J Anaesthesiol.* 2010;27:714.
96. Lequeux PY, et al. *Eur J Anaesthesiol.* 2010;27:295.
97. Lamia B, et al. *Minerva Anestesiol.* 2006;72:597.
98. Suter PM, et al. *Crit Care Med.* 1975;3:175.
99. Pond CG, et al. *J Cardiothorac Vasc Anesth.* 1992;6:280.
100. Maddirala S, Khan A. *Crit Care Clin.* 2010;26:323.
101. Scuderi PE, et al. *Anesthesiology.* 1994;81:245.
102. Baulig W, et al. *J Clin Monit Comput.* 2008;22:183.
103. Baulig W, et al. *Eur J Anaesthesiol.* 2010;27:720.
104. Schmidt CR, et al. *Crit Care Med.* 1984;12:523.
105. Routsi C, et al. *Anesth Analg.* 1993;77:1104.
106. Polonen P, et al. *Acta Anaesthesiol Scand.* 1997;41:810.
107. Pearse R, et al. *Crit Care.* 2005;9:R694.
108. Collaborative Study Group on Perioperative Scvo2 Monitoring. *Crit Care.* 2006;10:R158.
109. Polonen P, et al. *Anesth Analg.* 2000;90:1052.
110. Rivers E, et al. *N Engl J Med.* 2001;345:1368.
111. Donati A, et al. *Chest.* 2007;132:1817.
112. Dellinger RP, et al. *Crit Care Med.* 2008;36:296.
113. Otero RM, et al. *Chest.* 2006;130:1579.
114. Bellomo R, et al. *Crit Care.* 2008;12:130.
115. Peake SL, et al. *Resuscitation.* 2009;80:811.
116. Jones AE, et al. *JAMA.* 2010;303:739.
117. Suehiro K, et al. *J Cardiothorac Vasc Anesth.* 2014;28:528.
118. Bickler P, et al. *Anesth Analg.* 2017;124:72.
119. Ubbink R, et al. *J Clin Monit Comput.* 2017;31:1143.
120. Wahr JA, et al. *J Cardiothorac Vasc Anesth.* 1996;10:406.
121. Cui W, et al. *Opt Lett.* 1991;16:1632.
122. Schober P, Schwarte LA. *J Clin Monit Comput.* 2012;26:255.
123. Jobsis FF. *Science.* 1977;198:1264.
124. Watzman HM, et al. *Anesthesiology.* 2000;93:947.
125. Sakr Y, et al. *Eur J Anaesthesiol.* 2010;27:388.
126. Holzle F, et al. *Int J Oral Maxillofac Surg.* 2010;39:21.
127. Karliczek A, et al. *Colorectal Dis.* 2010;12:1018.
128. Pham TH, et al. *Ann Thorac Surg.* 2011;91:380.
129. Friedland S, et al. *Gastrointest Endosc.* 2003;57:492.
130. Friedland S, et al. *Gastrointest Endosc.* 2007;65:294.
131. Bludau M, et al. *Ann Thorac Surg.* 2010;90:1121.
132. Highton D, et al. *Curr Opin Anaesthesiol.* 2010;23:576.
133. Chan MJ, et al. *J Cardiothorac Vasc Anesth.* 2017;31:1155.
134. Murkin JM, et al. *Anesth Analg.* 2007;104:51.
135. Slater JP, et al. *Ann Thorac Surg.* 2009;87:36. discussion 44.
136. Yao FS, et al. *J Cardiothorac Vasc Anesth.* 2004;18:552.
137. Fischer GW, et al. *J Thorac Cardiovasc Surg.* 2011;141:815.
138. de Tournay-Jette E, et al. *J Cardiothorac Vasc Anesth.* 2011;25:95.
139. Ghosal S, et al. *J Cardiothorac Vasc Anesth.* 2018;32:1185.
140. Kirkpatrick PJ, et al. *J Neurosurg.* 1998;89:389.
141. Grubhofer G, et al. *Anesth Analg.* 2000;91:1339.
142. Vets P, et al. *Acta Anaesthesiol Belg.* 2004;55:215.
143. Al-Rawi PG, Kirkpatrick PJ. *Stroke.* 2006;37:2720.
144. Moritz S, et al. *Anesthesiology.* 2007;107:563.
145. de Letter JA, et al. *Neurol Res.* 1998;20(suppl 1):S23.
146. Hirofumi O, et al. *J Clin Neurosci.* 2003;10:79.
147. Rigamonti A, et al. *J Clin Anesth.* 2005;17:426.
148. Yamamoto K, et al. *Int Angiol.* 2007;26:262.
149. Jonsson M, et al. *Eur J Vasc Endovasc Surg.* 2017;53:783.
150. Samra SK, et al. *Anesthesiology.* 2000;93:964.
151. Mille T, et al. *Eur J Vasc Endovasc Surg.* 2004;27:646.
152. Boezeman RP, et al. *Ann Thorac Surg.* 2015;99:1267.
153. Casati A, et al. *Anesth Analg.* 2005;101:740.
154. Tang L, et al. *Br J Anaesth.* 2012;108:623.
155. Murphy GS, et al. *Anesth Analg.* 2010;111:496.
156. Moerman AT, et al. *Eur J Anaesthesiol.* 2012;29:82.
157. Tange K, et al. *Minerva Anestesiol.* 2010;76:485.
158. Crookes BA, et al. *J Trauma.* 2005;58:806. discussion 813.
159. Cohn SM, et al. *J Trauma.* 2007;62:44. discussion 54.
160. Ikossi DG, et al. *J Trauma.* 2006;61:780. discussion 788.
161. Yu Y, et al. *Cochrane Database Syst Rev.* 2018;1:CD010947.
162. Sun X, et al. *Br J Anaesth.* 2015;114:276.
163. Bohr C. *Skandinavisches Archiv Für Physiologie.* 1891;2:236.
164. Mogue LR, Rantala B. *J Clin Monit.* 1988;4:115.
165. Bhavani-Shankar K, et al. *J Clin Monit.* 1995;11:175.
166. Gravenstein JS, et al. *Capnography in Clinical Practice.* Boston: Butterworth; 1989.
167. Gravenstein JS, et al. *Gas Monitoring in Clinical Practice.* Boston: Butterworth-Heinemann; 1995.
168. Jaffe MB. *Anesth Analg.* 2008;107:890.
169. Raemer DB, Calalang I. *J Clin Monit.* 1991;7:195.
170. Hess D. *Respir Care.* 1990;35:557.
171. Brunner JX, Westenskow DR. *Br J Anaesth.* 1988;61:628.
172. Jaffe MB. *Mainstream or Sidestream Capnography? Technical Considerations.* Wallingford, Conn: Respironics Novametric; 2002.
173. Kaczka DW, et al. *J Appl Physiol.* 2011;110:1473.
174. Bhavani-Shankar K, Philip JH. *Anesth Analg.* 2000;91:973.
175. Moon RE, Camporesi EM. Respiratory monitoring. In: Miller RD, ed. *Miller's Anesthesia.* 6th ed. New York: Churchill Livingstone; 2005:1255–1295.
175a. Mondoñedo JR, et al. *ASME J of Medical Diagnostics.* 2018;1(031003):031003–031010.
176. Fletcher R, et al. *Br J Anaesth.* 1981;53:77.
177. McKenzie DC. *Br J Sports Med.* 2012;46:381.
178. Grocott MP, et al. *N Engl J Med.* 2009;360:140.

179. Wagner PD, et al. *J Clin Invest.* 1974;54:54.
180. Ravin MB, et al. *J Appl Physiol.* 1965;20:1148.
181. Brismar B, et al. *Anesthesiology.* 1985;62:422.
182. Rothen HU, et al. *Br J Anaesth.* 1998;81:681.
183. Riley RL, Cournand A. *J Appl Physiol.* 1949;1:825.
184. Whiteley JP, et al. *Br J Anaesth.* 2002;88:771.
185. Gould MK, et al. *Crit Care Med.* 1997;25:6.
186. McCahon RA, et al. *Br J Anaesth.* 2008;101:358.
187. Kathirgamanathan A, et al. *Br J Anaesth.* 2009;103:291.
188. Lilienthal JL Jr, Riley RL. *Am J Physiol.* 1946;147:199.
189. Mellemgaard K. *Acta Physiol Scand.* 1966;67:10.
190. Gowda MS, Klocke RA. *Crit Care Med.* 1997;25:41.
191. Definition Task Force ARDS, Ranieri VM, et al. *JAMA.* 2012;307:2526.
192. Rice TW, et al. *Chest.* 2007;132:410.
193. Khemani RG, et al. *Crit Care Med.* 2012;40:1309.
194. DesPrez K, et al. *Chest.* 2017;152:1151–1158.
195. Villar J, et al. *BMJ Open.* 2015;5. e006812,2014-006812.
196. Balzer F, et al. *BMC Anesthesiol.* 2016;16:108. 016-0272-4.
197. Ortiz RM, et al. *Pediatr Clin North Am.* 1987;34:39–46.
198. Trachsel D, et al. *Am J Respir Crit Care Med.* 2005;172:206–211.
199. Gajic O, et al. *Crit Care.* 2007;11:R53.
200. Kaczka DW, et al. *Anesthesiology.* 2015;123:1394.
201. Christiansen J, et al. *J Physiol.* 1914;48:244.
202. Severinghaus JW, Astrup PB. *J Clin Monit.* 1986;2:125.
203. Severinghaus JW. *Anesthesiology.* 2002;97:253.
204. Andritsch RF, et al. *Anesthesiology.* 1981;55:311.
205. Kern FH, Greeley WJ. *J Cardiothorac Vasc Anesth.* 1995;9:215.
206. Burrows FA. *J Cardiothorac Vasc Anesth.* 1995;9:219.
207. Patel RL, et al. *J Thorac Cardiovasc Surg.* 1996;111:1267.
208. Engelhardt W, et al. *Acta Anaesthesiol Scand.* 1996;40:457.
209. du Plessis AJ, et al. *J Thorac Cardiovasc Surg.* 1997;114:991. discussion 1000.
210. Bellinger DC, et al. *J Thorac Cardiovasc Surg.* 2001;121:374.
211. Kiziltan HT, et al. *Anesth Analg.* 2003;96:644.
212. Piccioni MA, et al. *Artif Organs.* 2004;28:347.
213. Sakamoto T, et al. *J Thorac Cardiovasc Surg.* 2004;127:12.
214. Hoover LR, et al. *Anesth Analg.* 2009;108:1389.
215. Nagy ZL, et al. *Circulation.* 2003;108:577.
216. Murkin JM, et al. *J Thorac Cardiovasc Surg.* 1995;110:349.
217. Svyatets M, et al. *J Cardiothorac Vasc Anesth.* 2010;24:644.
218. Biswas CK, et al. *Br Med J (Clin Res Ed).* 1982;284:923.
219. Kaczka DW, et al. Computational analyses of airway flow and lung tissue dynamics, image-based computational modeling of the human circulatory and pulmonary systems: methods and applications. In: Chandran KB, Udaykumar HS, Reinhardt JM, eds. *Image-based computational modeling of the human circulatory and pulmonary systems: Methods and applications.* 1st ed. New York: Springer; 2011:375,402; 10.
220. Kaczka DW, Smallwood JL. *Respir Physiol Neurobiol.* 2012;183:75.
221. Warner DO. *J Clin Monit Comput.* 2000;16:417.
222. Bates JHT. *Lung Mechanics: An Inverse Modeling Approach.* Cambridge: Cambridge University Press; 2009:220.
223. Pedley TJ, et al. *Respir Physiol.* 1970;9:387.
224. Rohrer F. *Pfluegers Arch Gesamte Physiol Menschen Tiere.* 1915;162:225.
225. Mora R, et al. *Am J Physiol Lung Cell Mol Physiol.* 2000;279:L342.
226. Fredberg JJ, Stamenovic D. *J Appl Physiol.* 1989;67:2408.
227. Fredberg JJ, et al. *Am J Respir Crit Care Med.* 1997;156:1752.
228. McIlroy MB, et al. *J Appl Physiol.* 1955;7:485.
229. Bachofen H. *J Appl Physiol.* 1968;24:296.
230. Hantos Z, et al. *J Appl Physiol.* 1992;72:168.
231. Kaczka DW, et al. *J Appl Physiol.* 1997;82:1531.
232. Hoppin FG Jr, Hildebrandt J. Mechanical properties of the lung. In: West JB, ed. *Bioengineering Aspects of the Lung.* New York: Marcel Dekker; 1977:83–162.
232a. Kano S, et al. *J Appl Physiol (1985).* 1994;77:1185.
232b. Amini R, et al. *IEEE Trans Biomed Eng.* 2017;64:681.
232c. Carvalho AR, et al. *Intensive Care Med.* 2008;34:2291.
232d. Carvalho AR, et al. *Anesth Analg.* 2013;116:677.
232e. D'Antini D, et al. *Anesth Analg.* 2018;126:143.
232f. Ranieri VM, et al. *Anesthesiology.* 2000;93:1320.
232g. Motulsky H, Christopoulos A. *Fitting Models to Biological Data using Linear and Nonlinear Regression. A Practical Guide to Curve Fitting.* New York: Oxford University Press; 2004:351.
232h. Huhle R, et al. *Anesth Analg.* 2018;126:725.
232i. Formenti P, et al. *Intensive Care Med.* 2011;37:561.
232j. Chiumello D, Gattinoni L. *Intensive Care Med.* 2011;37:561.
232k. Henzler D, et al. *Anesth Analg.* 2007;105(1072). table of contents.
233. Otis AB, et al. *J Appl Physiol.* 1956;8:427.
233a. Kaczka DW, et al. *Ann Biomed Eng.* 2011;39:1112.
233b. Suki B, Bates JHT. *J Appl Physiol (1985).* 2011;110:1111.
233c. Carvalho AR. *Crit Care.* 2007;11:R86.
233d. Dellacà RL. *Intensive Care Medicine.* 2011;37:1021.
233e. Zannin E, et al. *Crit Care.* 2012;16:R217.
233f. Writing Group for the Alveolar Recruitment for Acute Respiratory Distress Syndrome, Trial I, Cavalcanti AB, et al. *JAMA.* 2017;318:1335.
233g. Fumagalli J, et al. *Crit Care Med.* 2017;45(8):1374.
234. Mead J. *J Appl Physiol.* 1956;9:208.
235. Hager DN, et al. *Crit Care Med.* 2007;35:1522.
235a. Kaczka DW, et al. *Anesthesiology.* 2015;123:1394.
235b. Amini R, Kaczka DW. *Ann Biomed Eng.* 2013;41:2699.
236. Kaczka DW, et al. *Ann Biomed Eng.* 1995;23:135.
237. Peslin R, et al. *Eur Respir J.* 1992;5:871.
238. Ruiz-Ferron F, et al. *Intensive Care Med.* 2001;27:1487.
239. Kaczka DW, et al. *J Appl Physiol.* 2001;90:1833.
240. Kaczka DW, et al. *Ann Biomed Eng.* 2011;39:1112.
241. Downie JM, et al. *Am J Respir Crit Care Med.* 2004;169:957.
242. Lu Q, Rouby JJ. *Critical Care.* 2000;4:91.
243. Salazar E, Knowles JH. *J Appl Physiol.* 1964;19:97.
244. Venegas JG, et al. *J Appl Physiol.* 1998;84:389.
245. Mead J, et al. *J Appl Physiol.* 1957;10:191.
246. Bates JH, Irvin CG. *J Appl Physiol.* 2002;93:705.
247. Hildebrandt J. *J Appl Physiol.* 1970;28:365.
248. Otis AB, et al. *J Appl Physiol.* 1950;2:592.
249. Bates JHT, Milic-Emili J. *Ann Biomed Eng.* 1993;21:489.
249a. Moraes L, et al. *Front Physiol.* 2018;9:318.
249b. Cressoni M, et al. *Anesthesiology.* 2016;124:1100.
249c. Gattinoni L, et al. *Intensive Care Med.* 2016;42:1567.
249d. Santos RS, et al. *Anesthesiology.* 2018;128:1193.
250. Masselli GM, et al. *Conf Proc IEEE Eng Med Biol Soc.* 2006;1:5603.
251. Jensen A, Lutchen KR, Kaczka DW, et al. Estimation of respiratory dynamic mechanical properties during clinically used mechanical ventilation. In: *Proceedings of the first joint BMES/EMBS Conference.* Vol 1. Atlanta: IEEE; 1999:337.
252. Lancaster CT, Boyle PM, Kaczka DW. Delivered tidal volume from the Fabius GS depends upon breathing circuit configuration despite compliance compensation. In *Proceedings of the American Society of Anesthesiologists 2005 Annual Meeting,* Atlanta, 2005, abstract A863.
253. Loring SH, et al. *J Appl Physiol.* 2010;108:512.
253a. Akoumianaki E, et al. *Am J Respir Crit Care Med.* 2014;189:520.
254. Schuessler TF, et al. *Ann Biomed Eng.* 1998;26:260.
255. Hager DN, Brower RG. *Crit Care Med.* 2006;34:1544.
256. Talmor D, et al. *N Engl J Med.* 2008;359:2095.
256a. Eichler L, et al. *Obes Surg.* 2018;28:122.
257. Schultz MJ, et al. *Anesthesiology.* 2007;106:1226.
257a. Mauri T, et al. *Intensive Care Med.* 2016;42:1360.
257b. Yoshida T, et al. *Am J Respir Crit Care Med.* 2018;197(1018).
257c. Amato MB, et al. *N Engl J Med.* 2015;372:747.
257d. Bugedo G, et al. *Crit Care.* 2017;21:199.
258. Ladha K, et al. *BMJ.* 2015;351:h3646.
259. Neto AS, et al. *Lancet Respir Med.* 2016;4:272.
260. Laghi F, Goyal A. *Minerva Anestesiol.* 2012;78:201.
261. Brochard L. *Intensive Care Med.* 2002;28:1552.
262. McCall CB, et al. *J Appl Physiol.* 1957;10:215.
263. Lutchen KR, et al. *J Appl Physiol.* 1993;75:2549.
264. Jackson AC, Vinegar A. *J Appl Physiol.* 1979;47:462.
265. Schuessler TF, Bates JHT. *IEEE Trans Biomed Eng.* 1995;42:860.
266. Schuessler TF, Bates JHT, Maksym GN. Estimating tracheal flow in small animals: Engineering in Medicine and Biology Society, 1993. In: *Proceedings of the 15th Annual International Conference of the IEEE.* 1993:560–561.
267. Simon BA, Mitzner W. *IEEE Trans Biomed Eng.* 1991;38:214.
268. Sullivan WJ, et al. *Respir Care.* 1984;29:736.
269. Yeh MP, et al. *J Appl Physiol.* 1982;53:280.
270. Renzi PE, et al. *J Appl Physiol.* 1990;68:382.
271. Jaffe MB. *IEEE Eng Med Biol Mag.* 2010;29:44.
272. Plakk P, et al. *Med Biol Eng Comput.* 1998;36(17).

273. Ligeza P. *Rev Sci Instrum*. 2008;79(096105).
274. Al-Salaymeh A, et al. *Med Eng Phys*. 2004;26:623.
275. Ligeza P. *Rev Sci Instrum*. 2007;78(075104).
276. Hager DN, et al. *Crit Care Med*. 2006;34:751.
276a. Mondonedo JR, et al. *J Clin Monit Comput*. 2017;31:1263.
276b. Farre R, et al. *Medical & Biological Engineering & Computing*. 1991;29:18.
276c. Jandre FC, et al. *Respir Physiol Neurobiol*. 2005;148:309–314.
277. Schmolzer GM, et al. *Arch Dis Child Fetal Neonatal Ed*. 2010;95:F295.
278. Wolf GK, Arnold JH. *Crit Care Med*. 2005;33:S163.
279. Stick SM, et al. *Pediatr Pulmonol*. 1992;14:187.
280. van Vonderen JJ, et al. *Arch Dis Child Fetal Neonatal Ed*. 2015;100:F514.
281. Khemani RG, et al. *Am J Respir Crit Care Med*. 2016;193:198.
282. Atkins JH, et al. *Anesth Analg*. 2010;111:1168.
283. Greenstein YY, et al. *J Bronchology Interv Pulmonol*. 2017;24:206.
284. Mandel JE, Atkins JH. *Anesth Analg*. 2016;122:126.
285. Overdyk FJ, et al. *Anesth Analg*. 2007;105:412.
286. Walther-Larsen S, Rasmussen LS. *Acta Anaesthesiol Scand*. 2006;50:888.
287. Folke M, et al. *Med Biol Eng Comput*. 2003;41:377.
288. Al-Khalidi FQ, et al. *Pediatr Pulmonol*. 2011;46:523.
289. Wiklund L, et al. *J Clin Anesth*. 1994;6:182.
290. Lam T, et al. *Anesth Analg*. 2017;125:2019.
290a. Meade MO, et al. *Am J Respir Crit Care Med*. 2017;196:727.
291. Gaucher A, et al. *Br J Anaesth*. 2012;108:316.
292. Kasuya Y, et al. *Anesthesiology*. 2009;111:609.
293. Chang KC, et al. *J Clin Monit Comput*. 2016;30:169.
294. Cashman JN, Dolin SJ. *Br J Anaesth*. 2004;93(212).
295. Walder B, et al. *Acta Anaesthesiol Scand*. 2001;45:795.
296. Shapiro A, et al. *J Clin Anesth*. 2005;17:537.
297. Nassi N, et al. *Arch Dis Child*. 2008;93:126.
298. Lightdale JR, et al. *Pediatrics*. 2006;117:e1170.
299. Waisman D, et al. *Intensive Care Med*. 2011;37:1174.
300. Curry J, Lynn L. *APSF Newsletter*. 2011;26:32.
301. Gupta R, Edwards D. *APSF Newsletter*. 2018;32:70–72.
302. Gupta K, et al. *Curr Opin Anaesthesiol*. 2018;31:110.
303. Simon BA, et al. *J Appl Physiol*. 2012;113:647.
304. Harris RS, Schuster DP. *J Appl Physiol*. 2007;102:448.
305. Bodenstein M, et al. *Crit Care Med*. 2009;37:713.
306. Turner JP, Dankoff J. *Emerg Med Clin North Am*. 2012;30:451.
307. Volpicelli G, et al. *Intensive Care Med*. 2012;38:577.
308. Kruisselbrink R, et al. *Anesthesiology*. 2017;127:568.
309. Lichtenstein DA. *Chest*. 2015;147:1659.
310. Lichtenstein DA, et al. *Intensive Care Med*. 2004;30:276.
311. Lichtenstein D, et al. *Anesthesiology*. 2004;100:9.
312. Lichtenstein DA. *Crit Care Med*. 2007;35:S250.
313. Lichtenstein D. *Minerva Anestesiol*. 2009;75:313.
314. Lichtenstein D, et al. *Intensive Care Med*. 2000;26:1434.
315. Lichtenstein DA, Meziere GA. *Chest*. 2008;134:117.
316. Adler A, et al. *Physiol Meas*. 2012;33:679.
317. Costa EL, et al. *Curr Opin Crit Care*. 2009;15:18.
318. Hahn G, et al. *Physiol Meas*. 2006;27:S187.
319. Frerichs I, et al. *Thorax*. 2017;72:83.
320. Humphreys S, et al. *Paediatr Anaesth*. 2011;21:887.
321. Victorino JA, et al. *Am J Respir Crit Care Med*. 2004;169:791.
322. Radke OC, et al. *Anesthesiology*. 2012;116:1227.
323. Frerichs I, et al. *J Crit Care*. 2012;27:172.
324. Karsten J, et al. *Acta Anaesthesiol Scand*. 2011;55:878.
325. Costa EL, et al. *Intensive Care Med*. 2009;35:1132.
326. Nestler C, et al. *Br J Anaesth*. 2017;119:1194.
327. Costa EL, et al. *Crit Care Med*. 2008;36:1230.
328. Borges JB, et al. *J Appl Physiol*. 2012;112:225.
329. Kok J, et al. *Pathology*. 2015;47:405.
330. Leino A, Kurvinen K. *Clin Chem Lab Med*. 2011;49:1187.
331. Luukkonen AA, et al. *Clin Chem Lab Med*. 2016;54:585.
332. Hopfer SM, et al. *Ann Clin Lab Sci*. 2004;34:75.
333. Gayat E, et al. *Anesth Analg*. 2017;124:1820.
334. Allardet-Servent J, et al. *PLoS One*. 2017;12:e0169593.
335. Van de Louw A, et al. *Intensive Care Med*. 2007;33:355.
336. Seguin P, et al. *J Crit Care*. 2011;26:423.
337. Wax DB, Reich DL. *Anesth Analg*. 2007;105:1711.
338. Chang HK. *J Appl Physiol*. 1984;56:553.
339. Pillow JJ. *Crit Care Med*. 2005;33:S135.
340. Fredberg JJ. *J Appl Physiol*. 1980;49:232.
341. Hurst JM, et al. *Ann Surg*. 1990;211:486.
342. Venegas JG, et al. *J Appl Physiol*. 1986;60:1025.
342a. Herrmann J, et al. *J Appl Physiol (1985)*. 2016;121:1306.
343. Pillow JJ. *Eur Respir J*. 2012;40:291.
344. Courtney SE, et al. *N Engl J Med*. 2002;347:643.
345. Johnson AH, et al. *N Engl J Med*. 2002;347:633.
345a. Ferguson ND, et al. *N Engl J Med*. 2013;368:795.
345b. Young D, et al. *N Engl J Med*. 2013;368:806.
346. Fessler HE, Brower RG. *Crit Care Med*. 2005;33:S223.
347. Fessler HE, et al. *Crit Care Med*. 2007;35:1649.
348. Krishman JA, Brower RG. *Chest*. 2000;118:795.
349. Ali S, Ferguson ND. *Crit Care Clin*. 2011;27:487.
350. Ip T, Mehta S. *Curr Opin Crit Care*. 2012;18:70.
351. Custer JW, et al. *Pediatr Crit Care Med*. 2011;12:e176.
352. Pillow JJ, et al. *Am J Respir Crit Care Med*. 2001;164:1019.
353. Kaczka DW, Lutchen KR. *Ann Biomed Eng*. 2004;32:596.
354. Biro P. *Anesth Clin*. 2010;28:397.
355. Hess DR, et al. *Respir Care Clin North Am*. 2001;7:577.
356. Kalenga M, et al. *J Appl Physiol*. 1998;84:1174.
357. Pillow JJ, et al. *Pediatr Crit Care Med*. 2004;5:172.
358. Pillow JJ, et al. *Pediatr Res*. 2002;52:538.
358a. Harcourt ER, et al. *Pediatr Crit Care Med*. 2014.
358b. Tingay DG, et al. *Neonatology*. 2015;108:220.
359. Hager DN. *Curr Opin Anaesthesiol*. 2012;25:17.
360. Lucangelo U, et al. Capnography and adjuncts of mechanical ventilation. In: Gravenstein JS, et al., ed. *Capnography*. 2nd ed. Cambridge: Cambridge University Press; 2011:169–181.
361. Kil HK, et al. *Yonsei Med J*. 2002;43:20.
362. Kugelman A, et al. *Pediatr Pulmonol*. 2012;47:876.
363. Frietsch T, et al. *Acta Anaesthesiol Scand*. 2000;44:391.
364. Nishimura M, et al. *Chest*. 1992;101:1681.
365. Biro P, et al. *Anesth Analg*. 1998;87:180.
365a. Herrmann J, et al. *J Appl Physiol (1985)*. 2018;124:653.
365b. Mehta PP, et al. *Am J Gastroenterol*. 2016;111:395.
366. Evans KL, et al. *J Laryngol Otol*. 1994;108:23.
367. Miodownik S, et al. *Crit Care Med*. 1984;12:718.
368. Algora-Weber A, et al. *Crit Care Med*. 1986;14:895.
369. Sehati S, et al. *Br J Anaesth*. 1989;63:47S.
370. Simon M, et al. *Acta Anaesthesiol Scand*. 2003;47:861.
371. Wallen E, et al. *Crit Care Med*. 1995;23:1588.
372. Waydhas C, et al. *Intensive Care Med*. 1995;21:784.
373. Bercault N, et al. *Crit Care Med*. 2005;33:2471.
374. Nakamura T, et al. *Chest*. 2003;123:159.
375. Kue R, et al. *Am J Crit Care*. 2011;20:153.
376. Prodhan P, et al. *Pediatr Crit Care Med*. 2010;11:227.
377. Szem JW, et al. *Crit Care Med*. 1995;23:1660.
378. Tobias JD, et al. *Pediatr Emerg Care*. 1996;12:249.
379. Ansermino JM, et al. *Anesth Analg*. 2009;108:873.
380. Lee J, et al. *Conf Proc IEEE Eng Med Biol Soc*. 2011;2011:8315.
381. Saeed M, et al. *Crit Care Med*. 2011;39:952.
382. Imhoff M, Kuhls S. *Anesth Analg*. 2006;102:1525.
383. Melek WW, et al. *IEEE Trans Biomed Eng*. 2005;52:639.
384. Simons DJ, Rensink RA. *Trends Cogn Sci*. 2005;9:16.
385. Dosani M, et al. *Br J Anaesth*. 2009;102:686.
386. Schadler D, et al. *Am J Respir Crit Care Med*. 2012;185:637.
387. Blount M, et al. *IEEE Eng Med Biol Mag*. 2010;29:110.
388. Chatburn RL, Mireles-Cabodevila E. *Respir Care*. 2011;56:85.
389. Epstein RH, Dexter F. *Anesth Analg*. 2012;115:929.
390. Chiumello D, et al. *Crit Care*. 2008;12:R150.
391. Dellamonica J, et al. *Crit Care*. 2011;15:R294.
392. Pillow JJ, et al. *Pediatr Pulmonol*. 2006;41:105.
393. Tobias JD. *Paediatr Anaesth*. 2009;19:434.
394. Sorensen LC, et al. *Scand J Clin Lab Invest*. 2011;71:548.
395. Sandberg KL, et al. *Acta Paediatr*. 2011;100:676.
396. Xue Q, et al. *Anesth Analg*. 2010;111:417.
397. Klopfenstein CE, et al. *Acta Anaesthesiol Scand*. 2008;52:700.
398. De Oliveira GS Jr, et al. *Br J Anaesth*. 2010;104:774.
399. Chakravarthy M, et al. *J Cardiothorac Vasc Anesth*. 2010;24:451.
400. Kelly AM, Klim S. *Respir Med*. 2011;105:226.
401. Spelten O, et al. *J Clin Monit Comput*. 2017;31:153.
402. Yu M, et al. *Shock*. 2007;27:615.
403. Chakravarthy M, et al. *J Clin Monit Comput*. 2009;23:363.
404. He HW, et al. *Shock*. 2012;37:152.
405. Yu M, et al. *Shock*. 2006;26:450.

406. Michard F. *J Clin Monit Comput*. 2018.
407. Pistolesi M, Giuntini C. *Radiol Clin North Am*. 1978;16:551.
408. Rubenfeld GD, et al. *Chest*. 1999;116:1347.
409. Meade MO, et al. *Am J Respir Crit Care Med*. 2000;161:85.
410. Sakka SG, et al. *Intensive Care Med*. 2000;26:180.
411. Isakow W, Schuster DP. *Am J Physiol Lung Cell Mol Physiol*. 2006;291:L1118.
412. Martin GS, et al. *Crit Care*. 2005;9:R74.
413. Kuzkov VV, et al. *Crit Care Med*. 2006;34:1647.
414. Phillips CR, et al. *Crit Care Med*. 2008;36:69.
415. Fernandez-Mondejar E, et al. *J Trauma*. 2005;59:1420. discussion 1424.
416. Assaad S, et al. *J Cardiothorac Vasc Anesth*. 2017;31:1471.
417. Stephan F, et al. *Crit Care Med*. 2017;45:e409–e417.
418. Pottecher J, et al. *Transplantation*. 2017;101:112.
419. Michelet P, et al. *Anesthesiology*. 2006;105:911.
420. Mitchell JP, et al. *Am Rev Respir Dis*. 1992;145:990.
421. Mutoh T, et al. *Stroke*. 2009;40:2368.
422. von Spiegel T, et al. *Anesthesiology*. 2002;96:827.
423. Perkins GD, et al. *Am J Respir Crit Care Med*. 2006;173:281.
424. Licker M, et al. *Chest*. 2008;133:845.
425. Effros RM, et al. *Am J Physiol Lung Cell Mol Physiol*. 2008;294:L1023.
426. Easley RB, et al. *Anesthesiology*. 2009;111:1065.
427. de Prost N, et al. *J Appl Physiol*. 2011;111:1249.
428. Roch A, et al. *Crit Care Med*. 2004;32:811.
429. Carlile PV, Gray BA. *J Appl Physiol*. 1984;57:680.
430. Kuntscher MV, et al. *J Burn Care Rehabil*. 2003;24:142.
431. Saugel B, et al. *Scand J Trauma Resusc Emerg Med*. 2011;19:31.
432. Saugel B, et al. *J Clin Monit Comput*. 2018.
433. Rossi P, et al. *Crit Care Med*. 2006;34:1437.

42 Renal Pathophysiology and Treatment for Perioperative Ischemia and Nephrotoxic Injury

KATHLEEN D. LIU, DANIEL H. BURKHARDT III, and RUPERT M. PEARSE

KEY POINTS

- The incidence of perioperative acute kidney injury (AKI) (previously referred to as acute renal failure) varies, depending on the definition used.
- Although uncommon, AKI requiring dialysis is associated with extremely high morbidity and mortality rates.
- The mechanism for perioperative AKI is complex and commonly involves multiple factors including ischemia-reperfusion injury, inflammation, and toxins.
- Repeated direct perioperative assessments of renal hemodynamics or tubular function are impractical; therefore indirect assessments, such as trends of serum creatinine concentrations, are the best practical perioperative tools to assess renal function.
- Intraoperative urine formation depends on many factors and is not validated as a measure of the risk of postoperative renal dysfunction. Yet postoperatively, patients with low intraoperative urine output may develop renal dysfunction. Therefore urine output should be carefully monitored in the intraoperative setting.
- Early biochemical markers for kidney injury may soon become new tests that can provide prompt clinical information.
- As part of preoperative risk assessment, both serum creatinine and proteinuria can provide important and useful information.
- Intraoperative hypotension and hypovolemia are significant risk factors for AKI.
- With regard to fluid management, the use of balanced salt solutions may reduce the risk of AKI. Volume overload is a risk factor for adverse outcomes in patients with AKI and may influence concentrations of conventional markers of kidney function such as serum creatinine.
- Renal replacement therapy may be indicated for severe AKI: at present, data does not support the use of one modality over another.

Introduction and Acute Kidney Injury Definitions

Acute kidney injury (AKI) (previously known as acute renal failure) is characterized by rapid decline in the glomerular filtration rate (GFR) and the accumulation of nitrogenous waste products (blood urea nitrogen [BUN] and creatinine). AKI occurs in approximately 5% to 25% of all hospitalized patients, depending on the precise definition used for AKI, and with more frequent rates in patients who are critically ill in the intensive care unit (ICU) (also see Chapter 17). AKI is also a serious perioperative complication for patients undergoing major surgery.[1-4] As the incidence of AKI varies by the definition used, the mortality of AKI ranges from 10% to 35% for mild AKI, whereas AKI in the ICU setting is associated with a 50% to 80% mortality rate. However, supportive care with dialysis has reduced mortality from AKI. Whereas the mortality rate of oliguric AKI was 91% during World War II, mortality declined to 53% during the Korean War with the provision of dialysis.[5] AKI requiring dialysis develops in 1% to 7% of patients after cardiac or major vascular surgery and is strongly associated with morbidity and mortality in this context.[6-9]

Perioperative renal failure was long defined as a requirement for postoperative dialysis. However, this concept has evolved during the past several years. First, because the implications of requiring postoperative dialysis are quite different for a patient starting with a normal baseline renal function compared with one starting with advanced chronic kidney disease and because the criteria for the use of dialysis are not standardized, the usefulness of dialysis alone to define AKI has been questioned. Second, studies are difficult to compare because of the use of nonstandard definitions for AKI. For example, in one review of 28 studies,[10] definitions for perioperative AKI varied. Third, consensus definitions that focus on small changes in serum creatinine and on

TABLE 42.1 Comparison of the RIFLE, AKIN, and KDOQI Consensus Criteria for Acute Kidney Injury

RIFLE		AKIN		KDIGO		
Class	**SCr**	**Stage**	**SCr**	**Stage**	**SCr**	**Urine Output**[a]
Risk	Increase in SCr to >1.5× baseline	1	Increase in SCr ≥0.3 mg/dL or to ≥1.5×-2× baseline	1	Increase in SCr ≥0.3 mg/dL within 48 h or to ≥1.5×-2× baseline, which is known or presumed to have occurred within the past 7 days	Urine output <0.5 mg/kg/h for >6 h
Injury	Increase in SCr to >2× baseline	2	Increase in SCr to >2×-3× baseline	2	Increase in SCr to >2×-3× baseline	Urine output <0.5 mg/kg/h for >12 h
Failure	Increase in SCr to >3× baseline, or increase of ≥0.5 mg/dL to absolute value of ≥4 mg/dL	3	Increase in SCr to >3× baseline, or increase of ≥0.5 mg/dL to absolute value of ≥4 mg/dL, or need for RRT	3	Increase in SCr to >3× baseline, or increase to absolute value of ≥4 mg/dL, or need for RRT; in pediatric patients eGFR <35 mL/min/1.73 m^2	Urine output <0.3 mg/kg/h for >12 h or anuria for >12 h
Loss	Need for RRT >4 weeks					
End stage	Need for RRT >3 months					

[a]Is common to all three consensus criteria.
The three consensus criteria use the same urine output criteria, but slight differences in the creatinine criteria are used to define AKI.
AKI, Acute kidney injury; *AKIN,* acute kidney injury network; *eGFR,* estimated glomerular filtration rate; *KDIGO,* kidney disease: improving global outcomes; *RIFLE,* risk, injury, failure, loss, end-stage disease; *RRT,* renal replacement therapy; *SCr,* serum creatinine.

changes in urine output to define AKI have received widespread adoption. This last conclusion is based on the recognition that small changes in renal function directly relate to an increased risk of death.[11]

As a result, recent consensus criteria are being used to define AKI in both the perioperative and other medical settings. The first proposed consensus criteria were the RIFLE (**R**isk, **I**njury, **F**ailure, **L**oss, **E**nd-stage) kidney disease criteria developed by the Acute Dialysis Quality Initiative (Table 42.1).[12] These have subsequently undergone two modifications by the Acute Kidney Injury Network[13] and in the Kidney Disease: Improving Global Outcomes (KDIGO) AKI guidelines.[14] As detailed in Table 42.1, the central components of these criteria are the focus on relative and absolute changes in creatinine from a baseline value and the definition of several degrees of AKI severity. Consequently, milder AKI (e.g., KDIGO, stage 1 disease) will be more common than stage 3 disease and will also be associated with a lower mortality rate. These criteria have also proposed definitions for AKI based on urine output. Overall, although there are studies demonstrating that AKI defined based on urine output is associated with adverse outcomes in the critical care setting and is more common than AKI defined based on creatinine,[15] the urine output criteria are not as well validated. At present, there is no clear method to correct urine output for morbid obesity; in addition, urine output may be unmeasurable if a urinary bladder catheter is not present.[16] Not surprisingly, AKI by urine output criteria is substantially more common than AKI by creatinine-based criteria; in a study of more than 4000 subjects undergoing major noncardiac surgery, the incidence of AKI increased from 8% to 64% when urine output criteria were incorporated.[17] Although each AKI stage was associated with an increased risk of death, the association with mortality was attenuated in this analysis when urine output criteria for AKI were used. Finally, it should be noted that the importance of oliguria (<0.5 mL/kg/h) as a predictor of creatinine-based AKI is less well established in the perioperative setting than in other clinical settings.[18,19] In a recent large single-center observational study, urine output of less than 0.3 mL/kg/h during major abdominal surgery was associated with an increased risk of perioperative AKI (defined as a 0.3 mg/dL rise in serum creatinine within 48 hours or a 50% increase over 7 days from baseline).[20] However, urine output within the 0.3 to 0.5 mL/kg/h range was not associated with creatinine-based AKI.

Additional challenges for the identification of AKI in the intraoperative setting include large blood volume loss and fluid shifts, which may artificially dilute serum creatinine. Unlike the postoperative or critical care setting where renal monitoring can involve periodic evaluation of kidney function under relatively stable conditions, intraoperative renal monitoring involves a briefer unstable period, often involving significant blood loss, major fluid shifts, wide hemodynamic fluctuations, and even direct compromise to renal artery blood flow. Therefore the anesthesia provider is likely the first monitor (in a sense) required for preserving renal function by recognizing and treating factors that may contribute to or exacerbate AKI; for example, the toxic effects of aminoglycosides and iodinated contrast materials are exacerbated by intravascular volume depletion.

As medical populations shift toward older and more critically ill patients undergoing increasingly high-risk procedures, patients are at an increased risk of AKI in the perioperative setting, and the role of the anesthesia provider becomes even more critical. Indeed, a recent study of dialysis after elective major surgery suggests that the incidence of dialysis-requiring AKI is rising from 0.2% in 1995 to 0.6% in 2009, with the majority of the increase occurring after vascular and cardiac surgery.[21] Although ischemic causes may be primarily responsible for perioperative AKI,[22,23] the successful development of renoprotective strategies has not occurred. Furthermore, other pathophysiologic contributors to perioperative AKI may include contrast-induced nephropathy, pigment nephropathy (e.g., hemoglobin, myoglobin), cholesterol emboli (e.g., atheroembolic renal disease), aminoglycoside toxicity, and sepsis. Animal studies of such pure nephropathies treated

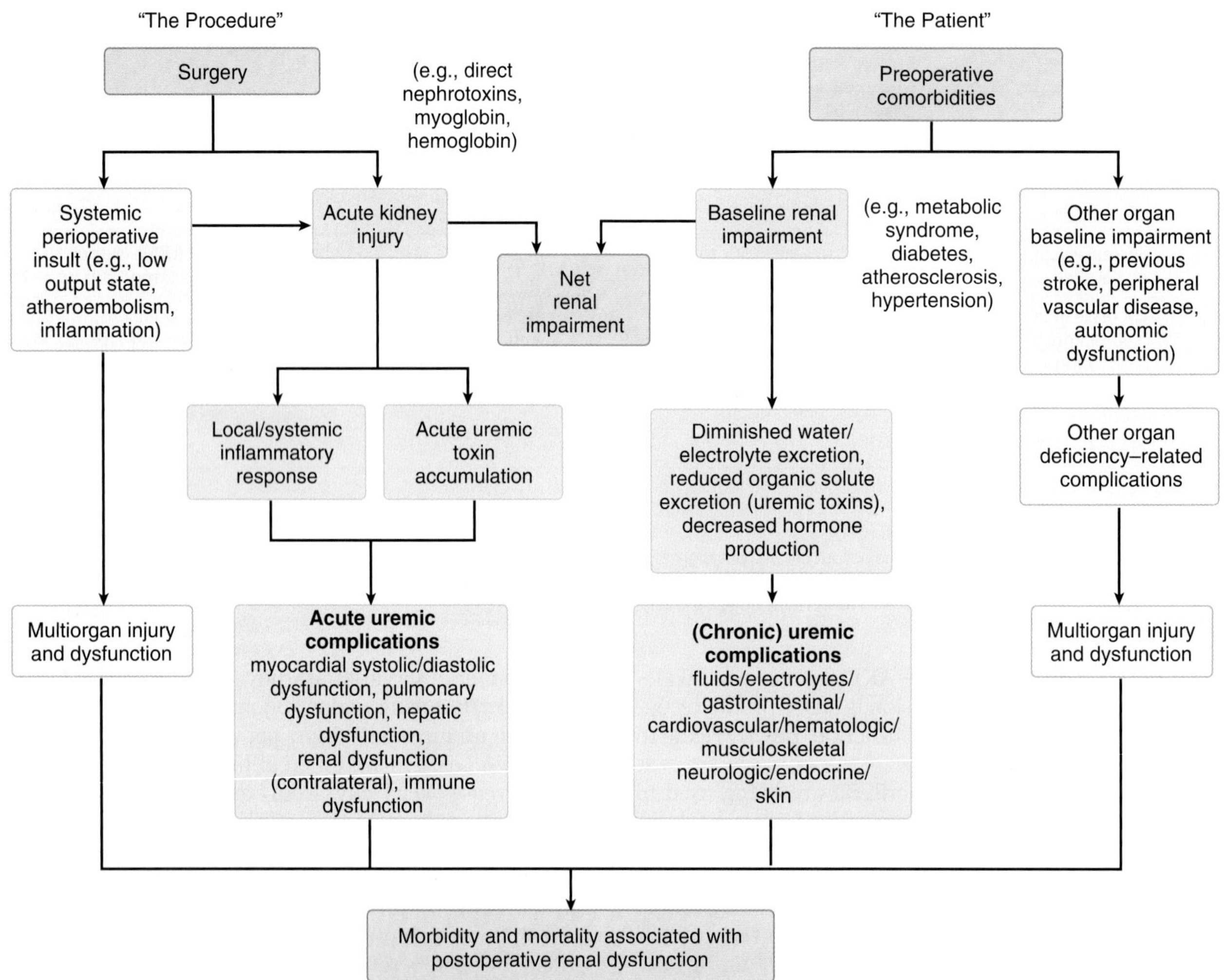

Fig. 42.1 Procedural and patient factors related to surgery contributing to the risk of perioperative acute kidney injury (AKI) and postoperative morbidity and mortality. Of note, although AKI contributes to the risk of morbidity and mortality, a significant part of this association must also be attributed to other very serious conditions, such as sepsis, that can cause injury and are also major sources of adverse outcomes. (Modified from Stafford-Smith M, Patel U, Phillips-Bute B, et al. Acute kidney injury and chronic kidney disease after cardiac surgery. *Adv Chronic Kid Dis.* 2008;15:157–177. Used with permission.)

with logical renoprotective interventions often demonstrate success; unfortunately, this success has not extended to equivalent renoprotection in humans. It may not be surprising that a specific treatment for a pure nephropathy nonselectively applied to a mixture of nephropathies, variably expressed in different patients, would be unsuccessful. Postoperative AKI, rather than being a single entity, is likely a mosaic of several pure nephropathies, each of varying importance for a particular patient and procedure (Fig. 42.1).

Pathophysiologic Processes of Ischemic Acute Kidney Injury

In general, the causes for AKI can be divided into prerenal, intrinsic renal, and postrenal sources. In the perioperative setting, patients may be at increased risk for prerenal AKI, either attributable to volume depletion or to exacerbation of associated chronic prerenal physiologic conditions, such as congestive heart failure, which may be exacerbated by volume overload. Intraoperatively, hypotension due to vasodilation and negative inotropy/chronotropy from anesthetic agents may lead to prerenal physiology. Depending on the nature of the surgical procedure, the patient may also be at increased risk of postrenal AKI attributable to obstruction of the ureters, bladder, or urethra. However, the primary cause of perioperative AKI is *acute tubular necrosis* (ATN). Defining the cause of AKI is also critical because treatment of the underlying cause is critical for the reversal of AKI and potential renal recovery.

The two primary mechanisms of ATN are ischemia-reperfusion and nephrotoxic effects, with three sources of insult common to many surgical procedures during which postoperative AKI is prevalent: hypoperfusion, inflammation, and atheroembolism. Other sources of renal insult in selected patients may include rhabdomyolysis and specific drug-related effects. Certain classes of medications may also contribute to hypoperfusion by virtue of their hemodynamic effects (notably angiotensin-converting enzyme [ACE] inhibitor 1, angiotensin-receptor blockers [ARBs], and nonsteroidal antiinflammatory drugs [NSAIDs]), and, consequently, the risk of ATN.

Ischemic renal failure related to shock or severe dehydration is always preceded by an early compensatory phase of normal renal adaptation (e.g., pre-prerenal failure),

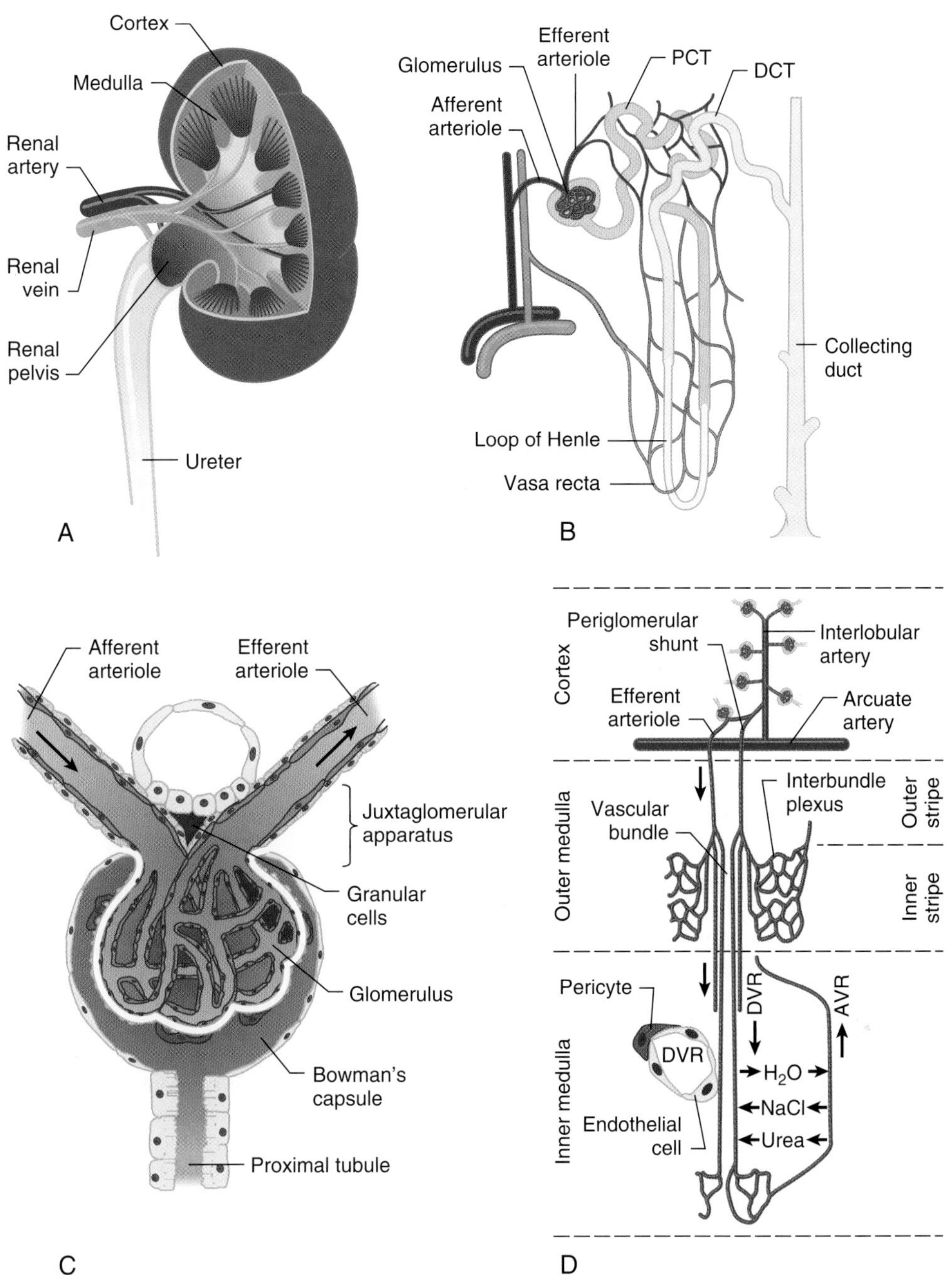

Fig. 42.2 (A) The internal structure of the kidney includes the vasculature, cortex and medulla regions, and urinary tract structures. (B) The functional unit of the kidney is the nephron. (C) The glomerulus is the site where plasma filtration occurs; approximately 20% of plasma entering the glomerulus will pass through the specialized capillary wall into the Bowman capsule and enter the tubule to be processed and to generate urine. (D) The vascular anatomy of the kidney is highly organized, and the medullary microcirculation is part of the mechanism that permits countercurrent exchange.[42] *AVR,* Ascending vasa recta; *DCT,* distal convoluted tubule; *DVR,* descending vasa recta; *NaCl,* sodium chloride; *PCT,* proximal convoluted tubule. (A, From http://www.nida.nih.gov/consequences/kidney/. Accessed February 17, 2008. B, From http://cnx.org/content/m44809/1.8/. Accessed February 24, 2014. C, From http://www.cixip.com/index.php/page/content/id/422/. Accessed June 26, 2014. D, From Pallone TL, Zhang Z, Rhinehart K. Physiology of the renal medullary microcirculation. *Am J Physiol Renal Physiol.* 2003;284:F253–F266. Used with permission.)

followed by a condition termed *prerenal azotemia* during which the kidney maximizes activities at the expense of the retention of nitrogenous end-products to preserve the internal environment through retention of solutes and water (Fig. 42.2). In studies of community-acquired AKI, the incidence of prerenal azotemia may be as frequent as 70%.[24] In contrast, in a classic study of hospital-acquired AKI, although hypoperfusion accounted for 42% of cases of AKI, only 41% of these cases of hypoperfusion were attributable to inadequate intravascular volume.[25]

Although prerenal azotemia is ominous and typically accompanied by oliguria (<0.5 mL/kg/h), it is reversible. At a critical tilting point, as conditions go beyond the compensatory mechanisms that maintain renal perfusion, ischemia leads to irreversible renal cell necrosis or ATN.[26] This represents the pure form of ischemic AKI. Other forms of ATN are due to toxins, including medications (e.g., aminoglycosides, cisplatinum), pigments (e.g., hemoglobin, myoglobin), and iodinated contrast dye. These forms of ATN do not involve the typical pattern of preceding prerenal azotemia with

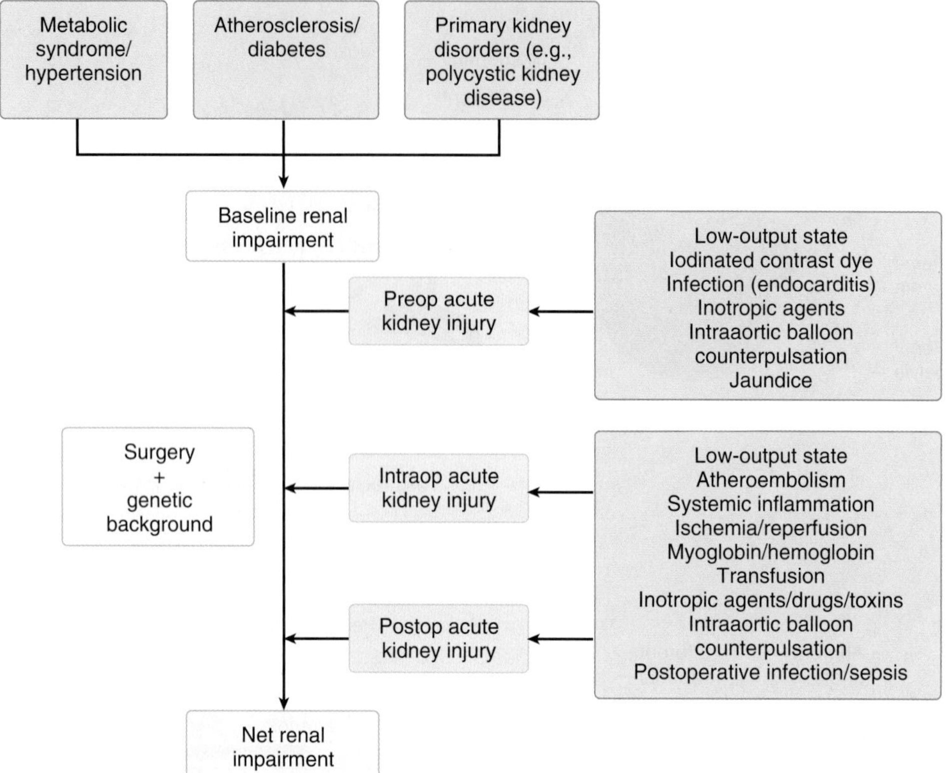

Fig. 42.3 Perioperative clinical risk factors associated with postoperative kidney injury.

associated oliguria, since the insult is sudden. Importantly, most cases of perioperative AKI are the result of numerous renal insults, rather than being attributable to one pure source (Fig. 42.3). In particular, patients with prerenal azotemia are likely at increased risk for toxic ATN.

Interruption of blood flow to the kidneys for more than 30 to 60 minutes results in ATN and irreversible cell damage. The kidneys receive 1000 to 1250 mL/min of blood or 3 to 5 mL/min/g of tissue for the average adult, and this amount far exceeds what is needed to provide the kidney's intrinsic oxygen requirement. Intracortical blood flow may not be evenly distributed.[27] Because the renal cortex contains most of the glomeruli and depends on oxidative metabolism for energy, ischemic hypoxia injures the renal cortical structures, particularly the pars recta of the proximal tubules. As ischemia persists, the supply of glucose and substrates continues to decrease; glycogen is consumed, and the medulla, which depends to a great extent on glycolysis for its energy sources, becomes more adversely affected. Early cell changes are reversible, such as the swelling of cell organelles, especially the mitochondria. As ischemia progresses, a lack of adenosine triphosphate interferes with the sodium pump mechanism, water and sodium accumulate in the endoplasmic reticulum of tubular cells, and the cells begin to swell. Onset of tubular damage usually occurs within 25 minutes of ischemia as the microvilli of the proximal tubular cell brush borders begin to change. Within an hour, they slough off into the tubular lumen, and membrane bullae protrude into the straight portion of the proximal tubule. After a few hours, intratubular pressure rises, and tubular fluid passively backflows. Within 24 hours, obstructing casts appear in the distal tubular lumen.

RENAL RESPONSE TO HYPOPERFUSION: AUTOREGULATION AND DISTRIBUTION OF CARDIAC OUTPUT TO THE KIDNEYS

A common intraoperative stress that puts patients at risk for AKI is hypoperfusion due to hypotension and/or hypovolemia. The fraction of cardiac output perfusing the kidneys depends on the ratio of renal vascular resistance to systemic vascular resistance.[26] In general, the response to renal hypoperfusion involves three major regulatory mechanisms that support renal function: (1) afferent arteriolar dilation increases the proportion of cardiac output that perfuses the kidney; (2) efferent arteriolar resistance increases the filtration fraction and preserves GFR; and (3) hormonal and neural responses improve renal perfusion by increasing intravascular volume, thereby indirectly increasing cardiac output.

The kidney produces vasodilator prostaglandins to counteract the effects of systemic vasoconstrictor hormones such as angiotensin II. In a state of low cardiac output when systemic blood pressure is preserved by the action of systemic vasopressors, RBF is not depressed because the effect of the vasopressors is blunted within the kidney. Studies using specific inhibitors of angiotensin II have shown that efferent arteriolar resistance largely results from the action of angiotensin II.[28] At low concentrations, norepinephrine has a vasoconstricting effect on efferent arterioles, indicating that the adrenergic system may also be important for maintaining the renal compensatory response.[29]

Reductions in cardiac output are accompanied by the release of vasopressin and by increased activity of the sympathetic nervous system and the renin-angiotensin-aldosterone system. These regulatory mechanisms to preserve RBF conserve salt and water. One study reported the normal response to hemorrhage in otherwise healthy patients, describing a 30% reduction in RBF with a decrease in mean perfusion pressure from 80 to 60 mm Hg.[30] Changes known to occur at the initiation of cardiopulmonary bypass (CPB) surgery include greater reduction in renal perfusion than systemic perfusion, loss of RBF autoregulation, and stress hormone and inflammatory responses known to be harmful to the kidney.[31,32] These effects may explain why the duration of CPB surgery independently predicts postcardiac surgery renal impairment.

Detection of Acute Kidney Injury

LABORATORY TESTS OF SERUM AND URINE AS MARKERS OF RENAL FUNCTION

Standard serum and urine markers of renal function are discussed in Chapter 17. It should be emphasized that at present, repeated serum creatinine determinations (relative or absolute changes), are most often used to identify AKI. An inherent limitation of almost all currently available tools to detect AKI is the obligate delay between the *onset* of AKI and the *diagnosis* of AKI. One striking difference between the management of AKI and acute myocardial infarction is the lack of early biomarkers for AKI in routine clinical practice to guide prompt recognition and intervention when tissue is threatened. Thus significant ongoing efforts are testing the value of early AKI biomarkers and of real-time measurement of GFR.

NOVEL (EARLY) BIOMARKERS OF ACUTE KIDNEY INJURY

Limited progress in the care for AKI has fueled an enormous interest in new early biomarkers.[33-36] Although a few of the new tools represent attempts to find a filtration marker that is better than creatinine (e.g., cystatin C), most novel AKI biomarkers take advantage of one of the three early consequences of AKI: (1) tubular cell damage, (2) tubular cell dysfunction, and (3) adaptive stress response of the kidney. The hope is that such biomarkers will allow timely AKI identification, diagnosis (e.g., prerenal azotemia vs. ATN), and prognosis. Some of the more promising biomarkers are presented here (Box 42.1).

BOX 42.1 Early Biomarkers of Acute Kidney Injury

Filtration-Based Markers of Renal Dysfunction

Cystatin C
β-trace protein
β-2 microglobulin

Biomarkers Reflecting Renal Tubular Cell Damage (Tubular Enzymuria)

α-Glutathione S-transferase
π-Glutathione S-transferase
β-*N*-Acetyl-β-D-glucosaminidase
γ-Glutamyl transpeptidase
Alkaline phosphatase
Sodium hydrogen exchanger isoform 3

Biomarkers Reflecting Renal Tubular Cell Dysfunction (Tubular Proteinuria)

α_1-Microglobulin
β_2-Microglobulin
Albumin
Retinol-binding protein
Immunoglobulin G
Transferrin
Ceruloplasmin
Lambda and kappa light chains

Biomarkers Reflecting Renal Tubular Cell Response to Stress

Neutrophil gelatinase–associated lipocalin
Urinary interleukin-18
Kidney injury molecule-1
Liver fatty acid–binding protein
Insulin-like growth factor binding protein 7
Tissue inhibitor of metallo-proteinase 2

New Filtration-Based Markers of Renal Dysfunction

Of the most novel filtration-based markers of renal dysfunction, the most advanced is cystatin C, a member of the cystatin superfamily of cysteine-proteinase inhibitors that is produced by all nucleated cells at a constant rate. Cystatin C has been clinically available for longer than 15 years and can be rapidly determined. Similar to creatinine, cystatin C accumulates in the circulation with renal impairment and can be used as a marker of glomerular filtration. Serum cystatin C has theoretical advantages over creatinine, particularly as an indicator of mild chronic kidney disease and its sequelae.[38] Several GFR estimating equations have been proposed, based on cystatin C alone or cystatin C and creatinine for use in chronic kidney disease.[39,40] Although these are commonly used in clinical research studies, in general these are not in widespread clinical use at present.

Although cystatin C outperformed creatinine in detecting AKI after cardiac surgery in some small studies,[41] this sensitivity has not consistently been the case. Indeed, a large multicenter prospective observational study of AKI after cardiac surgery suggested that serum cystatin C was less, not more, sensitive for the detection of AKI. This study, conducted by the Translational Research Investigating Biomarker Endpoints in Acute Kidney Injury (TRIBE-AKI) Consortium, prospectively enrolled more than 1200 adults undergoing cardiac surgery and has rapidly advanced the field of novel biomarkers in this context. Of note, the subset of patients who had AKI by cystatin C and creatinine had more frequent risk of dialysis and death than those who had AKI by creatinine alone.[42] Conditions such as malignancy, human immunodeficiency viral infection, or corticosteroidal or thyroid hormone therapy are associated with increased serum levels of cystatin C without changes in renal function. Other novel markers of filtration include β-trace protein and β-2-microglobulin; these markers may be novel markers of mortality in the general population, compared with creatinine-based eGFR.[42] However, the additional utility of these markers in estimating GFR above and beyond creatinine and cystatin C is unknown.

Biomarkers Reflecting Renal Tubular Cell Damage (Tubular Enzymuria)

Renal tubular cells contain enzymes that are highly specific to their location within the kidney and even tubule region. Under conditions of cellular stress, these enzymes are shed into the urine, making these potentially appealing markers of kidney dysfunction. These markers include α and π isomers of glutathione s-transferase (GST), which are cytosolic enzymes from proximal and distal tubular cells, respectively, and N-acetyl-β-D-glucosaminidase, a proximal tubule lysosomal enzyme. Of note, although enhanced urinary excretion of tubular enzymes can signal damaged tubular cells, it can also reflect an increased turnover of tubular cells or some other metabolic disturbance; thus the use of these markers may need to be applied with caution.

Biomarkers Reflecting Renal Tubular Cell Dysfunction (Tubular Proteinuria)

When small proteins are filtered by the glomerulus, binding and endocytic reuptake in the proximal tubule normally returns these substances to the body through a megalin-mediated transport system. So-called tubular proteinuria results from functional impairment of this process and the escape of small proteins into the urine. Endogenous low molecular weight proteins that are normally taken up in this way include β_2- and α_1-microglobulin, retinol-binding protein, lysozyme, ribonuclease, IgG, transferrin, ceruloplasmin, and lambda (λ) and kappa (κ) light chains. Appearance of any of these substances in the urine heralds abnormal proximal nephron function consistent with AKI. However, lysine and its analog (e.g., ε-aminocaproic acid, tranexamic acid) can cause a profound but reversible inhibition of low molecular weight protein reuptake[43] that is transient and apparently benign due to blocking renal-binding sites.[44,45]

Biomarkers Reflecting Renal Tubular Cell Response to Stress

Examples of markers that assess the response of the kidney to stress include neutrophil gelatinase–associated lipocalin (NGAL), kidney injury molecule–1 (KIM-1), liver fatty acid–binding protein, and interleukin-18 (IL-18). These have each been extensively reviewed in detail in recent literature.[33-36] Two markers of G1-cell cycle arrest have been shown to be upregulated in AKI, insulin-like growth factor–binding protein 7 (IGFBP-7) and tissue inhibitor of metalloproteinases–2 (TIMP-2).[46] A test that combines levels of IGFBP-7 and TIMP-2 has received U.S. Food and Drug Administration (FDA) clearance as a biomarker for the identification of patients at high risk of AKI.

NGAL is a protein with a critical role in iron scavenging. A transcriptome-wide interrogation for genes induced very early after renal ischemia identified NGAL as a protein generated by ischemic renal tubular cells.[47] Administration of exogenous NGAL in animal models attenuates renal injury.[48] Enthusiasm for NGAL as a biomarker of AKI was fueled by a study in pediatric patients who underwent cardiac surgery, suggesting that plasma and urinary NGAL could predict AKI before elevations in serum creatinine (Fig. 42.4).[49] Although increased NGAL levels are associated with adverse outcomes,[50,51] studies in the adult perioperative literature have not consistently shown NGAL to predict AKI before elevations in serum creatinine.

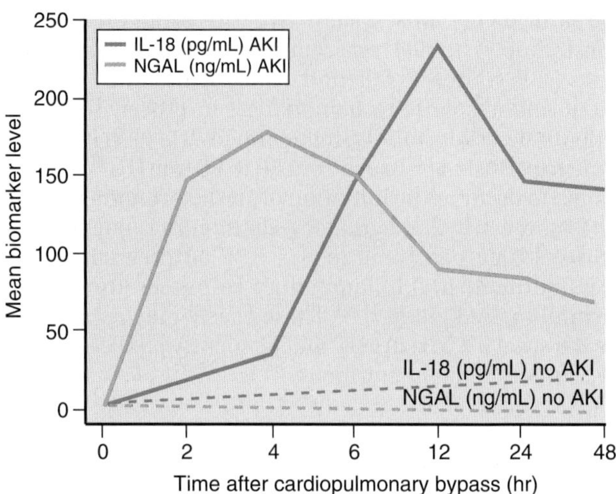

Fig. 42.4 Pattern of early biomarkers for urinary interleukin *(IL)*-18 and neutrophil gelatinase–associated lipocalin *(NGAL)* after cardiopulmonary bypass surgery in 55 patients with and without criteria for acute kidney injury *(AKI)* diagnosed 48 to 72 hours postoperatively (defined as a peak rise in serum creatinine concentration to >150% of baseline). (From Parikh CR, Mishra J, Thiessen-Philbrook H, et al. Urinary IL-18 is an early predictive biomarker of acute kidney injury after cardiac surgery. *Kidney Int.* 2006;70:199–203. Used with permission.)

KIM-1 is a transmembrane protein expressed at low levels under normal conditions that is significantly upregulated in proximal renal tubular cells in response to ischemic or nephrotoxic AKI.[52] In studies conducted by the Predictive Testing Safety Consortium, an academic-industrial partnership that has worked closely with the FDA to develop novel biomarkers of kidney injury for use in the preclinical setting (in particular, as markers of drug toxicity), KIM-1 outperformed a number of traditional markers of kidney injury in a variety of preclinical models.[53] More recently, assays have been developed to detect plasma KIM-1, which appears to correlate with urinary KIM-1 in the setting of both acute and chronic kidney disease.[54]

Finally, cell cycle arrest has been implicated in models of AKI; more recently, two proteins that induce cell cycle arrest, IGFBP-7 and TIMP-2, have both been shown in a multicenter study to predict the development of KDIGO stage 2 and 3 AKI in critically ill patients. In a validation cohort, these biomarkers had an impressive area under the ROC curve of 0.80 for subsequent AKI.[55] There has been tremendous interest in the use of these biomarkers for perioperative risk stratification,[56,57] with clinical trials enrolling patients based on elevated levels of IGFBP-7 and TIMP-2 (typically expressed as the product of these two biomarkers).[58]

Preoperative Evaluation of Renal Function and Risk Stratification

The greater the magnitude and duration of the surgical insult and the number of acute and chronic risk factors, the greater the likelihood of perioperative renal compromise and hence the need for preoperative identification of high-risk individuals.[58-61] Common risk factors for AKI include intravascular volume depletion, aminoglycoside use, radiocontrast dye exposure, use of NSAIDs, septic shock, and pigmenturia. ACE inhibitors and ARBs, respectively, may contribute to intraoperative hypotension and may exacerbate AKI in the setting of impaired hemodynamics (volume depletion, NSAID use). Patients with preexisting renal insufficiency are clearly at increased risk for AKI and should be identified in the perioperative evaluation through measurement of serum creatinine and urinalysis (to evaluate for albuminuria/proteinuria). Chronic kidney disease affects more than 10% of the United States population. Common risk factors for chronic kidney disease include advanced age, diabetes, and hypertension. The potential value of understanding the genetic makeup of patients has yet to be fully explored and is likely to be important. For example, several genetic polymorphisms known to affect inflammation and vasoconstriction demonstrate strong associations with AKI after cardiac surgery,[62] including the IL-6 572C and angiotensinogen 842C polymorphisms. In the future, identification of such polymorphisms may improve perioperative risk stratification.

Large multicenter epidemiologic studies have identified a relationship between markers of abnormal central aortic compliance, such as preoperative isolated systolic hypertension (>160 mm Hg) and wide pulse pressure hypertension (>40 mm Hg),[63,64] and postoperative AKI and dialysis, in particular in patients undergoing cardiac surgery. Pulse pressure is an index of the effects of large artery stiffness and the rate of pressure on propagation and reflection within the arterial tree. Early return of reflected arterial waves during late systolic rather than early diastolic pressure (from increased propagation velocity in stiff vessels) increases systolic blood pressure (i.e., afterload) and decreases diastolic blood pressure (i.e., perfusion pressure). Perfusion pressure and the risk of perioperative renal dysfunction are linked by the preexisting capacity of the vasculature to compensate for low pressure as it determines flow. Those with a predisposition to low flow attributable to abnormal central aortic compliance (e.g., those with wide pulse pressure) may represent patients who require higher pressure to maintain adequate flow and minimize renal risk compared with normotensive patients.

In the context of specific surgery types (e.g., cardiac surgery), perioperative risk prediction tools have been developed. In general, these tend to effectively identify low-risk populations, but discrimination for higher risk patients is more modest. This may reflect the fact that intraoperative factors play a major role in the pathogenesis of AKI in a vulnerable patient. In addition, a number of these risk prediction tools focus on dialysis-requiring AKI, which is only the "tip of the iceberg" with regard to disease burden.

Perioperative Acute Kidney Injury: Mechanisms and Treatment

As described in Chapter 17, anesthesia and surgery influence normal renal function primarily through changes in GFR and urine flow that are attributable to changes in blood pressure and cardiac output. Fluctuations in blood pressure have a major effect on RBF and glomerular filtration.[19,31,65] Here, we will briefly discuss considerations for several anesthetic techniques, followed by several specific perioperative considerations.

REGIONAL ANESTHESIA

Regional anesthetics and the kidneys interact in a complex manner that varies according to the underlying cardiovascular, renal, fluid, and electrolyte status of the patient.[66] In general, epidural and spinal anesthesia reduce systemic and renal vascular sympathetic tone.[67] Spinal cord segments T4 through L1 contribute to the sympathetic innervation of the renal vasculature, which is mediated by sympathetic fibers from the celiac and renal plexus.[67,68] Autonomic blockade above the fourth thoracic level also blocks cardioaccelerator sympathetic innervation to the heart. If neuraxial blockade reduces arterial blood pressure and cardiac output, then the RBF will be decreased with matching reductions in glomerular filtration and urine output.

Although controversial, intraoperative neuraxial blockade and postoperative epidural analgesia decrease rates of AKI. Rodgers and colleagues conducted a systematic review of 107 randomized clinical trials of intraoperative neuraxial blockade and demonstrated a 30% reduction in the odds of postoperative mortality.[69] This reduction was associated with decreases in the incidence of deep venous thrombosis, pulmonary embolism, transfusion, pneumonia, and respiratory depression, as well as renal failure, although the confidence limits for the renal failure estimates were very wide, in part due to the small number of cases of renal failure observed. Moraca and associates conducted a meta-analysis and reported on the association of thoracic epidural anesthesia with improved surgical outcomes attributable, in part, to a reduction of perioperative morbidity, including reductions in infection, ileus, blood loss, and AKI.[70] Other studies have examined the impact of epidural anesthesia during cardiac surgery and have suggested a benefit with regards to renal failure, although the confidence intervals were wide.[71] Unfortunately, renal failure was not an outcome of several recently published meta-analyses focused on epidural anesthesia during cardiac surgery.[72,73] Finally, with regard to postoperative analgesia, a recent Cochrane meta-analysis that focused on abdominal aortic surgery suggested better postoperative analgesia and a reduction in other complications including myocardial infarction and respiratory with epidural analgesia but no effect on AKI or postoperative mortality.[74]

EFFECTS OF INHALED ANESTHETICS

From a historic perspective, older volatile inhaled anesthetics including methoxyflurane and enflurane (no longer clinically used) when used for prolonged periods lead to significant generation of inorganic fluoride[74-77] and were associated with polyuric renal insufficiency. However, despite significant fluoride generation with sevoflurane and the generation of compound A (a metabolite associated with renal injury in experimental models), there is no reported association with AKI.[76] This may be due to the shorter duration of elevated fluoride levels with sevoflurane and the site of metabolism (intrarenal metabolism of methoxyflurane is fourfold greater than that of sevoflurane).

EFFECTS OF INTRAVENOUS ANESTHETICS

Propofol and dexmedetomidine may have antiinflammatory effects that are renoprotective. Propofol increases production of bone morphogenetic protein–7 (BMP-7), which suppresses the tumor necrosis factor α–induced inflammatory cascade during sepsis-induced AKI,[78] as well as decreased injury during ischemia-reperfusion[79,80] and unilateral ureteral obstruction.[81] Similarly, in addition to altering RBF and sodium and water handling, the α_2-adrenoreceptor agonists such as dexmedetomidine may stimulate BMP-7 production in the setting of sepsis and ischemia-reperfusion.[81-84] There has been significant interest in the use of dexmetomidine, in particular in the setting of cardiac surgery, with a recent meta-analysis suggesting a reduction in postoperative AKI with the use of dexmetomidine (OR 0.65; 95% confidence interval [CI], 0.45-0.92, $P = .02$).[85]

SPECIFIC PERIOPERATIVE PERTURBATIONS AND RENAL FUNCTION

Several surgical interventions can affect RBF and, consequently, renal function. Whereas aortic cross-clamping above the renal arteries has obvious influence on glomerular filtration, infrarenal aortic cross-clamping and unclamping also have significant indirect effects on glomerular filtration and urine formation through changes in myocardial function, sympathetic activity, neuronal and hormonal activity (e.g., renin and angiotensin production), intravascular volume, and systemic vascular resistance.[86] During standard CPB surgery, cardiorenal relationships are approximately as expected; RBF decreases to 12% to 13% of total pump flow and is predicted by flow rate and perfusion pressure; however, only mean pressure correlates with urine output.[31,87]

AKI after aortocoronary bypass surgery continues to be a devastating complication that is associated with multiorgan dysfunction, increased resource utilization, high cost, and increased mortality. Annually, approximately 350,000 patients in the United States undergo coronary artery bypass graft (CABG) surgery. In a multicenter observational study focused on AKI after cardiac surgery, 5% of participants developed AKI as defined by the need for acute dialysis or a doubling of serum creatinine from baseline.[88] The mechanism of perioperative AKI during cardiac surgery is multifactorial. Significant risk factors for AKI include underlying patient characteristics, such as age older than 75 years, history of diabetes, hypertension, pulse pressure, ventricular dysfunction, myocardial infarction, renal disease, perioperative medication exposures (e.g., aprotinin, hetastarch), and surgical characteristics such as intraoperative use of multiple inotropes, insertion of intraaortic balloon pump, and extended duration of the CPB surgery.[63,89-92]

The role of CPB surgery in postoperative AKI remains controversial. In their comprehensive guidelines on AKI, KDIGO reviewed the literature on postoperative AKI between patients undergoing off-pump and on-pump coronary revascularization surgeries and ultimately recommended that "off-pump CABG surgery not be selected solely for the purpose of reducing perioperative AKI or need for renal replacement therapy (RRT)."[14] However, patients with chronic kidney disease, who are at the highest risk for AKI after CPB surgery, have often been excluded from randomized clinical trials of off-pump versus on-pump CABG. For example, in the Randomized On/Off Bypass (ROOBY) trial, in which 2303 patients were randomized to off-pump versus on-pump CABG, approximately 7.5% of patients had a preoperative serum creatinine level ≥1.5 mg/dL.[93]

A large observational study of 742,909 nonemergent, isolated CABG cases (including 158,561 off-pump cases) from the Society of Thoracic Surgery Database suggests a benefit to off-pump CABG in those with chronic kidney disease.[94] Propensity methods were used to adjust for patient- and center-level imbalances. The primary endpoint was death or dialysis. In those with lower estimated GFR (eGFR), the risk difference (i.e., number of patients with the outcome per 100 patients in those who underwent CPB minus the number with the outcome in those who underwent off-pump CABG) for the primary endpoint was 0.66 (95% CI, 0.45-0.87) for eGFR 30 to 59 mL/min/1.73 m^2 and 3.66 (95% CI, 2.14-5.18) for eGFR 15 to 29 mL/min/1.73 m^2. Both component endpoints followed the same trend. Highlighting the importance of chronic kidney disease as a risk factor for AKI after cardiac surgery, whereas slightly less than 1% of the overall cohort received dialysis after cardiac surgery, 2% of those with eGFR 30 to 59 mL/min/1.73 m^2 and 12.5% of those with eGFR 15 to 29 mL/min/1.73 m^2 required dialysis. The risk difference for dialysis alone in the same groups was 0.47 (95% CI, 0.31-0.62) and 2.79 (95% CI, 1.37-4.20) with on-pump versus off-pump CABG, respectively (Fig. 42.5). Along the same lines, a 2932 patient-substudy of the CORONARY clinical trial followed patients after off- or on-pump CABG surgery and demonstrated an interaction between preoperative chronic kidney disease (defined as eGFR <60 mL/min/1.73 m^2) and AKI (defined as a 50% increase in serum creatinine from prerandomization baseline within 30 days). In those with chronic kidney disease, 19.2% of those in the off-pump arm had AKI, compared to 30.2% in those who had on-pump surgery. However, there was no difference in sustained renal dysfunction, defined as a 20% or greater loss in eGFR at 1 year between the two study arms (17.1% vs. 15.3% in the off- vs. on-pump arms, $P = .23$). However, when those with AKI were compared to those who did not have AKI (regardless of treatment arm), AKI was independently associated with an increased risk of sustained renal dysfunction, with an adjusted odds ratio of 3.37 (95% CI, 2.65-4.28, $P < .001$.[95] This study highlights the fact that in the setting of chronic kidney disease, AKI is only one of many risk factors for chronic kidney disease progression.

In the setting of CABG, there has been tremendous interest in prevention of AKI, and numerous pharmacologic interventions have been tested. As stated previously, one of the major challenges for AKI prevention is that both pre- and intraoperative factors impact the risk of AKI, so it is difficult to identify a priori those who are at highest risk of AKI. Interventions of recent interest where there is not a sufficient evidence base for wide-spread adoption include remote ischemic preconditioning, atrial natriuretic peptide, and fenoldopam, among others.[96,97]

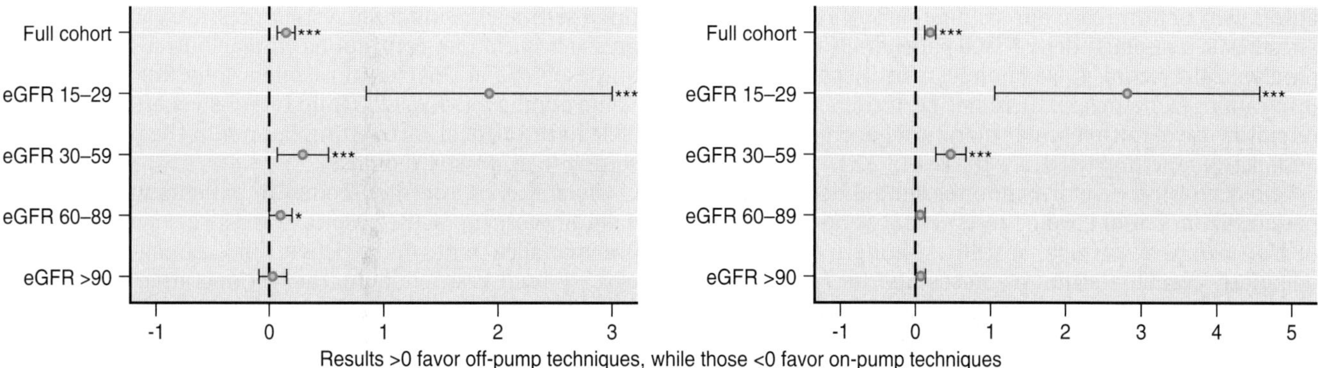

Fig. 42.5 Estimates of adverse outcomes associated with on-pump versus off-pump coronary artery bypass grafting by baseline estimated glomerular filtration rate *(eGFR)*. For both mortality *(left panel)* and renal replacement therapy *(right panel)*, off-pump CABG techniques appear to confer a benefit in those with lower eGFR. $^{*}P < .05$, $^{**}P < .01$, $^{***}P < .001$. (Redrawn from Chawla LS, Zhao Y, Lough FC, et al. Off-pump versus on-pump coronary artery bypass grafting outcomes stratified by preoperative renal function. *J Am Soc Nephrol*. 2012;23:1389–1397.)

INTRAOPERATIVE MANAGEMENT FOR AKI PREVENTION: OXYGEN DELIVERY: BLOOD GAS, ACID-BASE BALANCE, AND HEMATOCRIT

Severe arterial hypoxemia to a partial arterial pressure of oxygen (PaO_2) value of less than 40 mm Hg is associated with decreased RBF and renal vasoconstriction.[98,99] Inequalities in oxygen supply and demand are exaggerated and medullary hypoxia is extreme during CPB, effects that last well beyond separation from circulatory support in experimental models.[100]

The effects of anemia on the kidney have been studied mostly in the context of CPB management. When crystalloid and colloid solutions are used to prime an extracorporeal circuit, the initiation of CPB surgery obligates an acute decrease of approximately 30% in oxygen-carrying capacity. Animal studies endorse moderate hemodilution (hematocrit 20% to 30%) as renoprotective during CPB surgery through a reduction of blood viscosity and improved regional blood flow.[101] However, although hematocrit values less than 20% during CPB surgery are commonly accepted clinically (extreme hemodilution), very low hematocrit values are linked with adverse outcomes, including AKI.[102-104] The Society of Thoracic Surgeons and the Society of Cardiovascular Anesthesiologists guidelines suggest that transfusion triggers should be lower during CPB surgery and that a transfusion trigger of 6 g/dL is reasonable, except in those at risk for end-organ ischemia, in whom a higher trigger may be reasonable.[105] More recently, the European Association for Cardio-Thoracic Surgery and the European Association of Cardiothoracic Anesthesia have developed comprehensive guidelines and suggest that a target hematocrit of 21% to 24% during cardiopulmonary bypass is reasonable.[106]

The solution may not be as simple as transfusion because blood transfusions themselves have been linked to AKI. In a systematic review, Karkouti found 22 studies that examined the association between blood transfusions and AKI postcardiac surgery. An independent association between transfusions and AKI was found in 18 of the 22 studies.[107] The association of perioperative anemia with AKI was further examined in 14 studies, and 9 of the studies found an independent association of perioperative anemia with AKI. Proposed mechanisms for transfusion-associated AKI include exacerbation of inflammation and oxidative stress, which occur during the CPB surgery.

There has been tremendous interest in the impact of the age of stored blood on the risk of AKI. Old blood may result in higher circulating levels of free hemoglobin and free iron, and there has been interest in the impact of the "storage lesion" on AKI. However, at present, data does not support the selective use of fresh blood in the perioperative setting to reduce the risk of AKI.[108-110]

Perioperative Blood Pressure and Fluid Management

There has been significant interest in perioperative blood pressure targets and the impact on AKI. Several large observational cohort studies have suggested that even transient hypotension was associated with postoperative AKI.[111-115] One prospective randomized trial compared an individualized blood pressure management strategy targeted at maintaining systolic blood pressure within 10% of baseline versus a standard management strategy (treatment of systolic blood pressure <80 mm Hg or lower than 40% from baseline) and demonstrated a significant reduction in the primary composite endpoint (systemic inflammatory response and at least one organ dysfunction within 7 days). This modest sized clinical trial demonstrated a nonsignificant trend toward reduced postoperative AKI in the individualized blood pressure management arm.[116] Thus blood pressure targets, in particular in patients with chronic kidney disease, need to take into consideration preoperative blood pressure.

Intravascular volume depletion, which commonly occurs in fasting patients undergoing surgery, is a risk factor for AKI. For example, the combination of diabetes mellitus and intravascular volume depletion increases the chance of developing AKI by 100-fold.[117] The most practical preoperative methods to assess volume status are with preoperative patient history and physical examination and by assessing changes in arterial blood pressure in response to changing conditions and dynamic maneuvers. For example, an awake patient normally does not have significant orthostatic changes in arterial blood pressure unless an autonomic or intravascular volume deficit exists. During anesthesia, a similarly dehydrated patient may demonstrate paradoxical arterial pulse changes with positive-pressure inspiration. Nonetheless, there has been tremendous interest in the use of intravascular monitoring techniques in the perioperative setting to reduce the risk of AKI.

The decision to use any monitor should depend on the patient's functional cardiac reserve status and the extent of the proposed surgical insult. Although maintaining adequate cardiac output is necessary for maintaining adequate RBF, adequate flow may still not occur. The use of intravascular volume monitoring techniques must include cautious identification of physiologic conditions that influence their validity as a reflection of preload in a particular patient. For example, monitoring central venous pressure to assess preload involves assumptions about normal left and right ventricular function; pulmonary vascular resistance; and mitral, pulmonary, and tricuspid valve function. Similarly, monitoring pulmonary artery pressure or pulmonary capillary wedge pressure assumes normal left ventricular compliance, mitral valve function, and normal airway pressure.

Direct measurements of left atrial pressure may offer insight into the kidney pressure-flow relationship because left atrial hypotension is a powerful stimulus for renal vasoconstriction. Despite equivalent reductions in cardiac output and arterial blood pressure, RBF decreases significantly more when left atrial pressure is decreased (e.g., hemorrhagic shock), compared with left atrial pressure when it is increased (e.g., cardiogenic shock).[118] Left atrial pressure receptors modulate renal vasoconstriction through the release of ANP, a hormone secreted by the cardiac atria in response to intravascular volume expansion.[119] ANP acts on the arterial and venous systems, the adrenal glands, and the kidneys to reduce intravascular volume and decrease blood pressure.[120] Within the kidney, the hormone increases hydraulic pressure in the glomerular capillaries through afferent arteriolar dilation and efferent arteriolar vasoconstriction. ANP reduces arterial blood pressure by relaxing smooth muscle and reducing sympathetic vascular stimulation and also inhibits renin and aldosterone secretion, causing renal vasodilation, natriuresis, and diuresis.

Despite the direct relationship of left atrial pressure and renal vasoconstriction, static monitors of intravascular volume status are gradually being replaced by echocardiographic and dynamic monitors of intravascular volume status. Intraoperatively, one of the most direct ways to monitor intravascular volume may be by direct assessment of the left ventricular end-diastolic area with transesophageal echocardiography. However, monitoring with invasive devices, such as pulmonary artery catheters, arterial cannulas, and transesophageal echocardiography, has not been demonstrated to reduce the incidence of AKI.

Guided fluid optimization has recently garnered significant interest as a step beyond traditional, somewhat unreliable guides to fluid administration (e.g., central venous pressure).[121,122] The principle behind fluid optimization is to maximize tissue-oxygen delivery by achieving a maximum stroke volume. Intravascular fluid management is typically guided by the physiologic response to dynamic measures; proposed measures include systolic pressure variation, pulse pressure variation, continuous cardiac output monitoring, and esophageal Doppler ultrasonography fluid boluses.[123] Some maneuvers to assess fluid responsiveness may be feasible in the critical care setting but not in the perioperative setting (e.g., passive leg raise).

Given the improved outcomes in patients who are critically ill with the acute respiratory distress syndrome and are managed with a restrictive fluid management strategy,[124] fluid restriction in the perioperative setting has gained attention. A meta-analysis of seven randomized clinical trials in the setting of intraabdominal surgery suggested a restrictive fluid strategy offered no benefit; however, there was also no evidence of harm, including AKI.[125] In some studies, excessive fluid restriction was associated with harm, including an increased risk of anastomotic breakdown and sepsis, and should clearly be avoided.[126] However, more recently, the RELIEF clinical trial randomized 3000 patients undergoing major abdominal surgery to a restrictive or liberal fluid strategy during surgery and up to 24 hours afterward; the restrictive fluid strategy was designed to provide a net even fluid balance.[127] There was no difference in the primary endpoint of disability-free survival at 1 year. However, the restrictive fluid strategy was associated with an increased rate of AKI (8.6% vs. 5.0%, $P < .001$) and surgical site infections (16.5% vs. 13.6%, unadjusted $P = .02$), though the comparison for surgical site infections was not considered significant after adjustment for multiple comparisons. Thus at present, fluid management strategies should avoid markedly positive fluid balance, but also need to be wary of underresuscitation.

There has been considerable interest in the use of balanced salt solutions instead of chloride-rich solutions to prevent AKI; the rationale is that chloride-rich solutions reduce renal perfusion in animal models.[128] Subsequently, a pre-post study of chloride-rich versus balanced salt solutions demonstrated a reduced incidence of stage 2 and 3 AKI during the balanced salt solution period.[129] Similarly, a propensity-matched study of patients undergoing major abdominal surgery suggested that patients who received balanced salt solutions had fewer postoperative complications, including postoperative dialysis.[130] However, a subsequent clinical trial, the SPLIT trial, suggested that there was no decrease in AKI with the use of Plasma-Lyte 148 in ICU patients.[131] Of note, 72% of the trial population was enrolled after surgery, with 49% enrolled after cardiac surgery. More recently, the SALT-ED and SMART trials were pragmatic clinical trials that randomized patients to receive balanced salt solutions or normal saline in alternating months in the Emergency Department and Intensive Care Units, respectively, at a single clinical center.[132,133] Both studies demonstrated a statistically significant reduction in the rate of major adverse kidney events at 30 days, a composite endpoint of death, dialysis, and persistent doubling of creatinine. In SMART, approximately 20% of subjects were admitted in the postoperative setting; there was no evidence of an interaction between treatment effect and type of ICU, but the study was underpowered to observe a difference within this subgroup.

Finally, are these solutions safe in patients who are prone to hyperkalemia? Because balanced salt solutions contain a physiologic amount of potassium, there has been concern that the administration of balanced salt solutions might lead to hyperkalemia in patients with reduced renal function. However, in two randomized clinical trials of intraoperative fluid selection in end-stage kidney disease patients undergoing kidney transplantation, there was no increase in the incidence of hyperkalemia.[134] The median volume of intravenous solution administered in a the trial that compared normal saline to an acetate based buffer was 2625 mL (IQR 2000-3001 mL);[135] in a trial comparing normal saline to lactated Ringers, mean fluid volumes were 6.1 ± 1.2 L and 5.6 ± 1.4 L, respectively.[136] Thus at reasonable doses, balanced salt solutions appear safe across a wide variety of patient populations and are associated with a decreased risk of AKI.

EXCESSIVE INTRAVASCULAR VOLUME AND THE ABDOMINAL COMPARTMENT SYNDROME

The abdominal compartment syndrome was first defined in 1985; since then, it has been progressively recognized as a common contributor to renal dysfunction in the setting of excessive intravascular volume.[137-139] Not surprisingly, excessive intravascular volume and mechanical ventilation with high airway pressures are significant contributors to the abdominal compartment syndrome. Abdominal compartment syndrome is defined as a sustained increase in intraabdominal pressures to greater than 20 mm Hg that causes organ dysfunction; in contrast, intraabdominal hypertension is typically defined as intraabdominal pressures ≥12 mm Hg without organ dysfunction. This increase in intraabdominal pressure decreases abdominal perfusion pressure (which is mean arterial pressure − intraabdominal pressure), and results in a functional prerenal state attributable to reduced renal perfusion.

The intraabdominal pressure can easily be measured using an indwelling Foley catheter and the same pressure tubing setup used for arterial line blood pressure monitoring.[140] The Foley catheter is clamped distal to the instillation port, and up to 25 mL of saline is instilled into the bladder. The transducer should be zeroed at the midaxillary line, and the pressure should be measured at end-expiration approximately 30 to 60 seconds after fluid is instilled into the bladder to allow for detrusor muscle relaxation. Of note, intraabdominal pressure may be chronically elevated to as high as 12 mm Hg in the obese adult but is not associated with end-organ dysfunction in this context.[141] Prompt recognition of the abdominal compartment syndrome and treatment via decompression in the appropriate clinical context is critical.

Nephrotoxins and Acute Kidney Injury

Recently, there has been significant controversy regarding the impact of iodinated contrast on AKI, with a number of observational studies suggesting that at a population level, iodinated contrast is not associated with an increased risk of AKI.[142,143] However, iodinated contrast is associated with intense renal vasoconstriction and causes significant AKI in the vulnerable subject. There has been significant interest in pharmacologic prevention of contrast-associated AKI. Clinical trials have demonstrated that pharmacologic interventions, including fenoldopam, n-acetyl-cysteine, and sodium bicarbonate, do not reduce the incidence of contrast-associated AKI.[144,145] Volume depletion and concomitant exposure to other nephrotoxins are key, preventable risk factors for AKI.

Other nephrotoxins commonly encountered in the perioperative setting include aminoglycosides and NSAIDs. In addition, there has been increasing interest in antibiotic nephrotoxicity. Specifically, the combination of vancomycin and piperacillin-tazobactam has been associated with an increased rate of AKI.[146] When possible, avoiding combinations of nephrotoxins is likely beneficial for AKI prevention.[147]

Renal Replacement Therapy

Despite best supportive care, at times, AKI progresses, and RRT is indicated. Conventional indications for dialysis include acidosis, electrolyte abnormalities (in particular, hyperkalemia), ingestions, volume overload, and uremia. There has been considerable interest in the optimal timing of dialysis initiation in critically ill and postoperative patients. A provocative, single-center study suggested that after cardiac surgery, there was significant benefit to initiation of dialysis for stage 2 AKI (doubling of sCr from baseline or urine output <0.5 mL/kg/h for 12 hours) versus waiting until stage 3 AKI (tripling of sCr from baseline, sCr ≥4 mg/dL with an acute rise of ≥0.5 mg/dL, or urine output <0.3 mL/kg/h for 24 hours).[148] Early RRT was associated with a lower incidence of death (39.3% vs. 54.7%, $P = .03$) and a greater rate of renal recovery at 90 days (53.6% vs. 38.7%, $P = 0.02$). It should be noted 90% of patients in the delayed arm received RRT, and the median difference in time to dialysis initiation was only 21 hours, so this is a remarkably large effect size that should be interpreted with caution. This study is in marked contrast to two large randomized clinical trials in critically ill patients suggesting that dialysis can be safely delayed in a number of patients.[149,150] In these clinical trials, patients were randomized to receive dialysis when they met criteria for stage 3 AKI or to initiate dialysis only after prespecified electrolyte/metabolic criteria were met or after AKI exceeded a prespecified duration. There was no difference in mortality between the two treatment arms; in addition, a significant proportion of subjects in the delayed therapy arm recovered and never required dialysis (29% in the IDEAL-ICU trial). Additional clinical trials are ongoing to further test the hypothesis that in critically ill patients, dialysis can be safely delayed.[151]

There has also been considerable interest in dialysis modality and the impact on outcomes. At present, four modalities of dialysis are possible in the ICU. Peritoneal dialysis requires placement of a catheter in the intraabdominal space; this is typically performed laparoscopically, but can be inserted at the bedside if needed. Dextrose-containing fluids drive fluid and solute removal. Thus a significant risk of peritoneal dialysis is infection (e.g., peritonitis). Furthermore, this modality cannot be used in patients who have had recent intraabdominal surgery, so in general, its role is quite limited in the perioperative setting, with the exception of patients who are maintained on this therapy for end-stage renal disease preoperatively. With regard to hemodialysis, modalities are typically divided into: intermittent hemodialysis (IHD), prolonged intermittent RRT (PIRRT)/slow low efficiency dialysis (SLED), and continuous renal replacement therapies (CRRT). As the name implies, IHD is typically performed over a 3- to 4-hour period, 3 to 6 days/week. PIRRT/SLED is typically performed over 6 to 12 hours/day, 3 to 6 days/week; there is no standard dialysis machine for PIRRT/SLED so dialysis programs may use this therapy quite differently. CRRT is performed on a continuous, 24 hours/day basis.

With regard to modality and outcomes, it has been specifically hypothesized that intradialytic hypotension might prolong AKI and delay renal recovery. However, no randomized clinical trials have demonstrated clear benefit to continuous RRT with regards to mortality or renal recovery.[152] Clinical trials have also examined the impact of dialysis dose and membrane on outcomes. These studies have established that there is a minimum dose of dialysis that should likely be measured and delivered,[153,154] and that modern dialysis membranes are all relatively biocompatible and there is no benefit of one membrane over another.

To maintain circuit patency, anticoagulation is often needed. At present, the two most common forms of anticoagulation are low-dose heparin (100 to 500 units/h) and regional citrate. In both cases, the anticoagulant is infused prefilter to minimize systemic effects. Even though the goal of heparin anticoagulation is to not affect systemic coagulation parameters such as partial thromboplastin time, there is a small increase in bleeding risk.[155,156] The goal of regional citrate anticoagulation is to reduce the ionized calcium concentration in the dialysis filter, since calcium is a required cofactor in the coagulation cascade. Thus citrate is infused prefilter and titrated to maintain a low postfilter ionized calcium. One of the challenges in the United States to the routine use of citrate anticoagulation is the lack of a citrate solution approved by the Food and Drug Administration for use with RRT; thus each center typically has developed its own protocol for titration and monitoring. That said, regional citrate anticoagulation is typically recommended in favor of other forms of anticoagulation.[14,155,156]

Occasionally, RRT is indicated in the operating room, typically during prolonged cases with significant blood product transfusion (e.g., liver transplantation). Close coordination between the nephrologist and the anesthesiologist is needed.

Summary

In patients with or at risk for developing AKI, perioperative management continues to be challenging. Numerous factors contribute to the heterogeneous condition referred to as perioperative AKI, but insults collectively combine through ischemic and toxic mechanisms. Recent research efforts directed to the investigation of AKI will likely lead to rapid developments in the field of renal function monitoring. At present, serum creatinine continues to be the mainstay of most renal function monitoring strategies, along with urine output. Best supportive care for perioperative AKI includes preoperative risk stratification with quantitation of serum creatinine and proteinuria/albuminuria for moderate-high risk surgeries, avoidance of hypotension and hypovolemia, along with judicious use of nephrotoxins. In the setting of severe AKI, support with RRT may be needed. At present, the timing of dialysis initiation is controversial, but early initiation does not appear to be associated with improved outcomes in critically ill patients.

Acknowledgment

The editors, publisher, and authors, Drs. Kathleen D. Liu, Daniel H. Burkhardt III, and Rupert M. Pearse, would like to thank Drs. Mark Stafford-Smith and Andrew Shaw for their contribution to this chapter in the prior edition of this work. It has served as the foundation for the current chapter.

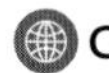 **Complete references available online at expertconsult.com.**

References

1. Thakar CV. *Adv Chronic Kidney Dis.* 2013;20(67).
2. Chaudery H, et al. *Anesth Analg.* 2018. https://doi.org/10.1213/ANE.0000000000003923.
3. O'Connor ME, et al. *Br J Surg.* 2017;104:868.
4. Zarbock A, et al. *Anesth Analg.* 2018;127:1236.
5. Smith Jr LH, et al. *Am J Med.* 1955;18:187.
6. Gaffney AM, Sladen RN. *Curr Opin Anaesthesiol.* 2015;28:50.
7. Hoste EAJ, Vandenberghe W. *Best Pract Res Clin Anaesthesiol.* 2017;31:299.
8. Fuhrman DY, Kellum JA. *Curr Opin Anaesthesiol.* 2017;30:60.
9. Hobson C, et al. *J Vasc Surg.* 2018;68:916.
10. Novis BK, et al. *Anesth Analg.* 1994;78(143).
11. Chertow GM, et al. *Am J Med.* 1998;104:343.
12. Bellomo R, et al. *Crit Care.* 2004;8:R204.
13. Mehta RL, et al. *Crit Care.* 2007;11:R31.
14. Group KDIGO KAKIW. *Kidney Int Suppl.* 2012;2(1).
15. Kellum JA, et al. *J Am Soc Nephrol.* 2015;26:2231.
16. Palevsky PM, et al. *Am J Kidney Dis.* 2013;61:649.
17. Quan S, et al. *Nephrol Dial Transplant.* 2016;31:2049.
18. Alpert RA, et al. *Surgery.* 1984;95:707.
19. Knos GB, et al. *J Clin Anesth.* 1989;1:181.
20. Mizota T, et al. *Br J Anaesth.* 2017;119:1127–1134.
21. Siddiqui NF, et al. *CMAJ.* 2012;184(1237).
22. Myers BD, Moran SM. *N Engl J Med.* 1986;314:97.
23. Myers BD, et al. *J Clin Invest.* 1984;73:329.
24. Kaufman J, et al. *Am J Kidney Dis.* 1991;17:191.
25. Hou SH, et al. *Am J Med.* 1983;74:243.
26. Badr KF, Ichikawa I. *N Engl J Med.* 1988;319:623.
27. Barger A, Herd J. In: Orlaff J, Berliner R, eds. *Handbook of Physiology.* Baltimore, MD: Williams and Wilkins; 1973.
28. Packer M, et al. *Circulation.* 1986;74:766.
29. Edwards RM. *Am J Physiol.* 1983;244:F526.
30. Stone AM, Stahl WM. *Ann Surg.* 1970;172:825.
31. Andersson LG, et al. *Eur J Cardiothorac Surg.* 1994;8:597.
32. Laffey JG, et al. *Anesthesiology.* 2002;97:215.
33. Mcmahon G, Waikar S. *Am J Kidney Dis.* 2013;61:165.
34. Parikh CR, Mansour SG. *J Am Soc Nephrol.* 2017;28:1677.
35. Waikar SS, Bonventre JV. *Nephron Clin Pract.* 2008;109:c192.
36. Chen L-X,C, Koyner JL. *Crit Care Clin.* 2015;31:633–648.
37. Shlipak MG, et al. *Am J Kidney Dis.* 2013;62:595–603.
38. Inker LA, et al. *N Engl J Med.* 2012;367:20.
39. Stevens LA, et al. *Am J Kidney Dis.* 2008;51:395.
40. Zhu J, et al. *Clin Chim Acta.* 2006;374:116.
41. Spahillari A, et al. *Am J Kidney Dis.* 2012;60:922.
42. Foster MC, et al. *Am J Kidney Dis.* 2013;62:42.
43. Mogensen CE. Sølling. *Scand J Clin Lab Invest.* 1977;37:477.
44. Smith MS. *Anesthesiology.* 1999;90:928.
45. Stafford-Smith M. *Am J Kidney Dis.* 2011;57:960; author reply, p1.
46. Kashani K, et al. *Crit Care.* 2013;17:R25.

47. Mishra J, et al. *J Am Soc Nephrol*. 2003;14:2534.
48. Mishra J, et al. *J Am Soc Nephrol*. 2004;15:3073.
49. Mishra J, et al. *Lancet*. 2005;365:1231.
50. Haase-Fielitz A, et al. *Ann Clin Biochem*. 2014;51:335.
51. Haase M, et al. *J Am Coll Cardiol*. 2011;57:1752.
52. Ichimura T, et al. *Am J Physiol Renal Physiol*. 2004;286:F552.
53. Vaidya VS, et al. *Nat Biotechnol*. 2010;28:478.
54. Sabbisetti VS, et al. *J Am Soc Nephrol*. 2014;25(2177).
55. Bihorac A, et al. *Am J Respir Crit Care Med*. 2014;189:932.
56. Gunnerson KJ, et al. *J Trauma Acute Care Surg*. 2016;80:243.
57. Meersch M, et al. *PLoS One*. 2014;9:e93460. 3968141.
58. Meersch M, et al. *Intensive Care Med*. 2017;43:1151.
59. Wang Y, Bellomo R. *Nat Rev Nephrol*. 2017;13:697.
60. Wilson T, et al. *Nephrol Dial Transplant*. 2016;31:231.
61. Hobson C, et al. *Crit Care Clin*. 2017;33(379).
62. Stafford-Smith M, et al. *Am J Kidney Dis*. 2005;45:519.
63. Aronson S, et al. *Circulation*. 2007;115:733.
64. Chertow GM, et al. *Circulation*. 1997;95:878.
65. Everett GB, et al. *Anesth Analg*. 1973;52:470.
66. Mark JB, Steele SM. *Int Anesthesiol Clin*. 1989;27:31.
67. Kennedy Jr WF, et al. *Anesthesiology*. 1969;31:414.
68. Kennedy Jr WF, et al. *Acta Anaesthesiol Scand Suppl*. 1969;37:163.
69. Rodgers A, et al. *BMJ*. 2000;321:1493.
70. Moraca RJ, et al. *Ann Surg*. 2003;238:663.
71. Bignami E, et al. *J Cardiothorac Vasc Anesth*. 2010;24:586.
72. Landoni G, et al. *Br J Anaesth*. 2015;115:25.
73. Svircevic V, et al. *Cochrane Database Syst Rev*. 2013;6:CD006715.
74. Guay J, Kopp S. *Cochrane Database Syst Rev*. 2016;1:CD005059.
75. Cousins MJ, Mazze RI. *JAMA*. 1973;225:1611.
76. Mazze RI. *Anesthesiology*. 2006;105:843.
77. Mazze RI, et al. *Anesthesiology*. 1977;46:265.
78. Hsing CH, et al. *Nephrol Dial Transplant*. 2011;26:1162.
79. Yuzbasioglu MF, et al. *Renal Fail*. 2010;32(578).
80. Sanchez-Conde P, et al. *Anesth Analg*. 2008;106:371; table of contents.
81. Dikmen B, et al. *J Anesth*. 2010;24:73.
82. Hsing CH, et al. *Am J Physiol Renal Physiol*. 2012;303:F1443.
83. Sugita S, et al. *J Nippon Med Sch*. 2013;80:131.
84. Gu J, et al. *Crit Care*. 2011;15:R153.
85. Liu Y, et al. *BMC Anesthesiol*. 2018;18(7).
86. Gamulin Z, et al. *Anesthesiology*. 1984;61:394.
87. Szabo G, et al. *Injury*. 1977;9(146).
88. Parikh CR, et al. *J Am Soc Nephrol*. 2011;22(1748):3171945.
89. Rioux JP, et al. *Crit Care Med*. 2009;37:1293.
90. Myburgh JA, et al. *N Engl J Med*. 2012;367:1901.
91. Rosner MH, Okusa MD. *Clin J Am Soc Nephrol*. 2006;1(19).
92. Mangano DT, et al. *N Engl J Med*. 2006;354:353.
93. Shroyer AL, et al. *N Engl J Med*. 2009;361:1827.
94. Chawla LS, et al. *J Am Soc Nephrol*. 2012;23:1389.
95. Garg AX, et al. *JAMA*. 2014;311:2191.
96. Deferrari G, et al. *Nephrol Dial Transplant*. 2018;33:813.
97. Romagnoli S, et al. *Curr Opin Anaesthesiol*. 2017;30:92.
98. Kilburn KH, Dowell AR. *Arch Intern Med*. 1971;127:754.
99. Pelletier CL, Shepherd JT. *Am J Physiol*. 1975;228:331.
100. Stafford-Smith M, et al. *Am J Kidney Dis*. 2005;45:519.
101. Utley JR, et al. *Ann Thorac Surg*. 1981;31:121.
102. Karkouti K, et al. *J Thorac Cardiovasc Surg*. 2005;129:391.
103. Swaminathan M, et al. *Ann Thorac Surg*. 2003;76(784):92; discussion.
104. Mehta RH, et al. *Ann Thorac Surg*. 2013;96:133.
105. Ferraris VA, et al. *Ann Thorac Surg*. 2011;91:944.
106. Pagano D, et al. *Eur J Cardiothorac Surg*. 2018;53(79).
107. Karkouti K. *Br J Anaesth*. 2012;109(suppl 1):i29.
108. Hovaguimian F, Myles PS. *Anesthesiology*. 2016;125:46.
109. Curley GF. *Crit Care Med*. 2014;42:2611.
110. Mazer CD, et al. *N Engl J Med*. 2017;377:2133.
111. Walsh M, et al. *Anesthesiology*. 2013;119(507).
112. Sun LY, et al. *Anesthesiology*. 2015;123:515.
113. Salmasi V, et al. *Anesthesiology*. 2017;126:47.
114. Hallqvist L, et al. *Eur J Anaesthesiol*. 2018;35:273.
115. Vernooij LM, et al. *Br J Anaesth*. 2018;120:1080.
116. Futier E, et al. *JAMA*. 2017;318(1346).
117. Shusterman N, et al. *Am J Med*. 1987;83:65.
118. Gorfinkel HJ, et al. *Am J Physiol*. 1972;222:1260.
119. Kahl FR, et al. *Am J Physiol*. 1974;226:240.
120. Cogan MG. *Annu Rev Physiol*. 1990;52:699.
121. Bednarczyk JM, et al. *Crit Care Med*. 2017;45(1538).
122. Vincent JL, et al. *Crit Care*. 2015;19(224).
123. Busse L, et al. *Adv Chronic Kidney Dis*. 2013;20:21.
124. Wiedemann HP, et al. *N Engl J Med*. 2006;354:2564.
125. Boland MR, et al. *World J Surg*. 2013;37:1193.
126. Futier E, et al. *Arch Surg*. 2010;145:1193.
127. Myles PS, et al. *N Engl J Med*. 2018;378:2263.
128. Wilcox CS. *J Clin Invest*. 1983;71(726).
129. Yunos NM, et al. *Crit Care*. 2010;14:226.
130. Shaw AD, et al. *Ann Surg*. 2012;255:821.
131. Young P, et al. *JAMA*. 2015;314:1701.
132. Self WH, et al. *N Engl J Med*. 2018;378:819.
133. Semler MW, et al. *N Engl J Med*. 2018;378:829.
134. Wan S, et al. *Cochrane Database Syst Rev*. 2016;CD010741.
135. Potura E, et al. *Anesth Analg*. 2015;120(123).
136. O'Malley CM, et al. *Anesth Analg*. 2005;100(1518); table of contents.
137. Mohmand H, Goldfarb S. *J Am Soc Nephrol*. 2011;22:615.
138. Carr JA. *J Am Coll Surg*. 2013;216:135.
139. Rogers WK, Garcia L. *Chest*. 2018;153:238.
140. Malbrain ML, et al. *Intensive Care Med*. 2006;32:1722.
141. Lambert D, et al. *Obes Surg*. 2005;15:1225.
142. Wilhelm-Leen E, et al. *J Am Soc Nephrol*. 2017;28:653.
143. Luk L, et al. *Adv Chronic Kidney Dis*. 2017;24:169.
144. Weisbord SD, et al. *Clin J Am Soc Nephrol*. 2013;8:1618.
145. Weisbord SD, et al. *N Engl J Med*. 2018;378:603.
146. Luther MK, et al. *Crit Care Med*. 2018;46(12).
147. Goldstein SL, et al. *Kidney Int*. 2016;90:212.
148. Zarbock A, et al. *JAMA*. 2016;315:2190.
149. Gaudry S, et al. *N Engl J Med*. 2016;375:122.
150. Barbar SD, et al. *N Engl J Med*. 2018;379:1431.
151. Wald R, et al. *Kidney Int*. 2015;88:897.
152. Nash DM, et al. *J Crit Care*. 2017;41:138.
153. Palevsky PM, et al. *N Engl J Med*. 2008;359(7).
154. Bellomo R, et al. *N Engl J Med*. 2009;361:1627.
155. Oudemans-van Straaten HM. *Semin Thromb Hemost*. 2015;41:91.
156. Brandenburger T, et al. *Best Pract Res Clin Anaesthesiol*. 2017;31:387.

43 Neuromuscular Monitoring

CASPER CLAUDIUS and THOMAS FUCHS-BUDER

KEY POINTS

- Good evidence-based practice dictates that clinicians always quantitate the extent of neuromuscular block by objective monitoring.
- The neuromuscular block should be adjusted to ensure optimal surgical conditions. In most procedures, one or two responses to train-of-four (TOF) stimulation will suffice. To avoid involuntary diaphragmatic movements, a deeper level of neuromuscular block is required (i.e., one to five responses to post-tetanic count [PTC]).
- Adequate recovery of postoperative neuromuscular function cannot be guaranteed without objective neuromuscular monitoring.
- Objective neuromuscular monitoring is essential for management of neuromuscular blockade intraoperatively and its reversal for postoperative care. Muscle relaxants should not be given in the intensive care unit without proper monitoring.
- It is impossible to exclude with certainty clinically significant residual neuromuscular block by clinical evaluation of recovery of neuromuscular function.
- Residual postoperative neuromuscular block causes decreased chemoreceptor sensitivity to hypoxia, functional impairment of the pharyngeal and upper esophageal muscles, impaired ability to maintain an open upper airway, and an increased risk of hypoxemic events, as well as the development of postoperative pulmonary complications.
- Absence of tactile fade in the response to TOF stimulation, tetanic stimulation, and double-burst stimulation does not exclude significant residual block.
- To exclude clinically significant residual neuromuscular block, the TOF ratio must exceed 0.9 when measured mechanically or electromyographically and 1.0 when measured acceleromyographically.
- Antagonism of the neuromuscular block with a cholinesterase inhibitor should not be initiated before at least two to four responses to TOF stimulation are observed.
- Antagonism of the neuromuscular block achieved by rocuronium and vecuronium can be initiated at all levels of block with the selective relaxant binding agent sugammadex.
- If adequate recovery (TOF ≥0.9-1.0) has not been documented objectively at the end of the surgical procedure, the neuromuscular block should be antagonized.

Our understanding of the pathophysiologic consequences of residual paralysis has improved over the last decades, and it is now generally accepted that even small degrees of residual paralysis (i.e., a train-of-four [TOF] ratio 0.7-0.9) may be clinically harmful.[1-4] As a consequence, the benchmark of adequate neuromuscular recovery has been revised several times; an adductor pollicis TOF ratio of 0.9 or greater is now required to exclude relevant residual neuromuscular block (i.e., paralysis). Clinically significant residual paralysis cannot be excluded using clinical criteria and it can persist postoperatively.[5,6] Objective monitoring of the degree of neuromuscular block associated with pharmacologic reversal reduces the incidence of residual paralysis and should be part of standard perioperative monitoring when neuromuscular blocking agents (NMBAs) are used.[7-13]

In awake patients, muscle power can be evaluated by tests of voluntary muscle strength, but this is impossible during anesthesia and recovery from anesthesia. Historically, anesthesiologists have used clinical tests to assess muscle power directly and to estimate neuromuscular function indirectly (muscle tone; feel of the anesthesia bag as an indirect measure of pulmonary compliance, tidal volume, and inspiratory force). All these tests are influenced by factors other than the degree of neuromuscular block and, therefore, should not be used to evaluate recovery from neuromuscular blockade. Whenever precise information regarding the status of neuromuscular functioning is desired, the response of muscle to nerve stimulation should be assessed. This procedure also takes into account the considerable variation in individual response and sensitivity to muscle relaxants.

This chapter reviews the basic principles of neuromuscular monitoring and the requirements for effective use of nerve stimulators for peripheral nerve stimulation. It also describes the response to nerve stimulation during depolarizing (phase I and phase II) and nondepolarizing neuromuscular block, provides information about the level of neuromuscular blockade, and discusses the consequences of residual paralysis. Moreover, methods of evaluating evoked neuromuscular responses with and without the availability of recording equipment are discussed.

Principles of Peripheral Nerve Stimulation

Neuromuscular monitoring is used to evaluate the effect of a NMBA. The muscle response after stimulation of its corresponding motor nerve is assessed. The most frequently assessed nerve-muscle unit is the ulnar nerve and the adductor pollicis muscle. The muscle response can be evaluated either qualitatively with a peripheral nerve stimulator or quantified with objective monitors. With the peripheral nerve stimulator, the observer evaluates the muscle response either tactically or visually, whereas with the monitor the response is objectively measured and displayed on a screen. Whatever method is used for neuromuscular monitoring, the clinician should be familiar with the following terms: supramaximal stimulation, calibration, impedance, and safety margin.

SUPRAMAXIMAL STIMULATION

The reaction of a single muscle fiber to a stimulus follows an all-or-none pattern. In contrast, the response (the force of contraction) of the whole muscle depends on the number of muscle fibers activated. If a nerve is stimulated with sufficient intensity, all fibers supplied by the nerve will react, and the maximum response will be triggered. After administration of a neuromuscular blocking drug, the response of the muscle decreases in parallel with the number of fibers blocked. The reduction in response during constant stimulation reflects the degree of neuromuscular block.

For the preceding principles to work, the stimulus must be truly maximal throughout the whole period of monitoring; therefore, the electrical stimulus applied is usually at least 15% to 20% greater than that necessary for a maximal response. For this reason, the stimulus is said to be supramaximal. This compensates for potential changes in skin resistance intraoperatively and assures constant maximal stimulation throughout the procedure.

However, supramaximal electrical stimulation can be painful, which is not a concern during anesthesia, but during recovery the patient may be awake enough to experience the discomfort of nerve stimulation. Therefore, some researchers advocate stimulation with submaximal current during recovery. Although several investigations indicate that testing of neuromuscular function can be reliably performed postoperatively with submaximal stimulation,[14,15] the accuracy of such monitoring is unacceptable with that low current.[15]

CALIBRATION

A device used for objective monitoring of the neuromuscular function should be calibrated before the NMBA is administered. Calibration adjusts the gain of the device to ensure that the observed response to supramaximal stimulation is within the measurement window of the device and as close as possible to the "100% control response." The calibration procedure varies with the type of device used, but most often it is done with 1.0 Hz single-twitch stimulation. It is especially important to calibrate when the onset and recovery of the neuromuscular block are established with single-twitch stimulation.

In the TOF mode of nerve stimulation, calibration is considered less important because all four responses are amplified equally. Consequently, the TOF ratio is rarely influenced by calibration; however, in patients with very weak or strong responses to nerve stimulation, one or more responses to TOF stimulation might be out of the recording window, and the displayed TOF response might be incorrect. In some devices, supramaximal stimulation is established concurrently with the calibration procedure.

IMPEDANCE

An alternative and novel option to ensure a constant maximum stimulus throughout the whole procedure is to control the impedance (resistance) of the skin. Indeed, as long as the resistance of the skin is below a threshold value, the neuromuscular monitoring device will stimulate with the same user-selected electrical current (i.e., 60 mA). For a maximum current of 60 mA, the maximal resistance of the skin should be equal to or lower than 5 kΩ. If the resistance of the skin is above this value, the monitor will not be able to stimulate the patient with the selected current. More recently, nerve stimulators have been introduced that indicate the level of skin impedance on the screen (e.g., TofScan by iDMed, Marseille, France). Using this approach, establishment of supramaximal stimulation is not needed to assure that nerve stimulation is effective and constantly maximal through the whole procedure.

SAFETY MARGIN

Neuromuscular transmission has a substantial margin of safety. Neuromuscular block only becomes evident when 70% to 80% of acetylcholine receptors at the neuromuscular endplate are occupied by nondepolarizing NMBDs and to produce complete block, 90% to 95% of receptors must be occupied. Thus, the currently available equipment and the currently applied stimulation patterns allow only insight to this 70% to 95% range of receptor occupancy. This should be kept in mind, especially during recovery of neuromuscular block, where 70% of the acetylcholine receptors at the neuromuscular endplate may still be occupied but no longer detectable with neuromuscular monitoring.

Types of Peripheral Nerve Stimulation

Neuromuscular function is monitored by evaluating the muscular response to supramaximal stimulation of a peripheral motor nerve. Theoretically, two types of stimulation can be used: electrical and magnetic. Electrical nerve stimulation is by far the most commonly used method in clinical practice, and it is described in detail in this chapter. In theory, magnetic nerve stimulation has several advantages over electrical nerve stimulation.[2,16] It is less painful and does not require physical contact with the body; however, the equipment required is bulky and heavy, it cannot be used for TOF stimulation, and it is difficult to achieve supramaximal stimulation with this method. As a result, magnetic nerve stimulation is not used in clinical anesthesia.

Basic Considerations

STIMULATING ELECTRODES

Electrical impulses are transmitted from stimulator to nerve by means of surface or needle electrodes. Normally, disposable pre-gelled silver or silver chloride surface electrodes are used. The conducting area should be small, approximately 7 to 11 mm in diameter (Fig.43.1). Otherwise, the current produced in the underlying nerve may not be adequate.[17] Ideally, the skin should be cleansed properly and preferably rubbed with an abrasive before application of the electrodes. When the selected current cannot be obtained with surface electrodes, needle electrodes can be used in a few exceptional cases. Although specially coated needle electrodes are commercially available, ordinary steel injection needles often suffice. A sterile technique should be used, and the needles should be placed subcutaneously to avoid direct injury to the underlying nerve.

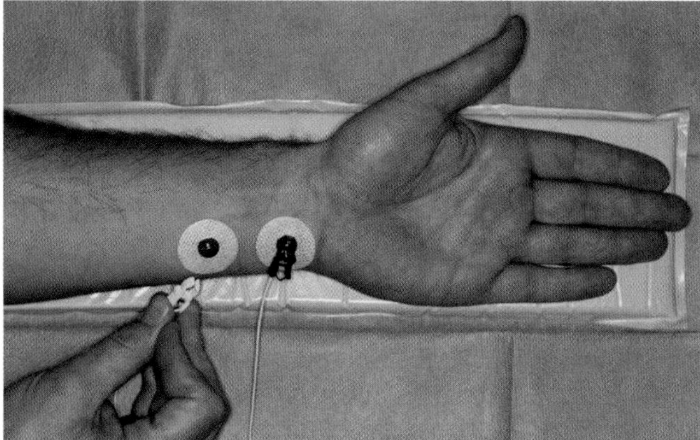

Fig. 43.1 Stimulating electrodes with the appropriate contact area in the correct position over the ulnar nerve of the left forearm.

Sites of Nerve Stimulation and Different Muscle Responses

In principle, any superficially located peripheral motor nerve can be stimulated and the response to corresponding muscle measured. Choosing the site of neuromuscular monitoring depends on several factors: the site should be easily accessible during surgery, it should allow quantitative monitoring and finally, direct muscle stimulation should be avoided. Direct muscle stimulation is characterized by weak contractions without fade persisting even at a deep level of neuromuscular blockade. The risk is increased when the stimulation electrodes are directly attached over the muscle to be assessed. To prevent direct muscle stimulation, the nerve-muscle unit should be chosen so that the site of nerve stimulation and the site of the subsequent evaluation of the twitch response are topographically (anatomically) distinct.

In clinical anesthesia, the ulnar nerve is the gold standard as a stimulation site, but the median, posterior tibial, common peroneal, and facial nerves are also sometimes used. For stimulation of the ulnar nerve, the electrodes are best applied to the volar side of the wrist (see Fig. 43.1). The distal electrode should be placed approximately 1 cm proximal to the point at which the proximal flexion crease of the wrist crosses the radial side of the tendon to the flexor carpi ulnaris muscle. The proximal electrode should preferably be placed so that the distance between the centers of the two electrodes is 3 to 6 cm (see Fig. 43.1). With this placement of the electrodes, electrical stimulation normally elicits only finger flexion and thumb adduction. If one electrode is placed over the ulnar groove at the elbow, thumb adduction is often pronounced because of stimulation of the flexor carpi ulnaris muscle. When this latter placement of electrodes (sometimes preferred in small children) is used, the active negative electrode should be at the wrist to ensure maximal response. Polarity of the electrodes is less crucial when both electrodes are close to each other at the volar side of the wrist; however, placement of the negative electrode distally normally elicits the greatest neuromuscular response.[18] When the temporal branch of the facial nerve is stimulated, the negative electrode should be placed over the nerve, and the positive electrode should be placed somewhere else over the forehead. When the posterior tibial nerve is stimulated, the electrodes should be placed close to the medial malleolus, with the same distance as described above and the negative electrode being placed distally.

NERVE-MUSCLE UNIT

Several nerve-muscle units may be chosen in clinical practice. Most often the ulnar nerve-adductor pollicis muscle is used.

Ulnar nerve-adductor pollicis muscle: This nerve-muscle unit is easily accessible intraoperatively if the arm is in the outstretched position and the hand in the supine position. The stimulatory response can be evaluated tactilely, visually, or by objective means. It has the lowest risk of direct muscle stimulation, because it ensures topographic separation of the stimulated nerve and the evaluated muscle by stimulating the ulnar nerve running along the median side of the arm and assessing the muscle response at the adductor pollicis muscle, which is indeed located on the lateral side of the hand.

Posterior tibial nerve-flexor hallucis brevis muscle: This nerve-muscle unit can be used for monitoring when the hands are inaccessible. The flexor hallucis brevis muscle produces flexion of the big toe following posterior tibial nerve stimulation. The characteristics (onset and recovery) of the neuromuscular block at the flexor hallucis brevis muscle is almost consistent with that of the adductor pollicis muscle.

Facial nerve-orbicularis oculi and facial nerve-corrugator supercilii muscle: When the arms are tucked under surgical drapes, quite often the only accessible site for monitoring is the head. Two facial muscles can be used as monitoring sites: the orbicularis oculi muscle and the corrugator supercilii muscle. The former encircles the orbital opening; its stimulation through the zygomatic branches of the facial nerve causes the eyelids to close. Stimulation by the temporal branch of the facial nerve of the latter one draws the medial end of the eyebrow downward, producing wrinkling of the brow. However, because the facial nerve is in direct proximity to the intrinsic mimic muscles, the risk of direct muscle stimulation is significant. Therefore, care must be

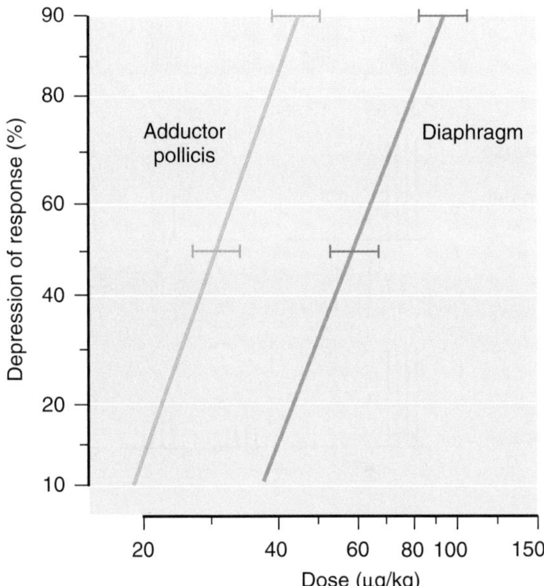

Fig. 43.2 The mean cumulative dose-response curve for pancuronium in two muscles shows that the diaphragm requires approximately twice as much pancuronium as the adductor pollicis muscle for the same amount of neuromuscular block. The depression in muscle response to the first stimulus in train-of-four nerve stimulation (probit scale) was plotted against dose (log scale). The force of contraction of the adductor pollicis was measured on a force-displacement transducer; response of the diaphragm was measured electromyographically. (From Donati F, Antzaka C, Bevan DR. Potency of pancuronium at the diaphragm and the adductor pollicis muscle in humans. *Anesthesiology.* 1986;65[1]:1–5.)

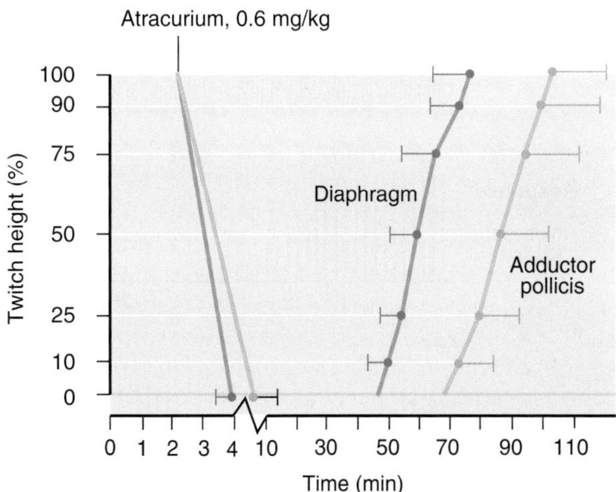

Fig. 43.3 Evolution of twitch height (mean ± SD) of the diaphragm *(blue circles)* and the adductor pollicis muscle *(yellow circles)* in 10 anesthetized patients after the administration of atracurium (0.6 mg/kg). (From Pansard J-L, Chauvin M, Lebrault C, et al. Effect of an intubating dose of succinylcholine and atracurium on the diaphragm and the adductor pollicis muscle in humans. *Anesthesiology.* 1987;67[3]:326–330.)

taken that the correct stimulatory response is assessed, and any other twitching muscle in the direct proximity of the stimulation electrodes is not falsely interpreted. Stimulation of the facial nerve can be accomplished with significantly lower currents: most often 25 to 30 mA are sufficient. Stimulation of these two muscles is technically difficult and the result often unsatisfactory in clinical practice.

Because different muscle groups have different sensitivities to neuromuscular blocking drugs, results obtained for one muscle cannot be automatically extrapolated to other muscles. However, most of the studies that are the base for dosing recommendations of NMBAs arise from measurement of the stimulation of the ulnar nerve. The diaphragm is among the most resistant of all muscles to both depolarizing[19] and nondepolarizing neuromuscular blocking drugs.[20] In general, the diaphragm requires 1.4- to 2.0-fold as much muscle relaxant as the adductor pollicis muscle for an identical degree of block (Fig. 43.2).[20] Also of clinical significance is that onset time is normally shorter for the diaphragm than for the adductor pollicis muscle, and the diaphragm recovers from paralysis more quickly than the peripheral muscles (Fig. 43.3).[21] The other respiratory muscles are less resistant than the diaphragm, as are the larynx and the corrugator supercilii muscles.[22-24] Most sensitive are the abdominal muscles, the orbicularis oculi muscle, the peripheral muscles of the limbs, and the geniohyoid, masseter, and upper airway muscles.[1,25-27] From a clinical point of view, the response of the corrugator supercilii to facial nerve stimulation reflects the extent of neuromuscular block of the laryngeal adductor muscles and abdominal muscles better than the response of the adductor pollicis to ulnar nerve stimulation.[24,28] Furthermore, the upper airway muscles seem to be more sensitive than the peripheral muscles.[25,26] Although some investigations using acceleromyography (AMG) have indicated small differences in the response to TOF nerve stimulation in the hand (adductor pollicis muscle) compared to the leg (flexor hallucis brevis muscle), these differences are probably of little clinical significance.[29,30] When comparing different sites of stimulation, there might be large differences between contralateral limbs (e.g., arm-to-arm variation of ± 20%).[31,32]

Although the precise source of these differences is unknown, possible explanations may be variations in acetylcholine receptor density, acetylcholine release, acetylcholinesterase activity, fiber composition, innervation ratio (number of neuromuscular junctions), blood flow, and muscle temperature.

Patterns of Nerve Stimulation

For the evaluation of the neuromuscular function, the most commonly used patterns are TOF stimulation, double-burst stimulation (DBS), and posttetanic count (PTC) stimulation. Single-twitch stimulation and tetanic stimulation are mainly used as a component in composite stimulation patterns (i.e., TOF, DBS, or PTC).

SINGLE-TWITCH STIMULATION

Background: Single-twitch stimulation is the earliest and simplest pattern. The first device specifically developed to monitor the neuromuscular block, the "St. Thomas's Hospital nerve stimulator," could only deliver a single twitch.[33] For decades it remained the only established stimulation pattern to assess neuromuscular blockade intraoperatively.

Stimulation pattern: In the single-twitch mode of stimulation, single electrical stimuli are applied to a peripheral motor nerve at frequencies ranging from 1.0 Hz (once every second) to 0.1 Hz (once every 10 seconds; Fig. 43.4) and

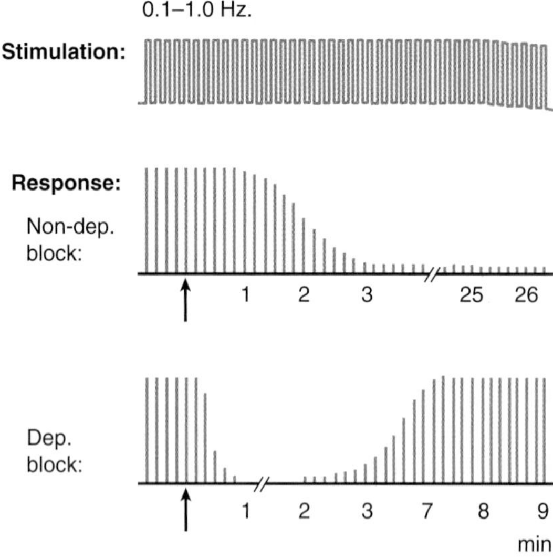

Fig. 43.4 Pattern of electrical stimulation and evoked muscle responses to single-twitch nerve stimulation (at frequencies of 0.1-1.0 Hz) after injection of nondepolarizing (Non-dep.) and depolarizing (Dep.) neuromuscular blocking drugs *(arrows)*. Note that except for the difference in time factors, no differences in the strength of the evoked responses exist between the two types of block.

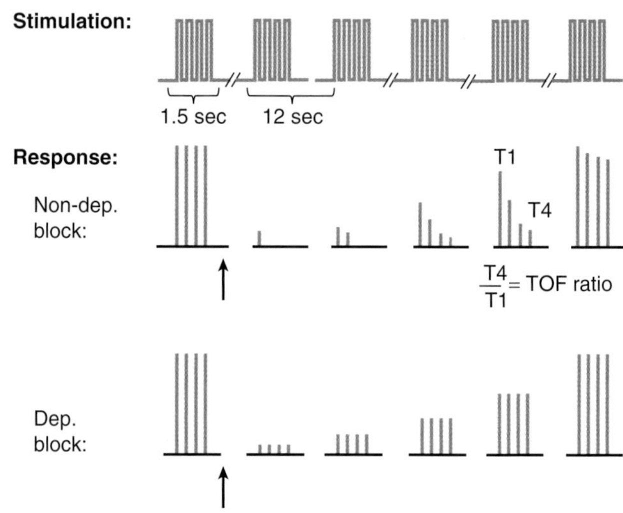

Fig. 43.5 Pattern of electrical stimulation and evoked muscle responses to train-of-four *(TOF)* nerve stimulation before and after injection of nondepolarizing (Non-dep.) and depolarizing (Dep.) neuromuscular blocking drugs *(arrows)*.

the subsequent muscle response is evaluated. The response to single-twitch stimulation depends on the frequency at which the individual stimuli are applied. If the rate of delivery is increased to greater than 0.15 Hz, the evoked response will gradually decrease and stabilize at a lower level. Therefore, results obtained with 1-Hz single-twitch stimulation cannot be compared with results obtained using, for example, 0.1-Hz single-twitch stimulation.[34] As a result, a frequency of 0.1 Hz is generally recommended.

Clinical application: To assess the degree of neuromuscular blockade after single-twitch stimulations, a comparison with a reference value recorded before administration of the NMBA is mandatory. Thus, without appropriate monitoring equipment, this stimulation pattern does not provide sufficient information of the level of block. In clinical practice, the single twitch stimulation has only limited value as a stand-alone stimulation pattern; it is mainly used as a component of the PTC stimulation and as 0.1 Hz single-twitch stimulation, it is sometimes used in scientific trials specifically to evaluate the time to onset of neuromuscular blockade. Moreover, it is the only stimulation pattern that allows, in conjunction with a monitoring device, assessing a depolarizing neuromuscular block after succinylcholine.

TRAIN-OF-FOUR STIMULATION

Background: The TOF stimulation pattern was introduced by Ali and associates[35,36] during the early 1970s. They aimed to develop a tool providing clinically reliable information throughout all phases of neuromuscular blockade with simple nerve stimulator and without the need for a monitoring device.

Stimulation pattern: TOF stimulation consists of four supramaximal stimuli given every 0.5 seconds (2 Hz; Fig.43.5) and each stimulus in the train causes the muscle to contract. The basis for evaluation is either the number of discernible responses after TOF stimulation (i.e., TOF count) or the "fade" in the train of responses—that is, dividing the amplitude of the fourth response by the amplitude of the first response (i.e., TOF ratio). Without prior administration of a muscle relaxant, all four responses are normally the same: the TOF ratio is 1.0. During a partial nondepolarizing block, the TOF ratio decreases (fades) and is inversely proportional to the degree of block. During a partial depolarizing block, no fade occurs in the TOF response and the TOF ratio remains 1.0, independently of the level of depolarizing neuromuscular blockade. Fade in the TOF response after injection of succinylcholine signifies the development of a phase II block (discussed later in the section on depolarizing neuromuscular block).

When used continuously, an interval of at least 10 seconds should be allowed between each set (train) of four stimuli to avoid fade during the measurement.

Application: TOF stimulation is still the most frequently used stimulation pattern. The advantages of TOF stimulation are most apparent during a nondepolarizing neuromuscular block because the degree of block can be read directly from the TOF response even though a preoperative value is lacking. Clinically relevant information about the onset, surgical relaxation, and neuromuscular recovery can be obtained with the same stimulation pattern by using a simple peripheral nerve stimulator; the TOF count allows reliable assessment of the onset of neuromuscular block, and moderate blockade. Moreover, the TOF ratio can be taken as a measure of neuromuscular recovery from nondepolarizing blockade. TOF stimulation has some advantages over DBS and PTC stimulation; it is less painful and, unlike tetanic stimulation, does not generally influence subsequent monitoring of the degree of neuromuscular block. There are major limitations of the TOF stimulation pattern. First, the subjective assessment of the TOF ratio overestimates neuromuscular recovery, as the tactile of visual estimation of fade is accurate only if the TOF ratio is less than 0.4; in other words, at a TOF ratio between 0.4 and 0.9, fade cannot be detected either visually or tactically. Therefore, objective monitoring devices are needed to further quantify neuromuscular recovery and to reliably exclude residual

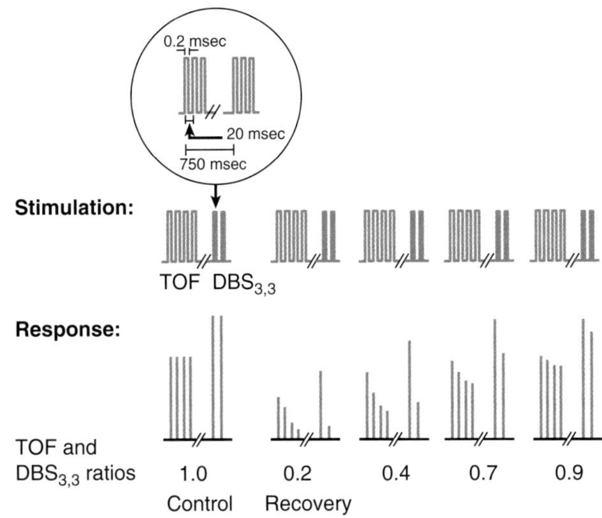

Fig. 43.6 Pattern of electrical stimulation and evoked muscle responses to train-of-four *(TOF)* nerve stimulation and double-burst nerve stimulation (i.e., three impulses in each of two tetanic bursts, *$DBS_{3,3}$*) before injection of muscle relaxants (control) and during recovery from nondepolarizing neuromuscular block. The TOF ratio is the amplitude of the fourth response to TOF divided by the amplitude of the first response. The $DBS_{3,3}$ ratio is the amplitude of the second response to $DBS_{3,3}$ divided by the amplitude of the first response. (See text for further explanation.)

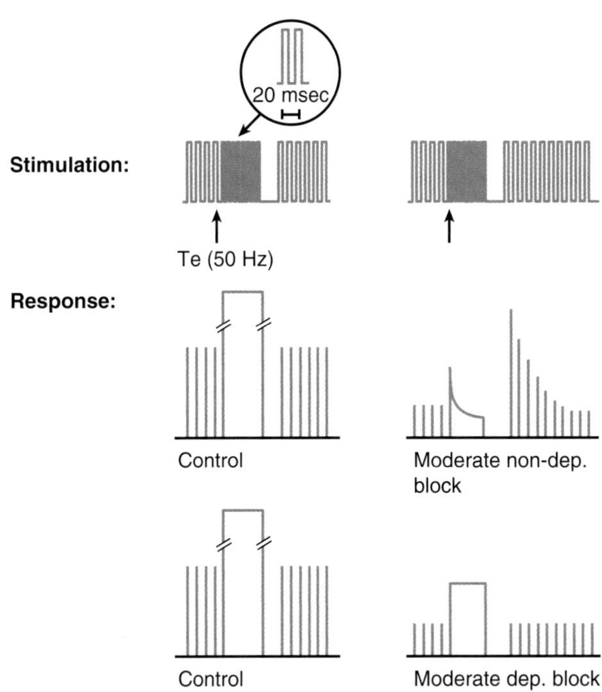

Fig. 43.7 Pattern of stimulation and evoked muscle responses to tetanic (50 Hz) nerve stimulation for 5 seconds *(Te)* and posttetanic twitch stimulation (1.0 Hz; *arrows*). Stimulation was applied before the injection of neuromuscular blocking drugs and during moderate nondepolarizing (non-dep.) and depolarizing (dep.) blocks. Note the fade in the response to tetanic stimulation, plus the posttetanic facilitation of transmission during nondepolarizing block. During depolarizing block, the tetanic response is well sustained, and no posttetanic facilitation of transmission occurs.

paralysis. Second, the TOF stimulation does not allow the clinician to quantify intense and deep levels of neuromuscular blockade (i.e., at no responses to TOF). Finally, the TOF stimulation does not allow monitoring of the depolarizing phase I blockade.

DOUBLE-BURST STIMULATION

Background: DBS was developed by Viby-Mogensen and associates in 1989 to improve the tactile or visual evaluation of recovery from nondepolarizing neuromuscular blockade.

Stimulation pattern: DBS consists of two short bursts of 50-Hz tetanic stimulation separated by 750 ms, with a 0.2-ms duration of each square wave impulse in the burst (Fig. 43.6). The number of impulses in each burst can vary: in the $DBS_{3,3}$ mode, there are three impulses in each of the two bursts, whereas in the $DBS_{3,2}$ mode, the first burst had three impulses and the second burst consisted of only two impulses.[37-39] The individual twitches elicited by each burst blend together and are felt as one single muscle contraction. Thus, the response to DBS is two short muscle contractions and fade in the second burst compared to the first one is the basis for evaluation. In nonparalyzed muscle, both muscle contractions are of equal strength. In a partially paralyzed muscle, the second response is weaker than the first and corresponds to the typical TOF fade (see Fig 43.6). When measured mechanically, the TOF ratio correlates closely with the $DBS_{3,3}$ ratio. Compared to $DBS_{3,3,}$ tactile detection of fade is slightly improved with the $DBS_{3,2}$ mode, especially at higher TOF ratios.

Clinical application: DBS was developed with the specific aim of improving manual (tactile or visual) detection of residual nondepolarizing block under clinical conditions,[38] or during recovery and immediately after surgery. Indeed, tactile evaluation of the response to DBS is more accurate in detecting fade compared to TOF. However, a DBS is still insufficient to exclude reliably residual paralysis corresponding to a TOF ratio between 0.6 and 0.9.[39-41] Accordingly, DBS cannot replace objective monitoring.

TETANIC STIMULATION

Background: Tetanic stimulation was proposed by Tassonyi in 1975[42] as an alternative method to evaluate residual neuromuscular blockade.

Stimulation pattern: Tetanic stimulation consists of high-frequency delivery of electrical stimuli (e.g., 50-100 Hz). The most commonly used pattern in clinical practice is 50-Hz stimulation given for 5 seconds, although some investigators have advocated the use of 100-Hz, or even 200-Hz stimulation for 1 second. In normal neuromuscular transmission, the observer detects one strong, sustained muscle contraction, and fade after tetanic stimulation is the basis for evaluation of nondepolarizing block. During a depolarizing block, the muscle response to 50-Hz tetanic stimulation for 5 seconds is sustained. In contrast, during a phase II block after the injection of succinylcholine, the response following tetanic stimulation is not sustained (i.e., fade occurs; Fig. 43.7).

Fade in response to tetanic stimulation is normally considered a presynaptic event. The traditional explanation is that at the start of tetanic stimulation, large amounts of acetylcholine are released from immediately available stores in the presynaptic nerve terminal. As these stores become depleted, the rate of acetylcholine release decreases until equilibrium between mobilization and synthesis of acetylcholine is achieved. Despite this equilibrium, the muscle response to tetanic nerve stimulation is maintained (given normal neuromuscular transmission) because the acetylcholine released is many times greater than the amount necessary to evoke a response. However, when the "margin of safety"[43] at the postsynaptic membrane (i.e., the number of free cholinergic receptors) is reduced by nondepolarizing neuromuscular blocking drugs, a typical reduction in twitch height is seen with a fade, especially during repetitive stimulation. In addition to this postsynaptic block, nondepolarizing neuromuscular blocking drugs can also block presynaptic neuronal subtype acetylcholine receptors, thereby leading to impaired mobilization of acetylcholine within the nerve terminal.[44] This effect substantially contributes to fade in the response to tetanic (and TOF) stimulation. Although the degree of fade depends primarily on the degree of neuromuscular block, fade also depends on the frequency (Hz), the length (seconds) of stimulation, and on how often tetanic stimuli are applied. Unless these variables are kept constant, results from different studies using tetanic stimulation cannot be compared.

Clinical application: Traditionally, tetanic stimulation was proposed to evaluate residual neuromuscular block. While the sensitivity of tetanic stimulation to detect residual paralysis is about 70%, its specificity is only about 50%. Especially when anesthesia was maintained with volatile anesthetics, a marked fade can be observed despite adequate neuromuscular recovery or even without prior administration of a nondepolarizing NMBA. Hence, this test is of limited value for assessing neuromuscular recovery. Furthermore, tetanic stimulation is very painful, which limits its use in unanesthetized patients. In the late phase of neuromuscular recovery, tetanic stimulation can produce lasting antagonism of neuromuscular block in the stimulated muscle such that the response of the tested site may no longer be representative of other muscle groups.[45] For all these reasons, tetanic stimulation has little, if any, use in everyday clinical anesthesia, except as a component in DBS and PTC stimulation.

POSTTETANIC COUNT STIMULATION

Background: PTC stimulation was developed by Viby-Mogensen to allow tactile or visual evaluation of profound nondepolarizing neuromuscular blockade that does not respond to TOF stimulation.[46]

Stimulation pattern: PTC is a composite stimulation pattern composed by a tetanic stimulation (50 Hz for 5 seconds) followed by 10 to 15 single twitches (i.e., PTC twitches) given at 1 Hz starting 3 seconds after the end of tetanic stimulation.[46] It is based on a phenomenon called "posttetanic potentiation": tetanic stimulation leads to a transient, exaggerated release of acetylcholine that briefly shifts the ratio of acetylcholine and NMBA at the motor endplate in favor of acetylcholine. Even if no twitch response has been discernible prior to the tetanic stimulation, noticeable muscle contractions might occur briefly after tetanic stimulation (see Fig. 43.7). The basis for evaluation of the PTC is the count of these discernible posttetanic twitches.

The response to PTC stimulation depends primarily on the degree of neuromuscular block. It also depends on the frequency and duration of tetanic stimulation, the length of time between the end of tetanic stimulation and the first posttetanic stimulus, the frequency of the single-twitch stimulation, and probably the duration of single-twitch stimulation before tetanic stimulation. When the PTC method is used, these variables should be kept constant. Because of interference between PTC stimulation and the actual neuromuscular block within the monitored hand, tetanic stimulation should ideally not be performed more often than every 6 minutes.[46]

Clinical application and limitation: Moderate levels of neuromuscular blockade (i.e., TOF count between 1 and 4) are not sufficient to reliably prevent reactions of the diaphragm and/or laryngeal muscles after stimulation. Both muscles are rather resistant to the effect of nondepolarizing NMBA. Therefore, more profound levels of neuromuscular blockade are needed in clinical situations where any bucking or coughing in response to tracheal stimulation or sudden diaphragmatic movements during surgery should be avoided. Only PTC stimulation allows assessment of these degrees of neuromuscular blockade. During intense block, there is no response to either tetanic or posttetanic stimulation (Fig. 43.8). As the period of intense neuromuscular block dissipates, the first response to posttetanic twitch stimulation occurs and is followed by a gradual return of posttetanic twitches until the first response to TOF stimulation reappears. The PTC should be 3 or less if a deep block is required for clinical reasons; at 6 to 10 PTC, the return of the first TOF response is most often imminent (Fig. 43.9).[46-50] Because tetanic stimulation should not be performed more often than every 6 minutes, this stimulation pattern cannot be applied continuously.

Equipment

Although many nerve stimulators are commercially available, not all meet the basic requirements for clinical use. The stimulus should produce a monophasic and rectangular waveform, and the length of the pulse should not exceed 0.2 to 0.3 ms. A pulse exceeding 0.5 ms may stimulate the muscle directly or cause repetitive firing. Stimulation at a constant current is preferable to stimulation at a constant voltage because current is the determinant of nerve stimulation. Furthermore, for safety reasons, the nerve stimulator should be operated by a rechargeable battery, include a battery check, and be able to generate 60 to 70 mA, but not more than 80 mA. Some commercially available stimulators can deliver just 25 to 50 mA and provide a constant current only when skin resistance ranges from 0 to 2.5 kΩ. This is a limitation, as skin resistance can increase to approximately 5 kΩ, especially during lower skin temperature. The high skin resistance can cause the current delivered to the nerve to decrease below the supramaximal level and lead to a decrease in the response to stimulation. Ideally, the nerve stimulator should have a built-in warning system, or a current level display that alerts the user when the selected current is not delivered to the nerve. Alternatively, the impedance should be indicated at the screen. The polarity of the electrodes should be indicated, and the

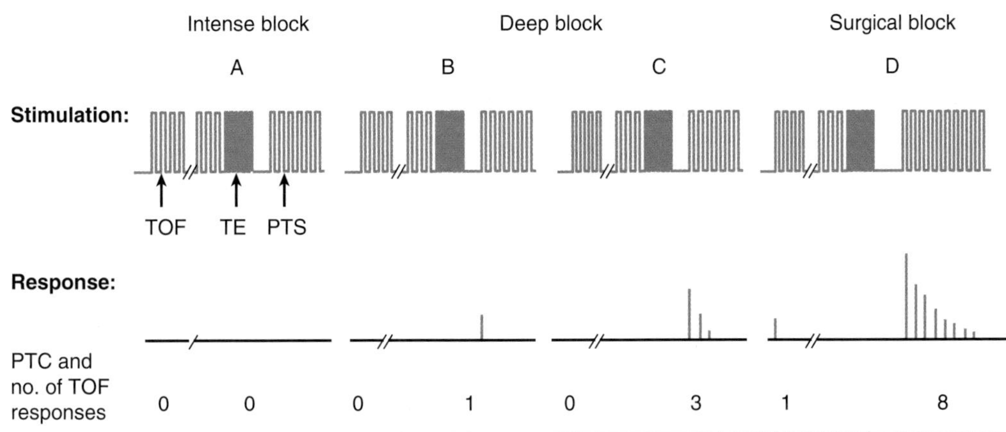

Fig. 43.8 Pattern of electrical stimulation and evoked muscle responses to train-of-four *(TOF)* nerve stimulation, 50-Hz tetanic nerve stimulation for 5 seconds *(TE)*, and 1.0-Hz posttetanic twitch stimulation *(PTS)* during four different levels of nondepolarizing neuromuscular block. During intense block of peripheral muscles (A), no response to any of the forms of stimulation occurs. During less pronounced block (deep block, B and C), there is still no response to TOF stimulation, but posttetanic facilitation of transmission is present. During surgical block (D), the first response to TOF appears and posttetanic facilitation increases further. The posttetanic count (see text) is 1 during very deep block (B), 3 during less deep block (C), and 8 during surgical (or moderate) block (D).

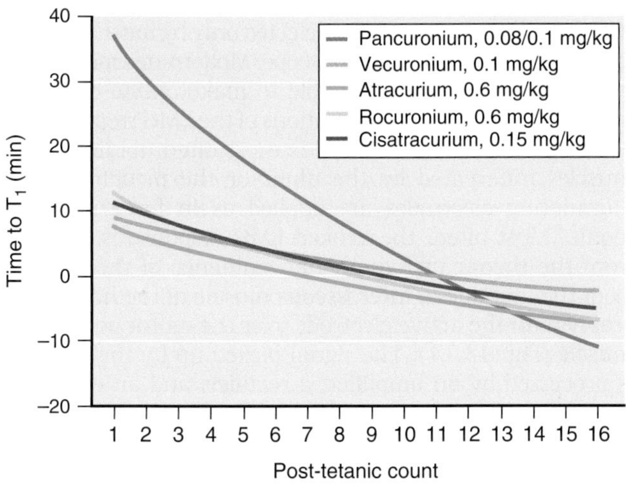

Fig. 43.9 Relationship between the posttetanic count and time when onset of train-of-four (T_1) is likely to be elicited for various neuromuscular blocking agents. (From El-Orbany MI, Joseph JN, Salem MR. The relationship of post-tetanic count and train-of-four responses during recovery from intense cisatracurium-induced neuromuscular block. *Anesth Analg.* 2003;97[1]:80–84.)

apparatus should be capable of delivering the following modes of stimulation: TOF (as both a single train and in a repetitive mode, with TOF stimulation being given every 10-20 seconds), and PTC. Some recent nerve stimulators switch automatically between TOF and PTC, depending on the level of neuromuscular blockade. If the nerve stimulator does not allow objective measurement of the response to TOF stimulation, at least one DBS mode should be available, preferably $DBS_{3,2}$.

Peripheral Nerve Stimulator

Peripheral nerve stimulators only allow stimulation of the target nerve; the subsequent muscular response is assessed subjectively either tactilely or visually. When applying TOF stimulation and evaluating the TOF count, the peripheral nerve stimulator may deliver clinically useful information about the onset of neuromuscular block or the need for an additional dose of relaxant. Moreover, the clinician could be guided for the timing and dosing of reversal agents. It is in the determination of full neuromuscular recovery these devices have clinical limitations. It is impossible to reliably exclude residual paralysis. A simple nerve stimulator acts only as a guide and should not be used as a diagnostic tool to exclude residual paralysis.

Objective Monitors

Objective monitors measure the evoked responses objectively and display it on a screen.

Several methods may be used for objective clinical monitoring of neuromuscular function: evoked mechanical response of the muscle (mechanomyography [MMG]), evoked electrical response of the muscle (electromyography [EMG]), acceleration of the muscle response (AMG), evoked electrical response in a piezoelectric film sensor attached to the muscle (kinemyography [KMG]), measurement of pressure changes in blood pressure cuff after contractions of the upper arm muscles (cuff pressure modality [CPM]), measurement of pressure change of a spherical balloon after hand contraction (compressomyography [CMG]), and measurement of low-frequency sounds evoked by the muscle contraction (phonomyography [PMG]). The different methods are described below. For further information on recording evoked responses, the reader is referred to guidelines for good clinical research practice in pharmacodynamic studies of neuromuscular blocking drugs.[17] The only objective monitors currently available are based on AMG, EMG, CPM, and KMG. The use of computer-guided administration of neuromuscular blocking drugs and "closed loop control" systems has been suggested, but no systems are commercially available.[51,52]

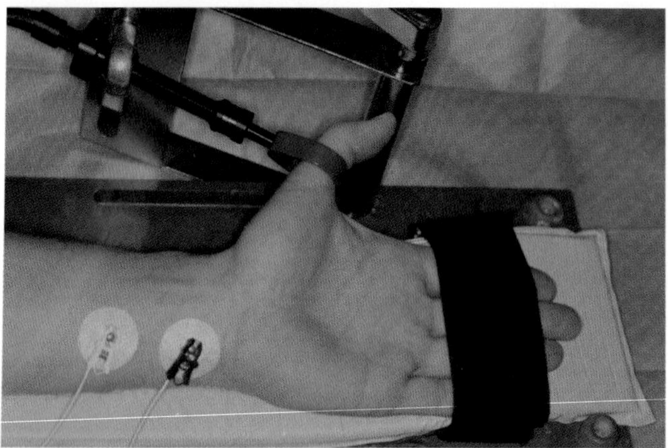

Fig. 43.10 The setup for mechanomyography. The response to nerve stimulation is measured using a force transducer (TD-100; Biometer, Odense, Denmark) placed at the proximal phalanx of the thumb.

MECHANOMYOGRAPHY

MMG measures the isometric contraction of a muscle after stimulation of the corresponding nerve. A transducer converts the force of an isometric contraction into an electrical signal. For correct and reproducible measurement, the muscle contraction needs to be isometric. In clinical anesthesia, this condition is most easily achieved by measuring the force of contraction of the thumb after the application of a resting tension of 200 to 300 g (a preload) to the thumb. When the ulnar nerve is stimulated, the thumb (the adductor pollicis muscle) acts on a force-displacement transducer (Fig. 43.10). The force of contraction is then converted into an electrical signal, which is amplified, displayed, and recorded. The arm and hand should be rigidly fixed, and care should be taken to prevent overloading of the transducer. In addition, the transducer should be placed in correct relation to the thumb (i.e., the thumb should always apply tension along the length of the transducer). It is important to remember that the response to nerve stimulation depends on the frequency with which the individual stimuli are applied and that the time used to achieve a stable control response may influence subsequent determination of the onset time and duration of block.[17] Generally, the reaction to supramaximal stimulation increases during the first 8 to 12 minutes after commencement of the stimulation (staircase phenomenon). Therefore, in clinical studies, recording of the control response (before injection of muscle relaxant) should not be made until the response has stabilized for 8 to 12 minutes or a 2- or 5-second 50-Hz tetanic stimulation has been given.[53] Even then, twitch response often recovers to 110% to 150% of the control response after paralysis with succinylcholine. This increase in response, possibly caused by a change in the contractile response of the muscle, normally disappears within 15 to 25 minutes.

Although there are numerous methods for mechanical recording of evoked mechanical responses, not all meet the criteria outlined. MMG is recognized as the gold standard of neuromuscular monitoring.[17]

Despite this status, there is no commercially available neuromuscular monitor for daily clinical use based on this principle. This type of monitor is relegated to research purpose only.

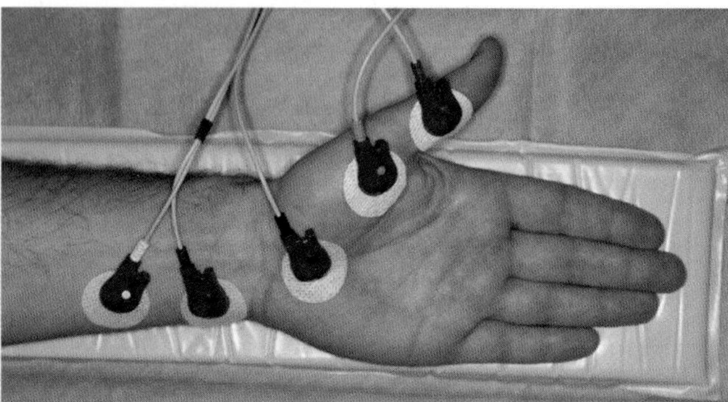

Fig. 43.11 The setup for electromyography (NMT ElectroSensor, Datex-Ohmeda, Helsinki, Finland) for recording the compound action potential from the adductor pollicis muscle.

ELECTROMYOGRAPHY

EMG is the oldest technique used for quantification of neuromuscular blockade. Evoked EMG records the compound muscle action potentials produced by stimulation of a peripheral nerve. The compound action potential is an electrical activity that for many years could be detected only by means of a preamplifier and a storage oscilloscope. Modern neuromuscular transmission analyzers are able to make online electronic analyses and graphic presentations of the EMG response.

The evoked EMG response is most often obtained from muscles innervated by the ulnar or the median nerves. Stimulating electrodes are applied as in force measurements. Most often, the evoked EMG response is obtained from the thenar or hypothenar eminence of the hand or from the first dorsal interosseous muscle of the hand, preferably with the active electrode over the motor point of the muscle (Fig. 43.11). The signal picked up by the analyzer is processed by an amplifier, a rectifier, and an electronic integrator. The results are displayed either as a percentage of control or as a TOF ratio.

Two new sites for recording the EMG response have been introduced: the larynx and the diaphragm.[54,55] Using a noninvasive disposable laryngeal electrode attached to the tracheal tube and placed between the vocal cords, it is possible to monitor the onset of neuromuscular block in the laryngeal muscles. However, the method is mainly of interest in clinical research when investigating onset times of the laryngeal muscles. In paravertebral surface diaphragmatic EMG, the recording electrodes are placed on the right of vertebrae T12/L1 or L1/L2 for monitoring the response of the right diaphragmatic crux to transcutaneous stimulation of the right phrenic nerve at the neck.[54-57] As is the case with surface laryngeal EMG, surface diaphragmatic EMG is mainly of interest in clinical research.

Evoked electrical and mechanical responses represent different physiologic events. Evoked EMG records changes in the electrical activity of one or more muscles, whereas evoked MMG records changes associated with excitation-contraction coupling and contraction of the muscle as well. For these reasons, the results obtained with these methods may differ.[57,58] Although evoked EMG responses generally correlate well with evoked mechanical responses,[38] marked differences can occur, especially in the response to succinylcholine and in the TOF ratio during recovery from a nondepolarizing block.[38,57,59]

In theory, recording of evoked EMG responses has several advantages over recording of evoked mechanical responses. Equipment for measuring-evoked EMG responses is easier to set up, the response reflects only factors influencing neuromuscular transmission, and the response can be obtained from muscles not accessible to mechanical recording. However, evoked EMG does entail some difficulties. Although high-quality recordings are possible in most patients, the results are not always reliable. For one thing, improper placement of electrodes can result in inadequate pickup of the compound EMG signal. If the neuromuscular transmission analyzer does not allow observation of the actual waveform of the compound EMG, determining optimal placement of the electrodes is difficult. Another source of unreliable results may be that fixation of the hand with a preload on the thumb might be more important than is generally appreciated, inasmuch as changes in the position of the electrodes in relation to the muscle can affect the EMG response. In addition, direct muscle stimulation sometimes occurs. If muscles close to the stimulating electrodes are stimulated directly, the recording electrodes can pick up an electrical signal even though neuromuscular transmission is completely blocked. Another difficulty is that the EMG response often does not return to the control value. Whether this situation is the result of technical problems, inadequate fixation of the hand, or changes in temperature is unknown (Fig. 43.12). Finally, the evoked EMG response is highly sensitive to electrical interference, such as that caused by diathermy.

Currently, to our knowledge, there are only a few EMG-based monitors available for clinical use, but more devices are under development.

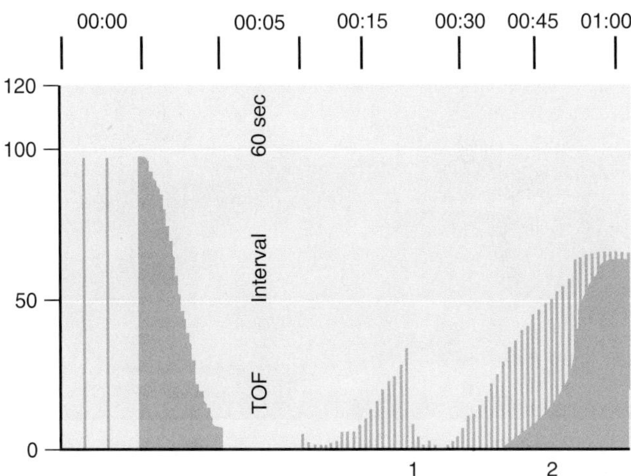

Fig. 43.12 Evoked electromyographic printout from a Relaxograph (Datex-Ohmeda, Helsinki, Finland). Initially, single-twitch stimulation was given at 0.1 Hz, and vecuronium (70 μg/kg) was administered intravenously for tracheal intubation. After approximately 5 minutes, the mode of stimulation was changed to train-of-four *(TOF)* stimulation every 60 seconds. At a twitch height (first twitch in the TOF response) of approximately 30% of control (marker 1), 1 mg of vecuronium was given intravenously. At marker 2, 1 mg of neostigmine was given intravenously, preceded by 2 mg of glycopyrrolate. The printout also illustrates the common problem of failure of the electromyographic response to return to the control level. (Courtesy Datex-Ohmeda, Helsinki, Finland.)

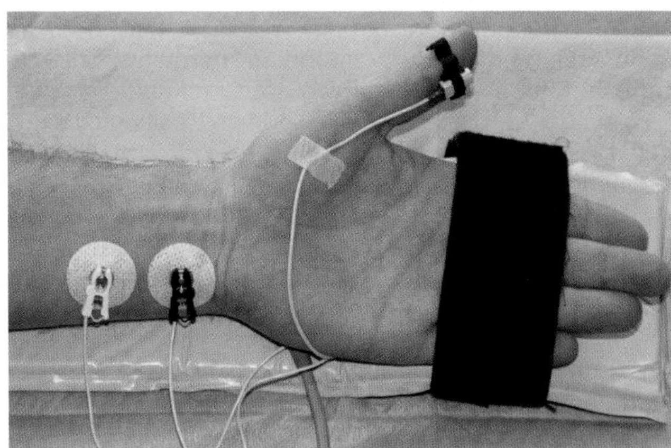

Fig. 43.13 The setup of acceleromyography without preload (TOF Watch, Biometer, Odense, Denmark). The response to nerve stimulation is measured with a small piezoelectric acceleration transducer placed distally on the volar site of the thumb.

ACCELEROMYOGRAPHY

AMG was developed specifically for clinical use and is widely practiced. The technique of AMG is based on Newton's second law: force = mass × acceleration, it measures the isotonic acceleration of the stimulated muscle.[60] If mass is constant, acceleration is directly proportional to force. Accordingly, after nerve stimulation, one can measure not only the evoked force but also acceleration of the thumb.

AMG uses a piezoelectric ceramic wafer with electrodes on both sides. Exposure of the electrode to a force generates an electrical voltage proportional to acceleration of the electrode. Consequently, when an accelerometer is fixed to the thumb and the ulnar nerve is stimulated, an electrical signal is produced whenever the thumb moves (Fig. 43.13). This signal can be analyzed in a specially designed analyzer[61] or displayed on a recording system.

AMG is a simple method of analyzing neuromuscular function, both in the operating room and in the intensive care unit. Although good correlation exists between the TOF ratio measured by this method and the TOF ratio measured with a force-displacement transducer or EMG,[60,62,63] measurements made via AMG are not directly comparable with results obtained by the other two methods.[63-69] When AMG is used with a free-moving thumb, as originally suggested,[60] wide limits of agreements in twitch height (T1) and TOF ratio and differences in the onset and recovery course of block between AMG and MMG have been found. Moreover, the AMG control TOF ratio is consistently higher than when measured with a force-displacement transducer. In accordance with this, several studies have indicated that when using AMG, the TOF ratio indicative of sufficient postoperative neuromuscular recovery is 1.0 rather than 0.90, as when measured by MMG or EMG in the adductor pollicis muscle.[6,68,70-72] In contrast to MMG and EMG, the control baseline TOF value before administration of a neuromuscular blocking drug is most often 1.1 to 1.2 when measured with AMG, and in some patients is as high as 1.4. A high control baseline value probably indicates that the TOF ratio necessary for excluding residual curarization is equally higher. For instance, in a patient with a high control baseline value (e.g., TOF = 1.2), it is to be expected that a higher TOF ratio during recovery is necessary to exclude residual

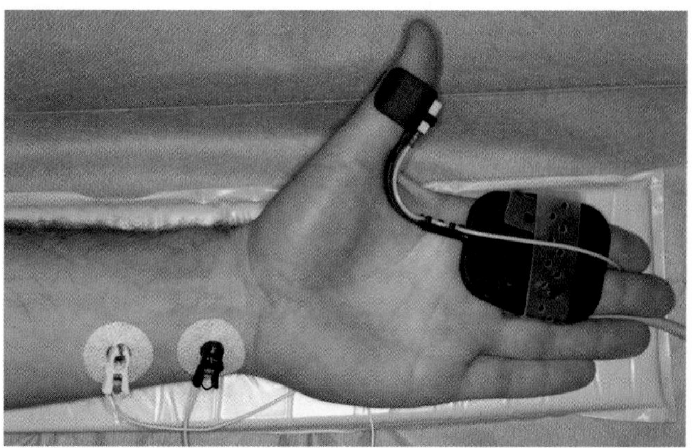

Fig. 43.14 The setup of acceleromyography with preload (TOF Watch with Hand Adapter, Biometer, Odense, Denmark). The piezoelectric acceleration transducer is placed in the Hand Adapter. The stretching wing ensures that the thumb does not touch the palm of the hand.

block compared with a patient with a low control baseline value (e.g., TOF = 0.95). It is generally accepted that the TOF ratio should be at least 0.90 to exclude clinically significant residual paralysis; using the preceding example, a TOF ratio of 1.08 (90% of 1.2) would represent safe recovery in the first patient, whereas a TOF ratio of 0.86 (90% of 0.95) would suffice in the other patient. To overcome such problems, it has been suggested to refer the actually obtained TOF ratios during recovery to the baseline control TOF ratio (normalization).[67,72-76] Currently, no commercially available monitors can "normalize" the TOF ratio automatically. Intuitively, for excluding residual block using AMG, a TOF ratio of at least 1.0 should be targeted to exclude residual block.[67,68,72,74]

One reason for the wide limits of agreement between AMG and MMG is probably and paradoxically connected with one of the originally claimed advantages of the method, that fixation of the hand could be reduced to a minimum as long as the thumb could move freely.[60] In clinical practice, it is often not possible to ensure that the thumb can move freely and that the position of the hand does not change during the surgical procedure. The evoked response can therefore vary considerably. Several solutions have been proposed, but the use of an elastic preload on the thumb improves the precision without compromising the agreement between results obtained with AMG and MMG (Fig. 43.14).[67,68] Several studies have indicated that objective monitoring with AMG reduces and almost eliminates the problem of postoperative residual neuromuscular block.[67,77-81]

When the thumb is not available for monitoring during surgery, some clinicians prefer to monitor the AMG response of the orbicularis oculi or the corrugator supercilii in response to facial nerve stimulation.[28] However, neuromuscular monitoring of both sites with AMG is subject to both large uncertainty regarding the extent of paralysis and high risk of direct muscle stimulation, and it cannot be recommended for routine monitoring. It provides only a rough estimate of the degree of block of the peripheral muscles.[82,83]

AMG was one of the first widely distributed commercially available monitors and has therefore become the standard for qualitative monitoring in the clinical setting. Today, AMG devices are available as portable monitors as well as integrated in the anesthesia monitor.

Recently, AMG monitors with three-dimensional piezoelectric transducers were introduced, which sense the motion of the thumb in all directions,[83a,83b] and not just in one plane. This might further improve the reliability of the AMG technology. This novel method has been compared to the TOF-Watch (one-dimensional AMG) in two small studies. Although both studies showed some disagreement between the two methods, the authors agreed that the three-dimensional monitor may be used in clinical practice. An advantage seems to be that the monitors' integrated internal check-up ensuring that all components including the piezoelectric element are functional is developed. The newest monitors also display the impedance and calculate automatically a modified normalized TOF ratio. Hopefully, the new generation of AMG monitors becomes even more user-friendly and more reliable.

KINEMYOGRAPHY

The technique of KMG is based on the principle that stretching or bending a flexible piezoelectric film (e.g., one attached to the thumb) in response to nerve stimulation generates a voltage that is proportional to the amount of stretching or bending.[84,85]

Few studies have evaluated the function of these monitors.[84-86] Limited data indicate not only a good relationship between results obtained with KMG, AMG, and MMG, but also wide limits of agreement between the methods. Therefore, although KMG may be a valuable clinical tool, the values obtained in an individual patient with this method can vary from those obtained with MMG or AMG. Only one device based on this principle is available commercially in two sizes (adult and pediatric): the NMT MechanoSensor (Datex-Ohmeda, Helsinki, Finland).

CUFF PRESSURE MODALITY (CPM)

The cuff modality detects changes in cuff pressure due to muscle contraction. Electrodes integrated into a blood pressure cuff stimulate the brachial plexus at the humeral level. The subsequent bulk contraction of the upper arm generates pressure change in the blood pressure cuff which is analyzed and displayed at the monitor. However, only limited data are currently available and further clinical investigations are needed to prove the reliability and reproducibility of the new monitoring modality. One monitor based on this technology is commercially available: the TOF-Cuff NMT monitor (RGB Medical devices, Madrid, Spain).

COMPRESSOMYOGRAPHY

CMG measures pressure changes in a hand-held balloon. Following ulnar nerve stimulation, the force of muscle contraction of the hand muscles is transmitted to a balloon secured in the patient's hand. Despite encouraging results of the only publication investigating the device,[49] this technique has not been further developed and is not commercially available.

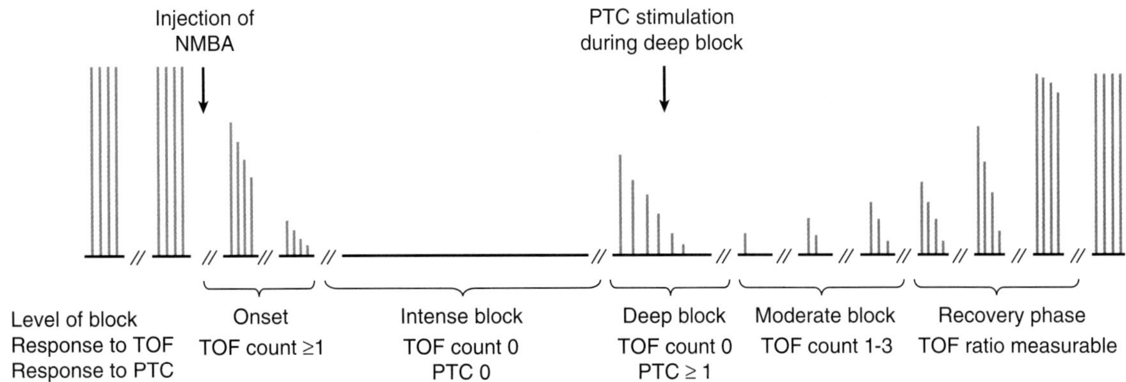

Fig. 43.15 Levels of block after a normal intubating dose of a nondepolarizing neuromuscular blocking agent *(NMBA)* as classified by posttetanic count *(PTC)* and train-of-four *(TOF)* stimulation. During intense (profound) block, there are no responses to either TOF or PTC stimulation. During deep block, there is response to PTC but not to TOF stimulation. Intense (profound) block and deep block together constitute the "period of no response to TOF stimulation." Reappearance of the response to TOF stimulation heralds the start of moderate block. Finally, when all four responses to TOF stimulation are present and a TOF ratio can be measured, the recovery period has started. (From Fuchs-Buder T, Claudius C, Skovgaard LT, et al. Good clinical research practice in pharmacodynamic studies of neuromuscular blocking agents II: The Stockholm revision. *Acta Anaesthesiol Scand*. 2007;51[7]:789–808.)

PHONOMYOGRAPHY

PMG measures the intrinsic low-frequency sounds of muscle contraction with special microphones following nerve stimulation. PMG has been evaluated for clinical and research purposes by one study group. This group reports good correlation between evoked acoustic responses and those obtained with more traditional methods of recording, such as MMG, EMG, and AMG.[31,87-92] A potential advantage of PMG, however, is that the method can be applied not only to the adductor pollicis muscle, but also to other muscles of clinical interest such as the diaphragm, larynx, and eye muscles. In addition, the ease of application is attractive. However, PMG-based monitors are not currently commercially available.

Evaluation of Recorded Evoked Responses

In daily clinical practice, the recorded response to TOF stimulation and PTC stimulation are typically used to explain how to evaluate the degree of neuromuscular block during clinical anesthesia.

NONDEPOLARIZING NEUROMUSCULAR BLOCK

After injection of a nondepolarizing neuromuscular blocking drug in a dose sufficient for smooth tracheal intubation, TOF recording demonstrates four phases, or levels, of neuromuscular block: intense block, deep block, moderate or surgical block, and recovery (Fig. 43.15).

Intense Neuromuscular Block

Intense or profound neuromuscular block occurs within 3 to 6 minutes of injection of an intubating dose of a nondepolarizing muscle relaxant, depending on the drug and the dose given. This phase is also called the "period of no response" because no response to any pattern of nerve stimulation occurs. The length of this period varies, again depending primarily on the duration of action of the muscle relaxant and the dose given. The sensitivity of the patient to the drug also affects the period of no response. An intense block cannot be antagonized with a cholinesterase inhibitor (e.g., neostigmine), and only a high dose of sugammadex (16 mg/kg) can antagonize an intense block caused by rocuronium or vecuronium.[93,94]

Deep Neuromuscular Block

Intense neuromuscular block is followed by a period of deep neuromuscular block, characterized by absence of response to TOF stimulation, but with the presence of at least one response to PTC stimulation (i.e., PTC ≥1; compare with Fig. 43.8). To avoid diaphragmatic movements and thus, to assure surgical stillness and improve surgical space conditions during laparoscopic abdominal procedures, deep neuromuscular blockade corresponding to ≤3 PTC responses is recommended.[49] Although prediction of the duration of a deep neuromuscular block is difficult, correlation usually exists between PTC stimulation and the time until reappearance of the first response to TOF stimulation (see Fig. 43.9). Attempts to reverse a deep neuromuscular block with neostigmine are usually impossible. However, a deep neuromuscular block caused by rocuronium or vecuronium can be antagonized completely within a few minutes using a dose of sugammadex of 4 mg/kg.[95-97]

Moderate Neuromuscular Block

Moderate neuromuscular block begins when the first response to TOF stimulation appears. This phase is characterized by a gradual return of the four responses to TOF stimulation. Furthermore, good correlation exists between the degree of neuromuscular block and the number of responses to TOF stimulation. When only one response is detectable, the degree of neuromuscular block (the depression in twitch tension) is 90% to 95%. When the fourth response reappears, neuromuscular block is usually 60% to 85%.[98,99] The presence of one or two responses in the TOF pattern normally indicates sufficient relaxation for most surgical procedures. During light anesthesia, however, patients may move, buck, or cough; therefore, a deeper block (or a deeper level of anesthesia) may be necessary when elimination of sudden movements or facilitation of surgery is necessary.

Antagonism of neuromuscular block with neostigmine should usually not be attempted when the block is intense or deep. Even if some reversal occurs, it will often be inadequate, regardless of the dose of neostigmine administered.[100] Furthermore, after the administration of large doses of muscle relaxants, reversal of the block with neostigmine to clinically normal activity is not always possible if only one TOF response is present. In general, antagonism with neostigmine should not be initiated before all four responses after TOF stimulation are observed. Even then, sufficient recovery may take time and cannot be guaranteed unless documented using objective monitoring.[101-103]

Antagonism of moderate block induced by rocuronium and vecuronium can be achieved with a small dose of sugammadex (2 mg/kg) within a few minutes.[104-106] However, the reappearance of neuromuscular blockade has been reported by anesthesiologists from Japan[107] when the 2 mg/kg dose has been used. However, they did not monitor the degree of neuromuscular blockade; did the reappearance of neuromuscular blockade occur because of inadequate monitoring or too small a dose of sugammadex? Although the antagonism of neuromuscular block from sugammadex seems to be fast and predictable, neuromuscular monitoring is mandatory for proper dosing, and objective monitoring should still be used until the TOF ratio is 0.9 to 1.0.

Recovery from Neuromuscular Block

Return of the fourth response in the TOF heralds the recovery phase. During neuromuscular recovery, a reasonably good correlation exists between the actual TOF ratio and clinical observation, but the relationship between the TOF ratio and signs and symptoms of residual block varies greatly among patients.[81,100] When the TOF ratio is 0.4 or less, the patient is generally unable to lift the head or arm. Tidal volume may be normal, but vital capacity and inspiratory force is reduced. When the ratio is 0.6, most patients are able to lift their head for 3 seconds, open their eyes widely, and stick out their tongue, but vital capacity and inspiratory force are often still reduced. At a TOF ratio of 0.7 to 0.75, the patient can normally cough sufficiently and lift the head for at least 5 seconds, but grip strength may still be as low as about 60% of control.[108] When the ratio is 0.8 and higher, vital capacity and inspiratory force are normal.[36,109-111] The patient may, however, still have diplopia, blurred vision, and facial weakness (Table 43.1).[81,108]

However, the TOF ratio must exceed 0.90 when recorded with MMG or EMG, and 1.0 when using AMG to exclude clinically important residual neuromuscular block.[1,3,38,67,68,70,112-116] Moderate degrees of neuromuscular block can impair carotid body chemosensitivity to hypoxia with absent ventilatory response to arterial desaturation.[3,112,114,116] Moreover, residual block (TOF < 0.90) is associated with functional impairment of the pharyngeal and upper esophageal muscles, which most probably predisposes to regurgitation and aspiration of gastric contents.[1] Eikermann and colleagues[4] have documented that partial neuromuscular block, even to a degree that does not evoke dyspnea or oxygen desaturation, can decrease inspiratory upper airway volume and can evoke partial inspiratory airway collapse.[4] Also, residual block (TOF < 0.70) caused by the long-acting muscle relaxant pancuronium is a significant risk factor for the development of postoperative pulmonary complications (Table 43.2 and Fig. 43.16).[113] Intraoperative neuromuscular monitoring, followed by appropriate pharmacological reversal, reduces the risk of residual neuromuscular block and results in fewer patients with hypoxemic events or airway obstruction in the postanesthesia care unit.[80] Even in volunteers without sedation or impaired consciousness, a TOF ratio of 0.90 or less can impair the ability to maintain the airway.[77,108,117] Even small degrees of residual block are unpleasant for patients, causing symptoms such as general weakness and blurred vision.[81] In summary, adequate recovery of neuromuscular function requires the return of an MMG or EMG TOF ratio to at least 0.90, and an AMG TOF ratio to at least 1.0 (or normalized to 0.90),[74] which cannot be guaranteed without objective neuromuscular monitoring.[78,79,81,118-121]

TABLE 43.1 Clinical Signs and Symptoms of Residual Paralysis in Awake Volunteers after Mivacurium-Induced Neuromuscular Block

Train-of-Four Ratio	Signs and Symptoms
0.70-0.75	Diplopia and visual disturbances
	Decreased handgrip strength
	Inability to maintain apposition of the incisor teeth
	"Tongue depressor test" negative
	Inability to sit up without assistance
	Severe facial weakness
	Speaking a major effort
	Overall weakness and tiredness
0.85-0.90	Diplopia and visual disturbances
	Generalized fatigue

From Kopman AF, Yee PS, Neuman GG. Relationship of the train-of-four fade ratio to clinical signs and symptoms of residual paralysis in awake volunteers. *Anesthesiology*. 1997;86(4):765–761.

DEPOLARIZING NEUROMUSCULAR BLOCK (PHASE I AND II BLOCKS)

Fade and posttetanic facilitation are the basis for evaluation of all stimulation patterns applied in clinical practice (i.e., TOF, DBS, and PTC stimulation). It is important to realize that during depolarizing neuromuscular phase I block, neither fade nor posttetanic facilitation occurred. Thus, the usually applied stimulation patterns do not allow assessment of depolarizing neuromuscular block. After TOF stimulation, all four responses are reduced at the same degree, no fade occurred, and all four disappear simultaneously. Thus, independently of the degree of depolarizing neuromuscular block, the TOF-ratio remains 1 and the TOF-count is either 4 or 0.

Patients with normal plasma cholinesterase activity who are given a moderate dose of succinylcholine (0.5-1.5 mg/kg) undergo a typical depolarizing neuromuscular block (phase I block; i.e., the response to TOF or tetanic stimulation does not fade, and no posttetanic facilitation of

TABLE 43.2 Relationship Between Train-of-Four Ratio at the First Postoperative Recording and Postoperative Pulmonary Complications

	PANCURONIUM (*n* = 226)			ATRACURIUM OR VECURONIUM (*n* = 450)		
		PATIENTS WITH POPC			PATIENTS WITH POPC	
	No. of patients	***n***	**%**	**No. of Patients**	***n***	**%**
TOF ≥ 0.70	167	8	4.8	426	23	5.4
TOF < 0.70	59	10	16.9*	24	1	4.2

*$P < .02$ versus patients in the same group with a train-of-four ratio of 0.70 or greater.

Results from a prospective, randomized, and blinded study of postoperative pulmonary complications (POPC) in a total of 691 adult patients undergoing abdominal, gynecologic, or orthopedic surgery and receiving either pancuronium, atracurium, or vecuronium.[82] In 4 of the 46 patients with POPC (1 in the pancuronium group and 3 in the atracurium and vecuronium groups), the train-of-four (TOF) ratio was not available. Because there were no significant differences in the two groups of patients given the intermediate-acting muscle relaxants, the data from these groups are pooled.

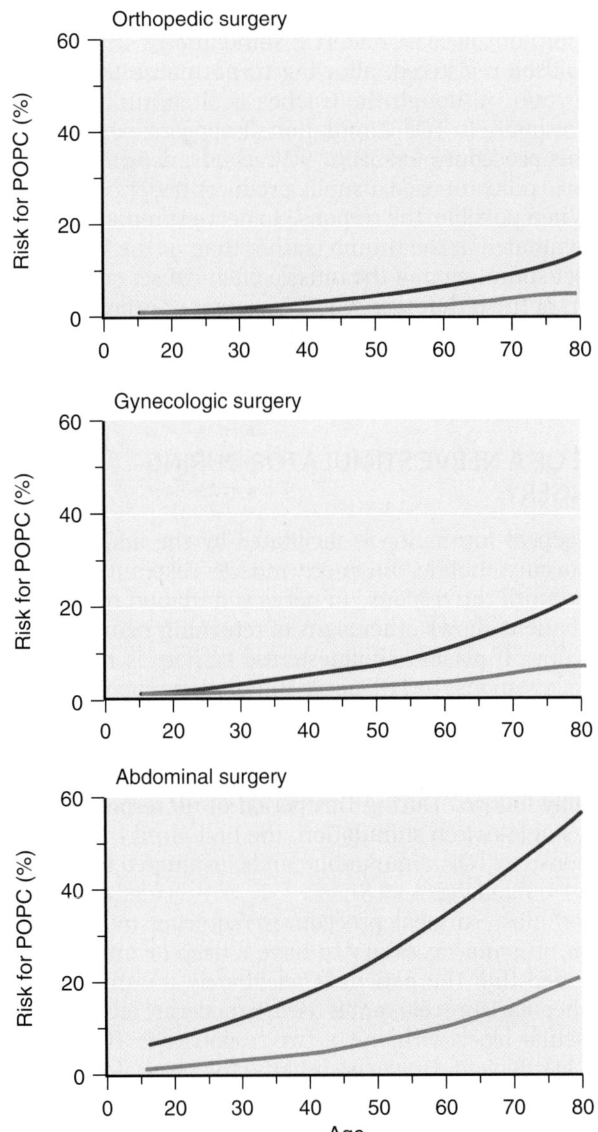

Fig. 43.16 Predicted probabilities of a postoperative pulmonary complication *(POPC)* in different age groups in orthopedic, gynecologic, and major abdominal surgery with duration of anesthesia of less than 200 minutes. The *red lines* represent patients with residual neuromuscular block (train-of-four [TOF] < 0.70) after the administration of pancuronium; the *blue lines* represent patients with a TOF of 0.70 or greater after the administration of pancuronium, as well as all patients after the administration of atracurium and vecuronium, independent of the TOF ratio at the end of anesthesia.[113]

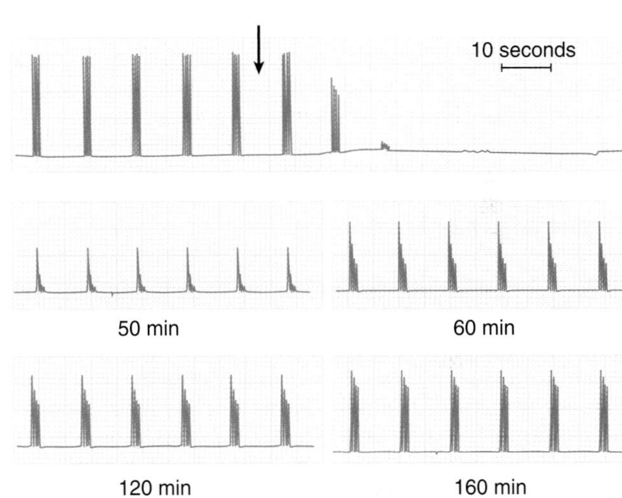

Fig. 43.17 Typical recording of the mechanical response to train-of-four ulnar nerve stimulation after injection of 1 mg/kg of succinylcholine *(arrow)* in a patient with genetically determined abnormal plasma cholinesterase activity. The prolonged duration of action and the pronounced fade in the response indicate a phase II block.

transmission occurs. All four responses are reduced at the same degree [TOF ratio is 1.0] or 0). In contrast, some patients with genetically determined abnormal plasma cholinesterase activity who are given the same dose of succinylcholine undergo a nondepolarizing-like block characterized by fade in the response to TOF and tetanic stimulation and the occurrence of posttetanic facilitation of transmission (Fig. 43.17). This type of block is called a *phase II block* (dual, mixed, or desensitizing block). In addition, phase II blocks sometimes occur in genetically normal patients after repetitive bolus doses or a prolonged infusion of succinylcholine. Therefore, in a clinical setting, TOF stimulation can be used to distinguish depolarizing phase I block and phase II block. Patients with normal plasma cholinesterase activity would recover from the neuromuscular block within a few minutes, showing four equally weak responses (TOF ratio 1.0), which quickly become stronger (still at TOF ratio 1.0). In contrast, patients with abnormal plasma cholinesterase activity and subsequent phase II block would not recover quickly and will return with a TOF count of 1, slowly increasing to 2, 3, and last 4 counts—then having a fade of TOF (TOF-ratio <1.0) during recovery as seen with nondepolarizing block.

From a therapeutic point of view, a phase II block in normal patients must be differentiated from a phase II block in patients with abnormal cholinesterase activity. In healthy patients, a phase II block can be antagonized by administering a cholinesterase inhibitor a few minutes after discontinuation of succinylcholine. In patients with abnormal genotypes, however, the effect of intravenous injection of a cholinesterase inhibitor (e.g., neostigmine) is unpredictable because it inhibits acetylcholinesterase and plasma-cholinesterase. For example, neostigmine can potentiate the block dramatically, temporarily improve neuromuscular transmission, and then potentiate the block or partially reverse the block, all depending on the time elapsed since administration of succinylcholine and the dose of neostigmine given. Therefore, unless the cholinesterase genotype is known to be normal, antagonism of a phase II block with a cholinesterase inhibitor should be undertaken with extreme caution. Even if neuromuscular function improves promptly, patient surveillance should continue for at least 1 hour.

Use of Nerve Stimulators in Daily Clinical Practice

Whenever a neuromuscular blocking drug is administered to a patient, objective monitoring of the evoked response using recording equipment is the best way to evaluate the neuromuscular block.[121a] However, tactile and visual evaluation are still common forms of clinical neuromuscular monitoring, not least when recording equipment is not available or considered unreliable. The following is a description of how to use nerve stimulators with or without recording equipment (objective monitoring).

PREPARATIONS BEFORE INDUCTION OF ANESTHESIA AND ADMINISTRATION OF THE NEUROMUSCULAR BLOCKING AGENT

First, for reliable stimulation, careful cleansing of the skin and proper placement and fixation of electrodes are essential. When the ulnar nerve is used for nerve stimulation, one should take advantage of the fact that the nerve follows the artery by placing the electrodes above the pulse. This placement gives the best response (see Fig. 43.1). Second, every effort should be taken to prevent central cooling, as well as cooling of the extremity being evaluated. Both central and local surface cooling of the adductor pollicis muscle can reduce twitch tension and the TOF ratio.[122-124] Peripheral cooling can affect nerve conduction, decrease the rate of release of acetylcholine and muscle contractility, increase skin impedance, and reduce blood flow to the muscles, thus decreasing the rate of removal of muscle relaxant from the neuromuscular junction. These factors might account for the occasional and pronounced difference in muscle response between a cold extremity and the contralateral warm extremity.[125]

USE OF A NERVE STIMULATOR DURING INDUCTION OF ANESTHESIA

The nerve stimulator should be attached to the patient before induction of anesthesia but should not be turned on until after the patient is unconscious.

Single-twitch stimulation at 1 Hz can be used initially when seeking supramaximal stimulation. However, after supramaximal stimulation has been ensured and before the muscle relaxant is injected, the recording equipment (when using objective monitoring) should be calibrated to ensure that the response is in the measurement window and the response to 1 Hz stimulation is set to 100%. Currently, all commercially available devices have an automatic calibration modus. Without calibration, the recorded response to nerve stimulation might differ significantly from the visual or tactile response throughout all levels of neuromuscular block; therefore, the mode of stimulation should be changed to TOF (or 0.1-Hz twitch stimulation). When the response to this stimulation is observed (the control response), the neuromuscular blocking drug is injected. However, devices with integrated impedance measurement do not need calibration, but at least one TOF stimulation without NMBA should be registered, allowing to normalize the recovery TOF-ratio. Although the trachea is often intubated when the response to TOF stimulation disappears, postponement of this procedure for 30 to 90 seconds, depending on the muscle relaxant used, usually produces better conditions.

When possible, the response to nerve stimulation should be evaluated at the thumb (rather than at the fifth finger). Direct stimulation of the muscle often causes subtle movement of the fifth finger when no response is present at the thumb. Finally, the different sensitivities of various muscle groups to neuromuscular blocking drugs should always be kept in mind.

USE OF A NERVE STIMULATOR DURING SURGERY

If tracheal intubation is facilitated by the administration of succinylcholine, no more muscle relaxant should be given until the response to nerve stimulation reappears or the patient shows other signs of returning neuromuscular function. If plasma cholinesterase activity is normal, the muscle response to TOF nerve stimulation reappears within 4 to 8 minutes.

When a nondepolarizing neuromuscular drug is used for tracheal intubation, a longer-lasting period of intense block usually follows. During this period of no response to TOF and single-twitch stimulation, the time until the return of response to TOF stimulation can be evaluated by PTC (see Fig. 43.9 and Fig. 43.18).

For most surgical procedures requiring muscle relaxation, it is not necessary to have a deep or intense block, provided that the patient is adequately anesthetized. If a nondepolarizing relaxant is used, a moderate level of neuromuscular block with one or two responses to TOF stimulation is sufficient. However, because the respiratory muscles (including the diaphragm) are more resistant to neuromuscular blocking drugs than the peripheral muscles are, the patient may breathe, hiccup, or even cough at this moderate level of block. Moreover, tonus of the diaphragm might impede the surgical conditions, especially during abdominal laparoscopic surgery. To ensure paralysis of the diaphragm, neuromuscular block of the peripheral muscles must be deep so that the PTC is 1-3 at the thumb.

The disadvantages of sustaining a deep or intense neuromuscular block is that at these levels of block, the muscles

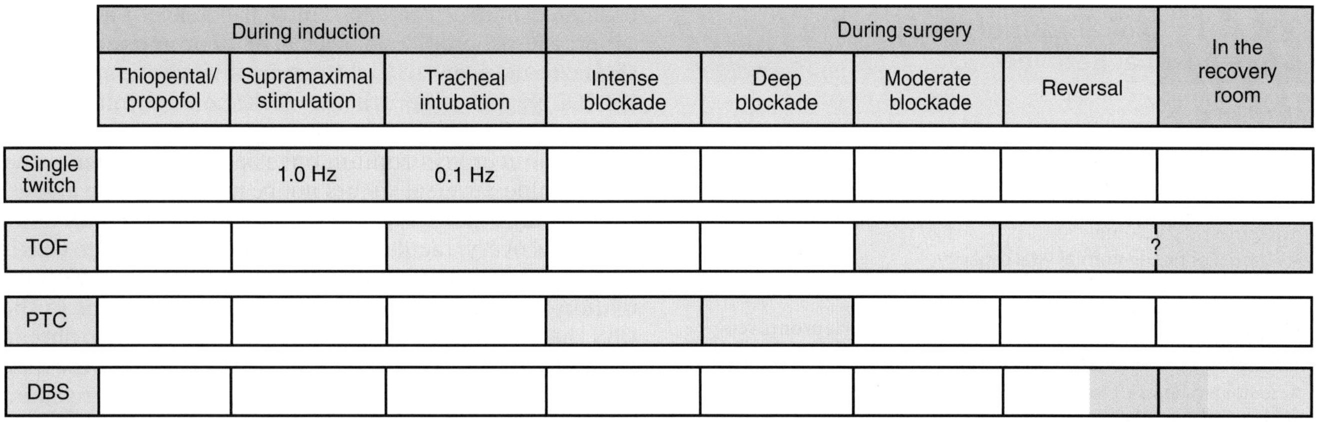

	During induction			During surgery				In the recovery room
	Thiopental/ propofol	Supramaximal stimulation	Tracheal intubation	Intense blockade	Deep blockade	Moderate blockade	Reversal	
Single twitch		1.0 Hz	0.1 Hz					
TOF								?
PTC								
DBS								

Fig. 43.18 Diagram showing when the different modes of electrical nerve stimulation can be used during clinical anesthesia. *Dark areas* indicate appropriate use and *light areas*, less effective use. Modes of nerve stimulation are train-of-four *(TOF)* stimulation; posttetanic count *(PTC)*; double-burst stimulation *(DBS)*; and the question mark (?), indicating that TOF is less useful in the recovery room unless measured with mechanomyography, electromyography, or acceleromyography. (See text for further explanation.)

are completely paralyzed and the patient cannot signal awareness with voluntary or involuntary movements. Another disadvantage is that deep or intense block cannot readily be reversed by neostigmine. Only sugammadex can reverse a deep or intense neuromuscular block (if caused by rocuronium or vecuronium).

USE OF A NERVE STIMULATOR DURING REVERSAL OF NEUROMUSCULAR BLOCK

Antagonism of nondepolarizing neuromuscular block is most often facilitated with a cholinesterase inhibitor, such as neostigmine, or with the selective relaxant binding agent sugammadex when the neuromuscular block is achieved using rocuronium or vecuronium.

Antagonism with neostigmine should not be initiated before at least all four responses to TOF stimulation are present. Reversal of neuromuscular block will not be hastened and can possibly be delayed by giving neostigmine when no response to peripheral nerve stimulation is present. Moreover, even when there are four responses to TOF stimulation, the reversal is slow and insufficient in some patients. With a large dose of neostigmine (e.g., 5 mg/70 kg), the median time to achieve a TOF ratio of 0.90 is 15 to 20 minutes, and it will take approximately 90 to 120 minutes to achieve a TOF ratio of 0.90 in 95% of the patients after an intermediate-acting neuromuscular blocking drug (e.g., rocuronium).[126] Conversely, a large dose of neostigmine after full recovery might give a paradoxical block with decreasing TOF ratio.[127-131]

When rocuronium or vecuronium is used, the selective relaxant binding drug sugammadex can be used for reversal.[104,105] Sugammadex encapsulates rocuronium and vecuronium with a high affinity, thereby antagonizing the neuromuscular blocking effect. Three different doses of sugammadex are recommended according to the level of block. A large dose (16 mg/kg) is given during intense block (no response to PTC stimulation),[93,94] a medium dose (4 mg/kg) during deep block (at least one response to PTC),[95-97] and a low dose (2 mg/kg) during moderate block (two or more responses to TOF stimulation).[104-106] In most patients,

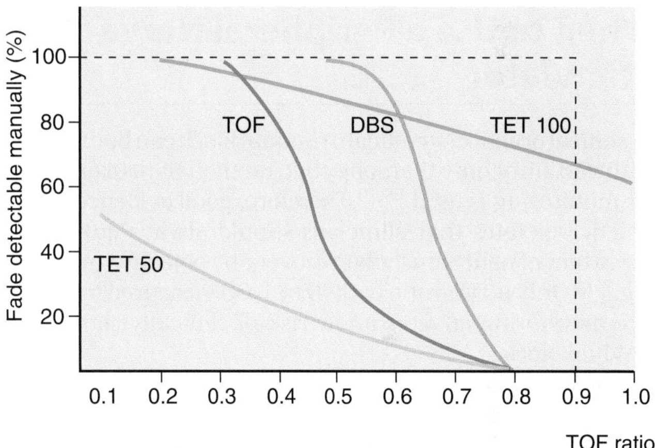

Fig. 43.19 Fade detectable by feel in the response to train-of-four *(TOF)*, double-burst stimulation *($DBS_{3,3}$)*, and 50- and 100-Hz tetanic stimulation (*TET* 50 and TET 100) in relation to the true TOF ratio, as measured mechanically. The axis indicates the percentage of instances in which fade can be detected at a given TOF ratio.[37,39,72] It appears that it is not possible to exclude residual neuromuscular block by any of the methods. (See text for further explanation.)

all levels of neuromuscular block are reversed within 2 to 5 minutes. However, appropriate dosing requires neuromuscular monitoring and residual neuromuscular block can be excluded only with objective monitoring (TOF ratio, 0.9-1.0), even after routine use of sugammadex.[107,132]

During recovery of neuromuscular function, when all four responses to TOF stimulation can be felt, an estimation of the TOF ratio can be attempted. However, manual (tactile) evaluation of the response to TOF stimulation (Fig. 43.19) is not sensitive enough to exclude the possibility of residual neuromuscular block.[37,72,118,133] Greater sensitivity is achieved with $DBS_{3,3}$, but even absence of manual fade in the $DBS_{3,3}$ response does not exclude clinically significant residual block (i.e., TOF 0.6-0.9).[41,72] Moreover, some patients might suffer from residual block, even after recovery to a TOF ratio of 0.9 to 1.0.[77,81] Therefore, manual evaluation of responses to nerve stimulation should always be considered in relation to reliable clinical signs and symptoms of residual neuromuscular block (Box 43.1).

BOX 43.1 Clinical Tests of Postoperative Neuromuscular Recovery

Unreliable

- Sustained eye opening
- Protrusion of the tongue
- Arm lift to the opposite shoulder
- Normal tidal volume
- Normal or nearly normal vital capacity
- Maximum inspiratory pressure less than 40-50 cm H_2O

More Reliable, But Still Not Excluding Residual Neuromuscular Block

- Sustained head lift for 5 s
- Sustained leg lift for 5 s
- Sustained handgrip for 5 s
- Sustained "tongue depressor test"
- Maximum inspiratory pressure

When to Use a Peripheral Nerve Stimulator

In clinical practice, significant residual block can be excluded with certainty only if an objective method of neuromuscular monitoring is used.[78,79] Therefore, good evidence-based practice dictates that clinicians should always quantitate the extent of neuromuscular recovery by objective monitoring.[7-13] Only a TOF ratio of 0.90 to 1.00 measured by objective monitoring ensures a low risk of clinically significant residual block.

However, in many departments, clinicians do not have access to equipment for measuring the degree of block.[134] How then to evaluate and, as far as possible, exclude a clinically significant postoperative block? First, long-acting neuromuscular blocking drugs should not be used. Second, the tactile response to TOF nerve stimulation should be evaluated during surgery. Third, if possible, total twitch suppression should be avoided. The neuromuscular block should be managed so that there are always one or two tactile TOF responses. Fourth, the block should be antagonized at the end of the procedure, preferably with sugammadex if rocuronium or vecuronium have been used. When using neostigmine, reversal should not be initiated before at least two to four responses to TOF stimulation are present. Fifth, during recovery, tactile evaluation of the response to DBS is preferable to tactile evaluation of the response to TOF stimulation because it is easier to manually assess fade in the DBS than in the TOF response. Sixth, the clinician should recognize that the absence of tactile fade in both the TOF and DBS responses does not exclude significant residual block. Finally, reliable clinical signs and symptoms of residual block (see Box 43.1) should be considered in relation to the response to nerve stimulation. Fig. 43.20 shows how to minimize the risk of residual block with or without objective monitoring.[135]

In view of the uncertainty connected with the use of clinical tests of postoperative neuromuscular recovery and tactile evaluation of the response to nerve stimulation, all patients receiving neuromuscular blocking drugs should be monitored with an objective monitor. Whether the functioning of such a neuromuscular transmission analyzer is based on EMG, MMG, AMG, CPM, CMG, or PMG is not crucial as long as the apparatus is used appropriately.

Acknowledgment

The editors, publisher, and Dr. Casper Claudius would like to thank Dr. Jorgen Viby-Mogensen for his contribution to this chapter in the prior edition of this work. It has served as the foundation of the current chapter.

Complete references available online at expertconsult.com.

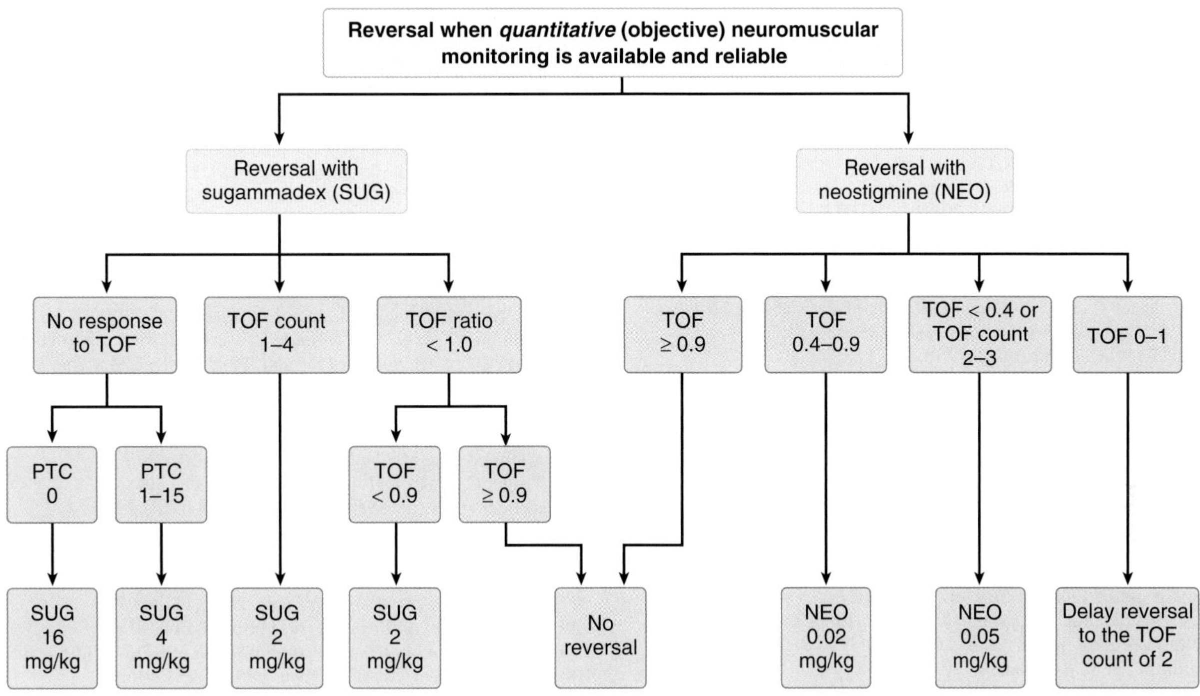

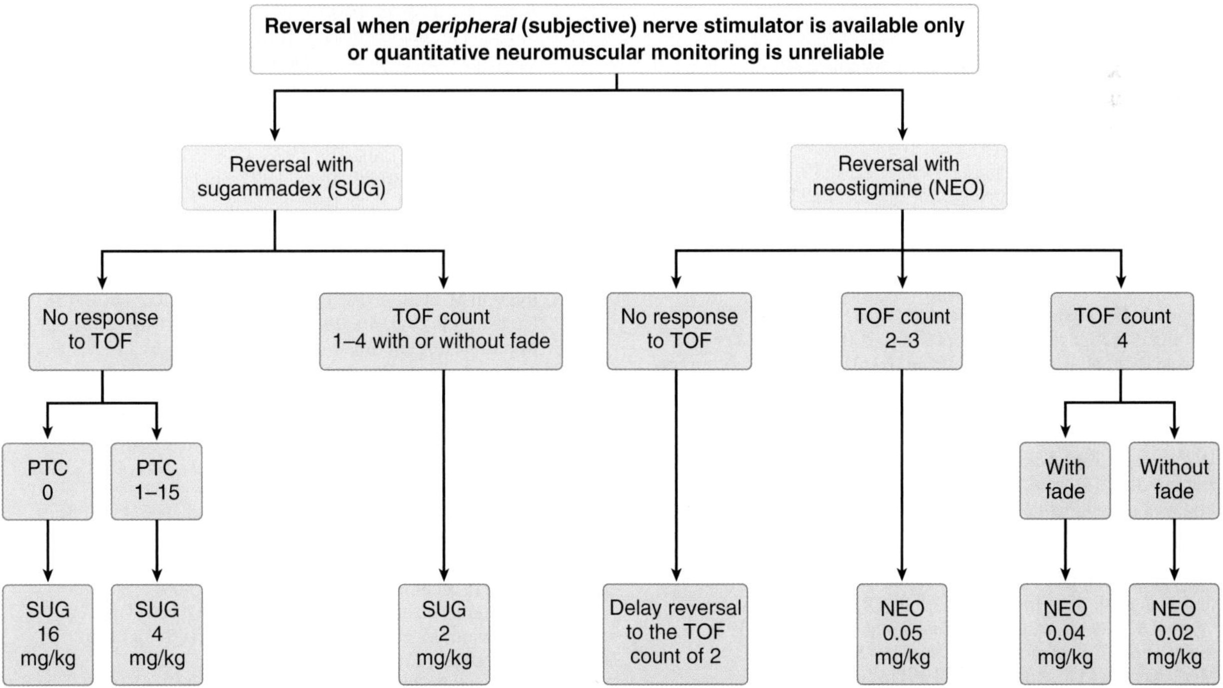

Fig. 43.20 Suggestion to diminish the incidence of residual curarization by neostigmine (NEO) or sugammadex (SUG) according to the level of block, determined with a nerve stimulator (quantitative or peripheral). Note that only a quantitative measured TOF ratio of 0.90 to 1.00 ensures low risk of clinically significant residual block. *PTC,* Posttetanic count; *TOF,* train-of-four. (Modified from Kopman AF, Eikermann M. Antagonism of non-depolarising neuromuscular block: current practice. *Anaesthesia.* 2009;64[Suppl 1]:22–30.)

References

1. Eriksson LI, et al. *Anesthesiology*. 1997;87(5):1035.
2. Moerer O, et al. *Eur J Anaesthesiol*. 2002;19(12):883.
3. Eriksson LI, et al. *Anesthesiology*. 1993;78(4):693.
4. Eikermann M, et al. *Am J Respir Crit Care Med*. 2007;175(1):9.
5. Viby-Mogensen J, et al. *Anesthesiology*. 1979;50:539.
6. Debaene B, et al. *Anesthesiology*. 2003;98:1042.
7. Viby-Mogensen J. *Br J Anaesth*. 2000;84:301.
8. Eriksson LI. *Anesthesiology*. 2003;98(5):1037.
9. Viby-Mogensen J, Claudius C. *Anesth Analg*. 2010;111(1):1.
10. Miller RD, Ward TA. *Anesth Analg*. 2010;111(1):3.
11. Donati F. *Anesth Analg*. 2010;111(1):6.
12. Kopman AF. *Anesth Analg*. 2010;111(1):9.
13. Futter M, Gin T. *Anesth Analg*. 2010;111(1):11.
14. Brull SJ, et al. *Anesthesiology*. 1990;72(4):629.
15. Brull SJ, et al. *Can J Anaesth*. 1991;38(2):164.
16. Iwasaki H, et al. *Anaesthesia*. 1994;49(9):814.
17. Fuchs-Buder T, et al. *Acta Anaesthesiol Scand*. 2007;51(7):789.
18. Brull SJ, Silverman DG. *Anesthesiology*. 1995;83(4):702.
19. Smith CE, et al. *Anesth Analg*. 1988;67(7):625.
20. Donati F, et al. *Anesthesiology*. 1986;65(1):1.
21. Pansard JL, et al. *Anesthesiology*. 1987;67(3):326.
22. Donati F, et al. *Anesthesiology*. 1990;73(5):870.
23. Rimaniol JM, et al. *Anesth Analg*. 1996;83(4):808.
24. Plaud B, et al. *Anesthesiology*. 2001;95(1):96.
25. Pavlin EG, et al. *Anesthesiology*. 1989;70(3):381.
26. Isono S, et al. *Anesthesiology*. 1991;75(6):980.
27. Dhonneur G, et al. *Br J Anaesth*. 2007;99(3):376.
28. Kirov K, et al. *Br J Anaesth*. 2007;98(5):611.
29. Kern SE, et al. *J Clin Anesth*. 1997;9(5):383.
30. Saitoh Y, et al. *Eur J Anaesthesiol*. 1998;15(6):649.
31. Michaud G, et al. *Anesth Analg*. 2005;100(3):718; table of contents.
32. Claudius C, et al. *Br J Anaesth*. 2010;105(3):310.
33. Christie Th, Churchill-Davidson HC. *Lancet*. 1958;21:776.
34. Curran MJ, et al. *Br J Anaesth*. 1987;59(8):989.
35. Ali HH, et al. *Br J Anaesth*. 1970;42(11):967.
36. Ali HH, et al. *Br J Anaesth*. 1971;43(5):478.
37. Viby-Mogensen J, et al. *Anesthesiology*. 1985;63(4):440.
38. Engbaek J, et al. *Anesthesiology*. 1989;71(3):391.
39. Drenck NE, et al. *Anesthesiology*. 1989;70(4):578.
40. Saddler JM, et al. *Anesthesiology*. 1990;73(3):401.
41. Fruergaard K, et al. *Acta Anaesthesiol Scand*. 1998;42(10):1168.
42. Tassonyi E. *Anaesthesist*. 1975;24:374.
43. Paton WD, Waud DR. *J Physiol*. 1967;191(1):59.
44. Jonsson M, et al. *Anesthesiology*. 2006;105(3):521.
45. Saitoh Y, et al. *Br J Anaesth*. 1994;73(3):416.
46. Viby-Mogensen J, et al. *Anesthesiology*. 1981;55(4):458.
47. Bonsu AK, et al. *Br J Anaesth*. 1987;59(9):1089.
48. Muchhal KK, et al. *Anesthesiology*. 1987;66(6):846.
49. Fernando PU, et al. *Acta Anaesthesiol Scand*. 1987;31(7):593.
50. Schultz P, et al. *Acta Anaesthesiol Scand*. 2001;45(5):612.
51. Eleveld DJ, et al. *Anesth Analg*. 2005;101(3):758; table of contents.
52. Gilhuly TJ, et al. *Anesth Analg*. 2008;107(5):1609.
53. Lee GC, et al. *Anesthesiology*. 1997;86(1):48.
54. Hemmerling TM, et al. *Anesth Analg*. 2000;90(2):494.
55. Hemmerling TM, et al. *Anesth Analg*. 2001;92(1):106.
56. Hemmerling TM, et al. *Can J Anaesth*. 2001;48(4):356.
57. Engbaek J, et al. *Acta Anaesthesiol Scand*. 1993;37(8):788.
58. Kopman AF. *Anesthesiology*. 1985;63(2):208.
59. Kopman AF, et al. *Anesthesiology*. 2002;96(3):583.
60. Viby-Mogensen J, et al. *Acta Anaesthesiol Scand*. 1988;32(1):45.
61. Jensen E, et al. *Acta Anaesthesiol Scand*. 1988;32(1):49.
62. Werner MU, et al. *Acta Anaesthesiol Scand*. 1988;32(5):395.
63. May O, et al. *Acta Anaesthesiol Scand*. 1988;32(3):239.
64. McCluskey A, et al. *Anaesthesia*. 1997;52(4):345.
65. Kirkegaard-Nielsen H, et al. *J Clin Monit Comput*. 1998;14(1):19.
66. Eikermann M, et al. *Acta Anaesthesiol Scand*. 2004;48(3):365.
67. Claudius C. *Viby-Mogensen J: Anesthesiology*. 2008;108(6):1117.
68. Claudius C, et al. *Anesthesiology*. 2009;110(6):1261.
69. Claudius C, et al. *Acta Anaesthesiol Scand*. 2009;53(4):449.
70. Eikermann M, et al. *Anesthesiology*. 2003;98(6):1333.
71. Capron F, et al. *Anesthesiology*. 2004;100(5):1119.
72. Capron F, et al. *Anesth Analg*. 2006;102(5):1578.
73. Kopman AF. *Acta Anaesthesiol Scand*. 2005;49(10):1575.
74. Suzuki T, et al. *Br J Anaesth*. 2006;96(1):44.
75. Heier T, et al. *Anesthesiology*. 2010;113(4):825.
76. Heier T, et al. *Br J Anaesth*. 2012;108(3):444.
77. Eikermann M, et al. *Anesth Analg*. 2006;102(3):937.
78. Gätke MR, et al. *Acta Anaesthesiol Scand*. 2002;46(2):207.
79. Mortensen CR, et al. *Acta Anaesthesiol Scand*. 1995;39(6):797.
80. Murphy GS, et al. *Anesthesiology*. 2008;109(3):389.
81. Murphy GS, et al. *Anesthesiology*. 2011;115(5):946.
82. Gätke MR, et al. *Acta Anaesthesiol Scand*. 2002;46(9):1124.
83. Larsen PB, et al. *Acta Anaesthesiol Scand*. 2002;46(9):1131.
83a. Colegrave N, et al. *Anaesth Crit Care Pain Med*. 2016;35(3):223.
83b. Murphy GS, et al. *Anesthesiology*. 2018;29(5):880.
84. Kern SE, et al. *Anesth Analg*. 1994;78(5):978.
85. Pelgrims K, Vanacker B. *Acta Anaesthesiol Belg*. 2001;52(3):297.
86. Dahaba AA, et al. *Anesth Analg*. 2002;94(3):591; table of contents.
87. Barry DT. *Arch Phys Med Rehabil*. 1991;72(8):573.
88. Dascalu A, et al. *Br J Anaesth*. 1999;83(3):405.
89. Hemmerling TM, et al. *Br J Anaesth*. 2002;88(3):389.
90. Hemmerling TM, et al. *Anesthesiology*. 2003;98(2):359.
91. Michaud G, et al. *Can J Anaesth*. 2005;52(8):795.
92. Trager G, et al. *Can J Anaesth*. 2006;53(2):130.
93. de Boer HD, et al. *Anesthesiology*. 2007;107(2):239.
94. Pühringer FK, et al. *Anesthesiology*. 2008;109(2):188.
95. Groudine SB, et al. *Anesth Analg*. 2007;104(3):555.
96. Sparr HJ, et al. *Anesthesiology*. 2007;106(5):935.
97. Duvaldestin P, et al. *Anesth Analg*. 2010;110(1):74.
98. O'Hara DA, et al. *Br J Anaesth*. 1986;58(11):1300.
99. Gibson FM, et al. *Acta Anaesthesiol Scand*. 1987;31(7):655–657.
100. Engbaek J, et al. *Anesthesiology*. 1990;72(5):803.
101. Kirkegaard H, et al. *Anesthesiology*. 2002;96(1):45.
102. Kopman AF, et al. *Anesth Analg*. 2004;98(1):102; table of contents.
103. Tajaate N, et al. *Eur J Anaesthesiol*. 2018;35:184.
104. Sorgenfrei IF, et al. *Anesthesiology*. 2006;104(4):667.
105. Suy K, et al. *Anesthesiology*. 2007;106(2):283.
106. Pühringer FK, et al. *Br J Anaesth*. 2010;105(5):610.
107. Kotake Y, Ochiai R, Suzuki T, et al. *Anesth Analg*. 2013;117:345.
108. Kopman AF, et al. *Anesthesiology*. 1997;86(4):765.
109. Ali HH, et al. *I. Br J Anaesth*. 1971;43(5):473.
110. Ali HH, et al. *Br J Anaesth*. 1975;47(5):570.
111. Brand JB, et al. *Anesth Analg*. 1977;56(1):55.
112. Eriksson LI, et al. *Acta Anaesthesiol Scand*. 1992;36(7):710.
113. Berg H, et al. *Acta Anaesthesiol Scand*. 1997;41(9):1095.
114. Wyon N, et al. *Anesthesiology*. 1998;89(6):1471.
115. Sundman E, et al. *Anesthesiology*. 2000;92(4):977.
116. Jonsson M, et al. *Acta Anaesthesiol Scand*. 2002;46(5):488.
117. Herbstreit F, et al. *Anesthesiology*. 2009;110(6):1253.
118. Kopman AF, et al. *Anesthesiology*. 1996;85(6):1253.
119. Naguib M, et al. *Br J Anaesth*. 2007;98(3):302.
120. Shorten GD, et al. *Can J Anaesth*. 1995;42(8):711.
121. Viby-Mogensen J, et al. *Br J Anaesth*. 2007;99(2):297; author reply 297.
121a. https://www.ncbi.nlm.nih.gov/pubmed/29200077.
122. Eriksson LI, et al. *Acta Anaesthesiol Scand*. 1991;35(3):247.
123. Heier T, et al. *Anesthesiology*. 1990;72(5):807.
124. Heier T, Caldwell JE. *Anesthesiology*. 2006;104(5):1070.
125. Thornberry EA, Mazumdar B. *Anaesthesia*. 1988;43(6):447.
126. Brull SJ, Kopman AF. *Anesthesiology*. 2017;126:173.
127. Payne JP, et al. *Br J Anaesth*. 1980;52(1):69.
128. Eikermann M, et al. *Anesthesiology*. 2007;107(4):621.
129. Eikermann M, et al. *Br J Anaesth*. 2008;101(3):344.
130. Caldwell JE. *J Crit Care*. 2009;24(1):21.
131. Herbstreit F, et al. *Anesthesiology*. 2010;113(6):1280.
132. Le Corre F, et al. *Can J Anaesth*. 2011;58(10):944.
133. Pedersen T, et al. *Anesthesiology*. 1990;73(5):835.
134. Naguib M, et al. *Anesth Analg*. 2010;111(1):110.
135. Kopman AF, Eikermann M. *Anaesthesia*. 2009;64(suppl 1):22.

44 Airway Management in the Adult

CARLOS A. ARTIME and CARIN A. HAGBERG

KEY POINTS

- One of the fundamental responsibilities of the anesthesiologist is to mitigate the adverse effects of anesthesia on the respiratory system by maintaining airway patency and ensuring adequate ventilation and oxygenation. The term *airway management* refers to this practice and is a cornerstone of anesthesia.
- Successful airway management requires a range of knowledge and skill sets—specifically, the ability to predict difficulty with airway management and to formulate an airway management strategy, as well as the skills to execute that strategy using the wide array of airway devices available.
- The American Society of Anesthesiologists' *Practice Guidelines for Management of the Difficult Airway* and the accompanying Difficult Airway Algorithm provide guidelines for the evaluation of the airway and preparation for difficult airway management and can guide clinical decision making when an anesthesiologist is faced with a known or potentially difficult airway. Cognitive aids, such as the Vortex approach, are useful to help implement airway algorithms in an emergency situation.
- A detailed understanding of airway anatomy is essential for the anesthesia provider.
- A complete evaluation of the airway and knowledge of difficult airway predictors can alert the anesthesiologist to the potential for difficulty with airway management and allow for appropriate planning.
- Apneic oxygenation can be used to prolong the duration of apnea without desaturation and is increasingly being adopted during the management of both difficult and routine airways.
- Application of local anesthesia to the airway or induction of general anesthesia is usually required to facilitate airway management, to provide comfort for the patient, and to blunt airway reflexes and the hemodynamic response to airway instrumentation.
- Over the past 30 years, the laryngeal mask airway (LMA) has emerged as one of the most important developments in airway devices.
- Tracheal intubation establishes a definitive airway, provides maximal protection against aspiration of gastric contents, and allows for positive-pressure ventilation with higher airway pressures than via a face mask or supraglottic airway.
- Flexible scope intubation of the trachea in an awake, spontaneously ventilating, and cooperative patient is the *gold standard* for the management of the difficult airway.
- Invasive airways are indicated as a rescue technique when attempts at establishing a noninvasive airway fail. The anesthesia practitioner should become proficient with techniques for transtracheal jet ventilation and cricothyrotomy.
- Extubation is a critical component of airway management with the potential for significant complications. The plan for extubation of the trachea must be preemptively formulated and includes a strategy for reintubation should the patient be unable to maintain an adequate airway after extubation.

Introduction

General anesthesia is associated with various effects on the respiratory system, including the loss of airway patency, loss of protective airway reflexes, and hypoventilation or apnea. Therefore one of the fundamental responsibilities of the anesthesiologist is to establish airway patency and to ensure adequate ventilation and oxygenation. The term *airway management* refers to the practice of establishing and securing a patent airway and is a cornerstone of anesthetic practice. Traditionally, ventilation via a mask and tracheal intubation have been the foundation of airway management; however, in the past 30 years, the laryngeal mask airway (LMA) has emerged as one of the most important developments in airway devices.

Because failure to secure a patent airway can result in hypoxic brain injury or death in only a few minutes, difficulty with airway management has potentially grave implications. Analysis of the American Society of Anesthesiologists (ASA) Closed Claims Project database has demonstrated that the development of an airway emergency increases the odds of death or brain damage by 15-fold.[1]

Although the proportion of claims attributable to airway-related complications has decreased over the past 3 decades, airway complications are still the second-most common cause of claims.[2] In 2011, the Royal College of Anaesthetists and the Difficult Airway Society (DAS) of the United Kingdom reported the results of the 4th National Audit Project (NAP4), a 1-year audit aimed at determining the incidence of major complications of airway management in anesthesia. NAP4 identified 133 major airway-related events in the perioperative period resulting in 16 deaths—a mortality incidence of 1 per 180,000 anesthetics—a number that could be as high as 1 per 50,000 anesthetics when underreporting is considered.[3] The most common airway problems in the NAP4 study were failure, delay, or difficulty in securing the airway; aspiration of gastric contents; and extubation-related complications. Poor assessment of the airway, poor planning, and a lack of personal and/or institutional preparedness for managing difficulty with airway management were the most common contributing factors.[4]

Studies such as these highlight the importance of successful airway management, which requires a range of knowledge and skill sets—specifically, the ability to predict difficulty with airway management, to formulate an airway management strategy, and to have the skills necessary to execute that strategy using the wide array of available airway devices.[5] Development of these skills should be an ongoing endeavor for all anesthesiologists. As with any manual skill, continued practice improves performance and may reduce the likelihood of complications. New airway devices are continually being introduced into the clinical arena, each with unique properties that may be advantageous in certain situations. Becoming familiar with new devices under controlled conditions is important for the anesthesia practitioner—the difficult airway is not an appropriate setting during which to experiment with a new technique.

ALGORITHMS FOR MANAGEMENT OF THE DIFFICULT AIRWAY

The American Society of Anesthesiologists Algorithm

In 1993, the ASA published the first *Practice Guidelines for Management of the Difficult Airway*, which was written with the intent to "facilitate the management of the difficult airway and to reduce the likelihood of adverse outcomes."[6] The most recent update to this report, published in 2013, defines the difficult airway as "the clinical situation in which a conventionally trained anesthesiologist experiences difficulty with ventilation of the upper airway via a mask, difficulty with tracheal intubation, or both" and provides guidelines for the evaluation of the airway and preparation for difficult airway management, including a Difficult Airway Algorithm (DAA) intended to guide clinical decision making when an anesthesiologist is faced with a known or potential difficult airway (Fig. 44.1).[7] The ASA DAA begins with a consideration of the relative clinical merits and feasibility of four basic management choices: (1) awake intubation versus intubation after induction of general anesthesia, (2) noninvasive techniques versus invasive techniques (i.e., surgical or percutaneous airway) for the initial approach to intubation, (3) video-assisted laryngoscopy (VAL) as an initial approach to intubation, and (4) preservation versus ablation of spontaneous ventilation.

The ASA DAA does not follow a linear decision-making tree, as the advanced cardiac life support (ACLS) algorithms do. It can be better understood and remembered by considering it as three separate scenarios: (1) predicted difficult airway (awake intubation), (2) difficult intubation with adequate oxygenation/ventilation (the "*non-emergency*" pathway), and (3) difficult intubation without adequate oxygenation/ventilation (the "cannot intubate, cannot oxygenate" [CICO] scenario or the "*emergency*" pathway).

Other Difficult Airway Algorithms

In addition to the ASA, several different national anesthesia societies have published their own guidelines for management of the difficult airway, including the Difficult Airway Society (DAS) from the United Kingdom,[8] the Canadian Airway Focus Group (CAFG),[9,10] the French Society of Anesthesia and Intensive Care (SFAR),[11] the German Society of Anesthesiology and Intensive Care Medicine (DGAI),[12] the Italian Society for Anesthesia and Intensive Care (SIAARTI),[13] and the Japanese Society of Anesthesiologists.[14] All of these include recommendations for the prediction of the difficult airway and suggest awake intubation as a management strategy (with the exception of the DAS guidelines) and all incorporate algorithms for both unanticipated difficult intubation with adequate oxygenation and the CICO scenario. Common elements include a focus on awakening the patient in the setting of a difficult intubation with adequate ventilation, the use of the LMA as a rescue for difficult mask ventilation, and emergency front of neck access (FONA) in the CICO scenario. The primary differences in these algorithms are in specific details, such as the number of intubation attempts suggested, the specific alternate devices recommended for difficult intubation, and the organization of the algorithm.[15]

Human Factors and Cognitive Aids

There has been growing attention to the influence of "human factors" on difficult airway management—namely, human behaviors, abilities, shortcomings, and biases as well as individual and team performance. Studies such as NAP4 have shown that these human factors contribute to an adverse airway outcome in over 40% of cases.[3] The use of airway checklists, preprocedural team briefings, and cognitive aids are all strategies for addressing human factor challenges.[16]

The Vortex approach, conceived by Dr. Nicholas Chrimes, a specialist anaesthetist in Melbourne, Australia, is one such cognitive aid designed to facilitate management of the unanticipated difficult airway.[17] Rather than relying on complex algorithms that are based on decision trees, the Vortex model utilizes a visual aid in the shape of a funnel or vortex (Fig. 44.2) to guide the airway practitioner through the three basic nonsurgical airway techniques (face-mask ventilation, supraglottic airway [SGA], and tracheal intubation). If after an "optimal attempt" at each of these nonsurgical modalities alveolar oxygen delivery has not been achieved, then one "travels down the vortex," and an emergency surgical airway is indicated. Because this strategic approach is more conceptual, it is simple enough to be utilized and recalled during a stressful airway emergency.

Functional Airway Anatomy

A detailed understanding of airway anatomy is essential for the anesthesiologist. Various aspects of airway

1. Assess the likelihood and clinical impact of basic management problems:
   - Difficulty with patient cooperation or consent
   - Difficult mask ventilation
   - Difficult supraglottic airway placement
   - Difficult laryngoscopy
   - Difficult intubation
   - Difficult surgical airway access

2. Actively pursue opportunities to deliver supplemental oxygen throughout the process of difficult airway management.

3. Consider the relative merits and feasibility of basic management choices:
   - Awake intubation *vs.* intubation after induction of general anesthesia
   - Noninvasive technique *vs.* invasive techniques for the initial approach to intubation
   - Video-assisted laryngoscopy as an initial approach to intubation
   - Preservation *vs.* ablation of spontaneous ventilation

4. Develop primary and alternative strategies:

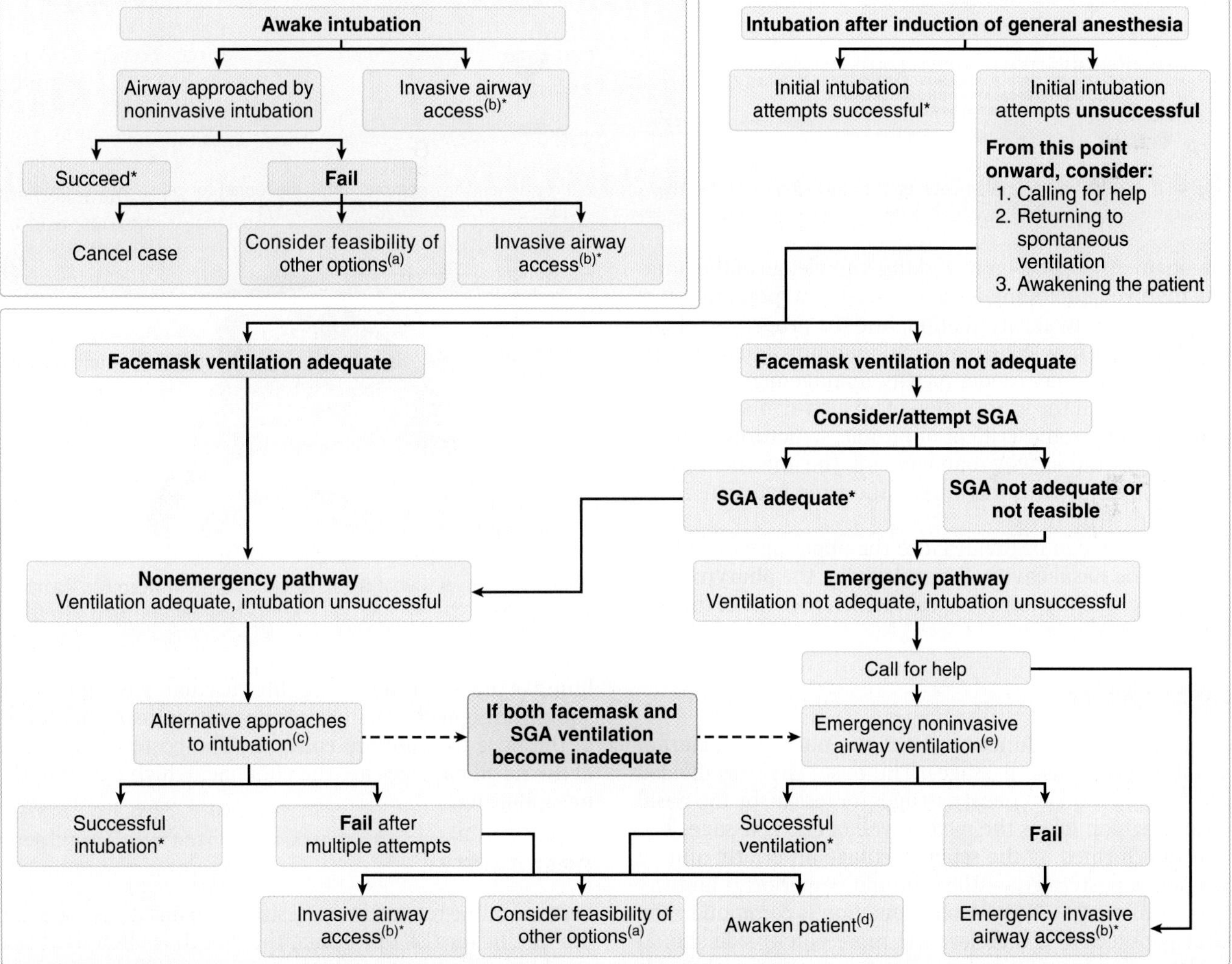

***Confirm ventilation, tracheal intubation, or SGA placement with exhaled CO_2.**

a. Other options include (but are not limited to): surgery using facemask or supraglottic airway (SGA) anesthesia (e.g., LMA, ILMA, laryngeal tube), local anesthesia infiltration, or regional nerve blockade. Pursuit of these options usually implies that mask ventilation will not be problematic. Therefore these options may be of limited value if this step in the algorithm has been reached via the Emergency Pathway.

b. Invasive airway access includes surgical or percutaneous airway, jet ventilation, and retrograde intubation.

c. Alternative difficult intubation approaches include (but are not limited to): video-assisted laryngoscopy, alternative laryngoscope blades, SGA (e.g., LMA or ILMA) as an intubation conduit (with or without fiberoptic guidance), fiberoptic intubation, intubating stylet or tube changer, light wand, and blind oral or nasal intubation.

d. Consider re-preparation of the patient for awake intubation or canceling surgery.

e. Emergency noninvasive airway ventilation consists of a SGA.

Fig. 44.1 **The American Society of Anesthesiologists' Difficult Airway Algorithm.** (From Apfelbaum JL, Hagberg CA, Caplan RA, et al. Practice guidelines for management of the difficult airway: an updated report by the American Society of Anesthesiologists Task Force on Management of the Difficult Airway. *Anesthesiology*. 2013;118:251–270.)

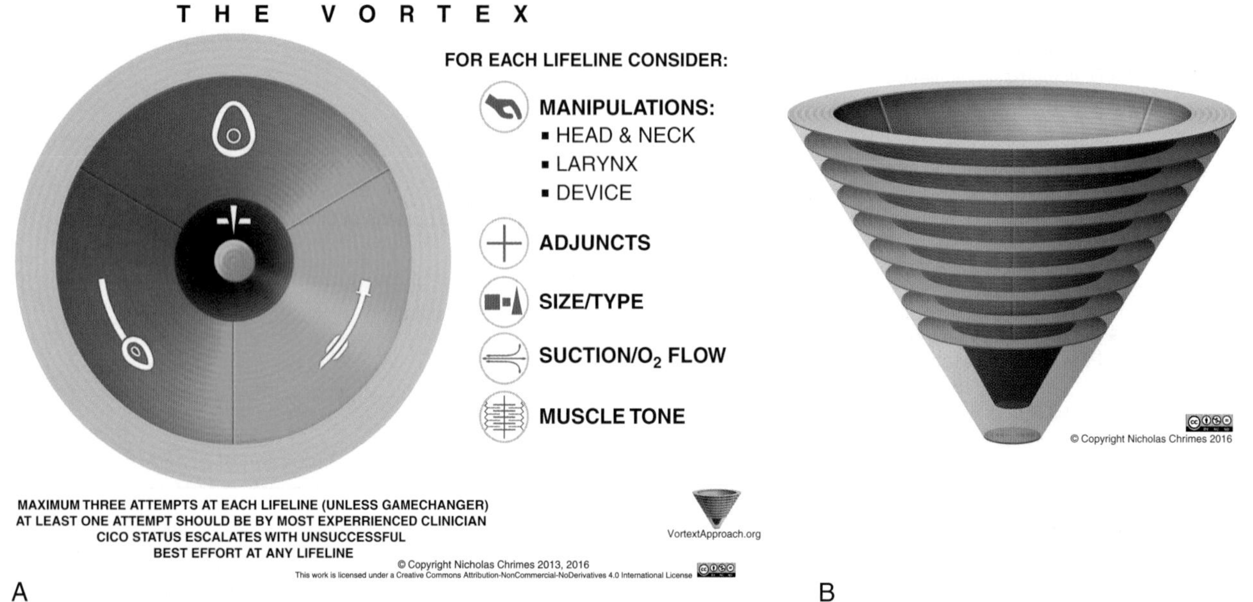

Fig. 44.2 (A) The Vortex implementation tool. (B) Lateral aspect of the Vortex in three dimensions, demonstrating the funnel concept. (From Chrimes N. The Vortex: a universal 'high-acuity implementation tool' for emergency airway management. *Br J Anaesth*. 2016;117:i20–i27.)

management depend on a working knowledge of the anatomy involved, including airway assessment, preparation of the airway for awake intubation, and the proper use of airway devices. Knowledge of normal anatomy and anatomic variations that may render airway management more difficult helps with the formulation of an airway management plan. Because some critical anatomic structures may be obscured during airway management, the anesthesiologist must be familiar with the interrelationship between different airway structures.

The airway can be divided into the upper airway, which includes the nasal cavity, the oral cavity, the pharynx, and the larynx; and the lower airway, which consists of the tracheobronchial tree.

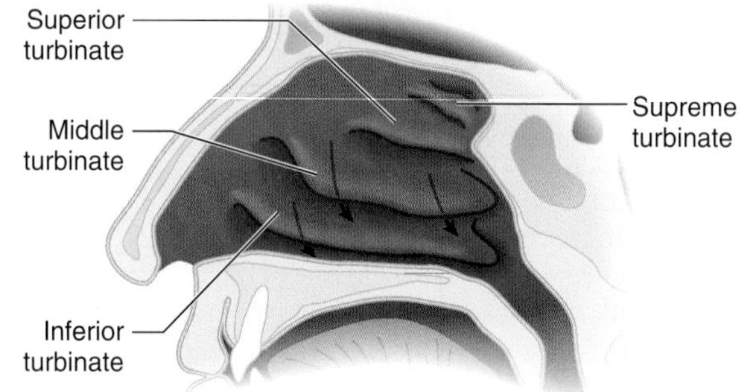

Fig. 44.3 Lateral wall of the nasal cavity. (From Redden RJ. Anatomic considerations in anesthesia. In: Hagberg CA, ed. *Handbook of Difficult Airway Management*. Philadelphia: Churchill Livingstone; 2000, p. 3, Fig. 1.2.)

NASAL CAVITY

The airway begins functionally at the naris, the external opening of the nasal passages. The nasal cavity is divided into the right and left nasal passages (or fossae) by the nasal septum, which forms the medial wall of each passage. The septum is formed by the septal cartilage anteriorly and by two bones posteriorly—\the ethmoid (superiorly) and the vomer (inferiorly). Nasal septal deviation is common in the adult population[18]; therefore the more patent side should be determined before passing instrumentation through the nasal passages. The lateral wall of the nasal passages is characterized by the presence of three turbinates (or conchae) that divide the nasal passage into three scroll-shaped meatuses (Fig. 44.3). The inferior meatus, between the inferior turbinate and the floor of the nasal cavity, is the preferred pathway for passage of nasal airway devices[19]; improper placement of objects in the nose can result in avulsion of a turbinate.[20,21] The roof of the nasal cavity is formed by the cribriform plate, part of the ethmoid bone. This fragile structure, if fractured, can result in communication between the nasal and intracranial cavities and a resultant leakage of cerebrospinal fluid. Because the mucosal lining of the nasal cavity is highly vascular, vasoconstrictor should be applied, usually topically, before instrumentation of the nose to minimize epistaxis. The posterior openings of the nasal passages are the choanae, which lead into the nasopharynx.

ORAL CAVITY

Because of the relatively small size of the nasal passages and the significant risk of trauma, the mouth is often used as a conduit for airway devices. Many airway procedures require adequate mouth opening, which is accomplished by rotation within the temporomandibular joint (TMJ) and subsequent opening by sliding (also known as *protrusion* or *subluxation*) of the condyles of the mandible within the TMJ.[22]

The oral cavity leads to the oropharynx and is inferiorly bounded by the tongue and superiorly by the hard and soft palates. The hard palate, formed by parts of the maxilla and the palatine bone, makes up the anterior two thirds of the roof of the mouth; the soft palate (velum palatinum), a fibromuscular fold of tissue attached to the hard palate, forms the posterior one third of the roof of the mouth.

BOX 44.1 Components of the Physical Examination of the Airway

- Visual inspection of the face and neck
- Assessment of mouth opening
- Evaluation of oropharyngeal anatomy and dentition
- Assessment of neck range of motion (ability of the patient to assume the sniffing position)
- Assessment of the submandibular space
- Assessment of the patient's ability to slide the mandible anteriorly (test of mandibular prognathism)

for difficulty with airway management. These include obvious facial deformities, neoplasms involving the face or neck, facial burns, a large goiter, a short or thick neck, or a receding mandible. The presence of a beard has been shown to be associated with difficult ventilation attributable to the difficulty in obtaining a mask seal.[32,33] Cervical collars or cervical traction devices can interfere with both mask ventilation and DL. A neck circumference greater than 43 cm (17 inches) is associated with difficulty with tracheal intubation[34]; Brodsky demonstrated that a large neck circumference is, in fact, more predictive of difficulty with tracheal intubation than a high body mass index (BMI).[35]

Assessment of mouth opening and inspection of the oropharyngeal anatomy is achieved by instructing the patient to open his or her mouth as wide as possible. An interincisor distance of less than 3 cm (or 2 fingerbreadths), as measured from the upper to the lower incisors with maximal mouth opening, can suggest the possibility of difficult intubation[7]; some studies have used 4 or 4.5 cm as the cutoff.[36] A thorough inspection of the oropharynx can help identify pathologic characteristics that may result in difficulty with intubation, such as neoplasm, a high arched palate, or macroglossia. In 1983, Mallampati and associates described a clinical sign to predict difficult tracheal intubation based on the size of the base of the tongue.[37] A Mallampati classification of I to III is assigned, based on the visibility of the faucial pillars, uvula, and soft palate when the patient is seated upright with the head neutral, the mouth open, the tongue protruded, and no phonation.[38] Higher scores on the Mallampati classification indicate poor visibility of the oropharyngeal structures attributable to a large tongue relative to the size of the oropharyngeal space, and, subsequently, a more difficult laryngoscopy. The modified Mallampati classification described by Samsoon and Young,[39] which adds a fourth classification, is the most commonly used airway assessment test in current anesthesia practice and is defined as follows (Fig. 44.8):

- Class I: Faucial pillars, uvula, and soft palate are visualized.
- Class II: Base of the uvula and soft palate are visualized.
- Class III: Soft palate only is visualized.
- Class IV: Hard palate only is visualized.

As a stand-alone test, the modified Mallampati classification is insufficient for accurate prediction of difficult intubation; however, it may have clinical utility in combination with other difficult airway predictors.[40] Some studies support obtaining a Mallampati score with the head in full extension to improve the predictive value of the test.[38,41]

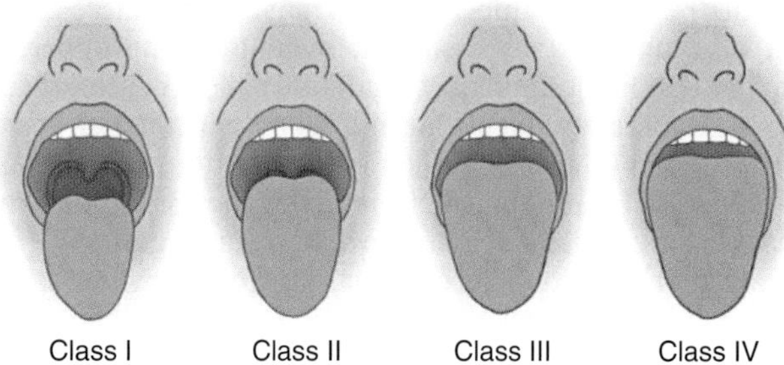

Fig. 44.8 Modified Mallampati classification as described by Samsoon and Young. Classes are differentiated on the basis of the structures visualized: class I—soft palate, fauces, uvula, tonsillar pillars; class II—soft palate, fauces, uvula; class III—soft palate, base of the uvula; class IV—soft palate not visible. (From Mallampati SR. Recognition of the difficult airway. In: Benumof JL, ed. *Airway Management Principles and Practice.* St Louis: Mosby; 1996, p. 132.)

A Mallampati *zero* classification has been proposed when the epiglottis can be visualized during examination of the oropharynx; this finding is usually associated with easy laryngoscopy,[42,43] although difficulty with airway management attributable to a large, floppy epiglottis in patients with a Mallampati zero classification can occur.[44,45]

An examination of dentition should be performed when the oropharyngeal anatomy is being evaluated.[7] Relatively long upper incisors can impair DL. Poor dentition and loose teeth increase the risk of dental trauma and present a risk of tooth dislodgment with subsequent aspiration; very loose teeth should be removed before laryngoscopy. Cosmetic dental work, such as veneers, caps, crowns, and bridges, are particularly susceptible to damage during airway management. Edentulousness is predictive of easy tracheal intubation but potentially difficult mask ventilation.[46]

The ideal positioning for DL is achieved by cervical flexion and atlantooccipital extension and is most commonly referred to as the *sniffing position*[47] (see Direct Laryngoscopy: Preparation and Positioning). Assessment of a patient's ability to assume this position should be included in the airway examination; an inability to extend the neck at the atlantooccipital joint is associated with difficult intubation.[48] Head and neck mobility can also be quantitatively assessed by measuring the sternomental distance between the sternal notch and the point of the chin with the head in full extension and the mouth closed. Distances less than 12.5 cm are associated with difficult intubation.[49] An assessment of overall neck range of motion can be performed by measuring the angle created by the forehead when the neck is fully flexed and then fully extended; a measurement of less than 80 degrees is predictive of difficult intubation.[50]

During DL, the tongue is displaced into the submandibular space; glottic visualization may be inadequate if this space is diminished because of a small mandible. This scenario is frequently referred to as an *anterior larynx*. A thyromental distance of less than 6.5 cm (3 fingerbreadths), as measured from the thyroid notch to the lower border of the mentum, is indicative of reduced mandibular space and may predict difficulty with intubation.[36,49] Compliance of this space should also be assessed; a lack of compliance or the presence of a mass is a nonreassuring finding.[7]

Tests of the ability for mandibular protrusion (prognathism) have predictive value and should be included in the airway assessment. The inability to extend the lower incisors beyond the upper incisors may be indicative of difficult laryngoscopy.[51] A similar evaluation, the upper lip bite test (ULBT) described by Khan and colleagues, has been shown to predict difficult laryngoscopy with higher specificity and less interobserver variability than the Mallampati classification; an inability of the lower incisors to bite the upper lip is associated with more difficult laryngoscopy.[52,53]

Although individual airway tests are limited by low sensitivity and positive predictive value, some multivariable assessments have been shown to have higher predictive power. The Mallampati score has been shown to have improved predictive value when combined with thyromental, sternomental, and/or interincisor distances.[49] Models that use several risk factors, such as the Wilson risk sum score (weight, head and neck movement, jaw movement, receding mandible, and buck teeth) and the El-Ganzouri risk index (mouth opening, thyromental distance, Mallampati class, neck movement, prognathism, weight, and history of difficult intubation) have been developed in an attempt to improve the predictive value of airway assessment.[50,54] On the other hand, a recent large database study of an airway risk index that utilizes seven independent risk factors found that it does not improve prediction of difficult intubation.[55] Langeron and associates developed a computer-assisted model that uses complex interactions among several risk factors (BMI, mouth opening, thyromental distance, Mallampati class, and receding mandible) to predict difficult intubation more accurately than other models based on simpler statistical analyses.[56]

NEW MODALITIES

Owing to the poor sensitivity and specificity of traditional metrics for airway assessment, a number of new modalities are being studied. The use of point-of-care ultrasonography for the prediction of difficult laryngoscopy and intubation has shown some promise in small studies, but its overall value has yet to be established.[57] Computed tomographic images of the head and neck can be used to create three-dimensional virtual endoscopic images that can be used for planning difficult airway management, particularly for patients with complex airway pathology.[58] Early studies of facial image analysis have also shown promise for the use of this technology in predicting difficult intubation.[59]

Physiologic Concepts for Airway Management

PREOXYGENATION

With the induction of anesthesia, hypoxemia can quickly develop as a result of hypoventilation or apnea in combination with decreases in functional residual capacity (FRC) attributable to the supine position, muscle paralysis, and the direct effects of the anesthetic agents themselves. Preoxygenation, the process of replacing nitrogen in the lungs with oxygen, provides an increased length of time before hemoglobin desaturation occurs in an apneic patient. This lengthened *apnea time* provides an improved margin of safety while the anesthesiologist secures the airway and resumes ventilation. Adequate preoxygenation is essential when mask ventilation after the induction of anesthesia is contraindicated or anticipated to be difficult, when intubation is anticipated to be difficult, and in patients with a smaller FRC (i.e., patients who are obese or pregnant).[60] Because difficulty with airway management can unexpectedly occur, routine preoxygenation before induction of general anesthesia is recommended.[61]

Preoxygenation is typically performed via a face mask attached to either the anesthesia machine or a Mapleson circuit. To ensure adequate preoxygenation, 100% oxygen must be provided at a flow rate high enough to prevent rebreathing (10 to 12 L/min), and no leaks around the face mask must be present. An end-tidal concentration of oxygen greater than 90% is considered to maximize apnea time. With maximal preoxygenation, the time to oxyhemoglobin desaturation below 80% can vary from 9 minutes in a healthy, nonobese adult to 3 minutes or less in children or obese adults.[62]

Two primary methods are used to accomplish preoxygenation. The first method uses tidal volume ventilation through the face mask for 3 minutes, which allows the exchange of 95% of the gas in the lungs.[60] The second method uses vital capacity breaths to achieve adequate preoxygenation more rapidly. Four breaths over 30 seconds is not as effective as the tidal volume method but may be acceptable in certain clinical situations; eight breaths over 60 seconds has been shown to be more effective.[60]

Transnasal humidified rapid-insufflation ventilatory exchange (THRIVE) at 60 L/min for 3 minutes has been demonstrated to be as effective as tidal volume preoxygenation by face mask (see Apneic Oxygenation).[63] Head-up positioning has been shown to improve the quality of preoxygenation in both obese[64] and nonobese patients.[65] The use of noninvasive positive-pressure ventilation (PPV) for preoxygenation also prolongs apnea time.[66,67]

APNEIC OXYGENATION

Apneic oxygenation is a physiologic phenomenon by which oxygen from the oropharynx or nasopharynx diffuses down into the alveoli as a result of the net negative alveolar gas exchange rate resulting from oxygen removal and carbon dioxide excretion during apnea. Assuming the airway is patent and oxygen is insufflated through the nose and/or mouth, oxygenation occurs, prolonging apnea time beyond that of standard face-mask preoxygenation.[68]

Oxygen can be insufflated at up to 15 L/min with nasal cannulae (nasal oxygen during efforts securing a tube [NO DESAT])[69] or with a catheter placed through the nose or mouth with the tip in the pharynx (pharyngeal oxygen insufflation).[70] Studies have demonstrated that these techniques are effective in delaying oxyhemoglobin desaturation in morbidly obese patients[71,72] and during emergency tracheal intubation.[73,74]

THRIVE involves the administration of warmed, humidified oxygen, allowing higher oxygen flow rates than the previously described techniques—up to 70 L/min. These higher flows extend the apnea time even further and improve the clearance of carbon dioxide, preventing the potential development of severe respiratory acidosis. In 25 patients with a difficult airway at risk for rapid desaturation, THRIVE was used to achieve a median apnea time of 14 minutes, with a range of 5 to 65 minutes, and an average rate of carbon dioxide rise of only 1.1 mm Hg per minute.[63]

PULMONARY ASPIRATION OF GASTRIC CONTENTS

In 1946, Mendelson was the first to describe aspiration pneumonitis attributable to the pulmonary aspiration of acidic gastric secretions in pregnant women undergoing anesthesia.[75] This potentially fatal complication, occasionally referred to as Mendelson syndrome, has since been the intense focus of preventive efforts among the anesthesia community. Prevention of aspiration of gastric contents is primarily accomplished by adherence to established preoperative fasting guidelines, premedication with drugs that may decrease the risk of aspiration pneumonitis, and specialized induction techniques, which are discussed later in this chapter.

Traditionally, patients who were scheduled for elective procedures requiring sedation, regional anesthesia, or general anesthesia were instructed to remain NPO (Latin for *nulla per os* or *nothing by mouth*) after midnight to ensure an empty stomach to decrease the risk of regurgitation. Based on evidence that allowing ingestion of clear liquids 2 to 4 hours before surgery resulted in lower gastric volumes and higher gastric pH, the ASA published *Practice Guidelines for Preoperative Fasting and the Use of Pharmacologic Agents to Reduce the Risk of Pulmonary Aspiration* in 1999 that liberalized the traditional NPO policy and allowed clear liquids up to 2 hours before beginning elective procedures requiring anesthesia. The guidelines, most recently updated in 2017, recommend 4 hours of fasting from breast milk and 6 hours of fasting from solid foods, infant formula, and nonhuman milk.[76] Fried or fatty foods may require longer fasting times (e.g., 8 hours or more).[76] Although the ASA guidelines do not specifically address chewing gum, hard candies, or smoking, guidelines published by the European Society of Anaesthesiology on the topic do not recommend delaying the start of anesthesia if a patient has consumed any of these immediately before the induction of anesthesia.[77]

The routine use of drugs as prophylaxis against aspiration pneumonitis is not recommended by the ASA guidelines[76] but may be beneficial in patients with specific risk factors for aspiration, such as a full stomach, symptomatic gastroesophageal reflux disease (GERD), hiatal hernia, presence of a nasogastric tube, morbid obesity, diabetic gastroparesis, or pregnancy.[78,79] The goal of aspiration prophylaxis is twofold: to decrease gastric volume and to increase gastric fluid pH. Commonly used agents include nonparticulate antacids (e.g., Bicitra), promotility drugs (e.g., metoclopramide), and H_2-receptor antagonists. These drugs may be used alone or in combination.[80]

AIRWAY REFLEXES AND THE PHYSIOLOGIC RESPONSE TO INTUBATION OF THE TRACHEA

One of the most important teleologic functions of the larynx is that of airway protection, which is primarily provided by the glottic closure reflex. This reflex is triggered by sensory receptors in the glottic and subglottic mucosa and results in strong adduction of the vocal cords.[81] An exaggerated, maladaptive manifestation of this reflex, referred to as *laryngospasm*, is a potential complication of airway management. Laryngospasm is usually provoked by glossopharyngeal or vagal stimulation attributable to airway instrumentation or vocal cord irritation (e.g., from blood or vomitus) in the setting of a light plane of anesthesia (stage II of the Guedel classification), but it can also be precipitated by other noxious stimuli and can persist well after the removal of the stimulus. Treatment of laryngospasm includes removal of airway irritants, deepening of the anesthetic, and the administration of a rapid-onset neuromuscular blocking drug (NMBD), such as succinylcholine.[82] Continuous positive airway pressure with 100% oxygen is commonly cited as a therapeutic maneuver, although the pressure may push the aryepiglottic folds closer together and may actually promote laryngospasm by acting as a mechanical stimulus.[83,84] Bilateral pressure at the *laryngospasm notch* between the condyle of the mandible and the mastoid process can be effective at treating laryngospasm by causing an intense, painful stimulus, which may function to terminate laryngospasm by arousing a semiconscious patient or by activating autonomic pathways.[82]

The tracheobronchial tree also possesses reflexes to protect the lungs from noxious substances. Irritation of the lower airway by a foreign substance activates a vagal reflex–mediated constriction of bronchial smooth muscle, resulting in bronchospasm. Untreated bronchospasm can result in an inability to ventilate because of an extremely elevated airway resistance. Treatment includes a deepening of anesthetic with propofol or a volatile agent and the administration of inhaled β_2-agonist or anticholinergic medications. Administration of intravenous (IV) lidocaine has been studied, but the evidence does not support its use for treatment of bronchospasm.[85]

Tracheal intubation, as well as laryngoscopy and other airway instrumentation, provides an intense noxious stimulus via vagal and glossopharyngeal afferents that results in a reflex autonomic activation, which is usually manifested as hypertension and tachycardia in adults and adolescents; in infants and small children, autonomic activation may result in bradycardia. Hypertension and tachycardia are usually of short duration; however, they may have consequences in patients with significant cardiac disease. Central nervous system activation as a result of airway management results in increases in electroencephalographic (EEG) activity, cerebral metabolic rate, and cerebral blood flow, which may result in an increase in intracranial pressure in patients with decreased intracranial compliance.[85]

Anesthesia for Airway Management

To facilitate airway management, some form of anesthesia is usually required to provide comfort for the patient, to blunt airway reflexes, and to blunt the hemodynamic response to airway instrumentation. Most commonly, airway management is performed after induction of general anesthesia. Alternatively, an *awake* technique, which entails establishing an airway (including tracheal intubation) by using local anesthesia of the airway and/or sedation, can be used to meet these goals when clinically indicated. In emergency scenarios where the patient is obtunded or comatose, such as in the event of acute respiratory or cardiac arrest, anesthetic drugs may not be required.

AIRWAY MANAGEMENT AFTER THE INDUCTION OF GENERAL ANESTHESIA

Airway management is usually performed after the induction of general anesthesia if the anesthesiologist determines that it is safe to do so. Several pharmacologic techniques are used for the induction of anesthesia, each with its own implications for airway management. The decision of which induction technique to use should be made with careful consideration of the specific clinical circumstances at hand.

Standard Intravenous Induction with Neuromuscular Blockade

The most common technique for induction of general anesthesia is the standard IV induction, which entails the administration of a rapid-acting IV anesthetic, followed by an NMBD. Muscle relaxation achieved by the administration of NMBDs improves intubating conditions by facilitating laryngoscopy, preventing both reflex laryngeal closure and coughing after intubation.[22,86]

Propofol is the most frequently used IV anesthetic drug; other options include etomidate, ketamine, thiopental, and midazolam. The choice of drug depends on a variety of factors including the patient's hemodynamic status, comorbidities, and allergies, as well as drug pharmacokinetics, side effects, physician preference, and availability.[87] Whether the choice of an anesthetic drug has any effect on the quality of intubating conditions when NMBDs are also administered is not well established. Studies comparing propofol, etomidate, and thiopental in combination with NMBDs showed no difference in intubating conditions between the different anesthetics.[88,89] On the other hand, one study, during which patients received cisatracurium, showed that larger doses of propofol were associated with improved intubating conditions, as compared with smaller doses.[90]

For many years, succinylcholine was the most frequently used NMBD for routine IV induction[87]; however, nondepolarizing NMBDs have gained greater popularity attributable to the risk of adverse effects from succinylcholine administration, including bradycardia, myalgia, hyperkalemia, increased intracranial pressure, and increased intragastric pressure.[91] Succinylcholine, the only depolarizing NMBD in clinical use, has the benefit of a rapid onset combined with a short duration of action, and it is currently used most often when those properties are desired. Most notably, succinylcholine is still commonly used in the setting of a suspected difficult airway; its short duration of action theoretically allows for the resumption of spontaneous ventilation before severe hypoxia develops in a preoxygenated patient, although evidence suggests that this may not predictably occur.[92]

Nondepolarizing NMBDs are the more frequently used relaxants for routine IV induction of anesthesia.[91] The most commonly used nondepolarizing NMBDs in current practice—rocuronium, vecuronium, and cisatracurium—are notable for having a favorable safety profile with relatively few side effects. The primary limitation of these drugs is a significantly longer duration of action; once administered, a functional airway must be established within minutes to avoid life-threatening hypoxia. Sugammadex is a selective relaxant-binding agent for rocuronium that has the ability to reverse profound neuromuscular blockade rapidly in a time comparable with spontaneous recovery from succinylcholine (also see Chapter 28).[93]

Traditional teaching in the United States has advocated withholding NMBDs until the ability to mask ventilate has been established. If ventilation via a mask cannot be achieved, a preoxygenated patient can then theoretically resume spontaneous ventilation or be awakened before the onset of hypoxia.[94] This practice has been increasingly questioned in the literature in part because of a number of studies demonstrating that ventilation via a mask is *not* rendered more difficult by muscle relaxation[95,96]; rather, mask ventilation is, in fact, facilitated by muscle relaxation.[97] One issue with the traditional paradigm is that the theoretical advantage of the practice—the ability to awaken the patient if mask ventilation fails—is rarely used.[98] The desire to preserve that ability may, in fact, result in giving an inadequate dose of anesthetic during induction, resulting in a difficult mask ventilation situation when one would not have otherwise occurred.[98] Delaying the administration of NMBDs can result in the onset of hypoxia before spontaneous recovery (with succinylcholine) or reversal (with sugammadex) is possible.

The authors do not recommend withholding NMBDs in patients who are predicted to be easy to mask ventilate and/or intubate. For patients in whom difficulty with both mask ventilation and intubation are predicted, awake intubation or inhalation induction of anesthesia should be considered, and the administration of NMBDs is best withheld until the ability to ventilate is proven.

Rapid-Sequence Induction and Intubation

Rapid-sequence induction and intubation (often simply referred to as *rapid sequence induction* [RSI] in the anesthesia literature) is a specialized method of IV induction commonly used when an increased risk of gastric regurgitation and pulmonary aspiration of gastric contents exists. After adequate preoxygenation and while cricoid pressure is applied, an induction dose of IV anesthetic is rapidly followed by 1 to 1.5 mg/kg of IV succinylcholine, and the trachea is intubated without attempts at PPV. The goal is to achieve optimal intubating conditions rapidly to minimize the length of time between the loss of consciousness (LOC) and securing of the airway with a cuffed endotracheal tube (ETT). Cricoid pressure, eponymously referred to as the Sellick maneuver after the physician who first described it, involves the application of pressure at the cricoid ring to occlude the upper esophagus, thereby preventing the regurgitation of gastric contents into the pharynx.[99] The recommended force to be applied is 10 Newtons (N) while the patient is awake, increased to 30 N after LOC. These values are based on esophageal manometry on patients undergoing induction of anesthesia and cadaver studies of safe amounts of pressure.[100] RSI is widely practiced and approaches a standard of care in patients with a full stomach (i.e., when NPO guidelines have not been observed) and in the setting of bowel obstruction.[101,102] RSI has historically been recommended for patients who are pregnant, starting in the second trimester,[103] but this dogma has been called into question.[104,105] Other clinical situations for which RSI may be considered due to a higher than normal risk for aspiration of gastric contents, include poorly controlled GERD, presence of a nasogastric tube, morbid obesity, and diabetic gastroparesis. RSI is also a useful induction technique when mask ventilation is predicted to be difficult, but intubation is not, such as with an edentulous, bearded patient with an otherwise reassuring airway examination.

Some common variations to RSI have developed from the technique first described in 1970.[106] When succinylcholine is contraindicated or its side effects are undesired, RSI can be accomplished using nondepolarizing NMBDs (rocuronium 1.0 to 1.2 mg/kg or vecuronium 0.3 mg/kg); these doses provide adequate intubating conditions in less than 90 seconds.[107,108] The primary disadvantage with the nondepolarizing NMBDs used to be the prolonged duration of neuromuscular blockade; however, since the introduction of sugammadex these agents are increasingly employed in place of succinylcholine for RSI (also see Chapters 27 and 28). Although traditional RSI calls for induction with a fixed dose of thiopental, the use of other anesthetics such as propofol, etomidate, or ketamine is common. Some advocate for the titration of the chosen anesthetic agent to LOC rather than the delivery of a fixed, predetermined dose.[101]

The application of cricoid pressure is the most controversial aspect of RSI.[101] Opponents point to studies demonstrating that cricoid pressure results in a decrease in lower esophageal sphincter tone, potentially increasing the risk for regurgitation,[109] and to magnetic resonance imaging (MRI) studies showing that cricoid pressure does not, in fact, result in compression of the esophagus, but rather a lateral displacement.[110] Cricoid pressure also worsens laryngeal visualization during DL, potentially lengthening the time to intubation and increasing the risk of pulmonary aspiration, and can result in occlusion of the subglottic airway, resulting in difficulty with tracheal intubation or mask ventilation.[111] On the other hand, advocates argue that properly applied cricoid pressure is effective in reducing the risk of aspiration and that reports of problems are due to incorrect application. The authors of an MRI study of cricoid pressure argue that the position of the esophagus is irrelevant because the effectiveness of cricoid pressure is due to occlusion of the hypopharynx.[112] In general, because of the relatively low risk of application of cricoid pressure, its use is encouraged for RSI unless glottic visualization proves difficult, in which case it can be easily released.

The term *modified RSI* is frequently used, but no standardized definition exists. A survey of anesthesia residents and attending anesthesiologists in the United States showed that the term was most commonly used to refer to the use of mask ventilation in conjunction with cricoid pressure.[113] Indications for this technique include patients at risk for rapid development of hypoxemia (e.g., patients who are obese, pregnant, or critically ill; pediatric patients) in emergent situations during which preoxygenation cannot be satisfactorily completed, or when a longer time to acceptable intubating conditions is required because of the use of standard doses of nondepolarizing NMBDs. Although the effect of PPV with cricoid pressure applied in terms of gastric insufflation of air is not definitively known, gentle PPV (inspiratory pressure <20 cm water [H_2O]) in conjunction with cricoid pressure may be acceptable in these clinical scenarios.[114]

Inhalational Induction of Anesthesia

Another option for the induction of general anesthesia is inhalational induction with volatile anesthetic. This technique is commonly used in pediatric anesthesia to provide a painless, needle-free experience for the child. In adults, an inhalational induction of anesthesia is used when IV access is not available or when the specific advantages of the technique are desirable. Advantages of an inhalational induction of anesthesia are the maintenance of spontaneous ventilation and the potential for gradual changes in the depth of anesthesia and associated respiratory and cardiovascular effects.[22] Inhalational induction of anesthesia has also been used for RSI, with a rapid-onset NMBD administered at LOC[115] (also see Chapter 27).

Sevoflurane is currently the most commonly used volatile anesthetic for inhalational induction because of its lack of pungency and low blood:gas solubility, allowing for a smooth induction of anesthesia that can provide suitable conditions for airway management with or without adjuvant drugs such as NMBDs or opioids.[116] The two principal techniques for sevoflurane induction of anesthesia are a *tidal volume induction*, in which patients are instructed to breathe normally through the face mask, and a *vital capacity induction*, in which patients are instructed to exhale to residual volume and then take a vital capacity breath from the face mask. High delivered concentrations of sevoflurane (8%) are used for vital capacity induction, whereas tidal volume inductions may start with lower sevoflurane concentrations before the concentration is increased. Nitrous oxide (N_2O) can be used with either method to speed induction via the second-gas effect.[117] Both methods are effective and can be used for either LMA placement or tracheal intubation.[116] Deep levels of anesthesia are required to achieve satisfactory intubating conditions when using sevoflurane as a sole induction agent, increasing the risk of adverse effects, such as hypotension. The administration of propofol,[118] rapid-onset opioids,[119,120] NMBDs,[121] and ketamine[122] have all been shown to improve intubating conditions and allow for lower end-tidal concentrations of sevoflurane.

Halothane, which is still used in developing countries, can also be used for inhalational induction of anesthesia.[123] One main disadvantage of halothane is its high blood:gas partition coefficient, which leads to relatively long induction times. It also can produce cardiac dysrhythmias, myocardial depression, and halothane-induced hepatitis. Because of the inability to achieve deep levels of anesthesia with halothane as a result of its side effects, the use of NMBDs, opioids, or both, is often required.[116] The use of desflurane for inhalational induction of anesthesia is limited by its tendency to cause airway irritation, although reports of its use for induction in combination with opioids has been reported.[124,125]

Intravenous Induction Without Neuromuscular Blocking Drugs

IV induction of general anesthesia without the use of NMBDs is commonly used for LMA placement but can be used to achieve satisfactory intubating conditions as well. This technique is useful when the use of succinylcholine is contraindicated and the prolonged recovery time from nondepolarizing NMBDs is undesirable and their reversal not possible (e.g., when sugammadex is not available). Of the commonly available IV anesthetics, propofol is the best suited for induction without muscle relaxation because of its unique ability to suppress airway reflexes and to produce apnea.[126,127] Larger doses are required, however, when propofol is used as a sole anesthetic, increasing the risk of significant hypotension. Improvement of intubating conditions and smaller doses of propofol are possible when rapid-onset opioids (e.g., alfentanil, remifentanil) or IV magnesium are administered.[128,129] Remifentanil is more effective than comparable doses of alfentanil[128]; in combination with propofol 2 mg/kg, remifentanil 4 to 5 μg/kg can reliably provide good-to-excellent intubating conditions.[130] When combined with cricoid pressure and an avoidance of mask ventilation, this induction technique can be used for RSI.[131]

Disadvantages of this technique include a potentially more frequent incidence of difficult intubation,[132] pronounced hemodynamic side effects such as bradycardia and hypotension, and an increased risk for laryngeal morbidity.[86,133] This technique also introduces the risk of opioid-induced muscle rigidity resulting in difficulty with mask ventilation. Although this risk is commonly attributed to chest wall rigidity, studies in intubated patients and patients with tracheostomies have shown that decreases in pulmonary compliance due to chest wall rigidity are not sufficient to explain an inability to mask ventilate after a large dose of an opioid.[134,135] Examination of the vocal cords during induction with opioids has shown that vocal cord closure is the primary cause of difficult ventilation after opioid-induced anesthesia.[136,137] Treatment with small doses of NMBD or topical lidocaine (laryngotracheal anesthesia [LTA]) can be effective in relaxing the vocal cords to allow for mask ventilation and/or intubation.[136]

AIRWAY MANAGEMENT IN AN AWAKE (NON-ANESTHETIZED) PATIENT

As noted in the ASA DAA, a consideration of whether the airway should be secured before or after induction of general anesthesia is one of the basic management choices that should be considered when an airway management plan is being devised.[7] The benefits of awake airway management include the preservation of pharyngeal muscle tone and patency of the upper airway, the maintenance of spontaneous ventilation, an ability to obtain a quick neurologic examination, and a safeguard against aspiration attributable to the preservation of protective airway reflexes.[138] In general, when difficult mask ventilation and difficult intubation are expected, the safest approach to airway management is to secure the airway while the patient remains awake.[7] Other indications for awake airway management include the risk of severe aspiration of gastric contents, facial or airway trauma, severe hemodynamic instability, and unstable cervical spine pathology.[139]

Because of the nature of these indications, tracheal intubation is most often chosen as the goal of awake airway management; however, awake placement of an LMA for diagnostic bronchoscopy has been described. The most useful technique for awake intubation is the flexible scope intubation (FSI),[138] although other techniques have been successfully used, including VAL,[140] optical stylets,[141] lighted stylets,[142] intubating LMAs,[143] and retrograde intubation (RI).[144]

Topical application of local anesthetic to the airway should, in most cases, be the primary anesthetic for awake airway management.[138] Lidocaine is the most commonly used local anesthetic for awake airway management because of its rapid onset, high therapeutic index, and availability in a wide variety of preparations and concentrations.[145,146] Benzocaine and Cetacaine (a topical application spray containing benzocaine, tetracaine, and butamben; Cetylite Industries, Pennsauken, NJ) provide excellent topical anesthesia of the airway, but their use is limited by the risk of methemoglobinemia, which can occur with as little as 1 to 2 seconds of spraying.[147] Topical cocaine is primarily used for anesthesia and vasoconstriction of the nasal mucosa during awake nasotracheal intubation.[148] A mixture of lidocaine 3% and phenylephrine 0.25%, which can be made by combining lidocaine 4% and phenylephrine 1% in a 3:1 ratio, has similar anesthetic and vasoconstrictive properties as topical cocaine and can be used as a substitute.[149]

Topical application of local anesthetic should primarily be focused on the base of the tongue (pressure receptors here act as the afferent component of the gag reflex), the oropharynx, the hypopharynx, and the laryngeal structures; anesthesia of the oral cavity is unnecessary. If a nasotracheal intubation is planned, then the nasal cavity should also be topicalized. Before topical application of local anesthetic to the airway, administration of an anticholinergic agent should be considered to aid in the drying of secretions, which helps improve both the effectiveness of the topical local anesthetic and visualization during laryngoscopy. Glycopyrrolate is usually preferred because it has less vagolytic effects than atropine at doses that inhibit secretions and does not cross the blood-brain barrier. It should be administered as early as possible to maximize its effectiveness.

Direct application of topical cocaine, lidocaine 4% with epinephrine, or lidocaine 3%/phenylephrine 0.25% solution via cotton swabs or cotton pledgets is effective for anesthesia of the nasal mucosa. Oropharyngeal anesthesia can be achieved by the direct application of local anesthetic or by the use of an atomizer or nebulizer. Topical application of local anesthetic to the larynx can be achieved by directed atomization of a local anesthetic or by the *spray-as-you-go* (SAYGO) method, which involves intermittently injecting local anesthetic through the suction port or working channel of a flexible intubation scope (FIS) or optical stylet, as it is advanced toward the trachea.

Topical application of local anesthetic to the airway mucosa using one or more of these methods is often sufficient. If supplemental anesthesia is required, then a variety of nerve blocks may be used. Three of the most useful are the glossopharyngeal nerve block, superior laryngeal nerve block, and translaryngeal block.

The glossopharyngeal nerve supplies sensory innervation to the posterior third of the tongue, vallecula, the anterior surface of the epiglottis, and the posterior and lateral walls of the pharynx, and is the afferent pathway of the gag reflex. To block this nerve, the tongue is displaced medially, forming a gutter (glossogingival groove). A 25-gauge spinal needle is inserted at the base of the anterior tonsillar pillar, just lateral to the base of the tongue, to a depth of 0.5 cm (Fig. 44.9). After negative aspiration for blood or air, 2 mL of 2% lidocaine is injected. The process is then repeated

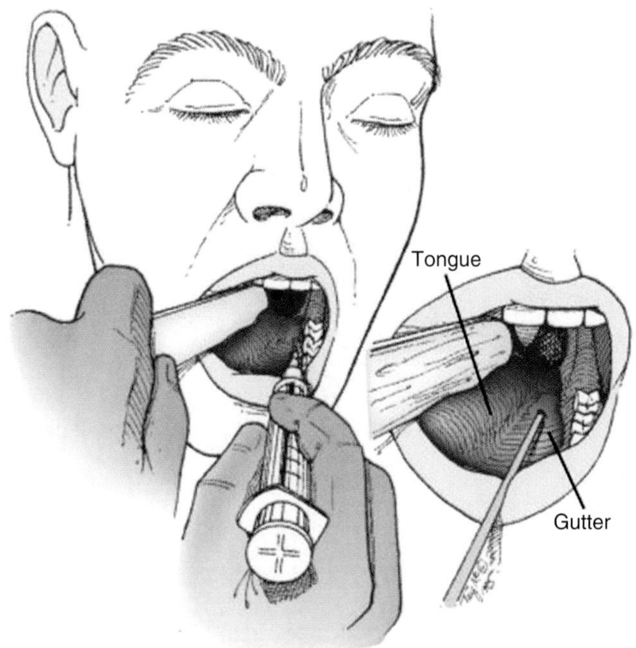

Fig. 44.9 Left glossopharyngeal nerve block. (Reprinted from Artime CA, Sanchez A. Preparation of the patient for awake intubation. In: Hagberg CA, Artime CA, Aziz M, eds. *Hagberg and Benumof's Airway Management*. 4th ed. Philadelphia: Elsevier; 2018. From Difficult airway teaching aids, Irvine, University of California, Department of Anesthesia.)

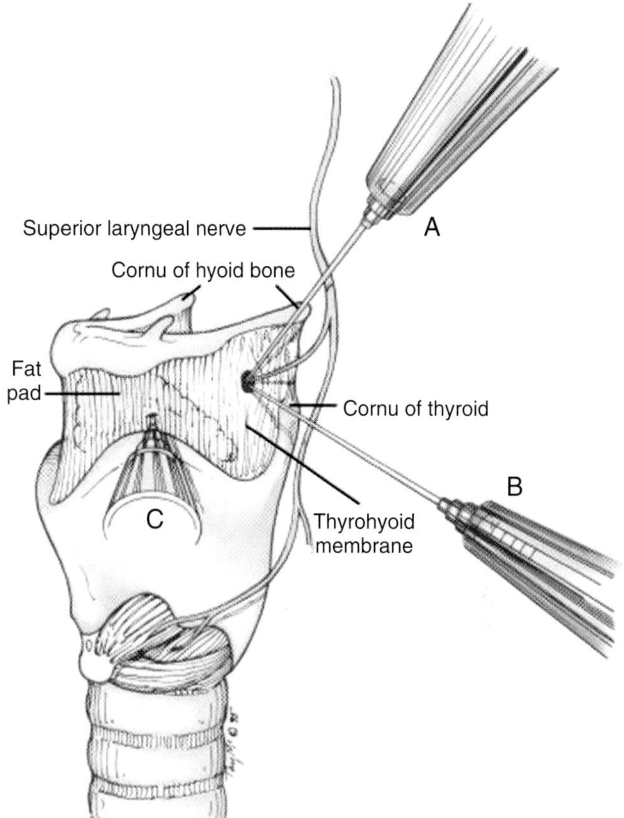

Fig. 44.10 **Superior laryngeal nerve block, external approach using as a landmark the greater cornu of the hyoid bone (A), the superior cornu of the thyroid cartilage (B), or the thyroid notch (C).** (Reprinted from Artime CA, Sanchez A. Preparation of the patient for awake intubation. In: Hagberg CA, Artime CA, Aziz M, eds. *Hagberg and Benumof's Airway Management*. 4th ed. Philadelphia: Elsevier; 2018. From Difficult airway teaching aids, Irvine, University of California, Department of Anesthesia.)

on the contralateral side.[138] The same procedure can be performed noninvasively with cotton-tipped swabs soaked in 4% lidocaine; the swabs are held in place for 5 minutes (Video 44.1).

The superior laryngeal nerve, a branch of the vagus nerve, provides sensory input from the lower pharynx and the upper part of the larynx, including the glottic surface of the epiglottis and the aryepiglottic folds. Blockade of this nerve may be achieved using one of three landmarks (Fig. 44.10). Using either the superior cornu of the hyoid or the superior cornu of the thyroid cartilage, a 25-gauge spinal needle is walked off the cornu anteriorly toward the thyrohyoid ligament. Resistance is felt as the needle is advanced through the ligament, usually at a depth of 1 to 2 cm. After negative aspiration for blood and air, 1.5 to 2 mL of 2% lidocaine is injected and then repeated on the opposite side.[146] The third landmark for the superior laryngeal nerve block is particularly useful in patients who are obese, in whom palpation of the hyoid or the superior cornu of the thyroid cartilage may be difficult or uncomfortable for the patient. In this approach, the needle is inserted 2 cm lateral to the superior notch of the thyroid cartilage and directed in a posterior and cephalad direction to 1 to 1.5 cm depth, where 2 mL of 2% lidocaine is infiltrated and, again, repeated on the contralateral side.[150]

Translaryngeal (or transtracheal) block provides anesthesia of the trachea and vocal cords. This block may be particularly useful in situations where a neurologic examination is needed after intubation; it makes the presence of the ETT in the trachea more comfortable. The CTM is identified, and a 20- to 22-gauge needle attached to 5-mL syringe is directly advanced posteriorly and slightly caudally until air is aspirated, at which point 4 mL of either 2% or 4% lidocaine is quickly injected. This causes the patient to cough, anesthetizing the vocal cords and the trachea. To minimize the risk of trauma, a catheter may first be placed over the needle and the local anesthetic then injected through the catheter (Fig. 44.11 and Video 44.2).[146]

These techniques may be used in various different combinations as long as the maximum dose of local anesthetic is not exceeded. The maximum dose of lidocaine for application to the airway is not well established; different sources suggest total doses in the range of 4 to 9 mg/kg.[146,151,152] Monitoring for signs and symptoms of lidocaine toxicity, including tinnitus, perioral tingling, metallic taste, lightheadedness, dizziness, and sedation is important. Severe lidocaine overdose can cause hypertension, tachycardia, seizures, and cardiovascular collapse.[153]

Depending on the clinical circumstance, IV sedation may facilitate airway management in an awake patient by providing anxiolysis, amnesia, and analgesia. Benzodiazepines, opioids, IV hypnotics, α_2 agonists, and neuroleptics can be used alone or in combination. A summary of common medications used for sedation can be found in Table 44.1. These drugs should be carefully titrated to effect; oversedation can render a patient uncooperative and make awake intubation more difficult. Spontaneous ventilation should always be maintained. Care should be taken in situations with critical airway obstruction since awake muscle tone is sometimes necessary in these patients to maintain airway patency.

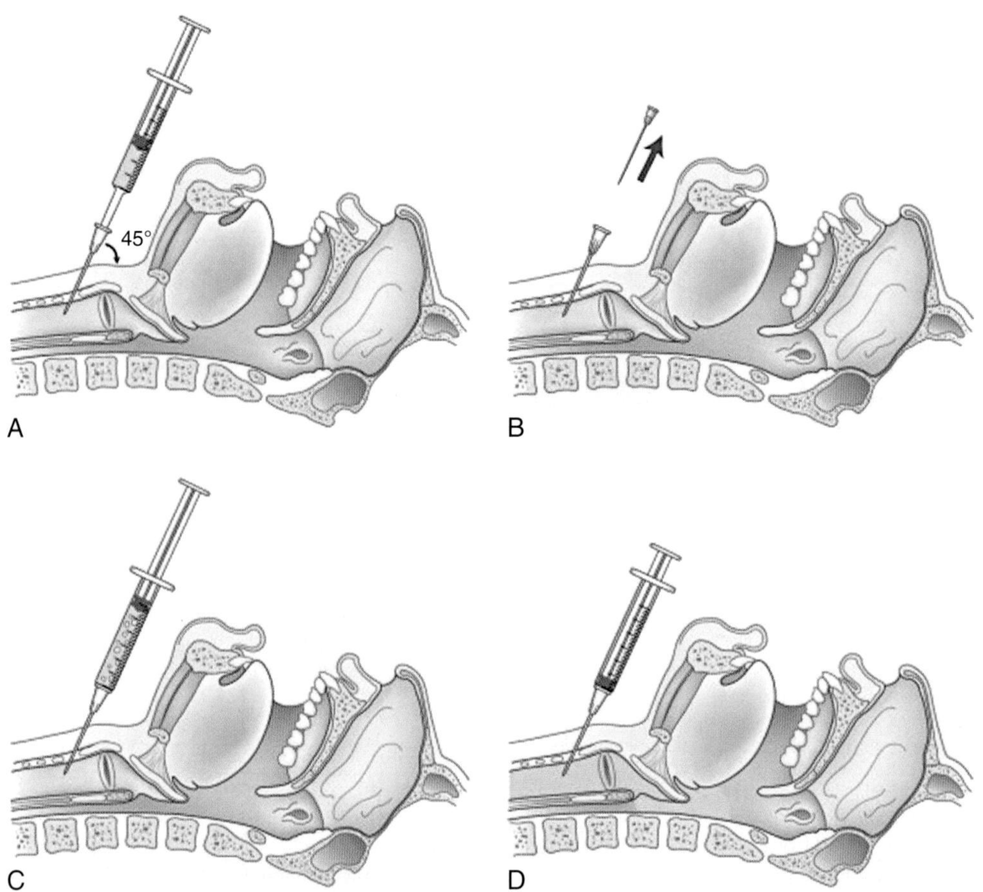

Fig. 44.11 Translaryngeal anesthesia, angiocatheter technique (midsagittal view of the head and neck). (A) The angiocatheter is inserted at the cricothyroid membrane, aimed caudally. An aspiration test is performed to verify the position of the tip of the needle in the tracheal lumen. (B) The needle is removed from the angiocatheter. (C) The syringe containing local anesthetic is attached, and the aspiration test is repeated. (D) Local anesthetic is injected, resulting in coughing and nebulization of the local anesthetic *(shaded blue area)*. (Reprinted from Artime CA, Sanchez A. Preparation of the patient for awake intubation. In: Hagberg CA, Artime CA, Aziz M, eds. *Hagberg and Benumof's Airway Management*. 4th ed. Philadelphia: Elsevier; 2018. From Difficult airway teaching aids, Irvine, University of California, Department of Anesthesia.)

TABLE 44.1 Sedative Drugs for Awake Airway Management

Drug	Class	Sedative Dose	Notes
Midazolam	Benzodiazepine	1-2 mg IV, repeated prn (0.025-0.1 mg/kg)	Frequently used in combination with fentanyl.
Fentanyl	Opioid	25-200 μg IV (0.5-2 μg/kg)	Usually used in combination with other agents (e.g., midazolam, propofol).
Alfentanil	Opioid	500-1500 μg IV (10-30 μg/kg)	Has a faster onset, shorter duration than fentanyl.
Remifentanil	Opioid	Bolus 0.5 μg/kg IV, followed by an infusion of 0.1 μg/kg/min	Infusion can be subsequently titrated by 0.025-0.05 μg/kg/min in 5-minute intervals to achieve adequate sedation.
Propofol	Hypnotic	0.25 mg/kg IV in intermittent boluses or Continuous IV infusion of 25-75 μg/kg/min, titrated to effect	Can also be used in combination with remifentanil (decrease dose of both drugs).
Ketamine	Hypnotic	0.2-0.8 mg/kg IV	Pretreat with an antisialagogue. Consider administration of midazolam to attenuate undesirable psychologic effects.
Dexmedetomidine	α_2 Agonist	Bolus 1 μg/kg IV over 10 minutes, followed by an infusion of 0.3-0.7 μg/kg/hr	Reduce dose in older adults and in patients with depressed cardiac function.

IV, Intravenous; *prn*, as needed, *pro re nata* (Latin).

Avoiding oversedation is also important in the patient at increased risk for aspiration of gastric contents, because an awake patient can protect his or her own airway if regurgitation should occur.[80]

Mask Ventilation

Mask ventilation is a straightforward, noninvasive technique for airway management that can be used as a primary mode of ventilation for an anesthetic of short duration or as a bridge to establish a more definitive airway. The use of a face mask is common for preoxygenation, inhalational induction of anesthesia, and as a means to provide oxygen and anesthetic gases to both a spontaneous ventilating patient and an anesthetized, apneic patient via PPV. Mask ventilation is not only used to ventilate and oxygenate before conditions for tracheal intubation have been achieved, but it is also a valuable rescue technique when tracheal intubation proves difficult. For this reason, mask ventilation is an important part of the ASA DAA and an essential skill for the anesthesia practitioner.[7]

Mask ventilation is relatively contraindicated when the risk for regurgitation is increased; no protection from pulmonary aspiration of gastric contents exists. Mask ventilation should also be performed with caution in patients with severe facial trauma and in patients in whom head and neck manipulation must be avoided (e.g., those with an unstable cervical spine fracture).

Anesthesia face masks are designed to form a seal around the patient's nose and mouth, allowing for PPV and the administration of anesthetic gases; they should not be confused with oxygen face masks, which are designed only to administer supplemental oxygen. Early anesthesia face masks were reusable and composed of black rubber. These have been almost entirely replaced in clinical use by disposable, clear plastic masks, which are less frightening for patients and have the added benefit of allowing for better visualization of cyanosis or the need for oral suctioning. Face masks are available in various styles and sizes but share a basic design: a main body, seal, and connector. The seal is the portion of the mask that comes in contact with the face, and in clear plastic masks is comprised of a plastic, air-filled, high-volume, low-pressure cushion that conforms to the facial anatomy while minimizing the chance for pressure ischemia; some models have a valve on the cushion to allow changing the volume of the air within. The connector is a standard 22-mm female adapter that allows a connection to a standard anesthesia circuit or a bag-valve device; pediatric masks usually have a 15-mm male adapter that allows the same connections.

The technique for mask ventilation is dependent on two key elements: (1) maintenance of a seal between the face mask and the patient's face, and (2) an unobstructed upper airway.[22] The mask is usually held with the left hand, with the thumb and index finger forming a "C" around the collar of the connector, the third and fourth digits on the ramus of the mandible, and the fifth digit on the angle of the mandible (Fig. 44.12). The thumb and index finger are used to produce downward pressure to ensure a tight mask seal, while the remaining digits provide upward displacement of the mandible (jaw thrust) to aid with airway patency. The right hand is free to provide manual ventilation. Ensuring that pressure from the digits is placed on the bony ridge of the mandible and not the soft tissue is important—compression of the submandibular space can cause obstruction of the airway and difficulty with mask ventilation. Many face masks have hooks around the collar for use with mask straps that can facilitate formation of a seal.

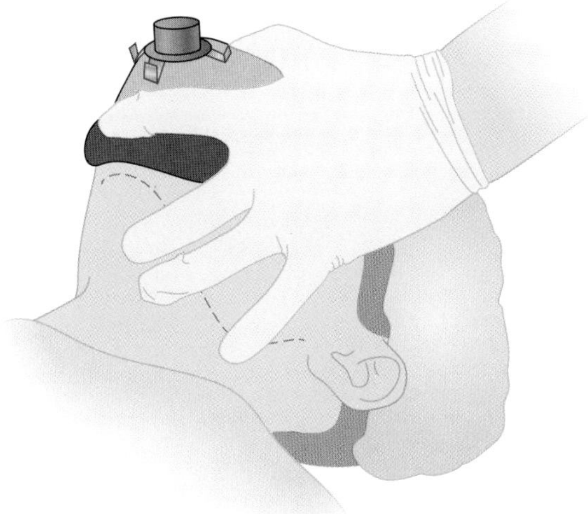

Fig. 44.12 Standard one-handed face-mask ventilation technique. The position of the fifth digit is at the angle of the jaw. (From Matioc AA. The adult ergonomic face mask: historical and theoretical perspectives. *J Clin Anesth.* 2009;21:300–304.)

The one-handed technique is occasionally ineffective, especially in patients who are obese or edentulous, attributable to the failure to maintain a seal and/or a patent upper airway. In these situations, a two-handed technique can be more successful. Two-handed techniques depend on either an assistant or the use of pressure-control ventilation (PCV) with the anesthesia machine to provide PPV. The use of PCV for mask ventilation results in lower peak airway pressures and reduced inspiratory flow rates when compared with manual ventilation, providing an additional measure of safety against gastric insufflation.[154] In one approach to the two-handed technique, the left hand is positioned as in the one-handed technique and the right hand is placed on the other side of the mask in an identical conformation. A more effective approach involves using the second and third digits to perform a jaw thrust while the mask is held in place with the thumbs (Video 44.3). A study in anesthetized patients showed that this technique improved upper airway patency, compared with the traditional one-handed technique, as measured by greater tidal volumes during PCV.[155] Additional techniques to improve the mask seal in difficult scenarios include leaving dentures in place in edentulous patients and placing an adhesive plastic dressing over facial hair.

Once a seal is established between the face mask and the patient's face, ventilation is achieved by either spontaneous ventilation or PPV. The effectiveness of mask ventilation should be ascertained by observing for chest rise, exhaled tidal volumes, pulse oximetry, and capnography. During controlled ventilation in patients with normal lungs and a

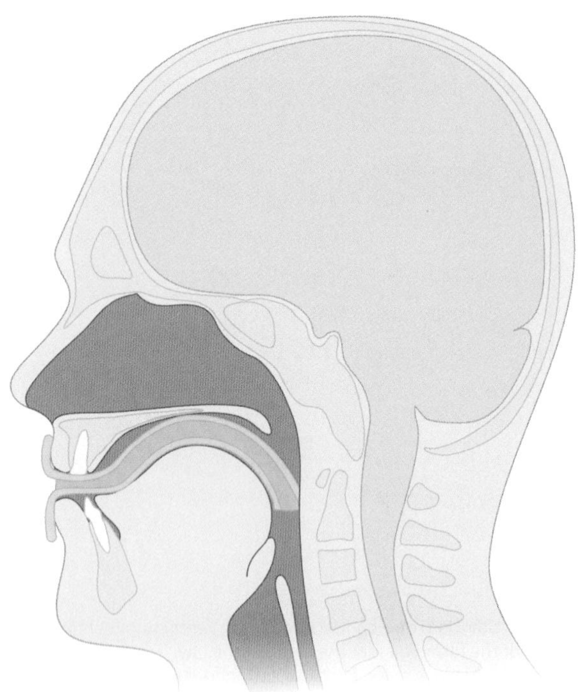

Fig. 44.13 Oropharyngeal airway in place. The airway follows the curvature of the tongue. It pulls the tongue and the epiglottis away from the posterior pharyngeal wall and provides a channel for the passage of air. (Modified from Dorsch JA, Dorsch SE. *Understanding Anesthesia Equipment*. 4th ed. Baltimore: Williams & Wilkins; 1999.)

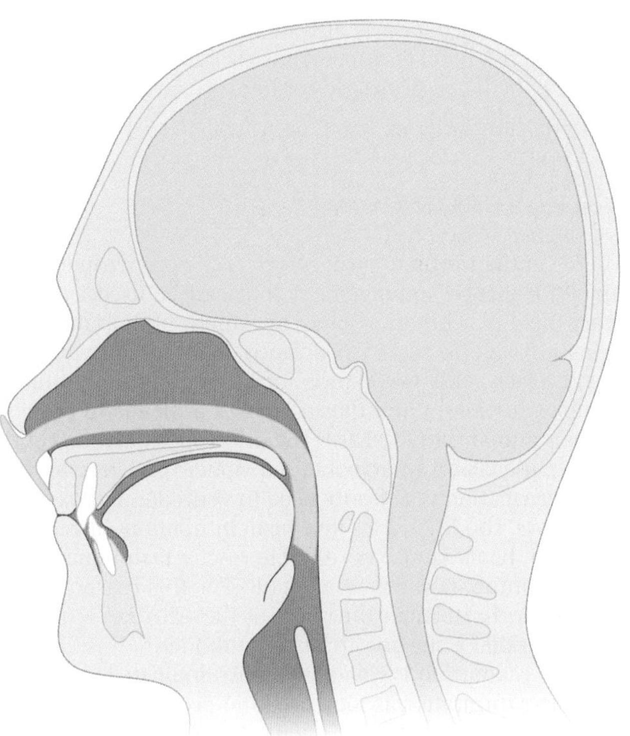

Fig. 44.14 Nasopharyngeal airway in place. The airway passes through the nose and ends at a point just above the epiglottis. (Modified from Dorsch JA, Dorsch SE. *Understanding Anesthesia Equipment*. 4th ed. Baltimore: Williams & Wilkins; 1999.)

patent airway, adequate tidal volumes should be achieved with peak inspiratory pressures less than 20 cm H_2O; higher pressures should be avoided to prevent gastric insufflation.[156] If PPV is inadequate at acceptable inspiratory pressures, then airway patency and pulmonary compliance should be assessed.

Because of a reduction in muscle tone as a result of general anesthesia, tissues fall backward under the influence of gravity in a supine patient and can obstruct the upper airway. Upper airway obstruction most commonly takes place at the level of the soft palate (velopharynx), epiglottis, and tongue.[22,26] To maximize airway patency, mask ventilation can be performed with maximal atlantooccipital extension in combination with the forward displacement of the mandible (jaw thrust) involved in the mask-holding techniques.[157] The addition of cervical flexion to head extension (i.e., placing the patient in the sniffing position) improves pharyngeal patency.[158] If the sniffing position and jaw thrust fail to relieve airway obstruction, then oropharyngeal or nasopharyngeal airways may be used to facilitate airway patency.

Oropharyngeal airways are the most commonly used. They follow the curvature of the tongue, pulling it away from the posterior pharynx (Fig. 44.13). Because they place pressure on the base of the tongue and may come in contact with the epiglottis, oropharyngeal airways can precipitate coughing, retching, or laryngospasm if laryngeal and pharyngeal reflexes are not sufficiently blunted; therefore they are not appropriate for use in conscious patients who have not had local anesthetic applied to the airway. The oropharyngeal airway is sized by measuring from the corner of a patient's mouth to the angle of the jaw or the earlobe. Inappropriately sized oropharyngeal airways can actually worsen airway obstruction; therefore correct size selection is important. Proper placement is accomplished by inserting the oropharyngeal airway with the curvature facing posteriorly and then rotating 180 degrees; alternatively, a tongue depressor can be used to displace the tongue anteriorly as the oropharyngeal airway is inserted with the curvature facing anteriorly. Complications from oropharyngeal airways include lingual nerve palsy and damage to the teeth.[159,160] Nasopharyngeal airways are less stimulating than oropharyngeal airways once in place and thus are more appropriate for conscious patients (Fig. 44.14). They should be well lubricated before insertion and inserted perpendicularly to the longitudinal axis of the body with the bevel facing the nasal septum. To avoid epistaxis, force should never be used during insertion of a nasopharyngeal airway.

Difficult mask ventilation occurs when ventilating via the face mask is not possible because of an inadequate mask seal, excessive gas leak, and/or excessive resistance to the ingress or egress of gas.[7] Predictors for difficult mask ventilation that can be identified during the preoperative airway assessment are listed in Box 44.2.

Supraglottic Airways

The term *supraglottic airway* or *extraglottic airway* refers to a diverse family of medical devices that are blindly inserted into the pharynx to provide a patent conduit for ventilation,

BOX 44.2 Predictors of Difficult Mask Ventilation

- Obstructive sleep apnea or history of snoring
- Age older than 55 years
- Male gender
- Body mass index of 30 kg/m^2 or greater
- Mallampati classification III or IV
- Presence of a beard
- Edentulousness

oxygenation, and delivery of anesthetic gases without the need for tracheal intubation. SGAs have the advantage of being less invasive than tracheal intubation while providing a more definitive airway than a face mask and can be used for either spontaneous ventilation or PPV. One of the first SGAs, the LMA, was described in 1983 by Dr. Archie Brain and introduced into clinical practice in 1988.[161] Since that time, the LMA has proved to be one of the single most important developments in both routine and difficult airway management and is a pivotal component of the ASA DAA. Various different designs of SGAs are now available and are widely used in current anesthesia practice as a primary airway management device, a rescue airway device, and a conduit for tracheal intubation.

The specific advantages of SGAs include the ease and speed of placement, improved hemodynamic stability, reduced anesthetic requirements, lack of a need for muscle relaxation, and an avoidance of some of the risks of tracheal intubation (e.g., trauma to the teeth and airway structures, sore throat, coughing on emergence, or bronchospasm).[162,163] The primary disadvantages are that SGAs have comparatively smaller seal pressures than ETTs, which can lead to ineffective ventilation when higher airway pressures are required, and they provide no protection from laryngospasm. First-generation SGAs also provide little protection from gastric regurgitation and aspiration, although newer devices have incorporated design elements to minimize this risk.

SGAs have many applications. They are considered the first choice for airway management for diagnostic and minor surgical procedures.[164] No standardized classification system exists for the different designs of SGAs, although several have been proposed. This chapter uses the terminology described by Donald Miller: perilaryngeal sealers; cuffless, anatomically preshaped sealers; and cuffed pharyngeal sealers.[165] Second-generation SGAs are differentiated from first-generation SGAs in that they incorporate features designed to reduce the incidence of aspiration.[166]

LARYNGEAL MASK AIRWAY

LMA Classic

The LMA (LMA North America, San Diego, CA) is the most widely used, well-studied SGA and is the archetype of the perilaryngeal sealer. The original version, the LMA Classic (cLMA), consists of an oval-shaped, silicone mask with an inflatable cuff that sits in the hypopharynx and forms a seal around the periglottic tissues (Fig. 44.15). An airway tube attached to the mask exits the mouth and has a standard 15-mm connector for attachment to an anesthesia circuit or to a bag-valve device. The seal around the laryngeal inlet allows for the delivery of oxygen and inhaled anesthetics during spontaneous ventilation and permits PPV at pressures up to 20 cm H_2O. The cLMA is reusable up to 40 times and is available in a variety of sizes from size 1 (neonate) to size 6 (large adult, >100 kg).

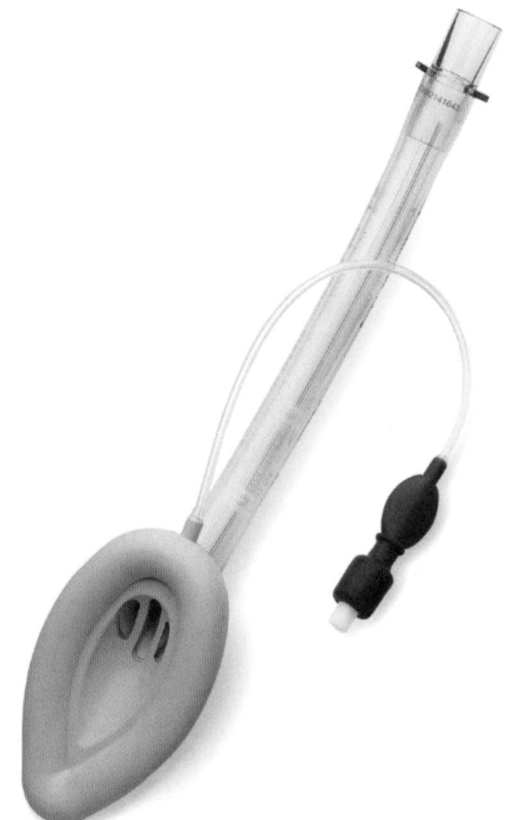

Fig. 44.15 LMA Classic. (Image provided courtesy LMA North America, San Diego, CA.)

The LMA Classic Excel is an updated version that incorporates design features to facilitate tracheal intubation through the device, including an epiglottic-elevating bar, a wider-bore airway tube, and a removable connector. A disposable, single-use version of the cLMA, the LMA Unique, is available with either a polyvinyl chloride (PVC) or silicone cuff and has gained popularity because of its lower cost and maintenance, as well as concerns over the perceived risk of cross-contamination and the transmission of infection with reusable medical devices. The LMA Flexible, available in reusable and single-use models, has a flexible, kink-resistant airway tube that can be positioned away from the surgical field for head and neck procedures.

To achieve a proper fit, the manufacturer of the LMA suggests placing the largest size LMA possible; an airtight seal is achieved more frequently with a size 5 LMA in the average adult man and a size 4 LMA in the average adult woman.[167] Using an undersized LMA can result in overinflation of the cuff to achieve a seal, which can predispose the patient to oropharyngolaryngeal morbidity and nerve damage.[168] Smaller LMA sizes have also been shown to be associated with placement failure.[169] Larger sizes, however, may be

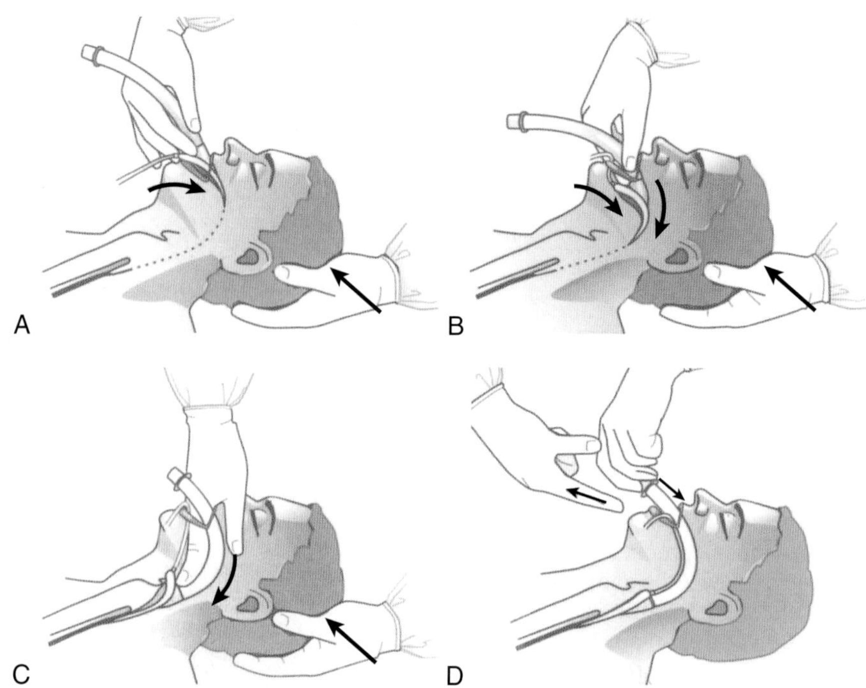

Fig. 44.16 Insertion of a laryngeal mask airway (LMA). (A) The tip of the cuff is pressed upward against the hard palate by the index finger while the middle finger opens the mouth. (B) The LMA is pressed backward in a smooth movement. The nondominant hand is used to extend the head. (C) The LMA is advanced until definite resistance is felt. (D) Before the index finger is removed, the nondominant hand presses down on the LMA to prevent dislodgment during removal of the index finger. The cuff is subsequently inflated. (Courtesy LMA North America, San Diego, CA.)

associated with a more frequent incidence of sore throat; therefore a smaller size may be appropriate when spontaneous ventilation through the LMA is planned.[170]

The manufacturer's instructions for the placement of the cLMA are summarized in Fig. 44.16. Adequate depth of anesthesia for LMA insertion can be achieved with propofol or sevoflurane[171]; short-acting opioids such as fentanyl, alfentanil, and remifentanil may be coadministered to facilitate placement and to decrease the incidence of coughing, gagging, and laryngospasm.[172,173] Before insertion, the LMA cuff should be deflated and the posterior aspect of the mask should be lubricated with a water-based lubricant. Once positioned (see Fig. 44.16), the cuff should be inflated with the minimum effective volume of air, with a target cuff pressure of 40 to 60 cm H_2O.[167] To allow the LMA to position itself correctly, the device should not be secured or attached to the anesthesia circuit until the cuff has been inflated. Confirmation of proper placement is performed by attempting gentle PPV while checking capnography and auscultation and by quantifying the inspiratory pressure at which a leak is audible, which should be 18 to 20 cm H_2O. Once proper positioning is confirmed, a roll of gauze is inserted as a bite block and the LMA is secured in place with tape. Several modifications to the recommended insertion technique have been described, including a *thumb insertion method* by the manufacturer (Video 44.4).[174,175] Cuff pressure should be periodically monitored if N_2O is being used; cuff pressures may increase above the recommended threshold of 60 cm H_2O as a result of diffusion of N_2O into the cuff.

Initial difficulty with ventilation after the placement of an LMA may be due to a down-folded epiglottis. The *up-down maneuver* described by Dr. Brain may help correct this problem; the LMA is withdrawn 2 to 4 cm and reinserted without deflating the cuff. Head extension and LMA repositioning may also improve ineffective ventilation. If these actions do not correct the problem, then a different size may be needed. Insufficient depth of anesthesia, resulting in laryngospasm or bronchospasm, may make ventilation through an LMA impossible; the administration of topical, inhaled, or IV anesthesia can help to correct this. Although not necessary, DL can also facilitate proper LMA placement.

Serious complications from LMA use are relatively rare. More commonly, minor oral, pharyngeal, or laryngeal injury occurs, expressed as complaints of a dry or sore throat.[176] The incidence of sore throat is approximately 10% to 20%,[163,177] and has been linked to higher cuff pressures and larger LMA sizes.[170,178] More serious cases of oropharyngolaryngeal injury have been described, such as trauma to the uvula and pharyngeal necrosis.[179,180] Injury to the lingual, hypoglossal, and recurrent laryngeal nerves has also been reported; these usually spontaneously resolve over a period of weeks to months.[168] Predisposing factors include high cuff pressures (often attributable to the use of N_2O), using too small of an LMA, and nonsupine positions.[168]

LMA ProSeal

The LMA ProSeal (PLMA, LMA North America, San Diego, CA) is a reusable second-generation SGA that incorporates a posterior cuff, improving the perilaryngeal seal and allowing for PPV at pressures up to 30 cm H_2O. It also incorporates a gastric drainage tube that allows for gastric access with an orogastric tube and channels any regurgitated gastric contents away from the airway, effectively isolating the respiratory and gastrointestinal tracts.[181] Additional features include an incorporated bite block and a softer cuff.

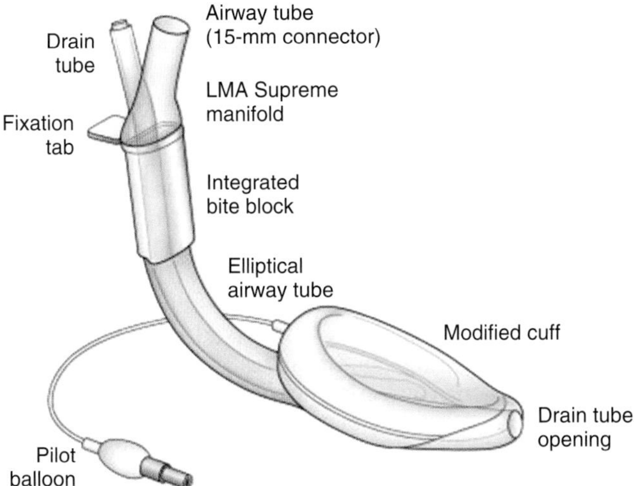

Fig. 44.17 **The LMA Supreme has a modified cuff design, a drainage tube that allows for gastric access, and an integrated bite block.** (From Verghese C, Mena G, Ferson DZ, Brain AIJ. Laryngeal mask airway. In: Hagberg CA, ed. *Benumof and Hagberg's Airway Management*. 3rd ed. Philadelphia: Saunders; 2013.)

The insertion technique is similar to the cLMA but requires deeper anesthetic levels.[181,182] An optional introducer can be used to facilitate insertion. As with the cLMA, cuff pressure should not exceed 60 cm H_2O. Once inserted, assessment of proper placement is accomplished by providing PPV; adequate tidal volumes should be accomplished with reasonable peak inspiratory pressures, leak pressure should be above 20 cm H_2O, and the capnography waveform should appear normal.[22] An additional test to confirm proper placement and separation of the airway and gastrointestinal tract is performed by placing a small layer (<5 mm) of water-based lubricant over the drainage tube orifice; PPV and suprasternal notch palpation should result in a small up-down movement of the gel meniscus. Easy passage of an orogastric tube through the gastric drainage tube confirms proper positioning.

LMA Supreme

The LMA Supreme (SLMA) is a single-use, second-generation SGA based on the PLMA design. Similar to the PLMA, the SLMA has an improved cuff design that produces higher airway leak pressures, a drainage tube that allows for gastric access, and an integrated bite block (Fig. 44.17). A fixation tab allows for determination of proper sizing (the tab should rest 1 to 2.5 cm above the upper lip) and provides an improved perilaryngeal seal when inward pressure is maintained by securing the mask into position by taping cheek to cheek across the fixation tab.

Although not clinically proven, evidence suggests that second-generation SGAs, such as the PLMA and the SLMA, reduce the risk of aspiration of gastric contents. This property, along with the improved airway seal and higher leak pressures, have enabled SGA devices to be used in various applications where the cLMA is potentially unsuitable, such as in nonsupine positions (e.g., lateral, prone),[183] in laparoscopic surgery (e.g., cholecystectomy, gynecologic surgery),[184,185] and in patients who are obese.[186] The successful, routine use of the SLMA in fasted, nonobese patients for cesarean section has also been reported.[187]

NEWER LMA MODELS

The LMA Protector is an all-silicone second-generation SGA with integrated Cuff Pilot Technology, which allows constant cuff pressure monitoring. Color-coded indicator bands alert the clinician to changes in cuff pressure attributable to temperature, N_2O, and movement within the airway, allowing the clinician to maintain the recommended cuff pressure of 40 to 60 cm H_2O. The LMA Protector is designed to channel fluids away from the airway in the unlikely event of regurgitation and allows for gastric suctioning. The airway channel is wide enough to allow intubation with a standard-sized ETT (see Tracheal Intubation Through a Supraglottic Airway Device). The LMA Gastro is a single-use silicone LMA designed for upper gastrointestinal endoscopy procedures, simultaneously protecting the airway and facilitating passage of an endoscope.

OTHER PERILARYNGEAL SEALERS

Over the past 15 years, a multitude of manufacturers have produced SGAs that incorporate the basic perilaryngeal sealing design of the cLMA. Because the term *LMA* is a protected trademark, these devices are referred to as *laryngeal masks* (LMs). Each has its own unique characteristics that may afford it specific advantages over other designs. Although an exhaustive description of every available LM is outside the scope of this chapter, some unique features merit mentioning.

Some design features address the issue of high cuff pressures, which can lead to oropharyngolaryngeal morbidity, nerve palsies, and improper device positioning. The line of LMs manufactured by AES, Inc. (Black Diamond, WA) incorporates a cuff pilot valve (CPV) that allows constant cuff pressure monitoring. The air-Q SP (Cookgas LLC, St. Louis, MO; distributed by Mercury Medical, Clearwater, FL) has a self-pressurizing cuff that uses the positive pressure that ventilates the patient to also pressurize the cuff, obviating the need for an inflation line and eliminating the possibility of cuff overinflation. On exhalation, the mask cuff deflates to the level of positive end-expiratory pressure (PEEP), decreasing the total mucosal pressure over the course of an anesthetic, thereby potentially reducing the incidence of cuff pressure–related complications.

CUFFLESS ANATOMICALLY PRESHAPED SEALERS

Cuffless anatomically preshaped sealers do not have a cuff; rather, they provide an airway seal by their anatomically preshaped design. Advantages include simplicity of insertion and positioning and the lack of a need to inflate a cuff. The first of these devices, the SLIPA (Curveair, London, UK), contains a hollow chamber that can trap regurgitated liquid and prevent aspiration. Other cuffless devices such as the i-gel (Intersurgical Inc., Wokingham, Berkshire, UK) and the Baska Mask (Strathfield, NSW, Australia) can also be included in this classification.

CUFFED PHARYNGEAL SEALERS

Cuffed pharyngeal sealers have an airway with a pharyngeal cuff that seals at the level of the base of the tongue and can be subclassified as to whether they also possess an esophageal sealing cuff.[165] SGAs with only a pharyngeal cuff include the Cobra Perilaryngeal Airway (CobraPLA; Engineered Medical Systems, Indianapolis, IN) and the Tulip Airway (Marshall Medical, Bath, UK); they are not detailed in this chapter. The following devices all have an esophageal sealing cuff.

The esophageal-tracheal combitube (ETC) (Covidien, Mansfield, MA) is a uniquely designed SGA with both a pharyngeal and esophageal sealing cuff and two lumina. The ETC is primarily designed for emergency intubation and is mostly used in the prehospital setting, although it has occasionally been used during general anesthesia as both a primary airway and as a rescue airway device.[188,189] It is inserted blindly through the mouth in a curved, downward motion until the printed ring marks lie between the teeth. Both the proximal, oropharyngeal cuff and the distal esophageal-tracheal cuff are inflated. Greater than 90% of the time, esophageal placement of the device occurs, in which ventilation should be performed via the longer, blue, #1 (esophageal) lumen.[190] This lumen has a closed distal end with eight small perforations located between the two cuffs, which allow oxygenation and ventilation. When the device is placed into the trachea, ventilation should occur via the shorter, clear, #2 (tracheal) lumen, which is open at its distal end. When the ETC is placed in the esophagus, an orogastric tube may be passed through the tracheal lumen to empty the stomach. Use of the ETC as a primary airway is limited by a higher risk of complications, compared with the LMA or tracheal intubation, including hoarseness, dysphagia, and bleeding.[191] Because the oropharyngeal cuff of the ETC contains latex, this device should not be used in latex-sensitive individuals.

The Rüsch EasyTube (Teleflex Medical, Research Triangle Park, NC) is a double-lumen SGA that is similar to the ETC. The primary differences are its nonlatex construction and a proximal lumen that ends just below the oropharyngeal balloon, allowing for the passage of a tube exchanger or FIS. The insertion technique and risks are similar to the ETC; a comparative study showed shorter insertion times with the EasyTube.[192]

The King LT series of SGAs (King Systems Corporation, Noblesville, IN) are similar in design to the ETC and EasyTube, with a ventilation port between the pharyngeal and esophageal cuffs. The King LT and the King LT-D (reusable and disposable, respectively) are single-lumen devices with a tapered distal tip that allows easy passage into the esophagus. The distal (esophageal) portion of the tube is occluded. The King LTS and the disposable King LTS-D, on the other hand, have an open distal tip with a secondary channel to allow suctioning of gastric contents. Although tracheal placement of a King LT device has not be reported, if it should occur, then the device should be removed and reinserted.

Tracheal Intubation

Tracheal intubation is the gold standard for airway management. It establishes a definitive airway, provides maximal protection against the aspiration of gastric contents, and allows for PPV with higher airway pressures than with a face mask or an SGA. Tracheal intubation is usually facilitated by DL; however, a wide variety of alternative intubation devices and techniques have been developed to circumvent the problems encountered when conventional DL is difficult.

In the fasted patient undergoing elective surgery with general anesthesia, an SGA is often suitable. Certain conditions or clinical situations, however, favor tracheal intubation, although the advent of second-generation SGAs has somewhat narrowed this list. Absolute indications for tracheal intubation include patients with a full stomach or who are otherwise at increased risk for aspiration of gastric secretions or blood, patients who are critically ill, patients with significant lung abnormalities (e.g., low lung compliance, high airway resistance, impaired oxygenation), patients requiring lung isolation, patients undergoing otorhinolaryngologic surgery during which an SGA would interfere with surgical access, patients who will likely need postoperative ventilatory support, and patients in whom SGA placement has failed. Other indications for intubation include a surgical requirement for NMBDs, patient positioning that would preclude rapid tracheal intubation (e.g., prone or turned away from the anesthesia provider), a predicted difficult airway, and prolonged procedures.[22]

ENDOTRACHEAL TUBES

The modern, standard ETT is a disposable, single-use, cuffed, plastic tube that is designed to be inserted through the nose or mouth and sit with its distal end in the mid-trachea, providing a patent airway to allow for ventilation of the lungs. A variety of different types of ETTs are available for use in specialized situations. Several features are commonplace among the different styles, however, including a universal 15-mm adapter that allows the attachment of the proximal end to different ventilating circuits and devices; a high-volume, low-pressure cuff; a beveled tip to facilitate passage through the vocal cords; and an additional distal opening in the side wall of the ETT known as a *Murphy eye*, which serves to provide an additional portal for ventilation should the distal end of the lumen become obstructed by either soft tissue or secretions.

Cuffed ETTs are routinely used for tracheal intubation in most patients; cuffless ETTs are used in neonates and infants. The high-volume, low-pressure cuff is inflated with air to provide a seal against the tracheal wall to protect the lungs from pulmonary aspiration and to ensure that the tidal volume delivered ventilates the lungs rather than escapes into the upper airway.[22] A pilot balloon with a one-way valve allows for the inflation of the cuff and an assessment of the cuff pressure. The cuff should be inflated to the minimum volume at which no air leak is present with positive pressure inspiration; the cuff pressure should be less than 25 cm H_2O.[193] Excessive cuff pressure may result in tracheal mucosal injury, vocal cord dysfunction from recurrent laryngeal nerve palsy, and sore throat. Monitoring the cuff pressure with a pressure gauge is recommended. When N_2O is used as part of the anesthetic, cuff pressure should be periodically measured throughout the surgery; N_2O diffusion into the cuff can result in increases in cuff pressure to potentially dangerous levels.

ETT size is normally described in terms of its internal diameter (ID); the relationship of the ID to the external diameter varies between different designs and manufacturers. Selection of the ETT size depends on the reason for placement and patient-specific factors such as gender and airway pathologic conditions. Smaller ETTs result in increased airway resistance and work of breathing, and ETTs with a smaller ID may preclude therapeutic fiberoptic bronchoscopy. Larger ETTs are more likely to be associated with laryngeal or tracheal mucosal trauma and have a higher incidence of sore throat after general anesthesia. Generally, in patients intubated only for the purposes of a general anesthetic, a smaller ETT may be used than on the patient who will remain intubated in the medium to long term as a result of respiratory failure; typically a 7-mm ETT is used for women and a 7.5- or 8-mm ETT is used for men.

A variety of specialized tracheal tubes are available for use in specific clinical situations. Preformed tubes, such as the nasal and oral Ring-Adair-Elwin (RAE) tubes, have a specific contour to maintain a low profile and to avoid surgical interference. Armored (reinforced) tubes have an embedded coil that minimizes kinking of the tube when it is subjected to angulation. Microlaryngeal tubes, which have small IDs with a longer length tube, are useful in laryngeal surgery or for specific applications, such as intubation through a cLMA. The VivaSight ETT (Ambu, Inc., Ballerup, Denmark) has an integrated video camera at the tip, useful during intubation and for confirming ETT position throughout the procedure. Other specialized tubes include laser-resistant tubes and both single- and double-lumen tubes that allow for one-lung ventilation.

ENDOTRACHEAL TUBE INTRODUCERS

ETT introducers are long, slender devices used to assist in guiding an ETT through the glottis. They are particularly useful for performing a blind intubation when the glottic opening cannot be visualized during laryngoscopy.

The original ETT guide was the Eschmann introducer, developed by Venn in 1973.[194] This device, also known as the *gum elastic bougie*, is long enough to allow advancement of an ETT over its distal end after being placed through the vocal cords. It also possesses an anterior angulation at the distal end (coudé tip) to facilitate maneuvering underneath the epiglottis toward the glottic opening, even when the glottic structures are not visualized. A variety of similar introducers with different sizes and features are available; some are hollow to allow for ventilation if the need arises.

Coudé-tip introducers are particularly useful when only a portion of the laryngeal structures, such as only the tip of the epiglottis, can be visualized. Proper placement of the stylet is indicated by the perception of *tracheal clicks* as the coudé tip passes along the tracheal rings and by a *distal hold-up* as it reaches the small bronchi. An ETT is subsequently advanced over the introducer into the correct position (Video 44.5).[195]

OROTRACHEAL VERSUS NASOTRACHEAL INTUBATION

Tracheal intubation can proceed via the orotracheal or nasotracheal route—this decision should be made before deciding which airway management technique will be used. Nasotracheal intubation is generally indicated when the orotracheal route is not possible (e.g., when the mouth opening is severely limited) or when the need for surgical access precludes an orotracheal route. In addition, certain intubation techniques, such as blind intubation, awake intubation, and FSI, are significantly easier when performed through the nose.

When the nasotracheal route is not specifically indicated, however, the orotracheal route is usually preferred for several reasons. The orotracheal route is potentially less traumatic and presents a lower risk of bleeding, it usually allows for the placement of a larger ETT, and it provides for more options in terms of airway management techniques. The major disadvantages include the potential for damage to the teeth and stimulation of the gag reflex during awake intubation, requiring denser airway anesthesia and potentially being less comfortable for the patient. Nasotracheal intubation, on the other hand, bypasses the gag reflex and is usually more easily tolerated by the awake patient. However, the risks of epistaxis, trauma to the nasal turbinates, and submucosal tunneling in the nasopharynx must be taken into account.[138] Nasotracheal intubation is relatively contraindicated in the setting of maxillary or skull base fractures.

DIRECT LARYNGOSCOPY

The most commonly used technique for tracheal intubation is DL, which involves direct visualization of the glottis with the assistance of a laryngoscope. The ETT is inserted through the glottic opening into the trachea under continuous observation.

Preparation and Positioning

Preparation for DL includes proper patient positioning, adequate preoxygenation, and ensuring the availability and proper functioning of all necessary equipment—laryngoscopes, tracheal tubes, tube stylets, an empty syringe for inflating the tracheal tube cuff, a suction apparatus, and the essential equipment for mask ventilation, including an oxygen source. A skilled assistant should be present to help with external laryngeal manipulation and stylet removal, among other tasks. Adequate preparation is of the utmost importance; as with any airway procedure, the first attempt should be the best attempt.

For DL to be successful, a line of sight from the mouth to the larynx must be achieved. The classical model used to describe the anatomic relationships necessary to achieve this was proposed in 1944 by Bannister and Macbeth and involves the alignment of three anatomic axes—oral, pharyngeal, and laryngeal.[196] Positioning the patient in the sniffing position approximates this alignment. Cervical flexion aligns the pharyngeal and laryngeal axes, and maximal head extension at the atlantooccipital joint brings the oral axis closer into alignment (Fig. 44.18). The accuracy of this model has been questioned,[197] and various alternative models to explain the anatomic advantage of the sniffing position have been proposed.[198,199] Regardless of the explanatory model, the evidence in the literature supports the assertion that the sniffing position is the optimal position for DL.[47,200]

Proper positioning in the sniffing position involves approximately 35 degrees of cervical flexion, which is accomplished by a 7- to 9-cm elevation of the head on a firm

Head and neck position and the axes of the head and neck upper airway

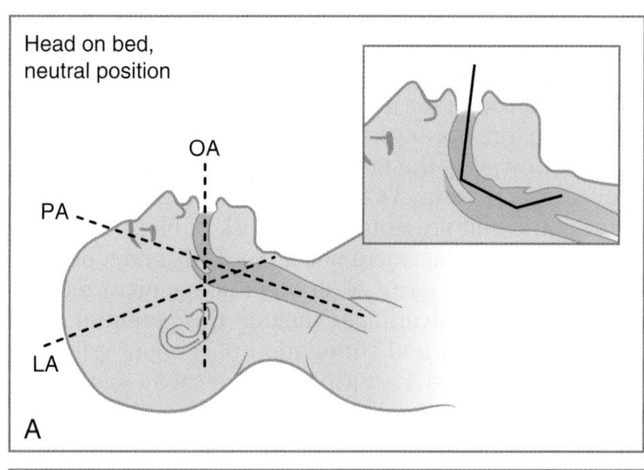

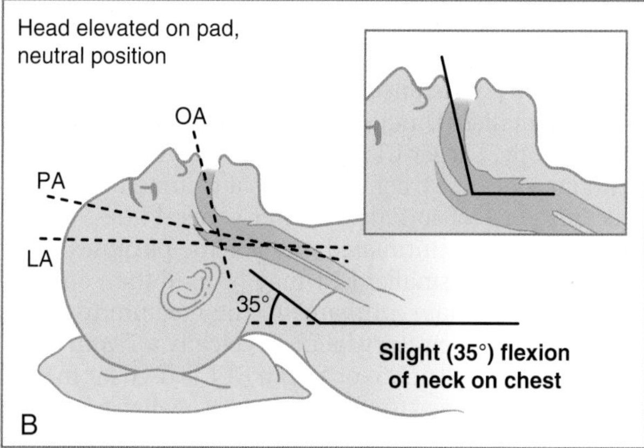

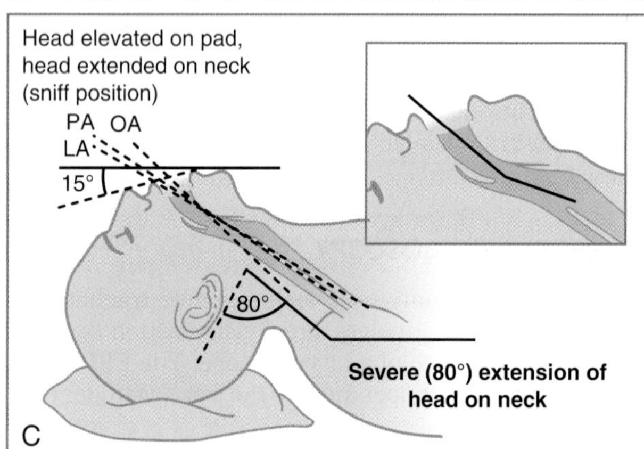

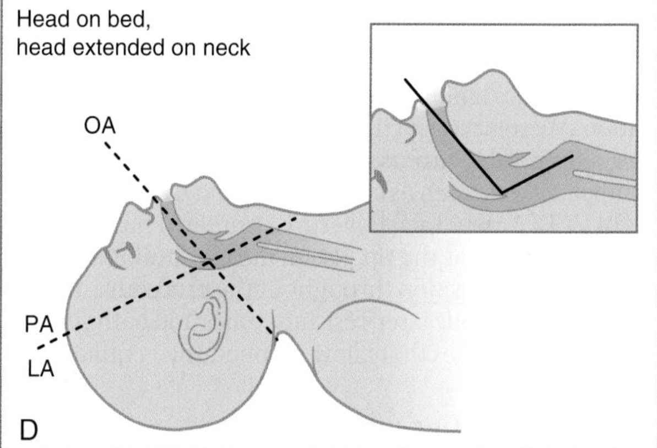

Fig. 44.18 Schematic diagrams show the alignment of the oral axis *(OA)*, pharyngeal axis *(PA)*, and laryngeal axis *(LA)* in four different head positions. Each head position is accompanied by an inset that magnifies the upper airway (oral cavity, pharynx, and larynx) and superimposes *(bold line)* the continuity of these three axes within the upper airway. (A) The head is in the neutral position with a marked degree of nonalignment of the LA, PA, and OA. (B) The head is resting on a large pad that flexes the neck on the chest and aligns the LA with the PA. (C) The head is resting on a pad (which flexes the neck on the chest). Concomitant extension of the head on the neck brings all three axes into alignment (sniffing position). (D) Extension of the head on the neck without concomitant elevation of the head on a pad, which results in nonalignment of the PA and LA with the OA. (From Baker PA, Timmermann A. Laryngoscopic tracheal intubation. In: Hagberg CA, Artime CA, Aziz M, eds. *Hagberg and Benumof's Airway Management*. 4th ed. Philadelphia: Elsevier; 2018.)

cushion; patients with shorter necks may require less head elevation.[47,201] Patients who are obese often require elevation of the shoulders and upper back to achieve adequate cervical flexion, which can be accomplished by placing the patient in the *ramped* position using either a specialized device, such as the Troop Elevation Pillow (Mercury Medical, Clearwater, FL), or folded blankets. Confirming horizontal alignment of the external auditory meatus with the sternal notch is useful for ensuring optimal head elevation in both obese and nonobese patients.[202] Adequate cervical flexion also facilitates maximal atlantooccipital extension, which provides optimal alignment of the oral and pharyngeal axes (the primary determinant for quality of laryngeal view) and enhanced mouth opening.[203]

Technique

The laryngoscope is a handheld instrument consisting of a blade attached to a handle containing a light source. Most are reusable and made of steel, although disposable, plastic versions are available. The curved blade and the straight blade are the two basic types of laryngoscope blades available for DL; multiple variations of both styles exist. The Macintosh is the most commonly used curved blade, whereas the Miller is the most commonly used straight blade. Both are designed to be held in the left hand, and both have a flange on the left side that is used to retract the tongue laterally. Each type of blade has its benefits and drawbacks and is associated with its own technique for use.

The technique for laryngoscopy consists of the opening of the mouth, inserting the laryngoscope blade, positioning of the laryngoscope blade tip, applying a lifting force exposing the glottis, and inserting a tracheal tube through the vocal cords into the trachea. Mouth opening is best achieved using the *scissors* technique; the right thumb pushes caudally on the right lower molars while the index or third finger of the right hand pushes on the right upper molars in the opposite direction (Fig. 44.19).

The decision of whether to use a Macintosh or a Miller blade is multifactorial; however, the personal preferences and experience of the laryngoscopist is a significant consideration. In general, the Macintosh is most commonly used for adults, whereas the straight blades are typically used in pediatric patients.[204] Curved blades provide greater room for passage of an ETT through the oropharynx, attributable to their larger flange, and are generally considered less likely to cause dental damage.[205] Straight blades are preferred in patients with a short thyromental distance or prominent incisors, and usually provide a better view of the glottis in patients with a long, floppy epiglottis. Often, when one style of laryngoscope does not provide an adequate view of the glottis, the other may be more effective. For most adults, a Macintosh size 3 or a Miller size 2 blade is usually the proper size; in larger patients or patients with a very long thyromental distance, a larger blade may be more appropriate.

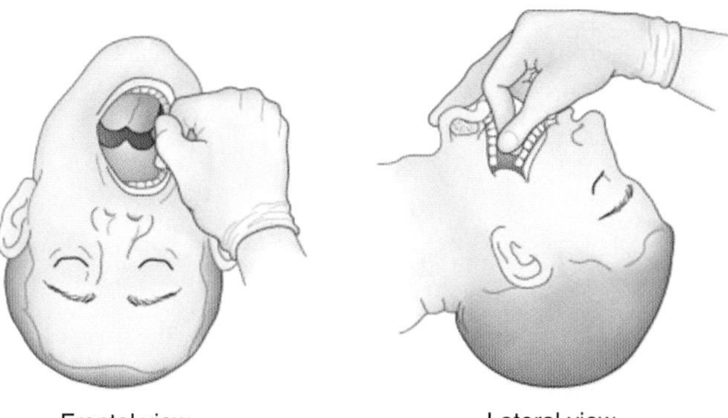

Fig. 44.19 The scissors technique for mouth opening. The thumb of the right hand is pressed on the right lower molars in a caudad direction while the index or third finger of the right hand presses on the right upper molars in a cephalad direction. (From Baker PA, Timmermann A. Laryngoscopic tracheal intubation. In: Hagberg CA, Artime CA, Aziz M, eds. *Hagberg and Benumof's Airway Management*. 4th ed. Philadelphia: Elsevier; 2018.)

The Macintosh blade is inserted in the right side of the mouth, and the flange is used to sweep the tongue to the left. Once the laryngoscope has been inserted in the mouth, the right hand can be used to ensure that the upper lip is not impinged between the laryngoscope and the upper incisors. The blade is advanced along the base of the tongue until the epiglottis is visualized; the tip of the blade is then advanced further and positioned in the vallecula. A force oriented at a 45-degree angle up and away from the laryngoscopist indirectly lifts the epiglottis by placing tension on the hyoepiglottic ligament, exposing the glottic structures (Fig. 44.20). The tip of the blade should not be lifted by using the laryngoscope as a lever, rocking back on the upper incisors, which can damage the teeth and provides an inferior view of the glottis. A properly oriented vector of force is achieved by using the anterior deltoid and triceps, not by radial flexion of the wrist. Once a complete view of the glottis is achieved, the ETT is grasped similar to a pencil with the right hand and guided through the vocal cords into the trachea. Passage of the ETT may be facilitated by an anterior angulation of the tip, which can be accomplished by shaping the ETT with a malleable stylet into a *hockey stick* shape, with approximately a 60-degree angle formed 4 to 5 cm from the distal end, or by accentuating the natural anterior curvature of the ETT by inserting the tip into the 15-mm connector, forming a circle, for several minutes before performing DL.

Conventional Laryngoscopy with a Curved Blade

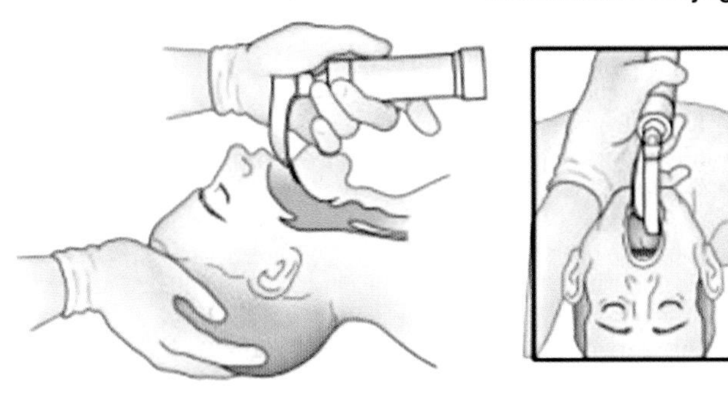
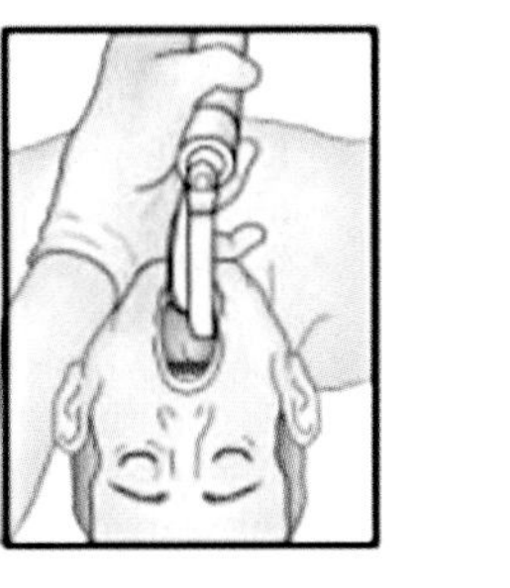

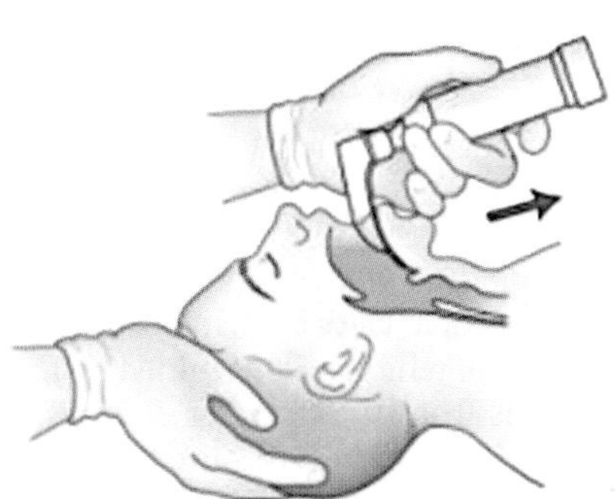
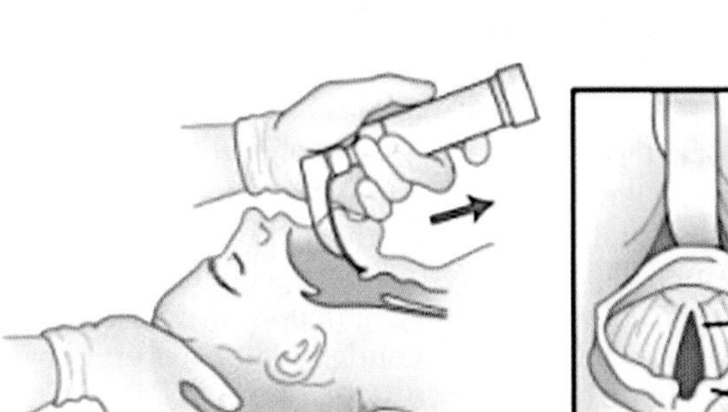

Fig. 44.20 Laryngoscopy technique with a Macintosh (curved) blade. (A) The laryngoscope blade is inserted into the right side of the mouth, sweeping the tongue to the left of the flange. (B) The blade is advanced toward the midline of the base of the tongue by rotating the wrist so that the laryngoscope handle becomes more vertical *(arrows)*. (C) The laryngoscope is lifted at a 45-degree angle *(arrow)* as the tip of the blade is placed in the vallecula. (D) Continued lifting of the laryngoscope handle at a 45-degree angle results in exposure of the laryngeal aperture. The epiglottis (1), vocal cords (2), cuneiform cartilage (3), and corniculate cartilage (4) are identified. (From Baker PA, Timmermann A. Laryngoscopic tracheal intubation. In: Hagberg CA, Artime CA, Aziz M, eds. *Hagberg and Benumof's Airway Management*. 4th ed. Philadelphia: Elsevier; 2018.)

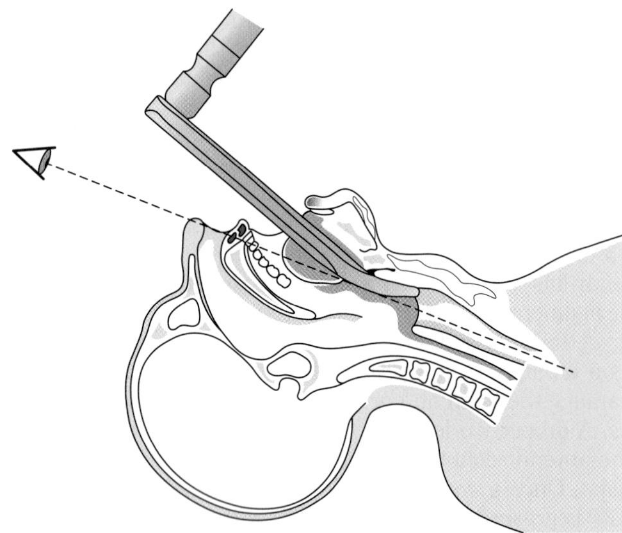

Fig. 44.21 Paraglossal laryngoscopy technique with a Miller (straight) blade. The blade is at the right side of the tongue. The line of sight over the molars is achieved by rotating the head to the left and moving the heel of the laryngoscope to the right. The tip of the blade is placed beneath the epiglottis and a 45-degree lifting force applied to expose the glottic aperture. (From Baker PA, Timmermann A. Laryngoscopic tracheal intubation. In: Hagberg CA, Artime CA, Aziz M, eds. *Hagberg and Benumof's Airway Management*. 4th ed. Philadelphia: Elsevier; 2018.)

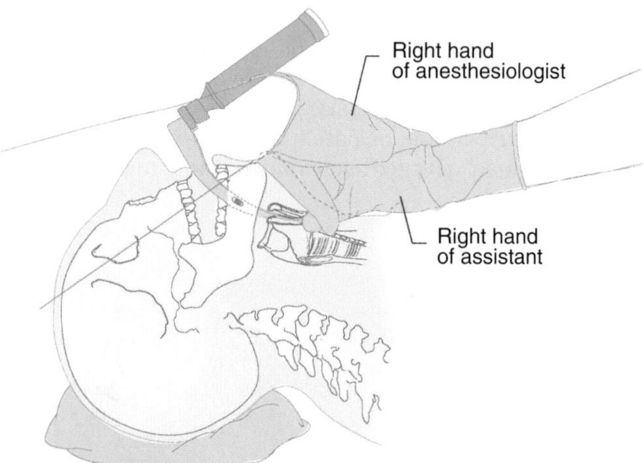

Fig. 44.22 Optimal external laryngeal manipulation. The laryngoscopist guides the position, and pressure is exerted by the assistant's hand on the larynx to maximize the view of the vocal cords. The left hand of the laryngoscopist, which holds the laryngoscope handle, is omitted. (From Henderson J. Airway management. In: Miller RJ, ed. *Anesthesia*. 7th ed. Philadelphia: Churchill Livingstone; 2009.)

The Miller laryngoscope blade is inserted using the paraglossal technique described by Henderson.[22] This method provides maximal tongue control and avoids contact of the laryngoscope with the maxillary incisors. The laryngoscope is inserted lateral to the tongue and carefully advanced along the paraglossal gutter between the tongue and tonsil. Application of continued moderate lifting force to the laryngoscope handle helps maintain lateral displacement of the tongue and reduces contact with the maxillary teeth. As the laryngoscope is advanced, the epiglottis comes into view and the tip of the laryngoscope is passed posterior to the epiglottis. The optimal position of the tip of the straight laryngoscope is in the midline of the posterior surface of the epiglottis, close to the anterior commissure of the vocal cords (Fig. 44.21).[22] This position achieves good control of the epiglottis and facilitates the passage of the tracheal tube. The direction of force applied to the handle is the same as when using the Macintosh blade.

The use of external laryngeal manipulation can improve the laryngeal view. Backward, upward, rightward pressure (the BURP maneuver) on the thyroid cartilage is most commonly used. Optimal external laryngeal manipulation (OELM) is achieved when the laryngoscopist uses his or her right hand to guide the position and pressure is exerted by an assistant's hand on the larynx (Fig. 44.22).

Difficulty with tracheal intubation by DL is primarily a function of an inadequate view of the glottis. Predictors for difficult laryngoscopy that can be identified during the preoperative airway assessment are listed in Box 44.3. Cormack and Lehane developed a grading scale in 1984 to describe laryngoscopic views.[206] The grades range from I to IV, beginning with grade I (the best view), in which the epiglottis and vocal cords are in complete view, and culminating with grade IV (the most difficult view), in which the epiglottis or larynx is not visualized (Fig. 44.23). A modified classification scheme with five different grades based on the Cormack-Lehane scoring system is described by Yentis, who proposed that grade II be differentiated into IIA (partial view of the glottis) and IIB (arytenoids or posterior vocal cords only are visible).[207] Intubation is rarely difficult when a grade I or IIA view is achieved; grades IIB and III are associated with a significantly higher incidence of failed intubation. A grade IV laryngoscopic view requires an alternate method of intubation. An alternate method of rating laryngoscopic view is the percentage of glottic opening (POGO) scale, which is determined by the percentage of the vocal cords from the anterior commissure to the arytenoid notch that can be visualized during laryngoscopy. This scale has been shown to have a higher interobserver reliability than the Cormack-Lehane scoring system and is potentially more useful for research studies in direct and indirect laryngoscopy.[208]

When the laryngeal view is inadequate, the laryngoscopist should verify that the patient is in an optimal position, that OELM is being provided, and that the laryngoscope has not been inserted too deeply. Whether a larger laryngoscope or an alternate style of blade would be beneficial should be

BOX 44.3 Predictors of Difficult Laryngoscopy

- Long upper incisors
- Prominent overbite
- Inability to protrude mandible
- Small mouth opening
- Mallampati classification III or IV
- High, arched palate
- Short thyromental distance
- Short, thick neck
- Limited cervical mobility

Modified from Apfelbaum JL, Hagberg CA, Caplan RA, et al. Practice guidelines for management of the difficult airway: an updated report by the American Society of Anesthesiologists Task Force on Management of the Difficult Airway. *Anesthesiology*. 2013;118:251–270.

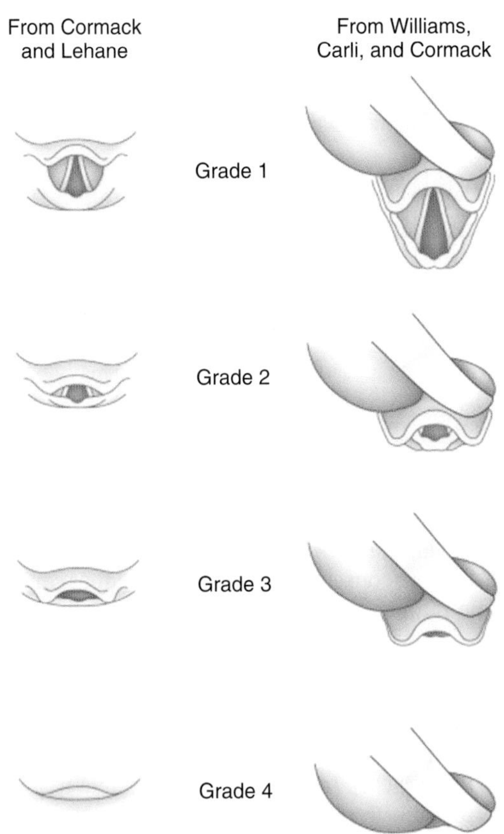

Fig. 44.23 The Cormack-Lehane grading system for laryngoscopic view. Grade 1 is visualization of the entire laryngeal aperture; grade 2 is visualization of only the posterior portion of the laryngeal aperture; grade 3 is visualization of only the epiglottis; and grade 4 is no visualization of the epiglottis or larynx. (Modified from Cormack RS, Lehane J. Difficult tracheal intubation in obstetrics. *Anaesthesia.* 1984;39:1105; and Williams KN, Carli F, Cormack RS. Unexpected difficult laryngoscopy: a prospective survey in routine general surgery. *Br J Anaesth.* 1991;66:38.)

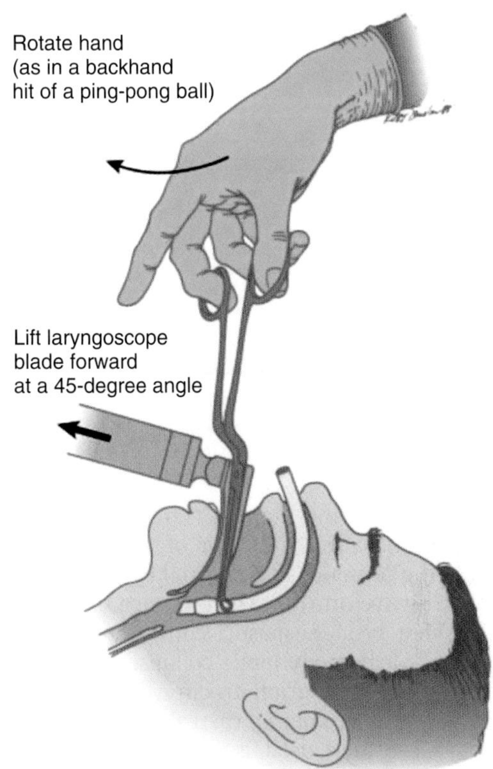

Fig. 44.24 Guiding a nasal endotracheal tube into the larynx with Magill forceps. (From Berry JM, Harvey S. Laryngoscopic orotracheal and nasotracheal intubation. In: Hagberg CA, ed. *Benumof and Hagberg's Airway Management.* 3rd ed. Philadelphia: Saunders; 2013, p. 357.)

considered. When the ETT cannot be passed into the trachea under direct visualization, the options include the following: (1) attempts at blind passage of the ETT, which risks laryngeal trauma, bleeding, and airway obstruction; (2) the use of an ETT introducer; and (3) alternative approaches to intubation as per the ASA DAA.

When the glottic view is adequate, the ETT should be inserted into the right corner of the mouth and advanced such that it intercepts the long axis of the laryngoscope blade at the glottis, rather than inserted midline and parallel to the long axis of the laryngoscope blade, ensuring that the view of the glottis is not obscured. The tip of the ETT is passed through the glottic inlet and advanced until the proximal portion of the cuff is approximately 2 cm past the vocal cords. If a stylet is being used, then the stylet should be removed when the tip of the ETT is at the level of the vocal cords while the ETT is firmly held stationary; this technique helps limit trauma to the tracheal mucosa from the semirigid stylet.

Nasotracheal Intubation Technique

Before nasotracheal intubation, the more patent nostril should be selected. This selection can be accomplished by separately occluding each nostril and having the patient inhale—the patient will usually be able to inhale more effectively through one of the nares. To reduce the risk of epistaxis, a nasal mucosal vasoconstrictor (e.g., cocaine, phenylephrine, oxymetazoline) should be administered. The nasal ETT should be lubricated and inserted into the naris with the bevel facing away from the midline, which decreases the risk of avulsion of a turbinate. Cephalad traction should be applied as the ETT is advanced through the nasal passage to ensure a trajectory along the floor of the nose, beneath the inferior turbinate.

Once the ETT enters the oropharynx (typically at a depth of 14 to 16 cm), standard DL is performed. The ETT can be guided into the laryngeal inlet by repositioning the head as the ETT is advanced or with the aid of Magill forceps (Fig. 44.24). Care should be taken to grasp the ETT proximal to the cuff to prevent cuff damage. Other techniques for nasotracheal intubation include blind nasal intubation, VAL, and FSI.

Confirmation of Endotracheal Tube Placement

Once the ETT is in place, the laryngoscope is removed from the mouth, the ETT cuff is appropriately inflated, and the patient is manually ventilated while the ETT is manually held in place. Immediate verification of endotracheal placement of the ETT is necessary; esophageal or endobronchial intubation is a significant source of avoidable anesthetic-related morbidity and mortality. Endotracheal placement can be determined by confirmation of chest rise, visible condensation in the ETT, equal breath sounds bilaterally over the chest wall, lack of breath sounds over the epigastrium, large exhaled tidal volumes, and appropriate compliance of

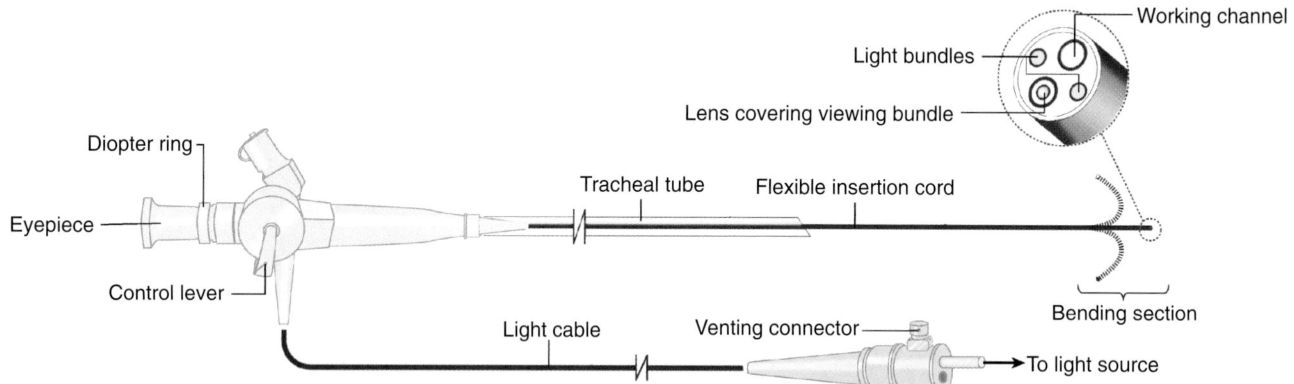

Fig. 44.25 Flexible fiberoptic bronchoscope. (From Henderson J. Airway management. In: Miller RJ, ed. *Anesthesia*. 7th ed. Philadelphia: Churchill Livingstone; 2009.)

the reservoir bag during manual ventilation.[209] The most important and objective indicator of tracheal intubation, however, is the presence of a normal capnogram (carbon dioxide [CO_2] waveform) for the presence of at least three breaths. Severe bronchospasm, equipment malfunction, cardiac arrest, or hemodynamic collapse may prevent the appearance of a capnogram tracing despite proper ETT placement. If doubt remains, then flexible bronchoscopy, although not routinely used, is very reliable at confirming ETT placement.

Hypoxemia, increased airway pressures, asymmetric chest expansion, and the absence of breath sounds over one lung, generally the left, are indicative of endobronchial intubation; pneumothorax can also produce this picture. Flexible bronchoscopy or chest radiography can be used if the clinical picture is unclear.

Securing the Endotracheal Tube

Once the proper depth of the ETT has been determined, the tube should be secured in place to prevent movement and inadvertent endobronchial intubation or extubation. The most common method is to tape the ETT to the skin of the face. Because it is less mobile, the skin of the maxilla is preferred. When tape cannot be used, such as in the case of a severe tape allergy, extensive facial burns, or epidermolysis bullosa, a surgical mask may be tied around the back of the head to secure the ETT. Other methods that may be used for intraoral or facial surgery include wire fixation to a tooth or suturing the ETT to the skin of the cheek.

INDIRECT LARYNGOSCOPY

Conventional DL requires wide mouth opening, cervical flexion, and atlantooccipital extension to create a direct line of vision from the mouth to the larynx. In certain conditions, this positioning is impossible or contraindicated. Other times, attributable to anatomic variations in the airway (e.g., redundant soft tissue, protruding incisors, anterior larynx), DL cannot be achieved, despite optimal positioning and technique. Indirect laryngoscopy entails the indirect visualization of the glottis by way of optical aids, such as fiberoptic bundles, video cameras, mirrors, prisms, or lenses. Various different devices that use indirect laryngoscopy are available, including FISs, video laryngoscopes (VLs), and intubating optical stylets. They are indispensable tools for the management of the known or predicted difficult airway. Because no direct line of sight is needed, visualization of the larynx can occur without tissue distortion; consequently, these techniques can be readily used with topical anesthesia in an awake patient.[22]

Flexible Intubation Scopes

The FIS is the most widely used, versatile, indirect laryngoscopy device. Since the first use of fiberoptics for airway management in 1967, FISs, including the flexible fiberoptic bronchoscope (FOB), have become invaluable tools for tracheal intubation in both awake and anesthetized patients. There are various clinical scenarios within which FSI provides a superior technique for airway management, as compared with DL or alternative airway devices. FSI of the awake and cooperative, spontaneously ventilating patient is considered the *gold standard* for the management of the difficult airway.[195]

The standard FOB (Fig. 44.25) consists of thousands of flexible glass fibers approximately 8 to 10 μm in diameter that are capable of transmitting reflected light along their length. Light is transmitted from an external light source to the distal end of the FOB; the light reflecting off the object to be viewed is transmitted back along the length of the FOB to an eyepiece or video camera at the proximal end of the scope. In recent years, FOBs have been replaced by modern FISs that use video chip and light-emitting diode (LED) technology instead of fiberoptics.

Indications for FSI essentially include any indication for tracheal intubation. However, FSI may be the airway management technique of choice in any one of the following clinical scenarios[195]:

- Known or anticipated difficult airway (i.e., cannot intubate or cannot ventilate [CICV])
- Contraindication to extension of the neck (e.g., unstable cervical fracture, severe cervical stenosis, vertebral artery insufficiency, Chiari malformation)
- Increased risk of dental damage (e.g., poor dentition, fragile dental work)
- Limited mouth opening (e.g., TMJ disease, mandibular-maxillary fixation, severe facial burns)

No specific contraindications exist for FSI; however, in certain clinical situations, successful FSI is unlikely. Severe airway bleeding can obscure anatomic landmarks and soil the tip of the FIS with blood, making visualization of the larynx extremely difficult. Obstruction or severe stenosis of the airway, resulting in the inability to pass an FIS, can also make FSI impossible.

FSI provides several advantages over DL[195]:

- Allows for a more complete visual examination of the airway before intubation.
- Provides confirmation of tube placement, avoiding esophageal and endobronchial intubation.
- Eliminates the need for three-axis alignment; therefore FSI is among the techniques least likely to result in cervical spine movement.
- Is well-tolerated in awake patients; results in less tachycardia and hypertension.
- Has less of a potential for airway and dental trauma.
- Can be performed in multiple positions.

FSI can be performed in the awake or anesthetized patient. Indications for an awake FSI are generally those situations in which ventilation via a mask is anticipated to be difficult, when a postintubation neurologic examination is needed, or when induction of general anesthesia could cause adverse hemodynamic or respiratory consequences. The major technical disadvantage to performing FSI under general anesthesia is the loss of pharyngeal muscle tone, which can lead to upper airway collapse and difficult fiberoptic laryngoscopy.[195]

Before its use, the anesthesia practitioner or skilled assistant must ensure that the FIS, light source, and video monitor are in proper working condition and that all components have been fully prepared for use. This preparation includes focusing the image if using a FOB, ensuring proper view orientation if using a video camera, lubricating the distal third of the flexible insertion cord, applying antifogging solution to the tip of the scope, and connecting a suction line or oxygen source to the suction port. The ETT should be prepared by placing it in a warm water bath, which softens the plastic, easing passage into the trachea and minimizing airway trauma.

FSI is usually performed in the supine or sitting (i.e., beach-chair) position, although emergency FSI in the lateral decubitus or even prone position has also been described.[210] When performing FSI in the supine position, the anesthesia provider stands at the head of the patient. Advantages to this position are that the laryngeal view through the FIS is in the same orientation as during DL, and the patient and physician are already in the optimal position to perform mask ventilation or other airway maneuvers, if necessary. When performing FSI with the patient in the sitting or beach-chair position, the practitioner should stand facing the patient at the patient's side. This position may be the position of choice in awake FSI because of improved ventilation and greater patient comfort. In addition, the sitting position optimizes airway anatomy and prevents airway collapse in patients who are obese, in patients with obstructive sleep apnea, and in patients with anterior extrinsic airway obstruction.[211]

Before FSI, unless contraindicated, an anti-sialagogue, such as glycopyrrolate 0.2-0.4 mg IV, may be administered to dry airway secretions. Both the orotracheal and nasotracheal routes can be used for FSI. While weighing the advantages and disadvantages, the clinician should determine which approach is best-suited for the clinical situation. Whichever route is chosen, however, essentially two steps to FSI must be taken[195]:

1. Indirect laryngoscopy and endoscopy are performed, obtaining a view of the glottis with the FIS and maneuvering the FIS through the vocal cords into the trachea.
2. The ETT is advanced over the FIS into its proper position in the trachea, and the FIS is removed.

When performing orotracheal FSI, navigating the FIS around the base of the tongue to achieve a satisfactory view of the larynx is one of the major challenges. The FIS has a tendency to stray off the midline, and, frequently, little to no airspace is found between the tongue and the palate through which to navigate the FIS. To mitigate this issue, several devices or techniques can be used. Specialized intubating oral airways can be used to protect the FIS from damage by biting, to prevent the tongue from falling back into the pharynx and obstructing the airspace, and to keep the FIS midline while it is guided to the larynx. Several types of intubating oral airways are available, each with unique design differences, and include the Ovassapian, Berman, and Williams airways. A disadvantage of these devices is that they place pressure on the base of the tongue, potentially causing gagging in awake patients. In both awake patients and those under general anesthesia, gentle traction on the tongue anteriorly is helpful in preventing the tongue from falling back into the pharynx if an intubating airway is not used. This traction can be easily accomplished by hand with the help of 4- × 4-inch gauze pads for traction or with Magill forceps. Care should be taken to not injure the tongue on the bottom teeth. As previously described, LMAs and intubating LMAs can also be used as conduits for oral FSI. Obtaining a laryngeal view during nasal FSI is often easier, as compared with the oral approach, as a result of the fact that the FIS stays midline and the tip of the FIS is usually directed at the glottis as it enters the oropharynx.

Once the FIS has been successfully positioned in the oropharynx, the epiglottis and vocal cords can usually be visualized with a slight anterior deflection of the tip of the FIS. The FIS is aimed toward the anterior commissure of the vocal cords and posteriorly flexed to enter into the trachea. The trachea is easily identifiable by the presence of the cartilaginous tracheal rings. The FIS is advanced distally until a point just above the carina, and the ETT is advanced over the FIS while continually visualizing the trachea through the FIS, providing confirmation that the FIS and ETT have not been accidentally dislodged into the oropharynx or esophagus (Video 44.6). Frequently, especially with orotracheal intubation, resistance is met as the tip of ETT reaches the glottic inlet. Often, this resistance has been shown to be attributable to the bevel of the ETT impinging on the right arytenoid.[212] A slight withdrawal of the ETT and a counterclockwise 90-degree turn, orienting the bevel posteriorly, usually resolves this issue. For nasotracheal intubation, a clockwise 90-degree turn, ensuring that the bevel is oriented anteriorly, can prevent the tip of the ETT from impinging on the epiglottis. Alternatively, the Parker Flex-Tip ETT (Parker Medical, Englewood, CO), which has a bull-nosed tip directed toward the center of the distal lumen, can be used. This ETT has been shown to have a high first-pass success rate when being advanced over an FIS.[213]

After successful passage of the ETT, proper depth (2 to 3 cm from the carina) is confirmed during the withdrawal of the FIS. On rare occasions, the FIS may prove difficult to remove from the ETT, which may be attributable to the FIS having passed through the Murphy eye rather than the distal lumen or a result of inadequate lubrication of the FIS. In these situations, forceful removal may damage the device; therefore the FIS and ETT should be removed as a unit and the procedure repeated.

Rigid Indirect Laryngoscopes

The first indirect laryngoscopes for intubation were based on modifications of the standard direct laryngoscope and used mirrors or prisms to project an image at an angle from the horizontal, facilitating visualization of the larynx. Modern indirect laryngoscopes based on the direct laryngoscope design that use optical lenses to project a refracted image of the glottis include the Viewmax (Rüsch, Duluth, GA) and the TruView EVO2 (Truphatek, Netanya, Israel).

The Airtraq SP (Prodol Meditec S.A., Guecho, Spain) is a disposable, portable, anatomically shaped, optical laryngoscope that provides a magnified view of the glottis without alignment of the oral, pharyngeal, and laryngeal axes. It includes a guiding channel to hold the ETT and direct it toward the vocal cords. It can be used for a variety of applications, including the known or predicted difficult airway, as well as for awake intubation. The Airtraq laryngoscope has been shown to result in more rapid tracheal intubation with a reduced incidence of esophageal intubation when compared to DL, especially when used by novices.[214] It is available in two adult and two pediatric sizes, as well as in specific designs for nasotracheal intubation and double-lumen tube placement. The Airtraq Avant is a newer model that features a reusable optic piece that is used in combination with disposable blades.

Lighted Optical Stylets

Lighted optical stylets are rigid or semirigid fiberoptic devices that incorporate the optical and light-transmitting components into a tubular, stainless steel sheath over which the ETT is loaded. A substantial body of evidence supports the use of these optical stylets in patients with limited neck mobility,[215] small mouth opening,[216] abnormal airway anatomy,[217] or anticipated difficult laryngoscopy.

The Bonfils retromolar intubation fiberscope (Karl Storz Endoscopy, Tuttlingen, Germany) is a 40-cm long, rigid optical stylet with a fixed anterior tip curvature of 40 degrees (Video 44.7).[218] The proximal eyepiece can be used with the naked eye or connected to a video monitor. It is available with a working channel that can be used for suction, SAYGO local anesthesia,[219] or oxygen insufflation (oxygen flow rates should be limited to 3 L/min to avoid barotrauma).[220] The Shikani optical stylet (Clarus Medical, Minneapolis, MN) is a similar device to the Bonfils fiberscope but with a malleable shaft. The Levitan FPS stylet (Clarus Medical, Minneapolis, MN) is a shorter version of the Shikani stylet intended for use in combination with DL, although usable on its own.[221] The Clarus Video System (Clarus Medical, Minneapolis, MN) is a newer version of the Shikani stylet that incorporates a liquid crystal display (LCD) screen (Video 44.8).

These optical stylets can be used on their own or in combination with DL or VAL[222] The ETT is mounted on the optical stylet and advanced under direct vision via a midline or right paraglossal route until it passes under the tongue. After indirect visualization of the tip of the stylet passing through the vocal cords (via the eyepiece or video monitor), the ETT is advanced over the stylet into the trachea. When these are not used in conjunction with DL or VAL, the left hand of the operator should lift the patient's jaw by gently grasping the mandible and displacing it anteriorly. This maneuver helps create more airspace in the oropharynx and lifts the epiglottis. Optical stylets can be used for awake intubation and have also been used for the transillumination technique (see Lighted Stylets).[218,223]

The SensaScope (Acutronic, Hirzel, Switzerland) is a hybrid rigid optical stylet that uses video chip technology. It has an S-shaped curvature and a 3-cm long steerable tip.[224] Visualization is achieved by a connection to a video monitor. The SensaScope is designed to be used in combination with DL and has been successfully used for awake intubation in patients with a predicted difficult airway.[225] The Video RIFL (AI Medical Devices, Williamston, MI) is a similar device with a rigid shaft and a flexible, steerable tip. This device features an LCD monitor attached to the handle that displays the video image.

Video Laryngoscopes

As with flexible bronchoscopes, video chip technology has begun to largely replace fiberoptic technology in rigid indirect laryngoscopes because of the advantages of a higher quality image, increased durability, and reduced maintenance costs. Over the past 15 years, VLs have revolutionized the practice of airway management, and their use may become standard not only for difficult airways, but also for routine airways as well. In fact, VAL is now included in the ASA DAA as an alternative approach to intubation and should be considered for patients with a known or predicted difficult airway.[7] A VL is also listed as a suggested piece of equipment on a portable difficult airway cart.[7]

VAL has been shown to result in improved glottic visualization, compared with DL, in both routine airway management and in the predicted difficult airway.[7,226] Although this improved visualization does not necessarily translate into increased success with intubation (particularly in the normal airway), studies have shown improved intubation success with VAL in patients with predicted difficult airways.[227,228] VLs are also useful in the unexpected difficult airway; intubation success rates of 94% and 99% have been reported for VAL as a rescue modality after failed DL.[229,230] These devices have also been successfully used for awake intubation.[231,232]

Various different VLs have been introduced, each with its own design and specific features. Generally, VLs can be divided into three groups: (1) those whose design is based on the Macintosh blade, (2) those that incorporate highly curved or distally angulated blades, and (3) those that incorporate an ETT-guiding channel.[233] Although no single design has been shown to be superior, there are certain clinical circumstances where one style may be preferable to another. Other features that vary among different VLs include the degree of portability and the size of the video monitor. Many VLs are available in both reusable and single-use models.

VLs based on the Macintosh blade design include the C-MAC laryngoscope (Karl Storz, Tuttlingen, Germany), the McGrath MAC laryngoscope (Aircraft Medical, Edinburgh, UK), and the GlideScope Titanium MAC (Verathon, Bothell, WA). These devices can be used for both DL and VAL, making them particularly useful for teaching the DL technique. The C-MAC laryngoscope is the most extensively studied of these and is associated with shorter intubation times and greater ease of use, compared with other VLs,[234,235] which is possibly due to laryngoscopists' familiarity with the use of a Macintosh-style blade (Fig. 44.26). The technique for using the C-MAC laryngoscope is identical to that of DL with a Macintosh blade; alternatively, the tip of the VL can be used to lift the epiglottis directly.[236] In contrast to other VLs, most intubations with the C-MAC laryngoscope can be performed without the use of a stylet[237,238]; the use of an oral RAE ETT can facilitate tracheal intubation.[239]

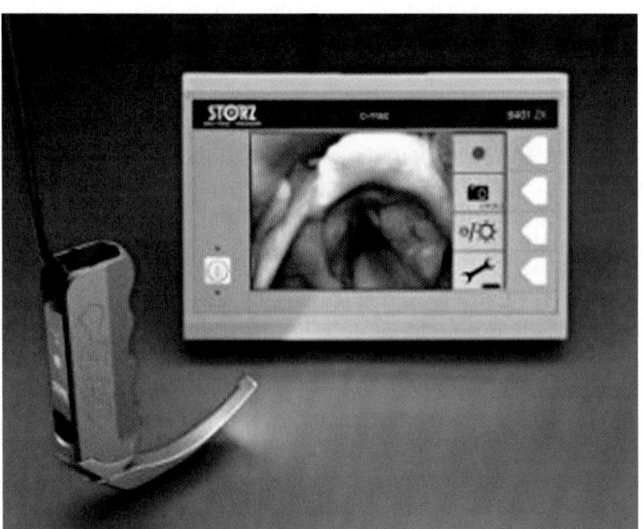

Fig. 44.26 **The Storz C-MAC videolaryngoscope.** (From Aziz M, Brambrink A. Video-assisted laryngoscopy. In: Hagberg CA, Artime CA, Aziz M, eds. *Hagberg and Benumof's Airway Management*. 4th ed. Philadelphia: Elsevier; 2018.)

VLs with a distally angulated or highly curved blade permit a "look around the corner," providing an improved laryngoscopic view without requiring manipulation of the cervical spine. These devices are therefore of particular utility in patients with cervical immobilization, micrognathia, or limited mouth opening.[233] The GlideScope Titanium LoPro (Verathon, Bothell, WA) is the updated version of the archetype for this subset of devices. It possesses a 60-degree blade angulation, an antifogging mechanism, a 6.4-inch video monitor, and is available in reusable and single-use models (Fig. 44.27). The McGrath Series 5 laryngoscope (Aircraft Medical, Edinburgh, UK) is a similar device in that it possesses a distally angulated blade; its primary difference is its greater portability and a disarticulating handle that can be useful in patients with limited mouth opening and limited movement of the head and neck. The X-Blade is a hyperangulated blade for the McGrath MAC, while the D-Blade (Karl Storz, Tuttlingen, Germany) is a highly curved VL blade for use with the C-MAC system. These devices are typically inserted in the mouth midline, without sweeping the tongue from right to left as in DL. Because of the high degree of angulation of the blade, an ETT stylet is almost always necessary; malleable stylets with a 60- to 90-degree bend, articulating stylets, and the GlideRite stylet (a rigid stylet with a 90-degree curve specifically designed for use with the GlideScope) have all been successfully used with these VLs.[240,241] The VL and the styletted ETT should be inserted into the oral cavity under direct vision to avoid oropharyngeal trauma (Video 44.9).[242]

Some VLs with highly curved blades have integrated tube-guiding channels to facilitate intubation without the use of a stylet, similar to the Airtraq. The King Vision (King Systems, Noblesville, IN) and the Pentax Airway Scope (AWS; Pentax Medical, distributed by Ambu Inc., Ballerup, Denmark) fall into this category. This type of VL has been shown to be useful in patients with cervical immobilization and has been successfully used for awake intubation.[243,244]

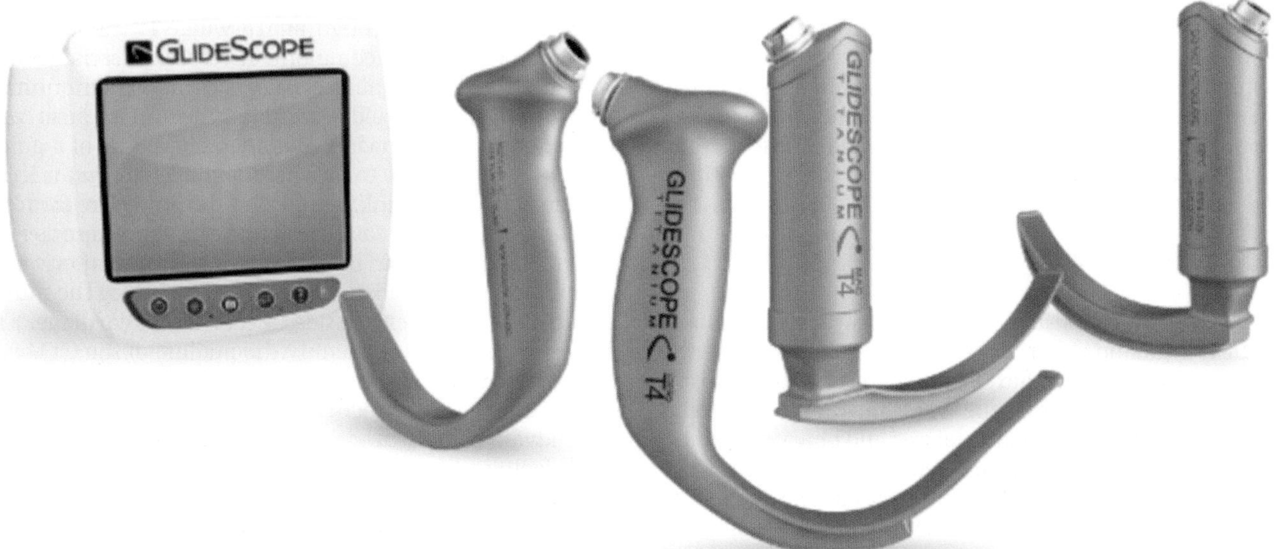

Fig. 44.27 **The GlideScope AVL videolaryngoscope system with titanium blades.** (From Aziz M, Brambrink A. Video-assisted laryngoscopy. In: Hagberg CA, Artime CA, Aziz M, eds. *Hagberg and Benumof's Airway Management*. 4th ed. Philadelphia: Elsevier; 2018.)

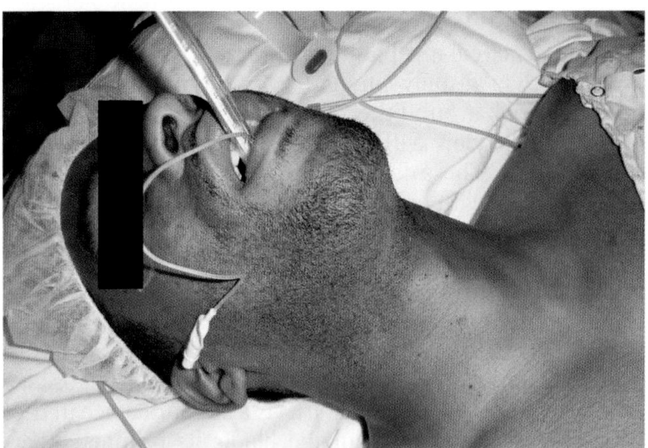

Fig. 44.28 When the tip of a lighted stylet is placed at the glottic opening, a well-circumscribed glow can be seen in the anterior neck just below the thyroid prominence.

The VividTrac (Vivid Medical, Palo Alto, CA) is a single-use, channeled VL with a Universal Serial Bus (USB) interface that works with any monitor.

Lighted Stylets

Lighted stylets make use of the transillumination technique to blindly intubate the trachea and have been described in the literature as an alternative or aid to DL, particularly in the predicted difficult airway. Lighted stylets may be particularly helpful when the presence of blood or heavy secretions limits visualization of the airway. However, because lighted stylet insertion is a blind technique, it is contraindicated in certain clinical situations, such as neoplasm of the airway or airway trauma. Because increased soft tissue leads to difficulty with transillumination, this technique is less useful in the patient who is morbidly obese.[245]

To perform the transillumination technique, an ETT is preloaded onto the stylet. The left hand of the operator lifts the supine patient's jaw by gently grasping the mandible and displacing it anteriorly to facilitate the insertion of the stylet under the tongue. The stylet should be inserted using a retromolar approach. Once inserted, the stylet should be kept midline and advanced under the tongue. A well-circumscribed *glow* (approximately the size of a quarter) should appear in the midline of the patient's neck at the level of the cricoid cartilage (Fig. 44.28), indicating correct positioning of the stylet within the trachea. Subsequently, the ETT can be advanced over the stylet into proper position (Video 44.10).[245]

RETROGRADE INTUBATION

RI is a well-described technique for orotracheal or nasotracheal intubation that involves guiding an ETT into the trachea with a narrow, flexible guide that has been percutaneously placed through the CTM into the trachea and passed retrograde through the larynx and pharynx, exiting the mouth or nose. The guide is typically a steel guidewire, although an epidural catheter can be used. This technique has several modifications, each with its own benefits and disadvantages, and can be successfully used in awake, sedated, obtunded, or apneic patients who have either an anticipated or unanticipated difficult airway.[246] Indications include failure of DL; obstruction of the view of the vocal cords by blood, secretions, or anatomic derangement; and difficult intubation scenarios such as unstable cervical spine, ankylosing spondylitis, maxillofacial trauma, or trismus. RI is also an alternative to FSI in developing countries where the availability of FISs is limited.[246]

The ASA DAA describes RI as an alternative approach to difficult intubation in the nonemergent pathway, when intubation is unsuccessful but mask ventilation is adequate. It is suggested that equipment for RI be included in a portable storage unit for difficult airway management. RI can take several minutes to accomplish; therefore this technique is contraindicated in an emergent CICV scenario.[246] Other contraindications are generally relative and include anatomic abnormalities (e.g., malignancy, goiter) that preclude access to the CTM, tracheal stenosis at the level of the CTM, coagulopathy, and local infection.

The ideal position for RI is supine with the neck in extension, allowing easy palpation of the cricoid cartilage and surrounding structures. If this position is not possible, then RI can also be performed with the patient in the sitting position or with the neck in a neutral position. If landmarks are difficult to identify, then ultrasound guidance may be used. The anterior neck should be cleansed before puncture, and aseptic technique should be used. The translaryngeal puncture site can be performed superior or inferior to the cricoid cartilage. The CTM (superior to the cricoid cartilage) has the advantage of being relatively avascular; however, a puncture at this site allows only 1 cm of space below the level of the vocal cords for the tip of the ETT. A puncture site inferior to the cricoid cartilage, at the cricotracheal ligament, allows the ETT to travel in a straight path with a long length of the ETT below the vocal cords; however, this site is associated with a greater potential for bleeding.[246]

The classic technique for RI involves using a Tuohy needle to puncture the CTM and an epidural catheter as the guide. More commonly, an IV catheter and a steel guidewire are used. The diameter of the guidewire should be small enough to fit through the IV catheter and should be at least twice as long as the ETT to be used; a guidewire with a .038-inch diameter (which passes through an 18-gauge IV catheter) and a length of 110 cm is commonly used. Commercial kits are available that include all necessary equipment. Performing a RI with a J-tip, steel guidewire rather than an epidural catheter provides the following advantages: the J-tip of a guidewire is less traumatic to airway, the guidewire has a lower tendency to coil or kink, retrieval of the guidewire from the oral or nasal cavity is easier, and the technique is quicker.[246]

Once the patient has been positioned, the operator's nondominant hand stabilizes the trachea by placing the thumb and third digit on either side of the cricoid cartilage. The index finger is used to identify the midline of the CTM and the upper border of the cricoid cartilage. A syringe half-filled with saline is attached to an 18-gauge angiocatheter and advanced at a 90-degree angle to the CTM with the bevel facing cephalad, aspirating for air bubbles to confirm the position inside the trachea. The angle of insertion is slightly lowered, and the needle is removed. At this stage, reconfirmation of a position within the trachea and instillation of a local anesthetic can be performed with a second syringe filled with 2 to 4 mL of 2% or 4% lidocaine. This transtracheal block can provide additional comfort to a patient who is awake or sedated and undergoing RI, or it can reduce the incidence of sympathetic stimulation and laryngospasm in a patient under general anesthesia.

The guidewire is then advanced through the angiocatheter until it exits the mouth or nose. DL can be used to facilitate the wire exiting the mouth, if necessary. The guidewire is clamped with a hemostat at the level of the skin of the neck to prevent migration. Although the ETT can then be directly advanced over the guidewire, a tapered guide catheter (e.g., Arndt airway exchange catheter) is useful to reduce the discrepancy in diameter between the guide-wire and the ETT, which can predispose the ETT to catch on the arytenoids or vocal cords rather than smoothly slide into the trachea. The guide catheter is placed over the portion of the wire exiting the mouth or nose and advanced until it contacts the CTM. The wire is then removed, and an ETT is advanced over the guide catheter (Fig. 44.29 and Video 44.11). Potential complications include bleeding (usually minimal), subcutaneous emphysema, pneumomediastinum, pneumothorax, and injury to the posterior trachea or esophagus.[246]

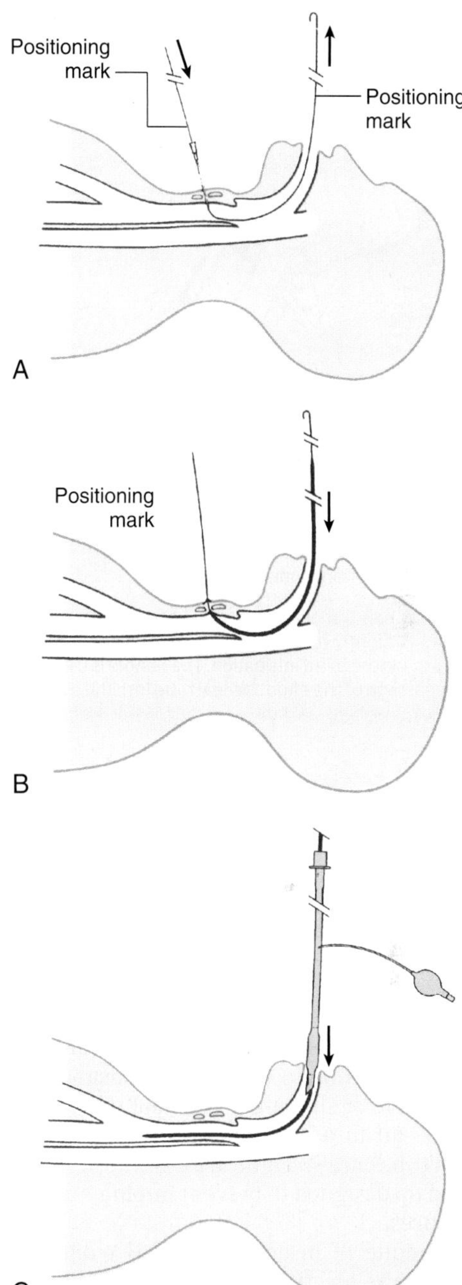

Fig. 44.29 The guidewire technique for retrograde intubation. (A) After the placement of an 18-gauge angiocatheter through the cricothyroid membrane, the J-tip of the guidewire is inserted in a cephalad direction until it exits the mouth or nose. (B) The guide catheter is threaded over the guidewire until it contacts the laryngeal access site. The guidewire is then removed from above. (C) After advancing the guide catheter 2 to 3 cm, the endotracheal tube is advanced into the trachea. (Courtesy Cook Critical Care, Bloomington, IN.)

DOUBLE-LUMEN TUBES AND BRONCHIAL BLOCKERS

Single-lung ventilation is required for certain clinical circumstances, including protective lung isolation from infection or hemorrhage, attaining adequate exposure for surgical procedures (e.g., video-assisted thoracoscopy), and for controlling the distribution of ventilation in the setting of major bronchial surgery, trauma, or fistula. Double-lumen tubes (DLTs) and bronchial blockers are two options that allow for ventilation of only one lung (also see Chapter 53).

DLTs have a bronchial lumen and a tracheal lumen. They are designated as left-sided or right-sided, depending on whether the bronchial lumen goes to the left or right main bronchus. Most commonly, a left-sided DLT is used to avoid blockage of the right upper lobe bronchus. DLTs are placed in a similar fashion to the standard ETT, although placement is usually more difficult because of their size and stiffness. Video laryngoscopy can facilitate DLT placement.[247] After placing the DLT into the trachea, verification of the location of the bronchial port with an FIS should be determined. The blue bronchial cuff should be positioned just below the carina in the appropriate bronchus. Inflation of the blue bronchial balloon under direct visualization helps verify proper placement. Care should be taken to ensure that the bronchial cuff does not herniate over the carina. The VivaSight-DL (Ambu Inc., Ballerup, Denmark) is a single-use left-sided DLT with an integrated camera located at the tip of the tracheal lumen and allows for accurate positioning of the DLT without the use of an FIS. Once a DLT is properly placed, isolating a lung is possible by inflating the bronchial cuff and clamping either the tracheal or bronchial connector.

Bronchial blockers are essentially hollow, balloon-tipped catheters that are endobronchially placed to isolate and deflate one lung. In some clinical situations, lung isolation is required, but the use of a DLT is not practical because of a difficult airway, decreased size of the tracheal lumen, or the need for postoperative mechanical ventilation. In these instances, the use of a modified single-lumen tube with an integrated bronchial blocker (e.g., the Univent [Fuji Systems, Tokyo, Japan]) or the use of a bronchial blocker in conjunction with a standard ETT is appropriate.

COMBINATION TECHNIQUES

Tracheal Intubation Through a Supraglottic Airway Device

The intubating LMA (ILMA), known as the LMA Fastrach (LMA North America, San Diego, CA), was first described

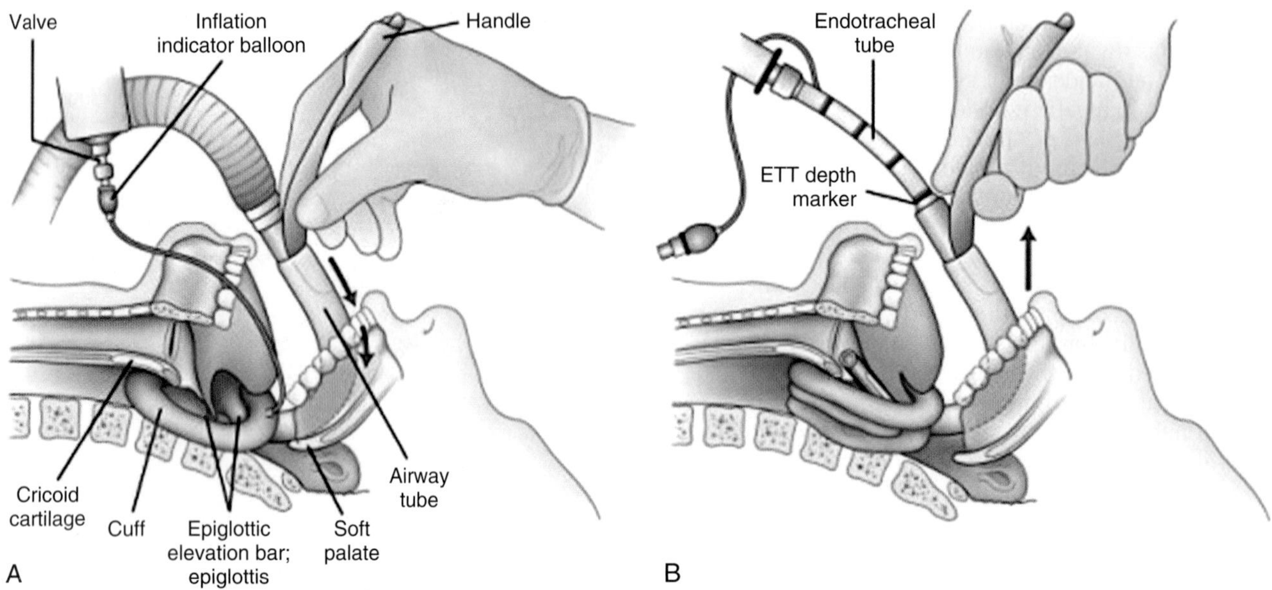

Fig. 44.30 The Chandy maneuver consists of two steps. (A) The first step is important for establishing optimal ventilation. The intubating laryngeal mask airway (ILMA) is slightly rotated in the sagittal plane using the handle until the least resistance to bag ventilation is achieved. (B) The second step is performed just before blind intubation. The handle is used to lift (but not tilt) the ILMA slightly away from the posterior pharyngeal wall, which facilitates the smooth passage of the endotracheal tube into the trachea. (From Lindsay HA, Cook TM, Russo SG, Hagberg CA. Supraglottic airway techniques: laryngeal mask airways. In: Hagberg CA, Artime CA, Aziz M, eds. *Hagberg and Benumof's Airway Management*. 4th ed. Philadelphia: Elsevier; 2018.)

by Dr. Archie Brain in 1997; it became available for commercial use in the United States shortly thereafter. The ILMA was designed as a conduit for tracheal intubation to facilitate ventilation between attempts at tracheal intubation. The rigid handle and airway tube enable a rapid and precise control of mask position. An epiglottic elevating bar is designed to elevate the epiglottis as the tube is advanced into the bowl. A disposable, single-use version is available in addition to the original reusable model. Specialized reusable or single-use tracheal tubes are designed to facilitate atraumatic blind intubation through the ILMA. The tubes are straight, wire-reinforced, and have a soft molded tip designed to prevent impingement on laryngeal structures.

The technique of inserting the ILMA differs in many respects from the insertion of the cLMA, and the learning curve is significant. A neutral head position (nonextended head on a support) is recommended. The ILMA handle is used to rotate the mask into the pharynx. Oxygenation, ventilation, and anesthesia are stabilized after insertion. If resistance to ventilation is encountered, then the position of the ILMA is adjusted. The *Chandy maneuver* consists of two separate maneuvers: (1) the ILMA is rotated in the sagittal plane until resistance to bag ventilation is minimal; and then (2) the ILMA is gently lifted from the posterior pharyngeal wall just before passage of the tracheal tube (Fig. 44.30). The original, reusable ILMA should be removed soon after tracheal intubation has been verified because its rigidity results in high pressure on adjacent tissues. Although the blind technique has a high rate of success, intubation under vision with an FIS through the ILMA achieves higher first-attempt and overall success rates.

Other SGAs can be used to facilitate tracheal intubation. The cLMA, although not designed for intubation, can be an effective conduit if used in conjunction with an FIS. Because of the long and narrow airway shaft, a microlaryngeal tube must be used. Alternatively, a cLMA can be exchanged for an ETT by using an FIS in conjunction with the Aintree intubation catheter (Cook Critical Care, Bloomington, IN), which is a hollow airway exchange catheter designed to fit over a standard FIS (Fig. 44.31 and Video 44.12). Most newer SGAs have airway shafts that are wide enough to allow intubation through the device with a standard-sized ETT (Video 44.13).

Combined Direct Laryngoscopy Techniques

DL can be used to expand the space available in the oral cavity to manipulate an FIS by displacing pharyngeal tissue, and the epiglottis can be elevated allowing the scope to be more easily directed underneath the epiglottis toward the glottic opening. This may be especially helpful in the morbidly obese patient or patients with soiled airways (e.g., with blood, secretions, or vomitus).[248]

When a Cormack-Lehane grade III view is encountered during DL, the coudé tip of an ETT introducer can be passed underneath the epiglottis, and tracheal positioning confirmed by the sensation of clicks as the bougie tip passes the tracheal rings.

While using an optical stylet as an adjunct to DL, the tip of the stylet can be guided just beneath the tip of the epiglottis under direct vision. While holding the ETT/fiberoptic stylet securely, the clinician transfers his/her vision to the eyepiece or monitor where the glottic opening can be visualized, and the ETT can be advanced through the vocal cords and into the trachea.[248]

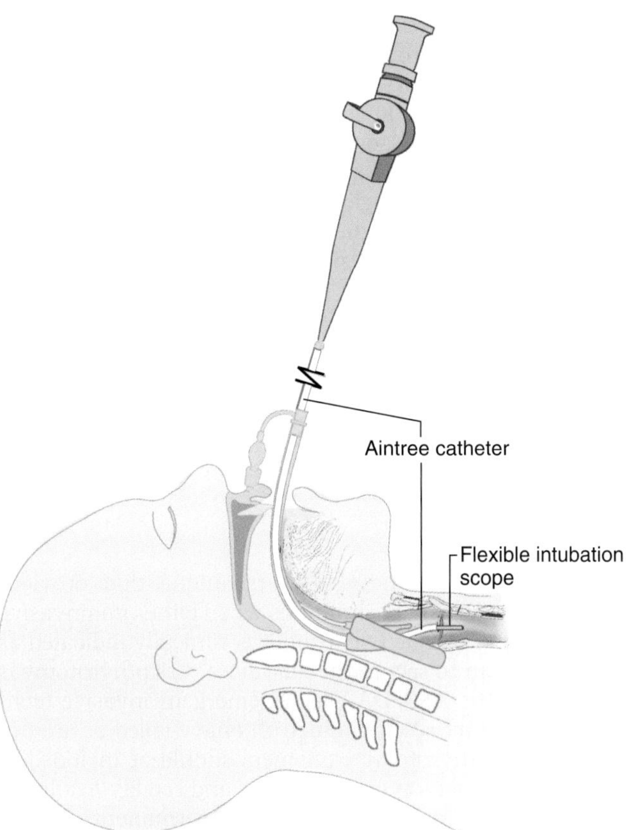

Fig. 44.31 Aintree intubating catheter within a flexible intubation scope, inserted through a laryngeal mask airway. (From Henderson J. Airway management. In: Miller RJ, ed. *Anesthesia.* 7th ed. Philadelphia: Churchill Livingstone; 2009.)

Combined Video-Assisted Laryngoscopy Techniques

Just as the bougie has been demonstrated to be an invaluable adjunct to DL, it may be used in combination with VAL in order to improve the success of tracheal intubation, and may offer additional advantages. In a trial featuring a simulated airway with vomitus, the use of a bougie improved intubation success rate and decreased the time to intubation with the Pentax-AWS and the McGrath MAC compared to DL.[249] A bougie may also facilitate advancement of the ETT into the trachea when an adequate view is obtained with VAL, but difficulty is encountered with intubation (Video 44.14).[250]

Optical stylets can also be used in combination with VAL. A study examining the use of the C-MAC VL and the Bonfils Intubation Scope in patients with a history of difficult intubation found that the combination of the two devices was superior in terms of glottic view than either device by itself.[251]

Certain circumstances may arise in which a combination of VAL and FSI may be beneficial. A patient with severely limited mouth opening and/or unstable cervical spine injury may preclude the use of DL in order to assist in FSI; using VAL in this situation may provide the ability to view the glottic opening and better guide the FIS into position. VAL can also diagnose difficulties with the passage of the ETT over the FIS into the glottis (Video 44.15).[248]

Combined Retrograde Intubation Techniques

To improve the success of retrograde intubation, it can be combined with DL or an FIS. DL can be used as an adjunct in order to improve success during retrograde guided intubation. During the classic technique of retrograde intubation, after a catheter is placed in the inferior cricothyroid membrane, the J-tip of a guidewire is directed upward until it can be retrieved from the mouth or nares. If orotracheal intubation is desired, DL can aid the clinician in opening the oropharynx and visualizing the wire so that it may be retrieved more easily through the mouth prior to entering the nasopharynx. In addition, after the guiding catheter is advanced anterograde over the wire until tenting is noted at the cricothyroid access point, DL may be used in order to lift the epiglottis and pharyngeal tissue, facilitating the passage of an ETT through the vocal cords.[248]

Alternatively, an FIS can be used to facilitate retrograde intubation. After the guidewire is retrieved from the mouth or naris, it is passed through the working channel of the FIS from distal to proximal. The FIS is then passed over the guidewire and into the glottis until resistance is met at the cricothyroid membrane. The hemostat that held the guidewire in place internally may now be released and the guidewire removed. The FIS may then be advanced until the carina is visualized and the ETT is passed into the trachea. In this fashion, the FOB reduces the likelihood that the ETT will become dislodged and the airway can be visualized throughout the procedure. There are several advantages to passing a FOB antegrade over a retrograde placed wire[248]:

- The outer diameter of the guidewire and the internal diameter of the fiberoptic suction port form a tight fit that allows the FOB to follow a straight path through vocal cords without impinging on anatomic structures.
- The FIS acts as large antegrade guide catheter and allows easy passage of the ETT.
- It allows placement of the ETT under direct visualization.
- The FIS may be advanced to the carina freely (past the puncture site) which eliminates the problem of distance between vocal cords and puncture site.

Emergency Front of Neck Access

Emergency FONA refers to rescue techniques used in a CICO situation when attempts at establishing a noninvasive airway have failed. These techniques may also be used as a primary airway in some difficult airway situations when attempts at securing a noninvasive airway are likely to fail, such as a patient with a laryngeal neoplasm and critical airway obstruction. Options for FONA include transtracheal jet ventilation (TTJV), cricothyrotomy, and tracheostomy. Whereas tracheostomy is usually performed by a surgeon, the anesthesia practitioner should become proficient with the techniques for TTJV and cricothyrotomy; the situation will inevitably arise in which an invasive airway will become necessary. An emergent situation is not the time to become familiar with a new technique.

TRANSTRACHEAL JET VENTILATION

Percutaneous TTJV is a relatively quick and effective but invasive method of oxygenation and ventilation in the CICV scenario when more conservative measures fail. The ASA DAA lists TTJV as an emergent invasive technique to be used in patients who cannot be conventionally ventilated or intubated.[7] TTJV is widely regarded as a life-saving procedure that can provide adequate, temporary oxygenation and ventilation with less training and complications than a surgical airway, the last resort for obtaining an airway in the algorithm.[252] Nonetheless, TTJV is an invasive technique, and its primary use is as an emergency airway. Occasionally, it is used on an elective basis for laryngeal surgery.

Inspiration during TTJV is achieved by insufflation of pressurized oxygen through a cannula placed by needle cricothyrotomy. Expiration is passive as a result of the elastic recoil of the lungs and the chest wall. Allowing sufficient time for passive expiration to avoid barotrauma from breath stacking is essential. Expiration occurs through the glottis and depends on a nonobstructed upper airway, which is imperative to avoid barotrauma and resulting pneumothorax. The egress of air through the glottic aperture can also provide bubbles to facilitate the placement of an ETT. In fact, several case reports have demonstrated that after the initiation of TTJV in an airway with little or no visualization of the glottis, successful intubation occurred because of the opening of the glottis and guidance from the bubbles with jet ventilation.

TTJV should not be performed in patients who have sustained direct damage to the cricoid cartilage or larynx or in patients with complete upper airway obstruction. Other relative contraindications to TTJV include coagulopathy, obstructive pulmonary disease, or distorted anatomy in which catheter placement might be difficult.

Typically, a 12- to 16-gauge kink-resistant catheter is used for TTJV. A coil-reinforced 6Fr catheter (Cook Critical Care, Bloomington, IN) is specifically designed for TTJV to prevent kinking, and its Teflon coating facilitates its passage through the CTM into the trachea. The technique for placement is similar to the technique for RI, with the exception that the needle is inserted with the bevel facing caudally. Confirmation of proper intratracheal placement of the catheter by testing for aspiration of air is imperative before initiating jet ventilation.

The minimum pressure required to drive a jet ventilator is 15 psi. The pipeline pressure for oxygen in hospitals in the United States is approximately 55 psi. Commercially available jet ventilators generally contain pressure regulators to lower the pipeline pressure to provide successful jet ventilation while avoiding higher pressures that might result in barotrauma. In most instances in the operating room, adequate pressure for jet ventilation can be achieved by connecting straight to the pipeline supply. Difficulty usually arises in locations outside of the surgical unit where TTJV may be needed but adequate driving pressure is not available.[252]

A major complication of TTJV is barotrauma with resulting pneumothorax from the use of high-pressure oxygen. To prevent this complication, ensuring that a path for air egress exists and that adequate time for passive expiration is available is an absolute necessity. The lowest possible pressure that will provide adequate oxygenation and ventilation should be used. Other complications associated with TTJV include subcutaneous or mediastinal emphysema, hemorrhage, aspiration, and perforation of the posterior wall of the trachea or esophagus.[252]

The Ventrain is a single-use, manually operated oxygen insufflation device designed to decrease the risk of barotrauma when compared to TTJV through a small-bore percutaneous catheter.[253] It uses the Bernoulli principle to provide expiratory ventilation assistance, meaning that negative pressure is generated that facilitates the egress of gas, and therefore can even be used when the upper airway is obstructed.[254] It is driven by oxygen from a high-pressure source with a controllable flow, e.g., a wall-mounted flowmeter or an oxygen cylinder with a flow regulator.

CRICOTHYROTOMY

Cricothyrotomy is an invasive technique that provides access to the airway in situations when either noninvasive maneuvers have failed or when it is clinically indicated as a primary plan to secure the airway.[255] Cricothyrotomy is included in the ASA DAA as an emergent invasive technique after other rescue maneuvers have failed or are not feasible. Cricothyrotomy equipment should be included in all emergency airway storage units and readily available. Cricothyrotomy is not considered a permanent airway, and, after placement, plans should be made for either the removal of the cricothyrotomy catheter or conversion to a formal tracheostomy.[255]

In children younger than 6 years of age (also see Chapter 77), the cricoid cartilage is the narrowest portion of the airway and the isthmus of the thyroid gland typically reaches the level of the CTM; therefore cricothyrotomy is contraindicated. Needle cricothyrotomy with TTJV is indicated in this pediatric population. Other contraindications to cricothyrotomy include laryngeal fractures, laryngeal neoplasm, subglottic stenosis, coagulopathy, and distorted or unidentifiable neck anatomy.

The two most common techniques for performing a cricothyrotomy are the percutaneous dilational cricothyrotomy and the surgical cricothyrotomy. For the anesthesiologist, the percutaneous technique has historically been preferred because of the familiarity of using the Seldinger technique for other procedures (e.g., central venous catheterization). Recently, however, surgical cricothyrotomy has been advocated as the preferred technique due to its faster speed and higher reliability.[8]

A number of surgical methods for cricothyrotomy have been described; however, the scalpel-bougie technique is the preferred technique in the Difficult Airway Society guidelines for management of the difficult airway. The process is outlined in Box 44.4 and Fig. 44.32. It is recommended that all anesthesiologists learn this technique and receive regular training to avoid fading of skill.[8]

A number of commercially available cricothyrotomy kits use the percutaneous dilational technique. The basis for this procedure is the insertion of an airway catheter over a dilator that has been inserted over a guidewire. The patient's neck is extended, and the cricothyroid groove is identified. If landmarks are difficult to identify, then

BOX 44.4 Surgical Cricothyrotomy

Equipment

- No. 10 scalpel
- Bougie with a coudé (angled) tip
- Cuffed endotracheal tube (ETT) with a 6-mm internal diameter

Technique

1. Stand on the patient's left-hand side if you are right handed (reverse if left handed).
2. Stabilize the larynx using the left hand.
3. Use the left index finger to identify the cricothyroid membrane (CTM). If the CTM is not palpable, make a 8-10 cm vertical incision in the midline and use blunt dissection with the fingers of both hands to separate tissues and identify and stabilize the larynx with the left hand.
4. Holding the scalpel in your right hand, make a transverse stab incision through the skin and cricothyroid membrane with the cutting edge of the blade facing toward you.
5. Keep the scalpel perpendicular to the skin and turn it through 90° so that the sharp edge points caudally (toward the feet).
6. Swap hands; hold the scalpel with your left hand.
7. Maintain gentle traction, pulling the scalpel toward you (laterally) with the left hand, keeping the scalpel handle vertical to the skin (not slanted).
8. Pick the bougie up with your right hand.
9. Holding the bougie at a right angle to the trachea, slide the coudé tip of the bougie down the side of the scalpel blade furthest from you into the trachea.
10. Rotate and align the bougie with the patient's trachea and advance gently up to 10-15 cm.
11. Remove the scalpel.
12. Stabilize trachea and tension skin with left hand.
13. Railroad a lubricated size 6.0 mm cuffed tracheal tube over the bougie.
14. Rotate the tube over the bougie as it is advanced. Avoid excessive advancement and endobronchial intubation.
15. Remove the bougie.
16. Inflate the cuff and confirm ventilation with capnography.

Modified from Frerk C, Mitchell VS, McNarry AF, et al. Difficult Airway Society 2015 guidelines for management of unanticipated difficult intubation in adults. *Br J Anaesth.* 2015;115(6):827–848.

ultrasound guidance may be used. A 1- to 1.5-cm vertical incision is made through the skin overlying the CTM. An 18-gauge needle-catheter attached to a fluid-filled syringe is passed through the incision at a 45-degree angle in the caudal direction with continuous aspiration. Because of the location of the cricothyroid artery and the proximity of the CTM to the vocal folds, puncture of the CTM should be made in the lower third of the membrane and directed inferiorly (Fig. 44.33).[255] Aspiration of free air confirms passage through the CTM. The catheter is advanced over the needle into the trachea. The needle is removed, and the catheter is left in place. The guidewire is inserted caudally to a depth of approximately 2 to 3 cm. The catheter is removed, and the curved dilator with the airway cannula is threaded over the guidewire. The dilator and cannula unit is advanced through the CTM while maintaining control of the guidewire. The dilator and guidewire are removed together while the cannula remains in place. The cuff is inflated, and ventilation is attempted. Proper placement is confirmed by capnography, and the airway cannula is secured in place (Video 44.16).[255]

Complications include hemorrhage, injury to the posterior tracheal wall or esophagus, vocal cord injury, laceration of the thyroid gland, and improper insertion of the cannula. Placement of the airway cannula in the subcutaneous tissue can result in subcutaneous or mediastinal emphysema. Late complications from cricothyrotomy include swallowing dysfunction, infection, voice changes, and tracheal stenosis. Tracheal stenosis has an incidence of approximately 2% to 8% in adults and is more likely if preexisting trauma or infection is present.

Extubation of the Trachea

A critical component of airway management is the process of extubation. Although considerable emphasis is placed on the problems that can arise during induction and intubation, the risk of complications can potentially be higher during extubation of the trachea.[256] Analysis of the ASA Closed Claims database has shown that although the number of claims for death and brain damage during intubation have decreased since the adoption of the ASA *Practice Guidelines for Management of the Difficult Airway*, the number of claims arising from injury at extubation and during recovery have not decreased.[1] In response to these trends and in the absence of any well-established strategies for the management of tracheal extubation, the DAS established a set of guidelines in 2012 to "discuss the problems arising during extubation and recovery" and to "promote a strategic, stepwise approach to extubation."[257]

A number of complications can arise during extubation (Box 44.5); although some of these complications are minor with no long-term sequelae, others can lead to a failed extubation. Failed extubation can result from the failure of oxygenation, failure of ventilation, inadequate clearance of pulmonary secretions, or loss of airway patency.[84] If an airway is not quickly reestablished, then serious complications, including death, may result. As such, the anesthesia practitioner needs to stratify extubation risk preemptively and establish an extubation plan before attempting extubation. Per the DAS guidelines, risk stratification can be accomplished by considering the following: (1) whether the airway was normal and uncomplicated at induction; (2) whether the airway has become difficult to manage as a result of surgical changes, trauma, or nonsurgical factors; and (3) whether the patient has general risk factors for an unsuccessful extubation.[257]

GENERAL CONSIDERATIONS FOR EXTUBATION OF THE TRACHEA

For both routine and difficult extubation scenarios, an extubation plan must be preemptively formulated, including a plan for reintubation that can be implemented should the patient be unable to maintain an adequate airway after extubation.[7] The decision of whether to extubate the trachea when the patient is fully awake versus a deep extubation before the return of consciousness should be made based on the risks and benefits of each technique. The awake patient can more easily maintain a patent airway, attributable to the recovery of awake pharyngeal muscle tone and airway reflexes. Deep extubation avoids coughing

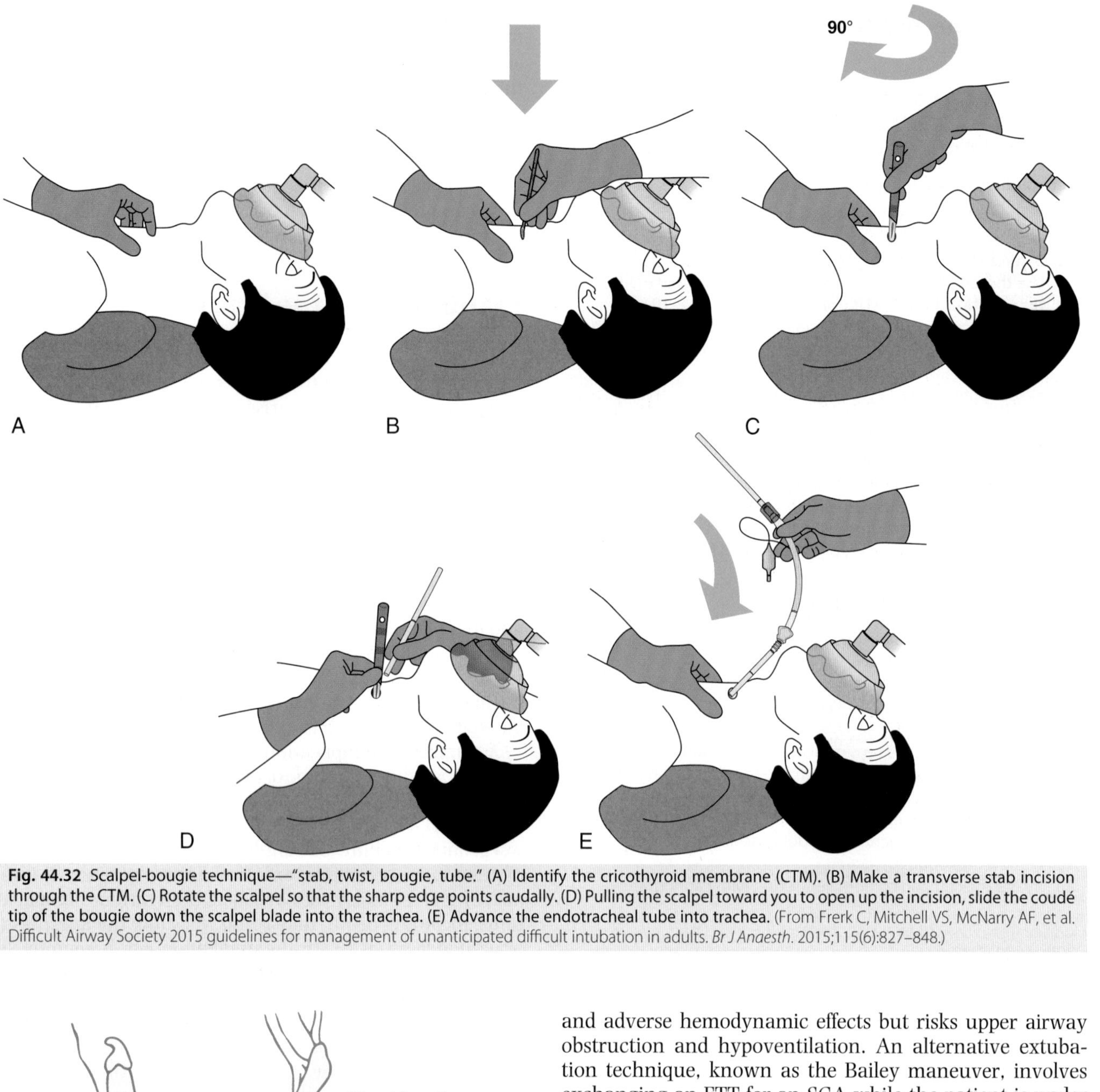

Fig. 44.32 Scalpel-bougie technique—"stab, twist, bougie, tube." (A) Identify the cricothyroid membrane (CTM). (B) Make a transverse stab incision through the CTM. (C) Rotate the scalpel so that the sharp edge points caudally. (D) Pulling the scalpel toward you to open up the incision, slide the coudé tip of the bougie down the scalpel blade into the trachea. (E) Advance the endotracheal tube into trachea. (From Frerk C, Mitchell VS, McNarry AF, et al. Difficult Airway Society 2015 guidelines for management of unanticipated difficult intubation in adults. *Br J Anaesth*. 2015;115(6):827–848.)

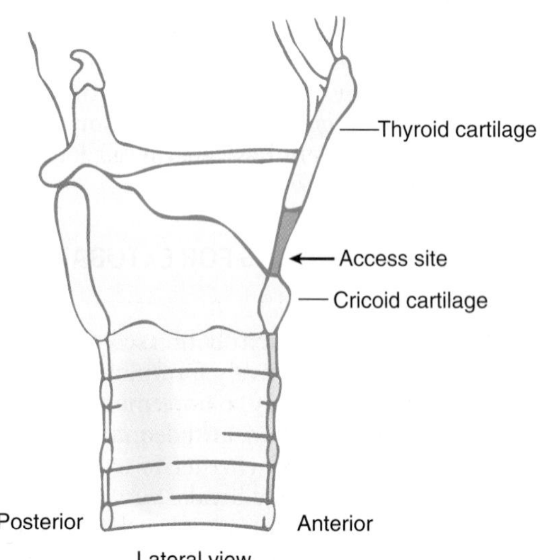

Fig. 44.33 Midsagittal anatomy of the larynx and trachea. The access point for percutaneous cricothyrotomy is in the lower third of the cricothyroid membrane. (Courtesy Cook Critical Care; Bloomington, IN.)

and adverse hemodynamic effects but risks upper airway obstruction and hypoventilation. An alternative extubation technique, known as the Bailey maneuver, involves exchanging an ETT for an SGA while the patient is under deep anesthesia.[258] Extubation during a light plane of anesthesia (stage II) can increase the risk for laryngospasm and other airway complications and should be avoided.

General preparations for extubation should include ensuring adequate reversal or recovery from neuromuscular blockade, hemodynamic stability, normothermia, and adequate analgesia. Patients should be preoxygenated with a 100% fraction of inspired oxygen concentration (FIO_2), and alveolar recruitment maneuvers should be considered if appropriate. Suctioning of the pharynx (and the trachea, if indicated), the removal of throat packs, and the placement of a bite block should be performed while the patient is under deep anesthesia.[22] Bite blocks are essential for an awake intubation to prevent biting of the tube during emergence, which can result in airway obstruction and the development of negative-pressure pulmonary edema. Oropharyngeal airways are not recommended for use as a

Box 44.5 Complications Associated with Extubation

- Laryngospasm and bronchospasm
- Upper airway obstruction
- Hypoventilation
- Hemodynamic changes (hypertension, tachycardia)
- Coughing and straining, leading to surgical wound dehiscence
- Laryngeal or airway edema
- Negative-pressure pulmonary edema
- Paradoxical vocal cord motion
- Arytenoid dislocation
- Aspiration

bite block because they can result in dental damage; rather, taped, rolled gauze securely inserted between the molars should be used.[259]

Gastric insufflation with air can increase the risk of pulmonary aspiration after extubation and can impede ventilation. Patients in whom mask ventilation with high pressures is necessary should have an orogastric tube placed and suctioned before extubation.

The sniffing position is the standard position for extubation; its major advantage is that the patient is optimally positioned for airway management, if necessary. Patients who are morbidly obese and other patients at risk for hypoventilation and airway obstruction can benefit from extubation in the head-up position. The lateral decubitus position may be the preferred option when the risk for pulmonary aspiration is high.[22]

Application of positive pressure immediately before cuff deflation may help expel secretions that have collected above the ETT cuff. Inspection of the pilot balloon to ensure complete cuff deflation before extubation is essential; extubation with an inflated cuff can cause vocal cord injury or arytenoid dislocation.

EXTUBATION AND REINTUBATION OF THE DIFFICULT AIRWAY

Many surgical and anesthetic factors can increase extubation risk. A summary of the most pertinent factors is listed in Box 44.6. Although several techniques can be used to manage extubation of the difficult airway, including the Bailey maneuver and remifentanil infusion,[257] the use of an airway exchange catheter (AEC) is most common and recommended by the ASA's Task Force on Management of the Difficult Airway. This hollow reintubation guide is passed through the ETT before extubation and kept in situ until the possible need for reintubation has passed. AECs have the additional capability of maintaining oxygenation or monitoring respiration by connection to a capnograph. Smaller AECs (11Fr) are generally well-tolerated by awake patients, who can breathe, talk, and cough around them. They should be secured with tape in place to prevent accidental dislodgement and labeled to distinguish them from traditional feeding tubes, which can have a similar appearance. Reintubation over an AEC, if necessary, can be facilitated by gentle DL to retract the tongue and oropharyngeal soft tissue.

Box 44.6 Factors Associated with Increased Extubation Risk

Airway Risk Factors

- Known difficult airway
- Airway deterioration (bleeding, edema, trauma)
- Restricted airway access
- Obesity and obstructive sleep apnea
- Aspiration risk

General Risk Factors

- Cardiovascular disease
- Respiratory disease
- Neuromuscular disease
- Metabolic derangements
- Special surgical requirements

Modified from Popat M, Mitchell V, Dravid R, et al. Difficult Airway Society guidelines for the management of tracheal extubation. *Anaesthesia.* 2012;67:318–340.

Dissemination of Critical Airway Information

As stated earlier, one of the most predictive factors for difficult intubation is a history of previous difficulty with intubation. Therefore it is crucial that critical airway information be documented and disseminated in such a way that clinicians who subsequently care for a patient with a difficult airway be alerted to the history and obtain the necessary information to safely manage the patient's airway. The ASA Practice Guidelines for Management of the Difficult Airway recommend the that clinicians document the difficulty with airway management and inform the patient or responsible person of the difficulty encountered.[7] Consideration of notification systems, such as a written report or letter to the patient, a written report in the medical chart, communication with the patient's surgeon or primary caregiver, a notification bracelet or equivalent identification device, and/or chart flags is recommended.

In 1992, the MedicAlert Foundation National Difficult Airway/Intubation Registry was created to standardize the documentation and dissemination of critical airway information. By 2010, more than 11,000 patients were included in the registry.[260] Patients with a difficult airway should be directed to the MedicAlert website.

Summary

Airway management is at the core of safe anesthetic practice. The anesthesia practitioner must have a fundamental knowledge of airway anatomy, physiology, and pharmacology, and well-developed skills in the use of a wide variety of airway devices. Although most airways are straightforward, management of the difficult airway remains one of the most relevant and challenging tasks for anesthesia care providers. Prediction and anticipation of the difficult airway and the formulation of an airway management plan are essential. Many airway problems can be solved with relatively simple devices and techniques; however, experience and good clinical judgment are necessary for their successful application. Newer airway devices with the potential to improve patient outcomes are continually being developed. Anesthesia providers must concurrently develop their skills and learn new techniques to be prepared when difficulty presents itself. Competency-based training with routine assessment of clinical ability with airway techniques is likely in the future for all practitioners involved in airway management. Expertise comes from dedicated practice and a commitment from the practitioner for career-long learning.

Complete references available online at expertconsult.com.

References

1. Peterson GN, et al. *Anesthesiology*. 103:33, 2005.
2. Metzner J, et al. *Best Pract Res Clin Anaesthesiol*. 2011;25:263.
3. Cook TM, et al. *Br J Anaesth*. 2011;106(5):617.
4. Cook TM, MacDougall-Davis SR. *Br J Anaesth*. 2012;109(suppl 1):i68.
5. Behringer EC. *Anesthesiol Clin North America*. 20:813, 2002.
6. *Anesthesiology*. 1993;78:597.
7. Apfelbaum JL, et al. *Anesthesiology*. 2013;118:251.
8. Frerk C, et al. *Br J Anaesth*. 2015;115(6):827.
9. Law JA, et al. *Can J Anaesth*. 2013;60(11):1119.
10. Law JA, et al. *Can J Anaesth*. 2013;60(11):1089.
11. Langeron O, *Anesthesiology Annales francaises d'anesthesie et de reanimation*. 2008;27(1):41.
12. Piepho T, et al. *Anaesthesist*. 2015;64(suppl 1):27.
13. Petrini F, et al. *Minerva anestesiologica*. 2005;71(11):617.
14. Japanese Society of Anesthesiologists. *J Anesth*. 2014;28(4):482.
15. Artime CA, et al. Airway algorithms and guidelines. In: Berkow LC, et al, eds. *Cases in Emergency Airway Management*. Cambridge, UK, 2015, Cambridge University Press; 10–18.
16. Kovacs G, et al. Human factors in airway management. In: Kovacs G, Law JA, eds. *Airway Management in Emergencies: aimeairway.ca*. 2018.
17. Chrimes N. *Br J Anaesth*. 2016;117(suppl 1):i20.
18. Reitzen SD, et al. *Ear Nose Throat J*. 2011;90:112.
19. Ahmed-Nusrath A, et al. *Br J Anaesth*. 2008;100:269.
20. Cavusoglu T, et al. *J Craniofac Surg*. 2009;20:566.
21. Zwank M. *Am J Emerg Med*. 2009;27:513.
22. Henderson J. Airway management. In: Miller RD, ed. *Miller's Anesthesia*. 7th ed. Philadelphia: Churchill Livingstone; 2010:1573.
23. Srirompotong S. Art-Smart T. *Eur Arch Otorhinolaryngol*. 2003;260:401.
24. Krebs MJ, Sakai T. *J Clin Anesth*. 2008;20:218.
25. Hirshoren N, et al. *J Trauma*. 2009;67:891.
26. Hillman DR, et al. *Br J Anaesth*. 2003;91:31.
27. Kuna ST. *Respir Physiol*. 2000;119:155.
28. Reber A, et al. *Anesthesiology*. 1999;90:1617.
29. Leder SB, et al. *Ann Otol Rhinol Laryngol*. 2010;119:795.
30. Coleman L, et al. Functional anatomy of the airway. In: Hagberg CA, ed. *Benumof's Airway Management: Principles and Practice*. 2nd ed. Philadelphia: Mosby; 2012:3.
31. Lundstrom LH, et al. *Anaesthesia*. 2009;64:1081.
32. Kheterpal S, et al. *Anesthesiology*. 2006;105:885.
33. Yildiz TS, et al. *J Anesth*. 2005;19:7.
34. Gonzalez H, et al. *Anesth Analg*. 2008;106:1132.
35. Brodsky JB, et al. *Anesth Analg*. 2002;94:732.
36. Shiga T, et al. *Anesthesiology*. 2005;103:429.
37. Mallampati SR. *Can Anaesth Soc J*. 1983;30:316.
38. Mashour GA, et al. *Anesth Analg*. 2008;107:1919.
39. Samsoon GL, Young JR. *Anaesthesia*. 1987;42:487.
40. Lundstrom LH, et al. *Br J Anaesth*. 2011;107:659.
41. Mashour GA, Sandberg WS. *Anesth Analg*. 2006;103:1256.
42. Hegde HV, et al. *Eur J Anaesthesiol*. 2012;29:338.
43. Ezri T, et al. *Anesth Analg*. 2001;93:1073.
44. Fang B, Norris J. *Anesth Analg*. 2004;98:870.
45. Grover VK, et al. *Anesth Analg*. 2003;96:911.
46. Racine SX, et al. *Anesthesiology*. 2010;112:1190.
47. El-Orbany M, et al. *Anesth Analg*. 2011;113:103.
48. Karkouti K, Rose DK, et al. *Can J Anaesth*. 2000;47(8):730.
49. Iohom G, et al. *Eur J Anaesthesiol*. 2003;20:31.
50. Wilson ME, et al. *Br J Anaesth*. 1988;61:211.
51. Calder I, et al. *Anaesthesia*. 1995;50:756.
52. Khan ZH, et al. *Anesth Analg*. 2003;96:595.
53. Eberhart LH, et al. *Anesth Analg*. 2005;101:284.
54. el-Ganzouri AR, et al. *Anesth Analg*. 1996;82:1197.
55. Norskov AK, et al. *Br J Anaesth*. 2016;116(5):680.
56. Langeron O, et al. *Anesthesiology*. 2012;117:1223.
57. Kristensen MS, Teoh WH. Ultrasonography in Airway Management. In: Hagberg CA, et al. eds. *Hagberg and Benumof's Airway Management*. 4th ed. Philadelphia, PA: Elsevier; 2018:74–91.
58. Ahmad I, et al. *J Clin Anesth*. 2015;27(6):508.
59. Cuendet GL, et al. *IEEE Trans Biomed Eng*. 2016;63(2):328.
60. Tanoubi I, et al. *Can J Anaesth*. 2009;56:449.
61. Benumof JL. *Anesthesiology*. 1999;91:603.
62. Dixon BJ, et al. *Anesthesiology*. 2005;102:1110.
63. Patel A, Nouraei SA. *Anaesthesia*. 2015;70(3):323.
64. Dixon BJ, et al. *Anesthesiology*. 2005;102(6):1110; discussion 1115A.
65. Ramkumar V, et al. *J Anesth*. 2011;25:189.
66. Futier E, et al. *Anesthesiology*. 2011;114:1354.
67. Herriger A, et al. *Anaesthesia*. 2004;59:243.
68. Levitan RM, et al. Preoxygenation. In: Hagberg CA, Artime CA, Aziz MF, eds. *Hagberg and Benumof's Airway Management*. 4th ed. Philadelphia, PA: Elsevier; 2018:249–264.
69. Levitan RM. NO DESAT! (Nasal oxygen during efforts securing a tube). *Emergency Physicians Monthly*. 2010.
70. Teller LE, et al. *Anesthesiology*. 1988;69(6):980.
71. Baraka AS, et al. *Anaesthesia*. 2007;62(8):769.
72. Ramachandran SK, et al. *J Clin Anesth*. 2010;22(3):164.
73. Binks MJ, et al. *Am J Emerg Med*. 2017;35(10):1542.
74. Pavlov I, et al. *Am J Emerg Med*. 2017;35(8):1184.
75. Mendelson CL. *Am J Obstet Gynecol*. 1946;52:191.
76. *Anesthesiology*. 2017;126(3):376.
77. Smith I, et al. *Eur J Anaesthesiol*. 2011;28:556.
78. Mahajan V, et al. *J Clin Anesth*. 2015;27(5):396.
79. Paranjothy S, et al. *Cochrane Database Syst Rev*. 2014;(2):CD004943.
80. Artime CA, Sanchez A. Preparation of the patient for awake intubation. In: Hagberg CA, et al. eds. *Hagberg and Benumof's Airway Management*. 4th ed. Philadelphia, PA: Elsevier; 2018:216–234.
81. Kim YH, et al. *Yonsei Med J*. 2009;50:380.
82. Al-alami AA, et al. *Curr Opin Anaesthesiol*. 2009;22:388.
83. Silva DA, Sanders I. *Ann Otol Rhinol Laryngol*. 1992;101(11):893.
84. Cooper RM. Extubation and Reintubation of the Difficult AIrway. In: Hagberg CA, et al. eds. *Hagberg and Benumof's Airway Management*. 4th ed. Philadelphia, PA: Elsevier; 2018:844–867.
85. Dorsey DP, Joffe AM. Physiologic and Pathophysiologic Responses to Intubation. In: Hagberg CA, et al. eds. *Hagberg and Benumof's Airway Management*. 4th ed. Philadelphia, PA: Elsevier; 2018:163–177.
86. Combes X, et al. *Br J Anaesth*. 2007;99:276.
87. Gal TJ. Airway management. In: Miller RD, ed. *Miller's Anesthesia*. ed 6. Philadelphia: Churchill Livingstone; 2005:1617.
88. El-Orbany MI, et al. *Br J Anaesth*. 2005;95:710.
89. El-Orbany MI, et al. *J Clin Anesth*. 2003;15:9.
90. Lieutaud T, et al. *Can J Anaesth*. 2003;50:121.
91. Naguib M, et al. *Anesth Analg*. 2010;111:110.
92. Heier T, et al. *Anesthesiology*. 2001;94:754.
93. Lee C, et al. *Anesthesiology*. 2009;110:1020.
94. Broomhead RH, et al. *Br J Anaesth*. 2010;104:313.
95. Goodwin MW, et al. *Anaesthesia*. 2003;58:60.
96. Ikeda A, et al. *Anesthesiology*. 2012;117:487.
97. Warters RD, et al. *Anaesthesia*. 2011;66:163.
98. Calder I, Yentis SM. *Anaesthesia*. 2008;63:113.
99. Sellick BA. *Lancet*. 1961;2:404.
100. Vanner RG, Asai T. *Anaesthesia*. 1999;54:1.
101. El-Orbany M, Connolly LA. *Anesth Analg*. 2010;110:1318.
102. Koerber JP, et al. *Anaesthesia*. 2009;64:54.
103. Rosen MA. *Anesthesiology*. 1999;91:1159.
104. de Souza DG, et al. *Anesth Analg*. 2010;110:1503.
105. Paech MJ. *Anaesth Intensive Care*. 2010;38:989.
106. Stept WJ, Safar P. *Anesth Analg*. 1970;49:633.
107. Deepika K, et al. *J Clin Anesth*. 1992;4:106.
108. Williamson RM, et al. *Acta Anaesthesiol Scand*. 2011;55:694.
109. Thorn K, et al. *Anesth Analg*. 2005;100:1200.
110. Smith KJ, et al. *Anesthesiology*. 2003;99:60.
111. Palmer JH, Ball DR. *Anaesthesia*. 2000;55:263.
112. Rice MJ, et al. *Anesth Analg*. 2009;109:1546.
113. Ehrenfeld JM, et al. *Anesth Analg*. 2012;115:95.

114. Clements P, et al. *Br J Hosp Med (Lond)*. 2009;70:424.
115. El-Orbany MI, et al. *J Clin Anesth*. 2002;14:115.
116. Wappler F, et al. *Eur J Anaesthesiol*. 2003;20:548.
117. Lee SY, et al. *Br J Anaesth*. 2012;110:81.
118. Kim SH, et al. *Anaesth Intensive Care*. 2011;39:899.
119. Kim JY, et al. *Acta Anaesthesiol Scand*. 2008;52:106.
120. Wei LX, et al. *Acta Academiae Medicinae Sinicae*. 2008;30:723.
121. Hung CT, et al. *Chang Gung Med J*. 2005;28:174.
122. Kim KS, et al. *J Anesth*. 2011;25:195.
123. Mahboobi N, et al. *East Mediterr Health J*. 2012;18:159.
124. Kong CF, et al. *Br J Anaesth*. 2000;85:364.
125. Lee J, Jung CW. *Korean J Anesthesiol*. 2011;60:12.
126. Erhan E, et al. *Can J Anaesth*. 2003;50:108.
127. Gore MS, Harnagale KD. *J Anaesthesiol Clin Pharmacol*. 2011;27:27.
128. Erhan E, et al. *Eur J Anaesthesiol*. 2003;20:37.
129. Aissaoui Y, et al. *Eur J Anaesthesiol*. 2012;29:391.
130. Bouvet L, et al. *Anaesthesia*. 2009;64:719.
131. Politis GD, Tobias JD. *Paediatr Anaesth*. 2007;17:285.
132. Lundstrom LH, et al. *Br J Anaesth*. 2009;103:283.
133. Mencke T, et al. *Anesthesiology*. 2003;98:1049.
134. Abrams JT, et al. *Anesth Analg*. 1996;83:629.
135. Scamman FL. *Anesth Analg*. 1983;62:332.
136. Bennett JA, et al. *Anesthesiology*. 1997;87:1070.
137. Kohno T, Ikoma M. *Masui*. 2008;57:1213.
138. Benumof JL. *Anesthesiology*. 1991;75:1087.
139. Thomas JL. *Anaesthesia*. 1969;24:28.
140. Rosenstock CV, et al. *Anesthesiology*. 2012;116:1210.
141. Xue FS, et al. *Eur J Anaesthesiol*. 2012;29:209; author reply 210–211.
142. Xue FS, et al. *Chin Med J (Engl)*. 2009;122:408.
143. Sarma J. *J Clin Anesth*. 2007;19:322.
144. Raval C, et al. *Saudi J Anaesth*. 2010;4:38.
145. Bekhit MH. Lidocaine for neural blockade. In: Sinatra RS, et al. eds. *The Essence of Analgesia and Analgesics*. New York: Cambridge University Press; 2011:279.
146. Simmons ST, Schleich AR. *Reg Anesth Pain Med*. 2002;27:180.
147. Novaro GM, et al. *J Am Soc Echocardiogr*. 2003;16:170.
148. Cara DM, et al. *Anaesthesia*. 2003;58:777.
149. Gross JB, et al. *Anesth Analg*. 1984;63:915.
150. Walsh ME, Shorten GD. *Yale J Biol Med*. 1998;71:537.
151. British Thoracic Society Bronchoscopy Guidelines Committee: a Subcommittee of Standards of Care Committee of British Thoracic Society. *Thorax*. 2001;56(suppl 1):i1.
152. Williams KA, et al. *Br J Anaesth*. 2005;95:549.
153. Reed AP. *Chest*. 1992;101:244.
154. von Goedecke A, et al. *Anesth Analg*. 2004;98:260.
155. Joffe AM, et al. *Anesthesiology*. 2010;113:873.
156. Weiler N, et al. *Prehosp Disaster Med*. 1995;10:101.
157. Safar P, et al. *J Appl Physiol*. 1959;14:760.
158. Isono S, et al. *Anesthesiology*. 2005;103:489.
159. Kok PH, et al. *Singapore Med J*. 2001;42:322.
160. Wang KC, et al. *Acta Anaesthesiol Taiwan*. 2006;44:119.
161. Brain AI. *Br J Anaesth*. 1983;55:801.
162. Brimacombe J. *Can J Anaesth*. 1995;42:1017.
163. Yu SH, Beirne OR. *J Oral Maxillofac Surg*. 2010;68:2359.
164. Lindsay HA, et al. Supraglottic Airway Techniques: Laryngeal Mask Airways. In: Hagberg CA, et al. eds. *Hagberg and Benumof's Airway Management*. 4th ed. Philadelphia, PA: Elsevier; 2018:328–348.
165. Miller DM. *Anesth Analg*. 2004;99:1553.
166. Vaida S, et al. Supraglottic Airway Techniques: Nonlaryngeal Mask Airways. In: Hagberg CA, et al. eds. *Hagberg and Benumof's Airway Management*. 4th ed. Philadelphia, PA: Elsevier; 2018:349–370.
167. Asai T, Brimacombe J. *Anaesthesia*. 2000;55:1179.
168. Brimacombe J, et al. *Br J Anaesth*. 2005;95:420.
169. Vannucci A, et al. *Anesth Analg*. 2018;126(6):1959.
170. Grady DM, et al. *Anesthesiology*. 2001;94:760.
171. Siddik-Sayyid SM, et al. *Anesth Analg*. 2005;100:1204.
172. Hui JK, et al. *Can J Anaesth*. 2002;49:508.
173. Bouvet L, et al. *Can J Anaesth*. 2010;57:222.
174. Jaffe RA, Brock-Utne JG. *J Clin Anesth*. 2002;14:462.
175. Nakayama S, et al. *Paediatr Anaesth*. 2002;12:416.
176. Weber S. *Anesthesiol Clin North America*. 2002;20:503.
177. Dingley J, et al. *Anaesthesia*. 1994;49:251.
178. Burgard G, et al. *J Clin Anesth*. 1996;8:198.
179. Brimacombe J, Costa e Silva L. *Eur J Anaesthesiol*. 2003;20:502.
180. Emmett SR, et al. *Br J Anaesth*. 2012;109:468.
181. Cook TM, et al. *Can J Anaesth*. 2005;52:739.
182. Handa-Tsutsui F, Kodaka M. *J Clin Anesth*. 2005;17:344.
183. Sharma V, et al. *Br J Anaesth*. 2010;105:228.
184. Abdi W, et al. *Acta Anaesthesiol Scand*. 2010;54:141.
185. Maltby JR, et al. *Can J Anaesth*. 2002;49:857.
186. Abdi W, et al. *Obes Surg*. 2009;19:1624.
187. Yao T, et al. *Zhonghua Yi Xue Za Zhi*. 2010;90:2048.
188. Gaitini LA, et al. *Anesthesiology*. 2001;94:79.
189. Mort TC. *Anesth Analg*. 2006;103:1264.
190. Ochs M, et al. *Prehosp Emerg Care*. 2000;4:333.
191. Oczenski W, et al. *Anaesthesia*. 1999;54:1161.
192. Gaitini LA, et al. *J Clin Anesth*. 2011;23:475.
193. Sultan P, et al. *J Perioper Pract*. 2011;21:379.
194. Sparrow KA, et al. Intubating Introducers and Lighted and Optical Stylets. In: Hagberg CA, et al. eds. *Hagberg and Benumof's Airway Management*. 4th ed. Philadelphia, PA: Elsevier; 2018:402–416.
195. Artime C. Flexible Fiberoptic Intubation. In: Hagberg CA, et al. eds. *The Difficult Airway: A Practical Guide*. Oxford: Oxford University Press; 2013:97–108.
196. Bannister FB, Macbeth RG. *Lancet*. 1944;2:651.
197. Adnet F, et al. *Anesthesiology*. 2001;94:83.
198. Chou HC, Wu TL. *Acta Anaesthesiol Scand*. 2001;45:261.
199. Greenland KB, et al. *Br J Anaesth*. 2010;105:683.
200. Isono S. *Anesthesiology*. 2001;95:825.
201. Park SH, et al. *J Anesth*. 2010;24:526.
202. Greenland KB, et al. *Br J Anaesth*. 2010;104:268.
203. Takenaka I, et al. *Can J Anaesth*. 2007;54:129.
204. Jain RR, Cameron SD. Airway Management in Pediatric Patients. In: Hagberg CA, et al. eds. *Hagberg and Benumof's Airway Management*. 4th ed. Philadelphia, PA: Elsevier; 2018:608–639.
205. Baker PA, Timmermann A. Laryngoscopic Tracheal Intubation. In: Hagberg CA, et al. eds. *Hagberg and Benumof's Airway Management*. 4th ed. Philadelphia, PA: Elsevier; 2018:371–390.
206. Cormack RS. *Lehane J: Anaesthesia*. 1984;39:1105.
207. Yentis SM, Lee DJ. *Anaesthesia*. 1998;53:1041.
208. Ochroch EA, et al. *Can J Anaesth*. 1999;46:987.
209. Straker T, Urdaneta F. Confirmation of Tracheal Intubation. In: Hagberg CA, et al. eds. *Hagberg and Benumof's Airway Management*. 4th ed. Philadelphia, PA: Elsevier; 2018:540.
210. Hung MH, et al. *Anesth Analg*. 2008;107:1704.
211. Cattano D, Cavallone L. *Anesthesiology News*. 2011;37:17.
212. Asai T, Shingu K. *Br J Anaesth*. 2004;92:870.
213. Kristensen MS. *Anesthesiology*. 2003;98:354.
214. Lu Y, et al. *Anaesthesia*. 2011;66:1160.
215. Rudolph C, et al. *Anaesthesia*. 2005;60:668.
216. Shollik NA, et al. *Case Rep Anesthesiol*. 2012;2012:297.
217. Mazeres JE, et al. *Eur J Anaesthesiol*. 2011;28:646.
218. Abramson SI, et al. *Anesth Analg*. 2008;106:1215.
219. Xue FS, et al. *J Clin Anesth*. 2009;21:154.
220. Sorbello M, et al. *Anesth Analg*. 2009;108:386.
221. Aziz M, Metz S. *Anaesthesia*. 2011;66:579.
222. Van Zundert AA, Pieters BM. *Br J Anaesth*. 2012;108:327.
223. Xue FS, et al. *Eur J Anaesthesiol*. 2009;26:261.
224. Biro P, et al. *Br J Anaesth*. 2006;97:255.
225. Greif R, et al. *Anaesthesia*. 2010;65:525.
226. Kaplan MB, et al. *J Clin Anesth*. 2006;18:357.
227. Aziz MF, et al. *Anesthesiology*. 2012;116:629.
228. Jungbauer A, et al. *Br J Anaesth*. 2009;102:546.
229. Asai T, et al. *Anesthesiology*. 2009;110:898.
230. Aziz MF, et al. *Anesthesiology*. 2011;114:34.
231. Moore AR, et al. *Anaesthesia*. 2012;67:232.
232. Xue FS, et al. *Anesthesiology*. 2013;118:462.
233. Aziz M, Brambrink A. Video-Assisted Laryngoscopy. In: Hagberg CA, et al. eds. *Hagberg and Benumof's Airway Management*. 4th ed. Philadelphia, PA: Elsevier; 2018:417–427.
234. McElwain J, et al. *Anaesthesia*. 2010;65:483.
235. Ng I, et al. *Br J Anaesth*. 2012;109:439.
236. Cavus E, et al. *Anesth Analg*. 2010;110:473.
237. Maassen R, et al. *Anesth Analg*. 2009;109:1560.
238. van Zundert A, et al. *Anesth Analg*. 2009;109:825.
239. Meininger D, et al. *Anaesthesist*. 2010;59:806.
240. Jones PM, et al. *Can J Anaesth*. 2011;58:256.
241. Cattano D, et al. *Intern Emerg Med*. 2012;7:59.
242. Dupanovic M. *J Clin Anesth*. 2010;22:152.

243. Komasawa N, et al. *J Anesth*. 2011;25:898.
244. Komasawa N, et al. *Masui*. 2011;60:84.
245. Ferrario L. Intubation stylets. In: Hagberg CA, et al. eds. *The Difficult Airway: A Practical Guide*. Oxford: Oxford University Press; 2013:83.
246. Normand KC, Aucoin AP. Retrograde intubation. In: Hagberg CA, et al. eds. *The Difficult Airway: A Practical Guide*. Oxford: Oxford University Press; 2013:109.
247. Hsu HT, et al. *Anaesthesia*. 2012;67:411.
248. Pinsky JR, Hagberg CA. Combination Techniques. In: Hagberg CA, et al. eds. *The Difficult Airway: A Practical Guide*. Oxford: Oxford University Press; 2013:143–154.
249. Ohchi F, et al. *Am J Emerg Med*. 2017;35(4):584.
250. Budde AO, Pott LM. *J Clin Anesth*. 2008;20(7):560.
251. Pieters BM, et al. *Anesth Analg*. 2018;126(3):988.
252. Normand KC. Percutaneous transtracheal jet ventilation. In: Hagberg CA, et al. eds. *The Difficult Airway: A Practical Guide*. Oxford: Oxford University Press; 2013:117.
253. Hamaekers AE, et al. *Br J Anaesth*. 2012;108(6):1017.
254. Fearnley RA, et al. *J Clin Anesth*. 2016;33:233.
255. Normand KC. Cricothyrotomy. In: Hagberg CA, et al. eds. *The Difficult Airway: A Practical Guide*. Oxford: Oxford University Press; 2013:125.
256. Asai T, et al. *Br J Anaesth*. 1998;80:767.
257. Popat M, et al. *Anaesthesia*. 2012;67:318.
258. Nair I, Bailey PM. *Anaesthesia*. 1995;50:174.
259. Falzon D, et al. *Anaesthesia*. 2012;67:919; author reply 921.
260. Foley L, et al. Dissemination of Critical Airway Information. In: Hagberg CA, et al. eds. *Hagberg and Benumof's Airway Management*. 4th ed. Philadelphia, PA: Elsevier; 2018:905–910.

45 Spinal, Epidural, and Caudal Anesthesia

RICHARD BRULL, ALAN J.R. MACFARLANE, and VINCENT W.S. CHAN

KEY POINTS

- The distal termination of the spinal cord varies from L3 in infants to the lower border of L1 in adults.
- The speed of neural blockade depends on the size, surface area, and degree of myelination of the nerve fibers exposed to the local anesthetic.
- Blockade of the peripheral (T1-L2) and cardiac (T1-T4) sympathetic fibers is responsible for the decrease in arterial blood pressure (cardiac output and systemic vascular resistance) associated with neuraxial techniques.
- Cerebrospinal fluid volume and local anesthetic baricity are the most important determinants for the spread (i.e., block height) of spinal anesthesia.
- The use of smaller-gauge spinal needles decreases the incidence of post–dural puncture headache.
- Serious neurologic complications associated with neuraxial blockade are rare, but the risk increases in the elderly and those with preexisting spinal pathology.
- The use of low-molecular-weight heparin and potent platelet inhibitors increases the risk of epidural hematoma from neuraxial blockade.
- Epidural blood patches are greater than 90% effective in relieving post–dural puncture headache.
- Local anesthetic systemic toxicity results from unintentional administration of the drug into an epidural vein.
- Use of neuraxial blockade, particularly when used as the sole anesthetic, can reduce perioperative morbidity and may reduce mortality.

Principles

Spinal, epidural, and caudal neuraxial blocks result in one or a combination of sympathetic blockade, sensory blockade, or motor blockade depending on the dose, concentration, or volume of local anesthetic administered. Despite these similarities, there are significant technical, physiologic, and pharmacologic differences. Spinal anesthesia requires a small mass (i.e., volume) of drug that is almost devoid of systemic pharmacologic effects to produce rapid (<5 minutes), profound, reproducible sensory analgesia. In contrast, epidural and caudal anesthesia progress more slowly (>20 minutes) after a large mass of local anesthetic that produces pharmacologically active systemic blood levels, which may be associated with side effects and complications unknown to spinal anesthesia. The introduction of combined spinal and epidural techniques blurs some of these differences, but also adds flexibility to clinical care.

Practice

Neuraxial blockade has a wide range of clinical applications for surgery, obstetrics, acute postoperative pain management, and chronic pain relief. Single-injection spinal or epidural anesthesia with local anesthetic is most commonly used for surgery to the lower abdomen, pelvic organs (e.g., prostate), and lower limbs, and for cesarean deliveries. Continuous catheter-based epidural infusions of dilute local anesthetics and opioids are used for obstetric labor analgesia and postoperative pain relief after major surgery (e.g., thoracic, abdominal, and less commonly lower limb) to provide analgesia for days if required. Evidence demonstrating that epidural analgesia can reduce pulmonary morbidity and mortality in high-risk patients undergoing major thoracic and abdominal surgery served to propel the practice of epidural analgesia at the beginning of the millennium.[1] Caudal blocks are mostly performed for surgical anesthesia and analgesia in children, and for therapeutic analgesia in adults with chronic pain. Indwelling spinal catheters can be applied long term (from months to years) for the treatment of chronic malignant and nonmalignant pain.

Historical Perspectives

The first case of spinal anesthesia in humans was performed by August Bier in 1898 using the local anesthetic cocaine.[2] Subsequently, spinal anesthesia was successfully performed using procaine by Braun in 1905, tetracaine by Sise in 1935, lidocaine by Gordh in 1949, chloroprocaine by Foldes and McNall in 1952, mepivacaine by Dhunér and

Sternberg in 1961, and bupivacaine by Emblem in 1966. Spinal anesthesia using ropivacaine and levobupivacaine was introduced in the 1980s. The year 1901 marked the first reported use of intrathecal morphine described by Racoviceanu-Pitesti, as well as the first description of caudal anesthesia reported by Cathleen. Lumbar epidural anesthesia in humans was first described by Pagés in 1921, the loss-of-resistance technique by Dogliotti in the 1930s, continuous caudal for obstetrics by Hingson in 1941, and lumbar epidural catheterization for surgery by Curbelo in 1947.[3] The use of epidural morphine analgesia was first reported by Behar in 1979.

Despite the extensive experience using neuraxial techniques throughout the past century, several events caused major setbacks along the way, including the Woolley and Roe case detailing paraplegia after spinal anesthesia in 1954,[4] the reports of persistent neurologic deficits and adhesive arachnoiditis with spinal chloroprocaine in the early 1980s, and cauda equina syndrome with continuous spinal lidocaine anesthesia in the early 1990s.[5] More recently, the potential for catastrophic epidural hematoma with newer potent anticoagulants (e.g., low-molecular-weight heparin [LMWH]) and antiplatelet agents (e.g., clopidogrel) has caused concern.[6]

Anatomy

The spinal cord is continuous with the brainstem proximally and terminates distally in the conus medullaris as the filum terminale (fibrous extension) and the cauda equina (neural extension). This distal termination varies from L3 in infants to the lower border of L1 in adults because of differential growth rates between the bony vertebral canal and the central nervous system.

Surrounding the spinal cord in the bony vertebral column are three membranes (from innermost to outermost): the pia mater, the arachnoid mater, and the dura mater (Fig. 45.1). The cerebrospinal fluid (CSF) resides in the space between the pia mater and the arachnoid mater, termed the *subarachnoid* (or *intrathecal*) *space*. The pia mater is a highly vascular membrane that closely invests the spinal cord and brain. Approximately 500 mL of CSF is formed daily by the choroid plexuses of the cerebral ventricles, with 30 to 80 mL occupying the subarachnoid space from T11 to T12 downward. The arachnoid mater is a delicate, nonvascular membrane that functions as the principal barrier to drugs crossing into (and out of) the CSF and is estimated to account for 90% of the resistance to drug migration.[7] As Liu and McDonald[8] and Bernards[9] emphasize, the functional proof of the arachnoid's role as the primary barrier to flow is the observation that spinal CSF resides in the subarachnoid, and not the subdural, space. The outermost layer is the dura.

Surrounding the dura mater is the epidural space, which extends from the foramen magnum to the sacral hiatus and surrounds the dura mater anteriorly, laterally, and posteriorly. The epidural space is bound anteriorly by the posterior longitudinal ligament, laterally by the pedicles and intervertebral foramina, and posteriorly by the ligamentum flavum. Contents of the epidural space include the nerve roots and fat, areolar tissue, lymphatics, and blood vessels including the well-organized Batson venous plexus.

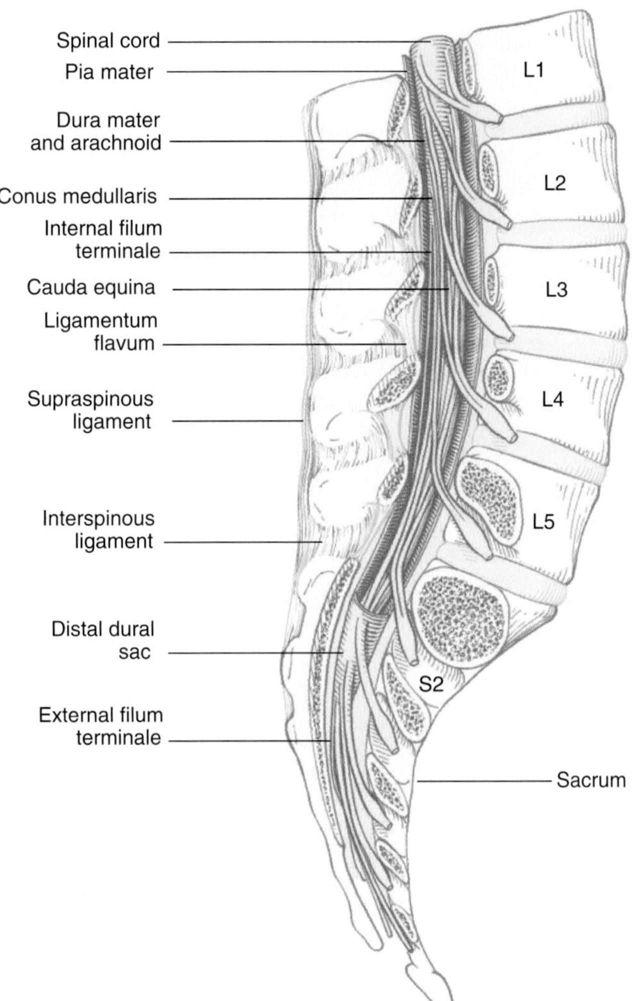

Fig. 45.1 Spinal cord anatomy. Notice the termination of the spinal cord (i.e., conus medullaris) at L1-L2 and termination of the dural sac at S2.

Posterior to the epidural space is the ligamentum flavum (the so-called yellow ligament), which extends from the foramen magnum to the sacral hiatus. Although classically portrayed as a single ligament, it is actually comprised of two ligamenta flava—the right and the left—which join in the middle and form an acute angle with a ventral opening (Fig. 45.2).[10,11] The ligamentum flavum is not uniform from skull to sacrum, nor even within an intervertebral space. Ligament thickness, distance to the dura, and skin-to-dura distance vary with the area of the vertebral canal. The vertebral canal is triangular and largest in area at the lumbar levels, and it is circular and smallest in area at the thoracic levels. The two ligamenta flava are variably joined (fused) in the midline, and this fusion or lack of fusion of the ligamenta flava occurs at different vertebral levels in individual patients.[10] Immediately posterior to the ligamentum flavum are the lamina and spinous processes of vertebral bodies or the interspinous ligaments. Extending from the external occipital protuberance to the coccyx posterior to these structures is the supraspinous ligament, which joins the vertebral spines (see Fig. 45.2).

There are 7 cervical vertebrae, 12 thoracic vertebrae, 5 lumbar vertebrae, and a sacrum. The vertebral arch, spinous process, pedicles, and laminae form the posterior

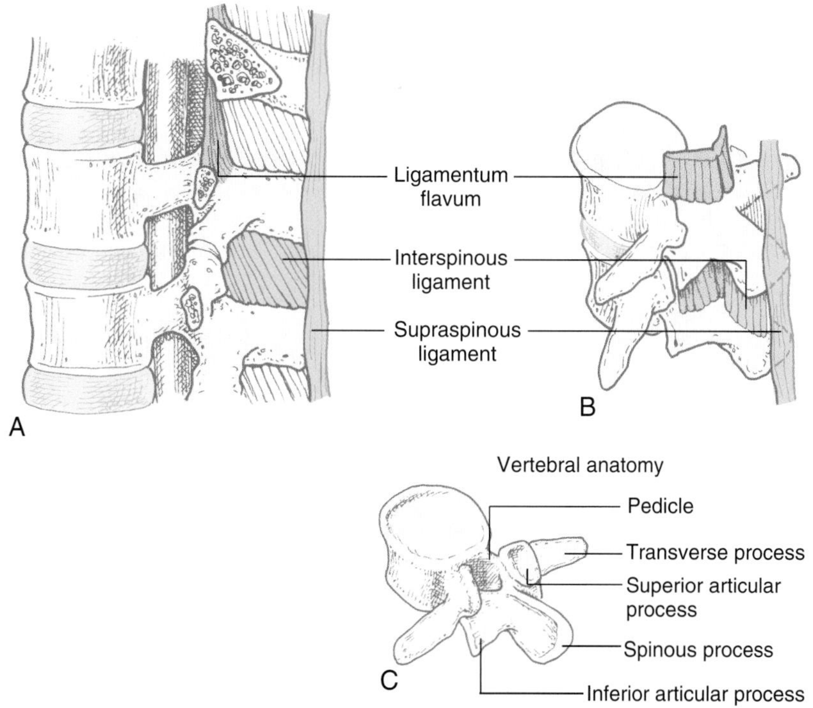

Fig. 45.2 Vertebral anatomy. (A) Sagittal view. (B) Oblique view of the lumbar vertebrae showing the ligamentum flavum thickening in the caudad extent of the intervertebral space and in the midline. (C) Oblique view of a single lumbar vertebra.

elements of the vertebra, and the vertebral body forms the anterior element. The vertebrae are joined together anteriorly by the fibrocartilaginous joints with the central disks containing the nucleus pulposus, and posteriorly by the zygapophyseal (facet) joints. The thoracic spinous process is angulated steeply caudad as opposed to the almost horizontal angulation of the lumbar spinous process. This is a clinically important distinction for needle insertion and advancement in the thoracic versus lumbar levels.

The sacral canal contains the terminal portion of the dural sac, which typically ends at S2. Variation is found in this feature as well, with the termination of the dural sac being lower in children. In addition to the dural sac, the sacral canal contains a venous plexus, which is part of the valveless internal vertebral venous plexus. The volume of the caudal canal in adults, excluding the foramina and dural sac ranges, is about 10 to 27 mL. Perhaps this wide variability in volume accounts for some of the variation in block height with caudal anesthesia (Fig. 45.3).[12]

BLOOD SUPPLY

Blood is supplied to the spinal cord from one anterior spinal artery (originating from the vertebral artery), two posterior spinal arteries (originating from the inferior cerebellar artery), and the segmental spinal arteries (originating from the intercostal and lumbar arteries).[13] The spinal arteries enter the spinal canal at each intervertebral foramen and give off branches to both the nerve roots and the medullary branches to the spinal cord; one of the major branches is the artery of Adamkiewicz, variably entering between T7 and L4 on the left, which supplies the lower thoracic and upper lumbar regions. The anterior two thirds of the spinal cord is supplied by the anterior arterial branches and the posterior one third by the posterior branches. The anterior and deep portion of the cord (gray matter) is most prone to ischemia (leading to anterior horn motor neuron injury, or anterior spinal syndrome) because there are fewer anterior medullary feeder vessels than posterior feeder vessels. Likewise, the midthoracic part of the spinal cord (from T3 to T9) is most at risk where segmental medullary feeder vessels are rare. Venous drainage of the spinal cord follows a similar distribution as the spinal arteries. There are three longitudinal anterior spinal veins and three posterior spinal veins that communicate with the segmental anterior and posterior radicular veins before draining into the internal vertebral venous plexus in the medial and lateral components of the epidural space. There are no veins in the posterior epidural space except those caudal to the L5-S1 disk.

Anatomic Variations

NERVE ROOTS

The spinal nerve roots are not uniform in size and structure. Specifically, Hogan and Toth[14,15] have shown that there is considerable interindividual variability in nerve root size. These differences may help to explain the interpatient differences in neuraxial block quality when equivalent techniques are used on seemingly similar patients. Another anatomic relationship may affect neuraxial blocks; although generally larger than the ventral (motor) roots, the dorsal (sensory) roots are often blocked more easily. This apparent paradox is explained by organization of the dorsal roots into component bundles, which creates a much larger surface area on which the local anesthetics act, possibly explaining why larger sensory nerves are blocked more easily than smaller motor nerves.[8]

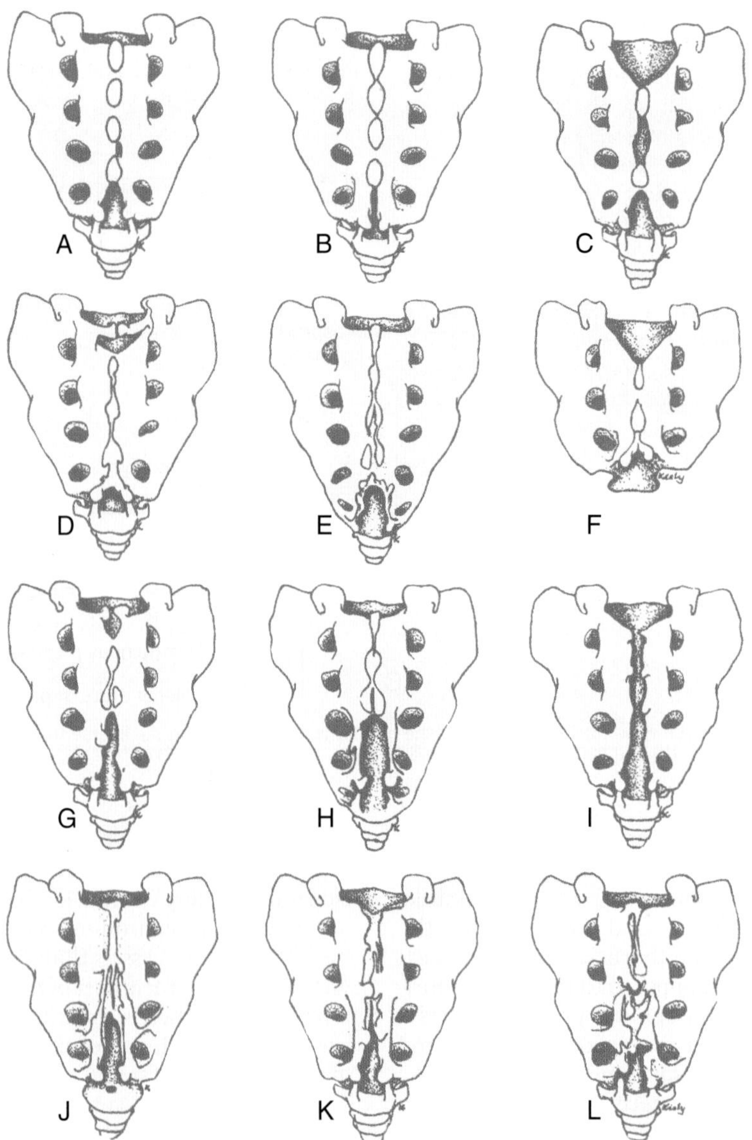

Fig. 45.3 Anatomic variants of the sacrum and sacral hiatus. (A) Normal. (B) Longitudinal slitlike hiatus. (C) Second midline hiatus. (D) Transverse hiatus. (E) Large hiatus with absent cornua. (F) Transverse hiatus with absent coccyx, two prominent cornua, and two proximal "decoy hiatuses lateral to the cornua." (G–I) Large midline defects contiguous with the sacral hiatus. (J–L) Enlarged longitudinal hiatuses, each with an overlying decoy hiatus. (From Willis RJ. Caudal epidural block. In: Cousins MN, Bridenbaugh PO, eds. *Neural blockade in clinical anesthesia and management of pain*. 2nd ed. Philadelphia: JB Lippincott; 1988:365.)

CEREBROSPINAL FLUID

Lumbosacral CSF has a constant pressure of approximately 15 cm H_2O, but its volume varies by patient, in part because of differences in body habitus and weight.[16] It is estimated that CSF volume accounts for 80% of the variability in peak block height and regression of sensory and motor blockade. Nevertheless, except for body weight (less CSF in subjects with high body mass index [BMI]), the volume of CSF does not correlate with other anthropomorphic measurements available clinically.[17] (See section, Factors Affecting Block Height, later in the chapter.)

EPIDURAL SPACE

Hogan's[10] study of frozen cryomicrotome cadaver sections suggests that the epidural space is more segmented and less uniform than previously believed from indirect anatomic analysis. Another study by Hogan[18] has also shown in cadavers that the spread of solution after epidural injection into the tissues of the epidural space is nonuniform, and he postulated that this accounts for the clinical unpredictability of epidural drug spread. This lack of uniformity also extends to age-related differences. There is evidence that adipose tissue in the epidural space diminishes with age,[19] and this decrease in epidural space in adipose tissue may dominate the age-related changes in epidural dose requirements (see Chapter 65).

Mechanism of Action

Local anesthetic binding to nerve tissue disrupts nerve transmission, resulting in neural blockade. For spinal and epidural anesthesia, the target binding sites are located within the spinal cord (superficial and deep portions) and on the spinal nerve roots in the subarachnoid and epidural spaces. The spinal nerve roots and dorsal root ganglia are considered the most important sites of action. Nerves in the subarachnoid space are highly accessible and easily anesthetized, even with a small dose of local anesthetic, compared with the extradural nerves, which are often ensheathed by dura mater (the "dural sleeve"). The speed of neural blockade depends on the size, surface area, and degree of myelination of the nerve fibers exposed to the local anesthetic. Anatomic studies show that the S1 and L5 posterior roots are the largest and thus most resistant to blockade during epidural anesthesia.[15] Smaller nerves are more sensitive to the effects of local anesthetics because of their relatively high membrane surface area to axon unit volume ratio. For example, the small preganglionic sympathetic fibers (B fibers, 1-3 μm, minimally myelinated) are most sensitive to local anesthetic blockade. Among the sensory nerves, the C fibers (0.3-1 μm, unmyelinated), which conduct cold temperature sensation, are blocked more readily or earlier than the A-delta fibers (1-4 μm, myelinated), which conduct pinprick sensation. The A-beta fibers (5-12 μm, myelinated), which conduct touch sensation, are the last to be affected among the sensory fibers. The larger A-alpha motor fibers (12-20 μm, myelinated) are more resistant than any of the sensory fibers. Regression of blockade ("recovery") follows in the reverse order: motor function followed first by touch, then pinprick, and finally cold sensation.[20] Another manifestation of relative sensitivity or susceptibility to the effects of local anesthetics is the observed differences in the peak block height (highest or most cephalad level of anesthesia) according to each sensory modality, which is termed *differential sensory block*. For example, the level of anesthesia to cold sensation (also an approximate level of sympathetic blockade) is most cephalad and is on average one to two spinal segments higher than the level of pinprick anesthesia, which in turn is one to two segments higher than the level of touch anesthesia.[21]

DRUG UPTAKE

When local anesthetic is injected directly into the subarachnoid space during spinal anesthesia, it diffuses through the pia mater and penetrates through the spaces of Virchow-Robin (extensions of the subarachnoid space accompanying the blood vessels that invaginate the spinal cord from the pia mater) to reach the deeper dorsal root ganglia.[22] Furthermore, a portion of the subarachnoid drug diffuses outward through the arachnoid and dura mater to enter the epidural space,[23] whereas some is taken up by the blood vessels of the pia and dura maters.[24]

Drug penetration and uptake is directly proportionate to the drug mass, CSF drug concentration, contact surface area, lipid content (high in spinal cord and myelinated nerves), and local tissue vascular supply, but is inversely related to nerve root size. The concentration of local anesthetic in the CSF is highest at the site of subarachnoid injection in the case of spinal anesthesia (generally L2-L4 levels).

For epidural anesthesia, drug uptake is more complex. Some of the injected local anesthetic will move from the epidural space through the meninges into the CSF to exert its neural blocking effect, whereas some will be lost through vascular absorption into the capillary vessels and into the systemic circulation and uptake into epidural fat. The bioavailability of local anesthetics found in the CSF after epidural administration is low (<20%).

DRUG DISTRIBUTION

Diffusion is the primary mechanism of local anesthetic distribution in the CSF from areas of high concentration (i.e., at the site of injection) toward other segments of the spinal cord with low drug concentration.[25] Rostral spread after the administration of a small local anesthetic dose, often evident within 10 to 20 minutes, is related to the CSF circulation time. Longitudinal oscillations generated by the pulsations of the arteries in the skull are believed to be responsible for CSF bulk flow. This likely facilitates the cephalad distribution of local anesthetic from the lumbar subarachnoid space to the basal cisterns within 1 hour of injection.

Drug distribution in the epidural space is more complex, with possible contributions from one, some, or all of the following mechanisms: (1) crossing the dura mater into the subarachnoid space, (2) rostral and caudal (longitudinal) spread within the epidural space, (3) circumferential spread within the epidural space, (4) exit of the epidural space through the intervertebral foramina, (5) binding to epidural fat, and (6) vascular absorption into the epidural vessels. Longitudinal spread of local anesthetic by bulk flow within the epidural space may occur after the administration of a larger dose (i.e., volume). Factors that may enhance the distribution of local anesthetic within the epidural space are small caliber (greater spread in the thoracic space), increased epidural space compliance, decreased epidural fat content, decreased local anesthetic leakage through the intervertebral foramina (e.g., in the elderly and with spinal stenosis), and increased epidural pressure (e.g., pregnancy).[26] Drug is also preferentially distributed from areas of high to low concentration. Finally, the direction of drug spread varies with the vertebral level—that is, epidural spread is mostly cephalad in the lumbar region, caudad after a high thoracic injection, and spread mostly cephalad after a low thoracic njection.[26]

DRUG ELIMINATION

Regression of neural blockade results from a decline in the CSF drug concentration, which in turn is caused by nonneural tissue uptake and, most importantly, vascular absorption. Time for block regression is also inversely correlated with CSF volume.[27] Drug is absorbed by the vessels in the pia mater or the epidural vessels through back diffusion before entering the systemic circulation. No drug metabolism takes place in the CSF. The rate of elimination is also dependent on the distribution of local anesthetic; greater spread will expose the drug to a larger area for vascular absorption and thus a shorter duration of action. Lipid-soluble local anesthetics (e.g., bupivacaine) bind to epidural fat to form a depot that can slow vascular absorption.

Physiologic Effects

Safe conduct of spinal, epidural, and caudal anesthesia requires an appreciation of their physiologic effects. Neuraxial anesthesia evokes blockade of the sympathetic and somatic (sensory and motor) nervous systems, along with compensatory reflexes and unopposed parasympathetic activity.[28] The physiologic effects of epidural anesthesia are similar to those of spinal anesthesia, with the exception that local anesthetic blood levels reach concentrations sufficient enough to produce systemic effects on their own.

CARDIOVASCULAR

The effects of neuraxial blocks on blood pressure are similar in some ways to the combined use of intravenous α_1- and β-adrenergic blockers on cardiac output: decreased stroke volume and heart rate (see Chapter 14) caused by blockade of the peripheral (T1-L2) and cardiac (T1-T4) sympathetic fibers as well as adrenal medullary secretion. The decrease in arterial blood pressure is believed to be more gradual and of less magnitude with epidural than with spinal anesthesia of comparable sensory block levels. However, when tetracaine (10 mg) spinal anesthesia was compared with lidocaine (20-25 mL of a 1.5% solution) epidural anesthesia, there was a larger decrease in arterial blood pressure (approximately 10%) with the epidural technique than with the spinal anesthetic.[29] Of prime importance, the extent to which arterial blood pressure decreases with either technique depends on multiple factors, including patient age and intravascular volume status.

Stroke Volume

Sympathectomy usually decreases stroke volume. Venous and arterial vasodilation reduces preload (venous return) and afterload (systemic vascular resistance), respectively. Because of the large amount of blood that resides in the venous system (approximately 75% of the total blood volume), the venodilation effect predominates, owing to the limited amount of smooth muscle in venules; in contrast, the vascular smooth muscle on the arterial side of the circulation retains a considerable degree of autonomous tone. Cardiac output is thought to be either maintained or slightly decreased during the onset of spinal anesthesia. Yet a biphasic response, characterized by an early transient increase followed by an eventual decrease in cardiac output,[30] has been observed. This initial increase is caused by a greater magnitude of decline in the systemic vascular resistance than by venous return, especially in elderly patients with preexisting hypertension and high baseline systemic vascular resistance (also see Chapter 65).

The vasodilatory changes after neuraxial blockade that can affect cardiac output depend on each patient's baseline sympathetic tone (i.e., higher sympathetic tone in the elderly equates to a greater hemodynamic change) and the extent of the sympathectomy (i.e., the height of the block). The extent of the sympathectomy is typically described as extending for two to six dermatomes above the sensory block level with spinal anesthesia and at the same level with epidural anesthesia.[31] If normal cardiac output is maintained, systemic vascular resistance should decrease only 15% to 18% after neuraxial blockade in healthy normovolemic patients, even with nearly total sympathectomy. In elderly patients with cardiac disease, systemic vascular resistance may decrease almost 25% after spinal anesthesia, whereas cardiac output decreases only 10%.[32] Determination of baseline autonomic nervous system activity (e.g., blood pressure variability signaled by low-frequency band power and near-infrared spectroscopy reduction) has been found to predict the risk of hypotension in the elderly.[30]

Heart Rate

Heart rate may decrease during a high neuraxial block as a result of blockade of the cardioaccelerator fibers arising from T1 to T4.

Heart rate may also decrease in the presence of extensive peripheral sympathectomy (T5-L2), with venous pooling in the lower extremity and the abdominal and pelvic viscera. Although hypotension will trigger a compensatory baroreceptor sympathetic response (vasoconstriction and increased heart rate) above the level of blockade, the reduction in venous return and right atrial filling causes a decrease in signal output from intrinsic chronotropic stretch receptors located in the right atrium and great veins,[31] leading to a marked increase in parasympathetic activity (vagal tone). The two opposing responses are usually in check with a minimal change in heart rate (or a slight reduction). However, when neuraxial anesthesia is extended to the T1 level, blockade of the cardioaccelerator fibers in addition to a marked reduction in venous return may result in severe bradycardia and even asystole because of unopposed parasympathetic activity. However rare, the likelihood of cardiac arrest appears to be more likely in young, healthy, and conscious patients.[33] The Bezold-Jarisch reflex may be a possible cause of profound bradycardia and circulatory collapse after spinal anesthesia, especially in the presence of hypovolemia, when a small end-systolic left ventricular volume may trigger a mechanoreceptor-mediated bradycardia.[34]

Coronary Blood Flow

When coronary artery blood flow and myocardial metabolism were determined in humans during spinal anesthesia to T4 in hypertensive and normotensive patients, decreases in coronary blood flow (153 to 74 mL/100 g per minute) paralleled the decrease in mean arterial blood pressure (119 to 62 mm Hg), and the percent extraction of myocardial oxygen was unchanged (75% to 72%). Extraction of oxygen was unchanged because myocardial work, as expressed by myocardial use of oxygen, paralleled the decrease in mean arterial blood pressure and coronary blood flow (16 to 7.5 mL/100 g per minute).[35] A high thoracic block in patients with ischemic heart disease can be beneficial, with improvement in global and regional myocardial function and reversal of ischemic changes likely a result of reduced myocardial oxygen demand and left ventricular afterload.[36] Both infarction size and ischemia-induced arrhythmias improved in coronary occlusion experiments in animals, with no apparent vasodilatory effect on the coronary vessels.[37] These data support the observations by Stanley and coworkers[38] but still do not provide a patient-by-patient indication of the organ most at risk for flow-related ischemia.

Treatment

The clinical question of what level of decrease in arterial blood pressure after a neuraxial block is acceptable without a significant decrease in organ perfusion (e.g., brain, liver, gut) remains to be answered, although some human and animal data are available (see respective sections). Once arterial blood pressure decreases to a level at which treatment is believed to be necessary, ephedrine, a mixed adrenergic agonist, provides more appropriate therapy for the noncardiac circulatory sequelae of neuraxial block than does a pure α-adrenergic agonist (see Chapter 14), unless the patient has a specific and defined arterial blood pressure requirement.[39]

That the decrease in arterial blood pressure after neuraxial block can be minimized by the administration of crystalloids intravenously is probably not a valid concept. Specifically, 250- to 2000-mL preblock hydration regimens may temporarily increase preload and cardiac output but do not consistently increase arterial blood pressure or prevent hypotension.[8] Useful techniques to prevent hypotension include the repeated low-dose local anesthetic boluses through a continuous spinal catheter,[40] small-dose unilateral spinal anesthesia, and selective small-dose spinal anesthesia.

CENTRAL NERVOUS SYSTEM

Spinal anesthesia–induced hypotension may decrease regional cerebral blood flow (CBF) in elderly patients and those with preexisting hypertension. In a study of elderly patients who had hypotension during bupivacaine spinal anesthesia, Minville and colleagues demonstrated a significant but transient decrease of middle cerebral artery blood flow velocity and an increase in cerebral vascular resistance, both of which suggest a decrease in cerebral perfusion.[41] There was no change in cognitive function after surgery in any of these patients. Both CBF and velocity decline as a result of changes in the cerebral vasculature, especially in the elderly. Whether cerebral autoregulation is impaired in the elderly is still debatable (see Chapter 65).

Kety and colleagues[42] demonstrated that producing spinal anesthesia to the midthoracic levels with procaine, even in patients with essential hypertension, results in a decrease in mean arterial blood pressure of 26% (155 to 115 mm Hg) accompanied by a 12% (52 to 46 mL/100 g per minute) decrease in CBF. When the level of spinal anesthesia was purposely increased to produce higher levels of block (T4) in normotensive and hypertensive patients, CBF was unchanged in the normotensive group (45-46 mL/100 g per minute), whereas a 19% decrease occurred in the apparently untreated hypertensive patients (46.5-37.5 mL/100 g per minute).[43]

RESPIRATORY

Alterations in pulmonary variables in healthy and even in elderly patients during neuraxial block are usually of little clinical consequence.[44] A decrease in vital capacity follows a reduction in expiratory reserve volume related to paralysis of the abdominal muscles necessary for forced exhalation rather than a decrease in phrenic or diaphragmatic function.[45] Blockade of the intercostal and abdominal muscles during neuraxial anesthesia is adequately compensated by unaltered function of the diaphragm and other accessory respiratory muscles (e.g., sternomastoid, scalenes), especially for forceful inspiration and expiration.[46] Nonetheless, neuraxial block should be used cautiously in the setting of severe respiratory disease because paralysis of the intercostal and abdominal muscles is common. However rare, respiratory arrest associated with spinal anesthesia is often unrelated to phrenic or inspiratory dysfunction but rather to hypoperfusion of the respiratory centers in the brainstem. Supportive evidence for this concept is observed after resuscitation, when apnea almost always disappears as soon as pharmacologic and intravascular fluid therapies have restored cardiac output and arterial blood pressure.

Pregnancy

In young healthy pregnant women undergoing cesarean delivery, spinal bupivacaine, ropivacaine, and levobupivacaine affect pulmonary function minimally (a reduction of 3% to 6% for forced vital capacity and 6% to 13% for peak expiratory flow rate), irrespective of the peak sensory block level.[47] However, in overweight pregnant women, vital capacity declines even more (24% vs. 11%) and recovers more slowly compared with normal-weight pregnant women after hyperbaric spinal bupivacaine administration (see also Chapter 62).[48]

Obesity (also see Chapter 58)

The impact of spinal anesthesia on lung volume variables is significantly reduced compared with general anesthesia[49] but is significantly more in overweight patients than in normal-weight patients.[48] The magnitude of decline in vital capacity is proportional to the BMI value (vital capacity 19% for BMI 30–40 kg/m^2 vs. 33% for BMI >40 kg/m^2).[50] Importantly, however, for obese patients undergoing laparotomy surgery, thoracic epidural anesthesia (TEA) lessens the extent of decline in postoperative vital capacity and hastens recovery when compared with parenterally administered opioids.[49]

GASTROINTESTINAL

Neuraxial blockade from T6 to L1 disrupts splanchnic sympathetic innervation to the gastrointestinal tract, resulting in a contracted gut and hyperperistalsis. Nausea and vomiting may be associated with neuraxial block in as much as 20% of patients and they are primarily related to gastrointestinal hyperperistalsis caused by unopposed parasympathetic (vagal) activity.[51] Atropine is effective in treating nausea associated with high (T5) subarachnoid anesthesia.[52]

TEA has a direct blood pressure–dependent effect on intestinal perfusion.[53] TEA improves anastomotic mucosal blood flow in patients undergoing esophagectomy when mean arterial blood pressure is minimally altered but worsens local perfusion when arterial blood pressure is decreased by about 50%. In colorectal surgery, TEA decreases anastomotic blood flow but improves gastric and transverse colonic blood flow.[54] Correction of systemic hypotension by vasopressor therapy (e.g., norepinephrine) has been found to reverse impaired colonic perfusion. TEA may also reduce the rate of anastomotic leak after emergency laparotomy, esophageal surgery,[55] and other gastrointestinal interventions.[56]

A reduction in hepatic blood flow parallels the reduction in mean systemic arterial pressure in the setting of spinal anesthesia.[57] Although lumbar epidural anesthesia also results in a decline in hepatic perfusion despite colloid preloading in young and elderly patients, hepatic perfusion can increase, though mildly (<10%), with TEA after major abdominal surgery.[57]

RENAL

Despite a predictable decrease in renal blood flow accompanying neuraxial blockade, this decrease is of little physiologic importance.[58,59] One aspect of genitourinary function of clinical importance is the belief that neuraxial blocks are a frequent cause of urinary retention, which delays discharge of outpatients and necessitates bladder catheterization in inpatients (see section Complications–Urinary Retention, later in the chapter). However, this belief is questionable. For example, in orthopedic patients undergoing hip replacement, bladder catheterization was no more frequent after spinal or epidural anesthesia than it was after general anesthesia and opioid analgesics. In any case, excessive volumes of intravenous crystalloid solutions should not be given to patients undergoing spinal anesthesia. The requirement for voiding before discharge in low-risk ambulatory surgery patients after short-acting spinal or epidural anesthetics should be encouraged.[60]

Indications

At the most basic level, neuraxial blockade is indicated when the surgical procedure can be accomplished with a sensory level of anesthesia that does not produce adverse patient outcomes. The level of anesthesia or analgesia required is of prime importance because the physiologic effects of a high-level block may be untenable.

NEURAXIAL ANESTHESIA

When considering neuraxial anesthesia, the nature and duration of surgery, patient comorbidities, the ease of spinal insertion (i.e., positioning and spinal pathology), and the relative benefits and risks to the individual are important. Spinal anesthesia is most commonly used for patients who require surgical anesthesia for procedures of known duration that involve the lower extremities, perineum, pelvic girdle, or lower abdomen. Descriptions of spinal anesthesia as the primary surgical anesthetic have more recently expanded to include lumbar spine surgery,[61] as well as upper abdominal procedures, such as laparoscopic cholecystectomy.[62] Spinal anesthesia may be useful when patients wish to remain conscious or when comorbidities such as severe respiratory disease or a difficult airway increase the risks of using general anesthesia. Epidural anesthesia can also be used for the lower extremities, perineum, pelvic girdle, or lower abdomen, but by virtue of intermittent or continuous catheter-based local anesthetic delivery, the duration of surgical anesthesia is not necessarily finite as it is with single-injection spinal anesthesia. Continuous catheter-based spinal anesthesia is both less conventional and less commonly used than either single-shot spinal anesthesia or catheter-based epidural anesthesia, but may be especially useful when insertion of an epidural catheter is challenging[63] or in the setting of severe cardiac disease when the reliability of a single-shot spinal anesthetic must be combined with more hemodynamically stable incremental dosing.

NEURAXIAL ANALGESIA

Local anesthetics (as well as other additives, discussed later) applied to the neuraxis in subanesthetic doses can provide potent, long-lasting analgesia for a variety of indications, including intraoperative analgesia, acute postsurgical pain,[64] and severe chronic pain associated with malignancy. The use of intrathecal and/or epidural opioids either alone or in combination with local anesthetics can provide excellent quality pain relief[65,66,66a] and are an analgesic mainstay in labor and delivery,[67,68] during and after hip[69] or knee replacement,[70] in laparotomy,[71] in thoracotomy,[72] and increasingly even in cardiac surgery.[73,74] Some of the most important benefits of epidural analgesia are realized in patients with preexisting respiratory disease undergoing abdominal surgery.[75] Neuraxial analgesia may have other beneficial outcomes beyond analgesia and these are reviewed later.

Contraindications

ABSOLUTE

There are few absolute contraindications to neuraxial blockade. Some of the most important include patient refusal, localized sepsis, and an allergy to any of the drugs planned for administration. A patient's inability to maintain stillness during needle puncture, which can expose the neural structures to traumatic injury,[76] as well as raised intracranial pressure, which may theoretically predispose to brainstem herniation,[77] should also be considered absolute contraindications to a neuraxial technique.

RELATIVE

Relative contraindications must be weighed against the potential benefits of neuraxial blockade. Relative contraindications can be approached by system.

Neurologic

Myelopathy or Peripheral Neuropathy. A preexisting neurologic deficit can in theory worsen the extent of any injury in this group of patients (so-called double-crush phenomenon). While many reports suggest central neuraxial techniques may be used safely, there is no definitive evidence.[76,78-80] Chronic low back pain without neurologic deficit is not a contraindication to neuraxial blockade. The association between neuraxial techniques and the exacerbation of back pain symptoms is not documented.

Spinal Stenosis. Patients with spinal stenosis appear to be at increased risk of neurologic complications after neuraxial blockade,[81] but the relative contribution of surgical factors and natural history of the spinal pathology itself is unknown. Using a lower mass of local anesthetic may in theory reduce the risk if spinal anesthesia is undertaken in the setting of spinal stenosis.

Spine Surgery. Previous spine surgery does not predispose patients to an increased risk of neurologic complications after neuraxial blockade.[81,82] However, depending on postsurgical anatomy and the presence of scar tissue, adhesions, hardware, and/or bone grafts, needle access to the CSF, or epidural space and/or epidural catheter insertion may be challenging or impossible. In addition, the resultant spread of local anesthetic in the CSF or epidural space can be unpredictable and incomplete.

Multiple Sclerosis. Patients with multiple sclerosis (MS) may be more sensitive to neuraxial local anesthetics and thus exhibit a prolonged duration of motor and sensory blockade; however, any association between neuraxial anesthesia and exacerbation of MS symptoms is not based in evidence.[83,84] Given that demyelinated fibers may be more prone to the toxic effects of local anesthetics, it is prudent to use a lower dose and concentration of spinal local anesthetic in this group of patients, or else consider epidural rather than spinal anesthesia.

Spina Bifida. Spina bifida comprises a wide spectrum of congenital spinal cord malformations. Depending on the severity of the neural tube defect, patients with spina bifida may have a tethered cord and the ligamentum flavum may be absent, thereby increasing the potential for traumatic needle injury to the spinal cord. In patients who have undergone repair of open spinal dysraphisms, the spread of local anesthetic in the CSF and epidural space (if present) can be highly variable. Neuraxial techniques have been successfully used in isolated spina bifida occulta patients, but are not advised in the setting of severe neural tube defects such as diastematomyelia or tethered cord.

If, after consideration of risks and benefits, a neuraxial technique is to be undertaken in a patient with a neural tube defect, a careful clinical and radiologic evaluation of neurologic status must first be undertaken and noted along with documentation of the discussion of the risks and benefits.

Cardiac (also see Chapter 54)

Aortic Stenosis or Fixed Cardiac Output. The unpredictable speed and extent to which systemic vascular resistance is reduced after spinal anesthesia may cause many providers to avoid spinal anesthesia in preload-dependent patients and try to prevent a dangerous decrease in coronary perfusion. This concern is borne of theoretic risk and a great deal of caution rather than evidence.[85] Clinical practice mandates that neuraxial anesthesia be considered individually for each patient with aortic stenosis in the context of their own disease severity, left ventricular function, and case urgency. A catheter-based neuraxial anesthetic, whether it is an epidural or intrathecal catheter, allows for the repeated administration of small doses of local anesthetic, with potentially more control over hemodynamic changes, and may be a logical alternative choice.

Hypovolemia. An extension of patients who are preload-dependent, hypovolemic patients may exhibit an exaggerated hypotensive response to the vasodilatory effects of neuraxial blockade.

Hematologic

Thromboprophylaxis. Borne of the catastrophic cases of spinal hematoma causing paralysis associated with the introduction and use of LMWH in the United States (US FDA public health advisory: reports of epidural or spinal hematomas with the concurrent use of low molecular weight heparin and spinal/epidural anesthesia or spinal puncture. US Department of Health and Human Resources, 1997), the American Society of Regional Anesthesia and Pain Medicine (ASRA) first published a practice advisory to guide the provision of neuraxial techniques in patients receiving antithrombotic or thrombolytic therapy in 2004. Now in its fourth iteration and addressing a myriad of novel potent oral anticoagulants, the ASRA practice advisory[6] is an invaluable resource for providers performing neuraxial techniques in this challenging and ever-growing patient population. A summary of the ASRA guidelines[1] is reproduced in Table 45.1.

Inherited Coagulopathy. The safety of neuraxial techniques in patients with common bleeding diatheses is not well documented. Hemorrhagic complications after neuraxial techniques in patients with known hemophilia, von Willebrand disease, or idiopathic thrombocytopenic purpura appear infrequently when factor levels are more than 0.5 IU/mL for factor VIII, von Willebrand factor, and ristocetin cofactor activity, or when the platelet count is greater than $50 \times 10^9/L$[1] before block performance.[86] The minimum safe factor levels and platelet count for neuraxial blockade, however, remain undefined in both the obstetric and general populations.[86]

Infection

Theoretic concerns based on animal data and laboratory and case reports in humans[87-89] suggest iatrogenic seeding of the neuraxis in the setting of a systemic infection. Some providers avoid neuraxial techniques in febrile patients. A definitive causative relationship between existing systemic infection and meningitis or epidural abscess after a neuraxial technique has never been shown. In fact, a lumbar puncture is a critical component of the investigation of fever of unknown origin, yet there are no definitive data linking lumbar puncture to increased risk of neuraxial infection in this setting.[90] Although the profound vasodilation may be sufficient reason to avoid neuraxial techniques in patients with profound bacteremia or septic shock, the theoretic risk of seeding the intrathecal or epidural spaces by performing neuraxial techniques in patients with untreated systemic infection further supports using another technique. Yet patients with evidence of systematic infection may safely undergo neuraxial anesthesia once antibiotic therapy has been initiated and the patient has demonstrated a response to the antibiotics.[90]

Spinal Anesthesia

FACTORS AFFECTING BLOCK HEIGHT

The dermatomal level required for various surgical procedures is outlined in Table 45.2. The provider must recall that intraabdominal structures such as the peritoneum (T4), bladder (T10), and uterus (T10) have a spinal segment innervation that may be much more cephalad compared with that of the corresponding skin incision used to operate on these structures.

Drug, patient, and procedural factors can all affect the distribution of local anesthetic spread within the intrathecal space, some of which are more clinically relevant than others.[25,91] Many of these factors are not controllable by the anesthesiologist, leading to significant interpatient variability (Table 45.3).

TABLE 45.1 ASRA Evidence-Based Guidelines for Neuraxial Anesthesia in the Patient Receiving Thromboprophylaxis

DRUG	NEURAXIAL NEEDLE/CATHETER PLACEMENT			NEURAXIAL CATHETER REMOVAL		COMMENTS
	Discontinuation prior to placement	**Restart following needle placement**	**Indwelling catheter placement**	**Discontinuation prior to removal**	**Restart following removal**	
Antiplatelet agents						
Aspirin	*Safe for all categories*					
NSAIDs	*Safe for all categories but caution with concomitant drugs that may affect coagulation*					
Clopidogrel	5-7 d		Catheters may be maintained for 1-2 days after restarting Clopidogrel or Ticlodipine			
Ticlodipine	10 d	Immediately			Immediately	
Prasugrel	7-10 d	*If loading dose*: 6 h	Avoid catheters		*If loading dose*: 6 h	
Ticagrelor	5-7 d					
Dipyridamole	24 h	6 h	Avoid catheters		6 h	
GP IIa/IIIb inhibitors Abciximab Eptifibatide Tirofiban	*Avoid until platelet function returns to normal*	*These drugs are generally contraindicated for 4 weeks post surgery*				
Unfractionated Heparin						
Intravenous	4-6 h and confirm normal coagulation	1 h	Safe	4-6 h and confirm normal coagulation	1 h	*Check platelet count before needle placement or catheter removal if duration of LMWH > 4 d*
Subcutaneous						
Low-dose prophylaxis	4-6 h or confirm normal coagulation		Safe	4-6 h and confirm normal coagulation		*5,000 U SC bid or tid*
Higher-dose prophylaxis	12 h and confirm normal coagulation	1 h	Safety of catheters not established		1 h	*7,500-10,000 U SC bid or ≤20,000 U/d*
Therapeutic	24 h and confirm normal coagulation		Avoid catheters			*>10,000 U SC/dose or >20,000 U/d*
Low molecular weight heparin						
Once daily prophylaxis	12 h	12 h	Safe	12 h	4 h	*Check platelet count before needle placement or catheter removal if duration of LMWH > 4 d*
Twice daily prophylaxis			Avoid catheters			
Therapeutic dose	24 h	24 - 72 h	Avoid catheters			
Oral anticoagulants						
Coumarins	Ideally 5 d and INR <1.5	No delay	Monitor INR daily and check sensory/motor function routinely	INR < 1.5	No delay	
Apixaban	72 h	6 h	Avoid catheters		6 h	*Refer to ASRA guidelines if unanticipated indwelling catheter*
Rivaroxaban		6 h				

Abbreviations: bid=twice a day, tid=three times a day, d=day(s), h=hour(s), SC=subcutaneous, U=unit(s). *Reg Anes Pain Med* 2018; 43: 263-309.

Drug Factors

The adjustable factors for any given local anesthetic solution are dose, volume, concentration, temperature, and baricity. Baricity and dose are most important.

Baricity. Baricity is the ratio of the density of a local anesthetic solution to the density of CSF. Density is defined as the mass per unit volume of solution (g/mL) at a specific temperature. Density may be compared between different substances by calculating the specific gravity, which is the ratio of the density of a solution to the density of water. Because density varies inversely with temperature, the baricity of a local anesthetic solution is conventionally defined at 37°C. The density of CSF is 1.00059 g/L.[92] Local anesthetic solutions that have the same density as CSF are termed *isobaric*, those that have a higher density than CSF are termed *hyperbaric*, and those with a lower density than CSF are termed *hypobaric*. The spread of hyperbaric solutions is more predictable,[93] with less interpatient variability.[94] To make a drug hyperbaric to CSF, it must be denser than CSF, with a baricity appreciably more than 1.0000 or a density appreciably more than 1.00059. The reverse is true for making a drug hypobaric to the CSF. Dextrose and sterile water are commonly added to render local anesthetic solutions either hyperbaric or hypobaric, respectively. The clinical importance of baricity is the ability to influence the distribution of local anesthetic spread based on gravity. Hyperbaric solutions will preferentially spread to the dependent regions of the spinal canal, whereas hypobaric solutions will spread to nondependent regions. Isobaric solutions tend not to be influenced by gravitational forces.[95] Anesthesiologists can capitalize on this phenomenon by altering the position of the patient. For example, the administration of hyperbaric local anesthetic to patients in the lateral decubitus position will result in a preferential anesthetic effect on the dependent side, whereas the opposite is true for the administration of a hypobaric solution. A thoughtful understanding of the natural curvatures of the vertebral column can help predict local anesthetic spread in patients placed in the horizontal supine position immediately after intrathecal administration. Hyperbaric local anesthetics injected, while sitting, at the L3-L4 or L4-L5 interspace will spread with gravity from the height of the lumbar lordosis down toward the trough of the thoracic kyphosis in the horizontal supine position, resulting in a higher level of anesthetic effect than isobaric or hypobaric solutions.[91] Hyperbaric solutions are also useful in small doses for a saddle block and to achieve unilateral anesthesia. CSF and local anesthetic density change with temperature. Plain bupivacaine 0.5%, for example, may be isobaric at 24°C but is slightly hypobaric at 37°C. A small volume of drug at room temperature injected intrathecally quickly equilibrates after injection and increases to the temperature of the CSF. Nevertheless, increasing temperature decreases density of a solution and warming of local anesthetic solution to body temperature, therefore making it more hypobaric, increases the block height in patients who remain seated for several minutes after injection.[96]

Dose, Volume, and Concentration. The dose, volume, and concentration are inextricably linked (Volume × Concentration = Dose), but dose is the most reliable determinant of local anesthetic spread (and thus block height) when compared with either volume or concentration for isobaric and hypobaric local anesthetic solutions.[97,98] Hyperbaric local anesthetic injections are primarily influenced by baricity.

The choice of local anesthetic itself does not influence spread if all other factors are controlled. Additive drugs, other than opioids, also do not affect spread. However, opioids do seem to increase mean spread,[91,99] possibly as a result of pharmacologic enhancement at the extremes of the spread where the local anesthetic block alone would have been subclinical.[100,101]

TABLE 45.2 Dermatomal Level Required for Various Common Surgical Procedures

Type of Surgery	Dermatomal Level
Upper abdominal surgery	T4
Cesarean delivery	T4
Transurethral resection of prostate	T10
Hip surgery	T10
Foot and ankle surgery	L2

TABLE 45.3 Factors Affecting Local Anesthetic Distribution and Block Height

	More Important	Less Important	Not Important
Drug factors	Dose Baricity	Volume Concentration Temperature of injection Viscosity	Additives other than opioids
Patient factors	CSF volume Advanced age Pregnancy	Weight Height Spinal anatomy Intraabdominal pressure	Menopause Gender
Procedure factors	Patient position Epidural injection post spinal	Level of injection (hypobaric more than hyperbaric) Fluid currents Needle orifice direction Needle type	

CSF, Cerebrospinal fluid. Modified from Greene NM. Distribution of local anesthetic solutions within the subarachnoid space. *Anesth Analg*. 1985;64(7):715–730.

Patient Factors

Patient characteristics that may influence block height include patient height, weight, age, sex, pregnancy, anatomic configuration of the spine, and the CSF properties (volume and composition). Within the range of "normal-sized" adults, patient height does not seem to affect the spread of spinal anesthesia. This is likely because the length of the lower limb bones rather than the vertebral column contributes most to adult height. A correlation has been found between the vertebral column length and local anesthetic spread[102] and, at extremes of height, consideration should be given to altering the dose accordingly.

The CSF volume is an important patient-related factor that significantly influences peak block height and regression of sensory and motor blockade.[17] Lumbosacral CSF has a fairly constant pressure of approximately 15 cm H_2O but its volume varies from patient to patient, in part because of differences in body habitus and weight.[16] In a small sample of patients, block height varied indirectly with CSF volume.[17] Unfortunately, CSF volume does not correlate well with anthropomorphic measurements available clinically other than body weight.[17] In theory, the increased abdominal mass in obese patients, and possible increased epidural fat, may decrease the CSF volume and therefore increase the spread of local anesthetic and block height. This has indeed been demonstrated using hypobaric solutions,[103,104] which are characterized by more variable spread anyway, but not hyperbaric solutions (see Chapter 58).[103,105]

CSF density can also vary between and within individuals depending on sex, menopausal status, and pregnancy (see Chapter 62).[92] The density of CSF is lower in women compared with men, premenopausal compared with postmenopausal women, and pregnant compared with nonpregnant women. Although this may affect relative baricity of local anesthetics, the clinical variation in spread is probably unimportant.

Advanced age is associated with increased block height (see Chapter 65).[106,107] In older patients, CSF volume decreases, whereas its specific gravity increases. Further, the nerve roots appear more sensitive to local anesthetic in the aged population.

Gender can theoretically affect block height by several mechanisms. CSF density is higher in males, thereby reducing the baricity of local anesthetic solution and possibly limiting the extent of cephalad spread. In the lateral position, the broader shoulders of males relative to their hips make the lateral position slightly more head-up. The reverse is true in females who have a slightly head-down tilt in the lateral position compared with males. Despite this, there is little objective data that males have a slightly less cephalad spread than females in the lateral position.

Variations of the spine may be an important contributor to block height. Scoliosis, although it possibly makes insertion of the needle more difficult, will have little effect on local anesthetic spread if the patient is turned supine. Kyphosis, however, in a supine patient may affect the spread of a hyperbaric solution. Spread of local anesthetic is enhanced by changes in the lumbar lordosis during pregnancy, as well as by the volume and density of CSF, by twin pregnancies compared with singletons, by intraabdominal pressure increases (possibly), and by a progesterone-mediated increase in neuronal sensitivity.

Procedure Factors

Patient position, needle type and alignment, and the level of injection are each procedure-related factors that can affect block height. Combined with the baricity and local anesthetic dose, patient position is the most important factor in determining the block height. Position should not affect the spread of a truly isobaric solution.[95] Intrathecal local anesthetic appears to stop spreading 20 to 25 minutes after injection, thus positioning of the patient is most important during this time period, but particularly in the initial few minutes. However, marked changes in patient posture up to two hours after injection can still result in significant changes in the block level, probably because of bulk movement of CSF.[108,109] Although a 10-degree head-up tilt can reduce the spread of hyperbaric solutions without hemodynamic compromise,[110] a head-down tilt does not always increase the spread of hyperbaric bupivacaine.[111] Flexion of the hips in combination with the Trendelenburg position flattens the lumbar lordosis and has been shown to increase cephalad spread of hyperbaric solutions.[112] A "saddle block" where only the sacral nerve roots are anesthetized can be achieved by using a small dose of hyperbaric local anesthetic while the patient remains in the sitting position for up to 30 minutes. When larger hyperbaric doses are administered, however, the block can still extend cephalad despite maintaining the sitting position for a prolonged period of time.[113] The reverse holds true for hypobaric solutions, where block height is greater (than hyperbaric solutions) if they are administered in a sitting position.[114]

The specific needle type and orientation of the orifice may affect block quality. With hypobaric solutions, cephalad alignment of the orifice of Whitacre, but not Sprotte, needles produces greater spread.[115-117] The orientation of the needle orifice does not appear to affect the spread of hyperbaric solutions. When directing the needle orifice to one side (and using hyperbaric anesthetic), a more marked unilateral block is achieved again when using a Whitacre, rather than a Quincke, needle.[118]

The level of injection affects block height. Most studies have demonstrated that, even when the difference is only one interspace more cephalad, the block height is greater[119-122] when using isobaric bupivacaine. The level of injection does not appear to influence the spread of hyperbaric solutions.[123,124] Injection rate and barbotage (repeated aspiration and reinjection of CSF) of isobaric and hyperbaric solutions have not consistently been shown to affect block height.[91] A slower injection may actually increase spread, and this is perhaps also safer because forceful injection may cause the syringe to disconnect from the needle. Other maneuvers that do not appear to affect block height are coughing and straining after local anesthetic injection. This is related to the physics of injecting drugs into a closed column of CSF, which instantaneously transmits pressure changes throughout the CSF column, such as those that occur with coughing or straining.[25] The injection of local anesthetic or even saline into the epidural space after a spinal anesthetic increases the block height. This is discussed separately in the combined spinal-epidural (CSE) section.

DURATION

The duration of a spinal anesthetic depends on how this variable is defined. For example, the duration of surgical anesthesia is less than the time for complete block resolution. In addition, surgical anesthesia depends on the surgical site because anesthesia is more prolonged at the lower lumbar and sacral levels than at those more cephalad from where the block regresses first. Duration is affected primarily by the dose,[97,125] the intrinsic properties of the local anesthetic (which affect elimination from the subarachnoid space), and the use of additives (if applicable). The latter two are described later. Hyperbaric solutions have a shorter duration of action than isobaric solutions.[125]

PHARMACOLOGY

The clinical effects of intrathecal local anesthetics are mediated by drug uptake and distribution within the CSF and elimination. These in turn are dictated in part by the p*K*a, lipid solubility, and protein binding of the local anesthetic solution. Rather than their pharmacologic structure (i.e., amide or ester), it is the duration of action—short-acting (i.e., procaine, chloroprocaine, articaine), intermediate-acting (i.e., lidocaine, prilocaine, mepivacaine), and long-acting (i.e., tetracaine, bupivacaine, levobupivacaine, ropivacaine)—that is most often used to classify local anesthetics in the clinical setting. The choice and dose of local anesthetic depend on both the expected duration and the nature (location, ambulatory) of surgery. Table 45.4 shows a range of local anesthetics used for spinal anesthesia with corresponding doses, onset times, and durations of action.[126-134]

Short- and Intermediate-Acting Local Anesthetics

Procaine. Procaine is a short-acting ester local anesthetic and one of the oldest spinal anesthetics, having originally replaced cocaine as the drug of choice for spinal anesthesia in the early 20th century. Procaine itself was then replaced by lidocaine, but with concerns about lidocaine and transient neurologic symptoms (TNS), procaine has recently been reexamined as an alternative fast-acting local anesthetic. However, it is not commonly used because of a more frequent failure rate than lidocaine, significantly more nausea, and a slower time to recovery.[135] If used, it is often administered as a hyperbaric drug in a dose ranging between 50 and 200 mg in a 10% concentration.

Chloroprocaine. Chloroprocaine is an ultra–short-acting ester local anesthetic that was introduced in the 1950s. Its initial popularity stemmed from its rapid metabolism by pseudocholinesterase, which translated into minimal systemic or fetal effects in the setting of epidural labor analgesia. However, its reputation as a spinal anesthetic has been tarnished because of reports of neurologic injury associated with the preservative once used in older preparations of the drug (see Complications, discussed later).[136-139] Recently, interest in chloroprocaine has increased for use in spinal anesthesia for ambulatory surgery (see Chapter 72). Modern, preservative-free preparations of chloroprocaine administered in small doses (30-60 mg) produce reliable, short-duration spinal anesthesia,[126] with a faster recovery time than procaine, lidocaine, and bupivacaine.[140-144] TNS can occur with modern chloroprocaine preparations, albeit at a considerably lesser rate (0.6%) than lidocaine (14%).[145-147]

Articaine. Articaine is a relatively novel amide local anesthetic that also has an ester linkage. The ester linkage allows for metabolism by nonspecific cholinesterases. It has been widely used since 1973 for dental nerve blocks with a good safety profile. Intrathecal articaine has not been extensively investigated, but studies do suggest that doses of 50 to 80 mg with or without glucose appear to provide rapid-onset spinal anesthesia for about 1 hour, with a recovery profile faster than bupivacaine.[148,149]

Lidocaine. Lidocaine is a hydrophilic, relatively poorly protein-bound amide local anesthetic. It has a rapid onset

TABLE 45.4 Dose, Block Height, Onset Times, and Duration of Commonly Used Spinal Anesthetics

	DOSE (MG)		DURATION (MIN)		
Local Anesthetic Mixture	**To T10**	**To T4**	**Plain**	**Epinephrine (0.2 mg)**	**Onset (min)**
Lidocaine 5% (with/without dextrose)*	40-75	75-100	60-150†	20%-50%	3-5
Mepivacaine 1.5% (no dextrose)	30-45‡	60-80§	120-180¶¶	—	2-4
Chloroprocaine 3% (with/without dextrose)	30-40	40-60	40-90¶	N/R	2-4
Bupivacaine 0.5%-0.75% (no dextrose)	10-15	12-20	130-230#	20%-50%	4-8
Levobupivacaine 0.5% (no dextrose)	10-15	12-20	140-230#	—	4-8
Ropivacaine 0.5%-1% (with/without dextrose)	12-18	18-25	80-210**	—	3-8

*Lidocaine is not commonly used now.
†Regression to T12.
‡Note peak with these doses was T12, and not in all cases.
§Median peak block height in this study with 60 mg was T5, not T4.
¶¶Regression to S1 for block duration.
¶Regression to L1.
#Regression to L2.
**Regression to S2.
N/R, Not recommended. Note that duration depends on how the regression of the block is measured, which varies widely between studies.

and intermediate duration and is used in doses of 50 to 100 mg for shorter procedures that can be completed in 1.5 hours or less. It was traditionally prepared as a 5% solution in 7.5% dextrose; this preparation has been associated with both permanent nerve injury and TNS (see section Complications, discussed later). Despite efforts to reduce the concentration of both the drug and dextrose,[150,151] the use of intrathecal lidocaine declined and has not yet recovered.

Prilocaine. Prilocaine is an amide local anesthetic based on the structure of lidocaine. Prilocaine was introduced in 1965 and has an intermediate duration of action that may lend itself to use in the ambulatory surgery setting.[152] A dose of 40 to 60 mg of 2% hyperbaric prilocaine can provide a block to T10 for 100 to 130 minutes, whereas as little as 20 mg combined with fentanyl has been successfully used for ambulatory arthroscopic knee surgery.[153] Prilocaine is rarely associated with TNS.[152,154,155] In large doses (>600 mg), prilocaine can result in methemoglobinemia. This should not be an issue with doses used for spinal anesthesia, but it has been reported after epidural infusions.[156]

Mepivacaine. Mepivacaine is another short-acting amide local anesthetic. It was first introduced for spinal anesthesia in 1962 and was initially prepared as a hyperbaric solution. The use of spinal mepivacaine has declined because the incidence of TNS after hyperbaric mepivacaine was similar to that of lidocaine,[147] although TNS were less frequent with the isobaric preparation of mepivacaine.[157-159] Doses of 30 to 80 mg with and without additives have been used (see Table 45.4) and, when compared with lidocaine, mepivacaine has a slightly longer duration of action.[160]

Long-Acting Local Anesthetics

Tetracaine. Tetracaine is an ester local anesthetic with a rate of metabolism one tenth that of chloroprocaine. It is packaged either as Niphanoid crystals (20 mg) or as an isobaric 1% solution (2 mL, 20 mg). When Niphanoid crystals are used, a 1% solution is obtained by adding 2 mL of preservative-free sterile water to the crystals. Mixing 1% solution with 10% dextrose produces a 0.5% hyperbaric preparation that may be used for perineal and abdominal surgery in doses of 5 and 15 mg, respectively. Tetracaine is usually combined with a vasoconstrictor additive because the duration of tetracaine alone can be unreliable. Although such combinations can provide up to 5 hours of anesthesia,[161-164] the addition of phenylephrine in particular has been associated with TNS.[165]

Bupivacaine. Bupivacaine was introduced in 1963 and is a highly protein-bound amide local anesthetic with a slow onset because of its relatively high p*K*a. It is appropriate for procedures lasting up to 2.5 to 3 hours (see Table 45.4).[166,167] Bupivacaine is available as 0.25%, 0.5%, and 0.75% clear isobaric solutions and also as a hyperbaric 0.5% (in Europe) and 0.75% solution containing 80 mg/mL glucose. At room temperature, plain bupivacaine is actually slightly hypobaric compared with CSF. Recovery profiles using small doses appear to be similar to that of lidocaine[168-170] and thus low-dose bupivacaine is used in ambulatory procedures. A recent systematic review[171] concluded that 4 to 5 mg of hyperbaric bupivacaine combined with unilateral positioning was adequate for short knee arthroscopy procedures. Bupivacaine is rarely associated with TNS.

Levobupivacaine. Levobupivacaine is the pure S (−) enantiomer of racemic bupivacaine. Although it is used in similar doses to bupivacaine and has a similar onset and duration, levobupivacaine potency appears to be slightly less than bupivacaine.[129] Nevertheless, the majority of clinical studies using identical doses of levobupivacaine and bupivacaine have found no significant difference in clinical efficacy for spinal anesthesia.[129,172-174] The main advantage of levobupivacaine is that it is less cardiotoxic than bupivacaine,[175,176,178] which is more of a theoretic than a real risk in the setting of spinal anesthesia.

Ropivacaine. Ropivacaine was introduced in 1996 and is another highly protein-bound amide local anesthetic. It is structurally related to bupivacaine, with the same p*K*a (8.1) and so it is also characterized by slow onset and a long duration of action. Compared to bupivacaine, the proposed advantages of spinal ropivacaine were less cardiotoxicity and greater motor-sensory block differentiation, resulting in less motor block. Subsequently, the potency of ropivacaine was found to be 0.6 that of bupivacaine.[179-181] When ropivacaine is given in an equivalent dose to bupivacaine, there is slightly less motor block and earlier recovery with ropivacaine.[8,182-184]

Spinal Additives

Whether administered into the CSF in conjunction with a local anesthetic or alone, a variety of medications may exert a direct analgesic effect on the spinal cord and nerve roots, or prolong the duration of sensory and motor blockade. As such, the coadministration of these agents often allows for a reduction in the required dose of local anesthetic, with the advantage of motor block sparing and faster recovery while still producing the same degree of analgesia.

Opioids. The effects of opioids within the CSF are complex, because of a combination of direct spinal cord dorsal horn opioid receptor activation, cerebral opioid receptor activation after CSF transport, and peripheral and central systemic effects after vascular uptake. The effect at each of these sites depends on both the dose administered and the physicochemical properties of the opioid, particularly lipid solubility. Highly lipid-soluble drugs such as fentanyl and sufentanil have a more rapid onset and shorter duration of action than more hydrophilic opioids. In addition to increasing uptake into neural tissue, greater lipid solubility results in rapid uptake into both blood vessels (with a resultant systemic effect) and fatty tissue. The spread of lipophilic opioids within the CSF is therefore more limited than hydrophilic opioids such as morphine, which demonstrate greater spread as a result of slower uptake and elimination from the CSF. As a result, hydrophilic opioids have a greater risk of late respiratory depression, which is one of the rare but most serious consequences of intrathecal opioid administration. The extent of neural tissue and vascular uptake also affects the potency of intrathecal opioids. For example, the relative intrathecal to intravenous potency of morphine is 200 to 300 to 1, whereas for fentanyl and sufentanil it is only 10 to 20 to 1.[185] In addition to respiratory depression, intrathecal opioids have other side effects including nausea and vomiting, pruritus, and urinary retention. These are discussed later in the Complications section.

Hydrophilic Opioids. Preservative-free morphine is the most widely used hydrophilic opioid in spinal anesthesia. It has a slow onset but provides analgesia for up to 24 hours.[186] Adequate analgesia is achieved with 100 μg, with minimal side effects for cesarean deliveries, whereas the most efficacious dose for major orthopedic surgery is less clear.[187] Doses as high as 1000 μg may be used for major abdominal surgery or thoracotomies, where it is becoming increasingly common to administer spinal opioids alone as a simple alternative to epidural local anesthetic–based analgesia. The magnitude of the analgesic response and the optimal dose remain unclear. Given adverse effects increase at higher doses it has been suggested that the lowest effective dose (<300 microg) should be used.[66a] Overall, the beneficial effects of intrathecal morphine seem most marked in abdominal surgery, and within the first 24 hours in particular.[186,188]

Diamorphine is available for use in the United Kingdom only. It is a lipid-soluble prodrug that crosses the dura faster than morphine and is cleared from the CSF more quickly than morphine. Once in the dorsal horn of the spinal cord, it is converted to morphine and 6-monoacetyl morphine, both of which are μ-agonists with a relatively long duration of action. It is recommended for use in doses of 0.3 to 0.4 mg for cesarean delivery[189] and is widely used instead of morphine in the United Kingdom.

There are only limited data related to the use of hydromorphone for spinal analgesia. It is more commonly used epidurally, as discussed later. Limited data suggest that intrathecal hydromorphone 50 to 100 μg provides comparable analgesia with similar side effects to 100 to 200 μg of morphine, with a similar duration of action. However, it has not undergone full neurotoxicity screening and does not provide any advantage compared with morphine.[190]

Meperidine is an opioid of intermediate lipid solubility, but it also has some local anesthetic properties and has been used as the sole intrathecal agent (doses ranging from 0.5 to 1.8 mg/kg) in both obstetric and general surgery.[191,192] Smaller doses are used in combination with local anesthetics. Both 10 mg and 20 mg improve analgesia compared with placebo after cesarean delivery,[193] although side effects were more frequent with the larger dose. However, this drug is used infrequently because of the availability of other opioids and its unknown neurotoxicity profile.

Lipophilic Opioids. Fentanyl and sufentanil are used frequently in obstetrics for labor analgesia and cesarean delivery as discussed elsewhere (also Chapter XX). Sufentanil 2 to 10 μg and fentanyl 25 μg provide comparable analgesia in early labor.[194-197] In transurethral prostatectomy surgery, when combined with low-dose bupivacaine, sufentanil 5 μg provides superior analgesia compared with fentanyl 25 μg.[198] Fentanyl in doses of 10 to 30 μg is commonly used in ambulatory surgery because of its rapid onset time of 10 to 20 minutes and relatively short duration of 4 to 6 hours. Although the local anesthetic dose can be reduced and analgesia prolonged,[199] the addition of fentanyl to bupivacaine may increase side effects and delay discharge.[171]

Vasoconstrictors. Vasoconstrictors, such as epinephrine and phenylephrine, prolong the duration of sensory and motor blockade when added to local anesthetics. The mechanism of action is reduced systemic local anesthetic uptake caused by an α_1-mediated vasoconstriction. Epinephrine may also enhance analgesia via a direct α_2-mediated effect. Traditionally, epinephrine 0.1 to 0.6 mg was thought to prolong tetracaine spinal anesthesia, but not bupivacaine or lidocaine spinal anesthesia.[22] This theory was postulated because of differences in the vasodilatory action of the local anesthetic drugs; plain lidocaine and bupivacaine cause vasodilation, whereas plain tetracaine does not. However, lidocaine spinal anesthesia can be prolonged by epinephrine when measured by both two-dermatome regression in the lower thoracic dermatomes and by occurrence of pain at the operative site for procedures carried out at the level of the lumbosacral dermatomes.[200,201] Similarly, bupivacaine spinal duration may be increased, but because of the already long duration, epinephrine is not generally added to bupivacaine. There is a concern that potent vasoconstrictive action places the blood supply of the spinal cord at risk. However, there are no human data supporting this theory, and in animal studies,[164,202-204] administering either subarachnoid epinephrine (0.2 mg) or phenylephrine (5 mg) does not decrease spinal cord blood flow. Phenylephrine 2 to 5 mg prolongs both lidocaine and tetracaine spinal anesthesia to a similar extent as epinephrine.[201,205] Bupivacaine spinal anesthesia is not prolonged by phenylephrine.[206,207] Concepcion and co-workers[208] compared epinephrine (0.2 and 0.3 mg) and phenylephrine (1 and 2 mg) added to tetracaine and did not find any differences in duration between the two vasoconstrictors. Caldwell and associates[163] used larger doses of vasoconstrictors, epinephrine at 0.5 mg and phenylephrine at 5 mg, and showed that phenylephrine prolonged tetracaine spinal anesthesia significantly more than did epinephrine. The addition of phenylephrine has declined in popularity because of its association with TNS.[165,209]

α_2-Agonists. Clonidine, dexmedetomidine, and epinephrine all act on prejunctional and postjunctional α_2 receptors in the dorsal horn of the spinal cord. Activation of presynaptic receptors reduces neurotransmitter release, whereas postjunctional receptor activation results in hyperpolarization and reduction of pulse transmission.[210] In doses of 15 to 225 μg, clonidine prolongs the duration of sensory and motor blockade by approximately 1 hour and improves analgesia, reducing morphine consumption by up to 40%.[211-215] It appears to cause less urinary retention than morphine but, as with intravenous clonidine administration, spinal clonidine can also cause hypotension. A systematic review concluded that the hypotension associated with spinal clonidine was not dose-related and that the risk of bradycardia with clonidine was not increased.[216] Sedation can also occur with spinal clonidine, peaking within 1 to 2 hours and lasting up to 8 hours.[210] Dexmedetomidine is approximately 10-fold more α_2-selective than clonidine is.[217] As little as 3 µg of dexmedetomidine can prolong motor and sensory block without hemodynamic compromise.[218,219]

Other Drugs. Neostigmine in doses of 10 to 50 µg has analgesic effects after intrathecal administration.[220,221] Intrathecal neostigmine has been shown to prolong motor and sensory blockade and reduce postoperative analgesic requirements. Neostigmine inhibits the breakdown of acetylcholine, therefore increasing acetylcholine concentration, which itself is antinociceptive. It also appears to stimulate the release of nitric oxide in the spinal cord. Its benefits, however, are limited by nausea, vomiting, bradycardia, and, in higher doses, lower extremity weakness,[222,223] and is therefore not in widespread use.[224] Midazolam is a γ-aminobutyric acid receptor agonist that in doses of 1 to 2 mg appears to increase sensory and motor block and decrease analgesic requirements postoperatively, without the adverse effects observed with α_2 agonists or opioids. Early work raised concerns of spinal cord toxicity, but more recent studies suggest that it is safe.[225] Ketamine, adenosine, tramadol, magnesium, and nonsteroidal antiinflammatory drugs have also all been administered intrathecally, but further work is required to establish safety and whether these drugs have any clinical value.

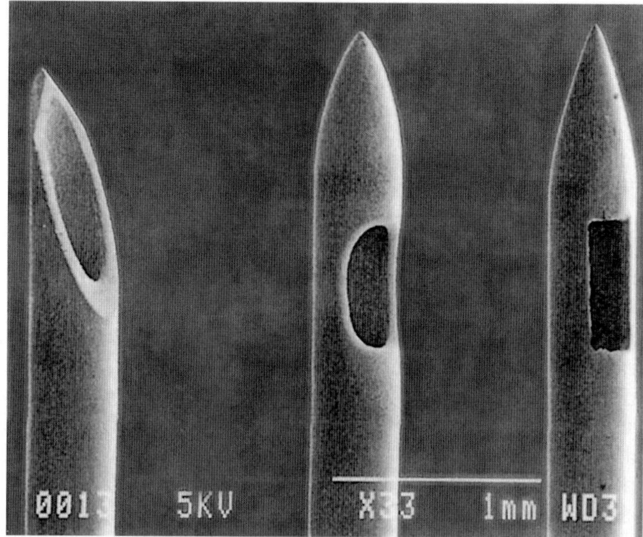

Fig. 45.4 Scanning electron micrographs of spinal needle tip designs: Quincke *(left)*, Sprotte *(middle)*, and Whitacre *(right)*. (Modified from Puolakka R, Andersson LC, Rosenberg PH. Microscopic analysis of three different spinal needle tips after experimental subarachnoid puncture. *Reg Anesth Pain Med.* 2000;25:163–169.)

Technique

Technique should be classified into a series of steps (i.e., the four Ps): preparation, position, projection, and puncture.

Preparation. Informed consent must be obtained, with adequate documentation of the discussion of risk (see Complications, discussed later). Resuscitation equipment must always be readily available whenever a spinal anesthetic procedure is performed. The patient should have adequate intravenous access and be monitored with pulse oximetry, noninvasive arterial blood pressure, and electrocardiogram. Preprepared packs are now commonly used and often contain fenestrated drapes, swabs and towels, syringes, needles, filters, spinal needles, sterilizing solution, and local anesthetic for skin infiltration. When the local anesthetic for subarachnoid injection is chosen, the duration of block should be matched with both the surgical procedure and patient variables (see Table 45.4).

The most important characteristics of a spinal needle are the shape of the tip and the needle diameter. Needle tip shapes fall into two main categories: those that cut the dura and those with a conical, pencil-point tip. The former include the Pitkin and the Quincke-Babcock needle, and the Whitacre and Sprotte needles belong to the latter group (Fig. 45.4). The orifice of the Whitacre needle is smaller. If a continuous spinal technique is chosen, use of a Tuohy or other thin-walled needle can facilitate passage of the catheter. The use of small needles reduces the incidence of post–dural puncture headache from 40% with a 22-G needle to less than 2% with a 29-G needle. The use of larger needles, however, improves the tactile sense of needle placement, and so although 29-G needles result in a very low rate of post–dural puncture headache, the failure rate is increased.[226,227] Pencil-point needles provide better tactile sensation of the different layers encountered during needle insertion but, more importantly, they reduce the incidence of post–dural puncture headache. Pencil-point needles of 25, 26, and 27-G probably represent the optimal needle choice. An introducer needle can assist with guidance of smaller-gauge spinal needles in particular. Special Luer-Lok needles and syringes for spinal kits are now also available. These have been designed to prevent inadvertent intrathecal injection but still rely on the correct drug being drawn up into the "special" connector syringe (see Fig. 45.4).

Sterility is an issue of utmost importance. One of the most common organisms responsible for postspinal bacterial meningitis is *Streptococcus viridans*, which is an oral commensal, emphasizing the purpose of wearing a mask as part of a full aseptic technique. Hands and forearms must be washed and all jewelry removed. A variety of solutions may be used to clean the patient's back prior to skin puncture, such as chlorhexidine or alcohol (alone or in combination), or iodine solutions. Chlorhexidine and alcohol together have been concluded to be most effective.[229-231] It is important that chlorhexidine is allowed to dry completely before skin puncture because chlorhexidine is neurotoxic.

The recently published Practice Advisory for the Prevention, Diagnosis, and Management of Infectious Complications Associated with Neuraxial Techniques by the American Society of Anesthesiologists (ASA) Task Force on Infectious Complications Associated with Neuraxial Techniques and the ASRA[229] recommends that to prevent infection, it is important to identify patients at increased risk of infection (e.g., known bacteremia, immunocompromised) and consider alternatives, consider pre-procedure antibiotics in patients with bacteremia, ensure full asepsis including masks and use antiseptic solution such as chlorhexidine, sterile occlusive dressings, and bacterial filters. Disconnection and reconnection of neuraxial catheters should be minimized and catheters should not remain in situ longer than clinically necessary. Patients should be evaluated daily for signs of infection and if suspected then this should be promptly investigated and treated appropriately.

Position (also see Chapter 34). The three primary patient positions include the lateral decubitus, sitting, and prone positions, each of which has advantages in specific situations. The superiority of any one particular position is unclear. In the obstetric population, there have been small studies demonstrating that block operator performance was faster in the sitting position, albeit this benefit was offset by a slower onset time compared with the lateral decubitus position (see Chapter 62).[232] Current consensus guidelines state that neuraxial blocks should not be routinely performed with the patient anesthetized or deeply sedated,[76] except in those circumstances where the physician and patient conclude that benefit outweighs the risk. General anesthesia or heavy sedation can prevent a patient from recognizing warning signs of pain or paresthesia if the needle is in close proximity to nervous tissue.

A patient in the lateral decubitus position facilitates the administration of sedative medication if required, is less dependent on a well-trained assistant than for a patient in the sitting position, and is arguably more comfortable. Patients are placed with their back parallel to the edge of the operating table nearest the anesthesiologist, thighs flexed onto the abdomen, with the neck flexed to allow the forehead to be as close as possible to the knees in an attempt to "open up" the vertebral spaces. The assistant may still be invaluable during this positioning by encouraging and assisting the patient in assuming the ideal lateral decubitus position. Because of the differing proportional sizes of hips and shoulders, the spine may slope down toward the head in females, with the opposite occurring in males. The patient should be positioned so that spread of hypobaric, isobaric, or hyperbaric solution to the operative site is optimized.

Identification of the midline may be easier when the patient is placed in the sitting position, especially when obesity or scoliosis renders midline anatomy difficult to examine. Ultrasound may also be used to identify the midline (see later discussion). When placing patients in this position, a stool can be provided as a footrest and a pillow placed in the lap, or a specially designed stand may be used. The assistant helps to maintain the patient in a vertical plane while flexing the patient's neck and arms over the pillow, relaxing the shoulders, and asking the patient to "push out" the lower back to open up the lumbar vertebral spaces. Care must be taken not to oversedate a patient in this position. Hypotension may also be more common for a person in the sitting position.

The prone position is rarely used but may be chosen when the patient is to be maintained in that position (often with the jack-knife modification) during the surgical procedure. Such cases may include rectal, perineal, or lumbar procedures. The anesthesiologist may have to aspirate for CSF because CSF pressure is minimized when insertion of the lumbar needle is carried out in this position.

Projection and Puncture. The midline approach relies on the ability of patients and assistants to minimize lumbar lordosis and allow access to the subarachnoid space between adjacent spinous processes, usually at the L2-L3, L3-L4, or the L4-L5 space. The spinal cord ends at the level of L1-L2 and so needle insertion above this level should be avoided. The intercristal line is the line drawn between the two iliac crests and traditionally corresponds to the level of the L4 vertebral body or the L4-L5 interspace, but the reliability of this landmark is questionable as demonstrated by recent ultrasonography studies.[233] Once the appropriate space has been selected, a subcutaneous skin wheal of local anesthetic is developed over this space, and the introducer is inserted at a slight cephalad angle of 10 to 15 degrees through skin, subcutaneous tissue, and supraspinous ligament to reach the substance of the interspinous ligament. The introducer is grasped with the palpating fingers and steadied while the other hand is used to hold the spinal needle like a dart, and the fifth finger is used as a tripod against the patient's back to prevent patient movement and unintentional insertion to a level deeper than intended. The needle, with its bevel parallel to the midline, is advanced slowly to heighten the sense of tissue planes traversed and to prevent skewing of nerve roots, until the characteristic change in resistance is noted as the needle passes through the ligamentum flavum and dura. On passing through the dura, there is often a slight "click" or "pop" sensation. The stylet is then removed, and CSF should appear at the needle hub. The smaller the needle diameter, the longer the wait for CSF flow, particularly if the patient is not in the sitting position. If the CSF does not flow, the needle might be obstructed and rotation in 90-degree increments can be undertaken until CSF appears. If CSF does not appear in any quadrant, the needle should be advanced a few millimeters and rechecked in all four quadrants. If CSF still has not appeared and the needle is at a depth appropriate for the patient, the needle and introducer should be withdrawn and the insertion steps should be repeated. A common reason for failure is insertion of the needle off the midline (Fig. 45.5).

After CSF is freely obtained, the dorsum of the anesthesiologist's nondominant hand steadies the spinal needle against the patient's back while the syringe containing the therapeutic dose is attached to the needle. CSF is again freely aspirated into the syringe, and the anesthetic dose is injected at a rate of approximately 0.2 mL/s. After completion of the injection, 0.2 mL of CSF can be aspirated into the syringe and reinjected into the subarachnoid space to reconfirm location and clear the needle of the remaining local anesthetic.

The paramedian approach exploits the larger "subarachnoid target" that exists if a needle is inserted slightly lateral to the midline (Fig. 45.6). The paramedian approach may be especially useful in the setting of diffuse calcification of the interspinous ligament. The most common error when using the paramedian technique is that the needle entry site is placed too far off midline, which makes the vertebral laminae barriers to insertion of the needle. In the paramedian approach, a skin wheal is raised 1 cm lateral and 1 cm caudad to the corresponding spinous process. A longer needle (e.g., 3-5 cm) is then used to infiltrate deeper tissues in a cephalomedial plane. The spinal introducer and needle are next inserted 10 to 15 degrees off the sagittal plane in a cephalomedial plane (see Fig. 45.6). Similar to the midline approach, the most common error is to angle the needle too far cephalad on initial insertion. Nevertheless, if the needle contacts bone, it is redirected slightly in a cephalad direction. If bone is again contacted, but at a deeper level, the slight cephalad angulation is continued because it is likely that the needle is being "walked up" the lamina. As

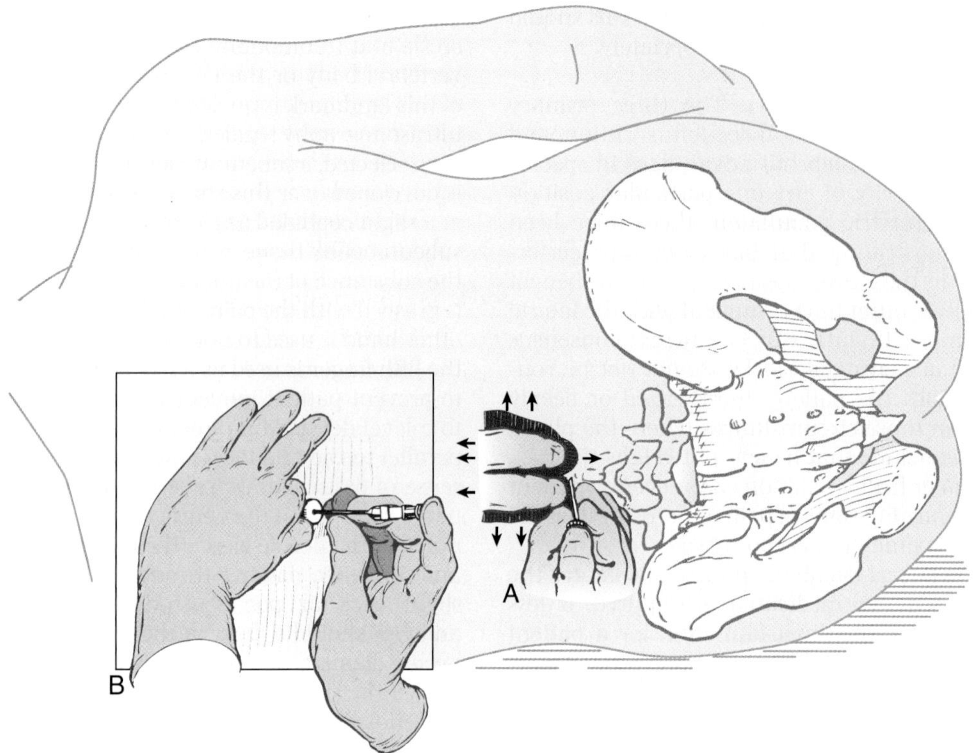

Fig. 45.5 Insertion of the spinal needle. (A) The palpating fingers are "rolled" in a side-to-side and a cephalad-to-caudad direction to identify the interspinous space. (B) During needle insertion, the needle should be stabilized in a tripod fashion while placed in the hand, similar to a dart being thrown.

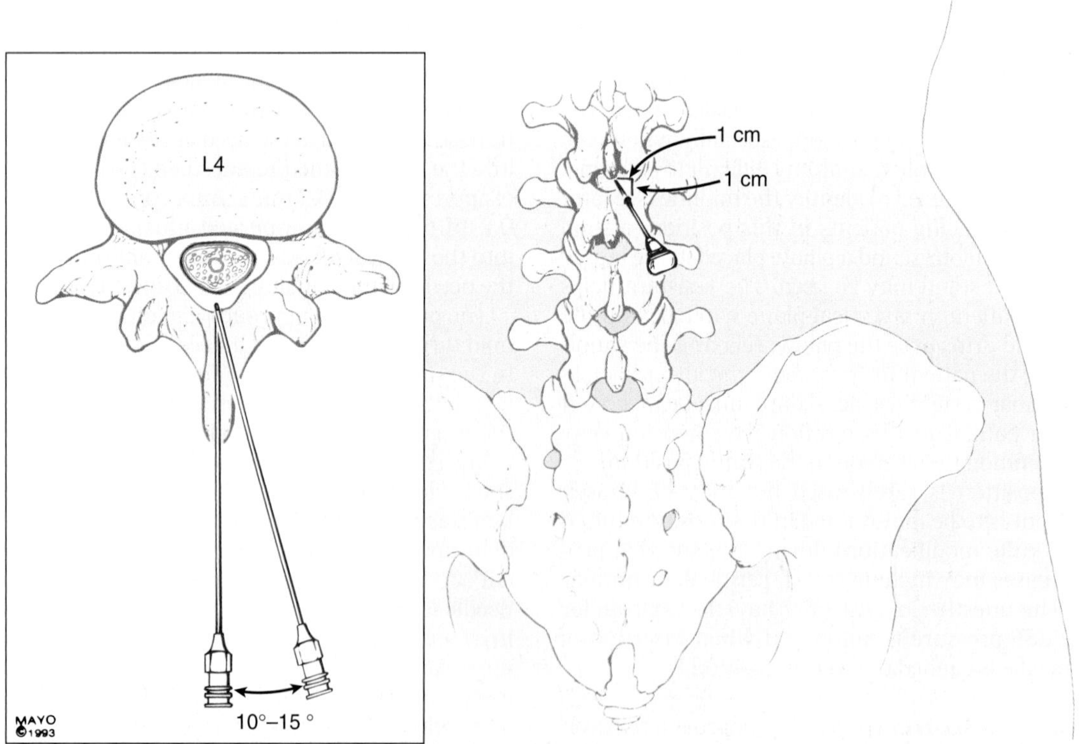

Fig. 45.6 Vertebral anatomy of the midline and paramedian approaches to centroneuraxis blocks. The midline approach highlighted in the inset requires anatomic projection in only two planes: sagittal and horizontal. The paramedian approach shown in the inset and in the posterior view requires an additional oblique plane to be considered, although the technique may be easier in patients who are unable to cooperate in minimizing their lumbar lordosis. The paramedian needle is inserted 1 cm lateral and 1 cm caudad to the caudad edge of the more superior vertebral spinous process. The paramedian needle is inserted approximately 15 degrees off the sagittal plane, as shown in the inset. (Courtesy the Mayo Foundation, Rochester, MN.)

in the midline approach, the characteristic feel of the ligaments and dura is possible, but only once the ligamentum flavum is reached because the needle this time is not passing through the supraspinous and interspinous ligaments. After CSF is obtained, the block is carried out in a manner similar to that described for the midline approach.

SPECIAL SPINAL TECHNIQUES

Continuous Spinal Anesthesia

Continuous spinal anesthesia allows incremental dosing of local anesthetic and therefore predictable titration of the block to an appropriate level, with better hemodynamic stability than a single-shot spinal.[40] It is useful in controlling arterial blood pressure in such patients with severe aortic stenosis or pregnant women with complex cardiac disease. In obstetrics, it may also be used in patients with morbid obesity and where previous spinal surgery may hinder epidural spread. Spinal catheters also serve as an alternative to the CSE technique for prolonged cases and have been used in selected patients for laparotomies where general anesthesia may be too great a risk.[234] If a continuous spinal anesthetic is undertaken, a needle with a laterally facing opening may be used to perform the lumbar puncture (Fig. 45.7). A midline or paramedian approach may be used, with some experts suggesting that use of the paramedian approach facilitates insertion of the catheter.[235] The catheter should be threaded 2 to 3 cm into the subarachnoid space and the needle withdrawn over the catheter. The catheter must never be withdrawn back into the needle shaft in case a piece of the catheter is sheared off and left in the subarachnoid space. Care must also be taken to ensure that the catheter is not inserted more deeply into the subarachnoid space when the needle is withdrawn over the catheter. Spinal microcatheters exist, but these have been associated with cauda equina syndrome,[5] probably because of lumbosacral pooling of local anesthetic. Catheter-over-the-needle devices are also available for use with continuous spinal anesthesia, with the advantage of minimizing leakage of CSF around the catheter,[236] but these may be more difficult to insert.[236] Finally, epidural doses of local anesthetic should not be infused or "bloused" into spinal catheters, and strict attention must also be paid to sterile technique.

Unilateral Spinal Anesthesia and Selective Spinal Anesthesia

The terms *unilateral spinal anesthesia* and *selective spinal anesthesia* overlap slightly, but both refer to small-dose techniques that capitalize on baricity and patient positioning to hasten recovery. A recent systematic review found that a dose of 4 to 5 mg of hyperbaric bupivacaine with unilateral positioning was adequate for knee arthroscopy.[171] This technique has also been used for unilateral inguinal hernia repair with a dose of 8 mg bupivacaine. In selective spinal anesthesia, minimal local anesthetic doses are used with the goal of anesthetizing only the sensory fibers to a specific area.[237,238] These doses are discussed in more detail in the chapter on anesthesia for ambulatory surgery (see Chapter 72).

BLOCK MONITORING

Once the spinal anesthetic has been administered, the onset, extent, and quality of the sensory and motor blocks must be assessed while heart rate and arterial blood pressure are also being monitored for any resultant sympathetic blockade. There are many methods of assessing sensory block, but cold sensation and pinprick representing C- and A-delta fibers, respectively, are used more often than mechanical stimuli such

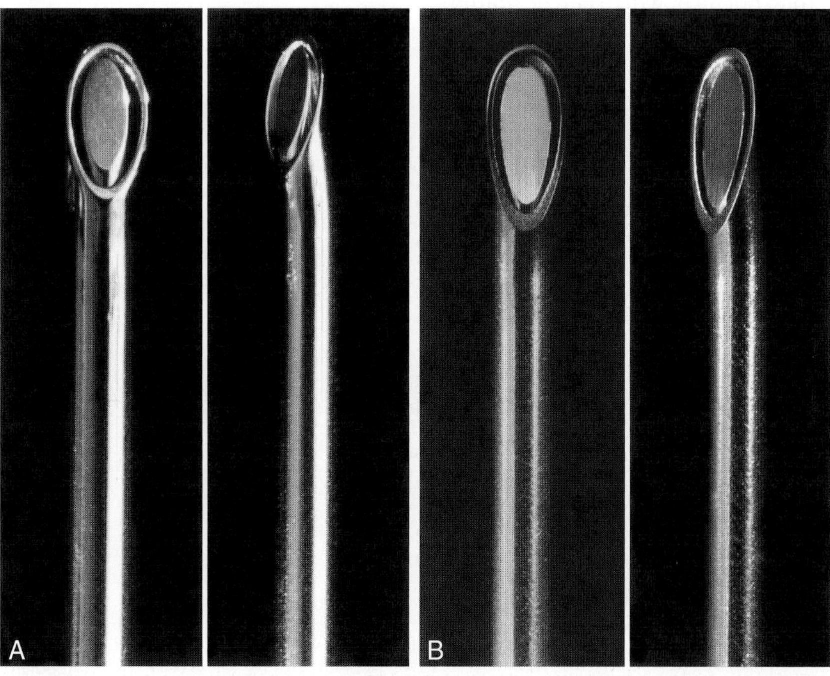

Fig. 45.7 Examples of continuous spinal needles, including a disposable, 18-G Hustead (A) and a 17-G Tuohy (B) needle. Both have distal tips designed to direct the catheters inserted through the needles along the course of the bevel opening; 20-G epidural catheters are used with these particular needle sizes.

as touch, pressure, and von Frey hairs, which reflect the A-beta nerves. Loss of sensation to cold usually occurs first, verified using an ethyl chloride spray, ice, or alcohol, followed by the loss of sensation to pinprick, verified using a needle that does not pierce the skin.[20] Finally, loss of sensation to touch occurs. Dermatomal block height also varies with the method of assessment, but in general, peak height is measured most cephalad using loss of cold, and is measured lower with pinprick, and lowest with touch.[239] Assessing dermatomal block height assumes that absence of sensation to these stimuli equates to blockade of the nociceptive fibers, but this is not necessarily the case.[240] Other electrical and experimental chemical methods of assessing pain have been used but gentle pinprick remains the simplest.[91,241] Motor block may also be measured in a variety of ways. The modified Bromage scale (Box 45.1) is most commonly used, although this represents only lumbosacral motor fibers.[242] Electromyography and pulmonary function tests have been used to measure abdominal and thoracic motor function, but these are neither practical nor specific.

In practice, the combination of sympathetic block with an adequate sensory level and motor block (inability to straight-leg raise ensures at least that lumbar nerves are blocked) is used to confirm spinal efficacy. Ensuring that the level of block using cold or pinprick is two to three segments above the expected level of surgical stimulus is commonly considered adequate.

Epidural Anesthesia

FACTORS AFFECTING EPIDURAL BLOCK HEIGHT

The epidural space is a collapsible, distensible reservoir through which drugs spread and are removed by diffusion, vascular transport, and leakage. Spread of anesthetic within the epidural space, and subsequent block height, is related to a variety of factors, not all of which can be manipulated by the anesthesiologist (Table 45.5).[26]

BOX 45.1 Modified Bromage Scale

- 0: No motor block
- 1: Inability to raise extended leg; able to move knees and feet
- 2: Inability to raise extended leg and move knee; able to move feet
- 3: Complete block of motor limb

Drug Factors

The volume and total mass of injectate are the most important drug-related factors that affect block height after the administration of local anesthetic in the epidural space. As a general principle, 1 to 2 mL of solution should be injected per segment to be blocked. Although additives such as bicarbonate, epinephrine, and opioids influence onset, quality, and duration of analgesia and anesthesia, these do not affect spread.

Patient Factors

Age can influence epidural block height.[26] There appears to be a stronger correlation with age and block height in thoracic epidurals, with one study suggesting that 40% less volume is required in the elderly (see Chapter 65).[243] Possible reasons include decreased leakage of local anesthetic through intervertebral foramina, decreased compliance of the epidural space in the elderly resulting in greater spread, or an increased sensitivity of the nerves in the elderly. As with spinal anesthesia, it appears that only the extremes of patient height influence local anesthetic spread in the epidural space. Weight is not well correlated with block height in the settings of either lumbar or TEA.[244] Less local anesthetic is required to produce the same epidural spread of anesthesia in pregnant patients. Although this may be in part a result of engorgement of epidural veins secondary to increased abdominal pressure, the effect also occurs in early pregnancy.[245] Also, continuous positive airway pressure increases the height of a thoracic epidural block.[246,247]

Procedure Factors

The level of injection is the most important procedure-related factor that affects epidural block height. In the upper cervical region, spread of injectate is mostly caudal, in the midthoracic region spread is equally cephalad and caudal, and in the low thoracic region spread is primarily cephalad.[248] After a lumbar epidural, spread is more cephalad than caudal. Some studies suggest that the total number of segments blocked is less in the lumbar region compared with thoracic levels for a given volume of injectate. Patient position has been shown to affect spread of lumbar epidural injections, with preferential spread and faster onset to the dependent side in the lateral decubitus position.[249] The sitting and supine positions do not affect epidural block height. However, the head-down tilt position does increase cephalad spread in obstetric patients.[250] Needle bevel direction

TABLE 45.5 Factors Affecting Epidural Local Anesthetic Distribution and Block Height

	More Important	Less Important	Not Important
Drug factors	Volume Dose	Concentration	Additives
Patient factors	Elderly age Pregnancy	Weight Height Pressure in adjacent body cavities	
Procedure factors	Level of injection	Patient position	Speed of injection Needle orifice direction

Modified from Visser WA, Lee RA, Gielen MJ. Factors affecting the distribution of neural blockade by local anesthetics in epidural anesthesia and a comparison of lumbar versus thoracic epidural anesthesia. *Anesth Analg*. 2008;107:708–721.

and speed of injection also do not appear to influence the spread of a bolus injection.

PHARMACOLOGY

Local anesthetics for epidural use may be classified into short-, intermediate-, and long-acting drugs. A single bolus dose of local anesthetic in the epidural space can provide surgical anesthesia ranging from 45 minutes up to 4 hours depending on the type of local anesthetic administered and the use of any additives (Table 45.6). Most commonly, an epidural catheter is left in situ so that local anesthetic–based anesthesia or regular analgesia can be extended indefinitely.

Short-Acting and Intermediate-Acting Local Anesthetics

Procaine. Similar to spinal anesthesia, procaine is not commonly used for epidural anesthesia. Five-percent procaine has a slow onset and the resultant block can be unreliable and of poor quality.

Chloroprocaine. Chloroprocaine is available preservative-free in 2% and 3% concentrations for epidural injection, with the latter preferable for surgical anesthesia because the former may not produce muscle relaxation. The 3% preparation has an onset time of 10 to 15 minutes and a duration of up to 60 minutes. Adding epinephrine prolongs the block for up to 90 minutes. Before the development of preservative-free preparations, large volumes (>25 mL) of chloroprocaine had been associated with deep, aching, burning lumbar back pain.[251] This was thought to be secondary to the ethylenediaminetetraacetic acid that chelated calcium and caused a localized hypocalcemia. In addition, chloroprocaine can antagonize the effects of epidural morphine.[242] This may be a result of opioid receptor antagonism by either the chloroprocaine or a metabolite. Antagonism of an intracellular messenger and decreased morphine availability caused by a reduction in perineural pH are also proposed mechanisms. However, morphine and chloroprocaine seem like an illogical combination because the beneficial ultrashort duration of action of chloroprocaine is offset by the addition of morphine.

Articaine. Articaine is not widely used for epidural anesthesia and has not been studied extensively. When 2% articaine was compared with epidural lidocaine in one study, it had a similar latency, spread, duration, and motor block.[252] It has also been used for obstetric epidural analgesia.[148]

Lidocaine. Lidocaine is available in 1% and 2% solutions; it has an onset time of 10 to 15 minutes and a duration of up to 120 minutes, which can be extended to 180 minutes with the addition of epinephrine. Unlike spinal anesthesia, TNS are not commonly associated with epidural lidocaine.[253]

Prilocaine. Prilocaine is available in 2% and 3% solutions. The 2% solution produces a sensory block with minimal motor block. Onset time is approximately 15 minutes, with a duration of approximately 100 minutes. When compared with lidocaine, prilocaine has a more marked sensory blockade and a longer duration (different from Cousins).[242] In large doses, prilocaine is associated with methemoglobinemia.[156,254]

Mepivacaine. Mepivacaine is available as 1%, 1.5%, and 2% preservative-free solutions. The 2% preparation has an onset time similar to lidocaine of approximately 15 minutes, but a slightly longer duration (up to 200 minutes with epinephrine), making it a preferred option by some centers for surgery of an intermediate duration.

Long-Acting Local Anesthetics

Tetracaine. Tetracaine is not widely used for epidural anesthesia because of unreliable block height and, in larger doses, systemic toxicity.

Bupivacaine. Bupivacaine is available in 0.25%, 0.5%, or 0.75% preservative-free solutions. The onset time is around 20 minutes with a duration of up to 225 minutes, which is prolonged only slightly by the addition of epinephrine (to 240 minutes). More dilute concentrations such as 0.125% to 0.25% can be used for analgesia. However, disadvantages include cardiac and central nervous system toxicity and the potential for motor block from larger doses. Solutions of 0.5% and 0.75% are used to provide surgical anesthesia.

TABLE 45.6 Comparative Onset Times and Analgesic Durations of Local Anesthetics Administered Epidurally in 20- to 30-mL Volumes

			DURATION (MIN)	
Drug	**Concentration (%)**	**Onset (min)**	**Plain**	**1:200,000 Epinephrine**
2-Chloroprocaine	3	10-15	45-60	60-90
Lidocaine	2	15	80-120	120-180
Mepivacaine	2	15	90-140	140-200
Bupivacaine	0.5-0.75	20	165-225	180-240
Etidocaine	1	15	120-200	150-225
Ropivacaine	0.75-1.0	15-20	140-180	150-200
Levobupivacaine	0.5-0.75	15-20	150-225	150-240

Modified from Cousins MJ, Bromage PR. Epidural neural blockade. In: Cousins MJ, Bridenbaugh PO, eds. *Neural Blockade in Clinical Anesthesia and Management of Pain*. Philadelphia: JB Lippincott; 1988;255.

Liposomal bupivacaine is currently under investigation for epidural use. An epidural bolus of liposomal 0.5% bupivacaine provided similar onset but longer-lasting analgesia to boluses of plain bupivacaine.[255] It does not appear to be more toxic than plain bupivacaine or to have a differing cardiac safety profile. The benefit, as with extended-release morphine (discussed later), is the lack of need for an epidural catheter. Conversely, such extended-release boluses are less titratable if for any reason the epidural needs to be terminated early.

Levobupivacaine. Levobupivacaine can be used as an epidural local anesthetic in 0.5% to 0.75% concentrations for surgical anesthesia, whereas analgesia can be achieved with concentrations of 0.125% to 0.25%. Levobupivacaine administered epidurally has the same clinical characteristics as bupivacaine.[129,256,257] The advantage of levobupivacaine is that it is less cardiotoxic compared with bupivacaine.[175,258]

Ropivacaine. Ropivacaine is available in 0.2%, 0.5%, 0.75%, and 1.0% preservative-free preparations. For surgical anesthesia, 0.5% to 1.0% is used, whereas 0.1% to 0.2% is used for analgesia. Ropivacaine is associated with a superior safety profile compared with bupivacaine.[259,260] Data from animal models suggest that bupivacaine has a 1.5 to 2.5 lower seizure threshold than ropivacaine. Ropivacaine is also less cardiotoxic. When compared with bupivacaine and levobupivacaine, ropivacaine at equivalent concentrations has a relatively similar clinical profile. Ropivacaine has a slightly shorter duration of action and less motor block, although the reduced motor block may in fact reflect different potencies of the drugs rather than a true motor-sparing effect of ropivacaine. Epidurally administered ropivacaine is 40% less potent than bupivacaine.[179,180,261]

Epidural Additives

Vasoconstrictors. Epinephrine reduces vascular absorption of local anesthetics in the epidural space. The local anesthetics vary in their responsiveness to epinephrine. The effect is the most with lidocaine,[262] mepivacaine, and chloroprocaine (up to 50% prolongation), with a lesser effect with bupivacaine, levobupivacaine, and etidocaine, and a limited effect with ropivacaine, which already has intrinsic vasoconstrictive properties (see Table 45.6). Epinephrine itself may also have some analgesic benefits because it is absorbed into the CSF, where it can act on dorsal horn α_2 receptors.[263] Phenylephrine has been used in epidural anesthesia less widely than in spinal anesthesia, perhaps because it does not reduce peak blood levels of local anesthetic as effectively as epinephrine does during epidural use.[264]

Opioids. Opioids synergistically enhance the analgesic effects of epidural local anesthetics, without prolonging motor block. A combination of local anesthetic and opioid reduces the dose-related adverse effects of each drug independently. The analgesic benefits of neuraxial opioids must be balanced against the dose-dependent side effects. As with intrathecal opioids, there appears to be a therapeutic ceiling effect above which only side effects increase. Opioids may also be used alone, particularly when there are concerns regarding hemodynamic instability. Epidural opioids work by crossing the dura and arachnoid membrane to reach the CSF and spinal cord dorsal horn. Lipophilic opioids, such as fentanyl and sufentanil, partition into epidural fat and therefore are found in lower concentrations in CSF than hydrophilic opioids, such as morphine and hydromorphone. Fentanyl and sufentanil are also readily absorbed into the systemic circulation, and several studies suggest that this is the principal analgesic mechanism.[265,266]

Epidural morphine is administered as a bolus of 1 to 5 mg, with an onset time of 30 to 60 minutes and duration of up to 24 hours. The optimal dose that balances analgesia while minimizing side effects is 2.5 to 3.75 mg.[267] Alternatively, morphine can be administered continuously in doses of 0.1 to 0.4 mg/h through an epidural catheter. Hydromorphone is more hydrophilic than fentanyl but more lipophilic than morphine. It can be administered as a bolus of 0.4 to 1.5 mg, with onset at 15 to 30 minutes and a duration of 18 hours. Hydromorphone used as an infusion is delivered at rates between 5 and 20 μg/h. The onset of epidural fentanyl and sufentanil is 5 to 15 minutes and lasts only 2 to 3 hours. Bolus doses of 10 to 100 μg may be used to provide analgesia. Diamorphine is available in the United Kingdom and used in doses of 2 to 3 mg as epidural boluses, or approximately 0.05 mg/mL in an infusion.

DepoDur is an extended-release liposomal formulation of morphine used as a single-shot lumbar epidural dose, thereby avoiding issues and side effects of a continuous local anesthetic infusion and indwelling catheters, particularly in patients receiving anticoagulants. When administered before surgery (or after clamping of the cord in cesarean deliveries), DepoDur can provide up to 48 hours of pain relief.[268,269] A dose of 10 to 15 mg is recommended for lower abdominal surgery, and 15 mg is recommended for major lower limb orthopedic surgery.

α_2-Agonists. Epidural clonidine can prolong sensory block to a greater extent than motor block. The mechanism appears to be mediated by the opening of potassium channels and subsequent membrane hyperpolarization[270] rather than an α_2-agonist effect. The addition of clonidine reduces both epidural local anesthetic and opioid requirements.[271-273] Other benefits of clonidine may include a reduced immune stress and cytokine response.[274] Epidural clonidine does have a variety of side effects including hypotension, bradycardia, dry mouth, and sedation. The cardiovascular effects may be greatest when clonidine is administered in the epidural space at the thoracic level.[275] In preliminary studies, epidural dexmedetomidine has also been shown to reduce intraoperative anesthetic requirements, improve postoperative analgesia, and prolong both sensory and motor block.[276]

Other Drugs. Conflicting reports exist regarding the benefit of epidural ketamine and whether it is neurotoxic.[277-279] Epidural neostigmine provides labor analgesia before local anesthetic infusion without causing respiratory depression, hypotension, or motor impairment.[280] Midazolam, tramadol, dexamethasone, and droperidol have also been studied but are not commonly used.

Carbonation and Bicarbonate. Many local anesthetic preparations have a pH between 3.5 and 5.5 for chemical stability and bacteriostasis. At these low pHs, a higher proportion of the drug is in the ionized form and is therefore unable to cross nerve membranes to reach the internal binding site on sodium channels. Both carbonation of the solution and adding bicarbonate have been used in an attempt to increase the solution pH, and therefore the nonionized free-base proportion of local anesthetic. Although carbonation may theoretically increase the speed of onset and quality of the block by producing more rapid intraneural diffusion and more rapid penetration of connective tissue surrounding the nerve trunk,[281,282] available data suggest that there are no clinical advantages for carbonated solutions.[235,283]

EPIDURAL TECHNIQUE

Preparation

Patient preparation as previously described for spinal anesthesia must equally be applied to epidural anesthesia, namely consent, monitoring, and resuscitation equipment, intravenous access, and choosing the patient and drugs appropriately depending on comorbidities and the nature of surgery. Sterility is arguably even more important than spinal anesthesia because a catheter is often left in situ. The extent of the surgical field must be understood so that the epidural may be inserted at the appropriate level—that is, the lumbar, low-, mid-, or high-thoracic, or less commonly, cervical.[26] A variety of epidural needles have been used for epidural anesthesia, but Tuohy needles are most common (Fig. 45.8). These needles are usually 16- to 18-g in size and have a 15- to 30-degree curved, blunt "Huber" tip designed to both reduce the risk of accidental dural puncture and guide the catheter cephalad. The needle shaft is marked in 1-cm intervals so that depth of insertion can be identified. The catheter is made of a flexible, calibrated, durable, radiopaque plastic with either a single end hole or multiple side orifices near the tip. Several investigators have found that multiple-orifice catheters are superior, with a reduced incidence of inadequate analgesia.[284-286] However, the use of multiorifice catheters in pregnant women resulted in a more frequent incidence of epidural vein cannulation.[287]

The method of identifying the epidural space must also be predetermined. Most practitioners use a loss-of-resistance technique to either air or saline, rather than the hanging drop technique, both of which are described later. If a loss-of-resistance technique is used, an additional decision about the type of syringe (i.e., glass vs. low-resistance plastic and Luer-Lok vs. friction hub) is required.

Position

The sitting and lateral decubitus positions necessary for epidural puncture are the same as those for spinal anesthesia (see also Chapter 62). As before, inadequate positioning of the patient can complicate an otherwise meticulous technique. Shorter insertion times occur in the sitting position for thoracic epidurals compared with the lateral decubitus position, but ultimately, success rates are comparable.[288] As with spinal anesthesia, epidurals are performed with the patient awake.[76]

Projection and Puncture

The level of needle insertion depends on the location of surgery (Table 45.7). Important surface landmarks include the intercristal line (corresponding to the L4-L5 interspace), the inferior angle of the scapula (corresponding to the T7 vertebral body), the root of the scapular spine (T3), and the vertebra prominens (C7). Ultrasonography may be useful to identify the correct thoracic space[233]; it is less commonly used for thoracic epidural insertion, however, because the acoustic shadows make visualization of landmarks such as the ligamentum flavum and intrathecal space more difficult.[289] A variety of different needle approaches exist: midline, paramedian, modified paramedian (Taylor approach), and caudal.

A midline approach is commonly chosen for lumbar and low thoracic approaches. After local anesthetic infiltration of the skin, the nondominant hand can be rested on the back of the patient, with the thumb and index finger holding the needle hub or wing. The angle of approach should be only slightly cephalad in the lumbar and low-thoracic regions, whereas in the midthoracic region, the approach should be more cephalad because of the significant downward angulation of the spinous processes (Fig. 45.9). In a controlled fashion, the needle should be advanced with the stylet in place through the supraspinous ligament and into the interspinous ligament, at which point the stylet can be removed and the syringe attached. If it is in the correct location, the needle should rest firmly in the tissues. Some advocate needle placement in the ligamentum flavum for both the loss-of-resistance and hanging-drop methods before attaching the syringe, but this may be difficult, particularly for novices; however, this may allow an improved appreciation of epidural anatomy for the operator. If the needle is merely inserted into the supraspinous ligament and then loss-of-resistance or hanging-drop insertion is begun, there is an increased chance of false loss-of-resistance, possibly because of defects in the interspinous ligament.[290] Such false-positive rates can be as high as 30%.

Air or saline are the two most common noncompressible media used to detect a loss-of-resistance when identifying the epidural space. Each involves intermittent (for air) or constant (for saline) gentle pressure applied to the bulb of the syringe with the dominant thumb while the needle is advanced with the nondominant hand. A combination of air and saline may also be used, incorporating 2 mL of saline and a small (0.25 mL) air bubble. Usually the ligamentum flavum is identified as a tougher structure with increased resistance, and when the epidural space is subsequently entered, the pressure applied to the syringe plunger allows the solution to flow without resistance into the epidural space. There are reports that air is less reliable in identifying the epidural space, results in a higher chance of incomplete block, and may also cause both pneumocephalus (which can result in headaches) and venous air embolism in rare cases. If air is chosen, the amount of air injected after loss-of-resistance should therefore be minimized. Evidence suggests that there is no difference in adverse outcome in the obstetric population when air or saline is used.[291] Another meta-analysis found that fluid inserted through the epidural needle before catheter insertion reduces the risk of epidural vein cannulation by the catheter.[287] One proposed disadvantage of using saline is that it may be more difficult to readily detect an accidental dural puncture.

An alternative method of identifying the epidural space is the hanging-drop technique. After the needle is placed into the ligamentum flavum, a drop of solution such as saline is placed within the hub of the needle. When the needle is advanced into the epidural space, the solution should be "sucked in." The theory behind this maneuver has traditionally been attributed to subatmospheric pressure in the epidural space, although recent experimental evidence in the cervical region suggests that using negative-pressure methods are poorly reliable and only useful in the sitting position.[292] The subatmospheric pressure has been related to expansion of the epidural space as the needle pushes the dura away from the ligamentum flavum.[293] The negative intrathoracic pressure may influence the pressure in the epidural space in the thoracic region and should be maximal during inspiration. Timing needle advancement to coincide with inspiration may be difficult, however.

When a lumbar midline approach is used, the depth from skin to the ligamentum flavum commonly reaches 4 cm, with the depth in most (80%) patients being between 3.5 and 6 cm; it can be longer or shorter in obese or very thin patients, respectively. Ultrasonography may be useful to predict the depth before needle insertion.[233] In the lumbar region, the ligamentum flavum is 5 to 6 mm thick in the midline. When a thoracic approach is chosen, needle control is of equal or greater importance because injury to the spinal cord is possible if the needle is advanced too far,

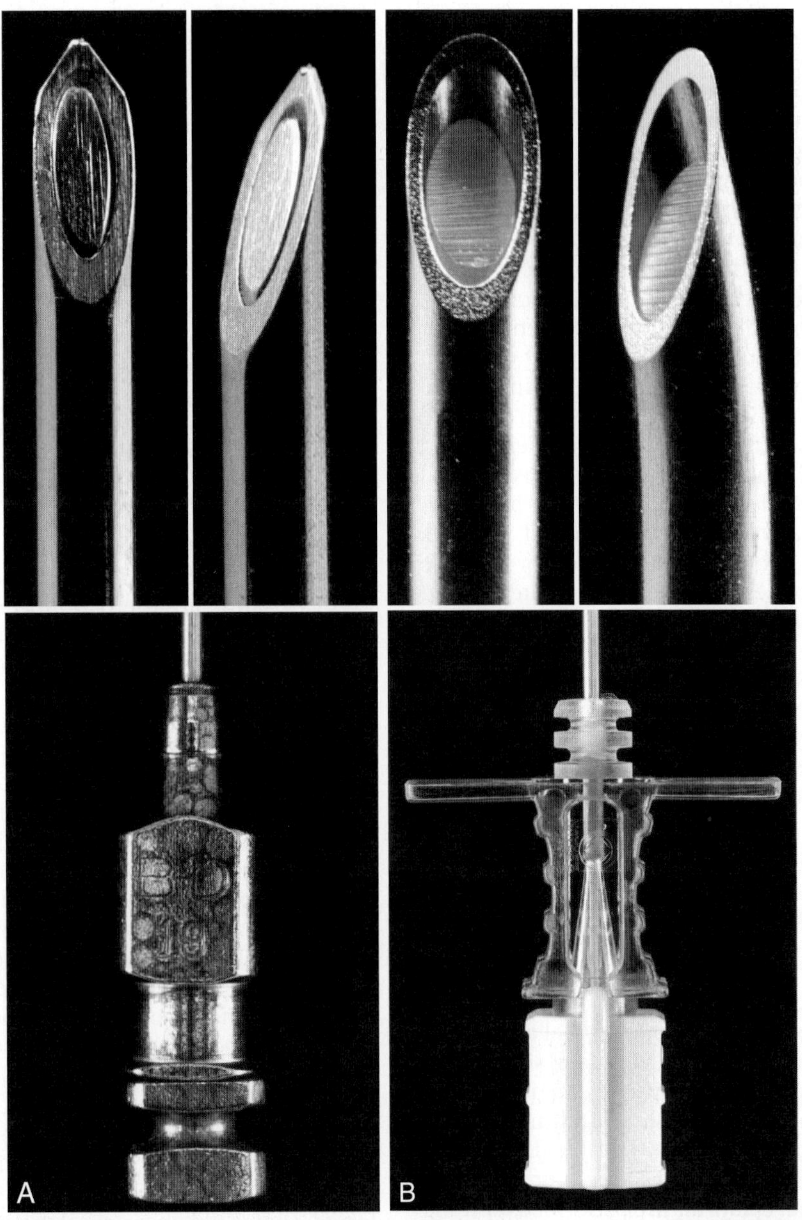

Fig. 45.8 Epidural needles with catheter assortment. (A) A 19-G reusable Crawford epidural needle. (B) A 19-G disposable Tuohy needle. (C) Single–end-hole epidural catheter. (D) Closed-tip, multiple–side-hole catheter. (E) Spring wire–reinforced, polymer-coated epidural catheter.

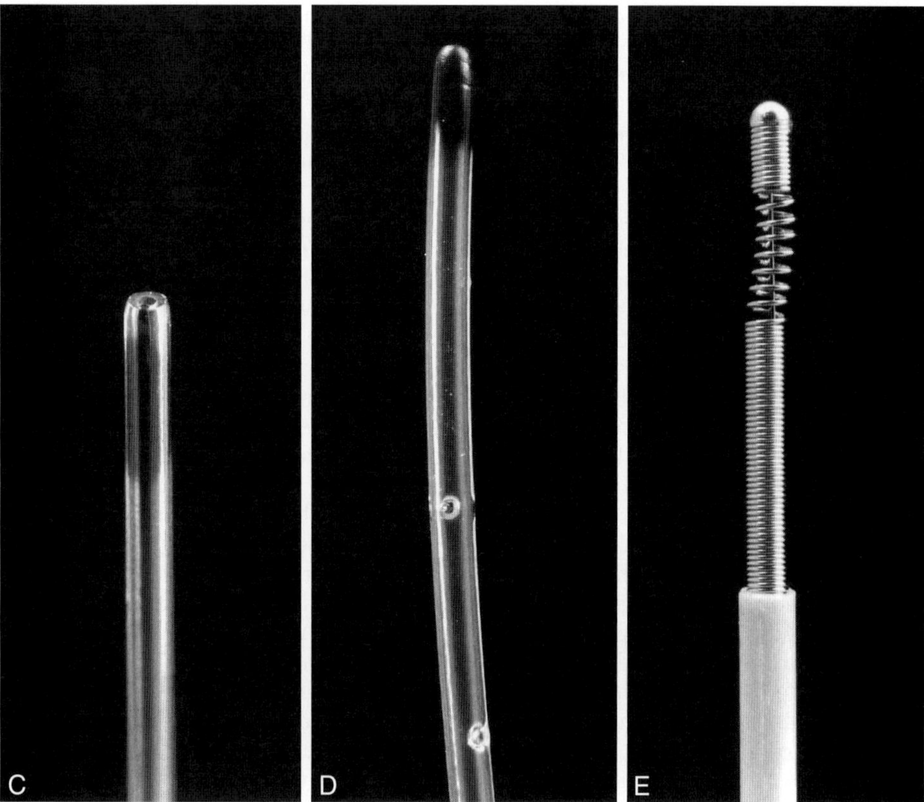

Fig. 45.8, cont'd

TABLE 45.7 Suggested Epidural Insertion Sites for Common Surgical Procedures

Nature of Surgery	Suggested Level of Insertion	Remarks
Hip surgery Lower extremity Obstetric analgesia	Lumbar L2-L5	
Colectomy, anterior resection Upper abdominal surgery	Lower thoracic T6-T8	Spread more cranial than caudal
Thoracic	T2-T6	Midpoint of surgical incision

Modified from Visser WA, Lee RA, Gielen MJ. Factors affecting the distribution of neural blockade by local anesthetics in epidural anesthesia and a comparison of lumbar versus thoracic epidural anesthesia. *Anesth Analg.* 2008;107:708–721.

although there are no data to suggest that approaching the epidural space at the lumbar level is any more or less safe than at the thoracic level. This may be partly because those using the thoracic technique are most often anesthesiologists with considerable experience in lumbar epidural anesthesia.[294] In addition, the increased angle of needle insertion in the thoracic region may theoretically provide an element of safety in that the more acute angle necessary to gain access to the epidural space provides some margin of safety (see Fig. 45.9).

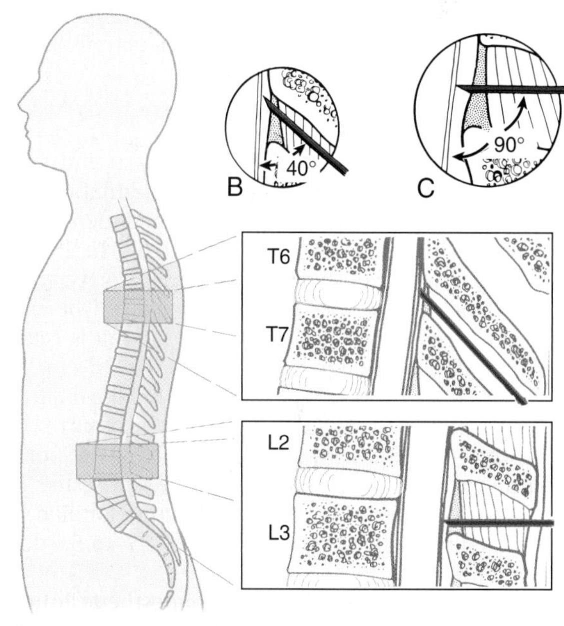

Fig. 45.9 (A) Lumbar and thoracic epidural technique. The increased angle of needle insertion during thoracic epidural cannulation may provide a slightly longer distance of "needle travel" before entering the subarachnoid space. In contrast to lumbar epidural cannulation (B), the distance traveled is modified by a more perpendicular angle of needle insertion (C).

When the epidural space is identified, the depth of the needle at the skin should be noted. The syringe can then be removed and a catheter gently threaded to approximately the 15- to 18-cm mark to ensure a sufficient length has entered the epidural space. The needle can then be carefully withdrawn, and the catheter is withdrawn to leave 4 to 6 cm in the space. Catheter space less than 4 cm in length in the epidural space may increase the risk of catheter dislodgement and inadequate analgesia, whereas threading more catheter may increase the likelihood of catheter malposition or complications.[295-298]

As described earlier, a false loss-of-resistance can occur and is one of the causes of a failed block. The Tsui test may be used to confirm the epidural catheter position.[299] This test stimulates the spinal nerve roots with a low electrical current conducted through normal saline in the epidural space and an electrically conducting catheter. A metal-containing catheter must be used, with the cathode lead of the nerve stimulator connected to the catheter via an electrode adapter, whereas the anode lead is connected to an electrode on the patient's skin. At currents of approximately 1 to 10 mA, corresponding muscle twitches (i.e., intercostal or abdominal wall muscles for thoracic epidural catheters) can be used to identify catheter tip location. Subarachnoid and subdurally positioned epidural catheters elicit motor responses at a much lower threshold current (<1 mA), because the stimulating catheter is in very close or direct contact with highly conductive CSF.[300,301]

When the catheter is positioned at the desired depth, it must be secured to the skin. Commercial fixation devices exist, and some are superior to tape alone.[302] Tunneling can reduce catheter migration and improve lasting block success.[303] However, tunneling has not been compared with noninvasive catheter fixation devices in a well-designed study.

Paramedian Approach

The paramedian approach is particularly useful in the mid- to high-thoracic region, where the angulation of the spine and the narrow spaces render the midline approach problematic. The needle should be inserted 1 to 2 cm lateral to the inferior tip of the spinous process corresponding to the vertebra above the desired interspace. The needle is then advanced horizontally until the lamina is reached and then redirected medially and cephalad to enter the epidural space. The Taylor approach is a modified paramedian approach via the L5-S1 interspace, which may be useful in trauma patients who cannot tolerate or are not able to maintain a sitting position. The needle is inserted 1 cm medial and 1 cm inferior to the posterior superior iliac spine and is angled medially and cephalad at a 45- to 55-degree angle.

Before initiating an epidural local anesthetic infusion, a test dose may be administered. The purpose of this is to exclude intrathecal or intravascular catheter placement. A small volume of lidocaine 1.5% with epinephrine is traditionally used for this purpose. A recent systematic review found reasonable evidence that 10 to 15 μg of epinephrine alone in nonpregnant adult patients was the best pharmacologic method of detecting intravascular placement, using endpoints of an increase in systolic blood pressure more than 15 mm Hg or an increase in heart rate more than 10 beats/min. The optimal method of detecting intrathecal or subdural placement, however, could not be ascertained.[304]

Combined Spinal-Epidural

CSE anesthesia was first described in 1937 but has subsequently been modified over the past 30 years[305-310] and the CSE technique is now seeing increasing popularity. A CSE allows flexibility in a number of clinical settings because the more rapid onset of spinal block compared with epidural anesthesia allows the operative procedure to begin earlier, whereas the epidural catheter still provides both effective postoperative analgesia and allows anesthesia to be extended as the spinal resolves. This is particularly useful during labor, where opioid and a small dose of local anesthetic may be injected through a small spinal needle to provide rapid analgesia, whereas the epidural catheter can be used thereafter for both analgesia and surgical anesthesia if an operative delivery becomes necessary. Another significant advantage of CSE in general is the ability to use a low dose of intrathecal local anesthetic, with the knowledge that the epidural catheter may be used to extend the block if necessary. The addition of either local anesthetic or saline alone to the epidural space via the catheter compresses the dural sac and increases the block height. This latter technique is called epidural volume extension (EVE) and has been shown in cesarean delivery to provide a comparable sensory block to larger doses of intrathecal local anesthetic (with no EVE) but with significantly faster motor recovery.[311] The principle of using a lower dose of spinal anesthetic and titrating the epidural dose after the spinal anesthetic to reach the appropriate block height is a reduction in side effects[312] with faster recovery, which can in turn potentially hasten discharge. This sequential technique also provides greater hemodynamic stability for high-risk patients using a lower initial mass of drug for spinal anesthetic, with subsequent gradual extension of the block if necessary using the epidural.

TECHNIQUE

The CSE technique most commonly involves placement of the epidural needle first, followed by either a "needle through needle" technique to reach the subarachnoid space or an altogether separate spinal needle insertion at either the same or different interspace. Some but not all studies have demonstrated greater success and lower failure rates with the separate needle insertion technique.[313-316] This method has the potential advantage of being able to confirm that the epidural catheter is functional before spinal anesthesia is administered, which, although it is time consuming, may be advantageous if the epidural catheter is to be relied upon for anesthesia when the spinal component resolves. Conversely, this method theoretically risks shearing the epidural catheter that is already in situ. If a needle-through-needle technique is chosen, special CSE kits are available with long spinal needles, some of which can be locked in place for the subarachnoid injection.

Caudal Anesthesia

Caudal anesthesia is popular in pediatric anesthesia (see Chapter 77), but the technique also can be used in adults, although it is unpredictable when upper abdominal or thoracic spread is required. Its indications in adults therefore are essentially the same as those for lumbar epidural anesthesia, although it may be particularly useful when sacral anesthetic spread is desired (e.g., perineal, anal, rectal procedures), where a spinal surgery scar may prevent a lumbar anesthetic technique and, more commonly, in chronic pain and cancer pain management (see Chapter 51). The use of fluoroscopic guidance and, more recently, ultrasonography can help guide correct needle placement and reduce the rate of a failed block.[317] Ultrasonography is of even greater benefit in children because the lack of bony ossification allows visualization of both local anesthetic spread and the position of caudal epidural catheters.[318,319]

PHARMACOLOGY

The local anesthetics used are similar to those described for epidural anesthesia and analgesia. However, in adults approximately twice the lumbar epidural dose is required to achieve a similar block with the caudal approach. The spread is also variable, making this technique in adults unreliable for procedures above the umbilicus.

TECHNIQUE

Patient preparation as described before for spinal and epidural anesthesia must be equally applied to caudal anesthesia, namely consent, monitoring and resuscitation equipment, intravenous access, and the same asepsis precautions. Caudal anesthesia requires identification of the sacral hiatus. The sacrococcygeal ligament (i.e., extension of ligamentum flavum) overlies the sacral hiatus between the two sacral cornua. To facilitate locating the cornua, the posterior superior iliac spines should be located and, by using the line between them as one side of an equilateral triangle, the location of the sacral hiatus should be approximated (Fig. 45.10). Ultrasonography can also be used to identify these landmarks,[317-319] as can fluoroscopy. Three positions (see Chapter 34) are available for caudal anesthesia, with the prone position most often chosen in adults, the lateral decubitus position most chosen in children, and the knee-chest position the most infrequently used. The lateral decubitus position is used in children because it is easier to maintain a patent airway in this position than in the prone position, and the landmarks are more easily palpable than they are in adults (see Chapter 76). This consideration is valuable because caudal anesthesia is often combined with general anesthesia in pediatric patients to decrease the amount of volatile agent used intraoperatively or to provide postoperative analgesia. In contrast, a caudal block is often administered during preoperative sedation in adults and when the prone position is applicable. When placing a patient in the prone position, a pillow should be inserted beneath the iliac crests to rotate the pelvis and make cannulation of the caudal canal easier. An additional aid is to spread the lower extremities about 20 degrees with the heels rotated laterally, which minimizes gluteal muscle contraction and eases needle insertion.

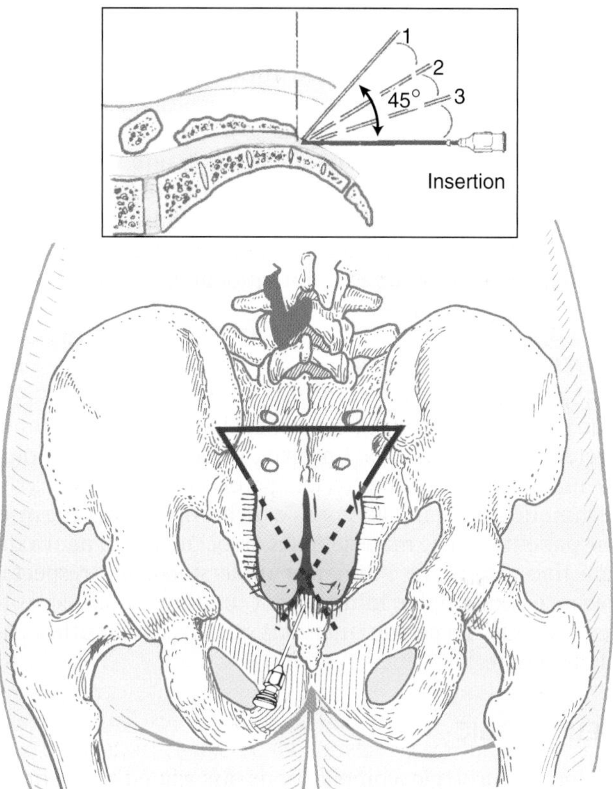

Fig. 45.10 Caudal technique. Palpating fingers locate the sacral cornua by using the equilateral triangle. Needle insertion is completed by insertion and withdrawal in a stepwise fashion (*inset,* so-called 1-2-3 insertion) until the needle can be advanced into the caudal canal and the solution can be injected easily (without creation of a subcutaneous "lump" of fluid).

After the sacral hiatus is identified, the index and middle fingers of the palpating hand are placed on the sacral cornua, and after local infiltration, the caudal needle (or Tuohy needle if a catheter is to be placed) is inserted at an angle of approximately 45 degrees to the sacrum. While the needle is advanced, a decrease in resistance to needle insertion should be appreciated as the needle enters the caudal canal. The needle is advanced until bone (i.e., the dorsal aspect of the ventral plate of the sacrum) is contacted and then is slightly withdrawn, and the needle is redirected so that the angle of insertion relative to the skin surface is decreased. In male patients, this angle is almost parallel to the coronal plane; in female patients, a slightly steeper angle (15 degrees) is necessary. During redirection of the needle, loss-of-resistance is sought to confirm entry into the epidural space, and the needle advanced no more than approximately 1 to 2 cm into the caudal canal. In adults, the tip should never be advanced beyond the S2 level (approximately 1 cm inferior to the posterior superior iliac spine), which is the level to which the dural sac extends. Additional advancement of the needle increases the risk of dural puncture, and unintentional intravascular cannulation becomes more likely. One method of increasing the likelihood of correct caudal needle placement is to inject 5 mL of saline rapidly through the caudal needle while palpating the skin overlying the sacrum. If no midline bulge is detected, the needle is probably positioned correctly. In contrast, if a midline bulge is detected during saline injection, the needle is positioned incorrectly.

After ensuring correct needle position and before injection of the therapeutic dose of caudal anesthetic, aspiration should be performed and a test dose administered because, as in lumbar epidural anesthesia, a vein or the subarachnoid space can be entered unintentionally.

Complications

The physiologic effects of neuraxial blocks may be misinterpreted as complications; however, clear distinction should be made between the physiologic effects of the neuraxial technique and complications, which imply some harm to the patient.[320] The material risks associated with neuraxial anesthesia must be intimately understood and respected because catastrophic injury is not unknown and serves to remind us that a person's nervous system is at the other end of the needle.[321]

NEUROLOGIC

Serious neurologic complications associated with neuraxial anesthesia are rare. As such, prohibitively large numbers of patients are required for study to estimate the frequency of these events. The true incidence of most neurologic injury after neuraxial anesthesia is unknown with published accounts of neurologic complications invariably influenced by the differing identification and reporting processes. The ASRA comprehensively addresses this important topic in their updated Practice Advisory on Neurologic Complications.[76]

Paraplegia

The frequency of paraplegia related to neuraxial anesthesia is reported to be approximately 0.1/10,000,[322,323] and the mechanism of such a severe injury is likely multifactorial and difficult to identify for certain.[324] Although injury resulting from direct needle trauma to the spinal cord[325-329] may be self-evident, historical cases highlight the fundamental danger that accompanies the injection of a foreign substance into the CSF. The highly publicized cases of Woolley and Roe, two healthy, middle-aged men who became paraplegic after spinal anesthesia by the same anesthesiologist using the same drug on the same day for minor surgery at the same hospital in the United Kingdom in 1947, arguably set back the practice of spinal anesthesia for decades despite evidence that contamination by the descaling liquid used to cleanse the procedure tray had most likely been responsible.[4] Another example of catastrophic injury related to intrathecal injectate was the chloroprocaine neurotoxicity experience in the early 1980s, during which several patients developed adhesive arachnoiditis, cauda equina syndrome, or permanent paresis thought to be related to a combination of low pH and the antioxidant sodium bisulfite preservative used in early (and discontinued) preparations of the short-acting ester local anesthetic chloroprocaine.[136-139,330]

Profound hypotension or ischemia of the spinal cord can be important contributing factors in cases of paraplegia associated with neuraxial anesthesia. Anterior spinal artery syndrome, characterized by painless loss of motor and sensory function, is associated with anterior cord ischemia or infarction with sparing of proprioception, which is carried by the posterior column. The anterior cord is believed to be especially vulnerable to ischemic insult because of its single and tenuous source of arterial blood supply (the artery of Adamkiewicz). Ischemia caused by any one or a combination of profound hypotension, mechanical obstruction, vasculopathy, or hemorrhage can contribute to irreversible anterior cord damage.[331-333]

Cauda Equina Syndrome

The rate of cauda equina syndrome is approximately 0.1/10,000 and invariably results in permanent neurologic deficit.[322] The lumbosacral roots of the spinal cord may be particularly vulnerable to direct exposure to large doses of local anesthetic, whether it is administered as a single injection of relatively highly concentrated local anesthetic (e.g., 5% lidocaine)[334] or prolonged exposure to a local anesthetic through a continuous catheter.[5,335,336] The US Food and Drug Administration withdrew approval for spinal catheters smaller than 24-g in size in 1992 because of concerns about a perceived association between the small-bore catheters and the development of cauda equina syndrome.[337] Although small-bore catheters can reduce the risk of headache, they can predispose to pooling of local anesthetic around the lumbosacral nerve roots, possibly because of slow injectate flow through the fine-bore catheter, thereby exposing them to high concentrations of local anesthetic. However, small-bore spinal catheters are being used effectively in Europe, and they are beginning to reappear in the United States, although it has taken nearly 15 years for them to emerge from the regulatory cloud of the early 1990s.[338] Another risk factor for cauda equine syndrome may be spinal stenosis wherein local anesthetic distribution may be limited, thus exposing the cauda equine to higher concentrations of local anesthetic.

Epidural Hematoma

Bleeding within the vertebral canal can cause ischemic compression of the spinal cord and lead to permanent neurologic deficit if not recognized and evacuated expeditiously. Many risk factors have been associated with the development of an epidural hematoma, including difficult or traumatic needle or catheter insertion,[339] coagulopathy, elderly age, and female gender.[340] Radicular back pain, prolonged blockade longer than the expected duration of the neuraxial technique, and bladder or bowel dysfunction are features commonly associated with a space-occupying lesion within the vertebral canal and should prompt magnetic resonance imaging on an urgent basis. Before the recently published United Kingdom National Health Service (NHS) audit, the largest contemporary studies reported rates of epidural hematoma of less than 0.06/10,000 after spinal anesthesia, whereas the reported rates of epidural hematoma after epidural blockade in the audit were as much as 10-fold higher.[294,341-345] The United Kingdom NHS audit arguably provides the most accurate rates of neurologic complications associated with neuraxial anesthesia in contemporary practice. This unique prospective nationwide audit found five cases of epidural hematoma among 707,455 neuraxial techniques (0.07/10,000), all of which occurred among 97,925 perioperative epidural techniques (0.5/10,000) performed over the course of 1 year.[323]

Nerve Injury

In 1955, Vandam and Dripps[346] were the first to capture data prospectively on nerve injury from more than 10,000 patients who underwent spinal anesthesia. No severe neurologic injuries occurred in this population. In 1969, Dawkins[347] published the classic review of neurologic complications after 32,718 epidural anesthetics and reported the frequency of transient and permanent nerve injury to be 0.1% and 0.02%, respectively. Despite interim advances in practice and research methodology, some of the largest contemporary studies available[341,344,348-350] suggest that the rate of neurologic injury related to neuraxial anesthesia is mostly unchanged compared with that reported nearly a half century ago. Most notable from these contemporary data are that epidural (including CSE) anesthesia is likely associated with a more frequent rate of radiculopathy or peripheral neuropathy compared with spinal anesthesia,[322] and that neuraxial anesthesia performed in adults for the purposes of perioperative anesthesia or analgesia is apparently associated with a higher likelihood of neurologic complications compared with that performed in the obstetric, pediatric, and chronic pain settings.[323,341,342,351,352] The rate of permanent nerve injury after neuraxial blockade is even more difficult to determine because methods of investigation and diagnosis, determination of causation, and reporting of outcomes are highly variable within the literature.[353] The United Kingdom NHS audit found the overall rate of permanent nerve injury to be 7 in 707,455 or 0.1/10,000,[323] which is remarkably similar to studies published a half century earlier by Dawkins. Three cases of nerve injury occurred among 293,050 epidurals (0.1/10,000), 3 among 324,950 spinal anesthetics (0.1/10,000), and 1 among 41,875 CSEs (0.2/10,000), mostly in young, healthy patients. Procedure-related risk factors traditionally associated with nerve injury after neuraxial anesthesia in the perioperative setting include radicular pain or paresthesia occurring during the procedure.[321,344,354,355]

Arachnoiditis

Arachnoiditis, an inflammatory reaction of the meninges, is rare after neuraxial anesthesia and its true incidence is unknown. The potential contributory effects of chlorhexidine disinfectant solution has led to the recommendation that chlorhexidine must dry fully before needle puncture,[76] and measures must also be taken to avoid splashing of any chlorhexidine solution onto the needles or syringes, and especially contamination of the injectate drugs.

Post–Dural Puncture Headache

A relatively common complication of neuraxial anesthesia is post–dural puncture headache. As the name implies, post–dural puncture headache is believed to result from unintentional or intentional puncture of the dura membrane in the setting of neuraxial anesthesia or after myelography and diagnostic lumbar puncture. There are two possible explanations for the cause of the headache, neither of which has ever been proven. First, the loss of CSF through the dura is proposed to cause traction on pain-sensitive intracranial structures as the brain loses support and sags. Alternatively, the loss of CSF initiates compensatory yet painful intracerebral vasodilation to offset the reduction in intracranial pressure.[356] The characteristic feature of a post–dural puncture headache is a frontal or occipital headache that worsens with the upright or seated posture and is relieved by lying supine. Associated symptoms can include nausea, vomiting, neck pain, dizziness, tinnitus, diplopia, hearing loss, cortical blindness, cranial nerve palsies, and even seizures. In more than 90% of cases, the onset of characteristic post–dural puncture headache symptoms will begin within 3 days of the procedure,[357] and 66% start within the first 48 hours.[358] Spontaneous resolution usually occurs within 7 days in the majority (72%) of cases, whereas 87% of cases resolve by 6 months.[359]

Post–dural puncture headache can occur in the setting of either spinal or epidural anesthesia, the former associated with certain modifiable risk factors during intentional dural puncture and the latter associated with unintentional puncture of the dura by advancing the Tuohy needle. Orienting a needle bevel parallel with the axis of the spine, such that the longitudinal fibers of the dura would more likely be separated than cut, results in a lower incidence of postspinal puncture headache.[360] This clinical observation is supported by laboratory investigations[361] showing that simulated spinal puncture with cone-shaped (pencil-point) spinal needle tips produces slower transdural loss of fluid than a similar puncture with cutting-tipped needles. Indeed meta-analysis has confirmed that noncutting needle tip designs have a lower frequency of post–dural puncture headache than do cutting spinal needle tip designs.[362] Other studies suggest that the collagen layers of the dura are oriented in a multidirectional fashion, not always in a cephalocaudad direction, and are variable in thickness, leading to the suggestion that damage to the longitudinal cells of the arachnoid membrane is more likely to be influenced by the type of bevel and may even be the predominant factor affecting post–dural puncture headache.[9] Reports vary as to whether the incidence of post–dural puncture headache is increased with the CSE technique compared with epidural alone.[363,364]

Aside from the type of needle tip (cutting vs. pencil-point) and the bevel direction, there are additional risk factors common to the performance of both spinal and epidural anesthesia that contribute to the likelihood of developing a post–dural puncture headache. These risk factors are listed in Box 45.2.[365]

Conservative management for post–dural puncture headache includes supine positioning, hydration, caffeine, and oral analgesics. Sumatriptan has also been used with varying effect but is not without side effects.[366,367] Epidural blood patch is the definitive therapy for post–dural puncture headache.[368] This therapy was introduced by Gormley[369]; its safety and efficacy have been well documented, and contemporary practice has validated that a single epidural blood patch continues to have up to a 90% initial improvement rate[370] and persistent resolution of symptoms in 61% to 75% of cases.[371]

Epidural blood patch is ideally performed 24 hours after dural puncture and after the development of classic

BOX 45.2 Relationships Among Variables and Post–Spinal Puncture Headache

Factors That Can Increase the Incidence of Headache After Spinal Puncture

- Age: Younger, more frequent
- Sex: Females > males
- Needle size: Larger > smaller
- Needle bevel: Less when the needle bevel is placed in the long axis of the neuraxis
- Pregnancy: More when pregnant
- Dural punctures: More with multiple punctures

Factors That Do Not Increase the Incidence of Headache After Spinal Puncture

- Insertion and use of catheters for continuous spinal anesthesia
- Timing of ambulation

post–dural puncture headache symptoms. The efficacy of prophylactic epidural blood patching is not supported by evidence.[372,373] By injecting radionuclide-labeled red blood cells epidurally, Szeinfeld and co-workers[374] demonstrated that approximately 15 mL of blood will spread over a mean distance of nine spinal segments, and that the direction of spread was preferentially cephalad relative to the level of blood injection. As a result, these authors recommend inserting the blood patch needle at or caudad to the level of the previous culprit dural puncture. These findings have since been validated by magnetic resonance imaging of epidural blood patch spread.[375] One multinational, multicenter, randomized, blinded trial suggested that 20 mL of blood is a reasonable starting target volume.[376] A second epidural blood patch may be performed 24 to 48 hours after the first in the case of ineffective or incomplete relief of symptoms.

Transient Neurologic Symptoms

Traditionally associated with lidocaine, TNS have been described after intrathecal administration of every local anesthetic used for spinal anesthesia. TNS, previously known as transient radicular irritation,[377] are usually characterized by bilateral or unilateral pain in the buttocks radiating to the legs or, less commonly, isolated buttock or leg pain. Symptoms occur within 24 hours of the resolution of an otherwise uneventful spinal anesthetic and are not associated with any neurologic deficits or laboratory abnormalities.[378] The pain can range from mild to severe and typically resolves spontaneously in 1 week or less.[379] The likelihood of TNS are highest after intrathecal lidocaine and mepivacaine, and are far less frequent with bupivacaine and other local anesthetics.[147,159,380] The phenomenon is not related to the concentration of lidocaine,[147] the addition of dextrose or epinephrine, or solution osmolarity. The type of needle can influence the likelihood of TNS, with the rate reduced by a double-orifice needle,[381] possibly because single-orifice needles increase the risk of injecting anesthetic caudally in the thecal sac. TNS are not commonly associated with epidural procedures but have occurred with epidural lidocaine and other local anesthetics.[253,382] Finally, TNS occur more commonly in patients who are placed in the lithotomy position for surgery. Nonsteroidal antiinflammatory drugs are the first line of treatment, but pain can be severe and may even require opioids.

CARDIOVASCULAR

Hypotension

Hypotension may be considered a complication of neuraxial blockade if the patient faces harm. Recent guidance has placed more emphasis on avoiding hypotension during neuraxial anesthesia (defined as 20%–30% below baseline) in order to reduce the possibility of spinal cord ischemia or infarction.[76] In the setting of spinal anesthesia, hypotension (defined as systolic blood pressure <90 mm Hg) is more likely to occur with a variety of factors including peak block height greater than or equal to T5, age older than or equal to 40 years, baseline systolic blood pressure less than 120 mm Hg, combined spinal and general anesthesia, spinal puncture at or above the L2-L3 interspace, and the addition of phenylephrine to the local anesthetic.[51] Hypotension (defined as a reduction in mean arterial blood pressure >30%) is independently associated with chronic alcohol consumption, history of hypertension, BMI, and the urgency of surgery.[383] Nausea is a common symptom of hypotension in the setting of neuraxial anesthesia, as are vomiting, dizziness, and dyspnea. Although prevention of hypotension caused by vasodilatation using a prophylactic ("preloading") infusion of colloid or crystalloid during the performance of the neuraxial block ("coloading") has been reported,[384] this is no longer recommended as a routine practice.[384]

Bradycardia

The development of severe bradycardia after spinal anesthesia has long been recognized as an important risk of spinal anesthesia.[385,386] Bradycardia stems from blockade of the thoracic sympathetic fibers (preganglionic cardiac accelerator fibers originating at T1-T5), as well as reflexive slowing of the heart rate as vasodilation reduces the venous return to the right atrium where stretch receptors respond by a compensatory slowing of the heart rate. Factors that may increase the likelihood of exaggerated bradycardia (40–50 beats/min) include baseline heart rate less than 60 beats/min, age younger than 37 years, male gender, nonemergency status, β-adrenergic blockade, and prolonged case duration. Severe bradycardia (<40 beats/min) is associated with a baseline heart rate less than 60 beats/min and male gender.[387]

Cardiac Arrest (also see Chapter 87)

In a review of closed insurance claims, Caplan and associates[388] identified 14 cases of sudden cardiac arrest in healthy patients receiving spinal anesthesia. The etiology of sudden cardiac arrest after spinal anesthesia is not understood. Whether these catastrophic events represented lack of vigilant monitoring and treatment as opposed to some mysterious physiologic explanation is not known.[389] The latter notwithstanding, it is clear that hypoxemia and oversedation are complicit in the severe bradycardia and asystole that can occur suddenly during well-conducted spinal anesthesia.[390,391] Curiously, these rare events seem to be preferentially associated with spinal anesthesia rather than epidural techniques. In their inaugural survey of French anesthesiologists, Auroy and colleagues reported the rate of cardiac arrest to be 6.4/10,000 after spinal anesthesia compared with 1/10,000 for all other neuraxial and peripheral regional anesthesia techniques combined.[344] In their larger follow-up survey of all anesthesiologists in France, Auroy and colleagues[350] reported 10 cases of cardiac arrest after 35,439 spinal anesthetics (2.5/10,000) and none after 5561 epidural techniques. Most recently, Cook and colleagues uncovered three cases of cardiovascular collapse among 707,425 neuraxial blocks (0.04/10,000) during their nationwide audit, two of which were during spinal anesthesia and one in the setting of CSE.[323]

RESPIRATORY

Neuraxial opioids are commonly added to local anesthetic solutions to improve the quality and duration of neuraxial anesthesia and analgesia. The risk of respiratory depression associated with neuraxial opioids is dose dependent, with a reported frequency that approaches 3% after the administration of 0.8 mg of intrathecal morphine.[392] Respiratory depression may stem from rostral spread of opioids within the CSF to the chemosensitive respiratory centers in the brainstem.[65] With lipophilic anesthetics, respiratory depression is generally an early phenomenon occurring within the first 30 minutes; respiratory depression has never been described more than 2 hours after the administration of intrathecal fentanyl or sufentanil.[225] With intrathecal morphine, there is a risk of late respiratory depression, occurring as much as 24 hours after injection. Respiratory monitoring for the first 24 hours after the administration of intrathecal morphine is therefore advisable. Patients with sleep apnea can be especially sensitive to the potent respiratory-depressant effects of opioid medications and although definitive safety data evidence is lacking, the decision to administer neuraxial opioids to these patients is made with considerable caution.[393,394] Older patients also have a higher risk of respiratory depression, and the dose of neuraxial opioids should be reduced in this population (see Chapter 65). Coadministration of systemic sedatives also increases this risk.

INFECTION

Bacterial meningitis and epidural abscess are rare, but potentially catastrophic, infectious complications of all neuraxial techniques. Sources of infection in neuraxial procedures include the equipment, the patient, or the practitioner. Staphylococcal infections arising from the patient's skin are one of the most common epidural-related infections, whereas oral bacteria such as *Streptococcus viridans* are a common cause of infection after spinal anesthesia, underscoring the need for the clinician to wear a facemask when performing neuraxial procedures. Other factors that may increase the likelihood of infection include the presence of a concomitant systemic infection, diabetes, immunocompromised states,[90] and prolonged maintenance of an epidural (or spinal) catheter. Large contemporary studies estimate the rate of serious neuraxial infection to be less than 0.3/10,000[341,348,350] for spinal anesthesia, whereas infectious complications after epidural techniques may be at least twice as common.[341,348,350,395-397] Obstetric patients are less likely to develop deep infections related to epidural analgesia. The recent United Kingdom NHS audit reported no cases of meningitis and eight cases of epidural abscess after 707,455 neuraxial techniques, five of which occurred among 293,050 epidural techniques, two among 324,950 spinal anesthetics, and one among 47,550 caudal blocks.[323]

In 2017, the ASA and ASRA published a practice advisory regarding infectious complications associated with neuraxial anesthesia,[229] specifically addressing (1) prevention, (2) diagnosis, and (3) management. Previous publications have addressed infectious risks of neuraxial anesthesia in the febrile or infected patient,[90] the immunocompromised patient,[398] and in the setting of chronic pain treatments.[399]

Aseptic meningitis occurred mostly in the early 20th century, likely secondary to chemical contamination and detergents, which are no longer present in modern preservative-free preparations.

BACKACHE

Back injury is perhaps the most feared complication of neuraxial anesthesia among patients. Evidence indicates that the incidence of back pain after spinal anesthesia is not different from general anesthesia.[400] Indeed, up to 25% of all surgical patients undergoing anesthesia, regardless of anesthetic technique, experience backache, the incidence of which increases to 50% when surgery lasts 4 to 5 hours.[401] There is also no association between epidural analgesia and new-onset back pain up to 6 months postpartum.[402,403] Preexisting back pain does appear to be a risk factor for persistent back pain after neuraxial anesthesia, although the severity of the pain does not appear to be worsened. Other risk factors include immobilization during surgery greater than 2.5 hours, lithotomy position, BMI greater than 32 kg/m^2, and multiple attempts at block placement.[400]

NAUSEA AND VOMITING

There are multiple possible mechanisms that contribute to nausea and vomiting in the setting of neuraxial anesthesia, including direct exposure of the chemoreceptive trigger zone in the brain to emetogenic drugs (e.g., opioids), as well as hypotension associated with generalized vasodilation and gastrointestinal hyperperistalsis secondary to unopposed parasympathetic activity (see also Chapter 80).[404] Although regional anesthesia is often recommended as an alternative to general anesthesia for patients at risk for postoperative nausea and vomiting, there are few studies that have primarily investigated the effects of neuraxial anesthesia on postoperative nausea and vomiting with sufficient statistical power. Factors associated with developing nausea or vomiting after spinal anesthesia include the addition of phenylephrine or epinephrine to the local anesthetic, peak block height greater than or equal to T5, baseline heart rate greater than 60 beats/min, use of procaine, history of motion sickness, and the development of hypotension during spinal anesthesia. Among the opioids commonly added to intrathecal or epidural local anesthetics, morphine administration has the most frequent risk of nausea or vomiting, whereas fentanyl and sufentanil carry the least frequent risk.[404] Neuraxial opioid-related nausea and vomiting appears to be dose dependent. Using less than 0.1 mg morphine reduces the risk of nausea and vomiting, without compromising the analgesic effect.[225]

URINARY RETENTION

Urinary retention can occur in as much as one third of patients after neuraxial anesthesia. Local anesthetic blockade of the S2, S3, and S4 nerve roots inhibits urinary function as the detrusor muscle is weakened. Neuraxial opioids can further complicate urinary function by suppressing detrusor contractility and reducing the sensation of urge.[405] Spontaneous return of normal bladder function is expected once the sensory level decreases to below S2-3.[406] Although male gender and age have been (albeit inconsistently) linked to urinary retention after neuraxial anesthesia, the administration of intrathecal morphine is strongly associated with this complication.[405,407,408]

PRURITUS

Pruritus can be distressing to the patient. It is the most common side effect related to the intrathecal administration of opioids, with rates between 30% and 100%.[225] Pruritus actually occurs more commonly after intrathecal opioid administration than after intravenous opioid administration and is not dependent on the type or dose of opioid administered. Reducing the dose of intrathecal sufentanil from 5 μg to as little as 1.5 μg can reduce the likelihood of pruritus without compromising analgesia when added to hyperbaric bupivacaine for cesarean delivery (see Chapter 62).[409] The mechanism of pruritus is unclear but is likely related to the central opioid receptor activation rather than histamine release because naloxone, naltrexone, or the partial agonist nalbuphine can be used for treatment. Ondansetron and propofol are also useful therapies. Some antiinflammatories have been shown to reduce pruritus (e.g., diclofenac and tenoxicam), while mirtazapine, an antidepressant with $5HT_3$ antagonism properties like ondansetron, may also be helpful if administered preoperatively.

SHIVERING

The rate of shivering related to neuraxial anesthesia is as frequent as 55%.[410] The intensity of shivering is likely related more to epidural anesthesia than spinal.[411] Although there are multiple possible explanations for the difference in shivering intensity, this observation may simply be related to the inability to shiver because of the profound motor block associated with spinal anesthesia compared with epidural techniques. Another explanation may be the relatively cold temperature of the epidural injectate, which can affect the thermosensitive basal sinuses.[410] The addition of neuraxial opioids, specifically fentanyl and meperidine, reduces the likelihood of shivering.[410] Recommended strategies to prevent shivering after neuraxial anesthesia include prewarming the patient with a forced air warmer for at least 15 minutes and avoiding the administration of cold epidural and intravenous fluids.

WRONG ROUTE ADMINISTRATION

Wrong route administration refers to the infusion or injection of a drug into the wrong body compartment. In addition to epidural catheter migration or inadvertent intravascular placement (described below), an epidural infusion may be mistakenly connected to an intravascular device. Using less cardiotoxic local anesthetics may reduce the risk of harm if this does occur. Prevention is paramount and devices have been developed to make regional anesthesia and intravenous connections technically incompatible.

COMPLICATIONS UNIQUE TO EPIDURAL ANESTHESIA

Intravascular Injection

Epidural anesthesia can produce local anesthetic–induced systemic toxicity (see Chapter 29), primarily through the unintentional administration of drug into an epidural vein. The frequency of vascular puncture with the needle or cannulation with the catheter can reportedly approach 10%, with the highest rates seen in the obstetric population, where these vessels are relatively dilated and more vulnerable to entry.[287,412] The rate of seizures related to epidural anesthesia may be as frequent as 1%.[294,344,350] In obstetrics (see also Chapter 62), the likelihood of intravascular injection is decreased by placing the patient in the lateral (as opposed to the sitting) position during needle and catheter insertion, administering fluid through the epidural needle before catheter insertion, using a single-orifice type rather than a multiorifice catheter or a wire-embedded polyurethane type compared with polyamide epidural catheter, and advancing the catheter less than 6 cm into the epidural space. The paramedian as opposed to the midline needle approach, and the use of a smaller-gauge epidural needle or catheter, does not reduce the risk of epidural vein cannulation.[287]

One of the most controversial issues related to epidural anesthesia has been the use of an epinephrine-containing test dose.[413] Epinephrine (15 μg) in 3 mL of local anesthetic remains the best pharmacologic method of detecting intravascular placement in nonpregnant adult patients.[304] However, controversy surrounds the use of epinephrine in obstetric patients, in whom uterine blood flow may be decreased by the intravascular injection, thereby putting the fetus at risk, and where the cardiovascular changes occurring in active labor may represent a false-positive response to epinephrine. Although epinephrine may place the fetus at risk in theory,[414] no such case has been described. The epidural epinephrine test dose can be unreliable in patients receiving β-adrenergic blockers[415] or if the test dose is administered during general anesthesia.[416] Because there is no fail-safe method of guaranteeing an extravascular location of an epidural local anesthetic, prevention of systemic toxicity should also involve aspiration of the catheter and incremental administration of the local anesthetic. The onset of block, quality of the block, and block height are unaffected by administration of the epidural drug in 5-mL fractions.[417]

Subdural Injection

Blomberg[418] used a fiberoptic technique to demonstrate that the subdural extra-arachnoid space is easily entered in 66% of autopsy attempts in humans. Despite this being an infrequent clinical problem with epidural anesthesia (<1%), it does allow a visual understanding of the subdural complications of epidural anesthesia.[419] This space, unlike the epidural space, also extends intracranially. When an epidural block is performed and a higher-than-expected block develops, but only after a delay of 15 to 30 minutes (unlike a total spinal), subdural placement of local anesthetic must be considered. With a subdural block, the motor block will be modest compared to the extent of the sensory block, and the sympathetic block may be exaggerated. The treatment is symptomatic.

COMPLICATIONS UNIQUE TO COMBINED SPINAL-EPIDURALS

The risk of metal toxicity from abraded spinal needle particles using the needle-through-needle technique has not been confirmed.[420]

Outcomes

Although the benefit of properly applied epidural anesthesia and analgesia as an excellent pain relief modality is unquestionable, its effect on postoperative morbidity and mortality is becoming more clear. Early meta-analysis showed a relative risk reduction in overall mortality in patients receiving neuraxial blockade, by as much as 30% in patients undergoing all types of surgery,[421] but these results included studies now over 40 years old, which may not reflect contemporary anesthetic practice. Recent work has focused on large prospective and retrospective database analyses as well as randomized controlled trials with some analyses including over 1 million patients.[422] Although these too must be treated with caution, there still appear to be benefits of neuraxial anesthesia beyond superior analgesia, particularly when neuraxial is used instead of, rather than combined with, general anesthesia.[422a] Furthermore, the specific surgical procedure may also influence outcome and it may be that any benefit is both procedure specific and technique specific (i.e., thoracic epidural may be more advantageous than lumbar epidural, and epidural local anesthetic may be more advantageous than epidural opioid).

As general anesthesia has become safer over the decades, demonstrating a mortality benefit is more challenging. Some large retrospective studies do show a reduction in mortality, but when present, the absolute difference is small. For cardiac surgery, meta-analyses have shown a reduced risk of mortality and myocardial infarction (composite endpoint); a reduced risk for acute renal failure, pulmonary complications, and supraventricular arrhythmia; and reduced duration of postoperative controlled ventilation in patients who received combined intraoperative general anesthesia and TEA.[74,423] For major thoracic and abdominal surgery, thoracic epidural analgesia can reduce mortality, along with reductions in respiratory complications and opioid consumption, and improvements in cough and time to ambulation.[422,424,425] Conversely, there is now some evidence that myocardial infarction rates may be increased when epidural and general anesthesia are combined.[422]

Mortality and morbidity aside, there are other important advantages of neuraxial blockade. For bilateral total knee arthroplasty, neuraxial anesthesia decreases the rate of blood transfusion.[426] In patients undergoing major vascular and abdominal surgery, thoracic epidural local anesthetic infusion can reverse postoperative paralytic ileus associated with pain-induced sympathetic overactivity and systemic opioid.[427] Lumbar epidural infusion or thoracic epidural opioid infusion alone does not speed intestinal function recovery. For fast-track laparoscopic colon resection, thoracic epidural analgesia provides superior pain relief but fails to speed intestinal function recovery or hospital discharge time. In a recent meta-analysis, which compared neuraxial to general anesthesia for all major limb and truncal surgery combined, there was a reduction in length of stay in hospital, but this was measured in hours rather than days.[422]

What are the potential effects of neuraxial anesthesia on stress response, the immune system, and cancer recurrence?[428-430a] Functional cell-mediated immunity is required for monitoring and eradicating cancer cell growth. Lymphocytes, such as the natural killer (NK) cells and the cytotoxic T lymphocytes, can lyse the cancer cell through the perforin and granzyme pathway or through secretion of cytokines (e.g., interferons) to induce cancer cell apoptosis. In addition, the helper T cells control tumor angiogenesis through interferons, inhibit oncogenic signaling, and stimulate tumor destruction by engaging macrophages and granulocytes through interleukin production. There is an inverse relationship between NK cell activity at the time of surgery and the development of metastatic disease. Systemic cancer cell seeding happens during surgical dissection and manipulation. Unfortunately, this happens at a time of significant immunosuppression. Surgically induced stress hormone (e.g., corticosteroids), as well as inhaled volatile anesthetics and systemic opioids (morphine and fentanyl), can diminish NK cell function. Morphine also has proangiogenic properties that may promote dissemination of angiogenesis-dependent tumors. TEA and analgesia may be beneficial by virtue of its opioid and general anesthetic sparing and surgical stress–alleviating properties. Some encouraging data indicate a reduction of cancer recurrence associated with the use of perioperative epidural anesthesia and analgesia in patients undergoing retropubic prostatectomy,[431,432] rectal cancer,[433] and ovarian cancer resection.[434,435] Volatile, but not intravenous, anesthetics have also been shown to have a negative effect on immune function and cancer spread and therefore any benefit of regional anesthesia may simply be due to a reduction or avoidance in the use of volatile anesthetic drugs. In the same manner, this potential effect on the immune system may explain why surgical site infection has been shown to be reduced when using neuraxial compared general anesthesia in some, but not all, studies.[422]

Recent Advances

ULTRASOUND

There is now considerable evidence to support the role of ultrasound imaging for neuraxial blockade, and for lumbar techniques in particular.[436] Ultrasound can accurately identify the intervertebral levels, the midline spinous process, the midline interspinous window, and the paramedian interlaminar window (see also Chapter 46).[233] Bone does not permit ultrasound beam transmission, thus casting a hypoechoic (dark) shadow on the image. Conversely, passage of the ultrasound beam through the interspinous and interlaminar windows allows visualization of the hyperechoic dura (a bright line), the subarachnoid space, and the posterior aspect of the vertebral body. Visualization of the ligamentum flavum and epidural space is often more difficult. Successful transverse or longitudinal scan facilitates identification of the optimal location for proper needle insertion during neuraxial block and an estimation of the skin-to-dura distance. This is particularly useful in patients with difficult surface anatomic landmarks (e.g., obesity), spine pathology (e.g., scoliosis), and previous spine surgery (e.g., laminectomy).[437]

Ultrasound-facilitated neuraxial block involves preprocedure scanning of the spine to determine the best possible intervertebral level and window for needle insertion without actual real-time guidance (a highly challenging technique). Imaging of the lumbar spine is significantly easier than that of the thoracic spine, which has narrow interspinous and interlaminar windows, especially at T5-T8 levels.[438] Ultrasonography in the pediatric population is impressive because the vertebral column with limited ossification not only permits visualization of the spinal canal sonoanatomy, but the inserted needle and catheter tip, dural displacement, and the extent of cranial spread can be visualized during a fluid bolus injection in young infants and children (also see Chapter 77).[439,440] Several outcome studies have confirmed the utility of ultrasonography when neuraxial block is performed by the novice and in patients with difficult anatomic landmarks.[441]

Acknowledgment

The authors thank Cyrus Tse for his assistance in preparing this chapter.

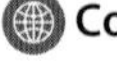 **Complete references available online at expertconsult.com.**

References

1. Rigg JRA, et al. *Lancet.* 2002;359(9314):1276.
2. Mandabach MG. *Int Cong Ser.* 2002;1242:163.
3. Franco A, Diz JC. *Curr Anaesth Crit Care.* 2000;11(5):274.
4. Maltby JR, et al. *Br J Anaesth.* 2000;84(1):121.
5. Rigler ML, et al. *Anesth Analg.* 1991;72(3):275.
6. Horlocker T, et al. *Reg Anesth Pain Med.* 2008;43:263-309.
7. Bernards CM, Hill HF. *Anesthesiology.* 1990;73(6):1214.
8. Liu SS, McDonald SB. *Anesthesiology.* 2001;94(5):888.
9. Bernards CM. *Reg Anesth Pain Med.* 2005;30(1):56.
10. Hogan QH. *Anesthesiology.* 1991;75(5):767.
11. Zarzur E. *Anesth Analg.* 1984;63(5):499.
12. Crighton IM, et al. *Br J Anaesth.* 1997;78(4):391.
13. Martirosyan NL, et al. *J Neurosurg Spine.* 2011;15(3):238.
14. Hogan Q, Toth J. *Reg Anesth Pain Med.* 1999;24(4):303.
15. Hogan Q. *Anesthesiology.* 1996;85(1):37.
16. Hogan QH, et al. *Anesthesiology.* 1996;84(6):1341.
17. Carpenter RL, et al. *Anesthesiology.* 1998;89(1):24.
18. Hogan Q. *Reg Anesth Pain Med.* 2002;27(2):150.
19. Igarashi T, et al. *Br J Anaesth.* 1997;78(2):149.
20. Liu S, et al. *Anesthesiology.* 1995;82(1):60.
21. Brull SJ, Greene NM. *Anesth Analg.* 1989;69(3):342.
22. Greene NM. *Anesth Analg.* 1983;62(11):1013.
23. Cohen EN. *Anesthesiology.* 1968;29(5):1002.
24. Vandenabeele F, et al. *J Anat.* 1996;189(Pt 2):417.
25. Greene NM. *Anesth Analg.* 1985;64(7):715.
26. Visser WA, et al. *Anesth Analg.* 2008;107(2):708.
27. Higuchi H, et al. *Anesthesiology.* 2004;100(1):106.
28. Butterworth J. *Reg Anesth Pain Med.* 1998;23(4):370; discussion 384.
29. Defalque RJ. *Anesthesiology.* 1962;23:627.
30. Meyhoff CS, et al. *Eur J Anaesthesiol.* 2007;24(9):770.
31. Greene NM. *Physiology of Spinal Anesthesia.* 3rd ed. Baltimore: Williams & Wilkins; 1981.
32. Rooke GA, et al. *Anesth Analg.* 1997;85(1):99.
33. Kopp SL, et al. *Anesth Analg.* 2005;100(3):855.
34. Crystal GJ, Salem MR. *Anesth Analg.* 2012;114(3):520.
35. Hackel DB, et al. *Circulation.* 1956;13(1):92.
36. Olausson K, et al. *Circulation.* 1997;96(7):2178.
37. Nygård E, et al. *Circulation.* 2005;111(17):2165.
38. Stanley GD, et al. *Reg Anesth.* 1997;22(1):53.
39. Butterworth JF, et al. *Anesth Analg.* 1986;65(6):612.
40. Moore JM. *Am J Ther.* 2009;16(4):289.
41. Minville V, et al. *Anesth Analg.* 2009;108(4):1291.
42. Kety SS, et al. *J Clin Invest.* 1950;29(4):402.
43. Kleinerman J, et al. *J Clin Invest.* 1958;37(2):285.
44. Sakura S, et al. *Anesth Analg.* 1996;82(2):306.
45. Greene NM. *Reg Anesth Pain Med.* 1982;7(2):55.
46. Groeben H. *J Anesth.* 2006;20(4):290.
47. Lirk P, et al. *Int J Obstet Anesth.* 2010;19(3):287.
48. von Ungern-Sternberg BS, et al. *Br J Anaesth.* 2005;94(1):121.
49. von Ungern-Sternberg BS, et al. *Acta Anaesthesiol Scand.* 2005; 49(7):940.
50. Regli A, et al. *Anaesthesia.* 2006;61(3):215.
51. Carpenter RL, et al. *Anesthesiology.* 1992;76(6):906.
52. Ward RJ, et al. *Anesth Analg.* 1966;45(5):621.
53. Freise H, Fischer LG. *Curr Opin Anaesthesiol.* 2009;22:644.
54. Sutcliffe NP, et al. *Anaesthesia.* 1996;51:37.
55. Michelet P, et al. *Chest.* 2005;128:3461.
56. Zügel N, et al. *Chirurgie.* 2002;73:262.
57. Greene N, et al. *Ann Surg.* 1954;140:641.
58. Suleiman MY, et al. *Anesth Analg.* 1997;84(5):1076.
59. Papper EM. *Acta Anaesthesiol Scand Suppl.* 1966;24:105.
60. Breebaart MB, et al. *Br J Anaesth.* 2003;90:309.
61. Jellish WS, et al. *Anesth Analg.* 1996;83:559.
62. van Zundert AAJ, et al. *Br J Anaesth.* 2007;98:682.
63. Denny NM, Selander DE. *Br J Anaesth.* 1998;81:590.
64. Block BM, et al. *JAMA.* 2003;290:2455.
65. Cousins MJ, Mather LE. *Anesthesiology.* 1984;61:276.
66. Wang JK, et al. *Anesthesiology.* 1979;50:149.

66a. Schug SA, et al. *Acute Pain Management: Scientific Evidence.* 4th ed. Melbourne, 2015, Australian and New Zealand College of Anaesthetists and Faculty of Pain Medicine.

67. American Society of Anesthesiologists Task Force on Obstetric Anesthesia. *Anesthesiology.* 2007;106:843.
68. Hawkins JL. *N Engl J Med.* 2010;362:1503.
69. Macfarlane AJR, et al. *Br J Anaesth.* 2009;103:335.
70. Macfarlane AJR, et al. *Clin Orthop Relat Res.* 2009;467:2379.
71. Nishimori M, et al. *Cochrane Database Syst Rev.* 2006;3:CD005059.
72. Joshi GP, et al. *Anesth Analg.* 2008;107:1026.
73. Svircevic V, et al. *Anesthesiology.* 2011;114:262.
74. Svircevic V, et al. *Anesthesiology.* 2011;114:271.
75. van Lier F, et al. *Anesthesiology.* 2011;115(2):315.
76. Neal JM, et al. *Reg Anesth Pain Med.* 2015;40:401.
77. Hilt H, et al. *Br J Anaesth.* 1986;58:676.
78. Upton AR, McComas AJ. *Lancet.* 1973;2:359.
79. Hebl JR, et al. *Anesth Analg.* 2006;103:223.
80. Vercauteren M, et al. *Acta Anaesthesiol Scand.* 2011;55(8):910.
81. Hebl JR, et al. *Anesth Analg.* 2010;111(6):1511.

82. Berkowitz S, Gold MI. *Anesth Analg*. 1980;59(11):881.
83. Bamford C, et al. *Can J Neurol Sci*. 1978;5(1):41.
84. Perlas A, Chan VWS. *Can J Anaesth*. 2005;52(5):454.
85. McDonald SB. *Reg Anesth Pain Med* 29(5):496.
86. Choi S, Brull R. *Anesth Analg*. 2009;109(2):648.
87. Ready LB, Helfer D. *Anesthesiology*. 1989;71(6):988.
88. Baker AS, et al. *N Engl J Med*. 1975;293(10):463.
89. Ericsson M, et al. *Scand J Infect Dis*. 1990;22(3):249.
90. Wedel DJ, Horlocker TT. *Reg Anesth Pain Med*. 2006;31(4):324.
91. Hocking G, Wildsmith JAW. *Br J Anaesth*. 2004;93(4):568.
92. Lui AC, et al. *Can J Anaesth*. 1998;45(4):297.
93. Tetzlaff JE, et al. *Reg Anesth*. 1995;20(6):533.
94. Brown DT, et al. *Br J Anaesth*. 1980;52(6):589.
95. Wildsmith JA, et al. *Br J Anaesth*. 1981;53(3):273.
96. Stienstra R, van Poorten JF. *Anesth Analg*. 1988;67(3):272.
97. Sheskey MC, et al. *Anesth Analg*. 1983;62(10):931.
98. Van Zundert AA, et al. *Reg Anesth*. 1996;21(2):112.
99. Henderson DJ, Jones G. *Br J Anaesth*. 1995;74(5):610.
100. Singh H, et al. *Can J Anaesth*. 1995;42(11):987.
101. Sarantopoulos C, Fassoulaki A. *Anesth Analg*. 1994;79(1):94.
102. Hartwell BL, et al. *Reg Anesth*. 1991;16(1):17.
103. Pitkänen MT. *Anesth Analg*. 1987;66(2):127.
104. Taivainen T, et al. *Br J Anaesth*. 1990;64(5):542.
105. Nossrin MC. *Anesthesiology*. 1990;72(3):478.
106. Pitkänen M, et al. *Br J Anaesth*. 1984;56(3):279.
107. Cameron AE, et al. *Anaesthesia*. 1981;36(3):318.
108. Niemi L, et al. *Br J Anaesth*. 1993;71(6):807.
109. Povey HM, et al. *Acta Anaesthesiol Scand*. 1989;33(4):295.
110. GPY Loke, et al. *Anaesthesia*. 2002;57(2):169.
111. Sinclair CJ, et al. *Br J Anaesth*. 1982;54(5):497.
112. Kim J-T, et al. *Br J Anaesth*. 2007;98(3):396.
113. Veering BT, et al. *Br J Anaesth*. 2001;87(5):738.
114. Loubert C, et al. *Anesth Analg*. 2011;113(4):811.
115. McShane FJ, et al. *AANA J*. 2000;68(1):67.
116. James KS, et al. *Br J Anaesth*. 1996;77(2):150.
117. Urmey WF, et al. *Anesth Analg*. 1997;84(2):337.
118. Casati A, et al. *Anesth Analg*. 1998;87(2):355.
119. Chin KW, et al. *Med J Malaysia*. 1994;49(2):142.
120. Logan MR, et al. *Br J Anaesth*. 1986;58(3):292.
121. Sanderson P, et al. *Br J Anaesth*. 1994;73(6):744.
122. Taivainen T, et al. *Br J Anaesth*. 1990;65(2):234.
123. Konishi R, et al. *Masui*. 1997;46(2):184.
124. Veering BT, et al. *Br J Anaesth*. 1996;77(3):343.
125. Malinovsky JM, et al. *Anesthesiology*. 1999;91(5):1260.
126. Goldblum E, Atchabahian A. *Acta Anaesthesiol Scand*. 2013;57:545.
127. Salinas FV, Liu SS. *Best Pract Res Clin Anaesthesiol*. 2002;16(2):195.
128. Urmey WF, et al. *Anesthesiology*. 1995;83(3):528.
129. Sanford M, Keating GM. *Drugs*. 2010;70(6):761.
130. Whiteside JB, et al. *Br J Anaesth*. 2001;86(2):241.
131. O'Donnell D, et al. *Can J Anaesth*. 2010;57(1):32.
132. Zayas VM, et al. *Anesth Analg*. 1999;89(5):1167.
133. Lee YY, et al. *Anesth Analg*. 2007;105:520.
134. McNamee DA, et al. *Br J Anaesth*. 2002;89(5):702.
135. Hodgson PS, et al. *Reg Anesth Pain Med*. 2000;25(3):218.
136. Ravindran RS, et al. *Anesth Analg*. 1980;59(6):447.
137. Reisner LS, et al. *Anesth Analg*. 1980;59(6):452.
138. Drasner K. *Anesth Analg*. 2005;100(2):549.
139. Taniguchi M, et al. *Anesthesiology*. 2004;100(1):85.
140. Gonter AF, Kopacz DJ. *Anesth Analg*. 2005;100(2):573.
141. Yoos JR, Kopacz DJ. *Anesth Analg*. 2005;100(2):566.
142. Casati A, et al. *Anesth Analg*. 2007;104(4):959.
143. Casati A, et al. *Anesth Analg*. 2006;103(1):234.
144. Hejtmanek MR, Pollock JE. *Acta Anaesthesiol Scand*. 2011;55(3):267.
145. Pollock JE. *Int Anesthesiol Clin*. 2012;50(1):93.
146. Vaghadia H, et al. *Acta Anaesthesiol Scand*. 2012;56(2):217.
147. Zaric D, Pace NL. *Cochrane Database Syst Rev*. 2009;2(2):CD003006.
148. Snoeck M. *Local Reg Anesth*. 2012;5:23.
149. Dijkstra T, et al. *Br J Anaesth*. 2008;100(1):104.
150. Douglas MJ. *Can J Anaesth*. 1995;42(3):181.
151. Liu S, et al. *Anesth Analg*. 1995;81(4):697.
152. Camponovo C, et al. *Anesth Analg*. 2010;111(2):568.
153. Black AS, et al. *Br J Anaesth*. 2011;106(2):183.
154. de Weert K, et al. *Anaesthesia*. 2000;55(10):1020.
155. Martínez-Bourio R, et al. *Anesthesiology*. 1998;88(3):624.
156. Climie CR, et al. *Br J Anaesth*. 1967;39(2):155.
157. Liguori GA, et al. *Anesthesiology*. 1998;88(3):619.
158. Salazar F, et al. *Acta Anaesthesiol Scand*. 2001;45(2):240.
159. Salmela L, Aromaa U. *Acta Anaesthesiol Scand*. 1998;42(7):765.
160. Pawlowski J, et al. *J Clin Anesth*. 2012;24(2):109.
161. Smith HS, et al. *Anesthesiology*. 1986;65(3A):A193.
162. Abouleish E. *Anesthesiology*. 1986;65:A375.
163. Caldwell C, et al. *Anesthesiology*. 1985;62(6):804.
164. Kozody R, et al. *Can Anaesth Soc J*. 1985;32(1):23.
165. Sakura S, et al. *Anesthesiology*. 1997;87(4):771.
166. Moore DC. *Anesth Analg*. 1980;59(10):743.
167. Casati A, Vinciguerra F. *Curr Opin Anaesthesiol*. 2002;15(5):543.
168. Ben-David B, et al. *Anesth Analg*. 1996;83(4):716.
169. Kuusniemi KS, et al. *Reg Anesth Pain Med*. 2001;26(1):30.
170. Fanelli G, et al. *Can J Anaesth*. 2000;47(8):746.
171. Nair GS, et al. *Br J Anaesth*. 2009;102(3):307.
172. Frawley G, et al. *Br J Anaesth*. 2009;103(5):731.
173. Alley EA, et al. *Anesth Analg*. 2002;94(1):188.
174. Glaser C, et al. *Anesth Analg*. 2002;94(1):194.
175. Bardsley H, et al. *Br J Clin Pharmacol*. 1998;46(3):245.
176. Gristwood RW. *Drug Saf*. 2002;25(3):153.
177. Deleted in proofs.
178. Groban L, et al. *Anesth Analg*. 2001;92(1):37.
179. Polley LS, et al. *Anesthesiology*. 1999;90(4):944.
180. Capogna G, et al. *Br J Anaesth*. 1999;82(3):371.
181. Camorcia M, et al. *Anesthesiology*. 2005;102(3):646.
182. Kallio H, et al. *Anesth Analg*. 2004;99(3):713.
183. Gautier P, et al. *Br J Anaesth*. 2003;91(5):684.
184. Whiteside JB, et al. *Br J Anaesth*. 2003;90(3):304.
185. Hamber EA, Viscomi CM. *Reg Anesth Pain Med*. 1999;24(3):255.
186. Meylan N, et al. *Br J Anaesth*. 2009;102(2):156.
187. Murphy PM, et al. *Anesth Analg*. 2003;97(6):1709.
188. Pöpping DM, et al. *Pain*. 2012;153(4):784.
189. National Institute for Health and Clinical Excellence. *Clinical Guideline*. 132 - Caesarean section. http://www.nice.org.uk/guidance/cg132/resources/guidance-caesarean-section.pdf. (Accessed 19.07.14.)
190. Quigley C. *Cochrane Database Syst Rev*. 2002;1:CD003447.
191. Nguyen TT, et al. *Reg Anesth Pain Med*. 1994;19:386.
192. Hansen D, Hansen S. *Anesth Analg*. 1999;88:827.
193. Yu SC, et al. *Br J Anaesth*. 2002;88:379.
194. Meininger D, et al. *Anesth Analg*. 2003;96:852.
195. Lee JH, et al. *Korean J Anesthesiol*. 2011;60(2):103.
196. Dahlgren G, et al. *Anesth Analg*. 1997;85(6):1288.
197. Bucklin BA, et al. *Reg Anesth Pain Med*. 2002;27(1):23.
198. Kim SY, et al. *Br J Anaesth*. 2009;103(5):750.
199. Liu S, et al. *Anesth Analg*. 1995;80(4):730.
200. Moore DC, et al. *Anesthesiology*. 1987;67(3):416.
201. Leicht CH, Carlson SA. *Anesth Analg*. 1986;65(4):365.
202. Kozody R, et al. *Can Anaesth Soc J*. 1985;32(5):472.
203. Kozody R, et al. *Can Anaesth Soc J*. 1984;31(5):503.
204. Porter SS, et al. *Acta Anaesthesiol Scand*. 1985;29(3):330.
205. Vaida GT, et al. *Anesth Analg*. 1986;65(7):781.
206. Chambers WA, et al. *Anesth Analg*. 1982;61(1):49.
207. Feldman HS, Covino BG, et al. *Reg Anesth*. 1986;10(3):133.
208. Concepcion M, et al. *Anesth Analg*. 1984;63(2):134.
209. Maehara Y, et al. *Hiroshima J Med Sci*. 2001;50(2):47.
210. Eisenach JC, et al. *Anesthesiology*. 1996;85(3):655.
211. Dobrydnjov I, et al. *Acta Anaesthesiol Scand*. 2002;46(7):806.
212. De Kock M, et al. *Anesthesiology*. 2001;94(4):574.
213. Dobrydnjov I, et al. *Anesth Analg*. 2003;96(5):1496.
214. Eisenach JC, et al. *Anesth Analg*. 1998;87(3):591.
215. Bedder MD, et al. *Can Anaesth Soc J*. 1986;33(5):591.
216. Elia N, et al. *Reg Anesth Pain Med*. 2008;33(2):159.
217. Kalso EA, et al. *Pharmacol Toxicol*. 1991;68(2):140.
218. Kanazi GE, et al. *Acta Anaesthesiol Scand*. 2006;50(2):222.
219. Abdallah FW, Brull R, et al. *Br J Anaesth*. 2013;110(6):915.
220. Liu SS, et al. *Anesthesiology*. 1999;90(3):710.
221. Xu Z, et al. *Anesthesiology*. 1996;85(1):107.
222. Eisenach JC, et al. *Anesth Analg*. 1997;85(4):842.
223. Habib AS, Gan TJ. *CNS Drugs*. 2006;20(10):821.
224. Lauretti GR, et al. *Anesthesiology*. 1998;89(4):913.
225. Rathmell JP, et al. *Anesth Analg*. 2005;101(suppl 5):S30.
226. Flaatten H, et al. *Anaesthesia*. 1989;44(2):147.
227. Morros-Viñoles C, et al. *Rev Esp Anestesiol Reanim*. 2002;49(9):448.
228. Deleted in proofs.
229. American Society of Anesthesiologists. *Anesthesiology*. 2017;126(4):585.
230. Scott M, et al. *Br J Anaesth*. 2009;103(3):456; author reply 456.

231. Sviggum HP, et al. *Reg Anesth Pain Med.* 2012;37(2):139.
232. Inglis A, et al. *Anaesthesia.* 1995;50(4):363.
233. Chin KJ, et al. *Anesthesiology.* 2011;114(6):1459.
234. Jaitly VK, Kumar CM. *Curr Anaesth Crit Care.* 2009;20(2):60.
235. Covino B, Scott D. *Handbook of Epidural Anaesthesia and Analgesia.*
236. Puolakka R, et al. *Reg Anesth Pain Med.* 2000;25(6):584.
237. Gudaityte J, et al. *Medicina (Kaunas).* 2005;41(8):675.
238. Vaghadia H, et al. *Can J Anaesth.* 2001;48(3):256.
239. Rocco AG, et al. *Anesth Analg.* 1985;64(9):917.
240. Liu SS, Ware PD. *Anesth Analg.* 1997;84(1):115.
241. Curatolo M, et al. *Anesthesiology.* 2000;93(6):1517.
242. Bromage PR. *Acta Anaesthesiol Scand Suppl.* 1965;16:55.
243. Hirabayashi Y, Shimizu R. *Br J Anaesth.* 1993;71(3):445.
244. Duggan J, et al. *Br J Anaesth.* 1988;61(3):324.
245. Fagraeus L, et al. *Anesthesiology.* 1983;58(2):184.
246. Visser WA, et al. *Anesth Analg.* 2006;102(1):268.
247. Visser WA, et al. *Anesth Analg.* 2007;105(3):868.
248. Visser WA, et al. *Anesth Analg.* 1998;86(2):332.
249. Seow LT, et al. *Anaesth Intensive Care.* 1983;11(2):97.
250. Setayesh AR, et al. *Can J Anaesth.* 2001;48(9):890.
251. Stevens RA, et al. *Anesthesiology.* 1993;78(3):492.
252. Brinklov MM. *Acta Anaesthesiol Scand.* 1977;21(1):5.
253. Wong CA, et al. *Reg Anesth.* 1996;21(6):600.
254. Konietzke D, et al. *Reg Anaesth.* 1985;8(4):67.
255. Chahar P, Cummings KC. *J Pain Res.* 2012;5:257.
256. Cox CR, et al. *Br J Anaesth.* 1998;80(3):289.
257. Kopacz DJ, et al. *Anesth Analg.* 2000;90(3):642.
258. Huang YF, et al. *Anesth Analg.* 1998;86(4):797.
259. McClure JH. *Br J Anaesth.* 1996;76(2):300.
260. Moller R, Covino BG. *Anesthesiology.* 1990;72(2):322.
261. Lacassie HJ, et al. *Anesth Analg.* 2002;95(1):204.
262. Marinacci AA. *Bull Los Angel Neuro Soc.* 1960;25:170.
263. Niemi G, Breivik H. *Anesth Analg.* 2002;94(6):1598.
264. Stanton-Hicks M, et al. *Anesthesiology.* 1973;39(3):308.
265. Loper KA, et al. *Anesth Analg.* 1990;70(1):72.
266. Miguel R, et al. *Anesthesiology.* 1994;81(2):346; discussion 25A.
267. Sultan P, et al. *Drugs.* 2011;71:1807.
268. Carvalho B, et al. *Anesth Analg.* 2007;105(1):176.
269. Hartrick CT, et al. *J Bone Joint Surg Am.* 2006;88(2):273.
270. Kroin JS, et al. *Anesthesiology.* 2004;101(2):488.
271. Dobrydnjov I, et al. *Acta Anaesthesiol Scand.* 2005;49(4):538.
272. Milligan KR, et al. *Anesth Analg.* 2000;91(2):393.
273. Farmery AD, Wilson-MacDonald J. *Anesth Analg.* 2009;108(2):631.
274. Wu C-T, et al. *Anesth Analg.* 2004;99(2):502.
275. De Kock M. *Anesthesiology.* 1991;75(4):715.
276. Grewal AJ. *Anaesthesiol Clin Pharmacol.* 2011;27(3):297.
277. Yanli Y, Eren A. *Anaesthesia.* 1996;51(1):84.
278. Himmelseher S, et al. *Anesth Analg.* 2001;92(5):1290.
279. Malinovsky JM, et al. *Anesthesiology.* 1993;78(1):109.
280. Roelants F, et al. *Anesthesiology.* 2005;102(6):1205.
281. Park WY, Hagins FM. *Reg Anesth Pain Med.* 11(3):128.
282. Bokesch PM, et al. *Anesth Analg.* 1987;66(1):9.
283. Morison DH. *Can J Anaesth.* 1995;42(12):1076.
284. Segal S, et al. *J Clin Anesth.* 1997;9(2):109.
285. Collier CB, Gatt SP. *Reg Anesth.* 1994;19(6):378.
286. D'Angelo R, et al. *Anesth Analg.* 1997;84(6):1276.
287. Mhyre JM, et al. *Anesth Analg.* 2009;108(4):1232.
288. Nishi M, et al. *J Cardiothorac Vasc Anesth.* 2006;20(5):656.
289. Grau T, et al. *Reg Anesth Pain Med.* 2002;27(2):200.
290. Sharrock NE. *Br J Anaesth.* 1979;51(3):253.
291. Schier R, et al. *Anesth Analg.* 2009;109(6):2012.
292. Moon JY, et al. *Anesthesiology.* 2010;113(3):666.
293. Zarzur E. *Anaesthesia.* 1984;39(11):1101.
294. Paech MJ, et al. *Int J Obstet Anesth.* 1998;7(1):5.
295. Afshan G, et al. *Anaesthesia.* 2011;66(10):913.
296. Beilin Y, et al. *Anesth Analg.* 1995;81(2):301.
297. D'Angelo R, et al. *Anesthesiology.* 1996;84(1):88.
298. Hamilton CL, et al. *Anesthesiology.* 1997;86(4):778; discussion 29A.
299. Tsui BC, et al. *Can J Anaesth.* 1998;45(7):640.
300. Tsui BC, et al. *Can J Anaesth.* 1999;46(7):675.
301. Tsui BC, et al. *Can J Anaesth.* 2000;47(5):471.
302. Clark MX, et al. *Anaesthesia.* 2001;56(9):865.
303. Burstal R, et al. *Anaesth Intensive Care.* 1998;26(2):147.
304. Guay J. *Anesth Analg.* 2006;102(3):921.
305. Curelaru I. *Prakt Anaesth.* 1979;14(1):71.
306. Brownridge P. *Anaesthesia.* 1981;36(1):70.
307. Carrie LE. *Acta Anaesthesiol Scand.* 1988;32(7):595.
308. Dennison B. *Can J Anaesth.* 1987;34(1):105.
309. Rawal N, et al. *Acta Anaesthesiol Scand.* 1988;32(1):61.
310. Soresi A. *Anesth Analg.* 1937;16:306.
311. Lew E, et al. *Anesth Analg.* 2004;98(3):810.
312. Fan SZ, et al. *Anesth Analg.* 1994;78(3):474.
313. McAndrew CR, Harms P. *Anaesth Intensive Care.* 2003;31(5):514.
314. Lyons G, et al. *Anaesthesia.* 1992;47(3):199.
315. Casati A, et al. *Reg Anesth Pain Med.* 1998;23(4):390.
316. Rawal N, et al. *Reg Anesth.* 1997;22(5):406.
317. Chen CPC, et al. *Anesthesiology.* 2004;101(1):181.
318. Roberts SA, Galvez I. *Paediatr Anaesth.* 2005;15(5):429.
319. Brenner L, et al. *Br J Anaesth.* 2011;107(2):229.
320. Mackey D. Physiologic effects of regional block. In: Brown DL, ed. *Regional Anesthesia and Analgesia.* Philadelphia: Saunders; 1996.
321. Fettes PDW, Wildsmith JAW. *Br J Anaesth.* 2002;88(6):760.
322. Brull R, et al. *Anesth Analg.* 2007;104(4):965.
323. Cook TM, et al. *Br J Anaesth.* 2009;102(2):179.
324. Skouen JS, et al. *Acta Neurol Scand.* 1985;72(4):437.
325. Reynolds F. *Anaesthesia.* 2000;55(11):1045.
326. Mayall MF, Calder I. *Anaesthesia.* 1999;54(10):990.
327. Katz N, Hurley R. *Anesth Analg.* 1993;77(5):1064.
328. Takii Y, et al. *Anesth Analg.* 2006;103(2):513.
329. Kasai T, et al. *Anesth Analg.* 2003;96(1):65.
330. Moore DC, et al. *Anesth Analg.* 1982;61(2):155.
331. Eastwood DW. *Anesth Analg.* 1991;73(1):90.
332. Hong DK, Lawrence HM. *Anaesth Intensive Care.* 2001;29(1):62.
333. Linz SM, et al. *Can J Anaesth.* 1997;44(11):1178.
334. Gerancher JC. *Anesthesiology.* 1997;87(3):687.
335. Drasner K, et al. *Anesthesiology.* 1994;80(4):847.
336. Lambert DH, Hurley RJ. *Anesth Analg.* 1991;72(6):817.
337. Benson J. *FDA Safety Alert: Cauda Equina Syndrome Associated with the Use of Small-Bore Catheters in Continuous Spinal Anesthesia.* Rockville, MD: Food and Drug Administration; 1992.
338. Förster JG, et al. *Br J Anaesth.* 2006;97(3):393.
339. Vandermeulen EP, et al. *Anesth Analg.* 1994;79(6):1165.
340. Horlocker TT. *Can J Anaesth.* 2004;51(6):527.
341. Moen V, et al. *Anesthesiology.* 2004;101(4):950.
342. Ruppen W, et al. *Anesthesiology.* 2006;105(2):394.
343. Horlocker TT, et al. *Anesth Analg.* 2003;96(6):1547.
344. Auroy Y, et al. *Anesthesiology.* 1997;87(3):479.
345. Giebler RM, et al. *Anesthesiology.* 1997;86(1):55.
346. Vandam L, Dripps R. *Surgery.* 1955;38(3):463.
347. Dawkins CJ. *Anaesthesia.* 1969;24(4):554.
348. Aromaa U, et al. *Acta Anaesthesiol Scand.* 1997;41(4):445.
349. Scott DB, Tunstall ME. *Int J Obstet Anesth.* 1995;4(3):133.
350. Auroy Y, et al. *Anesthesiology.* 2002;97(5):1274.
351. Lee LA, et al. *Anesthesiology.* 2004;101(1):143.
352. Wong CA, et al. *Obstet Gynecol.* 2003;101(2):279.
353. Price JM, Carpenter RL. *Anesthesiology.* 1998;89(3):790.
354. Cheney FW, et al. *Anesthesiology.* 1999;90(4):1062.
355. Reynolds F. *Anaesthesia.* 2001;56(3):238.
356. Turnbull DK, Shepherd DB. *Br J Anaesth.* 2003;91(5):718.
357. Reynolds F. *BMJ.* 1993;306(6882):874.
358. Leibold RA, et al. *Ann Emerg Med.* 1993;22:1863.
359. Vandam L, Dripps R. *J Am Med Assoc.* 1956;161(7):586.
360. Mihic DN. *Reg Anesth Pain Med.* 10(2):76.
361. Ready LB, et al. *Anesth Analg.* 1989;69(4):457.
362. Halpern S, Preston R. *Anesthesiology.* 1994;81(6):1376.
363. Rawal N, et al. *Anesthesiol Clin North America.* 2000;18(2):267.
364. Dunn SM, et al. *Anesth Analg.* 2000;90(5):1249.
365. Denny N, et al. *Anesth Analg.* 1987;66(8):791.
366. Connelly NR, et al. *Headache.* 2000;40(4):316.
367. Carp H, et al. *Anesth Analg.* 1994;79(1):180.
368. Harrington BE. *Reg Anesth Pain Med.* 2004;29:136.
369. Gormley JB. *Anesthesiology.* 1960;21:565.
370. Safa-Tisseront V, et al. *Anesthesiology.* 2001;95(2):334.
371. Duffy PJ, Crosby ET, et al. *Can J Anaesth.* 1999;46(9):878.
372. Scavone BM, et al. *Anesthesiology.* 2004;101(6):1422.
373. Boonmak P, Boonmak S. *Cochrane Database Syst Rev.* 2010;1:CD001791.
374. Szeinfeld M, et al. *Anesthesiology.* 1986;64(6):820.
375. Beards SC, et al. *Br J Anaesth.* 1993;71(2):182.

376. Paech MJ, et al. *Anesth Analg*. 2011;113(1):126.
377. Hampl KF, et al. *Reg Anesth*. 1995;20(5):363.
378. Pollock JE, et al. *Anesthesiology*. 1999;90(2):445.
379. Tarkkila P, et al. *Br J Anaesth*. 1995;74(3):328.
380. Gozdemir M, et al. *Acta Anaesthesiol Scand*. 2010;54(1):59.
381. Evron S, et al. *Anesth Analg*. 2007;105(5):1494.
382. Markey JR, et al. *Anesth Analg*. 2000;90(2):437.
383. Hartmann B, et al. *Anesth Analg*. 2002;94(6):1521.
384. Loubert C. *Can J Anaesth*. 2012;59(6):604.
385. Thompson KW, Cushing H. *Anesth Analg*. 1934;13:75.
386. Wetstone DL, Wong KC. *Anesthesiology*. 1974;41(1):87.
387. Lesser JB, et al. *Anesthesiology*. 2003;99(4):859.
388. Caplan RA, et al. *Anesthesiology*. 1988;68(1):5.
389. Zornow M, Scheller M. *Anesthesiology*. 1988;68:970.
390. Hogan QH, et al. *Anesthesiology*. 1998;88(3):761.
391. Mackey DC, et al. *Anesthesiology*. 1989;70(5):866.
392. Gwirtz KH, et al. *Anesth Analg*. 1999;88(3):599.
393. Gross JB, et al. *Anesthesiology*. 2006;104(5):1081; quiz 1117.
394. American Society of Anesthesiologists Task Force on Neuraxial Opioids, et al. *Anesthesiology*. 2009;110(2):218.
395. Phillips JMG, et al. *Br J Anaesth*. 2002;89(5):778.
396. Wang LP, et al. *Anesthesiology*. 1999;91:1928.
397. Kindler CH, et al. *Acta Anaesthesiol Scand*. 1998;42(6):614.
398. Horlocker TT, Wedel DJ. *Reg Anesth Pain Med*. 2006;31(4):334.
399. Rathmell JP, et al. *Reg Anesth Pain Med*. 2006;31(4):346.
400. Benzon HT, et al. *Anesth Analg*. 2016;122(6):2047.
401. Brown E, Elman D. *Anesth Analg*. 1961;40:683.
402. Dickinson JE, et al. *Aust N Z J Obstet Gynaecol*. 2002;42(1):59.
403. Breen TW, et al. *Anesthesiology*. 1994;81(1):29.
404. Borgeat A, et al. *Anesthesiology*. 2003;98(2):530.
405. Kuipers PW, et al. *Anesthesiology*. 2004;100(6):1497.
406. Kamphuis ET, et al. *Anesth Analg*. 2008;107(6):2073.
407. Izard JP, et al. *Can J Urol*. 2006;13(3):3158.
408. Griesdale DEG, et al. *Can J Anaesth*. 2011;58(12):1097.
409. Demiraran Y, et al. *J Anesth*. 2006;20(4):274.
410. Crowley LJ, Buggy DJ. *Reg Anesth Pain Med*. 2008;33(3):241.
411. Saito T, et al. *Reg Anesth Pain Med*. 1998;23(4):418.
412. Bell DN, Leslie K. *Anaesth Intensive Care*. 2007;35(3):335.
413. Moore DC, Batra MS. *Anesthesiology*. 1981;55(6):693.
414. Hood DD, et al. *Anesthesiology*. 1986;64(5):610.
415. Horn M, et al. *Anesthesiology*. 1987;67(3):A268.
416. Liu SS, Carpenter RL. *Anesthesiology*. 1996;84(1):81.
417. Okutumi T, Hashiba MM. *Reg Anes Pain Med*. 2001;26:450.
418. Blomberg R. *Anesth Analg*. 1986;65(7):747.
419. Blomberg RG. *Anesth Analg*. 1987;66(2):177.
420. Holst D, et al. *Anesth Analg*. 1999;88(2):393.
421. Rodgers A, et al. *BMJ*. 2000;321(7275):1493.
422. Smith LM, et al. *Anesth Analg*. 2017;125(6):1931.
422a. Perlas A, et al. *Anesthesiology*. 2016;125:724.
423. Bignami E, et al. *J Cardiothorac Vasc Anesth*. 2010;24(4):586.
424. Pöpping DM, et al. *Arch Surg*. 2008;143(10):990; discussion 1000.
425. Wu CL, et al. *J Clin Anesth*. 2006;18(7):515.
426. Stundner O, et al. *Reg Anesth Pain Med*. 2012;37(6):638.
427. Freise H, Van Aken HK. *Br J Anaesth*. 2011;107(6):859.
428. Tavare AN, et al. *Int J Cancer*. 2012;130(6):1237.
429. Heaney A, Buggy DJ. *Br J Anaesth*. 2012;109(suppl 1):i17.
430. Snyder GL, Greenberg S. *Br J Anaesth*. 2010;105(2):106.
430a. Sekandarzad MW, et al. *Anesth Analg*. 2017;124:1697.
431. Biki B, et al. *Anesthesiology*. 2008;109(2):180.
432. Wuethrich PY, et al. *Anesthesiology*. 2010;113(3):570.
433. Gupta A, et al. *Br J Anaesth*. 2011;107(2):164.
434. de Oliveira GS, et al. *Reg Anesth Pain Med*. 2011;36(3):271.
435. Lin L, et al. *Br J Anaesth*. 2011;106(6):814.
436. Perlas A, et al. *Reg Anesth Pain Med*. 2016;41(2):251.
437. Chin KJ, Chan V. *Anesth Analg*. 2010;110(1):252.
438. Avramescu S, et al. *Reg Anesth Pain Med*. 2012;37(3):349.
439. Triffterer L, et al. *Br J Anaesth*. 2012;108(4):670.
440. Tsui BCH, Suresh S. *Anesthesiology*. 2010;112(3):719.
441. Chin KJ, et al. *Anesthesiology*. 2011;115(1):94.

46 Peripheral Nerve Blocks and Ultrasound Guidance for Regional Anesthesia

REBECCA L. JOHNSON, SANDRA L. KOPP, JENS KESSLER, and ANDREW T. GRAY

KEY POINTS

- Regional anesthesia is only successful when local anesthetic is inserted in close proximity to the targeted nerves. From the inception of regional anesthesia over a century ago, several techniques have been designed and available to facilitate the correct placement of local anesthetic, including the paresthesia-seeking approach, peripheral nerve stimulator, and most recently ultrasound guidance.
- There are no data to support the superiority of one nerve localization technique—paresthesia, nerve stimulation, ultrasound—over another with regard to reducing the risk of nerve injury.
- Ultrasound imaging can elucidate the structure of peripheral nerves and adjacent anatomic structures for regional block. Peripheral nerves have a characteristic honeycomb echotexture, formed by the internal pattern of connective tissue and nerve fibers.
- Ultrasound provides real-time imaging for needle tip placement and drug injection. Successful local anesthetic injections clarify the border of the nerve and track along the nerve path and its branches. Ultrasound guidance results in more consistent procedure times for peripheral nerve blocks and can be applied to many regional anesthesia procedures. Anatomic variation in nerve position and course, which is a potential source of block failure, can be directly visualized.
- Lipid emulsion bolus and infusion improve the success of resuscitation from cardiac arrest because of local anesthetic toxicity if given immediately after a local anesthetic overdose.
- Prior to regional blocks checklists are now being performed in an effort to make rare adverse events even less common, thereby improving patient safety.

Introduction

Peripheral nerve blocks can be performed using a variety of guidance techniques. Recently, ultrasound has gained popularity for regional anesthesia because it allows direct imaging of peripheral nerves, the block needle, and injection distribution. This chapter is a focused update of two chapters on peripheral nerve blockade from the previous edition. The sections to follow contain a selective description of the more common peripheral nerve blocks utilized in clinical practice.

Techniques for Localizing Neural Structures

PARESTHESIA TECHNIQUES

The paresthesia-seeking technique has a long, successful history as a simple method that requires little specialized equipment. A paresthesia is elicited when a needle makes direct contact with a nerve. Paresthesia-seeking techniques are reliant on patient cooperation and participation to guide the needle and local anesthetic injection accurately; therefore only small doses of sedation medication are recommended. Paresthesia techniques have been criticized for causing patient discomfort, although clinical studies have not shown a significant increase in neurologic complications with this technique.[1] Caution should be used when initiating the injection of local anesthetic to ensure that the needle is not intraneural. There is controversy in the literature regarding the use of B-bevel (blunt bevel or short bevel) needles versus sharp needles regarding the incidence and severity of nerve injury if the needle inadvertently punctures or pierces the nerve. Because B-bevel needles have a blunt tip, which is likely to push the nerve aside, they are much less likely to penetrate the nerve; however, when an injury does occur, it appears to be more severe. In contrast, sharp needles are more likely to penetrate the nerve, but the injury appears to be less destructive.[2,3] Success with the paresthesia technique is highly dependent on the skill of the practitioner and requires a thorough understanding of anatomy. This technique was slowly replaced in the 1980s when peripheral nerve stimulation was introduced. Currently, no single technique has been shown to be superior with respect to incidence of neurologic complications.

PERIPHERAL NERVE STIMULATION

Peripheral nerve stimulators deliver small pulses of electric current to the end of a block needle to cause depolarization and muscle contraction when the tip of the needle is in close proximity to a neural structure. This technique allows for localization of a specific peripheral nerve without requiring the elicitation of a paresthesia, thus allowing patients to be more sedated during block placement. It is necessary to attach the cathode (negative terminal) to the stimulating needle and the anode (positive terminal) to the surface of the patient because cathodal stimulation is more efficient than anodal stimulation. Most current-stimulating needles are coated with a thin layer of electrical insulation along the needle shaft with the exception of the tip. This allows for higher current density at the tip of the needle. Higher current output (>1.5 mA) is more likely to stimulate neural structures through tissue or fascial planes and can be associated with painful, vigorous muscle contractions. After localization of the correct motor response, the current is gradually decreased to a current of 0.5 mA or less. A motor response at a current of approximately 0.5 mA is appropriate when used to facilitate the location for injection of local anesthetic or catheter placement.[4] Immediately following injection of local anesthetic or saline (ionic solutions), the current density at the needle tip will rapidly dissipate and the evoked motor response is eliminated (the Raj test)[5].

The stimulating current pulse can be modified to produce a sensory response. The short-duration impulse commonly used (0.1 ms) is effective in stimulating motor fibers, but a longer-duration pulse (0.3 ms) will also stimulate sensory fibers, a useful feature if a pure sensory nerve is being sought.

Ultrasound Guidance

Ultrasound imaging allows direct visualization of peripheral nerves, the block needle tip, and local anesthetic distribution.[6] This imaging modality has proven highly useful for guiding targeted drug injections and catheter placement. This section describes the general principles of ultrasound imaging for regional blocks.

FUNDAMENTAL ASSUMPTIONS AND ARTIFACTS

Ultrasound is sound with a frequency above the audible range (>20,000 cycles per second). The frequencies used in clinical imaging are within the range of 1 to 20 MHz. High-frequency ultrasound beams are well collimated and therefore can provide high resolution. For most regional blocks, the highest frequency is selected that adequately penetrates the depth of field. Sound waves reflected at the interface of two tissues with different acoustic impedances generate echoes. Ambient lighting has a large effect on visual discrimination; therefore dim lighting without glare is especially useful for imaging low-contrast targets such as peripheral nerves.

Ultrasound imaging is predicated on several common assumptions.[7] First, the speed of sound through soft tissue is 1540 m/s, meaning 13 μs elapse for each centimeter of soft tissue traversed back and forth for the total fly-back time of received echoes. This assumption allows interconversion of time and distance for echo ranging. Local heterogeneities in soft tissue can cause artifactual bending of the block needle on ultrasound scans, known as the bayonet artifact

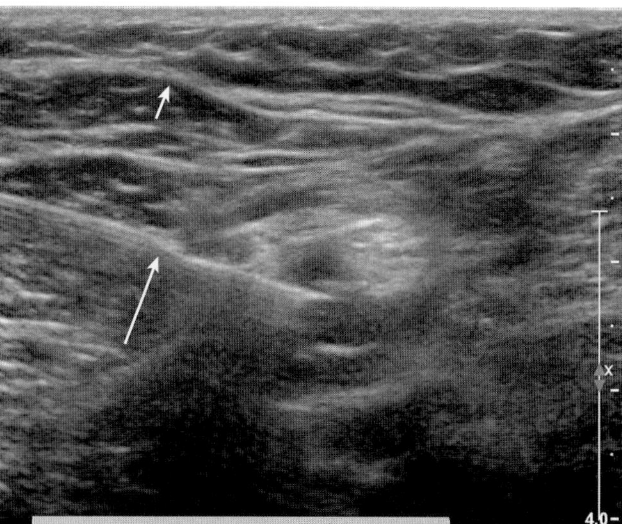

Fig. 46.1 Bayonet artifact is observed during popliteal block of the sciatic nerve. In this sonogram, the block needle appears to bend as it approaches the sciatic nerve in the popliteal fossa *(long arrow)*. The slower speed of sound in the overlying adipose tissue, compared with the adjacent muscle *(short arrow)*, produces this artifact.

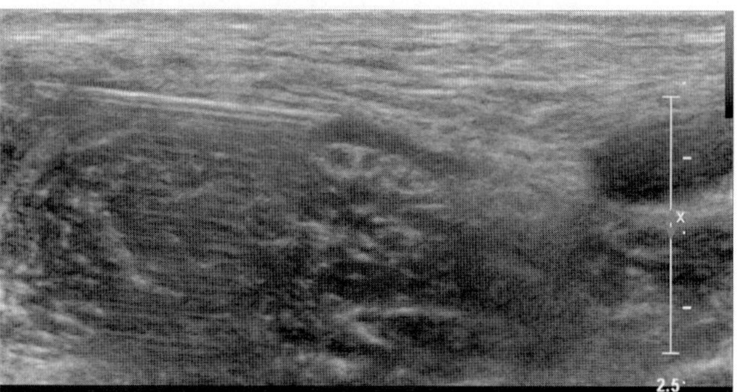

Fig. 46.2 Reverberation artifact is observed during femoral nerve block. Sound waves reverberate back and forth between the walls of the needle and then return later to the transducer. Because the sound waves return at a later time, they are displayed deep within the field of imaging. No reverberation artifact is observed from the needle tip because the bevel opening does not have opposing walls.

(Fig. 46.1).[8,9] Bayonet artifacts are commonly observed during the lateral in-plane approach to popliteal block (see Sciatic Nerve Blocks in the Popliteal Fossa) because more adipose tissue is present over the nerves near the posterior midline of the leg (adipose tissue has a slower speed of sound than the adjacent muscle). The speed of sound artifacts relate both to time-of-flight considerations and to refraction that occurs at the interface of tissues with different speeds of sound.

Second, ultrasound waves are assumed to take a straight path to and from tissue. When this does not occur, reverberation artifacts are displayed deep to the reflector. Reverberation artifacts are commonly observed from the block needle shaft at shallow angles of insertion because sound waves bounce back and forth between the walls of the needle before returning to the transducer (Fig. 46.2). Comet tail artifact is another type of reverberation artifact and helps identify strong reflectors such as the pleura during supraclavicular and intercostal blocks. At low receiver gain, the comet tail is seen as a tapering series of discrete echo bands just deep

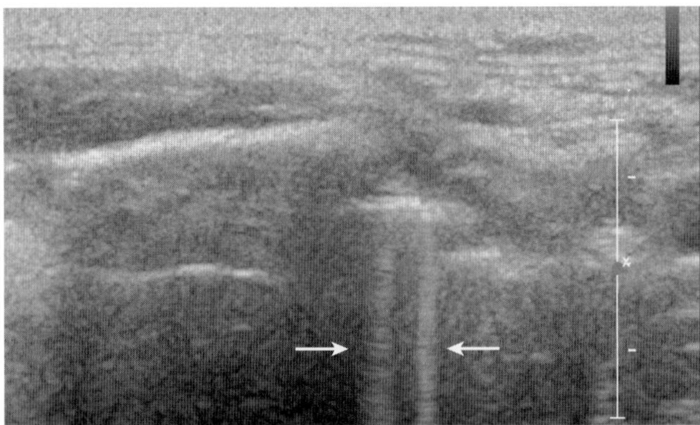

Fig. 46.3 Comet-tail artifact is observed during the scanning of the upper airway *(arrows)*. Small collections of water near the air interface, which also are seen during scanning of the pleura, generate this artifact.

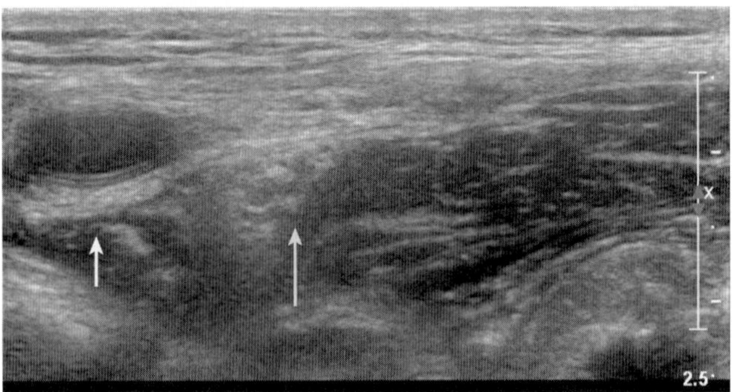

Fig. 46.4 Posterior acoustic enhancement artifact is observed during femoral nerve block. The echoes deep to the femoral artery are enhanced *(white arrow)* and may be incorrectly identified as the femoral nerve *(yellow arrow)*.

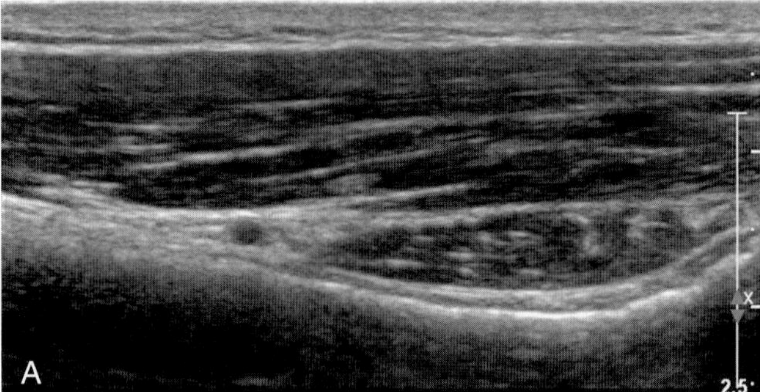

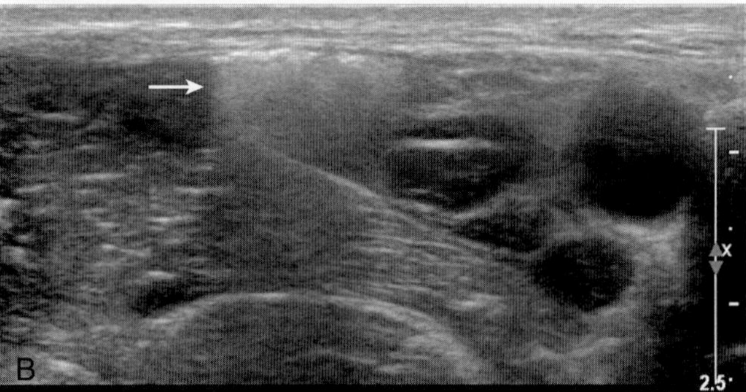

Fig. 46.5 Acoustic shadowing occurs during regional blocks. (A) During block of the axillary nerve in the proximal arm, the cortical surface of the humerus reflects and absorbs sound waves, thereby producing acoustic shadowing deep to the bone surface. (B) During femoral nerve block, air inadvertently injected into the field layers produces strong reflection and acoustic shadowing *(arrow)*.

to a strongly reflecting structure. The spacing between the bands represents the distance between the anterior and posterior walls of the object.[10] Internal reverberations (arising from within the object) cause the comet tail artifact, most intensely observed when the anatomic object is perpendicular to the beam. Comet tail artifact from the pleura relates to lung water content, because small collections of lung water lined by the strongly reflecting pleura can allow the sound beam to enter and then return at varying times to the transducer (Fig. 46.3).

Third, all reflectors are assumed to be on the central ray of the transducer beam. When this assumption is not true, out-of-plane artifacts are observed (slice thickness artifacts). Definitive proof of out-of-plane artifacts requires multiple views, which are recommended when such ambiguities arise.

Unlike adjacent soft tissue, most biologic fluids do not significantly attenuate the sound beam and therefore cause acoustic enhancement (sometimes referred to as posterior acoustic enhancement or increased through-transmission). Acoustic enhancement artifacts deep to blood vessels can be erroneously interpreted as peripheral nerves (Fig. 46.4). For example, acoustic enhancement deep to the second part of the axillary artery in the axilla can be mistaken for the radial nerve. In the infraclavicular region, acoustic enhancement deep to the axillary artery can be mistaken for the posterior cord of the brachial plexus (and similarly, for the femoral artery and the femoral nerve in the inguinal region).

Acoustic shadowing occurs deep to strong reflecting structures, such as the cortical surface of mature bone (Fig. 46.5). Acoustic shadows from refraction (also termed refractile shadowing or lateral edge shadowing) are often observed deep to the edges of blood vessels when the vessels are imaged in the short-axis view. Refractive edge shadows can be seen from the carotid artery during stellate ganglion block or from the second part of the axillary artery during infraclavicular block. Refraction artifacts (e.g., refractile shadowing) are less apparent when spatial compound imaging (for further information, see later in this chapter) is used to reduce angle-dependent artifacts.

Transducer Selection, Manipulation, and Modes of Imaging

Ultrasound transducers consist of piezoelectric crystals that emit and receive high-frequency sound waves by interconverting electrical and mechanical energy. Transducer selection is important to the success of ultrasound-guided regional anesthesia procedures. High-frequency sound waves provide the best resolution but will not penetrate far into tissue. The frequency range is therefore chosen to be the highest that will allow adequate insonation of the entire depth of field. A low-frequency transducer can be used to image large nerves that lie deep, such as the cords of the

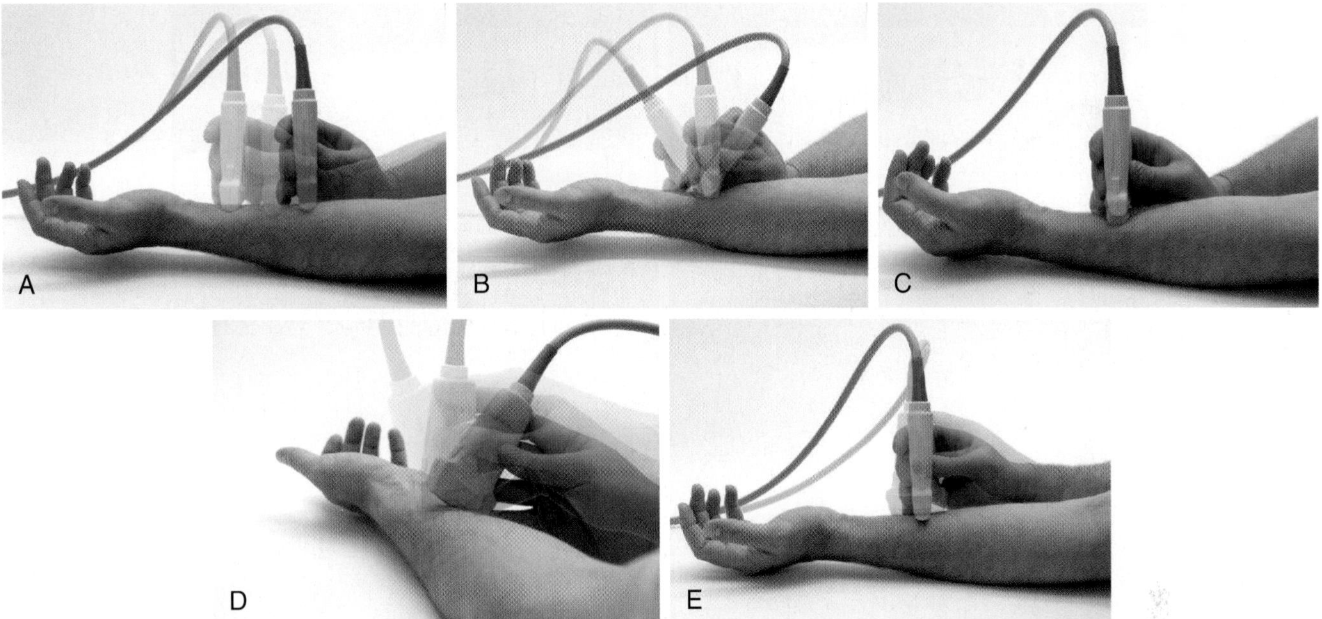

Fig. 46.6 Transducer manipulation. Sliding (A), tilting (B), compression (C), rocking (D), and rotation (E) of the transducer are shown.

brachial plexus that surround the second part of the axillary artery or the proximal sciatic nerve in the gluteal region.

The footprint size (i.e., the length of the active face transducer that contacts the skin) is chosen to provide a broad enough view of the structures of interest. As a general rule, the footprint should be at least as large as the anticipated depth of field. A square or landscape view is better than a keyhole view (i.e., depth greater than footprint) for guidance. As a rule of thumb, for in-plane technique (see Approaches to Regional Block With Ultrasound), every millimeter of the footprint is approximately a millimeter of guidance.

Linear-array transducers generally have a higher scan-line density than curved arrays and therefore produce the best image quality. Images from linear arrays are usually displayed in a rectangular format. When a linear transducer is needed but space at the site of block is limited by anatomic structures such as adjacent bone, a compact linear (hockey stick) transducer that has a smaller footprint can be very useful. Curved arrays provide a broad field of view for a given footprint size and are generally used when space is limited (e.g., infraclavicular region). Curved probes are easier to rock (see Infraclavicular Blocks) and produce images in sector format.

Universal precautions should be used when handling dirty equipment. External surface probes require disinfection between every use and after extended periods of nonuse, per instructions of the manufacturer. Do NOT drop any ultrasound transducer, because the active face of the transducer is especially sensitive to contact with hard surfaces.

One of the essential skills to acquire for regional block with ultrasound is transducer manipulation (Fig. 46.6). For this reason, standardized nomenclature has been established[11]:

- Sliding (moving contact) the transducer along the known course of the nerve using a short-axis view often helps.
- Tilting (cross-plane, side-to-side) will vary the echo brightness of peripheral nerves. Optimizing this angle is critical to promote nerve visibility.
- Compression is often used to confirm venous structures. To improve imaging, compression not only provides better contact, but it also brings the structures closer to the surface of the transducer. Soft tissue is subject to compression; therefore estimates of tissue distances will vary.
- Rocking (in-plane, toward, or away from the indicator) is often necessary to improve visibility of the needle and anatomic structures when the working room is limited.
- Rotation of the probe will produce true short-axis views rather than oblique or long-axis views.

Anisotropy is the change in echogenicity with inclination of the transducer. In general, when objects are obliquely imaged, they appear less echogenic (Fig. 46.7). This relationship is most pronounced for tendons but also occurs for muscle and nerves.[12] Although the term anisotropy was first used to describe changes in received echoes when rocking the transducer with structures viewed in long axis, it has also been used for short-axis views when tilting the transducer. With experience, operators learn to rock and tilt the transducer naturally to fill in the received echoes from peripheral nerves. Sliding and rotating the transducer achieves needle tip localization after optimizing peripheral nerve echoes by tilting.

Spatial compound imaging steers ultrasound beams in different, predetermined angles, typically within approximately 20 degrees from the perpendicular (Fig. 46.8). These multiple lines of insonation are then combined to produce a single composite image. Spatial compound imaging appears to reduce angle-dependent artifacts, anisotropic effects, and acoustic shadows. Another advantage for regional block is that the definition of tissue planes and the detection of nerve borders can be improved. In the systems that have been tested, spatial compound imaging improves needle tip visibility over a limited range of needle insertion angles (<30 degrees). The stray lines of sight (i.e., those that travel off the field underneath the transducer) can be used to form a wider field of view in a trapezoidal format.

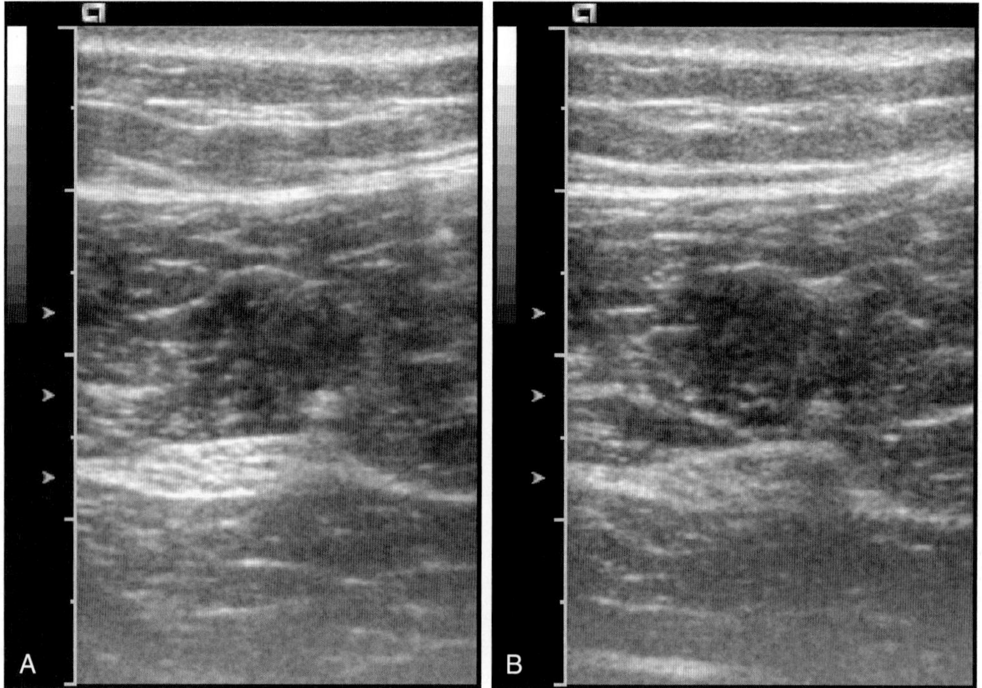

Fig. 46.7 (A) Sciatic nerve imaging in the subgluteal region. (B) The amplitude of the received echoes diminishes when the angle of insonation is changed away from perpendicular to the nerve path, thereby demonstrating anisotropy.

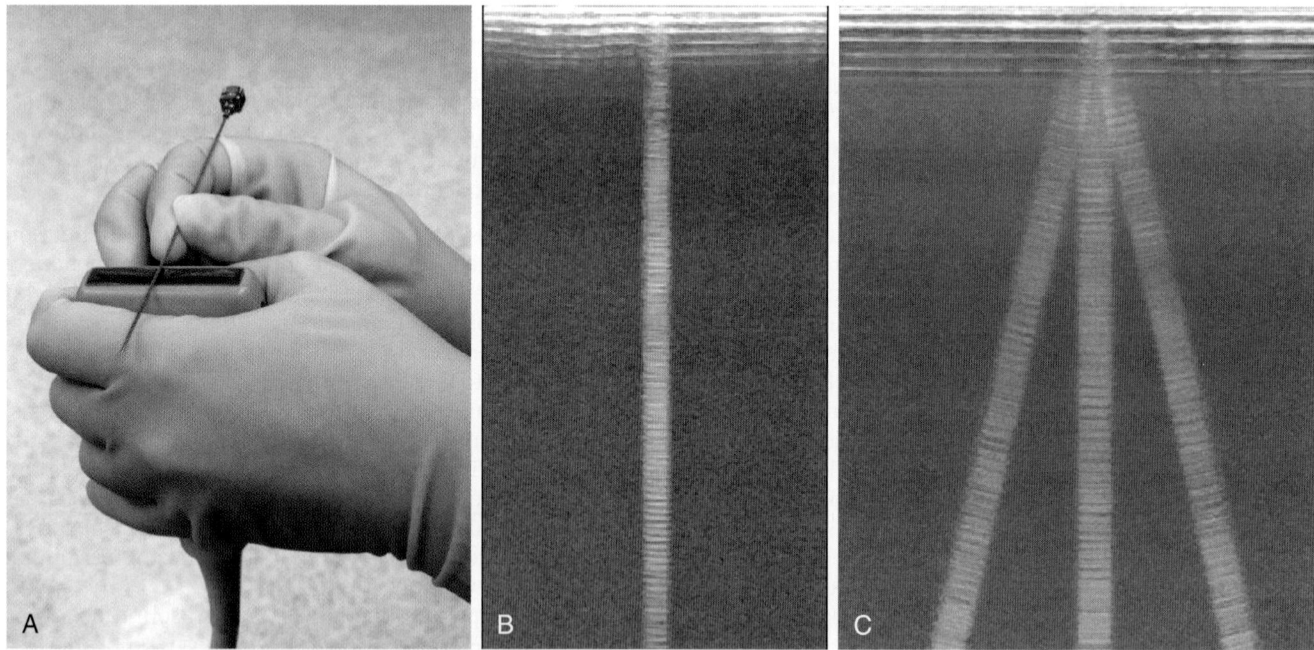

Fig. 46.8 Spatial compound imaging. Some forms of ultrasound imaging use multiple lines of sight by electronically steering the beam to different angles. These sonograms were obtained by placing a linear array test tool (the solid metal stylet of a 17-gauge epidural needle) over the active face of the transducer to isolate a single element. (A) External photograph demonstrates the linear array test tool applied to the active face of the ultrasound transducer. (B) Single-beam imaging is demonstrated. (C) Three lines of sight are used to form a compound image. The test tool images do not display the beam itself, but rather the transmit and receive apertures.

A Doppler shift occurs when a wave source and receiver are moving relative to each other, which produces a change in frequency such that the frequencies of the transmitted and reflected sound waves are not the same. When a wave source and receiver are moving toward each other, the observed frequency is greater than the source frequency; and when moving away from each other, the observed frequency is lower. The change in frequency is related to the velocity of moving reflectors and the angle of insonation. In clinical medicine, red blood cells are the primary reflectors that produce Doppler shifts.

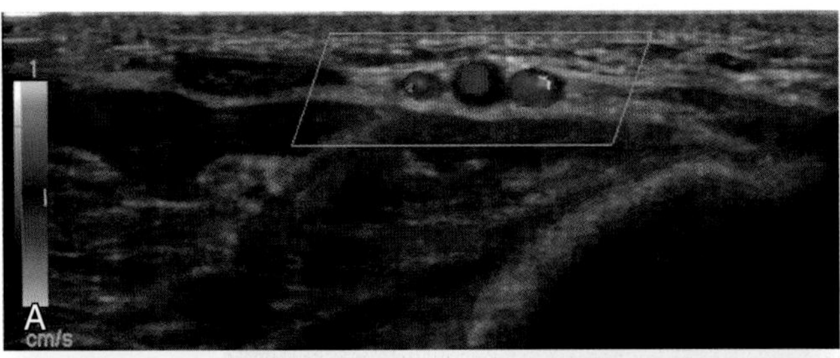

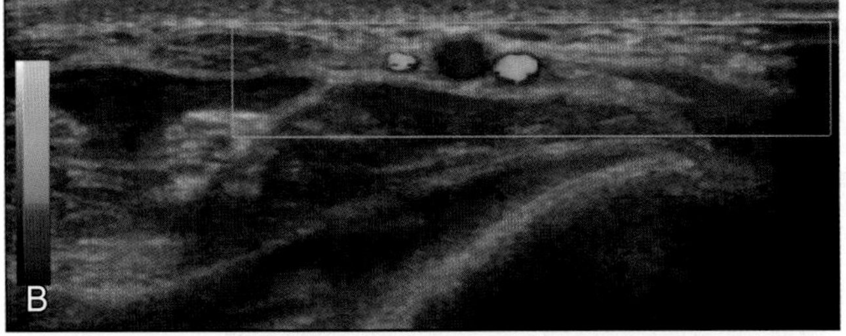

Fig. 46.9 Duplex sonograms illustrate the Doppler shift. (A) In color Doppler, color encoding is based on the mean frequency shift. (B) In power Doppler, color encoding is based on the power spectrum.

Box 46.1 Respective Advantages of Color and Power Doppler Imaging Modalities

Color Doppler

Directional information
Velocity estimates
Less motion artifact (flash artifact)

Power Doppler

More sensitive to detect the presence of flow (by a factor of 3-5 in some cases)
Less angle dependent
No aliasing

Doppler ultrasound imaging has different modes (Fig. 46.9). Traditional color Doppler encodes mean frequency shifts to provide directional velocity information; that is, conventional blue color indicates flow away from the transducer, whereas red color indicates flow toward the transducer. More recently, a more sensitive Doppler technology has been developed that encodes color based on the integration of the Doppler power spectrum.[13] Power Doppler is less angle dependent and not subject to aliasing. The disadvantages are that no directional information is provided and motion sensitivity (flash artifact) is high. Power Doppler is especially useful for detecting small arteries that accompany nerves (Box 46.1). Power Doppler can detect these small arteries and better delineate the course of tortuous vessels that have unfavorable angles to the ultrasound beam.

Needle Tip Visibility

A large number of factors influence needle tip visibility in clinical practice. Metal needles are hyperechoic and can cause reverberation artifact. Needle tip visibility is best when the needle path is parallel to the active face of the transducer. Under this condition, the needle is perpendicular to the sound beam; therefore strong specular reflections will be produced; that is, mirror-like reflections will be produced from a smooth surface. As the angle of incidence is increased, the mean brightness will decrease.[14] In this same study, the bevel angles were ground from 10 to 70 degrees but were found to have no effect on the needle tip echo. However, bevel orientation does influence the needle tip echo; visibility is best with the bevel either directly facing or averting the transducer.[15] Because needle diameters are smaller than the scan plane thickness, larger needles are more echogenic than finer ones.

Visualization of needles in echogenic tissue is difficult, particularly in bright adipose tissue. A number of strategies have been proposed to improve needle tip visibility.[16,17] A low-receiver gain can improve the detection of the needle tip echo. Spatial compound imaging can help identify the needle tip when the needle path is at an angle with respect to the transducer. However, one limitation of this strategy is that only a small triangular section of the field of imaging receives all the lines of sight and is therefore fully compounded. In addition, the range of angles for spatial compound imaging is limited and is usually exceeded by the desired needle insertion path. Rocking back the transducer can improve the angle between the ultrasound beam and needle during in-plane technique (see Approaches to Regional Block with Ultrasound). Most practitioners orient the needle so that the needle bevel faces the transducer.

Among needles originally developed for use in regional anesthesia, Hustead bevels tended to be more visible than side port needles that lack cutting bevels. Needles with echogenic modifications are now commercially marketed for peripheral nerve blocks. One engineering strategy has been to texture the needle surface so that echoes return to the transducer source, regardless of the angle of insonation (Fig. 46.10). One potential limitation of these needle designs is the finite size of the needle texturing. Low-frequency transducers produce longer wavelengths that may be too large to reflect strongly back from the textured surface of the needle.

Approaches to Regional Block With Ultrasound

Peripheral nerves can be directly detected with high-resolution ultrasound imaging.[18] The fascicular echotexture is the most distinguishing feature of nerves (honeycomb architecture) (Fig. 46.11). More central nerves, such as the cervical ventral rami, have fewer fascicles and can appear monofascicular on ultrasound scans. Ultrasound frequencies of 10 MHz or higher are required to distinguish tendons from nerves based on echotexture alone. One of the most powerful techniques to identify nerve fascicles is to slide a broad linear transducer over the known course of a peripheral nerve with the nerve viewed in short axis (transverse cross section).

Nerves can be round, oval, or triangular in shape. Although nerve shape can change along the nerve path, the cross-sectional nerve area is relatively constant in the absence of major branching (Fig. 46.12).[19] Peripheral

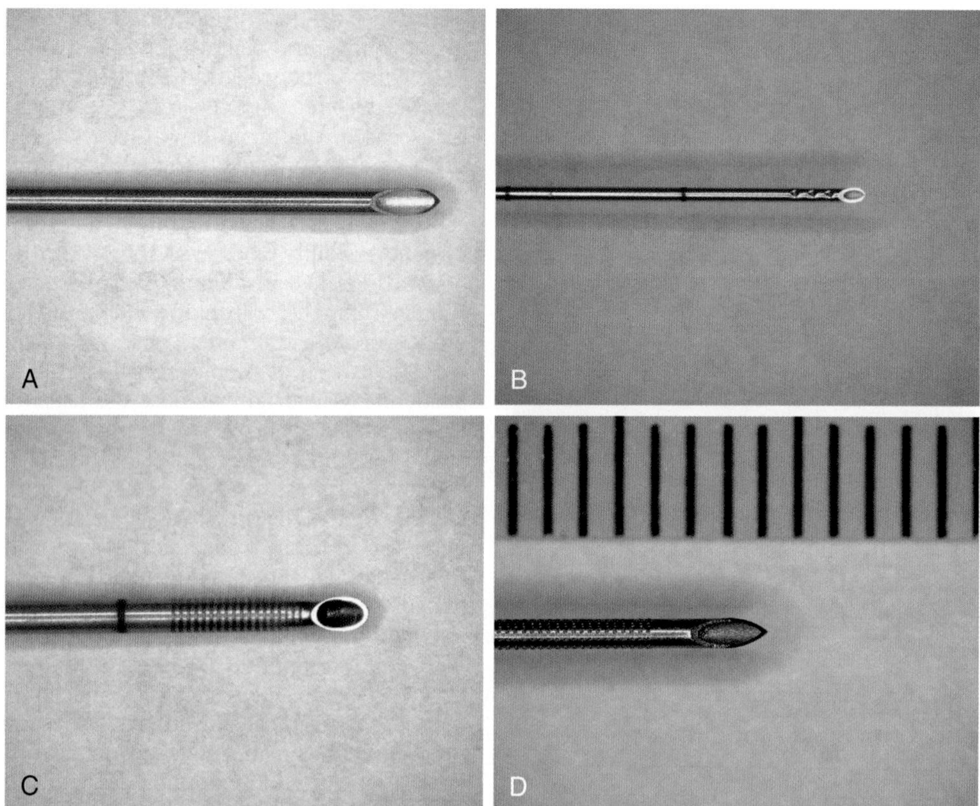

Fig. 46.10 Photomicrographs of needles are used for regional block. A plain conventional needle (A) and echogenic designs (B, C, D) are shown. A smooth needle may not generate a recordable echo because its rounded shaft reflects most incident sound away from the source. A variety of textured surfaces are manufactured and marketed to improve needle tip detection on acquired sonograms. (Modified from Gray AT. *Atlas of Ultrasound-Guided Regional Anesthesia*. 3rd ed. Philadelphia: Saunders; 2018.)

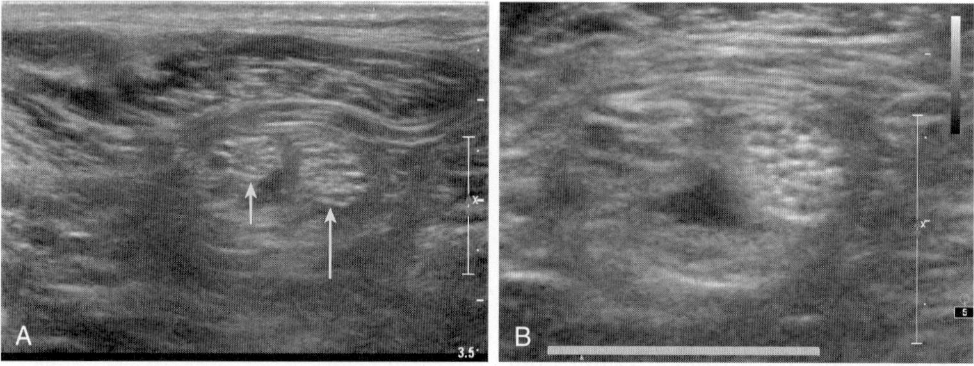

Fig. 46.11 Nerve echotexture. (A) Fascicles of the common peroneal *(short yellow arrow)* and tibial *(long yellow arrow)* nerves are visualized in the popliteal fossa. In this sonogram the honeycomb appearance of a polyfascicular peripheral nerve is observed. (B) Close-up view shows detailed echotexture of the two nerves.

nerves are pathologically enlarged either by entrapment or in certain neuromuscular disorders, such as Charcot-Marie-Tooth, type 1A, disease (Fig. 46.13). Some evidence suggests that patients with diabetic neuropathy also have enlarged peripheral nerves.

Although direct nerve imaging has led to a phenomenal increase in ultrasound-guided regional anesthesia, the identification of other nearby anatomic structures, such as the fascia and other connective tissue, is also critical in this endeavor. These layers permit favorable distribution of local anesthetic, making nerve contact with the block needle unnecessary.

Many approaches to regional blocks with ultrasound are available (Table 46.1). Peripheral nerves are usually viewed in short axis rather than long axis. The needle can approach within the plane of imaging (in-plane technique) or cross the plane of imaging as an echogenic dot (out-of-plane technique). For some regional blocks, offline markings (skin markings before needle insertion) are used instead of online imaging (i.e., imaging during needle insertion and injection). Most studies have suggested that adequate visualization and correct identification of the relevant structures (e.g., peripheral nerve, needle tip, local anesthetic, adjacent anatomic structures) is more important than the

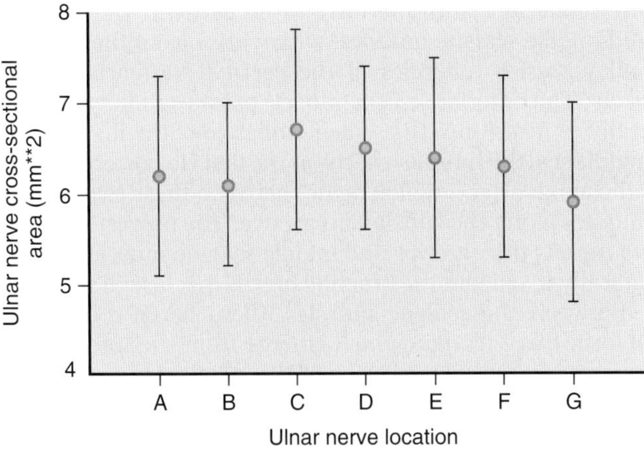

Fig. 46.12 Cross-sectional area of a peripheral nerve as a function of nerve path length. In this figure the cross-sectional area of the ulnar nerve is shown at various points in the upper extremity. Axilla (A); midhumerus (B); 2 cm proximal to medial epicondyle (C); medial epicondyle (D); 2 cm distal to medial epicondyle (E); arterial split (F); and wrist crease (G). Data are shown as mean values with standard deviations. Despite changes in shape that can occur, the cross-sectional area of nerves is relatively constant along the nerve path in the absence of major branching. (Modified from Cartwright MS, Shin HW, Passmore LV, Walker FO. Ultrasonographic findings of the normal ulnar nerve in adults. *Arch Phys Med Rehabil.* 288[3]:394–396, 2007.)

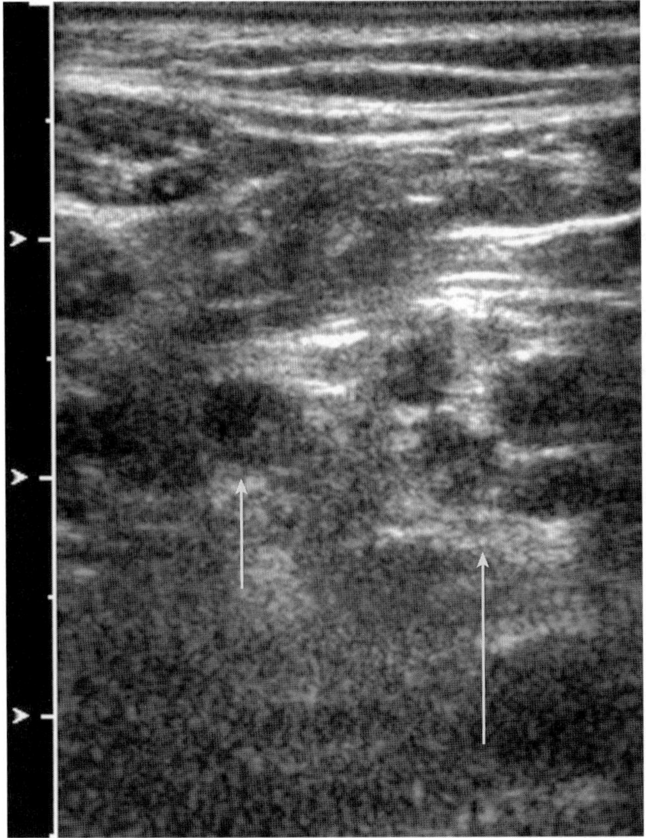

Fig. 46.13 Sonogram demonstrates the popliteal fossa of a patient with Charcot-Marie-Tooth, type 1A, disorder. The peripheral nerves are significantly enlarged because of the large fascicles *(yellow arrows)*. Nerves of the symptomatic and asymptomatic sides can appear similar in these patients. Large tick marks are 10 mm apart.

Table 46.1 Examples of Approaches to Regional Blocks With Ultrasound Guidance

Approach	Examples of Regional Block
Short-axis view, in-plane	Almost any peripheral nerve block Almost any peripheral catheter placement
Short-axis view, out-of-plane	Shallow blocks Interscalene catheter Lateral femoral cutaneous nerve block Femoral nerve catheter placement
Long-axis view, in-plane	Proximal fascia iliaca block Proximal obturator block Anterior sciatic block
Long-axis view, out-of-plane	Epidural placement (longitudinal paramedian view during midline approach) Transtracheal anesthesia

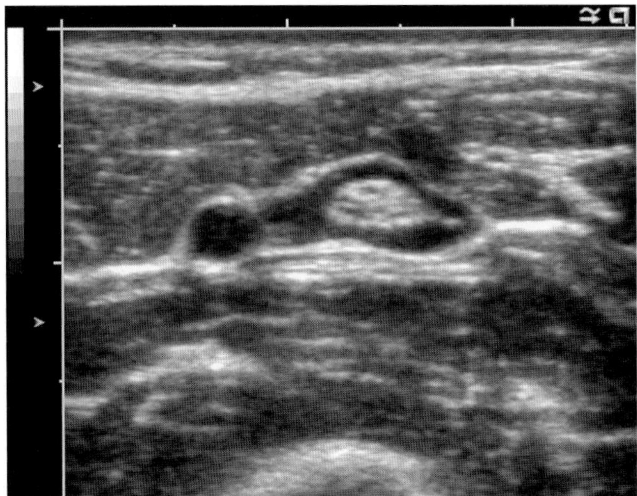

Fig. 46.14 Local anesthetic injection for successful peripheral nerve block. The ulnar nerve and ulnar artery are viewed in short axis in the forearm in this sonogram. The nerve is surrounded with anechoic local anesthetic.

approach, per se, for outcomes after regional blocks. Nevertheless, consistent practice patterns are developing among institutions and illustrate the underlying principles.

Successful injection for peripheral nerve block has typical characteristics (Fig. 46.14). Injections should distribute around the nerve (clarifying the nerve border), travel along the nerve path and branches, and separate the nerve from common anatomic structures such as adjacent arteries that are wrapped together in common fascia and connective tissue. Because anechoic fluid is typically injected, echoes received from the peripheral nerve will also be enhanced by increased through transmission (but not necessarily a sign of block success).

REGIONAL BLOCK TECHNIQUES

Cervical Plexus Blocks

The cervical plexus is derived from the C1, C2, C3, and C4 spinal nerves and supplies branches to the prevertebral muscles, strap muscles of the neck, and phrenic nerve. The deep cervical plexus supplies the musculature of the neck.

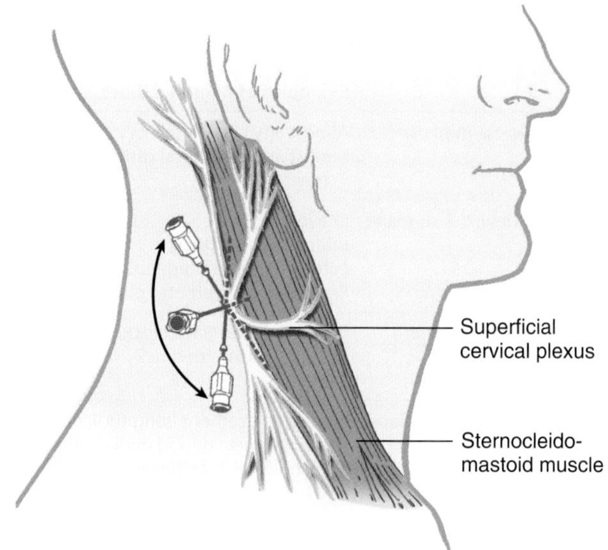

Fig. 46.15 Anatomic landmarks and method of needle placement for a superficial cervical plexus block.

The superficial cervical plexus provides cutaneous sensation of the skin between the trigeminal innervation of the face and the T2 dermatome of the trunk.

Clinical Applications

Blocks of the cervical plexus are easy to perform and provide anesthesia for surgical procedures in the distribution of C2 to C4, including lymph node dissections, plastic surgery repairs, and carotid endarterectomy.[20,21] The ability to continuously monitor the awake patient's neurologic status is an advantage of this anesthetic technique for the latter procedure and has resulted in an upsurge in the popularity of this technique. Bilateral blocks can be used for tracheostomy and thyroidectomy. A variety of approaches to cervical plexus block have been described, including some guided by ultrasound imaging.[22,23]

Superficial Cervical Plexus

The superficial cervical plexus is blocked at the midpoint of the posterior border of the sternocleidomastoid muscle. A skin wheal is made at this point, and a 22-gauge, 4-cm needle is advanced, injecting 5 mL of solution along the posterior border and medial surface of the sternocleidomastoid muscle (Fig. 46.15). It is possible to block the accessory nerve with this injection, resulting in temporary ipsilateral trapezius muscle paralysis. Deep cervical plexus blocks also are possible but have been associated with a higher incidence of respiratory complications.[24]

Brachial Plexus Blocks

BRACHIAL PLEXUS ANATOMY

The brachial plexus is derived from the anterior primary rami of the fifth, sixth, seventh, and eighth cervical nerves and the first thoracic nerve, with variable contributions from the fourth cervical and second thoracic nerves. After leaving their intervertebral foramina, these nerves course anterolaterally and inferiorly to lie between the anterior and middle scalene muscles, which arise from the anterior and posterior tubercles of the cervical vertebra, respectively. The anterior scalene muscle passes caudally and laterally to insert into the scalene tubercle of the first rib; the middle scalene muscle inserts on the first rib posterior to the subclavian artery, which passes between these two scalene muscles along the subclavian groove. The prevertebral fascia invests the anterior and middle scalene muscles, fusing laterally to enclose the brachial plexus in a fascial sheath.

Between the scalene muscles, these nerve roots unite to form three trunks, which emerge from the interscalene space to lie cephaloposterior to the subclavian artery as it courses along the upper surface of the first rib. The superior (C5 and C6), middle (C7), and inferior (C8 and T1) trunks are arranged accordingly and are not in a strict horizontal formation, as often depicted. At the lateral edge of the first rib, each trunk forms anterior and posterior divisions that pass posterior to the midportion of the clavicle to enter the axilla. Within the axilla, these divisions form the lateral, posterior, and medial cords, named for their relationship with the second part of the axillary artery. The superior divisions from the superior and middle trunks form the lateral cord, the inferior divisions from all three trunks form the posterior cord, and the anterior division of the inferior trunk continues as the medial cord.

At the lateral border of the pectoralis minor, the three cords divide into the peripheral nerves of the upper extremity. The lateral cord gives rise to the lateral head of the median nerve and the musculocutaneous nerve; the medial cord gives rise to the medial head of the median nerve, as well as the ulnar, the medial antebrachial, and the medial brachial cutaneous nerves; and the posterior cord divides into the axillary and radial nerves (Fig. 46.16).

Aside from the branches from the cords that form the peripheral nerves as described, several branches arise from the roots of the brachial plexus providing motor innervation to the rhomboid muscles (C5), the subclavian muscles (C5 and C6), and the serratus anterior muscle (C5, C6, and C7). The suprascapular nerve arises from C5 and C6, supplies the muscles of the dorsal aspect of the scapula, and makes a significant contribution to the sensory supply of the shoulder joint.

Sensory distributions of the cervical roots and the peripheral nerves are shown in Fig. 46.17.

Branches arising from the cervical roots were traditionally blocked with the interscalene approach to the brachial plexus. However, interscalene block has a well-documented risk of concomitant phrenic nerve block. This can result in symptomatic hemi-diaphragmatic paralysis and respiratory compromise, especially among those patients with obesity or moderate to severe obstructive pulmonary disease.[25,26] Recent evidence suggests diaphragm paresis may be avoidable with more distal "lung-sparing" block techniques that target the terminal nerves supplying the shoulder joint.

By design, brachial plexus blocks above the clavicle (e.g., interscalene and supraclavicular blocks) primarily target local anesthetic placement near the ventral rami, trunks, and divisions. Blocks below the clavicle (e.g., infraclavicular and axillary blocks) primarily target the cords and terminal nerves.

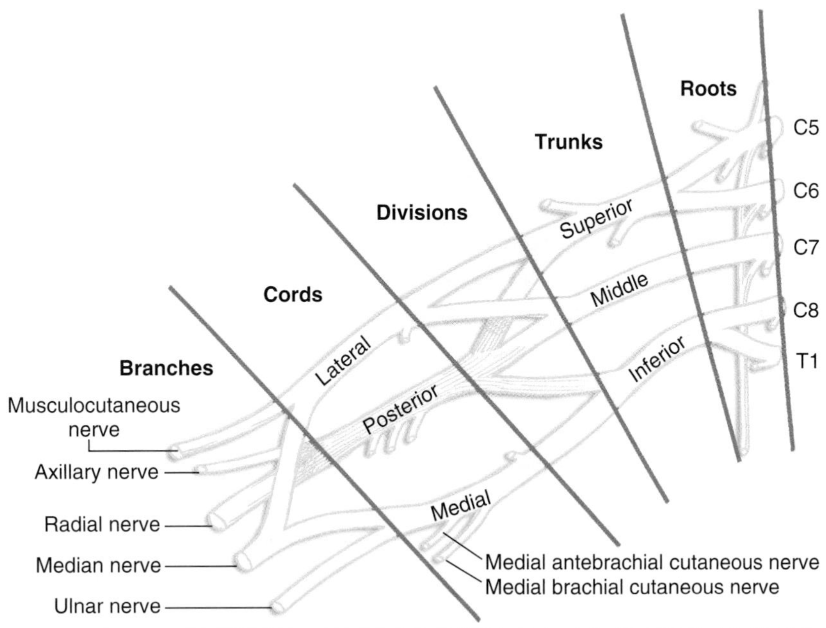

Fig. 46.16 Roots, trunks, divisions, cords, and branches of the brachial plexus.

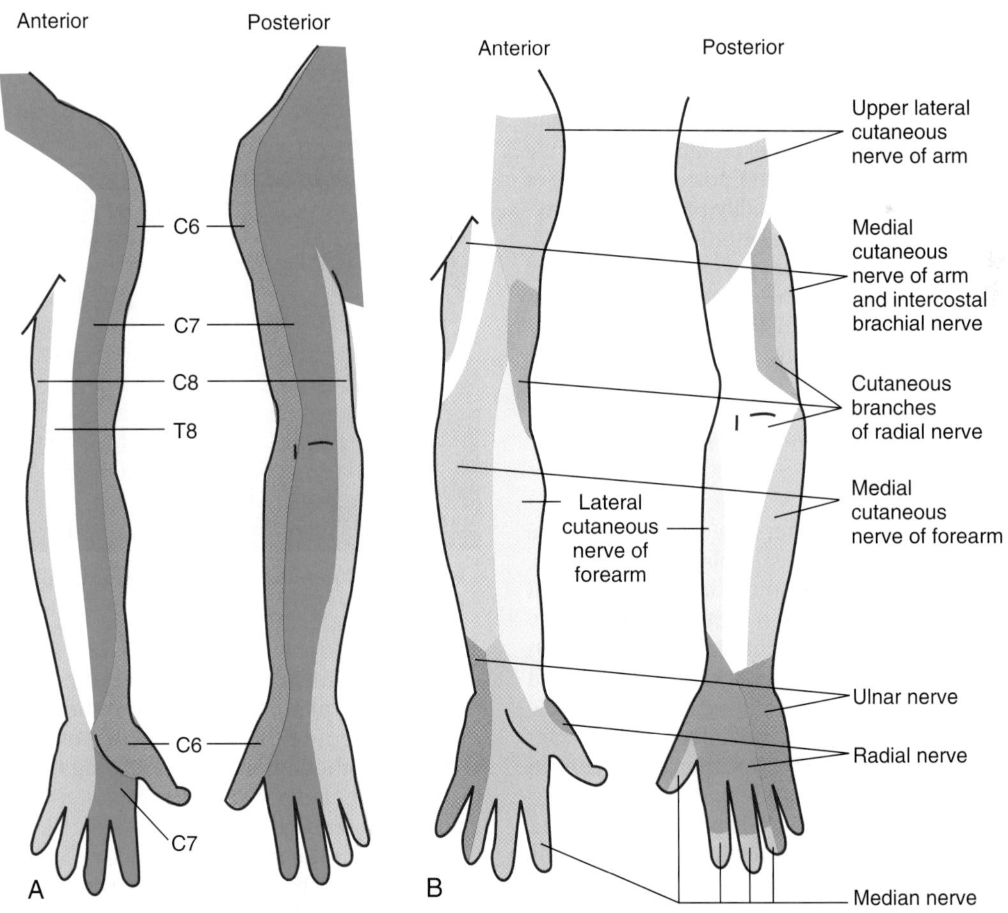

Fig. 46.17 (A) Cutaneous distribution of the cervical roots. (B) Cutaneous distribution of the peripheral nerves.

Interscalene Blocks

The interscalene block is often chosen for regional anesthesia technique of the shoulder[27] in those patients without significant pulmonary disease. Blockade occurs at the level of the superior and middle trunks of the brachial plexus. Although this approach can be used for forearm and hand surgery, blockade of the inferior trunk (C8 and T1) can be incomplete and may require supplementation of the ulnar nerve for adequate surgical anesthesia in that distribution.[28] Ultrasound guidance for interscalene block reduces the chance of inferior trunk sparing.[29]

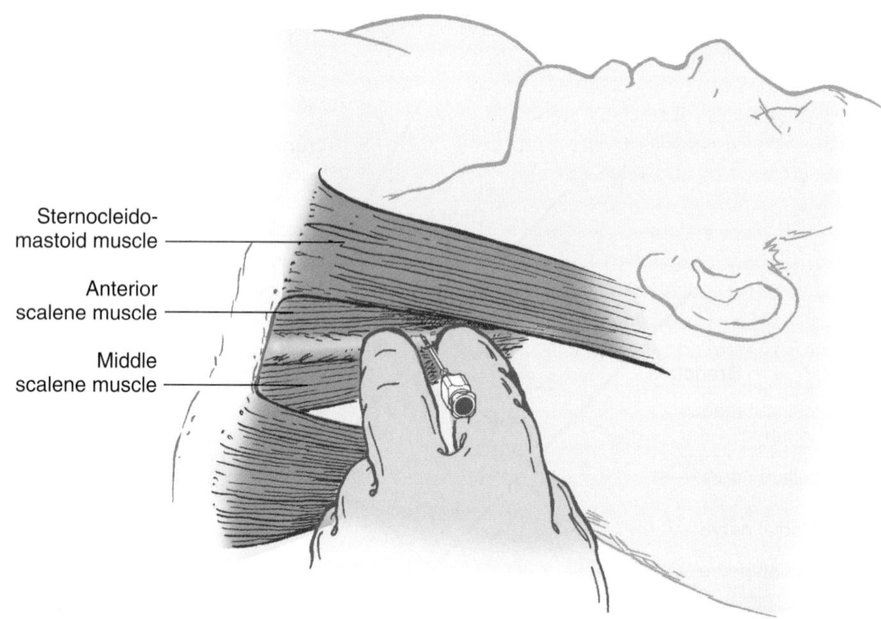

Fig. 46.18 Interscalene block guided by palpation. The fingers palpate the interscalene groove, and the needle is inserted with a caudad and slightly posterior angle.

Several adjacent anatomic structures can serve as important landmarks for performance of interscalene block. The patient should be in the supine position, with the head turned away from the side to be blocked and the patient's arm in any comfortable position. The posterior border of the sternocleidomastoid muscle is readily palpated by having the patient briefly lift the head. The interscalene groove can be palpated by rolling the fingers posterolaterally away from this border over the belly of the anterior scalene muscle into the groove (Fig. 46.18). A line is extended laterally from the cricoid cartilage to intersect the interscalene groove, indicating the level of the transverse process of C6. Although the external jugular vein often overlies this point of intersection, it is not a consistent landmark.

Ultrasound-Guided Technique

Traditional approaches to the interscalene block include paresthesia or peripheral nerve stimulation technique. However, this block is well suited to the use of ultrasound guidance. It is often easiest to obtain a supraclavicular view of the subclavian artery and brachial plexus (Fig. 46.19) and then trace the plexus up the neck with the ultrasound probe until the plexus trunks are visualized as hypoechoic structures between the anterior and medial scalene muscles (the "stoplight" sign[30]). The needle can then be advanced with either an in-plane or out-of-plane approach. After negative aspiration, a small test dose is administered, and local anesthetic spread around the brachial plexus confirms appropriate placement of the needle. Volumes as little as 5 mL may be successful and associated with a decreased frequency of diaphragmatic paresis.[31]

Side Effects and Complications

At the traditional (C6) level of interscalene block, ipsilateral phrenic nerve block and resultant diaphragmatic paresis are inevitable. This effect probably results from the proximity of the phrenic nerve at this level[32] and may cause subjective symptoms of dyspnea. Respiratory compromise can occur in patients with severe preexisting respiratory disease or contralateral phrenic nerve dysfunction.

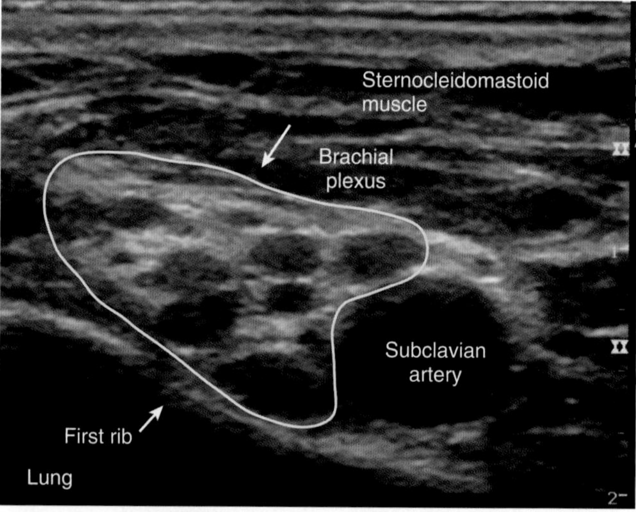

Fig. 46.19 Ultrasound image of the brachial plexus at the level of the first rib.

Involvement of the vagus, recurrent laryngeal, and cervical sympathetic nerves is rarely significant if unilateral, but the patient experiencing symptoms related to these side effects may require reassurance. The risk of pneumothorax is small when the needle is correctly placed at the C5 or C6 level because of the distance from the dome of the pleura.

Severe hypotension and bradycardia (i.e., Bezold-Jarisch reflex) can occur in awake, sitting patients undergoing shoulder surgery under an interscalene block. The cause is presumed to be stimulation of intracardiac mechanoreceptors by decreased venous return, producing an abrupt withdrawal of sympathetic tone and enhanced parasympathetic output. This effect results in bradycardia, hypotension, and syncope. The frequency is decreased when prophylactic β-adrenergic blockers are administered.[33]

Epidural and intrathecal injections can occur with this block. The proximity of significant neurovascular structures may increase the risk of serious neurologic complications when interscalene block is performed in heavily sedated or anesthetized patients. Accordingly, interscalene blocks are usually placed under light sedation in adult patients.

Supraclavicular Blocks. Indications for supraclavicular blocks include operations on the elbow, forearm, and hand. Blockade occurs at the distal trunk–proximal division level of the brachial plexus. At this point, the brachial plexus is relatively compact, and a small volume of local anesthetic produces rapid onset of reliable blockade.

Ultrasound-Guided Technique

The patient is placed in supine position, with the head turned away from the side to be blocked. The arm to be anesthetized is adducted against the side of the body. Similar to interscalene block, traditional approaches to the supraclavicular block include paresthesia or peripheral nerve stimulation. Given the widespread use and availability of ultrasound, this block is now more commonly performed with sonographic guidance. This allows the practitioner to visualize the brachial plexus, subclavian artery, pleura, and first rib. The inherent safety of this technique requires continuous visualization of the needle tip and adjacent anatomic structures during needle advancement.

A high-frequency (15-6 MHz) linear transducer is positioned just proximal to the supraclavicular fossa to obtain a supraclavicular view (see Fig. 46.19). The brachial plexus trunks and divisions are clustered vertically over the first rib on the lateral side of the subclavian artery. The first rib acts as a medial barrier to the needle reaching the pleural dome and is short, wide, and flat.

The needle can then be advanced under direct ultrasound guidance using an in-plane approach from lateral to medial.[34,35] The transducer rests near the clavicle so manipulation can be challenging. Thus advanced skills with needle control are required. After negative aspiration, a small test dose is administered, and local anesthetic spread around the brachial plexus confirms appropriate placement of the needle tip. Volumes as low as 15 to 30 mL may be successful.

Side Effects and Complications

The prevalence of pneumothorax after supraclavicular block is 0.5% to 6% and diminishes with increased experience. Importantly, although the use of ultrasound may decrease the incidence of pneumothorax, the risk has not been eliminated.[36] When this occurs, the onset of symptoms is usually delayed, and it can take up to 24 hours to develop. Thus routine chest radiography after the block is not justified. The supraclavicular approach is best avoided when the patient is uncooperative or cannot tolerate any degree of respiratory compromise. Other complications include phrenic nerve block (as high as 40%-60%), Horner's syndrome, and neuropathy. The presence of phrenic or cervical sympathetic nerve block usually requires only reassurance. Although nerve damage can occur, it is uncommon and usually self-limited.

Suprascapular Nerve Blocks. Suprascapular nerve (SSN) block above the clavicle (anterior approach) is a viable alternative to interscalene block for analgesia of the shoulder region.[37,38] The advantage of this more peripheral approach is that the chance of concomitant phrenic nerve block is significantly reduced. In addition, if the block is semi-selective then other nerves that contribute articular branches to the shoulder joint (e.g., axillary nerve, lateral pectoral nerve) also can be blocked. The anterior approach to SSN block is more shallow (5-10 mm depth) than the more traditional block of the SSN block at the suprascapular notch (20-40 mm depth). Furthermore, the suprascapular notch has variable morphology and in some subjects this landmark is absent. The SSN is the primary sensory innervation of the shoulder joint[39] and is not blocked with approaches to the brachial plexus below the clavicle. Selective low-volume approaches to SSN block above the clavicle also may be useful for pain medicine and rehabilitation.[40]

Indications

The SSN, a mixed-motor and sensory nerve originating from the superior trunk (C5 and C6 nerve roots and often C4 as well) makes a significant contribution to the sensory supply of the shoulder joint. The SSN root may be accessed from within the posterior cervical triangle of the neck where it passes underneath the omohyoid muscle toward the suprascapular notch. The SSN, unlike the suprascapular vessels that remain superficial, then passes deep to the superior transverse scapular ligament exiting through the scapular foramen into the supraspinous fossa finally providing nerve branches to muscles of the shoulder girdle.

Ultrasound-Guided Technique

The anterior SSN block is performed in the supine position with head turned to the contralateral side when accessing the nerve within the posterior cervical triangle (similar positioning as the interscalene nerve block). Alternatively, the patient would be in a seated position to access the scapula for a more distal and posterior SSN block. In the seated position, ask the patient to place his/her hand over to the contralateral shoulder (full shoulder adduction) to move the target (nerve) and scapula lateral from the thorax. Ultrasound guidance is the preferred technique, although a landmark-based method with nerve stimulation for neurolocalization is an option.

Proximal Suprascapular Nerve Block (Anterior Suprascapular Nerve Block). The anterior SSN block technique has emerged as the preferred lung-sparing block alternative to interscalene nerve block.[37,41] A high-frequency linear transducer (15-6 MHz) probe is positioned just proximal to the supraclavicular fossa. Under dynamic scanning, the SSN can be visualized as a round hypoechoic structure deep to the inferior belly of the omohyoid muscle and lateral to the superior trunk in the posterior cervical triangle of the neck (Fig. 46.20) Consider tracing the SSN from its origin (nerve root C5) to facilitate identification. The nerve is then traced more posterior-lateral to a distance away from the superior trunk. A 22-gauge, 5-cm needle is most often selected with shallow 2- to 3-cm depths to the target. Through an out-of-plane or in-plane approach approximately 5 to 15 mL of local anesthetic is deposited deep into omohyoid muscle, but shallow to the prevertebral fascia (higher volumes could result in phrenic nerve blockade). Color Doppler use is advised as the superficial cervical artery and the suprascapular artery, also hypoechoic structures, are strong mimickers of the SSN within the posterior cervical triangle. Auyong and colleagues have shown the anterior SSN block technique provides noninferior, yet lung-sparing, analgesia compared to interscalene nerve block without need for additional terminal nerve block supplementation (e.g., axillary or SSN block).[41]

Shoulder Block (Suprascapular Nerve Plus Axillary [Circumflex] Nerve Block)[42]

In contrast to the anterior suprascapular block, a more distal block of the SSN at the scapula requires the axillary (circumflex) nerve to be also blocked to be remotely comparable to more proximal brachial plexus blockade.[43,44] Unfortunately, the posterior SSN block even with the axillary (circumflex) nerve block will not provide complete anesthesia to the shoulder joint; therefore routinely general anesthesia with supplemental opioid medications would be expected for adequate analgesia.

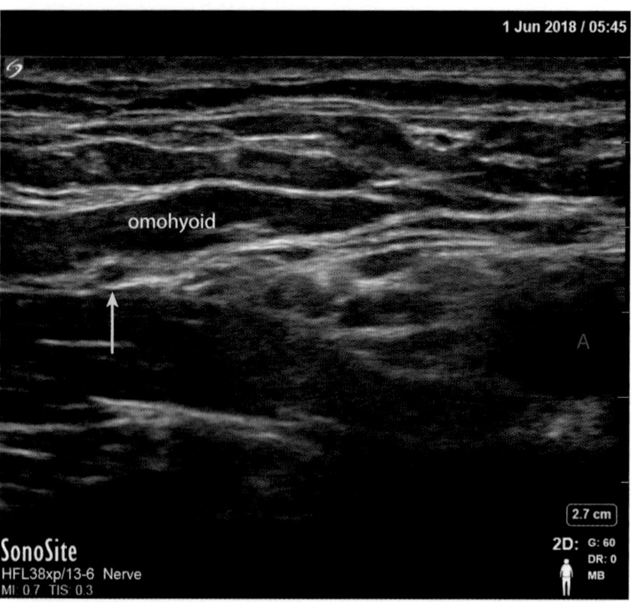

Fig. 46.20 Proximal suprascapular nerve block (anterior suprascapular nerve block). The suprascapular nerve is featured as a round hypoechoic structure deep to the inferior belly of the omohyoid muscle lateral to the superior truck of the brachial plexus within the posterior cervical triangle.

Side Effects and Complications

Serious side effects and complications are primarily due to insertion complications and side effects from local anesthesia use.

Avoid directly targeting the SSN in the suprascapular notch because accidental anterior needle advancement can puncture the pleura. Also, avoid intramuscular placement whether it be avoiding deposit of local anesthesia within the omohyoid (anterior) or within the supraspinatus muscle (posterior), which may result in myotoxicity/myonecrosis. Additionally, the axillary (circumflex) nerve and posterior circumflex artery lie only 2 to 3 mm below the inferior capsule within the neurovascular quadrangular space. Thus a more proximal injection on the posterior upper arm carries a risk of entering the glenohumeral joint space with the block needle and higher local anesthesia volumes have been associated with spread to the posterior cord resulting in radial nerve blockade.

INFRACLAVICULAR BLOCKS

The advantages of the infraclavicular block are that it usually results in complete brachial plexus anesthesia, it is a stable place for a catheter, and no manipulation of the arm is necessary.[45-47] The disadvantages are that the infraclavicular block is a deeper block; therefore needle or probe manipulations are necessary, along with steep angles of needle insertion that result in needle tip visibility issues. Although the arm can remain at the side of the patient, the block is easier when the arm is abducted to straighten the neurovascular bundle. The three arterial wall-hugging cords are named with respect to the second part of the axillary artery; therefore the expected positions are medial, lateral, and posterior. The artery is visualized in short-axis view deep to the pectoralis major and minor muscles (Fig. 46.21). Most practitioners use an in-plane approach from the head of the

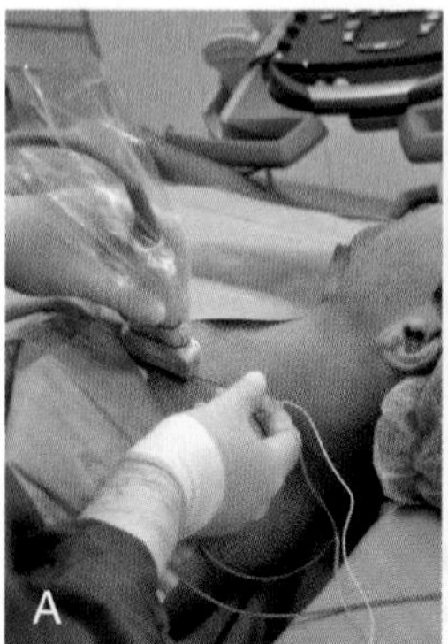

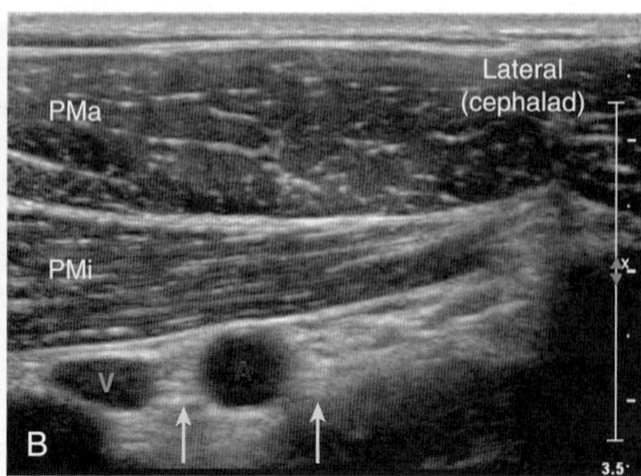

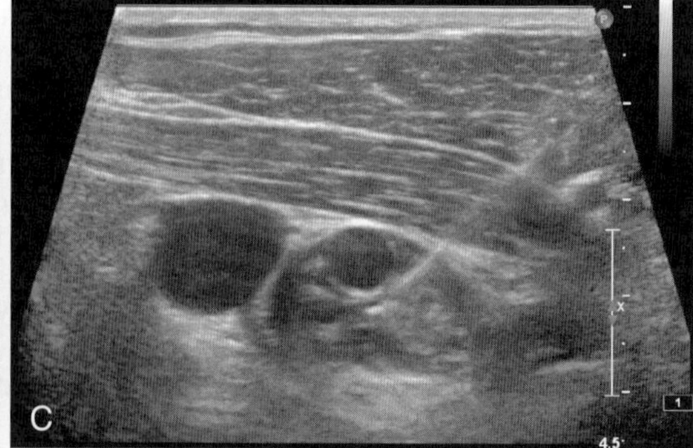

Fig. 46.21 Infraclavicular block with ultrasound imaging. (A) External photograph of the setup for infraclavicular block shows the arm has been abducted in this case. (B) Sonogram of the cords of the brachial plexus *(yellow arrows)* are adjacent to the axillary artery *(A)* and vein *(V)*. The neurovascular bundle lies deep to the pectoralis major *(PMa)* and pectoralis minor *(PMi)* muscles in this anatomic region. (C) Needle tip is in position for infraclavicular block and the resulting local anesthetic distribution.

Table 46.2 Examples of Sonographic Landmarks for Infraclavicular Block

Proximal	Optimal Location	Distal
Cephalic vein	Pectoralis minor muscle (midportion)	Subscapular artery
Thoracoacromial artery	Brachial plexus cords surround axillary artery	Coracobrachialis muscle
Chest wall and pleura	Posterior (or medial) cord underneath axillary artery	Anterior circumflex artery Posterior circumflex artery

Infraclavicular block is usually performed at the level of the second part of the axillary artery (deep to the pectoralis minor muscle). Proximal and distal landmarks along the course of the axillary artery are listed.

Box 46.2 **Sonographic Signs Indicating Infraclavicular Block Success**

- Reduction in axillary artery diameter during injection
- "U-shaped" distribution underneath the axillary artery
- Separation of cords from axillary artery
- *White wall* appearance to the axillary artery (free walls)
- *Dark layer* underneath the axillary artery (long-axis view)

Several studies of clinical block characteristics have validated the high predictive value of local anesthetic distribution underneath the axillary artery for three-cord anesthesia ("U-shaped" distribution).

table or side of the table. The ideal place for local anesthetic distribution to achieve complete infraclavicular block of the brachial plexus is posterior to the axillary artery for single-shot or catheter placement. Substantial evidence suggests that local anesthetic distribution posterior to the axillary artery produces complete brachial plexus block in the infraclavicular region (Table 46.2 and Box 46.2). The cords of the brachial plexus do not need to be directly visualized for successful block. Duplication of the axillary vein is one of the few anatomic variations in the infraclavicular region. The clinical problem is that the accessory vein lies adjacent to the lateral cord of the brachial plexus and near the usual desired position of the needle tip.

AXILLARY BLOCKS

The axillary block is a versatile block for upper extremity anesthesia. Although relatively safe and effective with classical approaches, the cardinal weakness has been the failure to block the musculocutaneous nerve. With the advent of ultrasound imaging, this limitation can be overcome by directly visualizing the musculocutaneous nerve.

The axillary block provides surgical anesthesia of the elbow and more distal upper extremity. The shallow depth of the neurovascular bundle (a 20-mm field is typical) and the large amount of working room make this block relatively easy with ultrasound guidance (Table 46.3). Usually, three arterial wall-hugging branches (median, ulnar, and radial) and one branch with a characteristic medial-to-lateral course in the axilla (musculocutaneous) are visualized. In addition, the musculocutaneous nerve has a characteristic change in shape as it moves from adjacent to the artery (round) to within the coracobrachialis muscle (flat) and then exiting the muscle (triangular).

Table 46.3 Comparison of the Infraclavicular and Axillary Approaches to Brachial Plexus Block

	Infraclavicular Block	Axillary Block
Depth	Deep (two overlying muscles)	Shallow
Onset	Slower	Faster
Tourniquet tolerance	Good	Fair
Catheter success	High	Low

Both in-plane (with needle approaching from the lateral side of the arm) and out-of-plane (with needle approaching from distal to proximal) techniques can be used (Figs. 46.22 and 46.23). The block is performed in the proximal axilla, with the transducer gently pressed against the chest wall to visualize the conjoint tendon of the latissimus dorsi and teres major.[48] A high-frequency linear probe with a small footprint (25–50 mm) with sterile cover can be used for axillary block. The ideal location for local anesthetic injection is between the nerves and the artery so that separation between the two structures occurs to ensure distribution within the neurovascular bundle. These injections result in excellent clinical sensory and motor blocks. The musculocutaneous nerve is usually blocked within the coracobrachialis, where its flat shape gives a large amount of surface area for rapid block. Duplication of the axillary artery and musculocutaneous-median nerve fusion (low-lying lateral cord) are common anatomic variations in the axilla.

Trunk Blocks

INTERCOSTAL NERVE BLOCKS

The intercostal nerves are the primary rami of T1 through T11. T12 is technically the subcostal nerve, and it can communicate with the iliohypogastric and ilioinguinal nerves. Fibers from T1 contribute to the brachial plexus; T2 and T3 provide a few fibers to the formation of the intercostobrachial nerve, which supplies the skin of the medial aspect of the upper arm. Each intercostal nerve has four branches: the gray ramus communicans, which passes anteriorly to the sympathetic ganglion; the posterior cutaneous branch, supplying skin and muscle in the paravertebral area; the lateral cutaneous branch, arising just anterior to the midaxillary line and sending subcutaneous branches anteriorly and posteriorly; and the anterior cutaneous branch, which is the termination of the nerve.

Medial to the posterior angles of the ribs, the intercostal nerves lie between the pleura and the internal intercostal fascia. At the posterior angle of the rib, the nerve lies in the costal groove accompanied by the intercostal vein and artery.

Clinical Applications

Few surgical procedures can be performed with an intercostal block alone, and the application of these blocks in combination with other techniques has largely been supplanted by epidural blockade. However, in patients with contraindications to neuraxial blockade, these techniques can be used alone or combined with other blocks and light

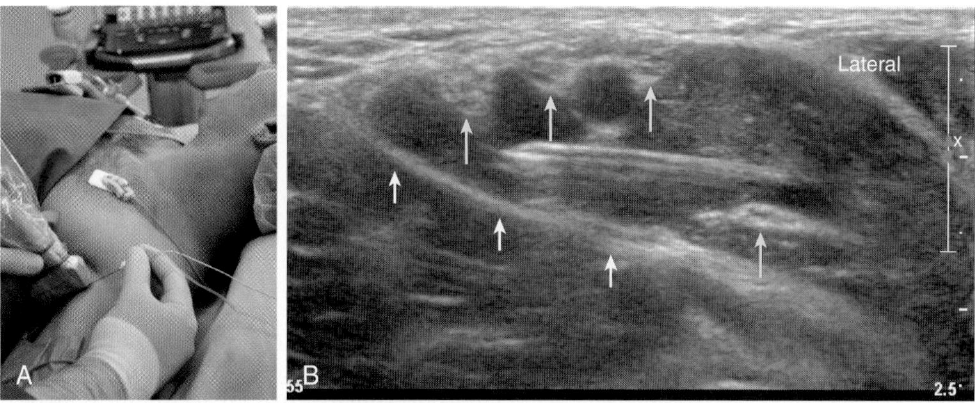

Fig. 46.22 Axillary block with ultrasound guidance. (A) External photograph demonstrates the in-plane approach. (B) Sonogram of the neurovascular bundle in the short-axis view shows the needle tip in-plane after injection of the local anesthetic. The probe compression is just sufficient to coapt the walls of the satellite veins. The block is performed at the level of the conjoint tendon of the latissimus dorsi and teres major *(white arrows)*, which lies under the neurovascular structures. The third part of the axillary artery (A) and nerves of the brachial plexus—radial, ulnar, median, and musculocutaneous—in order from medial to lateral *(yellow arrows)* are shown.

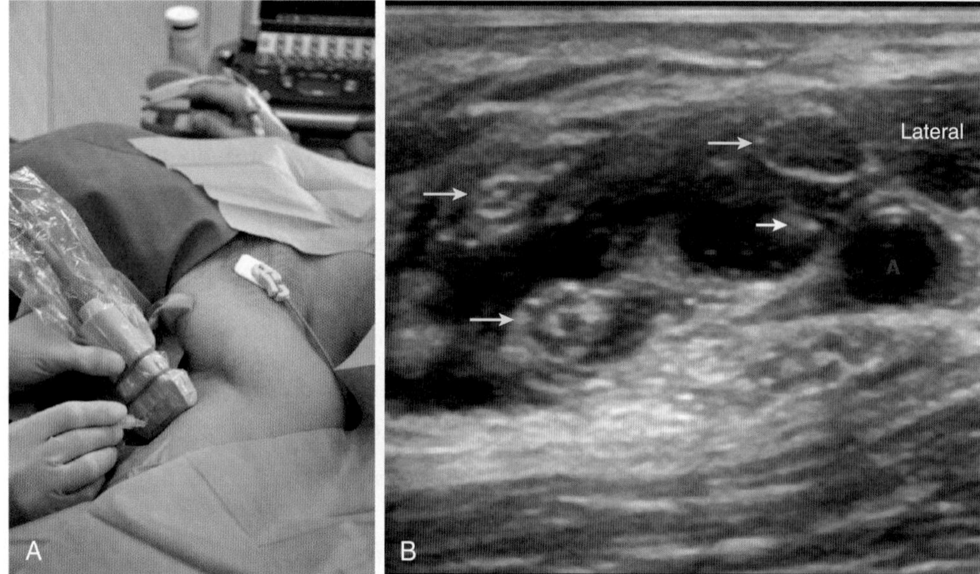

Fig. 46.23 Axillary block with ultrasound guidance. (A) External photograph demonstrates the out-of-plane approach. (B) Sonogram of the neurovascular bundle in the short-axis view shows the needle tip *(white arrow)* crossing the plane of imaging. The probe compression is just sufficient to coapt the walls of the satellite veins. The third part of the axillary artery (A) and nerves of the brachial plexus *(yellow arrows)* are shown.

general anesthesia to provide excellent surgical conditions for intraabdominal procedures. Although surgical applications are possible, the majority of indications are for postoperative analgesia. Intercostal blocks provide a viable alternative to epidural and paravertebral blocks, with a similar safety and efficacy profile.[49]

Intercostal Block Technique

The intercostal nerve can be blocked at the angle of the rib just lateral to the sacrospinalis muscle group. The patient is placed in the prone position with a pillow placed under the abdomen to reduce the lumbar curve (Fig. 46.24). A line is drawn along the posterior vertebral spines. Nearly parallel lines are drawn along the posterior angles of the rib, which can be palpated 6 to 8 cm from the midline. These lines angle medially at the upper levels to prevent overlying of the scapula. The inferior edge of each targeted rib is palpated and is marked on the line intersecting the posterior angle of the rib. After appropriate skin preparation, skin wheals are injected at each of these points. A 22-gauge, short-bevel, 4-cm needle is attached to a 10-mL syringe. Beginning at the lowest marked rib, the index finger of the left hand displaces the skin up over the patient's rib. The needle is inserted at the tip of the finger until it rests on the rib. The fingers of the left hand are shifted to grasp the needle hub firmly. The left hand then walks the needle 3 to 5 mm off the lower rib edge, where 3 to 5 mL of local anesthetic are injected (see Fig. 46.24B and C). This process is repeated at each marked rib. Appropriate intravenous sedation providing analgesia and some degree of amnesia is desirable for the patient's comfort.

Alternatively, intercostal block can be performed in the supine patient at the midaxillary line. Theoretically, the lateral cutaneous branch of the nerve can be missed, but computed tomography studies show that injected solutions spread several centimeters along the costal groove. Further injection of 1 to 2 mL of local anesthetic as the needle is withdrawn blocks the subcutaneous branches.

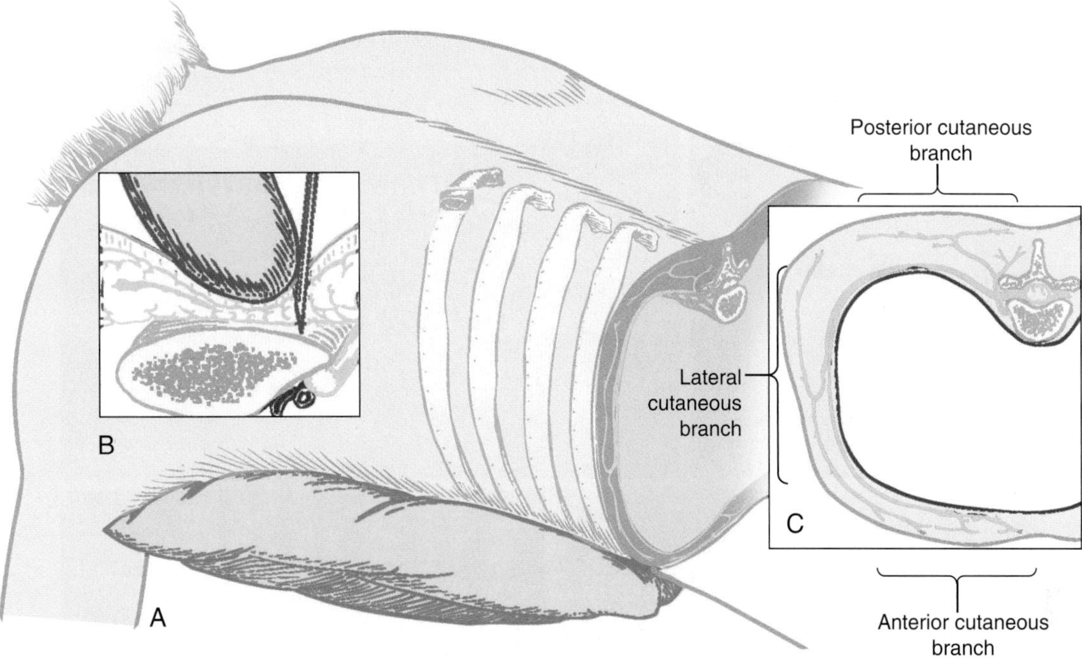

Fig. 46.24 (A) Patient positioning for an intercostal nerve block. (B) The index finger displaces the skin up over the rib. The needle is inserted at the tip of the finger and rests on the rib. The needle is walked off the lower rib edge and inserted 3 to 5 mm. (C) An intercostal nerve and its branches.

Alternative Techniques

Intercostal blocks are possible with ultrasound imaging for guidance. However, the intercostal nerves and vessels are small (about 1-2 mm in diameter) and run in the costal groove and can therefore be difficult to directly image. Similarly, the innermost intercostal muscle, which separates the intercostal nerves and vessels from the internal and external intercostal muscles, is incomplete in the posterior thorax and can be difficult to image.[50] When detected, the innermost intercostal muscle is thin and hypoechoic on ultrasound scans.[51] Intercostal arteries are most visible medially before they enter the costal groove.[52,53] Intercostal arteries are more tortuous in elderly patients, and therefore more exposed and vulnerable to injury.[54]

Intercostal injections dent the pleura, similar to the displacement seen with paravertebral injections.[55] Injections of local anesthetic at the angle of the rib can track medially along the intercostal vessels within the costal groove toward the paravertebral space.[56,57] While variations on ultrasound-guided intercostal nerve blocks have been developed, including anterior approaches to intercostal branches in the serratus plane[58,59] and parasternal region,[60] new technologies are now being developed to improve ultrasound imaging of intercostal nerves and vessels.[61]

Side Effects and Complications

The major complication with intercostal blockade is pneumothorax. The actual incidence, however, was as low as 0.07% in a large series performed by anesthesiologists at all levels of training. Routine postoperative chest radiographs showed an incidence of nonsymptomatic pneumothorax of 0.4% to 1.0%.[62,63] If this unusual complication occurs, treatment is usually limited to observation, administration of oxygen, or needle aspiration. Rarely, chest tube drainage is required.

The risk of systemic local anesthetic toxicity is present with multiple intercostal blocks because of the large volumes and rapid systemic absorption of the solutions. Use of epinephrine has been shown to decrease blood levels. Patients should be monitored and observed carefully during the block and for at least 20 to 30 minutes afterward. Patients with severe pulmonary disease who rely on their intercostal muscles can exhibit respiratory decompensation after bilateral intercostal blockade.

TRANSVERSUS ABDOMINIS PLANE BLOCKS

Four peripheral nerves, the subcostal, ilioinguinal, iliohypogastric, and genitofemoral, primarily innervate the lower abdominal wall. The extended course of the first three nerves through the abdominal wall within the layer between the transversus abdominis and the internal oblique muscles makes this the desired anatomic location for regional block. For ultrasound-guided transversus abdominis plane (TAP) block, the patient is usually in the supine position (Fig. 46.25). The transducer is placed between the iliac crest and costal margin in the midaxillary line. In this location, the muscle layers of the lateral abdominal wall (external oblique, internal oblique, and transversus abdominis) are well defined.

Injection is in the fascial layer that separates the internal oblique and the transversus abdominis muscles. Direct visualization and proximity to the nerves is not critical if 15 to 20 mL of dilute local anesthetic is injected in this layer. The needle approach is in-plane from the anterior side and directed toward the posterolateral corner of the transversus abdominis muscle. The respiratory motion of the peritoneal cavity and influence of muscle contraction makes general anesthesia an appealing option for performing this block. The transversus abdominis muscle is relatively thin; therefore careful placement of the needle tip is necessary.

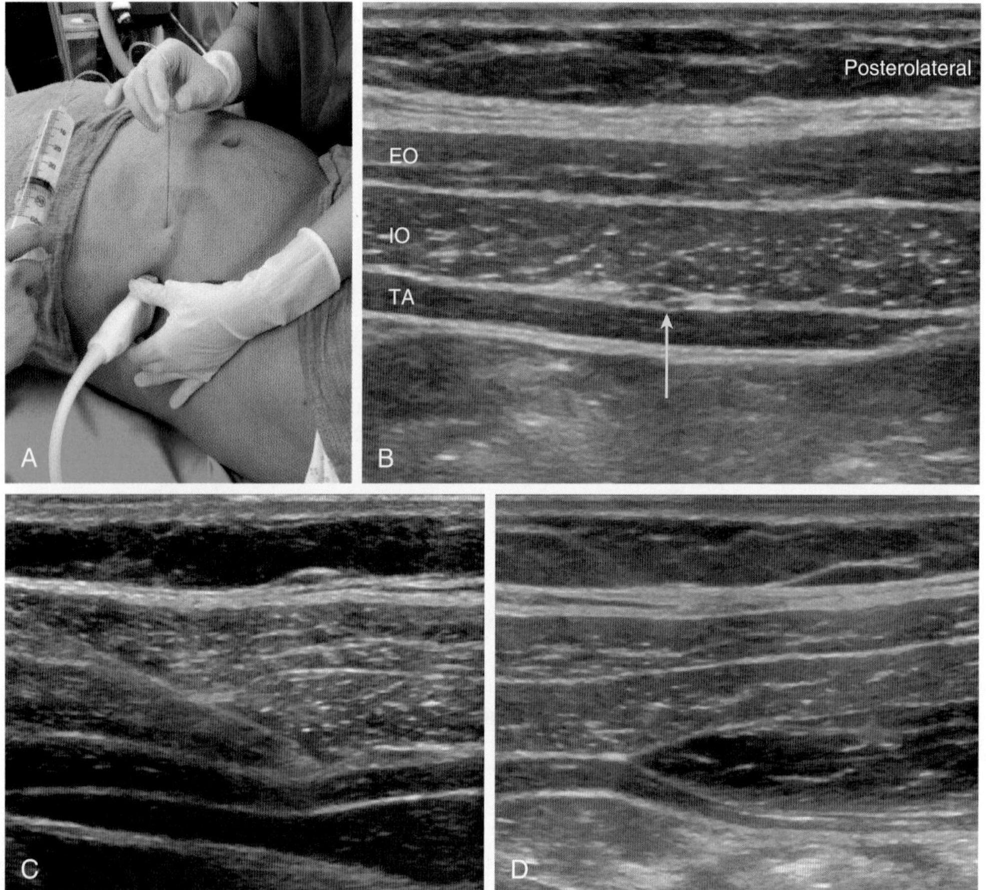

Fig. 46.25 Transversus abdominis plane (TAP) block with ultrasound guidance. (A) Abdominal wall image demonstrates the approach for TAP block. (B) In this sonogram the external oblique *(EO)*, internal oblique *(IO)*, and transversus abdominis *(TA)* muscles are identified (the three-layer-cake appearance). Nerves *(yellow arrow)* are seen entering the plane between the *IO* and *TA* muscles. (C) The needle approaches in-plane and is directed toward the posterolateral edge of the *TA* muscles. (D) The kayak sign demonstrates successful TAP injection. The fascia between the *IO* and *TA* muscles is split apart in the shape resembling a kayak.

ILIOINGUINAL AND ILIOHYPOGASTRIC NERVE BLOCKS

The ilioinguinal and iliohypogastric nerves arise from the first lumbar spinal root. They pierce the transversus abdominis muscle cephalad and medial to the anterior superior iliac spine to lie between the transversus abdominis and internal oblique muscles. After traveling a short distance caudally and medially, their ventral rami pierce the internal oblique muscle before giving off branches, which then pierce the external oblique and provide sensory fibers to the skin. The ilioinguinal nerve courses anteriorly and inferiorly to the inguinal ring, where it exits to supply the skin on the proximal, medial portion of the thigh. The iliohypogastric nerve supplies the skin of the inguinal region.

Indications

Ilioinguinal and iliohypogastric blocks are used for analgesia following inguinal hernia repair and for lower abdominal procedures utilizing a Pfannenstiel incision. These blocks have been shown to reduce pain associated with herniorrhaphy significantly, although they do not provide visceral analgesia, and they cannot be used as the sole anesthetic during surgery. Despite the relatively simple technique, a failure rate as frequent as 10% to 25% has been reported.

Landmark-Based Technique. These blocks can be performed using a loss-of-resistance technique. The local anesthetic should be injected between the transversus abdominis and the internal oblique and between the internal and external oblique muscles.

The anterior superior iliac spine is located and a mark is made 2 cm cephalad and 2 cm medial. A blunt needle is inserted perpendicular to the skin through a small puncture site. Increased resistance is noted as the needle passes into the external oblique muscle. A loss of resistance is then observed as the needle passes through the external oblique muscle to lie between it and the internal oblique muscle. After negative aspiration, 2 mL of local anesthetic is injected. The needle is then inserted further until another loss of resistance is noted as the needle passes out of the internal oblique to lie between it and the transversus abdominis muscle where another 2 mL of local anesthetic is injected. The needle is withdrawn, and the same procedure is repeated two more times in a fan-like distribution between the internal and external oblique and then between the internal oblique and the transversus abdominis muscles. Typically, a total volume of approximately 12 mL of local anesthetic is used.

It is often difficult to appreciate the loss of resistance. Given the potential complications of advancing the needle too far, ultrasound guidance is often used for these

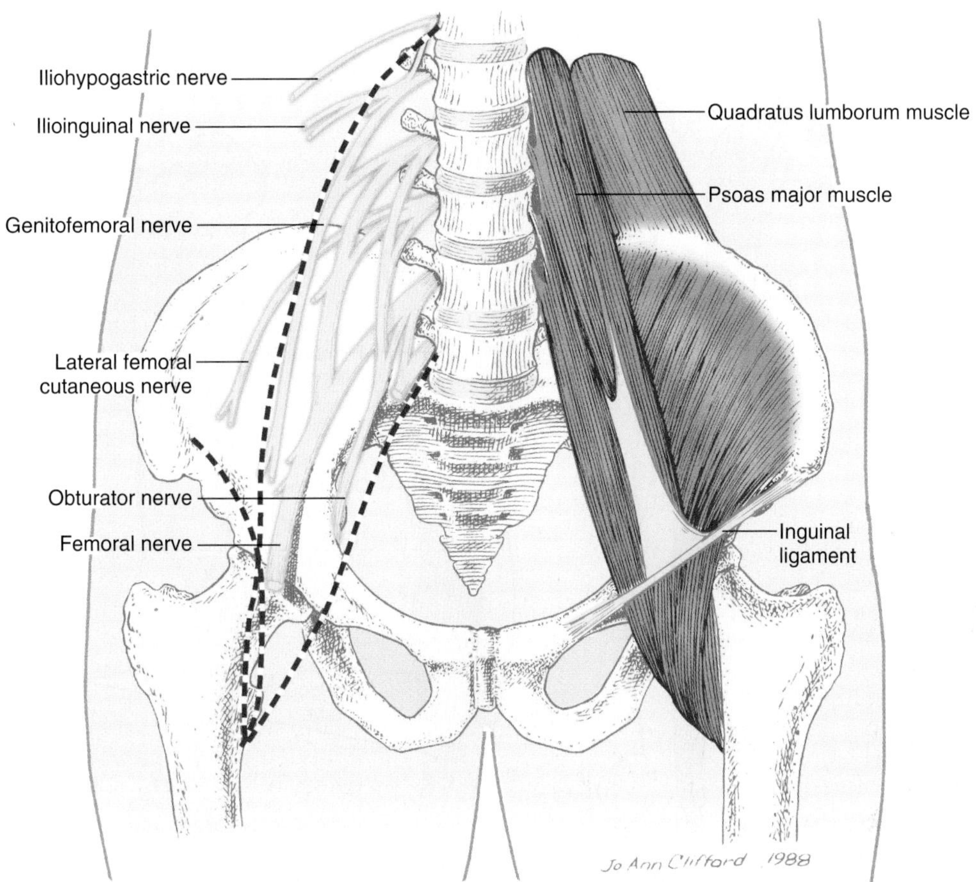

Fig. 46.26 The lumbar plexus lies in the psoas compartment between the psoas major and quadratus lumborum muscles.

blocks.[64,65] The ilioinguinal and iliohypogastric nerves cannot be selectively blocked, even if injection volumes of less than 1 mL are used.[66]

Side Effects and Complications

Blind injection can result in inadvertent injury to the intestine or blood vessels with perforation of the large and small bowel and pelvic hematoma. Lower extremity weakness owing to local anesthetic spread and subsequent femoral nerve blockade can also occur.[66]

Lower Extremity Blocks

LOWER EXTREMITY ANATOMY

The nerve supply to the lower extremity is derived from the lumbar and sacral plexuses. The lumbar plexus is formed by the anterior rami of the first four lumbar nerves, frequently including a branch from T12 and occasionally from L5 (Fig. 46.26). The plexus lies between the psoas major and quadratus lumborum muscles in the psoas compartment. The lower components of the plexus, L2, L3, and L4, primarily innervate the anterior and medial thigh. The anterior divisions of L2, L3, and L4 form the obturator nerve; the posterior divisions of the same components form the femoral nerve; and the lateral femoral cutaneous nerve is formed from posterior divisions of L2 and L3.

The sacral plexus gives off two nerves that are important for lower extremity surgery: the posterior cutaneous nerve of the thigh and the sciatic nerve. The posterior cutaneous nerve of the thigh and the sciatic nerve are derived from the first, second, and third sacral nerves plus branches from the anterior rami of L4 and L5, respectively. These nerves pass through the pelvis together and are blocked by the same technique. The sciatic nerve is a combination of two major nerve trunks, the tibial (i.e., ventral branches of the anterior rami of L4, L5, S1, S2, and S3) and the common peroneal (i.e., dorsal branches of the anterior rami of L4, L5, S1, S2, and S3), which form the sciatic nerve. The trunks separate at or above the popliteal fossa, with the tibial nerve passing medially and the common peroneal laterally. The cutaneous distributions of the lumbosacral and peripheral nerves are shown in Fig. 46.27.

FEMORAL NERVE BLOCKS

The advantages of using ultrasound to guide femoral nerve block include a more complete block, local anesthetic volume sparing, and fewer side effects such as vascular punctures. The femoral nerve usually lies lateral to the femoral artery in the groove formed by the iliacus and psoas muscles. The nerve can be oval or triangular in cross-sectional shape with an anteroposterior diameter of approximately 3 mm and a mediolateral diameter of 10 mm. The best depiction of the femoral nerve is from 10 cm proximal to 5 cm distal to the inguinal ligament. According to the pelvic

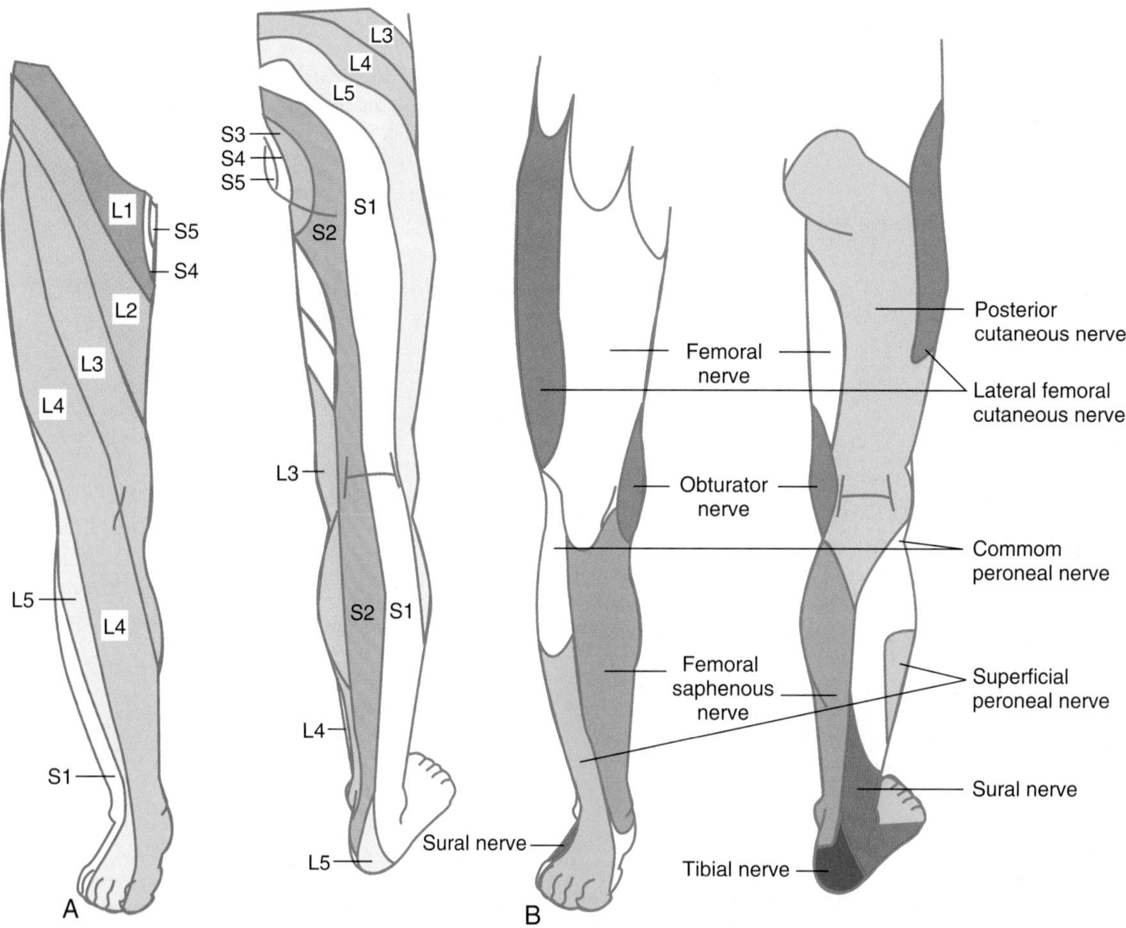

Fig. 46.27 (A) Cutaneous distribution of the lumbosacral nerves. (B) Cutaneous distribution of the peripheral nerves of the lower extremity.

inclination, some tilting of the ultrasound probe is necessary for the sound beam to meet the nerve perpendicularly for optimal scanning. In addition, the femoral nerve has a slight medial-to-lateral course; therefore some rotation of the probe is also necessary for the best view of the nerve. Because the femoral nerve is covered by echobright adipose tissue and fascia, the echogenic outer sheath of the nerve is difficult to establish. In some patients, the psoas tendon can appear similar to the femoral nerve. However, the psoas tendon lies deep within the muscle. If the profunda femoris artery (i.e., the deep branch of the femoral artery) is visualized, then the transducer is usually too distal for complete femoral nerve block. The femoral nerve is often identified as a slight indentation in the surface of the iliacus and psoas muscles.

For femoral nerve block, a broad (35-50 mm footprint) linear transducer is used (Fig. 46.28). Both in-plane (from lateral to medial) and out-of-plane (from distal to proximal) approaches can be used. The advantage of the in-plane approach is visualization of the approaching needle. The disadvantages are the longer needle path and a tendency of the needle to skim over the fascia iliaca by deforming it rather than puncturing it. The out-of-plane approach is often used for catheter placement.

For either approach, the needle tip is positioned between the fascia iliaca and the iliopsoas muscle near the lateral corner of the femoral nerve to avoid the femoral vessels, similar to the method for fascia iliaca block. The fascia iliaca has a characteristic mediolateral slant. The desired distribution is local anesthetic layering under or completely around the femoral nerve. When layering of local anesthetic is restricted over the nerve, the concern is that the fascia iliaca is intact and that block failure will result. In the obese patient, femoral nerve imaging is challenging and ultrasound can therefore be combined with nerve stimulation for successful block in these patients. After successful injection of a local anesthetic, distal branches of the femoral nerve can be appreciated by sliding the transducer along the known course of the nerve.

Fascia Iliaca (Modified Femoral Nerve) Blocks

Technique. The fascia iliaca block was originally described in children and involved detection of a double pop sensation as the needle traverses the fascia lata and fascia iliaca of the thigh (see also Chapter 77).[67] Penetration of both layers of fascia is important for block success. To facilitate the appreciation of the "clicks" or "pops," the use of a short-bevel or bullet-tipped needle has been advocated to provide more tactile feedback than with cutting needles.

Because the fascia iliaca invests the iliopsoas muscle and femoral nerve, high volumes of dilute long-acting local anesthetic can be injected to block nerves of the lumbar plexus via this anterior approach. The clinical applications for fascia iliaca block are similar as those for femoral nerve block.[68]

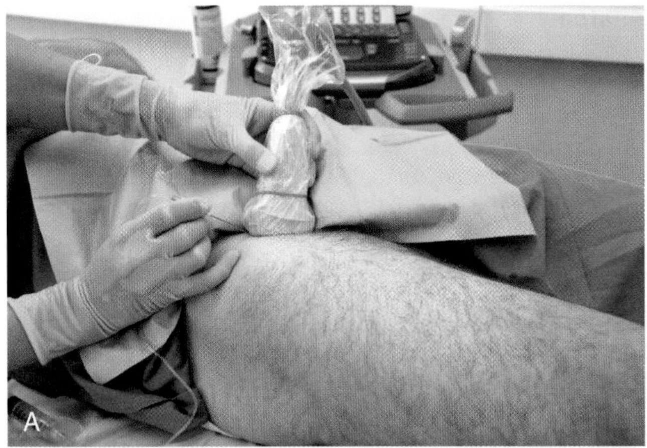

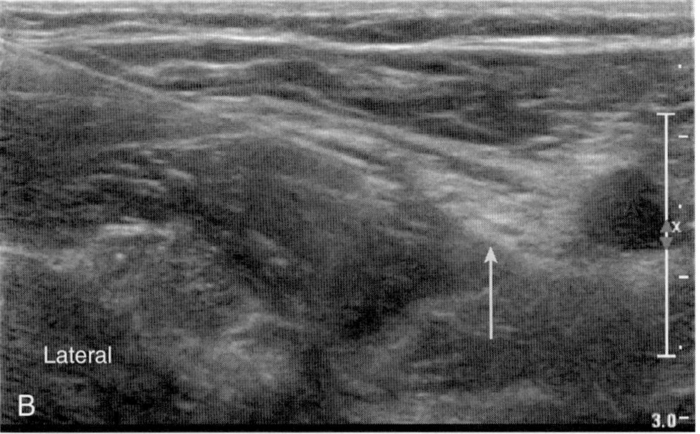

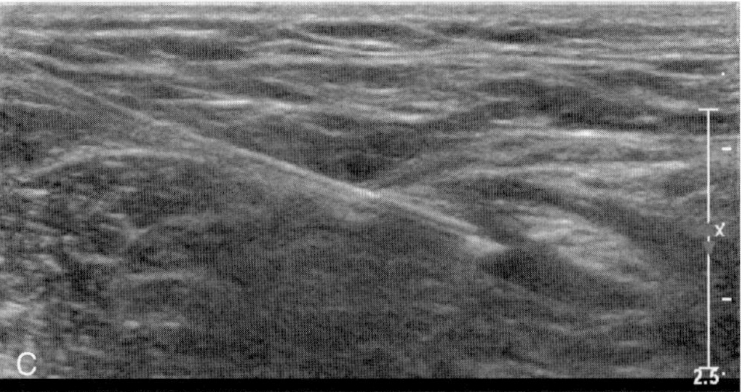

Fig. 46.28 Femoral nerve block with ultrasound imaging (in-plane approach). (A) External photograph shows the setup for femoral nerve block. (B) The needle tip is in position before injecting adjacent to the femoral nerve *(yellow arrow)*. The femoral nerve lies lateral to the femoral artery (A). (C) Local anesthetic surrounds the femoral nerve after injection. (Modified from Gray AT. *Atlas of Ultrasound-Guided Regional Anesthesia*. 3rd ed. Philadelphia: Saunders; 2018.)

The needle entry site for the fascia iliaca block is determined by drawing a line between the pubic tubercle and the anterior superior iliac spine and dividing this line into thirds. The needle entry point is 1 cm caudal to the intersection of the medial two thirds and lateral one third along this line. This site is well away from the femoral artery, which is useful for patients in whom femoral artery puncture is contraindicated. Ultrasound can also be used to visualize the two fascial layers and monitor the spread of local anesthetic beneath the fascia iliaca.[69,70]

Side Effects and Complications. Intravascular injection and hematoma are possible because of the proximity of the femoral artery. Anatomically, the femoral nerve and artery are located in separate sheaths approximately 1 cm apart. In most patients with normal anatomy, the femoral artery can be easily palpated, allowing correct, safe needle positioning lateral to the pulsation. The presence of femoral vascular grafts is a relative contraindication to these techniques, but these grafts are easily identified with ultrasound imaging in most cases. Because the injection is made between the femoral and lateral femoral cutaneous nerves, nerve damage is rare.

SAPHENOUS NERVE BLOCKS ABOVE THE KNEE (INCLUDING ADDUCTOR CANAL BLOCK)

Indications

Several approaches to the saphenous nerve block have been described using an above-the-knee approach. When used in combination with multimodal analgesia, a saphenous nerve block at or near the mid-thigh can be as effective or in some studies preferable to a femoral nerve block following knee surgery because of reduced rates of quadriceps weakness.[71-73] The correct "adductor canal block" location is a source of active debate even though the putative anatomic targets may be separated by mere inches. The "true" adductor canal block may best be determined with ultrasound by identifying the medial border of the sartorius muscle converging with the medial border of the adductor longus muscle.[74] A double contour is appreciated on the roof of the canal, which denotes the vastoadductor membrane. This anatomic distinction holds importance as the nerve to the vastus medialis often lies outside the adductor canal in a distinct fascial sheath. Hence a too distal adductor canal block within the "true" adductor canal may miss the nerve to the vastus medialis, a major contributor to knee joint pain following total knee arthroplasty. Jaeger and colleagues advocate for a periarterial injection of local anesthesia lateral to the femoral artery under the sartorius muscle deep to the vastoadductor membrane midway between the anterior superior iliac spine and the patella where local anesthetic is likely to bathe both the saphenous nerve and the nerve to the vastus medialis.[71]

Anatomy

As the saphenous nerve is a terminal sensory branch of the femoral nerve above the knee, it supplies innervation to the infrapatellar branches to the knee joint. It pierces the fascia lata between the tendons of the sartorius and gracilis muscles before it runs in the adductor canal along the posterior border of the sartorius muscle. The nerve emerges and divides at the level of the knee before continuing distally along the medial border of the lower leg.

Technique

Adductor canal block is performed in the supine position with thigh positioned in slight external rotation with leg extended to expose the inner thigh. Ultrasound guidance is the preferred neurolocalization technique, although nerve stimulation would also be an option or both used in combination.

Ultrasound-Guided Technique. A high-frequency linear transducer (15-6 MHz) probe is positioned transverse on the anteromedial thigh, which is scanned in short-axis beginning at the junction between the middle and distal thirds of the thigh. The thick vastoadductor membrane

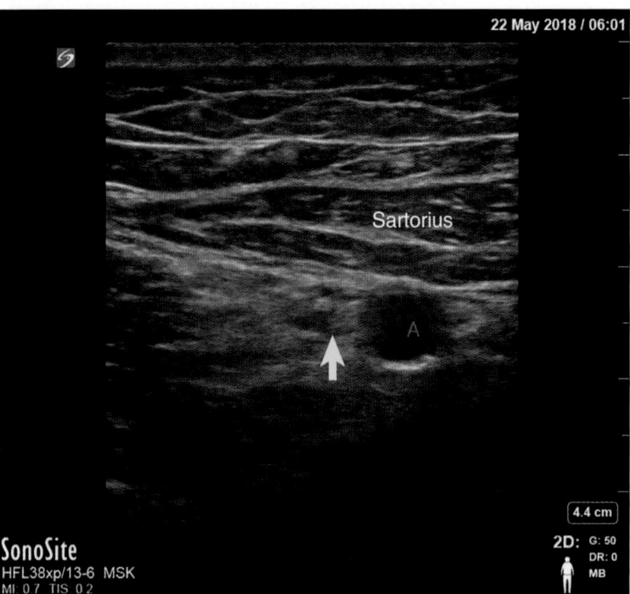

Fig. 46.29 Proximal saphenous nerve block (adductor canal block). Sonographically, the adductor canal block may best be determined by identifying the converging borders between the vastus medialis muscle (lateral), sartorius muscle (anterior), and femoral artery (most medial). Periarterial deposit of local anesthesia is desired lateral to the femoral artery midway between the anterior superior iliac spine and the patella.

defines the border between vastus medialis muscle (lateral), sartorius muscle (anterior), and femoral artery (most medial) (Fig. 46.29). A 22-gauge, 5-cm needle is most often selected with 2- to 3-cm depths to the target. Through an in-plane approach approximately 10 to 15 mL of local anesthetic (higher volumes may result in quadriceps paresis)[75] is injected lateral to the artery, deep to the sartorius muscle.

Side Effects and Complications

The risks of complications with this block are low, although the same theoretical risks with all regional anesthetic techniques apply to this block. Vascular injury leading to arterial pseudoaneurysm is possible. Intramuscular spread of local anesthetic should be avoided as cases of myonecrosis have been reported[76] and unexpected thigh weakness should prompt evaluation. Although adductor canal block is considered among the more selective "muscle-sparing" peripheral blocks of the lower extremity, caution is still advised and fall prevention strategies are important, including patient education on avoidance of unsupported ambulation.[77]

SAPHENOUS NERVE BLOCKS BELOW THE KNEE

Indications

The saphenous nerve provides innervation to the medial aspect of the lower extremity from the knee to the medial malleolus. Saphenous nerve blocks are commonly combined with popliteal and ankle blockade. Several approaches to the saphenous nerve block have been described, including a paravenous (below the knee) approach. Ultrasound guidance can be used for this technique. The saphenous nerve can be blocked at the level of the ankle and can be combined with other injections for ankle block.

Anatomy

The saphenous nerve emerges from the adductor canal hiatus and divides at the level of the knee before continuing distally along the medial border of the tibia, posterior to the great saphenous vein. The saphenous nerve is located approximately 1 cm medial and 1 cm posterior to the saphenous vein at the level of the tibial tuberosity.

Technique

The saphenous nerve at this point is purely sensory; therefore a field block technique is possible and likely equally effective to nerve stimulation. Ultrasound guidance has gained significant popularity as a tool to identify the neural and vascular structures that lie in close proximity to the saphenous nerve.

Paravenous Approach. At the level of the tibial tuberosity, approximately 5 to 10 mL of local anesthetic is infiltrated deep to the great saphenous vein.

Localized Field Block. Approximately 5 to 10 mL of local anesthetic may be infiltrated from the medial condyle of the tibia anteriorly to the tibial tuberosity and posteriorly to the medial head of the gastrocnemius muscle. Success rates for this technique range from 33% to 65%.

Side Effects and Complications

The risks of complications with this block are low, although the same risk pattern for all regional anesthetic techniques apply to this block; that is, nerve or tissue damage and vascular puncture with hematoma formation. Given that the great saphenous vein is used as a landmark for the field block technique, minor hematoma formation is not uncommon.

SCIATIC NERVE BLOCKS IN THE POPLITEAL FOSSA

The sciatic nerve can be blocked anywhere along its course from the gluteal region to the popliteal fossa.[78-80] Many approaches have been described, including those from the anterior aspect of the thigh.[81] One of the most common approaches is to block the sciatic nerve in the popliteal fossa using a lateral approach in supine position with the leg elevated.[82] In this anatomic location, the block can be performed close to the skin surface. The division of the sciatic nerve provides a broad target with large surface area to promote clinical block characteristics. For this technique, the needle tip is positioned between the tibial and common peroneal components of the sciatic nerve near the division so that a single injection distributes to both nerves (Fig. 46.30). By sliding the transducer along the known course of the sciatic nerve, its characteristic division in the popliteal fossa can be identified. This method of sliding assessment is also important to verify the local anesthetic distribution after injection. The tibial nerve has a straighter course than the common peroneal nerve and has approximately twice the cross-sectional area. The tibial nerve lies posterior to the popliteal artery and vein at the popliteal crease, and this location can be a useful starting point when imaging is difficult. When the foot is moved, the nerves of the popliteal fossa have characteristic motions that can be helpful for nerve identification in some patients. The advantages of this

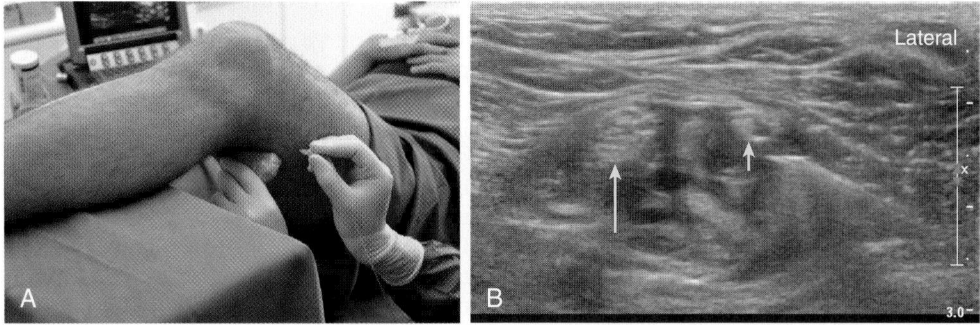

Fig. 46.30 Popliteal block with ultrasound imaging (in-plane approach). (A) External photograph shows the setup for popliteal nerve block in the supine position. The leg is elevated, and the transducer is applied to the posterior surface of the leg. (B) The needle approaches the bifurcation of the sciatic nerve in the plane of imaging from the lateral aspect of the leg. The needle tip is positioned between the tibial *(long yellow arrow)* and common peroneal *(short yellow arrow)* nerves.

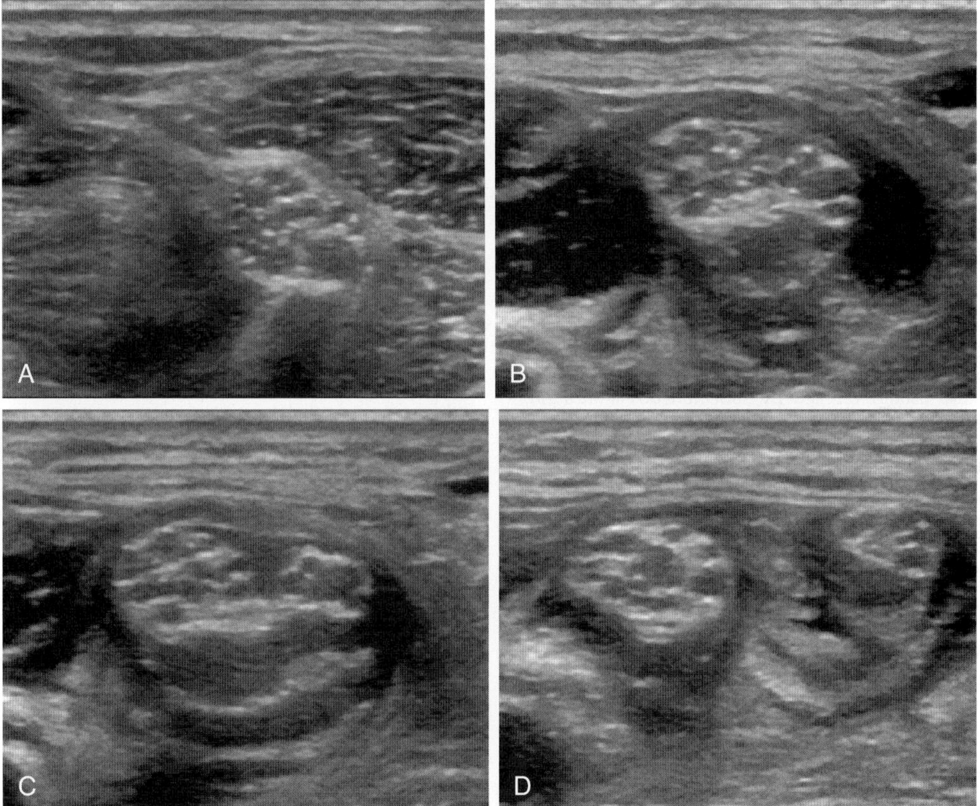

Fig. 46.31 Sciatic nerve imaging in the popliteal fossa before (A), during (B and C), and after (D) division into the tibial and common peroneal nerves. Local anesthetic tracks with both individual nerves, thereby confirming a successful block.

approach are the convenient position, the transducer position is remote from the site of needle entry, and the parallel in-plane approach of the block needle results in optimal needle tip visibility. After injection, following the local anesthetic distribution around and along the nerve path (Fig. 46.31) is relatively easy.

ALTERNATIVE APPROACHES TO SCIATIC NERVE BLOCK

The sciatic nerve can be blocked anywhere along its course. However, approaches proximal to the popliteal fossa are usually more difficult because the nerve lies deeper from the skin surface. The sciatic nerve is a mobile structure with position and orientation varying with extremity motion.[83,84] Because of the depth and variation in position, ultrasound guidance is useful for proximal sciatic nerve blocks in both adults and children.[85]

For procedures above the knee, the parasacral sciatic nerve block can provide an advantage over more distal approaches because the block of both the sciatic and posterior femoral cutaneous nerves is possible.[86-89] Alternatively, the posterior femoral cutaneous nerve can be blocked separately using ultrasound guidance.[90] The subgluteal approach to sciatic nerve block is useful when block of the hamstring muscles is indicated.[91] The anterior approach to sciatic nerve block is useful when the patient cannot be positioned for other approaches due to pain or leg traction.[92-94] These proximal approaches to sciatic nerve block may require multiple injections for rapid onset.[91] The

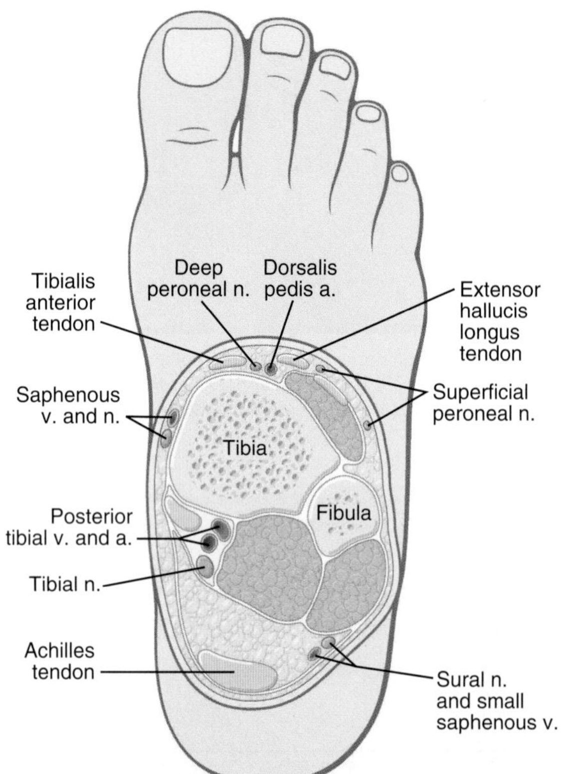

Fig. 46.32 Cross-sectional anatomy for an ankle block. An ankle block is performed by injecting local anesthetic solution at five separate nerve locations. The superficial peroneal nerve, sural nerve, and saphenous nerve are usually blocked by subcutaneous infiltration because they may have already branched as they cross the ankle joint. The tibial and deep peroneal nerves require deeper injection adjacent to the accompanying blood vessels (the posterior tibial and anterior tibial arteries, respectively). Because the block needle approaches the ankle from many angles, it is convenient to elevate the foot by supporting the calf. (Modified from Brown DL, Factor DA, eds. *Regional Anesthesia and Analgesia*. Philadelphia: WB Saunders; 1996.)

blood supply of the sciatic nerve in the gluteal region can be detected with ultrasound imaging, and this can help with nerve localization in some patients.[95]

NERVE BLOCKS AT THE ANKLE

Ankle blocks are relatively simple to perform and offer adequate anesthesia for surgical procedures of the foot. These blocks are traditionally performed at the level of the malleoli and guided by surface landmarks.

Four of the five individual nerves that can be blocked at the ankle to provide anesthesia of the foot are terminal branches of the sciatic nerve: the tibial, sural, superficial peroneal, and deep peroneal branches (Fig. 46.32). The sciatic nerve divides at or above the apex of the popliteal fossa to form the common peroneal and tibial nerves. The common peroneal nerve descends laterally around the neck of the fibula, where it divides into the superficial and deep peroneal nerves. The sural nerve forms in the leg from both tibial and common peroneal nerve contributions.

The saphenous nerve is the major descending sensory branch of the femoral nerve. The territory of this nerve is the medial leg and can extend as far as the base of the great toe and is included as part of the ankle block.[96]

Tibial Nerve Technique

The tibial nerve can be blocked with the patient in either the prone or the supine positions. The posterior tibial artery is palpated, and a 25-gauge, 3-cm needle is inserted posterolateral to the artery at the level of the medial malleolus (Fig. 46.33A and B). A paresthesia is often elicited; however, it is not necessary for a successful block. If a paresthesia is obtained, 3 to 5 mL of local anesthetic should be injected. Otherwise, 7 to 10 mL of local anesthetic should be injected as the needle is slowly withdrawn from the posterior aspect of the tibia. Blockade of the tibial nerve provides anesthesia of the heel, plantar portion of the toes, and the sole of the foot, as well as some motor branches in the same area. Ultrasound imaging of the tibial nerve can shorten onset time (Fig. 46.34).[97]

Sural Nerve Technique. The sural nerve is located superficially between the lateral malleolus and the Achilles tendon. A 25-gauge, 3-cm needle is inserted lateral to the tendon and is directed toward the malleolus as 5 to 10 mL of solution is injected subcutaneously (see Figs. 46.33 and 46.35). This block provides anesthesia of the lateral foot and the lateral aspects of the proximal sole of the foot.

Deep Peroneal, Superficial Peroneal, and Saphenous Nerve Techniques. The deep peroneal, superficial peroneal, and saphenous nerves can be blocked through a single needle entry site (see Fig. 46.35). A line is drawn across the dorsum of the foot connecting the malleoli. The extensor hallucis longus tendon is identified by having the patient dorsiflex the big toe. The anterior tibial artery lies between this structure and the tendon of the extensor digitorum longus muscle and is palpable at this level. A skin wheal is raised just lateral to the arterial pulsation between the two tendons on the intermalleolar line. A 25-gauge, 3-cm needle is advanced perpendicular to the skin entry site, and 3 to 5 mL of local anesthetic is injected deep to the extensor retinaculum to block the deep peroneal nerve. This technique anesthetizes the skin between the first and second toes and the short extensors of the toes.

The needle is directed laterally through the same skin wheal while injecting 3 to 5 mL of local anesthetic subcutaneously, blocking the superficial peroneal nerve and resulting in anesthesia of the dorsum of the foot, excluding the first interdigital cleft. The same maneuver can be performed in the medial direction, thereby anesthetizing the saphenous nerve, a terminal branch of the femoral nerve that supplies a strip along the medial aspect of the foot.

Side Effects and Complications

Multiple injections are required for this procedure, which can result in discomfort for the patient. Persistent paresthesias can occur, but they are generally self-limited. The presence of edema or induration in the area of the ankle block can make palpation of landmarks difficult. When this pathology is present, a more proximal block is usually performed (e.g., popliteal and saphenous nerves blocks in the distal thigh). Intravascular injection is possible but unlikely if aspiration for blood is negative.

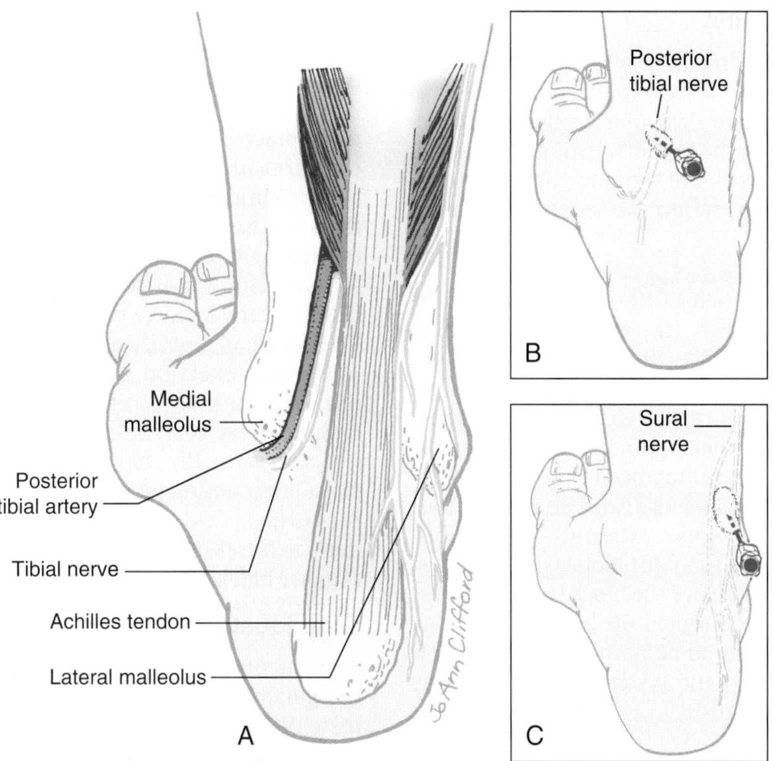

Fig. 46.33 (A) Anatomic landmarks for a block of the posterior tibial and sural nerves at the ankle. (B) Posterior tibial nerve and method of needle placement for a block at the ankle. (C) Sural nerve and method of needle placement for a block at the ankle.

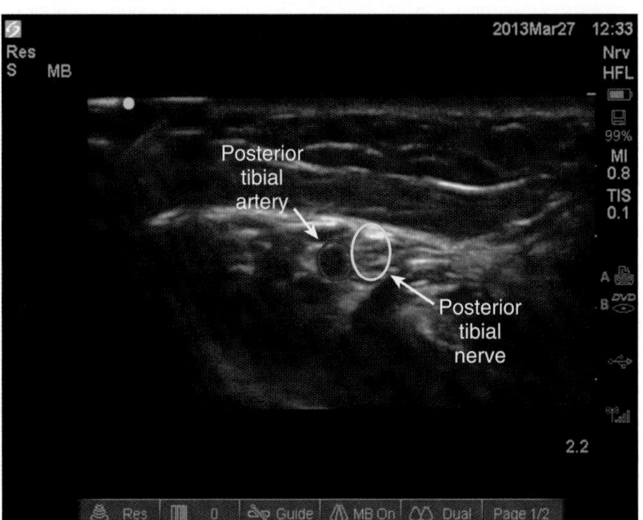

Fig. 46.34 Ultrasound image of the medial aspect of the ankle showing the posterior tibial artery *(red)* and the posterior tibial nerve *(yellow)*.

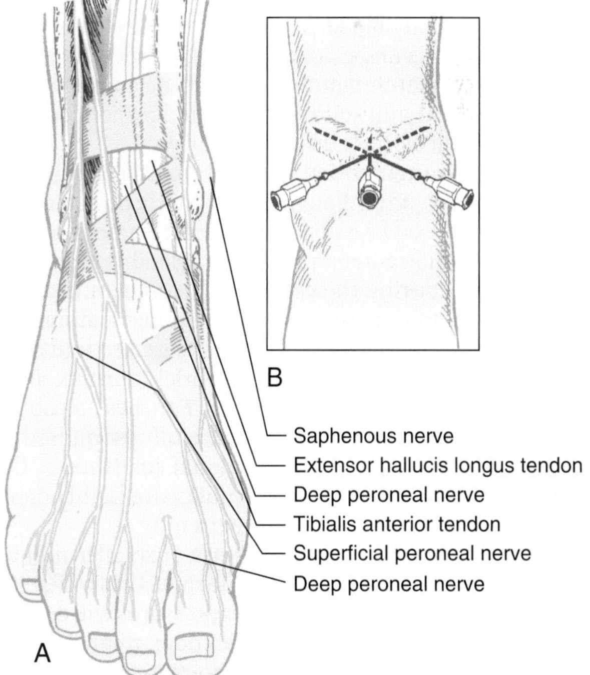

Fig. 46.35 (A) Anatomic landmarks for a block of the deep peroneal, superficial peroneal, and saphenous nerves at the ankle. (B) Method of needle placement for a block of the deep peroneal, superficial peroneal, and saphenous nerves through a single needle entry site.

INTRAVENOUS REGIONAL ANESTHESIA (OR BIER BLOCK)

Introduction and Clinical Applications

Intravenous regional blocks were first described in 1908 by the German surgeon, August Bier. The Bier block has multiple advantages, including ease of administration, rapid onset and recovery, muscular relaxation, and controllable duration of anesthesia. It is an excellent technique for short (<60 minutes) surgical procedures. Bier blocks are also used in the management of complex regional pain syndromes (for further details on intravenous regional analgesia in pain syndromes, see Chapter 51). Most commonly IVRA is used for upper extremity procedures such as excision of soft tissue masses or carpal tunnel release. Lower extremity blocks are also possible.

Technique (Upper Extremity)

With this technique blood is replaced with local anesthetic using a tourniquet to isolate the extremity from the central circulation. The duration of surgical anesthesia and analgesia for Bier block is essentially the time of tourniquet inflation. Contraindications to Bier block are the same as contraindications to tourniquet placement (limb ischemia, infection).

Prerequisites

Place a thin intravenous catheter (20 or 22 gauge) in the operative extremity (to reduce the amount of bleeding when the catheter is removed). Use only a minimal amount of dressing to secure the catheter. The intravenous catheter is usually placed distal or near the surgical site (although it is not clear if this influences block quality). If intravenous access is difficult, the procedure may need to be aborted.

Importantly, the patient should also have an intravenous cannula in the nonoperative upper extremity for administration of fluids and other drugs. If antibiotics are indicated they should be administered before the block (to allow these drugs to effectively reach the surgical site before tourniquet inflation). Lipid emulsion should be immediately available in the event that local anesthetic systemic toxicity occurs (see Chapter 29 for more details).

Extremity Exsanguination and Tourniquet Inflation

Raise the extremity above the level of the heart prior to exsanguination with an Esmarch bandage. This will passively drain venous blood from the extremity over one to two minutes (this can be done during the timeout). Stretch and wrap an Esmarch bandage around the extremity from distal to proximal in a spiral overlapping fashion, continuing until the cuff of the tourniquet is covered.

Following exsanguination with an Esmarch bandage, the tourniquet is typically inflated to 250 mm Hg or 100 mm Hg above systolic blood pressure. Therefore it is important that the patient be normotensive (systolic blood pressure 150 mm Hg or less) during the period of tourniquet inflation. If necessary, sedation or antihypertensive medications may be given. Another alternative is to increase the tourniquet inflation pressure to 275 mm Hg for brief tourniquet runs (usually <60 minutes for Bier blocks). For these reasons, it is important that blood pressure be carefully monitored and controlled during intravenous regional anesthesia. Both the surgical conditions and block quality are highly dependent on the exsanguination of the extremity.

Use of a single, wide cuff allows use of smaller inflation pressures during intravenous regional anesthesia. The postulated advantage is that the smaller pressures will decrease the incidence of neurologic complications related to high inflation pressures with the narrow double cuffs.[98]

Preservative free 2-chloroprocaine 0.5%, lidocaine 0.5%, or prilocaine 0.5% can be used for intravenous regional anesthesia (plain solution, without epinephrine).[99-101] For upper extremity anesthesia, an arm (about 0.6 mL/kg, maximum 50 mL) or forearm (about 0.4 mL/kg, maximum 25 mL) tourniquet can be used, depending on the surgical site.[102] Bupivacaine is not recommended for intravenous regional anesthesia because cases of severe local anesthetic toxicity have been reported.[103] However, dilute solutions of long-acting amides (0.125% levobupivacaine or 0.2% ropivacaine) have successfully been used to prolong sensory block and analgesia after tourniquet deflation.[104-106]

An additional temporary tourniquet (used for intravenous placement) can be placed immediately proximal to the surgical site while the first 10 or 20 mL of local anesthetic is injected via the catheter (the second tourniquet is then released). This will confine local anesthetic to the distal extremity and promote block onset.[107,108] Inject slowly so that venous pressures remain low. If the injection is at a distal site the leakage under the tourniquet will be reduced. The onset of anesthesia is usually within 5 to 10 minutes. After injection, the intravenous catheter is typically removed (although repeat injections using an indwelling catheter have been described).

Because the Bier block does not result in prolonged analgesia, long-acting local anesthetic should be infiltrated into the surgical field prior to tourniquet deflation. In this manner the onset of infiltrative analgesia matches the offset of the Bier block.

Tourniquet Deflation

The tourniquet can be safely released after 25 minutes, but the patient should be closely observed for local anesthetic toxicity for several minutes after the tourniquet release. Shorter tourniquet times (<25 minutes) are possible with 2-chloroprocaine because this local anesthetic is rapidly degraded by plasma esterases when blood re-enters the extremity upon tourniquet deflation. Rare cases of systemic toxicity from 2-chloroprocaine have been reported in patients with atypical esterases.[109]

Systemic plasma levels of local anesthetic will increase with venous return from the extremity following tourniquet deflation. This occurs when the tourniquet inflation pressure is less than venous levels (nearly 0 mm Hg). Cyclic deflation of the tourniquet at 10-second intervals for two or three cycles increases the time to peak arterial lidocaine levels, which may decrease potential toxicity.[110] It is recommended to not raise the extremity immediately after the tourniquet is removed, as this will promote venous return containing local anesthetic. Reinflate the tourniquet if any signs of systemic toxicity occur.

Comments

Double-Cuff Tourniquets. A double-cuff tourniquet can be used instead of a single-cuff tourniquet to extend the tourniquet tolerance time (Fig. 46.36). Both adjacent cuffs should have secure closures and reliable pressure gauges. After exsanguination of the arm, the proximal cuff is inflated to approximately 100 mm Hg greater than the systolic pressure, and absence of a radial pulse confirms adequate tourniquet pressure. When the patient complains of tourniquet pain, the distal tourniquet, which overlies anesthetized skin, is inflated, and the proximal tourniquet is released. However, if a long tourniquet time is anticipated it is usually best to choose other peripheral nerve block or provide a general anesthesia.

Additives and Adjuncts. Additives and adjuncts should be used with caution because prolonged exposure of these compounds to the venous endothelium during tourniquet

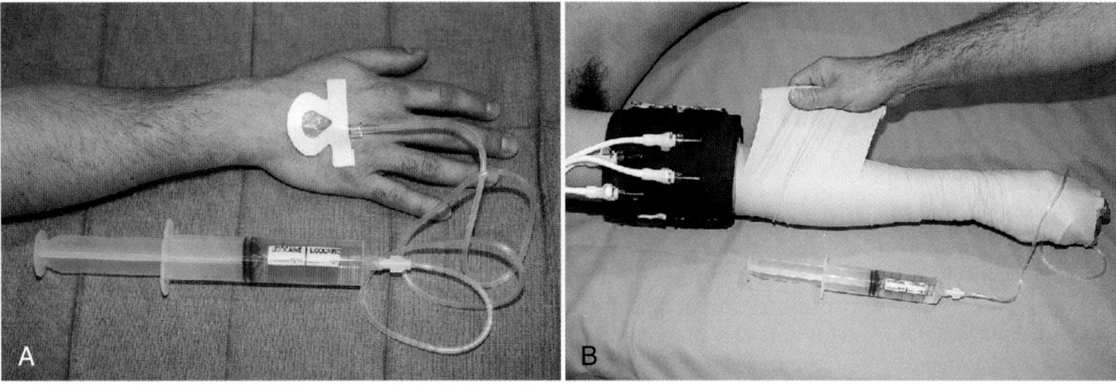

Fig. 46.36 (A) Placement and securing of a small intravenous catheter. (B) Exsanguination of the arm with an Esmarch bandage before inflation of the tourniquet and injection of the local anesthetic solution through the catheter. In this figure a double-cuff tourniquet is shown.

inflation may result in phlebitis (even if the compounds are considered safe for routine intravenous use).

Complications

Technical problems with this block include tourniquet discomfort, rapid resolution leading to postoperative pain, difficulty in providing a bloodless field, and the necessity of exsanguination in the case of a painful injury. Accidental or early deflation of the tourniquet or use of excessive doses of local anesthetics can result in systemic toxicity. Injection of the drug as distally as possible at a slow rate decreases blood levels and theoretically may increase safety. Nerve injury and compartment syndrome have been reported with long tourniquet times and high tourniquet inflation pressures. Hypertonic solutions can cause compartment syndrome and should never be used for intravenous regional anesthesia.[111]

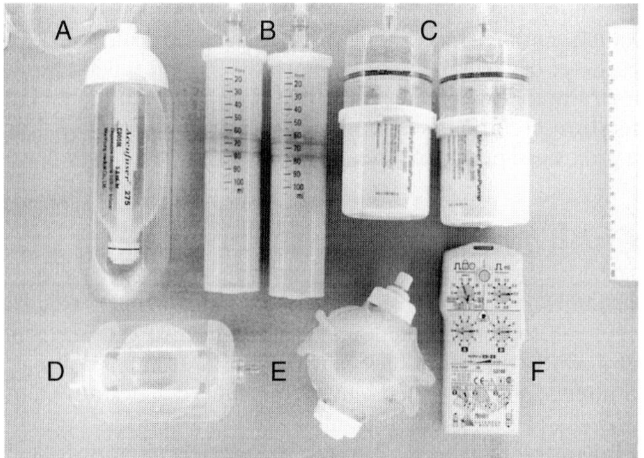

Fig. 46.37 Portable infusion pumps. (A) Accufuser (McKinley Medical, Wheat Ridge, Colo.). (B) Sgarlato (Sgarlato Labs, Los Gatos, Calif.). (C) Stryker PainPump (Stryker Instruments, Kalamazoo, Mich.). (D) MedFlo II (MPS Acacia, Brea, Calif.). (E) C-Bloc (I-Flow, Lake Forest, Calif.). (F) Microject PCA (Sorenson Medical, West Jordan, Utah). (From Ilfeld BM, Morey TE, Enneking FK. The delivery rate accuracy of portable infusion pumps used for continuous regional analgesia. *Anesth Analg*. 2002;95:1331–1336.)

Continuous Catheter Techniques

The advantages cited for continuous nerve blockade include prolongation of surgical anesthesia, decreased risk of systemic toxicity because of lower incremental doses, postoperative pain relief, and sympathectomy. Catheter placement using over-needle and through-needle methods have been described. Advances in equipment technology, including the development of stimulating needles and catheters and portable pumps allowing local anesthetic infusion after hospital dismissal, have increased the success rate and popularity of continuous peripheral blockade (Fig. 46.37). Although concern regarding accurate catheter placement and maintenance still exists, the use of stimulating catheters and radiographic confirmation may further improve the functionality. Ultrasound guidance appears to produce more consistent times for catheter placement.[112] Overall, continuous peripheral nerve block provides superior analgesia compared with conventional opioid therapy. Minor technical problems such as catheter kinking, displacement or leakage, and bacterial colonization are frequent, with no adverse clinical consequences in the large majority of cases. Major neurologic and infectious adverse events are rare.

Methods of providing continuous brachial plexus anesthesia have been described since the 1940s. These methods frequently offer ingenious solutions for the placing and securing of the needle or catheter. This technique is especially applicable to patients with upper extremity or digit replantation, total shoulder or elbow arthroplasty, or reflex sympathetic dystrophies, for which prolonged pain relief and sympathectomy are advantageous.

Continuous lower extremity techniques were also described decades ago, but until recently have remained underused compared with continuous upper extremity and neuraxial approaches. Reliable, improved success rates and the risk of spinal hematoma after neuraxial techniques led clinicians to reconsider continuous lower extremity blocks. Contemporary applications for continuous psoas compartment, sciatic, femoral, adductor canal, and popliteal fossa blockade have been reported. Compared with conventional systemic and neuraxial analgesic methods, continuous lower extremity blocks provide superior analgesia with fewer side effects, improve perioperative outcomes, and accelerate hospital dismissal after major joint replacement.

TESTING THE CATHETER

Test injections of saline, local anesthetic, or air with real-time ultrasound imaging can be used to assess catheter tip function. The overall success rate of peripheral nerve catheter placement with ultrasound guidance is high, so the additional value of these subsequent tests is still being established.[113,114]

SECURING THE CATHETER

Catheter migration and dislodgement are clinically relevant issues. Catheter threading distances do not seem to correlate with the chance of dislodgement.[115] Excessively large threading distances (>5 cm) may result in catheter knotting. If ultrasound guidance is used for catheter placement, sterile dry gauze can be used to remove excess gel prior to securing the catheter. Skin adhesive applied to the catheter at the skin exit site may reduce catheter dislodgment, fluid leakage at the site, and chance of catheter related infection.[116,117] Application of skin adhesive at more than one site along the catheter may improve fixation.[118] A partial loop or coiling the catheter at the exit site will help reduce catheter dislodgement, and a variety of strain relief devices are now commercially available. Some practitioners elect to use tunnel catheters that are intended to remain in place for a prolonged period of time.

Choice of Local Anesthetic

The choice of local anesthetic for a peripheral nerve block depends to some extent on the duration of the surgical procedure, although other factors are also important (see Chapter 29). Prolonged blockade for up to 24 hours often occurs with long-acting local anesthetics such as bupivacaine or ropivacaine. Although this feature often results in superb postoperative pain relief, it may be undesirable in some patients because of the possible risk of nerve or tissue injury in a partially blocked limb. A short- or medium-acting local anesthetic, such as lidocaine or mepivacaine, may be more appropriate for surgical anesthesia. Whatever drug is chosen, the total dosage should be calculated for each patient and should be kept within safe limits (see Chapter 29 for details).

The highest concentrations of local anesthetic drugs are not appropriate for peripheral neural blockade; therefore 0.75% bupivacaine or ropivacaine, 2% lidocaine, 2% mepivacaine, and 3% 2-chloroprocaine are not recommended. The lowest concentrations of the same local anesthetics (i.e., 0.25% bupivacaine or ropivacaine and 0.5% mepivacaine or lidocaine) might not provide complete motor blockade.

Vasoconstrictors, usually epinephrine, can be added to the chosen local anesthetic to improve onset of action, to decrease drug uptake, and to prolong action. A concentration of 1:200,000 epinephrine is usually recommended. Ideally, the epinephrine should be added to the local anesthetic at the time the block is to be performed. Commercially prepared solutions with epinephrine have a lower pH than those in which it is freshly added, resulting in a higher percentage of ionized drug molecules. These ionized molecules do not readily cross the neural membrane, delaying the onset of drug action after injection. Epinephrine should not be added to the local anesthetic for blocks of the digits or penis because tissue ischemia can result. Various other additives, including steroids, clonidine, dexmedetomidine, opioids, and ketamine have been reported to enhance or prolong local anesthetic peripheral nerve blockade. Liposomal bupivacaine, which slowly releases this local anesthetic, is now FDA approved for some peripheral nerve blocks.

Box 46.3 Recommendations: Needle Tip Location, Choice of Local Anesthetic, and Nerve Localization Techniques

Needle Tip Location, Choice of Local Anesthetic, and Paresthesia

- Intrafascicular needle insertion and injection should be avoided because it can cause histological and/or functional nerve injury.

Nerve Localization Techniques

- There are no human data to support the superiority of one nerve localization technique over another with regard to reducing the likelihood of peripheral nerve injury.
- Peripheral Nerve Stimulation
  - Presence of an evoked motor response at a current of <0.5 (0.1 ms) indicates intimate needle-nerve relationship, needle-nerve contact, or an intraneural needle placement.
- Injection Pressure Monitoring
  - Animal data have linked high injection pressures to subsequent fascicular injury, but there are no human data that confirm or refute the effectiveness of injection pressure monitoring for limiting PNI.
- Ultrasound
  - Ultrasound can detect intraneural injection.
  - Current ultrasound technology does not have adequate resolution to discern between an interfascicular and intrafascicular injection.
  - Adequate images of needle-nerve interface are not consistently obtained by all operators and in all patients.

Modified from Neal JM, Barrington MJ, Brull R, et al. The second ASRA practice advisory on neurologic complications associated with regional anesthesia and pain medicine: executive summary 2015. *Reg Anesth Pain Med.* 2015;40(5):401–430. PMID:26288034.

Complications and Safety

Nerve injury is a recognized complication of peripheral regional techniques (Box 46.3). Risk factors contributing to neurologic deficit after regional anesthesia include neural ischemia, traumatic injury to the nerves during needle or catheter placement, and infection. However, postoperative neurologic injury because of pressure from improper patient positioning, tightly applied casts or surgical dressings, and surgical trauma is often attributed to the regional anesthetic. Patient factors such as body habitus or a preexisting neurologic dysfunction can also contribute.[119-121]

Although needle gauge, type (i.e., short vs. long bevel), and bevel configuration can influence the degree of nerve injury after peripheral nerve block, the findings are conflicting, and there are no confirmatory human studies. Theoretically, localization of neural structures with a nerve stimulator or ultrasound guidance would allow a high success rate without increasing the risk of neurologic complications, but this has not been established. Likewise, prolonged

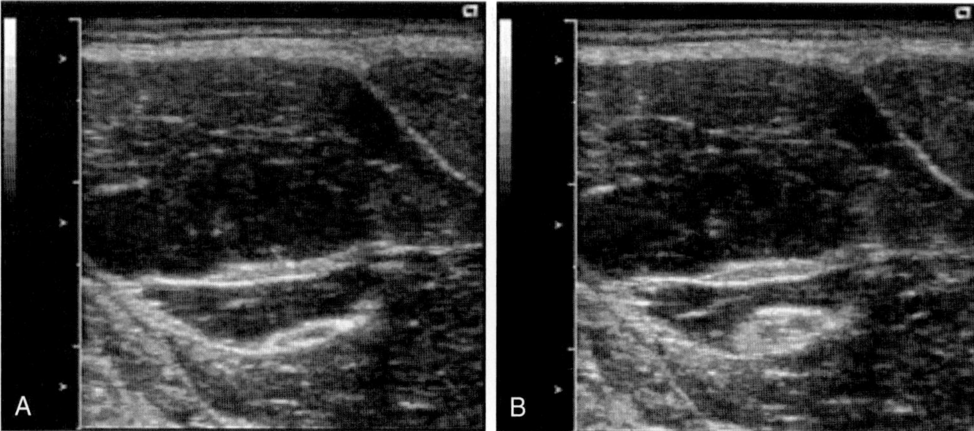

Fig. 46.38 Ultrasound image reveals intraneural injection. These sonograms were obtained in the axilla before (A) and after (B) injection in the musculocutaneous nerve. Nerve expansion is detected but with preservation of the overall integrity of the nerve borders. No paresthesias were observed during or after the procedure. Neurologic outcome was favorable after this low-volume, low-pressure injection.

exposure, high dose, or high concentrations of local anesthetic solutions can also result in permanent neurologic deficits. In laboratory models, the addition of epinephrine increases the neurotoxicity of local anesthetic solutions and decreases nerve blood flow; however, the clinical relevance of these findings in humans remains unclear. Nerve damage caused by traumatic needle placement, local anesthetic neurotoxicity, and neural ischemia during the performance of a regional anesthetic can worsen neurologic outcome in the presence of an additional patient factor or surgical injury.

Hemorrhagic complications have been described with nearly every peripheral technique and range from localized bruising and tenderness to severe hematomas or hemorrhagic complications. The placement of peripheral nerve blocks in patients with a coagulopathy should be performed with caution, especially in a deep, noncompressible site where an expanding hematoma could go unnoticed (e.g., lumbar plexus) or in a location where a hematoma could compress the airway (e.g., interscalene).[122]

Prevention of neurologic complications begins during the preoperative visit with a careful evaluation of the patient's medical history and appropriate preoperative discussion of the risks and benefits of the available anesthetic techniques. It is imperative that all preoperative neurologic deficits are documented to allow early diagnosis of new or worsening neurologic dysfunction postoperatively. Postoperative sensory or motor deficits must also be distinguished from residual (prolonged) local anesthetic effect. Imaging techniques, such as computed tomography and magnetic resonance imaging, are useful in identifying infectious processes and expanding hematomas. Although most neurologic complications resolve completely within several days or weeks, significant neural injuries necessitate neurologic consultation to document the degree of involvement and coordinate further workup. Neurophysiologic testing, such as nerve conduction studies, evoked potentials, and electromyography, are often useful in establishing a diagnosis and prognosis.

Infectious complications can be caused by exogenous (contaminated medication or equipment) or endogenous sources. Infection at the site of needle placement is an absolute contraindication to peripheral nerve blockade, although caution should be used in patients with nearby cellulitis or systemic blood infections (bacteremia or sepsis). Although bacterial colonization of peripheral nerve catheters is not uncommon, cellulitis, abscess, or bacteremia are extremely rare.[123-125]

Several large studies have established that severe systemic toxicity (seizures with or without cardiac arrest) occur on the order of 1:1000 for peripheral nerve blocks. Therefore practitioners of regional anesthesia must be familiar with the immediate detection and treatment of systemic local anesthetic toxicity. Systemic local anesthetic toxicity can occur immediately from an intravascular injection or it may be delayed because of rapid or excessive systemic absorption of local anesthetic. In addition to frequent aspiration during injection of local anesthetic, the addition of epinephrine can help alert the practitioner to potential intravascular injection. Attaching intravenous tubing to the needle allows immobility of the needle during injection. Typically, an assistant will aspirate with the syringe after each 5 mL injection of local anesthetic. Recent studies indicate that lipid emulsion rescue therapy improves success of resuscitation from cardiac arrest due to local anesthetic toxicity if given immediately after a local anesthetic overdose.[126-130]

For more details on treatment of local anesthesia toxicity, see Chapter 29.

Training

Interventional sonography is not without risks. Many studies have now demonstrated efficacy of ultrasound-guided regional blockade. Ultrasound has the potential to prevent and detect two important adverse events during peripheral nerve blocks: intravascular injection and intraneural injection of a local anesthetic.[131,132] The characteristic contrast from dissolved gas that is distributed within the vessel lumen can identify intravascular injection. The hallmark sign of intraneural injection is nerve expansion during injection (Fig. 46.38). Although ultrasound may have a profound impact on the safety of regional blockade,

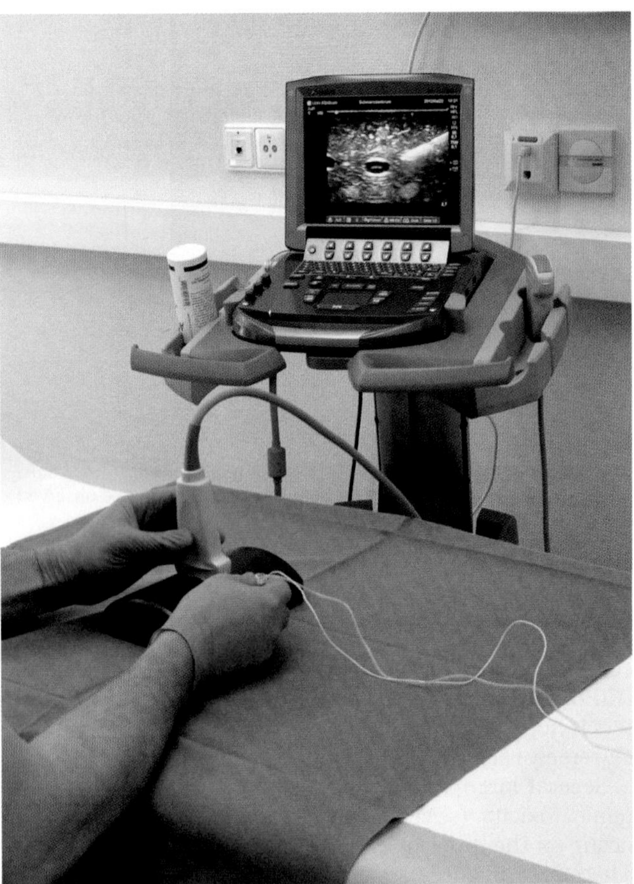

Fig. 46.39 Tissue equivalent phantom for training in ultrasound-guided interventions.

confirmatory studies of clinical practice are in progress. Many of these adverse events have only been recognized in retrospect by the review of recorded sonograms, which is a valuable training practice.

One of the original techniques developed for training novices in ultrasound-guided interventions was use of a tissue-equivalent phantom.[133] The phantom consisted of simulated tissue for needle placement practice (Fig. 46.39). To be realistic, the speed of sound must be similar as in soft tissue. In the first prototype, the phantom and container were clear; as a result, visual confirmation was possible. Several phantoms are now marketed for regional anesthesia purposes, and biologic tissue models that simulate nerve blocks have been developed.

A number of other effective teaching tools are being used. Cadavers have the advantage of realistic regional anatomic structures and can be used for simulated interventions.[134] The cost and use of specialized embalming methods that preserve nerve imaging and cadaver flexibility have limited this approach to a few specialized institutions. Most training studies have concluded that skills for ultrasound-guided procedures can be rapidly acquired.

One training study has identified common errors of novices while learning ultrasound-guided regional blocks.[135] These errors included advancing the needle when it was not visualized and unintentional probe movement. Novices often advance the needle even when it is not visualized, presumably because the natural inclination is to assume the needle has not reached the field of view. The potentially quality-compromising behaviors were largely eliminated by the end of the study period, which ranged from 66 to 114 blocks per training participant.

Summary and Conclusions

Peripheral nerve block techniques benefit the patient intraoperatively and postoperatively. Successfully mastering these techniques and applying them to the appropriate clinical situations add valuable options to the anesthetic care. Knowledge of regional anesthesia is also essential for the diagnosis and treatment of acute and chronic pain syndromes (see Chapters 51 and 82).

Ultrasound is a guidance tool that many people are electing to choose for regional anesthesia blocks. Once proficiency is established for a particular procedure, starting to use ultrasound for other interventional applications is relatively easy. Ultrasound imaging can prevent and detect critical events such as intravascular or intraneural injection that may improve safety during regional anesthesia procedures. However, if safety outcomes are to improve, then education and training play key roles in reducing these relatively uncommon adverse events.

Acknowledgments

The authors would like to thank Ram Jagannathan, MD, MBBS, for his help with imaging. Additionally, we would like to acknowledge Dr. Adam B. Collins for providing figure 46.36.

This chapter contains content from two chapters in the 8th edition text. The editors, publisher, and returning contributors, Drs. Sandra L. Kopp and Andrew T. Gray, would like to thank Drs. Terese T. Horlocker and Denise J. Wedel for their contribution in the prior edition of this work. It has served as a foundation for the current chapter.

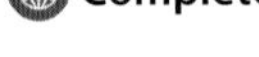

Complete references available online at expertconsult.com.

References

1. Selander D, et al. *Acta Anaesthesiol Scand.* 1979;23(1):27. PMID: 425811.
2. Selander D, et al. *Acta Anaesthesiol Scand.* 1977;21(3):182.
3. Rice AS, McMahon SB. *Br J Anaesth.* 1992;69:433.
4. Klein SM, et al. *Reg Anesth Pain Med.* 2012;37(4):383.
5. Tsui BC, et al. *Reg Anesth Pain Med.* 2004;29(3):189.
6. Gray AT, et al. *Anesthesiology.* 2006;104:368.
7. Goldstein A, et al. *J Clin Ultrasound.* 1981;9:365.
8. Fornage BD, et al. *AJR Am J Roentgenol.* 1995;164(4):1022.
9. Gray AT, et al. *Anesthesiology.* 2005;102(6):1291.
10. Ziskin MC, et al. *J Ultrasound Med.* 1982;1(1):1.
11. AIUM technical bulletin. *J Ultrasound Med.* 1999;18(2):169.
12. Soong J, et al. *Reg Anesth Pain Med.* 2005;30(5):505.
13. Rubin JM, et al. *Radiology.* 1994;190(3):853.
14. Bondestam S, et al. *Invest Radiol.* 1989;24(7):555.
15. Hopkins RE, et al. *Clin Radiol.* 2001;56(6):499.
16. Schafhalter-Zoppoth I, et al. *Reg Anesth Pain Med.* 2004;29(5):480.
17. Gray AT, et al. *Atlas of Ultrasound-Guided Regional Anesthesia.* 3rd ed. Saunders; 2018.
18. Silvestri E, et al. *Radiology.* 1995;197(1):291.
19. Cartwright MS, et al. *Arch Phys Med Rehabil.* 2007;88(3):394.
20. Roessel T, et al. *Reg Anesth Pain Med.* 2007;32(3):247.
21. Seidel R, et al. *Anaesthesist.* 2016;65(12).
22. Winnie AP, et al. *Anesth Analg.* 1975;54(3):370.

23. Choquet O, et al. *Anesth Analg*. 2010;111(6):1563.
24. Pandit JJ, et al. *Br J Anaesth*. 2007;99(2):159.
25. Urmey WF, et al. *Anesth Analg*. 1991;72:498.
26. Urmey WF, McDonald M. *Anesth Analg*. 1992;74:352.
27. Winnie AP, et al. *Anesth Analg*. 1970;49(3):455.
28. Lanz E, et al. *Anesth Analg*. 1983;62(1):55.
29. Kapral S, et al. *Reg Anesth Pain Med*. 2008;33(3):253.
30. Franco CD, et al. *Reg Anesth Pain Med*. 2016;41(4):452.
31. Gautier P, Williams JM. *Anesth Analg*. 2011;113(4):951.
32. Kessler J, et al. *Reg Anesth Pain Med*. 2008;33(6):545.
33. Liguori GA, et al. *Anesth Analg*. 1998;87(6):1320.
34. Soares LG, et al. *Reg Anesth Pain Med*. 2007;32(1):94.
35. Kang RA, et al. *Reg Anesth Pain Med*. 2018.
36. Bhatia A, et al. *Anesth Analg*. 2010;111(3):817.
37. Siegenthaler A, et al. *Reg Anesth Pain Med*. 2012;37(3):325.
38. Wiegel M, et al. *Reg Anesth Pain Med*. 2017;42(3):310.
39. Aszmann OC, et al. *Clin Orthop Relat Res*. 1996;(330):202.
40. Chang KV, et al. *J Ultrasound Med*. 2015;34(11):2099.
41. Auyong DB, et al. *Anesthesiology*. 2018. PMID:29634491.
42. Price DJ, et al. *Anaesth Intensive Care*. 2007;35(4):575.
43. Dhir S, et al. *Reg Anesth Pain Med*. 2016;41(5):564.
44. Lee JJ, et al. *Arthroscopy*. 2014;30(8):906.
45. Raj PP, et al. *Anesth Analg*. 1973;52:897.
46. Ootaki C, et al. *Reg Anesth Pain Med*. 2000;25(6):600.
47. Sandhu NS, et al. *Br J Anaesth*. 2002;89(2):254.
48. Gray AT. *Reg Anesth Pain Med*. 2009;34(2):179.
49. Perttunen K, et al. *Br J Anaesth*. 1995;75(5):541.
50. Im JG, et al. *Radiology*. 1989;171(1):125.
51. Sakai F, et al. *Rofo*. 1990;153:390.
52. Koyanagi T, et al. *Echocardiography*. 2010;27(1):17. Epub 2009 Aug 31.
53. Helm EJ, et al. *Chest*. 2012.
54. Choi S, et al. *J Med Imaging Radiat Oncol*. 2010;54(4):302.
55. Crossley AW, Hosie HE. *Br J Anaesth*. 1987;59(2):149.
56. Moore DC, et al. *Anesth Analg*. 1980;59(11):815.
57. Hord AH, et al. *Reg Anesth*. 1991;16(1):13.
58. Blanco R, et al. *Anaesthesia*. 2013;68(11):1107.
59. Mayes J, et al. *Anaesthesia*. 2016;71(9):1064.
60. Ohgoshi Y, et al. *J Anesth*. 2016;30(5):916.
61. Klingensmith JD, et al. *Ultrasound Med Biol*. 2018;(18):30114. pii: S0301.
62. Moore DC, Bridenbaugh LD. *Anesth Analg*. 1962;41:1.
63. Shanti CM, et al. *J Trauma*. 2001;51(3):536.
64. Eichenberger U, et al. *Br J Anaesth*. 2006;97(2):238.
65. Schmutz M, et al. *Br J Anaesth*. 2013;111(2):264.
66. Olsen D, et al. *A Case Rep*. 2016;6(11):362.
67. Dalens B, et al. *Anesth Analg*. 1989;69(6):705.
68. Guay J, et al. *Anesth Analg*. 2018;126(5):1695.
69. Hebbard P, et al. *Anaesthesia*. 2011;66(4):300.
70. Desmet M, et al. *Reg Anesth Pain Med*. 2017;42(3):327.
71. Jæger P, et al. *Reg Anesth Pain Med*. 2013;38(6):526.
72. Kim DH, et al. *Anesthesiology*. 2014;120(3):540.
73. Macrinici GI, et al. *Reg Anesth Pain Med*. 2017;42(1):10.
74. Wong WY, et al. *Reg Anesth Pain Med*. 2017;42(2):241.
75. Chen J, et al. *Reg Anesth Pain Med*. 2014;39(2):170.
76. Neal JM, et al. *Reg Anesth Pain Med*. 2016;41(6):723.
77. Johnson RL, et al. *Anesth Analg*. 2014;119(5):1113.
78. Gray AT, et al. *Anesth Analg*. 2003;97(5):1300.
79. Chan VW, et al. *Anesthesiology*. 2006;104(2):309.
80. Karmakar MK, et al. *Br J Anaesth*. 2007;98(3):390.
81. Tsui BC, et al. *Reg Anesth Pain Med*. 2008;33(3):275.
82. Gray AT, et al. *Reg Anesth Pain Med*. 2004;29(5):507.
83. Schafhalter-Zoppoth I, et al. *Anesthesiology*. 2004;101(3):808.
84. Balius R, et al. *Skeletal Radiol*. 2018;47(6):763.
85. Gray AT, et al. *Anesth Analg*. 2003;97(5):1300.
86. Fuzier R, et al. *Anesth Analg*. 2005;100(5):1511.
87. Valade N, et al. *Anesth Analg*. 2008;106(2):664.
88. Dillow JM, et al. *Paediatr Anaesth*. 2013;23(11):1042.
89. Bendtsen TF, et al. *Br J Anaesth*. 2011;107(2):278.
90. Johnson CS, et al. *J Ultrasound Med*. 2018;37(4):897.
91. Yamamoto H, et al. *Anesth Analg*. 2014;119(6):1442.
92. Beck GP. *Anesthesiology*. 1963;24:222.
93. Tsui BC, Ozelsel TJ. *Reg Anesth Pain Med*. 2008;33(3):275.
94. Ota J, et al. *Anesth Analg*. 2009;108(2):660.
95. Elsharkawy H, et al. *Reg Anesth Pain Med*. 2018;43(1):57.
96. Benzon HT. *Anesthesiology*. 2005;102(3):633.
97. Redborg KE, et al. *Reg Anesth Pain Med*. 2009;34(3):256.
98. Pedowitz RA. *Acta Orthop Scand Suppl*. 1991;245:1.
99. Pitkänen MT, et al. *Anaesthesia*. 1992;47(7):618.
100. Pitkänen M, et al. *Anaesthesia*. 1993;48(12):1091.
101. Marsch SC, et al. *Anesth Analg*. 2004;98(6):1789.
102. Chan VW, et al. *Anesthesiology*. 1999;90(6):1602.
103. Davies JA, et al. *Anaesthesia*. 1984;39(10):996.
104. Atanassoff PG, et al. *Anesthesiology*. 2002;97(2):325.
105. Atanassoff PG, et al. *Anesthesiology*. 2001;95(3):627.
106. Horn JL, et al. *Reg Anesth Pain Med*. 2011;36(2):177.
107. Tham CH, Lim BH, et al. *J Hand Surg Br*. 2000;25:575.
108. Fletcher SJ, et al. *Eur J Anaesthesiol*. 2011;28(2):133.
109. Smith AR, et al. *Anesth Analg*. 1987;66(7):677.
110. Sukhani R, et al. *Anesth Analg*. 1989;68(5):633.
111. Guay J. *J Clin Anesth*. 2009;21(8):585.
112. Mariano ER, et al. *Reg Anesth Pain Med*. 2009;34(5):480.
113. Swenson JD, et al. *Anesth Analg*. 2008;106(3):1015.
114. Johns J, et al. *J Ultrasound Med*. 2014;33(12):2197.
115. Ilfeld BM, et al. *Reg Anesth Pain Med*. 2011;36(3):261.
116. Klein SM, et al. *Anesthesiology*. 2003;98(2):590.
117. Auyong DB, et al. *Anesth Analg*. 2017;124(3):959.
118. Tadokoro T, et al. *Anesth Analg*. 2018. PMID 29533260.
119. Neal JM, et al. *Reg Anesth Pain Med*. 2015;40(5):401.
120. Sites BD, et al. *Reg Anesth Pain Med*. 2012;37(5):478.
121. Neal JM, et al. *Reg Anesth Pain Med*. 2017;42(5):681.
122. Horlocker TT, et al. *Reg Anesth Pain Med*. 2018;43(3):263.
123. Hebl JR. *Reg Anesth Pain Med*. 2006;31(4):311.
124. Provenzano DA, et al. *Reg Anesth Pain Med*. 2013;38(5):415.
125. Alakkad H, et al. *Reg Anesth Pain Med*. 2015;40(1):82.
126. Neal JM, et al. *Reg Anesth Pain Med*. 2018a;43(2):113.
127. Neal JM, et al. *Reg Anesth Pain Med*. 2018b;43(2):150.
128. Mulroy MF, et al. *Reg Anesth Pain Med*. 2014;39(3):195.
129. Barrington MJ, Kluger R. *Reg Anesth Pain Med*. 2013;38(4):289.
130. Weinberg GL. *Anesthesiology*. 2012;117(1):180.
131. Schafhalter-Zoppoth I, et al. *Anesth Analg*. 2004;99(2):627.
132. Fredrickson MJ, et al. *Can J Anaesth*. 2009;56(12):935.
133. Fornage BD, et al. *J Ultrasound Med*. 1989;8(12):701.
134. Kessler J, et al. *Surg Radiol Anat*. 2014;36(4):383.
135. Sites BD, et al. *Reg Anesth Pain Med*. 2007;32(2):107.

47 Perioperative Fluid and Electrolyte Therapy

MARK R. EDWARDS and MICHAEL P.W. GROCOTT

KEY POINTS

- Intravenous fluid therapy is a core part of perioperative practice, with the potential to influence patient outcomes.
- Water makes up approximately 60% of total body weight, varying widely with age and body composition. The ratio between the water volume within the intracellular and functional extracellular compartments is approximately 2:1.
- The endothelial glycocalyx forms a protein-poor intravascular fluid layer at the vessel perimeter; it has been integrated into a revised version of the Starling equation and updated model of capillary fluid movement.
- Sodium is the dominant extracellular cation and is responsible for much of extracellular fluid osmolality; dysnatremia is typically associated with disturbed extracellular fluid volume.
- Potassium is the dominant intracellular cation with a key role in the maintenance of transmembrane potentials; dyskalemia may be accompanied by impaired function of excitable tissues.
- Calcium is a key intracellular second messenger with roles in neuromuscular function, cell division, and oxidative pathways.
- Magnesium has a diverse range of physiologic effects, underlined by the increasing range of therapeutic applications of supplemental magnesium in the perioperative setting.
- Acid-base balance is relevant to fluid therapy because fluids containing supraphysiologic levels of chloride may cause an iatrogenic acidosis; the clinical relevance of this acidosis is debated.
- Intravenous fluids have a range of physiologic effects and should be considered drugs with indications, dose ranges, cautions, and side effects.
- The physiologic insult of the perioperative period may lead to a wide variety of disturbances in fluid and electrolyte balance.
- Clinical evidence to guide perioperative fluid therapy is lacking in many areas and cannot be directly extrapolated from general critical care trials.
- A balance must be found between inadequate fluid administration—allowing tissue hypoperfusion—and the adverse effects of excess intravenous fluids and toxicities related to fluid constituents.
- Goal-directed fluid therapy (GDT) may help in finding this balance for an individual patient in the perioperative setting, with evidence of reduced postoperative morbidity supporting its use in many surgical settings.
- No clear consensus exists on which intravenously administered fluid is associated with the best clinical outcomes in the perioperative setting. Comparisons of "balanced" with "unbalanced" and "crystalloid" with "colloid" fluids are being studied in many clinical settings; definitive conclusions are often lacking.
- The approach to fluid and electrolyte management may need adapting to numerous patient and surgical factors.

The administration of intravenous (IV) fluid is a core expertise for anesthesia providers and an area in which we have an important role in advising clinical colleagues. Alongside the traditional triad of maintenance of unconsciousness, pain relief, and neuromuscular relaxation, IV fluid therapy is a core element of the perioperative practice of anesthesia. The aims of perioperative fluid administration should be to avoid dehydration, maintain an effective circulating volume, and prevent inadequate tissue perfusion during a period when the patient is unable to achieve these goals through normal oral fluid intake.

Knowledge of the clinical effects of different fluids has increased substantially in recent years. The choice of fluid type in a variety of clinical situations can be rationally guided by an understanding of the physicochemical and biologic properties of the various crystalloid and colloid solutions available in combination with the available clinical trial data. Each clinical decision about fluid therapy has two key elements: which fluid to use and how much fluid to give. Recently, several clinical studies have changed our concepts regarding both these questions. However, we should be cautious about overinterpreting data from nonperioperative contexts. Despite recent high-quality "mega-trials" involving thousands of critically ill patients, key questions remain unresolved in the perioperative setting. Goal-directed fluid therapy (GDT) is a good example of an intervention that is effective in the perioperative phase, but ineffective in established critical illness, and this should alert us to other possible similar distinctions. This chapter will review the physiology and pharmacology of IV fluid therapy in humans and discuss the impact of fluid and electrolyte management and alternative approaches on clinical outcomes.

Physiology

FLUID COMPARTMENTS

Water makes up approximately 60% of total body weight in the average adult, varying with age, gender, and body composition. Adipose tissue contains little water compared with other tissues, leading to marked variability in total body water (TBW) proportion between lean (75%) and obese (45%) individuals. Variation in adipose tissue also contributes to differences in TBW between adult males and females; these differences are reduced in old age as adipose tissue is reduced. The variations in body composition with age lead to a wide variation in TBW (Table 47.1). TBW is divided between anatomic and functional fluid compartments within the body, with the major division between intracellular fluid (ICF) and extracellular fluid (ECF). The size of these compartments and their widely differing composition are shown in Fig. 47.1 and Table 47.2. The ECF can be subdivided into the following compartments:

- Interstitial fluid (ISF): Lymphatic fluid and protein-poor fluid occupying cell spaces.
- Intravascular fluid: Plasma volume, including a proportion contained within the subglycocalyx (see later discussion).
- Transcellular fluid: Includes gastrointestinal (GI) tract fluid, bile, urine, cerebrospinal fluid, aqueous humor, joint fluid, and pleural, peritoneal, and pericardial fluid. These are functionally important fluids of widely varying composition contained within epithelial-lined spaces and regulated by active cellular transport (Table 47.3).
- Water in bone and dense connective tissue: Constitutes a substantial proportion of TBW but not part of the *functional* ECF because of slow kinetics of water distribution between this and other compartments.[1]

Total *blood* volume comprises extracellular (plasma and subglycocalyx compartments) and intracellular (blood cells) elements. With the nonfunctional ECF compartment (bone and connective tissue) excluded, the ratio between ICF and functional ECF is approximately 2:1 (ICF 55% of body weight to ECF 27.5% of body weight).

PHYSICOCHEMICAL LAWS GOVERNING FLUID AND ELECTROLYTE MOVEMENT

The movement of water and solutes is governed by a variety of physicochemical and biologic processes, discussed in the following section.

Diffusion

Diffusion is the process by which solute particles fill the available solvent volume by motion from areas of high to low concentration. The speed of this equilibration is proportional to the square of the diffusion distance.

Diffusion also may occur across permeable membranes, according to Fick's law of diffusion:[1]

$$J = -DA\left(\frac{\Delta c}{\Delta x}\right)$$

where J is the net rate of diffusion, D is the diffusion coefficient, A is the cross-sectional area available for diffusion, and $\Delta c/\Delta x$ is the concentration (chemical) gradient.

Diffusion may also be driven by the tendency of charged solutes to move down electrical gradients.

Osmosis

If a semipermeable membrane (one that is permeable to water but not a solute) separates pure water from water in which solute is dissolved, water molecules will diffuse across the membrane into the region of higher solute concentration. The hydrostatic pressure required to resist the movement of solvent molecules in this way is osmotic pressure. This is one of the fundamental colligative properties of a solution—that is, it depends on the number rather than the type of osmotically active particles in a solution, which may be complete molecules or dissociated ions.

Osmotic pressure in an ideal solution is affected by temperature and volume[2]:

$$P = \frac{nRT}{V}$$

TABLE 47.1 Age-Related Variation in Total Body Water and Extracellular Fluid as Percent of Body Weight (MULTIPLY by 10 for mL/kg)

Age	TBW (%)	ECF (%)	Blood Volume (%)
Neonate	80	45	9
6 months	70	35	
1 year	60	28	
5 years	65	25	8
Young adult (male)	60	22	7
Young adult (female)	50	20	7
Elderly	50	20	

In pregnancy, blood and plasma volumes increase by 45% and 50%, respectively, by term.

ECF, Extracellular fluid; *TBW*, total body water.

Data from Jones JG, Wardrop CA. Measurement of blood volume in surgical and intensive care practice. *Br J Anaesth*. 2000;84(2):226–235; Chumlea WC, Guo SS, Zeller CM, et al. Total body water data for white adults 18 to 64 years of age: the Fels Longitudinal Study. *Kidney Int*. 1999;56(1):244–252; Baarsma R, Hof P, Zijlstra WG, et al. Measurement of total bodywater volume with deuterated water in newborn infants. *Biol Neonate*. 1992;62(2–3):108–112; and Ellis KJ, Shypailo RJ, Abrams SA, et al. The reference child and adolescent models of body composition. A contemporary comparison. *Ann N Y Acad Sci*. 2000;904:374–382.

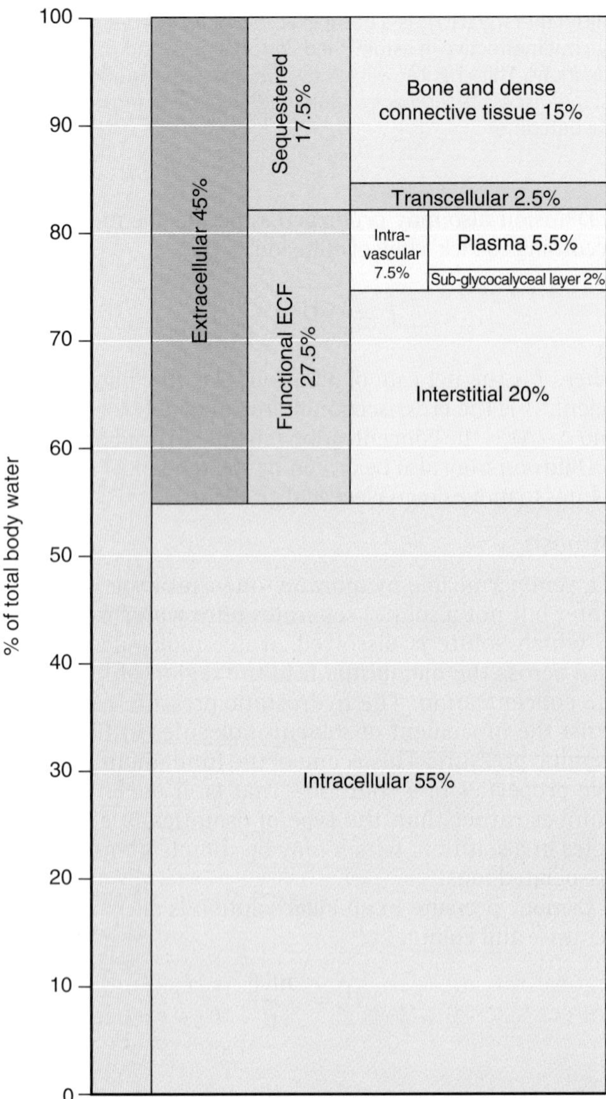

Fig. 47.1 Distribution of total body water between fluid compartments. "Sequestered" extracellular fluid *(ECF)* refers to water associated with bone and dense connective tissue or within the transcellular compartment and therefore not immediately available for equilibration with the other fluid compartments.

where *P* is the osmotic pressure, n is the number of particles, *R* is the gas constant, *T* the absolute temperature, and *V* the volume. The number of particles *(n)* can be calculated by multiplying (mass of solute/molecular weight of solute) by the number of particles into which the solute dissociates. However, body fluids are not ideal solutions, because interionic interactions reduce the number of particles free to exert an osmotic effect. The total osmotic pressure of plasma is approximately 5545 mm Hg.

Osmolality

Molality is the number of moles (each containing 6×10^{23} particles of *a specific substance*) present in 1 kg of solvent. Osmolality may be used to describe solutions containing many different types of particles and is the number of osmoles (each containing 6×10^{23} of *any type of particle present*) present in 1 kg of solvent. Normal body osmolality is 285 to 290 mOsm/kg and is the same in intracellular and extracellular compartments because of the free movement of water between compartments that consequently prevents the development of any osmotic gradients. The largest contribution to plasma osmolality is made by sodium and its related anions chloride and bicarbonate.

It can be estimated by[3]:

$$\text{Serum osmolality} = (2 \times \text{Na}) + (\text{glucose}/18) + (\text{urea}/2.8)$$

where Na is the serum sodium concentration (mEq/L), glucose is the serum glucose concentration (mg/dL), urea is the blood urea nitrogen concentration (mg/dL), and the (2 × Na) component reflects both Na and its associated anions (predominantly Cl^- and HCO_3^-). Alternatively, osmolality can be measured by depression of plasma freezing point.

Osmolarity is the number of osmoles of solute per liter of solution; unlike osmolality, this may be affected by temperature changes as a result of the volume-expanding effect of increasing temperature.

Tonicity

This is the *effective osmolality* of a solution with respect to a particular semipermeable membrane and takes into account solutes that do not exert an in vivo osmotic effect. For example, Na^+ and Cl^- do not cross cell membranes freely and therefore exert an effective osmotic force across these membranes, whereas urea freely diffuses across cell

TABLE 47.2 Composition of Intracellular and Extracellular Fluid Compartments (in mOsm/L Water)

		EXTRACELLULAR	
	Intracellular	**Intravascular**	**Interstitial**
CATIONS			
Na^+	10	142	145
K^+	157	4	4
Ca^{2+}	0.5*	2.5	2.5
Mg^{2+}	20	0.8	0.7
ANIONS			
Cl^-	10	103	117
HCO_3^-	7	25	27
$HPO_4^{2-}/H_2PO_4^-$	11	2	2
SO_4^{2-}	1	0.5	0.5
Organic acids		6	6
Protein	4	1.2	0.2

*Total intracellular Ca^{2+} concentration may be as high as extracellular levels; however, this is largely sequestered or buffered, such that the cytoplasmic ionized Ca^{2+} concentration is approximately 1000 times lower than extracellular fluid (0.3-2.6 μEq/L). The intracellular content of anions such as PO_4^{3-} has been difficult to establish for similar reasons.

Data from Campbell I. Physiology of fluid balance. *Anaesth Intensive Care Med.* 2009;10(12):593–596; Hoffer LJ, Hamadeh MJ, Robitaille L, et al. Human sulfate kinetics. *Am J Physiol Regul Integr Comp Physiol.* 2005;289(5):R1372–R1380; and Hall JE. The body fluid compartments. In: *Guyton and Hall Textbook of Medical Physiology.* 12th ed. Philadelphia: WB Saunders; 2010:285–300.

TABLE 47.3 Composition of Transcellular Fluids (mEq/L Unless Stated)

	Daily Volume (L)	Cations				Anions		pH
Fluid		Na^+	K^+	Ca^{2+}	Mg^{2+}	Cl^-	HCO_3^-	
Gastrointestinal tract								
Saliva	1-1.5	30-90	20-40	2.5	0.6	15-35	10-40	6-7
Gastric	1.5-2.5	20-60	10-20			20-160	0	1-3.5
Bile	0.7-1.2	130-150	5-12	10-50		25-100	10-45	7-8
Pancreatic	1-1.5	125-150	5-10			30-110	40-115	8-8.3
Small bowel (concentrations from proximal to distal)	1.8	140-125	5-9			110-60	100-75	7-8
Large bowel	0.2 (lost in feces)	20-40	30-90			0-15	40	7-8
Sweat	0.1-0.5	45-60	5-10			45-60	0	5.2
Cerebrospinal fluid		140	2.8	2.1	1.7	120		7.33

Data from Grădinaru I, Ghiciuc C-M, Popescu E, et al. Blood plasma and saliva levels of magnesium and other bivalent cations in patients with parotid gland tumors. *Magnes Res*. 2007;20(4):254–258; Sewón LA, Karjalainen SM, Söderling E, et al. Associations between salivary calcium and oral health. *J Clin Periodontol*. 1998;25(11 Pt 1):915–919; and Lentner C. *Geigy Scientific Tables. Vol. 1. Units of Measurement, Body Fluids, Composition of the Body, Nutrition*. 8th ed. Basle: Ciba-Geigy Ltd; 1981.

membranes and therefore does not exert an osmotic effect here. Similarly, glucose is normally taken into cells by insulin-stimulated facilitated diffusion, so it is an ineffective osmole. Tonicity is important in determining in vivo distribution of fluids across a cell membrane and is sensed by the hypothalamic osmoreceptors. It can be estimated by subtracting urea and glucose concentrations from measured osmolality.

Oncotic Pressure

Oncotic pressure is the component of total osmotic pressure that is due to the colloids, that is, large molecular-weight particles, predominantly proteins (albumin, globulins, fibrinogen). Of the total plasma osmotic pressure of 5545 mm Hg, 25 to 28 mm Hg is due to plasma oncotic pressure. The negative charge on proteins has the net effect of retaining a small excess of Na^+ ions within the plasma (the Gibbs-Donnan effect), which effectively increases the oncotic pressure above what would be predicted by calculations based purely on protein concentration. As the most abundant plasma protein, albumin is responsible for 65% to 75% of plasma oncotic pressure.

FLUID COMPARTMENT BARRIERS AND DISTRIBUTION

The volume and composition of each fluid compartment depends on the barriers separating it from neighboring compartments.

Cell Membrane

The cell membrane separates the intracellular and extracellular compartments and as a lipid bilayer is impermeable to large hydrophilic molecules and charged particles such as free ions. Other than by passive diffusion of certain molecules, solutes may cross cell membranes in several ways.

Carrier Proteins

PRIMARY ACTIVE TRANSPORT. Solute transport against a concentration gradient requires energy and is therefore directly coupled to adenosine triphosphate (ATP) hydrolysis—for example, by Na^+/K^+–adenosine triphosphatases (ATPases). This is the fundamental mechanism by which ionic concentration gradients are maintained, which in turn drive a variety of biologic processes, including water and solute movement and electrical impulse transmission in excitable tissues.

SECONDARY ACTIVE TRANSPORT. The process of secondary active transport uses concentration gradients set up by ATPases to transport a solute driven by an ion moving down its concentration gradient, typically Na^+. This process is termed cotransport when the solute is also moving down its concentration gradient or countertransport when the solute is being moved against its concentration gradient.

Solute Channels. The solute channels allow much faster transport of solutes than by ATPases or transmembrane diffusion. Examples include voltage-gated Na^+ channels and the glucose transporter GLUT1, which when inserted into the plasma membrane allows glucose to travel down its concentration gradient. This process is termed *facilitated diffusion.*

Endocytosis and Exocytosis. The processes of endocytosis and exocytosis are involved in the transport of large proteins and polypeptides across cell membranes.

Vascular Endothelium

The barrier function of the vascular endothelium is particularly relevant perioperatively because of its key role in maintaining intravascular fluid volume. Surgical tissue trauma typically leads to loss of intravascular volume through surgical blood loss or inflammation-related shifts to other tissue compartments. The physiologic effect of IV fluid administered to overcome these losses and maintain adequate tissue oxygen delivery is highly dependent on

TABLE 47.4 Capillary Characteristics

Capillary Type	Site	Large Pores	Basement Membrane	Glycocalyx Layer	Notes on Function
Nonfenestrated (continuous)	Muscle, connective tissue, lung, nervous tissue	None	Continuous	Continuous	Intercellular clefts are the main route for fluid filtration. These are partly occluded by junctional strands with multiple breaks. In the blood-brain barrier, these breaks are small (1 nm) and infrequent (zona occludens tight junctions), permitting passage of only the smallest non-lipid soluble molecules. In other tissues, the breaks are larger (5-8 nm) and more frequent (macula occludens loose junctions).
Fenestrated	Endocrine, gut mucosa, choroid plexus, lymph nodes	Pores within endothelial cells with covering diaphragm 6-12 nm size	Continuous	Continuous	Fenestrations allow capillary reabsorption of fluid from ISF, in contrast to other capillary types.
	Glomeruli	Endothelial pore size up to 65 nm	Continuous	Discontinuous over pores, reducing *effective* pore size	Numerous pores allow large-volume filtration at the glomerulus. The effective pore size is reduced further to 6 nm by podocytes; thus, proteins not usually filtered.
Sinusoidal	Liver, spleen, bone marrowd	Large intercellular gaps up to 120 nm	Discontinuous	No effective layer because of endothelial uptake of hyaluronic acid	Large fenestrations allow macromolecules (lipoproteins, chylomicrons) to pass between plasma and ISF; the result is no COP to oppose filtration, and the ISF in these tissues is effectively part of the plasma volume. Large volume filtration to the ISF here cannot be accommodated by tissue expansion because of fibrous capsules and is returned via lymphatics (e.g., liver lymph production accounts for 50% of total body lymph production)

COP, Colloid oncotic pressure; *ISF*, interstitial fluid.
Key:
Basement membrane/extracellular matrix
Endothelial cell
Endothelial glycocalyx layer
Erythrocyte

Modified from Woodcock TE, Woodcock TM. Revised Starling equation and the glycocalyx model of transvascular fluid exchange: an improved paradigm for prescribing intravenous fluid therapy. *Br J Anaesth.* 2012;108:384.

fluid handling at the capillary level. Our understanding of this area has been refined by experimental physiologic models and techniques.

Capillary Structure. As shown in Table 47.4, the structure of capillaries varies depending on the underlying organ function. The most common capillary type is the nonfenestrated capillary, comprising continuous basement membrane and a single layer of endothelial cells joined by junctions that are punctuated by breaks. These intercellular clefts are the primary channel for transcapillary fluid flow. The intravascular aspect of the endothelial cells is covered by a continuous network of glycosaminoglycan (GAG) chains, including syndecan-1, hyaluronic acid, and glypican, associated with membrane-bound proteoglycans; and glycoproteins, together forming the endothelial glycocalyx layer (EGL). The EGL covers fenestrations and intercellular clefts and has a thickness of up to 1 μm. In addition to its functions in preventing platelet and leukocyte adhesion, it has emerged as an important semipermeable layer contributing to endothelial barrier function.[2] Water and electrolytes can move freely across the vascular endothelial barrier through the EGL and then intercellular clefts or through fenestrations in the more specialized capillaries. Proteins were previously thought to be excluded from the ISF at the level of endothelial cells; however, it now appears that this occurs at the level of the glycocalyx. The subglycocalyceal layer (SGL) therefore contains protein-poor fluid; slower protein transport into the ISF may occur across the endothelial cells by endocytosis and exocytosis and by transport through a small number of large pores, forming a gradient in protein concentration from SGL to ISF compartments. The volume of the SGL may be as much as 700 to 1000 mL; this volume therefore forms part of the intravascular volume and has an electrolyte composition in equilibrium with the plasma but a much lower protein concentration because of the effective exclusion of larger molecules by the glycocalyx.

Capillary Function. The movement of fluid across the capillary membrane was initially described by Starling and then further refined. A hydrostatic pressure gradient at the arteriolar end of the capillary, greater than the inward oncotic pressure gradient, leads to net filtration of water into the ISF. Much of this water was previously thought to be reabsorbed into the vascular space toward the venular end of the capillary, where the outward hydrostatic pressure is lower and the inward oncotic pressure gradient is increased by exclusion of proteins from the capillary filtrate by the capillary endothelium. The water not reabsorbed by the capillary is removed from the ISF by the lymphatics.

More recent experimental and modeling techniques have integrated the role of the glycocalyx into a revised Starling equation and updated model of capillary fluid movement:[4]

$$J_v = K_f([P_c - P_i] - \sigma[\pi_c - \pi_{sg}])$$

where J_v is the transcapillary flow, K_f is the filtration coefficient, P_c is capillary hydrostatic pressure, P_i is the interstitial hydrostatic pressure, σ is the reflection coefficient (the degree to which the tendency of a macromolecule to cross the endothelial barrier is resisted), π_c is the capillary oncotic pressure, and π_{sg} is the subglycocalyx oncotic pressure.

The key differences and their clinical relevance are as follows[3]:

- At steady state, continuous capillaries *do not* exhibit fluid reabsorption toward the venous end of the capillary (the "no-absorption" rule). However, overall measured capillary filtration (J_v) is much less than predicted by the Starling principle, consistent with the larger colloid oncotic pressure (COP) gradient between SGL and capillary (opposing filtration) than between ISF and capillary. The smaller volume of filtrate is returned to the circulation by lymphatics.
- Plasma-SGL COP difference, not plasma-*ISF* COP difference, affects J_v. However, the no-absorption rule means that artificially raising COP (e.g., by albumin infusion) may reduce J_v but will not lead to reabsorption of fluid from the ISF into the plasma.
- An exception to the no-absorption rule occurs in acutely subnormal capillary pressures; a transient period of autotransfusion may occur, limited to approximately 500 mL. If subnormal pressures persist beyond this, J_v will approach zero, but ongoing reabsorption does not occur. Infusion of colloid in this setting will expand plasma volume, whereas infusion of crystalloid will expand total *intravascular* volume (plasma and EGL); J_v will remain close to zero in both cases until capillary pressure rises to normal or supranormal levels.
- At supranormal capillary pressures, COP difference is maintained and J_v is proportional to the hydrostatic pressure difference. In this setting, colloid infusion will maintain plasma COP but raise capillary pressure further and increase J_v. Crystalloid infusion will also increase capillary pressure but reduce plasma COP and therefore increase J_v to a greater extent than colloids.

The revised EGL model of fluid distribution, including the proposal that the intravascular volume effects of crystalloids and colloids are partly dependent on the preexisting capillary pressures (context sensitivity), helps explain some of the apparently conflicting findings in clinical fluid research.

Crystalloid versus Colloid Intravascular Volume Effects. Infused crystalloid has been thought to distribute evenly throughout the extracellular compartments as a result of capillary filtration (J_v), leaving approximately one fourth or one fifth of the original volume within the circulating blood volume, whereas colloids were presumed to initially remain largely within the intravascular volume. However, many studies of the effects of fluids on blood volume are based on red blood cell (RBC) dilution and changes in the hematocrit and do not account for the influence of the SGL volume, from which RBCs are excluded. Colloids are also excluded from the SGL; by remaining in the plasma volume, they will have a diluting effect on the hematocrit and appear to remain within the circulating volume. Crystalloids initially distribute throughout the plasma and SGL volumes. As a result, their RBC dilutional effects are less than those of colloids. This has previously been interpreted as crystalloid leaving the circulating compartment and entering the ISF; however, a proportion of the infused crystalloid will remain in the blood volume within the SGL. Furthermore, context sensitivity is responsible for the observation that clearance of crystalloid from its central compartment (the intravascular volume) is slower under anesthesia than in awake subjects.[4] It may also explain why the amount of crystalloid required to get intravascular volume effects similar to colloid is in the ratio 1.5:1 rather than the predicted 4:1.[5–7] The value of this ratio in the perioperative context is less clear and has been inferred from large clinical trials in critically ill patients. However, it is likely to be closer to the measured values in critical illness than the theoretic values traditionally used.

Failure to Reduce Edema by Increasing Capillary Colloid Oncotic Pressure. Hypoalbuminemia is well recognized as a marker of disease severity in critical illness. However, administering exogenous albumin or other colloids to increase capillary COP does not reduce peripheral or pulmonary edema, nor improve overall outcomes in sepsis. The no-absorption rule can provide a partial explanation, because even increasing COP gradient across the capillary wall by administration of albumin will not lead to reabsorption of fluid from edematous tissues. Again, previous studies showing apparent shifts of fluid from the interstitial to the intravascular compartment based on a reduced hematocrit after albumin infusion do not account for the potential role of compaction of the glycocalyx layer and transfer of fluid from the SGL to the plasma volume.

Finally, the importance of the endothelial glycocalyx is highlighted by studies showing that its degradation significantly impairs endothelial barrier function.[8] A range of physiologic insults may lead to glycocalyx injury and shedding, with the subsequent appearance of free heparin, chondroitin, and hyaluronic acid in the plasma. These include natriuretic peptides (which may be released in acute excessive increased intravascular volume),[9] hyperglycemia, and inflammatory mediators released during surgery, trauma, and sepsis, such as C-reactive protein, bradykinin, and tumor necrosis factor (TNF).[10] Glycocalyx degradation may make an important contribution to the already well-characterized endothelial dysfunction seen in inflammation, in which phenotypic changes occur in endothelial cells. Here, an increase in the number of large pores, and a reduction in interstitial hydrostatic pressure favor J_v, with an increase in edema in compliant tissues such as the lung, muscles, and loose connective tissue. Impaired glycocalyx function will further favor J_v and lead to endothelial platelet aggregation and leukocyte adhesion. Maintenance of glycocalyx integrity is therefore gaining interest as a therapeutic target in perioperative fluid management.[11]

PHYSIOLOGIC CONTROL OF OVERALL FLUID BALANCE

In health, 60% of daily water loss is through urinary excretion, although this proportion is less when sweating and insensible losses are increased. Integrated cardiovascular and renal neuroendocrine mechanisms attempt to maintain fluid volume homeostasis in response to perioperative challenges, such as reduced oral fluid intake, blood loss, and IV fluid administration.

TBW volume is controlled by a system of sensors, central control, and effectors. The sensors are (1) hypothalamic osmoreceptors that respond to changes in ECF tonicity, (2) low-pressure baroreceptors in the large veins and right atrium that sense central venous pressure (CVP), and (3) high-pressure baroreceptors in the carotid sinus and aortic arch that sense mean arterial pressure. The sensory inputs are integrated within the hypothalamus, which then triggers either increased water intake from thirst or increased water output via antidiuretic hormone (ADH, arginine vasopressin) secretion. Thirst and ADH release may be triggered by increased plasma tonicity, hypovolemia, hypotension, and angiotensin II. ADH release also may be stimulated by stress (including surgery and trauma) and certain drugs (e.g., barbiturates). Water intake does not usually depend on thirst because of social drinking behavior; thirst acts as a backup mechanism when the normal intake is inadequate. ADH, produced in the hypothalamus and released from the posterior pituitary, acts on the principal cells of the renal collecting ducts, which in the absence of ADH are relatively impermeable to water. ADH combines with the vasopressin 2 (V2) receptors on the basolateral membrane of the cells, triggering cyclic adenosine monophosphate (cAMP)-mediated insertion of aquaporin 2 water channels into the apical membrane. This results in water reabsorption down its osmotic gradient and formation of concentrated urine.

Acute Disturbances in Circulating Volume

Acute variation in the intravascular volume leads to compensatory mechanisms over minutes to hours in an attempt to correct the acute abnormality. The homeostatic processes occurring in response to rapid blood loss are aimed at minimizing the change in effective blood volume (venoconstriction and mobilization of venous reservoirs, limited autotransfusion from ISF to plasma, reduced urine production) and maintenance of cardiac output and arterial pressure (tachycardia, increased inotropy, and vasoconstriction). The sensor organs for the acute change are the low-pressure and high-pressure baroreceptors, and initial changes are mediated through increased sympathetic outflow. Renal vasoconstriction leads to a reduced volume of filtrate and activates the renin-angiotensin-aldosterone (RAA) axis. Renin is released from the juxtaglomerular cells and cleaves angiotensinogen to form angiotensin I, which is rapidly converted to angiotensin II. This induces further sympathetic activity, vasoconstriction, aldosterone release from the adrenal cortex, and hypothalamic ADH production. The overall result is increased renal salt and water retention, increased peripheral vascular resistance, and increased cardiac output. In the absence of ongoing loss, the delayed responses to major blood loss restore plasma volume within 12 to 72 hours, increase hepatic plasma protein synthesis, and restore RBC levels by erythropoiesis within 4 to 8 weeks.

Conversely, the rapid infusion of fluid to a normovolemic healthy adult leads to an initial rise in venous and arterial pressure and cardiac output. Several mechanisms act rapidly to bring these cardiovascular parameters toward normal, including pressure receptor-mediated venodilation and venous blood pooling and reduction in systemic vascular resistance. At a tissue level, autoregulatory responses lead to arteriolar vasoconstriction to maintain constant blood flow in the face of increased perfusion pressure. Multiple mechanisms then act to return circulating volume toward normal. A proportion of the infused fluid will be lost as a result of capillary filtration, particularly if the infused fluid reduces COP. Low-pressure baroreceptor stimulation leads to a decrease in pituitary ADH secretion, allowing diuresis, and atrial stretch leads to atrial natriuretic peptide (ANP) release, favoring natriuresis. Further ADH-independent renal mechanisms include glomerulotubular imbalance resulting from the marginal reduction in plasma COP; this rapidly increases the glomerular filtration rate (GFR) and reduces proximal tubule water and Na^+ reabsorption, increasing urine volume. Finally, increased arterial blood pressure promotes the excretion of excess water and salt (i.e., pressure natriuresis and pressure diuresis). This is the pressure-volume control mechanism, one of the key mechanisms for the long-term maintenance of normal blood volume. However, arterial blood pressure is only slowly restored by cardiovascular reflexes after acute hypervolemia. It may take several days for a 20 mL/kg dose of isotonic salt solution to be fully excreted. Excretion of excess Na^+ and water depends more on these passive processes and suppression of the RAA axis than on natriuretic peptide activity.[12] The contrast between this inefficiency and the rapid, effective mechanisms for dealing with reduced fluid volume and Na^+ content reflects the evolution of physiology in an environment with a paucity of salt and variable water availability; excess Na^+ intake is a feature of modern diets.

Long-Term Control of Circulating Intravascular Volume

The Guyton-Coleman model is the archetypal representation of the circulation. Despite calls to refine the mathematic modeling of the long-term control of arterial blood pressure, it remains the most widely used model to explain the chronic control of blood volume and arterial pressure.[13–15] In health, short-term variations in blood volume are very small and the cardiovascular system behaves as a closed system with arterial pressure a product of peripheral resistance, vascular compliance, and the Starling curve.[16] In the chronic setting or in acute alterations in blood volume, as described earlier, the circulating volume will vary and equality of input and output must be restored to avoid chronic fluid retention or dehydration; thus, the circulation acts as an open system. The kidneys are the primary organ regulating this equilibrium, largely through pressure natriuresis and diuresis. Indeed, in the chronic setting, arterial pressure subserves the renal requirement to excrete ingested Na^+ and water rather than simply being a product of cardiac output, vascular compliance, and resistance. A recent interpretation integrates the Guyton-Coleman model with experimental observations (Fig. 47.2).[16] In health, the pressure-natriuresis curve is relatively flat, and excess intake of salt and water can be excreted without long-term rises in circulating volume or blood pressure. In many models of chronic hypertension, the renal excretion mechanism is reset such that natriuresis occurs only at higher arterial pressures and excessive exogenous water and salt results in higher blood pressure.

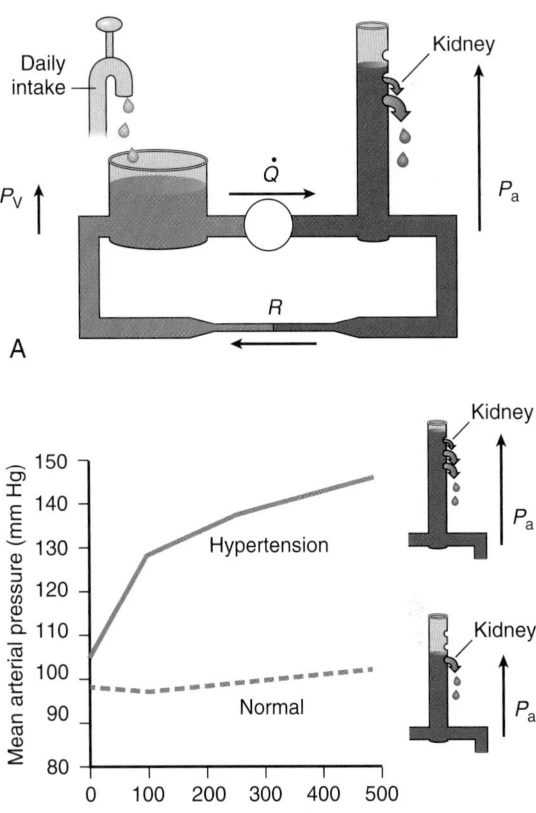

Fig. 47.2 Long-term control of blood volume in health and hypertension. (A) Representation of the open circulation model. In the chronic setting, arterial pressure (P_a) depends on daily water and sodium intake *(dripping tap)* and the renal pressure-natriuresis relationship *(represented by the height of the holes in the arterial column)* rather than cardiac output ($\dot{Q}$) and peripheral resistance *(R)*. (B) Experimental models of hypertension (e.g., long-term angiotensin II infusion) with controlled sodium intake (and therefore excretion) demonstrate a reset pressure-natriuresis curve in hypertension. This may be represented by kidney *holes* positioned further up the arterial column. Natriuresis occurs to a degree similar to that in normotension, so as to maintain a stable body water volume, but requires a higher arterial pressure to do so. P_v, Venous pressure. (A, Redrawn from Dorrington KL, Pandit JJ. The obligatory role of the kidney in long-term arterial blood pressure control: extending Guyton's model of the circulation. *Anaesthesia.* 2009;64:1218. B, Data from Hall JE. The kidney, hypertension, and obesity. *Hypertension.* 2003;41:625.)

ELECTROLYTE PHYSIOLOGY

Sodium Physiology

Na^+ is the dominant extracellular cation, and along with its associated anions accounts for nearly all the osmotically active solute in plasma and interstitial fluid. The relatively free movement of water throughout the fluid compartments means that Na^+ is therefore the prime determinant of ECF volume. Total body Na^+ content is approximately 4000 mmol, of which only 10% is intracellular. The concentration gradient between the intracellular and extracellular compartments (ratio 1:15) is maintained by ATPases and is vital for the function of excitable tissues, including action potentials and membrane potential, and for the handling of renal solute.

Na^+ intake is typically far in excess of minimum daily requirements, which are 2 to 3 mEq/kg/day at birth and decrease to 1 to 1.5 mEq/kg/day in adulthood.[17,18] Na^+ is actively absorbed from the small intestine and colon under the influence of aldosterone and the presence of glucose in the gut lumen. Loss is predominantly by the renal route, with minor contributions from feces, sweat, and skin (10 mEq/day each). Na^+ is freely filtered at the glomerulus, of which 99.5% is reabsorbed, mainly at the proximal convoluted tubule. Serum Na^+ concentrations are maintained within a tight range (138-142 mEq/L) despite wide variation in water intake by the systems involved in the control of circulating volume outlined previously:

- hypothalamic osmoreceptor: ADH release
- atrial volume sensing: ANP release
- juxtaglomerular apparatus (renal arteriolar baroreceptor and filtrate NaCl content sensing): RAA activation

The excretion of total body excess Na^+ relies on inefficient passive mechanisms, particularly the pressure-volume effect. Long-term ingestion of excess salt combined with low potassium ingestion contributes to hypertension, a condition not seen in populations with daily salt intake less than 50 mmol. The mechanism involves renal salt retention and initial extracellular volume expansion (later mitigated by pressure natriuresis), with release of an endogenous digitalis-like factor and stimulation of renal Na^+ pumps, furthering renal Na^+ retention. Low K^+ combined with the chronic action of digitalis-like factor inhibits vascular smooth muscle cell Na^+/K^+ ATPases, resulting in excess intracellular Na^+ content and reduced intracellular K^+, smooth muscle contraction, and increased peripheral vascular resistance.[19]

Potassium Physiology

K^+ is the dominant intracellular cation in the body, with a total body content of approximately 4000 mmol, 98% of which is intracellular, particularly in muscle, liver, and RBCs. The ratio of ICF to ECF K^+ balance is vital in the maintenance of cellular resting membrane potential, and K^+ therefore has a key role in the behavior of all excitable tissues. Daily requirements reflect age and growth, with more K^+ required at higher metabolic rates. Term infants require 2 to 3 mEq/kg/day and adults 1 to 1.5 mEq/kg/day. Nearly all ingested K^+ is absorbed by the intestine, and minimal amounts are excreted in feces. The acute and chronic handling of K^+ must therefore maintain a stable plasma K^+ concentration and resting membrane potential in the face of a daily K^+ intake of a similar magnitude to the entire ECF K^+ content. Transmembrane potentials particularly depend on K^+ permeability, with K^+ egress occurring through ion channels down its concentration gradient. This leaves behind intracellular anions, with a resultant negative transmembrane potential. The resting value of this potential is achieved when the tendency of K^+ to move extracellularly as a result of its concentration gradient is matched by the tendency of K^+ to move intracellularly because of the electrical gradient.

Acute K^+ distribution involves shifts in K^+ between the ECF and ICF, performed by ion transport systems under the influence of insulin, catecholamines, and ECF pH. The cell membrane Na^+/K^+ ATPase exports three Na^+ for every two K^+ imported and is the means by which the gradients of these ions are maintained. Insulin, released after ingestion of K^+-containing food, stimulates the Na^+/H^+ antiporter, increasing intracellular Na^+, which is then removed by Na^+/K^+ ATPase with the net cellular uptake of K^+. Conversely, in the presence of hypokalemia, skeletal muscle expression of Na^+/K^+ ATPase is reduced, allowing a "leak" of K^+ from the ICF to ECF.[20] Catecholamines activate β_2-adrenoceptors, which ultimately stimulate Na^+/K^+ ATPase activity, leading to increases in ICF K^+, a mechanism that counteracts the release of K^+ from muscle cells during exercise.[21] ECF pH also has a bearing on K^+ handling. The presence of mineral organic acids (where the acid anion is unable to diffuse into the cell) leads to increased cellular H^+ uptake in exchange for K^+ ions with consequent increases in ECF K^+. Organic acids (e.g., lactic acid and ketone bodies) are more able to diffuse across cellular membranes and H^+/K^+ exchange is much less. Hyperkalemia may be observed in the setting of organic acidemia resulting from alternative mechanisms, such as insulin deficiency and osmotic drag in diabetic ketoacidosis or a failure of ATP production for Na^+/K^+ ATPase in situations typified by anaerobic metabolism and lactic acidosis. Other factors that may influence ECF to ICF K^+ balance include aldosterone (which at high levels may induce intracellular K^+ shift, beyond its renal effects), hyperosmolar states (solvent drag of K^+ along with water efflux), and digoxin (inactivates Na^+/K^+ ATPase and may cause hyperkalemia).

Chronic K^+ distribution involves renal mechanisms. K^+ is freely filtered at the glomerulus, and undergoes extensive unregulated reabsorption along the proximal tubule, with only 10% to 15% reaching the distal nephron, where its reabsorption or secretion is tightly controlled. This occurs predominantly in two cell types found in the collecting ducts.

Principal Cells. The principal cells are able to secrete K^+ under the electrochemical gradients set up by basal Na^+/K^+ ATPases, which maintain low intracellular Na^+ concentrations (aiding Na^+ reabsorption from the tubule via Na^+ channels) and high intracellular K^+ concentrations (favoring K^+ secretion into the tubule via K^+ channels). Principal cell behavior is influenced by the following:

- Aldosterone, synthesized and released by the adrenal glands in response to raised K^+ concentrations. This mineralocorticoid increases the synthesis and activity of both basal Na^+/K^+ ATPases and luminal K^+ channels to drive urinary K^+ secretion.
- Tubular Na^+ delivery. Increased distal tubular Na^+ content leads to a steeper Na^+ concentration gradient and increased principal cell reabsorption of Na^+. To maintain electroneutrality of the tubular fluid, K^+ efflux into the tubule increases; this is partly responsible for the hypokalemia associated with diuretics that increase delivery of Na^+ to the cortical collecting ducts (thiazides and loop diuretics). In contrast, amiloride blocks the principal cell luminal Na^+ channel and therefore does not affect K^+ efflux here.

Intercalated Cells. In addition to basal Na^+/K^+ ATPases, these cells have luminal H^+/K^+ ATPases that excrete one hydrogen into the tubule for every K^+ reabsorbed. Low K^+ settings lead to up-regulation of this luminal antiporter, reabsorbing more K^+ at the expense of renal acid loss.

In addition to mechanisms involving aldosterone in a feedback loop, it is likely that feed-forward mechanisms also exist to rapidly modulate renal K^+ handling when K^+ is sensed in the GI system, even before plasma K^+ levels rise.[20]

Calcium Physiology

Beyond its role in bone structure, where 98% of body calcium (Ca^{2+}) is stored, Ca^{2+} is one of the body's most important intracellular second messengers, playing a key role in muscular contraction, neuromuscular transmission, cell division and movement, and oxidative pathways. Intracellular Ca^{2+} entry may have direct effects in cardiac and skeletal muscle contraction—for example, leading to neurotransmitter release or inducing further large-scale release of Ca^{2+} from intracellular stores (Ca^{2+}-induced Ca^{2+} release). A large ECF-to-ICF gradient of ionized Ca^{2+} is maintained by ATPases, and cytoplasmic free Ca^{2+} levels are kept low by pumping into the sarcoplasmic reticulum. Increases in cytoplasmic Ca^{2+} concentration occurring as a result of cellular energetic failure and impaired Ca^{2+} transport are a key mediator of cell death pathways.[22] Ca^{2+}also plays a key role in coagulation by linking coagulation factors to the negatively charged plasma membrane of activated platelets.

Homeostatic mechanisms maintain serum Ca^{2+} concentrations between 4.5 and 5 mEq/L (8.5-10.5 mg/dL), largely under the influence of vitamin D and parathyroid hormone (PTH). Ionized Ca^{2+} is sensed by the extracellular domain of a G-coupled receptor expressed on parathyroid cells (the Ca^{2+}/Mg^{2+}-sensing receptor), inhibiting PTH release.[23] When ionized Ca^{2+} levels decrease, PTH is rapidly released with the following actions:

- Stimulates osteoclast bone resorption, releasing Ca^{2+} into the ECF
- Stimulates distal tubule calcium reabsorption
- Stimulates the renal conversion of 25-(OH)-vitamin D to 1,25-$(OH)_2$-vitamin D (calcitriol, the most active vitamin D metabolite)

The manufacture of active vitamin D involves cholecalciferol formation in the skin during exposure to ultraviolet

TABLE 47.5 Physiologic Roles of Magnesium

System	Effect	Mechanism and Clinical Relevance
Neurologic	Reduction in pain transmission	NMDA antagonism. Mg^{2+} treatment provides effective perioperative analgesia.[254]
	Reduces neuromuscular transmission	Inhibition of neuronal Ca^{2+} influx reduces neuromuscular junction ACh release (and motor end-plate sensitivity to ACh). Hypermagnesemia potentiates the effects of neuromuscular blockade.
	Sympatholysis	Inhibition of neuronal Ca^{2+} influx reduces catecholamine release from adrenal medulla and adrenergic nerve endings. Pharmacologic use of Mg^{2+} in obtunding pressor response to intubation or during surgery for pheochromocytoma.
	Anticonvulsant	Mechanism may relate to NMDA antagonism or cerebral arteriolar vasodilation, possible mechanisms for its efficacy in eclampsia, in which vasospasm has been observed.[29]
	Cortical depression at high levels	
Cardiovascular	Vasodilation	Predominantly arteriolar, because of inhibition of Ca^{2+} influx-mediated vascular smooth muscle contraction. Mg^{2+} administration typically leads to a minor reflex increase in inotropy despite the direct action of Mg^{2+} on reducing cardiac contractility.[255]
	Antiarrhythmic effects	Mixed class IV (Ca^{2+} channel inhibition) and weak class I (Na^{+} channel inhibition) effects. Increases atrioventricular nodal conduction time and refractory periods, suppresses accessory pathway transmission, and inhibits early and delayed afterdepolarizations. Clinical use is in supraventricular tachycardias, atrial fibrillation rate control and postoperative prophylaxis, and tachyarrhythmias associated with dyskalemia, digoxin, bupivacaine, or amitriptyline.[29]
	Improved myocardial O_2 supply-to-demand ratio	Coronary vasodilation in combination with reductions in heart rate and contractility; however, no clear evidence of benefit in the setting of acute myocardial infarction.
Respiratory	Bronchodilation	Smooth muscle relaxation. Pharmacologic use of Mg^{2+} is in acute bronchospasm.
Renal	Renal vasodilation and diuresis	Ca^{2+} antagonism-related smooth muscle relaxation
Immune	Antiinflammatory	Pharmacologic doses of magnesium sulfate reduce monocyte inflammatory cytokine production.[256]
	Adaptive immunity	Mg^{2+} is required as a second messenger during T-lymphocyte activation.[257]
Obstetric	Tocolysis	May be due to smooth muscle relaxation

ACh, Acetylcholine; NMDA, N-methyl-D-aspartate.

light, which then undergoes hepatic hydroxylation to 25-hydroxy-calciferol, then renal hydroxylation under the influence of PTH to 1,25-dihydroxycalciferol (calcitriol). As with PTH, this stimulates osteoclastic bone resorption and additionally stimulates absorption of Ca^{2+} from the GI tract.

Ca^{2+} homeostasis is interlinked with that of other anions. In particular, magnesium is also able to modulate PTH levels, and hypocalcemia and hypomagnesemia frequently coexist. The homeostasis of phosphate (PO_4^{3-}) is effectively the converse of Ca^{2+} (e.g., renal hydroxylation of vitamin D is inhibited by hyperphosphatemia), and in health the (calcium × phosphate) product is kept relatively stable. An increase in the (calcium × phosphate) product may be seen in advanced chronic kidney disease and is associated with ectopic bone deposition.

Approximately 50% of circulating Ca^{2+} is in the biologically active ionized form (the remaining 40% are bound to proteins, predominantly albumin and globulins, and 10% are complexed to anions such as HCO_3^{-}, citrate, sulfate, PO_4^{3-}, and lactate). Hypoalbuminemia decreases the total serum Ca^{2+} but has less effect on the biologically important ionized form. To calculate the corrected total Ca^{2+} concentration, 0.8 mg/dL is added per 1 g/dL decrease in albumin concentration below 4 g/dL. The degree of albumin-protein binding is affected by pH, with acidemia reducing protein binding and increasing the ionized fraction. Ionized Ca^{2+} rises by approximately 0.1 mEq/L per 0.1 decrease in pH.[26] Given the approximate nature of corrected total Ca^{2+}, biologically active ionized Ca^{2+} should be measured when possible. Specimens should ideally be taken without tourniquet (uncuffed), because local acidosis increases the ionized fraction.

Magnesium Physiology

Mg^{2+} has a diverse range of cellular actions, including modulation of ion channel activity and as an essential component of ATP production and hydrolysis. It is primarily an intracellular anion, although most is sequestered within organelles, bound to phospholipids, proteins, and nucleic acids. Free ionized Mg^{2+} levels within the cytoplasm and ECF are therefore low (0.8-1.2 mM), and chemical concentration gradients are much less than for other anions. Of total body Mg^{2+}, 50% is within bone, 20% within muscle, and the rest in liver, heart, and other tissues. Only 1% is within the ECF, and normal plasma levels may be maintained in the face of total body Mg^{2+} depletion. Within the plasma, total Mg^{2+} concentration is 1.5 to 2.1 mEq/L, of which approximately 25% is protein (mostly albumin) bound, 65% is in the biologically active ionized form, and the remainder is complexed to phosphates, citrates, and other anions.[27] Measurement of ionized Mg^{2+} can be performed, although correction is required for interference from Ca^{2+} ions.[28] The key roles of Mg^{2+} (Table 47.5) highlight its diverse range of clinical applications when administered exogenously and stem from the following three main cellular actions:

1. Energy metabolism: Mg^{2+} is required for ATP phosphorylation reactions, interacting with the outer two PO_4^{3-}

groups of ATP. Intracellular Mg^{2+} deficiency therefore impairs any enzyme systems using high-energy PO_4^{3-} bonds, such as glucose metabolism.[27]

2. Nucleotide and protein production: Mg^{2+} acts as a cofactor in every step of DNA transcription and replication and messenger RNA (mRNA) translation.
3. Ion transport: by supporting the activity of ion-pumping ATPases, Mg^{2+} helps maintain normal transmembrane electrochemical gradients, effectively stabilizing cell membranes and organelles. In addition, effects on ion *channels* underlie one of the core functions of Mg^{2+}, namely physiologic competitive antagonism of Ca^{2+}. This is mediated through inhibition of L-type Ca^{2+} channels and extracellular local modification of membrane potential, preventing the intracytoplasmic influx of Ca^{2+} from both the ECF and intracellular sarcoplasmic reticulum stores. Mg^{2+} also effectively antagonizes *N*-methyl-D-aspartate (NMDA) receptors within the central nervous system, reducing Ca^{2+} entry by specific ion channels. These effects result in inhibition of a diverse array of excitable tissue cellular actions, including neurotransmitter release, muscular contraction, cardiac pacemaker and action potential activity, and pain signal transmission.

Mg^{2+} is absorbed from the GI tract by a saturable transport system and passive diffusion, in quantities inversely proportional to the amount ingested. Excretion is via the GI tract (~60% of the ingested amount) and kidneys. Seventy-five percent is freely filtered at the glomerulus, and proximal tubule reabsorption is minimal, with 60% to 70% being reabsorbed at the thick ascending loop of Henle and 10% reabsorbed under regulation in the distal tubule. The regulation of total body Mg^{2+} levels by GI uptake and control of renal excretion is not under the control of a well-defined hormonal feedback loop. Although many factors can influence Mg^{2+} reabsorption (particularly PTH but also calcitonin, glucagon, acid-base balance, Ca^{2+} and K^+ levels), the main determinant is the plasma Mg^{2+} concentration, sensed by Ca^{2+}/Mg^{2+}-sensor receptors present on the basal aspect of thick ascending loop cells. Other influences may alter the intracellular-extracellular balance of magnesium distribution. Catecholamines, acting by both α- and β-adrenoreceptors, and glucagon lead to extrusion of magnesium from intracellular stores. Although experimental models have shown that adrenergic stimulation may increase serum Mg^{2+} concentrations, decreases in serum Mg^{2+} concentrations actually occur after stressors such as surgery, trauma, burns, and sepsis.[27,29] This may be due to a later phase of catecholamine-driven cellular uptake after the initial Mg^{2+} efflux.[30]

Phosphate Physiology

PO_4^{3-} is the most abundant intracellular anion and helps form some of the most important biologic molecules, including ATP, DNA, and RNA, membrane phospholipids, 2,3-diphosphoglycerate (2,3-DPG), and hydroxyapatite in bone. PO_4^{3-} is therefore required for energy metabolism, cellular signaling through phosphorylation reactions, cellular replication and protein synthesis, membrane integrity, and O_2 delivery. In addition, the PO_4^{3-} buffer system is one of the key intracellular buffers. Of total body phosphorus, 80% to 90% is stored in bone, with the remainder in the intracellular (soft tissues and erythrocytes) and extracellular fluid compartments.[31] Normal plasma inorganic phosphates are maintained at 3 to 5 mg/dL, and at normal pH, 80% exists in the divalent (HPO_4^{2-}) rather than monovalent ($H_2PO_4^-$) form. Plasma phosphates also include lipid phosphates and organic ester phosphates. Most intracellular PO_4^{3-} is organic.[18]

The typical daily intake of PO_4^{3-} (~1 g) outweighs metabolic requirements, yet 70% is absorbed, leading to postprandial increases in serum PO_4^{3-} levels that are rapidly dealt with by increased renal excretion. GI uptake occurs predominantly by paracellular diffusion and is unregulated unless PO_4^{3-} ingestion is reduced, when vitamin D and PTH-stimulated active transport intervene.[32,33] Plasma inorganic PO_4^{3-} is freely filtered at the glomerulus, 80% of which is reabsorbed in the proximal tubule and a smaller amount in the distal tubule. Proximal tubule reabsorption is via Na^+-dependent cotransporters, the expression and activity of which are under the influence of PTH and PO_4^{3-} intake.

The regulation of normal PO_4^{3-} levels is mediated primarily by the PTH and vitamin D systems. Low plasma PO_4^{3-} levels stimulate 1-hydroxylase activity, with the formation of active vitamin D (1,25-dihydroxycalciferol), which increases GI and renal PO_4^{3-} absorption. Conversely, PTH release (stimulated by reduced plasma Ca^{2+}) reduces renal PO_4^{3-} reabsorption. PO_4^{3-} plasma levels also may be reduced in the short term by cellular uptake in response to dopamine and adrenergic activity and alkalosis and intestinal factors (phosphatonins) released in response to increased intestinal luminal PO_4^{3-}.[31]

Chloride Physiology

As the second most abundant electrolyte in the extracellular compartment, chloride (Cl^-) has a key role in the maintenance of plasma osmolality, preservation of electrical neutrality, and acid-base status (explained by the Stewart model, see later discussion). Normal plasma values are 97 to 107 mEq/L; Cl^- is therefore responsible for nearly a third of plasma osmolality and two thirds of plasma negative charge.[34] Most Cl^- intake is derived from dietary NaCl, and the GI tract absorbs and secretes large amounts of Cl^-, primarily as gastric hydrochloric acid, but also throughout the intestinal lumen. This cellular Cl^- secretion leads to paracellular movement of Na^+ into the lumen, with water moving down its osmotic gradient to form GI secretions. Cl^- excretion is primarily renal, largely in the proximal tubule by passive reabsorption or cotransport. More regulated control of Cl^- excretion is performed in the intercalated cells of the distal nephron under the influence of plasma acid-base balance by exchange of HCO_3^- for Cl^-.

ACID-BASE DISTURBANCES AND FLUID THERAPY

Acid-base balance in general is discussed in Chapter 48; however, the two key areas in which intravascular fluid therapy may affect acid-base balance are iatrogenic acidosis caused by the administration of Cl^--rich fluids and administration of sodium bicarbonate to correct acidosis. In summary, the interpretation of acid-base balance can be viewed in three main ways: by the Henderson-Hasselbach equation, by anion gap, or by Stewart's strong ion model.

The Henderson-Hasselbach equation represents the HCO_3^- buffer system and has plasma HCO_3^- concentration as an independent determinant of plasma pH. The anion gap model is consistent with the Henderson-Hasselbach equation, because it places changes in plasma HCO_3^- at the core of plasma acid-base balance. It represents a simple method for differentiating causes of metabolic acidosis and is defined as the difference between the most abundant *measured* cation and anion concentrations in the plasma ($[Na^+]$ + $[K^+]$) − ($[Cl^-]$ + $[HCO_3^-]$). The normal anion gap is 4 to 11 mEq/L, and this difference is represented by "unmeasured" anions (PO_4^{3-}, sulfate, and anionic proteins). In the presence of excess organic acids (e.g., lactic acid or ketoacid), the accumulation of unmeasured anions is accompanied by a reduction in HCO_3^- to buffer the excess H^+ ions, leading to an increase in the anion gap. In cases in which Cl^- is administered, even if HCO_3^- falls, the anion gap will remain normal.[35]

Stewart's model of acid-base balance has a different approach and proposes that plasma pH is dependent on the following three independent variables:

1. pCO_2 (the plasma CO_2 tension)
2. A_{tot}, the total plasma concentration of all nonvolatile buffers (albumin, globulins, and PO_4^{3-})
3. Strong ion difference (SID), the difference between the total charge of plasma-strong cations (Na^+, K^+, Mg^{2+}, and Ca^{2+}) and strong anions (Cl^-, lactate, sulfate, and others). In a more simplified approach, apparent SID is defined as ($[Na^+]$ + $[K^+]$) − ($[Cl^-]$ + [lactate]). Normal plasma SID is approximately 42 mEq/L, and reductions in SID will lead to a fall in plasma pH.

The Stewart model has caused some controversy by representing HCO_3^- as a dependent variable,[36] but it has utility in explaining acid-base disturbances caused by fluid administration.[37]

Hyperchloremic Acidosis

Administration of fluid with Cl^- concentration higher than that of plasma will in sufficient quantities (e.g., 30 mL/kg/h of 0.9% saline) cause a metabolic acidosis due to the Cl^- content.[38] This hyperchloremic acidosis may be explained by the Henderson-Hasselbach model of acidosis, where saline infusion causes dilution of bicarbonate and a resultant base deficit, or by the Stewart model. Here, the increasing plasma Cl^- concentration reduces apparent SID and therefore reduces plasma pH; the SID of completely ionized saline is zero, therefore its infusion progressively dilutes the normal plasma SID. Similar changes are not seen with solutions containing non-Cl^- anions which are metabolized after infusion, such as lactated Ringer solution. Although in vitro as an electroneutral solution it also has an SID of zero, following administration, the lactate undergoes metabolism in patients with intact hepatic function, giving it an effective in vivo SID of approximately 29 mEq/L. This is slightly less than the plasma SID and is enough to counteract any alkalosis caused by dilution of A_{tot}.

Saline-induced hyperchloremic acidosis has a variety of potentially deleterious physiological effects. These include renal vasoconstriction, reduced GFR and reduced renin activity in animal models,[39–41] and reduced renal cortical perfusion in healthy volunteers.[42] Coagulopathy and gastrointestinal dysfunction have also been suggested.[43] However, it is not clear that acidosis purely attributable to iatrogenic hyperchloremia leads to clinically important morbidity. A meta-analysis of studies comparing saline with balanced perioperative fluid regimes confirmed the presence of hyperchloremia and acidosis postoperatively in the saline groups, but typically these biochemical abnormalities were cleared by the first or second postoperative day.[38] There were no overall differences in markers of kidney injury or need for renal replacement therapy, nor in other morbidities such as clinically important coagulopathy or gastrointestinal symptoms. However, the available trials were relatively small, and higher-risk surgical groups (those with pre-existing impairment of acid-base status, emergency and major surgery) were under-represented. Interestingly, in one trial of patients undergoing renal transplant, saline administration was associated with significant hyperkalemia, presumably caused by cellular potassium extrusion due to extracellular acidosis.[44] It is therefore possible that the acidosis observed due to saline administration has a greater clinical effect on a selected high-risk group. Recent large trials in the emergency department and intensive care settings have shown an increase in a composite outcome of death or adverse renal event when patients are given saline rather than balanced crystalloid.[45,46] The effect seemed to be greatest in medical patients with sepsis. The difference in composite outcomes was small (15.4% in the saline group, 14.3% in the balanced group), but this should be taken in the context of the large number of hospitalized patients that receive intravenous fluids. Although these trials did not relate specifically to the perioperative setting, an increasingly cautious approach to saline administration seems appropriate.

Bicarbonate Administration

The administration of IV $NaHCO_3$ to treat metabolic acidosis should be reserved for the emergency treatment of select conditions, including severe hyperkalemia and arrhythmias associated with tricyclic antidepressant overdose. In many other situations, clinical benefit is not apparent, a finding that highlights an important pathophysiologic concept. Acidosis in itself may not be physiologically deleterious; indeed, it is a normal event during strenuous exercise, in which it may aid O_2 offloading to tissues. Perhaps acidosis serves as a marker for the severity of underlying disease processes, such as hypoxia, ischemia, or mitochondrial dysfunction, which cause morbidity without adequate correction.[43] HCO_3^- administration also has the following negative effects[18]:

1. Carbon dioxide production. Most of the HCO_3^- administered is converted to CO_2, with two important consequences. First, excess CO_2 requires excretion by hyperventilation. Converted HCO_3^- of 100 mEq represents an excess of 2.24 L of CO_2 to be exhaled, which may present a significant physiologic challenge to critically ill patients with preexisting ventilatory impairment. Although this is disputed, the excess CO_2 may also diffuse into the intracellular space, aggravating intracellular acidosis.[18]

2. IV HCO_3^- brings a significant Na^+ content and therefore osmotic load. This may lead to hyperosmolar hypernatremia, ECF expansion, and volume overload.
3. If renal HCO_3^- distribution is impaired, there may be an "overshoot" toward metabolic alkalosis once the underlying disease process causing the initial acidosis is resolved.

In situations in which HCO_3^- administration is required, the total dose required to correct the base deficit can be calculated using the equation:[5]

$$\text{Dose (mEq)} = 0.3 \times \text{weight(kg)} \times \text{base deficit(mEq/L)}$$

Although half this dose is usually given, because of the problems outlined above, treatment should stop once the pH rises above 7.2.

Fluid Pharmacology

Given the diverse range of physiologic effects of administered fluids, and the potentially large volumes which can be administered perioperatively, they should be considered as drugs with specific indications, cautions, and side effects. Many of the fluids available currently were developed several decades ago and entered clinical practice without rigorous analysis of their clinical benefits, or knowledge of their effects at an organ or cellular level. Newer colloid solutions have been approved by regulatory authorities and entered widespread clinical usage based on relatively small trials of efficacy. In some cases, safety concerns such as the impact of colloid-related renal dysfunction have only been highlighted by much later adequately powered trials.[47] The composition of available fluids is shown in Table 47.6, although not all fluids are available in all countries.

CRYSTALLOIDS

Crystalloids are solutions of electrolytes in water. They may be classified by their tonicity after infusion or their overall composition. Crystalloids containing electrolytes found in plasma and a buffer such as lactate or acetate may be referred to as balanced solutions. Crystalloids are indicated for replacement of free water and electrolytes but also may be used for volume expansion. Conventional concepts of fluid compartments dictate that infused electrolytes will distribute freely throughout the ECF, water will follow down osmotic gradients, and the net result is a distribution of infused crystalloids throughout the entire ECF, with only 20% remaining in the intravascular compartment. This is challenged by large clinical trials and current knowledge of microvascular fluid handling (see the Vascular Endothelium section), which suggest that isotonic crystalloids may have a larger intravascular volume expanding effect than this, particularly in patients with low capillary hydrostatic pressures. The study of volume kinetics has quantified the redistribution of crystalloids from the central (intravascular) volume to the larger peripheral (total extracellular) volume. Perhaps up to 70% of a crystalloid infusion remains in the intravascular compartment at the end of a 20-minute continuous infusion, decreasing to 50% after 30 minutes.[4] Nevertheless, more fluid will ultimately be filtered out of the capillary with crystalloids than with colloids, owing to colloids' effects on oncotic pressure. Patients resuscitated with crystalloids have a more positive fluid balance for the same volume expansion effect.[51] Tissue edema may increase in compliant tissues such as the lung, gut, and soft tissues, particularly when crystalloid solutions are infused into normovolemic subjects. Large-volume crystalloid infusions also may be associated with a hypercoagulable state caused by dilution of circulating anticoagulant factors; the clinical significance of this is not currently known.[52]

Saline Solutions

0.9% Sodium Chloride. One of the most commonly administered crystalloids is 0.9% NaCl solution, yet it is not clear historically how it entered routine clinical practice. Although many of the crystalloids being examined for in vivo clinical usage during the 1800s had a composition much closer to that of plasma, Hamburger ascertained using in vitro red cell lysis experiments that 0.9% was the NaCl concentration that was isotonic with human plasma. Therefore, 0.9% saline was not initially developed with the aim of in vivo administration, yet has entered widespread clinical use despite having a Na^+ and Cl^- concentration far in excess of that of plasma.[53] Its osmolarity, calculated as the sum of the solutes present, is slightly higher than that of plasma, although the osmolality (measured by freezing point depression) is 285 mOsm/kg, very similar to that of plasma. This discrepancy reflects the nonideal behavior of solutions. Both ions remain in the ECF after infusion, and it can be said to be isotonic—that is, of a similar *effective osmolarity* to that of plasma with respect to the cell membrane.

A 2-L infusion of 0.9% NaCl leads to an increase in ECF volume, dilutional decrease in hematocrit and albumin, increase in Cl^- and K^+ concentrations, and decrease in plasma HCO_3^-.[42] The expansion of the ECF is more persistent than with balanced crystalloid solutions. Although both fluids induce diuresis, 0.9% NaCl has a later onset and the excess salt and water load may take multiple days for even a healthy subject to excrete.[12]

A 0.9% NaCL infusion leads to a hyperchloremic metabolic acidosis and reduced renal perfusion. Although important differences in clinical outcomes in the surgical populations are not clear,[54] in the wider critical care population an increased incidence of kidney injury and requirement for renal replacement therapy are seen when compared with the use of lower Cl^- solutions.[46,55] In healthy volunteers, large-volume (50 mL/kg) saline infusions lead to abdominal discomfort, nausea, and vomiting.

These side effects mean that the volume of saline administered perioperatively should be limited, unless there are compelling indications such as the following:

- Situations in which increased plasma Na^+ may be beneficial, such as in the presence of cerebral edema.
- Preexisting Na^+ or Cl^- total body depletion, such as gastric outlet obstruction (see later discussion). However, 0.9% NaCl is not suitable for the treatment of acute severe hyponatremia, because it has little effect on plasma Na^+ levels in this situation.

TABLE 47.6 Composition of Fluids Available for Intravenous Administration*

Fluid	Sodium	Potassium	Chloride	Calcium	Magnesium	Bicarbonate	Lactate	Acetate	Gluconate	Glucose (g/L)$^{-1}$	Other	Osmolarity	Notes	pH (In Vitro)
Plasma	140	5	100	4.4	2	24	1	—	—	—	—	285	SID 42	7.4
0.9% NaCl	154	—	154	—	—	—	—	—	—	—	—	308	SID 0	6.0
1.8% NaCl	308	—	308	—	—	—	—	—	—	—	—	616		
0.45% NaCl	77	—	77	—	—	—	—	—	—	—		154		
5% dextrose	—	—	—	—	—	—	—	—	—	50		252		4.5
5% dextrose/0.45% NaCl	77	—	77	—	—	—	—	—	—	50		406		4.0
4% dextrose/0.18% NaCl	33	—	33	—	—	—	—	—	—	40		283		
Lactated Ringer solution (U.S. composition)	130	4	109	3	—	—	28	—	—	—		273		6.5
5% dextrose in lactated Ringer solution	130	4	109	3	—	—	28	—	—	50		525		5.0
Hartmann solution/compound Na$^+$ lactate	131	5	111	4	—	—	29	—	—	—		275	In vivo SID 27	6.5
Plasma-Lyte 148/ Normosol-R	140	5	98	—	3	—	—	27	23	—	—	294		4-6.5
Plasma-Lyte 56 and 5% dextrose/ Normosol M with 5% dextrose	40	13	40	—	3	—	—	16	—	50		389 / 363		3.5-6
Plasma-Lyte A pH 7.4	140	5	98	—	3	—	—	27	23	—	NaOH for pH	294		7.4
Sterofundin	140	4	127	5	2	—	—	24	—	—	Maleate 5	309		5.1-5.9
Plasma-Lyte R	140	10	103	5	3	—	8	47	—	—		312		
Hemosol	140	—	109.5	3.5	1	32	3	—	—	—			In vivo SID 33	
4%-5% albumin	†	—	†	—	—	—	—	—	—	—	Stabilizer: octanoate (caprylate)	†		7.4
20% albumin	†	—	†	—	—	—	—	—	—	—	Stabilizer: octanoate (caprylate)	†		
Plasmanate: Plasma protein fraction (human) 5%	145	0.25	100	—	—	—	—	—	—	—	88% human albumin, 12% α-/β-globulins		COP 20 mm Hg	7.4

Continued

TABLE 47.6 Composition of Fluids Available for Intravenous Administration*—cont'd

Fluid	Sodium	Potassium	Chloride	Calcium	Magnesium	Bicarbonate	Lactate	Acetate	Gluconate	Glucose $(g/L)^{-1}$	Other	Osmolarity	Notes	pH (In Vitro)
Gelofusine (4%)	154	—	125	—	—	—	—	—	—	—	MWw 30 kDa		Succinylated gelatin	
Plasmion/Geloplasma (3%)	150	5	100	—	3	—	30	—	—	—	MWw 30 kDa		Succinylated gelatin	
Isoplex (4%)	145	4	105	—	1.8	—	25	—	—	—	MWw 30 kDa		Succinylated gelatin	
Gelaspan (4%)	151	4	103	2	2	—	—	24	—	—	MWw 30 kDa			
Haemaccel (polygeline)	145	5.1	145	12.5	—	—	—	—	—	—	MWw 35 kDa			
Voluven: Waxy maize HES 6% (130/0.4)	154	—	154	—	—	—	—	—	—	—		308		
Venofundin: Potato HES 6% (130/0.42)	154	—	154	—	—	—	—	—	—	—				
Hetastarch: Waxy maize HES 6% (670/0.75)	154	—	154	—	—	—	—	—	—	—		309		5.5
Hextend: Waxy maize HES 6% (670/0.75)	143	3	124	5	1	—	28	—	—	—				
Pentaspan: Pentastarch 10%	154	—	154	—	—	—	—	—	—	—	MWw 264 kDa	326		5.0
Volulyte: Waxy maize HES 6% (130/0.4)	137	4	110	—	3	—	—	34	—	—		287		
Plasma volume: Potato HES 6% (130/0.42)	130	5.4	112	1.8	2	—	—	27	—	—				
Tetraspan: Potato HES 6% (130/0.42)	140	4	118	5	2	—	—	24	5	—				
10% Dextran 40	—	—	—	—	—	—	—	—	—	50		255		4.0

HES, Hydroxyethyl starch; *MWw,* weight-averaged mean molecular weight. Plasma-Lyte, PlasmaVolume, Baxter International, Deerfield, IL; Gelofusine, Gelaspan, Venofundin, Sterofundin, and Tetraspan, B Braun (Melsungen, Germany); Plasmion, Geloplasma, Voluven, and Volulyte, Fresenius-Kabi, Bad Homburg, Germany; Hextend, BioTime, Berkeley, Calif; Pentaspan from Bristol-Myers Squibb, Canada; Hemosol, Hospital, Rugby, United Kingdom.; Isoplex Beacon, Kent, United Kingdom; Normosol, Hospira, Lake Forest, IL.

*Presented as mEq/L, except where stated.

†The NaCl content and osmolarity of albumin solutions varies dependent on formulation. Osmolarity values are calculated in vitro.

Hypertonic Saline. Solutions of 1.8%, 3%, and 7.5% NaCl are available. Their uses include:

Plasma volume expansion: The hypertonic nature of these solutions draws water out of the intracellular compartment and into the extracellular (including plasma) volume and may therefore achieve plasma volume expansion while minimizing the volume of fluid administered. Although it has not been studied extensively, use of hypertonic saline for trauma resuscitation, particularly in the prehospital phase, has not shown convincing benefit. In fact, one large trial showed no improvement in outcome and was stopped early.[56]

- Correction of hypoosmolar hyponatremia (see later discussion)
- Treatment of increased intracranial pressure: The increased plasma osmolality reduces cerebral edema and decreases intracranial pressure. Hypertonic saline may be superior to mannitol in this regard.[57] However, hypertonic saline used early in traumatic brain injury without knowledge of intracranial pressure has not been shown to be beneficial in clinical trials.[58]

At NaCl concentration greater than 7.5%, these solutions may cause endothelial damage; indeed, 11.7% NaCl may be used as a sclerosant agent and should therefore be administered into a central vein.

Balanced Crystalloid Solutions

Intravenous crystalloid solutions were initially used clinically for the management of cholera in 1832 by O'Shaughnessy and Latta. The early solutions were more closely matched to physiologic plasma composition than NaCl solutions and contained 134 mEq/L Na^+, 118 mEq/L Cl^-, and 16 mEq/L HCO_3^-.[53] However, clinical interest in more balanced solutions waned until Hartmann in 1932 used a lactated modification of Ringer solution for pediatric patients with acidosis associated with hypovolemia and liver and renal failure.[59] By this time, NaCl solutions were already in use for resuscitation from hemorrhage and trauma.[53]

Currently available balanced crystalloid solutions have lower overall osmolarity than 0.9% NaCl, with a lower Na^+ concentration and much lower Cl^- concentration (see Table 47.6). The reduction in anionic content is compensated for by the addition of stable organic anionic buffers such as lactate, gluconate, or acetate. The measured osmolality of balanced solutions (265 mOsm/kg) is slightly lower than that of plasma, and they are therefore mildly hypotonic. Fluid compartment distribution of balanced solutions is resembles that of other crystalloids. After administration, the buffer is metabolized to produce HCO_3^- in equimolar quantities by entry into the citric acid cycle. Lactate undergoes predominantly hepatic oxidation or gluconeogenesis to yield HCO_3^- at a maximum rate of approximately 200 mmol/h.[60] Acetate is normally present in trace quantities in the plasma (0.2 mM), because it is rapidly oxidized by liver, muscle, and heart to yield HCO_3^- at a maximum turnover of 300 mmol/h, beyond which zero-order kinetics intervene.[61] A small proportion may be converted to the acetoacetate. The metabolism of gluconate is less well characterized in terms of location and kinetics, but it is converted to glucose with subsequent entry into the citric acid cycle.[62] Although balanced crystalloids can be constituted with HCO_3^- as a main anion, this is limited by two factors. First, HCO_3^- reacts with water to form CO_2, which can diffuse out of most packaging materials. This has been addressed by some products, although availability is limited.[63,64] Second, the pH shift induced by the presence of HCO_3^- can lead to precipitation of Ca^{2+} (and Mg^{2+}) if present.

The excretion of the excess water and electrolyte load with balanced crystalloids is more rapid than with isotonic saline.[65] This is due to the transient decrease in plasma tonicity after infusion, which suppresses ADH secretion and allows diuresis in response to the increased intravascular circulating volume. Balanced crystalloids do not reduce plasma SID to the same degree as NaCl solutions and therefore do not cause an acidosis; HCO_3^- concentration is maintained or slightly elevated.

Some potential negative effects have been identified with balanced crystalloid solutions. Lactated Ringer solutions contain racemic (D- and L-) lactate, although D-lactate is only found in trace quantities in vivo. Concerns that large doses of D-lactate may be associated with encephalopathy and cardiac toxicity in patients with renal failure[66,67] have not been confirmed in human studies at plasma levels achievable with racemic lactated Ringer solution. The metabolism of D-lactate appears to be nearly as rapid as that of L-lactate.[68] The reliance on hepatic metabolism of most of the infused lactate means that lactated solutions should be avoided in severe liver failure. Concerns over the negative effects of excess exogenous acetate have been raised in patients receiving dialysis with an acetate-based dialysate. The proinflammatory, myocardial depressant, vasodilatory, and hypoxemia-promoting effects of high acetate levels manifest as nausea, vomiting, headaches, and cardiovascular instability and have led to the removal of acetate from contemporary dialysis fluids.[61,69–73] Acetate turnover is limited in patients with end-stage kidney disease and by the presence of other substrates for oxidation—for example, during lactic acidosis or proteolysis. It is therefore possible that critically ill patients or those with advanced kidney disease may exhibit biochemical acetate intolerance, although this possibility has not been explored in patients receiving acetate-based balanced crystalloids. Unlike acetate, much less is known about the effects of gluconate-containing fluids.[74] Indeed, this area requires investigation at a cellular, organ, and whole organism level, particularly because data in animal studies suggest poorer outcome and late increases in lactate in a hemorrhage model when acetate/gluconate-containing crystalloids are compared to lactated Ringer solution or isotonic saline for resuscitation.[75]

Dextrose Solutions

Dextrose solutions have the following two main indications in the perioperative setting:

1. As a source of free water: An infusion of 5% dextrose effectively represents administration of free water. The in vitro osmolality resembles that of plasma so the infusion does not lead to hemolysis, but soon after administration, the dextrose is taken up into cells in the presence of insulin, leaving free water. These solutions are therefore hypotonic with respect to the cell membrane and

in excess can dilute plasma electrolytes and osmolality. They should therefore be used with care in the postoperative period, during which the relative syndrome of inappropriate secretion of antidiuretic hormone (SIADH) leads to water retention, increasing the risk for hyponatremia (see later discussion). Nevertheless, in carefully controlled volumes and with regular monitoring of serum electrolytes, they are a useful source of free water for maintenance requirements postoperatively, particularly if combined with a low concentration of NaCl. Dextrose solutions are less suitable for intravascular plasma volume expansion, because water can move between all fluid compartments, and a very small volume remains in the intravascular space.

2. Source of metabolic substrate: Although the caloric content of 5% dextrose is inadequate to maintain nutritional requirements, higher concentrations are adequate as a metabolic substrate, such as 4000 kCal/L for 50% glucose. Glucose solutions also may be coadministered with IV insulin to diabetic patients to reduce the risk for hypoglycemia, such as 10% dextrose at 75 mL/h.

COLLOIDS

Colloid is defined as large molecules or ultramicroscopic particles of a homogeneous noncrystalline substance dispersed in a second substance, typically isotonic saline, or a balanced crystalloid. These particles cannot be separated out by filtration or centrifugation. Although not all solutions are available in all countries, those in production include semisynthetic colloids and human plasma derivatives. Semisynthetic colloids have a range of molecular sizes (polydispersed) in contrast to human albumin solution, which contains more than 95% albumin molecules of a uniform size (monodispersed). Colloid molecules above 70 kDa are too large to pass through the endothelial glycocalyx and are excluded from the subglycocalyx layer, so their initial volume of distribution is the plasma (rather than the entire intravascular) volume (see discussion of vascular endothelium). In contrast to pure electrolyte solutions, colloids have a higher COP and minimize transcapillary filtration, particularly at low capillary hydrostatic pressures. This maximizes their potential intravascular plasma volume expansion effect. However, at normal or supranormal capillary pressures, hydrostatic pressure will be increased and transcapillary filtration will occur.[3] In addition, colloid molecules may be lost from circulation in several ways—by filtration across capillaries whose barrier function is impaired by glycocalyx shedding or endothelial cell pore formation in inflammation or other stressors, by renal filtration of smaller colloid molecules, or by removal from the circulation by metabolism. Therefore, colloids have variable effective plasma half-lives, as outlined later. Colloids alter blood rheology, improving blood flow by hemodilution which leads to reductions in plasma viscosity and red cell aggregation.[52] In contrast to their beneficial effects, the introduction of a large dose of semisynthetic molecules (typically 40-60 g/L) to a complex physiologic system may bring a variety of undesired effects on the immune, coagulation, and renal systems. To limit these toxicities, maximum dosages are recommended for most colloids, but adverse effects may still occur with lower doses. As the potential clinical relevance of toxicity is highlighted by large clinical trials, the use of colloids, at least in critical care, deserves increasing caution.[76] Whether these trials in critical care can be applied to the entire perioperative period has not been established. The evolving evidence base on the differential effects of isotonic saline or balanced crystalloid is also likely to focus more attention on the carrier solute used in colloids.

Semisynthetic Colloids

Gelatins. Gelatins are derived from the hydrolysis of bovine collagen, with subsequent modification by succinylation (Gelofusine, B Braun, Bethlehem, Pa; Geloplasma®, Fresenius, Waltham, MA) or urea-linkage to form polygeline (Haemaccel, Piramal, Orchard Park, NY). These forms have a similar molecular weight (MW), but the succinylated version undergoes conformational change as a result of increased negative charges, such that it is a larger molecule. The wide range of MWs means that much of an infused gelatin bolus will rapidly leave the circulation, predominantly by renal filtration. Despite this, a recent study suggests that 60 minutes after the end of infusion, 50% of the infused fluid volume remains in the intravascular space, similar to larger MW colloids.[77] Excretion is primarily by the renal route. In terms of negative effects, the gelatins have the least impact on clinically relevant hemostasis of all the semisynthetic colloids despite reductions in von Willebrand factor (vWF), factor VIIIc, and ex vivo clot strength,[78] but the highest estimated incidence of severe anaphylactic and anaphylactoid reactions (<0.35%).[52] The high Ca^{2+} content of Haemaccel is a contraindication to coadministration of citrated blood products in the same infusion set. No known cases of variant Creutzfeldt-Jakob disease transmission have occurred involving pharmaceutical gelatin preparations. Gelatins are commonly used in perioperative practice in Europe but are not approved by the U.S. Food and Drug Administration.

Hydroxyethyl Starches. Hydroxyethyl starches (HESs) are modified natural polymers of amylopectin derived from maize or potato. Substitution of hydroxyethyl radicals onto glucose units prevents rapid in vivo hydrolysis by amylase, and the degree of substitution both in terms of hydroxyethyl substitutions per glucose unit (maximum three) and total number of glucose units with substitutions is a determinant of HES elimination kinetics. The degree of substitution (DS) is expressed as the number of substituted glucose molecules present divided by the total number of glucose molecules present. An alternative measure of substitution is the molar substitution (MS) ratio, calculated as the total number of hydroxyethyl groups present divided by the quantity of glucose molecules. MS is used to define starches as hetastarches (MS 0.7), hexastarches (MS 0.6), pentastarches (MS 0.5), or tetrastarches (MS 0.4). The pattern of substitution may vary because hydroxyethylation can occur at carbon positions 2, 3, or 6 of the glucose unit. The substitution type is defined by the C2/C6 hydroxyethylation ratio, and a higher ratio leads to slower starch metabolism. Starches are also classified by in vitro MW into high (450-480 kDa), medium (200 kDa), and low (70 kDa). However, HES solutions are very polydispersed and the MW quoted is an average. The size of starch molecule is responsible for both the therapeutic volume effects and adverse side effects. After administration, smaller HES molecules (<50-60 kDa) are rapidly excreted and larger molecules are hydrolyzed to form a greater number of smaller molecules at a rate depending on the degree of substitution and C2/C6 hydroxyethylation ratio. The in vivo MW is therefore smaller and has a narrower distribution.[79] Ongoing renal excretion accounts for the elimination of smaller HES molecules, with medium-sized molecules being excreted in the bile and feces. A proportion of larger molecules, particularly those resistant to hydrolysis, is taken up by the mononuclear phagocyte (reticuloendothelial) system, where they may persist for several weeks or more.[80] The prolonged metabolism of HES means that their plasma volume effects typically last longer than those of gelatins or crystalloids. Larger MW starches can increase intravascular volume by approximately 70% to 80% of the infused dose even at 90 minutes.[81] Smaller MW starches with a low MS may have even larger volume effects as a result of the rapid initial metabolism with the formation of a large number of oncotically active molecules,[82] but studies in healthy human volunteers suggest only a similar volume effect to that of gelatins.[77]

For all fluids in this category, starch-related side effects have been associated with adverse outcomes in critical illness. Problems such as coagulopathy, accumulation, and renal dysfunction initially appeared to be related to larger MW starches, but now smaller tetrastarches are a concern as well. Despite this, study populations with critical illness, particularly sepsis, cannot be compared directly with elective perioperative patients. These trials should be interpreted with caution when considering the relevance of HES to surgical patients. Nevertheless, the official recommendations against the use of HES are clearly negative.

Coagulation. As with other synthetic colloids, HES products affect coagulation through dilutional effects in the circulation and MW-dependent reductions in vWF, factor VIII, and clot strength. The effect is most likely to occur with larger MW or slowly degraded medium MW (200 kDa/MS 0.62 or 200 kDa/MS 0.5/C2:C6 13) HES preparations and larger amounts of perioperative blood loss. This clinical effect is less marked with more rapidly degraded medium and small MW starches.[52] In patients with sepsis, even lower MW HES is associated with an increased risk of bleeding and blood transfusion, but it is unclear whether this also occurs in the perioperative setting.[83,84]

Accumulation. The accumulation of HES molecules in the mononuclear phagocyte system and skin, liver, muscle, and gut is a dose-dependent effect that gradually decreases over time. However, the accumulation may persist for several years, and larger amounts of tissue deposition are associated with pruritus.[80]

Anaphylactoid Reactions. The estimated incidence of severe anaphylactoid or anaphylactic reactions with HES products is less than with other colloids (<0.06%).[52]

Renal Dysfunction. HES products with medium-to-high MW are associated with oliguria, increased creatinine, and acute kidney injury in critically ill patients with preexisting renal impairment.[6,85] Although newer solutions with low MW (130 kDa/MS 0.4) were initially thought to be safer in this respect, recent large-scale trials have shown a similar effect on the need for renal replacement therapy in severe sepsis, particularly when compared with balanced crystalloids.[83,84] A recent large trial in a mixed critical care population comparing HES with isotonic saline also reported an increase in renal replacement therapy with the starch solution. This study is more difficult to interpret, given the potential renal effects of saline, and, as with previous studies, the possibility that patients were given study fluids after partial resuscitation had already been achieved.[51] Currently, no similar data are available from large-scale studies on the intraoperative use of HES solutions, and a recent meta-analysis examining perioperative use of 6% HES concluded that although no increase in mortality or kidney injury was seen, the available evidence lacked statistical power to definitively answer this question.[86] Meanwhile, the use of starch-based colloids has been restricted or even completely suspended by regulatory authorities in both the United States and Europe.

Dextrans. Dextrans are highly branched polysaccharide molecules produced by the bacterium *Leuconostoc mesenteroides* after conversion of sucrose in the growth medium by bacterial dextran sucrase. The large-MW dextrans produced undergo acid hydrolysis to yield smaller MW molecules, which are then separated by fractionation to produce a solution with a restricted range of MWs. Available dextrans have an average MW of 40 kDa or 70 kDa. As with other colloids, the polydisperse nature of dextran solutions means that a proportion of smaller MW molecules are present that are rapidly filtered at the glomerulus; 70% of a dextran dose is renally excreted within 24 hours. Higher MW molecules are excreted into the GI tract or taken up into the mononuclear phagocyte system, where they are degraded by endogenous dextranases.[52] Dextrans have a plasma volume effect similar to that of starches, with a duration of 6 to 12 hours. In addition to their use in volume expansion, dextran 40 may be used in microvascular surgery, where its dilutional effects on blood viscosity and anticoagulant effects (see later discussion) favor flow in the microcirculation. Overall, the use of dextrans is limited by their range of toxicities.

Antithrombotic effect: This is particularly marked in lower MW dextrans and is mediated through a range of mechanisms, including red cell coating and inhibition of aggregation, factor VIIIc and vWF reductions, and impaired activity of factor VIII. Platelet aggregation is also inhibited. The result is clinically impaired hemostasis and increased perioperative blood loss.[78]

- Blood cross-matching: Dextrans coat the erythrocyte cell membrane and may interfere with blood type cross-matching.
- Anaphylactoid reactions: Dextrans have an intermediate risk for serious anaphylactic and anaphylactoid reactions (<0.28%). Preemptive treatment with dextran 1, a hapten inhibitor, may reduce this incidence to less than 0.0015%.[52]
- Renal dysfunction: Renal dysfunction resulting from osmotic nephrosis is recognized after low-MW dextran infusion,[87] although the true incidence of this phenomenon in perioperative patients is difficult to estimate

because of the limited use of dextrans in contemporary practice.

Human Plasma Derivatives

The human plasma derivatives include human albumin solutions, plasma protein fractions, fresh frozen plasma, and immunoglobulin solution. Preparation techniques result in relatively purified solutions with the elimination of infective agents, although the theoretic risk for transmission of variant Creutzfeldt-Jakob disease and associated bovine spongiform encephalopathy remains. One U.K. case of presumed prion transmission has been described in association with factor VIII transfusion, although without clinical manifestation.[88] The ongoing transmission risk has been mitigated by sourcing many plasma derivatives from non-U.K. sources.

Solutions such as 5% albumin have a near-physiologic COP of 20 mm Hg and are used for volume expansion. Despite the association of hypoalbuminemia with worse outcomes from critical illness, the administration of exogenous albumin does not improve outcome in these situations. Early concerns that resuscitation with albumin may actually increase mortality in critical illness were not confirmed by a large controlled trial that found no difference in outcomes whether albumin or isotonic saline was used for resuscitation.[5] In this heterogeneous population, the albumin group required less fluid to attain similar endpoints (ratio 1:1.4), although in the subgroup of patients with trauma, and particularly brain injury, albumin may be associated with an increased incidence of mortality.[5,89] Conversely, in a subgroup analysis of patients with sepsis, albumin administration trended toward a decreased frequency of mortality that was supported by a subsequent meta-analysis.[90]

Clinical Fluid and Electrolyte Management

PATHOPHYSIOLOGIC FLUID ALTERATIONS IN THE PERIOPERATIVE PHASE

Before recommending practical approaches to administering fluid in the perioperative phase, it is important to consider the pathophysiologic processes, which affect not just the body's requirement for exogenous fluid and electrolytes but also the manner by which fluids are distributed by the body. The patient may enter the perioperative phase with abnormalities of intravascular fluid volume and distribution. Subsequent trauma (including surgery) induces a range of evolutionarily conserved neurohumoral and inflammatory changes, termed the stress response, which may have a significant impact on fluid and electrolyte responses and distribution. When the stress response is of an appropriate magnitude and duration, it can be a beneficial process for recovery from trauma; however, it could become pathologic if it is either exaggerated or prolonged or presents a physiologic burden to patients with limited baseline physiologic reserves.

Preoperative

Patients may enter the perioperative phase with established derangements of fluid and electrolyte balance. Hepatic, renal, and cardiac dysfunction are all associated with disordered Na^+ distribution (see later discussion), which has profound secondary effects on ECF volume. Patients with end-stage renal disease depend on dialysis for fluid removal, and the timing of dialysis relative to surgery is critical. Chronic treatment with diuretics may also lead to electrolyte depletion. Depending on the treatment, hypertensive patients may have a volume-contracted circulation, making them prone to intraoperative hypovolemia.

The effects of preoperative fasting also should be considered, although its influence on fluid balance has perhaps been overstated. Modern perioperative practice mandates cessation of oral fluids only 2 hours before elective surgery, and overnight fasting usually does not result in changes to normal blood volume when measured using robust experimental techniques.[91] Conversely, bowel preparation can cause a weight loss of 1.5 to 1.7 kg[92,93] with a high water and K^+ content. The potentially deleterious effects of this should be limited by restricting bowel preparations when possible and compensating for fluid loss with simultaneous IV infusion of 1 to 2 L of crystalloid with K^+ supplementation, which can improve hemodynamics and lower serum creatinine.[93]

More severe disturbances of fluid and electrolyte balance can occur in patients presenting with acute disease requiring surgical intervention:

- Direct intravascular depletion from bleeding.
- Loss of fluid from the GI tract. This results in ECF depletion and loss of electrolytes, depending on the GI tract location. Excess gastric loss because of obstruction, vomiting, or excess nasogastric suction results in loss of Na^+, K^+, Cl^-, and acid. Loss of small bowel secretions results in high losses of Na^+, Cl^-, and HCO_3^- with lesser K^+ losses. Large bowel losses, such as in diarrhea, deplete large quantities of K^+ with lesser losses of Na^+ and HCO_3^-. Pathologic fluid sequestration within the bowel lumen may have similar effects without external signs of fluid loss.
- Inflammation-related redistribution from the intravascular to the extracellular compartment (see later discussion).
- Fluid sequestration in the physiologic third space, with edema, pleural effusions, and ascites.

Intraoperative

Many factors influence intraoperative fluid balance, such as:

- Altered distribution of intravascular volume. Anesthetic agents lead to vasodilation, which can affect both the venous and arterial systems and may reduce cardiac preload and afterload. This reduction may be exacerbated by sympathetic blockade caused by central neuraxial blockade, and cardiac output may also be decreased by the negative inotropic effect of anesthetic drugs. The distribution of blood within the vascular system is also influenced by the differential blunting of autoregulatory responses within organ beds caused by anesthesia. Microcirculatory dysfunction related to the effects of anesthesia and the inflammatory response to surgery may result in impaired functional matching of local O_2 delivery with tissue O_2 requirements, which may not be responsive to intravascular fluid therapy.

- Direct loss of intravascular volume from hemorrhage. The clinical manifestation of surgical blood loss may vary greatly depending on the volume and time course of the blood loss.
- Insensible losses. The opening of anatomic compartments leads to evaporative fluid loss from mucosal surfaces, although estimating the extent of this loss may be difficult. Humidity chamber studies indicate that the loss may be as little as 1 mL/kg/h even during a major laparotomy with extensive bowel exposure.[94]
- Inflammation-related redistribution. Major surgery induces an inflammatory response that redistributes fluid from the intravascular to the extracellular compartment. This typically manifests in the postoperative phase (see later discussion), although it may become clinically apparent intraoperatively during surgery of sufficient magnitude and duration.
- Renal output. The suppression of renal urine production is related to perioperative ADH secretion and may also be influenced by the effects of positive-pressure ventilation. Increased intrathoracic pressure reduces venous return and cardiac output, which combine with a variety of neurohumoral responses such as sympathetic activation and suppression of ANP release to decrease GFR and urine output.[95] As a result, intraoperative urine output may be low regardless of the volume of IV fluid administered.[96]

The early phase of the stress response is triggered during major surgery. Absolute or relative (redistributive) hypovolemia during the intraoperative phase invokes a range of conservative responses—described in the section on Acute Disturbances in Circulating Volume—that are aimed at redistributing blood away from the periphery and toward vital organs and maintaining circulating volume by retaining salt and water. The tissue trauma of surgery also triggers a well-described inflammatory and immune response, and together these changes may persist into the postoperative phase. The inflammatory response elicited by tissue trauma may be aggravated by periods of hypotension and tissue hypoperfusion.

Postoperative

As a result of the preoperative and intraoperative factors outlined previously, patients may start the postoperative phase with significant derangements of intravascular volume and fluid compartment distribution. The stress response triggered by surgery may also have an ongoing influence on postoperative fluid balance.

Inflammation and Immune Response. Tissue injury leads to local vasodilation, increased endothelial permeability, and influx of leukocytes to the damaged area, with consequent production of proinflammatory cytokines for up to 72 hours, particularly interleukin-1 (IL-1), TNF-α, and IL-6. Cardiopulmonary bypass, extensive tissue trauma, or surgery in areas with subclinical preoperative inflammation, such as tumor or infection, may lead to a postoperative systemic inflammatory response syndrome (SIRS). An alternative trigger for SIRS is GI hypoperfusion. The physiologic response to hypovolemia is preservation of cardiac and brain perfusion at the expense of kidney, gut, and peripheral perfusion. The intestinal villi have a countercurrent blood supply that shunts blood away from the mucosa in this situation, leading to mucosal necrosis and further impairment of gut barrier function by luminal digestive enzymes and bacteria. This allows gut bacterial endotoxin to translocate into the systemic circulation, acting as a potent trigger for systemic inflammation.[97,98] The reactive O_2 species released on reperfusion of compromised bowel further aggravate the inflammatory cascade.

Systemic inflammation impairs endothelial barrier function through changes in endothelial cell phenotype, increases in endothelial large pores, and degradation of the endothelial glycocalyx.[2] Hypervolemia caused by excessive fluid infusion leads to the release of cardiac natriuretic peptides, which may further degrade the endothelial glycocalyx.[9,99] In severe cases, inflammation-related endothelial dysfunction leads to a capillary leak syndrome, with loss of water, electrolytes, and proteins into the interstitial space causing edema in the lungs, bowel, and connective tissue. Reduced plasma oncotic pressure facilitates ongoing capillary fluid filtration into the extravascular space and consequent hypovolemia.

Catabolic Metabolism. The response to tissue injury requires an increase in energy substrate delivery, particularly to leukocytes involved in the acute inflammatory and immune reaction. This metabolic shift is mediated by catecholamine and cortisol release and involves muscle protein catabolism, with associated hepatic gluconeogenesis and acute phase protein production, and increased substrate delivery to damaged tissues. An increase in basal metabolic rate and adequate circulating volume are required to meet the needs of increased fuel mobilization, processing, and delivery.

Regulation of Salt and Water Balance. As described in the section on physiologic control of overall fluid balance, ADH release is induced during surgery, leading to postoperative retention of water. This may be a direct result of the acute stress response, and IL-6 has been proposed as a key mediator.[100] In addition, periods of hypovolemia and hypotension further stimulate ADH release and activate the RAA system with further water and salt retention and amplified ADH production. This may lead to a temporary period of oliguria despite a restored circulating volume and the risk for postoperative fluid overload and sodium fluctuations. Na^+ retention postoperatively is more pronounced in the hypercatabolic state after major surgery, as excess nitrogen competes with Na^+ for renal excretion.

In addition to these processes, fluid may be lost from the circulating volume as a result of reaccumulation into third spaces drained intraoperatively (ascites or pleural effusions), sequestration into the bowel lumen or removal through vomiting, nasogastric drainage, or stoma losses. Intravascular fluid *distribution* is also a dynamic situation postoperatively because of changes in vascular tone caused by rewarming, evolving epidural sympathetic blockade, or systemic inflammation.

ASSESSMENT AND TREATMENT OF PERIOPERATIVE FLUID AND ELECTROLYTE IMBALANCE

Intravascular Volume

As a key variable influencing cardiac output (preload), and therefore tissue O_2 delivery, intravascular volume is at the core of adequate tissue perfusion. Although the assessment of intravascular volume is an important part of perioperative fluid therapy, it may be challenging. Clinical history suggesting abnormal volume status should be sought (see earlier discussion) and accompanied by frequent clinical examinations, although many of the conventional markers of volume status are not reliable when taken in isolation. Obvious hypovolemia may manifest with tachycardia, reduced pulse pressure, hypotension, and increased capillary refill time, but the abnormalities of these individual physiologic variables may have numerous causes in the perioperative phase. Conversely, loss of up to 25% of blood volume may not be accompanied by significant hemodynamic alterations in healthy patients.[101] Urine output, frequently taken as a measure of adequate end-organ perfusion, may also be reduced postoperatively, even in the presence of normal circulating volume, as a result of ADH and RAA activation. More invasive measures of intravascular volume also have limitations. CVP is used as a marker of central venous volume, but it is also influenced by venous compliance. CVP may be normal or high in venoconstricted states even when the absolute vascular volume is reduced. Furthermore, the relationship between right-heart and left-heart filling pressures is not reliable in the presence of cardiopulmonary pathologic processes. Trends in CVP values over time may be a more useful marker, because static CVP readings are poorly predictive of subsequent responses to intravascular fluid challenges.[102] Stroke volume (SV) and cardiac output may be measured using a variety of techniques, and targeting these variables has been widely investigated in perioperative fluid management, as described later. Alternatively, the adequacy of tissue perfusion may be assessed at a whole organism level using blood lactate concentrations, which may also be elevated during reperfusion of ischemic tissue or in advanced liver failure, or mixed venous O_2 saturation, which identifies a mismatch between global O_2 delivery (DO_2) and O_2 usage (VO_2). Techniques used to assess the perfusion of individual organs have the potential to detect clinically occult hypovolemia affecting those tissue beds or surgical sites most at risk for hypoperfusion, such as the gut. These include near-infrared spectroscopy,[103] microdialysis,[104] and GI CO_2 and pH measurement. The latter technique is gastric tonometry and is based on the association between inadequate gut perfusion and mucosal hypercarbia and acidosis.[105] It may detect hypovolemia of a magnitude not detectable by changes in systemic blood lactate, SV, or other cardiovascular parameters[101] that is nevertheless associated with increased postoperative morbidity.[106] Despite some encouraging findings in early research studies, none of these monitors is currently in routine use for guiding perioperative hemodynamic therapy.

Both excessive and inadequate intravascular volume can have adverse physiologic effects and achieving the fine balance between the two is a key goal of perioperative fluid administration. This concept of the "sweet spot" of fluid volume is backed up by large clinical datasets showing associations between both under- and over-resuscitation and postoperative morbidity.[107] Modest hypovolemia, through its effects on gut perfusion and stimulation of protective neurohumoral reflexes, may exacerbate the inflammatory and antidiuretic aspects of the surgical stress response. More severe hypovolemia reduces preload, cardiac output, and therefore DO_2. The result may be inadequate DO_2 to meet metabolic demands, with an increase in O_2 extraction ratio (reflected in reduced mixed venous O_2 saturation), progressing to inefficient anaerobic ATP production if mitochondrial oxidative phosphorylation cannot be sustained. This situation may be aggravated by insufficient compensatory increases in cardiac output, impaired microvascular blood flow, or failure of cellular O_2 usage. Lactate is a by-product of anaerobic metabolism and its accumulation leads to a metabolic acidosis. ATP production may be inadequate to support normal cell functions in tissues with poor perfusion, leading to cell death and organ dysfunction in the most extreme circumstances. Inadequate global O_2 delivery has been associated with a range of postoperative morbidities and increased mortality and has been the target of numerous clinical trials. At an individual organ level, specific areas that have been manipulated surgically, such as tissue flaps and bowel anastomoses, may be susceptible to poor healing and failure when local perfusion is insufficient.

Hypervolemia also has adverse effects and is often an iatrogenic problem in the perioperative setting. Crystalloids or colloids administered when capillary hydrostatic pressures are normal or increased lead to increased capillary filtration of fluid into the interstitial space. If this exceeds the capacity of the lymphatics to return the excess fluid to the circulation, edema will develop in compliant tissues such as the lungs, muscle, and bowel. The effect is more pronounced if inflammation or deterioration of the glycocalyx reduces the endothelial barrier function opposing the passage of large molecules into the interstitium. The correction of salt and water overload is a slow process because of inefficient renal handling of excess Na^+ loads, and the effects of postoperative ADH secretion. Clinically significant edema contributes to postoperative GI dysfunction, although this is not well defined by small clinical trials.[108,109] Further potential effects of excessive intravascular fluid include reduced tissue oxygenation with impaired healing, pulmonary congestion predisposing to pulmonary infection, and increased myocardial work resulting from ventricular filling beyond the optimum portion of the Starling curve.[110] Side effects may occur that are attributable to the amount of fluid given, such as hypercoagulability or hypocoagulability, hyperchloremic acidosis, or renal dysfunction. A positive fluid balance and weight gain in the early perioperative period increases postoperative morbidity.[111,112]

Electrolyte Imbalance

Sodium Disorders

HYPONATREMIA. Hyponatremia may be present preoperatively, develop as a consequence of perioperative events, or both. It is classified as mild (130-134 mEq/L), moderate (120-130 mEq/L), or severe (<120 mEq/L). Moderate-to-severe hyponatremia, particularly of acute onset, is associated with significant perioperative morbidity.

CAUSES. Assessment of serum osmolality, TBW status, and urinary Na^+ concentration is vital for the accurate diagnosis of the underlying cause of hyponatremia.[113,114] A diagnostic algorithm with common causes is shown in Fig. 47.3. Na^+ is normally the key determinant of serum osmolality, and hyponatremia is usually observed in conjunction with reduced osmolality. In some situations, however, osmolality is normal or raised by the presence of solutes that induce cellular dehydration and translocation of water from cells to

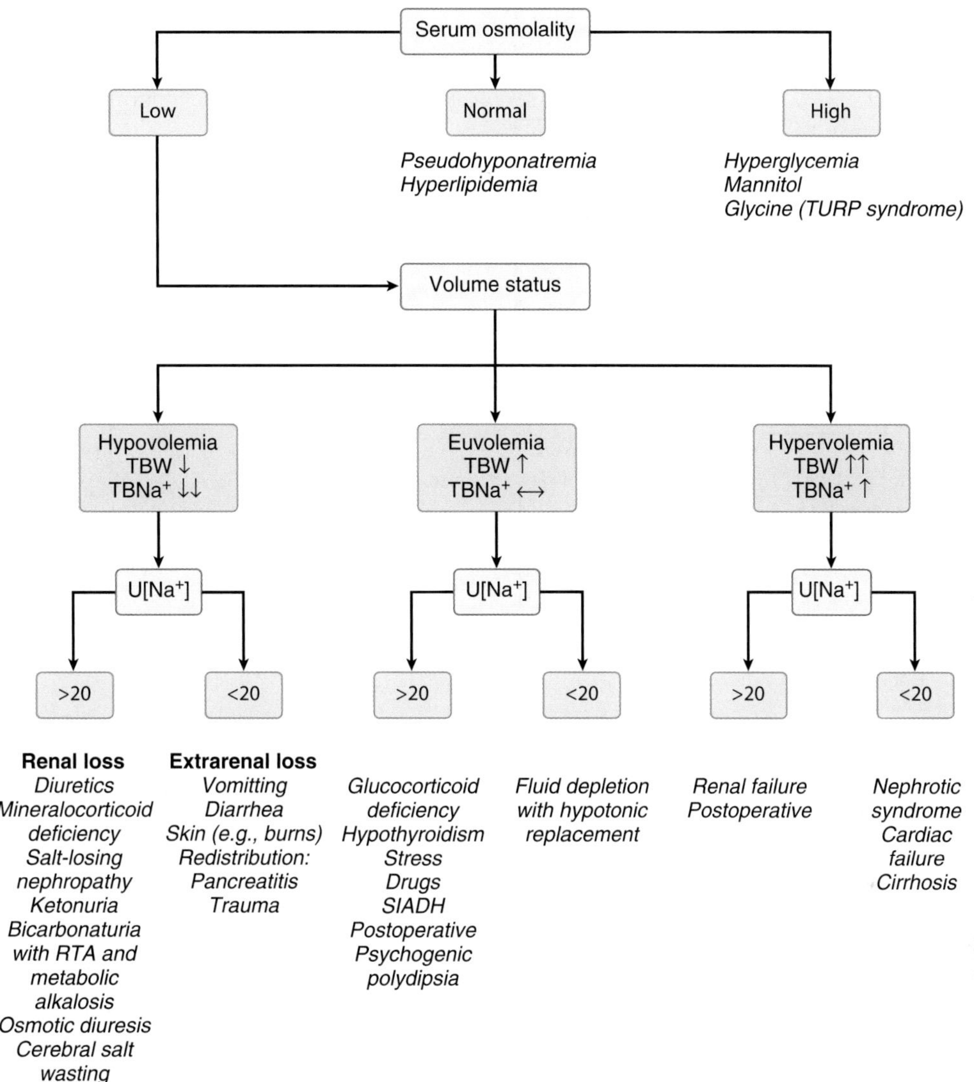

Fig. 47.3 Causes and diagnostic algorithm for hyponatremia. The diagnostic criteria for the syndrome of inappropriate antidiuretic hormone secretion *(SIADH)* include exclusion of adrenal, thyroid, and renal disease or diuretic usage, serum hypoosmolality (<270 mOsmol/kg), clinical euvolemia, increased urinary [Na^+] despite normal water and salt intake and inappropriate urinary concentration (>100 mOsmol/kg). A characteristic response to water restriction occurs, with a 2- to 3-kg fall in weight accompanied by a reduction in salt wasting over 2 to 3 days. *RTA,* Renal tubular acidosis; *TBW,* total body water; *TURP,* transurethral resection of the prostate; *U[Na⁺],* urinary sodium concentration in mEq/L. (Modified from Kumar S, Berl T. Sodium. *Lancet.* 1998;352:220; and Tisdall M, Crocker M, Watkiss J, et al. Disturbances of sodium in critically ill adult neurologic patients: a clinical review. *J Neurosurg Anesthesiol.* 2006;18:57.)

the ECF. These include glucose in the absence of adequate insulin, mannitol, maltose, and glycine. Alternatively, hyponatremia may be artifactual (pseudohyponatremia), caused by the presence of high lipid concentrations. In hypoosmolar hyponatremia, imbalanced gains or losses of TBW and Na^+ occur such that serum Na^+ concentration is reduced.

PREOPERATIVE HYPONATREMIA. Hyponatremia may be an incidental finding during preoperative assessment, with the underlying pathologic mechanisms identified in Fig. 47.3. Even mild preoperative hyponatremia is associated with increased 30-day mortality, major cardiac events, wound infection, and pneumonia.[115] Whether hyponatremia is a direct causal mechanism in postoperative adverse events or a marker of underlying overt or subclinical pathologic processes, such as cardiac failure, is not clear, although excess risk is seen even in American Society of Anesthesiologists (ASA) class 1 and 2 patients undergoing elective surgery. Interestingly, correcting preoperative hyponatremia does not clearly improve outcomes. The finding of preoperative hyponatremia should prompt a search for, and optimization of, potential underlying diseases. In moderate-to-severe hyponatremia, nonurgent surgery should probably be postponed to allow for gradual correction of hyponatremia (see later discussion).

POSTOPERATIVE HYPONATREMIA. As previously discussed, the surgical stress response, aggravated by periods of hypotension and pain-related or physiologic stress-related sympathetic activity, can lead to a state of Na^+ and water retention similar to SIADH. Avid water retention puts postoperative patients at risk for hyponatremia, particularly when administration of free water from IV dextrose-containing or other hypotonic solutions is ongoing. The incidence of postoperative hyponatremia is 1% to 5%, with children and premenopausal females at particularly high risk for neurologic

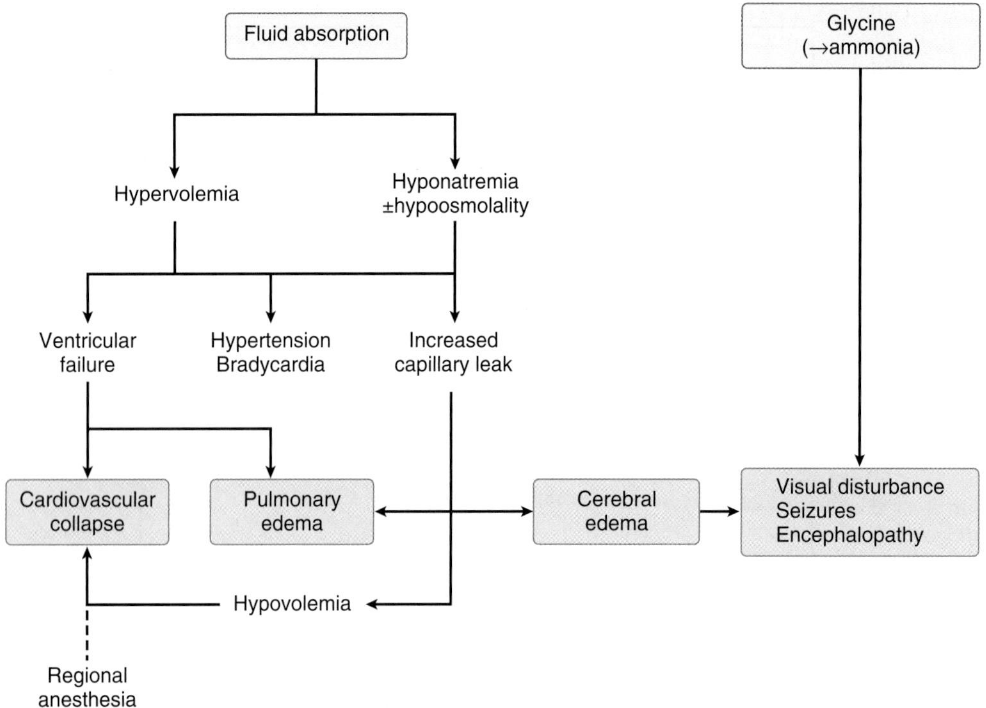

Fig. 47.4 The transurethral resection of the prostate (TURP) syndrome. Early hypervolemia-related hypertension may be followed by profound hypotension as a result of increased capillary filtration with hypovolemia, depressed cardiac function, and sympathetic blockade. Glycine itself may lead to seizures through allosteric activation of the *N*-methyl-D-aspartate receptor and is thought to cause the visual disturbance of the TURP syndrome. The hepatic deamination of glycine yields ammonia, which can further contribute to encephalopathy. (Modified from Gravenstein D. Transurethral resection of the prostate [TURP] syndrome: a review of the pathophysiology and management. *Anesth Analg.* 1997;84:438.)

symptoms. In these groups, symptoms and neurologic sequelae may occur at Na^+ levels as high as 128 mEq/L. Elderly women typically do not become symptomatic until 120 mEq/L, unless the decrease is particularly rapid. The potential impact of postoperative hyponatremia is considerable; 8% of hyponatremic patients may develop encephalopathy, of whom 52% suffer permanent neurologic sequelae or death.[116] Failure to recognize hyponatremia as a cause of postoperative symptoms (see later discussion) or inadequate treatment based on fears of causing osmotic demyelination may contribute to these poor outcomes.[117] Prevention of postoperative hyponatremia should be a key goal of postoperative fluid therapy, based on limiting free water administration to pure maintenance requirements (1-1.2 mL/kg/h), replacing losses of Na^+-containing fluids (e.g., GI) with an appropriate isotonic salt solution, stopping IV therapy as soon as the oral route can be used, and daily (or more frequent in high-risk groups) monitoring of serum electrolytes.

Transurethral Resection of the Prostate Syndrome. The transurethral resection of the prostate (TURP) syndrome describes symptomatic hyponatremia, excessive intravascular volume, and edema resulting from IV absorption of hypotonic nonconductive (electrolyte-free) irrigation fluid during TURP or, rarely, transurethral resection of the bladder[118] or during ureteroscopic or hysteroscopic procedures. The syndrome may complicate 10% to 15% of TURP procedures, with onset between 15 minutes and 24 hours after the onset of resection.[119] Risk factors include increased intravesical pressure, prolonged resection, hypotonic irrigants, and open prostatic sinuses. The clinical features (Fig. 47.4) are related to intravascular volume changes, hyponatremia, and absorption of irrigant solutes; the use of distilled water as an irrigant has largely been replaced by solutions of glycine, sorbitol, or mannitol because of the incidence of massive hemolysis. Hyponatremia resulting from free water absorption may lead to hypoosmolality, although the presence of glycine or other osmotically active solutes may maintain osmolality in the normal range. The following measures may help prevent the TURP syndrome:

- The use of conducting (isotonic saline) irrigant with bipolar diathermy.[120]
- Monitoring fluid absorption by comparing the amount instilled with the amount removed. Surgery should be halted if 750 mL (for females) or 1000 mL (for males) has been absorbed and the patient should be assessed for Na^+ levels and neurologic status (if awake). Surgery should be terminated if 1000 to 1500 mL (for females) or more than 2000 mL (for males) has been absorbed. If saline irrigant is used, surgery should be terminated after 2500 mL has been absorbed. Although the risk for hypoosmolar hyponatremia is removed, the risk for excessive intravascular volume remains.[121,122]
- Limiting the duration of irrigation: irrigation should continue only for longer than 1 hour after careful assessment of the patient for possible TURP syndrome.
- Limiting intravesical pressure to less than 15 to 25 mm Hg or 70 mm Hg for endometrial procedures.
- Monitoring the patient's neurologic status by using regional anesthetic techniques. Symptoms in the awake patient include nausea and vomiting, visual disturbance, reduced level of consciousness, agitation, confusion, and seizures.

Treatment of the TURP syndrome should take into account the patient's intravascular volume status, Na^+ level, and osmolality, but typically involves cessation of irrigation solutions and water restriction. A loop diuretic should be given to promote free water excretion if intravascular volume overload is present. In severe hypoosmolar hyponatremia with neurologic symptoms, hypertonic saline may be used. When osmolality is normal or marginally decreased, hemodialysis is preferred.[123] Mg^{2+} can be given for seizures, because its negative control of NMDA receptors counteracts dilutional hypomagnesemia and the excitatory effects of glycine.[119]

Presentation and Treatment of Hyponatremia. The symptoms of hyponatremia are related to cerebral edema and increased intracranial pressure and are highly dependent on how rapidly the hyponatremia occurred. In acute onset, symptoms typically occur when Na^+ concentrations are as low as 120 to 125 mEq/L (higher in children and premenopausal females) with headache, confusion, agitation, vomiting, and lethargy. At Na^+ concentrations less than 110 mEq/L, symptoms progress to seizures and coma. In the chronic setting, clinical features may be absent even at concentrations less than 120 mEq/L. In all cases of hyponatremia, potential underlying causes such as steroid deficiency, renal disease, and cardiac disease should be identified and treated. Treatment should be tailored to the patient's intravascular volume status, the chronicity of onset, and the presence of symptoms. Chronic hyponatremia (>48 hours or of unknown duration) should be treated cautiously because of cerebral compensation for the hypoosmolar state; sudden increases in osmolality lead to cerebral water loss and osmotic demyelination (e.g., central pontine myelinolysis). Treatment options for other scenarios are listed below:

- Hypovolemic hyponatremia: Symptoms are unusual because osmotic shifts in the brain are limited by the loss of both Na^+ and water. ECF volume should be restored with isotonic saline, which will also reduce ongoing ADH release.
- Hypervolemic hyponatremia: In chronic cases, this should focus on restriction of water intake and optimization of the underlying disease state, such as improving cardiac output with angiotensin-converting enzyme (ACE) inhibitors to reduce the neurohumoral influence on water retention in cardiac failure. Loop diuretics (rather than thiazides, which impair urinary dilution) can be used to excrete free water once a negative Na^+ balance has been achieved.
- Chronic, asymptomatic hyponatremia: No immediate correction of hyponatremia is required, and the underlying cause should be treated. Fluid restriction, ADH antagonists (lithium, demeclocycline), and loop diuretics may be used.
- Symptomatic hyponatremia (typically euvolemic or hypervolemic): In patients with moderate symptoms (confusion, lethargy, nausea, and vomiting), hypertonic 3% saline may be used at an initial rate of 1 mL/kg/h with the goal of increasing [Na^+] by 1 mEq/L/h for 3 to 4 hours, after which electrolytes should be rechecked. The infusion rate should be modified to ensure that [Na^+] is increased by no more than 10 mEq/L in the first 24 hours of treatment. Severely symptomatic hyponatremia (coma, seizures, often with [Na^+] <120 mEq/L) is typically of acute onset and the risks of undertreating are more than those of osmotic demyelination. A bolus of 100 mL of 3% saline should initially be given with the aim of acutely increasing [Na^+] by 2 to 3 mEq/L. If no improvement in neurologic status occurs, this approach may be repeated once or twice at 10-minute intervals. After this, treatment should continue as for moderately symptomatic patients, with a similar goal of increasing [Na^+] by no more than 10 mEq/L in the first 24 hours.[124] Electrolytes and osmolality should be rechecked every few hours, fluid balance should be carefully monitored, and patients reassessed regularly.

Hypernatremia. Hypernatremia ([Na] >145 mEq/L) is less common than hyponatremia but may affect up to 10% of critically ill patients. If severe ([Na] >160 mEq/L), a 75% mortality may occur depending on the severity of the underlying disease process (Fig. 47.5).[113,114] The major mechanisms are excessive water loss with inadequate compensatory intake, lack of ADH, or administration of exogenous sodium. Diabetes insipidus (DI) is caused by a lack of ADH action as a result of impaired production or release (central DI) or reduced renal sensitivity to ADH (nephrogenic DI) with consequent failure to concentrate urine and excretion of large quantities of inappropriately dilute urine. If the patient is unable to accept compensatory fluid orally (e.g., because of coma or in the elderly with impaired thirst reflexes), they may rapidly become hypovolemic. Central DI is seen after pituitary surgery, subarachnoid hemorrhage, traumatic brain injury (particularly skull base fractures), and brainstem death. Nephrogenic DI may be due to renal disease, electrolyte disorders, or drugs (lithium, foscarnet, amphotericin B, demeclocycline).

Clinical features of hypernatremia include altered mental status, lethargy, irritability, seizures, hyperreflexia, and spasticity. Diagnosis is based on assessment of intravascular volume status, urinary osmolality, and Na^+ concentration. In patients with persistent urine output of more than 100 mL/h and hypernatremia, DI should be considered. Diagnostic criteria include an inappropriately dilute urine (<300 mOsm/kg) in combination with hypernatremia and high serum osmolality (>305 mOsm/kg). Urine specific gravity (SG) may provide a rapid guide to urine osmolality where urgent treatment is being considered; urine SG less than 1.005 in the context of hypernatremia and a potential underlying cause is consistent with DI.

Treatment is tailored to the intravascular volume status, but as with hyponatremia, correction of the Na^+ concentration should be no more rapid than 10 mEq/L/day unless the onset has been very acute.

- Hypovolemic hypernatremia: correction of the intravascular volume deficit with isotonic saline and correction of the underlying cause (e.g., insulin to reduce hyperglycemia), then correction of the water deficit with 0.45% saline, 5% dextrose, or enteral water to cover the deficit and ongoing losses.
- Euvolemic hypernatremia: use of 0.45% saline, 5% dextrose, or enteral water to replace the deficit and ongoing losses. In central DI, in which urine output is greater than 250 mL/h and risk exists for hypovolemia, titrated

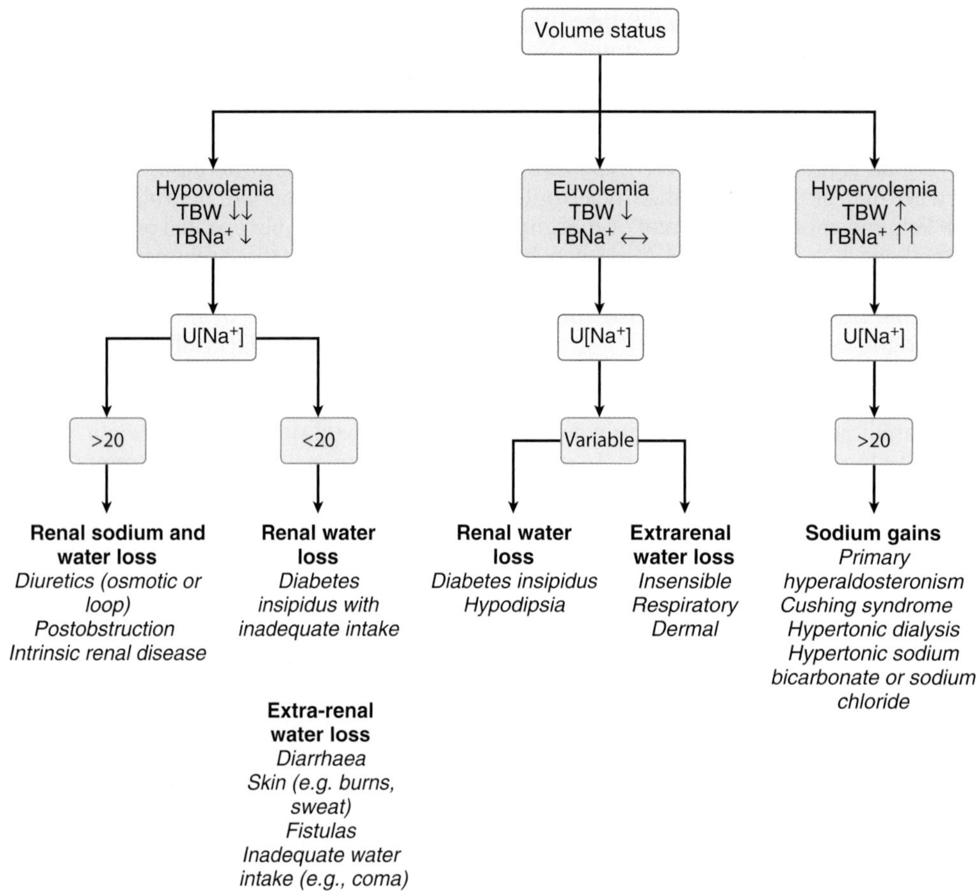

Fig. 47.5 Causes and diagnostic algorithm for hypernatremia. *TBW*, Total body water; *U[Na+]*, urinary sodium concentration in mEq/L. (Modified from Kumar S, Berl T. Sodium. *Lancet.* 1998;352:220.)

intravenous doses of desmopressin acetate 0.4 to 1 μg (1-deamino-8-D-arginine vasopressin [DDAVP], an ADH analogue) should be given to reduce the urine output. Higher acute doses may have a prolonged effect with the risk for water intoxication.[113,114]

- Hypervolemic hypernatremia: stop administration of exogenous Na^+, give furosemide with 5% dextrose or enteral water. Dialysis may be indicated in the presence of renal failure.

Potassium Disorders. Because of the key role of K^+ on excitable tissue resting membrane potential, dyskalemia can lead to life-threatening cardiac arrhythmias in the perioperative period. The normally predominant intracellular distribution of K^+ means that abnormal plasma K^+ levels may reflect abnormal ECF to ICF distribution, derangements of total body K^+ content, or both. Sampling artifacts may be introduced into laboratory tests of K^+; anticoagulated samples typically give results 0.4 to 0.5 mEq/L less than those from clotted samples because of erythrocyte K^+ release during clotting. Hemolysis also artificially increases K^+ levels and may be introduced by poor sampling technique or delayed processing of samples.

Hypokalemia. Hypokalemia (<3.5 mEq/L) may be caused by the conditions outlined in Table 47.7. Moderate-to-severe hypokalemia (2-2.5 mEq/L) leads to muscle weakness, electrocardiogram (ECG) abnormalities (ST segment depression, T wave depression, U wave elevation), and arrhythmias (atrial fibrillation and ventricular extrasystoles). All logic dictates that hypokalemia (e.g., as low as 2.6 mEq/L) should be associated with an increased rate of perioperative morbidity or mortality; however, no data support this conclusion.[18] Hypokalemia should be pragmatically corrected in the perioperative period to optimize neuromuscular function and reduce cardiac irritability. Such treatment is of prime importance when acute arrhythmias exist, and K^+ should be maintained at greater than 4 to 4.5 mEq/L. The speed of the infusion should be slow enough to allow equilibration throughout the entire ECF, typically no faster than 0.5 mEq/kg/h. K^+ solutions of concentration more than 40 mEq/L may be an irritant to veins and should be administered via a central venous catheter.

Hyperkalemia. Hyperkalemia (>5.5 mEq/L) may result from excess intake, failure of excretion, or shift from the intracellular to extracellular compartment (Table 47.8). Failure of renal secretion is mediated through impaired principal cell function in the cortical collecting duct, which depends on aldosterone-stimulated Na^+/K^+ exchange via basal Na^+/K^+ATPases and luminal Na^+ and K^+ channels. The features of hyperkalemia include muscle weakness, paralysis, and altered cardiac conduction (increased

TABLE 47.7 Causes and Mechanisms of Hypokalemia

Mechanism	Cause	Notes
Inadequate intake	Anorexia nervosa Alcoholism Malnutrition	
Gastrointestinal loss	Vomiting	
	Diarrhea	Especially secretory diarrhea
	Fistulas	
Excess renal loss	Mineralocorticoid excess	Primary and secondary hyperaldosteronism
	Glucocorticoid excess	High concentration of cortisol overwhelms mineralocorticoid receptor despite lower affinity
	Diuretics	Loop or thiazide diuretics deliver increased Na^+ load to principal cells
	Osmotic substances	Glucose, urea, and mannitol also lead to increased collecting duct Na^+ delivery
	Hypomagnesemia	Impairs thick ascending limb Na^+ reabsorption; therefore, increased distal N^+ delivery and K^+ loss via principal cells
	Renal tubular acidosis	Failure of principal cell H^+/K^+ exchange
	Bartter and Gitelman syndromes	Tubule ion transporter mutations mimicking loop or thiazide diuretic effect, respectively
Intracellular K^+ shift	β_2-Agonists	Also seen in sympathetic activity
	Insulin therapy Acute alkalosis Lithium overdose Hypokalemic periodic paralysis Vitamin B_{12} therapy	

Modified from Kaye AD, Riopelle JM. Intravascular fluid and electrolyte physiology. In: Miller RD, Eriksson LI, Fleisher LA, et al, eds. *Miller's Anesthesia.* 7th ed. New York: Churchill Livingstone; 2009:1705.

TABLE 47.8 Causes and Mechanisms of Hyperkalemia

Mechanism	Cause	Notes
Increased intake	Excessive K^+ treatment	
	Blood transfusion	Typically in patients who also have impaired excretion (i.e., severe chronic kidney disease)
	Antibiotics containing K^+ salts	
Failure of renal secretion	Mineralocorticoid deficiency	Hypoaldosteronism Hyporeninemic, hypoaldosteronemic state (diabetic nephropathy, tubulointerstitial disease)
	Drugs causing mineralocorticoid blockade	Spironolactone (blocks mineralocorticoid receptor) ACE-I and ARBs (reduce aldosterone production) Heparin (selective hypoaldosteronism)
	Collecting duct Na^+ channel blockade	Amiloride Trimethoprim Triamterene Pentamidine
	Tubulointerstitial nephritis Renal obstruction	Cause damage or destruction of the cortical collecting duct
Extracellular K^+ shift	Succinylcholine	
	Reperfusion of ischemic tissues	Cellular ischemia reduces ATP production with failure of Na^+/K^+ATPase activity and K^+ "leak" to the ECF. Cell lysis further releases K^+. On reperfusion, excess ECF K^+ is rapidly delivered to the systemic circulation. During solid organ transplantation, this may be combined with residual perfusing solution used for ex vivo organ preservation, which contains a high K^+ content
	Insulin deficiency Acute acidosis Malignant hyperpyrexia	

ACE-I, Angiotensin-converting enzyme inhibitor; *ARBs,* angiotensin II receptor blockers; *ATP,* adenosine triphosphate; *ECF,* extracellular fluid.

automaticity and enhanced repolarization) with consequent ECG changes as K^+ levels increase[125]:

- 5.5 to 6.5 mEq/L: tall, peaked T-waves
- 6.5 to 7.5 mEq/L: prolonged PR interval
- Greater than 7.5 mEq/L: widened QRS
- Greater than 9.0 mEq/L: sine wave pattern, bradycardia, ventricular tachycardia, increased risk for cardiac arrest

Chronically induced hyperkalemia (e.g., chronic renal failure) is better tolerated than acute increases in K^+ concentrations. Ratios between intracellular and extracellular K^+ concentrations may be very abnormal with acute hyperkalemia. With chronic hyperkalemia, these ratios are probably reestablished to normal. Acute hyperkalemia sufficient to induce electrocardiographic changes is a medical emergency that requires rapid treatment. The acute treatment of hyperkalemia involves shifting K^+ from the ECF to ICF, antagonizing its cardiac toxicity with Ca^{2+}, and increasing renal excretion. Elimination by GI resin exchange also may be used in more chronic cases (Table 47.9). Hyperkalemia greater than 6.5 mEq/L, in the context of anuric renal failure, is an indication for acute dialysis.

Calcium Disorders

HYPOCALCEMIA. The causes of hypocalcemia are related to reduced PTH and/or vitamin D activity, increased bone deposition, Ca^{2+} chelation, or changes in binding protein concentration or ionized fraction (Table 47.10). The

TABLE 47.9 Treatments for Hyperkalemia

Mechanism	Treatment	Indication	Notes
Antagonize cardiac toxicity	$CaCl_2$ 10% (10 mL) or Calcium gluconate	K^+ >6.5 mEq/L, particularly with ECG changes	Onset of action within a few minutes, duration 30-60 min
Intracellular potassium shift	Insulin 10-20 units (administered in 50 mL 50% glucose to avoid hypoglycemia)	K^+ >6.0 mEq/L	Onset within 10-20 min, duration 4-6 h
	β_2-Agonists (e.g., nebulized albuterol 2.5 mg)		
	Hyperventilation		Induce K^+ uptake by increasing extracellular pH
	$NaHCO_3$ 1 mEq/kg	K^+ >6.5 mEq/L	
Increase renal excretion	Furosemide 20-40 mg IV	Moderate-to-severe hyperkalemia	Increases Na^+ delivery to cortical collecting duct and exchange with K^+
	Volume expansion with isotonic saline		
	Fludrocortisone		Mineralocorticoid effect
Other routes of K^+ elimination	Gastrointestinal resin exchange: sodium polystyrene sulfonate (Kayexalate) 15-30 g PO or per rectum	Any sustained hyperkalemia	
	Hemodialysis	Moderate-to-severe hyperkalemia with oliguria	

Hyperkalemia can be defined as mild (5.5-5.9 mEq/L), moderate (6.0-6.4 mEq/L) or severe (>6.5 mEq/L), with or without ECG changes.[258]
ECG, Electrocardiogram.

TABLE 47.10 Causes and Mechanisms of Hypocalcemia

Mechanism	Cause	Notes
Reduced regulatory hormones	Hypoparathyroidism	Postparathyroid or thyroid surgery. May be acute effect of reduced PTH or more long-term hypocalcemia during remineralization of bone after surgery for hyperparathyroidism ("hungry bone syndrome")
		Hypomagnesemia (suppresses PTH secretion)
	Pseudohypoparathyroidism	Reduced receptor response to PTH
	Reduced vitamin D activity	Hyperphosphatemia (inhibits hydroxylation—e.g., in chronic kidney disease)
		Dietary/sunlight deficiency
		Anticonvulsants (increased turnover into inactive forms)
Ca^{2+} chelation	Massive transfusion	Caused by citrate in stored red blood cell solutions
	Cell lysis	Phosphate release as a result of tumor lysis syndrome, trauma, or rhabdomyolysis
	Pancreatitis	Intraperitoneal free fatty acids formed by the action of released pancreatic lipase, which chelate Ca^{2+} salts; further contributions from coexistent hypomagnesemia and hypoalbuminemia
Increased bone deposition	Prostate, breast cancer	Increased osteoclastic activity
Reduced ionized fraction	Alkalosis	For example, acute intraoperative hyperventilation
Reduced bound Ca^{2+}	Hypoalbuminemia	Critical illness (where ionized Ca^{2+} may be normal, and Ca^{2+} replacement not required), poor nutrition
Unknown mechanism	Endotoxemic shock	

PTH, Parathyroid hormone.

following are characteristic symptoms, some of which will be absent in the anesthetized patient:

- Neuromuscular irritability
  - Circumoral and peripheral paresthesia
  - Chvostek sign (facial twitching induced by tapping on the facial nerve)
  - Trousseau sign (forearm muscular spasm induced by inflating a pressure cuff)
  - Muscle cramps
  - Laryngospasm
  - Tetany
  - Seizures
- Cardiac
  - Impaired inotropy
  - Prolonged QT
  - Ventricular fibrillation
  - Heart block

After a rapid large volume transfusion of citrate-stored blood (>1.5 mL/kg/min) or fresh frozen plasma, ionized hypocalcemia may occur as a result of citrate chelation. This may be particularly severe and prolonged in patients with hepatic impairment, in whom citrate metabolism is reduced.[126] Citrate intoxication has been described for

TABLE 47.11 Causes and Mechanisms of Hypercalcemia

Mechanism	Cause	Notes
Increased PTH	Primary hyperparathyroidism	The most common cause typically manifests with mild hypercalcemia resulting from an isolated parathyroid adenoma
	Secondary and tertiary hyperparathyroidism	The hypocalcemia of kidney disease-related hyperparathyroidism may progress to hypercalcemia with prolonged disease
Malignancy	PTH-related peptide secretion	PTH-rP may be secreted by most solid tumors; mimics PTH effects
	Osteolytic metastases	Breast, lung, lymphoma, thyroid, kidney, prostate, and multiple myeloma
	Calcitriol production	Typical in lymphoma
Excess vitamin D	Ectopic production	Granulomatous disease (e.g., sarcoid), malignancy
	Excess intake	
Decreased renal excretion	Thiazide diuretics	
Increased bone turnover	Hyperthyroidism	
	Immobilization	
Increased Ca^{2+} intake	Milk-alkali syndrome	

PTH, Parathyroid hormone; *PTH-rP*, parathyroid hormone–related peptide.

many years but is rarely a clinical problem. Although Ca^{2+} plays an important role in coagulation, coagulopathy specifically attributable to hypocalcemia only occurs at ionized Ca^{2+} concentrations less than 1.2 mEq/L (0.625 mmol/L); rather, supplemental Ca^{2+} should be given in this situation to support cardiac inotropy and neuromuscular function, aiming for ionized Ca^{2+} more than 1.8 mEq/L (0.9 mmol/L).[127] Ca^{2+} also may be given during other situations in which myocardial contractility is impaired, such as during cardiac surgery, to optimize ventricular function. After parathyroidectomy, Ca^{2+} levels should be checked frequently until they have stabilized, because Ca^{2+} and vitamin D supplementation may be required in both the short and long term. In critical illness, total Ca^{2+} levels may be reduced because of hypoalbuminemia; however, Ca^{2+} supplementation should be required only if the ionized levels are low. Ca^{2+} may be given intravenously as 10% (weight/volume) calcium gluconate or 10% (weight/volume) $CaCl_2$. Although in these formulations calcium gluconate contains less elemental Ca^{2+} (0.45 mEq/mL vs. 1.36 mEq/mL for $CaCl_2$), they are equally efficacious as long as the total Ca content given is equal. Calcium gluconate may be preferable for peripheral administration because the tissue injury from inadvertent extravasation is less severe than with $CaCl_2$. Mg^{2+} levels are often low during hypocalcemia and should also be corrected, particularly when hypocalcemia has been caused by infusion of isotonic saline or colloids in large volumes.

HYPERCALCEMIA. Hypercalcemia occurs when ECF Ca^{2+} influx from the GI tract and/or bone outweighs efflux to bone or excretion via the kidneys (Table 47.11). The symptoms are related to the severity and speed of onset of the abnormality, so mild chronic hypercalcemia is usually asymptomatic. More severe hypercalcemia manifests with neurologic symptoms (drowsiness, weakness, depression, lethargy, coma), GI symptoms (constipation, nausea, vomiting, anorexia, peptic ulcers), renal manifestations (nephrogenic diabetes insipidus—which may further aggravate hypercalcemia through dehydration—and renal stones), electrocardiographic abnormalities (shortened QT interval, prolonged PR interval), and potentiation of digoxin toxicity. Treatment should address the underlying cause, including surgical parathyroidectomy in cases of severe hyperparathyroidism, or cessation of thiazide diuretics. In addition, the treatment of symptomatic hypercalcemia should aim to increase renal Ca^{2+} excretion by volume expansion with isotonic saline and possibly loop diuretics. This combination may reduce Ca^{2+} by 1 to 3 mg/dL in 1 to 2 days.[26] Bisphosphonates enhance osteoclastic bone deposition and are given if the hypercalcemia is severe or in milder cases in which response to hydration has been inadequate. A single IV dose of pamidronate 60 mg (moderate hypercalcemia, up to 13.5 mg/dL) or 90 mg (severe hypercalcemia) should return Ca^{2+} levels to normal within 7 days, and the effect may persist for up to 1 month. Zoledronic acid is a newer bisphosphonate that may be even more effective and is given intravenously at a dose of 4 mg.[128] Bisphosphonates should only be given when clinical dehydration has been treated to avoid calcium bisphosphonate precipitation and nephrotoxicity. Glucocorticoids may also be given for hypercalcemia associated with lymphoproliferative disease or ectopic vitamin D production.[129] Calcitonin increases renal Ca^{2+} excretion and reduces bone resorption for up to 48 hours when given intramuscularly or intravenously and may contribute to a mild reduction in Ca^{2+} levels during the rehydration phase.

Magnesium Disorders

HYPOMAGNESEMIA. Serum Mg^{2+} concentration may be a poor indicator of total body content because of its large distribution in the intracellular compartment and slow equilibration with bone stores. Intraerythrocyte or intralymphocyte Mg^{2+} levels may give a better approximation of total body and tissue stores, but are more complex to process.[130,131] Both chronic and acute hypomagnesemia are associated with cardiovascular morbidity[29] and are particularly prevalent in diverse hospitalized patients (12% of general inpatients, 19% of preoperative cardiac surgery patients, 65% of critical care patients). The causes

TABLE 47.12 Causes and Mechanisms of Hypomagnesemia

Mechanism	Cause
Inadequate gastrointestinal uptake	Malnutrition Prolonged vomiting or diarrhea Intestinal fistula Pancreatitis Prolonged nasogastric suction Malabsorption syndromes Small bowel syndrome Primary intestinal hypomagnesemia
Increased renal losses	Chronic parenteral fluid therapy Hypercalcemia and hypercalciuria Osmotic diuresis Drugs: Alcohol, loop and thiazide diuretics, aminoglycosides, cisplatin, amphotericin, cyclosporin, foscarnet Phosphate depletion Hungry bone syndrome Postobstructive nephropathy Renal transplantation Polyuric phase of acute kidney injury Primary hyperparathyroidism Bartter and Gitelman syndromes

are related to reduced Mg^{2+} intake from the GI tract or increased renal losses (Table 47.12), although relative depletion may occur in times of increased cell turnover and protein production (pregnancy, athletes, cold acclimatization). The clinical presentation of hypomagnesemia may be nonspecific; symptoms often relate to common coexisting hypocalcemia or hypokalemia[32]:

- Neuromuscular: Trousseau and Chvostek signs, vertigo, seizures, weakness
- Metabolic: Carbohydrate intolerance, hyperinsulinemia, atherosclerosis
- Cardiovascular: Wide QRS, prolonged PR, T-wave inversion, ventricular arrhythmias
- Musculoskeletal: Osteoporosis and osteomalacia

Treatment should be tailored to the severity of symptoms and degree of hypomagnesemia. Asymptomatic patients with moderate-severe hypomagnesemia should receive oral supplementation, as acute IV infusions will stimulate the renal Ca^{2+}/Mg^{2+}-sensing receptor, reducing Mg^{2+} reabsorption and leading to renal excretion of much of the acute dose. In the presence of symptoms or Mg^{2+} concentration of less than 1 mg/dL, IV Mg^{2+} should be administered (initial dose of 1-2 gm over 5 to 10 minutes in the presence of seizures or acute arrhythmias).[32] Coexistent hypocalcemia, hypokalemia, or both should also be treated, but they are unlikely to improve without replenishment of Mg^{2+}. Mg^{2+} has many other therapeutic indications, even in the absence of hypomagnesemia, as outlined earlier. A few of these patients are likely to have total body Mg^{2+} depletion that has not been detected by serum Mg^{2+} levels.

HYPERMAGNESEMIA. Limited GI absorption and efficient renal excretion mean that hypermagnesemia is typically iatrogenic. Symptoms reflect the effect of Mg^{2+} on neurologic and cardiac function and relate to the serum concentration[18]:

- 5 to 7 mg/dL: Therapeutic levels in the treatment of preeclampsia
- 5 to 10 mg/dL: Impaired cardiac conduction (widened QRS, long PR), nausea
- 20 to 34 mg/dL: Sedation, reduced neuromuscular transmission with hypoventilation, reduced tendon reflexes, and muscle weakness
- 24 to 48 mg/dL: Diffuse vasodilation with hypotension, bradycardia
- 48 to 72 mg/dL: Areflexia, coma, respiratory paralysis

Mg^{2+} administration should therefore be performed with several important caveats. First, serum Mg^{2+} levels should be monitored closely during therapeutic administration. Second, because excretion is renal, doses should be decreased for patients with kidney disease. Third, it should be used with extreme caution in patients with a background impairment of neuromuscular transmission (myasthenia gravis, Lambert-Eaton myasthenic syndrome). Fourth, coadministration of neuromuscular blockers during anesthesia should be performed in reduced doses titrated to neuromuscular monitoring, because Mg^{2+} potentiates the effects of both depolarizing and nondepolarizing neuromuscular blockers. Treatment of acute hypermagnesemia includes promoting renal excretion by administration of fluids intravenously and diuresis. IV Ca^{2+} is given to temporarily antagonize Mg^{2+} and avoid diuretic-induced hypocalcemia. Definitive treatment, particularly in the presence of renal disease, may require dialysis.

Phosphate Disorders

HYPOPHOSPHATEMIA. Hypophosphatemia may be related to impaired enteral uptake, increased renal excretion, or shifts to the cellular compartment or bone (Table 47.13). Symptoms of hypophosphatemia may be precipitated by hyperventilation in patients with chronic depletion. Refeeding syndrome may be observed on commencement of enteral or parenteral nutrition after a period of prolonged starvation and may manifest postoperatively. Insulin secretion is decreased during starvation. The consequent fat and protein catabolism results in intracellular electrolyte depletion despite normal plasma levels, particularly phosphate. On refeeding, a switch back occurs to carbohydrate metabolism, increased insulin secretion, and an increased cellular uptake of PO_4^{3-}, which may lead to profound hypophosphatemia. In the most severe forms (<1.5 mg/dL), features may include rhabdomyolysis, leukocyte dysfunction, cardiac and respiratory failure, seizures, hypotension, and coma. IV PO_4^{3-} replacement carries a risk for precipitating severe hypocalcemia, so should be reserved for moderate (<2.2 mg/dL) to severe or symptomatic cases and avoided in cases of ongoing hypocalcemia. Replacement protocols should be based on patient weight and serum PO_4^{3-}.[132]

HYPERPHOSPHATEMIA. The causes of hyperphosphatemia are shown in Table 47.13. The most common cause in clinical practice is renal failure, in which the filtered PO_4^{3-} load is reduced. This may be partly compensated for in mild chronic kidney disease by increased PTH secretion and inhibition of tubular PO_4^{3-} reabsorption, but in more severe kidney disease hyperphosphatemia must be controlled with

TABLE 47.13 Causes and Mechanisms of Phosphate Abnormalities

HYPOPHOSPHATEMIA		HYPERPHOSPHATEMIA	
Mechanism	**Cause**	**Mechanism**	**Cause**
Internal redistribution	Respiratory alkalosis Refeeding Hormones (insulin, glucagon, epinephrine, cortisol) Sepsis Hungry bone syndrome	Increased endogenous load	Tumor lysis syndrome Rhabdomyolysis Bowel infarction Malignant hyperthermia Hemolysis
Increased urinary excretion	Hyperparathyroidism Disorders of vitamin D metabolism Renal transplant Volume expansion Malabsorption Renal tubular defects Alcoholism Metabolic or respiratory acidosis	 Increased exogenous load Reduced urinary excretion	Acidosis Intravenous infusion Oral supplementation Vitamin D intoxication Renal failure Hypoparathyroidism Acromegaly Tumor calcinosis
Decreased intestinal absorption	Dietary restriction Excess antacids Vitamin D deficiency Chronic diarrhea	 Pseudohyperphosphatemia	Bisphosphonate therapy Magnesium deficiency Multiple myeloma In vitro hemolysis Hypertriglyceridemia

Data from Weisinger JR, Bellorín-Font E. Magnesium and phosphorus. *Lancet.* 1998;352:391.

oral PO_4^{3-} binders. The features of hyperphosphatemia may be related to symptomatic hypocalcemia caused by an acute elevation in PO_4^{3-} levels. Hypocalcemia is mediated via Ca^+ deposition in soft tissues when the calcium × phosphate product is elevated, and by inhibition of renal 1α-hydroxylase.[32]

Chloride Disorders. Disorders of Cl^- have the potential to affect acid-base balance, although this depends on the other constituents of the SID. As described, exogenous Cl^- administration from isotonic saline will increase the plasma Cl^- concentration with a lesser effect on Na^+ concentration, thus reducing the plasma SID and therefore pH. Conversely, disease states exemplified by both hyperchloremia and hypernatremia or by hypochloremia and hyponatremia will not affect the SID and therefore not alter pH. Many of the causes of Cl^- abnormalities (Table 47.14) are pathologic processes that also affect Na^+ levels. Investigation and treatment of these "matched" electrolyte imbalances should initially target the dysnatremia.

PRACTICAL MANAGEMENT OF PERIOPERATIVE FLUID THERAPY

At each stage in the perioperative journey, the physician must decide how much and what type of IV fluid is required. Unfortunately, a robust evidence base with answers to these questions is not always available, so a pragmatic approach based on sound physiologic knowledge and the best available evidence is required. To make the process more complicated, fluid and electrolyte requirements are a dynamic situation with great inter-individual variability. Different fluid requirements are encountered in the preoperative, intraoperative, and postoperative phases, and these vary depending on patient factors, including weight and comorbidity, and on surgical factors, such as the magnitude and site of surgery. Furthermore, the goals of fluid therapy vary depending on the severity of surgery and its associated morbidity. In "low-risk" minor surgery, fluid strategies may influence the incidence of relatively minor morbidity such as nausea and vomiting,[133,134] whereas in major surgery the focus is on the potential for fluid administration to affect postoperative morbidity, length of stay, and mortality.[111,135,136]

The goals of fluid therapy for major surgery are as follows:

- To ensure adequate circulating volume to support cellular O_2 delivery and avoid the deleterious effects of hypoperfusion on cellular function and survival, inflammation, and neurohumoral responses. This may involve manipulation of not just circulating volume but also of cardiac output and vascular resistance.
- To avoid the iatrogenic side effects of fluid administration; excessive intravascular volume (which may not be readily apparent clinically), edema, excess Na^+ or Cl^- load, toxicities related to synthetic compounds, or nonphysiologic quantities of anions (lactate, acetate, gluconate).

Large studies show that even during relatively standardized surgical procedures, there is a large variety in the volumes of fluid administered. This unexplained variability may be linked with postoperative morbidity, and regrettably appears to be more closely related to the approach of the individual anesthesia provider rather than justifiable patient or surgical factors.[107,137] A number of approaches are still being investigated in an effort to determine the optimum quantity and type of fluid that should be given in order to achieve these goals in perioperative care.

Quantity of Fluid

IV fluid quantities may be given in two main ways: (1) by estimating the requirements based on patient weight, the phase of surgery, and nature of losses to estimate the

TABLE 47.14 Causes and Mechanisms of Chloride Abnormalities

HYPOCHLOREMIA		HYPERCHLOREMIA	
Mechanism	**Cause**	**Mechanism**	**Cause**
Cl^- loss	Diuretics	Cl^- infusion	Cl^--rich fluids
	Gastric drainage		Parenteral nutrition
	Vomiting	Water loss	Skin
	Chronic respiratory acidosis		Fever
			Renal losses
Water balance in excess of Cl^-	Congestive cardiac failure		Diabetes insipidus
	Syndrome of inappropriate of antidiuretic hormone secretion	Water loss exceeding Cl^- loss (extrarenal)	Diarrhea
	Infusion of hypotonic fluids		Burns
		Water loss exceeding Cl^- loss (renal)	Osmotic diuresis
			Postobstructive diuresis
			Intrinsic renal disease
		Increased tubular chloride reabsorption	Renal tubular acidosis
			Recovery from diabetic ketoacidosis
			Early renal failure
			Acetazolamide
			Ureteral diversion
			Posthypocapnia

Data from Yunos NM, Bellomo R, Story D, et al. Bench-to-bedside review: chloride in critical illness. *Crit Care.* 2010;14:226.

required dose, or (2) by direct measurement of an individual's physiologic variables and administering fluid in sufficient quantities to achieve an improvement in these physiologic variables, so-called goal-directed therapy.

Targeting Overall Fluid Balance. Traditional approaches to perioperative fluid administration are based on historical estimates of fluid requirements during fasting (e.g., using the "4-2-1" calculation; Table 47.15[138]) and during episodes of excess loss, such as when body cavities are open or bleeding occurs. The fluid volumes prescribed are then based on perceived knowledge of the movement of fluids between compartments—for example, crystalloid being used to replace blood loss in a 3:1 ratio to account for crystalloid movement into the extravascular compartment.[18] However, much of the physiologic basis of this management approach has been questioned recently.[3,11]

An extension of the milliliter-per-kilogram approach to fluid administration has been to examine whether higher (e.g., 12-18 mL/kg/h of intraoperative crystalloid) or lower (5-7 mL/kg/h) fluid doses in the immediate perioperative phase are associated with benefit after major surgery. Unfortunately, this work has been hampered by widely varying definitions of restrictive/conservative, standard, and liberal, differing fluid types (colloids/crystalloids), and different time courses over which the fluid strategy is applied. Despite these differences, a common theme is that when fluid is given based on a milliliter-per-kilogram protocol and on clinical assessment rather than to target defined physiologic endpoints, the administration of more than 3500 to 5000 mL of crystalloid solution in the immediate perioperative period is associated with increased postoperative morbidity in contrast

TABLE 47.15 The 4-2-1 Estimation of Maintenance Water Requirements

Weight	Fluid Prescription
First 10 kg	4 mL/kg/h
Second 10 kg	2 mL/kg/h
All subsequent kilograms	1 mL/kg/h

Example: A 25-kg patient would require (4 × 10) + (2 × 10) + (1 × 5) = 65 mL/h "maintenance" water.

Data from Holliday MA, Segar WE. The maintenance need for water in parenteral fluid therapy. *Pediatrics.* 1957;19:823.

to administration of lower fluid volumes. This may be reflected in increased weight gain, cardiopulmonary dysfunction, impaired wound healing,[111,133] delayed GI function, and increased hospital length of stay.[139,140] One study gives apparently conflicting results,[141] although this may be partly accounted for by methodologic differences with the other studies here. In the recent pragmatic international RELIEF trial,[142] 3000 patients at increased risk for complications during major abdominal surgery were randomly assigned to receive a restrictive or liberal IV fluid regimen during and up to 24 hours after surgery. The restrictive group had a median IV fluid intake of 3.7 liters and a median weight gain of 0.3 kg as compared with 6.1 L and 1.6 kg in the liberal fluid group. There was no difference in the primary outcome of disability-free survival at 1 year, but the rates of surgical-site infection (16.5% vs. 13.6%) and renal-replacement therapy (0.9% vs. 0.3%) were increased in the restrictive group. This study provides an important warning of the consequences of excessive fluid restriction, a target for weight change after surgery (+1.5 kg), and a useful benchmark recipe.

Very few studies have robustly examined the specific effects of postoperatively administered fluid volumes. Of those tackling this area, one showed an earlier return to gut function and hospital discharge when postoperative infusions were limited to 2000 mL of water and less than 100 mEq Na^+/24 h,[108] whereas another showed no difference.[143] These represent very small studies with methodologic differences.

Although it seems likely that there exists an optimum fluid volume to be given to maximize perfusion while avoiding excessive intravascular volumes, the position of this curve likely varies widely across patients and in response to different insults. This is the rationale behind individualization of fluid therapy, where objective variables are measured and targeted with fluid therapy.

Goal-Directed Therapy. The practice of GDT is based on measuring key physiologic variables related to cardiac output or global O_2 delivery and administering fluids, and possibly inotropes, vasopressors, vasodilators, and RBCs to improved tissue perfusion and clinical outcome. This approach to fluid administration is a continuous dynamic process that targets defined physiologic endpoints rather than giving fluids without objective assessments of fluid status. GDT, used both in the perioperative and critical care setting, originated from observations that survivors of high-risk surgery achieved a particular elevation in global O_2 delivery and utilization in the perioperative period.[144] Subsequent trials used hemodynamic manipulation in an effort to replicate these supranormal "survivor values" in patients undergoing major surgery (cardiac index >4.5 L/min/m^2, O_2 delivery index (DO_2I) >600 mL/min/m^2, O_2 consumption index >170 mL/min/m^2).[145,146] The GDT approach has been studied in a wide variety of surgical settings and at various time points, including during preoperative optimization, intraoperative management, and the immediate postoperative period. Various tools to measure the physiologic targets of GDT are discussed below.

- Pulmonary artery catheter (PAC). Considered to be the gold standard hemodynamic monitor, providing measured and derived values for left-heart and right-heart filling pressures, mixed and central venous saturations, cardiac output, DO_2, and VO_2 while allowing access to the central circulation. This was the tool used in the earlier GDT trials targeting increases in cardiac index and DO_2I, but its use is declining because of concerns about catheter-associated morbidity, reduced expertise in insertion and data interpretation, and the availability of less invasive tools. In countries such as the United Kingdom, its use is typically restricted to cardiac, major liver, and transplant surgery.
- Esophageal Doppler monitor (EDM). This device uses transesophageal ultrasound measurement of descending aorta blood velocity, integrating this with estimated aortic cross-sectional area to derive SV. Other measurements include peak velocity, used as an indicator of ventricular contractility, and corrected flow time (FTc), and the duration of systolic aortic blood flow corrected for heart rate. FTc may be reduced (<330 ms) by increased systemic vascular resistance (SVR), reduced SV, or both. SVR may be calculated by inputting CVP and mean arterial pressure (MAP), helping to identify whether a low FTc is due to inadequate preload or excessive afterload. Variation in SV with positive pressure ventilation (stroke volume variation, SVV) is also measured by the latest EDM models.
- Arterial pressure and waveform analysis. These monitors analyze the invasive arterial blood pressure, continuous non-invasive blood pressure from a finger cuff, or plethysmograph trace to yield two types of measurement. First, an estimate of SV (and therefore cardiac output and index) based on the principle that pulse pressure is proportional to SV when arterial compliance is constant. Interpatient variation in arterial compliance may be accounted for by regular calibration steps using lithium dilution (LiDCO Plus, LiDCO, Lake Villa, IL) or thermodilution (PiCCO, Phillips, Andover, MA) or ignored in uncalibrated monitors (LiDCO Rapid, LiDCO; FloTrac, Edwards, Washington, DC), which represent SV trends rather than absolute estimates. Second, SVV, a predictor of fluid responsiveness based on systolic pressure variation with intermittent positive-pressure ventilation, can be measured.
- Thoracic bioimpedance, relatively underexplored in perioperative interventional trials.
- CVP: Despite one study that demonstrated improved outcomes from hip fracture surgery when CVP response to intravascular fluid challenges was compared to unmonitored control,[147] CVP readings are clearly poorly predictive of intravascular blood volume and fluid responsiveness.[148]
- Echocardiography: This advanced technique is used for guiding fluid therapy and yielding information on cardiac performance and filling, but requires operator expertise and a transesophageal approach in the intraoperative setting.
- Lactate: A reduction in elevated blood lactate concentrations is used clinically as a marker of successful resuscitation.[149]
- O_2 extraction and venous O_2 saturation (SvO_2) or central venous saturation ($ScvO_2$): Inadequate tissue O_2 delivery may be signaled by increased O_2 extraction and the resultant mixed or central venous O_2 desaturation. Low $ScvO_2$ is associated with poor outcomes after high-risk surgery,[150] although it has been targeted in only one interventional study in major noncardiac surgery.[151]

A typical approach to GDT is to rapidly administer 250 mL boluses of colloid or crystalloid, aiming to increase SV by 10% or more each time. This process is continued until there is no further rise in SV, at which point ventricular filling is taken to be on the flatter part of the Starling curve. One example is in Fig. 47.6. Trials have varied in terms of the period during which this intervention is used (intraoperative or intra- and postoperative) and whether fluid loading is combined with protocolized inotrope infusion. Recent meta-analyses have highlighted the potential benefits of the GDT process. One meta-analysis with the most

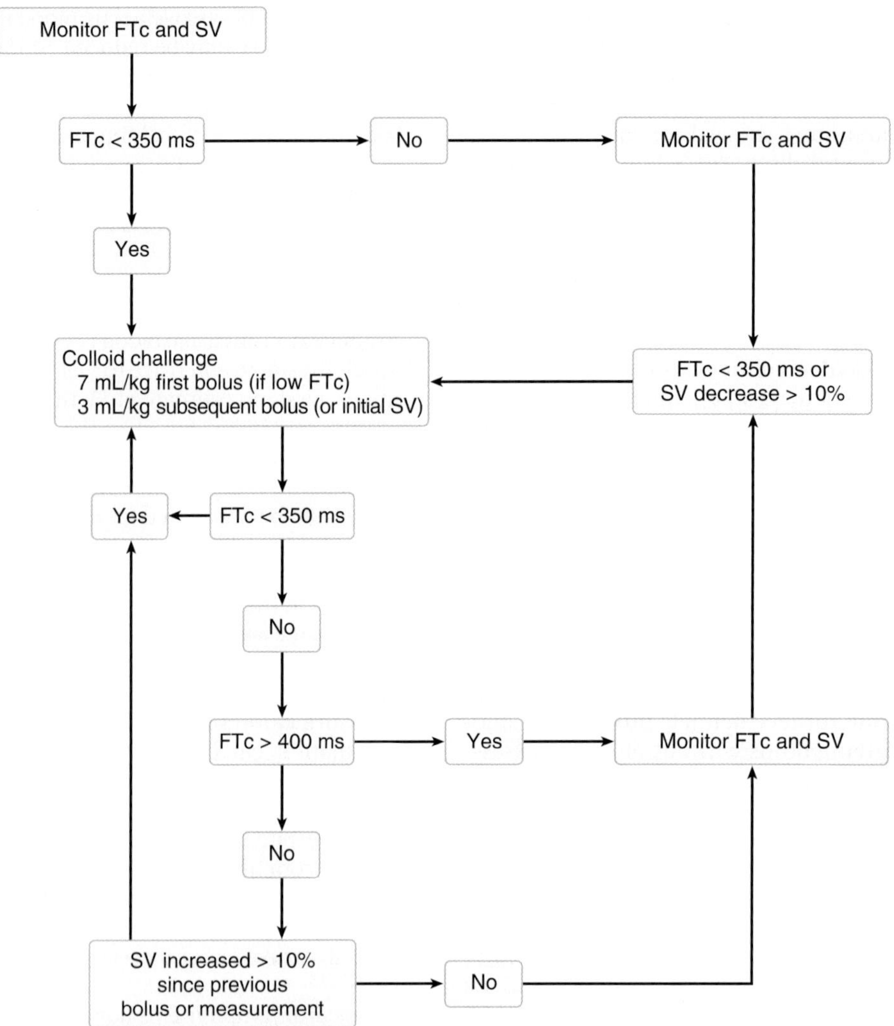

Fig. 47.6 Protocol for EDM-based intraoperative goal-directed fluid therapy. *FTc,* Heart rate-corrected descending aorta flow time; *SV,* stroke volume. (Redrawn from Noblett SE, Snowden CP, Shenton BK, et al. Randomized clinical trial assessing the effect of Doppler-optimized fluid management on outcome after elective colorectal resection. *Br J Surg.* 2006;93:1069.)

tightly defined patient group (surgery but not trauma or sepsis) and all time points (preoperative, intraoperative, and postoperative GDT) and GDT tools (PAC, EDM, and arterial waveform analysis), showed GDT to be associated with a reduction in postoperative morbidity and hospital length of stay.[136] Specifically, GDT leads to a reduction in the number of patients with postoperative renal impairment, respiratory failure, and postoperative wound infection. Many of the individual studies were not powered to detect a mortality difference; however, when analyzed rigorously in this Cochrane systematic review, excluding poorly controlled studies, hospital or 28-day mortality was reduced by GDT.[136]

The lack of more contemporary trials of adequate size to detect important outcome differences has been addressed in recent years. An increasing number of large, pragmatic clinical effectiveness trials using minimally invasive arterial waveform or Doppler devices have been completed or are in progress. Although the results of individual trials are mixed, most results appear to agree with the potential benefit of using these monitors in elective surgery suggested by the previous Cochrane meta-analysis.[152–154] Large trials aiming to give a definitive answer on this intervention are currently underway in both elective and emergency gastrointestinal surgery.

A frequent finding in GDT studies is that the intervention group receives more fluid, typically an extra 500 mL of colloid, a finding that has raised questions, as follows:

- This fluid excess may seem to be at odds with the potential benefits of a conservative fluid strategy. However, it should be noted that the fluid excess in the liberal groups of fluid balance studies is typically of greater magnitude and different type (~1500 mL of excess crystalloid overall) and is indiscriminate, in comparison to the targeted administration to some patients based on specific physiologic variables in GDT. This difference may be partly responsible for the finding that overall outcomes in "liberal" groups are worse than those in GDT groups in their respective trials.[112]
- The potential benefit of the GDT process is underlined by a failure to replicate the improved outcomes when these

fluid balance differences are used as therapeutic targets. This was shown in a study in which the intervention group subjects were uniformly administered an extra 500 mL of colloid compared with the control group, with no improvement in postoperative outcomes.[155] This suggests that it is the individualization of therapy supported by monitored variables that may bring the clinical benefit.
- Even in GDT trials with few overall differences in intravascular fluid balance between the control and intervention groups, the individualization of patient fluid requirements may be reflected in the timing of intraoperative fluid administration. In one study, early intraoperative EDM-guided fluid administration in the first quarter of surgery increased cardiac output above that of the control group, a difference that was sustained until the end of surgery and reduced postoperative morbidity.[156]

Despite the apparent benefit of GDT in the studies performed so far, further research is still required in large-scale multicenter trials to address the following:

- Although most of the GDT studies have used boluses of a variety of colloids, it is not clear if one colloid is superior or whether crystalloids could be used for boluses instead. This is particularly relevant given the cost and potential toxicities of colloids when examined in sufficiently powered studies in critical care populations.[51,84,157]
- Hemodynamic monitors are currently under rapid development, and newer devices should be compared with existing ones for their utility in guiding GDT. Ultimately, as newer technologies are evaluated, the potential benefits of GDT may relate to the process of administering fluids based on rational physiologic endpoints rather than to the specific GDT tool used. As previous evaluations of monitoring devices have shown, no benefit is gained from using a device per se, but rather from the therapeutic intervention that the device allows.[158]

Appropriate Fluid Selection

Crystalloids or Colloids for Intravascular Plasma Volume Expansion. Although crystalloids are the most rational choice of fluid for replacement of evaporative losses, maintenance fluid requirements, and expansion of the entire extracellular fluid volume, the choice of crystalloid or colloid for plasma volume replacement in the perioperative phase is not clear. This underlines the lack of adequately powered perioperative studies directly comparing the two fluid types when administered in a similar fashion. Although most GDT studies use colloid for their intravascular volume expansion, these studies are also comparisons of fluid administration guided by physiologic endpoints with nonguided therapy. Whether the same level of benefit can be achieved by crystalloid-based GDT merits further investigation. Crystalloid may be effective in plasma volume expansion (PVE) at amounts less than previously reported, although typically 40% to 50% more crystalloid than colloid must be administered to obtain the same clinical volume effect.[3] When combined with the increased propensity of crystalloid to filter across the capillary membrane, more extravascular volume expansion occurs, potentially causing tissue edema. When compared with colloids, crystalloids may lead to increased GI mucosal edema[159] and the potential for delayed postoperative GI function and bacterial translocation. The differential effect of crystalloids when compared to colloids on tissue O_2 tension has no clear consensus.[52] The limited data comparing colloid with crystalloid for perioperative PVE may lead clinicians to extrapolate findings from studies in critical care. A Cochrane review highlighted the lack of improvement in all-cause mortality when colloids were used for intravascular volume expansion in unselected critical care populations.[160] In studies specific to patients with sepsis, starch-based colloids, including smaller MW versions, are associated with an increased requirement for renal replacement therapy, blood transfusion, and an increase in severe adverse events.[83] These data should be interpreted cautiously. First, some critical care studies compared starches with saline in the control group, which may itself be associated with renal problems.[51] Second, the surgical population has a different physiologic phenotype to those in critical care; meta-analysis suggests that starch is not associated with excess mortality or kidney injury in surgical patients, although the available trials are limited.[86] Despite these limitations, it is reasonable to avoid starch colloids in perioperative patients with severe sepsis or at increased risk of renal failure, pending the necessary large-scale trials assessing their safety in the perioperative setting. This is reflected in license restrictions for these fluids in the United States. In the United Kingdom, the use of starches has been suspended in all settings. The potential toxicities of colloids must be weighed against the potential fluid overloading effects of PVE using crystalloids until more data are available informing the debate on crystalloids versus colloids for perioperative PVE.

Saline-Based or Balanced Solutions

TYPICAL PRACTICAL APPROACH. The following suggestions represent an assimilation of the physiology, fluid pharmacology, and available evidence presented in this chapter. However, in many areas of perioperative fluid management, the lack of robust evidence means that the choice of fluid and method of administration remains a clinician's choice informed by the balance of risks and benefits. The overall themes in prescribing fluids in moderate-to-major surgery are:

- The indication for giving a specific fluid should always be considered. Pure "maintenance" fluid should be given at a low fixed rate, with fluid required for replacement of losses or for resuscitation considered separately.
- Fluids administered should be individualized. This may be as simple as dosing postoperative maintenance fluids on a milliliter-per-kilogram basis or titrating intraoperative plasma volume expansion to objectively measured physiologic variables.
- Fluid status changes constantly throughout the perioperative period and should be frequently reassessed.
- The approach should be adapted to the patient and surgical factors outlined later.

Preoperative. In preparing for elective surgery, oral clear fluid intake should continue until 2 hours preoperatively and longer fasting discouraged. The use of preoperative bowel preparation should be restricted to carefully selected cases, and in these cases an infusion of 1 to 2 L of balanced crystalloid with K^+ supplementation should be given in the preoperative period. Chronic comorbidities should be assessed for their influence on fluid and electrolyte balance, as outlined later.

Emergency surgery patients are likely to have acute disturbances of fluid compartments. They require timely resuscitation guided by rational physiologic endpoints such as trends in blood pressure and heart rate, lactate, urine output, and mixed or central venous O_2 saturations. Although preoperative fluid administration using cardiac output monitoring makes clinical sense, often logistical implications are involved with this approach and in some cases (ongoing blood loss or early surgical control of sepsis) surgery should not be delayed. A pragmatic approach is required to provide ongoing fluid resuscitation without compromising early surgical intervention. Upper GI losses should be quantified and replaced with isotonic saline, and lower GI losses (fistula, ileus, or obstruction) with balanced crystalloid. K^+ should be supplemented as appropriate.

Intraoperative. A low background infusion (e.g., 1-1.5 mL/kg/h) of crystalloid should be used for maintenance requirements during surgery. Hypotension caused by general or regional anesthesia is related primarily to vasodilation and reduced inotropy, and unless the patient is hypovolemic because of preoperative factors, it is more rational to treat this with small doses of vasopressors and/or inotropes.[11] Fluid therapy in patients considered to be at higher risk should be guided by invasive pressure monitoring to allow for early recognition of overt hypovolemia and global tissue perfusion. Although no universally accepted definitions of a high-risk case exist,[161] factors such as major elective or emergency surgery, advanced age, comorbidities, and poor exercise tolerance, increase postoperative mortality risk to greater than 5%. In these cases and particularly in certain orthopedic and intraabdominal operations, where the evidence is strongest, cardiac output should be optimized by titrating boluses of a suitable colloid or balanced crystalloid to a measured variable such as SV and FTc, or cardiac output and O_2 delivery. Stroke volume variation may also be measured, although its ability to accurately predict fluid responsiveness may be limited.[162] Blood loss should be replaced with colloid or blood products depending on the volume lost and variables suggesting inadequate tissue O_2 delivery. Crystalloid may be used as an alternative for intravascular plasma volume expansion, but the increased volume required and potential for extravascular volume expansion should be considered. Overall, the goal should be to achieve euvolemia by the end of surgery or the early postoperative period.

Postoperative. High-risk surgical patients may benefit from an ongoing period of GDT targeting O_2 delivery in the early postoperative period.[163] In all other patients after major surgery, an assessment of fluid status should be made based on clinical examination and supporting physiologic measurements such as lactate, central or mixed venous saturations, and cardiac output variables, if available. If patients are euvolemic and able to return to oral fluid intake, this is the best way of avoiding the iatrogenic effects of postoperative fluid administration. Early oral intake is typically well tolerated and safe, and early oral nutrition may reduce the incidence of postoperative complications.[164]

The following should be done in patients requiring ongoing IV therapy:

- Electrolytes should be checked at least daily to monitor for hyponatremia and other electrolyte derangements.
- Fluid requirements should be strictly divided into three categories for their ongoing assessment and treatment
  - **"Pure" maintenance requirements.** These should be salt-poor and contain a modest volume of free water to account for the postoperative state of salt and water retention. Infusions should therefore consist of the following[164]: (1) 1500 to 2500 mL in 24 hours, depending on weight, or 1 to 1.2 mL/kg/h. Given the relative reduction in TBW in obesity (see previous discussions on crystalloids, fluid compartments), consideration should be given to dosing this fluid requirement based on ideal body weight in this setting. (2) 50 to 100 mEq Na^+ should be given in 24 hours, and (3) 40 to 80 mEq K^+ should be given in 24 hours.
  - It is likely that part of this minimal maintenance volume should comprise hypotonic fluids such as 5% dextrose or 0.18% saline with 4% dextrose. Because of the risk for postoperative hyponatremia, this maintenance intravascular fluid volume should not be increased if suspicion for hypovolemia exists. Rather, the source of the ongoing loss should be identified and treated separately. As oral fluid intake increases, this maintenance fluid should be reduced proportionately.
  - **Replacement of ongoing losses.** This fluid requirement requires frequent reassessment to appropriately titrate replacement fluids. Volumes given should reflect measured amounts lost and an assessment of intravascular volume status and adequacy of organ perfusion (mental state, lactate, hemodynamic trends). Losses from the GI tract (vomiting, nasogastric aspirates, stoma) should be replaced with an equal volume of isotonic saline or balanced crystalloid with K^+ as appropriate. Losses to third spaces, such as reaccumulation of ascites, should be treated with a mixture of colloid and crystalloid, and blood loss replaced with colloid, blood, or blood products.
  - **New requirements (resuscitation).** New requirements may relate to the development of postoperative complications such as hemorrhage (absolute hypovolemia) or acute sepsis (relative or absolute hypovolemia).

Postoperative oliguria should be interpreted cautiously, particularly in the first postoperative day. The patient should be carefully assessed for corroborative evidence of impaired end-organ perfusion and alternative causes of oliguria, including catheter obstruction and intraabdominal hypertension. In the absence of markers indicating hypovolemia and inadequate tissue perfusion, large volumes of fluid challenge are inappropriate and may aggravate postoperative positive fluid and Na^+ balance in the face of a normal surgical stress response.

Special Considerations

Patient Factors

HEART FAILURE. The diverse pathophysiologic effects of heart failure and their treatment may make perioperative fluid management particularly challenging. The hemodynamic effects of chronic heart failure are characterized by systolic and diastolic dysfunction of the left, right, or both ventricles with secondary maladaptive neurohumoral responses. These include persistent activation of the RAA axis, with consequent salt and water retention, and chronic sympathetic nervous system (SNS) activation, with persistent tachycardia and vasoconstriction. Undertreated patients may therefore present with edema in lungs and peripheral tissues and increased central blood volume in the face of poor myocardial function.

Treatments for heart failure attempt to correct many of the neurohumoral responses, and many have been shown to improve long-term prognosis in heart failure. In the perioperative phase, they may bring challenges to fluid management, including chronic volume depletion, blunting of normal sympathetic responses, and electrolyte disturbances. They include β-adrenoreceptor antagonists, diuretics, digoxin, and antagonists of aldosterone and angiotensin.

Perioperative fluid therapy in patients with heart failure has two goals. The first is to preserve cardiac output, bearing in mind the influence of preload, contractility, and afterload. The ventricles are typically poorly compliant and require adequate preload, which may be reflected in a relatively high CVP and adequate diastolic filling time to maintain good cardiac output. However, the flattened Starling curve of the failing heart means that excessive intravascular volume infusion and preload may lead to impaired contractility and worsening cardiac output. This leads to "forward failure," manifested as inadequate organ perfusion, and "backward failure," manifested as pulmonary and peripheral edema, particularly in the presence of aberrant salt and water excretion. The second goal is to minimize the cardiac work to avoid a vicious cycle of increased cardiac O_2 demand, inadequate O_2 supply, and worsening myocardial function. In particular, tachycardia triggered by hypovolemia and other stimuli should be avoided. Striking a balance between hypovolemia and hypervolemia is particularly important in patients with heart failure, but it may be difficult to assess clinically.

The practical approach to patients with heart failure involves careful preoperative assessment of fluid status and electrolytes and optimization of heart failure treatments when time allows. The complex cardiovascular situation often requires cardiac output monitoring for moderate or major surgery. Invasive modalities include transesophageal echocardiography or pulmonary artery catheterization,[165] although less invasive modalities may also be helpful. Measurement of cardiac filling and contractility is particularly important because the sources of intraoperative hypotension (reduced preload, contractility, or afterload) require different treatments. Infusion of large volumes of any fluid, including blood and products, should be undertaken only with objective evidence of intravascular volume loss.

The effects of heart failure therapies should be evaluated carefully in the perioperative phase. Diuretics may leave patients in a chronically volume-contracted state that worsens anesthesia-related hypotension. Loop diuretics frequently cause hypokalemia and hypomagnesemia, whereas aldosterone antagonists cause hyperkalemia, which may be severe when combined with ACE-inhibitor treatment or chronic kidney disease. Normalization of electrolytes is particularly important in patients taking digoxin, in whom hypokalemia may potentiate digoxin toxicity. ACE-inhibitors or angiotensin receptor antagonists themselves lead to a blunted sympathetic and angiotensin response to anesthesia-related vasodilation. The hypotension caused by these should be treated appropriately by small doses of inotropes or vasopressors, which may include vasopressin analogs.[165]

KIDNEY DISEASE. Patients with dialysis-dependent chronic kidney disease have multiple pathologic features that must be considered in perioperative fluid therapy. Overall fluid balance may be disturbed by reduced or absent native urine production, with reliance on dialysis to achieve the target "dry" weight, representing estimated euvolemia. Organ O_2 delivery may be impaired by various factors, including chronic anemia, endothelial dysfunction, and microvascular perfusion abnormalities. The frequent coexistence of heart failure and systemic or pulmonary hypertension and the bleeding tendency caused by platelet dysfunction further increase the perioperative risk.[166]

Preoperative assessment should focus on the adequacy of chronic dialysis in attaining euvolemia and estimating the normal volume of native urine output. Comorbidities should be assessed and optimized. Surgery should be undertaken in a facility where preoperative and postoperative dialysis or hemofiltration can be offered in case of intraoperative fluid overload or hyperkalemia. In elective surgery, preoperative dialysis should be timed such that the patient enters the intraoperative phase with a normal blood volume. Surgery in the presence of hypervolemia increases the risk for pulmonary and peripheral edema, hypertension, and poor wound healing, whereas hypovolemia increases the risk for anesthesia-related hypotension and inadequate tissue perfusion. Practically, this means performing dialysis the day before surgery to allow for equilibration of fluid and electrolyte compartments and time for dialysis anticoagulants to be metabolized. Electrolytes should be checked on the morning of surgery; sampling too soon after dialysis, before equilibration, may give an artificially low K^+ result leading to unnecessary exogenous supplementation. Conversely, fasting may actually favor a hyperkalemic state as a result of the reduced presence of insulin; the ideal K^+ value after dialysis is in the low-to-normal range. For emergency surgery, there may not be sufficient time to safely dialyze patients preoperatively. In this case, electrolyte abnormalities must be managed conservatively, with particular care paid to intraoperative fluid balance.

As with other major comorbidities with a critical impact on fluid and electrolyte balance, the importance of avoiding both hypovolemia and hypervolemia and the predisposition to inadequate tissue perfusion mean that detailed monitoring of hemodynamic variables, including invasive central venous and arterial pressure and cardiac output, should be considered for moderate-to-major surgery. The amount of fluid administered intraoperatively should be titrated to objective physiologic measurements, although the type of fluid given is open to debate. Large volumes of isotonic saline should be avoided, because the induced acidosis favors extrusion of K^+ from cells. In contrast, K^+-containing balanced crystalloids did not cause hyperkalemia in clinical trials.[44,167] An alternative crystalloid is a K^+-free HCO_3^--buffered dialysis solution such as Hemosol. Colloids may be used for intravascular volume replacement, although owing to their predominantly renal excretion, the volume effect and potential toxicities may be exaggerated in these patients. Liaising with the nephrologist is important before considering blood transfusion; if the patient is awaiting renal transplantation, human leukocyte antigen-matched blood may be required to minimize antibody formation and future difficulties with blood and tissue matching.

Upper Gastrointestinal Loss. Large volume gastric fluid loss may be caused by congenital or acquired gastric outlet obstruction and lead to a distinct pattern of fluid and acid-base abnormalities. Dehydration occurs as a result of water loss, reduced total body Cl^- content, and alkalosis caused by proton loss, with raised serum HCO_3^-. The initial renal response is formation of urine with low Cl^- and high HCO_3^- content. However, progressive dehydration leads to increased aldosterone secretion, aimed at retaining Na^+ and water. Na^+ is retained at the expense of K^+ and H^+ ions, leading to hypokalemia, and worsening metabolic alkalosis with a paradoxically acid urine. The alkalosis also reduces the circulating ionized fraction of Ca^{2+}.

Correction should include gradual rehydration with isotonic saline and K^+ supplementation, changing to dextrose-containing saline solutions depending on electrolyte analysis. Any surgery required to treat gastric outlet obstruction should be scheduled after correction of the volume and acid-base status.

Sepsis and Acute Lung Injury. Patients with infection and sepsis syndromes may be encountered early in their presentations, as surgical source control of infection (drainage of abscesses, debridement of necrotic tissues, removal of infected devices) forms a key part of early sepsis therapy.[168] Cardiovascular instability may be a particular problem, contributed to by endothelial dysfunction and intravascular fluid loss, vasodilation with fluid maldistribution, sympathetic redistribution of blood volume away from the peripheral circulation, and impairment of cardiac function. Fluid resuscitation, with the goal of maintaining adequate end organ perfusion, has historically been a key part of the first six hours of sepsis treatment, which may represent the perioperative period for some patients. Early trials suggested that protocolized fluid resuscitation targeting central venous oxygen saturation was more effective than resuscitation guided by only CVP, MAP, and urine output targets in reducing mortality from sepsis.[169] However, more recent large international trials have shown that this approach has similar outcomes to resuscitation based on standard or protocolized care without targeting central venous oxygen saturations.[170-172] The following approach is suggested for septic patients with evidence of tissue hypoperfusion:[173]

- At least 30 mL/kg of crystalloid should be given within the first three hours of resuscitation.
- Further fluids should be guided by frequent reassessment of hemodynamic status. This assessment may incorporate more detailed measurements such as cardiac output, in addition to routinely available physiological variables (heart rate, blood pressure, urine output).
- Dynamic tests of fluid responsiveness such as passive leg raise or stroke volume response to a fluid challenge are recommended over static targets such as a fixed CVP value.
- Other resuscitation targets may include a MAP >65 mm Hg in those requiring vasopressors, and normalization of lactate in patients with elevated levels.

These guidelines are based on a limited evidence base and further research is needed to refine this area. For example, some trials have suggested that a fluid bolus strategy may not be helpful in attaining hemodynamic targets[174] or may even be harmful in some settings.[175]

In established sepsis, fluid management becomes even more challenging due to the frequent presence of microvascular dysfunction, extravascular fluid overload, and disturbed neurohumoral responses to variations in intravascular volume.[176] There is uncoupling of the O_2 delivery and consumption relationship as a result of cellular inability to use O_2 (cytopathic hypoxia).[177,178] Because of this uncoupling, strategies to elevate global O_2 delivery may be of little benefit while exposing patients to potential side effects of excessive fluid and catecholamine administration.[179,180] At this stage, a less positive overall fluid balance is associated with improved outcomes.[181]

Patients with established acute respiratory distress syndrome (ARDS) may also present for surgical procedures. Here the focus of fluid therapy is the fine balance between avoiding an increase in lung edema while maintaining adequate tissue perfusion. ARDS is typified by increased pulmonary endothelial permeability, with extravasation of water and protein. The consequences are interstitial and alveolar edema, reduced pulmonary compliance, increased pulmonary artery pressures, and hypoxemia. Meanwhile, organ perfusion may be impaired by increased intrathoracic pressures and reduced cardiac filling pressures. Observational studies have highlighted an association between overall positive fluid balance and mortality in ARDS,[182] backed by a large randomized controlled trial demonstrating a reduction in ventilator and intensive therapy unit days in patients treated with a conservative fluid administration strategy.[183] The findings were similar in a subgroup of patients from this trial who had undergone surgery and were treated with lower fluid volumes. There was also no increased kidney injury seen in the low fluid volume group.[184] Extravascular lung water (EVLW) seems to be important in predicting the worse outcomes associated with a more positive fluid balance. Thermodilution studies showed excess EVLW to have reasonable sensitivity and specificity in predicting ICU mortality in patients with ARDS.[185] Assuming global organ perfusion appears adequate, as demonstrated by normal lactate levels, intraoperative losses should be replaced but otherwise be conservative in the volumes of fluid given to patients with ARDS intraoperatively. There is a lack of adequately powered studies on the choice of colloid or crystalloid for intravascular volume replacement in patients with ARDS.

BURNS. Extensive burns create a situation of copious fluid loss from the circulation combined with particular sensitivity to the effects of excess fluid administration. Thermal injury creates an area of necrotic tissue with surrounding ischemic areas. The combination of dead tissue with areas undergoing ischemia and subsequent reperfusion causes localized and systemic inflammatory reactions through histamine, prostaglandin, reactive O_2 species, and cytokine release. Local impairment of endothelial barrier function leads to the loss of oncotically active plasma constituents, increased capillary filtration into the interstitial compartment, and evaporative transcutaneous fluid loss as a result of loss of skin integrity. Through similar mechanisms, extensive burns may lead to the systemic inflammatory response syndrome, with its well-recognized effects on fluid compartments outlined previously. The deleterious role of this inflammatory response is underlined by the reduction in mortality seen with early burn excision compared with conservative care.[186] IV fluid therapy is generally instituted for burns of greater than 15% total body surface area in adults and 10% total body surface area in children.[187] However, increasing uncertainty exists about the volume and type of fluid that should be given to patients with burns. Fluid administration is largely still based on formulas such as the Parkland formula (Box 47.1) or the Muir and Barclay versions. Although these have given a starting point for resuscitation volumes based on patient weight and extent of burn, myriad other patient and pathologic factors put such a recipe-based approach at odds with modern perioperative fluid therapy based on objective physiologic goals. Although the approaches based on these formulas advocate down-titration of administered fluid volumes if urine output is adequate (0.5-1 mL/kg/h),[188] in reality this appears not to be practiced. Indeed, large studies have shown that the majority of burn patients receive fluid volumes in excess of those predicted by the Parkland formula, with a mean of 6 mL/kg/% burn compared with 4 mL/kg/% burn in 24 hours predicted by the formula.[189] Conversely, patients with inhaled and other nonburn injuries, electrical burns, or delayed resuscitation are considered to need increased resuscitation intravascular volumes, yet this is not taken into account by the formulas.

Excessive fluid administration in burned patients ("fluid creep") is not benign. As in all conditions typified by systemic inflammation, excess administered fluid will collect in compliant compartments. Pulmonary edema requiring ventilatory support, fasciotomies in muscle compartments, raised intraocular pressure, and conversion of superficial to deep burns have been observed and attributed to fluid resuscitation.[187] Intraabdominal hypertension and compartment syndrome are correlated to the volume of fluid administered, with a particular rise when more than 300 mL/kg is administered in 24 hours.[190] These concerns have led to renewed efforts to find the optimum regimen for burn resuscitation in terms of crystalloid versus colloid, newer formulas using lower volumes such as the Haifa formula, and targeting objective physiologic parameters such as SV or intrathoracic blood volume. Early trials have suggested that minimally invasive cardiac output monitoring may have a role, although there are no adequately sized trials to

BOX 47.1 Parkland Burn Fluid Resuscitation Formula

First 8 h: 2 mL/kg × % TBSA (lactated Ringer solution)
Next 16 h: 2 mL/kg × %TBSA (lactated Ringer solution)
Next 24 h: 0.8 mL/kg × %TBSA (5% dextrose) + 0.015 mL/kg × %TBSA (5% albumin)

%TBSA, Burn size as % of total body surface area. Time periods refer to the time since the burn occurred.

Data from Baxter CR. Problems and complications of burn shock resuscitation. *Surg Clin North Am.* 1978;58:1313.

show whether this approach improves outcomes.[191] Pending a consensus from this ongoing work, burn resuscitation should be commenced with one of the currently accepted formulas, but actively down-titrated if a urine output of 0.5 to 1 mL/kg/h is obtained. A combination of crystalloids and colloids may be used to reduce the total fluid volume administered,[192] although the early use of colloids is controversial due to the perceived risk of extravasation of oncotically active molecules in the presence of severe capillary leak. In addition, patients with burns were included in recent license restrictions on the use of starches.[191] Intraabdominal pressure should be monitored, and consideration given to assessing resuscitation endpoints, such as lactate and cardiac output, in addition to urine output.

PEDIATRICS. Perioperative fluid therapy in pediatric patients has for many years been based on traditional approaches that are increasingly being reexamined. Holliday and Segar[138] proposed a quantity and composition of maintenance fluid in hospitalized children in 1957 based on water requirements to sustain average metabolic activity and the electrolyte composition of milk. This developed into the 4-2-1 volume calculation for maintenance fluid requirements aimed at replacing insensible and urinary losses with hypotonic crystalloids containing glucose to maintain isoosmolality. These concepts were translated into the perioperative phase and glucose-based solutions were administered intraoperatively to reduce the apparently high risk for preoperative hypoglycemia after prolonged fasting,[193] and postoperative maintenance fluids were prescribed based on the 4-2-1 calculation using hypotonic crystalloids. Furthermore, the pediatric population was thought to be at risk for clinically significant preoperative dehydration by fasting, as a result of limited urinary concentrating ability and ongoing insensible losses because of the relatively large body surface area. Intraoperative replenishment of these volumes using 25 mL/kg of isotonic salt solution for those 3 years of age and younger or 15 mL/kg for those 4 years of age and older has been recommended.[194]

Multiple factors have led to a reevaluation of this approach. First, the modern approach to preoperative fasting, such that children may take clear—and potentially carbohydrate-containing—fluids up to 2 hours before surgery, reduces the risk for hemodynamically significant preoperative dehydration.[195] Second, the incidence of preoperative hypoglycemia is infrequent (<2.5%) and related to inappropriately prolonged fasting or other risk factors, such as prematurity, small for gestational age, or poor nutritional status.[196,197] Surgery itself increases blood glucose concentration, and administering glucose-containing solutions intraoperatively may cause hyperglycemia,[198] with the potential for osmotic diuresis and electrolyte abnormalities, or even adverse neurologic outcomes in the event of an ischemic or hypoxic event.[197] Glucose-free balanced crystalloid solutions should therefore be used intraoperatively, except in those at particularly high risk for hypoglycemia. Third, increasing awareness of the incidence and potentially disastrous neurologic outcomes from postoperative hyponatremia in pediatric populations has led to a reappraisal of postoperative hypotonic crystalloid maintenance fluids in 4-2-1 volumes. The effective SIADH induced by surgical stress and aggravated by the presence of pain and hypovolemia causes water retention and the risk for hypoosmolar hyponatremia if hypotonic solutions continue to be infused in significant volumes. Proposed strategies to avoid this include using one half to two thirds of the calculated 4-2-1 formula for maintenance fluids,[195] avoiding the most hypotonic fluids (4% dextrose with 0.18% NaCl),[197] using balanced isotonic crystalloids (containing glucose if available).[199,200] General measures that should be applied to all patients include:

- returning to oral fluids as early as possible
- ensuring euvolemia to minimize the ADH response[201]
- clearly dividing *maintenance* requirements from the variable amounts of fluid required because of *ongoing losses* (e.g., GI or blood), which should typically be replaced by isotonic crystalloids, colloids, or blood
- checking electrolytes at least daily in those still receiving IV fluids

Although isotonic saline has been advocated as a "safer" fluid for postoperative maintenance, this brings the risk for Na^+ overload and hyperchloremic acidosis.

More recent developments in perioperative fluid management remain underexplored in pediatric populations. In particular, there is little data on whether colloid volume expansion is beneficial or harmful in pediatrics when compared with crystalloids, or whether goal-directed fluid therapy may confer the advantages that have been suggested in adult populations.

Hepatic failure. Progressive liver disease and cirrhosis cause a distinctive pattern of abnormal fluid balance. The combination of peripheral vasodilation and relative intravascular depletion can mimic a decrease in intravascular volume. Yet, total body Na^+ and water are retained with ascites and edema.[202]

The widely accepted pathophysiologic mechanisms are that progressive disruption of liver architecture combines with decreased hepatic nitric oxide (NO) bioavailability and increased vasoconstrictor production, leading to sinusoidal hypertension. Compensatory vasodilatory mechanisms, including NO overproduction, lead to splanchnic and systemic vasodilation, relative hypovolemia, and reduced systemic arterial pressure. This triggers baroreceptor-mediated activation of the RAA, SNS, and ADH release. Although cardiac output increases, reduced systemic vascular resistance persists despite these compensatory mechanisms. The state of hyperaldosteronism causes salt and water retention, but hyponatremia occurs because of a relative excess of water retention. Splanchnic vasodilation and vascular permeability combine with decreased lymphatic drainage to favor the formation of ascites. The neurohumoral response also induces renal artery vasoconstriction, reducing renal blood flow and increasing the risk for hepatorenal syndrome. A range of therapies to maintain patients in a compensated state include: dietary fluid and salt restriction, diuretics (particularly spironolactone and loop diuretics), and intermittent or continuous drainage of ascites. However, the perioperative period presents considerable potential for disturbance of this fine balance. Excessive administration of isotonic saline will aggravate the preexisting salt and water overload, leading to further ascites and edema formation. Conversely, periods of hypovolemia are poorly tolerated, leading to a significant deficit in organ perfusion, further stimulation of the RAA, SNS, and ADH axes, and increasing risk for kidney injury. The approach should therefore be to assess volume status carefully, considering cardiac output monitoring, and to replace losses with appropriate volumes of isotonic crystalloid, colloid, or blood but to avoid salt and water overload. In instances of large-volume (>6 L) paracentesis, hemodynamic instability is a risk. Albumin appears to be a more effective prophylactic treatment for this than saline, abrogating the stimulated increase in plasma renin activity and maintaining more stable hemodynamics.[203] Lactate and other buffered fluids may be used in hepatic failure, although their metabolism may be slowed in advanced liver disease.

In decompensated liver disease with encephalopathy, raised intracranial pressure may be present and osmotherapy, such as hypertonic saline, should be used to bring plasma Na^+ into the high-normal range.[204] This is in contrast to chronic compensated liver disease, in which a degree of hyponatremia is well tolerated and does not require acute correction unless it is severe or symptomatic (see earlier discussion).

Obstetrics: preeclampsia. Preeclampsia is a multisystem disease of pregnancy characterized by hypertension, proteinuria, and multiorgan involvement that may affect the kidneys, liver, pulmonary, and central nervous systems. In contrast to the usual volume-expanded status in pregnancy, patients with preeclampsia have reduced plasma volume, combined with endothelial dysfunction and hypoalbuminemia. Previously IV volume expansion was thought to be beneficial in treating hypertension in preeclampsia; however, this has not been borne out by later studies.[205,206] Furthermore, a clear association exists between positive fluid balance and the incidence of pulmonary edema in this condition.[207] Acute pulmonary edema occurs in between 5% and 30% of cases of preeclampsia. It is associated with increased hospital length of stay and is a leading cause of death in preeclamptic patients. Most cases present in the postpartum period, perhaps reflecting the autotransfusion into a vasoconstricted circulation that occurs after delivery. Low COP also contributes.

Patients with preeclampsia should receive restricted volumes of IV crystalloid (80 mL/h, including that received as drug diluents[208]), and fluid balance should be observed carefully. Oliguria should not be treated by administration of large volumes of fluids in the presence of normal renal function. This conservative strategy has not been associated with an increase in kidney injury.[209] Any blood loss in the peripartum or perioperative period should be replaced with an appropriate volume of crystalloid, colloid, or blood, depending on magnitude. Invasive monitoring should be used to direct fluid therapy in cases of severe preeclampsia.

Surgical Factors

NEUROSURGERY. Multiple physiologic factors mean that fluid and electrolyte therapy are a key component in the perioperative management of intracranial pathology. This management may be complicated by disturbances of water and Na^+ balance caused by neurosurgical diseases themselves. Much of the current fluid management in this area is based on knowledge of this physiology, experimental models, and gradual evolution of interventions investigated in small trials rather than large randomized studies.

The intact blood-brain barrier (BBB) excludes electrolytes and large molecules but allows passage of water. Extravascular brain water is therefore related to plasma osmolality, with cerebral edema a feature of hypoosmolar hyponatremic conditions. Intracranial diseases may compromise the integrity of the BBB, increasing the predisposition to edema. Cerebral perfusion also may be impaired if systemic blood pressure is inadequate in the face of increased intracranial pressure, particularly in pathologic conditions in which autoregulation is impaired. Rational management of fluids in neurosurgical patients should start with maintaining baseline blood volume and cerebral perfusion and avoiding significant decreases in serum Na^+, osmolality, and oncotic pressure. Several situations may require more specific management:

1. Increased intracranial pressure: Increasing serum osmolality may reduce total brain water and therefore intracranial pressure by creating brain-blood osmotic gradients. Mannitol and hypertonic saline given by bolus have been the pharmacologic mainstays in this area. The osmotic action of these drugs may be reduced if the BBB is disrupted by brain injury; however, they also have therapeutic benefits beyond simple osmotic effects.[210] A meta-analysis of the small studies available suggests that hypertonic saline may be superior to mannitol in reducing intracranial hypertension, but large-scale controlled studies are required to confirm this.[57] Conversely, using hypertonic saline in all patients with early traumatic brain injury without intracranial pressure monitoring has not been shown to improve outcomes.[58] Similarly, continuous infusion of hypertonic saline to induce persistent hypernatremia in the presence of cerebral edema also lacks evidence of benefit.[211] Restrictive fluid strategies have been advocated to minimize intracranial hypertension in severe traumatic brain injury. Although retrospective data analysis suggests that positive fluid balance is not associated with refractory intracranial hypertension, an association between hypervolemia and pulmonary edema was observed.[212]
2. Cerebral vasospasm: Manipulation of hemodynamics and hematocrit is traditionally used in the treatment of vasospasm after subarachnoid hemorrhage. This "triple-H" therapy (hypervolemia, hemodilution, hypertension) has entered practice based on small studies of efficacy rather than randomized trials.[213,214] Some workers, using extensive animal models, have advocated a hematocrit no lower than 30%, below which the benefits of reducing blood viscosity are outweighed by a reduction in O_2 delivery. They also caution against hypervolemia, both for its potentially injurious effects in the presence of a dysfunctional BBB and for the extracranial effects such as pulmonary edema.[215] "Prophylactic" hypervolemia aiming to prevent vasospasm is not recommended.[216]
3. An intracranial pathologic condition may itself be a cause of disturbances of both water and Na^+ balance through diabetes insipidus, cerebral salt wasting, or SIADH. This should be assessed and treated as described in the section on electrolyte imbalance.

Clear comparisons of crystalloid and colloid in a variety of neurosurgical settings are lacking. Of the available evidence, albumin is associated with an increase in mortality in traumatic brain injury compared with isotonic saline.[5] In the absence of more robust evidence, a mixture of isotonic crystalloids and colloids is advocated in other neurosurgical settings.[214,217]

TRAUMA. In patients with evidence of major traumatic hemorrhage, the key goals are to avoid clot disruption until definitive control of bleeding, to treat the acute coagulopathy of trauma, to maximize tissue O_2 delivery by the early use of packed red cell transfusion, and to avoid hypothermia and acidosis. This approach is termed hemostatic resuscitation. In the prehospital setting, restrictive fluid therapy may improve outcomes, particularly in penetrating trauma.[218] The approach should initially be one of permissive hypovolemia, with fluid administered to achieve cerebration rather than normotension in awake patients, systolic blood pressure of 70 to 80 mm Hg in penetrating trauma, or 90 mm Hg in blunt trauma.[219] The duration of organ hypoperfusion that may be involved with this approach should be minimized by rapid transfer for damage control intervention to stop bleeding, whether radiologic or surgical. Large volumes of IV crystalloids or colloids in early resuscitation will cause hemodilution and dilute clotting factors, and saline-based fluids may aggravate the acidosis associated with major blood loss. Rather, packed RBCs (PBRCs), clotting factors (e.g., fresh frozen plasma [FFP]) and platelets should be replaced early. Limited evidence, particularly from military populations and retrospective analyses, suggests "high" ratios of FFP to PRBC (e.g., 1:1-1:2) are associated with the best outcomes in massive transfusion compared with lower ratios (e.g., 1:9)[219,220]. Active warming should be used and clot stability improved with tranexamic acid.[221] Once hemostasis has been achieved, restoration of normal circulating volume and tissue perfusion is the goal, with ongoing blood, clotting factors, platelet, and fluid infusions targeting normalization of cardiac output and O_2 delivery, lactate levels, and blood clotting (best checked using near-patient whole-blood tests of clotting, such as thromboelastography). A small number of trials support the practice of GDT in the immediate perioperative trauma setting, but larger controlled trials are required. After surgery and initial resuscitation, much of the evidence for ongoing fluid approaches is derived from unselected critical care populations. As outlined previously, the evidence suggests that in established critical illness, aggressive GDT may be harmful.[218]

Patients with traumatic brain injury in addition to major hemorrhage present a dilemma because the raised cerebral perfusion pressure required for adequate cerebral blood flow in the face of raised intracranial pressure is at odds with the hypotensive resuscitation approach. In isolated head injuries, using fluids and vasopressors to achieve a mean arterial pressure *above* 90 mm Hg is recommended, with avoidance of hyponatremia and hypoosmolality to minimize cerebral edema.[210,217] Little evidence exists to inform resuscitation treatment in patients with mixed intracranial and extracranial trauma, so the strategy should be based on clinical judgment, prioritizing the requirements of the most severe injuries. Control of bleeding is particularly important to allow subsequent normalization of systemic blood pressure to meet the need for adequate cerebral perfusion. Even in general trauma, much of the evidence supporting current resuscitation approaches is derived from animal models and limited randomized trials, predominantly in young otherwise healthy subjects in the prehospital setting.[218] The needs of individual patients should therefore be taken into account, particularly because older patients with comorbidities may tolerate periods of hypoperfusion very poorly.

Free Tissue Flap Surgery. Free tissue flaps are frequently used during oncoplastic surgery, typically for breast reconstruction or after resection of head and neck tumors and involve the autologous transplantation of tissue to fill a defect, complete with arterial supply and venous drainage. Transplanted vessels are denervated and lack intrinsic sympathetic tone, but the feeding vessels are not; vasoconstriction in these feeding vessels related to cold and excessive doses of vasopressor must be avoided because it may threaten the perfusion of the flap. Flap blood flow depends on systemic blood pressure and blood viscosity, and hypervolemic hemodilution has traditionally been used to address these requirements. However, given the reduction in O_2 carrying capacity and potential for flap edema that this entails, a more conservative fluid strategy should be used, which may improve flap outcome.[219] The use of dextrans to improve blood flow is not currently favored, because no benefit has been demonstrated and the risks for medical complications is relatively high.[220] Free tissue flaps have disrupted lymphatics, which take several weeks to reconnect, making them particularly prone to interstitial edema. Large volumes of crystalloid—favoring increased capillary filtration—should be avoided and colloids used for blood volume expansion.[221]

Intrathoracic Procedures. Any procedure within the thorax, including upper GI and thoracic surgery, can lead to postoperative respiratory problems, including ARDS and acute lung injury (ALI). The development of ARDS and ALI is partly due to the proinflammatory nature of one-lung ventilation,[222,223] modified by a host of other patient and surgical risk factors. In esophagogastrectomy, retrospective studies and case series have suggested reduced pulmonary complications with restrictive fluid strategies.[224-227] One retrospective observational study of esophagectomy patients found a cumulative fluid balance greater than 1900 mL from surgery to the second postoperative day to be an independent risk factor for other adverse outcomes, including death.[228] The use of diuretics to actively target fluid balance, degree of cardiovascular support, and presence or absence of epidurals was not explored in this study. More controlled trials of different fluid balance approaches are required in this population. However, the potential benefit of conservative fluid administration in this group is consistent with the large randomized study of patients with ARDS demonstrating improved pulmonary outcomes in those treated with a restrictive rather than liberal fluid regimen.[183] While maintaining adequate tissue perfusion, a cautious approach to fluid administration is recommended, both to minimize pulmonary complications and to avoid anastomotic edema.

Hepatic Resection. Blood loss during liver parenchymal resection, a risk factor for worse outcomes, is associated with high venous pressure and backflow of blood through the valveless hepatic veins. One study has shown that a CVP of 5 cm H_2O or lower is associated with significantly lower blood loss and transfusion requirements.[229] Several techniques are used to maintain a low CVP, including conservative fluid management, at least until the hepatic resection is completed. Despite evidence that using a low CVP technique does not have adverse effects on renal or liver function,[230] a pragmatic compromise must be sought for each patient. Inducing hypovolemia during liver resection risks hemodynamic instability and end-organ hypoperfusion, increases the risk for air embolism, and reduces the physiologic reserve should massive blood loss occur. Once the liver resection is finished, a more generous fluid approach can be taken to ensure adequate circulating volume. This may be guided by invasive hemodynamic monitoring and minimally invasive cardiac output monitoring to provide a rational endpoint to fluid therapy in this phase.

Major Intraabdominal Surgery. Major intraabdominal operations, particularly those involving multiple organ resections for tumor, require careful perioperative fluid management. Major gynecologic operations such as pelvic exenteration or ovarian debulking and urologic procedures including cystectomy, radical nephrectomy, and major retroperitoneal lymph node dissection can involve dramatic fluid shifts in the perioperative period. Fluid losses during surgery are caused by prolonged peritoneal exposure, significant blood loss, and acute drainage of tumor-related ascites. The total volume lost is difficult to quantify, so cardiac output monitoring is valuable when combined with CVP and arterial pressure monitoring and serial blood gas analysis.[231,232] Intraoperative drainage of ascites is followed by fluid shift from the vascular space, as this reaccumulates postoperatively and may require large volumes to replace the ongoing loss. Another consequence of fluid redistribution is electrolyte abnormalities; hypokalemia and hypomagnesemia are frequently seen.

Renal Transplant. The key goals of fluid therapy in the perioperative management of renal transplant are to ensure adequate renal perfusion to support early graft function and avoid fluid therapy side effects to which patients with impaired renal function may be susceptible. Traditionally, CVP-guided intraoperative fluid therapy has been advocated, using large volumes of crystalloid (up to 60-100 mL/kg) to achieve a CVP of 10 to 12 mm Hg or higher before reperfusion.[233] Recently, more conservative goals have been advocated, limiting crystalloid infusion to 15 mL/kg/h, aiming for a CVP of 7 to 9 mm Hg with no apparent increase in graft failure.[234] The role of alternative tools such as esophageal Doppler or pulse contour analysis to supplement or replace CVP-guided fluid therapy in this area also has been suggested, but so far only exploratory trials have been conducted.[235,236] Patients with renal failure may develop acidosis-related hyperkalemia when isotonic saline is infused during transplant,[44] so balanced crystalloid solutions, or even K^+-free, buffered dialysate solutions, should be used. The role of colloids in this population requires further study, although concerns over renal toxicity of starches may limit their use.[235] Postoperative fluid therapy should take into account the baseline maintenance requirements and the ongoing losses resulting from urine production.

LIVER TRANSPLANT. Liver transplantation involves a series of major physiologic disruptions that have direct relevance to fluid and electrolyte management.[237] Therapy should be guided by data from invasive monitoring, possibly including pulmonary artery catheterization. During phase I (preanhepatic), large volume blood loss and further fluid shifts resulting from drainage of ascites may occur. During phase II (anhepatic), a major reduction in venous return and therefore cardiac output may occur if a bicaval approach is used. Crystalloid and colloid infusion may be required along with vasopressors to maintain arterial pressure during this phase, although excessive volume administration risks right heart failure after unclamping. Absent citrate and lactate metabolism during this phase contributes to acidosis, hypocalcemia, and hypomagnesemia. On reperfusion and unclamping, cold, acidotic, hyperkalemic fluid is released into the circulation. Preparation for this must include normalizing pH and maintaining plasma K^+ in the low-normal range during phase II. This may require Ca^+, insulin-dextrose, hyperventilation, and even $NaHCO_3$ treatment. Phase III (reperfusion) leads to an acute rise in CVP, possibly with hepatic congestion and right heart strain. Systemic vasodilation and cardiac arrest may occur, leading to hypotension requiring vasopressor or inotrope support. If not given already, a bolus of $CaCl_2$ should be used to prevent hyperkalemia-related arrhythmias. Subsequent uptake of K^+ by a working graft may then require aggressive replacement. Ongoing infusion of fluids, red cells, and blood products should be guided by clinical blood loss. Other goals are to maintain a hematocrit of 26% to 32% and to correct the coagulopathy as guided by coagulation testing. There is increasing interest in the role of cardiac output-guided fluid in the perioperative care of patients undergoing liver transplantation.[238]

Complete references available online at expertconsult.com.

References

1. Brandis K. Fluid & electrolyte physiology. In: *The Physiology Viva: Questions & Answers*. Queensland, Australia, Southport: Author; 2003. Author.
2. Levick JR, et al. *Cardiovasc Res*. 2010;87:198.
3. Woodcock TE, et al. *Br J Anaesth*. 2012;108:384.
4. Hahn RG. *Anesthesiology*. 2010;113:470.
5. Finfer S, et al. *N Engl J Med*. 2004;350:2247.
6. Brunkhorst FM, et al. *N Engl J Med*. 2008;358:125.
7. James MFM, et al. *Br J Anaesth*. 2011;107:693.
8. Rehm M, et al. *Anesthesiology*. 2004;100:1211.
9. Bruegger D, et al. *Am J Physiol Heart Circ Physiol*. 2005;289:H1993.
10. Henry CB, et al. *Am J Physiol Heart Circ Physiol*. 2000;279:H2815.
11. Chappell D, et al. *Anesthesiology*. 2008;109:723.
12. Drummer C, et al. *Acta Physiol Scand Suppl*. 1992;604:101.
13. Montani J-P, et al. *Exp Physiol*. 2009;94:382.
14. Hall JE, et al. *Fed Proc*. 1986;45:2897.
15. Guyton AC. *Am J Physiol*. 1990;259:R865.
16. Dorrington KL, et al. *Anaesthesia*. 2009;64:1218.
17. Committee on Medical Aspects of Food Policy. *Rep Health Soc Subj (Lond)*. 1991;41:1.
18. Kaye AD, et al. Intravascular fluid and electrolyte physiology. In: Miller RD, et al., ed. *Miller's Anesthesia*. 7th ed. New York: Churchill Livingstone; 2009:1705.
19. Adrogué HJ, et al. *N Engl J Med*. 2007;356:1966.
20. Greenlee M, et al. *Ann Intern Med*. 2009;150:619.
21. Clausen T. Role of Na+,K+-pumps and transmembrane Na+,K+-distribution in muscle function. The FEPS lecture - Bratislava 2007. *Acta Physiol (Oxf)*. 2008;192(3):339–349.
22. Kroemer G, et al. *Annu Rev Physiol*. 1998;60:619.
23. Brown EM, et al. *N Engl J Med*. 1995;333:234.
24. Pondel M. Calcitonin and calcitonin receptors: bone and beyond. *Int J Exp Pathol*. 2000;81(6):405–422.
25. Olsen HS, Cepeda MA, Zhang QQ, Rosen CA, Vozzolo BL. Human stanniocalcin: a possible hormonal regulator of mineral metabolism. *Proc Natl Acad Sci USA*. 1996;93(5):1792–1796.
26. Bushinsky DA. *Lancet*. 1998;352:306.
27. Dubé L, Granry J-C. *Can J Anaesth*. 2003;50:732.
28. Dimeski G, et al. *Clin Chim Acta*. 2010;411:309.
29. Gomez MN. *Anesthesiology*. 1998;89:222.
30. Günther T, et al. *FEBS Lett*. 1992;307:333.
31. Shaikh A, et al. *Pediatr Nephrol*. 2008;23:1203.
32. Weisinger JR, et al. *Lancet*. 1998;352:391.
33. Sabbagh Y, et al. *J Am Soc Nephrol*. 2009;20:2348.
34. Yunos NM, et al. *Crit Care*. 2010;14:226.
35. Kraut JA, et al. *Clin J Am Soc Nephrol*. 2007;2:162.
36. Morgan TJ. *Clin Biochem Rev*. 2009;30:41.
37. Guidet B, et al. *Crit Care*. 2010;14:325.
38. Bampoe S, et al. *Cochrane Database Syst Rev*. 2017;21:9. CD004089.
39. Wilcox CS. *J Clin Invest*. 1983;71:726.
40. Wilcox CS, et al. *Am J Physiol*. 1987;253:F734.
41. Quilley CP, et al. *Br J Pharmacol*. 1993;108:106.
42. Chowdhury AH, et al. *Ann Surg*. 2012;256:18.
43. Handy JM, et al. *Br J Anaesth*. 2008;101:141.
44. O'Malley CMN, et al. *Anesth Analg*. 2005;100:1518.
45. Self WH, et al. *N Engl J Med*. 2018;378(9):819.
46. Semler MW, et al. *N Engl J Med*. 2018;378(9):829.
47. Reinhart K, Takala J. *Anesth Analg*. 2011;112(3):507.
48. Lobo DN, Dube MG, Neal KR, Simpson J, Rowlands BJ, Allison SP. Problems with solutions: drowning in the brine of an inadequate knowledge base. *Clin Nutr*. 2001;20(2):125–130.
49. Walsh SR, Walsh CJ. Intravenous fluid-associated morbidity in postoperative patients. *Ann R Coll Surg Engl*. 2005;87(2):126–130.
50. Stoneham MD, Hill EL. Variability in post-operative fluid and electrolyte prescription. *Br J Clin Pract*. 1997;51(2):82–84.
51. Myburgh JA, et al. *N Engl J Med*. 2012;367:1901.
52. Grocott MPW, et al. *Anesth Analg*. 2005;100:1093.
53. Awad S, et al. *Clin Nutr*. 2008;27:179.
54. Burdett E, et al. *Cochrane Database Syst Rev*. 2012;12:CD004089.
55. Yunos NM, et al. *JAMA*. 2012;308:1566.
56. Bulger EM, et al. *Ann Surg*. 2011;253:431.
57. Kamel H, et al. *Crit Care Med*. 2011;39:554.
58. Bulger EM, et al. *JAMA*. 2010;304:1455.
59. Hartmann AF, et al. *J Clin Invest*. 1932;11:345.
60. Kreisberg RA. *Ann Intern Med*. 1980;92:227.
61. Vinay P, et al. *Am J Nephrol*. 1987;7:337.
62. Stetten MR, et al. *J Biol Chem*. 1953;203:653.
63. Satoh K, et al. *Eur J Anaesthesiol*. 2005;22:703.
64. Ruttmann TG, et al. *Anesth Analg*. 2007;104:1475.
65. Reid F, et al. *Clin Sci*. 2003;104:17.
66. Htyte N, et al. *Nephrol Dial Transplant*. 2011;26:1432.
67. Chan L, et al. *Integr Physiol Behav Sci*. 1994;29:383.
68. Kuze S, et al. *Anesth Analg*. 1992;75:702.
69. Bingel M, et al. *Lancet*. 1987;1:14.
70. Thaha M, et al. *Acta Med Indones*. 2005;37:145.
71. Veech RL, et al. *Adv Enzyme Regul*. 1988;27:313.
72. Jacob AD, et al. *Kidney Int*. 1997;52:755.
73. Selby NM, et al. *ASAIO J*. 2006;52:62.
74. Davies PG, et al. *Crit Care*. 2011;15:R21.
75. Traverso LW, et al. *J Trauma*. 1986;26:168.
76. Reinhart K, et al. *Intensive Care Med*. 2012;38:368.
77. Lobo DN, et al. *Crit Care Med*. 2010;38:464.
78. De Jonge E, et al. *Crit Care Med*. 2001;29:1261.
79. Treib J, et al. *Intensive Care Med*. 1999;25:258.
80. Sirtl C, et al. *Br J Anaesth*. 1999;82:510.
81. Lamke LO, et al. *Resuscitation*. 1976;5:93.
82. James MFM, et al. *Anaesthesia*. 2004;59:738.

83. Haase N, et al. *BMJ*. 2013;346:f839.
84. Perner A, et al. *N Engl J Med*. 2012;367:124.
85. Dart AB, et al. *Cochrane Database Syst Rev*. 2010;1:CD007594.
86. Gillies MA, et al. *Br J Anaesth*. 2014;112:25.
87. Dickenmann M, et al. *Am J Kidney Dis*. 2008;51:491.
88. Peden A, et al. *Haemophilia*. 2010;16:296.
89. Choi PT, et al. *Crit Care Med*. 1999;27:200.
90. Delaney AP, et al. *Crit Care Med*. 2011;39:386.
91. Jacob M, et al. *Acta Anaesthesiol Scand*. 2008;52:522.
92. Ackland GL, et al. *Anesth Analg*. 2008;106:924.
93. Sanders G, et al. *Br J Surg*. 2001;88:1363.
94. Lamke LO, et al. *Acta Chir Scand*. 1977;143:279.
95. Koyner JL, et al. *Blood Purif*. 2010;29:52.
96. Mackenzie AI, et al. *Br Med J*. 1969;3:619.
97. Mythen MG, et al. *Br J Anaesth*. 1993;71:858.
98. Deitch EA. *Arch Surg*. 1990;125:403.
99. Lewis H, et al. *Adv Exp Med Biol*. 1989;247A:281.
100. Swart RM, et al. *Nephron Physiol*. 2011;118:45.
101. Hamilton-Davies C, et al. *Intensive Care Med*. 1997;23:276.
102. Osman D, et al. *Crit Care Med*. 2007;35:64.
103. Thorniley MS, et al. *Br J Plast Surg*. 1998;51:218.
104. Edsander-Nord A, et al. *Plast Reconstr Surg*. 2002;109:664.
105. Hameed SM, et al. *Chest*. 2003;123:475S.
106. Mythen MG, et al. *Arch Surg*. 1995;130:423.
107. Thacker JKM, et al. *Ann Surg*. 2016;263(3):502.
108. Lobo DN, et al. *Lancet*. 2002;359:1812.
109. Mythen MG. *Anesth Analg*. 2005;100:196.
110. Holte K, et al. *Br J Anaesth*. 2002;89:622.
111. Brandstrup B, et al. *Ann Surg*. 2003;238:641.
112. Corcoran T, et al. *Anesth Analg*. 2012;114:640.
113. Kumar S, et al. *Lancet*. 1998;352:220.
114. Tisdall M, et al. *J Neurosurg Anesthesiol*. 2006;18:57.
115. Leung AA, et al. *Arch Intern Med*. 2012;172:1474.
116. Ayus JC, et al. *Neurology*. 1996;46:323.
117. Lane N, et al. *BMJ*. 1999;318:1363.
118. Dorotta I, et al. *Anesth Analg*. 2003;97:1536.
119. Gravenstein D. *Anesth Analg*. 1997;84:438.
120. Mamoulakis C, et al. *BJU Int*. 2012;109:240.
121. Olsson J, et al. *Acta Anaesthesiol Scand*. 1995;39:252.
122. American College of Obstetricians and Gynecologists. *Obstet Gynecol*. 2005;106:439.
123. Agarwal R, et al. *Am J Kidney Dis*. 1994;24:108.
124. Sterns RH, et al. *Semin Nephrol*. 2009;29:282.
125. Alfonzo AVM, et al. *Resuscitation*. 2006;70:10.
126. Chung HS, et al. *J Int Med Res*. 2012;40:572.
127. Lier H, et al. *J Trauma*. 2008;65:951.
128. Major P, et al. *J Clin Oncol*. 2001;19:558.
129. Aguilera IM, et al. *Anaesthesia*. 2000;55:779.
130. Huijgen HJ, et al. *Am J Clin Pathol*. 2000;114:688.
131. Saris NE, et al. *Clin Chim Acta*. 2000;294:1.
132. Taylor BE, et al. *J Am Coll Surg*. 2004;198:198.
133. Holte K, et al. *Anesth Analg*. 2007;105:465.
134. Maharaj CH, et al. *Anesth Analg*. 2005;100:675.
135. Rhodes A, et al. *Intensive Care Med*. 2010;36:1327.
136. Grocott MPW, et al. *Cochrane Database Syst Rev*. 2012;11:CD004082.
137. Lilot M, et al. *Br J Anaesth*. 2015;114(5):767.
138. Holliday MA, et al. *Pediatrics*. 1957;19:823.
139. Nisanevich V, et al. *Anesthesiology*. 2005;103:25.
140. Hübner M, et al. *J Surg Res*. 2012;173:68.
141. Futier E, et al. *Arch Surg*. 2010;145:1193.
142. Myles PS, et al. *N Engl J Med*. 2018;378(24):2263.
143. MacKay G, et al. *Br J Surg*. 2006;93:1469.
144. Shoemaker WC, et al. *Arch Surg*. 1973;106:630.
145. Shoemaker WC, et al. *Chest*. 1988;94:1176.
146. Boyd O, et al. *JAMA*. 1993;270:2699.
147. Venn R, et al. *Br J Anaesth*. 2002;88(1):65.
148. Marik PE, et al. *Chest*. 2008;134:172.
149. Polonen P, et al. *Anesth Analg*. 2000;90:1052.
150. Pearse R, et al. *Crit Care*. 2005;9:R694.
151. Donati A, et al. *Chest*. 2007;132:1817.
152. Pearse RM, et al. *JAMA*. 2014;311(21):2181.
153. Calvo-Vecino JM, et al. British Journal of Anaesthesia [Internet]. 2018 Feb [cited 2018 Mar 11]; Available from: http://linkinghub.elsevier.com/retrieve/pii/S0007091217542075
154. Pestaña D, et al. *Anesth Analg*. 2014;119(3):579.
155. Parker MJ, et al. *Br J Anaesth*. 2004;92:67.
156. Noblett SE, et al. *Br J Surg*. 2006;93(9):1069.
157. Morris C, et al. *Anaesthesia*. 2011;66:819.
158. Harvey S, et al. *Lancet*. 2005;366:472.
159. Prien T, et al. *J Clin Anesth*. 1990;2:317.
160. Perel P, et al. *Cochrane Database Syst Rev*. 2012;6:CD000567.
161. Ackland GL, et al. *Curr Opin Crit Care*. 2010;16:339.
162. MacDonald N, et al. *Br J Anaesth*. 2015;114(4):598.
163. Pearse R, et al. *Crit Care*. 2005;9:R687.
164. Lewis S, et al. *J Gastrointest Surg*. 2009;13:569.
165. NICE. *Intravenous Fluid Therapy in Adults in Hospital (Clinical Guidance 174) [Internet]*. 2014 [cited 2014 Apr 16]. Available from: http://www.nice.org.uk/.
166. Groban L, et al. *Anesth Analg*. 2006;103:557.
167. Trainor D, et al. *Semin Dial*. 2011;24:314.
168. Khajavi MR, et al. *Ren Fail*. 2008;30:535.
169. Dellinger RP, et al. *Intensive Care Med*. 2013;39:165.
170. Rivers E, et al. *N Engl J Med*. 2001;345(19):1368.
171. The ProCESS Investigators. *N Engl J Med*. 2014;370:1683.
172. ARISE Investigators, et al. *N Engl J Med*. 2014;371(16):1496.
173. Mouncey PR, et al. *N Engl J Med*. 2015;372(14):1301.
174. Rhodes A, et al. *Crit Care Med*. 2017;45(3):486.
175. Bihari S, et al. *Shock*. 2013;40(1):28.
176. Maitland K, et al. *N Engl J Med*. 2011;364(26):2483.
177. Godin PJ, et al. *Crit Care Med*. 1996;24(7):1117.
178. Krafft P, et al. *Chest*. 1993;103:900.
179. Singer M. *Clin Chest Med*. 2008;29:655.
180. Hayes MA, et al. *N Engl J Med*. 1994;330:1717.
181. Gattinoni L, et al. *N Engl J Med*. 1995;333:1025.
182. Boyd JH, et al. *Crit Care Med*. 2011;39:259.
183. Rosenberg AL, et al. *J Intensive Care Med*. 2009;24:35.
184. Wiedemann HP, et al. *N Engl J Med*. 2006;354:2564.
185. Stewart RM, et al. *J Am Coll Surg*. 2009;208:725.
186. Neamu RF, et al. *Curr Opin Crit Care*. 2013;19:24.
187. Ong YS, et al. *Burns*. 2006;32:145.
188. Tricklebank S. *Burns*. 2009;35:757.
189. Baxter CR. *Surg Clin North Am*. 1978;58:1313.
190. Cartotto R, et al. *J Burn Care Res*. 2010;31:551.
191. Oda J, et al. *Burns*. 2006;32:151.
192. Guilabert P, et al. *Br J Anaesth*. 2016;117(3):284.
193. O'Mara MS, et al. *J Trauma*. 2005;58:1011.
194. Thomas DK. *Br J Anaesth*. 1974;46:66.
195. Berry F. Practical aspects of fluid and electrolyte therapy. In: Berry F, ed. *Anesthetic Management of Difficult and Routine Pediatric Patients*. New York: Churchill Livingstone; 1986:107.
196. Murat I, et al. *Paediatr Anaesth*. 2008;18:363.
197. Phillips S, et al. *Br J Anaesth*. 1994;73:529.
198. Bailey AG, et al. *Anesth Analg*. 2010;110:375,.
199. Welborn LG, et al. *Anesthesiology*. 1986;65:543.
200. Sümpelmann R, et al. *Pediatric Anesthesia*. 2017;27(1):10.
201. McNab S, et al. *Cochrane Database Syst Rev*. 2014;(12):CD009457.
202. Holliday MA, et al. *Arch Dis Child*. 2007;92:546.
203. Kashani A, et al. *QJM*. 2008;101:71.
204. Sola-Vera J, et al. *Hepatology*. 2003;37:1147.
205. Stravitz RT, et al. *Crit Care Med*. 2007;35:2498.
206. Ganzevoort W, et al. *BJOG*. 2005;112:1358.
207. Duley L, et al. *Cochrane Database Syst Rev*. 2000;2:CD001805.
208. Thornton CE, et al. *Hypertens Pregnancy*. 2011;30:169.
209. National Institute for Health and Clinical Excellence. 2010. NICE clinical guideline no. 107.
210. Thornton C, et al. *J Obstet Gynaecol Can*. 2007;29:794.
211. Wijayatilake DS, et al. *Curr Opin Anaesthesiol*. 2012;25:540.
212. Ryu JH, et al. *Neurocrit Care*. 2013;19:222.
213. Fletcher JJ, et al. *Neurocrit Care*. 2010;13:47.
214. Velat GJ, et al. *World Neurosurg*. 2011;76:446.
215. Sen J, et al. *Lancet Neurol*. 2003;2:614.
216. Tummala RP, et al. *Clin Neurosurg*. 2006;53:238.
217. van der Jagt M. *Critical Care*. 2016;20:126.
218. Van Aken HK, Kampmeier TG, Ertmer C, Westphal M. Fluid resuscitation in patients with traumatic brain injury: what is a SAFE approach? *Curr Opin Anaesthesiol*. 2012;25(5):563–565.
219. Levett D, Vercueil A, Grocott M. Resuscitation fluids in trauma 1: why give fluid and how to give it. *Trauma*. 2006;8(1):47–53.

220. Harris T, et al. *BMJ*. 2012;345:e5752.
221. Johansson PI, Oliveri RS, Ostrowski SR. Hemostatic resuscitation with plasma and platelets in trauma. *J Emerg Trauma Shock*. 2012;5(2):120–125.
222. Roberts I, Shakur H, Coats T, Hunt B, Balogun E, Barnetson L, et al. The CRASH-2 trial: a randomised controlled trial and economic evaluation of the effects of tranexamic acid on death, vascular occlusive events and transfusion requirement in bleeding trauma patients. *Health Technol Assess*. 2013;17(10):1–79.
223. Brain Trauma Foundation, *J Neurotrauma*. 2007;24(suppl 1):S1.
224. Sigurdsson GH. *J Reconstr Microsurg*. 1995;11:57.
225. Disa JJ, et al. *Plast Reconstr Surg*. 2003;112:1534.
226. Shetty PS, et al. *Curr Anaesth Crit Care*. 2009;20:18.
227. Ojima H, et al. *Hepatogastroenterology*. 2007;54:111.
228. Michelet P, et al. *Anesthesiology*. 2006;105:911.
229. Low D, et al. *J Gastrointest Surg*. 2007;11:1395.
230. Kita T, et al. *J Clin Anesth*. 2002;14:252.
231. Neal JM, et al. *Reg Anesth Pain Med*. 2003;28:328.
232. Tandon S, et al. *Br J Anaesth*. 2001;86:633.
233. Wei S, et al. *Ann Thorac Surg*. 2008;86:266.
234. Jones RM, et al. *Br J Surg*. 1998;85:1058.
235. Redai I, et al. *Surg Clin North Am*. 2004;84:401.
236. Moore J, et al. *Curr Anaesth Crit Care*. 2009;20(8).
237. Shenoy S, et al. *Curr Anaesth Crit Care*. 2009;20(22).
238. Rabey PG. *BJA CEPD Reviews*. 2001;1:24.
239. De Gasperi A, et al. *Transplant Proc*. 2006;38:807.
240. Schmid S, et al. *Eur J Anaesthesiol*. 2012;29:552.
241. Calixto Fernandes MH, et al. 2018. Available from: https://www.ncbi.nlm.nih.gov/pmc/articles/PMC5784708/
242. Fabbroni D, et al. *Crit Care Pain*. 2006;6:171.
243. Froghi F, et al. 2018. Available from: https://www.ncbi.nlm.nih.gov/pmc/articles/PMC5842525/
244. Jones JG, et al. *Br J Anaesth*. 2000;84:226.
245. Chumlea WC, et al. *Kidney Int*. 1999;56:244.
246. Baarsma R, et al. *Biol Neonate*. 1992;62:108.
247. Ellis KJ, et al. *Ann N Y Acad Sci*. 2000;374:904.
248. Campbell I. *Anaesth Intensive Care Med*. 2009;10:593.
249. Hoffer LJ, et al. *Am J Physiol Regul Integr Comp Physiol*. 2005;289:R1372.
250. Hall JE. The body fluid compartments. In: *Guyton and Hall Textbook of Medical Physiology*. Philadelphia: Saunders; 2010:285.
251. Grădinaru I, et al. *Magnes Res*. 2007;20:254.
252. Sewón LA, et al. *J Clin Periodontol*. 1998;25:915.
253. Lentner C. Units of measurement, body fluids, composition of the body, nutrition. In: *Geigy Scientific Tables*. Basel: Ciba-Geigy Ltd; 1981.
254. Albrecht E, et al. *Anaesthesia*. 2013;68:79.
255. Rasmussen HS, et al. *Clin Cardiol*. 1988;11:541.
256. Sugimoto J, et al. *J Immunol*. 2012;188:6338.
257. Li F-Y, et al. *Nature*. 2011;475:471.
258. Soar J, et al. *Resuscitation*. 2010;81:1400.

48 Perioperative Acid-Base Balance

PATRICK J. NELIGAN

KEY POINTS

- The presence of a significant acid-base abnormality often signals a sinister underlying problem.
- All acid-base abnormalities result from alterations in the dissociation of water.
- Only three factors independently affect acid-base balance—the arterial partial pressure of carbon dioxide (PaCO2), the strong ion difference (SID), and the total concentration of weak acids (A_{TOT}).
- Respiratory acidosis and alkalosis are caused by hypercarbia and hypocarbia, respectively.
- Metabolic acidosis is caused by decreased SID or increased A_{TOT}. Decreased SID results from accumulation of metabolic anions (shock, ketoacidosis, and renal failure), hyperchloremia, and free water excess. Increased A_{TOT} results from hyperphosphatemia.
- Metabolic alkalosis is caused by increased SID or decreased A_{TOT}. SID increases due to sodium gain, chloride loss, or free water deficit. A_{TOT} decreases in hypoalbuminemia and hypophosphatemia. This is particularly common in critical illness.
- Most acid-base disorders are treated by reversal of the cause.

Introduction—Why Is Acid-Base Balance Important?

Blood gas and pH analyses have been the most robust laboratory and bedside tools for identifying and monitoring critical illness since the advent of modern medicine. There is good reason to believe that understanding acid-base chemistry will continue to be important for physicians for decades to come.[1]

The human body is composed principally of water, partitioned into intracellular and extracellular compartments. The electrolyte composition of each of these spaces is tightly controlled to maintain homeostasis. Alterations in the relative concentrations of electrolytes and of carbon dioxide (CO_2) impact the tendency of water to auto-ionize into its component parts: hydrogen and hydroxyl ions.[2] Alterations in the water, gas, and electrolyte composition of the fluid compartments manifests as changes in the chemistry profile of body water and acid-base balance.

The hydrogen ion concentration is conventionally measured as pH (literally the "power of hydrogen"), the negative logarithmic value of its concentration. Deviations in extracellular pH away from the resting value of 7.4 have long been associated with acute and critical illness. Such deviations are known as "acid-base abnormalities."[3] All acid-base abnormalities result from changes in the local concentration of strong ions, weak acids, and CO_2.[2,4,5]

This chapter first looks at the basic science behind acid-base abnormalities. Subsequently, we explore the detection and treatment of acid-base conundrums, with specific reference to perioperative medicine and critical care.

What Are Acids and Bases?

The concept of acids and bases is relatively new in medicine,[6] and arose with the development of laboratory science in the early part of the 20th century. However, as early as 1831, O'Shaughnessy identified loss of "carbonate of soda" from the blood as a fundamental disturbance in patients dying of cholera.[7] This led directly to the development of crystalloid replacement therapy for hypovolemic shock. In 1909, L.J. Henderson coined the term "acid-base" balance.[8] He was able to define this process in terms of carbonic acid equilibrium. Henderson's work was later refined by Hasselbalch in 1916.[9] Their method described acid-base balance in terms of the hydration equation for CO_2[10]:

$$CO_2 + H_2O \rightarrow H_2CO_3 \rightarrow H^+ + HCO_3^-$$

$$pH = pK_a + \log\ [HCO_3^-] / [H_2CO_3]$$

$$[\text{Total } CO_2] = [HCO_3^-] + [\text{Dissolved } CO_2] + [\text{Carbamino } CO_2] + [H_2CO_3]$$

$$\approx P_{CO_2} \times 0.03 \text{ mmol } CO_2/\text{L/mm Hg}$$

So, substituting into the foregoing equation:

$$pH = 6.1 + \log\ [HCO_3^-] / PCO_2 \times 0.03$$

This is the Henderson-Hasselbalch equation.

The introduction of this concept into clinical practice became possible with the development of volumetric CO_2 analysis by Van Slyke and others in 1919.[11] This led to

60 years of research and interest in CO_2 and its derivative, bicarbonate, as the principle agents that impact acid-base chemistry, despite the knowledge in the 1920s of the importance of chloride in acid-base equilibria.[12]

An understanding of acid-base chemistry in the human body requires familiarity with physical chemistry. Because the body contains a large quantity of water, the physical properties of water have enormous implication for maintenance of homeostasis. Water is a simple triatomic molecule. Its chemical formula is H_2O and its structural formula is H-O-H. The charge distribution of each covalent bond is unequal, and the molecule has a polar conformation and an H-O-H bond angle of 105 degrees. Water molecules attract and form hydrogen bonds with one another. Consequently, water has a high surface tension, a low vapor pressure, a high specific heat capacity, a high heat of vaporization, and a high boiling point.

Water molecules are in continual motion. Occasionally a collision generates sufficient energy to transfer a proton from one water molecule to another. Thus, water is always slightly dissociated into a negatively charged hydroxyl (OH^-) ion and a positively charged hydronium (H_3O^+) ion. Conventionally, this self-ionization of water is written as follows:

$$[H_2O] \leftrightarrow H^+ + OH^-$$

The symbol H^+ is convenient because, although protons dissociating from water have many aliases (such as H_3O^+ and $H_9O_4{}^+$), most physicians and chemists refer to them as hydrogen ions.

The self-ionization of water is miniscule. In pure water at 25°C, the $[H^+]$ and $[OH^-]$ are 1.0×10^{-7}mmol/L. The tendency for water to dissociate into its component parts is represented by the expression

$$K_{eq}H_2O = [H^+][OH^-]$$

The molarity of water is extremely high—55.5 M ("there is a lot of water in water"). As the concentration of water and the K_{eq} are constants, the ion-product dissociation constant (pKa) for water can be expressed as follows:

$$K_{eq}H_2O = K_{eq}(55.5) = K_w' = [H^+][OH^-]$$

The implication is that the product of the concentrations of hydroxyl and hydrogen is constant, so when there is an increase in the concentration of hydrogen ions, there is a concomitant decrease in the concentration of hydroxyl ions, and vice versa.

Pure water is considered neutral because the relative concentrations of hydrogen and hydroxyl are equal at 1.0×10^{-7}mmol/L. A solution is considered *acidic* if the concentration of hydrogen ions exceeds that of hydroxyl ions ($[H^+] > 1.0 \times 10^{-7}$mmol/L, $[OH^-] < 1.0 \times 10^{-7}$ mmol/L). A solution is considered *alkaline* if the hydroxyl ion concentration exceeds the hydrogen ion concentration.

In 1903, Svante Arrhenius (1859-1927) established the foundations of acid-base chemistry. In an aqueous solution, an Arrhenius acid is any substance that delivers a hydrogen ion into the solution.[5] A base is any substance that delivers a hydroxyl ion into the solution. Because of its high dielectric constant, water is a highly ionizing solution. Therefore, substances with polar bonds will dissociate into their component parts (dissolve) in water. Brønsted and Lowry (BL) independently advanced this concept using slightly different terminology: an acid is a proton donor, a base a proton acceptor. Water itself is amphoteric and can act as either an acid or as a base. Thus, when hydrochloric acid (HCl) is dissolved in water, chloride, the acid, donates a proton to water, the base. Similarly, when potassium hydroxide (KOH) is dissolved in water, potassium, the base, receives a hydrogen ion from water, the acid or proton donor.

The degree of dissociation of substances in water determines whether they are strong acids or strong bases. Lactic acid, which has an ion pKa of 3.4, is completely dissociated at physiologic pH, and is a strong acid. Conversely, carbonic acid, which has a pKa of 6.4, is incompletely dissociated, and is a weak acid. Similarly, ions such as sodium (Na^+), potassium (K^+), and chloride (Cl^-), which do not easily bind other molecules, are considered *strong ions*—they exist free in solution. As each Na^+ delivers a hydroxyl moiety into extracellular fluid (ECF), it is functionally a base, as are all cations. As each Cl^- delivers a hydrogen moiety into ECF, it is functionally an acid, as are all anions. The hydrogen and hydroxyl ions delivered in this way bind to one another, forming water molecules, and relatively few free hydrogen or hydroxyl ions remain free in solution.

$$HCL + H_2O \rightarrow H_3O^+ + Cl^-$$

In this reaction, hydrogen chloride acts as a BL acid and water as a BL base.

$$NaOH + H_2O \rightarrow H_2O + OH^- + Na^+$$

In this reaction, water acts as a BL acid and sodium as a BL base.

$$OH^- + Na^+ + H_3O^+ + Cl^- = Na^+ + Cl^- + H_2O$$

Because of electrical neutrality, the hydrogen and hydroxyl ions delivered by chloride and sodium become water.

In summary, all acid-base reactions in the human body relate to the presence of charged particles within an aqueous environment. In the following section, how the components of ECF influence the acid-base status of the body, as measured by clinicians, is discussed. This is followed by an explanation of different acid-base abnormalities, and the tools used to identify them. These approaches are neither distinct from one another nor scientifically incompatible.

What Determines the Acidity or Alkalinity of a Solution?

Because all acid-base reactions are based on the principles of physical chemistry, three simple rules must be followed:[2]

1. *Electrical neutrality*: in aqueous solutions, in any compartment, the sum of all the positive charged ions must equal the sum of all the negative charged ions.

2. *Dissociation equilibria*: the dissociation equilibria of all incompletely dissociated substances, as derived from the law of mass action, must be satisfied at all times.
3. *Mass conservation*: the amount of a substance in a given compartment remains constant unless it is added, removed, generated, or destroyed. Therefore, the total concentration of an incompletely dissociated substance is the sum of concentrations of its dissociated and undissociated forms.

To determine the acid-base status of a fluid, all substances to which these rules could be applied must be accounted for. Fundamentally this involves counting up all the charges (and hence hydrogen and hydroxyl ions) delivered by strong cations (bases) and strong anions (acids), weak acid buffers, and CO_2.[13] A discussion of key groups follows.

STRONG IONS

The first group of ions, the strong ions, dissociate completely. The most abundant strong ions in the extracellular space are Na^+ and Cl^-. Other important strong ions include K^+, sulfate (SO_4^{2-}), magnesium (Mg^{2+}), and calcium (Ca^{2+}). These are occasionally referred to as "mineral" acids or bases because they cannot be metabolized.[6] Organic acids are generated from metabolism and accumulate when there is metabolic dysfunction—such as kidney failure, splanchnic hypoperfusion, or hormonal deficiency.

In a solution containing strong ions, created, for example, using specified concentrations of sodium hydroxide (NaOH) and HCL, the hydrogen ion concentration can be calculated by solving for electric neutrality:

$$(Na^+ - Cl^-) + (H^+ - OH^-) = 0$$

This creates two separate simultaneous equations[14]:

$$H^+ = \sqrt{K_W' + \frac{([Na^+] - [Cl^-])^2}{4}} - \frac{([Na]^+ - [Cl^-])}{2}$$

and

$$OH^- = \sqrt{K_W' + \frac{([Na^+] - [Cl^-])^2}{4}} + \frac{([Na^+] - [Cl^-])}{2}$$

These equations tell us that hydrogen and hydroxyl concentrations are determined by the Kw′ (water pKa), and the difference in charge between Na^+ and Cl^-. Because the former is constant, in this system ($[Na^+] - [Cl^-]$) must determine $[H^+]$ and $[OH^-]$. Given that the concentration of both Na+ and Cl^- are known, the net positive charge minus net negative charge can be quantified. It is the *strong ion difference* (SID).[14] Logically, in any solution, the sum total of the charges imparted by strong cations minus the charges from strong anions will represent the SID. SID independently influences hydrogen ion concentration (Fig. 48.1). In human ECF, SID is always positive.

$$SID = ([Na^+] + [K^+] + [Ca^{2+}] + [Mg^{2+}]) - ([Cl^-] + [A^-]) = 40 - 44 mEq/L$$

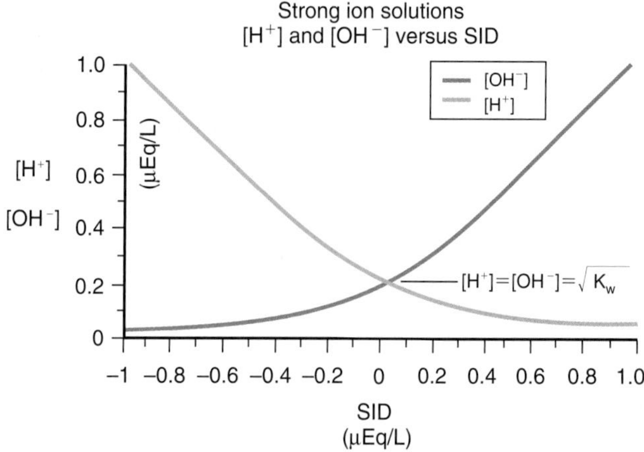

Fig. 48.1 Effect of Changes in the Strong Ion Difference (*SID*) on Hydrogen and Hydroxyl Ion Concentration. (Modified from Stewart PA. Modern quantitative acid-based chemistry. *Can J Physiol Pharmacol.* 1983;61:1444–1461.)

Hydroxyl ions almost always exceed hydrogen ions quantitatively in solution. The relationship between SID and $[H^+]$ is nonlinear in these conditions. Any change in SID will change both $[H^+]$ and $[OH^-]$ concentrations. Because of the Kw′, this relationship is inverse: as $[H^+]$ increases, $[OH^-]$ decreases (see Fig. 48.1). SID is an independent variable, and $[H^+]$ and $[OH^-]$ are dependent, meaning that the addition of hydrogen ions alone (without strong corresponding anions) cannot influence the pH of the solution.

WEAK ACID "BUFFER" SOLUTIONS

The degree of water dissociation, and thus the hydrogen ion concentration, is also influenced by charges derived from weak acids. These acids are partially dissociated compounds whose degree of dissociation is determined by the prevailing temperature and pH. The predominant molecules in this group are albumin and phosphate. Stewart used the term A_{TOT} to represent the total concentration of weak anions or acids that influence acid-base balance.[2]

The acid HA will only partly dissociate, represented by the equilibrium

$$[H^+] \times [A^-] = K_A \times [HA]$$

K_A is the weak acid pKa. If we assume that HA and A^- play no further part in this reaction (the law of mass conservation), the amount of A^- present in the solution must equal the amount initially present, so:

$$[HA] + [A^-] = [A_{TOT}]$$

where $[A_{TOT}]$ is the total weak acid concentration.

In order to calculate the effect of weak acid dissociation on $[H^+]$, we must take into account water dissociation and electrical neutrality:

$$[H^+] + [OH^-] = K_w' \text{ (water dissociation).}$$

$$[SID] + [H^+] - [A^-] - [OH^-] = 0 \text{ (electrical neutrality).}$$

These four simultaneous equations determine the $[H^+]$ in this solution containing strong ions and weak acids. SID and A_{TOT} are independent variables. Kw′ and KA are constants. Consequently, the other variables [HA], $[H^+]$, $[OH^-]$, and $[A^-]$ must adjust to satisfy the foregoing equations. They are dependent variables.

CARBON DIOXIDE

Along with strong ions and weak bases, ECF contains CO_2. The concentration of CO_2 in ECF is determined by tissue production and alveolar ventilation. CO_2, when in solution, exists in four forms: CO_2 (denoted $CO_2[d]$), carbonic acid (H_2CO_3), bicarbonate ions (HCO_3^-), and carbonate ions CO_3^{2-}.

The concentration of $CO_2(d)$ is determined by the solubility coefficient of CO_2 (SCO_2), which depends on body temperature, PCO_2, and other factors. Several equilibrium equations can be derived from the hydration of CO_2:

$$[CO_2\,(d)] = [Sco_2] \times Pco_2$$

The tendency for CO_2 to hydrate to H_2CO_3, and subsequently dissociate to H^+ and HCO_3^-, is reflected by the equation:

$$[CO_2\,(d)] \times [OH^-] = K_1 \times [HCO_3^-]$$

These equations can be combined together and with water equilibrium to the following:

$$[H^+] \times [HCO_3^-] = K_c \times pCO_2$$

HCO_3^- also dissociates to release hydrogen ions and carbonate, the equilibrium reaction which is represented by this equation:

$$[H^+] \times [CO_3^{2-}] = K_3[HCO_3^-]$$

FACTORS INDEPENDENTLY INFLUENCING WATER DISSOCIATION

Now that we have looked at the different factors that may influence the concentration of hydrogen ions in a solution—strong ions, weak acids, and CO_2—we can combine the derived equations to a solve for $[H^+]$:

1. Water dissociation equilibrium:

$$[H^+] \times [OH^-] = K_W'$$

2. Weak acid dissociation equilibrium:

$$[H^+] \times [A^-] = K_A \times [HA]$$

3. Conservation of mass for weak acids:

$$[HA] + [A^-] = [A_{TOT}]$$

4. HCO_3^- formation equilibrium:

$$[H^+] \times [HCO_3^-] = K_C \times pCO_2$$

5. Carbonate ion formation equilibrium:

$$[H^+] \times [CO_3^{2-}] = K_3 \times [HCO_3^-]$$

6. Electrical neutrality:

$$[SID] + [H^+] - [HCO_3^-] - [A^-] - [CO_3^{2-}] - [OH^-] = 0$$

There are six independent simultaneous equations, and just six unknown, dependent variables determined by them: [HA], $[A^-]$, $[HCO_3^-]$, $[CO_3^{2-}]$, $[OH^-]$, and $[H^+]$. There are three known independent variables: [SID], $[A_{TOT}]$, and PCO_2

Solving the equations for $[H^+]$:

$$[SID] + [H^+] - K_C \times P_C / [H^+] - K_A \times [A_{TOT}] / (K_A + [H^+]) - K_3 \times K_C P_C / [H^+]^2 - K_W' / [H^+] = 0$$

In other words, $[H^+]$ is a function of SID, A_{TOT}, PCO_2, and a number of constants. All other variables, most notably $[H^+]$, $[OH^-]$, and $[HCO_3^-]$ are dependent and cannot independently influence acid-base balance.

Acid-Base Abnormalities

The value of the physical chemistry ("Stewart") approach is that it allows us to use a simple model for understanding acid-base disturbances, as all abnormalities can be explained in terms of SID, A_{TOT}, or PCO_2.[2,14] Traditionally, acid-base disturbances have been classified as resulting from either alterations in arterial carbon dioxide ($PaCO_2$) tension (respiratory acidosis or alkalosis) or alterations in blood chemistry (metabolic acidosis or alkalosis).[16] This remains a useful classification, although it must be remembered that respiratory or metabolic abnormalities rarely occur independent of one another.

RESPIRATORY ACID-BASE ABNORMALITIES

Respiratory Alkalosis

The normal $PaCO_2$ is 40 mm Hg (5.3 kPa). Respiratory alkalosis occurs when there is an acute decrease in $PaCO_2$ as a result of hyperventilation. Acute respiratory alkalosis is characterized by a pH > 7.45, a low $PaCO_2$, and a low HCO_3^-. A simple rule of thumb for this reaction is as follows:

Acute respiratory alkalosis:

$$\Delta HCO_3^- = 0.2\ \Delta PaCO_2$$

The hyperventilating patient will present with symptoms and signs of vasoconstriction: lightheadedness, visual disturbances, dizziness, and hypocalcemia from increased binding of calcium to albumin. The hypocalcemia is caused by an increase in the available negative charge on albumin in alkaline states. Acute hypocalcemia is associated with paresthesia and tetany. In anesthesia practice, patients may hyperventilate preoperatively as a consequence of anxiety, and postoperatively secondary to pain, agitation, or a full bladder. More commonly, hyperventilation results from poor mechanical ventilation strategy and may result in significant systemic and, in particular, cerebral vasoconstriction. Therapeutic hyperventilation is no longer used to treat intracranial hypertension because of significant concerns regarding cerebral hypoperfusion and ischemia.

Respiratory Acidosis

Respiratory acidosis occurs when there is an acute rise in $PaCO_2$ usually associated with respiratory failure. This may result from problems with

- Central ventilator control—such as toxicity from anesthetic agents, benzodiazepines, or opioids, stroke, spinal cord injury;
- Peripheral ventilator control—such as myasthenia gravis, poliomyelitis, polymyopathy, or neuromuscular blockade;
- Ventilation-perfusion mismatch—associated with pneumothorax, pleural effusion, atelectasis, pneumonia, or pulmonary edema.

Clinically, patients have signs of CO_2 retention: cyanosis, vasodilatation, and narcosis.

Respiratory acidosis causes a rapid increase in $[H^+]$. Compensation for hypercarbia is slow, requiring increased urinary excretion of Cl^-,[8] and pH falls rapidly. A concomitant increase in the plasma HCO_3^- occurs and reflects a higher total CO_2 load. In the mid-1960s, Brackett, Cohen, and Schwartz elegantly described the relative changes in HCO_3^- in response to acute and chronic elevations in $PaCO_2$, providing us with extremely useful "rules of thumb":[17]

In acute hypercarbia, the bicarbonate concentration of plasma rises slowly

- An increase in $PaCO_2$ by 10 mm Hg (1.3 kPa) results in an increase in HCO_3^- by 1 mmol/L (1 mEq/L)

A patient returning to the intensive care unit from the operating room who has been under ventilation for several hours may be hypercapnic, for example, with a $PaCO_2$ of 80 mm Hg (10.5 kPa). Using this rule, the expected HCO_3 will be 28 mmol/L (Table 48.1).

In chronic respiratory failure, the total CO_2 load in the body increases substantially, reflected by relatively high levels of plasma $HCO3^-$. There is a concomitant fall in plasma chloride, reflecting compensation for elevated levels of carbonic acid.

In chronic respiratory acidosis:

- ΔH^+ (nEq/L) $= 0.8$ (ΔPCO_2)
- An increase in $PaCO_2$ by 10 mm Hg (1.3 kPa) will increase plasma $[HCO_3^-]$ by 3 mmol/L (3 mEq/L)

A patient returning to the intensive care unit from the operating room, ventilated to a $PaCO_2$ of 40 mm Hg (5.3 kPa) but with high total CO_2, secondary to chronic respiratory failure (for example, from COPD), may fail to liberate from mechanical ventilation, due to acute metabolic alkalosis. Using the "rule" the patient's preoperative total CO_2 of 33 mEq/L (mmol/L) will indicate a baseline $PaCO_2$ of 70 mm Hg (9.3 kPa) for that patient (see Table 48.1).

For anesthesiologists, who routinely administer mechanical ventilation to patients with various levels of CO_2 retention, it is important to consider goals for both arterial and end tidal carbon dioxide ($etCO_2$) in the operating room. This should also include consideration of the impact of drugs, such as opioids and benzodiazepines, on respiratory function and on the effect of intravenous fluids on overall acid-base dynamics. For example, both isotonic saline (0.9%) solution and Ringer's Lactate (or Hartmann's) solution will cause progressive increase in extracellular chloride in a dose-dependent manner. This does not occur with truly balanced solutions such as Plasmalyte-148 or Normosol-R. In theory, this may impact postoperative CO_2-HCO_3^- homeostasis and respiratory function.

In critical illness, in particular in patients with acute respiratory distress syndrome (ARDS), there is general consensus among intensivists that aggressive mechanical ventilation to normalize pH and $PaCO_2$ is more harmful than "permissive" hypercapnia. Data support that such an approach—a "lung protective" strategy— is well tolerated,[18,19] and may indeed be beneficial.[20]

TABLE 48.1 Changes in Bicarbonate HCO_3^- and $PaCO_2$ in Acute and Chronic Hypercarbia

ACUTE HYPERCARBIA		
Measured Bicarbonate	**Expected $PaCO_2$ in Acute Respiratory Failure**	
HCO_3^- mEq/L or mmol/L	$PaCO_2$ mm Hg	$PaCO_2$ kPa
24	40	5.3
25	50	6.6
26	60	8.0
27	70	9.3
28	80	10.5
29	90	11.8
30	100	13
CHRONIC HYPERCARBIA		
Measured Bicarbonate	**Expected $PaCO_2$ in Chronic Respiratory Failure**	
HCO_3^- mEq/L or mmol/L	$PaCO_2$ mm Hg	$PaCO_2$ kPa
24	40	5.3
27	50	6.6
30	60	8.0
33	70	9.3
36	80	10.5
39	90	11.8
42	100	13

METABOLIC ACID-BASE DISTURBANCES

Metabolic acid-base disturbances are caused by abnormalities of extracellular water and electrolyte composition and serum protein levels. Using the terminology described above, metabolic acid-base abnormalities are caused by alterations in the SID or A_{TOT}, or both. An increase in the SID causes alkalemia; a decrease in the SID causes acidemia. The alternation may be caused by a change in the total or relative concentration of strong ions. For example, a decrease in the SID (i.e., more anions relative to cations)

TABLE 48.2 Classification of Primary Acid-Base Abnormalities

Abnormalities	Acidosis	Alkalosis
Respiratory	Increased PCO_2	Decreased PCO_2
Metabolic		
ABNORMAL SID		
Caused by water excess or deficit	Water excess = dilutional	Water deficit = contraction
	↓ SID + ↓ [Na⁺]	↑ SID ↑ [Na⁺]
Caused by electrolytes	Chloride excess	Chloride deficit
Chloride (measured)	↓ SID ↑ [Cl⁻]	↑ SID + ↓ [Cl⁻]
Other (unmeasured) anions, such as lactate and keto acids	↓ SID ↑ [UMA⁻]	—
ABNORMAL A_{TOT}		
Albumin [Alb]	↑ [Alb] (rare)	↓ [Alb]
Phosphate [Pi]	↑ [Pi]	

[Alb], Concentration of serum albumin; *A_{TOT}*, to represent the total concentration of weak ions; *[Cl⁻]*, concentration of chloride ions; *[Na⁺]*, concentration of sodium ions; *PCO_2*, partial pressure of carbon dioxide; *[Pi]*, concentration of inorganic phosphate; *SID*, strong ion difference; *[UMA⁻]*, unmeasured anions; ↑, increased; ↓, decreased.

(Modified from Fencl V, Jabor A, Kazda A, Figge J. Diagnosis of metabolic acid-base disturbances in critically ill patients. *Am J Respir Crit Care Med.* 2000;162:2246–2251.)

causes acidosis; this may occur because of a net increase in anions: mineral acids such as chloride or organic acids lactate or ketones (organic acids can be metabolized). In addition, SID can fall due to an increase in the volume of distribution of the same quantity of ions (Table 48.2). A useful rule of thumb is that for every 1 mEq/L fall in the SID, there is a 1 mEq/L fall in the [HCO_3^-] from baseline (although the "normal" level varies with respiratory function; see Table 48.1)—and this approach is widely used to characterize metabolic acidosis. Likewise, for every 1 mEq/L increase in the SID, there is a 1 mEq/L increase in the [HCO_3^-] from baseline—and this approach is widely used to characterize metabolic alkalosis. Note that, in all scenarios, [HCO_3^-] is a *dependent* variable—dependent on changes in SID or A_{TOT}.

Metabolic acidosis is of clinical significance for two reasons: pathologies arising from the acidosis itself and pathologies arising from the cause of the acidosis. Acidosis is associated with alterations in transcellular ion pumps and increased ionized calcium. The result is vasodilation, diminished muscular performance (particularly myocardial), and arrhythmias. The oxyhemoglobin dissociation curve shifts rightward to increase oxygen offload into the tissues. Rapid-onset metabolic acidosis may be associated with profound hypotension, cardiac arrhythmias, and death. The malignancy of the acidosis is strongly related to the underlying disease process; lactic acidosis caused by circulatory shock is more malevolent than hyperchloremic acidosis.[13] The body is hyperresponsive to acidosis. Increasing hydrogen ion content in cerebrospinal fluid activates the respiratory center to stimulate respiration. Alveolar ventilation increases, reducing arterial CO_2 content, hence reducing the total body [H^+]. Bicarbonate concentration simultaneously falls, due to buffering activity, and due to the reduction in total CO_2. As a result, the blood pH falls less in metabolic acidosis compared with respiratory acidosis.

Metabolic alkalosis rarely occurs as a result of acute illness. Symptoms and signs of metabolic alkalosis include widespread vasoconstriction, lightheadedness, tetany, and paresthesia. The main compensatory mechanism is hypoventilation that may delay weaning from mechanical ventilation in critically ill patients.

In normal ECF, the SID is 40 to 44 mEq/L, this positive charge being balanced principally by weak acids (without which the pH of blood would be 11.9). Anything that increases the SID will increase the relative concentration of cations to anions and alkalinize the solution. Anything that decreases the SID will decrease the relative concentration of cations to anions and will acidify the solution. Hence, if the extracellular compartment volume is expanded with free water (no electrolytes), the components of the system are diluted, with relatively more dilution of more abundant moieties (sodium rather than chloride); the result is a reduction in SID and "dilutional acidosis." This is rarely seen in clinical practice, due to the renal water clearance. Conversely, if free water is removed from the ECF, for example from increased evaporative losses, there is an increase in the relative concentration of charged moieties, and this concentration effects more abundant ions and compounds (sodium rather than chloride). The SID increases and the patient develops a "contraction alkalosis" (see Table 48.2). This is commonly seen in clinical practice, in particular following the administration of loop diuretics that have a greater impact on water removal over salt.

In hospital medicine, "normal saline" (NaCl 0.9%—NS), containing 154 mEq (3.5 g) of sodium and 154 mEq (5.5 g) of chloride, is commonly used. The SID of this solution is 0. As each liter of fluid delivers relatively more chloride than sodium (as the baseline proportions in ECF are 1.4:1—SID 40), progressive hyperchloremia results. This reduces SID and results in "hyperchloremic acidosis."[21]

Any process that removes chloride without sodium, such as vomiting or aggressive nasogastric suctioning with a loss of HCl, causes metabolic alkalosis (hypochloremic alkalosis) due to an increase in SID. The alkalosis is caused by chloride loss, which obeys the law of conservation of mass (i.e., there is a finite quantity available in the ECF), not hydrogen ions, whose source—water—is unlimited. Severe diarrhea, which is associated with loss of both potassium and sodium, reduces the SID, and is associated with metabolic acidosis. Aggressive use of diuretics causes a net loss of free water over sodium and chloride and causes contraction alkalosis.

The most significant form of metabolic acidosis is associated with a net gain of "unmeasured" (organic—that is electrolytes not conventionally measured on serum chemistry analysis) anions and, consequently, a decreased SID.

1. In dysoxia, liver dysfunction, and, in particular, states of severe stress, lactate is produced, reducing the SID and causing acidosis
2. In out-of-control diabetes (ketoacidosis) or during starvation or liver disease, β-hydroxybutyrate and acetoacetate are produced, reducing SID and causing acidosis
3. In severe renal failure, Cl^-, SO_4^{2-}, PO_4^{3-} ("fixed renal acids"), and various other metabolic intermediaries are not excreted, causing acidosis.

The total weak acid pool, principally serum albumin and phosphate, is also an important determinant of acid-base status. Hyperphosphatemia has long been associated with the acidosis of renal failure. Hypoalbuminemia is common in critical care. Hypoalbuminemia decreases A_{TOT} and is associated with metabolic alkalosis.[22,23] There is a strong association between hypoalbuminemia and severity of critical illness. Albumin deficits result from four different homeostatic changes: reprioritization of hepatic protein production favoring production of acute phase reactants and limiting albumin synthesis; capillary leak with loss of albumin into the interstitium; breakdown of pre-existing albumin so that its constituent amino acids can be used for protein synthesis; and replacement of plasma with protein-free fluids.

The impact of hypoalbuminemia on acid-base balance has been grossly underestimated. Stewart's original theory has been subsequently modified by Fencl and Figge.[24] The serum albumin concentration is the core negative charge offsetting the net positive charge of the SID.[22] Consequently, the presence of hypoalbuminemia may mask the detection of acidosis[25] caused, for example, by unmeasured anions (UMA), when using conventional tools of acid-base chemistry: pH, bicarbonate, base deficit, and the anion gap (AG).[26] Indeed, the presence of hypoalbuminemia has significant implications, not least for its association with adverse outcomes.[27] Hyperalbuminemia is very unusual; in cholera, when associated with hemoconcentration, it results in acidosis.[28]

Regulation of Acid-Base Balance

Extracellular hydrogen ion concentration appears to be tightly controlled by the body. In all probability this regulation reflects a need to prevent rapid changes in extracellular electrochemical balance from interfering with the function of transcellular ion pumps. To prevent fluctuation a variety of intracellular and extracellular buffering systems have evolved. A *buffer* is a solution of two or more chemicals that minimizes changes in pH in response to the addition of an acid or base. Ideally, a buffer has a pK_a that is equal to the pH, and an ideal body buffer has a pK_a between 6.8 and 7.2. Most biologically salient buffers are weak acids.

It is valuable to view control of hydrogen ion concentration in terms of volatile and metabolic acids (mineral and organic). The major source of acid in the body is the volatile acid CO_2, which produces 12,500 mEq of H^+ a day, mostly excreted by the lungs. In contrast, only 20 to 70 mEq of hydrogen ion-promoting anions are excreted daily thru the kidney. Volatile acid is principally buffered by hemoglobin (Hb). Deoxygenated Hb is a strong base and there would be a huge rise in the pH of venous blood if Hb did not bind the hydrogen ions produced in oxidative metabolism.

Carbon dioxide easily passes through cell membranes. Within the erythrocyte CO_2 combines with H_2O, under the influence of the enzyme carbonic anhydrase, to form H_2CO_3, which ionizes to hydrogen and bicarbonate. Hydrogen ions bind to histidine residues on deoxyhemoglobin (the "Haldane" effect), and bicarbonate is actively pumped out of the cell. Chloride moves inward to maintain electroneutrality (the chloride shift) and to ensure the continued production of carbonic acid. CO_2 is also buffered directly by Hb (carbaminohemoglobin) and by plasma proteins (carbamino proteins). Venous blood contains 1.68 mmol/L extra CO_2 over arterial blood: 65% as HCO_3^- and H^+ bound to Hb, 27% as carbaminohemoglobin (CO_2 bound to Hb), and 8% dissolved.

When respiratory failure occurs, the principal CO_2 buffering system, Hb, becomes overwhelmed, leading to the rapid development of acidosis. In response, the kidney excretes an increased chloride load, using NH_4^+, a weak cation, for electrochemical balance. Thus ECF osmolality is maintained. This process is conventionally referred to as "metabolic compensation." Chronic respiratory acidosis is associated with increase in total body CO_2 content, reflected principally by an increase in serum bicarbonate (see Table 48.1). Hypercapnia is associated with a progressive increase in CSF bicarbonate, reflecting an overall increase in total CO_2 load. Compensation for this hypercarbia is a reduction in CSF chloride[29] and an increase in CSF SID.[30-32] This is probably controlled by active transport mechanisms across the blood-brain barrier or at the level of the choroid plexus and can be blocked by furosemide and acetazolamide.[33-36] The result is a rightward shift in the PCO_2 response curve: the respiratory center responds to hypercarbia by increasing respiratory drive at a higher PCO_2 level than under normal conditions.

Bicarbonate is a dependent variable that increases or decreases with PCO_2.[37] The rate of conversion of CO_2 to HCO_3^- is dependent on carbonic anhydrase activity and occurs slowly. Thus, it is possible to mathematically determine whether a rise in $PaCO_2$ is acute or longstanding (see Table 48.1). Metabolic acid is buffered principally by increased alveolar ventilation, producing respiratory alkalosis, and extracellular weak acids. These weak acids include plasma proteins, phosphate, and bicarbonate. The bicarbonate buffering system (92% of plasma buffering and 13% overall) is probably the most important extracellular buffer. The pK_a of bicarbonate is relatively low (6.1), but the system derives its importance from the enormous quantity of CO_2 present in the body. The coupling of bicarbonate and H_2O produces CO_2, which is then excreted through the lungs, increasing alveolar ventilation. Physicians must be aware of the importance of this compensatory mechanism. For example, anesthetized or critically ill patients on controlled mechanical ventilation lose the capacity to regulate their own PCO_2. Consequently, the combination of acute metabolic and respiratory acidosis can cause a devastating reduction in pH.

The major effect of the kidney on acid-base balance relates to renal handling of sodium and chloride ions. As dietary intake of sodium and chloride is roughly equal, the kidney excretes a net chloride load, using NH_4^+, a weak cation, to electrochemically neutralize urinary chloride.[38]

In metabolic acidosis, the kidneys preferentially excrete chloride. In metabolic alkalosis, chloride is retained and sodium and potassium are excreted. The presence of bicarbonate in the urine reflects the need to maintain electrical neutrality. Abnormalities in the renal handling of chloride may be responsible for several inherited acid-base disturbances. In renal tubular acidosis, there is inability to excrete Cl^- in proportion to Na^+.[39] The diagnosis can be made by observing a hyperchloremic metabolic acidosis, with inappropriately low levels of Cl^- in the urine: the urinary SID is positive. If the urinary SID is negative, the process is not of renal origin. Similarly, pseudohypoaldosteronism appears to be due to high reabsorption of chloride.[40] Bartter syndrome is caused by a mutation in the gene encoding the chloride channel—CLCNKB—that regulates the Na-K-2Cl cotransporter (NKCC2).[41]

The other causes of hyperchloremic metabolic acidosis are gastrointestinal losses (diarrhea, small bowel or pancreatic drainage), parenteral nutrition, excessive administration of saline, and the use of carbonic anhydrase inhibitors.

Analytic Tools Used in Acid-Base Chemistry

Acid-base balance is a core component of the clinical evaluation of the acutely and critically ill. Arterial blood gas (ABG) analysis provides immediate information on the status of the patient's respiratory system and whether or not a state of acidosis or alkalosis is present. By applying a variety of empiric rules, the information contained in an ABG is often sufficient to allow one to identify the presence, cause, and progression of a disease. The diagnostic sensitivity of blood gas analysis is augmented when a blood chemistry panel, glucose and lactate, and blood and urinary ketones measurements are added.

Several different approaches to acid-base balance are in widespread use.[42] These can be described as descriptive, based on changes in the Henderson Hasselbalch equation; semi-quantitative, based on calculations and nomograms; or quantitative, based on physical chemistry. These may be used interchangeably—and I would suggest that there is no best or worst approach, merely different methods of analyzing the data. The descriptive approach utilizes the inter-relationship between $PaCO_2$ and $[HCO_3^-]$ to detect and diagnose acid-base abnormalities. An extension of this is the anion gap (AG). The semi-quantitative approach includes the buffer base (BB) concept, the standardized base excess (BE), and the base-deficit gap (BDG). The quantitative approach utilizes SID and A_{TOT} and is quantified using the strong ion gap (SIG).

Over time, quantitative analyses are likely to dominate the clinical approach to acid-base chemistry. Many of the early approaches were developed at a time when only total CO_2 levels could be measured. Indeed, the continued popularity of the AG is curious given that serum lactate and blood ketones can now be easily measured at the bedside.

THE DESCRIPTIVE (CO_2-BICARBONATE [BOSTON]) APPROACH

Schwartz, Brackett, Relman, and colleagues at Tufts University in Boston developed the most popular descriptive approach to acid-base chemistry in the 1960s. Their formulation uses acid-base maps and the mathematical relationship between CO_2 tension and plasma bicarbonate (or total CO_2), derived from the Henderson-Hasselbalch equation, to classify acid-base disturbances in term of two independent variables: $PaCO_2$ and $[HCO_3^-]$.[43,44] To validate

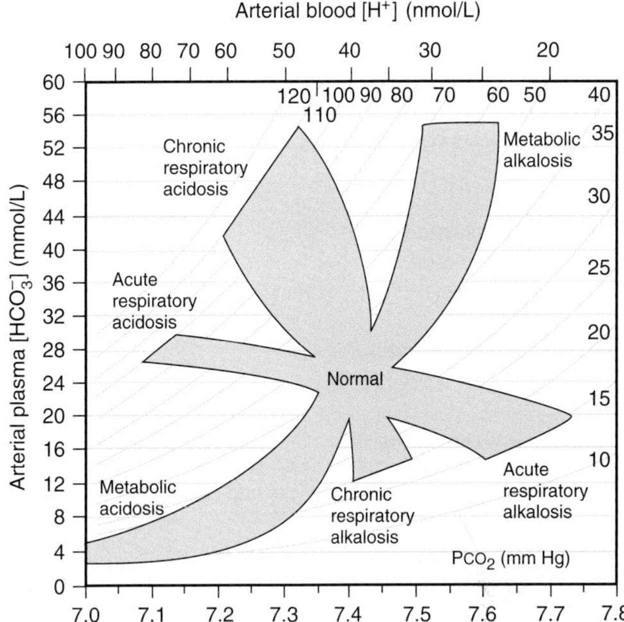

Fig. 48.2 Acid-Base Nomogram Using the Boston Approach. Different acid-base disturbances can be distinguished based on the relative values of PCO_2 and HCO_3^-. (Modified from Brenner BM, Rector FC. *The Kidney*. 3rd ed. Philadelphia, PA: WB Saunders; 1986:473.)

this approach, a number of patients with known acid-base disturbances, at steady states of compensation, were evaluated. The degree of compensation, relative to what was considered normal, was measured for each disease state. The investigators were able to describe six primary states of acid-base imbalance, using linear equations or maps, relating hydrogen ion concentration to PCO_2 for respiratory disturbances, and PCO_2 to HCO_3^- concentration for metabolic disturbances (Fig. 48.2). For any given acid-base disturbance, an expected HCO_3^- concentration was determined. These were then compiled into a series of mathematical rules (see Table 48.1 and Box 48.1). For most simple disturbances, this is a reasonable approach. As discussed above, in acute respiratory acidosis, the $[HCO_3^-]$ will increase by 1 mmol/L (mEq/L) for every 10 mm Hg (1.3 kPa) elevation in $PaCO_2$ above 40 mm Hg (5.3 kPa). In chronic respiratory acidosis, the $[HCO_3^-]$ will increase by 3 mEq/L for every 10 mm Hg (1.3 kPa) elevation in $PaCO_2$ above 40 mm Hg (5.3 kPa).

In acute metabolic acidosis, the $[HCO_3^-]$ falls by 1 mEq/L for every 1 mEq/L in strong anions. The respiratory center is activated, resulting in a predictable fall in the $PaCO_2$. This was neatly characterized by Winters in a pediatric population in 1967 and remains robust.[45] In acute metabolic acidosis, the $PaCO_2$ (in mm Hg) falls predictably, using the $1.5 \times [HCO_3^-]$ plus 8 rule. For example, if the $[HCO_3^-]$ is 12 mmol/L (mEq/L), then the expected $PaCO_2$ is $1.5 \times 12 + 8 = 26$ mm Hg. If the $PaCO_2$ is higher than this, then compensation is inadequate and there is a concomitant respiratory problem (for example, ketoacidosis in the presence of a respiratory tract infection). Winters also described expected compensation using the BE approach (see next section): for every 1 mEq/L reduction in the BE the $PaCO_2$ is expected to fall by 1 mm Hg—otherwise "compensation" is inadequate.

BOX 48.1 The Descriptive (CO_2–HCO_3^-) Approach to Acid-Base

Respiratory Disorders

Acute Respiratory Acidosis

$$\text{Expected } [HCO_3^-] = 24 + [(\text{measured } PaCO_2 - 40)/10]$$

Chronic Respiratory Acidosis

$$\text{Expected } [HCO_3^-] = 24 + 4\,[(\text{measured } PaCO_2 - 40)/10]$$

Acute Respiratory Alkalosis

$$\text{Expected } [HCO_3^-] = 24 - 2\,[(40 - \text{measured } PaCO_2)/10]$$

Chronic Respiratory Alkalosis

$$\text{Expected } [HCO_3^-] = 24 - 5\,[(40 - \text{measured } PaCO_2)/10] \text{ (range: } \pm 2)$$

Metabolic Disorders

Metabolic Acidosis

$$\text{Expected } PaCO_2 = 1.5 \times [HCO_3^-] + 8 \text{ (range: } \pm 2)$$

Metabolic Alkalosis

$$\text{Expected } PaCO_2 = 0.7\,[HCO_3^-] + 20 \text{ (range: } \pm 5)$$

In metabolic alkalosis, in order to restore pH to homeostatic levels, it is necessary to retain carbonic acid, and hypoventilation occurs, ultimately resulting in increased [HCO_3^-]. The expected $PaCO_2$ equals $0.7 \times [HCO_3^-] + 20$ (in mm Hg). So if a patient has a [HCO_3^-] of 34 mEq/L (mmol/L), then the $PaCO_2$ should be 44 mm Hg.

Using these maps, equations, and rules, physicians can determine the nature of most respiratory and metabolic acid-base disturbances and in a manner that is usually accurate. Although there is a mathematical relationship in place, alterations in [H^+] and [HCO_3^-] do not reflect cause and effect. For example, chronic hypoventilation is associated with an increase in PCO_2 and [HCO_3^-]. Many physicians have incorrectly assigned the increase in [HCO_3^-] as compensation for raised PCO_2. It is not. The increased HCO_3^- concentration reflects increased total CO_2 in the body.

Although the PCO_2-HCO_3^- approach is relatively accurate for most disturbances, and is particularly useful for respiratory problems, there are several inherent pitfalls, particularly in relation to the metabolic component. First, the approach is not as simple as it seems, requiring the clinician to refer to confusing maps or to learn formulas and perform mental arithmetic. Second, the system neither explains nor accounts for many of the complex acid-base abnormalities seen in perioperative and critically ill patients, such as those with acute acidosis in the setting of hypoalbuminemia, free water deficit or excess, hyperchloremia, hyperphosphatemia, or concurrent metabolic acidosis and alkalosis.

ANION GAP APPROACH

The most widely used tool for investigating metabolic acidosis is the AG, developed by Emmett and Narins in 1977.[46] It is based on the law of electrical neutrality. It is entirely consistent with the physical chemistry approach, described in the next section, and is usually used alongside the Boston approach to acid-base. Again, the system is based on data that were not easily available or known at the time of publication: the contribution to electrical neutrality ascribed to weak acids (phosphate and albumin) and UMA. The sum of the difference in charge of the common extracellular ions reveals an unaccounted for "gap" of −10 to −12 mEq/L. There are three widely used variants of the AG (Fig. 48.3), depending on whether or not potassium and lactate are included:

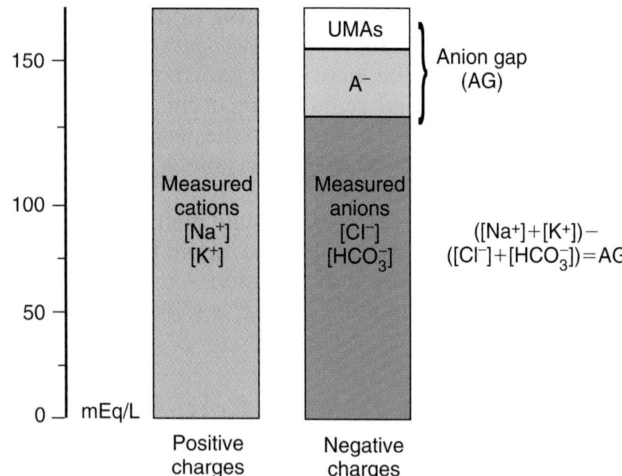

Fig. 48.3 The Anion Gap Represents the Difference in Charge Between Measured Cations and Measured Anions. The missing negative charge is made up of weak acids *(A^-)*, such as albumin and phosphate, and strong unmeasured anions *(UMAs)*, such as lactate.

$$\text{Anion gap (simple)} = ([Na^+] - [Cl^-] + [HCO_3^-]) = 12 \text{ to } 14 \text{ mEq/L}$$

$$\text{Anion gap (conventional)} = ([Na^+] + [K^+] - ([CL^-] + [HCO_3^-])) = 14 \text{ to } 18 \text{ mEq/L}$$

$$\text{Anion gap (modern)} = ([Na^+] + [K^+] - ([Cl^-] + [HCO_3^-] + [\text{lactate}^-])) = 14 \text{ to } 18 \text{ mEq/L}$$

If the patient develops a metabolic acidosis, and the gap widens to, for example, >20 mEq/L, then the acidosis is caused by UMA (usually renal acids or ketones). If the gap does not widen, then the anions are being measured, and the acidosis has been caused by hyperchloremia (bicarbonate cannot independently influence acid-base status) or lactate (if used). While this is a useful tool, it is weakened by the assumption of what is or is not a "normal gap."[47] The AG frequently underestimates the extent of the metabolic disturbance.[26] The majority of critically ill patients are hypoalbuminemic, and many are also hypophosphatemic. Consequently, the gap may be normal in the presence of UMA. This has been extensively studied by Fencl and Figge, who have provided us with a variant known as the "corrected AG":[26]

$$\text{Anion gap corrected (for albumin)} = \text{calculated anion gap} + 0.25\left(\text{normal albumin}^* - \text{observed albumin g/L}\right).$$

*which may vary between populations/labs; if g/dL used the factor is 2.5.

In this corrected form the AG accurately quantifies metabolic acidosis, and it is useful in discriminating an acidosis due to UMA from one reflecting hyperchloremia, in a previously healthy patient (e.g., in acute trauma). Moviat and colleagues have demonstrated that the AG corrected for albumin accurately detects complex acid-base abnormalities in intensive care.[48]

Another version of the AG is the delta AG (delta ratio DR—Box 48.2), an approach that has successfully predicted adverse outcomes in critical illness.[49] Simply, if the AG is normal, or unchanged, and the bicarbonate level falls, then the delta ratio will be less than 0.4, and a hyperchloremic acidosis is present. A DR between 1 and 2 is what one would expect from metabolic acidosis due to UMA or lactate. If the ratio is greater than 2, mixed acid-base abnormalities are present. Although on the surface, this process is relatively simple, it assumes that the clinician knows the normal AG and bicarbonate for that particular patient. In addition, it does not result in a clear diagnosis other than hyperchloremia.

Fig. 48.4 is a decision tree that uses this descriptive approach to acid-base.

BOX 48.2 The Delta Anion Gap (Delta Ratio)

$$\text{Delta ratio} = \Delta\text{Anion gap}/\Delta\,[HCO_3^-] \text{ or } \uparrow\text{anion gap}/\downarrow[HCO_3^-]$$

$$= \frac{\text{Measured anion gap} - \text{Normal anion gap}}{\text{Normal }[HCO_3^-] - \text{Measured }[HCO_3^-]}$$

$$= \frac{(AG - 12)}{(24 - [HCO_3^-])}$$

THE SEMI-QUANTITATIVE (BASE DEFICIT/EXCESS [COPENHAGEN]) APPROACH

In metabolic acidosis, the addition of UMA to the ECF results in a net gain of one hydrogen ion for each anion. This is buffered, principally by bicarbonate, such that each anion gained results in an equivalent fall in the bicarbonate concentration. Thus, the change in the bicarbonate concentration from baseline should reflect the total quantity of net

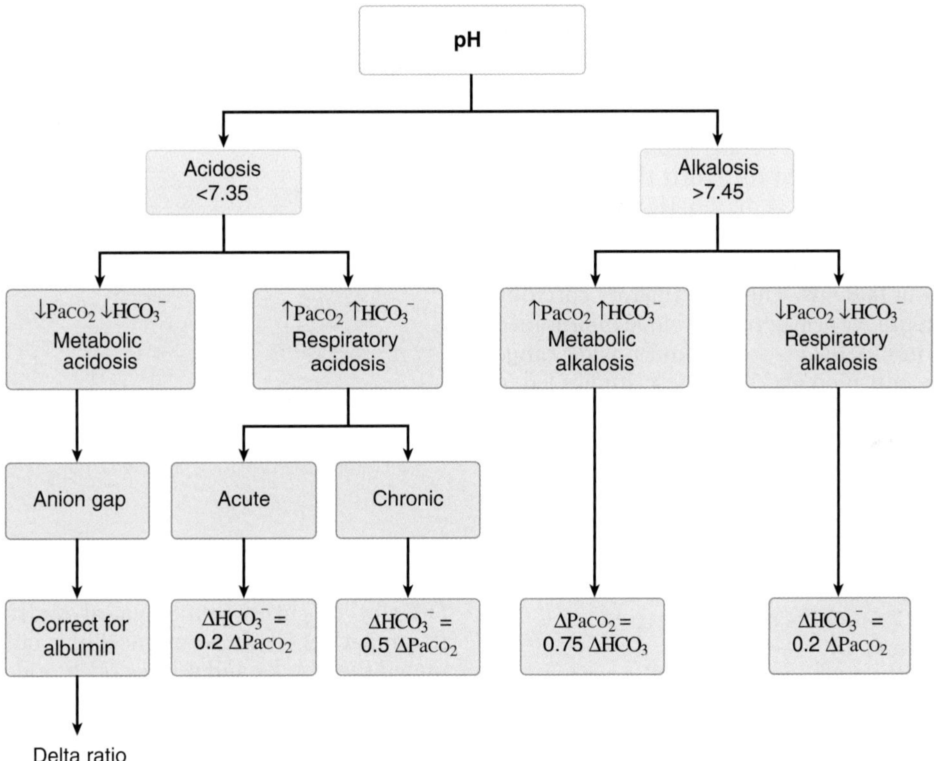

Delta ratio	Clinical assessment
<0.4	Hyperchloremic normal AG acidosis
<1	High AG and normal AG acidosis
1 to 2	Pure anion gap acidosis Lactic acidosis: average value 1.6 DKA more likely to have a ratio closer to 1 because of urine ketone loss
>2	High AG acidosis and concurrent metabolic alkalosis or preexisting compensated respiratory acidosis

Fig. 48.4 The Descriptive ("Boston") Approach to Acid-Base Balance. *DKA*, Diabetic ketoacidosis; *AG*, Anion gap.

anions gained. Adherents to the descriptive approach to acid-base refer to this as the "delta" bicarbonate. However, this is problematic, as it does not separate out the effect of CO_2 metabolism on the [HCO_3^-].

In 1948, Singer and Hastings[50] proposed that changes in the whole blood BB could be used to quantify the metabolic component independent of Henderson-Hasselbalch. The BB represented the sum of the bicarbonate and the nonvolatile buffer ions (essentially the serum albumin, phosphate, and Hb). Applying the law of electrical neutrality, the BB was forced to equal the electrical charge difference between strong (fully dissociated) ions. Thus, normally BB = [Na^+] + [K^+] − [Cl^-]. Alterations in BB represented changes in strong ion concentrations (which could not be easily measured in 1948). BB increases in the presence of a metabolic alkalosis and decreases in metabolic acidosis. The major drawback of BB measurements is the potential for changes in buffering capacity associated with alterations in Hb concentration and pH.

Following the development of sophisticated electrodes for measuring CO_2 tension in Copenhagen in the early 1950s,[51] Astrup and Jorgensen developed the standard bicarbonate—the bicarbonate concentration at 37°C and at a $PaCO_2$ of 40 mm Hg (5.3 kPa).[52] Building upon this work, Siggaard-Anderson and Astrup[53] recognized that PCO_2 and [HCO_3^-] were not independent variables. As a result, they derived the BE as a measure that could differentiate respiratory from metabolic acid-base disturbances. As defined, the BE is the amount of strong acid (strong anion) or base (strong cation) required to return the pH to 7.4, assuming that PCO_2 is constant at 40 mm Hg (5.3 kPa) and that the temperature is 37°C.[54] Like the Boston group, the Siggaard-Anderson data were derived from observations on a large population of patients. The investigators carefully titrated known amounts of acid or base to blood maintained by tonometry at various $PaCO_2$ values and a wide range of hemoglobin concentration at 37°C. These studies led to the development of an alignment nomogram (Fig. 48.5 and Table 48.3) that allowed for the determination of BE from a single measurement of pH, $PaCO_2$, and Hb concentration at 37°C. Current algorithms for computing the BE are derived from the Van Slyke equation (1977).[55]

$$BE = (HCO_3^- - 24.4 + [2.3 \times Hb + 7.7] \times [pH - 7.4] \times (1 - 0.023 \times Hb))$$

The most commonly used estimation of BE uses just the bicarbonate and pH by the following equation:

$$BE = 0.93 \times ([HCO_3^-] - 24.4 + 14.83 \times [pH - 7.4])$$

There is a very high level of agreement between this calculation and the empirical data that were used to construct the original nomogram. The calculation is accurate in vitro, but not in vivo because of the dynamic buffering activity of Hb within the acid-base paradigm of gas and electrolyte exchange. Moreover, weak acids such as phosphate and albumin also contribute to nonbicarbonate buffering. Hence the following formula is now used to calculate the standard base excess (SBE) or the BE of ECF:

$$SBE = ((HCO_3^- \text{ actual mEq/L}) - 24.8 + (16.2 \times (pH - 7.40))$$

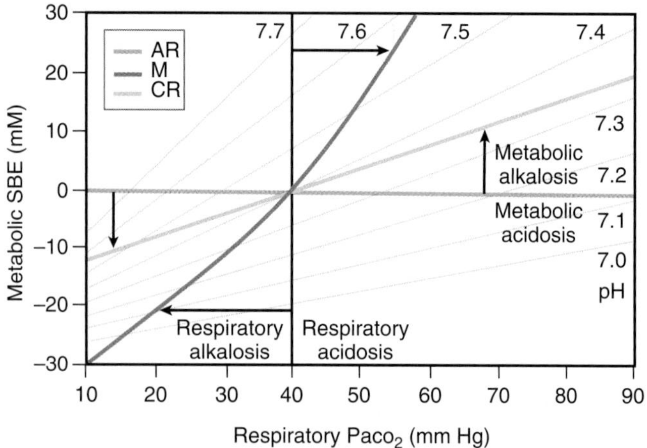

Fig. 48.5 Acid-Base Nomogram Using the Copenhagen Approach as Revised by Schlichtig. The various acid-base disturbances can be distinguished based on PCO_2 and base deficit or excess, here referred to as standard base excess *(SBE)*. *Arrows* represent changes as the body compensates for acute acidosis or alkalosis. *AR*, Acute respiratory acidosis or alkalosis; *CR*, chronic respiratory acidosis or alkalosis; *M*, metabolic acidosis or alkalosis. (From Schlichtig R, Grogono AW, Severinghaus JW. Human $Paco_2$ and standard base excess compensation for acid-base imbalance. *Crit Care Med.* 1998;26:1173–1179.)

TABLE 48.3 Changes in Standard Base Deficit or Excess in Response to Acute and Chronic Acid-Base Disturbances

Disturbance	SBDE vs. $PaCO_2$
Acute respiratory acidosis	$\Delta BDE = 0$
Acute respiratory alkalosis	$\Delta BDE = 0$
Chronic respiratory acidosis	$\Delta BDE = 0.4\ \Delta PaCO_2$
Metabolic acidosis	$\Delta PaCO_2 = \Delta BDE$
Metabolic alkalosis	$\Delta PaCO_2 = 0.6\ \Delta BDE$

Δ, Change in value; *BDE*, base deficit or excess; *$PaCO_2$*, partial pressure of arterial carbon dioxide.

Modified from Narins RB, Emmett M. Simple and mixed acid-base disorders: a practical approach. *Medicine (Baltimore).* 1980;59:161–187.

The value of 16.2 mEq/L approximates all of the nonbicarbonate buffers in ECF (albumin, phosphate, and mean ECF Hb). It is likely that Siggaard-Andersen overestimated the impact of Hb as an extracellular buffer and underestimated the uptake and release of chloride into erythrocytes in the peripheries and lungs respectively.[56]

Although various descriptions of this approach to acid-base chemistry refer to the *BE*—and that term is reported on blood gas forms, when a negative base excess (1-BE) is reported—the correct terminology refers to it as the *base deficit*.[57] For simplicity, in the following discussion, I will refer to the BE, keeping in mind that it may be positive (metabolic alkalosis) or negative (metabolic acidosis).

Application of simple mathematical rules allows for use of the BE in each of the common acid-base disturbances (Box 48.3 and Fig. 48.6). For example, in acute respiratory acidosis or alkalosis, BE does not change. Conversely, in acute metabolic acidosis, the magnitude of change of the $PaCO_2$ (in millimeters of mercury) is the same as that of the BE (in mmol/L or mEq/L).

BOX 48.3 Calculation of the Base Excess Gap[12,58,59]

$$BE_{NaW} \text{ (water and sodium effect)} = 0.3\ ([Na^+{}_{meas}]\ \text{-}140)\ mEq/L$$

$$BE_{Cl} \text{ (chloride effect)} = 102 - [Cl^- \text{ effective}]\ (mEq/L)$$

$$BE_{Pi} \text{ (phosphate effect)} = (0.309 \times (pH - 0.47)) \times Pi\ mEq/$$

$$BE_{prot} \text{ (protein effect)} = (42 - [\text{Albumin g/L}]) * (0.148 \times pH - 0.818)$$

$$BE_{calc} = NE_{NaW} + BE_{Cl} + BE_{PO4} + BE_{prot}$$

$$BE_{Gap} = BE_{calc} - BE_{actual} - [\text{lactate mEq/L}]$$

A Simplified Calculation of the Base Excess Gap[60]

$$BE_{NaCl} = ([Na^+] - [Cl^-]) - 38$$

$$BE_{Alb} = 0.25\ (42 - \text{albumin g/L})$$

$$BE_{NaCl} - BE_{Alb} = BDE_{calc}$$

$$BE_{actual} - BE_{calc} - [\text{lactate}] = BEG = \text{the effect of unmeasured anions or cations}$$

*This approach involves calculating the base deficit excess for sodium, chloride, and free water (BE_{NaCl}), and that for albumin (BE_{Alb}). The result is the calculated BE (BE_{calc}). This is subtracted from the measured BE to find the BE gap.

There has been considerable discussion over the past 60 years about the merits and demerits of the BE, as compared to the CO_2-HCO_3^- system. In reality, there is little difference between the two; both equations and nomograms were derived from patient data and abstracted backward. Calculations use bicarbonate as measured on a blood gas analyzer. Consequently, for most patients, either approach is relatively accurate but may be misleading because they do not allow the clinician to distinguish between, for example, acidosis due to lactate or chloride, or alkalosis due to dehydration or hypoalbuminemia. These measures may miss the presence of an acid-base disturbance entirely; for example, a hypoalbuminemic (metabolic alkalosis) critically ill patient with a lactic acidosis (metabolic acidosis) may have a normal range pH, bicarbonate, and BE. This lack of precision may lead to inappropriate or inadequate therapy.

Changes in the BE occur secondary to alterations in the relative concentrations of sodium, chloride, free water, albumin, phosphate, and UMA. By calculating the contribution of the individual components of the BE it is possible to identify: (1) contraction alkalosis, (2) hypoalbuminemic alkalosis, (3) hyperchloremic acidosis, (4) dilution acidosis (if indeed it exists), and (5) acidosis secondary to UMA. This approach, which can be labelled the base-deficit gap, has been proposed by Gilfix and Magder (see Box 48.3)[58] and simplified subsequently by Balasubramanyan and associates[59] and Story and associates.[60] The BDG should mirror the SIG (below) the corrected AG.

The simplified calculation as proposed by Story et al. is very easy to calculate at the bedside and in the majority of situations (see Box 48.3) replicates the more complex calculations originally proposed by Gilfix and Magder.[58]

STEWART APPROACH

A more accurate reflection of true acid-base status can be derived using the Stewart or physical chemical approach, subsequently updated by Fencl.[5,15] This approach is based on the concept of electrical neutrality, a small advance from the AG. There exists, in plasma, a SIDa $[(Na^+ + Mg^{2+} + Ca^{2+} = K^+) - (Cl^- + A^-)]$ of 40 to 44 mEq/L, balanced by the negative charge on bicarbonate and A_{TOT} (the BB—SIDe). There is a small difference between SIDa (apparent SID) and BB (SIDe—effective SID) that represents a SIG and quantifies the amount of UMA present (Fig. 48.7).

$$\text{SIDa (apparent SID)} = ([Na^+] + [K^+] + [Mg^{2+}] + [Ca^{2+}]) - [Cl^-]$$

$$\text{SIDe (effective)} = [HCO_3^-] + [\text{charge on albumin}] + [\text{charge on Pi}]\ (\text{in mmol/L})$$

Weak acids' degree of ionization is pH dependent, so one must calculate for this:

$$[alb^-] = [\text{alb g/L}] \times (0.123 \times pH - 0.631)$$

$$Pi\ (mmol/L) = [PO_4] \times (0.309 \times pH - 0.469)$$

$$\text{Strong Ion Gap (SIG)} = SIDa - SIDe$$

Unfortunately, the SIG may not represent unmeasured strong anions but only all anions that are unmeasured. For example, if a patient has been resuscitated with gelatin, his/her SIG will increase. Further, SID changes quantitatively in absolute and relative terms when there are changes in plasma water concentration. Fencl has addressed this by correcting the chloride concentration for free water (Cl^-corr) using the following equation[5]:

$$[Cl^-]corr = [Cl^-]\text{observed} \times ([Na^+]\text{normal} / [Na^+]\text{observed}).$$

This corrected chloride concentration may then be inserted into the SIDa equation above. Similarly, the derived value for UMA can also be corrected for free water by substituting UMA for Cl^- in the above equation.[25] In a series of nine normal subjects, Fencl estimated the "normal" SIG as 8 ± 2 mEq/L.[25]

Calculation of SIG is cumbersome. The data required are more extensive and thus more expensive than other approaches and there is much confusion about the normal range of SIG. It is unclear, in standard clinical practice, that SIG has any advantage over AGc (which is SIG without calcium, magnesium, and phosphate—which usually cancel out each other's charges).

In all likelihood no single number will ever allow us to make sense of complex acid-base disturbances. Fencl[25] has suggested that, rather than focusing on AG or BDE, physicians should address each blood gas in terms of all alkalinizing and acidifying effects: respiratory acidosis/alkalosis, the presence or absence of abnormal SID (due to

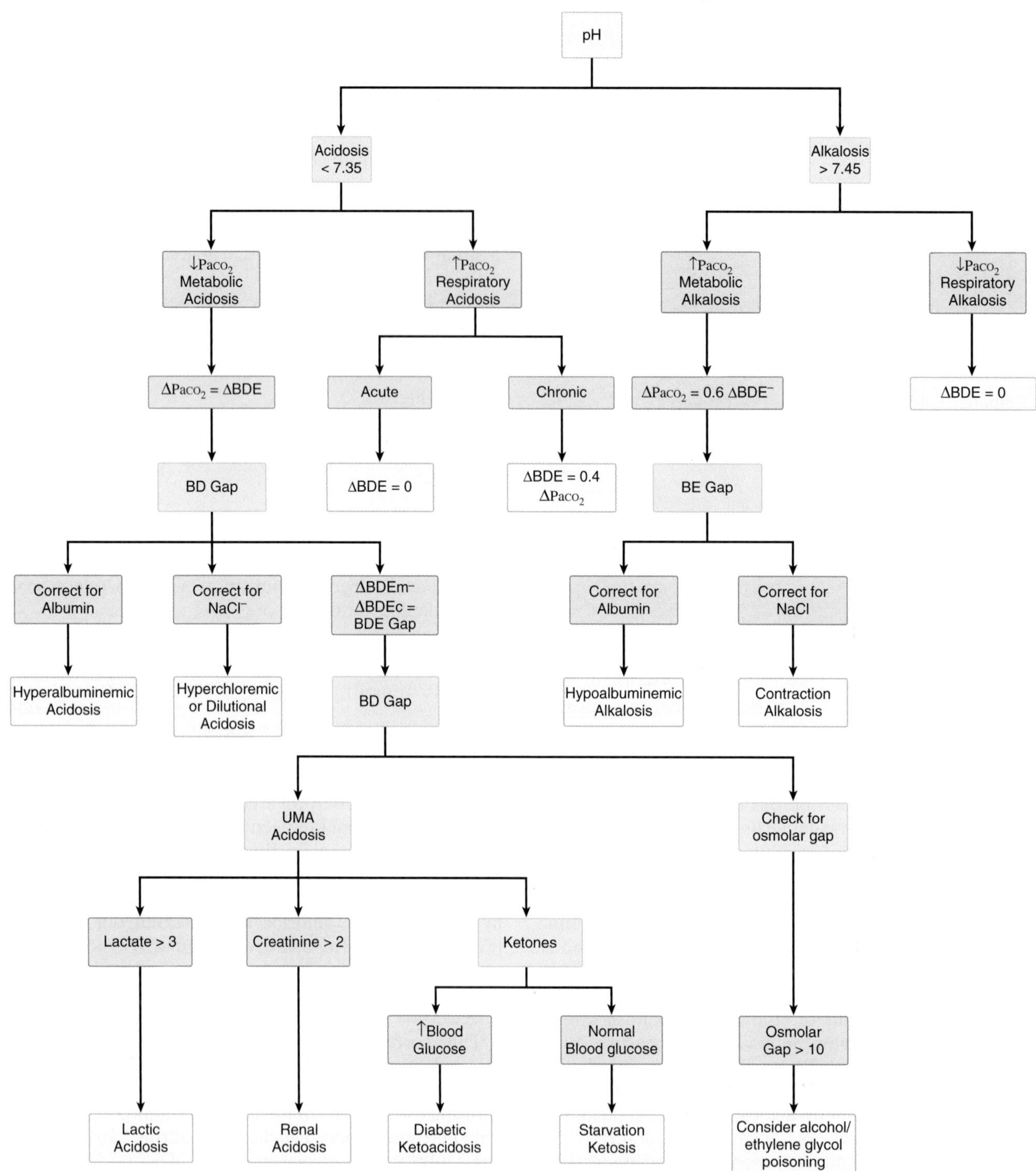

Fig. 48.6 The Semi-Quantitative ("Copenhagen") Approach to Acid-Base Balance. *BD*, Base deficit, *BE*, base excess, *BDEm*, measured base deficit or excess, *BDEc*, Base deficit or excess corrected for albumin, sodium, chloride, and free water (see Box 48.3); *UMA*, unmeasured anions; lactate in mmol/L, creatinine in mg/dL, osmolar gap in mOsm.

water excess/deficit, measured electrolytes, or unmeasured electrolytes), and abnormal A_{TOT}. Consider the following patient, described by Fencl[25](data in mEq/L unless otherwise stated):

Na 117, Cl 92, Ca 3.0, Albumin 6.0 g/L
K 3.9, Mg 1.4, Pi 0.6 mmol/L

ABG: pH 7.33, PCO_2 30 mm Hg, HCO3 15

Derived values would be:

AG 13, $AG_{corrected}$ 23, BE −10, SID 18, $Cl_{corrected}$ 112, $UMA_{corrected}$ 18.

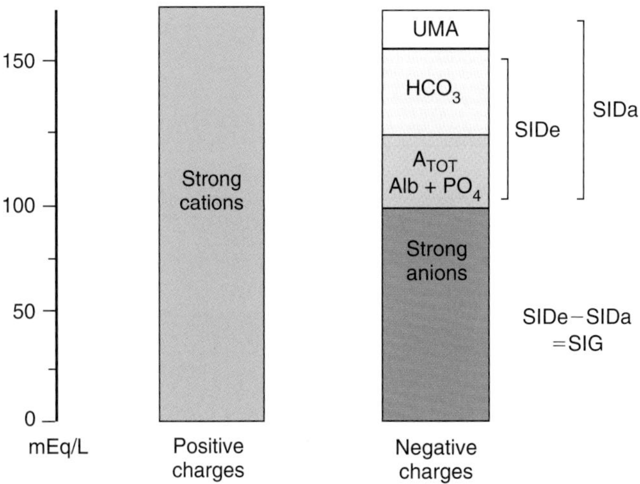

Fig. 48.7 The Strong Ion Gap: SID Apparent is the Sum of ATOT plus $[HCO_3^-]$. SID effective is the real SID. The difference between the two is made up of unmeasured anions (*UMA*). *SID*, Strong ion difference; *SIG*, strong ion gap.

Using traditional methodology, one would describe this as a nongap metabolic acidosis and look for causes of bicarbonate wasting such as renal tubular acidosis or gastrointestinal losses. The degree of respiratory alkalosis is appropriate for the degree of acidosis ($\Delta BD = \Delta PCO_2$). However, the Fencl-Stewart approach reveals a much more complex situation. SID is reduced to 18 mEq/L, caused by free water excess, UMA, and, surprisingly, hyperchloremia (see the corrected chloride). However, the degree of acidosis does not mirror the metabolic disturbance because of the alkalizing force of hypoalbuminemia. The corrected AG mirrors the change in SID, but this alteration is grossly underestimated by the base deficit. This patient has a dilutional acidosis, a hyperchloremic acidosis, and a lactic acidosis!

In conclusion, for the majority of patients presenting to the emergency room or operating suite who have been previously healthy, the use of tools such as the base deficit or AG to assess metabolic disturbances remains reasonable, particularly if corrected for albumin. However, for critically ill patients, the most effective method of interpreting acid-base conundrums involves unraveling simultaneous acidifying and alkalinizing processes and using calculations to distinguish between the various forces at play. Unfortunately, a clinician's ability to interpret such information is dependent on the amount of available data. A simple blood gas alone may camouflage a significant acid-base disturbance.

In the next section, we will look at the causes of many commonly seen acid-base disturbances in different clinical settings.

Acid-Base Problems in Perioperative and Critical Care Medicine

RESPIRATORY ACIDOSIS AND ALKALOSIS

In perioperative medicine respiratory acid-base abnormalities are an uncommon complication of prolonged spontaneous breathing under anesthesia, inadequate mechanical ventilation (both acute respiratory acidosis) or excessive mechanical ventilation (respiratory alkalosis) (Table 48.4). Acute respiratory acidosis results from hypoventilation or increased dead space ventilation. Patients may manifest respiratory distress characterized by respiratory acidosis in the recovery room PACU or surgical ICU. Assessment begins with an examination of the patient's breathing pattern (Fig. 48.8): slow shallow breathing indicates impaired respiratory drive, rapid shallow breathing suggests chest wall or lung pathology, and obstructed breathing signifies airway obstruction. Blood gas analysis of acute respiratory acidosis will reflect a dramatic fall in pH, an elevated $PaCO_2$, and a slight rise in HCO_3^- (by 1 mEq/L [mmol/L] for every 10 mm Hg [or 1.2 kPa] rise in $PaCO_2$). The BE should be zero. Respiratory acidosis as a complication of anesthesia is relatively common—excessive sedation (particularly opioids), partial neuromuscular blockade, intraoperative hypoventilation, pneumothorax, etc. It may also complicate CO_2 insufflation during laparoscopy—the patients' minute ventilation should be dynamically adjusted intraoperatively to maintain $etCO_2$ levels near baseline.

TABLE 48.4 Acid-Base Disturbances Commonly Seen Perioperatively

Disorder	Cause
Respiratory acidosis	Hypoventilation; narcosis, incomplete reversal of neuromuscular blockade
Respiratory alkalosis	Hyperventilation; anxiety, pain
Metabolic acidosis due to unmeasured anions (widened gap acidosis)	Hypoperfusion—lactic acidosis; diabetic ketoacidosis; renal failure
Metabolic acidosis due to measured anions (non-gap hyperchloremic acidosis)	Hyperchloremia—"normal" saline and saline-containing fluids; renal tubular acidosis; bladder reconstructions
Metabolic acidosis due to free water excess (hyponatremia, dilution acidosis)	Hypotonic fluid administration; sodium loss—diarrhea; administration of hyperosmolar fluids—mannitol, alcohol, hyperproteinemia
Metabolic alkalosis	Hyperventilation of patient with history of CO_2 retention (COPD); sodium gain (sodium bicarbonate, massive blood transfusion); chloride loss—nasogastric suctioning

For patients with COPD (or other causes of chronic respiratory failure), it is worthwhile, preoperatively, to calculate the baseline $PaCO_2$ on a patient from the total CO_2 on blood chemistry panel. As discussed earlier, the total CO_2 (HCO_3^-) rises by 3 mEq/L (mmol/L) for every 10 mm Hg (1.3 kPa) rise in $PaCO_2$. A patient, for example, with a baseline total CO_2 of 33 mEq/L (mmol/L) would be expected to have a baseline $PaCO_2$ of 70 mm Hg (9.3 kPa). For intraoperative management, the $etCO_2$ should be maintained, if the patient is undergoing mechanical ventilation, between 3 and 5 mm Hg (0.5 –1 kPa) of baseline (the $PaCO_2$-$etCO_2$ gradient increases with age and nonsupine positioning).

If the patient is hypoventilating, perioperatively, the pH falls, the $PaCO_2$ rises, but the rise in the total CO_2 (HCO_3^-) is lower than expected. If this patient's $PaCO_2$, postoperatively, is 90 mm Hg (12 kPa) and the total CO_2 (HCO_3^-) is

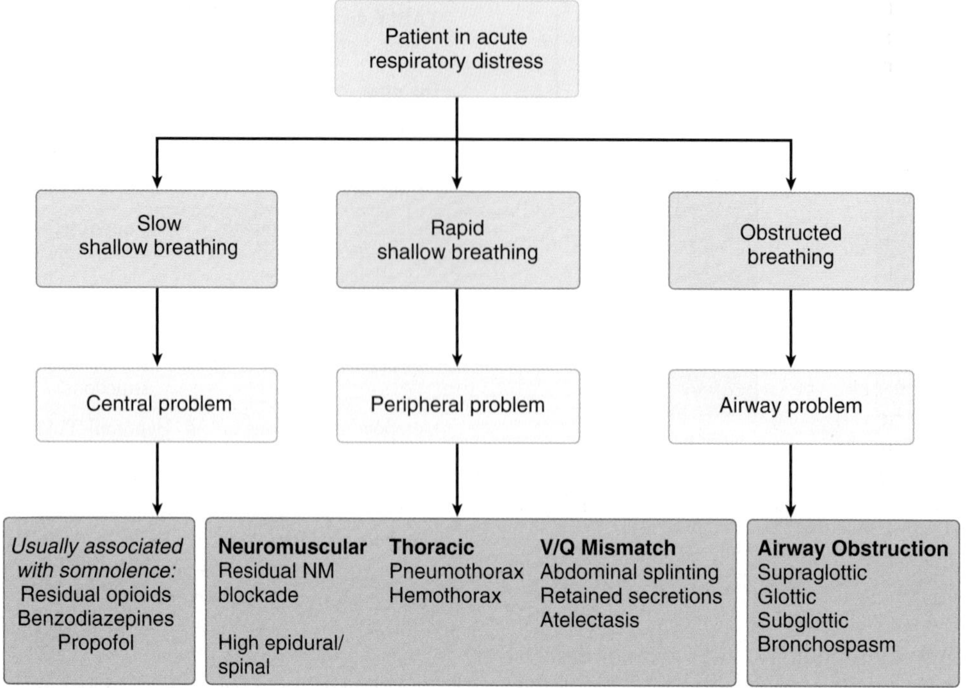

Fig. 48.8 Using the Breathing Pattern to Determine the Cause of Acute Respiratory Distress and Respiratory Acidosis.

35 mmol/L (mEq/L), then the patient has acute or chronic respiratory acidosis. This problem may be compounded by the patient's lack of pulmonary reserve and the negative impact on the respiratory center by opioids and other anesthetic agents. Consideration should be given to administration of noninvasive ventilation to restore $PaCO_2$ to what is normal for that patient.

In emergency medicine and critical illness, respiratory acidosis complicates a wide variety of pathologies. Most commonly, these cause a problem of the patient "can't breathe"—a neuromuscular or anatomical problem—or the patient "won't breathe"—a central nervous system pathology. The latter includes neurologic injury (stroke, spinal cord injury, botulism, tetanus, and toxic suppression of the respiratory center [opioids, barbiturates, benzodiazepines]). Patients "can't breathe" due to a variety neuromuscular disorders (Guillain-Barré syndrome, myasthenia gravis), flail chest, hydro-hemo-pneumo-thorax, pulmonary edema, and pneumonia. Failure to ventilate, as manifest by respiratory acidosis, may result from abdominal hypertension and abdominal compartment syndrome, where diaphragmatic excursion is impeded by high intra-abdominal pressures, often with associated oliguria and hypotension.

Acute respiratory alkalosis is caused by hyperventilation, either due to anxiety or pain, central respiratory stimulation (as occurs early in salicylate poisoning), or excessive artificial ventilation. In acute respiratory alkalosis the pH is above 7.45, the $PaCO_2$ below 40 mm Hg (5.3 kPa), and the $[HCO_3^-]$ falls by 2 mEq/L (mmol/L) for every 10 mm Hg (1.3 kPa) fall in $PaCO_2$. There is no change in the BE. So, if a patient has a $PaCO_2$ of 30 mm Hg, the $[HCO_3^-]$ should be 22 mEq/L (mmol/L).

Acute respiratory alkalosis usually accompanies acute metabolic acidosis, in which case the reduction in PCO_2 from baseline (usually 40 mm Hg) is equal to the magnitude of the base deficit (see Table 48.3). The fall in bicarbonate, from baseline, is significantly greater than that seen in primary respiratory alkalosis, due to the consumption of bicarbonate as extracellular buffer (the $[HCO_3^-]$ falls 1 mEq/L for every 1 mEq/L gain in strong anions). For example, in a patient with a lactic acidosis whose lactate is 10 mEq/L, the BE should be −10, the $[HCO_3^-]$ 10 mEq/L (mmol/L) lower than baseline, and the PCO_2 30 mm Hg. If the PCO_2 is higher than expected, then there is a concomitant problem with the respiratory apparatus. An example would be a multi-trauma patient, where massive blood loss leads to lactic acidosis and a flail chest causes respiratory acidosis.

Metabolic Acidosis and Alkalosis

METABOLIC ACIDOSIS

Acute metabolic acidosis is caused by an alteration in SID or A_{TOT}. SID is changed by an alteration in the relative quantity of strong anions to strong cations. Anions, mineral or organic, can be gained, as occurs with lactic-, renal-, keto-, and hyperchloremic acidosis, or cation can be lost, as occurs with severe diarrhea or renal tubular acidosis.

Acute metabolic acidosis is characterized by a pH of < 7.35 and a fall in both $PaCO_2$ and (HCO_3^-) below the patient's baseline. For patients without COPD or chronic CO_2 retention, this represents a $PaCO_2$ < 40 mm Hg (5.3 kPa) and a $[HCO_3^-]$ below 24 mEq/L (mmol/L), there is a negative BE (base deficit) whose magnitude represents the net strong anion gain. This simple approach indicates that an acidosis is present, and that it is metabolic in origin. To further investigate the acidosis, one or more of the analytical tools described above may be employed. The most widely used tool is the AG, which should be adjusted for albumin. This differentiates hyperchloremic acidosis from acidosis caused by other measured and UMA. In the setting of metabolic acidosis, where possible, these anions should be directly measured—lactate, ketones, phosphate, albumin or surrogate markers of anion accumulation—serum creatinine and the osmolar gap. Causes of metabolic acidosis that are commonly encountered by anesthesiologists are discussed below.

LACTIC ACIDOSIS

The presence of lactic acidosis is an excellent marker of acute critical illness, the magnitude of which often reflects the degree of hyperlactatemia. Lactic acidosis occurs when the production of lactate in the body is greater than the liver's capacity to clear it—there is a problem of overproduction or inadequate clearance.

Lactic acid is produced physiologically as a degradation product of glucose metabolism. In nature it exists as two isoforms: L-lactate which is produced by the human body and is measured by blood gas analyzers, and D-lactate which can only be produced by fermentation by bacteria. The formation of L-lactate (lactate) from pyruvate is catalyzed by lactate dehydrogenase. Lactate is used as a "buffer" in isotonic fluids, principally lactated Ringer's solution and Hartmann's solution; these contain a racemic mixture of both D and L lactate at a concentration of 14 mmol/L each.

Under normal conditions, the ratio of lactate to pyruvate ratio is less than 20:1. In anaerobic conditions, for example following vigorous exercise, lactate levels increase dramatically, and high levels of circulating lactate are frequently interpreted as evidence of increased glycolytic activity. However, lactate is often produced under aerobic conditions. Activation of β-adrenergic receptors in skeletal muscle by stress (increased circulating catecholamines) or exogenous infusion (epinephrine/norepinephrine infusions) increases [lactate], resulting in aerobic glycolysis. Lactate is metabolized to pyruvate and then into glucose (gluconeogenesis) in the liver and subsequently to CO_2 and H_2O (the Cori cycle). Hence the lactate in Ringer's lactate (or Hartmann's) solution is considered to be a source of bicarbonate. This is only the case if the liver is capable of handling the lactate load.

Plasma lactate and arterial pH should be measured early in any critically ill patient—it is now a diagnostic component of the definition of septic shock.[61] A lactate concentration > 2 mEq/L (mmol/L) is clinically significant and a level of 5 mEq/L(mmol/L) in the presence of metabolic acidosis is severe.[62] Isolated hyperlactatemia in the absence of acidosis is of unclear clinical significance.[63]

Traditionally, lactic acidosis has been described as taking one of two forms: type 1 (may also be termed type A, global inadequate oxygen delivery) is seen in hypovolemic/hemorrhagic shock while type 2 (type B) occurs despite normal global oxygen delivery and tissue perfusion. Lactic acidosis may also develop in situations where there is significant regional hypoperfusion. Examples include bowel ischemia, where lactate is produced in large quantity due to glycolysis despite global oxygen delivery that is normal. Type 2 lactic acidosis is associated with any state in which circulating catecholamines (endogenous or exogenous) are in excess. Examples include simple exercise and the hyperinflammatory state of trauma or sepsis. Type 2 lactic acidosis may also be seen in cyanide poisoning (associated with sodium nitroprusside), with biguanides (metformin, which blocks hepatic gluconeogenesis), and in hypercatabolic diseases such as lymphoma, leukemia, AIDS, or diabetic ketoacidosis (DKA). In critical illness, type 1 and type 2 lactic acidosis frequently coexist.

It is universally accepted that lactic acidosis is a sensitive marker of disease severity.[64] Persistence of lactic acidosis strongly predicts poor outcomes in acute illness.[65-67] Rapid clearance (i.e., reduced plasma concentration presumably due to reduced production and increased metabolism) of lactate has been associated with improved outcomes.[68,69] It remains controversial whether it is possible to institute therapy that improves outcomes and simultaneously increases lactate clearance. Simplistically, improved overall perfusion consequent of blood or isotonic fluid administration should reduce glycolysis and reduce lactate production, increasing hepatic blood flow and increasing metabolism. However, not all patients who are under-resuscitated are hyperlactatemic, and probably the minority of patients who are hyperlactatemic are under-resuscitated. Although fluid resuscitation with the goal of normalizing serum lactate may be associated with improved outcomes, excessive or late fluid resuscitation increases mortality.[70] It is important to note that, following fluid bolus, plasma lactate rapidly falls, perhaps due to hemodilution, and then falls slowly, at 10% to 20% per hour, due to rate-limited hepatic clearance. If plasma lactate does not fall, fluid resuscitation should be discontinued.[71]

The presence of evidence of good overall oxygen delivery and normal consumption, as measured by cardiac output monitors and mixed venous oxygen saturation, in lactic acidosis is not reassuring. Indeed, bowel ischemia may be indicated by otherwise unexplained lactic acidosis, and the availability heuristic associated with sepsis may result in delayed diagnosis and inappropriate fluid resuscitation (Fig. 48.9).

Metformin is associated with severe lactic acidosis, a phenomenon that appears more likely when the patient has liver dysfunction, is dehydrated, is in heart failure, has suffered acute kidney injury (AKI), or is septic.[72] The mechanism of harm is unknown, although metformin is thought to impair oxidative metabolism in hepatocyte mitochondria, and block gluconeogenesis. Renal impairment appears to be a significant risk factor. The patient presenting with metformin-associated lactic acidosis frequently looks reasonably well, despite serum lactate that may exceed 10 mmol/L. There is no specific treatment except for withdrawal of the drug, gentle rehydration, and patience.

D-lactate-induced acidosis can occur, typically in patients with short bowel syndrome and bacterial overgrowth. It manifests as a widened AG acidosis where no other potential source of metabolic acid is identified. Crucially, point-of-care blood gas analyzers do not measure D-lactate. However, many laboratories are able to measure the molecule, and this test should be considered in a high-risk patient (post major abdominal surgery) with unexplained acidosis.

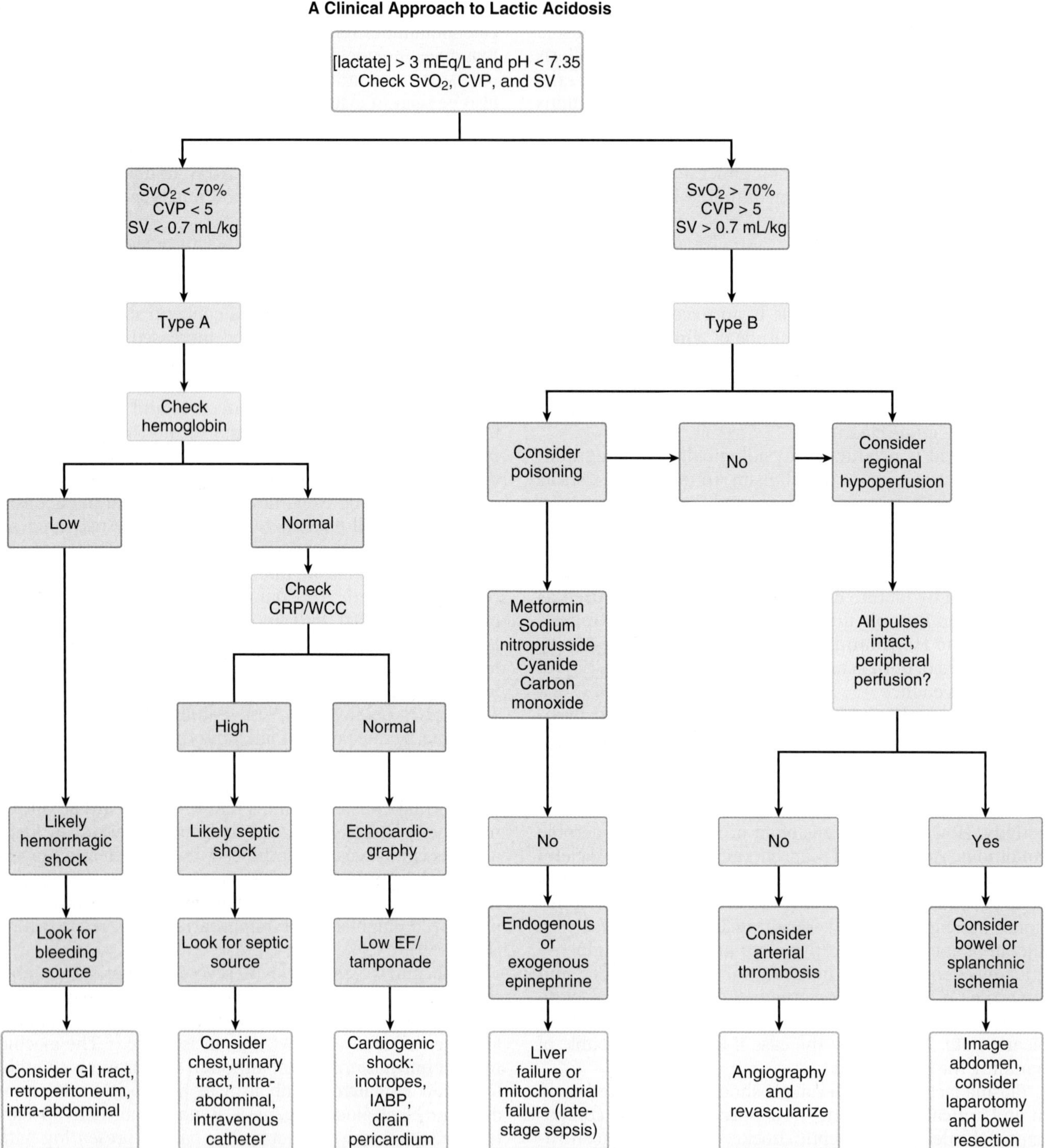

Fig. 48.9 Evaluation of a Patient with Lactic Acidosis. *CRP,* C-Reactive protein; *CVP,* central venous pressure; *EF,* ejection fraction; *GI,* gastrointestinal; *IABP,* intra-aortic balloon counterpulsation; *SV,* stroke volume; *SvO_2,* mixed venous oxygen saturation; *WCC,* white cell count.

Ketoacidosis

Ketone bodies—acetone (<2%), acetoacetate (20%), and 3-β-hydroxybutyrate (βOHB) (78%)—are normal by-products of fat metabolism. They are produced when fatty acids are metabolized by the liver, when glucose is unavailable as an energy source. During ketogenesis, acetoacetate is generated from acetyl co-enzyme A. This either enters mitochondria to be converted to βOHB or it spontaneously decarboxylates to acetone. Ketones are transported by blood to the tissues, in particular the brain, where they are used as energy sources. Under normal dietary conditions, ketones are undetectable in blood and urine. However, in situations where fat becomes the primary source of energy (for example in starvation or low-carbohydrate diets), ketones can be measured in blood (principally βOHB) and urine (principally acetoacetate). In a variety of clinical situations, such as prolonged starvation, alcoholism, alcoholic- or obesity-related steatohepatitis, and, most commonly, insulin deficiency (diabetes mellitus), a dramatic increase in circulating ketones occurs. As these are strong anionic compounds, ketones reduce SID, resulting in metabolic acidosis. When this occurs in type-1 diabetes (T1D), it is known as diabetic ketoacidosis (DKA).

DKA may be the first manifestation of T1D, or may result from poor glycemic control or specific stress triggers, such as infection, trauma, or surgery. Typically there is an imbalance between the relative quantity of insulin and glucose-promoting hormones (cortisol, epinephrine, and glucagon). Blood glucose increases, exceeding the renal reabsorption threshold. This results in glycosuria, osmotic diuresis, dehydration, and the vicious cycle of activation of stress hormones. This leads to increased metabolism of fatty acids and, in the absence of insulin, or consequent of severe insulin resistance, there is unrestrained oxidation of fatty acids to ketones in the liver. Regardless of the cause, there is usually elevated blood glucose, significant dehydration, and depletion of potassium, phosphorous, and magnesium.

The diagnosis of DKA is relatively simple. Usually there is a clear history of either diabetes or polyuria and polydipsia: the patient presents to the emergency room with hyperglycemia and glycosuria, and, usually, positive urinary ketones. Ketoacidosis is confirmed by performing ABG analysis. Every hospital has a protocol for the management of DKA. Insulin is administered by an infusion (with or without an initial bolus). This may be a weight-based fixed-rate infusion (0.1 units of insulin per kilo per hour) or more traditional infusion based on blood glucose.[73] The patient is resuscitated with several liters of isotonic crystalloid (usually isotonic saline [0.9%] solution), and when blood glucose falls within a "controlled" range, intravenous dextrose is administered. Insulin suppresses ketone production. Glucose is required to assist ketone metabolism, which can take some time. Two major mistakes are made in the management of DKA. Administration of 0.9% NaCl results in an entirely predictable hyperchloremic acidosis; this may or may not be harmful but may be perceived incorrectly as persistence of ketoacidosis. A small study that compared NS with Plasmalyte-148 (a balanced salt solution [BSS]) reported that patients receiving the balanced solution instead of NS had more rapid resolution of metabolic acidosis, less hyperchloremia, improved blood pressure profile, and greater urinary output.[74]

The second error is very important for anesthesiologists. As noted above, the majority of ketones in the body are in the form of βOHB. These can only be identified by measuring "blood" ketones. Urinary ketone sticks measure only acetoacetate.[75] The absence of ketones in the urine does not eliminate the diagnosis of ketoacidosis (particularly if it is not associated with diabetes). Blood ketones are easily measured using handheld devices (although these may be hard to find in hospitals due to the current disenfranchisement of point-of-care testing). Interestingly, as βOHB must be metabolized to acetoacetate, urinary ketones may actually increase during the time that the whole body ketone load is falling and ketosis is resolving.

Patients presenting for emergency surgery may have multiple simultaneous acid-base abnormalities, and physicians often miss ketoacidosis due to availability bias—the presence of elevated lactate may result in search satisficing—and a major metabolic abnormality is missed.[76] Despite fluid resuscitation and source control, the acidosis may not resolve. This in turn may lead to inappropriate therapy such as renal replacement therapy (RRT) and sodium bicarbonate administration, neither of which are of any value in ketoacidosis. All forms of ketoacidosis require insulin therapy and, eventually, glucose administration. Ketoacidosis of non-diabetic origin may take many hours, and occasionally days, to resolve.

Renal Acidosis

The kidney excretes water and a variety of metabolic byproducts, principally derived from proteins. The kidney also excretes surplus electrolytes, some of which are strong ions, including chloride, sulfate, formate, urate citric acid cycle metabolites (fumarate, citrate), and phosphate. These accumulate in AKI and cause "renal acidosis." Early in AKI, hyperchloremia is the principle source of acidosis; subsequently, 50% to 60% of acidosis is caused by UMA and up to 30% is associated with hyperphosphatemia.[77] Fifty percent of patients with AKI in critical illness have a normal AG.[77]

AKI, in perioperative medicine, may accompany hypotension, hypovolemia, renal hypoperfusion (from aortic cross clamping or intraabdominal hypertension), rhabdomyolysis, sepsis, or urinary obstruction. Irrespective of the cause, patients develop oliguria, volume overload, and hyperkalemia secondary to metabolic acidosis.

The identification of metabolic acidosis in AKI is key to the diagnosis, severity, and therapeutic strategy in AKI. Although serum creatinine is the most widely used marker of renal function, isolated readings are unhelpful. Fluid resuscitation can artificially lower the creatinine concentration, by dilution; diuresis can artificially elevate it. Metabolic acidosis, particularly in the presence of hyperkalemia with elevated creatinine, should always prompt the clinician to determine the extent of renal acidosis. This is not easy. Hyperchloremia typically accompanies renal acidosis, but isotonic saline solution is frequently administered to patients with elevated creatinine under the mistaken belief that patients are less likely to develop hyperkalemia compared with BSSs.[78] A study of anephric patients undergoing renal transplantation demonstrated that patients treated with NS were more acidotic and hyperkalemic than patients treated with lactated Ringer's solution.[78] Hyperphosphatemia is a minor contributor to renal acidosis, and currently no tests are available to clinically identify the UMA, except by a process of exclusion. Hence, renal acidosis is usually diagnosed by identifying a widened AG, base deficit gap, or SIG, and excluding ketones and lactate. Usually the key decision step regarding RRT involves uncontrolled hyperkalemia. Renal acidosis can be temporarily controlled by administration of sodium bicarbonate (assuming the patient can clear CO_2), by increasing the SID. This may be necessary if the risk of delaying surgery exceeds the risk of delaying RRT. Note, however, in critical illness, delaying RRT was associated with a 4.7% increase in mortality at 90 days.[79]

Hyperchloremic Acidosis

Hyperchloremia has been a known cause of metabolic acidosis since the dawn of acid-base chemistry,[12] but due to difficulty in measuring serum Cl^- during most of the 20th century, hyperchloremia was largely ignored until recent decades. The extracellular space contains 110 to 130 g of salt. For a 70 kg male (ECF volume 18 L), this is approximately 58 g of Na^+ (3.22 g/L) and 65 g (3.62 g/L) of Cl^-. The average American ingests approximately 3 g or more of salt (NaCl) each day (2.3 g is recommended). To maintain the normal ratio of Na^+ to Cl^- (1.4:1 approximately), the body needs to excrete 30% more Cl^- than Na^+, and this is one of the major excretory roles of the kidney. This approximates to 15 to 20 mmol of Cl^- excretion per day; to maintain electrical neutrality Cl^- is excreted with ammonium (NH_4^+), a byproduct of nitrogen metabolism. In renal failure, Cl^- accumulates, and this is often the cause of the early metabolic acidosis associated with AKI. For decades, it has been hypothesized that elevated circulating levels of Cl^-, usually as a consequence of intravenous administration, may actually be nephrotoxic, due, presumably, to increased metabolic demands on the kidney. One liter of isotonic saline solution (0.9%, normal saline, NS) contains 9 g of salt, 3.5 g Na^+, and 5.5 g Cl^- (154 mmol/L of each). For a euchloremic patient (the human body does not store chloride, unlike, for example, calcium), this means that if 1 L of NaCl 0.9% is administered, most or all of the Cl^- must be excreted—an 8- to 10-fold increase in metabolic load for the kidney. Moreover, as NS has a SID of 0, elevated serum chloride is usually associated with a non-AG (hyperchloremic) metabolic acidosis.[80]

Hyperchloremic acidosis is a complication of renal tubular acidosis, which is caused by a defect in chloride excretion. The urine is relatively alkaline. Hyperchloremia also occurs when ureters have been re-implanted in the bowel after, for example, cystectomy, and excreted chloride is reabsorbed.

Are hyperchloremia and hyperchloremic acidosis clinically significant? As a cause of acidosis, hyperchloremia is less sinister than other causes: in a study of critically ill patients with various acid-base disorders, mortality was highest for lactic acidosis (56%); for SIG acidosis it was 39% and for hyperchloremic acidosis 29% ($P < .001$).[81] Nevertheless, hyperchloremia may result in clinically significant organ dysfunction. An observational study of 31,000 surgical patients comparing intravenous saline to intravenous BSS demonstrated significant outcome differences, favoring BSS.[82] Complications enhanced by the use of normal saline included postoperative infections, blood transfusions, and kidney injury requiring dialysis.

A hyperchloremic state may be associated with nephrotoxicity; saline infusion has been associated with reduced renal blood flow, renal vasoconstriction, reduced glomerular filtration, and splanchnic hypoperfusion.[83] In a relatively large before-and-after cohort study of patients treated in an Australian ICU, the use of chloride-rich fluids was associated with a 3.7% absolute increase in the risk for need in RRT relative to BSS.[84]

Two large randomized controlled trials looked at the use of isotonic saline solution versus BSS in emergency medicine patients[85] and critically ill patients.[86] Although the volume of fluid administered intravenously was relatively low, certainly in comparison with perioperative patients, in both studies there was approximately a 1% increase in renal complications. Whether this effect scales up with larger volumes will presumably be the subject of further study and meta-analysis.

NS solution, originally introduced by Hamburger in the 19th century and labelled "normal" due to flawed research, has been the most widely used intravenous fluid for over a century, despite minimal research demonstrating its clinical efficacy and safety.[87] As mounting research demonstrates that this particular fluid may be harmful, and with a variety of other balanced solutions available for clinical practice, the role of NS in perioperative medicine is highly questionable.

Perioperative Metabolic Alkalosis

Perioperative metabolic alkalosis is usually of iatrogenic origin. Overventilation of patients with chronic respiratory failure results in acute metabolic alkalosis because the presence of chronic compensatory alkalosis associated with chloride loss in urine has not been taken into account (Fig. 48.10). More frequently, metabolic alkalosis is associated with increased SID due to sodium gain. This abnormality results from the administration of fluids in which sodium is buffered by weak ions, citrate (in blood products), acetate (in parenteral nutrition), and, of course, bicarbonate. It is important to recognize that buffer ions such as citrate, acetate, gluconate, and lactate are, under normal conditions, rapidly cleared by the liver and do not contribute to acid-base balance. Sodium and chloride obey the law of conservation of mass. Sodium gain is "chloride sensitive" alkalosis, treated by administration of net loads of chloride—0.9% NaCl, potassium chloride, calcium chloride, and, occasionally, hydrogen chloride. It is important to correct chloride-sensitive alkalosis, as the normal compensatory measure is hypoventilation, increasing $PaCO_2$, which may lead to CO_2 narcosis and failure to liberate from mechanical ventilation.

Large volumes of BSSs are likely to cause metabolic alkalosis, due to dilution of A_{TOT} (principally hypoalbuminemia), a process that is curtained when using lactated Ringer's solution (Hartmann's) due to lower SID (20 mEq/L). The acquired hypoalbuminemic alkalosis is of undetermined clinical significance.

Another cause of metabolic alkalosis in perioperative patients reflects loss of chloride-rich fluids from the gastrointestinal tract. Gastric juice contains HCl, which, when lost as a result of continuous suctioning or vomiting, obeys the law of conservation of mass and leads to alkalosis.

Perioperative fluid therapy remains highly controversial. Isotonic fluids are usually administered due to fear of cerebral edema associated with stress-induced water retention. However, this results in large amounts of solute, in particular sodium and chloride, accumulating in the extravascular space. Acquired hypernatremia is associated with adverse clinical outcomes and is very difficult to treat.[88] BSSs appear safer than NS, but large-volume administration of these resuscitation fluids are also associated with worse outcomes.[89]

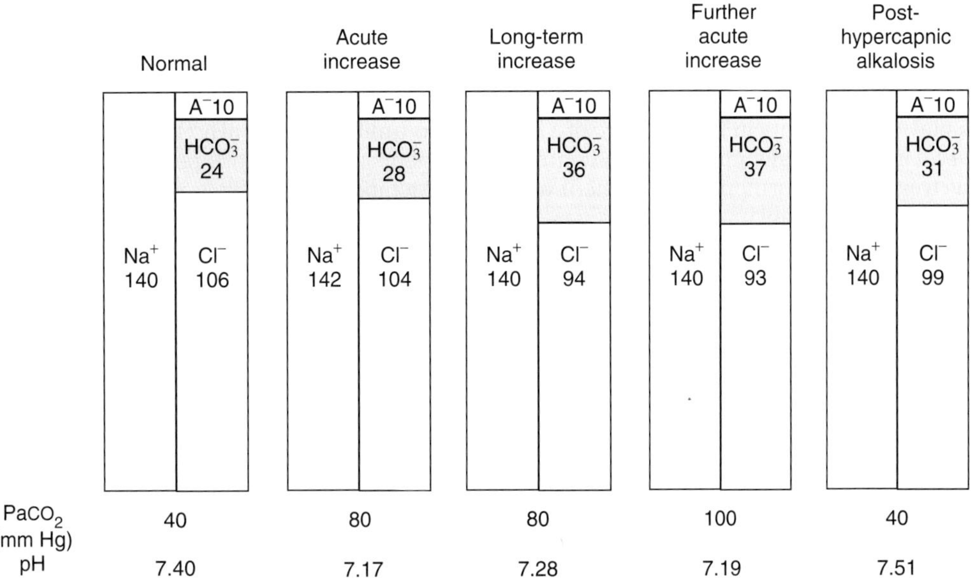

Fig. 48.10 Changes in Acid-Based and Electrolyte Composition in Patients With Respiratory Acidosis. *Left to right*, the panels depict normal acid-base status; adaptation to an acute rise in the partial pressure of arterial carbon dioxide ($PaCO_2$) to 80 mm Hg; adaptation to a long-term rise in $PaCO_2$ to 80 mm Hg; superimposition of an acute further increment in $PaCO_2$ (to a level of 100 mm Hg) in the same patient; and post-hypercapnic alkalosis resulting from an abrupt reduction in $PaCO_2$ to the level of 40 mm Hg in the same patient. A^- denotes unmeasured plasma anions, and the numbers within the bars give ion concentrations in millimoles per liter. (Modified from Adrogué HJ, Madias NE. Management of life-threatening acid-base disorders. First of two parts. *N Engl J Med*. 1998;338[1]:26–34.)

ACID-BASE DISTURBANCES IN CRITICAL ILLNESS

Critically ill patients may have many confounding acid-base disturbances that are not evident when only a single quantitative measure, such as base deficit, is employed. Patients will frequently have perturbations of PCO_2, SID, and A_{TOT}, and significant pathology may be overlooked due to apparently normal blood gas results.[90]

The most common single disturbance in acid-base chemistry in critically ill patients is hypoalbuminemia.[24] This abnormality is ubiquitous and causes a metabolic alkalosis of unpredictable magnitude. Hypoalbuminemia may mask significant alterations in SID, for example lactic or renal acidosis. Therefore, when the AG is used in critically ill patients it should be corrected for albumin.[26] Similarly, the use of base deficit to predict lactate is unreliable in critical illness, particularly in patients undergoing secondary deterioration.[25] Further, prolonged respiratory failure, with associated hypercarbia, leads to additional metabolic alkalosis due to chloride loss in urine (see Fig. 48.10)[91] Kidney injury is associated with accumulation of metabolic by-products, phosphate, renal anions, chloride, and other UMA, leading initially to metabolic acidosis. However, late polyuric renal failure may be associated with significant contraction alkalosis, due to loss of sodium, potassium, and free water.

Critically ill patients are vulnerable to significant changes in SID and free water. Nasogastric suctioning causes chloride loss, diarrhea leads to sodium and potassium deficits. Surgical drains placed in tissue beds may remove fluids with varying electrolyte concentrations (the pancreatic bed, for example, secretes fluid rich in sodium). Fever, sweating, evaporation from denuded tissue, and inadequately humidified ventilator circuits all can lead to large-volume insensible loss and contraction alkalosis.

Infusions administered to patients may be responsible for unrecognized alterations in serum chemistry. Many antibiotics, for example piperacillin-tazobactam, are diluted in sodium-rich solutions. Others, such as vancomycin, are administered in large volumes of free water (5% dextrose). Lorazepam is diluted in propylene glycol, large volumes of which will cause metabolic acidosis similar to that seen with ethylene glycol.[92]

Continuous renal replacement therapy (CRRT) is used in critical illness to hemofilter and hemodialysis patients who are hemodynamically unstable. Rocktaschel[93] and colleagues have demonstrated that CRRT resolved the acidosis of acute renal failure by removing strong ions and phosphate. However, in the presence of hypoalbuminemia, use of dialysis to correct a metabolic acidosis may unmask a metabolic alkalosis due to hypoalbuminemia. CRRT is not an effective treatment for lactic acidosis or ketoacidosis.

Other seemingly innocuous therapies may cause significant disturbances to acid-base balance. Loop diuretics, such as furosemide, are often administered to critically ill patients. These agents preferentially excrete water over electrolytes and provoke a contraction alkalosis. Similarly, carbonic anhydrase inhibitors such as acetazolamide may be used to treat patients with hypochloremic metabolic alkalosis or respiratory alkalosis by decreasing the plasma SID. This effect is completely explained by the increased renal excretion ratio of sodium to chloride, resulting in an increase in serum chloride.[94]

Neurosurgical patients are vulnerable to a variety of acid-base disturbances as a result of osmotherapy or from disturbances caused by brain injury. Most commonly, NS solution is administered to these patients and results in hyperchloremic acidosis.[95] Diabetes insipidus (DI) is a frequent complication of severe head injury, particularly when the patient is progressing toward brain death. DI is caused by damage to the pituitary and/or the hypothalamus and results in a loss of antidiuretic hormone (ADH) secretion. Absent ADH, the kidney is unable to concentrate the urine and a massive diuresis follows. The disorder is characterized by an increase in plasma osmolality in the presence of a low urinary osmolality. DI will typically manifest as a contraction alkalosis. The treatment is hormonal replacement with either vasopressin or desmopressin.

TREATING ACID-BASE DISTURBANCES

In general, in acute illness and perioperative medicine, acid-base disturbances are clinical indicators of disease processes that are more harmful than hydrogen ion abnormalities themselves. Correcting the pH is usually unlikely to resolve the problem, except in certain circumstances, such as hyperkalemia in AKI, where acidosis is the major cause of the problem.

The treatment of acid-base abnormalities is determined by whether the acids, in particular, are organic or mineral acids. Organic acids can be metabolized, excreted, or dialyzed from the body. Diabetic and nondiabetic ketoacidosis are treated primarily with insulin, intravenous fluid, and glucose. The ketoacids causing metabolic acidosis are metabolized by the liver. AKI is treated with dialysis and ultrafiltration, which directly removes UMA. Surprisingly, there are no clear guidelines regarding the optimal timing of initiation of RRT,[79,96] particularly in the perioperative period.[97]

For decades, sodium bicarbonate ($NaHCO_3^-$) has been used to "correct" acidosis. The sodium component, as a strong anion, widens the SID and is alkalizing. Simultaneously, the bicarbonate moiety provides buffer for hydrogen ions, generating CO_2, which is presumably excreted from the body by increased alveolar ventilation. In respiratory failure, sodium bicarbonate will worsen respiratory acidosis despite increased SID. CO_2 also enters cells and may cause intracellular acidosis, the clinical significance of which is unclear.[98]

$NaHCO_3^-$ is commonly used to treat hyperchloremic acidosis. For patients with renal tubular acidosis, this involves long-term treatment with sodium bicarbonate tablets and chloride restriction. In acquired hyperchloremic acidosis, intravenous sodium bicarbonate corrects the base deficit,[99] but the benefit is unclear. The major drawbacks of $NaHCO_3^-$ therapy include sodium and volume overload, metabolic alkalosis, hypertension, and hypocalcemia.

Sodium bicarbonate therapy has been extensively studied in lactic acidosis and circulatory shock.[100] A recent randomized trial of 389 critically ill patients with metabolic acidosis compared the administration of 4.2% (hypertonic) $NaHCO_3^-$ to keep pH above 7.3, up to a maximum of 1000 mL in the first 24 hours, versus no intervention.[101] Although there were no differences in the primary outcome—28-day mortality—the patients who received $NaHCO_3^-$ had a lower incidence of AKI and requirement for RRT. It is unclear why there was a reduction in the need for RRT. Perhaps the reduction in acidosis delayed the decision to start RRT and resulted in the intervention being avoided completely,[96] or reversal of acidosis reduced vasopressor requirement and improved kidney blood flow; but this is merely speculation. Previous meta-analyse have failed to demonstrate benefit from $NaHCO_3^-$ therapy,[102] presumably due to the paucity of available research. Until larger multicenter trials have been conducted, $NaHCO_3^-$ therapy should be used with caution for treatment of metabolic acidosis, due to circulatory shock or ketoacidosis. It is also unlikely that $NaHCO_3^-$ therapy benefits perioperative patients at risk for postoperative kidney failure.[103]

Metabolic alkalosis is rarely seen in elective perioperative care. It is most likely encountered when unmasked by overventilation of patients who chronically retain CO_2. Minute ventilation should be reduced. Critically ill patients may have metabolic alkalosis due to chloride deficit, free water deficit, or hypoalbuminemia. Contraction alkalosis is treated by correcting the free water deficit using the formula below:

$$\text{Free water deficit} = 0.6 \times \text{patient's weight in kg} \times (\text{patient's sodium}/140 - 1)$$

Hypochloremic alkalosis should be treated by correcting the chloride deficit using NS or LR.

There is no evidence that correcting hypoalbuminemia is of clinical benefit for the majority of patients.[104] Respiratory alkalosis usually results from anxiety or pain. Short-term therapy, such as CO_2 rebreathing, should be followed by treating the underlying problem—for example with opioids or benzodiazepines.

Hypercarbic acidosis may be encountered in the perioperative period due to deliberate[105] or inadvertent hypoventilation. It is also associated with elevated dead space ventilation as seen in ARDS. In general, acute respiratory acidosis is well tolerated and can be easily reversed by increasing minute ventilation. However, in ARDS, a high tidal volume and transpulmonary pressures result in ventilator induced lung injury (VILI) and increased mortality.[106] Consequently, hypercarbia must be tolerated by the physician and patient ("permissive hypercarbia") or CO_2 removed by an extracorporeal circuit.[107]

Summary

Much of the confusion regarding acid-base chemistry relates to the attempt to apply observational approaches, such as that of Henderson-Hasselbalch and Schwartz and Brackett, to the entire spectrum of pathophysiologic processes. The use of physical chemistry principles has permitted easier explanation of acid-base balance, and tools to apply to a wide variety of clinical situations. This does not suggest that the "traditional" approach is incorrect, merely that it looks at a mirror image of that proposed by Stewart, Fencl, and others. All acid-base disorders can be explained in terms of SID, A_{TOT}, and PCO_2. This is important to anesthesiologists, who may significantly impact acid-base balance with our choice of fluids and mechanical ventilation strategy.

Acknowledgment

The editors, publisher, and Dr. Patrick Neligan would like to thank Dr. Clifford S. Deutschman for his contribution to previous editions of this chapter.

 **Complete references available online at expertconsult.com.**

References

1. Berend K, et al. *N Engl J Med.* 2014;371:1434.
2. Stewart PA. *Can J Physiol Pharmacol.* 1983;61:1444.
3. Gomez H, Kellum JA. *Crit Care Clin.* 2015;31:849.
4. Adrogue HJ, Madias NE. *Am J Kidney Dis.* 2016;68:793.
5. Fencl V, Leith DE. *Respir Physiol.* 1993;91:1.
6. Aiken CGA. *JCDR.* 2013;7:2038.
7. Moon JB. *N Engl J Med.* 1967;276:283.
8. Henderson LJ. *Ergebn Physiol.* 1909;8:254.
9. Hasselbalch KA. *Biochem Z.* 1916;78:112.
10. Sirker AA, et al. *Anaesthesia.* 2002;57:348.
11. Van Slyke DD. *Proc Natl Acad Sci USA.* 1921;7:229.
12. Henderson LH. Blood as a physiochemical system. *J Biol Chem.* 1921;46:411.
13. Corey HE. *Kidney Int.* 2003;64:777.
14. Stewart PA. Modern quantitative acid-base chemistry. *Can J Physiol Pharmacol.* 1983;61:1444–1461.
15. Deleted in proofs.
16. Severinghaus JW. *Anesthesiology.* 1976;45:539.
17. Brackett NC, Cohen JJ, Schwartz WB. Carbon dioxide titration curve of normal man. *N Engl J Med.* 1965;272:6–12.
18. Hickling KG. *Respir Care Clin North Am.* 2002;8:155.
19. Laffey JG, Kavanagh BP. *Lancet.* 1999;354:1283.
20. Contreras M, et al. *Crit Care Med.* 2012;40:2622.
21. Scheingraber S, et al. *Anesthesiology.* 1999;90:1265.
22. Figge J, et al. *J Lab Clin Med.* 1992;120:713.
23. Story DA, et al. *Br J Anaesth.* 2004;92:54.
24. Figge J, et al. *J Lab Clin Med.* 1991;117:453.
25. Fencl V, et al. *Am J Respir Crit Care Med.* 2000;162:2246.
26. Figge J, et al. *Crit Care Med.* 1998;26:1807.
27. Goldwasser P, Feldman J. *J Clin Epidemiol.* 1997;50:693.
28. Wang F, et al. *N Engl J Med.* 1986;315:1591.
29. Bleich HL, et al. *J Clin Invest.* 1964;43:11.
30. Kazemi H, Johnson DC. *Physiol Rev.* 1986;66:953.
31. Bondoli A, et al. *Resuscitation.* 1981;9:99.
32. Javaheri S, et al. *Am J Respir Crit Care Med.* 1994;150:78.
33. Johnson DC, et al. *Respir Physiol.* 1984;56:301.
34. Johnson DC, et al. *J Appl Physiol.* 1987;63:1591.
35. Smith QR, Johanson CE. *Brain Res.* 1991;562:306.
36. Javaheri S. *J Appl Physiol.* 1987;62:1582.
37. Narins R, Emmett M. *Medicine (Baltimore).* 1980;59:161.
38. Kellum JA. *Diagnosis and Treatment of Acid Base Disorders, Textbook of Critical Care Medicine.* 4th ed. Shoemaker, ed. Saunders; 2000: 839–853.
39. Rodriguez-Soriano J. *Pediatr Nephrol.* 2000;14:1121.
40. Choate KA, et al. *Proc Natl Acad Sci U S A.* 2003;100:663.
41. Shaer AJ. *Am J Med Sci.* 2001;322:316.
42. Kellum JA. *Crit Care.* 2005;9:500.
43. Schwartz WB, et al. *J Clin Invest.* 1965;44:291.
44. Brackett NC, et al. *N Engl J Med.* 1965;272:6.
45. Albert MS. *Ann Intern Med.* 1967;66:312.
46. Emmett M, Narins RG. *Medicine (Baltimore).* 1977;56:38.
47. Salem MM, Mujais SK. *Arch Intern Med.* 1992;152:1625.
48. Moviat M, et al. *Crit Care.* 2003;7:R41.
49. Lipnick MS, et al. *Crit Care Med.* 2013;41:49.
50. Singer RB, Hastings AB. *Medicine (Baltimore).* 1948;10:242.
51. Severinghaus JW. The invention and development of blood gas analysis apparatus. *Anesthesiology.* 2002;97:253.
52. Jorgensen K. *Scand J Clin Lab Invest.* 1957;9:122.
53. Astrup P, Siggard-Andersen O. *Adv Clin Chem.* 1963;69:1.
54. Wooten EW. *J Appl Physiol.* 2003;95:2333.
55. Siggaard-Andersen O. *Scand J Clin Lab Invest Suppl.* 1977;37:15.
56. Prange HD, et al. *J Appl Physiol.* 2001;91(1985):33.
57. Siggaard-Andersen O. *Scand J Clin Lab Invest.* 1971;27:239.
58. Gilfix BM, et al. *J Crit Care.* 1993;8:187.
59. Balasubramanyan N, et al. *Crit Care Med.* 1999;27:1577.
60. Story DA, et al. *Br J Anaesth.* 2004;92:54.
61. Singer M, et al. *JAMA.* 2016;315:801.
62. Fall PJ, Szerlip HM. *J Intensive Care Med.* 2005;20:255.
63. Lee SW, et al. *Emerg Med J.* 2008;25:659.
64. Mikkelsen ME, et al. *Crit Care Med.* 2009;37:1670.
65. Abramson D, et al. *J Trauma.* 1993;35:584.
66. Arnold RC, Shapiro NI, et al. *Shock.* 2009;32:35.
67. McNelis J, et al. *Am J Surg.* 2001;182:481.
68. Jones AE, et al. *JAMA.* 2010;303:739.
69. Jansen TC, et al. *Am J Respir Crit Care Med.* 2010;182:752.
70. Liu V, et al. *Ann Am Thorac Soc.* 2013;10:466.
71. Bakker J, et al. *Intensive Care Med.* 2016;42:472.
72. DeFronzo R, et al. *Metabolism.* 2016;65:20.
73. Tran TTT, et al. *Front Endocrinol.* 2017;8:106.
74. Chua HR, et al. *J Crit Care.* 2012;27:138.
75. Brewster S. *Practical Diabetes.* 2017;34:13.
76. Saposnik G, et al. *BMC Med Inform Decis Mak.* 2016;16:138.
77. Rocktaeschel J, et al. *Crit Care.* 2003;7:R60.
78. O'Malley, et al. *Anesth Analg.* 2005;100:1518.
79. Zarbock A. *JAMA.* 2016;315(20):2190.
80. Myles PS, et al. *World J Surg.* 2017;41:2457.
81. Gunnerson KJ, et al. *Crit Care.* 2006;10:R22.
82. Shaw AD, et al. *Ann Surg.* 2012;255:821.
83. Wilkes NJ, et al. *Anesth Analg.* 2001;93:811.
84. Yunos N. *JAMA.* 2012;308:1566.
85. Self WH, et al. *N Engl J Med.* 2018;378:819.
86. Semler MW, et al. *N Engl J Med.* 2018;378:829.
87. Awad S. The history of 0.9% saline. *Clin Nutr.* 2008;27(2):179.
88. Tsipotis E, et al. *Am J Med.* 2018;131:72.
89. Simoes CM, et al. *BMC Anesthesiol.* 2018;18:49.
90. Moviat M, et al. *Crit Care Med.* 2008;36:752.
91. Adrogue HJ, et al. *Kidney Int.* 1984;(25):591.
92. Tayar J, et al. *N Engl J Med.* 2002;346:1253.
93. Rocktaeschel J, et al. *Int J Artif Organs.* 2003;26:19.
94. Moviat M, Pickkers P, et al. *Crit Care.* 2006;10:R14.
95. Lima MF, et al. *J Neurosurg Anesthesiol.* 2018.
96. Gaudry S, et al. *N Engl J Med.* 2016;375:122.
97. Romagnoli S, et al. *Nephron.* 2018:1.
98. Swenson ER. *Anesthesiology.* 2018;128:873.
99. Rehm M, Finsterer U. *Anesth Analg.* 2003;96:1201.
100. Forsythe SM, Schmidt GA. *Chest.* 2000;117:260.
101. Jaber S, et al. *Lancet.* 2018;392:31.
102. Velissaris D, et al. *Crit Care Res Pract.* 2015;2015:605830.
103. McGuinness SP, et al. *Crit Care Med.* 2013;41:1599.
104. Caironi P, et al. *N Engl J Med.* 2014;370:1412.
105. Lyons C, Callaghan M. *Anaesthesia.* 2017;72:1379.
106. Slutsky AS, Ranieri VM. *N Engl J Med.* 2013;369:2126.
107. Barrett NA, Camporota L. *Crit Care Resusc.* 2017;19(suppl 1):62.

49 Patient Blood Management: Transfusion Therapy

MATTHEW DUDLEY, RONALD D. MILLER, and JOHN H. TURNBULL

KEY POINTS

- Blood transfusion is safer now than at any other time in history. Advances in donor screening, improved testing, automated data systems, and changes in transfusion medicine practices account for these increases in safety.
- Although the overall condition of the patient is of prime importance, hemoglobin (Hb) values remain a primary component for transfusion decisions with the use of either a restrictive or liberal strategy. In general, a transfusion trigger of 6 to 8 g/dL Hb (restrictive strategy) can be tolerated by patients.
- Preoperative anemia is an independent, and potentially modifiable, risk factor for postoperative morbidity and mortality.
- The term *patient blood management* has become synonymous with appropriate transfusion strategy.
- The addition of plasma and sometimes platelets to packed red blood cells (PRBCs) is described by the term *transfusion ratios.* For example, 2 units of plasma with 1 unit of platelets with 1 unit of PRBCs would be 2:1:1.
- Infectivity of blood is no longer a major cause of transfusion-related morbidity and mortality. Transfusion-related acute lung injury is the leading cause of transfusion-related mortality.
- Fresh whole blood has gained renewed interest as a choice in patients with major blood loss and related coagulopathy (see also Chapter 50).
- Although storage lesions of red blood cells increase over time, there is no evidence that blood stored for short periods compared with moderately long periods of time contributes to worse clinical outcomes. However, as newer solutions extend the shelf-life of blood, this may need continued evaluation, particularly in high-risk groups.

Transfusion of human-derived blood products is one of the most common procedures in modern medicine, often proving life-saving. In a recent analysis of electronic medical records from hospitals in the United States, blood transfusion occurred for 12.5% of hospitalized inpatient encounters, with red blood cells (RBCs) being the most commonly transfused component, followed by platelets and plasma.[1] Transfusion is not without risk, and the anesthesiologist must weigh the risks and benefits of providing or withholding transfusion therapy for individual patients in specific clinical settings. This chapter focuses on the physiology and pathology of transfusion medicine with particular attention to the acquisition, processing, storage, indication for, and risk of blood therapy in the perioperative period.

Evolution and Recent History of Blood Transfusion Therapy

THE 1960S

Transfusion medicine has undergone enormous changes in the last 60 years, but the consensus of whether to use whole blood, its components, or both has vacillated every decade or so. In the 1960s, most blood given was in the form of whole blood, whereas fresh frozen plasma (FFP) was available for the treatment of coagulopathies.[2,3]

THE 1970S THROUGH THE 1980S

Transfusion therapy was characterized in this period by "giving the patient only the component of blood that was needed." Component transfusion therapy rather than whole blood transfusion was the standard of care. For example, if the patient was anemic, only packed red blood cells (PRBCs) would be transfused, or if thrombocytopenia existed, only platelet concentrates would be given. Caution regarding administration of blood transfusions increased during this time period in part because of concern regarding the infectivity of blood (e.g., hepatitis and human immunodeficiency virus [HIV]). Furthermore, individual clinical decisions regarding blood transfusions were and continue to be monitored by local hospital transfusion committees (as required by regulatory agencies of various countries including the United States). These committees have the responsibility of monitoring the individual and institutional transfusion practices by evaluating clinical appropriateness of transfusion triggers.[4]

1990S THROUGH THE 2000S

With improved screening techniques for HIV and other blood-borne pathogens during this decade, the incidence of blood transfusion–related infectious disease transmission decreased 10,000-fold. The focus of blood product safety now shifted to *noninfectious serious hazards of transfusion*.[5] These hazards include hemolytic transfusion reactions, transfusion-related acute lung injury (TRALI), and transfusion-associated circulatory overload (TACO), to name a few. With an increased awareness of the potential morbidity and mortality associated with blood product administration, research focused on the concept of liberal versus restrictive blood transfusion strategy. Attention now turned to balancing the threats posed by two independent (yet related) risk factors of patient outcome—anemia and transfusion.

Although the strategy of specific component therapy was still prominent, the concept of reconstituted "whole blood" was introduced during this decade. Led by trauma hospitals and the military, FFP and platelets were transfused along with PRBCs, resulting in a transfusion ratio that was similar to that of whole blood.[6,7] Because the concept of transfusing components that reconstitute whole blood rouses the prior practice of transfusing whole blood, that concept is being reexamined[8] again in the literature and may yet prove beneficial in patients with life-threatening bleeding.[9,10]

2010 TO THE PRESENT

The 2010s saw a shift away from simply correcting anemia and coagulopathy, to a more patient-centered, multipronged approach to transfusion medicine. As a result, the term *patient blood management (PBM)* has become synonymous with modern, evidence-based transfusion medicine.[11] The Society for the Advancement of Blood Management defines PBM as "the timely application of evidence-based medical and surgical concepts designed to maintain hemoglobin concentration, optimize hemostasis and minimize blood loss in an effort to improve patient outcome." [12] PBM recognizes transfusions are but a temporary solution to an often complex, multifactorial process that requires attention to the underlying cause of anemia.[13]

Integration of PBM into clinical pathways has reduced the reliance on allogenic blood product transfusion as the only means to avoid anemia and likely explains the continued decrease in transfusions noted in U.S. hospitals over the last decade.[14] In a recent retrospective analysis, implementation of a PBM system with a reduced transfusion threshold from 8 g/dL to 7 g/dL Hb in orthopedic surgical patients reduced the use of erythrocytes by 32% while improving clinical outcomes. Most notably, patients 65 years and older demonstrated the most improved clinical outcomes, including 30-day readmission rates.[15] Comprehensive PBM programs also can include evaluation of preoperative anemia, clinical decision support, educational efforts, improved surgical techniques, and blood conservation strategies.

PBM in many countries has been facilitated by computerized data systems[16] and supply guidelines.[17] A limitation of most of the PBM publications is that they describe mostly nonbleeding, anemic patients and the decision to initiate transfusion. Very little information addresses what guidelines should be used for repetitive transfusions. The anesthesia provider offers insight into these issues and can provide guidance as to how PBM fits into the perioperative clinical environment.

Blood Procurement

SOURCE OF DONORS

Significant global disparities exist regarding access to "safe" blood, or blood that is properly collected and tested. According to World Bank definitions, low- and middle-income countries collect 53% of all blood donations worldwide, yet represent 81% of the world's population. In addition, the prevalence of transfusion-transmissible infections in blood donations from low- and middle-income countries is significantly higher than those from high-income countries, yet low-income countries have less access to basic quality screening procedures.[18] Another issue, particularly in low-income countries, is incentivized donors. The World Health Organization's (WHO) decision-making body, the World Health Assembly, has issued resolutions and consensus statements that emphasize the need for all member states to develop national blood systems based on voluntary, unpaid donations as a means to ensure a safe, secure, and sufficient supply of blood products.[19] Some experts have suggested that offering economic incentives or rewards to donors should be seriously considered,[20] because limited empirical research exists to support the assumption that incentivized donations, including noncash incentives, either improve recruitment of donors or pose a risk to blood product safety.[21] However, the WHO strongly defends voluntary nonremunerated blood donation as a vehicle to a safer blood supply and increased donor participation.[22]

In the United States, the Food and Drug Administration's (FDA) Center for Biologics Evaluation and Research provides the regulatory oversight for blood banks and donation centers, with most voluntarily obtaining accreditation from the AABB (formerly, American Association of Blood Banks). In Europe, the European Commission sets standards for blood products and their components in the European Blood Directive (Directive 2002/98/EC). These regulatory and professional societies set standards with regard to the donation, collection, testing, processing, storage, and distribution of products.

In the United States, those over the age of 16 and who weigh at least 110 pounds are eligible for screening for potential blood donation. Vital signs are assessed, including temperature, heart rate, and blood pressure. Hb levels are measured, with minimum cutoffs of 13 g/dL for men and 12.5 g/dL for women. Blood is collected either as whole blood and separated by centrifugation or by apheresis, in which only specific components are collected while other components are returned to the donor. An outline of the separation scheme by which various blood components are derived is shown in Fig. 49.1. Apheresis is particularly helpful in donors with blood type AB, as they represent a rare blood type yet serve as the universal plasma donor. As recipients, patients with blood type AB rarely require AB specific blood, as they can be transfused with any type of red cell. Therefore, if plasma is collected from AB donors while

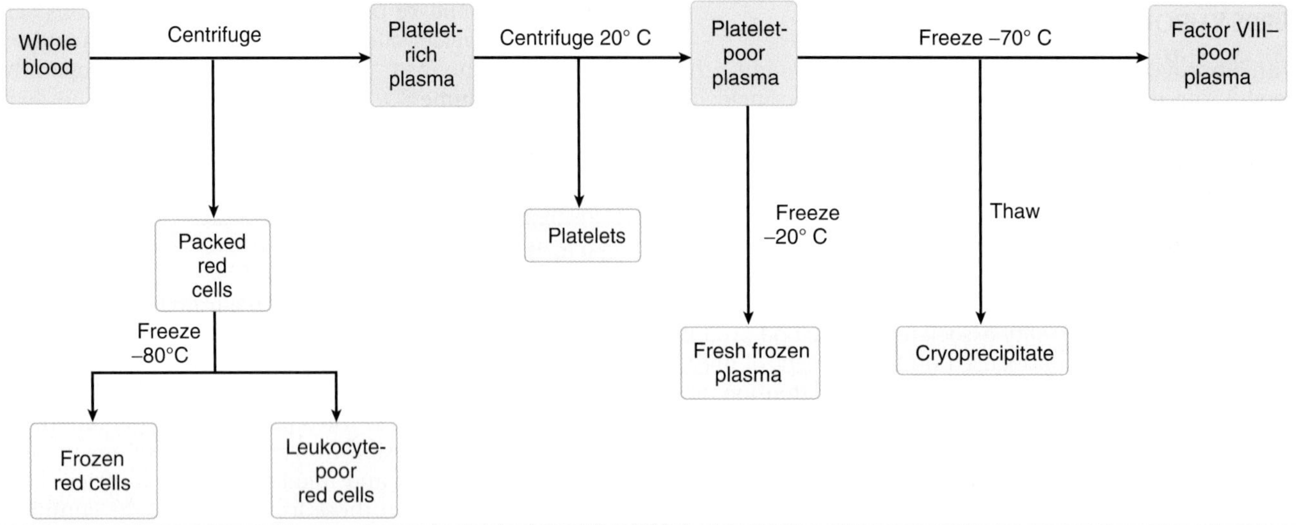

Fig. 49.1 Scheme for separation of whole blood for component therapy.

red cells are immediately returned, this may allow for more frequent plasma donation from this small but vitally important group of donors.

TRANSFUSION-TRANSMISSIBLE INFECTIONS

Donor screening attempts to reduce the risk of a transfusion-transmissible disease and to protect the donor from an adverse reaction due to donation. Deferment based on medical history includes those considered to be in high-risk categories for potential transmission of an infectious agent, including those with a significant travel history, history of injection drug use, recent tattoos, or men who have had sex with men (MSM) in the previous 12 months. The latter deferment category has been controversial in recent years, given the changing epidemiology of the HIV epidemic and improved screening methods. In this population, some advocate for reducing the time interval between potential exposure and donation to 3 months.[23]

The use of more sensitive screening tests in conjunction with changes in transfusion medicine practices have made infectious risks quite rare. The FDA requires blood products to be tested for hepatitis B and C, HIV (types 1 and 2), human T-lymphotropic virus (HTLV; types 1 and 2), and *treponema pallidum* (syphilis), West Nile virus, and Zika virus. Testing is recommended for *Trypanosoma cruzi* (Chagas disease) for first-time donors. Historically, the FDA has published tables on the risks for infectivity, Table 49.1 but because the rates are so infrequent, the last tables published were for data from 2011.

Several blood-safety changes made between the years of 1982 and 2008 have decreased the risk for disease transmission by allogenic blood so that the demand for autologous blood has declined as well. The West Nile virus story illustrates how rapidly our blood banks can respond. In 2002, West Nile virus caused the largest outbreak of arboviral encephalitis ever recorded in the United States (i.e., approximately 4200 patients). Twenty-three cases of transfusion-transmitted infections resulted in seven deaths. In 2003, testing became available that now makes that infection very rare (see Table 49.1). The FDA's response to the 2015 to 2016 Zika virus outbreak was similarly swift—the blood supply was immediately shifted from areas with low risk of infections to areas of known infection; authorization for screening tests was issued within months, and universal screening with a qualitative nucleic acid test (NAT) for the detection of Zika virus ribonucleic acid (RNA) was mandated.[24]

The changes in blood transfusion testing can be appreciated when comparing tests used in 1998 (Box 49.1) with those used in 2018 (Table 49.2. The use of nucleic acid technology has decreased the window of infectivity (i.e., time from being infected to a positive test result), which is a major reason for the decrease in infectivity with hepatitis, HIV, West Nile virus, and Zika virus.

TABLE 49.1 Percentage Risk of Transfusion-Transmitted Infection With a Unit of Screened Blood in the United States

Infection	Risk	Window Period (Days)
Human immunodeficiency virus-1 and -2	1:1,476,000	5-6
Human T-lymphotropic virus (HTLV-II)	1:2,993,000	51
Cytomegalovirus (CMV)	Infrequent with leukocyte-reduced components	
Hepatitis C virus (HCV)	1:1,149,000	3-4
Hepatitis B virus (HBV)	1: 280,000	24
Hepatitis A virus (HAV00)	1:1,000,000	
Bacteria red blood cells	1:1,000 with septic reaction in 1:500,000	
Pheresis platelets (with early aerobic culture)		
Parasites: Babesia and malaria	<1:4,000,000	7-14
West Nile virus (WNV)	1/1,100,000	?
Acute hemolytic transfusion reactions	1:38,000-1:70,000	

Data from AABB: *AABB Technical Manual,* 17th ed. 2011, AABB; and Fiebig ER, Busch MP. Infectious risks of transfusions. In: Spiess BD, Spence RK, Shander A, eds. *Perioperative Transfusion Medicine.* Philadelphia: Lippincott Williams & Wilkins; 2006.

BOX 49.1 Infectious Disease Testing for Blood Transfusions

1. Discontinue serum alanine aminotransferase testing
2. Hepatitis C antibody testing
3. Antibody to hepatitis B core antigen
4. Human immunodeficiency virus (HIV) type 1
5. HIV-2
6. HIV Ag (p24 antigen)
7. Human T-cell lymphotropic virus (HTLV) types 1 and 2
8. Serologic test for syphilis

Modified from National Institutes of Health, Consensus Development Panel on Infectious Disease Testing for Blood Transfusions. Infectious disease testing for blood transfusions. *JAMA.* 1995;274:1374–1379.

TABLE 49.2 Tests Used for Detecting Infectious Agents in All Units of Blood: 2018

Virus	Genetic Testing	Antibody To
Human immunodeficiency virus (HIV)	Nucleic acid technology	HIV-1, HIV-2
Hepatitis C virus (HCV)	Nucleic acid technology	HCV
Hepatitis B virus (HBV)	Nucleic acid technology	Anti-HBc, HBsAg
Human T-cell lymphotropic, virus (HTLV)		HTLV-1, HTLV-2
West Nile virus	Nucleic acid technology	
Zika virus	Nucleic acid technology	

Posttransfusion Hepatitis

When blood transfusions became a reality in the 1940s, viral hepatitis was recognized as a major complication. The concern is primarily with hepatitis B, C, and, rarely, D, which are parenterally transmitted viruses. Before 1985, the overall incidence of posttransfusion hepatitis ranged from a low of 3% to a high of 19%, depending on the institution and the location (e.g., donors from large cities have a more frequent incidence of the hepatitis virus). In most areas, the incidence of hepatitis has ranged from 3% to 10%. Ninety percent of posttransfusion hepatitis is caused by the hepatitis C virus. Fewer than a third of these patients develop jaundice.[25] To determine their ultimate fate, Tong and colleagues[25] monitored 131 patients with chronic posttransfusion hepatitis C for several years and found the following incidence of signs, symptoms, and conditions:

- Fatigue (67%)
- Hepatomegaly (67%)
- Chronic hepatitis (23%)
- Chronic active hepatitis (51%)
- Hepatocellular carcinoma (11%)

It was found that 20 patients had died of the following:

- Complications of cirrhosis (8 patients)
- Hepatocellular carcinoma (11 patients)
- Chronic active hepatitis-pneumonia (1 patient)

Even today, patients with hepatitis C and apparent recovery from the acute infection may go on to develop cirrhosis and hepatocellular carcinoma. Several antiviral therapies, such as Mavyret (glecaprevir-pibrentasvir), Harvoni (ledipasvir-sofosbuvir), Epclusa (sofosbuvir-velpatasvir), and Vosevi (sofosbuvir-velpatasvir-voxilaprevir), now exist that may stop progression and even cure infection from certain genotypes of hepatitis C. However, any person who has ever tested positive for hepatitis B or hepatitis C, at any age, is currently ineligible to donate blood.[26]

Cytomegalovirus

Asymptomatic chronic infection with cytomegalovirus (CMV), a double-stranded DNA virus belonging to the herpesviridae family, is common enough in healthy adults that some view CMV as normal flora. Infection with the CMV virus is limited to humans, requires contact with the body fluids of a previously infected individual, survives best within cells, and persists in its latent form in the monocytes of people with antibody evidence of previous exposure infection. Fortunately, the primary concern is recipients who are at risk because of pregnancy (multiple), immaturity, or immunosuppression. CMV seroconversion usually occurs in subsets of patients receiving multiple transfusions. CMV causes a heterophil antibody-negative response that closely resembles infectious mononucleosis in many respects. An infectious mononucleosis–like syndrome that can occur 1 to 2 months after open-heart surgery is known as the *postperfusion syndrome* or *posttransfusion mononucleosis*.[27] The evidence for transmission of CMV is most convincing when the recipient changes from a seronegative state before transfusion to a seropositive state accompanied by the mononucleosis-like illness several weeks after transfusion.

Transfusion-transmitted CMV can cause significant clinical problems in certain patient populations, such as premature neonates, allograft recipients, and patients post splenectomy.[28] To prevent infection in high-risk populations, use of leukocyte-reduced blood, use of frozen deglycerolized RBCs, and screening for CMV antibody negative donors have been recommended (see the section on leukoreduction and irradiation of blood transfusions). Wilhelm and associates[29] concluded that it is not necessary to provide blood products from CMV-seronegative donors for most patients who receive blood transfusions, because the risk for seroconversion is approximately 0.14% overall, or 0.38% per unit of seropositive donor blood. They do recommend continuing to use CMV-seronegative blood to prevent CMV infection in preterm and newborn infants. Plasma components, such as FFP and cryoprecipitate, and leukoreduced components from seropositive donors are considered to be CMV safe.

Zika Virus

More recently, transfusion-transmissible Zika virus infection has been of concern.[30] Transmitted by mosquitos, Zika virus infection is associated with Guillain-Barre syndrome[31] and microcephaly in newborns whose mothers were infected during pregnancy.[32] Although these manifestations of Zika virus infection are striking, 80% of infected persons are asymptomatic, and thus pose a potential threat to the blood supply. As a result, the FDA issued guidance that all donations collected in the United States be tested for Zika virus using NAT.[33]

TABLE 49.3 Infectious Diseases Theoretically Transmissible by Blood Transfusion for Which No Test Is Available: 2004

Disease	Risk
Malaria	<1 million in the United States
Severe acute respiratory syndrome (SARS)	Unknown
Variant Creutzfeldt-Jakob disease	Three potential cases in the United Kingdom

Other Transfusion-Associated Infectious Diseases

Although many other infectious diseases can theoretically be transmitted by blood transfusion, only a few are of real concern. They include *Yersinia enterocolitica* infection, syphilis, malaria, Chagas disease, variant Creutzfeldt-Jakob disease, parvovirus B19, and severe acute respiratory syndrome (SARS; Table 49.3).

During the late 1980s, Tripple and colleagues[34] described seven cases of fatal transfusion-associated *Y. enterocolitica* sepsis. These investigators also reviewed the literature and found 26 cases of gram-negative bacterial sepsis with whole blood or PRBCs. *Y. enterocolitica* is a bacterium that can cause mostly mild gastrointestinal problems. However, in severe cases, sepsis and death can occur. Unfortunately, storage of blood at 4°C in phosphate buffer enhances its growth.

Fortunately, posttransfusion syphilis is unlikely because the infective agent cannot survive during storage at 1°C to 6°C. Platelet concentrates are the blood component most likely to be implicated because they commonly are stored at room temperature.

Posttransfusion malaria has never been a significant cause of blood recipient morbidity. Nevertheless, malaria can occur, especially if blood donors at risk for harboring parasites are not excluded. Consequently, blood banks thoroughly question donors for history of travel or migration from areas where malaria is endemic.

Even though there are no cases of variant Creutzfeldt-Jakob disease from blood transfusions, the virus can be transmitted by blood in animal models and stringent donor policies based on travel and residence in England or other countries in Europe are in place.

Like malaria, there are other infectious agents that can transmit disease through blood transfusions, but there are no available blood testing methods for these cases (see Table 49.3). Without a specific diagnostic test, screening with restrictive donor criteria is used. For example, in 2003 in the United States, donors with suspected SARS or who traveled to certain countries in Southeast Asia would not be accepted.

BIOCHEMICAL CHANGES IN STORED BLOOD

Units of blood collected from donors are usually separated into components (e.g., RBCs, plasma, cryoprecipitate, and platelets; see Fig. 49.1). Citrate phosphate dextrose adenine-1 (CPDA-1) is an anticoagulant preservative that is used for blood stored at 1°C to 6°C. Citrate prevents clotting by binding Ca^{2+}. Phosphate serves as a buffer, and dextrose is a red cell energy source, allowing the RBCs to continue glycolysis and maintain sufficient concentrations of high-energy nucleotides (adenosine triphosphate [ATP]) to ensure continued metabolism and subsequent viability during storage. The addition of adenine prolongs storage time by increasing the survival of RBCs, allowing them to resynthesize the ATP needed to fuel metabolic reactions. This extends the storage time from 21 to 35 days.[35] Without adenine, RBCs gradually lose their ATP and their ability to survive after transfusion. Finally, storage at 1°C to 6°C assists preservation by reducing the rate of glycolysis approximately 40 times the rate at body temperature.

The shelf life of PRBCs can be extended to 42 days when AS-1 (Adsol), AS-3 (Nutricel), or AS-5 (Optisol) is used.[36,37] Adsol contains adenine, glucose, mannitol, and sodium chloride (NaCl). Nutricel contains glucose, adenine, citrate, phosphate, and NaCl. Optisol contains only dextrose, adenine, NaCl, and mannitol. On a national level, 85% of RBCs are collected in AS-1. In Europe, a solution similar to AS-1 containing saline, adenine, glucose, and mannitol is used. As of 2015, the FDA approved a new additive solution, AS-7, which increases storage time to at least 56 days; however, the solution is not yet commercially available in the United States.[38]

The hematocrit (Hct) of the transfused product depends on the storage method. When CPDA is the anticoagulant used, the Hct is greater than 65%, because most of the plasma is removed, and the resulting volume is approximately 250 mL. When AS-1 is used, most of the plasma is also removed, but 100 mL of storage solution is added, resulting in an Hct of 55% to 60% and volume of 310 mL.[39] The duration of storage is set by U.S. federal regulation and is based on the requirement that at least 70% of the transfused RBCs remain in circulation for 24 hours after infusion.

During storage of whole blood and PRBCs, a series of biochemical reactions occur that alter the biochemical makeup of blood and account for some of the complications. Collectively, these are known as *red cell storage lesions* and may be responsible for the organ injury associated with red cell transfusion. During storage, RBCs metabolize glucose to lactate; hydrogen ions accumulate, and plasma pH decreases, while increases in oxidative damage to lipids and proteins are noted. The storage temperature of 1°C to 6°C inhibits the sodium-potassium pump, resulting in a loss of potassium ion (K^+) from the cells into the plasma and a gain of intracellular sodium.[40] Although K^+ concentrations appear elevated in 35-day stored RBC concentrates, the total plasma volume in the concentrates is only 70 mL, so total K^+ is not markedly elevated. Over time, there are progressive decreases in RBC concentrations of ATP, nitric oxide (NO), and 2,3-diphosphoglycerate (2,3-DPG).

The osmotic fragility of RBCs increases during storage, and some cells undergo lysis, resulting in increased plasma Hb levels. In addition, deformability of RBCs appears impaired in patients who receive allogenic blood cell transfusion, potentially resulting in micro-occlusive events.[41] Frank and associates[42] studied the blood of patients undergoing posterior spinal fusion surgery and found that increased duration of blood storage was associated with decreased RBC deformability, which was not "readily" reversible after transfusion. They speculated that these deformed cells may be defective in delivering oxygen (O_2) to

TABLE 49.4 Properties of Whole Blood and Packed Red Cell Concentrates Stored in CPDA-1

	DAYS OF STORAGE		
Variable	**0**	**35 (Whole Blood)**	**35 (Packed Cells)**
pH	7.55	6.73	6.71
Plasma hemoglobin (mg/dL)	0.50	46.00	246.00
Plasma potassium (mEq/L)	4.20	17.20	76.00
Plasma sodium (mEq/L)	169.00	153.00	122.00
Blood dextrose (mg/dL)	440.00	282.00	84.00
2,3-Diphosphoglycerate (µM/mL)	13.20	1.00	1.00
Percent survival*	—	79.00	71.00

*Percent recovery of O_R-tagged red blood cells at 24 h.
CPDA-1, Citrate phosphate dextrose adenine-1.

the cells and concluded that both the "age of blood storage" and "amount" of blood given should be considered when giving blood (Table 49.4).

CHANGES IN OXYGEN TRANSPORT

RBCs are transfused primarily to increase transport of O_2 to tissues. Theoretically, an increase in the circulating red cell mass will produce an increase in O_2 uptake in the lungs and a corresponding increase in O_2 delivery to tissues, but RBC function may be impaired during preservation, making it difficult for them to release O_2 to the tissues immediately after transfusion.

The O_2 dissociation curve is determined by plotting the partial pressure of O_2 (Po_2) in blood against the percentage of Hb saturated with O_2 (Fig. 49.2). As Hb becomes more saturated, the affinity of Hb for O_2 also increases. This is reflected in the sigmoid shape of the curve, which indicates that a decrease in the arterial partial pressure of oxygen (Pao_2) makes considerably more O_2 available to the tissues. Shifts in the O_2 dissociation curve are quantitated by the P_{50}, which is the partial pressure of O_2 at which Hb is half saturated with O_2 at 37°C and pH 7.4. A low P_{50} indicates a left shift in the O_2-dissociation curve and an increased affinity of Hb for O_2. The left shift of the curve indicates that a lower than normal O_2 tension saturates Hb in the lung, but the subsequent release of O_2 to the tissues is more difficult, as it occurs at a lower than normal capillary O_2 tension compared with an unshifted curve. In other words, the increased affinity of Hb for O_2 makes it more difficult for Hb to release O_2 to hypoxic tissues. This leftward shift is likely a result of decreased levels of 2,3-DPG in stored RBCs, which can remain low for up to 3 days posttransfusion.[43]

Many of the advances in blood processing and storage are centered on the material of the collections and storage containers.[44] Innovative methods of storing blood are being developed. For example, storing blood in an electrostatic field of 500 to 3000 V decreases hemolysis and attenuates the decrease in pH associated with prolonged storage.[45] Current blood collection and storage systems are made of disposable plastic; these materials must have properties compatible with collection, processing, storage, and administration. Polyvinylchloride (PVC) with use of different plasticizers is commonly used because it is nontoxic, has flexibility, mechanical strength, water impermeability, resistance to temperature extremes for sterilization and freezing, compatibility with blood components, and selective permeability for cellular gas exchange.

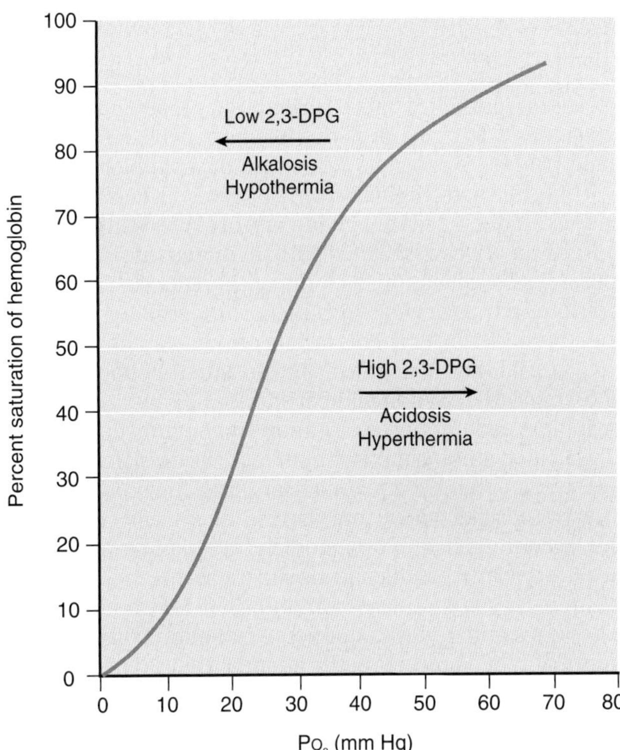

Fig. 49.2 Factors that shift the oxygen dissociation curve. ***2,3-DPG*, 2,3-Diphosphoglycerate.** (From Miller RD. The oxygen dissociation curve and multiple transfusions of ACD blood. In: Howland WS, Schweizer O, eds. *Management of Patients for Radical Cancer Surgery: Clinical Anesthesia Series.* Vol. 9. Philadelphia: FA Davis; 1972:43.)

Recent animal data suggest that red cells in stored blood can be rejuvenated with solutions of inosine prior to administration, reversing storage lesions and mitigating the potential for organ damage. This could be a promising technique to restore ATP and 2,3-DPG levels, while reducing a recipient's immune response and transfusion-associated organ injury.[46] However, small clinical trials in humans demonstrating clinical benefit are lacking.[47] Larger trials are ongoing.

CLINICAL IMPLICATIONS: DURATION OF BLOOD STORAGE

The fact that blood can be stored for 42 days is a mixed blessing. The obvious advantage is the increased availability of blood, but the clinical evidence regarding safety has not been consistent, reflecting the difficulty of conducting a systematic study of patients in varied clinical settings. For decades, many clinicians have tried to establish a firm relationship between the 2,3-DPG levels associated with stored blood and patient outcome. In 1993, Marik and Sibbald[48] found that the administration of blood that had been stored for more than 15 days decreased intramucosal pH, suggesting that splanchnic ischemia had occurred. In addition, an increased incidence of postoperative pneumonia in cardiac patients has been associated with the use of older blood.[49] Yet prolonged storage of blood was not associated with increased morbidity after cardiac surgery.[50] Purdy and colleagues[51] found that patients who received 17-day-old blood (range, 5-35 days) versus 25-day-old blood (range, 9-36 days) had higher survival rates. Koch and colleagues[52] concluded that giving erythrocytes (PRBCs) older than 14 days was associated with an increased risk for postoperative complications, along with reduced short-term and long-term survival in patients undergoing coronary artery bypass surgery. This article also had an accompanying editorial that concluded, "to the extent possible, newer blood might be used in clinical situations that seem to call for it."[53] In addition, a meta-analysis concluded that older stored blood is associated with an increased risk for death.[54]

However, there is equal data arguing the contrary, and other researchers have not arrived at a clear conclusion and recommended more studies. Weiskopf and associates[55] performed studies in healthy volunteers who were evaluated by a standard computerized neuropsychologic test 2 days and 1 week after acute isovolumic anemia was induced. When correcting the anemia, they concluded that erythrocytes stored for 3 weeks are as efficacious as those stored for 3.5 hours. Spahn[4] wrote an accompanying editorial agreeing with Weiskopf and associates[55] and, furthermore, postulated that 2,3-DPG levels may not be the key factor in determining the delivery of O_2 (i.e., 2,3-DPG levels are reduced in older blood, but the blood still delivers O_2). Cata and associates[56] also concluded that no change in outcome occurred in patients undergoing radical prostatectomy and receiving older blood. Saager and colleagues[57] also found no relationship between duration of blood storage and mortality in nearly 7000 patients undergoing noncardiac surgery.

Since the publication of the eighth edition of this text, several randomized control trials evaluating the influence of the duration of blood storage have been published. In 2016, Heddle and colleagues[58] published results from the INFOMR trial, a large, pragmatic, randomized controlled trial enrolling adult hospitalized patients in six centers from four countries. Patients were randomized to receive either blood that had been stored for the shortest duration (mean duration of storage 13 days) versus blood stored for the longest duration (mean duration of storage 23 days). Only patients with A and O blood types were included as the less common blood types could not achieve an appropriate difference in mean duration of storage. More than 20,000 patients were included in the primary analysis. No significant differences in mortality were noted between the two groups. In prespecified high-risk categories, including patients undergoing cardiovascular surgery, patients admitted to the intensive care unit (ICU), and those with cancer, the results remained the same.

Similarly, the results of the recent RECESS trial published in 2015[59] revealed similar mortality rates among those transfused with blood stored less than 10 days (median storage time 7 days) compared with those transfused with blood stored for more than 21 days (median storage time 28 days). Changes in preoperative to 7 days postoperative Multiple Organ Dysfunction Score (MODS) were similar between the two groups, as well. Finally, two randomized controlled trials in critically ill adults evaluating the age of transfused blood on mortality and other outcomes, such as new bloodstream infections, duration of mechanical ventilation, and the use of renal replacement therapy, failed to demonstrate differences between groups transfused with fresher blood compared with those transfused with older blood.[60,61]

These recent randomized controlled trials demonstrate the safety and noninferiority of "older" versus "younger" blood, but the complete answer may still need further data. First, the measures of outcome may be insufficiently sensitive to detect important and meaningful clinical outcomes. Many studies use mortality as their primary outcome measure. Although this is obviously a critical benchmark, it may not be sensitive enough to detect clinical differences regarding the safe or optimal length of time for the storage of blood. Important adverse clinical outcomes could occur without a change in mortality per se (e.g., duration of hospitalization, cardiovascular events, quality of life, neurocognitive decline). Second, these studies compare moderately young with moderately old blood. Ethical and logistical issues preclude a trial comparing "very" young and "very" old blood or even comparing moderately aged blood to very old blood (e.g., stored for 35-42 days).[62-64] Because the quality of blood decreases with length of storage, increased morbidity with exposure to more aged red cells is physiologically plausible, but the debate regarding the effectiveness of a blood transfusion and its duration of storage continues. More prospective studies are likely required.

Blood Component Therapy: Indications for Transfusion

A major advance in the field of blood banking has been the development of blood component therapy. The basic philosophy is that patients are best treated by administration of the specific fraction of blood that they lack. This concept has presented problems to the surgical team, who often desire the physiologic effects of whole blood.

ALLOGENEIC (HOMOLOGOUS) BLOOD

PRBCs contain the same amount of Hb as whole blood, but much of the plasma has been removed. The Hct value of PRBCs is approximately 60% (Table 49.5). Other than severe hemorrhage, most indications for RBCs can be effectively treated with PRBCs, conserving the plasma and the components for other patients (see Fig. 49.1). Many blood banks have conscientiously followed this principle, and whole blood is not available or only available in trauma centers or by special arrangement.

The administration of PRBCs is facilitated by utilizing crystalloid or colloid as a carrier; however, not all crystalloids are suitable. Solutions containing Ca^{2+} may precipitate clotting. Lactated Ringer solution is not recommended for use as a diluent or carrier for PRBCs because of the Ca^{2+} (Table 49.6), although several experimental studies found lactated Ringer solution and normal saline to be equally acceptable.[65,66] A more important factor may be whether the diluent is hypotonic with respect to plasma. In hypotonic solutions, the RBCs will swell and eventually lyse.

TABLE 49.5 Metabolic Characteristics of Packed Red Blood Cells

Value	Packed Red Blood Cells
Hematocrit (%)	57
pH	6.79
pCO_2 (mm Hg)	79
Bicarbonate (mmol/L)	11
Plasma sodium (mmol/L)	126
Plasma potassium (mmol/L)	20.5
Glucose (mmol/L)	24
Lactic acid (mmol/L)	9.4

From Sumplemann R, Schürholz T, Thorns E, et al. Acid-base, electrolyte and metabolite concentration in packed red blood cells for major transfusion in infants. *Paediatr Anaesth*. 2001;11:169–173.

TABLE 49.6 Compatibility of Blood With Intravenous Solutions

	HEMOLYSIS AT 30 MIN	
Blood to Intravenous Solution (1:1 Ratio)	**Room Temperature**	**37°C**
5% Dextrose in water	1+	4+
Plasmanate*	1+	3+
5% Dextrose in 0.2% saline	0	3+
5% Dextrose in 0.45% saline	0	0
5% Dextrose in 0.9% saline	0	0
0.9% Saline	0	0
Normosol-R, pH 7.4†	0	0
Lactated Ringer solution	0 (clotted)	0 (clotted)

*Cutter Laboratories, Berkeley, CA.
†Abbott Laboratories, Chicago, IL.

Solutions that cause hemolysis are listed in Table 49.6. Recommended solutions compatible with packed erythrocytes are 5% dextrose in 0.45% saline, 5% dextrose in 0.9% saline, 0.9% saline, and Normosol-R with a pH of 7.4.

RBC transfusions are given to increase O_2-carrying capacity. Increasing intravascular volume in the absence of significant anemia is not an indication for blood transfusion because volume can be augmented with administration of intravascular fluids that are not derived from human blood (e.g., crystalloids). As such, a sole Hb value should not be the only basis for a transfusion decision. It should be the overall status of the patient that prompts transfusion therapy (e.g., hemodynamics, organ perfusion and oxygen delivery, and anticipated surgical needs).[67] Even so, the Hb value has become the basis for many transfusion strategies. It is the prime criterion for defining restrictive versus liberal transfusion strategies.

When a patient is hemorrhaging, the goals should be to restore and maintain intravascular volume, cardiac output, and organ perfusion to normal levels. By using crystalloids, colloids, or both to treat hypovolemia, normovolemic dilutional anemia may be created. Increasing cardiac output enhances O_2 delivery to the tissues only to a limited extent. In fact, during normovolemic anemia, Mathru and colleagues[68] found inadequate splanchnic and preportal O_2 delivery and consumption when the Hb level decreased to 5.9 g/dL. Although the current PBM emphasis is on fewer or even avoidance of blood transfusions, clearly an Hb value exists below which a blood transfusion should be given.

The basis for using the Hb or Hct value as the initial consideration for defining transfusion requirements followed a 1988 National Institutes of Health (NIH) Consensus Conference that concluded that otherwise healthy patients with Hb value more than 10 g/dL rarely require perioperative blood transfusions, whereas patients with acute anemia with a Hb value of less than 7 g/dL frequently require blood transfusions.[69] They also recognized that patients with chronic anemia (as in renal failure) might tolerate an Hb concentration of less than 6 to 7 g/dL. Amazingly, despite many studies, publications, and debates, the fundamental guidelines have not changed substantially in the 30 plus years since this conference.

An excellent editorial by LeManach and Syed[70] outlines key questions that should be considered regarding transfusion triggers, including what we need to learn and the role of databases. Of prime importance is identifying the variables that predict the need for erythrocyte transfusion and the approach that can most accurately estimate the impact of transfusions. Many studies use death rate as their main indicator. Although clearly an important indicator, there are additional obvious factors in between the extremes of life and death, including vital signs, key laboratory values, and other indicators used in critical care units. Several groups working with patients in ICUs have attempted to define the point at which blood transfusions should be given by measures of tissue oxygenation and hemodynamics (e.g., increase in O_2 consumption in response to added O_2 content).[71-73] The O_2 extraction ratio has been recommended as an indicator for transfusions;[74] however, this technique requires invasive monitoring, and the results were not dramatic between groups who were or were not transfused. No specific measure can consistently predict when a patient will benefit from a blood transfusion. The ultimate determination of the Hb or Hct value at which blood should be given is a clinical judgment based on many factors, such as cardiovascular status, age, anticipated additional blood loss, arterial oxygenation, mixed venous O_2 tension, cardiac output, and intravascular blood volume (Table 49.7).

ADDITIONAL BLOOD TRANSFUSIONS

To determine whether subsequent units of blood are indicated after the initial administration, the overall condition of the patient and the clinical situation need to be reassessed. The following key components of information to consider include:

1. Measurement and trend of vital signs
2. Measurement of blood loss and assessment of anticipated blood loss
3. Quantitation of intravenous fluids given
4. Determination of Hb concentration
5. Surgical concerns.

TABLE 49.7 American College of Surgeons Classes of Acute Hemorrhage

Factors	Class I	Class II	Class III	Class IV
Blood loss (mL)	750	750-1500	1500-2000	2000 or more
Blood loss (% blood volume)	15	15-30	30-40	40 or more
Pulse (beats/min)	100	100	120	140 or higher
Blood pressure	Normal	Normal	Decreased	Decreased
Pulse pressure (mm Hg)	Normal or increased	Decreased	Decreased	Decreased
Capillary refill test	Normal	Positive	Positive	Positive
Respirations per minute	14-20	20-30	30-40	35
Urine output (mL/h)	30	20-30	5-10	Negligible
Central nervous system: mental status	Slightly anxious	Mildly anxious	Anxious, confused	Confused, lethargic
Fluid replacement (3-1 rule)	Crystalloid	Crystalloid	Crystalloid + blood	Crystalloid + blood

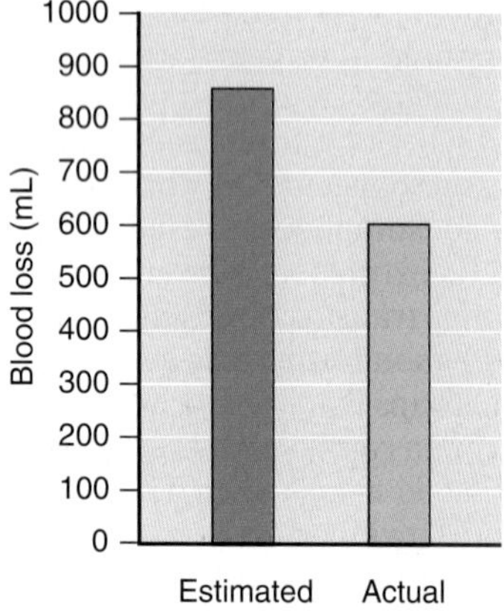

Fig. 49.3 Discrepancy between estimated and actual blood loss. (From Stovener J. Anesthesiologists vastly overstate bleeding. *Anesthesiol News*, May 14, 2012.)

Measurement of Blood Loss

Measuring blood loss is obviously important when assessing the need for both the initial and subsequent blood transfusions (see Table 49.7). A standard approach includes a combination of visualization and gravimetric measurements based on weight differences between dry and blood-soaked gauze pads. A study in patients undergoing spine surgery found that anesthesiologists tended to overestimate blood loss by as much as 40% (Fig. 49.3). On the other hand, optical scanners tended to underestimate blood loss compared with the standard gravimetric calculations.[75] The accuracy of measurements is not uniformly consistent and no "gold standard" for blood loss quantification exists.

Predicting surgical blood loss is also an important component to intraoperative transfusion medicine. As part of the WHO preoperative guidelines to improve the safety of patients undergoing surgery, the anesthesiologist must consider the possibility of a large-volume blood loss prior to the induction of anesthesia.[76] In a prospective trial evaluating both surgeons' and anesthesiologists' ability to predict the estimated blood loss prior to incision, members of both these medical professions underestimated the blood loss by greater than 500 mL in 10% of intermediate or major surgeries, which potentially placed those patients at risk for being without adequate intravenous access or appropriate resuscitative volume.[77]

Determination of Hemoglobin Concentration

While transfusion decisions depend on many clinical factors, the blood Hb value is an important measurement that is fraught with confounding variables. With regard to measurement of blood loss, clinical investigators at Duke University emphasized that "interpretation of intermittent measurements of Hb levels is often complicated by fluid shifts, intravenous volume infusions, and actual transfusions,"[78] yet these values are critical to transfusion decisions.

Continuous blood Hb monitoring has become available on a noninvasive basis using spectrophotometric finger technology (Masimo SpHb, Masimo, Irvine, CA). Numerous studies have been performed in a variety of clinical situations with emphasis on assessment of blood loss and/or the need for transfusions. Although measurements are relatively accurate (i.e., SpHb correlate within 1.0-1.5 g/dL with laboratory Hb measurements), the appearance of inaccurate values is not uncommon.[79,80] SpHb appears to perform worse in patients with moderately to severely low Hb levels or in patients being actively resuscitated.[81,82]

Accuracy also depends on finger blood flow and temperature. The monitor displays a value for perfusion index (PI), which can be helpful in assessing the accuracy of the SpHb value. The accuracy of SpHb can be improved with a PI greater than 4% to 5%. A bupivacaine digital nerve block decreases the number of inaccurate values and increases the number of accurate values for several hours.[83,84] Although not specifically studied, warming the finger should also increase the PI and, therefore, the accuracy of SpHb.

SpHb monitoring can still be valuable even though its accuracy is not consistent. Observation of the trend is often recommended to help clinicians detect a changing Hb level when it is suspected to be stable. For example, Giraud and colleagues[85] concluded that SpHb is less invasive and less accurate than other measurements but provides valuable data on a continuous basis. They then concluded that none of the results would have led to transfusion errors as identified by the American Society of Anesthesiologists (ASA) Task Force on Perioperative Blood Transfusion and Adjuvant Therapies' practice guidelines. If the SpHb value suddenly changes 1 or 2 g/dL, the reasons for this change should be explored, even if the absolute value is satisfactory. For example, if the SpHb reading is 11 g/dL, but rapidly decreases to 9.5 g/dL, the clinical situation needs to be reassessed. Although an attractive concept and possibly accurate, more definitive studies are necessary.[86] SpHb could become very valuable with transfusion decision making in the future.[87]

Invasive point-of-care testing, such as HemoCue (HCue; Hemocue America, Brea, CA), provides a quick and efficient method to accurately determine Hb value. This point-of-care test allows for the determination of Hb levels at the bedside in less than 5 minutes. If the person performing the test is properly trained, HCue measurements are extremely accurate.[80,85] Several other point-of-care Hb tests exist, including RapidLab (Siemens, Malvern, PA) and I-Stat (Abbot Inc, Princeton, NJ). Comparative testing of these three modalities demonstrates favorable intertest reliability.[88]

Preoperative Anemia

Preoperative anemia (i.e., low Hb value in women <12 g/dL; in men <13 g/dL) is a common comorbidity among patients undergoing major surgery with an incidence up to 40% and is an independent risk factor for increased perioperative mortality,[89] and postoperative acute kidney injury (AKI).[90] In patients with a moderate to high risk of significant blood loss (defined as >500 mL), the Hb value ideally should be obtained 3 to 8 weeks prior to surgery.[91] This provides sufficient time for the patient to undergo iron therapy or to correct nutritional deficiencies. Erythropoiesis-stimulating agents, especially intravenously administrated iron therapy, may be beneficial for treatment of preoperative anemia. The concept of treating anemia preoperatively as a means to decrease the need for intraoperative transfusions is widely accepted. For example, intravascular iron therapy in patients undergoing abdominal surgery significantly increased preoperative Hb levels, reduced the need for transfusion, and shortened hospital length of stay.[92] PREVENTT, a large phase III randomized controlled trial investigating preoperative intravenous iron therapy, is ongoing to further characterize this intervention. Oral therapy, if given with sufficient time preoperatively and tolerated by the patient, may be just as effective at correcting the anemia as intravenous therapy.[93]

Erythropoiesis-stimulating agents (ESAs), such as darbepoetin alfa, act by stimulating red cell progenitor cells in the bone marrow and inducing erythropoiesis. They are frequently prescribed for patients with anemia who have end-stage renal disease or who are undergoing chemotherapy treatment to increase their Hb levels and reduce the incidence of transfusion. The evidence has been mixed on the utility and safety of ESAs as a means to increase Hb levels and decrease transfusions in various perioperative patient populations. This may be a result of the heterogeneity of study protocols. A more recent randomized controlled trial in patients undergoing cardiac surgery found a decreased incidence of transfusion in patients with preoperative anemia who were treated with a single dose of erythropoietin administered 2 days prior to surgery.[94] Although no difference in adverse events was noted, the study was underpowered, leaving the question of safety due to the association of ESAs with hypertension and thrombotic events unanswered.[95]

If limited preoperative time is available, Karkouti and associates[96] suggested that prophylactic erythrocyte transfusion should be used to reduce perioperative anemia. This suggestion met with controversy, and many editorials and letters to the editor were written supporting[97] and condemning[98] such an approach. Recent retrospective data suggest that preoperative transfusion, even in severely anemic patients, offers no benefit and may be an independent predictor of complications in some patients.[99]

Liberal Versus Restrictive Transfusion Strategy

The terminology of liberal versus restrictive has become completely indoctrinated into the transfusion therapy vocabulary. Several medical and surgical organizations have provided documents regarding their own definition of liberal and restrictive approaches. Some of these organizations include the American Association of Blood Banks,[100] International Conference on Transfusion Outcomes Group,[6] and Surgical Hip Fracture Repair (FOCUS).[101] In fact, many of these studies were supported by the NIH, which is an indication of how important this topic is for patient care.

Liberal versus restrictive transfusion strategy is based on the Hb value when a transfusion decision is made. A restrictive policy is the administration of blood transfusion when the Hb value is 7 to 8 g/dL or less. In contrast, a liberal policy is the administration of blood transfusion when the Hb value is 9 to 10 g/dL or greater. Many studies have been performed in multiple clinical situations, with varying patient conditions and acuity. The most recent randomized controlled studies continue to show no benefit to a liberal strategy compared with a restrictive strategy. One conclusion is that if no clinical advantages are associated with the liberal transfusion policy, perhaps the restrictive approach should be used. Certainly, fewer transfusion reactions would be expected with the restrictive approach.[101]

How liberal should the transfusion trigger be in critically ill patients? Some critical care physicians have suggested that administration of blood transfusions is related to the incidence of ventilator-assisted pneumonia[102] and nosocomial infections.[103] Although this possibility cannot be excluded, these are complicated outcomes with many confounding variables. Despite the difficulty with identifying a specific transfusion trigger, Ely and Bernard[104] have generally confirmed the conclusions discussed earlier: better outcomes have not consistently occurred with liberal transfusion triggers (i.e., 9.0 to 10.0 g/dL).[105,106] Subsequent editorials have leaned toward a lower transfusion trigger even for critically ill patients.[107,108]

Recent data from prospective, randomized controlled trials in high-risk cardiac surgery patients and critically ill patients with septic shock continue to show the noninferiority of restrictive transfusion thresholds.[109,110] In addition, a meta-analysis of randomized trials of liberal versus restrictive transfusion approaches concluded, "restrictive strategies may decrease the incidence of healthcare-associated infections."[111]

Perhaps a one-value, one-size-fits-all approach to a liberal versus restrictive transfusion strategy is too simplistic of an approach for transfusion decision making. In an editorial, Beattie and Wijeysundera[67] advocated for a more context-specific approach to appropriate transfusion triggers. That is, the transfusion trigger for an otherwise healthy young adult patient should be different than that for an elderly patient with significant cardiovascular comorbidities. The American College of Surgeons attempted to categorize patient characteristics and blood loss as a basis for transfusion decisions (see Table 49.7). Small aggregate data support this theory of customized transfusion thresholds, but the results have yet to be proven in a prospective, randomized trial.[112] Hb values are important, but the overall condition of the patient may be of prime importance.

In addition to a dichotomized one-size-fits-all approach, the liberal versus restrictive strategy associated with PBM has some additional limitations. This strategy primarily addresses the indications for administering an initial unit of blood.[113] Most of this strategy is directed toward anemia in stable patients who are not actively bleeding. It does not describe what the indications for administration of subsequent units of blood should be. The need for repetitive transfusions in a bleeding patient is not addressed in the liberal versus restrictive discussion. Yet it is a very important topic for anesthesia providers. Patients with active bleeding, especially those with cardiovascular disease, should probably be subjected to a more liberal transfusion strategy.[114]

General Conclusions

The emphasis on Hb levels for transfusion decisions needs some caution. There can be variability from one patient to another regarding the need for increased O_2-carrying capacity via blood transfusions. Also, an individual patient's Hb level may vary markedly in the perioperative period independent of and in addition to transfusions of RBCs. During acute bleeding, Hb values are only slightly decreased initially because the intravascular volume has not been repleted and the Hb level has not been diluted.[114] The development of more sensitive indicators of tissue oxygenation (e.g., intramucosal pH) may provide indicators for transfusion in the future. As concluded by Weiskopf,[115] "we merely await advances in technology that will enable us to measure directly the value of concern and thereby free us from arguments over which surrogate (e.g., hemoglobin) to measure and what value indicates the need for augmented oxygen delivery." Although Weiskopf wrote this opinion in 1998, surrogate indicators are still used for transfusion decisions today.

In the presence of incomplete data, the ASA's 2015 updated practice guidelines offer these recommendations:[116]

1. Transfusion is rarely indicated when the Hb concentration is more than 10 g/dL and is almost always indicated when it is less than 6 g/dL, especially when the anemia is acute.
2. A restrictive transfusion strategy (Hb <8 g/dL) should be employed to reduce the patient's transfusion requirements and decrease the potential harmful effects of transfusions.
3. Multimodal protocols and algorithms should be employed to reduce intraoperative blood loss and transfusion requirements. These pathways include point-of-care testing to direct care.
4. The use of a single Hb trigger for all patients and other approaches that fail to consider all important physiologic and surgical factors affecting oxygenation is not recommended.
5. When appropriate, intraoperative and postoperative blood recovery, acute normovolemic hemodilution (ANH), and measures to decrease blood loss (i.e., deliberate hypotension and pharmacologic drugs) may be beneficial.

PLATELET CONCENTRATES

Platelet concentrates are obtained either as pooled concentrates from 4 to 6 whole-blood donations or as apheresis concentrates obtained from one donor.[117] If platelets are stored at room temperature, they can be used up to 7 days after collection with constant and gentle agitation. Bacterial contamination, mainly from platelet concentrates, is the third leading cause of transfusion-related deaths (Table 49.8), although the incident rate has steadily declined over the last 15 years.[118] In a report of 10 contaminated platelet transfusions between 1982 and 1985, half were platelets stored for 5 days or more. A prospective analysis from 1987 to 1990 resulted in seven cases of sepsis in patients receiving platelets for thrombocytopenia secondary to bone marrow failure.[119] Because the use of multidonor platelet products stored for 5 days results in an incidence of sepsis five times higher than use of those stored for 4 days, shorter storage times are being emphasized. In studies that actively survey transfused platelets,[120] a rate of bacterial contamination has been identified of approximately 1 per 2500 units (Table 49.9). Twenty-five percent of the patients exposed to contaminated platelet products developed a septic transfusion reaction, although these cases were only identified by active surveillance. Prior to this study, septic transfusion reactions associated with platelet transfusions were reported at a rate of 1 per 100,000 transfused platelets, suggesting this is likely an underreported event.[121]

TABLE 49.8 Transfusion-Related Fatalities in the United States, 2012 Through 2016

Complication	FY 2012-2015 (Number)	FY 2012-2015 (Percent)	FY 2016 (Number)	FY 2016 (Percent)
Anaphylaxis	6	4	5	12
Contamination	14	10	5	12
HTR (ABO)	10	7	4	9
HTR (non-ABO)	18	13	1	2
Hypotensive Reaction	2	1	1	2
TACO	37	26	19	44
TRALI	56	39	8	19

TACO, Transfusion-associated circulatory overload; *TRALI*, transfusion-related acute lung injury.
From Fatalities reported to FDA following blood collection and transfusion: annual summary for fiscal year 2016. These reports are available online at https://www.fda.gov/media/111226/download

TABLE 49.9 History of Platelet Concentrates Shelf Life in Relationship to Key Events

Year	Shelf Life	Practical Shelf Life*
1984-1986	7 days	6-7 days†
1986-1999	5 days	3 days‡
1999-2004	5 days	3 days§
2004-present	5 days	2.5-3 days

*Days that platelet concentrates are actually available to clinicians.
†Reports of bacterial contamination.
‡Nucleic acid technology testing, centralized blood donor testing.
§Bacterial detection implemented.

At present, platelet concentrates are routinely tested for bacteria and are the only blood product stored at room temperature.[122] For any patient who develops a fever within 6 hours after receiving platelets, sepsis from platelets should be considered.

Indications for the use of platelets are somewhat difficult to define. The most recent guidelines published in 2015 by the ASA Task Force on Perioperative Blood Management[116] provide the following recommendations regarding management for platelet transfusions:

1. Monitor platelet count, except in situations of massive transfusion.
2. Monitor platelet function, if available.
3. Consider use of desmopressin in patients with excessive bleeding or suspected platelet dysfunction.
4. Platelet transfusion may be indicated despite an adequate platelet count if there is known or suspected platelet dysfunction (e.g., cardiopulmonary bypass, bleeding, recent use of antiplatelet therapy, congenital platelet dysfunction).
5. Prophylactic platelet transfusion is rarely indicated in surgical or obstetric patients when the platelet count is greater than 100 × 10^9/L and is usually indicated when the platelet count is less than 50 × 10^9/L. The determination of whether patients with intermediate platelet counts (50-100 × 10^9/L) require therapy should be based on the patient's risk for bleeding.

Many institutions have strict thresholds targeted to the patient's condition that outline the minimum platelet count needed for the categories of (1) prophylaxis, (2) periprocedural (based on type of procedure), and (3) active bleeding. In the first category, a required platelet count may be 10 × 10^9/L in patients receiving chemotherapy.[123] In the second category, patients undergoing bone marrow biopsy or lumbar puncture should have platelet counts between 20 and 30 × 10^9/L. For neurosurgery, a platelet count of 100 × 10^9/L may be targeted. Such thresholds are often guided by professional societies. The American Society of Regional Anesthesia and Pain Medicine guidelines also include recommendations in the setting of therapy that may alter platelet function.[124] A clinician's institution will likely have precise platelet recommendations for most procedures.

Patients with severe thrombocytopenia (<20 × 10^9/L) and clinical signs of bleeding usually require platelet transfusion. However, patients may have very low platelet counts (much lower than 20 × 10^9/L) and not have clinical bleeding. These patients probably do not need platelet transfusions (Table 49.10). The recent PATCH trial evaluated patients receiving antiplatelet therapy who presented with intracerebral hemorrhage (ICH).[125] Such patients often receive platelet transfusions due to concern about the irreversible inhibition of platelet function and the high risk of morbidity and mortality associated with ICH. Study participants were excluded if their Glasgow Coma Scale score was less than 8 or if their treatment plan included expected surgical intervention within the first 24 hours of presentation. Platelet transfusion increased the risk of death or dependence at 3 months and the risk of a serious adverse event during the hospital stay compared with standard medical therapy without transfusion. Although this study excluded patients who were deemed surgical candidates at presentation, even in this high-risk patient population, platelet transfusions are not indicated unless there is active bleeding.

TABLE 49.10 Correlation Between Platelet Count and Incidence of Bleeding

Platelet Count (cells/mm³)	Total No. Patients	No. Patients With Bleeding
>100,000	21	0
75,000-100,000	14	3
50,000-75,000	11	7
<50,000	5	5

Data from Miller RD, Robbins TO, Tong MJ, et al. Coagulation defects associated with massive blood transfusions. *Ann Surg*. 1971;174:794.

When possible, ABO-compatible platelets should be used. The need to use them, however, is not well documented, and specific testing is difficult. Aggregation cannot be used for matching, because platelets cause clumping. The platelet membrane has immunoglobulins, and any additional deposit of recipient antibodies is difficult to detect. Despite the fact that platelets can be destroyed by antibodies directed against class I human leukocyte antigen (HLA) proteins on their membranes and by antibodies against ABO antigens, platelets will continue to be chosen without regard to antigen systems for the majority of patients.[126] ABO-incompatible platelets produce very adequate hemostasis.

The effectiveness of platelet transfusions is difficult to monitor. Under ideal circumstances, one platelet concentrate usually produces an increase of approximately 7 to 10 × 10^9/L at 1 hour after transfusion in the 70-kg adult. Ten units of platelet concentrates are required to increase the platelet count by 100 × 10^9/L. However, many factors, including splenomegaly, previous sensitization, fever, sepsis, and active bleeding, may lead to decreased survival and decreased recovery of transfused platelets.

Other various different types of platelet concentrates have been proposed, including leukocyte-depleted platelets and ultraviolet–irradiated platelets. The use of these products is reviewed by Kruskall.[127]

FRESH FROZEN PLASMA

FFP is the most frequently used plasma product. It is processed shortly after donation, generally frozen within 8 hours or 24 hours (PF24). It contains all the plasma proteins, particularly factors V and VIII, which gradually decline during the storage of blood. PF24 is comparable to FFP, except for a slight reduction in factor V and approximately 25% decrease in factor VIII.[128,129] Thawed plasma is stored at 1 °C to 6 °C for up to 5 days. The use of FFP carries with it the same inherent risks that are observed with the use of any blood product, such as sensitization to foreign proteins.

Although FFP is a reliable solution for intravascular volume replacement in cases of acute blood loss, alternative therapies are equally satisfactory and considerably safer. The risks of FFP administration include TRALI, TACO, and allergic or anaphylactic reactions.

In 2015 the ASA Task Force recommended the following guidelines regarding the administration of FFP:

1. Prior to the administration of FFP, coagulation studies should be obtained when feasible.
2. For the correction of coagulopathy when the international normalized ratio (INR) is greater than 2, in the absence of heparin.
3. For the correction of coagulopathy due to coagulation deficiencies in patients transfused with more than one blood volume (approximately 70 mL/kg) when coagulation studies cannot be easily or quickly obtained.
4. Replacement of known coagulation factor deficiencies with associated bleeding, disseminated intravascular coagulation (DIC), or both, when specific components are not available.
5. Reversal of warfarin anticoagulation when severe bleeding is present and prothrombin complex concentrations are not available.

FFP or plasma is often given to critical care patients before insertion of an intravascular catheter. Hall and associates[130] studied 1923 patients admitted to 29 ICUs in the United Kingdom who underwent intravascular catheterization. They compared patients who did and did not receive FFP. Chronic liver disease and more abnormal coagulation tests increased the frequency of patients receiving FFP, but the severity of the prothrombin time (PT) alone was not a factor. Whether prophylactic FFP should be given in this situation is not well defined. In 2015, Muller and associates[131] published results from a randomized, open-label trial of prophylactic FFP use prior to an invasive procedure in critically ill patients with an INR of 1.5 to 3. The trial ended before reaching target enrollment, because of slow recruitment. The occurrence of bleeding did not differ between the two groups, but the trial may not have had enough power to distinguish a statistical significance between groups. Also, an INR reduction below 1.5 only occurred in 54% of patients in the intervention group.

In an effort to "expedite" the availability of plasma for patients who require massive transfusions, some trauma centers keep thawed plasma readily available. In one study, patients with severe trauma who had already received 1 unit of RBCs and plasma were then divided into two groups, one of which immediately received 4 units of thawed plasma. The patients who received the plasma had a reduction in overall blood product use and 30-day mortality.[132] More recently, Sperry and colleagues[133] randomized prehospital injured patients in flight transport who were at risk for hemorrhage to standard of care versus empiric administration of 2 units FFP. By 3 hours, Kaplan-Meier curves revealed early separation of the two groups, favoring empiric administration of FFP in the prehospital setting that persisted until their prespecified end point of 30 days following randomization.

CRYOPRECIPITATE

Cryoprecipitate is prepared when FFP is thawed, and the precipitate is reconstituted. The product contains factor VIII:C (i.e., procoagulant activity), factor VIII:vWF (i.e., von Willebrand factor), fibrinogen, factor XIII, and fibronectin, which is a glycoprotein that may play a role in reticuloendothelial clearance of foreign particles and bacteria from the blood. All other plasma proteins are present in only trace amounts in cryoprecipitate.

Cryoprecipitate is frequently administered as ABO compatible; however, this probably is not very important because the concentration of antibodies in cryoprecipitate is extremely low. Cryoprecipitate may contain RBC fragments, and cryoprecipitate prepared from Rh-positive donors can possibly sensitize Rh-negative recipients to the Rh antigen. Cryoprecipitate should be administered through a filter and as rapidly as possible. The rate of administration should be at least 200 mL/h, and the infusion should be completed within 6 hours of thawing.

According to the 2015 ASA Task Force on Perioperative Blood Management,[116] transfusion of cryoprecipitate is rarely indicated when the fibrinogen levels are greater than 150 mg/dL in nonobstetric patients. The following indications were provided regarding the administration of cryoprecipitate:

1. When testing of fibrinogen activity reveals evidence for fibrinolysis
2. When fibrinogen concentrations are less than 80 to 100 mg/dL in patients experiencing excessive bleeding
3. Obstetrical patients who are experiencing excessive bleeding despite a measured fibrinogen concentration greater than 150 mg/dL
4. In patients undergoing massive transfusion when the timely assessment of fibrinogen concentrations cannot be determined
5. In patients with congenital fibrinogen deficiencies and when possible, in consultation with the patient's hematologist
6. In bleeding patients with von Willebrand disease types 1 and 2A who fail to respond to desmopressin or vWF/FVIII concentrates (or if not available)
7. In bleeding patients with von Willebrand disease types 2B, 2M, 2N, and 3 who fail to respond to vWF/FVIII concentrates (or if concentrates are not available)

Fibrin glue may be used by surgeons to create local hemostasis. It is prepared in a manner similar to that of cryoprecipitate. With added thrombin, it is applied locally to the surgical site. The efficacy of this product has been difficult to demonstrate in clinical trials.

MASSIVE TRANSFUSION AND TRANSFUSION RATIOS

The transition from administration of whole blood to component therapy in the 1970s created new challenges in transfusion medicine, especially in patients undergoing trauma or any type of surgery associated with significant blood loss. FFP was not usually required as a separate component with the administration of whole blood, and significant thrombocytopenia usually occurred only after 15 to 20 units of blood.[5] With the change from whole blood to PRBCs, the incidence of coagulopathies increased, especially in units responsible for trauma patients. Rather than basing transfusion decisions on clinical judgment or laboratory tests, the concept of developing ratios of FFP and/or platelet concentrates with PRBCs evolved. For example, a 1:1:1 ratio would be transfusion of 1 unit of plasma, and one-sixth unit of platelets to 1 unit of RBCs. A 1:1:2 ratio would be transfusion of 1 unit of plasma, and one-sixth unit of platelets to every 2 units of RBCs. The convention of one-sixth unit of platelets results from the common allocation of platelet products in 1 unit (apheresis) from a single donor or 1 pool (pooled) from six donors in a "six pack." In review of the literature, ratios may be expressed as plasma/platelets/RBCs or RBCs/plasma/platelets.

Holcomb and associates[134] concluded that increased platelet ratios were associated with improved survival after massive blood transfusions. Subsequently, Kornblith and associates[135] concluded that the laboratory clotting profile of 1:1:1 plasma/platelets/RBC was significantly more hemostatic when examining activity of factors II, V, VII, VIII, IX, and X; antithrombin III, as well as protein C and higher fibrinogen levels when compared with a 1:1:2 ratio. Results of the Prospective Observational Multicenter Major Trauma Transfusion (PROMMTT) study supported this idea. With data from 10 U.S. level-I trauma centers, the conclusion of the study[136] was that higher plasma and platelet ratios early in resuscitation were associated with decreased mortality in patients who received transfusions of at least 3 units of blood products during the first 24 hours after admission.[136] Among survivors at 24 hours, the subsequent risk for death by day 30 was not associated with plasma or platelet ratios. When comparing groups of patients with similar Injury Severity Scores, only a survival benefit was seen in ratios with high plasma to RBC resuscitation. However, no additional morbidity benefit of 1:1 over 1:2 ratios was identified.[137]

More recently in the randomized control trial Pragmatic Randomized Optimal Platelet and Plasma Ratios (PROPPR) study, Holcomb and associates[138] found that among patients with severe trauma and major bleeding, early administration of plasma, platelets, and red blood cells in a 1:1:1 ratio versus a 1:1:2 ratio did not result in significant differences in mortality at 24 hours or at 30 days.

These aggressive uses of FFP, platelets, and other blood products have only been shown to be beneficial in response to coagulopathies from massive blood transfusions. Aggressive plasma administration to other transfused patients was associated with an increased rate of serious complications, including acute respiratory distress syndrome (ARDS) and organ dysfunction.[126] A retrospective study showed that a higher FFP-PRBC ratio was associated with the need for advanced interventional procedures in patients with postpartum hemorrhage.[139]

Synthetic Oxygen-Carrying Substances

HB-BASED OXYGEN CARRIERS

Various other substances that carry or facilitate the transport of O_2 have been made. Oxygen therapeutics are labeled as Hb-based O_2 carriers (HBOCs). HBOCs have advantages over human blood of not requiring type and crossmatch and not transmitting infectious viruses, typical characteristics of most synthetic blood products (Table 49.11).

Two approaches have dominated attempts to develop synthetic blood. The first approach uses linear binding kinetics, unlike the nonlinear binding of Hb. The most notable is the perfluorochemical emulsion called Fluosol-DA. Fluosol-DA was initially approved by the FDA for perfusion of ischemic tissues in the setting of percutaneous coronary intervention.[140] However, it had little use because it carried O_2 only when the PaO_2 was more than 300 mm Hg.[141] Fluosol was withdrawn from the market in 1994. Another perfluoro compound, perfluorooctyl bromide, carries three to four times more O_2, has a longer half-life, and presumably fewer problems than are associated with Fluosol-DA, but it is not available on the market.[142]

TABLE 49.11 Comparison of General Synthetic Blood With Allogeneic Blood

Parameter	Synthetic	Allogeneic
Oxygen delivery	Rapid and consistent	Dependent on 2,3-DPG
Risk for disease transmission	None	See Table 49.2
Storage	Room temperature	Refrigeration
	Stable efficacy	Loss of efficacy
Shelf life	1-3 year	42 days
Preparation	Ready to use	Crossmatch
Compatibility	Universal	Type specific
Duration of action	1-3 days	60-90 days

2,3-DPG, 2,3-Diphosphoglycerate.

Most HBOCs modify the Hb molecule from humans, animals, or recombinant technology. Original efforts required Hb to be stroma free to prevent nephrotoxicity. The stroma-free Hb needed to be modified to have a favorable O_2 affinity (i.e., decreased O_2 affinity/right shift in the O_2 dissociation curve) and to extend its relatively short intravascular half-life. A variety of approaches have been used, including crosslinking, pyridoxylation and polymerization, and conjugation and encapsulation to accomplish this. Stroma-free Hb causes severe arteriolar vasoconstriction of microvascular structures from NO scavenging, which is not beneficial for organ perfusion. A human recombinant hemoglobin (rHb 1.1) was made in *Escherichia coli* and functions as normal Hb in terms of O_2-carrying capacity, but it, too, was plagued by microvascular vasoconstriction. Although a subsequent iteration, rHbg 2.0, minimized NO scavenging and caused little arteriolar vasoconstriction when compared with rHb 1.1 and diaspirin crosslinked Hb,[143,144] vasoconstriction may still prove to be their ultimate downfall.

Most clinical trials have shown increased use of allogeneic blood transfusions;[145] however, the outcome of the HBOCs have been similar: failure in clinical trials due to increased adverse events. Natanson and colleagues[146] performed a cumulative meta-analysis on 16 trials involving 5 different products and 3711 patients. They concluded that there was a significant increased risk for myocardial infarction and death when HBOCs were given, an outcome that was found among all the technologies (e.g., cross-linked, polymerized, or conjugated). An accompanying editorial concluded that a 30% increased risk for death and a threefold increase in the risk for myocardial infarction should preclude any additional studies.[147]

Several HBOCs are available clinically under the FDA's Expanded Access (compassionate use) program. HBOC-201 hemoglobin glutamer-250 (bovine), Hemopure (Biopure Corporation) is developed from ultrapurified bovine RBCs that have been glutaraldehyde polymerized. It has a higher P_{50} (i.e., 43 instead of 26 mm Hg), which means that it may deliver O_2 to the tissues at least as well, if not better, than human RBCs.[148] A recent case series reported three cases of HBOC–201, under the FDA's Expanded Access to patients in severe sickle cell crisis (SCC) with multiorgan failure, who refused RBCs (Jehovah's Witnesses) or for whom compatible RBCs were not available.[149] A recent case report described use of bovine pegylated carboxyhemoglobin (Sanguinate) in a Jehovah's Witness with a lymphoproliferative disorder, gastrointestinal bleeding, and resultant severe anemia who was bridged to hemostatic interventions.[150] For now, HBOCs are likely to be reserved for situations in which RBC transfusion is not an option or as a bridge to stabilizing therapy.

Autologous Blood

Autologous blood transfusion constitutes three distinct procedures (1) preoperative autologous donation (PAD), (2) acute normovolemic hemodilution (ANH), and (3) intraoperative and postoperative blood salvage. Although the advantages and disadvantages vary with each technique, autologous transfusion aims to decrease the incidence and severity of complications associated with allogenic transfusions and conserve the supply of banked blood. Autologous blood may also be an acceptable solution in patients with rare blood phenotypes or alloantibodies.[151]

PREOPERATIVE AUTOLOGOUS DONATION

It is assumed that preoperative autologous blood transfusion is safer than allogeneic blood, mainly because of the decreased risk for transfusion-transmissible infections, such as HIV and hepatitis C. However, as blood safety has improved with a marked decrease in infectivity from allogeneic blood, the difference in safety compared with autologous blood is much less. Not surprisingly, the proportion of autologous blood collected has significantly decreased since the peak in the mid-1990s.[152]

To be eligible, the AABB requires that most donor's Hb be no less than 11 g/dL prior to donation. Repeated donations should be separated by a week with 72 hours between the last donation and the time of surgery. The latter recommendation is to ensure restoration of intravascular volume and appropriate testing and preparation of the donated blood.[153] At 72 hours postdonation, while intravascular volume may be restored, red cell mass is not. According to the Hemoglobin and Iron Recovery Study (HEIRS), recovery of 80% red cell mass varies from 25 to more than 168 days.[154] On average, for those who undergo PAD, Hb is 1.1 g/dL less than those who do not donate preoperatively. In a meta-analysis incorporating data from multiple surgical patient populations, while PAD decreased the absolute risk of receiving allogenic blood by 44%, the risk of receiving a transfusion from any source (i.e., allogenic or PAD), increased by 24%, which questions the procedure's use as a transfusion-sparing practice.[155]

BOX 49.2 Contradictions to Participation in Autologous Blood Donation Programs

1. Evidence of infection and risk of bacteremia
2. Scheduled surgery to correct aortic stenosis
3. Unstable angina
4. Active seizure disorder
5. Myocardial infarction or cerebrovascular accident within 6 months of donation
6. High-grade left main coronary artery disease
7. Cyanotic heart disease
8. Uncontrolled hypertension

Donation itself is not without risk. In a study of American Red Cross donors, PAD was associated with nearly 12 times the postdonation hospitalization rate as allogenic donors.[156] The criteria for autologous donation are less stringent than those for allogenic donors, as historically 15% of autologous donors do not meet safety criteria for allogenic donation.[157] As such, certain patient populations are poor candidates for PAD because of their underlying comorbidities. These populations include patients with severe cardiopulmonary disease (e.g., severe aortic stenosis, recent myocardial infarction, or cerebrovascular event) and those with bacteremia (Box 49.2).

ACUTE NORMOVOLEMIC HEMODILUTION

ANH is a procedure initiated before the start of significant blood loss, by which the anesthesiologist removes whole blood from a patient while simultaneously restoring intravascular volume with either crystalloid (3 mL/1 mL of blood removed) or colloid (1 mL/1 mL of blood removed) solutions to maintain adequate hemodynamics. Blood is collected in standard blood bags containing citrate anticoagulant and maintained at room temperature in the operating room for up to 8 hours or at 4°C for 24 hours. Bleeding that occurs following ANH sheds a lower percentage of RBCs per unit of total blood volume lost, constituting the presumed major benefit of this procedure.[158]

When major bleeding has stopped or when clinically appropriate, the sequestered blood is then reinfused into the patient in the reverse order of collection because the first unit collected has the highest concentration of coagulation factors and platelets and the highest Hb level.[159] Although some providers advocate that stored blood be gently agitated to preserve platelet function, most practitioners do not do this, and no formal recommendations exist requiring this procedure. Reassuringly, no differences in thromboelastography (TEG) measurements have been noted between samples agitated during storage compared with those left stationary.[160]

The amount of blood saved by ANH is both of a function of the postdilutional Hb achieved and the amount of blood volume lost intraoperatively, the latter hopefully occurring after the blood salvage. Patients undergoing minimal ANH—less than 15% of a patient's blood volume—would only save 100 mL of RBCs, equaling 0.5 units of PRBCs. However, increasing the ANH to target postdilutional Hct of 28% in the setting of 2600 mL blood loss resulted in savings of 215 mL of RBC compared with blood loss without prior hemodilution (Fig. 49.4).[161]

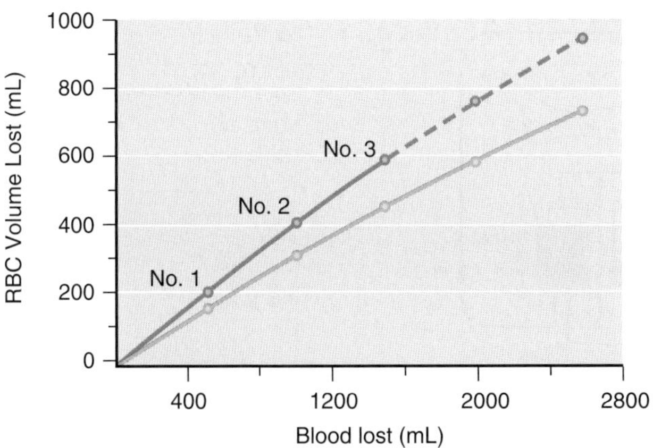

Fig. 49.4 The relationship between whole blood volume *(mL)* lost (abscissa) and red blood cell *(RBC)* volume lost *(ordinate)* in a 100-kg patient undergoing hemodilution: RBC volume lost with 2800 mL whole blood intraoperatively after hemodilution of 1500 mL whole blood *(solid blue line)*; RBC volume lost with 2800 mL whole blood lost during hemodilution at each of three 500 mL volumes *(solid orange line)*; cumulative RBC volume lost intraoperatively, derived for 2800 mL whole blood lost if hemodilution had not been performed *(blue dashed line)*. A net of 215 mL reduction in RBC volume lost with hemodilution is illustrated by the divergence of the two curves. (From Goodnough LT, Grishaber JE, Monk TG, et al. Acute preoperative hemodilution in patients undergoing radical prostatectomy: a case study analysis of efficacy. *Anesth Analg*. 1994;78:932–937, with permission.)

Although larger volumes of hemodilution provide the largest benefit in terms of RBC mass saved and allogenic transfusions avoided,[162] retrospective data suggest that even mild ANH may help to improve outcomes.[163] Prospective, randomized trials demonstrate ANH as a means to decrease transfusion requirements in multiple types of surgeries, including hip replacement,[164] hepatic resection,[165] and vascular surgery.[166] A recent meta-analysis evaluated 29 randomized controlled trials involving 1252 patients undergoing ANH (and 1187 controls) during cardiac surgery.[167] They found patients who underwent ANH were transfused less frequently than those in the control groups, receiving on average three-fourths fewer allogenic blood units than those in the control groups. Not surprisingly, patients undergoing ANH experienced less postoperative blood cell mass loss with a mean loss of 388 mL in the ANH groups and 450 mL in the control groups. Another meta-analysis demonstrated similar findings in a broader patient population that included multiple surgical specialties, but the findings were criticized due to the heterogeneity of the studies included and the potential for publication bias, which would likely overestimate any true benefit.[168] ANH has also been shown to decrease the need for other component therapy, because the removal of whole blood also removes and stores platelets and plasma.[162] In cardiac surgery specifically, ANH may protect the sequestered blood from the effects of cardiopulmonary bypass and the platelet dysfunction that occurs.[169]

Decisions regarding the use of ANH should be made with consideration given to the patient's vital signs, Hct, blood volume, and the estimation of surgical blood loss and risk of transfusion (Box 49.3). ANH is not without potential risk. A recent study in porcine animal models demonstrated significant adverse effects of ANH transfusions particularly in the adult compared with infant animal models. These effects included the development of bronchoconstriction and acute lung injury as a result of extravasation of fluid and deterioration of cardiopulmonary hemodynamics.[170] Similarly, in dog models, ANH to a Hct of 30% demonstrated decreased oxygen delivery to the kidneys with preserved delivery to other organs, including the heart, brain, and spinal cord, suggesting ANH may place the kidneys at risk.[171] Most studies evaluating ANH have focused on a reduction in RBC mass loss and the use of allogenic blood cell transfusions as the primary outcomes. Fewer studies have reported favorable findings with respect to end-organ damage in patients treated with ANH compared with those not treated, but studies in the future should look more closely at these important outcomes.[162]

BOX 49.3 Criteria for Selection of Patients for Acute Normovolemic Hemodilution

1. Likelihood of transfusion exceeding 10% (i.e., blood requested for crossmatch according to a maximum surgical blood order schedule)
2. Preoperative Hb of at least 12 g/dL
3. Absence of clinically significant coronary, pulmonary, renal, or liver disease
4. Absence of severe hypertension
5. Absence of infection and risk of bacteremia

INTRAOPERATIVE CELL SALVAGE

The term *intraoperative blood collection* or *cell salvage* describes the technique of collecting, processing, and reinfusing blood lost by a patient during surgery. It is a perioperative blood conservation technique to reduce use of allogenic blood and the risks associated with allogeneic blood exposure. It may be acceptable for use in patients that do not consent to allogeneic or preoperative autologous blood transfusions, such as Jehovah's Witnesses. This technique should be discussed with such patients and acceptability should be determined on a case-by-case basis.[172]

The AABB continues to recommend the following general indications for cell salvage use in their 2016 guidelines:[173]

1. Anticipated blood loss is 20% or more than the patient's estimated blood volume.
2. Crossmatch-compatible blood is unobtainable.
3. Patient is unwilling to accept allogeneic blood but will consent to receive blood from intraoperative blood salvage.
4. The procedure is likely to require more than one unit of RBCs.

Cell salvage involves the collection of blood from the surgical field through a specialized double-lumen suction tubing that delivers anticoagulant, commonly heparin or citrate, to the tip of the suction catheter (Fig. 49.5). This prevents suctioned blood from clotting within the collection system. Blood from the surgical field is collected in a reservoir until enough fluid accumulates for processing. Processing involves specialized centrifugation that causes the lower density plasma and anticoagulant fluid to rise up and separate from the higher density RBCs, which are collected at the bottom of a conical- or cylindrical-shaped bowl. In general,

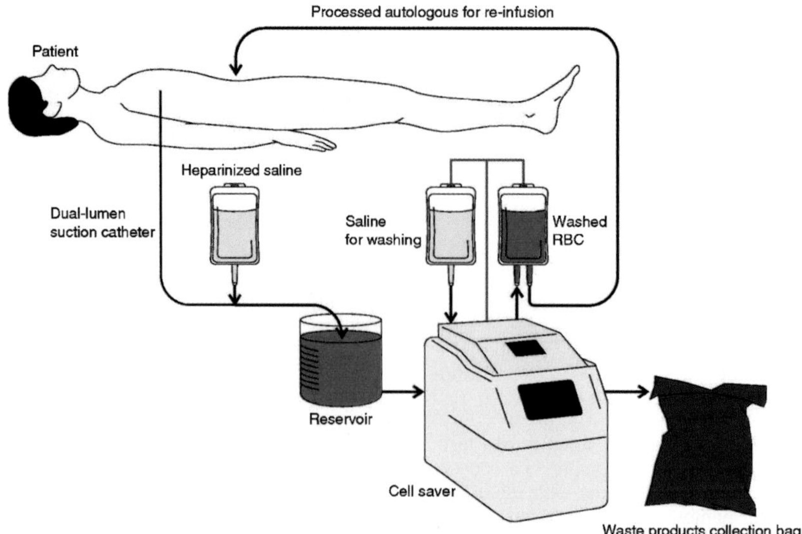

Fig. 49.5 Diagram of the setup of a standard cell salvage circuit. *RBC*, Red blood cell. (From Ashworth A, Klein A. Cell salvage as part of a blood conservation strategy in anaesthesia. *Br J Anaesth.* 2010;105[4]:401–416. https://doi.org/10.1093/bja/aeq244.)

500 to 700 mL of collected blood is required for processing to produce 225 to 250 mL of salvaged saline-suspended PRBCs with a Hct of 50% to 60%.[174] At this point, the salvaged PRBCs are ready for immediate or delayed transfusion. Microaggregate filters (40 μm) are most often employed during reinfusion because recovered and processed blood may contain tissue debris, small blood clots, or bone fragments. Some systems are able to continually process blood and can provide the equivalent of 12 units/h of banked blood to a massively bleeding patient.[175]

The oxygen transport properties and survival of recovered RBCs appears to be equivalent to those of stored allogeneic RBCs. Levels of 2,3-DPG appear to be present at near normal levels in salvaged blood compared with stored allogenic blood cells, which have up to 90% reduction in 2,3-DPG levels.[43] Similarly, the P50 of salvaged blood is similar to that of fresh venous blood drawn from the same patient and significantly higher than that of 2-week old banked blood, suggesting better oxygen-offloading capabilities.[176] RBC deformability also appears improved compared with PRBCs.[41]

Some practical considerations for cell recovery programs are listed in (Box 49.4). If collected under aseptic conditions with a saline-wash device and if properly labeled, blood may be stored at room temperature for up to 4 hours or at 1°C to 6°C for up to 24 hours, provided storage at 1°C to 6°C is begun within 4 hours of ending the collection.[173] The allowable interval of room temperature storage is shorter for recovered blood (4 hours) than for ANH blood (8 hours). Storage times are the same for recovered blood regardless of whether unwashed or washed.

BOX 49.4 Practical Considerations for Intraoperative Cell Recovery, Storage, and Reinfusion

1. If not transfused immediately, units collected from a sterile operating field and processed with a device for intraoperative blood collection that washes with 0.9% saline should be stored under one of the following conditions before initiation of transfusion:
   a. At room temperature for up to 4 h after terminating collection
   b. At 1°C-6°C for up to 24 h, provided storage at 1°C-6°C is begun within 4 h of ending the collection
2. Transfusion of blood collected intraoperatively by other means should begin within 6 h of initiating the collection.
3. Each unit collected intraoperatively should be labeled with the patient's first name, last name, and hospital identification number; the date and time of initiation of collection and of expiration; and the statement "For Autologous Use Only."
4. If stored in the blood bank, the unit should be handled like any other autologous unit.
5. The transfusion of shed blood collected under postoperative or posttraumatic conditions should begin within 6 h of initiating the collection.

Reinfusion of salvaged blood is not without risk (Box 49.5).[177] Air embolism is a serious, potentially fatal problem, but this risk is now mitigated with newer systems that do not allow for the system's direct connection to the patient's intravenous tubing. Collection systems that neither concentrate nor wash shed blood before reinfusion increase the risk of adverse effects. Shed blood has undergone varying degrees of coagulation or fibrinolysis and hemolysis, and infusion of large volumes of washed or unwashed blood has been associated with disseminated intravascular coagulation (DIC).[178] In general, blood collected at low flow rates or during slow bleeding from patients who are not systemically anticoagulated will have undergone coagulation and fibrinolysis and will not contribute to hemostasis on reinfusion. The high suction pressure and surface skimming during aspiration and the turbulence or mechanical compression that occurs in roller pumps and plastic tubing make some degree of hemolysis inevitable.[179] Patients exhibit a level of plasma-free hemoglobin that is usually higher than after allogeneic transfusion. High concentrations of free hemoglobin can be nephrotoxic to patients and free hemoglobin causes severe arteriolar vasoconstriction of microvascular structures from NO scavenging.[180] However, the clinical importance of this phenomenon in

BOX 49.5 Types of Adverse Reactions That May Be Seen With Blood Transfusion from Intraoperative Cell Salvage

Hypervolemia
Bacterial contamination
Hypotension
Nonimmune hemolysis
Immune hemolysis
Febrile nonhemolytic reactions
Allergic reactions
Disseminated intravascular coagulation
Coagulopathies
Air embolus
Reactions secondary to reinfusion of anticoagulants or other contaminants
Nonspecific temperature increases, chills, skin flushing, etc.

From Domen R. Adverse reactions associated with autologous blood transfusion: evaluation and incidence at a large academic hospital. *Transfusion*. 1998;38:296–300. https://doi.org/10.1046/j.1537-2995.1998.38398222875.x

intraoperative cell salvage has not been established. Many programs limit the quantity of recovered blood that may be reinfused without processing. To minimize hemolysis, the vacuum level should ordinarily not exceed 150 mm Hg, although higher levels of suction may occasionally be needed during periods of rapid bleeding. One study found that vacuum settings as high as 300 mm Hg could be used, when necessary, without causing excessive hemolysis.[181]

Positive bacterial cultures from recovered blood are sometimes observed, but clinical infection is rare[182] and may be mitigated with the use of a leukocyte filter in the system[183] Intraoperative collection is contraindicated when certain procoagulant materials (e.g., topical collagen) are applied to the surgical field because systemic activation of coagulation may result. Other instances that may preclude use of cell savage include: use of parenterally incompatible chemicals (e.g., chlorhexidine, betadine, hydrogen peroxide) in the surgical field, and use of hypotonic solutions in the surgical field, which may lyse red blood cells.

Clinical Studies

As with PAD and ANH, collection and recovery of intraoperative autologous blood should undergo scrutiny with regard to both safety and efficacy.[184] A meta-analysis of 75 studies evaluating the utility for cell salvage to minimize allogeneic blood transfusion found that cell salvage reduced the need for allogeneic blood transfusion in adult-elective surgeries by 38%.[185] The greatest benefit was seen in orthopedic procedures but cardiac surgery patients also benefited. On average, intraoperative blood salvage saved an average of 0.68 units of allogenic banked blood. Of note, two randomized controlled trials published in 2014 of patients undergoing hip and knee arthroplasty with either preoperative hemoglobin concentration between 10 to 13 g/dL or more than 13 g/dL failed to show cell salvage as an effective means to reduce allogenic blood requirements.[186,187] However, both studies combined intraoperative and postoperative cell salvage and did not separate patients who received one technique (or both techniques) from those who received another.

TABLE 49.12 Procedures Where Intraoperative Cell Salvage May Be Indicated

General Surgery	Hepatic resection
	Splenectomy
Neurosurgery	Basilar Aneurysm
Transplant Surgery	Liver transplant
	Kidney transplant
Cardio/Thoracic	Cardiac transplant/VAD implant
	Pulmonary transplant
	Coronary artery bypass grafting
	Cardiac valve repair/replacement
	Aortic arch Aneurysm
	Thoracic trauma
Vascular	Aortic Aneurysm repair
	Femoral bypass grafting
Orthopedic	Total shoulder replacement
	Total hip replacement or revision
	Bilateral knee replacement
	Open reduction/internal fixation pelvic or long bone fracture
	Multilevel spine surgery
Urology	Nephrectomy
	Radical prostatectomy
Gynecology	Hysterectomy
Obstetrics	Placenta accreta, increta, or percreta

Adapted from Esper SA, Waters JH. Intra-operative cell salvage: a fresh look at the indications and contraindications. *Blood Transfus*. 2011;9(2):139–147.

In some cases, the value of blood salvage may not be in terms of patient outcome or reduction of transfusion requirements, but instead in cost savings. The value of intraoperative blood collection was recently demonstrated for high-risk cesarean surgeries but not for routine procedures.[188] A list of surgeries where intraoperative cell salvage may be indicated are provided in Table 49.12. As comprehensive PBM pathways continue to evolve and improve patient outcomes, future studies regarding the efficacy and cost-effectiveness of cell salvage will be needed.

POSTOPERATIVE CELL SALVAGE

Postoperative blood collection denotes the recovery of blood from surgical drains followed by reinfusion, with or without processing.[166] In some programs, postoperative shed blood is collected into sterile canisters and reinfused, without processing, through a microaggregate filter. Recovered blood is dilute, is partially hemolyzed, and may contain high concentrations of cytokines. For these reasons, most programs set an upper limit on the volume (e.g., 1400 mL) of unprocessed blood that can be reinfused. If transfusion of blood has not begun within 6 hours of initiating the

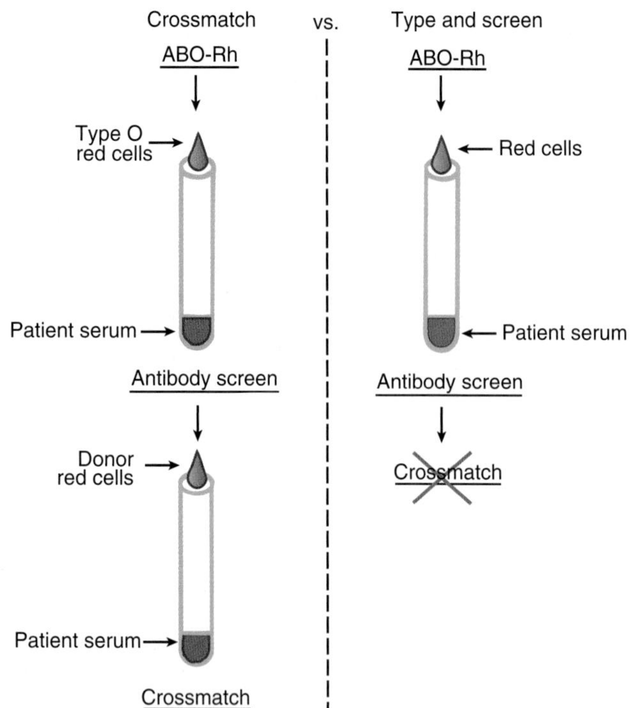

Fig. 49.6 Outline of the tests used for a crossmatch. The X over the word *crossmatch* means that the crossmatch is not included in the type and screen.

collection, the blood must be discarded. Although this technique gained popularity for total joint arthroplasties, the technique is being used less frequently because of a number of factors, including improved PBM programs, lack of evidence for effectiveness, and care pathways that lead to earlier hospital discharge.[174]

Compatibility Testing

GENERAL PRINCIPLES

The ABO-Rh type, antibody screen, and crossmatch are frequently referred to as compatibility tests. These tests were designed to demonstrate harmful antigen-antibody interactions in vitro so that harmful in vivo antigen-antibody interactions can be prevented. Donor blood used for emergency transfusion of type-specific blood must be screened for hemolytic anti-A and/or anti-B antibodies, and Rh antibodies. Similarly, recipient blood must also undergo ABO-Rh typing, as well as testing for unexpected antibodies. Once this has been completed, proper selection of donor blood requires a crossmatch to test for compatibility between recipient blood and donor blood (Fig. 49.6). All approved blood banks have redundant processes in place to ensure that the patient receives the correct unit of blood. Most will require a second confirmatory specimen drawn on a separate occasion from the first type and screen to reduce the risk of a crossmatch error and a hemolytic blood transfusion reaction.[189]

ABO-RH TYPING

Determination of the patient's correct blood type is exceedingly important because the most serious and tragic reactions are usually caused by accidental transfusion of ABO-incompatible blood. In fact, 15% of all transfusion-related deaths are related to hemolytic reactions due to antibody incompatibility.[190] These reactions result from naturally occurring antibodies (i.e., anti-A and anti-B), which activate complement and lead to rapid intravenous hemolysis. Anti-A or anti-B antibodies are formed whenever the individual lacks either or both of the A and B antigens. ABO typing is performed by testing RBCs for the A and B antigens and the serum for the A and B antibodies before transfusion (Table 49.13).

TABLE 49.13 ABO Compatibility Testing

	RED CELLS TESTED WITH		SERUM TESTED WITH	
Blood Group	**Anti-A**	**Anti-B**	**A Cells**	**B Cells**
A	+	–	–	+
B	–	+	+	–
AB	+	+	–	–
O	–	–	+	+

The second most important testing is that for the Rh(D) antigen. Antigen D is very common, and, except for the A and B antigens, the one most likely to produce immunization. Of Rh(D)-negative recipients, 60% to 70% of patients given Rh(D)-positive blood produce anti-D antibodies. Anti-D antibodies may also be formed in the Rh(D)-negative parturient. Approximately 85% of individuals possess the D antigen and are classified as Rh(D) positive; the remaining 15%, who lack the D antigen, are classified as Rh(D) negative. Transfusion of Rh(D)-positive blood to a Rh(D)-negative patient with Rh(D) antibodies may produce a hemolytic transfusion reaction. Table 49.14 identifies compatible donor/recipient blood types.

TABLE 49.14 Donor Blood Groups That Patients Can Receive

Donor	**Recipient**
O	O, A, B, AB
A	A, AB
B	B, AB
AB	AB

ANTIBODY SCREENING

Antibody screens are performed to identify unexpected RBC alloantibodies. The patient's serum is combined with commercially supplied RBCs that are specifically selected due to their expression of RBC antigens for which clinically significant alloantibodies are formed.[191] The reagent RBCs are type O so they do not react to anti-A or anti-B antibodies that may be present in the patient's serum. Alloantibodies are typically immunoglobulin (Ig)G, and thus do not readily produce agglutination in vitro, but do so in vivo. As a result, an indirect antiglobulin test (formerly an indirect Coombs test) is undertaken to evaluate for the presence of IgG alloantibodies. The patient's serum is combined with the reagent RBCs with an additive that promotes binding of antibodies to the RBCs. The mixture is incubated at 37°C, washed and mixed with reagent containing antibodies to IgG and complement. The reagent binds to any IgG attached to the RBCs, crosslinking the RBCs and producing agglutination in vitro. If the test is positive, follow-up testing must be undertaken to identify the target antigen.

The screen for unexpected antibodies is also used on donor serum and is performed shortly after withdrawal of blood from the donor. It is necessary to screen donor serum for unexpected antibodies to prevent their introduction into the recipient's serum.

Daratumumab, a human monoclonal antibody targeting the CD38 glycoprotein was recently approved for the treatment of multiple myeloma, and has been noted to interfere with antibody screening. The drug binds to CD38 expressed on reagent RBCs, leading to a potentially false positive result.[192] Treatment of reagent RBCs with dithiothreitol negates the interference but also leads to denaturing Kell antigens; therefore, K^- RBC units should be allocated in this circumstance unless the patient is known to be K^+.[193] As immunotherapeutic agents and their indications expand, anesthesiologists should be aware of their implications to antibody screening to allow for appropriate testing to avoid delays in the allocation of blood products.[194]

CROSSMATCHING

A crossmatch is a trial transfusion within a test tube in which donor RBCs are mixed with recipient serum to detect a potential for transfusion reaction. The full crossmatch can be completed in 45 to 60 minutes and is performed in three phases: an immediate spin (IS) phase, an incubation phase, and an indirect antiglobulin phase.

First, the IS phase is conducted at room temperature and is a check against errors in ABO typing. It detects ABO incompatibilities and those caused by naturally occurring antibodies in the MN, P, and Lewis systems, but is insensitive to the presence of other RBC alloantibodies. This takes 1 to 5 minutes to complete. In the setting of a negative antibody screen or during emergency situations when an abbreviated crossmatching process is required, this step may serve as the sole confirmatory process to eliminate reactions that may result from human errors in ABO-Rh typing alone. Blood given after this test is more than 99% safe in terms of avoiding incompatible transfusion reactions caused by unexpected antibodies.[195]

Next, the incubation and indirect globulin or "indirect Coombs" phases primarily detect antibodies in the Rh system and other non-ABO blood group systems.[196] This two-step process involves incubation of the test tube at 37°C in albumin or low–ionic strength salt solution, which aids in the detection of incomplete antibodies or antibodies able to attach to a specific antigen (i.e., sensitization) but are unable to cause agglutination in a saline suspension of RBCs. An incubation period of 30 to 45 minutes in albumin and 10 to 20 minutes in low–ionic strength salt solution in this phase is of sufficient duration to allow antibody binding to cells so that incomplete antibodies missed in this phase can be detected in the subsequent antiglobulin phase. The RBCs are centrifuged, resuspended, and observed for hemolysis and agglutination. The RBCs are then washed and resuspended in solution to remove unbound immunoglobulins. Antiglobulin sera is added to the test tubes. The antihuman antibodies present in the sera become attached to the antibody on the RBCs, causing agglutination. This antiglobulin phase detects most incomplete antibodies in the blood group systems, including the Rh, Kell, Kidd, and Duffy blood group systems.

The incubation and antiglobulin phases are important because the antibodies appearing in these phases are capable of causing serious hemolytic reactions. Except for hemolytic reactions involving anti-A and anti-B, reactions caused by antibodies appearing in the immediate phase are frequently less severe as many are naturally occurring, present in low titers, and not reactive at physiologic temperatures.

ELECTRONIC CROSSMATCH

In previously transfused or pregnant patients, only 1 patient in 100 may have an irregular antibody other than the anti-A and anti-B antibodies. However, some of these irregular antibodies are reactive only at temperatures below 30°C and therefore are insignificant in most transfusions. Others that are reactive at approximately 30°C can produce serious reactions if the transfused cells contain the appropriate antigen. In order of probable significance, anti-Rh(D), Kell, C, E, and Kidd are the most common of clinically significant antibodies. If the correct ABO and Rh blood type is given, the possibility of transfusing incompatible blood is less than 1 in 1000. ABO-Rh typing alone results in a 99.8% chance of a compatible transfusion, the addition of an antibody screen increases the safety to 99.94%, and a crossmatch increases this to 99.95%.[197] Complete transfusion testing for compatibility between donor and recipient blood ensures optimal safety and therapeutic effect of transfused blood, but the process is time-consuming and costly.

Once a serologic crossmatch is complete, blood is allocated and set aside for that patient for up to 72 hours. If unused, the product is returned to circulation for other potential recipients. This practice leads to the loss of use for that blood product and increases the chance for outdating of unused products. Eliminating the serologic crossmatch and replacing it with a type and screen followed by a computerized or electronic crossmatch improves the efficiency of the blood banking system, while maintaining, if not improving, patient safety.[198] According to FDA guidance in the United States, a computerized match requires that software determine if incompatibility exists between donor and recipient. Decisions are made based on two separate ABO/Rh typing results from separate specimens from both the donor and the recipient. Under usual perioperative circumstances, measuring the two results from a single specimen should be avoided, as a major cause of ABO errors is a mislabeled specimen.[199] Mislabeling of specimens occurs with an incidence of more than 7 per 1000 specimens with "wrong blood in tube" occurring at a rate of 0.4 instances per 1000 specimens.[200] Interestingly, in this study by Novis and associates, the incident error rate did not decrease between the years of 2007 and 2015, despite the institution of barcode scanning.

A clinically significant current or previously detected positive antibody screen excludes the use of the electronic crossmatch and a serologic crossmatch should be performed.[201]

Patients with a history of a clinically significant antibody despite a current negative antibody screen should continue to be excluded from the electronic crossmatch. The concern is that low titers of circulating antibodies can produce a falsely negative antibody screen.[202]

The type and screen without the serologic crossmatch does not protect against reactions caused by antibodies reactive against lower incidence antigens. These are antigens not represented on the screening cells but present on the donor RBCs. In general, antibodies that are not detected in the type and screen are weakly reactive antibodies that do not result in serious hemolytic transfusion reactions. In a study of 13,950 patients, Oberman and associates[203] discovered only eight "clinically significant" antibodies after complete crossmatch that were not detected during the antibody screening. The antibodies were all in lower titer and were believed to be unlikely to cause serious hemolytic reactions.

Maximal Surgical Blood Order Schedule

In the 1960s and 1970s, the number of crossmatched units ordered for certain surgical procedures frequently far exceeded the number actually transfused. This led to blood being set aside and potential outdating. To better quantify this problem, the crossmatch-to-transfusion (C/T) ratio has been used. If the C/T ratio is high, a blood bank is burdened with keeping a large blood inventory, using excessive personnel time, and having a high incidence of outdated units. Sarma[204] recommended that for surgical procedures in which the average number of units transfused per case is less than 0.5, determination of the ABO-Rh type and a screen of the patient serum for unexpected antibodies (type and screen) should be used. This would be in lieu of a complete crossmatch for patients with negative antibody screens. More recently, Dexter and associates[205] established that using the estimated blood loss reported in an anesthesia information system is more efficacious at predicting the need for transfusions. Their data indicated that for surgical procedures with less than 50 mL expected blood loss, a type and screen is not required.

To increase the rate of use and lower the C/T ratio, blood banks attempt to decrease the emphasis on crossmatching of blood through such programs as the maximal surgical blood order schedule (MSBOS).[206] Ideally, blood banks aim to maintain C/T ratio of less than 2.[207] The MSBOS consists of a list of surgical procedures and the maximal number of units of blood that the blood bank will crossmatch for each procedure. This schedule is based on the blood transfusion experience for surgical cases in a hospital. Each hospital's MSBOS is unique to that practice. The implementation of the MSBOS resulted in a decrease of blood unit expiration from 6.5% to 4.5% at the University of Michigan.[208] Subsequently, patients were categorized into one of three groups: (1) requiring a crossmatch, (2) requiring a type and screen, or (3) no sample required. Preoperative blood orders decreased by 38% with a C/T ratio that decreased by 27%. However, the authors noted the rate of emergency release RBC units increased from 2.2 to 3.1 patients per 1000, but 60% of those patients requiring emergency release blood were undergoing emergency surgery. Of the patients in the "no sample required" category, only a marginal increase of 0.4 to 1 per 1000 patients requiring emergency release blood was noted.[209]

Instead of the blood bank examining the next day's surgical schedule and allocating blood as described in the previous paragraph, now information technology systems have the capability of displaying the surgical schedule along with the MSBOS's recommendation regarding blood preparation. The night before, the blood bank examines the surgical schedule and MSBOS recommendations to see whether blood is needed. The blood bank also uses the MSBOS information to see if additional testing should be performed. Missing tests are communicated to the primary team so that appropriate orders can be placed.

Emergency Transfusion

In many situations, urgent need for blood occurs before completion of compatibility testing (ABO-Rh typing, antibody screen, or crossmatch; see also Chapter 66, which describes transfusion challenges in patients who require surgery and anesthesia after injury from trauma). In essence, for those situations that do not allow time for complete testing, an abbreviated format for testing can be used or uncrossmatched group O blood can be allocated. The procedures described in the following paragraphs aim to provide the potentially life-saving blood product, while minimizing the risk for acute, intravascular hemolytic transfusion reactions.

TYPE-SPECIFIC, PARTIALLY CROSSMATCHED BLOOD

When using uncrossmatched blood, it is best to obtain at least an ABO-Rh typing and an immediate-phase crossmatch. This incomplete crossmatch is accomplished by adding the patient's serum to donor RBCs at room temperature, centrifuging it, and then reading it for macroscopic agglutination. This takes 1 to 5 minutes and eliminates serious hemolytic reactions resulting from errors that may occur in ABO typing. Only a few unexpected antibodies outside the ABO systems are detected, such as those directed against antigens in the MN, P, and Lewis systems, most of which are not clinically significant.

TYPE-SPECIFIC, UNCROSSMATCHED BLOOD

For proper use of type-specific blood, the ABO-Rh type must be determined during the patient's hospitalization. Reports of blood type from patients, relatives, outside medical records may be inaccurate. For those who have never been exposed to foreign RBCs, most ABO type-specific transfusions are successful. Caution should be used for patients who have previously received transfusions or have been pregnant. Historically, in the military, type-specific uncrossmatched blood has been used in emergencies with no serious consequence. In the civilian setting, using 1 year's experience with 56 patients, uncrossmatched, type-specific blood for emergency transfusion produced no adverse effects.[210] The investigators concluded that although the use of uncrossmatched blood is usually safe, the potential for serious reaction still exists, and they cautioned against its indiscriminate use. For those who have previously been exposed to RBC antigens, transfusion of the ABO-Rh type-specific, uncrossmatched blood may be more hazardous.

TYPE O RH-NEGATIVE (UNIVERSAL DONOR), UNCROSSMATCHED BLOOD

Type O blood lacks A and B antigens and consequently cannot be hemolyzed by anti-A or anti-B antibodies in the recipient's plasma (see Tables 49.13 and 49.14). Type O blood can be used for transfusions when typing or crossmatching is not available. However, some type O donors produce high titers of hemolytic IgG, IgM, anti-A, and anti-B antibodies. High titers of these hemolysins in donor units are capable of causing destruction of A or B RBCs of a non–type O recipient. Type O Rh-negative, uncrossmatched PRBCs should be used in preference to type O Rh-negative whole blood because packed erythrocytes have smaller volumes of plasma and are almost free of hemolytic anti-A and anti-B antibodies. If type O Rh-negative whole blood is to be used, the blood bank must supply type O blood that is previously determined to be free of hemolytic anti-A and anti-B antibodies.

Some hospitals have an emergency-release pack of uncrossmatched O negative RBCs. This blood usually can be provided in approximately 5 minutes for urgent situations. Also available in some hospitals is a massive transfusion protocol (MTP), which provides 4 units uncrossmatched O negative RBCs, 4 units thawed AB plasma, and 1 unit of platelet concentrates. Use of MTP blood is determined by physician judgment, but that decision is reviewed after the emergency situation. Although uncrossmatched blood appropriately causes great concern, the risks for complication appear to be quite infrequent.[211] Boisen and associates describe only a 0.1% occurrence of detectable hemolysis in the transfusion of 10,916 uncrossmatched units in 2906 patients.[212] Also, in patients transfused with uncrossmatched blood with antigens for which they are later found to have antibodies against, only 7 out of 262 patients experienced hemolytic reactions.[213]

If emergency transfusion of more than 2 units of type O Rh-negative, uncrossmatched whole blood is used, the patient cannot be switched to his or her blood type (A, B, or AB) once that is determined. Switching could cause major intravascular hemolysis of donor RBCs because of high titers of transfused anti-A and anti-B. Continued use of O Rh-negative whole blood results only in minor hemolysis of recipient RBCs and hyperbilirubinemia. The patient must not be transfused with his or her correct blood type until the blood bank determines that the transfused anti-A and anti-B has decreased to levels that permit safe transfusion of type-specific blood.

Fresh Whole Blood

The definition of fresh whole blood is based on storage time, which varies widely in the literature.[214] Some investigators[215] define fresh blood as blood stored at 1°C to 6°C within 8 hours after collection and used within 24 hours, while other investigators define it as fresh if it has been stored less than 48 hours at 2°C to 5°C. The degree to which fresh blood regains its various functions is directly related to the length of storage and whether it has been cooled. The longer blood is stored, the less effective it becomes, especially regarding coagulation. Whole blood stored for 24 hours at 4°C has less hemostatic effects than blood stored for less than 6 hours because of decreased platelet aggregability.[216] Whole blood that has been typed and crossmatched, but not cooled, retains most of the factors of normal in vivo blood. The difference between 1 hour and 2 days of storage can be tremendous and may impact clinical outcomes.

Numerous studies have examined the use and safety of fresh whole blood, particularly by the U.S. military in Iraq and Afghanistan.[217] Whole blood has been a component of transfusion for over 70 years.[9] Experience in Vietnam showed that typed and crossmatched warm whole blood was extremely effective in treating the coagulopathy from massive transfusions.[2,3,218]

Complications

COAGULATION ABNORMALITIES

Major trauma or blood loss will initiate a cascade of coagulation abnormalities, including a consumptive coagulopathy from tissue hypoperfusion as manifested by increased protein C levels.[219] This coagulopathy is caused by a combination of factors, of which the most important are the dilution of coagulation factors by volume administration (e.g., crystalloid, colloid, PRBC), and the duration of hypotension and hypoperfusion. Various protocols have been developed for approaches to massive blood transfusion administration (Fig. 49.7). Patients who have adequate perfusion and are not hypotensive for a long period (e.g., 1 hour or less) may tolerate administration of multiple units of blood without developing a coagulopathy. The patient who is hypotensive and has received many units of RBCs will develop a coagulopathy that resembles DIC. When such bleeding occurs, the differential diagnosis is dilutional thrombocytopenia, deficiency of factors V and VIII, a DIC-like syndrome, or a transfusion reaction. Clinical signs include oozing into the surgical field, hematuria, gingival bleeding, petechia, bleeding from venipuncture sites, and ecchymosis.

THROMBOCYTOPENIA

Thrombocytopenia is defined as a platelet count less than 150×10^9/L or more than 50% decrease compared with the previous measurement. Clinical bleeding usually does not occur during surgery until platelet counts are less than 50×10^9/L and for spontaneous bleeding until platelet counts are less than 10×10^9/L.[220] Independent of whether whole blood or PRBCs are given, few viable platelets exist in a unit of blood stored for more than 24 hours. For whole blood stored at 4°C, platelets are damaged sufficiently to be readily trapped and absorbed by the reticuloendothelial system soon after infusion. Even platelets that are not immediately stored have a reduced survival time.

Thrombocytopenia can trigger a hemorrhagic diathesis in a patient who has received multiple units of bank blood.

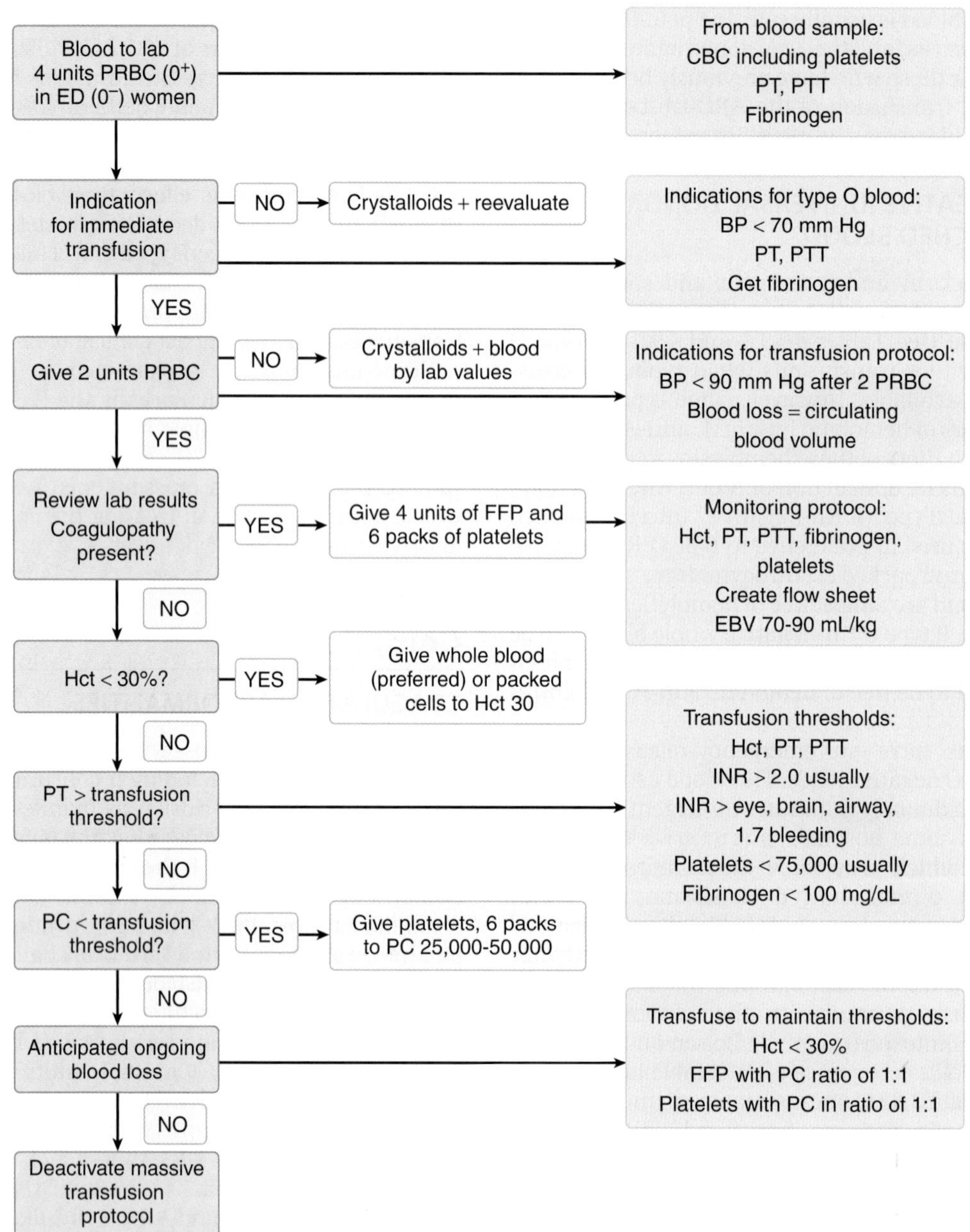

Fig. 49.7 This algorithm for diagnosing and treating a massive transfusion was modified from the massive transfusion protocol used at the San Francisco General Hospital. This protocol suggests how to approach a patient with major blood loss. *BP*, Blood pressure; *CBC*, complete blood cell count; *EBV*, effective blood volume; *ED*, emergency department; *FFP*, fresh frozen plasma; *Hct*, hematocrit; *INR*, international normalized ratio; *PC*, platelet count; *PRBCs*, packed red blood cells; *PT*, prothrombin time; *PTT*, partial thromboplastin time.

Platelet counts decreased to less than 100×10^9/L when 10 to 15 units of blood were given to acutely wounded, previously healthy soldiers.[219] Miller and colleagues[2] found that platelet counts less than 75×10^9/L are a reasonably accurate guide as to when patients will develop a bleeding problem from dilutional thrombocytopenia (see Table 49.10). One trauma group suggests that a higher than normal platelet count may be required in severely injured trauma patients[222] to maintain adequate hemostasis because damaged capillaries require platelets to "plug the holes." The military and trauma hospitals tend to follow transfusion ratios and do not follow strict platelet thresholds for transfusion.

Several investigators[223,224] have questioned the role of dilutional thrombocytopenia in the coagulopathy of massively transfused patients. They point out that the platelet count rarely decreases to as low a level as would be predicted from dilution alone (Fig. 49.8). It may be that platelets are released into the circulation from the spleen and bone marrow but that some of the platelets present function poorly. Patients with chronic thrombocytopenia or leukemia often do not have a hemorrhagic diathesis with a platelet count lower than 15×10^9/L. For unexplained reasons, patients with an acute induced thrombocytopenia (e.g., from blood transfusions) develop a hemorrhagic diathesis at a much higher platelet count than patients with chronic thrombocytopenia (e.g., idiopathic thrombocytopenic purpura).

Most would agree that platelets should not be given to treat laboratory evidence of thrombocytopenia unless

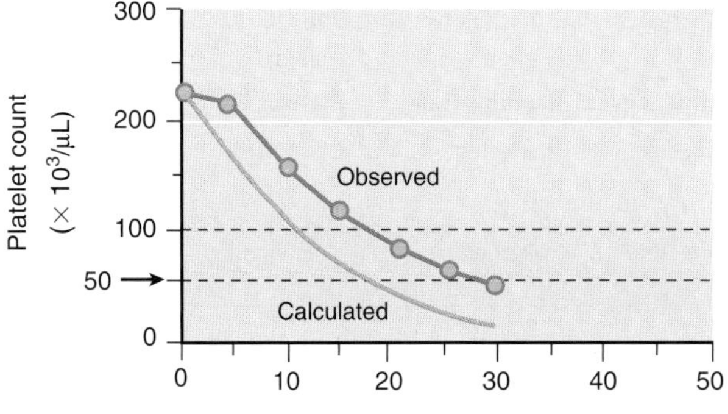

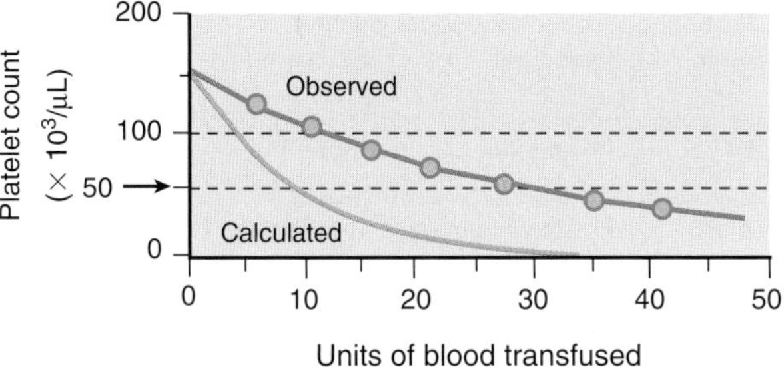

Fig. 49.8 Mean platelet counts after massive transfusions in relation to number of units of blood transfused. Observed versus predicted values calculated on the basis of 2 blood exchange models. (From Myllylä G. New transfusion practice and haemostasis. *Acta Anaesthesiol Scand. Suppl.* 1988;89:76.)

clinical coagulopathy is also present. Treating laboratory numbers without correlation with the clinical status is fundamentally contrary to good medical practice. When the platelet count is less than 50 to 70 × 10^9/L, coagulation is likely impaired due to a combination of dilutional thrombocytopenia and DIC. In many cases, certainly with a concomitant medical condition (e.g., DIC, sepsis), the platelet count as a result of dilutional thrombocytopenia cannot be predicted,[225] nor can the actual impact on clinical bleeding. This is just one of the reasons why efficacy of blood product administration is often difficult to assess. Growing use of point-of-care viscoelastic tests such as tTEG and rotational thromboelastometry instead of platelet count to guide hemostatic therapy is becoming more common.[226]

LOW LEVELS OF FIBRINOGEN AND FACTORS V AND VIII

Considerable attention has been paid to the decreases in blood fibrinogen concentrations that occur during blood loss and blood replacement, likely due to the availability of a lyophilized fibrinogen concentrate for clinical use. Fibrinogen supplementation was previously provided by administration of FFP and cryoprecipitate. Levy and colleagues[227] provided an excellent scholarly review of fibrinogen and hemostasis and concluded that fibrinogen is critical for effective clot formation, and its monitoring and supplementation as the treatment of major bleeding should be recognized. Many prospective studies of fibrinogen supplementation in acquired bleeding report that it is the most effective method of supplementation, and a comprehensive safety profile of fibrinogen concentrate is beginning to appear.

Factors V and VIII may also be affected during storage and significant transfusion.[228] These factors decrease to 50% and 30% of normal, respectively, in whole blood after 21 days of storage[229] and are not present in units of PRBCs. By 35 days of storage, factor V and factor VIII fall further to approximately 20% activity of normal.[230]

Administration of FFP, which contains all the factors, has been recommended. However, this practice is of questionable benefit because only 5% to 20% of factor V and 30% of factor VIII are needed for adequate hemostasis during surgery, and even during massive blood transfusion, factors V and VIII rarely decrease below those levels.

DISSEMINATED INTRAVASCULAR COAGULATION–LIKE SYNDROME

The coagulation system consists of clotting and fibrinolytic mechanisms. The function of the former is to prevent excessive blood loss, and that of the latter is to ensure circulation within the vasculature. With this DIC-like syndrome, the clotting system is deranged, leading to disseminated fibrin deposition, which renders the blood unclottable. The deposited fibrin may severely alter the microcirculation and lead to ischemic necrosis in various organs, particularly the kidney. Table 49.15 displays the interchange between various medical conditions and their impact on various measures of the coagulation system.[231]

The specific reasons for the development of DIC syndrome are usually not apparent. However, hypoxic acidotic tissues with stagnant blood flow probably release tissue thromboplastin directly or through the protein C pathway.[219] The release of tissue plasminogen activator from damaged tissue may cause fibrinolysis. The coagulation system is activated by tumor necrosis factor and endotoxins, resulting in consumption of factors I, II, V, and VIII, and platelets. In an attempt to counteract the hypercoagulable state, the fibrinolytic system is activated to lyse the excessive fibrin. If enough thromboplastin lodges in the circulating blood, the result is massive focal necrosis or more generalized activation of the coagulation system.

DIAGNOSIS AND TREATMENT OF A HEMORRHAGIC DIATHESIS AFTER BLOOD TRANSFUSIONS

Although treatment is more likely to be successful when the cause of the bleeding problem has been identified, precise diagnosis is often difficult. In addition to clinical examination of the patient, various coagulation laboratory tests may be helpful. One traditional approach has been to obtain a blood sample for platelet count, PTT, and plasma fibrinogen level; observation of a clot for size, stability, and lysis; and observation of the plasma for evidence of hemolysis. If the PTT is 1.5 times normal or more and other tests are normal, the bleeding is probably a result of very low levels of factors V and VIII. This can be treated with FFP or with cryoprecipitate (Fig. 49.9).

Whether platelets are administered in the form of fresh blood, platelet-rich plasma, or platelet concentrates depends on intravascular volume replacement requirements, personal preference, and availability of laboratory personnel. Fresh blood (<6 hours old) supplies the

TABLE 49.15 Laboratory Findings in Various Platelet and Coagulation Disorders in the Intensive Care Unit

Condition	Prothrombin Time	Activated Partial Thromboplastin	Fibrinogen Level	D-Dimer Level	Bleeding Time	Platelet Count	Findings on Blood Smear
Vitamin K deficiency or use of vitamin K antagonist	Prolonged	Normal or mildly prolonged	Normal	Unaffected	Unaffected	Unaffected	
Aspirin or thienopyridines	Unaffected	Unaffected	Unaffected	Unaffected	Prolonged	Unaffected	
Liver failure							
Early stage	Prolonged	Unaffected	Unaffected	Unaffected	Unaffected	Unaffected	
End stage	Prolonged	Prolonged	Low	Increased	Prolonged	Decreased	
Uremia	Unaffected	Unaffected	Unaffected	Unaffected	Prolonged	Unaffected	
DIC	Prolonged	Prolonged	Low	Increased	Prolonged	Decreased	Fragmented red cells
TTP	Unaffected	Unaffected	Unaffected	Unaffected	Prolonged	Very low	Fragmented red cells
Hyperfibrinolysis	Prolonged	Prolonged	Low	Very high	Possibly prolonged	Unaffected	

DIC, Disseminated intravascular coagulation; *TTP*, thrombotic thrombocytopenic purpura.
From Hunt BJ. Bleeding and coagulopathies in critical care. *N Engl J Med*. 2014;370;847–859.

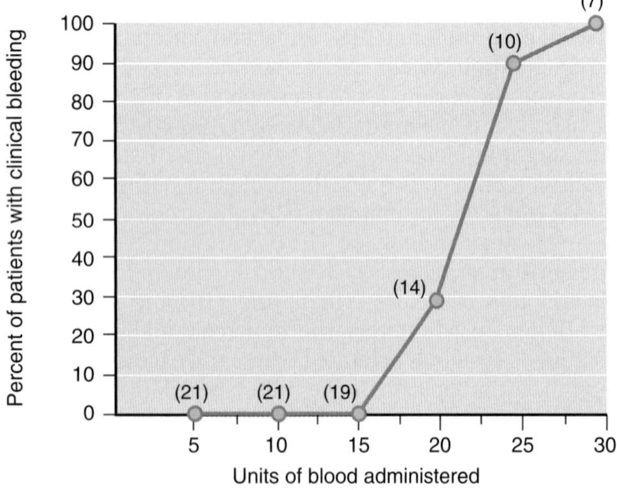

Fig. 49.9 Correlation between units of blood administered and percent of patients who had a hemorrhagic diathesis. The numbers in parentheses represent the number of patients at each data point. (From Miller RD. Transfusion therapy and associated problems. *Reg Refresher Courses Anesthesiol*. 1973;1:101.)

largest number of platelets per donation. More than 80% of the platelets can be given by platelet-rich plasma, which has half of the volume of a unit of blood. However, because most blood banks only have components, platelet concentrates are frequently recommended. Platelet concentrates are contained in a 50-mL unit and provide approximately 70% of the platelets in a unit of blood. In a 70-kg person, approximately 10 units of platelet concentrates are required to increase the platelet count by 10 × 10^9/L in absence of a consumptive process. Although logistically difficult to obtain, fresh blood is extremely effective in treating transfusion-induced coagulopathies. Lavee and associates[232] found that 1 unit of fresh whole blood was as effective as, if not superior to, 8 to 10 platelet units.

Determining the plasma fibrinogen level is useful because this coagulation factor does not decrease in whole blood. If the in vivo plasma fibrinogen level is low (<150 mg/dL), it is not a result of a dilutional coagulopathy and strongly suggests DIC or a DIC-like syndrome. DIC is likely with thrombocytopenia, hypofibrinogenemia, and lysis of clot.[228] With much less plasma, dilution of certain coagulation values may be more profound with the use of PRBCs rather than whole blood. With use of PRBCs, fibrinogen levels decreased significantly in contrast to use of whole blood, in which fibrinogen levels remained unchanged unless DIC is present (Fig. 49.10).[233]

An algorithm for the evaluation and initial therapy of a patient with a suspected coagulopathy is given in Fig. 49.11 (see also the section on blood transfusions, pharmacology, and hemostasis).

Citrate Intoxication and Hyperkalemia

Citrate intoxication leads to hypocalcemia, dysrhythmia, and hypotension due to the sequestration of ionized calcium by citrate. The probability of citrate intoxication is increased in pediatric populations[234] and in the setting of hyperventilation, liver disease, and liver transplantation. Infusion of more than 1 unit of blood every 10 minutes can lead to decreasing ionized Ca^{2+} levels. Even at these rates of infusion, ionized calcium levels do not decrease enough to cause bleeding. Citrate reactions in the setting of apheresis for donation of blood components, however, are more common and in one study occurred in more than 5% of donations.[235]

Similar to citrate intoxication, hyperkalemia as a result of transfusion is relatively rare. Although hyperkalemia is occasionally reported,[234,236] large amounts of blood must be given. Even though serum K^+ levels may be as high as 19 to 50 mEq/L in blood stored for 21 days,[237] the net gain of K^+ is

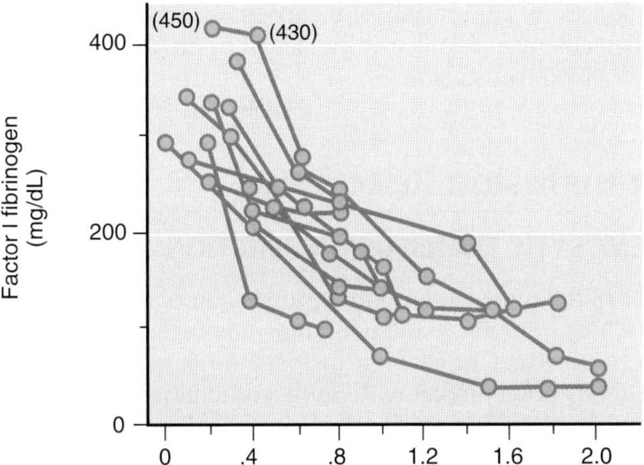

Fig. 49.10 Decreases in fibrinogen level as blood volume is replaced with Adsol-packed red blood cells and crystalloid solutions. Each patient is represented by a solid line. (From Murray DJ, Olson J, Strauss R, et al. Coagulation changes during packed red cell replacement of major blood loss. *Anesthesiology*. 1988;69:839.)

approximately only 10 mEq/L when the loss of K^+ via blood loss is taken into account. For clinically significant hyperkalemia to occur, banked blood must be given at a rate of 120 mL/minute or more. Although still rare, hyperkalemia can occur more frequently in patients with impaired renal function.[238]

Temperature

Administration of blood that has been stored at 4°C can decrease the recipient's temperature and should be avoided if possible due to complications from hypothermia. Hypothermia can interfere with the coagulation process. Even small decreases in body temperature can significantly impair coagulation factors and platelet function.[239] If the temperature decreases to less than 30°C, ventricular irritability and cardiac arrest may occur. Shivering from even mild hypothermia increases metabolic demands and is counterproductive to tissue perfusion, especially in settings where anemia or hypoperfusion is contributing to tissue ischemia.[240]

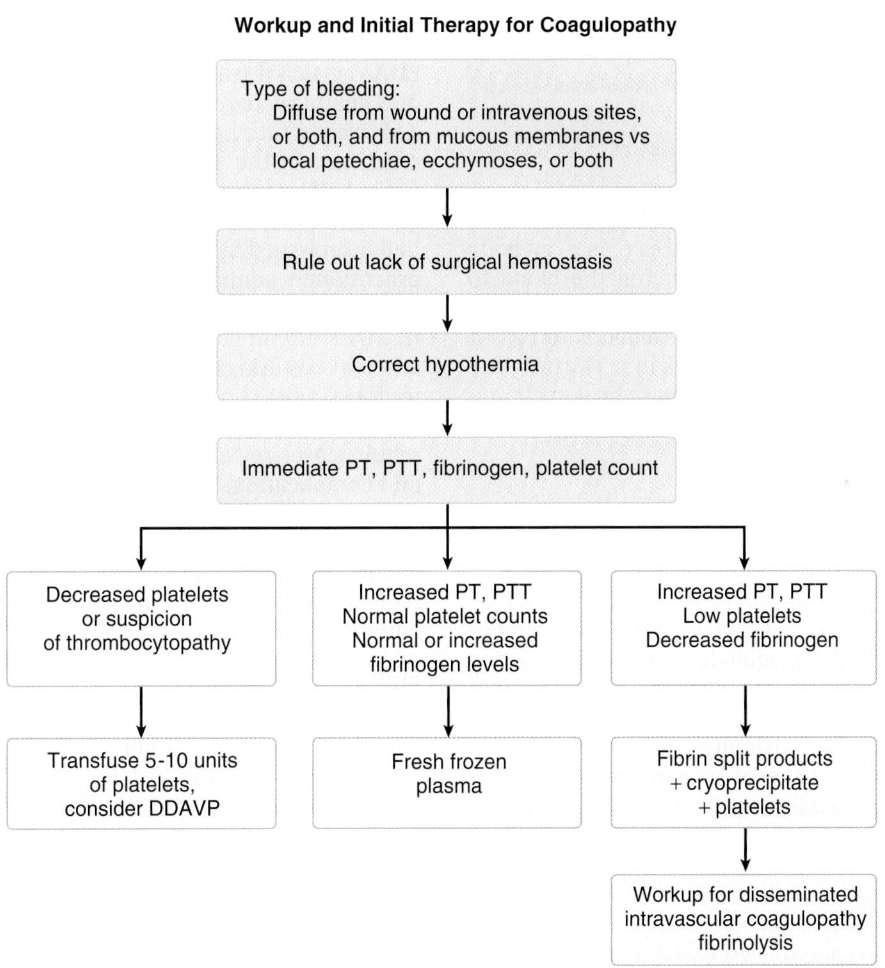

Fig. 49.11 Algorithm for the evaluation and initial therapy of a patient with suspected perioperative coagulopathy. The evaluation is based on the clinical scenario and is affected by the type and location of injury, the amount of fluid administered, and the age and body temperature of the patient. *DDAVP*, 1-Deamino-8-D-arginine vasopressin, a vasopressin analogue also known as desmopressin acetate; *PT*, prothrombin time; *PTT*, partial thromboplastin time. (Modified from Habibi S, Corrsin DB, McDermott JC, et al. Trauma and massive hemorrhage. In: Muravchick S, Miller RD, eds. *Atlas of Anesthesia: Subspecialty Care*. New York: Churchill Livingstone; 1998.)

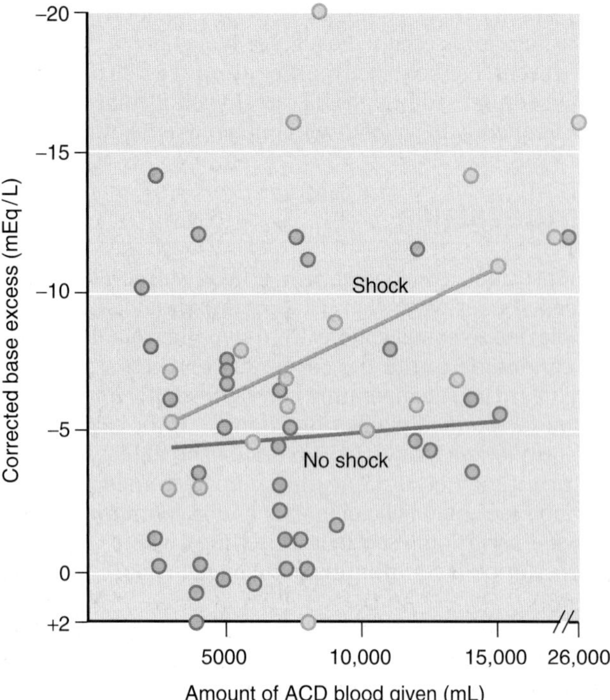

Fig. 49.12 Correlation between the amount of blood administered (milliliters) and intraoperative base excess. *ACD,* Acid citrate dextrose. (From Miller RD, Tong MJ, Robbins TO. Effects of massive transfusion of blood on acid-base balance. *JAMA.* 1971;216:1762.)

Maintaining a patient's normal temperature is considered to be increasingly important. Decreases in body temperature can be prevented by warming the blood to body temperature before transfusing. Perhaps the safest and most common method of warming blood is to pass it through plastic coils or plastic cassettes in a warm water (37°C-38°C) bath or warming plates. These heat exchangers should have upper (e.g., 43°C) and lower (e.g., 33°C) temperature limits.

Acid-Base Abnormalities

The pH of most storage media is very acidic (e.g., pH 5.5 for CPD). When this solution is added to a unit of freshly drawn blood, the pH of the blood immediately decreases from 7.4 to 7.1. As a result of accumulation of lactic and pyruvic acids by RBC metabolism and glycolysis, the pH of bank blood continues to decrease to approximately 6.9 after 21 days of storage. A large portion of the acidosis can be accounted for by the carbon dioxide partial pressure (P_{CO_2}) of 150 to 220 mm Hg. P_{CO_2} is high mainly because the plastic container of blood does not provide an escape mechanism for carbon dioxide. With adequate ventilation in the recipient, the high P_{CO_2} should be of little consequence.

Even when the P_{CO_2} is returned to 40 mm Hg, a metabolic acidosis can be still present in blood (see Table 49.4). The metabolic acid-base response to blood transfusion can be quite variable (Fig. 49.12).[241] The empirical administration of sodium bicarbonate is not indicated because of these unpredictable acid-base changes, but administration should be guided by analyses of arterial blood gases.[242] Blood transfusions provide citrate, which can lead to the endogenous generation of bicarbonate. In some patients, this leads to a significant incidence of metabolic alkalosis after blood transfusions.[242]

Transfusion Reactions

HEMOLYTIC TRANSFUSION REACTION

One of the most catastrophic transfusion reactions is intravascular hemolysis. Intravascular hemolysis occurs when there is a direct attack on transfused donor cells by recipient antibody and complement. Such a reaction can occur from infusion of as little as 10 mL of blood.[243] If properly treated, death is rare.[244] However, prevention of renal failure and DIC is crucial. Hemolytic transfusion reactions involving extravascular RBC destruction are generally less serious than those of the intravascular variety. In these cases, recipient antibody coats but does not immediately hemolyze the transfused RBCs and destruction occurs primarily in the reticuloendothelial system.

Since 1975, the FDA has required that all fatal reactions occurring in blood recipients or donors be reported within 24 hours by telephone or within 7 days in writing by all FDA-registered transfusion services. From 1976 to 1985, 328 deaths were reported and analyzed.[245] Of these deaths, 159 were acute hemolytic reactions and 23 from delayed reactions. Of the 159 deaths from acute hemolytic reactions, 137 were caused by errors involving ABO incompatibility. More than half of these errors occurred after the blood had been issued by the blood bank and were committed by practitioners administering blood products to the patient in the operating room, emergency department, ICU, or ward. In 2011, the incidence of an acute hemolytic transfusion reaction resulting from ABO incompatibility was 1:1200 to 1:190,000.[246] The incidence of hemolytic transfusion reactions is sufficient enough that The Joint Commission[244] requires peer-review programs to reduce transfusion errors and complications. Specifically, two patient identifiers and confirmation of the correct blood product are required before a blood product can be given. New technologies are being used to facilitate a decreased incidence of transfusion-related errors such as barcode scanning of blood prior to administration.

Signs and Symptoms

The classic signs and symptoms (Table 49.16) of a hemolytic transfusion reaction—chills, fever, chest and flank pain, and nausea—are masked by anesthesia. Under general anesthesia, hemoglobinuria, bleeding diathesis, or hypotension may be the only clue. The presenting sign is usually hemoglobinuria. As little as 50 mL of incompatible blood may exceed the binding capacity of haptoglobin, which is a protein that can bind approximately 100 mg of Hb/100 mL of plasma. Usually, free hemoglobin circulates as a complex with haptoglobin, which is cleared by the reticuloendothelial system (Fig. 49.13). A sample of plasma that contains 2 mg/dL of Hb is faintly pink or light brown. When the level of Hb reaches 100 mg/dL, the plasma is red. When the level of plasma Hb reaches 150 mg/dL, hemoglobinuria occurs. In general, the quantity of the free Hb in the plasma correlates with the volume of incompatible blood transfused.

TABLE 49.16 Frequency and Signs and Symptoms of Hemolytic Transfusion Reactions in 40 Patients

Sign or Symptom	No. Patients
Fever	19
Fever and chills	16
Chest pain	6
Hypotension	6
Nausea	2
Flushing	2
Dyspnea	2
Hemoglobinuria	1

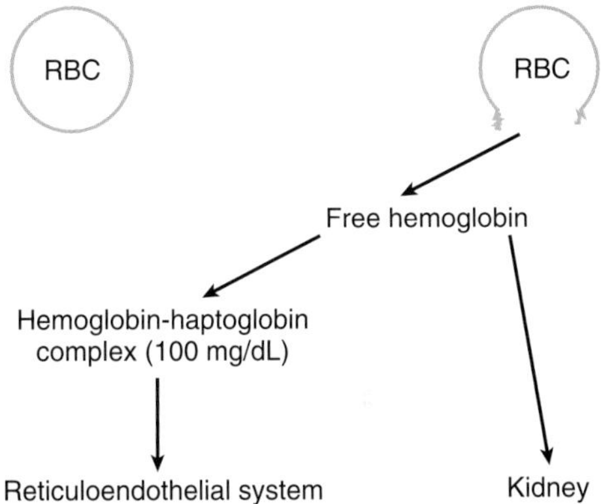

Fig. 49.13 Schematic representation of the effect on hemolyzed erythrocytes *(RBC)* due to the administration of incompatible blood.

Complement activation also causes release of various substances, including histamines and vasoactive amines. The symptoms can be so alarming that cessation of blood is indicated, even if Hb is not seen in plasma. Laboratory tests that should be performed if a hemolytic transfusion reaction is suspected include serum haptoglobin, plasma and urine Hb, bilirubin, and direct antiglobulin determinations. The direct antiglobulin test can confirm the presence of hemolytic transfusion reaction because it shows that antibody is attached to transfused donor RBCs.

Treatment

Although several consequences of intravascular hemolysis are possible, the renal and coagulation systems are affected the most. The cause of acute renal failure from intravascular hemolysis is likely due to precipitation of Hb in the form of acid hematin in the distal tubule causing mechanical tubular blockage. The magnitude of the precipitation probably is inversely related to the pH and volume of urine flow. Therapy should be directed toward maintaining urinary output in excess of 75 mL/h by generous administration of intravenous fluids and diuretics. One approach is summarized in Box 49.6 and includes the administration of crystalloids to maintain adequate intravascular volume while initially administering mannitol. If this is ineffective, the dose of mannitol may be increased or the use of more potent diuretics, such as furosemide may be required to maintain adequate urinary output. Alkalization of the urine to prevent precipitation of acid hematin in the distal tubules is of questionable value but is easy and therefore recommended. DIC commonly occurs with hemolytic transfusion reactions, probably because RBC stroma is severed, releasing erythrocytin, which activates the intrinsic system of coagulation and leads to fibrin formation. Subsequently, platelets and factors I, II, V, and VII are consumed. As soon as a hemolytic transfusion reaction is recognized, platelet count, PT, and PTT should be obtained to provide baseline values with which subsequent laboratory values can be compared. Hypotension during a hemolytic transfusion reaction may result from activation of the kallikrein system.[247]

BOX 49.6 Steps in the Treatment of a Hemolytic Transfusion Reaction

1. Stop the transfusion.
2. Maintain the urine output at a minimum of 75-100 mL/h by the following methods:
   a. Administer fluids intravenously and possibly mannitol
   b. Administer furosemide if intravenous fluids and mannitol are ineffective
3. Alkalinize the urine
4. Assay urine and plasma hemoglobin concentrations.
5. Determine platelet count, prothrombin time, partial thromboplastin time, and serum fibrinogen level.
6. Return unused blood to blood bank for repeat crossmatch.
7. Send patient's blood and urine sample to blood bank for examination.
8. Prevent hypotension to ensure adequate renal blood flow.

DELAYED HEMOLYTIC TRANSFUSION REACTION (IMMUNE EXTRAVASCULAR REACTION)

An immediate hemolytic transfusion reaction often is a dramatic event because the concentration of the antibody is high enough to cause immediate and appreciable RBC destruction. In many cases of hemolytic transfusion reaction, the transfused donor cells may survive initially, but after a variable delay (2-21 days), they are hemolyzed.[248] This type of reaction occurs mainly in recipients sensitized to RBC antigens by previous blood transfusions or pregnancy. As a result, this delayed reaction is more common in females with a known disposition for alloimmunization. These delayed hemolytic transfusion reactions occur when the level of antibody at the time of transfusion is too low to be detected. RBC destruction occurs only when the level of antibody is increased after a secondary stimulus (i.e., anamnestic response). These delayed reactions are often manifested only by a decrease in the posttransfusion Hct. Jaundice and hemoglobinuria can occur in these patients and can cause some impairment in renal function, but only rarely do they lead to death. Unlike immediate reactions, antibodies most commonly involved in delayed hemolytic reactions are those in the Rh and Kidd systems rather than the ABO system. Although improved blood-banking procedures have decreased the incidence of immediate hemolytic transfusion reactions, the delayed hemolytic reaction may not be preventable, because pretransfusion testing is unable to detect very low levels of antibody present in potential blood recipients.

The surgical team should include in their differential diagnosis a delayed hemolytic transfusion reaction in any patient who has an unexplained decrease in Hb 2 to 21 days after a transfusion, even without obvious manifestation of hemolysis. This is especially important in a postoperative patient when the decrease in Hb may be attributed to postoperative bleeding and lead to a return to the operative room for additional surgery.

TRANSFUSION-RELATED ACUTE LUNG INJURY

When a blood transfusion is implicated as the cause of ARDS, it is classified as TRALI. From 2012 to 2016, TRALI was the most common cause of transfusion-related mortality reported to the FDA[118] (see Table 49.8). Although it is underdiagnosed and underreported,[249-251] the incidence of TRALI varies from 1.3% to 3%, depending on the surgical procedures. In addition, larger transfused blood volumes appear to be associated with an increased incidence.[252] TRALI occurs in the absence of excessive intravascular volume and cardiac failure[253] and manifests as noncardiogenic pulmonary edema. Symptoms and signs usually appear within 6 hours after transfusion with a clear temporal relationship to the transfusion.[249] Fever, dyspnea, fluid in the endotracheal tube, and severe hypoxia are typical. During anesthesia, a persistent decrease of oxygen saturation can herald its insidious onset. Although the chest radiograph reveals pulmonary edema, excessive circulatory volume (i.e., left atrial hypertension) is not present. All blood components, especially FFP, are implicated as inciting factors. The only specific therapy is to stop the transfusion and institute supportive measures. The blood bank should be notified to provide blood components from a different donor and to quarantine all units from the donor in question. All records should be reexamined, and the results of the patient's HLA testing should be evaluated if possible. Although most patients recover within 96 hours, TRALI remains the leading cause of transfusion-related death.

Identified risk factors include higher interleukin-8 (IL-8) levels, liver surgery, chronic alcohol abuse, shock, higher peak airway pressures while being mechanically ventilated, smoking, and positive fluid-balance.[254] As far as blood products are concerned, receipt of plasma or whole blood from female donors, especially multiparous donors, was identified as the most common risk factor. The decreased use of plasma from female donors has markedly reduced the incidence of TRALI.

TRANSFUSION ASSOCIATED CIRCULATORY OVERLOAD

Unlike TRALI, TACO refers to an excessive administration volume of blood leading to pulmonary edema with evidence for increased left-sided cardiac filling pressures (e.g., elevated B-type natriuretic peptide/protein, elevated central venous pressure, new or worse left heart failure). TRALI and TACO have overlapping clinical findings and can be easily confounded (Table 49.17). In 2016 the FDA noted an increase in the case fatalities attributable to TACO, perhaps as a result of the increased reporting and improved understanding of the two entities.[118]

Recently, a retrospective analysis demonstrated a decreasing incident rate—with a rate of 5.5% in 2004 and 3% in 2011.[254a] Reasons for the decline are unclear but may be related to a more restrictive transfusion practice, thus limiting the exposure of a patient to potential volume overload; although this latter statement is purely conjecture and not supported by the findings of Clifford and associates. Besides volume transfused, other risk factors included advancing age and intraoperative fluid balance. Interestingly, leukoreduction may play a role in the reduced incidence of TACO, suggesting additional mechanisms of this entity's pathophysiology.[255] Diuretics may be helpful, but in both cases supportive measures such as lung protective ventilation should be instituted.

TABLE 49.17 Comparison of definitions of TACO and TRALI per CDC Guidelines.

TACO	TRALI
New onset or exacerbation of 3 or more of the following within 6 h of cessation of transfusion: ▪ Acute respiratory distress (dyspnea, cough, orthopnea) ▪ Elevated brain natriuretic peptide (BNP) ▪ Elevated central venous pressure (CVP) ▪ Evidence of left heart failure ▪ Evidence of positive fluid balance ▪ Radiographic evidence of pulmonary edema	No evidence of acute lung injury prior to transfusion AND ALI onset during or within 6 h of cessation of transfusion AND Hypoxemia defined by any of these methods ▪ PaO2/FiO2 less than or equal to 300 mm Hg ▪ Oxygen saturation less than 90% on room air ▪ Other clinical evidence AND Radiographic evidence of bilateral infiltrates without evidence of left atrial hypertension (i.e., circulatory overload)

Adapted from the CDC, National Healthcare Safety Network Biovigilance Component. Hemovigilance Surveillance Protocol v2.5.2. April 2018.

NONHEMOLYTIC TRANSFUSION REACTIONS

Nonhemolytic reactions to blood transfusions usually are not serious and are categorized into febrile or allergic. The most common adverse reactions to blood transfusions are febrile reactions. The symptoms consist of chills, fever, headache, myalgia, nausea, and nonproductive cough occurring shortly after a blood transfusion and are caused by pyrogenic cytokines and intracellular contents released by donor leukocytes. Use of leukoreduced blood has lowered the incidence of febrile reactions.[256] Less frequently, the patient may have other symptoms such as hypotension, chest pain, vomiting, and dyspnea. Even pulmonary infiltrations with radiographic evidence of prehilar nodule formation and lower lung infiltrates along with overt pulmonary edema have been reported.[256] A direct antiglobulin test readily differentiates a hemolytic reaction from a febrile reaction because this test rules out the attachment of antibody to transfused donor RBCs. More serious complications may need to be ruled out (e.g., hemolytic or septic reactions), which may also be associated with fever and chills. No clear consensus exists on whether the transfusion should be terminated when a febrile reaction occurs.[257,258]

Allergic reactions can be minor, anaphylactoid, or anaphylactic. An anaphylactoid reaction is clinically similar to anaphylaxis, but it is not mediated by IgE. Most allergic transfusion reactions are minor and caused by the presence of foreign protein in the transfused blood. The most common symptom is urticaria associated with itching. Occasionally, the patient has facial swelling. The transfusion usually does not need to be discontinued. Antihistamines are used to relieve the symptoms of the allergic reaction. Infrequently, a more severe form of allergic reaction involving anaphylaxis occurs in which the patient has dyspnea, hypotension, laryngeal edema, chest pain, and shock. These are anaphylactic reactions caused by the transfusion of IgA to patients who are IgA deficient and have formed anti-IgA. This type of reaction does not involve red cell destruction and occurs very rapidly, usually after the transfusion of only a few milliliters of blood or plasma. Patients who experience anaphylactic reactions should be given transfusions with washed RBCs so that all traces of donor IgA have been removed or with blood that lacks the IgA protein.

OTHER ADVERSE EFFECTS OF BLOOD TRANSFUSION

Transfusion-Associated Graft-Versus-Host Disease

Transfusion-associated graft-versus-host disease (GVHD) is caused by engraftment of donor lymphocytes from transfused blood products, initiating an immune reaction against recipient tissues. Severely immunocompromised patients are at risk. Also, directed donations from first- or second-degree relatives are at risk because transfused lymphocytes with shared HLA haplotypes cannot be recognized and eliminated.[259] A generalized rash, leukopenia, and thrombocytopenia occur. Sepsis and death usually result. Irradiation of blood can prevent transfusion-associated GVHD from occurring, although one case reported it occurring despite leukocyte filtering.[260]

Transfusion-Related Immunomodulation

Homologous (allogeneic) blood transfusion exerts a nonspecific immunosuppressive action on the recipient. More than 150 clinical studies have tried to relate allogeneic blood transfusions to recurrence of resected cancers, postoperative infections, and virus activation, with the conclusion that adverse effects may be caused by transfusion-related immunomodulation. Although the conclusions of these studies are contradictory and inconclusive, universal leukocyte reduction of RBCs is moving forward.[261,262]

OTHER NONINFECTIOUS RISKS OF BLOOD TRANSFUSIONS

Table 49.18 lists some of the less common noninfectious risks of blood transfusions.

1. Microchimerism: Chimerism refers to more than one cell line in an individual organism. Specifically, donor lymphocytes may persist in a patient. The outcome of patients with microchimerism is not known.
2. Posttransfusion purpura: This refers to recipient alloantibodies attacking donor platelet antigens and is treated with intravenous immunoglobulin.
3. Hypotensive transfusion reactions: Activation of the coagulation pathway activates production of bradykinin and allergic reactions.
4. Transfusion-related AKI.
5. Alloimmunization: Only 2% to 8% of recipients who are chronically transfused develop RBC alloantibodies.[5]
6. HLA alloimmunization and human platelet antigen (HPA) alloimmunization: HLA alloimmunization refers to patients whose platelet counts become refractory to transfusions because of antibodies directed against HLA class I antibodies. HPA alloimmunization is platelet refractoriness from antibodies against platelet antigens (HPA antibodies).
7. Iron overload: This complication is the result of chronic transfusion therapy. Iron begins to deposit into vital organs. In the absence of adequate chelation of iron, fatal liver or heart dysfunction, or both, can occur.
8. Adverse ocular reaction: In 1997, 112 cases of bilateral conjunctival erythema occurred within 24 hours of transfusion. The Centers for Disease Control and Prevention (CDC) studied 49 other cases in 1997 and 1998 and concluded that they were toxic reactions to a chemical or material used in the blood collection filtration system, most likely a leukocyte-reducing filter system.[263]

Leukoreduction and Irradiation of Blood Transfusions

GENERAL CONSIDERATIONS

Universal leukoreduction has been implemented because of some anticipated benefits. The chances of a febrile reaction can be reduced, especially in patients who are already alloimmunized from pregnancy. The risk for HLA alloimmunization from blood transfusions can be reduced, minimizing refractoriness to platelet transfusions, and the risk for CMV can be reduced. Leukoreduction can also decrease transmission of variant Creutzfeldt-Jakob disease, leukocyte-induced immunomodulation, and even postoperative mortality. In 2001, the case for and against universal leukoreduction was debated.[264,265] As of 2004, these anticipated benefits were not confirmed, despite numerous studies attempting to do so,[266] but a “may help, won’t hurt” approach has been used to justify universal leukoreduction.[264]

IRRADIATED BLOOD PRODUCTS

Blood products are irradiated to prevent the proliferation of donor T lymphocytes in blood, which are the immediate cause of transfusion-associated GVHD.[267] Fewer than one per million transfusions result in transfusion-associated GVHD, but this disease has a fatality rate greater than 90%. Only cellular products (RBCs, platelets, and granulocytes), but not noncellular products (thawed frozen plasma and cryoprecipitate), need be irradiated. Indications for irradiation include:

1. Fetal recipients of intrauterine transfusions
2. Infants younger than 4 months of age
3. Critically ill children
4. Children younger than 1 year of age undergoing extracorporeal membrane oxygenation/extracorporeal cardiac life support
5. Recipients of cellular components known to be from a blood relative
6. Recipients of cellular components whose donor is selected for HLA compatibility
7. Recipients who have undergone marrow or peripheral blood progenitor cell transplantation

TABLE 49.18 Noninfectious Hazards of Transfusion

Transfusion Reaction	Incidence (per 10^5 Transfusions)	Etiology	Therapy	Prevention
Febrile	All components: 70-6800	Storage-generated proinflammatory cytokines Patient antileukocyte antibodies bind to donor leukocytes	Stop transfusing Give antipyretics Supportive care	Prestorage leukoreduction
TACO	All components: 16.8-8000 Practice-dependent	Circulatory overload Patients with cardiac or renal disease, infants, and the critically ill are at increased risk	Stop transfusing Give diuretics Oxygen	Identify patients at high risk Transfuse slowly
TRALI	Erythrocytes: 10-20 Platelets/plasma: 50-100	Passive transfusion of donor antibodies Storage-generated toxic lipids	Supportive care	Remove high-risk donors from the donor pool
Allergic	All components: 3000 mild, 2 anaphylactic	Mild reactions: Transfusion of soluble antigens in donor plasma Anaphylaxis: IgA deficiency or other recipient protein deficiency	Stop transfusing ASA monitors Large-bore IV access Epinephrine Antihistamines Supportive care	Pretransfusion antihistamine use remains common practice despite limited evidence
Hemolytic	Erythrocytes: 1.1-9.0	Donor antibodies bind to patient erythrocytes Patient antibodies bind to donor erythrocytes	Stop transfusing Repeat matching Supportive care Treat DIC	Standard operating procedures
TRIM	Unknown	The mechanism is unknown but may depend on the presence of donor leukocytes	Treat complications (e.g., infection, malignancy)	Prestorage leukocyte reduction may be beneficial, but this approach is controversial
Microchimerism	All components: 5000-10,000 massive transfusion	Permanent residence of donor cells in recipient	Unknown	Unknown
Posttransfusion purpura	All components: 2	Recipient alloantibodies attack donor platelet antigens	IVIG	Avoid units positive for implicated HPA antigens in patients with a history of PTP
Hypotensive	Unknown	Production of kinins by the activation of the contact system Patients on ACE inhibitors are at increased risk	Stop transfusing ASA monitors Large-bore IV access Supportive care	Avoid the use of negatively charged leukocyte reduction filters
Graft-versus-host	Varies by patient population	Transfusion into immunocompromised host Transfusion of donor cells closely matching HLA type	No consensus exists Consider bone marrow transplant	Gamma irradiation of cellular products

ACE, Angiotensin converting enzyme; *ASA*, American Society of Anesthesiologists; *DIC*, disseminated intravascular coagulation; *HLA*, human leukocyte antigen; *HPA*, human platelet alloantigen; *IgA*, immunoglobulin A; *IV*, intravenous; *IVIG*, intravenous immunoglobulin; *PTP*, posttransfusion purpura; *TACO*, transfusion associated circulatory overload; *TRALI*, transfusion-related acute lung injury; *TRIM*, transfusion-related immunomodulation.

Reprinted from Hillyer CD, Silberstein LE, Ness PM, et al. *Blood Banking and Transfusion Medicine: Basic Principles and Practice*. 2nd ed. Philadelphia: Elsevier; 2007:678–679.

Irradiation is not necessary for patients undergoing routine nonmyeloablative chemotherapy for solid tumors and solid organ transplant patients receiving routine posttransplant immunosuppressive therapy.

Informed Consent

Before any transfusion is given, informed consent should be obtained from the patient or guardian. What constitutes consent varies across the United States and is still changing. If a patient is injured by a transfusion administered without a valid consent, damages may be recovered even though the defendant did everything properly.[146] Many years ago, the *Paul Gann Blood Safety Act* was passed in California. This law mandated that patients be informed of the risks of blood transfusions and of any alternatives. The changes in transfusion medicine should lead to additional education for clinicians who administer blood products to ensure they are compliant with current laws and regulations. Local hospital transfusion medicine committees can provide clinicians with such information.

Acknowledgment

This chapter incorporates portions of the 8th edition Chapter 63, "Patient Blood Management: Autologous Blood Procurement, Recombinant Factor VIIa Therapy, and Blood Utilization." The editors and publisher would like to thank Drs. Lawrence T. Goodnough and Terri Monk for contributing content on this topic in the prior edition of this work.

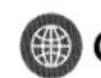 **Complete references available online at expertconsult.com.**

References

1. Karafin MS, et al. *Transfusion*. 2017;57(12):2903–2913.
2. Miller RD, et al. *Ann Surg*. 1971;174:794.
3. Miller RD. *Anesthesiology*. 2009;110:1412–1416.
4. Spahn DR. *Anesthesiology*. 2006;104:905.
5. Hendrickson JE, Hillyer CD. *Anesth Analg*. 2009;108:759–769.
6. Shander A, et al. *Transfus Med Rev*. 2011;25:232–246.
7. Lelubre C, et al. *Transfusion*. 2009;49:1384.
8. Yazer MH, et al. *J Trauma Acute Care Surg*. 2016;81:21.
9. Miller RD. *Anesth Analg*. 2013;116:1392.
10. Spinella PC, Cap AP. *Curr Opin Hematol*. 2016;23:536.
11. Desai N, et al. *Anesth Analg*. 2018;127:1211.
12. Society for the Advancement of Blood Management. *A Guide to Patient Blood Management*; 2016. https://www.sabm.org/wp-content/uploads/2018/08/Guide-to-PBM-2016.pdf. Accessed 28 March 2019.
13. Shander A, Goodnough LT. *Annals of Internal Med*. 2019;170:125–126.
14. Ellingson KD, et al. *Transfusion*. 2017;57(suppl 2):1588–1598.
15. Gupta PB, et al. *Anesthesiology*. 2018;129:1082.
16. Mukhtar SA, et al. *Anaesth Intensive Care*. 2013;41:207.
17. Liebscher K, et al. *Anästh Intensivmed*. 2013;54:295.
18. WHO. *Global Status Report on Blood Safety and Availability 2016*. Geneva: World Health Organization; 2017. License: CC BY-NC-SA 3.0 IGO.
19. WHO Expert Group. *Vox Sang*. 2012;103:337–342.
20. Lacetera N, et al. *Science*. 2013;342:692.
21. Chell K, et al. *Transfusion*. 2018;58:242–254.
22. Dhingra N. *Science*. 2013;342:691–692.
23. Haire B, et al. *Transfusion*. 2018;58:816–822.
24. https://www.fda.gov/%20EmergencyPreparedness/Counterterrorism/MedicalCountermeasures/MCMIssues/ucm485199.htm. Accessed 10 December 2018.
25. Tong MJ, et al. *N Engl J Med*. 1995;332:1463–1466.
26. Centers for Disease Control and Prevention. Hepatitis C FAQs for the Public. https://www.cdc.gov/hepatitis/hcv/cfaq.htm. Accessed 16 March 2019.
27. Preiksaitis VK, et al. *J Med Virol*. 1985;15:283–290.
28. Preiksaitis JK, et al. *J Infect Dis*. 1988;157:523–529.
29. Wilhelm JA, et al. *J Infect Dis*. 1986;154:169–171.
30. Goodnough LT, Marques MB. *Anesthesia Analg*. 2017;124:282.
31. Peterson LR, et al. *N Eng J Med*. 2016;374:1552–1563.
32. Schuler-Faccini L, et al. *MMWR Morb Mortal Wkly Rep*. 2016;65:59–62.
33. U.S. Food and Drug Administration. *Revised recommendations for reducing the risk of Zika virus transmission by blood and blood components;* 2018. https://www.fda.gov/downloads/BiologicsBloodVaccines/GuidanceComplianceRegulatoryInformation/Guidances/Blood/UCM518213.pdf. Accessed 8 November 2018.
34. Tripple MA, et al. *Transfusion*. 1990;30:207–213.
35. Moore GL, et al. *Transfusion*. 1981;21:135–137.
36. Valeri CR. *N Engl J Med*. 1985;312:377–378.
37. Lovric VA, et al. *Vox Sang*. 1985;49:181–186.
38. Cancelas JA, et al. *Transfusion*. 2015;55:491–498.
39. Kleinman S. et al. *UpToDate*. https://www.uptodate.com/contents/practical-aspects-of-red-blood-cell-transfusion-in-adults-storage-processing-modifications-and-infusion. Accessed Feb 7, 2019.
40. Nagababu E, et al. *Transfusion*. 2016;56:1101–1111.
41. Salaria ON, et al. *Anesth Analg*. 2014;118:1179–1187.
42. Frank SM, et al. *Anesth Analg*. 2013;116:975–981.
43. Scott AV, et al. *Anesth Analg*. 2016;122:616–623.
44. Tsoi W. *VOXS*. 2016;11:49–54.
45. Nishiyama T, Hayashi D. *J Anesth*. 2007;21:42–46.
46. Wozniak MJ, et al. *Anesthesiology*. 2018;128:375–385.
47. Wozniak MJ, et al. *Br J Anaesth*. 2017;118:689–698.
48. Marik PE, Sibbald WJ. *JAMA*. 1993;269:3024–3029.
49. Vamvakas EC, Carven JH. *Transfusion*. 1999;39:701–710.
50. Leal-Noval SR, et al. *Anesthesiology*. 2003;98:815–822.
51. Purdy RF, et al. *Can J Anaesth*. 1997;44:1256–1261.
52. Koch CG, et al. *N Engl J Med*. 2008;358:1229–1239.
53. Adamson JW. *N Engl J Med*. 2008;358:1295–1296.
54. Wang D, et al. *Transfusion*. 2012;52:1184–1195.
55. Weiskopf RB, et al. *Anesthesiology*. 2006;104:911–920.
56. Cata JP, et al. *Mayo Clin Proc*. 2011;86:120–127.
57. Saager L, et al. *Anesthesiology*. 2013;118:51–58.
58. Heddle NM, et al. *N Eng J Med*. 2016;375:1937.
59. Steiner ME, et al. *N Eng J Med*. 2015;372:1419.
60. Cooper DJ, et al. *N Eng J Med*. 2017;377:1858.
61. Lacroix J, et al. *N Eng J Med*. 2015;372:1410.
62. Garraud O. *J Thoracic Dis*. 2017;9:E146–E148.
63. Tobian A, et al. *N Eng J Med*. 2016;375:1995–1997.
64. Goel R, et al. *Transfusion*. 2016;56:1690–1698.
65. Cull DL, et al. *Surg Gynecol Obstet*. 1991;173:9–12.
66. Albert K, et al. *Can J Anaesth*. 2009;56:352–356.
67. Beattie WS, Wijeysundera DN. *Anesthesiology*. 2016;125(1):11–13.
68. Mathru M, et al. *Anesthesiology*. 2006;105:37.
69. Consensus conference. *JAMA*. 1988;260:2700–2703.
70. Le Manach Y, Syed S. *Anesthesiology*. 2012;117:1153–1155.
71. Corwin HL, et al. *Chest*. 1995;108:767–771.
72. Hébert PC, et al. *JAMA*. 1995;273:1439–1444.
73. Bishop MH, et al. *J Trauma*. 1995;38:780–787.
74. Frank SM, et al. *Anesthesiology*. 2012;117:99–106.
75. McNamara D. *Anesthesiology News32*. 2012.
76. World Alliance for Patient Safety. *WHO Guidelines for Safe Surgery*; 2008.
77. Solon JG, et al. *J EvalClin Prac*. 2013;19:100–105.
78. Stovener J. *Anesthesiology News 14*. 2012.
79. Berkow L, et al. *Anesth Analg*. 2011;113:1396–1402.
80. Miller RD, et al. *Anesth Analg*. 2011;112:858–863.
81. Xu T, et al. *Crit Care Med*. 2016;44:e344–e352.
82. Bridges E, et al. *Shock*. 2016;46:55–60.
83. Miller RD, et al. *J Anesth*. 2012;26:845–850.
84. Miller RD, et al. *Anesth Analg*. 2014;118:766–771.
85. Giraud B, et al. *Br J Anaesth*. 2013;111:946–954.
86. Barker SJ, et al. *Anesth Analg*. 2016;122:565–572.
87. Frasca D, et al. *Anaesthesia*. 2015;70:803–809.
88. Kolotiniuk NV, et al. *J Cardiothor Vasc Anesthesia*. 2018;32:1638–1641.
89. Musallam KM, et al. *Lancet*. 2011;3278:1396–1407.
90. Karkouti K, et al. *Can J Anesth*. 2015;62:377–384.
91. Kozek-Langenecker SA, et al. *Eur J Anaesthesiology*. 2017;34:332–395.
92. Froessler B, et al. *Ann Surg*. 2016;264:41–46.
93. Keeler BD, et al. *Br J Surg*. 2017;104:214–221.
94. Weltert L, et al. *Transfusion*. 2015;55:1644–1654.
95. Unger EF, et al. *N Engl J Med*. 2010;362:189–192.
96. Karkouti K, et al. *Anesthesiology*. 2011;115:523–530.
97. Goodnough LT, Shander A. *Anesth Analg*. 2013;116:15–34.
98. Levy JH. *Anesthesiology*. 2011;114:1016–1018.
99. Papageorge CM, et al. *Surgery*. 2017;161:1067–1075.
100. Carson JL, et al. *JAMA*. 2016;316:2025–2035.
101. Carson JL, et al. *N Engl J Med*. 2011;365:2453–2462.
102. Shorr AF, et al. *Crit Care Med*. 2004;32:666–674.
103. Taylor RW, et al. *Crit Care Med*. 2006;34:2302–2308.
104. Ely EW, Bernard GR. *N Engl J Med*. 1999;340:467–468.
105. Hébert PC, Fergusson DA. *JAMA*. 2002;288:1525–1526.
106. Vincent JL, et al. *JAMA*. 2002;288:1499–1507.
107. Walsh TS, McClelland DBL. *Br J Anaesth*. 2003;90:719–722.
108. McCrossan L, Masterson G. *Br J Anaesth*. 2002;88:6–9.
109. Mazer CD, et al. *N Eng J Med*. 2017;377:2133–2144.
110. Holst LB, et al. *N Engl J Med*. 2014;371:1381–1391.
111. Rohde HM, et al. *JAMA*. 2014;311:1317–1326.
112. Hovaguimian F, Myles PS. *Anesthesiology*. 2016;125:46–61.
113. Villanueva C, et al. *N Engl J Med*. 2013;368:11–21.
114. Laine L. *N Engl J Med*. 2013;368:75–76.
115. Weiskopf RB. *Transfusion*. 1998;38:517–521.
116. American Society of Anesthesiologists Task Force on Perioperative Blood Management. Practice Guidelines for Perioperative Blood Management. *Anesthesiology*. 2015;122:241.
117. Thiel T, et al. *New Engl J Med*. 2013;368:487–489.
118. https://www.fda.gov/downloads/BiologicsBloodVaccines/SafetyAvailability/ReportaProblem/TransfusionDonationFatalities/UCM598243.pdf. Accessed 22 March 2019.
119. Morrow JF, et al. *JAMA*. 1991;266:255–258.
120. Hong H, et al. *Blood*. 2016;127:496.
121. Benjamin RJ. *Blood*. 2016;127:380.
122. Dunne WM, et al. *Transfusion*. 2005;45:1138–1142.
123. Rebulla R, et al. *N Engl J Med*. 1997;337:1870–1875.
124. Horlocker TT, et al. *Reg Anesth Pain Med*. 4th ed. 2018;43:263–309.
125. Baharoglu MI, et al. *Lancet*. 2016;387:2605.
126. Teixeira PG, et al. *J Trauma*. 2009;66:693–697.
127. Kruskall MS. *N Engl J Med*. 1997;337:1914–1915.
128. Scott E, et al. *Transfusion*. 2009;49:1584–1591.
129. Cardigan R, et al. *Transfusion*. 2005;45:1342–1348.
130. Hall DP, et al. *Br J Anaesthesia*. 2012;109:919–927.
131. Muller MC, et al. *Transfusion*. 2015;55:26.
132. Radwan ZA, et al. *JAMA*. 2013;148:170–175.

133. Sperry JL, et al. *N Engl J Med.* 2018;379:315.
134. Holcomb JB, et al. *J Trauma.* 2011;71:S315–S317.
135. Kornblith LZ, et al. *J Trauma Acute Care Surg.* 2014;77:818.
136. Holcomb JB, et al. *JAMA Surg.* 2013;148:127–136.
137. Bhangu A, et al. *Injury.* 2013;44:1693–1699.
138. Holcomb JB, et al. *JAMA.* 2015;313(5):471–482.
139. Pasquier P, et al. *Anesth Analg.* 2013;116:155–161.
140. Kerins DM. *Am J Med Sci.* 1994;307:218.
141. Tremper KK, et al. *N Engl J Med.* 1982;307:277–283.
142. Spahn DR, et al. *Anesthesiology.* 2002;97:1338–1349.
143. Hermann J, et al. *Anesthesiology.* 2007;107:273–280.
144. Crawford MW, et al. *Anesthesiology.* 2007;107:281–287.
145. Wahr JA. *Anesth Analg.* 2002;94:799–808.
146. Natanson C, et al. *JAMA.* 2008;299:2304–2312.
147. Fergusson DA, McIntyre SL. *JAMA.* 2008;299:2324–2326.
148. Levy J. *Expert Opin Biol Ther.* 2003;3:509–517.
149. Davis JM, et al. *Transfusion.* 2018;58:132.
150. DeSimone, RA, et al. 2018; 58:2297-2300.
151. Goodnough LT, et al. *Transfusion.* 2003;43:668.
152. Vassallo R, et al. *Transfusion Med Reviews.* 2015;29:268–275.
153. AABB. *Standards for Blood Banks and Transfusion Services.* 29th ed. Bethesda MD: AABB Press; 2014.
154. Kiss JE, et al. *JAMA.* 2015;313:575–583.
155. Henry DA, et al. *Cochrane Database Syst Rev.* 2002;(2):CD003602.
156. Popovsky MA, et al. *Transfusion.* 1995;35:734–737.
157. AuBuchon JP, et al. *Transfusion.* 1991;31:513–517.
158. Messmer K, et al. *Eur Surg Res.* 1986;18:254–263.
159. Goodnough LT, et al. *Transfusion.* 1998;38:473–476.
160. Lu SY, et al. *Anesth Analg.* 2014;118:264–268.
161. Goodnough LT, et al. *AnesthAnalg.* 1994;78:932–937.
162. Goldberg J, et al. *Ann Thoracic Surg.* 2015;100:1581–1587.
163. Zhou Z, et al. *BMC Anesthesiology.* 2017;17:13.
164. Roberts, et al. *Am J Surg.* 1991;162:477.
165. Jarnagin, et al. *Ann Surg.* 2008;248:360.
166. De Haan, et al. *Ann Thoracic Surg.* 1995;59:901.
167. Barile L, et al. *Anesth Analg.* 2017;124:743.
168. Sniecinksi RM, Mascha EJ. *AnesthAnalg.* 2017;124:726.
169. Sebastian R, et al. *PedAnesth.* 2017;27:85–90.
170. Albu G, et al. *AnesthAnalg.* 2018;126:995.
171. Crystal GJ. *J Cardiothorac Vasc Anesth.* 2015;29:320–327.
172. Kisilevksy AE, et al. *J ClinAnesth.* 2016;35:434–440.
173. AABB. *Standards for Perioperative Autologous Blood Collection and Administration.* 7th ed. AABB; 2016.
174. Sikorski RA, et al. *Vox Sanguinis.* 2017;112:499–510.
175. Williamson KR, Taswell HF. *Transfusion.* 1991;31:662.
176. Li, et al. *J Cardiothoracic Surg.* 2015;10:126.
177. Domen RE. *Transfusion.* 1998;38:296.
178. Konig G, et al. *Transfus Altern Transfus Med.* 2012;12:78–87.
179. Yazer MH, et al. *Transfusion.* 2008;48:1188–1191.
180. Tsai AG, et al. *Blood.* 2006;108(10):3603–3610.
181. Gregoretti S. *Transfusion.* 1996;36:57.
182. Bell K, et al. *Transfusion Med.* 1992;2:295.
183. Waters JH, et al. *Anesthesiology.* 2003;99(3):652–655.
184. Esper SA, Waters JH. *Blood Transfusion Med.* 2011;9:139.
185. Carless PA, et al. *Cochrane Database Syst Rev.* 2010;(3):CD001888.
186. So-Osman C, et al. *Anesthesiology.* 2014;120:839–851.
187. So-Osman, et al. *Anesthesiology.* 2014;120:852–860.
188. Lim G, et al. *Anesthesiology.* 2018;128:328–337.
189. Gilsch C, et al. *BMJ Open Quality.* 2018;7:e000270.
190. Hendrickson JE, et al. *Transfusion Med Rev.* 2014;28:137–144.
191. American Society of Anesthesiologists. *Transfusion Practices: Questions and Answers.* 3rd ed. Chicago: American Society of Anesthesiologists; 1998:8–9.
192. Chapuy CI, et al. *Transfusion.* 2015;55:1545–1554.
193. Chapuy CI, et al. *Transfusion.* 2016;56:2964–2972.
194. Murphy MF. *N Eng J Med.* 2016;375(3):295–296.
195. Boyd PR, et al. *Am J Clin Pathol.* 1980;74:694–699.
196. Coombs RR, et al. *Br J Exp Pathol.* 1945;26:255–266.
197. Walker RH. In: Polesky HF, Walker RH, eds. *Safety and Transfusion Practices.* Skokie, Ill: College of American Pathologists; 1982:79.
198. Butch SH, et al. *Transfusion.* 1994;34:105–109.
199. Daurat A, et al. *Transfus Clin Biol.* 2017;24:47–51.
200. Novis DA, et al. *Arch Pathol Lab Med.* 2017;141:255–59.
201. U.S. Food and Drug Administration. *Guidance for Industry: Computer Crossmatch.* April 2011.
202. Mazepa MA. *Am J Clin Pathol.* 2014;141:618–624.
203. Oberman AJ, et al. *Transfusion.* 1978;18:137–141.
204. Sarma DP. *JAMA.* 1980;243:1536–1538.
205. Dexter F, et al. *Anesthesiology.* 2012;116:768–778.
206. Friedman BA. *Transfusion.* 1979;19:268–278.
207. Krier DB. *Am J Med Qual.* 1996;11:68–72.
208. Frank SM, et al. *Anesthesiology.* 2013;118:1286–1297.
209. Frank SM, et al. *Anesthesiology.* 2014;121:501–509.
210. Gervin AS, Fischer RP. *J Trauma.* 1984;24:327–331.
211. Mulay SB, et al. *Transfusion.* 2013;53:1416–1420.
212. Boisen et al. *Anesthesiology.* 2015;122:191–195.
213. Goodell PP, et al. *Am J Clin Pathol.* 2010;134:202–206.
214. Fergusson DA, et al. *JAMA.* 2012;308:1443–1451.
215. Spinella PC, et al. *Anesth Analg.* 2012;115:571–578.
216. Weiskopf RB. *Anesthesiology.* 2012;116:518–521.
217. Auten JD, et al. *J Trauma Acute Care Surg.* 2015;79:790-611.
218. Erber WN, et al. *Med J Aust.* 1996;165:11–13.
219. Brohi K, et al. *Ann Surg.* 2007;245:812–818.
220. Kaufman RM, et al. *Ann Intern Med.* 162:205–213.
221. Deleted in proofs.
222. Brown LM, et al. *J Trauma.* 2011;71(suppl 3):S337–S342.
223. Counts RB, et al. *Ann Surg.* 1979;190:91–99.
224. Reed RL, et al. *Ann Surg.* 1986;203:40–48.
225. Wang HL, et al. *J Intensive Care Med.* 2013;28:268–280.
226. Gorlinger K, et al. *Br J Anaesth.* 2012;110:222–230.
227. Levy JH, et al. *Anesth Analg.* 2012;114:261–274.
228. Miller RD. *Anesthesiology.* 1973;39:82–93.
229. Hondow JA, et al. *TANZ J Surg.* 1982;52:265–269.
230. Simon TL. *Plasma Ther Transfus Technol.* 1988;9:309–315.
231. Hunt BJ. *N Engl J Med.* 2014;370:847–859.
232. Lavee J, et al. *J Thorac Cardiovasc Surg.* 1989;97:204–212.
233. Murray DJ, et al. *Anesthesiology.* 1988;69:839–845.
234. Parshuram CS, Jaffe AR. *Pediatr Crit Care Med.* 2003;4:65–68.
235. Robillard P, Grégoire Y. *Comparison of vasovagal and citrate reaction rates in donors according to type of apheresis procedure.* Abstract Presented at American Association of Blood Banks. 09 October 2017.
236. Linko K, Tigerstedt I. *Acta Anaesthesiol Scand.* 1984;28:220–221.
237. Kleinman, S. Red blood cell transfusion in adults: Storage, specialized modifications, and infusion parameters. *UpToDate.* Available at: www.uptodate.com/contents/red-blood-cell-tranfusion-in-adults-storage-specialized-modifications-and-infusion-parameters? Accessed April 14, 2013.
238. Smith HM, et al. *Anesth Analg.* 2008;106:1062–1069.
239. Van Poucke S, et al. *Thromb J.* 2014;12(1):31.
240. De Witte J, Sessler D. *Anesthesiology.* 2002;96(2):467–484.
241. Miller RD, et al. *JAMA.* 1971;216:1762–1765.
242. Collins JA, et al. *Ann Surg.* 1971;173:6–18.
243. Seyfried H, Walewska I. *World J Surg.* 1987;11:25–29.
244. Linden JV, et al. *Transfusion.* 2000;40:1207–1213.
245. Capon SM, Sacher RA. *J Intensive Care Med.* 1989;4:100–111.
246. *AABB Technical Manual.* 17th ed. AABB; 2011.
247. Lopas H. *Am J Physiol.* 1973;225:372–379.
248. Schonewille H, et al. *Transfusion.* 2006;46:630–635.
249. Toy P, et al. *Crit Care Med.* 2005;33:721–726.
250. Zhou L, et al. *Transfusion.* 2005;45:1056–1063.
251. Kleinman S, et al. *Transfusion.* 2004;44:774–789.
252. Clifford L, et al. *Anesthesiology.* 2015;122:12–20.
253. Triuli DJ. *Anesth Analg.* 2009;108:770–776.
254. Toy P, et al. *Blood.* 2012;119:1757–1767.
254a. Clifford L, et al. *Anesthesiology.* 2015;122:21–28.
255. Blumberg, et al. *Transfusion.* 2010;50:2738–2744.
256. King KE, et al. *Transfusion.* 2004;44:25–29.
257. Oberman HA. *Transfusion.* 1994;34:353–355.
258. Widman FK. *Transfusion.* 1994;34:356–358.
259. Ohto H, Anderson KC. *Trans Med Rev.* 1996;10:31–43.
260. Hayashi H, et al. *Anesthesiology.* 1992;79:1419–1421.
261. Vamvakas EC. *Transfus Altern Transfus Med.* 2002;4:48–52.
262. Youssef LA, Spitalnik SL. *Curr Opin Hematol.* 2017;24(6):551–557.
263. Centers for Disease Control and Prevention. *JAMA.* 1998;279:576–578.
264. Corwin HL, AuBuchon JP. *JAMA.* 2003;289:1993–1995.
265. Vamvakas EC, Blajchman MA. *Transfusion.* 2001;41:691–712.
266. Hébert PC, et al. *JAMA.* 2003;289:1941–1949.
267. *American Association of Blood Banks Technical Manual.* 19th ed. AABB; 2017.
268. Kleinman S, et al. *Transfus Med Rev.* 2003;17:120–162.

50 Patient Blood Management: Coagulation

ANIL K. PANIGRAHI and LINDA L. LIU

KEY POINTS

- Normal hemostasis is a balance between generation of a localized hemostatic clot and uncontrolled thrombus formation.
- The extrinsic pathway of coagulation begins with exposure of blood plasma to tissue factor and represents the initiation phase of plasma-mediated hemostasis.
- The intrinsic pathway amplifies and propagates the hemostatic response to maximize thrombin generation.
- The common pathway generates thrombin, forms fibrin, and crosslinks fibrin strands to produce an insoluble fibrin clot.
- Routine preoperative coagulation testing of all surgical patients is costly and lacks predictive value for detection of hemostatic abnormalities. Testing should be based on the preoperative history and physical examination and the planned surgery.
- Antiplatelet agents and anticoagulants are used to reduce the formation of blood clots in the setting of coronary or cerebral atherosclerosis or after vascular thrombosis.
- Thrombolytic therapy is used to break up or dissolve blood clots.
- Procoagulant drugs (antifibrinolytics, factor replacements, prothrombin complex concentrate) help control blood loss during surgery.
- Perioperative management of patients who require chronic anticoagulation or antiplatelet therapy involves balancing the risk of surgical bleeding against the risk of developing postoperative thromboembolism.

Introduction

Hemostasis is an ordered enzymatic process involving cellular and biochemical components that function to preserve the integrity of the circulatory system after injury. The ultimate goal of this process is to limit blood loss secondary to vascular injury, maintain intravascular blood flow, and promote revascularization after thrombosis. As such, normal physiologic hemostasis is a constant balance between procoagulant pathways responsible for generation of a stable localized hemostatic clot and counter-regulatory mechanisms inhibiting uncontrolled thrombus propagation or premature thrombus degradation. Vascular endothelium, platelets, and plasma coagulation proteins play equally important roles in this process. Derangements in this delicate system can lead to excessive bleeding or pathologic thrombus formation. This chapter will examine normal and abnormal hemostasis, mechanisms to monitor coagulation, medications to manipulate coagulation, and management options for the perioperative anticoagulated patient.

Normal Hemostasis

Vascular endothelial injury—mechanical or biochemical—leads to platelet deposition at the injury site, a process often referred to as primary hemostasis. Although this initial platelet plug may prove adequate for a minor injury, control of more significant bleeding necessitates stable clot formation incorporating crosslinked fibrin—a process mediated by activation of plasma clotting factors and often referred to as secondary hemostasis. Although the terms primary and secondary hemostasis remain relevant for descriptive and diagnostic purposes, advances in understanding cellular and molecular processes underlying hemostasis suggest a far more complex interplay between vascular endothelium, platelets, and plasma-mediated hemostasis than is reflected in this model.[1]

VASCULAR ENDOTHELIAL ROLE IN HEMOSTASIS

In order to maintain blood flow throughout the circulatory system, the vascular endothelium employs several strategies to inhibit unprovoked thrombus formation. Healthy endothelial cells possess antiplatelet, anticoagulant, and profibrinolytic effects to inhibit clot formation.[2] The negatively charged vascular endothelium repels platelets, and endothelial cells produce potent platelet inhibitors such as prostacyclin (prostaglandin I_2,) and nitric oxide (NO).[3,4] An adenosine diphosphatase (CD39) expressed on the surface of vascular endothelial cells also serves to block platelet activation via degradation of adenosine diphosphate (ADP), a potent platelet activator.[5] Given these endogenous antiplatelet effects, quiescent platelets normally do not adhere to healthy vascular endothelial cells.

The vascular endothelium also plays a pivotal anticoagulant role through expression of several inhibitors of plasma-mediated hemostasis. Endothelial cells increase activation of protein C, an anticoagulant, via surface glycoprotein thrombomodulin (TM), which acts as a cofactor for thrombin-mediated activation of protein C, making its activation 1000 times faster. Endothelial cells also increase endothelial cell protein C receptor, which further enhances protein C activation by an additional 20-fold.[6] Endothelial-bound glycosaminoglycans, such as heparan sulfate, function to accelerate the protease activity of antithrombin (AT), which degrades factors IXa, Xa, and thrombin.[7] Endothelial cells also produce tissue factor pathway inhibitor (TFPI), which inhibits the procoagulant activity of factor Xa as well as the TF-VIIa complex.[8] Finally, the vascular endothelium synthesizes tissue plasminogen activator (t-PA), which is responsible for activating fibrinolysis, a primary counter-regulatory mechanism limiting clot propagation.

Despite these natural defense mechanisms to inhibit thrombus generation, a variety of mechanical and chemical stimuli may shift the balance such that the endothelium instead promotes clot formation. Damage to vascular endothelial cells exposes the underlying extracellular matrix (ECM), which contains collagen, von Willebrand factor (vWF), and other platelet-adhesive glycoproteins.[9,10] Platelets bind to and are activated by exposure to ECM components. Exposure of tissue factor, constitutively expressed by fibroblasts in the ECM, activates plasma-mediated coagulation pathways to generate thrombin and fibrin clot.[11] Certain cytokines (i.e., interleukin-1, tumor necrosis factor, and γ-interferon) and hormones (i.e., desmopressin acetate [DDAVP] or endotoxin) induce prothrombotic changes in vascular endothelial cells by increasing synthesis and expression of vWF, tissue factor, and plasminogen activator inhibitor-1 (PAI-1), and down-regulating normal antithrombotic cellular and biochemical pathways.[12,13] Finally, thrombin, hypoxia, and high fluid shear stress can also induce prothrombotic vascular endothelial changes such as increased synthesis of PAI-1. This associated inhibition of fibrinolysis has been implicated in the prothrombotic state and high incidence of venous thrombosis after surgery.[14,15]

PLATELETS AND HEMOSTASIS

Platelets contribute a critical role in hemostasis. Derived from bone marrow megakaryocytes, nonactivated platelets circulate as discoid anuclear cells with a lifespan of 8 to 12 days.[16] Under normal conditions, approximately 10% of platelets are consumed to support vascular integrity with $1.2–1.5 \times 10^{11}$ new platelets formed daily.[17] The platelet membrane is characterized by numerous receptors and a surface-connected open canalicular system serving to increase platelet membrane surface area and provide rapid communication between the platelet interior and exterior environment.[18] Under normal circumstances, platelets do not bind the vascular endothelium. However, when injury occurs, platelets contribute to hemostasis by adhering to the damaged vasculature, aggregating with one another to form a platelet plug, and facilitating generation of fibrin crosslinks to stabilize and reinforce the plug. Initially, upon exposure of the ECM, platelets undergo a series of biochemical and physical alterations characterized by three major phases: adhesion, activation, and aggregation. Exposure of subendothelial matrix proteins (i.e., collagen, vWF, fibronectin) allows for platelet adhesion to the vascular wall. vWF proves particularly important as a bridging molecule between ECM collagen and platelet glycoprotein Ib/factor IX/factor V receptor complexes.[19] Absence of either von Willebrand disease (vWF) or glycoprotein Ib/factor IX/factor V receptors (Bernard-Soulier syndrome) results in a clinically significant bleeding disorder.

In addition to promoting their adhesion to the vessel wall, the platelet interaction with collagen serves as a potent stimulus for the subsequent phase of thrombus formation, termed platelet activation. The generation of thrombin resulting from exposure of tissue factor, functions as a second pathway for platelet activation. Platelets contain two specific types of storage granules: α granules and dense bodies.[18] α granules contain numerous proteins essential to hemostasis and wound repair, including fibrinogen, coagulation factors V and VIII, vWF, platelet-derived growth factor, and others. Dense bodies contain the adenine nucleotides ADP and adenosine triphosphate, as well as calcium, serotonin, histamine, and epinephrine. During the activation phase, platelets release granular contents, resulting in recruitment and activation of additional platelets and propagation of plasma-mediated coagulation.[20] During activation, platelets undergo structural changes to develop pseudopod-like membrane extensions and to release physiologically active microparticles, which serve to dramatically increase platelet membrane surface area. Redistribution of platelet membrane phospholipids during activation exposes newly activated glycoprotein platelet surface receptors and phospholipid binding sites for calcium and coagulation factor activation complexes, which is critical to propagation of plasma-mediated hemostasis.[1]

During the final phase of platelet aggregation, activators released during the activation phase recruit additional platelets to the site of injury. Newly active glycoprotein IIb/IIIa receptors on the platelet surface bind fibrinogen, thereby promoting cross-linking and aggregation with adjacent platelets.[20] The importance of these receptors is reflected by the bleeding disorder associated with their hereditary deficiency, Glanzmann thrombasthenia.

PLASMA-MEDIATED HEMOSTASIS

Plasma-mediated hemostasis was originally described as a cascade or waterfall sequence of steps involving the serial activation of enzymes and cofactors to accelerate and amplify fibrin generation by thrombin.[21] Trace plasma proteins, activated by exposure to tissue factor or foreign surfaces, initiate this series of reactions culminating in conversion of soluble fibrinogen to insoluble fibrin clot.[22] Thrombin generation, the "thrombin burst," represents the key regulatory step in this process. Thrombin not only generates fibrin but also activates platelets and mediates a host of additional processes affecting inflammation, mitogenesis, and even down-regulation of hemostasis.[23]

Traditionally, the coagulation cascade describing plasma-mediated hemostasis has been depicted as extrinsic and intrinsic pathways, both of which culminate in a common pathway in which fibrin generation occurs.[24] This cascade model has proven to be an oversimplification,

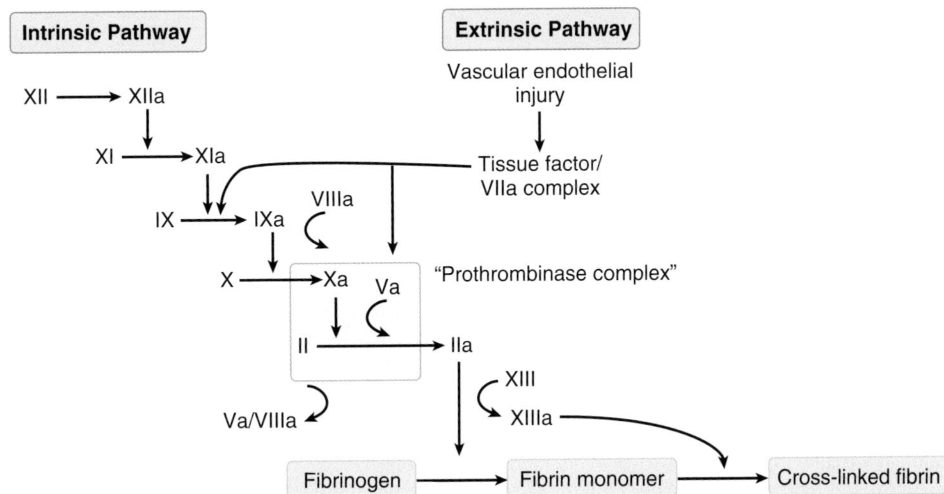

Fig. 50.1 Depiction of the Classic Coagulation Cascade Incorporating Extrinsic and Intrinsic Pathways of Coagulation. (From Slaughter TF. The coagulation system and cardiac surgery. In: Estafanous FG, Barasch PG, Reves JG, eds. *Cardiac Anesthesia: Principles and Clinical Practice*. 2nd ed. Philadelphia: Lippincott Williams & Wilkins; 2001: 320, with permission.)

as it does not fully reflect in vivo hemostasis. For instance, individuals with deficiencies in the intrinsic pathway (factor XII, prekallikrein, or high molecular weight kininogen) exhibit prolongations of the activated partial thromboplastin time (aPTT), but do not actually experience an increased bleeding risk. Nevertheless, the cascade model remains a useful descriptive tool for organizing discussions of plasma-mediated hemostasis (Fig. 50.1). Coagulation factors are, for the most part, synthesized by the liver and circulate as inactive proteins termed zymogens. The somewhat confusing nomenclature of the classic coagulation cascade derives from the fact that inactive zymogens were identified using Roman numerals assigned in order of discovery. As the zymogen is converted to an active enzyme, a lower-case letter "a" is added to the Roman numeral identifier. For example, inactive prothrombin is referred to as factor II and active thrombin is identified as factor IIa. Some numerals were subsequently withdrawn or renamed as our understanding of the coagulation pathway evolved.

The cascade characterizes a series of enzymatic reactions in which inactive precursors—zymogens—undergo activation to amplify the overall reaction. Each stage of the cascade requires assembly of membrane-bound activation complexes, each composed of an enzyme (activated coagulation factor), substrate (inactive precursor zymogen), cofactor (accelerator or catalyst), and calcium.[25] Assembly of these activation complexes occurs on platelet or microparticle phospholipid membranes that localize and concentrate reactants. Coagulation factor activation slows dramatically in the absence of these phospholipid membrane anchoring sites. This requirement functionally confines clot formation to sites of injury.

Extrinsic Pathway of Coagulation

The extrinsic pathway of coagulation is now understood to represent the initiation phase of plasma-mediated hemostasis and begins with exposure of blood plasma to tissue factor.[26] Tissue factor is prevalent in subendothelial tissues surrounding the vasculature. Under normal conditions, the vascular endothelium minimizes contact between tissue factor and plasma coagulation factors. After vascular injury, small concentrations of factor VIIa circulating in plasma form phospholipid-bound activation complexes with tissue factor, factor X, and calcium to promote conversion of factor X to Xa.[22] Additionally, the tissue factor/factor VIIa complex also activates factor IX of the intrinsic pathway, further demonstrating the key role of tissue factor in initiating hemostasis.[27]

Intrinsic Pathway of Coagulation

Classically, the intrinsic or contact activation system was described as a parallel pathway for thrombin generation initiated by factor XII activation after contact with negatively charged surfaces such as glass, dextran sulfate, or kaolin. However, the rarity of bleeding disorders resulting from contact activation factor deficiencies led to our current understanding of the intrinsic pathway as an amplification system to propagate thrombin generation initiated by the extrinsic pathway.[28] Recent cell-based models of coagulation suggest that thrombin generation by way of the extrinsic pathway is limited by a natural inhibitor, TFPI,[29] but the small quantities of thrombin generated do activate factor XI and the intrinsic pathway. The intrinsic pathway then subsequently amplifies and propagates the hemostatic response to maximize thrombin generation (Fig. 50.2). Although factor XII may be activated by foreign surfaces (i.e., cardiopulmonary bypass [CPB] circuits or glass vials), the intrinsic pathway plays a minor role in the initiation of hemostasis. Proteins of the intrinsic pathway may, however, contribute to inflammatory processes, complement activation, fibrinolysis, kinin generation, and angiogenesis.[28]

Common Pathway of Coagulation

The final pathway, common to both extrinsic and intrinsic coagulation cascades, depicts thrombin generation and subsequent fibrin formation. Signal amplification results from activation of factor X by both intrinsic (FIXa, FVIIIa, Ca^{2+}) and extrinsic (tissue factor, FVIIa, Ca^{2+}) tenase complexes. The tenase complexes in turn facilitate formation of the

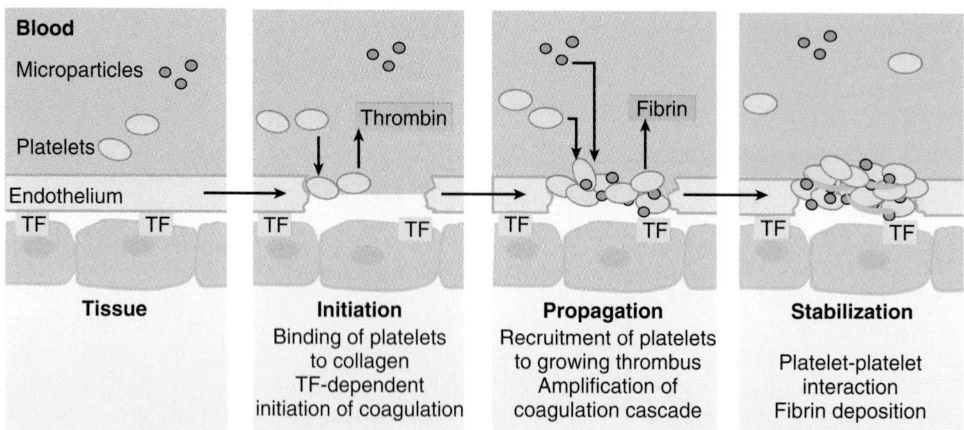

Fig. 50.2 Clot Formation at Vascular Injury Site. Vascular injury exposes subendothelial tissue factor *(TF)* initiating plasma-mediated hemostasis via the extrinsic pathway. The intrinsic pathway further amplifies thrombin and fibrin generation. Platelets adhere to exposed collagen to undergo activation, resulting in recruitment and aggregation of additional platelets. (From Mackman N, Tilley RE, Key NS. Role of extrinsic pathway of blood coagulation in hemostasis and thrombosis. *Arterioscleros Thromb Vasc Biol.* 2007;27:1687–1693, with permission.)

prothrombinase complex (FXa, FII [prothrombin], FVa [cofactor], and Ca^{2+}), which mediates a surge in thrombin generation from prothrombin.[30] Thrombin proteolytically cleaves fibrinopeptides A and B from fibrinogen molecules to generate fibrin monomers, which polymerize into fibrin strands to form clot.[30] Finally, factor XIIIa, a transglutaminase activated by thrombin, covalently crosslinks fibrin strands to produce an insoluble fibrin clot resistant to fibrinolytic degradation.[31]

Both fibrinogen and factor XIII have been implicated in acquired bleeding disorders. Reduced concentrations of either protein may promote excess postoperative hemorrhage and transfusion requirements. Recent availability of plasma concentrates for both fibrinogen and factor XIII suggest the potential for randomized controlled trials to determine efficacy of these biologics in treatment of acquired coagulopathies.[32]

Thrombin generation remains the key enzymatic step regulating hemostasis. Not only does thrombin activity mediate conversion of fibrinogen to fibrin, but it also has a host of other actions. It activates platelets and factor XIII, converts inactive cofactors V and VIII to active conformations, activates factor XI and the intrinsic pathway, up-regulates expression of tissue factor, stimulates vascular endothelial expression of PAI-1 to down-regulate fibrinolytic activity, and suppresses uncontrolled thrombosis through activation of protein C.[33]

Intrinsic Anticoagulant Mechanisms

Once activated, regulation of hemostasis proves essential to limit clot propagation beyond the injury site. One simple, yet important, anticoagulant mechanism derives from flowing blood and hemodilution. The early platelet and fibrin clot proves highly susceptible to disruption by shear forces from flowing blood. Blood flow further limits localization and concentration of both platelets and coagulation factors such that a critical mass of hemostatic components may fail to coalesce.[30,34] However, later in the clotting process, more robust counter-regulatory mechanisms are necessary to limit clot propagation. Four major counter-regulatory pathways have been identified that appear particularly crucial for down-regulating hemostasis: fibrinolysis, TFPI, the protein C system, and serine protease inhibitors (SERPINs).

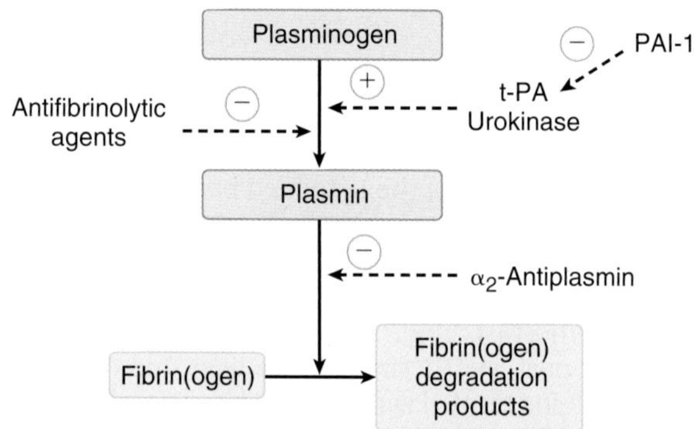

Fig. 50.3 Principal Mediators of Fibrinolysis. Dashed lines depict sites of action for promoters and inhibitors of fibrinolysis. *PAI,* Plasminogen activator inhibitor; *tPA,* tissue plasminogen activator. (From Slaughter TF. The coagulation system and cardiac surgery. In: Estafanous FG, Barasch PG, Reves JG, eds. *Cardiac Anesthesia: Principles and Clinical Practice.* 2nd ed. Philadelphia: Lippincott Williams & Wilkins; 2001:320, with permission.)

The fibrinolytic system comprises a cascade of amplifying reactions culminating in plasmin generation and proteolytic degradation of fibrin and fibrinogen. As with the plasma-mediated coagulation cascade, inactive precursor proteins are converted to active enzymes, necessitating a balanced system of regulatory controls to prevent excessive bleeding or thrombosis (Fig. 50.3). The principal enzymatic mediator of fibrinolysis is the serine protease, plasmin, which is generated from plasminogen.[35] In vivo, plasmin generation is most often accomplished by release of t-PA or urokinase from the vascular endothelium. Activity of t-PA and urokinase is accelerated in the presence of fibrin, which limits fibrinolysis to areas of clot formation. Factor XIIa and kallikrein of the intrinsic pathway also contribute to fibrinolysis through activation of plasminogen after exposure to foreign surfaces.[36] Fortunately, fibrinolytic activity is limited by the rapid inhibition of free plasmin. In addition to enzymatic degradation of fibrin and fibrinogen, plasmin inhibits hemostasis by degrading essential cofactors V and VIII and reducing platelet glycoprotein surface receptors essential to adhesion and aggregation.[37] Fibrin degradation products also possess mild anticoagulant properties.

TFPI and factor Xa form phospholipid membrane-bound complexes that incorporate and inhibit tissue factor/factor VIIa complexes.[38] This inhibition leads to downregulation of the extrinsic coagulation pathway.[39] As TFPI rapidly extinguishes tissue factor/VIIa activity, the critical role of the intrinsic pathway to continued thrombin and fibrin generation becomes apparent.[28]

The protein C system proves particularly important in down-regulating coagulation through inhibition of thrombin and the essential cofactors Va and VIIIa. After binding to TM, thrombin's procoagulant function decreases and instead its ability to activate protein C is augmented.[40] Protein C, complexed with the cofactor protein S, degrades both cofactors Va and VIIIa. Loss of these critical cofactors limits formation of tenase and prothrombinase activation complexes essential to formation of factor Xa and thrombin, respectively. Additionally, once bound to TM, thrombin is rapidly inactivated and removed from circulation, providing another mechanism by which the protein C pathway down-regulates hemostasis.[40]

The most significant SERPINs regulating hemostasis include AT and heparin cofactor II. AT inhibits thrombin, as well as factors IXa, Xa, XIa, and XIIa. [41] Heparin binds AT causing a conformational change that accelerates AT-mediated inhibition of targeted enzymes. Heparin cofactor II is a more recently discovered SERPIN that inhibits thrombin alone.[42] Although the precise physiologic role for heparin cofactor II remains unclear, when bound by heparin, its inhibitory activity is dramatically increased.

Disorders of Hemostasis

EVALUATION OF BLEEDING DISORDERS

The perioperative period presents significant challenges to the hemostatic system; therefore, identification and correction of hemostatic disorders can be of vital importance. Unfortunately, assessment of bleeding risk continues to be a challenge and the optimal methods for preoperative evaluation remain controversial. Although routine preoperative coagulation testing of all surgical patients may seem prudent, such an approach is costly and lacks predictive value for detection of hemostatic abnormalities. Standard coagulation tests such as the prothrombin time (PT) and aPTT were designed as diagnostic tests to be used when a bleeding disorder is suspected based on clinical evaluation. As a result, when used as screening tests, these in vitro assays are limited in their ability to reflect the in vivo hemostatic response.[43] For example, because of the nature of establishing normal value ranges for these tests, 2.5% of healthy individuals will have abnormal PT or aPTT values. Meanwhile, those with mild hemophilia A, vWD, and factor XIII deficiency may experience clinically significant bleeding despite having normal values on standard testing.[44] Consequently, a carefully performed bleeding history remains the single most effective predictor of perioperative bleeding.

A thorough history should focus on prior bleeding episodes.[45] In particular, patients should be asked whether they have experienced excessive bleeding after hemostatic challenges such as dental extractions, surgery, trauma, or childbirth and whether blood transfusions or reoperation were required to control the bleeding. Common presentations suggestive of a bleeding disorder may include frequent epistaxis necessitating nasal packing or surgical intervention. Oral surgery and dental extractions prove particularly good tests of hemostasis because of increased fibrinolytic activity on the mucous membranes of the oral cavity. Women with platelet disorders or vWD may experience menorrhagia, and postpartum hemorrhage commonly occurs in those with underlying disorders of hemostasis.[46] A history of spontaneous nontraumatic hemorrhage proves particularly concerning when associated with hemarthroses or deep muscle bleeding. Identification of a bleeding disorder at an early age or in family members suggests an inherited condition. A careful medication history including direct questions relating to consumption of aspirin and nonsteroidal antiinflammatory drugs (NSAIDs), as well as supplements such as ginkgo and vitamin E.[47] Finally, inquiries regarding coexisting diseases should be included (i.e., renal, hepatic, thyroid, and bone marrow disorders and malignancy).

For most patients, a thoughtfully conducted bleeding history will eliminate the need for preoperative laboratory-based coagulation testing. Should the preoperative history or physical examination reveal signs or symptoms suggestive of a bleeding disorder, further laboratory testing is indicated. Preoperative coagulation screening tests may be indicated, despite a negative history, in cases in which the planned surgery is commonly associated with significant bleeding (i.e., CPB). Finally, preoperative testing may prove justified in settings in which the patient is unable to provide an adequate preoperative bleeding history. Should evidence of a bleeding disorder be detected, underlying etiologies should be clarified if possible before proceeding with surgery.

INHERITED BLEEDING DISORDERS

Von Willebrand Disease

Inherited disorders of hemostasis include those involving platelet quantity and function, coagulation factor deficiencies, or disorders of fibrinolytic pathways. Among these inherited bleeding disorders, vWD is the most common and is characterized by quantitative or qualitative deficiencies of vWF resulting in defective platelet adhesion and aggregation.[48] Affecting up to 1% of the population, vWD is categorized into three main types (types 1, 2, and 3), with most cases demonstrating an autosomal dominant inheritance pattern.[49] Types 1 and 3 lead to varying quantitative vWF deficiencies, while type 2 encompasses four subtypes expressing qualitative defects that affect vWF function. Under normal conditions, vWF plays a critical role in platelet adhesion to the ECM and prevents degradation of factor VIII by serving as a carrier molecule.[50] Classically, patients with vWD describe a history of easy bruising, recurrent epistaxis, and menorrhagia, which are characteristic of defects in platelet-mediated hemostasis. In more severe cases (i.e., type 3 vWD), concomitant reductions in factor VIII may lead to serious spontaneous hemorrhage, including hemarthroses.

Routine coagulation studies are generally not helpful in the diagnosis of vWD, as the platelet count and PT will be normal in most patients and the aPTT may demonstrate mild-to-moderate prolongation depending on the level of factor VIII reduction.[51] Instead, initial screening tests involve measurement of vWF levels (vWF antigen) and vWF platelet binding activity in the presence of the ristocetin cofactor, which leads to platelet agglutination. Measurable reductions in factor VIII activity may occur in severe cases.[52] Increasingly, platelet function tests have replaced bleeding times in assessing for vWD.[53,54] Mild cases of vWD often respond to DDAVP, which results in the release of vWF from endothelial cell. Use of vWF:factor VIII concentrates (Humate-P, CSL Behring, King of Prussia, PA) may be indicated in the perioperative period if there is a significant bleeding history.[55]

Hemophilias

Although less common than vWD, the hemophilias merit consideration given their diverse clinical presentation. Hemophilia A, factor VIII deficiency, and hemophilia B, factor IX deficiency, are both X-linked inherited bleeding disorders most frequently presenting in childhood as spontaneous hemorrhage involving joints, deep muscles, or both. Hemophilia A occurs with an incidence of 1:5000 males and hemophilia B in 1:30,000 males. While most cases are inherited, nearly one third of cases represent new mutations with no family history.[56] The severity of the disease depends on an individual's baseline factor activity level.[57] In mild cases, patients with hemophilia may not be identified until later in life, often after unexplained bleeding with surgery or trauma. Classically, laboratory testing in patients with hemophilia reveals prolongation of the aPTT, whereas the PT, bleeding time, and platelet count remain within normal limits. However, a normal aPTT may also be seen in mild forms of hemophilia; therefore, specific factor analyses need to be performed to confirm the diagnosis and determine the severity of the factor deficiency. In most cases, perioperative management of patients with hemophilia A or B necessitates consultation with a hematologist and administration of recombinant or purified factor VIII or factor IX concentrates, respectively.[58] Mild cases of hemophilia A may be treated with desmopressin. An increasingly common complication of hemophilia, particularly in the case of hemophilia A, has been the development of alloantibodies directed against the factor VIII protein.[59] Administration of factor VIII concentrates will fail to control bleeding in patients with high-titer antibodies. Several approaches to reduce bleeding in these patients include: substitution of porcine factor VIII, administration of activated (FEIBA, Shire Inc., Lexington, MA) or non-activated prothrombin complex concentrates (PCCs), or treatment with recombinant factor VIIa (NovoSeven, Novo Nordisk Inc., Bagsvaerd, Denmark).[60]

ACQUIRED BLEEDING DISORDERS

Drug Induced

Medications represent the most significant cause of acquired coagulopathy in perioperative patients. In addition to anticoagulants such as heparin and warfarin, the increasing number of direct oral anticoagulants(DOACs) and antiplatelet drugs have further complicated perioperative management. An understanding of the effect of these agents and strategies for reversal can be critical to reduce bleeding complications during urgent and emergent procedures. Additionally, there are several classes of medications that may unintentionally increase bleeding risk due to side effects, primarily via platelet inhibition. β-Lactam antibiotics impair platelet aggregation that can result in clinically significant bleeding in patients with higher baseline risk.[61] Nitroprusside,[62] nitroglycerin,[63] and NO[64] also result in decreased platelet aggregation and secretion. Similarly, selective-serotonin reuptake inhibitors, such as paroxetine, decrease platelet serotonin storage, which inhibits platelet aggregation and may have clinical consequences in individuals with preexisting coagulopathies.[65] These medications should be considered in patients with an otherwise unexplained coagulopathy.

Liver Disease

Hemostatic defects associated with hepatic failure prove complex and multifactorial. Severe liver disease impairs synthesis of coagulation factors, produces quantitative and qualitative platelet dysfunction, and impedes clearance of activated clotting and fibrinolytic proteins. The liver is the primary site for the production of procoagulant factors including fibrinogen, prothrombin (factor II), factors V, VII, IX, X, XI, XII, as well as the anticoagulants protein C and S, and AT. Laboratory findings commonly associated with liver disease include a prolonged PT and possible prolongation of the aPTT, suggesting that these individuals are at increased risk of bleeding. However, the abnormal values only reflect the decrease in procoagulant factors and do not account for the concomitant decrease in anticoagulant factors.[66] As a result, patients with chronic liver disease are thought to have a rebalanced hemostasis and actually generate amounts of thrombin equivalent to healthy individuals.[67]

Similarly, thrombocytopenia from splenic sequestration is often observed in patients with liver disease and portal hypertension[68] and is accompanied by platelet dysfunction due to increased production of endothelial NO and prostacyclin resulting in platelet inhibition.[69] Despite these alterations, increases in vWF commonly observed in these patients may serve to restore platelet function. Also, levels of the plasma metalloprotease ADAMTS13, responsible for cleaving vWF multimers, are decreased in chronic liver disease and result in high circulating levels of large vWF multimers that promote platelet aggregation.[70] This increase in vWF may in part correct for thrombocytopenia and platelet dysfunction but also can result in a prothrombotic state and increased clotting risk.

Fibrinolysis of formed clot is also aberrant in patients with liver disease. Normally, fibrin clot is degraded by plasmin, which is converted to its active form by t-PA and urokinase plasminogen activator (u-PA). Excessive fibrinolysis is prevented by thrombin-activatable fibrinolysis inhibitor (TAFI), which blocks activation of plasmin from plasminogen. TAFI is synthesized by the liver and as levels are decreased in patients with chronic liver disease, it was believed that such individuals are at increased bleeding risk due to hyperfibrinolysis.[71] However, levels of PAI-1, a SERPIN of t-PA and u-PA, are also increased in liver disease, which may in actuality normalize fibrinolysis.[72]

In summary, procoagulant and anticoagulant hemostatic mechanisms are rebalanced in patients with chronic liver disease, but this balance is easily disrupted and these patients are at risk for both bleeding and inappropriate clotting.[73] Traditional coagulation testing does not correlate with bleeding risk in these patients, which has led to studies looking at the use of viscoelastic coagulation testing using thromboelastography (TEG) or rotational thromboelastometry (ROTEM) as a means of assessing functional coagulation and guiding perioperative blood product transfusion and administration of antifibrinolytic agents.[73,74]

Renal Disease

Platelet dysfunction commonly occurs in association with chronic renal failure and uremia, as reflected by a prolonged bleeding time and propensity for bleeding associated with surgery or trauma. The underlying mechanisms are multifactorial but have mostly been attributed to decreased platelet aggregation and adhesion to injured vessel walls. Impaired adhesion is likely due to defects of the glycoprotein IIb/IIIa, which facilitates platelet binding of fibrinogen and vWF.[75,76] Additionally, accumulation of guanidinosuccinic acid and the resulting increase in endothelial NO synthesis further decreases platelet responsiveness.[77] Red blood cell (RBC) concentration has also been speculated to contribute to platelet dysfunction, as correction of anemia results in shortened bleeding times, presumably related to the role of RBCs in causing platelet margination along the vessel wall under laminar flow conditions.[78] Both dialysis and correction of anemia have been reported to shorten bleeding times in patients with chronic renal failure. Treatment of platelet dysfunction related to chronic renal disease includes transfusion of cryoprecipitate (rich in vWF) or administration of desmopressin (0.3 μg/kg), which stimulates release of vWF from endothelial cells.[79] Additionally, conjugated estrogens (0.6 mg/kg intravenously for 5 days) have been demonstrated to shorten bleeding times,[80] perhaps via decreased generation of NO.[81]

Disseminated Intravascular Coagulation

Disseminated intravascular coagulation (DIC) is a pathologic hemostatic response to tissue factor/factor VIIa complex that leads to excessive activation of the extrinsic pathway, which overwhelms natural anticoagulant mechanisms and generates intravascular thrombin. Numerous underlying disorders may precipitate DIC, including trauma, amniotic fluid embolus, malignancy, sepsis, or incompatible blood transfusions.[82] Most often, DIC presents clinically as a diffuse bleeding disorder associated with consumption of coagulation factors and platelets during widespread microvascular thrombotic activity, which results in multiorgan dysfunction. Laboratory findings typical of DIC include reductions in platelet count; prolongation of the PT, aPTT, and thrombin time (TT); and elevated concentrations of soluble fibrin and fibrin degradation products. However, DIC is both a clinical and laboratory diagnosis; hence, laboratory data alone do not provide sufficient sensitivity or specificity to confirm a diagnosis.[83] For example, chronic DIC states have been identified with relatively normal screening coagulation tests accompanied by elevated concentrations of soluble fibrin and fibrin degradation products.[84] Management of DIC requires management of the underlying condition precipitating hemostatic activation. Otherwise, treatment is mostly supportive and includes selective blood component transfusions to replete coagulation factors and platelets consumed in the process. The use of anticoagulants such as heparin remains controversial with recommendations that its use be limited to conditions with the highest thrombotic risk.[85] Antifibrinolytic therapy generally is contraindicated in DIC, owing to the potential for catastrophic thrombotic complications.[86]

CARDIOPULMONARY BYPASS-ASSOCIATED COAGULOPATHY

Institution of CPB by directing blood flow through an extracorporeal circuit causes significant perturbations to the hemostatic system. Initial priming of the bypass circuit results in hemodilution and thrombocytopenia.[87] Adhesion of platelets to the synthetic surfaces of the bypass circuit further decreases platelet counts and contributes to platelet dysfunction.[88] During CPB, expression of platelet surface receptors important for adhesion and aggregation (GPIb, GPIIb/IIIa) are downregulated and the number of vWF-containing α granules are decreased, thereby impairing platelet function.[89] Furthermore, induced hypothermia during CPB results in reduced platelet aggregation and plasma-mediated coagulation by decreasing clotting factor production and enzymatic activity.[90] Hyperfibrinolysis may also occur as a result of CPB, supporting the use of antifibrinolytic drugs to decrease intraoperative blood loss.[91]

TRAUMA-INDUCED COAGULOPATHY

Uncontrolled hemorrhage is a frequent cause of trauma-related deaths. Coagulopathy in this setting may be due to acidosis, hypothermia, and hemodilution from resuscitation; however, an independent acute coagulopathy is also experienced by these individuals.[92] Termed trauma-induced coagulopathy (TIC) or acute traumatic coagulopathy, this process involves disordered hemostasis and increased fibrinolysis observed early after injury.[93] The anticoagulant effect of activated protein C (APC) is thought to play a primary role in TIC by decreasing thrombin generation via inhibition of factor Va and VIIIa and promoting fibrinolysis through inhibition of PAI-1. The relevance of APC in the development of TIC is supported by the association of hypoperfusion and increasing injury severity with increased levels of APC activity.[94] Hypoperfusion is thought to be the stimulus for APC activation.[95] Additionally, degradation of the endothelial glycocalyx (EG), a gel-like matrix lining the vascular endothelium, is linked to factors associated with trauma, including tissue damage, hypoperfusion, elevated catecholamines, and inflammation. The EG has anticoagulant properties and contains proteoglycans such as syndecan-1, hyaluronic acid, heparan sulfate, and chondroitin sulfate which are shed during endothelial injury. Shedding of proteoglycans results in an "autoheparinization" phenomenon that contributes to TIC. Markers of EG degradation have been found to be associated with inflammation, coagulopathy, and increased mortality in trauma patients.[96]

Although platelet counts appear to be normal, platelet dysfunction contributes to increased bleeding in TIC. Significant platelet hypofunction in response to various agonists, including ADP, arachidonic acid, and collagen, has

BOX 50.1 Hypercoagulable States and Risk for Perioperative Thrombosis

High Risk

Heparin-induced thrombocytopenia
Antithrombin deficiency
Protein C deficiency
Protein S deficiency
Antiphospholipid antibody syndrome

Moderate Risk

Factor V Leiden genetic polymorphism
Prothrombin G20210A genetic polymorphism
Hyperhomocysteinemia
Dysfibrinogenemia
Postoperative prothrombotic state
Malignancy
Immobilization

been observed acutely in trauma patients prior to resuscitation.[97,98] It is hypothesized that trauma patients experience "platelet exhaustion" as a result of activation from widespread release of ADP from injured tissues. This diffuse activation renders platelets unresponsive to subsequent stimulation.[98] Platelet insensitivity to ADP is also associated with increased susceptibility of clots to tPA-mediated fibrinolysis.[99] The importance of early treatment to reduce hyperfibrinolysis in trauma is supported by the findings of the Clinical Randomisation of an Antifibrinolytic in Significant Haemorrhage 2 (CRASH-2) trial, which demonstrated a mortality benefit from early administration of tranexamic acid (TXA).[100,101]

PROTHROMBOTIC STATES

Thrombophilia, a propensity for thrombotic events, commonly manifests clinically in the form of venous thrombosis (frequently deep venous thrombosis [DVT] of the lower extremity).[102] As with bleeding disorders, thrombophilia may result from inherited or acquired conditions (Box 50.1). The pathogenesis of thrombosis is thought to be due to Virchow's triad (blood stasis, endothelial injury, and hypercoagulability).[9] In the majority of cases, a risk factor or precipitating event is identified; however, a single factor generally does not result in clinically significant thrombosis.[103] Instead, multiple factors act synergistically to increase risk.[104] For example, thrombotic complications often occur after surgery or during pregnancy in association with obesity, underlying malignancy, or an inherited thrombophilia.[105] Random screening of asymptomatic patients for thrombotic risk has not proven cost effective or clinically efficacious.[106,107] As with bleeding disorders, a history focusing on prior thrombotic events, family history of thrombosis, and concurrent drug therapy offers greater predictive value than random screening.

INHERITED THROMBOTIC DISORDERS

Improvements in biochemical and molecular testing have dramatically improved our understanding of blood coagulation and the prevalence of prothrombotic disorders.[108] Because of more specific testing, an inheritable thrombotic predisposition is identified in as many as 50% of patients presenting with venous thromboembolism.[109] The most common inherited prothrombotic conditions include single point mutations in genes for factor V (factor V Leiden) or prothrombin (prothrombin G20210A). In the case of the factor V Leiden, the mutation results in APC resistance whereby the essential cofactor Va is no longer susceptible to APC-mediated degradation. This simple alteration in balance between hemostasis and the APC counter-regulatory system induces a prothrombotic condition present in approximately 5% of the Caucasian population.[110] In the case of the prothrombin gene mutation, increased prothrombin concentrations in plasma generate a hypercoagulable state. Less common inherited forms of thrombophilia include deficiencies of AT, protein C, or protein S.[108] Inherited forms of thrombophilia are characterized by highly variable penetrance affected by blood type, sex, and other confounding variables. Environmental factors such as oral contraceptive use, pregnancy, immobility, infection, surgery, or trauma greatly affect the incidence of thrombosis in those with an inherited predisposition.[111] In the absence of coexisting precipitating conditions, presence of a family history, test abnormality suggesting thrombophilia, or history of thrombosis, risks associated with long-term preventive anticoagulation may outweigh potential benefits.[106] After a thrombotic complication, however, these patients most often are managed with life-long anticoagulation.

ACQUIRED THROMBOTIC DISORDERS

Antiphospholipid Syndrome

Antiphospholipid syndrome (APS) describes an acquired autoimmune disorder characterized by venous or arterial thromboses, or both, and recurrent pregnancy loss. This syndrome may occur in association with autoimmune disorders such as systemic lupus erythematosus or rheumatoid arthritis, or it may occur in isolation. APS results from development of autoantibodies directed against phospholipid-binding proteins, which affect the coagulation system and is associated with up to 10% of cases of DVT and 6% of pregnancy-associated morbidity.[112] Characteristically, APS results in mild prolongation of the aPTT and positive testing for lupus anticoagulant, anticardiolipin or anti-β2-glycoprotein I antibodies.[113] Antibodies associated with APS interfere with phospholipids common to many laboratory-based tests of coagulation. Despite the prolonged aPTT, APS poses no increased bleeding risk but rather increases the potential for thrombosis. Isolated prolongation of an aPTT in a preoperative patient merits consideration of the diagnosis of APS. Patients with this syndrome who have experienced a thrombotic complication are at increased risk for recurrent thrombosis and most often are managed by life-long anticoagulation.[114]

HEPARIN-INDUCED THROMBOCYTOPENIA

Heparin-induced thrombocytopenia (HIT) describes an autoimmune-mediated drug reaction occurring in as many as 5% of patients receiving heparin therapy. Patients with HIT experience a mild-to-moderate thrombocytopenia. As opposed to other drug-induced thrombocytopenias, HIT

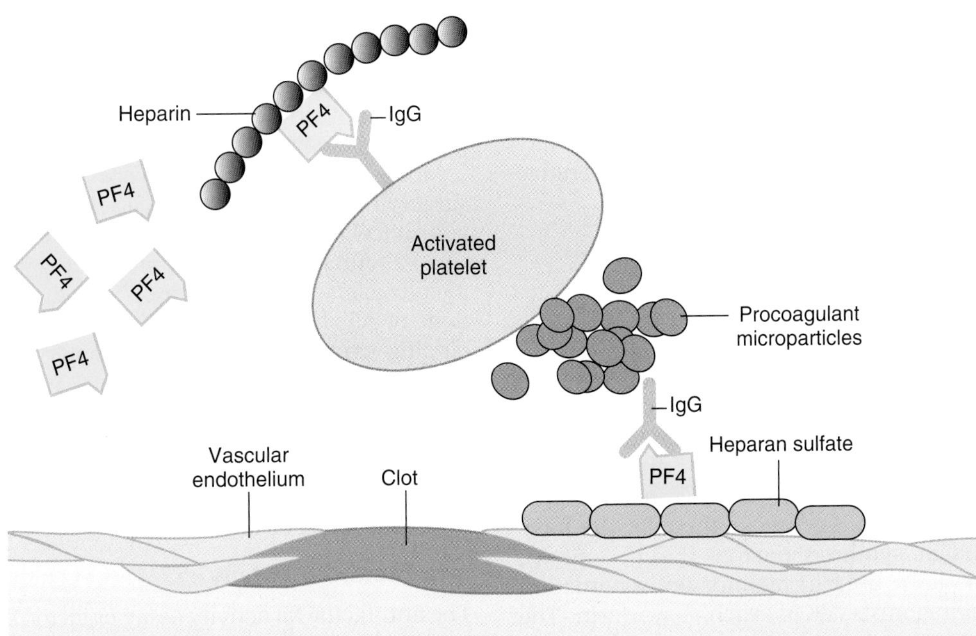

Fig. 50.4 Mechanisms Underlying Thrombosis in Heparin-Induced Thrombocytopenia. Immune complexes composed of heparin, platelet factor 4 *(PF4)*, and antibodies bind to platelet surface Fcγ receptors to activate platelets. PF4/heparin immune complexes further activate vascular endothelium, monocytes, and macrophages to increase tissue factor expression. *IgG,* Immunoglobulin G. (From Slaughter TF, Greenberg CS. Heparin-associated thrombocytopenia and thrombosis: Implications for perioperative management. *Anesthesiology.* 1997;87:669, with permission.)

results in platelet activation and potential for venous and arterial thromboses.[115] Evidence suggests that HIT is mediated by immune complexes (composed of immunoglobulin G [IgG] antibody, platelet factor 4 [PF4], and heparin) that bind platelet Fcγ receptors to activate platelets. Anti-PF4/heparin antibodies may "activate" vascular endothelium, monocytes, and macrophages by up-regulating tissue factor expression (Fig. 50.4). Risk factors for development of HIT include patient population, gender, and heparin formulation used. Women are at increased risk of HIT (odds ratio [OR] 2.37; 95% CI 1.37-4.09) as are surgical patients compared to medical patients (OR 3.25; 95% CI 1.98-5.35). [116] Given the high doses of heparin administered during cardiac surgery with CPB, these patients have a higher incidence of anti-PF4 antibody development (up to 50%); however, the incidence of HIT in this population appears to be similar to other surgical groups.[117] Use of unfractionated heparin (UFH) carries a greater risk of HIT development than low-molecular-weight heparin (LMWH) (absolute risk 2.6% vs. 0.2%).[118] Patients developing HIT during heparin therapy experience substantially increased risk for thrombosis (OR 20:40, absolute risk 30% to 75%).[115]

HIT manifests clinically as thrombocytopenia occurring 5 to 14 days after initiating heparin therapy. With prior heparin exposure, thrombocytopenia or thrombosis may occur within 1 day. A diagnosis of HIT should be entertained for any patient experiencing thrombosis or thrombocytopenia (absolute or relative ≥ 50% reduction in platelet count) during or after heparin administration. Although HIT remains a clinical diagnosis, HIT antibodies testing should be undertaken to confirm the diagnosis. The enzyme-linked immunosorbent assay (ELISA) is sensitive, but not as specific as the serotonin release assay (SRA), because the SRA indicates heparin-induced platelet activation. For many intensive care patients, a positive ELISA test does not lead to a positive SRA, which means these patients are unlikely to have HIT.[119]

In cases where HIT is suspected, heparin must be discontinued immediately (including UFH, LMWH, heparin-bonded catheters, heparin flushes). Alternative nonheparin anticoagulation must be administered concurrently. In most cases, a direct thrombin inhibitor (DTI, e.g., bivalirudin, lepirudin, or argatroban) is substituted for heparin until adequate prolongation of the international normalized ratio (INR) can be achieved with warfarin. Initiation of warfarin alone is contraindicated for HIT treatment because the initial decreased synthesis of proteins C and S enhances the patient's prothrombotic state. Platelet transfusions should be held unless the patient is severely thrombocytopenic ($<20 \times 10^9$/L) with signs of bleeding. Use of DOACs (e.g., rivaroxaban, apixaban, dabigatran, edoxaban) is being investigated.[120]

Typically, PF4/heparin immune complexes are cleared from the circulation within 3 months. If possible, patients experiencing HIT should avoid future exposure to UFH; however, several reports describe subsequent limited perioperative reexposure to UFH after laboratory testing to ensure absence of PF4/heparin immune complexes. If titers remain high, treatment with plasmapheresis for rapid antibody clearance is an alternative plan, but risks and benefits should be discussed with the hematologists.[121] Otherwise, bivalirudin, the shortest acting DTI, is the alternative agent for anticoagulation while on CPB.

MONITORING COAGULATION

Traditionally, perioperative coagulation monitoring has focused on (1) preoperative testing to identify patients at increased risk for perioperative bleeding and (2) intraoperative monitoring of heparin therapy during cardiac and vascular surgery. The ideal test for perioperative coagulation should be simple to perform, accurate, reproducible, diagnostically specific, and cost effective. No current coagulation monitor meets these expectations; however, integrating results from multiple forms of monitoring may provide valuable diagnostic insight into perioperative coagulopathies.

COMMON LABORATORY-BASED MEASURES OF COAGULATION

Prothrombin Time

The PT assesses the integrity of the extrinsic and common pathways of plasma-mediated hemostasis. It measures time required in seconds for clot formation to occur after mixing a sample of patient plasma with tissue factor (thromboplastin) and calcium. It is sensitive to deficiencies in fibrinogen, and factors II, V, VII, or X. As three of these factors have vitamin K-dependent synthesis (factors II, VII, and X), the PT assay has been used to monitor anticoagulation with vitamin K antagonists (VKAs) such as warfarin. The thromboplastin reagent, derived from animal or recombinant sources, can vary in its ability to bind factor VII and initiate coagulation, which limits interlaboratory comparisons. Given the importance of monitoring PT results for patients on long-term warfarin therapy, the INR was introduced as a means of normalizing PT results among different laboratories.[122]

Thromboplastin reagents are tested against an international recombinant standard and assigned an international sensitivity index (ISI) based on the results. The INR subsequently is calculated as INR = $(\text{patient PT/standard PT})^{ISI}$, in which the standard PT represents the geometric mean of multiple normal samples from the testing laboratory. Institution of the INR substantially reduced interlaboratory variations. The PT is more sensitive at detecting decreases in factors VII and X than levels of fibrinogen and factors II and V; however, due to variations in thromboplastin reagents, factor levels as low as 40% to 50% may not prolong the PT.[123]

Any prolongation of the PT should be assessed further with mixing studies to determine whether delayed clot formation is attributable to a coagulation factor deficiency or an inhibitor (e.g., antiphospholipid antibody, fibrin degradation products). The mixing study is performed by mixing the patient's plasma sample with "normal" donor plasma. In the case of a coagulation factor deficiency, time to clot formation will correct whereas time to clot formation will not correct in the presence of an inhibitor.

Activated Partial Thromboplastin Time

The aPTT assesses integrity of the intrinsic and common pathways of plasma-mediated hemostasis. It measures the time required in seconds for clot formation to occur after mixing a sample of patient plasma with phospholipid, calcium, and an activator of the intrinsic pathway of coagulation (e.g., celite, kaolin, silica, or ellagic acid). The aPTT is more sensitive to deficiencies in factors VIII and IX than other factors in the intrinsic and common pathways. In most cases, coagulation factor levels below 30% to 40% of normal are detectable; however, aPTT reagents vary in their sensitivity to factor concentrations and may not be prolonged until levels drop below 15% for some factors.[124] Additionally, as there is no reference standard reagent for the aPTT analogous to the INR for PT, individual institutions must set their own normal ranges and aPTT values cannot be compared between laboratories.

Monitoring anticoagulation during cardiac and vascular surgery remains necessary given the widely acknowledged pharmacokinetic and pharmacodynamic response to heparin. Patient-specific factors affecting response to heparin include age, weight, intravascular volume, and concentrations of AT, heparin cofactor II, PF4, and other heparin-binding proteins. Therefore, patients experience widely divergent anticoagulant responses to identical weight-based doses of heparin. In situations where heparin therapy must be initiated in patients with a baseline aPTT prolongation (lupus anticoagulant or factor inhibitors), alternative tests such as anti-factor Xa activity or heparin level measurements must be used.

Anti-Factor Xa Activity

The anti-factor Xa activity assay or factor Xa inhibition test is being used with increasing frequency to monitor heparin anticoagulation instead of, or in addition to, the aPTT assay. The assay involves combining patient plasma with reagent factor Xa and an artificial substrate that releases a colorimetric signal after factor Xa cleavage, thereby providing a functional assessment of heparin anticoagulant effect.[125] While aPTT values can be affected by several patient factors such as coagulation factor deficiencies, factor inhibitors, or the presence of lupus anticoagulant, measurement of the heparin-bound AT inhibition of factor Xa activity is not influenced by these variables. Anti-factor Xa testing can also be used to measure the effect of other anticoagulants such as LMWH, fondaparinux, and factor Xa inhibitors. As with the aPTT assay, the anti-factor Xa test lacks adequate standardization, and activity levels vary based on the type of assay used, and patient population assayed.[126] Furthermore, significant discordance between aPTT and anti-factor Xa results can be observed in hospitalized patients receiving heparin therapy.[127] Data supporting the use of anti-factor Xa over aPTT is sparse; however, it may be helpful to use anti-factor Xa testing in combination with the aPTT to monitor both heparin effect and generalized coagulation status, respectively.

Platelet Count and Bleeding Time

The platelet count remains a standard component in screening for coagulation abnormalities. Automated platelet counts are performed in bulk using either optical-based or impedance-based measurements. Recommendations regarding optimal platelet counts prove somewhat arbitrary, but platelet counts exceeding 100,000 μL commonly are associated with normal hemostasis. Abnormally low platelet counts merit further assessment, including a visual platelet count from a blood smear. Sample hemodilution and platelet clumping are common etiologies for falsely low platelet counts.

With the growth of point-of-care platelet function monitors, the bleeding time has declined in popularity. Limitations of the bleeding time include poor reproducibility, time needed to perform the test, and potential for scarring. Furthermore, the bleeding time is affected by numerous confounding variables, including skin temperature, skin thickness, age, ethnicity, anatomic test location, and a host of other factors.[128] In general, the bleeding time is not predictive of bleeding and for that reason its use as a preoperative screening test to assess bleeding risk is not recommended.[129]

COMMON POINT-OF-CARE MEASURES OF COAGULATION

Although laboratory-based measures of coagulation remain the mainstay of preoperative coagulation testing, increasing availability of sensitive and specific point-of-care coagulation monitoring may soon offer opportunities to direct blood component and hemostatic drug therapy more specifically without delays inherent to standard laboratory testing. Commercially available point-of-care tests applicable in the perioperative setting may be considered in four broad categories: (1) functional measures of coagulation that measure the intrinsic ability of blood to generate clot, (2) heparin concentration monitors, (3) viscoelastic measures of coagulation, and (4) platelet function monitors.

Activated Clotting Time

The activated clotting time (ACT), described by Hattersley in 1966 as a variation of the Lee-White whole blood clotting time, employs a contact activation initiator, typically celite (diatomaceous earth) or kaolin, to accelerate clot formation and reduce time for assay completion.[130] Current commercial ACT monitors automate clot detection. One of the more widely available ACT monitors uses a glass test tube containing a small magnet (Hemochron Response Whole Blood Coagulation System, ITC, Edison, NJ). After adding sample blood, the tube is placed into the analyzer and the tube is rotated slowly at 37°C, allowing the magnet to maintain contact with a proximity detection switch. As fibrin clot forms, the magnet becomes entrapped and dislodged from the detection switch, thereby triggering an alarm to signal completion of the ACT. Another ACT device uses a "plumb bob" flag assembly that is raised and released repeatedly to settle in the sample vial containing blood and contact activator (Hepcon HMS Plus, Medtronic, Minneapolis, MN). With clot formation, the flag descent slows, which triggers an optical detector and sets off an alarm to signal completion of the ACT.

The ACT in normal individuals is 107 ± 13 seconds. Because the ACT measures clot formation by way of intrinsic and common pathways, heparin and other anticoagulants prolong time to clot formation. The ACT proves somewhat resistant to platelet dysfunction and thrombocytopenia. ACT testing remains a popular perioperative coagulation monitor because of its simplicity, low cost, and linear response at high heparin concentrations. Limitations of ACT monitoring include lack of sensitivity at low heparin concentrations and poor reproducibility.[131] Further limitations of the ACT include artefactual prolongation of results with hemodilution or hypothermia, and values beyond 600 seconds exceed the linear response range for the assay. Although duplicate measurements improve results, newer electrochemically based ACT analyzers (i-STAT, Abbott, Princeton, NJ) improve reproducibility such that single ACT determinations may prove adequate.

Heparin Concentration Measurement

Protamine titration remains the most popular point-of-care method for determining heparin concentration in perioperative settings. Protamine, a strongly basic polycationic protein, directly inhibits heparin in a stoichiometric manner. In other words, 1 mg of protamine will inhibit 1 mg (~100 units) of heparin, thereby forming the basis for protamine titration as a measure of heparin concentration. As increasing concentrations of protamine are added to a sample of heparin-containing blood, time to clot formation decreases until the point at which the protamine concentration exceeds heparin concentration to delay clot formation. If a series of blood samples with incremental doses of protamine are analyzed, the sample in which the protamine and heparin concentrations are most closely matched will clot first. This methodology allows for an estimate of heparin concentration. Assuming that the heparin-protamine titration curve for an individual patient remains constant throughout the operative period, protamine titration methods may estimate heparin doses required to achieve a desired plasma heparin concentration or the protamine dose needed to reverse a given heparin concentration in blood.[132] Current point-of-care heparin concentration monitoring employs automated measurement techniques (Hepcon HMS Plus, Medtronic, Minneapolis, MN). The advantages of measuring heparin concentration include sensitivity for low heparin concentrations as well as relative insensitivity to hemodilution and hypothermia. A major limitation of heparin concentration monitoring is failure to assess directly for an anticoagulant effect. For example, consider a patient with a homozygous deficiency of AT; in this case, heparin concentration determination alone would fail to identify the lack of anticoagulant effect after heparin administration.

Viscoelastic Measures of Coagulation

Initially developed in the 1940s, viscoelastic measures of coagulation have undergone a resurgence in popularity. The unique aspect of viscoelastic monitors lies in their ability to measure the entire spectrum of clot formation in whole blood from early fibrin strand generation through clot retraction and fibrinolysis. The early TEG developed by Hartert in 1948 has evolved into two independent viscoelastic monitors: the modern TEG (TEG 5000 Thromboelastograph Hemostasis Analyzer System, Haemoscope, Braintree, MA) and ROTEM (TEM Systems, Durham, NC).[133] In the case of the TEG 5000, a small (0.35-mL) sample of whole blood is placed into a disposable cuvette within the instrument. The cuvette is maintained at a temperature of 37°C and continuously rotates around an axis of approximately 5 degrees. A sensor "piston" attached by a torsion wire to an electronic recorder is lowered into the blood within the cuvette. Addition of an activator, most often kaolin or celite, initiates clot formation. As the fibrin-platelet plug evolves, the piston becomes enmeshed within the clot, transferring rotation of the cuvette to the piston, torsion wire, and electronic recorder.[134]

Although variables derived from the TEG tracing do not coincide directly with laboratory-based tests of coagulation, the TEG depicts characteristic abnormalities in clot formation and fibrinolysis. Various parameters describing clot formation and lysis are identified and measured by the TEG.

For example, the R value (reaction time) measures time to initial clot formation. The R value may be prolonged by a deficiency of one or more plasma coagulation factors or inhibitors such as heparin. Maximum amplitude provides a measure of clot strength and may be decreased by either qualitative or quantitative platelet dysfunction or decreased fibrinogen concentration. The α angle and K (BiKoatuguli-erung or coagulation) values measure rate of clot formation and may be prolonged by any variable slowing clot generation such as a plasma coagulation factor deficiency or heparin anticoagulation. Modification of clotting activators may be incorporated to assess platelet or fibrin contributions to clot strength.

In a somewhat analogous manner, ROTEM measures viscoelastic changes in a sample of whole blood subjected to coagulation activation. Specific activators differ from that of the TEG with resulting quantitative measures termed (1) coagulation time (seconds), (2) α angle (clot formation time; seconds), (3) maximal clot firmness (MCF; millimeter), and (4) lysis time (LT; second)(Fig. 50.5 on TEG in attached file).

In contrast to TEG and ROTEM, an alternative viscoelastic measure of coagulation (Sonoclot Analyzer, Sienco Inc., Arvada, CO) immerses a rapidly vibrating probe into a 0.4-mL sample of blood. As clot formation proceeds, impedance to probe movement through the blood increases to generate an electrical signal and characteristic clot signature. The analyzer signature may be used to derive the ACT and to provide information regarding clot strength and presence of fibrinolysis.

Viscoelastic monitors generate characteristic diagrams by translating mechanical resistance to sensor movement within a sample of whole blood to an electronic waveform subject to quantitative analysis.[133] One of the more common applications for viscoelastic monitoring has been real-time detection of excess fibrinolysis during liver transplantation or cardiac surgery. Evidence suggests that viscoelastic monitoring may prove beneficial in differentiating surgically related bleeding from that due to a coagulopathy. When used as one component of a diagnostic algorithm, both TEG and ROTEM have been demonstrated to reduce blood administration.[135,136] More widespread application of viscoelastic monitoring has been hindered by lack of specificity associated with abnormal findings and qualitative assay interpretation.[137] Digital automation of these instruments has simplified interpretation and improved reproducibility.

Platelet Function Monitors

Assessment of platelet function has proved challenging for several reasons. Historically, tests of platelet function are costly, time consuming, and technically demanding. Platelet dysfunction may occur as a result of diverse inherited or acquired disorders affecting surface receptors involved in adhesion or aggregation, storage granules, internal activation pathways, phospholipid membranes, or other mechanisms.[138] Lack of standardized quality controls necessitates use of local donor blood to establish normal control ranges. Complicating assessment further is the fact that platelets are highly susceptible to activation or desensitization during sample collection, transport, storage, and processing.

The technique for platelet aggregometry was developed in the 1960s and soon became the gold standard for assessment of platelet function.[139] The classic method involves centrifugation of patient blood to obtain platelet-rich plasma, which is then analyzed in a cuvette at 37°C placed between a light source and photocell. Addition of platelet agonists such as ADP, epinephrine, collagen, and ristocetin, stimulates platelet aggregation, which in turn results in a decrease in turbidity of the solution and an increase in light transmission. Patterns based upon the kinetics and amplitude of response to these various agonists are associated with specific platelet disorders and aid in diagnosis.[140] In an effort to decrease the labor required to prepare the platelet rich plasma solution as well as to include the effect of RBCs and plasma proteins on platelet function, a technique for whole blood aggregometry was developed.[141] Whole blood aggregometry uses platinum electrodes onto which platelets adhere. Platelet aggregation induced by agonists results in increased adhesion of aggregates to the electrodes, raising the impedance which is measured over time. A multichannel system (Multiplate Analyzer, Roche Diagnostics, Indianapolis, IN) is available and is used to diagnose platelet dysfunction as well as monitor anti-platelet therapy.[142] Flow cytometry employing fluorescent-labeled antibodies provides another sensitive method for quantitating platelet activation, responsiveness, and surface receptor availability.[143] Despite representing standards of care, these measurements remain technically challenging, costly, and time-consuming laboratory-based assays.

Although viscoelastic measures of coagulation (i.e., TEG or ROTEM) may detect platelet dysfunction, the sensitivity and specificity are limited. Incorporation of a platelet mapping assay into TEG provides a method for viscoelastic measurement of drug-induced platelet inhibition with reasonable correlation to optical aggregometry.[134]

Fortunately, an increasing array of platelet function assays specifically designed as point-of-care instruments are becoming available.[140] As a measure of primary hemostasis, a platelet function analyzer (PFA-100, Siemens, Tarrytown, NY) increasingly has replaced the bleeding time in assessment of hemostasis. The PFA-100 incorporates high-shear conditions to simulate small vessel injury in the presence of either ADP or epinephrine, both potent platelet activators.[144] Time to clot-mediated aperture occlusion is reported as closure time. The PFA-100 has proven effective in detecting vWD and aspirin-mediated platelet dysfunction. This instrument, as a component of a standardized screening protocol, reduces time to identify and classify platelet dysfunction. Limitations of the PFA-100 include interference by thrombocytopenia and hemodilution.

Many other different point-of-care platelet function testing devices are on the market today. It is important to keep in mind that monitors from different manufacturers measure differing aspects of platelet-mediated or plasma-mediated hemostasis. When using different instruments, results may vary from "severe" platelet dysfunction to "no platelet dysfunction" in a single sample of blood. Before adopting any point-of-care monitoring, an understanding of the quality assurance requirements, test methodology, and concomitant strengths and weaknesses are essential to inform patient care. Also, in considering any point-of-care coagulation testing, it must be recognized that results will not necessarily mirror those reported from laboratory-based

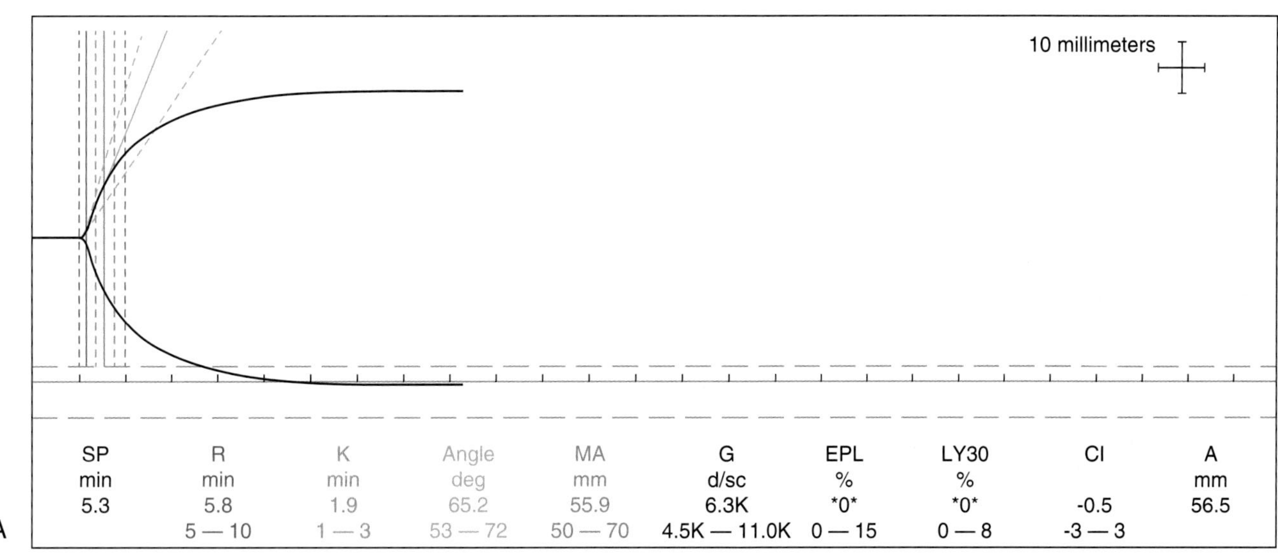

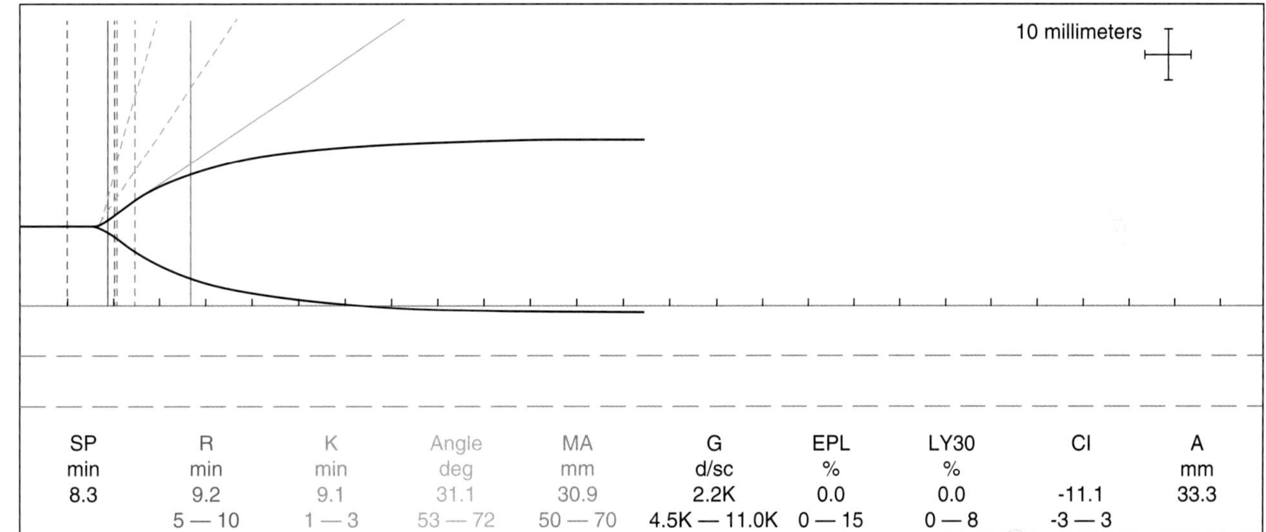

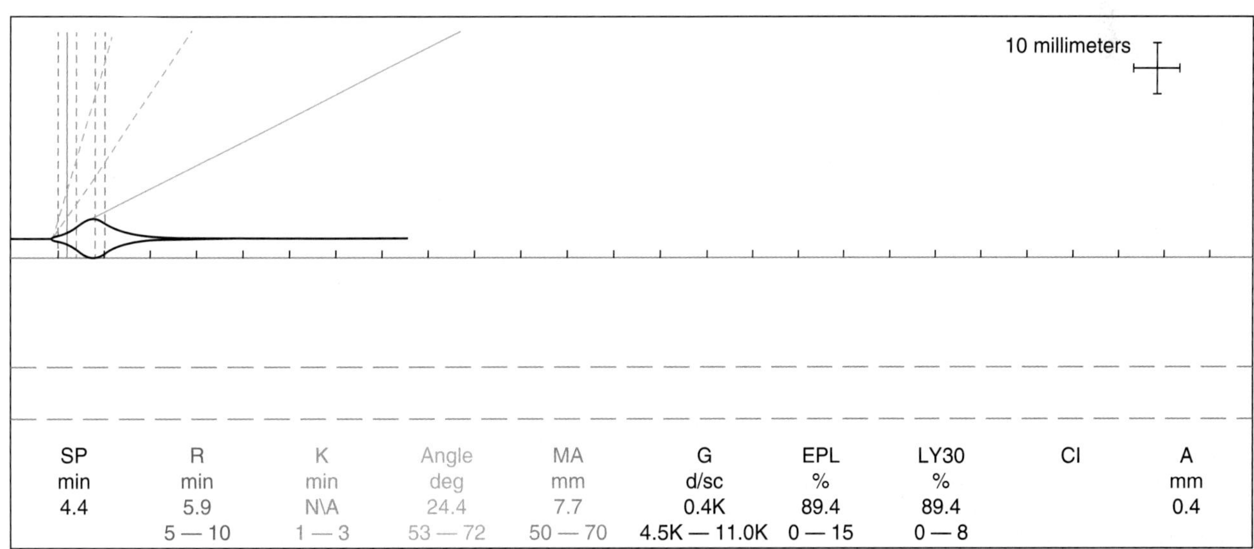

Fig. 50.5 Thromboelastographs from kaolin-activated samples analyzed using a TEG 5000 system depicting (A) normal coagulation, (B) hypofibrinogenemia, and (C) hyperfibrinolysis .

testing because of differences between using whole blood samples for testing as opposed to plasma or processed platelets. Reagent sensitivities can vary across manufacturers and lots. Hopefully, further advances in point-of-care coagulation monitoring will offer the opportunity for clinicians to make informed, bedside decisions about transfusion therapy and hemostatic drug administration to minimize perioperative bleeding and adopt effective patient blood management practices.

Antithrombotics, Thrombolytics, and Procoagulant Drugs

In the following sections, we will briefly review some common medications used to decrease or increase clot formation and then examine perioperative management strategies to reverse anticoagulants. This is not intended to be an exhaustive list of all FDA-approved drugs, so only more commonly used medications are discussed here.

Starting with antithrombotic drugs, these drugs are usually used to reduce the formation of blood clots in the setting of coronary or cerebral atherosclerosis or after vascular thrombosis. They can be further subdivided into antiplatelet agents and anticoagulants (Table 50.1).

TABLE 50.1 Common Classes of Antithrombotics, Thrombolytics, and Procoagulants

Category	Subcategory	Generic Drug Names
Antiplatelet agents	Cyclooxygenase inhibitors	Aspirin, NSAIDS
	P2Y12 receptor antagonists	Ticlopidine, clopidogrel, prasugrel, cangrelor, and ticagrelor
	Platelet GPIIb/IIIa antagonists	Abciximab, eptifibatide, and tirofiban
Anticoagulants	Vitamin K antagonists	Warfarin
	Heparin	UFH, LMWH, fondaparinux
	Direct thrombin inhibitors	Argatroban, bivalirudin (IV) Desirudin (SQ) Dabigatran (PO)
	Factor Xa inhibitors	Rivaroxaban, apixaban, edoxban
Thrombolytics	Fibrin-specific agents	Alteplase, reteplase, tenecteplase
	Non-fibrin-specific agents	Streptokinase
Antifibrinolytics	Lysine analogs	Tranexamic acid, epsilon-aminocaproic acid
Factor Replacements	Recombinant Factor VIIa	
	Factor VIII-vWF	
	Prothrombin complex concentrates	3-factor PCC; 4-factor PCC, activated PCC, FEIBA
	Fibrinogen concentrates	

FEIBA, Factor VIII Bypass Activity; *IV,* intravenous; *LMWH,* low-molecular-weight heparin; *NSAIDS,* nonsteroidal antiinflammatory drugs; *PCC,* prothrombin complex concentrate; *PO,* per os, by mouth; *SQ,* subcutaneous; *UFH,* unfractionated heparin; *vWF,* von Willebrand factor.

ANTIPLATELET AGENTS

Antiplatelet agents inhibit thrombus formation by inhibiting platelet aggregation and/or adhesion to clot or damaged endothelium. Depending on the drug, they can work either reversibly or irreversibly. Most common antiplatelet agents can be divided into: (1) cyclooxygenase (COX) inhibitors, (2) P2Y12 receptor antagonists, and (3) platelet GPIIb/IIIa antagonists, although there are several other classes available such as phosphodiesterase inhibitors, protease-activated receptor-1 antagonists, adenosine reuptake inhibitors, and thromboxane inhibitors.

Cyclooxygenase Inhibitors

Aspirin and NSAIDS are the two primary members of this class. There are two forms of the cyclooxygenase enzyme: COX-1 and COX-2. COX-1 maintains the integrity of the gastric lining and renal blood flow and initiates the formation of thromboxane A_2 (TxA_2), which is important for platelet aggregation. COX-2 is responsible for synthesizing the prostaglandin mediators in pain and inflammation.

Aspirin

Aspirin is a non-selective and irreversible COX inhibitor. It acetylates a serine residue on COX-1 and prevents the production of TxA_2 in platelets.[145] COX-2, which leads to antiinflammatory and analgesic effects, is 170 times less sensitive than COX-1 to aspirin so only at high doses can aspirin irreversibly inhibit both COX-1 and COX-2.[146] Because platelets are anuclear, they are unable to synthesize new COX-1 once aspirin has irreversibly inhibited the enzyme. Consequently, despite its short half-life of approximately 15 to 20 minutes, aspirin's inhibitory effect persists through the platelet lifespan of 7 to 10 days.[147]

The recovery of platelet function after aspirin depends on platelet turnover. Generally, megakaryocytes generate 10% to 12% of platelets daily, so near normal hemostasis is expected in 2 to 3 days after the last dose of aspirin with typical platelet turnover. High platelet turnover diseases, which result from increased production (e.g., essential thrombocythemia) or increased consumption (e.g., inflammation), may require more frequent than once daily aspirin dosing.[148] Immediate reversal of aspirin for emergencies can be achieved with platelet transfusions.

NONSTEROIDAL ANTIINFLAMMATORY DRUGS

Most NSAIDS are nonselective, reversible COX inhibitors and therefore provide antipyretic, analgesic, and antiplatelet aggregation effects.[149] Platelet function normalizes 3 days after discontinuing the use of NSAIDS. Selective COX-2 antagonists such as celecoxib were introduced in the late 1990s to provide antiinflammatory, analgesic, and antipyretic activity without the gastrointestinal complications,[150] but clinical trials with selective COX-2 antagonists have reported increased risks for cardiovascular complications.[151] COX-2 specific inhibitors do not affect platelet function because platelets do not express COX-2. The increased cardiovascular risk is thought to be due to inhibition of PGI_2 without inhibition of TxA_2, thus tipping the balance toward thrombosis. Current recommendations are to use COX-2 inhibitors only when necessary for pain and then with the lowest effective dose possible after weighing the risks and benefits.[152]

P2Y12 RECEPTOR ANTAGONISTS

These drugs (ticlopidine, clopidogrel, prasugrel, cangrelor, and ticagrelor) interfere with platelet function by inhibiting the P2Y12 receptor, which inhibits platelet adhesion and aggregation by preventing the expression of GPIIb/IIIa on the surface of activated platelets.[153] Ticlopidine, clopidogrel, and prasugrel are members of a class known as thienopyridines, and are pro-drugs requiring hepatic metabolism to generate the active metabolite that then irreversibly inactivates the ADP-binding site of the P2Y12 receptor.[154] Ticagrelor and cangrelor are reversible inhibitors.

Clopidogrel (Plavix) is the most commonly prescribed agent in this class. Platelet functions normalize 7 days after discontinuing clopidogrel and 14 to 21 days after discontinuing ticlopidine. Because clopidogrel is a pro-drug and requires CYP2C19 for activation, it has wide interindividual variability in inhibiting ADP-induced platelet function. Although many factors may be involved in this variability, genetic polymorphism of CYP2C19 along with ABCB1, which affects the intestinal permeability and oral bioavailability of clopidogrel, are thought to play a significant role.[155] Patients treated with clopidogrel who have decreased CYP2C19 and ABCB1 activity were shown to have increased risk of major cardiovascular events.[156] The FDA put a black box warning on clopidogrel to make patients and healthcare providers aware that CYP2C19-poor metabolizers, representing up to 14% of patients, are at high risk of treatment failure and that genotype testing may be helpful prior to drug initiation.[157]

Ticagrelor binds to the P2Y12 receptor at a different site than the thienopyridines, and causes a conformational change of the receptor.[158] While ticagrelor needs to undergo metabolism to an active metabolite, both the parent drug and the active metabolite have anti-platelet effects.[159] Genetic polymorphisms do not appear to be clinically relevant for this drug.[160] Because it is much shorter acting than clopidogrel, ticagrelor must be dosed twice daily, which may be of benefit prior to surgery.

The newest drug in this group is cangrelor. It is the only one available for intravenous administration, and like ticagrelor, it changes the conformation of the P2Y12 receptor, resulting in inhibition of ADP-induced platelet aggregation.[158] It received FDA approval in 2015 for adult patients undergoing percutaneous coronary intervention (PCI). This drug has the fastest onset of action (seconds), and platelet function normalizes within 60 minutes after drug discontinuation.[161] This rapid onset may allow for bridging therapy in patients with drug-eluting stents who require surgery.

GLYCOPROTEIN IIB/IIIA INHIBITORS

Glycoprotein IIb/IIIa inhibitors (GPI) (abciximab, eptifibatide, and tirofiban) work to prevent platelet aggregation by decreasing the binding of fibrinogen and vWF to glycoprotein IIb/IIIa receptors on the surface of activated platelets.[162] They are given intravenously in order to: (1) stop ongoing arterial thrombosis or (2) eliminate excessive platelet reactivity in diseased vessels so that occlusive thrombi and restenosis do not occur. Their use was highly touted in the past with balloon angioplasty where acute closure was a feared complication. Now with the introduction of stents and P2Y12 receptor antagonists, GPI have become less popular in routine PCI because of the associated bleeding risk and their use is only recommended in a subset of patients with high risk angiographic features or those not loaded adequately with dual antiplatelet agents.[163] Although abciximab has a short plasma half-life (approximately 10 minutes), its effects on platelet function can be seen for much longer, even after the infusion has been stopped. One rare, but serious side effect to be aware of, abciximab can produce thrombocytopenia immediately after drug administration in a small proportion of patients. Mild thrombocytopenia (platelet count $<100 \times 10^9$/L) developed more frequently in patients treated with the drug than control subjects (4.2% vs. 2.0%; $P < .001$).[164]

ANTICOAGULANTS

Vitamin K Antagonists

Warfarin, the most frequently used oral VKA in the United States, inhibits the vitamin K-dependent carboxylation of coagulation factors II, VII, IX, and X and proteins C and S. Warfarin is highly effective in reducing the risk of venous and arterial thromboemboli, and is still the anticoagulant of choice for patients with valvular atrial fibrillation and mechanical heart valves despite the popularity and increased utilization of DOACs for nonvalvular atrial fibrillation.[165]

Warfarin has a long half-life (40 hours) and the complete anticoagulant effect can take 3 to 4 days to emerge because of the long half-lives of the preexisting coagulation factors. Prothrombin (factor II) has the longest half-life (~60 hours). Factor VII and protein C have the shortest half-lives (3-6 hours).[166] Because of this long initiation period, patients at high risk for thromboembolism must be bridged with another anticoagulant (usually UFH or LMWH) until the target INR is achieved. Also, early reductions in the anticoagulant protein C can cause an imbalance toward a hypercoagulable state if warfarin is started alone, resulting in thrombosis or warfarin-induced skin necrosis.

Warfarin is monitored using the INR, and the therapeutic range for warfarin anticoagulation is generally an INR of 2.0 to 3.0, except for patients with mechanical heart valves, where higher values are necessary (INR 2.5-3.5). The INR is not calibrated to evaluate non-warfarin deficiencies such as liver disease and should not be used to evaluate therapeutic effects of other anticoagulants. Warfarin has a very narrow therapeutic window and can be easily affected by drug-drug interactions and patient variability. The need for frequent laboratory monitoring makes warfarin a difficult drug for patients to maintain compliance and the reported time in therapeutic range is only about 65% ± 20% in patients with atrial fibrillation.[167]

Warfarin's pharmacology can be affected by genetic variations in the metabolism of the drug (CYP2C9) and in the production of a vitamin K epoxide reductase enzyme (VKORC1), which reduces vitamin K after it has been oxidized. Recent meta-analyses of randomized trials found that pharmacogenetics testing for polymorphisms unfortunately did not reduce rates of bleeding or thromboembolism.[168] Current recommendations are to only perform pharmacogenetics testing in patients who consistently have INRs outside the therapeutic range or who have an adverse event while on therapy.[169]

Unfractionated Heparin

UFH can be isolated from porcine or bovine intestines and is a mixture of different length polysaccharides with a high molecular weight (mean molecular weight around 15,000 daltons or 35-45 polysaccharide units).[170] UFH binds to AT and indirectly inhibits thrombin (factor IIa) and factor Xa. Benefits of heparin are its short half-life and full reversibility with protamine. Heparin does not have any fibrinolytic activity, so it will not lyse an existing clot.

Full-dose heparin for cardiac surgery is administered as an intravenous bolus of 300 to 400 U/kg. An ACT greater than 400 to 480 seconds is usually considered safe for initiation of CPB. Patients may be resistant to UFH if they have a hereditary deficiency of AT or an acquired deficiency of AT from prolonged heparin administration. The incidence of heparin resistance during CPB is reported at approximately 21%.[171] Simply increasing the dose of heparin in patients with an AT deficiency is often not effective. For these patients, treatment should be with fresh frozen plasma (FFP) transfusions or AT concentrate, which will replenish AT levels and restore heparin response.[172] Other causes of heparin resistance can be due to increased heparin clearance, increased levels of heparin-binding proteins, or elevations of fibrinogen and factor VIII levels.

Low Molecular Weight Heparin and Fondaparinux

LMWH, produced by cleaving UFH into shorter fragments (mean molecular weight approximately 4000 daltons, approximately 15 saccharide units)[173] and fondaparinux, a synthetic pentasaccharide (mean molecular weight 1700 daltons) of the AT binding region of heparin, act more specifically via AT to inhibit factor Xa. LMWH and fondaparinux do not affect the aPTT assay, and coagulation testing is usually not needed. Anti-factor Xa activity levels may be necessary in patients who may have unpredictable drug levels (e.g., renal failure, pregnancy, and body weight less than 50 kg or more than 80 kg).

LMWH has a longer half-life than heparin and can be administered subcutaneously either once or twice daily. LMWH is primarily excreted by the kidney, so its half-life is prolonged in patients with renal failure. Approximately 25% to 50% of LMWH molecules contain 18 or more saccharide units and can inhibit factor Xa and thrombin, while the remaining 50% to 75% of LMWH molecules contain <18 saccharide units and only inhibit factor Xa. [174] Protamine requires more than 14 saccharide units in the heparin molecule for interaction. [175] Therefore, protamine is only partially effective in reversing LMWH. It does not completely abolish the anti-Xa activity, but it may neutralize the higher molecular weight fractions of LMWH.

Fondaparinux has a much longer half-life (17-21 hours) and can be dosed daily.

Because it is only 5 saccharide units, protamine is not effective for reversing fondaparinux.[176] Because antigen formation by the PF4/heparin complex requires a polysaccharide chain of at least 8 to 10 saccharides, fondaparinux-associated HIT is unlikely to occur,[177] and only eight cases of possible fondaparinux-associated HIT have been reported in the literature.[178] Currently, fondaparinux is not FDA approved for use in HIT, but there is considerable positive anecdotal experience in the literature (e.g., decreased bleeding risk) when compared with DTIs.[179]

Direct Thrombin Inhibitors

DTIs bind directly to thrombin and do not require a cofactor such as antithrombin to exert their effect. All DTIs inhibit thrombin in its free (soluble) and fibrin-bound (insoluble) states, unlike heparin, which only has effect on free thrombin. Other advantages over heparin include: lack of binding to other plasma proteins that leads to a more predictable anticoagulant effect, and no concern for developing an immune-mediated thrombocytopenia.

Hirudin is a naturally occurring anticoagulant found in leeches, while argatroban and bivalirudin are synthetic agents. Argatroban, with a half-life of 45 minutes, is the preferred DTI in patients with renal insufficiency because it is eliminated by the liver. It reversibly binds to the active site on thrombin. Argatroban is FDA approved for the prophylaxis and treatment of thrombosis and for PCI anticoagulation in patients with HIT. Clinical effects are usually monitored with aPTT or ACT in the operating room. Dosing goals are to maintain an aPTT 1.5 to 3 times baseline. Because argatroban prolongs thrombin-dependent coagulation, the PT and INR will be prolonged as well, which can complicate transition to warfarin therapy for long-term anticoagulation.[180]

Bivalirudin, a 20-amino acid synthetic analogue of hirudin, is a reversible DTI, and is metabolized by proteolytic cleavage and hepatic metabolism.[181] It has the shortest half-life among the intravenous DTIs and is the drug of choice for patients with both renal and hepatic dysfunction, although dose adjustments are still necessary. In studies, bivalirudin has been shown to have better efficacy in preventing primary outcomes with lower bleeding rates when compared with UFH for percutaneous transluminal coronary angioplasty for unstable or postinfarction angina,[182] and for use as an alternative to heparin in patients with HIT undergoing PCI.[183]

Desirudin was approved in 2010 and is the only DTI available for subcutaneous administration. An early, small, open label study (16 patients) showed that desirudin may be a potentially cost-effective alternative to argatroban for patients with suspected HIT.[184] Desirudin also has more predictable pharmacokinetics, and dosage adjustments and aPTT monitoring may be unnecessary in patients with a creatinine clearance greater than 30 mL/min.[185]

Direct Oral Anticoagulants

Several new oral anticoagulants have been introduced into the market over the past 10 years. These new drugs have more predictable pharmacokinetics and pharmacodynamics and fewer drug-drug interactions, allowing them to be dosed without daily laboratory monitoring. The drawback has been the lack of specific antidotes for anticoagulation reversal, but this is slowly changing with the introduction of idarucizumab.

Most DOACs are approved for prevention of venous thromboembolism after hip or knee replacement surgery, treatment and secondary prevention of venous thromboembolism, and prevention of stroke in nonvalvular atrial fibrillation. Many are also being studied for use in secondary prevention of coronary events after acute coronary syndrome, prevention of thrombosis in elective PCI, and prevention of thrombus formation on mechanical heart valves. The results from early preclinical trials have been positive and encourage further randomized trials, so increased impact of these agents in the future is expected.[186] The DOACs have a shorter half-life than warfarin and have demonstrated noninferior efficacy to warfarin. A meta-analysis of phase II and phase III randomized clinical trials comparing DOACs with VKAs in patients with atrial fibrillation showed that use of DOACs was associated with a significant reduction in major bleeding (Relative risk [RR] 0.86, 95% CI 0.72-1.02) and a significantly decreased risk of intracranial hemorrhage (RR 0.46, 95% CI 0.39-0.56).[187]

Dabigatran (Pradaxa), an oral DTI, was the first new antithrombotic agent approved for the prevention of ischemic stroke in patients with non-valvular atrial fibrillation since warfarin. When given at a dose of 150 mg twice daily, dabigatran was shown to reduce the risk of stroke while having a similar bleeding risk as warfarin at an INR of 2.0 to 3.0.[188] Although the bleeding risk is similar, the bleeding profile does differ between the two drugs. Dabigatran increases the risk of major gastrointestinal bleeding but lowers the risk of intracranial bleeding when compared with warfarin.[189] Dabigatran is predominantly eliminated by the kidneys, so the dose should be reduced in patients with a creatinine clearance less than 30 mL/min.

Monitoring of dabigatran therapy is difficult because the perfect laboratory test does not exist. The aPTT does not become linear until dabigatran concentrations are quite high (>200 ng/mL).[190] The TT is very sensitive to dabigatran, so while it is useful to detect any presence of the drug, it cannot be used to quantify the amount of drug present.[191] If available, dilute TT or ecarin clotting time are both linear at clinically relevant dabigatran concentrations and are the tests of choice if monitoring is necessary.[192]

Direct Xa inhibitors, rivaroxaban (Xarelto), apixaban (Eliquis), and edoxaban (Savaysa) are agents whose activity is directed against the active site of factor Xa. Factor Xa inhibitors have been associated with fewer strokes and embolic events, fewer intracranial hemorrhages, and lower all-cause mortality compared with warfarin.[193] A comparison of apixaban versus warfarin in patients with atrial fibrillation showed a reduction in stroke risk along with a significant reduction in major bleeding.[194] The anti-factor Xa assays are the tests best suited for monitoring the effects of the direct Xa inhibitors, but assays must be individually calibrated for each drug.[192]

THROMBOLYTICS

Thrombolytic therapy is used to break up or dissolve blood clots. These medications are most commonly used during acute myocardial infarctions, strokes, massive pulmonary embolus, arterial thromboembolism, and venous thrombosis. Thrombolytics may be given through an intravenous line systemically or directly to the site of the blockage. Most thrombolytic agents are serine proteases that work by converting plasminogen to plasmin. Plasmin then lyses the clot by breaking down fibrinogen and fibrin. Fibrinolytic agents are divided into two categories: (1) fibrin-specific agents and (2) non–fibrin-specific agents. Fibrin-specific agents are alteplase (tPA), reteplase, and tenecteplase. They theoretically produce less plasminogen conversion in the absence of fibrin and result in less fibrinogen depletion. Non–fibrin-specific agents (e.g., streptokinase) catalyze systemic fibrinolysis. Streptokinase, produced by beta-hemolytic streptococci, is highly antigenic and can cause immunologic sensitization and allergic reactions, particularly with repeat administration even several years after previous exposure.[195] Streptokinase is not widely used in the United States but is still used internationally because of its lower cost.

t-PAs are both thrombolytics and anticoagulants because as mentioned earlier, fibrinolysis generates increased amounts of circulating fibrin degradation products, which inhibit platelet aggregation. Surgery or puncture of noncompressible vessels is contraindicated within a 10-day period after the use of thrombolytic drugs.

Time is usually of the essence when administering these drugs. Medical providers should quickly obtain a history and physical exam, review absolute and relative contraindications, (Table 50.2), order relevant laboratory tests, request necessary consultations, and proceed with decision making. Many studies have investigated the use of thrombolytics in acute pulmonary embolus, ST-elevation myocardial infarction (STEMI), and ischemic stroke. Thrombolytics are indicated in the setting of hemodynamic instability due to acute pulmonary embolus.[196] A meta-analysis in patients with massive pulmonary embolism found that systemic thrombolytic therapy decreased the composite endpoint of death and recurrent thromboembolism (9.4% vs. 19%, odds ratio 0.45, 95% CI 0.22-0.92).[197] Primary PCI is the preferred treatment for patients with acute STEMI if it can be performed by an experienced operator within 2 hours from presentation to the emergency department, but fibrinolytic therapy remains an important modality in hospitals with limited primary PCI

TABLE 50.2 Absolute and Relative Contraindications for Thrombolytics

Absolute Contraindications	Relative Contraindications
Vascular lesions	Ischemic stroke >3 months prior
Severe, uncontrolled hypertension (SBP > 185 or DBP > 110)	Active peptic ulcer
Recent cranial surgery or trauma	Current use of anticoagulant drugs
Brain tumor	Pregnancy
Ischemic stroke <3 months prior	Prolonged/traumatic CPR <3 weeks prior
Active bleeding	Major surgery <3 weeks prior

CPR, Cardiopulmonary resuscitation; *DBP*, diastolic blood pressure; *SBP*, systolic blood pressure.

availability. Early thrombolysis was associated with a lower mortality rate. When compared between less than 2 hours versus greater than 4 hours from time of symptom presentation to thrombolysis administration, 30-day mortality was decreased with earlier administration (5.5% vs. 9%).[198] For stroke care, the primary goal is to restore blood flow to ischemic regions in order to reduce stroke-related disability and mortality. Alteplase is the recommended therapy for treatment of acute ischemic stroke if treatment can be initiated within 4.5 hours of symptom onset.[199] Mechanical thrombectomy should still be considered even if thrombolysis has been administered for ischemic stroke.

PROCOAGULANT DRUGS

Anesthesiologists may use procoagulant drugs for individuals at risk of bleeding to help control blood loss during surgery. These drugs can be divided into two different classes: antifibrinolytics and factor replacements. (see Table 50.1).

Antifibrinolytics

There are two types of antifibrinolytics, the lysine analogs, epsilon-aminocaproic acid (EACA) and TXA, and a SERPIN, aprotinin. Aprotinin was removed from the US market due to concerns of renal and cardiovascular toxicity and is now only available in Europe and Canada. The lysine analogs act by competitively inhibiting the binding site on plasminogen, leading to inhibition of plasminogen activation as well as preventing plasminogen binding of fibrin, therefore impairing fibrinolysis.[200] TXA has been more thoroughly studied than EACA, but aside from subtle differences, both agents appear to have similar efficacy and have been shown to decrease perioperative blood loss.

TXA has been studied in the large CRASH-2 trial of patients admitted after trauma and was associated with a reduction in all-cause mortality (14.5% vs. 16%, P = .0035), including the risk of death due to bleeding (4.9% vs. 5.8%, P = .0077), without an increase in vascular occlusive events.[100] Subgroup analysis of the CRASH-2 data showed that early treatment (≤1 hour) after traumatic injury significantly reduced the risk of death due to bleeding events in the TXA group (RR 0.68; 95% CI, 0.57-0.82; P < .0001). RR was also lower 0.79 (95% CI, 0.64-0.97; P = .03) if TXA was administered between 1 and 3 hours; however, treatment after 3 hours seemed to increase death due to bleeding, with a RR of 1.44 (95% CI, 1.12-1.84; P = .004).[101]

Aside from trauma, there are also trials studying use of TXA in cardiac surgery, orthopedic surgery, neurosurgery, hepatic surgery, and obstetric and gynecology surgery. The World Maternal Antifibrinolytic Trial (WOMAN) found that administration of TXA reduced death due to bleeding in women with postpartum hemorrhage, especially if given within 3 hours of birth, and was not associated with an increase in adverse effects.[201] In a recent meta-analysis in surgical patients, TXA reduced the probability of receiving a blood transfusion by a third (risk ratio 0.62; 95% CI, 0.58-0.65; P < .001). [202] Fewer deaths occurred in the TXA group (risk ratio 0.61; 95% CI, 0.38-0.98; P = .04), but the effect of TXA on myocardial infarction (risk ratio 0.68; 95% CI, 0.43-1.09; P = .11), stroke (risk ratio 1.14; 95% CI, 0.65-2.00; P = .65), deep vein thrombosis (risk ratio 0.86; 95% CI, 0.53-1.39; P = .54), and pulmonary embolism (risk ratio 0.61; 95% CI, 0.25-1.47; P = .27) was inconclusive. A Cochrane review also found that TXA significantly reduced blood transfusions by 39%; however, TXA was not associated with decreased mortality in all surgeries in their analysis.[203]

Overall, the lysine analogs (TXA and EACA) appear to be inexpensive and low risk adjunctive agents that should be considered for use in major surgery or critical bleeding. The rate of thrombosis does not appear to be elevated, but further studies are necessary before this can be definitively concluded. In terms of side effects, there is a reported dose-response relationship of high-dose TXA and seizures in patients undergoing cardiac surgery.[204] The reported mechanism is TXA binding to $GABA_A$ receptors, subsequently blocking $GABA_A$-mediated inhibition in the central nervous system.[205]

Factor Replacements

Recombinant Factor VIIa. Recombinant factor VIIa (rFVIIa) increases the generation of thrombin via the intrinsic and extrinsic pathways to enhance hemostasis. The drug was originally FDA approved for use in hemophilia patients. It binds to tissue factor at the site of vessel injury and to the surface of the activated platelet, leading to activation of factor X. Both mechanisms result in a "burst" of thrombin and fibrin generation, which leads to clot formation. The half-life of rFVIIa is only 2 to 2.5 hours, so the initial dose may require repeating until the bleeding is controlled.

Successful use of rFVIIa in hemophilia patients with inhibitors generated a great deal of interest in the drug's ability to enhance hemostasis in hemorrhaging patients without a preexistent coagulation disorder. This off-label use of rFVIIa had been quite varied, and included patients with intracranial hemorrhage,[206,207] trauma,[208,209] and traumatic brain injury,[210] and patients undergoing cardiac surgery[211] and liver transplantation.[212,213] While treatment with rFVIIa reduced the progression of the hematoma following intracranial hemorrhage and reduced the risk of acute respiratory distress syndrome (risk reduction, −0.05; 95% CI, −0.02 to −0.08) in trauma patients, mortality or functional outcomes were not improved in any patient subset.[211]

As the off-label use of rFVIIa increased, there were more troubling reports of arterial and venous thromboses. A review studying the safety of off-label rFVIIa reported a higher rate of arterial thromboembolic events with the use of rFVIIa compared with placebo (5.5% vs. 3.2%, P = .003), and an increased observed rate for coronary events (2.9% vs. 1.1%, P = .002). [214] This rate was noted to be increased with age (for patients aged 65-74 years, OR 2.12; 95% CI: 0.95-4.71 and for those ≥75 years, OR 3.02, 95% CI: 1.22-7.48), as well as higher doses. Considering that no randomized controlled trial has been able to demonstrate a significant benefit in terms of intensive care stay, hospital stay, or mortality, guidelines currently recommend that rFVIIa no longer be used for the off-label indications of prevention and treatment of bleeding in patients without hemophilia.[215] Each clinician will have to weigh the risk of thromboembolic events against the benefit for the refractory bleeding patient where the "last ditch" use of rFVIIa in massive hemorrhage has not been formally assessed.

Prothrombin Complex Concentrate. PCCs are commercially available purified concentrates containing varying amounts of vitamin K-dependent coagulation factors. Three-factor PCCs differ from 4-factor PCCs in that they do not contain significant amounts of factor VII. Most of the factors are preserved in the inactive state, with the aim of decreasing thrombogenic risk; however, FEIBA is a 4-factor PCC that contains activated factor VII. The products may also contain coagulation inhibitors such as heparin, AT, protein C, and protein S to mitigate the thrombotic risk by providing more balanced replacement of procoagulant factors and anticoagulant proteins.

While PCCs are derived from human plasma, they are treated with at least one viral reduction process, reducing the risk of transfusion-transmitted infection and the lower administration volume decreases the risk of transfusion-associated circulatory overload (TACO).[216] While PCCs appear to be safe and have low risk of thrombosis, there is accumulating evidence that the level of factor II and its balance with the coagulation inhibitors may be the important key.[217]

Fibrinogen Concentrate. Fibrinogen concentrate is produced from pooled human plasma, but viral inactivation steps are incorporated into the manufacturing. It can be used to correct hypofibrinogenemia with the goals of reducing coagulopathy, bleeding, and transfusion requirements. Fibrinogen concentrate offers benefits over FFP and cryoprecipitate in terms of standardized fibrinogen content, low infusion volume, and faster time to administration due to rapid reconstitution. Alternatively, cryoprecipitate and FFP are cheaper, and they also provide additional procoagulant factors that could be beneficial during massive bleeding. In a recent meta-analysis, seven randomized controlled trials showed a significant reduction in bleeding and transfusion requirements with the use of fibrinogen concentrates, but data on mortality were lacking and there was significant heterogeneity among the trials.[218] While the data are inconclusive, some hospitals have incorporated fibrinogen concentrate into algorithms based on viscoelastic coagulation tests with the goal of reducing transfusion requirements.

Perioperative Management of Anticoagulation

The perioperative management of patients who require chronic anticoagulation or antiplatelet therapy involves balancing the risk of surgical bleeding against the risk of developing postoperative thromboembolism. Patients should be evaluated with enough time prior to elective surgery to perform these necessary risk assessments and make management decisions regarding discontinuation and reinstitution of anticoagulation or antiplatelet therapy.

VITAMIN K ANTAGONISTS

For patients taking VKAs, the current recommendation is to stop VKAs 5 days prior to surgery for those who are at low risk for perioperative thromboembolism (Table 50.3). VKAs should be restarted 12 to 24 hours postoperatively if there is adequate hemostasis. For patients at high risk of thromboembolism, bridging anticoagulation with UFH or LMWH after discontinuation of VKAs should occur. The difficulty arises in defining a plan for patients who are at moderate risk. No definitive evidence exists, so the approach chosen should be based on individual patient and surgical risk factors.[219]

TABLE 50.3 Perioperative Thromboembolism Risk Stratification

Risk	Indication
High	Mechanical heart valve
	Rheumatic valvular heart disease
	CHADS score ≥ 5
	VTE within 3 months or h/o VTE when VKAs are discontinued
Moderate	CHADS score of 3 or 4
	VTE between 3 and 12 months or h/o recurrence
	Active cancer
Low	CHADS score 0-2
	VTE > 12 months prior and no other risk factors

CHADS, Congestive heart failure, hypertension, age ≥ 75, diabetes mellitus, prior stroke; *VKA*, vitamin K antagonists; *VTE*, venous thromboembolism.

HEPARINS

For those patients receiving bridging therapy with UFH, the infusion should be stopped 4 to 6 hours prior to surgery[220] and resumed without a bolus dose no sooner than 12 hours postoperatively. In surgeries with high postoperative bleeding risk, resumption of UFH should be delayed 48 to 72 hours until adequate hemostasis has been achieved. In patients receiving bridging therapy with LMWH, the last dose of LMWH should be administered 24 hours prior to surgery and dosing should be resumed 24 hours postoperatively in low bleeding risk surgery and delayed until 48 to 72 hours postoperatively for surgeries with high bleeding risk.[219]

ASPIRIN

For patients receiving aspirin therapy, risk assessment is based on (1) the patient's risk of a perioperative cardiovascular event; (2) whether the surgery is a minor procedure, major procedure, or cardiac procedure; and (3) the timing and type of stent placement for those patients who have undergone recent PCI. Low-dose aspirin (acetylsalicylic acid, ASA) has been shown to reduce the risk of stroke and myocardial infarction by 25% to 30%,[221,222] and studies report significant increased risk with the withdrawal of low-dose aspirin because of a platelet rebound phenomenon that leads to increased thrombus stability, improved fibrin crosslinking, and decreased fibrinolysis.[223] The decision to discontinue low-dose aspirin must weigh the risks of bleeding versus the benefits of cardiovascular risk reduction. Studies suggest that perioperative aspirin use may lead to a small increase in the risk for major bleeding (2.9% vs. 2.4%, $P = .04$), [222,224] but continuation of perioperative aspirin may confer a significant reduction in myocardial infarction and other major cardiovascular events (1.8% vs. 9.0%, $P = .02$). [225]

Recommendations currently are to continue aspirin for patients who are at moderate to high risk for cardiovascular events requiring noncardiac surgery and only stop aspirin use 7 to 10 days prior to surgery for patients at low risk for cardiovascular events.[226] Patients who are having minor procedures (e.g., minor dental, dermatologic procedures, or cataract surgery) and are on aspirin for the secondary prevention of cardiovascular disease should continue taking it in the perioperative period.

Patients with coronary stents presenting for surgery are problematic because of the concerns for in-stent thrombosis that can occur with stopping antiplatelet therapy. Surgery should be delayed if possible for at least 6 weeks after bare-metal stent placement and for at least 6 months after drug-eluting stent placement.[227] If surgery is required before this time has passed, dual anti-platelet therapy should be continued unless the risk of bleeding is thought to outweigh the risk of stent thrombosis.

Many studies have examined management of aspirin therapy perioperatively; however, there is much less data for management of clopidogrel in the perioperative setting. In most clinical situations, aspirin provides benefit that outweighs the bleeding risk and should be continued unless the patient is undergoing intracranial procedures, transurethral prostatectomy, intraocular procedures, or surgeries with extremely high bleeding risk.[228] The data are inconclusive about use of bridging therapy for patients with coronary stents who require noncardiac surgery. For patients with a very high risk of stent thrombosis, bridging therapy with intravenous, reversible glycoprotein inhibitors or a reversible intravenous P2Y12 inhibitor have been suggested, but concomitant parenteral anticoagulation therapy is not recommended.

NEURAXIAL ANESTHESIA AND ANTICOAGULATION

In addition to surgical bleeding risk assessment, many patients who are on anticoagulant or antiplatelet therapy can potentially benefit from neuraxial anesthetics. Management of perioperative anticoagulation is becoming increasingly more complex with the advent of the DOACs and the number of patients who are now receiving chronic anticoagulation. There is a lack of randomized controlled trials showing safety in the timing of surgical procedures and regional anesthesia because a broad clinical experience with these drugs along with neuraxial techniques does not exist. Most guidelines in the literature are based exclusively on the pharmacokinetics and pharmacodynamics of these drugs.[229] These guidelines and recommendations will continue to be updated as evidence emerges on the bleeding risk and pharmacologic profiles of the newer anticoagulants. In the absence of concrete data, many hospital committees are setting local practice guidelines (Table 50.4). Early preoperative assessment of patients receiving anticoagulation and a multidisciplinary team approach between the patient, primary care physician, surgeon, anesthesiologist, and hematologist is essential to ensure the perioperative safety of these patients. Continued research on thromboembolic events and bleeding risk in the setting of these novel therapies is needed before official recommendations can be made regarding management.

TABLE 50.4 UCSF Guidelines for the Use of Antithrombotic Agents in the Setting of Neuraxial Procedures

Anticoagulant	Minimum Time Between the Last Dose and When Neuraxial Catheter can Occur	Minimum Time After Catheter Placement to Drug Start	Minimum Time Between Last Dose of Drug and Catheter Removal	Minimum Time Between Neuraxial Catheter Removal and When Next Dose can be Given
NSAIDs/ASA	No restrictions for catheter placement or removal			
Heparin SQ BID	No restrictions for catheter placement or removal			
Heparin SQ TID	4 h	2 h	4 h	2 h
Lovenox qD	12 h	6 h	12 h	4 h
Warfarin	5 days and INR < 1.5	Contraindicated while catheter in place		2 h
Clopidogrel	7 days	Contraindicated while catheter in place		2 h
Ticlodipine	14 days	Contraindicated while catheter in place		2 h
Dabigatran	5 days	Contraindicated while catheter in place		6 h
Rivaroxaban	3 days	Contraindicated while catheter in place		6 h
Apixaban	3 days	Contraindicated while catheter in place		6 h
Abciximab	48 h	Contraindicated while catheter in place		2 h
Eptifibatide	8 h	Contraindicated while catheter in place		2 h
Alteplase*	10 days	Contraindicated while catheter in place		10 days

*Full dose for stroke or myocardial infarction. No time restrictions for catheter placement or removal with low dose (2 mg) for catheter clearance

ASA, acetylsalicylic acid; *BID*, two times a day; *INR*, international normalized ratio; *NSAIDs*, nonsteroidal antiinflammatory drugs; *qD*, once a day; SQ, subcutaneous; *TID*, three times a day. Adapted from UCSF Guidelines for the use of antithrombotic agents in the setting of neuraxial procedures and Horlocker TT, Wedel DJ, Rowlingson JC, et al. Regional anesthesia in the patient receiving antithrombotic or thrombolytic therapy: American Society of Regional Anesthesia and Pain Medicine Evidence-Based Guidelines (third edition). *Reg Anesth Pain Med.* 2010; 35:64–101.

Emergent Reversal of Anticoagulants

VITAMIN K ANTAGONISTS

The incidence of VKA-associated major bleeding is between 1.1% and 8.1% per year depending on the study design.[230,231] Some of these patients will require warfarin reversal for bleeding and other patients will require warfarin reversal prior to emergency surgery. Four-factor PCCs as opposed to three-factor PCCs are now the drug of choice for emergent reversal of oral VKA in place of FFP or rFVIIa,[232] but PCCs only provide a transient correction due to the short half-life of these factors relative to the long half-life of warfarin. Concomitant administration of vitamin K is required to restore carboxylation of the vitamin K dependent factors (VKDFs) by the liver and provide a more sustained correction after the factors in the PCC infusion have been metabolized. Intravenous administration of vitamin K gives a more rapid response than subcutaneous or oral administration.[233] The dose required depends on the clinical situation and the need to be able to re-establish anticoagulation after surgery. For instance, lower doses (3 mg) may allow for warfarin reversal during the acute event, while avoiding warfarin resistance if rapid re-establishment of a therapeutic INR is required.[234]

Rapid reversal of VKA with FFP is difficult and often unrealistic. Time to thaw ABO-compatible units is a concern, but the large volume required to raise the VKDF by 50% is often untenable, especially in a patient population prone to pulmonary, renal, and cardiac disease.[235] There are also concerns for transmission of viral diseases, and transfusion-related complications such as volume overload, TACO, and lung injury (transfusion-related acute lung injury). In a recent randomized controlled trial using 4-factor PCC to reverse VKA prior to surgery or invasive interventions, effective hemostasis was higher (90% PCC vs. 75% FFP), fluid overload was lower (3% PCC vs. 13% FFP), and thromboembolic events were similar compared with patients who received FFP (7% PCC vs. 8% FFP).[236]

DIRECT THROMBIN INHIBITORS

There are no direct reversal agents for intravenous DTIs; however, their half-lives are relatively short, so time and supportive medical care are often sufficient to manage their anticoagulant effect in acute clinical situations. For the DOACs, idarucizumab, a specific antidote for dabigatran, is a humanized antibody fragment that binds to dabigatran with an affinity 350 times greater than thrombin. The drug received FDA approval in 2015 and can completely reverse the anticoagulant effect of dabigatran in minutes.[237] Andexanet alfa, a recombinant derivative of factor Xa, was developed to reverse the factor Xa inhibitors by acting as a decoy. It has a higher affinity for factor Xa inhibitors than intrinsic factor Xa. The drug was recently approved by the FDA for patients who present with an acute hemorrhage while receiving apixaban or rivaroxaban. The indication currently does not cover edoxaban, or enoxaparin.[238,239]

EMERGING AGENTS

There are additional reversal agents in development that may be approved by the FDA soon. Ciraparantag (PER977), a small, synthetic, water-soluble, cationic molecule, binds and neutralizes UFH, LMWH, fondaparinux, dabigatran, and factor Xa inhibitors through hydrogen bonding and charge-charge interactions. Phase I trials have been completed in healthy volunteers.[240] Common anticoagulants and possible reversal agents for emergencies are listed for reference in Table 50.5.

TABLE 50.5 Common Anticoagulants Along with the Required Laboratory Monitoring and Possible Reversal Agents for Emergencies

Antithrombotic Agent	Drug Name	Stop Before Procedure	Monitoring	Reversal Agents
Antiplatelet agents	ASA P2Y12 receptor antagonists GPIIb/IIIa antagonists	7 days 7-14 days 24-72 h	None	Platelet transfusion
Vitamin K antagonists	Warfarin	2-5 days	PT, INR	PCC, FFP, vitamin K
Heparins	Unfractionated heparin (UFH)(IV)	6 h	aPTT	Protamine
	Low-molecular weight heparin (LMWH)	12-24 h	None required, but fXa levels can monitor levels	Partially reversed by protamine
Pentasaccharide	Fondaparinux	3 days (prophylactic dosing)	None required, but fXa levels can monitor levels	None
Direct thrombin inhibitors	Argatroban, Bivalirudin	4-6 h 3 h	aPTT or ACT	None
	Dabigatran	2-4 days (longer if renal impairment)	None required, thrombin time can monitor levels	Idarucizumab
FXa inhibitors	Rivaroxaban, Apixaban, Edoxaban	2-3 days 2-3 days 2-3 days	None required, but fXa levels can monitor levels	Andexanet alfa for rivaroxaban and apixaban

ACT, activated clotting time; *aPTT*, activated partial thromboplastin time; *ASA*, acetylsalicylic acid; *FFP*, fresh frozen plasma; *INR*, international normalized ratio; *IV*, intravenous; *PCC*, prothrombin complex concentrate; *PT*, prothrombin time.

Conclusion

The coagulation system remains exceedingly complex, but an understanding of the fundamental principles of hemostasis will allow the anesthesia provider to identify patients at risk of bleeding preoperatively, and safely manage blood loss and treat acquired coagulopathy both intraoperatively and postoperatively. Given the abundance of different antithrombotic and anticoagulant medications, perioperative management is becoming increasingly challenging. Early preoperative assessment of patients receiving anticoagulation and a multidisciplinary team approach between the patient, primary care physician, hematologist, surgeon, and anesthesiologist is essential to ensure the perioperative safety of these patients.

 **Complete references available online at expertconsult.com.**

Acknowledgment

The editors and publisher would like to thank Drs. Thomas F. Slaughter, Lawrence T. Goonough, and Terri G. Monk for their contributions in the prior edition of this work. Excerpts of their chapters were incorporated and serve as the foundation for the current chapter.

References

1. Furie B, et al. *N Engl J Med*. 2008;359(9):938–949.
2. van Hinsbergh VW, et al. *Semin Immunopathol*. 2012;34(1):93–106.
3. Moncada S, et al. *Nature*. 1976;263(5579):663–665.
4. Broekman MJ, et al. *Blood*. 1991;78(4):1033–1040.
5. Marcus AJ, et al. *J Clin Invest*. 1997;99(6):1351–1360.
6. Esmon CT, et al. *Semin Thromb Hemost*. 2006;32(suppl 1):49–60.
7. Mertens G, et al. *J Biol Chem*. 1992;267(28):20435–22043.
8. Wood JP, et al. *Blood*. 2014;123(19):2934–2943.
9. Wolberg AS, et al. *Anesth Analg*. 2012;114(2):275–285.
10. Chiu JJ, et al. *Physiol Rev*. 2011;91(1):327–387.
11. Stern D, et al. *Proc Natl Acad Sci U S A*. 1985;82(8):2523–2527.
12. Margetic S. *Biochem Med (Zagreb)*. 2012;22(1):49–62.
13. Van De Craen B, et al. *Thromb Res*. 2012;130(4):576–585.
14. Achneck HE, et al. *Vascular*. 2008;16(suppl 1):S6–13.
15. Kassis J, et al. *Blood*. 1992;80(7):1758–1764.
16. Broos K, et al. *Thromb Res*. 2012;129(3):245–249.
17. Hanson SR, et al. *Blood*. 1985;66(5):1105–1109.
18. Broos K, et al. *Blood Rev*. 2011;25(4):155–167.
19. Wu YP, et al. *Arterioscler Thromb Vasc Biol*. 2000;20(6):1661–1667.
20. Brass L. *Hematology Am Soc Hematol Educ Program*. 2010;2010: 387–396.
21. Macfarlane RG. *Nature*. 1964;202:498–499.
22. Hoffman. *J Thromb Thrombolysis*. 2003;16(1-2):17–20.
23. Coughlin SR. *J Thromb Haemost*. 2005;3(8):1800–1814.
24. Schenone M, et al. *Curr Opin Hematol*. 2004;11(4):272–277.
25. Mann KG, et al. *Blood Cells Mol Dis*. 2006;36(2):108–117.
26. Furie B, et al. *N Engl J Med*. 1992;326(12):800–806.
27. Osterud B, et al. *Proc Natl Acad Sci U S A*. 1977;74(12):5260–5264.
28. Renne T. *Semin Immunopathol*. 2012;34(1):31–41.
29. Hoffman M. *Blood Rev*. 2003;17(suppl 1):S1–5.
30. Furie B, et al. *J Thromb Haemost*. 2007;5(suppl 1):12–17.
31. Pisano JJ, et al. *Science*. 1968;160(3830):892–893.
32. Levy JH, et al. *Transfusion*. 2013;53(5):1120–1131.
33. Crawley JT, et al. *J Thromb Haemost*. 2007;5(suppl 1):95–101.
34. Barshtein G, et al. *Expert Rev Cardiovasc Ther*. 2007;5(4):743–752.
35. Kolev K, et al. *Thromb Haemost*. 2003;89(4):610–621.
36. Woodruff RS, et al. *J Thromb Thrombolysis*. 2011;32(1):9–20.
37. Andrews RK, et al. *Arterioscler Thromb Vasc Biol*. 2007;27(7):1511–1520.
38. Crawley JT, et al. *Arterioscler Thromb Vasc Biol*. 2008;28(2):233–242.
39. Broze GJ, et al. *Proc Natl Acad Sci U S A*. 1987;84(7):1886–1890.
40. Esmon CT. *Chest*. 2003;123):26S–32S.
41. Perry DJ. *Blood Rev*. 1994;8(1):37–55.
42. Tollefsen DM, et al. *J Biol Chem*. 1982;257(5):2162–2169.
43. Segal JB, et al. *Transfusion*. 2005;45(9):1413–1425.
44. Chee YL, et al. *Br J Haematol*. 2008;140(5):496–504.
45. Greaves M, et al. *J Thromb Haemost*. 2007;5(suppl 1):167–174.
46. Sadler JE. *Annu Rev Med*. 2005;56:173–1791.
47. Dinehart SM, et al. *Dermatol Surg*. 2005;31(7 Pt 2):819–826. discussion 26.
48. Leebeek FW, et al. *N Engl J Med*. 2016;375(21):2067–2080.
49. Rodeghiero F, et al. *Blood*. 1987;69(2):454–459.
50. Brinkhous KM, et al. *Proc Natl Acad Sci U S A*. 1985;82(24):8752–8756.
51. Lippi G, et al. *Blood Coagul Fibrinolysis*. 2007;18(4):361–364.
52. Roberts JC, et al. *Int J Lab Hematol*. 2015;37(suppl 1):11–17.
53. Posan E, et al. *Thromb Haemost*. 2003;90(3):483–490.
54. Castaman G, et al. *Br J Haematol*. 2010;151(3):245–251.
55. Miesbach W, et al. *Thromb Res*. 2015;135(3):479–484.
56. Kasper CK, et al. *Haemophilia*. 2007;13(1):90–92.
57. Franchini M, et al. *J Thromb Haemost*. 2010;8(3):421–432.
58. Srivastava A, et al. *Haemophilia*. 2013;19(1):e1–47.
59. Franchini M, et al. *Blood*. 2008;112(2):250–255.
60. Hoffman M, et al. *J Thromb Haemost*. 2012;10(8):1478–1485.
61. Sattler FR, et al. *Am J Surg*. 1988;155(5A):30–39.
62. Hines R, et al. *Anesthesiology*. 1989;70(4):611–615.
63. Schafer AI, et al. *Blood*. 1980;55(4):649–654.
64. Hogman M, et al. *Lancet*. 1993;341(8861):1664–1665.
65. Hergovich N, et al. *Clin Pharmacol Ther*. 2000;68(4):435–442.
66. Tripodi A, et al. *N Engl J Med*. 2011;365(2):147–156.
67. Tripodi A, et al. *Hepatology*. 2005;41(3):553–558.
68. Afdhal N, et al. *J Hepatol*. 2008;48(6):1000–1007.
69. Lisman T, et al. *J Hepatol*. 2002;37(2):280–287.
70. Lisman T, et al. *Hepatology*. 2006;44(1):53–61.
71. Leebeek FW, et al. *Semin Thromb Hemost*. 2015;41(5):474–480.
72. Lisman T, et al. *Gastroenterology*. 2001;121(1):131–139.
73. Forkin KT, et al. *Anesth Analg*. 2018;126(1):46–61.
74. Yates SG, et al. *Transfusion*. 2016;56(4):791–798.
75. Benigni A, et al. *Am J Kidney Dis*. 1993;22(5):668–676.
76. Gawaz MP, et al. *J Am Soc Nephrol*. 1994;5(1):36–46.
77. Noris M, et al. *Blood*. 1999;94(8):2569–2574.
78. Turitto VT, et al. *Science*. 1980;207(4430):541–543.
79. Kim JH, et al. *Ann Hematol*. 2015;94(9):1457–1461.
80. Liu YK, et al. *Lancet*. 1984;2(8408):887–890.
81. Zoja C, et al. *Lab Invest*. 1991;65(4):479–483.
82. Gando S, et al. *Nat Rev Dis Primers*. 2016;2:16037.
83. Toh CH, et al. *Ann Lab Med*. 2016;36(6):505–512.
84. Thachil J. *Anesthesiology*. 2016;125(1):230–236.
85. Kitchens CS. *Hematology Am Soc Hematol Educ Program*. 2009: 240–246.
86. Levi M, et al. *Br J Haematol*. 2009;145(1):24–33.
87. Woodman RC, et al. *Blood*. 1990;76(9):1680–1697.
88. Gluszko P, et al. *Am J Physiol*. 1987;252(3 Pt 2):H615–621.
89. Harker LA, et al. *Blood*. 1980;56(5):824–834.
90. Weidman JL, et al. *Anesthesiology*. 2014;120(4):1009–1014.
91. Brown JR, et al. *Circulation*. 2007;115(22):2801–2813.
92. Brohi K, et al. *J Trauma*. 2003;54(6):1127–1130.
93. Chang R, et al. *Blood*. 2016;128(8):1043–1049.
94. Cohen MJ, et al. *Ann Surg*. 2012;255(2):379–385.
95. Brohi K, et al. *Ann Surg*. 2007;245(5):812–818.
96. Johansson PI, et al. *Ann Surg*. 2011;254(2):194–200.
97. Kutcher ME, et al. *J Trauma Acute Care Surg*. 2012;73(1):13–19.
98. Wohlauer MV, et al. *J Am Coll Surg*. 2012;214(5):739–746.
99. Moore HB, et al. *J Thromb Haemost*. 2015;13(10):1878–1887.
100. CRASH Trial collaborators, et al. *Lancet*. 2010;376(9734):23–32.
101. CRASH Trial collaborators, et al. *Lancet*. 2011;377(9771):1096–1101. 101 e1–e2.
102. Esmon CT, et al. *Blood Rev*. 2009;23(5):225–229.
103. Piazza G, et al. *Circulation*. 2010;121(19):2146–2150.
104. Spencer FA, et al. *J Gen Intern Med*. 2006;21(7):722–727.
105. Douketis J, et al. *BMJ*. 2011;342:d813.
106. Middeldorp S. *Hematology Am Soc Hematol Educ Program*. 2011;2011:150–155.

107. Wu O, et al. *Health Technol Assess.* 2006;10(11):1–110.
108. Dahlback B. *Blood.* 2008;112(1):19–27.
109. Heit JA. *Am J Hematol.* 2012;87(suppl 1):S63–67.
110. Ridker PM, et al. *JAMA.* 1997;277(16):1305–1307.
111. Goldhaber SZ, et al. *J Am Coll Cardiol.* 2010;56(1):1–7.
112. Andreoli L, et al. *Arthritis Care Res (Hoboken).* 2013;65(11):1869–1873.
113. Giannakopoulos B, et al. *Blood.* 2009;113(5):985–994.
114. Lim W, et al. *JAMA.* 2006;295(9):1050–1057.
115. Kelton JG, et al. *Blood.* 2008;112(7):2607–2616.
116. Warkentin TE, et al. *Blood.* 2006;108(9):2937–2941.
117. Warkentin TE, et al. *Blood.* 2000;96(5):1703–1708.
118. Martel N, et al. *Blood.* 2005;106(8):2710–2715.
119. Berry C, et al. *J Am Coll Sur.* 2011;213(1):10–17.
120. Warkentin TE, et al. *Blood.* 2017;130(9):1104–1113.
121. Welsby IJ, et al. *Anesth Analg.* 2010;110(1):30–35.
122. Poller L. *J Thromb Haemost.* 2004;2(6):849–860.
123. Massignon D, et al. *Thromb Haemost.* 1996;75(4):590–594.
124. Burns ER, et al. *Am J Clin Pathol.* 1993;100(2):94–98.
125. Teien AN, et al. *Thromb Res.* 1976;8(3):413–416.
126. Ignjatovic V, et al. *Thromb Res.* 2007;120(3):347–351.
127. Price EA, et al. *Ann Pharmacother.* 2013;47(2):151–158.
128. Rodgers RP, et al. *Semin Thromb Hemost.* 1990;16(1):1–20.
129. Lind SE. *Blood.* 1991;77(12):2547–2552.
130. Hattersley PG. *JAMA.* 1966;196(5):436–440.
131. Paniccia R, et al. *Anesthesiology.* 2003;99(1):54–59.
132. Enriquez LJ, et al. *Br J Anaesth.* 2009;103(suppl 1):i14–22.
133. Ganter MT, et al. *Anesth Analg.* 2008;106(5):1366–1375.
134. Bolliger D, et al. *Transfus Med Rev.* 2012;26(1):1–13.
135. Shore-Lesserson L, et al. *Anesth Analg.* 1999;88(2):312–319.
136. Weber CF, et al. *Anesthesiology.* 2012;117(3):531–547.
137. Bolliger D, et al. *Semin Thromb Hemost.* 2017;43(4):386–396.
138. Hayward CP. *Blood Rev.* 2011;25(4):169–173.
139. Born GV. *Nature.* 1962;194:927–929.
140. Harrison P. *Br J Haematol.* 2000;111(3):733–744.
141. Cardinal DC, et al. *J Pharmacol Methods.* 1980;3(2):135–158.
142. Jambor C, et al. *Anesth Analg.* 2011;113(1):31–39.
143. Panzer S, et al. *Vox Sang.* 2011;101(1):1–9.
144. Kundu SK, et al. *Semin Thromb Hemost.* 1995;21(suppl 2):106–112.
145. Roth GJ, et al. *J Clin Invest.* 1975;56(3):624–632.
146. Mitchell JA, et al. *Proc Natl Acad Sci U S A.* 1993;90(24).
147. Costello PB, et al. *Arthritis Rheum.* 1982;25(5):550–555.
148. Pascale S, et al. *Blood.* 2012;119(15):3595–3603.
149. Diaz-Gonzalez F, et al. *Eur J Immunol.* 2015;45(3):679–686.
150. Silverstein FE, et al. *JAMA.* 2000;284(10):1247–1255.
151. Solomon SD, et al. *N Engl J Med.* 2005;352(11):1071–1080.
152. Coxib and Traditional NSAID Trialists' (CNT) Collaboration. *Lancet.* 2013;382(9894):769–779.
153. Ferri N, et al. *Drugs.* 2013;73(15):1681–1709.
154. Savi P, et al. *Thromb Haemost.* 2000;84(5):891–896.
155. Taubert D, et al. Impact of P-glycoprotein on clopidogrel absorption. *Clin Pharmacol Ther.* 2006;80(5):486–501.
156. Mega JL, et al. *Lancet.* 2010;376(9749):1312–1319.
157. Mega JL, et al. *JAMA.* 2010;304(16):1821–1830.
158. Wallentin L. *Eur Heart J.* 2009;30(16):1964–1977.
159. Floyd CN, et al. *Clin Pharmacokinet.* 2012;51(7):429–442.
160. Wallentin L, et al. *Lancet.* 2010;376(9749):1320–1328.
161. Akers WS, et al. *J Clin Pharmacol.* 2010;50(1):27–35.
162. Subban V, et al. *Indian Heart J.* 2013;65(3):260–263.
163. Hanna EB, et al. *JACC Cardiovasc Interv.* 2010;3(12):1209–1219.
164. Dasgupta H, et al. *Am Heart J.* 2000;140(2):206–211.
165. Yates SG, et al. *J Thromb Haemost.* 2015;13(suppl 1):S180–186.
166. Benzon HT, et al. *Anesthesiology.* 2010;112(2):298–304.
167. Pokorney SD, et al. *Am Heart J.* 2015;170(1):141–148.
168. Stergiopoulos K, et al. *JAMA Intern Med.* 2014;174(8):1330–1338.
169. Shaw K, et al. *Ther Drug Monit.* 2015;37(4):428–436.
170. Johnson EA, et al. *Carbohydr Res.* 1976;51(1):119–127.
171. Ranucci M, et al. *Perfusion.* 2002;17(3):199–204.
172. Finley A, et al. *Anesth Analg.* 2013;116(6):1210–1222.
173. Li G, et al. *Anal Chem.* 2014;86(13).
174. Hirsh J, et al. *Circulation.* 1998;98(15):1575–1582.
175. Harenberg J, et al. *Thromb Res.* 1985;38(1):11–20.
176. van Veen JJ, et al. *Blood Coagul Fibrinolysis.* 2011;22(7):565–570.
177. Greinacher A, et al. *Thromb Haemost.* 1995;74(3):886–892.
178. Bhatt VR, et al. *Eur J Haematol.* 2013;91(5):437–441.
179. Schindewolf M, et al. *J Am Coll Cardiol.* 2017;70(21):2636–2648.
180. Hursting MJ, et al. *Clin Appl Thromb Hemost.* 2005;11(3):279–287.
181. Robson R, et al. *Clin Pharmacol Ther.* 2002;71(6):433–439.
182. Bittl JA, et al. *Am Heart J.* 2001;142(6):952–959.
183. Mahaffey KW, et al. *J Invasive Cardiol.* 2003;15(11):611–616.
184. Boyce SW, et al. *Am J Ther.* 2011;18(1):14–22.
185. Nafziger AN, et al. *J Clin Pharmacol.* 2010;50(6):614–622.
186. Lee CJ, et al. *Br J Clin Pharmacol.* 2011;72(4):581–592.
187. Dentali F, et al. *Circulation.* 2012;126(20):2381–2391.
188. Connolly SJ, et al. *N Engl J Med.* 2009;361(12):1139–1151.
189. Wallentin L, et al. *Lancet.* 2010;376(9745):975–983.
190. Garcia D, et al. *J Thromb Haemost.* 2013;11(2):245–252.
191. Miyares MA, et al. *Am J Health Syst Pharm.* 2012;69(17):1473–1484.
192. Tripodi A. 2013;121(20):4032–4035.
193. Bruins Slot KM, et al. *JAMA.* 2014;311(11):1150–1151.
194. Granger CB, et al. Apixaban versus warfarin in patients with atrial fibrillation. *N Engl J Med.* 2011;365(11):981–992.
195. Squire IB, et al. *Eur Heart J.* 1999;20(17):1245–1252.
196. Kearon C, et al. *Chest.* 2012;141(suppl 2):e419S–e96S.
197. Wan S, et al. *Circulation.* 2004;110(6):744–749.
198. Boersma E, et al. *Lancet.* 1996;348(9030):771–775.
199. Powers WJ, et al. *Stroke.* 2015;46(10):3020–3035.
200. Astedt B, et al. *Scand J Gastroenterol Suppl.* 1987;137:22–25.
201. WOMAN Trial Collaborators. *Lancet.* 2017;389(10084):2105–2116.
202. Ker K, et al. *BMJ.* 2012;344:e3054.
203. Henry DA, et al. *Cochrane Database Syst Rev.* 2011;(3):CD001886.
204. Manji RA, et al. *Can J Anaesth.* 2012;59(1):6–13.
205. Lecker I, et al. *Can J Anaesth.* 2012;59(1):1–5.
206. Mayer SA, et al. *N Engl J Med.* 2005;352(8):777–785.
207. Mayer SA, et al. *N Engl J Med.* 2008;358(20):2127–2137.
208. Boffard KD, et al. *J Trauma.* 2005;59(1):8–15; discussion -8.
209. Hauser CJ, et al. *J Trauma.* 2010;69(3):489–500.
210. Narayan RK, et al. *Neurosurgery.* 2008;62(4):776–786.
211. Yank V, et al. *Ann Intern Med.* 2011;154(8):529–540.
212. Lodge JP, et al. *Liver Transpl.* 2005;11(8):973–979.
213. Planinsic RM, et al. *Liver Transpl.* 2005;11(8):895–900.
214. Levi M, et al. *N Engl J Med.* 2010;363(19):1791–1800.
215. Lin Y, et al. *Transfus Med.* 2012;22(6):383–394.
216. Sorensen B, et al. *Crit Care.* 2011;15(1):201.
217. Dusel CH, et al. *Blood Coagul Fibrinolysis.* 2004;15(5):405–411.
218. Lunde J, et al. *Acta Anaesthesiol Scand.* 2014;58(9):1061–1074.
219. Douketis JD, et al. *Chest.* 2012;141(suppl 2):e326S–e50S.
220. Hirsh J, et al. *Chest.* 2004;126(suppl 3):188S–203S.
221. Antithrombotic Trialists' Collaboration. *BMJ.* 2002;324(7329):71–86.
222. Burger W, et al. *J Intern Med.* 2005;257(5):399–414.
223. Lordkipanidze M, et al. *Pharmacol Ther.* 2009;123(2):178–186.
224. Pulmonary Embolism Prevention Trial Collaborative Group. *Lancet.* 2000;355(9212):1295–1302.
225. Oscarsson A, et al. *Br J Anaesth.* 2010;104(3):305–312.
226. Biondi-Zoccai GG, et al. *Eur Heart J.* 2006;27(22):2667–2674.
227. Levine GN, et al. *J Am Coll Cardiol.* 2016;68(10):1082–1115.
228. Valgimigli M, et al. *Eur Heart J.* 2018;39(3):213–260.
229. Horlocker TT, et al. *Reg Anesth Pain Med.* 2010;35(1):64–101.
230. Palareti G, et al. *Lancet.* 1996;348(9025):423–428.
231. Levine MN, et al. *Chest.* 1992;102(suppl 4).
232. Sarode R, et al. *Circulation.* 2013;128(11):1234–1243.
233. Dezee KJ, et al. *Arch Intern Med.* 2006;166(4):391–397.
234. Burbury KL, et al. *Br J Haematol.* 2011;154(5):626–634.
235. Hickey M, et al. *Circulation.* 2013;128(4):360–364.
236. Goldstein JN, et al. *Lancet.* 2015;385(9982):2077–2087.
237. Pollack CV, et al. *N Engl J Med.* 2015;373(6):511–520.
238. Connolly SJ, et al. *N Engl J Med.* 2016;375(12):1131–1341.
239. Connolly SJ, et al. *N Engl J Med.* 2019;Feb 7. [Epub ahed of print].
240. Ansell JE, et al. *Thromb Haemost.* 2017;117(2):238–245.

Index

A

Note: Page numbers followed by "f" indicate figures, "t" indicate tables and "b" indicate boxes.

B

E

G

H

I

J

K

L

N

O

P

U

W

X

Y

Z